$FiCO_2$	fractional inspired carbon dioxide
FIF	forced inspiratory flow
F_iO_2	fractional inspired oxygen
FIVC	forced inspiratory vital capacity
FRC	functional residual capacity
FVC	forced vital capacity
FVS	full ventilatory support
f/V_T	rapid shallow breathing index (frequency divided by tidal volume)
G_{aw}	airway conductance
g/dl	grams per deciliter
$[H^+]$	hydrogen ion concentration
HAP	hospital-acquired pneumonia
Hb	hemoglobin
HBO	hyperbaric oxygen (therapy)
HCAP	health care–associated pneumonia
HCH	hygroscopic condenser humidifier
HCO_3^-	bicarbonate
H_2CO_3	carbonic acid
He	helium
He/O_2	helium/oxygen mixture; heliox
HFFI	high-frequency flow interrupter
HFJV	high-frequency jet ventilation
HFNC	high-flow nasal cannula
HFO	high-frequency oscillation
HFOV	high-frequency oscillatory ventilation
HFPV	high-frequency percussive ventilation
HFPPV	high-frequency positive pressure ventilation
HFV	high-frequency ventilation
HHb	reduced or deoxygenated hemoglobin
HMD	hyaline membrane disease
HME	heat and moisture exchanger
HMEF	heat and moisture exchange filter
H_2O	water
HR	heart rate
ht	height
Hz	hertz
IBW	ideal body weight
I	inspired
IC	inspiratory capacity
ICP	Intracranial pressure
ICU	intensive care unit
ID	inner diameter
I:E	inspiratory-to-expiratory ratio
ILD	interstitial lung disease
IMPRV	intermittent mandatory pressure release ventilation
IMV	intermittent mandatory ventilation
INO	inhaled nitric oxide
IPAP	inspiratory positive airway pressure
IPPB	intermittent positive pressure breathing
IPPV	intermittent positive pressure ventilation
IR	infrared
IRB	institutional review board
IRDS	infant respiratory distress syndrome
IRV	inverse ratio ventilation
IRV	inspiratory reserve volume
IV	intravenous
IVC	inspiratory vital capacity
IVH	intraventricular hemorrhage
IVOX	intravascular oxygenator
kcal	kilocalorie
kg	kilogram
kg-m	kilogram-meters
kPa	kilopascal
KPI	key performance indicator
L	liter
LAP	left atrial pressure
lb	pound
LBW	low birth weig[illegible]
LED	light emitting d[illegible]
$LFPPV\text{-}ECCO_2R$	low-frequency p[illegible] ventilation with extracorporeal carbon dioxide removal
LMS	learning management system
LTACH	long term acute care hospital
LV	left ventricle
LVEDP	left ventricular end-diastolic pressure
LVEDV	left ventricular end-diastolic volume
LVSW	left ventricular stroke work
m^2	meters squared
MABP	mean arterial blood pressure
MAlvP	mean alveolar pressure
MAP	mean arterial pressure or mean airway pressure
MAS	meconium aspiration syndrome
max	maximal
MDI	metered dose inhaler
MDR	multidrug resistant
mEq/L	milliequivalents per liter
MEP	maximum expiratory pressure
metHb	methemoglobin
mg	milligram
mg%	milligram percent
mg/dl	milligrams per deciliter
MI	myocardial infarction
MICP	mobile intensive care paramedic
MI-E	mechanical insufflation-exsufflation
MIF	maximum inspiratory force
MIGET	multiple inert gas elimination technique
min	minute
MIP	maximum inspiratory pressure
ml	milliliter
mm	millimeter
MMAD	median mass aerodynamic diameter
mm Hg	millimeters of mercury
mmol	millimole
MMV	mandatory minute ventilation
mo	month
MOV	minimal occluding volume
$mP_{aw} - P_{\overline{aw}}$	mean airway pressure
MRI	magnetic resonance imaging
msec	millisecond
MV	mechanical ventilation
MVV	maximum voluntary ventilation
NaBr	sodium bromide
NaCl	sodium chloride
NAVA	neurally adjusted ventilatory assist
NBRC	National Board of Respiratory Care
NEEP	negative end expiratory pressure
nHFOV	nasal high-frequency oscillatory ventilation
NICU	neonatal intensive care unit
NIF	negative inspiratory force (also see MIP and MIF)
NIH	National Institutes of Health
NIV	noninvasive ventilation
nM	nanomole
nm	nanometer
NMBA	neuromuscular blocking agent
nM/L	nanomole per liter
NO	nitric oxide
NO_2	nitrous oxide
NP	nasopharyngeal
NPO	nothing by mouth
NPV	negative pressure ventilation
NPPV	noninvasive positive pressure ventilation
NSAIDs	nonsteroidal antiinflammatory drugs
nSIMV	nasal synchronized intermittent mandatory ventilation

EGAN'S
Fundamentals OF Respiratory Care

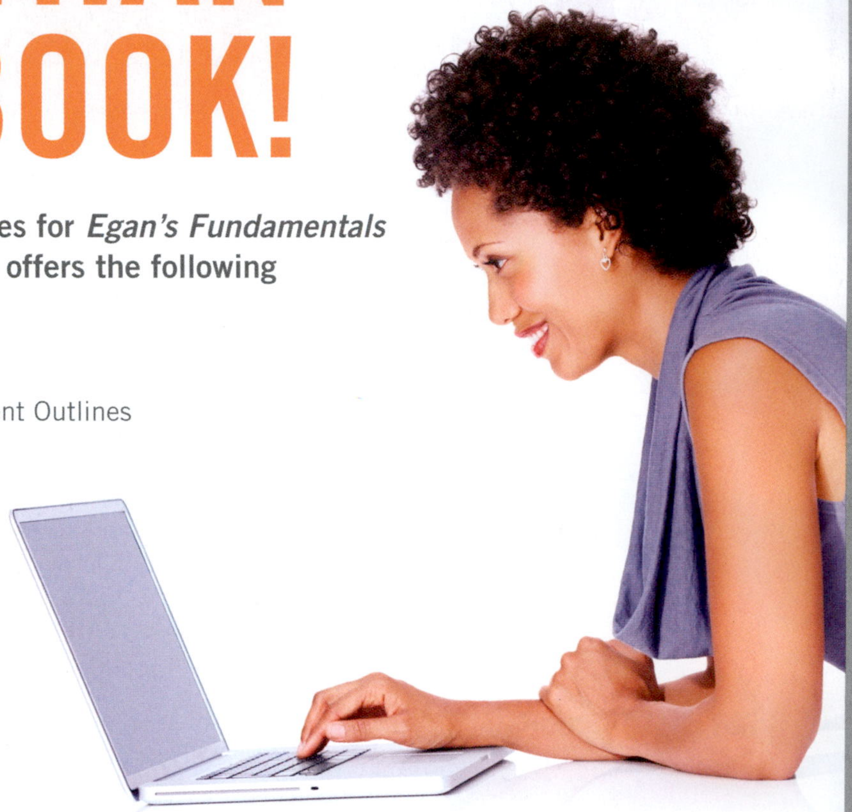

EGAN'S

Fundamentals OF Respiratory Care

EDITION 11

Robert M. Kacmarek, PhD, RRT
Professor of Anesthesiology
Department of Anesthesia, Critical Care and Pain Medicine
Harvard Medical School;
Director of Respiratory Care
Respiratory Care Services
Massachusetts General Hospital
Boston, Massachusetts

James K. Stoller, MD, MS, FAARC, FCCP
Jean Wall Bennett Professor of Medicine
Cleveland Clinic Lerner College of Medicine;
Chair, Education Institute
Cleveland Clinic
Cleveland, Ohio

Albert J. Heuer, PhD, MBA, RRT, RPFT
Program Director and Professor
Masters of Science in Health Care Management & Respiratory Care Program
Rutgers, School of Health Related Professions
Newark, New Jersey

Consulting Editors

Robert L. Chatburn, MHHS, RRT-NPS, FAARC
Adjunct Professor
Department of Medicine
Cleveland Clinic Lerner College of Medicine;
Clinical Research Manager
Department of Respiratory Therapy
Cleveland Clinic
Cleveland, Ohio

Richard H. Kallet, MS, RRT
Director of Quality Assurance
Respiratory Care Division
Department of Anesthesia
University of California, San Francisco;
San Francisco General Hospital
San Francisco, California

ELSEVIER

ELSEVIER

3251 Riverport Lane
St. Louis, Missouri 63043

EGAN'S FUNDAMENTALS OF RESPIRATORY CARE, ELEVENTH EDITION ISBN: 978-0-323-34136-3

Notices

Knowledge and best practice in this field are constantly changing. As new research and experience broaden our understanding, changes in research methods, professional practices, or medical treatment may become necessary.

Practitioners and researchers must always rely on their own experience and knowledge in evaluating and using any information, methods, compounds, or experiments described herein. In using such information or methods they should be mindful of their own safety and the safety of others, including parties for whom they have a professional responsibility.

With respect to any drug or pharmaceutical products identified, readers are advised to check the most current information provided (i) on procedures featured or (ii) by the manufacturer of each product to be administered, to verify the recommended dose or formula, the method and duration of administration, and contraindications. It is the responsibility of practitioners, relying on their own experience and knowledge of their patients, to make diagnoses, to determine dosages and the best treatment for each individual patient, and to take all appropriate safety precautions.

To the fullest extent of the law, neither the Publisher nor the authors, contributors, or editors, assume any liability for any injury and/or damage to persons or property as a matter of products liability, negligence or otherwise, or from any use or operation of any methods, products, instructions, or ideas contained in the material herein.

Previous editions copyrighted 2013, 2009, 2003, 1999, 1995, 1990, 1982, 1977, 1973, and 1969.

Library of Congress Cataloging-in-Publication Data

Egan's fundamentals of respiratory care / [edited by] Robert M. Kacmarek, James K. Stoller, Albert J. Heuer ; consulting editors, Robert L. Chatburn, Richard H. Kallet.—Eleventh edition.
p. ; cm.
Fundamentals of respiratory care
Includes bibliographical references and index.
ISBN 978-0-323-34136-3 (hardcover : alk. paper)
I. Kacmarek, Robert M., editor. II. Stoller, James K., editor. III. Heuer, Albert J., editor. IV. Chatburn, Robert L., editor. V. Kallet, Richard H., editor. VI. Title: Fundamentals of respiratory care.
[DNLM: 1. Respiratory Therapy–methods. 2. Respiratory Tract Diseases–therapy. WF 145]
RM161
615.8′36–dc23

2015036692

Content Strategist: Sonya Seigafuse
Content Development Manager: Billie Sharp
Content Development Specialist: Heather Yocum
Publishing Services Manager: Catherine Jackson
Senior Project Manager: Rachel E. McMullen
Design Direction: Renee Duenow

Printed in Canada

Last digit is the print number: 9 8 7 6 5 4

For Robert, Julia, Katie, and Callie, who all make it worthwhile, and for Cristina who has made me whole again.

RMK

I dedicate this work to the memory of my parents, Norma and Alfred Stoller, who instilled the values of rigor and commitment that inform this book; to my wife, Terry Stoller, whose love and support have been the foundation upon which my contribution to this book is possible; to our son, Jake Fox Stoller, whose shining promise gives purpose and illuminates the world; and to generations of Respiratory Therapists, whose daily activities and commitment better our health and give hope.

JKS

To my mother, who is long gone from this earth, but continues to be the most dominant, positive influence in my life. Mom taught me many lessons, including that failure is to be expected on the way to success, and excellence can only be achieved through hard work, sacrifice, and perseverance. These lessons have proven invaluable and, hence, my work on this text is dedicated to my mother, Edith; as well as my wife, Laurel; my faculty and students; fellow respiratory therapists; and the patients we tirelessly serve.

AJH

Contributors

Loutfi S. Aboussouan, MD
Staff
Respiratory Institute
Cleveland Clinic
Cleveland, Ohio

Neila Altobelli, BA, RRT
Respiratory Therapist, Clinical Scholar, Clinical Educator
Department of Respiratory Care
Massachusetts General Hospital
Boston, Massachusetts

Arzu Ari, PhD, RRT, PT, CPFT, FAARC
Associate Professor
Department of Respiratory Therapy
Georgia State University
Atlanta, Georgia

Rendell W. Ashton, MD
Pulmonary and Critical Care Fellowship Program Director
Department of Critical Care Medicine
Cleveland Clinic
Cleveland, Ohio

Joseph T. Azok, MD
Staff Radiologist
Section of Thoracic Imaging, Imaging Institute
Cleveland Clinic
Cleveland, Ohio

Jami E. Baltz, RD, CNSC
Clinical Dietitian
Department of Clinical Nutrition
Stanford Health Care
Stanford, California

Lorenzo Berra, MD
Assistant Professor of Anesthesia
Department of Anesthesia
Harvard Medical School;
Anesthesiologist and Intensivist
Department of Anesthesia, Critical Care and Pain Medicine
Massachusetts General Hospital
Boston, Massachusetts

Thomas A. Barnes, EdD, RRT, FAARC
Professor Emeritus of Cardiopulmonary Sciences
Master of Science in Respiratory Care Leadership Program
Northeastern University
Boston, Massachusetts

Will Beachey, PhD, RRT, FAARC
Professor and Chair
Department of Respiratory Therapy
University of Mary/CHI St. Alexius Health
Bismarck, North Dakota

Jason Bordelon, MHA, RRT
Director
Department of Respiratory & Clinical Diagnostics
Cleveland Clinic Abu Dhabi
Abu Dhabi, United Arab Emirates

Jeffrey T. Chapman, MD
Chief
Respiratory & Critical Care Institute
Cleveland Clinic Abu Dhabi
Abu Dhabi, United Arab Emirates

Robert L. Chatburn, MHHS, RRT-NPS, FAARC
Adjunct Professor
Department of Medicine
Cleveland Clinic Lerner College of Medicine;
Clinical Research Manager
Department of Respiratory Therapy
Cleveland Clinic
Cleveland, Ohio

Daniel W. Chipman, BS, RRT
Assistant Director
Respiratory Care
Massachusetts General Hospital
Boston, Massachusetts

Zaza Cohen, MD, FCCP
Medical Director, Respiratory Care Program—North
Rutgers School of Health Related Professions
Newark, New Jersey;
Director, Intensive Care Unit
Hackensack University Medical Center—Mountainside
Montclair, New Jersey

Douglas D. Deming, MD
Professor and Chief
Division of Neonatology
Department of Pediatrics
Loma Linda University School of Medicine
Loma Linda, California

Anthony L. DeWitt, RRT, CRT, BHA, JD
Partner
Bartimus, Frickleton, Robertson & Goza, PC
Jefferson City, Missouri

Enrique Diaz-Guzman, MD
Associate Professor of Medicine
Division of Pulmonary, Critical Care and Sleep Medicine
University of Alabama at Birmingham
Birmingham, Alabama

Patrick J. Dunne, MEd, RRT, FAARC
President/CEP
HealthCare Productions, Inc.
Fullerton, California

Raed A. Dweik, MD, FACP, FRCP(C), FCCP, FCCM, FAHA
Professor of Medicine
Cleveland Clinic Lerner College of Medicine;
Director, Pulmonary Vascular Program
Departments of Pulmonary and Critical Care Medicine/ Respiratory Institute
Cleveland Clinic
Cleveland, Ohio

Patricia English, MS, RRT
ECMO Program Coordinator
Department of Respiratory Care
Massachusetts General Hospital
Boston, Massachusetts

Matthew C. Exline, MD, MPH
Assistant Professor; Medical Director, Medical Intensive Care Unit
Division of Pulmonary, Allergy, Critical Care, and Sleep Medicine
The Ohio State University
Columbus, Ohio

James B. Fink, RRT, NPS, PhD, FAARC, FCCP
Adjunct Professor
Division of Respiratory Therapy
Georgia State University
Atlanta, Georgia

Daniel F. Fisher, MS, RRT
Assistant Director
Respiratory Care Services
Massachusetts General Hospital
Boston, Massachusetts

Crystal L. Fishman, BS, RRT
Faculty Instructor
Respiratory Care Program
Rutgers School of Health Related Professions
Newark, New Jersey

Thomas G. Fraser, MD
Vice Chairman
Department of Infectious Disease
Cleveland Clinic
Cleveland, Ohio

Douglas S. Gardenhire, EdD, RRT-NPS, FAARC
Chair and Clinical Associate Professor
Department of Respiratory Therapy
Georgia State University
Atlanta, Georgia

Donna D. Gardner, Dr(c)PH, RRT, FAARC
Chair, Department of Respiratory Care
Interim Chair, Department of Clinical Laboratory Sciences
University of Texas Health Science Center at San Antonio
San Antonio, Texas

Michael A. Gentile, RRT, FAARC, FCCM
Associate in Research
Department of Critical Care Medicine
Duke University Medical Center
Durham, North Carolina

Umur Hatipoğlu, MD
Quality Improvement Officer
Respiratory Institute
Cleveland Clinic
Cleveland, Ohio

Albert J. Heuer, PhD, MBA, RRT, RPFT
Program Director and Professor
Masters of Science in Health Care Management & Respiratory Care Program
Rutgers, School of Health Related Professions
Newark, New Jersey

R. Duncan Hite, MD
Chairman
Department of Critical Care Medicine
Respiratory Institute
Cleveland Clinic
Cleveland, Ohio

Robert M. Kacmarek, PhD, RRT
Professor of Anesthesiology
Department of Anesthesia, Critical Care and Pain Medicine
Harvard Medical School;
Director of Respiratory Care
Respiratory Care Services
Massachusetts General Hospital
Boston, Massachusetts

Richard H. Kallet, MS, RRT
Director of Quality Assurance
Respiratory Care Division
Department of Anesthesia
University of California, San Francisco;
San Francisco General Hospital
San Francisco, California

Danai Khemasuwan, MD, MBA
Fellow
Department of Interventional Pulmonary Medicine
Henry Ford Hospital
Detroit, Michigan

Euhan John Lee, MD
Clinical Assistant Professor of Medicine
Division of Pulmonary, Allergy, and Critical Care Medicine
University of Pittsburgh Medical Center
Pittsburgh, Pennsylvania

David L. Longworth, MD
Lahey Health System and Lahey Hospital and Medical Center
Division of Primary Care
Lahey Health System
Burlington, Massachusetts

Sarah A. Longworth, MD
Clinical Fellow
Department of Infectious Disease
Hospital of University of Pennsylvania
Philadelphia, Pennsylvania

Scott P. Marlow, BA, RRT
Pulmonary Rehabilitation Coordinator
Respiratory Institute
Cleveland Clinic
Cleveland, Ohio

Peter J. Mazzone, MD, MPH, FCCP
Director of Lung Cancer Program
Respiratory Institute
Cleveland Clinic
Cleveland, Ohio

Atul C. Mehta, MBBS, FACP, FCCP
Professor of Medicine
Cleveland Clinic Lerner College of Medicine;
Staff Physician
Department of Pulmonary Medicine, Respiratory Institute
Cleveland Clinic
Cleveland, Ohio;
Senior Editor
Journal of Bronchology and Interventional Pulmonology

Michele Messam, BSMT(ASCP), CIC
Infection Preventionist
Infection Prevention, Quality and Patient Safety Institute
Cleveland Clinic
Cleveland, Ohio

Eduardo Mireles-Cabodevila, MD
Assistant Professor of Medicine
Department of Pulmonary, Allergy and Critical Care Medicine
Cleveland Clinic Lerner College of Medicine;
Program Director, Critical Care Medicine Fellowship
Department of Critical Care Medicine, Respiratory Institute
Cleveland Clinic
Cleveland, Ohio

Ariel M. Modrykamien, MD, FACP, FCCP
Clinical Associate Professor of Medicine
Department of Medicine
Texas A&M University—Health Science Center;
Medical Director, Respiratory Therapy and Pulmonary Function Laboratory
Department of Pulmonary and Critical Care Medicine
Baylor University Medical Center
Dallas, Texas

Kimberly N. Otsuka, MD
Assistant Professor of Pediatrics
Division of Allergy, Immunology, and Pulmonology
Loma Linda University School of Medicine
Loma Linda, California

Hilary Petersen, MPAS, PA-C
Physician Assistant
Respiratory Institute
Cleveland Clinic
Cleveland, Ohio

Thomas Piraino, RRT
Assistant Clinical Professor (Adjunct)
Department of Anesthesia, Division of Critical Care
McMaster University;
Best Practice Clinical Educator
Department of Respiratory Therapy Services
St. Joseph's Healthcare
Hamilton, Ontario, Canada

Narciso E. Rodriguez, BS, RRT-NPS, ACCS, RPFT, AE-C
Adjunct Faculty
Respiratory Care Program
Rutgers, School of Health Related Professions
Newark, New Jersey

Madhu Sasidhar, MBBS, FCCP
Section Head
Department of Respiratory Therapy
Respiratory Institute
Cleveland Clinic
Cleveland, Ohio

Steven K. Schmitt, MD
Associate Professor of Medicine
Cleveland Clinic Lerner College of Medicine;
Staff Physician
Department of Infectious Diseases, Medicine Institute
Infectious Disease
Cleveland Clinic
Cleveland, Ohio

James K. Stoller, MD, MS, FAARC, FCCP
Jean Wall Bennett Professor of Medicine
Cleveland Clinic Lerner College of Medicine
Chair, Education Institute
Cleveland Clinic
Cleveland, Ohio

Charlie Strange, MD
Professor of Pulmonary and Critical Care, Allergy, and Sleep Medicine
Department of Medicine
Medical University of South Carolina
Charleston, South Carolina

Patrick J. Strollo, Jr, MD
Professor of Medicine and Clinical and Translational Science
Division of Pulmonary, Allergy and Critical Care Medicine
University of Pittsburgh
Pittsburgh, Pennsylvania

Clorinda Suarez, BS, RRT-NPS
Senior Registered Respiratory Therapist
Department of Respiratory Care
Massachusetts General Hospital
Boston, Massachusetts

Adriano R. Tonelli, MD
Staff
Respiratory Institute
Cleveland Clinic
Cleveland, Ohio

David L. Vines, MHS, RRT, FAARC
Chair, Respiratory Care Program Director
Department of Cardiopulmonary Science
Rush University Medical Center
Chicago, Illinois

Teresa A. Volsko, MHHS, RRT, FAARC
Director, Respiratory Care and Transport
Department of Nursing Administration
Akron Children's Hospital
Akron, Ohio

Purris F. Williams, BS, RRT
Respiratory Therapist, Senior Clinician
Respiratory Care Services
Massachusetts General Hospital
Boston, Massachusetts

Kenneth A. Wyka, MS, RRT, AE-C, FAARC
Director of Clinical Education and Associate Dean
Respiratory Therapy Program
Independence University
Salt Lake City, Utah

Reviewers

Catherine Bitsche EdS, RRT-NPS,RCP
Program Director
Catawba Valley Community College
Respiratory Therapy
Hickory, North Carolina

Greg Carter BS, RRT
Program Chair/Director
Tacoma Community College
Respiratory Care
Tacoma, Washington

Donna Davis, BS, RRT
Program Director
Butte Glenn Community College
Respiratory Care
Oroville, California

Kathleen Geier, M.Ed, RRT
Instructor
Southeast Community College
Health Science Division
Lincoln, Nebraska

Robert L. Joyner, Jr., PhD, RRT, RRT-ACCS, FAARC
Professor of Health Sciences
Associate Dean, Henson School of Science & Technology
Director, Respiratory Therapy Program
Salisbury University
Department of Health Sciences
Salisbury, Maryland

Stephen F. Wehrman RRT, RPFT
Professor Emeritus
University of Hawaii
Kapi'olani Community College
Health Sciences
Honolulu, Hawaii

Peggy Wells, RRT, RCP, MAED
Program Director
Respiratory Therapy Program
Grossmont College
Respiratory Therapy
El Cajon, California

Preface

Donald F. Egan, MD, the original author of *Egan's Fundamentals of Respiratory Care,* sought to provide a foundation of knowledge for respiratory students learning the practice in 1969. However, the scope of the respiratory care profession is ever-expanding, and the skills and information needed to be an effective respiratory therapist have expanded with it. With improved technology and vast scientific and medical advances, the body of knowledge required for respiratory therapists has increased greatly since the first edition of the text was published.

Now in its eleventh edition, *Egan's Fundamentals of Respiratory Care* encompasses the most relevant information to date and has provided a comprehensive knowledge base for students and professionals for more than 45 years. While these updated editions of *Egan's Fundamentals of Respiratory Care* still accomplish Dr. Egan's original goal—"to present what is felt to be the minimum knowledge for the safe and effective administration of inhalation therapy"—this text also goes far beyond the minimum, delving into important concepts and providing detailed information and resources to enhance student comprehension.

Every editor, guest editor, and contributor to the book is a leading figure in respiratory care, and the vast experience of these individuals ensures that critical content is covered accurately. Using the combined knowledge of these individuals, *Egan's Fundamentals of Respiratory Care* covers the role of respiratory therapists, the scientific bases for treatment, and clinical application skills. With 56 detailed chapters all focused on a unique aspect of respiratory care, *Egan's Fundamentals of Respiratory Care* is without equal in providing the prerequisite information required of a respiratory therapist today.

ORGANIZATION

This edition of the text is organized in a logical sequence of sections and chapters that build on each other to facilitate comprehension of the material. The earlier sections provide a basis for the profession and cover the physical, anatomic, and physiologic principles necessary to understand succeeding chapters. The later chapters address specific cardiopulmonary diseases and the diagnostic and therapeutic techniques that accompany them. Details on preventive and long-term care are also provided in the later chapters. In order of presentation, the seven sections are:

I. Foundations of Respiratory Care
II. Applied Anatomy and Physiology
III. Assessment of Respiratory Disorders
IV. Review of Cardiopulmonary Disease
V. Basic Therapeutics
VI. Acute and Critical Care
VII. Patient Education and Long-Term Care

FEATURES

There are many characteristic features throughout the book designed with the student in mind, making *Egan's Fundamentals of Respiratory Care* unique and engaging as a primary textbook. Each chapter begins in a similar manner, outlining the content and drawing attention to what should be mastered through the use of:

- Chapter Objectives
- Chapter Outlines
- Key Terms

The most important features within each chapter are accented by the ample use of figures, boxes, and tables containing key information and by the use of:

- "Rules of Thumb"—"pearls" of information highlighting rules, formulas, and key points necessary to the study of respiratory therapy and to future clinical practice
- "Mini-Clinis"—critical thinking case studies illustrating potential problems that may be encountered during patient care
- Clinical Practice Guidelines—statements of care extracted from the AARC list of guidelines defining evidence-based practice
- Therapist-Driven Protocols—examples of decision trees developed by hospitals and used by respiratory therapists to assess patients, initiate care, and evaluate outcomes

Also, each chapter concludes with:

- A "Summary Checklist" of key points that the student should have mastered on completion of the chapter
- A complete list of references

NEW TO THIS EDITION

This edition has been updated to reflect the most current information in the National Board for Respiratory Care (NBRC) Therapist Exam Content Outline. Also featured is an expanded role for the NBRC Exam Matrix Correlation chart within all of the student and instructor offerings. Several chapters have been added, including Fundamentals of Respiratory Care Research; Flexible Bronchoscopy and the Respiratory Therapist;

Extracorporeal Life Support (ECLS); Patient Ventilator Interaction; and Trauma, Obesity, Burns, and Near Drowning; and many other chapters have been substantially revised or completely rewritten to reflect the dynamic and expanding field of respiratory care. Furthermore, the content of the entire text has been refined and simplified to be more easily understood and relevant to our key audiences: respiratory therapy students, faculty, and therapists throughout the world.

LEARNING AIDS

Workbook

The *Workbook for Egan's Fundamentals of Respiratory Care* is an exceptional resource for students. Offering a wide range of activities, it allows students to apply the knowledge they have gained using the core text. Presented in an engaging format, the workbook breaks down the more difficult concepts and guides students through the most important information. Beyond the many NBRC-style multiple-choice questions in the workbook, students are challenged with exercises such as fill-in-the-blanks, matching, case studies, short answers, and more. Answers to the Workbook are available on the Evolve site.

FOR THE INSTRUCTOR

Evolve Resources

Evolve is an interactive learning environment designed to work in coordination with this text. Instructors may use Evolve to provide an Internet-based course component that expands the concepts presented in class. Evolve can be used to publish the class syllabus, outlines, and lecture notes; set up "virtual office hours" and e-mail communication; and encourage student participation through chatrooms and discussion boards. Evolve also allows instructors to post exams and manage their grade books.

The intuitive and comprehensive Evolve Learning Resources associated with this text provide instructors with valuable resources to use as they teach, including:

- More than 3000 test bank questions available in ExamView
- Comprehensive PowerPoint presentations for each chapter
- An image collection of the figures in the book
- Lesson plans
- Workbook answer key

For more information, visit http://evolve.elsevier.com/Egans or contact an Elsevier sales representative.

Contents

SECTION I

FOUNDATIONS OF RESPIRATORY CARE

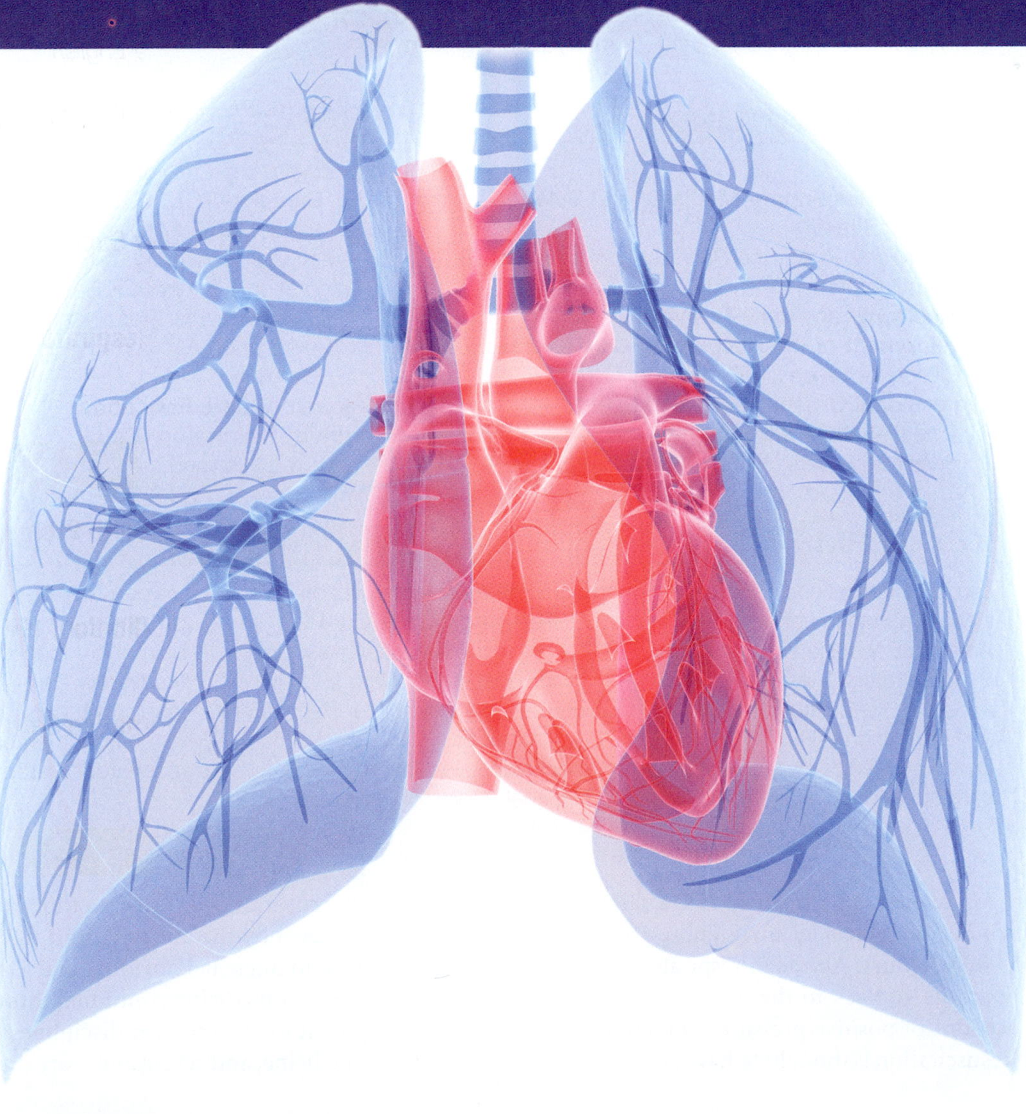

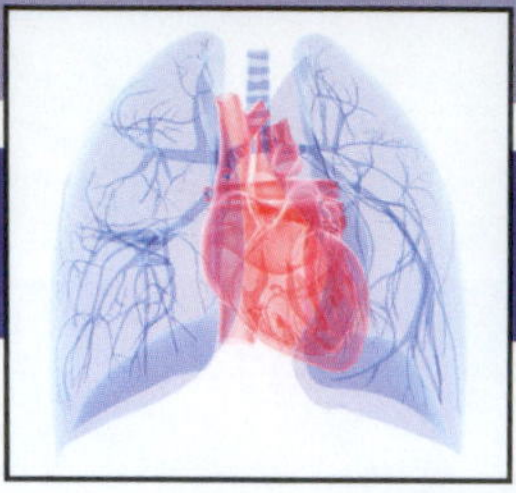

CHAPTER 1

History of Respiratory Care

PATRICK J. DUNNE

CHAPTER OBJECTIVES

After reading this chapter you will be able to:

- Define *respiratory care.*
- Summarize some of the major events in the history of science and medicine.
- Explain how the respiratory care profession began.
- Describe the historical development of the major clinical areas of respiratory care.
- Name some of the important historical figures in respiratory care.
- Describe the major respiratory care educational, credentialing, and professional associations.
- Explain how the important respiratory care organizations began.
- Describe the development of respiratory care education.
- Predict future trends for the respiratory care profession.

CHAPTER OUTLINE

Definitions
History of Respiratory Medicine and Science
- Ancient Times
- The Middle Ages, the Renaissance, and the Enlightenment Period
- Nineteenth and Early Twentieth Centuries

Development of the Respiratory Care Profession
- Clinical Advances in Respiratory Care

Professional Organizations and Events
- American Association for Respiratory Care (AARC)
- Respiratory Care Week
- Fellow of the American Association for Respiratory Care (FAARC)
- Board of Medical Advisors (BOMA)
- American Respiratory Care Foundation (ARCF)
- International Council for Respiratory Care (ICRC)
- National Board for Respiratory Care (NBRC)
- Committee on Accreditation for Respiratory Care (CoARC)

Respiratory Care Education
Future of Respiratory Care
- 2015 and Beyond

KEY TERMS

aerosol medications
airway management
American Association for Respiratory Care (AARC)
American Respiratory Care Foundation (ARCF)
Board of Medical Advisors (BOMA)
cardiopulmonary system
Committee on Accreditation for Respiratory Care (CoARC)
Fellow of the American Association for Respiratory Care (FAARC)
International Council for Respiratory Care (ICRC)
mechanical ventilation
National Board for Respiratory Care (NBRC)
oxygen therapy
physician assistant
pulmonary function testing
respiratory care
respiratory care practitioner(s)
respiratory therapist(s) (RTs)
respiratory therapy

The history of science and medicine is a fascinating topic, which begins in ancient times and progresses to the twenty-first century. Although respiratory care is a newer discipline, its roots go back to the dawn of civilization. The first written account of positive pressure ventilation using mouth-to-mouth resuscitation is thought to have been recorded more than 28 centuries ago.[1] Air was thought to be one of the four basic elements by the ancients, and the practice of medicine dates back to ancient Babylonia and Egypt. The progression of science and medicine continued through the centuries, and development of the modern disciplines of anesthesiology, pulmonary medicine, and respiratory care during the twentieth century depended on the work of many earlier scientists and physicians. This chapter describes the history and development of the field of respiratory care and possible future directions for the profession.

DEFINITIONS

Respiratory care, also known as **respiratory therapy**, has been defined as the health care discipline that specializes in the promotion of optimal cardiopulmonary function and health.[2] **Respiratory therapists (RTs)** apply scientific principles to prevent, identify, and treat acute or chronic dysfunction of the **cardiopulmonary system**.[2] Respiratory care includes the assessment, treatment, management, control, diagnostic evaluation, education, and care of patients with deficiencies and abnormalities of the cardiopulmonary system.[2] Respiratory care is increasingly involved in the prevention of respiratory disease, the management of patients with chronic respiratory disease, and the promotion of health and wellness.[2]

RTs, also known as **respiratory care practitioners**, are health care professionals who are educated and trained to provide respiratory care to patients. Approximately 75% of all RTs work in hospitals or other acute care settings.[3] However, many RTs are employed in clinics, physicians' offices, skilled nursing facilities, cardiopulmonary diagnostic laboratories, and public schools. Others work in research, disease management programs, home care, and industry. RTs also are employed by colleges and universities to teach students the skills they need to become RTs. Regardless of practice setting, all direct patient care services provided by RTs must be done under the direction of a qualified physician. Medical directors are usually physicians who are specialists in pulmonary medicine, anesthesiology, and/or critical care medicine.

A human resources survey conducted in 2014 by the American Association for Respiratory Care (AARC) revealed that there were approximately 172,000 RTs practicing in the United States[3]; this represented a 19% increase over a similar study conducted 4 years earlier in 2009. As the incidence of chronic respiratory diseases continues to increase, the demand for RTs is expected to be even greater in the years ahead. Although the RT as a distinct health care provider was originally a uniquely North American phenomenon, since the 1990s there has been a steady increase in interest of other countries in having specially trained professionals provide respiratory care. This trend is referred to as the *globalization of respiratory care.*

HISTORY OF RESPIRATORY MEDICINE AND SCIENCE

Several excellent reviews of the history of respiratory care have been written, and the reader is encouraged to review these publications.[1,4-6] Summaries of notable historical events in science, medicine, and respiratory care are provided in Tables 1-1 and 1-2. A brief description of the history of science and medicine follows.

Ancient Times

Humans have been concerned about the common problems of sickness, disease, old age, and death since primitive times. Early cultures developed herbal treatments for many diseases, and surgery may have been performed in Neolithic times. Physicians practiced medicine in ancient Mesopotamia, Egypt, India, and China.[1,4,7] However, the foundation of modern Western medicine was laid in ancient Greece with the development of the Hippocratic Corpus.[1,4,7,8] This ancient collection of medical treatises is attributed to the "father of medicine," Hippocrates,

TABLE 1-1
Major Historical Events in Science, Medicine, and Respiratory Care from Ancient Times to the Nineteenth Century

Dates	Historical Event
Ancient Period	
1550 BC	What may be the world's oldest medical document, known as *Ebers Papyrus,* describes an ancient Egyptian inhalational treatment for asthma.
800 BC	Biblical reference to what may be the first recorded episode of mouth-to-mouth resuscitation.
500-300 BC	Hippocrates (460-370 BC; Greece) describes diseases as "humoral disorders" and speculates that an essential substance in air enters the heart and is distributed throughout the body.
304 BC	Erasistratus of Alexandria describes the pneumatic theory of respiration, in which air travels through the lungs to the heart and then through the air-filled arteries to the tissues of the body.
100-200 AD	Galen (130-199 AD) in Asia Minor identifies "pneuma" as the vital substance in inspired air that enters the heart and then the blood.
Middle Ages (500-1500 AD) and Renaissance (1450-1600)	
500-1500 AD	The Middle Ages brings a period of little scientific progress in the West; however, this period coincides with the Golden Age of Arabian medicine (850-1050 AD).
1400s-1500s	da Vinci (1452-1519; Italy) performs human dissections and physiologic experiments on animals, learning that subatmospheric intrapleural pressures inflate the lungs and that there is a vital substance in air that supports combustion.
1542	Vesalius (1514-1564; Belgium), one of the great early pioneers in human anatomy, performs a thoracotomy on a pig, placing a reed tracheotomy tube for ventilation of the animal, and resuscitates an apparently dead person.

Continued

TABLE 1-1
Major Historical Events in Science, Medicine, and Respiratory Care from Ancient Times to the Nineteenth Century—cont'd

Dates	Historical Event
Seventeenth Century (1600s)	
1628	Harvey (1578-1657; England) describes the arterial and venous circulatory systems.
1643	Torricelli (1608-1647; Italy) builds the world's first barometer for measurement of atmospheric pressure.
1648	Pascal (1623-1662) describes the relationship between altitude and barometric pressure.
1662; 1666	Boyle (1627-1691; England) explains the inverse relationship between gas pressure and volume (Boyle's law: pressure [P] × volume [V] = k or $[P_1V_1] = [P_2V_2]$). Boyle also describes a mysterious substance in air that supports combustion.
1683	van Leewenhoek (1632-1723; Holland) improves the microscope and begins the science of microbiology.
Eighteenth Century (1700s)	
1738	Bernoulli (1700-1782; Switzerland) determines that as the velocity of a liquid or gas increases, the pressure decreases (Bernoulli principle). Bernoulli also proposed that gases are composed of tiny particles in rapid, random motion. This idea became the basis of the modern kinetic theory of gases, which was developed further by Maxwell (1831-1879; Scotland) in 1860.
1744	Fothergill (1712-1780; England) reports successful resuscitation methods.
1754	Black (1728-1799; Scotland) rediscovers carbon dioxide, which he calls "fixed air" (prior work had been done by van Helmot in the 1600s).
1771	Scheele (1742-1786; Sweden) makes "fire air" (oxygen) by heating magnesium oxide; Scheele's findings are published in June 1774.
1774	Priestley (1733-1804; England), usually credited with the discovery of oxygen, publishes his work on "dephlogisticated air" (oxygen) 3 months after Scheele's report.
1775	Lavosier (1743-1794; France) renames "dephlogisticated air" "oxygen," or "acid maker" and shows that oxygen is absorbed by the lungs and consumed by the body, producing carbon dioxide and water vapor, which are exhaled.
1776	Hunter (1728-1793; England) recommends use of a fireplace bellows for artificial ventilation.
1787	Charles (1746-1823; France) describes the relationship between gas temperature and volume; Charles' law: volume (V)/temperature (T) = constant; or $(V_1/T_1) = (V_2/T_2)$.
1794	Lavosier (1743-1794; France) describes oxygen absorption by the lungs and carbon dioxide production.
1798	Beddoes (1760-1808; England) establishes the Pneumatic Institute in Bristol and uses oxygen to treat various disorders.
Nineteenth Century (1800s)	
1800	Henry (1774-1836; England) determines that the amount of gas dissolved in a liquid is directly proportioned to its partial pressure (Henry's law).
1800s	Fick (1829-1911) describes a method to calculate cardiac output based on oxygen consumption and arterial and venous oxygen content: $Qt = (\dot{V}O_2)/(CaO_2 - CvO_2)$.
1801-1808	Dalton (1766-1844; England) describes his atomic theory and the relationship between the partial pressures and total pressure of a gas mixture; Dalton's law: $P_1 + P_2 + P_3 \ldots P_N = P_{Total}$, where P = pressure.
1806	de LaPlace (1749-1827; France) describes the relationship between pressure and surface tension in fluid droplets.
1808	Gay-Lussac (1778-1850; France) describes the relationship between gas pressure and temperature; Gay-Lussac's law: pressure (P)/temperature (T) = constant; or $(P_1/T_1) = (P_2/T_2)$.
1811	Avogadro (1776-1856; Italy) describes "Avogadro principle," in which equal volumes of all gases (at the same temperature and pressure) contain the same number of molecules.
1816	Laennec (1781-1826; France) invents the stethoscope for chest auscultation and lays the foundation for modern pulmonology with his book *Diseases of the Chest.*
1831	Graham (1805-1869; Scotland) describes diffusion of gases (Graham's law).
1837	Magnus (1802-1870; Germany) measures arterial and venous blood oxygen and carbon dioxide content.
1846	Hutchinson (1811-1861; England) develops the spirometer and measures the vital capacity of more than 2000 human subjects.
1864	Jones (United States) patents a negative pressure device to support ventilation.
1865	Pasteur (1822-1895; France) describes his "germ theory" of disease.
1876	Woillez develops the spirophore negative pressure ventilator.
1878	Bert (1833-1886; France) shows that low inspired oxygen levels cause hyperventilation.
1880	MacEwen reports success with oral endotracheal intubation.
1885	Miescher-Rusch demonstrates that carbon dioxide is the major stimulus for breathing.
1886; 1904	Bohr (1855-1911; Danish) describes the oxyhemoglobin dissociation curve.
1888	The Fell-O'Dwyer device combines a foot-operated bellows with a laryngeal tube for ventilatory support.
1895	Roentgen (1845-1923; Germany) discovers the "x-ray." A direct vision laryngoscope is introduced by Jackson in the United States and Kirstein in Germany.

Data from references 1, 3-9, 11-14, and 17.

TABLE 1-2

Major Historical Events in Science, Medicine, and Respiratory Care in the Twentieth and Twenty-First Centuries

Twentieth Century	
Early 1900s	Bohr (1855-1911; Denmark), Hasselbach (1874-1962; Denmark), Krogh (1874-1940; Denmark), Haldane (1860-1936; Scotland), Barcroft (1872-1947; Ireland), Priestly (1880-1941; Britain), Y. Henderson (1873-1944; United States), L. J. Henderson (1878-1942; United States), Fenn (1893-1971; United States), Rahn (1912-1990; United States), and others make great strides in respiratory physiology and the understanding of oxygenation, ventilation, and acid-base balance.
1904	Bohr, Hasselbach, and Krogh (1874-1940) describe the relationships between oxygen and carbon dioxide transport. Sauerbruch (1875-1951; Germany) uses a negative pressure operating chamber for surgery in Europe.
1907	von Linde (1842-1934; Germany) begins large-scale commercial preparation of oxygen.
1909	Melltzer (1851-1920; United States) introduces oral endotracheal intubation.
1910	Oxygen tents are in use, and the clinical use of aerosolized epinephrine is introduced.
1911	Drager (1847-1917; Germany) develops the Pulmotor ventilator for use in resuscitation.
1913	Jackson develops a laryngoscope to insert endotracheal tubes.
1918	Oxygen mask is used to treat combat-induced pulmonary edema.
1919	Strohl (1887-1977; France) suggests the use of forced vital capacity as a measure of pulmonary function.
1920	Hill develops an oxygen tent to treat leg ulcers.
1926	Barach develops an oxygen tent with cooling and carbon dioxide removal.
1928	Drinker develops his "iron lung" negative pressure ventilator.
1938	Barach develops the meter mask for administering dilute oxygen. Boothby, Lovelace, and Bulbulian devise the BLB mask at the Mayo Clinic for delivering high concentrations of oxygen.
1940	Isoproterenol, a potent beta-1 and beta-2 bronchodilator administered via aerosol, is introduced. Most common side effects are cardiac (beta-1).
1945	Motley, Cournand, and Werko use intermittent positive pressure breathing to treat various respiratory disorders.
1947	The ITA is formed in Chicago, Illinois. The ITA later becomes the AARC.
1948	Bennett introduces the TV-2P positive pressure ventilator.
1948	FEV_1 is introduced as a pulmonary function measure of obstructive lung disease.
1951	Isoetherine (Bronkosol), a preferential beta-2 aerosol bronchodilator with fewer cardiac side effects, is introduced.
1952	Mørch introduces the piston ventilator.
1954	The ITA becomes the AAIT.
1958	Bird introduces the Bird Mark 7 positive pressure ventilator.
1960	The Campbell Ventimask for delivering dilute concentrations of oxygen is introduced.
1961	Jenn becomes the first registered respiratory therapist. Also, metaproterenol, a preferential beta-2 bronchodilator, is introduced
1963	Board of Schools is formed to accredit inhalation therapy educational programs.
1964	The Emerson Postoperative Ventilator (3-PV) positive pressure volume ventilator is introduced.
1967	The Bennett MA-1 volume ventilator is introduced, ushering in the modern age of mechanical ventilatory support for routine use in critical care units.
1967	Combined pH-Clark-Severinghaus electrode is developed for rapid blood gas analysis.
1968	Fiberoptic bronchoscope becomes available for clinical use. The Engström 300 and Ohio 560 positive pressure volume ventilators are introduced.
1969	ARDS and PEEP are described by Petty, Ashbaugh, and Bigelow.
1970	Swan-Ganz catheter developed for measurement of pulmonary artery pressures. The ARCF is incorporated. The JRCITE is incorporated to accredit respiratory therapy educational programs.
1971	Continuous positive airway pressure is introduced by Gregory. *Respiratory Care* journal is named.
1972	Siemens Servo 900 ventilator is introduced.
1973	IMV is described by Kirby and Downs. The AAIT becomes the AART.
1974	IMV Emerson ventilator is introduced.
1974	NBRT is formed.
1975	Bourns Bear I ventilator is introduced.
1977	The JRCITE becomes the JRCRTE.
1978	Puritan Bennett introduces the MA-2 volume ventilator. The *AAR Times* magazine is introduced.
1979	AIDS is recognized by the Centers for Disease Control (CDC [later, Centers for Disease Control and Prevention]).
1982	Siemens Servo 900C and Bourns Bear II ventilators are introduced.
1983	The NBRT becomes the NBRC.
1983	President Reagan signs proclamation declaring National Respiratory Care Week
1984	Bennett 7200 microprocessor controlled ventilator is introduced.
1984	The AART is renamed the AARC.
1991	Servo 300 ventilator is introduced.
1992, 1993	The AARC holds national respiratory care education consensus conferences.
1994	The CDC publishes the first guidelines for the prevention of ventilator-associated pneumonia.
1998	The CoARC is formed, replacing the JRCRTE.

Continued

TABLE 1-2
Major Historical Events in Science, Medicine, and Respiratory Care in the Twentieth and Twenty-First Centuries—cont'd

Twenty-First Century	
2002	The NBRC adopts a continuing competency program for respiratory therapists to maintain their credentials.
2002	The Tripartite Statements of Support are adopted by the AARC, NBRC, and CoARC to advance respiratory care education and credentialing.
2003	The AARC publishes its white paper on the development of baccalaureate and graduate education in respiratory care. Asian bird flu appears in South Korea.
2004	The Fiftieth AARC International Congress is held in New Orleans.
2005	Number of working respiratory therapists in the United States reaches 132,651.
2006	The National Heart, Lung and Blood Institute (NHLBI) of the U.S. Department of Health and Human Services begins national awareness and education campaign for COPD. The AARC works with government officials to recruit and train respiratory therapists for disaster response
2007	The first AARC president to serve a 2-year term begins term of office.
2008	First of three conferences held for 2015 and Beyond strategic initiative of the AARC.
2010	The *Patient Protection and Affordable Care Act* is signed into law by President Barak Obama.

Data from references 1, 3-9, 11-14, and 17.

a Greek physician who lived during the fifth and fourth centuries BC.[1,7,8] Hippocratic medicine was based on four essential fluids, or "humors"—phlegm, blood, yellow bile, and black bile—and the four elements—earth (cold, dry), fire (hot, dry), water (cold, moist), and air (hot, moist). Diseases were thought to be humoral disorders caused by imbalances in these essential substances. Hippocrates believed there was an essential substance in air that was distributed to the body by the heart.[1] The Hippocratic Oath, which admonishes physicians to follow certain ethical principles, is given in a modern form to medical students at graduation.[1,8]

Aristotle (384-322 BC), a Greek philosopher and perhaps the first great biologist, believed that knowledge could be gained through careful observation.[1,8] Aristotle made many scientific observations, including observations obtained by performing experiments on animals. Erasistratus (~330-240 BC), regarded by some as the founder of the science of physiology, developed a pneumatic theory of respiration in Alexandria, Egypt, in which air *(pneuma)* entered the lungs and was transferred to the heart.[1,7] Galen (130-199 AD) was an anatomist in Asia Minor whose comprehensive work dominated medical thinking for centuries.[1,6,7] Galen also believed that inspired air contained a vital substance that somehow charged the blood through the heart.[1]

The Middle Ages, the Renaissance, and the Enlightenment Period

The Romans carried on the Greek traditions in philosophy, science, and medicine. With the fall of the Western Roman Empire in 476 AD, many Greek and Roman texts were lost and Europe entered a period during which few advances were made in science or medicine. In the seventh century AD, the Arabians conquered Persia, where they found and preserved many of the works of the ancient Greeks, including the works of Hippocrates, Aristotle, and Galen.[1,7] A Golden Age of Arabian medicine (850-1050 AD) followed.

An intellectual rebirth in Europe began in the twelfth century.[1,7] Medieval universities were formed, and contact with the Arabs in Spain and Sicily reintroduced ancient Greek and Roman texts. Magnus (1192-1280) studied the works of Aristotle and made many observations related to astronomy, botany, chemistry, zoology, and physiology. The Renaissance (1450-1600) ushered in a period of scientific, artistic, and medical advances. Leonardo da Vinci (1452-1519) studied human anatomy, determined that subatmospheric intrapleural pressures inflated the lungs, and observed that fire consumed a vital substance in air without which animals could not live.[1,4] Vesalius (1514-1564), considered to be the founder of the modern field of human anatomy, performed human dissections and experimented with resuscitation.[1] In 1543, the date commonly given as the start of the modern Scientific Revolution, Copernicus observed that the Earth orbited the sun.[8] Before this time, it had been accepted that the Earth was the center of the universe.

The seventeenth century was a time of great advances in science. Accomplished scientists from this period include Kepler, Bacon, Galileo, Pascal, Hooke, and Newton. In 1628, Harvey fully described the circulatory system.[4,8] In 1662, the chemist Boyle published what is now known as Boyle's law, governing the relationship between gas volume and pressure.[8] Torricelli invented the barometer in 1650, and Pascal showed that atmospheric pressure decreases with altitude.[1,4] van Leeuwenhoek (1632-1723), known as the "father of microbiology," improved the microscope and was the first to observe and describe single-celled organisms, which he called "animalcules."[7]

The eighteenth-century Enlightenment Period brought further advances in the sciences. In 1754, Black described the properties of carbon dioxide, although the discovery of carbon dioxide should be credited to van Helmont, whose work occurred approximately 100 years earlier.[1] In 1774, Priestley described his discovery of oxygen, which he called "dephlogisticated air."[1,4] Before 1773, Scheele performed the laboratory synthesis of oxygen, which he called "fire air"; a general description of his discovery appeared in 1774, and a more thorough description appeared in 1777.[1,4] Shortly after the discovery of oxygen, Spallanzani worked out the relationship between the consumption of oxygen and tissue respiration.[1] In 1787, Charles described the relationship between gas temperature and volume now known as Charles' law.[8] In experiments performed between 1775 and 1794, Lavoisier showed that oxygen was absorbed by the lungs and that carbon dioxide and water were exhaled.[1,4] In 1798, Beddoes began using oxygen to treat various conditions at his Pneumatic Institute in Bristol.[1,4]

Nineteenth and Early Twentieth Centuries

During the nineteenth century, important advances were made in physics and chemistry related to respiratory physiology. Dalton described his law of partial pressures for a gas mixture in 1801 and his atomic theory in 1808.[8] Young in 1805 and de LaPlace in 1806 described the relationship between pressure and surface tension in fluid droplets.[8] Gay-Lussac described the relationship between gas pressure and temperature in 1808; in 1811, Avogadro determined that equal volumes of gases at the same temperature and pressure contain the same number of molecules.[1,8] In 1831, Graham described his law of diffusion for gases (Graham's law).[8]

In 1865, Pasteur advanced his "germ theory" of disease, which held that many diseases are caused by microorganisms.[8] Medical advances during this time included the invention of the spirometer and ether anesthesia in 1846, antiseptic techniques in 1865, and vaccines in the 1880s.[1,4,7] Koch, a pioneer in bacteriology, discovered the tubercle bacillus, which causes tuberculosis, in 1882, and the vibrio bacterium, which causes cholera, in 1883.[7] He also developed Koch's postulates, which are criteria designed to establish a causative relationship between a microbe and a disease. Respiratory physiology also progressed with the measurement in 1837 of blood oxygen and carbon dioxide content, description around 1880 of the respiratory quotient, demonstration in 1885 that carbon dioxide is the major stimulant for breathing, and demonstration in 1878 that oxygen partial pressure and blood oxygen content were related.[1,4,9] In 1895, Roentgen discovered the x-ray, and the modern field of radiologic imaging sciences was born.[8] Pioneering respiratory physiologists of the early twentieth century described oxygen diffusion, oxygen and carbon dioxide transport, the oxyhemoglobin dissociation curve, acid-base balance, and the mechanics of breathing and made other important advances in respiratory physiology (see Table 1-2).

DEVELOPMENT OF THE RESPIRATORY CARE PROFESSION

Clinical Advances in Respiratory Care

The evolution of the respiratory care profession depended in many ways on developments in the various treatment techniques that matured in the twentieth century. As the scientific basis for oxygen therapy, mechanical ventilatory support, and administration of medical aerosols became well established, the need for a health care practitioner to provide these services became apparent. Concurrent with this need was the continuing development of specialized cardiopulmonary diagnostic tests and monitoring procedures, which also required health care specialists to perform.

The first health care specialists in the field were oxygen technicians in the 1940s.[1,4,5] The first inhalation therapists were oxygen technicians or oxygen orderlies who could haul cylinders of oxygen and related equipment around the hospital and set up oxygen tents, masks, and nasal catheters. The development of positive pressure breathing during World War II for breathing support of high-altitude pilots led to its use as a method to treat pulmonary patients and deliver aerosol medications during the 1950s, expanding the role of the inhalation therapist. Inhalation therapists began to be trained in the 1950s, and formal education programs began in the 1960s.[1,4,5] The development of sophisticated mechanical ventilators in the 1960s naturally led to a further expansion in the role of RTs, who soon also found themselves responsible for arterial blood gas and pulmonary function laboratories. In 1974, the designation *respiratory therapist* became standard, and the RT became the allied health professional primarily concerned with the assessment, diagnostic testing, treatment, education, and care of patients with deficiencies and abnormalities of the cardiopulmonary system. The historical development of several clinical areas of respiratory care is described next, followed by an overview of the establishment of the major professional organizations in the field. The evolution of respiratory care education is also described.

RULE OF THUMB

When looking for information about the respiratory care profession, the best place to look is the AARC (see www.AARC.org). The AARC's newly constructed *Virtual Museum* can be accessed through the AARC Web site.

Oxygen Therapy

The therapeutic administration of oxygen first occurred in 1798, and in 1878 Bert showed that lack of oxygen caused hyperventilation. But the physiologic basis and indications for **oxygen therapy** were not well understood until the twentieth century.[1,4] Large-scale production of oxygen was developed by von Linde in 1907. The use of a nasal catheter for oxygen administration was introduced by Lane in the same year.[1,4] Oxygen tents were in use in 1910, and an oxygen mask was used to treat combat gas–induced pulmonary edema in 1918.[1] In 1920, Hill developed an oxygen tent to treat leg ulcers, and in 1926, Barach introduced a sophisticated oxygen tent for clinical use. Oxygen chambers and whole oxygen rooms were designed.[1,4] In 1938, a meter mask was developed by Barach to administer dilute oxygen.[1,4] The BLB mask (named for Boothby, Lovelace, and Bulbulian) to administer 80% to 100% oxygen to pilots was introduced during World War II and later used on patients.[1,4] By the 1940s, oxygen was widely prescribed in hospitals, although there was still no good way to measure blood oxygen levels routinely until the mid-1960s, with the introduction of the Clark electrode, followed by the clinical use of the ear oximeter in 1974 and the pulse oximeter in the 1980s.[1,4,5] The Campbell Ventimask, which allowed the administration of 24%, 28%, 35%, or 40% oxygen, was introduced in 1960, and modern versions of the nasal cannula, simple oxygen mask, partial rebreathing mask, and nonrebreathing mask were available by the late 1960s. Portable liquid oxygen systems for long-term oxygen therapy in the home were introduced in the 1970s, and the oxygen concentrator soon followed. Oxygen-conserving devices, including reservoir cannulas, demand pulse oxygen systems, and transtracheal oxygen catheters, were introduced in the 1980s.

The 2000s saw further advances in home oxygen therapy equipment with the introduction of oxygen concentrators used in conjunction with a pressure booster to allow for the transfilling of small, portable oxygen cylinders in the home. Smaller, lightweight portable oxygen concentrators were also introduced. Both of these advances have greatly enhanced the ability of patients receiving long-term oxygen therapy to ambulate beyond the confines of their home. Furthermore, the National Institutes of Health launched the Long-Term Oxygen Treatment Trial (LOTT) as a randomized trial to explore the benefits of supplemental oxygen in patients with chronic obstructive pulmonary disease (COPD) and only mild resting hypoxemia (SpO_2 89% to 93%) or with exercise desaturation.[10]

Aerosol Medications

Aerosol therapy is defined as the administration of liquid or powdered aerosol particles via inhalation to achieve a desired therapeutic effect. Bland aerosols (sterile water, saline solutions) or solutions containing pharmacologically active drugs may be administered. In 1802, the use of inhaled *Datura* leaf fumes, which contain atropine, to treat asthma was described.[11] Early use of **aerosol medications** dates to 1910, when the first use of aerosolized epinephrine was reported. Later, other short-acting bronchodilators such as isoproterenol (1940), isoetharine (1951), metaproterenol (1961), albuterol sulfate (1980), and levalbuterol (2000) were introduced, primarily for the emergency treatment of acute asthma attacks.[11] In the late 1990s, long-acting bronchodilators—administered twice daily—were introduced for the maintenance treatment of COPD. Oral and injectable steroids were first used in the treatment of asthma in the early 1950s, and the use of aerosolized steroids for the maintenance of patients with moderate to severe asthma began in the 1970s.[11] Newer medications continued to be developed for aerosol administration, including even longer acting bronchodilators (once every 24 hours), mucolytics, antibiotics, antiinflammatory agents, and combination drugs such as long-acting bronchodilators and antiinflammatories in a single dose. Along with newer respiratory drugs, newer delivery devices such as dry powder inhalers and innovative designs for small-volume nebulizers have been introduced.

Mechanical Ventilation

Mechanical ventilation refers to the use of a mechanical device to provide ventilatory support for patients. In 1744, Fothergill advocated mouth-to-mouth resuscitation for drowning victims.[1,6] During the mid to late 1700s, there was a great deal of interest in resuscitation and additional procedures for cardiopulmonary resuscitation were developed.[1,4,6] Positive pressure ventilation using a bag-mask system or bellows was suggested. However, the observation that a fatal pneumothorax may result caused this technique to be rejected around 1827.[1,4] Interest in negative pressure ventilation developed, and the first negative pressure tank ventilator was described in 1832.[6] Other negative pressure ventilators began to appear in the mid-1800s; in 1928, the iron lung was developed by Drinker, an industrial hygienist and faculty member at Harvard University.[1] Emerson developed a commercial version of the iron lung that was used extensively during the polio epidemics of the 1930s and 1950s (Figure 1-1).[1,12] The chest cuirass negative pressure ventilator was introduced in the early 1900s, and a negative pressure "wrap" ventilator was introduced in the 1950s.[13] Other early noninvasive techniques to augment ventilation included the rocking bed (1950) and the pneumobelt (1959).[13]

Originally, positive pressure ventilators were developed for use during anesthesia and later were altered for use on hospital wards.[14] Early positive pressure ventilators included the Drager Pulmotor (1911), the Spiropulsator (1934), the Bennett TV-2P (1948), the Morch Piston Ventilator (1952), and the Bird Mark 7 (1958) (Figure 1-2).[1,14] More sophisticated positive pressure volume ventilators were developed in the 1960s and included the Emerson Postoperative Ventilator, MA-1 (Figure 1-3), Engstrom 300, and Ohio 560.[1,14] A new generation of volume ventilators appeared in the 1970s that included the Servo 900, Bourns Bear I and II, and MA-II. By the 1980s, microprocessor-controlled ventilators began to appear, led by the Bennett 7200 in 1984; in 1988, the Respironics bilevel positive airway pressure (BiPAP) device was introduced for providing noninvasive positive pressure ventilation in a wide variety of settings.[1] During

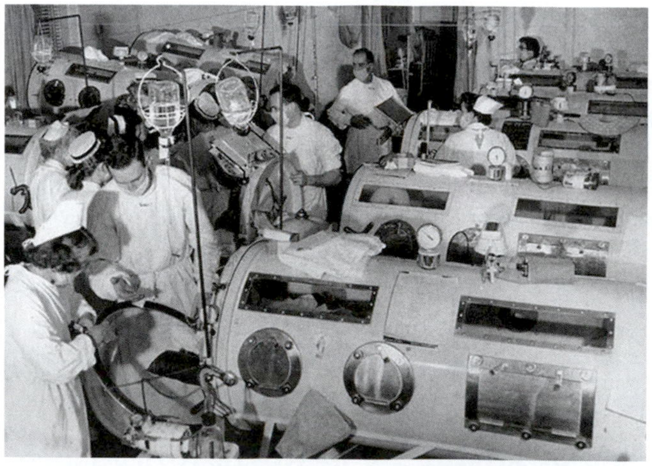

FIGURE 1-1 Iron lung patients in a 1950s polio ward. (From the Associated Press and Post-Gazette.com Health, Science and Environment. http://www.post-gazette.com/pg/05094/482468.stm.)

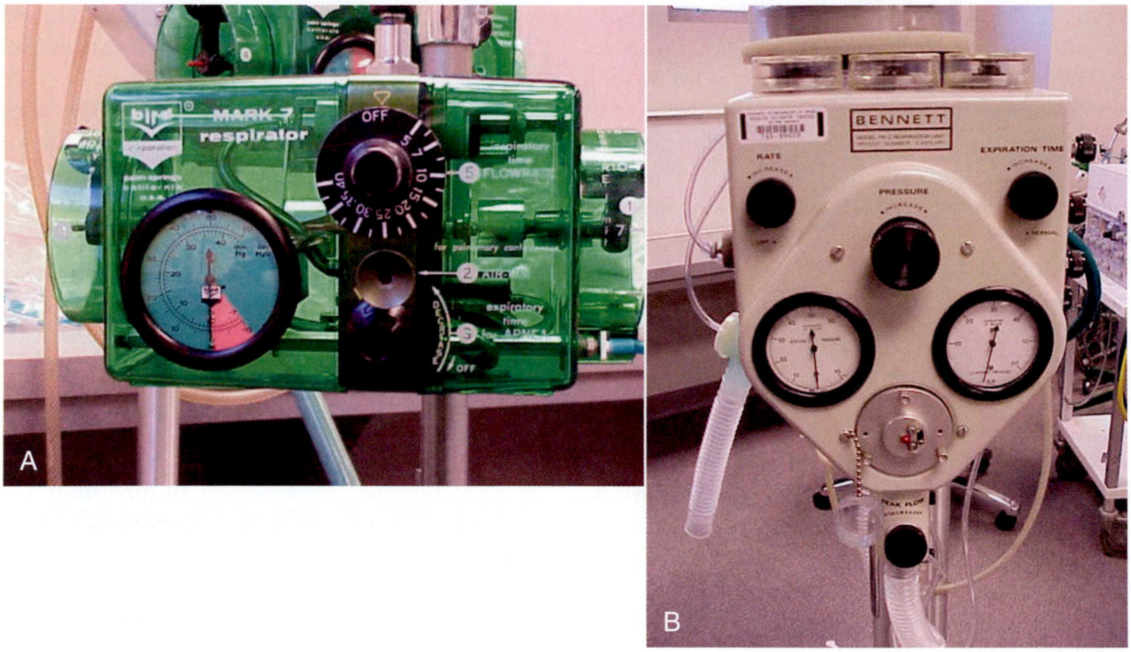

FIGURE 1-2 Bird Mark 7, introduced in 1958 by Bird **(A),** and Bennett PR-2, introduced in 1963 by Bennett **(B),** were pneumatically powered, pressure-limited positive pressure ventilators that could provide assist-control ventilation and were used to deliver intermittent positive pressure breathing treatments.

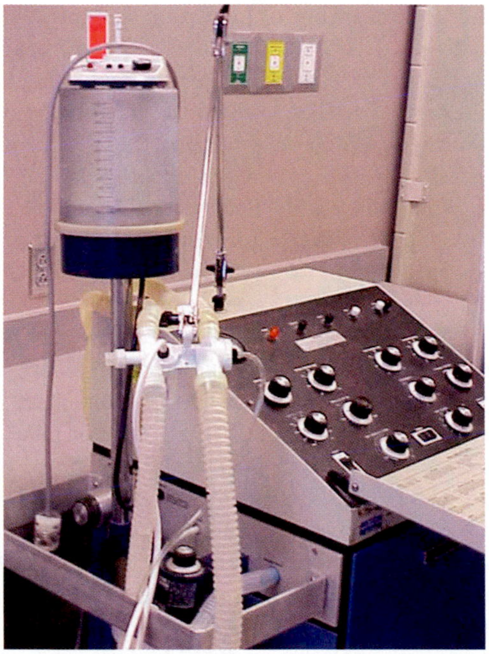

FIGURE 1-3 Bennett MA-1 ventilator, introduced in 1967, played a major role in making mechanical ventilatory support routinely available in intensive care units throughout the world.

the 1990s and early 2000s, new ventilators have continued to be developed, including the Hamilton G5, Servo-i, PB 980, and Drager V500 and VN500 series (see Chapter 45). Between 1970 and 2004, more than 50 new ventilators with various characteristics were introduced for clinical use.[15,16]

Early mechanical ventilators provided modes for which breaths were delivered according to a preset frequency and inspiratory time, regardless of any inspiratory effort on the part of the patient (what anesthesiologists of the time called "controlled" ventilation). The early Bird and Bennett ventilators invented in the 1950s allowed for initiating inspiration by detecting the patient' inspiratory effort, called "assist." This feature was incorporated in later modes that also had preset breath frequency (called *assist/control,* a term that is anachronistic but persistent to this day). The terminology related to modes of ventilation has evolved along with the complexity of ventilator technology (see Chapter 45). In 1967, the addition of positive end expiratory pressure (PEEP) as a mode feature was introduced for use in patients dying from the newly described acute respiratory distress syndrome (ARDS). The use of PEEP helped stabilize and keep alveoli from collapsing at the end of exhalation. Other forms of modern ventilation include intermittent mandatory ventilation (IMV), introduced in 1971, followed by synchronized IMV, in 1975, and mandatory minute volume ventilation in 1977.[1,4] Pressure support ventilation and pressure-controlled ventilation were introduced in the 1980s, followed by airway pressure release ventilation and inverse ratio ventilation. In the 1990s, volume support ventilation, pressure-regulated volume control, and adaptive support ventilation were introduced. Automatic tube compensation, proportional assist ventilation, neutrally adjusted ventilatory assist, and other modes of ventilation occurred in the twenty-first century. In fact, there are now hundreds of names of modes of ventilation, making a classification system essential for understanding ventilator technology (see Chapter 45).

Because traditional short-term mechanical ventilation, regardless of mode, necessitates using an endotracheal tube, there is always the potential for one or more serious complications known as ventilator-associated events (VAEs). The most common (but preventable) VAE is an infection known as ventilator-associated pneumonia (VAP). VAP is a deadly and very costly complication of invasive mechanical ventilation that develops when external microorganisms accidentally enter the airway. There has been a concerted effort to try to support inadequate ventilation noninvasively, by using a nasal or full-face mask, to avoid the need for endotracheal intubation. When noninvasive ventilation does not work and endotracheal or tracheostomy tubes are necessary, RTs must be constantly vigilant in their efforts to prevent VAP and all other VAEs.

Airway Management

Airway management refers to the use of various techniques and devices to establish or maintain a functional air passageway. Tracheotomies may have been performed to relieve airway obstruction in 1500 BC.[6] Galen, the Greek anatomist, described a tracheotomy and laryngeal intubation in 160 AD. Vesalius, the anatomist, described a tracheotomy in an animal in 1555.[1,6] In 1667, Hooke described a tracheotomy and use of a bellows for ventilation.[6] In 1776, tracheal intubation was suggested for resuscitation.[6] In 1880, MacEwen reported success with oral endotracheal intubation in patients.[6] O'Dwyer further described the technique for endotracheal tube placement. By 1887, Fell had developed a bellows–endotracheal tube system for mechanical ventilation, and this system was used in 1900 to deliver anesthesia.[6]

In 1913, the laryngoscope was introduced by Jackson. Additional early laryngoscopes were designed by Kirstein, Janeway, and others.[1,6] Endotracheal intubation for anesthesia administration was firmly established by World War I. After the war, Magill introduced the use of soft rubber endotracheal tubes, and this made blind nasal intubation possible, as described by Magill in 1930.[6] In 1938, Haight advocated nasotracheal suctioning for secretion removal, and in 1941, Murphy described the ideal suction catheter, which included side holes known as "Murphy eyes."[6] The double-lumen Carlen tube for independent lung ventilation was introduced in 1940, followed by a double-lumen tube developed by Robertshaw in 1962. Damage to the trachea by the tube cuff was reduced with the introduction of low-pressure cuffs in the 1970s.[6]

Cardiopulmonary Diagnostics and Pulmonary Function Testing

Pulmonary function testing refers to a wide range of diagnostic procedures to measure and evaluate lung function. The volume of air that can be inhaled in a single deep breath was first measured in 1679, and the measurement of the lung's residual volume was first performed in 1800.[9] In 1846, Hutchinson developed a water seal spirometer, with which he measured the vital capacity of more than 2000 subjects.[9,17] Hutchinson observed the relationship between height and lung volume and that vital capacity decreases with age, obesity, and lung disease. Hering and Breuer described the effects of lung inflation and deflation on breathing—the Hering-Breuer reflex—in 1868.[4] In 1919, Strohl suggested the use of forced vital capacity (FVC), and in 1948, forced expiratory volume in 1 second (FEV_1) was suggested as a measure of obstructive lung disease by Tiffeneau.[9]

Arterial and venous oxygen and carbon dioxide contents were measured in 1837, and methods to measure blood oxygen and carbon dioxide levels were available in the 1920s. These early methods for measuring blood oxygen, carbon dioxide, and pH were slow and cumbersome. In 1967, the combined pH, Clark, and Severinghaus electrodes produced a rapid and practical blood gas analyzer for routine clinical use.[1,4] The ear oximeter was introduced in 1974, and the pulse oximeter was introduced in the 1980s. Sleep medicine became well established in the 1980s, and polysomnography became a routine clinical test, often performed by RTs.

PROFESSIONAL ORGANIZATIONS AND EVENTS

American Association for Respiratory Care (AARC)

Founded in 1947 in Chicago, the Inhalational Therapy Association (ITA) was the first professional association for the field of respiratory care.[1,4,5] The purpose of the ITA was to provide for professional advancement, foster cooperation with physicians, and advance the knowledge of inhalation therapy through educational activities.[5] The ITA provided a forum to discuss the clinical application of oxygen therapy, improve patient care, and advance the art and science of the field.[1] There were 59 charter members of the ITA.[1] The ITA became the American Association for Inhalation Therapists (AAIT) in 1954, the American Association for Respiratory Therapy (ARRT) in 1973, and the **American Association for Respiratory Care (AARC)** in 1982.[4,5] By 2014, membership in the AARC had reached 50,000 RTs, RT students, physicians, nurses, and others interested in respiratory care. The AARC also has a formal affiliation with all 50 state respiratory societies (known as *Chartered Affiliates*), as well as with similar organizations in several foreign countries.[17]

During the 1980s, the AARC began a major push to introduce state licensure for RTs based on the National Board for Respiratory Care (NBRC) credentials.[18] As of 2014, 49 states, the District of Columbia, and Puerto Rico have state licensure or some other form of legal credentialing required for the practice of respiratory care. State licensing laws set the minimum educational requirements and the method of determining competence to practice. Competency is typically determined by obtaining a passing grade on a credentialing examination (administered by the NBRC) after graduation from an approved training program. State licensing boards also set the number of continuing education credits required to keep a license active.

The stated mission of the AARC is to "encourage and promote professional excellence, advance the science and practice of respiratory care, and serve as an advocate for patients, their families, the public, the profession and the respiratory therapist."[19] The AARC serves as an advocate for the profession to legislative and regulatory bodies, the insurance industry, and

MINI CLINI

Preparing a Presentation for Respiratory Care Week

PROBLEM: You are a staff therapist in a 300-bed hospital. Your supervisor asks you to prepare a 20-minute presentation on the history and development of the respiratory care profession to be presented at the department's annual Respiratory Care Week luncheon. How would you gather the information needed and develop your presentation?

SOLUTIONS: First, review this chapter to get an overview of the history and development of the respiratory care profession. You may also want to read one or two of the supplemental references that are cited. Next, go to the AARC Web site (see www.AARC.org) and review the "Resources" and "Site Map" sections, which list many helpful resources. You should be able to find sections on "The History of the AARC," "Strategic Plan of the AARC," "Position Statements," and "White Papers." There will also be a portal to AARC's Virtual Museum. You should also find a section on Respiratory Care Week. Review the material that the AARC has provided and develop an outline for your presentation. Your outline may include a brief overview of the history of science and medicine, the development of the respiratory care profession, and the future of respiratory care in the twenty-first century. After you have your outline, decide on your delivery method. PowerPoint slides are easy to make and use. If you choose to do a PowerPoint presentation, a good rule of thumb is about one slide per minute, so you would need about 20 slides. Using your outline, begin to develop your presentation.

the general public. To fulfill its mission, the AARC sponsors many continuing educational activities, including international meetings, conferences and seminars, publications, and a sophisticated Web site (see www.AARC.org).[18] In addition to the monthly science journal *Respiratory Care*, the AARC publishes the monthly news magazine *AARC Times* and numerous electronic newsletters. In the fall of each year, the AARC also sponsors the International Respiratory Congress, the largest respiratory care scientific meeting in the world. Finally, in an effort to ensure that the unique practice interests of AARC members are addressed (e.g., neonatal/pediatrics, adult acute care, management, home care, diagnostics), members are invited to join one or more of 10 Specialty Sections (Box 1-1) within the AARC, designed to facilitate networking and the free exchange of ideas.

The leadership and direction of the AARC is provided by a Board of Directors, which comprises members who volunteer their time and services. The executive officers of the Board of Directors include the president, immediate past-president, president-elect, vice-president for internal affairs, vice-president for external affairs, and secretary-treasurer. The remainder of the Board of Directors consists of a minimum of six members-at-large plus the chairpersons of the Specialty Sections having at least 1000 members. At the present time, 6 of the 10 Specialty Sections meet this requirement. All members of the Board of Directors, including Specialty Section chairpersons, are elected directly by the AARC membership. The AARC Board of Directors meets three times per year to conduct the official business of the association.

Box 1-1 AARC Specialty Sections

Adult Acute Care
Continuing Care/Rehabilitation
Diagnostics
Education
Home Care
Long-Term Care
Management
Neonatal/Pediatrics
Sleep
Surface and Air Transport

Each year, the incoming AARC president assigns interested members to chair or serve on more than 50 standing or temporary AARC committees. Many of the initiatives of the AARC are undertaken and eventually brought to completion through committee work. The AARC Board of Directors also receives input from each of the 50 Chartered Affiliates that constitute the House of Delegates. Each Chartered Affiliate elects two of their members to represent the interests of their state affiliate in the meetings of the House of Delegates. The 100 delegates elect their own leaders so that they can conduct the business of the House of Delegates. The House of Delegates meets twice per year. The efforts of the Board of Directors, the House of Delegates, and the numerous committees of the AARC are supported by a staff of more than 35 employees of the AARC who work full time in the association's executive offices, which are located in Irving, Texas.

Many volunteers who have been elected to the AARC or House of Delegates leadership positions or have been asked to chair important committees started by volunteering at the affiliate level. Student members of the AARC are always welcomed as volunteers, especially at the affiliate level. Student members of the AARC have access to a wide array of resources that can greatly enhance the experience of becoming a professional RT.

Respiratory Care Week

In November 1982, President Reagan signed a proclamation declaring the third week of each October as National Respiratory Care Week. Since then, Respiratory Care Week has become a yearly event to promote lung awareness and the work of RTs in all care settings. RTs (and students) around the United States use Respiratory Care Week to celebrate their profession and dedication to high-quality patient care. Many respiratory care departments use the opportunity to conduct special events in their hospitals to help raise awareness of the vital role the RT plays as a member of the health care team. Other departments plan community activities to help the public understand the importance of good lung health and the role RTs play in diagnosing and treating breathing disorders. Respiratory Care Week is also an excellent opportunity for respiratory therapy students to become ambassadors of the profession to the rest of the student body. Some respiratory therapy classes conduct free breathing tests on campus, in shopping malls, or in community centers.

Fellow of the American Association for Respiratory Care (FAARC)

In any given profession, there are always individuals who go above and beyond what is expected of the average practitioner. To recognize RTs and physician members who have achieved such distinction, in 1998, the AARC established the **Fellow of the American Association for Respiratory Care (FAARC)** award. To be considered for FAARC status, nominees must be either a registered RT or a licensed physician and have a minimum of 10 consecutive years of membership in the AARC. Of greater importance, nominees for FAARC demonstrate superior achievement, not only in patient care and research, but as a volunteer serving the profession. Individuals selected to receive this prestigious award are so noted by having "FAARC" appear after their name following educational degrees and credentials.

Board of Medical Advisors (BOMA)

Because RTs can practice only under medical direction, it is essential that the AARC leadership receive formal input from physicians on all matters and questions pertaining to patient care. The **Board of Medical Advisors (BOMA)** is the group of physicians who provide this valuable input. The BOMA comprises approximately 18 physicians who are appointed by their respective professional medical associations (e.g., American College of Chest Physicians, American Thoracic Society, Society for Critical Care Medicine) to serve this cause voluntarily. The BOMA meets annually, but the chairperson of the BOMA attends all meetings of the AARC Board of Directors. Individual members of the BOMA are assigned by the AARC president to serve as a medical liaison to each of the 10 Specialty Sections of the AARC and to standing committees. Effective medical direction at the hospital level is indispensable for the practice of safe, high-quality respiratory care.

American Respiratory Care Foundation (ARCF)

Established in 1970 by the AARC, the **American Respiratory Care Foundation (ARCF)** is a not-for-profit charitable foundation that helps promote and further the mission of the AARC. Commonly known as the Foundation, the ARCF collects and manages contributions from individuals, corporations, and other foundations to recognize individual achievements of excellence in clinical practice, chronic disease management, public respiratory health, scientific research, and literary excellence. A current focus of the ARCF is to promote the attainment of more advanced training among RTs to advance scientific inquiry in respiratory care. The ARCF also provides research grants to establish the scientific basis of respiratory care further. Finally, the ARCF oversees and distributes numerous scholarships for respiratory therapy students who are student members of the AARC. The ARCF awards and scholarships are presented at the awards ceremony held in conjunction with the annual International Respiratory Congress of the AARC. Respiratory therapy students who are interested in applying for an ARCF scholarship should visit the ARCF Web site (see www.arcfoundation.org) to learn more about this great opportunity.

International Council for Respiratory Care (ICRC)

The **International Council for Respiratory Care (ICRC)** is an AARC-sponsored organization dedicated to the globalization of high-quality respiratory care. As mentioned previously, having formally trained professionals working in a dedicated department to assume full responsibility for providing respiratory care under medical direction was a uniquely North American phenomenon (i.e., the United States and Canada). However, during the 1970s and 1980s, when many foreign physicians came to the United States to study, they became aware of what an RT was and the important role RTs played in hospitals nationwide. When these physicians returned to their native countries, they wished to have their own specialized team able to provide the same level of high-quality respiratory care. However, because the health care delivery system is structured differently in each country, the specially trained teams were most often nurses, physicians, or physical therapists, not RTs.

Formed in 1991, the ICRC (in close collaboration with the International Committee of the AARC) began to offer fellowships to interested foreign clinicians that provide the opportunity to visit the United States for 2 weeks before the annual International Respiratory Congress to observe how respiratory care is practiced in various settings. The idea is to allow these international fellows to observe how the various components of respiratory care are practiced in several cities. The international fellows can then take back to their home countries ideas and practices that can be integrated into their unique health care delivery systems. The program has been so successful that many countries (e.g., Mexico, Costa Rica, Taiwan) are starting to establish respiratory therapy training programs similar to the American model. As of 2014, participants in this program have included 142 international fellows from 54 countries.

National Board for Respiratory Care (NBRC)

The credentialing body for registered RTs began in 1960 as the American Registry of Inhalation Therapists (to test and credential registered therapists), and a certification board was established in 1968 to certify technicians.[1,4] These two groups merged in 1974 as the National Board for Respiratory Therapy, which became the **National Board for Respiratory Care (NBRC)** in 1983.[1,4] Also in 1983, the National Board for Cardiopulmonary Technologists joined the NBRC, and the credentialing examinations for pulmonary function technology were brought in under the respiratory care umbrella.[1,4] Currently, there are two levels of clinical practice credentialing examinations in the United States: the certified respiratory therapist (CRT) and the registered respiratory therapist (RRT) (see www.NBRC.org). The NBRC also offers several specialty credentialing examinations for RRTs who satisfy additional requirements through experience in a specialized area of practice.

> **RULE OF THUMB**
>
> For requirements for testing, examination schedules, study guides, and requirements for maintaining your CRT or RRT credential, check with the NBRC (see www.NBRC.org).

In 1998, the NBRC renamed the lower level *certified respiratory therapist* (*CRT,* or *entry-level respiratory therapist*); the advanced level remained registered respiratory therapist (RRT, or advanced-level respiratory therapist).[20] The NBRC began offering specialty examinations for pulmonary function technology in 1984 and neonatal/pediatrics in 1991. Because of the proliferation of new technology and innovative medical practice, additional specialty credentialing examinations have been proposed in the areas of adult acute care and polysomnography.

Committee on Accreditation for Respiratory Care (CoARC)

In 1956, the first guidelines for respiratory care educational programs were published, followed by the formation of the Board of Schools to accredit programs in 1963.[1] The Board of Schools was replaced by the Joint Review Committee for Inhalation Therapy Education (JRCITE) in 1970, led by its first chairman, Helmholtz.[1,4] The JRCITE became the Joint Review Committee for Respiratory Therapy Education (JRCRTE) in 1977 and then the **Committee on Accreditation for Respiratory Care (CoARC)** in 1996 (see www.COARC.com).[4] Today, respiratory care educational programs in the United States are accredited by the CoARC in collaboration with the Association of Specialized and Professional Accreditors.[21,22]

RESPIRATORY CARE EDUCATION

The first formal educational course in inhalation therapy was offered in Chicago in 1950.[1] In the 1960s, numerous schools were developed to prepare students to become RTs. Early programs concentrated on teaching students the proper application of oxygen therapy, oxygen delivery systems, humidifiers, and nebulizers and the use of various intermittent positive pressure breathing (IPPB) devices. The advent of sophisticated critical care ventilators, blood gas analyzers, and monitoring devices in the 1960s and 1970s helped propel the RT into the role of cardiopulmonary technology expert.

Respiratory care educational programs in the United States are offered at technical and community colleges, 4-year colleges, and universities. These programs are designed to prepare competent RTs to care for patients. The minimum degree required to become an RT has traditionally been an associate degree.[21] However, many associate degree graduates see great opportunity in pursuing their bachelor's degree and some even higher degrees. There are approximately 300 associate, 50 baccalaureate, and 3 graduate-level degree programs in the United States; 19 programs in Canada; and a handful of respiratory care educational programs in Mexico, South America, Japan, India, Taiwan, and other countries.[23,24]

> **RULE OF THUMB**
>
> Jobs in management, education, research, or advanced clinical practice may require bachelor or graduate level educational preparation.

The AARC completed a Delphi study and held two important Education Consensus Conferences in the early 1990s to assess the status of respiratory care education and recommend future direction for the field.[25-28] The first conference suggested that major trends affecting the field were advances in technology; demographic trends and the aging of the population; a need to provide better assessment, outcome evaluation, problem solving, and analytic skills; use of protocol-based care; and the need to increase the focus on patient education, prevention, and wellness, to include tobacco education and smoking cessation.[27] The conference concluded that the curriculum should encompass a broad scope of clinical practice, a significant arts and science component, emphasis on communication skills, and a minimum of an associate degree to enter practice. The second Educational Consensus Conference, held in the fall of 1993, focused on strategies to implement the recommendations made at the first conference.[28] Both conferences identified the need for more baccalaureate and graduate education in respiratory care. The view that programs should prepare students better in the areas of patient assessment, care plan development, protocols, disease management, pulmonary rehabilitation, research, and geriatrics/gerontology became well accepted.[29,30]

In 1997, Mishoe and MacIntyre[31] described a profession as "a calling or vocation requiring specialized knowledge, methods, and skills as well as preparation, in an institution of higher learning, in the scholarly, scientific, and historical principles underlying such methods and skills." These authors noted that professional roles are different and more complex than technical roles, which are oriented to performing specific tasks as ordered by the physician. Examples of professional roles in respiratory care include patient assessment and care plan development, ventilator management, disease management, pulmonary rehabilitation, and respiratory care consulting services. Technical roles may include basic task performance (e.g., oxygen, aerosol therapy, bronchial hygiene), routine diagnostic testing (e.g., electrocardiography, phlebotomy), and other routine tasks in which little or no assessment is required and decisions are limited to device selection and fine-tuning therapy.[31] In professional practice, the therapist may function as a physician extender who applies protocols or guidelines.[31] Examples include making protocol-based ventilator adjustments, applying assessment-based care plans, and performance of advanced procedures such as arterial line insertion and management, intubation and extubation of patients, application of ventilator weaning protocols, and application of advanced cardiopulmonary technologies (e.g., extracorporeal membrane oxygenation, nitric oxide therapy, aortic balloon pumps).

According to Mishoe and MacIntyre,[31] economic, educational, and institutional forces may limit respiratory care in certain settings to a task-oriented, technical role. There are many opportunities, however, for the RT to function as a physician extender, in a role similar to that of the **physician assistant**. Working under the supervision of a physician, the physician assistant may perform many medical procedures that might otherwise be performed by a physician. In a similar way, the respiratory physician extender could improve the quality of care while controlling costs and minimizing unnecessary care. Many authorities believe that the critical thinking, assessment, problem-solving, and decision-making skills needed for advanced practice in the twenty-first century require advanced levels of education.[31]

In 1998, Hess[32] observed that a task orientation has coincided with a pattern of overordering and misallocation of respiratory care services. Therapist-driven protocols and the increasing use of the RT as a consultant may allow physicians to order protocols as opposed to specific therapies. The therapist assesses the patient, develops a care plan, implements the plan, and evaluates and modifies care as appropriate.[32] Protocol-based care has been shown to be safe and effective, while reducing misallocation of care and helping to control costs.[33,34] Acceptance by physicians of RTs as consultants depends on the professionalism, education, and skill of the therapists at the bedside.[32]

In 2001, a report of the Conference Proceedings on Evidence-Based Medicine in Respiratory Care was published.[34] Evidence-based practice requires careful examination of the evidence for diagnosis, treatment, prognosis, and, in turn, practice using a formal set of rules.[35] The best evidence is used for clinical decision making, which should lead to optimal respiratory care.[35] Evidence-based practice has been advocated for all respiratory care delivered.

In 2002, the AARC, NBRC, and CoARC published their "Tripartite Statements of Support," which suggested that all RTs seek and obtain the RRT credential.[36] An AARC white paper followed in 2003, which encouraged the continuing development of baccalaureate and graduate education in respiratory care.[37]

FUTURE OF RESPIRATORY CARE

In 2001, David Pierson, MD, a prominent pulmonary physician and one of the many physician supporters of RTs, set out to describe the future of respiratory care.[38] Among other responsibilities, Pierson predicted a much greater use of patient assessment and protocols in chronic disease state management in all clinical settings. He also envisioned a more active role for RTs in palliative and end-of-life care, increasing emphasis on smoking COPD. Pierson also predicted an increase in the use of RTs acting as coordinators and caregivers in home care.

MINI CLINI

Educational Program Advisory Committee

PROBLEM: You are asked to serve on your respiratory care educational program advisory committee. The committee wants to know how respiratory care education has developed and where it should be headed. You are appointed as a member of a subcommittee to research these issues. What should you do?

SOLUTIONS: You may want to read the sections in this chapter that cover the history and development of respiratory care education to get an overview. You may wish to obtain copies of some of the reference materials that are cited. Items that may be helpful are the AARC Delphi Study,[26] reports of the AARC education consensus conferences,[27,28] and articles about the future of respiratory care.[30-33,37-41] You may wish to review the AARC strategic plan (see www.AARC.org) and AARC statements regarding respiratory care education and credentialing.[11,40,41] By reviewing these materials, you should be well-prepared to discuss the future direction of your educational program.

2015 and Beyond

In 2005, recognizing that many national politicians were beginning to call for an overhaul of the U.S. health care delivery system, the AARC Board of Directors began to think strategically, which led to the formation in 2007 of a special task force called "2015 and Beyond." The task force was charged with the envisioning potential new roles and responsibilities of RTs by 2015 and beyond. The leadership of the task force decided to convene three strategic conferences to answer the following five key questions about the profession[39]:

1. How will most patients receive health care services in the future?
2. How will respiratory care services be provided?
3. What new knowledge, skills, and attributes will RTs need to be able to provide care that is safe, efficacious, and cost-effective in 2015?
4. What education and credentialing systems will be needed to ensure RTs acquire the new knowledge, skills, and attributes?
5. How should the profession transition from traditional practice to the newer system without adversely affecting the existing workforce?

The initial 2015 and Beyond conference was held in the spring of 2008, and a consensus was reached that there were likely to be[40]:

- Eleven significant changes in how health care would be delivered (Box 1-2)
- Nine changes likely to occur in the U.S. health care workforce (Box 1-3)
- Five expected changes in how respiratory care services would be provided (Box 1-4)

Box 1-2 2015 and Beyond: *11 Predicted Changes in Health Care*

1. More patients will receive diagnoses of chronic and acute respiratory diseases.
2. Cost increases will continue to grow, creating challenges for all payers of health care services.
3. Personal electronic health records will become more widely used in all health care settings.
4. Health care consumers will pay a greater percentage of costs but will have new options for obtaining care.
5. Retail storefront health care and the Internet will stimulate consumer-driven cost competition.
6. Acute care hospitals will continue to provide episodic, cutting-edge respiratory life support technology; however, subacute and home care providers will continue to play important roles.
7. Subacute and long-term care will increase in volume and complexity.
8. The disconnect between prevention and acute care treatment will lessen but not disappear.
9. All health care delivery will undergo increasing scrutiny for quality that will be linked to reimbursement under a new system called *Pay for Performance.*
10. New models for the delivery of health care will emerge, such as *Accountable Care Organizations* and *Medical Home.*
11. Reimbursement and costs will influence the development and success of these new models.

From Bunch D: 2015 and beyond. AARC Times 33:50, 2009.

Box 1-3 2015 and Beyond: *Nine Likely Changes in the Health Care Workforce*

1. There will be national and regional shortages of certain providers in all sectors of health care.
2. There will be long-term competition for all health care professionals.
3. The clinical demand will increase at a faster pace than the workforce will be able to expand.
4. The imbalance in jobs and available workforce will be aggravated by the retirement of current providers.
5. Brutal work hours requiring 24/7 staffing will dissuade many individuals from pursuing health care careers.
6. Shortages of teaching faculty and a limited number of training programs will limit the number of entrants into allied health professional schools.
7. Traditional clinical sites will be limited in number and variety and will need to be expanded to alternative sites, such as physicians' offices and patients' homes.
8. Newer educational technologic resources will challenge traditional education.
9. Health care delivery organizations will find reinvestment in education an attractive way to secure competent and loyal workers.

From Bunch D: 2015 and beyond. AARC Times 33:50, 2009.

Box 1-4 2015 and Beyond: *Five Changes Expected in Respiratory Care*

1. The science of respiratory care will continue to evolve and increase in complexity, and clinical decisions will increasingly be data-driven.
2. Patient care teams will become the standard throughout health care.
3. New respiratory life-support technologies will be developed and deployed.
4. Reimbursement changes will be the most important impetus for more recognition of the importance of health promotion and disease state management.
5. Concerns over public health issues and military and disaster response will continue and require new skill sets for all respiratory care providers.

From Bunch D: 2015 and beyond. AARC Times 33:50, 2009.

Box 1-5 Seven Major Competencies Required by Respiratory Therapists by 2015

1. Diagnostics
2. Chronic disease state management
3. Evidence-based medicine and respiratory care protocols
4. Patient assessment
5. Leadership
6. Emergency and critical care
7. Therapeutics

From Barnes TA, Gale DD, Kacmarek RM, et al: Competencies needed by graduate respiratory therapists in 2015 and beyond. Respir Care 55:601, 2010.

In the words of one conference organizer, "the take home message was that indeed the scope and depth of respiratory care practice will increase by 2015."[39] The second conference was held in the spring of 2009 and built on the findings of the 2008 conference by identifying the competencies needed by graduate RTs and the educational content and curriculum that would be needed to practice in 2015 and beyond. Conference participants agreed that there would be seven major competencies (Box 1-5) that future RTs would need to practice effectively by 2015.[40,41] The third conference was held in the summer of 2010 to determine how the educational programs for entry-level RTs would have to be structured to accomplish the seven major competencies identified during the 2009 conference. The recommendations of the third conference were published in 2011.[42]

Although the respiratory care profession is undergoing substantial change, there will be a continuing demand for respiratory care services well into the future because of advances in treatment and technology, increases in the general population, and increases in the elderly population (the baby boomers). A growing population will result in increases in asthma, COPD, and other chronic respiratory diseases. There will also be a continuing demand for controlling costs and ensuring that care provided is evidence-based, safe, and effective. Respiratory care will need to be provided using carefully designed protocols to ensure that patients get the appropriate care at the right time and that unnecessary care is reduced or eliminated. Aggressive steps to prevent disease and control the cost of chronic respiratory disease will be essential. Effective smoking cessation and tobacco education programs and aggressive disease management and pulmonary rehabilitation for patients with moderate to severe asthma, COPD, and other chronic respiratory disease will continue to be needed.

As exemplified by the 2015 and Beyond project, the knowledge, skills, and attributes needed by RTs will continue to expand, and it will become increasingly difficult to prepare RTs for expanded practice within the credit hour limitations of many existing programs. To alleviate this situation, associate degree programs may develop articulation agreements with 4-year colleges and universities to allow their graduates to complete the bachelor degree in respiratory care without leaving their home campus; distance education technology will play an important role and allow this to occur at minimal cost.

Bachelor degree programs often seek to provide students with a foundation for leadership in the profession in the areas of management, supervision, research, education, or clinical specialty areas. To meet the leadership needs of the profession, some baccalaureate programs have already implemented post-baccalaureate certificates or master degree programs. Clinical areas in which more graduate education programs could be beneficial include critical care, cardiopulmonary diagnostics, clinical research, sleep medicine, rehabilitation, and preparation as a pulmonary physician assistant. There also will be an increasing demand for RTs with master and doctoral degrees to serve as university faculty, educators, and researchers.

SUMMARY CHECKLIST

- RTs apply scientific principles to prevent, identify, and treat acute or chronic dysfunction of the cardiopulmonary system.
- Respiratory care includes the assessment, treatment, management, control, diagnostic evaluation, education, and care of patients with deficiencies and abnormalities of the cardiopulmonary system.
- The AARC is the professional association for the profession.
- RTs work under the direction of a physician who is specially trained in pulmonary medicine, anesthesiology, and critical care medicine.
- The NBRC, the credentialing board for RTs, was founded in 1974. The American Registry of Inhalation Therapists was founded in 1960.
- The CoARC accredits respiratory care educational programs. The first Board of Schools was established in 1963.
- As the physiologic basis for oxygen therapy became understood, use of oxygen to treat respiratory disease became established by the 1920s, and oxygen was used routinely in hospitals by the 1940s.
- Use of aerosolized medications for the treatment of asthma began in 1910, with numerous new drugs being developed in the twentieth century and continuing up to the present.
- Mechanical ventilation was explored in the 1800s. In 1928, Drinker developed his iron lung; this was followed by the Emerson iron lung in the 1930s, which was used extensively during the polio epidemics of the 1940s and 1950s, and the modern critical care ventilator, which became available in the 1960s.
- The ITA was founded in 1947, becoming the AAIT in 1954, the AART in 1973, and the AARC in 1982.
- The AARC now has 10 Specialty Sections to provide resources to members based on where they are employed and practice.
- The ARCF offers many scholarships and grants to respiratory therapy students and is promoting advanced training for RTs.
- Although originally found only in the United States and Canada, the practice of respiratory therapy is quickly expanding around the world.
- Respiratory Care Week is a yearly event to promote the profession and raise awareness of the importance of good lung health.
- In the future, there will be an increase in demand for respiratory care because of advances in treatment and technology; increases in and aging of the population; and increases in the number of patients with asthma, COPD, and other cardiopulmonary diseases.

The RT of the future will be focused on patient assessment, care plan development, protocol administration, disease management and rehabilitation, and patient and family education, to include tobacco education and smoking cessation.

References

1. Ward JJ, Helmholtz HF: Roots of the respiratory care profession. In Burton GG, Hodgkin JE, Ward JJ, editors: *Respiratory care: a guide to clinical practice*, ed 4, Philadelphia, 1997, Lippincott.
2. American Association for Respiratory Care: *Definition of respiratory care.* <http://www.aarc.org/resources/position_statements/defin.html>, December 2006 (Accessed October 5, 2014.)
3. Dubbs WH: AARC's 2009 human resources survey. *AARC Times* 33, 2009.
4. Smith GA: *Respiratory care: evolution of a profession*, Lenexa, KS, 1989, AMP.
5. Weilacher RR: History of the respiratory care profession. In Hess DR, MacIntyre NR, Mishoe SC, et al, editors: *Respiratory care: principles and practice*, Philadelphia, 2002, Saunders.
6. Stoller JK: The history of intubation, tracheotomy and airway appliances. *Respir Care* 44:595, 1999.
7. *Medicine, history of.* Encyclopaedia Britannica Premium Service. <http://www.britannica.com/eb/article-9110313>, 2006 (Accessed October 5, 2014.)
8. Verma S: *The little book of scientific principles, theories and things*, New York, 2005, Sterling.
9. Cotes JE: *Lung function assessment and application in medicine*, ed 4, Oxford, 1979, Blackwell Scientific.
10. Stoller JK, Panos R, Krachman S, et al: Oxygen therapy for patients with COPD: evidence for current therapy and the Long-term Oxygen Treatment Trial (LOTT). *Chest* 138:179, 2010.

11. Rau JL: *Respiratory care pharmacology*, ed 5, St Louis, 1998, Mosby.
12. Branson RD: A tribute to John H Emerson. *Respir Care* 43:567, 1998.
13. Hill NS: Use of negative pressure ventilation, rocking beds and pneumobelts. *Respir Care* 39:532, 1994.
14. Mushin WW, Rendell-Baker L, Thompson PW, et al: *Automatic ventilation of the lungs*, ed 3, Oxford, 1980, Blackwell Scientific, pp 184–249.
15. Chatburn RL: Mechanical ventilators. In Branson RD, Hess DR, Chatburn RL, editors: *Respiratory therapy equipment*, ed 2, Philadelphia, 1999, Lippincott Williams & Wilkins, pp 395–525.
16. Cairo JM, Pilbeam SP: *Mosby's respiratory care equipment*, ed 7, St. Louis, 2004, Mosby.
17. Petty TL: John Hutchinson's mysterious machine revisited. *Chest* 121:219S, 2002.
18. American Association for Respiratory Care: *Member services.* <www.aarc.org/member_services>, (Accessed October 10, 2014.)
19. American Association for Care: *Strategic plan.* <www.aarc.org/members_area/resources/strategic.asp>, (Accessed October 10, 2014.)
20. Wilson BG: Delivering "the promise." *NBRC Horizons* 25:1, 3, 5, 1999.
21. Commission on Accreditation of Allied Health Education Programs: *Standards and guidelines for the profession of respiratory care*, Bedford, TX, 2003, Committee on Accreditation for Respiratory Care.
22. Committee on Accreditation for Respiratory Care: *Respiratory care accreditation handbook*, Bedford, TX, 2001, Committee on Accreditation for Respiratory Care.
23. American Association for Respiratory Care: *Accredited programs.* <http://www.aarc.org/education/accredited_programs/>, (Accessed October 10, 2014.)
24. Canadian Society for Respiratory Therapy: *Education: respiratory therapy programs approved by a CSRC.* <http://www.csrt.com/en/coarte/index.asp>, (Accessed October 10, 2014.)
25. O'Daniel C, Cullen DL, Douce FH, et al: The future educational needs of respiratory care practitioners: a Delphi study. *Respir Care* 37:65, 1992.
26. Douce HF: A critical analysis of respiratory care scope of practice and education: past, present, and future. In *American Association for Respiratory Care: Delineating the educational direction for the future respiratory care practitioner: proceedings of a National Consensus Conference on Respiratory Care Education*, Dallas, 1992, AARC.
27. American Association for Respiratory Care: *Delineating the educational direction for the future respiratory care practitioner: proceedings of a National Consensus Conference on Respiratory Care Education*, Dallas, 1992, AARC.
28. American Association for Respiratory Care: *An action agenda: proceedings of the Second National Consensus Conference on Respiratory Care Education*, Dallas, 1993, AARC.
29. Meredith RL, Pilbeam SP, Stoller JK: Is our educational system adequately preparing respiratory care practitioners for therapist-driven protocols? (editorial). *Respir Care* 39:709, 1994.
30. Kester L, Stoller JK: Respiratory care education: current issues and future challenges (editorial). *Respir Care* 41:98, 1996.
31. Mishoe SC, MacIntyre NR: Expanding professional roles for respiratory care practitioners. *Respir Care* 42:71, 1997.
32. Hess DR: Professionalism, respiratory care practice and physician acceptance of a respiratory care consult service (editorial). *Respir Care* 43:546, 1998.
33. Stoller JK, Mascha EJ, et al: Randomized controlled trial of physician-directed versus respiratory therapy consult service-directed respiratory care to adult non-ICU inpatients. *Am J Respir Crit Care Med* 158:1068, 1998.
34. Mishoe SC, Hess DR: Forward: evidence-based medicine in respiratory care. *Respir Care* 46:1200, 2001.
35. Montori VM, Guyatt GH: What is evidence-based medicine and why should it be practiced? *Respir Care* 46:1201, 2001.
36. American Association for Respiratory Care: *Respiratory care: advancement of the profession tripartite statements of support.* <http://www.aarc.org/resources/cpgs_guidelines_statements/>, (Accessed April 4, 2007.)
37. American Association for Respiratory Care, Barnes TA, Black CP, et al: A white paper from the AARC Steering Committee of the Coalition for Baccalaureate and Graduate Respiratory Therapy Education: development of baccalaureate and graduate degrees in respiratory care. *Respir Care Educ Annu* 12:29, 2003.
38. Pierson DJ: The future of respiratory care. *Respir Care* 46:705, 2001.
39. Bunch D: 2015 and beyond. *AARC Times* 33:50, 2009.
40. Kacmarek RM, Durbin CG, Barnes TA, et al: Creating a vision for respiratory care in 2015 and beyond. *Respir Care* 54:375, 2009.
41. Barnes TA, Gale DD, Kacmarek RM, et al: Competencies needed by graduate respiratory therapists in 2015 and beyond. *Respir Care* 55:601, 2010.
42. Barnes TA, Kacmarek RM, Kageler WV, et al: Transitioning the respiratory therapy workforce for 2015 and beyond. *Respir Care* 56:2011.

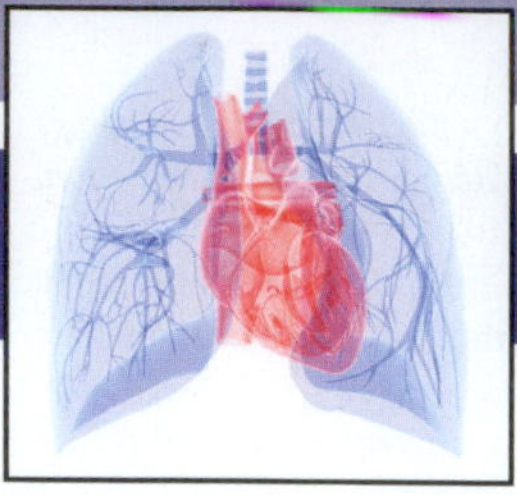

CHAPTER 2

Delivering Evidence-Based Respiratory Care

JAMES K. STOLLER AND ARIEL M. MODRYKAMIEN

CHAPTER OBJECTIVES

After reading this chapter you will be able to:

- Understand the elements for delivering high-quality respiratory care.
- Explain how respiratory care protocols improve the quality of respiratory care services.
- Understand evidence-based medicine.

CHAPTER OUTLINE

Elements of a Hospital-Based Respiratory Care Program: Roles Supporting Quality Care
- Medical Direction
- Respiratory Therapists
- Designations and Credentials of Respiratory Therapists
- Professionalism
- Technical Direction
- Respiratory Care Protocols

Evidence-Based Medicine

Summary Checklist

KEY TERMS

algorithms
Committee on Accreditation for Respiratory Care (CoARC)
evidence-based medicine
The Joint Commission (TJC)
misallocation
National Board for Respiratory Care (NBRC)
performance improvement
quality
respiratory care protocols
respiratory therapy consult service
therapist-driven protocols

Quality is defined as a characteristic reflecting a high degree of excellence, fineness, or grade. Ruskin, a nineteenth-century British author, stated, "Quality is never an accident. It is always the result of intelligent effort." Conclusions drawn from the assessment of quality are only temporary because the components of quality are constantly changing. Specifically, quality, as applied to the practice of respiratory care, has many dimensions. It encompasses the people who administer the respiratory care, the equipment used, and the manner in which the care is provided. Determining the quality of services provided by a respiratory care department requires intelligent efforts to establish guidelines for delivering high-quality care and a method for monitoring the care. The conclusions about how respiratory care has been delivered change as clinical practice and expectations change. In the current cost-attentive era of health care, quality can be challenged by pressures to minimize cost, making the measurement and monitoring of quality even more important. There is a new emphasis on the value of the care that is provided, where value is defined as quality/cost. The higher the quality and the lower the cost, the higher the value will be of the care delivered.

This chapter reviews systems for delivering respiratory care and the evidence that supports providing high-quality respiratory care. In particular, we review the elements of a hospital-based respiratory care program, focusing on medical direction, practitioners, and technical direction. With the goal of high quality being the competent delivery of care that is appropriate, we then discuss respiratory care protocols as an important way to deliver high-quality respiratory care. Finally, we review the concept of evidence-based medicine as it applies to the practice of respiratory care. Other aspects of measuring and monitoring quality and patient safety are discussed in Chapter 3.

ELEMENTS OF A HOSPITAL-BASED RESPIRATORY CARE PROGRAM: ROLES SUPPORTING QUALITY CARE

Medical Direction

The medical director of respiratory care is professionally responsible for the clinical function of the department and provides oversight of the clinical care that is delivered (Box 2-1). Medical direction for respiratory care is usually provided by a pulmonary/critical care physician or an anesthesiologist. Whether the role of a respiratory care service medical director is designated as a full-time or part-time position, it is a full-time responsibility; the medical director must be available on a 24-hour basis for consultation with and to give advice to other physicians and the respiratory care staff. The current philosophy of cost containment and cost-effectiveness, dictated by medical care market forces, poses a challenge to the medical and technical leadership of respiratory care services to provide increasingly high-quality patient care at low cost. A medical director must possess administrative, leadership, and medical skills.[1]

Perhaps the most essential aspect of providing high-quality respiratory care is to ensure that the care being provided is appropriate (i.e., is clinically indicated) and that it is delivered competently. Traditionally, the physician has evaluated patients for respiratory care and has written the specific respiratory therapy orders for the respiratory therapist (RT) to follow. However, such traditional practices often have been associated with what has been called "misallocation of respiratory care."[2-4] Such **misallocation** may consist of ordering therapy that is not indicated, ordering therapy to be delivered by an inappropriate method, or failing to provide therapy that is clinically indicated.[5] Table 2-1 reviews studies evaluating the allocation of respiratory care services and the frequency of misallocated care.[3,6-12] These studies provide much evidence that misallocation of respiratory care occurs frequently. Such misallocation has led to the use of respiratory care protocols that are implemented by RTs (as described in the section on Methods for Enhancing the Quality of Respiratory Care).

Box 2-1 Responsibilities of a Medical Director of Respiratory Care

- Medical supervision of respiratory therapist in the following areas:
  - General medical, surgical, and respiratory nursing wards
  - Intensive care units
  - Ambulatory care (including rehabilitation)
  - Pulmonary function laboratory
- Development and approval of department clinical policies and procedures
- Supervision of ongoing quality assurance activities
- Medical direction for respiratory care in-service and training programs
- Education of medical and nursing staffs regarding respiratory therapy
- Participation in the selection and promotion of technical staff
- Participation in preparing the department budget

Respiratory Therapists

In addition to competent medical direction and using well-constructed respiratory care protocols (see Fig. 2-1), capable RTs are an indispensable element in delivering high-quality respiratory care. The quality of RTs depends primarily on their training, education, experience, and professionalism. Training teaches students to perform tasks at a competent level, whereas clinical education provides students with the knowledge they can use in evaluating a situation for making appropriate decisions.[13] Both adequate training and clinical education are required to produce qualified RTs for assessing patients and implementing respiratory care protocols.[14]

Designations and Credentials of Respiratory Therapists

The two levels of general practice credentialing in respiratory care are (1) certified respiratory therapists (CRTs) and (2) registered respiratory therapists (RRTs). Students eligible to become CRTs and RRTs are trained and educated in colleges and universities. After completion of an approved respiratory care educational program, a graduate may become credentialed by taking the entry-level examination to become a CRT. A CRT may be eligible to sit for the registry examinations to become a credentialed RRT. Students who complete a 2-year program graduate with an associate degree, and students who complete a 4-year program receive a baccalaureate degree. Some RTs go on to complete a graduate degree (e.g., master or doctorate) with additional study in the areas of respiratory care, education, management, or health sciences. The further development of graduate education in respiratory care has been encouraged by the American Association for Respiratory Care (AARC), and several masters-level RT programs are currently available.[15]

Respiratory care education programs are reviewed by the **Committee on Accreditation for Respiratory Care (CoARC).** This committee is sponsored by four organizations: the AARC, the American College of Chest Physicians (ACCP), the American Society of Anesthesiologists (ASA), and the American Thoracic Society (ATS). The CoARC is responsible for ensuring that respiratory therapy educational programs follow accrediting standards or essentials as endorsed by the American Medical Association (AMA). Members of the CoARC visit respiratory therapy educational programs to judge applications for accreditation and make periodic reviews. The mission of the CoARC, in collaboration with the Association of Specialized and Professional Accreditors, is to promote high-quality respiratory therapy education through accreditation services. An annual listing of accredited respiratory therapy programs is published.

TABLE 2-1
Frequency of Misallocation of Respiratory Care Services in Selected Series

Type of Service	Author	Date	Patient Type	No. Patients	Frequency of Overordering	Frequency of Underordering
Supplemental oxygen	Zibrak et al[6]	1986	Adults	NS	55% reduction in incentive spirometry after therapist supervision began	NA
	Brougher et al[7]	1986	Adult, non-ICU inpatients	77	38% ordered to receive O_2 despite adequate oxygenation	NA
	Small et al[8]	1992	Adult, non-ICU inpatients	47	72% of patients checked had PaO_2 > 60 mm Hg or SaO_2 > 90% but were prescribed O_2	NA
	Kester and Stoller[3]	1992	Adult, non-ICU inpatients	230	28% for supplemental O_2	8% for supplemental O_2
	Albin et al[9]	1992	Adult, non-ICU inpatients	274	61% ordered to receive supplemental O_2 despite $SaO_2 \geq 92\%$	21% underordered, including 19% prescribed to receive inadequate O_2 flow rates
	Shelledy et al[12]	2004	Adults	75	0	5.3% indicated but not ordered
Bronchial hygiene techniques	Zibrak et al[6]	1986	Adults	NS	55% reduction in incentive spirometry after therapist supervision began	NA
	Shapiro et al[10]	1988	Adult, non-ICU inpatients	3400 evaluations	61% reduction of bronchial hygiene after system implemented	NA
	Kester and Stoller[3]	1992	Adult, non-ICU inpatients	230	32%	8%
	Shelledy et al[12]	2004	Adults	75	37.5%	8%
Bronchodilator therapy	Zibrak et al[6]	1986	Adults	NS	50% reduction in incentive aerosolized medication after therapist supervision began	NA
	Kester and Stoller[3]	1992	Adult, non-ICU inpatients	230	12%	12%
	Shelledy et al[12]	2004	Adults	75	34.4%	5.3%
	Kester and Stoller[3]	1992	Adult, non-ICU inpatient	230	40%	6.7%
ABGs	Browning et al[11]	1989	Surgical ICU inpatients	724 ABGs	42.7% inappropriately ordered before guidelines implemented	NA

Modified from Stoller JK: The rationale for therapist-driven protocols. Respir Care Clin N Am 2:1, 1996.
ABGs, Arterial blood gases; *ICU,* intensive care unit; *NS,* Not stated; *NA,* not assessed.

As of May 2014, there were approximately 453 CoARC-approved respiratory care programs.

Credentialing is a general term that refers to recognizing individuals in particular occupations or professions. Generally, the two major forms of credentialing in the health fields are state licensure and voluntary certification. Licensure is the process in which a government agency gives an individual permission to practice an occupation. Typically, a license is granted only after verifying that the applicant has demonstrated the minimum competency necessary to protect the public health, safety, or welfare. Licensure laws are normally made by state legislatures and enforced by specific state agencies, such as medical, nursing, and respiratory care boards. In states where licensure laws govern an occupation, practicing in the field without a license is considered a crime punishable by fines or imprisonment or both. Licensure regulations are based on a practice act that defines (and limits) what activities the professional can perform. Two other forms of state credentialing are less restrictive. States that use title protection simply safeguard the use of a particular occupational or professional title. Alternatively, states may request or require practitioners to register with a government agency (registration). Neither title protection nor state registration constitutes a true practice act, and because both title protection and registration are voluntary, neither provides strong protection against unqualified or incompetent practice.

Certification is a voluntary, nongovernment process whereby a private agency grants recognition to an individual who has met certain qualifications. Examples of qualifications are graduating from an approved educational program, completing a specific amount of work experience, and performing acceptably on a qualifying examination. The term *registration* is often used interchangeably with the term *certification,* but it also may refer to a type of government credentialing. As a voluntary process, certification involves standards that are often higher than the minimum standards specified for entry-level competency. A major difference between certification and licensure is that certification generally does not prevent others from working in that occupation, as do most forms of licensure. Both types of credentialing apply in respiratory care.

The primary method of ensuring quality in respiratory care is voluntary certification or registration conducted by the **National Board for Respiratory Care (NBRC).** The NBRC is an independent national credentialing agency for individuals who work in respiratory care and related services. The NBRC is cooperatively sponsored by the AARC, ACCP, ASA, ATS, and National Society for Pulmonary Technology. Representatives of these organizations make up the governing board of the NBRC, which assumes the responsibility for all examination standards and policies through a standing committee. The NBRC provides the credentialing process for both the entry-level CRT and the advanced-practitioner RRT. As established in January 2006, to be eligible for either the CRT or the RRT examination, all candidates must have an associate degree or higher. An additional advanced-practitioner credential, the neonatal/pediatric specialist (NPS), has been established for the field of pediatrics. The NBRC also encourages professionals in the field to maintain and upgrade their skills through voluntary recredentialing. Both CRTs and RRTs may demonstrate ongoing professional competence by retaking examinations. Individuals who pass these examinations are issued a certificate recognizing them as "recredentialed" practitioners. In addition to the certification and registration of RTs, the NBRC provides credentialing in the area of pulmonary function testing for certified pulmonary function technologists (CPFTs) and registered pulmonary function technologists (RPFTs). Since its inception, the NBRC has issued more than 350,000 professional credentials to more than 209,000 individuals. According to United States Bureau of Labor Statistics data from 2012, there were approximately 119,300 active RTs, many of whom hold more than one credential. Table 2-2 shows the distribution of these credentialed individuals.

At the time of publication, 48 states, the District of Columbia, and Puerto Rico have some form of state licensure. Many states use the NBRC entry-level respiratory care examination for state licensing, whereas others simply verify NBRC credentials. Most licensure acts require the RT to attain a specified number of continuing education credits to maintain his or her license. Continuing education helps practitioners keep up to date and aware of the changes and advances that occur in their health care field.

TABLE 2-2
Distribution of Credentialed Practitioners

Credential Type	No. Credentialed Practitioners
CRT	219,830
RRT	130,375
CPFT	12,711
RPFT	4279
NPS	11,491

Note: As of February 2013. Practitioners may hold more than one credential (i.e., RRTs are also CRTs and NPS are also CRTs or RRTs).

Licensure and certification help ensure that only qualified RTs participate in the practice of respiratory care. Many institutions conduct annual skills checks or competency evaluations in compliance with The Joint Commission (TJC, formerly the Joint Commission on Accreditation of Healthcare Organizations [JCAHO]) requirements. Beyond TJC-required skills checks, experience with respiratory care protocols suggests the need to develop and monitor additional skills among RTs (Box 2-2). Ensuring and maintaining these skills require ongoing training and quality review programs, which are discussed in Chapter 3 (see section on Monitoring Quality in Respiratory Care).

Professionalism

By definition, professionalism is a key attribute to which all RTs should aspire and that must guide respiratory care practice. *Webster's New Collegiate Dictionary* defines a *profession* as "a calling that requires specialized knowledge and often long and intensive academic preparation." A professional is characterized as an individual conforming to the technical and ethical standards of a profession. RTs demonstrate their professionalism by maintaining the highest practice standards, engaging in ongoing learning, conducting research to advance the quality of respiratory care, and participating in organized activities through professional societies such as the AARC and associated state societies. Box 2-3 lists the professional attributes of the RT. We emphasize the importance of these attributes because the continued value and progress of the field depend critically on the professionalism of each practitioner.[16]

Box 2-2 Additional Respiratory Therapist Skills Required for Implementing Protocols

- Assess and evaluate patients regarding indications for therapy and for the most appropriate delivery method
- Be cognizant of age-related issues and how they affect the patient's ability to understand and use various treatments
- Adapt hospital policies and procedures to alternative care sites
- Conduct and participate in research activities to ensure a scientific basis for advances in respiratory care technology
- Communicate effectively with all members of the health care team, and advance knowledge in the field of respiratory care

Box 2-3 Professional Characteristics of a Respiratory Therapist

- Completes an accredited respiratory therapy program
- Obtains professional credentials
- Participates in continuing education activities
- Adheres to the code of ethics put forth by the institution or state licensing board or both
- Joins professional organizations

Box 2-4 *Health Insurance Portability and Accountability Act of 1996*

The use and disclosure of protected health information (PHI) by a covered entity are prohibited by the *Health Insurance Portability and Accountability Act* unless it is a permitted use or disclosure for purposes of treatment, payment, or health care operations or is authorized by the patient. When disclosure or use of PHI is permitted, ensure that only the minimum necessary information is disclosed.

DEFINITION OF TERMS

Use: Release of PHI within the institution
Disclosure: Release of PHI outside the institution
PHI: Individually identifiable health information
Covered entity: Health care provider, health plan, health care clearinghouse
Permitted: As long as there are reasonable safeguards in place regarding the Privacy Rule and the information given is the "minimum necessary"
Treatment: Necessary information can be disclosed to all involved in treatment (physicians, nurses, allied health personnel)
Payment: To allow for billing, for insurance purposes and third-party payers
Authorized: Patient's written agreement for permitted use
Minimum necessary: Reasonably necessary to accomplish intended purpose

In the highly regulated careers of health care, professionalism also requires compliance with external standards, such as the standards set by TJC and the government. One such standard is defined by the *Health Insurance Portability and Accountability Act* (HIPAA) of 1996. HIPAA sets standards regarding the way personal health information is communicated and revealed in the transmission of medical records and in the written and verbal communication in the hospital. Some specific provisions of HIPAA are presented in Box 2-4. As with all hospital and health care personnel, standards of respiratory therapy professionalism require knowledge of HIPAA and compliance with its terms.

Technical Direction

Another important element for delivering quality respiratory care is technical direction. Technical direction is often the responsibility of the manager of a respiratory care department, who must ensure the equipment and the associated protocols and procedures have sufficient quality to ensure the safety, health, and welfare of the patient using the equipment. Medical devices are regulated under the *Medical Device Amendment Act* of 1976, which comes under the authority of the U.S. Food and Drug Administration (FDA). The FDA also regulates the drugs that are delivered by RTs. The purpose of the FDA is to establish safety and effectiveness standards and to ensure that these standards are met by equipment and pharmaceutical manufacturers.

Procedures and protocols related to the use of equipment and medications must be written to provide a guide for the respiratory care staff. In addition, equipment must be safety checked and specific maintenance procedures must be performed on a regular basis. Because of rapidly changing respiratory care technology, the job of the technical director poses significant challenges. Circuit boards and computers have replaced simpler mechanical devices. New medications and delivery devices for the treatment of asthma and newer strategies for treating other respiratory diseases (e.g., low-stretch ventilatory approaches for acute respiratory distress syndrome [ARDS]) continue to evolve. Individuals responsible for technical direction must ensure that these new devices, methods, and strategies not only are effective but also have value.

Respiratory Care Protocols

In an effort to improve the delivery and allocation of respiratory care services, **respiratory care protocols** (also known as **therapist-driven protocols**) have been developed and are in use in many hospitals in the United States, Canada, and other countries. Respiratory care protocols are guidelines for delivering appropriate respiratory care treatments and services (i.e., treatments and services that are clinically indicated, delivered by the correct method, and discontinued when no longer needed). Protocols may be written in outline form or may use **algorithms** (an example of which is a branching logic flow diagram [Figures 2-1 and 2-2]).

Gaylin and colleagues[17] conducted a telephone survey in 1999 of 371 RT members of the AARC, of whom 51% were practitioners, 26% were clinical supervisors, and 23% were administrators. When asked if their organizations used guidelines or protocols, 98% of the respondents indicated that they did. Of the 2% who did not, 53% were planning their use. A survey conducted by the AARC in 2005 indicated that of 681 responding hospitals, 73% were providing care by means of at least one protocol.[18] More recently, the 2009 AARC Human Resources Survey showed that of 2764 responders, approximately two-thirds (65.7%) indicated that they have delivered respiratory care by protocol.[19] Finally, in a survey of 348 RT program directors, more than 95% reported teaching RT students how to treat using RT protocols.[20] The use of respiratory care protocols by qualified RTs is a logical practice because well-trained RTs possess extensive knowledge of respiratory care modalities and have the assessment and communication skills required to implement the protocols effectively.[21]

The success of a respiratory care protocol program requires several key elements, including active and committed medical direction, capable RTs, collaboration with physicians and nurses, careful monitoring, and a responsive hospital environment (Box 2-5). As further evidence that RT protocols have been widely adopted, the ACCP has identified the elements of an acceptable respiratory care protocol (Box 2-6). This document may serve as a guide for developing protocols. Protocols may be constructed for individual therapies, such as aerosol therapy, bronchopulmonary hygiene, bronchodilators, O_2 therapy, hyperinflation techniques, suctioning, and pulse oximetry. Protocols also can be written for a specific purpose, such as arterial blood gas (ABG) sampling, weaning from mechanical ventilation, decannulating a tracheostomy, and titrating O_2 therapy.

MINI CLINI

A Specific Treatment Protocol: Aerosolized Bronchodilator Therapy

PROBLEM: A 54-year-old woman is admitted to the hospital with an exacerbation of chronic obstructive pulmonary disease (COPD). She has a history of smoking one and one-half pack of cigarettes per day for 32 years. She is alert and oriented, and her respiratory rate is 32 breaths/min. On auscultation, she has bilateral wheezes on inspiration and exhalation. Her vital capacity (1.3 L) is greater than the predicted minimal volume for effective incentive spirometry, but she is unable to take in a slow, deep breath and hold it for longer than 5 seconds, which is the criterion sometimes used for appropriate metered dose inhaler (MDI) use. What should the RT do now?

SOLUTION: Following the aerosol therapy protocol algorithm, this patient would receive an aerosolized bronchodilator treatment from a small-volume nebulizer with a mouthpiece. An algorithm for aerosolized bronchodilator therapy is shown in Figure 2-1.

MINI CLINI

A Specific Treatment Protocol: Aerosolized Bronchodilator Therapy

PROBLEM: A 70-year-old woman is admitted from the emergency department with an asthma exacerbation. She is a nonsmoker and has advanced dementia. She is alert and calm, and her respiratory rate is 24 breaths/min. She has bilateral wheezes on exhalation. The patient is able to take deep breaths, but she cannot follow simple directions. What would be the bronchodilator device of choice for this patient?

SOLUTION: This patient should receive a small-volume nebulizer, because she does not fulfill MDI criteria (because of her advanced dementia). The aerosolized bronchodilator therapy algorithm that guides this decision is shown in Figure 2-1.

MINI CLINI

A Specific Purpose Protocol: Oxygen Therapy Titration

PROBLEM: A 42-year-old man has returned to a medical-surgical nursing unit from the recovery room after a cholecystectomy. He has no history of lung disease and is wearing a nasal cannula at 2 L/min. He is alert and oriented; his respiratory rate is 18 breaths/min and heart rate is 82 beats/min. When the RT arrives to check his oxygen setup and pulse oximeter reading, his SpO_2 (pulse oximeter reading) is 97% on the 2 L/min nasal cannula. What should the RT do next?

SOLUTION: Following the O_2 therapy titration protocol algorithm, the RT removes the nasal cannula and returns in 15 minutes to recheck the patient's SpO_2 reading, which is now 93% on room air. The RT discontinues the O_2 therapy. An O_2 therapy titration algorithm is shown in Figure 2-2.

Box 2-5 Key Elements of a Respiratory Care Protocol Program

- Strong and committed medical direction
- Capable respiratory therapists (RTs)
- Active quality monitoring
- Collaborative environment among RTs, physicians, and nurses
- Responsiveness of all participants to address and correct problems

Box 2-6 Elements of an Acceptable Respiratory Care Protocol as Described by the American College of Chest Physicians

- Clearly stated objectives
- Outline that includes an algorithm
- Description of alternative choices at decision and action points
- Description of potential complications and corrections
- Description of end points and decision points at which the physician must be contacted
- Protocol program

Successful implementation of protocols requires acceptance by various stakeholders in the hospital, including the hospital administrators, physicians, nurses, and RTs. Hospital administrators are likely to accept RT protocols if they are convinced that protocols enhance patient care, improve allocation of respiratory care services, and reduce costs. Physicians are likely to accept RT protocols if they are convinced that protocols will enhance their patients' care, preserve the physician's ability to specify orders if desired, and maintain the physician's awareness of changes in a patient's condition and changes in the respiratory care plan. Physicians' acceptance also requires their having trust in the quality, professionalism, and competence of the respiratory therapy staff. Nurses are likely to accept protocols if they are persuaded that protocols will enhance the efficiency of care, help relieve sometimes excessive nursing workloads, and preserve communication with the bedside nurse regarding the patient's plan of treatment. Finally, successful implementation and acceptance of protocols by RTs requires a desire to be progressive, confidence in their own assessment and communication skills, "ownership" of the protocol process (e.g., by participating in drafting the protocol policies and strategies by which protocols are put in place), and willingness to change and to abandon outdated task-driven practices in respiratory care.

Features of RT departments that are ready for and embrace change have been studied[22] and are presented in Box 2-7. Steps and tactics to ensure successful implementation of respiratory care protocols are described in Box 2-8. Selecting a planning team with broad membership that includes physicians, nurses, and administrators is a key element in developing a protocol implementation process that avoids potential barriers and satisfies the institution's specific and unique requirements. Once

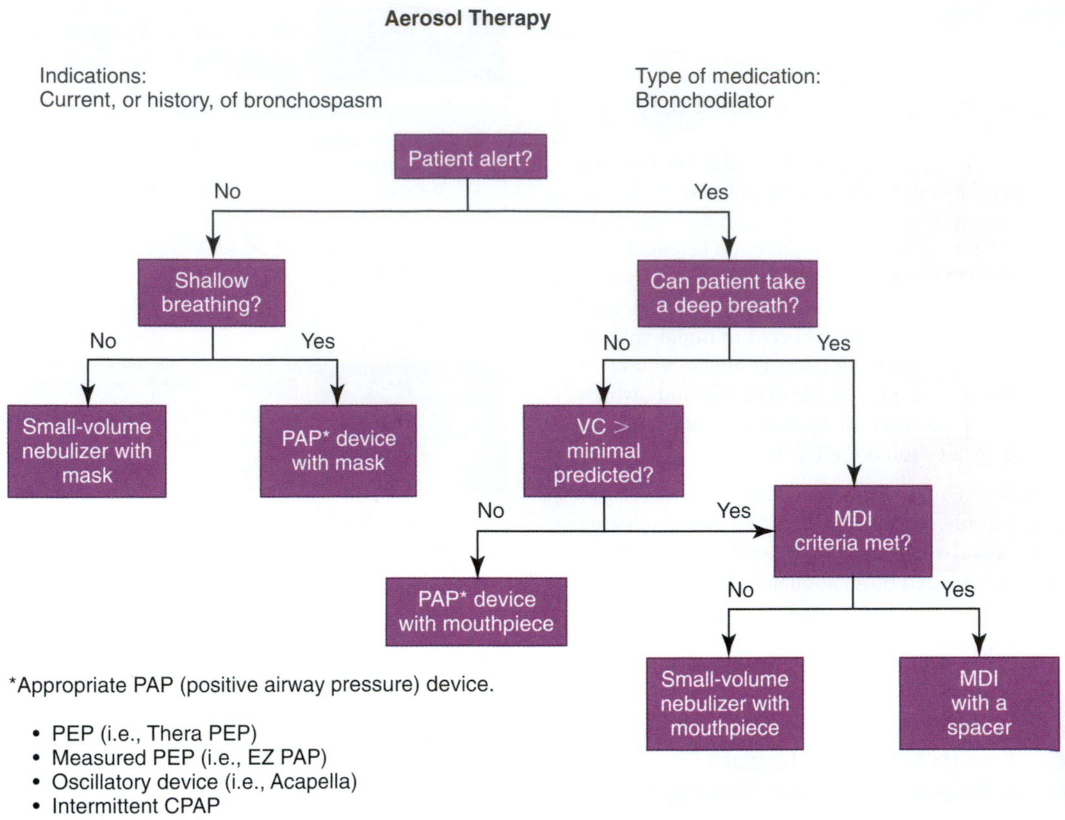

FIGURE 2-1 Respiratory care protocol. Aerosolized bronchodilator therapy algorithm for current or history of bronchospasm. *CPAP,* Continuous positive airway pressure; *MDI,* metered dose inhaler; PAP, positive airway pressure; *PEP,* positive expiratory pressure; *VC,* vital capacity.

Box 2-7 "Highly Desired" Features of a Change-Avid Respiratory Therapy Department

1. Having a close and collegial working relationship between the medical director and the respiratory therapists (RTs)
2. Having a strong and supportive champion for change in the hospital administrative structure (e.g., hospital leaders, medical director)
3. Using data and other evidence to define problems and measure the effectiveness of proposed solutions
4. Using multiple and redundant types of communication to cascade information throughout the respiratory therapy department
5. Being attentive to the forces of resistance and obstacles to change and being able to navigate within institutional systems and people to achieve change
6. Being willing to confront, engage, and gain closure on tough issues
7. Having and maintaining a culture of internal, self-imposed, systematic, ongoing education and knowledge acquisition
8. Consistently rewarding and recognizing change-avid behavior among respiratory therapy department members
9. Fostering ownership for change rather than just complying with external policies and demands and, as part of this ownership, taking the time to identify and involve stakeholders (e.g., physicians, nurses, hospital thought leaders and decision makers) in change
10. Paying attention to leadership development and succession planning in the RTs
11. Having and communicating a vision in the department

From Stoller JK, Kester L, Roberts VT, et al: An analysis of features of respiratory therapy departments that are avid for change. Respir Care 53:871, 2008.

protocols have been designed, it is often advisable to do pilot studies, either of each protocol individually or of a group of protocols on a single hospital floor or unit. By using this staged rollout with an initial pilot trial, unexpected problems can be worked out and helpful feedback can be gathered from protocol users before the protocols are implemented on a hospital-wide basis.

A comprehensive approach for using protocols is to combine specific protocols to form a **respiratory therapy consult service** or an evaluate-and-treat program, which is used in institutions such as the Cleveland Clinic and the University of California at San Diego. With the use of a respiratory therapy consult service, the sequence of events for a respiratory therapy consult may occur as shown in Box 2-9.

A carefully structured assessment tool and care plan form (Figures 2-3 and 2-4) are essential elements for a comprehensive protocol program. These tools help ensure consistency among therapist evaluators. The following Mini Clini on Writing a

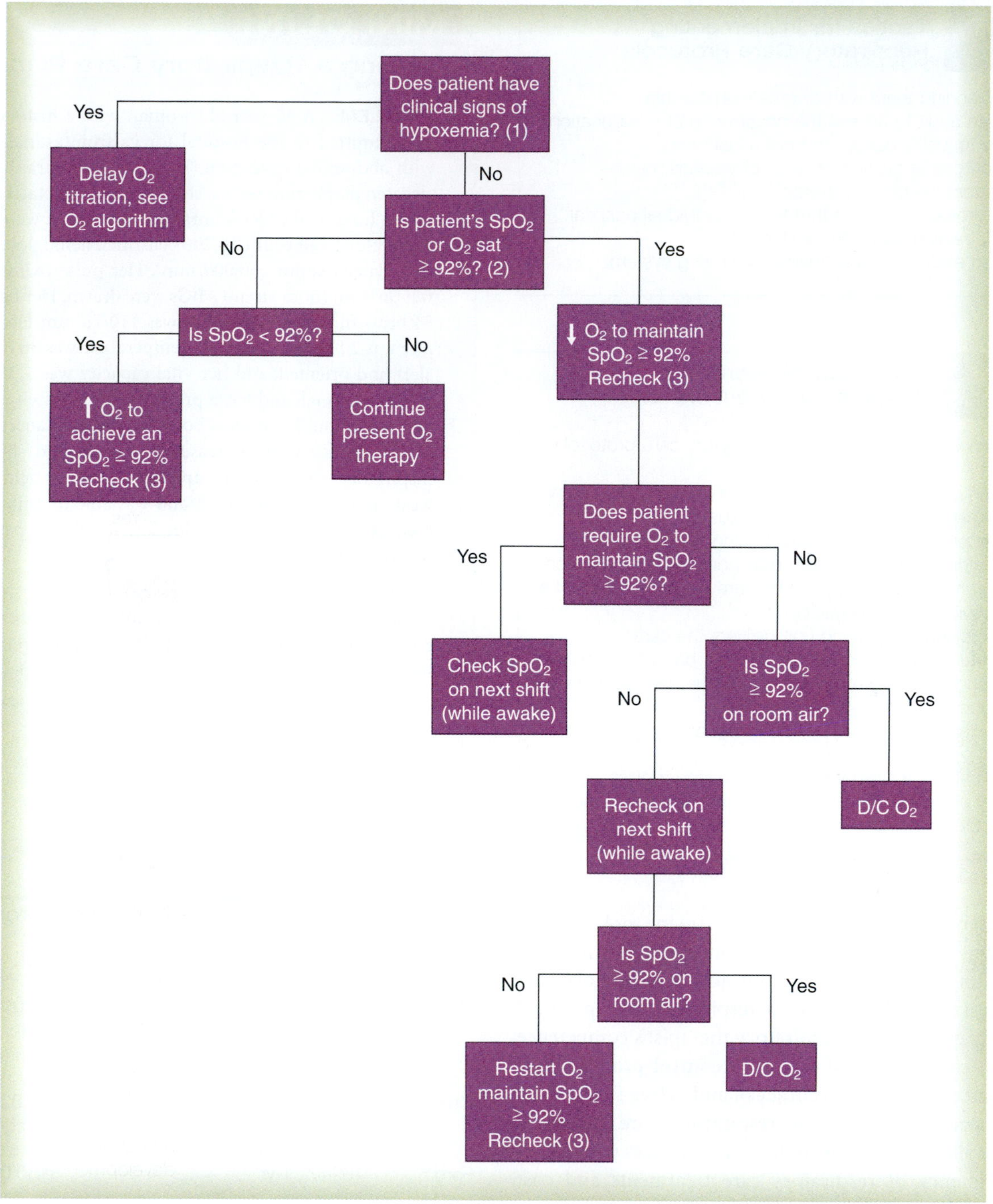

FIGURE 2-2 Respiratory care protocol to determine when oxygen concentration should be increased or decreased or when the therapy should be discontinued. *(1)* Shortness of breath, tachycardia, diaphoresis, confusion. *(2)* O_2 saturation measured by pulse oximeter (SpO_2) criteria may be modified with documented evidence of preexisting chronic hypoxemia. *(3)* Appropriate time lapse for recheck: 10 minutes for patients without pulmonary history; 20 minutes for patients with pulmonary history. *NOTE:* O_2 concentration should not be decreased more than once per shift. *D/C,* Discontinue.

Box 2-8 Tactics for Implementing Respiratory Care Protocols

1. Select a planning team with diverse membership.
2. Conduct an audit to assess the occurrence of misallocation of therapy to justify departure from usual care.
3. Identify sources of resistance (e.g., physicians, nurses, administrators, respiratory therapists [RTs]).
4. Design a protocol program that fits the individual hospital.
5. Develop a training program for RTs.
6. Develop an evaluation and quality monitoring system.

Box 2-9 Sequence of Events for a Respiratory Care Consult

1. A physician writes an order for a respiratory care protocol or consult.
2. A physician order entry system or the nursing unit secretary notifies a respiratory therapist (RT) evaluator.
3. The evaluator assesses the patient using specific guidelines.
4. The evaluator writes a care plan using designated indications and algorithms and documents the care plan in the patient's chart for review by the physician.
5. The RT covering the nursing unit delivers the care.
6. The patient is assessed on a shift-by-shift basis for changes in status and indicated modifications for the care plan, which are also documented.
7. The physician is notified of any deterioration in the patient's status.
8. When indications for respiratory care no longer exist, respiratory care treatment is discontinued, and notification is placed in the patient's chart.

Respiratory Care Plan shows how an assessment tool and care plan document, used along with corresponding algorithms, can guide therapists in developing an appropriate respiratory care plan. Other essential elements of a respiratory care protocol service include ensuring the respiratory therapist's competence to deliver the care as part of a quality control program (see Figure 2-5) and assessing the accuracy of audits (see Figure 2-6).

Demonstrated advantages of respiratory care protocols include better allocation of respiratory care services without an increased frequency of respiratory care treatments and cost savings (Tables 2-3 and 2-4). Other advantages include more responsive respiratory care with more adjustment of respiratory care services to keep pace with patients' changing clinical status and more versatile use of respiratory care services (Table 2-5).[12,23-26]

RULE OF THUMB

Respiratory care protocols have been shown to help ensure that the correct respiratory care treatments are delivered to the patients who are likely to benefit from the therapy (i.e., improved allocation of respiratory care).

MINI CLINI

Writing a Respiratory Care Plan

PROBLEM: A 40-year-old woman with a history of asthma was admitted to the hospital for gastrointestinal dysmotility with abdominal distention. Her chest radiograph showed an elevated diaphragm with accompanying atelectasis in the bases of the lung fields. Her laboratory test results were as follows: white blood cell count 10,200 cells/mcl, hemoglobin 11.6 g/dl, and platelet count 260,000/mm^3. Her pulse oximetry reading was 96% on room air; no ABGs were drawn. Her heart rate was 84 beats/min, blood pressure was 110/78 mm Hg, respiratory rate was 20 breaths/min, and temperature was 36.8° C. She was alert and oriented, and her vital capacity was 1.35 L. She is 5 feet 7 inches tall and has a predicted minimal vital capacity of 0.927 L (15 ml/kg of ideal body weight). On auscultation, her breath sounds were decreased bilaterally and she had slight inspiratory wheezes in the apices of her lung fields. She had a weak, nonproductive cough and was able to ambulate on her own. A respiratory care evaluation should be performed for this patient.

SOLUTIONS: The patient's assessment score sheet and her respiratory therapy care plan, using the respiratory therapy consult protocol and treatment algorithms currently in use at the Cleveland Clinic, are shown (see Figures 2-3 and 2-4).

TABLE 2-3 Cost Savings Associated With Respiratory Care Protocols

Author	Date	Duration of Study	Cost Savings
Hart et al[36]	1989	3 mo	$4316 (decrease in actual costs)
Walton et al[37]	1990	6 yr	9.7% (decrease in charges)
Orens[38]	1993	1 yr	$81,826 (decrease in costs for one nursing unit)
Ford[39]	1994	1 yr	$150,000 (decrease in costs)
Komara and Stoller[40]	1995	40 postsurgical patients; oxygen use up to 6 days	53.3% (decrease in costs)
Shrake et al[41]	1996	2 years, 4420 patients; cost comparisons: 3 months after protocol	$15,337 for 3 study months, annualized to $61,348/year
Stoller et al[25]	1998	1 year, 145 patients	$20 (decrease in true costs/patient)
Kollef et al[26]	2000	9 months, 694 patients	$186 (decrease in charges/patient)
Shelledy et al[12]	2004	3 months, 75 patients	$75,395 (estimated annual decrease)

Modified from Haney DJ: Therapist-driven protocols for adult non-intensive care unit patients: availability and efficacy. Respir Care Clin N Am 2:93, 1996.

The Cleveland Clinic Foundation
Department of Pulmonary Disease
Respiratory Therapy Evaluation

Date: ___ /___ /___ Age: 40

Time: ______________ Ht: 5' 7"

Diagnosis: ______________

Respiratory therapist ______________

Inpatient ID label

Chart Assessment

Clinical findings	0	X	1	X	2	X	3	X	4	X	Points
Pulmonary status	(−) History (−) Smoking		Smoking history <1 pk a day		Smoking history ≥1 pk a day		Pulmonary impairment (acute or chronic)	X	Severe or chronic with exacerbation		3
Surgical status	No surgery	X	General surgery		Lower abdominal		Thoracic or upper abdominal		Thoracic with pulmonary disease		0
Chest x-ray	Clear or not indicated		Chronic changes or x-ray pending		Infiltrates, atelectasis or pleural effusions	X	Infiltrations in more than one lobe		Infiltrate + atelectasis ±pleural effusion		2

Lab test: Date: ___/___/___ WBC 10.2 Hb 11.6 Plts 260k

Date: ___/___/___ | pH | $PaCO_2$ | PaO_2 | HCO_3 | Sat/FIO_2

Pulmonary function test: Minimal pred. VC 0.927L VC 1.35L Peak flow ______

SpO_2/FIO_2 96% RA

Vital signs: HR 84 BP 110/70 RR 20 Temperature (24 hr max)

Patient Assessment

Clinical findings		X		X		X		X		X	Points
Respiratory pattern	Regular pattern RR 12-20	X	Increased RR 21-25		Dyspnea on exertion, irregular pattern RR 26-30		Decreased vital capacity* RR 31-35		Severe SOB, use of accessory muscles RR > 35		0
Mental status	Alert, oriented, cooperative	X	Lethargic, follows commands		Confused, does not follow commands		Obtunded		Comatose		0
Breath sounds	Clear to auscultation		Decreased unilaterally		Decreased bilaterally	X	Crackles in the bases		Wheezing and/or rhonchi	X	4
Cough effectiveness	Strong, spontaneous, nonproductive		Strong, productive		Weak, nonproductive	X	Weak, productive or weak with rhonchi		No spontaneous cough or may require suctioning		2
Level of activity	Ambulatory	X	Ambulatory with assistance		Temporarily nonambulatory		Bed rest, able to position self		Bed rest, unable to position self		0
Oxygen required for $SpO_2 < 92\%$	No oxygen	X	1-3 liters		4-6 liters		>50% <100%		100%		0

Total points 11

*VC × 10 minimal predicted:

Predicted ideal body weight
(males: 50 + 2.54 x inches >60)
(females: 45 + 2.54 × inches >60)
Multiply above ideal body wt. × 15 cc for min. pred. VC

Triage 1	Triage 2	Triage 3	Triage 4	Triage 5
>20	(16-20)	(11-15)	(6-10)	(0-5)

Triage # 3

FIGURE 2-3 Evaluation form for guiding a standardized patient assessment and assigning a severity of respiratory illness score. The score for the greatest degree of dysfunction for each assessment category is written in the right-hand column and tallied to determine the severity of respiratory illness (triage) score. *RR,* Respiratory rate; *VC,* vital capacity. (Courtesy Cleveland Clinic Respiratory Institute, Cleveland, Ohio.)

Respiratory Therapy Consult/Evaluation

Your patient has been evaluated by the Respiratory Therapy Consult Service. Based on the patient's clinical indicators, the Care Plan designated below will be implemented.

IMPRINT/LABEL

Date of Evaluation ____________________

Time of Evaluation ____________________

Diagnosis(es) GI dysmotility

Hx asthma

Post Thoracic Surgery Protocol ☐

Clinical Indications

Aerosol Therapy	Broncho/Pulm Hygiene	Hyperinflation	Oxygen Therapy	Respiratory Monitoring	Suctioning
☒ Bronchospasm	☐ Productive cough	☒ Atelectasis	☐ $SpO_2 < 92\%$ on room air	☐ O_2 titration (pulse ox.)	☐ Presence of secretions
☒ History of bronchospasm	☐ Rhonchi on auscultation	☐ Upper abdominal or thoracic surgery, or COPD & surgery	☐ $PaO_2 <$ 55 mm Hg on room air	☐ Unstable resp. status	☐ Unable to cough effectively
☐ Inflammation/ mucosal edema	☐ History of mucous prod. disease	☐ Restrictive disease associated with quadriplegia and/ or dysfunctional diaphragm	☐ Clinical signs of hypoxemia	☐ $SpO_2 < 92\%$ on room air or 4 Lpm O_2 (ABGs)	☐ Altered consciousness
☐ Proteinaceous secretions	☐ Patient unable to deep breathe and cough spontaneously			Oximetry sat/FIO_2: 96%/RA	Vital capacity: 1.35 l
☐ Home regimen					
☐ Physician order					

Care Plan

Aerosol Therapy

	DPI	Neb.	MDI	Frequency
Albuterol			X	QID and prn
				at night

				Frequency
bph	☐ Pos. drainage	☐ Percussion/vibration	☐ Coughing techniques	
Hyperinflation	☒ Incen. spiro.	☐ CPAP/PEP	☐ IPPB	To be used q1hr
Oxygen Therapy	☐ FIO_2 % ____	☐ Liters/minute________		
Monitoring	☐ Pulse oximetry	☐ ABGs	☐ Resp. mechanics	
Suctioning	☐ Nasal-tracheal	☐ Tracheal		

Comments Patient needs encouragement to cough effectively.

Triage Number 3

Signature: Respiratory Therapy Evaluator

Print Name: ____________________ /Beeper: __________

Care plan modifications, made in response to changes in the patient's condition, are available for your review through the Phamis Last Word computer system.

FIGURE 2-4 Care plan form for recording a patient's indications for therapy and the therapeutic modalities for treating the indications. *ABGs,* Arterial blood gases; *COPD,* chronic obstructive pulmonary disease; *CPAP,* continuous positive airway pressure; *GI,* gastrointestinal; *Hx,* history; *IPPB,* intermittent positive pressure breathing; *Incen. spiro.,* incentive spirometer; *PEP,* positive expiratory pressure; *RA,* room air. (Courtesy Cleveland Clinic Respiratory Institute, Cleveland, Ohio.)

Skills Checklist

Suctioning

Date ________ (mm/dd/yyyy) First name ________ Last name ________ Employee number ________
Use your employee number only, Do NOT use any letters.

Supervisor ________ Observed by ________ (Last name, first name)

Patient or simulation? ☐ Patient ☐ Simulation Last 4 digits of patient MRN ________ (If applicable) Unit ________ (Enter as unit-bed number ex. H81-15 or G111-09)

Age (If applicable) ☐ Neonate/infant (0-18 mos.) ☐ Child (19 mos.-8 yrs.) ☐ Adolescent (9-18 yrs.) ☐ Adult (19-69 yrs.) ☐ Geriatric (70+yrs.)

Did the RT interact appropriately with the patient with regard to the specific age category listed above? (If applicable)	☐ Yes	☐ No
According to section standards		
Prepare equipment and assess patient 1. Verify order, verifies patient using at least 2 patient identifiers (Name, MRN, DOB) 2. Introduce self and explains procedure (If applicable) 3. Correctly assemble the equipment per procedure manual, suction kit, manual resuscitator, oxygen, saline for lavage, suction source (wall outlet: 80-120 mm Hg portable: 3-5 inches Hg), lubricating jelly for nasotracheal route	☐ Yes	☐ No
Observe OSHA standards for universal precautions	☐ Yes	☐ No
Pre-assesses patient 1. Heart rate 2. Respiratory rate 3. Breath sounds 4. Pulse oximetry	☐ Yes	☐ No
Perform suctioning procedure 1. Maintain sterile technique 2. Pre-oxygenate 3. Hyper-inflate at least 5-6 times with artificial airways 4. Suction 5. Lubricate catheter for nasotracheal route 6. Insert catheter smoothly as far as possible, careful to stop on encountering resistance 7. Apply suction intermittently as catheter is withdrawn 8. Suction period should not exceed 15 seconds 9. Oxygenate and hyper-inflate after each pass with the catheter 10. Lavage as needed 11. Repeat until airways are clear or as the patient tolerates 12. Note amount, color, and consistency of any secretions	☐ Yes	☐ No
Post treatment assessment 1. Heart rate 2. Respiratory rate 3. Breath sounds 4. Cough 5. Sputum 6. Mental status 7. Activity	☐ Yes	☐ No
Assures patient safety and clean environment 1. Removes all other trash from bed and area 2. Verifies medical support systems are intact (ex. oxygen) 3. Ensures patient safety (ex. bedrails are up)	☐ Yes	☐ No
Charts appropriately 1. Charts correctly in Mediserve in a timely manner 2. Includes any complications and/or adverse events and informs physician	☐ Yes	☐ No
Comments		

FIGURE 2-5 Example of a skills checklist for suctioning. *DOB,* Date of birth; *MRN,* medical record number.

Stamp Here

Care Plan Audit

Date:__________________________
Auditor:________________________
Therapist:_______________________

Diagnosis:____________________________________

A = Auditor
T = Therapist

Triage Score

	0	1	2	3	4
Pulmonary Status					
Surgical Status					
Chest X-Ray					
Respiratory Pattern					
Mental Status					
Breath Sounds					
Cough					
Level of Activity					
Oxygen Requirement					

The triage score was __________% correct.* Total A___ T___

*"% Correct" defined as the percent of auditor's scores (for each of the eight axes) with which the therapist's score agrees.

Care Plan

	Aerosol	bph	Hyperinflation	Oxygen	Pulse Ox	Suctioning
A = Auditor						
T = Therapist						

The care plan was _____% correct.*

*"% Correct" defined as (number of agreements)/six (total items for therapy).

Care plan complete? Yes No

Evaluation on time? Yes No

Frequencies correct? Yes No

Comments:____

FIGURE 2-6 Form for providing feedback to therapist evaluators on their patient assessment and care plan writing performance. Agreement is indicated by an *A* (auditor) and a *T* (therapist) in the same triage scoring box or therapeutic category. (Courtesy Cleveland Clinic Respiratory Institute, Cleveland, Ohio.)

EVIDENCE-BASED MEDICINE

Another important concept regarding high-quality care is evidence-based medicine. **Evidence-based medicine** refers to an approach to determining optimal clinical management based on several practices, as follows[28-32]: (1) a rigorous and systematic review of available evidence, (2) a critical analysis of available evidence to determine which conclusions are most sound and applicable, and (3) a disciplined approach to incorporating the literature with personal practice and experience. In a broader context, evidence-based medicine can be thought of as understanding and using the best quality evidence available (i.e., the best-designed, most rigorous clinical trials) to support the most appropriate and correct possible clinical decisions.

In rating the quality of scientific evidence, it is important to recognize the various designs and types of study designs from which scientific evidence comes.[32] This section reviews these designs. The simplest and least rigorous design is a single case

TABLE 2-4

Summary of Available Randomized Trials on the Effectiveness of Respiratory Care Protocols

Clinical Activity	Author	Date	No. Patients	Findings
Weaning from mechanical ventilation	Kollef et al[43]	1997	357	Use of protocols was associated with shorter duration of mechanical ventilation
	Ely et al[44]	1996	300	Routine daily trials of spontaneous breathing trials were associated with shorter duration of mechanical ventilation
	Marelich et al[45]	2000	253	Use of protocols shortened duration of mechanical ventilation
Respiratory care protocol service	Stoller et al[25]	1998	145	Use of respiratory therapy consult service was associated with improved allocation of respiratory care service with lower costs and no adverse events
	Kollef et al[26]	2000	694	Use of respiratory protocol service was associated with fewer orders discordant with guidelines and lower charges

From Stoller JK: Are respiratory therapists effective? Assessing the evidence. Respir Care 46:56, 2001.

TABLE 2-5

Changes in Modalities After Protocol Implementation

Author	Date	Observed Reductions in Misallocated Therapy After Implementation of Protocols (%)	Change from Before Protocol to Current Status
Hart et al[36]	1989	37 (aerosol, hyperinflation)	48%-11%
Walton et al[37]	1990	49.1 (aerosol, chest physiotherapy)	
Beasley et al[46]	1992	11.9% (blood gas use)	42.7%-30.8%
Ford,[39] 1994		57% (aerosol, chest physiotherapy)	7000-4000 treatments
Orens,[38] 1993		35% (aerosol, bronchopulmonary, hygiene, hyperinflation oxygen, oximetry)	

From Haney DJ: Therapist-driven protocols for adult non-intensive care unit patients: availability and efficacy. Respir Care Clin N Am 2:93, 1996.

report, in which a new clinical issue or problem is described in a single patient. A description of the favorable outcome of using a new mode of mechanical ventilation in one patient with refractory hypoxemia is an example of a single case report. Although single case reports have value in pointing out new insights and new possibilities for treatment, disease associations, or disease causation, they cannot prove the effectiveness of a treatment or the causality of a risk factor because, by nature, they lack a control or comparison group (i.e., a group that is similar to the patient or patients described, differing only in whether the risk factor of interest was present or the treatment of interest was applied). Collecting a group of patients with similar clinical features is called a case series and may have greater impact than a single case report because it suggests that the issue is more general than in a single patient alone. However, like a single case report, a case series cannot prove the efficacy of a treatment or the causality of a risk factor because no comparison or control group is included.

Cohort studies, which compare the clinical outcomes in two compared groups (or cohorts), generally have greater scientific rigor than case studies or case series and consist of two broad types of study designs: observational cohort studies and randomized controlled trials. In trying to establish whether a treatment works (i.e., has efficacy), an observational cohort study compares the outcomes between two groups of patients when the treatment is allocated to one group but not the other. More specifically, an observational cohort study of a new mode of mechanical ventilation would compare the outcomes between two groups of similar patients (i.e., especially similar with regard to their risk for developing the outcome measure that is being studied) when the mode of mechanical ventilation is determined either by physician choice (i.e., the physician decided to use this treatment in this patient) or by patient choice. In contrast to an observational cohort study, in a randomized controlled trial, sometimes regarded as the most methodologically rigorous study design (when well conducted), the outcomes of two similar groups of patients are compared when the use of the new mode of mechanical ventilation is determined not by patient or physician choice but rather by chance alone (randomization). When ideally designed and conducted, a randomized controlled treatment trial eliminates all sources of bias that would prevent attributing differences in outcomes between the compared groups to anything other than the treatment that is being studied. In this way, randomization can "isolate" the effect of the treatment. Said differently, at its best, a randomized controlled treatment trial provides rigorous evidence about the efficacy of the treatment because all other potential biases and confounding variables (e.g., features of the compared patient groups, other medications, or other treatments that the study participants are receiving) are eliminated from consideration. This allows the investigators and the readers of the clinical trial results to confidently attribute outcome differences between the compared groups to the treatment that is being studied.

Different types of the randomized controlled trials exist and include the parallel-control study and the crossover study (Figure 2-7). Parallel-control treatment studies compare two groups: one receives the treatment being studied, and the other receives the control treatment. Sometime after the end of the treatment, outcomes in the two groups are assessed and compared, especially regarding the main outcome of interest in the study. For example, a parallel-control randomized trial of low-stretch ventilation for ARDS would compare one group of patients receiving low-stretch ventilation with another (otherwise similar) group receiving higher stretch ventilator settings, and the two groups would be compared after a prespecified period with regard to key outcomes, such as survival, discharge from the intensive care unit, and organ system failures. This very design was used in the ARDSNet parallel-control randomized controlled trial that showed the superiority of using a tidal volume of 6 ml/kg (ideal body weight) in managing patients with acute lung injury or ARDS.[33]

In the other type of randomized controlled trial—the crossover trial—the study treatment is first administered to one group of study subjects while the other group receives the control or comparison treatment, and then, after measuring outcomes and a subsequent "washout period" (in which the effects of the initial treatment decay and wear off fully), the group initially given the study treatment receives the control treatment and the group initially given the control treatment receives the study treatment. The crossover study design offers a statistical advantage of greater power to detect a difference between the compared groups, which means that fewer study participants are required to find a statistically significant difference, if one exists. However, crossover studies can be performed only when the effects of the initial treatment administered to the first study group can wear off completely (or so-called washout), allowing the study group to return to its baseline state before the alternative treatment is administered. When the effects of treatment are permanent (e.g., surgery, radiation therapy), a crossover trial involving that treatment cannot be done because washout of the treatment effect is not possible.

Evidence-based medicine requires knowledge of how to analyze carefully the results of clinical trials (e.g., randomized controlled trials and observational cohort studies) and how to apply the results of such research to high-quality clinical practice. Other tools of evidence-based medicine include systematically reviewing the available literature, or what is called *meta-analysis* of the literature.[29,30] A meta-analysis of a clinical question (e.g., does a low-stretch mechanical ventilation strategy improve survival in ARDS?)[33] identifies, analyzes, and summarizes the body of literature about this topic by assessing the quality of the available evidence and giving greater weight to better designed, more rigorous studies. Sometimes, meta-analyses pool the actual data from different trials together when pooling is scientifically and statistically permissible. In other instances (called *narrative analyses*), the meta-analysis simply evaluates the quality of the data from each available trial (based on explicit methodologic criteria) to offer a conclusion about the clinical issue.

A meta-analysis performed as part of an evidence-based approach to determining the optimal ventilatory approach for ARDS might weigh the results of large randomized clinical trials of low-stretch versus conventional tidal volume approach mechanical ventilation more heavily than the results of small observational studies. As an example of a narrative meta-analysis, a 2003 evidence-based review of the management of individuals with alpha-1 antitrypsin deficiency issued graded recommendations for testing for this genetic cause of COPD.[34]

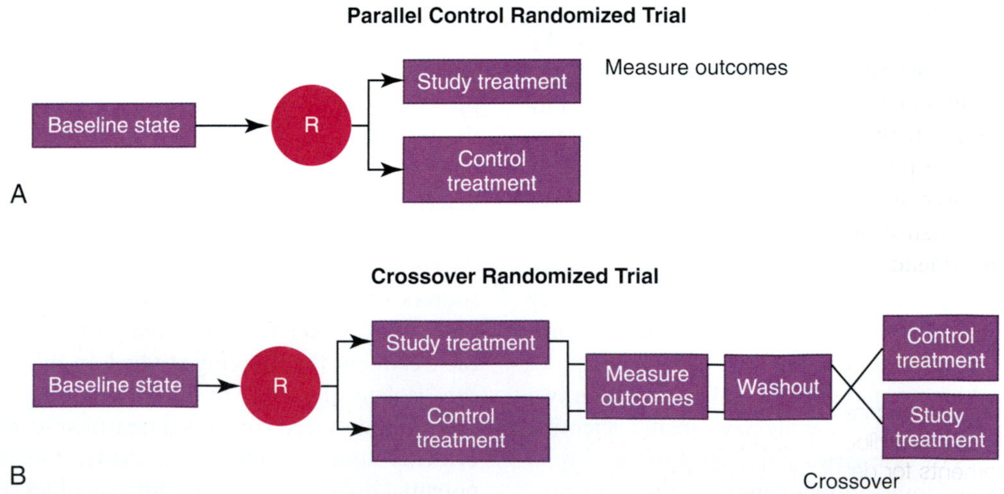

FIGURE 2-7 Study design of the two types of randomized controlled trial: parallel-control and crossover. In a parallel-control trial, after randomization *(R)*, one group receives the study treatment, while the control group receives the comparison treatment (possibly a placebo). At the end of the subsequent observation period, study outcomes are measured, and the trial is over. In a crossover trial, one group initially receives the study treatment and the other group receives the comparison treatment; outcomes are measured; and after a washout period (see text), each group receives the alternative treatment for another period, after which outcomes are measured again.

A level A recommendation (i.e., that testing should be performed) was issued to test all symptomatic adults with airflow obstruction on pulmonary function tests (whether carrying the diagnosis of emphysema, COPD, or asthma in which airflow obstruction fails to reverse completely with bronchodilators), asymptomatic individuals with persistent airflow obstruction on pulmonary function tests with identifiable risk factors (e.g., cigarette smoking, occupational exposure), individuals with unexplained liver disease, and adults with the skin condition necrotizing panniculitis.[34] Although the hope is that issuing such evidence-based guidelines will improve the care that such individuals receive by allowing clinicians to access efficiently the best available information, experience suggests that clinicians may sometimes be slow to adopt the best available evidence in caring for their patients.[35]

RULE OF THUMB

The randomized controlled clinical trial is often considered to be the most rigorous type of study design to prove the efficacy of a treatment. The optimal randomized controlled clinical trial is designed to be free from bias that can confuse the study results and is well-conducted.

Although some authors point out that evidence-based medicine does not differ from prior practice in which clinicians were always called on to analyze carefully available data and make clinical judgments based on the best quality information available, evidence-based medicine does specify precise methods for analyzing available information and allowing the clinician to judge best the available evidence. As a measure of the importance of evidence-based medicine in respiratory care, several articles in *Respiratory Care* considered the effectiveness of RTs and of various respiratory care treatment modalities using an evidence-based approach.[28-30] The Clinical Practice Guidelines of the AARC are being systematically reviewed to reflect the rigorous techniques of evidence-based medicine and to ensure that guidelines for respiratory care management reflect the best available evidence.[30] The proof that low-stretch ventilation is associated with improved survival in patients with ARDS and the methods used to enhance awareness of this best practice are further examples of evidence-based medical practice.

SUMMARY CHECKLIST

- High-quality respiratory care can be defined as the competent delivery of indicated respiratory care services.
  - Essential elements for delivering quality respiratory care include:
    - Energetic and competent medical direction
    - Methods for providing indicated and appropriate respiratory care
    - Educated, competent respiratory care personnel
    - Adequate, well-maintained equipment
    - Intelligent system for monitoring **performance improvement**
- Delivery of high-quality respiratory care requires the combined activities of a qualified and committed medical director and capable RTs and can be enhanced by well-constructed respiratory care protocols.
- Respiratory care protocols are guidelines for delivering appropriate respiratory care services and are widely used in current respiratory care practice.
- Available evidence suggests that use of respiratory care protocols can improve allocation of respiratory care services. In doing so, the use of respiratory care protocols lessens misallocation of respiratory care.
  - Misallocation of respiratory care services, which hinders the delivery of high-quality respiratory care, can be defined as overordering or underordering of respiratory care services and is common in current practice.
- Practitioner credentialing is important in respiratory care; the RRT represents the highest credential and is based on successful completion of the NBRC examination.
- Maintaining and improving quality requires ongoing monitoring, as may be accomplished by quality audits and repeated competence testing of RTs.
- Evidence-based medicine is an approach to determining the best possible patient management based on critically assessing the available evidence. It is recommended that RTs use this approach as they assess the information that is available regarding respiratory care management strategies.

References

1. Stoller JK: Medical direction of respiratory care: past and present. *Respir Care* 43:217, 1998.
2. Stoller JK: Misallocation of respiratory care services: time for a change (editorial). *Respir Care* 38:263, 1993.
3. Kester L, Stoller JK: Ordering respiratory care services for hospitalized patients: practices of overuse and underuse. *Cleve Clin J Med* 59:581, 1992.
4. Kallam A, Meyerink A, Modrykamien A: Physician-order aerosol therapy versus respiratory therapy-driven protocol: the effect on resource utilization. *Respir Care* 58:431, 2013.
5. Stoller JK: Why therapist-driven protocols? A balanced view (editorial). *Respir Care* 39:706, 1994.
6. Zibrak JD, Rossetti P, Wood E: Effect of reductions in respiratory therapy on patient outcomes. *N Engl J Med* 315:292, 1986.
7. Brougher LI, Blackwelder AK, Grossman GD, et al: Effectiveness of medical necessity guidelines in reducing cost of oxygen therapy. *Chest* 39:646, 1986.
8. Small D, Duha A, Weiskopf B, et al: Uses and misuses of oxygen in hospitalized patients. *Am J Med* 92:591, 1992.
9. Albin RJ, Criner GJ, Thomas S, et al: Pattern of non-ICU inpatient supplemental oxygen utilization in a university hospital. *Chest* 102:1992, 1672.
10. Shapiro BA, Cane RD, Peterson J, et al: Authoritative medical direction can assure cost-beneficial bronchial hygiene therapy. *Chest* 93:1038, 1988.
11. Browning JA, Kaiser DL, Durbin CG: The effect of guidelines on the appropriate use of arterial blood gas analysis in the intensive care unit. *Respir Care* 34:269, 1989.
12. Shelledy DC, LeGrand TS, Peters JI: An assessment of the appropriateness of respiratory care delivered at a 450 bed acute care Veterans Affairs hospital. *Respir Care* 49:907–916, 2004.
13. Kester L, Stoller JK: Respiratory care education: current issues and future challenges (editorial). *Respir Care* 41:98, 1996.

14. Stoller JK: Are respiratory therapists effective? Assessing the evidence. *Respir Care* 46:56, 2001.
15. Stoller JK: The future of respiratory therapy (RT) research and scholarship: when you're finished changing, you're finished. *Can J Respir Therapy* 46:8, 2010.
16. Beachey WD: A comparison of problem-based learning and traditional curricula in baccalaureate respiratory therapy education. *Respir Care* 52: 1497, 2007.
17. Gaylin DS, Shapiro JR, Mendelson DN, et al: The role of respiratory care practitioners in a managed healthcare system: emerging areas of clinical practice. *Am J Manag Care* 5:749, 1999.
18. Dubbs W: By the numbers: results from the AARC's 2005 human resources study. *AARC Times* 30:37, 2005.
19. American Association for Respiratory Care: *2009 human resources survey of respiratory therapists*. American Association for Respiratory Care, 2009. <http://www.aarc.org>. Accessed May 1, 2015.
20. Barnes TA, Kacmarek RM, Durbin CG, Jr: Survey of respiratory therapy education program directors in the United States. *Respir Care* 56:2011, 1906.
21. Stoller JK: The rationale for therapist-driven protocols. *Respir Care Clin N Am* 2:1, 1996.
22. Stoller JK, Kester L, Roberts VT, et al: An analysis of features of respiratory therapy departments that are avid for change. *Respir Care* 53:871, 2008.
23. Stoller JK, Haney D, Burkhart J, et al: Physician-ordered respiratory care vs. physician-ordered use of a respiratory therapy consult service: early experience at the Cleveland Clinic Foundation. *Respir Care* 38:1143, 1993.
24. Stoller JK, Skibinski C, Giles D, et al: Physician-ordered respiratory care vs. physician-ordered use of a respiratory therapy consult service: results of a prospective observational study. *Chest* 110:422, 1996.
25. Stoller JK, Mascha EJ, Kester L, et al: Randomized controlled trial of physician-directed versus respiratory therapy consult service-directed respiratory care to adult non-ICU inpatients. *Am J Respir Crit Care Med* 158:1068, 1998.
26. Kollef MH, Shapiro SD, Clinkscale D, et al: The effect of respiratory therapist-initiated treatment protocols on patient outcomes and resource utilization. *Chest* 117:467, 2000.
27. Elrodt G, Cook DJ, Lee J, et al: Evidence-based disease management. *JAMA* 278:1997, 1687.
28. Stoller JK: Donald F. Egan Scientific Lecture: are respiratory therapists effective? Assessing the evidence. *Respir Care* 46(56):2001, 2000.
29. Respiratory Care Special Issue: Evidence-based medicine in respiratory care, Part I. *Respir Care* 46:11, 2001.
30. Respiratory Care Special Issue: Evidence-based medicine in respiratory care, Part II. *Respir Care* 46:12, 2001.
31. Hess DR: Evidence-based clinical practice guidelines: where's the evidence and what do I do with it? *Respir Care* 48:838, 2003.
32. Feinstein AR: Randomized clinical trials. In Feinstein AR, editor: *Clinical epidemiology: the architecture of clinical research*, Philadelphia, 1985, Saunders, pp 683–718.
33. The ARDS Network: Ventilation with lower tidal volumes as compared with traditional tidal volumes for acute lung injury and the ARDS. *N Engl J Med* 342:1301, 2000.
34. American Thoracic Society/European Respiratory Society: Standards for the diagnosis and management of individuals with alpha-1 antitrypsin deficiency. *Am J Respir Crit Care Med* 168:816, 2003.
35. Carlbom DJ, Rubenfeld GD: Barriers to implementing protocol-based sepsis resuscitation in the emergency department: results of a national survey. *Crit Care Med* 35:2525, 2007.
36. Hart SK, Dubbs W, Gil A, et al: The effects of therapist-evaluation of orders and interaction with physicians on the appropriateness of respiratory care. *Respir Care* 34(3):185–190, 1989.
37. Walton JR, Shapiro BA, Harrison EH: Review of a bronchial hygiene evaluation program. *Respir Care* 35:1214, 1990.
38. Orens DK: A manager's perspective on a respiratory therapy consult service (editorial). *Respir Care* 38:884, 1993.
39. Ford R: *The University of California San Diego experience with patient-driven protocols*. Presented at AARC State-of-the-Art Conference: therapist-driven protocols, Dallas, May 1994.
40. Komara JJ, Stoller JK: The impact of a postoperative oxygen therapy protocol on use of pulse oximetry and oxygen therapy. *Respir Care* 40:1125, 1995.
41. Shrake KL, Scaggs JE, England KR, et al: A respiratory care assessment-treatment program: results of a retrospective study. *Respir Care* 41:703, 1996.
42. Epstein RS, Sharwood LM: From outcomes research to disease management: a guide for the perplexed. *Ann Intern Med* 124:832, 1996.
43. Kollef MH, Shapiro SD, Silver P, et al: A randomized, controlled trial of protocol-directed versus physician-directed weaning from mechanical ventilation. *Crit Care Med* 25(4):567–574, 1997.
44. Ely EW, Baker AM, Dunagan DP, et al: Effect on the duration of mechanical ventilation of identifying patients capable of breathing spontaneously. *N Engl J Med* 335(25):1864–1869, 1996.
45. Marelich GP, Murin S, Battistella F, et al: Protocol weaning of mechanical ventilation in medical and surgical patients by respiratory care practitioners and nurses: effect on weaning time and incidence of ventilator-associated pneumonia. *Chest* 118(2):459–467, 2000.
46. Beasley K, Darin J, Durbin C: The effect of respiratory care department management of a blood gas analyzer on the appropriateness of arterial blood gas utilization. *Respir Care* 37:343, 1992.

CHAPTER 3

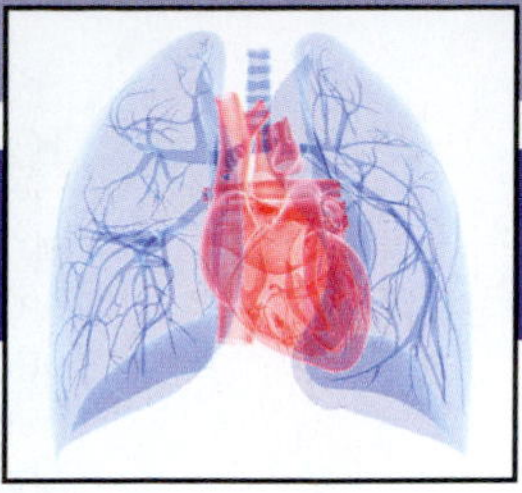

Quality, Patient Safety, Communication, and Recordkeeping

SCOTT P. MARLOW AND UMUR HATIPOĞLU

CHAPTER OBJECTIVES

After reading this chapter you will be able to:

- Define the meaning of *quality* in health care services.
- Understand the basic tools used in quality improvement projects.
- Describe established methods of quality improvement such as Six Sigma and Lean Management.
- Understand the importance of monitoring quality to promote better patient outcomes.
- Identify impediments to care and risk in the direct patient environment.
- State how communication can affect patient care.
- Describe the two-patient identifier system.
- List the factors associated with the communication process.
- Describe how to improve your communication effectiveness.
- Describe how to recognize and help resolve interpersonal or organizational sources of conflict.
- List the common components of a medical record.
- State the legal and practical obligations involved in recordkeeping.
- Describe how to maintain a problem-oriented medical record.
- Describe how to apply good body mechanics and posture to moving patients.
- Describe how to ambulate a patient and the potential benefits of ambulation.
- Write definitions of key terms associated with electricity, including voltage, current, and resistance.
- Identify the potential physiologic effects that electrical current can have on the body.
- State how to reduce the risk for electrical shock to patients and yourself.
- Identify key statistics related to the incidence and origin of hospital fires.
- List the conditions needed for fire and how to minimize fire hazards.

CHAPTER OUTLINE

Quality Considerations
- What Is Quality?
- The Methods of Quality Improvement
- Plan-Do-Study-Act Cycle
- Six Sigma
- Lean Management
- What Is Quality in Health Care?
- Monitoring Quality in Respiratory Care
- Peer Review Organizations

Safety Considerations
- Patient Movement and Ambulation
- Electrical Safety
- Fire Hazards
- General Safety Concerns

Communication
- Communication in Health Care
- Factors Affecting Communication
- Improving Communication Skills

Conflict and Conflict Resolution
- Sources of Conflict
- Conflict Resolution

Recordkeeping
- Components of a Traditional Medical Record
- Legal Aspects of Recordkeeping
- Practical Aspects of Recordkeeping
- Problem-Oriented Medical Record

KEY TERMS

ambulation
ampere
attending
auditory
channel
competencies
cross-training
current
disease management
feedback
ground
macroshock
microshock
ohm
performance improvement
problem-oriented medical record (POMR)
process control
quality assurance
quality improvement
resistance
SOAP
voltage

Provision of high-quality care in a safe environment is the focus of today's health care industry. Achieving this goal requires the integration of multiple disciplines, including respiratory therapy. Consequently, respiratory therapists (RTs) should be familiar with the concepts of **quality improvement** as it relates to health care.

This chapter will define quality and how it relates to health care. Through a narrative review, we will outline how quality is measured, monitored, and adapted to our health care environment. Discussions regarding quality in health care will demonstrate how RTs share the general responsibilities for providing a safe and effective health care environment with nurses and other members of the health care team. RTs are also required to have specific technical knowledge of the environment of direct patient care. In addition to technical skills, all health care professionals must be able to communicate effectively with each other and with patients and patients' families and to document pertinent information. Figure 3-1 shows this relationship for patient safety. This chapter aims to provide the foundational knowledge needed to understand the general aspects of patient safety considerations, communication in health care, conflict resolution, and recordkeeping that comprise essential components of high-quality patient care.

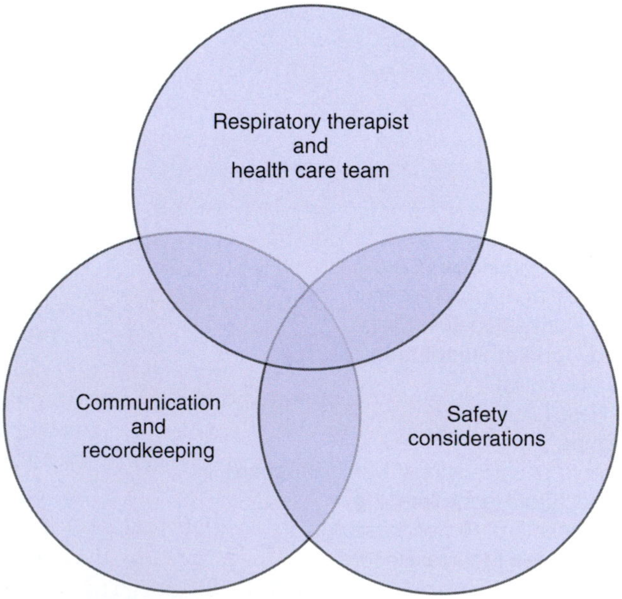

FIGURE 3-1 Patient safety continuum.

QUALITY CONSIDERATIONS

What Is Quality?

The quality of a service or product refers to the sum of its properties that serve to satisfy the needs of its consumer. High-quality services get high demand and also become a source of pride and financial success for the producer.

The Methods of Quality Improvement

Methods of attaining and ensuring quality were born in the automobile manufacturing industry in Japan, led by American engineers and scientists. These principles were only later adopted in the United States. William Edwards Deming (1900-1993), an electrical engineer and statistician, is credited for laying the foundations of quality control and management. Working first with the Japanese automobile industry and later with Ford Motor Company, Deming believed that high quality can be obtained only by a major culture change promoting a continuous improvement cycle in an organization. In essence, Deming suggested that the purpose of an organization is to constantly seek improvement of its product or service aligned with customer needs.[1] Rather than relying on constant inspection, quality should be built into the product from the beginning by design of the process or structure. Emphasis must be placed on the quality of the product and pride in the workmanship rather than on sheer quantitative productivity. Quality improvement must be everyone's job, starting from executive management to the front-line worker. Deming heavily relied on statistical quality control techniques, established by Walter A. Shewhart (1891-1967), another American engineer and scientist. Through statistical **process control** charts (SPCs), Shewhart pointed out that in every process associated with production, there was a variability, which he termed common cause variation. Common cause variation in a process can be quantitated by monitoring over time. Using sound statistical principles, an upper confidence limit (UCL) and a lower confidence limit (LCL) could be determined that define the range of common cause variation. A continuous monitoring of the process is possible by taking a small but representative sample and charting

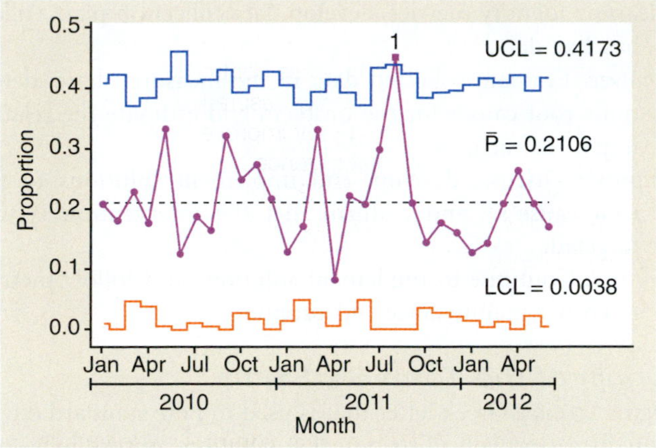

FIGURE 3-2 Statistical process control chart showing proportion of patients having to be readmitted to the hospital after discharge. Upper *(UCL)* and lower *(LCL)* control limits are marked with *gray lines.* At approximately September 2011, there appears to be a spike in readmissions to the hospital outside of the UCL that may require investigation.

numerical values on the SPC. Should the sample for any given time interval reveal values outside of the range—for example, higher or lower than UCL and LCL, respectively—then special cause variation is suspected (Figure 3-2). This unnatural pattern will then need to be investigated for a cause. Shewhart's SPCs continue to form the backbone of continuous quality improvement. Another important contribution to the practice of quality improvement by this brilliant engineer is the Plan-Do-Study-Act (or Plan-Do-Check-Act) cycle, also known as the Shewhart cycle.

Plan-Do-Study-Act Cycle

The Plan-Do-Study-Act Cycle (PDSA) can be seen visualized as the wheels of the car that is continuous quality improvement. As the wheels of PDSA turn, one gets closer to that difficult-to-achieve "perfect" product or service.

Plan Phase

In the *Plan* phase, clear goals are set for the quality improvement process. These goals are best stated in the form of hard numbers such as "a 20% increase in referrals to pulmonary rehabilitation on discharge for patients with chronic obstructive pulmonary disease (COPD." The planned intervention should be stated clearly. For instance, "respiratory therapist stationed on the nursing floor will distribute pulmonary rehabilitation program pamphlets to clinical team and remind clinicians to place the order for patients with COPD." A time limit should be specified, for example "a 20% increase in referrals to pulmonary rehabilitation on discharge over the next 3 months." During the planning phase, it is also helpful to create a diagram or a flow chart of the process that needs to be improved. The project team may choose to use tools such as the fishbone (or Ishikawa) diagram to systematically evaluate the different factors that affect the process and contribute to the problem, that is, people, technology, environment, materials, equipment, and methods (see Mini Clini and Figure 3-3).

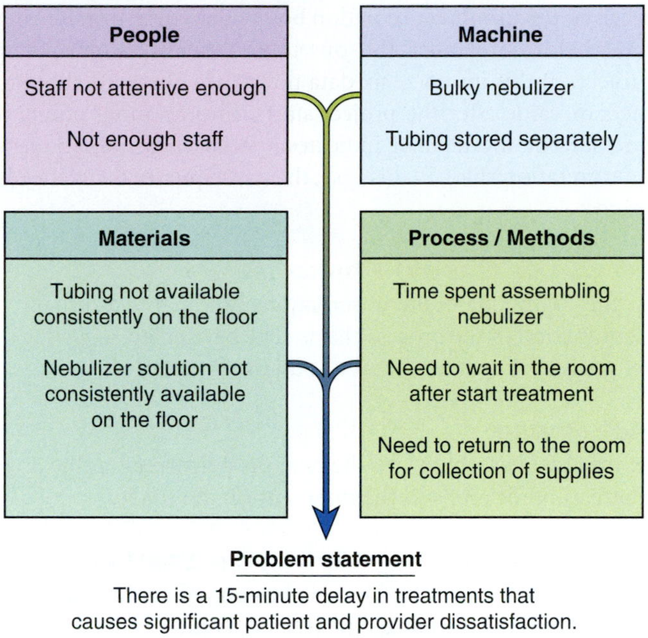

FIGURE 3-3 Fishbone diagram.

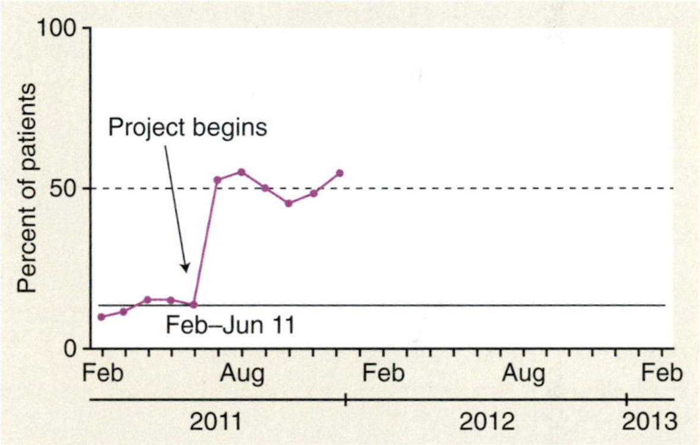

FIGURE 3-4 Run chart showing percentage of patients who received pneumonia vaccination over time.

Do Phase

In the *Do* phase, the intervention is begun and observations are recorded. On occasion, observations may need to be made on a limited sample that is representative of the entire process. The size of that sample should be determined by statistical methods that may require the help of a quality improvement professional or biostatistician. The observations are plotted on a statistical process chart or its simpler version, a so-called *run chart,* for analysis (Figure 3-4).

Run charts are graphic representations of data over a period of observation. In contrast to SPCs, there are no defined upper and lower limits. Rather, movement of the data points around the median value (the gray line) is visualized and interpreted. Rules of interpretation are based on statistical principles. A consistent change in the placement of data points on either side of the median indicates special cause variation. The run chart in Figure 3-4 displays the percentage of patients who have received pneumonia vaccination before discharge from the hospital before and after the onset of a quality improvement project. In this instance, six data points are observed above the median value after the project starts. Five or more points on one side of the median indicates special cause variation (an interpretation rule), in this case, the consequence of an effective project.

Study (or Check) Phase

In the *Study* phase, the observations are analyzed, usually by examination of the process charts. The barriers to achieving the set goals are considered and discussed.

Act Phase

In the *Act* phase, based on the analysis performed in the Study phase, modifications to the intervention are made.

The Plan-Do-Study-Act Cycle Starts Over

The paradigm of the PDSA cycle has served as the foundation for modern quality management systems such as the lean management system and Six Sigma, which are discussed in the following section.

RULE OF THUMB

The crucial components of a quality improvement project are summarized in the PDSA cycle:

Plan: Determine the specific aim, duration, data collection strategy, and team that will run the quality improvement project.
Do: Collect data and record the observations.
Study: Analyze results and derive conclusions.
Act: Change the process for improvement, plan the next cycle.

Six Sigma

By the mid-twentieth century, it had become obvious to the leading industrial companies that the rate of defective products had to be lowered to maintain market competitiveness and customer loyalty. Developed by the American telecommunications company Motorola, the Six Sigma method for quality improvement recognizes that there is a natural variation in process output that can be measured and monitored over time. Controlling and reducing this variation are the keys to business success. Statistical methods are used to calculate acceptable variation. There has to be a strong commitment on the part of management, from top to bottom, to these principles. The Six Sigma method also is based on the belief that improvement to existing processes is always possible and has to be achieved systematically. Analogous to the PDSA cycle, Six Sigma adopts the (Define-Measure-Analyze-Improve-Control (DMAIC) cycle for continuous quality improvement.

Define: Describe and validate the problem, create solutions, create a process map, and create a timeline for completion of the project.
Measure: Identify metrics, develop data collection plan, collect baseline data.
Analyze: Evaluate collected data in the measure phase, determine root causes for the problem and estimate the relative impact of each.
Improve: Discuss, develop, and implement solutions to the root cause(s), and confirm that the intervention is well targeted.
Control: Continue to implement solutions and follow metrics to ensure maintenance and adoption.

Origin of the Term Six Sigma

Sigma (σ) is a Greek letter that is used to note standard deviation in a normally distributed population. Accordingly, one standard deviation from the mean in each direction, that is, ± 1 σ, contains approximately 68% of the population. Similarly, 2 times σ contains 95% and 3 times σ contains 99%. If one considers a process to operate at 1 σ, then one would have to accept a 68% rate of successful product (or a failure rate of 32%). At the 2 σ level of acceptance, the failure rate would be 5% and at 3 σ, it would be 1%. At 6 Sigma, the rate of failure would be 3 in 1 million (or 0.000003). Thus, the Six Sigma process has a goal of a very, very small error rate (Figure 3-5).

Lean Management

Lean management is a business management philosophy that focuses on eliminating waste or non–value added activities. The origins of lean management are in the Japanese automobile maker, Toyota Motor Company. Lean management is analogous to ergonomics; eliminating waste of time, excess work, and unevenness of product are the goals. This goal is achieved by broadly using the principles of "just in time" (i.e., having equipment, personnel, supplies at the right place at the right time, Figures 3-6 and 3-7) and "Jidoka" (a joining of automation and human intelligence that results in a higher level of quality control). According to the Jidoka principle, any person involved in a service or manufacturing of product can stop the process if he or she sees a defect.

Lean management uses tools similar to those in PDSA and Six Sigma, with emphasis on waste elimination. These have been collectively termed the *lean toolbox.* The main instrument is value stream mapping, which is essentially a flow chart with emphasis on identifying value-added activities versus those that are not.

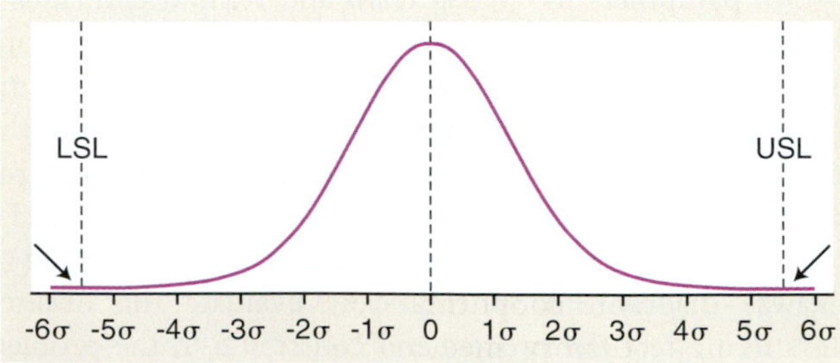

FIGURE 3-5 Normal (Gaussian) distribution. *LSL,* Lower specific limit; USL, upper specific limit.

MINI CLINI

Case Study

Michael Breathewell, an RRT, is the respiratory therapy manager in the respiratory care department of a 300-bed unit in Our Lady of Sacred Lungs Hospital. Over the past 6 months, he has been made aware, through the newly implemented serious event reporting system (SERS), of the time delay in delivery of scheduled inhaled bronchodilator treatments to patients. There is increasing pressure from physicians, nursing, and administration to fix this problem. After careful review of the cases, Michael determines that the problem occurs throughout all shifts and with different RTs and services involved. He believes that the problem may be due to a system issue and not special cause variation.

There are over 200 scheduled treatments given per day at the hospital. Tracking each treatment delay on a daily basis would be a huge job. Therefore, Michael has to select a sample that represents the time delay for the entire population. He asks the hospital biostatistician for help. Based on several assumptions, the biostatistician determined that 16 randomly sampled events were needed to have a fair idea of the average time delay between scheduled treatments and actual delivery.

Next, Michael asks for the help of a quality improvement professional in choosing the appropriate statistical process control chart for studying and monitoring the process of bronchodilator administration. He then begins collecting and graphing the data.

After a 3-month period of observation, he determines that there is an average of 15 minutes of delay between scheduled time and delivery time per patient see (Figure 3-6).

Michael decides to apply the Plan-Do-Study-Act cycle (PDSA) to tackle the issue.

PLAN: Michael calls a brainstorming session with floor respiratory managers and the medical director of respiratory care at this hospital. During the meeting, Michael and the group identify and analyze the problem and map the process. To facilitate the discussion, he uses an Ishikawa fishbone diagram to explore potential causes. Figure 3-6 shows the completed fishbone diagram. The fishbone allows a systematic discussion of possible contributors to the problem by considering factors related to machines, people, material, and process. The attendees overwhelmingly feel that the bulk of the time is spent getting the nebulizer and tubing, setting up the patient, and then returning back to the room. They also research best practices and conduct a literature review to understand reasons for delay in delivering nebulized treatments.

An attendee points out that administration of bronchodilators via metered dose inhalers (MDIs) has been found to be equivalent in efficacy across different diseases and disease severity.[2-4]

After some deliberation, weighing the balancing measures such as cost difference, the group decides to switch to bronchodilator administration via MDIs with a spacer and to follow time delay between scheduled time of bronchodilator delivery and actual time of delivery. The group decides that a 3-month observation should be enough to determine the effect of the intervention and meet monthly to review results. Michael and the team also identify the measures of success, including monitoring time delay between order entry and administration of the medication and employee satisfaction. Michael meets with hospital administration and with the chief financial officer, getting their support and ensuring financial feasibility of the switch.

DO: The group begins to administer scheduled short-acting bronchodilators by MDI with a spacer throughout the hospital floors. At least 16 observations of bronchodilator administration are made randomly throughout the day and recorded on the statistical process chart. Although the literature provides strong support for this intervention, Michael carefully reviews patient outcomes (e.g., treatment failure that results in a higher level of care or intensive care unit admission) to ensure that the switch to MDIs does not have unintended consequences.

STUDY: Michael measures the effect of the intervention and sees a trend toward reduction in delay times after 1 month and is pleased. However, some RTs suggest that further reduction in delays might be possible if patients' MDIs and spacers are kept at the bedside.

ACT: The suggestion to switch to delivery by MDI is discussed with the committee for pharmacy and therapeutics and is approved. MDIs with the patient's name stamp and spacer are kept at the bedside.

At the end of 3 months, Michael studies the process chart (Figure 3-7) and notes that delays have been consistently below the LCL of the original process. He congratulates the entire team and continues to monitor progress. Michael and colleagues plan to refine the intervention through iterative cycles, going back to the plan phase if future results are not as expected or yield unintended consequences.

What Is Quality in Health Care?

As the reader can see, there are common themes in all quality improvement approaches: Identification of process components, increasing efficiency (reducing waste), standardization (reducing common variation), and a teamwork approach in implementing solutions. Broadly speaking, health care delivery systems were slow to adopt these principles, with the possible exception of laboratory medicine. Rising health care costs, however, have brought about a revolution in how health care is delivered in the United States. In line with the *Patient Protection and Affordable Care Act*, the Centers for Medicare and Medicaid Services (CMS) began the Hospital Value-Based Purchasing Program, which rewarded or penalized hospitals based on their performance in the domains of process measures (also called *core measure compliance*), outcomes, patient experience, and efficiency. The Hospital Value-Based Purchasing Program is budget neutral, meaning that superior performance is rewarded and poor performers have to pay a penalty. Funds from the penalties provide the money for the rewards to hospitals that perform well. The federal government also enacted the Hospital Readmissions Reduction Program, which is strictly a penalty

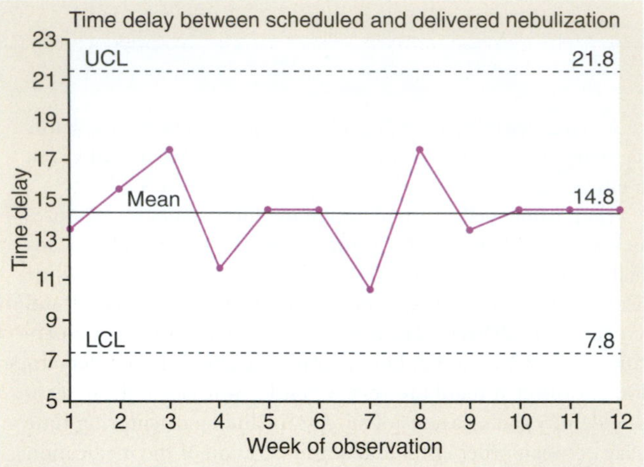

FIGURE 3-6 Time delay between scheduled and delivered nebulization. LCL, Lower control limit; UCL, upper control limit.

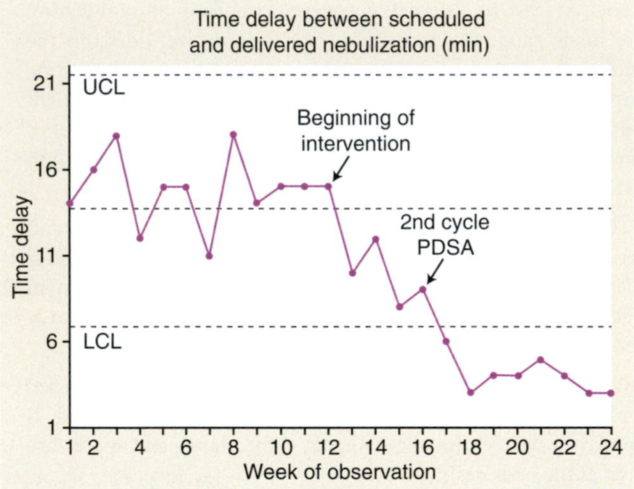

FIGURE 3-7 Time delay between scheduled and delivered nebulization. *LCL,* Lower control limit; *PDSA,* Plan-Do-Study-Act; *UCL,* upper control limit.

program that withholds a certain percentage of entire CMS reimbursements if the hospital has excess readmissions within 30 days of index discharge, compared to the national mean. With these incentives and threats of penalties, the health care industry is now adopting principles of quality improvement quickly.

The National Academy of Medicine (formerly the Institute of Medicine), the health arm of the National Academy of Sciences, suggests the following dimensions in health care quality: Safety, Timeliness, Effectiveness, Efficiency, Equity, Patient-centeredness (STEEP). These elements also define the starting points for quality improvement projects in health care.

Adoption of clinical guidelines and protocols are also important steps toward standardizing care and thereby driving improvement and reducing variation in outcomes (see Chapter 2). This satisfies the effectiveness and efficiency dimensions of health care quality. The patient safety dimension is addressed by adopting the "Jidoka" principle—stopping the process when any team member sees a defect in delivery of the care. Comprehensive and effective handoffs, as discussed later, between RTs are also critical for patient safety. RT-run education programs fulfill the patient centeredness principle. RTs also play a vital role in implementation of the guideline-based RT protocols and disease management programs, which represent a holistic approach to patient care across the continuum of health care settings. Disease management is discussed in the following section, and protocols are discussed in more detail in Chapter 2.

Disease Management

Disease management refers to an organized strategy of delivering care to a large group of individuals with chronic disease to improve outcomes and reduce cost. Disease management has been defined as a systematic population-based approach to identify persons at risk, intervene with specific programs of care, and measure clinical and other outcomes.[5,6] Disease management programs comprise four essential components: (1) an integrated health care system that can provide coordinated care across the full range of patient needs; (2) a comprehensive knowledge base regarding the prevention, diagnosis, and treatment of disease that guides the plan of care; (3) sophisticated clinical and administrative information systems that can help assess patterns of clinical practice; and (4) a commitment to continuous quality improvement. Disease management programs may be developed for chronic conditions such as asthma, diabetes, COPD, and congestive heart failure.

A disease management program for COPD might be adopted by a health care provider, insurance company, or health maintenance organization in defining its practice approach to individuals with COPD. The disease management program might contain algorithms addressing when to suspect COPD, tests to perform (e.g., spirometry, $alpha_1$-antitrypsin level, diffusing capacity), medications to prescribe based on disease severity, management of exacerbations, and indications for rehabilitation. Disease management programs are often outlined in documents containing branched logic algorithms that specify care, similar to respiratory care protocols (see Chapter 2); however, disease management protocols often address large groups and are based on an underlying diagnosis rather than on individual signs and symptoms. Other dimensions of the COPD management program include a data collection activity regarding the number of patients served, the outcomes of care, and, perhaps, the associated costs. In addition, as with quality monitoring in general, ongoing review and periodic updating and revision of the care algorithms are important dimensions of the program.

Monitoring Quality in Respiratory Care

Beyond ensuring that all elements of a high-quality respiratory care program are in place, quality must be monitored to ensure that it is being maintained. Strategies to monitor quality include intrainstitutional monitoring practices, centralized government monitoring bodies, such as the Centers for Medicare and Medicaid Services (CMS), and independent agencies such as The Joint Commission (TJC).

Intrainstitutional quality assurance often uses skills checks or **competencies**. Competence, or the quality of being competent, can be defined as having suitable or sufficient skill, knowledge, and experience for the purposes of a specific task.[7] Competence for a specific skill is frequently determined by observation of the practitioner's performance of the skill according to a prescribed checklist. Annual competency checks are documented for skills and procedures that carry some degree of patient risk (e.g., arterial puncture, aerosol therapy, bilevel positive airway pressure setup). An example of a skills checklist is shown in Figure 2-5.

Although skills checks have traditionally been done in person or with direct supervision of patient care activities, a new dimension of skills training and certification that is being widely implemented is the use of clinical simulation, using either low-fidelity or high-fidelity simulation trainers. Such simulation training, in which RTs use technology that attempts to reproduce reliably a true patient or true patient scenario, is similar to the flight simulator training that commercial airline pilots undergo to achieve certification to fly various airplanes. Uses of simulation training in respiratory therapy involve intubation, ventilator management, arterial line placement, and optimizing teamwork in acute resuscitation scenarios.[8]

Many health care organizations, including hospitals, subacute care facilities, and outpatient clinics, seek voluntary accreditation as a way to improve their service and assure the public that they maintain high standards. In health care, TJC is a very important organization. TJC (as the Joint Commission on the Accreditation of Healthcare) was formed in 1951 by the American College of Surgeons, the American Hospital Association, and the American Medical Association. Accreditation by TJC is based on satisfying specific standards established by professional and technical advisory committees.

TJC requires a hospital service to have a **quality assurance** plan to provide a system for controlling quality. Nine generally recognized steps for a quality assurance plan are used as the basis for quality assurance programs (Box 3-1).

Current standards of TJC for accreditation emphasize organization-wide efforts for **performance improvement**. Despite increased emphasis on cost containment, quality care remains the first goal of hospitals and respiratory care services. Performance improvement, also commonly called *continuous quality improvement,* is an ongoing process designed to detect and correct factors hindering the provision of quality and cost-effective health care. This process crosses department boundaries and follows the continuum of the patient's care. In 2009, TJC set forth three standards for monitoring performance improvement along with associated elements of performance detailing how the monitoring is to be conducted. These standards are listed in Box 3-2. Meeting quality goals is increasingly being tied to reimbursement rates by the CMS and insurers to hospitals; this phenomenon has been called "pay for performance."[9] Beyond general monitoring goals for respiratory therapy, use of respiratory care protocols creates the need for additional quality monitoring benchmarks regarding correctness, consistency, efficacy, and effectiveness (Box 3-3, Chapter 2).

At the present time, specific methods to monitor the quality of respiratory care protocol programs include conducting care plan audits in real time and ensuring practitioner training by using case study exercises. Evolving innovations include using simulation exercises to enhance and to measure the performance of RTs.

Monitoring correctness of respiratory care plans can be accomplished by using a care plan audit system. Care plan auditors must be therapists who are experienced in providing respiratory care and patient assessment. The auditors must also be practiced in using the institution's protocol system and in writing care plans. With an auditing system, the auditor writes a care plan for a patient and compares it with the care plan written by the therapist evaluator to determine correctness. A specified number of audits should be performed monthly, with results tabulated and reported monthly or quarterly, depending on the size of the hospital. Feedback must be provided to the evaluators whose care plans are being audited to show their proficiency or to indicate areas that require improvement. Figure 2-6 shows a form used at the Cleveland Clinic to provide feedback to evaluators.

Box 3-1 Nine Steps for a Quality Assurance Plan

1. Identify problem
2. Determine cause of problem
3. Rank problem
4. Develop strategy for resolving problem
5. Develop appropriate measurement techniques
6. Implement problem-resolution strategy
7. Analyze and compile results of intervention
8. Report results to appropriate personnel
9. Evaluate intervention outcome

Box 3-2 The Joint Commission Standards for Performance Improvement

- The hospital collects data to monitor its performance.
- The hospital compiles and analyzes data.
- The hospital improves performance on an ongoing basis.

Compiled from The Joint Commission, Oakbrook Terrace, IL.

Box 3-3 Quality Monitoring Benchmarks

- Monitoring the correctness of respiratory care plans
- Monitoring the consistency of formulating respiratory care plans among therapist evaluators
- Evaluating the efficacy of algorithms or protocols
- Evaluating the overall effectiveness of the protocol program

Another monitoring method found useful for respiratory therapy consult services is the case study exercise (or simulated patient scenario exercise). Simulated patient exercises can help determine the consistency of respiratory care plans among therapist evaluators. The scores of individual RTs may be tracked over time to identify problems and assess improvement.

Simulated patient exercises may consist of a set of three or four patient scenarios. All RTs working under the protocol system, whether or not they are evaluators, complete an assessment sheet and, following the associated algorithms, write a care plan for each scenario. The assessment sheets and the care plans are compared with the gold standard, or correct assessments and care plans, as determined by the consensus of the education coordinator and the supervisors. Scores are tabulated for the individual RTs, and the number of errors for each therapy is examined. If a particular therapy consistently has a large number of associated errors, the algorithm is reviewed for errors or vagueness. To facilitate administering and grading patient simulation exercise results, a computer-based system that scores the assessments and care plans and provides feedback to the RT has been used.[10] Performance data of individual RTs are maintained in a database to calculate and track aggregate performance statistics.

Peer Review Organizations

In addition to the voluntary accreditation process that health care organizations use to help ensure patients are receiving quality care, the federal government has established an elaborate system of peer review organizations (PROs) to evaluate the quality and appropriateness of care given to Medicare beneficiaries. PROs evaluate care provided to individual patients in real time to assess and ensure compliance with federal guidelines.

In recent years, health care organizations have attempted to improve the quality of patient care while reducing costs by implementing several innovative health care models. Historically, models that were commonly implemented were hospital restructuring and redesign and patient-focused care. Protocols and disease management represent continuing solutions. Accountable care organizations (ACOs)[11] have been proposed as a solution to enhance quality and lessen cost. An ACO can be broadly thought of as an emerging model in which a group of health care providers aligns and agrees together to try to meet quality and care targets and to receive payments as a collective entity, from which individual payments then can be disbursed. The ACO can benefit as a group from its success and can absorb losses as a group related to its failure to meet the targets.

Restructuring and redesign involved changing the basic organization of health care services in an attempt to do more with less, thereby increasing value. Approaches for restructuring have commonly included cross-training employees, using unlicensed assistive staff, and decentralizing services.[12] In one of these approaches, when respiratory therapy departments are decentralized and respiratory care management is eliminated, RTs are deployed to individual nursing units and report to nursing supervisors. When complete decentralization occurs, the responsibilities of equipment purchase and maintenance, continuing education, and quality improvement may be assigned to nursing personnel. Some experience suggests that nurses may be uncomfortable with these additional burdens,[13] so careful planning and stakeholder assessment is needed before decentralization could be implemented.

Although less commonly practiced, another aspect of restructuring and redesign is **cross-training** personnel and using assistive staff. Cross-training among professional health care workers can be attempted by teaching activities normally performed by a specific discipline but not restricted by licensing to personnel of another discipline. Nurses might cross-train RTs to perform phlebotomy, whereas RTs might cross-train nurses to perform metered dose inhaler (MDI) therapy. Although theoretically appealing, this strategy has fallen into disfavor because of the substantial associated challenges in implementation.

Cross-training assistive personnel involves on-the-job training of unlicensed personnel, who may not have an educational background in health care, to perform basic technical functions. These assistive personnel may learn to perform some nursing functions, such as taking vital signs, measuring intake and output, and inserting urinary catheters; laboratory technician activities, such as phlebotomy and simple urinalysis; and respiratory therapy activities, such as incentive spirometry follow-up and O_2 checks. The intent of using cross-trained assistive personnel, whose compensation is lower than that of licensed health care workers, is to enable an institution to reduce the number of nurses, laboratory technicians, and RTs they employ, thereby reducing costs. Although some aspects of hospital restructuring and redesign have been implemented and persist, others (e.g., cross-training and decentralization) have been abandoned.

SAFETY CONSIDERATIONS

Safety is a very important part of ensuring high-quality care. Importantly, patient safety must always be the first consideration in respiratory care. Although the RT usually does not have full control over the patient's environment, efforts must be made to minimize potential hazards associated with respiratory care. The key areas of potential risk for patients, RTs, and co-workers are patient movement and ambulation, electrical hazards, fire hazards, and general safety concerns. Each of these will be discussed as part of attention to providing high-quality, safe care.

Patient Movement and Ambulation

Basic Body Mechanics

Posture involves the relationship of the body parts to each other. A person needs good posture to reduce the risk for injury when lifting patients or heavy equipment. Poor posture may place inappropriate stress on joints and related muscles and tendons. Figure 3-8 illustrates the correct body mechanics for lifting a heavy object. The correct technique calls for a straight spine and use of the leg muscles to lift the object.

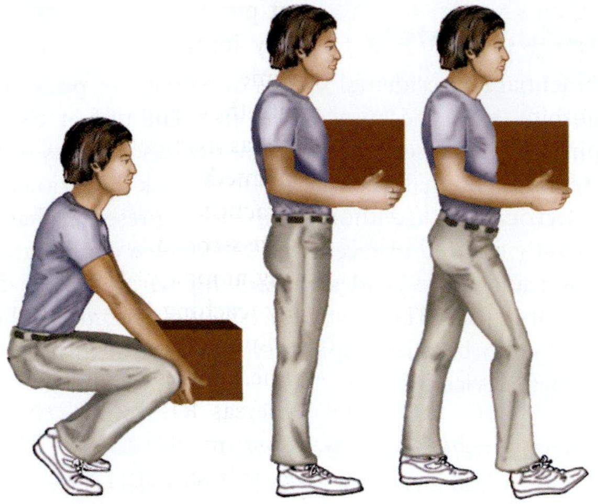

FIGURE 3-8 Body mechanics for lifting and carrying objects.

Moving the Patient in Bed

Conscious people assume positions that are the most comfortable. Bedridden patients with acute or chronic respiratory dysfunction often assume an upright position, with their arms flexed and their thorax leaning forward. This position helps decrease their work of breathing. In other cases, patients may have to assume certain positions for therapeutic reasons such as when postural drainage is applied.

Figure 3-9 shows the correct technique for lateral movement of a bed-bound patient. Figure 3-10 illustrates the ideal method for moving a conscious patient toward the head of a bed. Figure 3-11 shows the proper technique for assisting a patient to the bedside position for dangling his or her legs or transfer to a chair.

Ambulation

Ambulation (walking) helps maintain normal body function. Extended bed rest can cause numerous problems, including bed sores and atelectasis (low lung volumes). Ambulation should begin as soon as the patient is physiologically stable and free of severe pain. Ambulation has been shown to reduce the length of hospital stay after hip surgery and in patients recovering from community-acquired pneumonia.[13,14] RTs may assist to ambulate patients while they are on a mechanical ventilator or while on O_2. Safe patient movement includes the following steps:

1. Place the bed in a low position and lock its wheels.
2. Place all equipment (e.g., intravenous [IV] equipment, nasogastric tube, surgical drainage tubes) close to the patient to prevent dislodgment during ambulation.
3. Move the patient toward the nearest side of bed.
4. Assist the patient to sit up in bed (i.e., arm under nearest shoulder and one under farthest armpit).
5. Place one hand under the patient's farthest knee, and gradually rotate the patient so that his or her legs are dangling off the bed.
6. Let the patient remain in this position until dizziness or lightheadedness lessens (encouraging the patient to look forward rather than at the floor may help).

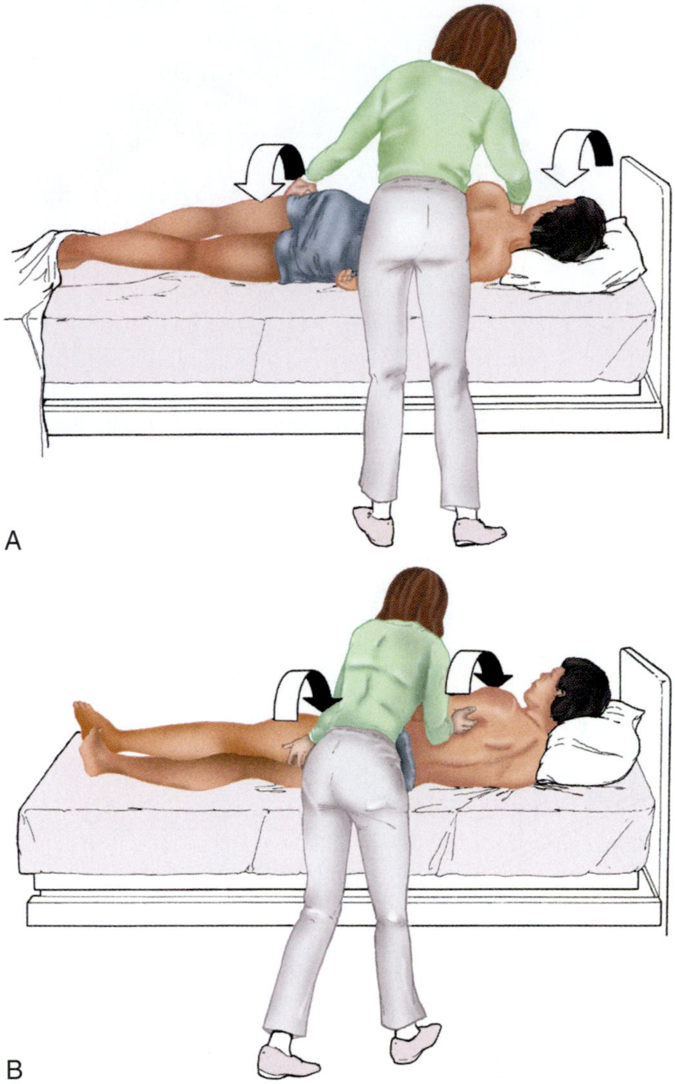

A

B

FIGURE 3-9 **A,** Method to pull a bed-bound patient. **B,** Method to push a bed-bound patient.

7. Assist the patient to a standing position.
8. Encourage the patient to breathe easily and unhurriedly during this initial change to a standing posture.
9. Walk with the patient using no, minimal, or moderate support (moderate support requires the assistance of two practitioners, one on each side of the patient).
10. Limit walking to 5 to 10 minutes for the first exercise.

Monitor the patient during ambulation. Note the patient's level of consciousness, color, breathing, strength or weakness, and complaints such as pain or shortness of breath throughout the activity. Ask the patient about his or her comfort level frequently during the ambulation period. Ensure that chairs are present so emergency seats are available if the patient becomes distressed. Ambulation is increased gradually until the patient is ready to be discharged. Each ambulation session is documented in the patient chart and includes the date and time of ambulation, length of ambulation, and degree of patient tolerance.

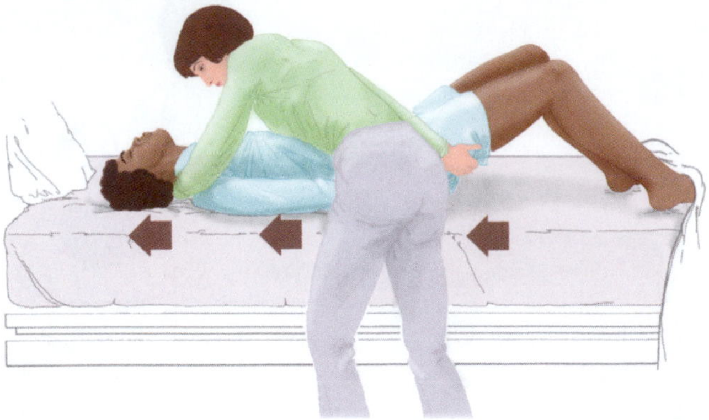

FIGURE 3-10 Method to move a patient up in bed with the patient's assistance.

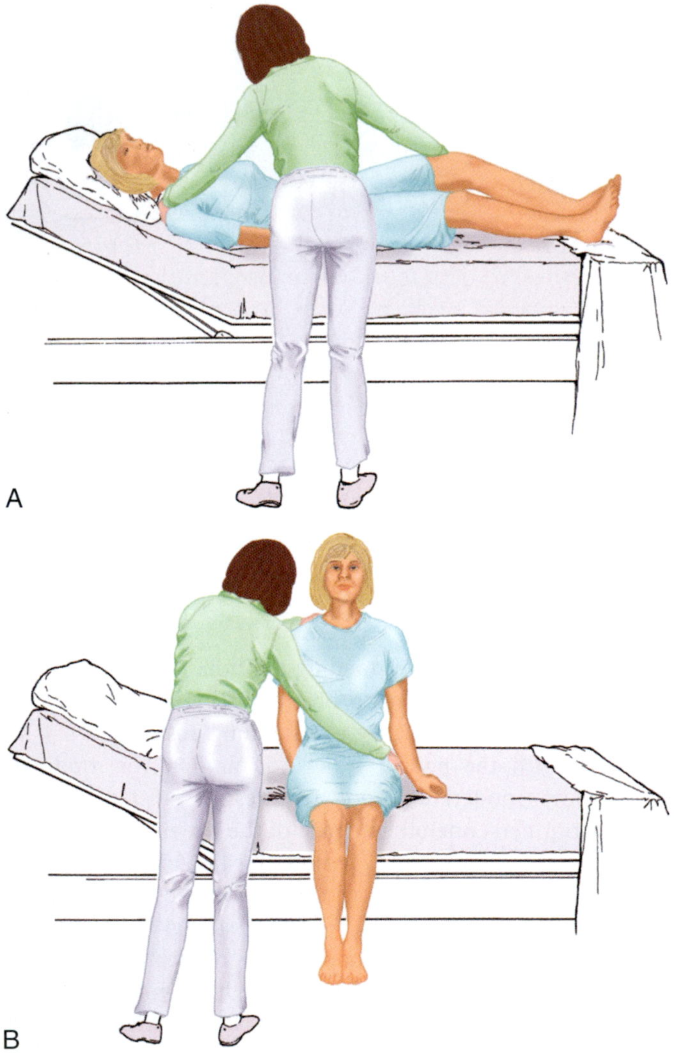

FIGURE 3-11 Method to assist a patient in dangling the legs at the side of the bed.

Electrical Safety

The potential for accidental shocks of patients or personnel in the hospital exists because of the frequent use of electrical equipment. The presence of invasive devices, such as internal catheters and pacemakers, may add to the risk for serious harm from electrical shock. Although this risk is present, it has been significantly reduced in recent years through a combination of education and more rigid standards for wiring, especially in patient care areas. RTs must understand the fundamentals of electrical safety because respiratory care often involves the use of electrical devices.

Fundamentals of Electricity

The ability of humans to create and harness electricity is one of the most important developments in modern times. Because controlled electricity is available on a 24-hour-a-day basis, we can depend on it to power the equipment and appliances that make modern life comfortable and productive. Despite the fact that electricity is one of the most popular sources of power, most people who use it have a poor understanding of it. This lack of knowledge is often a major factor in cases of electrocution.

MINI CLINI

"Tingling" Equipment

PROBLEM: An RT is caring for a patient on a mechanical ventilator that requires both electrical and pneumatic power for operation. When the RT touches the metal housing of the ventilator, a shock is felt. How should the RT handle the situation based on this observation?

DISCUSSION: All therapeutic instruments used in patient care, including mechanical ventilators, should be connected to grounded outlets (three-wire). Because the ground wire is a protection device only and not part of the main circuit, equipment may continue to operate without the clinician being aware that a problem exists. Because the RT felt a tingling sensation when touching the ventilator, this could represent an improper ground and possible serious current leakage. In this situation, the RT should immediately take the equipment out of service and get it replaced (while providing backup ventilation). All electrical equipment used in patient care should be routinely checked for appropriate grounding.

Electricity moves from point *A* to point *B* because of differences in voltage. **Voltage** is the power potential behind the electrical energy. Low-voltage batteries (e.g., 9 V) are sufficient to power a small flashlight but inadequate to power a major appliance such as a microwave oven. Most homes and hospitals are powered with 120-V power sources. Power sources that have high voltage have the potential to generate large amounts of electrical current. The current that moves through an object is directly related to the voltage difference between point *A* and point *B* and inversely related to the resistance offered by the makeup of the object. Objects with low resistance (e.g., copper wires) allow maximum current to flow through the object. Objects with high resistance (e.g., rubber tubing) allow minimal or no current to flow through the object despite higher levels of voltage.

The simple analogy of water flowing through a piping system is useful to understand electricity. The water pressure level at the source is equivalent to the voltage. Higher water pressure provides the potential for greater water flow or current. The friction (**resistance**) offered by the pipe across the length of the pipe influences the flow exiting the other end. Pipes with lots of friction reduce the water flow (current) greatly. If the friction (resistance) is minimal, the water flow (current) is maximal. Similarly, when voltage is high and resistance is low, electrical current flows easily through the object.

The difference in resistance between two people or two objects explains why the same voltage applied to both can seriously damage one and cause no effect to the other. Two people accidentally touching a "hot" wire with 120 V can experience two completely different sensations. A person with wet skin offers little resistance, and the 120 V passes through the person with high current and can cause serious injury or death. A person with dry skin, which offers high resistance, may not even feel a shock and experiences no injury. The degree of resistance offered by the skin varies from person to person based on the chemistry of the person's skin, the cleanliness of the skin, and the amount of moisture on the surface. For this reason, it is never wise to touch a potentially hot wire even though your skin is dry.

As stated before, voltage is the energy potential from an electrical source, and it is measured with a voltmeter. **Current** is the flow of electricity from a point of higher voltage to one of lower voltage and is reported in **amperes** (amps). Current is measured with an ampmeter. The resistance to electrical current is reported in **ohms**. We can determine the resistance to current for any object by the following equation:

$$\text{Resistance (ohms }[\Omega]) = \text{Voltage (V)/Current (amps [A])}$$

Current represents the greatest danger to you or your patients when electrical shorts occur. Voltage and resistance are important only because they determine how much current potentially can pass through the body. High voltage provides greater potential for high currents, but if resistance is also very high, current would be minimal or nonexistent. Current represents the potential danger to the patient. The harmful effects of current depend on: (1) the amount of current flowing through the body, (2) the path it takes, and (3) the duration the current is applied. Higher currents (>100 milliamps [mA]) that pass through the chest can cause ventricular fibrillation, diaphragm dysfunction (owing to severe, persistent contraction), and death.

Because current is most important, you should be familiar with the equation used to calculate it:

$$\text{Current (A)} = \text{Voltage (V)/Resistance } (\Omega)$$

For example, as long as a person is insulated by normal clothing and shoes and is in a dry environment, a 120-V shock may hardly be felt because the resistance is high in this situation (10,000 Ω). Current can be calculated as:

$$\text{Current (A)} = 120\ \text{V}/10{,}000\ \Omega = 0.012\ \text{A or } 12\ \text{mA}$$

Currents of 12 mA would cause a tingling sensation but no physical damage.

However, if the same person is standing without shoes on a wet floor, a much higher current occurs because the resistance is much lower (1000 Ω). The current is then calculated as:

$$\text{Current (A)} = 120\ \text{V}/1000\ \Omega = 0.12\ \text{A or } 120\ \text{mA}$$

Because the heart is susceptible to any current level greater than 100 mA, 120 mA represents a potentially fatal shock; this is in sharp contrast to the first example, in which the same voltage caused only a tingling sensation.

A shock hazard exists only if the electrical "circuit" through the body is complete, meaning that two electrical connections to the body are required for a shock to occur. In the previous example, the person standing in water with no shoes has "grounded" himself. The finger touching the hot wire provides the input source while the feet standing in water provide the exit to ground. If the same person is wearing rubber boots, the connection to ground does not exist and the current cannot flow through the individual.

In electrical devices, these two connections typically consist of a "hot" wire and a "neutral" wire. The neutral wire completes the circuit by taking the electrical current to a ground. A **ground** is simply a low-resistance pathway to a point of zero voltage, such as the earth (hence the term *ground*).

Figure 3-12 shows how current can flow through the body. In this case, a piece of electrical equipment is connected to an AC line power via a standard three-prong plug. However, unknown to the practitioner, the cord has a broken ground wire. Normally, current leakage from the equipment would flow back to the ground through the ground wire. However, this pathway is unavailable. Instead, the leakage current finds a path of low resistance through the practitioner to the damp floor (an ideal ground).

Current can readily flow into the body, causing damage to vital organs when the skin is bypassed via conductors such as pacemaker wires or saline-filled intravascular catheters (Figures 3-13 and 3-14). Even urinary catheters can provide a path for current flow. The heart is particularly sensitive to electrical shock. Ventricular fibrillation can occur when currents of 20 μA (20 microamperes, or 20 millionths of 1 ampere) are applied directly to the heart.

Electrical shocks are classified into two types: macroshock and microshock. A **macroshock** exists when a high current (usually >1 mA) is applied externally to the skin. A **microshock** exists when a small, usually imperceptible current (<1 mA) bypasses the skin and follows a direct, low-resistance path into the body. Patients susceptible to microshock hazards are termed *electrically sensitive* or *electrically susceptible*. Table 3-1 summarizes the different effects of these two types of electrical shock.

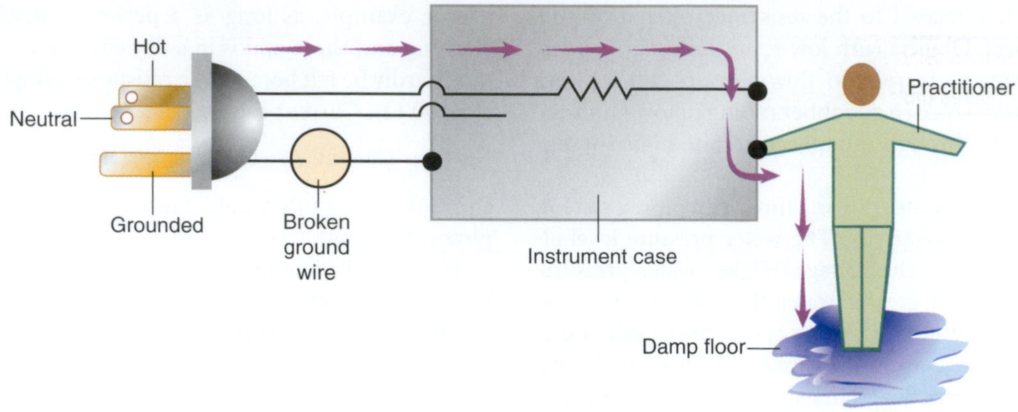

FIGURE 3-12 Hazard created by broken ground wire.

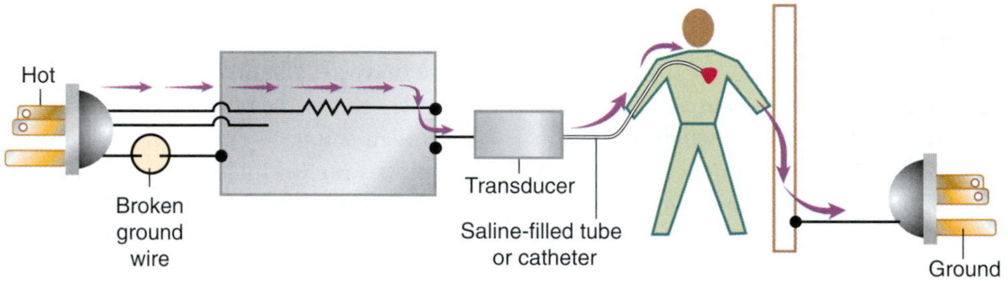

FIGURE 3-13 Possible microshock hazard caused by patient grounding.

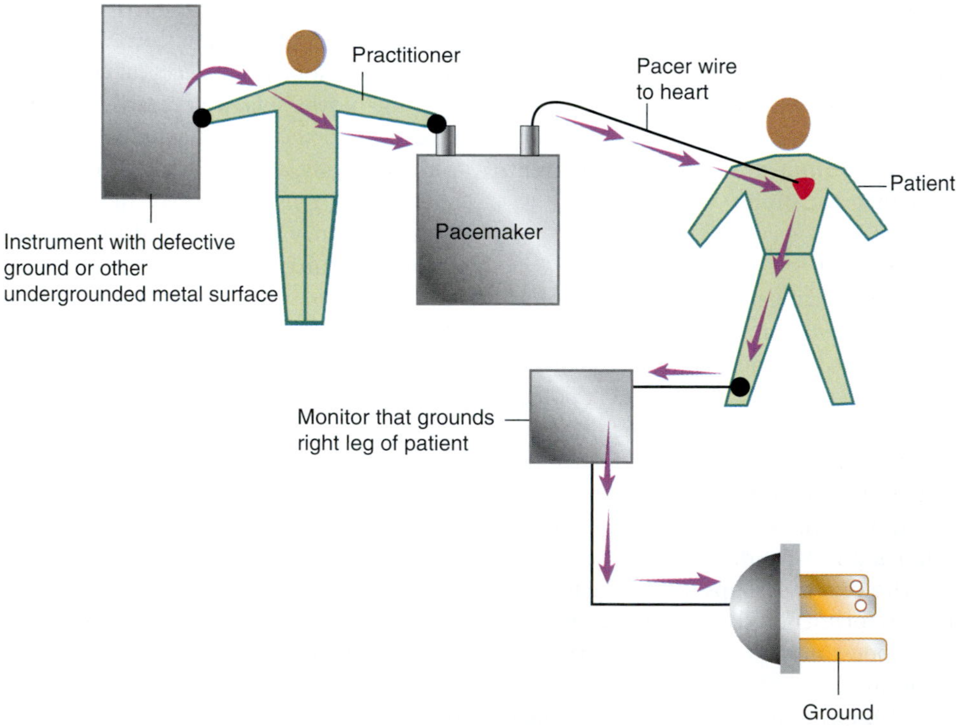

FIGURE 3-14 Possible hazard through use of certain cardiac monitors and a pacemaker.

TABLE 3-1

Effects of Electrical Shock*

Amperes (A)	Milliamperes (mA)	Microamperes (μA)	Effects
Applied to Skin (Macroshock)			
≥6	>6000	>6,000,000	Sustained myocardial contraction followed by normal rhythm; temporary respiratory paralysis; burns, if small area of contact
0.1-3	100-3000	100,000	Ventricular fibrillation; respiratory center intact
0.050	50	50,000	Pain; fainting; exhaustion; mechanical injury; heart and respiratory function intact
0.016	16	16,000	"Let go" current; muscle contraction
0.001	1	1000	Threshold of perception; tingling
Applied to Myocardium (Microshock)			
0.001	0.1	100	Ventricular fibrillation

Duration of exposure and current pathway are major determinants of human response to electrical shock.
*Physiologic effects of AC shocks applied for 1 second to the trunk or directly to the myocardium.

Preventing Shock Hazards

Most shock hazards are caused by inappropriate or inadequate grounding. Shock hazards can be eliminated or minimized if wiring in patient care areas is appropriate and if all equipment brought into the patient care area has been Underwriters Laboratories (UL) approved and checked on a regular basis by a qualified person.

Ground Electrical Equipment Near the Patient

All electrical equipment (e.g., lights, electrical beds, ventilators, monitoring or therapeutic equipment) should be connected to grounded outlets with three-wire cords. In these cases, the third (ground) wire prevents the dangerous buildup of voltage that can occur on the metal frames of some electrical equipment.

Modern electrical devices used in hospitals are designed so their frames are grounded, but their connections to the patient are not. In this manner, all electrical devices in reach of the patient are grounded, but the patient remains isolated from ground. Because the ground wire is simply a protection device and not part of the main circuit, equipment continues to operate normally even if the ground wire is broken. All electrical equipment, particularly devices used with electrically susceptible patients, must be checked for appropriate grounding on a regular basis by a qualified electrical expert.

Fire Hazards

In 1980, approximately 12,000 health care facility fires were officially reported in the United States.[15] During the period of 2006 to 2010, the average annual number of fires in health care facilities was 6240.[14] These health care facilities include hospitals, hospice facilities, nursing homes, mental health facilities, and doctors' offices or clinics. This significant reduction in health care facility fires is primarily due to education and enforcement of strict fire codes.

Approximately 23% of fires in health care facilities occur in hospitals or hospice, and 46% occur in nursing homes; the most common site of origin of the fire is the kitchen.[15] Medical facility fires cause an annual average of 6 civilian deaths, 171 civilian injuries, and approximately $52.1 million in damage.[15]

Hospital fires can be very serious, especially when they occur in patient care areas and when supplemental O_2 is in use. Fires in O_2-enriched atmospheres (OEAs) are larger, more intense, faster burning, and more difficult to extinguish. In addition, some material that would not burn in room air would burn in O_2-enriched air. Hospital fires are also more serious because evacuation of critically ill patients is difficult and slow. For these reasons, hospital fires often cause more injuries and deaths per fire than do residential fires. For a fire to start, three conditions must exist: (1) flammable material must be present, (2) O_2 must be present, and (3) the flammable material must be heated to or above its ignition temperature. When all three conditions are present, a fire starts. Conversely, removing any one of the conditions can stop a fire from starting or extinguish it after it has begun. Fire is a serious hazard around respiratory care patients using supplemental O_2. Although O_2 is nonflammable, it greatly accelerates the rate of combustion. Burning speed increases with an increase in either the concentration or the partial pressure of O_2.

Flammable material should be removed from the vicinity of O_2 use to minimize fire hazards. Flammable materials include cotton, wool, polyester fabrics, bed clothing, paper materials, plastics, and certain lotions or salves such as petroleum jelly. Removal of flammable material is particularly important whenever O_2 enclosures, such as O_2 tents or croupettes, are used.

Ignition sources, such as cigarette lighters, should not be allowed in rooms where O_2 is in use. In addition, the use of electrical equipment capable of generating high-energy sparks, such as exposed switches, must be avoided. All appliances that transmit house current should be kept out of O_2 enclosures. Children should not play with toys that may create a spark when O_2 is in use. RTs must be diligent in educating patients and visitors about the dangers associated with spark-producing items, open flames, and burning cigarettes in the hospital environment, especially in areas with O_2-enriched air.

A frequent source of concern is the presence of static electrical sparks generated by friction. Even in the presence of high O_2 concentrations, the overall hazard from static sparks with the materials in common use is very low. Solitary static sparks generally do not have sufficient heat energy to raise common materials to their flash points. The minimal risk that may be present can be reduced further by maintaining high relative humidity (>60%).

If you identify a fire in a patient care area, you must know what to do. Each hospital must have a core fire plan that identifies the responsibilities of hospital personnel. The plan should be taught to all hospital personnel and practiced with fire drills to reinforce the education. Requirements may include routinely walking the fire exits and reviewing proper fire extinguisher training. Fire extinguisher training includes following the acronym PASS:

*P*ull the pin. There may be an inspection tag attached.

*A*im the nozzle. Aim low at the bottom of the fire.

*S*queeze the handle. The extinguisher has less than 30 seconds of spray time.

*S*weep the nozzle across the base of the fire.

The core fire plan follows the acronym *RACE:*

*R*escue patients in the immediate area of the fire. The person discovering the fire should perform the rescue.

*A*lert other personnel about the fire so they can assist in the rescue and can relay the location of the fire to officials. This step also involves pulling the fire alarm.

*C*ontain the fire. After rescuing patients, shut doors to prevent the spread of the fire and the smoke. In patient care areas, follow your hospital policy regarding turning off O_2 zone valves.

*E*vacuate other patients and personnel in the areas around the fire who may be in danger if the fire spreads.

RTs are frequently key participants in successful handling of hospital fires. First, they know where the O_2 zone valves are located and how to shut them off. Second, they have the knowledge and skills needed to evacuate patients receiving mechanical ventilation or supplemental O_2 to sustain life. Third, they know how to treat and resuscitate victims of smoke inhalation. For these reasons, RTs should be included in all hospital evacuation planning and practices.

General Safety Concerns

In addition to electrical and fire safety, RTs need to be aware of general safety concerns, including the direct patient environment, disaster preparedness, magnetic resonance imaging (MRI) safety, and medical gas safety. Medical gas safety is discussed in more detail in Chapter 40.

Direct Patient Environment

The immediate environment around the patient can create risk for patient safety. Because RTs use medical equipment and participate in direct patient care, it is necessary for RTs to be cognizant of the patient's immediate environment.

To reduce the risk for patient falls and allow easy access to care, the patient care environment should be as free of impediments to care as possible. Use of respiratory supplies and medical equipment by the RT creates an environment that could impede access to care and create a fall risk. It is the responsibility of the RT to position equipment, tubing, and treatments in a way that does not impede access to care and that reduces risk for falls. In addition, when care is completed, the RT should ensure that the patient has easy access to the patient call system.

Disaster Preparedness

A key component of disaster preparedness involves learning to transport and transfer critically ill patients safely. Another component includes preparing for a loss of electricity, whether it is due to an internal or external disaster. In these emergencies, hospitals have backup generators to power essential equipment. All electrical outlets may not function on the backup generator. Some hospitals designate emergency outlets with a red outlet or red dot on an outlet, whereas others may power an entire wing, such as a medical intensive care unit, with the backup generator power. It is important for the RT to know the specific hospital policy for power failures and other potential disasters.

Magnetic Resonance Imaging Safety

MRI exposes the body to powerful magnetic fields and a small amount of radiofrequency. This powerful magnetic field can create a risk to patients, health care workers, and equipment if metal objects are brought within specified proximity to the field. There are safe proximity areas referred to as *safety zones* or *Gauss lines*. Metal objects can be so forcefully attracted to the magnetic field that they can mimic a missile, causing physical harm. Reports of accidents associated with MRI have involved O_2 cylinders, stethoscopes, scissors, and IV poles. Deaths have been described when O_2 cylinders were pulled into the magnetic area where a patient was lying to undergo an MRI examination. RTs need to become familiar with MRI-compatible ventilators, O_2 supplies, and ancillary equipment. Each radiology department has specific rules and safety precautions that need to be communicated to all patients, caregivers, and health care personnel.

Medical Gas Cylinders

Use of compressed gas cylinders by RTs requires special handling. The physical hazards resulting from improper storage or handling of cylinders include increased risk for fire, explosive release of high-pressure cylinders, and the toxic effect of some gases. It is important to store and transport cylinders in appropriate racks or chained containers. Compressed gas cylinders should never be stored without support.

Storage of medical-grade gases is regulated by National Fire Protection Association Standards 99 Healthcare Facilities Code (2014 edition) and monitored by TJC. Quantities of O_2 or nitrous oxide of 300 cubic feet or less (about 12 E-cylinders) in a patient care area not to exceed 2100 m^2 are required to be secured properly but do not have special storage room requirements.[16] Storing 300 to 3000 cubic feet of O_2 or N_2O requires noncombustible or limited combustible storage rooms with self-closing doors and at least a 30-minute fire rating.[16] Cylinders must be stored 20 feet from any combustibles (5 feet if room is equipped with a sprinkler system).[16] Follow your hospital policies and procedures when handling, transporting, or storing medical gas cylinders.

COMMUNICATION

Because the delivery of safe, high-quality health care requires interactions among many contributors from different disciplines (e.g., physicians, RTs, nurses, etc.), communication is essential to the quality mission of a health care organization. Strategies to enhance communication are critical to organizational success.

Communication is a dynamic human process involving sharing of information, meanings, and rules. Communication has five basic components: sender, message, channel, receiver, and feedback (Figure 3-15).

The sender is the individual or group who transmits the message. The message is the information or attitude that is communicated by the sender. Messages may be verbal or nonverbal. Verbal messages are voiced or written. Examples of different kinds of messages are lectures, letters, and e-mail memos. Nonverbal communication is any communication that is not voiced or written. Nonverbal communication includes gestures, facial expressions, eye movements and contact, voice tone, space, and touch.

The **channel** of communication is the method used to transmit messages. The most common channels involve sight and hearing, such as written and oral messages. However, other sensory input, such as touch, may be used with visual or **auditory** communication. In addition, communication channels may be formal (memos or letters) or informal (conversation).

The receiver is the target of the communication and can be an individual or a group. One-on-one communication is often more effective because both parties can respond to each other. Communication with a group can be more challenging but is a more efficient way to get information to numerous individuals.

The last essential part of communication is **feedback**. Human communication is a two-way process in which the receiver serves an active role. Feedback from the receiver allows the sender to measure communication success and provide additional information when needed.

Communication in Health Care

Effective communication is the most important aspect of providing safe patient care. The first two 2010 National Patient Safety Goals of TJC are to improve accuracy of patient identification and effectiveness of communicating critical test values among caregivers.[17] All health care personnel must correctly identify patients before initiating care using a two–patient identifier system. The patient identifiers can include any two of the following: name, birth date, and medical record number. Effectively communicating critical test values should include a "read back" scenario verifying the reporter and the receiver of the information and accurate reporting and recording of test values. Each institution may have specific values as critical test values; for example, RTs may be expected to report blood gas values of a pH less than 7.2 or a PaO_2 less than 50 mm Hg. The process of the read back scenario is described in Box 3-4.

Box 3-4 "Read Back" Process to Ensure Accurate Communication of Information

PRESCRIBER/REPORTER
- Orders or critical test results are read and clearly enunciated, using two patient identifiers.
- Avoid abbreviations.
- Ask receiver to "read back" the information if this is not done voluntarily.
- Verify with the receiver that the information is correct.

RECEIVER
- Record the order or value.
- Ask "prescriber/reporter" to repeat if information is not understood.
- "Read back" the information, including two patient identifiers.
- Receive confirmation from the "prescriber/reporter" that the information is correct; if incorrect, repeat the process.

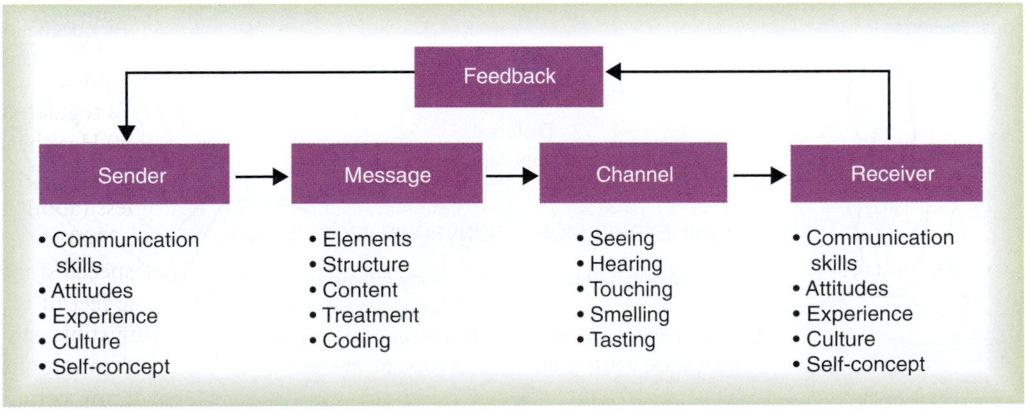

FIGURE 3-15 Elements of human communication. (See text on pp. 49 to 50.)

Another setting for improving communication between RTs regards transitions of care or "hand-off" of care; that is, when one RT is telling a colleague about the care of a patient who will be passed to the incoming RT for care. An effective communication tool in this instance may be an SBAR (Situation, Background, Assessment, and Recommendation).[18] An example of this would be an RT discussing a patient's intolerance to noninvasive ventilation. The *situation* is the patient is prescribed noninvasive ventilation but is not tolerating the device. The *background* is the patient has COPD and was admitted with a high $PaCO_2$ and would benefit from the noninvasive ventilation. The *assessment* is the patient feels "claustrophobic" in the current full-face mask. Finally, the *recommendation* would be to try a smaller, less-confining mask to improve patient comfort.

As an RT, you will have many opportunities to communicate with patients, other RTs, nurses, physicians, and other members of the health care team. Success as an RT depends on your ability to communicate with these key people. Poor communication skills can limit your ability to treat patients, work well with others, and find satisfaction in your employment.

Factors Affecting Communication

Many factors affect communication in the health care setting (Figure 3-16). The uniquely human or "internal" qualities of sender and receiver (including their prior experiences, attitudes, values, cultural backgrounds, and self-concepts and feelings) play a large role in the communication process.

Generally, the verbal and nonverbal components of communication should enhance and reinforce each other. Other factors that can affect communication include the patient's direct health care environment and their sensory or emotional state. The RT who considers all of these factors will become a better communicator. One example of this would the RT who combines a compassionate-toned verbal message such as, "You're going to be all right now," with a confirming touch of the hand is sending a much stronger message to an anxious patient than the message provided by either component alone. Several key purposes of communication are summarized in Box 3-5.

Improving Communication Skills

To enhance your ability to communicate effectively, focus on improving sending, receiving, and feedback skills. In addition, identify and overcome common barriers to effective communication.

Box 3-5 Purposes of Communication in the Health Care Setting

- To establish rapport with another individual, such as a colleague, a patient, or a member of the patient's family
- To comfort an anxious patient by explaining the unknown
- To obtain information, such as during a patient interview
- To relay pertinent information, as when charting the results of a patient's treatment
- To give instructions, as when teaching a patient how to perform a lung function test
- To persuade others to take action, as when attempting to convince a patient to quit smoking
- To educate and confirm understanding as in a "teach back" scenario

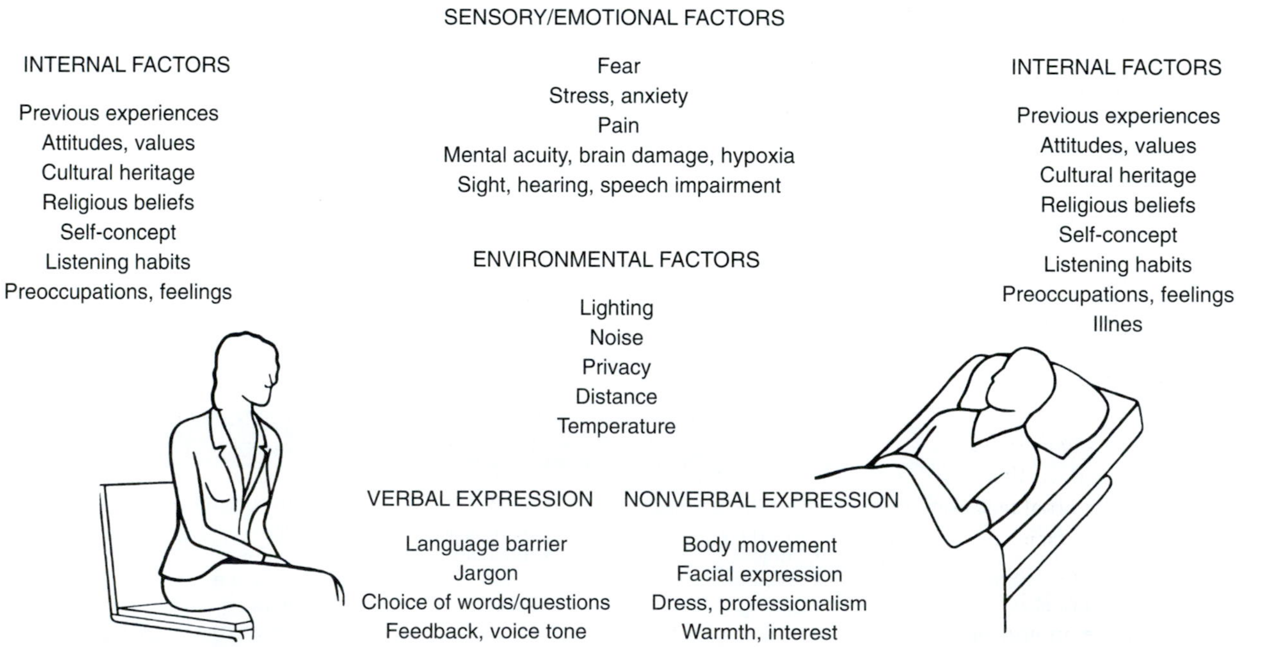

FIGURE 3-16 Factors influencing communication. (Modified from Wilkins RL, Sheldon RL, Krider SJ: Clinical assessment in respiratory care, ed 6, St. Louis, 2010, Mosby.)

MINI CLINI

Patient Communication

PROBLEM: A 73-year-old man with COPD is admitted to the emergency department for acute shortness of breath that is not relieved with rest. The patient has been admitted more than eight times during the past year for various respiratory problems. The patient's physician thinks that this episode may reflect a worsening of his disease process and orders an inhaled bronchodilator via an MDI. After the RT enters the room and introduces herself, the patient becomes quite defensive, stating that he does not need any assistance with treatments and that she should just leave the medication in the room. The RT has not treated the patient in the past and has to decide how to respond to the patient's request.

DISCUSSION: Although this patient exhibited reluctance in allowing the RT to administer the therapy, enough verbal and perhaps nonverbal communication (message) was expressed by the patient (sender) for the RT (receiver) to determine a plan of action. Because human communication is a two-way process, the RT serves an active role for further messages and interaction. This is a key concept for RTs to master because it helps in identifying a patient's problems, evaluating progress, and recommending further respiratory care. The RT must recognize that when an individual verbalizes disagreement with a treatment order and exhibits defensive behavior, the RT must attempt to understand what the patient is saying and must not overreact. The RT could try to put the patient at ease by making eye contact, gesturing effectively, and maintaining a safe distance from the patient when talking. The RT should seek feedback from the patient to ensure that the message was understood as it was intended. In this situation, it may be appropriate for the RT to review and demonstrate MDI use, ask the patient to "teach back" proper inhaler use, and observe the patient self-administer the medication. This process (message) can be repeated until the patient can demonstrate proper technique. Allowing the patient to participate actively in medical care when feasible may serve to help him maintain a sense of control over his disease process.

Practitioner as Sender

Your effectiveness as a sender of messages can be improved in several ways. These suggestions may be applied to the clinical setting as follows:

- *Share information rather than telling.* Health professionals often provide information in an authoritative manner by telling colleagues or patients what to do or say. This approach can cause defensiveness and lead to uncooperative behavior. Conversely, sharing information creates an atmosphere of cooperation and trust.
- *Seek to relate to people rather than control them.* This is of particular significance during communication with patients. Health care professionals often attempt to control patients. Few people like to be controlled. Patients feel much more important if they are treated as an equal partner in the relationship. Explaining procedures to patients and asking their permission to proceed is a way to make them feel a part of the decision making regarding their care.
- *Value disagreement as much as agreement.* When individuals express disagreement, make an attempt to understand what they are saying and do not become defensive. Be prepared for disagreement and be open to the input of others.
- *Use effective nonverbal communication techniques.* The nonverbal communication that you use is just as important as what you say. Nonverbal techniques may include eye contact, effective gesturing, facial expressions, and voice tone. It is important that your nonverbal communication matches what you are saying. It is also important to be cognizant of cultural differences in nonverbal contact. Some cultures may view direct eye contact as inappropriate, whereas in our country most find it an effective communication tool.

Practitioner as Receiver and Listener

Receiver skills are just as important as sender skills. Messages sent are of no value unless they are received as intended. Active listening on the part of the receiver is required. Learning to listen requires a strong commitment and great effort. A few simple principles can help improve your listening skills, as follows:

- *Work at listening.* Listening is often a difficult process. It takes effort to hear what others are saying. Focus your attention on the speaker and on the message.
- *Stop talking.* Practice silent listening and avoid interrupting the speaker during an interaction. Interrupting the patient is a sure way to diminish effective communication.
- *Resist distractions.* It is easy to be distracted by surrounding noises and conversations. This is particularly true in a busy environment such as a hospital. When you are listening, try to tune out other distractions and give your full attention to the person who is speaking.
- *Keep your mind open; be objective.* Being open-minded is often difficult. All people have their own opinions that may influence what they hear. Try to be objective in your listening so that you treat everyone fairly.
- *Hear the speaker out before making an evaluation.* Do not just listen to the first few words of the speaker. This is a common mistake made by listeners. Often, listeners hear the first sentence and tune out the rest, assuming they know what is being said. It is important to listen to the entire message; otherwise, you may miss important information.
- *Maintain composure; control emotions.* Allowing emotions, such as anger or anxiety, to distort your understanding or drawing conclusions before a speaker completes his or her thoughts or arguments is a common error in listening.

- Active listening is a key component in health care communication. Many of the messages being sent are vital to patient care. If you do not listen effectively, important information may be lost and the care of your patients may be jeopardized.

Providing Feedback

To enhance communication with others, effective feedback needs to be provided. Examples of effective feedback mechanisms in oral communication with patients include attending, paraphrasing, requesting clarification, perception checking, and reflecting feelings:

- *Attending.* **Attending** involves the use of gestures and posture that communicates one's attentiveness. Attending also involves confirming remarks, such as, "I see what you mean."
- *Paraphrasing.* Paraphrasing, or repeating the other's response in one's own words, is a technique that is useful in confirming that understanding is occurring between the parties involved in the interaction. However, overuse of paraphrasing can be irritating.
- *Requesting clarification.* Requesting clarification begins with an admission of misunderstanding on the part of the listener, with the intent being to understand the message better through restating or using alternative examples or illustrations. Overuse of this technique, as with paraphrasing, can hamper effective communication, especially if it is used in a condescending or patronizing manner. Requests for clarification should be used only when truly necessary and always should be nonjudgmental in nature.
- *Perception checking.* Perception checking involves confirming or disproving the more subtle components of a communication interaction, such as messages that are implied but not stated. For example, the RT might sense that a patient is unsure of the need for a treatment. In this case, the RT might check this perception by saying, "You don't seem to be sure that you need this treatment. Is that correct?" By verifying or disproving this perception, both the health care professional and the patient understand each other better.
- *Reflecting feelings.* Reflecting feelings involves the use of statements to determine better the emotions of the other party. Nonjudgmental statements, such as, "You seem to be anxious about (this situation)," provide the opportunity for patients to express and reflect on their emotions and can help them confirm or deny their true feelings.

Minimizing Barriers to Communication

There are many potential barriers to effective communication. A skillful communicator tries to identify and eliminate or minimize the influence of these barriers in all interactions. By minimizing the influence of these barriers, the sender can help ensure that the message will be received as intended. Key barriers to effective communication are the following:

- *Use of symbols or words that have different meanings.* Words and symbols (including nonverbal communication) can mean different things to different people. These differences in meaning derive from differences in the background or culture between the sender and receiver and the context of the communication. For example, RTs often use the letters COPD to refer to patients with chronic obstructive pulmonary disease caused by long-term smoking. Patients may hear COPD used in reference to them and be confused about the meaning and interpret COPD to mean a fatal lung disease. Never assume that the patient has the same understanding as you in the interpretation of commonly used symbols or phrases.
- *Different value systems.* Everyone has his or her own value system, and many people do not recognize the values held by others. A large difference among the values held by individuals can interfere with communication. A clinical supervisor may inform students of the penalties for being late with clinical assignments. If a student does not value timeliness, he or she may not take seriously what is being said.
- *Emphasis on status.* A hierarchy of positions and power exists in most health care organizations. If superiority is emphasized by individuals of higher status, communication can be stifled. Everyone has experienced interactions with professionals who make it clear who is in charge. Emphasis on status can be a barrier to communication not only among health care professionals but also between health care professionals and patients.
- *Conflict of interest.* Many people are affected by decisions made in health care organizations. If people are afraid that a decision will take away their advantage or invade their territory, they may try to block communication. An example might be a staff member who is unwilling to share expertise with students. This person may feel that a student is invading his or her territory.
- *Lack of acceptance of differences in points of view, feelings, values, or purposes.* Most of us are aware that people have different opinions, feelings, and values. These differences can thwart effective communication. To overcome this barrier, an effective communicator allows others to express their differences. Encouraging individuals to communicate their feelings and points of view benefits everyone. Most of us think we are always correct. Accepting input from others promotes growth and cooperation.
- *Feelings of personal insecurity.* It is difficult for people to admit feelings of inadequacy. Individuals who are insecure do not offer information for fear they appear ignorant or they may be defensive when criticized, blocking clear communication. Many of us have worked with individuals who are insecure, realizing the difficulty in communicating with them.

To become an effective communicator, identify the purpose of each communication interaction and your role in it. Use specific sending, receiving, and feedback skills in each interaction. Finally, minimize any identified barriers to communication with patients or peers, to ensure that messages are received as intended.

CONFLICT AND CONFLICT RESOLUTION

Conflict is sharp disagreement or opposition among people over interests, ideas, or values. Because no two people are exactly alike in their backgrounds or attitudes, conflict can be found in every organization. Health care professionals experience a great deal of conflict in their jobs. Rapid changes occurring in health care have made everyone's jobs more complex and often more stressful. Because conflict is inevitable, all health care professionals must be able to recognize its sources and help resolve or manage its effect on people and on the organization.

Sources of Conflict

The first step in conflict management is to identify its potential sources. The four primary sources of conflict in organizations are (1) poor communication, (2) structural problems, (3) personal behavior, and (4) role conflict.

Poor Communication

Poor communication is the primary source of conflict in organizations. The previously discussed barriers to communication all are potential sources of conflict. If a supervisor is unwilling to accept different points of view for dealing with a difficult patient, an argument may occur. The importance of good communication cannot be overemphasized.

Structural Problems

The structure of the organization itself can increase the likelihood of conflict. Conflict tends to grow as the size of an organization increases. Conflict is also greater in organizations whose employees are given less control over their work and in organizations in which certain individuals or groups have excessive power. Structural sources of conflict are the most rigid and are often difficult to control.

Personal Behavior

Personal behavior factors are a major source of conflict in organizations. Different personalities, attitudes, and behavioral traits create the possibility of great disagreement among health care professionals and between health care professionals and patients.

Role Conflict

Role conflict is the experience of being pulled in several directions by individuals who have different expectations of a person's job functions. A clinical supervisor is often expected to function both as a staff member and as a student supervisor. Trying to fill both roles simultaneously can cause stress and create interpersonal conflict.

Conflict Resolution

Conflict resolution or management is the process by which people control and channel disagreements within an organization. The following are five basic strategies for handling conflict:

1. Competing
2. Accommodating
3. Avoiding
4. Collaborating
5. Compromising

Competing

Competing is an assertive and uncooperative conflict resolution strategy. Competing is a power-oriented method of resolving conflict. A supervisor who uses rank or other forces to attempt to win is using the competing strategy. This strategy may be useful when an unpopular decision must be made or when one must stand up for his or her rights. However, because it often causes others to be quiet and feel inferior, competing should be used cautiously.

Accommodating

Accommodating is the opposite of competing. Accommodating is being unassertive and cooperative. When people accommodate others involved in conflict, they neglect their own needs to meet the needs of the other party. Accommodation is a useful strategy when it is essential to maintain harmony in the environment. Accommodation is also appropriate when an issue is much more important to one party or the other in a dispute.

Avoiding

Avoiding is both an unassertive and an uncooperative conflict resolution strategy. In avoiding conflict, one or both parties decide not to pursue their concerns. Avoidance may be appropriate if there is no possibility of meeting one's goals. In addition, if one or both of the parties are hostile, avoidance may be a good strategy, at least initially. However, too much avoidance can leave important issues unattended or unresolved.

Collaborating

As a conflict resolution strategy, collaborating is the opposite of avoiding. Collaborating is assertive and cooperative. In collaboration, the involved parties try to find mutually satisfying solutions to their conflict. Collaboration usually takes more time than other methods of conflict management and cannot be applied when the involved parties harbor strong negative feelings about each other.

Compromising

Compromising is a middle-ground strategy that combines assertiveness and cooperation. People who compromise give up more than individuals who compete but give up less than individuals who accommodate. Compromise is best used when a quick resolution is needed that both parties can accept. However, because both parties often feel they are losing, compromise should not be used exclusively.

Deciding which type of conflict resolution strategy to use requires knowledge of the context, the specific underlying problem, and the desires of the involved parties.

RECORDKEEPING

By 2015, the U.S. government would like all medical recordkeeping to be done electronically. The electronic medical record (EMR) is changing the way health care practitioners document care, but the overall content and concept of what we record remains the same (see Chapter 7 for a full discussion of the EMR). A medical record or chart presents a written picture of occurrences and situations pertaining to a patient throughout his or her stay in a health care institution. Medical records are the property of the institution and are strictly confidential. This information is protected under the *Health Insurance Portability and Accountability Act* (HIPAA) of 1996. The content of a patient's medical records, health insurance, or billing are not to be read or discussed by anyone except for the individuals directly caring for the patient in a hospital or medical care facility. In addition, the medical record is a legal document.

MINI CLINI

Legal Aspects of Recordkeeping

PROBLEM: A patient was given a respiratory treatment by a respiratory care student, who forgot to chart that the therapy was given. The student reasoned that because he did not observe any adverse effects during or immediately after the treatment and he knew that the treatment was given, not documenting the treatment in the medical record this one time would be acceptable. What are the problems associated with this student's judgment and subsequent actions?

DISCUSSION: The medical record is a legal document intended to identify types of care given to a patient and serve as a source of information to the physician, RT (including the student), and other health care providers in developing an individualized plan of care. It further serves as a tool for evaluating the effectiveness in reaching the goals of therapy. Hospitals and other health care agencies critically evaluate the medical records of patients to maintain high-quality patient care. Failure to document care rendered, such as a respiratory treatment, hinders the process of providing high-quality care in several ways.

First, information that is important to the physician and other caregivers interested in the patient's respiratory status is missing from the medical record. In this situation, although the student observed a lack of response by the patient during and immediately after the treatment, a delayed effect still could have occurred. Consequently, the physician or RT would have difficulty in establishing the cause of a condition change in the patient related to the respiratory treatment. From a legal perspective, patient care not documented may be viewed as care not rendered, making the hospital or institution vulnerable to charges of patient neglect, which would be difficult to defend in a court of law.

Because the law requires that a record be kept of the patient's care, a patient's chart is also a legal document. For this reason, charting or recordkeeping must be done so that it is meaningful for days, months, or years.

Components of a Traditional Medical Record

Each health care facility has its own specification for the medical records it keeps. Although the forms themselves vary among institutions, most acute care medical records share common sections (Box 3-6). Documentation sheets are designed to report data briefly and to decrease time spent in documentation. Entries can include many measurements, and review of a sequence of entries can reveal trends in patient status.

Legal Aspects of Recordkeeping

Legally, documentation of the care given to a patient means that care was given; no documentation means that care was not given. Hospital accreditation agencies critically evaluate the medical records of patients. If the RT does not document care given (i.e., patient assessment data, interventions, and evaluation of care rendered), the practitioner and the hospital may be accused of patient neglect.

Adequate documentation of care is valuable only in reference to standards and criteria of care. Similar to all departments in health care facilities, respiratory care departments must generate their own standards of patient care. For each standard, criteria must be outlined so that the adequacy of patient care can be measured. Documentation must reflect these standards.

Practical Aspects of Recordkeeping

Recordkeeping is one of the most significant duties that a health care professional performs. Documentation is required for each medication, treatment, or procedure. Accounts of the patient's condition and activities must be charted accurately and in clear terms. Brevity is essential, although a complete account of each patient encounter is needed. The use of standardized terms and abbreviations is acceptable; however, TJC had published a "Do Not Use" abbreviation list developed to reduce potential errors (Table 3-2).[19] Documentation of consultations with the attending physician that include the date and time of the conversation is recommended.

Accounts of care and the patient's condition can be handwritten, but with increasing frequency, EMRs facilitate data entry by selection from menus of choices or direct typing (see section on EMR in Chapter 7). In either case, you must document only what is—not an interpretation or a judgment. Assessments of data must be clearly within one's professional domain. When a practitioner cannot interpret the data obtained, he or she should state so in the record and contact another health care professional for advice or referral and document the referral in the patient's medical record. Other general rules for medical recordkeeping are listed in Box 3-7. In addition to these general rules, each institution has its own policies governing medical recordkeeping.

Box 3-6 General Sections Found in a Patient Medical Record

ADMISSION DATA
Records pertinent patient information (e.g., name, address, religion, nearest of kin), admitting physician, and admission diagnosis

HISTORY AND PHYSICAL EXAMINATION
Records the patient's admitting history and physical examination, as performed by the attending physician or resident

HEALTH MAINTENANCE AND IMMUNIZATIONS
Records the dates of administration

PHYSICIAN'S ORDERS
Records the physician's orders and prescriptions

PROGRESS NOTES
Keeps a continuing account of the patient's progress for the physician

NURSES' NOTES
Describes the nursing care given to the patient, including the patient's complaints (subjective symptoms), the nurses' observations (objective signs), and the patient's response to therapy

MEDICATION RECORD
Notes drugs and IV fluids that are given to the patient

ALLERGIES
Notes reaction, severity, type, and date

VITAL SIGNS FLOWSHEET
Records the patient's temperature, pulse, respirations, and blood pressure over time

I/O SHEET
Records patient's fluid intake (I) and output (O) over time

LABORATORY RESULTS
Summarizes the results of laboratory tests

CONSULTATION NOTE
Records notes by physicians who are called in to examine a patient to make a diagnosis

SURGICAL OR TREATMENT CONSENT
Records the patient's authorization for surgery or treatment

ANESTHESIA AND SURGICAL RECORD
Notes key events before, during, and immediately after surgery

SPECIALIZED THERAPY RECORDS AND PROGRESS NOTES
Records specialized treatments or treatment plans and patient progress for various specialized therapeutic services (e.g., respiratory care, physical therapy)

SPECIALIZED FLOW DATA
Records measurement made over time during specialized procedures (e.g., mechanical ventilation, kidney dialysis)

ADVANCED DIRECTIVES
Records wishes and documents regarding living wills, power of attorney, and do-not-resuscitate orders

TABLE 3-2
The Joint Commission "Do Not Use" List*

Do Not Use	Potential Problem	Use Instead
U (unit)	Mistaken for 0 (zero), the number 4 (four) or cc	Write "unit"
IU (international unit)	Mistaken for IV (intravenous) or the number 10 (ten)	Write "international unit"
Q.E., QD, q.d., qd (daily); Q.O.D., POD, q.o.d, qod (every other day)	Mistaken for each other; period after the Q mistaken for I and the O mistaken for I	Write "daily" or "every other day"
Trailing zero (X.0 mg)†; lack of leading zero (.X mg)	Decimal point is missed	Write "X mg" or "0.X mg"
MS	Can mean morphine sulfate or magnesium sulfate	Write "morphine sulfate"
MSO_4, $MgSO_4$	Confused for one another	Write "magnesium sulfate"
Additional Abbreviations, Acronyms, and Symbols for *Possible* Future Inclusion in the Official "Do Not Use" List		
> (greater than); < (less than)	Misinterpreted as the number 7 (seven) or the letter L; confused for one another	Write "greater than" or "less than"
Abbreviations for drug names	Misinterpreted owing to similar abbreviations for multiple drugs	Write drug names in full
Apothecary units	Unfamiliar to many practitioners; confused with metric units	Use metric units
@	Mistaken for the number "2" (two)	Write "at"
cc	Mistaken for U (units) when poorly written	Write "mL" or "ml" or "milliliters" ("mL" is preferred)
µg	Mistaken for mg (milligrams) resulting in 1000-fold overdose	Write "mcg" or "micrograms"

From Joint Commission on Accreditation of Healthcare Organizations: 2010 JCAHO "Do Not Use" list. http://www.jointcommission.org/hospitals. Accessed September 17, 2014.
*Applies to all orders and all medication-related documentation that is hand-written (including free-text computer entry) or on preprinted forms.
†*Exception:* A "trailing zero" may be used only where required to show the level of precision of the value being reported, such as for laboratory results, imaging studies that report size of lesions, or catheter/tube sizes. It may not be used in medication orders or other medication-related documentation.

Box 3-7 General Rules for Medical Recordkeeping

- Entries on the patient's chart should be printed or handwritten unless the institution is using an electronic medical record. After completing the account in the handwritten record, sign the chart with one initial and your last name and your title (CRT, RRT, Resp Care Student; e.g., S. Smith, CRT). Institutional policy may require that supervisory personnel countersign student entries in the hand-written record.
- Do not use ditto marks.
- Do not erase. Erasures provide reason for question if the chart is used later in a court of law. If a mistake is made, a single line should be drawn through the mistake and the word *error* printed above it. Then continue your charting in a normal manner.
- Record after completing each task for the patient, and sign your name correctly after each entry.
- Be exact in noting the time, effect, and results of all treatments and procedures.
- Chart patient complaints and general behavior. Describe the type, location, onset, and duration of pain. Describe clearly and concisely the character and amount of secretions.
- Leave no blank lines in the charting. Draw a line through the center of an empty line or part of a line. This prevents charting by someone else in an area signed by you.
- Use standard abbreviations. (Follow the "Do Not Use" list.[18])
- Use the present tense. Never use the future tense, as in "Patient to receive treatment after lunch."
- Spell correctly. If you are unsure about the spelling of a word, look it up in a dictionary.
- Document conversations with the patient or other health care providers that you think are important (e.g., you informed the patient's physician or nurse that the patient seems confused or more short of breath).

Problem-Oriented Medical Record

The **problem-oriented medical record (POMR)** is an alternative documentation format used by some health care institutions. The POMR contains four parts: (1) the database, (2) the problem list, (3) the plan, and (4) the progress notes. Whether electronic or written, the precise forms these records take vary among institutions but will share common information.

The database contains routine information about the patient. A general health history, physical examination results, and results of diagnostic tests are included.

In the POMR, a problem is something that interferes with a patient's physical or psychologic health or ability to function. The patient's problems are identified and listed on the basis of the information provided by the database. The list of problems is dynamic; new problems are added as they develop, and problems are removed as they are resolved.

The POMR progress notes contain the findings (subjective and objective data), assessment, plans, and orders of the physicians, nurses, and other practitioners involved in the care of the patient. The format used is often referred to as **SOAP** (*S* = subjective information, *O* = objective information, *A* = assessment, *P* = plan of care). Figure 3-17 shows a representative SOAP form for respiratory care progress notes. Box 3-8 provides a handwritten example of a SOAP entry. Table 3-3 lists common objective data gathered by RTs and examples of applicable assessments and plans. In many institutions, all caregivers chart on the same form, using the SOAP format.

TABLE 3-3

Examples of Objective Data, Assessments, and Plans Typical for Documentation Using SOAP Notes

Objective Data	Assessment	Plan
Sputum Production		
Thick, purulent	Respiratory infection	Humidity therapy, antibiotics
Auscultation		
Expiratory wheezing	Bronchospasm	Bronchodilator
Stridor	Upper airway obstruction	Racemic epinephrine, possible intubation
Late-inspiratory crackles	Atelectasis	Lung expansion therapy
Breathing Pattern		
Prolonged expiratory time	Bronchospasm	Bronchodilators
Prolonged inspiratory time	Upper airway obstruction	Racemic epinephrine; consider need for intubation
Rapid and shallow	Restrictive lung disease	Notify physician, perform additional assessment, consider lung expansion therapy
Vital Signs		
Acute tachycardia/tachypnea	Acute respiratory failure	Obtain ABGs, chest x-ray films; call physician
Abnormal sensorium	Acute hypoxia	Assess patient further; oxygen therapy
ABGs		
PaO_2 40-60 mm Hg	Moderate hypoxemia	Give O_2 via cannula or mask
PaO_2 < 40 mm Hg	Severe hypoxemia	Give high concentration O_2 as needed and consider positive pressure ventilation with PEEP or CPAP
Chest Radiograph		
Low lung volumes or infiltrates	Atelectasis	Lung expansion therapy
Air in pleural space	Pneumothorax	Insert chest tube

ABGs, Arterial blood gas analysis; *CPAP,* continuous positive airway pressure; *PEEP,* positive end-expiratory pressure.

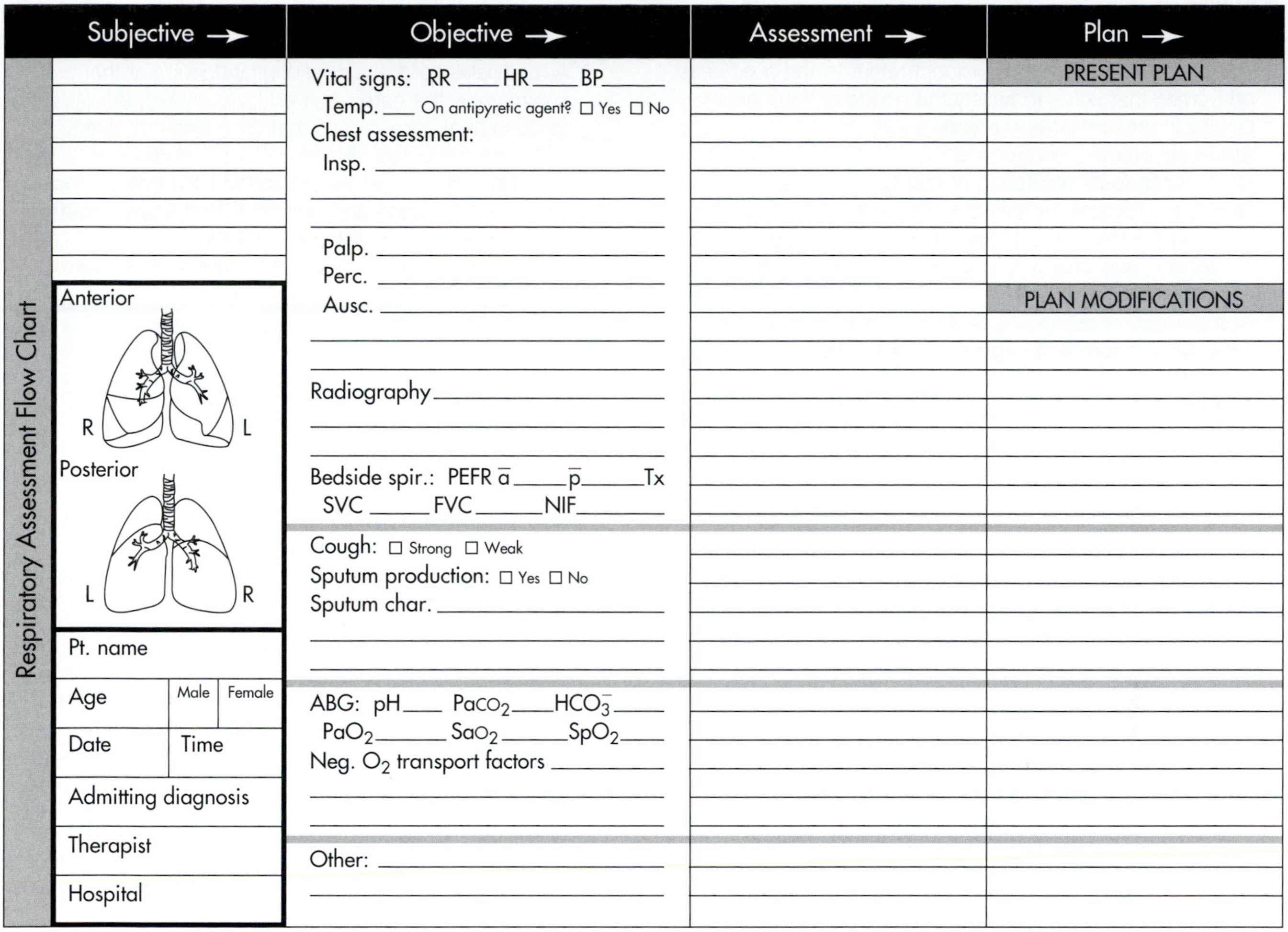

Respiratory Assessment Flow Chart

Subjective → | Objective → | Assessment → | Plan →

Vital signs: RR ___ HR ___ BP ___
Temp. ___ On antipyretic agent? ☐ Yes ☐ No
Chest assessment:
Insp. ___
Palp. ___
Perc. ___
Ausc. ___
Radiography ___
Bedside spir.: PEFR ā ___ p̄ ___ Tx
SVC ___ FVC ___ NIF ___
Cough: ☐ Strong ☐ Weak
Sputum production: ☐ Yes ☐ No
Sputum char. ___
ABG: pH ___ $PaCO_2$ ___ HCO_3^- ___
PaO_2 ___ SaO_2 ___ SpO_2 ___
Neg. O_2 transport factors ___
Other: ___

PRESENT PLAN

PLAN MODIFICATIONS

Anterior
R L
Posterior
L R

Pt. name
Age | Male | Female
Date | Time
Admitting diagnosis
Therapist
Hospital

FIGURE 3-17 Example of a SOAP form for respiratory care progress notes. (From Des Jardins T, Burton GG: Clinical manifestations and assessment of respiratory disease, ed 6, St. Louis, 2011, Mosby.)

Box 3-8 Example of SOAP Entry

PROBLEM 1
Difficult breathing.

SUBJECTIVE
"I can't catch my breath."

OBJECTIVE
Awake; alert; oriented to time, place, and person; sitting upright in bed with arms leaning over the bedside stand; pale, dry skin; respirations 26 breaths/min and shallow; pulse 98 beats/min, regular and faint to palpation; blood pressure 112/68 mm Hg, left arm, sitting position; body temperature 101°F; bronchial breath sounds in lower posterior lung fields; occasionally expectorating small volumes of mucopurulent sputum. Chest x-ray film shows left lower lung infiltrate.

ASSESSMENT
Retained mucus and possible infection.

PLAN
Therapeutic: Assist with coughing and deep breathing at least every 2 hours; postural drainage and percussion every 4 hours; assist with ambulation as per physician orders and patient tolerance.
Diagnostic: Continue to monitor lung sounds before and after each treatment.
Education: Teach patient to cough and deep breathe and evaluate return demonstration.

RULE OF THUMB

Charting Progress Notes Using the SOAP Format

SOAP stands for Subjective, Objective, Assessment, Plan.

- Subjective information obtained from the patient, his or her family members, or a similar source
- Objective information based on caregivers' observations of the patient, the physical examination, or diagnostic or laboratory tests such as arterial blood gases or pulmonary function tests
- Assessment, which refers to the analysis of the patient's problem
- Plan of action to be taken to resolve the problem

SUMMARY CHECKLIST

- The quality of a service or product refers to the sum of its properties that serve to satisfy the needs of its consumer.
- Quality improvement is everyone's job.
- Statistical process control and run charts are tools that allow continuous monitoring of quality of service.
- Quality improvement projects involve different phases: Planning the project, implementing the project, analyzing the results, and changing course of action based on analysis.
- Competency is defined as having suitable or sufficient skills, knowledge, and experience for the purposes of the specific task.
- Annual competency checks need to be documented for skills and procedures that pose potential risk to patient safety.
- The Joint Commission (TJC) is an independent, non-for-profit organization that strives to continuously improve quality and safety of health care services by setting high standards and evaluating health care organizations for adherence.
- TJC requires hospitals to have quality assurance plans and encourages performance improvement efforts.
- Hospital accreditation by TJC is based on satisfying specific standards established by professional and technical advisory committees.
- Good posture is needed when lifting patients or heavy equipment to avoid injury.
- Electrical current (flow) is the dangerous element of electricity. Current is directly related to voltage and inversely related to resistance.
- A microshock is a small, imperceptible current (<1 mA) that enters the body through external wires or catheters; microshocks can cause ventricular fibrillation.
- To avoid electrical hazards, always ground equipment and use only equipment that has been checked for proper wiring.
- Fires in health care facilities most often start in the kitchen, but when they occur in patient care areas, loss of life and serious injuries are likely.
- Maintain a safe and clutter-free direct patient care environment.
- Store and transport medical grade gases in a safe and effective manner.
- Communication skills play a key role in the ability to identify a patient's problems, to evaluate the patient's progress, to make recommendations for respiratory care, and to achieve desired patient outcomes.
- Individuals' prior experiences, attitudes, values, cultural backgrounds, self-concepts, and feelings play a large role in the communication process.
- To enhance communication ability, focus on improving sending, receiving, and feedback skills; in addition, be able to identify and overcome common barriers to effective communication.
- Choose the best strategy for handling conflict considering knowledge of the context, the specific underlying problem, and the desires of the involved parties.
- The EMR is transforming the way we document care but not the concept and content of what is documented.
- A medical record is a confidential document that summarizes the care received by a patient; legally, a failure to document care means that care was not given.
- Following accepted standards, each medication, treatment, or procedure provided to the patient, including his or her condition and response to therapy, must be documented in accurate and clear terms.
- When entering notes in a POMR, use a SOAP format.

References

1. Deming WE: *Out of the crisis*, Cambridge, MA, 2009, Massachusetts Institute of Technology Center for Advanced Engineering Study.
2. Turner MO, Patel A, Ginsburg S, et al: Bronchodilator delivery in acute airflow obstruction: a meta-analysis. *Arch Intern Med* 157:1736, 1997.
3. Cates C: Spacers and nebulisers for the delivery of beta-agonists in non-life-threatening acute asthma. *Respir Med* 97:762, 2003.
4. Cates CC, Welsh EJ, Rowe BH: Holding chambers versus nebulisers for beta-agonist treatment of acute asthma. *Cochrane Database Syst Rev* (9): CD000052, 2013.
5. Epstein RS, Sharwood LM: From outcomes research to disease management: a guide for the perplexed. *Ann Intern Med* 124:832, 1996.
6. Elrodt G, Cook DJ, Lee J, et al: Evidence-based disease management. *JAMA* 78:1997, 1687.
7. Mish FC, Gilman WW, editors: *Webster's ninth new collegiate dictionary*, Springfield, MA, 1985, Merriam-Webster.
8. Harder BN: Use of simulation in teaching and learning in health sciences: a systematic review. *J Nurs Educ* 49:23, 2010.
9. Van Herck P, De Smedt D, Annemans L, et al: Systematic review: effects, design choices, and context of pay-for- performance in healthcare. *BMC Health Serv Res* 10:247, 2010.
10. Kester EL, Stoller JK: A computer-aided audit system for respiratory therapy consult evaluations: description of a method and early results. *Respir Care* 58:790, 2013.
11. Lowell KH, Bertko J: The accountable care organization (ACO) model: building blocks for success. *J Ambul Care Manage* 33:81, 2010.
12. Kester L, Stoller JK: Respiratory care in the adult non-ICU setting. *Respir Care* 42:101, 1997.
13. Siu AL, Penrod JD, Boockvar KS, et al: Early ambulation after hip fracture: effects on function and mortality. *Arch Intern Med* 166:766, 2006.
14. Mundy LM, Leet TL, Darst K, et al: Early mobilization of patients hospitalized with community-acquired pneumonia. *Chest* 124:883, 2003.
15. Ahrens M: *U.S. Fires in healthcare facilities*, Quincy, MA, 2012, National Fire Protection Association. <http://www.nfpa.org>. Accessed May 15, 2015.
16. National Fire Protection Association: *Healthcare facilities 99, standard for healthcare facilities*, ed 2015, Quincy, MA, 2014, National Fire Protection Association.
17. Joint Commission: *National Patient Safety Goals 2014*. http://www.jointcommission.org/assets/1/6/HAP_NPSG_Chapter_2014.pdf. Accessed September 17, 2014.
18. Haig K, Sutton S, Whittington J: SBAR: a shared mental model for improving communication between clinicians. *Jt Comm J Qual Patient Saf* 32:171, 2006.
19. Joint Commission on Accreditation of Healthcare Organizations: *2010 JCAHO "Do Not Use" list*. http://www.jointcommission.org/hospitals. Accessed September 17, 2014.

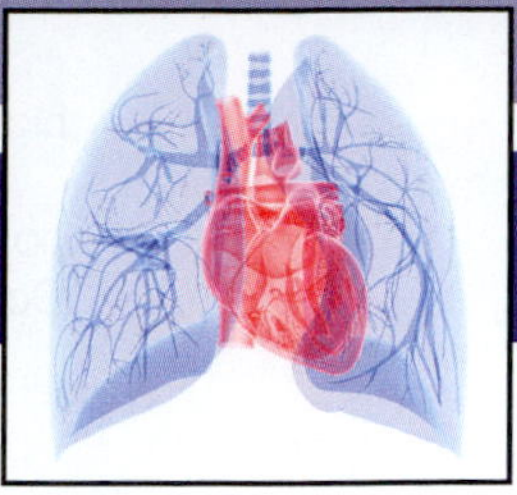

CHAPTER 4

Principles of Infection Prevention and Control

MICHELE MESSAM AND THOMAS G. FRASER

CHAPTER OBJECTIVES

After reading this chapter you will be able to:

- Define health care–associated infections and state how often they occur.
- Describe why infection prevention is important in respiratory care.
- Identify and describe the three elements that must be present for transmission of infection within a health care setting.
- List the factors associated with an increased risk for a patient acquiring a hospital-acquired infection.
- State the three major routes for transmission of human sources of pathogens in the health care environment.
- Describe strategies to control the spread of infection in the hospital.
- Describe how to select and apply chemical disinfectants for processing respiratory care equipment.
- Describe equipment-handling procedures that help prevent the spread of pathogens.
- State when to use personal protective equipment during patient care.
- Describe surveillance with regard to infection control.

CHAPTER OUTLINE

KEY TERMS

antiseptic
bactericidal
bacteriostatic
cohorting
contact precautions
disinfection
droplet nuclei
droplet precautions
fomites
health care–associated infection
Healthcare Infection Control Practices Advisory Committee

high-efficiency particulate air/aerosol filters
hospital-acquired infections
Occupational Safety and Health Administration
respiratory hygiene/cough etiquette
sporicidal
standard precautions
sterilization
surveillance
virucidal

Patients are at risk for developing infections during their hospital stay. A recent study estimated that 4% of hospitalized patients in the United States develop a health care–associated infection.[1] To help better understand preventive measures, infections can be categorized by where they originate. Those that develop outside the hospital are called *community onset.* Those that develop in the hospital are called *hospital-onset* or *nosocomial* infections. However, in the current era, patients can receive care in many different settings—the home, the hospital, a skilled nursing facility, or an outpatient treatment center. Patients who are at home but getting care in a nonhospital setting can develop community-onset infections that are related to health care and are not community acquired. The term **health care–associated infection** (HAI) refers to infections that develop in a patient during the course of medical treatment. This classification system is not arbitrary, because there are unique risks for HAIs such as the presence of an endotracheal tube or a central venous catheter. HAIs also can be related to certain pathogens that are more likely to be resistant to one or more classes of antimicrobial agents. For example, *Pseudomonas aeruginosa* is commonly seen as a cause of HAI pneumonia; however, it is not routinely seen as a cause of community-acquired disease.

Efforts to decrease **hospital-acquired infection** and HAIs are commonly organized and coordinated by a hospital's Infection Prevention (IP) program. IP programs are charged with reducing the risk for HAIs and thereby protecting patients, employees, and visitors. They do this by providing guidance to their organizations so that they can break the chain of events leading to HAIs. Guidance and prevention efforts are directed at overall organizational structure and systems ("this is what we do as an institution to prevent infection") and at the individual caregiver level ("this is what I do to prevent infection").

Protecting patients and health care professionals against HAIs requires strict adherence to IP procedures. These procedures aim to eliminate the sources of infectious agents, create barriers to their transmission, and monitor and evaluate the effectiveness of control. IP departments coordinate activities and provide guidance to their institutions. Decreasing the risk for HAIs is a major and ongoing responsibility of all health care workers, including respiratory therapists (RTs). To fulfill this responsibility, RTs must be able to select and consistently apply a full spectrum of daily competencies. This chapter provides the foundation needed to assume this important responsibility.

SPREAD OF INFECTION

Three elements must be present for transmission of infection within a health care setting: (1) a *source* (or reservoir) of pathogens, (2) a *susceptible host,* and (3) a *route* of transmission for the pathogen (Figure 4-1).[2]

Sources of Infectious Agents

Humans (patients, personnel, or visitors) are the primary source for infectious agents in the health care setting, but inanimate objects (e.g., contaminated medical equipment, linen, medications) also have been implicated in transmission. Patients quickly contaminate their local hospital environment, particularly high-touch surfaces, such as call lights, bed rails, tray tables, and bathrooms. People also may serve as their own source of infection, via endogenous flora. This latter process is called *autogenous infection.*

Susceptible Hosts

Susceptibility and resistance to infection vary greatly. Host factors in the acute setting that predispose to HAI can be considered modifiable and nonmodifiable. Host factors, such as poorly controlled diabetes mellitus, extremes of age, and underlying acquired (human immunodeficiency virus [HIV] infection) or iatrogenic (through chemotherapy or anti–tumor necrosis factor inhibitors) immunodeficiency, can enhance susceptibility to infection and are not readily modifiable in the acute setting. Surgical incisions and radiation therapy impair defenses of the skin and organ space. Medical devices, such as urinary tract catheters, central venous catheters, and endotracheal tubes, increase the risk for infection by impeding local host defenses and providing a surface for the development of biofilms. The need for the medical device may be unavoidable. However, the risk for infection associated with it can be modified by employing appropriate techniques for insertion, maintenance, and removal.

Modes of Transmission

The three major routes for transmission of human pathogens in the health care environment are *contact* (direct and indirect), *respiratory droplets,* and *airborne droplet nuclei* (respirable particles <5 μm). Table 4-1 provides examples of the common transmission routes for selected microorganisms.[3]

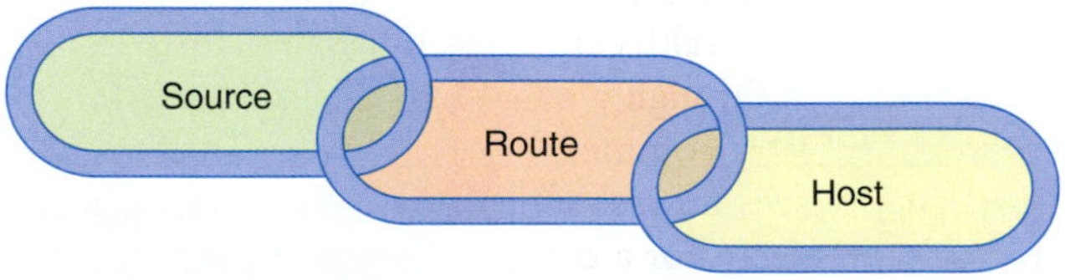

FIGURE 4-1 Elements that must be present for infection to spread.

TABLE 4-1

Routes of Infectious Disease Transmission

Mode	Type	Examples
Contact	Direct	Hepatitis A HIV *Staphylococcus* Enteric bacteria
	Indirect	*Pseudomonas aeruginosa* Enteric bacteria Hepatitis B and C HIV
Droplet		*Haemophilus influenzae* (type B) pneumonia and epiglottitis *Neisseria meningitidis* pneumonia Diphtheria Pertussis Streptococcal pneumonia Influenza Mumps Rubella Adenovirus Rhinovirus
Vehicle	Water-borne	Shigellosis Cholera
	Food-borne	Salmonellosis Hepatitis A
Airborne	Aerosols	Legionellosis
	Droplet nuclei	Tuberculosis Varicella Measles Smallpox
Vector-borne	Ticks and mites	Rickettsia Lyme disease
	Mosquitoes	Malaria
	Fleas	Bubonic plague

HIV, Human immunodeficiency virus.

Contact Transmission

Contact transmission is the most common route of transmission and is divided into two subgroups: direct and indirect. *Direct contact transmission* occurs when a pathogen is transferred directly from one person to another. Direct contact transmission occurs less frequently than indirect contact in the health care environment but is more efficient. An example of direct contact transmission would be development of respiratory syncytial virus bronchiolitis in a bone marrow transplant recipient owing to transmission of the virus from an ill health care worker who did not perform appropriate hand hygiene before providing care.

Indirect contact transmission is the most frequent mode of transmission in the health care environment and involves transfer of a pathogen through a contaminated intermediate object or person. The most common indirect contact transmission in health care involves unwashed hands of health care personnel that touch an infected or a colonized body site on one patient, or a contaminated inanimate object, and subsequently touch another patient. Inanimate objects that may serve to transfer pathogens from one person to another are called **fomites.** Indirect contact transmission involving fomites can occur when instruments have been inadequately cleaned between patients before disinfection or sterilization.

Droplet Transmission

Droplet transmission is a form of contact transmission, but the mechanism of transfer of the pathogen is distinct and additional prevention measures are required. Organisms that are transmitted by respiratory droplets include influenza and *Neisseria meningitidis.* Respiratory droplets are generated when an infected individual discharges large contaminated liquid droplets into the air by coughing, sneezing, or talking. Respiratory droplets are also generated during procedures such as suctioning, bronchoscopy, and cough induction. Transmission occurs when infectious droplets are propelled (usually ≤3 feet through the air) and are deposited on another person's mouth or nose. Using the distance of 3 feet or less as a minimum threshold for donning a mask has been effective in preventing transmission of infectious agents. However, experimental studies with smallpox and investigations of outbreaks of severe acute respiratory syndrome (SARS) suggest that droplets from infected patients rarely are able to reach a person 6 feet away.[4] A distance of 3 feet or less around the patient is considered a short distance and is not used as a criterion for deciding when a mask should be donned to protect from exposure. **Healthcare Infection Control Practices Advisory Committee** (HICPAC) guidelines state it may be prudent to don a mask when within 6 to 10 feet of a patient or on entry into the room of a patient who is on droplet isolation.[3]

Airborne Transmission

Airborne transmission occurs via the spread of airborne **droplet nuclei.** These are small particles (≤5 μm) of evaporated droplets containing infectious microorganisms that can remain suspended in air for long periods. Microorganisms carried in this manner may be dispersed widely by air currents because of their small size and inhaled by susceptible hosts over a longer distance from the source patient compared with droplet transmission. Examples of pathogens transmitted via the airborne route include *Mycobacterium tuberculosis,* varicella-zoster virus (chickenpox), and rubeola virus (measles).[4]

Special air handling and ventilation and respiratory protection are required to prevent airborne transmission because microorganisms may remain suspended in air and be widely dispersed by air currents before contacting a susceptible host. In addition to airborne infection isolation rooms, personal respiratory protection with National Institute for Occupational Safety and Health (NIOSH)–approved N-95 or higher respirators is required to prevent airborne transmission.[3] A surgical mask, used for droplet precautions, is insufficient.

Miscellaneous Types of Aerosol Transmission

The separation of organisms that are transmitted by aerosols into the categories of droplet and airborne is based on the usual manner in which disease is transmitted. In-depth investigations of outbreaks have demonstrated that the line between these two categories of transmission is sometimes blurry. In certain circumstances, such as during endotracheal intubation and aerosol-generating procedures, there is some evidence that organisms such as influenza and SARS can be transmitted via droplet nuclei. Similarly, norovirus, the most common cause of infectious diarrhea transmitted mainly by contact, probably also can be transmitted by swallowing aerosolized virus from vomitus. Based on these examples, aerosol transmission of droplet nuclei can be further refined as follows[3]:

- *Obligate transmission:* Under natural conditions, disease occurs after transmission of the microorganism only through airborne (droplet nuclei) aerosols. An example of obligate transmission is tuberculosis.
- *Preferential transmission:* Natural infection results from transmission through multiple routes, but airborne transmission predominates. Measles is an example of preferential airborne transmission.
- *Opportunistic transmission:* Microorganisms that cause disease through other routes—droplet or contact—but under certain environmental conditions may be transmitted via airborne transmission. An example of this is SARS transmission via an aerosol plume that originated from sewage in the Amoy Gardens housing complex in the Kowloon section of Hong Kong in 2003.[4]

Awareness of these nuances of transmission informs health care workers to wear the appropriate personal protective equipment depending on the clinical circumstances. For example, during a bronchoscopy for a patient infected with influenza, the possibility of opportunistic airborne transmission of the virus would cause one to consider wearing an N95 mask as opposed to a regular surgical mask.

Other Sources of Infection Not Involving Person-to-Person Transmission

Common vehicle transmission occurs via exposure to pathogens in contaminated food, water, or medications (e.g., heparin solution). Vector-borne transmission of infectious diseases from insects and rats and other vermin occurs but is of less significance in U.S. health care facilities.

INFECTION PREVENTION STRATEGIES

Creating a Safe Culture

From an organizational perspective, a crucial first step to decrease the risk for HAIs is the creation by leadership, at all levels, of a culture of safety in which there is a shared commitment to patient and health care worker safety. Creating a culture of safety is also the responsibility of each individual health care worker. It is important that each person is empowered and willing to speak up and "stop the line" if the person has a concern that a patient or employee is in an unsafe situation.

Organizations also endorse best practices for infection prevention by ensuring that the bedside caregiver has the appropriate time, equipment, and training to provide the best possible care. Competent health care workers execute appropriate practice, such as attention to hand hygiene and adherence to infection prevention bundles of care on a daily basis with every patient. Failure to perform these basics is a deviation from good practice and cannot be tolerated. The presence of appropriate systems to deliver care and a committed workforce consistently executing best practice are necessary for an organization to reliably prevent infections.[6]

Maintaining a Healthy Workforce

The day-to-day care of hospitalized patients relies on people. A sick health care worker not only has difficulty executing assignments but could also serve as a source of infection for vulnerable patients. There are multiple different components to maintaining a healthy workforce. The standard and transmission-based precautions described later not only prevent transmission of pathogens from patient to patient but also protect health care workers. Other efforts employed to protect health care workers are employee immunization and chemoprophylaxis. Certain immunizations are recommended for susceptible health care personnel to decrease the risk for infection and the potential for transmission to patients and co-workers within the health care facility.[5] The **Occupational Safety and Health Administration** (OSHA) mandates that employers offer hepatitis B vaccination. Vaccinations of health care workers in the absence of evidence of immunity against varicella, rubella, and measles should be strongly encouraged. In addition, health care personnel should receive the adult acellular pertussis vaccine, particularly those who care for young infants and children. Health care personnel without medical contraindications should receive an annual influenza vaccination.[5] Health care worker influenza vaccination is the single most effective way to prevent health care–associated influenza. A vaccinated population decreases the risk for presenteeism (health care workers being at work when sick). The importance of receiving an influenza vaccine is reflected in the recent requirement that health care facilities publicly report vaccination rates of their employees, licensed independent practitioners, volunteers, and adult students.[7] To improve health care worker vaccination adherence, many organizations have made receiving a flu vaccine mandatory.

Uncommonly, health care workers are recommended to take antibiotics in addition to standard and transmission-based precautions and vaccination, to prevent disease. Examples of these situations include postexposure prophylaxis after close contact with a patient with meningococcal meningitis or exposure to blood or body fluid of a patient with HIV. One specific situation in which vaccination and chemoprophylaxis are combined is exposure to a patient with *Bordetella pertussis* (whooping cough). Infants can develop severe complications from whooping cough, including death. If health care workers have had close contact with an active case of whooping cough, and have contact with infants younger than 1 year of age or women in the third trimester of pregnancy, they should receive prophylaxis in addition to having their vaccination status updated.[3,5]

> **RULE OF THUMB**
> All health care workers with patient contact should undergo immunization for hepatitis B and varicella (if not immune), pertussis booster, and annual influenza vaccination.

Eliminating the Source of Pathogens

Elimination of all pathogens from any working environment is impossible. Nonetheless, standard infection prevention procedures always include efforts to eliminate pathogens, and recommended practices for cleaning and disinfecting noncritical surfaces in patient care areas should be followed. Procedures designed to remove environmental pathogens fall into two major categories: *general sanitation measures* and *specialized equipment processing.*

General sanitation measures help keep the overall environment clean. General sanitation aims to reduce the number of pathogens to a safe level. This reduction is achieved through sanitary laundry management, food preparation, and housekeeping. Environmental control of the air (using specialized ventilation systems) and water complements these efforts.

The goal of specialized equipment processing is to decontaminate equipment capable of spreading infection. Equipment processing involves cleaning, disinfection, and sterilization (when necessary). Methods that kill bacteria are **bactericidal,** whereas methods and techniques that inhibit the growth of bacteria are **bacteriostatic.** Methods that destroy spores are **sporicidal,** and methods that destroy viruses are **virucidal.**

Interrupting Transmission

General sanitation measures and equipment processing have limits. To prevent the spread of infections between patients and to keep themselves healthy, health care personnel must take measures to stop infection. Best practices to limit transmission of pathogens in the hospital have been put forth by HICPAC and the Centers for Disease Control and Prevention (CDC). These recommendations include standard precautions and transmission-based precautions.[3]

Standard Precautions

The term **standard precautions** refers to the simplest level of infection control based on the recognition that all blood, body fluids, secretions, and excretions (with the exception of sweat) may contain transmissible infectious agents. Standard precautions are intended to be applied to the care of all patients in all health care settings all the time. This is the primary strategy for the prevention of health care–associated transmission of infections among patients and health care personnel. To reduce risk for infection, a health care worker should employ personal protective equipment (PPE). PPE refers to various barriers used alone or in combination to protect mucous membranes, skin, and clothing from contact with infectious agents. Gloves, gowns, masks, eye protection, and face shields should be employed depending on the anticipated exposure.

The application of standard precautions by health care personnel during patient care depends on the nature of the interaction and the potential for blood, body fluid, or pathogen contact. For some patient care situations, only gloves are required. In other cases, gloves, gowns, and face shield may be required. Box 4-1 describes standard precautions, including hand hygiene; use of gloves, masks, and eye protection; equipment handling; and patient placement.

Hand Hygiene

The importance of hand hygiene to reduce the transmission of infectious agents cannot be overemphasized and is an essential element of standard precautions.[8] Hand hygiene includes handwashing with either plain or **antiseptic**-containing soap and water for at least 15 seconds or the use of alcohol-based products (gels, rinses, and foams). In the absence of visible soiling of hands, approved alcohol-based products are preferred over antimicrobial or plain soap and water because of their superior microbicidal activity, reduced drying of skin, and convenience. The quality of performing hand hygiene can be affected by the type and length of fingernails and by wearing jewelry. Artificial fingernails and extenders should not be worn by health care workers because of their association with infections.[8] Figure 4-2 illustrates the proper technique for handwashing.

Gloves

Gloves protect both patients and health care workers. Gloves protect patients from exposure to pathogens that may be carried on the hands of health care workers. Gloves protect caregivers from contamination when contacting blood, body fluids, secretions, excretions, mucous membranes, and nonintact skin of patients and when handling or touching visibly or potentially contaminated patient care equipment and environmental surfaces.[8]

Caregivers should wear sterile gloves whenever performing invasive procedures. A single pair of nonsterile disposable gloves (e.g., latex, vinyl, nitrile) may be used for routine patient care. Hand hygiene always should be performed before donning gloves. Gloves should be changed between each patient contact and after any direct contact with infectious material, even if in the middle of a procedure. After removing the gloves, caregivers always must clean their hands. Gloves may have small, invisible defects or may be torn during use. The hands also can be contaminated during removal of the gloves. For these reasons, the wearing of gloves should never be used as a substitute for hand hygiene.

Mouth, Nose, Eye, and Face Protection

Face protection is an important component of standard precautions because the mucous membranes of the eyes, nose, and mouth are particularly vulnerable to some types of pathogens. Masks protect mucosal surfaces against splashes or sprays, but should not be confused with particulate respirators that are recommended for protection from small particles (as described subsequently for airborne isolation [AI]). The wearing of masks,

Box 4-1 Standard Precautions

HAND HYGIENE
- Perform hand hygiene before and after patient contacts, immediately after removing gloves, and when otherwise indicated to avoid cross contamination.
- Perform hand hygiene after touching blood, body fluids, secretions, excretions, and contaminated items, even if wearing gloves.
- Perform hand hygiene between tasks and procedures on the same patient if cross contamination of different body sites is possible (e.g., tracheostomy care after assistance with a bedpan).
- Use an approved alcohol-based product for routine hand hygiene. If hands are visibly soiled, use soap and water.

GLOVES
- Perform hand hygiene before and after removing gloves.
- Wear clean gloves when touching blood, body fluids, secretions, excretions, and contaminated items.
- Don clean gloves just before touching mucous membranes and nonintact skin.
- Change gloves between tasks and procedures on the same patient after contact with infectious material.
- Remove gloves promptly after use, before touching noncontaminated items and environmental surfaces, and before going to another patient.

MASKS, EYE PROTECTION, FACE SHIELDS
- Wear a mask and eye protection or a face shield to protect mucous membranes of the eyes, nose, and mouth during procedures and patient care activities that are likely to generate splashes or sprays of blood, body fluids, secretions, and excretions.

GOWNS
- Wear a clean gown to protect skin and prevent soiling of clothing during procedures and patient care activities that are likely to generate splashes or sprays of blood, body fluids, secretions, or excretions.
- Remove a soiled gown as promptly as possible and perform hand hygiene to avoid transfer of microorganisms to other patients or environments.

PATIENT CARE EQUIPMENT
- Handle used patient care equipment soiled with blood, body fluids, secretions, and excretions in a manner that prevents skin and mucous membrane exposures, contamination of clothing, and transfer of microorganisms to other patients and environments.
- Do not use reusable equipment to care for another patient unless it has been cleaned and reprocessed appropriately.
- Discard single-use items properly.

OCCUPATIONAL HEALTH AND BLOOD-BORNE PATHOGENS
- Exercise extreme caution when handling needles, scalpels, and other sharp instruments or devices; when cleaning used instruments; and when disposing of used needles.
- Never recap used needles, handle them using both hands, or point toward any part of the body.
- Do not remove used needles from disposable syringes by hand, and do not bend, break, or otherwise manipulate used needles by hand.
- Place used disposable syringes and needles, scalpel blades, and other sharp items in appropriate puncture-resistant containers; place reusable syringes and needles in a puncture-resistant container for transport to the reprocessing area.
- Use mouthpieces, resuscitation bags, or other ventilation devices as an alternative to mouth-to-mouth resuscitation methods in areas where the need for resuscitation is predictable.

PATIENT PLACEMENT
- Place patients who contaminate the environment or who do not (or cannot be expected to) assist in maintaining appropriate hygiene or environmental control in a private room.
- If a private room is unavailable, consult with infection preventionist regarding patient placement.

eye protection, and face shields in specified circumstances when exposures are likely to occur (e.g., bronchoscopy suite) is mandated by the OSHA Bloodborne Pathogen Standard.

Respiratory Protection

Respiratory protection (use of NIOSH-approved N-95 or higher level respirator) is intended for diseases (e.g., *M. tuberculosis*) that could be transmitted through the airborne route.[3] The term *respiratory protection* has a regulatory context that includes components of a program required by OSHA to protect workers: (1) medical clearance to wear a respirator, (2) provision and use of appropriate NIOSH-approved fit-tested respirators, and (3) education in respirator use.

Gowns, Aprons, and Protective Apparel

Isolation gowns and other apparel (aprons, leg coverings, boots, or shoe covers) also provide barrier protection and can prevent the contamination of clothing and exposed body areas from blood and body fluid contact and transmissible pathogens (e.g., respiratory syncytial virus and *Clostridium difficile*). Selection of protective apparel is dictated by the nature of the interaction of the health care worker with the patient, including anticipated degree of body contact with infectious material.[3] In most instances, gowns are worn only if contact with blood and body fluid is likely. Clinical coats and jackets worn over clothing are not considered protective apparel. Isolation gowns always should be donned with gloves and other protective equipment as indicated. As with gloves and masks, a gown should be worn only once and then discarded. In most situations, aseptically clean, freshly laundered, or disposable gowns are satisfactory.

Cough Etiquette

The emergence of novel respiratory viruses such as SARS and Middle East respiratory syndrome (MERS) along with pandemic H1N1 influenza have reinforced the need for a strategy for preventing transmission of respiratory infections at the first point of contact within a health care setting (e.g., physician's office), termed **respiratory hygiene/cough etiquette.** This concept is a component of standard precautions.[3] The elements of respiratory hygiene/cough etiquette include (1) education of health care personnel, patients, and visitors; (2) posted signs in language appropriate to the population served with instructions for patients and accompanying family members or friends; (3) source control measures (covering the mouth and nose with a tissue when coughing or placing a surgical mask on a coughing person when possible); (4) hand hygiene after contact with respiratory secretions; and (5) spatial separation (≥3 feet from persons with respiratory infections in common waiting areas).

Transmission-Based Precautions

Transmission-based precautions are for patients who are known or suspected to be infected with pathogens that require additional control measures to prevent transmission. There are three categories of transmission-based precautions based on the predominant manner in which the pathogen is transmitted: contact

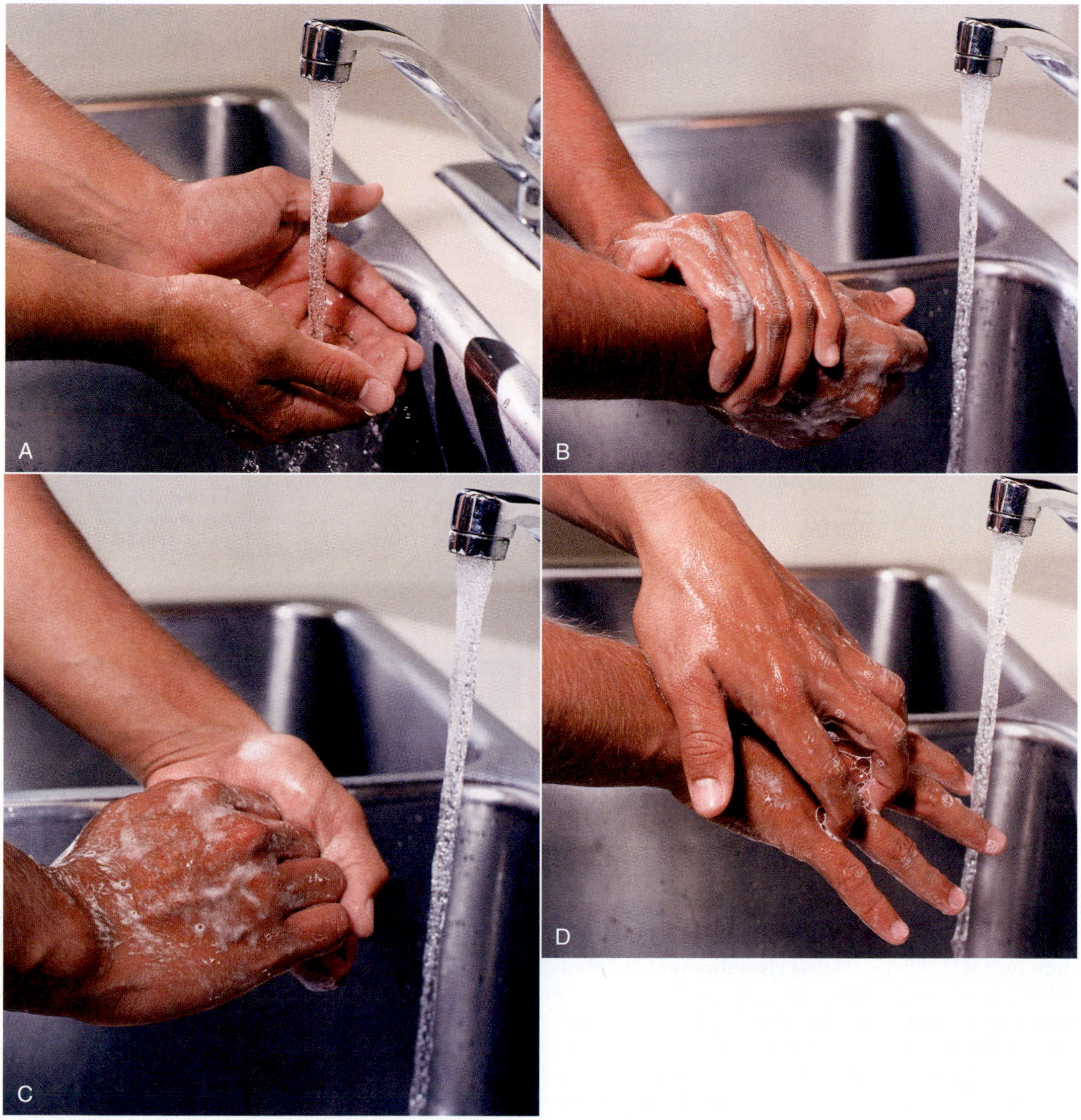

FIGURE 4-2 Steps for handwashing. **A,** Thorough wetting of hands. **B,** Washing around wrist and forearm. **C,** Scrubbing palm of hand. **D,** Washing between digits on back of hand.

Continued

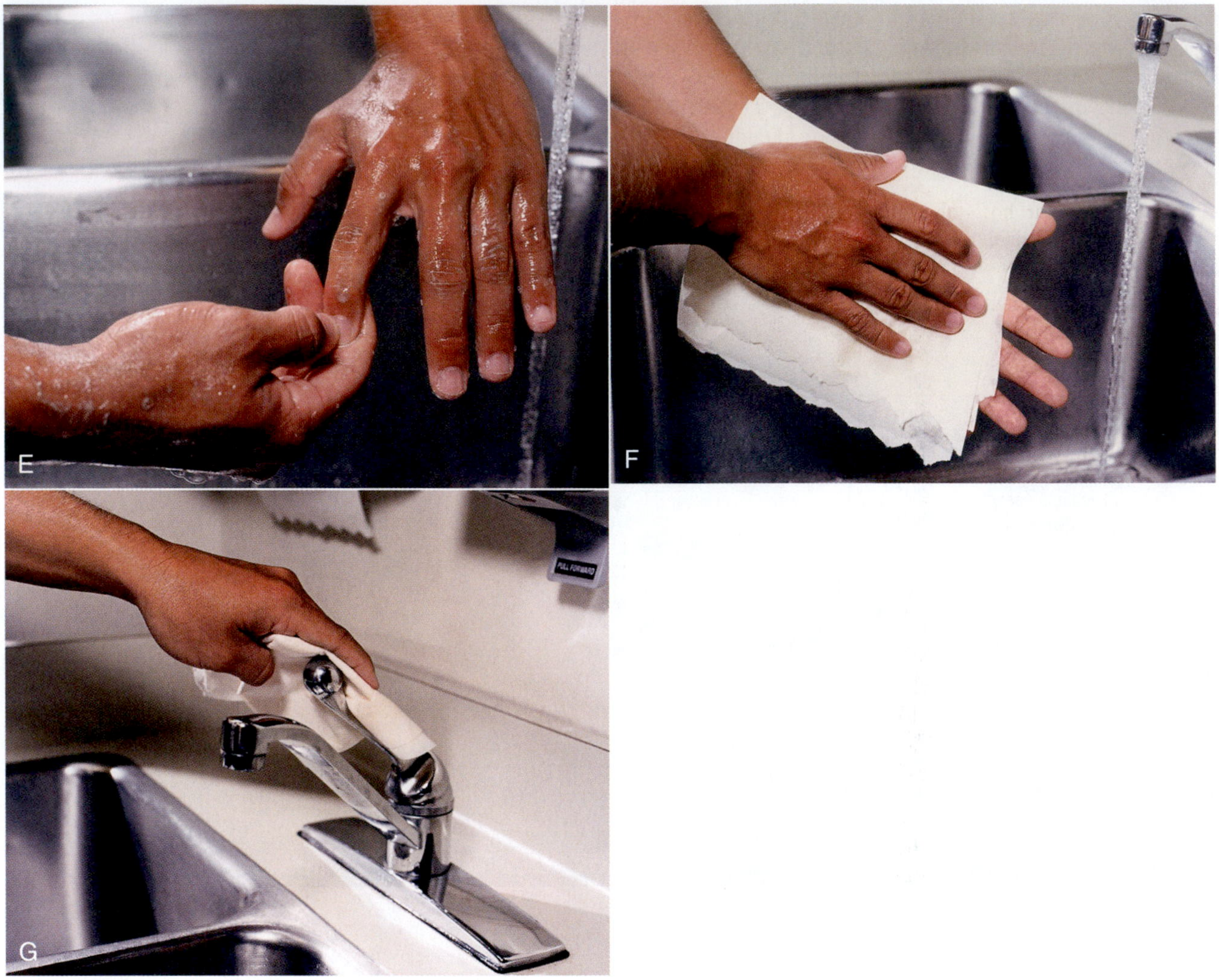

FIGURE 4-2, cont'd **E,** Washing around the cuticle. **F,** Drying hands with clean towel. **G,** Using towel to turn off faucet.

precautions, droplet precautions, and airborne infection isolation (see earlier section on Modes of Transmission). Whether used singularly or in combination, these precautions are always used in addition to standard precautions.[3]

Contact precautions are intended to reduce the risk for transmission by direct or indirect contact with the patient or the patient's environment. Contact precautions require health care personnel and visitors to wear gowns and gloves for all interactions that may involve contact with the patient or the patient's environment. Contact precautions are most commonly employed to decrease the spread of multidrug-resistant organisms such as *C. difficile*. Contact precautions are described in Box 4-2.

Droplet precautions are used to prevent a form of contact transmission that occurs when droplets are propelled short distances (≤3 feet through the air). Droplets are often generated with coughing, sneezing, suctioning, bronchoscopy, and cough induction. Health care personnel and visitors should don a mask during all interactions that may involve contact with such patients. Droplet precautions are employed for patients with

Box 4-2 Contact Precautions (Used *in Addition to* Standard Precautions)

- Place the patient in a private room; if a private room is unavailable, cohorting is acceptable.
- Perform hand hygiene and don gown and gloves to enter room whether or not direct patient contact is anticipated. Wear clean gloves when entering the room.
- Remove gown and gloves before leaving the patient's environment and perform hand hygiene.
- After glove removal and hand hygiene, ensure that hands do not touch potentially contaminated environmental surfaces or items in the patient's room.
- Limit transport of the patient from the room to essential purposes only.
- When possible, dedicate the use of noncritical patient care equipment to a single patient or patient cohort.
- If use of common equipment or items cannot be avoided, ensure that it is adequately cleaned and disinfected before use on another patient.

MINI CLINI

Isolation Methods

PROBLEM: A serious influenza outbreak occurs in a local long-term care facility. You are called to the emergency department (ED) because four of the sickest patients are being admitted together to your hospital for treatment. Currently, no private rooms are available for these patients. Outline the key isolation methods you would apply to help prevent the spread of influenza in your institution.

DISCUSSION: Influenza spreads via the droplet route. Both standard and droplet precautions must be applied for these patients. When transporting these patients out of the ED, you must be sure they wear surgical masks. Because private rooms are unavailable, these patients need to be grouped together. If this is not feasible, the patients must be separated from other patients by at least 3 feet. Special air handling and ventilation are unnecessary, and the door may remain open. In addition to following standard precautions, all caregivers and visitors should wear surgical masks when within 3 feet of these patients (or entering the room). All remaining patients at the long-term care facility should be immunized with the flu vaccine (if not already) and be given antiviral prophylaxis.

Box 4-3 Droplet Precautions (Used *in Addition to* Standard Precautions)

- Place the patient in a private room; if a private room is unavailable, cohorting is acceptable.
- Special air handling and ventilation are unnecessary, and the door may remain open.

MASK

- Perform hand hygiene and put on a surgical mask before entering the room.
- Remove mask before exiting the room and perform hand hygiene.
- Limit movement and transport of the patient from the room to essential purposes only.
- If transport or movement is necessary, minimize droplet transmission by having the patient wear a surgical mask.

presumed or confirmed infection with organisms known to be transmitted by respiratory droplets such as influenza. Droplet precautions are described in Box 4-3. Precautions for use when performing cough-inducing and aerosol-producing procedures are described in Box 4-4. Airborne infection isolation (AII) refers to isolation techniques intended to reduce the risk for selected infectious agents transmitted by "small droplets" of aerosol particles (e.g., *M. tuberculosis*).[5] Persons who enter an AII room must wear respiratory protection (an NIOSH-approved N-95 or higher respirator). Patients should be placed in a single-patient AII room that is equipped with special air handling and ventilation capacity that meets the American Institute of Architects/Facility Guidelines Institute standards (monitored negative pressure relative to surrounding area, minimum of two outdoor air changes per hour, minimum of 12 total air changes per hour for new construction or 6 air changes per hour for existing buildings, and air exhausted directly to the outside).[9] In settings where AII cannot be implemented because of limited resources, physical separation, mask patients, and respiratory protection for health care personnel should be implemented to reduce the likelihood of airborne transmission. Box 4-5 describes airborne precautions that should be used in addition to standard precautions.

Box 4-4 Guidelines for Cough-Inducing and Aerosol-Generating Procedures

- Cough-inducing procedures include endotracheal intubation and suctioning, diagnostic sputum induction, aerosol treatments (e.g., pentamidine therapy), and bronchoscopy.
- Cough-inducing procedures should not be performed on patients who may have infectious tuberculosis, unless the procedures are essential and can be performed with appropriate precautions.
- All cough-inducing procedures performed on patients who may have infectious tuberculosis should be performed using booths or special enclosures; if this is not feasible, a room that meets the ventilation requirements for airborne infection isolation can be used.
- After completion of cough-inducing procedures, patients who may have infectious tuberculosis should remain in their isolation rooms or enclosures until coughing subsides. They should be required to cover their mouths and noses with tissues when coughing.
- Before the enclosure or room is used for another patient, enough time should be allowed to pass for at least 99% of airborne contaminants to be removed (this time varies according to the efficiency of the ventilation or filtration system).

Box 4-5 Airborne Precautions (Used *in Addition to* Standard Precautions)

- Place the patient in a private negative-pressure room that has 6 to 12 air changes per hour and either safe external air discharge or HEPA filtration of recirculated air.
- Keep the room door closed and the patient in the room.
- If a private room is unavailable, cohorting is acceptable.
- Perform hand hygiene and don respiratory protection when entering the room of a patient with known or suspected infectious pulmonary tuberculosis.
- Remove respiratory protection and perform hand hygiene after leaving the room.
- Susceptible persons should not enter the room of patients known or suspected to have measles (rubeola) or varicella (chickenpox) if other immune caregivers are available; individuals who are immune to measles or varicella need not wear respiratory protection.
- Limit transport of the patient from the room to essential purposes only.
- If transport or movement is necessary, minimize patient dispersal of droplet nuclei by having the patient wear a surgical mask.

Protective Environment

A specialized engineering approach to protect highly immunocompromised patients is a protective environment. A protective environment is used for patients with allogeneic hematologic stem cell transplants to minimize fungal spore counts in the air.[3] The rationale for such controls has been studies showing outbreaks of aspergillosis associated with construction. Air quality for patients with hematologic stem cell transplants is improved through a combination of environmental controls that include (1) high efficiency particulate air (HEPA) filtration of incoming air, (2) directed room airflow, (3) positive room air pressure relative to the corridor, (4) well-sealed rooms to prevent infiltration of outside air, (5) ventilation to provide 12 or more air changes per hour, (6) strategies to reduce dust, and (7) prohibition of dried and fresh flowers and potted plants in rooms.

Transport of Infected Patients

By limiting the transport of patients with contagious disease, the risk for cross infection can be reduced. However, infected patients sometimes do need to be transported and, when that occurs, the patient needs to wear appropriate barrier protection (mask, gown, impervious dressings) consistent with the route and risk for transmission.[3] Health care personnel receiving the patient need to be notified of the patient's impending arrival and what infection control measures are required.

RULE OF THUMB

Apply standard precautions when caring for all patients.

1. Wash your hands after touching blood, body fluids, or contaminated items (even if gloves were worn).
2. Wear fresh, clean gloves for all tasks and procedures involving potential contact with blood, body fluids, or contaminated items.
3. Exercise extreme caution when handling "sharps."
4. Handle soiled equipment in a manner that prevents skin and mucous membrane exposures, contamination of clothing, and transfer of microorganisms to other patients and environments.[5]

Medical Devices and Bundles

A large percentage of HAIs are device-related infections, including ventilator-associated pneumonia (VAP), catheter-related bloodstream infection, and catheter-associated urinary tract infection. The best way to decrease host susceptibility to a device-related infection is first to limit device use and second to ensure that devices are placed and maintained appropriately. Prevention bundles—defined as the use of multiple different evidence-based best practices to prevent device-related infection—have been shown to decrease the incidence of HAIs significantly.[10,11] Exactly how much each component of a bundle contributes to a reduction in infection is often difficult to determine. There are bundles for placement of central vascular catheters, placement and maintenance of urinary catheters, and for the management of patients on ventilators. There are several different permutations of VAP bundles described. Common components to most include maintaining the head of the bed above 30 degrees, routine mouth care with chlorhexidine, and minimizing sedation (daily sedation vacation).[11] Other practices commonly included in VAP bundles are venous thromboembolism prophylaxis and stress ulcer prophylaxis, even though these practices do not have a direct effect on the risk for pneumonia. Institutions should be committed to these processes of care, and individual health care workers should be familiar with these practices and execute them on a routine basis.[11–13] Compliance with bundles can be tracked over time as part of process improvement projects. Each individual component can be tracked, or all components can be tracked in an all or none, total appropriateness of care manner.

MINI CLINI

Spread of Infection

PROBLEM: You work in the neonatal intensive care unit (NICU) of a large urban hospital. Over the last 2 days, many infants in the unit have developed serious *Staphylococcus aureus* infections. Identify the most likely source and route of transmission and suggest ways to prevent spread of this serious infection.

DISCUSSION: In hospitals, *S. aureus* commonly colonizes the skin of both health care professionals and visitors. Neonates are very susceptible hosts because of their poor immunity. *Staphylococcus* infections spread mainly via direct contact transmission (see Table 4-1). To help prevent the spread of this infection to the newborn infants, you should try to disrupt the transmission route. Meticulous attention to hand hygiene and use of gloves would help. In addition, you could isolate the infected neonates from uninfected infants (**cohorting**) and, in an effort to identify patients who may be colonized, begin *S. aureus* screening of the umbilicus and nares of all infants in the NICU and all new admissions.

DISINFECTION AND STERILIZATION

Medical instruments are used in tens of millions of procedures in the United States every year. When properly performed, cleaning, disinfection, and sterilization procedures can reduce the risk for infection associated with the use of invasive and noninvasive medical instruments. Although a detailed review of disinfection and sterilization is beyond the scope of this chapter, overall principles are discussed, particularly as they pertain to the use of bronchoscopes. The interested reader is referred to detailed guidance available from the CDC.[14] Table 4-2 lists definitions of the steps involved in equipment reprocessing.

Spaulding Approach to Disinfection and Sterilization of Patient Care Equipment

In 1968, Spaulding published his approach to disinfection and sterilization, which was based on the degree of risk for infection involved in the use of the item in patient care.[15] The three categories he described were critical, semicritical, and noncritical (Table 4-3). *Critical* items are categorized based on the high risk for infection if such an item is contaminated with pathogens, including bacterial spores (e.g., items that enter sterile tissue or the vascular system). Critical devices enter normally sterile tissues. Most of these items should be purchased sterile or be sterilized with steam if possible. *Semicritical* items come into contact with mucous membranes or nonintact skin; this includes most respiratory equipment. These items should be free of all microorganisms before use (bacterial spores may be present). Semicritical items require at least high-level disinfection using chemical disinfectants. *Noncritical* items come into contact with intact skin (an effective barrier to most microbes) but not mucous membranes. Most noncritical reusable devices may be decontaminated where they are used (e.g., bedpans, patient bed rails).

Bronchoscopes routinely become contaminated with high levels of organisms during a procedure because of the body cavities in which they are used. The benefits of these medical devices are numerous; however, proper reprocessing is crucial because numerous outbreaks and pseudo-outbreaks owing to improper procedures have been described. Individuals responsible for bronchoscope reprocessing should receive initial and annual training, and their competency should be ensured. The five key components to bronchoscope reprocessing are cleaning, disinfecting, rinsing, drying, and storage (Box 4-6).[14] Automated bronchoscope reprocessors (ABRs) offer many advantages over manual disinfection because they automate several of these steps. Regardless of whether disinfection is done manually or with an ABR, personnel responsible for this task need to ensure reprocessing is done per device manufacturer and reprocessor guidelines with products registered with U.S. Environmental Protection Agency (EPA) or cleared by the U.S. Food and Drug Administration (FDA). Health care workers should wear appropriate PPE while cleaning, disinfecting, or sterilizing medical equipment to protect themselves from potentially infectious material and chemical products used in the process.

TABLE 4-2

Equipment Processing Definitions

Term	Definition
Cleaning	Removal of all foreign material (e.g., soil, organic material) from objects
Disinfection (general term)	Inactivation of most pathogenic organisms, excluding spores
Disinfection, low level	Inactivation of most bacteria, some viruses, and fungi, without destruction of resistant microorganisms such as *Mycobacterium tuberculosis* or bacterial spores
Disinfection, intermediate level	Inactivation of all vegetative bacteria, most viruses, most fungi, and *M. tuberculosis,* without destruction of bacterial spores
Disinfection, high level	Inactivation of all microorganisms *except* bacterial spores (with sufficient exposure times, spores may also be destroyed)
Sterilization	Complete destruction of all forms of microbial life

Cleaning

Medical equipment must be cleaned and maintained according to the manufacturer's instructions. Cleaning is the first step in all equipment processing, including those undergoing low-level or high-level disinfection and sterilization. Cleaning involves removing all dirt and organic material from equipment, usually by washing (see Table 4-3).[14] Failure to clean

TABLE 4-3

Processing of Medical Equipment According to Infection Risk Categories

Category	Description	Examples	Processing
Critical	Devices introduced into the bloodstream or other parts of the body	Surgical devices Intravascular catheters Implants Heart-lung bypass components Dialysis components Bronchoscope forceps/brushes	Sterilization
Semicritical	Devices that directly or indirectly contact mucous membranes	Bronchoscopes Oral, nasal, and tracheal airways Ventilator circuits/humidifiers Pulmonary function testing mouthpieces and tubing Nebulizers and their reservoirs Resuscitation bags Laryngoscope blades/stylets Pressure, gas, or temperature probes	High-level disinfection
Noncritical	Devices that touch only intact skin or do not contact patient	Face masks Blood pressure cuffs Ventilators	Detergent washing Low- to intermediate-level disinfection

Modified from Chatburn RL, Kallstrom TJ, Bajasouzian S: A comparison of acetic acid with a quaternary ammonium compound for disinfection of hand-held nebulizers. Respir Care 34:98–109, 1989.

Box 4-6 Key Components of Bronchoscope Sterilization or Disinfection

Clean: Mechanically clean external surfaces, including brushing internal channels and flushing each internal channel with water and a detergent or enzymatic cleaner.

1. *Disinfect:* Immerse bronchoscope in high-level disinfectant and perfuse disinfectant into the suction/biopsy channel and air/water channel and expose for at least 20 minutes (or FDA-cleared exposure time).
2. *Rinse:* The bronchoscope and all channels should be rinsed with sterile water, filtered water, or tap water.
3. *Dry:* Rinse insertion tube and inner channels with alcohol, and dry with forced air after disinfection and before storage.
4. *Store:* The bronchoscope should be stored in a way that prevents recontamination (e.g., hung vertically in an enclosed cabinet, the bronchoscope should not touch any surface of the cabinet).

Data from Rutala WA, Weber DJ, and the Healthcare Infection Control Practices Advisory Committee (HICPAC), Centers for Disease Control and Prevention: Guidelines for sterilization and disinfection in healthcare facilities, Atlanta, 2008. http://www.edu.gov./hicpac/.pdf/guidelines.

equipment properly can render all subsequent processing efforts ineffective. Cleaning should occur in a designated facility with separate dirty and clean areas. Before being cleaned, the equipment should be disassembled per manufacturer's recommendations and examined for worn parts. Disassembly helps ensure good exposure to the cleaning agent.

Because water alone cannot dissolve organic matter, detergents or enzymatic cleaners and brushes should be used to clean all internal and external surfaces of equipment. Enzymatic cleaners are neutral detergents with enzymes added that help remove organic (proteinaceous) material from equipment. Some EPA-registered products combine a germicide with a detergent, providing the dual action of cleaning and disinfection. This product type is generally appropriate for use on noncritical items. Noncritical items, such as stethoscopes, intravenous pumps, and ventilator surfaces, must be cleaned and low-level disinfected using an appropriate EPA-registered product before use on another patient.

Although careful cleaning removes most pathogens from the equipment, it cannot eliminate the risk for infection. For this reason, semicritical and critical medical equipment must then undergo either high-level disinfection or sterilization.

Disinfection

Disinfection describes a process used on medical equipment that destroys the vegetative form of all pathogenic organisms on an inanimate object, except bacterial spores. By definition, *disinfection* differs from *sterilization* by its lack of sporicidal activity.[14] However, a few disinfectants kill spores with prolonged exposure times (hours) and are called *chemical sterilants*. Disinfection can involve either physical or chemical methods. The most common physical method of disinfection is *pasteurization*. Many chemical methods are used to disinfect respiratory care equipment.

Chemical Disinfection

Chemical disinfection involves the application of chemical solutions to contaminated surfaces or equipment. The EPA groups disinfectants based on whether the product label claims "limited," "general," or "hospital" disinfection.[14] Numerous disinfectants are used alone or in combination in the health care setting, including alcohol, chlorine and chlorine products, glutaraldehyde, iodophors, phenolics, quaternary ammonium compounds, peracetic acid, and hydrogen peroxide. In most cases, a given product is designed for a specific purpose and should be used in a certain manner; the label should be read carefully. Table 4-4, excerpted from the CDC guideline for sterilization and disinfection, summarizes common chemical disinfectants and their activity against various pathogens.[14] Health care facilities should select disinfectant agents that best meet their overall needs. Product manufacturer's recommendations for the amount, dilution, and contact time of disinfectants should be followed. A comprehensive overview of disinfectants in the hospital can be found in the updated CDC guidelines for disinfection and sterilization in health care facilities.[14]

For high-level disinfection to be effective, cleaned equipment must be completely immersed in the disinfectant solution. The FDA provides a list of cleared chemical disinfectants that can be used for high-level disinfection of medical devices. Cleared agents include 2.4% or greater glutaraldehyde, 0.55% orthophthaldehyde (OPA), 0.95% glutaraldehyde with 1.64% phenylphenate, 7.35% hydrogen peroxide with 0.23% peracetic acid, 1.0% hydrogen peroxide with 0.08% peracetic acid, and 7.5% hydrogen peroxide.[16] The choice of agent used in high-level disinfection is dictated by the device manufacturer.

After a set "contact" time, the equipment is removed, rinsed in sterile water (to remove toxic residues), and thoroughly dried. Equipment must be handled and stored carefully, to prevent recontamination during subsequent reassembly, packaging, and storage.

Sterilization

Sterilization destroys all microorganisms on the surface of an article or in a fluid, which prevents transmission of pathogens associated with the use of that item. Both physical and chemical means can achieve sterilization. Physical methods include various forms of heat (steam) and ionizing radiation. Chemical methods of sterilization include low-temperature sterilization technologies such as ethylene oxide (EtO) gas. Table 4-5, excerpted from the CDC guideline for sterilization and disinfection, compares and contrasts the major methods of sterilization.[14]

Medical devices that have contact with sterile body tissues or fluids are critical items and should be sterile before use. If the object is heat resistant, steam sterilization is usually recommended. However, increases in the use of medical devices that are heat and moisture sensitive have necessitated the development of low-temperature sterilization technology. These include, but are not limited to, EtO, hydrogen peroxide gas plasma, and peracetic acid. A review of the commonly used sterilization technologies with a summary of advantages and

TABLE 4-4

Comparison of the Characteristics of Selected Chemicals Used as High-Level Disinfectants or Chemical Sterilants

	HP (7.5%)	PA (0.2%)	Glut (≥2.0%)	OPA (0.55%)	HP/PA (7.35%/0.23%)
HLD claim	30 min at 20° C	NA	20-90 min at 20°-25° C	12 min at 20° C, 5 min at 25° C in AER	15 min at 20° C
Sterilization claim	6 hr at 20° C	12 min at 50°-56° C	10 hr at 20°-25° C	None	3 hr at 20° C
Activation	No	No	Yes (alkaline glut)	No	No
Reuse life[a]	21 days	Single use	14-30 days	14 days	14 days
Shelf life stability[b]	2 yr	6 mo	2 yr	2 yr	2 yr
Disposable restrictions	None	None	Local[c]	Local[c]	None
Materials compatibility	Good	Good	Excellent	Excellent	No data
Monitor MEC[d]	Yes (6%)	No	Yes (≥1.5%)	Yes (0.3% OPA)	No
Safety	Serious eye damage (safety glasses)	Serious eye and skin damage (conc soln)[e]	Respiratory	Eye irritant, stains skin	Eye damage
Processing	Manual or automated	Automated	Manual or automated	Manual or automated	Manual
Organic material resistance	Yes	Yes	Yes	Yes	Yes
OSHA exposure limit	1 ppm TWA	None	None[f]	None	HP-1 ppm TWA
Cost profile (per cycle)[g]	+ (manual), ++ (automated)	++++ (automated)	+ (manual), ++ (automated)	++ (manual)	++ (manual)

Data from Rutala WA, Weber DJ, and the Healthcare Infection Control Practices Advisory Committee (HICPAC), Centers for Disease Control and Prevention: Guidelines for sterilization and disinfection in healthcare facilities, Atlanta, 2008, *http://www.edu.gov./hicpac/.pdf/guidelines.*

glut, Glutaraldehyde; HLD, high level-disinfectant; *HP,* hydrogen peroxide; *NA,* not applicable; *OPA,* orthophthalaldehyde (FDA cleared as a high-level disinfectant, included for comparison with other chemical agents used for high-level disinfection); *PA,* peracetic acid; *PA/HP,* peracetic acid and hydrogen peroxide; *TWA,* time-weighted average for a conventional 8-hour workday.

[a]Number of days a product can be reused as determined by reuse protocol.

[b]Time a product can remain in storage (unused).

[c]No U.S. Environmental Protection Agency regulations, but some states and local authorities have additional restrictions.

[d]Minimum effective concentration is the lowest concentration of active ingredients at which the product is still effective.

[e]Conc soln, concentrated solution.

[f]The ceiling limit recommended by the American Conference of Governmental Industrial Hygienists is 0.05 ppm.

[g]Per cycle cost profile considers cost of the processing solution (suggested list price to health care facilities in August 2001) and assumes maximum use life (e.g., 21 days for hydrogen peroxide, 14 days for glutaraldehyde), five reprocessing cycles per day, 1-gallon basin for manual processing, and 4-gallon tank for automated processing.

+, Least expensive; ++++, most expensive.

MINI CLINI

Selection of a Disinfectant

PROBLEM: You work in the pulmonary function laboratory of a community hospital. Immediately after performing spirometry on a patient, you learn that he has been admitted and tests positive for pulmonary tuberculosis. You also remember him coughing into the spirometry tubing. You have four more patients scheduled for spirometry testing, beginning in 45 minutes. How should you process the spirometry tubing to prevent transmission of the tuberculosis?

DISCUSSION: Ideally, you would have a backup set of tubing to deal with this type of problem. If not, you need to disinfect or sterilize the tubing quickly. Because permanent spirometry tubing is made from heat-labile plastics, you cannot use steam (damage). Ethylene oxide (EtO) gas is an option, but aeration would take too long. Instead, you should select a broad-spectrum, quick-acting disinfectant solution that works well in the presence of organic matter and does not damage rubber or plastic. Glutaraldehyde is a good choice, with a minimum exposure time of 20 minutes. A stabilized hydrogen peroxide–based compound or a 1:50 sodium hypochlorite solution also might be considered.

disadvantages can be found in the updated CDC guidelines for disinfection and sterilization in health care facilities.[14] Following is an overview of a few of these technologies.

Steam Sterilization

Moist heat in the form of steam under pressure is the most common, most efficient, and easiest sterilization method. Steam sterilization is the application of steam under pressure. Steam sterilization is efficient, quick, cheap, clean, and reliable. Equipment always must be thoroughly cleaned before sterilization because materials that remain on the surfaces of equipment interfere with the effectiveness of the sterilization process. Clean equipment is wrapped in muslin, linen, or paper or placed in specially designed rigid containers, all of which are easily penetrated by steam. Items must be properly packed in the autoclave to ensure exposure. The higher the temperature and pressure of the sterilizer, the shorter is the time needed for sterilization. The combination most commonly used for autoclaving is 15 psi at 121° C for a minimum of 30 minutes. After sterilization, the packaging prevents recontamination during handling and storage. Numerous quality control monitors (mechanical, chemical, and biological) are employed to ensure adequate sterilization has taken place.

TABLE 4-5
Advantages and Disadvantages of Accepted Methods for Equipment Sterilization

Sterilization Method	Advantages	Disadvantages
Steam	Nontoxic to patient, staff, environment Cycle easy to control and monitor Rapidly microbial Least affected by organic/inorganic soils among sterilization processes listed Rapid cycle time Penetrates medical packing, device lumens	Deleterious for heat-sensitive instruments Microsurgical instruments damaged by repeated exposure May leave instruments wet, causing them to rust Potential for burns
Hydrogen peroxide gas plasma	Safe for the environment Leaves no toxic residuals Cycle time is 28-75 min (varies with model type) and no aeration necessary Used for heat- and moisture-sensitive items because process temperature <50° C Simple to operate, install (208 V outlet), and monitor Compatible with most medical devices Requires electrical outlet only	Cellulose (paper), linens, and liquids cannot be processed Sterilization chamber size from 1.8-9.4 ft^3 total volume (varies with model type) Some endoscopes or medical devices with long or narrow lumens cannot be processed at this time in the United States (see manufacturer's recommendations for internal diameter and length restrictions) Requires synthetic packaging (polypropylene wraps, polyolefin pouches) and special container tray Hydrogen peroxide may be toxic at levels >1 ppm TWA
100% Ethylene oxide (EtO)	Penetrates packaging materials, device lumens Single-dose cartridge and negative pressure chamber minimizes potential for gas leak and EtO exposure Simple to operate and monitor Compatible with most medical materials	Requires aeration time to remove EtO residue Sterilization chamber size 4.0-7.9 ft^3 total volume (varies with model type) EtO is toxic, a carcinogen, and flammable EtO emission regulation by states but catalytic cell removes 99.9% of EtO and converts it to CO_2 and H_2O EtO cartridges should be stored in flammable liquid storage cabinet Lengthy cycle/aeration time
EtO mixtures: 8.6% EtO/91.4% HCFC; 10% EtO/90% HCFC; 8.5% EtO/91.5% CO_2	Penetrates medical packaging and many plastics Compatible with most medical materials Cycle easy to control and monitor	Some states (e.g., California, New York, Michigan) require EtO emission reduction of 90%-99.9% CFC (inert gas that eliminates explosive hazard) banned in 1995 Potential hazards to staff and patients Lengthy cycle/alteration time EtO is toxic, a carcinogen, and flammable
Peracetic acid	Rapid cycle time (30-45 min) Low temperature (50°-55° C) liquid immersion sterilization Environmentally friendly by-products Sterilant flows through endoscope, which facilitates salt, protein, and microbe removal	Point-of-use system, no sterile storage Biologic indicator may be unsuitable for routine monitoring Used for immersible instruments only Some material incompatibility (e.g., aluminum anodized coating becomes dull) One scope or a small number of instruments processed in a cycle Potential for serious eye and skin damage (concentrated solution) with contact

Data from Rutala WA, Weber DJ, and the Healthcare Infection Control Practices Advisory Committee (HICPAC), Centers for Disease Control and Prevention: Guidelines for sterilization and disinfection in healthcare facilities, Atlanta, 2008, http://www.edu.gov./hicpac/.pdf/guidelines.
CFC, Chlorofluorocarbon; *HCFC,* hydrochlorofluorocarbon; TWA, time-weighted average.

Immediate Use Sterilization

Immediate-use (previously referred to as *flash* sterilization) "steam sterilization" is a modification of conventional steam sterilization in which the item is placed in an open tray or a specially designed container to allow for rapid penetration of steam.[14] It is considered an acceptable practice for processing cleaned patient care items that cannot be packaged, sterilized, and stored before use. Its use only for reasons of convenience (e.g., to save time) should be discouraged.

Low-Temperature Sterilization Technologies

Low-temperature (<60° C) sterilants are needed for sterilizing temperature-sensitive and moisture-sensitive medical devices and equipment. Low-temperature sterilant technology includes EtO, hydrogen peroxide gas plasma, ozone, vaporized hydrogen peroxide, and peracetic acid.[14] We review the most commonly used process—EtO.

EtO is a colorless, toxic gas and potent sterilizing agent. Because it is active at ambient temperatures and is harmless to rubber and plastics, EtO is a good sterilant for items that cannot be autoclaved. Similar to steam, EtO penetrates most packaging materials, permitting prewrapping. Were it not for its many hazards, EtO would be the ideal sterilant.[16] Acute exposure to EtO gas can cause airway inflammation, nausea, diarrhea, headache, dizziness, and seizures. Chronic exposure to the gas is associated with respiratory infections, anemia, and altered behavior. Residual EtO left on processed equipment can cause tissue inflammation and hemolysis. When combined with water, EtO forms ethylene glycol, which also can irritate tissues. Other potential problems include carcinogenic, mutagenic, and teratogenic effects. EtO concentrations greater than 3% are explosive.

EtO requires special attention to general safety precautions, equipment preparation, and sterilization cycle parameters. In addition, because of its toxicity, residual EtO must be removed from equipment after sterilization via a process called *aeration*. EtO is used to sterilize critical (and sometimes semicritical) items that cannot be steam sterilized.

EQUIPMENT HANDLING PROCEDURES

Equipment handling procedures that help prevent the spread of pathogens include maintenance of in-use equipment, processing of reusable equipment, application of one-patient-use disposables, and fluid and medication precautions.

Maintenance of In-Use Equipment

In-use respiratory care equipment that can spread pathogens includes nebulizers, ventilator circuits, bag-valve-mask devices (manual resuscitators), and suction equipment. Oxygen therapy and pulmonary function equipment are also implicated as potential sources of HAIs.

Nebulizers

Small-volume medication nebulizers (SVNs) also can produce bacterial aerosols. SVNs have been associated with health care–associated pneumonia, including Legionnaires disease, resulting from either contaminated medications or contaminated tap water used to rinse the reservoir. Procedures designed to prevent nebulizers from spreading pathogens are presented in Box 4-7.

Box 4-7 Procedures to Minimize Infection Risk With Nebulizers

LARGE-VOLUME NEBULIZERS AND MIST TENTS

- Always fill nebulizers with sterile distilled water.
- Fill fluid reservoirs immediately before use; do not add fluid to replenish partially filled reservoirs. If fluid is to be added, discard the remaining old fluid first.
- Drain tubing condensate away from the patient and discard as contaminated waste; do not allow condensate to drain back into reservoir.
- Sterilize or high-level disinfect large-volume nebulizers between patients and after every 24 hours of use on the same patient.
- Use mist tent nebulizer and reservoirs that have undergone sterilization or high-level disinfection, and replace them between patients.
- Do not use large-volume room air humidifiers that create aerosols unless they can be sterilized or subjected to high-level disinfection at least daily and filled only with sterile water.

SMALL-VOLUME NEBULIZERS

- Between treatments on the same patient, disinfect, rinse with sterile water, and air dry small-volume nebulizers.
- Between patients, replace small-volume nebulizers with sterile or high-level disinfected units.
- Use only sterile fluids for nebulization, and dispense these fluids aseptically.
- When possible, use single-use medication vials; if using multidose vials, handle, dispense, and store them according to manufacturer's instructions and checking expiration dates.

Ventilators and Ventilator Circuits

The internal workings of ventilators are uncommon sources for infection; this is partly a result of the widespread use of **high-efficiency particulate air/aerosol (HEPA) filters,** which have an efficiency rate of 99.97%, and the use of sheathed suction catheters, which help reduce endotracheal tube contamination. An inspiratory HEPA filter (placed between the machinery and the external circuit, proximal to any humidifier) can eliminate bacteria from the driving gas and prevent retrograde contamination back into the machine. An expiratory filter using a heated thermistor to prevent condensation performs the same function and still protects the internal ventilator components. Expiratory filters also prevent pathogens from being expelled into the surroundings from the patient's expired air.

The external ventilator circuitry poses the most significant contamination risk, particularly in systems using heated humidifiers. The humidifiers themselves are rarely the problem. Bubble or wick designs produce little or no aerosol and pose minimal infection risk. In addition, heating the humidifier reduces or eliminates growth of most bacterial pathogens. However, because tap water or distilled water may harbor heat-resistant pathogens, sterile water should still be used to fill bubble-type humidifiers.

The primary problem stems from contaminated condensate in the inspiratory limb of the ventilator circuit. Most often, the source of this contamination is the patient. Spillage of contaminated condensate into the patient circuit and the patient occurs when moving the tubing or the patient, increasing the risk for self-infection. In addition, microorganisms in this condensate can be transmitted to other patients via the hands of the health care worker handling the fluid, if he or she is negligent. This is another reason why it is crucial for RTs to practice hand hygiene before and after contact with every ventilated patient. Contact with the patient's ventilator is considered contact with the patient's body.

One way to address this problem is by reducing or eliminating circuit condensation. This reduction or elimination is easily achieved using heated wire circuits or a *heat-and-moisture exchanger (HME)*. Available guidance does not recommend daily changing of HMEs. These devices should be inspected daily and replaced if contaminated with patient secretions or if flow resistance has increased. HMEs can be used safely for 48 hours, and with some patient populations they may be able to be used for up to 7 days.[17]

Based on current knowledge, both the CDC and the American Association for Respiratory Care (AARC) have developed guidelines addressing ventilator-associated infection control. Box 4-8 provides general procedures for minimizing HAIs

Box 4-8 Procedures to Minimize Infection Risk With Mechanical Ventilators

- Do not routinely sterilize or disinfect the internal workings of ventilators.
- Do not routinely change ventilator circuit more often than every 48 to 72 hours with HME.
- Sterilize or high-level disinfect reusable breathing circuits and humidifiers.
- Periodically drain tubing condensate away from patient and discard.
- Wash hands after draining tubing condensate or handling the fluid.
- Do not place bacterial filters distal to humidifier reservoirs.
- Use sterile water to fill bubble humidifiers.
- Use sterile, distilled water to fill wick humidifiers.
- Change HMEs according to manufacturer's recommendation and when you observe evidence of gross contamination or mechanical dysfunction.
- Do not routinely change HME breathing circuits while in use.

HME, Heat-and-moisture exchanger.

associated with ventilator use. Mechanical ventilation exposes the patient to the risk for VAP, and the frequency of circuit changes and the relationship to VAP have been investigated.[11] Current guidelines suggest that ventilator circuits should not be changed routinely for infection control purposes; however, they should be changed when visibly soiled or malfunctioning.[18]

Bag-Mask Devices

Bag-mask devices are a source for colonizing both the airways of intubated patients and the hands of medical personnel.[19] Nondisposable bag-mask devices should be sterilized or high-level disinfected between patients. In addition, the exterior surface of any bag-mask device should be cleaned of visible debris and disinfected at least once a day.

Suction Systems

Tracheal suctioning increases the risk for infection. Proper hand hygiene and gloving help minimize this risk. Although much has been made of the infection prevention advantages of sheathed suction systems over open tracheal suction systems, evidence is mixed as to whether it is clearly superior. However, guidance recommends in-line suctioning as part of VAP reduction program.[18] There is no need to change a closed system suction catheter daily. To minimize the risk for cross contamination during suctioning with an open system, a fresh, sterile, single-use catheter should be used on each patient. In addition, only sterile fluid should be used to remove secretions from the catheter. Last, both the suction collection tubing and collection canister should be changed between patients except in short-term care units, where only the collection tubing needs to be changed.

Oxygen Therapy Apparatus

O_2 therapy devices pose much less risk than other in-use equipment but are still a potential infection hazard. In-use nondisposable O_2 humidifiers have a contamination rate of 33%. Conversely, prefilled, sterile disposable humidifiers present a negligible infection risk.[20] On the basis of this knowledge, procedures that can help prevent O_2 therapy apparatus from spreading pathogens are outlined in Box 4-9.

Box 4-9 Procedures to Minimize Infection Risk With Oxygen Therapy Apparatus

- Humidifiers are not needed with flows less than 4 L/min.
- When needed and whenever possible, prefilled, sterile disposable humidifiers should be used.
- With reusable humidifiers, fluid reservoirs should be filled immediately before use with sterile distilled water.
- Fluid must not be added to replenish partially filled reservoirs. If fluid is to be added, discard the remaining old fluid first, then clean and dry reservoir before refilling.
- The tubing and oxygen delivery device should be changed between patients; prefilled, sterile, disposable humidifiers do not need to be changed between patients in high-use areas such as the recovery room.
- Prefilled, disposable humidifiers can be used safely for 30 days.

Pulmonary Function Equipment

The inner parts of pulmonary function testing equipment are not a major source for spread of infection. However, contamination of external tubing, connectors, rebreathing valves, and mouthpieces can occur during testing. These components should be cleaned and subjected to high-level disinfection or sterilization between patients.[21,22] The common practice of using HEPA filters to isolate the spirometer from the patient makes sense logically but has yet to be proved either effective or necessary in preventing HAI.

Other Respiratory Care Devices

Use of other respiratory care equipment, including O_2 analyzers, the hand-held bedside spirometer, and circuit probes, has been linked with hospital outbreaks of gram-negative bacterial infections.[21] The most likely transmission route is direct patient-to-patient contact via either the device itself or the contaminated hands of caregivers. The best way to control this problem is with proper hand hygiene and sterilization or high-level disinfection of the devices between patients.

Processing Reusable Equipment

Improperly processed reusable equipment is another potential source for pathogens. General principles for cleaning, disinfection, and sterilization were provided previously. This section presents specific guidelines for processing reusable respiratory care equipment and a special section on bronchoscope disinfection.

Respiratory Care Equipment

Several factors must be considered in selecting a processing method for reusable respiratory care equipment (Box 4-10).

4-1 Care of the Ventilator Circuit and Its Relationship to Ventilator-Associated Pneumonia

AARC Clinical Practice Guideline (Excerpts)*

INTRODUCTION

A concern related to the care of a mechanically ventilated patient is the development of VAP. For many years, this concern focused on the ventilator circuit and humidifier. The circuit and humidifier have been changed on a regular basis in an attempt to decrease the VAP rate. However, as the evidence evolved, it became apparent that the origin of VAP is more likely from sites other than the ventilator circuit, and the prevailing practice has become one of changing circuits less frequently. If this practice is safe, it would offer substantial cost savings. Other issues related to the components of the circuit and VAP also have become more important. Humidification systems can be either active or passive. Increasingly, in-line suction is used and this becomes part of the ventilator circuit.

QUESTIONS

A systematic review of the literature was conducted with the intention of making recommendations for change frequency of the ventilator circuit and additional components of the circuit. Specifically, the Writing Committee wrote these evidence-based clinical practice guidelines to address the following questions:

1. Do ventilator circuits need to be changed at regular intervals?
2. What is the economic impact of decreasing the frequency of ventilator circuit changes?
3. What are the issues related to circuit type?
4. Does the choice of active versus passive humidification affect ventilator circuit change frequency?
5. Do passive humidifiers need to be changed at regular intervals?
6. Do in-line suction catheters need to be changed at regular intervals?
7. Are there specific populations for which the recommendations should be altered?

RECOMMENDATIONS

Recommendation #1

Ventilator circuits should not be changed routinely for infection control purposes. The available evidence suggests no patient harm and considerable cost savings associated with extended ventilator circuit change intervals. The maximum duration of time that circuits can be used safely is unknown. (Evidence Grade A)

Recommendation #2

Evidence is lacking related to VAP and issues of heated versus unheated circuits, type of heated humidifier, method for filling the humidifier, and technique for clearing condensate from the ventilator circuit. It is prudent to avoid excessive accumulation of condensate in the circuit. Care should be taken to avoid accidental drainage of condensate into the patient's airway and to avoid contamination of caregivers during ventilator disconnection or during disposal of condensate. Care should be taken to avoid breaking the ventilator circuit, which could contaminate the interior of the circuit. (Evidence Grade D)

Recommendation #3

Although the available evidence suggests a lower VAP rate with passive humidification than with active humidification, other issues related to the use of passive humidifiers (e.g., resistance, dead space volume, airway occlusion risk) preclude a recommendation for the general use of these devices. The decision to use a passive humidifier should not be based solely on infection control considerations. (Evidence Grade A)

Recommendation #4

Passive humidifiers do not need to be changed daily for reasons of infection control or technical performance. They can be safely used for at least 48 hours, and with some patient populations, some devices may be able to be used for up to 1 week. (Evidence Grade A)

Recommendation #5

The use of closed suction catheters should be considered part of a VAP prevention strategy. When closed suction catheters are used, they do not need to be changed daily for infection control purposes. The maximum time that closed suction catheters can be used safely is unknown. (Evidence Grade A)

Recommendation #6

Clinicians (e.g., respiratory therapists, nurses, and physicians) caring for mechanically ventilated patients should be aware of risk factors for VAP (e.g., nebulizer therapy, manual ventilation, and patient transport). (Evidence Grade B)

EVIDENCE GRADES

Grade A: Scientific evidence provided by randomized, well-designed, well-conducted, controlled trials with statistically significant results that consistently support the guideline recommendation; supported by Level 1 or 2 evidence

Grade B: Scientific evidence provided by well-designed, well-conducted observational studies with statistically significant results that consistently support the guideline recommendation; supported by Level 3 or 4 evidence

Grade C: Scientific evidence from bench studies, animal studies, and case studies; supported by Level 5 evidence

Grade D: Expert opinion provides the basis for the guideline recommendation, but scientific evidence either provided inconsistent results or was lacking

**For the complete guidelines, see AARC Clinical Practice Guidelines, Care of the ventilator circuit and its relation to ventilator-associated pneumonia. Respir Care 48:569–879, 2003.*

Box 4-10 Factors to Consider in Processing Reusable Equipment

- Infection risk (critical, semicritical, noncritical)
- Material and equipment configuration
- Available hospital disinfection resources
- Relative cost (labor and materials)

When a device's risk category is known, its composition must be matched to the resources available for hospital disinfection and sterilization. In this manner, each reusable device undergoes the most effective and least costly processing approach available.

MINI CLINI

Selection of Equipment Processing Methods

PROBLEM: A patient is discharged from the intensive care unit after extubation from mechanical ventilatory support. The following contaminated nondisposable items are returned to the respiratory care department for processing: the ventilator, the ventilator circuit and humidifier, a resuscitation bag, a mechanical (vane-type) respirometer, and a laryngoscope with blades. Outline what processing you would select for each item and why.

DISCUSSION: First, the circuit, humidifier, and resuscitation bag should be disassembled and cleaned using a detergent or enzymatic cleaner combined with a low-level or intermediate-level disinfectant. Because the ventilator, respirometer, and laryngoscope and blades cannot be immersed in water, they should immediately undergo surface disinfection, using an appropriate EPA-registered product.

After cleaning and initial disinfection, you should sort the items according to risk category and heat sensitivity. No items from this patient pose a critical infection risk. The ventilator circuit, humidifier, resuscitation bag, respirometer, and laryngoscope are semicritical items, whereas the ventilator itself is a noncritical item. The ventilator circuit, humidifier, and resuscitation bag are also plastic and probably heat labile. The respirometer and laryngoscope are heat stable.

When possible, semicritical items should be sterilized between patients; the heat-stable items should be autoclaved, and heat-labile items should undergo EtO sterilization. The ventilator (a noncritical item) need undergo only low-level to intermediate-level surface disinfection. The inner parts of the ventilator need not be sterilized or disinfected between patients.

HAIs associated with bronchoscopes have been most commonly reported with *M. tuberculosis*, nontuberculosis mycobacteria, and *P. aeruginosa*.[22] The most common reasons for transmission include failure to adhere to recommended cleaning and disinfection procedures, failure of automated endoscope reprocessors, and flaws in design. Flexible endoscopes are particularly difficult to disinfect, and meticulous cleaning must precede any sterilization or high-level disinfection process.

Disposable Equipment

An important alternative to reprocessing equipment continually is employing single-patient-use disposable devices. In the past, only O_2 therapy devices (i.e., masks, cannulas), suction apparatus (i.e., catheters, tubing), and some supplies were disposable. Today, manufacturers provide a range of disposable devices, including humidifiers, nebulizers, incentive spirometers, ventilator circuits, bag-valve-masks, and monitoring transducers.

Three major issues are involved in using disposable devices: *cost, quality,* and *reuse*. Cost issues boil down to straightforward dollar comparisons between purchasing and processing reusable devices versus stocking and distributing disposable devices. Good comparisons take into account direct and indirect costs (e.g., personnel, inventory, maintenance) and risk factors. Most recent findings support the cost-effectiveness of disposable devices over reusable devices in respiratory care.

Cost savings notwithstanding, many quality issues persist. Although disposable devices generally perform well, poor quality control remains a problem.[20] Respiratory care managers need to evaluate carefully disposable devices being considered for bulk purchase before actual clinical use. To ensure reliability, this evaluation should include physical testing of multiple units of each model being assessed. Finally, bedside clinicians need to inspect carefully and confirm the operation of any disposable device before use.

Reusing high-cost, high-volume disposable equipment saves hospitals money. The practice of reusing devices labeled by the manufacturer for "single-use only" raises significant safety concerns and issues of negligence. The FDA provides stringent regulations for reprocessing and reusing single-use devices.[23] A reused single-use device must comply with the same regulatory requirements of the original manufactured device, including, but not limited to, submitting documents for premarket notification or approval, submitting adverse event reports, and meeting manufacturing and labeling requirements. The U.S. Centers for Medicare and Medicaid Services recommends that the reprocessing of single-use devices be performed by an FDA-approved third-party reprocessor and not by hospitals.

Fluids and Medications Precautions

Unit dosing has decreased but has not eliminated the infection hazard associated with medications. Box 4-11 outlines several simple procedures designed to help prevent cross contamination while using fluids and medications.

Handling Contaminated Articles and Equipment

Contaminated items, whether reusable or disposable, should be enclosed in an impervious bag before removal from a patient's room. Bagging helps prevent accidental exposure of both personnel and the environment to contaminated articles. A single bag is satisfactory if (1) the bag is strong and impervious, and

Box 4-11 Fluids and Medications Precautions

- Sterile fluids should always be used for tracheal suctioning and to fill nebulizers and bubble humidifiers. These fluids should be dispensed aseptically.
- Sterile water should be used when rinsing equipment. If tap water must be used, either an alcohol rinse must follow or the equipment must thoroughly air dry before use.
- If a large stock bottle of sterile fluid must be reused, the container must be resealed and dated after opening. Remaining fluid should be discarded within 24 hours.
- When multidose medication vials are being used, they must be handled, dispensed, and stored according to manufacturer's instructions (on the label or package insert). Medication must not be used after its expiration date.

(2) the contaminated items can be bagged without contaminating the outer surface of the bag. Otherwise, the contaminated items should be double-bagged. Bags used for contaminated articles or waste materials should be clearly labeled or color-coded for this purpose.

After bagging, reusable patient care equipment must be returned to the applicable processing area. Contaminated reusable equipment should remain bagged until ready for decontamination or sterilization. When contaminated waste is being discarded, both OSHA procedures and any applicable local, state, or federal regulations must be followed.

Handling Laboratory Specimens

When gathering laboratory specimens (e.g., sputum), extreme care needs to be taken to prevent contamination of the external surface of the container. If the outside of the container is contaminated, the caregiver must either disinfect it or place it in an impervious bag. To minimize the likelihood of laboratory specimens leaking during transport, they always should be placed in a sturdy container with a secure lid. When gathering a specimen from a patient on isolation precautions, the container must be placed in an appropriately labeled, impervious bag before it is removed from the room.

SURVEILLANCE FOR HOSPITAL-ACQUIRED INFECTIONS

Surveillance is an ongoing process of monitoring patients and health care personnel for acquisition of infection, colonization of pathogens, or both. It is one of the five key recommended components of an infection prevention program; the others are *investigation, prevention, control,* and *reporting*.[2] Surveillance is a tool to provide HAI data on patients to provide outcome measurements either to ensure there is no ongoing problem or detect problems and intervene to prevent transmission of pathogens in the health care environment.

Generally, an infection prevention committee establishes surveillance policies and an infection preventionist or epidemiologist administers them. The surveillance program may be centralized or decentralized (to the various service departments). The following principles should be a part of any infection prevention surveillance program[2]: (1) use of standard definitions for HAIs; (2) use of microbiology-based data (when available), including resistance patterns for pathogens of significance (e.g., *S. aureus*); (3) establishment of risk stratification for infection risk when available (e.g., ventilator days, device days); (4) monitoring of results prospectively and identifying trends that indicate unusual rates of infection or transmission within the facility; and (5) provision of feedback to stakeholders within the institution (e.g., surgical site infection rates reported back to individual surgeons). It is also common for infection prevention programs to oversee hand hygiene and standard precautions adherence observations.

Most hospitals perform surveillance for device-related infections: central line-associated bloodstream infections (CLABSI), catheter-associated urinary tract infections (CAUTI), and VAPs. It is also commonplace to track certain organisms, including *C. difficile* infection and methicillin-resistant *S. aureus* infection. Surveillance is performed by applying National Healthcare Safety Network (NHSN) definitions. Increasingly, there are regulatory mandates for the public reporting of surveillance results.

Traditionally, VAP was tracked and a standardized definition was employed. The VAP surveillance definition has significant limitations, including a lack of sensitivity and specificity that limits its usefulness.[11] Recently, a new construct for evaluating the development of complications in ventilated adult patients has been developed and publicized by NHSN.[24] Instead of following patients only for the development of VAP, surveillance is performed to look for ventilator-associated events (VAE). VAEs are broken down into three tiers: ventilator-associated conditions (VAC), infection-related ventilator-associated conditions (IVAC), and possible and probable VAP (Figure 4-3). VAE surveillance starts with the identification of a VAC defined as an increase in the daily minimum positive end expiratory pressure (PEEP) or daily minimum fraction of inspired oxygen (FiO_2) for 2 calendar days or longer after a period of stability. An IVAC is considered present if a VAC has been identified and there is an elevated temperature or white blood cell count and new antibiotics have been started and administered for 4 or more days. Possible VAP is identified in a patient with an IVAC who has purulent sputum by Gram stain or a positive sputum culture. Probable VAP is an IVAC in a patient with purulent sputum by Gram stain and a positive semiquantitative or quantitative sputum culture. The cultures need to be positive for a known respiratory pathogen. VAE surveillance is a new paradigm in surveillance in that it tries to examine the overall safety of ventilator therapy and not focus just on infection-related outcomes. Conduct of this surveillance requires a partnership among infection prevention, critical care physicians, and respiratory therapists.

The surveillance activities of an infection prevention program are most effective when they generate actionable data that are communicated to the bedside caregiver in a timely fashion. These data can become the springboard for continuous

Device-associated Module
VAE

Figure 1: Ventilator-Associated Events (VAE) Surveillance Algorithm*

Patient has a baseline period of stability or improvement on the ventilator, defined by ≥2 calendar days of stable or decreasing daily minimum* FiO_2 or PEEP values. The baseline period is defined as the 2 calendar days immediately preceding the first day of increased daily minimum PEEP or FiO_2.
*Daily minimum defined by lowest value of FiO_2 or PEEP during a calendar day that is maintained for at least 1 hour.

↓

After a period of stability or improvement on the ventilator, the patient has at least one of the following indicators of worsening oxygenation:
1) Increase in daily minimum* FiO_2 of ≥0.20 (20 points) over the daily minimum FiO_2 in the baseline period, sustained for ≥2 calendar days.
2) Increase in daily minimum* PEEP values of ≥3 cmH_2O over the daily minimum PEEP in the baseline period,† sustained for ≥2 calendar days.
*Daily minimum defined by lowest value of FiO_2 or PEEP during a calendar day that is maintained for at least 1 hour.
†Daily minimum PEEP values of 0-5 cmH_2O are considered equivalent for the purposes of VAE surveillance.

↓

Ventilator-Associated Condition (VAC)

↓

On or after calendar day 3 of mechanical ventilation and within 2 calendar days before or after the onset of worsening oxygenation, the patient meets both of the following criteria:

1) Temperature >38 °C or <36°C, **OR** white blood cell count ≥12,000 cells/mm^3 or ≤4,000 cells/mm^3.
AND
2) A new antimicrobial agent(s) (see Appendix for eligible antimicrobial agents) is started, and is continued for ≥4 calendar days.

↓

Infection-Related Ventilator-Associated Complication (IVAC)

↓

On or after calendar day 3 of mechanical ventilation and within 2 calendar days before or after the onset of worsening oxygenation, ONE of the following criteria is met (**taking into account organism exclusions specified in the protocol**):

1) Criterion 1: Positive culture of one of the following specimens, meeting quantitative or semi-quantitative thresholds as outlined in protocol, without requirement for purulent respiratory secretions:
   - Endotracheal aspirate, ≥10^5 CFU/ml or corresponding semi-quantitative result
   - Bronchoalveolar lavage, ≥10^4 CFU/ml or corresponding semi-quantitative result
   - Lung tissue, ≥10^4 CFU/g or corresponding semi-quantitative result
   - Protected specimen brush, ≥10^3 CFU/ml or corresponding semi-quantitative result
2) Criterion 2: Purulent respiratory secretions (defined as secretions from the lungs, bronchi, or trachea that contain ≥25 neutrophils and ≤10 squamous epithelial cells per low power field [lpf, x100])† plus a positive culture of one of the following specimens (qualitative culture, or quantitative/semi-quantitative culture without sufficient growth to meet criterion #1):
   - Sputum
   - Endotracheal aspirate
   - Bronchoalveolar lavage
   - Lung tissue
   - Protected specimen brush

   † If the laboratory reports semi-quantitative results, those results must correspond to the above quantitative thresholds. See additional instructions for using the purulent respiratory secretions criterion in the VAE Protocol.
3) Criterion 3: One of the following positive tests:
   - Pleural fluid culture (where specimen was obtained during thoracentesis or initial placement of chest tube and NOT from an indwelling chest tube)
   - Lung histopathology, defined as: 1) abscess formation or foci of consolidation with intense neutrophil accumulation in bronchioles and alveoli; 2) evidence of lung parenchyma invasion by fungi (hyphae, pseudohyphae or yeast forms); 3) evidence of infection with the viral pathogens listed below based on results of immunohistochemical assays, cytology, or microscopy performed on lung tissue
   - Diagnostic test for *Legionella* species
   - Diagnostic test on respiratory secretions for influenza virus, respiratory syncytial virus, adenovirus, parainfluenza virus, rhinovirus human metapneumovirus coronavirus

↓

Possible Ventilator-Associated Pneumonia (PVAP)

*According to Centers for Disease Control (CDC).

January 2015 (Modified April 2015)

FIGURE 4-3 Ventilator-associated events (VAE) surveillance algorithm.

improvement in the delivery of care. Infection preventionists must communicate the results of surveillance activities to bedside caregivers in a meaningful way so that continuous improvements in care occur based on local data. Health care workers need to be willing to accept surveillance data in the way it is intended, not as a punitive grade, but as a tool to encourage reflection on current processes for delivering care. All health care workers should be aware of the rates of adherence in their area to bundles, hand hygiene, and HAI and should seek out their infection preventionist with any questions, observations, and suggestions on how care could be improved.

SUMMARY CHECKLIST

- The five major routes for transmission of pathogens are contact, droplet, airborne, common vehicle, and vector-borne.
- Infection prevention procedures involve (1) eliminating the sources of infectious agents, (2) creating barriers to their transmission, and (3) monitoring and evaluating the effectiveness of control.
- Failure to clean equipment properly can render all subsequent processing efforts ineffective.
- Physical or chemical disinfection destroys the vegetative form of pathogenic organisms but cannot kill bacterial spores.
- Glutaraldehyde (20 minutes) is the most common option for high-level disinfection of semicritical respiratory care equipment.
- EtO is best suited for sterilization of critical moisture-sensitive or heat-sensitive items; heat-stable critical items should be steam-sterilized.
- Among respiratory care equipment, large-volume nebulizers have the greatest potential to spread infection.
- Ventilator circuits should be changed when visibly soiled or malfunctioning.
- HMEs may be used up to 96 hours before they need to be changed.
- Single-use items should be reused only if there is hard documented evidence that reprocessing poses no threat to the patient, it does not alter the function of the device, and FDA guidelines are followed. The use of a third-party reprocessor is recommended.
- Sterile fluids always must be used for tracheal suctioning and filling nebulizers and humidifiers.
- Hands need to be thoroughly cleaned after any patient contact, even when gloves are used.
- Standard precautions must be used in caring for all patients, regardless of their diagnosis or infection status.
- The use of gloves is part of routine basic care when there is skin contact with a patient.
- Masks, goggles, or a face shield must be worn during any procedure that can generate splashes or sprays of blood, body fluids, secretions, or excretions.
- RTs must be familiar with the overall infection prevention program, including surveillance policies and procedures.

References

1. Magill SS, Edwards JR, Bamberg W, et al: Multistate point-prevalence survey of healthcare associated infections. *New Engl J Med* 370:1198–1208, 2014.
2. Centers for Disease Control and Prevention, Healthcare Infection Control Practices Advisory Committee: *Guidelines for environmental infection control in healthcare facilities*, Atlanta, 2003, Centers for Disease Control and Prevention.
3. Siegel JD, Rhinehart E, Jackson M, et al: Healthcare infection control practices advisory committee: 2007 guideline for isolation precautions: preventing transmission of infectious agents in healthcare settings. <http://www.cdc.gov/ncidod/dhap/pdf/isolation2007pdf>. Accessed August 19, 2015.
4. Yu I, Li Y, Wong TW, et al: Evidence of airborne transmission of the severe acute respiratory syndrome virus. *N Engl J Med* 350:1731–1739, 2004.
5. Reason J: Human error: models and management. *BJM* 320:768–770, 2000.
6. Advisory Committee on Immunization Practices, Centers for Disease Control and Prevention: Immunization of health-care personnel: recommendations of the Advisory Committee on Immunization Practices. *MMWR Recomm Rep* 60:1–45, 2011.
7. Centers for Disease Control and Prevention: NHSN healthcare personnel safety component protocol: healthcare personnel vaccination module: influenza vaccination summary, Atlanta, Centers for Disease Control and Prevention.
8. Boyce JM, Pittet D, Healthcare Infection Control Practices Advisory Committee, Society for Healthcare Epidemiology of America, Association for Professionals in Infection Control, Infectious Diseases Society of America, Hand Hygiene Task Force: Guideline for hand hygiene in health-care settings: recommendations of the Healthcare Infection Control Practices Advisory Committee and the HICPAC/SHEA/APIC/IDSA hand hygiene task force. *MMWR Recomm Rep* 51(RR–16):1–56, 2002.
9. Facility Guideline Institute: *Guidelines for design and construction of hospitals and outpatient facilities*, Chicago, 2014, American Society for Healthcare Engineering of the American Hospital Association.
10. Pronovost P, Needham D, Berenholtz S, et al: An intervention to decrease catheter-related bloodstream infections in the ICU. *N Engl J Med* 355:2725–2732, 2006.
11. Klompas M, Branson R, Eichenwald EC, et al: Strategies to prevent ventilator-associated pneumonia in acute care hospitals: 2014 update. *Infect Control Hosp Epidemiol* 35:915–936, 2014.
12. O'Grady NP, Alexander M, Burns LA, et al: Healthcare Infection Control Practices Advisory Committee: Guidelines for the prevention of intravascular catheter-related infections. *Am J Infect Control* 39(4 Suppl):S31–S34, 2011.
13. Marschall J, Mermel LA, Fakih M, et al: Strategies to prevent central line–associated bloodstream infections in acute care hospitals: 2014 update. *Infect Control Hosp Epidemiol* 35:753–771, 2014.
14. Rutala WA, Weber DJ: *Healthcare Infection Control Practices Advisory Committee: Guideline for disinfection and sterilization in healthcare facilities, 2008*, Atlanta, 2008, Centers for Disease Control and Prevention, pp 38–52.
15. Spaulding EH: Chemical disinfection of medical and surgical materials. In Lawrence C, Block SS, editors: *Disinfection, sterilization, and preservation*, Philadelphia, 1968, Lea & Febiger, pp 517–531.
16. Haney PE, Raymond BA, Lewis LC: Ethylene oxide: an occupational health hazard for hospital workers. *AORN J* 51:480–481, 1990.
17. Restrepo RD, Walsh BK: American Association of Respiratory Care: Humidification during invasive and noninvasive mechanical ventilation: 2012. *Respir Care* 57:782–788, 2012.
18. Hess DR, Kallstrom TJ, Mottram CD: Care of the ventilator circuit and its relation to ventilator-associated pneumonia. *Respir Care* 48:869–879, 2003.
19. Weber DJ, Wilson MB, Rutala WA, et al: Manual ventilation bags as a source for bacterial colonization of intubated patients. *Am Rev Respir Dis* 142:892–894, 1990.

20. Kallstrom TJ: American Association for Respiratory Care: AARC guideline: oxygen therapy for adults in acute care facilities. *Respir Care* 47:717–720, 2002.
21. Centers for Disease Control and Prevention: Guideline for preventing health-care associated pneumonia, 2003. *MMWR Morb Mortal Wkly Rep* 53(RR03):1–36, 2003.
22. Miller MR, Crapo R, Hankinson J, et al: General considerations for lung function testing. *Eur Respir J* 26:153–161, 2005.
23. U.S. Food and Drug Administration: Reprocessing of single-use devices. <http://www.fda.gov/MedicalDevices/DeviceRegulationandGuidance/ReprocessingofSingle-UseDevices/default.htm>. Accessed August 19, 2015.
24. National Health and Safety Network, Device associated module: ventilator associated event. <http://www.cdc.gov/nhsn/acute-care-hospital/index.html>. Accessed December 1, 2014.

CHAPTER 5

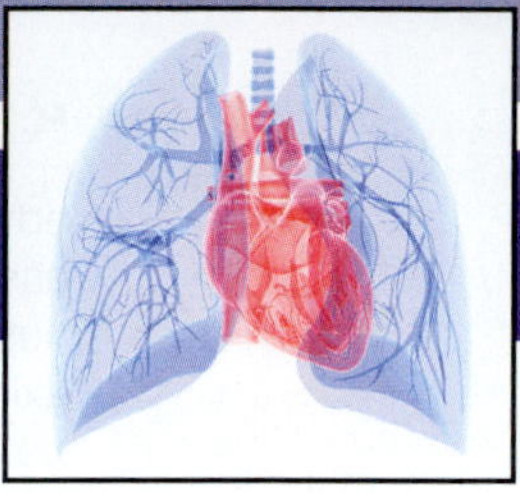

Ethical and Legal Implications of Practice

ANTHONY L. DEWITT

CHAPTER OBJECTIVES

After reading this chapter you will be able to:

- Summarize the philosophical foundations of ethics.
- Explain what constitutes an ethical dilemma and how such dilemmas arise in health care.
- Describe how professional codes of ethics apply to ethical decision making.
- Explain how traditional ethical principles are useful in resolving ethical dilemmas.
- Describe the information that should be gathered before making an ethical decision.
- Explain how the systems of civil and criminal law differ.
- Describe what constitutes professional malpractice and negligence.
- Explain how a respiratory therapist can become liable for wrongful acts.
- List the elements that constitute a practice act.
- Explain how licensing affects legal responsibility and liability.
- Describe how changes in health care delivery have shaped the ethical and legal aspects of practice.
- Summarize the basic elements of the *Health Insurance Portability and Accountability Act* of 1996 (HIPAA).
- Describe the role of advance directives and living wills in health care.

CHAPTER OUTLINE

Philosophical Foundations of Ethics
Ethical Dilemmas of Practice
Codes of Ethics
Ethical Theories and Principles
  Autonomy
  Veracity
  Nonmaleficence
  Beneficence
  Confidentiality
  Justice
  Role Duty
Ethical Viewpoints and Decision Making
  Formalism
  Consequentialism
  Mixed Approaches
  Virtue Ethics
  Intuitionism
  Comprehensive Decision-Making Models
Legal Issues Affecting Respiratory Care
  Systems of Law
  Health Insurance Portability and Accountability Act of 1996
  Medical Supervision
Interaction of Ethics and the Law
Professional Licensure Issues
  Licensure Statute
  Understanding the Causes of Discipline
  Engaging Counsel
Respiratory Therapists Who Speak Out About Wrongdoing
  Patient Protection and Affordable Care Act
  National Labor Relations Act
  False Claims Act
Health Care and Change
  Health Care Advance Directives

KEY TERMS

advance directives	defendant	nonmaleficence
assault	distributive justice	plaintiff
autonomy	double effect	*res ipsa loquitur*
axiology	formalism	*respondeat superior*
battery	informed consent	rule utilitarianism
beneficence	intuitionism	slander
benevolent deception	justice	strict liability
breach of contract	libel	tort
compensatory justice	living will	veracity
confidentiality	malpractice	virtue ethics
consequentialism	negligence	

An effective respiratory therapist (RT) must possess excellent clinical skills and an understanding of the business of health care. The health care industry, similar to all industries, must deliver services in an atmosphere in which ethical and legal considerations are an integral part of the organizational culture. RTs regularly encounter circumstances that require them to make choices or take actions that have ethical and legal implications. In society, ethics and law help maintain order, stability, and accountability. In professional practices, ethics guide RTs in carrying out their duties in a morally defensible way. Law establishes the minimum legal standards to which practitioners must adhere. Although not always the case, ethical practice may require a standard above that of legal practice. The tension between these two competing values can sometimes be problematic.

The force behind law is threefold: (1) state statutes regulate individual conduct by imposing criminal and sometimes civil penalties on those whose actions are considered to be against public policy by the legislative branch of government. The sanctions range from reparations and fines to imprisonment; (2) state statutes and professional boards regulate the practice of therapists and set minimum standards for competent practice as well as requirements for continuing education. Violation of licensing statutes and regulations can result in fines or discipline or revoking of the individual practitioner's license; and (3) the common law of civil liability for negligent and intentional acts imposes a duty to pay compensation to individuals who are injured. Civil judgments are usually monetary—they do not affect personal liberty.

Sanctions for ethical misconduct range from a loss of professional standing to expulsion from the profession or professional societies. In some cases, ethical misconduct and legal misbehavior may result from the same incident. The distinction between illegal acts and unethical behavior is not always obvious but is straightforward. *An illegal act violates the standards of conduct set down for all citizens (e.g., domestic assault), whereas ethical misconduct usually relates to violations of professional and ethical norms established by the profession as a whole.* A given act may fit any one of the following categories, depending on the circumstances and the ethical orientation of the person involved: ethical and legal, unethical but legal, ethical but illegal, or unethical and illegal.

For example, a therapist who spends 30 minutes after clocking out visiting with a patient because the patient has no family is performing an act that is both ethical and legal. If the purpose of the visit, however, is to encourage the patient to offer her monetary gratuities for this extra visitation, the act would be *legal but unethical* because it seeks to exploit the emotional vulnerability of a patient. If the same patient, however, was a prisoner subject to a restriction on their right to visitation by the state, and the therapist knowingly violated the prohibition against visitation in violation of a state statute, the act *would not be unethical* (because the act does not violate the standards of the profession) *but may well be illegal* under state law. Finally, if the purpose of the visit was to rummage through a demented patient's valuables for the purpose of taking their credit card and checkbook, the act would be *both unethical* (because it would be exploiting the patient's mental vulnerabilities in violation of professional norms) *and illegal* (because it would be theft in violation of state criminal laws).

This chapter provides a foundation of principles related to the ethical and legal practice of respiratory care.

PHILOSOPHICAL FOUNDATIONS OF ETHICS

Although an in-depth discussion of philosophy is beyond the scope of this chapter, you should realize that ethics has its origins in philosophy. *Philosophy* may be defined as the love of wisdom and the pursuit of knowledge concerning humankind, nature, and reality.[1] *Ethics* is one of the disciplines of philosophy, which include ontology (the nature of reality), metaphysics (the nature of the universe), epistemology (the nature of knowledge), **axiology** (the nature, types, and criteria of values), logic, and aesthetics. Ethics is primarily concerned with the question of how we should act. Although ethics may share common origins with the disciplines of law, theology, and economics, as an applied practice, ethics is clearly different from these disciplines.[1] Ethics can be described philosophically as a moral principle that supplements the golden rule and can be summed up by a commitment to "respect the humanity in persons."[2]

ETHICAL DILEMMAS OF PRACTICE

The growth of respiratory care has paralleled the development of advanced medical technology and treatment protocols. At the same time, during the 1970s and through the 1990s, the medical community has experienced rising expectations about acceptable standards of care. This is due to an ever-growing and sophisticated patient population fueled by medical benefit packages from the government and employers. In the latter part of the 1990s, managed care strategies and other cost-containment methods adopted by most third-party payers slowed the growth of the health care industry. The ethical and legal issues faced by practitioners, although changed in many cases, continued to grow. In the earlier period, RTs faced ethical dilemmas and legal issues associated with patient expectations, staffing, and quality of care, among others. RTs continue to face ethical dilemmas and legal issues; however, such dilemmas may now include the rationing of care, dealing with conflicts associated with third party–imposed standards of care, and delivery of the appropriate standard of care in the face of cost constraints and corporate influence. Staffing issues continue to be a problem and are at the root of many of the ethical and legal concerns faced by RTs. As respiratory care continues to mature as a profession, these challenges are likely to increase. The twenty-first century has brought one particular challenge, although not new to health care or to RTs: a heightened awareness of the patient's right to privacy. The *Health Insurance Portability and Accountability Act* of 1996 (HIPAA), discussed later in this chapter, is now a major consideration for RTs as they perform their jobs. It also has brought new opportunities in the form of the *Patient Protection and Affordable Care Act* of 2010 (PPACA). The PPACA has improved access to health care and increased reimbursement for patient care services, as well as creating disease management opportunities for RTs.

RTs work in complex health care settings. As a result, there is a large range of ethical dilemmas that may face the RT on a regular basis. The clinical aspects and the management aspects of health care are full of possibilities for ethical dilemmas. In addition, the ethical orientation of the RT plays a role in recognition and identification of ethical dilemmas. The health care industry continues to be in a period of dynamic change, bringing many new challenges. New technologic and management methodologies are continuously being introduced to accomplish the missions and goals of health care organizations. Over the past decade, there has been an almost complete change from a relatively open fee-for-service system to one in which care is managed in some fashion and the fees are in some form of capitated payment. These changes often pose serious ethical dilemmas.

For example, managed care uses a concept known as "restrictive gatekeeping." Restrictive gatekeeping requires patients to obtain prior approval from their third-party payer, usually an insurance company, before hospitalization and before certain procedures. When the hospital admission or procedure is approved, specific requirements or limitations are usually associated with the patient's care. As a result, health care workers, including RTs, may find themselves engaged in clinical processes that are dictated more by the third-party payers than by patient needs. Under these circumstances, health care workers may feel frustrated and helpless if they believe a patient needs care beyond that approved by the third-party payer. Ethics may impose a duty on professionals to interact with and press for change with the third party.

The rationing of care continues to be a side effect of staffing patterns created by managed care. Although all businesses must carefully balance staffing patterns against productivity, managed care has brought this concept home in a major way to health care facilities. An RT working in an understaffed department may decide that Patient A can really forego therapy because the department is short staffed and Patient A is really not going to get better anyway. Although this may sound at first like a case of simple neglect of duty, it is also an ethical dilemma. Unless this behavior is endorsed by a treatment protocol approved by the medical director and medical staff, it may violate professional norms and be unethical to effectively prefer one patient over another on the basis of factors beyond the patient's control.

The approaches used to address ethical issues in health care range from the specific to the general. Specific guidance in resolving ethical dilemmas is usually provided by a professional code of ethics. General approaches involve the use of ethical theories and principles to reach a decision.[3]

CODES OF ETHICS

A *code of ethics* is an essential part of any profession that claims to be self-regulating. The adoption of a code of ethics is one way in which an occupational group establishes itself as a profession. A code may try to limit competition, restrict advertisement, or promote a particular image in addition to setting forth rules for conduct.[4]

The first American medical code of ethics (established in 1847) was as much concerned with separating orthodox practitioners from nontraditional ones as it was with regulating behavior. Even modern codes tend to be vague regarding what is prescribed and what is to be avoided.

The American Association for Respiratory Care (AARC) has adopted a Statement of Ethics and Professional Conduct. The current code appears in Box 5-1. This code represents a set of general principles and rules that have been developed to help ensure that the health needs of the public are provided in a safe, effective, and caring manner. Codes for different professions might differ from the code governing respiratory care because they may seek different goals. However, all codes of ethics seek to establish parameters of behavior for members of the chosen profession. Professional codes of ethics often represent overly simplistic or prohibitive notions of how to deal with open misbehavior or flagrant abuses of authority.

The most difficult ethical decisions arise from situations in which two or more right choices are incompatible, in which the

Box 5-1 American Association for Respiratory Care Statement of Ethics and Professional Conduct (Revised July, 2004)

In the conduct of professional activities, the respiratory therapist shall be bound by the following ethical and professional principles. Respiratory therapists shall:

- Demonstrate behavior that reflects integrity, supports objectivity, and fosters trust in the profession and its professionals. Actively maintain and continually improve their professional competence and represent it accurately.
- Perform only those procedures or functions in which they are individually competent and that are within the scope of accepted and responsible practice.
- Respect and protect the legal and personal rights of patients they treat, including the right to informed consent and refusal of treatment.
- Divulge no confidential information regarding any patient or family unless disclosure is required for responsible performance of duty or required by law.
- Provide care without discrimination on any basis, with respect for the rights and dignity of all individuals.
- Promote disease prevention and wellness.
- Refuse to participate in illegal or unethical acts and refuse to conceal illegal, unethical, or incompetent acts of others.
- Follow sound scientific procedures and ethical principles in research.
- Comply with state or federal laws that govern and relate to their practice.
- Avoid any form of conduct that creates a conflict of interest and shall follow the principles of ethical business behavior.
- Promote health care delivery through improvement of the access, efficacy, and cost of patient care.
- Encourage and promote appropriate stewardship of resources.

choices represent different priorities, or in which limited resources exist to achieve a desired end. Ethicists readily admit that reducing these issues to simple formulations is not an easy task. The number and complexity of ethical dilemmas continue to grow as the complexity of life and health care increases. For health care, difficult ethical dilemmas continue to involve concerns about the practical limits on financial resources, the growing emphasis on individual autonomy, and more research advances such as cloning and stem cell research. Resolution of these more complex problems requires a more general approach than that provided by a code of ethics. This more general perspective is provided by ethical theories and principles.

In addition to the moral obligations that ethical duties impose on RTs, ethical obligations are often cited in legal proceedings as a tool of cross-examination. If an RT expresses opinions or is accused of actions that would violate the ethical duties of the profession, the RT's ignorance of ethical standards during cross-examination can have a powerful effect on a jury.

ETHICAL THEORIES AND PRINCIPLES

Ethical theories and principles provide the foundation for all ethical behavior. Contemporary ethical principles have evolved from many sources, including Aristotle's and Aquinas' natural law, Judeo-Christian morality, Kant's universal duties, and the values characterizing modern democracy.[5,6] Although controversy exists, most ethicists agree that autonomy, veracity, nonmaleficence, beneficence, confidentiality, justice, and role fidelity are the primary guiding principles in contemporary ethical decision making.[1,5]

Each of these ethical principles, as applied to professional practice, consists of two components: a *professional duty* and a

MINI CLINI

Conflicting Obligations

PROBLEM: Mary Smith, a registered RT with 18 years' experience, has worked for a large regional medical center for the past 10 years. She is generally happy with her work but is concerned about the financial stability of the hospital. As a result, she has signed on with a temporary agency to ensure that she will have work if the hospital decides to initiate a reduction in force. On one of her scheduled days off, Mary Smith agrees to work a shift for the temporary agency at another hospital. Two hours before her shift is scheduled to begin, she receives a telephone message from the medical center where she is employed. Her supervisor asks Mary Smith to report to work at the medical center because the only experienced therapist on the shift has been in an automobile accident. Mary Smith is torn between her obligation to the medical center where she has worked for 10 years and the agency.

DISCUSSION: Professionalism and ethics generally require a commitment to one's duties. In this situation, Mary Smith must consider not only her duty but also the consequences of each decision that she might make. In either case, there is the possibility that her decision will leave a staffing shortage at one of the hospitals.

DISCUSSION QUESTIONS: Should Mary Smith cancel her shift with the agency, although she has agreed to give the agency a 4-hour notice except in an emergency? Should she work the shift at the agency as scheduled, using the rationale that she did not create the staffing problem at the medical center? Should she call her supervisor, explain the situation, and ask for help in making the right decision, realizing that the final decision would still be hers? Should she call her supervisor and tell the supervisor that she is ill and cannot come in and report to the agency job?

GUIDANCE: Generally, a therapist's loyalty should be to the primary institution that employs her. In this situation the hospital has invested time, money, and benefits, as well as training, in the therapist, and the therapist owes the institution a duty of loyalty. Saying "I didn't create the problem" does not solve the problem; it merely passes the buck. The agency may be annoyed at the change of plans, but likely has others to call. The same does not appear to be true of the hospital. Calling the supervisor makes the problem a shared problem, and that is probably not fair to the supervisor because the supervisor did not seek outside employment. Thus this situation requires the therapist to consider her duty of loyalty to her employer and do the right thing.

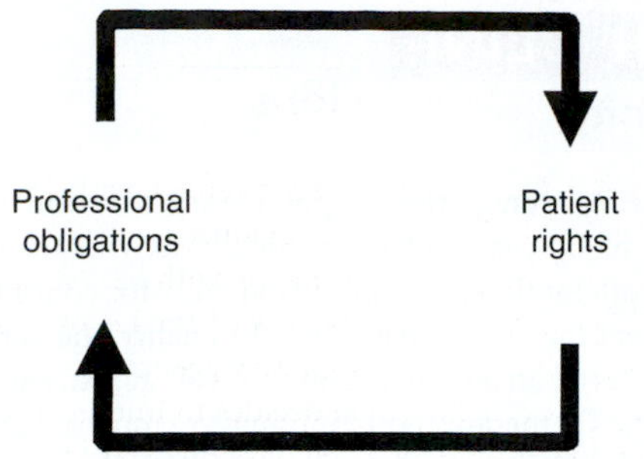

FIGURE 5-1 Reciprocal relationship between professional obligations and patient rights.

patient right (Figure 5-1). The principle of autonomy obliges health care professionals to uphold the freedom of will and freedom of action of others. The principle of beneficence obliges health care professionals to further the interests of others, either by promoting their good or by actively preventing their harm. The principle of justice obliges health care professionals to ensure that others receive what they rightfully deserve or legitimately claim.

Expressed in each duty is a reciprocal patient right. Reciprocal patient rights include the right to autonomous choice, the right not to be harmed, and the right to fair and equitable treatment. More specific rules can be generated from these general principles of rights and obligations, such as those included in a code of ethics.

Autonomy

The principle of **autonomy** acknowledges the personal liberty of patients and their right to decide their own course of treatment and follow through on a plan on which they freely agree. It is from this principle that rules about **informed consent** are derived. Under the principle of autonomy, the use by an RT of deceit or coercion to get a patient to reverse the decision to refuse a treatment is considered unethical. Likewise, it is unethical and illegal to threaten a patient who is unwilling to sign a consent form.

Veracity

The principle of **veracity** (accuracy or truthfulness) is often linked to autonomy, especially in the area of informed consent. Generally, veracity binds the health care provider and the patient to tell the whole truth about the choices inherent in medical care. This means providing not only information about the benefits of a particular course of action but also what might go wrong and what kinds of frequent complications occur. The nature of the health care delivery process is such that both parties involved are best served in an environment of trust and mutual sharing of all information. Problems with the veracity principle revolve around such issues as benevolent deception. In actions of **benevolent deception**, the truth is withheld from the patient for, supposedly, his or her own good.

When the physician decides to withhold the truth from a conscious, well-oriented adult, the decision affects the interactions between health care providers and the patient and has a chilling effect on the rapport that is so necessary for good care. In a poll conducted by the Louis Harris group, 94% of Americans surveyed indicated that they wanted to know everything about their cases, even the dismal facts. Other than with pediatrics and rare cases in which there is evidence that the truth would lead to a harm (e.g., suicide), the truth, provided in as pleasant a manner as possible, is probably the best policy.[7]

Truth telling also can involve documentation and medical recordkeeping. This type of dilemma is occurring more frequently under strict managed care reimbursement protocols.

MINI CLINI

Patient Rights

PROBLEM: An RT working at a hospital receives a physician order to administer an aerosolized bronchodilator treatment to a 26-year-old female patient with asthma admitted for suspected pneumonia. The patient refuses the treatment on entering the room, stating that she is having a "bad day" today and does not want to be bothered by anyone. The patient is regarded as being competent and fully capable of making health care decisions for herself. How should the RT handle this situation?

DISCUSSION: The RT must acknowledge and respect the patient's right to decide freely whether or not to allow the respiratory care treatment. According to the principles of ethical theory and conduct, health care professionals have an obligation to promote patient autonomy by permitting freedom of will and freedom of action. It is also important that neither coercion nor deceit be used to get a patient to reverse his or her decision to refuse a treatment. According to the American Hospital Association statement called "The Patient Care Partnership," the patient has the right to refuse treatment and to be informed of the medical consequences of her action.

The RT could talk to the patient and explore what the term "bad day" meant to her. It might be that she is not feeling well because of breathing problems from her asthma condition and worsening symptoms of possible pneumonia. The RT has an important role in ensuring that the patient understands the benefits of the respiratory treatment and the health consequences of refusal so that the patient can make a well-informed decision. If the RT approaches the patient in a professional, nonthreatening manner, she may feel more at ease and be willing to discuss in greater depth why she does not want to take the treatment. It is common for a patient to refuse therapy initially only to change his or her mind after discussion with the RT. Should the patient still refuse the treatment after discussion with the RT, the RT should remain nonjudgmental, even if he or she disagrees with the patient's decision. Appropriate documentation in the medical record and physician notification should then occur.

Nonmaleficence

The principle of **nonmaleficence** requires that health care providers avoid harming patients and prevent harm actively where possible. It is sometimes difficult to uphold this principle in modern medicine because in many cases, drugs and procedures have secondary effects that may be harmful in varying degrees. Procedures carry risks for complications, not all of which can be predicted. For example, an RT might ask whether it is ethical to give a high dose of steroids to an asthmatic patient, knowing the many harmful consequences of these drugs. One solution to these dilemmas is based on the understanding that many helping actions inevitably have both a good and a bad effect, or *double effect*. The key is the *first intent*. If the first intent is good, the harmful effect is viewed as an unintended result. The **double effect** brings us to the essence of the definition of the word *dilemma*. The word comes from the Greek terms *di*, meaning "two," and *lemma*, meaning "assumption" or "proposition."[8]

Consideration of intent alone, however, does not settle the issue. Nonmaleficience and veracity cannot always be separated; effects must be explained, even if this may lead the patient to pass up the intended benefits of the treatment.

Beneficence

The principle of **beneficence** raises the "do no harm" requirement to an even higher level. Beneficence requires that health care providers go beyond doing no harm and contribute actively to the health and well-being of their patients. Many quality-of-life issues are included within this dictum. Practitioners of medicine today possess the technology to keep some individuals alive well beyond any likelihood of meaningful recovery. This technology presents dilemmas for practitioners who have the ability to prolong life but not the ability to restore any uniquely human qualities.

One approach in this situation is for the RT to tell the patient that the physician will interpret the studies and provide a full report at the next office visit. All final discussion of results must ultimately go through the physician.

Some individuals interpret the principle of beneficence to mean that they must do everything to promote a patient's life, regardless of how useful the life might be to that individual. Other professionals in the same situation might believe they are allowing the principle to be better served by doing nothing and allowing death to occur without taking heroic measures to prevent it. In an attempt to allow patients to participate in resolving this dilemma, legal avenues, called **advance directives**, have been developed.[9] Advance directives allow a patient to give direction to health care providers about treatment choices in circumstances in which the patient may no longer be able to provide that direction. The two types of advance directives available at the present time and widely used are the *living will* and the *durable power of attorney for health care*. A durable power of attorney for health care allows the patient to identify another person to carry out his or her wishes with respect to health care, whereas a **living will** states a patient's health care preferences in writing. As a result of the *Patient Self-Determination Act* of 1990, most states require that all health care agencies receiving federal reimbursement under Medicare/Medicaid legislation provide adult clients with information on advance directives.[9,10]

MINI CLINI

Veracity

PROBLEM: Jon performs pulmonary function testing, including blood gases, for his hospital. Many of the patients he sees are attempting to qualify or requalify for continuous reimbursement for home oxygen use. To qualify, the patient's PaO_2 must be less than 60 mm Hg on room air at rest. Patient A, who has home O_2 therapy, is attempting to requalify, although her condition has improved from what it was 1 year earlier. Her blood gas results show a PaO_2 of 63 mm Hg. The patient's husband asks Jon if there is anything he can do, while relating how greatly his wife benefits from the O_2. Jon tells the husband that there is nothing he can do and assists the husband in taking the patient out to her car. At the car, the husband pulls out his wallet, shows it to Jon, and repeats the question.

DISCUSSION POINTS: RTs have an obligation to carry out their duties in the most competent and professional manner possible. Failure to do so may constitute both an ethical dilemma and a legal issue. Similarly, RTs have a duty to be truthful with third parties who may rely on their clinical results.

DISCUSSION QUESTIONS: What is the potential ethical dilemma in this situation? What ethical principles are involved here? What other ways could Jon have chosen to handle this situation?

GUIDANCE: The ethical dilemma here is whether to accept cash to change a blood gas result, and there should be no question about the right answer. It is never okay to accept money from patients for doing your job. It creates a situation in which a clinician feels obligated to perform additional or, in this case, unlawful acts for the patient. That is a slippery slope, and once a therapist starts down that path, there is frequently no turning back. Falsification of medical records can result in both civil and criminal liability. Accepting money to change the test result could be viewed as receiving a kickback under the federal Anti-Kickback statute, which carries criminal penalties. It could be viewed as an unlawful and unethical act by the state board, and result in license discipline. Worse, it erodes the trust of other professionals—including physicians and nurses—in the scientific objectivity and professional status of all the other therapists who will be tarred with the same brush.

This Mini Clini involves the ethical principles of veracity and the duty of candor to third parties. Therapists have fought hard for professional recognition, and selling test results undermines the entire profession. The ethical principle of veracity is among the most important of the ethical principles because it has the potential to do the most damage if it is violated.

Confidentiality

The principle of **confidentiality** is founded in the Hippocratic Oath; it was later reiterated by the World Medical Association in 1949. It obliges health care providers to "respect the secrets which are confided even after the patient has died."[11] Confidentiality, as with the other axioms of ethics, often must be balanced against other principles, such as beneficence. Notably, state laws require a breach of confidence under certain conditions (e.g., reporting gunshot wounds or child abuse) in which risk to other parties may result from not disclosing events or results.

The main ethical issue surrounding confidentiality is whether more harm is done by occasionally violating its mandate or by always upholding it regardless of the consequences. This limitation to confidentiality is known as the *harm principle.* This principle requires that practitioners refrain from acts or omissions in which foreseeable harm to others could result, especially when the others are vulnerable to risk. This principle would require that confidentiality be maintained for a patient with acquired immunodeficiency syndrome (AIDS) in matters involving his or her landlord. In this case, confidentiality is justified because the landlord is not particularly vulnerable. However, if the patient was planning to marry, the harm principle would require that confidentiality be broken because of the special vulnerability of the future spouse.

Confidentiality is usually considered a qualified, rather than an absolute, ethical principle in most health care provider–patient relationships. These qualifications are often written into codes of ethics. The American Medical Association Code of Ethics, Section 9, provides the following guidelines: "A physician may not reveal the confidences entrusted to him in the course of medical attendance or the deficiencies he may observe in the character of patients, unless he is required to do so by law or unless it becomes necessary in order to protect the welfare of the community or a vulnerable individual." Under the requirements of public health and community welfare, there is often a legal requirement to report such things as child abuse, poisonings, industrial accidents, communicable diseases, blood transfusion reactions, narcotic use, and injuries caused with knives or guns.[12] In many states, child abuse statutes protect the health care practitioner from liability in reporting even if the report should prove false as long as the report was made in good faith. Failure to report a case of child abuse can leave the practitioner legally liable for additional injuries that the child may sustain after being returned to the hostile environment.

Breaches of confidentiality more often result from careless slips of the tongue than from decision making or purposeful actions. Trading gossip about patients is unprofessional, unethical, and, in certain cases, illegal. Risks for inadvertent disclosure increase markedly when RTs may exchange information on social networks such as Facebook and LinkedIn. Such information should never be placed in such social media networks, because doing so violates the rights of individual patients.

RULE OF THUMB

Patient information should be discussed **only** in private and with persons who have a legitimate reason and need to know.

Because of the widespread use of computerized databases, confidential information, previously highly protected, is now relatively easy to obtain. Clinical data are available for close scrutiny by the clerical staff, laboratory personnel, and other health care providers. The widespread use of these data systems also threatens patient confidentiality. In an attempt to reduce this threat, most clinical databases are restricted to use by only the health care workers who have a need to know. In addition to being unethical, an RT who reads the file of a patient whom he or she is not treating would likely be in violation of institutional policy. The accompanying Mini Clini below provides an example.

MINI CLINI

Confidentiality

PROBLEM: Mary, an RT, is working the evening shift at a large urban medical center when she receives a telephone call from a friend telling her that her next door neighbor has been admitted to the medical center. Mary's first thought is to check the neighbor's file on the computer system to see why her neighbor has been hospitalized.

DISCUSSION POINT: Mary knows that the medical center has a policy that employees are to access only the charts for which they have a reason to do so.

DISCUSSION QUESTIONS: Should Mary access this chart via the computer system? If she does, what kind of violation will she be committing—ethical, legal, or both? What ethical principles, if any, would apply here? What is the harm in simply checking the computer on this patient? Is anyone likely to know if Mary accesses this patient's information?

GUIDANCE: The answer here is straightforward. She should absolutely not access the computer. The policy is there to keep the facility compliant with HIPPA and with state laws regarding privacy. Mary runs the risk for being fired because this action violates hospital policy. What harm does looking at the computer do? It erodes the confidentiality that patients expect. The far greater harm will be to Mary's reputation and future employability. If Mary does this, she will certainly be found out because the electronic medical record system has an "audit trail" that indicates who accessed the record and when. Mary will face hospital discipline for the policy violation (likely termination) and she may face criminal charges or civil administrative penalties under state and federal law for breaches of patient confidentiality. This action also places Mary at risk for a civil lawsuit for invasion of privacy.

The only exception to the rule of confidentiality regarding Mary's neighbor is if Mary is assigned to provide care to her as a treating RT. Only then does she have a need to know what is in the chart and what is wrong with her neighbor. But even then, the wiser course, because of the close relationship, would be for Mary to ask that she be excused from this case and that someone else handle the clinical duties for the patient.

Why? If the patient has an illness that carries any stigma with it (human immunodeficiency virus [HIV] infection, pediculosis capitis, etc.), the patient will likely be very embarrassed if her neighbor knows about it. And, if the patient's other neighbors learn about the condition from another source, Mary will be suspected. This will have consequences at work. For this reason, Mary should steer clear of this patient's medical record.

Despite medical and sociologic advances, potential violations of the individual's right to privacy in certain populations, such as patients with AIDS, pose a special risk because disclosure may result in economic, psychologic, or physical harm to the patient. RTs should adhere to the dictum found in the Hippocratic Oath: "What I may see or hear in the course of the treatment or even outside of treatment of the patient in regard to the life of men, which on no account one must spread abroad, I will keep to myself, holding such things to be shameful to be spoken about."[13]

Justice

The principle of **justice** involves the fair distribution of care. Rising health care expectations, coupled with the decreased availability of care because of cost, is making this principle an important one for health care workers. Population trends and the financial shortfalls in programs such as Medicaid and Medicare will contribute to the continuing importance of this principle.

The United States is rapidly approaching the point at which a balance must be found between health care expenses and the revenue available to pay for them. Efforts to achieve this balance may lead to some form of rationing of the delivery of health care services. This type of justice is properly referred to as **distributive justice**.

A second form of justice seen in health care is **compensatory justice**. This form of justice calls for the recovery for damages that were incurred as a result of the action of others. Damage awards in civil cases of medical malpractice or negligence are examples of compensatory justice. Compensatory justice often has been cited as playing a major role in increasing the cost of health care. However, the Congressional Budget Office estimates that less than 2% of the cost of health care is related to medical malpractice. Studies by Zurich Insurance Company,[14] Harvard University, and Dartmouth College showed little to no impact on the cost of health care and generally debunk the myth that physicians always practice defensive medicine. The Harvard study showed that patients were not compensated in the presence of actual malpractice more frequently than physicians were held accountable in the absence of actual malpractice. Other studies generally confirm that the civil justice system does a good job of protecting the rights of health care workers and patients in negligence litigation. There is a general bias, fueled in part by media reports, against medical liability. Nationally, 75% of medical negligence cases that go to trial are won by the medical provider.

Role Duty

Because no single individual can be solely responsible for providing all of a patient's health care needs, modern health care is necessarily a team effort. There are more than 100 allied health professions, and allied health workers (excluding nursing and physicians) provide approximately 60% of all patient care. Each of the allied health professions has its own practice niche, defined by tradition or by licensure law. Practitioners have a duty to understand the limits of their role and to practice with fidelity. For example, because of differences in *role duty,* an RT might be ethically obliged not to tell a patient's family how critical the situation is, instead having the attending physician do so.[3] The previous Mini Clinis addressed role duty, and the accompanying Mini Clini presents another example of the ethics of role duty.

ETHICAL VIEWPOINTS AND DECISION MAKING

In deciding ethical issues, some practitioners try to strictly interpret one or more of the aforementioned ethical principles. Other practitioners seek to decide the issue solely on a case-by-case basis, considering only the potential good (or bad) consequences. Still other practitioners would appeal to the image of a "good practitioner," asking themselves what a virtuous person would do in a similar circumstance. Finally, many practitioners acknowledge that they largely follow their intuition for making ethical decisions. These different viewpoints represent the four dominant theories underlying modern ethics.[5,15] The viewpoint that relies on rules and principles is called **formalism**, or duty-oriented reasoning. The viewpoint in which decisions are based on the assessment of consequences is called **consequentialism**. The viewpoint that asks what a virtuous person would do in a similar circumstance is called **virtue ethics**. When intuition is involved in the decision-making process, the approach is called **intuitionism**.

Formalism

Formalist thought asserts that certain features of an act determine its moral rightness. In this framework, ethical standards of right and wrong are described in terms of rules or principles. These rules function apart from the consequences of a particular act. An act is considered morally justifiable only if it upholds the rules or principles that apply.

The major objection to this duty-oriented approach lies in its potential for inconsistency. Critics of formalist reasoning insist that no principle or rule can be framed that does not have exceptions. These critics claim that no principle or rule can be framed that does not conflict with other rules.

Consequentialism

For the consequentialist, an act is judged to be right or wrong based on its consequences. Each possible act is assessed in terms of the relative amount of good (over evil) that it would cause. The most common application of consequentialism judges acts according to the *principle of utility*. The principle of utility, in its simplest form, aims to promote the greatest general good for most people.

Critics of this approach claim that it has two fundamental flaws. First, the analyzing and weighing the amount of good over evil that might occur is not always possible. Second, reliance on the principle of utility to the exclusion of all else can result in actions that are incompatible with ordinary judgments about right and wrong. A classic example of this problem can be seen in the true World War II case of the battle for

MINI CLINI

Role Duty

PROBLEM: Sue, an RT, receives a request to perform a blood gas analysis for a patient on a ventilator because, as reported by the nurse, the patient's oxygen saturation is only 61%. The patient has an order to obtain blood gas values as needed. As the nurse and RT look at the blood gas results, they both are surprised because the saturation is now 93%. The nurse suggests repeating the blood gas examination. The RT is about to comply until she notes the oximeter display on which the nurse is relying shows the patient with an O_2 saturation of 93% and a pulse rate of 61 beats/min.

DISCUSSION POINT: Teamwork and role delineation are both essential components of good patient care. Each practitioner also has an obligation to perform his or her duties in the most competent and professional manner possible.

DISCUSSION QUESTIONS: What kind of issue or dilemma exists here—legal, ethical, or both? What should the RT do at this point? Should an incident report be written and, if so, by whom?

GUIDANCE: The dilemma here is to explain the nurse's mistake in a way that does not jeopardize the working relationship with the nurse, while at the same time protecting the patient and the facility. Clearly a second blood gas value should not be obtained. Placement of the oximeter should be checked, and, if the oximeter is functioning properly, then it should be believed.

There are both legal and ethical components to the problem. The nurse had a good-faith belief that blood gas levels were required based on her understanding of the pulse oximeter. Her belief was wrong but reasonable. It is easily corrected with some training, and it is far better to discover this problem with an error that does not harm a patient as opposed to an error in which patient harm might have resulted.

The first issue is to explain the way the oximeter works and the meaning of the readings. Many nurses fail to understand the oxyhemoglobin dissociation curve, and as a result, interpret data from oximeters incorrectly. A therapist's job is to educate both patients and other caregivers and to do so in a professional and nonjudgmental manner.

The second issue is to evaluate the level of risk. There is very limited legal risk in this situation because the patient simply was not harmed by the error. The ethical duty of veracity and the duty of loyalty to the employer create a tension, however, regarding the filing of an incident report. Incident reports are necessary to protect the institution.

The nurse may be very reluctant to write an incident report about this event because it makes her look bad. Sadly, in some institutions incident reports are used incorrectly as a disciplinary tool instead of as a method of reporting errors from which systems can be improved. So the nurse may not wish to write an incident report, but the therapist must insist in this case. In the current era ensuring high-quality care is so important that hospitals must establish a culture in which reporting errors is encouraged and, in fact, expected as every caregiver's obligation to use the experience of errors and "near miss" errors to improve care.

Why must a report be filed regarding the current event? First, the incident carried with it a strong presumption that risk to patients was present because the nurse did not understand the limits of the technology. Second, although a bad outcome was averted, at least one unnecessary blood gas level was obtained and a second was advocated. Third, the therapist is involved because she should have checked the oximeter before doing the first blood gas measurement to determine that the equipment was operating within specifications. So there is error on both sides of the issue. Even if the nurse does not write an incident report, the incident report should be written by the therapist and the mistake disclosed to the physician. Teamwork and a commitment to high-quality care for patients requires honesty and full disclosure. Hospitals must ensure that reporting such events causes a focus on the process of care and opportunities to improve rather than on punishing the caregivers involved.

North Africa. In this scenario, there were two groups of soldiers but only enough antibiotics for one group. One group required the medication for syphilis contracted in the local brothels; the other group needed antibiotics for wounds sustained in battle. The dilemma arose as to who should receive the antibiotics. Formalist or duty-oriented reasoning would base the decision about who should receive the antibiotics on some concept of justice, such as giving priority to the sickest or to the individuals most in need. However, the actual decision in this case was a consequentialist one, based not on the desire to distribute the drug justly but rather on the need to obtain a quick victory with as few casualties as possible. The scarce medication was given to the soldiers who were "wounded" in the brothels rather than in battle because these soldiers could be restored quickly and returned to the frontlines to aid the war effort.

Mixed Approaches

Mixed approaches to moral reasoning try to capitalize on the strengths of two major lines of ethical thought. One approach, called **rule utilitarianism**, is a variation of consequentialism. Under this framework, the question is not which act has the greatest utility but which rule would promote the greatest good if it were generally followed.

The rule utilitarian would agree with the formalist that truth telling is a necessary ethical principle but for a different reason. To the rule utilitarian, truth telling is a needed principle not because it has any underlying moral rightness but because it promotes the greatest good in professional-patient relationships. Specifically, if truth telling were not followed consistently, trusting relationships between patients and health care professionals would be impossible.

MINI CLINI

Role Duty

PROBLEM: Courtney is the lone RT on duty on the midnight shift in a small, 65-bed rural hospital. She likes working at the small hospital and knows most of the patients and their conditions by memory. The night is quiet and uneventful until 2:00 AM, when a code is called for a patient in the intensive care unit (ICU). Courtney immediately heads for the ICU while mentally noting the condition of the patient on whom the code has been called. She remembers that the patient is 78 years old and has COPD. Just as she nears the ICU, a second code is called for a patient in a room just outside of the ICU. Courtney quickly jogs her memory and remembers that this patient is a 25-year-old woman with diabetes who has just given birth to a baby girl.

DISCUSSION POINT: The lone RT can attend to only one code, although she has an obligation to provide the best care possible to all patients. There is no protocol of which the RT is aware that would provide guidance about which patient she should help first. At the time the second code is called, she is at an equal distance from both patients.

DISCUSSION QUESTIONS: Is this RT facing an ethical dilemma? If so, what guiding principle or principles should be relied on to determine the best course of action? Which patient should the RT help first?

GUIDANCE: The ethical dilemma here is one that arises more frequently than most clinicians realize. Fortunately, however, because it is not new there are certain principles that can be used to help guide decision making.

First of all, there is no "right" answer. The life of a 78-year-old man is no less valuable than the life of a 25-year-old woman. They are both equal under the law and from an ethical point of view. But the therapist cannot be in two places at once. So, irrespective of whether it is fair, a choice must be made. Triage is the principle that guides the approach to these situations. According to the 2014 Unabridged *Webster's Third New International Dictionary,* the term *triage* comes from the French verb *trier,* meaning to separate, sift, or select. In this situation, the therapist has to sift through two choices. Triage originated from the need to treat multiple wounded soldiers with limited resources. Wounded soldiers were initially assigned into three categories: (1) those who would likely live without medical aid, (2) those who would likely die no matter what was done, and (3) those for whom immediate treatment would likely be lifesaving.

Between the two patients, there is a strong likelihood that no matter what is done for the 78- year-old patient, that patient will expire given his diagnosis and comorbidities. The young woman likely has the greatest chance for survival, so that lifesaving care will likely benefit her more than the 78-year-old patient. These are the factors that could be used to make the decision, but ultimately, the decision belongs to the therapist. No one can say whether one choice is better than the other. Ethics rarely involves the choice between good and evil, it usually involves a choice between good and better, or better and best. Because the lines are so gray, it is easy to cross them.

The rule utilitarian approach is probably the most appealing and useful to health care professionals. This approach is appealing because it addresses both human rights and obligations and the consequences of actions. Rule utilitarianism seems best able to account for the modern realities of human experience that so often affect the day-to-day practice of health care. However, although it has some value as an ethical framework, it has the disadvantage of being quite variable among caregivers. Where caregivers have different values and different educational levels, ethical decision making using this tool frequently is inconsistent.

Virtue Ethics

A theory of virtue ethics has evolved based in part on the limits of both formalism and consequentialism. Virtue ethics is founded not in rules or consequences but in personal attributes of character or virtue. Under this formulation, the first question is not, "How do I act in this situation?" but rather, "How should I carry out my life if I am to live well?" or "How would the good RT act?"

Virtue-oriented theory holds that professions have historical traditions. Individuals entering a profession enter into a relationship not only with current practitioners but also with the practitioners who have come before them. With these traditions comes a history of character standards set by the individuals who have previously distinguished themselves in that profession.

According to this perspective, the established practices of a profession can give guidance, without an appeal to either the specific moral principles or the consequences of an act.[3] When the professional is faced with an ethical dilemma, he or she need only envision what the "good practitioner" would do in a similar circumstance. It is hard to imagine the good RT stealing from the patient, charging for services not provided, or smothering a patient with a pillow.

Rapidly changing fields such as respiratory care pose some problems for virtue ethics. What might be considered good ethical conduct at one time might be deemed wrong the next time. An example of this change over time is an RT who is asked not only to disconnect a brain-dead patient from a ventilator but also to remove the feeding tubes and intravenous lines.

In addition to the difficulty with changing values in virtue ethics, it provides no specific directions to aid decision making. The heavy reliance of virtue ethics on experience rather than on reason makes creative solutions less likely. Finally, practitioners often find themselves in conflicting role situations for which virtue ethics has no answers. A good example is an RT who practices the virtue of being a good team player but is confronted with the need to "blow the whistle" on a negligent or incompetent team member.[3] Despite these limitations, virtue ethics is probably the way most practitioners make their ethical decisions.

Intuitionism

Intuitionism is an ethical viewpoint that holds that there are certain self-evident truths, usually based on moral maxims such

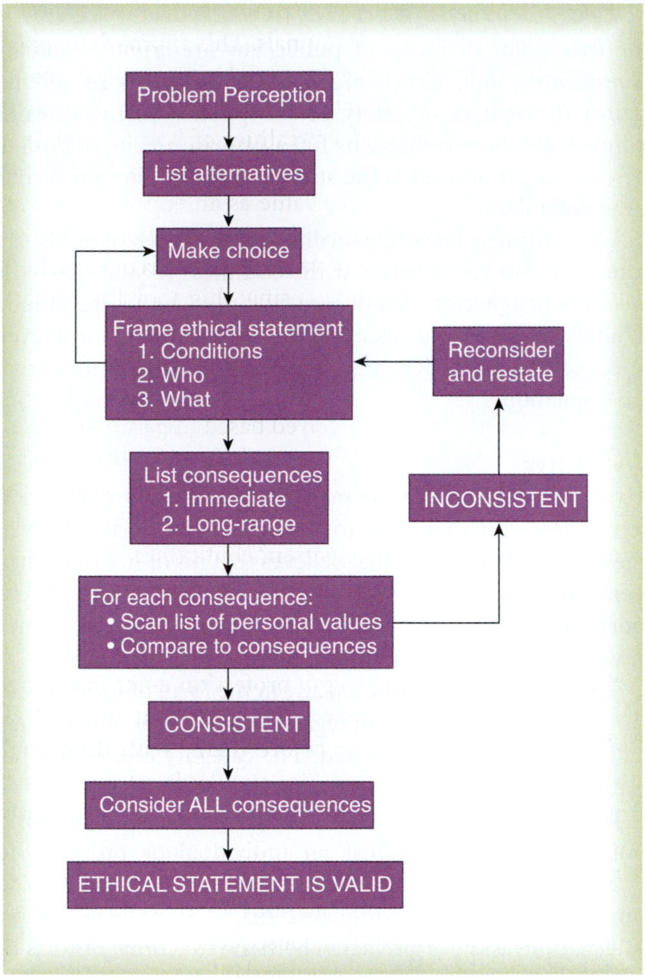

FIGURE 5-2 Comprehensive ethical decision-making model. (Redrawn from Brody H: Ethical decisions in medicine, ed 2, Boston, 1981, Little, Brown.)

as "treat others fairly." The easiest way to understand intuitionism is to think of as many timeless maxims as you can, which form the basis for intuitionism. These maxims may range from "do not kill" to "look before you cross the street."[6] As a decision-making tool, intuitionism is not helpful, mostly because it depends on the intuitional abilities of the specific caregiver.

Comprehensive Decision-Making Models

To aid in the process of decision making in bioethics, several comprehensive models have been developed. Figure 5-2 depicts one example of a comprehensive decision-making model that combines the best elements of formalism, consequentialism, and virtue ethics. As is evident in this approach, the ethical problem is framed in terms of the conditions and who is affected. Initially, an action is chosen based on its predicted consequences. The potential consequences of this decision are compared with the human values underlying the problem. The short test of this comparison is a simple restatement of the golden rule, that is, "Would I be satisfied to have this action performed on me?" The initial decision is considered ethical if, and only if, it passes this test of human values. A simpler but nonetheless comprehensive model is used by many ethicists. The model uses eight key steps (Box 5-2).

Box 5-2 Ethical Decision-Making Model

1. Identify the problem or issue.
2. Identify the individuals involved.
3. Identify the ethical principle or principles that apply.
4. Identify who should make the decision.
5. Identify the role of the practitioner.
6. Consider the alternatives (long-term and short-term consequences).
7. Make the decision (including the decision not to act).
8. Follow the decision to observe its consequences.

With or without these models, RTs are often at a double disadvantage in ethical decision making because RTs not only must live with their own decisions but also must support (and act on) the decisions of their physician colleagues. Unless excellent communication exists, misunderstandings can occur. Such misunderstandings may be an essential factor in the high job stress, burnout, and attrition in respiratory care.

Classes in ethics, decision making, and communication skills are crucial components of the preparation of RTs for the often confusing and frustrating practice in today's medical settings. The specialty requires practitioners who can go beyond simple assertions of right or wrong and provide justifications that are both right and reasoned. Many hospitals have ethics boards or committees to review and set policy and to assist in making informed ethical decisions. In addition to administrators and medical staff members, these committees may include a member of the lay public, a chaplain, and one or more experts in bioethics.

A major factor in the disciplinary decisions of professional boards is frequently whether the acts of the RT conformed to the ethical standards of the profession. Nearly every respiratory care practice act has ethical principles embedded in the statute and codified in state regulations. Every RT should be aware of what the particular state dictates in terms of ethical practice.

RULE OF THUMB

Never attempt to make ethical decisions for others. You can only make them for yourself.

LEGAL ISSUES AFFECTING RESPIRATORY CARE

Not all decisions can be made in the confines of the medical community. The patient comes from outside this community of professionals, and with expectations different from those of the professionals who will care for her. Sometimes there is a conflict in the expectations and the results. Other times, there are medical errors or acts by professionals that fail to meet professional standards. When the result of those errors is patient injury or death, the possibility of professional liability results.

Recently, some hospitals and health care organizations have adopted a model that attempts to subvert the medical liability process. It involves the rapid investigation of sentinel events, and, where errors are made, the disclosure of those errors to the patient followed by an immediate apology. In those instances where there is compensable injury, immediate compensation is offered. This process has reduced medical liability costs for some providers.*

Unfortunately for professionals, in the absence of a system designed to address errors within the professional community, these problems often go to the courts. The problem of professional liability in the delivery of health care is significant. Professional liability may contribute to increasing health care costs. Limits on medical liability have been key factors in recent legislation; however, these limits often suffer from constitutional flaws.†

Practitioners are caught in the middle. On one hand, they are required to keep costs down by avoiding overuse of technology and therapeutics. On the other hand, they are faced with a level of consumerism that holds them accountable when medical errors result from scarcity of resources. The costs, losses, frustration, and distraction brought about by the current level of legal intervention in health care practice are a concern, but a manageable one. Very few cases actually wind up going to court, and most therapists will practice their entire career without ever seeing the inside of a courtroom.

Systems of Law

Under our legal system, the law is divided into two broad classes: *public law* and *civil law.* Public law deals with the relationships of private parties and the government. Civil law is concerned with the recognition and enforcement of the rights and duties of private individuals and organizations.

*See, for example, Health Affairs, January 2014—Communication-and-resolution programs: the challenges and lessons learned from six early adopters; American Journal of Gastroenterology, November 2013—Effect of a health system's medical error disclosure program on gastroenterology-related claims rates and costs; Bulletin of the American College of Surgeons, March 2013—The University of Michigan's Early Disclosure & Offer Program; Milbank Quarterly, December 2012—Disclosure, apology, and offer programs: stakeholders' views of barriers to and strategies for broad implementation; Press release: Doing the right thing when things go wrong; Frontiers in Health Services Management, April 2012—Nurturing a culture of patient safety and achieving lower malpractice risk through disclosure: lessons learned and future directions; Press release: Honesty is the best policy: UMHS approach to medical error & malpractice spreads beyond Michigan; Annals of Internal Medicine, August 2010—liability claims and costs before and after implementation of a medical error disclosure program; Press release: U-M's efforts to encourage disclosure of medical errors decreased claims; Journal of Health and Life Sciences Law, January 2009—A better approach to medical malpractice claims? The University of Michigan experience.

†See, for example, S. Okeson, Missouri Supreme Court overturns 2005 cap on liability lawsuits, Springfield News-Leader, August 1, 2012; available online at http://archive.news-leader.com/article/20120801/NEWS12/308010053/Missouri-Supreme-Court-liability-lawsuits-Springfield-Cox.

Public (Criminal and Administrative) Law

The two major divisions of public law are *criminal law* and *administrative law.* Criminal law deals with acts or offenses against the welfare or safety of the public. Offenses against criminal law are punishable by fines, imprisonment, or both. In these cases, the accuser is the state, and the person prosecuted is the **defendant**.

Administrative law is the second major branch of public law. Administrative law consists of the countless regulations set by government agencies. Health care facilities face a large number of administrative and agency rules that affect almost every aspect of operation. RTs are obligated to abide by these rules and regulations.

Civil Law

Private or civil law protects private citizens and organizations from others who might seek to take unfair and unlawful advantage of them. If an individual believes that his or her rights have been compromised, the individual can seek redress in the civil courts. In these cases, the individual bringing the complaint is known as the **plaintiff**, and the individual accused of wrong is the **defendant**. Civil courts, usually in the form of juries, decide between the two parties with regard to the degree of wrong and the level of reparation required. The category of civil law best related to respiratory care is tort law.

Tort Law. A **tort** is a civil wrong, other than a breach of contract, committed against an individual or property, for which a court provides a remedy in the form of an action for damages. Causes for the complaints may range from assault and battery to invasion of privacy. The basic functions of torts are to keep the peace between individuals and to substitute a compensatory remedy for personal injury instead of allowing individuals to seek vengeance.

There are three basic forms of torts: *negligent torts, intentional torts,* and torts in which liability is assessed regardless of fault (as in the case of manufacturers of defective products). The basic difference between negligent and intentional torts is the element of intent. An intentional tort always involves a willful act that violates another's interest. A negligent tort does not have to involve any action at all. Instead, a negligent tort can consist of an omission of an action or a failure to carry out a professional duty.

Professional Negligence. Negligence, in its simplest terms, is the failure to perform one's duties competently. For example, to clarify negligence to juries in Missouri, the state's jury instructions state:

The term *negligent* or *negligence* as used in this [these] instruction[s] means the failure to use that degree of skill and learning ordinarily used under the same or similar circumstances by the members of defendant's profession.‡

Negligence may involve acts of commission or omission. The tort of negligence is concerned with the compensation of an individual for loss or damages arising from the unreasonable behavior of another. The normal standard for the claim, for

‡Missouri Approved Instruction 11.06 (1990 Revision).

example, in an automobile accident, is the duty imposed on individuals not to cause risk or harm to others, the standard being what a reasonable and prudent person should have foreseen and avoided. Professional negligence is different because the duty is defined by other professionals, and for that reason, requires expert testimony to establish.

In negligence cases, the breach of duty often involves the matter of foreseeability. Cases in which the patient falls, is burned, is given the wrong medication, or is harmed by defects in an apparatus often revolve around the duty of the health care provider to anticipate the harm. Duty is imposed by law. Courts tell us the following about duty:

> *For purposes of determining whether a duty exists, this Court has defined foreseeability as the presence of some probability or likelihood of harm sufficiently serious that ordinary persons would take precautions to avoid it. [citation omitted] The existence of a mere possibility is insufficient. Id. The test is not the balance of probabilities, but of the existence of some probability of sufficient moment to induce the reasonable mind to take the precautions which would avoid it.*
>
> *Lopez v. Three Rivers Elec. Co-op., 26 S.W.3d 151, 156 (Mo. 2000)*

For the tort of negligence to be a valid claim, the four conditions listed in Box 5-3 must be met.

The assessment of what is reasonable and prudent for an RT can be determined by guidelines established by a professional group (e.g., the AARC), by direct expert testimony, or by circumstantial evidence. The legal principle ***res ipsa loquitur*** (the thing speaks for itself) may apply where a court determines under the facts that the circumstantial evidence rises to a level to permit its assertion. *Res ipsa loquitur* is sometimes invoked to show that the harm would not ordinarily have happened if the individuals in control had used appropriate care. In these cases, negligence is established by inference.

For a claim of *res ipsa loquitur* to be supported, three basic conditions must be met: (1) The harm was such that it would not normally occur without someone's negligence. (2) The action responsible for the injury was under the control of the defendant. (3) The injury did not result from any contributing negligence or voluntarily assumed risk on the part of the injured party. An example of *res ipsa loquitur* might be the failure to recognize that a patient's right main stem bronchus had been intubated with a resultant pneumothorax. For negligence to occur, the breach in duty also must cause damage or injury to the individual. The injured party must file the lawsuit within the time frame set by the statute of limitations. The term *injury,* in this sense, may include not only physical harm but also mental anguish and other invasions of the patient's rights and

Box 5-3 Elements of Negligence

- The practitioner owes a duty to the patient.
- The practitioner breaches that duty.
- The breach of duty was the cause of damages.
- Damage or harm came to the patient.

privileges. The claim must be established by a preponderance of the evidence to prevail. Essentially this means that a jury must be convinced that it is more likely than not that negligence occurred.

For the tort of negligence to cause liability, the breach of duty must be shown to be the cause of the injury. *Causation* revolves around whether the acts of negligence were the cause in fact and the legal cause of the damages. *Causation in fact* means simply that the negligent act of the caregiver caused the damages. *Proximate causation* or *legal causation* usually turns on foreseeability and whether it is fair to impose damages on a defendant.

Factual causation usually is a question for the jury. It is best illustrated in the context of a motor vehicle accident. If a car runs a stop sign but does not hit anyone, the driver may well be negligent, but no one could sue because the driver did not cause any harm. If there is a collision, there is harm flowing directly from the failure to stop. For that reason, the mere failure to provide the appropriate standard of care is insufficient to necessitate payment of damages unless injury occurs as a result of the action or omission. In most states, the act of negligence does not have to be the only cause; it only has to be one cause. Sometimes this is referred to in jury instructions as a requirement that the defendant's actions "caused or contributed to cause" the injury. Ordering O_2 turned off on a severely hypoxemic patient might be the direct cause of the patient's injury, but the therapist's acting on that order instead of questioning it could be thought of as a contributing cause.

Proximate causation turns on foreseeability. It tends to be a retrospective analysis. If an RT fails to check a ventilator as required, it is foreseeable that the patient could develop a compromised airway and sustain brain damage or die. The RT's failure would be both the factual and the legal cause of the injury. Proximate causation also comes into play, however, when there are multiple wrongdoers. For example, a nurse requests a therapist's help to place a patient on the bedside commode. The therapist is unaware that the patient's systolic blood pressure is 60 mm Hg by Doppler. The patient bears down, experiences a cardiac arrest, and dies. Although the actions of the therapist in helping to move the patient to the commode are the cause in fact, the therapist might escape liability because it was not foreseeable that helping the nurse move the patient would result in the patient's death.

Most medical negligence lawsuits are defended by claiming that no matter what the medical error was, it was not the cause in fact of the patient's death. This is frequently possible because only a very limited number of patients actually get autopsies. There may be no demonstrative evidence or pathology report detailing what caused the patient's death.

For example, in a situation in which the leads were reversed in a patient receiving a dual-chamber pacemaker, the heart, on autopsy, showed focal areas of inflammation. The defendant had a pathologist testify that the most likely cause of death was not the failure to place the pacemaker leads in the correct position, but rather, a particularly virulent virus (never identified) that caused rhythm disturbances and death. In nearly every case, one of the primary defenses will always be a lack of medical causation.

Damages are another factor in negligence lawsuits. There are three kinds of damages: economic, noneconomic, and punitive. Economic damages are awarded for economic loss. For example, a working wife and mother killed in a vehicular accident leaves a family without a caregiver for the children and without the $45,000 a year salary she earned. Her economic damages include both the salary figure (adjusted for inflation and wage increases over her work life) and the cost of replacing the home care she rendered to her family.

Noneconomic damages include pain, suffering, disability, disfigurement, and loss of the enjoyment of life. Although economic damages can be guided by hard numbers, juries are often left to decide the value of a person's pain or suffering. Many states have limited the amounts that can be awarded for these elements of damage, as noted earlier, but in some states those caps have been overturned.

Punitive damages are damages that are awarded to punish wrongful conduct and discourage future unlawful conduct. Punitive damages are quite rare in medical negligence cases except where alcohol or drug use by caregivers is involved or where there is overwhelming negligence that is equivalent to intentional conduct. Some states also limit these damages.

Malpractice. **Malpractice**, as a form of negligence, can involve professional misconduct, unreasonable lack of skill or fidelity in professional duties, evil practice, or unethical conduct. There are three classifications of malpractice: (1) *Criminal* malpractice includes crimes such as assault and battery or euthanasia (handled in criminal court). (2) *Civil* malpractice includes negligence or practice below a reasonable standard (handled in civil court). (3) *Ethical* malpractice includes violations of professional ethics and may result in censure or disciplinary actions by licensure boards.

Intentional Torts. An intentional tort is a wrong perpetrated by someone who intends to do the act and, possibly, intends to do the harm. In contrast, in negligence, the professional fails to exercise adequate care in doing what is otherwise permissible. The acts must be intentionally performed to produce the harm or must be performed with the belief that the result was likely to follow. These torts are more serious than the tort of negligence, in that the defendant intended to commit the wrong. Consequently, punitive and actual damages may be awarded. Examples of intentional torts are acts that involve fraud, defamation of character, invasion of privacy, deceit, infliction of mental distress, and assault and battery.

In the hospital, the unwarranted discussion of the patient's condition, diagnosis, or treatment for purposes other than the exchange of information is always deemed suspect in regard to defamation of character. Under the general title of defamation of character are the torts of libel and slander. **Slander** is the verbal defamation of an individual by false words by which his or her reputation is damaged. **Libel** is printed defamation by written words, cartoons, and such representations to cause the individual to be avoided or held in contempt. Libel and slander do not exist unless they are seen or heard by a third person. If the practitioner directed such remarks only to the individual involved, it would not be slanderous; if the remark was made in the presence of a third party, it might constitute slander. Torts involving defamation are subject to short statutes of limitation and are generally disfavored in the law. The First Amendment to the Constitution may even provide a shield against slander or libel in many cases.

Caution to avoid unauthorized disclosure of patient information is especially critical in cases involving diseases such as AIDS, which often carries a high degree of medical and social stigma. Patients have the legal right to expect that all information about their illness will be held in strict confidence. Several states now have civil liability and criminal penalties for the release of confidential HIV test results in which the breach of confidence results in economic, psychologic, or bodily harm to the patient.

An **assault** is an intentional act that places another person in fear of immediate bodily harm. Threatening to injure someone through some overt act (e.g., swinging a bat at a person, even if it misses) is considered an act of assault. **Battery** represents unprivileged, nonconsensual physical contact with another person. In the classic act of assault and battery, one individual threatens injury through some overt act (throws a punch) and injures another through an overt act (connects with the punch).

Although battery is an unusual charge against a clinician (because of the nature of the work), it creates special problems. The major element of battery is physical contact without consent. When a practitioner performs a procedure without the patient's consent, this contact may be considered battery. In most instances, there is an implied consent, created when the patient seeks care from the physician. This implied consent allows the performance of ordinary procedures without written consent. In all cases of unusual, difficult, or dangerous procedures, such as surgery, the courts require written consent. For this reason, to avoid being accused of battery, RTs should always explain all procedures involving physical contact to their patients before they proceed. If a patient refuses something like a blood gas test, in the absence of some other factor that makes it unreasonable to do so, the patient's refusal should be honored.

There are two general defenses against intentional torts. The first defense is that there was a lack of intent to harm and that only clinicians who engage in intentional conduct are liable. For example, if a practitioner fainted during a procedure and caused the patient injury, he or she would not be liable because the action was involuntary. The second defense is that the patient gave consent for the procedure. If the patient consented to the action, knowing the risks involved, the practitioner would not be liable. Consent by the patient for both nonroutine and routine procedures should be obtained in writing before care is rendered.

Strict Liability. **Strict liability** is a theory in tort law that can be used to impose liability without fault, even in situations in which injury occurs under conditions of reasonable care. The most common cases of strict liability are cases involving the use of dangerous products or techniques. Courts have imposed this principle on medical equipment manufacturers and on hospitals. However, strict liability generally has not been extended to professional services.

Breach of Contract. **Breach of contract** is a more unusual legal claim than negligence. This claim is based on the theory that when a health care professional renders care, an implicit or explicit professional-patient "contract" is established. Essentially, the contract binds the health care professional to place the patient's welfare as the foremost concern, to act only in the patient's behalf, to protect the patient's life, to preserve the patient's health, to relieve suffering, and to protect privacy. When the patient is injured as a result of the services rendered under this contract, the patient may claim that the failure of the health care professional to perform the service competently is a breach of the contract. Most state laws do not permit this kind of action, and those that do require high standards for proof.

RTs are responsible for their actions, as are members of all other professions. When these actions result in the injury of another, the injured party may turn to the courts for redress. If the RT, while acting for the physician, injures the patient through some negligent act, the patient may sue both the RT and the physician.

Civil Suits. Civil action can be brought for many reasons, such as to challenge a law or to prevent an activity. However, as in the case of malpractice suits, most civil suits seek monetary damages. The following scenario is an example of a situation that might involve the RT. The physician intends to order 0.5 ml of a bronchodilator for a 3-year-old asthmatic patient but inadvertently prescribes 5.0 ml of the drug. Because of the overdose given by the RT, the child dies.

A clearly articulated legal principle in negligence is that the duty owed to the patient is commensurate with the patient's needs. In short, the more vulnerable the patient, the greater is the caregiver's duty to protect. When the order is unclear or seems inappropriate under this principle, clinicians have an obligation to clarify rather than risk harm.

The suit could be brought against the physician for negligence for ordering the overdose, against the nurses and RT for failing to recognize that the dose was incorrect for the child, and, possibly, against the pharmacist for failing to gain adequate information as to the nature of the patient so that an appropriate dosage could be calculated. The plaintiff would base the secondary charges against the nurses and allied health practitioners on the theory that liability would be incurred by the individuals who missed an opportunity to correct the first wrongdoer's mistake. The hospital's risk management department and legal counsel can sometimes provide direction and counsel to the RT in the case of a civil suit. If the hospital in which the RT works does not provide malpractice insurance for the RT, then he or she should carry his or her own policy of malpractice insurance.

Professional liability insurance is available through the AARC's preferred provider, and it provides RTs with an attorney not only to represent them in the case of a malpractice lawsuit but also in those rare instances in which a professional board questions the conduct of the RT. Should a judgment result, it protects the RT not only from the plaintiff but also from any settling defendant who attempts to point the finger at the RT. It is crucial that the RT adhere to professional legal advice and not try to "go it alone" in a malpractice case. Sometimes well-meaning but poorly informed risk professionals tell therapists that having their own insurance is likely to get them sued. This is simply untrue.

There is no central registry or online resource where an attorney can look up an individual and determine if she has malpractice insurance. As therapists exercise greater discretion about what treatments to give and under what circumstances, that discretion is likely to increase rather than decrease their malpractice liability risk. It is the negligent act that determines who will be sued, not the insurance status of that individual. Decisions about whom to sue are made early, before any opportunity is developed for discovery, and the presence or absence of insurance is unlikely to have any impact on the person suing. Whether the person being sued has malpractice insurance can have a huge impact, because the defendant may stand to risk losing her home and everything she has worked for in the event of an unsuccessful defense. For this reason, malpractice insurance is an essential element of every RT's professional responsibility. No therapist should practice without it.

Avoiding Lawsuits

There is no foolproof formula for avoiding lawsuits; the right to bring suit is protected by the United States Constitution and guarded by the U.S. legal system. But the simplest and most effective way of avoiding lawsuits is both providing excellent care that meets professional standards and documenting that care carefully. Documenting the care that was given is a skill that every RT should develop, because it is what prevents, in most cases, lawsuits for professional negligence.

Practitioners should always deliver care in a professional manner and document care in a way that proves professional standards were met. For example, in the case of routine ventilator care, frequent documentation of tube position and suctioning is vital to show that the patient's airway was protected and that therapists were aware of the patient's condition. Documentation of an Allen's test before an arterial blood gas measurement shows attention to detail and documents that the patient's circulation was assessed. Knowing both what to do and how to document it are critical to avoiding litigation.

A key step to avoid litigation is being aware of and conforming to all professional standards regarding the care that is being delivered. All professionals should adhere to the legal requirements of professional licensure, and institutions should have policies and procedures that require the licensure status be verified upon employment and regularly thereafter.

Being aware of professional standards also includes keeping pace with institutional practice policies and procedures and the facility's own internal standards of care.

Moreover, risk management is a job requirement for every clinician. It should be an ongoing component of departmental operation and professional development and should always address documentation standards and risk management.

Even if everyone does every possible thing right, there is no guarantee that the plaintiff or her attorney will understand this if the patient meets an untimely or unexpected death because of things outside the control of the clinicians. Just as there are "professionals" with medical degrees who will testify that everything was done properly when standards of care were violated, so too are there people who are willing to say anything on behalf of a plaintiff in a lawsuit. Once a professional meets the baseline requirements of an expert witness (skill and expertise in the field and exposure to the facts of the case sufficient to form an opinion), in most cases his or her opinion will become evidence in the case. For this reason, malpractice insurance as well as having a good legal team to defend the case are the best safeguards a clinician has to protect against liability.

Not all cases wind up in court. Sometimes, when the parties are willing, a lawsuit can be avoided with mediation. However, when any potential legal claim or lawsuit surfaces, decisions about how to proceed should be made only with full input of institutional risk management and legal counsel experienced in professional negligence defense.

In recent years, the experience of several large hospital systems has suggested that active risk management practices and appropriate guest relations policies are two of the most effective tools to prevent malpractice litigation. Unhappy patients are identified quickly, and corrective action is implemented immediately. Good guest relations programs encourage listening that often results in better clinical decision making, preventing the malpractice that is at the heart of every medical malpractice lawsuit. The best way to avoid a malpractice suit is to develop a good, sound relationship with the patient that communicates to the patient that he or she is important and valued.

Health Insurance Portability and Accountability Act of 1996

In August 1996, the U.S. Congress enacted HIPAA, which required, among other things, the establishment of Standards for Privacy of Individually Identifiable Health Information. These standards, which have become known as simply the Privacy Rule, added a major dimension to the need to treat medical records and information as confidential. The Privacy Rule was developed, with public comment and input, in the years after enactment of HIPAA. The final rule was issued in March 2002. Updates to the Privacy Rule are likely to continue, making it imperative that the practitioner remain up to date with the latest requirements of the rule. The primary goal of the rule was to strike a balance between protecting individuals' health information and not impeding the exchange of information needed to provide quality health care and protect the public's health and well-being.[16]

The Privacy Rule applies to all health care providers, health plan providers (with some exceptions, such as small employer plans with fewer than 50 participants administered solely by the employer), and health care clearinghouses. An example of a health care clearinghouse is an entity that processes insurance claims for payment. Some of the exceptions are complex and beyond the scope of this chapter. The practitioner in clinical practice need not be concerned with particular exceptions because, in most cases, basic patient confidentially requires a standard at least equal to the strictest interpretation of the Privacy Rule.[16]

The basic goal of the Privacy Rule is to protect all "individually identifiable health information," commonly referred to as *protected health information*. Protected information includes any record or information that would or could identify or reveal (1) an individual's past, present, or future physical or mental health or condition; (2) the provision of health care to the individual; or (3) the past, present, or future payment for the provision of health care to the individual. Protected health information includes information in any format, which may include patient charts (electronic or paper), faxes, e-mails, or other records. The Privacy Rule provides avenues for the normal and appropriate conduct of health care treatment and business for all "covered entities," individuals, and organizations that have a legitimate need to access and use the information. Consent of the individual is not required for these covered entities.[16]

Medical Supervision

RTs are required by their scope of practice to work under competent medical supervision. This requirement creates not only a professional relationship but also a legal one. If the RT is employed by the physician, the physician is liable for the RT's actions. If the RT is employed by the hospital, the hospital is liable for the RT's actions. Under the laws of some states, the supervising physician may still be liable even if the RT is employed by the hospital where the legal theory involves a failure to supervise. The legal basis for this liability is rooted in centuries-old common law. When tradesmen had apprentices and masters had servants, the negligence of the apprentice or servant was applied to the master who controlled the action of the servants. Under modern law, an employer is deemed a master, and an employee is deemed a servant. This principle, sometimes called *vicarious liability,* is premised on this centuries-old concept expressed in Latin as ***respondeat superior*** ("let the master answer").

Under the doctrine of medical supervision, the physician assumes responsibility for the wrongful actions of the RT as long as such negligence occurred in the course of the employer-employee relationship. For this liability to apply, two conditions must be met: (1) the act must be within the scope of employment, and (2) the injury caused must be the result of an act of negligence. If the RT acted outside of his or her scope of practice, as outlined by licensure laws or by institutional regulations, the court would have to decide whether the physician would still be liable. If the RT, while in the patient's room to deliver an aerosol treatment, went beyond the normal scope of practice and adjusted cervical traction, causing injury, it is doubtful that the physician could be held fully responsible. However, under the principle of *respondeat superior,* the hospital, as a corporate entity, could be held responsible for the actions of its employees.

MINI CLINI

Health Insurance Portability and Accountability Act

PROBLEM: You, the RT, are in Ms. Smith's room tending to her respiratory equipment when the telephone rings. Ms. Smith and some of her family members are well known to you because of her many previous hospitalizations. During this hospitalization, Ms. Smith's condition has progressively worsened and today has been a particularly bad day for her. At this point, she is having serious difficulty moving and even talking. As the telephone rings, she looks at you and in a barely audible voice asks you to please answer the telephone. You do so, and the person on the other end identifies herself as Ms. Smith's granddaughter. You tell Ms. Smith that her granddaughter is on the telephone, but Ms. Smith simply looks away. You tell the granddaughter that Ms. Smith cannot talk right now and to call back later. The granddaughter asks you why Ms. Smith cannot talk, along with a series of specific questions about her condition.

DISCUSSION: As the RT, how should you handle this situation?

1. What HIPAA guidelines, if any, are applicable in this case?
2. Because you know Ms. Smith and her family, is it permissible to answer the granddaughter's questions?
3. To avoid alarming the granddaughter, should you say Ms. Smith is asleep or in the bathroom?

GUIDANCE: The first question is whether HIPAA applies. HIPAA pertains to "the individual's past, present or future physical or mental health or condition."* HIPAA requires that protected health care information never be disclosed to those who are not authorized to receive it, and the rule requires a written authorization of who can receive protected health information by the patient. Until you verify that the person on the other end of the phone is authorized in writing to receive information, you cannot disclose anything. You also may have no way of knowing whether this really is the daughter of the patient, even if you think you recognize the voice. The hospital has specific policies regarding the release of information, and you must follow those to protect yourself from any allegation of wrongdoing.

Simply because you know Mrs. Smith and her family, it is not sufficient to disclose information. Information must be given only to those on the written authorization. Verbal authorizations are not permitted because (1) you have no way to prove that it happened and (2) the patient may later change his or her mind or forget who was authorized. Thus, until you know that the person is authorized in writing to receive the information, you may not disclose protected health information.*

Even though it may be difficult to tell a family member of a patient that you cannot share information over the phone, that is the answer that you must give. You may not say that Mrs. Smith is in the bathroom because it is not true. There is no ethical exception that permits lying to family members. Lying erodes trust in the health care system.

*See, for example, "What information is protected" on the Department of Health and Human Services website: http://www.hhs.gov/ocr/privacy/hipaa/understanding/summary/index.html.

Historically, RTs have not been named individually as defendants in malpractice cases because the law generally has not focused on their role as specialized health care providers separate from the health care facility. Either the hospital or the physician is usually named as the defendant for the acts of the practitioner. RTs in these cases have been viewed simply as employees, merely carrying out the orders of a superior. However, with the increased application of state licensure regulations governing respiratory care, and especially with the development of respiratory care protocols giving RTs more autonomy, this relative protection from liability is changing rapidly. As RTs are given more discretion and are permitted to exercise independent judgment, their decision making is likely to be more frequently called into question in court.

Scope of Practice

One measure of professionalism is the extent to which the group is willing to direct its own development and regulate its own activities. This self-direction is carried out mainly through professional associations and state licensure boards, which attempt to ensure that professionals exhibit minimum levels of competence.

Basic Elements of a Practice Act. Some practice acts emphasize one area over another, but most acts address the following elements:

- Scope of professional practice
- Requirements and qualifications for licensure
- Exemptions
- Grounds for administrative action
- Creation of examination board and processes
- Penalties and sanctions for unauthorized practice

Licensure Laws and Regulations. In licensure legislation, there is always a clause specifying a scope of practice. The scope-of-practice statutes give general guidelines and parameters for the clinician's practice. Deviation from these statutes could be a source of legal problems as the specialty seeks to add new duties. Practitioners must know the limits of their scope of care and seek amendments to the licensure regulations as they expand their practice. Ideally, the original language of a licensure law should be broad enough to account for changes in practice without requiring continual amendment. Continuing education and regular review of the practice act are essential to ensure compliance with both the statute and evolving rules of the practice act.

Providing Emergency Care Without Physician Direction. One unique area that allows practice without the direction of a competent physician is that of rendering emergency medical care to injured persons. Good Samaritan laws protect citizens from civil liability for any errors they make while attempting to give emergency aid. Most states have legislated Good Samaritan statutes to encourage individuals to give needed emergency medical assistance. It is necessary for this aid to be given in good faith and free of gross negligence or willful misconduct. However, it is unlikely that the RT would be protected for giving aid that went beyond the expected skills of the individual or aid that went beyond that which could be defined as first aid, such as performing a tracheostomy. Good Samaritan rules generally apply only to roadside accidents and emergency situations outside the hospital, although this is not always the case. The doctrine has sometimes been used by physicians inside a health care organization who respond to an emergency on a patient who is not their own. However, in California, the statute for RTs specifically extends protection only where the acts of the RT are "outside both the place and the course of employment."[||]

INTERACTION OF ETHICS AND THE LAW

A good example of the interaction of ethics and the law in respiratory care is the diversification of the field into home care and durable medical equipment supply. This diversification has led to new relationships between these elements of the health care system and has created the potential for unethical and unlawful activity. If a practitioner accepts some payment, such as a finder's fee or percentage of the total lease costs for referring patients to a particular home care company or equipment service, he or she should be prepared to face charges of unethical and perhaps illegal practice.

Several federal and many state statutes address the legality of these types of transactions. Generally, these statutes say that anyone who knowingly or willfully solicits, receives, offers, or pays directly or indirectly any payment in return for Medicare business is guilty of a criminal offense. Violation of these statutes carries the potential for prison, a substantial fine, or both. In addition, violation of the statutes by an organization can result in exclusion from Medicare and other federal health care programs.

In recent years, hospitals have been encouraged to appoint a corporate compliance officer (CCO) to oversee the hospital's business practices and ensure that the hospital conforms to the law. In most hospitals with a working compliance plan, the CCO is freely available to discuss legal or ethical issues arising in the course of care. Appointed by the board of directors and reporting both to the hospital administration and to the board, the CCO often can address legal issues quickly and competently. Most hospitals use a toll-free anonymous number to allow employees who wish to remain anonymous to report wrongful activity. If the practitioner is aware of others who are engaged in these practices, he or she should report these activities to the appropriate state or federal health care agency. To aid the clinician in maintaining an ethical stance on these new issues, the AARC has established a position statement about ethical performance of respiratory home care.

PROFESSIONAL LICENSURE ISSUES

Because nearly every state has now passed some form of licensure for respiratory care practitioners, more RTs are being disciplined for various offenses related to the practice of respiratory care. Most RTs serve their entire professional careers and never have a problem with their professional boards. There are four significant things that RTs can be aware of now that would help prevent problems with their professional boards later.

Licensure Statute

All RTs should know in detail the requirements of their respiratory care practice act. They should know what is expected of them in terms of obtaining licensure and in the requirements to remain licensed. After receiving licenses, many professionals never look at their statute and never evaluate what actions are mandated by the rules and regulations enacted by their board. Some states by statute require that RTs report certain behavior.

Section 3758.5. Reporting Violations

If a licensee has knowledge that another person may be in violation of, or has violated, any of the statutes or regulations administered by the board, the licensee shall report this information to the board in writing and shall cooperate with the board in furnishing information or assistance as may be required.

California Respiratory Care Practice Act

Some states also require that employers make reports not only on individuals terminated for cause but also on the supervisors of the RTs.

Section 3758.6. Report on Supervisor

1. In addition to the reporting required under Section 3758, an employer shall also report to the board the name, professional licensure type and number, and title of the person supervising the licensee who has been suspended or terminated for cause, as defined in subdivision (b) of Section 3758. If the supervisor is a licensee under this chapter, the board shall investigate whether due care was exercised by that supervisor in accordance with this chapter. If the supervisor is a health professional, licensed by another licensing board under this division, the employer shall report the name of that supervisor and any and all information pertaining to the suspension or termination for cause of the person licensed under this chapter to the appropriate licensing board.
2. The failure of an employer to make a report required by this section is punishable by an administrative fine not to exceed $10,000 per violation.

The second thing all RTs should do to protect themselves against licensure issues is to purchase an insurance policy that covers professional discipline. Most policies available for purchase by RTs provide for coverage of both malpractice liability and professional discipline.

Understanding the Causes of Discipline

A review of professional discipline cases available from publicly available sources, including the California Board for

[||]Cal. Bus. & Prof. Code § 3706.

Respiratory Care, reveals that the most frequent causes of professional discipline are as follows:

- Substance abuse
- Domestic violence
- Sexual abuse
- Gross incompetence

Even in cases in which the cause of discipline is rooted in domestic violence or sexual abuse of another person, some form of substance abuse is often a contributing factor. Alcohol violations (driving while intoxicated, driving while impaired) are often the most frequent violation that brings an RT face to face with his or her professional board. RTs with alcoholism or a significant drug habit are almost certain to come before their professional board. Sometimes employers and supervisors take the position that as long as such a problem does not affect a person's work at the facility, they should not address it. However, even in cases in which an RT does not use drugs or alcohol at work, the disease process is affecting their judgment and decision making and should be addressed. A supervisor who fails to report a substance abuser of any kind is asking for legal trouble, in the form of either a damages lawsuit or a visit from the professional board. Academic RTs should be especially vigilant with students and should insist on substance abuse counseling for any student who appears to have such a problem.

Sometimes human resources personnel and administrators do not see the value in addressing these kinds of problems and may counsel against discipline for impaired workers. Sometimes supervisors ignore the behaviors that should be red flags. Sometimes the human resources department may have made exceptions for other workers and fears that these exceptions may permit an inference of discrimination. None of these excuses sounds good to a jury.

Any good attorney will tell you that it is far better to defend a wrongful termination lawsuit than a wrongful death lawsuit. If you are wrong about the termination, the employee can be rehired. There is no remedy for the patient when an employee's substance abuse leads to that patient's death.

Engaging Counsel

If approached by the professional board, an RT should never talk to investigators without an attorney present. Every investigation is by its nature oppressive and burdensome, and an attorney ensures that the RT's rights are respected and protected. Often in cases in which an RT has violated the professional code or engaged in conduct that merits discipline, an attorney can help negotiate a better resolution than the RT could without the help of a professional.

RESPIRATORY THERAPISTS WHO SPEAK OUT ABOUT WRONGDOING

RTs are in a unique position to help protect patients from multiple harms. Sometimes they have a duty to speak out about problems or issues in the department. Usually working with a CCO is the most effective way to effect change inside an organization. However, sometimes the person who speaks out and identifies a problem still faces retaliation. Several federal laws protect RTs who, because of their respect for ethical issues, speak out about wrongdoing.

Patient Protection and Affordable Care Act

In 2010, Congress passed the PPACA in an attempt to reform health care. Challenges to the PPACA are still finding their way through the state and federal courts, and results to date have been mixed. One thing that the statute did was improve whistleblower protections for hospital workers. Section 1558 of the PPACA amends the *Fair Labor Standards Act* of 1938 (FLSA) by adding Section 18C, which provides that an employer cannot discriminate "against any employee with respect to his or her compensation, terms, conditions, or other privileges of employment" because the employee, among other things:

1. Provided, caused to be provided, or is about to provide or cause to be provided to the employer, the Federal Government, or the attorney general of a State information relating to the violation of, or any act or omission the employee reasonably believes to be a violation of, any provision of this title;
2. Actually did or is about to assist, participate, or testify in a proceeding about such violation; or
3. Objected to or refused to participate in any activity or task that the employee "reasonably believed" to be in violation of the statute or any rule or regulation promulgated under the statute.

Any employee who believes that he or she has been discharged or discriminated against in violation of Section 18C of the FLSA is entitled to seek relief using the same procedures provided in 15 U.S.C. §2087(b), which contains the extensive whistleblower protections contained in the *Consumer Product Safety Improvement Act* of 2008. These procedures include filing a complaint concerning discrimination or retaliation with the Department of Labor, going through an administrative process to determine whether the employee's conduct protected by Section 18C was "a contributing factor in the unfavorable personnel action" alleged by the employee, and providing for the filing of a civil action in federal court after exhaustion of the administrative remedies provided by the statute.

Section 1558 explicitly limits application of Section 18C only to violations of the statute's central provisions related to medical care in hospital and clinic settings. Employees who report fraud, waste, or violations in traditional health care settings fall under the protections afforded by Section 1558. In most cases, an employee needs legal advice to pursue remedies under this section of the FLSA.

National Labor Relations Act

Although the *National Labor Relations Act* (NLRA) is usually thought of as a "union" statute, the NLRA provides protections to hospital workers whether they are organized into a union or not. Specifically, the NLRA provides for protection where a worker engages in actions for the benefit of all employees. For example, when an RT approaches the supervisor on behalf of all the workers on the second shift to request that shift differentials be increased, that RT—who is engaged in what is called "protected concerted activity"—cannot be discharged for acting on behalf of the other RTs in the department. When an RT is discharged for such an offense, the RT has 180 days in which to make a complaint to the local office of the National Labor Relations Board. No attorney is necessary to make such a complaint.

False Claims Act

Buried in the banking section of the United States Code is a little-known statute called the *False Claims Act* (FCA) (31 USC §3729). The statute forbids making false claims against the government and provides for severe sanctions for people who do. Someone making a false claim against a government health care program can be made to repay three times the amount of the false claim plus a civil penalty of $5500 to $11,000 per false claim. Similar to the whistleblower protections built into the PPACA, the FCA contains language that prevents retaliation against an employee who gathers information or supports a government case against his or her employer. Remedies may include reinstatement and back pay.

Perhaps the most powerful part of the statute is the part that permits an employee with knowledge of fraud or false billing to file a lawsuit against the company or organization engaging in fraud. For example, when an emergency medical technician (EMT) knows that his employer is giving away free ambulance services to nursing homes in exchange for the Medicare business of the nursing homes, the EMT could file an FCA case against the employer.

The government investigates such lawsuits and frequently intervenes in them. Where the government intervenes, the employee who blows the whistle stands to receive an award of up to 25% of the amount the government recovers. In recent years, the United States has recovered greater than $3 billion in fraudulently paid claims, most of which came from employees who blew the whistle on the fraud of their employers or competitors.

HEALTH CARE AND CHANGE

The health care industry is experiencing rapid change relating to how services are funded and how patients and health care workers interact. These changes are occurring at the same time that ethical considerations are reemerging as significant components of how health care should be structured and delivered. Managed care affects the ethical decision-making process. Although the effect is not negative, it forces health care workers to take a new look at ethical dilemmas to arrive at both the best ethical outcome and the best managed care outcome. Patients no longer freely choose who will deliver health care services to them. Health care practitioners must consider not only the best services to deliver to patients but also the best managed care outcome.

If ethical reasoning is to be of any value, it must account for the reality of human experience and take into account changes in the health care system. Specific considerations include (1) factual premises and beliefs, such as the definition of death; (2) legal concepts, such as tort laws; (3) externally imposed mandates or expectations, such as hospital accreditation standards; and (4) the best managed care outcome. In many instances, such considerations uphold our moral convictions and provide support for a given action. The real challenge to RTs arises when moral principles dictate one course of action and factual knowledge, legal concepts, or external expectations dictate another.

Socrates demanded that professionals acknowledge the social context of their activities and recognize their obligations toward the segment of society that they profess to serve. As our analysis of ethical reasoning and the law has made clear, only by identifying, justifying, and prioritizing basic principles of human values can the RT resolve the difficult questions of professional behavior consistently. To the extent that clearly articulated principles guide our choices and actions, all involved will be well served.

RULE OF THUMB

The letters RCP are used to indicate respiratory care practitioner. They also suggest three important characteristics of the RT when confronted with ethical dilemmas:
*R*espect
*C*ompassion
*P*rofessionalism

Health Care Advance Directives

In recognition of the right of competent adults to exercise choices concerning their health care, all 50 states and the District of Columbia have adopted some form of health care advance directives. Although the federal government acknowledged the need for advance directives with the 1991 *Patient Self-Determination Act* by requiring that all hospitals receiving Medicaid or Medicare funds ascertain whether patients have or wish to have advance directives, the advance directive instruments are state regulated.

SUMMARY CHECKLIST

- Ethical dilemmas occur when there are two equally desirable or equally undesirable choices. Ethical dilemmas may involve situations that are either legal or illegal.
- Ethical dilemmas in respiratory care involve scope of practice, confidentiality, working within levels of professional responsibility, professional development issues, staffing patterns, or recordkeeping.
- Professional codes of ethics are general guidelines established to identify ideal behavioral parameters by members of a professional group. These codes are often simplistic and tend to deal with behavior over which there is little disagreement.
- Traditional ethical principles are rooted in philosophical thought and include autonomy, beneficence,

confidentiality, role fidelity, justice, nonmaleficence, and veracity. These principles are used in the ethical decision-making process.

- There are two basic ethical theories: formalism and consequentialism. The most commonly used ethical decision-making model is the mixed approach. The mixed approach combines components of formalism, consequentialism, and modern decision-making theory.
- The basic information that must be identified before a reasoned ethical decision is made includes the problem or issue, the individuals involved, and the ethical principle or principles that apply; a determination of who should make the decision; and the role of the practitioner.
- Public law deals with the relationships of private parties and the government. Civil law is concerned with the recognition and enforcement of the rights and duties of private individuals and organizations.
- Professional malpractice is negligence in which a professional has failed to provide the care expected, resulting in harm to someone. Examples of situations that RTs might encounter include attempting procedures beyond the practitioner's skill level, failure to perform a duty as assigned, or failure to perform the duty correctly.
- Like members of other professions, RTs are responsible for their actions. If their actions result in injury to others, the injured party or parties are entitled to seek redress in the courts.
- A professional license provides a framework under which a licensee carries out his or her duties. Because licensure acts define who can perform specified duties, it is expected that the duties will be performed in a responsible manner and the professional will be responsible for his or her actions. The purpose of licensure is to provide for the public's safety. Practitioners must carry out their duties with an eye toward defending themselves in the case of legal action.
- Patients today are better educated and hold higher expectations from health care practitioners. Many patients are assuming responsibility for their own health care, placing the health care practitioner into the role of consultant.

References

1. Brincat CA, Wike VS: *Morality and the professional life: values at work*, Upper Saddle River, NJ, 2000, Prentice Hall.
2. Bowie NE: Respecting the humanity in a person. In Ciulla JB, et al, editors: *Honest work: a business ethics reader*, New York, 2007, Oxford University Press.
3. Carroll C: *Legal issues and ethical dilemmas in respiratory care*, Philadelphia, 1996, FA Davis.
4. Edge R, Groves R: *The ethics of health care: a guide for practice*, Albany, NY, 1994, Delmar.
5. Beauchamp TL, Childress JF: *Principles of biomedical ethics*, ed 4, New York, 1994, Oxford University Press.
6. Boylan M: *Business ethics: basic ethics in action*, Upper Saddle River, NJ, 2001, Prentice Hall.
7. Husted GL, Husted JH: *Ethical decision-making in nursing*, St Louis, 1991, Mosby.
8. Pickett JP, et al: *The American heritage dictionary of the English language*, ed 4, Boston, 2000, Houghton Mifflin.
9. Logue B: *Rights: death control and the elderly in America*, New York, 1993, Macmillan.
10. Hill TP, Shirley D: *A good death: taking more control at the end of your life*, Reading, MA, 1992, Addison-Wesley.
11. World Medical Association: *Code of medical ethics*, <http://www.wma.net/en/30publications/10policies/c8/index.html>. Accessed June 22, 2015.
12. Pozgar G: *Legal aspects of health care administration*, Gaithersburg, MD, 1990, Aspen.
13. Hippocrates: The oath. In Jones WHS, translator: *The Loeb classical library: Hippocrates, no. 147–150*, Cambridge, MA, 1948, Harvard University Press.
14. Sernick TH, Knight AP: *An integrated and forward-looking approach to risk management in healthcare, published in The Risk Management Quarterly*, Spring 2010 Edition, p 7.
15. Ross WD: *The right and the good*, Oxford, 1930, Clarendon Press.
16. U.S. Department of Health and Human Services: *Summary of the HIPAA privacy rule*. Revised 2003. <http://www.hhs.gov/ocr/privacysummary.pdf>. Accessed June 22, 2015.

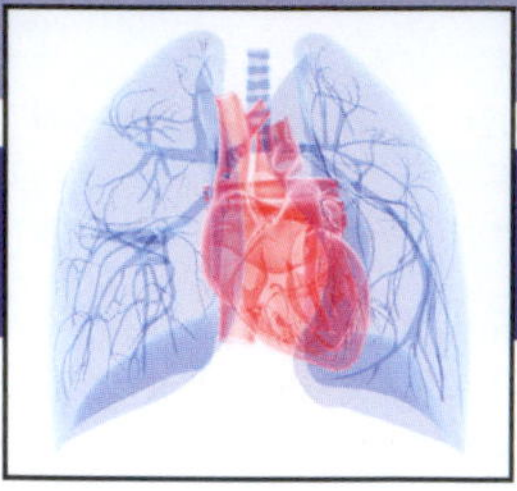

CHAPTER 6

Physical Principles of Respiratory Care

DANIEL F. FISHER

CHAPTER OBJECTIVES

After reading this chapter you will be able to:

- Describe the properties that characterize the three states of matter.
- Describe how heat transfer occurs among substances.
- Identify the three common temperature scales and explain how to use them.
- Describe how substances undergo change of state.
- Describe how water vapor capacity, absolute humidity, and relative humidity are related.
- Describe how to predict gas behavior under changing conditions, including at extremes of temperature and pressure.
- Describe the principles that govern the flow of fluids.

CHAPTER OUTLINE

States of Matter
- Internal Energy of Matter
- Laws of Thermodynamics

Change of State
- Liquid-Solid Phase Changes (Melting and Freezing)
- Properties of Liquids
- Liquid-Vapor Phase Changes
- Properties of Gases

Gas Behavior Under Changing Conditions
- Gas Laws
- Effect of Water Vapor
- Properties of Gases at Extremes of Temperature and Pressure
- Critical Temperature and Pressure

Fluid Dynamics
- Pressures in Flowing Fluids
- Patterns of Flow
- Flow, Velocity, and Cross-Sectional Area
- Bernoulli Principle
- Fluid Entrainment
- Fluidics and the Coanda Effect

KEY TERMS

absolute humidity
adhesion
ATPS
Avogadro's law
BTPS
Coanda effect
cohesion
condensation
conduction
convection
critical temperature
Dalton's law
dew point
evaporation
flow resistance
Graham's law
Henry's law
jet entrainment
kinetic energy
laminar flow
Laplace's law
latent heat of fusion
latent heat of vaporization
law of continuity
laws of thermodynamics
melting point
Pascal's principle
Poiseuille's law
potential energy
radiation
relative humidity (RH)
solubility coefficient
specific gravity
STPD
strain-gauge pressure transducers
surface tension
thermal conductivity
thermodynamics
turbulent flow
vaporization
viscosity
water vapor pressure

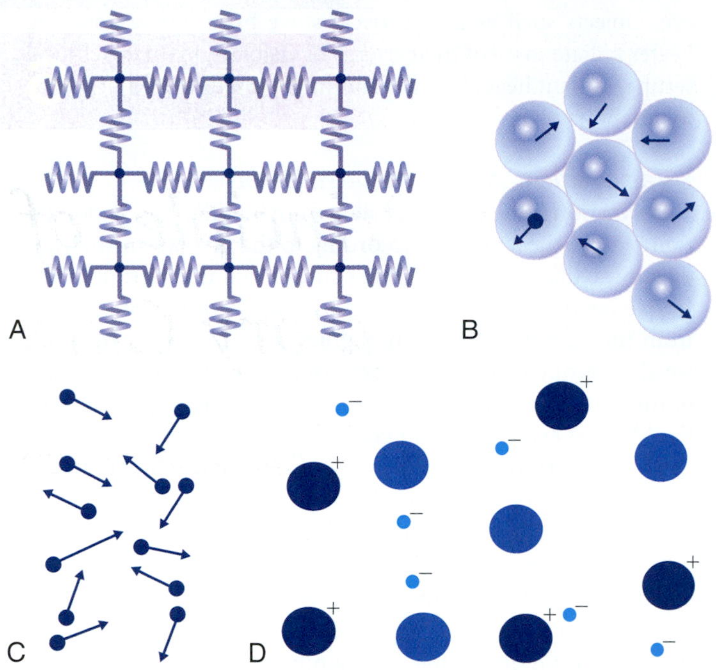

FIGURE 6-1 Simplified models of the four states of matter. **A,** Solid (rigid network of interconnected springs). **B,** Liquid (freely moving spheres with no space among them). **C,** Gas (small rapidly moving particles with a lot of space among them). **D,** Plasma (small rapidly moving charged particles with a lot of space among them).

STATES OF MATTER

There are three primary states of matter: solid, liquid, and gas. Figure 6-1, *A to C* depicts simplified models of these states of matter.

Solids have a fixed volume and shape. The molecules that make up the solid have the shortest distance to travel until they collide with one another. This motion has been referred to as a "jiggle." Solids have a high degree of internal order; their atoms or molecules are limited to back-and-forth motion about a central position, as if held together by springs (see Figure 6-1, *A*). Solids maintain their shape because their atoms are kept in place by strong mutual attractive forces, called *van der Waals forces.*[1]

Liquids have a fixed volume, but adapt to the shape of their container. If a liquid is not held within a container, the shape is determined by numerous internal and external forces. Liquid molecules exhibit mutual attraction. However, because these forces are much weaker in liquids than in solids, liquid molecules can move about freely (see Figure 6-1, *B*). This freedom of motion explains why liquids take the shape of their containers and are capable of flow. However, similar to solids, liquids are dense and cannot be compressed easily.

In a *gas,* molecular attractive forces are very weak. Gas molecules, which lack restriction to their movement, exhibit rapid, random motion with frequent collisions (see Figure 6-1, *C*). Gases have no inherent boundaries and are easily compressed and expanded. Similar to liquids, gases can flow. For this reason, both liquids and gases are considered fluids. Gases have no fixed volume or shape. Both of these qualities depend on local conditions for the gas.

Plasma has been referred to as a fourth state of matter. Plasma is a combination of neutral atoms, free electrons, and atomic nuclei. Plasmas can react to electromagnetic forces and flow freely similar to a liquid or a gas (see Figure 6-1, *D*). Although mentioned here for the sake of completeness, plasmas are not discussed further because at this time they are not known to be relevant to the practice of respiratory care.

Internal Energy of Matter

The atoms that make up all matter are in constant motion at normal temperature.[2] This motion is resulting from *internal energy*. There are two major types of internal energy: (1) **potential energy**, and (2) **kinetic energy**. Potential energy is referred to as the energy of position—that is, object balanced on a shelf. Potential energy is a result of the strong attractive forces between molecules. These intermolecular forces are why solids are rigid and liquids have viscosity and cohesiveness. These same intermolecular forces are not as strong in gases. Kinetic energy is the energy of motion, such as a falling object. Most internal energy in gases is in the form of kinetic energy.

Laws of Thermodynamics

The term **thermodynamics** can refer to either the science studying the properties of matter at various temperatures or the kinetics (speed) of reactions of matter at various temperatures. From the study of physics, we take special notice of the **laws of thermodynamics**. The laws describe how fundamental physical quantities (temperature, energy, and entropy) behave under various circumstances and forbid certain phenomena (such as perpetual motion). A basic knowledge of these principles is helpful in understanding many aspects of respiratory care. Of particular interest is the first law of thermodynamics, one version of which states that an increase in the internal energy of a closed system can be the result only of work performed on the system. Work can be viewed as the process of transferring energy to or from a system. The increase in internal energy of a system can be observed as an increase in heat (as with a humidifier) or pressure (as during mechanical ventilation).

Heat Transfer

When two objects exist at different temperatures, the first law of thermodynamics tells us that heat will move from the hotter object to the cooler object until the objects' temperatures are equal. This is an example of transitioning from a higher state of energy to a lower state. Two objects with the same temperature exist in thermal equilibrium. Heat can be transferred in four ways: (1) *conduction,* (2) *convection,* (3) *radiation,* and (4) *evaporation and condensation.*

Conduction

Heat transfer in solids occurs mainly via conduction. **Conduction** is the transfer of energy by direct contact between hot and cold molecules. How well heat transfers by conduction depends

TABLE 6-1

Thermal Conductivities in (cal/sec)/(cm² °C/cm)

Material	Thermal Conductivity (k)
Silver	1.01
Copper	0.99
Aluminum	0.50
Iron	0.163
Lead	0.083
Ice	0.005
Glass	0.0025
Concrete	0.002
Water at 20°C	0.0014
Asbestos	0.0004
Hydrogen at 0°C	0.0004
Helium at 0°C	0.0003
Snow (dry)	0.00026
Fiberglass	0.00015
Cork board	0.00011
Wool felt	0.0001
Air at 0°C	0.000057

From Nave CR, Nave BC: Physics for the health sciences, ed 3, Philadelphia, 1985, WB Saunders.

on both the number and the force of molecular collisions between adjoining objects.

Heat transfer between objects is quantified by using a measure called **thermal conductivity**. Table 6-1 lists the thermal conductivities of selected substances in centimeter-gram-second (cgs) system units. As is evident, solids (especially metals) tend to have high thermal conductivity. This is why metals feel cold to the touch even when at room temperature. In this case, the high thermal conductivity of metal quickly draws heat away from the skin, creating a feeling of "cold." In contrast, with fewer molecular collisions than in solids and liquids, gases exhibit low thermal conductivity.

Convection

Heat transfer in both liquids and gases occurs mainly by convection. **Convection** involves the mixing of fluid molecules at different temperatures. Although air is a poor heat conductor (see Table 6-1), it can efficiently transfer heat by convection. To do so, the air is first warmed in one location and then circulated to carry the heat elsewhere; this is the principle behind forced-air heating in houses and convection heating in infant incubators. Fluid movements carrying heat energy are called *convection currents.*

Radiation

Radiation is another mechanism for heat transfer. Conduction and convection require direct contact between two substances, whereas radiant heat transfer occurs without direct physical contact. Heat transfer by radiation occurs even in a vacuum, such as when the sun warms the earth.

The concept of radiant energy is similar to that of light. Radiant energy given off by objects at room temperature is mainly in the infrared range, which is invisible to the human eye. Objects such as an electrical stove burner or a kerosene heater radiate some of their energy as visible light. In the clinical setting, radiant heat energy is commonly used to keep newborn infants warm.

Evaporation and Condensation

Vaporization is the change of state from liquid to gas. Vaporization requires heat energy. According to the first law of thermodynamics, this heat energy must come from the surroundings. In one form of vaporization, called **evaporation,** heat is taken from the air surrounding the liquid, cooling the air. In warm weather or during strenuous exercise, the body takes advantage of this principle of *evaporative cooling* by producing sweat. The liquid sweat evaporates and cools the skin.

Condensation is the opposite of evaporation. In condensation, gases become liquids. Because vaporization takes heat from the air around a liquid (cooling), condensation must give heat back to the surroundings (warming). A refrigerator (or air conditioner) works on the principle of repeated vaporization cycles. The food cools as it passes energy through the walls of the refrigerator into pipes containing condensed refrigerant. The refrigerant warms, vaporizes, and expands. Then a compressor condenses the refrigerant again, releasing heat that is carried away to the atmosphere by a radiator. The condensed refrigerant is then passed by the food and the cycle repeats. The whole system is basically a heat pump transferring thermal energy from the food to the atmosphere. The next section expands on the concept of change of state and provides more detail on the processes of vaporization and condensation.

Temperature

Temperature and kinetic energy are closely related.[2] Temperature is a measurement of heat. Heat is the result of molecules colliding with one another. The temperature of a gas, with most of its internal energy spent keeping molecules in motion, is directly proportional to its kinetic energy. In contrast, the temperatures of solids and liquids represent only part of their total internal energy.

Absolute Zero

In concept, absolute zero is the lowest possible temperature that can be achieved. That is the temperature at which there is no kinetic energy. Because there is no energy, the molecules cease to vibrate and the object has no heat that can be measured. This temperature is defined to be absolute zero. Although researchers have come close to attaining absolute zero, no one has actually achieved it; this is due to the third law of thermodynamics, which states absolute zero is impossible to achieve.

Temperature Scales

Multiple scales can be used to measure temperature. The Fahrenheit and Celsius scales are based on properties of water (freezing and boiling). A third scale, the Kelvin scale, is based on molecular motion. Absolute zero provides a logical zero point on which to build a temperature scale. The International System of Units (SI) units for temperature is measured in Kelvin (K)

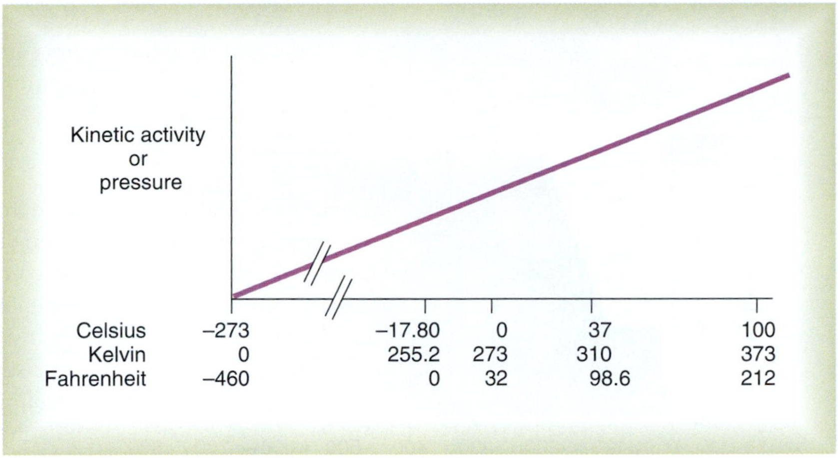

FIGURE 6-2 Linear relationship between gas molecular activity, or pressure, and temperature. The graph shows comparable readings on three scales for five temperature points.

with a zero point equal to absolute zero (0° K).[3-7] Because the Kelvin scale has 100 degrees between the freezing and boiling points of water, it is a centigrade, or 100-step, temperature scale. The Kelvin scale has the unique quality of being based on the triple-point definition for water (the temperature at which all three phases of water exist). This temperature happens to be approximately 273° K (0.0° C).[5-7]

The cgs temperature system is based on Celsius (C) units. Similar to the Kelvin scale, the Celsius scale is a centigrade scale (100 degrees between the freezing and boiling points of water). However, 0° C is not absolute zero but instead is the freezing point of water.

In Celsius units, kinetic molecular activity stops at approximately −273° C. Therefore 0° K equals −273° C, and 0° C equals 273° K. To convert degrees Celsius to degrees Kelvin, simply add 273:

$$°K = °C + 273$$

For example:

$$25°\,C = 25 + 273 = 298°\,K$$

Conversely, to convert degrees Kelvin to Celsius, you simply subtract 273. For example:

$$310°\,K = 310 - 273 = 37°\,C$$

The Fahrenheit scale is the primary temperature scale in the foot, pound, and second (fps) or British system of measurement. Absolute zero on the Fahrenheit scale equals −460° F.

To convert degrees Fahrenheit to degrees Celsius, use the following formula:

$$°C = (°F - 32)/1.8$$

For example:

$$°F = 98.6$$
$$°C = (98.6 - 32)/1.8$$
$$°C = 37$$

To convert degrees Celsius to degrees Fahrenheit, simply reverse this formula:

$$°F = (1.8 \times °C) + 32$$

For example:

$$°C = 100$$
$$°F = (1.8 \times 100) + 32$$
$$°F = 212$$

Figure 6-2 shows the relationship between the kinetic activity of matter and temperature on all three common temperature scales. For ease of reference, four key points are defined: (1) the zero point of each scale, (2) the freezing point of water (0° C), (3) body temperature (37° C), and (4) the boiling point of water (100° C).

CHANGE OF STATE

All matter can change state. Because respiratory therapists work extensively with both liquids and gases, they must have a good understanding of the key characteristics of these states and the basic processes underlying their phase changes.

Liquid-Solid Phase Changes (Melting and Freezing)

When a solid is heated, its molecular kinetic energy increases. This added internal energy increases molecular vibrations. If enough heat is applied, these vibrations eventually weaken the intermolecular attractive forces. At some point, molecules break free of their rigid structure, and the solid changes into a liquid.

Melting

The changeover from the solid to liquid state is called *melting*. The temperature at which this changeover occurs is the **melting point.**[2] The range of melting points is considerable. For example, water (ice) has a melting point of 0° C, carbon has a melting

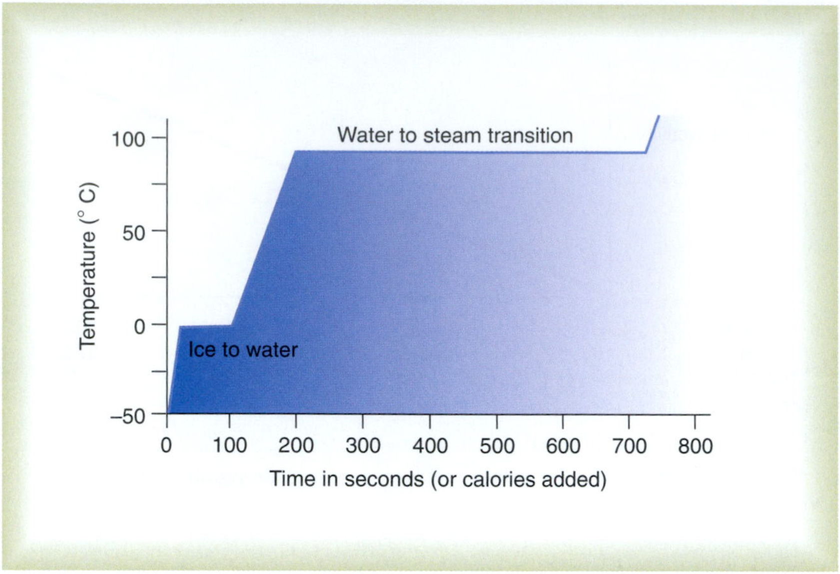

FIGURE 6-3 Temperature as a function of time for 1 g of water heated at the rate of 1 cal/sec. (Modified from Nave CR, Nave BC: Physics for the health sciences, ed 3, Philadelphia, 1985, WB Saunders.)

point of greater than 3500° C, and helium has a melting point of less than −272° C.

Figure 6-3 depicts the phase change caused by heating water. At the left origin of −50° C, water is solid ice. As the ice is heated, its temperature increases. At its melting point of 0° C, ice begins to change into liquid water. However, the full change to liquid water requires additional heat. This additional heat energy changes the state of water but does not immediately change its temperature.

The extra heat needed to change a solid to a liquid is the **latent heat of fusion**. In cgs units, the latent heat of fusion is defined as the number of calories required to change 1 g of a solid into a liquid without changing its temperature. The latent heat of fusion of ice is 80 cal/g, whereas the latent heat of fusion of oxygen is 3.3 cal/g. This change of state, compared with simply heating a solid, requires enormous energy.

Freezing

Freezing is the opposite of melting. Because melting requires large amounts of externally applied energy, you would expect freezing to return this energy to the surroundings, and this is exactly what occurs. During freezing, heat energy is transferred from a liquid back to the environment, usually by exposure to cold.

As the kinetic energy of a substance decreases, its molecules begin to regain the stable structure of a solid. According to the first law of thermodynamics,[4] the energy required to freeze a substance must equal that needed to melt it. The freezing and melting points of a substance are the same.

Sublimation is the term used for the phase transition from a solid to a vapor without becoming a liquid as an intermediary form. An example of sublimation is dry ice (frozen carbon dioxide). Dry ice sublimates from its solid form into gaseous CO_2 without first melting and becoming liquid CO_2. This sublimation occurs because the vapor pressure is low enough for the intermediate liquid not to appear.

Properties of Liquids

Liquids exhibit flow and assume the shape of their container. Liquids also exert pressure, which varies with depth and density. Variations in liquid pressure within a container produce an upward supporting force, called *buoyancy*.

Although melting weakens intermolecular bonding forces, liquid molecules still attract one another. The persistence of these cohesive forces among liquid molecules helps explain the physical properties of viscosity, capillary action, and surface tension.

Pressure in Liquids

Liquids exert pressure, which has the dimensions of force per unit area. The *pressure* exerted by a liquid depends on both its *height* (depth) and *weight density* (weight per unit volume), which is shown in equation form:

$$P_L = h \times d_w$$

where P_L is the static pressure exerted by the liquid, h is the height of the liquid column, and d_w is the liquid's weight density.

For example, to compute the pressure at the bottom of a 33.9-ft (1034-cm)-high column of water (density = 1 g/cm^3), you would use this equation:

$$\begin{aligned} P_L &= h \times d_w \\ &= 1034\ \text{cm} \times (1\ \text{g/cm}^3) \\ &= 1034\ \text{g/cm}^2 \end{aligned}$$

The answer (1034 g/cm^2) also equals 1 atmosphere of pressure (atm), or approximately 14.7 lb/in^2. This figure does not account for the additional atmospheric pressure (P_B) acting on the top

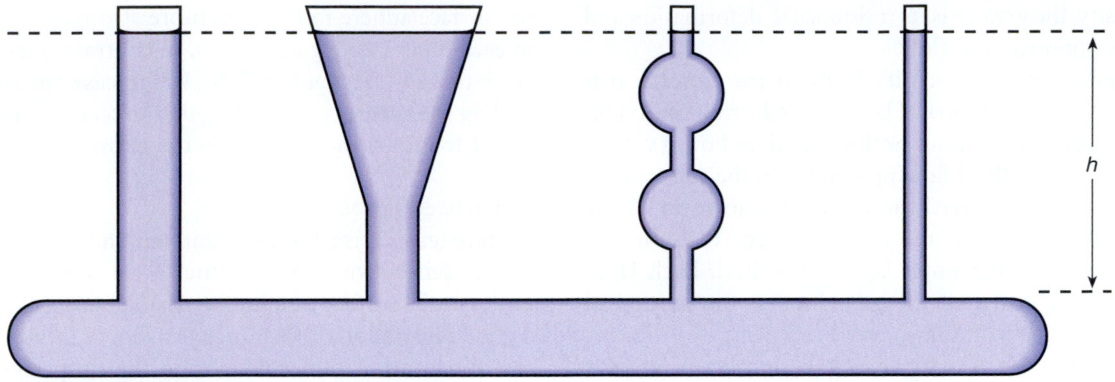

FIGURE 6-4 Pascal's principle. Liquid pressure depends only on the height (h) and not on the shape of the vessel or the total volume of liquid. (Modified from Nave CR, Nave BC: Physics for the health sciences, ed 3, Philadelphia, 1985, WB Saunders.)

of the liquid. The total pressure at the bottom of the column equals the sum of the atmospheric and liquid pressures. In this case, the total pressure is 2068 g/cm², equal to 29.4 lb/in², or 2 atm.

As shown in Figure 6-4, the pressure of a given liquid is the same at any specific depth (h), regardless of the container's shape. This is because the pressure of a liquid acts equally in all directions. This concept is called **Pascal's principle**.

Buoyancy (Archimedes' Principle)

Thousands of years ago, Archimedes showed that an object submersed in water appeared to weigh less than in air. This effect, called *buoyancy*, explains why certain objects float in water. Liquids exert buoyant force because the pressure below a submerged object always exceeds the pressure above it. This difference in liquid pressure creates an upward or supporting force. According to Archimedes' principle, this buoyant force must equal the weight of the fluid displaced by the object. The buoyant force (B) may be calculated as follows:

$$B = d_w \times V$$

where d_w is weight density (weight/unit volume) and V is volume of displaced fluid. If the weight density of an object is *less* than that of water (1 g/cm³), it will displace a weight of water greater than its own weight. In this case, the upward buoyant force will overcome gravity, and the object will float. Conversely, if an object's weight density exceeds the weight of water, the object will sink.

Clinically, Archimedes' principle is used to measure the specific gravity of certain liquids. The term **specific gravity** refers to the ratio of the density of one fluid compared with the density of another reference substance, which is typically water. Figure 6-5 shows the use of a hydrometer to measure the specific gravity of urine. The specific gravity of gases also can be measured. In this case, O_2 or hydrogen is used as the standard instead of water.

Gases also exert buoyant force, although much less than that provided by liquids. Buoyancy helps keep solid particles suspended in gases. These suspensions, called *aerosols*, play an important role in respiratory care. More detail on the characteristics and use of aerosols is provided in Chapters 38 and 39.

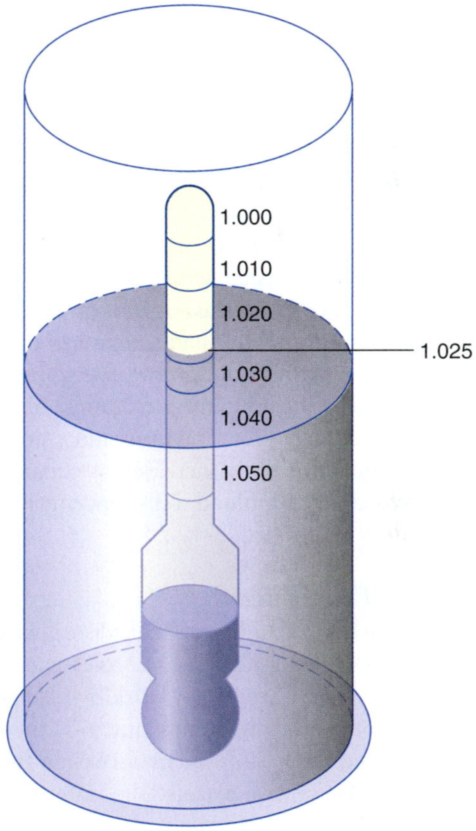

FIGURE 6-5 Using a hydrometer to measure the specific gravity of a urine specimen. The scale value of 1.025 indicates that this urine sample has a weight density 1.025 times greater than that of water.

Viscosity

Viscosity is the force opposing a fluid's flow and is similar to friction in solids. The viscosity of a fluid is directly proportional to the cohesive forces between its molecules. The stronger these cohesive forces are, the greater the fluid's viscosity. The greater a fluid's viscosity, the greater is its resistance to deformation and the greater its opposition to flow.

The understanding of viscosity leads to the concept that fluids move in discrete cylindrical layers, called *streamlines.* This pattern of motion is called **laminar flow**. Laminar flow is viewed as concentric layers of fluid flowing parallel to the tube wall at velocities that increase toward the center. As shown in Figure 6-6, frictional forces between the streamlines and the tube wall impede movement of the outer layers of a fluid. Each layer, moving toward the center of the tube, hinders the motion of the next inner layer less and less.

The difference in the velocity among these concentric layers is called the *shear rate* and is simply a measure of how easily these layers separate. Shear rate depends on two factors: (1) the pressure pushing or driving the fluid, called the *shear stress,* and (2) the viscosity of the fluid. Shear rate is directly proportional to shear stress and inversely proportional to viscosity.

In uniform fluids such as water or oil, viscosity varies with temperature. Because higher temperatures weaken the cohesive forces between molecules, heating a uniform fluid reduces its viscosity. Conversely, cooling a fluid increases its viscosity. This is why a car's engine is so hard to start on a cold winter morning. The oil becomes so viscous that it impedes movement of the engine's parts.

Blood, in contrast to water or oil, is a complex fluid that contains not only liquid (plasma, which is 90% water) but also cells in suspension. For this reason, blood has a viscosity approximately five times greater than the viscosity of water. The greater the viscosity of a fluid, the more energy is needed to make it flow. The heart works harder to pump blood than it would if it were pumping water. The heart must perform even more work when blood viscosity increases, as occurs in *polycythemia* (an increase in red blood cell concentration in the blood).

Cohesion and Adhesion

The attractive force between like molecules is called **cohesion**. The attractive force between unlike molecules is called **adhesion**. These forces can be observed at work by placing a liquid in a small-diameter tube. As shown in Figure 6-7, the top of the liquid forms a curved surface, or *meniscus*. When the liquid is water, the meniscus is concave because the water molecules at the surface adhere to the glass more strongly than they cohere to each other (see Figure 6-7, *A*). In contrast, a mercury meniscus is convex (see Figure 6-7, *B*). In this case, the cohesive forces pulling the mercury atoms together exceed the adhesive forces trying to attract the mercury to the glass.

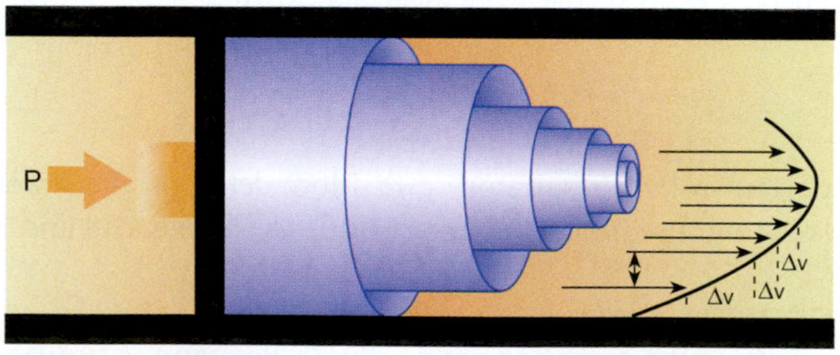

FIGURE 6-6 Effects of shear stress or pressure *(P)* on shear rate (velocity gradient *[v]*) in a Newtonian fluid. (Modified from Winters WL, Brest AN, editors: The microcirculation, Springfield, IL, 1969, Charles C Thomas.)

Surface Tension

Surface tension is a force per unit length (equivalent to surface energy density with units of $Nm^{-1} = Jm^{-2}$) exerted by like molecules at the surface of a liquid. A small drop of fluid provides a good illustration of this force. As shown in Figure 6-8, cohesive forces affect molecules inside the drop equally from all

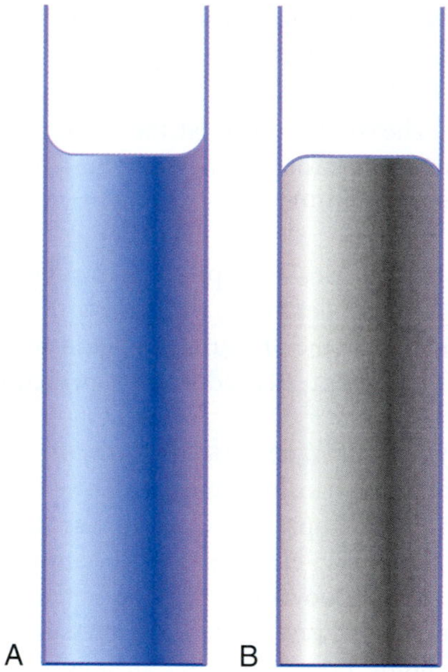

FIGURE 6-7 The shape of the meniscus depends on the relative strengths of adhesion and cohesion. **A,** Water: Adhesion stronger than cohesion. **B,** Mercury: Cohesion stronger than adhesion.

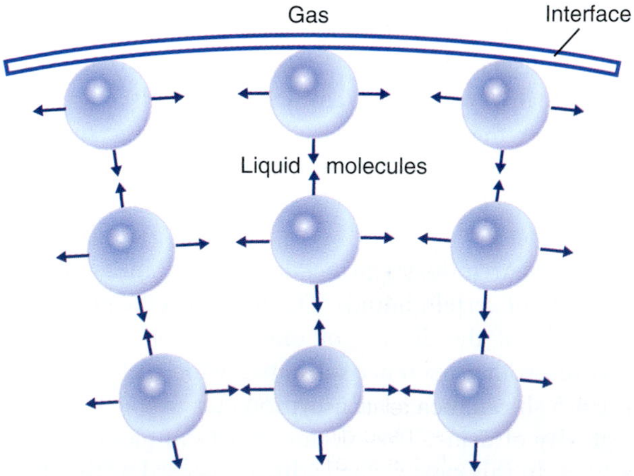

FIGURE 6-8 The force of surface tension in a drop of liquid. Cohesive force *(arrows)* attracts molecules inside the drop to one another. Cohesion can pull the outermost molecules inward only, creating a centrally directed force that tends to contract the liquid into a sphere.

directions. However, only inward forces affect molecules on the surface. This imbalance in forces causes the surface film to contract into the smallest possible surface area, usually a sphere or curve (meniscus). This phenomenon explains why liquid droplets and bubbles retain a spherical shape.

Surface tension is quantified by measurement of the force needed to produce a "tear" in a fluid surface layer. Table 6-2 lists the surface tensions of selected liquids in dynes per centimeter (cgs). For a given liquid, surface tension varies inversely with temperature: The higher the temperature, the lower is the surface tension. Surface tension plays an important role in determining the relative sizes of connected alveoli (Figure 6-9). To understand this, consider a spherical bubble of air in a liquid (analogous to an alveolus). According to **Laplace's law**, the pressure inside the bubble varies directly with the surface tension of the liquid and inversely with its radius. Internal surface tension (T) will attempt to contract the bubble but is opposed by the resulting pressure inside the bubble (P). To increase the radius by an amount dR, we must perform work, dW (where d represents an infinitesimal change as used in calculus). The work, $dW = PdV = TdA$, where dV is the change in volume and dA is the change in surface area. Because the area of a sphere is $4\pi R^2$, $dA = d(4\pi R^2)$. From calculus, the differential of the expression $4\pi R^2$ is $8\pi RdR$. The volume of a sphere is $4\pi R^3/3$, so $dV = d(4\pi R^3/3)$. Again taking the differential of this expression gives $dV = 4\pi R^2dR$. Returning to dW, we now see that because $PdV = TdA$, it follows that $P(4\pi R^2dR) = T(8\pi RdR)$. Rearranging and solving for P with simple algebra we get the common expression for the law of Laplace:

$$P = \frac{2T}{R}$$

For a structure such as a soap bubble, which has two liquid-air surfaces (and hence twice the surface tension) the equation is:

$$P = \frac{4T}{R}$$

TABLE 6-2

Examples of Surface Tension

Substance	Temperature (°C)	Surface Tension (dynes/cm)
Water	20	73
Water	37	70
Whole blood	37	58
Plasma	37	73
Ethyl alcohol	20	22
Mercury	17	547

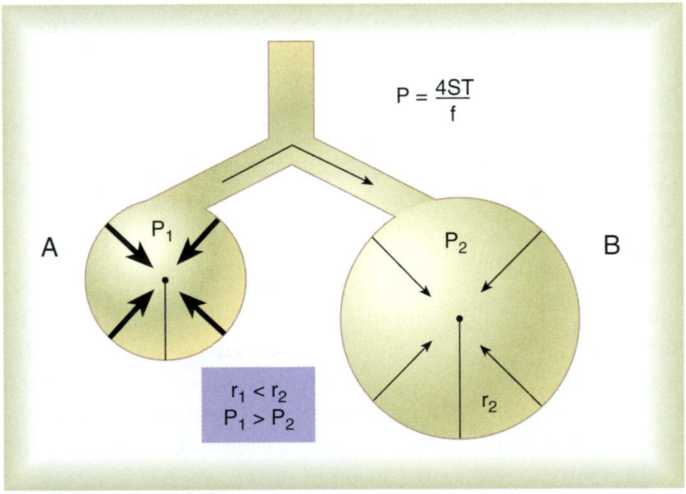

FIGURE 6-9 Laplace relationship. Two bubbles in a liquid matrix (models of alveoli). They have different sizes but the same surface tension. Bubble *A*, with the smaller radius, has the greater inward or deflating pressure and is more prone to collapse than the larger bubble, *B*. Because the two bubbles are connected, bubble *A* would tend to deflate and empty into bubble *B*. Conversely, because of the greater surface tension of bubble *A*, it would be harder to inflate than bubble *B*.

Figure 6-9 suggests that if two alveoli of different sizes are connected, the smaller one will tend to empty into the larger one. However, this does not happen because, in reality, the two alveoli would have different surface tensions. This is because of the thin layer of surfactant inside the alveoli that counteracts the surface tension. As the radius of the alveoli decreases, its internal surface area also increases but the volume of surfactant stays the same. Hence the thickness of the layer of surfactant increases, which decreases the surface tension. Therefore all other factors being equal, the two alveoli will reach equilibrium, at which point they have the same radius. Abnormalities in alveolar surface tension occur in certain clinical conditions, such as *prematurity*. These abnormalities may result in collapse of alveoli secondary to high surface tension.

Capillary Action

Capillary action is a phenomenon in which a liquid in a small tube moves upward, against gravity. Capillary action involves both adhesive and surface tension forces. As shown in Figure 6-10, *A*, the adhesion of water molecules to the walls of a thin tube causes an upward force on the edges of the liquid and produces a concave meniscus.

Because surface tension acts to maintain the smallest possible liquid-gas interface, instead of just the edges of the liquid moving up, the whole surface is pulled upward. The strength of this force depends on the amount of liquid that contacts the tube's surface. Because a small capillary tube creates a more concave meniscus and a greater area of contact, liquid rises higher in tubes with smaller cross-sectional areas (see Figure 6-10, *B*).

Capillary action is the basis for blood samples obtained by use of a capillary tube. The absorbent wicks used in some gas humidifiers are also an application of this principle, as are certain types of surgical dressings.

Liquid-Vapor Phase Changes

Only after ice completely melts does additional heat increase the temperature of the newly formed liquid (see Figure 6-3). As

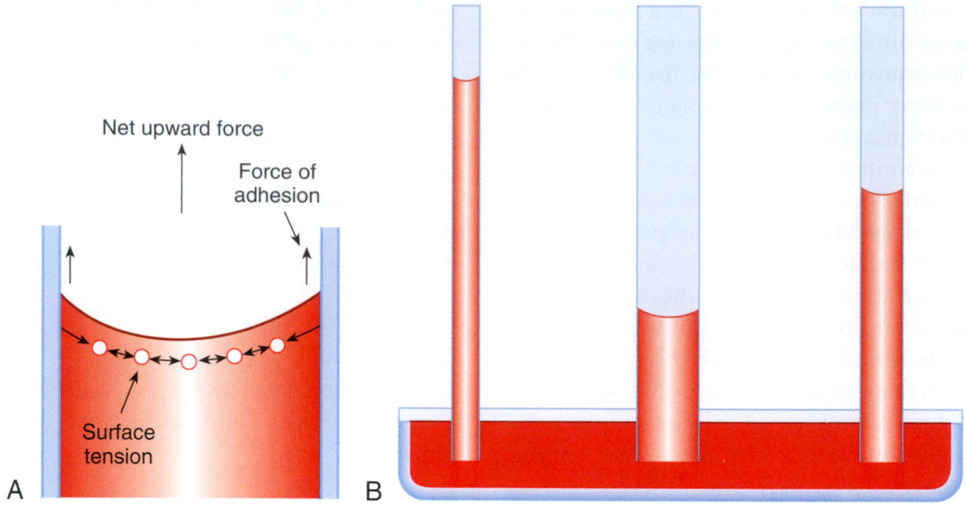

FIGURE 6-10 Capillary action. **A,** Adhesion and surface tension contribute to capillary action (capillarity). **B,** The liquid rises highest in the smallest tube. (Modified from Nave CR, Nave BC: Physics for the health sciences, ed 3, Philadelphia, 1985, WB Saunders.)

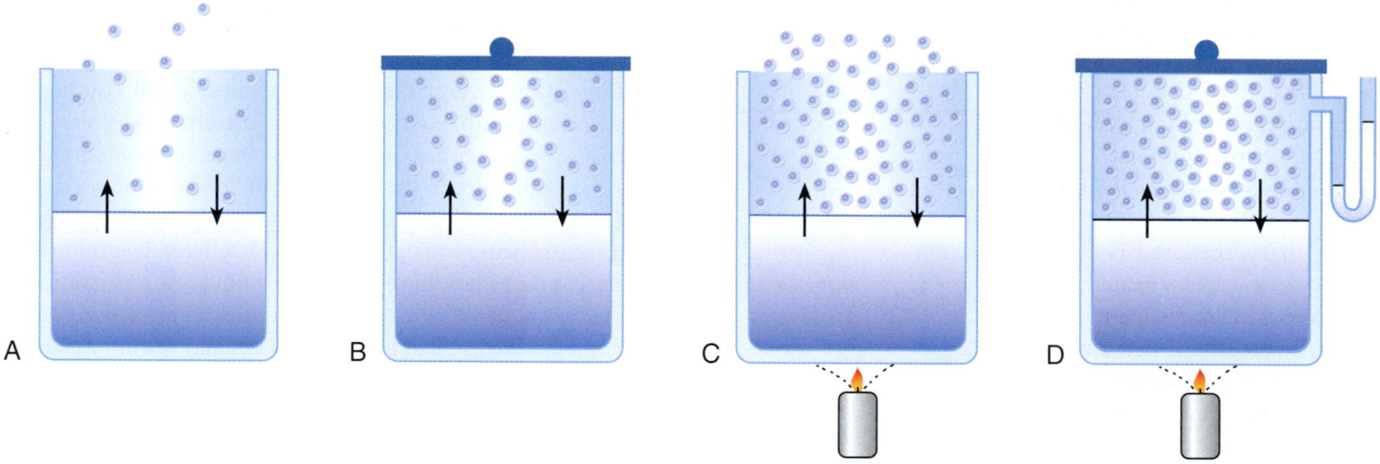

FIGURE 6-11 Factors influencing vaporization of water. See text for details.

the water temperature reaches 100°C, a new change of state begins—from liquid to vapor. This change of state is called *vaporization.* There are two different forms of vaporization: *boiling* and *evaporation.*

Boiling

The *boiling point* of a liquid is the temperature at which its vapor pressure exceeds atmospheric pressure. When a liquid boils, its molecules must have enough kinetic energy to force themselves into the atmosphere against the opposing pressure. Because the weight of the atmosphere retards the escape of vapor molecules, the greater the ambient pressure, the greater is the boiling point. Conversely, when atmospheric pressure is low, liquid molecules escape more easily and boiling occurs at lower temperatures. This is why cooking times must be increased at higher altitudes.

Although boiling is associated with high temperatures, the boiling points of most liquefied gases are very low. At 1 atm, O_2 boils at −183°C.

Energy is also needed to vaporize liquids, as with other phase changes. The energy required to vaporize a liquid is the **latent heat of vaporization.** In cgs units, the latent heat of vaporization is the number of calories required to vaporize 1 g of a liquid at its normal boiling point.

Melting weakens attractive forces between molecules, whereas vaporization eliminates them. Elimination of these forces converts essentially all of the internal energy of a substance into kinetic energy. For this reason, vaporization requires substantially more energy than melting. As shown in Figure 6-3, almost seven times more energy is needed to convert water to steam (540 cal/g) than is needed to melt ice.

Evaporation, Vapor Pressure, and Humidity

Boiling is only one type of vaporization. A liquid also can change into a gas at temperatures lower than its boiling point through a process called *evaporation.* Water is a good example (Figure 6-11). When at a temperature lower than its boiling point, water enters the atmosphere via evaporation. The liquid molecules are in constant motion, as in the gas phase. Although this kinetic energy is less intense than in the gaseous state, it allows some molecules near the surface to escape into the surrounding air as water vapor (see Figure 6-11, *A*).

After water is converted to a vapor, it acts like any gas. Not to be confused with visible particulate water, such as mist or fog, this invisible gaseous form of water is called *molecular water.* Molecular water obeys the same physical principles as other gases and exerts a pressure called **water vapor pressure**. This pressure needs to be considered when calculating gas exchange (Chapter 13).

Evaporation requires heat. The heat energy required for evaporation comes from the air next to the water surface. As the surrounding air loses heat energy, it cools. This is the *principle of evaporative cooling,* which was previously described.

If the container is covered, water vapor molecules continue to enter the air until it can hold no more water (see Figure 6-11, *B*). At this point, the air over the water is saturated with water vapor. However, vaporization does not stop when saturation occurs. Instead, for every molecule escaping into the air, another returns to the water reservoir. These conditions are referred to as a *state of equilibrium.*

Influence of Temperature. No other factor influences evaporation more than temperature. Temperature affects evaporation in two ways. First, the warmer the air, the more vapor it can hold. Specifically, the capacity of air to hold water vapor increases with temperature. The warmer the air contacting a water surface, the faster is the rate of evaporation.

Second, if water is heated, its kinetic energy is increased, and more molecules are helped to escape from its surface (see Figure 6-11, *C*). Last, if the container of heated water is covered, the air again becomes saturated (see Figure 6-11, *D*). However, the heated saturated air, compared with the unheated air (see Figure 6-11, *B*), now contains more vapor molecules and exerts a higher vapor pressure (as shown by the manometer in Figure 6-11, *D*). The temperature of a gas affects both its capacity to hold molecular water and the water vapor pressure.

The relationship between water vapor pressure and temperature is shown graphically in Figure 6-12. The left vertical axis plots water vapor pressure in both millimeters of mercury (mm Hg) and (kilopascals (kPa). The horizontal axis plots temperatures between 0° and 70° C. This graph shows that the greater the temperature, the greater is the saturated water vapor pressure *(bold red dots).* Table 6-3 lists actual water vapor pressures in saturated air in the clinical range of temperatures (20° to 37° C).

Humidity. Water vapor pressure represents the kinetic activity of water molecules in air. For the actual amount or weight of water vapor in a gas to be determined, the water vapor content or absolute humidity must be measured.

Absolute humidity can be measured by weighing the water vapor extracted from air using a drying agent. The common unit of measure for absolute humidity is milligrams of water vapor per liter of gas (mg/L). Absolute humidity values for saturated air at various temperatures are plotted against the right vertical axis of Figure 6-12. The middle column of Table 6-3

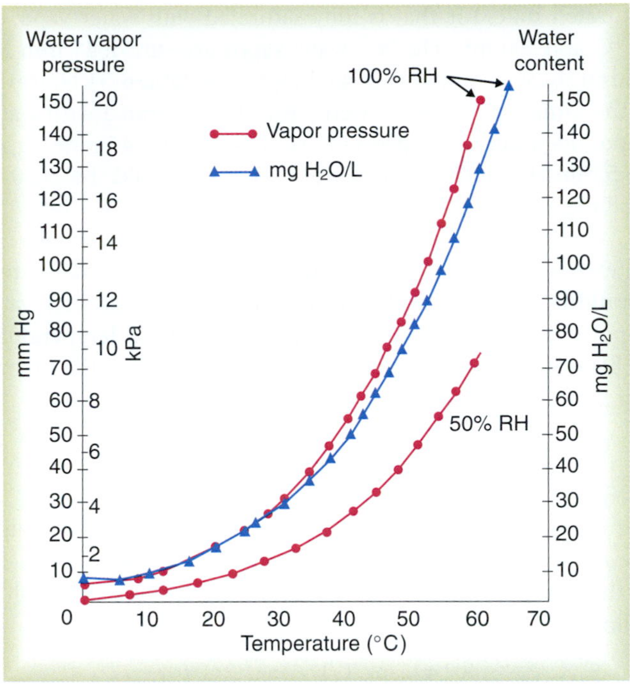

FIGURE 6-12 Water vapor pressure (P_{H_2O}) and absolute humidity (mg H_2O/L) curves for gas that is fully saturated (relative humidity [RH] = 100%) and gas that is half saturated (RH = 50%).

TABLE 6-3

Vapor Pressure and Absolute Humidity for Air Saturated with Water Vapor

Temperature (°C)	Vapor Pressure (mm Hg)	Water Vapor Content (mg/L)	ATPS to BTPS Correction Factor*
20	17.50	17.30	1.102
21	18.62	18.35	1.096
22	19.80	19.42	1.091
23	21.10	20.58	1.085
24	22.40	21.78	1.080
25	23.80	23.04	1.075
26	25.20	24.36	1.068
27	26.70	25.75	1.063
28	28.30	27.22	1.057
29	30.00	28.75	1.051
30	31.80	30.35	1.045
31	33.70	32.01	1.039
32	35.70	33.76	1.032
33	37.70	35.61	1.026
34	39.90	37.57	1.020
35	42.20	39.60	1.014
36	44.60	41.70	1.007
37	47.00	43.80	1.000

ATPS, Ambient temperature and pressure saturated; *BTPS,* body temperature and pressure saturated.
*Correction factors are based on 760 mm Hg pressure.

lists these absolute humidity values for saturated air between 20° and 37° C.

A gas does not need to be fully saturated with water vapor. If a gas is only half saturated with water vapor, its water vapor pressure and absolute humidity are only half that in the fully saturated state. Air that is fully saturated with water vapor at 37° C, and 760 mm Hg has a water vapor pressure of 47 mm Hg and an absolute humidity of 43.8 mg/L (see Table 6-3). However, if the same volume of air were only 50% saturated with water vapor, its water vapor pressure would be 0.50 × 47 mm Hg, or 23.5 mm Hg and its absolute humidity would be 0.50 × 43.8 mg/L, or 21.9 mg/L.

When a gas is not fully saturated, its water vapor content can be expressed in relative terms using a measure called **relative humidity (RH)**. The RH of a gas is the ratio of its actual water vapor content to its saturated capacity at a given temperature. RH is expressed as a percentage and is derived with the following simple formula:

$$RH\,(\%) = \frac{\text{content}}{\text{capacity}} \times 100\%$$

For example, saturated air at a room temperature of 20° C has the capacity to hold 17.3 mg/L of water vapor (see Table 6-3). If the absolute humidity is 12 mg/L, the RH is calculated as follows:

$$RH = 12\ mg/L / 17.3\ mg/L \times 100\%$$
$$RH = 0.69 \times 100\%$$
$$RH = 69\%$$

Actual water vapor content does not have to be measured for RH to be computed. Instruments called *hygrometers* allow measurement of RH using a wide variety of ingenuous mechanisms based on the effects of humidity on, for example, temperature through evaporation (psychrometers), the length of a human hair, or electrical capacitance and resistance.

When the water vapor content of a volume of gas equals its capacity, the RH is 100%. When the RH is 100%, a gas is fully saturated with water vapor. Under these conditions, even slight cooling of the gas causes its water vapor to turn back into the liquid state, a process called *condensation*.

Condensed moisture deposits on any available surface, such as on the walls of a container or delivery tubing or on particles suspended in the gas. Condensation returns heat to and warms the surrounding environment, whereas vaporization of water cools the adjacent air.

If air that is at an RH of 90% is cooled, its capacity to hold water vapor decreases. Although the water vapor capacity of the air decreases, its content remains constant. With a lower capacity but the same content, the RH of the air must increase. Continued cooling decreases the air's water vapor capacity until it eventually equals the water vapor content (RH = 100%). When content equals capacity, the air is fully saturated and can hold no more water vapor.

Because RH never exceeds 100%, any further decrease in temperature causes condensation. The temperature at which condensation begins is called the **dew point**. Cooling a saturated gas below its dew point causes increasingly more water vapor to condense into liquid water droplets.

Figure 6-13 provides a useful analogy of the relationship among water vapor content, capacity, and RH. The various-sized glasses represent the capacity of a gas to hold water vapor. The larger the glass, the greater is its capacity. The water in the glasses represents the actual water vapor content. A glass that is half full is at 50% capacity, or 50% RH. A full glass represents the saturated state, which is equivalent to 100% RH.

Figure 6-13, *A*, shows what happens when a saturated gas is heated. Warming a gas increases its capacity to hold water vapor but does not change its content. This is equivalent to pouring the contents of the full glass on the *left* in Figure 6-13, *A* into

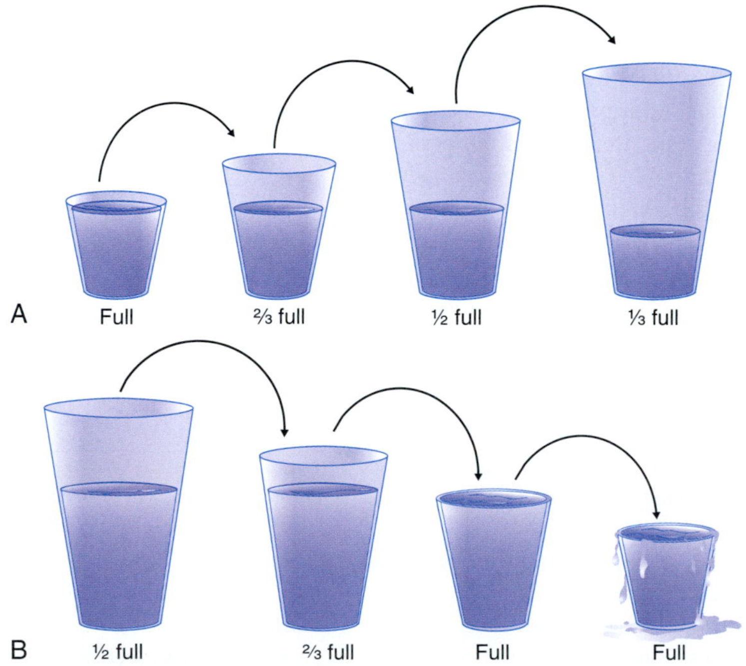

FIGURE 6-13 Relative humidity analogy. **A,** The effect of increasing capacity without changing content, as when heating a saturated gas. **B,** The effect of decreasing capacity, as when cooling a gas. See text for details.

progressively larger glasses. The amount of water does not change, but as the glasses get larger, they become less full. We started with a full glass (100% RH) but end up with one that is only one-third full (33% RH).

A decrease in capacity would have the opposite effect. In Figure 6-13, *B*, we start with a large glass, which is half full (50% RH). The capacity of the glass is decreased by pouring the water into progressively smaller glasses (equivalent to decreasing the gas temperature). Eventually, the water volume is enough to fill a smaller glass (100% RH). What happens if we try to empty this full glass into an even smaller one? Because the smaller glass has less capacity, the excess content must spill over. This spillover is analogous to the condensation occurring when a saturated gas cools below its dew point. However, although condensation has removed the excess moisture from the air, the smaller glass is still full (100% RH).

MINI CLINI

Condensation and Evaporation

A good clinical example of condensation and evaporation is the hygroscopic condenser humidifier, a form of artificial nose (Figure 6-14). These devices consist of layers of water-absorbent material encased in plastic. When a patient exhales into an artificial nose, the warm, saturated expired gas cools, causing condensation on the absorbent surfaces. As condensation occurs, heat is generated in the device. When the patient inhales through the device, the inspired gases are warmed and the previously condensed water evaporates, aiding in airway humidification. Chapter 38 provides more detail on humidification devices, including the artificial nose.

In clinical practice, two additional measures of humidity are used: *percent body humidity* (BH) and *humidity deficit*. The BH of a gas is the ratio of its actual water vapor content to the water vapor capacity in saturated gas at body temperature (37° C). The BH is the same as RH except that the capacity (or denominator) is fixed at 43.8 mg/L:

$$\text{BH}\,(\%) = \frac{\text{content (mg/L)}}{43.8} \times 100\%$$

The humidity deficit associated with a BH less than 100% represents the amount of water vapor the body must add to the inspired gas to achieve saturation at body temperature (37° C).

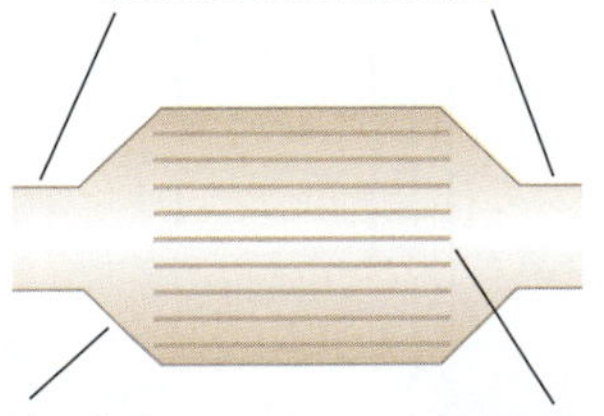

FIGURE 6-14 Hygroscopic condenser humidifier.

To compute the humidity deficit, simply subtract the actual water vapor content from its capacity at 37° C (43.8 mg/L).

Influence of Pressure. High temperatures increase vaporization, whereas high pressures impede this process. Water molecules trying to escape from a liquid surface must push their way out against the opposing air molecules. If the surrounding air pressure is high, there are more opposing air molecules and vaporization decreases. Alternatively, low atmospheric pressures increases vaporization.

Influence of Surface Area. The greater the available surface area of the gas in contact with air, the greater is the rate of liquid evaporation. This statement can be easily proved by comparing how quickly equal volumes of water evaporate under dry conditions from a flat plate versus from a tall, narrow glass. The water spread over a flat plate evaporates more quickly compared with the same amount of liquid in a tall, narrow glass. This principle is applied to the design of certain humidifiers to increase their ability to put water vapor in the passing gas.

Properties of Gases

Gases share many properties with liquids. Specifically, gases exert pressure, are capable of flow, and exhibit the property of viscosity. However, in contrast to liquids, gases are readily compressed and expanded and fill the spaces available to them through diffusion.

Kinetic Activity of Gases

Because the intermolecular forces of attraction of a gas are so weak, most of the internal energy of a gas is kinetic energy. *Kinetic theory* says that gas molecules travel about randomly at very high speeds and with frequent collisions.

The velocity of gas molecules is directly proportional to temperature. As a gas is warmed, its kinetic activity increases, its molecular collisions increase, and its pressure increases. Conversely, when a gas is cooled, molecular activity decreases, particle velocity and collision frequency decrease, and the pressure decreases.

Molar Volume and Gas Density

A major principle governing chemistry is **Avogadro's law**. This law states that the 1-g atomic weight of any substance contains exactly the same number of atoms, molecules, or ions. This number, 6.023×10^{23}, is *Avogadro's constant.* In SI units, this quantity of matter equals 1 mole.

Molar Volume. Avogadro's law states that equal volumes of gases under the same conditions must contain the same number of molecules. At a constant temperature and pressure, 1 mole of a gas should occupy the same volume as 1 mole of any other gas. This ideal volume is termed the *molar volume.*

At standard temperature (0.0° C) and pressure (760 mm Hg), dry (**STPD**); the ideal molar volume of any gas is 22.4 L. In reality, there are small deviations from this ideal. For example, although the molar volumes of both O_2 and nitrogen are 22.4 L at STPD, the molar volume of CO_2 is closer to 22.3 L. These values are used to calculate gas densities and convert dissolved gas volumes into moles per liter.

Density. Density is the ratio of the mass of a substance to its volume. A dense substance has heavy (high atomic weight) particles packed closely together. Uranium is a good example of a dense substance. Conversely, a low-density substance has a low concentration of light atomic particles per unit volume. Hydrogen gas is a good example of a low-density substance.

In clinical practice, weight is often substituted for mass, and weight density (weight per unit volume [d_w]) is actually measured. Solid or liquid weight density is commonly measured in grams per cubic centimeter. For gases, the most common unit is grams per liter. Because weight density equals weight divided by volume, the density of any gas at STPD can be computed easily by dividing its molecular weight (gmw) by the universal molar volume of 22.4 L (22.3 for CO_2). Box 6-1 provides examples of gas density calculations.

For the density of a gas mixture to be calculated, the percentage or fraction of each gas in the mixture must be known. To calculate the density of air at STPD, the following equation is used:

$$d_w \text{ air} = (\text{FN} \times \text{gmw N}) + (\text{FO}_2 \times \text{gmw O}_2)/22.4\text{ L}$$
$$d_w \text{ air} = (0.79 \times 28) + (0.21 \times 32)/22.4$$
$$d_w \text{ air} = 1.29\text{ g/L}$$

FN and FO_2 equal the fractional concentrations of N and O_2 in air.

Gaseous Diffusion

Diffusion is the process whereby molecules move from areas of high concentration to areas of lower concentration. *Kinetic energy* is the driving force behind diffusion. Because gases have high kinetic energy, they diffuse most rapidly. However, diffusion also occurs in liquids and can occur in solids. Gas diffusion rates are quantified using **Graham's law**. Mathematically, the rate of diffusion of a gas (D) is inversely proportional to the square root of its gram molecular weight:

$$D_{gas} \propto \frac{1}{\sqrt{\text{gmw}}}$$

According to this principle, light gases diffuse rapidly whereas heavy gases diffuse more slowly. Because diffusion is based on kinetic activity, anything that increases molecular activity quickens diffusion. Heating and mechanical agitation speed diffusion.

Gas Pressure

Whether free in the atmosphere, enclosed in a container, or dissolved in a liquid such as blood, all gases exert pressure. In physiology, the term *tension* is often used to refer to the pressure exerted by gases when dissolved in liquids. The pressure or tension of a gas depends mainly on its kinetic activity. In addition, gravity affects gas pressure. Gravity increases gas density, increasing the rate of molecular collisions and gas tension; this explains why atmospheric pressure decreases with altitude.

Pressure is a measure of force per unit area. The SI unit of pressure is the N/m^2, or Pascal (Pa). Pressure in the cgs system is measured in $dynes/cm^2$, whereas pounds per square inch (lb/in^2 or psi) is the British foot-pound-second (fps) pressure unit. Pressure can also be measured indirectly as the height of a column of liquid, as is commonly done to determine atmospheric pressure.

Measuring Atmospheric Pressure. Atmospheric pressure is measured with a barometer. A barometer consists of an evacuated glass tube approximately 1 m long. This tube is closed at the top end, with its lower, open end immersed in a mercury reservoir (Figure 6-15). The pressure of the atmosphere on the mercury reservoir forces the mercury up the vacuum tube a distance equivalent to the force exerted. In this manner, the height of the mercury column represents the downward force of atmospheric pressure and is measured in either inches (British) or millimeters (metric). Barometer pressure is reported with readings such as 30.4 inches of mercury (Hg) or 772 mm Hg; this means that the atmospheric pressure is great enough to support a column of mercury 30.4 inches or 772 mm in height.

Alternatively, the term *torr* may be used in pressure readings. Torr is short for Torricelli, the seventeenth-century inventor of the mercury barometer. At sea level, 1 torr equals 1 mm Hg. A pressure reading of 772 torr is the same as 772 mm Hg.

Box 6-1 Examples of Gas Densities d_w at Standard Temperature and Pressure, Dry

$d_w\ O_2$ = gmw/22.4 = 32/22.4 = 1.43 g/L
$d_w\ N_2$ = gmw/22.4 = 28/22.4 = 1.25 g/L
d_w He = gmw/22.4 = 4/22.4 = 0.179 g/L
$d_w\ CO_2$ = gmw/22.4 = 44/22.4 = 1.97 g/L

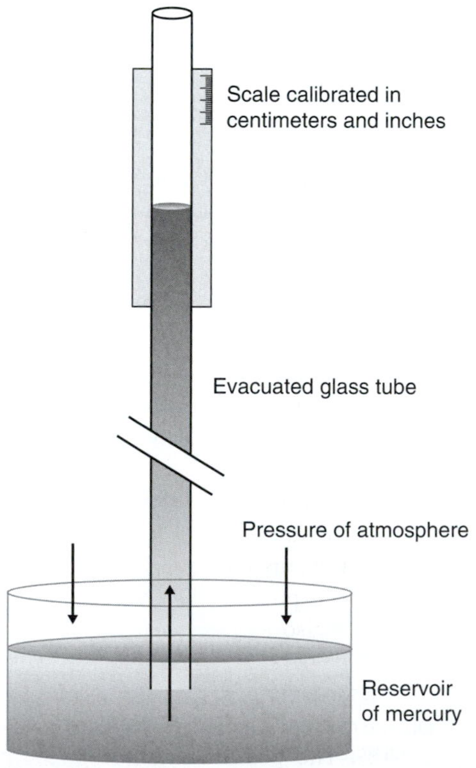

FIGURE 6-15 Major components of a mercury barometer.

The height of a column of mercury is not a true measure of pressure. Height is a linear measure, whereas pressure represents force per unit area. The pressure exerted by a liquid is directly proportional to its depth (or height) times its density:

$$\text{Pressure} = \text{Height} \times \text{Density}$$

At sea level, the average atmospheric pressure supports a column of mercury 76 cm (760 mm) or 29.9 inches in height. If we also know that mercury has a density of 13.6 g/cm^3 (0.491 lb/in^3), the average atmospheric pressure (P_B) is calculated as follows:

$$\text{cgs units: } P_B = 76\,\text{cm} \times 13.6\,\text{g/cm}^3 = 1034\,\text{g/cm}^2$$
$$\text{fps units: } P_B = 29.9\,\text{in} \times 0.491\,\text{lb/in}^3 = 14.7\,\text{lb/in}^2$$

These two measures, 1034 g/cm^2 and 14.7 lb/in^2, are considered standards in the cgs and British fps systems, each being equivalent to 1 atm.[4-7]

Similar to any solid material, a barometer's housing reacts to temperature changes by expanding and contracting. In addition, the mercury column acts like a large thermometer. Both pressure and temperature affect the mercury level of a barometer. For accuracy, the reading must be corrected for temperature changes.

Clinical Pressure Measurements. Mercury is the most common fluid used in pressure measurements both in barometers and at the bedside. Because of the high density (13.6 g/cm^3) of mercury, it assumes a height that is easy to read for most pressures in the clinical range. Water columns also can be used to measure pressure (in centimeters of water [cm H_2O]) but only low pressures. Because water is 13.6 times less dense than mercury, 1 atm would support a water column 33.9 feet high or about as tall as a two-story building.

Both mercury and water columns are still used in clinical practice, especially when vascular pressures are being measured. However, these traditional tools are rapidly being replaced by mechanical or electronic pressure-measuring devices. Even so, these new instruments must be calibrated against a mercury or water column before making measurements.

The simplest mechanical pressure gauge is the *aneroid barometer,* which is common in homes. An aneroid barometer consists of a sealed evacuated metal box with a flexible, spring-supported top that responds to external pressure changes (Figure 6-16). This motion activates a geared pointer, which provides a scale reading analogous to pressure.

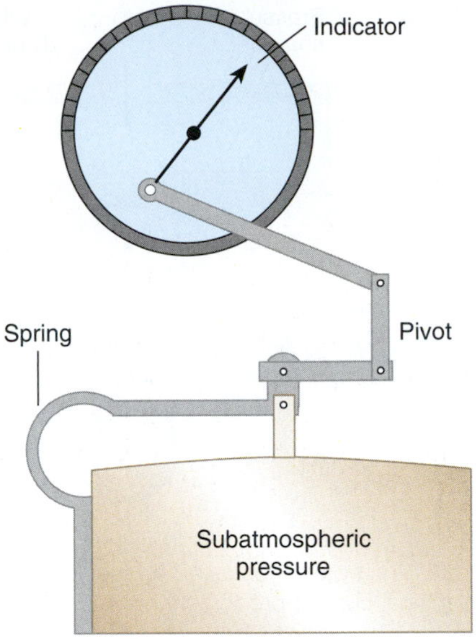

FIGURE 6-16 Aneroid barometer.

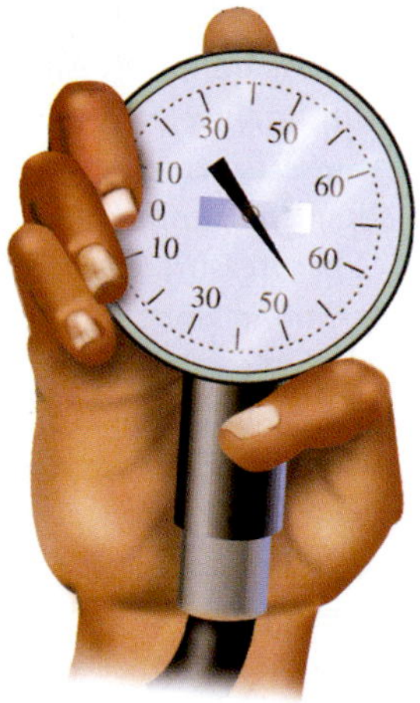
FIGURE 6-17 Mechanical manometer used to measure a patient's airway pressure.

This same concept underlies the simple mechanical manometers used to measure blood or airway pressure at the bedside (Figure 6-17). However, rather than the pressure acting externally on the sealed chamber, the inside is connected to the pressure source. In this manner, the flexible chamber wall expands and contracts as pressure increases or decreases.

A flexible chamber also can be used to measure pressure electronically. These devices are called **strain-gauge pressure transducers.** In these devices, pressure changes expand and contract a flexible metal diaphragm connected to electrical wires (Figure 6-18). The physical strain on the diaphragm changes the amount of electricity flowing through the wires. By measuring this change in electrical voltage, we are indirectly measuring changes in pressure. Most modern medical devices use small, solid-state, piezoelectric pressure sensors. These devices work on the principle that certain materials generate an electric charge in response to applied mechanical stress.

Although millimeters of mercury and centimeters of water are still the most common pressure units used at the bedside, they do not represent the SI standard. The SI unit of pressure is the kPa; 1 kPa equals approximately 10.2 cm H_2O or 7.5 torr. To convert between these pressure units accurately, use the factors provided in the rear inside cover of this book.

RULE OF THUMB

One kilopascal equals approximately 10.2 cm H_2O. A pressure of 10 kPa equals approximately 100 cm H_2O. Conversely, a pressure of 60 cm H_2O equals approximately 6 kPa.

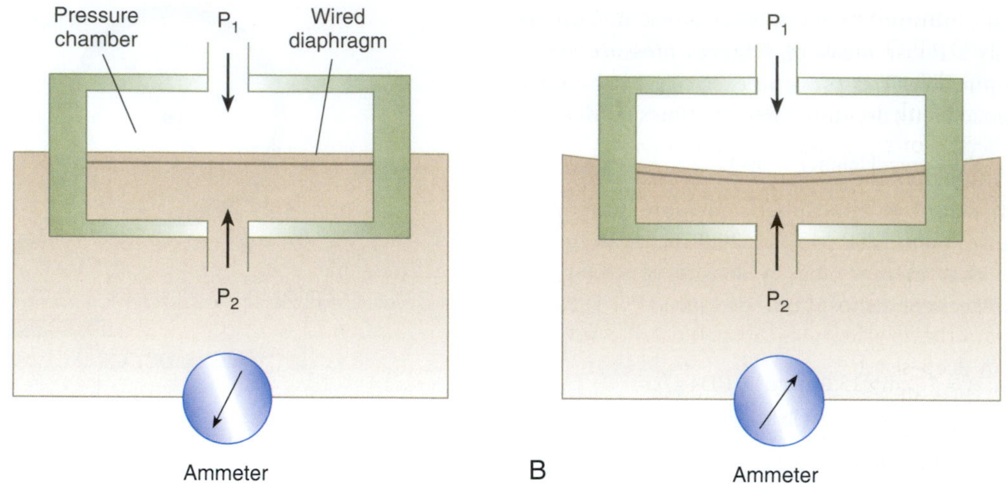

FIGURE 6-18 Strain-gauge pressure transducer. **A,** No pressure is applied. **B,** Pressure is applied to the transducer. An ammeter shows a change in electrical current proportional to the magnitude of pressure applied.

Partial Pressures (Dalton's Law)

Many gases exist together as mixtures. Air is a good example of a gas mixture, consisting mainly of O_2 and N. A gas mixture, similar to a solitary gas, exerts pressure. The pressure exerted by a gas mixture must equal the sum of the kinetic activity of all its component gases. The pressure exerted by a single gas in a mixture is called its *partial pressure.*

Dalton's law describes the relationship between the partial pressure and the total pressure in a gas mixture. According to this law, the total pressure of a mixture of gases must equal the sum of the partial pressures of all component gases. The principle states that the partial pressure of a component gas must be proportional to its percentage in the mixture.[8]

A gas making up 25% of a mixture would exert 25% of the total pressure. For consistency, the percentage of a gas in a mixture is usually expressed in decimal form, using the term *fractional concentration.* A gas that is 25% of a mixture has a fractional concentration of 0.25. For example, air consists of approximately 21% O_2 and 79% N. To compute the partial pressure of each component, simply multiply the fractional concentration of each component by the total pressure. Assuming a normal atmospheric pressure of 760 torr, the individual partial pressure is computed as follows:

$$\text{Partial pressure} = \text{Fractional concentration} \times \text{Total pressure}$$
$$PO_2 = 0.21 \times 760 \text{ torr} = 160 \text{ torr}$$
$$PN = 0.79 \times 760 \text{ torr} = 60 \text{ torr}$$

As predicted by Dalton's law, the sum of these partial pressures equals the total pressure of the gas mixture.

What if the total pressure changed? Barometric pressure changes, in addition to minor fluctuations caused by weather, are mainly a function of altitude. Considering only O_2, we know that its fractional concentration, or fractional inspired O_2 (FiO_2), remains constant at approximately 0.21. At a P_B of 760 torr, the PO_2 is equal to 0.21 × 760, or 160 torr. At 25,000 feet, the FiO_2 of air is still 0.21. However, the P_B is only 282 torr, and the resulting PO_2 is 0.21 × 282, or 59 torr, just more than one-third of that available at sea level. Because the PO_2 (not its percentage) determines physiologic activity, high altitudes can impair O_2 uptake by the lungs. Mountain climbers must sometimes use supplemental O_2 at high altitudes for this reason. By increasing the amount of O_2 more than 0.21, we can raise its partial pressure and increase uptake by the lungs. For a practical application of this principle, see the accompanying Mini Clini.

MINI CLINI

Why Are Oxygen Masks Needed on Airplanes?

PROBLEM: People who have traveled by air are familiar with the safety instructions given by the crew before flight. Instructions are included on how to use the O masks. When and why are these masks needed?

DISCUSSION: At a typical cruising altitude of 30,000 feet, the P_B outside the airplane cabin is approximately 226 torr. The inspired partial pressure of O_2 (PiO_2) is calculated as follows:

$$PiO_2 = 0.21 \times 226 \text{ torr} = 47 \text{ torr}$$

If the cabin were to depressurize, travelers inside would be exposed to this low PiO_2. At this PiO_2, most people become unconscious within seconds and eventually die of lack of O_2 (anoxia).

To overcome this problem, emergency O_2 masks are available when the cabin depressurizes. These masks, assuming a tight fit, probably provide approximately 70% O_2, or an FiO_2 of 0.70. The PiO_2 of a person wearing a mask under these conditions is calculated as follows:

$$PiO_2 = 0.70 \times 226 \text{ torr} = 158 \text{ torr}$$

This PiO_2 (about the same as at sea level) is sufficient to keep the passengers alive until the crew can bring the plane down to a safe altitude.

In contrast, high atmospheric pressures increase the partial pressure of inspired O_2 (PiO_2) in an air mixture. Pressures above atmospheric are called *hyperbaric pressures.*[9] Hyperbaric pressures commonly occur only in underwater diving and in special hyperbaric chambers.[9] For example, at a depth of 66 feet under the sea, water exerts a pressure of 3 atm, or 2280 mm Hg (3×760). At this depth, the O_2 in an air mixture breathed by a diver exerts a PO_2 of 0.21×2280, or approximately 479 mm Hg. This is nearly three times the PO_2 at sea level.

The same conditions can be created on dry land in a *hyperbaric chamber.* Hyperbaric chambers are used for controlled depressurization of deep-sea divers and to treat certain types of diving accidents. Clinically, hyperbaric chambers and O_2 are used together to treat various conditions, including carbon monoxide poisoning and gangrene. Chapter 41 provides more details on this use of high-pressure O_2.

Solubility of Gases in Liquids (Henry's Law)

Gases can dissolve in liquids. Carbonated water and soda are good examples of a gas (CO_2) dissolved in a liquid (water). **Henry's law** states that at a constant temperature, the amount of a given gas that dissolves in a given type and volume of liquid is directly proportional to the partial pressure of that gas in equilibrium with that liquid. For O_2 dissolved in blood, the equation is

$$C_{dO_2} = kP_{O_2}$$

where C_{dO_2} is the concentration of O_2 of dissolved O_2 in the blood at standard temperature and pressure dry conditions (milliliters per deciliter of blood, equivalent to mL/100 mL, also called volume percent), k is the constant of proportionality, or **solubility coefficient** (for blood k = 0.0031 mL/mm Hg/dL blood at 37°C). Note that this term shows up in the equation for the total O_2 content of blood (see Chapter 12). For example, if the PaO_2 is 100 mm Hg, the concentration of dissolved O_2 is:

$$C_{dO_2} = 0.0031 \times 100 = 0.3\ \text{mL/dL}$$

Temperature plays a major role in gas solubility. High temperatures decrease solubility, and low temperatures increase solubility. This is why an open can of soda may still fizz if left in the refrigerator but quickly goes flat when left out at room temperature. The effect of temperature on solubility is a result of changes in kinetic activity. As a liquid is warmed, the kinetic activity of any dissolved gas molecules is increased. This increase in kinetic activity increases the escaping tendency of the molecules and partial pressure. As an increasing number of gas molecules escape, the amount left in a solution decreases rapidly. For a practical application of this principle, see the accompanying Mini Clini, which discusses blood gases and patient temperature.

MINI CLINI

Blood Gases Versus Patient Temperature

PROBLEM: Respiratory therapists (RTs) frequently need to sample and measure the partial pressures of O_2 and CO_2 in patients' arterial blood. These samples are called *arterial blood gas* (ABG) samples. Typically, ABG samples are measured in analyzers kept at a normal body temperature of 37°C. However, not all patients have normal body temperatures. Many are feverish (hyperpyrexia), and some have low body temperatures (hypothermia). What effect does this have on the measurements?

DISCUSSION: The direct relationship between temperature and partial pressure causes higher arterial PO_2 and PCO_2 readings at higher temperatures. At 37°C, the arterial PO_2 in a normal adult is approximately 100 torr. However, at 47°C, the PO_2 would be nearly twice as high. A smaller increase from 37° to 39°C increases the arterial PO_2 less markedly from 100 torr to approximately 110 torr. Likewise, an increase in temperature increases the arterial PCO_2. Arterial PCO_2 values increase approximately 5% per degree Celsius. An increase in temperature from 37° to 39°C increases the PCO_2 by approximately 10%, from 40 torr to 44 torr.

The reverse is also true. Decreased temperatures decrease the arterial partial pressures of O_2 and CO_2. Correction equations are available to help compute these corrections; however, they correct only for the relationship between temperature and pressure and do not take into account metabolic and cardiovascular changes that accompany a change in a patient's temperature. For this reason, the use of corrected PO_2 and PCO_2 readings remains controversial.

GAS BEHAVIOR UNDER CHANGING CONDITIONS

Gases, with large distances between their molecules, are easily compressed and expanded. When a gas is pressurized, the molecules are squeezed closer together. If a gas-filled container could be enlarged, the gas would expand to occupy the new volume. Figure 6-19 illustrates the concepts of gas compression and expansion.

Gas Laws

Several laws help define the relationships among gas pressure, temperature, mass, and volume (Table 6-4). Using these laws,[10,11] the behaviors of gases under changing conditions can be predicted. Underlying all these laws are three basic assumptions: (1) No energy is lost during molecular collisions, (2) the volume of the molecules themselves is negligible, and (3) no forces of mutual attraction exist between these molecules. These three assumptions describe the behavior of an "ideal gas." Under normal conditions, most gases exhibit ideal behavior.

Effect of Water Vapor

In clinical practice, most gas law calculations must take into account the presence of water vapor. Water vapor, similar to any gas, occupies space. The dry volume of a gas at a constant pressure and temperature is always smaller than its saturated volume. The opposite is also true. Correcting from the dry state to the saturated state always yields a larger gas volume.

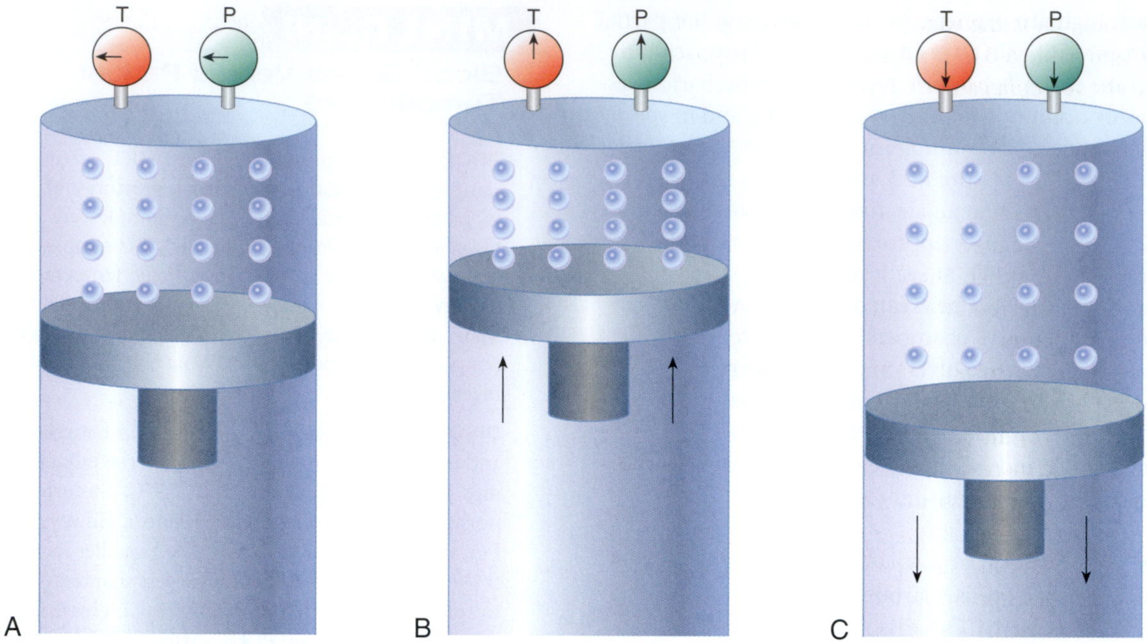

FIGURE 6-19 A mass of gas in the resting state exerts a given pressure *(P)* at a given temperature *(T)* in cylinder **A.** In cylinder **B,** as the piston compresses the gas, the molecules are crowded closer together, and the increased energy of molecular collisions increases both the temperature and the pressure. Conversely, as the gas expands in cylinder **C,** molecular interaction decreases and the temperature and pressure decrease.

TABLE 6-4
Laws Describing Gas Behavior Under Changing Conditions

Gas Law	Basic Relationship	Constants	Description	Working Formula*	Clinical Applications
Boyle's law	$P \times V = k$	Temperature, mass	Volume of a gas varies inversely with its pressure	$P_1V_1 = P_2V_2$	Ventilation (see Chapter 11) Body plethysmography (see Chapter 19) Compressed volume (see Chapter 38)
Charles' law	$\frac{V}{T} = k$	Pressure, mass	Volume of gas varies directly with changes in its temperature (°K)	$\frac{V_1}{T_1} = \frac{V_2}{T_2}$	ATPS to BTPS corrections (see this chapter)
Gay-Lussac's law	$\frac{P}{T} = k$	Volume, mass	Pressure exerted by a gas varies directly with its absolute temperature	$\frac{P_1}{T_1} = \frac{P_2}{T_2}$	Cylinder pressures (see Chapter 38)
Combined gas law	$PV = nRT$	—	Interaction of above (none held constant)	$\frac{P_1V_1}{nT_1} = \frac{P_2V_2}{nT_2}$	Complex interactions of variables

*Use the working formulas to calculate the new value of a parameter when a gas undergoes a change in P, V, n, or T. For example, to solve for a new volume (V_2) using Boyle's law, you would simply rearrange its working equation as follows:

$$V_2 = V_1 \times P_1/P_2$$

n, Mass; *P,* pressure; *R,* the gas constant (a combined constant of proportionality); *T,* temperature (°K); *V,* volume.

The pressure exerted by water vapor is independent of the other gases with which it mixes, depending only on the temperature and RH. The addition of water vapor to a gas mixture always lowers the partial pressures of the other gases present. This fact becomes relevant when discussing the partial pressure of gases in the lung, where the gases are saturated with water vapor at body temperature.

Corrected Pressure Computations

To compute the new or corrected partial pressure of a gas after saturation with water vapor, the following formula is applied:

$$P_C = F_{gas} \times (P_T - P_{H_2O})$$

P_C is the corrected gas pressure, F_{gas} is the fractional concentration of the gas in the gas mixture, P_T is the total gas pressure of the mixture, and P_{H_2O} is the water vapor pressure at the given temperature (see Table 6-3). If only a single gas is present, F_{gas} equals 1, and the formula can be simplified:

$$P_C = (P_T - P_{H_2O})$$

Correction Factors

Correction factors can be used to convert gas volumes from one set of conditions to another. Such computations are common in pulmonary function laboratories. But they are also common to mechanical ventilators. For example, suppose you set a tidal volume on a ventilator to 500 mL. If the ventilator's output control valve metered out 500 mL, and if the gas was heated and humidified to body conditions (fully saturated at 37° C), then the gas volume would increase because of the heat and addition of water vapor. But how much would it increase? To find out, we need to use conversion equations. As it turns out, the volume increases to 562 (assuming ambient barometric pressure of 760 mm Hg) which is a significant increase of 12%. The current standard of care for mechanical ventilation places emphasis on accurately dosing tidal volume to approximately 6 mL/kg. To maintain the desired accuracy, most intensive care unit ventilator manufacturers correct the set tidal volume to convert from ambient temperature and pressure dry conditions (ATPD) to body temperature and pressure saturated conditions (BTPS), which in this case would mean decreasing the volume exiting the control valves by 62 mL. Such conversions are important for research when evaluating the performance of mechanical ventilators in terms of volume delivery accuracy. In that case, the experiment generally involves measuring gas at (ATPD) and then converting to BTPS to make a fair comparison to the ventilator's display (which is corrected to BTPS).

In gas volume conversions, the four most common computations are as follows (P_B in millimeters of mercury and temperature in °C):

1. Correction from ambient temperature and pressure dry **(ATPD)** to body temperature and pressure saturated **(BTPS)**, as is done in some mechanical ventilators.

$$\text{Correction factor} = \frac{P_B}{P_B - 47} \times \frac{310}{273 + T}$$

2. Correction from ambient temperature and pressure saturated **(ATPS)** to body temperature and pressure saturated **(BTPS)**.

$$\text{Correction factor} = \frac{P_B - P_{H_2O}}{P_B - 47} \times \frac{310}{273 + T}$$

3. Correction from ATPS to standard temperature and pressure dry, **STPD** (0° C and 760 torr)

$$\text{Correction factor} = \frac{P_B - P_{H_2O}}{760} \times \frac{273}{273 + T}$$

4. Correction from STPD to BTPS:

$$\text{Correction factor} = \frac{760}{P_B - 47} \times \frac{310}{273 + T}$$

In each case, the new volume equals the original volume times the correction factor.

Properties of Gases at Extremes of Temperature and Pressure

Most gases exhibit ideal behavior under normal conditions. However, gases can deviate from these expectations, especially at the extremes of pressure and temperature. The accompanying Mini Clini (page 6-19) provides two good clinical examples of how gas behavior can deviate from the ideal.

Weak attractive forces (van der Waals forces) between gas molecules oppose their kinetic activity. Both temperature and pressure affect these forces. At high temperatures, the increased kinetic activity of gas molecules far overshadows these forces. However, at very low temperatures, kinetic activity lessens and these forces become more important. Likewise, very low pressures permit gas molecules to move freely about with little mutual attraction. In contrast, high pressures crowd molecules together, increasing the influence of these forces.

The actual space occupied by gas molecules also can influence their behavior. At low pressure, the total mass of matter in a gas is a negligible fraction of the total volume. However, at very high pressures, molecular density becomes important, altering the expected relationship between pressure and volume.

Critical Temperature and Pressure

For every liquid, there is a temperature above which the kinetic activity of its molecules is so great that the attractive forces cannot keep them in a liquid state. This temperature is called the **critical temperature**. The critical temperature is the highest temperature at which a substance can exist as a liquid. The pressure needed to maintain equilibrium between the liquid and gas phases of a substance at this critical temperature is the *critical pressure*. Together, the critical temperature and pressure represent the critical point of a substance.

The critical temperature of water is 374° C. At this temperature, a pressure of 218 atm is needed to maintain equilibrium between the liquid and gaseous forms of water. No pressure can return water vapor to its liquid form at a temperature greater than 374° C.

Compared with liquids, gases have much lower critical points. Table 6-5 lists the critical points of four gases used in clinical practice: O_2, helium, CO_2, and nitrous oxide. The critical temperatures of O_2 and He are well below the normal room temperature of 20° C (68° F).

TABLE 6-5

Critical Points of Three Gases

Gas	°C	°F	Atmosphere
Helium (He)	−267.9	−450.2	2.3
Oxygen (O_2)	−118.8	−181.1	49.7
Carbon dioxide (CO_2)	31.1	87.9	73.0
Nitrous oxide (N_2O)	36.5	97.7	71.8

MINI CLINI

Variations from Ideal Gas Behavior: Expansion Cooling and Adiabatic Compression

Boyle's law describes gas behavior under constant temperature, or isothermal conditions.[10] During isothermal conditions, the temperature of an ideal gas should not change with either expansion or contraction. For example, if an ideal gas were to escape rapidly from a high-pressure cylinder into the atmosphere, its temperature should not change. The rapid expansion of real gases causes substantial cooling. This phenomenon of expansion cooling is called the *Joule-Thompson effect.*

A rapidly expanding gas cools because the attractive force between its molecules is broken. Because the energy needed to break these forces must come from the gas itself, the temperature of the gas must decrease. This decrease in temperature, depending on the pressure drop that occurs, can be large enough to liquefy the gas. This is the primary method used to liquefy air for the production of O_2.

Isothermal processes keep gas temperature constant. The internal energy will remain constant. In an *adiabatic process,* the container is insulated, resulting in no heat transfer into or out from the system. If the volume increases, the internal energy decreases to perform the work and thus the temperature decreases. If the volume is increased the internal energy is also increased, resulting in a higher temperature. Adiabatic processes are used in liquefying gases.

Lung simulators are often constructed from rigid-walled containers such that the compressibility of the gas in the container represents the compliance of the lungs (particularly useful for neonatal lung simulators). Such containers are often filled with very fine strands of copper (called copper wool) to absorb the heat generated when the gas is compressed, approximating isothermal conditions. However, this is not essential and adiabatic conditions can be assumed instead. The volume of the container (V in liters) required to simulate a given compliance (C in cm H_2O/L) is given by the equations:

$$V = 1.35 \times P_B \times C_I \text{ (isothermanal)}$$
$$V = 1.9 \times P_B \times C_A \text{ (adiabatic)}$$

The derivation of these equations is described elsewhere.[12]

The concept of critical temperature can be applied to distinguish between a true gas and a vapor. A true gas, such as O_2, has a critical temperature so low that at room temperature and pressure it cannot exist as a liquid. In contrast, a vapor is the gaseous state of a substance coexisting with its liquid or solid state at room temperature and pressure. This is why molecular water is referred to as *water vapor.*

The concept of critical temperature and pressure also helps explain how gases are liquefied. A gas can be liquefied by being cooled to below its boiling point. Alternatively, a gas can be liquefied by being cooled to less than its critical temperature and then being compressed. The more a gas is cooled below its critical temperature, the less pressure will be needed to liquefy it. However, under no circumstances can pressure alone liquefy a gas existing above its critical temperature.

According to these principles, any gas with a critical temperature above ambient should be able to be liquefied simply by having pressure applied. Both CO_2 and N_2O have critical temperatures above normal room temperature (see Table 6-5). Both gases can be liquefied by simple compression and stored as liquids at room temperature without cooling. However, both liquefied gases still need to be stored under pressure, usually in strong metal cylinders.

Liquid O_2 is produced by separating it from a liquefied air mixture at a temperature below its boiling point (−183° C or −297° F). After it is separated from air, the O_2 must be maintained as a liquid by being stored in insulated containers below its boiling point. As long as the temperature does not exceed −183° C, the O_2 remains liquid at atmospheric pressure. If higher temperatures are needed, higher pressures must be used. If at any time the liquid O_2 exceeds its critical temperature of −118.8° C, it converts immediately to a gas.

FLUID DYNAMICS

So far, liquids and gases have been presented under static, or nonmoving, conditions. However, both liquids and gases can flow. Flow is the bulk movement of a substance through space. The study of fluids in motion is called *hydrodynamics.* Because many respiratory care devices use hydrodynamic principles, the RT must have a good understanding of the basic concepts governing fluids in motion.

Pressures in Flowing Fluids

As we have seen, the pressure of a static liquid depends solely on the depth and density of the fluid. In contrast, the pressure exerted by a liquid in motion depends on the nature of the flow itself. As shown in Figure 6-20, *A,* the pressure exerted by a static fluid is the same at all points along a horizontal tube, depending only on the height (h) of the liquid column. However, when the fluid flows out through the bottom tube, the pressure progressively decreases all along the tube length (see Figure 6-20, *B*). In addition, the decrease in pressure between each of the equally spaced vertical tubes is the same.

The decrease in fluid pressure along the tube reflects a cumulative energy loss, as predicted by the second law of thermodynamics.[4] Available energy decreases because frictional forces (flow resistance) oppose fluid flow. Frictional resistance to flow exists both within the fluid itself (viscosity) and between the fluid and the tube wall. Generally, the greater the viscosity of the fluid and the smaller the cross-sectional area of the tube, the greater is the decrease in pressure along the tube.

For any given tube length, **flow resistance** is defined as the constant of proportionality for an assumed linear relation between the pressure difference between the two points along the tube and the flow. The constant of proportionality (R) is simply the slope of the straight line relation:

$$R = \frac{\Delta(P_1 - P_2)}{\Delta\dot{V}}$$

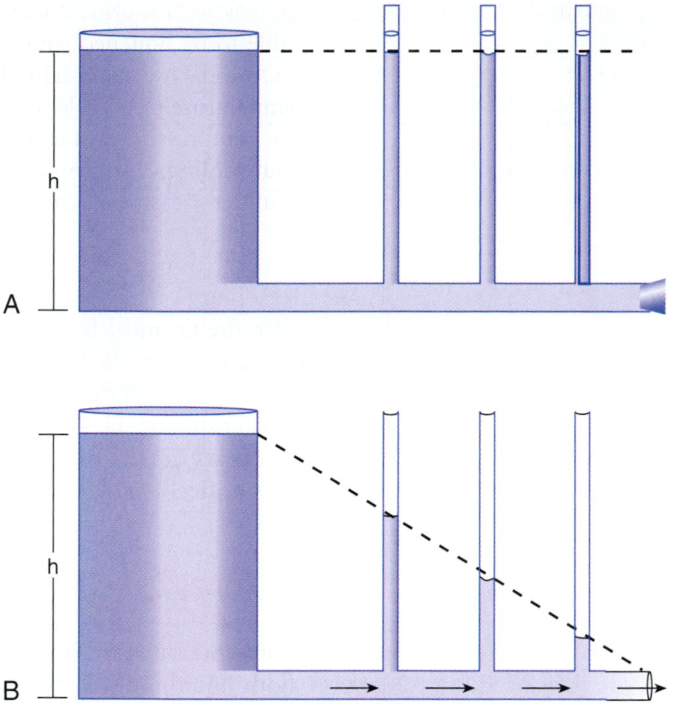

FIGURE 6-20 **A,** The pressure is the same at all points along the horizontal tube when there is no flow. **B,** A progressive decrease in pressure occurs as the fluid flows. (Modified from Nave CR, Nave BC: Physics for the health sciences, ed 3, Philadelphia, 1985, WB Saunders.)

where R is resistance (cm H_2O/L/sec, the most common units in pulmonary physiology), P_1 is the pressure (cm H_2O) at the upstream point (point 1), P_2 is the pressure at the downstream point (point 2), and $\dot{V}$ is the flow (L/sec). This equation has wide application in pulmonary physiology and respiratory care. The accompanying Mini Clini provides a good example of such application.

MINI CLINI

Differential Pressure Pneumotachometer

PROBLEM: It is often necessary to measure and record changes in airflow as a patient breathes. How can we apply the formula for resistance to measure and record airflow?

DISCUSSION: Airflow can be measured using a device called a *pneumotachometer*. One of the simplest designs is the differential pressure pneumotachometer. A differential pressure pneumotachometer incorporates a flow tube with a known and constant resistance. If the formula for resistance is rearranged to solve for flow, it appears as follows:

$$\Delta\dot{V} = k \times \Delta(P_1 - P_1)$$

Patterns of Flow

The pressure difference that results from flow also varies with the pattern of flow. There are three primary patterns of flow through tubes: laminar, turbulent, and transitional (Figure 6-21).

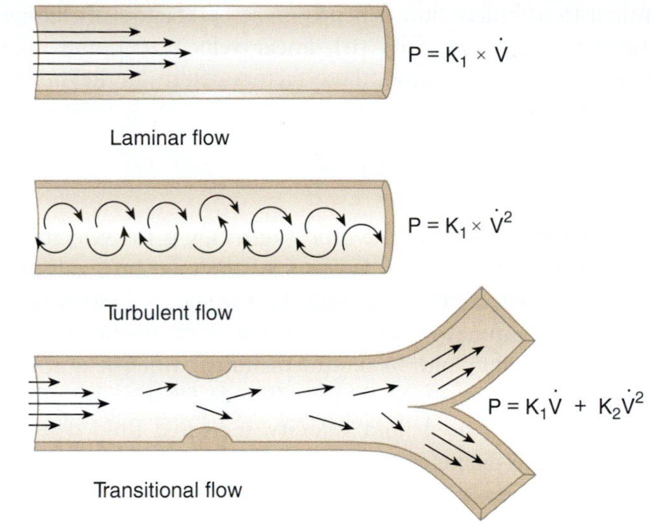

FIGURE 6-21 Three patterns of flow—laminar, turbulent, and transitional. (Modified from Moser KM, Spragg RG: Respiratory emergencies, ed 2, St Louis, 1982, Mosby.)

Laminar Flow

As discussed earlier, during laminar flow, a fluid moves in discrete cylindrical layers or streamlines (see Figure 6-6). The difference in pressure required to produce a given flow, under conditions of laminar flow through a smooth tube of fixed size, is defined by **Poiseuille's law**[12]:

$$P_1 - P_2 = \frac{8nL\dot{V}}{\pi r^4}$$

where P_1 is the pressure (dyne/cm^2; equal to 0.001 cm H_2O) at the upstream point (point 1), P_2 is the pressure at the downstream point (point 2), n is viscosity (dyne • sec/cm^2, called poise), L is length (cm), r is radius (cm) and $\dot{V}$ is the flow (cm^3/min = mL/min). The viscosity of air is approximately 1.9×10^{-4} poises; for water it is approximately 8.90×10^{-3} poises. A pressure of 1 cm H_2O is about 980 dyne/cm^2.

Occasionally flow resistance is expressed in terms of the Poiseuille equation as:

$$R = \frac{\Delta P}{\dot{V}} = \frac{8nL}{\pi r^4}$$

which indicates that resistance is very sensitive to changes in tube radius (e.g., doubling the tube radius decreases the resistance by a factor or $2^4 = 8$). Another way to view this is that increasing the tube radius by 19% will increase the flow by 100% (i.e., double the flow; $1.19^4 = 2.0$).

Turbulent Flow

Under certain conditions, the pattern of flow through a tube changes significantly, with a loss of regular streamlines. Instead, fluid molecules form irregular eddy currents in a chaotic pattern called **turbulent flow** (see Figure 6-21). This changeover from laminar to turbulent flow depends on several factors, including fluid density (d), viscosity (n), linear velocity (v), and tube radius (r). In combination, these factors determine **Reynold's number** (Re).

$$Re = \frac{\rho v d_h}{\mu}$$

where ρ is the density of the fluid (kg/m^3), v is the velocity of the fluid (m/sec), d_h is the diameter of the tube (m), and μ is the dynamic viscosity of the fluid [kg/(m • sec)]. Flow is considered to be laminar when Re is less than 2000, transient when it is between 2000 and 3000, and turbulent when it is above 3000. The equation shows that conditions favoring turbulent flow include increased fluid velocity, increased fluid density, increased tube diameter, and decreased fluid viscosity. In the presence of irregular tube walls, turbulent flow can occur when Re is less than 2000.

Flow through a tube with constant resistance is directly proportional to the pressure difference ($P_1 - P_2$) across the tube. By measuring this pressure difference we can measure flow. To ensure linearity between pressure and flow, the pneumotachometer is usually designed so that the flow pattern through the tube remains laminar, which simplifies calibration and use by having only one constant value for k.[13] The pneumotachometer is calibrated by measuring ($P_1 - P_2$) at different flows, plotting flow on the vertical axis and ($P_1 - P_2$) on the horizontal axis. Then, using linear regression, the calibration factor k is derived (this is essentially drawing a straight line through the data points and calculating the slope). When using the pneumotachometer, the pressure difference is multiplied by k to get the flow. This technique is at the heart of many pulmonary function laboratory procedures and is also used by some mechanical ventilators that have flow sensors at the airway opening portion of the patient circuit.

When flow becomes turbulent, Poiseuille's law no longer applies. Instead, the pressure difference across a tube is defined as follows:

$$P_1 - P_2 = \frac{fL\dot{V}^2}{4\pi^2 r^5}$$

where ΔP is the driving pressure, f is a friction factor based on the density and viscosity of the fluid and the tube wall roughness, L is the tube length, and $\dot{V}$ is the fluid flow.

Figure 6-22 compares the relationship between pressure and flow under laminar and turbulent conditions. As can be seen, when flow is laminar (Poiseuille's law), the relationship between driving pressure and flow is linear. However, when flow becomes turbulent, driving pressure varies with the square of the flow ($\dot{V}^2$). To double flow under laminar conditions, it is necessary to only double the driving pressure. To double flow under turbulent conditions, the driving pressure would be increased fourfold.

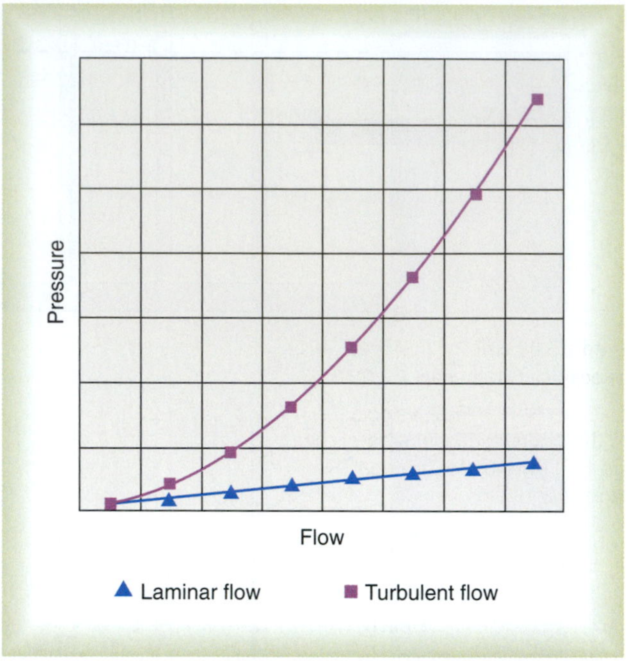

FIGURE 6-22 Relationship between driving pressure and flow under laminar and turbulent conditions.

Transitional Flow

Transitional flow is a mixture of laminar and turbulent flow. Flow in the respiratory tract is mainly transitional. When flow is transitional, the total driving pressure equals the sum of the pressures resulting from laminar and turbulent flow:

$$P_1 - P_2 = (k_1 \times \dot{V}) + (k_2 \times \dot{V}^2)$$

where k_1 and k_2 are factors indicating the respective contribution of laminar and turbulent flow to overall driving pressure. When flow is mainly laminar, the pressure varies linearly with the flow. When flow is mainly turbulent, driving pressure varies exponentially with the flow. With all else equal, pressures generated during laminar flow are most affected by fluid viscosity, whereas fluid density is the key factor when flow is turbulent.

Flow, Velocity, and Cross-Sectional Area

Clinically, the most common units of measurement describing flow are liters per minute (L/min) or liters per second (L/sec). In contrast, velocity is a measure of linear distance traveled by the fluid per unit of time. Centimeters per second (cm/sec) is a common velocity unit used in pulmonary physiology.

Although fluid flow and velocity are different measures, the two concepts are closely related. The key factor relating velocity to flow is the cross-sectional area of the conducting system. Figure 6-23 shows this relationship.

Throughout the tube, the fluid flows at a constant rate of 5 L/min. At *point A*, with a cross-sectional area of 5.08 cm^2, the velocity of the fluid is 16.4 cm/sec. At *point B*, the cross-sectional area of the tube decreases to 2.54 cm^2, half its prior value. At this point, the velocity of the fluid doubles to 32.8 cm/sec. At *point C*, the passage divides into eight smaller tubes. Although each tube is smaller than its "parent," together they provide a

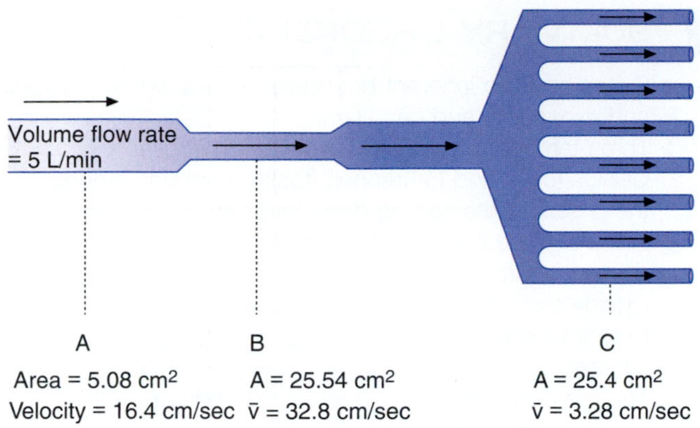

FIGURE 6-23 Fluid velocity, at a constant flow, varies inversely with the cross-sectional area of the tube. (Modified from Nave CR, Nave BC: Physics for the health sciences, ed 3, Philadelphia, 1985, WB Saunders.)

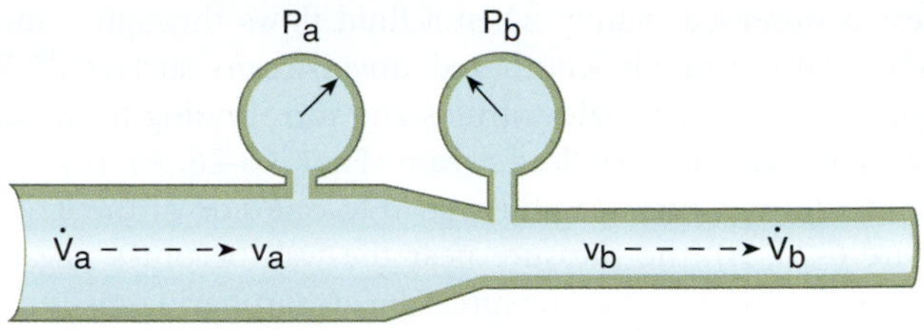

FIGURE 6-24 According to the Bernoulli theorem, lateral pressure of a flowing fluid must vary inversely with its velocity. $\dot{V}_a$, flow in tube "a"; v_a, velocity in tube "a"; v_b, velocity in tube "b"; $\dot{V}_b$, flow in tube "b"; P_a, lateral wall pressure in tube "a"; P_b, lateral wall pressure after restriction (see text).

10-fold increase in the cross-sectional area available for flow compared with *point B*. The velocity of the fluid decreases proportionately, from 32.8 cm/sec to 3.28 cm/sec.

These observations show that the velocity of a fluid moving through a tube at a constant flow varies inversely with the available cross-sectional area. This relationship is called the **law of continuity**. Mathematically, the equation is as follows:

$$(A_1 \times v_1) + (A_2 \times v_2) + (A_n \times v_n) = k$$

where A is the cross-sectional area of the tube; v is the velocity of the fluid; 1, 2, and n are different points in the tube; and k is a constant value.

Although the principle holds true only for incompressible liquids, the qualitative features are similar for gas flow. This principle also underlies the application of nozzles or jets in fluid streams. Nozzles and jets are simply narrow passages in a tube designed to increase fluid velocity. A garden-hose nozzle is a good example of this principle in action. Clinically, jets are used in many types of respiratory care equipment, including pneumatic nebulizers (see Chapter 39) and gas entrainment or mixing devices (see Chapter 41).

Bernoulli Principle

In a steady flow, the sum of all forms of energy in a fluid is the same at all points along the path of flow. Consequently, the sum of kinetic energy, potential energy, and internal energy remains constant. The Bernoulli principle states that an increase in the velocity of the fluid results in a decrease in the sum of its static pressure, potential energy, and internal energy.[11] The Bernoulli equation is:

$$p + \frac{1}{2}\rho v^2 + \rho g y = \text{constant}$$

where p = pressure at some point in a tube, ρ = fluid density, v = fluid velocity, g = acceleration due to gravity, and y = elevation of the pressure point above a reference plane. Figure 6-24 shows this relationship. Fluid is flowing through a tube at a point with a certain velocity (v_a) and a lateral pressure (P_a). According to the law of continuity, as the fluid moves into the narrow or constricted portion of the tube, its velocity must increase ($v_b > v_a$). According to the Bernoulli theorem, the higher velocity at point b should result in a lower lateral pressure at that point ($P_b < P_a$). As a fluid flows through the constriction, its velocity increases and its lateral pressure decreases.

This equation also helps demonstrate how heliox therapy works. The equation implies that the lower the density, the higher is the velocity (and hence flow) for the same inspiratory effort (driving pressure) or the lower is the pressure for the same velocity—either way that is a good effect for someone struggling to breathe.

Fluid Entrainment

Jet entrainment is the design principle used in simple O_2 masks with variable FiO_2 settings, although they are often mistakenly called *Venturi masks*. In this case, a pressurized gas, usually O_2, serves as the primary flow source. This pressurized gas passes through a nozzle or jet, beyond which is an air entrainment port (Figure 6-25, *A*). In this case, air entrainment occurs as a consequence of fluid viscosity. The viscous shearing force that exists between moving and static layers of gas causes the nonmoving gas (room air) to be dragged into the moving stream of O_2.[14] The amount of air entrained depends on both the diameter of the jet orifice and the size of the air entrainment ports. For a fixed jet size, the larger the entrainment ports, the greater is the volume of air entrained, the higher is the total flow, and the lower is the FiO_2 (see Figure 6-25, *B*). The entrained volume can still be altered, with fixed entrainment ports, by changing the jet diameter (see Figure 6-25, *C*). A large jet results in a lower gas velocity and less entrainment, whereas a small jet boosts velocity, entrained volume, and total flow.

Fluidics and the Coanda Effect

Fluidics is a branch of engineering that applies hydrodynamic principles in flow circuits for purposes such as switching, pressure and flow sensing, and amplification. Because fluidic devices have no moving parts, they are very dependable and require little maintenance.

The primary principle underlying most fluidic circuitry is a phenomenon called *wall attachment*, or the **Coanda effect**. This effect is observed mainly when a fluid flows through a small orifice with properly contoured downstream surfaces.[15] We know that a jet or nozzle entrains any surrounding fluid, such as air, into the primary flow stream (Figure 6-26, *A*). If a carefully contoured curved wall is added to one side of the jet (see Figure 6-26, *B*), the pressure near the wall becomes negative relative to atmospheric pressure. The atmospheric pressure on the other side of the gas stream pushes it against the wall, where it remains "locked" until interrupted by some counterforce. By carefully extending the wall contour, we can deflect the fluid stream through a full 180-degree turn.

Various fluidic devices can be designed using this principle, including on/off switches, pressure and flow sensors, and flow amplifiers. These individual components can be combined into *integrated fluidic logic circuits,* which function much like electronic circuit boards but without the need for electrical power.

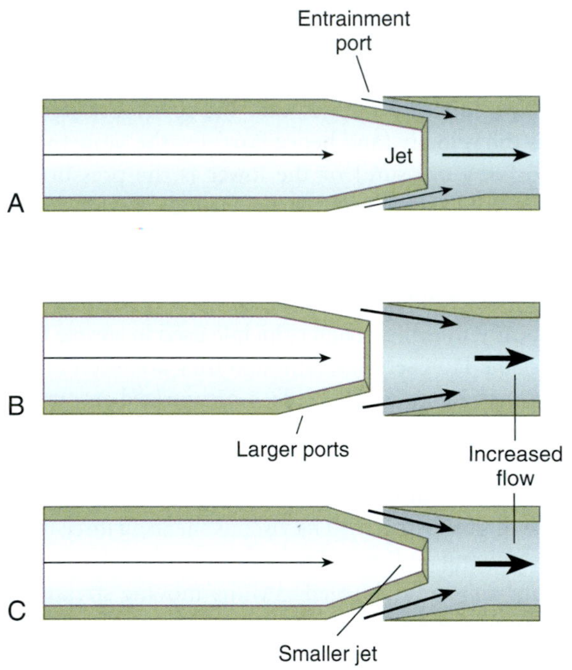

FIGURE 6-25 Air injector. **A,** Basic design. **B,** Greater entrainment and total flow occurs with larger entrainment ports. **C,** Alternatively, a smaller jet increases source gas velocity and entrains more air.

SUMMARY CHECKLIST

- Gases have no inherent boundary, are readily compressed and expanded, and can flow.
- Three temperature scales are in common use: Kelvin (SI), Celsius (cgs), and Fahrenheit (fps); conversion among these scale units can be done by using simple formulas.
- Transfer of heat energy can occur by conduction, convection, radiation, and evaporation.
- Liquids exert pressure and exhibit the properties of flow, buoyant force, viscosity, capillary action, and surface tension.
- The pressure exerted by a liquid depends on both its height (depth) and weight density.
- Surface tension forces increase the pressure inside a liquid drop or bubble; this pressure varies directly with the surface tension of the liquid and varies inversely with the radius.
- A liquid can vaporize by either boiling or evaporation; in evaporation, the required heat energy is taken from the air surrounding the liquid, cooling the air.
- Vaporization causing cooling and condensation causes warming of the surroundings.
- The capacity of air to hold water vapor increases with temperature.
- Relative humidity (RH) is the ratio of water vapor content (absolute humidity) to saturated water vapor capacity; for a constant content, cooling increases RH and warming decreases RH.
- The rate of diffusion of a gas is inversely proportional to its molecular weight.
- The total pressure of a mixture of gases must equal the sum of the partial pressures of all component gases.
- The volume of a gas that dissolves in a liquid equals its solubility coefficient times its partial pressure; high temperatures decrease gas solubility, and low temperatures increase gas solubility.
- Volume and pressure of a gas vary directly with temperature; however, with constant temperature, gas volume and pressure vary inversely.
- The critical temperature of a substance is the highest temperature at which it can exist as a liquid; gases with critical temperatures higher than room temperature can be stored under pressure as liquids without cooling.
- Under conditions of laminar flow, the difference in pressure required to produce a given flow is defined by Poiseuille's law.

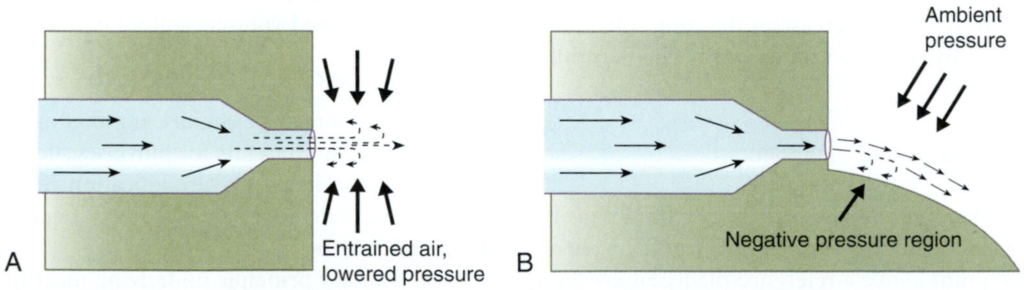

FIGURE 6-26 Coanda wall effect. **A,** Entrainment into the fluid stream. **B,** Wall attachment initiated by negative pressure near wall.

References

1. McNaught AD, Wilkinson A: *Compendium of chemical terminology, IUPAC Gold Book*, Oxford, 2010, Blackwell Scientific.
2. Debenedetti PG, Stillinger FH: Supercooled liquids and the glass transition. *Nature* 410:259–267, 2001.
3. Ojovan MI: Configurons: thermodynamic parameters and symmetry changes at glass transition. *Entropy* 10:334–364, 2008.
4. Leland TW, Jr: *Basic principles of classical and statistical thermodynamics*. https://www.uic.edu/labs/trl/1.OnlineMaterials/BasicPrinciplesByTWLeland.pdf. Accessed September 1, 2014.
5. International System of Units (SI), *Bureau International des Poids et Mesures (BIPM)*; 2006.
6. Cohen ER, Cvitas T, Frey JG, et al: *Quantities, units and symbols in physical chemistry, IUPAC Green Book*, ed 3, Cambridge, 2008, IUPAC & RSC.
7. Mohr PJ, Taylor BN, Newell DB: CODATA recommended values of the fundamental physical constants. *Rev Mod Phys* 84:1527–1605, 2012.
8. National Aeronautics and Space Administration (NASA) Animated Gas Lab: http://www.grc.nasa.gov/WWW/K-12/airplane/Animation/frglab.html. Accessed February 2011.
9. Thom SR: Hyperbaric oxygen: its mechanisms and efficacy. *Plast Reconstr Surg* 127:131S–141S, 2011.
10. West JB: Robert Boyle's landmark book of 1660 with the first experiments on rarified air. *J Appl Physiol* 98:31–39, 2004.
11. Eastlake CN: An aerodynamicist's view of lift, Bernoulli, and Newton. *Phys Teach* 40:166–176, 2002.
12. Chatburn RL, Craig KC: *Fundamentals of respiratory care research*, Norwalk, CT, 1988, Appleton & Lange, pp 91–97.
13. Comroe JH, Forster RE, DuBoise AB, et al: *The lung*, Chicago, 1977, Year Book Medical, pp 360–361.
14. Scacci R: Air entrainment masks: jet mixing is how they work—the Bernoulli and Venturi principles are how they don't. *Respir Care* 24:928–931, 1977.
15. Ginghina C: The Coanda effect in cardiology. *J Cardiovasc Med* 8:411–413, 2007.

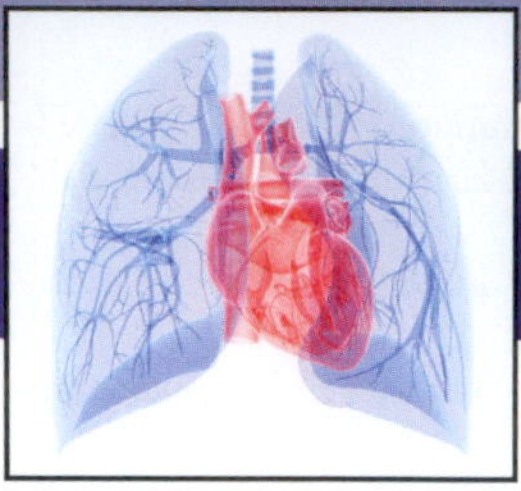

CHAPTER 7

E-Medicine in Respiratory Care

NARCISO E. RODRIGUEZ, ALBERT J. HEUER, AND MADHU SASIDHAR

CHAPTER OBJECTIVES

After reading this chapter you will be able to:

- Define electronic health records and their major uses in respiratory care.
- State the differences between the electronic health records and the electronic medical record.
- Identify the value of E-medicine applications in informatics and clinical decision support.
- Describe E-medicine applications in clinical care and management.
- Evaluate the trustworthiness and accuracy of health information sources.
- Describe major uses of E-medicine applications in health care administration.
- Outline steps to maintain security and confidentiality of electronic health records.
- Describe major E-medicine applications in respiratory care education and training.

CHAPTER OUTLINE

The Electronic Health Record and the Electronic Medical Record
- Computerized Physician Order Entry
- Enterprise Software Packages

Applications in Patient Care
- Applications in Diagnostics
- Applications in Treatment
- Applications in Disease Prevention

Informatics and Clinical Decision Support
- Business Intelligence
- Clinical Decision Support
- American Association for Respiratory Care Benchmarking System

Telemedicine and Telemonitoring

Sources of Health Information
- Health Information Sources for Respiratory Therapists and Other Clinicians
- Health Information Sources for Consumers

Applications in Health Care Administration
- Documentation, Workload, Staffing, and Scheduling
- Financial Management
- Quality Assurance
- Regulatory Compliance
- Web Analytics
- Human Resources
- Privacy and Confidentiality

Application in Training and Education
- Clinical Simulations
- Full-Scale Physiologic Clinical Simulators
- Clinical Education Applications
- National Board for Respiratory Care Credentialing
- Learning Management Systems

Future of E-Medicine

KEY TERMS

benchmarking
business intelligence
clinical decision support
clinical simulation
computerized physician order entry
continuing respiratory care education
continuous quality improvement
electronic health record
electronic medical record
enterprise software packages
E-medicine
health informatics
Health Information Technology for Economic and Clinical Health Act
information retrieval
key performance indicators
learning management systems
picture archiving and communication systems
point-of-care testing
root-cause analysis
telemedicine
telemonitoring
value-based purchasing

E-*Medicine* is the term that relates to the use of computerized or digital technology to enhance efficiency and effectiveness of health care in general and more specifically in patient care. E-Medicine was initially used to describe the use of basic computer applications in clinical care, recordkeeping, and health education. However, because of significant and wide-spread technologic advancements, the term *E-medicine* now refers to a wide array of hardware and software applications used in essentially every facet of health care. As a vital part of the patient care team, respiratory therapists (RTs) need to have an understanding of, and be proficient in, many aspects of E-medicine. This chapter describes digital applications related to electronic health records, direct clinical care, disease management, health care administration, health information sources, and training and education.

THE ELECTRONIC HEALTH RECORD AND THE ELECTRONIC MEDICAL RECORD

A transformation has taken place in the recent past whereby medical records formerly maintained primarily in paper form are now almost exclusively computerized and are maintained as part of the patient's **electronic health record** (EHR). A closely related but different term is the **electronic medical record** (EMR), which represents the computerized record produced every time the patient (or consumer) uses health services. The EHR is the sum of all EMRs produced by a patient during the different encounters with various health care entities throughout a lifetime. Unlike the EHR, which is owned by the patient, the EMR (the "chart") is owned by the hospital or health care delivery organization.[1] The terms EHR and EMR are so closely related that for simplicity we will use the term EHR to describe both concepts for the rest of this chapter.

Nonclinical information is also now electronic, such as patient demographics (e.g., age, gender, religion) and health insurance, as well as clinical information, including the patient's history and physical examination information, progress notes, physician orders, laboratory and other testing results, vital signs trending, and other information formerly found only in the hard-copy chart. This information is now readily available to authorized clinicians via secured personal computers and mobile devices. In addition to being able to access existing medical information, new records can be more readily entered making most EHRs more current than paper records. Medical imaging and laboratory tests generally become a part of the EHR immediately as the results are finalized. The net impact of these factors is that the EHR has helped make disease diagnosis quicker and more accurate by facilitating the efficient access of medical records.[2,3] EHRs are also proving to be a significant asset in the realm of patient treatment. When coupled with other computerized tools such as clinical decision support applications, EHRs have enhanced treatment and disease management, as discussed in more detail later. The core functions of EHRs are shown in Box 7-1.

Box 7-1 Core Functions of Electronic Health Records

- Medical records
- Results reporting
- Computerized physician order entry
- Clinical decision support
- Electronic communication
- Channels between health care providers and patients
- Patient-entered data

EHRs are more than a repository for medical records and patient-related information. EHRs are also a rich source of information that can be used in a variety of applications, including quality improvement and regulatory compliance, as detailed later in this chapter. EHRs also can serve as a vital source of data for conducting research, as discussed in Chapter 7 of this text.

Computerized Physician Order Entry

A subset of EHRs is the **computerized physician order entry** (CPOE) system. Through CPOEs, orders can be electronically transmitted to the EHR, saving time and reducing transcription errors resulting from handwriting clarity issues. Built in stopgaps and prescribing templates alert physicians about potential dosing problems and drug interaction concerns. The interfacing of CPOE systems with other hospital computer systems also alerts RTs and other clinicians of new, expired, or changed orders. Thus the CPOE has helped facilitate patient care and reduce medical errors.[4] All of these factors combined make both EHR and CPOE systems value-added features for health care organizations, clinicians, and patients alike. Indeed, EHRs and other computerized applications are helping transform medicine and enhancing both efficiency and effectiveness in essentially all aspects of health care and respiratory care.[5]

Enterprise Software Packages

An issue that had plagued health care organizations and our health care system involves the use of separate software packages for individual organizational functions, including but not limited to EHRs. In the past, the need for one such system to interface or "talk" to another was dealt with on an as-needed basis through ad-hoc software "patches." Over time these separate software packages, which were originally designed to stand alone or provide a specific or limited number of functions, became inefficient and much less able to meet the increasingly sophisticated and numerous requirements of health care organizations, including hospitals and departments within them. At about the same time that this problem was reaching critical proportions, the U.S. government (as part of a larger legislative initiative) passed the ***Health Information Technology for Economic and Clinical Health Act***, or the HITECH Act, as part of a national strategy for building a national health information infrastructure (Figure 7-1). Among other things, HITECH began providing incentives to hospitals, physicians, and other

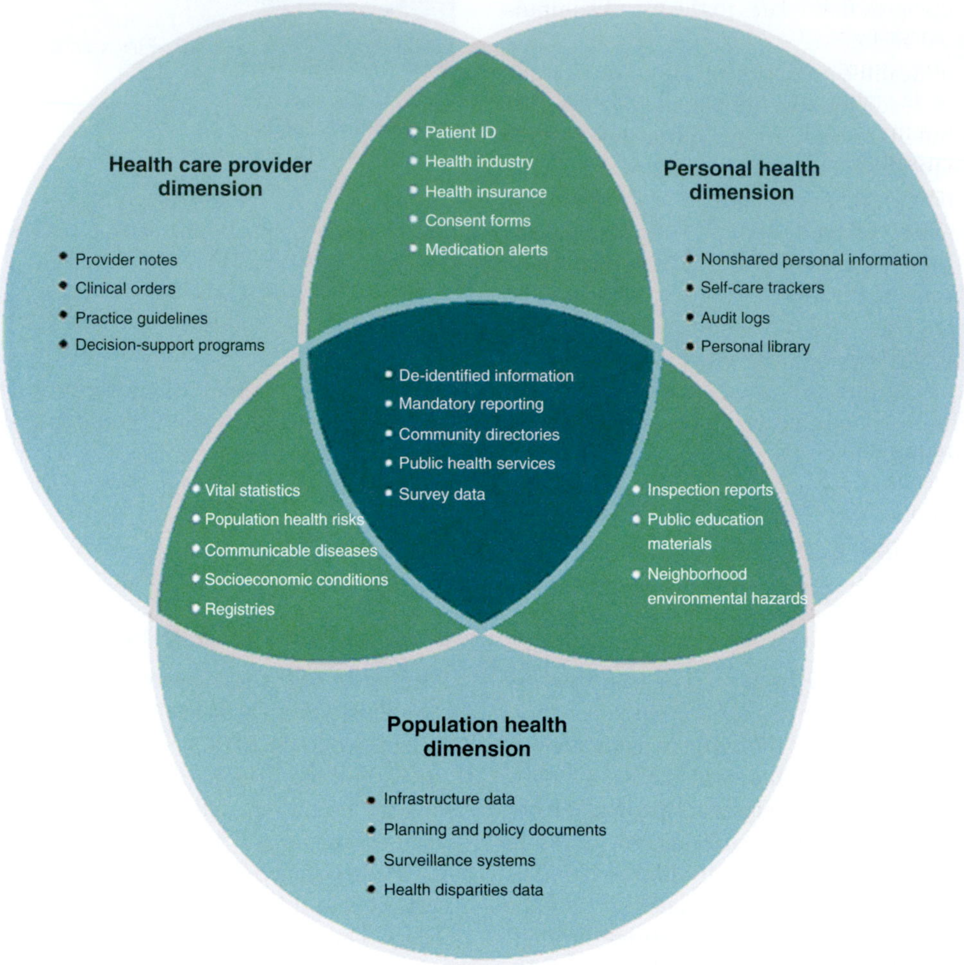

FIGURE 7-1 Electronic health records: dimensions of the national health information structure. (From U.S. Department of Health and Human Services. Information for health: a strategy for building the national health information infrastructure. http://aspe.hhs.gov/sp/NHII/Documents/NHIIReport2001/default.htm. Accessed September 25, 2006.)

health service providers who demonstrated that they are meaningfully using their EHRs by meeting predefined standards for a number of objectives. These objectives relate to the submission of patient data to authorized third-party surveillance registries, making clinical data more easily available to patients via secure Internet sources, including vital sign changes and office visit summaries, as well as interfacing multiple functions together, such as EHRs with CPOE.[6-8]

To address these issues, hospitals and other health care providers often now use a single comprehensive software system or **enterprise software package** designed to provide integrated functionality to enhance both efficiency and effectiveness, as well as comply with the HITECH Act. A variety of such software packages are available to health care organizations (Table 7-1). These include McKesson, Cerner, Epic, Meditech, Siemens, which are major vendors of integrated software for health care organizations.[7] In addition to serving as a secure repository for EHRs, these software packages provide integrated functionality for the use of EHR data for a multitude of purposes. Some purposes are for data input, such as what occurs when a

TABLE 7-1

Top Vendors of Enterprise Electronic Health Record Systems (February 2010 to February 2011)

Vendor	Location	Website
Cerner	Kansas City, MO	http://www.cerner.com
CPSI	Mobile, AL	http://www.cpsinet.com
Eclipsys	Atlanta, GA	http://www.allscripts.com
Epic Systems	Verona, WI	http://www.epic.com
Healthcare Management Systems	Nashville, TN	http://www.hmstn.com
Healthland	Minneapolis, MN	http://www.healthland.com
McKesson Provider Technologies	Alpharetta, GA	http://www.mckesson.com
Meditech	Westwood, MA	http://www.meditech.com
Siemens Healthcare	Malvern, PA	http://www.medical.siemens.com

Modified from Top vendors of enterprise EMR systems. Modern Healthc 41:35, 2011.

physician enters an order into a CPOE or an RT documents therapy given. Other purposes are for the retrieval, review, and interpretation of existing records, such as those used to provide direct patient care, or for nondirect care functions, such as billing, process improvement, regulatory reporting, or other similar functions discussed later in this chapter.[4] In addition, enterprise software systems that interface the EHRs with functions relevant to respiratory care and other clinical departments are almost universally in use.

APPLICATIONS IN PATIENT CARE

Applications in Diagnostics

Because the EHR contains an abundance of important clinical information, the RT needs to be able to promptly access and interpret key elements of it to assist the patient care team in accurately diagnosing the patient's condition. This may involve hemodynamic monitoring, blood gas and point-of-care testing, medical imaging applications, and pulmonary function testing (PFT), among others.

Hemodynamic Monitoring

In hemodynamic monitoring computers calculate cardiac output (CO), monitor intravascular fluid volume, and provide cardiac parameters and indices using both invasive and noninvasive applications. However, invasive methods using a pulmonary artery catheter (see Chapter 51) have a multitude of complications, including the risk for infection and death.

As a result, the rapid evolution of E-medicine has allowed for the development of safer noninvasive continuous cardiac output monitoring applications in perioperative and intensive care medicine. Some of these applications include thoracic electrical bioimpedance, thoracic bioreactance, vascular unloading technique, pulse wave transit time, and radial artery applanation tonometry. According to clinical studies, these technologies are capable of providing cardiac output readings noninvasively and continuously with minimal complications. Like most new technologies, their performance and accuracy needs further validation. These new applications might prove to be innovative tools for the assessment of advanced hemodynamic monitoring without the drawbacks of invasive techniques.[8] However, further discussion of these techniques is beyond the scope of this chapter.

Blood Gas Laboratories and Point-of-Care Applications

The accuracy and precision of blood gas data influence clinical decisions and patient safety. Computerized blood gas analyzers and computer-assisted quality assurance measures in a blood gas laboratory are crucial functions in a respiratory care department. Quality assurance data are necessary for accreditation of blood gas laboratories by the College of American Pathologists (CAP), the Clinical Laboratory Improvement Amendments (CLIA), and The Joint Commission (TJC). Blood gas laboratory applications interface analyzers with the patient's EHR to make blood gas results immediately available at the point of care and alert the clinician of critical results. Additionally, this interfacing enables the storage, retrieval, billing, and quality assurance of the blood gas analyzer data.

Point-of-care testing (POCT) refers to blood gas analysis performed at or near the site of a patient, in a setting that is different from a normal hospital clinical laboratory. POCT testing reduces the time required to produce blood gas test results (turnaround time) and thus improves clinical care and decision making for the clinician. POCT applications integrate seamlessly with the EHR allowing for immediate reporting of results and flagging of critical values. POCT applications can be used in a variety of clinical settings, including the operating room, critical care unit, emergency department (ED), maternity unit, and outpatient clinic.[9]

Medical Imaging and Picture Archiving and Communication Systems

Chest imaging (see Chapter 21), is critical in the practice of pulmonary and critical care medicine. Likewise, remote access of a patient's imaging studies has become an important element in the delivery of care. Clinical integration of all these imaging modalities with the EHR is essential for the RT and other clinicians to help in the diagnosis of the pulmonary patient and to improve patient care and safety. A **picture archiving and communication system** (PACS) is an application that allows for imaging storage, portability, communication, and clinical integration of all imaging modalities with the EHR.[10] Technologic advances in E-medicine and computer applications have allowed for PACS enterprise systems to flourish. In addition to the advantages mentioned earlier, current PACS applications have enhanced medical treatment and research by providing a variety of digital tools for the manipulation and interpretation of radiologic images, including three-dimensional imaging and three-dimensional printing technology.

Pulmonary Function Testing and Interpretation

Essentially all of the older volume displacement and spirograph pulmonary function test (PFT) systems have been replaced by those that use computer interfaces to measure and interpret the results. Similarly, most hospitals interface their PFT systems with the EHR, which allows clinicians to access reports and graphics from multiple workstations and remote devices.

Interpretation of Pulmonary Function Tests

Computer algorithms use standard reference predicted values to aid in the interpretation of PFTs, including spirometry, lung volume, diffusing capacity, and bronchodilator response. The algorithms compare the patterns of the patient's measured values with reference values based on age, height, gender, and race. The computer classifies the patterns of the patient's measured values as either normal or abnormal with degrees of severity. However, qualified interpreters must consider the effect of patient effort and other factors on the computer-assisted interpretation of PFTs.

The American Thoracic Society has recommended pulmonary function reference standards based on the National Health and Nutrition Examination Survey. These standards for prediction of normal PFT values may differ from other reference values. This difference can confound the interpretation of successive PFTs in an individual patient when clinicians focus on the computer-assisted interpretation of percent-of-predicted values, rather than the actual observed values.[11] Clinicians should have a clear understanding of which reference values were used for each test and interpret PFT results accordingly.

MINI CLINIC

Computer-Assisted Interpretations of Pulmonary Function Tests in an Individual Patient

PROBLEM: A patient with alpha$_1$-antitrypsin deficiency has repeat PFTs, including a diffusing capacity of the lung for carbon monoxide (DLCO). Based on a computer-assisted interpretation, there appears to be a remarkable decrease in the percent-of-predicted value for DLCO. It was previously normal; now it is 68% of predicted, indicative of emphysema. An effective therapy, pooled human plasma alpha$_1$-antitrypsin, is available but expensive. What additional information should the clinician evaluate?

DISCUSSION: The clinician should determine (1) the actual observed DLCO values of the previous and repeat test and (2) whether the computer-assisted interpretations are based on different reference values among the tests. If the computer-assisted percent-of-predicted values for each test were based on different sets of reference values, it could account for the change in DLCO. Further investigation of the results is warranted.

Applications in Treatment

Many current devices, therapies, and protocols developed in the last decade rely on technologic advances generated by E-medicine applications. These applications can be used in acute or nonacute settings by RTs to provide support and care for the pulmonary patient.

Applications in the Acute Care Setting

Mechanical Ventilators. Conventional mechanical ventilators use microprocessors to deliver and monitor modes of ventilation.[12] A "mode" of ventilation is a predetermined pattern of patient-ventilator interaction. Modes can be quite complex, as explained in detail in Chapter 45. Newer modes, such as neurally adjusted ventilatory assist (NAVA), aim to enhance the patient-ventilator synchrony via automation that is highly responsive to the patient.[13]

Microprocessors perform additional functions. They provide for graphic outputs and touch screens and interfaces; they also control ventilator alarms and archive the history of set and measured values, which can be uploaded to a computer. Current conventional ventilators allow for updating and adding new modes of ventilation via software updates, rather than purchasing new ventilators.

Protocols for ventilator weaning and management of certain respiratory conditions (e.g., acute respiratory distress syndrome) coupled with the trending capabilities of today's microprocessor ventilators can improve patients' outcomes and decrease length of stay. Complete, accurate, and consistent documentation of ventilator settings is key to achieve these goals. However, manual ventilator charting is frequently incomplete, inaccurate, and inconsistent, particularly regarding nomenclature.[14] Computerized ventilator charting applications have the potential to improve the quality and consistency of ventilator charting, especially when fully integrated with the patient's EHR. Automated ventilator charting, verified by RTs, takes ventilator charting a step further, with the potential to improve completeness, accuracy, consistency, and efficiency.[15] Figure 7-2 is an example of a computer screen for automated charting.

Therapist-Driven Protocols. Evidence-based, therapist-driven protocols can improve health outcomes.[16] Under medical supervision and based on patient assessment, RTs use protocols to allocate and titrate respiratory care. Consistency and timeliness of implementation are keys to the effectiveness of protocols. Automation of protocols at the point of care can help RTs address these concerns. An automated protocol for discontinuation of the mechanical ventilation program on hand-held devices can decrease the time to the first spontaneous breathing trial and the length of stay in the intensive care unit (ICU) compared with a protocol without automation.[17] These protocols allow the RTs to enter information about each mechanically ventilated patient via a hand-held device throughout the shift. When the patients meet preset criteria, the computer application prompts the RTs to conduct a spontaneous breathing trial to help determine the patient's readiness for ventilator discontinuation.

Applications in Nonacute Care Settings and Chronic Diseases

Management of chronic diseases presents a serious challenge to the U.S. health care system. As of 2012, approximately half of all adults—117 million people—have one or more chronic health conditions. One of four adults has two or more chronic health conditions.[18] Of the top 10 causes of death in 2010, 7 were chronic diseases. Two of these chronic diseases—heart disease and cancer—together accounted for nearly 48% of all deaths.[19] Chronic disease is present in 8 of 10 Americans on Medicare, and 84% of all health care spending in 2006 was for the 50% of the population who have one or more chronic medical conditions.[20] As baby boomers continue to age, the proportion of the U.S. population 65 years old and older is expected to double. There is much interest in optimizing chronic disease management through advances in E-medicine technologies to improve health outcomes in a cost-effective manner. This is particularly noteworthy given the focus by the U.S. government on reducing short-term (within 30 days) hospital readmissions. Hospitals have begun being penalized for

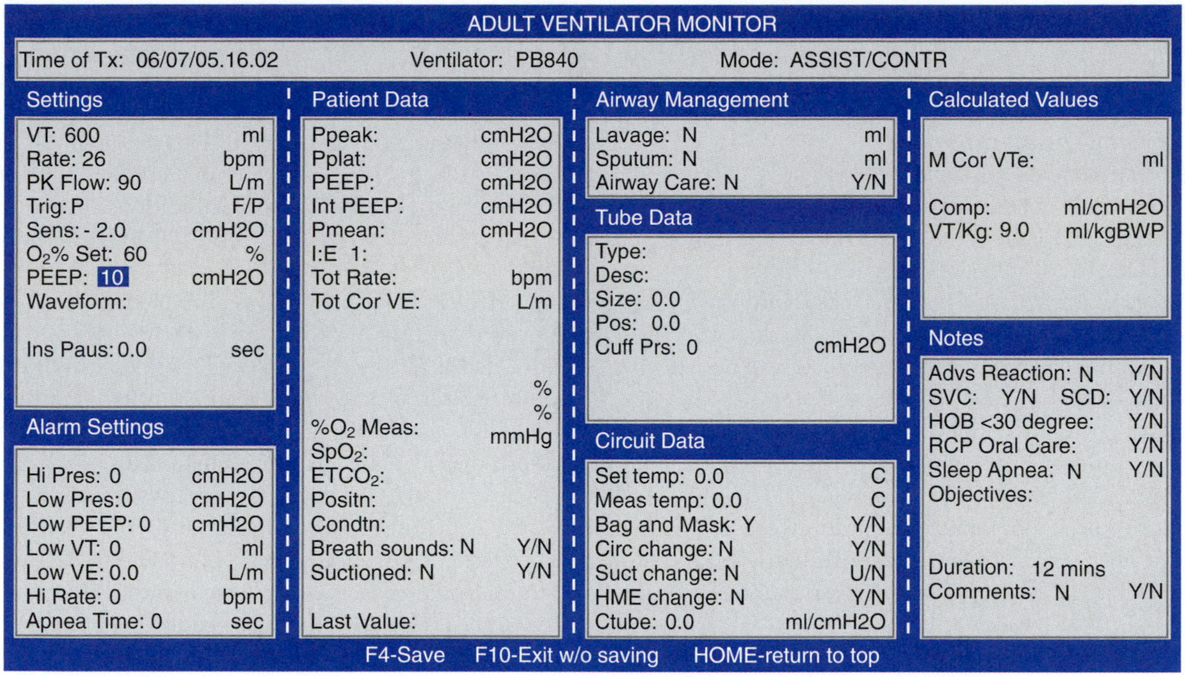

FIGURE 7-2 Automated ventilator charting.

excessive short-term readmissions for their patients with certain conditions, including chronic obstructive pulmonary disease (COPD). To address this initiative, hospitals and other health care providers have developed an array of protocols to address the main reasons for such readmissions. These protocols often emphasize patient and family education and follow-up and often use computer applications to help accomplish this.[21,22]

Asthma. E-Medicine applications for asthma include interactive Internet applications, such as games for children, web applications linked to cell phones for personalized or automated voice or text messaging, and other telemonitoring applications. Many of these applications use monitored patient data to tailor the adjustment to the plan of care. Some provide for personalized goals, calendars, and reminders. Educational tools include audiovisuals, games, and quizzes. In patients with persistent asthma, evidence from research studies shows that these E-medicine applications can result in an improvement in asthma knowledge, self-management skills, peak flow rates, and adherence to inhaled corticosteroid controller medications and fewer symptoms, missed school days, nighttime awakenings, activity limitations, ED visits, and hospitalizations.[23-26] These applications are generally well received by patients.[24]

Chronic Obstructive Pulmonary Disease. Increasingly, COPD is being managed in the home. Web-based telemonitoring systems, smartphones, and mobile phones with computer applications extend the reach of health care providers into the home. E-Medicine applications for patients with COPD facilitates education, self-management, and timely feedback from health care providers (Figure 7-3). Patients generally have a positive attitude about the role of this technology, and the quality of the transmitted data is generally good.[27] Improved outcomes include earlier identification of deteriorating symptoms, better response to exacerbations, increased rate of sustained exercise after pulmonary rehabilitation and decreased ED visits and hospitalizations.[27-29] Additionally, E-medicine applications can help detect comorbidities, such as sleep apnea.[27]

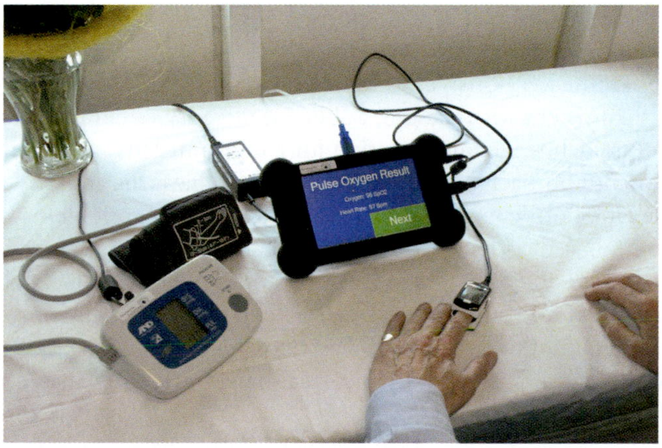

FIGURE 7-3 Telehealth Homepod. (Courtesy Tele Health Ltd. Dublin, Ireland.)

Applications in Disease Prevention

As explained earlier, through HITECH, the federal government has committed unprecedented resources to supporting the adoption and use of EHRs.[30] HITECH's goal is not adoption alone but "meaningful use" of EHRs—that is, their use by providers to achieve significant improvements in care. Payments by third-party payers to health service providers are specifically tied to the achievement of advances in health care processes and outcomes. Disease prevention and patient education are intrinsically part of these processes.

Treatment of Tobacco Use and Dependence

In the United States, tobacco use and dependence is the leading preventable cause of death and chronic diseases.[31] Health care costs attributable to tobacco use are quite significant. Effective evidence-based treatments are available, but their implementation by health care providers is lagging.[32] RTs can play a vital role in the treatment of tobacco-related diseases and are now using E-medicine as an aid to help tobacco users.

E-Medicine, including phone-based applications, provides exciting new components of treatment for tobacco use and dependence. With the extensive reach of the Internet and the demonstrated efficacy of some applications, the potential impact on health outcomes is immense. More than 10 million Internet users have searched for online information about how to quit smoking.[33]

Internet-based treatment programs can recruit tobacco users via search engines, or they can be an adjunct to telephone *quitline* counseling. Figure 7-4 shows the smokefree.gov tobacco treatment website. When E-medicine applications are tailored to individual tobacco users, with frequent automated contacts via e-mail or text messages, rates of long-term abstinence from tobacco use are similar to those with traditional evidenced-based interventions.[33-36]

Consistent with the U.S. Public Health Service clinical practice guideline recommendation for a high-intensity, multicomponent approach, web-based applications have the capacity to provide both counseling that promotes tailored quit strategies and tobacco cessation medications that have been approved by the U.S. Food and Drug Administration.[37] These applications can provide sustained access to virtually limitless numbers of participants and are therefore very cost-effective. Table 7-2 lists some websites related to the treatment of tobacco use and dependence.

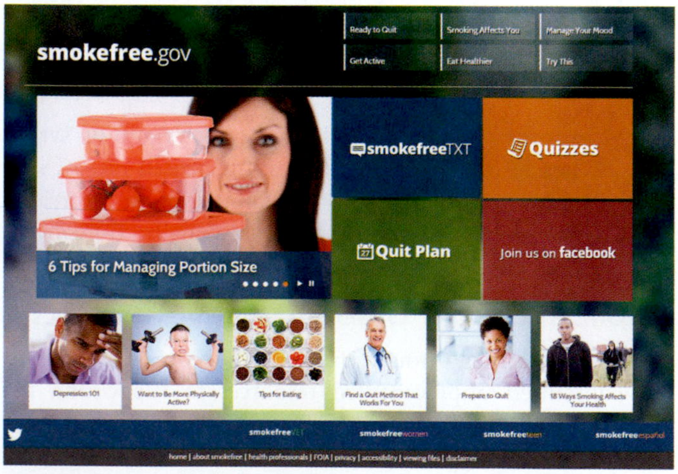

FIGURE 7-4 Example of a web-based tobacco cessation resource. (From http://smokefree.gov.)

Education of the Public and Health Care Consumer

Today's savvy health care consumers understand that access to good information is essential to health-related decision making. The Pew Internet and American Life Project found that more than 80% of Internet users report seeking health information online; for those with chronic conditions, the rate is 86%.[38] Those percentages will most likely increase over the coming years.

E-Medicine applications offer unique public access to health education materials through the use of a variety of interactive tools such as websites, videos and graphics, chat rooms, e-mail, games, social media, and so on, through any web-enabled device. RTs should not underestimate the impact of these applications on public health education and disease prevention.

The amount of data available on health-related and wellness-related issues increases exponentially each year. RTs play an important role in helping their pulmonary patients assess accurate information found on E-medicine applications. Box 7-2 lists the factors to consider when educating pulmonary patients on evaluating the worthiness of E-medicine sources.[39]

INFORMATICS AND CLINICAL DECISION SUPPORT

Health informatics, which refers to the use of information technology in health care, combines advances in computer science and technology to improve clinical care, manage the health of populations, and accelerate research.

Business Intelligence

Business intelligence refers to a set of tools that permit capture, storage, and transformation of data into useful and actionable information. In health care, business intelligence tools are used to capture and integrate clinical data with relevant financial and

TABLE 7-2
Websites Related to the Treatment of Tobacco Use and Dependence

Organization	Website
Association for the Treatment of Tobacco Use and Dependence	http://www.ATTUD.org
Centers for Disease Control and Prevention	http://www.cdc.gov/tobacco/quit_smoking/
International Tobacco Control Policy Evaluation Project	http://www.ITCProject.org
QuitNet	http://www.quit.com/
U.S. Department of Health and Human Services	http://www.SmokeFree.gov
U.S. Surgeon General's Office	http://www.Surgeongeneral.gov/initiatives/tobacco/
Society for Research on Nicotine and Tobacco	http://www.TreaTobacco.net
Tobacco Free Kids	http://www.TobaccoFreeKids.org
World Health Organization, Tobacco Free Initiative	http://www.WHO.int/tobacco

Box 7-2 Factors to Consider When Reviewing E-Medicine Sources

- Web address:
  - .com—A website most likely to a for-profit company
  - .org—A website most likely from a nonprofit organization
  - .edu—A website published by an educational institution such as a university
  - .go—A web page that belongs to a governmental organization
- When assessing credibility, consider the following:
  - Who are the authors?
  - What are their credentials?
  - Is there a hidden agenda?
  - Who published the information?
  - Is the information peer reviewed?
- When assessing accuracy, consider the following:
  - Is the information current?
  - Is the information supported by facts?
  - Is the information based on scientific evidence?
  - Is the original source listed?
  - Do other sources back up the information?
- Red flags to consider:
  - Anonymous information.
  - There appears to be a conflict of interest.
  - The information presented is one-sided or biased.
  - The information is outdated.
  - There is a claim of a miracle or secret cure.
  - No evidence is cited.
  - The grammar is poor and words are misspelled.

operational data. **Key performance indicators** (KPIs) are indicators of quality and efficiency that are selected based on reporting or operational requirements. Commercially available business intelligence systems allow KPIs to correlate with dimensions that typically include person, time, place, and so forth. For example, a hospital may be interested in ventilator-associated pneumonia (VAP) events. In this case, KPIs may include daily ventilator census and incidence of VAP, which are then correlated with dimensions such as practitioners involved in the care of the patient before the event, hospital unit, date of VAP, and so on. This allows an institution to not only report on the aggregate rate of VAP but also recognize patterns relating to specific units and caregivers. Business intelligence also can be quite useful in research, especially in accessing data for retrospective clinical studies, as discussed in Chapter 8.

Clinical Decision Support

Clinical decision support (CDS) has been defined as "Health information technology functionality that builds upon the foundation of an EHR to provide persons involved in care processes with general and person-specific information, intelligently filtered and organized, at appropriate times, to enhance health and health care."[40,41] Examples of CDS include computerized alerts and reminders, such as notification to a therapist that the selected tidal volume exceeds the recommended range for a patient, based on ideal weight and calculated using a previously recorded height measurement. CPOE systems, discussed elsewhere in this chapter, frequently incorporate decision support alerts for drug-drug interactions and drug-allergy reactions. More advanced implementations may include examples of drug-disease interactions, such as when the selected drug dose is high for a patient whose latest creatinine value indicates renal impairment. More complex clinical guidelines, such as for weaning from mechanical ventilation, may be embedded within the EHR system. Condition-specific order sets, such as "care paths" for patients admitted with COPD, can guide the caregivers to ensure provision of evidence-based care.

Documentation templates are frequently used for decision support where rules are embedded into the logic behind the templates. As an example, a template for charting may direct the therapist to chart breath sounds and then subsequently direct them to record the type of sounds and location in the chest. Similar directions also may be used to prompt the RT for volume and flow settings for volume control modes of ventilation versus pressure and inspiratory time for pressure control modes.

Summaries of patient data and patient lists created based on specific criteria are other examples of decision support. For example, a work list may summarize patients who have been on noninvasive ventilation longer than a specified time and are therefore appropriate candidates for evaluation for skin breakdown. There is also increasing use of contextual reference information within the EHR, using links to internal or external resources for additional information. Examples of this include reference links to internally hosted protocol documents from order sets and links to external web-based content providers such as UpToDate.

Evidence Supporting Clinical Decision Support

Several studies have evaluated the usefulness of CDS in patient care. CDS has demonstrated value in identifying high-risk patients using blood gas and laboratory results,[42-44] as a diagnostic aid and in early identification of patients for intervention.[45,46] Knowledge-based systems have been shown to improve outcomes such as length-of-stay after myocardial infarction[47] and weaning from mechanical ventilation.[48]

Mobile Applications

Increasingly, mobile applications are being used to not only provide information to users but also capture health care data. Applications such as AirStrip allow remote users to visualize streaming vitals sign data and graphics. At the consumer level, mobile applications are driving consumer engagement via telehealth, consumer education, and health applications that use mobile devices as a data collection tool.

Administrative Decision Support

Administrative decision support using electronic data takes two main forms, which could be considered as external and internal benchmarking. External benchmarking is most prominently represented by the American Association for Respiratory Care (AARC) Benchmarking System, which facilitates identification and adoption of best practices among similar respiratory care departments. Internal benchmarking is exemplified by the hospital business review process. This form of benchmarking involves the creation and tracking of relevant quality and productivity metrics to inform internal process improvement activities.

American Association for Respiratory Care Benchmarking System

In the 1950s, the Xerox corporation invented a process called **benchmarking** as a way to identify and adopt best practices that have developed among similar organizations.[49] In 1989 Robert Camp wrote one of the first textbooks on benchmarking,[50] outlining four basic steps (1) know your operation, (2) know the industry leaders or competitors, (3) incorporate the best, and (4) gain superiority.

Early in 2006, the leadership of the AARC, recognizing the need to establish a valid benchmarking resource for respiratory care, created an official benchmarking website designed for respiratory care department managers (http://www.respiratorybenchmarking.org). Anyone can visit the site and take advantage of educational resources (from the Site Navigation drop-down menu). Department managers who are members (i.e., have a paid subscription to the AARC benchmarking system) may enter their department's profile, including information on structure and function as well as personal contact information, although an anonymous option is provided.[51] Next, managers enter productivity data on a monthly basis. This activity builds the communal database from which benchmarking reports are generated by all members.

Best practices are identified using reports. A manager creates a report based on a "compare group" comprising several other departments that are similar in structure and function. This compare group is identified by performing searches on the database using various criteria from the profile and studying the profiles of the departments matching those criteria. The report has two sections. The first section gives numeric values for various productivity metrics[52] (definitions are available on the AARC benchmarking website) that indicate the department's percentile ranking. The manager is given the option of entering a desired percentile ranking, and the report will then calculate the opportunity (both in terms of dollars and number of staff positions) associated with improving the percentile ranking. The second section of the report is a list of all the departments in the compare group ranked according to percentile[53] on each of the productivity metrics. This section of the report allows the department manager to identify the top performers. The next step for the manager is to study the profiles and monthly productivity data of the top performers to find clues about how they are achieving best practices. The manager is also encouraged to contact the top performers personally to ask questions.

The AARC Benchmarking System has grown and evolved since its inception and continues to provide essential information to forward-thinking managers. It is a valuable tool for maintaining a completive advantage in the ever more demanding economic environment of U.S. health care.

Research

Research is based on data (facts) that can be transformed into information (facts that answer questions). Thus any of the sources of data described earlier are potential research tools. Online databases provide both the framework and content for designing research studies (e.g., PubMed). Private databases (e.g., productivity and hospital business review resources) support internal process improvement initiatives.[54,55] These issues are discussed in more detail in Chapter 8.

TELEMEDICINE AND TELEMONITORING

Telemedicine refers to the use of electronic and telecommunication technologies to support health care at a geographically different location from the patient, increasing access to specialty and patient care. Telemedicine can allow for the evaluation, diagnosis, treatment, monitoring, triage, consultation, and follow-up of patients without travel.[56,57] According to the Centers for Medicare and Medicaid Services (CMS), telemedicine seeks to improve a patient's health by permitting two-way, real-time interactive communication between the patient and the physician or practitioner at the distant site. This electronic communication means the use of interactive computerized telecommunications equipment that generally includes audio and video equipment. Telemedicine is viewed as a cost-effective alternative to the more traditional in-person way of providing medical care, such as face-to-face consultations or examinations between the clinician and patient.[58] A form of telemedicine is **telemonitoring,** which involves the use of telecommunications and information technology to provide access to health assessment, diagnosis, intervention, consultation, supervision, and information across distance.

Although best-practices in this area are still emerging, telemedicine and telemonitoring are gaining ground in respiratory care and in the overall management of all type of patients, including those with pulmonary disease. In some cases, it has facilitated the timely diagnosis and treatment of patients with limited access to health care facilities. In particular, patients in remote geographic locations or those with limited mobility such as ventilator-dependent individuals with severe neuromuscular disease have benefited from telemedicine.[59] Computer interfaces for telemonitoring facilitate patient assessment through the two-way transmission of key clinical data such as vital signs, pulmonary function measures, and patient-ventilator data and even the patient's physical appearance captured by computer web cameras. Similar monitoring also can facilitate the early detection of and intervention for any deterioration in a patient's condition. Such inventions have been shown to be helpful in reducing doctor visits and hospital admissions, a benefit to the patient and to the economics of health care.[60]

In addition, telemedicine has proved useful in facilitating the patient's participation in computer-based disease management programs. In particular, selected telemedicine applications have been created that bundle patient education, disease management, interactive communication, and other features. Such multipronged systems have been shown to be effective in helping reduce chronic disease exacerbations and enhance the daily functioning and quality of life of patients with asthma and COPD, as discussed earlier in this chapter.[61] Other telemedicine programs have shown promise in helping overcome logistical barriers such as transportation and scheduling that too often prevent individuals from participating in valuable disease management programs. In particular, telemedicine has helped facilitate the participation of COPD patients in remote access pulmonary rehabilitation programs in which they otherwise would not have been able to participate. Furthermore, their participation in such computer-aided rehabilitation programs has permitted these patients to achieve similar benefits associated with traditional rehabilitation programs (see Chapter 55), such as demonstrable enhancement in their tolerance for activities of daily living.[62]

Like many aspects of E-medicine, telemedicine seems to be in its infancy. As health care resource limitations and cost-containment pressures continue, as well as improvements in the applications and the efficiencies they offer, it appears inevitable that use of this and related technologies will expand and become commonplace in health care and more specifically in respiratory care.

SOURCES OF HEALTH INFORMATION

Considering that almost half of adults in the United States have limited health literacy, E-medicine applications have the potential to improve our patients' level of health literacy if used appropriately.[63] Low health literacy compromises patient safety, limits the overall quality of health care, and accounts for increased health care costs. When patients have poor knowledge about their disease and the management of it, positive outcomes become more difficult to achieve.[64]

Health Information Sources for Respiratory Therapists and Other Clinicians

Effective **information retrieval** is essential to evidence-based respiratory care. It enhances clinical expertise by providing information for the development of evidence-based, therapist-driven protocols, and it aids in clinical decision making for the clinician. Although assessment skills of RTs generally sharpen with experience, their knowledge of the most up-to-date therapies may diminish over time.[65] However, the best available medical evidence is dynamic rather than static and the amount of available information is staggering. RTs need to be knowledgeable about efficient ways to access, filter, and retrieve relevant information effectively. They also must be prepared to guide increasingly sophisticated patients, many of whom actively seek medical information on the Internet.

E-Medicine applications are a far-reaching, rich source of information. RTs can use search engines such as PubMed, MEDLINE, and Google Scholar to access, filter, and retrieve information effectively. RTs can "bookmark" helpful websites, manuscripts and other sources for clinical practice guidelines, evidence-based systematic reviews of clinical questions, accrediting agencies, or other relevant sources of important information (Table 7-3).

TABLE 7-3
Helpful websites for Respiratory Therapists

Organization	Website
American Academy of Allergy, Asthma, and Immunology	http://www.aaaai.org
American Academy of Pediatrics	http://www.aap.org
American Academy for Sleep Medicine	http://www.aasmnet.org
American College of Allergy, Asthma, and Immunology	http://www.acaai.org
American Association for Respiratory Care	http://www.aarc.org
American Cancer Society	http://www.cancer.org
American College of Chest Physicians	http://www.chestnet.org
American Heart Association	http://www.heart.org
American Lung Association	http://www.lung.org
American Thoracic Society	http://www.thoracic.org
ARDS Network	http://www.ardsnet.org
Centers for Disease Control and Prevention	http://www.cdc.gov
Cochrane Collaboration	http://www.cochrane.org
Committee on Accreditation for Respiratory Care	http://www.coarc.com
Cystic Fibrosis Foundation	http://www.cff.org
Global Initiative for COPD	http://www.goldcopd.com
National Board for Respiratory Care	http://www.nbrc.org
National Heart, Lung, and Blood Institute	http://www.nhlbi.nih.gov/health-pro
Society for Critical Care Medicine	http://www.sccm.org
U.S. Surgeon General	http://www.surgeongeneral.gov

Health Information Sources for Consumers

As discussed earlier, patients increasingly seek knowledge about diseases and treatments on their own. However, many users neglect to scrutinize the quality or source of the information, which is largely unregulated. Selected resources for pulmonary patients are listed in Table 7-4 and include the AARC website for patients (http://www.yourlunghealth.org), the websites of the National Lung Health Education Program (http://www.nlhep.org) dedicated to COPD patients, and MedlinePlus.gov of the National Library of Medicine. MedlinePlus features online interactive tutorials, practical instructional handouts for patients, a medical encyclopedia, and videos of surgical procedures.

APPLICATIONS IN HEALTH CARE ADMINISTRATION

E-Medicine applications also play an integral role in helping respiratory care managers and leaders maximize the value they

TABLE 7-4
Helpful Websites for Pulmonary Patients

Organization	Website
Medical Associations	
American Academy of Allergy, Asthma, and Immunology	http://www.aaaai.org
American Academy for Sleep Medicine	http://www.aasmnet.org
American College of Chest Physicians	http://www.chestnet.org
American Thoracic Society	http://www.thoracic.org
Society of Critical Care Medicine	http://www.sccm.org
Patient Education and Support Organizations	
American Association for Respiratory Care	http://www.aarc.org http://www.yourlunghealth.org
American Heart Association	http://www.heart.org/heartorg
American Lung Association	http://www.lungusa.org
Cystic Fibrosis Foundation	http://www.cff.org
COPD Foundation	http://www.copdfoundation.org/
Global Initiative for COPD	http://www.goldcopd.com
Healthways	http://www.QuitNet.com
National Lung Health Education Program	http://www.nlhep.org
SmokeFree: U.S. Department of Health and Human Services	http://www.SmokeFree.gov
Government Agencies	
Centers for Disease Control and Prevention	http://www.cdc.gov
Food and Drug Administration (FDA)	http://www.fda.gov
National Heart, Lung, and Blood Institute (NHLBI)	http://www.nhlbi.nih.gov
National Institutes of Health (Medline)	http://www.nlm.nih.gov/medlineplus/
National Library of Medicine	http://www.nlm.nih.gov/

add to their health care organizations. In addition to the benchmarking resources and business intelligence concepts described earlier in this chapter, there are other highly useful digital applications related to documentation, workload, and staffing; financial and quality management; human resources; regulatory compliance; and similar tools related to management and administration.

Documentation, Workload, Staffing, and Scheduling

Increasingly, the comprehensive software systems used by health care organizations, provide features that support department-specific functions, including those essential to respiratory care departments. These software packages enable respiratory care department managers and other authorized personnel to retrieve, sort, and use information-relevant managing strategic functions such as resource use, staffing, and financial management. In addition, such software systems can link these strategic functions with day-to-day operations, such as using hospital census (e.g., percentage occupancy) and acuity (e.g., average severity of illness) data, with how many RTs are needed during a given shift or other period to adequately handle such a patient load. These same data can be used by most such systems to calculate productivity of an individual RT or the department as a whole. Often such productivity results are expressed as a percentage of a certain benchmark or reference range. For example, if the productivity expectation for an RT to complete 24 aerosol treatments for an 8-hour shift (assuming no other workload), but because of several call-outs, the RT is assigned and completes 30 such treatments, then that therapist would have a productivity percentage of 30 (actual)/24 (assigned) or 125%. Figure 7-5 shows an example of a worksheet for workload calculation. These software packages also facilitate computerized documentation, including ventilator-patient monitoring or charting the delivery of all forms of respiratory therapy, through computers or remote devices interfaced with the EHR. These documentation systems not only provide a record of the care provided and patient's response, but are also interfaced with other facets of the comprehensive software platform, including those for billing and quality assurance.[66]

Financial Management

Computer hardware and software are universally used in the financial aspects of health care. The more predominant uses relate to financial accounting applications, including billing and accounts receivable, as well as managerial accounting functions, which encompass financial statement reporting, budgeting, and forecasting. A detailed description of each of these functions is beyond the scope of this text. Briefly, however, under the category of financial accounting, *accounts receivable* is a fancy term for billing for and monitoring of the reimbursement for services provided. Most of the billing to CMS and private health insurance providers and monitoring of such payments by hospitals is done through electronic software platforms. Often this process is facilitated by features within the health care organization's EHR system, which accesses a portal to the payment system of CMS, the health insurance providers, or a subcontractor acting on their behalf.[66]

The financial accounting systems facilitate billing and interface closely with the managerial platforms used for financial statement and budgeting. For example, once the software recognizes that a payment has been made by CMS, higher level financial statements such as the income statement can be immediately updated to show an increase in revenue received. These and other computerized functions permit almost immediate updating and real-time viewing of the financial condition of the health care organizations. Software applications have enhanced managerial accounting functions in other ways, by facilitating the budgeting process, which ensure the health care organizations and respiratory departments have adequate resources to provide their services and perform their functions. Likewise, computer software permits faster and often more accurate financial forecasting, as well as the ability to make predictions under various economic and environmental scenarios.[67]

Quality Assurance

Computer software applications are a vital tool in health care quality assurance. Chapter 3 of this text provides some detail

Bennett Memorial Hospital

Workload Estimate for 3 Shifts by Zone

Procedure Name	Time Standard	Number of Orders	------Shift One------		------Shift Two------		------Shift Three------	
			# of Txs	Work Units	# of Txs	Work Units	# of Txs	Work Units
CCU								
ABG	20	3	3	60	3	60	3	0
AIRWAY CARE	25	1	1	0	1	0	1	0
ASSESSMENT	30	1	1	30	1	0	1	0
CPAP	5	1	1	5	1	5	1	5
EKG	22	1	1	22	1	22	1	0
EQUIPMENT CHANGE	10	1	1	10	1	0	1	0
MED NEB	13	2	2	26	2	26	2	26
METER DOSE INHALER	7	3	3	42	3	35	3	35
O2/LPM	5	1	1	15	1	10	1	10
O2/VENTI MASK	5	1	1	5	1	5	1	5
SPONTANEOUS MECHS	25	1	1	25	1	25	1	0
VENT CARE/ADULT	12	2	2	0	2	0	2	0
Total by Zone		18	18	240	18	188	18	81
# of Therapists Required for Zone				0.53		0.42		0.18
PEDS								
MED NEB	13	1	1	26	1	26	1	26
Total by Zone		1	1	26	1	26	1	26
# of Therapists Required for Zone				0.06		0.06		0.06
RICU								
AIRWAY CARE	25	1	1	0	1	0	1	0
CPT	20	1	1	40	1	40	1	0
EKG	22	1	1	22	1	22	1	0
MED NEB	13	1	1	26	1	26	1	26
METER DOSE INHALER	7	1	1	0	1	0	1	0
O2/AEROSOL	5	1	1	5	1	5	1	5
O2/LPM	5	1	1	5	1	5	1	5
Total by Zone		7	7	98	7	98	7	36
# of Therapists Required for Zone				0.22		0.22		0.08
SICU								
ABG	20	2	2	40	2	40	2	0
AIRWAY CARE	25	2	2	0	2	0	2	0
CPR	30	1	1	30	1	30	1	0
CPT	20	1	1	40	1	40	1	40
INCENT SPIROMETER	10	1	1	20	1	20	1	0
METER DOSE INHALER	7	3	3	49	3	42	3	14
O2/AEROSOL	5	1	1	5	1	5	1	5
O2/LPM	5	1	1	5	1	5	1	5
VENT CARE/ADULT	12	2	2	0	2	0	2	0
Total by Zone		14	14	189	14	182	14	64
# of Therapists Required for Zone				0.42		0.40		0.14

FIGURE 7-5 Clinivision Mobile Patient Charting (MPC). Workload estimate for 3 shifts by zone. This report is grouped by zone and then procedure to show the estimate for the number of procedures, work units, and therapists required. (Image used by permission from Nellcor Puritan Bennett LLC, Boulder, Colorado, doing business as Covidien.)

on the principles of and tools used for quality assurance in respiratory care and health care in general. However, it is important to note that many tools used in the **continuous quality improvement** (CQI) model, for both enhancing and monitoring quality, are computer-based. For example, a **root-cause analysis** is a process by which the underlying primary, secondary, and other notable causes of a medical error or other safety issues are identified, and then an action plan is created and implemented. Finally, an ongoing monitoring system is put in place to evaluate the plan's effectiveness. Software applications exist and are commonly used to perform such an analysis. More broadly, hospital quality assurance, risk management, and even respiratory care departments use software applications that track quality data such as unplanned extubations and noninvasive mask-induced facial sores, to examine trends and the potential impact of corrective action.[68]

Regulatory Compliance

In a similar way that accounts payable systems of health care organizations use portals to facilitate reimbursement of services rendered; shared applications exist for the reporting of key compliance and regulatory data. For example, compliance with the meaningful-use objectives HITECH ACT discussed earlier in this chapter is done in this manner. In addition, CMS has introduced the **value-based purchasing** system, whereby reimbursement by CMS to hospitals and health care providers is partially based on their ability to meet a predefined set of standards. Reporting by hospitals to CMS for this program and other similar ones, such as 30-Day Short-Term Readmission Rates, are monitored through similar computer-based reporting systems.[69]

Web Analytics

Web analytics is a generic term that encompasses the study of the impact of a website on its users. It employs software to measure trends such as how many people visited a website, how many of those visitors were first-time or repeat visitors, how they came to the site (i.e., if they followed a link to get to the site or came there directly), what keywords they searched within the site's search engine, how long they stayed on one or more web pages, what links they clicked on when they left the site, and other similar trends. Health care organizations have begun to use web analytics software for many purposes. In the realm of business management and administration, health care organizations are using web analytics to measure trends of current and potential customers, to help make predictions about future market conditions and as an aid in strategic business decisions. Many clinical applications for web analytics are gaining popularity, including to track usage of educational websites that are designed as patient resources—for example, those used to for patients with chronic disorders such as COPD, cystic fibrosis, and neuromuscular diseases.[70]

Human Resources

In addition to their use in staffing and scheduling described earlier in this chapter, computer databases have proved to be invaluable tools for human resource functions of heath care facilities and those more specific to respiratory care departments by enabling them to maintain employee records, track training and education, and keep abreast of licensure and credentialing renewals, among many other similar applications. In addition, web resources have proved invaluable in helping recruit talented staff. The AARC website has a "Job Bank" feature that enables employers to post openings and furnishes qualified candidates with instructions on how to apply. Many state societies for respiratory care offer similar resources, and there are many proprietary recruitment websites, including Monster.com, Indeed.com, and ZipRecruiter.com.

Beyond this, many health care organizations are using web resources to help evaluate job candidates. In addition to being able to search state agencies to confirm a candidates' licensure and the National Board for Respiratory Care (NBRC) websites to determine credentialing status, pre-employment criminal background checks can be easily done through services offered on the web for a fee-for-service basis. Furthermore, although it is controversial, employers are increasingly performing credit checks and reviewing the social media profiles and patterns in the screening process of candidates.[71]

Privacy and Confidentiality

The *Health Insurance Portability and Accountability Act* (HIPAA) of 1996 established standards and safeguards to protect the confidentiality of medical records, including those maintained on computers and other similar devices. Essentially all EHR software offered by reputable sources must be HIPAA compliant, and health care organizations are required to have their staff trained on performing their functions within the guidelines of this law. However, in some ways technologic advancements are threatening the protections offered by HIPAA. Increasingly, health information maintained and transmitted on portable devices such a laptop computers, tablets, and smartphones is circulating outside the HIPAA-protected zone. Such information is increasingly kept on, or downloaded to, storage devices such as "thumb drives" or in remote computerized servers known as "the cloud." Furthermore, clinical datasets and databases originally intended for one purpose, such as regulatory compliance reporting or for clinical purposes, are being acquired by other organizations for different purposes, such as research and marketing. The required protection of all protected health information within such datasets is not always properly done, which poses further threats to patient confidentiality. Patient information on social media is another area of concern. Although it will take some time for our governmental regulators to enact updated legislation to address the impact that such technology has had on HIPAA compliance and patient privacy and confidentially, the general sense is that such regulation will eventually be adopted. In the meantime, RTs need to be ever mindful to protect and respect the confidentiality of patient information. Whether communicating patient information verbally, in writing, or with the combined use of computerized hardware and software, RTs should apply the HIPPA principles in protecting such data and using it only for its intended purpose (see Rule of Thumb). Failure to comply with HIPAA is a federal violation of the law with financial and legal consequences for those involved.[72]

RULE OF THUMB

Users can take steps to help prevent computer infiltration by malicious software by doing the following:

- Users should never share or use their password on public unsecured devices.
- Users should regularly update their computers with security patches from authorized sources. For example, patches for Windows operating systems are available on the Microsoft website (see http://www.update.microsoft.com).
- Users should install a virus scanning program and regularly update it.
- Most importantly, users should be careful when opening e-mail file attachments and refrain from downloading applications from unknown sources.

APPLICATIONS IN TRAINING AND EDUCATION

Computing plays a central role in the education of respiratory care students, credentialing of graduates of educational programs, and continuing education for RTs.

Clinical Simulations

Computerized **clinical simulations** are a powerful learning tool. Computer-based simulation is a long-standing educational method for hazardous occupations that have shown remarkably low rates of failure (e.g., airline pilots, members of the military, astronauts, and nuclear power plant operators). Health care education has progressed to include the use of computer-based, full-body manikins and high-fidelity clinical simulators. These devices feature software to program clinical scenarios and simulated vital signs and physical examination findings that either improve or deteriorate in response to the actions of the learners. The simulators can reproduce situations requiring complex airway management or advanced life support. In virtual surgical simulators, certain devices allow learners to exert force against simulated tissue that offers realistic resistance, and in virtual bronchoscopy simulators, vocal cord movements are exhibited that are synchronous with the phases of breathing and cough.

Learners are able to better immerse themselves in carefully planned case scenarios and performing in a manner similar to that of real clinical situations (Figure 7-6). They develop psychomotor, critical thinking, decision-making, and team-building skills. In contrast, traditional methods of didactic education in combination with clinical apprenticeships can result in increased knowledge, but limited, inconsistent experiential learning opportunities. Clinical simulators, allow for more in-depth evaluation of learners' competencies in a safe environment. They are an excellent tool to help respiratory care departments meet The Joint Commission (TJC) requirement of demonstrating the competencies of respiratory care staff in an ongoing manner.[73] Recommended steps in clinical simulation education are diagrammed in Figure 7-7.

Clinical simulators are particularly valuable for learning how to function in rare but high-risk clinical situations. Training via simulators has resulted in improved performance of health care providers in emergency airway management, advanced life support, bronchoscopy, and surgery. Computer-based simulators also have become a useful tool in promoting and optimizing the use of interprofessional teams within clinical settings.[74,75] Clinical simulators have the potential to reduce medical errors and improve patient safety. Simulations promote relatively comprehensive learning (Box 7-3) and allow for performance in clinical settings to become more refined and automatic.

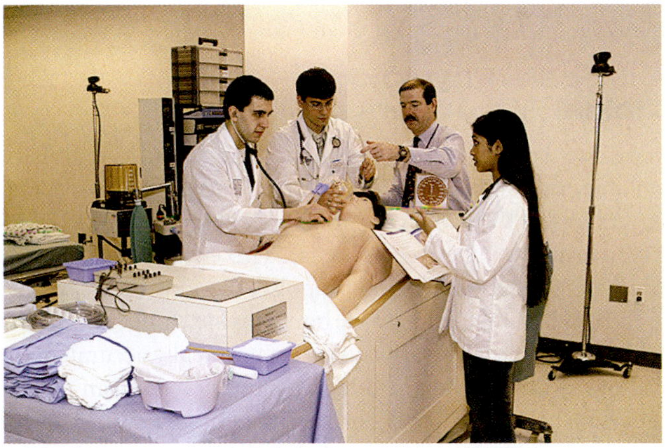

FIGURE 7-6 Clinical simulation benefits students. (From Cummings CW, et al: Cummings otolaryngeal: head and neck surgery, ed 2, St Louis, 2005, Mosby.)

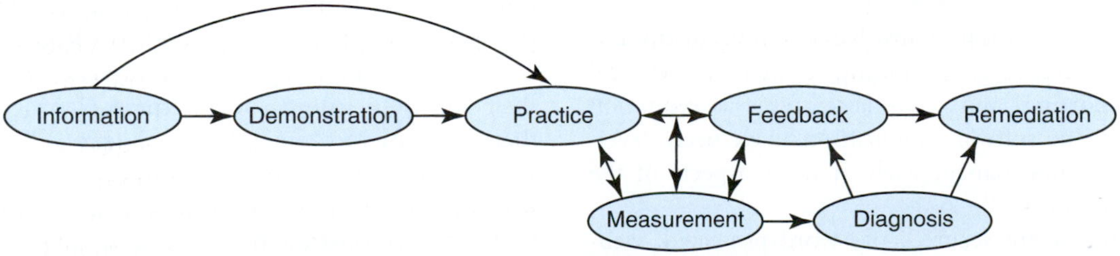

FIGURE 7-7 Steps in clinical simulation education.

Student name and initiator name	Date and IP address View record	Submission date Delete record	Patient and competency and summary	Clinical instructor	Clinical site and location	Area device
Kumar Patel Tonya Cook	Wednesday, December 16, 2009 144.30.0.221	Wednesday, January 6, 2010 at 1:42 PM 144.30.0.221	Adult vital signs Satisfactory	Tonya Cook	Baptist Health Clinic	Adult floor web
Kumar Patel Heather Neal-Rice	Saturday, April 3, 2010 144.30.0.221	Saturday, April 3, 2010 at 4:37 PM 144.30.0.221	Adult x-ray interpretation Satisfactory	Michael Anders	St. Vincent Infirmary Medical Center Clinic	Medical ICU web
Kumar Patel Tonya Cook	Tuesday, October 20, 2009 144.30.0.221	Tuesday, January 5, 2010 at 3:57 PM 144.30.0.221	Adult nasal cannula Satisfactory	Tonya Cook	Baptist Health Clinic	Adult floor web

FIGURE 7-8 DataArc documentation of clinical competencies. (Courtesy DataArc LLC, League City, TX.)

Box 7-3 Learner Objectives in Clinical Simulation

- Interpret data
- Recognize and prioritize problems
- Make decisions
- Observe consequences of decisions
- Develop leadership skills
- Develop interpersonal communication skills
- Develop team-building skills
- Use available resources
- Manage stress and crisis

Full-Scale Physiologic Clinical Simulators

There are several full-scale, physiologic, clinical simulators available, two of which are SimMan (Laerdal Medical, Wappingers Falls, NY) and the Human Patient Simulator (HPS) (CAE Healthcare, Quebec, Canada). These simulators generate physiologic functions, including pulse, blood pressure, cardiac rhythm, breathing, exhaled carbon dioxide, lung compliance, and bowel sounds. The airways are anatomically accurate to the level of the lung segments. Interdisciplinary teams can practice scenarios such as cardiac defibrillation, hemodynamic monitoring, apnea, right main stem intubations, tension pneumothoraces, anesthesia administration, occluded endotracheal tubes, high-pressure alarm limits during mechanical ventilation, and loss of medical gas.

Clinical Education Applications

Management of clinical education involves a significant amount of documentation, tracking, scheduling, evaluations, clinical competencies, reporting, and compliance with accreditation standards. E-Medicine software applications have been developed to help educators manage each of these aspects of the clinical education process.

These applications are secured, password-protected, web-based database management systems for documenting and reporting clinical educational activities for allied health professions, including respiratory care programs. The records help both students and faculty members track student progress in completing required competencies as they progress through their clinical rotation assignments (Figure 7-8). Functions may include the following:

- Streamlined data entry process minimizing data entry duplication that can occur between clinical sites, students, and the academic program
- A daily log for completed procedures and activities, which instructors validate
- Competency evaluations
- Automated surveys to accommodate questionnaires for students, graduates, and clinical affiliates as required by accrediting agencies
- Cloud-based data and backup storage

A variety of such as software applications are available to educational institutions. These include DataArc (http://www.dataarc.ws/), E*Value (http://evaluehealthcare.com), and Typhoon Group (http://www.typhongroup.com/), among others. Students and faculty can use any web-enabled device, including smart phones, to access these applications.

National Board for Respiratory Care Credentialing

The NBRC uses computerized credentialing examinations for both the written and clinical simulation examinations. Candidates must go to a designated testing center, sit at a monitored computer terminal, and take the examination during the designated timeframe. Once candidates are done with the examination, they receive their score immediately. In addition, to achieve the advanced credentialing level, or Registered Respiratory Therapist (RRT) designation, candidates must demonstrate their ability to gather and interpret clinical information and then make or recommend clinical actions based on a clinical scenario. In the computerized simulation examination (CSE), RRT candidates must complete a series of case-based simulations and demonstrate that they have adequately mastered the management of major respiratory diseases (Figure 7-9).

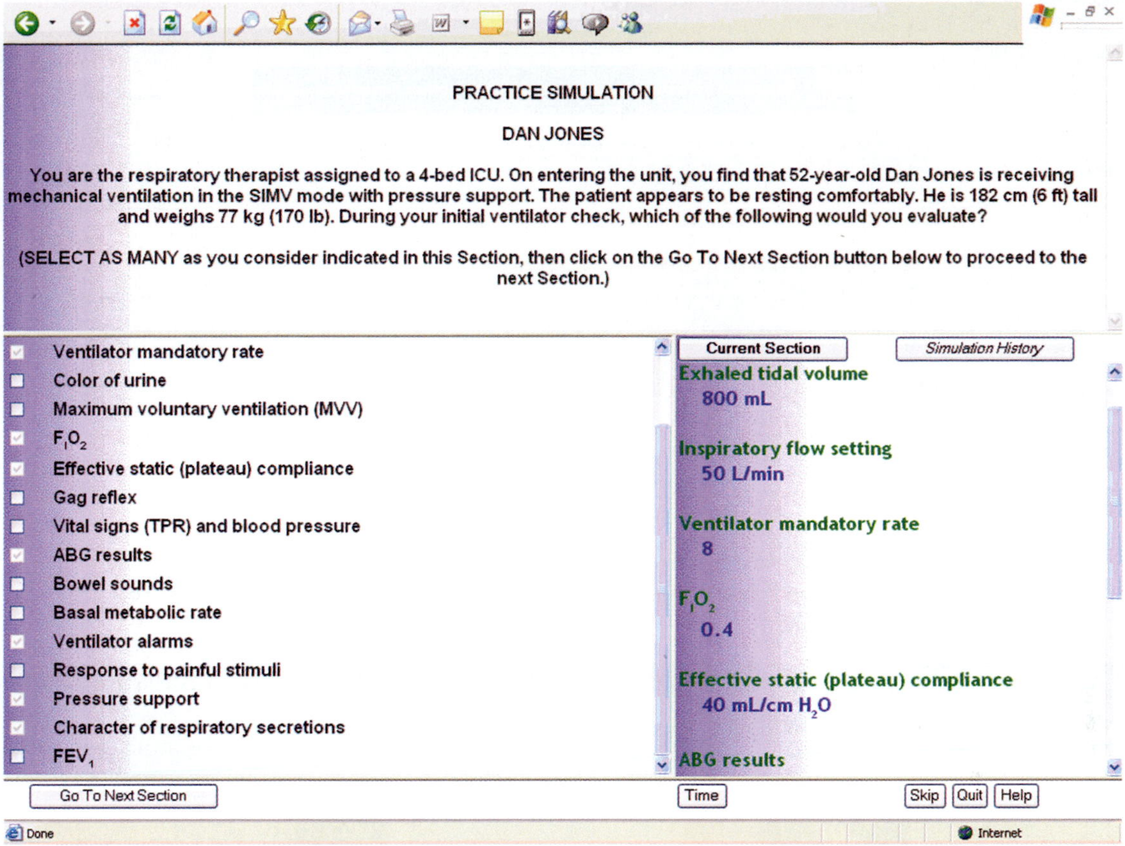

FIGURE 7-9 National Board for Respiratory Care. Practice simulation problem. (Courtesy NBRC, Olathe, KS.)

Continuing education is mandatory for national credentialing for the NBRC and often a requirement for state licensure. Credentials awarded by the NBRC are valid for a period of 5 years and are subject to renewal through the Continuing Competency Program (CCP) requirements. RTs are required to provide evidence to the NBRC that they are continuing to meet current standards of practice and have all the requirements for renewal. Web-based **continuing respiratory care education** (CRCE) courses, which have been preapproved or outright sponsored by the AARC, offer RTs an easily accessible, efficient, and cost-effective means of meeting continuing education requirements for CCP and state licensure purposes, as well as keeping current in their profession.

Learning Management Systems

To an increasing extent, respiratory care educators use online, web-based **learning management systems** platforms such as Moodle or Blackboard to augment traditional classroom courses known as web-enhanced courses or deliver entirely web-based courses (Figure 7-10). This technology improves access and management of course content for web-enhanced courses. Web-delivered courses make respiratory care education possible for students who might not otherwise be able to attend respiratory care programs such as those requiring flexible schedules or students in remote rural areas. Other adjunctive applications, such as Adobe Connect, permit live interaction between the student and faculty. Students can talk to their instructors and classmates via live audiovisual platforms. Participants also can have asynchronously access to archived classes and related course content and other material by the use of podcasts or recorded sessions.

American Association for Respiratory Care

The AARC provides many continuing education opportunities on the web (see http://www.aarc.org). Webinars and text-based courses are available in both live and asynchronous formats. RTs may earn CRCE credits by completing these courses (Figure 7-11). The AARC also provides web-based CRCE credits through the *Respiratory Care* journal. RTs can read the journal, use a copy of the test that appears in the journal to draft answers, and then complete the web-based test on the journal website (http://www.rcjournal.com/crce_ttj.cfm). The AARC maintains a transcript of members' CRCE credits, which RTs can access on the AARC website.

Additionally, to facilitate electronic networking among RTs, the AARC offers Specialty Sections and Roundtables. Each Specialty Section features an e-mail listserv for discussions, e-newsletters, e-bulletins, and a website.

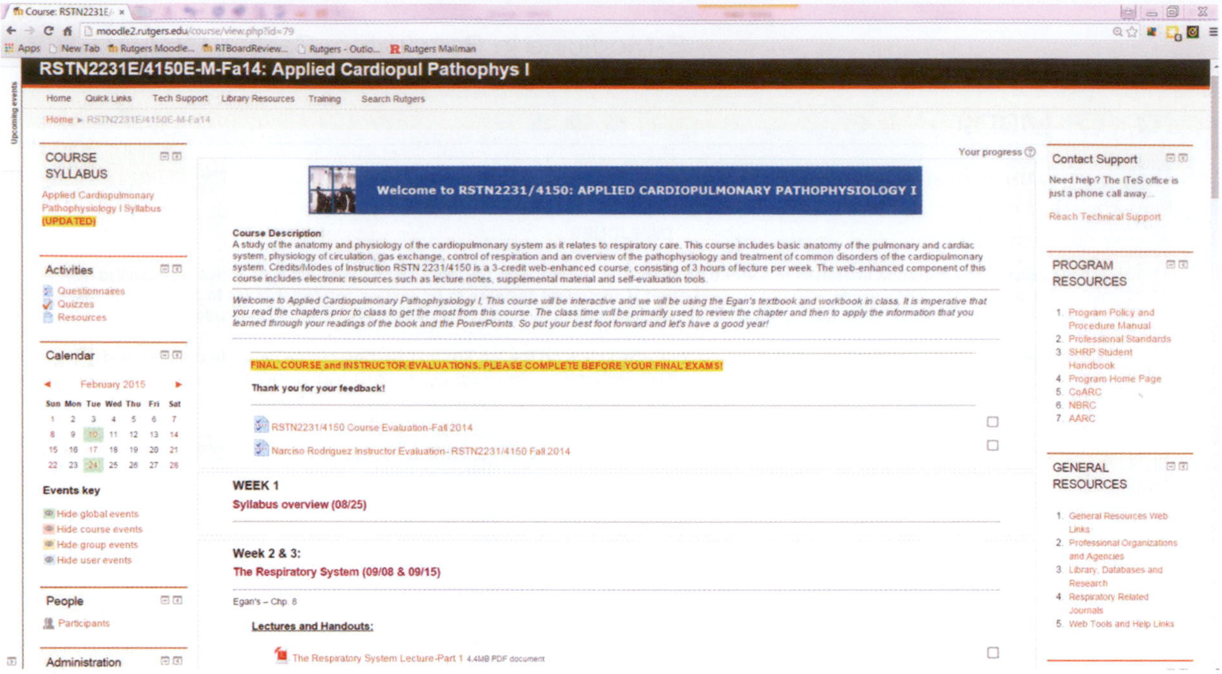

FIGURE 7-10 Moodle Learning Management System course homepage. (Courtesy Rutgers School of Health Related Professions, Respiratory Care Program–North, Newark, NJ.)

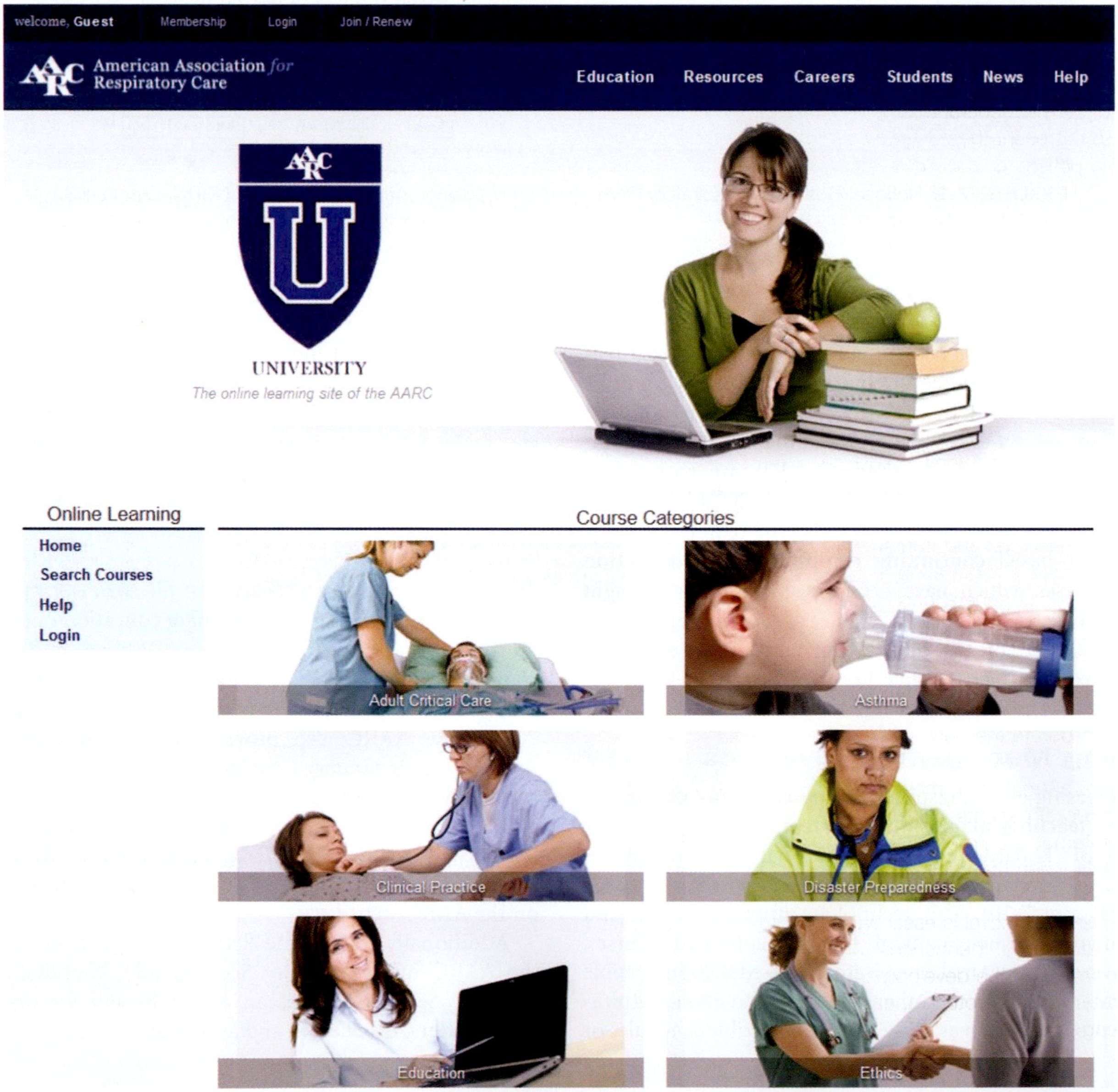

FIGURE 7-11 America Association for Respiratory Care, Continuing respiratory care education, web-based courses. (Courtesy AARC, Irving, TX.)

FUTURE OF E-MEDICINE

If the recent degree of changes in E-Medicine is a predictor of future developments, this chapter in the next edition of this book will look very different from this one. In the future, computerized technologic applications described in this chapter, such as telemedicine and closed-loop decision-making on mechanical ventilators, will be more widespread, as well as refined and improved and most likely able to do more in much less time. In addition, new digital applications will emerge, including a vast assortment of diagnostic, treatment, educational, and disease management applications available to patients and clinicians alike. The current technology coupled with new developments hold great promise for helping optimize the large-scale effectiveness and efficiency our health care system, as well as providing notable benefits to health care organizations and clinicians, including the RTs operating within it.

SUMMARY CHECKLIST

- E-Medicine relates to the use of computerized or digital technology to enhance efficiency and effectiveness of health care in general and more specifically patient care.
- EMRs represent the computerized records produced every time a patient (or consumer) uses health services.
- The EHR is the sum of all EMRs produced by the different encounters of the consumer with various health care entities throughout a lifetime.
- Enterprise software packages are designed to provide integrated functionality for health care organizations to enhance both efficiency and effectiveness of patient care.
- E-Medicine applications can be used in acute or nonacute settings by RTs to provide support and care for the pulmonary patient.
- Health informatics combines advances in computer science and technology to improve clinical care, manage the health of populations, and accelerate research.
- Business intelligence refers to a set of tools that permit capture, storage, and transformation of data into useful and actionable information.
- CDS provides general and person-specific information, intelligently filtered and organized, at appropriate times, to enhance health and health care.
- Benchmarking includes four basic steps (1) know your operation, (2) know the industry leaders or competitors, (3) incorporate the best, and (4) gain superiority.
- Telemedicine and telemonitoring allow for the evaluation, diagnosis, treatment, monitoring, triage, consultation, and follow up of patients without travel.
- The Internet is a rich source of information for RTs and patients when the quality and source of information are appropriate.
- Information retrieval is essential to practice evidence-based respiratory care. It enhances clinical expertise by providing information for the development of evidence-based, therapist-driven protocols, and it aids in clinical decision making for the RT.
- Computers and digital information can be useful to clinicians in optimizing quality of care and to patients and their families participating in care plans.
- Common sense is the best prevention against infiltration by malicious software.
- Emerging computer applications are expected to support management of chronic disease and potentially reduce medical errors.
- The role of computer applications in clinical care, diagnostics, management, and education is essential and will continue to expand.

References

1. Garets D, Mike D: *Electronic medical records vs. electronic health records: yes, there is a difference. Policy white paper*, Chicago, 2006, HIMSS Analytics.
2. Nguyen L, Bellucci E, Nguyen LT: Electronic health records implementation: an evaluation of information system impact and contingency factors. *Int J Med Inform* 83:779–796, 2014.
3. Struik MH, Koster F, Schuit AJ, et al: The preferences of users of electronic medical records in hospitals: quantifying the relative importance of barriers and facilitators of an innovation. *Implement Sci* 9:69, 2014.
4. Schiff GD, Amato MG, Eguale T, et al: Computerized physician order entry-related medication errors: analysis of reported errors and vulnerability testing of current systems. *BMJ Qual Saf* 24:264–271, 2015.
5. Weis JM, Levy PC: Copy, paste, and cloned notes in electronic health records: prevalence, benefits, risks, and best practice recommendations. *Chest* 145:632–638, 2014.
6. U.S. Department of Health and Human Services, Centers of Medicare and Medicaid Services: Eligible professional meaningful use: core and menu set objectives, stage 1-(2014 definition). <http://www.cms.gov/Regulations-and-Guidance/Legislation/EHRIncentivePrograms/>. Updated May 2014.
7. Top vendors of enterprise EMR systems. *Mod Healthc* 41:35, 2011.
8. Saugel B, Cecconi M, Wagner JY, et al: Noninvasive continuous cardiac output monitoring in perioperative and intensive care medicine. *Br J Anaesth* 114:562–575, 2015.
9. Pribul V, Woolley T: Point of care testing. *Surgery (Oxford)* 31:84–86, 2013.
10. Duncan LD, Gray K, Lewis GM, et al: Clinical integration of picture archiving and communication systems with pathology and hospital information system in oncology. *Am Surg* 76:982–986, 2010.
11. Stoller JK, McCarthy K: On the power and risks of the percent of predicted. *Respir Care* 51:722–725, 2006.
12. Chatburn RL, Mireles-Cabodevila E: Closed-loop control of mechanical ventilation: description and classification of targeting schemes. *Respir Care* 56:85–102, 2011.
13. Kacmarek RM: Proportional assist ventilation and neurally adjusted ventilatory assist. *Respir Care* 56:140–148, 2011.
14. Chatburn RL, Volsko TA: Documentation issues for mechanical ventilation in pressure-control modes. *Respir Care* 55:1705–1716, 2010.
15. Vawdrey DK, Gardner RM, Evans RS, et al: Assessing data quality in manual entry of ventilator settings. *J Am Med Inform Assoc* 14:295–303, 2007.
16. Blackwood B, Alderdice F, Burns KE, et al: Protocolized versus non-protocolized weaning for reducing the duration of mechanical ventilation in critically ill adult patients. *Cochrane Database Syst Rev* (5):CD006904, 2010.
17. Hadjitodorov S, Lyudmila T: Consultation system for determining the patients' readiness for weaning from long-term mechanical ventilation. *Comput Meth Progr Biomed* 100:59–68, 2010.
18. Ward BW, Schiller JS, Goodman RA: Multiple chronic conditions among US adults: a 2012 update. *Prev Chronic Dis* 11:E62, 2014.
19. Centers for Disease Control and Prevention: Death and mortality. NCHS FastStats website. <http://www.cdc.gov/nchs/fastats/deaths.htm>. Accessed January 20, 2015.

20. Robert Wood Johnson Foundation: *Chronic care: making the case for ongoing care*, Princeton, NJ, 2010, Robert Wood Johnson Foundation. <http://www.rwjf.org/content/dam/farm/reports/reports/2010/rwjf 54583>. Accessed January 20, 2015.
21. Verhaegh KJ, MacNeil-Vroomen JL, Eslami S, et al: Transitional care interventions prevent hospital readmissions for adults with chronic illnesses. *Health Aff* 33:1531–1539, 2014.
22. Sadatsafavi M, Lynd LD, De Vera MA, et al: One-year outcomes of inhaled controller therapies added to systemic corticosteroids after asthma-related hospital discharge. *Respir Med* 14:452–458, 2015.
23. Minard J, Dostaler SM, Taite AK, et al: Development and implementation of an electronic asthma record for primary care: integrating guidelines into practice. *J Asthma* 51:58–68, 2014.
24. Jan RL, Wang JY, Huang MC, et al: An internet-based interactive telemonitoring system for improving childhood asthma outcomes in Taiwan. *Telemed J E Health* 13:257–268, 2007.
25. Krishna S, Boren SA, Balas EA: Healthcare via cell phones: a systematic review. *Telemed J E Health* 15:231–240, 2009.
26. McLean S, Chandler D, Nurmatov U, et al: Telehealthcare for asthma. *Cochrane Database Syst Rev* 10:007717, 2010.
27. Jaana M, Paré G, Sicotte C: Home telemonitoring for respiratory conditions: a systematic review. *Am J Manag Care* 15:313–320, 2009.
28. Nguyen HQ, Donesky-Cuenco D, Wolpin S, et al: Randomized controlled trial of an internet-based versus face-to-face dyspnea self-management program for patients with chronic obstructive pulmonary disease: pilot study. *J Med Internet Res* 10:e9, 2008.
29. Polisena J, Tran K, Cimon K, et al: Home telehealth for chronic obstructive pulmonary disease: a systematic review and meta-analysis. *J Telemed Telecare* 16:120–127, 2010.
30. Blumenthal D, Tavenner M: The "meaningful use" regulation for electronic health records. *N Engl J Med* 363:501–504, 2010.
31. U.S. Department of Health and Human Services: *The health consequences of smoking—50 years of progress. A Report of the Surgeon General*, Atlanta, 2014, U.S. Department of Health and Human Services, Centers for Disease Control and Prevention, National Center for Chronic Disease Prevention and Health Promotion, Office on Smoking and Health.
32. Tong EK, Strouse R, Hall J, et al: National survey of US health professionals' smoking prevalence, cessation practices, and beliefs. *Nicotine Tob Res* 12: 724–733, 2010.
33. Civljak M, Sheikh A, Stead LF, et al: Internet-based interventions for smoking cessation. *Cochrane Database Syst Rev* 9:007078, 2010.
34. Whittaker R, Borland R, Bullen C, et al: Mobile phone-based interventions for smoking cessation. *Cochrane Database Syst Rev* 4:006611, 2009, 2009.
35. Shahab L, McEwen A: Online support for smoking cessation: a systematic review of the literature. *Addiction* 104:1792–1804, 2009.
36. Graham AL, Cobb NK, Papandonatos GD, et al: A randomized trial of Internet and telephone treatment for smoking cessation. *Arch Intern Med* 171:46–53, 2011.
37. Fiore MC, Jaén CR, Baker TB, et al: *Treating tobacco use and dependence: 2008 update—clinical practice guideline, U.S. Department of Health and Human Services*, Rockville, MD, 2008, Public Health Service.
38. Fox S: *E-patients with a disability or chronic disease*, Washington, DC, 2007, Pew Internet and American Life Project.
39. University of California–San Francisco Medical Center. Evaluating health information. <http://www.ucsfhealth.org/education/evaluating_health_information/>. Accessed February 13, 2015.
40. Wu HW, Davis PK, Bell DS: Advancing clinical decision support using lessons from outside of healthcare: an interdisciplinary systematic review. *BMC Med Inform Decis Mak* 12:90, 2012.
41. Medicare and Medicaid Programs: *Electronic health record incentive program. Vol 75 FR 44313; 4435*, Washington, DC, 2010, Centers for Medicare and Medicaid Services.
42. Shabot MM, LoBue M, Leyerle BJ, et al: Decision support alerts for clinical laboratory and blood gas data. *Int J Clin Monit Comput* 7:27–31, 1990.
43. Scheepers-Hoeks A-MJ, Grouls RJ, Neef C, et al: Physicians' responses to clinical decision support on an intensive care unit-Comparison of four different alerting methods. *Artif Intell Med* 59:33–38, 2013.
44. Norris PR, Dawant BM: Closing the loop in ICU decision support: physiologic event detection, alerts, and documentation. *Proc AMIA Annu Symp AMIA Symp* 498–502, 2001.
45. Schmickl CN, Shahjehan K, Li G, et al: Decision support tool for early differential diagnosis of acute lung injury and cardiogenic pulmonary edema in medical critically ill patients. *Chest* 141:43–50, 2012.
46. Sasidhar M, Green K, Stilphen M, et al: Computerized clinical decision support system for early identification of patients appropriate for rehabilitation services improves functional status in survivors of critical illness. In *B104. ICU weakness on the run: exercise, electrical stimulation, and pharmacotherapy*, New York, 2013, American Thoracic Society, pp A3621.
47. Lau F, Vincent DD: A knowledge-based care protocol system for ICU. *Medinfo* 8(Pt 2):979–983, 1995.
48. Jouvet P, Farges C, Hatzakis G, et al: Weaning children from mechanical ventilation with a computer-driven system (closed-loop protocol): a pilot study. *Pediatr Crit Care Med J Soc Crit Care Med World Fed Pediatr Intensive Crit Care Soc* 8:425–432, 2007.
49. Ford R: Benchmarking and best practice. *AARC Times* 1:24–27, 2007.
50. Camp R: *Benchmarking: the search for industry best practices that lead to superior performance*, New York, 1989, American Society for Quality Control.
51. Chatburn RL: Benchmarking for success: the AARC benchmarking project. I. Overview. *AARC Times* 6:26–28, 2006.
52. Chatburn RL: AARC benchmarking project: understanding the metrics. I. *AARC Times* 8:20–21, 2006.
53. Chatburn RL: AARC benchmarking project: understanding the metrics. II. *AARC Times* 9:30–36, 2006.
54. Chatburn RL, Gole S, Schenk P, et al: Respiratory care work assignment based on work rate instead of work load. *Respir Care* 56:1785–1790, 2011.
55. Stoller JK, Roberts V, Matt D, et al: Radio-frequency tracking of respiratory equipment: Rationale and early experience at the Cleveland Clinic. *Respir Care* 58:2069–2075, 2013.
56. Wootton R: Twenty years of telemedicine in chronic disease management: an evidence synthesis. *J Telemed Telecare* 18:211–220, 2012.
57. Swanson KA, McLeod AC, Wager KA: Telemedicine in an international context: definition, use, and future. *Adv Health Care Manag* 12:143–169, 2012.
58. Kahn JM, Cicero BD, Wallace DJ, et al: Adoption of ICU telemedicine in the United States. *Crit Care Med* 42:362–368, 2014.
59. Zamarrón C, Morete E, González F: Telemedicine system for the care of patients with neuromuscular disease and chronic respiratory failure. *Arch Med Sci* 10:1047–1051, 2014.
60. Thijssing L, van der Heijden JP, Chavannes NH, et al: Telepulmonology: effect on quality and efficiency of care. *Respir Med* 108:314–318, 2014.
61. Brown W, Odenthal D: The uses of telemedicine to improve asthma control. *J Allergy Clin Immunol Pract* 8:2014. pii: S2213-2198(14)00443-7.
62. Segrelles CG, Gómez-Suárez C, Soriano JB, et al: A home telehealth program for patients with severe COPD: the PROMETE study. *Respir Med* 108:453–462, 2014.
63. Institute of Medicine: *Health literacy, ehealth, and Communication putting the consumer first: workshop summary*, Washington, DC, 2009, Institute of Medicine.
64. Sarkar U, Karter AJ, Liu JY, et al: The literacy divide: health literacy and the use of an internet-based patient portal in an integrated health system: results from the Diabetes Study of Northern California (DISTANCE). *J Health Commun* 15(Suppl 2):183–196, 2010.
65. Timmermans S, Marc B: *The gold standard: the challenge of evidence-based medicine and standardization in health care*, Philadelphia, 2010, Temple University Press.
66. Sockolow PS, Bowles KH, Adelsberger MC, et al: Impact of homecare electronic health record on timeliness of clinical documentation, reimbursement, and patient outcomes. *Appl Clin Inform* 5:445–462, 2014.
67. Fleming NS, Becker ER, Culler SD, et al: The impact of electronic health records on workflow and financial measures in primary care practices. *Health Serv Res* 49(1 Pt 2):405–420, 2014.
68. Curcin V, Woodcock T, Poots AJ, et al: Model-driven approach to data collection and reporting for quality improvement. *J Biomed Inform* 52:151–162, 2014.

69. U.S. Department of Health and Human Services, Centers of Medicare and Medcaid Services: CMS data show gains in key quality indicators through Physician Quality Reporting System and ePrescribing Incentive Program. *Md Med* 12:16–17, 2011.
70. McAfee A, Brynjolfsson E: Big data: the management revolution. *Harv Bus Rev* 90:60–68, 2012.
71. Cerinus M, Shannon M: Improving staff selection processes. *Nurs Stand* 29:37–44, 2014.
72. Terry N: Health privacy is difficult but not impossible in a post-HIPAA data-driven world. *Chest* 146:835–840, 2014.
73. Tuttle RP, Cohen MH, Augustine AJ, et al: Utilizing simulation technology for competency skills assessment and a comparison of traditional methods of training to simulation-based training. *Respir Care* 52:263–270, 2007.
74. Wayne DB, Didwania A, Feinglass J, et al: Simulation-based education improves quality of care during cardiac arrest team responses at an academic teaching hospital: a case-control study. *Chest* 133:56–61, 2008.
75. Figueroa M, Sepanski R, Goldberg SP, et al: Improving teamwork, confidence, and collaboration among members of a pediatric cardiovascular intensive care unit multidisciplinary team using simulation-based team training. *Pediatr Cardiol* 34:612–619, 2013.

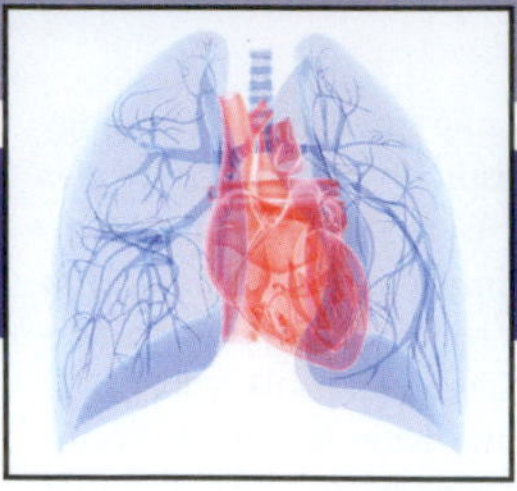

CHAPTER 8

Fundamentals of Respiratory Care Research

ROBERT L. CHATBURN

CHAPTER OBJECTIVES

After reading this chapter you will be able to:

- Explain why research activities are important in health care.
- Describe several sources of information that are commonly used during a literature search.
- Give examples of how to develop a study idea and write a research protocol.
- Describe the three basic formats for publishing a research study.

CHAPTER OUTLINE

Overview of Respiratory Care Research
- The Importance of Research in Health Care

How to Review the Literature
- Bibliographic Databases
- Synthesized Databases
- Portals
- Electronic Journals and Books
- General Internet Resources
- Suggestions for Conducting Searches

How to Be a Scientist
- How to Develop a Study Idea
- How to Write a Study Protocol
- How to Analyze the Data

How to Get a Scientific Paper Published
- How to Write the Abstract
- How to Make a Poster
- How to Write a Paper
- How to Respond to Reviews

Summary

KEY TERMS

bibliographic database
synthesized database
portals
PubMed
hypothesis
research protocol

OVERVIEW OF RESPIRATORY CARE RESEARCH

The chances that any of us will become a famous researcher may be slim. For example, more than 100,000 people are practicing respiratory therapy in the United States. Of those, maybe half are members of the American Association for Respiratory Care (AARC). Of those people, fewer than 1 in 100 are involved in presenting their research at the annual AARC Congress. Yet, every one of the 100,000 people in the respiratory care field needs to know how to read and understand scientific articles in medical journals. The same holds true for all health care workers. Even if you never conduct a study, you must be familiar with the basic concepts of research to practice as a professional whose understanding grows from a scientific basis for respiratory care practice and from continuing education.

The main purpose of this chapter is to help you become an educated consumer of medical research. It will present a brief overview[1] of the specific steps in conducting research and presenting your results. But if you want to actually perform research, to be a respiratory care scientist, the best thing you can do is find a mentor—someone who has experience conducting scientific studies and publishing the results. A mentor can help you turn the ideas in this chapter into practical realities.

The Importance of Research in Health Care

Academic medicine has three basic missions: to heal, to teach, and to discover. Scientific research is the underlying theme that ties these activities together. These activities imply several classes of stakeholders: clinicians (who need the ability to assess the usefulness of new equipment and treatments), educators (who need the ability to find, summarize, and present evidence for clinical activities), administrators (who need to evaluate the quality of services and the validity of policies/procedures), and finally researchers (who need to be able to generate new ideas that inform the other stakeholders). *The one skill that is common to all these stakeholders is the ability to read and critically evaluate published scientific reports.* Without this skill, no meaningful evaluation of current practices can be made and no research can be planned.

HOW TO REVIEW THE LITERATURE

Students who have grown up in the digital age are quite familiar with finding information on the Internet. Practically everybody has a smart phone, and, in my experience, it is not uncommon for a therapist or medical resident to look up the answer to a clinical question in a matter of seconds during bedside rounds. Here is a true story: An experienced colleague and I were helping a young physician write a **research protocol.** One of his outcome variables was some measure of atelectasis. I asked him how he would quantitate that outcome. He suggested that maybe he could create some kind of score. I said that I had done that a number of years ago in a paper by me and a co-author named Deakins. Almost before I had completed the sentence, my colleague had entered our names into a Google Scholar[2] search and had the paper on the screen with the method for creating an atelectasis score. All this took less than 60 seconds. That is the power of knowledge in the information age!

Unfortunately, not all sources of information are equally reliable. Let's take a look at what is available.[3,4]

Bibliographic Databases

A database is a structured collection of facts. A list of names and phone numbers on a piece of paper is a database. A spreadsheet containing a business profit and loss statement is a database. And of course, a project created with a software database design program (e.g., Microsoft Access) is a database. A bibliographic, or library database, contains books, book chapters, reports, citations, abstracts, and either the full text of the articles indexed or links to the full text. Perhaps the most popular **bibliographic database** is **PubMed**, a service of the U.S. National Library of Medicine that includes over 18 million citations from MEDLINE and other life science journals for biomedical articles back to 1948.[5] PubMed (Figure 8-1) includes links to full text articles and other related resources in medicine, nursing, dentistry, veterinary medicine, health care systems, and preclinical sciences. It provides a *Clinical Queries* search filters page as well as a *Special Queries* page. The site also provides automatic e-mailing of search updates, the ability to save records, and filters for search results using "My NCBI." The My NCBI feature is particularly useful because it will periodically e-mail you results of automatic searches on subjects and authors of interest to you, saving you a lot of time in just keeping up to date, aside from any focused research. Another free bibliographic medical database you should know about is SearchMedica. According to the website,

> *SearchMedica . . . (delivers) only the most clinically reputable content intended for practicing medical clinicians. With guidance from our advisory board of specialty physicians and our staff editors, SearchMedica scans well-known, credible journals, systematic reviews, and evidence-based articles that are written and edited for clinicians practicing in primary care and all major specialties. Using similar expertise, SearchMedica also selects and scans patient-directed websites, online CME courses,*

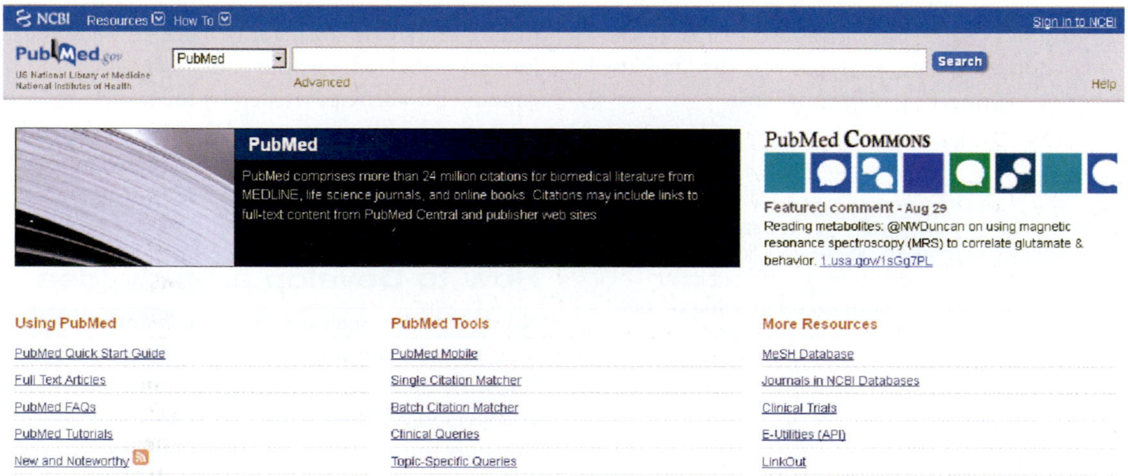

FIGURE 8-1 PubMed screenshot.

and government databases of clinical trials and practice guidelines.[6]

Synthesized Databases

Synthesized databases are prefiltered records for particular topics. They are usually subscription-based with relatively large fees. This type of database may provide the "best" evidence without extensive searches of standard bibliographic databases. The leading database in this category is the Cochrane Collaboration.[7] UpToDate is another subscription-based service.[8] It claims to be the largest clinical community in the world dedicated to synthesizing knowledge for clinicians and patients.

Portals

Portals are web pages that act as a starting point for using the Web or web-based services. One example of a subscription based service is ClinicalKey,[9] which provides links to books, journals, Clinics in Medicine, patient education resources, and images. Another example is Ovid,[10] which provides links to books, journals, evidence-based medicine databases (e.g., Cochrane Collaboration), and the Cumulative Index to Nursing and Allied Health Literature (CINAHL). Most medical libraries will have subscriptions to both of these services.

Electronic Journals and Books

We are rapidly reaching the point at which all medical journals are available online. Some are available *only* online. You should already be reading Respiratory Care journal.[11] Full text versions of Respiratory Care journal articles are available online back to January 2003. Open Forum abstracts (i.e., abstracts presented at the annual AARC Congress) are also available.

There are many sources of electronic versions of textbooks available on the Internet. From the PubMed homepage, select Books (instead of PubMed) from the drop down menu in the upper left-hand corner of the page. Enter a search term, and you will get a results page with links for books and figures from books. Subscription services include Oxford Reference Online,[12] STAT!Ref (great source for nursing and drugs),[13] and Safari Books Online (excellent source of technical reference books).[14] Again, your medical library will probably have subscriptions to these services. Another great book resource is Amazon.[15] Amazon sells new books, but many times you can find used editions for a small fraction of their original cost.

RULE OF THUMB

If you don't want to buy a book on Amazon.com, just use the website to get ideas before you go to the library. This is also a quick way to get the publisher information if you need to reference a book you do not have.

General Internet Resources

Google.com is perhaps the most popular of the general Internet search engines. Other options come and go, and, ironically, the best way to find new ones is to do a Google search on "search engines." But remember, these sites generally use proprietary search algorithms rather than controlled vocabularies like PubMed. As a result, you are likely to get unexpected results.

Suggestions for Conducting Searches

The first and most important suggestion I can offer is to talk to a professional librarian. These people can show you all the tricks of the trade—things you never imagined could be done. And in some cases, they will even do the search for you. Some libraries offer free courses on how to use all kinds of software tools for conducting searches.

Finally, buy and use bibliographic software such as EndNote[16] or RefWorks.[17] These programs let you import the results of your reference searches into your own database for future use. If you are an author, they will also help you manage the references in your manuscripts. Programs like these will save you a lot of time and effort. A great free alternative is Zotero.[18]

Before moving on, I want to call your attention to another challenge. Just finding a source of research information is not enough. You must know how to read it. A great resource on this topic is a comprehensive book called "Studying a Study and Testing a Test: Reading Evidence-based Health Research" by Richard Riegelman MD, MPH, PhD.

HOW TO BE A SCIENTIST

OK, so just being an educated consumer of research is not enough for you. You want to do your own research projects. Perhaps you need an abstract to advance on your career ladder. Maybe you are involved in a quality improvement project and need to know the basics of research methodology. Hopefully, you have decided to be the next leading scientist in the Respiratory Care field. Whatever your motivation, I remind you that your first task is to find a mentor. After that, find a good textbook. There have been only two textbooks on respiratory care research. One is fairly new,[19] and the other is out of print (but still very useful if you can find a used one on Amazon.com).[20] Of course, there are many other fine textbooks on health care research and I suggest you consider as many as you can find (again, search Amazon.com). Back in 2004, Respiratory Care journal dedicated a whole issue to research and publication. It contained 19 articles written by the leaders in Respiratory Care research. I highly recommend that you find it and read it (Respiratory Care, October 2004, Volume 49, Number 10).

In the next sections, we will look briefly at the major skills required to design, conduct, and report health care research.

How to Develop a Study Idea

No doubt, the biggest hurdle for someone new to research is how to generate an idea worth studying. You need passion. Those outside the research community often say that emotion and personal belief play no part in the scientific method and that only through detached objectivity can the truth be revealed. If this were in fact the case, there would be no human scientists. Without passion, there could be no **hypothesis**, without a hypothesis there could be no experiment, and without experimentation there would be no science. Choosing and defining a research topic are the first steps in applying the scientific method to a clinical research problem. This process implies concern or doubt about some concept or observation, usually based on the observer's experience from clinical practice. Indeed, the scientific method itself can be viewed as nothing more than organized curiosity. Curiosity about the details of one's everyday activity provides the motivation for finding out how or why events are related. Curiosity and the creative energy it produces are vital ingredients of a productive research effort. The scientific method simply provides a standardized and efficient technique for describing relationships among events in a way that can be verified by other observers. You can think of the scientific method as a way of creating beliefs based on evidence.

RULE OF THUMB

Richard Feynman, who received the Nobel Prize in Physics in 1965, once said that *"Science is the belief in the ignorance of experts."*

Your interest may be stimulated in a number of ways. One of the most obvious ways is to read medical journals. Often one investigator's results will not completely answer the questions that another investigator seeks to answer. Perhaps the authors themselves suggest areas in which further work needs to be done (usually found in the Discussion section of a scientific paper). Occasionally, the results of an article contradict those of a previous study, creating the need for yet another look at the research problem. Review articles that cover the state of the art in some area of research are especially useful in helping you generate ideas along these lines. The basic concept to remember is that research breeds more research and that the truth in scientific research is defined when the results of earlier experiments and studies can be reproduced consistently by others.

RULE OF THUMB

One of the best study ideas for a beginning respiratory therapy researcher is to do a device evaluation (particularly a new device).[21] This kind of study is usually very inexpensive (vendors often donate or loan equipment and supplies) and does not require approval by the institutional review board (IRB) (as is required for studies of human subjects).

Trying to develop research topics from personal experience is often the most frustrating approach for the beginning researcher. The natural tendency is to choose a general problem that everyone seems to recognize but no one does anything about. The difficulty lies in trying to narrow the general idea to a specific problem statement.[22] There are at least two reasons for this. First, a general problem, by its nature, is often spoken about in vague, undefined terms. Second, in attempting to explicitly describe the problem, it may appear to be overwhelming. One may easily become frustrated to the point of not being able to write anything.

Box 8-1 Factors Affecting the Feasibility of a Research Project

1. Significance or potential benefits of study results
2. Measurability of research variables
3. Duration and timing of study
4. Availability of research subjects
5. Availability of equipment and funds
6. Knowledge and experience of investigators

One way to avoid this situation is to start small. Begin with a specific incident that stimulated either curiosity or irritation. *Simply state what you see happening and why it is important.* Write a narrative, first-person account of the incident. Now you can begin reviewing the literature, using key definitions related to your study idea to speed the search. Try to find similar problems in other disciplines to create original experimental approaches. For example, many problems concerning clinical measurement (e.g., airway pressure measurement) have been solved in the context of electrical or mechanical engineering. Keep in mind that not all ideas you have will be practical to study. When searching the literature, consider whether the experimental methods you will use are feasible for your situation (Box 8-1).

Once you have clarified your study purpose through your literature review, the next step is to develop a formal problem statement. This problem statement is the foundation of the actual study design. It dictates the concepts and methods used to gather data. It also determines the theoretical context in which the conclusion will be interpreted. From the problem statement comes either a brief statement of the study purpose(s) or a hypothesis statement. A hypothesis is a supposition or proposed explanation for an observation. For example, here is an actual problem statement from a published abstract:

> *Protective lung ventilation requires calculation of predicted body weight from gender and height. Thus, inaccuracy of height data in the electronic health record (EHR) is a risk factor for volutrauma. A study showed that bedside tape measurements or visual estimates of height in ventilated patients may be highly inaccurate but that height predicted by ulnar length might be an alternative. In our institution, height records are often based on patient self-reporting, with uncertain accuracy. The purposes of this study were: (1) to evaluate the difference between patient height of unknown origin recorded in the EHR and predicted height from ulnar length, and (2) to determine the effect of height difference in setting V_T during ventilation.*[23]

This is a descriptive study. There are no predetermined hypotheses. But such a study might generate hypotheses to test in future studies (e.g., error in height determination is associated with increased duration of mechanical ventilation).

Here is an example of another published abstract with explicit hypotheses:

> *The FiO_2 for constant flow (CF) oxygen therapy via nasal cannula depends on a combination of factors, including breathing frequency and the anatomic reservoir (AR). Patients with COPD have end expiratory flows which do not reach zero, potentially eliminating the AR and decreasing FiO_2. Pulsed flow (PF) devices that do not depend on the AR and FiO_2 should not be affected by loss of the AR. The purpose of this study was to test 2 hypotheses: (1) loss of AR reduces FiO_2 for CF, and (2) loss of AR does not affect FiO_2 for PF.*[24]

Creating clear statements of study purpose or hypotheses is a key element for success in research. The purpose or hypothesis makes clear what the experimental method should be. The Methods section of your study protocol is related to the purpose or hypothesis because it dictates what the outcome variables are and how to measure them, as well as how to analyze the data and what statistical tests to use.

How to Write a Study Protocol

Whether you are doing a small process improvement project, a device evaluation, or a major randomized controlled trial, you need a written study plan. Here are three reasons why: First, the process of writing it out will help you clarify the goals of the study and methods of investigation. The realization that problems in approach or analysis exist may not become clear until ideas are committed to paper. Second, you often must present a plan to obtain permission or approval to proceed with the study. Permission may need to be sought from a funding source, IRB, department manager, or student advisor before a study may begin. Third, the research plan, or research protocol, as it is often called, provides an operational guide for the entire research team. Successful coordination of study personnel is all but impossible without a detailed protocol. For these reasons, a properly formulated proposal is an essential first step in the research process. An example of a protocol outline, as might be required for review before gaining permission from an IRB for human studies, is shown in Box 8-2. The outline in Box 8-2 might seem like overkill, but you can simplify it to fit your needs and it will impose discipline in the planning stages of your project. Another reason to do this is that it serves as the outline for any publication you may consider once the study is completed.

Box 8-2 Elements of a Protocol for Submission to an Institutional Review Board

1. Name of investigator/co-investigator
2. Title of project
3. Introduction
4. Purpose, specific aims, and hypotheses
5. Study design
   a. Specific procedures
   b. Population
   c. Financial considerations
      - Compensation to subjects.
      - Extra costs incurred for purposes of the study
   d. Risks and benefits
6. Consent form
   a. Purpose of the study and individual participation
   b. Study and procedures
   c. Risks and benefits
   d. Alternatives and withdrawal
   e. Treatment after the study
   f. Financial considerations (cost responsibility statement)
   g. Confidentiality statement
   h. Identification of persons obtaining consent

Box 8-3 Basic Concepts for Making Experimental Measurements

Basic measurement theory
- Accuracy
- Precision
- Inaccuracy, bias, and imprecision
- Linearity
- Calibration
- Sources of bias (systematic error)
- Sources of imprecision (random error)

Measuring specific variables
- Pressure
- Flow
- Volume
- Humidity

Computerized data acquisition
- Sensors
- Analogue to digital conversion
- Signal processing software

How to Analyze the Data

You don't have to be a statistician to conduct research. However, you do need to understand some basic concepts, even if only to be able to communicate with a statistician consultant. Of course, you also have to understand at least some of the terminology just to be able to read a scientific paper. Space does not permit us to explore this topic to any useful extent, so I will leave you with some suggestions for self-study in a series of boxes. If you are not familiar with any of the terms or topics in the boxes, study those. Textbooks are a good resource, and the Internet is a rich source of online texts, tutorials, and even statistical calculators. Box 8-3 lists some basic concepts for making experimental measurements. Box 8-4 lists some basic concepts in statistics.

There are hundreds, perhaps thousands, of statistical procedures used to analyze data once they are collected. Fortunately, there are only a handful of procedures that are used most of the time in the medical literature. If you learn nothing else, you should be familiar with calculating the mean and standard deviation of a set of numbers. You should know what a *p*-value is, that a t-test is used to compare two mean values (i.e., to test the hypothesis that they are from the same population of data), and that analysis of variance (ANOVA) is used to compare more than two mean values. A chi-square (χ^2) or Fisher exact test is

Box 8-4 Basic Concepts in Statistics

- Levels of measurement
  - Nominal
  - Ordinal
  - Continuous
- Significant figures
- Rounding off
- Descriptive statistics
  - Data representation
    - Graphs
    - Tables
  - Measures of the typical value of a set of numbers
    - Mean, median, mode
  - Measures of dispersion
    - Standard deviation, variance, coefficient of variation
  - Correlation and regression
- Inferential statistics
  - The concept of probability
  - The normal distribution and standard scores
  - Sampling distributions
  - Confidence intervals
  - Error intervals
  - Data analysis for device evaluation studies
  - Interpreting manufacturers' error specifications
  - Hypothesis testing
  - Type I and II errors
  - Power analysis and sample size
  - Rules of thumb for estimating sample size
  - Clinical importance versus statistical significance
  - Matched versus unmatched data

used to compare proportions. You do not need special statistical software; for many purposes, a Microsoft Excel spreadsheet functions quite well both for creating data collection forms and doing simple statistical procedures. Again, the Internet has many tutorials showing how to do these things. Finally, Figure 8-2 is an algorithm showing how to select the most appropriate statistical procedure for a given set of data.

RULE OF THUMB

Although you should be somewhat skeptical about what you read in Wikipedia (http://www.wikipedia.org), I have found it to be a rich and very detailed source of information about statistical concepts.

HOW TO GET A SCIENTIFIC PAPER PUBLISHED

Once you have completed a research project, you need to communicate the results. As a health care researcher, you will encounter three basic ways to formally present your findings: the abstract, the poster, and the paper. Abstracts and papers are published in electronic and/or printed form in medical journals. Posters are presented in person at medical conventions. All three venues share the same basic outline structure: Introduction, Methods, Results, and Discussion (or Conclusions [see the previous Rule of Thumb]). As with conducting the research itself, publishing your results requires much practice under the tutelage of an experienced mentor.

How to Write the Abstract

An abstract is a condensed version of a research paper that appears at the beginning of the publication. Many readers skim the abstract to see if they are interested enough to read the whole paper. Some readers do not have enough time to read anything more than abstracts. For these reasons, the abstract is an important element of a published paper. Furthermore, abstracts are sometimes published alone. For example, Respiratory Care journal devotes one issue each year (usually the November issue) to abstracts describing studies that were presented at the AARC Congress, the profession's annual scientific meeting.

Writing a good abstract is an art.[25] Most journals restrict the length of the abstract (e.g., 300 words or 2500 characters), so the challenge is to balance brevity with explicitness. My approach is to start with the text I wrote for the research protocol, including the Introduction, (study purpose, hypothesis) and Methods (outcome measures, procedures, data analysis). Then, because most journals restrict your abstract to having a single graphic (if any), I create one illustration (table or graph) that summarizes the data. Next, I simply describe that illustration in the Results section of the abstract. After that, I look again at the study purpose and/or hypothesis statements in the Introduction to the abstract. These are the key ideas that must be included in the Discussion/Conclusion section of the abstract. I explain how the results address the hypothesis and how I interpret the data. I may even provide a speculation or suggestion for further study.

My first draft of an abstract may be 800 words or more, which is way too long. Now the process of shortening or redaction begins. I read each word of every sentence and see which I can eliminate or replace with shorter ones or with abbreviations. If abbreviations are used, they should be placed in parentheses after the full word the first time they are used in the paper, to indicate the meaning of the abbreviation. *The idea is to decrease word count while increasing clarity*. It usually takes three or four passes through the entire abstract before the number of words is within the limit specified in the instructions to authors provided by the journal publisher. Needless to say, this process goes much more smoothly if you have an experienced mentor by your side. I find that if I have everything I need from the study, including the illustration, writing an abstract takes about 2 hours (but this is after 30 years of practice).

Once completed, the abstract is usually submitted online for peer review by the editors and reviewers of the medical journal. Figure 8-3 shows what such an abstract looks like after submitting online and conversion to a PDF format.

How to Make a Poster

If your abstract is accepted for publication, you may be invited to present a poster version at a medical convention, along with all the other studies from other authors that have been accepted.

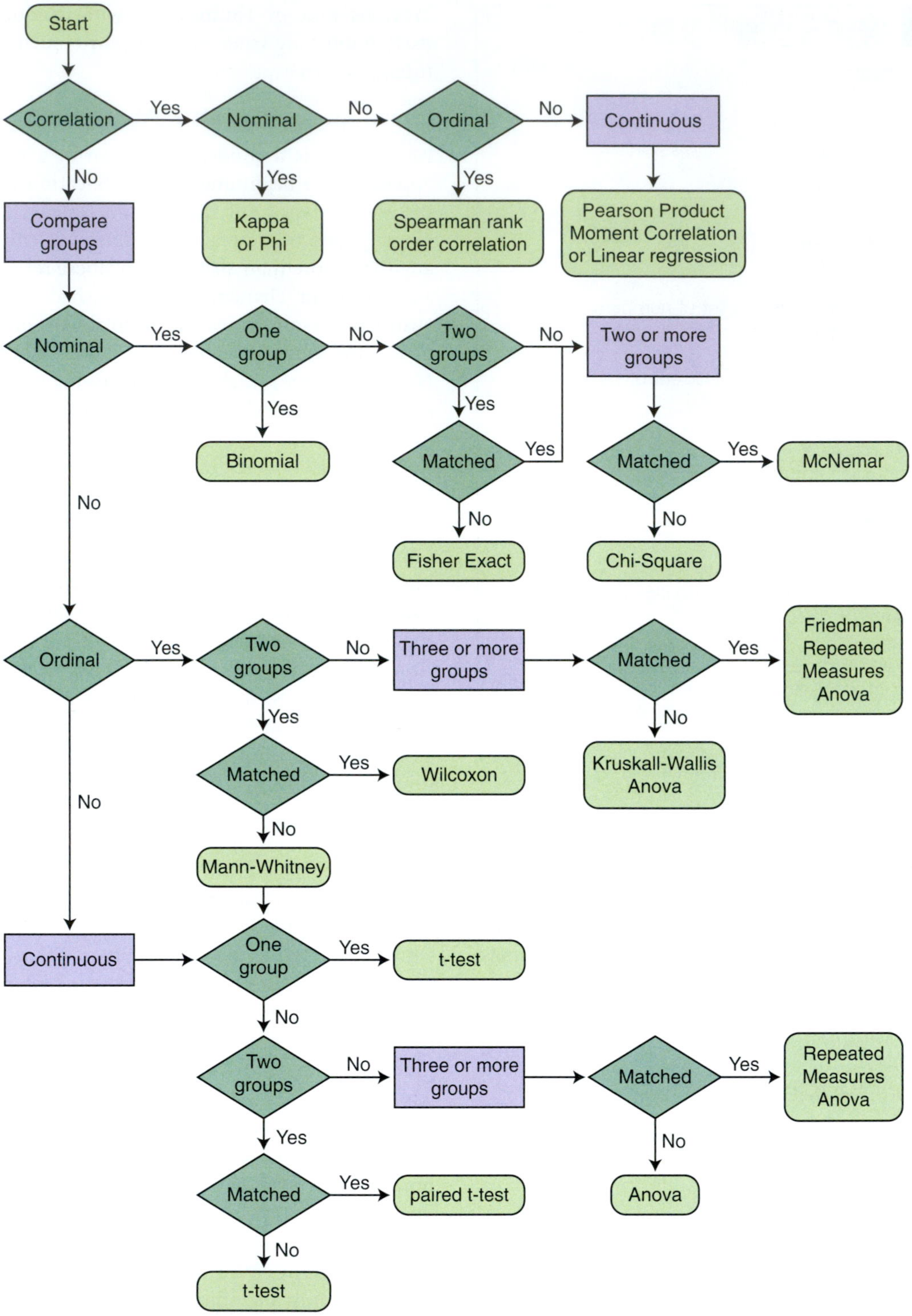

FIGURE 8-2 Statistics selector algorithm.

A poster allows a bit more freedom in terms of space.[26] You generally are allowed to create a paper or cardboard poster fitting a space of approximately 4 feet tall by 6 feet long. The way I do it is to create a template in Microsoft PowerPoint (Figure 8-4). On this template there are text boxes and graphics. Make sure the graphics are at least 300 dots per inch (dpi), usually TIFF files. If the graphics are not in the right format or have a resolution less than 200 dpi, they may look grainy when printed. Once the poster is created in PowerPoint (Figure 8-5), the file is taken to a printer (university or hospital art department or commercial establishment like Kinkos) and printed on a very large piece of poster paper (I use 42 by 74 inches). You can then roll it up and transport it in a special tube (cardboard—cheap; plastic—less cheap) made for the purpose (available at

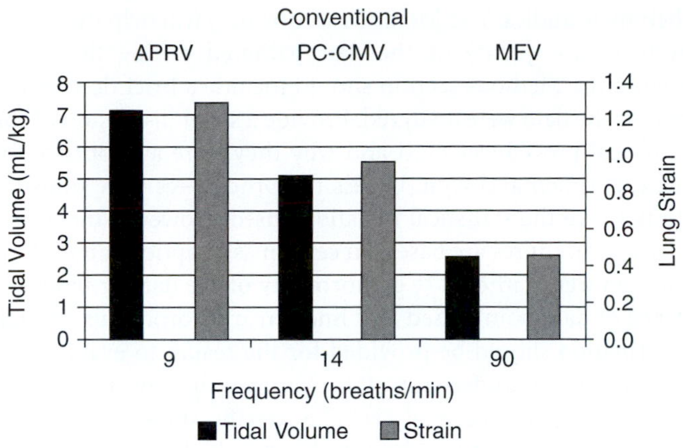

FIGURE 8-3 Abstract examination.

art supply stores). Such a tube is small enough to take as a carryon on a plane. Posters are usually presented in a group of maybe 10 to 15 in small rooms. The paper posters are hung on stands, and visitors walk around reading them and discussing them with the authors. In some cases, each author is given a few minutes at a podium to verbally summarize the study and answer questions.[27]

How to Write a Paper

If writing an abstract takes an experienced researcher 2 hours, then a full paper takes 20 to 100 hours. A paper has the same basic outline as an abstract or poster (Introduction, Methods, Results, Discussion or Conclusions) but goes into much greater detail. It also has an extra component, the References section.[28]

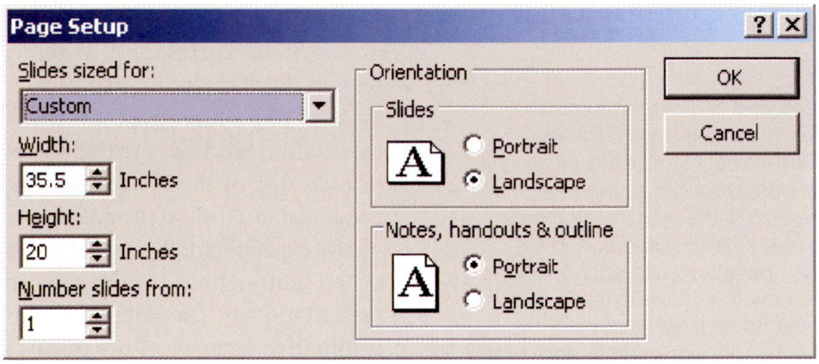

FIGURE 8-4 PowerPoint poster template.

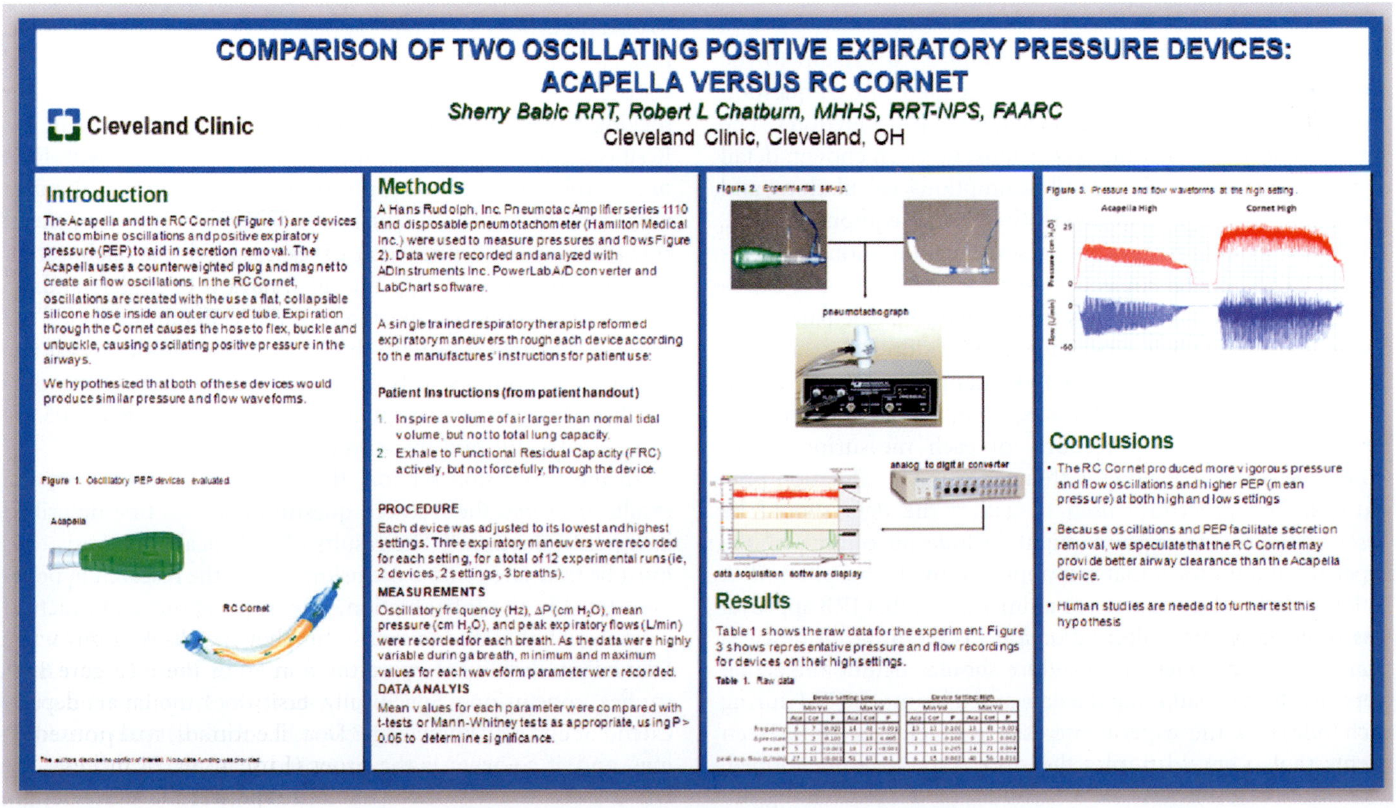

FIGURE 8-5 Example poster created in PowerPoint.

The Introduction of the paper can start with the full text of the Introduction from your research protocol. There is no word limit for the Introduction (within reason), but most journals have a maximal word count for the full text of the paper (usually in the range of 2000 to 3000 words, depending on the journal). The purpose of the Introduction is to provide a brief background explaining why the study was conducted and why it is of interest. A statement of the research problem or hypothesis should be included. The references cited in the Introduction (if any) should support the theoretical framework of the hypothesis, although an in-depth explanation should be saved for the Discussion section. The Introduction should also contain definitions of the general concepts discussed in the manuscript. Frequently used terms can be abbreviated after first being spelled out fully in the opening paragraphs.

RULE OF THUMB

Not including the hypothesis is a common mistake among beginners. Describing the hypothesis or research problem in the Introduction of the paper sets the stage for the Methods (which must describe how the hypothesis was tested), the Results (which must correspond to all the methods described), and the Discussion (which tells how the results addressed the hypothesis, discusses how this paper extends existing knowledge, and comments about limitations of the paper and further research opportunities to answer the questions posed in the paper).

The purpose of the Methods section is to explain to the reader exactly what was done to answer the research question and/or test the hypotheses described in the Introduction.[29] The key concept here is that the reader must be given enough detail to repeat the study, including all assumptions, calculations, and statistical procedures and descriptions of all equipment used. The Methods section may contain several subdivisions; description of experimental subject population, inclusion and exclusion criteria by which subjects are selected to participate in the research study, explicit experimental procedures, data analysis procedures, etc. An essential component of the Methods section is a complete description of any equipment used to gather the data. The calibration procedure for each measuring device should be described, along with any pertinent validation procedures. The procedure used to gather the data should be described. This description might include an outline of the experimental protocol that was approved by the hospital's IRB. If the study involves humans or animals, state that IRB approval was received before collecting data (as is required). A description of the experimental procedure should include the actual steps involved in gathering the data and the time elapsed during each phase of the experiment. Any problems or unforeseen events that occurred during the study should be mentioned. The information in this section should be detailed enough to guide other researchers who might wish to verify the results in their own studies. The Methods section also will help the reader evaluate the quality of the data gathered during the study. Finally, the Methods section should include a brief description of how the data were analyzed. Provide a short discussion of the statistical procedures used and why they were appropriate for the experimental design. Unless the procedures were unusual, do not give the statistical equations used. However, many statistical procedures are based on certain assumptions about how the data were gathered (e.g., normality of the data or independence of data points used in a linear regression). Thus enough information should be provided for the reader to evaluate the validity of any underlying statistical assumptions and, hence, the adequacy of the analysis. The specific statistical software that was used (if any) should also be cited in the Methods section.

The Results section of the paper presents the data gathered from the experiments. The order in which the information is given should correspond to the organization of the Methods section. In that section, the reader was introduced to the step-by-step procedure used to study a particular problem. An expectation has been created in the reader's mind for the result of each step of the procedure. Therefore the results should be presented in a logical progression from the beginning to the end of the experiment. This progression helps to assure the reader of the thoroughness of the experimental technique. The actual presentation of the data can take many forms. Use tables to summarize large amounts of raw data.[30] Each table should be constructed so that its meaning is clear without having to refer to the text. The idea is to summarize and guide the interpretation of large amounts of data and to reduce the time necessary to read the article. If the table appears to be too large or complex, make use of figures or graphs. Again, you do not need special statistical software; Microsoft Excel is an excellent tool for making tables and graphs. The information presented in the Results section is usually in the form of "bare facts," with little or no explanation of its significance. Interpretation of the data is presented in the Discussion section. Of course, this is a general rule and may be suspended at times if it is felt that elaboration of some point would help the reader's flow of understanding. The responsibility for interpreting the generalizability of the results ultimately rests with the reader. The significance of any statistical hypothesis tests is usually reported in terms of a *p*-value. Differences associated with *p*-values less than 0.05 are considered significant by convention in medical studies.

In the Discussion section, the author must show how the results answered the research question that was first described in the Introduction.[31] The results of statistical hypothesis tests must be translated into conclusions about the research hypotheses stated in the Introduction. The implications and practical meaning of the study results should be explained. Also, the Discussion should interpret the results in the face of earlier studies' conclusions. Specifically, how does the current study extend or add new knowledge? Does it contradict previous findings, and, if so, what is the proposed reason? In addition, the Discussion should describe the limitations of the study design, any problems encountered, and any recommendations for future studies. The process of interpreting the results concerns not only the data generated by the study but also relates that data to other studies and theoretical frameworks. The Discussion is the appropriate place to include detailed reviews of other related research, including references, which would help to develop the reader's perspective and appreciation for the significance of the study.

Some journals require a separate Conclusion statement at the end of the paper. The conclusions made should be briefly explained, including reasons for rejecting alternative interpretations. In addition, there should be a statement regarding the population to which the results can be generalized. Because the implications of a given study are usually speculative, it is appropriate to use words that are somewhat tentative in nature. For example, "The results of this study suggest that . . . ." or "Because of the significant differences found, it may be possible to . . . ." Such language emphasizes the fact that your interpretation is itself a hypothesis that may be tested by further research.

How to Respond to Reviews

Once your paper is completed and submitted to a journal for review, it will be given to two or three "peer reviewers." These are your scientist peers who have expertise in the area of research described in your paper. They are invited by the editor of the journal to review the paper you submitted and will read and critique everything about your paper, from what words you use, to what measurements you made, to what statistical procedures you used. They will then recommend to the journal editor one of three outcomes: that your paper should not be considered for publication; that, with luck, your paper is rejected with an opportunity to revise and resubmit; or that the paper should be accepted as is. Rarely does a paper get accepted without any suggested revisions. The main reasons that papers get rejected are given in Box 8-5.[32]

Having a paper rejected is like being told your child is ugly and stupid. Most people react with negative emotions and give up. But if you can get past that phase, you have several options. First, examine whether the reviewers' comments are justified. Sometimes they have just misunderstood what you did. If the comments are justified, see what you can do to make the required changes. Generally, you will be given a list of reviewers' comments. In your response, you need to repeat each of the reviewer's comments and then give your explicit answers and what you did to achieve the requested change in the manuscript (I use a numbered list to keep track of everything in this so-called *point-by-point response* that must accompany any resubmission). Keep three things in mind: (1) The time spent in revision is generally only a small fraction of the time already invested—you should not give up if you receive a rejection with an opportunity to revise. (2) Most manuscripts require revision and you are not being singled out. (3) Authors have the right to overrule a reviewer's objection, but they must adequately support their points of view and convince the editor that they are right and that the reviewer's point is in error. When the revision is complete, resubmit the manuscript. Depending on the journal, it may take as many as three rounds of revisions before a manuscript is accepted and ready for publication.

Box 8-5 The 10 Most Frequent Reasons for Manuscript Rejections

1. Inappropriate statistics
2. Inappropriate interpretation of results
3. Instrumentation insufficient for the study purpose
4. Inadequate or biased sampling of experimental subjects
5. Unclear, poorly written, or overly complex text
6. Insufficient (or absent) problem statement
7. Inaccurate or inconsistent data
8. Incomplete, inaccurate, or outdated literature review
9. Insufficient data
10. Defective tables or figures

Modified from Pierson DJ: The top 10 reasons why manuscripts are not accepted for publication. Respir Care 49:1246, 2004.

SUMMARY

Hopefully, this chapter has introduced you to the importance and methods of scientific research and has helped you become an educated consumer of medical research. Not everybody is cut out to be a scientist. But, as professionals, everyone practicing respiratory care has the responsibility to intelligently evaluate what they are doing in light of scientific evidence. Unfortunately, most of the things we do in medicine are not supported by strong evidence, despite the wealth of information in printed medical journals and on the Internet (in the form of databases, portals, and electronic media). And even when evidence is available, it is often controversial. We rarely know anything for sure, and we only have varying degrees of confidence. On the one hand, this situation is frustrating. On the other hand, there is no doubt that we are progressing. Which would you prefer, your least favorite health maintenance organization today or the best medicine of 100 years ago? Our current situation provides infinite possibilities for anyone who has an interest in research and the willingness to help clarify the confusion just a bit. If you have enough interest (and hopefully a mentor) you can begin to create basic study ideas and conduct experiments. With perseverance, it is quite possible for you to get your abstract accepted in Respiratory Care journal and present your poster at the Annual AARC Congress. Even if your personal goals do not include becoming a scientist, you should publish at least one abstract in your career to understand what is involved with moving the profession forward as a clinician, educator, or administrator.

RULE OF THUMB

Even after doing research, we may still be confused, but we believe we are confused at a higher level about more important things.

SUMMARY CHECKLIST

- All health care professionals have the responsibility to intelligently evaluate what they are doing in light of scientific evidence.
- Information required to evaluate professional practice can be found in printed medical journals and on the Internet (in the form of databases, portals, and electronic media).
- Research ideas can be obtained from reading research and from simply observing daily practice. General ideas can be turned into statements of study purpose by describing what you see happening and why it is important.
- Research results can be disseminated in three main ways: abstracts, posters, and papers in peer-reviewed medical journals.

References

1. Chatburn RL: Overview of respiratory care research. *Respir Care* 49:1149, 2004.
2. Google scholar: <http://scholar.google.com/>, Accessed June 30, 2015.
3. Chatburn RL: How to find the best evidence. *Respir Care* 54:1360, 2009.
4. Rau JL: Searching the literature and selecting the right references. *Respir Care* 49:1242, 2004.
5. PubMed: <http://www.ncbi.nlm.nih.gov/pubmed?dr=Abstract&holding=ohccalib_fft_ndi&otool=ohccalib>, Accessed June 30, 2015.
6. Search Medica: <http://www.searchmedica.com/>, Accessed June 30, 2015.
7. Cochrane: <http://www.cochrane.org/>, Accessed June 30, 2015.
8. UpToDate: <http://www.uptodate.com/contents/search>, Accessed June 30, 2015.
9. ClinicalKey: <http://www.clinicalkey.com>, Accessed June 30, 2015.
10. Ovid: <http://www.ovid.com/site/index.jsp>, Accessed June 30, 2015.
11. Respiratory Care: <http://www.rcjournal.com>, Accessed June 30, 2015.
12. Oxford Reference: <http://oxfordreference.com>, Accessed June 30, 2015.
13. STAT!Ref: <http://statref.com>, Accessed June 30, 2015.
14. Safari: <http://safaribooksonline.com>, Accessed June 30, 2015.
15. Amazon: <http://www.amazon.com>, Accessed June 30, 2015.
16. ENDNOTE: <http://www.endnote.com>, Accessed June 30, 2015.
17. RefWorks: <http://www.refworks.com>, Accessed June 30, 2015.
18. Zotero: <https://www.zotero.org/>, Accessed June 30, 2015.
19. Chatburn RL: *Handbook for health care research*, ed 2, Boston, 2009, Jones and Bartlett.
20. Chatburn RL, Craig KC: *Fundamentals of respiratory care research*, Norwalk, CT, 1988, Appleton & Lange.
21. Fink JB: Device and equipment evaluations. *Respir Care* 49:1157, 2004.
22. Durbin CG: How to come up with a good research question: framing the hypothesis. *Respir Care* 49:1195, 2004.
23. Jurecki M, Chatburn RL, Sasidhar M: Accuracy of the electronic health record: patient height. *Respir Care* 2015 (in press).
24. Zhou S, Chatburn RL: The effect of anatomic reservoir on FiO2 for constant flow versus pulse flow oxygen delivery devices. *Respir Care* 59(10): OF26, 2014.
25. Pierson DJ: How to write an abstract that will be accepted for presentation at a national meeting. *Respir Care* 49:1206, 2004.
26. Shelledy DC: How to make an effective poster. *Respir Care* 49:1213, 2004.
27. Campbell RS: How to present, summarize, and defend your poster at a meeting. *Respir Care* 49:1217, 2004.
28. Branson RD: Anatomy of a research paper. *Respir Care* 49:1222, 2004.
29. Kallet RH: How to write the methods section of a research paper. *Respir Care* 49:1229, 2004.
30. Durbin CG: Effective use of tables and figures in abstracts, presentations, and papers. *Respir Care* 49:1233, 2004.
31. Hess DR: How to write an effective discussion. *Respir Care* 49:1238, 2004.
32. Pierson DJ: The top 10 reasons why manuscripts are not accepted for publication. *Respir Care* 49:1246, 2004.

SECTION II

APPLIED ANATOMY AND PHYSIOLOGY

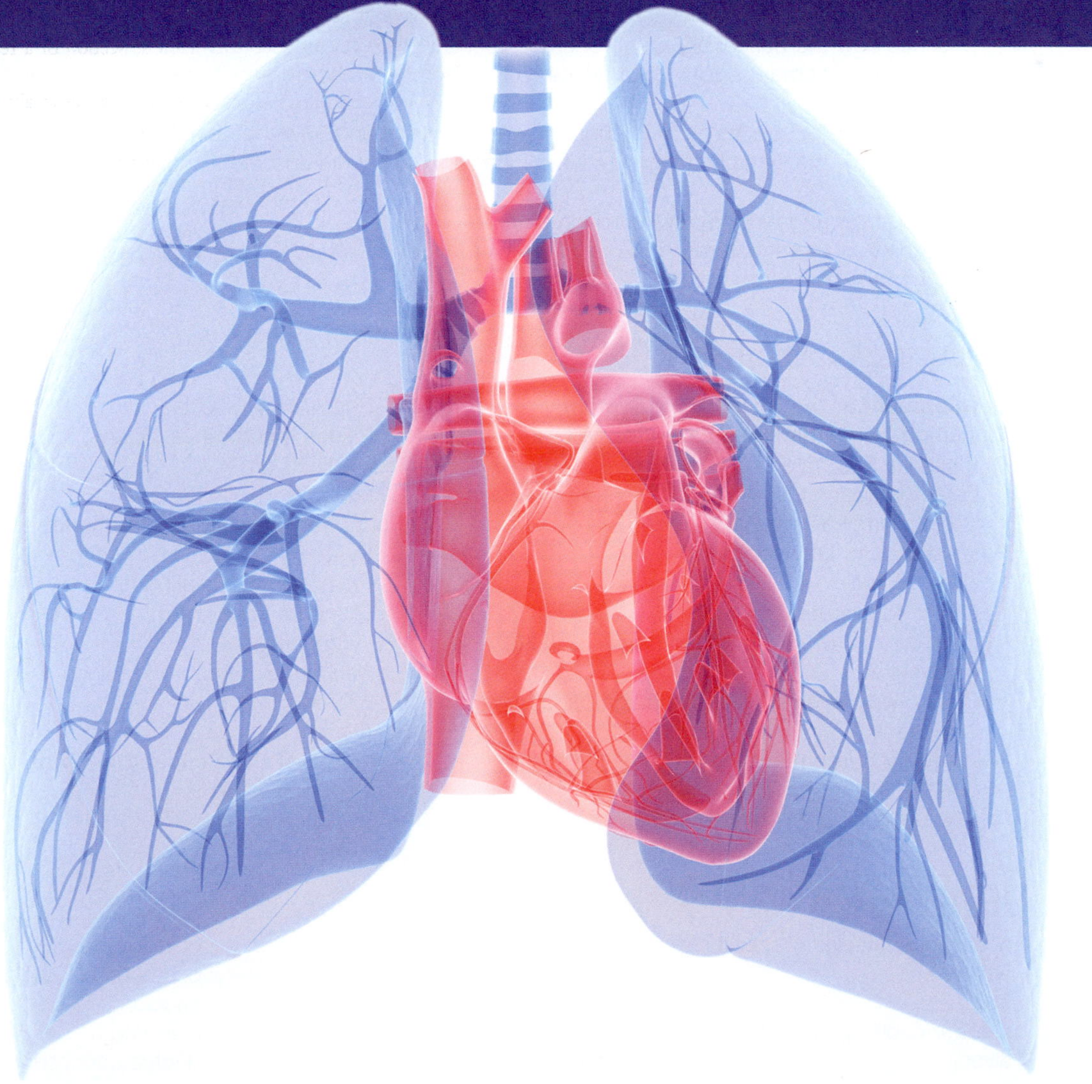

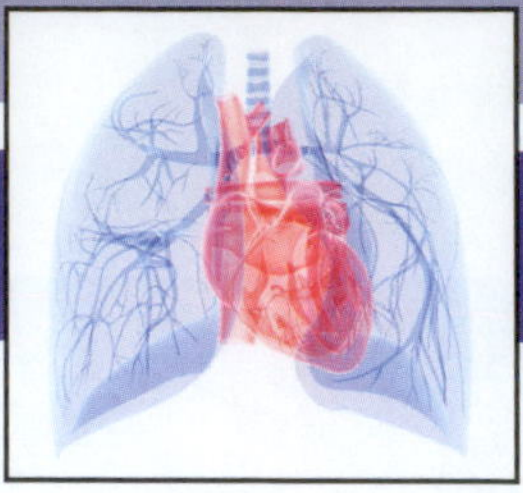

CHAPTER 9

The Respiratory System

CRYSTAL L. FISHMAN AND NARCISO E. RODRIGUEZ

CHAPTER OBJECTIVES

After reading this chapter you will be able to:

- State the major developmental events of the respiratory system.
- Describe how genes control lung development.
- Describe the key elements of normal fetal circulation.
- State what happens to the respiratory system at birth.
- Describe the developmental events in the respiratory system that continue after birth.
- Identify the main structures in the thorax and describe their functions.
- Identify and describe the primary and accessory muscles of breathing.
- Describe how the pulmonary and bronchial circulations are organized and their functions.
- Describe how somatic and autonomic nervous systems connect to and control the lungs and respiratory muscles.
- Identify the major structures of the upper respiratory tract and how they function.
- Describe how the lungs are organized into lobes and segments and the airways that supply them with ventilation.
- Describe how and why airways produce and move mucus.
- Describe how the structures in the respiratory bronchioles and alveoli are organized.
- Describe the blood-gas barrier.

CHAPTER OUTLINE

KEY TERMS

accessory muscles of breathing
acinus
alae
alveolar-capillary membrane
alveoli
angle of Louis
anterior nares
apexes
carina
cilia
costal cartilage
costophrenic angle
cricoid cartilage
diaphragm
ductus arteriosus

ductus venosus
epiglottis
epistaxis
eustachian tubes
external nares
external oblique
external respiration
false ribs
fissures
floating ribs
foramen ovale
gladiolus
glottis
hilum
hypopharynx
intercostal muscles
intercostal nerves
internal oblique
internal respiration
laryngopharynx
larynx
lobes
manubrium
mediastinum
mucociliary escalator
nasopharynx
oropharynx
palate
parietal pleura
pharynx
phrenic nerves
pores of Kohn
primary lobule
pseudostratified epithelia
pulmonary surfactant
rectus abdominis muscles
scalene muscles
segments
soft palate
sternal angle
sternocleidomastoid muscles
sternum
suprasternal notch
trachea
true ribs
turbinates
type I pneumocyte
type II pneumocyte
uvula
vallecula
visceral pleura
xiphoid process

The primary function of the respiratory system is the continuous absorption of oxygen and the excretion of carbon dioxide. This exchange between the gas of the atmosphere and blood is termed **external respiration.** This process supports **internal respiration,** which is the exchange of gases between blood and tissues. To carry out external respiration, the system brings gas into close proximity with the flowing blood in the pulmonary circulatory system. This close "match" of gas and blood across a large but extremely thin blood-gas barrier membrane enables efficient gas exchange to occur via simple diffusion.

The respiratory system includes the upper airways, chest wall, respiratory muscles, lower airways, pulmonary blood vessels, support nerves, and lymphatics. These organs support gas exchange and form early in the developing human. They undergo dramatic functional changes at the time of birth, beginning its primary role of breathing and external respiration at that moment.

From the moment of conception the human body undergoes tremendous growth and development—from embryo to fetus to infant and child, through puberty, and into young adulthood. A gradual loss of lung tissue and functional changes continue through the elderly years until the time of death. During the life span of a human, the respiratory system maintains external respiration by matching phenomenal amounts of air with a similar amount of blood flow. Approximately 250 million liters of each are moved and matched during an average 75-year life span. The respiratory system normally moves this amount of air and blood flow with a minimal amount of work. This system humidifies and warms inspired air while removing inhaled contaminants and filtering out chemicals and small blood clots deposited or formed in the blood. The respiratory system is regulated by the nervous system. It is capable of increasing function in response to elevated demands brought on by stressful conditions such as exercise and disease.

A functional understanding of the "normal" anatomy and physiology of the respiratory system is crucial to proper understanding of pulmonary disease and its treatment. The role of the respiratory care therapist in assessment and treatment of cardiopulmonary disorders requires an in-depth understanding of the structural and functional nature of the respiratory system.

DEVELOPMENT OF THE RESPIRATORY SYSTEM

The developing human undergoes a remarkable transformation from a single cell to an individual with a nearly complete set of organ systems. The developmental phases of a fertilized egg are divided into the *embryonic* and *fetal periods.* The embryonic period occurs during the first 8 weeks of pregnancy. Major organs will develop during this period. The fetal period occurs during the remaining 32 weeks of pregnancy. During this period, the organs continue to develop and refine their structure and function.

The respiratory system develops during these periods as a fluid-filled structure playing no role in gas exchange, yet must be developed sufficiently to assume this crucial activity at the time of birth. Its development is a continuous process that begins in the early stages of the embryonic period and extends for years after birth. The embryo is made up of three distinct germinal tissue layers that ultimately form all tissues and organs: *endoderm, mesoderm,* and *ectoderm.* From these layers the organs and systems will arise (Table 9-1).

The development of the respiratory system has been categorized into various stages.[1] Figure 9-1 shows the various stages of lung development, and Table 9-2 summarizes the major developmental events in each phase. Respiratory development begins in the embryonic period on or approximately day 22 after fertilization. A primitive laryngotracheal tube forms from a groove in the fourth pharyngeal pouch. From that groove a tracheal bud forms by the end of the fourth week of life (Figure 9-2). During week 5 of development, the tracheal bud continues to develop and bifurcates into left and right primary bronchial buds.

Injury to the embryo or genetic dysregulation during this crucial phase of development can lead to many congenital anomalies, including tracheoesophageal fistulas, esophageal atresia, choanal atresia, pulmonary hypoplasia, and complex heart and vascular anomalies discussed later in this text.

At approximately 6 weeks of development, lung and airway growth has the appearance of a glandular structure—hence the name of the second phase of development, the *pseudoglandular stage* (Figure 9-3). For the next 10 weeks, the growth and branching of the tracheobronchial tree and pulmonary vasculature continue and culminate with formation of the terminal and respiratory bronchioles. The distinction between these two types of bronchioles is important. Terminal bronchioles are conducting airways only and do not participate in gas exchange with blood. Respiratory bronchioles have more superficial capillaries and are capable of gas exchange with blood, becoming more elaborate as development continues.

Branching and dividing of the tracheobronchial tree occurs in several ways as the result of differential gene expression. The epithelial lining of the airways begins to differentiate into columnar epithelia in the proximal airways and differentiates into cuboidal epithelia in the more distal bronchioles (Figure 9-4, *A*). Development of *cilia, mucous glands,* and *goblet cells* occur at this time and line most of the conducting airways.

Beginning with the trachea and moving distally, the amount of cartilage supporting the airway decreases as smooth muscle cells in the middle layer of the airway increase. Altered development of smooth muscle, cartilage, and vascular structures can lead to other congenital pulmonary disorders, such as tracheomalacia and anomalous pulmonary arteries, causing the vascular rings to pinch the airway.

The *canalicular stage* (see Figure 9-4, *B*) begins at week 16 and continues until week 26. The canalicular stage overlaps with the pseudoglandular stage because the superior regions are developing slightly faster than the inferior regions. During this phase, primary changes include the development of two to four more generations of respiratory bronchioles from each terminal bronchiole. In the last several weeks of this stage, the region beyond each terminal bronchiole forms the functional structure called the **acinus,** the basic gas-exchanging unit of the lung. At this time, the two principal epithelial cell types that cover the gas-exchange surface begin to appear, *type I* and *type II* pneumocytes. At the end of the canalicular period (24 to 26 weeks of gestation), the fetus, if born, is capable of sufficient gas exchange and viable if supported with supplemental O_2, ventilatory support, and surfactant administration.

During the *terminal saccular stage* (see Figure 9-4, *C*), more terminal bronchioles and their associated acini form and develop from 26 weeks to birth. The formation of the total number of terminal bronchioles is complete at the end of this phase. The cuboidal epithelia that line the blind tubules of the acinus continue to differentiate into rounded secretory cells **(type II pneumocytes)** and flatter squamous epithelial cells **(type I pneumocytes).** Capillaries continue to form near and bulge from the surface of the acinus. Although some type II pneumocytes form by 20 weeks of gestation, they are in such small numbers and of such primitive function that their impact on lung function is marginal. From this point until birth, there

TABLE 9-1
Structures Arising from the Three Germ Layers

Endoderm	Mesoderm	Ectoderm
Respiratory tract	Dermis and muscles	Epidermis, hair, and nails
Digestive tract, bladder and thyroid	Bone, connective and lymph tissue	Lens of eyes and skin glands
Liver and pancreas	Reproductive and cardiovascular system	Central and peripheral nervous system

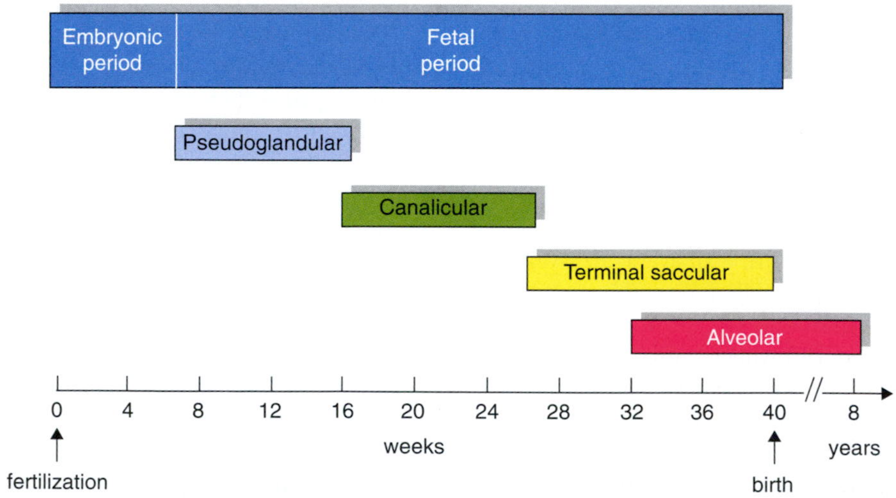

FIGURE 9-1 Major phases of respiratory development.

TABLE 9-2
Developmental Events of the Cardiopulmonary System

Gestational Age	Developmental Event
Embryonic Period	
20-22 days	Primordial pharyngeal arches form
21-23 days	Primordial respiratory cells form on fourth pharyngeal pouch, primordial heart starts forming
26th day	Laryngotracheal bud forms
4th wk	Primitive trachea develops
5th wk	Primary bronchial buds form, laryngeal structures develop
Fetal Period	
Pseudoglandular Stage	
6th wk	Segmental and subsegmental bronchioles form
7th wk	Diaphragm complete
8th wk	Heart complete, fetal circulatory pattern begins to develop
10th wk	Pulmonary lymphatic structures develop
12th wk	Major arteries formed
13th wk	Major airway epithelia and mucus-producing cells formed, smooth muscle cells developing
14th wk	Principal arteries formed
16th wk	Terminal bronchioles and associated pulmonary vessels form
Canalicular Stage	
16th-17th wk	Respiratory bronchioles and immature acini begin to form
20th-24th wk	Type I and II pneumocytes begin to appear and replicate
24th-26th wk	Pulmonary capillaries develop at surface of acinus, immature surfactant begins to appear in lung fluid
Terminal Saccular Stage	
26th wk–birth	Terminal saccules increase in number, pulmonary capillary density and proximity increase, type I and II pneumocytes continue to multiply, surfactant production increases, extrauterine life possible with support
Alveolar Stage	
32th-40th wk	Immature alveoli begin to form and increase in number; surfactant production matures
40th week	50 million immature alveoli formed
Period After Birth	
Birth	First breath and lung fluid cleared, adult circulatory pattern established
8-10 yr	470 million mature alveoli formed

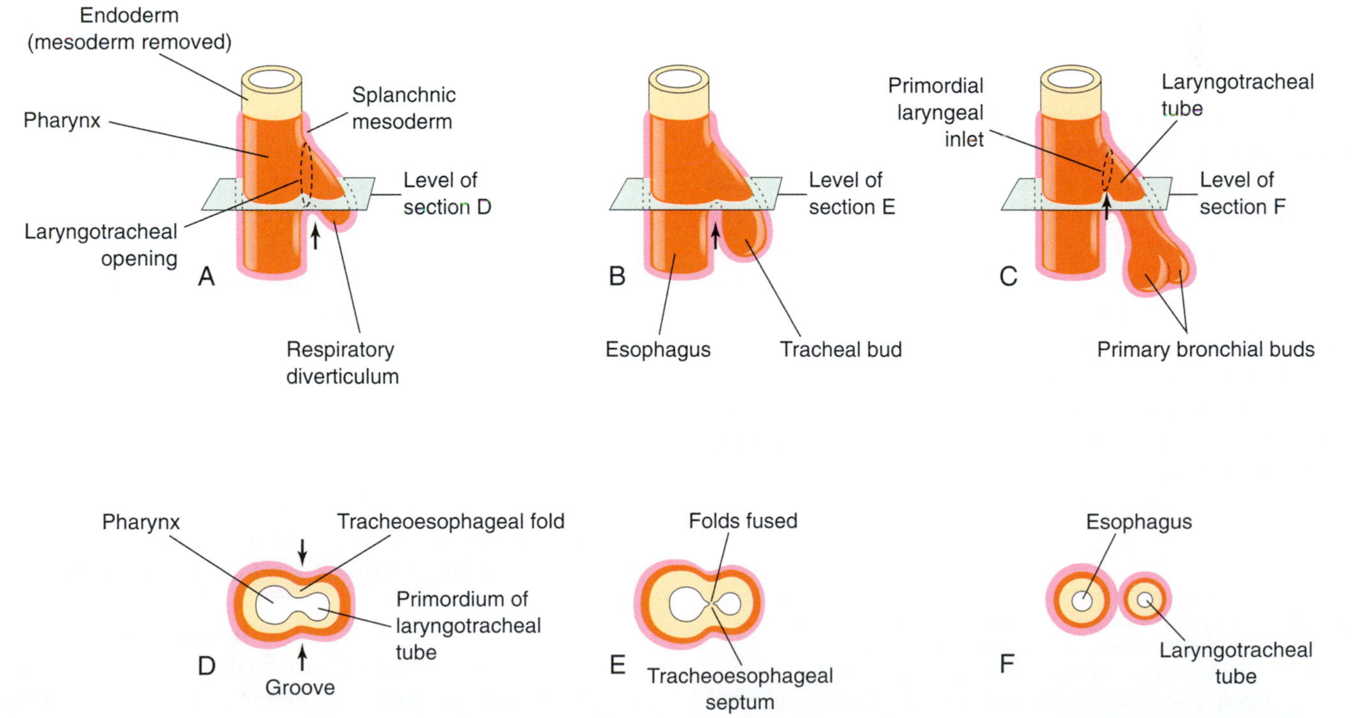

FIGURE 9-2 Successive stages in the development of the respiratory system from the primitive foregut. **A-C,** Lateral views of the caudal part of the primordial pharynx showing the respiratory diverticulum and partitioning of the foregut into the esophagus and laryngotracheal bud. **D-F,** Transverse sections illustrating the formation of the tracheoesophageal septum and showing how it separates the foregut into the laryngotracheal bud and esophagus. (From Moore KL, Persaud TVN: The respiratory system. In Moore KL, Persaud TVN, editors: The developing human: clinically oriented embryology, ed 8, Philadelphia, 2008, WB Saunders.)

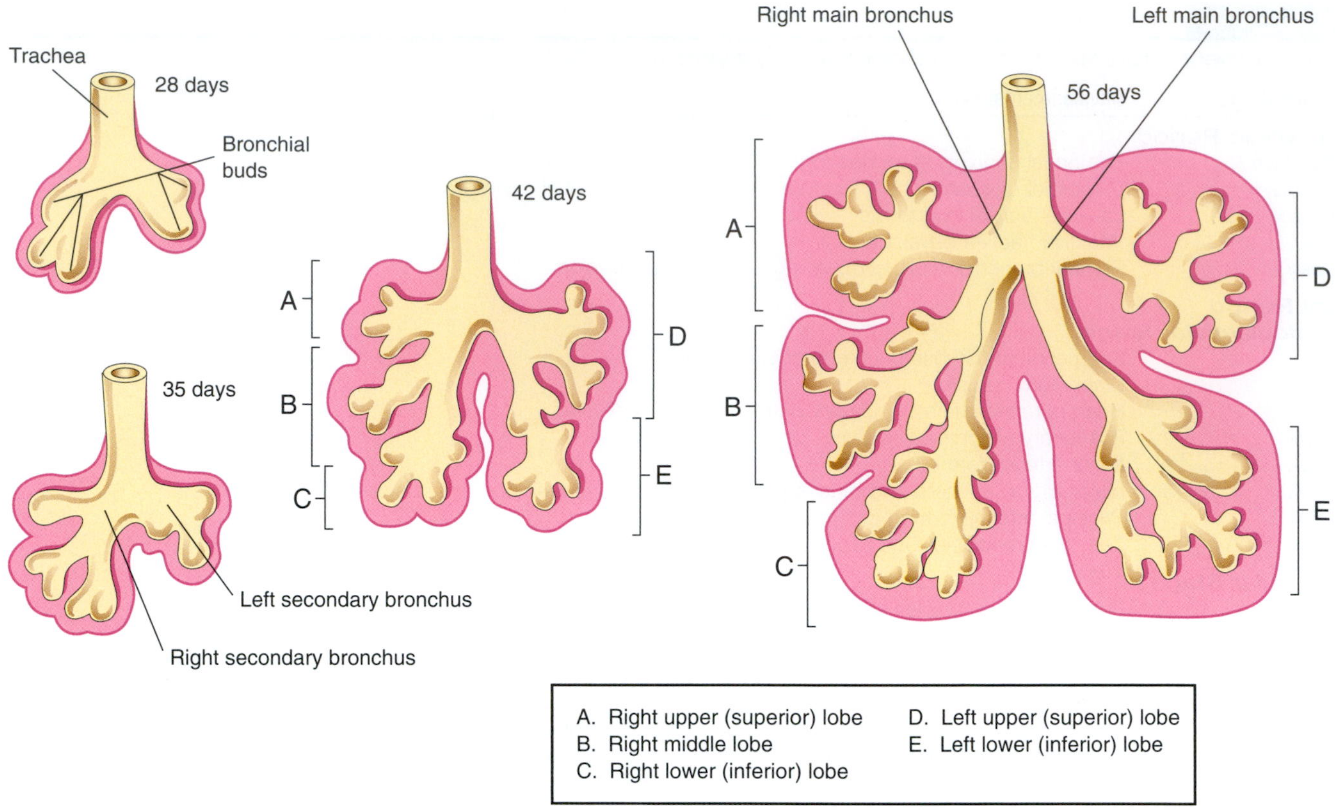

FIGURE 9-3 A-E, Various stages in the growth of the bronchi as the lungs enter the pseudoglandular period of development. (From Moore KL, Persaud TVN: The respiratory system. In Moore KL, Persaud TVN, editors: The developing human: clinically oriented embryology, ed 8, Philadelphia, 2008, WB Saunders.)

is rapid proliferation of alveolar ducts and sacs formed from the respiratory bronchioles.

The type I pneumocytes of the saccule walls thin and elongate to cover the walls of this region. Type I cells become the primary gas-exchange cells in the lung with close approximation to developing pulmonary capillaries. Type II pneumocytes form and secrete the vital pulmonary surfactants that are necessary to alter surface tension and help keep the lungs inflated.

The development of mature alveoli, accompanied by capillary proliferation within the walls, marks the final phase of lung development and is known as the *alveolar period* (see Figure 9-4, *D*). This phase begins at about week 32 of gestation and continues for years after birth. During this phase the terminal saccules develop hexagonal pouchlike regions called *alveoli* within their walls, resulting in greater numbers of alveoli that enlarge to a mature state over time.

RULE OF THUMB

The development of mature alveoli marks the final stage of lung development, known as the *alveolar period*. This period begins at approximately 32 weeks of gestation and continues for years after birth. As a result, premature infants younger than 32 weeks are at greater risk for developing respiratory distress.

A full-term newborn infant has approximately 50 million alveoli, this number continues to increase for approximately 2 to 3 years after birth.[2,3] The alveoli are lined with type I and II pneumocytes covering the pulmonary capillaries forming just below the basement membrane.

Human **pulmonary surfactant,** which promotes lung inflation and protects the alveolar surface, begins to be produced around 24 to 25 weeks of development by type II pneumocytes. It is composed primarily of phospholipids, a small amount of protein (types SP-A, SP-B, and SP-C), and a trace of carbohydrates.[4] Early research in pulmonary surfactants centered on the phospholipid components, mainly phosphatidylcholine (lecithin [L] and sphingomyelin [S]) and phosphatidylglycerol (PG). The amount of these phospholipids (the *L/S ratio* and *PG concentration*) provides a predictive index of the lung maturity in a fetus before birth and the risks for the development of respiratory distress.[5] An L/S ratio of 2 or more indicates a relatively low risk for the development of respiratory distress syndrome, whereas an L/S ratio of less than 1.5 is associated with a high risk.

Surfactant synthesis is regulated by numerous hormones, genes, and factors, including glucocorticoids.[6] Glucocorticosteroid production increases at the end of gestation and stimulates receptors in type II pneumocytes, increasing surfactant production and improving the L/S ratio.

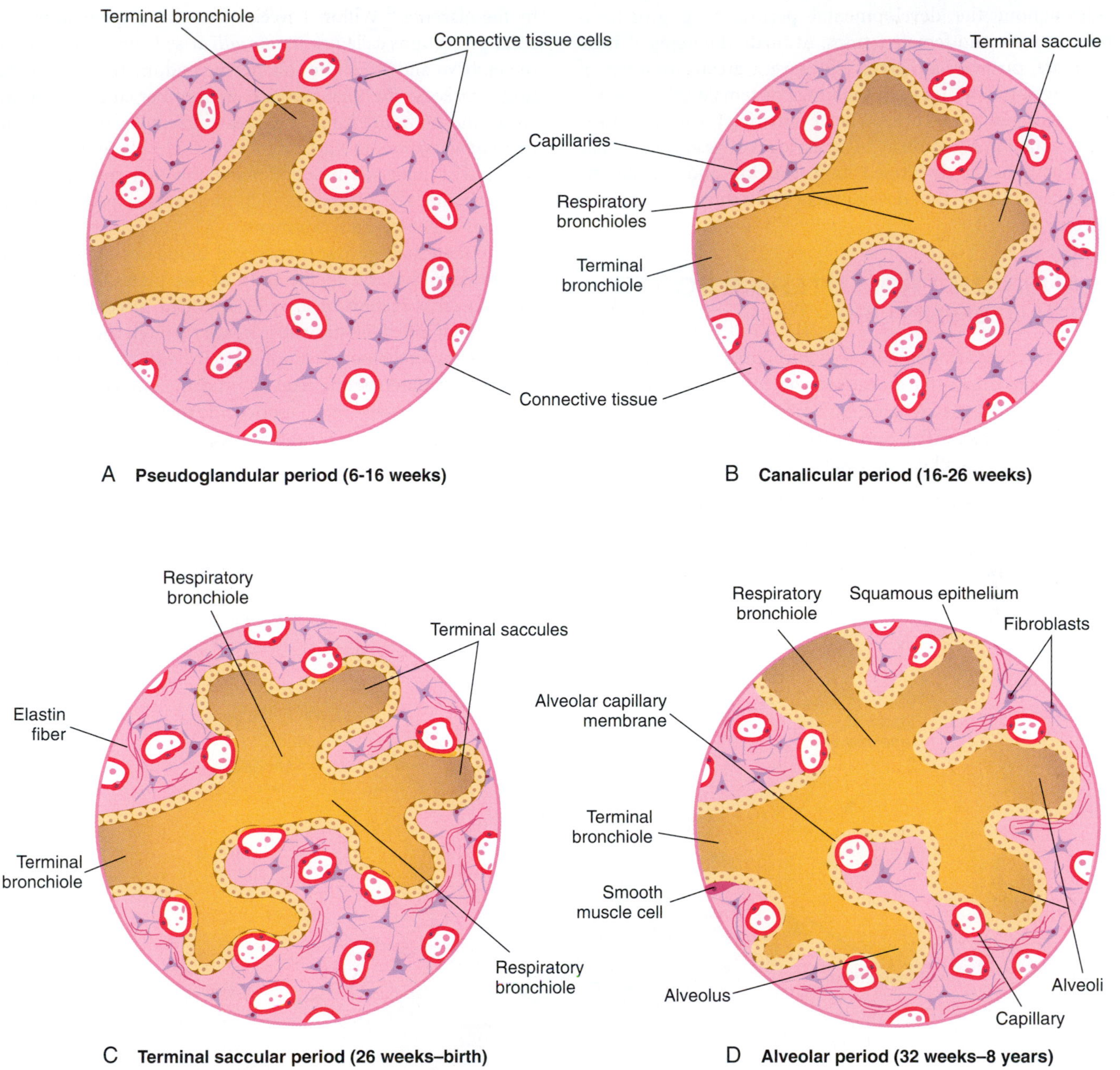

FIGURE 9-4 Histologic changes that illustrate various periods of airway development. **A and B,** There is considerable distance between the air within the airways and blood within the capillaries. **C and D,** The air-blood distance is considerably thinner and more supportive of effective air breathing. (From Moore KL, Persaud TVN: The respiratory system. In Moore KL, Persaud TVN, editors: The developing human: clinically oriented embryology, ed 8, Philadelphia, 2008, WB Saunders.)

A distinctive function of the developing lung is the formation of relatively large amounts of fetal lung fluid that passes into amniotic fluid. Fetal lung fluid is a unique combination of plasma ultrafiltrate from the fetal pulmonary microcirculation, components of pulmonary surfactant, and other fluids from pulmonary epithelial cells.[7] This fluid is constantly produced and replaced, keeping the fetal lung inflated at a slight positive pressure with respect to amniotic fluid pressure. This phenomenon is important in stimulating normal lung development.[8] At term, the fetal lung is filled with approximately 40 ml of fluid. Conditions that lead to inadequate fetal breathing and low amounts of amniotic fluid formation (oligohydramnios) are linked to incomplete inflation and poorly developed (hypoplastic) lungs.

A developing fetus begins to make respiratory efforts midgestation and continues these efforts until birth. During these efforts, the fetus moves little or no fluid in and out of the lungs. The rhythm and depth of fetal breathing are periodic and irregular, reflecting the development of the respiratory centers in the brain and respiratory muscles.

Throughout the developmental period, lung growth is similar in male and female fetuses. At birth, the lungs of male infants are, on average, larger and have a greater number of respiratory bronchioles than the lungs of female infants when adjusted for gestational age.[9] When evaluating breathing efforts and surfactant production at 26 to 36 weeks of gestation, female fetuses have better developed lung function and are slightly less susceptible to the development of respiratory distress syndrome.[10,11]

TRANSITION FROM UTERINE TO EXTRAUTERINE LIFE

At birth, the lungs undergo a rapid and remarkable transition. A liquid-filled organ that possesses very little circulation incapable of sufficient gas exchange becomes an air-filled organ that receives the entire cardiac output from the right heart. It then carries and delivers all gas necessary to sustain life.

Placental Structure and Function

Survival of the embryo/fetus requires an effective circulatory interface with the circulation of the mother, which is provided by the placenta.[12] Within 1 week of uterine implantation, vascular projections called *chorionic villi* arise from the chorion of the embryo and penetrate the uterine endometrium. As gestation proceeds, the villi increase in number and complexity, erode the endometrium, and create irregular pockets called *intervillous spaces* in the placenta, which fill with maternal blood. The maternal blood flowing through the intervillous spaces bathes the embryonic villi and creates an O_2-rich and nutrient-rich blood environment.

The maternal uterine tissues and blood vessels of the fetal chorionic villi make up the bulk of the placenta. Figure 9-5 shows a cross section of a well-developed placenta. Maternal blood flows into the intervillous space through the spiral arteries, whereas fetal blood is supplied to the villi from two umbilical arteries. Maternal and fetal blood come into close proximity but remain separated by an embryonic membrane that permits the exchange of O_2, CO_2, water, ions, various metabolic molecules, and hormones.

Various chemicals, hormones, bacteria, and viruses can also cross the intervillous space and cause a variety of fetal developmental problems. Oxygenated fetal blood leaves the chorionic villi capillaries through placental venules and returns to the

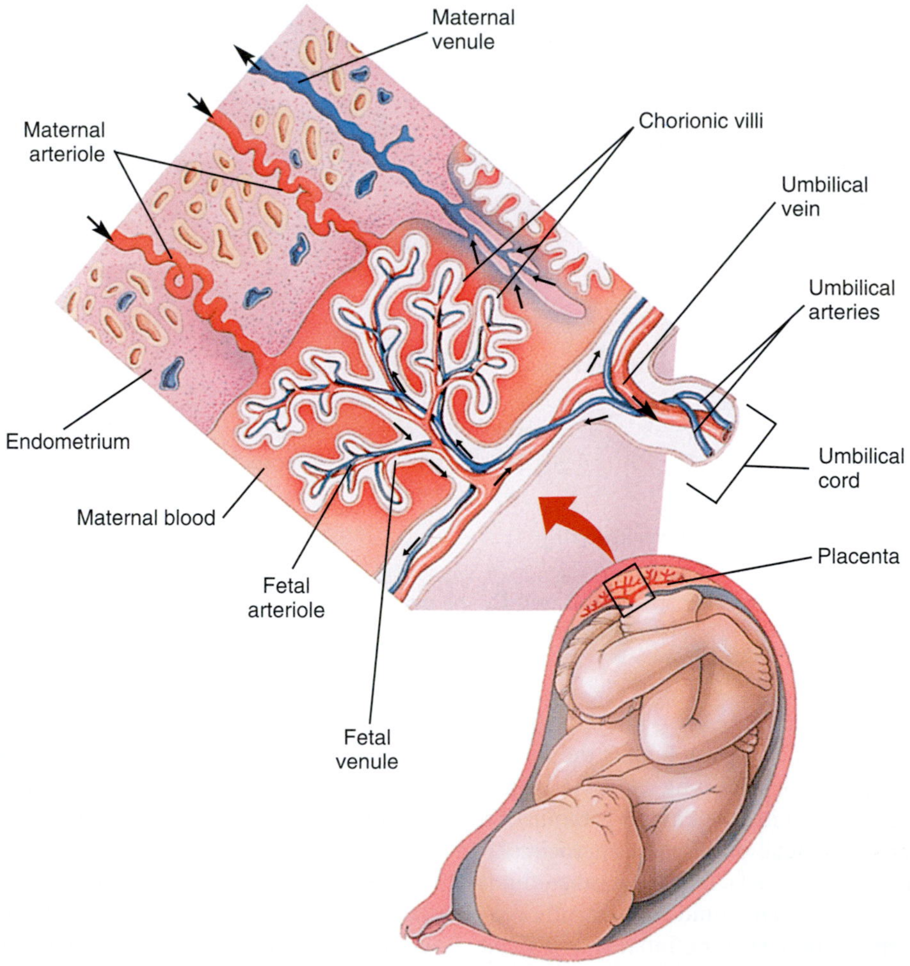

FIGURE 9-5 Cross-sectional view through the placenta showing the spiral arteries that supply maternal blood to the intervillous spaces. The fetal villi, immersed in maternal blood, are supplied with blood from the umbilical arteries and drain their blood back through the umbilical vein. (From Thibodeau GA, Patton KT: Anatomy and physiology, ed 7, St Louis, 2010, Mosby.)

TABLE 9-3

Approximate Normal Values of Blood Gases and Acid-Base in Fetal and Maternal Blood

Value	Maternal Intervillous Blood	Fetal Umbilical Artery Blood	Fetal Umbilical Venous Blood
pH	7.38	7.36	7.39
PCO_2 (mm Hg)	42	47	43
PO_2 (mm Hg)	50	19	30

fetus through a single umbilical vein. Abnormal implantation of the placenta, tearing of the placenta from the uterine wall, or decreased placental blood flow can stunt intrauterine growth. In severe cases this can cause fetal asphyxia, increasing the risk for brain damage and respiratory distress in the immediate postnatal period.

Many factors enhance the delivery of O_2 to fetal tissues. The partial pressure gradient for O_2 between maternal blood and fetal blood drives the diffusion of O_2 into fetal blood within the chorionic villi capillaries.[13,14] Maternal arterial blood has a partial pressure of O_2 (PaO_2) of approximately 100 mm Hg and mixes with the blood in the intervillous space, producing a mean PO_2 of approximately 50 mm Hg. Fetal blood that enters the villi has a PO_2 of approximately 19 mm Hg, and the pressure gradient between maternal and fetal blood PO_2 ($50 - 19 = 31$ mm Hg) causes O_2 to diffuse into fetal blood. Blood leaving the villi and entering the umbilical vein has a PO_2 of approximately 30 mm Hg. Table 9-3 summarizes the normal gas and acid-base values in normal fetal umbilical arteries and veins and maternal intervillous blood. Assessment of umbilical vein blood gas data (cord blood gas) shortly after birth is a method of determining the degree of fetal asphyxiation during the birth process.

The O_2 content and delivery by fetal blood are almost the same as adult blood despite the much lower PO_2. This is due to several factors, including relatively higher content of hemoglobin (18 g/dL) and hematocrit (54%) in fetal blood and the presence of fetal hemoglobin (HbF), which has an increased affinity for O_2 and a more pronounced Bohr effect (reduced oxyhemoglobin affinity with acidosis) to enhance O_2 release.[14] Figure 9-6 illustrates how the increased O_2 affinity is manifested by a leftward shift of the fetal oxyhemoglobin dissociation curve. The P_{50} (PO_2 that saturates 50% of the hemoglobin) is 6 to 8 mm Hg less than the P_{50} for adult hemoglobin (HbA), which indicates the degree of the shift toward higher affinity. At birth, approximately 70% of circulating hemoglobin is HbF. HbA gradually replaces HbF during the first 6 months of extrauterine life as HbA genes in bone marrow switch on and HbF genes in the liver (major site of fetal erythrocyte development) are switched off.

Fetal Circulation

Fetal circulation is different from the circulation of the neonate after birth.[15] Three important bypass pathways (shunts) function in the developing fetus to enhance the flow of blood to the developing organs: **ductus venosus, ductus arteriosus,** and **foramen ovale.** Oxygenated blood from the placenta is carried in the umbilical vein back to the fetal circulation via the hepatic circulatory system (Figure 9-7). Approximately one-third of this blood flows to the lower trunk and extremities. The other two-thirds flows through the *ductus venosus,* bypassing the liver's circulation, and flows to the inferior vena cava. This better oxygenated blood in the inferior vena cava mixes with the venous blood returning from the lower trunk and extremities entering the right atrium. Approximately 50% of this blood is shunted from the right atrium into the left atrium through an opening in the interatrial septum called the *foramen ovale.* Left atrial blood flows to the left ventricle and then to the ascending aorta, where it continues on to the brain, brachiocephalic trunk, and descending aorta. Venous blood from the superior vena cava is directed downward through the right atrium into the right ventricle and then into the main pulmonary artery.

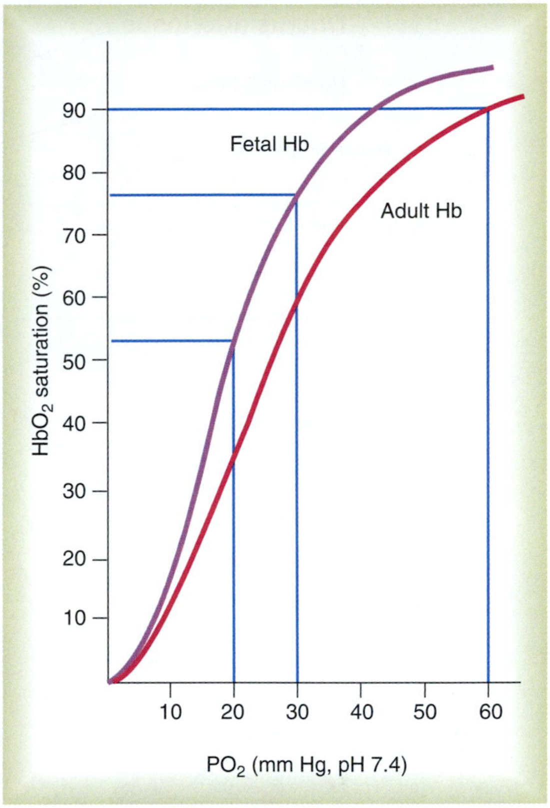

FIGURE 9-6 Fetal hemoglobin (Hb) has a leftward shift of the oxyhemoglobin (HbO_2) dissociation curve compared with adult Hb, indicating greater affinity for O_2. (Modified from Koff PB, Eitzman DV, Neu J: Neonatal and pediatric respiratory care, St Louis, 1988, Mosby.)

The relatively low PO_2 and various prostaglandins in fetal blood cause the *ductus arteriosus* (a muscular vessel attached to the trunk of the pulmonary artery and the aorta) to dilate and the pulmonary arteries to constrict. This leads to an increase in pulmonary vascular resistance, resulting in pulmonary artery pressure higher than aortic blood pressure. As a result, 90% of

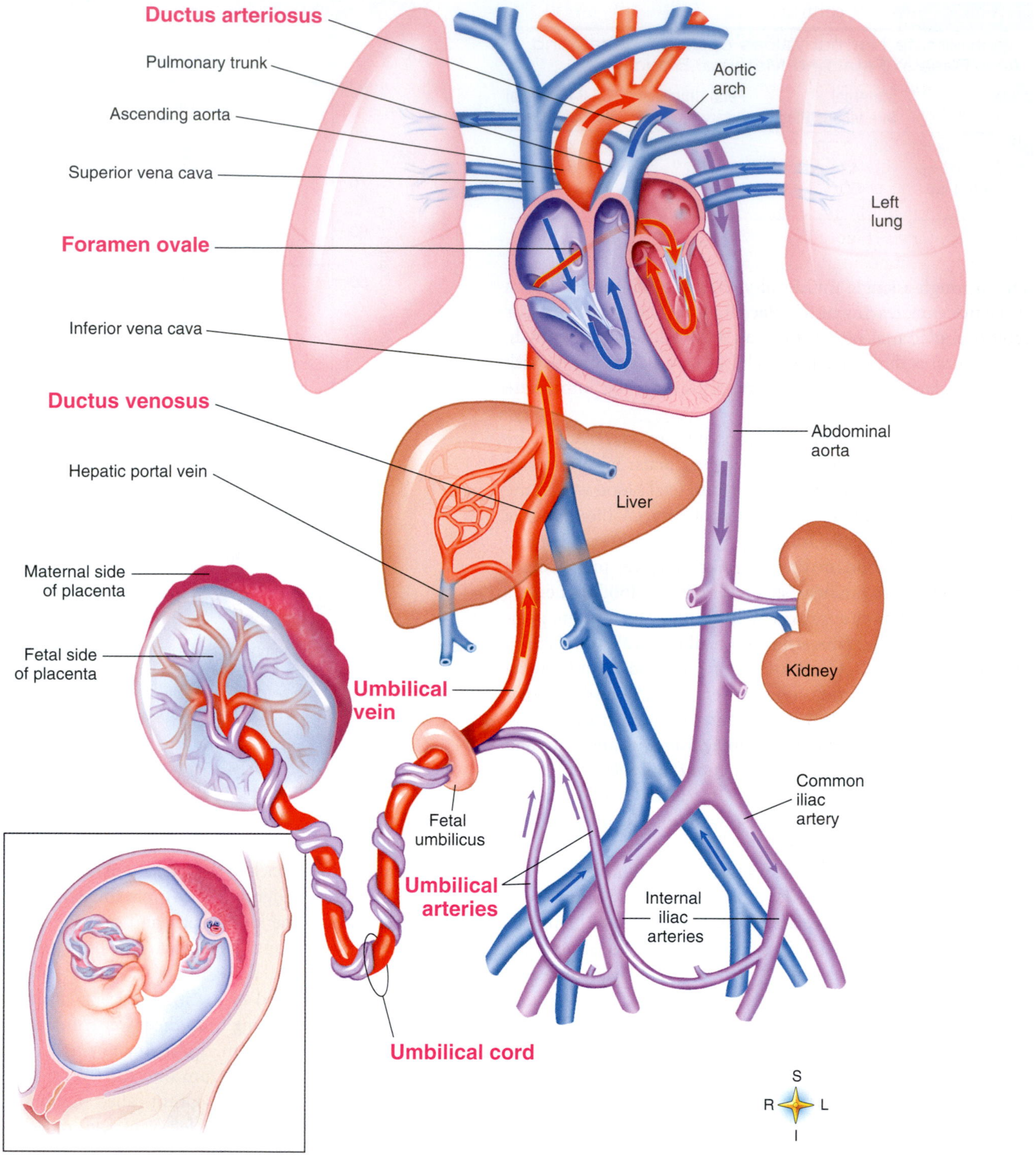

FIGURE 9-7 Fetal circulation before birth. Special features (shown in *red*) include the umbilical cord, two umbilical arteries, one umbilical vein, ductus venosus, foramen ovale, and ductus arteriosus. (From Thibodeau GA, Patton KT: Anatomy and physiology, ed 7, St Louis, 2010, Mosby.)

the blood flow entering the pulmonary artery takes the path of least resistance by shunting through the ductus arteriosus and flowing to the aorta. Only 10% flows into the lungs. Blood flowing through the ductus arteriosus mixes with blood flowing through the aorta, routing into the systemic circulation. Some of this blood flows to the gut, lower extremities, and placenta. Two umbilical arteries carry blood from the fetal aorta to the placenta, carrying out fetal-maternal gas and nutrient exchange.

Cardiopulmonary Events at Birth

Various mechanisms work together to reduce and clear the amount of lung fluid at birth in preparation for air inflation.[16]

Days before birth, the epithelia of the lung stop the production of lung fluid, which is actively absorbed back into fetal circulation. During normal vaginal delivery, approximately one-third of the lung fluid is cleared through compression of the thorax in the birth canal. The pulmonary capillaries and lymphatics clear the remaining fluid.

A newborn must develop very high transpulmonary pressure gradients during the first few breaths to open and replace the remaining lung fluid with air and establish a stable lung volume for gas exchange (Figure 9-8). These large pressure gradients overcome the opposing forces of fluid viscosity in the airways and surface tension in the alveoli. The stimulus for these initial respiratory efforts is sent via peripheral and central chemoreceptors and augmented further by skin thermoreceptors.

The first breath is triggered by new tactile and thermal stimuli. In addition, as placental gas transfer is suddenly interrupted, the newborn becomes hypoxemic, hypercapnic, and acidotic, triggering strong inspiratory efforts. The pressure-volume changes occurring during these first breaths are depicted in Figure 9-8. At first, no air enters the newborn lung until the transpulmonary pressure gradient exceeds 40 cm H_2O. As lung volume increases with each breath, decreasing amounts of pressure are needed to overcome the opposing forces. The volume trapped in the lung stabilizes quickly and is crucial to adequate gas exchange.

Figure 9-9 summarizes the major cardiopulmonary changes that occur during the transition from a fluid-filled lung to an air-filled lung. As the lung expands with air, and gas exchange starts within the lung, pulmonary blood PO_2 increases, PCO_2 decreases, and pH increases; this results in pulmonary vasodilation, lower pulmonary vascular resistance, and constriction of the ductus arteriosus, which facilitates greater blood flow through the pulmonary circulation. Ductus arteriosus closure is stimulated further by the loss of maternal prostaglandins. The combination of increasing alveolar air content and constriction

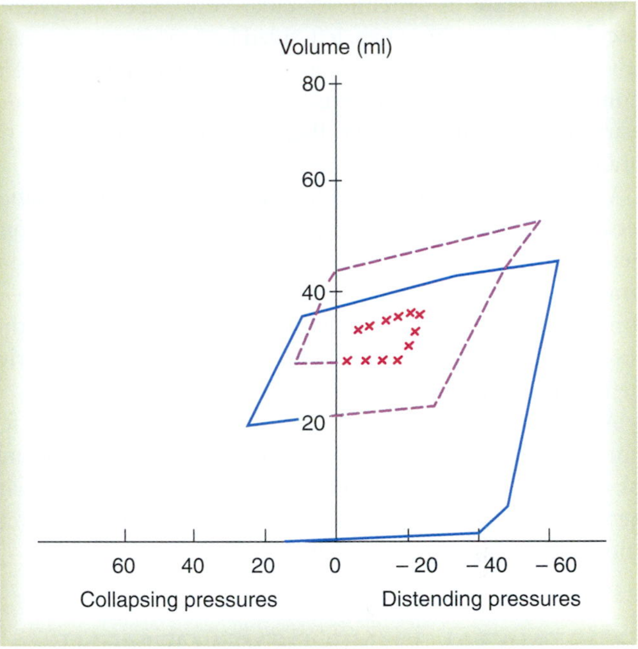

FIGURE 9-8 Pressure-volume changes in the human neonate during the first three breaths after birth: first breath (—), second breath (—), and third breath (xxx). (Modified from Taeusch WH, Ballard RA, Gleason, CA: Avery's diseases of the newborn, ed 8, Philadelphia, 2005, WB Saunders.)

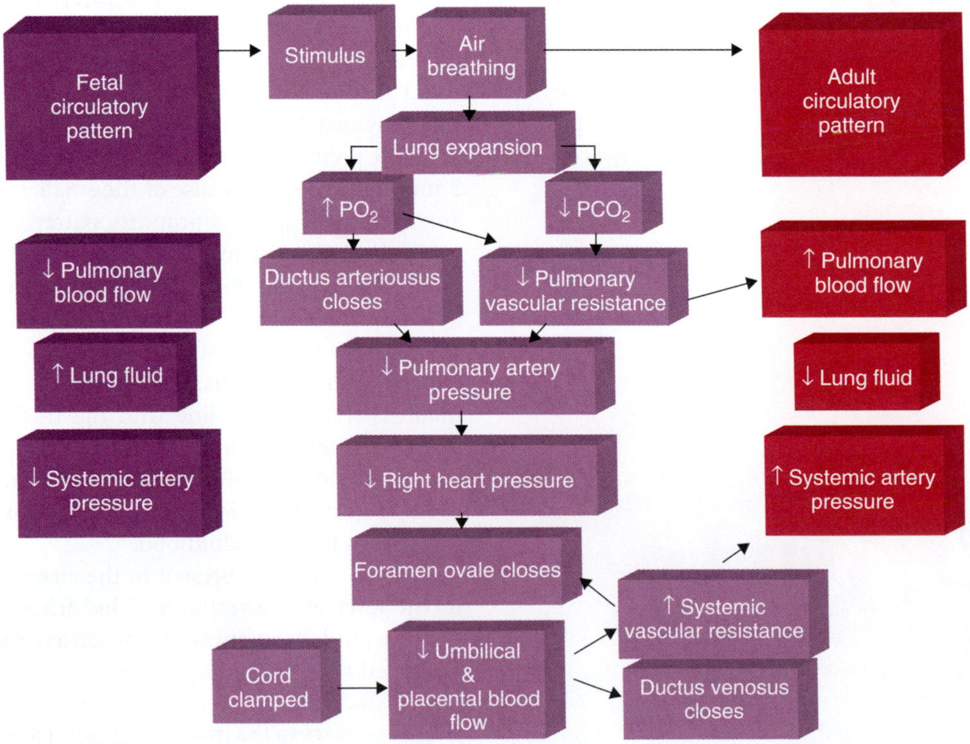

FIGURE 9-9 Major cardiopulmonary changes during the transition from the fetal to the adult circulatory pattern.

of the ductus arteriosus promotes progressive improvement in the matching of ventilation and blood flow, which increases the PO_2 and decreases the PCO_2 of blood leaving the lungs. After the clamping of the umbilical cord, cessation of umbilical and placental blood flow causes closure of the ductus venosus and a rapid increase in systemic vascular resistance. As systemic vascular resistance increases, left-sided heart pressures increase. Left atrial pressures also increase as a result of increased pulmonary blood flow that returns from the lungs. With left-sided heart pressures now higher than right-sided pressures, the foramen ovale closes.

When this last right-to-left shunt closes, the transition between fetal and extrauterine circulations is functionally complete. Full transition occurs later as the ductus arteriosus and foramen ovale close anatomically through the formation of fibrosis. Anatomic closure of the ductus normally occurs within 3 weeks of birth. Permanent closure of the tissue flap covering the foramen ovale may take several months.

All of these changes normally occur during the first few minutes after birth and allow the newborn to achieve normal gas exchange. Many abnormal conditions can interfere with these transition events, leading to persistence of the fetal circulation and cardiorespiratory failure.

POSTNATAL LUNG DEVELOPMENT

Upper Airway

The infant lung is a unique structure and not a mere miniaturization of the adult lung. The airways, distal lung tissue, and pulmonary capillary bed all continue to grow and develop after birth. Although the general pattern is well developed at birth, both the upper and the lower airways continue to change and are relatively unique in each person.

Figure 9-10 shows the relative differences of the upper airway in relation to body size in an infant and an adult. The greater relative weight of the head can cause acute flexion of the cervical spine in infants with poor muscle tone. Infant neck flexion causes acute airway obstruction. Although the head is larger, an infant's nasal passages are proportionately smaller than those of an adult. In addition, the infant's jaw is much rounder and the tongue is much larger relative to the size of the oral cavity.[17] These anatomic differences increase the likelihood of airway obstruction when an infant becomes unconscious and loses muscle tone.

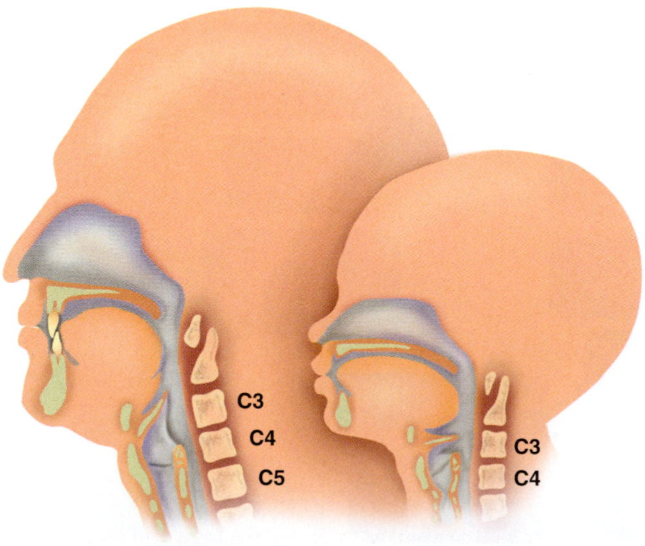

FIGURE 9-10 Adult and pediatric upper airways.

Most infants breathe preferentially through the nose. However, most term newborn infants shift to oral breathing in response to nasal occlusion and hypoxia.[18] As normal infants mature, they begin to use the oral breathing route more with increased capability of shifting to oral breathing when nasal obstruction is present.[19] At approximately 4 to 5 months of age, most infants are capable of full oral ventilation.

A newborn's larynx lies higher in the neck than the larynx of an adult, with the glottis located between C3 and C4, and is more funnel-shaped than that of an adult. In a child, the narrowest region of the upper airway is through the **cricoid cartilage,** rather than the **glottis,** as in adults. The **epiglottis** of an infant is longer and less flexible than the epiglottis of an adult and lies higher and in a more horizontal position. During swallowing, the infant's larynx provides a direct connection to the nasopharynx. This connection creates two nearly separate pathways, one for breathing and one for swallowing, allowing infants to breathe and suckle at the same time. Anatomic descent of the epiglottis begins at 2½ to 3 months of age. Mechanical and chemical irritant laryngeal reflexes develop at birth and can initiate protective laryngeal closure; these reflexes can trigger prolonged apnea in some and may be a cause of sudden infant death syndrome.[20] In addition, infections in this area, repeated attempts at intubation, or suctioning can easily cause swelling, leading to obstruction.

The large conducting airways of infants are shorter and narrower than the airways of adults. The normal newborn trachea is approximately 5 to 6 cm long and 4 mm in diameter, whereas in small preterm infants, it may be only 2 cm long and 2 to 3 mm in diameter. Because of the smaller airways, a newborn's anatomic dead space is proportionately smaller than the anatomic dead space of an adult, being approximately 1.5 ml/kg of body weight. Figure 9-11 compares the tracheal anatomy in an adult and newborn. The main stem bronchi branch off from the trachea in the infant at less acute angles than in the adult. Similar to that in adults, the right main stem bronchus of the infant is still more in line with the trachea, promoting right main stem intubation when airways or suction catheters are inserted too deeply. Mean airway diameter, from main bronchi to respiratory bronchioles, increases approximately two to three times from birth to adulthood.[21]

Smooth muscle is present in the airways of a neonate down to the level of the respiratory bronchioles and continues to increase until the infant is approximately 8 months old. Distinct C-shaped rings of cartilage are found in the trachea and main stem bronchi of the neonate. The amount of cartilage progressively decreases in the more distal bronchi and eventually disappears in airways smaller than 2 mm in diameter.

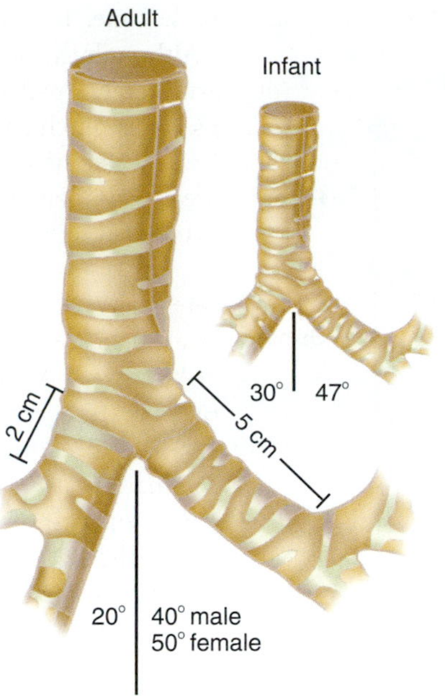

FIGURE 9-11 Adult and infant tracheas showing the different angles of main stem bifurcation.

Despite the presence of cartilage in the central airways of an infant, the trachea and larger bronchi of a neonate lack the rigidity of adult central airways. The compliant nature of these airways makes them prone to collapse and compression.

Lower Airway and Alveoli

The human lung continues to develop alveoli for years until it reaches a stable stage, at which the total number has increased to approximately 480 million alveoli.[22] All development is generally complete by 10 years of age, with most occurring in the first 1½ postnatal year.[23] By adulthood, the alveolar-capillary membrane has a gas exchange surface area of approximately 140 m^2.[24]

Compensatory lung growth can occur rapidly in the lung when part (or all) of the other lung is removed.[25-27] Stem cell activation in the lungs, in response to gene and mechanical stretch, appears to be responsible for alveolar development well into adulthood after loss of lung tissue.[28]

Development of Vascular, Lymphatic, and Nervous Systems

The basic architecture of the pulmonary circulation is complete at birth. The main pulmonary arterial trunk arises from the right ventricle and divides into left and right pulmonary arteries, which supply each lung. These arteries divide further to form direct or conventional arteries and supernumerary arteries. Both types of pulmonary arteries come together to supply blood to large clusters of alveoli that are supplied by a single bronchiole. Most of the growth in the vascular system that occurs after birth includes further smooth muscle growth within the walls of arteries and arterioles and greater density and refinement of the arterioles and capillaries in the distal airway region.[23,29]

The respiratory system is a unique organ in that it receives a double blood supply: one from the left ventricle and one from the right ventricle. The right heart supplies the bulk of the flow to the pulmonary circulation. The left heart supplies a smaller amount of flow (approximately 1% to 2% of cardiac output) to the bronchial arteries, which arise from the aorta and supply oxygenated blood to the tracheobronchial tree. The bronchial arteries supply O_2 to the airway tissue, blood vessels, nerves, lymphatics, and visceral pleura. In addition, O_2 is directly absorbed across the airway lumen. Although the pulmonary and bronchial circulations have entirely different origins and purposes, they mix and supply blood flow to the microcirculation of the alveoli; this provides some collateral circulation and allows the shunting of blood. The lung's double circulation benefits the entire lung in health and helps compensate for deficiencies or disease processes that can affect either circulation.

The lymphatic vessels located in the connective tissue tracts of the lung surround the bronchi, bronchioles, blood vessels, nerves, and pleural membrane. They play a central role in the control of fluid and protein balance within the lung and house various defensive cells. Fluid collected from the pleural space and interstitium is carried by the pleural capillaries and vessels through the lymphatic system back to the root of the lung **(hilum),** where numerous lymph nodes are located.

Before birth, neuronal centers in the brainstem (medulla oblongata and pons) form for the automatic control of breathing, and various afferent and efferent nerves form to sense and control different aspects of the respiratory system. The **phrenic nerves** and **intercostal nerves** are the primary components of the somatic (motor) nervous system that carry nervous signals from the brainstem to the respiratory muscles. They innervate the diaphragm (phrenic nerves) and intercostal muscles (intercostal nerves). These muscles are primarily responsible for enlarging the thorax during inspiration and allow exhalation by relaxing, letting the thorax and lungs recoil back to their preinspiratory position.

Visceral control of the smooth muscle of the respiratory system is carried out by branches of the sympathetic and parasympathetic nervous systems and mediators transported to the lungs via the pulmonary circulation. Nerve fibers from the brainstem and spinal cord enter the lungs and grow in the same connective tissue tracts that surround the airways and house the blood and lymphatic vessels long before birth. These nervous fibers innervate the smooth muscles of the bronchioles to cause bronchodilation (sympathetic fibers), the mucous glands to produce mucus (parasympathetic), and the blood vessels to cause vasoconstriction (sympathetic). Cranial nerve X (*vagus* nerve) carries motor and sensory signals of the parasympathetic system. Branches from each thoracic spinal nerve carry sympathetic motor and sensory signals to and from the lungs.

Chest Wall Development, Diaphragm, and Lung Volume

The thoracic wall in infants is more compliant and their muscles are less developed than the muscles of adults, providing little

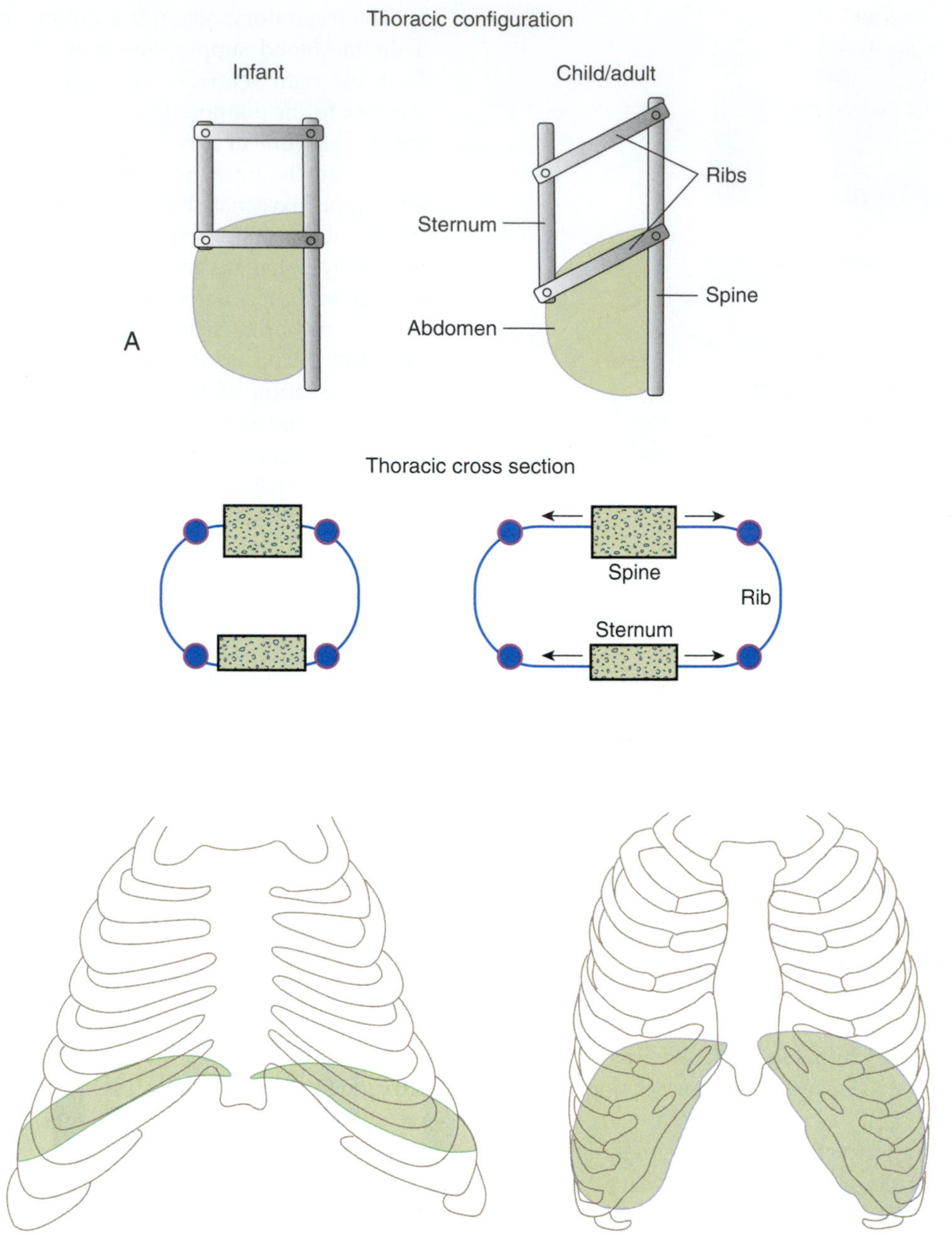

FIGURE 9-12 A, Changes in angularity of ribs and spine and cross-sectional shape of the thorax from an infant to an older child and adult. **B,** Anterior views of a newborn *(left)* and adult *(right)* rib cage and the relative position of the diaphragm *(shaded portions).* (Modified from Taussig LM, Landau LI, editors: Pediatric and respiratory medicine, ed 2, St Louis, 2008, Mosby.)

structural support. The infant thoracic cage is also more box-like, with the ribs being horizontally oriented or elevated (Figure 9-12). In addition, the diaphragm inserts into the thoracic cage in a horizontal plane decreasing the effective ability to enlarge the thorax.

As an infant inhales, the diaphragm moves down but the flexible chest wall moves very little in the anteroposterior dimension as the chest wall muscles attempt to pull it upward and outward. Compounding this situation is a proportionately larger abdominal visceral content that restricts the vertical motion of the diaphragm. The ribs take on a progressively downward slope as a child grows, and by 10 years of age the rib cage has the configuration seen in adults. Ossification of the ribs and sternum normally complete by 25 years of age, and this, combined with muscular development, results in a stiffer chest wall that moves more in the anteroposterior dimension with inspiratory effort.

The balance of these static forces results in reduced lung volume within this compliant thorax in an infant. Proportionately lower lung volumes can lead to early airway closure, widespread alveolar collapse (atelectasis), ventilation/perfusion ($\dot{V}/\dot{Q}$) mismatch, and resultant hypoxemia. The combination of a reduced lung volume and high O_2 consumption renders the infant more susceptible to profound hypoxemia in situations disturbing ventilation, lung volume, or $\dot{V}/\dot{Q}$ matching. Infants possess a remarkable ability to elevate their lung volume dynamically. Infants in distress can actively increase lung volume by trapping gas, improving $\dot{V}/\dot{Q}$ matching and gas exchange. Infants actively accomplish gas trapping by using the diaphragm during exhalation. This slows expiration that adducts (closes) the vocal cords and narrows the glottis. The combination of these two maneuvers effectively regulates volume in the lung and dynamically elevates lung volume. The narrowing of the glottis or larynx during exhalation is referred to as "laryngeal braking" or "grunting." Infants in respiratory distress commonly grunt, a manifestation of laryngeal braking. A more compliant chest wall contributes to suprasternal, substernal, intercostal, and subcostal retractions in distressed infants and young children (see Mini Clini).

MINI CLINI

Significance of Thoracic Soft Tissue Retractions

Supraclavicular and intercostal retractions are inward movements of the soft tissues above the clavicle and between the ribs of the chest wall during inspiration. This inward movement causes the clavicle and ribs to stand out prominently during inspiratory efforts.

PROBLEM: Why do infants and adults in respiratory distress with severe airway obstruction or reduced compliant ("stiff") lungs exhibit thoracic soft tissue retractions?

ANSWER: The pressure within the intrapleural space is slightly negative (e.g., –5 cm H_2O) as a result of the tendency of the lung to recoil inward and the rib cage to recoil outward. This pressure becomes more negative (e.g., –8 cm H_2O) during inspiration. The respiratory muscles enlarge the chest as the diaphragm descends and the intrathoracic volume increases. During these conditions, a much greater inspiratory effort is required. This increased effort translates into a much greater decrease in intrathoracic and pleural pressures (e.g., –40 cm H_2O). This greater decrease in intrathoracic and pleural pressure "sucks" the soft tissues inward and causes soft tissue retractions. These retractions significantly increase work of breathing.

RESPIRATORY SYSTEM IN THE ADULT

Surface Features of the Thorax

Thoracic shape and dimension vary from individual to individual and are linked to age, gender, and race. At birth, the thorax has a smaller transverse (side to side) dimension, widening with the onset of walking. Thoracic size and volume continue to increase throughout childhood and especially during the adolescent growth spurt. When evaluating lung size and volume throughout puberty and into adulthood, boys and men are consistently found to have larger lungs than age-matched and height-matched girls and women.[30]

Imaginary lines are commonly used to establish reference points and identify landmarks on the thorax. These lines and points help identify the location of underlying structures and the location of abnormal findings. On the anterior chest, the *midsternal line* divides the thorax into equal halves. The left and right *midclavicular lines* are parallel to the *midsternal line.* These are drawn through the midpoints of the left and right clavicles (Figure 9-13). The *midaxillary line* divides the lateral chest into equal halves. The *anterior axillary* line is parallel to the midaxillary line. It is situated along the anterolateral chest. The posterior axillary line is also parallel to the midaxillary line. It is located on the posterolateral chest wall (Figure 9-14). Three imaginary vertical lines are located on the posterior thorax. The midspinal line divides the posterior chest into two equal halves. The left and right midscapular lines are parallel to the midspinal line. They pass through the inferior angles of the scapulae in a relaxed upright subject (Figure 9-15).

RULE OF THUMB

Anatomic Directions

Descriptions of various anatomic structures often use the following terms:

Anterior, anteriorly	Front of the body, toward the front
Posterior, posteriorly	Back of the body, toward the back
Anteroposterior	In a direction from the front to the back
Lateral, laterally	Side of the body, toward the side
Medial, medially	Midline of the body, toward the midline

Components of the Thoracic Wall

The thoracic cavity is formed by the tissues of the chest, upper back, and diaphragm.[31] It is a cone-shaped cavity that houses the lungs, heart, and the contents of the mediastinum (Figure 9-16). It protects the vital organs within and is capable of changing shape to enable air to be moved into and out of the lungs. The thoracic cavity is formed from epithelial, connective, and muscle tissues.

The various parts of the thoracic wall are shown in Figure 9-17. The outer covering of the thorax is formed by the integumentary system, which includes skin, hair, subcutaneous fat, and breast tissues. Skeletal muscle tissue forms the various muscles of the chest and back and lies over and between the ribs. The ribs lie in the inner portion of the thoracic wall. The inner layer of the thoracic wall is lined with a serous membrane called the **parietal pleura.** It is opposite to another serous membrane called the **visceral pleura,** which covers the lung. A thin, fluid-filled pleural space forms between the parietal and visceral pleural membranes.

The rigidity of the thorax is provided by the bone tissue of the rib cage. The bony parts of the rib cage include the sternum, ribs, thoracic vertebral bones, scapula, and clavicle (Figure 9-18). The **sternum** is a long, vertical flat bone found on the anterior side that is composed of three bones: the **manubrium,**

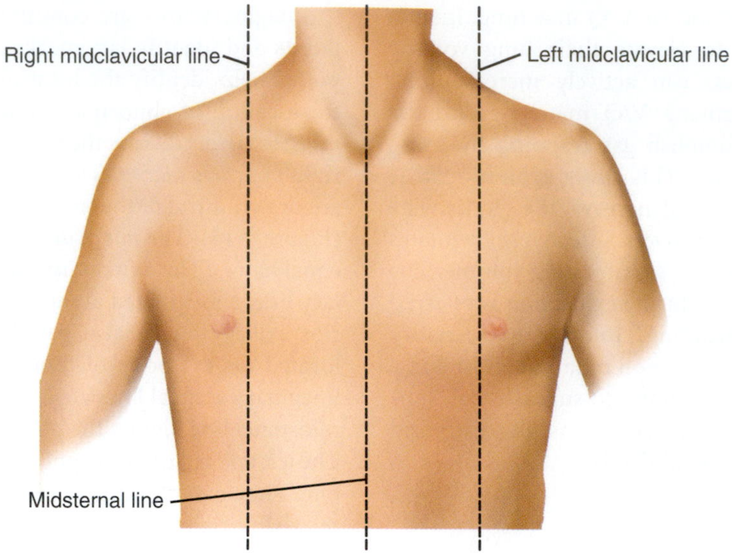

FIGURE 9-13 Anatomic reference lines on the anterior chest wall.

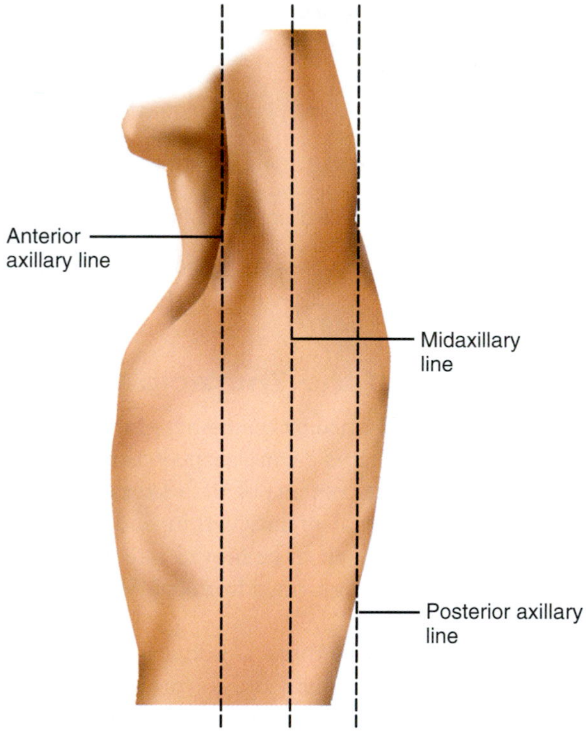

FIGURE 9-14 Anatomic reference lines on the lateral chest wall.

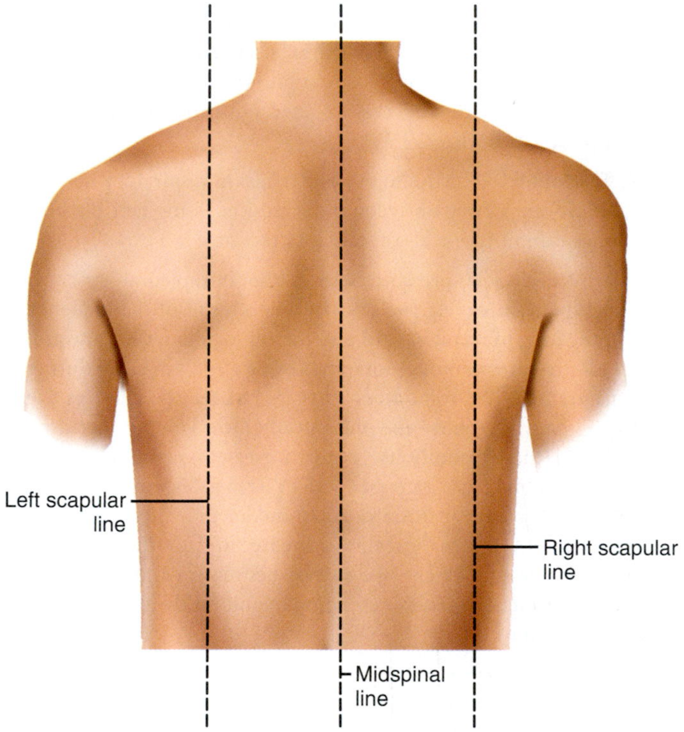

FIGURE 9-15 Anatomic reference lines on the posterior chest.

the body (or **gladiolus**), and the **xiphoid process.** The superior edge of the manubrium forms a shallow depression that is known as the **suprasternal notch** (or jugular notch). The fused connection between the manubrium and the body is known as the **sternal angle;** it is also known as the **angle of Louis.** The sternal angle is an external marker of the point where the trachea divides into the left and right main stem bronchi. A cartilaginous joint called the **costal cartilage** is on the lateral edges of the manubrium and sternal body and forms the attachment between the ribs and sternum. This joint allows the rib cage to bend and permits the thorax to increase and decrease in size.

RULE OF THUMB

Where the manubrium and body of the sternum meet, the anterior chest wall shows a slight depression that forms an oblique angle (when viewed from the side). This depression is referred to as the *angle of Louis*. Beneath this important landmark, the trachea divides into the right and left main stem bronchi.

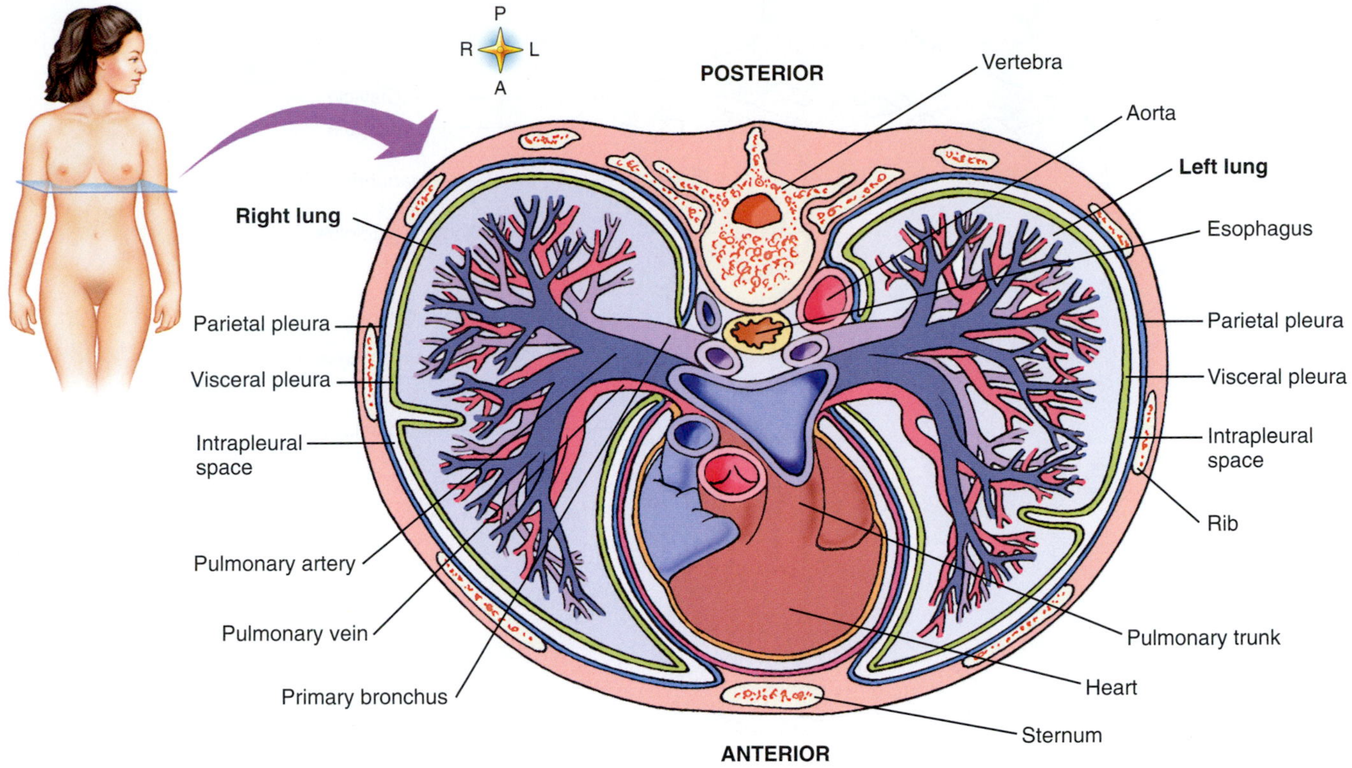

FIGURE 9-16 Transverse sectional view of the thorax showing its contents. (From Thibodeau GA, Patton KT: Anatomy and physiology, ed 7, St Louis, 2011, Mosby.)

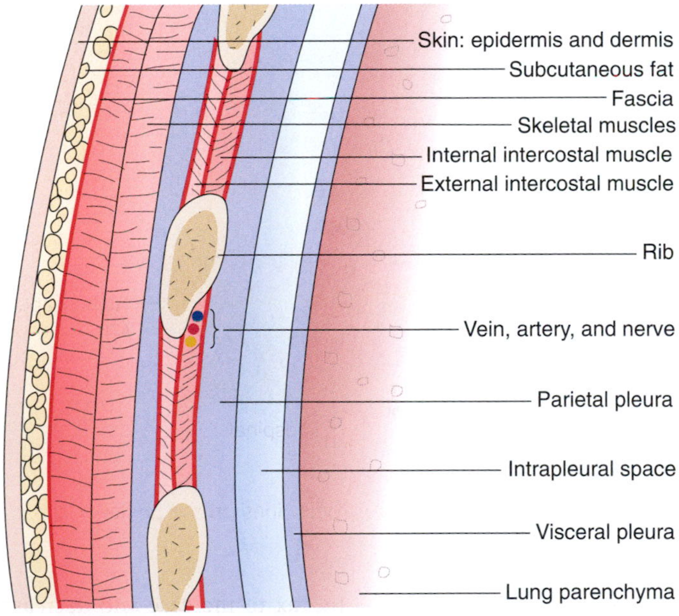

FIGURE 9-17 Sectional view of the thoracic wall. (From Hicks GH: Cardiopulmonary anatomy and physiology, Philadelphia, 2000, WB Saunders.)

The rib cage is formed by 12 pairs of ribs.[31] Rib pairs 1 through 7 are known as the **true ribs** because they are attached directly to the sternum. The first ribs and the upper sternum form the opening into the thorax that is called the *thoracic inlet,* or *operculum.* Ribs 8 through 12 are called **false ribs** because they are neither directly nor indirectly attached to the sternum. The vertebrochondral rib pairs 8, 9, and 10 are indirectly attached to the sternum through a common cartilaginous strap. Rib pairs 11 and 12 are called **floating ribs** because they are not attached to the sternum. Each rib has a sternal end; a long, curved, and relatively flat body; and a head that articulates with the thoracic vertebrae (Figure 9-19). Intercostal muscles lie between the ribs and hold them together. Just below each rib, in the costal groove, is a thoracic artery, vein, and nerve, supplying blood flow and nerve communications to that region of the chest wall (see Figure 9-17).

RULE OF THUMB

Numerous procedures require entry into the pleural cavity, such as thoracentesis or chest tubes. Insertions made during these procedures are always done directly above a selected rib to avoid injuring important structures. The intercostal nerves, veins, and arteries all lie in a groove below each rib.

The upper and lateral regions of the thorax house the bones of the pectoral girdles. The pectoral girdle on each side is formed by the clavicle and scapula.[31] The scapula forms the socket for the shoulder joint and is stabilized or moved by skeletal muscles of the upper back. The clavicle supports and stabilizes the shoulder joint through a flexible attachment to the manubrium of the sternum.

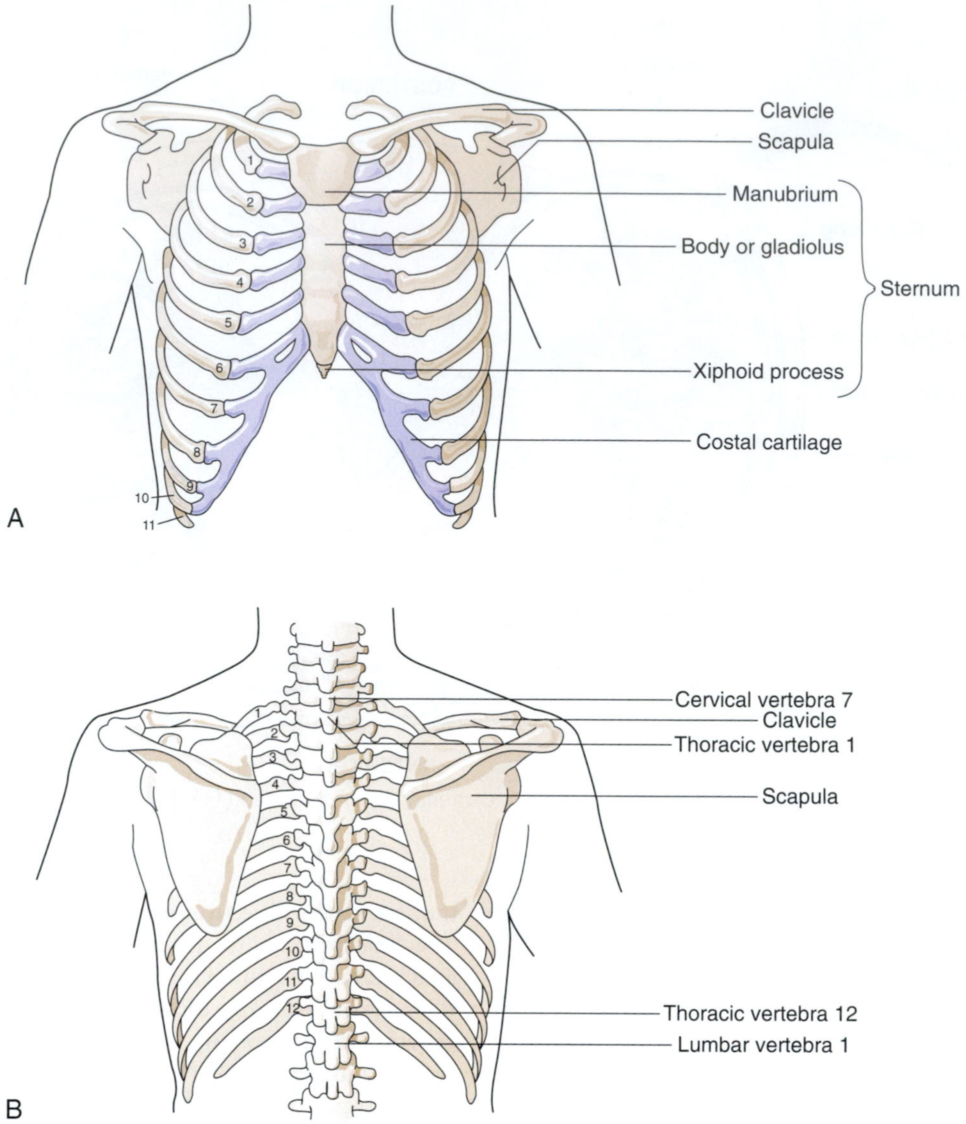

FIGURE 9-18 Anterior **(A)** and posterior **(B)** views of the bones of the thorax. (From Hicks GH: Cardiopulmonary anatomy and physiology, Philadelphia, 2000, WB Saunders.)

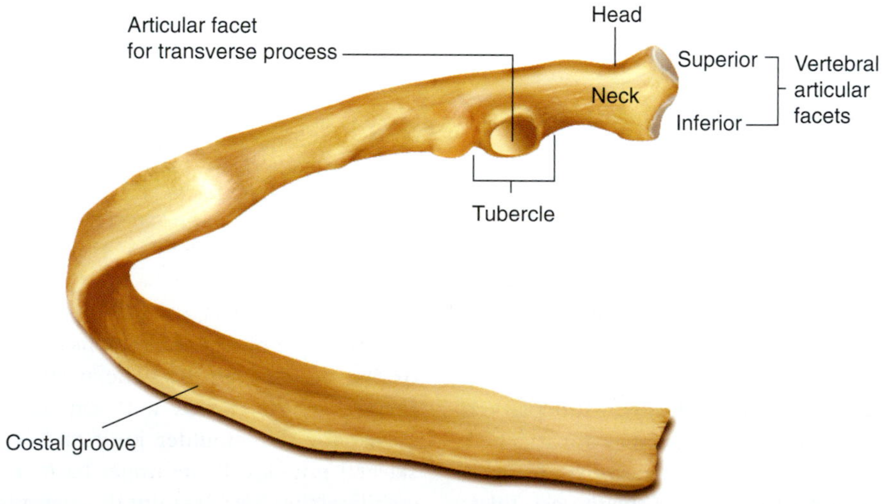

FIGURE 9-19 Typical middle rib as viewed from the posterior. The head end articulates with the vertebral bones, and the distal end is attached to the costal cartilage of the sternum.

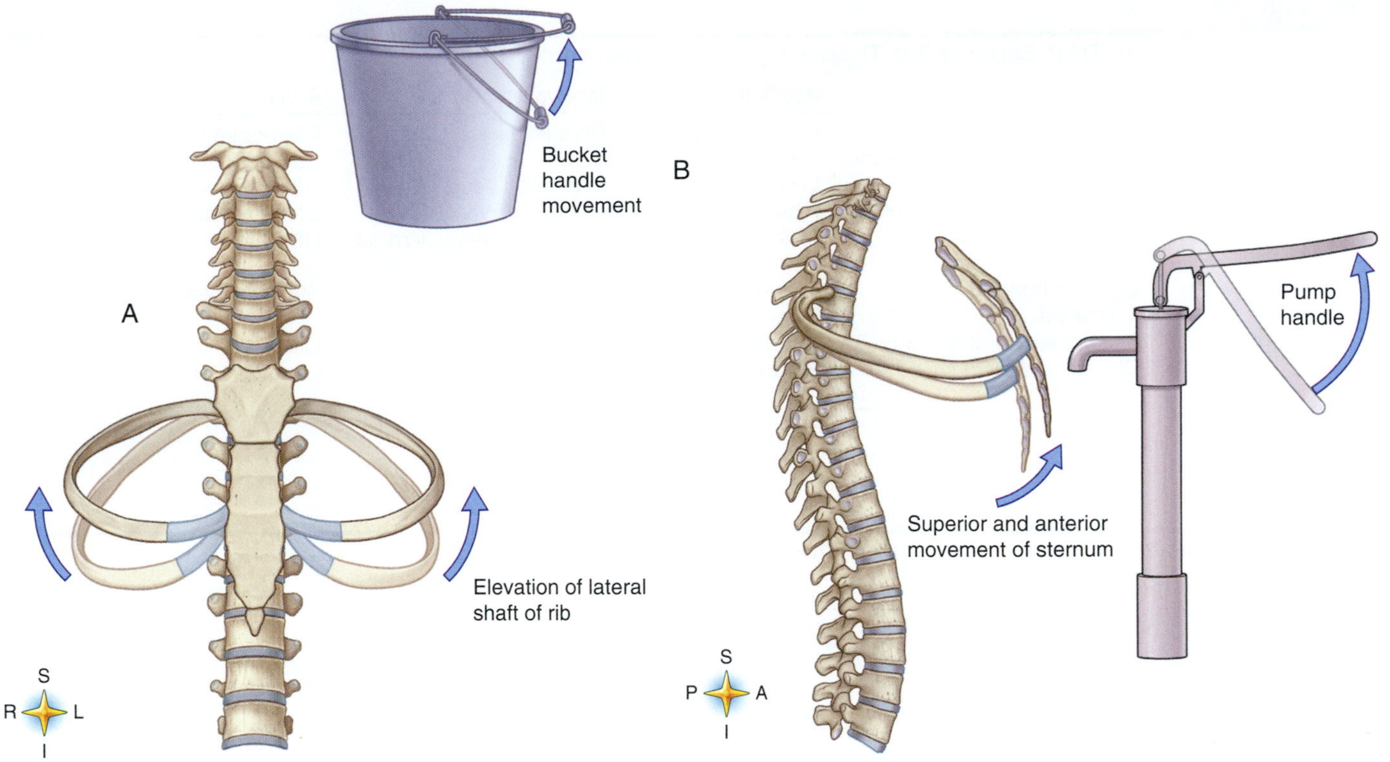

FIGURE 9-20 "Bucket handle" type and "pump handle" type of rib motions. (From Thibodeau GA, Patton KT: Anatomy and physiology, ed 7, St Louis, 2011, Mosby.)

Rib Movement

The various ribs move in different ways, and some may move more than others at different times. The first rib moves slightly, raising and lowering the sternum. Its slight motion increases the anteroposterior diameter of the chest. This action is not used during quiet breathing and becomes active only under conditions that require increased ventilation or deep breathing. Ribs 2 through 7 can move simultaneously about two axes (Figure 9-20). As each rib rotates about the axis of its neck its sternal end rises and falls. This movement increases the anteroposterior thoracic diameter in what is commonly referred to as a "pump handle" motion. At the same time, the rib moves about its long axis from its angle at the sternum. This motion causes the middle part of the rib to move up and down in what is commonly described as a "bucket handle." The compound action of ribs 2 through 7 changes both the anteroposterior and the transverse dimensions in an upward and outward motion. Ribs 8 through 10 rotate in a pattern similar to that of ribs 2 through 7. However, elevation of the anterior ends of these ribs produces a small backward movement of the lower sternum that slightly reduces the thoracic anteroposterior diameter. Outward rotation of the middle section of these ribs increases the transverse diameter of the thorax. Ribs 11 and 12 participate in changing the contour of the chest in a minor way as they are pulled upward and outward in a "caliper" motion.

Respiratory Muscles

Changes in thoracic cavity dimension during breathing are the product of tension developed by various skeletal muscles known as the *respiratory muscles.*[32] Their origins, insertions, somatic nervous supply, and actions are summarized in Tables 9-4 and 9-5. The **diaphragm** and **intercostal muscles** are the primary muscles of ventilation. They are active both while at rest and when the individual exhibits stress-induced increases in breathing. The accessory muscles of ventilation assist the diaphragm and intercostal muscles when ventilatory demand increases. The scalene, sternocleidomastoid, pectoral, and abdominal wall muscles are the predominant accessory muscles. Other abdominal and chest wall muscles may function as accessory muscles when needed.

The diaphragm is a thin, musculotendinous, dome-shaped structure that separates the thoracic and abdominal cavities (Figure 9-21).[33] It originates from the chest and abdominal wall and converges in a central tendon at the top of its dome. The diaphragm is a highly aerobic and fatigue-resistant muscle compared with other skeletal muscles and more capable of long-term rhythmic contraction.

In an upright position and with the diaphragm relaxed, the liver forces the dome of the right hemidiaphragm upward approximately 1 cm higher than the left hemidiaphragm at the end of a quiet exhalation. The highest portion of the right dome sits at the eighth or ninth thoracic vertebra posteriorly and at the fifth rib anteriorly. The left diaphragmatic dome sits at the ninth or tenth thoracic vertebra posteriorly and the sixth rib anteriorly. Movements of the hemidiaphragms are synchronous in healthy subjects. When lying down in a supine position, the weight of the abdominal contents forces the diaphragm farther up into the thoracic cavity. During quiet breathing, the

TABLE 9-4
Respiratory Muscles That Expand the Thorax During the Inspiratory Phase

Muscle	Origin	Insertion	Innervation	Action
Diaphragm	Xiphoid process, lower lateral ribs, lumbar vertebra	Central tendon of dome	Phrenic nerves (C3-5)	Diaphragm moves downward, abdominal wall forced outward
External intercostals	Upper ribs	Lower ribs	Intercostal nerves (T1-12)	Lift ribs upward
Scalene	Lower five cervical vertebrae	Ribs 1 and 2	Cervical nerves (C5-8)	Lifts ribs 1 and 2
Sternocleidomastoids	Manubrium and clavicle	Mastoid process of occipital bone	Accessory nerves (cranial nerve XI)	Lift sternum
Trapezius	Occipital bone, C7-T12 vertebrae	Scapula and clavicle	Accessory nerves (cranial nerve XI)	Stabilizes head
Pectoralis minor	Anterior region of ribs 3-5	Scapula	Pectoral nerves (C6-8)	Lifts upper ribs
Pectoralis	Clavicle and sternum	Humerus	Pectoral nerves (C5-C8)	Lifts sternum

TABLE 9-5
Respiratory Muscles That Compress the Thorax During the Expiratory Phase

Muscle	Origin	Insertion	Innervation	Action
Internal intercostals	Lower ribs	Upper ribs	Intercostal nerves (T1-12)	Pull ribs down
External oblique	Anterior lower eight ribs	Linea alba and iliac crest	Lower intercostal and iliohypogastric nerves (T7-12)	Pulls abdominal wall inward
Internal oblique	Lumbar vertebrae, iliac crest, and inguinal ligaments	Costal region of ribs and pubis	Lower intercostal and iliohypogastric nerves (T10-12 and L1)	Pulls abdominal wall inward
Transverse abdominis	Costal region of lower ribs, iliac crest, and inguinal crest	Linea alba	Lower intercostal and iliophypogastric (T7-L1)	Pulls abdominal wall inward
Rectus abdominis	Costal region and ribs 5-7	Pubis	Lower intercostal and iliophypogastric (T7-12)	Pulls abdominal wall inward
Serratus anterior	Costal region of upper eight ribs	Scapula	Long thoracic nerves (T5-7)	Compresses thorax when arm is stabilized
Serratus, posterior superior	Lower cervical and upper thoracic vertebrae	Posterior ribs 2-5	Intercostal nerves	Pulls ribs downward
Serratus, posterior inferior	Lower thoracic and upper lumbar vertebrae	Posterior ribs 9-12	Thoracic nerves	Pulls ribs downward
Latissimus dorsi	Lower thoracic, lumbar, sacral vertebrae, ilium, and lower ribs	Humerus	Thoracodorsal nerve (C6-8)	Compresses thorax when arm is stabilized

diaphragm is responsible for approximately 75% of the change in thoracic volume.[34] When the muscle fibers of the diaphragm are tensed during inspiration, the dome of the diaphragm is pulled down 1 to 2 cm; this results in enlargement of the thoracic cavity and compression of the abdominal contents. During maximal inspiration, the diaphragm can be pulled down approximately 10 cm. Exhalation results when diaphragmatic tension decreases and the diaphragm returns to its relaxed position.

Increased lung volume causes the diaphragm to flatten out. Contraction of a flattened diaphragm can result in tension on the lower ribs that causes them to be pulled inward, resulting in compression of the thoracic cavity. This condition can occur in individuals with severe gas trapping as a result of emphysema or asthma. To compensate, these individuals must recruit other muscles to enlarge the thorax. Less efficient breathing and excessive muscle work results. Nonpulmonary diseases also can affect diaphragm function. Abdominal wall muscle tensioning *(splinting)* owing to pain, abdominal distention with fluid *(ascites)*, or other causes of rigidity of the abdominal wall can interfere with diaphragmatic descent during inspiration.

Functionally, the diaphragm is divided into a right and a left hemidiaphragm. Each hemidiaphragm is innervated by a phrenic nerve that arises from branches of spinal nerves C3, C4, and C5.[33] Spinal cord injuries at or above the level of the third cervical vertebrae result in diaphragmatic paralysis. In this situation, the individual has lost *all* nervous control of the respiratory muscles and is unable to spontaneously breathe. Unilateral phrenic nerve injury or disease to one side can spare the other nerve and permit unilateral ventilation.

Although the diaphragm is the primary ventilatory muscle, it is not essential for survival. Limited, short-term ventilation is possible using accessory muscles even if the diaphragm is paralyzed. If either or both of the hemidiaphragms are paralyzed, the affected hemidiaphragm remains in a resting position. During deep inspiration, the paralyzed diaphragm rises as other ventilatory muscles reduce the intrathoracic pressure. During quiet breathing, the paralyzed diaphragm may remain

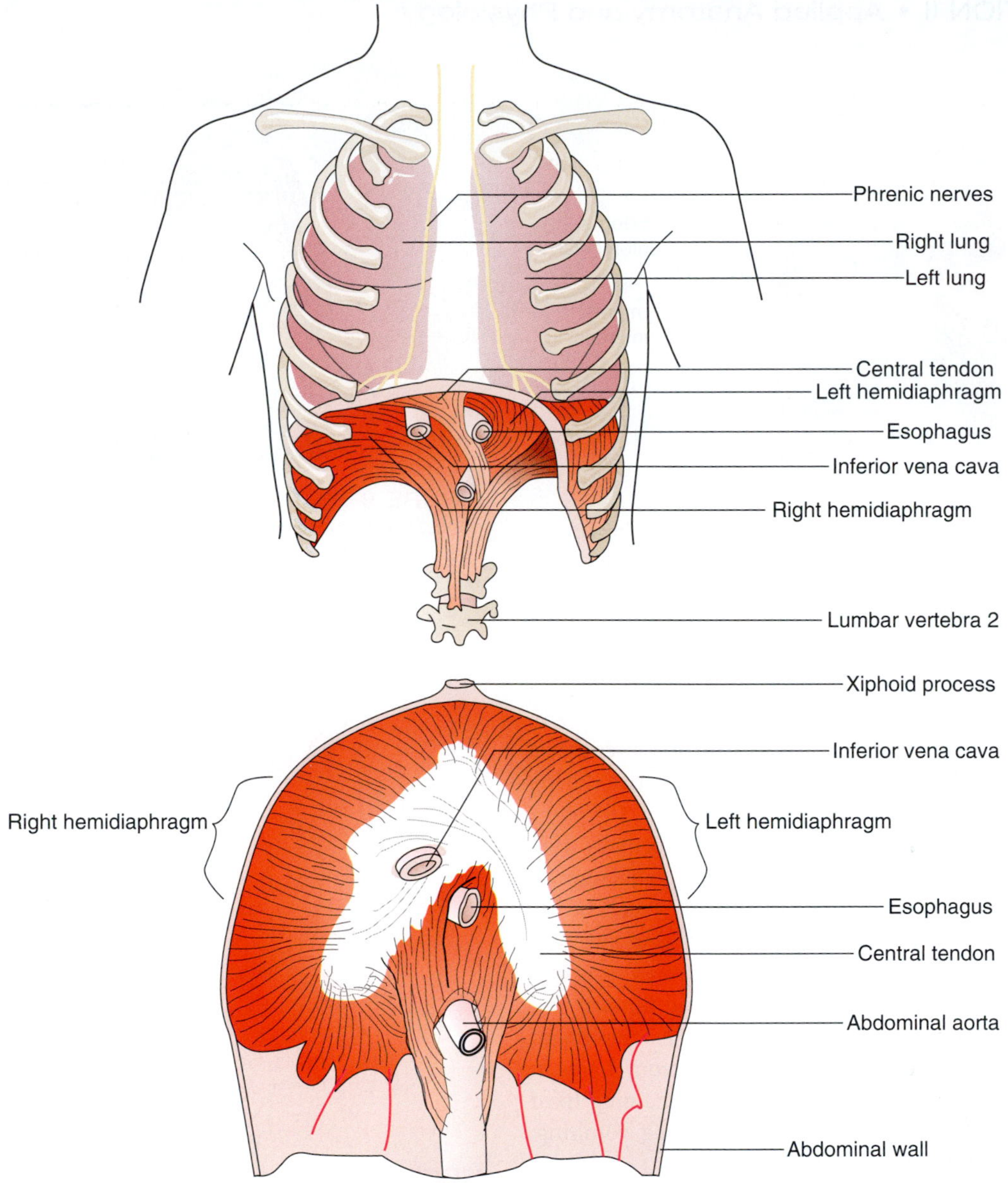

FIGURE 9-21 The diaphragm originates from the lumbar vertebrae, lower ribs, xiphoid process, and abdominal wall and converges in a central tendon. Note the locations of the phrenic nerves and openings for the inferior vena cava, esophagus, and abdominal aorta. (From Hicks GH: Cardiopulmonary anatomy and physiology, Philadelphia, 2000, WB Saunders.)

MINI CLINI

Lung Hyperinflation in Emphysema

Emphysema is a disease characterized by the destruction of the alveolar region of the lungs. This destruction causes the emphysematous lung to have less elastic recoil than a normal lung.

PROBLEM: Why do patients with severe emphysema have enlarged or overinflated lungs? How does hyperinflation interfere with breathing? What can be done to alleviate the problem?

ANSWER: The pathologic findings of emphysema include the destruction of elastic fibers in the alveolar region, reduced lung recoil, and expansion of the remaining lung tissue. As the disease progresses, the tendency of the lungs to collapse (because of their inherent elasticity) becomes less than the normal outward expanding force of the rib cage (because of its higher elasticity). The stronger outward expanding force of the rib cage expands the lungs, increases their volume, and results in overinflated lungs at the end of a normal, resting exhalation.

Hyperinflation "flattens" the diaphragm for similar reasons, making it less effective during inspiration, increasing work of breathing. Loss of elastic tissues allows small airways to collapse, resulting in air trapping and exaggerating hyperinflation.

Therapy for emphysema is directed at reducing the effects of air trapping. Administration of bronchodilators and corticosteroids may improve airway opening, reducing trapped gas and the work of breathing. Maneuvers such as pursed-lip exhaled breathing also may assist in reducing gas trapping by splinting open the airways and facilitating exhalation. Surgical removal of overdistended lung tissue (bullae) is known as *lung volume reduction surgery* and also may be beneficial. Surgical removal of nonfunctional hyperexpanded tissue may allow the remaining lung tissue to be better ventilated and improve gas exchange at the alveolar level.

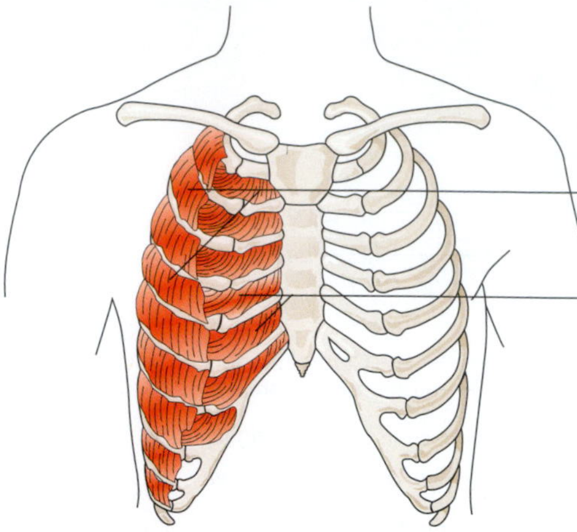

FIGURE 9-22 The external intercostal muscles lift the inferior ribs and enlarge the thoracic cavity. The internal intercostal muscles compress the thoracic cavity by pulling the ribs together. (From Hicks GH: Cardiopulmonary anatomy and physiology, Philadelphia, 2000, WB Saunders.)

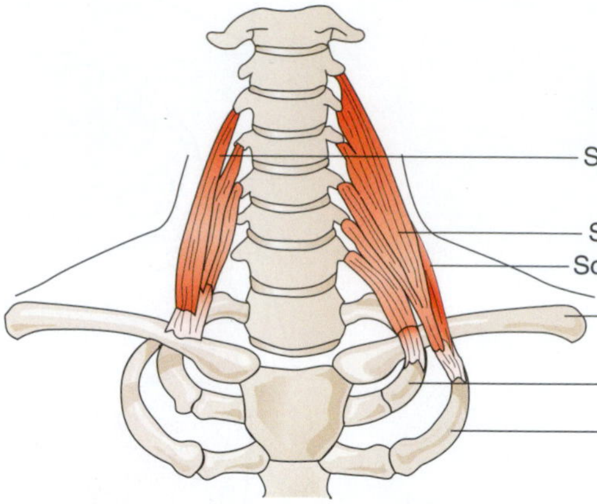

FIGURE 9-23 The scalene muscles originate from the lower cervical vertebrae and lift the clavicle and first two ribs. (From Hicks GH: Cardiopulmonary anatomy and physiology, Philadelphia, 2000, WB Saunders.)

immobile or may move in either direction. The pressures above and below a paralyzed diaphragm tend to make it rise during inspiration.

Because exhalation is *passive,* the diaphragm normally does not actively participate in exhalation. During exhalation it returns to its resting position during the passive recoil of the lungs and thorax. During forced exhalation, abdominal wall muscles compress the abdominal cavity and increase pressure in the abdominal cavity. The diaphragm is forced upward and the lungs compress, forcing gas from them. The diaphragm performs important functions other than ventilation; it aids in generating high intraabdominal pressures by remaining fixed while the abdominal muscles contract, facilitating vomiting, coughing, sneezing, defecation, and parturition.

During quiet breathing, the diaphragm does most of the work. Other muscles are slightly active during quiet breathing and become more active with forceful breathing. These other muscles are generally known as the **accessory muscles of breathing.**

The accessory muscles of inspiration include various muscles in the neck, chest, and upper back. The external intercostal muscles (Figure 9-22) originate on the upper ribs and attach to the lower ribs. The fibers of these muscles run at an oblique angle between the ribs. When they generate tension the ribs lift upward and cause the thoracic cavity to enlarge the thorax (Hamberger mechanism). Nerve signals are received from the intercostal nerves that arise from thoracic spinal nerves (T1 to 12). They are more active during the inspiratory phase of forceful breathing and are thought to play a role in stabilizing excessive rib motion during forceful breathing.[35]

Three pairs of **scalene muscles** (scalenus anterior, scalenus medius, and scalenus posterior) arise from the lower five or six cervical vertebrae and insert on the clavicle and first two ribs (Figure 9-23). They lift the upper chest when active. The scalene muscles are slightly active during resting inhalation and become more active with forceful inspiration, especially when ventilatory demands increase.[36] Such instances may occur in healthy subjects during exercise or in patients who have pulmonary disease. In healthy subjects, inspiratory efforts against a closed glottis or obstructed airway activate the scalene muscles. When alveolar pressure decreases to −10 cm H_2O, scalene muscles are active in all subjects. The scalene muscles are largely inactive during expiratory efforts but can become active to fixate the ribs as abdominal muscles contract during forceful exhalation such as coughing.

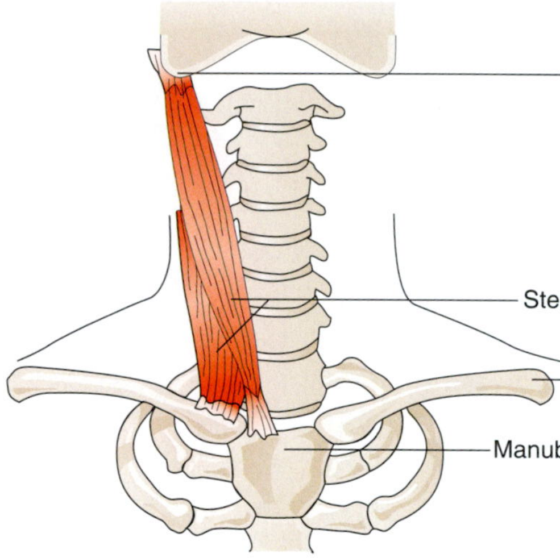

FIGURE 9-24 The sternocleidomastoid muscles originate from the manubrium and clavicle and insert on the mastoid process of the temporal bone. They lift the upper thorax when the trapezius stabilizes the head. (From Hicks GH: Cardiopulmonary anatomy and physiology, Philadelphia, 2000, WB Saunders.)

Sternocleidomastoid muscles (Figure 9-24) originate from the manubrium and clavicle and insert on the mastoid process of the temporal bone. Normally, this muscle flexes and rotates the head and is active during shoulder shrugging. When the head is held in an upright position by tensing the trapezius

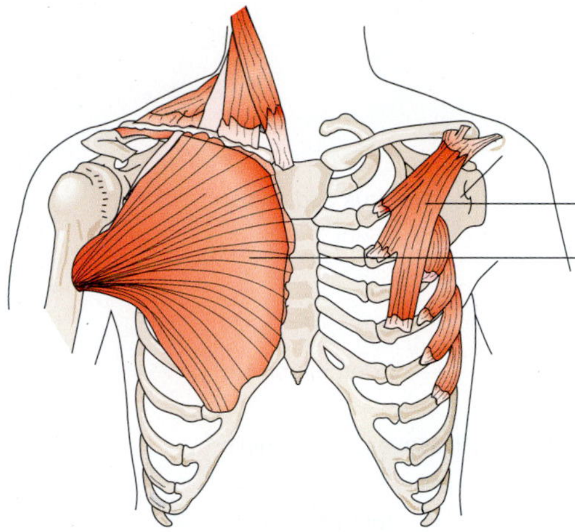

FIGURE 9-25 The pectoralis major and minor can lift and enlarge the thorax when the arms are braced by leaning forward on the elbows (tripod position). (From Hicks GH: Cardiopulmonary anatomy and physiology, Philadelphia, 2000, WB Saunders.)

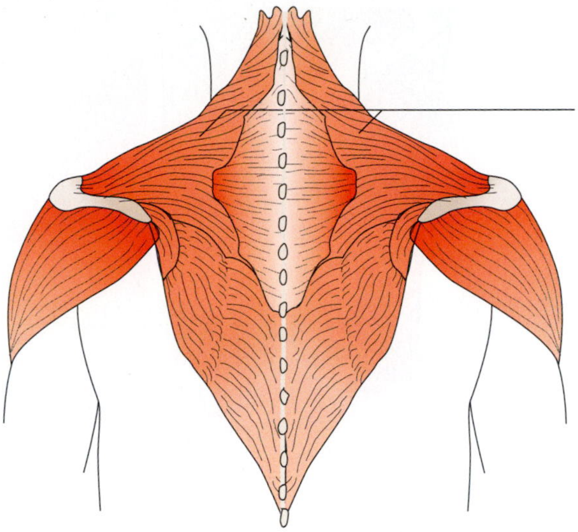

FIGURE 9-26 The trapezius assists forceful inspiration primarily by stabilizing the head, which allows the sternocleidomastoid to lift the anterior thorax. (From Hicks GH: Cardiopulmonary anatomy and physiology, Philadelphia, 2000, WB Saunders.)

muscle of the upper back and neck, the sternocleidomastoid muscles can function to lift the upper chest. These muscles are active during forceful inspiration and become visible as thick bands on either side of the neck during the inspiratory phase in an individual who is in respiratory distress. This motion increases the anteroposterior diameter of the chest.[37]

RULE OF THUMB

Patients with advanced chronic obstructive pulmonary disease (COPD) often use accessory muscles to assist the flattened diaphragm, helping relieve their work of breathing. The muscle groups used include the shoulder and neck muscles. To use these muscles, the shoulder girdle must be stabilized. Patients with COPD often do this by supporting their arms on a stationary object in front of them, forming a "tripod" position. This immobilizes the shoulders and allows the accessory muscles to raise the anterior chest wall.

The major and minor pectoralis muscles are broad fan-shaped muscles of the upper anterior chest (Figure 9-25). The pectoralis major originates on the humerus and inserts onto the clavicle and sternum. The pectoralis minor originates from the anterior region of the ribs 3 through 5 and inserts onto the scapula. They normally function to adduct the arms in a hugging motion. They are also capable of generating some anterior thoracic lift when the arms are braced on a surface in front of a subject. Individuals who have chronic shortness of breath often use these muscles by sitting in the "tripod" position (see Rule of Thumb).

The trapezius muscles are flat, triangular muscles located on the upper back and neck (Figure 9-26). Their action is to rotate the scapulae, lift the shoulders, and flex the head up and back. During forceful inspiration, they become more active by helping brace the head and allowing the sternocleidomastoid muscles to lift the thorax.

The accessory muscles of exhalation become active during forceful breathing (see Table 9-5). Generally, these muscles compress the thoracic cavity and facilitate exhalation. The internal intercostal muscles (see Figure 9-22) lie between the ribs and just behind the external intercostal muscles. The muscle fibers of the internal intercostal muscles run downward and less obliquely than the external intercostal muscle fibers. This orientation causes these muscles to pull the ribs together, which results in compression of the thoracic cavity. They are stimulated by branches of the intercostal nerves and are most active during forceful exhalation. They also become active toward the end of deep inhalation and antagonize the lifting effect of the external intercostal muscles, which effectively stabilizes rib motion during forceful exhalation.[37]

When the abdominal wall muscles contract, they compress the abdominal cavity. This compression forces the diaphragm upward, compressing the thoracic cavity. The abdominal muscles include pairs of **external oblique, internal oblique,** transverse abdominis, and **rectus abdominis muscles** (Figure 9-27).[38] The external oblique muscles are the outermost layer of abdominal wall muscle and lie over the lateral aspects of the abdominal cavity. The internal oblique muscles lie just underneath the external oblique muscles. They originate on the lumbar vertebrae, iliac crest, and inguinal ligaments, inserting into the pubis and costal region of the lower ribs; this results in a fiber orientation that is at right angles to the external oblique muscles. The transverse abdominis muscles lie below the internal oblique muscles. Muscle fibers of the transverse abdominis run around the lateral wall of the abdomen. The rectus abdominis muscles are a pair of muscular bands that run vertically on the anterior surface of the abdomen. These muscular bands arise from the pubis, travel upward over the abdominal cavity, and insert into the costal region of ribs 5, 6, and 7 and the xiphoid process of the sternum.

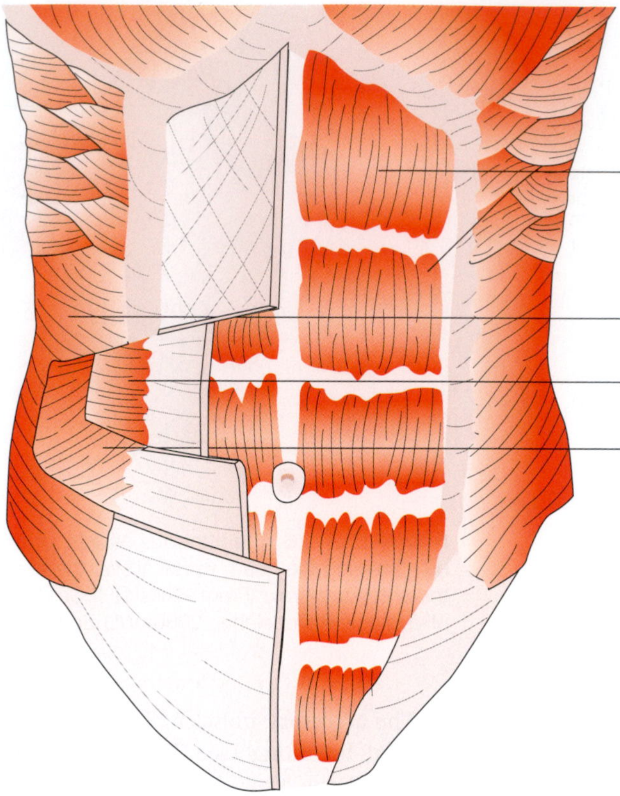

FIGURE 9-27 The abdominal wall muscles compress the thoracic cavity by compressing the abdominal wall and forcing the diaphragm upward. (From Hicks GH: Cardiopulmonary anatomy and physiology, Philadelphia, 2000, WB Saunders.)

Forceful contraction of the abdominal wall muscle group results in increasing intraabdominal pressure, forcing the diaphragm upward and compressing the thorax.

Abdominal wall muscles are active during resting and forceful exhalation.[39] They become more active when the elastic recoil of the lung and thorax cannot provide the needed expiratory flow during forceful exhalation, such as coughing, sneezing, talking loudly, and playing wind-powered musical instruments.[40] The most active muscle of the group during resting and forceful exhalation in most body positions is the transverse abdominis. The least active muscles are the rectus abdominis. The abdominal muscles also can contribute to inspiration by contracting at end-exhalation. This contraction reduces end-expiratory lung volume so the chest wall can recoil outward, assisting the next inspiratory effort.[41] Elevating abdominal pressure increases both the length and the radius of curvature of the diaphragm. Both of these effects result in greater transdiaphragmatic pressure for a given contractile tension. In patients with chronic obstructive pulmonary disease (COPD), any increase in ventilatory demand significantly increases the use of the abdominal muscles. Loss of effective use of the abdominal wall muscles results in a marked inability to exhale forcefully and to cough effectively.

Pleural Membranes, Space, and Fluid

The thoracic cavity is subdivided into the mediastinum and the left and right pleural cavities. The centrally located mediastinum contains the trachea, esophagus, heart, great vessels, and other organs.[42] The left and right pleural cavities contain the lungs. The surfaces of the inner thoracic wall, mediastinum, and lungs are covered with serous membranes called the *pleural membranes* (see Figure 9-17). The parietal pleural membrane lines the chest wall and mediastinum, whereas the lungs are covered by the visceral pleura. Both membranes are constructed from a thin surface layer of mesothelial cells, and below the layer of mesothelial cells is a layer of connective tissue that houses blood vessels, lymphatic vessels, and nerve fibers.[43] Numerous microscopic openings, called *stomata,* are found in the surface of the pleura and are surrounded by mesothelial cells. The stomata open into the lymphatic drainage system of the pleural membrane. The parietal pleura contain sensory fibers that are responsible for the painful sensation that is associated with inflammation of the pleura—a condition called *pleurisy*.

The space between the membranes is called the *pleural space* and is filled with approximately 0.26 ml/kg, or about 18 ml in a 70-kg adult, of pleural fluid.[44] Pleural fluid is a clear fluid with a pH of 7.60 to 7.65 that has few cells, a small amount of protein (about 1 g/dl), and glucose and electrolytes in concentrations that approximate those of plasma. The small volume of pleural fluid is spread out over the entire surface of both lungs and functions as a lubricant to reduce friction as the lungs move within the thorax. It acts as an airtight seal that adheres together the two pleural membranes. Pleural fluid is secreted and reabsorbed by the two pleural membranes. A little more than half of the pleural fluid is thought to be produced by the parietal pleura. Pleural fluid is formed from the systemic blood flow to each pleura. Blood pressure–driven filtration is supplied to the parietal pleura by blood flow from the intercostal arteries. The bronchial circulation of the lung supplies most of the blood flow to the visceral pleura.

It is estimated that the pleurae produce 150 to 250 ml of pleural fluid per day.[45] Most of the fluid is thought to be absorbed by the visceral pleura capillaries. The rest is cleared by drainage through the lymphatic stomata of parietal pleura by solute-coupled liquid absorption and through some transcytosis. Fluid and solutes or cells cleared by lymphatic drainage are carried by the pulmonary lymphatics to the hilar region. There they enter the major lymphatic vessels draining back to the subclavian veins and right heart.

The angle where the costal parietal pleura join the diaphragmatic parietal pleura is known as the **costophrenic angle.** It is located in the right and left lateral and inferior regions of the thoracic cavities. This angle is clearly visible and is an important landmark in the normal chest radiograph. Normally it is a sharp angle of approximately 30 to 45 degrees. Abnormal excess of fluids between the visceral and parietal pleura tend to pool here in an upright individual. This pooling of fluid causes the angle to appear blunted or flattened to 90 degrees when viewed in the chest radiograph.

MINI CLINI

Penetrating Chest Injury

Normally, the parietal and visceral pleurae are in physical contact with one another and are separated by only a thin liquid film or fluid. This liquid film allows these two pleural membranes to slide over one another with little friction. This film also provides a cohesive force that resists separation of the membranes. When the respiratory muscles move the rib cage outward in an inspiratory effort, the lung is literally pulled by the cohesive forces between the parietal and visceral pleurae. The elastic recoil forces of the lung resist this outward movement.

PROBLEM: A person sustains blunt force traumatic injury to the left chest. The fractured ribs are forced through the chest wall and parietal pleura, puncture the visceral pleura, and lacerate the lung. What happens to the lungs?

ANSWER: The lung on the affected side collapses as air and blood leak from the lacerated lung. As air and blood enter the pleural space (hemopneumothorax), the parietal and visceral pleurae separate. The chest wall expands outward, and the elastic recoil of the lung causes it to collapse. Both structures recoil in opposite directions as the pleural space between them separates, creating paradoxical movement. Treatment of a hemopneumothorax involves inserting a chest tube into the chest cavity and applying vacuum to remove the air and blood, reexpanding the lung.

Mediastinum

The **mediastinum** lies between the left and right pleural cavities that contain the lungs (see Figure 9-16). The mediastinum is bounded on either side by the pleural cavities, anteriorly by the sternum, posteriorly by the thoracic vertebrae, inferiorly by the diaphragm, and superiorly by the thoracic inlet. The mediastinum can be subdivided into three subcompartments. Between the sternum and pericardium is an anterior compartment containing the thymus gland and lymph nodes. The middle compartment contains the pericardium, heart, great vessels, phrenic and upper portions of the vagus nerves, trachea, portions of the right and left main stem bronchi, and lymph nodes. The posterior compartment contains the thoracic aorta, esophagus, and thoracic duct. Also found in the posterior mediastinum are the sympathetic nervous system ganglionic chains and lower portions of the vagus nerve and lymph nodes.

Lungs

The lungs are multilobed, cone-shaped, spongelike organs that lie within the pleural cavities (Figure 9-28). They are pink at birth and develop a gray coloration with age. Average adult lungs are hollow, low-density organs that occupy a volume of approximately 3.5 L and weigh approximately 900 g.[43] The organs within the mediastinum bulge into the left hemithorax, resulting in a narrower and slightly smaller left lung. The liver below the right lung elevates the right diaphragm and results in a slightly shorter right lung.

The lungs extend from the diaphragm to a point 1 to 2 cm above the medial third of the clavicles. The uppermost regions are called the **apexes.** At end-expiration, the anterior lower lung borders extend to approximately the sixth rib at the midclavicular line. Laterally, the lower lung border is at the eighth rib at the midaxillary line. The top of the lungs, viewed posteriorly, extend upward from the eighth or ninth thoracic vertebra to the first thoracic vertebra. The diaphragm rises and falls, with resting breathing between the ninth and twelfth thoracic vertebrae.

The anterior, lateral, and posterior lung surfaces lie and move against the thoracic inner wall. The medial surfaces of the lungs lie in close contact to the mediastinal surfaces. Figure 9-29 shows the medial surfaces of the lungs and the opening in this region known as the *hilum.* The main stem bronchi, blood vessels, lymphatics, and nerves that enter or exit the lung all pass through the hilum.

Each lung is divided into two or three **lobes** (see Figure 9-28) separated by one or more **fissures.** The right lung has upper, middle, and lower lobes. The left lung has only an upper and a lower lobe. Both lungs have an oblique fissure beginning on the anterior chest at approximately the sixth rib at the midclavicular line. These fissures extend laterally and upward until they cross the fifth rib on the lateral chest in the midaxillary line. The fissures continue to the posterior chest to approximately the third thoracic vertebra. The right lung also has a horizontal or "minor" fissure that separates the upper and middle lobes. This horizontal fissure extends from the fourth rib at the sternal border to the fifth rib at the midaxillary line.

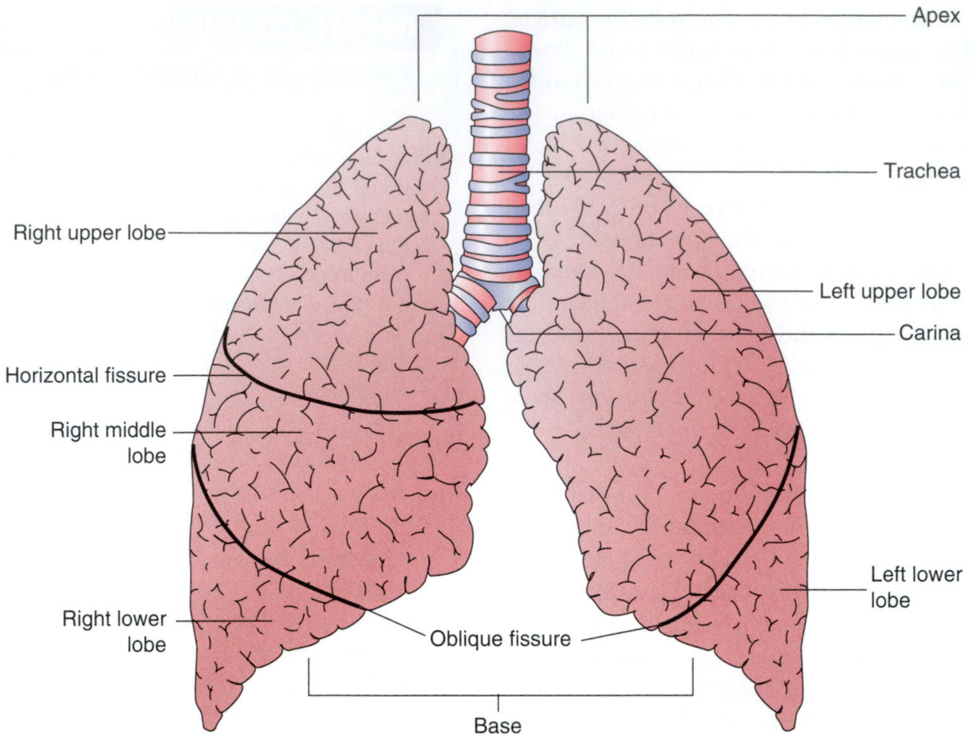

FIGURE 9-28 Anterior view of the lungs showing the lobes and fissures. (From Hicks GH: Cardiopulmonary anatomy and physiology, Philadelphia, 2000, WB Saunders.)

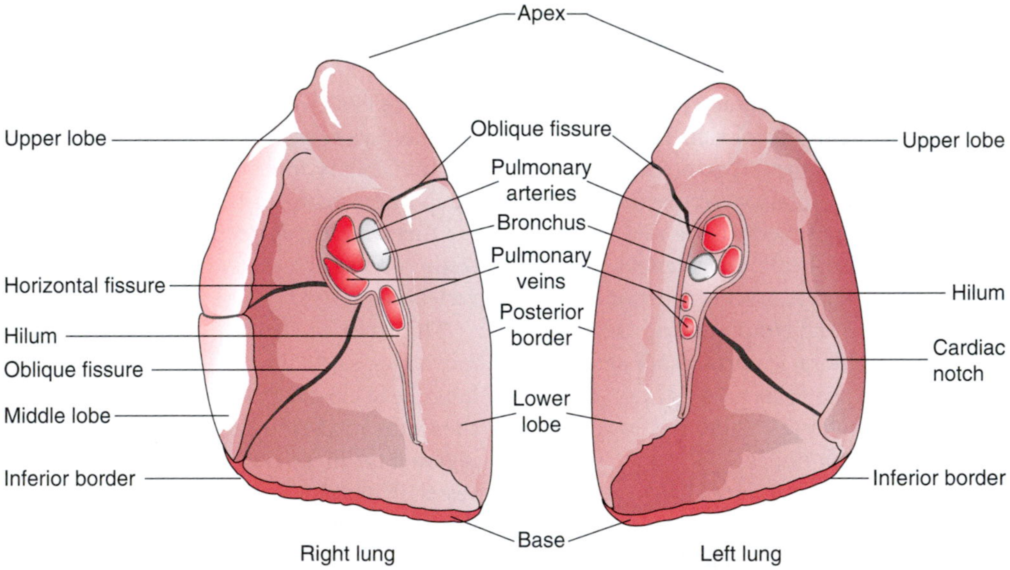

FIGURE 9-29 The medial surfaces of the lungs. (From Hicks GH: Cardiopulmonary anatomy and physiology, Philadelphia, 2000, WB Saunders.)

The lungs are elastic organs that can expand when inflated with air and recoil back to their resting volume when exhalation occurs. Lung elasticity stems from surface tension forces in the alveoli, elastic properties of the tissues, and various connective tissue fibers. Three different fiber systems form a scaffold that supports the structure of the lungs as tension develops in them with inflation.[46] The axial system, primarily composed of collagen and reticulin fibers, originates in the hilum and extends outward in all of the airway walls almost all the way to the alveolar region. The septal fiber system composed of collagen, reticulin, and elastin, supports the alveolar walls and capillaries. The peripheral fiber system, primarily composed of collagen, originates in the outer viscera and extends into the lung tissue to divide the lung tissue effectively into interlobular regions.

Collectively, these connective tissue fibers provide support to the airway walls, lungs, and effective gas-exchange membrane as it is stretched during inflation. When a lung is removed from the chest cavity, the lung quickly collapses to a smaller size. The same occurs if air or fluid enters into the pleural space; it is possible that individual lobes can collapse as the result of airway obstruction and gradual diffusion of air from the lobe. This tendency of the lung to collapse is counteracted by the tendency of the thoracic wall to spring outward and hold the lung inflated. The "tension" developed by these two opposing tendencies results in the development of subatmospheric (negative) intrapleural pressure.

PULMONARY VASCULAR, LYMPHATIC, AND NERVOUS SYSTEMS

The vascular supply of the lungs is composed of the pulmonary and bronchial circulations. The pulmonary circulation carries mixed venous blood from the systemic circuit to the lungs to increase O_2 and reduce CO_2 content of blood. The bronchial circulation provides systemic arterial blood to the airways and pleura supporting their metabolic needs. A network of lymphatics is also involved in fluid transport from the lungs. The lymphatic system removes fluid from the lung tissue and pleural space and returns it to the systemic circulation. The nervous system of the lungs acts to sense and modify lung function, helping defend while improving function.

Pulmonary Circulation

Pulmonary circulation is supplied with blood from the right heart (Figure 9-30). O_2-reduced systemic venous blood flows to the right heart via the inferior and superior venae cavae. This blood is pumped to the lungs by the right ventricle through the pulmonic semilunar valve and into the trunk of the pulmonary artery. The trunk of the pulmonary artery passes upward and divides into right and left pulmonary arteries just below the point of tracheal bifurcation into left and right main stem bronchi (the **carina**). The pulmonary arteries accompany the right and left main stem bronchi through the hilar opening into the lungs and continue dividing along with the airways. These divide to form two types of arteries: conventional, which continue to follow the airway branching, and supernumerary, which branch at 90-degree angles from the conventional arteries and travel outside the common path. Both sets of arteries form arterioles, connecting to and supplying blood to the microcirculation of the respiratory zone of the lung.

The pulmonary arterial system continues to divide into increasing numbers all the way to the distal airspaces. They subdivide, forming dense "sheetlike" beds of alveolar capillaries located within the walls of the alveoli, just below approximately 90% of the alveolar surface (Figure 9-31). The wall of the pulmonary capillary is formed by endothelial cells. At rest, the pulmonary capillary bed contains 60 to 80 ml of blood and can expand to 200 ml through dilation and recruitment of collapsed capillaries during conditions of higher cardiac output (e.g., exercise).[47] Pulmonary blood is collected from the capillaries by the pulmonary venules, combining into larger veins. Similar to their arterial counterparts, the veins also form conventional and supernumerary types of veins that drain blood from the pulmonary capillary beds. The pulmonary veins possess less smooth muscle in their medial walls and have thinner walls than similar-sized pulmonary arteries. The veins follow the same connective tissue path that houses the bronchi and arteries, merging into larger and fewer vessels. Four major pulmonary veins (superior and inferior veins from each lung) exit through the hila and return arterialized blood to the left atrium of the heart for delivery to the systemic circulation (Figure 9-32).

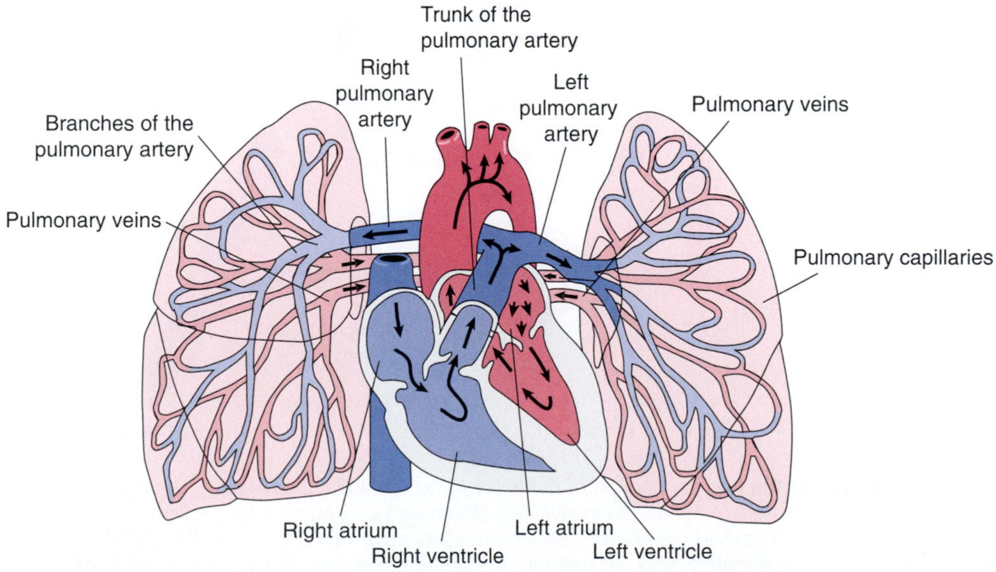

FIGURE 9-30 The pulmonary circulation. (From Hicks GH: Cardiopulmonary anatomy and physiology, Philadelphia, 2000, WB Saunders.)

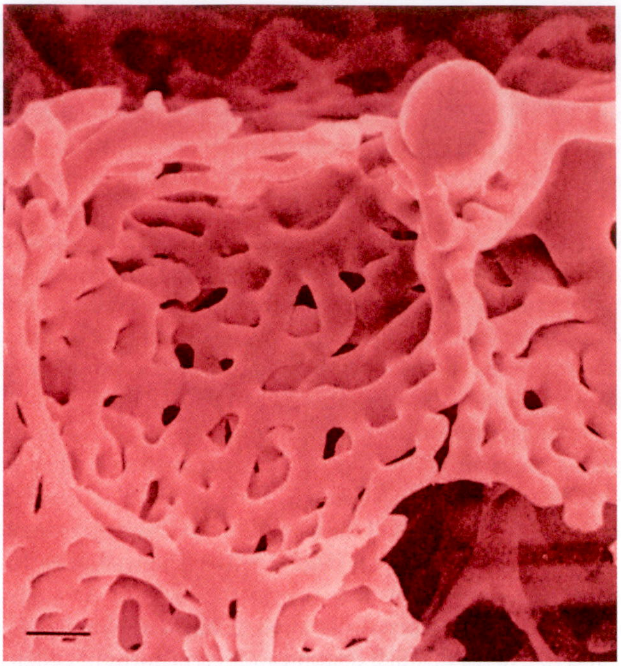

FIGURE 9-31 Scanning electron photomicrograph at high magnification of plastic cast of alveolar capillaries of the pulmonary circulation (black bar, 10 μm). (From Thibodeau GA, Patton KT: Anatomy and physiology, ed 7, St Louis, 2010, Mosby.)

RULE OF THUMB

The pulmonary artery and its branches are the only arteries in the body to carry deoxygenated blood. The pulmonary veins are the only veins that carry oxygenated blood back to the left side of the heart.

Respiratory Function of Pulmonary Circulation

The pulmonary circulation has several different functions.[48] Primary function of the pulmonary circulation is to deliver blood to the alveolar-capillary bed for the exchange of O_2 and CO_2 with alveolar gas, delivering it to the left heart. The second function is to serve as a barrier between the interstitial spaces and airspaces of the lung on one side and the blood within the capillaries on the other. Less than 0.3 μm thick, the endothelial capillary membrane is an active barrier that controls the exchange of fluid and solutes crossing it. In doing so, it plays a crucial role in the regulation of the fluid balance within the lungs. Injury to the pulmonary capillary often disrupts the fluid balance, resulting in excessive fluid leaks and the formation of pulmonary edema. The third function is nonrespiratory, involving the production, processing, and clearance of various chemicals and blood clots.

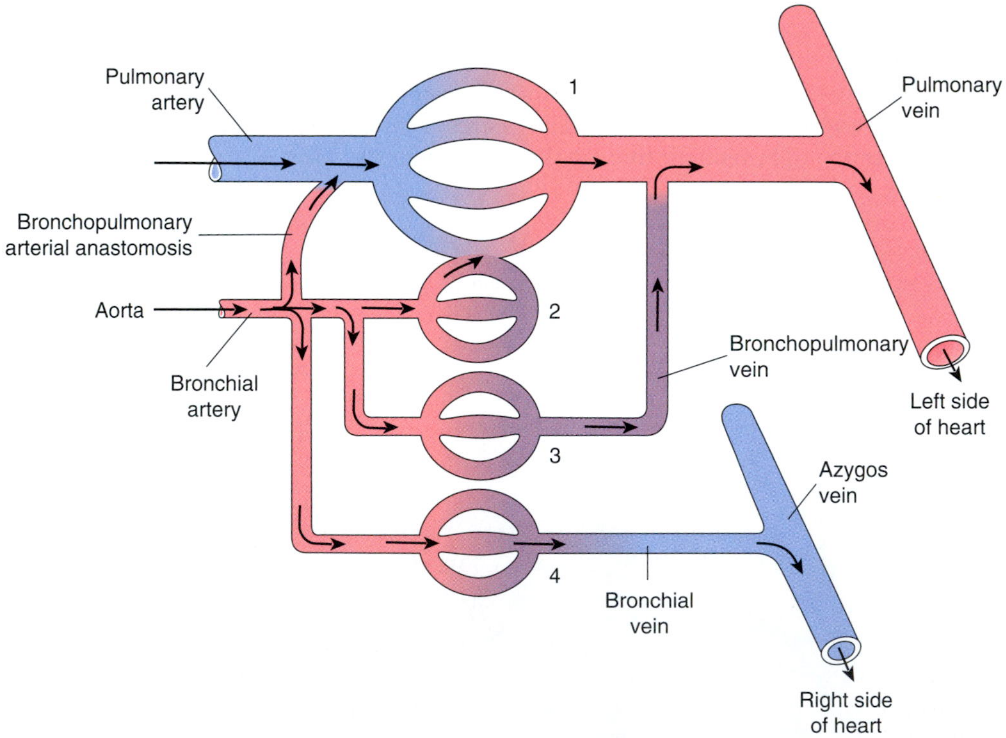

FIGURE 9-32 Schematic depiction of the interconnection of pulmonary and bronchial circulations. Bronchial blood flows to the pulmonary artery *(1),* through the capillary bed of the large airways and pleura and into pulmonary capillaries *(2),* through the bronchopulmonary veins and into the pulmonary veins *(3),* and through the bronchial vein and on to the azygos vein *(4).* The route through the bronchopulmonary vein allows less oxygenated blood to mix with the better oxygenated blood, which returns to the left side of the heart. (From Hicks GH: Cardiopulmonary anatomy and physiology, Philadelphia, 2000, WB Saunders.)

TABLE 9-6

Resting Hemodynamic Values in Adult Systemic and Pulmonary Vascular Systems

Parameter	Systemic Circuit	Pulmonary Circuit
Blood flow (cardiac output, L/min)	5	5
Arterial blood pressure (mm Hg)	120/80	25/10
Vascular resistance (dynes/sec/cm^{-5})	1200	120

Table 9-6 compares hemodynamic parameters of the systemic and pulmonary circulatory systems.[49] Although the entire cardiac output passes through both pulmonary and systemic circuits, the pulmonary circulation offers much lower resistance and consequently has a much lower blood pressure. The low vascular pressures within the pulmonary circuit are essential in maintenance of fluid balance at the alveolar-capillary interface. The pulmonary capillaries are exposed to vascular pressures of approximately 7 to 10 mm Hg. Increased pressure in the pulmonary circulation can occur with mitral valve disease or congestive (left) heart failure, disrupting fluid balance and leading to excessive fluid leakage, fluid accumulation, and alveolar congestion, which can impair gas exchange and lead to hypoxia.

The low vascular pressures of the pulmonary circulation result in regional blood flow within the lungs that is highly influenced by gravity, airway pressure, and gas exchange.[48] In the upright lung, blood pressure in the pulmonary arteries increases approximately 1 cm H_2O for each 1 cm traversed downward from the apex to the base. A consequence of having a low blood pressure in the pulmonary circulation and being susceptible to gravity, blood flow is much higher in the lung bases in resting upright subjects. Gravity-related effects also occur in recumbent positions but are less pronounced. The distribution of pulmonary blood flow is also closely related to local airway gas pressure and pulmonary gas exchange. Areas experiencing higher airway pressure (e.g., during positive pressure ventilation) that equals or exceeds local arteriole and capillary pressure have reduced blood flow as a result of the opposing airway pressure (zone 1 airways). Regions where blood pressure is greater than the surrounding air pressure, such as in the bases of the upright lung during spontaneous breathing, have greater blood flow (zone 3 airways). Areas of regional lung hypoxia, because of reduced ventilation, congestion, or airway obstruction, can result in local pulmonary arterial vasoconstriction and cause blood flow to shift from these areas toward areas of higher O_2 content and pulmonary vasodilation.[47]

Nonrespiratory Function of the Pulmonary Circulation

The pulmonary circulation also serves as a blood reservoir for the left ventricle.[47,48] This reservoir maintains stable left ventricular volumes despite small changes in cardiac output. The pulmonary blood volume (approximately 600 ml) is sufficient to maintain normal left ventricle filling for several cardiac cycles. This reservoir is important if filling of the right heart is temporarily decreased or interrupted.

The pulmonary circulation also acts as a filter for the systemic circulation. The capillaries have an inner diameter of approximately 7 to 10 μm and theoretically trap particles (e.g., blood clots) down to this size before they enter the systemic circulation, where blockages could be life-threatening.

The lungs also play an active role in the clearance, activation, and release of various biochemical factors.[47,48] They are responsible for synthesis, activation, inactivation, and detoxification of many bioactive substances. Angiotensin I is converted to its active form (angiotensin II) as it circulates through the lung. Various proinflammatory cytokines are also released from the lung when it is injured or repetitively overinflated during mechanical ventilation.[50]

Bronchial Circulation

A separate arterial supply called the *bronchial circulation* supplies blood to the airways from the trachea to the bronchioles and to most of the visceral pleurae.[51] The metabolic needs of the lung are comparatively low, and much of the lung parenchyma is oxygenated by direct contact with inspired gas. The bronchial circulation is a branch of the systemic circuit and is supplied with blood from the aorta via minor thoracic branches. Blood flow through the bronchial circulation constitutes approximately 1% to 2% of the total cardiac output.

A single right bronchial artery supplying the right lung arises from the upper intercostal artery, the right subclavian artery, or an internal mammary artery. Two bronchial arteries supply the left lung and branch directly from the upper thoracic aorta. Bronchial arteries follow their respective bronchi. The bronchial arterial circulation terminates in a plexus of capillaries joining the alveolar-capillary bed. Bronchial venous blood drains through the *azygos, hemiazygos,* and *intercostal* veins to the right atrium. Some drains through the pulmonary capillaries to the pulmonary veins and to the left atrium. Figure 9-32 shows the interrelationship and comingling of the pulmonary and bronchial circulatory systems.

The bronchial and pulmonary circulations share an important compensatory relationship.[52] Decreased pulmonary arterial blood pressure tends to cause an increase in bronchial artery blood flow to the affected area. This compensation minimizes the danger of pulmonary infarction, as sometimes occurs when a blood clot (pulmonary embolus) enters the lung. Similarly, loss of bronchial circulation can be partially offset by increases in pulmonary arterial perfusion. The adult lung does not require the bronchial circulation to remain viable, as evidenced by the success of lung transplantation, which does not preserve the bronchial circulation. However, this circulation apparently plays a more important role in lung development, helps to preserve gas exchange during various congenital cardiac conditions, and appears to compensate in certain pulmonary diseases (e.g., pulmonary fibrosis) for the gradual obstruction of the pulmonary circulation.

Lymphatics

The lymphatic system of the lungs is an extensive system of lymphatic vessels, lymph nodes, the tonsils, and the thymus gland.[53] The primary function of the lymphatic system is to clear fluid from the interstitial and pleural spaces to help maintain the fluid balance in the lungs. The lymphatic system also plays an important role in the specific defenses of the immune system. It removes bacteria, foreign material, and cell debris via the lymph fluid and through the action of various phagocytic cells (e.g., macrophages), providing defense against foreign material and cells that are able to penetrate deep into the lung. It also produces various lymphocytes and plasma cells to aid in defense. Both roles are essential for maintaining normal function of the respiratory system.

Most of the pulmonary lymphatic system consists of superficial and deep vessels.[54] The superficial (pleural) vessels that drain the lung surface and the deep (peribronchovascular) conduit-like vessels that travel through the connective tissue tracts. Both drain the blind lymphatic capillaries in the respective regions. The deeper lymph vessels are closely associated with the small airways but do not extend into the walls of the alveolar-capillary membranes. The lymphatic vessels are thin-walled vessels that contain little connective and muscle tissue in their walls.

Lymph fluid is collected by the loosely formed lymphatic capillaries and drains through the lymph vessels toward the hilum. The fluid is propelled through the lymphatic system by the collective actions of valves that direct flow toward the hilum. The combined milking actions of smooth muscle contractions in the deeper conduit-like vessels and the cycle of ventilation act as a pump and squeezes the lymphatic vessels.[55] Lymph fluid flow from the lungs can be increased after an injury to the pulmonary capillaries that results in increased leakage (e.g., acute respiratory distress syndrome) or from pulmonary capillary hypertension secondary to heart disease (e.g., left-sided heart failure).

The lymph vessels emerge from the hilum of each lung and drain lymph fluid through a series of lymph nodes clustered about each hilum and the mediastinum. From there, lymph fluid travels through various lymph nodes within the mediastinum (Figure 9-33). The lymph fluid rejoins the general circulation after passing through the right lymphatic or thoracic duct, draining into the jugular, subclavian, or innominate veins. The lymph fluid mixes with blood and returns back to the heart.

Lymphatic channels are not usually visible on chest radiographs. They may be detected if distended or thickened by disease. The "butterfly" pattern that radiates from the hilar region of both lungs during acute development of pulmonary edema is thought to be the result of interstitial and lymph vessel distention with fluid. In this situation, the lymphatic drainage system has been overwhelmed by a sudden and excessive surge of fluid from the circulation. The development of a pleural effusion is also evidence that the lymphatic system is unable to remove excess fluid in the lung.

Nervous Control of the Lungs

All of the major structures of the respiratory system are innervated by branches of the peripheral nervous system: the autonomic and somatic branches (Figure 9-34).[56] The somatic

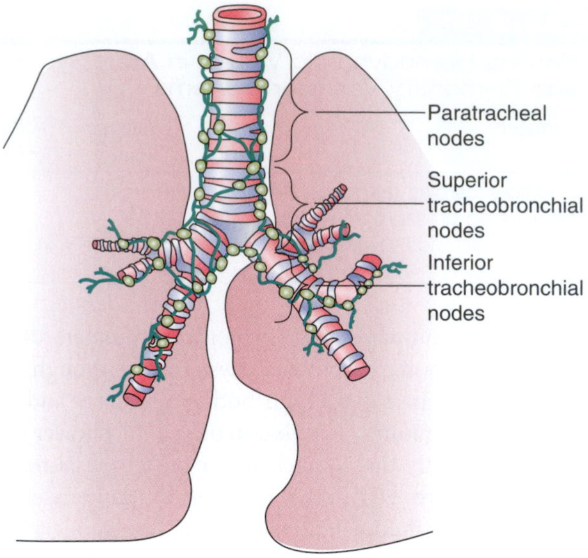

FIGURE 9-33 Mediastinal and paratracheal pulmonary lymph nodes. (From Hicks GH: Cardiopulmonary anatomy and physiology, Philadelphia, 2000, WB Saunders.)

system provides voluntary and automatic motor control and sensory innervation to the chest wall and respiratory muscles. Most of the major motor nerves that carry nervous signaling to the respiratory muscles are summarized in Tables 9-4 and 9-5. The autonomic nervous system signaling to and from the lungs is carried through efferent and afferent pathways. These pathways carry unconscious autonomic nervous system motor signals to smooth muscles and glands and various sensory signals back to the brain.

Autonomic innervation of the lungs is carried from the brainstem through branches of the right and left vagus nerves (cranial nerve X) and from the spinal cord to four or five thoracic sympathetic ganglia that lie just laterally to the spinal cord.[57] Both contribute fibers to the anterior and posterior pulmonary plexus at the root of each lung. From these plexuses, sympathetic and parasympathetic fibers enter the lung through the hilum and innervate various structures.

Efferent Pathways

The parasympathetic nervous preganglionic fibers exit the brainstem via the two vagus nerves. On entry into the chest, the vagus nerve branches to the larynx. This branch is called the *recurrent laryngeal nerve.* Each vagus nerve also develops a branch called the *superior laryngeal nerve.* The external branch of this nerve supplies the cricothyroid muscle. The internal branch provides sensory fibers to the larynx. The recurrent laryngeal nerves provide the primary motor innervation to the larynx. Damage to laryngeal nerves can cause unilateral or bilateral vocal cord paralysis, depending on which branches are involved. Hoarseness, loss of voice, and an ineffective cough may result.

After forming ganglia and postganglionic nerve fibers, parasympathetic and sympathetic nerve fibers enter the lung through the hilum and run parallel to the airways as they branch (Figure 9-35). Parasympathetic fibers form their ganglia much closer to

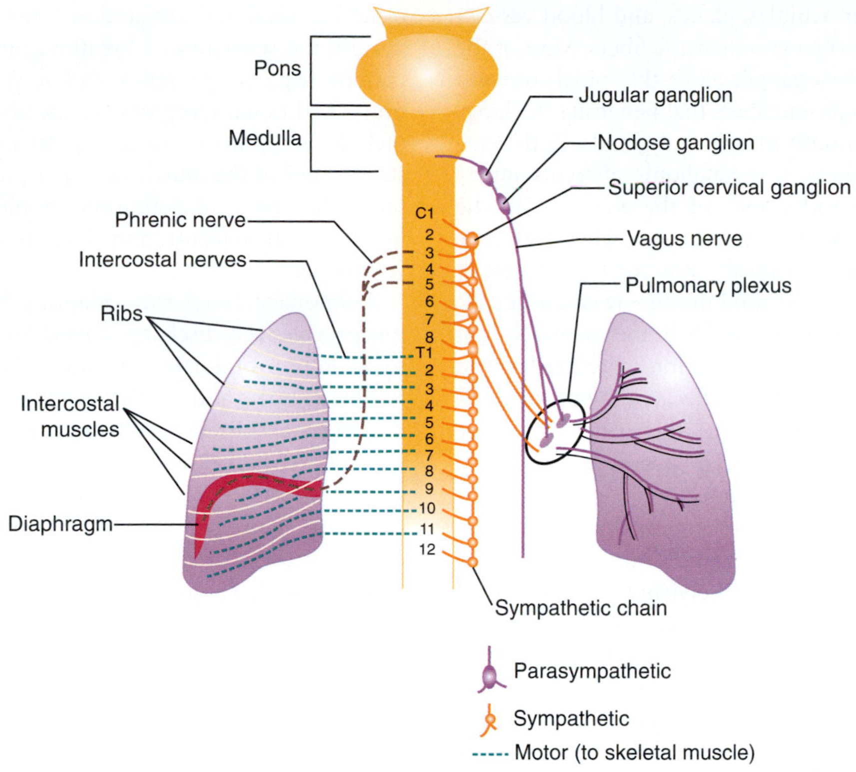

FIGURE 9-34 Schematic of the autonomic innervation (motor and sensory) of the lung and the somatic (motor) nerve supply to the intercostal muscles and diaphragm. (Modified from Murray JF: The normal lung, ed 2, Philadelphia, 1986, WB Saunders.)

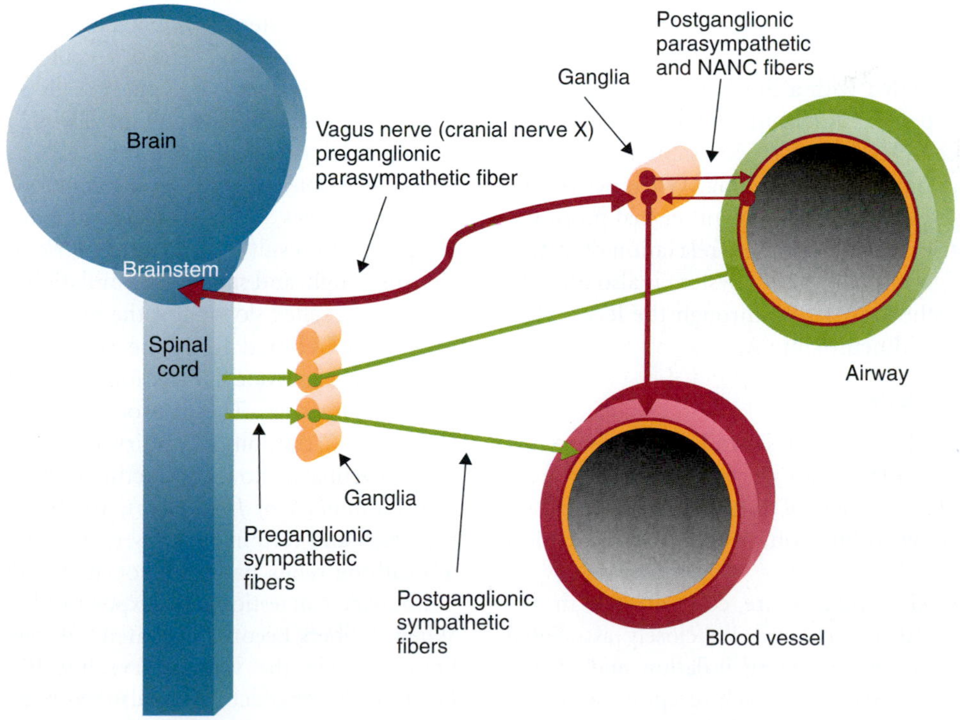

FIGURE 9-35 Schematic of sympathetic, parasympathetic, and nonadrenergic, noncholinergic *(NANC)* neural fiber connections to the airways and blood vessels of the lungs.

the target tissues (e.g., bronchioles, glands, and blood vessels) and have much shorter postganglionic nerve fibers. Most of the sympathetic fibers form their ganglia along the spinal cord and then form longer postganglionic fibers that penetrate the lungs and end on the airway smooth muscle and glands. Both sympathetic and parasympathetic postganglionic efferents innervate the smooth muscle and glands of the airways and the smooth muscles of the pulmonary arterioles. They influence the diameter of the airway by causing more or less tension in the smooth muscles that wrap around the airway and influence glandular secretion. The smooth muscles in the medial wall of the pulmonary arterioles cause constriction when tensed and dilation when relaxed. The combined effects of the parasympathetic and sympathetic nervous activity, which generally oppose each other's action, result in a balanced control of airway and vessel diameter and glandular secretion.

The parasympathetic postganglionic fibers generally secrete acetylcholine as their primary neurotransmitter when they receive signals from the brainstem. Acetylcholine binds to M_3 muscarinic cholinergic receptors, causing airway smooth muscle constriction, blood vessel dilation, and glandular secretion. The sympathetic postganglionic fibers are much less developed in comparison. The sympathetic postganglionic fibers in the lung primarily secrete norepinephrine. The adrenal glands release epinephrine into the circulation when they receive sympathetic signals from the spinal cord. Epinephrine and norepinephrine bind to alpha-adrenergic and beta-adrenergic receptors of blood vessels. This binding causes constriction in the alpha-adrenergic receptors and dilation and relaxation in the beta-adrenergic receptors of the bronchial airway and vessel smooth muscles.

The airways are provided with a third autonomic pathway that is neither parasympathetic nor sympathetic in action.[46] The nonadrenergic, noncholinergic (NANC) system nerve fibers travel within the vagus nerve to each lung. When active, the NANC nerve endings release a neurotransmitter that promotes the production of nitric oxide, causing the relaxation of airway smooth muscle and dilation. The NANC system is also thought to be capable of bronchoconstriction through the local reflex release of substance P and neurokinin A.

Afferent Pathways

Most afferent fibers follow pathways from the lungs to the central nervous system in the vagus nerve. The vagus afferent pathways are activated by a variety of different receptors within the lung that are sensitive to inflation, deflation, and chemical stimulation.[58]

Slow-adapting stretch receptors are concentrated in the small and medium-sized airways and are closely associated with the airway smooth muscle. Lung inflation and airway stretch stimulate the slow-adapting stretch receptors, and they continue to signal and do not adapt and drop their signaling rate—hence their name. In the mucosal layer of the airway, rapid-adapting receptors sense changes in tidal volume, respiratory rate, and lung compliance, responding to a wide variety of mechanical and chemical irritants. In addition, a variety of other chemical and congestion sensors, when active, seem to modify the sensation of breathing and modify the breathing pattern (e.g., cough reflex and response to alveolar congestion). Additional receptors are located outside the lungs; they include respiratory muscle proprioceptors that sense the stretch state of the muscles and peripheral chemoreceptors that sense the chemical condition of blood (e.g., O_2, CO_2, and hydrogen ion concentration) that are involved in the control of ventilation.

Pulmonary stretch slow-adapting and rapid-adapting receptors progressively discharge during lung inflation and are linked to inhibition of further inflation. This is a type of negative feedback known as the *inflation reflex*. It was originally described by Hering and Breuer and continues to bear their names. The inflation reflex is thought to be actively involved with controlling the depth of breathing and may affect the duration of the expiratory pause between breaths. The inflation reflex is probably very weak or absent during quiet breathing in healthy adults, but there appears to be evidence of its activity in newborns.[59]

Another reflex associated with slow-adapting and rapid-adapting receptor activity is the Head paradoxical reflex.[60] This reflex stimulates a deeper breath rather than inhibiting further inspiration. It may be the basis for occasional deep breaths or gasps. Deep breaths or sighs occur with normal breathing, presumably preventing alveolar collapse. The Head reflex also may be responsible for gasping in newborn infants as they progressively inflate their lungs.

Irritant or mechanical rapid-reacting receptors are found mainly in the posterior wall of the trachea and at bifurcations of the larger bronchi. These receptors respond to various mechanical, chemical, and physiologic stimuli and behave as irritant receptors. The stimuli include physical manipulation or irritation, inhalation of noxious gases, histamine-induced bronchoconstriction, asphyxia, and microembolization of the pulmonary arteries. Stimulation of the irritant rapid-adapting receptors can result in bronchoconstriction, hyperpnea, glottic closure, cough, and sneeze.[61] Stimulation of these receptors also can cause a reflex slowing of the heart rate (bradycardia). This response is referred to as the *vasovagal reflex*. It may occur during tracheobronchial suctioning, intubation of the airway, or bronchoscopy. These procedures can cause significant mechanical irritation of the airway.

Unmyelinated slow-conducting *C-fiber endings* (also known as *juxtacapillary* or *J receptors*), are present in the walls of the bronchial and terminal airway region and have been linked to a breathing reflex pattern associated with mechanical stretch, pulmonary congestion, and exposure to various chemicals.[62,63] When C-fibers become activated, signals are sent back to the brainstem via the vagus nerve, resulting in rapid, shallow breathing. C-fiber activation also has been shown to cause bradycardia, hypotension, bronchoconstriction, mucus production, and apnea in experimental animals.[64] Stimulation of these receptors may contribute to the sensation of dyspnea and, in severe cases, the vagovagal reflex, which can complicate pulmonary edema, pulmonary embolism, and pneumonia.

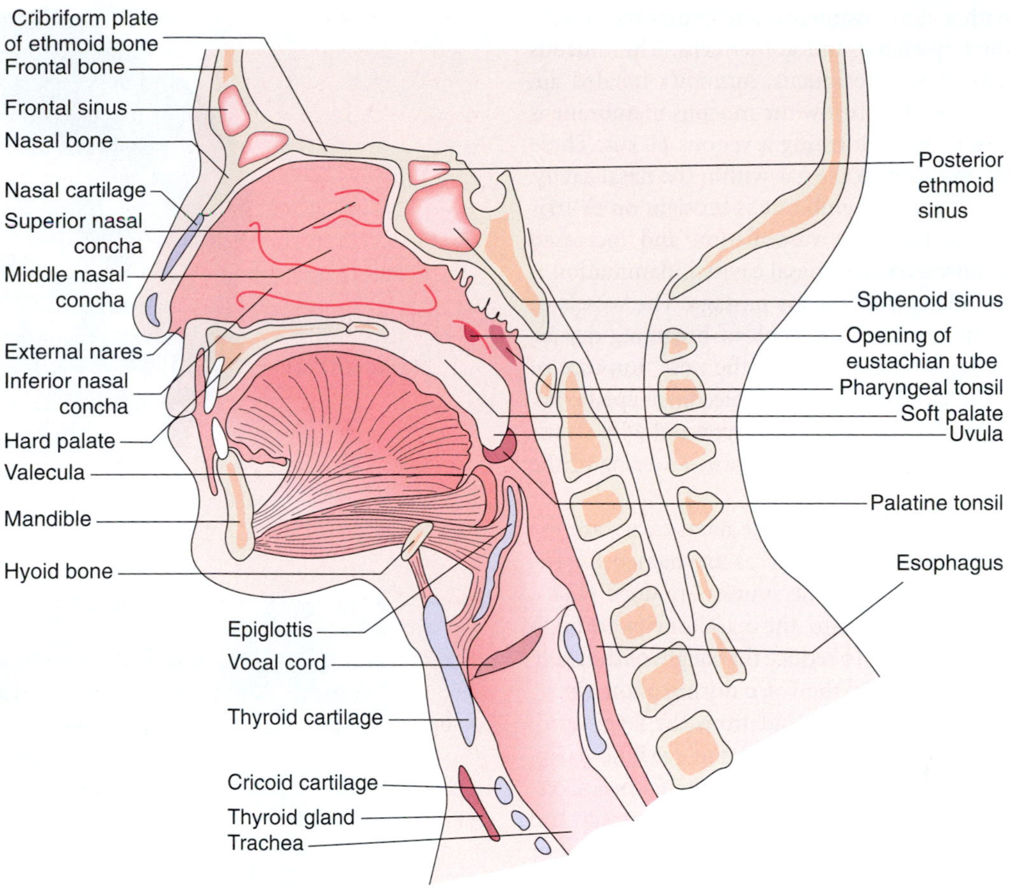

FIGURE 9-36 Midsagittal section through the upper airway. (From Hicks GH: Cardiopulmonary anatomy and physiology, Philadelphia, 2000, WB Saunders.)

ANATOMY OF THE RESPIRATORY TRACT

Upper Respiratory Tract

The *upper respiratory tract* is defined as the airways that start at the nose and mouth and extend down to the trachea (Figure 9-36).[65,66] The upper airway is open to the outside environment through the external nares, or nostrils, of the nose and the mouth of the oral cavity. Most of the air moved through the respiratory tract during resting breathing enters through the nares and nasal cavity. Mouth breathing is used during exercise to reduce the resistance to gas flow at higher ventilation rates. The functions of the upper airway are summarized in Box 9-1.

Box 9-1 Functions of the Upper Airway

- Passageway for gas flow
- Filter
- Heater
- Humidification
- Sense of smell and taste
- Phonation
- Protection of the lower airways

Nasal Cavity and Sinuses

There are two flared openings called **alae** that form the **external nares.** The alae enclose a space on each side called the *vestibule.* The vestibules have hairs that act as a gross filter. Located posterior to the vestibules are the openings to the internal nose, or the **anterior nares.** The left and right nasal cavities are formed by cartilage and numerous skull bones. The roof is formed by the nasal, frontal, sphenoid, and ethmoid bones. The septum separating the two cavities is formed by cartilage and the ethmoid and vomer bones. The lateral walls are created by the maxilla, lacrimal, and palatine bones. The floor of the cavity, or **palate,** is primarily formed by the maxilla. Three shelflike bones protrude into the cavity from the lateral walls. These bony shelves are called the superior, middle, and inferior *conchae,* or **turbinates.**

The conchae function to increase the surface area and complexity of the nasal cavity, enabling the nasal cavity to work as a passageway, filter, humidifier, and heater of inhaled airway. The posterior openings of the nasal cavity are called the *internal nares* and are formed in part by the flexible soft palate.

The surface of the nasal cavity is covered with epithelia. The anterior portion is covered with stratified squamous cells and possesses hair follicles and hair. This is the same type of tissue that forms the epidermis of skin. The middle portion of the cavity is covered with a mucous membrane composed of ciliated **pseudostratified epithelia** and goblet cells. The mucous membrane functions to secrete mucus, humidify inhaled air, and trap inhaled particles. Just below the mucous membrane is an extensive network of veins forming a venous plexus. These vessels supply water and heat to the gas within the nasal cavity. Inflammation of this mucous membrane is brought on by irritation or infection produced by vasodilation and increased vessel leakage. The consequence of nasal cavity inflammation is partial or complete blockage of the air passage. The vessels of the venous plexus can rupture as a result of breathing dry air or the passage of foreign bodies through the nose. Rupture of these vessels can cause considerable nasal bleeding (**epistaxis**). The posterior portion of the nasal cavity is covered with stratified squamous epithelium similar to the tissue covering of the nearby oral cavity.

Within the skull bones and around the nasal cavity are the *sinuses* (Figure 9-37). These hollow spaces are named for the bones in which they are found.[67] The sinuses are lined with a mucous membrane and drain into the nasal cavity through numerous ducts. They function to reduce the weight of the skull, strengthen the skull, and modify the voice during phonation.

The nasal cavity conducts air to and from the respiratory tract, conditions inhaled gas, acts as a sinus and eye fluid drain, and contains olfactory sensors for the sensation of smell. Conditioning inhaled gas helps defend the respiratory tract and involves filtering, heating, and humidifying air. Filtration of inhaled air is carried out by the hair in the anterior portion of the cavity and the sticky mucous membrane that covers the complex surface of the cavity. Filtration is enhanced by the flow pattern through the nasal cavity. Inspired gas is accelerated to a high velocity through the anterior nares. It changes direction sharply as it enters the internal nasal cavity. This pattern causes particles larger than 10 μm in diameter to have an impact on the nasal mucosa. Ciliary action or nose blowing clears these particles. Past the external nares, the cross-sectional area increases; this results in a decrease in gas velocity. Turbulence increases because of the narrow convolutions of the passages. Low velocity and turbulence combine to remove any remaining particles. Filtration is based on impaction, sedimentation, and diffusion of various-sized particles.

Surface fluids originate from the goblet cells and submucosal glands. This fluid lining has mild antibacterial properties. Ciliary activity in the nasal mucous membranes helps transport the mucus produced so it can be cleared. Foreign matter is typically cleared from the nasal cavity by sniffing and swallowing. During exhalation, the heated and moist expired air passes over the concha and is cooled. The excess moisture deposits on the concha as condensation to help retain and recycle water. These defense/conditioning mechanisms help ensure inspired air is free from particulate and bacterial contamination and is heated and humidified to 37° C and 100% relative humidity by the time it reaches the trachea. In addition, the mucous membrane contains chemoreceptors that send signals to the olfactory nerve for the sensation of smell in the superior portion of the cavity just above each of the superior conchae.

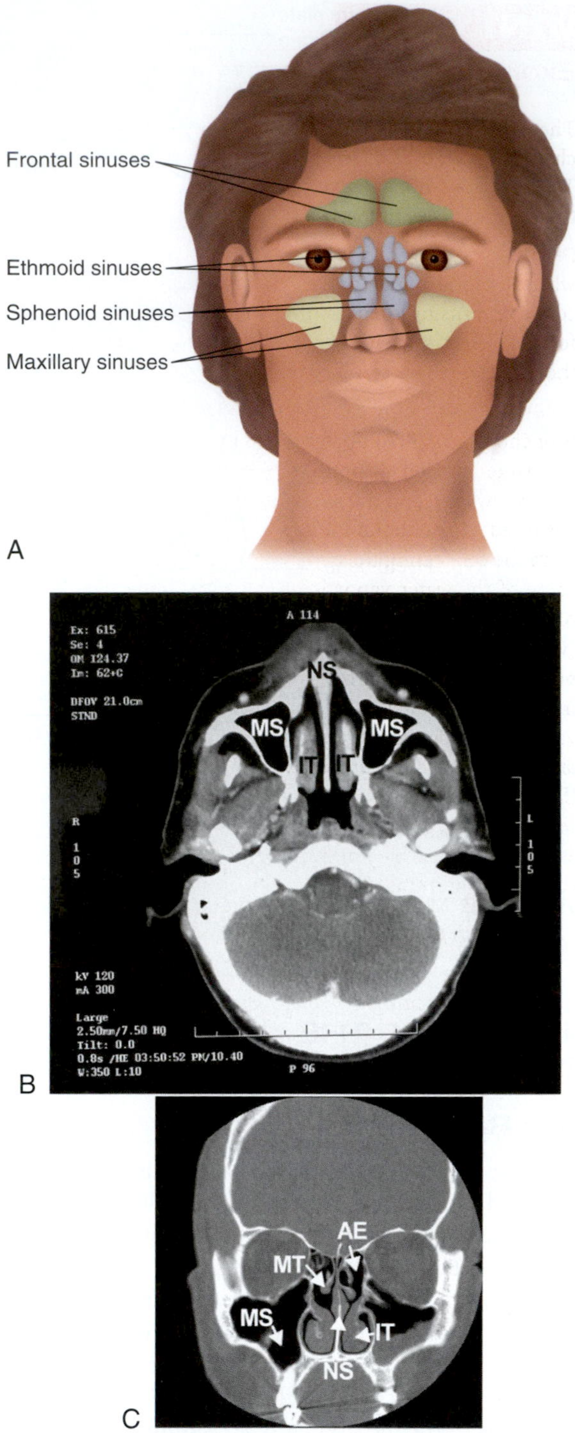

FIGURE 9-37 A, Positions of the frontal, maxillary, sphenoid, and ethmoid sinuses; the nasal sinuses are named for the bones in which they occur. **B,** Axial computed tomography (CT) scan at the approximate level of the inferior turbinates *(IT)* and maxillary sinuses *(MS)*. The nasal septum *(NS)* is also well defined. **C,** Coronal CT scan showing the anterior ethmoid sinuses *(AE)* and the middle turbinates *(MT)* in addition to the structures seen in **B**.

MINI CLINI

Exercise-Induced Asthma

The upper airway, along with the trachea and main stem bronchi, play crucial roles in conditioning the air being breathed. These airways not only conduct gas from the atmosphere to the lower airways but also warm, humidify, and filter it.

PROBLEM: Some individuals develop shortness of breath, wheezing, and coughing when they exercise outdoors. What could be causing their asthma attack? Is there an alternative form of exercise that could reduce the symptoms and allow them to receive an aerobic workout?

ANSWER: In many cases, exercise-induced asthma (EIA) or bronchospasm (EIB) appears to be triggered by reflexes from the large airways (upper airway, trachea, bronchi). These airways warm and humidify inspired gas. Water vapor is absorbed from the fluid lining of the airways and replenished from the cells lining the airways. As gas is expired, it cools, and some of the water vapor is reabsorbed. Only a small amount of water is lost from the body via this mechanism. Exercise (with its increased ventilatory demands) causes an increase in heat and water loss from the airways. The airways in some individuals are especially sensitive (hyperresponsive) to a wide variety of triggering agents. When these individuals exercise and increase their ventilation, the loss of heat or water from the large airways can trigger an asthmatic reaction (i.e., coughing, wheezing, and shortness of breath). This phenomenon is especially noticeable when susceptible individuals exercise in cold, dry conditions. Asthma is sometimes diagnosed by having patients hyperventilate breathing cold, dry gas and then measuring how much airflow decreases.

Swimming usually involves exercise in a warm, high-humidity environment. The preconditioned air breathed during swimming often reduces or eliminates EIB. Many asthmatic children can swim vigorously with few symptoms, even though other sports trigger their bronchospasm.

Oral Cavity

Air also can enter and exit from the respiratory tract through the oral cavity (Figure 9-38). The anterior roof of the oral cavity is called the *hard palate* and is formed by the maxillary bone. The posterior portion is known as the **soft palate.** Its soft tissue composition has the ability to move upward and seal off the nasal cavity. The end of the soft palate hangs down into the posterior portion of the oral cavity. This part of the soft palate is called the **uvula.** The walls of the oral cavity are formed by the cheeks, and the floor is dominated by the tongue.

The uvula and the surrounding walls control the flow of air, fluid, and food during eating, drinking, sneezing, coughing, and vomiting. The tongue is involved in mechanical digestion, taste, and phonation. The posterior surface of the tongue is supplied with many sensory nerve endings. These nerves produce a vagal gag reflex when stimulated, protecting the lungs from aspiration. This reflex must be considered when passing tubes or instruments through the mouth in conscious or semiconscious patients.

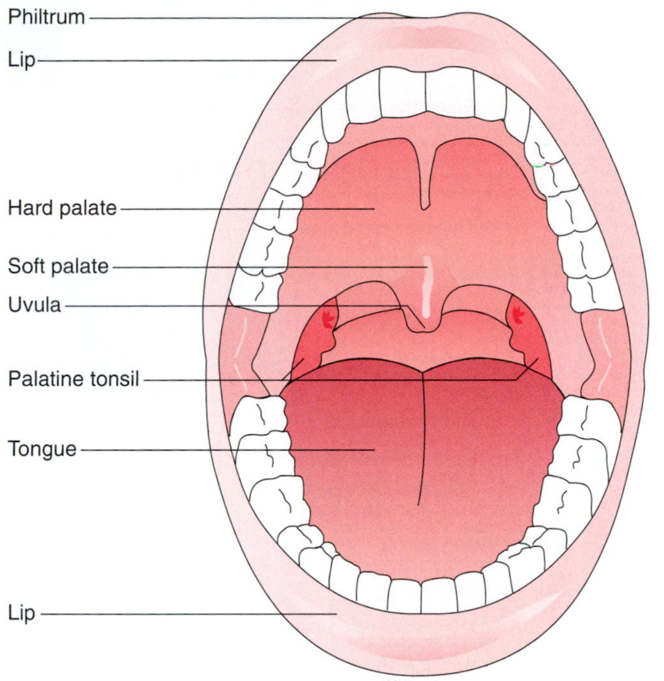

FIGURE 9-38 Frontal view into the open mouth showing the major structures within. (From Hicks GH: Cardiopulmonary anatomy and physiology, Philadelphia, 2000, WB Saunders.)

The mucosal surfaces of the oral cavity also provide humidification and warming of inspired air. These surfaces are much less efficient than the nose. Saliva is produced by major and minor salivary glands. Saliva functions primarily as a wetting and digestive agent for food but provides some humidification of inspired gas. The oral cavity ends at a double web on each side, called the *palatine folds.* The palatine tonsils sit between these folds on each side (see Figure 9-38). The palatine tonsils are vascularized lymphoid tissues that play an immunologic role, especially in childhood.

Reflexes of the mouth, pharynx, and larynx help protect the lower respiratory tract during swallowing.[68] These protective functions can be severely compromised during anesthesia or unconsciousness. Loss or compromise of these important reflexes can result in aspiration of bacteria-colonized saliva or food causing pulmonary infection and asphyxiation in severe cases.

Pharynx

The posterior portion of the nasal and oral cavities opens into a region called the **pharynx.** The entire pharynx is lined with stratified squamous epithelium. The pharynx is subdivided into the **nasopharynx, oropharynx,** and **hypopharynx,** or **laryngopharynx.** The nasopharynx lies at the posterior end of the nasal cavity and extends to the tip of the uvula. Numerous foreign particles impact the surface of the nasopharynx. Located in this region are two pharyngeal tonsils (also called the *adenoids*) on either side of the lateral and posterior walls of the pharynx. They monitor and interact with the particles inhaled through the actions of the lymphoid cells located there. In the same

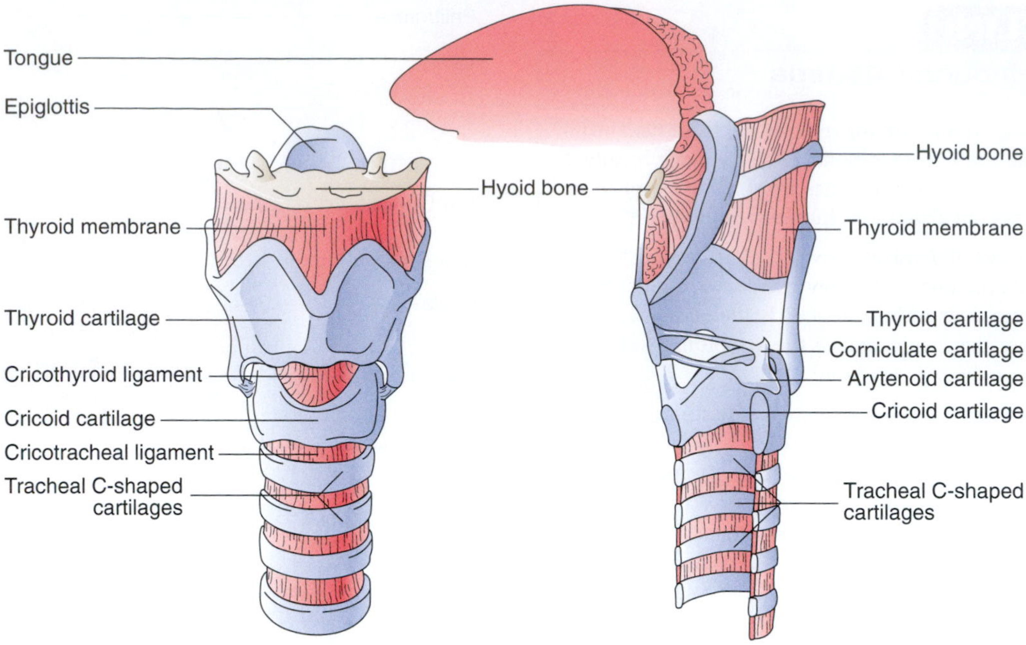

FIGURE 9-39 Anterior and lateral views of the larynx. (From Hicks GH: Cardiopulmonary anatomy and physiology, Philadelphia, 2000, WB Saunders.)

region are two openings into the left and right **eustachian tubes** that link the upper airway with the middle ear (see Figure 9-36). The eustachian tubes drain fluid out of the middle ear and allow gas to move in or out, equalizing pressure on either side of the tympanic membrane.

The oropharynx is located in the posterior region of the oral cavity that spans the space between the uvula and the upper rim of the epiglottis. This region is also equipped with a pair of palatine tonsils that are located on the lateral walls of the oropharynx. These tonsils can become chronically swollen causing partial airway obstruction. If swelling is excessive and the individual has numerous repeat throat and ear infections, the tonsils can be removed by the surgical procedure known as a *tonsillectomy.*

The region below the oropharynx is known as the *hypopharynx.* It extends from the upper rim of the epiglottis to the opening between the vocal cords. The tissues of the nasopharynx and hypopharynx can move and undergo large changes of shape during speech and swallowing. Immediately below the hypopharynx the digestive and respiratory tracts separate.

During unconsciousness, the muscles of the tongue and hypopharynx can relax and allow the tongue and other soft tissues to collapse and occlude the opening of the hypopharynx. This condition can result in partial to complete blockage of the upper airway and limit air movement to and from the respiratory tract. This condition is a primary cause of obstructive sleep apnea (OSA), discussed later in this text.

Larynx

The **larynx** lies below the hypopharynx and is formed by a complex arrangement of nine cartilages and numerous muscles (Figure 9-39).[69] It protects the respiratory tract during eating and drinking and in phonation. The *thyroid cartilage* forms most of the upper portion of the larynx and is generally referred to as the *Adam's apple.* This cartilage is named for the thyroid gland that lies over its outer surface. Just below the thyroid cartilage is the *cricoid cartilage.* It is the only laryngeal structure that forms a complete ring of cartilage around the airway and is the narrowest region of the upper airway in infants. A membrane of connective tissue called the *cricothyroid ligament* spans the space between the thyroid and cricoid cartilage. This membrane is occasionally used as the location for placement of an emergency prosthetic artificial airway in patients who have a life-threatening blockage of the upper airway.

Sleep studies can document partial and complete airflow obstruction. Management of OSA includes weight loss (to reduce anatomic narrowing of the airway), nasal continuous positive airway pressure (CPAP) to hold open the airway, surgical correction (uvulopalatopharyngoplasty) to remove obstructing tissue, and oral appliances that modify the shape of the oropharynx.

The cartilaginous and leaf-shaped epiglottis lies within and is attached to the thyroid cartilage by a flexible joint. In adults, it is 2 to 4 cm long, 2 to 3 cm wide, and 2 to 5 mm deep. It is not easily visualized in adults, but it can be seen in small children and crying infants because of its higher position. During breathing, the thyroid cartilage slides down and remains apart from the epiglottis, allowing air to move in and out of the respiratory tract. The *epiglottis* helps prevent liquids and food entering the respiratory tract by forming a tight seal with the thyroid cartilage during swallowing. The act of swallowing is a complex series of muscular contractions. It results in early

MINI CLINI

Snoring and Sleep Apnea

The upper airway in adults and children primarily functions as an open pathway to convey gas to and from the respiratory zone for gas exchange. The position, size, and shape of the upper airway also contribute to "protect" the lower airways.

PROBLEM: Can abnormalities of upper airway anatomy lead to obstructive sleep apnea (OSA), sleep disturbances, chronic fatigue, and hypertension?

ANSWER: Snoring and breath holding during sleep are often associated with OSA. Snorers usually exhibit narrowing of the oropharyngeal, retropalatal, or hypopharyngeal airways. This narrowing is often observed in obese people; people with short, thick necks; people with large tongues and soft palates; and people with small, receding jaws (micrognathia). During sleep, the upper airway muscles relax and the tissues of the upper airway can partially or completely obstruct the airway. This obstruction can lead to apnea, the development of hypoxia, gasping, and sudden waking after 10 to 20 seconds. This cycle can be repeated multiple times to the point of disturbing the quality and quantity of sleep, inducing stress-related hypertension.

closure of the vocal cords, upward motion of the thyroid cartilage, and movement of the epiglottis down and back to form a tight seal as food is propelled to the back of the mouth and toward the esophagus.[69,70]

The inlet to the larynx lies below and behind the base of the tongue. Figure 9-40 shows the inlet as it appears when viewed with a laryngoscope. The base of the tongue is attached to the epiglottis by three folds. These folds form a space between the tongue and the epiglottis called the **vallecula,** which is a key landmark in oral intubation (see Figure 9-36).

Within the thyroid cartilage and just above the cricoid cartilage are the arytenoid cartilages. The vocal ligaments or true cords span the opening in the larynx by attachments to the thyroid and movable arytenoid cartilages that lie posteriorly. Just above and laterally are the vestibular folds, or false cords. The true vocal cords are composed of connective tissue and muscle and covered with a mucous membrane. They have poor lymphatic drainage and are susceptible to inflammation, which can result in airway obstruction. In the same region are the *corniculate* and *cuneiform cartilages* that function to support the soft tissue on either side of the vocal cords. The opening formed between the vocal cords is called the *glottis*. During swallowing, the vocal cords close to help protect the lower airways. Damage to the cricoarytenoid joint, which allows the *arytenoid cartilages* to rotate, can result in inability to open the vocal cords properly and cause difficulties in speaking and breathing. Laryngeal spasm and resultant partial or total temporary airway closure is brought about by laryngeal stimulation and reflex spasm of various laryngeal muscles that cause closure of the false and true vocal cords.

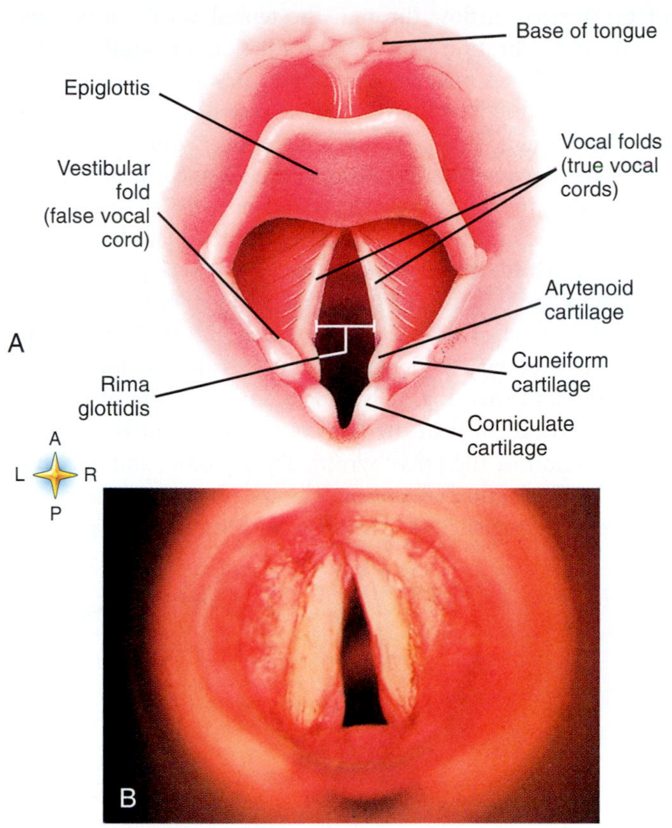

FIGURE 9-40 **A,** Superior view of true vocal cords, glottis (rima glottidis), epiglottis, and other structures within the larynx. **B,** Endoscopic photograph showing vocal cords in the open position. (From Thibodeau GA, Patton KT: Anatomy and physiology, ed 7, St Louis, 2011, Mosby.)

The muscles of the larynx are innervated by the *inferior laryngeal nerve,* also known as the *recurrent laryngeal nerve.* It is a motor nerve that branches from the vagus nerve. Impulses carried by this nerve are important in phonation and swallowing. Injuries to this nerve can cause partial or complete paralysis of the vocal cords and inability to swallow correctly. This nerve injury results in difficulty with speech and in severe cases can cause airway obstruction as a result of vocal cord closure.

Speech. The laryngeal component of speech is called *phonation*. It requires the adjustment of vocal cord tension and position relative to one another.[71] The action of the posterior cricoarytenoid muscles causes the arytenoid cartilages to rotate and opens the vocal cords. Closure of the vocal cords is accomplished by rotating the arytenoids in the opposite direction through the action of the lateral cricoarytenoid and oblique arytenoid muscles. On closure of the vocal cords, the expiratory muscles of breathing (e.g., abdominal wall muscle group) compress the thoracic cavity and can increase intrapulmonary pressures to 35 cm H_2O during forceful speech. To form sound, the cricothyroid muscles tilt the cricoid and arytenoid cartilages posteriorly with respect to the thyroid cartilage, elongating and tensing the vocal cords. Simultaneously, this action is opposed by the thyroarytenoid muscles, which pull the arytenoid cartilages anteriorly and relax vocal cord tension. Release of pressurized airflow through the tensed vocal cords causes vocal cord vibration and the production of audible sound waves, which resonate in the upper airway and sinuses. By careful adjustment of thyroarytenoid muscle tension and mandible and tongue position, fine control over sound production or speaking is achieved. Swelling of the vocal cords or the adjacent tissues increases their mass and disturbs their ability to vibrate; this can result in hoarseness and the inability to speak.

Breath Hold, Effort Closure, and Cough. Tight closure of the larynx and the buildup of intrapulmonary pressure through muscular effort are called *effort closure.* Effort closure of the larynx is necessary to generate loud sounds and for effective coughing and sneezing. It is generated by closure of the false and true vocal cords of the larynx. The vocal cords are closed by the action of the cricothyroid, aryepiglottic, and arytenoid muscles. This action effectively "clamps" the airway closed and enables the intraairway pressures to climb to greater than 100 cm H_2O when the various expiratory muscles compress the thorax. Sudden opening of the larynx results in the immediate release of high-flow gas that is necessary for coughing and sneezing. Patients who have artificial airways have difficulty producing an effective cough because the artificial airway prevents closure of the larynx.

Patent Upper Airway

The relative positions of the oral cavity, pharynx, and larynx are crucial to the patency of the upper airway in unconscious patients. In upright subjects, the head and neck form a 90-degree angle with the axis of the pharynx and larynx (Figure 9-41, *B*). With loss of consciousness, the head flexes forward and decreases this angle (see Figure 9-41, *A*). This positional change can partially or completely obstruct the upper airway. Extension of the head and lower jaw into the "sniff" position alleviates this obstruction (see Figure 9-41, *C*). Extension of the head moves

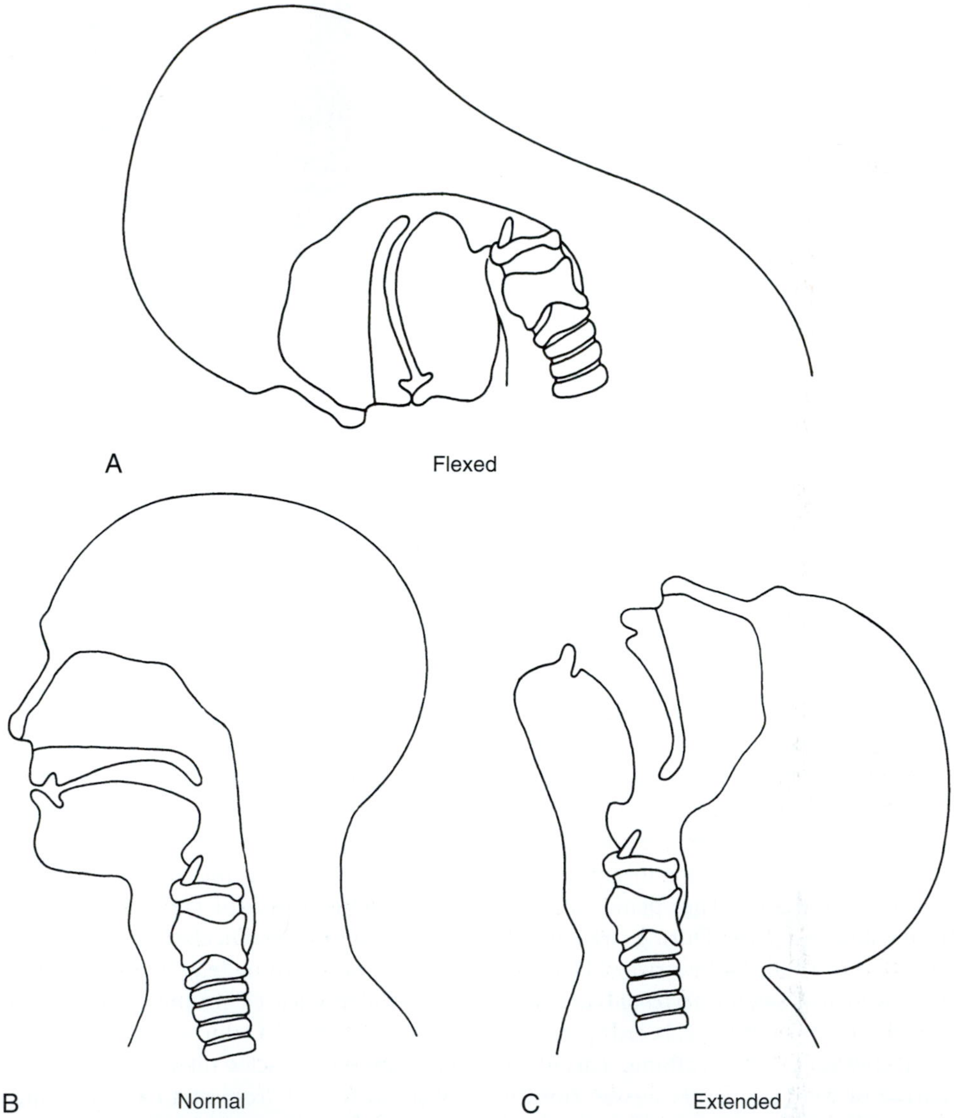

FIGURE 9-41 The position of the head affects patency of airway. **A,** With the head flexed, the airway may be kinked, making breathing or intubation difficult. **B,** Normal upright relationship of the head and neck to the chest. **C,** Extension of the head straightens the airway, making breathing, clearance of material, or intubation easier.

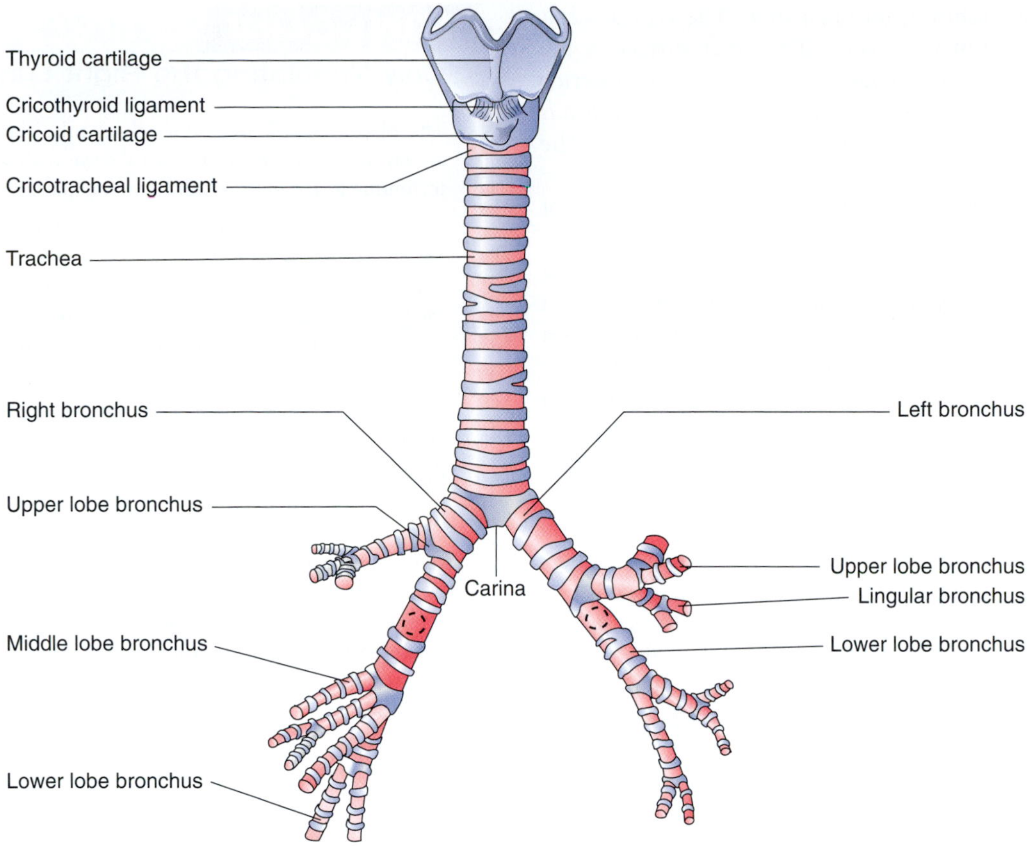

FIGURE 9-42 Major airways of the tracheobronchial tree. (From Hicks GH: Cardiopulmonary anatomy and physiology, Philadelphia, 2000, WB Saunders.)

the tongue away from the rear of the pharynx. This technique is used to maintain the airway in unconscious patients and facilitates placement of artificial airways.

Lower Respiratory Tract

The airways of the tracheobronchial tree extend from the larynx down to the airways participating in gas exchange. Each branching of an airway produces subsequent generations of smaller airways. The first 15 generations are known as *conducting airways* because they convey gas from the upper airway to the structures that participate in gas exchange with blood. The microscopic airways beyond the conducting airways that carry out gas exchange with blood are classified as the *respiratory airways.*

Trachea and Bronchi

The **trachea** extends from its connection to the cricoid cartilage down through the neck and into the thorax to the articulation point between the manubrium and body of the sternum (angle of Louis). At this point, it divides into two main stem bronchi (Figure 9-42). The adult trachea is approximately 12 cm long and has an inner diameter of about 2 cm. Figure 9-43 shows the different layers of tissue that form the trachea. The outermost layer is a thin connective tissue sheath. Below the sheath are numerous C-shaped cartilaginous rings that provide support

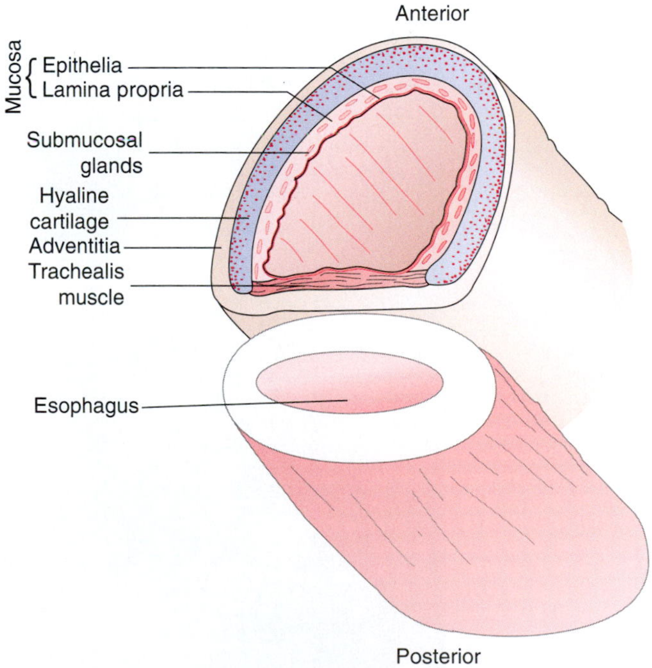

FIGURE 9-43 Cross-sectional view through the trachea and esophagus. (From Hicks GH: Cardiopulmonary anatomy and physiology, Philadelphia, 2000, WB Saunders.)

and maintain the trachea as an open tube. The typical adult trachea has 16 to 20 of these rings. The inner surface of the trachea is covered with a mucous membrane. In the posterior wall of the trachea is a thin band of tissue, called the *trachealis muscle* that supports the open ends of the tracheal rings. The esophagus lies just behind the trachea.

The cartilaginous rings support the trachea so it does not collapse during exhalation. Some compression occurs when the pressure around the trachea becomes positive. During a strong cough, the trachea is capable of some compression and even collapse. The negative pressure generated around the trachea during inhalation causes it to expand and lengthen slightly.

The trachea is positioned midline in the upper mediastinum and branches into right and left main stem bronchi (see Figure 9-42). At the base of the trachea, the last cartilaginous ring that forms the bifurcation for the two bronchi is called the *carina*. The carina is an important landmark used to identify the level where the two main stem bronchi branch off from the trachea; this is normally at the base of the aortic arch. The right bronchus branches off from the trachea at an angle of approximately 20 to 30 degrees, and the left bronchus branches with an angle of about 45 to 55 degrees (Figure 9-44). The lower angle branching (closer to mid-line) of the right bronchus results in a greater frequency of foreign body passage into the right lung because of the more direct pathway.

MINI CLINI

Only Ventilating the Right Lung

The placement of an endotracheal tube through the upper airway and into the trachea is a common airway management technique to facilitate artificial airway placement.

PROBLEM: After placement of an endotracheal tube in a patient with a 70-kg predicted body weight (PBW), it is noted that breath sounds are heard in the right chest only and that the patient's oxygenation is deteriorating. Is the airway placement the cause of the problem? How can this problem be avoided?

ANSWER: An endotracheal tube (ET) of proper diameter should be placed in the trachea so the tip is 3 to 5 cm above the carina. If the ET is advanced too far, it often enters the right main stem bronchus because of the straighter path this bronchus offers. A right main stem intubation results in right lung ventilation only. The left lung continues to receive pulmonary blood flow but does not oxygenate adequately. To avoid this problem the ET generally should not be advanced more than 24 cm past the lips in a 70-kg PBW patient. At this point, auscultation is done with a stethoscope to confirm breath sounds in both lungs. A chest radiograph can be taken to confirm the ET position.

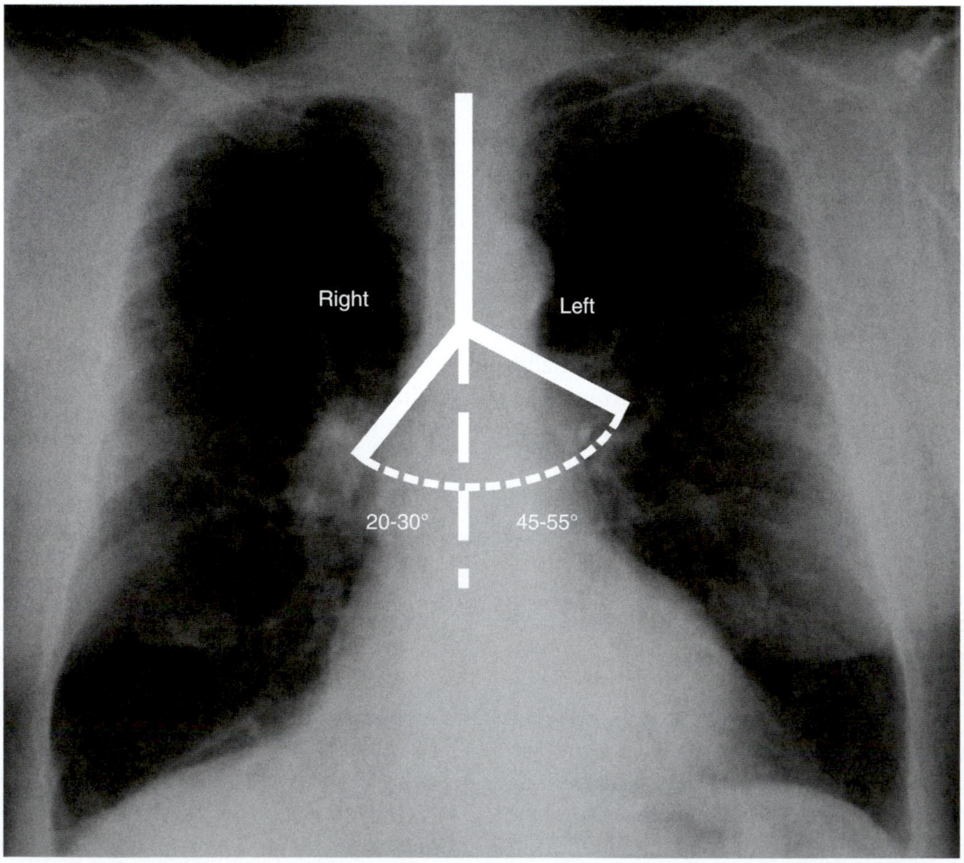

FIGURE 9-44 Course of trachea and right and left main stem bronchi, superimposed on a standard chest radiograph. The right main stem bronchus continues on a straighter course from midline than the left main stem bronchus.

TABLE 9-7
Bronchopulmonary Segments*

Segment	Number	Segment	Number
Right Upper Lobe		**Left Upper Lobe**	
Apical	1	Upper division	
Posterior	2	Apical-posterior	1 and 2†
Anterior	3	Anterior	3
Right Middle Lobe		**Lower Division (Lingula)**	
Lateral	4	Superior lingula	4
Medial	5	Inferior lingula	5
Right lower lobe		Left lower lobe	
Superior	6	Superior	6
Medial basal	7	Anterior basal	7 and 8
Anterior basal	8	Lateral basal	9
Lateral basal	9	Posterior basal	10
Posterior basal	10		

*The subdivisions of the lung and bronchial tree are fairly constant. Slight variations between right and left sides are noted by combined names and numbers.
†Some authors believe that the left lung should be numbered so that there are eight segments, where the apical-posterior is numbered 1 and the anteromedial is numbered 6.

Each bronchus carries gas to and from one lung. It enters the lung with the pulmonary vessels, lymph vessels, and nerves through the hilum. The bronchus branches repeatedly within each lung to supply gas to separate regions of each lung.

Lobar and Segmental Pulmonary Anatomy

The lungs have an apex and a base and are subdivided by fissures into lobes.[43] The lobes are subdivided further into bronchopulmonary **segments** (Table 9-7 and Figure 9-45). Each segment is supplied with gas from a single segmental bronchus. Controversy exists over the exact number of segments; some anatomists accept that each lung has 10 segments, whereas others maintain that the right has 10 and the left has 8. Knowledge of segmental anatomy is important in the physical examination of a patient to identify the location of a defect such as an infection site or a tumor mass in the lungs.

> **RULE OF THUMB**
>
> **The 60-to-40 Rule**
>
> The right lung is slightly larger than the left lung because of the location of the heart. The right lung has a sizable middle lobe and the left lung has a smaller lingular segment in the left upper lobe. For purposes of estimating the contribution of the right and left lungs to ventilation and gas exchange, the 60-to-40 rule is sometimes used. The right lung is assumed to provide 60% of the ventilation/gas–exchange capacity, and the left lung is assumed to provide the remaining 40%. If a patient requires removal of the entire left lung (pneumonectomy), a 40% decrease in lung volume would be expected.

The airways continue to divide as they penetrate deeper into the lungs. The segmental bronchi bifurcate into approximately 40 subsegmental bronchi, and these divide into hundreds of smaller bronchi. Thousands of bronchioles branch from the smaller bronchi. Bronchioles do not possess cartilage in their walls. Tens of thousands of terminal bronchioles arise from the bronchioles. *Terminal bronchioles* are the smallest conducting airways and function to supply gas to the respiratory zone of the lung.

With further divisions, the number of airways increases tremendously. The cross-sectional area of the conducting system increases exponentially. At the level of the terminal bronchioles, the cross-sectional area is approximately 20 times greater than that at the trachea. Gas flow in these airways conforms to the laws of fluid physics. Increased cross-sectional area reduces the velocity of gas flow during inspiration. When inspired gas reaches the level of the terminal bronchiole, its average velocity has fallen to about the same rate as the speed of diffusing gas molecules.[72] Low-velocity gas movement at the level of the terminal bronchiole and beyond is physiologically important for two reasons. First, laminar flow develops minimizing resistance in the small airways and decreases the work associated with inspiration. Second, low gas velocity facilitates rapid mixing of alveolar gases. This mixing provides a stable partial pressure of O_2 and CO_2 in the alveolar environment that supports stable diffusion and gas exchange.[73]

Histology of the Airway Wall

All of the conducting airways from the trachea to the bronchioles have walls that are constructed of three layers (Figures 9-46 and 9-47): an inner layer that forms a mucous membrane called the *mucosa,* which is primarily composed of epithelia; a submucosa composed of connective tissue, bronchial glands, and smooth fibers that wrap around the airway; and an outer covering of connective tissue called the *adventitia.*[74] The cartilaginous rings and plates found in larger airways are located in the adventitia.

The mucosa is composed of many different types of specialized epithelial cells that sit on top of a basement membrane. The most common type of epithelia are the numerous pseudostratified, ciliated, columnar epithelia.[75] The pseudostratified epithelial cells are held together toward their surface or apical end through three types of junctions—apical tight junctions, zonal adherens junctions, and desmosome-type junctions—and they are anchored in place to the basement membrane.[76] The junctions, especially the tight junctions, play an important role in the maintenance of fluid and electrolyte (e.g., chloride ions) transport across the mucous membrane. These junctions prevent the movement of fluids and electrolytes between the apical surface and basal surfaces of the airway. Disturbances in this transport (e.g., Cl^- transport malfunction in cystic fibrosis transport receptor membrane channels) lead to mucus and mucus transport abnormalities.

Near the base of the pseudostratified cells are large numbers of basal cells. The basal cells contribute to the appearance of a "pseudostratified" cellular layer. Basal cells mature into pseudostratified cells and are thought to play an important role in repair of the mucous membrane after diseases and injury.

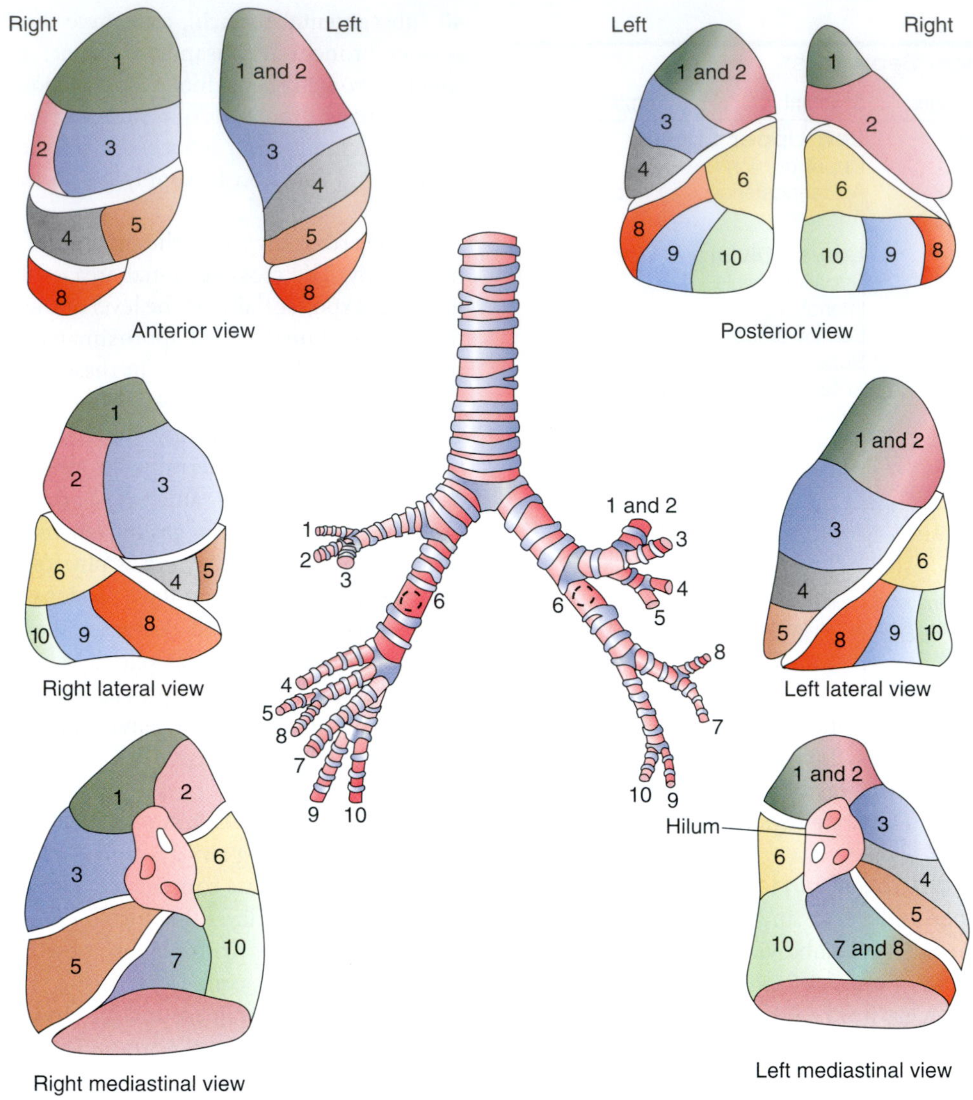

FIGURE 9-45 Bronchopulmonary segmental divisions of the lungs (see Table 9-7). (From Hicks GH: Cardiopulmonary anatomy and physiology, Philadelphia, 2000, WB Saunders.)

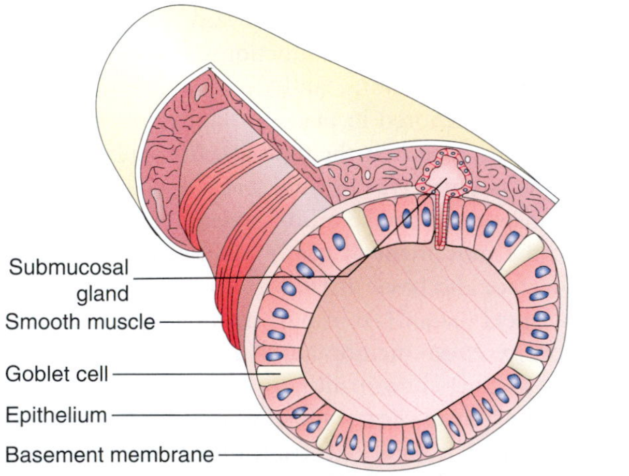

FIGURE 9-46 Cross-sectional view through a bronchiole. (From Hicks GH: Cardiopulmonary anatomy and physiology, Philadelphia, 2000, WB Saunders.)

Dispersed between the pseudostratified epithelia are mucus-producing goblet cells and serous cells (in newborns) and the openings of submucosal bronchial glands. The bronchial glands are exocrine glands formed by secretory epithelial cells that sit on the basement membrane, extending down into the lamina propria and the submucosa. In this region are also neuroendocrine cells (also known as *Kulchitsky cells*), which often are organized into small clusters called *neuroepithelial bodies*.[77] Neuroendocrine cells are connected to the vagus nerve and are thought to function during lung development, are hypoxia and stress-strain sensors, and secrete various bioactive chemicals (e.g., serotonin, calcitonin, and gastrin-releasing peptide). Lymphocytes are found intermixed with these cells, and it is thought they may be migratory.

Below the epithelial and basement membrane of the mucosa is the *lamina propria*.[76] It is composed of loose fibroelastic connective tissue, lymphoid tissue, and a dense layer of elastic

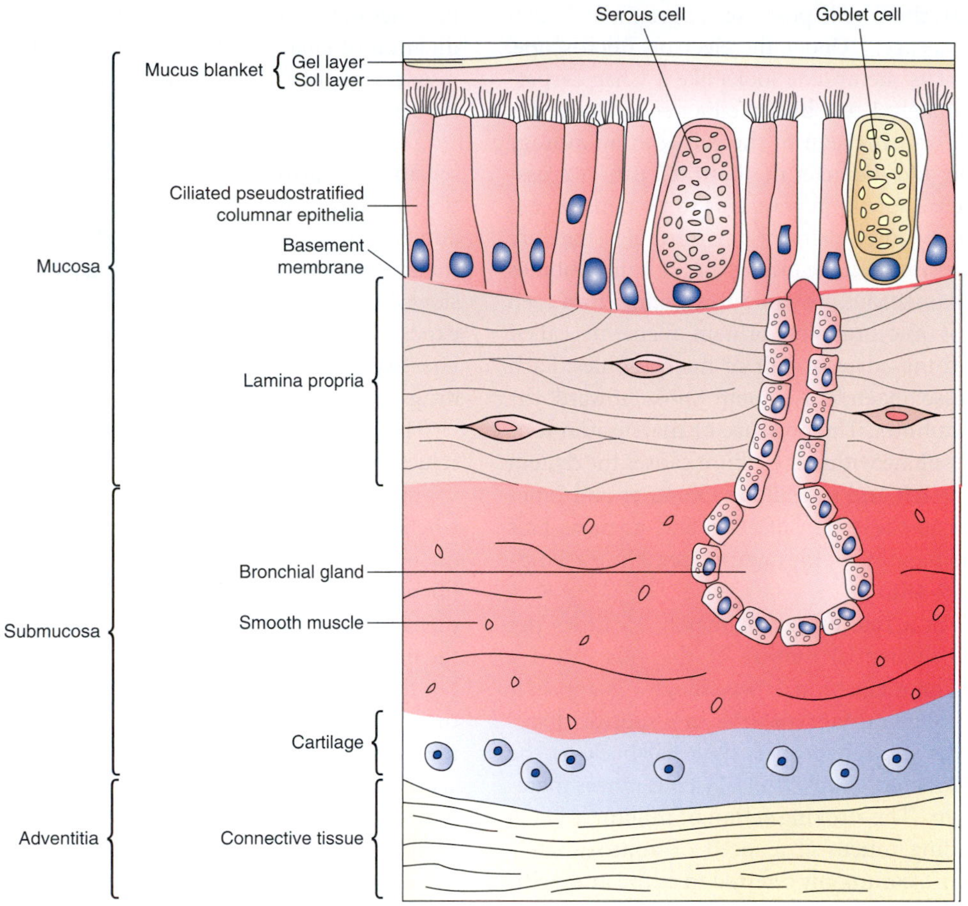

FIGURE 9-47 Microscopic view of mucous membrane. (From Hicks GH: Cardiopulmonary anatomy and physiology, Philadelphia, 2000, WB Saunders.)

fibers. Below the lamina propria lies the submucosa. The submucosa of large airways contains bronchial glands, a capillary network, smooth muscle, some elastic tissue, and cartilage in larger airways. Bronchial glands vary in size up to 1 mm in length and connect to the bronchial surface via long, narrow ducts. The number of these glands increases significantly in diseases such as chronic bronchitis. Mast cells are also found in the submucosa and release numerous and potent vasoactive and bronchoactive substances such as histamine.[78] Histamine causes vasodilation and bronchoconstriction, acting directly on smooth muscle. The triggering of mast cell release of its various substances and the resultant inflammation and bronchospasm of the airway are characteristic of the pathologic changes of asthma.

The various secretory cells (primarily goblet cells) of the mucosa and bronchial glands of the submucosa contribute to the production of mucus.[79] Normally, the respiratory tract produces approximately 100 ml of mucus per day. Most of the mucus formed in the larger airways is produced by the bronchial glands. Goblet cells contribute more in the smaller airways. The amount and composition of mucus produced can increase and change with airway irritation and diseases such as chronic bronchitis and asthma.[80] Mucus is spread over the surface of the mucus membrane to a depth of approximately 7 μm and is propelled by the ciliated epithelia toward the pharynx. The outer layer of mucus is more gelatinous and is called the *gel layer*. The inner layer is much more fluid-like and is referred to as the *sol layer*. The mucus normally produced is a nearly clear fluid with greater viscosity than water. It is a mixture of 97% water and 3% solute.[79] The solute portion is produced primarily by goblet cells and bronchial glands; it is called *mucin* and is composed of protein and minerals. The glycoprotein, lipid, and water content of mucus provide its viscoelastic gel properties. *Viscoelastic* refers to the ability of mucus to deform and spread when force is applied.

Mucus functions to protect the underlying tissue. It helps prevent excessive amounts of water moving into and out of the epithelia.[79] It shields the epithelia from direct contact with potentially toxic materials and microorganisms. It acts like sticky flypaper to trap particles that make contact with it. This makes mucus an important part of the pulmonary defenses. The production of mucus is stimulated by local mechanical and chemical irritation, release of proinflammatory mediators (e.g., cytokines), and parasympathetic (vagal) stimulation.

The ciliated pseudostratified epithelia play a crucial role in the defense of the respiratory tract by propelling mucus toward the pharynx. Ciliated cells are found in the nasal cavity and all the airways from the larynx to the terminal bronchioles.

Each of the pseudostratified cells possesses approximately 200 **cilia** on its luminal surface.[76] Under the electron microscope, the surface of the mucus membrane looks like a "shag carpet" of cilia with approximately 1 to 2 billion cilia per square centimeter. Each cilium is an extension of the cell with an average length of about 6 μm and diameter of about 0.2 μm. A cross-sectional view through the cilium reveals it to be constructed of one inner and nine outer pairs of microtubules that are encased in the cell membrane. The outer pairs of microtubules are interlinked by a filamentous protein called *nexin.* From each of the outer pairs of microtubules, protein filaments called *dynein* extend toward the adjacent pair of microtubules. Each of the outer pairs also extends a protein spoke toward the central pair of microtubules. The presence of magnesium ions and adenosine triphosphate within the cilium causes the dynein arms and spokes to attach and slide along the outer and inner microtubules, similar to the action of actin and myosin. This action results in rapid bending of the cilium resembling a whipping motion (Figure 9-48).

The cilia "stroke" at a rate of approximately 15 times per second, producing a sequential motion of the cilia called a *metachronal wave.*[81] The metachronal "wavelength" is approximately 20 μm and propels surface material in a specific direction. In the nose, this motion propels material back to the pharynx. From the bronchioles up to the larynx, it moves material toward the pharynx. The stroking action of millions of cilia propels the surrounding mucus at a speed of approximately 2 cm/min. This action is commonly referred to as the **mucociliary escalator.** In healthy lungs, this mechanism allows inhaled

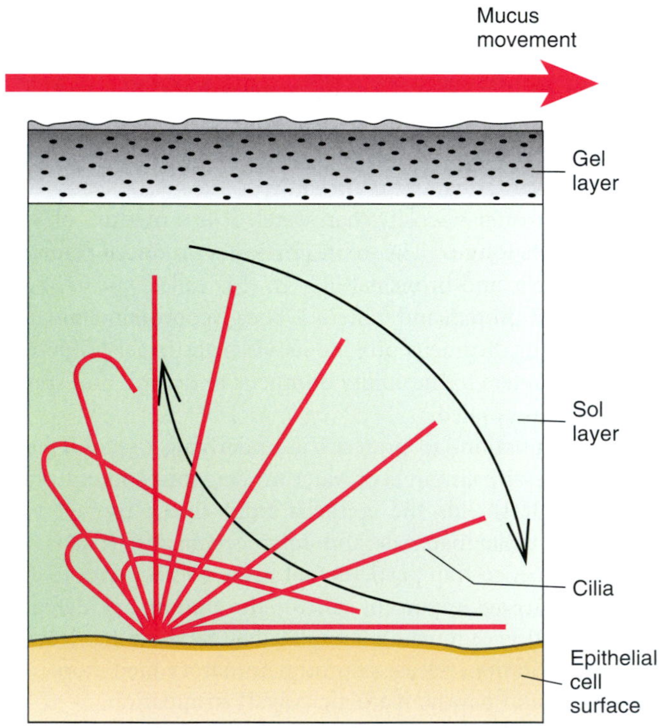

FIGURE 9-48 Whipping action of the cilium within the sol layer of mucus produces a metachronal wave motion. (From Hicks GH: Cardiopulmonary anatomy and physiology, Philadelphia, 2000, WB Saunders.)

particles to be removed within 24 hours. The control and coordination of ciliary motion are not totally understood and represent some of the many fascinating properties of pulmonary tissues.

The production of mucus and the rate of ciliary beating are sensitive to various conditions and chemicals. Mucus production increases when the respiratory tract is irritated by particles and by various chemicals and during increased parasympathetic nervous stimulation.[80] Ciliary beating can be effectively slowed or stopped if the viscosity of the sol layer is increased by exposure to dry gas. Ciliary motion is also slowed or stopped after exposure to smoke, high concentrations of inhaled O_2, and drugs such as atropine.

The smooth muscle of the airways varies in location and structure. In the large airways (e.g., the trachea), smooth muscle is bundled in sheets. In smaller airways, smooth muscle forms a helical pattern that wraps the airway in bundles in decreasing quantities as the airways branch and become smaller. Muscle fibers crisscross and spiral around the airway walls. This placement reduces the diameter of the airway and shortens it when the muscle contracts. This pattern of smooth muscle continues but thins out on reaching the smallest bronchioles. The tone of the smooth muscle is increased and results in bronchospasm by the activity of the parasympathetic nervous system (release of acetylcholine) and proinflammatory mediator release from mast cells, inflammatory cells, and neuroendocrine cells.

The adventitia is a sheath of connective tissue that surrounds the airways. It is interspersed with bronchial arteries, veins, nerves, lymph vessels, and adipose tissue. Between the submucosa and adventitia of the large airways are incomplete rings or plates of hyaline cartilage, providing structural support for the larger airways. The small airways depend on transmural pressure gradients and the "traction" of surrounding elastic tissues to remain open. During a forced expiration, pressures across the walls of the small airways exceed the supporting forces of the elastic tissues. As a result, the small airways can collapse. The cartilage in the larger airways prevents their collapse during such maneuvers.

The cells of the respiratory mucosa change as they progress into the smaller airways (Figure 9-49). As the thickness of the airway walls decreases, bronchial glands become fewer in number. At the bronchiolar level, the number of ciliated cells decreases. Simple columnar and cuboidal epithelial cells begin to predominate and are interspersed with goblet cells. In this region, large numbers of *Clara cells,* nonciliated cuboidal cells with apical granules, are found. It is thought that these cells play a role in degrading various oxidants, contribute proteins for surfactant production, synthesize various lipids, and play a role in lung repair by being able to differentiate into other important epithelial cells in the mucosa after injury.[82]

Respiratory Zone Airways

The terminal bronchioles begin about 12 to 15 generations beyond the trachea (Figure 9-50).[83] There are about 16,000 terminal bronchioles with airway opening diameters of approximately 700 μm. This yields a combined cross-sectional area

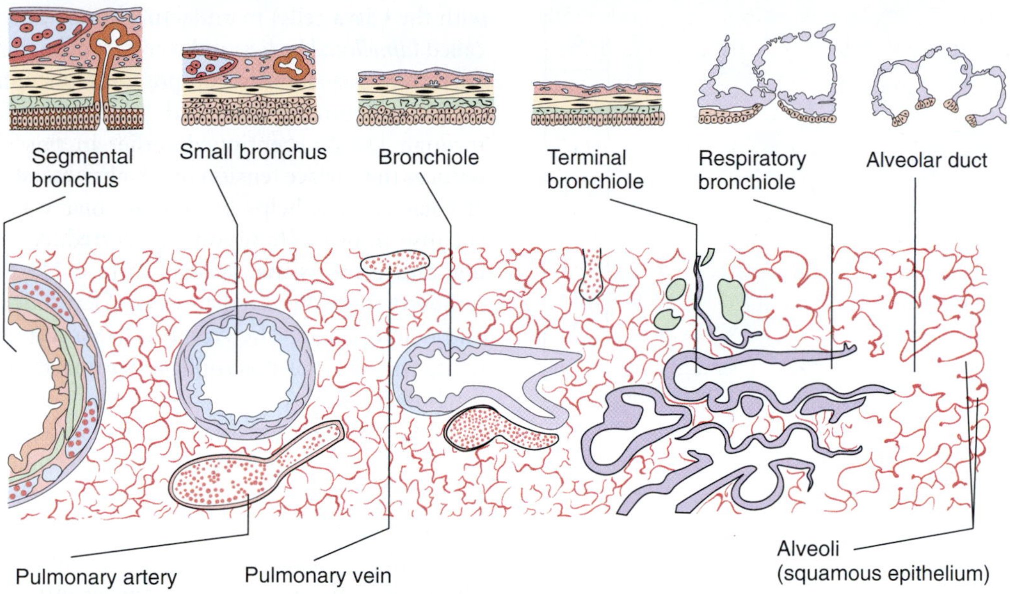

FIGURE 9-49 Histologic diagram of airways from the segmental bronchus to the alveolus. (Modified from Freeman WH, Bracegridle B: An atlas of histology, London, 1966, Heinemann Educational.)

opening that is almost 100 times that of the main stem bronchi. All of the airways down to and including the terminal bronchioles carry or conduct gas flow to and from the airways participating in gas exchange with blood. The airways from the nares to and including the terminal bronchioles constitute the *conducting zone airways,* which do not participate in gas exchange. These airways constitute the anatomic dead space of the respiratory system, which is rebreathed with each breath. In an adult human, the volume filling the airways of the anatomic dead space is approximately 2.2 ml/kg (1 ml/lb) of PBW, or about 150 ml in a typical adult.

Branching of the terminal bronchioles gives rise to unique airways called *respiratory bronchioles.* Respiratory bronchioles are approximately 0.4 mm in diameter and have walls formed largely from flattened squamous epithelia and a thin outer layer of connective tissue. They have some ciliated cells at the connection with the terminal bronchiole, generally lack mucus-producing cells, and have rings of smooth muscles where they branch to form alveolar ducts. Respiratory bronchioles have a dual function. Similar to conducting airways, they not only conduct gas flow but also have small outpouchings known as *alveoli* in their walls. The alveoli and their pulmonary capillary bed enable the respiratory bronchioles to carry out gas exchange. The respiratory bronchioles constitute a transitional zone type of airway.

A single terminal bronchiole supplies a cluster of respiratory bronchioles. Collectively, this unit is referred to as the *acinus,* or **primary lobule.** Each acinus comprises numerous respiratory bronchioles, alveolar ducts, and approximately 10,000 alveoli (Figure 9-51). The adult lung is thought to contain more than 30,000 acini. Each acinus is supplied with pulmonary blood flow from a pulmonary arteriole, and blood is drained away from several acini through a pulmonary venule. In addition, each acinus is equipped with a lymphatic drainage vessel and nervous fibers. These features make the primary lobule the functional unit of the lungs. Gas molecule movement in this region is largely via diffusion rather than convective flow, which occurs in larger airways.

Millions of alveolar ducts branch off the respiratory bronchioles (Figure 9-52). Alveolar ducts are tiny airways only 0.3 mm in diameter, and their walls are composed entirely of alveoli. Each alveolar duct ends in a cluster of alveoli, which is frequently referred to as an *alveolar sac.* Each alveolar sac opens into about 16 or 17 **alveoli,** and about one-half the total number of alveoli are found in this region.

Alveoli

More recent estimates suggest the number of alveoli in adult lungs range from 270 to 790 million, with an average of about 480 million.[22] The number of alveoli increases with an individual's height. Figure 9-53 shows alveoli in a normal rat lung at different states of inflation and how their shapes change. When inflated at and beyond the functional residual volume (see Figure 9-53, *A* to *C*), alveoli have a polyhedral shape resulting from numerous flat walls rather than a curved spherical structure. Alveoli found in the apical regions of the vertical lung have greater diameters than alveoli in the basal regions as a result of the gravitational effects. Alveoli in the basal regions are partially collapsed as a result of the weight of the organ.

The alveolar walls, or septa, are formed by various cell types that are arranged to provide a thin surface for gas exchange and strength.[84] The alveolar septa are covered with extremely flat squamous epithelia called *type I pneumocytes* (Figure 9-54). Although they represent only approximately 8% of all the cells found in the alveolar region, type I cells cover about 93% of the alveolar surface.[85] These cells form a "patchwork"-like surface

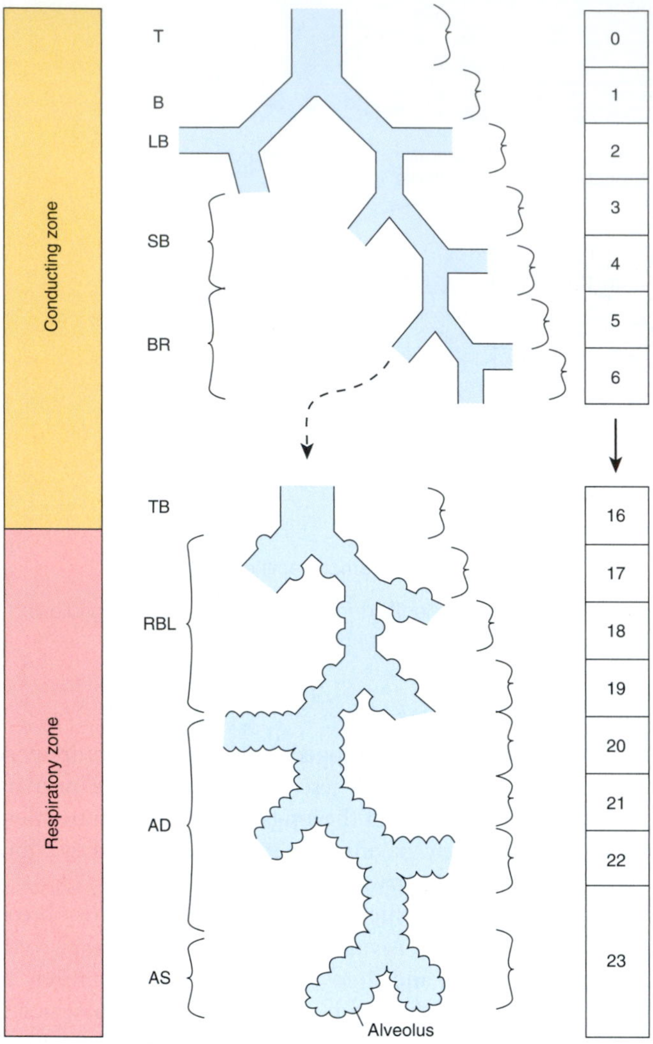

FIGURE 9-50 Airways of the conducting (generation *0* through *16*) and respiratory (generation *17* through *23*) zones: *T,* trachea; *B,* right and left bronchi; *LB,* lobar bronchi; *SB,* segmental and subsegmental bronchi; *BR,* bronchioles; *TB,* terminal bronchioles; *RBL,* respiratory bronchioles; *AD,* alveolar ducts; and *AS,* alveolar sacs. (From Hicks GH: Cardiopulmonary anatomy and physiology, Philadelphia, 2000, WB Saunders.)

that covers the alveolar capillaries and forms the gas-exchange surface of the alveolus. At the edges where they meet one another, they form tight junctions. This helps to limit the movement of material into the alveolar airspace from the interstitial space just below. They are held in place and supported from below by a network of collagen and elastin fibers. They are susceptible to injury and apoptosis (programmed cell death) from inhaled particles (e.g., cigarette smoke), bacterial infection, and high concentrations of inhaled O_2.

Interspersed on the alveolar surface and concentrated in the corners of the alveolar septa are type II pneumocytes, which are cuboidal epithelia with apical microvilli (Figure 9-55). These cells are twice as numerous as the type I cells, but they occupy only 7% of the alveolar surface.[85] Type II cells do not function as gas-exchange membranes as the type I cells do. They (along with the Clara cells) manufacture surfactant, store it in vesicles called *lamellated bodies,* and secrete it onto the alveolar surface.[86] Surfactant is primarily composed of phospholipids (dipalmitoylphosphatidylcholine) and proteins (surfactant proteins A through D). As mentioned earlier in this chapter, surfactant reduces the surface tension of the alveolus, sheds water from the alveolar surface, helps prevent alveolar surface tension-driven collapse, improves lung compliance, reduces the work of breathing, and protects the alveolar surface. Normally, surfactant is removed from the alveolar space continuously by type II cells and macrophages. The type II cells recycle approximately 50% of it, whereas the macrophages primarily remove it through catabolism.[87]

Although the lungs do not have stem cells in the classic sense, the type II cells do have a "stem cell"–like action. They can proliferate and differentiate into type I cells to repopulate and repair the alveolar surface after injury.[88] They are also involved in alveolar defense through surfactant production and the release of some cytokines that trigger inflammation.

Macrophages are another common cell found in the alveolar region.[85] They can move from the pulmonary capillary circulation by squeezing through openings in the alveolar septa and then move out onto the alveolar surface. They are defensive cells that patrol the alveolar region and phagocytize foreign particles and cells (e.g., bacteria). They can present portions of the foreign particles and bacteria to lymphocytes as part of the immune response and contain various digestive enzymes (e.g., trypsin) that break down the material they engulf.

Within the interalveolar septum is an interstitial space that contains matrix material and the pulmonary capillaries. Also found in the interstitial space are bands of elastin fibers and a collagen fiber matrix.[46] These fibers support the alveolar cells and the shape of the alveolus. Small openings are located in the alveolar septa. Some of the openings allow gas to move from one alveolus to another. These are called the **pores of Kohn.** Other openings connect alveoli with secondary respiratory bronchioles. These passageways are called the *canals of Lambert.* All of these alveolar openings and passageways facilitate the collateral movement of gas and help maintain alveolar volume.[89]

Blood-Gas Barrier

Gas exchange between alveolar gas and pulmonary capillary blood occurs across the **alveolar-capillary membrane.** In a typical adult, this blood-gas barrier stretches over a surface area of approximately 140 m^2 and is less than 1 μm thick.[90] This makes the membrane more than 50 times larger than the area covered by skin and more than 2000 times thinner.

The blood-gas barrier is composed of many different layers through which O_2 and CO_2 diffuse (Figure 9-56). The outermost layer is a very thin film of fluid composed primarily of surfactant that forms into a tubular myelin matrix. Below the surfactant fluid layer is the thinly stretched type I cell. The delicate structure of type I cells makes them highly susceptible to injury from toxins carried to them by either airborne or bloodborne routes. The interstitial space and its contents lie below. Within this space are basement membranes, matrix material

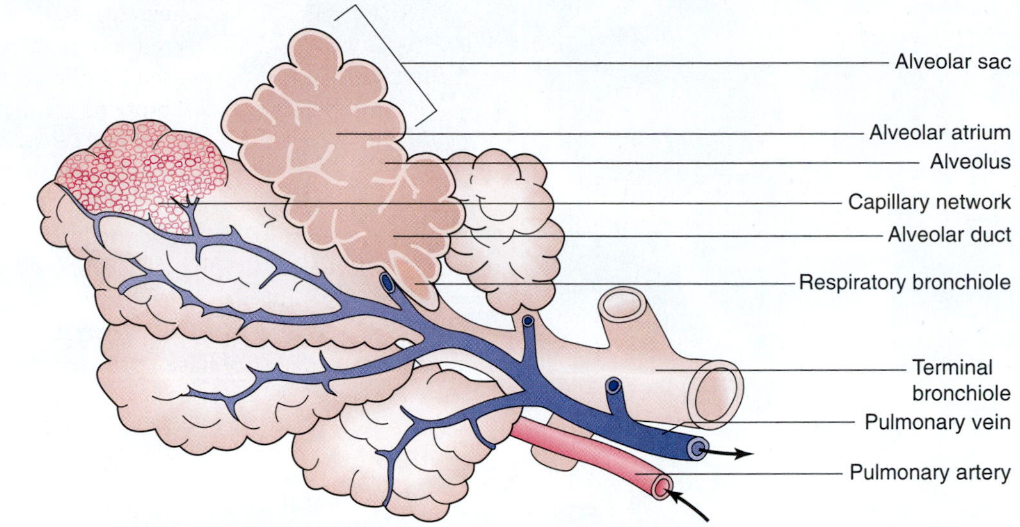

FIGURE 9-51 The acinus (primary lobule) of the lung is composed of a single terminal bronchiole, numerous respiratory bronchioles, alveolar ducts, sacs of alveoli, and about 10,000 alveoli. Pulmonary blood flow is delivered to the acinus by a pulmonary arteriole and drained from it by a pulmonary venule. (From Hicks GH: Cardiopulmonary anatomy and physiology, Philadelphia, 2000, WB Saunders.)

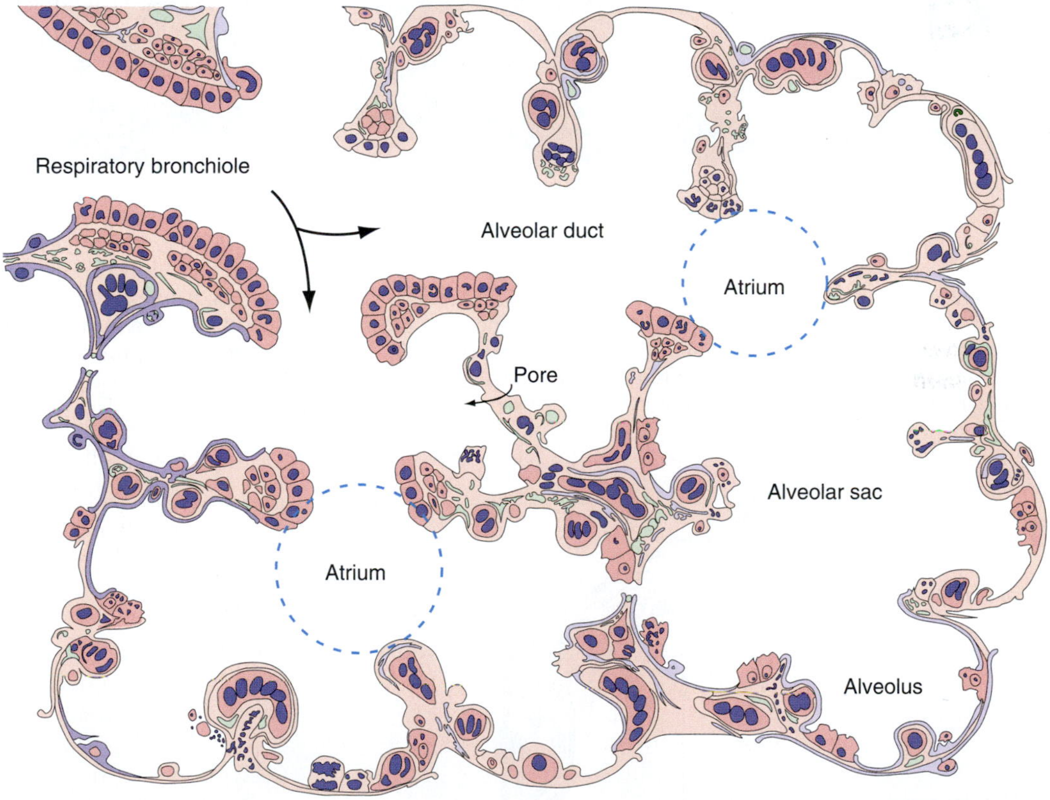

FIGURE 9-52 Microscopic view of respiratory zone airways. (Modified from Sorokin SP: The respiratory system. In Greep RO, Weiss L, editors: Histology, New York, 1973, McGraw-Hill.)

connective tissue fibers, and the alveolar capillary.[46] The capillary wall is formed from thin, flat squamous epithelia called *endothelial cells* that form a thin tube by connecting together at their edges with tight junctions. Within the capillary lie the plasma and, finally, the erythrocytes. Both O_2 and CO_2 cross through the membrane via partial pressure-driven diffusion.

The blood-gas barrier is not equal in thickness and chemical content from side to side (see Figure 9-56). On one side of the alveolar wall the type I cells and capillary endothelial cells lie close together, with a thin interstitial space. This part of the blood-gas barrier is, on average, 0.2 to 0.3 μm thick, and it is where the alveolar capillary bulges into the alveolar space.[90] On

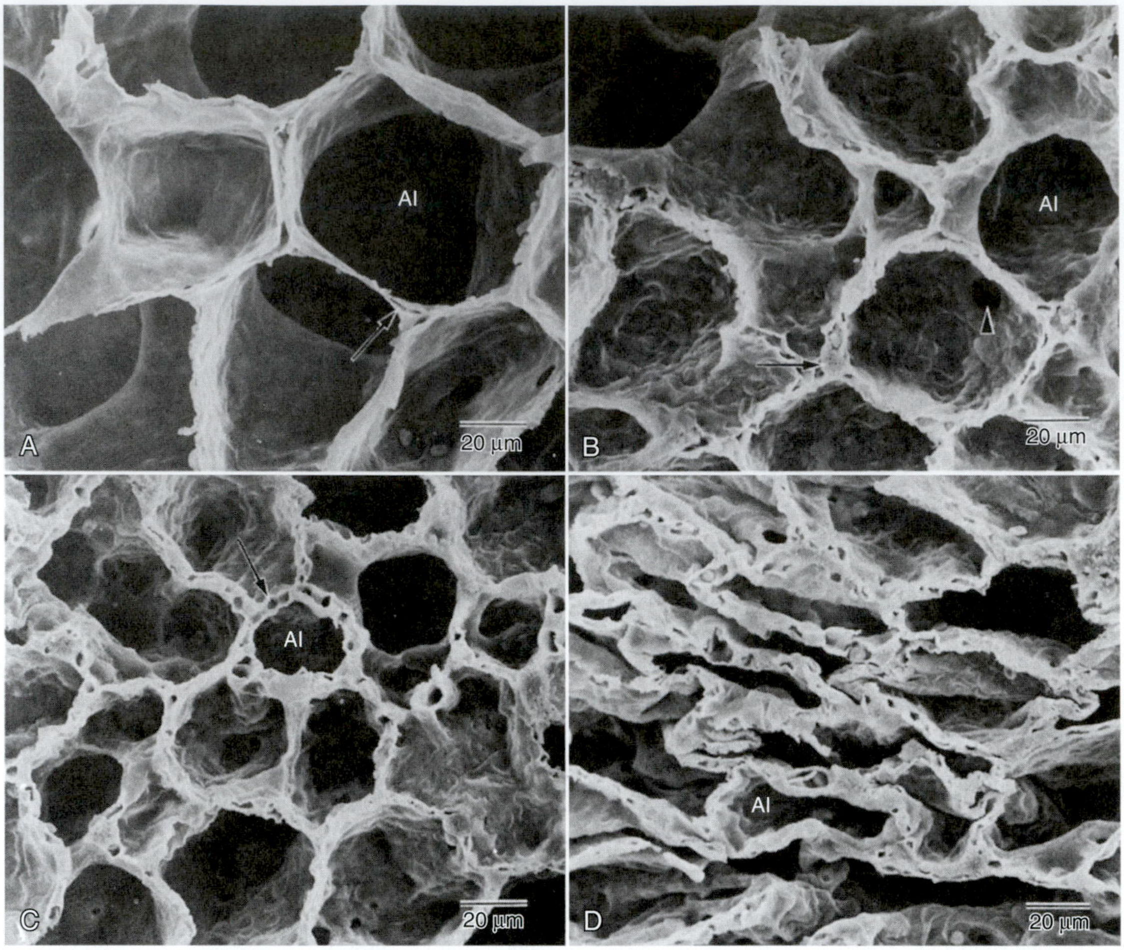

FIGURE 9-53 Scanning electron photomicrographs at the same magnification of perfusion-fixed normal rat lung at different degrees of inflation pressure. **A,** 30 cm H_2O (total lung capacity [TLC]). **B,** 8 cm H_2O (approximately 50% TLC). **C,** 4 cm H_2O (near resting inflation or functional residual capacity [FRC]). **D,** 0 cm H_2O (minimum volume). Pulmonary artery pressure was held constant at 25 cm H_2O, and left atrial pressure was held at 6 cm H_2O. Intrinsic shape of alveoli *(Al)* is maintained from FRC to TLC **(A-C).** Alveolar walls are flat with sharp corners where the adjacent walls meet. Note the flat shape of the alveolar capillaries *(arrow)* at TLC (**A,** lung zone 1 conditions, air pressure > blood pressure) compared with their round shape *(arrow)* at FRC (**C,** lung zone 3 conditions, blood pressure > air pressure). The alveolar walls are folded, and the alveolar shape is distorted at the minimum lung volume **(D).** The *arrow* in **B** identifies a type II pneumocyte at an alveolar corner. The *arrowhead* in **B** identifies a pore of Kohn through an alveolar wall. (From Mason RJ, Broaddus VC, Martin T, et al, editors: Murray and Nadel's textbook of respiratory medicine, ed 4, Philadelphia, 2011, WB Saunders.)

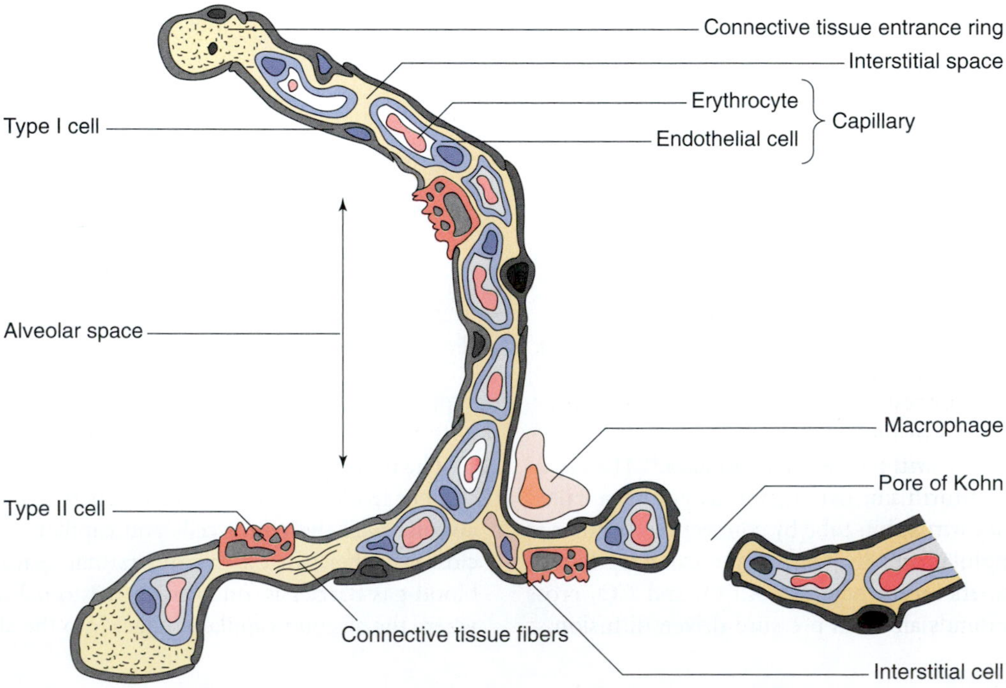

FIGURE 9-54 Highly magnified cross-sectional sketch of the cells and organization of the alveolar septa. (From Hicks GH: Cardiopulmonary anatomy and physiology, Philadelphia, 2000, WB Saunders.)

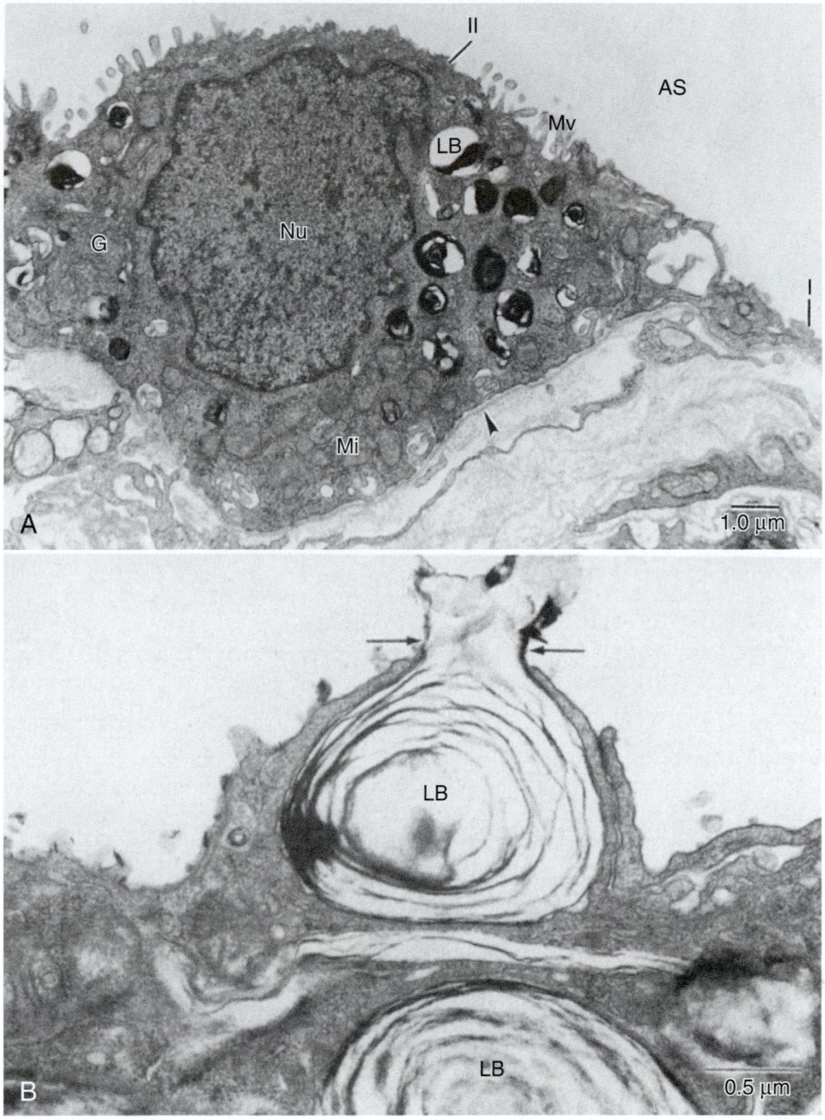

FIGURE 9-55 Transmission electron photomicrograph of human lungs at high magnification. **A,** Type II pneumocytes are cuboidal epithelial cells that contain characteristic lamellar bodies *(LB)* in their cytoplasm and have stubby microvilli *(Mv)* that extend from their apical surface into the alveolar airspace *(AS)*. Other prominent organelles within the type II cells are mitochondria *(Mi)*, a single nucleus *(Nu)*, and a Golgi apparatus *(G)*, which forms the lamellar bodies. Adjacent to the type II cell is a portion of a type I pneumocyte (I). The abluminal side of the epithelial cells of the alveolus rests on a continuous basal lamina *(arrowhead)*. **B,** Apical region of a type II cell contains two lamellar bodies *(LB)*, one of which has been fixed in the process of secreting its contents *(arrows)*. The lamellar bodies are believed to be the source of surfactant. Type II cells are more often found in the corners of the alveolar walls. (From Mason RJ, Broaddus VC, Martin, T, et al, editors: Murray and Nadel's textbook of respiratory medicine, ed 4, Philadelphia, 2011, WB Saunders.)

the other side, where there is a thicker interstitial space with greater fiber, matrix, and nuclear material content, the barrier can be more than 3 to 10 times thicker. This difference between the two sides functionally results in "faster-weaker" and "slower-stronger" diffusion sides of the blood-gas barrier.

The interstitial space within the alveolar septum contains a network of fibers that form a kind of connective tissue skeleton holding the alveolar structures in place and together.[91] The fibers within the alveolar septum are part of the continuum of connective tissue fibers found in the pleural surface and in the airway walls that extends all the way to the root of the lung in the hilar region. Elastin and collagen fiber bands are formed by fibroblasts into a network within the interstitial space into which the capillaries are woven. Also around the fibers and capillaries is a nonliving matrix of fluid and solutes. The weaving path taken by the capillaries passes them from the thick to the thin sides of the blood-gas barrier as they extend through the septum. In the thin side, the basement membranes of the endothelial and type I cells fuse into a structure called the *lamina densa,* which is formed from collagen.[92] In the thick side, thick bands of collagen and elastin are found. The collagen and endothelial cells are attached to either side of the *lamina densa* by a

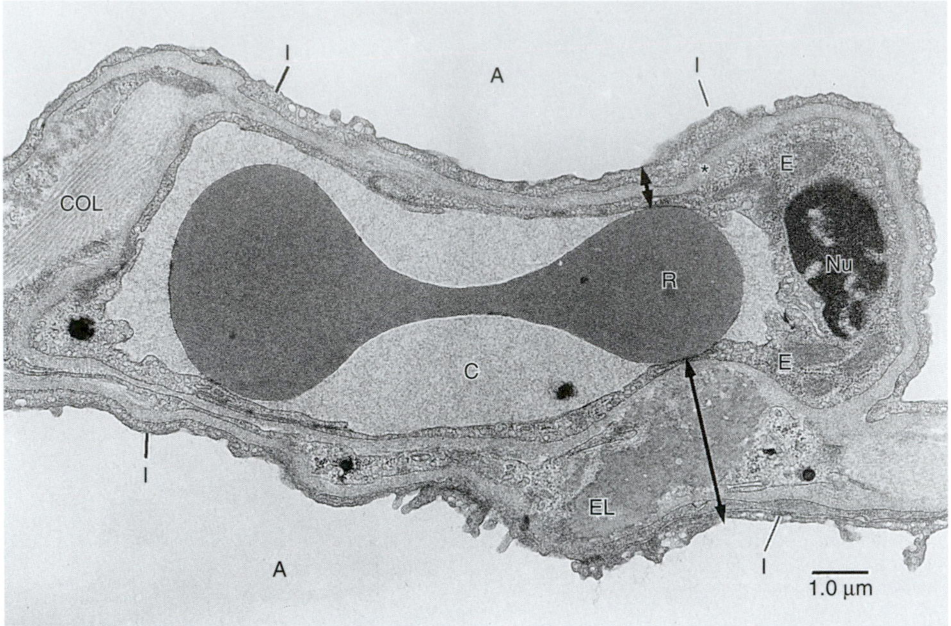

FIGURE 9-56 High-magnification transmission electron photomicrograph of a human lung showing a cross section of an alveolar wall through which O_2 and CO_2 diffuse. Air *(A)* in the alveolar space is seen on either side of the wall. The thin side of the alveolar-capillary membrane *(short double arrow)* consists of type I pneumocytes *(I),* interstitium *(*)* formed by the fused basement membranes of the type I cell and the endothelial cells *(E),* and its nucleus *(Nu)* that forms the pulmonary capillary wall. Within the capillary *(C)* is the erythrocyte *(R).* The thick side of the membrane *(long double arrows)* has an accumulation of elastin *(EL),* collagen *(COL),* and matrix material that jointly separates the type I cell from the capillary endothelial cell. Greater diffusion occurs across the thin side. (From Mason RJ, Broaddus VC, Martin T, et al, editors: Murray and Nadel's textbook of respiratory medicine, ed 4, Philadelphia, 2011, WB Saunders.)

series of protein fibers collectively known as *laminins.* Laminins effectively bind together the blood-gas barrier into a three-part laminate that results in a relatively strong and thin structure that can normally, with the additional support offered by the capillary network, withstand the everyday stress of alveolar and capillary stretch.[93]

However, conditions of pulmonary hypertension (e.g., capillary pressure >30 mm Hg during congestive heart failure and high-altitude pulmonary edema) and excessive tidal volume and airway pressure during positive pressure ventilation (e.g., tidal volume >6 to 8 ml/kg and airway pressures >30 cm H_2O) can result in stress failure of the blood-gas membrane. Stress failure results in endothelial or type I cell stretching and shearing injuries. Extreme examples are known to occur in racehorses that experience exercise-induced pulmonary hemorrhaging as a result of developing excessively high pulmonary vascular pressures (e.g., pulmonary capillary pressures 100 mm Hg).

RULE OF THUMB

The 30:30 Rule

Pulmonary hypertension (e.g., capillary pressure >30 mm Hg) and excessive tidal volume and airway pressure during positive pressure ventilation (e.g., tidal volume >6 to 8 ml/kg and airway pressures >30 cm H_2O) can result in stress failure of the blood-gas membrane.

SUMMARY CHECKLIST

- Many different genes regulate the development of the respiratory system from conception through adult life. Many pulmonary diseases are caused by genetic abnormalities.
- The development of the respiratory system follows a well-defined schedule; interruptions or insults in the course of development can result in respiratory disease at birth and in adulthood.
- Fetal circulation and respiration differ markedly from circulation and respiration in the postnatal period.
- The transition from intrauterine to extrauterine life involves a nonaerated, fluid-filled lung converting to an efficient air-filled organ of gas exchange.
- Closure of the foramen ovale and ductus arteriosus are important events in the transition to extrauterine life.
- The thorax houses and protects the lungs; it is also a movable shell that makes ventilation possible.
- The diaphragm is the primary muscle of ventilation; together with the accessory muscles and thoracic structures, it provides the ability to move large volumes of gas into and out of the lungs.
- The lungs receive blood flow from the pulmonary circulation for gas exchange and the bronchial circulation to support airway and pleural tissue metabolism.
- The pulmonary circulation is capable of acting as a reservoir, removing blood clots and numerous mediators, as well as activating important vasoactive agents.

- Motor and sensory neurons innervate the muscles of ventilation and various lung tissues. Autonomic neurons conduct motor and sensory signaling to control various tissues and sense various activities.
- The upper respiratory tract heats and humidifies inspired air. Its various structures also protect the lungs against foreign substances.
- The lower respiratory tract conducts respired gases from the upper airway to the respiratory zones of the lung. It contains many structures that help clear and defend the lung.
- The airways branch into lobes in both the right and the left lungs; these lobes consist of various segments.
- The respiratory bronchioles, alveolar ducts, and alveoli provide a large, yet extremely thin, membrane for the exchange of O_2 and CO_2 between air and blood. Disruption of the blood-gas barrier can occur from excessive capillary pressures, lung inflation, and exposure to various toxins (e.g., 100% O_2).

References

1. Moore KL, Persaud TVN, Torchia MG: The respiratory system. In Moore KL, Persaud TVN, editors: *The developing human: clinically oriented embryology*, ed 9, Philadelphia, 2011, Elsevier.
2. Langston C, Kida K, Reed M, et al: Human lung growth in late gestation and in the neonate. *Am Rev Respir Dis* 129:607, 1984.
3. Burri PH: Development and growth of the human lung. *Compr Physiol* Supplement 10: Handbook of Physiology, The Respiratory System, Circulation and Nonrespiratory Functions 1–46, 2011. doi: 10.1002/cphy.cp030101.
4. Perez-Gil J, Weaver TE: Pulmonary surfactant pathophysiology: current models and open questions. *Physiology (Bethesda)* 25:132, 2010.
5. Yarbrough ML, Grenache DG, Grownosky AM: Fetal lung maturity testing: the end of an era. *Biomark Med* 8:509, 2014.
6. Mendelson CR, Boggaram V: Hormone control of the surfactant system in fetal lung. *Annu Rev Physiol* 53:415, 1991.
7. Walsh BK: Neonatal and pediatrics respiratory care. In Walsh BK, editor: *Neonatal and pediatrics respiratory care*, ed 4, St Louis, 2015, Elsevier.
8. Morrisey EE, Hogan BLM: Preparing for the first breath: genetic and cellular mechanisms in lung development. *Dev Cell* 18:8, 2010.
9. Thurlbeck WM: Postnatal growth and development of the lung. *Am Rev Respir Dis* 111:803, 1975.
10. Hepper PG, Dornan JC, Lynch C: Sex differences in fetal habituation. *Dev Sci* 15:373, 2012.
11. Torday JS, Nielsen HC: The sex difference in fetal lung surfactant production. *Exp Lung Res* 12:1, 1987.
12. Taeusch WH, Ballard RA, Gleason CA, et al: *Avery's diseases of the newborn*, ed 9, Philadelphia, 2012, Elsevier.
13. Blackburn S: Fetal assessment. In Mattson S, Smith JE, editors: *Maternal, fetal, and neonatal physiology: a clinical perspective*, ed 4, Philadelphia, 2013, WB Saunders.
14. Davis L: Placental respiratory gas exchange. In Ginosar Y, Reynolds F, Halpern S, et al, editors: *Anesthesia and the fetus*, Oxford, UK, 2013, Wiley-Blackwell.
15. Czervinske MP: Fetal gas exchange and circulation. In Walsh B, Czervinske MP, DiBlasi R, editors: *Perinatal and pediatric respiratory care*, ed 3, Philadelphia, 2009, WB Saunders.
16. Katz C, Bentur L, Elias N: Clinical implication of lung fluid balance in the perinatal period. *J Perinatol* 31:230, 2011.
17. Stack CG, Dobbs P: *Differences between the child, the neonate and the adults: essentials of pediatric intensive care*, ed 4, New York, 2008, Cambridge University Press.
18. Cozzi F, Morini F, Tozzi C, et al: Effect of pacifier use on oral breathing in healthy newborn infants. *Pediatr Pulmonol* 33:36, 2002.
19. Bradley T, Thach MD: Maturation and transformation of reflexes that protect the laryngeal airway from liquid aspiration from fetal to adult life. *Am J Med* 111:69, 2001.
20. Praud JP, Reix P: Upper airways and neonatal respiration. *Respir Physiol Neurobiol* 149:131, 2005.
21. Gaultier C, Denjean A: Developmental anatomy and physiology of the respiratory system. In Taussig LM, Landau LI, editors: *Pediatric respiratory medicine*, ed 2, St Louis, 2008, Mosby.
22. Ochs M, Nyengaard JR, Jung L, et al: The number of alveoli in the human lung. *Am J Respir Crit Care Med* 169:120, 2004.
23. Zeltner TB, Burri PH: The postnatal development and growth of the human lung: II. Morphology. *Respir Physiol* 67:269, 1987.
24. Gehr P, Bachofen M, Weibel ER: The normal human lung ultrastructure and morphometric estimation of diffusion capacity. *Respir Physiol* 32:121, 1978.
25. Brown LM, Rannels SR, Rannels DE: Implications of post-pneumonectomy compensatory lung growth in pulmonary physiology and disease. *Respir Res* 2:340, 2001.
26. Hsia CC: Signals and mechanisms of compensatory lung growth. *J Appl Physiol* 97:1992, 2004.
27. Hsia CC, Johnson RL: Further examination of alveolar septal adaptation to left pneumonectomy in the adult lung. *Respir Physiol Neurobiol* 151:167, 2006.
28. Warburton D, Perin L, Defilippo R, et al: Stem/progenitor cells in lung development, injury repair, and regeneration. *Proc Am Thorac Soc* 5:703, 2008.
29. Burri PH: Structural aspects of postnatal lung development: alveolar formation and growth. *Biol Neonate* 89:313, 2006.
30. Hibbert M, Lannigan A, Raven J, et al: Gender differences in lung growth. *Pediatr Pulmonol* 19:129, 1995.
31. Gatzoulis M, Tsiridis E: Chest wall and breast. In Standring S, editor: *Gray's anatomy: the anatomic basis of clinical practice*, ed 40, St Louis, 2009, Elsevier.
32. De Troyer A: Respiratory muscle function. In Brewis RAL, Corrin B, Gedded DM, et al, editors: *Respiratory medicine*, London, 1995, WB Saunders.
33. Gatzoulis M, Pepper J: Diaphragm and phrenic nerve. In Standring S, editor: *Gray's anatomy: the anatomic basis of clinical practice*, ed 40, St Louis, 2009, Elsevier.
34. Celli B: The diaphragm and respiratory muscles. *Chest Surg Clin N Am* 8:207, 1998.
35. DeTroyer A, Boriek AM: Mechanics of respiratory muscles. *Compr Physiol* 1:1273, 2011.
36. DeTroyer A, Estenne M: Coordination between ribcage muscles and diaphragm during quiet breathing in humans. *J Appl Physiol* 57:899, 1984.
37. Celli BR: Clinical and physiologic evaluation of respiratory muscle function. *Clin Chest Med* 10:199, 1989.
38. Borley NR: Anterior abdominal wall. In Standring S, editor: *Gray's anatomy: the anatomic basis of clinical practice*, ed 40, St Louis, 2009, Elsevier.
39. Ishida H, Hirose R, Watanabe S: Comparison of changes in the contraction of the lateral abdominal muscles between the abdominal drawing-in maneuver and breathe held at the maximum expiratory level. *Man Ther* 17:427, 2012.
40. Iscoe S: Control of abdominal muscles. *Prog Neurobiol* 56:433, 1998.
41. Mier A, Brophy C, Estenne M, et al: Action of the abdominal muscles on the ribcage in humans. *J Appl Physiol* 58:1438, 1985.
42. Gatzoulis M, Padley S, Shah P, et al: Mediastinum. In Standring S, editor: *Gray's anatomy: the anatomic basis of clinical practice*, ed 40, St Louis, 2009, Elsevier.
43. Gatzoulis M, Padley S, Shah P, et al: Pleura, lungs and bronchi. In Standring S, editor: *Gray's anatomy: the anatomic basis of clinical practice*, ed 40, St Louis, 2009, Elsevier.
44. Noppen M: Normal volume and cellular contents of pleural fluid. *Curr Opin Pulm Med* 7:180, 2001.

45. Agostoni E, Zocchi L: Pleural liquid and its exchanges. *Respir Physiol Neurobiol* 159:311, 2007.
46. Weibel ER: What makes a good lung? *Swiss Med Wkly* 139:375, 2009.
47. Murray JF: Pulmonary circulation. In Murray JF, editor: *The normal lung: the basis for diagnosis and treatment of pulmonary disease*, ed 2, Philadelphia, 1986, WB Saunders.
48. Lumb AB: The pulmonary circulation. In Lumb AB, editor: *Nunn's applied respiratory physiology*, ed 7, Philadelphia, 2010, Elsevier.
49. Berne RM, Mathew LN: *Cardiovascular physiology*, ed 8, St Louis, 2001, Mosby.
50. Halbertsma FJ, Vaneker M, Scheffer GJ, et al: Cytokines and biotrauma in ventilator-induced lung injury: a critical review of the literature. *Neth J Med* 63:382, 2005.
51. McCullagh A, Rosenthal M, Wanner A, et al: The bronchial circulation: worth a closer look—a review of the relationship between the bronchial vasculature and airway inflammation. *Pediatr Pulmonol* 45:1, 2010.
52. Deffebach ME, Charan NB, Lakshminarayan S, et al: The bronchial circulation: small, but a vital attribute of the lung. *Am Rev Respir Dis* 135:463, 1987.
53. Murray JF: Lymphatics and nervous systems. In Murray JF, editor: *The normal lung: the basis for diagnosis and treatment of pulmonary disease*, ed 2, Philadelphia, 1986, WB Saunders.
54. Fraser RS, Müller NL, Colman N, et al: *Fraser and Pare's diagnosis of diseases of the chest* (vol 1), ed 4, Philadelphia, 1999, WB Saunders.
55. Drake RE, Dhother S, Oppenlander VM, et al: Lymphatic pump function curves in awake sheep. *Am J Physiol* 270:R486, 1996.
56. Jordan D: Central nervous pathways and control of the airways. *Respir Physiol* 125:67, 2001.
57. Canning BJ, Fischer A: Neural regulation of airway smooth muscle tone. *Respir Physiol* 125:113, 2001.
58. Widdicombe J: Airway receptors. *Respir Physiol* 125:3, 2001.
59. Rabbette PS, Fletcher ME, Dezateux CA, et al: Hering-Breuer reflex and respiratory system compliance in the first year of life: a longitudinal study. *J Appl Physiol* 76:650, 1994.
60. Coleridge HM, Coleridge JC: Pulmonary reflexes: neural mechanisms of pulmonary defense. *Annu Rev Physiol* 56:69, 1994.
61. Canning BJ: Functional implications of the multiple afferent pathways regulating cough. *Pulm Pharmacol Ther* 24:295, 2011.
62. Coleridge JCG, Coleridge HM: Afferent vagal C fiber innervation of the lungs and airways and its functional significance. *Rev Physiol Biochem Pharmacol* 99:1, 1984.
63. Kubin L, Alheid GF, Zuperku EJ, et al: Central pathways of pulmonary and lower airway vagal afferents. *J Appl Physiol* 101:618, 2006.
64. Carr MJ, Undem BJ: Bronchopulmonary afferent nerves. *Respirology* 8:291, 2003.
65. Proctor DF: The upper airways: I. Nasal physiology and defense of the lung. *Am Rev Respir Dis* 115:97, 1977.
66. Proctor DF: The upper airways: II. The larynx and trachea. *Am Rev Respir Dis* 115:315, 1977.
67. Jafeck B, Jones N: Nose, nasal cavity, and paranasal sinuses. In Standring S, editor: *Gray's anatomy: the anatomic basis of clinical practice*, ed 40, St Louis, 2009, Elsevier.
68. Strohl KP, Butler JP: Mechanical properties of the upper airway. *Compr Physiol* 2:1853, 2012.
69. Standring S: Larynx. In Standring S, editor: *Gray's anatomy: the anatomic basis of clinical practice*, ed 40, St Louis, 2009, Elsevier.
70. Shaker R, Dodds WJ, Dantas RO, et al: Coordination of deglutitive glottic closure with oropharyngeal swallowing. *Gastroenterology* 98:1478, 1990.
71. Bannister LH: Anatomy of speech. In Williams PL, editor: *Gray's anatomy*, London, 1995, Churchill Livingstone.
72. Fisher S, Dubois AE: *The lung: physiologic basis of pulmonary function tests*, ed 3, St Louis, 2000, Mosby.
73. Engle LA: Gas mixing within the acinus of the lung. *J Appl Physiol* 54:609, 1983.
74. Rhodin JA: Ultrastructure and function of the human tracheal mucosa. *Am Rev Respir Dis* 93(Suppl):1, 1966.
75. Breeze RG, Wheeldon EB: The cells of the pulmonary airways. *Am Rev Respir Dis* 116:705, 1977.
76. Albertine KH, Williams MC, Hyde DM: Anatomy of the lungs. In Mason RJ, Broaddus VC, Murray JF, et al, editors: *Murray and Nadel's textbook of respiratory medicine*, ed 5, Philadelphia, 2010, WB Saunders.
77. Cutz E, Yeger H, Pan J, et al: Pulmonary neuroendocrine cell system in health and disease. *Curr Respir Med Rev* 4:174, 2008.
78. Schulman ES: The role of mast cells in inflammatory responses in the lung. *Crit Rev Immunol* 13:35, 1993.
79. Fahy JV, Dickey BF: Airway mucus function and dysfunction. *N Engl J Med* 363:2233, 2010.
80. Rogers DF: Physiology of airway mucus secretion and pathophysiology of hypersecretion. *Respir Care* 52:1134, 2007.
81. Salathe M: Regulation of mammalian ciliary beating. *Annu Rev Physiol* 69:401, 2007.
82. Reynolds SD, Malkinson AM: Clara cell: progenitor for the bronchiolar epithelium. *Int J Biochem Cell Biol* 42:1, 2010.
83. Haefeli-Bleurer B, Weibel ER: Morphometry of the human pulmonary acinus. *Anat Rec* 220:401, 1988.
84. Johnson D, section editor: Microstructure of trachea, bronchi and lungs. In Standring S, editors: *Gray's anatomy: the anatomic basis of clinical practice*, ed 40, St Louis, 2009, Elsevier.
85. Crapo JD, Barry BE, Gehr P, et al: Cell number and cell characteristics of the normal human lung. *Am Rev Respir Dis* 125:740, 1982.
86. Tzortzaki EG, Vlachaki E, Siafakas NM: Pulmonary surfactant. *Pneumon* 4:364, 2007.
87. Ikegami M: Surfactant catabolism. *Respirology* 11:S24, 2006.
88. Crowther JA, Vijay KK, et al: Pulmonary surfactant protein a inhibits macrophage reactive intermediate production in response to stimuli by reducing NADPH oxidase activity. *J Immunol* 172:6866, 2004.
89. Topol M: Collateral respiratory pathways of pulmonary acini in man. *Folia Morphol* 54:61, 1995.
90. Weibel ER: *The pathway for oxygen*, Cambridge, 1984, Harvard University Press.
91. Dudek SM, Garcia JGN: Cytoskeletal regulation of pulmonary vascular permeability. *J Appl Physiol* 91:1487, 2001.
92. West JB: Thoughts on the pulmonary blood-gas barrier. *Am J Physiol Lung Cell Mol Physiol* 285:L501, 2003.
93. Maina JN, West JB: Thin and strong! The bioengineering dilemma in the structural and functional design of the blood-gas barrier. *Physiol Rev* 85:811, 2005.

CHAPTER 10

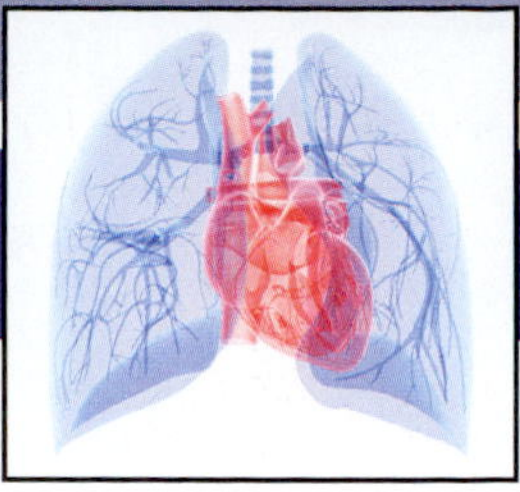

The Cardiovascular System

NARCISO E. RODRIGUEZ

CHAPTER OBJECTIVES

After reading this chapter you will be able to:

- Describe the anatomy of the heart and vascular systems.
- State the key characteristics of cardiac tissue.
- Describe the local and central control mechanisms of the heart and vascular systems.
- Describe how the cardiovascular system functions under normal and abnormal conditions.
- Calculate cardiac output given stroke volume and heart rate.
- Calculate ejection fraction given stroke volume and end-diastolic volume.
- Identify the electrical and mechanical events in relation to the normal cardiac cycle.

CHAPTER OUTLINE

KEY TERMS

afterload
arteriovenous anastomosis
automaticity
baroreceptors
cardiac output
cardiac tamponade
chemoreceptors
congestive heart failure (CHF)
contractility
end-diastolic volume (EDV)
end-systolic volume (ESV)
Frank-Starling law
heart rate (HR)
negative feedback loop
negative inotropism
pericardium
positive inotropism
preload
regurgitation
stenosis
stroke volume (SV)
vasoconstriction
vasodilation

FUNCTIONAL ANATOMY

Heart

Anatomy of the Heart

The heart is a hollow, four-chambered muscular organ approximately the size of a fist. It is positioned obliquely in the middle compartment of the mediastinum of the chest, just behind the sternum (Figure 10-1). Approximately two-thirds of the heart lies to the left of the midline of the sternum between the 2nd through the 6th ribs. The apex of the heart is formed by the tip of the left ventricle and lies just above the diaphragm at the level of the 5th intercostal space to the left. The base of the heart is formed by the atria and projects to the right, lying just below the 2nd rib. Posteriorly, the heart rests on the bodies of the 5th to the 8th thoracic vertebrae. Because of its position between the sternum and the spine, compression of the heart can maintain blood flow during cardiopulmonary resuscitation.[1]

Externally, surface grooves called *sulci* mark the boundaries of the heart chambers. Compared with the ventricles, the atria are small, thin-walled chambers that contribute little to the total pumping activity of the heart.

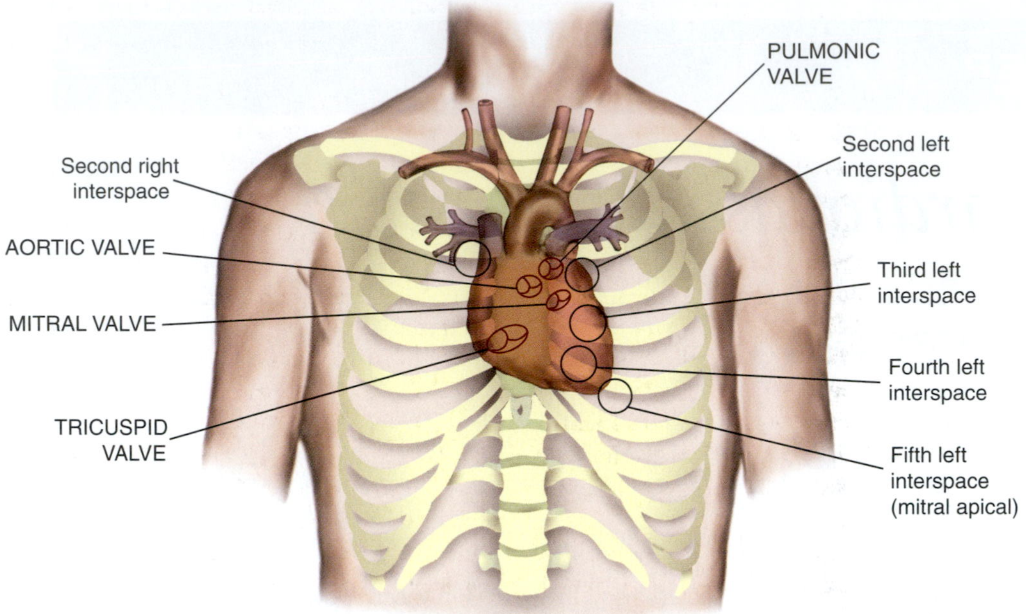

FIGURE 10-1 Anterior view of the thorax showing the position of the heart in relation to the ribs, sternum, diaphragm, and position of the heart valves. (From Seidel HM, et al: Mosby's guide to physical examination, ed 2, St Louis, 1991, Mosby.)

The heart is enclosed in a sac called the **pericardium.**[2] The structure of the pericardium can be summarized as follows:

1. *Fibrous pericardium:* Tough, loose-fitting, and inelastic sac surrounding the heart
2. *Serous pericardium:* Consisting of two layers:
   a. *Parietal layer:* Inner lining of the fibrous pericardium
   b. *Visceral layer or epicardium:* Covering the outer surface of the heart and great vessels

A thin layer of fluid called the *pericardial fluid* separates the two layers of the serous pericardium. This layer of fluid helps minimize friction within the pericardium. Inflammation of the pericardium results in a clinical condition called *pericarditis*. An abnormal amount of fluid can accumulate between the layers, resulting in a *pericardial effusion*. A large pericardial effusion may affect the pumping function of the heart, resulting in a **cardiac tamponade**. A cardiac tamponade compresses the heart muscle, leading to a serious decrease in blood flow to the body, which ultimately may lead to shock and death.[1,3]

The heart wall consists of three layers: (1) outer epicardium, (2) middle myocardium, and (3) inner endocardium. The myocardium composes the bulk of the heart muscle and consists of bands of involuntary striated muscle fibers. The contraction of these muscle fibers creates the pumplike action needed to move blood throughout the body.

Support for the four interior chambers and valves of the heart is provided by four atrioventricular (AV) rings, which form a fibrous "skeleton." Each ring is composed of dense connective tissue termed *annulus fibrosus cordis.* This connective tissue electrically isolates the atria from the ventricles. No impulses can be transmitted through the heart tissue from the atria to the ventricles.[1]

The two atrial chambers are thin-walled "cups" of myocardial tissue, separated by an interatrial septum. On the right side of the interatrial septum is an oval depression called the *fossa ovalis cordis,* the remnant of the fetal foramen ovale. In addition, each atrium has an appendage, or auricle, the function of which is unknown. In the presence of cardiac dysrhythmias (like atrial fibrillation), blood flow can pool on these appendages, leading to the formation of thrombi.

The two lower heart chambers, or ventricles, make up the bulk of the heart's muscle mass and do most of the pumping that circulates the blood (Figure 10-2). The mass of the left ventricle is normally approximately two-thirds larger than the mass of the right ventricle and has a spherical appearance when viewed across anteriorly.[4] The right ventricle is thin-walled, forming a pocket-like attachment to the left ventricle. Because of this relationship, contraction of the left ventricle pulls in the right ventricular wall, aiding its contraction. The effect, termed *left ventricular aid,* explains why some forms of right ventricular failure are less harmful than might be expected. The right and left ventricles are separated by a muscle wall termed the *interventricular septum* (see Figure 10-2).[4]

The valves of the heart are flaps of fibrous tissue firmly anchored to the *annulus fibrosus cordis* (Figure 10-3). Because they are located between the atria and ventricles, they are called *atrioventricular valves,* or AV valves. The valve in the right side is called the *tricuspid valve.* The valve on the left is the *bicuspid,* or *mitral, valve.* The AV valves close during systole (contraction of the ventricles), preventing backflow of blood into the atria. The free ends of the AV valves are anchored to papillary muscles of the endocardium by the *chordae tendineae cordis* (see Figure 10-2). During systole, papillary muscle contraction prevents the

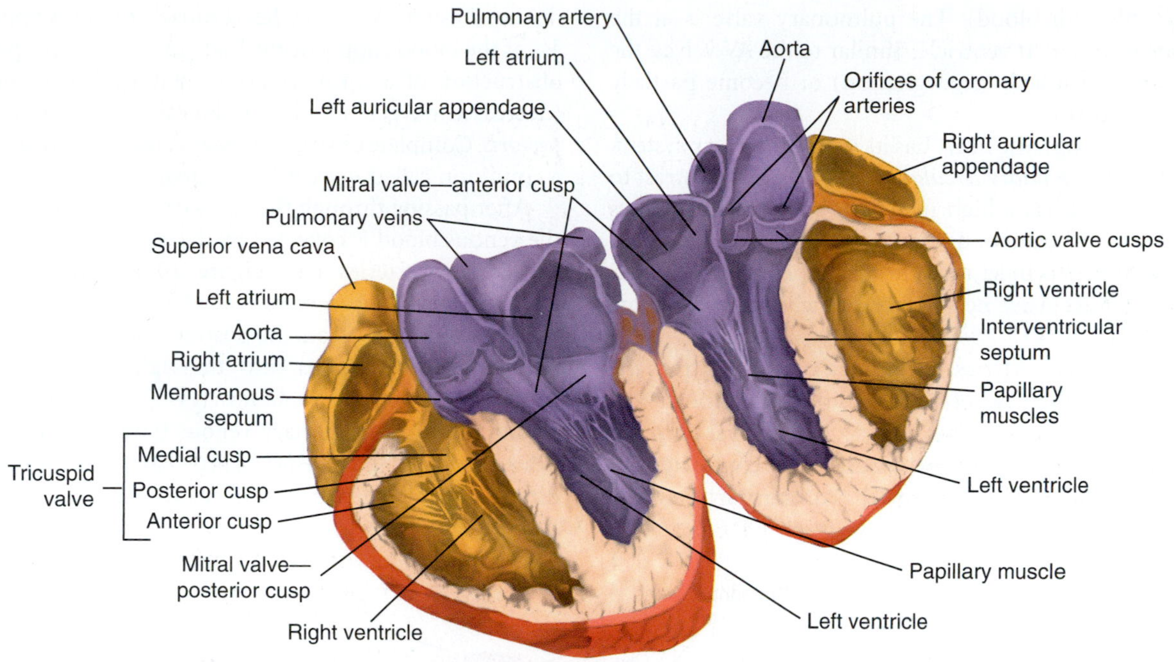

FIGURE 10-2 Drawing of the heart split perpendicular to the interventricular septum to illustrate anatomic relationships of the heart. (From Berne RM, Levy MN, editors: Physiology, ed 5, St Louis, 2004, Mosby.)

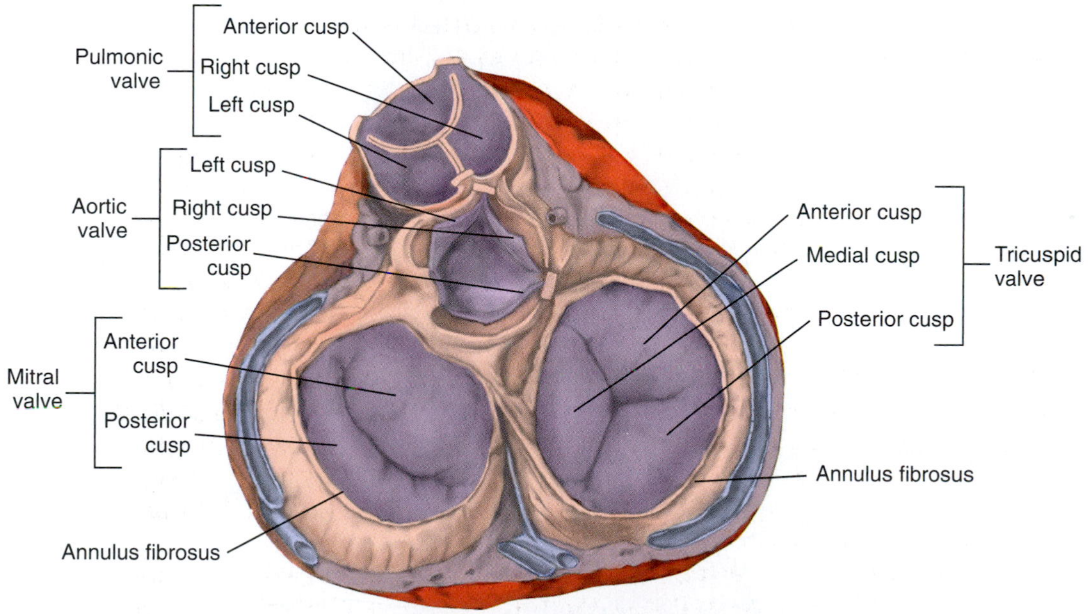

FIGURE 10-3 Four cardiac valves as viewed from the base of the heart. Note how the leaflets overlap in the closed valves.

AV valves from swinging upward into the atria. Damage to either the chordae tendineae cordis or the papillary muscles can impair function of the AV valves and cause leakage upward into the atria.[1]

Common valve problems include regurgitation and stenosis. **Regurgitation** is the backflow of blood through an incompetent or a damaged valve. **Stenosis** is a pathologic narrowing or constriction of a valve outlet, which causes increased pressure in the proximal chamber and vessels. Both conditions affect cardiac performance. In mitral stenosis, high pressures in the left atrium back up into the pulmonary circulation. This can cause pulmonary edema and a diastolic murmur (see Chapter 16).[3,5]

A set of semilunar valves separates the ventricles from their arterial outflow tracts, the pulmonary artery and the aorta (see Figure 10-3). Consisting of three half-moon–shaped cusps attached to the arterial wall, these valves prevent backflow of blood into the ventricles during diastole (or when the chambers of the heart fill with blood). The pulmonary valve is at the outflow tract of the right ventricle. Similar to the AV valves, the semilunar valves can leak (regurgitation) or become partially obstructed (stenosis).[1]

Similar to the lungs, the heart has its own circulatory system, which is called the *coronary circulation.* However, in contrast to the lungs, the heart has a high metabolic rate, which requires more blood flow per gram of tissue weight than any other organ except the kidneys. To meet these needs, the coronary circulation provides an extensive network of branches to all myocardial tissue (Figure 10-4).

Two main coronary arteries, a left and a right, arise from the root of the aorta. Because of their position underneath the aortic semilunar valves (see Figure 10-4), the coronary arteries get the maximal pulse of pressure generated by contraction of the left ventricle. Blood flows through the coronary arteries only during diastole. A healthy heart muscle requires approximately $\frac{1}{20}$ of the blood supply of the body to function properly. Partial obstruction of a coronary artery may lead to tissue ischemia (decreased oxygen supply), a clinical condition called *angina pectoris*. Complete obstruction may cause tissue death or infarct, a condition called *myocardial infarction (MI)*.[3]

After passing through the capillary beds of the myocardium, the venous blood is collected by the coronary veins that closely parallel the arteries (see Figure 10-4). These veins gather together into a large vessel called the *coronary sinus,* which passes left to right across the posterior surface of the heart. The coronary sinus empties into the right atrium between the opening of the inferior vena cava (IVC) and the tricuspid valve.[1] In addition, some coronary venous blood flows back into the heart through the *thebesian veins.*[1] The thebesian veins empty directly into all the heart chambers. Any blood coming from the

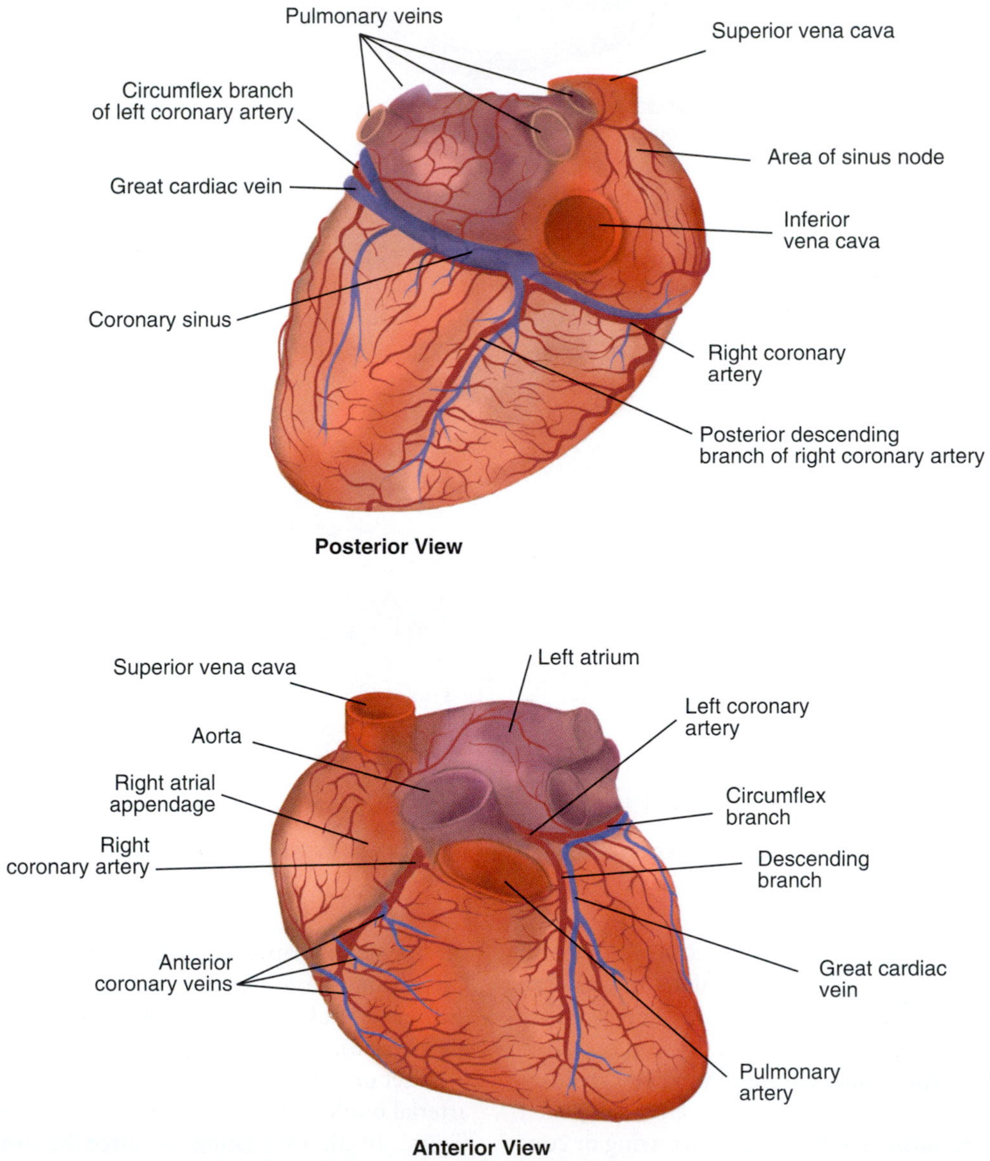

FIGURE 10-4 Coronary circulation as seen on anterior and posterior surfaces of the heart, illustrating the location and distribution of the principal coronary vessels.

MINI CLINI

Mitral Stenosis, Poor Oxygenation, and Increased Work of Breathing

The mitral valve lies between the left atrium and left ventricle. A stenotic mitral valve is one that is narrowed and offers high resistance to the blood flowing into the left ventricle from the left atrium. Pulmonary edema is a condition in which fluid collects in the alveoli and *interstitial spaces* in the lungs affecting oxygenation.

PROBLEM: Why does a patient with mitral stenosis have poor oxygenation of the blood and increased work of breathing?

DISCUSSION: Blood flows from the lungs into the left atrium, where it may encounter high resistance through a narrowed, stenotic mitral valve; this causes high pressure to build in the left atrium. Pressure in the pulmonary veins and eventually in the pulmonary capillaries also increases. This high pressure within the capillaries engorges them and forces fluid components of the blood plasma out of the vessels and into the interstitial spaces of the lungs and inside the alveoli, creating pulmonary edema. This collection of fluid interferes with O_2 diffusion from the lung into the blood. Engorged capillaries surrounding the alveoli create a stiff "web" around each alveolus, which makes expanding the lungs difficult. Some areas of the lung expand more easily than others, which causes inhaled air to be preferentially directed into these compliant regions, whereas "stiffer," more noncompliant regions are underventilated. The underventilated regions do not properly oxygenate the blood. Mitral stenosis, a cardiac problem, has significant pulmonary consequences.

MINI CLINI

Heart Rate and Coronary Perfusion

PROBLEM: Why might an extremely high heart rate decrease blood flow through the coronary arteries?

DISCUSSION: Blood flow through the coronary arteries occurs only during ventricular diastole when the aortic semilunar valves close. During systole, the myocardium contracts with such force that coronary artery pressures increase to values greater than aortic pressures. As the **heart rate (HR)** increases, both systolic and diastolic times must decrease. As diastolic time decreases, increasingly less time is available for coronary artery perfusion that occurs during diastole, until finally coronary blood flow is significantly reduced. This is critically important in an individual who already has reduced coronary circulation caused by arteriosclerotic heart disease. Not only is coronary artery perfusion compromised with severe tachycardia but also decreased ventricular filling time causes decreased **stroke volume (SV)** and decreased **cardiac output (CO).**

thebesian veins that enters the left atrium or ventricle mixes with arterial blood coming from the lungs. Whenever venous blood mixes with arterial blood, the overall O_2 content decreases. Because the thebesian veins bypass or shunt around the pulmonary circulation this phenomenon is called an *anatomic shunt.* When combined with a similar bypass in the bronchial circulation (see Chapter 9), these normal anatomic shunts account for approximately 2% to 3% of the total CO.[1,5]

Properties of the Heart Muscle

The performance of the heart as a pump depends on its ability to (1) initiate and conduct electrical impulses and to (2) contract synchronously the heart's muscle fibers quickly and efficiently.[5] These actions are possible only because myocardial tissue possesses the following four key properties:

- Excitability
- Inherent rhythmicity or automaticity
- Conductivity
- Contractility

Excitability is the ability of cells to respond to electrical, chemical, or mechanical stimulation. The myocardial property of *excitability* is the same as that exhibited by other muscles and tissues. Electrolyte imbalances and certain drugs can increase myocardial excitability and produce abnormalities in electrical conduction that may lead to cardiac arrhythmias.

Inherent rhythmicity, or **automaticity**, is the unique ability of the cardiac muscle to initiate a spontaneous electrical impulse. Although such impulses can arise from anywhere in the cardiac tissue, this ability is highly developed in specialized areas called *heart pacemaker,* or *nodal tissues.* The sinoatrial (SA) node and the atrioventricular (AV) node are the heart primary pacemakers (see Chapter 18). An electrical impulse from any source other than a normal heart pacemaker is considered abnormal and represents one of the many causes of *cardiac arrhythmias.*

Conductivity is the ability of myocardial tissue to spread and conduct electrical impulses. This property is similar to that of smooth muscle in that it allows the myocardium to contract without direct neural innervation (as required by skeletal muscle). The rate at which electrical impulses spread throughout the myocardium is variable. These differences in conduction rates are needed to ensure synchronous contraction of the cardiac chambers. Abnormal conductivity can affect the timing of chamber contractions and decrease cardiac efficiency.

Contractility, in response to an electrical impulse, is the primary function of the myocardium. In contrast to the contractions of other muscle tissues, cardiac contractions cannot be sustained or tetanized because myocardial tissue exhibits a prolonged period of inexcitability after contraction. The period during which the myocardium cannot be stimulated is called the *refractory period,* and it lasts approximately 250 msec, nearly as long as the heart contraction or systole.

Microanatomy of the Heart Muscle

Understanding how cardiac muscle contracts requires knowledge of the microanatomy of the heart. Unlike skeletal muscle

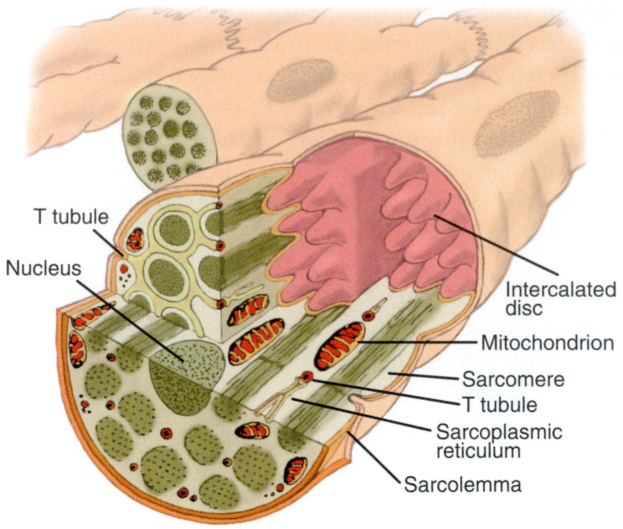

FIGURE 10-5 Major structural features of cardiac muscle fibers. Note the presence of intercalated discs connecting successive sarcomeres. (Modified from Moffett DF, Moffett SB, Schauf CL: Human physiology: foundations and frontiers, ed 2, St Louis, 1993, Mosby.)

fibers, cardiac cells are short, fat, branched, and interconnected. Individual cardiac fibers are enclosed in a membrane called the *sarcolemma,* which is surrounded by a rich capillary network (Figure 10-5).

Cardiac fibers are separated by irregular transverse thickenings of the sarcolemma called *intercalated discs.* These discs provide structural support and aid in electrical conduction between fibers. Each fiber consists of many smaller units called *myofibrils,* which contain repeated structures approximately 2 μm in size termed *sarcomeres.* Within the sarcomeres are contractile protein filaments responsible for shortening the myocardium during systole. These proteins are of two types: thick filaments composed mainly of myosin and thin filaments composed mostly of actin. Myocardial cells contract when actin and myosin combine to form reversible bridges between these thick and thin filaments.[2,5]

In principle, the tension developed during myocardial contraction is directly proportional to the number of cross-bridges between the actin and myosin filaments. This principle underlies Starling's law of the heart, also known as the **Frank-Starling law**. According to this law, the more a cardiac fiber is stretched (up to a point), the greater the tension it generates when contracted. This relationship is extremely important and is explored later in the discussion of the heart as a pump.[6]

Vascular System

The vascular system has two major subdivisions: the *systemic circulation* and the *pulmonary circulation*. The systemic circulation begins with the aorta on the left ventricle and ends in the right atrium. The pulmonary circulation begins with the pulmonary artery out of the right ventricle and ends in the left atrium. The blood flow to and from the heart is depicted in Figure 10-6.[1]

Venous, or deoxygenated blood from the head and upper extremities enters the right atrium from the superior vena cava (SVC), and blood from the lower body enters from the inferior vena cava (IVC). From the right atrium, blood flows into the right ventricle. The right ventricle pumps the blood into the pulmonary arteries, and on to the lungs.

Arterial, or oxygenated, blood returns to the left atrium through the pulmonary veins. The left atrium pumps blood into the left ventricle. The blood is then pumped to the body through the aorta. From the capillary network of the various body tissues, the deoxygenated venous blood returns to the right ventricle through the SVC and IVC.[1]

Systemic Circulation

The systemic circulation has three major components: (1) arterial system, (2) capillary system, and (3) venous system. These vessels regulate not only the amount of blood flow per minute (cardiac output) but also the distribution of blood to organs and tissues (perfusion). To achieve these functions, each component has a unique structure and plays a different role in the circulatory system as a whole.[2]

The *arterial system* consists of large, highly elastic, low-resistance arteries and small, muscular arterioles of varying resistance. With their elasticity, the large arteries help transmit and maintain the head of pressure generated by the heart. Together, the large arteries are called *conductance vessels.* Just as faucets control the flow of water into a sink, the smaller arterioles control blood flow into the capillaries. Arterioles provide this control by varying their flow resistance. Arterioles play a major role in the distribution and regulation of blood pressure and are referred to as *resistance vessels.*

The vast *capillary system,* or microcirculation, maintains a constant exchange of nutrients and waste products for the cells and tissues of the body. For this reason, the capillaries are commonly referred to as *exchange vessels.* Figure 10-7 shows the structure of a typical capillary network. Blood flows into the network by an arteriole and out through a venule. A direct communication between these vessels is called an **arteriovenous anastomosis**. When open, these anastomoses allows arterial blood to shunt around the capillary bed and flow directly into the venules. Downstream the arteriole divides into terminal arterioles, which branch further into thoroughfare channels and true capillaries.

Capillaries have smooth muscle rings at their proximal ends, called *precapillary sphincters.* Contraction of these sphincters decreases blood flow locally, whereas relaxation increases perfusion. In combination, these various channels, sphincters, and bypasses allow precise control over the direction and amount of blood flow to a given area of tissue.

The *venous system* consists of small, expandable venules and veins and larger, more elastic veins. Besides conducting blood back to the heart, these vessels act as a reservoir for the circulatory system. At any given time, the veins and venules hold approximately three-quarters of the body's total blood volume.

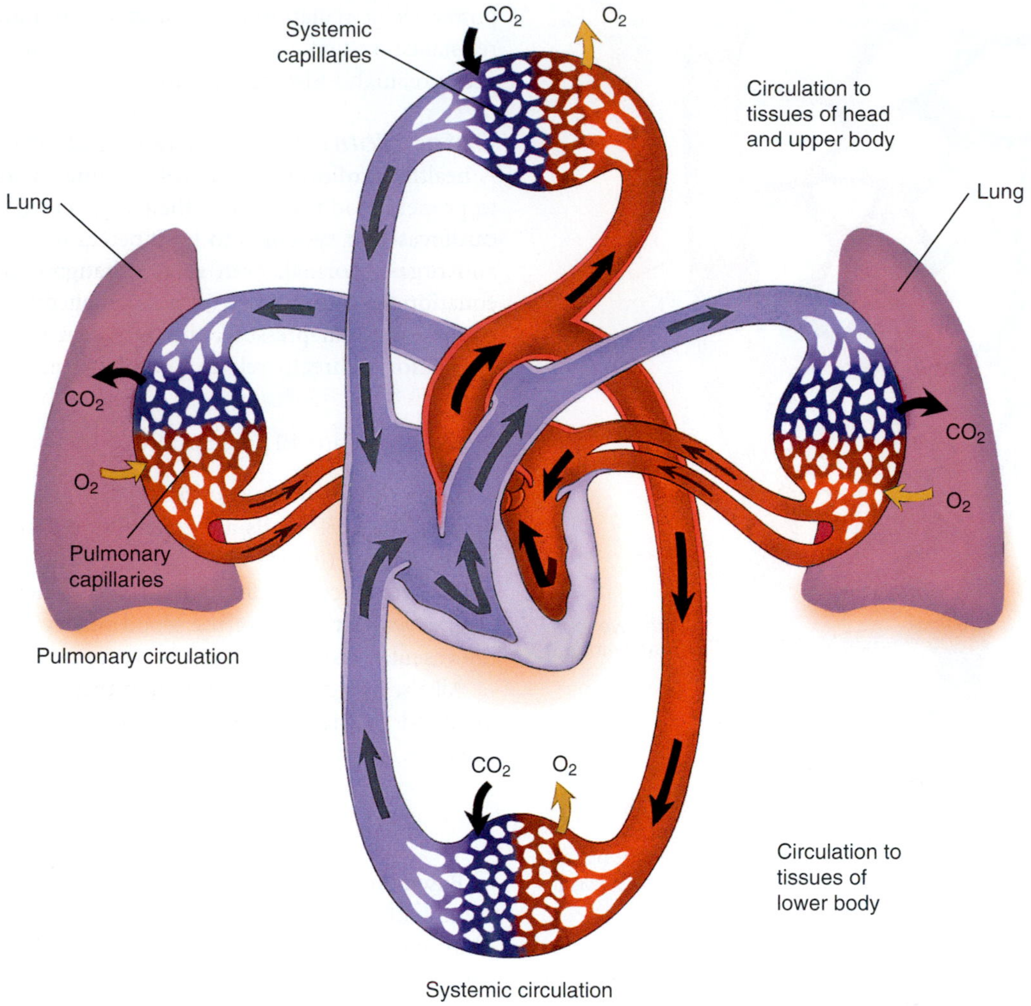

FIGURE 10-6 Generalized circulatory pathways between the heart, lung, and extremities.

The volume of blood held in this reservoir can be rapidly changed as needed simply by altering the tone of these vessels. By quickly changing its holding capacity, the venous system can match the volume of circulating blood to that needed to maintain adequate tissue perfusion. The components of the venous system, especially the small, expandable venules and veins, are termed *capacitance vessels.*

The venous system must overcome gravity to return blood to the heart. The following four mechanisms combine to aid venous return to the heart: (1) sympathetic venous tone; (2) skeletal muscle pumping, or "milking" (combined with venous one-way valves); (3) cardiac suction; and (4) thoracic pressure differences caused by respiratory efforts.[4]

The last mechanism is often called the *thoracic pump.* The thoracic pump is particularly important to respiratory therapists (RTs) because artificial ventilation with positive pressure reverses normal thoracic pressure gradients. Positive pressure ventilation (PPV) impedes, rather than assists, venous return. As long as blood volume, cardiac function, and vasomotor tone are adequate, PPV has a minimal effect on venous return. Patients who are hypovolemic or in cardiac failure are vulnerable to a reduction in CO when PPV is applied to the lungs.[6]

Although the heart is a single organ, it functions as two separate pumps. The right side of the heart generates a pressure of approximately 25 mm Hg to drive blood through the low-resistance, low-pressure pulmonary circulation. The left side of the heart generates pressures of approximately 120 mm Hg to propel blood through the higher pressure, high-resistance systemic circulation.

Vascular Resistance

Similar to the movement of any fluid through tubes, blood flow through the vascular system is opposed by frictional forces. The sum of all frictional forces opposing blood flow through the systemic circulation is called *systemic vascular resistance (SVR).* SVR must equal the difference in pressure between the beginning and the end of the circuit, divided by the flow. The beginning pressure for the systemic circulation is the mean aortic pressure; ending pressure equals right atrial pressure or *central venous pressure (CVP).* Flow for the system as a whole equals the CO. SVR can be calculated by the following formula:

$$\text{SVR} = \frac{\text{Mean aortic pressure} - \text{Right atrial pressure}}{\text{Cardiac output}}$$

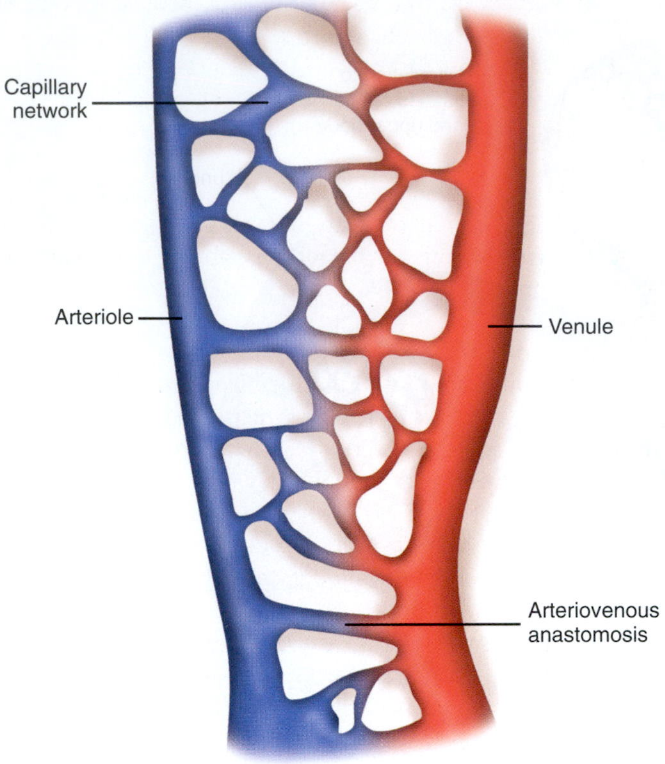

FIGURE 10-7 Components of a microcirculatory network. Blood flows from arteriolar to venular vessels through a network of capillaries. Opening of the arteriovenous anastomosis directs blood flow out of the capillary network. (Modified from Stevens A, Lowe J: Human histology, ed 2, St Louis, 1997, Mosby.)

Given a normal mean aortic pressure of 90 mm Hg, a mean right atrial pressure of approximately 4 mm Hg, and a normal CO of 5 L/min, normal SVR is computed as follows:

$$SVR = \frac{90\text{ mm Hg} - 4\text{ mm Hg}}{5\text{ L/min}}$$
$$= 17.2\text{ mm Hg/L/min}$$

The same concepts can be used to compute resistance in the pulmonary circulation. Beginning pressure for the pulmonary circulation is the mean pulmonary artery pressure; ending pressure equals left atrial pressure. Flow for the pulmonary circulation is the same as it is for the systemic system, which equals the CO. *Pulmonary vascular resistance (PVR)* can be calculated by using the following formula:

$$PVR = \frac{\text{Mean pulmonary artery pressure} - \text{Left atrial pressure}}{\text{Cardiac output}}$$

Given a normal mean pulmonary artery pressure of approximately 16 mm Hg and a normal mean left atrial pressure of 8 mm Hg, normal PVR is computed as follows:

$$PVR = \frac{16\text{ mm Hg} - 8\text{ mm Hg}}{5\text{ L/min}}$$
$$= 1.6\text{ mm Hg/L/min}$$

Resistance to blood flow in the pulmonary circulation is approximately one-tenth of the systemic circulation. The pulmonary circulation is characterized as a low-pressure, low-resistance system, and the systemic circulation as a high-pressure, high resistance system.

Determinants of Blood Pressure

A healthy cardiovascular system maintains sufficient pressure to propel blood throughout the body.[5] The first priority of the cardiovascular system is to keep perfusion pressures to tissues and organs normal, even under changing conditions. If the equation for computing SVR is rearranged by deleting the normally low atrial pressure, the average blood pressure in the circulation is directly related to both CO and flow resistance, as follows:

$$\text{Mean arterial pressure (MAP)} = (\text{CO} \times \text{SVR}) + \text{CVP}$$

Some MAP formulas disregard the CVP contribution because the CVP levels are generally negligible under normal circumstances (0 to 6 mm Hg). It is important to note that under many conditions, vascular resistance tends to vary inversely with the size of the blood vessels (i.e., the capacity of the vascular system).

All else being constant, MAP is directly related to the volume of blood in the vascular system and inversely related to its capacity:

$$MAP = \frac{\text{Volume}}{\text{Capacity}}$$

Based on this relationship, MAP is regulated by changing the volume of circulating blood, changing the capacity of the vascular system, or changing both. Volume changes can reflect absolute changes in total blood volume, such as changes resulting from hemorrhagic shock or blood transfusion. Alternatively, changes in "relative" volume can occur when vascular space increases or decreases. Vascular space decreases when **vasoconstriction** (constriction of the smooth muscles in the peripheral blood vessels) occurs; this causes blood pressure to increase even though blood volume is the same. Vascular space increases when **vasodilation** (relaxation of the smooth muscles in the arterioles) occurs; this causes blood pressure to decrease even though blood volume has not changed.

In a normal adult, MAP ranges from 80 to 100 mm Hg. When MAP decreases below 60 mm Hg, perfusion to the brain and the kidneys is severely compromised and organ failure may occur in minutes.[3]

To avoid organ and tissue damage and maintain adequate perfusion pressures under changing conditions, the cardiovascular system balances relative volume and resistance. When a person exercises, the circulating blood volume undergoes a relative increase, but blood pressure remains near normal; this is because the skeletal muscle vascular beds dilate, causing a large increase in system capacity. However, when blood loss occurs, as with hemorrhage, the system capacity is decreased by constriction of the peripheral vessels. Perfusion pressures are kept near normal until the volume loss is extreme.

Regulation of blood flow and pressure is much more complex than is suggested by these simplified equations. Cardiovascular control is achieved by a complex array of integrated functions. Some of these functions are explained subsequently.

CONTROL OF THE CARDIOVASCULAR SYSTEM

The cardiovascular system is responsible for transporting metabolites to and from the tissues under various conditions and demands. It must act in a highly coordinated fashion. Coordination is achieved by integrating the functions of the heart and vascular system. The goal is to maintain adequate perfusion to all tissues according to their needs.[6]

The cardiovascular system regulates blood flow mainly by altering the capacity of the vasculature and the volume of blood it holds. The heart plays only a secondary role in regulating blood flow. In essence, the vascular system tells the heart how much blood it needs, rather than the heart dictating what volume of blood the vascular system will receive.

These integrated functions involve local and central neural control mechanisms. Local, or *intrinsic,* controls operate independently, without central nervous system control. Intrinsic control alters perfusion under normal conditions to meet metabolic needs. Central, or *extrinsic,* control involves both the central nervous system and circulating *humoral agents.* Extrinsic control mechanisms maintain a normal level of vascular tone. However, central control mechanisms take over when the competing needs of local vascular beds must be coordinated. Knowledge of vascular regulatory mechanisms and factors controlling CO is essential to understanding how the cardiovascular system responds under both normal and abnormal conditions.[2]

Regulation of Peripheral Vasculature

A normal level of vascular muscle tone is normally maintained throughout the vascular system at all times. Normal muscle tone must be present to allow for effective regulation. If blood vessels remained in a completely relaxed state, further dilation would be impossible and local increases in perfusion could not occur.

Local vascular tone is maintained by the smooth muscle of the precapillary sphincters of the microcirculation and can function independently of neural control at the local tissue level according to metabolic needs. Central control of vasomotor tone involves either direct central nervous system innervation or circulation hormones. Central control mainly affects the high-resistance arterioles and capacitance veins.

Local Control

Local regulation of tissue blood flow includes both myogenic and metabolic control mechanisms. *Myogenic control* involves the relationship between vascular smooth muscle tone and perfusion pressure. Myogenic control ensures relatively constant flows to the capillary beds despite changes in perfusion pressures.

Metabolic control involves the relationship between vascular smooth muscle tone and the level of local cellular metabolites. High amounts of carbon dioxide (CO_2) or lactic acid, low pH levels, low partial pressures of O_2 levels, histamines (released during inflammatory response), endothelium-derived relaxing factor, and some prostaglandins all cause relaxation of the smooth muscle and vasodilation, increasing flow to the affected area.

The influence of myogenic and metabolic control mechanisms varies in different organ systems, with the brain being the most sensitive to changes in the local metabolite levels, particularly CO_2 and pH.[1]

Central Control

Central control of blood flow is achieved primarily by the sympathetic division of the autonomic nervous system. Smooth muscle contraction and increased flow resistance are mostly caused by adrenergic stimulation and the release of norepinephrine. Smooth muscle relaxation and vessel dilation occur as a result of stimulation of either *cholinergic* or specialized *beta-adrenergic* receptors. Although the contractile response is distributed throughout the entire vascular system, dilation response appears to be limited to the precapillary vessels. In addition to the sympathetic control, blood flow through the large veins can also be affected by abdominal and intrathoracic pressure changes.

Regulation of Cardiac Output

The heart, similar to the vascular system, is regulated by both intrinsic and extrinsic factors. These mechanisms act together, along with vascular control, to ensure that the output of the heart matches the different needs of the tissues.

The total amount of blood pumped by the heart per minute is called the *cardiac output* (CO). CO is simply the product of the HR and the volume ejected by the left ventricle on each contraction, or stroke volume (SV):

$$CO = HR \times SV$$

A normal resting CO of approximately 5 L/min can be calculated by substituting a normal HR (70 contractions/min) and SV (75 ml, or 0.075 L, per contraction):

$$CO = 70\ \text{beats/min} \times 0.075\ \text{L/beat} = 5.25\ \text{L/min}$$

This is a hypothetical average because actual CO varies considerably in health and disease states and according to a person's sex, height, and weight.

Regardless of an individual's state of health or disease, a change in CO must involve a change in SV, a change in HR, or both. SV is affected primarily by intrinsic control of three factors: (1) preload, (2) afterload, and (3) contractility (all three factors are discussed subsequently). HR is affected primarily by extrinsic or central control mechanisms.[3,6]

Changes in Stroke Volume

The heart does not eject all of the blood it contains during systole. Instead, a small volume, called the **end-systolic volume (ESV)**, remains behind in the ventricles. During the resting phase, or diastole, the ventricles fill to a volume called the

end-diastolic volume (EDV). SV equals the difference between the EDV and the ESV, as follows:

$$SV = EDV - ESV$$

In a healthy man at rest, the EDV ranges from 110 to 120 ml. Given a normal SV of approximately 70 ml, a normal ejection fraction (EF), or proportion of the EDV ejected on each stroke, can be calculated as follows:

$$EF = \frac{SV}{EDV} \times 100$$
$$= \frac{70\ ml}{110\ ml} \times 100$$
$$= 64\%$$

On each contraction, a healthy heart ejects approximately two-thirds of its stored volume. Decreases in EF are normally associated with a weakened myocardium (heart failure), decreased contractility, or both. When the EF decreases below 30%, a person's exercise tolerance becomes severely limited.[6]

As shown in Figure 10-8, an increase in SV occurs when either the EDV increases or the ESV decreases. Conversely, a decrease in SV occurs when either the EDV decreases or the ESV increases. This relationship is key to understanding regulation of CO.

The heart's ability to change SV solely according to the EDV is an intrinsic regulatory mechanism. The force of the ventricle can generate results from the length of the myocardial fibers just before contraction. As the ventricle fills with blood, the myocardial fibers are stretched. As stretch increases, the tension (force) within the walls of the heart increases (analogous to stretching a rubber band). This relationship between cardiac muscle length and tension is called the *Frank-Starling law of the heart.*[7]

The concepts of tension or force and filling volume are often described in term of **preload** and **afterload**. As with many terms in medicine, the definitions of preload and afterload vary considerably in the literature.[8] This variability seems to be related to the term *load,* which in general means "a force against which something that causes motion (a pump or motor) acts." In the context of the cardiovascular system, the heart is analogous to a pump and force in this sense is related to stretch of the cardiac muscle according to the Frank-Starling Law.

Using this description of load, preload therefore represents the combined force of all the factors that contribute to ventricular wall stretch at the end of diastole. Preload may be calculated in a manner that recognizes the force that stretches the resting cardiac muscle to a given length before contraction. Many factors determine preload, including venous return, total blood volume and distribution, and atrial activity. These and the other factors that influence preload are summarized in Table 10-1.[8]

In a similar fashion, afterload can be described as the combined force of all of the factors the left ventricle encounters and must overcome when stimulated to contract and achieve the

TABLE 10-1

Factors Affecting Preload

Factor	Affect
End-diastolic filling pressure	Total blood volume Blood volume distribution Atrial contraction Venous compliance Total peripheral resistance Venous return
End-diastolic stretch	End-diastolic filling pressure Compliance of ventricle and pericardium
Myocardial wall thickness	Normal physiology Compensatory hypertrophy

Data from Chiumello D, Carlesso E, Cadringher P, et al: Lung stress and strain during mechanical ventilation for acute respiratory distress syndrome. Am J Respir Crit Care Med 15;178:346, 2008.

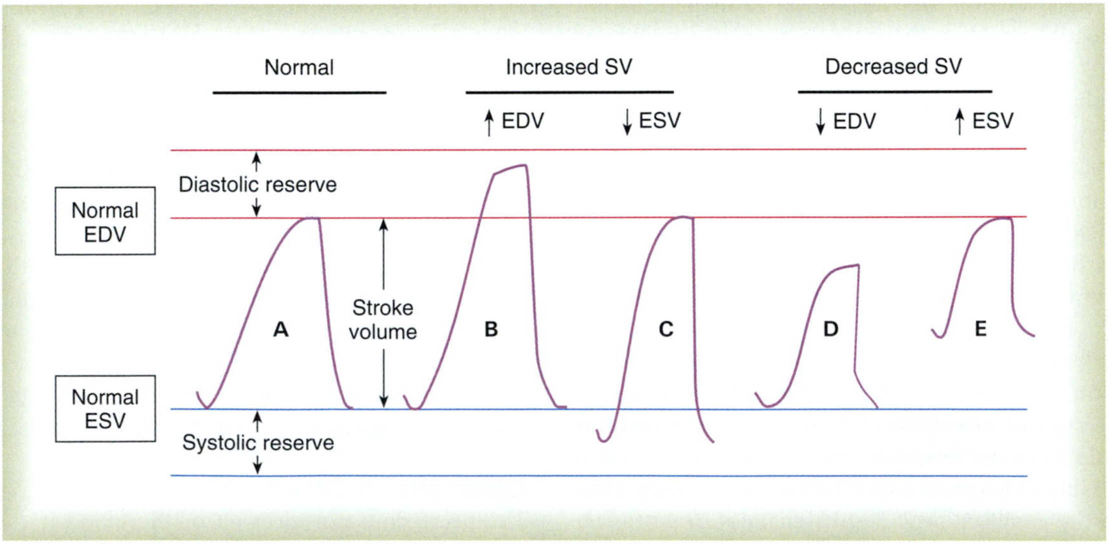

FIGURE 10-8 Relationship between stroke volume *(SV),* end-diastolic volume *(EDV),* and end-systolic volume *(ESV).* Normal relationship between EDV, ESV, and SV *(A);* increased SV resulting from increased EDV *(B);* increased SV resulting from decreased ESV *(C);* decreased SV resulting from decreased EDV (hypovolemia) *(D);* and decreased SV resulting from increased ESV (poor contractility) *(E).*

TABLE 10-2
Factors Affecting Afterload

Ventricular systolic pressure	Output impedance	Output flow resistance	Valvular resistance	
			Obstructive cardiomyopathy	
	Systemic arterial pressure	Arterial diastolic pressure	Blood volume	
			Total peripheral resistance	
		Arterial systolic pressure	Pulse pressure	Stroke volume
				Arterial compliance
Ventricular systolic stretch	End-diastolic volume			
Myocardial wall thickness	Normal physiology			
	Compensatory hypertrophy			

Data from Chiumello D, Carlesso E, Cadringher P, et al: Lung stress and strain during mechanical ventilation for acute respiratory distress syndrome. Am J Respir Crit Care Med 15;178:346, 2008.

end of systole.[8] Several factors determine afterload; most notably peripheral vascular resistance and the physical characteristics of arterial blood. These and the other factors that determine afterload are summarized in Table 10-2.[8]

It should be noted that an increased preload or afterload caused by an abnormal increased downstream resistance over time can be "normalized" (up to a point) by increasing the wall thickness of the heart, which the body attempts to do by increasing muscle mass (hypertrophy), leading to cardiomyopathy and heart failure.[8]

RULE OF THUMB

Increases in preload result in increased SV in the healthy heart.

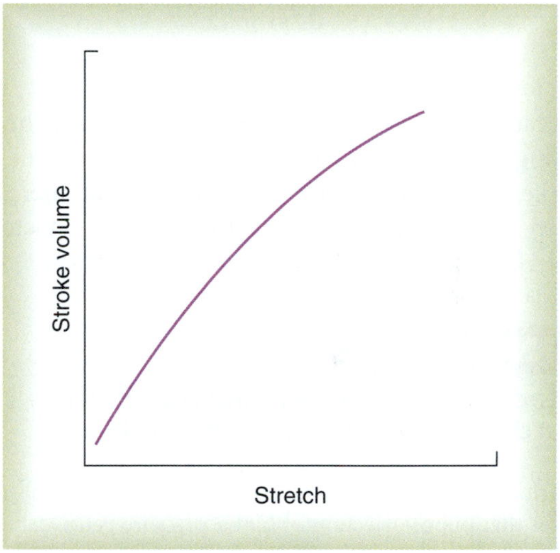

FIGURE 10-9 The Frank-Starling law: SV as a function of ventricular end-diastolic stretch. An increase in the stretch of the ventricles immediately before contraction (end-diastole) results in an increase in SV. Ventricular end-diastolic stretch is synonymous with the concept of preload.

All else being constant, the greater the afterload on the ventricles, the harder it is for the ventricles to eject their volume. For a given EDV, an increase in afterload means the ESV increased. If the EDV remains constant while the ESV increases, the SV (EDV − ESV) decreases (see Figure 10-8). Normally, however, the healthy heart muscle responds to increased afterload by altering its contractility.

RULE OF THUMB

Increases in afterload can decrease SV, especially in the failing heart.

Contractility represents the amount of systolic force exerted by the heart muscle at any given preload. At a given preload (or EDV), an increase in contractility results in an increased EF, a decreased ESV, and an increased SV. Conversely, a decrease in contractility results in a decreased EF, an increased ESV, and a decreased SV.

Changes in contractility affect the slope of the ventricular function curve (Figures 10-9 and 10-10). A higher SV for a given preload (increased slope) indicates a state of increased contractility, often referred to as **positive inotropism**. The opposite is also true. A lower SV for a given preload indicates decreased contractility, referred to as **negative inotropism**. Drugs that increase contractility of the heart muscle are called

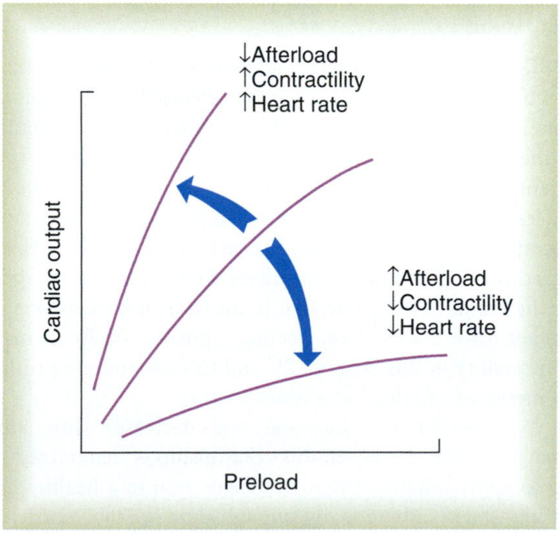

FIGURE 10-10 Effects of preload, afterload, contractility, and heart rate on cardiac output function curve. (Modified from Green JF: Fundamental cardiovascular and pulmonary physiology, ed 2, Philadelphia, 1987, Lea & Febiger.)

positive inotropes; drugs that decrease contractility are *negative inotropes.*[6]

In addition to local mechanisms, cardiac contractility is influenced by neural control, circulating hormonal factors, and certain medications. Typically, neural or drug-mediated *sympathetic* stimulation has a positive inotropic effect. Conversely, *parasympathetic* stimulation exerts a negative inotropic effect. *Profound hypoxia* and *acidosis* impair myocardial function and decrease cardiac contractility.

RULE OF THUMB

Hypoxia and acidosis decrease cardiac contractility and output.

Changes in Heart Rate

The last factor influencing CO is HR. In contrast to the factors controlling SV, the factors affecting HR are mainly of central origin (i.e., neural or hormonal). Factors that increase HR are called *positive chronotropic* factors. Likewise, factors that decrease HR are called *negative chronotropic* factors.

MINI CLINI

Effect of Increased Afterload on Cardiac Output in a Normal Heart

Afterload is the resistance the ventricle has to overcome, or the forces that oppose ejection of blood pressure generated as the heart works to eject its SV. As afterload increases, the SV ejected by the ventricle decreases, assuming that the contractility of the heart (force with which the heart contracts) remains constant.

PROBLEM: During exercise, a healthy person's blood pressure increases considerably, indicating that the afterload has increased. Yet the SV and CO in a healthy heart do not decrease. Why is this so?

DISCUSSION: When afterload increases, the initial ventricular contractions that experience the increased afterload produce smaller SVs; this causes more blood to remain in the ventricle at the end of systole (i.e., ESV is increased). During the subsequent diastole, blood rushes in from the atria to fill the ventricles, and because of the higher than normal ESV, the ventricle becomes more distended and stretched than before. Healthy heart muscle responds to increased stretch in a way described by the Frank-Starling law; that is, the heart now contracts with greater force than before, ejecting a greater SV. By increasing contractility in this fashion, SV and CO are not compromised by increased afterload in a healthy heart.

As expected, CO increases and decreases with similar changes in HR. However, this relationship is maintained only up to approximately 160 to 180 beats/min in a healthy heart. At higher HRs, there is not enough time for the ventricles to fill completely between each heartbeat, causing a decrease in EDV, SV, and CO. This phenomenon often occurs at significantly less than 160 beats/min in the failing heart.

RULE OF THUMB

Increase in HR increases CO in a healthy heart up to a rate of 160 to 180 beats/min.

The combined effects of preload, afterload, contractility, and HR on cardiac performance are graphically portrayed in Figure 10-10. The middle curve represents the normal state. The upper, steeper curve represents a hyperdynamic heart. In the hyperdynamic heart, a given preload results in a greater than normal CO. Factors contributing to this state include decreased afterload, increased contractility (decreased ESV), and increased HR. The bottom curve has a lower slope than normal, indicating a hypodynamic heart. Factors contributing to this state include increased afterload, decreased contractility (increased ESV), and decreased rate. When the pumping efficiency of the heart is so low that CO is inadequate to meet tissues needs, the heart is said to be in **congestive heart failure (CHF)**.[3,6]

Cardiovascular Control Mechanisms

Cardiovascular control is achieved by integrating local and central regulatory mechanisms that affect both the heart and the vasculature. The goal is to ensure that all tissues receive sufficient blood flow to meet their metabolic needs. However, when demands are increased or abnormal, such as during exercise or massive bleeding, central mechanisms take over primary control.

RULE OF THUMB

Blood flow to a specific vascular bed is primarily regulated by local mechanisms.

Central control of cardiovascular function occurs by interaction between the brainstem and selected peripheral receptors (Figure 10-11). The brainstem constantly receives feedback from these receptors about the pressure, volume, and chemical status of the blood. The brainstem also receives input from higher brain centers, such as the hypothalamus and cerebral cortex. These inputs are integrated with the inputs coming from the heart and blood vessels to maintain adequate blood flow and pressure in all but the most abnormal conditions.[2]

Cardiovascular Control Centers

Figure 10-11 is a simplified diagram of the cardiovascular regulatory centers. Areas in the medulla receive input from higher brain centers, peripheral pressure, and chemical receptors. Stimulation of the vasoconstrictor area within the medulla causes vasoconstriction and increased vascular resistance.

Closely associated with the vasoconstrictor center is a cardioaccelerator area. Stimulation of this center increases HR by increasing sympathetic discharge to the SA and AV nodes of the heart. A cardioinhibitory area plays the opposite role. Stimulation of this center decreases HR by increasing vagal (parasympathetic) stimulation to the heart.

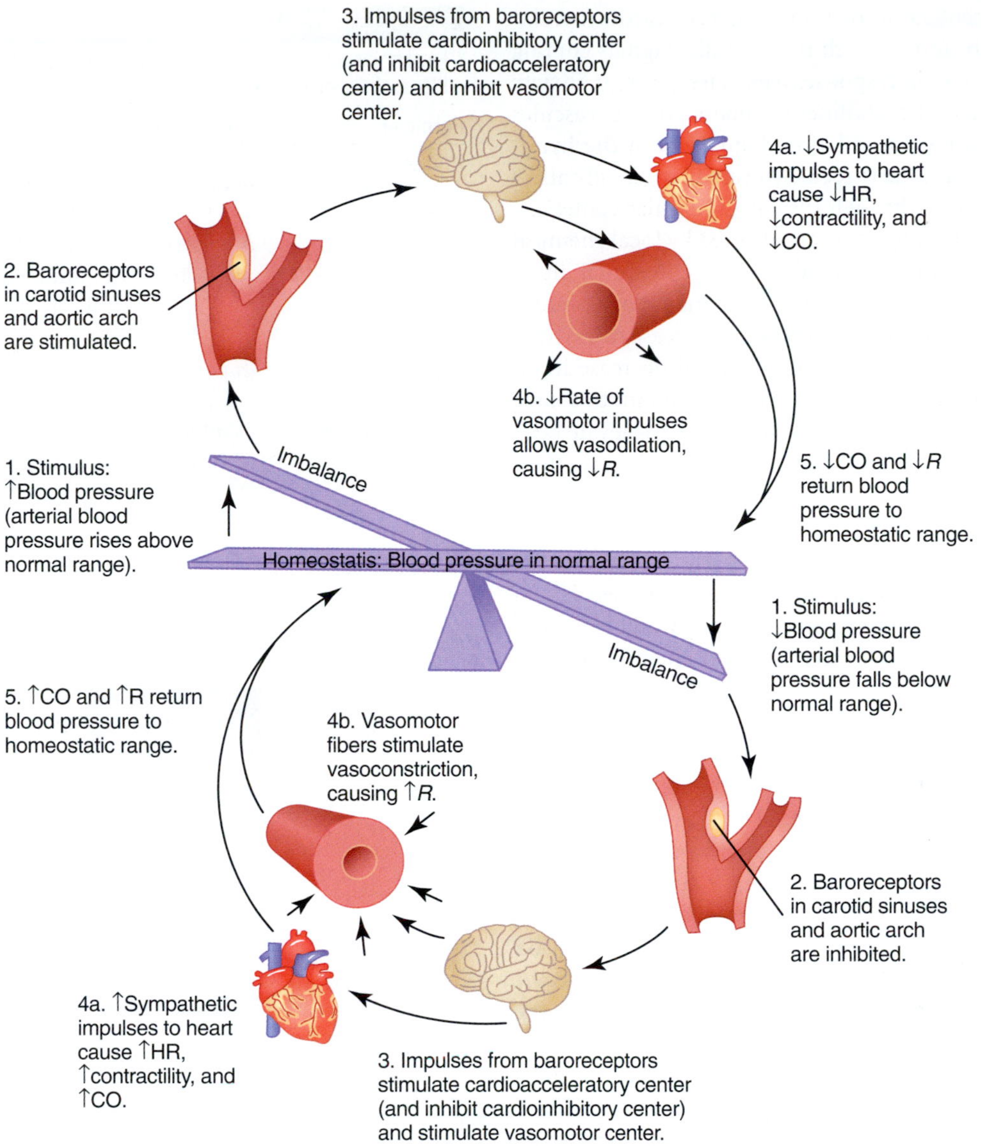

FIGURE 10-11 Simplified diagram of cardiovascular regulatory centers. *CO,* Cardiac output; *HR,* heart rate; *R,* respiration. (Modified from Marieb EN, Hoehn KN: Anatomy and physiology, ed 4, San Francisco, 2011, Pearson Benjamin Cummings.)

MINI CLINI

Heart Rate and the Administration of Bronchodilator Drugs

PROBLEM: You are giving a bronchodilator aerosolized drug to a patient, and you notice a significant increase in the patient's HR. Would you expect increased HR to be a common side effect of drugs that cause bronchodilation?

DISCUSSION: The discharge rate of the sinus node and the HR are increased by sympathetic nervous stimulation and decreased by parasympathetic nervous stimulation. The airways of the lung are dilated by sympathetic nervous stimulation and constricted by parasympathetic stimulation. Drugs that cause bronchodilation either mimic sympathetic stimulation (sympathomimetic) or block parasympathetic stimulation (parasympatholytic). Both of these drug actions also cause the HR to increase. Parasympatholytic drugs bring about effects similar to those of sympathetic stimulation; by inhibiting parasympathetic activity, they allow sympathetic impulses to predominate.

Higher brain centers also influence the cardiovascular system, both directly and through the medulla. Signals coming from the cerebral cortex in response to exercise, pain, or anxiety pass directly through the cholinergic fibers to the vascular smooth muscle, causing vasodilation. Signals from the hypothalamus, in particular its heat-regulating areas, indirectly affect HR and vasomotor tone through the cardiovascular centers.

The cardiovascular centers also are affected by local chemical changes in the surrounding blood and cerebrospinal fluid. Decreased levels of CO_2 tend to inhibit the medullary centers. General inhibition of these centers causes a decrease in vascular tone and a decrease in blood pressure. A local decrease in O_2 tension has the opposite effect. Mild hypoxia in this area increases sympathetic discharge rates; this tends to elevate both HR and blood pressure. Severe hypoxia has a depressant effect.

Peripheral Receptors

In addition to high-level and local input, the cardiovascular centers receive signals from peripheral receptors (see Figure 10-11). There are two types of peripheral cardiovascular receptors: **baroreceptors**, or stretch receptors, and **chemoreceptors**. Baroreceptors respond to pressure changes, whereas chemoreceptors respond to changes in blood chemistry.[3]

The cardiovascular system has two different sets of baroreceptors. The first set is located in the aortic arch and carotid sinuses. These receptors monitor arterial pressures generated by the left ventricle. The second set is located in the walls of the atria and the large thoracic and pulmonary veins. These low-pressure sensors respond mainly to changes in vascular volumes. Baroreceptor output is directly proportional to the stretch on the vessel wall. The greater the blood pressure, the greater is the stretch and the higher the rate of neural discharge to the medulla.

Together with the cardiovascular regulatory centers, these receptors form a **negative feedback loop**. In a negative feedback loop, stimulation of a receptor causes an opposite response by the effector. In the case of the arterial receptors, an increase in blood pressure increases aortic and carotid receptor stretch and their neuronal discharge rates. The increased discharge rates cause an opposite response by the medullary centers (i.e., depressor response decreasing blood pressure). Decreased blood pressure (decreased baroreceptor output) has the opposite effect, causing peripheral vessel constriction and increased HR and contractility. This mechanism usually restores blood pressure to normal (see Figure 10-11).[2,3]

Although the high-pressure arterial receptors constantly control blood pressure, the low-pressure sensors are responsible for long-term regulation of plasma volume. The low-pressure atrial and venous baroreceptors regulate plasma volume mainly by activating several chemical and hormonal mechanisms. Table 10-3 provides a detailed description of some of these mechanisms.

The major pathways for plasma volume control are outlined in Figure 10-12. Combined with a central nervous system–mediated increase in renal filtration, these humoral mechanisms decrease the overall plasma volume. A decrease in blood volume has the opposite effect (i.e., sodium and water retention and an increase in plasma volume).

TABLE 10-3

Hormonal Control Mechanisms Affecting Blood Pressure

Hormone	Place of Action	Effect
Angiotensin II	Arterioles	↑ SVR (vasoconstriction)
Antidiuretic hormone	Kidneys	↑ Blood volume (↑ water retention)
	Arterioles	↑ SVR (vasoconstriction)
Atrial natriuretic peptide	Arterioles	↓ SVR (vasodilation)
Aldosterone	Kidneys	↑ Blood volume (↑ water and salt retention)
Cortisol	Kidneys	↑ Blood volume (↑ water and salt retention)
Norepinephrine	Heart (beta-1 receptors)	↑ Cardiac output (HR and contractility)
	Arterioles (alpha receptors)	↑ SVR (vasoconstriction)

HR, Heart rate; *SVR,* systemic vascular resistance.

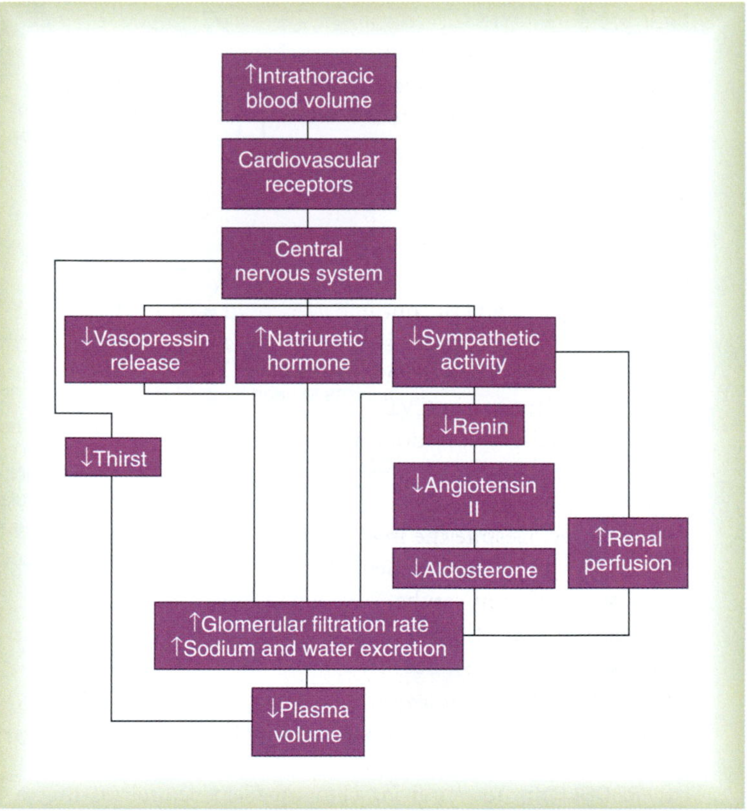

FIGURE 10-12 Major pathways for plasma volume control. See text for details. (Modified from Smith JJ, Kampine JP: Circulatory physiology: the essentials, ed 3, Baltimore, 1990, Williams & Wilkins.)

Chemoreceptors are small, highly vascularized tissues located near the high-pressure sensors in the aortic arch and carotid sinus that are sensitive to changes in blood chemistry. They are strongly stimulated by decreased O_2 tensions, although low pH or high levels of CO_2 also can increase their discharge rate. Simply put, the major cardiovascular effects of chemoreceptor stimulation are vasoconstriction and increased HR.

Because these changes occur only when the cardiopulmonary system is overtaxed, the chemoreceptors probably have little influence under normal conditions. However, their influence on respiration is clinically important. For this reason, the peripheral chemoreceptors are discussed in greater detail in Chapter 9.

Response to Changes in Overall Volume

The coordinated response of the cardiovascular system is best shown under abnormal conditions. Among the most common clinical conditions in which all essential regulatory mechanisms come into play is the large blood loss that occurs with hemorrhage. Figure 10-13 illustrates changes in these key factors during progressive blood loss in an animal model.

With 10% blood loss, the immediate decline in the CVP causes a 50% decrease in the discharge rate of the low-pressure (atrial) baroreceptors. There is little change in the activity of the high-pressure (arterial) receptors. The initial response, mediated through the medullary centers, is an increase in sympathetic discharge to the sinus node; this causes a progressive increase in HR. At the same time, plasma levels of antidiuretic hormone (vasopressin) begin to increase, thus maintaining normal arterial blood pressure.

As the blood loss becomes more severe (20%), atrial receptor activity decreases further; this increases the intensity of sympathetic discharge from the cardiovascular centers. Plasma antidiuretic hormone and HR continue to increase, as does peripheral vasculature tone. An increase in vascular tone occurs through constriction of the capacitance vessels in the venous system, slowing the decrease in CVP.[3]

The arterial pressure does not start to decrease until blood loss approaches 30%. At this point, arterial receptor activity begins to decrease, resulting in a marked increase in systemic vascular tone. Despite the magnitude of blood loss, CVP levels off. As long as no further hemorrhage occurs, blood pressure and tissue perfusion can be maintained at adequate levels.

If blood loss continues, central control mechanisms begin to take over. Massive vasoconstriction occurs in the resistance vessels, shunting blood away from skeletal muscle to maintain blood flow to the brain and heart. Increasing levels of local metabolites in these areas, especially CO_2 and other acids, override central control and cause further vessel dilation and increased blood flow. As these metabolites build up and as the tissues become hypoxic, cardiac function becomes impaired and vasodilation occurs throughout the body. This vasodilation signals the onset of irreversible shock, after which death ensues.

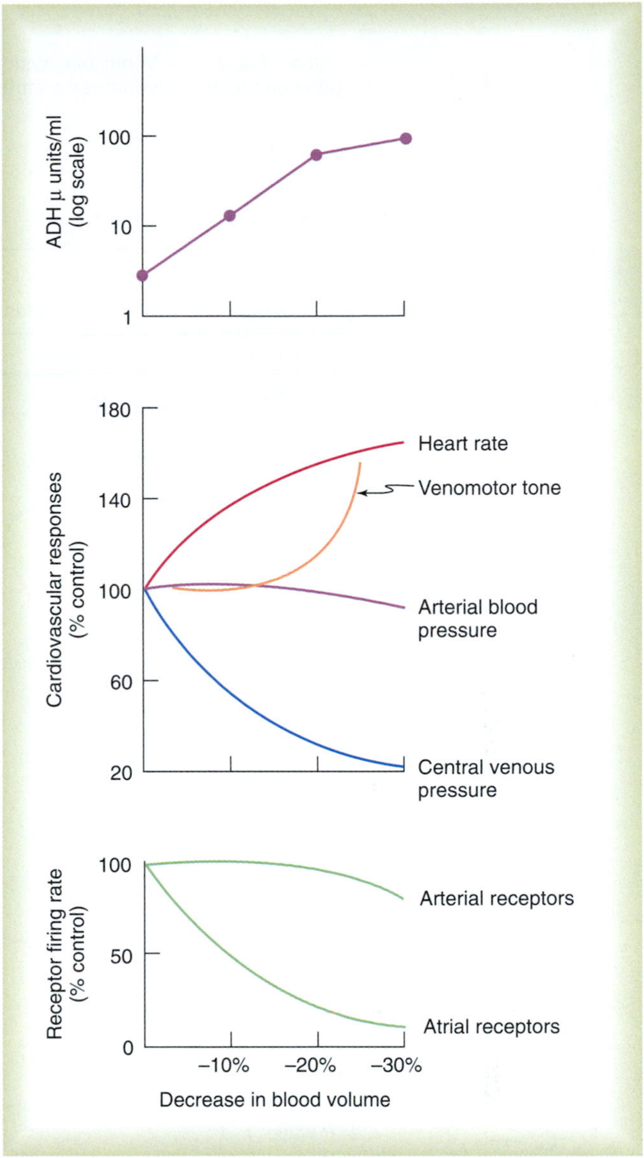

FIGURE 10-13 Plasma levels of antidiuretic hormone *(ADH)*, cardiovascular responses, and receptor firing rates in response to graded hemorrhage in the dog. See text for details. (From Richardson DR: Basic circulatory physiology, Boston, 1976, Little, Brown; venomotor tone data are those of W. Sears J, as cited in Gauer OH, Henry JP, Behn C: The regulation of extracellular fluid volume. Annu Rev Physiol 32:547, 1970. All other data are from Henry JP, et al: Can J Physiol Pharmacol 46:287, 1968.)

EVENTS OF THE CARDIAC CYCLE

This chapter has focused on the mechanical properties of the heart; the electrical activities of the heart are discussed in Chapter 18. Although they are discussed separately, the mechanical and electrical events are interdependent. Given the role of RTs in dealing with cardiovascular problems, an in-depth knowledge of how these events relate is essential.[2]

The events of the cardiac cycle are depicted in Figure 10-14. The top of the figure shows a time axis scaled in tenths of a second. Next are the timing bars for ventricular systole and diastole and pressure events in the atria, ventricles, and aorta. These are followed by an electrocardiogram (ECG), heart sounds, and ventricular flow (see Chapter 18 for an explanation of the ECG waves).

Going from left to right, the P wave (atrial depolarization) begins the ECG. Earlier, the ventricles have been passively filling

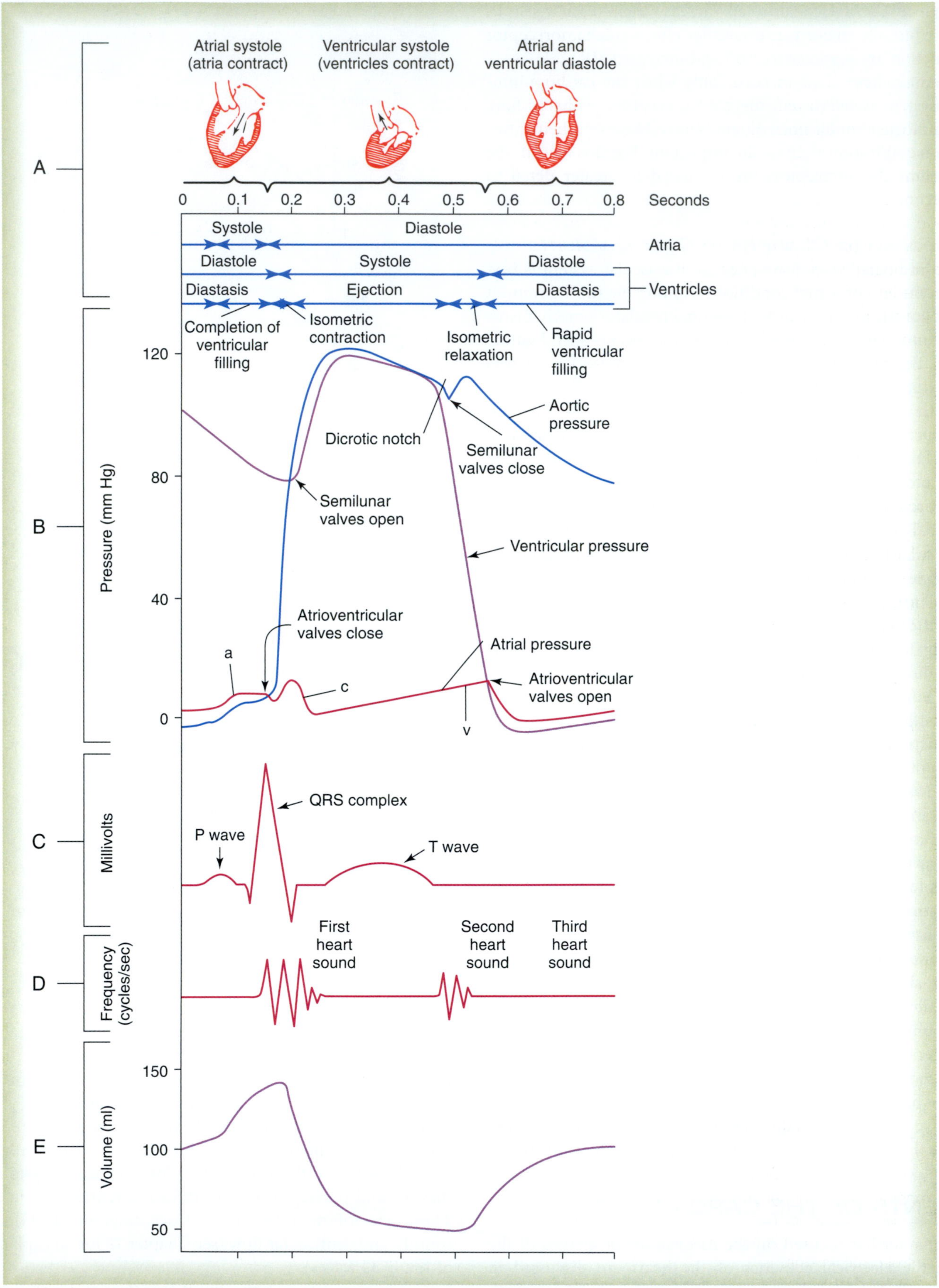

FIGURE 10-14 Cardiac cycle. **A,** Timing of cardiac events. **B,** Simultaneous pressures created in the aorta, left ventricle, and right atrium during the cardiac cycle. **C,** Electrical activity during the cardiac cycle. **D,** Heart sounds corresponding to the cardiac cycle. **E,** Ventricular blood volume during the cardiac cycle. (Modified from Moffett DF, Moffett SB, Schauf CL: Human physiology: foundations and frontiers, ed 2, St Louis, 1993, Mosby.)

with blood through the open AV valves. Within 0.1 second, the atria contract, causing a slight increase in both atrial and ventricular pressures *(a waves)*. This atrial contraction helps preload the ventricles, increasing their volume by 25%. This help from the atria to ventricular filling is called the *atrial kick*. Toward the end of diastole, the electrical impulses from the atria reach the AV node and bundle branches and ventricular depolarization (QRS complex) is initiated. Within a few hundredths of a second after depolarization, the ventricles begin to contract. As soon as ventricular pressures exceed pressures in the atria, the AV valves close. Closure of the mitral valve occurs first, followed immediately by closure of the tricuspid valve. This closure marks the end of ventricular diastole, producing the first heart sound on the phonocardiogram.[2]

Immediately after AV valve closure, the ventricles become closed chambers. During this short isovolemic phase of contraction, ventricular pressures increase rapidly. Upward bulging of the AV valves during this phase causes a slight upswing in atrial pressure graphs, called the *c wave*. Within 0.05 second, ventricular pressures increase to exceed the pressures in the aorta and pulmonary artery and opening the semilunar valves.

Toward the end of systole, as repolarization starts (indicated by the T wave), the ventricles begin to relax. Consequently, ventricular pressures decrease rapidly. When arterial pressures exceed pressures in the relaxing ventricles, the semilunar valves shut. Closure of the semilunar valves generates the second heart sound. Rather than immediately dropping off, aortic and pulmonary pressures increase again after the semilunar valves close. The *dicrotic notch* is caused by the elastic recoil of the arteries. This recoil provides the extra "push" that helps maintain the pressure created by the ventricles.

As the ventricles continue to relax, their pressures decrease to less than the pressures in the atria. This decline in pressure reopens the AV valves. As soon as the AV valves open, the blood collected in the atria rushes to fill the ventricles, causing a rapid decrease in atrial pressures (the *v wave*). Thereafter, ventricular filling slows as the heart prepares for a new cycle.

Knowledge of these events can help in understanding many of the diagnostic and monitoring procedures used for patients with cardiopulmonary disorders, including balloon-directed pulmonary artery catheterization and direct arterial pressure monitoring.

SUMMARY CHECKLIST

- The cardiovascular system consists of the heart and a vascular network that account for normal distribution and regulation of blood flow throughout the body to ensure tissue perfusion.
- Mechanical and electrical properties of cardiac tissue, combined with internal and external control mechanisms, provide the basis for coordinated cardiac function.
- The vascular system is regulated by local and central control mechanisms.
- CO is primarily determined by four factors: preload, afterload, contractility, and HR and is equivalent to the product of the SV × HR.
- Increased HR decreases CO by decreasing filling times (decreasing EDV) and decreasing contraction times, hence increasing ESV.
- Blood pressure is regulated by changing the volume of circulating blood, changing the capacity of the vascular system, or both.
- During increased demand, special compensatory mechanisms are called on to maintain stable blood flow.
- EF is the proportion of the EDV ejected on each stroke (SV/EDV).
- Failure of cardiovascular control mechanisms often requires clinical the intervention to help restore normal function.

References

1. Thibodaux GA, Patton KT: *Anatomy and physiology*, ed 7, St Louis, 2011, Mosby.
2. Marieb EN, Hoehn KN: *Anatomy and physiology*, ed 7, San Francisco, 2014, Pearson Benjamin Cummings.
3. Des Jardins T: *Cardiopulmonary anatomy and physiology*, ed 6, New York, 2013, Delmar Cengage Learning.
4. Berne RM, Levy MN, editors: *Physiology*, ed 6, St Louis, 2010, Mosby.
5. Barret KE, Barman SM, Boitano S, et al: *Ganong's review of medical physiology*, ed 24, New York, 2012, McGraw-Hill.
6. Wilkins RL, Sheldon RL, Krider SJ: *Clinical assessment in respiratory care*, ed 7, St Louis, 2013, Elsevier.
7. Michie DD, Kline J: The heart as a muscle and a pump. In Kline J, editor: *Biological foundations of biomedical engineering*, Boston, 1976, Little, Brown and Company, p 111.
8. Norton JM: Toward consistent definitions for preload and afterload. *Adv Physiol Educ* 25:53, 2001.

Bibliography

Andreoli TE, Benjamin I, Griggs RC, et al: *Cecil essentials of medicine*, ed 8, Philadelphia, 2010, WB Saunders.

Guyton AC, Hall JE: *Textbook of medical physiology*, ed 12, Philadelphia, 2010, WB Saunders.

Hess DR, MacIntyre NR, Mishoe SC, et al: *Respiratory care principles and practice*, ed 2, Boston, 2011, Jones & Bartlett Learning.

Moses KP, Nava P, Banks J, et al: *Atlas of clinical gross anatomy*, ed 2, St Louis, 2012, Mosby.

Stevens A, Lowe J: *Human histology*, ed 4, St Louis, 2014, Mosby.

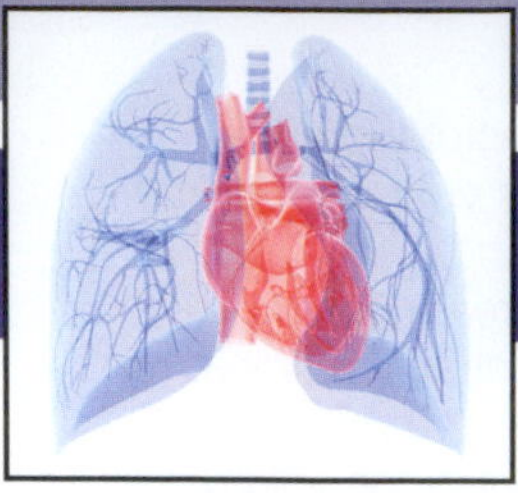

CHAPTER 11

Ventilation

EDUARDO MIRELES-CABODEVILA, ROBERT L. CHATBURN

CHAPTER OBJECTIVES

After reading this chapter you will be able to:

- Describe the physiologic functions provided by ventilation.
- Describe the pressure gradients responsible for gas flow, diffusion, and lung inflation.
- Identify the forces that oppose gas movement into and out of the lungs.
- Describe how surface tension contributes to lung recoil.
- Describe how lung, chest wall, and total compliance are related.
- State the factors that affect resistance to breathing.
- Describe how various lung diseases affect the work of breathing.
- State why ventilation is not evenly distributed throughout the lung.
- Describe how the time constants affect alveolar filling and emptying.
- Identify the factors that affect alveolar ventilation.
- State how to calculate alveolar ventilation, dead space, and the V_D/V_T ratio.

CHAPTER OUTLINE

KEY TERMS

airway resistance
alveolar dead space
compliance
dynamic compression
dynamic hyperinflation (air trapping)
elastance
elasticity
equal pressure point (EPP)
hyperventilation
hypoventilation
hysteresis
minute ventilation
physiologic dead space
plethysmograph
pneumotachometer
pressure gradient
sub-atmospheric
surface tension
tidal volume (V_T)
time constant
transairway pressure gradient
transairway pressure (P_{TAW})
transalveolar pressure (P_{TA})
trans–chest wall pressure (P_{TCW})
transpulmonary pressure difference (P_{TP})
transpulmonary pressure gradient
transrespiratory pressure (P_{TR})
transthoracic pressure difference (P_{TT})

The main functions of the lungs are to supply the body with oxygen and to remove carbon dioxide. To perform these functions, the lungs must be adequately ventilated. **Ventilation** is the process of moving gas (usually air) in and out of the lungs. Ventilation is to be distinguished from respiration, which refers to the physiologic processes of O_2 use at the cellular level.

In health, ventilation is regulated to meet the body's needs under a wide range of conditions. In disease, this process can be markedly disrupted and often results in inadequate ventilation and/or increased work of breathing. Respiratory care is directed toward restoring and supporting adequate and efficient ventilation. To provide effective respiratory care we need to have a solid understanding of the normal ventilation processes and of how diseases may affect it.

MECHANICS OF VENTILATION

Ventilation is a cycle. This cycle has two phases: inspiration and expiration. During each cycle, a volume of gas moves in and out of the respiratory tract. This volume, measured during either inspiration or expiration, is called the **tidal volume (V_T).** The V_T refreshes the gas present in the lung, removing CO_2 and supplying O_2 to meet metabolic needs. The V_T must be able to meet changing metabolic demands, such as during exercise or sleep. To achieve ventilation the respiratory muscles (and/or a mechanical ventilator) have to generate changes in pressure (a pressure gradient, see later discussion) so that gas will flow on in or out of the lungs. To better understand the forces that the muscles (or/and the machine) have to overcome to generate ventilation, we use a formula. This formula is a simplified version of the equation of motion for the respiratory system:

$$\Delta\text{Pressure} = (\text{Elastance} \times \Delta\text{Volume}) + (\text{Resistance} \times \Delta\text{Flow})$$

where:

ΔPressure = Force generated by the respiratory muscles or a mechanical ventilator, or both, during inspiration. This "pressure" is actually a pressure difference (see next section).

Volume = Volume change (e.g., V_T)

Elastance = Distensibility of the lungs and thorax (Δpressure/Δvolume); elastance is the reciprocal of compliance (Δvolume/Δpressure)

Resistance = Airflow and tissue resistance (Δpressure/Δflow)

Flow = Volume change per unit of time

In this equation, the terms *(elastance × volume)* and *(resistance × flow)* represent the loads (elastic and resistive) against which the respiratory muscles or ventilator must work to achieve gas movement. Thus you can now see that in patients with high elastance or/and high resistance the pressure needed to achieve ventilation will be high. In healthy lungs, this work is minimal and is performed during the inspiratory phase. Expiration is normally passive (i.e., no muscle force involved) and the result of the elastic recoil of the lung.

In discussing ventilation, it may be helpful to review some details about the equation of motion. First remember it is a mathematical model. This model lumps all the resistances of the many airways into a single flow-conducting tube and lumps *all* the elastances of the alveoli and airways into a single elastic compartment (see later discussions about elastance, compliance, and resistance). The graphic model is shown in Figure 11-1.[1] Surrounding the "lungs" is another elastic compartment representing the chest wall. This graphic depiction of the respiratory system allows us to define points in space where pressures may be measured (or inferred) as defined in Table 11-1.

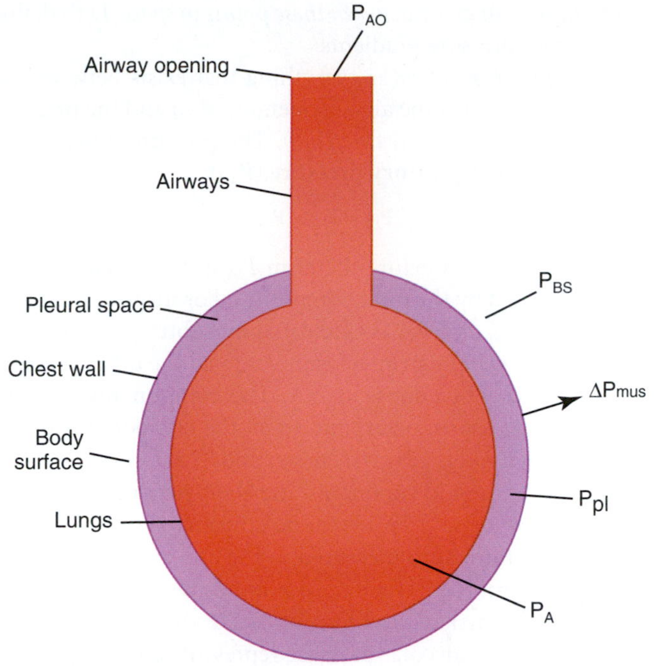

FIGURE 11-1 Schematic diagram of the respiratory system consisting of a flow-conducting tube (representing the airways) connected to a single elastic compartment (representing the lungs) surrounded by another elastic compartment (representing the chest wall). *ΔP_{mus}*, Muscle pressure difference; *P_A*, alveolar pressure; *P_{AO}*, pressure at the airway opening; *P_{BS}*, pressure on the body surface; *P_{pl}*, pressure in the intrapleural space. (From Primiano FP Jr, Chatburn RL: Zen and the art of nomenclature maintenance: a revised approach to respiratory symbols and terminology. Respir Care 51:1458, 2006.)

TABLE 11-1
Measurable Pressures Used in Describing Respiratory System Mechanics

Name	Symbol	Definition
Pressure at the airway opening	P_{AO}	Pressure measured at the opening of the respiratory system airway (e.g., mouth and nose, tracheostomy opening, and endotracheal tube opening)
Pleural pressure	P_{pl}	Pressure measured in the pleural space, changes that are often estimated by measuring pressure changes in the esophagus
Alveolar pressure	P_A	Pressure in the alveolar (gas space) region of the lungs
Body surface pressure	P_{BS}	Pressure measured at the body surface

Pressure Differences During Breathing

A pressure gradient is needed to achieve gas flow from one place to another. Using the equation of motion we can recognize the pressure gradients or differences in pressure between two points in space. in each of the components of the model. The components of the model (airways, lungs, and chest wall) are *defined as everything that exists between these points in space.* Let's define each of these pressure gradients.

The *respiratory system* is everything that exists between the pressure measured at the airway opening (P_{AO}) and the pressure measured at the body surface (P_{BS}). The pressure difference is called the **transrespiratory pressure (P_{TR}):**

$$P_{TR} = P_{AO} - P_{BS}$$

The term P_{AO} comes before the term P_{BS} in the equation. This order is dictated by the direction of flow. For inspiration, P_{AO} is higher than P_{BS}, and P_{TR} is calculated by subtracting P_{BS} from P_{AO}. The same general principle applies to all the other pressure differences described subsequently. The components of transrespiratory pressure correspond to all the components of the graphic model (i.e., airways, lungs, and chest wall). We can further divide these components and their pressure gradients. Starting at the airways in this model, the airways are whatever exists between pressure measured at the airway opening (P_{AO}) and pressure measured in the alveoli of the lungs (P_A). The graphic model makes the lungs look like one giant alveolus, which means that alveolar pressure represents an average pressure over all alveoli in real lungs. The pressure difference is called the **transairway pressure (P_{TAW}):**

$$P_{TAW} = P_{AO} - P_A$$

Thus P_{TAW} represents all the airways (real and artificial).

The alveolar region is whatever exists between pressure measured in the alveolus and pressure measured in the pleural space (P_{pl}). The associated pressure difference is **transalveolar pressure (P_{TA}):**

$$P_{TA} = P_A - P_{pl}$$

The P_{TA} represents all the alveoli as if they were one single alveolus.

We also take into account the chest wall. The chest wall exists between pressure measured in the pleural space and the pressure on the body surface. The pressure difference is called **trans–chest wall pressure (P_{TCW}):**

$$P_{TCW} = P_{pl} - P_{BS}$$

Some of these components can be combined to encompass structures that are of clinical importance. One of the most used combinations joins the airways (P_{TAW}) and alveolar region (P_{TA}) to assess the pulmonary system, and this is called the **transpulmonary pressure difference (P_{TP}):**

$$P_{TP} = P_{AO} - P_{pl}$$

What may be confusing is that there are other definitions of transpulmonary pressure in the literature. Some authors define P_{TP} as $P_A - P_{pl}$. The confusion arises from the fact that $P_{TA} = P_A - P_{pl}$, *but only under static conditions.* Static conditions can be imposed during mechanical ventilation by using an inspiratory or expiratory hold maneuver. This situation should be considered a special case of P_{TP}; however, the general case is $P_{TP} = P_{AO} - P_{pl}$, which shows what pressures must be measured to derive the mechanical properties of the pulmonary system under either static or dynamic (breathing) conditions. If we want to evaluate the elastance and resistance of *the pulmonary system,* we substitute P_{TP} for P in the equation of motion. Alternatively, if we want to evaluate the *total respiratory system* elastance and resistance, we substitute P_{TR} for P.

TABLE 11-2

Pressure Differences Used in Describing Respiratory System Mechanics

Definition	Name	Symbol
$P_{AO} - P_{BS}$	Transrespiratory pressure difference	ΔP_{TR}
$P_{AO} - P_A$	Transairway pressure difference	ΔP_{TAW}
$P_{AO} - P_{pl}$	Transpulmonary pressure difference	ΔP_{TP}
$P_A - P_{pl}$	Transalveolar pressure difference	ΔP_{TA}
$P_A - P_{BS}$	Transthoracic pressure difference	ΔP_{TT}
$P_{pl} - P_{BS}$	Trans–chest wall pressure difference	ΔP_{TCW}
	Global muscle pressure difference	ΔP_{mus}

Sometimes it may be useful to define the pressure required to expand the lung and chest wall components; to do this we use the **transthoracic pressure difference (P_{TT}),** which is defined as:

$$P_{TT} = P_A - P_{BS}$$

We use the transrespiratory **pressure gradient** and the other gradients to understand the gas flow into and out of the alveoli during breathing. Table 11-2 summarizes these equations. For a spontaneously breathing person, P_A is **sub-atmospheric** in the beginning of inspiration compared with P_{AO}, causing air to flow into the alveoli. The opposite happens in the beginning of exhalation; P_A is higher than P_{AO}, causing air to flow out of the airway opening. During a normal breathing cycle, the glottis remains open. The P_{BS} and P_{AO} remain at zero (i.e., atmospheric) throughout the cycle; only changes in P_A and P_{pl} are of interest. It is often helpful to use these to describe the changes in pressures during a breathing cycle.

Before inspiration, pleural pressure is approximately −5 cm H_2O (i.e., 5 cm H_2O below atmospheric pressure), and alveolar pressure is 0 cm H_2O. The **transpulmonary pressure gradient** is also approximately 5 cm H_2O in the resting state, that is, $P_{TP} = P_{AO} - P_{pl} = 0 - (-5) = 5$. This positive end-expiratory P_{TP} maintains the lung at its resting volume, functional residual capacity (FRC). Airway opening and alveolar pressures are both zero, so the **transairway pressure gradient** also is zero. No gas moves into or out of the respiratory tract.

Inspiration begins when muscular effort expands the thorax. Thoracic expansion causes a *decrease* in pleural pressure. This decrease in pleural pressure causes a positive change to P_{TP} and P_{TA}, which induces flow into the lungs. The inspiratory flow is proportional to the positive change in transairway pressure difference; the higher the change in P_{TA}, the higher is the flow.

Pleural pressure continues to decrease until the end of inspiration. Alveolar filling slows when alveolar pressure approaches equilibrium with the atmosphere, and inspiratory flow decreases to zero (Figure 11-2). At this point, called *end-inspiration,* alveolar pressure has returned to zero, and the intrapleural

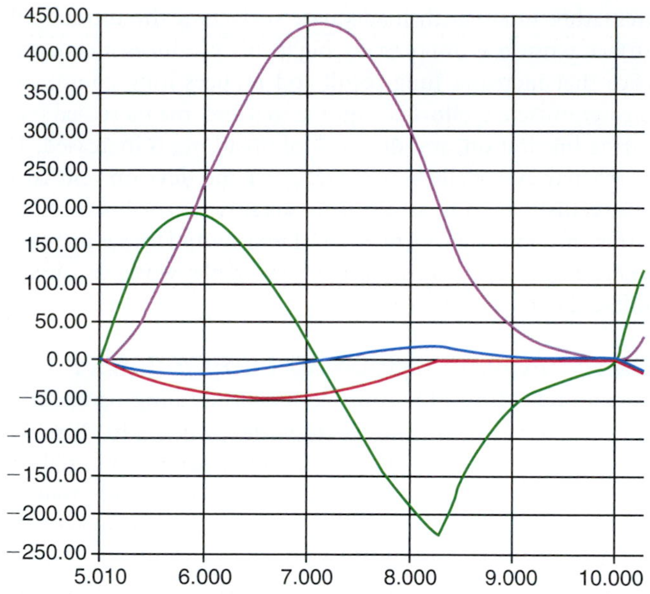

FIGURE 11-2 Waveforms for normal breathing. *Red,* Change in pleural pressure relative to end-expiratory value (cm H_2O, scaled times 10); *blue,* alveolar pressure (cm H_2O, scaled times 10); *green,* flow (L/min, scaled times 10); *purple,* volume (ml).

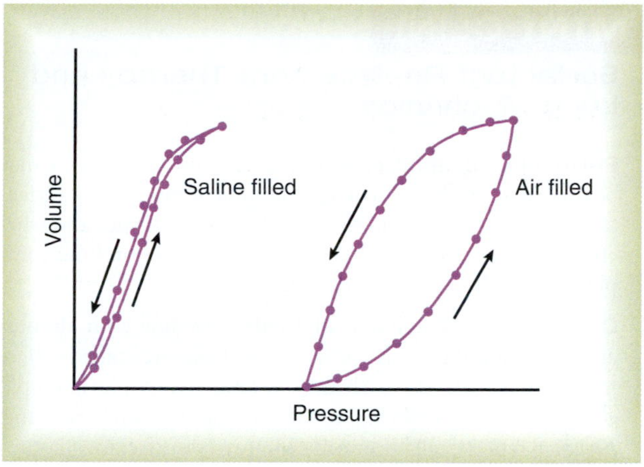

FIGURE 11-3 Static pressure-volume curves of saline-filled and air-filled excised lungs. In the saline-filled lung, the distending pressure is the same during inflation and deflation. The air-filled lung shows hysteresis (i.e., higher pressure for a given volume on inflation compared with deflation). The hysteresis results in part from the effects of surface tension forces caused by the air-liquid interface in the alveoli. (Modified from Slonim NB, Hamilton LH: Respiratory physiology, ed 5, St Louis, 1987, Mosby.)

pressure—and hence transpulmonary pressure gradient—reaches the maximal value (for a normal breath) of approximately 10 cm H_2O.

At end inspiration the muscle pressure relaxes and now alveolar pressure is higher than pressure at the airway opening, driving flow in the expiratory direction. The equation of motion shows this, setting the driving pressure, P_{mus}, to zero:

$$P_{mus} = 0 = (\text{Elastance} \times \text{Volume}) + (\text{Resistance} \times \text{Flow})$$

Rearranging the formula, we get:

$$\begin{aligned}(\text{Elastance} \times \text{Volume}) &= -(\text{Resistance} \times \text{Flow}) \\ &= \text{Resistance} \times (-\text{Flow})\end{aligned}$$

This equation says two important things: (1) Flow is negative, indicating expiration, and (2) the driving force (transthoracic pressure, equal to elastance × volume) for expiratory flow is the energy stored in the combined elastances of lungs and chest wall (the total elastance is the sum of the chest wall and lung elastances).

These events occur during normal V_T excursions. Similar pressure changes accompany deeper inspiration and expiration. The magnitude of the pressure changes is greater with deeper breathing. Pleural pressures are always negative (subatmospheric) during normal inspiration and exhalation. During forced inspiration with a big downward movement of the diaphragm, the pleural pressure can decrease to −50 cm H_2O, whereas during a forced expiration, pleural pressure may increase above atmospheric pressure to 50 to 100 cm H_2O.

Forces Opposing Inflation of the Lung

The lungs have a tendency to recoil inward, whereas the chest wall tends to move outward; these opposing forces keep the lung at its resting volume (i.e., FRC). To generate the previously described pressure gradients, the lungs must be distended. This distention requires several opposing forces to be overcome for inspiration to occur. As indicated in the equation of motion, the forces opposing lung inflation may be grouped into two categories: *elastic forces* and *frictional forces.* Elastic forces involve the tissues of the lungs, thorax, and abdomen, along with surface tension in the alveoli. Frictional forces include resistance caused by gas flow through the airways (natural and artificial) and tissue movement during breathing.

Surface Tension Forces

Part of the hysteresis (difference between inspiratory and expiratory pressure-volume curves) exhibited by the lung is a result of **surface tension** forces in the alveoli. If a lung is filled with fluid such as saline, the pressure-volume curves look much different than the pressure-volume curves of an air-filled lung (Figure 11-3). Less pressure is needed to inflate a fluid-filled lung to a given volume. This phenomenon indicates that a gas-fluid *interface* in the air-filled lung changes its inflation-deflation characteristics.

The recoil of the lung is a combination of tissue elasticity and the surface tension forces in the alveoli. During inflation, additional pressure is needed to overcome surface tension forces. During deflation, surface tension forces are reduced, resulting in altered pressure-volume characteristics (i.e., the leftward shift seen in Figure 11-3). In the intact lung (i.e., within the chest), the volume history also affects the degree of hysteresis that occurs. Factors such as the initial volume, the tidal excursion, and whether the lungs have been previously inflated or deflated help determine the volume history and the shape of the pressure-volume curves of the lung.

MINI CLINI

Surfactant Replacement Therapy and Lung Mechanics

PROBLEM: If an infant is born prematurely, the lungs may be unable to produce adequate amounts of pulmonary surfactant. How does this condition affect lung mechanics and what effect does surfactant replacement therapy have on lung compliance and the work of breathing?

DISCUSSION: The liquid molecules that line each alveolus attract one another. This attraction creates a force called *surface tension,* which tends to shrink the alveolus. A phospholipid called *pulmonary surfactant* reduces surface tension in the lung. Alveolar type II cells produce pulmonary surfactant. In contrast to typical surface-active agents, pulmonary surfactant changes surface tension according to its area.[2] The ability of pulmonary surfactant to reduce surface tension decreases as surface area (i.e., lung volume) increases. Conversely, when surface area decreases, the ability of pulmonary surfactant to reduce surface tension increases. This property of changing surface tension to match lung volume helps stabilize the alveoli. Any disorder that alters or destroys pulmonary surfactant can cause significant changes in the work of distending the lung.

The mechanism of action of pulmonary surfactant molecules is based on its weak intramolecular attractive forces. When surfactant molecules are mixed with other liquid molecules that have higher intramolecular attraction, the surfactant molecules are pushed to the surface of the liquid, where they form the air-liquid interface. Because of the weak intramolecular attraction between these surfactant molecules at the surface, the liquid lining of the alveoli exhibits much less surface tension than it would in the absence of pulmonary surfactant. In a premature infant with inadequate surfactant the intraalveolar surface tension is abnormally high; this produces a collapsing force that increases lung recoil and reduces lung compliance. Greater muscular effort is required to overcome increased recoil during inspiration, and the work of breathing is increased. The infant may eventually become fatigued and develop ventilatory failure. Instillation of artificial surfactant into the lungs reduces surface tension to its normal level. Lung compliance is increased, elastic recoil is reduced, and the muscular work required to inflate the lung is reduced.

Elastic Forces Opposing Lung Inflation

Elastin and *collagen* fibers are found in the lung parenchyma. These tissues give the lung the property of elasticity. **Elasticity** is the physical tendency of an object to return to an initial state after deformation. When stretched, an elastic body tends to return to its original shape. The tension developed when an elastic structure is stretched is proportional to the degree of deformation produced (Hooke's law). An example is a simple spring (Figure 11-4). When tension on a spring is increased, the spring lengthens. However, the ability of the spring to stretch is limited. When the point of maximal stretch is reached, further tension produces little or no increase in length. Additional tension may break the spring.

In the respiratory system, inflation stretches tissue. The elastic properties of the lungs and chest wall oppose inflation. To increase lung volume, pressure must be applied. This property may be shown by subjecting an excised lung to changes in transpulmonary pressure and measuring the associated changes in volume (Figure 11-5). To simulate the pressures during breathing, the lung is placed in an airtight jar. The force to inflate the lung is provided by a pump that varies the pressure around the lung inside the jar, simulating P_{pl}. This action mimics the pleural pressure changes associated with thoracic

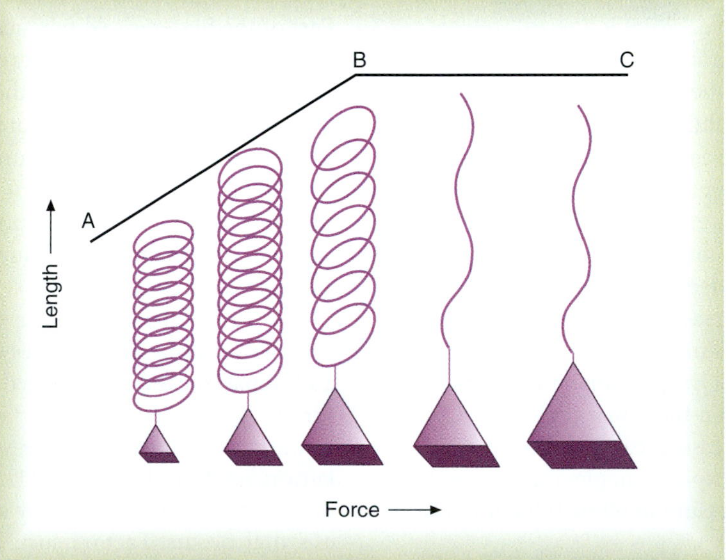

FIGURE 11-4 Graphic representation of the force-length relationship applied to a simple spring (increase in length with increase in force). With increasing force, or weight in this example, the spring lengthens from *A* to *B,* but at the point of maximal stretch, further force produces no additional increase in length (*B* to *C*).

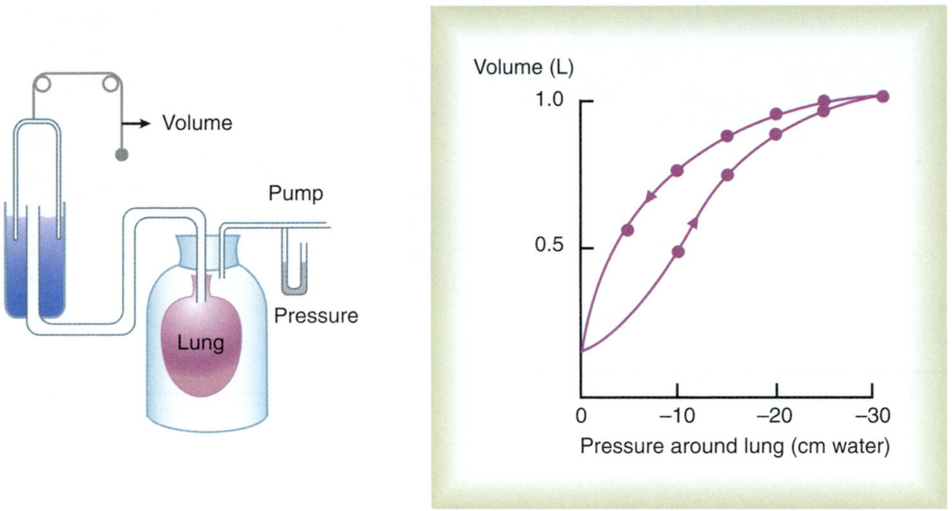

FIGURE 11-5 Measurement of the pressure-volume curve of an excised lung. The lung is placed in a sealed jar and connected to a spirometer (to measure volume). A pump generates sub-atmospheric pressure around the lung while its volume is measured. The curve plotting the relationship between pressure and volume is nonlinear and flattens at high expanding pressures (sub-atmospheric). The inflation and deflation curves are not the same. This difference is called *hysteresis.* (Modified from West JB: Respiratory physiology: the essentials, ed 7, Baltimore, 2005, Williams & Wilkins.)

expansion and contraction. The changes in transpulmonary pressure are made in discrete steps, allowing the lungs to come to rest in between so that all of the applied pressure opposes elastic forces and none of it opposes resistive forces (i.e., flow is zero when the measurements are made). The amount of stretch (inflation) is measured as volume by a spirometer. Changes in volume resulting from changes in transpulmonary pressure are plotted on a graph.

During inspiration in this model, increasingly greater negative pleural pressures are required to stretch the lung to a larger volume. As the lung is stretched to its maximum (total lung capacity [TLC]), the inflation curve becomes flat. This flattening indicates *increasing* opposition to expansion (i.e., for the same change in transpulmonary pressure, there is less change in volume).[3]

As with a spring when tension is removed, deflation occurs passively as pressure in the jar is allowed to return toward atmospheric pressure. Deflation of the lung does not follow the inflation curve exactly. During deflation, lung volume at any given pressure is slightly greater than it is during inflation. This difference between the inflation and deflation curves is called **hysteresis.**[3] Hysteresis indicates that factors other than simple elastic tissue forces are present. The major factor, particularly in sick lungs, is the opening of collapsed alveoli during inspiration that tend to stay open during expiration until very low lung volumes are reached.

Compliance

Compliance (C, the reciprocal of elastance, E) is caused by the tissue elastic forces and surface tension that oppose lung inflation. Compliance is defined as the constant of proportionality between volume (V) and pressure (P) in an elastic system and is usually expressed in units of ml/cm H_2O:

$$C = \frac{\Delta V}{\Delta P} = \frac{1}{E}$$

To calculate lung compliance, ΔP_{TP} is substituted for ΔP. To calculate respiratory system compliance, use ΔP_{TR}. To calculate chest wall compliance, use ΔP_{TCW}.

A graph of change in lung volume versus change in transpulmonary pressure (Figure 11-6, *A*) is called the *compliance curve of the lungs.* Figure 11-6, *B* compares a normal lung compliance curve with curves that might be observed in patients who have emphysema (obstructive lung disease) or pulmonary fibrosis (restrictive lung disease). The curve from a patient with emphysema is steeper and displaced to the left. The shape and position of this curve represent large changes in volume for small pressure changes (increased compliance). Increased compliance results primarily from loss of elastic fibers, which occurs in emphysema. The lungs become more distensible so that a normal transpulmonary pressure results in a larger lung volume. The term *hyperinflation* is used to describe an abnormally increased lung volume. A distinctly opposite pattern is seen in pulmonary fibrosis. Interstitial fibrosis is characterized by an increase in connective tissue. The compliance curve of a patient with pulmonary fibrosis is flatter than the normal curve, shifted down and to the right. As a result, there is a smaller volume change for any given pressure change (decreased compliance). Consequently, the lungs become stiffer, usually with a reduced volume.

Inflation and deflation of the lung occur with changes in the dimensions of the chest wall. The relationship between the lungs and the chest wall can be illustrated by plotting their relaxation pressure curves separately and combined (Figure 11-7). In the intact thorax, the lungs and chest wall recoil against each other. The point at which these opposing forces balance determines the resting volume of the lungs, or FRC.

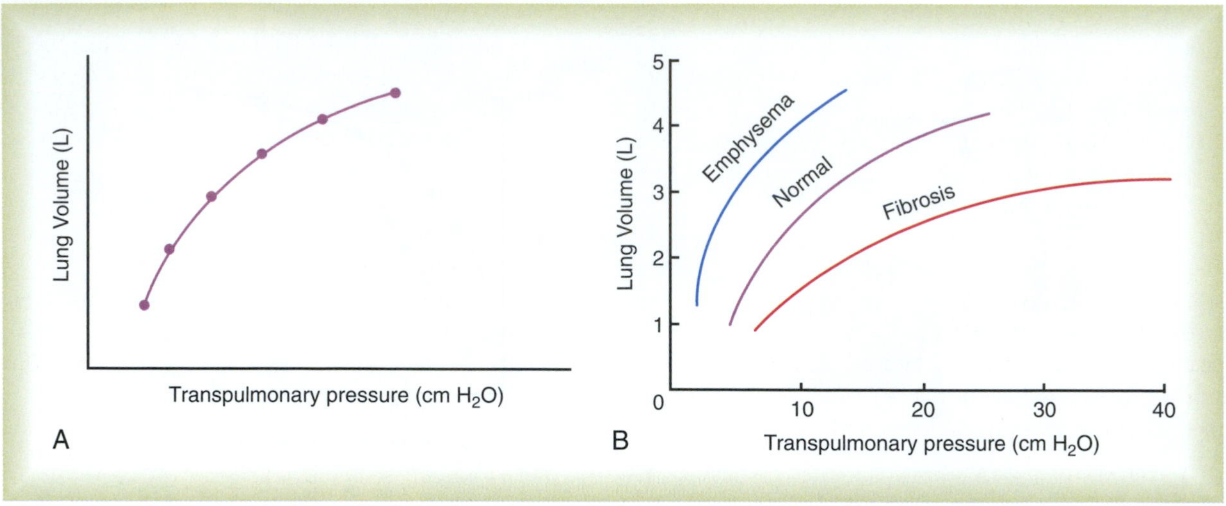

FIGURE 11-6 **A,** Compliance measurement (deflation curve). After swallowing an esophageal balloon, the person inhales a full breath and then exhales slowly. At specific lung volumes, he holds his breath with the glottis open, ensuring an alveolar pressure of zero. Lung volume is plotted against transpulmonary pressure (esophageal pressure is assumed to reflect pleural pressure) generating a compliance curve. **B,** Compliance curves. Normal lung compliance is approximately 0.2 L/cm H_2O (measured from the lower portion of the curve, near resting lung volume). Compliance is increased in emphysema because of the destruction of elastic tissue; conversely, it is decreased in pulmonary fibrosis because of increased elastic recoil. (Modified from Martin L: Pulmonary physiology in clinical practice: the essentials for patient care and evaluation, St Louis, 1987, Mosby.)

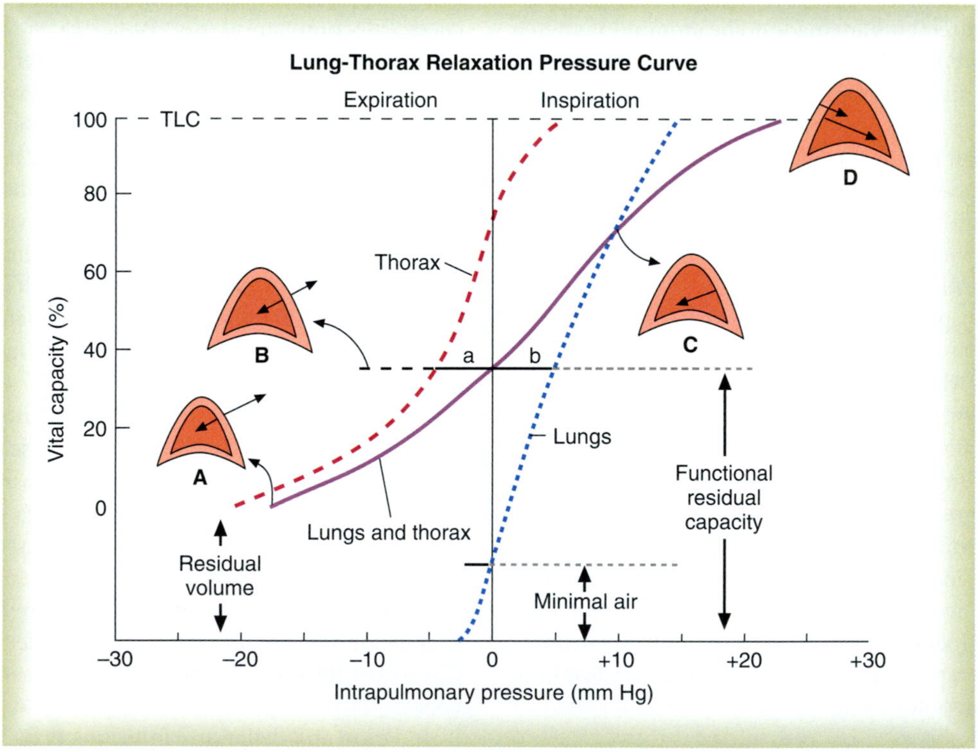

FIGURE 11-7 Relationship between the lungs and chest wall. Volumes of the lungs, thorax, and lungs and thorax combined are plotted as a percentage of vital capacity against intrapulmonary pressure (recoil pressure). The combined lung-thorax relaxation curve *(solid line)* is the sum of the individual lung and thorax curves. Equilibrium (zero pressure) occurs where the lung and thoracic recoil forces balance (a + b = 0). This point determines the functional residual capacity (lung *B*). Lung *A* represents low lung volume with greater recoil pressure exerted by the chest wall. Lung *C* shows a chest wall recoil of zero at approximately 70% of TLC. When lung volume is greater than 70% of TLC, greater pressures are required to distend both the lungs and the thorax (lung *D*). (Modified from Beachey W: Respiratory care anatomy and physiology, ed 2, St Louis, 2007, Mosby.)

This is also the point at which alveolar pressure equals atmospheric pressure. The normal FRC is approximately 40% of the TLC. The opposing forces between the chest wall and lungs are partially responsible for the sub-atmospheric pressure in the intrapleural space. Diseases that alter the compliance of either the chest wall or the lung often disrupt the balance point, usually with a change in lung volume.

Combined Compliances

The two lungs have their own (usually different) compliances. However, the muscles (or ventilator) see a combined compliance. Because the lungs have the same driving pressure but different flows, they are said to be connected in parallel. Parallel compliances combine by simple addition:

$$\text{Parallel compliances: } C_{total} = C_{right} + C_{left}$$

The total compliance of a parallel connection is more than any of the components.

The total lung compliance is connected in series with the chest wall compliance, meaning they have different driving pressures but the same flow. Series compliances combine as follows:

$$\text{Series compliances: } C_{total} = \frac{C_{chestwall} \times C_{lungs}}{C_{chestwall} + C_{lungs}}$$

The total compliance of a series connection is less than any of the components.

RULE OF THUMB

The lungs and chest wall each have their own compliance, or distensibility. In healthy adults, the compliance of the lungs and chest wall are each equal to approximately 0.2 L/cm H_2O. However, because the lungs are contained within the thorax, the two systems act as springs pulling against the driving force. This reduces the compliance of the system to approximately half that of the individual components, or 0.1 L/cm H_2O. This rule has many practical implications, particularly for mechanical ventilation of the lungs. Compliance of the chest wall, similar to lung compliance, is a measure of distensibility. Any disease process that alters the compliance of the lungs or chest wall can seriously disrupt the normal mechanics of ventilation. Obesity, kyphoscoliosis, ankylosing spondylitis, and many other abnormalities can reduce chest wall compliance and lung volumes.

Inhalation occurs when the balance between the lungs and chest wall shifts. Energy from the respiratory muscles (primarily the diaphragm) overcomes the contractile force of the lungs. At the beginning of the breath, the tendency of the chest wall to expand facilitates lung expansion. When lung volume nears 70% of the total lung capacity, the chest wall reaches its natural resting level. To inspire to a lung volume greater than approximately 70% of total lung capacity (TLC), the inspiratory muscles must overcome the recoil of both the lungs and the chest wall (see Figure 11-7).

For exhalation, potential energy "stored" in the stretched lung (and chest wall at high volumes) during the preceding inspiration causes passive deflation. To exhale below the resting level (FRC), muscular effort is required to overcome the tendency of the chest wall to expand. The expiration provides this energy.

Resistive Forces Opposing Lung Inflation

Frictional forces also oppose ventilation. Frictional opposition forces differ from the elastic properties of the lungs and thorax. Frictional opposition occurs only when the system is in motion. Frictional opposition to ventilation has the two components tissue viscous resistance and airway resistance.

Tissue Viscous Resistance. Tissue viscous resistance is the impedance of motion (opposition to flow) caused by displacement of tissues during ventilation. Displaced tissues include the lungs, rib cage, diaphragm, and abdominal organs. The frictional resistance is generated by the movement of each organ surface sliding against the other (e.g., the lung lobes sliding against each other and against the chest wall). Tissue resistance accounts for only approximately 20% of the total resistance to lung inflation. However, in conditions such as obesity, pleural fibrosis, and ascites, the tissue viscous resistance will increase the total impedance to ventilation.

Airway Resistance. Gas flow through the airways also causes frictional impedance, called *flow resistance.* Resistance to ventilation by the movement of gas through the airways is called **airway resistance.** Airway resistance accounts for approximately 80% of the frictional resistance to ventilation.

Resistance is defined as the constant of proportionality between pressure (P) and flow ($\dot{V}$) in a flow-conducting system and is usually expressed in units of cm H_2O/L/sec:

$$R = \frac{\Delta P}{\Delta \dot{V}}$$

To calculate airway resistance, R_{aw}, use ΔP_{TA} instead of ΔP. To calculate respiratory system resistance, use ΔP_{TR}.

Airway resistance in healthy adults ranges from approximately 0.5 to 2.5 cm H_2O/L/sec. To cause gas to flow into or out of the lungs at 1 L/sec, a healthy person needs to lower his or her alveolar pressure only 0.5 to 2.5 cm H_2O below atmospheric pressure.

R_{aw} in nonventilated patients is usually measured in a pulmonary function laboratory. Flow is measured with a **pneumotachometer.** Alveolar pressures are determined in a body **plethysmograph,** an airtight box in which the patient sits. By momentarily occluding the patient's airway and measuring the pressure at the mouth, alveolar pressure can be estimated (i.e., mouth pressure equals alveolar pressure under conditions of no flow). By relating flow and alveolar pressure to changes in plethysmograph pressure, airway resistance can be calculated.

Combined Resistances

The right and left main stem bronchi have their own (usually different) resistances. However, the muscles (or ventilator) see a combined resistance. Because these airways have the same driving pressure but different flows, they are said to be connected in parallel. Parallel compliances combine like compliances in series, as follows:

$$\text{Parallel resistances: } R_{total} = \frac{R_{right} \times R_{left}}{R_{right} + R_{left}}$$

The total resistance of a parallel connection is less than that of any of the components.

The bronchial airway resistance is connected in series with upper airway (and artificial airway, if any), meaning that they have different driving pressures but the same flow. Series resistances combine like compliances in parallel:

$$\text{Series resistance: } R_{total} = R_{upper\ airway} + R_{bronchi}$$

The total resistance of a series connection is more than that any of the components.

MINI CLINI

Helium and Oxygen Therapy for Large Airway Obstruction

PROBLEM: Patients with significant obstruction in the upper airway, trachea, or main stem bronchi expend a large amount of energy overcoming the resistance to breathing. What type of gas therapy would be most advantageous in this situation?

DISCUSSION: Because most (approximately 80%) of the resistance to breathing occurs in the upper and large airways, disease processes that increase resistance in these airways cause tremendous increases in the work of breathing. Vocal cord edema, tumors in the trachea, and foreign bodies in main stem bronchi are examples of the types of clinical conditions that can markedly increase the work of breathing. Patients who must breathe against high levels of resistance are prone to respiratory muscle fatigue and failure. Gas flow in the upper and large airways is predominantly turbulent. Turbulent flow is highly influenced by gas density. Patients with large airway obstruction often can be treated with a mixture of helium and O_2 (heliox or HeO_2). HeO_2, usually an 80/20 or 70/30 mixture, can be administered to reduce the work of breathing until the obstructive process can be treated. HeO_2 mixture does little for patients with small airway obstruction, as occurs in emphysema or asthma. Flow in the small airways is mainly laminar and largely independent of the density of the gas breathed. However, heliox therapy can be used for patients with small airway obstruction to allow them to exercise longer and more strenuously with less dyspnea and dynamic hyperinflation.

Factors Affecting Resistance. The two main patterns that characterize the flow of gas through the respiratory tract are *laminar flow* and *turbulent flow* (see Chapter 6). A third pattern, *tracheobronchial flow,* is a combination of laminar and turbulent flow. Laminar flow requires less driving pressure than turbulent flow.

Poiseuille's equation (see Chapter 6) describes laminar flow through a smooth, unbranched tube of fixed dimensions (i.e., length and radius). This equation says that for gas flow to remain constant, the pressure is *inversely proportional* to the fourth power of the airway's radius. That is, by reducing the radius of a tube by half requires a 16-fold pressure increase to maintain a constant flow ($2^4 = 16$)! Clinically this means that to maintain ventilation in the presence of narrowing airways, large increases in driving pressure may be needed, resulting in marked increases in the work of breathing.

RULE OF THUMB

A change in the radius of an airway by a factor of 2 causes a 16-fold change in resistance. This rule applies to human airways and artificial airways (i.e., endotracheal and tracheostomy tubes). If the size of a patient's airway is reduced from 2 mm to 1 mm, airway resistance increases by a factor of 16. Similarly, if a 4.5-mm endotracheal tube is replaced with a 9-mm tube, the pressure required to cause a flow of 1 L/sec through the tube decreases 16-fold. This rule has many practical consequences. It is the basis for bronchodilator therapy and for using the largest practical size of artificial airway.

Distribution of Resistance. Approximately 80% of the resistance to gas flow occurs in the nose, mouth, and large airways, where flow is mainly turbulent. Only approximately 20% of the total resistance to flow is attributable to airways smaller than 2 mm in diameter, where flow is mainly laminar. This fact seems to contradict the fact that resistance is inversely related to the radius of the conducting tube.

Branching of the tracheobronchial tree increases the cross-sectional area with each airway generation (Figure 11-8). As gas moves from the mouth to the alveoli, the combined cross-sectional area of the airways increases exponentially. Turbulent flow predominates in the mouth, trachea, and primary bronchi (Table 11-3). Gas velocity is high in the bigger airways, favoring turbulent flow patterns. As we move deeper into the lung segments, the airways branch into smaller, but more, airways and more cross-sectional area. At the level of the terminal bronchioles, the cross-sectional area increases more than 30-fold. The arrangement of the branches at the same bronchial generation is in parallel (compared to in series), thus decreasing the total resistance. According to the laws of fluid dynamics, this increase in cross-sectional area causes a decrease in gas velocity. The velocity of gas flow and resistance in a branching system arranged in parallel is inversely related to the cross-sectional area of the airways. The decrease in gas velocity promotes a

TABLE 11-3

Distribution of Airway Resistance

Location	Total Resistance (%)
Nose, mouth, upper airway	50
Trachea and bronchi	30
Small airways (<2 mm)	20

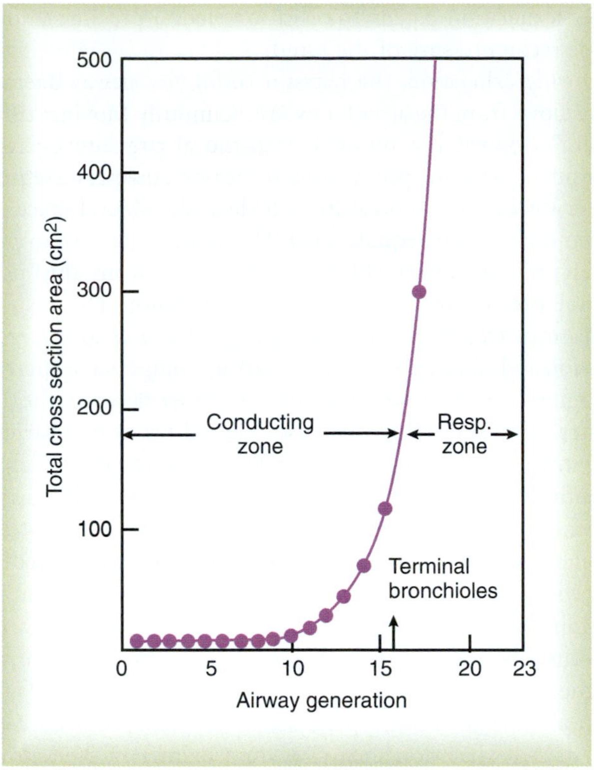

FIGURE 11-8 Cross-sectional area of the airways plotted against airway generation. The first 15 or 16 airway generations represent a conducting zone in which gas moves primarily by bulk flow, and no gas exchange takes place. These airways make up the anatomic dead space (see Chapter 9). The gas-exchange surface increases markedly at the level of the terminal bronchiole. (Modified from West J: Respiratory physiology: the essentials, ed 7, Baltimore, 2005, Williams & Wilkins.)

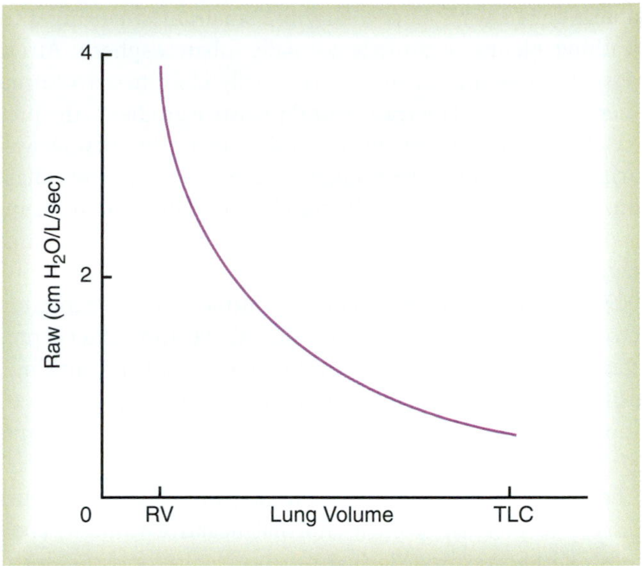

FIGURE 11-9 Change in airway resistance (R_{aw}) related to lung volume. Resistance to airflow is highly dependent on lung volume. At low lung volumes, near residual volume *(RV)*, the airways are compressed and resistance increases markedly. At high lung volumes, near total lung capacity *(TLC)*, the airways are distended and resistance decreases. See text for discussion.

laminar flow pattern, particularly in smaller (i.e., <2 mm) airways. The resistance to flow in these small airways is then very low. The driving pressure across these airways is less than 1% of the total driving pressure for the system.

We must remember that the diameter of the airways is not constant during the ventilatory cycle. During inspiration, the stretch of surrounding lung tissue and widening transpulmonary pressure gradient increase the diameter of the airways. The increase in airway diameter with increasing lung volume decreases airway resistance (Figure 11-9). As lung volume decreases toward residual volume, airway diameters also decrease and airway resistance dramatically increases; this explains why wheezing is most often heard during exhalation.

STATIC VERSUS DYNAMIC MECHANICS

Resistance and compliance can be evaluated under static or dynamic conditions.[4] The term *static* implies that flow throughout the respiratory system has ceased and all ventilatory muscle activity is absent ($P_{mus} = 0$). Static conditions can be imposed with an inspiratory pause when a patient is sedated and being mechanically ventilated. In contrast, the term *dynamic* (in this context) means that flow at the airway opening is zero. Mechanics are evaluated under dynamic conditions, for example, when a nonintubated patient breathes spontaneously. In this case, the pressure difference used to calculate lung resistance and elastance is P_{TP} and the driving pressure is P_{mus} instead of the ventilator.

In a single-compartment model (see Figure 11-1), estimation of resistance and compliance under static and dynamic conditions yields the same values. However, in a real respiratory system, composed of multiple compartments with different time constants (each compartment being a resistance in series with a compliance), mechanics estimated during static conditions yield different values than when evaluated during dynamic conditions. For a multiple-compartment system, when flow is zero at the airway opening, there may still be flow between compartments (pendelluft). As a result, dynamic mechanics become dependent on the respiratory frequency.[5,6] Typically, both compliance and resistance decrease as frequency increases.

MECHANICS OF EXHALATION

Airway caliber is determined by several factors, including anatomic (i.e., physical) support provided to the airways and pressure differences across their walls. Anatomic support comes from cartilage in the wall of the airway and from "traction" provided by surrounding tissues. The larger airways depend mainly on cartilaginous support. Because smaller airways lack cartilage, they depend on support provided by surrounding lung parenchyma.[7]

The airways are also supported by the pressure difference across their walls. This transpulmonary pressure gradient helps stabilize the airways, particularly the small ones. During quiet breathing, pleural pressure is normally subatmospheric. Airway pressure varies minimally and is usually close to zero (atmospheric pressure). The **transmural pressure** gradient (the pressure difference between inside and outside the airway wall) during normal quiet breathing is negative, even during exhalation. It ranges from −5 to −10 cm H_2O. This negative transmural pressure gradient helps maintain the caliber of the small airways.

During a forced exhalation, contraction of expiratory muscles can increase pleural pressure above atmospheric pressure; this reverses the transmural pressure gradient, making it positive. If the positive transmural pressure gradient exceeds the supporting force provided by the lung parenchyma, the small airways may collapse.

Forceful contraction of the expiratory muscles causes pleural pressure to increase from its normal negative value to above atmospheric pressure (Figure 11-10). Alveolar pressure during forced exhalation equals the sum of pleural pressure and the elastic recoil pressure of the lung.[8]

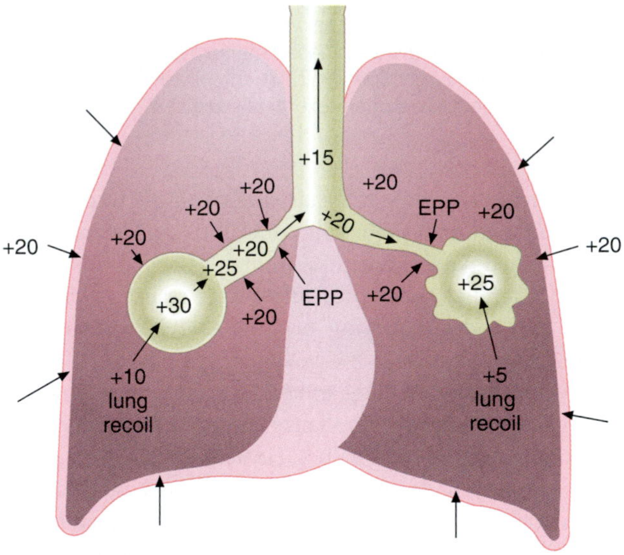

FIGURE 11-10 Generation of equal pressure point *(EPP)* in normal and diseased lungs during a forceful exhalation. In a normal lung *(left)*, pleural pressure (P_{pl}) increases to approximately +20 cm H_2O when a maximal expiratory effort is performed. Alveolar pressure is the sum of P_{pl} (+20 cm H_2O) and lung elastic recoil pressure (+10 cm H_2O), or +30 cm H_2O. Airway pressure falls along the airway from the alveolus to the mouth from +30 to 0 cm H_2O. At some point along the airway, pressure within the airway equals P_{pl}; this is the EPP. Further toward the mouth (downstream), airway pressure falls below P_{pl}, resulting in a narrowed airway and limitation of airflow. This narrowed airway normally occurs in healthy individuals only during forced exhalation. The EPP moves upstream from larger airways toward smaller airways as the lung empties. In lung diseases such as emphysema *(right)*, the same forces come into play. P_{pl} is still +20 cm H_2O, but lung elastic recoil pressure is only +5 cm H_2O. As a result, driving pressure is only +25 cm H_2O. This causes the EPP to occur in smaller airways (i.e., farther upstream) than normal; airways narrow or collapse at a higher lung volume than in healthy lungs. In patients with emphysema, airway collapse is complicated further by loss of support for the small airways. (Modified from Martin L: Pulmonary physiology in clinical practice: the essentials for patient care and evaluation, St Louis, 1987, Mosby.)

During exhalation, the pressure along the airway decreases as gas flows from the alveoli toward the mouth. Moving "downstream" (toward the mouth), transmural pressure decreases continually. At some point along the airway, the pressure inside the airway equals the pressure outside in the pleural space (i.e., transmural pressure equals zero). This point is referred to as the **equal pressure point (EPP).** Downstream from this point, pleural pressure exceeds the airway pressure. The resulting increase in transmural pressure gradient causes airway compression and can lead to collapse. Airway compression increases expiratory airway resistance and decreases flow. At the EPP, greater expiratory effort increases pleural pressure, restricting flow further.[9] Once the transmural pressure has increased sufficiently to cause this flow limitation (at the EPP), airflow becomes effort independent with airway caliber and elastic recoil pressure determining flow. **Dynamic compression** of the airways (narrowing of the airways owing to an increase in surrounding pressures) is responsible for the characteristic flow patterns observed in forced expiratory tests of pulmonary function.

In airways of healthy persons, airway collapse occurs only with forced exhalation and at low lung volumes. Tissue support opposes the collapsing force created by negative transmural pressure gradients. In pulmonary emphysema, the elastic tissue supporting the small airways is damaged.[9] Destruction of elastic tissue, such as occurs in emphysema, has multiple outcomes. It increases the compliance of the lung (i.e., elastic recoil decreases). The combination of decreased elastic recoil and loss of support for the small airways allows the airways to collapse during exhalation. Airway collapse causes air trapping and increase in the resting volume of the lung. Expiratory flow is reduced by airway collapse during exhalation (called *flow limitation*) and can occur during tidal breathing when emphysematous changes in the lung are severe.[10]

RULE OF THUMB

Patients who have emphysema can directly influence the EPP in their airways to reduce airway collapse and closure. Airway collapse may occur in patients who have emphysema because the normal support structure for small airways has been destroyed. By exhaling through "pursed lips," a patient with emphysema changes the pressure at the airway opening. The gentle back pressure created counters the tendency for small airways to collapse by moving the EPP toward larger airways.

WORK OF BREATHING

The respiratory muscles do the work for normal breathing. This work requires energy to overcome the elastic and frictional forces opposing inflation. Assessment of mechanical work involves measurement of the physical parameters of force and distance as they relate to moving air into and out of the lung. Assessment of metabolic work involves measurement of the O_2 cost of breathing.

During normal quiet breathing, inhalation is active and exhalation is passive. The work of exhaling is recovered from potential energy "stored" in the expanded lung and thorax during inhalation. However, forced exhalation requires additional work by the expiratory muscles. The actual work of forced expiration depends on the mechanical properties of the lungs and thorax.

Mechanical Work

Work done on an object is the result of the force exerted on the object and the distance it is moved.

Work may be expressed in units of either dyne • centimeters (dyne • cm) or joules (J). For a constant applied force, the equation for work is:

$$\text{Work} = \text{Force} \times \text{Distance}$$

In physiology, work is expressed in terms of pressure difference across a structure (P) and the volume change of the structure (V). Because pressure is equal to force/area and volume is equal to area multiplied by distance, work can have the dimensions of P × V:

$$\begin{aligned}\text{Pressure} \times \text{Volume} &= \frac{\text{Force}}{\text{Area}} \times (\text{Area} \times \text{Distance}) \\ &= \text{Force} \times \text{Distance} \\ &= \text{Work}\end{aligned}$$

Graphically, the work is expressed as the area between the pressure-volume curve and the volume axis (Figure 11-11). Pressure, of course, is actually a pressure difference across a structure (i.e., inside pressure minus outside pressure), and the pressure difference *defines the structure* for which work is evaluated. For example, if we want to evaluate the work the muscles do to inflate the pulmonary system we use the transpulmonary pressure, P_{TP}. Similarly, if we want to evaluate the work done by a ventilator to inflate the respiratory system we use the transrespiratory system pressure (P_{TR}).

Also, because of the equivalence of work and energy, the energy stored in a rigid wall container holding compressed gas is simply the product of the volume of the container and the pressure inside the container (relative to the outside). The higher the pressure, the more energy stored in the container. When the pressure is released, useful work can be recovered. This is the principle used in air rifles.

Figure 11-11 shows a graph of transpulmonary pressure versus lung volume derived from measurements taken during dynamic conditions (e.g., during a normal inspiration). The line *AB* connects two points in time when flow is zero. The work done overcoming purely elastic forces opposing inflation is represented by the triangular area 1 in Figure 11-11. The work required to overcome flow resistive forces is represented by area 2. The total mechanical work for one breath is the sum of the work overcoming both the elastic and the resistive forces opposing inflation; this is represented as the sum of areas 1 and 2. In healthy adults, approximately two-thirds of the work of breathing can be attributed to elastic forces opposing ventilation. The remaining one-third is a result of frictional resistance to gas and tissue movement.

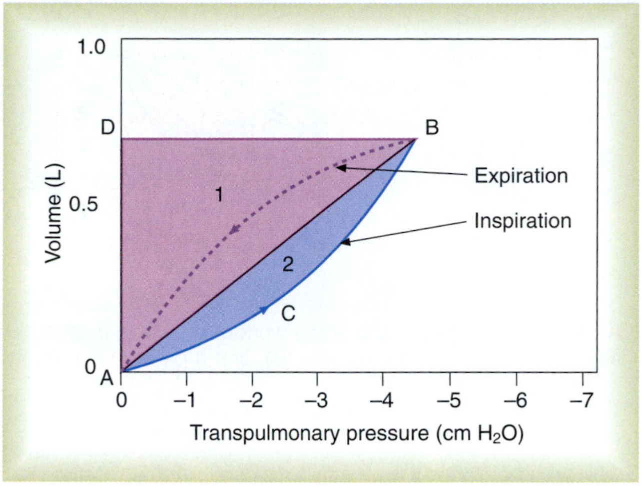

FIGURE 11-11 Factors involved in the work of breathing. Point *A* is the resting lung volume (functional residual capacity), and *B* is end-inspiration. The *straight solid line A-B* represents the pressure required to overcome simple elastic forces, and the *curved line A-C-B* represents the additional pressure required to overcome frictional resistance (airway and tissue). At *B,* where airflow momentarily ceases, frictional resistance is inactive. Area *1* represents the work (P × V) required to overcome elastic forces; area *2* represents the work required to overcome frictional forces. The work of breathing (inspiration) is the sum of these two areas. The *curved dashed line* within area *1* represents the pressure-volume curve of passive exhalation using energy stored during inspiration.

Traditionally, static pressure-volume curves have been created by injecting the lungs with discreet volume steps using a large calibrated syringe ("super syringe").[11] Alternatively, the line *AB* can be approximated under clinical conditions using a very slow inspiratory flow (with the patient heavily sedated) producing what is called a *quasistatic* pressure-volume curve.[12] Evaluation of this type of pressure-volume curve can be useful for setting optimal positive end-expiratory pressure (PEEP).[13] Ventilators made by Hamilton Medical (Reno, NV) offer the PV Tool, which generates a quasistatic pressure-volume curve using a slow pressure ramp rather than a slow inspiratory flow. This method allows evaluation of both compliance and lung recruitability.[14]

In the presence of pulmonary disease, work of breathing can increase dramatically (Figure 11-12). The areas of the volume-pressure curves for patients with obstruction or restriction are greater than in healthy persons.[15] The reasons for these increases in the mechanical work are quite different. In restrictive lung disease, the area of the volume-pressure curve is greater because the slope of the static component (compliance) is less than normal. The area of the volume-pressure curve in obstructive lung disease is increased because the portion associated with resistance is markedly widened. The leftward "bulge" of the loop

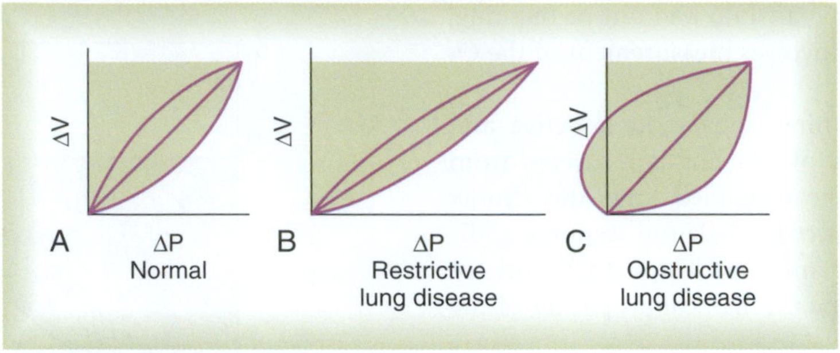

FIGURE 11-12 Comparison of the work of breathing *(shaded areas)* for a healthy person **(A),** a patient with restrictive ventilatory impairment (e.g., pulmonary fibrosis) **(B),** and a patient with airway obstruction (e.g., emphysema) **(C).**

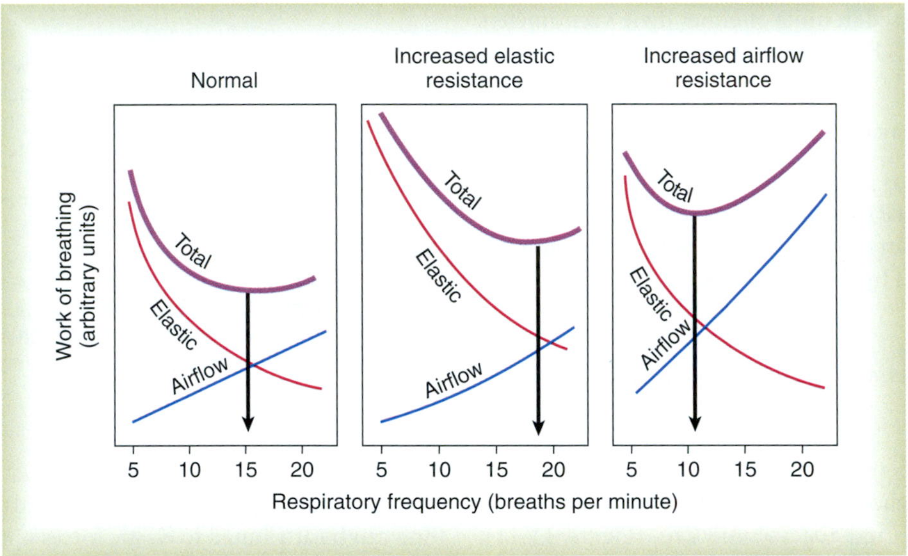

FIGURE 11-13 Work required to overcome airflow plus elastic resistance equals total work. In normal lungs, total work of breathing is minimal at approximately 15 breaths/min *(left).* To achieve the same minute volume with stiff lungs (increased elastic resistance), minimum work is performed at higher frequencies *(middle).* However, with increased airflow resistance (obstructive lung disease), minimum work requires lower rates of breathing *(right).* (Modified from Nunn JF: Applied respiratory physiology, ed 2, London, 1977, Butterworth.)

indicates positive pleural pressure that can occur during expiration, notably when lung compliance is increased (see Figure 11-12, *C*).

In healthy individuals, the mechanical work of breathing depends on the pattern of ventilation. Large V_T increases the elastic component of work. High breathing rates (and high flows) increase frictional work. When changing from quiet breathing to exercise ventilation, a healthy person adjusts V_T and breathing frequency to minimize the work of breathing.[5]

Similar adjustments occur in individuals who have lung disease (Figure 11-13). Patients with "stiff lungs" (i.e., increased elastic work of breathing), such as in pulmonary fibrosis, often assume a rapid, shallow breathing pattern. This pattern minimizes the mechanical work of distending the lungs but at the expense of more energy to increase breathing rate. Patients who have airway obstruction may assume a ventilatory pattern that reduces the frictional work of breathing. Breathing slowly and using pursed-lip breathing during exhalation minimize airway resistance.

Increased work of breathing is often complicated by *respiratory muscle weakness,* which may result from electrolyte imbalance, *acidemia,* shock, *sepsis,* or diseases affecting the muscles themselves.[16] When increased work of breathing occurs with respiratory muscle weakness, inspiratory muscles can fatigue. V_T decreases and respiratory rate increases as the muscles fatigue and fail.

Metabolic Work

To perform work, the respiratory muscles consume O_2. The rate of O_2 consumption ($\dot{V}_{O_2}$) by the respiratory muscles reflects their energy requirements. It also provides an indirect measure of the work of breathing.

The O_2 cost of breathing is assessed by measuring $\dot{V}_{O_2}$ at rest and at increased levels of ventilation. If no other factors increase O_2 consumption, the additional O_2 uptake is a result of respiratory muscle metabolism. The O_2 cost of breathing in healthy individuals averages 0.5 to 1 ml of O_2 per liter of increased ventilation. This range represents less than 5% of the O_2

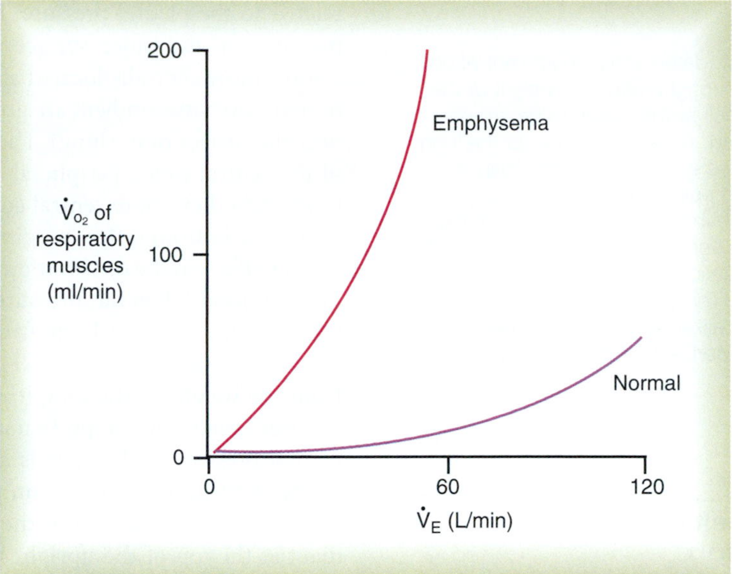

FIGURE 11-14 Relationship of oxygen cost of breathing to minute ventilation during maximum exercise for a healthy person and for a patient with emphysema. O_2 consumption ($\dot{V}O_2$) of the respiratory muscles is minimal at levels of ventilation up to approximately 100 L/min in normal persons. The metabolic demand is significantly higher in obstructive lung disease (e.g., emphysema), even at low and moderate levels of ventilation.

consumption of the body. At high levels of ventilation (i.e., >120 L/min), the O_2 cost of breathing increases tremendously and may exceed 30% of the O_2 consumption of the body.

The $\dot{V}_{O_2}$ of the respiratory muscles is closely related to the inspiratory pressures generated by the diaphragm. This transdiaphragmatic pressure can be measured by a technique similar to that used for measuring intrapleural pressure. A thin catheter with two small balloons is advanced into the esophagus. One balloon remains in the esophagus (above the diaphragm), and the balloon at the tip is placed in the stomach. The pressure difference between the balloons measures the pressure across the diaphragm. The greater the pressure required, the higher is the O_2 consumption of the respiratory muscles.

In the presence of pulmonary disease (either obstructive or restrictive), the O_2 cost of breathing may increase dramatically with increasing ventilation (Figure 11-14). In an obstructive disease such as emphysema, increased ventilation causes the O_2 consumption of the respiratory muscles to increase rapidly. This abnormally high O_2 cost of breathing is one factor that limits exercise in such patients. Increased O_2 consumption by the respiratory muscles may also contribute to the failure to wean patients from mechanical ventilation.[17] Intubation and mechanical ventilation in cases of shock may be indicated to decrease the excess O_2 consumption of the respiratory muscles and preserve the limited O_2 delivery (DO_2) for other vital body organs.

MINI CLINI

Oxygen Cost of Breathing During Weaning from Mechanical Ventilation

PROBLEM: During weaning from mechanical ventilation, O_2 cost of breathing may predict weaning failure. How can you simply detect O_2 cost of breathing at the bedside?

DISCUSSION: O_2 cost of breathing is the difference in O_2 consumption ($\dot{V}_{O_2}$) between unassisted breathing and passive assisted breathing during mechanical ventilation. Although O_2 consumption requires complicated equipment (indirect calorimetry or metabolic cart), simply looking at the mixed venous O_2 saturation (S_vO_2) before and after initiation of weaning may be a good surrogate for O_2 cost of breathing. If the S_vO_2 was 75% (normal) before initiation of weaning, and after 30 minutes of spontaneous breathing trial the value is 60% without other reason for increased O_2 consumption, it is fair to assume that the O_2 cost of breathing has increased significantly, and failure of weaning or extubation is possible. However, remember that a drop in S_vO_2 also may point toward cardiac dysfunction, clinical examination may help clarify this as the cause.

DISTRIBUTION OF VENTILATION

Neither ventilation nor perfusion is distributed evenly in healthy lungs, resulting in uneven ventilation-perfusion ($\dot{V}/\dot{Q}$) ratio (0.8). Regional and local factors account for this unevenness in the distribution of ventilation. Uneven ventilation helps explain why the lung is imperfect for gas exchange. In disease, the distribution of ventilation can worsen dramatically. The resulting deficiencies in gas exchange can be life-threatening. The maldistribution of ventilation in disease represents a primary cause of impaired O_2 and CO_2 exchange.

RULE OF THUMB

Gravity, to a large extent, determines where ventilation goes in the lungs. In an upright lung, the weight of the lung tissues causes alveoli at the bases to be smaller but more easily distended. Alveoli at the top of the lung are larger but distend less easily. Gravity also causes most blood flow through pulmonary capillaries to go to the bases. The pressure-volume characteristics of the upright lung direct most ventilation to these dependent portions, matching ventilation and blood flow to promote gas exchange. This phenomenon can be useful clinically when localized lesions (e.g., lobar pneumonia) cause $\dot{V}/\dot{Q}$ perfusion abnormalities.

MINI CLINI

Altering Patient Position to Improve Oxygenation

Altering patient position can improve oxygenation in some pulmonary diseases.[18]

PROBLEM: In patients with severe pulmonary disease causing hypoxemia, how can altering body position improve such hypoxemia?

DISCUSSION: In patients with unilateral lung disease (e.g., pneumonia), having the patient lie on his or her side with the good lung down may improve hypoxemia by altering the gravity-dependent ventilation distribution and the gravity-dependent perfusion distribution. Similarly in patients with severe bilateral pulmonary disease (e.g., acute respiratory distress syndrome [ARDS]), placing the patient in the prone position alters the ventilation and the perfusion, favoring the anterior areas of the lungs and improving the hypoxemia.

Regional Factors Affecting Distribution

Two factors interact with the effects of gravity to affect regional distribution of gas in the healthy lung: (1) relative differences in thoracic expansion and (2) regional transpulmonary pressure gradients. In upright individuals, these factors direct more ventilation to the bases and periphery of the lungs than to the apexes and central zones.

Differences in Thoracic Expansion

The conical configuration of the thorax and the action of the respiratory muscles cause proportionately greater expansion at the lung bases than at the apexes. Expansion of the lower chest is approximately 50% greater than expansion of the upper chest.[16] The action of the normal diaphragm preferentially inflates the lower lobes of the lung.

Transpulmonary Pressure Gradients

The transpulmonary pressure gradient is not uniform throughout the thorax. It varies substantially within the lung and from the top to the bottom of the lung. At a given level of alveolar inflation, the transpulmonary pressure gradient is directly related to the pleural pressure. Pleural pressure represents the pressure on the outer surface of the lung. Its effect lessens toward more centrally located alveoli. Changes in the transpulmonary pressure gradient are greatest in peripheral alveoli (i.e., near the surface of the lung). The changes are least in the alveoli of the central zones. Peripheral alveoli expand proportionately more than their more central counterparts.

Top-to-bottom differences in pleural pressure have an even greater effect on the distribution of ventilation, especially in the upright lung.[3] Pleural pressure increases by approximately 0.25 cm H_2O for each 1 cm, from the lung apex to its base for the average-sized adult lung. This increase in pressure results from the weight of the lung itself and the effect of gravity. In an adult-sized lung (approximately 30 cm from apex to base), pleural pressure at the apex is approximately −10 cm H_2O. At the base, pleural pressure is only approximately −2.5 cm H_2O. Because of these differences, the transpulmonary pressure gradient at the top of the upright lung is greater than it is at the bottom. As a result, alveoli at the apexes have a larger resting volume than do alveoli at the bases.

Because of their larger volume, alveoli at the apexes expand less during inspiration than alveoli at the bases. Apical alveoli rest on the upper portion of the lung's pressure-volume curve (Figure 11-15). This part of the curve is relatively flat. Each unit

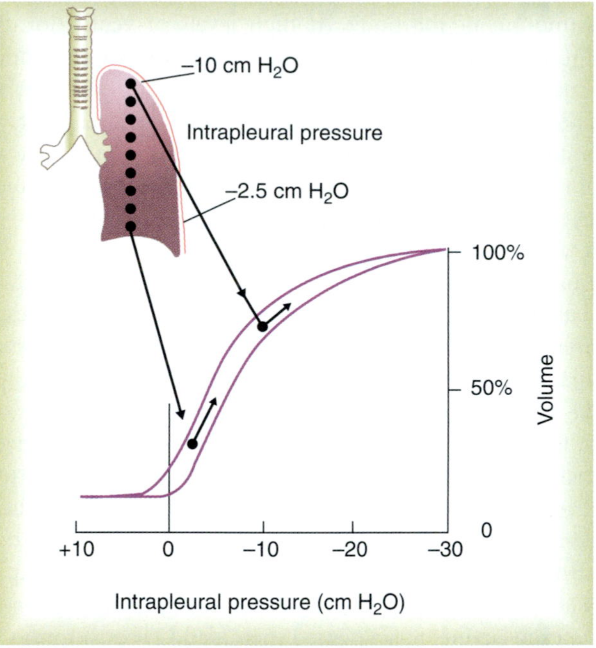

FIGURE 11-15 Causes of regional differences in ventilation from the apex to the base of an upright lung. Because of the weight of the lung and the influence of gravity, intrapleural pressure at the apex is more negative (sub-atmospheric) than at the base. Alveoli at the apex are maintained at a higher resting inflation volume than are further at the base. However, alveoli at the apex reside on the flatter upper portion of the pressure-volume curve. Alveoli at the base are positioned on the lower, steeper portion. For an equal change in intrapleural pressure, alveoli at the base expand more during inspiration than alveoli at the apex. This causes more ventilation to go to the bases in the upright lung. (Modified from West JB: Respiratory physiology: the essentials, ed 7, Baltimore, 2005, Williams & Wilkins.)

of pressure change causes only a small change in volume. Alveoli at the lung bases are positioned on the steeper middle portion of the pressure-volume curve. For each unit of pressure change, there is a larger change in volume (greater compliance). For a given transpulmonary pressure gradient, alveoli at the bases expand more than alveoli at the apexes. The bases of the upright lung receive approximately four times as much ventilation as the apexes.

These gravity-dependent differences also are observed in individuals lying down. The magnitude of the differences is less than in the upright lung because the top-to-bottom distance is less. Ventilation is still greatest in the dependent zones of the lung. In recumbent persons, the posterior regions are dependent. Lying on the side causes more ventilation to go to whichever lung is lower. This gravity dependence can be exploited to direct ventilation toward healthy lung segments or away from diseased segments by appropriate positioning of the patient.

Local Factors Affecting Distribution

Alveolar filling and emptying are affected by local factors. Individual respiratory units and their associated airways may differ from each other. These local factors contribute to uneven ventilation in healthy lungs. Their influence on gas distribution becomes particularly important in disease.

Each respiratory unit has an elastic element, the alveolus, and a resistive element, the airway. Change in alveolar volume and the time required for the change to occur depend on the compliance and resistance of each respiratory unit.[3] In terms of compliance, the more distensible the lung unit, the greater is the volume change at a given transpulmonary pressure. Lung units with high compliance have less elastic recoil than normal. These units fill and empty more slowly than normal units. Lung units with low compliance (high elastic recoil) increase their volume less. They fill and empty faster than normal. Alveolar surfactant helps to stabilize alveoli of different sizes and even out the filling and emptying times.

Airway resistance also affects emptying and filling. The size of the airway influences how much driving pressure reaches distal lung units. In healthy airways, the pressure decrease between the airway opening (i.e., the mouth) and the alveolus is minimal. Most of the driving pressure is available for alveolar inflation. If the airway is obstructed, high resistance to gas flow can occur in a local area. The pressure decrease across the obstruction may be substantial. Less driving pressure is available for alveolar inflation; there is less alveolar volume change.

Time Constants

Compliance and resistance determine local rates of alveolar filling and emptying. The time constant helps us understand these rates. The time constant is calculated as the product of resistance and compliance and is expressed in units of time (usually seconds). It is referred to as a "constant" because for any value of resistance and compliance, the time constant always equals the time necessary for the lungs to fill or empty by 63% in response to a sudden change in driving pressure. For unit of inspiratory or expiratory time equal to the time constant, lung volume changes by 63%. After two time constants, lung volume has changed 86%; after three time constants, it has changed 95%.

Time constants affect local distribution of ventilation within the lung. Areas having different time constants will have different volumes and pressures. Furthermore, the effects of unequal time constants within the lung are different for volume control ventilation (with constant inspiratory flow) compared with pressure-controlled ventilation (with constant inspiratory pressure).[19]

RULE OF THUMB

Understanding of the time constant is essential when setting mechanical ventilators (discussed later in this text). In pressure control modes, inspiratory time must be at least three time constants long to deliver 95% of the volume that is possible with the given pressure settings and lung mechanics. For any mode, expiratory time must be set to at least three time constants for the lungs to empty passively to 95% (i.e., 5% of inspired volume still remains). A lung unit has a long time constant if resistance or compliance is high. Units with long time constants take longer to fill and to empty than units with normal compliance and resistance. Lung units have a short time constant when resistance or compliance is low. Lung units with short time constants fill and empty more rapidly than lung units with normal compliance and resistance (see Figure 11-16).

Frequency Dependence of Compliance

Variations in time constants can affect ventilation throughout the lung. Abnormal ventilation is characteristic of obstruction in the small airways. This type of obstruction occurs in emphysema, asthma, and chronic bronchitis.[20] The time constants of many lung units are increased in obstructive lung disease. These long time constants are mainly caused by increased resistance to flow in the small airways. Loss of normal tissue elastic recoil, such as in emphysema, also contributes to slowed filling and emptying.

At increased breathing rates, units with long time constants fill less and empty more slowly than units with normal compliance and resistance. Increasingly more inspired gas goes to lung units with relatively normal time constants. When more inspired volume goes to a smaller number of lung units, higher transpulmonary pressures must be generated to maintain alveolar ventilation. Compliance of the lung seems to decrease as breathing frequency increases. This phenomenon is called *frequency dependence of compliance*.[5] If dynamic compliance decreases as the respiratory rate increases, some lung units must have abnormal time constants. Any stimulus to increase ventilation, such as exercise, may redistribute inspired gas. Mismatching of ventilation and perfusion can result in hypoxemia, severely limiting an individual's ability to perform daily activities.

Abnormal time constants in lung units and frequency dependence of compliance can have significant effects on patients

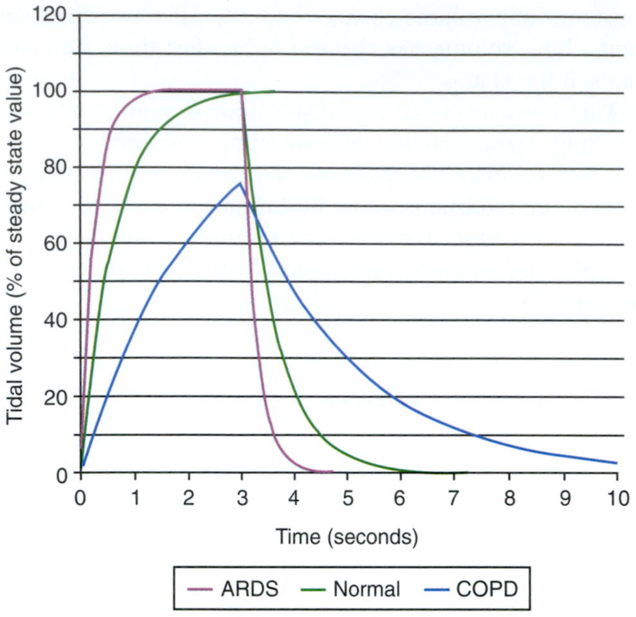

FIGURE 11-16 Graph illustrates the effect of the time constant on volume change in the lungs during passive ventilation with constant inspiratory pressure. The time constant for a ventilated patient with acute respiratory distress syndrome *(ARDS)* is short (in this example, 0.26 second) owing to normal resistance but low compliance. A person with normal lungs has a longer time constant (e.g., 0.65 second) owing to normal resistance and normal compliance. A patient with chronic obstructive pulmonary disease *(COPD)* has the longest time constant (e.g., 2.13 seconds) owing to high resistance and high compliance. The horizontal axis shows the expiratory time, and the vertical axis shows the percent of the V_T that remains at each moment. The curve representing the COPD time constant indicates significant gas trapping even after an expiratory time of 5 seconds.

requiring mechanical ventilation. When ventilation is controlled in terms of volume or inspiratory-expiratory times, **dynamic hyperinflation (air trapping)** can result. Lung volume can increase with mechanical ventilation in a manner similar to that occurring during exercise. Increased ventilation (i.e., breathing rates, flows, or both) exaggerates the differences between lung units with long or short time constants.

MINI CLINI

Breathlessness and Dynamic Hyperinflation in Obstructive Airway Disease

PROBLEM: Patients who have obstructive airway disease often complain of breathlessness (dyspnea). This breathlessness cannot be easily predicted from simple tests of lung function. Some patients with mild obstruction have debilitating dyspnea, whereas other patients with severe obstruction often have little sensation of breathlessness. Why does expiratory flow limitation cause dyspnea of varying degrees in patients who have obstructive lung disease?

DISCUSSION: Dynamic hyperinflation is an acute increase in the end-expiratory lung volume (EELV) as a result of insufficient expiratory time. This increase in EELV occurs because the rate of lung emptying, which is determined by the time constant, is prolonged while the expiratory time is shortened by the increase in ventilatory frequency. As a result, the inspiratory capacity decreases. Breathing at higher EELV increases the loading on the respiratory muscles and restricts the normal V_T expansion during exercise. There is a strong correlation between the sensation of dyspnea and the EELV. Patients with obstructive lung disease describe the sensation of dyspnea differently than normal exercising persons. Terms such as "difficulty inspiring" and "can't get the air in" are commonly used to identify the breathlessness associated with airflow limitation. These specific sensations suggest that patients with airway obstruction receive discordant sensory information from the receptors in the lungs and chest wall. The intensity of these sensations depends on the degree of dynamic hyperinflation that occurs. The use of bronchodilators and lung volume reduction surgery both relieve dyspnea by "deflating" the lungs and reducing hyperinflation. Both therapies improve dynamic airway function by improving lung emptying (more normal time constants). Patients are able to achieve the required ventilation at a lower operating lung volume with a lower O_2 cost of breathing.

EFFICIENCY AND EFFECTIVENESS OF VENTILATION

To be effective, ventilation must meet the body's needs for O_2 uptake and CO_2 removal. To be efficient, ventilation should consume little O_2 and should produce the minimum amount of CO_2.

Efficiency

Even in healthy lungs, ventilation is not entirely efficient. A substantial volume of inspired gas is wasted with each breath; this wasted ventilation is referred to as *dead space.* Gases must move in and out through the same airways leading to the gas-exchange units (alveoli). For each inspiration, the gas left in the conducting airways *(anatomic dead space)* does not participate in gas exchange and is, in effect, wasted. Alveoli that are ventilated but have no perfusion contribute what is called *alveolar dead space.* The sum of anatomic and alveolar dead space is called *physiologic dead space.* The relationship between V_T, dead space volume (V_D), and alveolar volume (V_A) is expressed as:

$$V_T = V_A + V_D$$

Because only alveolar volume participates in gas exchange, this equation shows that the larger the dead space, the less efficient the V_T would be in eliminating CO_2. That is, if efficiency is defined as output/input, CO_2 output would be less for a given input V_T as dead space increases.

Minute Ventilation

Ventilation is usually expressed in liters per minute of fresh gas entering the lungs. The total volume moving in or out of the lungs per minute is called *minute ventilation.* Minute ventilation (exhaled) is denoted by $\dot{V}_E$, which is calculated as the product of frequency of breathing (f_B) times the expired tidal volume (V_T):

$$\dot{V}_E = f_B \times V_T$$

For a healthy adult breathing 12 breaths/min and having a V_T of 500 ml:

$$\dot{V}_E = \left(12\frac{\text{breaths}}{\text{min}}\right) \times \left(500\frac{\text{ml}}{\text{breath}}\right) = 6000\ \text{ml/min} = 6\ \text{L/min}$$

Minute ventilation is normally driven by the production of CO_2 and depends on the size of the person and his or her metabolic rate. Minute ventilation values range from 5 to 10 L/min in healthy adults at rest.

Alveolar Ventilation

The efficiency of ventilation depends on the volume of fresh gas reaching the alveoli (V_A):

$$V_A = V_T - V_D$$

Alveolar ventilation, $\dot{V}_A$, is the product of breathing frequency (f_B) and alveolar volume per breath (V_A):

$$\dot{V}_E = f_B \times V_A$$

In a healthy adult with a respiratory rate of 12, V_T of 500 ml, and dead space (V_D) of 150 ml, alveolar ventilation is calculated as follows:

$$\dot{V}_A = \left(12\frac{\text{breaths}}{\text{min}}\right) \times \left(500\frac{\text{ml}}{\text{breath}} - 150\frac{\text{ml}}{\text{breath}}\right)$$
$$= 4200\ \text{ml/min} = 4.2\ \text{L/min}$$

Compare this volume with that described for minute ventilation. $\dot{V}_A$ is always less than $\dot{V}_E$ because of the effect of dead space.

Anatomic Dead Space

The volume of the conducting airways (including the nasopharynx and oropharynx) is called the *anatomic dead space,* or $V_{D\ anat}$. $V_{D\ anat}$ averages approximately 1 ml/lb of ideal body weight (2.2 ml/kg). For a person who weighs 150 lb (68 kg), $V_{D\ anat}$ is approximately 150 ml. $V_{D\ anat}$ does not participate in gas exchange because it is rebreathed. During exhalation of a 500-ml tidal breath, the first 150 ml of gas exhaled comes from the $V_{D\ anat}$. The remaining 350 ml is alveolar gas. At the end of exhalation, the airways contain 150 ml of alveolar gas. During the next inhalation, this 150-ml volume is rebreathed. Only approximately 350 ml of fresh gas reaches the alveoli per breath.

Alveolar Dead Space

In addition to the ventilation wasted on the conducting airways, some alveoli may not participate in gas exchange. These alveoli are ventilated but not perfused with mixed venous blood. Without perfusion, gas exchange cannot occur. Any gas that ventilates alveoli with no blood flow (unperfused) is also wasted *(dead space effect)*. Some alveoli have ventilation out of proportion to their perfusion (high $\dot{V}/\dot{Q}$ ratios). These alveoli also contribute to the inefficiency of ventilation because ventilation in excess of what is needed to arterialize the blood in an alveolus is wasted.

The volume of gas ventilating unperfused alveoli is called **alveolar dead space,** or $V_{D\ alv}$. $V_{D\ alv}$ is usually related to defects in the pulmonary circulation. A common clinical example of such a defect is a pulmonary embolism. A pulmonary embolus blocks a portion of the pulmonary circulation; this obstructs perfusion to ventilated alveoli, creating alveolar dead space. Alveolar dead space occurs in addition to the anatomic dead space. In a normal upright person at rest, alveoli at the apexes of the lungs have minimal or no perfusion and contribute to the total volume of dead space ventilation.

Physiologic Dead Space

The sum of anatomic and alveolar dead space is called **physiologic dead space** ($V_{D\ phy}$):

$$V_{D\ phy} = V_{D\ anat} + V_{D\ alv}$$

The total volume of wasted ventilation, or physiologic dead space, equals the sum of the conducting airways and the alveoli that are ventilated but not perfused (Figure 11-17).

Physiologic dead space includes both the normal and the abnormal components of wasted ventilation. $V_{D\ phy}$ is the preferred clinical measure of ventilation efficiency. Measuring $V_{D\ phy}$ more accurately assesses alveolar ventilation:

$$\dot{V}_A = f_B(V_T - V_{D\ phys})$$

or

$$\dot{V}_A = \dot{V}T_E - \dot{V}_{D\ phys}$$

Physiologic dead space is measured clinically by using a modified form of the Bohr equation (see later).

The common estimation of $V_{D\ phy}$ based on body weight goes back to a study published in 1955.[21] More recent research has shown poor agreement between an individual patient's measured dead space and dead space estimated by this and other "rule of thumb" equations.[22] The dead space to tidal volume ratio (V_D/V_T) can be more accurately estimated for mechanically ventilated adult patients using more data available at the bedside[23]:

$$V_D/V_T = 0.32 + 0.0106\,(PaCO_2 - P_{ET}CO_2)$$
$$+ 0.003\,(RR) + 0.0015\,(age)$$

where $PaCO_2$ is arterial O_2 tension (mm Hg), $P_{ET}CO_2$ is end-tidal CO_2 tension (mm Hg), RR is respiratory rate (breaths/min), and age is in years.

Ratio of Dead Space to Tidal Volume

In clinical practice, $V_{D\ phy}$ is often expressed as a ratio to V_T. This ratio (V_D/V_T) provides an index of the wasted ventilation (anatomic plus alveolar dead space) per breath. Measurement of the V_D/V_T ratio requires measurement (or estimation) of the arterial CO_2 (P_aCO_2) and the *mixed expired* CO_2 ($P_E - CO_2$). P_aCO_2 is usually measured by obtaining an arterial blood gas specimen

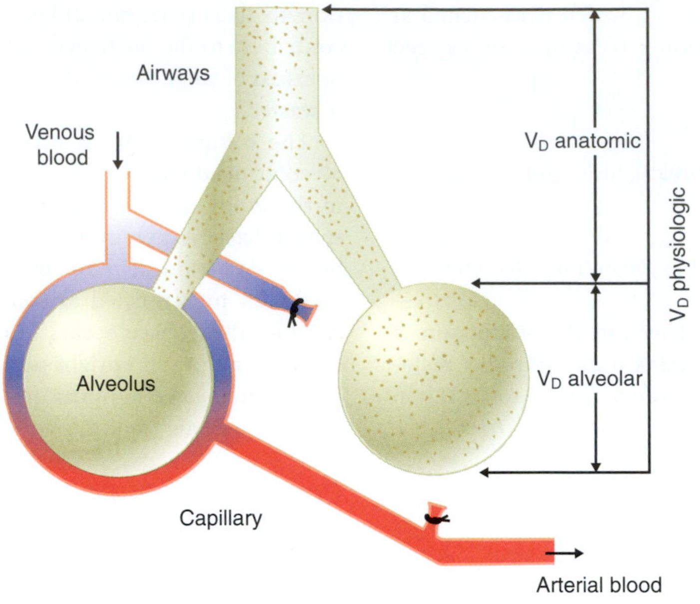

FIGURE 11-17 Three types of dead space. Anatomic dead space is composed of the conducting tubes leading to both alveoli. *Left,* Alveolus is normally perfused and ventilated. *Right,* Alveolus is ventilated but not perfused. The volume represents alveolar dead space. Physiologic dead space is the sum of the two components.

TABLE 11-4

Changes in Alveolar Ventilation Associated with Changes in Rate, Volume, and Physiologic Dead Space

Ventilatory Pattern	Rate of Breathing (breaths/min)	Tidal Volume (ml)	Minute Ventilation (ml)	Physiologic Dead Space (ml)	Alveolar Ventilation (ml)
Normal	12	500	6000	150	4200
High rate, low volume	24	250	6000	150	2400
Low rate, high volume	6	1000	6000	150	5100
Increased dead space	12	500	6000	300	2400
Compensation for increased dead space	12	650	7800	300	4200

but can be estimated from an end-tidal gas sample ($P_{ET}CO_2$). $P_E - CO_2$ may be collected in a sampling bag or balloon or estimated by means of capnography. The ratio is calculated using a modified form of the Bohr equation, which assumes that there is no CO_2 in inspired gas:

$$V_D/V_T \approx (P_aCO_2 - \bar{P}_ECO_2)/P_aCO_2$$

where $PaCO_2$ is arterial CO_2 tension and $\bar{P}_ECO_2$ is the average CO_2 tension in exhaled gas.

In a normal adult who has a P_aCO_2 of 40 mm Hg and an average expired (mixed expired) CO_2 of 28 mm Hg,

$$V_D/V_T = (40-28)/40 = 0.30$$

The equation indicates that the normal dead space ratio is approximately 30%. This equation assumes that all of the CO_2 in expired gas comes from ventilated alveoli. If all lung units contributed CO_2 equally to the expired gas and there was no anatomic dead space, P_ECO_2 would equal $PaCO_2$, and the V_D/V_T ratio would be zero. Because of anatomic and alveolar dead space, the P_ECO_2 is always less than P_aCO_2. In a healthy adult, physiologic dead space is approximately one-third of the V_T, with a normal range of 0.2 to 0.4. The V_D/V_T ratio normally decreases with exercise. Both V_T and V_D increase with increased ventilation during exertion, but the V_T normally increases to a greater degree; the ratio decreases (in healthy persons). V_D/V_T increases with diseases that cause significant dead space, such as pulmonary embolism.

Table 11-4 lists the effects of changes in the parameters that determine alveolar ventilation ($\dot{V}_A$). In healthy individuals, $\dot{V}_A$ changes with breathing rate and V_T because dead space is relatively fixed. High respiratory rate and low V_T result in a high proportion of wasted ventilation per minute (low $\dot{V}_A$). Generally, the most efficient breathing pattern is slow, deep breathing.

In pulmonary disease, increased $V_{D\ phy}$ causes a decrease in $\dot{V}_A$, unless compensation occurs. An increased breathing rate by itself worsens the problem. Effective compensation for increased $V_{D\ phy}$ requires an increased V_T. Elevating V_T increases the elastic work of breathing; however, this increases O_2 consumption by the respiratory muscles. In some patients, these increased

MINI CLINI

Minute Ventilation, Dead Space, and P_aCO_2

PROBLEM: A patient breathing at a rate of 12 breaths/min has a V_T of 600 ml and a measured physiologic dead space ($V_{D\ phy}$) of 200 ml. This ventilatory pattern produces a P_aCO_2 of 40 mm Hg with a pH of 7.39. Several hours later, the patient has a breathing rate of 24 breaths/min, but the minute ventilation ($\dot{V}_E$) has remained the same as before. Arterial blood gas analysis reveals a P_aCO_2 of 72 mm Hg with a pH of 7.20. Why has the P_aCO_2 increased even though the $\dot{V}_E$ remained constant?

DISCUSSION: The initial $\dot{V}_E$ and alveolar ventilation ($\dot{V}_A$) were as follows:

$$\begin{aligned}\dot{V}_E &= 600 \times 12\\ &= 7200\ \text{ml/min}\\ \dot{V}_A &= (600-200)\times 12\\ &= 4800\ \text{ml/min}\end{aligned}$$

The $\dot{V}_A$ of 4800 ml/min was responsible for maintaining a P_aCO_2 of 40 mm Hg. When respiratory rate increased to 24 breaths/min and $\dot{V}_E$ remained at 7200 ml/min, V_T must have decreased:

$$\begin{aligned}\dot{V}_T &= 7200 \div 24\\ &= 300\ \text{ml}\end{aligned}$$

However, if dead space remained at 200 ml, $\dot{V}_A$ subsequently decreased:

$$\begin{aligned}\dot{V}_A &= (300-200)\times 24\\ &= 2400\ \text{ml/min}\end{aligned}$$

The reduction from 4800 ml/min to 2400 ml/min explains the increase in $PaCO_2$ from 40 to 72 mm Hg. $PaCO_2$ is inversely proportional to $\dot{V}_A$. Because $\dot{V}_A$ was reduced by half, P_aCO_2 should have doubled. This approximates the data actually observed. Normally, increased CO_2 tension in the blood resulting in acidemia causes an increase in $\dot{V}_A$. This patient, although tachypneic, is hypoventilating.

demands cannot be met. In such cases, $\dot{V}_A$ may be inadequate to meet body needs, and CO_2 is not removed as rapidly as it is produced. CO_2 retention causes respiratory acidosis, often requiring mechanical support of ventilation.

Effectiveness

Ventilation is effective when it removes CO_2 at a rate that maintains a normal pH. Under resting metabolic conditions, a healthy adult produces approximately 200 ml of CO_2 per minute. Alveolar ventilation must match CO_2 production per minute to ensure acid-base balance.

The equilibrium between CO_2 production ($\dot{V}CO_2$) and $\dot{V}_A$ determines the PCO_2 in the lungs and arterial blood. This balance also plays a key role in determining the pH of arterial blood. The partial pressure of CO_2 in the alveoli and blood is directly proportional to its production ($\dot{V}CO_2$) and inversely proportional to its rate of removal by alveolar ventilation:

$$P_ACO_2 = \frac{\dot{V}CO_2 \times (P_B - P_{H_2O})}{\dot{V}_A} \approx P_aCO_2$$

where P_ACO_2 is alveolar CO_2 tension, $\dot{V}CO_2$ is CO_2 production), $\dot{V}_A$ is alveolar ventilation, P_B is barometric pressure, P_{H_2O} is the water vapor tension in the alveoli, and P_aCO_2 is arterial CO_2 tension.

Alveolar and arterial partial pressures of CO_2 are normally in equilibrium at approximately 40 mm Hg. If $\dot{V}_A$ decreases, $\dot{V}CO_2$ exceeds the rate at which the lungs are removing it. The P_aCO_2 increases to greater than its normal value of 40 mm Hg, and the arterial pH level decreases. Ventilation that does not meet metabolic needs (resulting in respiratory acidosis) is termed **hypoventilation.** Hypoventilation is indicated by the presence of an elevated P_aCO_2 and a pH level below the normal range (7.35 to 7.45).

If alveolar ventilation increases, the lungs may remove CO_2 faster than it is being produced. In this case, P_aCO_2 decreases to less than its normal value of 40 mm Hg, and pH increases (i.e., respiratory alkalosis). Ventilation that exceeds metabolic needs is termed **hyperventilation.** Hyperventilation is indicated by a lower than normal P_aCO_2 and a pH above the normal range.

Hyperventilation is often confused with the increased ventilation that occurs in response to increased metabolism. The changes observed during low or moderate levels of exercise are an example. Ventilation increases in proportion to the increased $\dot{V}CO_2$ from exercise. The P_aCO_2 remains in the normal range of 35 to 45 mm Hg, and the pH level remains near 7.4. The increase in ventilation that occurs with increased metabolic rates is termed *hyperpnea.*

Effectiveness of ventilation is determined by the partial pressure of CO_2 and the resulting pH, specifically in arterial blood. Ventilation is effective when the $PaCO_2$ is maintained at a level that keeps the pH within normal limits.

SUMMARY CHECKLIST

- Ventilation occurs because of pressure differences across the lung during breathing. Gas flows into the lung when the diaphragm creates a sub-atmospheric pressure in the lung; gas flows out of the lung when the recoil properties of the lung create a slight positive pressure.
- The forces that oppose lung inflation may be grouped into two categories: elastic forces and frictional forces.
- Resting lung volume is determined by the opposing elastic forces of the lungs and chest wall.
- Frictional forces opposing ventilation include airway and tissue resistance.
- Airway resistance accounts for 80% of the frictional resistance to ventilation in a healthy adult lung.
- Exhalation is normally passive but may become active when airway resistance is abnormally high.
- The work of breathing is performed by the muscles of breathing.
- Obstructive lung disease increases the frictional work of breathing, whereas restrictive lung disease increases the elastic work of breathing.

- Respiratory muscle fatigue causes a decrease in the tidal volume and an increase in the respiratory rate.
- Even a healthy lung does not distribute ventilation evenly throughout the lungs; greater ventilation normally occurs in the bases.
- The total volume of gas moving in and out of the lungs each minute is called the *minute volume or minute ventilation.* It is determined by multiplying the V_T times the breathing frequency.
- Homeostasis is present when the alveolar ventilation matches CO_2 production.
- The portion of the V_T that does not come into contact with pulmonary blood flow is called *dead space ventilation.*
- Normally approximately 30% of the V_T is dead space. Most of this is called *anatomic dead space* because it is made up of the larger airways that serve to conduct gas to the alveolar sacs.
- Alveoli that are ventilated but have no blood perfusion are called *alveolar dead space.* Normally, alveolar dead space is minimal.
- The combination of anatomic and alveolar dead space is called *physiologic dead space.*

References

1. Primiano FP, Jr, Chatburn RL: Zen and the art of nomenclature maintenance: a revised approach to respiratory symbols and terminology. *Respir Care* 51:1458, 2006.
2. West JB: *Respiratory physiology: the essentials*, ed 7, Baltimore, 2007, Lippincott Williams & Wilkins.
3. Harris RS: Pressure-volume curves of the respiratory system. *Respir Care* 50:78, 2005.
4. Lucangelo U, Bernabé F, Blanch L: Respiratory mechanics derived from signals in the ventilator circuit. *Respir Care* 50:55, 2005.
5. Otis AB, McKerrow CB, Bartlett RA, et al: Mechanical factors in distribution of pulmonary ventilation. *J Appl Physiol* 8:427, 1956.
6. Chatburn RL: Dynamic respiratory mechanics. *Respir Care* 31:703, 1986.
7. Lumb AB: *Nunn's applied respiratory physiology*, ed 6, London, 2005, Butterworth-Heinemann Medical.
8. Zach MS: The physiology of forced expiration. *Paediatr Respir Rev* 1:36, 2000.
9. Thurlbeck WM: Pathophysiology of chronic obstructive pulmonary disease. *Clin Chest Med* 11:389, 1990.
10. O'Donnell DE: Hyperinflation, dyspnea, and exercise intolerance in chronic obstructive pulmonary disease. *Proc Am Thorac Soc* 3:180, 2006.
11. Venegas JG, Harris RS, Simon BA: A comprehensive equation for the pulmonary pressure-volume curve. *J Appl Physiol* 84:389, 1998.
12. Hata JS, Simmons JS, Kumar AB, et al: The acute effectiveness and safety of the constant-flow, pressure-volume curve to improve hypoxemia in acute lung injury. *J Intensive Care Med* 27:129, 2012.
13. Caramez MP, Kacmarek RM, Helmy M, et al: A comparison of methods to identify open-lung PEEP. *Intensive Care Med* 35:740, 2009.
14. Grooms DA, Sibole SH, Tomlinson JR, et al: Customization of an open lung ventilation strategy to treat a case of life threatening acute respiratory distress syndrome. *Respir Care* 56:514, 2011.
15. Rochester DF: Respiratory muscles and ventilatory failure: 1993 perspective. *Am J Med Sci* 305:394, 1993.
16. Martin L: *Pulmonary physiology in clinical practice: the essentials for patient care and evaluation*, St Louis, 1987, Mosby.
17. Mitsuoka M, Kinninger KH, Jacobson KL, et al: Utility of measurements of oxygen cost of breathing in predicting success or failure in trials of reduced mechanical ventilatory support. *Respir Care* 6:902, 2001.
18. Charron C, Bouferrache K, Caille V, et al: Routine prone positioning in patients with severe ARDS: feasibility and impact on prognosis. *Intensive Care Med* 37:785, 2011.
19. Chatburn RL, El Khatib M, Smith P: Respiratory system behavior with constant inspiratory pressure or flow. *Respir Care* 39:979, 1994.
20. Hogg JC: Pathophysiology of airflow limitation in chronic obstructive pulmonary disease. *Lancet* 364:709, 2004.
21. Radford EP, Jr: Ventilation standards for use in artificial respiration. *J Appl Physiol* 7:451, 1955.
22. Brewer LM, Orr JA, Pace NL: Anatomic dead space cannot be predicted by body weight. *Respir Care* 53:885, 2008.
23. Frankenfield DC, Alam S, Bekteshi E, et al: Predicting dead space ventilation in critically ill patients using clinically available data. *Crit Care Med* 38:288, 2010.

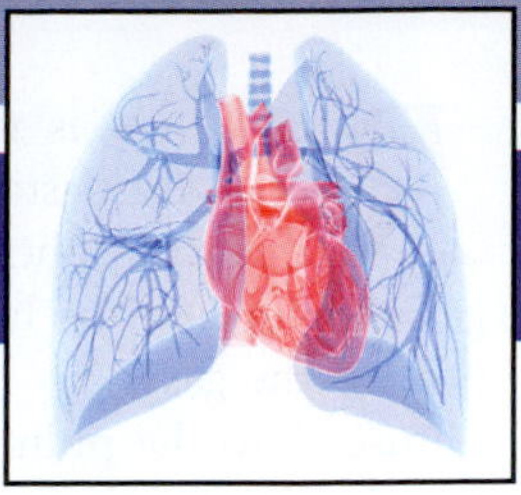

CHAPTER 12

Gas Exchange and Transport

ZAZA COHEN

CHAPTER OBJECTIVES

After reading this chapter you will be able to:

- Describe how oxygen and carbon dioxide move between the atmosphere and tissues.
- Identify what determines alveolar oxygen and carbon dioxide pressures.
- Calculate the alveolar partial pressure of oxygen at any given barometric pressure and fraction of inspired oxygen.
- State the effects that normal regional variations in ventilation and perfusion have on gas exchange.
- Describe how to compute total oxygen content for arterial blood.
- State the factors that cause the arteriovenous oxygen content difference to change.
- Identify the factors that affect oxygen loading and unloading from hemoglobin.
- Describe how carbon dioxide is carried in the blood.
- Describe how oxygen and carbon dioxide transport are interrelated.
- Describe the factors that impair oxygen delivery to the tissues and how to distinguish among them.
- State the factors that impair carbon dioxide removal.

CHAPTER OUTLINE

Diffusion
- Whole-Body Diffusion Gradients
- Determinants of Alveolar Gas Tensions
- Mechanism of Diffusion
- Systemic Diffusion Gradients

Variations from Ideal Gas Exchange
- Anatomic Shunts
- Ventilation-Perfusion Ratio

Oxygen Transport
- Chemically Combined Oxygen (Oxyhemoglobin)
- Total Oxygen Content of the Blood
- Normal Loading and Unloading of Oxygen (Arteriovenous Differences)
- Factors Affecting Oxygen Loading and Unloading
- Measurement of Hemoglobin Affinity for Oxygen

Carbon Dioxide Transport
- Transport Mechanisms
- Carbon Dioxide Dissociation Curve

Abnormalities of Gas Exchange and Transport
- Impaired Oxygen Delivery
- Dysoxia
- Impaired Carbon Dioxide Removal

KEY TERMS

acute chest syndrome
alveolar dead space
alveolar shunts
Bohr effect
carboxyhemoglobin (HbCO)
dead space
dysoxia
fetal hemoglobin (HbF)
Fick equation
Fick's first law of diffusion
Haldane effect
Hamburger phenomenon
hypoxemia
hypoxia
methemoglobin
methemoglobinemia
oxyhemoglobin
P_{50}
right-to-left anatomic shunts
sickle cell hemoglobin
venous admixture
ventilation/perfusion ratio ($\dot{V}/\dot{Q}$)

Respiration is the process of getting oxygen into the body for tissue use and removing carbon dioxide into the atmosphere. This complex process involves both gas exchange (at the lungs and at the cellular level) and transport of the gases. O_2 must be moved into the lungs, where it diffuses into the pulmonary circulation and is transported in the blood to the tissues. CO_2 builds up in the tissues because of metabolism and diffuses into the capillary blood before being carried to the lung for exchange with alveolar gases. Normally, these processes are well integrated. However, in disease states, impaired gas exchange or transport can cause physiologic imbalances, which can alter function or threaten survival. At such times, respiratory care intervention may be the only way to maintain or restore a level of function consistent with life. This chapter provides the background knowledge that respiratory therapists (RTs) need to understand and treat patients with diseases that affect gas exchange.

DIFFUSION

Whole-Body Diffusion Gradients

Gas movement between the lungs and tissues occurs via simple diffusion (see Chapters 6 and 9). Figure 12-1 shows the normal diffusion gradients for O_2 and CO_2. For O_2, there is a stepwise downward "cascade" of partial pressures from the normal atmospheric inspired partial pressure of O_2 (PiO_2) of 159 mm Hg to a low point of 40 mm Hg or less in the capillaries. The intracellular PO_2 (approximately 5 mm Hg) provides the final gradient for O_2 diffusion into the cell.

The diffusion gradient for CO_2 is the opposite of the diffusion gradient for O_2. The partial pressure of CO_2 (PCO_2) is highest in the cells (approximately 60 mm Hg) and lowest in room air (1 mm Hg). This reverse cascade causes CO_2 movement from the tissues into the venous blood, which is transported to the lungs and—with the aid of ventilation—out to the atmosphere.[1]

Determinants of Alveolar Gas Tensions

Alveolar Carbon Dioxide

The alveolar partial pressure of CO_2 (P_ACO_2) varies directly with the body's production of CO_2 ($\dot{V}CO_2$) and inversely with alveolar ventilation ($\dot{V}_A$). The relationship is expressed by the following formula:

$$P_ACO_2 = \frac{\dot{V}_{CO_2}}{\dot{V}_A} \times K$$

where:

P_ACO_2 = Alveolar CO_2 tension (mm Hg)
$\dot{V}CO_2$ = CO_2 production (in ml/min standard temperature and pressure, dry [STPD])
$\dot{V}_A$ = Alveolar ventilation (L/min body temperature and pressure, saturated [BTPS])

Because $\dot{V}CO_2$ and $\dot{V}_A$ are measured under different conditions (STPD and BTPS, respectively), a correction factor of K is used. When conventional units are used for $\dot{V}CO_2$ (ml/min), and $\dot{V}_A$ (L/min), K = 0.863.

As an example, given $\dot{V}CO_2$ of 200 ml/min and alveolar ventilation of 4.315 L/min, application of this formula yields a P_ACO_2 of approximately 40 mm Hg:

$$P_ACO_2 = 0.863 \times 200 \div 4.315$$
$$= 40\,(\text{mm Hg})$$

P_ACO_2 increases above this level if CO_2 production increases while alveolar ventilation remains constant or if alveolar ventilation decreases while $\dot{V}CO_2$ remains constant. An increase in **dead space,** the portion of inspired air that is exhaled without being exposed to perfused alveoli, also can lead to an increased P_ACO_2:

$$\dot{V}_A = f \times (V_D - V_D)$$

where:

$\dot{V}_A$ = Alveolar ventilation (L/min)
V_T = Tidal volume (L)

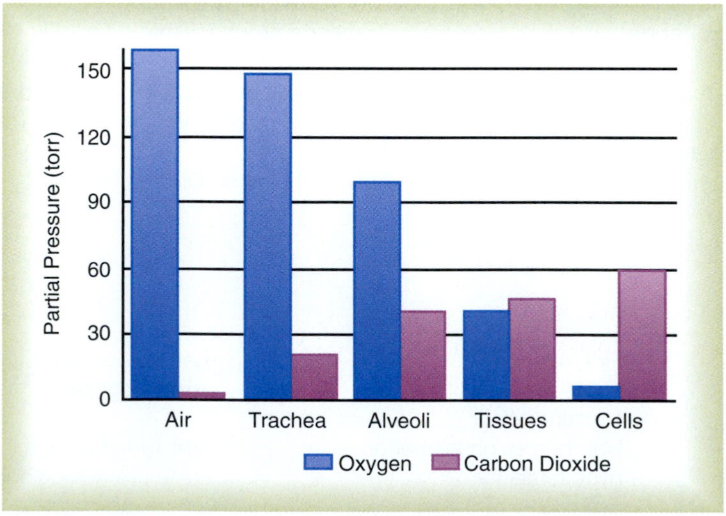

FIGURE 12-1 Normal diffusion gradients for O_2 and CO_2. There is a downward cascade for O_2 from air to cells, with a reverse gradient for CO_2.

V_D = Dead space volume (L)

f = Ventilatory frequency (breaths/min)

Likewise, P_ACO_2 decreases if CO_2 production decreases or alveolar ventilation increases. Normally, complex respiratory control mechanisms maintain P_ACO_2 within a range of 35 to 45 mm Hg under various conditions. If CO_2 production increases, as with exercise or fever, ventilation automatically increases to maintain P_ACO_2 within normal range.

Alveolar Oxygen Tensions

Many factors determine the alveolar partial pressure of O_2 (P_AO_2). The mathematical model relating these factors and applied here is called the *alveolar air equation*. One version of it is:

$$P_AO_2 = FiO_2 \times (P_B - P_{H_2O}) - (P_ACO_2 \div RQ)$$

where:

FiO_2 = Fraction of inspired O_2 (expressed in decimals)

P_B = Barometric pressure (mm Hg)

P_{H_2O} = Water vapor tension. At BTPS, a value of 47 mm Hg is usually used.

P_ACO_2 = Alveolar PCO_2 (mm Hg)

RQ = Respiratory quotent, usually estimated at 0.8.

In addition, $FiO_2 \times (P_B - P_{H_2O})$ represents the partial pressure of O_2 in the inspired air and is the most important determinant of P_AO_2. The expression ($P_ACO_2 \div RQ$) accounts for the alveolar CO_2. However, P_ACO_2 cannot simply be subtracted, as was done for water vapor. Instead, the equation must be corrected for the difference between O_2 and CO_2 movement into and out of the alveoli, which is done by dividing the P_ACO_2 by RQ. RQ is the ratio of CO_2 excretion to O_2 uptake, which normally averages 0.8 throughout the lung. In addition, because P_aCO_2 nearly equals P_ACO_2, P_aCO_2 can be substituted for P_ACO_2. For example, if FiO_2 is 0.21, P_B is 760 mm Hg, and $PaCO_2$ is 40 mm Hg, the normal alveolar partial pressure of O_2 can be estimated as follows:

$$P_AO_2 = 0.21 \times (760 - 47) - (40 \div 0.8)$$
$$= 99.73 \text{ (mm Hg)}$$

For patients at room air, sea level (FiO_2 = 0.21, P_B = 760), the equation can be simplified as:

$$P_AO_2 = 150 - P_aCO_2 \div 0.8$$

The accompanying Mini Clini provides an example of how to use the alveolar air equation.

Changes in Alveolar Gas Partial Tensions

In addition to CO_2, O_2, and water vapor, alveoli normally contain nitrogen. Nitrogen is inert and plays no role in gas exchange; however, it occupies space and exerts pressure. According to Dalton's law, the partial pressure of alveolar nitrogen (P_AN_2) must equal the pressure it would exert if it alone were present. To compute P_AN_2, subtract the pressures exerted by all the other alveolar gases, as follows:

$$P_AN_2 = P_B - (P_AO_2 + P_ACO_2 + P_{H_2O})$$

MINI CLINI

Alveolar-Arterial PO_2 Difference and P/F Ratio

Not all of the O_2 from the alveoli gets into the blood. Why this occurs is discussed later in this chapter. This Mini Clini considers how the efficiency of O_2 transfer from the alveoli to the blood can be computed.

Several bedside computations can be used to estimate the efficiency of pulmonary O_2 transfer. The most common computation is the difference between the alveolar and arterial PO_2, called the *A–a gradient* ($D_{A-a}O_2$). Normally, this difference is small—only 5 to 10 mm Hg. The reason for this slight difference in normal individuals is discussed later in this chapter. An increase in A–a gradient is often indicator of pulmonary parenchymal disease.

Another common bedside computation is the ratio of P_aO_2 to FiO_2, sometimes simplified to P/F (pronounced "PF") ratio. The P/F ratio has units of millimeters of mercury (because P_aO_2 has units of millimeters of mercury and FiO_2 is dimensionless). It is frequently used for ventilated patients as a measure of oxygenation abnormality and is one of the main criteria for diagnosing acute respiratory distress syndrome (ARDS). Mild ARDS is associated with a P/F ratio greater than 200 mm Hg and up to 300 mm Hg. Moderate ARDS is associated with a P/F ratio greater than 100 mm Hg and up to 200 mm Hg. Severe ARDS is associated with a P/F ratio of 100 mm Hg or less.

PROBLEM: Compute and interpret the $D_{A-a}O_2$ and P/F ratio for a 45-year-old woman breathing 70% O_2 at sea level, with the following blood gas values: P_aO_2, 50 mm Hg; P_aCO_2, 40 mm Hg.

SOLUTION: 1. Compute P_AO_2 using one form of the alveolar O_2 equation as follows:

$$P_AO_2 = FiO_2 \times (P_B - 47) - (P_ACO_2 \div 0.8)$$
$$P_AO_2 = 0.7 \times (760 - 47) - 40 \div 0.8$$
$$P_AO_2 = 449 \text{ mm Hg}$$

2. Compute $D_{A-a}O_2$ as follows:

$$D_{A-a}O_2 = P_AO_2 - PaO_2$$
$$D_{A-a}O_2 = 449 - 50$$
$$D_{A-a}O_2 = 399 \text{ mm Hg}$$

3. Compute P/F ratio as follows:

$$P_aO_2/FiO_2 = 50/0.7 = 71.4 \text{ mm Hg}$$

DISCUSSION: Both the $D_{A-a}O_2$ and the P/F ratio are abnormal. Compared with a normal value, the $D_{A-a}O_2$ of nearly 400 mm Hg is very high. This $D_{A-a}O_2$ indicates a large difference between the alveolar and arterial PO_2 values (i.e., inefficient O_2 transfer). Likewise, the P/F ratio of 71.4 indicates severe **hypoxemia.** Although the patient is receiving a high FiO_2 (0.70), she has a severe problem getting O_2 into her blood and needs immediate evaluation by a critical care physician.

$$P_AN_2 = 760\ \text{mm Hg} - (100\ \text{mm Hg} + 40\ \text{mm Hg} + 47\ \text{mm Hg})$$
$$P_AN_2 = 760\ \text{mm Hg} - 187\ \text{mm Hg}$$
$$P_AN_2 = 573\ \text{mm Hg}$$

Because both water vapor tension and P_AN_2 remain constant, the only partial pressures that change in the alveolus are O_2 and CO_2. Based on the alveolar air equation, if FiO_2 remains constant, P_AO_2 must vary inversely with P_ACO_2.[2-4]

RULE OF THUMB

When the patient is breathing room air, the sum of P_AO_2 and P_ACO_2 is approximately140 mm Hg (100 mm Hg + 40 mm Hg). This equation assumes a constant value for RQ. Changes in ventilation that affect P_ACO_2 will also alter P_AO_2 to keep the total at 140 mm Hg. If P_ACO_2 of a patient breathing room air decreases from 40 mm Hg to 20 mm Hg (a decrease of 20 mm Hg), P_AO_2 should increase by approximately 20 mm Hg. It is important to note that although hyperventilation will allow halving the PC_AO_2 (from 40 to 20), it will result only in modest increase of P_AO_2 (from 100 to 120; Figure 12-2).

Mechanism of Diffusion

Diffusion is the process whereby gas molecules move from an area of high partial pressure to an area of low partial pressure. To diffuse into and out of the lung and tissues, O_2 and CO_2 must move through significant barriers.

Barriers to Diffusion

The barrier to gaseous diffusion in the lung is the alveolar-capillary membrane. For CO_2 or O_2 to move between the alveoli and the pulmonary capillary blood, the following three barriers must be penetrated: (1) alveolar epithelium, (2) interstitial space, and (3) capillary endothelium. In addition, to pass into and out of the red blood cells (RBCs), these gases also must traverse the erythrocyte membrane.[5,6]

Fick's First Law of Diffusion

The bulk movement of a gas through a biologic membrane ($\dot{V}_{gas}$) is described by **Fick's first law of diffusion:**

$$\dot{V}_{gas} = \frac{A \times D \times (P_1 - P_2)}{T}$$

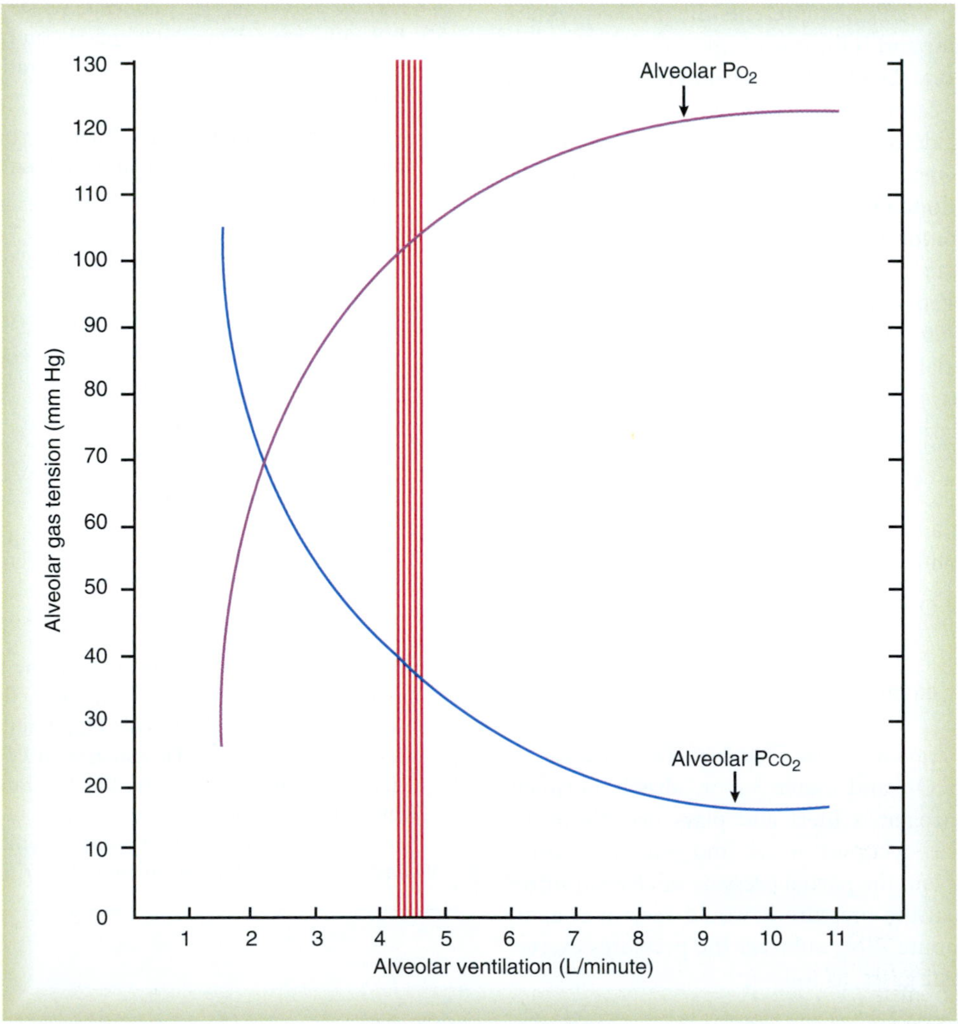

FIGURE 12-2 Effect of alveolar ventilation on alveolar gases. (Modified from Pilbeam SP: Mechanical ventilation, ed 4, St Louis, 2006, Mosby.)

In this formula, A is the cross-sectional area available for diffusion, D is the diffusion coefficient of the gas, T is the thickness of the membrane, and $(P_1 - P_2)$ is the partial pressure gradient across the membrane. According to Fick's law, the greater the surface area, diffusion constant, and pressure gradient, the more is the diffusion that occurs. Conversely, with greater the distance across the membrane (thickness), less diffusion occurs. Given that the area of and distance across the alveolar-capillary membrane are constant in healthy people, diffusion in the normal lung mainly depends on gas pressure gradients.

In clinical practice, it is impossible to measure the area and the thickness of the membrane, so the formula is often rewritten as:

$$\dot{V}_{gas} = D_L \times (P_1 - P_2)$$

where D_L (the diffusing capacity of the lungs) combines the area, thickness, and diffusion properties of the gas and the membrane and can be helpful in evaluating certain diseases. For various reasons, carbon monoxide is the gas is used to measure the diffusing capacity. Chapter 20 provides details on the technique for measuring D_L and its diagnostic use.

Pulmonary Diffusion Gradients

For gas exchange to occur between the alveoli and pulmonary capillaries, a difference in partial pressures $(P_1 - P_2)$ must exist. Figure 12-3 shows the size and direction of these gradients for O_2 and CO_2. In the normal lung, the alveolar PO_2 averages approximately 100 mm Hg, whereas the mean PCO_2 is approximately 40 mm Hg. Venous blood returning to the lungs has a lower PO_2 (40 mm Hg) than alveolar gas. The pressure gradient for O_2 diffusion into the blood is approximately 60 mm Hg (100 mm Hg – 40 mm Hg). As blood flows past the alveolus, it takes up O_2 and moves to the left atrium with a PO_2 close to 100 mm Hg in healthy people.

Because venous blood has higher PCO_2 than alveolar gas (46 vs. 40 mm Hg), the pressure gradient for CO_2 causes it to diffuse in the opposite direction, from the blood into the alveolus. This diffusion continues until capillary PCO_2 equilibrates with the alveolar level, at approximately 40 mm Hg. Although the pressure gradient for CO_2 is approximately one-tenth of the pressure gradient for O_2, CO_2 has little difficulty diffusing across the alveolar-capillary membrane. CO_2 diffuses approximately 20 times faster across the alveolar-capillary membrane than O_2 because of its much higher solubility in plasma.

Time Limits to Diffusion

For blood leaving the pulmonary capillary to be adequately oxygenated, it must spend sufficient time in contact with the alveolus to allow equilibration.[5,8] If the time available for diffusion is inadequate, blood leaving the lungs may not be fully oxygenated. As depicted in Figure 12-4, blood normally takes approximately one-third of the time it spends in the capillary to be fully oxygenated. If blood flow increases, such as during heavy exercise, capillary transit time can decrease to 0.25 second. This short period is still adequate to ensure that equilibration occurs as long as no other factors impair diffusion. However, in the presence of a diffusion limitation, it would take longer than 0.25 second for the blood to be fully oxygenated and rapid blood flow through the pulmonary circulation can result in

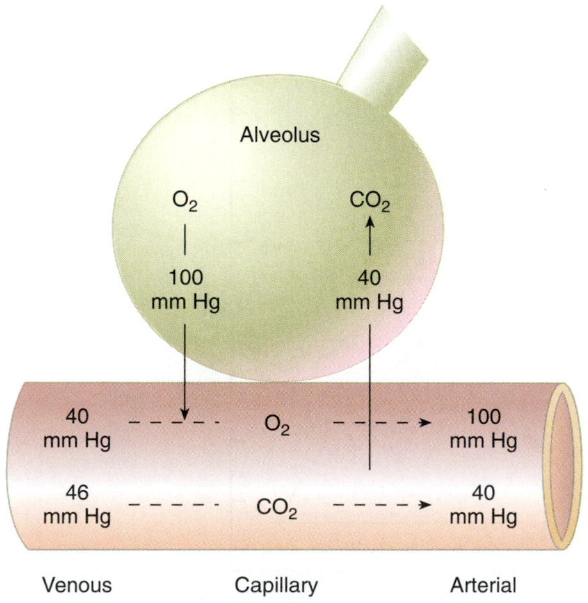

FIGURE 12-3 Ventilation maintains mean alveolar gas pressures for O_2 and CO_2 at approximately 100 mm Hg and 40 mm Hg. As blood enters the venous end of the capillary, it gives up CO_2 and loads O_2 until these two gases are in equilibrium with alveolar pressures. At this point, the blood is "arterialized."

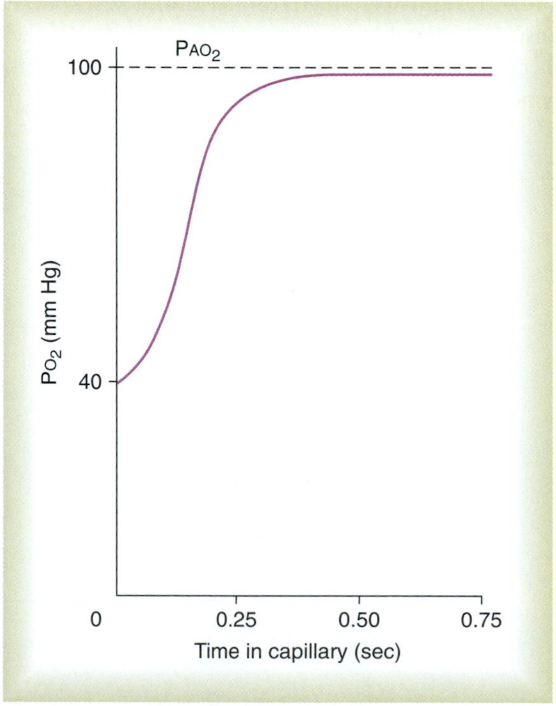

FIGURE 12-4 Alveolar-capillary PO_2 gradient. Normal transit time for RBC in the pulmonary capillary is approximately 0.75 second. Normally, blood PO_2 equilibrates with the alveolar PO_2 well before it reaches the end of the capillary.

inadequate oxygenation. For this reason, many patients with lung disease will have normal O_2 saturation at rest, but will quickly desaturate even on minimal exertion.

Systemic Diffusion Gradients

Partial pressure gradients in the tissues are the opposite of the partial pressure gradients in the lung. As cellular metabolism depletes its O_2, intracellular PO_2 decreases below PaO_2. O_2 diffuses from the tissue capillary blood ($PO_2 = 100$ mm Hg) to the cells ($PO_2 < 40$ mm Hg). Simultaneously, CO_2 diffuses from the cells ($PCO_2 > 46$ mm Hg) into the capillary blood ($PCO_2 = 40$ mm Hg). After equilibration, blood leaves the tissue capillaries with a PO_2 of approximately 40 mm Hg and PCO_2 of approximately 46 mm Hg.

Just as arterial blood reflects pulmonary gas exchange, venous blood reflects events occurring in the tissues. The use of venous blood to assess tissue oxygenation is discussed in Chapter 51.

VARIATIONS FROM IDEAL GAS EXCHANGE

As discussed previously in this chapter, there is a slight difference between alveolar and arterial PO_2 (normally 5 to 10 mm Hg). Two factors account for this difference: (1) right-to-left shunts in the pulmonary and cardiac circulation and (2) regional differences in pulmonary ventilation and blood flow.

Anatomic Shunts

A shunt is the portion of the cardiac output that returns to the left heart without being oxygenated by exposure to ventilated alveoli. Two **right-to-left anatomic shunts** exist in normal humans: (1) bronchial venous drainage and (2) thebesian venous drainage (see Chapters 9 and 10). A right-to-left shunt causes poorly oxygenated venous blood to move directly into the arterial circulation, reducing the O_2 content of arterial blood. Together, these normal shunts account for approximately three-fourths of the normal difference between P_AO_2 and P_aO_2. The remaining difference is a result of normal inequalities in pulmonary ventilation and perfusion.[5]

Inequalities in Ventilation and Perfusion

The normal respiratory exchange ratio of 0.8 assumes that ventilation and perfusion in the lung are in balance, with every liter of alveolar ventilation ($\dot{V}_A$) matched by approximately 1 L of pulmonary capillary blood flow ($\dot{Q}$). Any variation from this perfect balance alters gas tensions in the affected alveoli. The **ventilation/perfusion ratio** ($\dot{V}/\dot{Q}$) is one of the key concepts in pulmonary physiology because it plays a major role in gas exchange in health and disease.

Ventilation-Perfusion Ratio

Changes in $\dot{V}_A$ and $\dot{Q}_c$ are expressed as a ratio called the *ventilation-perfusion ratio* ($\dot{V}/\dot{Q}$). An ideal ratio of 1 indicates that ventilation and perfusion are in perfect balance. A high $\dot{V}_A/\dot{Q}$ indicates that ventilation is greater than normal, perfusion is less than normal, or both. Conversely, a low $\dot{V}_A/\dot{Q}$ indicates that ventilation is less than normal, perfusion is greater than normal, or both.

Effect of Alterations in Ventilation-Perfusion Ratio

Figure 12-5 shows graphs of the effect of $\dot{V}_A/\dot{Q}$ changes on the respiratory exchange ratio (R), plotting all possible values of P_AO_2 and P_ACO_2. When ventilation and perfusion are in perfect balance ($\dot{V}_A/\dot{Q} = 1$), R equals 0.8. At this point, P_AO_2 and P_ACO_2 values equal the ideal values of 100 mm Hg and 40 mm Hg.

As the $\dot{V}_A/\dot{Q}$ increases above 1 (see Figure 12-5, following the *curve* to the right), less blood reaches O_2-rich, CO_2-poor inspired gas. The result is a higher P_AO_2 and lower P_ACO_2. At

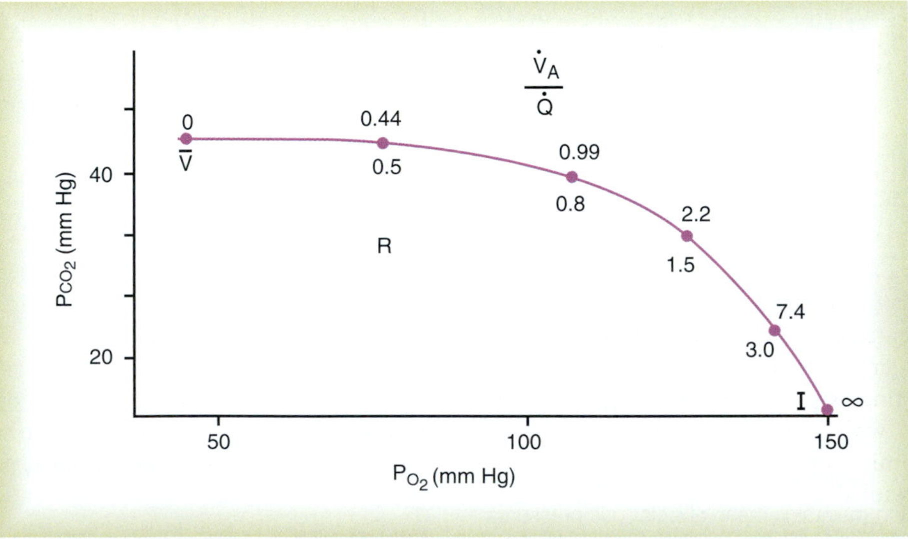

FIGURE 12-5 Relationship between alveolar PO_2 and PCO_2 with changes in $\dot{V}_A/\dot{Q}$ and respiratory exchange ratio. (From Cherniak RM, Cherniak L: Respiration in health and disease, ed 3, Philadelphia, 1983, Saunders.)

the extreme right of the graph, perfusion is zero ($\dot{V}_A/\dot{Q} = \infty$). Areas with ventilation but no blood flow essentially represent dead space. The makeup of gases in these areas is similar to that of inspired air (PO_2 = 150 mm Hg; PCO_2 = 0 mm Hg).

Dead space, mentioned earlier, has two components: **Alveolar dead space** is the portion of the tidal volume that enters into alveoli that are without any perfusion or without adequate perfusion. Conditions that can lead to alveolar dead space include pulmonary emboli, partial obstruction of the pulmonary vasculature, destroyed pulmonary vasculature (as can occur in chronic obstructive pulmonary disease [COPD]), and reduced cardiac output. Anatomic dead space is the portion of the tidal volume that never reaches the alveoli for gas exchange (upper airways, trachea, bronchi and so on until the respiratory bronchiole). The sum of alveolar and anatomic dead space is often referred to as physiologic dead space (V_D). The dead space to tidal volume ratio (V_D/V_T) affects alveolar ventilation:

$$\dot{V}_A = \dot{V}_E\left(1 - \frac{V_D}{V_T}\right)$$

where

$\dot{V}_A$ = alveolar ventilation (L/min)

$\dot{V}_E$ = minute ventilation (L/min)

V_D = dead space volume (ml)

V_T = tidal volume (ml)

The clinical significance of increased dead space, or V_D/V_T ratio, is that it decreases alveolar ventilation and hence increases P_aCO_2. This can happen by the addition of extra tubing to the ventilator (exogenous V_D), lung disease (increased alveolar V_D), or shallow breathing (decreased V_T that leads to increased V_D/V_T ratio). In the face of increased dead space, minute ventilation must increase to achieve normal $\dot{V}_A$ and P_aCO_2. This additional ventilation comes at a cost with an increase in the work of breathing, which consumes additional O_2 and further adds to the burden of external ventilation. Similarly, patients with rapid shallow breathing will often have ineffective ventilation with increased P_aCO_2 despite elevated minute ventilation.

As the $\dot{V}_A/\dot{Q}$ decreases below 1.0 (Figure 12-5, following the *curve to the left*), more O_2-poor, CO_2-rich blood reaches alveolar air. The result is a lower P_AO_2 and higher P_ACO_2. At the extreme left of the graph, there is perfusion but no ventilation ($\dot{V}_A/\dot{Q}$ = 0). With no ventilation to remove CO_2 and restore fresh O_2, the makeup of gases in these areas is similar to that of mixed venous blood ($P_{\bar{V}}O_2$ = 40 mm Hg; $P_{\bar{V}}O_2$ = 46 mm Hg).

Venous blood entering areas with $\dot{V}_A/\dot{Q}$ values of zero cannot pick up O_2 or unload CO_2 and leave the lungs unchanged. As this venous blood returns to the left side of the heart, it mixes with well-oxygenated arterial blood, diluting its O_2 contents in a manner similar to that described for a right-to-left anatomic shunt. To distinguish such areas from true anatomic shunts, exchange units with $\dot{V}_A/\dot{Q}$ values of zero are called **alveolar shunts.** Anatomic and alveolar shunts together cause venous blood to mix with the arterial blood, a phenomenon called **venous admixture.** Alveolar shunts can be caused by COPD, restrictive disorders, or any condition resulting in hypoventilation.

In addition to blood that perfuses anatomic and alveolar shunts, a portion of venous blood travels from the right heart to the left heart without being involved in adequate gas exchange with ventilated portions of the lung. Together, they are called *physiologic shunt.* The shunt equation quantifies the portion of blood included in the $\dot{V}_A/\dot{Q}$ mismatch, in which $\dot{V}_A/\dot{Q}$ is less than 1. It is usually expressed as a percentage of the total cardiac output:

$$\frac{Q_s}{Q_t} = \frac{C_cO_2 - C_aO_2}{C_cO_2 - C_vO_2}$$

where:

Q_s = Shunt flow; blood entering systemic blood without being oxygenated in the lungs

Q_t = Total cardiac output

C_cO_2 = O_2 content at the end of the ventilated and perfused pulmonary capillaries

C_aO_2 = Arterial O_2 content

C_vO_2 = Mixed venous O_2 content

Although arterial O_2 content can be directly measured from a systemic artery and mixed venous O_2 content can be directly measured from the pulmonary artery, the end capillary content must be derived from an additional calculation requiring use of the alveolar air equation and the Hb concentration. A more practical *estimation* of the shunt fraction is as follows: each increase of $D_{A\text{-}a}O_2$ by 100 mm Hg corresponds to 5% increase in shunt fraction.

Causes of Regional Differences in Ventilation-Perfusion Ratio

Regional variations in $\dot{V}_A/\dot{Q}$ for a normal lung are mainly caused by gravity and are most evident in the upright posture. Because the pulmonary circulation is a low-pressure system, blood flow in the upright lung varies considerably from top to bottom (see Chapter 9). Farther down the lung, perfusion increases linearly in proportion to the hydrostatic pressure so that the lung bases receive nearly 20 times as much blood flow as the apexes.

Regional differences in ventilation throughout the lung also occur, but they are less drastic than the differences in perfusion. Similar to perfusion, ventilation also is increased in the lung bases, with approximately four times as much ventilation going to the bases than to the apexes of the upright lung. These regional differences in ventilation are caused by the effect of gravity on pleural pressures (see Chapter 11).

Table 12-1 summarizes the relationships between ventilation and perfusion by lung region.[8] At the lung apexes, ventilation exceeds blood flow, resulting in a high $\dot{V}_A/\dot{Q}$ (approximately 3.3), high PO_2 (132 mm Hg), and low PCO_2 (32 mm Hg). Farther down the lung, blood flow increases more than ventilation owing to gravity. Toward the middle, the two are approximately equal ($\dot{V}_A/\dot{Q}$ = 1.0). At the bottom of the lung, blood flow is greater than ventilation, resulting in a low $\dot{V}_A/\dot{Q}$ (approximately 0.66), low PO_2 (89 mm Hg), and slightly higher PCO_2 (42 mm Hg).

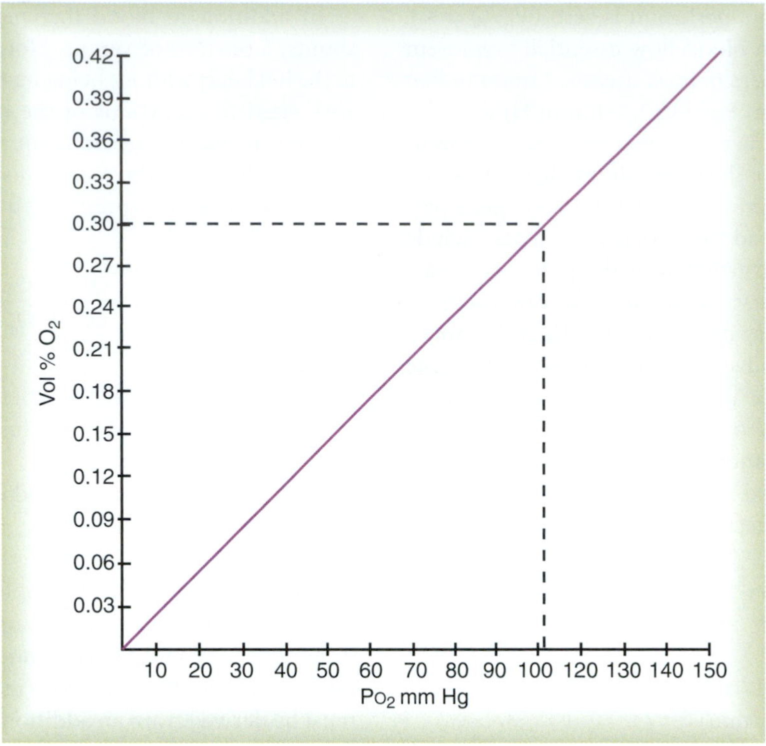

FIGURE 12-6 Relationship between PO_2 and dissolved O_2 contents of plasma at 37° C. The *dashed line* emphasizes the fact that arterial blood, with average PO_2 of 100 mm Hg, has 0.3 ml of O_2 dissolved in each deciliter (100 ml).

TABLE 12-1

Summary of Variations in Gas Exchange in the Upright Lung by Region

Lung Region	$\dot{V}_A/\dot{Q}$ Ratio	Mean P_AO_2 (mm Hg)	Mean P_ACO_2 (mm Hg)	Blood Flow
Apexes	3.3	132	32	Low
Middle	1.0	100	40	Moderate
Bases	0.66	89	42	High

As shown in Table 12-1, because of gravity, most blood flows to the lung bases, where PO_2 is less than normal and PCO_2 is greater than normal. After leaving the lung, this large volume of blood combines with the smaller volume coming from the middle and apical regions. The result is a mixture of blood with less O_2 and more CO_2 than would come from an ideal gas-exchange unit.

OXYGEN TRANSPORT

Blood carries O_2 in two forms. A small amount of O_2 exists in a simple physical solution, dissolved in the plasma and erythrocyte intracellular fluid. However, most O_2 is carried in a reversible chemical combination with hemoglobin (Hb) inside the RBC. As gaseous O_2 diffuses into the blood, it immediately dissolves in the plasma and erythrocyte fluid. By applying Henry's law (see Chapter 6), the amount of dissolved O_2 in the blood (at 37°C) can be computed with the following simple formula:

$$\text{Dissolved } O_2\ (\text{ml/dl}) = PO_2\ (\text{mm Hg}) \times 0.003$$

This equation is plotted in Figure 12-6, which shows that the relationship between partial pressure and dissolved O_2 is direct and linear. In normal arterial blood with PaO_2 of approximately 100 mm Hg, there is approximately 0.3 ml/dl of dissolved O_2. However, if an individual with normal arterial blood breathes pure O_2, PaO_2 increases to approximately 670 mm Hg. In this case, the dissolved O_2 would increase to approximately 2.0 ml/dl. The blood of someone breathing pure O_2 in a hyperbaric chamber at 3 atmospheres (2280 mm Hg) would carry nearly 6.5 ml/dl dissolved O_2 in the plasma. Despite such extreme conditions ($FiO_2 = 1$, barometric pressure = 3 atmospheres), the amount of dissolved O_2 is still a small fraction of the amount carried by hemoglobin under normal conditions.

Chemically Combined Oxygen (Oxyhemoglobin)

Hemoglobin and Oxygen Transport

Most blood O_2 is transported in chemical combination with Hb in the erythrocytes. Hb is a conjugated protein, consisting of four linked polypeptide chains (the *globin* portion), each of which is combined with a porphyrin complex called *heme*. The four polypeptide chains of Hb are coiled together into a ball-like structure, the shape of which determines its affinity for O_2.[5,8]

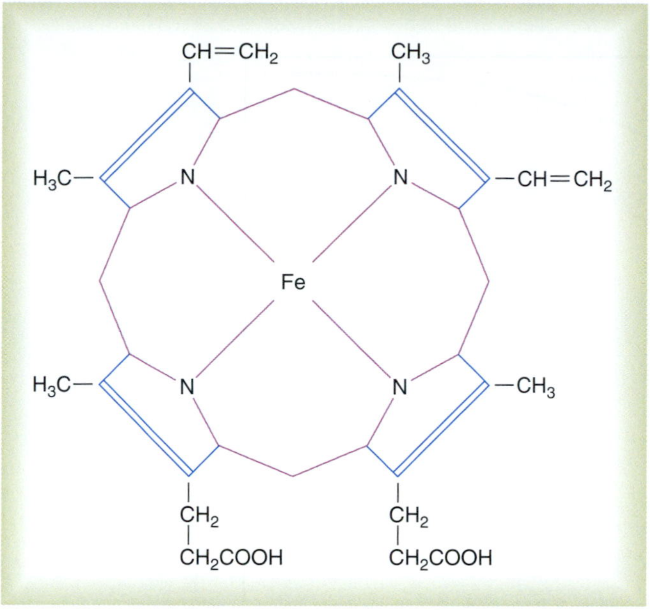

FIGURE 12-7 Structure of heme.

As shown in Figure 12-7, each heme complex contains a centrally located ferrous iron ion. When Hb is not carrying O_2, this ion has four unpaired electrons. In this deoxygenated state, the molecule exhibits the characteristics of a weak acid. Deoxygenated Hb serves as an important blood buffer for H+, a crucial factor in CO_2 transport.

When fully saturated, 4 O_2 molecules bind to the iron ion of Hb, one for each protein chain. With complete O_2 binding, all electrons become paired, and Hb is converted to its oxygenated state (**oxyhemoglobin** [HbO_2]).

In whole blood, 1 g of normal Hb can carry approximately 1.34 ml of O_2. Given an average blood Hb content of 15 g/dl, the O_2-carrying capacity of the blood can be calculated as follows:

$$1.34\ \text{ml/g} \times 15\ \text{g/dl} = 20.1\ \text{ml/dl}$$

The addition of Hb increases the O_2-carrying capacity of the blood nearly 70-fold compared with plasma alone. The amount of O_2 bound to Hb depends on its level of saturation with O_2 (see later).

Hemoglobin Saturation

Saturation is a measure of the proportion of available Hb that is carrying O_2. Saturation is computed as the ratio of HbO_2 (content) to total Hb (capacity). Hb arterial O_2 saturation (SaO_2) is usually expressed as a percentage of this ratio and calculated according to the following formula:

$$SaO_2 = (HbO_2 \div \text{Total Hb}) \times 100$$

where HbO_2 equals the oxyhemoglobin content. If there were a total of 15 g/dL Hb in the blood, of which 7.5 g was HbO_2, the SaO_2 would be calculated as follows:

$$SaO_2\ (\%) = (7.5 \div 15) \times 100 = 50\%$$

In this example, Hb is said to be 50% saturated: Only half of the available Hb is carrying O_2, and the remainder is unoxygenated. In clinical practice, both SaO_2 and total Hb content are measured directly to derive the HbO_2. Normal SaO_2 is 95% to 100% depending on the age of the patient.

Total Oxygen Content of the Blood

Total O_2 content of the blood equals the sum of O_2 dissolved and chemically combined with Hb.[2,7] For total O_2 content to be calculated, the following three values must be known: (1) PO_2, (2) total Hb content (g/dL), and (3) Hb saturation. Given these values, the following equation can be applied:

$$CaO_2 = (0.003 \times PaO_2) + (1.34 \times Hb \times SaO_2)$$

where:

CaO_2 = Total O_2 content (ml/dl)
PaO_2 = Partial pressure of O_2 in the blood
Hb = Hb content (in g/dl)
SaO_2 = Hb saturation with O_2 (as a decimal)

Typically, clinicians want to know the O_2 content of arterial blood (CaO_2). The ($0.003 \times PO_2$) component of the equation represents dissolved O_2, whereas the ($Hb \times 1.34 \times SO_2$) component represents the chemically combined oxyhemoglobin. For example, to compute the total O_2 content of normal arterial blood (assuming PaO_2 = 100, Hb = 15g/dl, SaO_2= 0.97):

$$CaO_2 = (0.003 \times PaO_2) + (1.34 \times Hb \times SaO_2)$$
$$CaO_2 = (0.003 \times 100) + (1.34 \times 15 \times 0.97)$$
$$CaO_2 = 0.3 + 19.5$$
$$CaO_2 = 19.8\ (\text{ml/dl})$$

The normal CaO_2 concentration is 16 to 20 ml/dl. Note that dissolved O_2 contributes a small fraction of blood's total O_2 carrying capacity (0.3/19.8 = 1.5%) and is often omitted from the practical discussions and calculations.

Oxyhemoglobin Dissociation Curve

Hb saturation with O_2 varies with changes in PO_2. Plotting the saturation (*y*-axis) against PO_2 (*x*-axis) yields the HbO_2 dissociation curve (Figure 12-8). In contrast to dissolved O_2, Hb saturation is not linearly related to PO_2.[4] Instead, the relationship forms an S-shaped curve. The flat upper part of this curve represents the normal operating range for arterial blood. Because the slope is minimal in this area, major changes in PaO_2 have little effect on SaO_2, indicating a strong affinity of Hb for O_2. With a normal PaO_2 of 100 mm Hg, SaO_2 is approximately 97%. If some abnormality (e.g., lung disease) reduced PaO_2 to 65 mm Hg, SaO_2 would still be approximately 90%.

However, with PO_2 less than 60 mm Hg, the curve steepens dramatically, which is why it is beneficial to keep PaO_2 greater than 60 mm Hg in clinical practice. With PO_2 less than 60 mm Hg, a small decrease in PO_2 causes a large decrease in SaO_2, indicating a lessening affinity for O_2. This normal decrease in the affinity of Hb for O_2 helps release large amounts of O_2 to the tissues, where PO_2 is low.

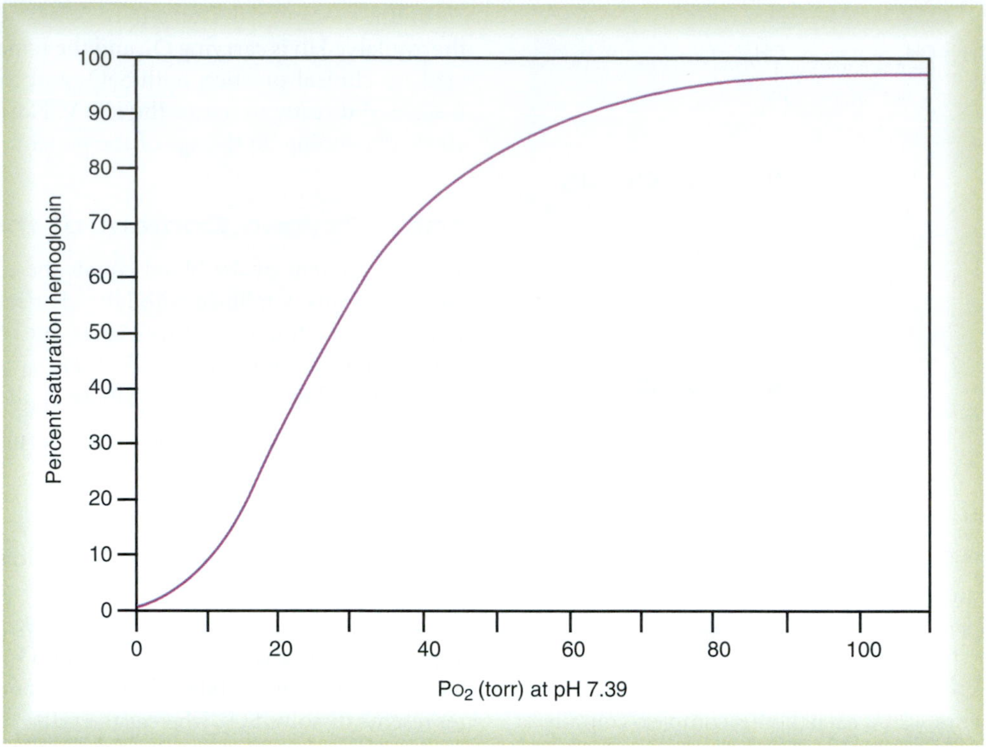

FIGURE 12-8 O_2 dissociation curve plots the relationship between plasma PO_2 (*x*-axis) and Hb saturation (*y*-axis).

MINI CLINI

Relating Hemoglobin Saturation and PaO_2

PROBLEM: Pulse oximeters are simple bedside devices that measure Hb saturation by way of a noninvasive probe taped to the patient's finger or forehead. Although oximeters measure Hb saturation percentage, blood oxygenation still tends to be quantified according to PaO_2. Is there a simple way to relate these two measures without carrying around an HbO_2 dissociation curve?

DISCUSSION: First, although extremely useful, pulse oximeters are relatively inaccurate (compared to other types of clinical measurement device) and they measure only normal Hb saturation. This limitation should be understood. The value of oximetry is in its ability to display trends and provide warning of significant changes in Hb saturation with O_2.

Even so, RTs often need to estimate PaO_2 from oximeter readings. The following simple rule, called the *40-50-60/70-80-90 rule,* should be helpful. Assuming normal pH, PCO_2, and Hb values, saturations of 70%, 80%, and 90% are roughly equivalent to PO_2 values of 40 mm Hg, 50 mm Hg, and 60 mm Hg:

Hb Saturation (%)	Approximate PaO_2 (mm Hg)
70	40
80	50
90	60

A patient with a pulse oximeter reading of 90% has a PaO_2 of approximately 60 mm Hg. If the saturation decreased to 80%, the PaO_2 would decrease to approximately 50 mm Hg. This rule works only in the middle range of PO_2 values, where the curve is most linear; it should not be applied with saturations greater than 90% or less than 70%.

Although SaO_2 plays a greater part in total blood O_2 content than PaO_2, it is often important to consider both when evaluating a patient's oxygenation. First, PaO_2 is a more accurate measurement than SaO_2, which is usually derived from pulse oximetry. In addition, a patient with an SaO_2 of 100% may have a PaO_2 between 100 and 600 mm Hg and the knowledge of exact PaO_2 value gives a clinician a better understanding of the patient's gas-exchange status.

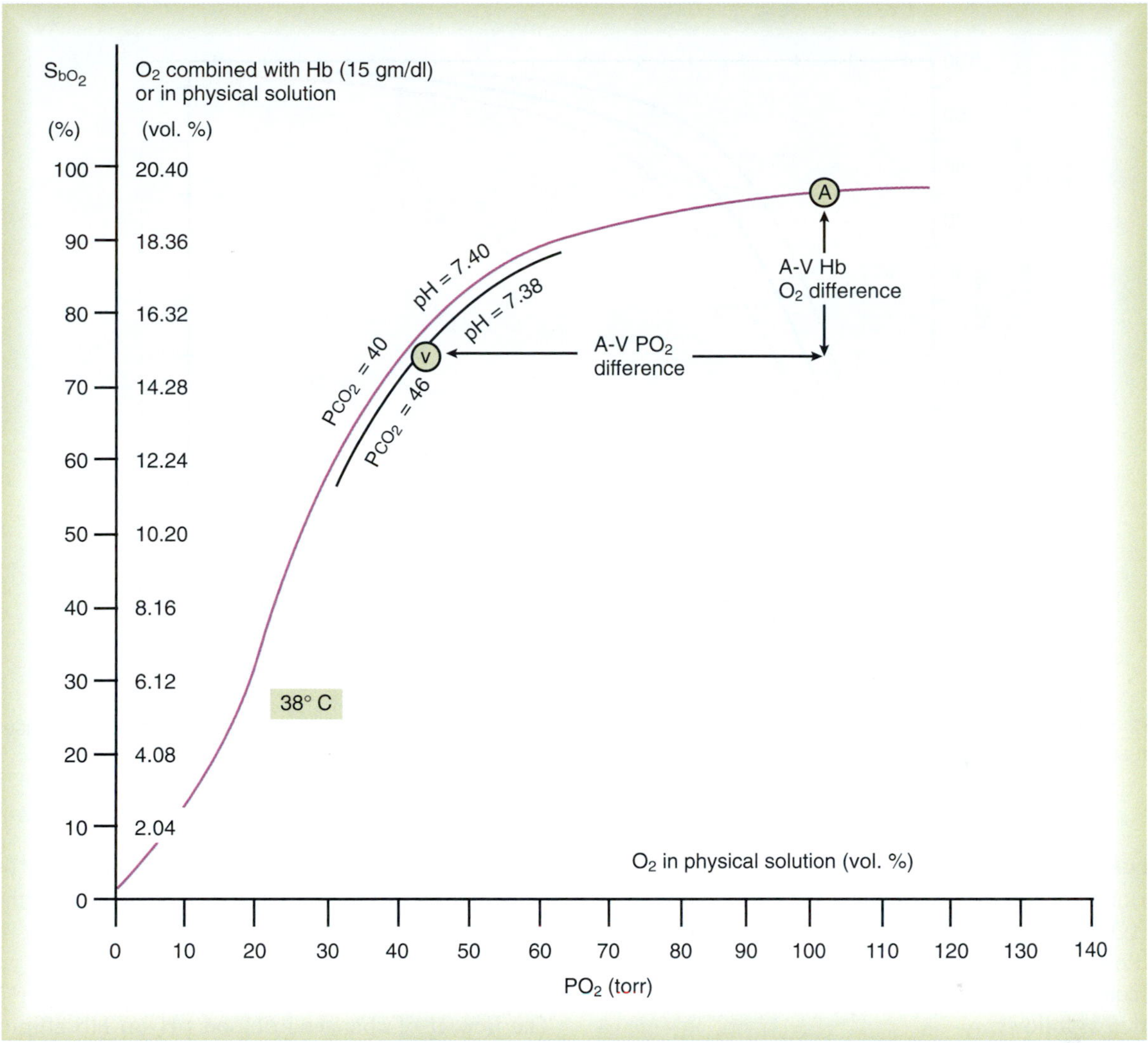

FIGURE 12-9 Normal oxyhemoglobin dissociation curve, showing the basic relationship of blood O_2 transport. Point *sA* represents normal values for arterial blood leaving the lungs (loading point). Point *sV* represents normal values for venous blood leaving the tissues (unloading point). The slight difference in curve position resulting from pH and CO_2 changes helps O_2 unloading at the tissues. Differences between O_2 content at these two points represent the amount of O_2 taken up by the tissues on one pass through the systemic circulation. (Modified from Slonim NB, Hamilton LH: Respiratory physiology, ed 5, St Louis, 1987, Mosby.)

Normal Loading and Unloading of Oxygen (Arteriovenous Differences)

Figure 12-9 uses the HbO_2 dissociation curve to show the effects of O_2 loading and unloading in the lungs and tissues. *Point A* represents freshly arterialized blood leaving the pulmonary capillaries, with PO_2 of approximately 100 mm Hg and Hb saturation of approximately 97%. As blood perfuses body tissues, O_2 uptake causes a decrease in both PO_2 and saturation, such that venous blood leaving the tissues *(point V)* has a PO_2 of approximately 40 mm Hg, with Hb saturation of approximately 75%.

Using a normal Hb content of 15 g/dl and knowing the saturation at each possible PO_2, the total O_2 content can be calculated at any PO_2 in the manner previously described. The *y*-axis of Figure 12-9 provides this information in SaO_2 increments of 10%. Table 12-2 summarizes the difference between the O_2 content of these normal arterial and venous points.

TABLE 12-2

Oxygen Content of Arterial and Venous Blood

O_2 Content	Arterial O_2 (ml/dl)	Venous O_2 (ml/dl)
Combined O_2 ($1.34 \times 15 \times SO_2$)	19.5	14.7
Dissolved O_2 ($PO_2 \times 0.003$)	0.3	0.1
Total O_2 content	19.8	14.8

As indicated in Table 12-2, the difference between the arterial and venous O_2 contents is normally approximately 5 ml/dl. This is the arterial-to-venous O_2 content difference ($C_{a-v}O_2$). It is the amount of O_2 given up by every 100 ml of blood on each pass through the tissues.

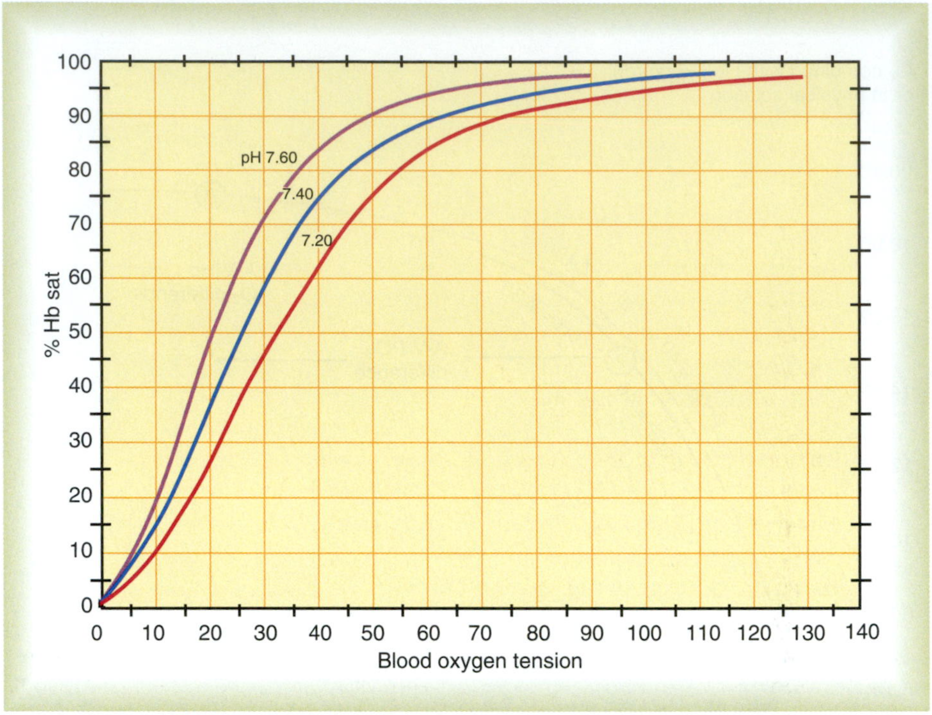

FIGURE 12-10 O_2 dissociation curve of blood at 37° C, showing variations at three pH levels. A right shift (lower pH) decreases Hb affinity for O_2, whereas a left shift (higher pH) increases Hb affinity for O_2.

Fick Equation

The Fick principle states that the total O_2 uptake by the peripheral tissues (O_2 consumption, or $\dot{V}_{O_2}$) is equal to the product of the blood flow to the peripheral tissues and the arterial-to-venous O_2 content difference ($C_{a-v}O_2$). The classic **Fick equation** is written as follows:

$$\dot{V}_{O_2} = CO \times (C_aO_2 - C_vO_2) \times 10$$

where

CO = cardiac output (ml/min)
$\dot{V}_{O_2}$ = whole-body O_2 consumption (ml/min)
C_aO_2 = arterial O_2 content (ml/dl)
C_VO_2 = venous O_2 content (ml/dl)

According to the Fick equation, if a patient becomes hypoxic (C_aO_2 falls), total-body O_2 consumption can be maintained by either increasing cardiac output. Also, hypoxic tissues compensate by vasodilation (increased blood flow to the tissues) or increasing O_2 extraction (C_aO_2 − C_vO_2). Although the Fick equation for calculating cardiac output has been replaced by other techniques, the principle relating O_2 extraction to perfusion is used to monitor tissue oxygenation at the bedside. More details on these methods are provided in Chapter 51.

Factors Affecting Oxygen Loading and Unloading

In addition to the shape of the HbO_2 curve, many other factors affect O_2 loading and unloading. Among the most important factors in clinical practice are blood pH, body temperature, and erythrocyte concentration of certain organic phosphates.[5] Variations in the structure of Hb also affect O_2 loading and unloading, as can chemical combinations of Hb with substances other than O_2, such as CO.

pH (Bohr Effect)

The impact of changes in blood pH on Hb affinity for O_2 is called the **Bohr effect.** As shown in Figure 12-10, the Bohr effect alters the position of the HbO_2 dissociation curve. A low pH (acidity) shifts the curve to the right, whereas a high pH (alkalinity) shifts it to the left. These changes are a result of variations in the shape of the Hb molecule caused by fluctuations in pH.

As blood pH decreases and the curve shifts to the right, the Hb saturation for a given PO_2 decreases. This is important for the tissue O_2 delivery because acidic environment of the tissues allows O_2 to dissociate from Hb into the tissues. Conversely, as blood pH increases and the curve shifts to the left, the Hb saturation for a given PO_2 increases (increased affinity of Hb for O_2).[4,5,8] Therefore, when venous blood returns to the lungs, the pH increases and higher pH shifts the HbO_2 curve back to the left, increasing the affinity of Hb for O_2 and enhancing its uptake from the alveoli.

Body Temperature

Variations in body temperature also affect the HbO_2 dissociation curve. As shown in Figure 12-11, a decrease in body temperature shifts the curve to the left, increasing Hb affinity for O_2. Conversely, as body temperature increases, the curve shifts to the right, and the affinity of Hb for O_2 decreases. As with the

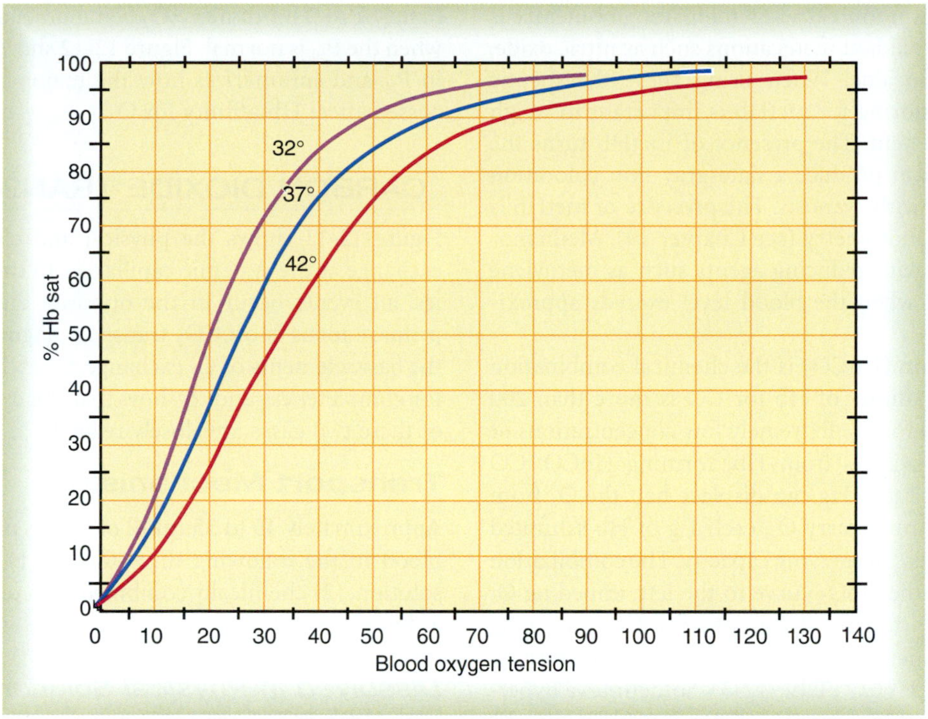

FIGURE 12-11 O_2 dissociation curve of blood at pH of 7.40, showing variations at three temperatures. For a given O_2 tension, the lower the temperature, the more the Hb holds onto O_2, maintaining a higher saturation.

Bohr effect, these changes enhance normal O_2 uptake and delivery. At the tissues, metabolic activity increases the temperature, which allows more O_2 to be released into the tissues.

Organic Phosphates (2,3-Diphosphoglycerate)

The organic phosphate 2,3-diphosphoglycerate (2,3-DPG) is found in abundance in the RBCs, where it forms a loose chemical bond with the globin chains of deoxygenated Hb. In this configuration, 2,3-DPG stabilizes the molecule in its deoxygenated state, reducing its affinity for O_2.[5-7] Without 2,3-DPG, Hb affinity for O_2 would be so great that normal O_2 unloading would be impossible. Increased 2,3-DPG concentrations shift the HbO_2 curve to the right, promoting O_2 unloading. Conversely, low 2,3-DPG concentrations shift the curve to the left, increasing Hb affinity for O_2.

Alkalosis, chronic hypoxemia, and anemia all tend to increase 2,3-DPG concentrations and promote O_2 unloading. Conversely, acidosis results in a lower intracellular level of 2,3-DPG and a greater affinity of Hb for O_2.

Erythrocyte concentrations of 2,3-DPG in banked blood decrease over time. After 1 week of storage, the 2,3-DPG level may be less than one-third of the normal value. This change shifts the HbO_2 curve to the left, decreasing the availability of O_2 to the tissues. Large transfusions of banked blood that is more than a few days old can severely impair O_2 delivery, even in the presence of normal PO_2. Improved maintenance levels of 2,3-DPG can be achieved with newer blood storage techniques.

Abnormal Hemoglobin

Structural or chemical abnormalities within the Hb also affect O_2 affinity. More than 120 abnormal HbS have been identified. In healthy individuals, 15% to 40% of the circulating Hb may be abnormal.

HbS (**sickle cell hemoglobin**) is less soluble than normal Hb, which causes it to become susceptible to polymerization and precipitation when deoxygenated. Certain events such as dehydration, hypoxia, and acidosis cause HbS to crystallize and the RBC to become hardened and curved like a sickle. Erythrocyte fragility is increased (leading to hemolysis), and the risk for thrombus formation is increased. Patients with sickle cell disease are prone to vasoocclusive disease and anemia. Some patients with sickle cell anemia develop **acute chest syndrome.** Acute chest syndrome is the most common cause of death in patients with sickle cell anemia. Patients usually complain of acute chest pain, cough, and shortness of breath. A new infiltrate is usually seen on the chest radiograph, and the patient often develops progressive anemia and hypoxemia. The causes of acute chest syndrome are multiple; the term *acute chest syndrome* does not indicate a definite diagnosis but rather indicates the clinical difficulty of defining a specific cause in most of such episodes.

Methemoglobin (metHb) is an abnormal form of the molecule, in which the heme-complex normal Fe^{++} loses an electron and is oxidized to its ferric state (Fe^{++}). In the ferric state, the iron ion cannot combine with O_2. This is called **methemoglobinemia.** As with HbCO, clinical abnormalities come from the associated increased affinity for O_2 and loss of O_2-binding capacity. The most common cause of methemoglobinemia is the therapeutic use of oxidant medications such as nitric oxide, nitroglycerin, and lidocaine. When using these therapeutic agents, frequent monitoring for metHb is important to weigh the risk against the benefit. The presence of metHb turns the blood brown, which can produce a slate-gray skin coloration that is often confused with cyanosis. The presence of metHb is confirmed by spectrophotometry (see Chapter 19). Methemoglobinemia is treated with reducing agents such as methylene blue or ascorbic acid when the blood level exceeds approximately 30%.

Carboxyhemoglobin (HbCO) is the chemical combination of Hb with CO. The affinity of Hb for CO is more than 200 times greater than it is for O_2. Extremely low concentrations of CO can quickly displace O_2 from Hb, forming HbCO. CO partial pressure of 0.12 mm Hg can displace half the O_2 from Hb. Because HbCO cannot carry O_2, each 1 g of Hb saturated with CO represents a loss in carrying capacity. The combination of CO with Hb shifts the HbO_2 curve to the left, impeding O_2 delivery to the tissues further. Treatment for CO poisoning involves giving the patient as much O_2 as possible because O_2 reduces the half-life of HbCO (Table 12-3). Sometimes a hyperbaric chamber is required to reverse rapidly the binding of CO with Hb.

During fetal life and for up to 1 year after birth, the blood has a high proportion of an Hb variant called **fetal hemoglobin (HbF).** HbF has a greater affinity for O_2 than normal adult Hb, as manifested by a leftward shift of the HbO_2 curve. Given the low PO_2 values available to the fetus in utero, this leftward shift aids O_2 loading at the placenta. Because of the relatively low pH of the fetal environment, O_2 unloading at the cellular level is not greatly affected. However, after birth, this enhanced O_2 affinity is less advantageous. Over the first year of life, HbF is gradually replaced with normal Hb.

Measurement of Hemoglobin Affinity for Oxygen

Variations in the affinity of Hb for O_2 are quantified by a measure called the **P50.**[2,8] The P_{50} is the partial pressure of O_2 at which the Hb is 50% saturated, standardized to a pH level of 7.40. A normal P_{50} is approximately 26.6 mm Hg. Conditions that cause a decrease in Hb affinity for O_2 (a shift of the HbO_2 curve to the right) increase the P_{50} to a value higher than normal. Conditions associated with an increase in affinity (a shift of the HbO_2 curve to the left) decrease the P_{50} to lower than normal. With 15 g/dl Hb, a 4-mm Hg increase in P_{50} results in approximately 1 to 2 ml/dl more O_2 being unloaded in the tissues than when the P_{50} is normal. Figure 12-12 shows the effect of changes in P_{50} and summarizes how the major factors previously discussed affect Hb affinity for O_2.

TABLE 12-3

Half-Life of Carboxyhemoglobin (HbCO) at Different Oxygen Exposures

HbCO Half-Life (min)	Inhaled FiO_2	PaO_2 (mm Hg)
280-320	0.21 at 1 atm	100
80-90	1.0 at 1 atm	673
20-30	1.0 at 3 atm	2193

CARBON DIOXIDE TRANSPORT

Figure 12-13 shows the physical and chemical events of gas exchange at the systemic capillaries. In the pulmonary capillaries, all events occur in the opposite direction. Although the primary focus is on CO_2 transport, Figure 12-13 also includes the basic elements of O_2 exchange. O_2 exchange is included here for completeness and to show that the exchange and transport of these two gases are closely related.

Transport Mechanisms

Approximately 45 to 55 ml/dl of CO_2 is normally carried in the blood in the following three forms: (1) dissolved in physical solution, (2) chemically combined with protein, and (3) ionized as bicarbonate.[5,7]

Dissolved in Physical Solution

As with O_2, CO_2 produced by the tissues dissolves in the plasma and erythrocyte intracellular fluid. However, in contrast to O_2, dissolved CO_2 plays an important role in transport, accounting for approximately 8% of the total released at the lungs; this is because of the higher solubility of CO_2 in plasma.

Chemically Combined With Protein

Molecular CO_2 has the capacity to combine chemically with free amino groups (NH_2) of protein molecules (Prot), forming a carbamino compound:

$$\text{Prot-NH}_2 + CO_2 = \text{Prot-NHCOO}^- + H^+$$

A small amount of the CO_2 leaving the tissues combines with plasma proteins to form these carbamino compounds. A larger fraction of CO_2 combines with erythrocyte Hb to form a carbamino compound called *carbaminohemoglobin*. As indicated in the previous equation, this reaction produces hydrogen ions. These H^+ ions are buffered by the reduced Hb, which is made available by the concurrent release of O_2.

The availability of additional sites for H^+ buffering increases the affinity of Hb for CO_2. Because reduced Hb is a weaker acid than HbO_2, pH changes associated with the release of the H^+ ions in the formation of carbaminohemoglobin are minimized. Carbaminohemoglobin constitutes approximately 12% of the total CO_2 transported.

Ionized as Bicarbonate

Approximately 80% of CO_2 in the blood is transported as bicarbonate. Of the CO_2 that dissolves in plasma, a small portion combines chemically with water in the process *hydrolysis*. Hydrolysis of CO_2 initially forms carbonic acid, which quickly ionizes into H^+ and bicarbonate ions:

$$CO_2 + H_2O = H_2CO_3 = HCO_3^- + H^+$$

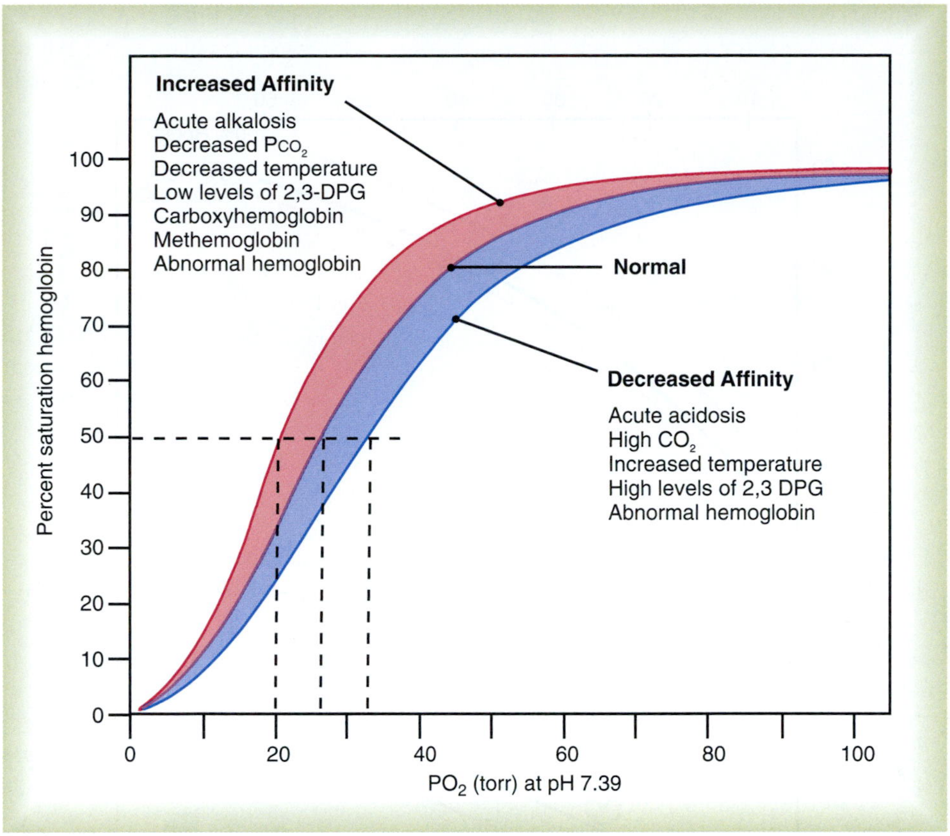

FIGURE 12-12 Conditions associated with altered affinity of Hb for O_2. P_{50} is PaO_2 at which Hb is 50% saturated (normally 26.6 mm Hg). A lower than normal P_{50} represents increased affinity of Hb for O_2. A high P_{50} is seen with decreased affinity. *2,3-DPG,* 2,3-Diphosphoglycerate. (Modified from Lane EE, Walker JF: Clinical arterial blood gas analysis, St Louis, 1987, Mosby.)

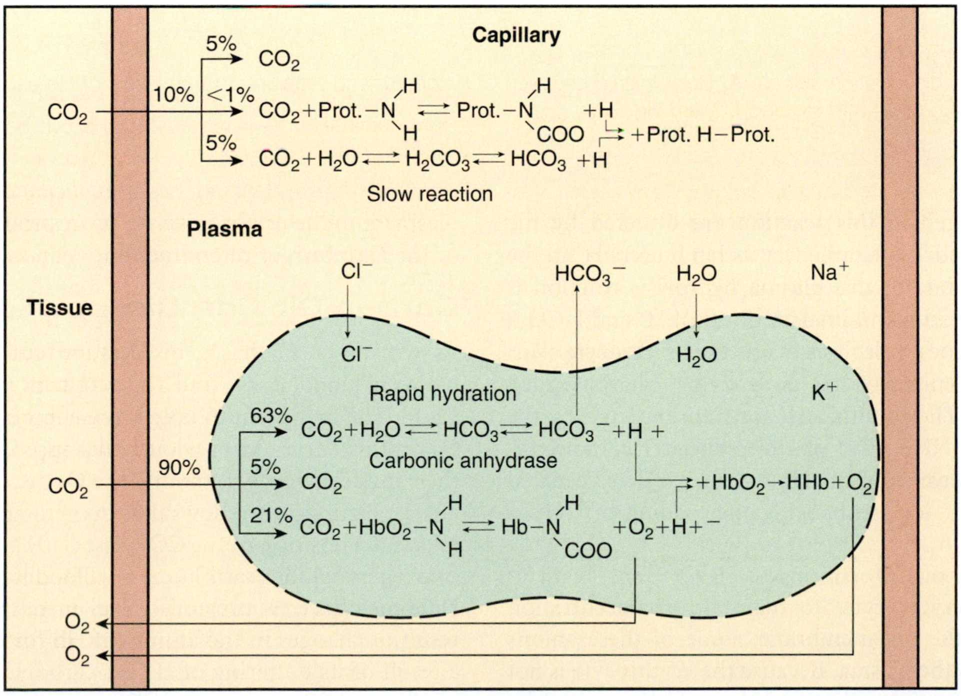

FIGURE 12-13 Summary diagram of various fates of CO_2 as it diffuses from the cells and interstitial spaces into the peripheral capillaries before its transport toward the venous circulation. (Modified from Martin DE, Youtsey JW: Respiratory anatomy and physiology, St Louis, 1988, Mosby.)

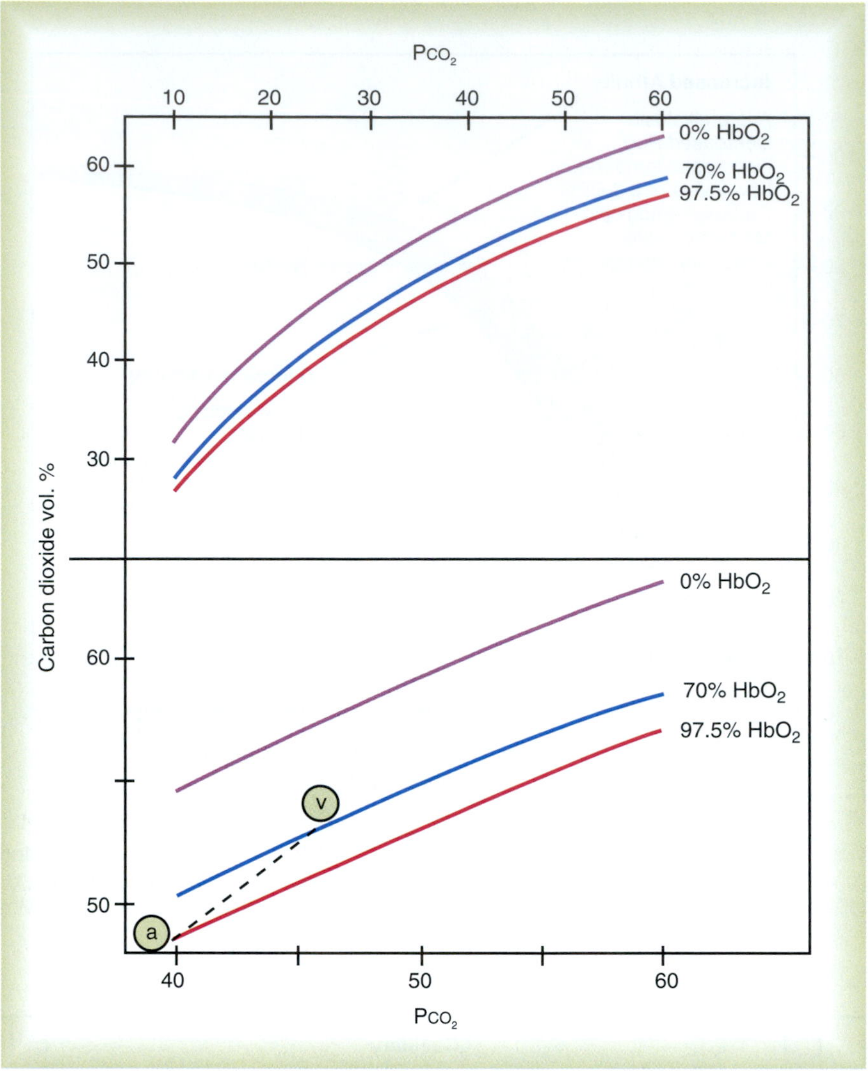

FIGURE 12-14 CO_2 dissociation curves. **A,** Relationship between CO_2 content and tension at three levels of Hb saturation. **B,** Close-up of curves between PCO_2 of 40 mm Hg and 60 mm Hg.

The H^+ ions produced in this reaction are buffered by the plasma proteins in much the same way as Hb buffers H^+ in the RBC. However, the rate of this plasma hydrolysis reaction is extremely slow, producing minimal amounts of H^+ and HCO_3^-.

Most CO_2 undergoes hydrolysis inside the erythrocyte. This reaction is greatly enhanced by an enzyme catalyst called *carbonic anhydrase.* The resulting H^+ ions are buffered by the imidazole group (R-$NHCOO^-$) of the reduced Hb molecule. The concurrent conversion of HbO_2 to its deoxygenated form helps buffer H^+ ions, enhancing the loading of CO_2 as carbaminohemoglobin.

As the hydrolysis of CO_2 continues, HCO_3^- ions begin to accumulate in the erythrocyte. To maintain a concentration equilibrium across the cell membrane, some of these anions diffuse outward into the plasma. Because the erythrocyte is not freely permeable by cations, electrolytic equilibrium must be maintained by way of an inward migration of anions. This migration is achieved by the shifting of chloride ions from the plasma into the erythrocyte—a process called the *chloride shift,* or the **Hamburger phenomenon.**

Carbon Dioxide Dissociation Curve

As with O_2, CO_2 has a dissociation curve. The relationship between blood PCO_2 and CO_2 content is depicted in Figure 12-14. The first point to note is the effect of Hb saturation with O_2 on this curve. As previously discussed, CO_2 levels, through their influence on pH, modify the O_2 dissociation curve (Bohr effect). Figure 12-14 shows that oxyhemoglobin saturation also affects the position of the CO_2 dissociation curve. The influence of oxyhemoglobin saturation on CO_2 dissociation is called the **Haldane effect.** As previously explained, this phenomenon is a result of changes in the affinity of Hb for CO_2, which occur as a result of its buffering of H^+ ions.[4-7]

Figure 12-14, *A* shows CO_2 dissociation curves for three levels of blood O_2 saturation. The first two are physiologic values, and the third extreme value is provided for contrast.

Figure 12-14, *B* amplifies selected segments of these curves in the physiologic range of PCO_2. Note first the arterial point *a* lying on the curve representing an SaO_2 of 97.5%. At this point, PCO_2 is 40 mm Hg and CO_2 content is approximately 48 ml/dl. The venous point *v* falls on the curve, representing SaO_2 of approximately 70%. At this point, PCO_2 is 46 mm Hg and CO_2 content is approximately 52 ml/dl. Because O_2 saturation changes from arterial to venous blood, the true physiologic CO_2 dissociation curve must lie somewhere between these two points. This physiologic curve is represented as the *dashed line* in Figure 12-14, B. At point *a*, the high SaO_2 decreases the capacity of the blood to hold CO_2, helping unload this gas at the lungs. At point *v*, the lower mixed venous O_2 saturation (S_vO_2) increases the capacity of the blood for CO_2, aiding uptake at the tissues.

The total CO_2 content of arterial and venous blood is compared in Table 12-4. The amounts of CO_2 are expressed in gaseous volume equivalents (milliliters per deciliter) and as millimoles per liter (mmol/L). This latter measure of the chemical combining power of CO_2 in solutions is critical in understanding the role of this gas in acid-base balance.

TABLE 12-4

Carbon Dioxide Content of Arterial and Venous Blood

Unit of Measure	Arterial	Venous
mmol/L	21.53	23.21
ml/dl	48.01	51.76

ABNORMALITIES OF GAS EXCHANGE AND TRANSPORT

Gas exchange is abnormal when either tissue O_2 delivery or CO_2 removal is impaired.

Impaired Oxygen Delivery

O_2 delivery (DO_2) to the tissues is a product of arterial O_2 content (CaO_2) and cardiac output (CO).

$$DO_2 = CaO_2 \times CO$$

When O_2 delivery is inadequate for cellular needs, **hypoxia** occurs. According to the preceding equation, hypoxia occurs if (1) the arterial blood O_2 content is decreased (*hypoxemia*), (2) cardiac output or perfusion is decreased (*shock* or *ischemia*). Table 12-5 summarizes causes, common clinical indicators, mechanisms, and examples of hypoxia.

Hypoxemia

Hypoxemia occurs when the partial pressure of O_2 in the arterial blood (PaO_2) is decreased to less than the predicted normal value based on the age of the patient. Impaired O_2 delivery also occurs in the presence of abnormalities that prevent saturation of Hb with O_2 (see subsequent discussion).

Decreased Partial Pressure of Oxygen in Arterial Blood. Decreased PaO_2 may be caused by a low ambient PO_2, hypoventilation, impaired diffusion, $\dot{V}_A/\dot{Q}$ imbalances, and right-to-left anatomic or physiologic shunting. PaO_2 also decreases normally with aging. The normal predicted PaO_2 decreases steadily with age, and the average is approximately 85 mm Hg at age 60 years (see later discussion).

TABLE 12-5

Causes of Hypoxia

Cause	Primary Indicator	Mechanism	Example
Hypoxemia			
Low PiO_2	Low P_AO_2 Low PaO_2	Reduced P_B	Altitude
Hypoventilation	High $PaCO_2$	Decreased $\dot{V}_A$	Drug overdose
$\dot{V}_A/\dot{Q}$ imbalance	Low PaO_2 High $D(A–a)O_2$; resolves with O_2	Decreased $\dot{V}_A$ relative to perfusion	COPD, aging
Anatomic shunt	Low PaO_2 High $D(A–a)O_2$; does not resolve with O_2	Blood flow from right to left side of heart	Congenital heart disease
Physiologic shunt	Low PaO_2 High $D(A–a)O_2$; does not resolve with O_2	Perfusion without ventilation	Atelectasis
Diffusion defect	Low PaO_2 High $D(A–a)O_2$; resolves with O_2	Damage to alveolar-capillary membrane	ARDS
Hb deficiency			
Absolute	Low Hb content Reduced CaO_2	Loss of Hb	Hemorrhage
Relative	Abnormal SaO_2 Reduced CaO_2	Abnormal Hb	Carboxyhemoglobin
Low blood flow	Increased $C(a–\bar{v})O_2$	Decreased perfusion	Shock, ischemia
Dysoxia	Normal CaO_2 Decreased $C(a–\bar{v})O_2$	Disruption of cellular enzymes	Cyanide poisoning

ARDS, Acute respiratory distress syndrome; *COPD,* chronic obstructive pulmonary disease.

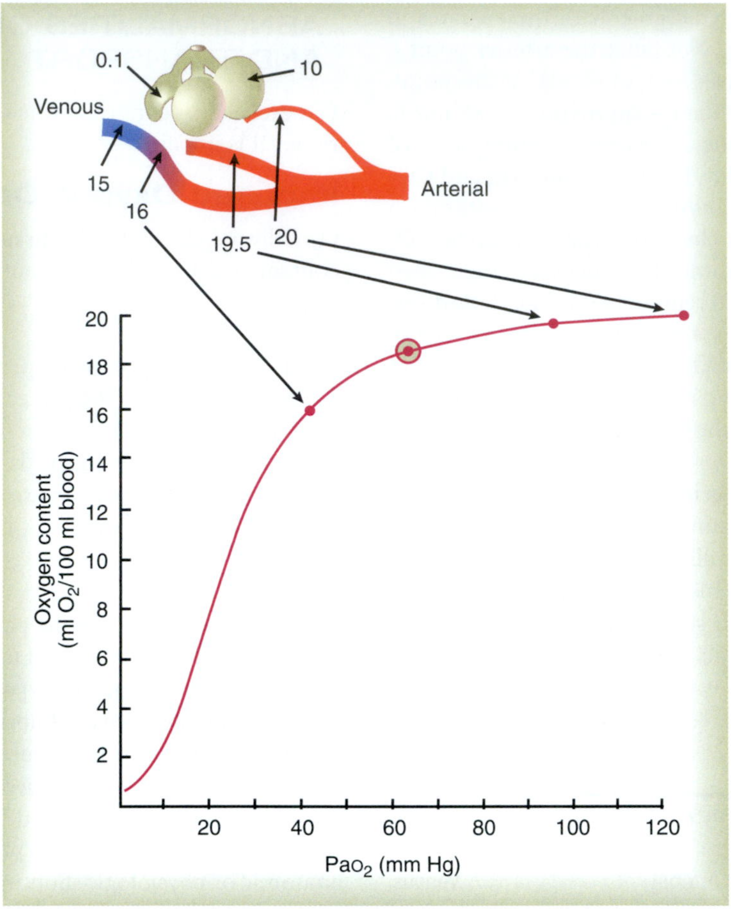

FIGURE 12-15 O_2 dissociation curve. PaO_2 versus O_2 content. O_2 content from alveolar-capillary units with $\dot{V}/\dot{Q}$ of 0.1, 1, and 10 is 16 ml/dl, 19.5 ml/dl, and 20 ml/dl. Lines are drawn for each O_2 content to its point on the dissociation curve. The average O_2 content, 18.5 ml/dl, is represented by a *circle* on the dissociation curve. (Modified from Martin L: Pulmonary physiology in clinical practice: the essentials for patient care and evaluation, St Louis, 1987, Mosby.)

Breathing gases with a low O_2 concentration (hypoxia chamber) or at pressures less than atmospheric (high altitude) lowers PiO_2, thus decreasing P_AO_2 and P_aO_2. A common example of this problem occurs during travel to high altitudes, where the visitor often experiences the ill effects of hypoxia for several days. This condition is called *mountain sickness.* In such cases, although P_aO_2 is reduced, the pressure gradient between the alveoli and the arterial blood for O_2 ($D_{A-a}O_2$) remains normal.

Assuming a constant FiO_2, P_AO_2 varies inversely with $PACO_2$. An increase in P_ACO_2 (hypoventilation) is always accompanied by a proportionate decrease in P_AO_2. $D_{A-a}O_2$ is normal in such cases. Conversely, hyperventilation decreases P_ACO_2 and helps compensate for hypoxemia (but only modestly, as discussed earlier in this chapter).

Even when P_AO_2 is normal, disorders of the alveolar-capillary membrane may limit diffusion of O_2 into the pulmonary capillary blood, decreasing P_aO_2. Examples are pulmonary fibrosis and interstitial edema. However, as previously noted, a pure diffusion limitation is an uncommon cause of hypoxemia at rest.

$\dot{V}_A/\dot{Q}$ imbalances are the most common cause of hypoxemia in patients with lung disease. A $\dot{V}_A/\dot{Q}$ imbalance is an abnormal deviation in the distribution of ventilation to perfusion in the lung. The normal lung has some $\dot{V}_A/\dot{Q}$ mismatch; however, in disease states, the degree of $\dot{V}_A/\dot{Q}$ imbalances becomes much greater. To understand how $\dot{V}_A/\dot{Q}$ imbalance causes hypoxemia, reinspect the normal oxyhemoglobin dissociation curve, with PO_2 plotted against O_2 content (Figure 12-15). The curve is nearly flat in the physiologic range of PaO_2 (>70 mm Hg) but falls steeply when PaO_2 is less than 60 mm Hg. Points representing O_2 content of three separate lung units also are shown. These units have $\dot{V}_A/\dot{Q}$ of 0.1, 1.0, and 10.0.

Blood leaving the normal unit ($\dot{V}_A/\dot{Q} = 1$) has a normal O_2 content (19.5 ml/dl). Blood leaving the unit with poor ventilation ($\dot{V}_A/\dot{Q} = 0.1$) has a low O_2 content (16.0 ml/dl). Because Hb is almost fully saturated at a normal PO_2 of 100 mm Hg, blood leaving the over ventilated unit ($\dot{V}_A/\dot{Q} = 10$) has an O_2 content that is just slightly greater than normal (20.0 ml/dl). When the blood from all three units mixes together, the result is O_2 content that is reduced (18.5 ml/dl). The decrease in oxygenation caused by the poorly ventilated unit is not fully compensated for by the high $\dot{V}_A/\dot{Q}$ unit.

$\dot{V}_A/\dot{Q}$ of zero represents a special type of imbalance. When $\dot{V}_A/\dot{Q}$ is zero, there is blood flow but no ventilation. The result is equivalent to a right to left anatomic shunt, shown at the *bottom* of Figure 12-16. Here, venous blood bypasses ventilated alveoli and mixes with freshly oxygenated arterial blood, resulting in venous admixture.

RULE OF THUMB

Although $\dot{V}_A/\dot{Q}$ imbalances are the most common cause of hypoxemia in patients with respiratory diseases, physiologic shunting also can occur commonly, especially in patients who are critically ill. To differentiate between hypoxemia caused by a $\dot{V}_A/\dot{Q}$ imbalance and hypoxemia caused by shunting, apply the following 50/50 rule: If FiO_2 is greater than 50 (%) and P_aO_2 is less than 50 (mm Hg), significant shunting is present; otherwise, the hypoxemia is mainly caused by a simple $\dot{V}_A/\dot{Q}$ imbalance.

When a low P_aO_2 is observed, the RT must take into account the normal decrease in arterial O_2 tension that occurs with aging. As shown in Figure 12-17, for an individual breathing air at sea level, the "normal" $P_{A-a}O_2$ increases in a near-linear fashion with increasing age *(shaded area)*. This increase in $P_{A-a}O_2$ results in a gradual decline in P_aO_2 over time and is probably caused by reduced surface area in the lung for gas exchange

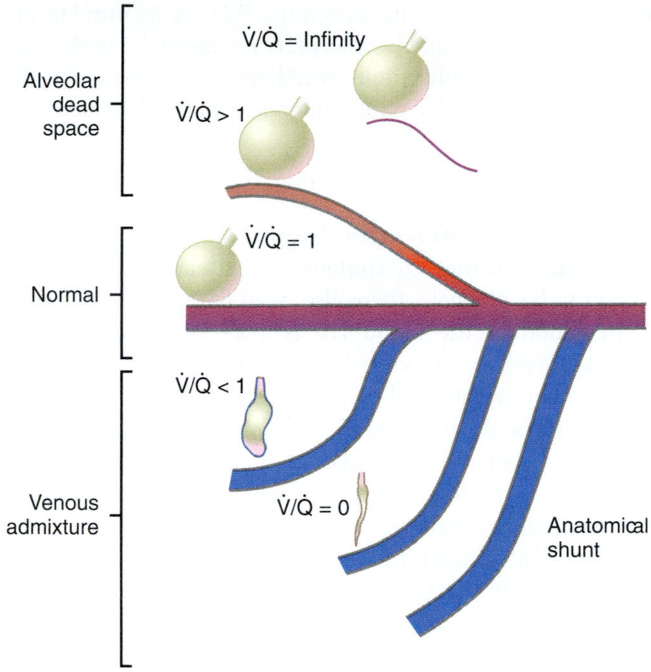

FIGURE 12-16 Range of $\dot{V}_A/\dot{Q}$ ratios. (Modified from Martin L: Pulmonary physiology in current practice: the essentials for patient care and evaluation, St Louis: 1987, Mosby).

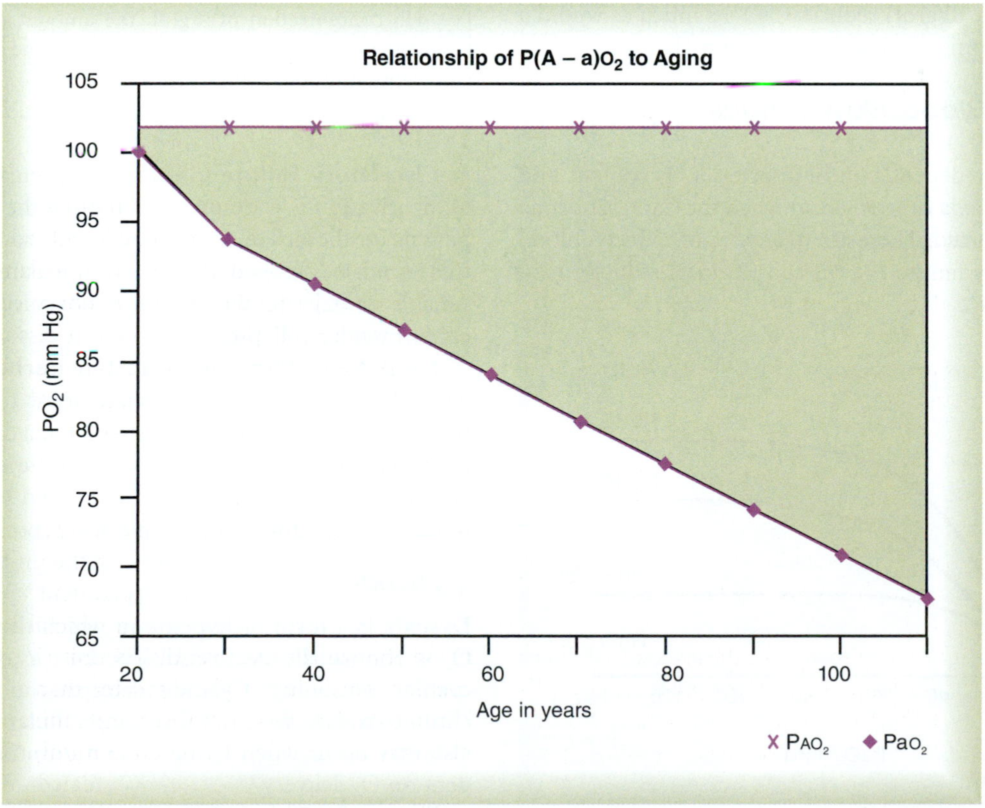

FIGURE 12-17 Relationship between $PA_{-a}O_2$ and aging. As P_aO_2 naturally decreases with age, $PA_{-a}O_2$ increases at the rate of approximately 3 mm Hg each decade beyond 20 years. (Modified from Lane EE, Walker JF: Clinical arterial blood gas analysis, St Louis, 1987, Mosby.)

and increases in $\dot{V}_A/\dot{Q}$ mismatching. P_aO_2 of 85 mm Hg in a 60-year-old adult would be interpreted as normal, but the same P_aO_2 in a 20-year-old adult would indicate hypoxemia. The expected P_aO_2 in older adults may be estimated by using the following formula:

$$\text{Expected } P_aO_2 = 100 - (0.323 \times \text{Age in years})$$

Hemoglobin Deficiencies. Normal P_aO_2 does not guarantee adequate arterial O_2 content or delivery. For arterial O_2 content to be adequate, there also must be enough normal Hb in the blood. If the blood Hb is low—even when PaO_2 is normal—hypoxia can occur because of low O_2 content in the arterial blood. Relative Hb deficiencies are caused by abnormal forms of Hb and have been discussed earlier in this chapter.

Hb deficiencies, or anemias, can be either absolute or relative. Absolute Hb deficiency occurs when the Hb concentration is lower than normal. Relative Hb deficiencies are caused by either the displacement of O_2 from normal Hb or the presence of abnormal Hb variants. A low blood Hb concentration may be caused either by a loss of RBCs, as with hemorrhage, or by inadequate erythropoiesis (formation of RBCs in the bone marrow). Regardless of the cause, a low Hb content can seriously impair the O_2-carrying capacity of the blood, even in the presence of a normal supply (P_aO_2) and adequate diffusion.[5]

Figure 12-18 plots the relationship between arterial O_2 content and PaO_2 as a function of Hb concentration. As can be seen, progressive decreases in blood Hb content causes large decreases in arterial O_2 content (CaO_2). A 33% decrease in Hb content (from 15 to 10 g/dl) reduces CaO_2 as much as would a decrease in PaO_2 from 100 mm Hg to 40 mm Hg.

Reduction in Blood Flow (Shock or Ischemia)

Because O_2 delivery depends on both arterial O_2 content and cardiac output, hypoxia can still occur when the CaO_2 is normal if blood flow is reduced. There are two types of reduced blood flow: (1) circulatory failure *(shock)* and (2) local reductions in perfusion *(ischemia)*.

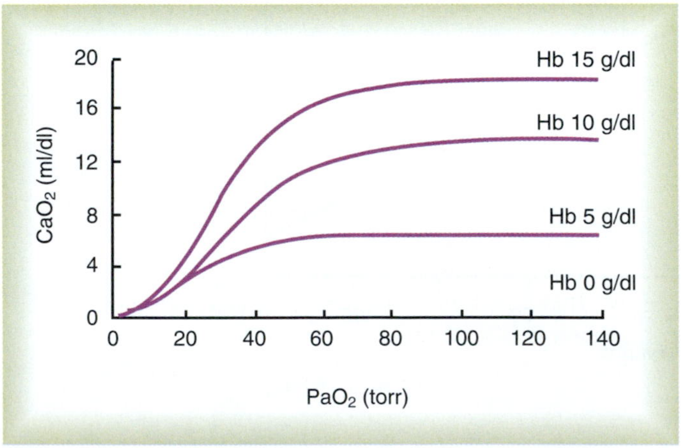

FIGURE 12-18 Relationship between CaO_2 and PaO_2 as a function of blood Hb concentration. Progressive decreases in Hb cause large decreases in CaO_2.

MINI CLINI

Effect of Anemia on Oxygen Content

In its most common form, anemia is a clinical disorder in which the number of RBCs is decreased. Because RBCs carry Hb, anemia decreases the amount of this O_2-carrying protein.

PROBLEM: What effect would anemia that causes a progressive decrease in Hb from (a) 15 g/dl, to (b) 12 g/dl, to (c) 8 g/dl, to (d) 4 g/dl, have on the amount of O_2 carried in a patient's blood? Assume that PO_2 and saturation stay normal at 100 mm Hg and 97%.

DISCUSSION: 1. Calculate dissolved O_2 the same way for all four examples as follows:

$$\text{Dissolved } O_2 = 100 \times 0.003 = 0.30 \text{ ml/dl}$$

2. Compute chemically combined O_2 as follows: Chemically combined O_2 = Hb (g/dl) × 1.34 ml/g × SaO_2
   a. 15 g/dl × 1.34 ml/g × 0.97 = 19.50 ml/dl
   b. 12 g/dl × 1.34 ml/g × 0.97 = 15.60 ml/dl
   c. 8 g/dl × 1.34 ml/g × 0.97 = 10.40 ml/dl
   d. 4 g/dl × 1.34 ml/g × 0.97 = 5.20 ml/dl
3. Compute total O_2 content as follows:

$$CaO_2 = \text{Dissolved } O_2 + \text{Chemically combined } O_2$$

   a. 0.30 + 19.50 = 19.80 ml/dl
   b. 0.30 + 15.60 = 15.90 ml/dl
   c. 0.30 + 10.40 = 10.70 ml/dl
   d. 0.30 + 5.20 = 5.50 ml/dl

Loss of Hb decreases the amount of O_2 carried in a patient's blood, even though PO_2 and saturation remain normal. With Hb concentration of 4 g/dl, the amount of O_2 carried in a patient's blood is only approximately one-fourth the normal concentration (5.50 vs. 19.80 ml/dl).

Circulatory Failure (Shock). In circulatory failure, tissue O_2 deprivation is widespread. Although the body tries to compensate for the lack of O_2 by directing blood flow to vital organs, this response is limited. Prolonged shock ultimately causes irreversible damage to the central nervous system and eventual cardiovascular collapse.

Local Reductions in Perfusion (Ischemia). Even when whole-body perfusion is adequate, local reductions in blood flow can cause localized hypoxia. Ischemia can result in anaerobic metabolism, metabolic acidosis, and eventual death of the affected tissue. Myocardial infarction and stroke are examples of ischemic conditions that can cause hypoxia and tissue death.

Dysoxia

Dysoxia is a form of hypoxia in which the cellular uptake of O_2 is abnormally decreased. The best example of dysoxia is cyanide poisoning. Cyanide disrupts the intracellular cytochrome oxidase system, preventing cellular use of O_2. Dysoxia also may occur when tissue O_2 consumption becomes dependent on O_2 delivery.

Figure 12-19 plots tissue O_2 consumption ($\dot{V}_2$) against O_2 delivery (DO_2) in both normal and pathologic states. Normally, the tissues extract as much O_2 as they need from what is

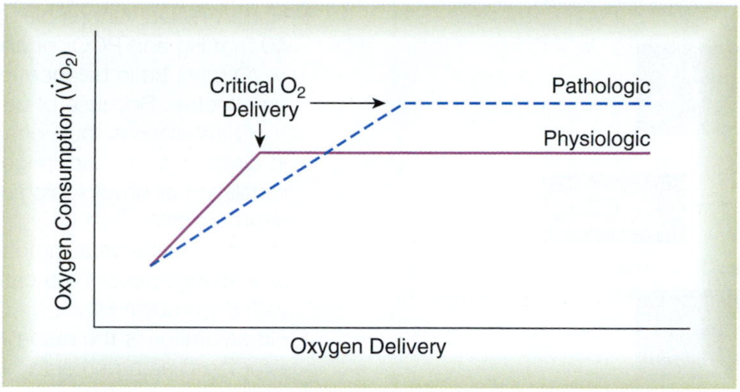

FIGURE 12-19 Physiologic versus pathologic O_2 consumption–delivery relationship. Critical O_2 delivery occurs at higher O_2 delivery in a pathologic state. The slope of the pathologic consumption curve below the critical delivery point reflects the decrease in O_2 extraction ratio that exists in these situations. (Modified from Pasquale MD, Cipolle MD, Cerra FB: Oxygen transport: does increasing supply improve outcome? Respir Care 38:800, 1993.)

delivered and O_2 consumption equals O_2 demand (flat portion of *solid line*). However, if delivery decreases, conditions begin to change *(solid line)*. At a level called the *point of critical delivery,* tissue extraction reaches a maximum. Further decreases in delivery result in an O_2 "debt," which occurs when O_2 demand exceeds O_2 delivery. Under conditions of O_2 debt, O_2 consumption becomes dependent on O_2 delivery *(sloped line)*. This dependence leads to lactic acid accumulation and metabolic acidosis.

In pathologic conditions such as septic shock and ARDS *(dotted line)*, this critical point may occur at levels of O_2 delivery considered normal. In addition, the slope of the curve below the point of critical delivery may be less than normal, indicating a decreased extraction ratio ($\dot{V}_2/DO_2$).[6] In combination, these findings indicate that O_2 demands are not being met and that a defect exists in the cellular mechanisms regulating O_2 uptake.

Impaired Carbon Dioxide Removal

Any disorder that decreases alveolar ventilation ($\dot{V}_A$) relative to metabolic need impairs CO_2 removal. Impaired CO_2 removal by the lung causes hypercapnia and respiratory acidosis (see Chapter 14). A decrease in alveolar ventilation occurs when (1) the minute ventilation is inadequate, (2) the dead space ventilation per minute is increased, or (3) a $\dot{V}_A/\dot{Q}$ imbalance exists.[4-8]

Inadequate Minute Ventilation

Clinically, inadequate minute ventilation is caused by decreased tidal volume, or respiratory rate. Inadequate minute ventilation occurs in restrictive conditions, such as atelectasis, neuromuscular disorders, or impeded thoracic expansion (e.g., kyphoscoliosis). A decrease in respiratory rate is less common but may be present with respiratory center depression, as in drug overdose.

Increased Dead Space Ventilation

An increase in dead space ventilation, or V_D/V_T, is caused by either (1) decreased tidal volume (as with rapid, shallow breathing) or (2) increased physiologic dead space as in various lung diseases. In either case, wasted ventilation increases. Without compensation, alveolar ventilation per minute is decreased, and CO_2 removal is impaired.

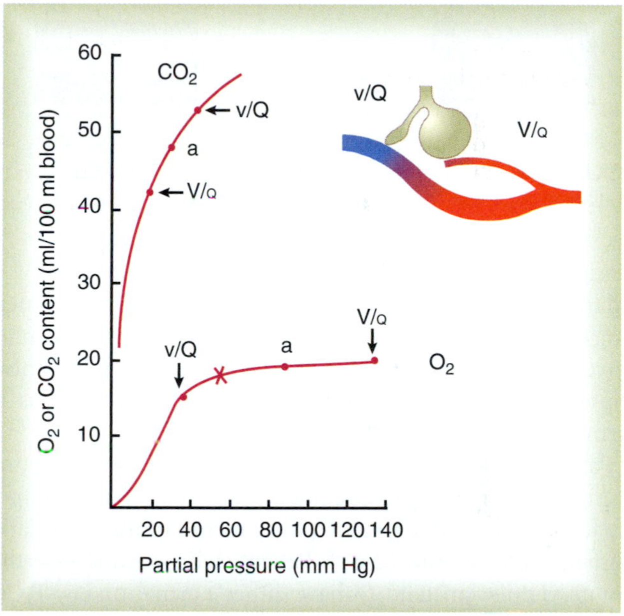

FIGURE 12-20 $\dot{V}_A/\dot{Q}$ imbalance and dissociation curves for CO_2 and O_2. v/Q represents low $\dot{V}_A/\dot{Q}$ units, and V/Q represents high $\dot{V}_A/\dot{Q}$ units. See text for discussion.

Ventilation-Perfusion Imbalances

Theoretically, any $\dot{V}_A/\dot{Q}$ imbalance should cause an increase in P_aCO_2. However, P_aCO_2 does not always increase in these cases. Many patients who are hypoxemic because of a $\dot{V}_A/\dot{Q}$ imbalance have a low or normal P_aCO_2. This common clinical finding suggests that $\dot{V}_A/\dot{Q}$ imbalances have a greater effect on oxygenation than on CO_2 removal.

Careful inspection of the O_2 and CO_2 dissociation curves supports this finding. The O_2 and CO_2 dissociation curves are plotted on the same scale in Figure 12-20. The upper CO_2 curve is nearly linear in the physiologic range. The lower O_2 curve is almost flat in the physiologic range. Point *a* on each curve is the normal arterial point for both content and partial pressure. To

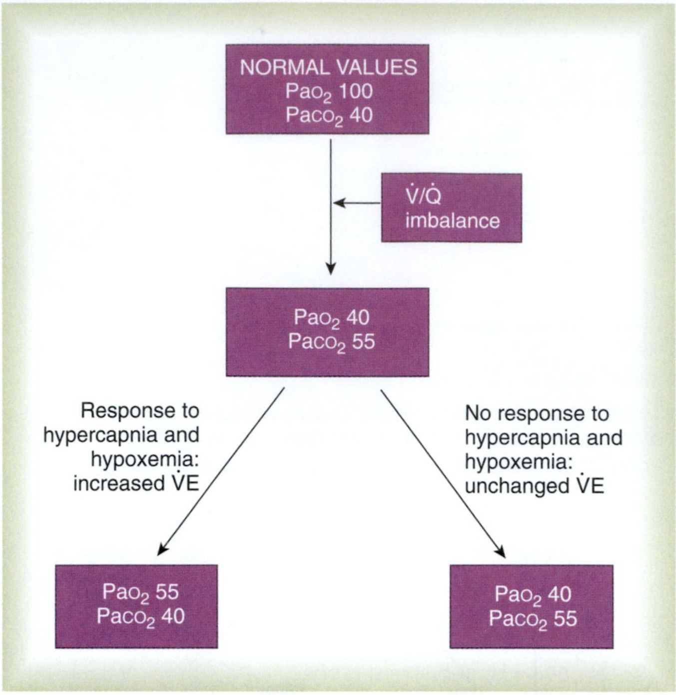

FIGURE 12-21 Changes in PaO_2 and $PaCO_2$ caused by $\dot{V}_A/\dot{Q}$ imbalance. All values are given in millimeters of mercury (mm Hg).

the right of the graph are two lung units, one with a low $\dot{V}_A/\dot{Q}$ and the other with a high $\dot{V}_A/\dot{Q}$. The blood O_2 and CO_2 contents from each unit are plotted on the curves. The final CO_2 content, arrived at by averaging the high and low $\dot{V}_A/\dot{Q}$ points, is shown as point *a* on the CO_2 curve. This point is the same as the normal arterial point for CO_2.

Patients with significant $\dot{V}_A/\dot{Q}$ imbalances must compensate for high PCO_2 coming from underventilated units. To compensate for these high PCO_2 values, the patient's minute ventilation must increase (Figure 12-21). Patients who can increase their minute ventilation tend to have either normal or low P_aCO_2, combined with hypoxemia.

Conversely, patients with $\dot{V}_A/\dot{Q}$ imbalance who cannot increase their minute ventilation are hypercapnic. Hypercapnia generally occurs only when the $\dot{V}_A/\dot{Q}$ imbalance is severe and chronic, as in COPD. Such a patient must sustain a higher than normal minute ventilation just to maintain normal $PaCO_2$. If the energy costs required to sustain a high minute ventilation are prohibitive, the patient opts for less work—and hence elevated P_aCO_2.

SUMMARY CHECKLIST

- Movement of gases between the lungs and the tissues depends mainly on diffusion.
- P_ACO_2 varies directly with CO_2 production and inversely with alveolar ventilation.
- P_AO_2 is computed using the alveolar air equation.
- With a constant FiO_2, P_AO_2 varies inversely with P_ACO_2.
- Normal P_AO_2 averages 100 mm Hg, with mean P_ACO_2 of approximately 40 mm Hg.
- Normal mixed venous blood has PO_2 of approximately 40 mm Hg and PCO_2 of approximately 46 mm Hg.
- $\dot{V}_A/\dot{Q}$ must be in balance for pulmonary gas exchange to be effective. Because of normal anatomic shunts and $\dot{V}_A/\dot{Q}$ imbalances, pulmonary gas exchange is imperfect.
- In disease, $\dot{V}_A/\dot{Q}$ can range from zero (perfusion without ventilation or physiologic shunting) to infinity (pure alveolar dead space).
- Blood carries a small amount of O_2 in physical solution, and larger amounts are carried in chemical combination with erythrocyte Hb.
- Hb saturation is the ratio of oxyhemoglobin to total Hb, expressed as a percentage.
- To compute total O_2 contents of the blood, add the dissolved O_2 content ($0.003 \times PO_2$) to the product of Hb content × Hb saturation × 1.34.
- Arteriovenous O_2 content difference, $C_{a-v}O_2$, is the amount of O_2 given up by every 100 ml of blood on each pass through the tissues. All else being equal, $C_{a-v}O_2$ varies inversely with cardiac output.
- Hb affinity for O_2 increases with high PO_2, high pH, low temperature, and low levels of 2,3-DPG.
- Hb abnormalities can affect O_2 loading and unloading and can cause hypoxia.
- Most CO_2 (approximately 80%) is transported in the blood as ionized bicarbonate; other forms include carbamino compounds in physical solution.
- Changes in CO_2 levels modify the O_2 dissociation curve (Bohr effect). Changes in Hb saturation affect the CO_2 dissociation curve (Haldane effect). These changes are mutually beneficial, assisting in gas exchange at the lung and the cellular level.
- Hypoxia occurs if (1) the arterial blood O_2 content is decreased, (2) blood flow is decreased, or (3) abnormal cellular function prevents proper uptake of O_2.
- Decreased PaO_2 level may be a result of a low ambient PO_2, hypoventilation, impaired diffusion, $\dot{V}_A/\dot{Q}$ imbalances, and right-to-left anatomic or physiologic shunting.
- A decrease in alveolar ventilation occurs when (1) the minute ventilation is inadequate, (2) dead space ventilation is increased, or (3) a $\dot{V}_A/\dot{Q}$ imbalance exists.

References

1. Mottram C: *Ruppel's manual of pulmonary function testing*, ed 10, St Louis, 2012, Elsevier.
2. Hennessey I, Japp A: *Arterial blood gases made easy*, ed 1, St Louis, 2007, Churchill Livingstone.
3. Rose BD, Post TW, Stakes J: *Clinical physiology of acid-base and electrolyte disorders*, ed 6, New York, 2014, McGraw-Hill.
4. Malley WJ: *Clinical blood gases: assessment and intervention*, ed 2, St Louis, 2005, Saunders.
5. Lump A, Pearl RG: *Nunn's applied respiratory physiology*, ed 7, St Louis, 2010, Elsevier.
6. West JB: *Pulmonary physiology and pathophysiology: an integrated, case-based approach*, ed 2, Philadelphia, 2007, Lippincott Williams and Williams.
7. Des Jardins T: *Cardiopulmonary anatomy and physiology, essentials for respiratory care*, ed 5, Clifton Park, NY, 2008, Delmar Publications.
8. Beachey W: *Respiratory care anatomy and physiology*, ed 3, St Louis, 2012, Elsevier.

CHAPTER 13

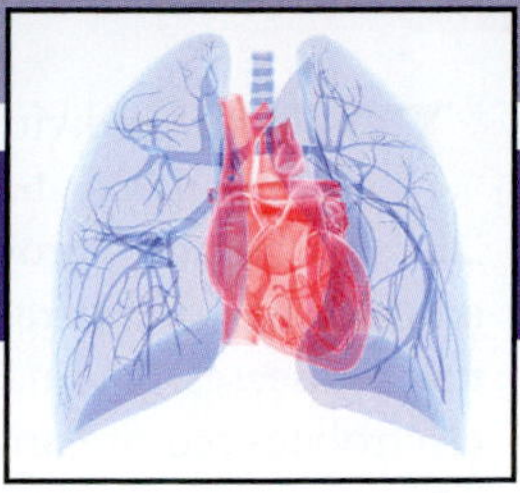

Solutions, Body Fluids, and Electrolytes

DANIEL F. FISHER

CHAPTER OBJECTIVES

After reading this chapter you will be able to:

- Describe the characteristics of and key terms associated with solutions, colloids, and suspensions.
- Describe the five factors that influence the solubility of a substance in a solution.
- Describe how osmotic pressure functions and what its action is in relation to cell membranes.
- Describe how to calculate the solute content of a solution using ratio, weight/volume, and percent methods.
- State the ionic characteristics of acids, bases, and salts.
- Describe how proteins can function as bases.
- Describe how to calculate the pH of a solution when given the $[H^+]$ in nanomoles per liter.
- Identify where fluid compartments are located in the body and their volumes.
- Describe how water loss and replacement occur.
- Define the roles played by osmotic and hydrostatic pressure in edema.
- Identify clinical findings associated with excess or deficiency of the seven basic electrolytes.

CHAPTER OUTLINE

KEY TERMS

acid
active transport
anions
base
buffering
cations
colloids
diluent
dilute solution
dilution equation
equivalent weight
hydrostatic pressure
hyperkalemia
hypertonic
hypotonic
ionic
interstitial fluid
isotonic
nanomole
normal solution
osmolality
osmotic pressure (oncotic pressure)
plasma colloid osmotic pressure (oncotic pressure)
saturated solution
solute
solution
solvent
Starling equilibrium
suspensions

In healthy individuals, body water and various chemicals are regulated to maintain an environment in which biochemical processes can continue. Imbalances in the amount or concentration of chemicals in the body occur in many diseases. The nature and importance of body fluids and electrolytes require an understanding of physiologic chemistry. This chapter provides the reader with the background knowledge needed to understand body chemistry.

SOLUTIONS, COLLOIDS, AND SUSPENSIONS

Definition of a Solution

The body is based on liquid water chemistry and the interaction of various substances either dissolved or suspended within the fluid. Water itself is a polar (having two sides with positive and negative charges) covalent (capable of forming bonds by sharing electrons) molecule and is referred to in chemistry as a *universal solvent*. Water is the primary component of any liquid within the body and has a great influence on the behavior of other materials as they are introduced. These substances and particles combine with water in the following three ways: as (1) colloids, (2) suspensions, or (3) solutions.

A **solution** is a stable mixture of two or more substances in a single phase that cannot be separated using a centrifuge. One substance is evenly distributed between the molecules of the other. The substance that dissolves is called the **solute.** The medium in which it dissolves is called the **solvent.** Gases, liquids, and solids can dissolve to become solutes; for example, carbon dioxide, alcohol, and salt can be dissolved in water. The process of dissolving involves breaking the (relatively weak) bonds between the solute-solute molecules and the solvent-solvent molecules. These intermolecular forces must be broken before a new solute-solvent bond can be formed. A solute dissolves in a solvent if the solute-solvent forces of attraction are great enough to overcome the solute-solute and solvent-solvent forces of attraction. If the solute-solvent force is less than the solute-solute or solvent-solvent force, the solute does not dissolve. When all three sets of forces are approximately equal, the two substances typically are soluble in each other.

In electrochemical terms, there are three basic types of physiologic solutions. Depending on the solute, solutions are **ionic** (electrovalent), *polar covalent,* or *nonpolar covalent* (Table 13-1). In ionic and polar covalent solutions, some of the solute ionizes into separate particles known as *ions.* A solution in which this dissociation occurs is called an *electrolyte solution* (Figure 13-1). If an electrode is placed in such a solution, positive ions migrate to the negative pole of the electrode (the cathode). These ions are called **cations.** Negative ions migrate to the positive pole of the electrode (the anode); they are called **anions.** In nonpolar covalent solutions, molecules of solute remain intact and do not carry electrical charges; these solutions are referred to as *nonelectrolytes.* These nonelectrolytes are not attracted to either the positive or the negative pole of an electrode (hence the designation *nonpolar*). All three types of solutions coexist in the body. These solutions also serve as the media in which colloids and simple suspensions are dispersed. Gases such as oxygen and CO_2

TABLE 13-1
Types of Physiologic Solutions

Type	Characteristics	Physiologic Example
Ionic (electrovalent)	Ionic compounds dissolved from crystalline form, usually in water (hydration); form strong electrolytes with conductivity dependent on concentration of ions	Saline solution (0.9% NaCl)
Polar covalent	Molecular compounds dissolved in water or other solvents to produce ions (ionization); electrolytes may be weak or strong, depending on degree of ionization; solutions polarize and are good conductors	Hydrochloric acid (HCl) (strong electrolyte); acetic acid (CH_3COOH) (weak electrolyte)
Nonpolar covalent	Molecular compounds dissolved into electrically neutral solutions (do not polarize); solutions are not good conductors; nonelectrolytes	Glucose ($C_6H_{12}O_6$)

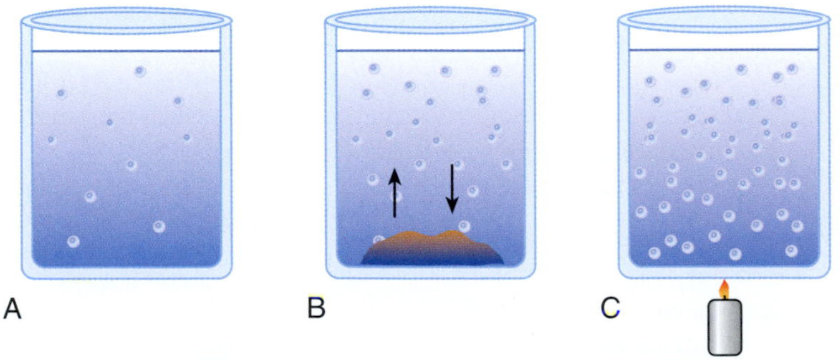

FIGURE 13-1 **A,** In the dilute solution, there are relatively few solute particles. **B,** In the saturated solution, the solvent contains all the solute it can hold in the presence of excess solute. **C,** Heating the solution dissolves more solute particles, which may remain in the solution if cooled gently, creating a state of supersaturation.

are nonpolar molecules (along with nitrogen) and do not dissolve very well in water, which is a polar solvent.

Colloids (sometimes called *dispersions* or *gels*) consist of large molecules that attract and hold water (*hydrophilic:* "water loving"). These molecules are uniformly distributed throughout the dispersion, and they tend not to settle. The protoplasm inside cells is a common example of a colloid. Physiologically, colloids provide very little free water to the patient's system, and care should be taken not to create a hypotonic environment.[1]

Suspensions are composed of large particles that float in a liquid. Suspensions can be physically separated by centrifugation and do not possess the same interactions between solvent and solute that are found in a true solution. Red blood cells in plasma are an example of a suspension. Dispersion of suspended particles depends on physical agitation. Particles settle because of gravity when the suspension is motionless.

The ease with which a solute dissolves in a solvent is its *solubility,* which is influenced by the following five factors:

1. *Nature of the solute.* The ease with which substances go into a solution (dissociation) in a given solvent depends on the forces of the solute-solute molecules and varies widely.
2. *Nature of the solvent.* The ability of a solvent to dissolve a solute depends on the bonds of the solvent-solvent molecules and varies widely. The electrical properties of the solvent molecules determine how soluble a substance is for a particular solvent. Polar solvents, such as water, dissolve other polar covalent bonds; nonpolar solvents dissolve nonpolar solutes: "Like dissolves like."
3. *Temperature.* The solubility of most solids increases with increased temperature. However, the solubility of gases varies inversely with temperature.
4. *Pressure.* The solubility of solids and liquids is not greatly affected by pressure. However, the solubility of gases in liquids varies directly with pressure.
5. *Concentration.* The concentration of a solute or available solvent affects how much of the substance goes into solution.

The effects of temperature and pressure on the solubility of gases are important. More gas dissolves in a liquid at lower temperatures. As the temperature of a liquid increases, gas dissolved in that liquid comes out of solution. Henry's law describes the effect of pressure on solubility of a gas in a liquid. At a given temperature, the volume of a gas that dissolves in a liquid is proportional to the solubility coefficient of the gas and the partial pressure of gas to which the liquid is exposed. O_2 and CO_2 transport can change significantly with changes in body temperature or atmospheric pressure (see Chapter 6).

Concentration of Solutions

The term *concentration* refers to the amount of solute dissolved into the solvent. Concentration can be described either qualitatively or quantitatively. Calling something a **dilute solution** is an example of a qualitative description. Stating that a specific container holds 50 ml of 0.4 molar solution of sodium hydroxide is a quantitative description (Figure 13-2, *A*). **Saturated solutions** occur when the solvent has dissociated the maximal amount of solute into itself. Additional solute added to a saturated solution does not dissociate into solution but remains at the bottom of the container (see Figure 13-2, *B*). Solute particles precipitate into the solid state at the same rate at which other particles go into solution. This equilibrium characterizes a saturated solution.

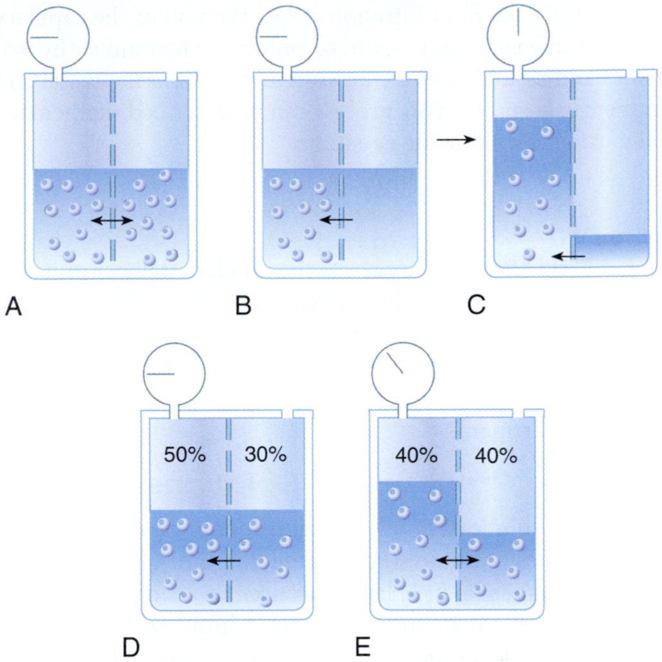

FIGURE 13-2 Osmotic pressure is illustrated by the solutions in the five containers. Each container is divided into two compartments by a semipermeable membrane, which permits passage of solvent molecules but not solute *(circles).* The number of solute particles represents relative concentrations of the solutions. Solute particles are fixed in number and are confined by the membranes. Volume changes are a function of the diffusible solvent. Solvent movement is indicated by *arrows* through the membranes. Container **A** shows a state of equilibrium, in which solute and solvent are equally distributed on either side of the membrane. Containers **B** and **C** show diffusion of solvent through the membrane as a result of solvent on only one side of the membrane and the resulting pressure change (osmotic pressure indicated by the gauge). Containers **D** and **E** show what happens when different concentrations exist on either side of a semipermeable membrane. Solvent moves from the lower concentration toward the higher concentration to establish an equilibrium because of osmotic pressure.

A solution is characterized as being *supersaturated* when the solvent contains more solute than a saturated solution at the same temperature and pressure. If a saturated solution is heated, the solute equilibrium is disturbed and more solute goes into solution. This is because of the space between the solvent molecules increases. If undissolved solute is removed and the solution is cooled gently, there is an excess of dissolved solute (see Figure 13-2, *C*). The excess solute of supersaturated solutions may be precipitated out if the solution is vibrated or if a "seed crystal" is introduced.

Starling Forces

Ernest Starling, a nineteenth-century British physiologist studied fluid transport across membranes. He described that the driving force for fluid filtration across the wall of the capillary is determined by four separate pressures: hydraulic (hydrostatic) and colloid osmotic pressure both within the vessel and in the tissue space.[2] This process can be described mathematically using the following equation:

$$Jv = Lp[Pc - Pi - s(pc - pi)]$$

where:

J_v = Fluid filtration flux across the capillary wall per unit area
L_p = Permeability of the capillary wall
s = Oncotic reflection coefficient
P_c, P_i, p_c, p_i = Global values for the hydrostatic and colloid osmotic pressures in the capillary and interstitial compartments

Osmotic Pressure of Solutions

Most of the solutions of physiologic importance in the body are dilute. Solutes in dilute solution resemble gases. This behavior results from the relatively large distances between the molecules of solute in dilute solutions. The most important physiologic characteristic of solutions is their ability to exert pressure.

Osmotic pressure (oncotic pressure)[3] is the force produced by solvent particles under certain conditions. A membrane that permits passage of solvent molecules but not solute is called a *semipermeable membrane*. If such a membrane divides a solution into two compartments, molecules of solvent can pass (diffuse) through it from one side to the other (Figure 13-3, *A*). The number of solvent molecules diffusing in one direction must equal the number of solute molecules passing in the opposite direction. An equal ratio of solute to solvent particles (i.e., the concentration of the solution) is maintained on both sides of the membrane. A capillary wall is an example of a semipermeable membrane.[4,5]

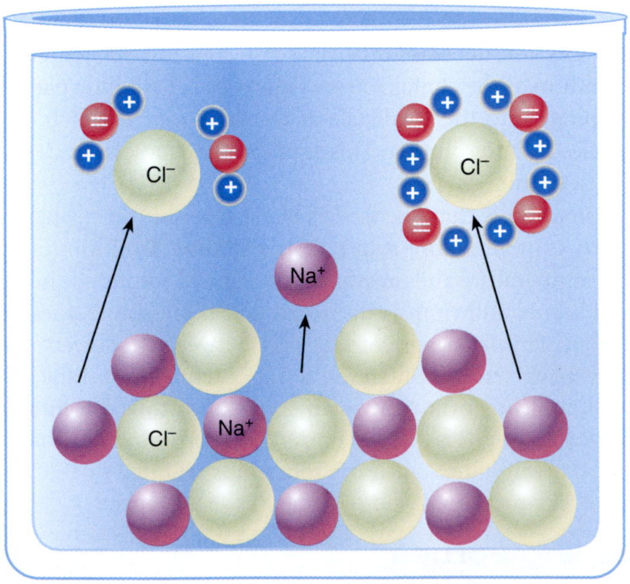

FIGURE 13-3 Sodium chloride (NaCl) is shown as a crystalline mass of ions being dissociated by the attraction of water dipoles.

If a solution is placed on one side of a semipermeable membrane and pure solvent is placed on the other, solvent molecules move through the membrane into the solution. The force driving solvent molecules through the membrane is called *osmotic pressure*. Osmotic pressure tries to redistribute solvent molecules so that the same concentration exists on both sides of the membrane. Osmotic pressure may be measured by connecting a manometer to the expanding column of the solution (see Figure 13-3, *B* and *C*).

Osmotic pressure also can be visualized as an attractive force of solute particles in a concentrated solution. If 100 ml of a 50% solution is placed on one side of a membrane and 100 ml of a 30% solution is placed on the other side, solvent molecules move from the dilute to the concentrated side (see Figure 13-3, *D* and *E*). The particles in the concentrated solution attract solvent molecules from the dilute solution until equilibrium occurs. Equilibrium exists when the concentrations (i.e., ratio of solute to solvent) in the two compartments are equal (40% in Figure 13-3).

Osmolality is defined as the ratio of solute to solvent. In physiology, the solvent is water.[1,4,6] Osmotic pressure depends on the number of particles in solution but not on their charge or identity. A 2% solution has twice the osmotic pressure of a 1% solution under similar conditions. For a given amount of solute, osmotic pressure is inversely proportional to the volume of solvent. Most cell walls are semipermeable membranes. Through osmotic pressure, water is distributed throughout the body within certain physiologic ranges. Tonicity is the relative concentration of solutions that determine the direction and extent of diffusion. Tonicity is a way of describing the response of cells immersed in an external solution. Tonicity is influenced by the concentration of solutes that cannot cross the membrane. Average body cellular fluid has a tonicity equal to a 0.9% solution of sodium chloride (sometimes referred to as *physiologic* or *normal saline*). Solutions with similar tonicity are called **isotonic.** Compared to body fluid, solutions with more tonicity (more oncotic pressure and higher concentration as a result of less water) are **hypertonic,** and solutions with less tonicity (less oncotic pressure and lower concentration as a result of more water) are **hypotonic.** For example, a hypotonic solution has a lower concentration of solutes outside the cell than inside the cell. In an attempt to balance the concentrations of solutes inside and outside the cell, water will move into the cell, causing it to enlarge. Pressure increases inside the cell to counteract osmotic pressure. This pressure is called *turgor*. Some cells have selective permeability, allowing passage not only of water but also of specific solutes. Through these mechanisms, nutrients and physiologic solutions are distributed throughout the body.

Quantifying Solute Content and Activity

The amount of solute in a solution can be quantified in two ways: (1) by actual weight (grams or milligrams) and (2) by chemical combining power *(electronegativity)*. The weight of a solute is easy to measure and specify. However, it does not indicate chemical combining power. The sodium ion (Na^+) has a gram ionic weight of 23. The bicarbonate ion (HCO_3^-) has a

RULE OF THUMB

Solutions that have osmotic pressures equal to the average intracellular pressure in the body are called *isotonic*. This is roughly equivalent to a saline solution (NaCl) of 0.9%. Solutions with higher osmotic pressure are called *hypertonic,* whereas solutions with lower osmotic pressure are called *hypotonic*. Administration of isotonic solutions usually causes no net change in cellular water content. Hypertonic solutions draw water out of cells. Hypotonic solutions usually cause water to be absorbed from the solution into cells.

MINI CLINI

Sputum Induction and Hypertonic Saline

PROBLEM: To obtain samples of respiratory secretions, aerosol therapy is sometimes used to increase the volume of secretions and promote coughing to recover sputum or cells or both from the respiratory tract. Sputum induction combines the effect of hypertonic aerosols on the lining of the respiratory tract and with the normal cough reflex.

DISCUSSION: Sputum induction is usually performed by having the patient inhale a sterile hypertonic saline solution. Isotonic saline is approximately 0.9% (i.e., normal saline); concentrations greater than 0.9% are considered hypertonic. In clinical practice, concentrations of 3% to 10% have been used. When the particles of hypertonic saline are deposited in the airway, osmotic pressure is thought to play a key role. When hypertonic saline comes into contact with the respiratory mucosa, water moves from the cells lining the airway into the sol-gel matrix that lines the airways, increasing its volume. The combination of increased volume of respiratory secretions with irritation of the epithelial cells themselves promotes reflex coughing. The volume of sputum and the rate of clearance from the lungs seem to depend on the osmolarity of the inhaled aerosol. Exposure of mast cells normally present in the airways to hypertonic aerosols results in the release of mediators (e.g., histamine) and bronchospasm. These effects may be related to the stimulation of the cough reflex. For the same reason, hypertonic saline is also sometimes used for bronchial challenge testing.

gram ionic weight of 61. Both ions have equal electronegativities (+1 for Na^+, −1 for HCO_3^-). The number of chemically reactive units is usually more meaningful than their weight.

Equivalent Weights

In medicine, it is customary to refer to physiologic substances in terms of chemical combining power. The measure commonly used is **equivalent weight.** Equivalent weights are amounts of substances that have equal chemical combining power. For example, if chemical *A* reacts with chemical *B*, by definition, 1 equivalent weight of *A* reacts with exactly 1 equivalent weight of *B*. No excess reactants of *A* or *B* remain.

Two magnitudes of equivalent weights are used to calculate chemical combining power: gram equivalent weight (gEq) and milligram equivalent weight, or milliequivalent (mEq). One milliequivalent (1 mEq) is $\frac{1}{1000}$ of 1 gEq.

Gram Equivalent Weight Values. A gram equivalent weight of a substance is calculated as its gram molecular (formula) weight divided by its valence. *Valence* refers to the number of electrons that need to be added or removed to make the substance electrically neutral. The valence signs (+ or −) are disregarded.

$$\text{gEq} = \text{Gram molecular weight/Valence}$$

The gram equivalent weight of N^+, with a valence of 1, equals its gram atomic weight of 23 g. The gram equivalent weight of calcium (Ca^{++}) is its atomic weight (i.e., 40) divided by 2, or 20 g. The gram equivalent weight of ferric iron (Fe^{+++}) is its atomic weight (i.e., 55.8) divided by 3, or approximately 18.6 g.

For radicals such as sulfate (SO_4^{2-}), the formula for sulfuric acid (H_2SO_4) shows that one SO_4^{2-} group combines with two atoms of H_2. Half (0.5) of a mole of SO_4^{2-} is equivalent to 1 mole of H atoms. The gram equivalent weight of SO_4^{2-} is half its gram formula weight, or 48 g. If an element has more than one valence, the valence must be specified or must be apparent from the observed chemical combining properties.

Gram Equivalent Weight of an Acid. The gram equivalent weight of an acid is the weight of the acid (in grams) that contains 1 mole of replaceable H. The gram equivalent weight of an acid may be calculated by dividing its gram formula weight by the number of H^+ atoms in its formula, as shown in the following reaction:

$$HCl + Na^+ \rightarrow NaCl + H^+$$

The single H^+ of hydrochloric acid (HCl) is replaced by Na^+. In 1 mole of HCl, there is 1 mole of replaceable H^+. By definition, the gram equivalent weight of HCl must be the same as its gram formula weight, or 36.5 g. The two H_2 of H_2SO_4 are both considered to be replaceable. In 1 mole of H_2SO_4, there are 2 moles of replaceable H^+, and the gram equivalent weight of H_2SO_4 is half its gram formula weight, or 48 g.

Acids in which H^+ atoms are not completely replaceable are exceptions to the rule. In some acids, H^+ replacement varies according to specific reactions. Carbonic acid (H_2CO_3) and phosphoric acid (H_3PO_4) are examples of such exceptions. Their equivalent weights are determined by the conditions of their chemical reactions.

For example, H_2CO_3 has two H^+ atoms. In physiologic reactions, only one is considered replaceable:

$$H_2CO_3 + Na^+ \rightarrow NaHCO_3 + H^+$$

Only one H^+ atom is released; the other remains bound. In 1 mole of H_2CO_3, there is only 1 mole of replaceable H^+. The gram equivalent weight of H_2CO_3 is the same as its gram formula weight, or 61 g.

Gram Equivalent Weight of a Base. The equivalent weight of a base is its weight (grams) containing 1 mole of replaceable hydroxyl (OH^-) ions. Similar to acids, the gram equivalent weight of bases is calculated by dividing gram formula weight by the number of OH^- groups in its formula.

Conversion of Gram Weight to Equivalent Weight. To determine the number of gram equivalent weights in a substance, the gram weight is divided by its calculated equivalent weight, as shown in the following example:

$$58.5\ \text{g NaCl/gEq } 58.5\ \text{g} = 1\ \text{gEq}$$
$$29.25\ \text{g NaCl/gEq } 58.5 = 0.5\ \text{gEq}$$

Milligram Equivalent Weights. The concentrations of most chemicals in the body are quite small. The term *milligram equivalent weight (milliequivalent)* is preferred for expressing these minute values; 1 mEq is simply 0.001 gEq:

$$\text{mEq} = \text{gEq}/1000$$

The normal concentration of potassium in plasma ranges from 0.0035 to 0.005 gEq/L. These values may be converted to milliequivalents by multiplying by a factor of 1000. The normal concentration of K^+ in the plasma would be expressed as ranging from 3.5 to 5.0 mEq/L.

Solute Content by Weight

The measurement of many electrolytes is based on actual weight rather than on milliequivalents. This weight is often expressed as milligrams per 100 ml of blood or body fluid. The units for this measurement are abbreviated as mg% (milligram percent) or mg/dl (milligrams per deciliter). This text uses the modern designation *mg/dL*. Some substances present in blood or body fluid are present in extremely small amounts and are expressed in *micrograms* ($\frac{1}{1000}$ of a milligram) per deciliter (µg/dl or mcg/dl).

Values stated in milligrams per deciliter may be converted into their corresponding equivalent weights and reported as milliequivalents per liter. Conversion between mEq/L and mg/dl may be calculated as follows:

$$\text{(1)} \qquad \text{mEq/L} = \frac{\text{mg/dl} \times 10}{\text{Equivalent weight}}$$

$$\text{(2)} \qquad \text{mEq/L} = \frac{\text{mEq/L} \times \text{Equivalent weight}}{10}$$

To convert a serum Na^+ value of 322 mg/dl to mEq/L, the equation is used as follows:

$$\begin{aligned}\text{mEq/L} &= \text{mg/dl} \times 10/\text{Equivalent weight}\\ &= 322 \times 10/23\\ &= 140\ \text{mEq/L}\end{aligned}$$

In clinical practice, electrolyte replacement is common when a laboratory test identifies a significant deficiency. The electrolyte content of intravenous solutions is usually stated in milligrams per deciliter or in milliequivalents per liter. Lactated Ringer's solution is one such infusion used for electrolyte replacement (Table 13-2).

Calculating Solute Content

In addition to gEq, mEq, mg/dl, and µg/dl (mcg/dl), several other methods of calculating solute content exist. These common chemical standards are used to compute solute content and dilution of solutions.

TABLE 13-2
Concentration of Ingredients in Lactated Ringer's Solution

Substance	mg/dl	Approximate mEq/L
NaCl (sodium chloride)	600 Na	130
	310 Cl	109
$NaC_3H_5O_3$ (sodium lactate)	30 $C_3H_5O_3$	28
KCl (potassium chloride)	30 K	4
$CaCl_2$ (calcium chloride)	20 Ca	27

Quantitative Classification of Solutions

The amount of solute in a solution may be quantified by the following six methods:

1. *Ratio solution.* The amount of solute to solvent is expressed as a proportion (e.g., 1:100). Ratio solutions are sometimes used in describing concentrations of drugs.
2. *Weight-per-volume (W/V) solution.* The W/V solution is commonly used for solids dissolved in liquids. It is defined as weight of solute per volume of solution. This method is sometimes erroneously described as a percent solution. W/V solutions are commonly expressed in grams of solute per 100 ml of solution. For example, 5 g of glucose dissolved in 100 ml of solution is properly called a *5% solution,* according to the W/V scheme. A liquid dissolved in a liquid is measured as volumes of solute to volumes of solution.
3. *Percent solution.* A percent solution is weight of solute per weight of solution. For example, 5 g of glucose dissolved in 95 g of water is a true percent solution. The glucose is 5% of the total solution weight of 100 g.
4. *Molal solution.* A molal solution contains 1 mole of solute per kilogram of solvent, or 1 mmol/g solvent. The concentration of a molal solution is independent of temperature.
5. *Molar solution.* A molar solution has 1 mole of solute per liter of solution, or 1 mmol/ml of solution. The solute is measured into a container, and solvent is added to produce the solution volume desired.
6. *Normal solution.* A **normal solution** has 1 gEq of solute per liter of solution, or 1 mEq/ml of solution. For all monovalent solutes, normal and molar solutions are the same. The equivalent weights of their solutes equal their gram formula weights. Equal volumes of solutions of the same normality contain chemically equivalent amounts of their solutes. If the solutes react chemically with one another, equal volumes of the solutions react completely. Neither substance remains in excess. In the analytic process of titration, normal solutions are often used as standards to determine the concentrations of other solutions.

Dilution Calculations

Dilute solutions are made from a stock preparation. Preparation of medications often involves dilution. Dilution calculations are based on the weight-per-unit volume principle (the aforementioned W/V solution method).

Diluting a solution increases its volume without changing the amount of solute it contains, and this reduces the concentration of the solution. The amount of solute in a solution can be expressed as volume times concentration. For example, 50 ml of a 10% solution (10 g/dl) contains 50 × 0.1, or 5 g. In the dilution of a solution, initial volume (V_1) multiplied by initial concentration (C_1) equals final volume multiplied by final concentration. This can be expressed as follows:

$$V_1C_1 = V_2C_2$$

This equation is sometimes referred to as the **dilution equation.** Whenever three of the variables are known, the fourth can be calculated as in the following examples:

1. Diluting 10 ml of a 2% (0.02) solution to a concentration of 0.5% (0.005) requires finding the new volume (V_2) by rearranging the dilution equation as follows:

$$V_2 = V_1C_1/C_2$$
$$V_2 = 10\ \text{ml} \times 0.02/0.005$$
$$V_2 = 40\ \text{ml}$$

2. If 50 ml of water is added to 150 ml of a 3% (0.03) solution, the new concentration is calculated by rearranging the dilution equation to find C_2 as follows:

$$C_2 = V_1C_1/V_2$$
$$C_2 = 150\ \text{ml} \times 0.02/(50\ \text{ml} + 150\ \text{ml})$$
$$C_2 = 0.0225\ \text{or}\ (2.25\%)$$

3. To dilute 50 ml of a 0.33 normal (N) solution to a 0.1 N concentration, concentration is given as normality, but it can be used similar to a percentage. The new volume (V_2) can be calculated by rearranging the dilution equation as follows:

$$V_2 = V_1C_1/C_2$$
$$V_2 = 50\ \text{ml} \times 0.33/0.1$$
$$V_2 = 165\ \text{ml}$$

In the last example, the volume needed to produce a 0.1 N solution would be 165 ml – 50 ml (the original volume), or 115 ml. In other words, 115 ml of solvent would have to be added to the original 50 ml of 0.33 N solution to produce the desired concentration. The added solvent is called the **diluent** because it dilutes the original concentration to a lower concentration.

ELECTROLYTIC ACTIVITY AND ACID-BASE BALANCE

Acid-base balance depends on the concentration and activity of electrolytic solutes in the body. Clinical application of acid-base homeostasis is discussed in detail in Chapter 14.

Characteristics of Acids, Bases, and Salts

Acids

The term **acid** refers to either compounds that can donate [H^+] (Brönsted-Lowry acid) or any compound that accepts an electron pair (Lewis acid). Although these two theories of acids differ in which is being transferred, both theories attempt to describe how reactive groups perform within an aqueous solution[7,8]:

$$NH_4Cl + NaOH \rightarrow NH_3 + NaCl + HOH$$

In this reaction, Na^+ and Cl^- ions are not involved in the proton transfer. The equation can be rewritten ionically as follows to show the acidity of the ammonium ion:

$$NH_4^+ + OH^- \rightarrow NH_3 + HOH$$

The ammonium ion donates a H^+ ion (proton) to the reaction. The H^+ combines with the hydroxide ion (OH^-), and this converts the former into ammonia gas and the latter into water.

Acids With Single Ionizable Hydrogen. Simple compounds such as hydrochloric acid (HCl) ionize into one cation and one anion:

$$HCl \rightarrow H^+ + Cl^-$$

Acids With Multiple Ionizable Hydrogens. The H^+ ions in an acid may become available in stages. The degree of ionization increases as an electrolyte solution becomes more dilute. Concentrated sulfuric acid ionizes only one of its two H^+ atoms per molecule, as follows:

$$H_2SO_4 \rightarrow H^+ + HSO_4^-$$

With further dilution, second-stage ionization occurs:

$$H_2SO_4 \rightarrow H^+ + H^+ + SO_4^-$$

Bases

A **base** is a compound that yields hydroxyl ions (OH^-) when placed into aqueous solution. A substance capable of inactivating acids is also considered a base. These compounds, called *hydroxides,* consist of a metal that is ionically bound to a OH^- ion or ions. The OH^- may also be bound to an ammonium cation (NH_4^+). An example of this type of base is sodium hydroxide (NaOH). The Brönsted-Lowry definition of a base is any compound that accepts a proton; bases are paired with acids that donate the proton, and these are called *conjugate pairs.* This definition includes substances other than hydroxides, such as ammonia, carbonates, and certain proteins.

Hydroxide Bases. In aqueous solution, the following are typical dissociations of hydroxide bases:

$$Na^+OH \rightarrow Na^+ + OH^-$$
$$K^+OH \rightarrow K^+ + OH^-$$
$$Ca^{++}\,(OH^-)2 \rightarrow Ca^{++} + 2(OH^-)$$

Inactivation of an acid is part of the definition of a base. This inactivation is accomplished by OH^- reacting with H^+ to form water:

$$NaOH + HCl \rightarrow NaCl + HOH$$

Nonhydroxide Bases. Ammonia and carbonates are examples of nonhydroxide bases. Proteins, with their amino groups, also can serve as nonhydroxide bases.

MINI CLINI

Methacholine Dilution

The dilution equation ($V_1C_1 = V_2C_2$) is commonly used to calculate volumes or concentrations of medications when a specific dosage needs to be administered to a patient. If three of the variables are known, the fourth can be determined.

PROBLEM: Methacholine is a drug used to induce airway constriction in patients suspected of having. In healthy subjects, only higher doses of methacholine cause bronchospasm. In asthmatics, very low doses can precipitate a 20% decrease in the forced expiratory volume in 1 second (FEV_1). The methacholine challenge test begins with a low dose and increases the concentration (either doubling or quadrupling) until the patient has a significant change in FEV_1 or the highest dose has been given. Methacholine is supplied in vials that contain 100 mg of the active substance to which 6.25 ml of diluent (saline) can be added to produce a concentration of 16 mg/ml. This is the highest dosage administered to the patient. How can you make serial dilutions of the drug so that five different dosages are available and each one is four times more concentrated than the previous dose?

SOLUTION: Starting with a 16 mg/ml stock solution of methacholine, how much diluent needs to be added to 3 ml of the stock to make a 4 mg/ml dose (one-fourth of the original concentration)?

Using the dilution equation:

$$C_1V_1 = C_2V_2$$

$$(16)(3.0) = (4)V_2$$

$$48/4 = V_2$$

$$12 = V_1$$

Because there was 3 ml of the stock solution to begin with, the amount of diluent to add is the difference between 12 (V_2) and 3, or 9 ml. Adding 9 ml of diluent to the original 3 ml of stock (16 mg/ml) provides 12 ml of methacholine with a concentration of 4 mg/ml, exactly one-fourth of the highest dose. Additional dilutions can be prepared using 3 ml of solution according to the following table:

Start With		To Make
3 ml of 4 mg/ml	9 ml	1 mg/ml
3 ml of 1 mg/ml	9 ml	0.25 mg/ml
3 ml of 0.25 mg/ml	9 ml	0.0625 mg/ml

Each of these dilutions uses the same proportions used in the first dilution as determined by the dilution equation. Methacholine is administered by nebulizer to the patient, starting with the lowest concentration (0.0625 mg/ml) and increasing until a change in FEV_1 is observed. (See Chapter 20 for additional information on pulmonary function testing.)

Ammonia. Ammonia qualifies as a base because it reacts with water to yield OH^-:

$$NH_3 + HOH \rightarrow NH_4^+ + OH^-$$

and neutralizes H^+ directly:

$$NH^3 + H^+ \rightarrow NH_4^+$$

In both instances, NH_3 accepts a proton to become NH_4^+. Ammonia plays an important role in renal excretion of acid (see Chapter 14).

Carbonates. The carbonate ion (CO_3^{2-}), can react with water in the following way to produce OH^-:

(1) $$Na_2CO_3 \rightleftharpoons 2Na^+ + CO_3^{2-}$$

(2) $$CO_3^{2-} + HOH \rightleftharpoons HCO_3^- + OH^-$$

In this reaction, CO_3^{2-} accepts a proton from water, becoming the HCO_3^- ion. It simultaneously produces a hydroxide ion. The CO_3^{2-} ion also can react directly with H^+ to inactivate it:

$$CO_3^{2-} + H^+ \rightleftharpoons HCO_3^-$$

Protein Bases. Proteins are composed of amino acids bound together by peptide links. Physiologic reactions in the body occur in a mildly alkaline environment. This environment allows proteins to act as H^+ receptors, or bases. Cellular and blood proteins acting as bases are transcribed as $prot^-$.

The imidazole group of the amino acid histidine is an example of an H^+ acceptor on a protein molecule (Figure 13-4). The ability of proteins to accept H^+ ions limits H^+ activity in solution, which is called **buffering.** The buffering effect of hemoglobin (Hb) is produced by imidazole groups in the protein. Each Hb molecule contains 38 histidine residues. Each O_2-carrying component (heme group) of Hb is attached to a histidine residue. The ability of Hb to accept (i.e., buffer) H^+ ions depends on its oxygenation state. Deoxygenated (reduced) Hb is a stronger base (i.e., a better H^+ acceptor) than oxygenated Hb. This difference partially accounts for the ability of reduced Hb to buffer more acid than oxygenated Hb can (see Chapter 14). Plasma proteins also act as buffers, although with less buffering power than Hb, which contains more histidine.

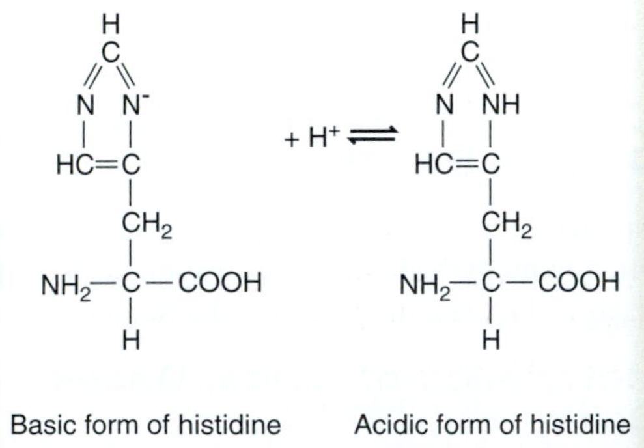

FIGURE 13-4 Histidine portion of a protein molecule (at *top*) serving as a proton acceptor (base).

Designation of Acidity and Alkalinity

Pure water can be used as a reference point for determining acidity or alkalinity. The concentration of both H^+ and OH^- in pure water is 10^{-7} mol/L. A solution that has a greater H^+ concentration or lower OH^- concentration than water acts as an acid. A solution that has a lower H^+ concentration or a greater OH^- concentration than water is alkaline, or basic.

The H^+ concentration $[H^+]$ of pure water has been adopted as the standard for comparing reactions of other solutions. Electrochemical techniques are used to measure the $[H^+]$ of unknown solutions. Acidity or alkalinity is determined by variation of the $[H^+]$ greater than or less than 1×10^{-7}. For example, a solution with a $[H^+]$ of 89.2×10^{-4} has a higher $[H^+]$ than water and is acidic. A solution with a $[H^+]$ of 3.6×10^{-8} has fewer H^+ ions than water and is by definition alkaline. Two related techniques are used for expressing the acidity or alkalinity of solutions using the $[H^+]$ of water (i.e., 10^{-7}) as a neutral factor: (1) the $[H^+]$ in nanomoles per liter and (2) the logarithmic pH scale.

Nanomolar Concentrations

The acidity or alkalinity of solutions may be reported using the molar concentration of H^+ compared with that of water. The $[H^+]$ of water is 1×10^{-7} mol/L, or 0.0000001 (one ten-millionth of a mole). The unit for one-billionth of a mole is a **nanomole** (nmol). The $[H^+]$ of water can be expressed as 100 nmol/L. A solution that has a $[H^+]$ of 100 nmol/L is neutral. A solution with an $[H^+]$ greater than 100 nmol/L is acidic; one with an $[H^+]$ less than 100 nmol/L is alkaline. This system is limited because of the wide range of possible $[H^+]$ but is applicable in clinical medicine because the physiologic range of $[H^+]$ is narrow. $[H^+]$ in healthy individuals is usually 30 to 50 nmol/L.

pH Scale

The pH scale is used to describe the concentration of H^+, ($[H^+]$), (i.e., Brönsted-Lowry acid) in a solution. Rather than expressing the $[H^+]$ in nanomoles, it is more convenient to describe it in terms of the negative logarithm of the nanomolar $[H^+]$. The equation for calculating pH is:

$$pH = -\log[H^+]$$

The pH of pure water is 7.0: The $[H^+]$ of water is 1×10^{-7} mol/L. The logarithm of 1×10^{-7} is −7, so the negative logarithm of 1×10^{-7} is 7.

Using this scheme, in a solution with a pH of 7.00, the $[H^+]$ is the same as would be seen in pure water, so by convention this is called "neutral." As the pH decreases below 7.00, the solution is termed *acidic.* When the pH increases above 7.00, the solution is considered to be *basic.* With a whole number change in pH (i.e., pH decreasing from 7.00 to 6.00), the $[H^+]$ is a factor of 10 less. With a pH increase from 7.00 to 8.00, the $[H^+]$ is 10 times greater (Figure 13-5). A pH of 7.00 is equivalent to a $[H^+]$ of 100 nmol. A pH of 8.00 is equivalent to a $[H^+]$ concentration of 10 nmol. Similarly, a change in pH of 0.3 units equals a twofold change in $[H^+]$.

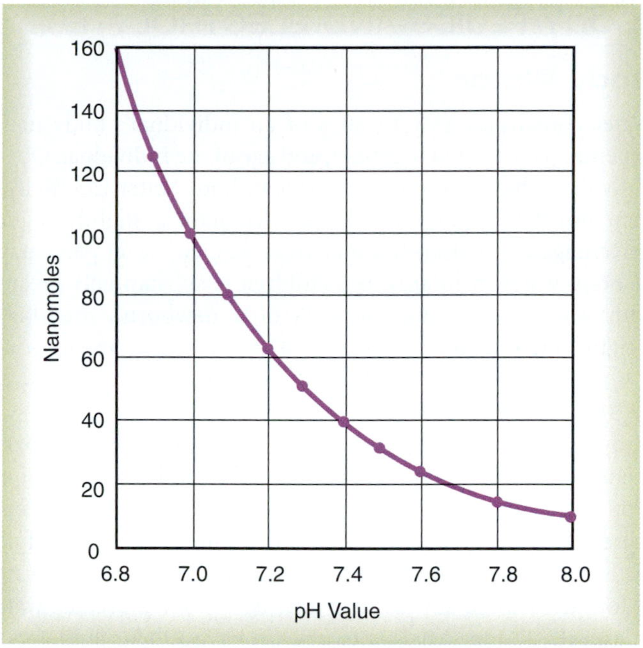

FIGURE 13-5 Relationship between pH scale and $[H^+]$ concentrations in nanomoles per liter (nmol/L). pH of 7.00 equals 100 nmol/L H^+, whereas the normal human pH (arterial blood) of 7.40 is equal to about 40 nmol/L.

Applying these concepts in an example pertinent to clinical medicine yields the following:

$$
\begin{aligned}
[H^+]\text{ in blood} &= 4.0 \times 10^{-8}\text{ mol/L} \\
pH &= -\log(4.0 \times 10^{-8}) \\
&= -\log 4.0 + -\log 10^{-8} \\
&= -\log 4.0 + \log 10^{8} \\
&= -0.602 + 8 \\
&= 7.40
\end{aligned}
$$

In this example, the $[H^+]$ in arterial blood of a healthy adult is approximately 4.0×10^{-8} mol/L, or 40 nmol/L.

RULE OF THUMB

The pH scale is logarithmic. pH is a positive number representing the negative log of the hydrogen ion concentration $[H^+]$ of a solution. To visualize changes in acidity or alkalinity, the following two rules are helpful:

1. A pH change of 0.3 unit equals a 2-fold change in $[H^+]$.
2. A pH change of 1 unit equals a 10-fold change in $[H^+]$.

For example, if a patient's blood pH decreased from 7.40 (normal) to 7.10, the $[H^+]$ concentration would be twice as high. If a patient's urine pH decreased from 7.00 to 6.00, the $[H^+]$ would have increased by 10 times.

BODY FLUIDS AND ELECTROLYTES

Body Water

Water constitutes 45% to 80% of an individual's body mass, depending on the mass, gender, and age of the individual. Obese individuals have a lower percentage of body water (≤30% less) than normal-weight individuals. Men have a slightly higher percentage of total-body water than women. Total percentage of body water in infants and children is substantially greater, with water accounting for 80% of a newborn's total-body weight (Table 13-3).

Distribution

Body water is divided into the following two major compartments: (1) *intracellular* ("within the cells") and (2) *extracellular* ("outside the cells"). Intracellular water accounts for approximately two-thirds of the total-body water, and extracellular water accounts for the remaining one-third. Extracellular water is found in three sub-compartments: (1) intravascular water (plasma), (2) interstitial water, and (3) transcellular fluid. Intravascular water constitutes approximately 5% of the body weight. Interstitial water is water in the tissues between the cells. It constitutes approximately 15% of the body weight. The proportion of *transcellular fluid* is quite small in proportion to plasma and **interstitial fluid.** Interstitial fluid is a matrix—a collagen/gel substance that allows the interstitium to provide structural support during times of extracellular volume depletion.[10] Examples of transcellular fluid include cerebrospinal fluid, digestive juices, and mucus. Transcellular fluid can become an important third space in some pathologic conditions, such as *ascites* (excess fluid in the peritoneal cavity) or *pleural effusion* (fluid collection in the pleural space).

Composition

The concentration of ionic solutes in intracellular and extracellular fluids differs significantly. Sodium (Na^+), chloride (Cl^-), and bicarbonate (HCO_3^-) are predominantly extracellular electrolytes. Potassium (K^+), magnesium (Mg^{++}), phosphate (PO_4^{3-}), sulfate (SO_4^{2-}), and protein constitute the main intracellular electrolytes. Although protein does not dissociate ionically, it can create H^+ and other weak bonds and distribute net extra charge within its molecule. Intravascular and interstitial fluids have similar electrolyte compositions. Plasma contains substantially more protein than interstitial fluid. Proteins, chiefly albumin, account for the high osmotic pressure of plasma. Osmotic pressure is an important determinant of fluid distribution between vascular and interstitial compartments.

TABLE 13-3
Distribution of Body Fluids

Body Water	Man (% Body Weight)	Woman (% Body Weight)	Infant (% Body Weight)
Total body Water	60 ± 15	50 ± 15	80
Intracellular	45	40	50
Extracellular	15-20	15-20	30
Interstitial	11-15	11-15	24
Intravascular	4.5	4.5	5.0
Transcellular	<1	<1	<1

Regulation

As discussed, movement of certain ions and proteins between body compartments is restricted yet water diffuses freely. Control of total-body water occurs through regulation of water intake (thirst) and water excretion (urine production, insensible loss, and stool water). The kidneys are mainly responsible for water excretion. If water intake is low, the kidneys reduce urine volume. Solutes in the urine can be concentrated up to four times the concentration of solutes in the plasma. If water intake is high, the kidneys can excrete large volumes of dilute urine.

The kidneys maintain the volume and composition of body fluids via two related mechanisms. First, filtration and reabsorption of Na^+ adjust urinary Na^+ excretion to match changes in dietary intake. Second, water excretion is regulated by osmoreceptors that are located in the hypothalamus and modulate secretion of antidiuretic hormone (ADH, also known as *vasopressin*).[6,11,12] These receptors are exceptionally sensitive; in vivo studies have shown that a single neuron can respond to either an osmotic or a nonosmotic baroreceptor simulus.[12] These mechanisms allow the kidneys to maintain the volume and concentration of body fluid despite variations in salt and water intake. Analysis of the urine (urinalysis) often provides diagnostic clues in disorders of body fluid volume.

Water Losses. Water may be lost from the body through the skin, lungs, kidneys, and gastrointestinal (GI) tract. Water loss can be *insensible,* such as evaporation of water from the skin and lungs, or *sensible,* such as losses from urine and the GI tract (Table 13-4).[13] Fluid losses from the body also may occur during vomiting, diarrhea, or suctioning from the stomach. Fever, in conjunction with sweating, also can cause significant losses.

The GI tract manufactures 8 to 10 L of fluid per day. More than 98% of this volume is reclaimed in the large intestine. In

TABLE 13-4
Daily Water Exchange

Regulation	Average Daily Volume (ml)	Maximum Daily Volume
Water Losses		
Insensible		
Skin	700	1500 ml
Lung	200	
Sensible		
Urine	1000-1200	>2000 ml/hr
Intestinal	200	8000 ml
Sweat	0	>2000 ml/hr
Water Gain		
Ingestion		
Fluids	1500-2000	1500 ml/hr
Solids	500-600	1500 ml/hr
Body metabolism	250	1000 ml

patients who are vomiting or have diarrhea, water losses through the GI tract can be considerable. Individuals with severe burns or open wounds can lose large quantities of water.

Other causes of abnormal fluid loss include certain renal and respiratory disorders. Patients with renal disease may have to excrete larger quantities of urine to get rid of extra nitrogenous wastes. Patients with increased ventilation also have increased water losses through increased evaporation from the respiratory tract. Patients with artificial airways are prone to evaporative water loss if inspired air is not adequately humidified. Infants have a greater proportion of body water than adults, particularly in the extracellular compartments (see Table 13-3). Water loss in infants may be twice the water loss in adults. Infants also have a greater body surface area (in proportion to body volume) than adults, making their basal heat production twice as high. Higher metabolic rates in infants necessitate greater urinary excretion. Infants turn over approximately half of their extracellular fluid volume daily versus one-seventh for adults. Fluid loss or lack of intake can rapidly deplete an infant of water.

Water Replacement. Water is replenished in two major ways: ingestion and metabolism (see Table 13-4).

Ingestion. Water is replaced mainly by ingestion, through the consumption of liquids. An average adult drinks 1500 to 2000 ml of water per day. An additional 500 to 600 ml of water is ingested from solid food.

Metabolism. Water also is gained from the oxidation of fats, carbohydrates, and proteins in the body; the destruction of cells also releases some water. During total starvation, 2000 ml of water can be produced daily by the metabolism of 1 kg of fat. Recovery after surgery or trauma may be similar to starvation; under such conditions, approximately 500 mg of protein and a similar amount of fat are metabolized. This metabolism yields approximately 1 L of water per day.

Transport Between Compartments

Homeostasis depends largely on the total volume of body fluids and on fluid transport between body compartments. The first stage of homeostasis is fluid exchange between systemic capillaries and interstitial fluid via passive diffusion. Capillary walls are permeable to crystalline electrolytes. This allows equilibrium between the two extracellular compartments to occur quickly. Except for the large protein molecules, plasma also can move through capillary walls into the tissue spaces. Because water and small molecules can cross the capillary membranes, they produce little or no osmotic effect.

Movement of fluid and solutes from capillary blood to interstitial spaces is enhanced by the difference in **hydrostatic pressure** (pressure exerted by a liquid at rest with respect to adjacent bodies) between compartments. Hydrostatic pressure difference depends on blood pressure, blood volume, and the vertical distance of the capillary from the heart (i.e., the effects of gravity). Hydrostatic pressure tends to cause fluid to leak out of capillaries into the interstitial spaces.

Osmotic pressure differences between interstitial and intravascular compartments oppose hydrostatic pressure; that is, osmotic pressure tends to keep fluid in the capillaries. Proteins with molecular weights greater than approximately 70,000 in colloidal suspension in the plasma cause this difference in osmotic pressure. Proteins such as albumin are too large to pass through the pores of the capillary. Instead, these proteins remain in the intravascular compartment and exert osmotic pressure, which draws water and small solute molecules back into the capillaries; this is called **plasma colloid osmotic pressure (oncotic pressure).** Because these large proteins are negatively charged, they attract (but do not bind) an equivalent amount of cations to the intravascular compartment. These cations have the effect of increasing osmotic pressure within the capillary *(Donnan effect)*.

In a typical capillary, blood pressure is approximately 30 mm Hg at the arterial end and approximately 20 mm Hg at the venous end (Figure 13-6). Colloid osmotic pressure of the intravascular fluid remains constant at approximately 25 mm Hg. Hydrostatic pressure along the capillary continually decreases. At the arterial end, hydrostatic pressure normally exceeds osmotic pressure, and water flows out of the vascular space into the interstitial space. At the venous end, colloidal osmotic pressure exceeds hydrostatic forces. Water is pulled back into the vascular compartment.

The outflow of water and electrolytes from the capillary at the arterial end is not completely balanced by the return on the venous end. Slightly more water diffuses out than is reabsorbed. This slight outward excess is balanced by fluid return through the lymphatic circulation (see Chapter 9). Fluid return via lymphatic channels also depends on pressure differences. The pressure in the interstitial space is determined by the volume of interstitial fluid and its electrolyte content. Interstitial fluid moves from a region of higher pressure (interstitial space) to a region of lower pressure (lymphatic channels). This lymph fluid moves into larger lymphatic spaces, where the pressure is continuously decreasing.

Three examples of the forces in Starling's equation are fluid return from gravity-dependent areas of the body, fluid exchange in the lung, and tissue edema.

Because of hydrostatic effects, capillary pressure in the feet can reach 100 mm Hg when an individual is standing. Reabsorption of tissue fluid can be accomplished, although hydrostatic pressure greatly exceeds colloidal osmotic pressure. Three factors favor reabsorption under these circumstances:

1. High intravascular hydrostatic pressure is balanced by a proportionally greater interstitial pressure.
2. The "pumping" action of the skeletal muscles surrounding leg veins reduces venous pressures.
3. Lymph flow back to the thorax is enhanced via a similar mechanism; this facilitates clearance of excess interstitial fluid.

However, when an imbalance results from changes in the basic pressures (e.g., arterial hypertension), edema tends to occur in the dependent limbs.

The lungs present a different situation. In systemic tissues, a constant exchange of interstitial fluid is essential. In the lungs, the alveoli must be kept relatively dry. Otherwise, interstitial

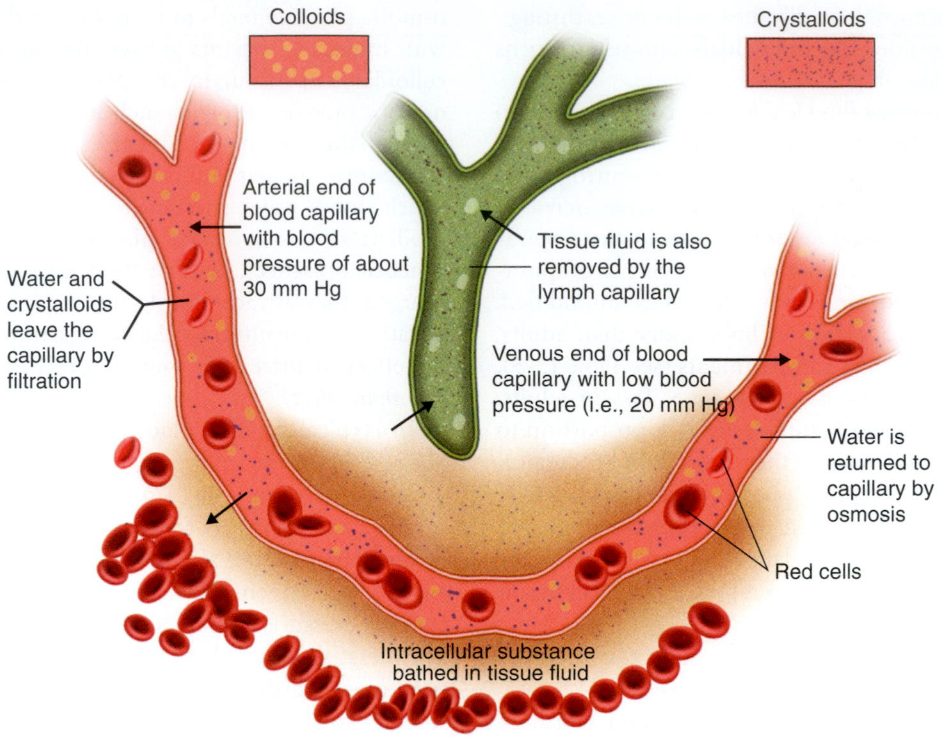

FIGURE 13-6 Tissue fluid is formed by a process of filtration at the arterial end of a systemic capillary *(left),* in which blood pressure exceeds colloid osmotic pressure. The fluid is absorbed by the blood capillaries and lymphatic vessels. It returns to the venous end of the capillary *(right)* when colloid osmotic pressure exceeds blood pressure. Fluid is absorbed into the lymphatic capillary system when interstitial fluid pressure is greater than the pressure within the lymphatic capillary. Normally, little colloid escapes from the capillary. Colloid that does escape is returned to the blood circulation by the lymphatic vessels. (Modified from Burke SR: The composition and function of body fluids, ed 3, St Louis, 1980, Mosby.)

fluid in the alveolar-capillary spaces would impede the diffusion of gas. Colloid osmotic pressure in pulmonary blood vessels is the same as it is in the systemic circulation. To minimize interstitial fluid in the alveolar-capillary region, the hydrostatic pressure difference must be kept low. The pulmonary circulation is a low-pressure system. The mean pulmonary vascular pressures are approximately one-sixth of those in the systemic circulation. Colloid osmotic pressure exceeds hydrostatic forces across the entire length of the pulmonary capillaries in healthy individuals. The alveoli are relatively free of excess interstitial water.

If hydrostatic pressure increases in the pulmonary circulation, this balance can be upset. This causes fluid movement into the alveolar-capillary spaces. Excess fluid in the interstitial space is called *edema*. In the lungs, edema caused by increased hydrostatic pressure often is a result of backpressure from a failing left ventricle (e.g., in congestive heart failure).

Edema can be caused by other factors. The **Starling equilibrium** equation given earlier shows that edema can be caused by a decrease in colloid osmotic pressure or an increase in capillary permeability. If albumin is depleted in the blood, the balance of forces is upset, favoring increased movement of fluid into the interstitium. Likewise, an increase in capillary permeability results in more fluid leaving the capillaries. Increased capillary permeability is a major factor in certain types of acute lung injuries (see Chapter 29).[14]

Electrolytes

Electrolytes in the various body fluids are not passive solutes. Electrolytes maintain the internal environment while making possible essential chemical and physiologic events. There are seven major electrolytes: sodium, chloride, bicarbonate, potassium, calcium, magnesium, and phosphorus (phosphate).

Sodium (Na^+)

Na^+ is the major circulating cation within the body.[15] Regulation of Na^+ concentration in plasma and urine is related to regulation of total-body water. Of the total-body stores of Na^+, 50% is extracellular. The remaining Na^+ is found in bone (40%) and in cells (10%). The normal serum concentration of Na^+ is 136 to 145 mEq/L. In cells, the Na^+ concentration is much lower, averaging only 4.5 mEq/L.

The average adult ingests and excretes approximately 100 mEq of Na^+ every 24 hours. Children require approximately half this amount, and infants typically exchange 20 mEq of Na^+ per day. Most Na^+ is reabsorbed through the kidney. Approximately 80% of the Na^+ in the body is reclaimed passively in the proximal tubules. The remainder is actively reabsorbed in the distal tubules. Na^+ reabsorption in the kidneys is governed mainly by the level of aldosterone, which is secreted by the adrenal cortex. Na^+ reabsorption in the distal tubules of the

TABLE 13-5
Electrolyte Disorders and Clinical Findings

Electrolyte	Imbalance	Causes	Symptoms
Sodium (Na^+)	Hyponatremia	GI loss, sweating, fever, diuretics, ascites, congestive heart failure, kidney failure	Weakness, lassitude, apathy, headache, orthostatic hypotension, tachycardia
	Hypernatremia	Net sodium gain, net water loss, increased aldosterone, steroid therapy	Tremulousness, irritability, ataxia, confusion, seizures, coma
Chloride (Cl^-)	Hypochloremia	GI loss, diuretics	Metabolic alkalosis, muscle spasm, coma (severe cases)
	Hyperchloremia	Dehydration, metabolic acidosis, respiratory alkalosis	(Minimal)
Potassium (K^+)	Hypokalemia	Diuretics, steroid therapy, renal tubular disease, vomiting, diarrhea, malnutrition, trauma	Muscle weakness, paralysis, ECG abnormalities, supraventricular arrhythmias, circulatory failure, cardiac arrest
	Hyperkalemia	Chronic renal disease, hemorrhage, tissue necrosis, nonsteroidal antiinflammatory drugs, ACE inhibitors, cyclosporine, K^+-sparing diuretics	ECG changes, ventricular arrhythmias, cardiac arrest
Calcium (Ca^{++})	Hypocalcemia	Hyperparathyroidism, pancreatitis, renal failure, trauma	Hyperactive tendon reflexes, muscle twitching, spasm, abdominal cramps, ECG changes, seizures (rarely)
	Hypercalcemia	Hyperthyroidism, hyperparathyroidism, metastatic bone cancer, sarcoidosis	Fatigue, depression, muscle weakness, anorexia, nausea, vomiting, constipation
Magnesium (Mg^{++})	Hypomagnesemia	Inadequate intake/impaired absorption of Mg^{++}, pancreatitis, alcoholism	Muscle weakness, irritability, tetany, ECG changes, arrhythmias, delirium, seizures
	Hypermagnesemia	Dehydration, renal insufficiency, tissue trauma, lupus erythematosus	ECG changes (along with hyperkalemia, cardiac arrest, respiratory muscle paralysis)
Phosphate (HPO_4^{2-})	Hypophosphatemia	Starvation, malabsorption, hyperparathyroidism, hyperthyroidism, uncontrolled diabetes mellitus	Diaphragmatic weakness
	Hyperphosphatemia	Endocrine disorders, acromegaly, chronic renal insufficiency, acute renal failure, tissue trauma	(Minimal)

ACE, Angiotensin-converting enzyme; *ECG,* electrocardiogram.

kidney occurs in exchange for other cations. Na^+ balance is involved in acid-base homeostasis (i.e., H^+ exchange) and the regulation of K^+. Abnormal losses of Na^+ can lead to *hyponatremia* (low Na^+ concentration in the plasma) and may occur for numerous reasons, as shown in Table 13-5.

Hyponatremia, which is the most common electrolyte imbalance found in hospitalized patients, is defined as having serum Na^+ levels less than 135 mEq/L.[6] Previously considered to be benign, mild hyponatremia has been shown in more recent studies to have a significant impact on a patient's cognitive function and gait stability, and it is thought to be a contributing factor in falls.[16] Hyponatremia can lead to cerebral edema owing to a change in osmotic pressure; the two most common causes for acute hyponatremia are postoperative iatrogenic and self-induced secondary to water intoxication.[16] One type of normal-volume (euvolemic) hyponatremia is known as the *syndrome of inappropriate antidiuretic hormone secretion* (SIADH).[15-17]

Treatment of hypovolemic hyponatremia can have dire consequences as well. If fluid is administered too quickly, damage to the central nervous system occurs. With significant fluid shifts in Na^+ concentrations, rapid changes in cellular volume can lead to cell damage and cell death (apoptosis).[6] Osmotic demyelination syndrome occurs when serum Na^+ concentration changes more than 10 mEq/L in chronic hyponatremia or 18 mEq/L over 48 hours.[16]

Chloride (Cl^-)

Cl^- is the most prominent anion in the body. Two-thirds of the body's store of Cl^- is extracellular; the remainder is intracellular. Intracellular Cl^- is present in significant amounts in red and white blood cells. It also is present in cells that have excretory functions, such as the GI mucosa.

Normal serum levels of Cl^- are 98 to 106 mEq/L. The concentration of extracellular Cl^- is inversely proportional to the concentration of the other major anion, HCO_3^-. Cl^- is regulated by the kidney in much the same manner as Na^+ (80% reabsorbed in the proximal tubules and 20% reabsorbed in the distal tubules). Cl^- is usually excreted with K^+ in the form of KCl. An imbalance in one of these electrolytes usually affects both. Replacement therapy usually includes both K^+ and Cl^-. The stomach and the small bowel also affect the balance of Cl^-, and sweat contains hypotonic quantities of Cl^-. Abnormal Cl^- levels may occur for various reasons (see Table 13-5).

Bicarbonate (HCO_3^-)

After Cl^-, HCO_3^- is the most important body fluid anion. It plays an important role in acid-base homeostasis and is the strong base in the HCO_3–H_2CO_3 buffer pair (see Chapter 14). HCO_3^- is the primary means for transporting CO_2 from the tissues to the lungs. The ratio of HCO_3^- to H_2CO_3 in healthy individuals is maintained near 20 : 1; this results in a pH of close to 7.40. HCO_3^- stores are evenly divided between intracellular and extracellular compartments. Normal serum HCO_3^- levels in arterial blood range from 22 to 26 mEq/L. HCO_3^- levels are slightly higher in venous blood as CO_2 is being transported to the lungs.

In acid-base disorders, the kidneys regulate HCO_3^- levels to maintain a near-normal pH. In healthy individuals, more than 80% of blood HCO_3^- is reabsorbed in the proximal tubules of the kidneys. The remainder is reclaimed in the distal tubules. In respiratory acidosis, the kidneys retain or produce HCO_3^- to buffer the additional acid caused by CO_2 retention. In respiratory alkalosis, the opposite occurs. A reciprocal relationship exists between Cl^- and HCO_3^- concentrations. HCO_3^- retention is associated with Cl^- excretion, and vice versa (Chapter 14).

MINI CLINI

Water, Salt, and Congestive Heart Failure

PROBLEM: Why do patients who have congestive heart failure (CHF) need to adhere to a low-salt diet?

SOLUTION: CHF occurs when the left ventricle cannot pump all of the blood presented to it. This situation leads to pooling of blood in the lungs and venous circulation and an increase in peripheral venous pressure. Normally, the ventricle pumps most of the blood entering it. This volume is the "preload" of the heart. The volume of extracellular water partially determines the preload of the ventricle.

The ventricle can fail as a pump either because of intrinsic heart disease, such as infarction or ischemia, or because of elevated distal pressures against which it must pump (hypertension). In addition to pooling of blood in the systemic venous circulation, blood can back up in the lungs, resulting in congestion and edema.

The most important determinant of the extracellular water volume is its Na^+ content. Changes in extracellular water are dictated by the net gain or loss of Na^+, with an accompanying gain or loss of water. To reduce the work of the heart, fluid volume must be carefully regulated. By restricting Na^+ intake, extracellular fluid volume can be reduced, allowing the heart to function more effectively as a pump. Treatment of CHF must address not only excess fluid volume but also the underlying cause.

Diuretics are often used to help reduce fluid volume. Many diuretics cause the kidney to excrete Na^+, causing water to follow and reducing the extracellular fluid load. Because some diuretics also cause K^+ to be excreted, care must be taken in the management of CHF not to cause electrolyte imbalances. K^+ supplements may be used so that diuresis does not result in hypokalemia. Because of the central role of extracellular water in CHF, weighing the patient is a simple yet sensitive means of detecting excess fluid volume.

Potassium (K^+)

K^+ is the main cation of the intracellular compartment. Most of the K^+ (98%) in the body is found in cells. **Active transport** of K^+ into the cells occurs through an ionic pump mechanism. An electrical differential across the cell membrane also facilitates K^+ movement into the cell. For every three K^+ ions that enter a cell, two Na^+ ions and one H^+ ion must leave. This transfer maintains electrical neutrality in the cell.

The difference in K^+ distribution is evident when comparing concentrations between fluid compartments. Intracellular K^+ concentration is approximately 150 mEq/L, whereas serum K^+ concentration normally ranges from 3.5 to 5.0 mEq/L. Serum K^+ is an indirect indicator only of the total-body K^+. Serum K^+ is usually analyzed by assessing both intake and excretion.

The average adult excretes 40 to 75 mEq of K^+ in the urine every 24 hours. An additional 10 mEq is excreted in the stool. The average dietary intake of K^+ ranges from 50 to 85 mEq/day. Patients who have undergone surgery, have sustained trauma, or have renal disease often have greater K^+ losses. Consequently, such patients may need K^+ replacement averaging 100 to 120 mEq/day.

Serum K^+ concentration is determined primarily by the pH of extracellular fluid and the size of the intracellular K^+ pool. In extracellular acidosis, excess H^+ ions are exchanged for intracellular K^+. Movement of K^+ from intracellular to extracellular spaces may produce dangerous levels of *hyperkalemia* (elevated K^+). Alkalosis has the opposite effect. When pH increases, K^+ moves into cells. In the absence of acid-base disturbances, serum K^+ reflects total-body K^+. With excessive loss of K^+ from the GI tract, serum K^+ decreases. A 10% loss of total-body K^+ causes the serum K^+ level to decrease approximately 1 mEq/L.

Renal excretion of K^+ is controlled by aldosterone levels.[18] Aldosterone inhibits the enzyme responsible for K^+ transport in the distal renal tubular cells of the kidney. Metabolic acidosis also inhibits the transport system. Na^+ and H^+ ions enter cells at the expense of increased K^+ excretion. Alkalosis has the reverse effect. It stimulates cellular retention of K^+. Kidney failure results in K^+ retention and hyperkalemia.

Hypokalemia (reduced serum K^+) disturbs cellular function in numerous organ systems, including the GI, neuromuscular, renal, and cardiovascular systems (see Table 13-5), and is one of the most common electrolyte abnormalities within the hospital environment.[18] Management of hypokalemia involves replacement of K^+ losses and treatment of the underlying disorder. To manage the associated Cl^- deficit, K^+ is given with Cl^-. Caution is required in the administration of intravenous K^+ because cardiac muscle is very sensitive to extracellular concentrations of this electrolyte.

Hyperkalemia (elevated serum K^+) is most common in patients with renal insufficiency (see Table 13-5). The primary treatment of hyperkalemia is restriction of K^+ intake. The processes that precipitated the hyperkalemia also must be controlled. Temporary measures for reducing serum K^+ levels include administration of insulin, calcium gluconate, Na^+ salts, or large volumes of hypertonic glucose. Cation exchange resins may be given orally or rectally. If these measures fail, peritoneal or renal dialysis can aid in K^+ removal.

Calcium (Ca^{++})

Ca^{++} is an important mediator of neuromuscular function and cell enzyme processes. Most of the Ca^{++} in the body is contained in the bones. The normal serum calcium is 8.7 to 10.4 mg/dl, or approximately 4.5 to 5.25 mEq/L. This concentration is maintained by the interaction of parathyroid hormone, vitamin D (calcitriol), and calcitonin.

Ca^{++} is present in the blood in the following three forms: ionized, protein bound, and complex. The proportion of Ca^{++} in each form is affected by blood pH, concentration of plasma proteins, and presence of Ca^{++}-combining anions (e.g., HCO_3^- and hydrogen phosphate [HPO_4^{2-}]). Approximately 50% of serum Ca is ionized (Ca^{++}) and is physiologically active. An additional 10% forms Ca-anion complexes. The remaining 40% is bound to plasma proteins, primarily albumen. Ionized Ca^{++} is physiologically active in processes such as enzyme activity, blood clotting, neuromuscular irritability, and bone calcification. Acidemia increases the concentration of Ca^{++} in the serum, and alkalemia decreases the concentration.

Abnormal levels of Ca^{++} can cause various serious symptoms (see Table 13-5). Treatment of *hypocalcemia* (low serum levels of Ca^{++}) consists of correcting the underlying cause and replacing Ca^{++} either orally or intravenously. *Hypercalcemia* (increased levels of Ca^{++}) can result from numerous disorders. The most common causes are hyperparathyroidism and malignancies (e.g., multiple myeloma, lung cancer). Acute hypercalcemia requires emergency treatment because death may occur quickly if serum Ca^{++} increases to more than 17 mg/L (8.5 mEq/L). In such cases, there is usually an associated deficit of extracellular fluid. Volume replacement reduces serum Ca^{++} by dilution.

Magnesium (Mg^{++})

Mg^{++} is the second most abundant intracellular cation after K^+. Mg^{++} plays an important role in cellular functions, including energy transfer; metabolism of protein, carbohydrate, and fat; and maintenance of normal cell membrane function (see Table 13-5). Systemically, Mg^{++} decreases blood pressure and alters peripheral vascular resistance. Abnormalities of Mg^{++} levels can result in disturbances in nearly every organ system and can cause potentially fatal complications (e.g., ventricular arrhythmia, coronary artery vasospasm, sudden death). Hypomagnesemia is also associated with multiple neuromuscular symptoms, such as muscular weakness, tetany, coma, and seizures. There is some evidence that intercellular Mg^{++} levels may be related to bronchial hyperresponsiveness.

Normal values for serum Mg^{++} range from 1.7 to 2.1 mg/dl (1.7 to 1.4 mEq/L) in healthy adults. Most (99%) of the Mg^{++} in the body is intracellular. Of the small portion in extracellular spaces, 80% is ionized or bound to other ions (e.g., phosphate) and the remaining 20% bound to proteins. Extracellular Mg^{++} is in equilibrium with Mg^{++} in the bone, kidneys, intestine, and other soft tissues. In contrast to most electrolytes, Mg^{++} excretion in urine is not regulated hormonally, and circulating Mg^{++} in the extracellular fluid does not exchange readily with its main repository—the bones. Serum levels of Mg^{++} may remain normal even if total-body stores are depleted by 20%. Conversely, when there is a negative Mg^{++} balance, most of the losses come from the extracellular spaces.

Phosphorus (P)

An average adult has approximately 1 kg (1000 g) of P, of which 80% to 90% is in bone and teeth in the form of apatite. The remaining P is mostly present in the viscera and skeletal muscle, with a very small amount (<0.1%) in the extracellular fluids.[19] Of this total, 10% to 17% is combined with proteins, carbohydrates, and lipids in muscle tissue and blood, and the remainder is incorporated into complex organic compounds. Only about 1% of the total-body P is available as free serum compounds, so the serum level (1.2 to 2.3 mEq/L) does not reflect total-body content. Serum P levels are influenced by several factors (see Table 13-5), including the serum Ca^{++} concentration and the pH of blood.

Organic phosphate (HPO_4^{2-}) is the main anion within cells, with 20% present in the mitochondria. Approximately 30% of cellular HPO_4^{2-} is stored in the endoplasmic reticulum and is used in the phosphorylation of various proteins.[19] Inorganic phosphate plays a primary role in the metabolism of cellular energy, being the source from which adenosine triphosphate is synthesized. In acid-base homeostasis, phosphate is the main urinary buffer for titratable acid excretion (see Chapter 14).

P homeostasis depends on balance between GI absorption and urinary excretion. The parathyroid hormone provides hormonal regulation. *Hyperphosphatemia* (elevated serum levels of P) can occur when the load (e.g., GI absorption, cellular release) exceeds renal excretion and tissue uptake. Hyperphosphatemia precipitates Ca^{++}, causing hypocalcemia, which can be life-threatening if severe. Central nervous system symptoms such as altered mental status, paresthesias, and seizures can result from hyperphosphatemia. Prolonged hyperphosphatemia can result in abnormal deposition of calcium phosphate in previously healthy connective tissues, such as cardiac valves, and in solid organs, such as muscles.

SUMMARY CHECKLIST

- The body is a water-based organism in which chemical substances and particles exist in solution or suspension.
- The concentration of solutes in a solution may be quantified (1) by actual weight (grams, milligrams, or micrograms) or (2) by chemical combining power (equivalents or milliequivalents). The weight of a solute does not give an indication of its chemical combining power, but gram equivalent weights do.
- Solutions commonly involve the action of osmotic pressure. Body cell membranes are semipermeable, and osmotic pressure maintains the distribution of water and solutes in physiologic ranges.
- Concentrations of solutions may be calculated using ratio, weight/volume, or percent methods.
- Physiologically active compounds in the body are mostly weak electrolytic covalent substances. In aqueous solutions, some molecules ionize, leaving the remainder

intact. Equilibrium is maintained between the ions and un-ionized molecules.

- Proteins made up of amino acids can function as bases in the mildly alkaline environment of the body; this allows Hb and plasma proteins to function as buffers.
- Acidity or alkalinity is determined by variation of $[H^+]$ greater than or less than 1×10^{-7} mol/L. Two methods for recording acidity or alkalinity use H^+ concentration of water as the neutral standard: (1) the actual measured molar concentration of H^+ in nanomoles per liter and (2) the logarithmic pH scale.
- Water makes up 45% to 80% of an individual's body weight. Percentage of total-body water depends on weight, gender, age, and adipose tissue. Total-body water is divided into intracellular and extracellular water. Extracellular water is divided further into intravascular and interstitial water, with a small component of transcellular fluids.
- Control of total-body water is regulated by water intake and excretion. The kidneys maintain the volume and composition of body fluids by two related mechanisms: (1) filtration and reabsorption of Na^+ and (2) regulation of water excretion in response to changes in secretion of ADH.
- A balance between hydrostatic and osmotic pressure keeps water in the appropriate body compartments. Plasma proteins account for the high colloid osmotic pressure of plasma. Colloid osmotic pressure determines distribution of fluid between vascular and interstitial compartments. Imbalances in osmotic and hydrostatic pressures can result in edema.
- Electrolytes help maintain the internal environment and make important chemical and physiologic events possible. The concentrations of electrolytes in the intracellular and extracellular fluid compartments differ markedly. Increased or decreased concentrations of any electrolytes can result in disease and sometimes death.

References

1. Kaplan LJ, Kellum JA: Fluids, pH, ions and electrolytes. *Curr Opin Crit Care* 16:323, 2010.
2. Fine LG: Ernest Henry Starling (1866-1927) on the formation and reabsorption of lymph. *Nephron Physiol* 126:9, 2014.
3. Kramer GC: Hypertonic resuscitation: physiologic mechanisms and recommendations for trauma care. *J Trauma* 54:S89, 2003.
4. Lewis CA, Martin GS: Understanding and managing fluid balance in patients with acute lung injury. *Curr Opin Crit Care* 10:13, 2004.
5. Levick JR, Michel CC: Microvascular fluid exchange and the revised Starling principle. *Cardiovasc Res* 87:198, 2010.
6. Cowen LE, Hodak SP, Verbalis JG: Age-associated abnormalities of water homeostasis. *Endocrinol Metab Clin North Am* 42:349–370, 2013.
7. McNaught AD, Wilkinson A: *Compendium of chemical terminology*, Oxford, 2010, IUPAC.
8. Borkum MI, Frey JG: Usage and applications of semantic web techniques and technologies to support chemistry research. *J Cheminform* 6:18, 2014.
9. Brogioli D: Violation of mass action law in dilute chemical systems. *J Chem Phys* 139:184, 2013.
10. Friedman A: Fluid and electrolyte therapy: a primer. *Pediatr Nephrol* 25:843, 2009.
11. Schrier RW, Bansal S: Diagnosis and management of hyponatremia in acute illness. *Curr Opin Crit Care* 14:627, 2008.
12. Bekheirnia M, Schrier R: Pathophysiology of water and sodium retention: edematous states with normal kidney function. *Curr Opin Pharmacol* 6:202, 2006.
13. Van Haren F, Zacharowski K: What's new in volume therapy in the intensive care unit. *Best Pract Res Clin Anaesthesiol* 28:275, 2014.
14. Morissette MP: Colloid osmotic pressure: its measurement and clinical value. *Can Med Assoc J* 116:897, 1977.
15. Bockenhauer D, Zieg J: Electrolyte disorders. *Clin Perinatol* 41:575, 2014.
16. Sterns RH, Hix JK, Silver S: Treatment of hyponatremia. *Curr Opin Nephrol Hypertens* 19:493, 2010.
17. Adrogue HJ, Madias NE: Hyponatremia. *N Engl J Med* 342:1581, 2000.
18. Buckley MS, LeBlanc JM, Cawley MJ: Electrolyte disturbances associated with commonly prescribed medications in the intensive care unit. *Crit Care Med* 38:S253, 2010.
19. Razzaque MS: Phosphate toxicity: new insights into an old problem. *Clin Sci* 120:91, 2011.

CHAPTER 14

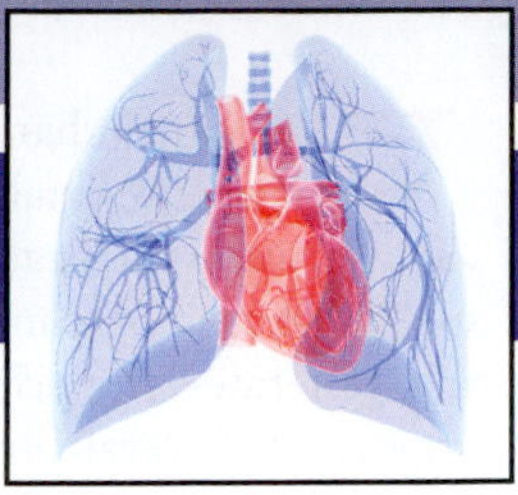

Acid-Base Balance

WILL BEACHEY

CHAPTER OBJECTIVES

After reading this chapter you will be able to:

- Describe how the lungs and kidneys regulate volatile and fixed acids.
- Describe how the equilibrium constant of an acid is related to its ionization and strength.
- Define open and closed buffer systems.
- Explain why open and closed buffer systems differ in their ability to buffer fixed and volatile acids.
- Explain how to use the Henderson-Hasselbalch equation in hypothetical clinical situations.
- Describe how the kidneys and lungs compensate for each other when the function of one is abnormal.
- Explain how renal absorption and excretion of electrolytes affect acid-base balance.
- Classify and interpret arterial blood acid-base results.
- Explain how to use arterial acid-base information to decide on a clinical course of action.
- Explain why acute changes in the carbon dioxide levels of the blood affect plasma bicarbonate ion concentration.
- Calculate the anion gap and use it to determine the cause of metabolic acidosis.
- Describe how standard bicarbonate and base excess measurements are used to identify the nonrespiratory component of acid-base imbalances.

CHAPTER OUTLINE

Hydrogen Ion Regulation in Body Fluids
- Strong and Weak Acids and Bases: Equilibrium Constants
- Buffer Solution Characteristics
- Bicarbonate and Nonbicarbonate Buffer Systems
- pH of a Buffer System: Henderson-Hasselbalch Equation
- Physiologic Roles of Bicarbonate and Nonbicarbonate Buffer Systems

Acid Excretion
- Lungs
- Kidneys

Acid-Base Disturbances
- Normal Acid-Base Balance
- Primary Respiratory Disturbances
- Primary Metabolic (Nonrespiratory) Disturbances
- Compensation: Restoring pH to Normal

Clinical Acid-Base States
- Systematic Acid-Base Classification
- Respiratory Acidosis
- Respiratory Alkalosis
- Metabolic (Nonrespiratory) Acidosis
- Metabolic Alkalosis
- Metabolic Acid-Base Indicators
- Mixed Acid-Base States
- Stewart's Strong Ion Approach to Acid-Base Balance

KEY TERMS

acidemia
alkalemia
base excess (BE)
buffer base
closed buffer system
conjugate base
equilibrium constant
fixed (nonvolatile) acids
Henderson-Hasselbalch (H-H) equation
hypercapnia
hypocapnia
isohydric buffering
metabolic acidosis
metabolic alkalosis
open buffer system
paresthesia
respiratory acidosis
respiratory alkalosis
standard bicarbonate
volatile acid

Even small changes in hydrogen ion concentration $[H^+]$ can cause vital metabolic processes in the body to fail. Note that brackets [ ] around the abbreviation for a substance indicate concentration. Normal metabolism continually generates H^+, which means H^+ regulation is extremely important. Several physiologic mechanisms work together to keep $[H^+]$ of body fluids in a range that supports life. This chapter will help respiratory therapists (RTs) understand how these mechanisms work and how to spot abnormalities in their function. This knowledge will help RTs and other members of the patient care team make informed decisions about treating the underlying causes of acid-base disturbances.

HYDROGEN ION REGULATION IN BODY FLUIDS

Acid-base balance refers to physiologic mechanisms that keep $[H^+]$ of body fluids in a range that supports life. H^+ ions react readily with the protein molecules of important cellular catalytic enzymes. These reactions change the physical shape of the protein molecule, which may inactivate enzymes. Body fluids must be kept in a narrow pH range of 7.35 to 7.45 to function normally. This corresponds to $[H^+]$ of 45 to 35 nmol/L.

H^+ ions formed in the body come from either *volatile* or *fixed* (nonvolatile) acids. **Volatile acids** are in equilibrium with a dissolved gas. The only volatile acid of physiologic importance in the body is carbonic acid (H_2CO_3), which is in equilibrium with dissolved carbon dioxide. Normal aerobic metabolism generates approximately 13,000 mmol/L of CO_2 each day, which produces an equal amount of H^+ as shown by the CO_2 hydration reaction:

$$\begin{array}{l} CO_2 + H_2O \rightarrow H_2CO_3 \rightarrow HCO_3^- + H^+ \\ \uparrow \\ \text{Aerobic metabolism} \end{array}$$

As CO_2 diffuses into the blood at the tissue level, this reaction occurs mostly in the erythrocyte, where it is catalyzed by carbonic anhydrase, an intracellular enzyme. In a process called **isohydric buffering**,[1] most H^+ produced in this way causes no change in pH because hemoglobin (Hb) in the erythrocyte immediately buffers the H^+. When blood reaches the lungs, Hb releases H^+ to form CO_2 as shown:

$$\begin{array}{l} \text{Ventilation} \\ \uparrow \\ CO_2 + H_2O \leftarrow H_2CO_3 \leftarrow HCO_3^- + H^+ \\ \qquad\qquad\qquad\qquad\qquad\quad \uparrow \\ \qquad\qquad\qquad\qquad HHb \rightarrow H^+ + Hb^- \end{array}$$

In this way, ventilation gets rid of H_2CO_3 just as fast as it is produced. Isohydric buffering and ventilation are the two major ways the body keeps the blood's pH constant regardless of how much CO_2 is produced.

Catabolism—the breakdown of proteins—continually produces **fixed (nonvolatile) acids** such as sulfuric and phosphoric acids. In addition, anaerobic metabolism produces lactic acid, another fixed acid. In contrast to H_2CO_3, these nonvolatile acids are not in equilibrium with a gas. However, the H^+ of fixed acids can be buffered by bicarbonate ions (HCO_3^-), which produce CO_2 and water (H_2O) (see the previous CO_2 hydration reaction); the CO_2 formed is removed from the body in exhaled gas. Compared with daily CO_2 production, fixed acid production is small, averaging only approximately 50 to 70 mEq/day.[2] Certain diseases, such as untreated diabetes, increase fixed acid production. H^+ ions produced in this way stimulate respiratory centers in the brain, increasing ventilation; this eliminates more CO_2, which pulls the CO_2 hydration reaction to the left and removes H^+ from the blood (refer to the CO_2 hydration reaction). In this way, the respiratory system *compensates* for increases in fixed acid; that is, it prevents $[H^+]$ from rising as sharply as it otherwise would when fixed acids are produced.

$$\begin{array}{l} \text{Increased ventilation} \\ \uparrow \\ CO_2 + H_2O \leftarrow H_2CO_3 \leftarrow HCO_3^- + H^+ \\ \qquad\qquad\qquad\qquad\qquad\quad \uparrow \\ \qquad\qquad\qquad\qquad\quad \text{Fixed acid } H^+ \end{array}$$

Strong and Weak Acids and Bases: Equilibrium Constants

Strong acid and base molecules dissociate or ionize almost completely in an aqueous (liquid) solution. Weak acids and bases ionize only to a small extent. An example of a strong acid is hydrochloric acid. Nearly 100% of the HCl molecules dissociate to form H^+ and Cl^-:

(1) $$HCl \rightarrow H^+ + Cl^-$$

At *equilibrium*, when all dissociation stops, the concentration of HCl is extremely small compared with either $[H^+]$ or $[Cl^-]$. There is no arrow pointing to the left in Reaction 1, emphasizing that HCl ionizes almost completely in solution. In contrast, H_2CO_3 is an example of a relatively weak acid:

(2) $$H_2CO_3 \rightleftharpoons HCO_3^- + H^+$$

The long arrow pointing to the left indicates that at *equilibrium*, the concentration of undissociated H_2CO_3 molecules is far greater than the concentration of either HCO_3^- or H^+.

The **equilibrium constant** of an acid is a measure of the extent to which the acid molecules dissociate (ionize). At equilibrium, the number of dissociating H_2CO_3 molecules in Reaction 2 is equal to the number of associating HCO_3^- and H^+, even though the concentrations of reactants and products are unequal. In this state, no further change occurs in $[H_2CO_3]$, $[HCO_3^-]$, or $[H^+]$. The following reaction expresses the state of affairs at equilibrium:

(3) $$\frac{[H^+] \times [HCO_3^-]}{[H_2CO_3]} = K_A \ (\textit{Small})$$

where K_A is the equilibrium constant for H_2CO_3. (K_A is also known as the acid's *ionization* or *dissociation* constant.)

K_A is a small number because $[H_2CO_3]$ is quite large with respect to the numerator of Reaction 3 ($[H^+] \times [HCO_3^-]$). The value of K_A is always the same for H_2CO_3 at equilibrium, regardless of the initial concentration of H_2CO_3.

A strong acid, such as HCl, has a *large* K_A because the denominator [HCl] is extremely small compared with the numerator ($[H^+] \times [Cl^-]$):

$$\textbf{(4)}\qquad \frac{[H^+]\times[Cl^-]}{[HCl]} = K_A\ (\textit{Large})$$

As shown by Equations 3 and 4, K_A is a measure of the strength of an acid—that is, how much the acid molecule dissociates.

Buffer Solution Characteristics

A buffer solution resists changes in pH when an acid or a base is added to it. Buffer solutions are aqueous mixtures of acids and bases. The acid component is the H^+ cation (positively charged ion), formed when a weak acid dissociates in solution. The base component is the remaining anion (negatively charged ion) portion of the acid molecule, known as the **conjugate base**. An important blood buffer system is a solution of carbonic acid and its conjugate base, HCO_3^-:

$$H_2CO_3(\text{Acid}) \rightleftharpoons HCO_3^-\ (\text{Conjugate base}) + H^+$$

In the blood, HCO_3^- combines with sodium ions to form sodium bicarbonate ($NaHCO_3$). If hydrogen chloride, a strong acid, is added to the $H_2CO_3/NaHCO_3$ buffer solution, HCO_3^- reacts with the added H^+ to form weaker H_2CO_3 molecules and a neutral salt:

$$HCl + H_2CO_3/Na^+HCO_3^- \rightarrow 2H_2CO_3 + NaCl$$

The strong acidity of HCl is converted to the relatively weak acidity of H_2CO_3, preventing a large decrease in pH.

Similarly, if sodium hydroxide, a strong base, is added to this buffer solution, it reacts with the H_2CO_3 molecule to form the weak base, $NaHCO_3$, and H_2O:

$$NaOH + H_2CO_3/NaHCO_3 \rightarrow 2NaHCO_3 + H_2O$$

The strong alkalinity of NaOH is changed to the relatively weak alkalinity of $NaHCO_3$. Again, pH change is minimized.

Bicarbonate and Nonbicarbonate Buffer Systems

Blood buffers are classified as bicarbonate or nonbicarbonate buffer systems. The bicarbonate buffer system consists of H_2CO_3 and its conjugate base, HCO_3^-. The nonbicarbonate buffer system consists mainly of phosphate and protein molecules, including the Hb molecule. The blood buffer base is the sum of bicarbonate and nonbicarbonate bases measured in millimoles per liter of blood.

The bicarbonate system is called an **open buffer system** because H_2CO_3 is in equilibrium with dissolved CO_2, which is readily removed by ventilation. That is, when H^+ is buffered by HCO_3^-, the product, H_2CO_3, is broken down into H_2O and CO_2 as long as ventilation removes CO_2. The removal of CO_2 from the reaction prevents the reaction from reaching equilibrium among its reactants. For this reason, buffering activity can continue without being slowed or stopped, as long as ventilation continues:

$$HCO_3^- + H^+ \rightarrow H_2CO_3 \rightarrow H_2O + CO_2\ (\text{Exhaled gas})$$

A nonbicarbonate buffer system is called a **closed buffer system** because all the components of acid-base reactions remain in the system. (In the following discussions, all nonbicarbonate buffer systems are grouped together and represented as *Hbuf/Buf*$^-$, where Hbuf is the weak acid, and Buf^- is the conjugate base.) When H^+ is buffered by Buf^-, the product, HBuf, builds up and eventually reaches equilibrium with the reactants, preventing further buffering activity:

$$Buf^- + H^+ \leftrightarrow Hbuf$$

Box 14-1 Classification of Whole Blood Buffers

OPEN SYSTEM
Bicarbonate
Plasma
Erythrocyte

CLOSED SYSTEM
Nonbicarbonate
Hemoglobin
Organic phosphates
Inorganic phosphates
Plasma proteins

From Beachey W: Respiratory care anatomy and physiology: foundations for clinical practice, ed 2, St Louis, 2007, Mosby.

Box 14-1 summarizes the characteristics and components of bicarbonate and nonbicarbonate buffer systems.

Open and closed buffer systems play different roles in buffering fixed and volatile acids, and they differ in their ability to function in wide-ranging pH environments. Volatile acid (H_2CO_3) accumulates in the body only if ventilation cannot eliminate CO_2 fast enough to keep up with the body's CO_2 production. In such a case, CO_2 builds up, continually pushing the hydration reaction (the reaction between CO_2 and H_2O) to the right, creating more H_2CO_3 and, ultimately, more H^+ and HCO_3^-. Because the HCO_3^- is co-produced with the H^+, the only buffer system that can buffer the H^+ of volatile acid is the nonbicarbonate buffer system. However, both nonbicarbonate and bicarbonate buffer systems can buffer the H^+ produced by fixed acids; this is true of the bicarbonate buffer system only if ventilation is normal and CO_2 can be adequately eliminated. Both systems are physiologically important, each playing a unique and essential role in maintaining pH homeostasis. Table 14-1 summarizes the approximate contributions of various blood buffers to the total buffer base. Bicarbonate buffers have the greatest buffering capacity because they function in an open system.

Of course, bicarbonate and nonbicarbonate buffer systems do not function in isolation from one another because they are intermingled in the same solution (whole blood) and are in equilibrium with the same $[H^+]$ (Figure 14-1). Increased ventilation increases the CO_2 removal rate, causing blood $[H^+]$ to fall, which causes nonbicarbonate buffers (Hbuf) to release more H^+. By the same token, decreased ventilation ultimately causes Hbuf to accept more H^+.

pH of a Buffer System: Henderson-Hasselbalch Equation

Buffer solutions in body fluids consist of mostly undissociated acid molecules and only a small amount of H^+ and conjugate base anions. The $[H^+]$ of a buffer solution can be calculated if the concentrations of the buffer's components and each acid's equilibrium constant are known. Consider the bicarbonate buffer system. As described earlier, the equilibrium constant (K_A) for H_2CO_3 is as follows:

$$K_A = \frac{[H^+]\times[HCO_3^-]}{[H_2CO_3]}$$

TABLE 14-1

Individual Buffer Contributions to Whole Blood Buffering

Buffer Type	Total Buffering (%)
Bicarbonate	
Plasma bicarbonate	35
Erythrocyte bicarbonate	18
Total bicarbonate buffering	*53*
Nonbicarbonate	
Hemoglobin	35
Organic phosphates	3
Inorganic phosphates	2
Plasma proteins	7
Total nonbicarbonate buffering	*47*
Total	*100*

From Beachey W: Respiratory care anatomy and physiology: foundations for clinical practice, ed 2, St Louis, 2007, Mosby.

$[H^+]$ can be calculated by algebraic rearrangement of this equation, as follows:

$$[H^+] = K_A \times \frac{[H_2CO_3]}{[HCO_3]}$$

This equation shows that $[H^+]$ is determined by the ratio between undissociated acid molecules $[H_2CO_3]$ and base anions $[HCO_3^-]$. This equation is the basis for deriving the **Henderson-Hasselbalch (H-H) equation**:

$$pH = 6.1 + \log\frac{[HCO_3^-]}{PaCO_2 \times 0.03}$$

pH is a logarithmic expression of $[H^+]$, and the term 6.1 is the logarithmic expression of the H_2CO_3 equilibrium constant. Because dissolved CO_2 ($PCO_2 \times 0.03$) is in equilibrium with and directly proportional to blood $[H_2CO_3]$, and because blood PCO_2 is more easily measured than $[H_2CO_3]$, dissolved CO_2 is used in the denominator of the H-H equation. The H-H equation is specific for calculating the pH of the bicarbonate buffer system of the blood. The calculation of this pH is important because it equals the pH of blood plasma; because all buffer systems in the blood are in equilibrium with the same pH, the pH of one buffer system is the same as the pH of the entire plasma solution (the isohydric principle).[1]

Clinical Use of Henderson-Hasselbalch Equation

The H-H equation allows the pH, $[HCO_3^-]$, or PCO_2 to be computed if two of these three variables are known (shown as follows for PCO_2 and HCO_3^-):

$$[HCO_3^-] = \text{antilog}(pH - 6.1)\times(PCO_2 \times 0.03)$$

$$PCO_2 = \frac{[HCO_3^-]}{(\text{antilog}[pH - 6.1]\times 0.03)}$$

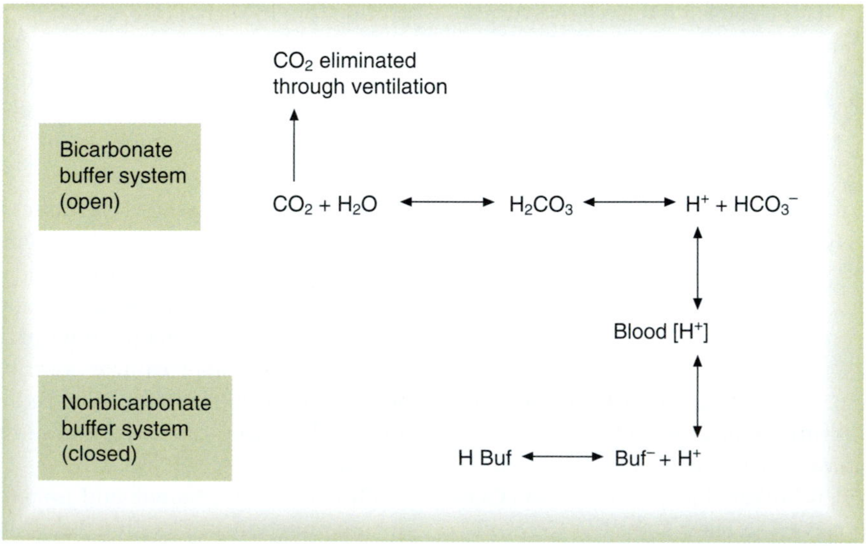

FIGURE 14-1 The bicarbonate and nonbicarbonate buffer systems exist in equilibrium in the plasma. (Modified from Beachey W: Respiratory care anatomy and physiology: foundations for clinical practice, ed 2, St Louis, 2007, Mosby.)

Blood gas analyzers *measure* pH and PCO_2 but *compute* $[HCO_3^-]$. Assuming a normal arterial pH of 7.40 and a $PaCO_2$ of 40 mm Hg, arterial $[HCO_3^-]$ can be calculated as follows:

$$pH = 6.1 + \log\left(\frac{[HCO_3^-]}{PCO_2 \times 0.03}\right)$$

$$7.40 = 6.1 + \log\left(\frac{[HCO_3^-]}{[40 \times 0.03]}\right)$$

$$7.40 = 6.1 + \log\left(\frac{[HCO_3^-]}{1.2}\right)$$

Solving for $[HCO_3^-]$:

$$\begin{aligned}[HCO_3^-] &= \text{antilog}\,(7.40 - 6.1) \times 1.2 \\ &= \text{antilog}\,(1.3) \times 1.2 \\ &= 20 \times 1.2 \\ &= 24\ \text{mEq/L}\end{aligned}$$

The H-H equation is useful for checking a clinical blood gas report to see if the pH, PCO_2, and $[HCO_3^-]$ values are compatible with one another. In this way, transcription errors and analyzer inaccuracies can be detected. It is also clinically useful to predict what effect changing one H-H equation component will have on the other components. For example, a clinician may want to know how low the arterial blood pH will fall for a given increase in $PaCO_2$.

Physiologic Roles of Bicarbonate and Nonbicarbonate Buffer Systems

The functions of bicarbonate and nonbicarbonate buffer systems are summarized in Table 14-2.

TABLE 14-2
Buffering Functions

Buffer	Type of System	Acids Buffered
Bicarbonate	Open	Fixed (nonvolatile)
Nonbicarbonate	Closed	Volatile (carbonic)
		Fixed

From Beachey W: Respiratory care anatomy and physiology: foundations for clinical practice, ed 2, St Louis, 2007, Mosby.

Bicarbonate Buffer System

The bicarbonate buffer system is particularly effective in the body because it is an open system—that is, one of its components (CO_2) is continually removed through ventilation:

$$(\text{Exhaled gas}) \leftarrow CO_2 + H_2O \leftarrow H_2CO_3 \leftarrow HCO_3^- + H^+$$

In this way, HCO_3^- continues to buffer H^+ as long as ventilation continues. Hypothetically, this buffering activity can continue until all body sources of HCO_3^- are used up in binding H^+.

The bicarbonate buffer system can buffer only fixed acid. An increased fixed acid load in the body (e.g., lactic acid) reacts with HCO_3^- of the bicarbonate buffer system:

$$\begin{array}{ccc} & & \text{Ventilation} \\ & & \uparrow \\ H^+ + HCO_3^- & \rightarrow H_2CO_3 \rightarrow & H_2O + CO_2 \\ \uparrow & & \\ \text{Fixed acid} & & \end{array}$$

As shown, the process of buffering fixed acid produces CO_2, which is eliminated in exhaled gas. Large amounts of acid are

MINI CLINI

Applying the Henderson-Hasselbalch Equation in a Clinical Setting

PROBLEM: The RT is caring for a mechanically ventilated patient. The patient has a tidal volume (V_T) of 800 ml and a breathing frequency of 10/min, yielding a minute ventilation ($\dot{V}_E$) of 8 L/min. The patient's $PaCO_2$ is 55 mm Hg, pH is 7.30, and bicarbonate is 26 mEq/L, and the RT wishes to maintain a pH of 7.35. How much does the RT need to change the $PaCO_2$ to achieve this desired pH, and what change in the patient's V_T does this require?

SOLUTION: First, the therapist needs to calculate the $PaCO_2$ required to achieve a pH of 7.35 using the known values:

$$PaCO_2 = \frac{26\ \text{mEq/L}}{1.003 \times \text{antilog}\,(7.35 - 6.1)}$$

$$PaCO_2 = \frac{26}{0.53}$$

$$PaCO_2 = 49\ \text{mm Hg}$$

Next, the RT must calculate the $\dot{V}_E$ required to produce a $PaCO_2$ of 49 mm Hg. Because $\dot{V}_E$ is inversely proportional to $PaCO_2$ (assuming that tidal volume remains constant), the following can be stated:

$$(\dot{V}_E)_1 \times (PaCO_2)_1 = (\dot{V}_E)_2 \times (PaCO_2)_2$$

where subscripts 1 and 2 represent current and future values. The RT then solves for $(\dot{V})_2$ as follows:

$$(8\ \text{L/min}) \times 55\ \text{mm Hg} = (\dot{V}_E)_2 \times 49\ \text{mm Hg}$$

$$\frac{(8 \times 55)}{49} = (\dot{V}_E)_2$$

$$8.98\ \text{L/min} = (\dot{V}_E)_2$$

Increasing the patient's $\dot{V}_E$ from 8 L/min to approximately 9 L/min yields a $PaCO_2$ of 49 mm Hg and a pH of approximately 7.35. Now the RT divides the new $\dot{V}_E$ of 9 L/min by the respiratory frequency to calculate the new V_T required:

$$9\ \text{L/min}/10 = 900\ \text{ml}$$

A V_T of 900 ml at a rate of 10 breaths/min should produce an arterial pH of 7.35, according to the H-H equation.

normally buffered in this fashion. If ventilation cannot keep up with the body's CO_2 production, this type of buffering cannot occur.

The bicarbonate buffer system cannot buffer carbonic (volatile) acid, which accumulates in the blood whenever ventilation fails to eliminate CO_2 as fast as it is produced (hypoventilation). The resulting accumulation of CO_2 drives the hydration reaction in the direction that produces more carbonic acid, H^+, and HCO_3^-, as shown:

$$\begin{array}{c}\text{Hypoventilation}\\ \downarrow \\ CO_2 + H_2O \rightarrow H_2CO_3 \rightarrow HCO_3^- + H^+\end{array}$$

H^+ produced by dissociating H_2CO_3 molecules cannot be buffered by the simultaneously produced HCO_3^- because hypoventilation prevents the reaction from reversing its direction. The closed nonbicarbonate buffer systems are the only buffers that can buffer H_2CO_3.

Nonbicarbonate Buffer System

Table 14-1 lists the nonbicarbonate buffers in the blood. Of these, Hb is the most important simply because it is the most abundant. As mentioned, these buffers are the only ones available to buffer H_2CO_3. However, they can buffer H^+ produced by any acid, fixed or volatile. Because nonbicarbonate buffers (Buf^-/HBuf) function in closed systems, the products of their buffering activity eventually accumulate and approach equilibrium, slowing or stopping further buffering activity:

$$H^+ + Buf^- \leftrightarrow HBuf$$

This slowing or stopping of buffering activity means that not all of the Buf^- reserves are available for buffering activity. At equilibrium (denoted by the *double arrow*), Buf^- still exists in solution but cannot combine further with H^+. In contrast, most of the HCO_3^- in the bicarbonate buffer system is available for buffering activity because it functions in an open system in which equilibrium between reactants and products does not occur as long as ventilation continues. Both open and closed systems function in a common fluid compartment (blood plasma), as illustrated in the following equation:

$$\begin{array}{c}(CO_2 \text{ removed by ventilation}) \quad (\text{from body's } HCO_3^- \text{ stores})\\ \uparrow \qquad\qquad\qquad \downarrow \\ \text{Open system: } CO_2 + H_2O \leftarrow H^+ + HCO_3^- \\ \uparrow \\ \text{Added fixed acid} \\ \downarrow \\ \text{Closed system: } HBuf \leftrightarrow H^+ + Buf^- \\ \uparrow \\ (\text{from body's } Buf^- \text{ stores})\end{array}$$

Most of the added fixed acid is buffered by HCO_3^- because ventilation continually pulls the reaction to the left. Smaller amounts of H^+ react with Buf^- because equilibrium is approached, slowing the reaction.

ACID EXCRETION

Bicarbonate and nonbicarbonate buffer systems are the immediate defense against the accumulation of H^+. However, if the body fails to eliminate the remaining acids, these buffers are soon exhausted and the pH of body fluids quickly decreases to life-threatening levels.

The lungs and kidneys are the primary acid-excreting organs. The lungs can excrete only volatile acid (i.e., the CO_2 from dissociating H_2CO_3). However, as discussed previously, bicarbonate buffers effectively buffer the H^+ originating from fixed acid, converting it to H_2CO_3 and to CO_2 and H_2O. By eliminating the CO_2, the lungs can rapidly remove large quantities of fixed acid from the blood. The kidneys also remove fixed acids but at a slow pace. In healthy individuals, the acid excretion mechanisms of lungs and kidneys are delicately balanced. In individuals affected by disease, failure of one system can be partially offset by a compensatory response of the other.

Lungs

Because the volatile acid H_2CO_3 is in equilibrium with dissolved CO_2, the lungs can decrease blood H_2CO_3 concentration through ventilation. The elimination of CO_2 is crucial because normal aerobic metabolism produces large quantities of CO_2, which reacts with H_2O to form large quantities of H_2CO_3. The reaction between fixed acids and bicarbonate buffers also produces H_2CO_3. H_2CO_3 generated by both pathways is eliminated as CO_2 through the lungs. Approximately 24,000 mmol/L of CO_2 is removed from the body daily through normal ventilation. CO_2 excretion of the lungs does not remove H^+ from the body. Instead, the chemical reaction that breaks down H_2CO_3 to form CO_2 binds H^+ in the harmless H_2O molecule:

$$H^+ + HCO_3^- \rightarrow H_2CO_3 \rightarrow H_2O + CO_2$$

Kidneys

The kidneys physically remove H^+ from the body. The following terms refer to certain kidney functions:

- *Excretion* is the elimination of substances from the body in the urine.
- *Secretion* is the process by which renal tubule cells actively transport substances into the fluid inside the tubule lumen (i.e., the *filtrate*).
- *Reabsorption* is the active or passive transport of filtrate substances back into the tubule cell and into the blood of nearby capillaries.

The amount of H^+ the kidney tubules secrete into the filtrate depends on the blood's pH. Secreted H^+ may originate from H_2CO_3 (when the blood PCO_2 is increased) or from fixed acids. The kidneys excrete less than 100 mEq of fixed acid per day, which is a small amount compared with volatile H_2CO_3 elimination by the lungs.[3] In addition to excreting H^+, the kidneys influence blood pH by reabsorbing or excreting HCO_3^-. If the blood PCO_2 is high, creating high levels of H_2CO_3, the kidneys excrete greater amounts of H^+ and reabsorb all of the tubule filtrate's HCO_3^- back into the blood. The opposite happens when the blood PCO_2 is low. The kidneys excrete less H^+ and more HCO_3^-. Compared with the ability of the lungs to change blood PCO_2 in seconds, the renal process is slow, requiring hours to days.

Basic Kidney Function

To understand how the kidneys determine whether to excrete acidic or basic urine, some fundamental facts about renal function must be understood. The *glomerulus* is the component of the renal nephron responsible for filtering the blood. Hydrostatic blood pressure forces water, electrolytes, and other nonprotein substances through semipermeable glomerular capillary endothelium. The resulting filtrate is greatly modified in volume and composition as it flows through the nephron tubules. Excreted filtrate is called *urine.*

HCO_3^- is one of the electrolytes filtered from the blood at the glomerulus to become part of the tubular filtrate. In this way, base (HCO_3^-) is removed from the blood. This loss of base is offset by the nephron's simultaneous secretion of H^+ into the filtrate of the tubular lumen. Under normal conditions, the rate of H^+ secretion is almost the same as the rate of HCO_3^- filtration.[4] In this way, the kidneys titrate H^+ and HCO_3^- against each other to form CO_2 and H_2O.

H^+ secretion begins with the diffusion of blood CO_2 into the tubule cell (Figure 14-2). Aided by the enzyme carbonic anhydrase, CO_2 reacts with H_2O to form H_2CO_3, which instantly forms HCO_3^- and H^+. The tubule cell actively secretes H^+ into the filtrate by means of *counter-transport,* in which Na^+ and H^+ are simultaneously transported in opposite directions. That is, Na^+ and H^+ combine with opposite ends of a carrier protein in the luminal border of the tubule cell membrane. Sodium ions move from the filtrate into the cell down its high concentration gradient, providing the energy to secrete H^+ back into the tubular filtrate (see Figure 14-2).[4]

The rate of tubular H^+ secretion increases if the concentration of H^+ in the blood plasma increases. Conversely, the rate of H^+ secretion decreases if blood plasma $[H^+]$ decreases (Figure 14-3). Any factor that increases $PaCO_2$, such as hypoventilation, increases $[H^+]$ in the blood and thus $[H^+]$ secretion; any factor that decreases $PaCO_2$, such as hyperventilation, decreases H^+ secretion.

HCO_3^- formed in the tubule cell from the reaction between CO_2 and H_2O (see Figure 14-2) diffuses back into the blood plasma because the luminal side of the tubule cell is relatively impermeable to HCO_3^-. HCO_3^- and Na^+ are reabsorbed whenever H^+ is secreted into the tubular filtrate.

Reabsorption of Bicarbonate Ion

Because the luminal side of the renal tubule cell is relatively impermeable to HCO_3^-, these ions are reabsorbed indirectly, as

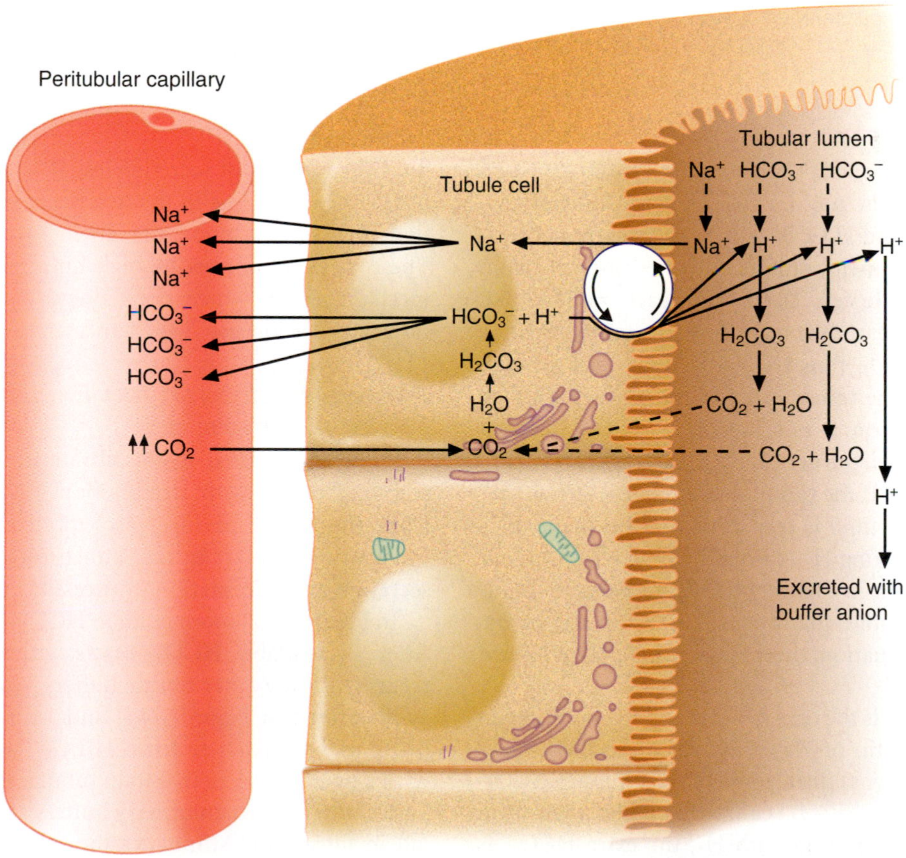

FIGURE 14-2 Renal response to respiratory acidosis. Filtrate HCO_3^- is reabsorbed by first reacting with secreted H^+. (Modified from Beachey W: Respiratory care anatomy and physiology: foundations for clinical practice, ed 2, St Louis, 2007, Mosby.)

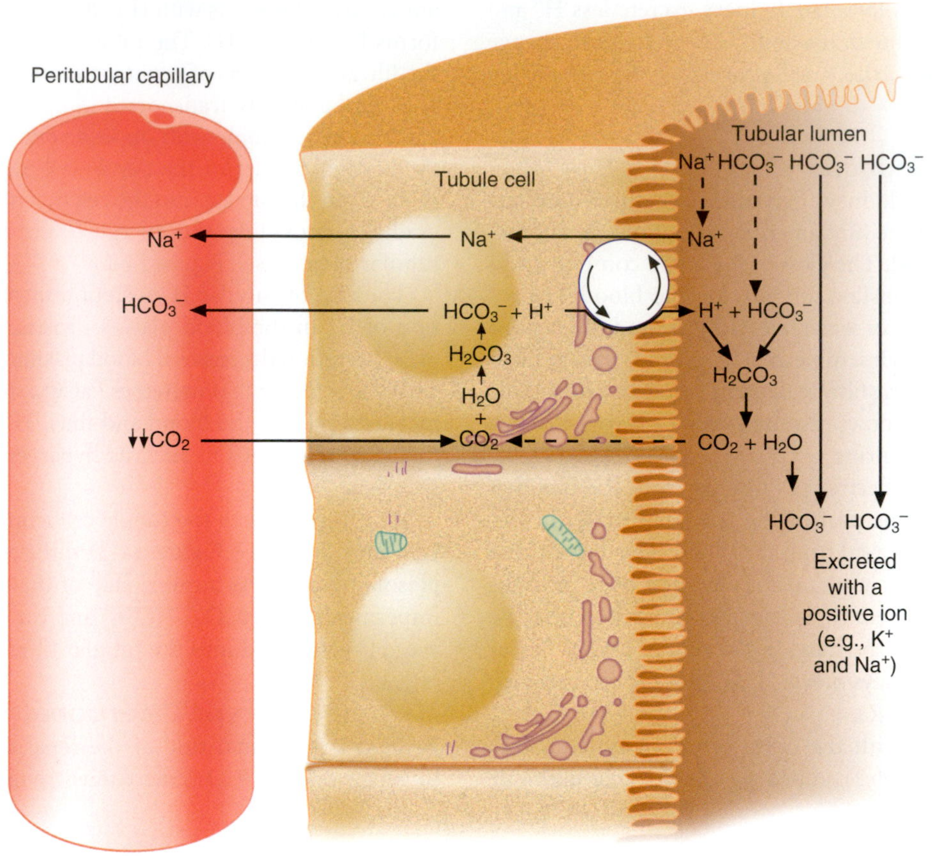

FIGURE 14-3 Renal response to respiratory alkalosis. Excess HCO_3^- is excreted in the urine with a positive ion. (Modified from Beachey W: Respiratory care anatomy and physiology: foundations for clinical practice, ed 2, St Louis, 2007, Mosby.)

shown in Figure 14-2. The HCO_3^- in the tubular filtrate reacts with the H^+ secreted by the tubular cells. The resulting H_2CO_3 breaks down into CO_2 and H_2O. Because CO_2 is extremely diffusible through biologic membranes, it diffuses instantly from the filtrate into the tubule cell. There CO_2 reacts rapidly with H_2O in the presence of carbonic anhydrase, instantly forming HCO_3^- and H^+. The HCO_3^- thus created diffuses back through the nonluminal side of the tubule cell into the blood. Although the reabsorbed HCO_3^- ion is not the same HCO_3^- ion that existed in the tubular fluid, the net result is the same as if HCO_3^- were directly reabsorbed. If the tubule cells secrete sufficient H^+, all HCO_3^- in the tubular fluid is reabsorbed in this manner.

The net effect of secreting H^+ (caused by high blood CO_2 or *hypoventilation,* as shown in Figure 14-2) is to reabsorb all filtrate HCO_3^-, increasing the quantity of HCO_3^- in the blood. According to the H-H equation, this brings blood pH up toward the normal range.

If blood CO_2 is low, as is the case in a state of *hyperventilation* (see Figure 14-3), the ratio of HCO_3^- to dissolved CO_2 molecules increases, and the renal filtrate ends up with more HCO_3^- than secreted H^+. Because HCO_3^- cannot be reabsorbed from the filtrate without first reacting with H^+, the extra HCO_3^- is excreted in the urine, which requires positive ions such as Na^+ or K^+ to also be excreted to maintain tubular electrical neutrality. The net effect of secreting less H^+ is to increase the quantity of HCO_3^- (base) lost in the urine. According to the H-H equation, this brings blood pH down toward the normal range. These renal responses to high and low blood PCO_2 are the mechanisms by which the kidneys compensate for or offset respiratory acid-base disturbances.

Excess Hydrogen Ion Excretion and Role of Urinary Buffers

If no buffers existed in the filtrate to react with H^+, the H^+-secreting mechanism would soon cease to function because when the filtrate pH decreases to 4.5, H^+ secretion stops.[4] In other words, buffers in the tubular filtrate are essential for the secretion and elimination of excess H^+ in acidotic states.

In Figure 14-2, more H^+ than HCO_3^- is present in the filtrate. After all available HCO_3^- reacts with H^+, the remaining H^+ reacts with two other filtrate buffers, phosphate and ammonia, as illustrated in Figures 14-4 and 14-5. In Figure 14-4, phosphate and H^+ react to form $H_2PO_4^-$, which must be excreted with a positive ion to maintain tubular electroneutrality. Figure 14-5 shows that when urinary buffers are depleted, the resulting fall in filtrate pH stimulates the tubules to secrete ammonia. The NH_3 molecule buffers H^+ by reacting with it to form the positively charged ammonium ion (NH_4^+). To maintain

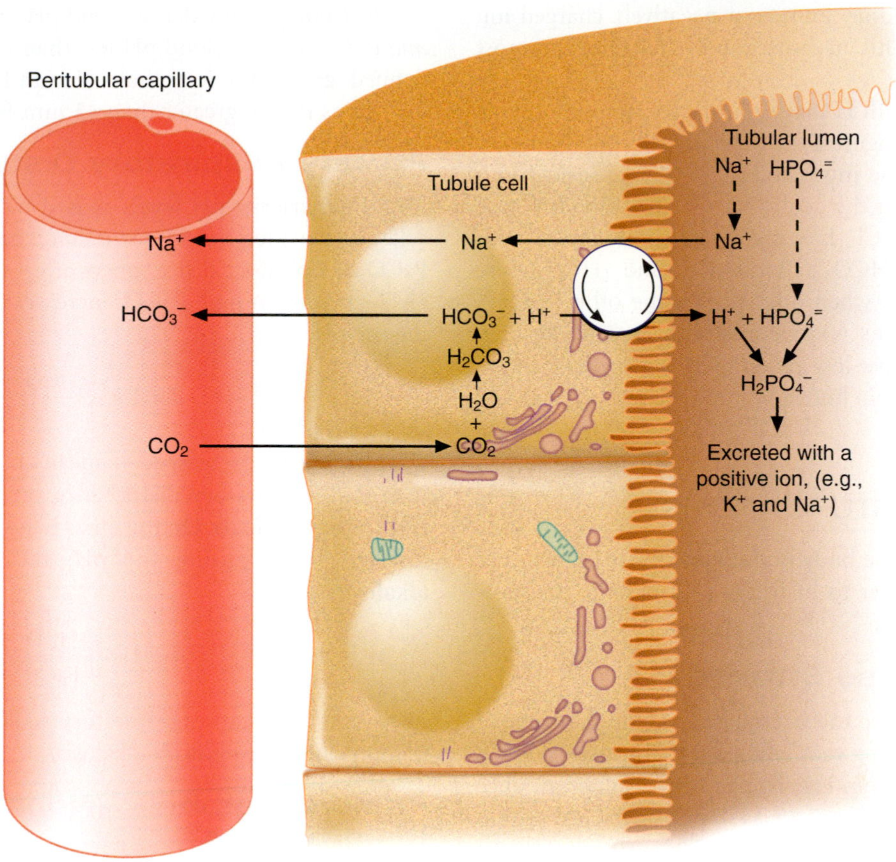

FIGURE 14-4 Phosphate buffer system. After HCO_3^- buffers are exhausted, the remaining H^+ reacts with urinary phosphate buffers. (Modified from Beachey W: Respiratory care anatomy and physiology: foundations for clinical practice, ed 2, St Louis, 2007, Mosby.)

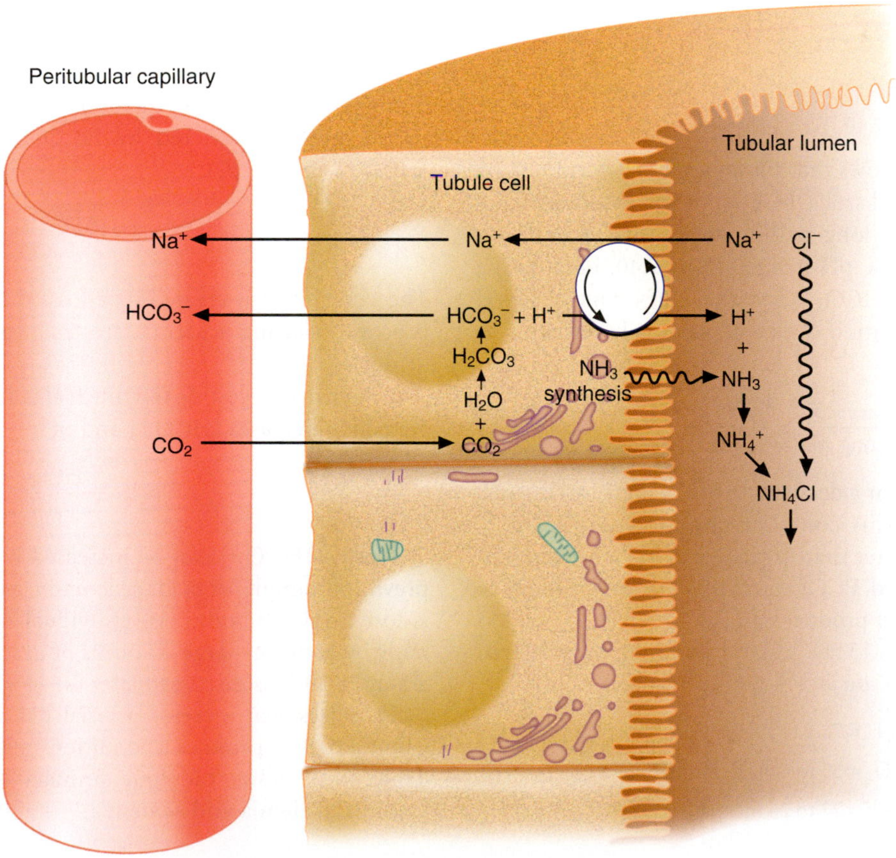

FIGURE 14-5 Tubule cells secrete ammonia in response to low-filtrate pH. NH_3 molecules buffer H^+, forming NH_4^+, which is excreted with Cl^-. (Modified from Beachey W: Respiratory care anatomy and physiology: foundations for clinical practice, ed 2, St Louis, 2007, Mosby.)

electroneutrality, the kidney excretes a negatively charged ion to accompany NH_4^+. This negative ion is chloride, the most abundant filtrate anion.

When NH_4^+ reacts with H^+, HCO_3^- diffuses from the tubule cell into the blood (see Figure 14-5). The net effect of ammonia buffer activity is to cause more HCO_3^- to be reabsorbed into the blood, counteracting the acidic state of the blood. Figure 14-5 shows that when Cl^- is excreted in combination with NH_4^-, the blood gains HCO_3^-. Blood $[Cl^-]$ and $[HCO_3^-]$ are reciprocally related (i.e., when one is high, the other is low). This relationship explains why people with chronically high blood PCO_2 tend to have low blood $[Cl^-]$ or *hypochloremia*. Activation of the ammonia buffer system enhances Cl^-loss and HCO_3^- gain.

ACID-BASE DISTURBANCES

In healthy individuals, the body buffer systems, the lungs, and the kidneys work together to maintain acid-base homeostasis under various conditions.

Normal Acid-Base Balance

Normally, the kidneys keep the arterial $[HCO_3^-]$ in the range of 22 to 26 mEq/L, while lung ventilation keeps the arterial PCO_2 in the range of 35 to 45 mm Hg. These normal values produce an arterial pH range of 7.35 to 7.45; as shown by the H-H equation, when $[HCO_3^-]$ is 24 mEq/L and $PaCO_2$ is 40 mm Hg, the pH is exactly 7.40:

$$pH = 6.1 + \log\frac{[HCO_3^-]}{PCO_2 \times 0.03}$$
$$pH = 6.1 + \log\frac{24}{1.2}$$
$$pH = 6.1 + \log[20]$$
$$pH = 7.40$$

The H-H equation shows that plasma pH is determined by the *ratio* of $[HCO_3^-]$ to dissolved CO_2, not the absolute values of these components. As long as the ratio of HCO_3^- buffer to dissolved CO_2 is 20:1, the pH is normal, or 7.40. Because the kidneys control blood $[HCO_3^-]$ and the lungs control blood CO_2 levels, the H-H equation can be conceptually rewritten as follows:

$$pH \propto \frac{\text{Kidney control of } [HCO_3^-]}{\text{Lung control of } PCO_2}$$

An increase in $[HCO_3^-]$ or a decrease in PCO_2 increases the pH, leading to **alkalemia**. This condition produces an $[HCO_3^-]/(PCO_2 \times 0.03)$ ratio greater than 20:1 (e.g., 25:1). A decreased $[HCO_3^-]$ or an increased PCO_2 decreases the pH, leading to **acidemia**. This condition produces an $[HCO_3^-]/(PCO_2 \times 0.03)$ ratio less than 20:1 (e.g., 15:1). The normal ranges for arterial pH, PCO_2, and $[HCO_3^-]$ are as follows:

$$pH = 7.35 \text{ to } 7.45$$
$$PaCO_2 = 35 \text{ to } 45 \text{ mm Hg}$$
$$[HCO_3^-] = 22 \text{ to } 26 \text{ mEq/L}$$

Alkalemia is defined as a blood pH greater than 7.45. *Acidemia* is defined as a blood pH less than 7.35. *Hyperventilation* is defined as $PaCO_2$ less than 35 mm Hg. *Hypoventilation* is defined as $PaCO_2$ greater than 45 mm Hg.

Primary Respiratory Disturbances

Abnormal arterial pH levels caused by changes in $PaCO_2$ are called *primary respiratory disturbances* because the lungs control $PaCO_2$. Respiratory disturbances affect the denominator of the H-H equation. A high $PaCO_2$ increases dissolved CO_2, decreasing the pH:

$$\downarrow pH \propto \frac{\rightarrow HCO_3^-}{\uparrow PaCO_2}$$

where ↓ means decreased, → means no change, and ↑ means increased. Respiratory disturbance causing acidemia is called **respiratory acidosis**. On the other hand, a low $PaCO_2$ decreases dissolved CO_2, raising the pH; this is called **respiratory alkalosis**:

$$\uparrow pH \propto \frac{\rightarrow HCO_3^-}{\downarrow PaCO_2}$$

*Hypo*ventilation causes respiratory acidosis, whereas *hyper*ventilation causes respiratory alkalosis.

Primary Metabolic (Nonrespiratory) Disturbances

Nonrespiratory processes change arterial pH, manifested by changes in $[HCO_3^-]$. These are called *primary metabolic disturbances*. Although the term *nonrespiratory* is more accurate, the term *metabolic* is, by convention, used to refer to all nonrespiratory acid-base disturbances. These kinds of disturbances involve a gain or loss of fixed acids or HCO_3^-. Such processes affect the numerator of the H-H equation. The build-up of a fixed acid in the body is buffered by HCO_3^-, decreasing the plasma $[HCO_3^-]$ and the pH:

$$\downarrow pH \propto \frac{\downarrow HCO_3^-}{\rightarrow PaCO_2}$$

The same effect is created by a loss of HCO_3^-. Nonrespiratory processes causing acidemia are traditionally called **metabolic acidosis**.

In contrast, ingesting too much alkali (e.g., $NaHCO_3$ or other antacids) increases $[HCO_3^-]$ and pH:

$$\uparrow pH \propto \frac{\uparrow HCO_3^-}{\rightarrow PaCO_2}$$

Plasma $[HCO_3^-]$ can be increased by its *addition*, as in the previous example, or by its *generation*, as occurs when fixed acid is lost from the body.[5] An individual may lose HCl from the body by vomiting large amounts of gastric juice. This loss generates HCO_3^-, as discussed later (see Figure 14-8, later).

Processes that increase arterial pH by losing fixed acid or gaining HCO_3^- produce a condition called **metabolic alkalosis**. Table 14-3 shows the four primary acid-base disturbances causing alkalemia and acidemia.

TABLE 14-3

Primary Acid-Base Disorders and Compensatory Responses

Acid-Base Disorder	Primary Defect	Compensatory Response
Respiratory acidosis	[→ HCO_3^-, ↑ **$PaCO_2$**] = ↓ pH	[↑ **HCO_3^-**, ↑ $PaCO_2$] = → pH
Respiratory alkalosis	[→ HCO_3^-, ↓ **$PaCO_2$**] = ↑ pH	[↓ **HCO_3^-**, ↓ $PaCO_2$] = → pH
Metabolic acidosis	[↓ **HCO_3^-**, → $PaCO_2$] = ↓ pH	[↓ HCO_3^-, ↓ **$PaCO_2$**] = → pH
Metabolic alkalosis	[↑ **HCO_3^-**, → $PaCO_2$] = ↑ pH	[↑ HCO_3^-, ↑ **$PaCO_2$**] = → pH

From Beachey W: Respiratory care anatomy and physiology: foundations for clinical practice, ed 2, St Louis, 2007, Mosby.

Note: Primary defects and compensatory responses appear in boldface type.

→, No change; ↓, decrease; ↑, increase.

Compensation: Restoring pH to Normal

When any primary acid-base defect occurs, the body immediately reacts to make up for the defect; that is, the body initiates a *compensatory* response. If a person hypoventilates (respiratory acidosis), the kidneys bring the pH back toward normal by returning the filtrate's HCO_3^- ions back to the blood, a process called *reabsorption*. In contrast, the compensatory renal response to hyperventilation (respiratory alkalosis) is urinary elimination of HCO_3^- (bicarbonate diuresis).

Similarly, if a nonrespiratory (metabolic) process decreases or increases [HCO_3^-], the lungs compensate by hyperventilating (eliminating CO_2) or hypoventilating (retaining CO_2), restoring the pH to near normal. Consider the following example of pure (uncompensated) respiratory acidosis in which the PCO_2 level increases to 60 mm Hg:

$$pH = 6.1 + \log \frac{(24\ mEq/L)}{(60\ mm\ Hg \times 0.03)}$$

$$pH = 6.1 + \log(13.3)$$

$$pH = 7.22$$

The kidneys compensate by reabsorbing HCO_3^- from the filtrate into the blood, returning the plasma HCO_3^-/dissolved CO_2 ratio to almost 20 : 1, as shown:

$$pH = 6.1 + \log \frac{(34\ mEq/L)}{(60\ mm\ Hg \times 0.03)}$$

$$pH = 6.1 + \log(18.9)$$

$$pH = 7.38$$

pH is restored to the normal range of 7.35 to 7.45, although the PCO_2 level remains abnormally high. This compensatory response of the kidney produces a high plasma [HCO_3^-], *not to be confused with primary metabolic alkalosis;* compensatory renal HCO_3^- retention is a normal secondary response to the primary event of respiratory acidosis.

The lungs normally compensate quickly for metabolic acid-base defects because ventilation can change the $PaCO_2$ within seconds. The kidneys require more time to retain or excrete significant amounts of HCO_3^- and compensate for respiratory defects at a much slower pace. Table 14-3 summarizes the four primary acid-base disturbances and the body's compensatory responses.

Effect of the Carbon Dioxide Hydration Reaction on [HCO_3^-]

In the previous examples of pure (uncompensated) respiratory acidosis and alkalosis, it was assumed that [HCO_3^-] did not change when the $PaCO_2$ level increased or decreased. However, arterial [HCO_3^-] does increase slightly as the $PaCO_2$ increases because the CO_2 hydration reaction generates HCO_3^-. This reaction occurs primarily in the red blood cell because the catalytic enzyme, carbonic anhydrase, is present:

$$CO_2 + H_2O - (\text{carbonic anhydrase}) \rightarrow H_2CO_3 \rightarrow H^+ + HCO_3^-$$

As H^+ and HCO_3^- are rapidly produced in the erythrocyte, Hb immediately buffers H^+, pulling the reaction to the right, generating more plasma HCO_3^-.

The amount of HCO_3^- generated by this buffering action depends on the amount of buffer available to accept the H^+ produced by the hydration reaction. Generally, when the nonbicarbonate buffer concentration is normal, and the PCO_2 increase is acute, the hydration reaction increases the plasma [HCO_3^-] approximately 1 mEq/L for every 10-mm Hg increase in PCO_2 higher than 40 mm Hg. Figure 14-6 illustrates this hydration reaction effect. Normal status is represented by point *A:* $PaCO_2$ of 40 mm Hg, pH of 7.40, and plasma HCO_3^- of 24 mEq/L. An acute increase in $PaCO_2$ from 40 to 80 mm Hg proceeds from point *A*, moving to the left, up the normal blood buffer line (line *BAC*) to point *D*, where the buffer line intersects the $PaCO_2$ = 80 mm Hg isopleth. Point *D* indicates an HCO_3^- of approximately 28.5 mEq/L and a pH of approximately 7.18. This small change in [HCO_3^-] is a natural result of the Hb buffering action and should not be wrongly interpreted as early renal compensation.

RULE OF THUMB

For an acute increase in PCO_2, the plasma [HCO_3^-] increases by approximately 1 mEq/L for every 10 mm Hg PCO_2 rise above 40 mm Hg.

CLINICAL ACID-BASE STATES

Systematic Acid-Base Classification

In analyzing an acid-base problem, it is helpful to use a series of systematic steps. Consistently applying them to all acid-base disturbances helps one avoid the tendency to jump to conclusions. Four steps in arterial blood acid-base classification are outlined in Box 14-2. After the pH is categorized, the order of

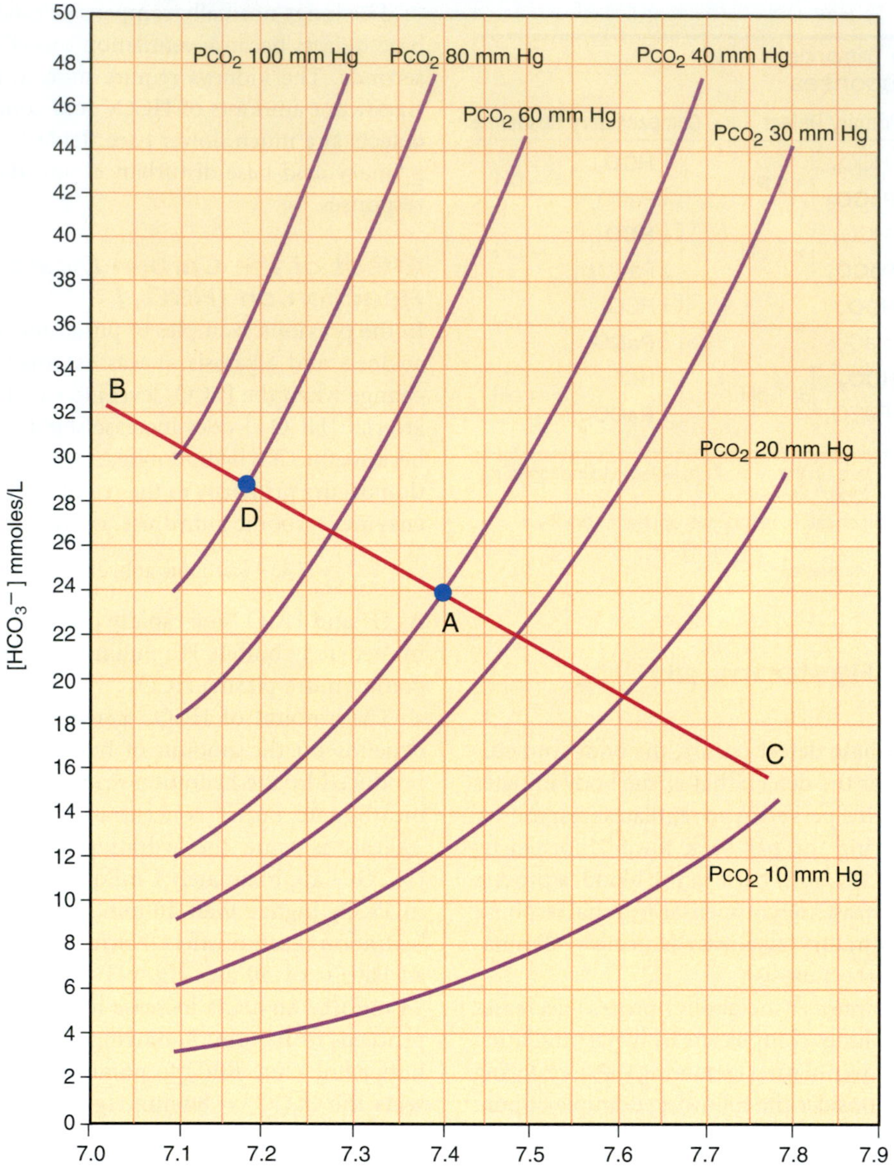

FIGURE 14-6 pH-PCO_2 diagram. Because of the hydration reaction between CO_2 and H_2O, acute increases in PCO_2 increase the plasma HCO_3^- concentration along line *CADB*. An acute increase in PCO_2 from 40 mm Hg to 80 mm Hg (point *A* to point *D*) increases [HCO_3^-] from 24 mEq/L to approximately 29 mEq/L. (Modified from Masoro EJ, Siegel PD: Acid-base regulation: its physiology and pathophysiology, Philadelphia, 1971, Saunders.)

Box 14-2 Systematic Acid-Base Classification

- Inspect the pH (acidemia, alkalemia, or normal).
- Inspect $PaCO_2$ (respiratory component). Can it explain the pH?
- Inspect HCO_3^- (metabolic component). Can it explain the pH?
- Check for compensation. Did the noncausative component respond appropriately?

From Beachey W: Respiratory care anatomy and physiology: foundations for clinical practice, ed 2, St Louis, 2007, Mosby.

the steps is not as important as following the same procedure for each situation.

Step 1: Categorize pH

If the arterial pH is greater than 7.45, a state of alkalemia exists. If the pH is less than 7.35, a state of acidemia exists. Steps 2 through 4 help the clinician determine whether an acid-base abnormality is of respiratory or metabolic (nonrespiratory) origin.

Step 2: Determine Respiratory Involvement

$PaCO_2$ is the marker for respiratory involvement because the lungs control the level of CO_2 in the arterial blood. (The normal range for $PaCO_2$ is 35 to 45 mm Hg.) If the arterial pH is abnormal, the clinician should determine whether the observed $PaCO_2$ could cause the abnormality by itself. If the pH was less than 7.35 (denoting an acidosis) and $PaCO_2$ was greater than 45 mm Hg, according to the H-H equation, the high $PaCO_2$ would lower the pH (i.e., produce an acidemia). In this case, the respiratory system would be at least partly, if not entirely, responsible for the acidemia. If the pH is less than 7.35 and $PaCO_2$ is in the normal range, the acidemia is of nonrespiratory, or metabolic origin.

Step 3: Determine Metabolic (Nonrespiratory) Involvement

Plasma $[HCO_3^-]$ is the marker for metabolic involvement because $[HCO_3^-]$ is controlled by nonrespiratory factors. (The normal plasma $[HCO_3^-]$ of arterial blood is 22 to 26 mEq/L.) If the arterial pH is abnormal, the clinician must determine whether the observed $[HCO_3^-]$ could cause the abnormality by itself. If the pH was less than 7.35 (denoting an acidemia) and the $[HCO_3^-]$ was less than 22 mEq/L, according to the H-H equation, the low $[HCO_3^-]$ would produce an acidosis. Nonrespiratory (metabolic) factors would be partly, if not entirely, responsible for the acidemia. If $[HCO_3^-]$ is in the normal range in the presence of this acidemia, the acidemia is of respiratory origin.

Step 4: Assess for Compensation

The system (respiratory or nonrespiratory) that is not primarily responsible for the acid-base imbalance usually attempts to return the pH to the normal range. Compensation may be complete (pH is brought into the normal range) or partial (pH is still out of the normal range but is in the process of moving toward the normal range). In a pure respiratory acidosis, the kidneys compensate by reabsorbing more $[HCO_3^-]$, restoring the pH to normal. Similarly, respiratory alkalosis elicits a compensatory loss of $[HCO_3^-]$, decreasing its plasma concentration. A pure metabolic acidosis normally stimulates a compensatory increase in ventilation, decreasing the $PaCO_2$. A pure metabolic alkalosis causes a compensatory decrease in ventilation, increasing the $PaCO_2$. All compensatory responses work to restore the pH to the normal range.

In cases in which compensation has occurred, if the pH is on the acidic side of the normal range (7.35 to 7.39), the event that would cause an acidosis (either increased $PaCO_2$ or decreased plasma HCO_3^-) is generally the primary cause of the original acid-base imbalance. If compensation is present but pH is on the alkalotic side of the normal range (7.41 to 7.45), the component that would cause an alkalosis (either decreased $PaCO_2$ or increased HCO_3^-) is generally the primary cause of the original acid-base disturbance.

Complete compensation refers to any case in which the compensatory response returns the pH to the normal range (7.35 to 7.45). *Partial compensation* refers to instances in which the expected compensatory response has begun but has not had sufficient time to return the pH into the normal range. For example, suppose a patient has a partially compensated respiratory acidosis. This condition is characterized by high $PaCO_2$ (>45 mm Hg), pH less than 7.35, and plasma $[HCO_3^-]$ greater than 26 mEq/L. The compensatory response (increased HCO_3^-) is not yet sufficient to return the pH into the normal range, although the expected compensatory activity has begun. By comparison, a completely compensated respiratory acidosis might be shown by the same patient several hours later, when the kidneys have had enough time to retain sufficient plasma HCO_3^- to bring the pH into the normal range. This completely compensated respiratory acidosis is characterized by the same originally observed high $PaCO_2$, pH that is in the 7.35 to 7.39 range, and plasma $[HCO_3^-]$ that is greater than it was before *complete compensation* took place. The pH remains on the acidic side of 7.40 because the primary disturbance (high $PaCO_2$) originally created an acidotic environment. Generally, the body does not overcompensate for an acid-base disturbance. Table 14-4 summarizes acid-base and ventilatory classification. Table 14-5 classifies the degree of compensation for acid-base disturbances.

Respiratory Acidosis

Any physiologic process that increases $PaCO_2$ (>45 mm Hg) with an accompanying decreased arterial pH (<7.35) produces respiratory acidosis. Increased $PaCO_2$ (**hypercapnia**) lowers the arterial pH because dissolved CO_2 produces H_2CO_3:

$$CO_2 + H_2O \rightarrow H_2CO_3 \rightarrow HCO_3^- + H^+$$

TABLE 14-4
Acid-Base and Ventilatory Classification

Component	Classification	Range
pH (arterial)	Normal status	7.35-7.45
	Acidemia	<7.35
	Alkalemia	>7.45
$PaCO_2$ (mm Hg)	Normal ventilatory status	35-45
	Respiratory acidosis (hypoventilation)	>45
	Respiratory alkalosis (hyperventilation)	<35
HCO_3^- (mEq/L)	Normal metabolic status	22-26
	Metabolic acidosis	<22
	Metabolic alkalosis	>26

From Beachey W: Respiratory care anatomy and physiology: foundations for clinical practice, ed 2, St Louis, 2007, Mosby.

TABLE 14-5
Degrees of Acid-Base Compensation

Compensating (Noncausative Component)	pH	Classification
Within normal range	Abnormal	Noncompensated (acute)
Out of normal range in the expected direction	Abnormal	Partially compensated
Out of normal range in the expected direction	Normal	Compensated (chronic)

From Beachey W: Respiratory care anatomy and physiology: foundations for clinical practice, ed 2, St Louis, 2007, Mosby.

MINI CLINI

Acute (Uncompensated) Respiratory Acidosis

PROBLEM: A 35-year-old woman was admitted to the emergency department with a diagnosis of heroin overdose. Her breathing was shallow and slow. Arterial blood gas analysis showed a pH of 7.30, PCO_2 of 55 mm Hg, and HCO_3^- of 26 mEq/L. How would the RT assess this patient's respiratory condition?

SOLUTION: The RT should follow these steps:

1. Categorize the pH. The pH is below normal, indicating the presence of acidemia.
2. Determine respiratory involvement. $PaCO_2$ is elevated above normal (hypercapnea), consistent with a low pH, indicating hypoventilation as a contributing factor to acidemia (respiratory acidosis).
3. Determine metabolic involvement. HCO_3^- is elevated slightly above normal. However, this is in the expected range for acute respiratory acidosis (1 mEq for each 10-mm Hg increase in PCO_2).
4. Assess for compensation. As explained in step 3, HCO_3^- is within the expected range for acute respiratory acidosis. There is no evidence of metabolic compensation. Therefore the condition is interpreted as an uncompensated respiratory acidosis.

Causes

Any process in which alveolar ventilation fails to eliminate CO_2 as rapidly as the body produces it causes respiratory acidosis. This acidosis could occur in two different ways. A person's ventilation may be decreased from a drug-induced central nervous system depression, or a person with limited ventilatory reserve may have a normal $PaCO_2$ at rest but cannot accommodate the increased CO_2 production associated with increased physical activity. Box 14-3 summarizes causes of respiratory acidosis.

If hypercapnia is uncompensated, respiratory acidosis occurs with decreased pH, increased $PaCO_2$, and normal or slightly increased [HCO_3^-].

Box 14-3 Common Causes of Respiratory Acidosis

NORMAL LUNGS

Central Nervous System Depression
Anesthesia
Sedative drugs
Narcotic analgesics

Neuromuscular Disease
Poliomyelitis
Myasthenia gravis
Guillain-Barré syndrome

Trauma
Spinal cord
Brain
Chest wall
Severe restrictive disorders
Obesity (pickwickian syndrome)
Kyphoscoliosis

ABNORMAL LUNGS
Chronic obstructive pulmonary disease
Acute airway obstruction (late phase)

Compensation

Renal compensation for respiratory acidosis begins as soon as $PaCO_2$ increases. The kidney reabsorbs HCO_3^- from the renal tubular filtrate, bringing the arterial pH into the normal range (see Figure 14-2). However, this process is slow and cannot keep pace with an acutely increasing $PaCO_2$. Full compensation may take several days.

Partly compensated respiratory acidosis is characterized by increased $PaCO_2$, increased [HCO_3^-], and an acid pH—still not quite up in the normal range. *Fully compensated* respiratory acidosis is characterized by a pH on the acidic side of the normal (<7.40 but >7.35), increased $PaCO_2$, and increased [HCO_3^-]. Increased [HCO_3^-] in the presence of increased $PaCO_2$ is a sign that the $PaCO_2$ has been elevated for a considerable time (i.e., the kidneys have had sufficient time to compensate). The underlying pathologic process that produced hypercapnia is still present; the kidneys simply mask the problem by maintaining a normal-range pH. Because hypercapnia is still present, the term *acidosis* is retained in classifying this condition (fully compensated respiratory *acidosis*). This terminology emphasizes that lung function is still abnormal, and, if it were unopposed by the renal compensatory mechanism, it would still produce an acidosis.

Correction

The main goal in correcting respiratory acidosis is to treat the underlying problem—to improve alveolar ventilation. Various respiratory care modalities may be used, ranging from bronchial hygiene and lung expansion techniques to mechanical ventilation. If hypoventilation is chronic and compensation has restored pH to the normal range, action aimed at decreasing $PaCO_2$ to the normal range is inappropriate and possibly harmful, because the high level of [HCO_3^-] in the blood created by the kidney's compensation would produce an alkalosis (Table 14-6).

Respiratory Alkalosis

Any physiologic process that decreases $PaCO_2$ (<35 mm Hg) and increases arterial pH (>7.45) produces respiratory alkalosis. A low $PaCO_2$ (**hypocapnia**) forces the hydration reaction to the left, decreasing H_2CO_3 concentration and increasing the pH:

$$CO_2 + H_2O \leftarrow H_2CO_3 \leftarrow HCO_3^- + H^+$$

Hypocapnia is synonymous with respiratory alkalosis.

Causes

Any process in which ventilatory elimination of CO_2 exceeds the body's production of CO_2 causes respiratory alkalosis. The

TABLE 14-6

Expected Effect of Acute Changes in $PaCO_2$ on Arterial pH

$PaCO_2$ Change	pH Change
Decrease	*Increase*
1 mm Hg	0.01
10 mm Hg	0.10
Increase	*Decrease*
1 mm Hg	0.006
10 mm Hg	0.06
Expected pH when measured $PaCO_2 < 40$ mm Hg	
Expected pH = 7.40 + (40 mm Hg – Measured $PaCO_2$)0.01	
Expected pH when measured $PaCO_2 > 40$ mm Hg	
Expected pH = 7.40 – (Measured $PaCO_2$ – 40 mm Hg)0.006	

MINI CLINI

Chronic (Compensated) Respiratory Acidosis

PROBLEM: A 73-year-old man is being treated on an outpatient basis for pulmonary emphysema, which was diagnosed 7 years earlier. His breathing is labored at rest, with marked use of accessory muscles. Arterial blood gas analysis showed a pH of 7.36, PCO_2 of 64 mm Hg, and HCO_3^- of 35 mEq/L. How would the RT assess this patient's arterial blood gas results?

SOLUTION: The RT should follow these steps:

1. Categorize the pH. The pH is on the acidic side of the normal range, but it is still normal.
2. Determine respiratory involvement. $PaCO_2$ is higher than normal, indicating hypoventilation as a contributing factor to the low-normal pH (respiratory acidosis).
3. Determine metabolic involvement. HCO_3^- is substantially elevated. By itself, this would cause alkalemia, but because pH is on the acidic side of normal, primary metabolic alkalosis is ruled out. Compensation for the respiratory acidosis has occurred.
4. Assess for compensation. HCO_3^- is approximately 8 to 10 mEq higher than normal. This is consistent with a compensatory response by the kidneys to offset the acidosis. In addition, the expected pH for a $PaCO_2$ of 64 mm Hg is [7.40 − (64 mm Hg − 40 mm Hg) × 0.006], or 7.26 (see Table 14-6). Because the actual pH is 7.36, metabolic compensation (retention of HCO_3^-) must have occurred. Therefore the interpretation is a fully compensated respiratory acidosis.

most common cause of hyperventilation in patients with pulmonary disease is decreased PaO_2 (hypoxemia). Hypoxemia causes specialized neural structures to signal the brain, increasing ventilation (see Chapter 15). Anxiety, fever, stimulatory drugs, pain, and central nervous system injuries are possible causes of hyperventilation. Other possible causes include stimulation of irritant receptors in the lung parenchyma, which may occur in pneumonia or pulmonary edema.

Box 14-4 Common Causes of Respiratory Alkalosis

NORMAL LUNGS
Anxiety
Fever
Stimulant drugs
Central nervous system lesion
Pain
Sepsis

ABNORMAL LUNGS
Hypoxemia-causing conditions
Acute asthma
Pneumonia
Stimulation of vagal lung receptors
Pulmonary edema
Pulmonary vascular disease

EITHER NORMAL OR ABNORMAL LUNGS
Iatrogenic hyperventilation

MINI CLINI

Acute (Uncompensated) Respiratory Alkalosis

PROBLEM: A distraught 77-year-old man experiencing anxiety of apparent psychosomatic origin was brought to the hospital by his wife. The patient exhibited rapid and deep breathing, had slurred speech, and complained about tingling in his extremities. Arterial blood gas analysis showed a pH of 7.57, PCO_2 of 23 mm Hg, and HCO_3^- of 22 mEq/L. How would the RT interpret this patient's acid-base condition?

SOLUTION: The RT should follow these steps:

1. Categorize the pH. The pH is substantially higher than normal, indicating the presence of an alkalemia.
2. Determine respiratory involvement. $PaCO_2$ is well below normal, which is consistent with the high pH, indicating hyperventilation as a contributing factor in alkalemia (respiratory alkalosis).
3. Determine metabolic involvement. HCO_3^- is slightly lower than normal. However, this is within the expected range for acute respiratory alkalosis (CO_2 hydration reaction's effect).
4. Assess for compensation. The decrease in HCO_3^- is within the expected range for acute respiratory alkalosis (1 mEq for each 5-mm Hg decline in PCO_2). Therefore the interpretation is an uncompensated respiratory alkalosis.

Hyperventilation and respiratory alkalosis also may be *iatrogenically* induced (induced by medical treatment). Iatrogenic hyperventilation is most commonly associated with overly aggressive mechanical ventilation. It may also be associated with aggressive deep breathing and lung expansion respiratory care procedures. Decreased $PaCO_2$, increased pH, and normal-range [HCO_3^-] characterize acute respiratory alkalosis. A slight decrease in [HCO_3^-] is expected from the effect of the hydration reaction. Box 14-4 summarizes causes of respiratory alkalosis.

Clinical Signs

An early sign of respiratory alkalosis is **paresthesia** (numbness or a tingling sensation in the extremities). Severe hyperventilation is associated with hyperactive reflexes and possibly tetany (seizures). The low $PaCO_2$ may constrict the brain's cerebral vessels enough to reduce cerebral circulation, causing lightheadedness and dizziness.

Compensation

The kidneys compensate for respiratory alkalosis by excreting more HCO_3^- in the urine (HCO_3^- diuresis; see Figure 14-3). This activity brings arterial pH down toward the normal range. As with respiratory acidosis, renal compensation is a slow process. Complete compensation may take days.

Partly compensated respiratory alkalosis is characterized by decreased $PaCO_2$, decreased $[HCO_3^-]$, and a high pH—still not quite down to the normal range. Fully compensated respiratory alkalosis is characterized by decreased $PaCO_2$, decreased $[HCO_3^-]$, and pH on the alkaline side of normal (pH > 7.40 but ≤ 7.45). Compensated respiratory alkalosis is sometimes called *chronic respiratory alkalosis* or *chronic alveolar hyperventilation*. The underlying hyperventilation and hypocapnia are still present. The terminology *respiratory alkalosis* is retained in classifying this condition, because although the pH is within the normal range, the $PaCO_2$ is still below normal.

Correction

Correcting respiratory alkalosis involves removing the stimulus that caused the hyperventilation. If hypoxemia is the stimulus, oxygen therapy is needed.

MINI CLINI

Compensated (Chronic) Respiratory Alkalosis

PROBLEM: A 27-year-old man was admitted to the hospital with a persistent case of bacterial pneumonia, which had not responded to 6 days of ambulatory care with antimicrobial drugs. He exhibited mild cyanosis and labored breathing. Arterial blood gas analysis (with the patient breathing room air) showed a pH of 7.44, $PaCO_2$ of 26 mm Hg, HCO_3^- of 17 mEq/L, and PaO_2 of 53 mm Hg. How would the RT interpret this patient's acid-base condition?

SOLUTION: The RT should follow these steps:

1. Categorize the pH. The pH is on the alkalotic side of the normal range, but it is still normal.
2. Determine respiratory involvement. PCO_2 is well below normal, indicating hyperventilation as a contributing factor to the high-normal pH (respiratory alkalosis).
3. Determine metabolic involvement. HCO_3^- is substantially lower than normal, but because the pH is on the alkalotic side of normal, primary metabolic acidosis is ruled out. Compensation for the respiratory alkalosis has occurred.
4. Assess for compensation. HCO_3^- is approximately 7 mEq below normal. This is consistent with a compensatory response by the kidneys. In addition, the expected pH for $PaCO_2$ of 26 mm Hg is [7.40 + (40 mm Hg − 26 mm Hg) × 0.01], or 7.54 (see Table 14-6). Because the actual pH is 7.44, metabolic compensation (excretion of HCO_3^-) must have occurred. Therefore the interpretation is a fully compensated respiratory alkalosis.

Alveolar Hyperventilation Superimposed on Compensated Respiratory Acidosis

Consider a patient with a compensated respiratory acidosis who has an arterial pH of 7.38, $PaCO_2$ of 58 mm Hg, and HCO_3^- of 33 mEq/L. If this patient becomes severely hypoxic, the hypoxia may stimulate increased alveolar ventilation if lung mechanics are not too severely impaired. If increased alveolar ventilation acutely lowers the $PaCO_2$ from 58 to 50 mm Hg, the pH could possibly increase to the alkalotic side of the normal range. For example, the patient's blood gas values might now be pH of 7.44, $PaCO_2$ of 50 mm Hg, and HCO_3^- of 33 mEq/L.

The inexperienced clinician might wrongly interpret these values as compensated metabolic alkalosis. This example shows that blood gas data alone are not enough to make an accurate acid-base assessment. Knowledge of the patient's medical history and the nature of the current problem are essential to evaluate this problem accurately. The blood gas values in this example would be properly classified as acute alveolar hyperventilation (even though the $PaCO_2$ is >45 mm Hg) superimposed on chronic alveolar hypoventilation (i.e., compensated respiratory acidosis).

Metabolic (Nonrespiratory) Acidosis

Any nonrespiratory process that decreases plasma $[HCO_3^-]$ causes metabolic acidosis. A reduction in $[HCO_3^-]$ decreases blood pH because it decreases the amount of base compared to the amount of acid in the blood.

Causes

Metabolic acidosis can occur in one of the following two ways: (1) fixed (nonvolatile) acid build-up in the blood or (2) an excessive loss of HCO_3^- from the body. An example of fixed acid build-up is a state of low blood flow in which tissue hypoxia and anaerobic metabolism produce lactic acid. The resulting H^+ accumulates and reacts with HCO_3^-, which reduces blood $[HCO_3]$. On the other hand, an example of HCO_3^- loss is severe diarrhea, in which large stores of HCO_3^- are eliminated from the body, also producing a nonrespiratory (metabolic) acidosis.

Because these two kinds of metabolic acidosis are treated differently, it is important to identify the underlying cause. Analysis of the plasma electrolytes is helpful in distinguishing between these two types of metabolic acidosis. Specifically, measuring the anion gap is helpful in making this distinction.

Anion Gap

The *law of electroneutrality* states that the total number of positive charges must equal the total number of negative charges in the body's fluids. *Cations* (positively charged ions) in the plasma produce a charge exactly balanced by plasma *anions* (negatively charged ions). Plasma electrolytes (cations and anions) *routinely* measured in clinical medicine are Na^+, potassium, Cl^-, and HCO_3^-. Normal plasma concentrations of these electrolytes are such that the cations (Na^+ and K^+) outnumber the anions (Cl^- and HCO_3^-), which leads to what seems to be an *anion gap.* Generally, K^+ is ignored in calculating this apparent anion gap:

$$\text{Anion gap} = [Na^+] - ([Cl^-] + [HCO_3^-])$$

Figure 14-7, *A* shows that normal concentrations of these ions in the plasma are as follows: 140 mEq/L for Na^+, 105 mEq/L for Cl^-, and 24 mEq/L for HCO_3^-, yielding an "anion gap" of 11 mEq/L (140 mEq/L − [105 mEq/L + 24 mEq/L] = 11 mEq/L). The normal anion gap range is 9 to 14 mEq/L.[6]

An increased anion gap (>14 mEq/L) is caused by a metabolic acidosis in which abnormal fixed acids accumulate in the body. The H^+ of these acids reacts with plasma HCO_3^-, lowering its concentration; this leads to a further increase in the anion gap (i.e., an increase in *unmeasured anions*) (see Figure 14-7, *B*). (When the H^+ of fixed acids is buffered by HCO_3^-, the anion portion of the fixed acid remains in the plasma, increasing unmeasured anion concentration.) A high anion gap indicates that fixed acid concentration in the body has increased.

Metabolic acidosis caused by HCO_3^- loss from the body does not cause a further increase in the anion gap. HCO_3^- loss is accompanied by Cl^- gain, which keeps the anion gap within normal limits (see Figure 14-7, *C*). The law of electroneutrality helps explain the reciprocal nature of $[HCO_3^-]$ and $[Cl^-]$ in this instance. With a constant cation concentration, losing HCO_3^- means that another anion must be gained to maintain electroneutrality. In this case, the kidney increases its reabsorption of the most abundant anion in the tubular filtrate, the Cl^- ion. The kind of metabolic acidosis in which HCO_3^- is lost from the body is sometimes called *hyperchloremic acidosis* because of the characteristic increase in plasma $[Cl^-]$. Box 14-5 summarizes causes of anion gap and non–anion gap metabolic acidosis.

Box 14-5 Causes of Anion Gap and Non–Anion Gap Metabolic Acidosis

HIGH ANION GAP

Metabolically Produced Acid Gain

Lactic acidosis
Ketoacidosis
Renal failure (e.g., retained sulfuric acid)

Ingestion of Acids

Salicylate (aspirin) intoxication
Methanol (formic acid)
Ethylene glycol (oxalic acid)

NORMAL ANION GAP (HYPERCHLOREMIC ACIDOSIS)

Gastrointestinal Loss of HCO_3^-

Diarrhea
Pancreatic fistula

Renal Tubular Loss: Failure to Reabsorb HCO_3^-

Renal tubular acidosis

Ingestion

Ammonium chloride
Hyperalimentation intravenous nutrition

From Beachey W: Respiratory care anatomy and physiology: foundations for clinical practice, ed 2, St Louis, 2007, Mosby.

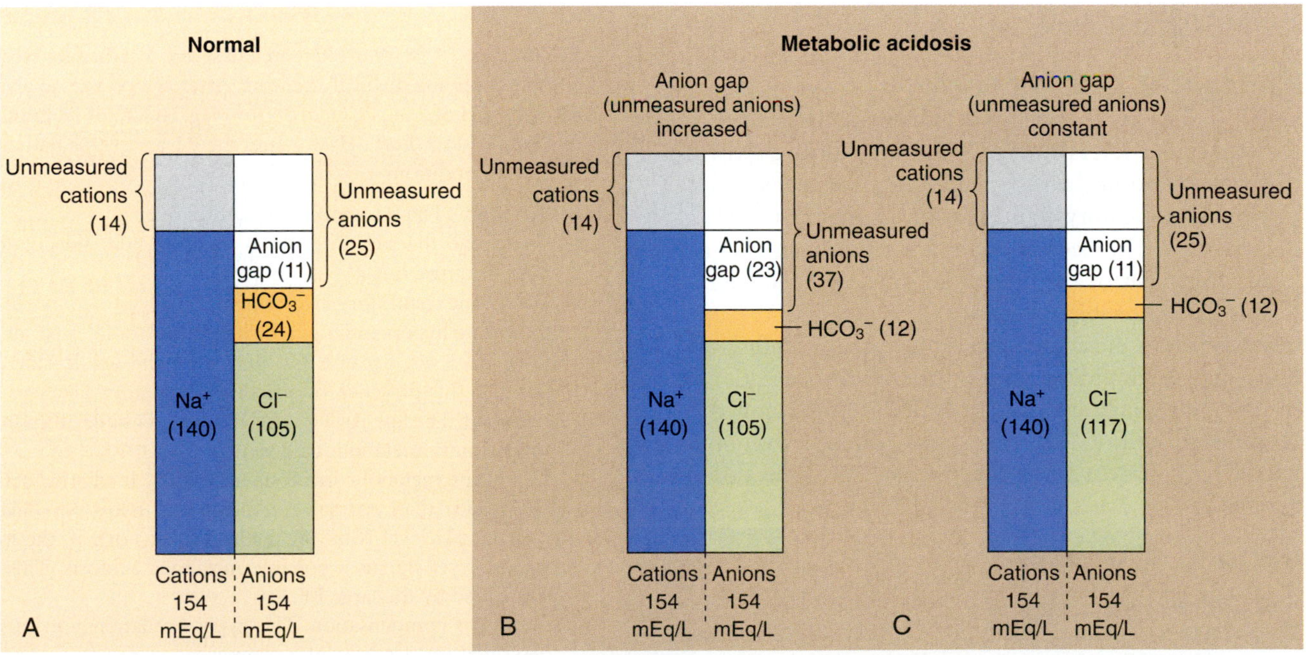

FIGURE 14-7 The anion gap in normal **(A)** and metabolic acidosis (**B** and **C**). Fixed acid accumulation increases the anion gap **(B)**, whereas HCO_3^- loss is accompanied by an equal Cl^- gain, keeping the anion gap within the normal range. (Modified from Beachey W: Respiratory care anatomy and physiology: foundations for clinical practice, ed 2, St Louis, 2007, Mosby.)

RULE OF THUMB

Metabolic acidosis accompanied by a higher than normal anion gap means that the body has accumulated an unusual fixed acid. A metabolic acidosis accompanied by a normal anion gap means that the body has lost a greater than normal amount of base.

Compensation

Hyperventilation is the main compensatory mechanism for metabolic acidosis. The increased plasma [H^+] of metabolic acidosis is buffered by plasma HCO_3^-, which reduces plasma [HCO_3^-] and pH. The low pH activates sensitive receptors in the brain that signal the respiratory muscles to increase ventilation. This increased ventilation lowers the blood's CO_2 levels, and thus it's volatile acid (H_2CO_3), which returns the pH toward the normal range. Uncompensated metabolic acidosis suggests that a ventilatory defect must be present, because ventilation usually responds to this stimulus immediately. Metabolic acidosis accompanied by $PaCO_2$ of 40 mm Hg means that something prevents the lungs from responding appropriately to the brain's stimulation. The defect may lie in nerve impulse transmission, the respiratory muscles, or the lungs.

Symptoms

Respiratory compensation in metabolic acidosis means there is a great increase in minute ventilation, which may cause patients to report dyspnea. Hyperpnea (increased tidal volume depth) is a common finding during physical examination of patients with metabolic acidosis. In patients with severe diabetic ketoacidosis, a very deep, fast breathing develops, called *Kussmaul respiration.* Neurologic symptoms of severe metabolic acidosis range from lethargy to coma.

Correction

The initial goal in severe acidemia is to increase the arterial pH greater than 7.20, a level below which serious cardiac arrhythmias become more likely, and treating them becomes more challenging. If respiratory compensation maintains the pH at or above this level, immediate corrective action is usually not indicated. Treatment of the underlying cause of acid gain or base loss is the reasonable approach.

In cases of severe metabolic acidosis, intravenous infusion of $NaHCO_3$ may be indicated. If respiratory compensation is under way, only small amounts of $NaHCO_3$ are required to attain an arterial pH of 7.20. In any case, rapid correction of an arterial pH greater than 7.20 by $NaHCO_3$ infusion is undesirable.

Metabolic Alkalosis

Metabolic alkalosis is characterized by increased plasma [HCO_3^-] or a loss of H^+ and a high pH. One must keep in mind that increased [HCO_3^-] is not always diagnostic of a primary metabolic alkalosis because it may be caused by renal compensation for respiratory acidosis.

MINI CLINI

Partially Compensated Metabolic Acidosis

PROBLEM: A 42-year-old woman in a diabetic coma was taken to the emergency department. She exhibited fast and deep respirations. Arterial blood gas analysis showed a pH of 7.22, PCO_2 of 20 mm Hg, HCO_3^- of 8 mEq/L, and base excess (BE) of −16 mEq/L. How would the RT interpret this patient's acid-base condition?

SOLUTION: The RT should follow these steps:

1. Categorize the pH. The pH is below the normal range, indicating the presence of acidemia.
2. Determine respiratory involvement. $PaCO_2$ is well below normal, indicating severe hyperventilation. By itself, this would cause alkalosis, but the presence of acidemia rules out primary respiratory alkalosis. The low $PaCO_2$ is probably a compensatory response to primary metabolic acidosis, although this response is currently insufficient to restore pH to the normal range.
3. Determine metabolic involvement. HCO_3^- is severely reduced, consistent with the low pH. In the presence of low pH and low $PaCO_2$, a low HCO_3^- signals primary metabolic acidosis. This is confirmed by the large BE.
4. Assess for compensation. The severe hyperventilation represents a compensatory response to primary metabolic acidosis, although compensation is far from complete. Nevertheless, the pH level would be even lower if the $PaCO_2$ were normal. Hence, the interpretation is a partially compensated metabolic acidosis.

MINI CLINI

Fully Compensated Metabolic Acidosis

PROBLEM: A 38-year-old man had severe diarrhea for weeks without receiving medical attention. Arterial blood gas analysis showed a pH of 7.36, PCO_2 of 24 mm Hg, HCO_3^- of 13 mEq/L, and BE of −11 mEq/L. How would the RT assess this patient's acid-base condition?

SOLUTION: The RT should follow these steps:

1. Categorize the pH. The pH is on the acidic side of the normal range, but it is still normal.
2. Determine respiratory involvement. $PaCO_2$ is below normal, indicating hyperventilation. By itself, this would cause alkalosis; however, because the pH is on the acidic side of normal, the presence of primary respiratory alkalosis is ruled out. The low $PaCO_2$ is likely a compensatory response to a primary metabolic acidosis.
3. Determine metabolic involvement. HCO_3^- level is substantially lower than normal, consistent with a low pH. Given that the pH level is on the acidic side of normal, the low HCO_3^- level signals a possible metabolic acidosis. This is confirmed by the large BE.
4. Assess for compensation. The hyperventilation previously described must represent a compensatory response to primary metabolic acidosis. The pH is in the normal range. Hence, the interpretation is a fully compensated metabolic acidosis.

MINI CLINI

Metabolic Alkalosis

PROBLEM: An 83-year-old woman with heart disease had been taking a powerful diuretic to remove excess edematous fluid from her legs and help keep her free of pulmonary edema. Blood gas and serum electrolyte analyses showed a pH of 7.58, $PaCO_2$ of 46 mm Hg, HCO_3^- of 44 mEq/L, BE of +19 mEq/L, serum K^+ of 2.5 mEq/L, and serum Cl^- of 95 mEq/L. How would the RT assess this patient's acid-base condition?

SOLUTION: The RT should follow these steps:

1. Categorize the pH. The pH level is substantially above normal, indicating the presence of alkalemia.
2. Determine respiratory involvement. $PaCO_2$ is slightly higher than normal, indicating mild hypoventilation. However, because alkalemia is present, the existence of primary respiratory acidosis is ruled out. The elevated $PaCO_2$ may be a compensatory response to a primary metabolic alkalosis.
3. Determine metabolic involvement. HCO_3^- is substantially higher than normal. Given the high pH, the elevated HCO_3^- signals a metabolic alkalosis. This is confirmed by the large BE. In addition, the low serum K^+ and Cl^- values indicate hypokalemic/hypochloremic metabolic alkalosis.
4. Assess for compensation. Although $PaCO_2$ is slightly elevated, compensation for metabolic alkalosis is minimal and the interpretation would be an uncompensated metabolic alkalosis.

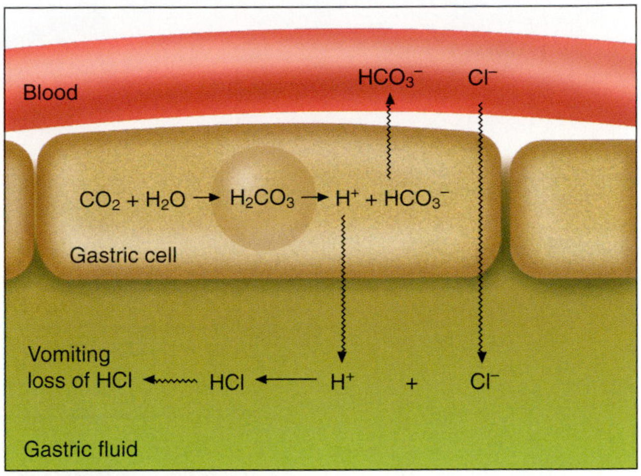

FIGURE 14-8 Gastric H^+ loss generates HCO_3^-, creating metabolic alkalosis. (Modified from Beachey W: Respiratory care anatomy and physiology: foundations for clinical practice, ed 2, St Louis, 2007, Mosby.)

Causes

Metabolic alkalosis can occur in one of the following two ways: (1) loss of fixed acids or (2) gain of blood buffer base. Both processes increase plasma $[HCO_3^-]$. To explain why losing fixed acid increases the plasma $[HCO_3^-]$, consider a situation in which vomiting removes gastric HCl from the body (Figure 14-8). In response to HCl loss, H^+ diffuses out of the gastric cell into the gastric fluid, where Cl^- accompanies it; this forces the CO_2 hydration reaction in the gastric cell to the right, which generates HCO_3^-. The HCO_3^- enters the blood in exchange for the Cl^-. The plasma gains an HCO_3^- for each Cl^- (or H^+) that is lost (see Figure 14-8).[6]

The causes of metabolic alkalosis are summarized in Box 14-6. Metabolic alkalosis is common in acutely ill patients and is probably the most complicated acid-base imbalance to treat because it involves fluid and electrolyte imbalances. Metabolic alkalosis is often iatrogenic, resulting from the use of diuretics, low-salt diets, and gastric drainage.

To understand how the loss of Cl^-, K^+, and fluid volume may cause alkalosis, one needs to understand how the kidney regulates Na^+. Approximately 26,000 mEq of Na^+ passes through the glomerular membrane daily, but the body's daily Na^+ intake averages only approximately 150 mEq.[4] The kidney's main job is to reabsorb Na^+, not to excrete it. For this reason, and because Na^+ has a major role in maintaining fluid balance, the kidney places a greater priority on reabsorbing Na^+ than on maintaining Cl^-, K^+, or acid-base balance.

Box 14-6 Causes of Metabolic Alkalosis (Increased Plasma HCO_3^-)

LOSS OF HYDROGEN IONS

Gastrointestinal

Vomiting
Nasogastric drainage

Renal

Diuretics (loss of Cl^-, K^+ fluid volume)
Hypochloremia (increased H^+ secretion and HCO_3^- reabsorption)
Hypokalemia (increased H^+ secretion and HCO_3^- reabsorption)
Hypovolemia (increased H^+)

RETENTION OF BICARBONATE ION

$NaHCO_3$ infusion or ingestion

From Beachey W: Respiratory care anatomy and physiology: foundations for clinical practice, ed 2, St Louis, 2007, Mosby.

Normally, Na^+ is reabsorbed through *primary active transport* (Figure 14-9), in which the sodium-potassium–adenosine triphosphatase (Na^+,K^+-ATPase) pump actively transports Na^+ out of the renal tubule cell into the blood. This process causes Na^+ to diffuse continually from the filtrate into the tubule cell. Cl^- (the most abundant anion in the filtrate) accompanies Na^+ because of electrostatic forces—that is to maintain electroneutrality in the filtrate. If blood Cl^- concentration is much below normal (hypochloremia), less Cl^- is available for reabsorption with Na^+, which means that the kidney relies more on other mechanisms to reabsorb Na^+. These other mechanisms, called *secondary active secretion,* require the kidney to secrete either H^+ or K^+ into the filtrate in exchange for Na^+. In this way, Na^+ is reabsorbed, and filtrate electroneutrality is preserved. Figures 14-10 and 14-11 illustrate the secondary active secretion process for H^+ and Na^+, which may lead to loss of plasma H^+ (alkalemia)

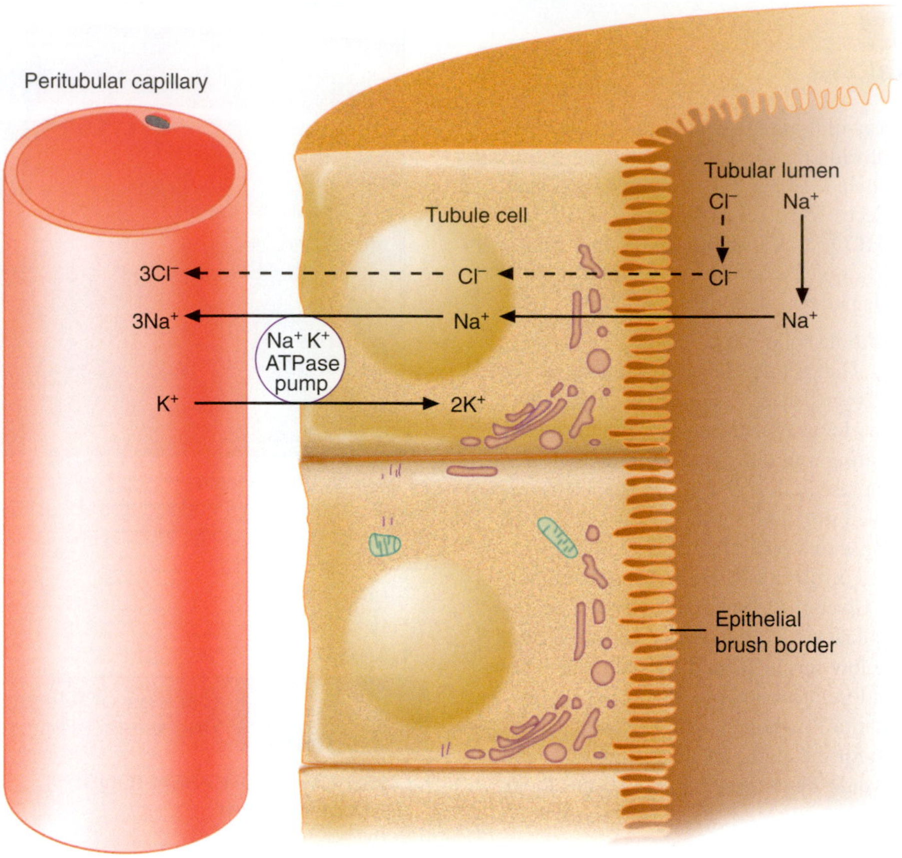

FIGURE 14-9 N^+ reabsorption through primary active transport. The sodium-potassium-adenosine triphosphatase (Na^+,K^+-ATPase) pump generates tubular cell electronegativity by pumping out more Na^+ than it pumps in K^+. This creates both electrostatic and concentration gradients favoring Na^+ diffusion from the filtrate into the tubular cell. Normally, negatively charged Cl^- passively follows Na^+ (cotransport). (Modified from Beachey W: Respiratory care anatomy and physiology: foundations for clinical practice, ed 2, St Louis, 2007, Mosby.)

and K^+ (hypokalemia). Preexisting hypokalemia (e.g., from inadequate K^+ intake) in the presence of hypochloremia places an even greater demand on the kidney to secrete H^+ to reabsorb Na^+; that is, hypokalemia leads to alkalosis. Dehydration (fluid volume depletion or hypovolemia) further aggravates alkalosis and hypokalemia because hypovolemia profoundly increases the kidney's stimulus to reabsorb Na^+, which means the kidney depends even more on these secondary mechanisms for Na^+ reabsorption.

Compensation

The expected compensatory response to metabolic alkalosis is hypoventilation (CO_2 retention). Traditionally, it was thought that the hypoxemia accompanying hypoventilation greatly limited respiratory compensation for metabolic alkalosis (i.e., hypoxemia itself stimulates ventilation and should prevent compensatory hypoventilation). However, metabolic alkalosis blunts the hypoxemic stimulus to ventilation; that is, neurologic receptors sensitive to hypoxemia become less sensitive in the presence of alkalemia. Individuals with PaO_2 levels of 50 mm Hg may still hypoventilate to $PaCO_2$ levels of 60 mm Hg to compensate for metabolic alkalosis.[6] Nevertheless, significant CO_2 retention is not seen often in cases of metabolic alkalosis, probably because metabolic alkalosis commonly coexists with other conditions that may cause hyperventilation, such as anxiety, pain, infection, fever, or pulmonary edema.

Correction

Correction of metabolic alkalosis is aimed at restoring normal fluid volume and electrolyte concentrations, especially K^+ and Cl^- levels. Inadequate fluid volume, especially if coupled with hypochloremia, causes excessive secretion and loss of H^+ and K^+ because of the great need to reabsorb Na^+. In treating this type of alkalosis, it is important to supply adequate fluids containing Cl^-. If hypokalemia is a primary factor, potassium chloride (KCl) is the preferred corrective agent. In rare cases of very severe metabolic alkalosis, acidifying agents, such as dilute HCl may be infused directly into a large central vein.[7]

Metabolic Acid-Base Indicators

Standard Bicarbonate

To eliminate the influence of the hydration reaction on plasma bicarbonate concentration, some laboratories report **standard bicarbonate**. The standard bicarbonate is the plasma concentration of HCO_3^- (in mEq/L) obtained from a blood sample that has been equilibrated (at body temperature) with a PCO_2

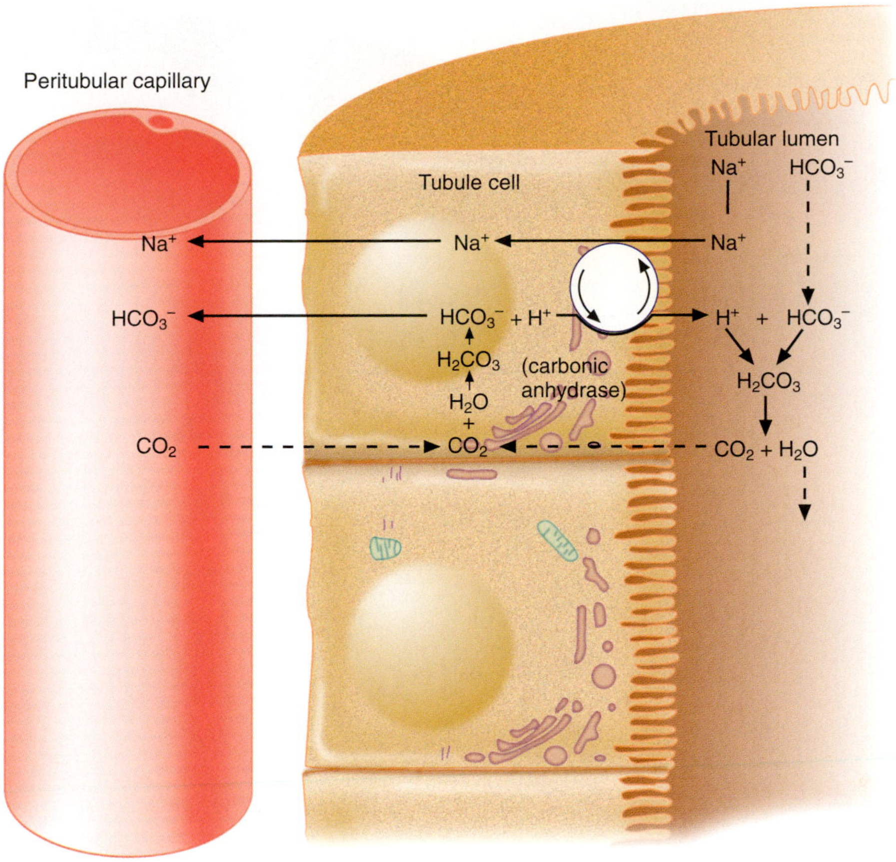

FIGURE 14-10 Na^+ reabsorption through secondary active H^+ secretion. Through the countertransport process, Na^+ is reabsorbed as H^+ is secreted into the filtrate. HCO_3^- ion is reabsorbed with Na^+ instead of Cl^-. This process becomes more predominant when Cl^- is scarce, and it leads to alkalosis. (Modified from Beachey W: Respiratory care anatomy and physiology: foundations for clinical practice, ed 2, St Louis, 2007, Mosby.)

of 40 mm Hg. This HCO_3^- measurement presumably reflects only the metabolic component of acid-base balance, unhampered by the influence that CO_2 changes have on HCO_3^-. However, the process of standardizing the bicarbonate under in vitro laboratory conditions creates an artificial situation not present in the patient's body. The blood in the patient's vascular system is separated from the extravascular fluid (fluid outside of the vessels) by a thin capillary endothelial membrane, readily permeable to HCO_3^-. When a patient hypoventilates and the blood $PaCO_2$ increases, the plasma HCO_3^- also increases because of the hydration reaction. Consequently, plasma HCO_3^- diffuses out of the capillary into the extravascular fluid until HCO_3^- equilibrium is established between the blood and extravascular fluid. If the patient were now to hyperventilate so that the $PaCO_2$ again was 40 mm Hg, blood HCO_3^- would decrease, and extravascular HCO_3^- would diffuse down its concentration gradient back into the blood until an HCO_3^- equilibrium was established again. This diffusion of HCO_3^- between vascular and extravascular spaces cannot occur in a laboratory blood sample when the blood PCO_2 of a hypercapnic patient is artificially lowered to 40 mm Hg. Thus, even the standard bicarbonate is not a perfect measure of purely nonrespiratory factors that influence blood pH.

Base Excess

Base excess (BE) is determined by equilibrating a blood sample in the laboratory to a PCO_2 of 40 mm Hg (at 37° C) and recording the amount of acid or base needed to titrate 1 L of blood to a pH of 7.40. A normal BE is ±2 mEq/L. A positive BE (>+2 mEq/L) indicates a gain of base or loss of acid from nonrespiratory causes. A negative BE (<−2 mEq/L) indicates a loss of base or a gain of acid from nonrespiratory causes. The BE measurement suffers from the same limitation as the standard bicarbonate because it is an in vitro, rather than in vivo, measurement. That is, in hypercapnia, the **buffer base** that diffused into the extravascular fluid in vivo cannot be recovered during laboratory in vitro titrations.

Further, the reliance on BE to quantify metabolic acid-base abnormalities can be misleading. In cases of acute (uncompensated) respiratory acidosis, the BE commonly would be within the normal range, indicating correctly that the disturbance is purely respiratory in origin. However, when renal compensation has occurred to offset chronic hypercapnia, the BE measurement is elevated above the normal range because of the compensatory increase in plasma HCO_3^-.

To illustrate, consider the accompanying Mini Clini in which the patient has respiratory acidosis for which the body has

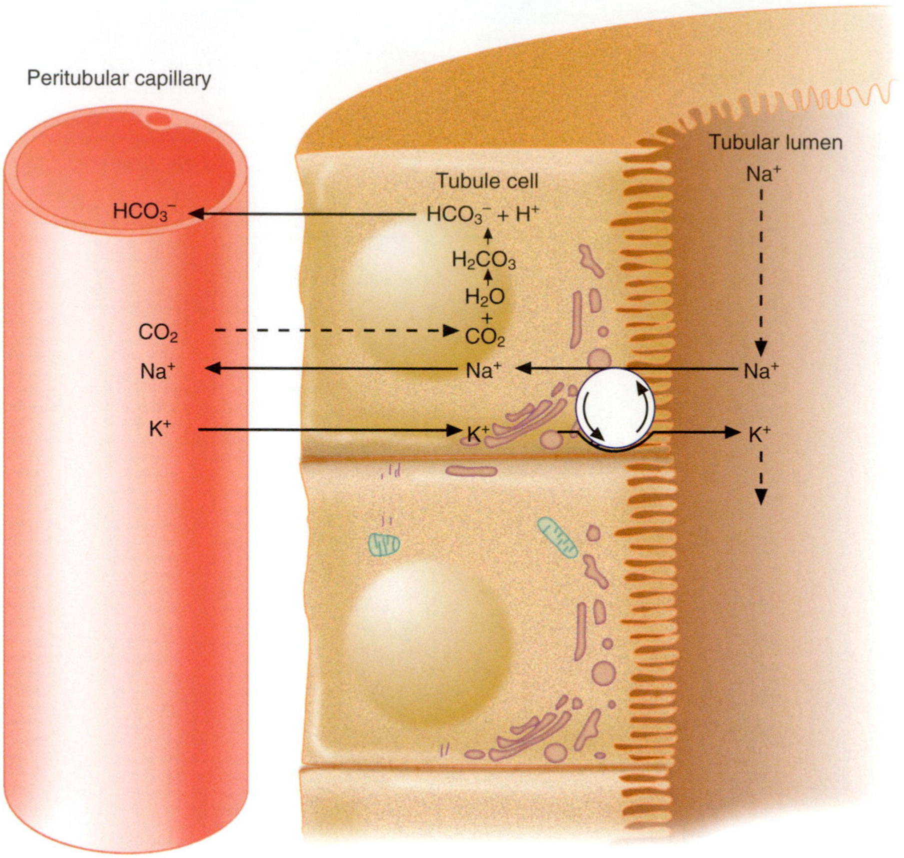

FIGURE 14-11 Na^+ reabsorption through secondary active K^+ secretion. This mechanism is more likely to occur when Cl^- is scarce and an alkalemia (low H^+) exists. In such instances, hypokalemia develops. (Modified from Beachey W: Respiratory care anatomy and physiology: foundations for clinical practice, ed 2, St Louis, 2007, Mosby.)

compensated by renal retention of HCO_3^-. If this patient's blood were equilibrated in vitro to a $PaCO_2$ of 40 mm Hg, the HCO_3^- would decrease by only 2 to 3 mEq/L to 32 to 33 mEq/L and the pH would increase to much greater than 7.45. This patient's BE would be well above normal. The high BE may lead the clinician to conclude incorrectly that this patient has a primary metabolic alkalosis. However, in this instance, the high BE does not indicate the presence of a pathologic process; it merely reflects the fact that renal compensation has occurred.

Mixed Acid-Base States

Combinations of acid-base disorders may occur in the same patient. A combined disturbance is one in which both respiratory and metabolic disturbances exist and promote the same acid-base disturbance. For example, consider the following arterial blood gas results: a pH of 7.62, $PaCO_2$ of 32 mm Hg, and HCO_3^- of 29 mEq/L. The pH indicates alkalemia, consistent with both the low $PaCO_2$ and the elevated HCO_3^-. This is a combined alkalosis, which means that the patient has two primary acid-base problems (i.e., respiratory and metabolic alkalosis combined); compensation cannot occur in this case. Further, consider the patient in cardiopulmonary arrest whose arterial blood gas results are pH of 7.09, $PaCO_2$ of 77 mm Hg, and HCO_3^- of 11 mEq/L, in all likelihood a result of cessation of breathing resulting in hypercapnia, an uncompensated respiratory acidosis, and moderate to severe hypoxemia, which lead to anaerobic metabolism, which produce a lactic (metabolic) acidosis and thus a combined respiratory and metabolic acidosis.

SUMMARY CHECKLIST

- The lungs regulate the volatile acid content (CO_2) of the blood, and the kidneys control the fixed acid concentration of the blood.
- The larger the equilibrium constant of an acid, the more the acid molecule dissociates and yields H^+.
- In the *open* bicarbonate buffer system, H^+ is buffered to form the volatile acid, H_2CO_3, which dissociates to form H_2O and CO_2; the CO_2 is exhaled into the atmosphere. In the *closed* nonbicarbonate buffer system, H^+ is buffered to form fixed acids, which accumulate in the body.
- Bicarbonate buffers can buffer only fixed acids, but nonbicarbonate buffers can buffer both fixed and volatile acids.
- The ratio between the plasma [HCO_3^-] and dissolved CO_2 determines the blood pH, according to the H-H equation; a ratio of 20:1 [HCO_3^-] to dissolved CO_2 always yields a normal arterial pH of 7.40.

- The kidneys respond to hypoventilation by reabsorbing HCO_3^-, and they respond to hyperventilation by excreting HCO_3^-.
- The lungs respond to metabolic acidosis by hyperventilating, and they respond to metabolic alkalosis by hypoventilating.
- $PaCO_2$ abnormalities characterize respiratory acid-base disturbances, and $[HCO_3^-]$ abnormalities characterize metabolic acid-base disturbances.
- Hypochloremia forces the kidneys to excrete increased amounts of H^+ and K^+ to reabsorb Na^+, causing alkalosis and hypokalemia.
- Hypokalemia forces the kidneys to excrete increased amounts of H^+ to reabsorb Na^+, causing alkalosis.
- Standard bicarbonate and BE measurements are made under conditions of a normal $PaCO_2$ (40 mm Hg), which means that any abnormality in these measurements reflects only nonrespiratory influences.

References

1. Masoro EJ, Siegel PD: *Acid-base regulation: its physiology and pathophysiology*, Philadelphia, 1971, Saunders.
2. Levitsky M: *Pulmonary physiology*, ed 10, New York, 2013, McGraw Hill.
3. West JB: *Respiratory physiology: the essentials*, ed 9, Baltimore, 2011, Lippincott Williams & Wilkins.
4. Hall JE: *Guyton and Hall textbook of medical physiology*, ed 12, Philadelphia, 2010, Saunders.
5. Keyes JL: *Fluid, electrolyte and acid-base regulation*, ed 1, Burlington MA, 2007, Jones & Bartlett.
6. Rose BD: *Clinical physiology of acid-base and electrolyte disorders*, ed 5, New York, 2001, McGraw-Hill.
7. DuBose TD: Disorders of acid-base balance. In Taal MW, Chertow GM, Marsden PA, et al, editors: *Brenner and Rector's the kidney*, ed 9, Philadelphia, 2012, Saunders.

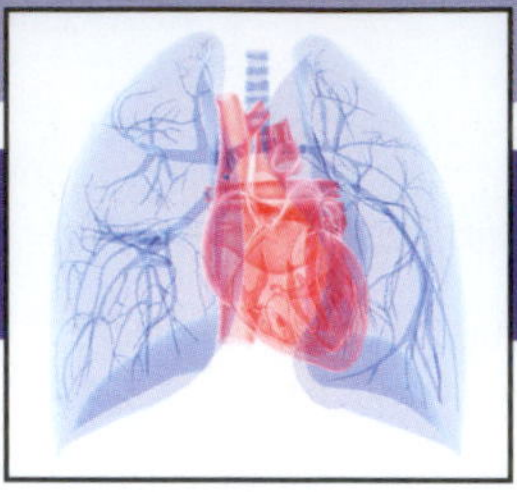

CHAPTER 15

Regulation of Breathing

WILL BEACHEY

CHAPTER OBJECTIVES

After reading this chapter you will be able to:

- Identify where the structures that regulate breathing are located.
- Explain how the inspiratory and expiratory neurons in the medulla establish the basic pattern of breathing.
- Describe the effect that impulses from the pneumotaxic and apneustic centers in the pons have on the medullary centers of breathing.
- Describe the effect of various reflexes on breathing.
- Explain how the central and peripheral chemoreceptors differ in the way they regulate breathing.
- Compare and contrast central chemoreceptors response to respiratory and nonrespiratory acid-base disorders.
- Contrast the regulation of breathing in individuals with chronic hypercapnia with the regulation of breathing in healthy individuals.
- Explain why administering high concentrations of oxygen to patients with chronic hypercapnia poses a special risk that is not present in healthy individuals.
- Describe why ascending to a high altitude has different immediate and long-term effects on ventilation.
- Explain why mechanically ventilated patients with head injuries may benefit from deliberate hyperventilation.
- Characterize various abnormal breathing patterns.

CHAPTER OUTLINE

Medullary Respiratory Center
- Dorsal Respiratory Groups
- Ventral Respiratory Groups
- Inspiratory Ramp Signal

Pontine Respiratory Centers
- Apneustic Center
- Pneumotaxic Center

Reflex Control of Breathing
- Hering-Breuer Inflation Reflex
- Deflation Reflex
- Head Paradoxical Reflex
- Irritant Receptors
- J-Receptors
- Peripheral Proprioceptors
- Muscle Spindles

Chemical Control of Breathing
- Central Chemoreceptors
- Peripheral Chemoreceptors
- Control of Breathing in Chronic Hypercapnia
- Oxygen-Associated Hypercapnia

Ventilatory Response to Exercise

Abnormal Breathing Patterns

Carbon Dioxide and Cerebral Blood Flow

KEY TERMS

apnea
apneustic breathing
apneustic center
Biot respiration
blood-brain barrier
chemoreceptors
Cheyne-Stokes respiration
dorsal respiratory groups (DRGs)
Hering-Breuer inflation reflex
J-receptors
pneumotaxic center
vagovagal reflexes
ventral respiratory groups (VRGs)

Breathing, similar to the heartbeat, is an automatic activity requiring no conscious awareness. In contrast to the heartbeat, breathing patterns can be consciously changed, although powerful neural control mechanisms overwhelm conscious control soon after one willfully stops breathing. The normal unconscious cycle of breathing is regulated by complex mechanisms that are still not completely understood. The rhythmic cycle of breathing comes from the brainstem, mainly from neurons located in the medulla. Higher brain centers and many systemic receptors and reflexes change the output of the medulla. These different structures function in harmony, precisely controlling ventilatory rate and depth to meet the gas exchange needs of the body. This chapter helps the respiratory therapist (RT) understand basic physiologic mechanisms that regulate breathing. With this knowledge, the RT and other members of the patient care team can help predict the effects that various therapies and disease processes have on ventilation.

MEDULLARY RESPIRATORY CENTER

Animal experiments show that cutting through the brainstem just below the medulla (Figure 15-1, *level IV*) stops all ventilatory activity. However, breathing continues rhythmically after the brainstem is cut just above the pons (see Figure 15-1, *level I*). Physiologists used to believe that separate inspiratory and expiratory neuron "centers" in the medulla were responsible for the cyclic pattern of breathing. Researchers believed that inspiratory and expiratory neurons fired by self-excitation and that they mutually inhibited one another. More recent evidence shows that inspiratory and expiratory neurons are anatomically mixed together and do not inhibit one another.[1] No clearly separate inspiratory and expiratory centers exist. Instead, the medulla contains widely scattered groups of respiratory-related neurons, as shown in Figure 15-1. The **dorsal respiratory groups (DRGs)** contain mainly inspiratory neurons, whereas the **ventral respiratory groups (VRGs)** contain both inspiratory and expiratory neurons.

Dorsal Respiratory Groups

As shown in Figure 15-1, DRG neurons are mainly inspiratory neurons located on both sides of the medulla. These neurons send the major inspiratory stimuli to the motor nerves of the diaphragm and external intercostal muscles.[1] Many DRG nerves extend into the VRGs, but few VRG nerve fibers extend into the DRGs. Mutual inhibition is an unlikely explanation for rhythmic, spontaneous breathing.[1]

The vagus and glossopharyngeal nerves transmit many sensory impulses to the DRGs from the lungs, airways, peripheral chemoreceptors, and joint proprioceptors. These impulses change the basic breathing pattern generated in the medulla.

Ventral Respiratory Groups

VRG neurons are located bilaterally in the medulla in two different nuclei and contain inspiratory and expiratory neurons (see Figure 15-1). Some inspiratory VRG neurons send motor impulses through the vagus nerve to the laryngeal and pharyngeal muscles, abducting the vocal cords and increasing the diameter of the glottis. Other VRG inspiratory neurons transmit impulses to the diaphragm and external intercostal muscles. Still other VRG neurons have mostly expiratory discharge patterns and send impulses to the internal intercostal and abdominal expiratory muscles.

The exact origin of the basic rhythmic pattern of ventilation is unknown. No single group of pacemaker cells has been identified. Two predominant theories of rhythm generation are

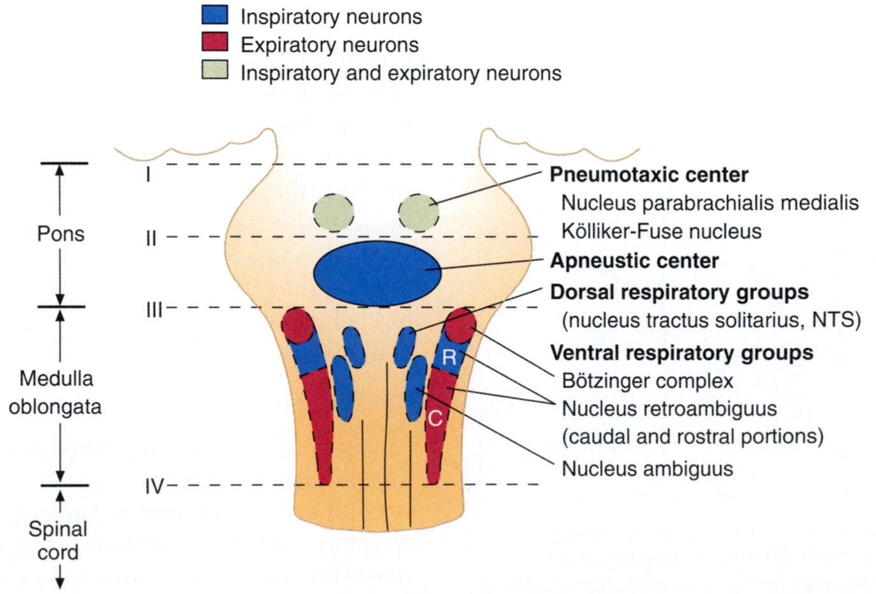

FIGURE 15-1 Dorsal view of the brainstem. Dashed lines *I* to *IV* refer to transections at different levels. (Modified from Beachey W: Respiratory care anatomy and physiology: foundations for clinical practice, ed 2, St Louis, 2007, Mosby.)

the *pacemaker hypothesis* and the *network hypothesis*.[2] The pacemaker hypothesis holds that certain medullary cells have intrinsic pacemaker properties (i.e., rhythmic self-exciting characteristics) and that these cells drive other medullary neurons. The network hypothesis suggests that rhythmic breathing is the result of a particular pattern of interconnections between neurons dispersed throughout the upper part of the VRG, the pre-Bötzinger complex, and the Bötzinger complex. This hypothesis assumes that certain populations of inspiratory and expiratory neurons inhibit one another and that one of the neuron types fires in a self-limiting way, such that it becomes less responsive the longer it fires. There is no definitive proof of either hypothesis; the precise origin of respiratory rhythm generation remains mysterious.[2]

Inspiratory Ramp Signal

The inspiratory muscles do not receive an instantaneous burst of signals from the dorsal and ventral inspiratory neurons. Rather, the firing rate of DRG and VRG inspiratory neurons increases gradually at the end of the expiratory phase, creating a ramp signal (Figure 15-2). The inspiratory muscles contract steadily and smoothly, gradually expanding the lungs rather than filling them in an abrupt inspiratory gasp. During exercise, various reflexes and receptors influence the medullary neurons, making the ramp signal much steeper, filling the lungs more rapidly.

During quiet breathing, inspiratory neurons fire with an increasing rate for approximately 2 seconds and then abruptly switch off, allowing expiration to proceed for approximately 3 seconds.[3] At the start of expiration, inspiratory neurons again fire briefly, holding back the early phase of expiration (see Figure 15-2). The inhibitory neurons that switch off the inspiratory ramp signal are controlled by the pneumotaxic center and pulmonary stretch receptors, which are discussed later in this chapter.

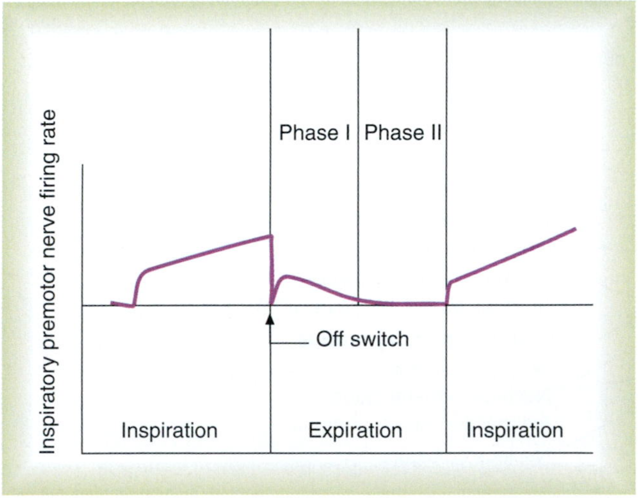

FIGURE 15-2 Inspiratory neural activity during breathing. Note the inspiratory ramp signal *(left)* and the braking action of inspiratory signals in the early part *(phase I)* of expiration. (Redrawn from Leff AR, Shumacher PT: Respiratory physiology: basics and applications, Philadelphia, 1993, Saunders.)

PONTINE RESPIRATORY CENTERS

If the brainstem is cut above the medulla (see Figure 15-1, *level III*), spontaneous respiration continues, although in an irregular pattern. The pons does not make breathing rhythmic; rather, it modifies the output of the medullary centers. Figure 15-1 shows two groups of neurons in the pons: (1) the apneustic center and (2) the pneumotaxic center.

Apneustic Center

The **apneustic center** does not occupy a well-defined anatomic location; its existence and function can be shown only if its connections to the higher pneumotaxic center and vagus nerves are severed. Under such circumstances, the DRG inspiratory neurons fail to switch off, causing prolonged inspiratory gasps interrupted by occasional expirations **(apneustic breathing).** Vagal and pneumotaxic center impulses hold the apneustic center's stimulatory effect on DRG neurons in check.

Pneumotaxic Center

The **pneumotaxic center** is a group of neurons located on both sides of the upper pons (see Figure 15-1). The pneumotaxic center controls the "off-switch" point of the inspiratory ramp, controlling inspiratory time. Strong pneumotaxic signals increase the respiratory rate, and weak signals prolong inspiration and increase tidal volumes. The exact nature of the interaction between the pneumotaxic and apneustic centers is poorly understood. They apparently work together to control the depth of inspiration.[3]

REFLEX CONTROL OF BREATHING

Hering-Breuer Inflation Reflex

The **Hering-Breuer inflation reflex,** described by Hering and Breuer in 1868, is generated by stretch receptors located in the smooth muscle of both large and small airways. When lung inflation stretches these receptors, they send inhibitory impulses through the vagus nerve to the DRG neurons, stopping further inspiration. In this way, the Hering-Breuer reflex has an effect similar to that of the pneumotaxic center. In adults, the Hering-Breuer reflex is activated only at large tidal volumes (≥800 to 1000 ml) and apparently is not an important control mechanism in quiet breathing.[2] This reflex is important, however, in regulating respiratory rate and depth during moderate to strenuous exercise.

Deflation Reflex

Sudden collapse of the lung stimulates strong inspiratory effort. This inspiratory effort may be the result of decreased stretch receptor activity, or it may be caused by the stimulation of other receptors, such as the irritant receptors and J-receptors (discussed later). Although it is unclear which receptors are involved, it is clear that the vagus nerve is the pathway (as it is for the Hering-Breuer reflex) and that the effect is hyperpnea.[1] The deflation reflex is probably responsible for the hyperpnea observed with pneumothorax (air in the pleural space).

Head Paradoxical Reflex

In 1889, Head observed that if the Hering-Breuer reflex is blocked by cooling the vagus nerve, lung hyperinflation causes a further increase in inspiratory effort—the opposite of the Hering-Breuer reflex. The receptors for this reflex are called *rapidly adapting receptors* because they stop firing promptly after a volume change occurs. The Head reflex may help maintain large tidal volumes during exercise and may be involved in periodic deep sighs during quiet breathing. Periodic sighs help prevent alveolar collapse, or atelectasis. The Head reflex also may be responsible for the first breaths of a newborn.[1]

Irritant Receptors

Rapidly adapting irritant receptors in the epithelium of the larger conducting airways have vagal sensory nerve fibers. Their stimulation, whether by inhaled irritants or by mechanical factors, causes reflex bronchoconstriction, coughing, sneezing, tachypnea, and narrowing of the glottis. Some of these reflexes, called **vagovagal reflexes,** have both sensory and motor vagal components; they are responsible for laryngospasm, coughing, and slowing of the heartbeat. Endotracheal intubation, airway suctioning, and bronchoscopy readily elicit vagovagal reflexes. Physical stimulation of the conducting airways, as with suctioning or bronchoscopy, may cause a severe case of bronchospasm, coughing, and laryngospasm.

J-Receptors

C fibers in the lung parenchyma near the pulmonary capillaries are called *juxtacapillary receptors,* or **J-receptors.** Alveolar inflammatory processes (pneumonia), pulmonary vascular congestion (congestive heart failure), and pulmonary edema stimulate these receptors. This stimulation causes rapid, shallow breathing; a sensation of dyspnea; and expiratory narrowing of the glottis.

Peripheral Proprioceptors

Proprioceptors in muscles, tendons, and joints and pain receptors in muscles and skin send stimulatory signals to the medullary respiratory center. Such stimuli increase medullary inspiratory activity and cause hyperpnea.[4] For this reason, moving the limbs, slapping or splashing cold water on the skin, and other painful stimuli stimulate ventilation in patients with respiratory depression.

Proprioceptors in joints and tendons may be important in initiating and maintaining increased ventilation at the beginning of exercise. Passive limb movement around a joint increases breathing rate in both anesthetized animals and unanesthetized humans.[4]

Muscle Spindles

Muscle spindles in the diaphragm and intercostal muscles are part of a reflex arc that helps the muscles adjust to an increased load. Muscle spindles are sensing elements located on intrafusal

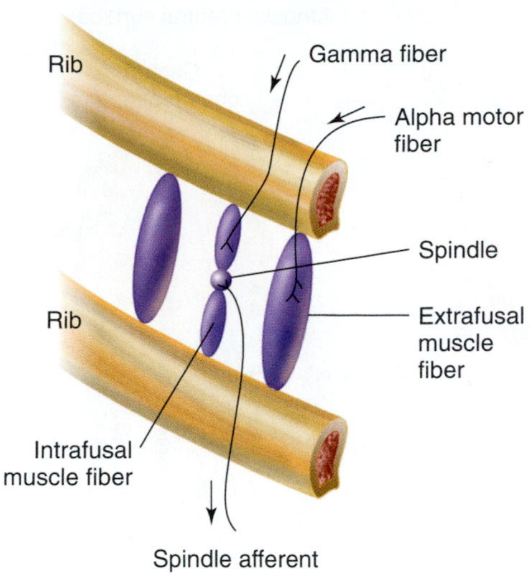

FIGURE 15-3 Stretch-sensitive muscle spindle located on the intrafusal fibers of intercostal muscles. Motor innervation for intrafusal fibers (gamma nerve fibers) is different than for extrafusal fibers (alpha nerve fibers). Spindle afferent nerve fibers synapse with alpha motor neurons in the spinal cord, creating a single synapse reflex arc.

muscle fibers, arranged parallel to the main extrafusal muscle fibers (Figure 15-3). The extrafusal fibers that elevate the ribs are innervated by motor fibers (alpha fibers) different from the fibers that innervate the intrafusal spindle fibers (gamma fibers). When the main extrafusal muscle fiber and the intrafusal fibers contract simultaneously, the sensing element *(spindle)* of the intrafusal muscle fiber stretches and sends impulses over spindle afferent nerves directly to the spinal cord (see Figure 15-3). The spindle's afferent (sensory) nerve synapses directly with the alpha motor neuron in the spinal cord, sending impulses back to the main extrafusal muscle. A single synapse reflex arc is created. Alpha motor neuron impulses cause the main extrafusal muscle fibers to contract with greater force, shortening the nearby intrafusal fibers. The stretch-sensitive spindle is thus unloaded, and its impulses cease. In this way, inspiratory muscle force adjusts to the load imposed by decreased lung compliance or increased airway resistance.

CHEMICAL CONTROL OF BREATHING

The body maintains the proper amounts of oxygen (O_2), carbon dioxide (CO_2), and hydrogen ions (H^+) in the blood mainly by regulating ventilation. Physiologic mechanisms that monitor these substances in the blood allow ventilation to respond appropriately to maintain homeostasis. An increase in blood H^+ concentration stimulates specialized nerve structures called **chemoreceptors.** As a result, the chemoreceptors transmit impulses to the medulla, increasing ventilation. Centrally located chemoreceptors in the medulla respond to H^+, which normally arises from dissolved CO_2 in the cerebrospinal fluid (CSF). Peripherally located chemoreceptors in the fork of the common carotid arteries and the aortic arch are also sensitive

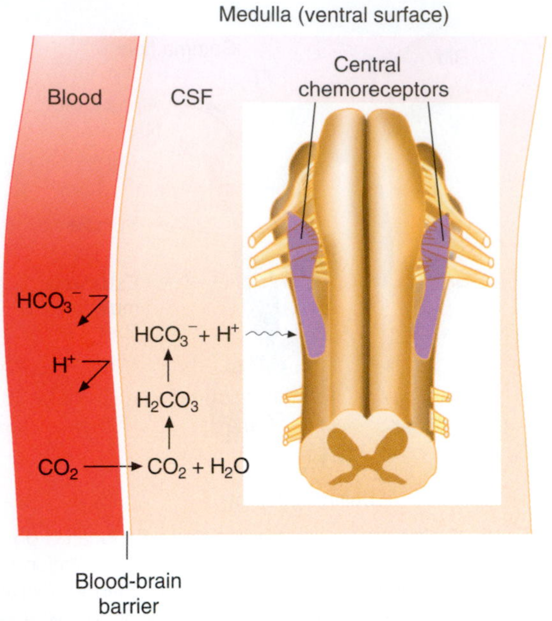

FIGURE 15-4 CO_2 stimulates the medullary chemoreceptors by forming H^+ in the cerebrospinal fluid (CSF). The blood-brain barrier is almost impermeable to H^+ and HCO_3^- but is freely permeable to CO_2. (Modified from Beachey W: Respiratory care anatomy and physiology: foundations for clinical practice, ed 2, St Louis, 2007, Mosby.)

to H^+ and indirectly to CO_2. These receptors are also indirectly sensitive to hypoxemia because hypoxemia increases the sensitivity of the peripheral chemoreceptors to H^+.[2]

Central Chemoreceptors

H^+ ions, not CO_2 molecules, stimulate highly responsive chemosensitive nerve cells, located on both sides of the medulla. Nevertheless, these central chemoreceptors are extremely sensitive to CO_2 in an indirect fashion. These chemoreceptors are not in direct contact with arterial blood (Figure 15-4). Instead, they are bathed in the CSF, separated from the blood by a semipermeable membrane called the **blood-brain barrier.** This membrane is almost impermeable to H^+ and HCO_3^-, but it is freely permeable to CO_2. When $PaCO_2$ increases, CO_2 diffuses rapidly through the blood-brain barrier into the CSF. In the CSF, CO_2 reacts with water (H_2O) to form H^+ and HCO_3^- (see Figure 15-4). The H^+ ions generated in this fashion stimulate the central chemoreceptors, which stimulate the medullary inspiratory neurons. In this way, $PaCO_2$ is indirectly the primary minute-to-minute controller of ventilation. CO_2 diffusing from the blood into the CSF increases $[H^+]$ almost instantly, exciting the chemoreceptors within seconds. Alveolar ventilation increases by approximately 2 to 3 L/min for each 1-mm Hg increase in $PaCO_2$.[5]

The stimulatory effect of chronically high CO_2 on the central chemoreceptors gradually declines over 1 or 2 days because the kidneys reabsorb HCO_3^- ions in response to respiratory acidosis, bringing the blood pH level back toward normal. The increased number of HCO_3^- ions in the blood eventually diffuses across the blood-brain barrier into the CSF, where they buffer H^+ and bring the CSF pH level back to normal. This activity removes the stimulus to the chemoreceptors, and ventilation decreases. Thus an acute increase in $PaCO_2$ has a powerful effect on ventilation, which is greatly weakened after 1 or 2 days of adaptation.

Peripheral Chemoreceptors

The peripheral chemoreceptors are small, highly vascular structures known as the *carotid* and *aortic bodies.* The carotid bodies are located bilaterally in the bifurcations of the common carotid arteries. The aortic bodies are found in the arch of the aorta. These neural structures increase their firing rates in response to increased arterial $[H^+]$ regardless of its origin (i.e., whether from fixed acid accumulation or increased CO_2). The carotid bodies send their impulses to the respiratory centers in the medulla via the glossopharyngeal nerve, whereas the aortic bodies send their impulses over the vagus nerve. The carotid bodies exert much more influence over the respiratory centers than the aortic bodies do, especially with respect to arterial hypoxemia and acidemia.[1]

Because the carotid bodies receive an extremely high rate of blood flow, they have little time to remove O_2 from the blood. Therefore venous blood leaving the carotid bodies has almost the same O_2 content as the arterial blood entering them. The carotid bodies are exposed at all times to arterial blood, not venous blood, and they sense arterial (not venous) $[H^+]$.

Response to Decreased Arterial Oxygen

Traditionally, it was believed that the carotid bodies directly sense low PaO_2, implying that arterial hypoxemia is an independent stimulus to breathe—the so-called *hypoxic drive.* Although the peripheral chemoreceptors fire more frequently in the presence of arterial hypoxemia, they do so only because hypoxemia makes them more sensitive to H^+.[2] In other words, when PaO_2 is low, carotid body sensitivity to a given $[H^+]$ increases; in this way, hypoxia increases ventilation for any given pH. On the other hand, elevated PaO_2 (hyperoxia) decreases carotid body sensitivity to $[H^+]$. The carotid bodies respond to arterial hypoxemia only because hypoxia makes them more sensitive to $[H^+]$. This means that if the arterial $[H^+]$ is extremely low (high pH), as in severe alkalemia, hypoxemia has little effect on the carotid bodies.[2] Simply stated, the ultimate effect of hypoxemia is to increase the sensitivity of the peripheral chemoreceptors to the given blood $[H^+]$, which increases their firing rate and brings about increased ventilation.

Because of their extremely high blood flow rates, the carotid bodies respond to decreased arterial *partial pressure* of O_2 (in the indirect way just described) rather than to an actual decrease in arterial O_2 *content.* That is, the amount of O_2 the carotid bodies extract from each unit of rapidly flowing blood is so small that their O_2 needs are met entirely by dissolved O_2 in the plasma—which depends on the PaO_2. This is why conditions associated with low arterial O_2 content but normal PaO_2 (e.g., anemia and carbon monoxide poisoning) do not stimulate ventilation.[5]

When pH and $PaCO_2$ are normal (pH = 7.40 and $PaCO_2$ = 40 mm Hg), the nerve-impulse transmission rate of the carotid bodies does not increase significantly until the PaO_2 decreases to approximately 60 mm Hg.[5] If PaO_2 decreases further from 60 mm Hg to 30 mm Hg, the rate of impulse transmission increases sharply because hypoxemia makes the carotid bodies much more sensitive to a pH of 7.40. A decrease in PaO_2 from 60 mm Hg to 30 mm Hg corresponds to the sharpest decrease in O_2 content on the O_2-Hb equilibrium curve (i.e., the steepest part of the curve). Arterial hypoxemia does not stimulate ventilation greatly until the PaO_2 decreases to less than 60 mm Hg.

O_2 plays no role in the drive to breathe in healthy individuals at sea level. High altitude causes a healthy person's ventilation to increase because low barometric pressure decreases the inspired PO_2 and the arterial PO_2, which increases the sensitivity of peripheral chemoreceptors to their H^+ environment. The resulting increase in ventilation is less than expected, however, because hyperventilation decreases $PaCO_2$ and increases arterial pH. The increased pH depresses the medullary respiratory center, counteracting the excitatory effect of a low PaO_2 on peripheral chemoreceptors. Hypoxemia-induced hyperventilation may be impossible in certain conditions, such as severe chronic obstructive pulmonary disease (COPD), in which lung mechanics are so deranged that the stimulatory effect of hypoxemia on ventilation fails to decrease $PaCO_2$ regardless of the patient's effort. In such instances, there is no alkalosis to counteract the stimulatory effects of hypoxemia on ventilation.

RULE OF THUMB

Hypoxemia is not associated with an increased drive to breathe until PaO_2 is less than 60 mm Hg, after which the drive to breathe increases proportionally with the decrease in PaO_2.

Response to Increased $PaCO_2$ and Hydrogen Ions

For a given increase in $PaCO_2$ or [H^+], the carotid bodies are less responsive than the central chemoreceptors. The peripheral chemoreceptors account for only 20% to 30% of the ventilatory response to hypercapnia.[5] However, they respond to increased arterial [H^+] more rapidly than the central chemoreceptors. The explanation is that, in contrast to the central chemoreceptors, the carotid bodies are exposed directly to arterial blood. The body's initial ventilatory response to metabolic acidosis is fairly quick, even though H^+ crosses the blood-brain barrier with difficulty.

As stated earlier, hypoxemia increases the sensitivity of the peripheral chemoreceptors to H^+ and indirectly to $PaCO_2$. Conversely, high PaO_2 (hyperoxia) *decreases* the peripheral chemoreceptors' PCO_2 sensitivity to almost zero.[2] This means that when the PaO_2 is high, the ventilatory response to $PaCO_2$ is mainly due to the central chemoreceptors, which are unaffected by hypoxemia.

Because the only effect of hypoxia on the peripheral chemoreceptors is to increase their sensitivity to arterial [H^{++}]—and indirectly to $PaCO_2$—the following statements are true: (1) High PO_2 renders the peripheral chemoreceptors almost unresponsive to PCO_2, and (2) low $PaCO_2$ renders the peripheral chemoreceptors almost unresponsive to hypoxemia.[2] Coexisting arterial hypoxemia, acidemia, and high $PaCO_2$ (i.e., asphyxia) maximally stimulate the peripheral chemoreceptors.

MINI CLINI

Delayed Hyperventilation at High Altitude

PROBLEM: If a person ascends to an elevation of 10,000 feet above sea level, his or her inspired PO_2 decreases because of low barometric pressure; this excites the peripheral chemoreceptors and causes an increase in ventilation. Why must a day or so pass at this altitude before ventilation increases to its maximal level?

SOLUTION: Hypoxia-induced hyperventilation reduces $PaCO_2$ and creates alkalemia. This condition produces an alkalotic CSF because the blood-brain barrier is nearly impermeable to HCO_3^- ions; that is, as CO_2 diffuses out of the CSF in response to the low arterial blood PCO_2, HCO_3^- remains behind in the CSF. The central chemoreceptors are exposed to an alkalotic environment, diminishing the effect of the hypoxic ventilatory stimulus on peripheral chemoreceptors. In other words, the development of respiratory alkalosis limits the degree of hypoxia-induced hyperventilation. Over the first 24 hours or so of hyperventilation, HCO_3^- gradually diffuses out of the CSF across the blood-brain barrier, restoring the CSF pH level to normal. In addition, the kidneys excrete HCO_3^- to compensate for the respiratory alkalemia. Consequently, the blood pH level decreases toward normal, and the hypoxic ventilatory stimulus keeps the $PaCO_2$ low. As the CSF pH level returns to normal, the progressively unrestrained hypoxic stimulus increases ventilation further. It takes approximately 24 hours of high-altitude exposure before ventilation increases to its maximal level.

Individuals with chronic hypercapnia secondary to advanced COPD have depressed ventilatory responses to acute increases in arterial CO_2, partly because of their altered acid-base status and partly because their deranged lung mechanics prevents them from increasing their ventilation adequately.[1] The altered acid-base status arises from the preexisting high levels of blood buffer base, a compensatory response to chronic respiratory acidosis (see Chapter 14).

RULE OF THUMB

The ventilatory response to hypoxemia is greatly enhanced by hypercapnia and acidemia.

Control of Breathing in Chronic Hypercapnia

A sudden increase in arterial PCO_2 causes an immediate increase in ventilation because CO_2 rapidly diffuses from the blood into

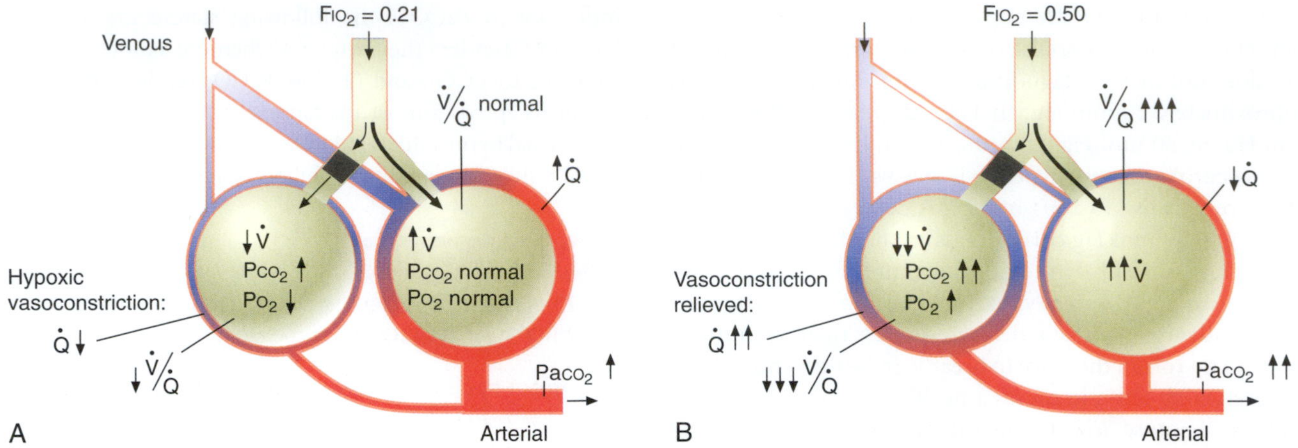

FIGURE 15-5 Proposed mechanism whereby O_2 administration in chronically hypercapnic individuals induces further hypercapnia by creating $\dot{V}/\dot{Q}$ mismatches. **A,** Low $\dot{V}/\dot{Q}$ unit *(left)* is hypoxic and hypercapnic while breathing ambient air; this induces pulmonary vasoconstriction. **B,** Breathing 50% O_2 predisposes the poorly ventilated unit to absorption atelectasis, further decreasing its ventilation, and simultaneously relieves hypoxic vasoconstriction, increasing its blood flow. These events (1) lower the poorly ventilated unit's $\dot{V}/\dot{Q}$ ratio further and (2) divert blood flow away from and ventilation toward already well-ventilated units. The latter increases alveolar dead space (high $\dot{V}/\dot{Q}$). (Modified from Beachey W: Respiratory care anatomy and physiology: foundations for clinical practice, ed 2, St Louis, 2007, Mosby.)

the CSF, increasing the $[H^+]$ surrounding central chemoreceptors. If $PaCO_2$ increases gradually over many years, as might occur in the development of severe COPD and worsening lung mechanics, the kidneys compensate by increasing the plasma $[HCO_3^-]$, which keeps arterial pH within normal limits. As plasma HCO_3^- levels increase, HCO_3^- ions slowly diffuse across the blood-brain barrier, keeping CSF pH within its normal range. Because the central chemoreceptors respond to $[H^+]$, not the CO_2 molecule, they sense a normal pH environment, even though the $PaCO_2$ is abnormally high.

This adaptation explains why the chronically high $PaCO_2$ of people with severe COPD does not overly stimulate their ventilation. Instead, the hypoxemia that accompanies chronic hypercapnia becomes a major part of the minute-to-minute breathing stimulus in the roundabout way discussed previously; hypoxemia increases the sensitivity of the peripheral chemoreceptors to $[H^+]$, increasing the nerve impulses they transmit to the medulla, which stimulates ventilation. Patients with severe COPD are invariably hypoxemic when breathing room air because their lungs have ventilation and blood flow mismatches. It stands to reason that breathing supplemental O_2 would increase the PaO_2 and make the carotid bodies less sensitive to $[H^+]$, which would decrease ventilation further and increase the $PaCO_2$.

Oxygen-Associated Hypercapnia

The $PaCO_2$ of chronically hypercapnic patients with COPD sometimes increases acutely after these patients are given supplemental O_2. The reason for this phenomenon has been a subject of much debate and misunderstanding. The traditional explanation for this phenomenon has been that O_2 breathing removes the hypoxic ventilatory stimulus and induces hypoventilation, but this explanation is probably overly simplified. The reduction in minute ventilation after O_2 breathing in patients with advanced COPD is generally severe enough to account for the increased $PaCO_2$. The most significant reason for hypercapnia following O_2 breathing in severe COPD is that it worsens the ventilation-perfusion ($\dot{V}/\dot{Q}$) relationships in the lungs.

When patients with severe COPD breathe supplemental O_2 it abolishes the hypoxic pulmonary vasoconstriction present in poorly ventilated lung regions. As a result, vascular resistance of underventilated regions decreases, and these areas receive more blood flow, drawing blood away from well-ventilated regions (Figure 15-5). At the same time that poorly ventilated regions receive more blood flow, they become even less ventilated as O_2-rich inspired gas washes out resident nitrogen gas, making these alveoli more subject to absorption atelectasis (i.e., O_2 may be absorbed by the pulmonary circulation more rapidly than the slowed ventilation can replenish it—notice the further decreased $\dot{V}$ in Figure 15-5, *B*). As a result, inspired gas flows preferentially to the compliant, already well-ventilated alveoli (see Figure 15-5, *B*), increasing their $\dot{V}/\dot{Q}$. The increased $\dot{V}/\dot{Q}$ in these alveoli is exaggerated further as a greater proportion of the cardiac output than before is redirected to poorly ventilated alveoli, because their vascular resistance was reduced by O_2 breathing.

To summarize, O_2 breathing causes more blood flow to be directed to poorly ventilated alveoli, which takes blood flow away from well-ventilated alveoli. The key point is that already underventilated alveoli receive additional blood flow, which causes blood PCO_2 to increase further. These events can occur without a decrease in overall minute ventilation.

It is important to keep in mind that the diagnosis of COPD on a patient's medical record does not mean the patient has a chronically high $PaCO_2$ or that O_2 administration may be associated with hypercapnia. These characteristics are present only in severe end-stage disease, which includes only a small percentage of patients with a COPD diagnosis. Concern about

O_2-associated hypercapnia and acidemia is not justifiable in most patients with a diagnosis of COPD. O_2 should never be withheld from acutely hypoxemic patients with COPD for fear of inducing hypoventilation and hypercapnia. Tissue oxygenation is the overriding priority; O_2 must never be withheld from exacerbated, hypoxemic patients with COPD for any reason. The clinician must be prepared to support ventilation mechanically if O_2 administration is accompanied by severe hypoventilation.

Central Chemoreceptor Response to Acute Carbon Dioxide Increase in Chronic Hypercapnia

As discussed earlier, the kidneys compensate for the acidic effects of chronic hypercapnia by increasing the plasma HCO_3^- level, keeping the medullary chemoreceptor pH environment in the normal range. This does not mean that the medullary chemoreceptors cannot respond to further *acute* increases in $PaCO_2$. A sudden elevation in $PaCO_2$ immediately crosses the blood-brain barrier into the CSF, generating H^+ that then stimulates the medullary chemoreceptors. The resulting ventilatory response is depressed, however, for chemical and mechanical reasons: (1) The blood's increased buffering capacity (high HCO_3^- level) in chronic hypercapnia prevents arterial pH from decreasing as sharply as it would in normal conditions, and (2) abnormal breathing mechanics hamper the lung's ability to increase ventilation appropriately. To illustrate the blood's changed buffering capacity, compare a healthy person (pH = 7.40, $PaCO_2$ = 40 mm Hg, HCO_3^- = 24 mEq/L) with a chronically hypercapnic person (pH = 7.38, $PaCO_2$ = 60 mm Hg, HCO_3^- = 34 mEq/L). A sudden increase of 30 mm Hg in $PaCO_2$ of both individuals causes the healthy person's arterial pH to decrease to 7.21 and the hypercapnic person's pH to decrease to only 7.24. (These values are calculated using the Henderson-Hasselbalch equation, assuming a 1-mEq/L increase in plasma HCO_3^- concentration for each acute increase of 10 mm Hg in $PaCO_2$.) The central chemoreceptors of a chronically hypercapnic patient experience less stimulation than the central chemoreceptors of normal individuals for the same increase in $PaCO_2$.

> **RULE OF THUMB**
>
> Tissue oxygenation is of overriding importance and must not be sacrificed because of concern about hypercapnia and acidemia in a patient with exacerbated COPD.

VENTILATORY RESPONSE TO EXERCISE

Strenuous exercise can increase CO_2 production and O_2 consumption by 20-fold.[3] Ventilation normally keeps pace with CO_2 production, keeping $PaCO_2$, PaO_2, and arterial pH constant. Because arterial blood gases do not change during normal exercise, some other mechanism must be responsible for the increased ventilation in healthy individuals during exertion.

The exact mechanism responsible for this increase in ventilation is not well understood. Especially mysterious is the abrupt increase in ventilation at the onset of exercise, long before any chemical or humoral changes can occur in the body. Two predominating theories for this phenomenon are: (1) When the cerebral motor cortex sends impulses to exercising muscles, it apparently sends collateral excitatory impulses to the medullary respiratory centers; (2) exercising limbs moving around their joints stimulate proprioceptors, which transmit excitatory impulses to the medullary centers.[1,3] Evidence also suggests that the sudden increase in ventilation at the onset of exercise is a learned response.[1,3] With repeated experience, the brain may learn to anticipate the proper amount of ventilation required to maintain normal blood gases during exercise.

ABNORMAL BREATHING PATTERNS

Commonly described abnormal breathing patterns include Cheyne-Stokes respiration, Biot respiration, apneustic breathing, and central neurogenic hypoventilation and hyperventilation. In **Cheyne-Stokes respiration,** respiratory rate and tidal volume gradually increase and then gradually decrease to complete **apnea** (absence of ventilation), which may last several seconds. Tidal volume and breathing frequency gradually increase again, repeating the cycle. This pattern occurs when cardiac output is low, as in congestive heart failure, delaying the blood transit time between the lungs and the brain.[4] In this instance, changes in respiratory center PCO_2 lag behind changes in arterial PCO_2.

For example, when an increased $PaCO_2$ from the lungs reaches the respiratory neurons, ventilation is stimulated; this lowers the $PaCO_2$ level. By the time the reduced $PaCO_2$ reaches the medulla to inhibit ventilation, hyperventilation has been in progress for an inappropriately long time. When blood from the lung finally does reach the medullary centers, the low $PaCO_2$ greatly depresses ventilation to the point of apnea. $PaCO_2$ increases, but an increase in respiratory center PCO_2 is delayed because of low blood flow rate. The brain eventually does receive the high $PaCO_2$ signal, and the cycle is repeated. Cheyne-Stokes respiration may also be caused by brain injuries in which the respiratory centers over-respond to changes in the PCO_2 level.

Biot respiration is similar to Cheyne-Stokes respiration except that tidal volumes are of identical depth. It occurs in patients with increased intracranial pressure (ICP), but the mechanism for this pattern is unclear.[4]

Apneustic breathing indicates damage to the pons. Central neurogenic hyperventilation is characterized by persistent hyperventilation driven by abnormal neural stimuli. It is related to midbrain and upper pons damage associated with head trauma, severe brain hypoxia, or lack of blood flow to the brain.[6] Conversely, central neurogenic hypoventilation means the respiratory centers do not respond appropriately to ventilatory stimuli, such as CO_2. It also is associated with head trauma and brain hypoxia as well as narcotic suppression of the respiratory center.[6]

CARBON DIOXIDE AND CEREBRAL BLOOD FLOW

CO_2 plays an important role in regulating cerebral blood flow. Its effect is mediated through the formation of H^+ by CO_2.[7] Increased PCO_2 dilates cerebral vessels, increasing cerebral blood flow, whereas decreased PCO_2 constricts cerebral vessels and reduces cerebral blood flow. In patients with traumatic brain injury (TBI), the brain swells acutely; this increases the ICP in the rigid skull to such high levels that blood supply to the brain might be cut off, causing cerebral hypoxia *(ischemia)*. That is, high ICP may exceed cerebral arterial pressure and stop blood flow to the brain.

Although controversial, mechanical hyperventilation has been used for many years in selected patients with TBI to decrease $PaCO_2$ and reduce the cerebral blood flow and ICP. In patients with TBI, a cerebral blood volume reduction of only 0.5 to 0.7 ml reduces the ICP by 1 mm Hg; for every 1-mm Hg acute reduction in $PaCO_2$ (between 20 mm Hg and 60 mm Hg), there is a 3% reduction in cerebral blood flow. Although an acute reduction in $PaCO_2$ reduces ICP, it also reduces cerebral blood flow and potentially causes cerebral ischemia. For this reason, the practice of inducing mechanical hyperventilation in patients with TBI is debatable primarily because it may well reduce blood flow and O_2 to an injured organ. On the other end of the spectrum; however, *hypoventilation* in a head trauma patient with an already high ICP is especially dangerous because hypercapnia dilates cerebral vessels and elevates the ICP even more.

The debate centers around the question of whether a hyperventilation-induced decrease in cerebral blood flow creates an additional hypoxic insult to the already ischemic brain and whether patients managed in this way have better clinical outcomes than patients in whom hyperventilation is not instituted. A comprehensive review of the subject published in 2005 concluded that hyperventilation produced no advantage in long-term clinical outcome of TBI compared with ventilation that maintained $PaCO_2$ in the normal range.[7] The authors concluded that in TBI, hyperventilation therapy should be considered only for patients with high ICPs; no benefit can be expected if ICP is normal. They further concluded that hyperventilation is most appropriate in the second or third day after injury because cerebral blood flow is lowest in the first 24 hours after injury, and the risk for inducing ischemia through hyperventilation is greatest during this time. The authors advise against the hyperventilation of patients with TBI to $PaCO_2$ less than 30 mm Hg because of the increased danger of cerebral ischemia. Finally, hyperventilation is effective for only approximately 24 to 48 hours because compensatory renal elimination of HCO_3^- in the face of alkalemia restores the acid-base balance, negating the vasoconstrictive effect of hypocapnia. In any case, *hypoventilation* in patients with head trauma and increased ICP is especially dangerous because hypercapnia dilates cerebral vessels and increases ICP further. Even opponents of hyperventilation generally maintain $PaCO_2$ of patients with TBI in the low to normal range at approximately 35 mm Hg.[8]

MINI CLINI

Mechanical Hyperventilation of a Patient With Traumatic Brain Injury

PROBLEM: An automobile accident victim, previously healthy, sustained a closed head injury with accompanying high ICP. Mechanical ventilation in the intensive care unit is required, and the physician asks the RT for input regarding ventilator strategies and what $PaCO_2$ should be targeted?

DISCUSSION: More than 40 years ago, clinical investigators showed that the volume of the swollen brain could be reduced by decreasing the $PaCO_2$. Since then, mechanical hyperventilation has been a cornerstone in managing increased ICP associated with TBI.[7] Hyperventilation decreases ICP by causing cerebral vasoconstriction, ultimately reducing cerebral blood volume. This subject is not without controversy because hyperventilation-induced cerebral vasoconstriction has the potential to reduce cerebral blood flow to levels that cause cerebral hypoxia *(ischemia)*. This concern has dampened enthusiasm for hyperventilation in TBI. Both the proponents and the opponents of hyperventilation recognize that TBI poses an ischemic threat to the brain; proponents believe that the reduction of cerebral blood flow ultimately improves cerebral oxygenation by reducing the ICP, which helps sustain the cerebral perfusion pressure. Opponents point out that no other hypoxic organ in the body is treated by reducing its blood flow and O_2 supply. (Hyperventilation in this context is generally defined as $PaCO_2 < 35$ mm Hg.[7])

SUMMARY CHECKLIST

- The DRGs and VRGs of neurons in the medulla generate the basic cyclic breathing pattern.
- Apneustic center impulses prevent medullary inspiratory neurons from switching off, creating a prolonged, gasping inspiration.
- Impulses from the pneumotaxic center inhibit the apneustic center and inspiratory neurons of the DRGs, shortening inspiratory time and increasing respiratory rate.
- Various reflexes from peripheral sources affect the breathing pattern by altering the output of the medullary center.
- Central chemoreceptors in the medulla are bathed in the CSF, separated from arterial blood by a semipermeable membrane called the *blood-brain barrier*.
- The blood-brain barrier is almost impermeable to arterial H^+ and HCO_3^- ions, but it is freely permeable to arterial CO_2.
- Central chemoreceptors stimulate increased ventilation in response to the H^+ formed in the CSF by the reaction between arterial CO_2 and H_2O.
- Peripheral chemoreceptors, located mainly in the carotid bodies, respond to arterial $[H^+]$; hypoxemia increases the sensitivity of chemoreceptors to a given arterial pH.
- The peripheral chemoreceptors are indirectly stimulated by arterial CO_2 to the extent that CO_2 reacts with H_2O to form H^+.

- The primary stimulus for breathing in healthy individuals is arterial CO_2, mediated through the central chemoreceptors via H^+ formed by the reaction between H_2O and CO_2 molecules.
- The secondary stimulus for breathing in healthy individuals is arterial hypoxemia, which is not clinically significant until PaO_2 is less than 60 mm Hg.
- Breathing of patients with chronic, compensated hypercapnia is driven more by the hypoxic stimulus than when acid-base status is normal.
- O_2 therapy is associated with acute arterial CO_2 retention and acidosis in patients with chronic hypercapnia.
- O_2 should never be withheld for any reason from patients with severe hypoxemia.
- CO_2 dilates cerebral blood vessels and increases ICP; reducing arterial CO_2 constricts cerebral vessels and decreases ICP.

References

1. Levitzky MG: *Pulmonary physiology*, ed 8, New York, 2013, McGraw-Hill Medical.
2. Philipson EA, Duffin J: Hypoventilation and hyperventilation syndromes. In Mason RJ, Broaddus VC, Martin TR, et al, editors: *Murray and Nadel's textbook of respiratory medicine*, ed 5, Philadelphia, 2010, Saunders.
3. Hall JE: *Guyton and Hall: textbook of medical physiology*, ed 12, Philadelphia, 2010, Saunders.
4. Comroe JH: *Physiology of respiration*, ed 2, Chicago, 1974, Year Book.
5. West JB: *Respiratory physiology: the essentials*, ed 9, Philadelphia, 2011, Lippincott Williams & Wilkins.
6. Bleck TP: Levels of consciousness and attention. In Goetz CG, editor: *Textbook of clinical neurology*, ed 2, Philadelphia, 2003, Saunders.
7. Stocchetti N, Maas AI, Chieregato A, et al: Hyperventilation in head injury: a review. *Chest* 127:1812, 2005.
8. Korbakis G, Bleck TP: The evolution of neurocritical care. *Crit Care Clin.* 30:657–671, 2014.

SECTION III

ASSESSMENT OF RESPIRATORY DISORDERS

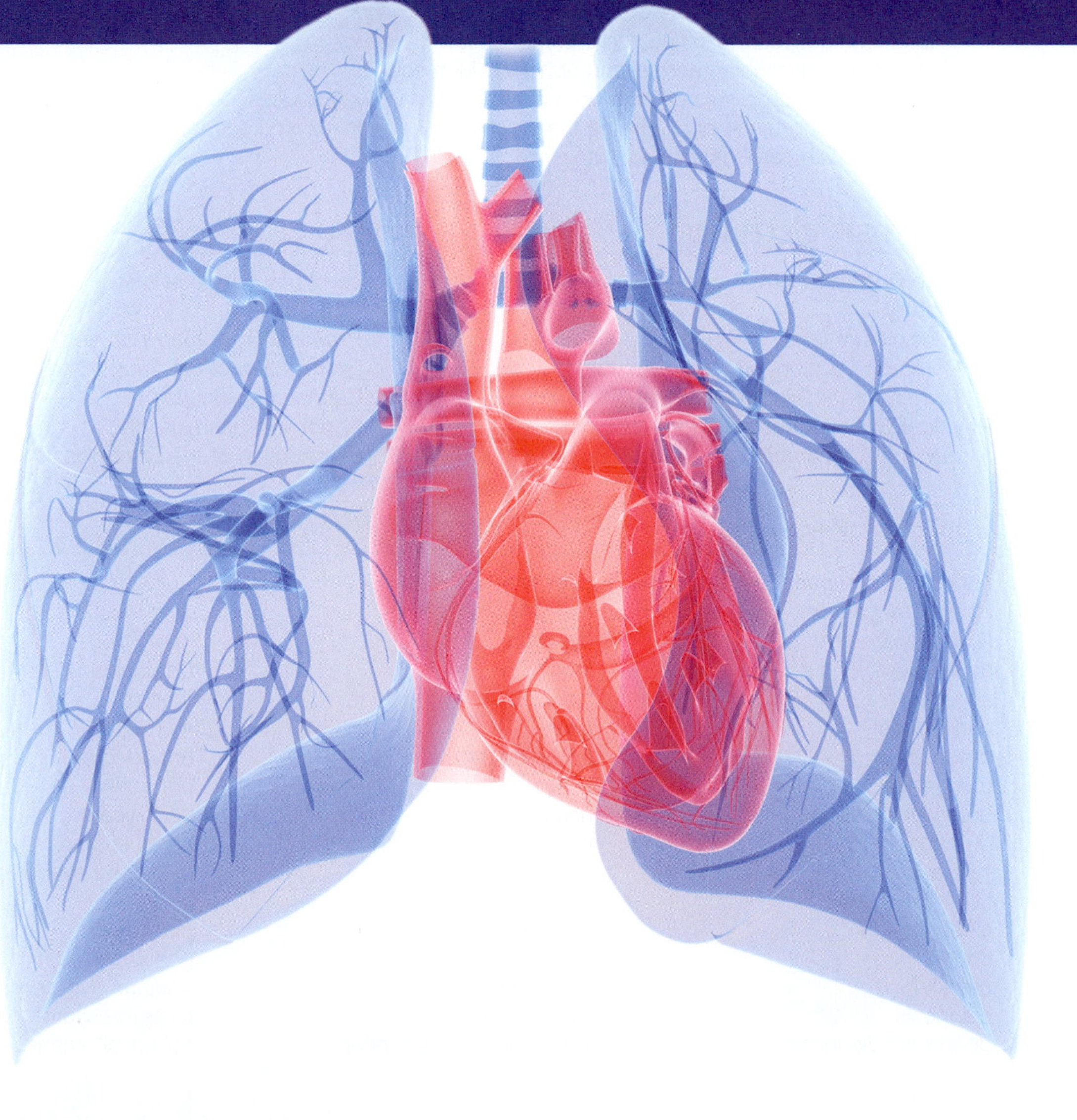

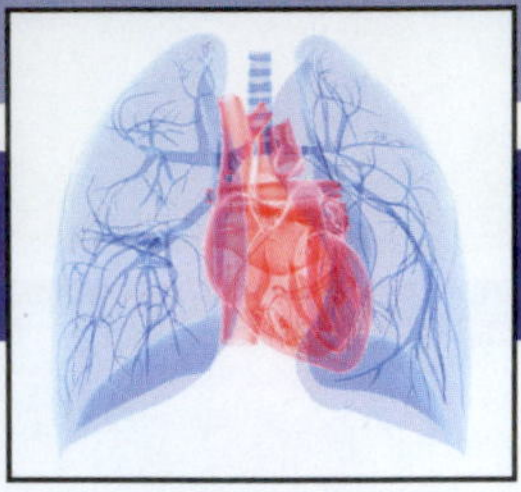

CHAPTER 16

Bedside Assessment of the Patient

RICHARD H. KALLET

CHAPTER OBJECTIVES

After reading this chapter you will be able to:

- Describe why patient interviews are necessary and the appropriate interview techniques.
- Identify abnormalities in lung function associated with common pulmonary symptoms.
- Identify breathing patterns associated with pulmonary disease.
- Differentiate between dyspnea and breathlessness.
- Identify terms describing normal and abnormal lung sounds.
- Describe the mechanisms causing normal and abnormal lung sounds.
- Review the importance of examining the precordium, abdomen, and extremities to identify abnormalities associated with cardiopulmonary disease.

CHAPTER OUTLINE

Interviewing the Patient and Taking a Medical History
- Principles of Interviewing
- Common Cardiopulmonary Symptoms
- Format for the Medical History

Physical Examination
- General Appearance
- Level of Consciousness
- Vital Signs
- Examination of the Head and Neck
- Examination of the Thorax and Lungs
- Cardiac Examination
- Abdominal Examination
- Examination of the Extremities

KEY TERMS

abdominal compartment syndrome
abdominal paradox
advance directive
adventitious lung sounds
angina
barrel chest
bradycardia
bradypnea
breathlessness
bronchophony
cachexia
central cyanosis
clubbing
cough
crackles
diagnosis
differential diagnosis
diaphoresis
diastolic pressure
dyspnea
febrile
fetid
fever
gallop rhythm
heave
hematemesis
hemoptysis
hepatomegaly
Hoover sign
hypertension
hypotension
hypothermia
hypovolemia
jugular venous distention
Kussmaul breathing
Kussmaul sign
loud P_2
lymphadenopathy
mucoid
murmurs
orthodeoxia
orthopnea
pack-years
pedal edema
peripheral cyanosis
phlegm
platypnea
pneumothorax
postural hypotension
pulse pressure
pulsus alternans

pulsus paradoxus
purulent
rales
respiratory alternans
retractions
sensorium
shock
signs
sputum
stridor
subcutaneous emphysema
symptoms
syncope
systolic pressure
tachycardia
tachypnea
thrills
tracheal tugging
trepopnea
tripodding
wheezes

Decisions regarding when to initiate, change, or discontinue therapy depend on accurate clinical assessments. The physician is ultimately responsible for these decisions. But because respiratory therapists (RTs) often participate in clinical decision making, they must develop competent bedside assessment skills. To do this effectively, the RT must assume responsibility for gathering and interpreting relevant bedside patient data.

Bedside assessment is the process of interviewing and examining a patient for signs and symptoms of disease, as well as evaluating the effects of treatment. Very often bedside assessment provides initial evidence that something is wrong. In contrast to some diagnostic tests, bedside assessment techniques are of little risk to the patient.

Two key sources of patient data are the medical history and the physical examination. Data gathered during the initial interview and physical examination help identify the need for subsequent diagnostic tests. After a tentative diagnosis is made, these assessment skills help the clinician in selecting the best therapy. These assessment skills are used repeatedly to monitor the patient's response to therapy, and make any necessary adjustments.

The patient initially is assessed to identify the correct diagnosis. **Diagnosis** (from the Greek *to know thoroughly*), is the process of identifying the nature and cause of illness. It is a disciplined, systematic approach based on careful history taking, physical examination and testing (e.g., laboratory analysis of blood or tissue samples, radiologic examinations, etc.). **Differential diagnosis** is the term used when signs and symptoms are shared by many diseases and the exact cause is unclear. For example a cough can be a symptom of a common cold, pneumonia, bronchitis, or congestive heart failure (CHF). **Signs** refer to the *objective manifestation* of illness (e.g., increased respiratory rate) whereas **symptoms** refer the sensation or *subjective experience* of some aspect of an illness (e.g., breathlessness). Symptoms must always be stated by the patient and never inferred from observed signs. Common symptoms and signs associated with cardiopulmonary disease are discussed in this chapter.

Diagnosis is performed primarily by a physician. Exceptions may occur in emergency situations when a physician is unavailable. In such cases, nurses and RTs may evaluate the patient to rapidly implement appropriate lifesaving therapy (e.g., cardiopulmonary resuscitation).

The mastery of bedside assessment skills described here requires practice. Initially, students should practice these skills on healthy individuals. This helps improve technique and provides an understanding of normal variations. The ability to discriminate abnormal findings from the range of normal findings is an important skill that requires experience to master.

INTERVIEWING THE PATIENT AND TAKING A MEDICAL HISTORY

Interviewing furnishes unique information because it provides the patient's perspective. It serves the following three related purposes:

1. To establish a rapport between the clinician and patient.
2. To obtain information essential for making a diagnosis.
3. To help monitor changes in the patient's symptoms and response to therapy.

MINI CLINI

Bedside Assessment of the Postoperative Patient

PROBLEM: The RT is called to see a 54-year-old woman who underwent abdominal surgery 2 days earlier. She is currently afebrile, alert, and oriented but is complaining of dyspnea. Her resting respiratory rate is 34 breaths/min, and the breaths are shallow. Her heart rate is 110 beats/min. She is 5 feet tall and weighs approximately 185 lb. During the brief interview, the RT identifies that the dyspnea has gradually increased over the past 12 hours and increases with exertion. The RT auscultates diminished breath sounds in the bases, with some fine, late inspiratory crackles. The remainder of the physical examination is normal. What is the most likely cause of this patient's dyspnea, and what should be done?

SOLUTION: The findings indicate a loss of lung volume as the cause of the sudden dyspnea. The rapid, shallow breathing; fine, late inspiratory crackles; and history of recent abdominal surgery suggest atelectasis. Patients who undergo abdominal surgery are prone to developing atelectasis in the postoperative period. The differential diagnosis would include CHF and pulmonary thromboembolism. The RT should ask the attending physician to order a chest radiograph and begin lung expansion therapy if the chest film confirms the presence of atelectasis.

Principles of Interviewing

Interviewing is the process of gathering relevant information from a patient, an essential element of which involves establishing rapport. Building rapport with a patient requires basic human skills of communicating concern, warmth, and empathy. Illness serious enough to require hospitalization causes stress. Meaningful human contact lessens a patient's sense of isolation and helps reduce stress. Factors affecting communication between the RT and the patient include the following:

- Sensory and emotional factors
- Environmental factors
- Verbal and nonverbal components of the communication process
- Cultural and other internal values, beliefs, feelings, habits, and preoccupations of *both* the RT and the patient.

Because of these factors, no two interviews are the same. Developing interview skills takes time and experience. This requires adherence to some basic interview techniques and becoming knowledgeable about the causes and characteristics of common cardiopulmonary symptoms. The following discussion provides some guidelines for interviewing and discusses common symptoms associated with diseases of the chest.

Structure and Technique for Interviewing

The ideal interview makes the patient feel secure enough to talk openly about important personal matters. Each interview should begin with the RT introducing himself or herself to the patient, and stating the purpose of the visit. To begin the process of establishing rapport, the introduction is done from the nonthreatening position referred to as *social space,* approximately 4 to 12 feet from the patient. Bear in mind that the perception of "appropriate" space varies across individuals and particularly those of different cultural backgrounds. Pulling the curtain between the beds of a semiprivate room also may be helpful in making the patient feel more at ease with the interview (Box 16-1).

Next, the RT might be able to move into what is considered *personal space* (2 to 4 feet from the patient) to begin the interview. In this space, the patient does not have to speak loudly in response to questions. The RT should assume a physical position at the same level with the patient (e.g., by sitting in a chair) before beginning the formal interview. Avoid standing over the patient, because this may feel intimidating and foster uneasiness. Appropriate eye contact with the patient is essential for a high-quality interview. Eye contact gives the patient more confidence in the interviewer. It also allows the interviewer to observe facial expressions that may communicate a patient's confusion, fear, frustration, or other emotions in response.

Use neutral questions and avoid leading questions during the interview. For example, asking the patient, "Is your breathing better now?" leads the patient toward a desired response and may elicit false information. Rather ask the patient, "How is your breathing now?" Often this gets more accurate information (Box 16-2).

Common characteristics of symptoms can be identified by asking the following questions during the interview:

- When did the symptom start?
- How severe is it? (This can be rated on a scale of 1 to 10.)
- Where on the body is it? (This is especially important for chest pain.)

Box 16-1 Guidelines for Effective Patient Interviewing

PROJECT A SENSE OF UNDIVIDED INTEREST IN THE PATIENT

- Provide for privacy and do not permit interruptions.
- Review records and prepare materials before entering the room.
- Listen and observe carefully.
- Use appropriate eye contact.
- Be attentive and respond to the patient's priorities, concerns, feelings, and comfort.

ESTABLISH YOUR PROFESSIONAL ROLE DURING THE INTRODUCTION

- Dress and groom professionally.
- Enter the room with a smile and unhurried manner.
- Make immediate eye contact.
- If the patient is well enough, introduce yourself with a firm handshake.
- State your role and the purpose of your visit, and define the patient's involvement in the interaction.
- Address adult patients by title (e.g., Mr., Mrs., Ms.) and their last name. Using these formal terms of address alerts the patient to the importance of the interaction.

SHOW YOUR RESPECT FOR THE PATIENT'S BELIEFS, ATTITUDES, AND RIGHTS

- Ensure the patient is appropriately covered.
- Position yourself so that eye contact is comfortable for the patient. (Ideally, patients should be sitting up, with their eye level at or slightly above yours.)
- Avoid standing at the foot of the bed or with your hand on the door because this may send the nonverbal message that you do not have time for the patient.
- Ask the patient's permission before moving any personal items or making adjustments in the room.
- Remember that the patient's dialogue with you and his or her medical record are confidential. Share this information only with other health care providers who need to know about it, and do not share the information in a place where others can overhear the conversation.
- Be honest; never guess at an answer or information that you do not know; do not provide information beyond your scope of practice; providing new information to the patient is the privilege and responsibility of the attending physician.
- Make no moral judgments about the patient; set your values for patient care according to the patient's values, beliefs, and priorities.
- Expect the patient to have an emotional response to illness and the health care environment.
- Listen, and then clarify and teach, but never argue.
- Adjust the time, length, and content of the interview to the patient's needs.

USE A RELAXED, CONVERSATIONAL STYLE

- Ask questions and make statements that communicate empathy.
- Encourage the patient to express his or her concerns.
- Expect and accept some periods of silence.
- Close even the briefest interview by asking whether there is anything the patient needs or wants to discuss.
- Tell the patient when you will return.

Box 16-2 Types of Questions Used in Patient Interviews

- *Open-ended questions* encourage patients to describe events and priorities as they see them, helping to bring out concerns and attitudes and to promote understanding. Questions such as "What brought you to the hospital?" or "What happened next?" encourage conversational flow and rapport, while giving patients enough direction to know where to start.
- *Closed questions,* such as "When did your cough start?" or "How long did the pain last?" focus on specific information and provide clarification.
- *Direct questions* can be open-ended or closed and always end in a question mark. Although they are used to obtain specific information, a series of direct questions or frequent use of the question "Why?" can be intimidating and cause the patient to minimize his or her responses to questions.
- *Indirect questions* are less threatening than direct questions because they sound like statements (e.g., "I gather your doctor told you to take the treatments every 4 hours"). Inquiries of this type also work well to confront discrepancies in the patient's statements (e.g., "If I understood you correctly, it is harder for you to breathe now than it was before your treatment").
- *Neutral questions* and statements are preferred for all interactions with the patient. "What happened next?" and "Can you tell me more about … ?" are neutral, open-ended questions. A neutral, closed question may give the patient a choice of responses, while focusing on the type of information desired (e.g., "Would you say there was a teaspoon, a tablespoon, or a half cup?"). Leading questions, such as "You didn't cough up blood, did you?" should be avoided because they imply an answer.

- What seems to make it better or worse?
- Has it occurred before? (If so, how long did it last?)

Identifying characteristics of any new symptom may be helpful in determining the cause and selecting appropriate therapy. Once therapy is started, further questions are used to evaluate the changes in the symptoms over the course of treatment. For example, the clinician may ask, "Has the symptom changed in any way since admission?" or, "Does the therapy seem to make a difference?"

The best interview techniques are worthless if the interviewer lacks knowledge about the pathophysiology and characteristic symptoms of common cardiopulmonary diseases. Essentially the interview is a series of focused questions pursuing specific information related to a tentative diagnosis. The ability to ask key questions at the right time comes from experience and familiarity with the signs and symptoms of lung disease.

Common Cardiopulmonary Symptoms

Dyspnea

Dyspnea is a *general term* describing the sensation of breathing discomfort. It is the most important symptom that the RT is called upon to assess and treat. Dyspnea is a *subjective experience* and should never be inferred from observing a patient's breathing pattern. Dyspnea and pain are similar in that both sensations possess qualitatively distinct features and have varying intensity. Similar to pain, dyspnea causes suffering. *As breathing is the primordial sensation of life,* dyspnea often is perceived as life-threatening and may provoke a profound sense of dread.

The term *dyspnea* also is used *specifically* to describe *difficulty in the mechanical act of breathing*. In essence, dyspnea occurs when the effort to breathe is disproportionately greater than the tidal volume achieved. The perception of breathing is a complex balance among three factors:

1. The neural drive to breathe emanating from the respiratory centers in the brainstem
2. The tension developed in the respiratory muscles
3. The corresponding displacement of the lungs and chest wall

When the neuronal signals governing these sensations become unbalanced, breathing is perceived to be abnormal and unpleasant. The technical name for this imbalance is *neuromechanical dissociation*. A normal individual experiences dyspnea only in unusual circumstances, such as trying to breathe through a straw or when wearing a restrictive garment.

Breathlessness. In contrast, **breathlessness** is an *unpleasant urge to breathe*. It is believed to be the conscious perception of intense neural discharge from the brainstem to the respiratory muscles. Breathlessness can be triggered by acute hypercapnia, acidosis, or hypoxemia. A normal experience of breathlessness is the unpleasant "throbbing" sensation induced by breath holding, or feeling "winded" during strenuous exercise. However, it is unknown whether these normal encounters with breathlessness actually resemble the sensation that arises in patients with cardiopulmonary disease. This is because dyspnea and breathlessness are influenced by other stimuli, including those arising from irritant receptors in the lungs and airways, as well as receptors in the blood vessels and heart. These various stimuli shape both the quality and intensity of the sensation.

Moreover, dyspnea and breathlessness are perpetuated and magnified by the emotional distress that accompanies them. This emotional distress is influenced by the situation, knowledge, and control. For example, a healthy person can quickly identify the source of breathlessness and arrest the symptom simply by stopping exercise or the breath hold. But a patient with cardiopulmonary disease often cannot control the symptom, let alone identify the source. This has a profound emotional impact that must be appreciated.

Positional Dyspnea. Dyspnea that is triggered when the patient assumes the reclining position is called **orthopnea** and is common in patients with CHF, mitral valve disease, and superior vena cava syndrome. **Platypnea** is dyspnea triggered by assuming the upright position. It typically occurs after pneumonectomy and in patients with chronic liver disease (hepatopulmonary syndrome). It is sometimes observed during hypovolemia and in some neurologic diseases. Platypnea may be accompanied by **orthodeoxia,** which is oxygen desaturation on assuming an upright position. **Trepopnea** is when lying on one side relieves dyspnea, It is usually associated with either CHF or pleural effusion.

Language of Dyspnea. Because dyspnea is a subjective experience, patients possess a nuanced language to describe their sensations. RTs should ask specific questions about the quality and characteristics of the patient's dyspnea. In this way, the RT might gain insight into the mechanism provoking dyspnea. The RT should try to categorize each sensation according to a particular aspect of breathing: inspiration, expiration, respiratory drive, or lung volume. A remark such as, "I feel that my breath stops," reflects a problem with inspiration, whereas the remark, "my breath does not go all the way out," suggests a problem with expiration. Statements such as, "I can't catch my breath," suggest elevated respiratory drive (i.e., breathlessness).

Different lung diseases often evoke unique sensations. Patients with asthma frequently complain of chest tightness, whereas, patients with interstitial lung disease tend to focus on the sensations of increased work of breathing, shallow breathing, and gasping. Unique to patients with CHF is the feeling of suffocation. However, the RT should keep in mind that many lung diseases evoke common sensations.

Patients with cardiopulmonary disease frequently experience several unpleasant breathing sensations simultaneously. A particular sensation may be more prominent than others and may change over time. For example, patients with asthma typically complain first about the sensation of chest tightness. As bronchoconstriction worsens and the lungs become more hyperinflated, patients often begin to focus more on the sensation of excessive work of breathing, air hunger, and the inability to take a deep breath.

Assessing Dyspnea in the Interview. Assessing dyspnea is largely determined by the situation. During the interview, the RT should pay particular attention to whether the patient can speak in full sentences. Patients with severe dyspnea often cannot speak more than a few words at a time. In this situation, the initial interview should be curtailed, and treatment should be initiated as soon as possible. Questions should be brief and when possible structured to elicit a yes or no response. Questions should be limited to the quality and intensity of dyspnea, the circumstances surrounding the onset, and current duration of dyspnea. The assessment of dyspnea should occur simultaneously with a gross examination of the patient's breathing pattern (see later section of this chapter). Assessment of acute dyspnea in patients without a prior history of cardiopulmonary disease does not require the same detail as in patients with longstanding cardiopulmonary or neurologic disease.

In patients with chronic cardiopulmonary disease, a detailed and systematic history should cover four major areas, as follows:

1. The RT should ask what activities of daily living tend to trigger episodes of dyspnea. For example, is dyspnea triggered by walking on flat surfaces, by climbing stairs, by bathing, by dressing?
2. The RT should ask how much exertion makes the patient to stop to catch his or her breath with different activities. Does the patient need to stop after walking up one flight of stairs or one step? Dyspnea provoked by less strenuous activities indicates more advanced disease.

Modified Borg Scale

Number	Verbal Description
10	Severe
9	
8	Moderately severe
7	
6	
5	Moderate
4	
3	
2	Slight
1	
0	None

A

Visual Scale

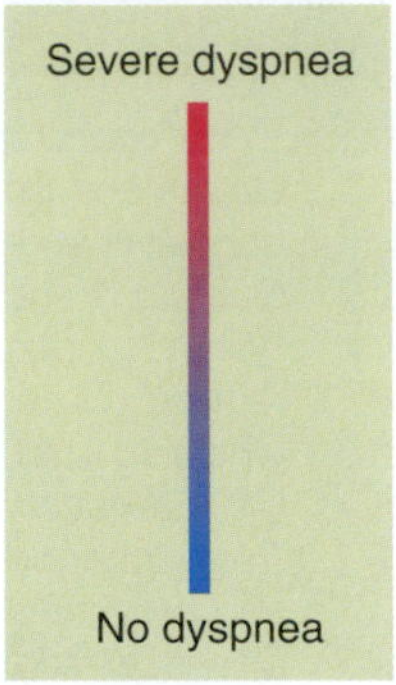

B

FIGURE 16-1 A, Modified Borg scale. **B,** Visual analogue scale for measuring the degree of dyspnea.

3. The RT should ask whether the quality or the sensation of breathing discomfort varies with different activities.
4. To gain a better understanding of the patient's history, ask the patient to recall when dyspnea first began and how it has evolved over time. Has dyspnea progressed slowly or rapidly? How long has this progression taken place: over a period of months or years? Has there been a dramatic change in the intensity of dyspnea over the recent past?

Beyond the information gleaned, a detailed conversation about patients' dyspnea allows them to share their experience and may decrease their sense of isolation.

The intensity of dyspnea can be documented using a numeric intensity or visual analogue scale (Figure 16-1). Such scales provide a way to evaluate the patient's response to treatment over time. These scales are important because, in many patients, objective measurements of lung function (e.g., pulmonary function tests, PaO_2) seldom correlate with the degree of dyspnea.

Psychogenic Dyspnea: Panic Disorders and Hyperventilation. There are perplexing situations in which a patient with normal cardiopulmonary function complains of dyspnea or suffocation. This is known as *psychogenic hyperventilation syndrome* and is associated with panic disorders. Hyperventilation may coincide with other symptoms such as chest pain, anxiety, palpitations, and *paresthesia* (the sensation of tingling and numbness in the extremities that accompanies respiratory alkalosis). This syndrome may be either sporadic or chronic and often is self-perpetuating.

Anxiety often is accompanied by breathlessness and hyperventilation. The resulting respiratory alkalosis amplifies the sensation of breathlessness and provokes more anxiety. This in turn increases the intensity of hyperventilation. The classic homespun remedy of slowly rebreathing into a paper bag holds merit, because this arrests respiratory alkalosis and helps break the cycle. However, rebreathing techniques may require formal behavioral therapy and may not be appropriate in the hospital setting. This condition usually is treated clinically by administering judicious amounts of anxiolytic agents.

The RT *always* must approach any situation involving hyperventilation or dyspnea as if it had a pathogenic basis. The first priority is to measure the vital signs, including SaO_2, and perhaps a 12-lead electrocardiogram and arterial blood gases. A psychogenic source is considered *only* after a pathogenic source for hyperventilation or dyspnea has been ruled out. Intense pain or fear often provokes anxiety and hyperventilation. The RT must work in concert with nurses and the physician to determine the root-cause of any hyperventilation syndrome.

Cough

A **cough** is the most common, yet nonspecific symptom observed in patients with pulmonary disease. Coughing is a forceful expiratory maneuver that expels mucus and foreign material from the airways. It usually occurs when cough receptors are stimulated by inflammation, mucus, foreign materials, or noxious gases. Cough receptors are located primarily in the larynx, trachea, and larger bronchi. The effectiveness of a cough depends on (1) the ability of the individual to take a deep breath, (2) lung elastic recoil, (3) expiratory muscle strength, and (4) level of airway resistance. The ability to take a deep breath and exhale forcefully is often impaired in patients with cardiopulmonary, neurologic, or neuromuscular diseases.

Effective coughing also is impaired in the early postoperative period after upper abdominal surgery or thoracic surgery or after trauma because of pain. Often, expiratory flow is limited by factors such as bronchospasm (e.g., asthma), reduced lung elastic recoil (as in emphysema) and muscle weakness. Patients with an inadequate ability to cough often have problems with atelectasis, retained secretions, and therefore are more prone to developing pneumonia and/or hypoxemia.

It is important for the RT to note several characteristics of the patient's cough. This includes whether it is dry or loose, productive or nonproductive, acute or chronic, and whether it occurs more frequently at particular times (i.e., day or night). Knowledge of such details may help in determining the cause of the cough. A dry, nonproductive cough is typical for restrictive lung diseases such as CHF or pulmonary fibrosis. A loose, productive cough is more often associated with inflammatory obstructive diseases such as bronchitis and asthma. The most common cause of an acute, self-limited cough is a viral infection of the upper airway.

A **chronic cough** is one lasting 8 weeks or longer.[1] It carries with it considerable frustration and anxiety for patients, with decreased quality of life and depression commonly reported. When a thorough examination and history fail to find evidence of disease (e.g., cancer, human immunodeficiency virus [HIV] disease) and the chest radiograph is normal, more than 90% of chronic cough cases are accounted for by upper airway cough syndrome (formerly called postnasal drip), asthma, and gastroesophageal reflux. Chronic coughing has numerous common and uncommon causes that sometimes may have multiple sources (Box 16-3).[1]

Box 16-3 Evaluating Chronic Cough in the Adult (>8 Weeks Duration)[1]

COMMON SOURCES

- Upper airway cough syndrome (formerly known as "postnasal drip")
- Asthma
- Gastroesophageal reflux
- Chronic bronchitis associated with cigarette smoking
- Angiotensin-converting enzyme–1 cough (caused by the antihypertensive drug angiotensin-converting enzyme inhibitor)
- Nonasthmatic eosinophilic bronchitis

LESS COMMON SOURCES

- Postinfection (e.g., pertussis, mycoplasma)
- Interstitial lung disease
- Bronchiectasis
- Obstructive sleep apnea
- Primary lung cancer
- Heart failure
- Pulmonary tuberculosis
- Environmental exposures

UNCOMMON SOURCES

- Sarcoidosis
- Recurrent aspiration
- Chronic tonsillar enlargement
- Chronic auditory canal irritation
- Foreign body aspiration
- Endemic fungi
- Peritoneal dialysis
- Cystic fibrosis
- Tracheomalacia
- Habit or "tic cough"

Sputum Production

Healthy airways produce mucus daily. Normally, the quantity of this mucus is minimal, and it is not enough to stimulate the cough receptors. Mucus is gradually moved to the hypopharynx by the mucociliary escalator, where it is either swallowed or expectorated. Disease of the airways (e.g., bronchitis or acute asthma attacks), may cause mucous glands located in the airways to produce abnormal amounts of mucus. This stimulates the cough receptors and causes a loose, productive cough.

RULE OF THUMB

Ineffective coughing is common in patients with cardiopulmonary, neurologic, or neuromuscular diseases, as well as in the early postoperative period after thoracic and upper abdominal surgery or trauma. Ineffective coughing places patients at increased risk for developing atelectasis, retained secretions, pneumonia, and hypoxemia.

RTs need to be aware of the terminology associated with sputum. Mucus from the tracheobronchial tree, *uncontaminated* by oral secretions, is called **phlegm.** Mucus from the lungs that passes through the mouth as it is expectorated is **sputum.** Because this is how most mucus samples from the lung are obtained, the term *sputum* is used in this chapter. Sputum that contains pus cells is said to be **purulent,** suggesting a bacterial infection. Purulent sputum appears thick, colored, and sticky. Sputum that is foul-smelling is said to be **fetid.** Sputum that is *clear and thick* is **mucoid** and commonly is seen in patients with asthma. Changes in the color, viscosity, or quantity of sputum produced are often signs of infection and must be documented and reported to the physician.

Hemoptysis

Coughing up blood or blood-streaked sputum from the lungs is common in patients with pulmonary disease and is called **hemoptysis.** *Frank hemoptysis* is the *primary* presence of blood in the expectorant. *Massive hemoptysis* is when more than 300 ml of blood is expectorated over 24 hours and represents a medical emergency. Common causes include bronchiectasis, lung abscess, and acute or chronic tuberculosis.

Nonmassive hemoptysis is observed in many conditions such as airway infections, pneumonia, lung cancer, tuberculosis, blunt or penetrating chest trauma, and pulmonary embolism. Infection-associated hemoptysis usually presents as blood-streaked, purulent sputum. Hemoptysis from bronchogenic carcinoma often is chronic and may be associated with a monophonic wheeze and cough.

Hemoptysis must be distinguished from **hematemesis,** which is vomiting blood from the gastrointestinal tract and is a common finding in patients with gastrointestinal disease. Whereas blood from the lungs often is mixed with sputum, blood from the stomach may be mixed with food particles.

Chest Pain

Chest pain is categorized as either pleuritic or nonpleuritic. *Pleuritic chest pain* usually is located *laterally or posteriorly* and typically worsens when taking a deep breath. Patients often describe it as a *sharp, stabbing* type of pain. It manifests primarily in chest diseases that cause the pleural lining of the lung to become inflamed (such as pneumonia, empyema, pleural effusion), but also is a common symptom in pulmonary embolism.

Nonpleuritic chest pain is located typically in the *center* of the anterior chest and may *radiate* to the shoulder, neck, or back. It is *not affected by breathing,* and is often described as a *dull ache* or *pressure* type of pain. A common cause of nonpleuritic chest pain is **angina.** It is classically described as a pressure sensation with exertion or stress that results from coronary artery occlusion. Other common causes of nonpleuritic chest pain include gastroesophageal reflux, esophageal spasm, chest wall pain (e.g., costochondritis), and gallbladder disease.

Fever

Fever is an elevated body temperature greater than 38.3°C (101°F),[2] with the most common sources being a bacterial, viral, or fungal infection. There are, however, numerous noninfectious causes of fever such as drug reaction (e.g., sulfa drugs), malignancies (e.g., lymphomas, metastatic cancer), head trauma (e.g., damage to the hypothalamus), burns, alcoholic cirrhosis, thromboembolic disorders (e.g., pulmonary embolism), and noninfectious inflammatory diseases (e.g., rheumatoid arthritis, systemic lupus erythematosus).[3] Therefore all patients with fever need further assessment to determine the cause. Sustained (e.g., >3 weeks), unexplained fever despite a comprehensive work-up is called a **fever of unknown origin (FUO)** and is a common finding in patients with HIV disease.[3]

The magnitude of temperature elevation during fever may indicate the type and virulence of the infection. Low-grade fever typically accompanies common upper respiratory tract infections, whereas a high fever occurs with viral influenza infection.

Fever that occurs with a cough suggests a respiratory tract infection. An infection is even more likely to be the cause of the fever if the patient is producing purulent sputum. In this situation, a persistent fever of 38.9°C (102°F) or greater for 2 days accompanied by chills is suggestive of pneumonia. However, the absence of coughing or sputum production does not rule out lung infection.

For many years it was believed that a link existed between fever and atelectasis in postoperative surgical patients. However, we now know that no such link exists.[4]

Patients with a significant fever have an increased metabolic rate that increases both O_2 consumption and carbon dioxide production and may cause tachypnea. Fever is particularly dangerous for patients with severe chronic cardiopulmonary disease because the increased ventilatory demand may induce acute respiratory failure.

Pedal Edema

Swelling of the lower extremities is known as **pedal edema** and often most occurs with heart failure. The diminished ability of the heart to effectively pump blood causes venous congestion. Increased hydrostatic pressure from blood pooling in the gravity-dependent lower extremities causes fluid to leak into the interstitial spaces. Afflicted patients often complain of "swollen ankles" in such cases. The degree of pedal edema depends on the severity of heart failure. There are two subtypes of pedal edema. *Pitting edema* is when finger pressure applied on a swollen extremity leaves an indentation mark on the skin. The height at which pitting edema occurs can indicate the severity of heart failure. Pitting edema that extends to the knee signifies a more significant problem than edema limited to the ankles. Furthermore, a standard scale may be used to quantify the severity of pitting edema, with "1" equating to a trace with rapid refill and "4" meaning severe pitting with refill time in excess of 2 minutes. Any patient who is suspected to have right-sided or left-sided heart failure is examined for pedal edema. *Weeping edema* occurs when the applied finger pressure causes a small fluid leak.

Patients with chronic hypoxemic lung disease are especially prone to right-sided heart failure (cor pulmonale) that also causes pedal edema. Chronic hypoxia causes severe pulmonary vasoconstriction and pulmonary hypertension. This places a heavy demand on the thin-walled right ventricle, which can eventually fail, resulting in venous congestion.

Format for the Medical History

All health care practitioners must be familiar with the medical history of the patients they are treating, even if their reason for contact is simply to provide intermittent therapy. The medical history familiarizes clinicians with the signs and symptoms the patient exhibited on admission and the reason the therapy is being administered.

The first priority of the RT reviewing the medical record is to ensure that all respiratory care procedures are supported by a physician order that is current, clearly written, and complete. Afterward, the RT should review the patient's medical record by reading about the patient's current medical problems. This information is found under the headings of *chief complaint* and *history of present illness*. This presents a detailed, systematic account of the patient's major complaints written by a physician after the postadmission interview with the patient.

The next step is to review the patient's *past medical history*, which describes all past major illnesses, injuries, surgeries, hospitalizations, allergies, and health-related habits. This information provides a basic understanding of the patient's previous experiences with illness and the health care system. The nature of past history may influence decisions made during the current hospitalization.

The *past medical history* is where the interviewer records the patient's cigarette and alcohol consumption. Accurate determination of a patient's smoking history is extremely important in assessing pulmonary health. The smoking history is often recorded in **pack-years.** This is determined by *multiplying the number of packs smoked per day by the number of years smoked.* Typically, a patient is asked how many cigarettes (on average) he or she smokes per day. If a patient states that he or she has smoked a pack of cigarettes a day for 20 years, the patient has a 20 pack-year smoking history.

If patients describe their smoking in terms of the number of cigarettes, or fractions of a pack, the calculation is slightly more difficult. Two examples may help illustrate how to calculate pack-years of smoking. There are 20 cigarettes per pack. If a patient states he or she has smoked a pack and a half of cigarettes per day for 20 years, the smoking history is calculated as follows:

$$\begin{aligned}30\text{ cigarettes}/20\text{ cigarettes per pack} &= 1.5\text{ packs} \times 20\text{ years}\\ &= 30\text{ pack years smoking history}\end{aligned}$$

If the patient states that he or she has smoked 15 cigarettes per day for 20 years:

$$\begin{aligned}15\text{ cigarettes}/20\text{ cigarettes per pack} &= 0.75\text{ packs} \times 20\text{ years}\\ &= 15\text{ pack years smoking history}\end{aligned}$$

Next, the *family* and *social/environmental history* should be reviewed. This focuses on potential genetic or occupational links to disease and the patient's current life situation. In many cases, there is a genetic predisposition to pulmonary disorders such as asthma, lung cancer, and cystic fibrosis. A detailed occupational history is important in establishing acquired pulmonary disorders resulting from inhaling dusts in the workplace, either organic (i.e., containing protein) or nonorganic (e.g., asbestos, silica). There is a strong link between many chronic pulmonary diseases and air pollution which predominantly effects those living in urban poverty.[5]

The *review of systems* is designed to uncover problem areas the patient forgot to mention or may have omitted. This information is usually obtained in a head-to-toe review of all body systems. For each body system, the interviewer obtains information about current, pertinent symptoms. During a review of the respiratory system, questioning would determine the presence or history of cough, hemoptysis, sputum production, chest pain, shortness of breath, and fever (Box 16-4).

Finally, the medical record should be examined for information indicating any limits on the extent of care to be provided in the event of cardiac or respiratory arrest. This information is known as an **advance directive,** whereby the patient (or a legally authorized representative) has formalized his or her wishes for resuscitative efforts; this is typically referred to as the *DNR status* ("do not resuscitate") or may be expressed as DNI ("do not intubate"). A less ambiguous acronym *AND* ("allow for natural death") is used to emphasize that care is primarily focused on patient comfort. This information may be found either in the admission note or within the body of the physician progress notes. In addition to this descriptive note, there must be an order written by the physician clearly specifying how care should be limited in the event of a medical emergency.

PHYSICAL EXAMINATION

A careful physical examination of the patient is essential for evaluating the patient's problem(s) and determining the effects of therapy. The physical examination consists of the following four general steps: (1) inspection (visually examining), (2) palpation (touching), (3) percussion (tapping), and (4) auscultation (listening with a stethoscope).

General Appearance

The first moments of an encounter with the patient may reveal the severity of the current problem. These initial impressions determine the course of subsequent assessment. If the patient's general appearance indicates an acute problem, the examination may be abbreviated and focused until the patient's condition is stabilized. When the initial impression indicates that the patient is stable, a more complete assessment can be conducted (Box 16-5). Several indicators are important in assessing the patient's overall appearance, including the patient's level of consciousness (see later discussion), facial expression, level of anxiety or distress, positioning, and personal hygiene.

The RT should look for specific characteristics when observing the patient's body. Does the patient appear well nourished or emaciated? Weakness and emaciation **(cachexia)** are signs of general ill health and malnutrition that increases susceptibility to infection. Is the patient sweating? **Diaphoresis** (sweating) can indicate fever, pain, severe stress, increased metabolism, or acute anxiety.

Box 16-4 Outline of a Complete Health History

Demographic data (obtained from admission interview): Name, address, age, birth date, place of birth, race, nationality, marital status, religion, occupation, and source of referral
Date and source of history and estimate of the reliability of the historian
Brief description of the patient's condition at the time the history or patient profile was taken
Chief complaint and reason for seeking treatment
History of present illness: Chronologic description of each symptom
- Onset: Time, type, source, setting
- Frequency and duration of symptoms
- Location and radiation of pain
- Severity (quantity)
- Quality (character)
- Aggravating and alleviating factors
- Associated manifestations

Past medical history
- Childhood diseases and development
- Hospitalizations, surgeries, injuries, accidents, and major illnesses
- Allergies
- Medications

Family history
- Familial disease history
- Marital history
- Family relationships

Social and environmental history
- Education
- Military experience
- Occupational history
- Religious and social activities
- Alcohol and cigarette consumption
- Living arrangements
- Hobbies and recreation
- Satisfaction with and stresses of life situation, finances, and relationships
- Recent travel or other event that might affect health

Review of systems: Respiratory system
- Cough
- Hemoptysis
- Sputum (amount and consistency)
- Chest pain
- Shortness of breath
- Hoarseness or changes in voice
- Dizziness or fainting
- Fever or chills
- Peripheral edema

Patient's printed name and signature

The general facial expression may help reveal pain or anxiety, as well as in evaluating alertness, mood, and mental capacity. Simple observation of the patient's anxiety level can indicate the severity of the current problem and whether cooperation can be expected. The patient's position also may be useful in assessing the severity of the problem and the patient's response to it. For example, a patient with severe pulmonary hyperinflation tends to sit upright while bracing his or her elbows on a table. This position helps the accessory muscles gain a mechanical advantage for breathing and is called **tripodding.** Finally, personal hygiene indicators may help determine both the duration and severity of the illness.

Box 16-5 Typical Format for Recording the Physical Examination

INITIAL IMPRESSION
- Age, height, weight, sensorium, and general appearance

VITAL SIGNS
- Pulse rate, respiratory rate, temperature, and blood pressure

HEAD, EARS, EYES, NOSE, AND THROAT
- Inspection findings

NECK
- Inspection and palpation findings

THORAX
- Lungs: Inspection, palpation, percussion, and auscultation findings
- Heart: Inspection, palpation, and auscultation findings

ABDOMEN
- Inspection, palpation, percussion, and auscultation findings

EXTREMITIES
- Inspection and palpation findings

Level of Consciousness

While observing the patient's overall appearance, the RT should assess the patient's level of consciousness (alertness). Evaluating the patient's alertness is a simple but important task (Box 16-6). If the patient appears conscious, the RT should assess the patient's orientation to time, place, person, and situation. This assessment often is called evaluating the **sensorium.** The sensorium is considered normal if the patient can correctly tell the interviewer his or her name, the current date, location, and situation (e.g., "I'm in the hospital because I fell and broke my hip") and this is typically documented as "oriented × 4." If the patient is not alert, the level of consciousness is assessed. The simple rating scale shown in Box 16-6 allows clinicians to describe the patient's level of consciousness objectively, using common clinical terms.

Depressed consciousness may occur with poor cerebral blood flow (e.g., hypotension, neurovascular lesion) or when poorly oxygenated blood perfuses the brain. As cerebral oxygenation acutely decreases, the patient initially becomes restless, confused, or disoriented. If hypoxia worsens, the patient may become comatose. However, patients with chronic hypoxia may adapt well and may have normal mental status despite significant hypoxemia. Abnormal consciousness also may occur in chronic degenerative brain disorders, as a side effect of certain medications, and in cases of drug overdose. The Glasgow Coma Scale score is used to assess the level of consciousness and neurologic function (see Chapter 51).

Vital Signs

Vital signs—the body temperature, pulse rate, respiratory rate, and blood pressure—are the most frequently used clinical

Box 16-6 Levels of Consciousness

CONFUSED
The patient
- Exhibits slight decrease of consciousness
- Has slow mental responses
- Has decreased or dulled perception
- Has incoherent thoughts

DELIRIOUS
The patient
- Is easily agitated
- Is irritable
- Exhibits hallucinations

LETHARGIC
The patient
- Is sleepy
- Arouses easily
- Responds appropriately when aroused

OBTUNDED
The patient
- Awakens only with difficulty
- Responds appropriately when aroused

STUPOROUS
The patient
- Does not awaken completely
- Has decreased mental and physical activity
- Responds to pain and exhibits deep tendon reflexes
- Responds slowly to verbal stimuli

COMATOSE
The patient
- Is unconscious
- Does not respond to stimuli
- Does not move voluntarily
- Exhibits possible signs of upper motor neuron dysfunction, such as Babinski reflex or hyperreflexia
- Loses reflexes with deep or prolonged coma

measurements because they are easy to obtain and provide useful information about the patient's clinical condition. Abnormal vital signs may reveal the first clue of adverse reactions to treatment. In addition, improvement in a patient's vital signs is strong evidence that a treatment is having a positive effect. For example, a decrease in the patient's breathing and heart rate toward normal after the application of O_2 therapy suggests a beneficial effect.

Body Temperature

The average body temperature for adults is approximately 37° C (98.6° F), with daily variations of approximately 0.5° C (1° F). Body temperature normally is lowest in the early morning and highest in the late afternoon. Body temperature is kept normal by balancing heat production with heat loss. The hypothalamus regulates heat loss by initiating peripheral vasodilation and sweating *(diaphoresis)* to dissipate body heat or vasoconstriction to preserve it. The respiratory system also helps remove excess heat through ventilation by warming the inspired air, which is subsequently exhaled.

Box 16-7 Key Characteristics of the Pulse

- Is the pulse rate normal, high, or low?
- Is the rhythm regular, consistently irregular, or irregularly irregular?
- Are there any changes in the amplitude (strength) of the pulse in relation to respiration? Are there changes in amplitude from one beat to another?
- Are there any other abnormalities, such as palpable vibrations (thrills or bruits)?

Elevated body temperature (*hyperthermia* or *hyperpyrexia*) can result from disease or from normal activities such as exercise. Temperature elevation caused by disease is called *fever,* and the patient is said to be **febrile.** Fever increases metabolism, causing both increased O_2 consumption and CO_2 production. Increased metabolism induces both increased circulation and ventilation to maintain homeostasis. This is why febrile patients often have increased heart and breathing rates. Fever increases the demand placed on the heart and lungs. This often complicates clinical management because some patients have limited ability to increase their circulation and ventilation. Thus respiratory failure can result.

A body temperature below normal is called **hypothermia.** The most common cause of hypothermia is prolonged exposure to cold, to which the hypothalamus responds by initiating shivering (to generate heat) and vasoconstriction (to conserve heat). Other, less common causes of hypothermia include head injury or stroke, causing dysfunction of the hypothalamus; decreased thyroid activity; and overwhelming infection, such as sepsis.

Because hypothermia reduces O_2 consumption and CO_2 production, patients with hypothermia may exhibit slow, shallow breathing and reduced pulse rate.

Body temperature is measured most often at one of the following four sites: mouth, axilla, ear (tympanic membrane), or rectum. The oral site is the most acceptable for an alert, adult patient, but it cannot be used with infants, comatose patients, or orally intubated patients. If a patient ingests hot or cold liquid or has been smoking, oral temperature measurement should be delayed for 10 to 15 minutes for accuracy. The axillary site is acceptable for infants or small children who do not tolerate rectal thermometers, but this site may underestimate core temperature by 1° to 2° C. The body temperature can also be assessed accurately with the use of a hand-held device to measure the temperature of the eardrum (tympanic membrane). Rectal temperatures are closest to actual core body temperature.

Pulse Rate

The peripheral pulse is evaluated for rate, rhythm, and strength (Box 16-7). The normal adult pulse rate is 60 to 100 beats/min, with a regular rhythm. A condition in which the pulse rate is greater than 100 beats/min is called **tachycardia.** Common causes of tachycardia are exercise, fear, anxiety, low blood pressure, anemia, fever, reduced arterial blood O_2 levels *(hypoxemia),* elevated CO2 (*hypercapnia*) and certain medications. A condition in which the pulse rate is less than 60 beats/min is called **bradycardia.** Bradycardia is less common than tachycardia but can occur with hypothermia, as a side effect of medications, with certain cardiac arrhythmias, and with traumatic brain injury.

The radial artery is the most common site used to palpate the pulse. The second and third fingertip pads (but not the thumb) are used to palpate the radial pulse. Ideally, the pulse rate is counted for 1 minute, especially if the pulse is irregular. Essential pulse characteristics that should be noted and documented are described in Box 16-7.

Spontaneous ventilation can influence pulse strength, or amplitude. A slight decrease in pulse pressure is normally present with each inspiratory effort. This decrease is caused by negative intrathoracic pressure from inspiratory muscle contraction. The decrease in blood pressure is the result of decreased left ventricular filling. This occurs by two mechanisms. First, negative intrathoracic pressure causes blood to pool in the pulmonary circulation, thereby reducing left heart filling. Second, negative intrathoracic pressure simultaneously increases both venous return and right ventricular volume. The engorged right ventricle limits left ventricular expansion and filling during diastole. The end result is a brief reduction in left ventricular stroke volume and decreases systolic blood pressure during inspiration.

Pulse pressure normally decreases slightly with inspiration (<10 mm Hg) and may not be noticeable with palpation. **Pulsus paradoxus** *("paradoxical pulse")* is a *significant* decrease in pulse strength (>10 mm Hg) during spontaneous inspiration. Pulsus paradoxus can be quantified with a blood pressure cuff (see later section) and is common in patients with acute obstructive pulmonary disease, especially patients experiencing an asthma attack. During respiratory distress, vigorous inspiratory efforts decrease stroke volume by impeding the strength of left ventricular contraction.[6] Pulsus paradoxus also may signal a mechanical restriction of the pumping action of the heart, as can occur with constrictive pericarditis or cardiac tamponade. **Pulsus alternans** is an alternating succession of strong and weak pulses. Pulsus alternans suggests left-sided heart failure and usually is not related to respiratory disease.

The pulse also may be assessed by palpating the carotid, brachial, femoral, temporal, popliteal, posterior tibial, and dorsalis pedis pulses. The more centrally located pulses (e.g., the carotid and femoral) should be used when the blood pressure is abnormally low. If the carotid site is used, great care must be taken to avoid the carotid sinus area. Pressure on the carotid sinus area may cause strong parasympathetic stimulation resulting in bradycardia.

Respiratory Rate

The normal resting adult rate of breathing is 12 to 18 breaths/min. **Tachypnea** is defined as a respiratory rate greater than 20 breaths/min. Rapid respiratory rates are associated with exertion, fever, hypoxemia, hypercarbia, metabolic acidosis, anxiety, pulmonary edema, lung fibrosis, and pain. A respiratory rate less than 10 breaths/min is called **bradypnea,** and may occur with traumatic brain injury, severe myocardial infarction, hypothermia, anesthetics, opiate narcotics, and recreational drug overdoses.

The respiratory rate is counted by watching the abdomen or chest wall move out and in. In some cases, the RT may need to place a hand on the patient's abdomen to confirm the breathing rate. Ideally, the patient should be unaware that the respiratory rate is being counted. One method to accomplish this is to count the respiratory rate immediately after evaluating the patient's pulse, while keeping the fingers on the patient's wrist. This gives the impression that the pulse rate is still being counted.

Blood Pressure

The arterial blood pressure is the force exerted against the wall of the arteries as the blood moves through them. Arterial **systolic pressure** is the peak force exerted in the major arteries during contraction of the left ventricle. Arterial blood pressure typically increases with age. The normal range for systolic blood pressure in an adult is 90 to 140 mm Hg. **Diastolic pressure** is the force in the major arteries remaining after relaxation of the ventricles; it is normally 60 to 90 mm Hg. **Pulse pressure** is the difference between the systolic and diastolic pressures. A normal pulse pressure is 30 to 40 mm Hg. When the pulse pressure is less than 30 mm Hg, the peripheral pulse is difficult to detect.

Blood pressure is determined by the interaction of the force of left ventricular contraction, the systemic vascular resistance, and the blood volume (see Chapter 10). The blood pressure is recorded by listing systolic pressure over diastolic pressure (e.g., 120/80 mm Hg).

Hypertension is an arterial blood pressure *persistently* greater than 140/90 mm Hg. Hypertension is a common medical problem in adults, and in approximately 90% of cases the cause is unknown (primary hypertension). There are two subcategories of hypertension.[7] *Stage I* hypertension occurs when the systolic blood pressure is 140 to 159 mm Hg or the diastolic blood pressure is 90 to 99 mm Hg. *Stage II* hypertension occurs when the systolic blood pressure is 160 mm Hg or greater or the diastolic blood pressure is 100 mm Hg or above. In addition, there is a third category known as *prehypertension,* which is a systolic blood pressure between 120 and 139 mm Hg or a diastolic blood pressure between 80 and 89 mm Hg. Prehypertension is not a disease state and does not require treatment but is used to assess the risk for eventually developing hypertension.

Mechanically, hypertension results from increased systemic vascular resistance or an increased force of ventricular contraction. Sustained hypertension can cause central nervous system abnormalities, such as headaches, blurred vision, and confusion. Other potential consequences of hypertension include uremia (renal insufficiency), CHF, and cerebral hemorrhage. Acute, severe elevation of blood pressure can cause acute neurologic, cardiac, and renal failure and is called an *acute hypertensive crisis.*

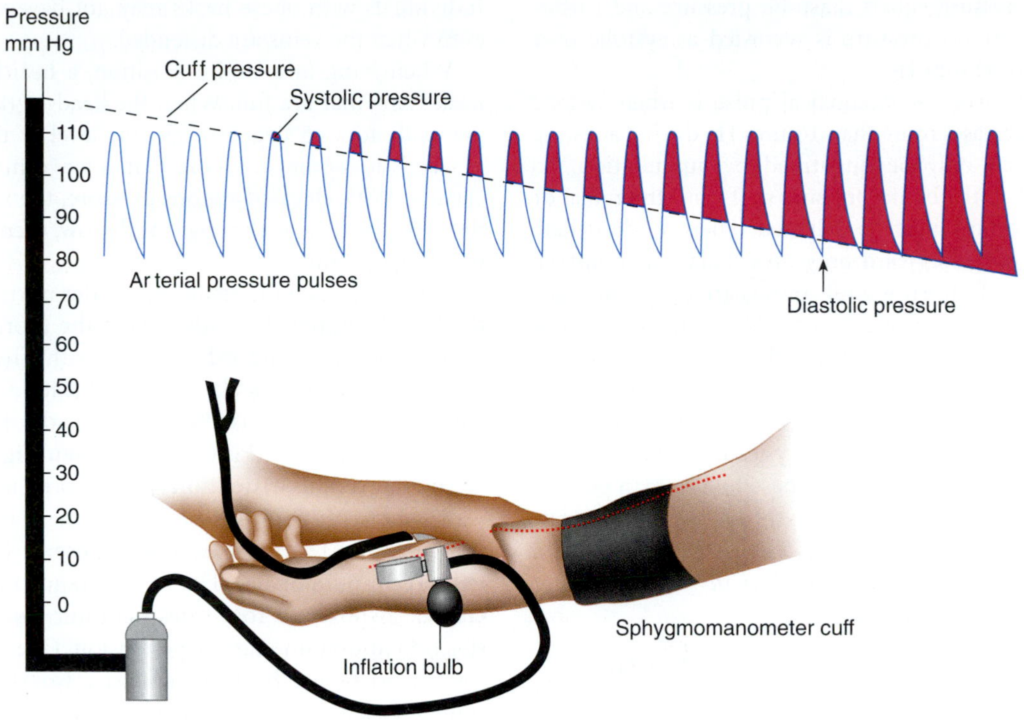

FIGURE 16-2 Auscultatory method for measuring arterial blood pressure, using a sphygmomanometer and a stethoscope. (Redrawn from Rushmer RR: Structure and functions of the cardiovascular system, ed 2, Philadelphia, 1976, WB Saunders.)

Hypotension is defined as a systolic arterial blood pressure less than 90 mm Hg or a mean arterial pressure less than 65 mm Hg.[8] Hypotension also can be defined as a decrease of more than 40 mm Hg from baseline. This expanded definition acknowledges that patients with baseline hypertension may have inadequate tissue perfusion at a blood pressure that may be considered normal for most patients.

Shock is defined precisely as the inadequate delivery of O_2 and nutrients to the vital organs relative to their metabolic demand.[9] Hypotension is not synonymous with shock. In shock, vital body organs are in imminent danger of receiving inadequate blood flow (underperfusion) and impaired O_2 delivery to the tissues (i.e., tissue hypoxia). For this reason, shock is usually treated aggressively with fluids, blood products, or vasoactive drugs, or a combination of these, depending on the cause and severity of shock.

There are two broad categories of hypotension and shock based on whether they are caused by a *hypodynamic* or *hyperdynamic* cardiovascular state.[10] Hypodynamic states include left ventricular failure *(cardiogenic)* and reduced blood volume (**hypovolemia** or *hypovolemic*) caused by either hemorrhage or severe fluid loss. Hyperdynamic states occur with profound systemic vasodilation *(peripheral vascular failure)* associated with overwhelming infection *(septic shock),* systemic allergic reaction *(anaphylaxis),* or severe liver failure.

Healthy individuals, when sitting or standing up, experience little change in blood pressure. However, similar postural changes may produce abrupt hypotension in hypovolemic patients. This condition is called **postural hypotension** and generally is treated with fluid administration. Postural hypotension is confirmed by measuring blood pressure with the patient supine and then measuring with the patient in the sitting (or standing) position. Postural hypotension may reduce cerebral blood flow and lead to **syncope** (fainting).

A common technique for measuring arterial blood pressure requires a blood pressure cuff (sphygmomanometer) and a stethoscope (Figure 16-2). When the cuff is applied to the upper arm and pressurized to exceed systolic blood pressure, the brachial artery blood flow stops. As the cuff pressure is slowly released to a point just below the systolic pressure, blood flows intermittently past the obstruction. Partial blood flow obstruction creates turbulence and vibrations called *Korotkoff sounds.* These sounds are heard with a stethoscope over the brachial artery distal to the cuff.

To measure the blood pressure, a deflated cuff is wrapped snugly around the patient's upper arm, with the lower edge of the cuff 1 inch above the antecubital fossa. While palpating the brachial pulse, the clinician inflates the cuff approximately 30 mm Hg above the point at which the pulse can no longer be felt. Then the diaphragm of the stethoscope is placed over the artery and the cuff is slowly deflated (2 to 3 mm Hg/sec) while observing the manometer.

The systolic pressure is recorded when the first Korotkoff sounds are heard. The point at which the sounds become muffled is the diastolic pressure. This muffling is the final change in the Korotkoff sounds just before they disappear. At this point, cuff pressure equals diastolic pressure and turbulence ceases. The blood pressure is recorded as systolic over diastolic (e.g., 120/60 mm Hg).

As mentioned earlier, a paradoxical pulse is when systolic blood pressure decreases more than 10 mm Hg during a resting inhalation and can only be quantified by auscultation. To measure this, inflate the blood pressure cuff until the radial or brachial pulse can no longer be palpated. Then slowly deflate the cuff until sounds are heard only on exhalation (point 1). Next, reduce the cuff pressure until sounds are heard throughout respiration (point 2). The difference between points 1 and 2 indicates the degree of paradoxical pulse.

Most hospitals and clinics now use digital blood pressure measuring devices that do not require clinicians to listen for the Korotkoff sounds. These devices are very accurate and eliminate variances in recorded blood pressures based on human perception. The clinician need only to apply the blood pressure cuff correctly and press the start button. The device inflates and deflates the cuff automatically and displays the blood pressure and pulse rate on a digital screen.

Examination of the Head and Neck

Head

The patient's face is inspected for abnormal signs that indicate respiratory problems. The most common facial signs are nasal flaring, cyanosis, and pursed-lip breathing. Nasal flaring occurs when the external nares flare outward during inhalation. This flaring is prevalent in respiratory distress and indicates an increased work of breathing.

Cyanosis is a bluish discoloration of the skin or tissues as a result of respiratory or cardiac disease. Cyanosis is discussed in more detail later in this chapter. Patients with chronic obstructive pulmonary disease (COPD) may use pursed-lip breathing during exhalation. Breathing through pursed lips during exhalation creates resistance to flow. The increased resistance creates a slight back pressure in the small airways during exhalation. This back-pressure prevents premature airway collapse and allows more complete emptying of the lung.

Neck

Inspection and palpation of the neck help determine the position of the trachea and the jugular venous pressure (JVP). Normally, when the patient faces forward, the trachea is located in the middle of the neck. The midline of the neck can be identified by palpating the suprasternal notch. The midline of the trachea should be directly below the center of the suprasternal notch.

The trachea can shift away from the midline in certain thoracic disorders. Generally, the trachea shifts *toward* an area of collapsed lung and shifts *away* from areas with increased air or fluid (e.g., tension pneumothorax or large pleural effusion).

JVP is estimated by determining how high the jugular vein extends above the level of the sternal angle. JVP reflects the volume and pressure of venous blood in the right heart. Typically, the internal vein is assessed because it is more reliable. Individuals with obese necks may not have visible neck veins, even when the veins are distended.

When lying in a supine position, a healthy individual has neck veins that are full. When the head of the bed is elevated gradually to a 45-degree angle, the level of the blood column descends to a point no more than a few centimeters above the clavicle. With elevated venous pressure, the neck veins may be distended as high as the angle of the jaw, even when the patient is sitting upright.

JVP may vary with breathing. Under normal circumstances, the blood column descends toward the thorax during inhalation and ascends with exhalation. For this reason, JVP should always be estimated at the end of exhalation. Under abnormal conditions (e.g., cardiac tamponade), the JVP may increase during inhalation and is called **Kussmaul sign.**

Jugular venous distention (JVD) is present when the jugular vein is enlarged and can be seen more than 4 cm above the sternal angle. The most common cause of JVD is right heart failure (cor pulmonale). This occurs frequently in patients with chronic hypoxemia that causes chronic pulmonary vasoconstriction and pulmonary hypertension. Over time this leads to right heart failure from the excessive workload. Other conditions associated with JVD include left heart failure, cardiac tamponade, tension pneumothoraces, and mediastinal tumors.

The neck is a common place for the physician to palpate for enlarged lymph nodes, which is known as **lymphadenopathy.** Lymphadenopathy occurs with various medical disorders, including infection, malignancy, and sarcoidosis. Tender lymph nodes in the neck suggest a nearby infection. The lymph nodes are not tender when malignancy is the cause.

Examination of the Thorax and Lungs

Inspection

The chest should be inspected visually to assess the thoracic configuration, expansion, and the pattern and effort of breathing. For adequate inspection, the room must be well lit and the patient should be sitting upright. When the patient is too ill to sit up, the clinician should carefully roll the patient to one side to examine the posterior chest. Inspection, palpation, percussion, and auscultation of the patient's chest require that the patient be disrobed. Consequently, the clinician should make every effort to respect the patient's modesty (especially for female patients) and drape the chest whenever possible.

Thoracic Configuration. The anteroposterior (AP) diameter of the average adult thorax is less than the transverse diameter. Normally, the AP diameter increases gradually with age but may prematurely increase in patients with COPD. This abnormal increase in AP diameter is called **barrel chest** and is associated with emphysema. When the AP diameter increases, the normal 45-degree angle of articulation between the ribs and spine is increased, becoming more horizontal (Figure 16-3). Other abnormalities of the thoracic configuration are listed in Table 16-1.

Thoracic Expansion. The diaphragm is the primary muscle of (and power source for) breathing. As the diaphragm contracts it pushes the ribs outward and upward. The diaphragm

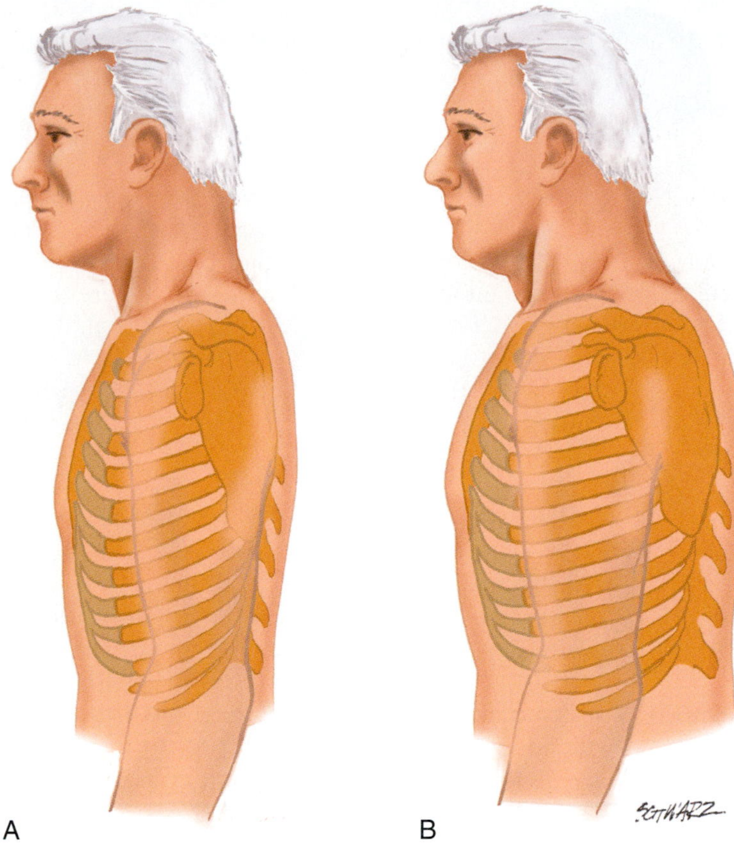

FIGURE 16-3 **A,** Patient with normal thoracic configuration. **B,** Patient with increased anteroposterior diameter. Note contrasts in the angle of slope of the ribs and development of accessory muscles.

TABLE 16-1

Abnormalities of Thoracic Configuration

Name	Condition
Pectus carinatum	Abnormal protrusion of sternum
Pectus excavatum	Depression of part or entire sternum, which can produce a restrictive lung defect
Kyphosis	Spinal deformity in which the spine has an abnormal anteroposterior curvature
Scoliosis	Spinal deformity in which the spine has a lateral curvature
Kyphoscoliosis	Combination of kyphosis and scoliosis, which may produce a severe restrictive lung defect as a result of poor lung expansion

also pushes downward on the abdominal organs, causing the abdominal wall to protrude. Therefore, when palpating the chest wall, both the chest and abdomen should expand synchronously during inspiration. However, the relative expansion of the chest and abdominal compartments depend on body position. In the supine position, the primary motion during *normal tidal breathing* is outward abdominal expansion with little noticeable chest excursion. In the upright position rib cage motion becomes more pronounced.[10]

The normal chest wall expands symmetrically and can be evaluated on the anterior and posterior chest. Anterior expansion is evaluated by placing the hands over the anterolateral chest; with the thumbs extended along the costal margin toward the xiphoid process. To evaluate posteriorly, position the hands over the posterolateral chest with the thumbs meeting at the T8 vertebra (Figure 16-4). Instruct the patient to exhale slowly and completely. When the patient has exhaled maximally, gently secure the fingertips against the sides of the patient's chest and extends the thumbs toward the midline until the tip of each thumb meets at the midline. Next instruct the patient to take a full, deep breath and note the distance the tip of each of the thumbs moves from midline. Normally, each thumb moves an equal distance of approximately 3 to 5 cm.

Diseases that affect the expansion of both lungs cause a bilateral reduction in chest expansion. Reduced expansion commonly is seen in neuromuscular disorders and COPD. Unilateral reduction in chest expansion occurs with respiratory diseases that reduce the expansion of one lung or a major part of one lung. This condition can occur with lobar consolidation, atelectasis, pleural effusion, or pneumothorax.

Breathing Pattern and Effort. At rest, a healthy adult has a consistent rate and rhythm of breathing. Breathing effort is minimal on inhalation and passive on exhalation. Abnormal breathing patterns can be broken down into two broad

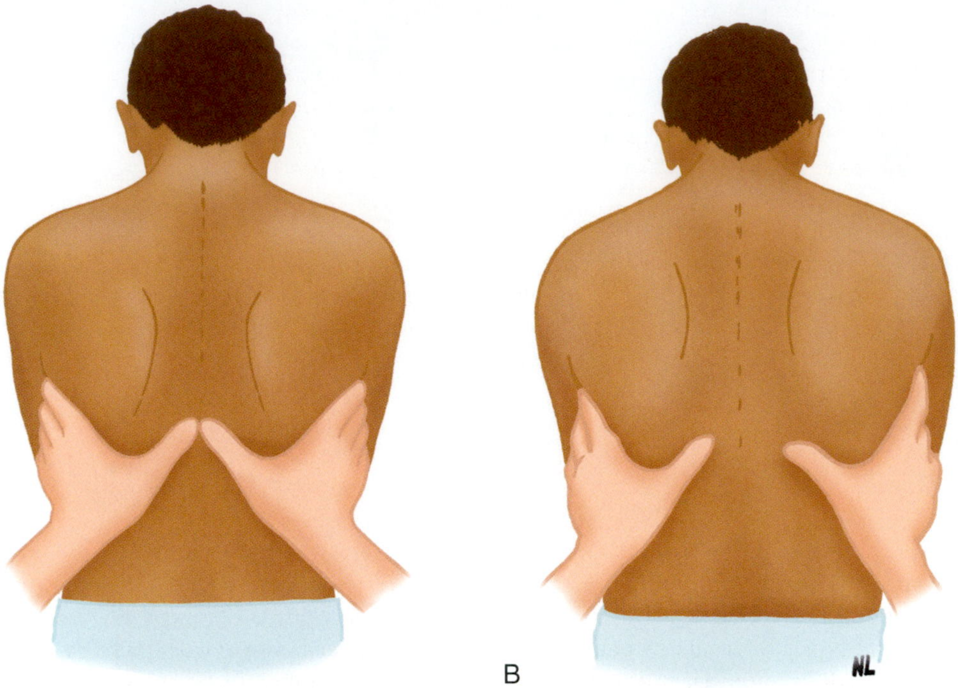

FIGURE 16-4 Estimation of thoracic expansion. **A,** Exhalation. **B,** Maximal inhalation.

TABLE 16-2
Abnormal Breathing Patterns

Breathing Pattern	Characteristics	Causes
Apnea	No breathing	Cardiac arrest, narcotic overdose, severe brain trauma
Apneustic breathing	Deep, gasping inspiration with brief, partial expiration	Damage to upper medulla or pons caused by stroke or trauma; sometimes observed with hypoglycemic coma or profound hypoxemia
Ataxic breathing	Completely irregular breathing pattern with variable periods of apnea	Damage to medulla
Asthmatic breathing	Prolonged exhalation with recruitment of abdominal muscles	Obstruction to airflow out of the lungs
Biot respiration	Clustering of rapid, shallow breaths coupled with regular or irregular periods of apnea	Damage to medulla or pons caused by stroke or trauma; severe intracranial hypertension
Cheyne-Stokes respiration	Irregular type of breathing; breaths increase and decrease in depth and rate with periods of apnea; variant of "periodic breathing"	Most often caused by severe damage to bilateral cerebral hemispheres and basal ganglia (usually infarction); also seen in patients with CHF owing to increased circulation time and in various forms of encephalopathy
Kussmaul breathing	Deep and fast respirations	Metabolic acidosis
Paradoxical breathing	*Abdominal paradox:* Abdominal wall moves inward on inspiration and outward on expiration	*Abdominal paradox:* Diaphragmatic fatigue or paralysis
	Chest paradox: Part or all of the chest wall moves in with inhalation and out with exhalation	*Chest paradox:* Typically observed in chest trauma with multiple rib or sternal fractures Also found in patients with high spinal cord injury with paralysis of intercostal muscles
Periodic breathing	Breathing oscillates between periods of rapid, deep breathing and slow, shallow breathing *without* periods of apnea	Same causes as Cheyne-Stokes respiration

categories: (1) those directly associated with cardiopulmonary or chest wall diseases that increase work of breathing and (2) those associated with neurologic disease (see Chapter 15). Table 16-2 describes common abnormal patterns of breathing.

Increased work of breathing causes accessory muscle recruitment to maintain ventilation. Common causes of an increase in the work of breathing include narrowed airways (e.g., COPD, asthma), "stiff lungs" (e.g., acute respiratory distress syndrome [ARDS], cardiogenic pulmonary edema), or a stiff chest wall (e.g., ascites, anasarca, pleural effusions). One sign of severely increased work of breathing is visable distortions in chest wall called *retractions*.

Retractions are an inward sinking of the chest wall during inspiration. This occurs when inspiratory muscle contractions generate very large negative intrathoracic pressures. The respiratory muscles can generate negative inspiratory pressures of approximately 150 cm H_2O (112 mm Hg) at maximal effort.[11] Retractions may be seen between the ribs, above the clavicles, or below the rib cage. These are called *intercostal, supraclavicular,* or *subcostal retractions.* Retractions are difficult to see in obese patients. Another form of retraction is **tracheal tugging**, which is the downward movement of the thyroid cartilage toward the chest during inspiration. Typically, this movement occurs in concert with recruitment of the accessory muscles of inspiration, primarily the sternocleidomastoid muscles of the neck.

Generally, two archetypal abnormal breathing patterns exist that provide clues about the underlying pulmonary problem. These are characterized by (1) a rapid, shallow breathing pattern and (2) a relatively brief inspiratory phase with an abnormally prolonged exhalation characterized by pronounced, sustained abdominal muscular contraction.

Rapid, shallow breathing typically occurs in patients with increased lung stiffness (e.g., ARDS, pulmonary fibrosis). Intrathoracic airways obstruction slows lung emptying and prolongs the expiratory phase as patients attempt to minimize gas trapping inside the lungs. The inspiratory-to-expiratory time ratio decreases from a normal value of 1 : 2 to 1 : 4 or greater. In contrast, extrathoracic upper airway obstruction (e.g., epiglottitis or croup) results in a prolonged inspiratory time because airways outside the thorax tend to narrow more on inhalation. Patients with severe metabolic acidosis exhibit a deep, rapid pattern called **Kussmaul breathing.**

RULE OF THUMB

Lung diseases that cause loss of lung volume (e.g., pulmonary fibrosis, ARDS) cause the patient to take rapid, shallow breaths.

RULE OF THUMB

Lung diseases that cause intrathoracic airways to narrow (e.g., asthma, bronchitis) also cause the patient to breathe with a prolonged expiratory phase.

RULE OF THUMB

Lung diseases that cause the upper airway to narrow (e.g., croup, epiglottitis) also cause the patient to breathe with a prolonged inspiratory phase.

The diaphragm may be nonfunctional in patients with spinal injuries or neuromuscular disease and may be severely limited in patients with COPD. When the diaphragm is nonfunctional or limited, the accessory muscles of ventilation become active to maintain adequate gas exchange. Heavy use of accessory muscles is reliable evidence of significant cardiopulmonary disease.

In patients with emphysema, the lungs lose their elastic recoil and become hyperinflated. Over time, hyperinflation forces the diaphragm into a low, flat position. Contraction of a flat diaphragm tends to draw in the lateral costal margins (**Hoover sign**) instead of normal expansion and greatly limits its effectiveness in moving air. Eventually, the accessory muscles assist ventilation by raising the anterior chest in an effort to increase thoracic volume. The severity of emphysema is often reflected by the magnitude of accessory muscle activity.

Diaphragmatic fatigue is found in many types of chronic and acute pulmonary diseases. Fatigue is the inability of a contracting muscle(s) to achieve a target pressure. This is distinguished from muscle weakness, the inability to achieve a target pressure in a rested muscle. For the respiratory muscles, the target pressure is that needed to maintain normal ventilation as assessed by the arterial CO_2 partial pressure ($PaCO_2$).

Acute diaphragmatic fatigue often manifests with distinctive breathing patterns; the first sign is tachypnea.[9] Sometimes tachypnea is followed by a breathing pattern in which the diaphragm and rib cage muscles alternately power breathing in an attempt to rest each muscle group (**respiratory alternans**). This pattern is noted by the upward motion of the diaphragm during inspiration on a *series of breaths,* followed by diaphragmatic contractions and outward movement of the abdominal wall on the following series of breaths. When the diaphragm is relaxed, contraction of the rib cage muscles sucks the diaphragm upward and the abdomen inward during inspiration. The opposite phenomenon occurs on breaths when the diaphragm is active. When the rib cage muscles are relaxed, the chest wall may appear to sink in as the abdomen protrudes during diaphragmatic contraction; this often gives the impression that the chest has a rocking motion. **Abdominal paradox** occurs with complete diaphragmatic fatigue, as the diaphragm is drawn upward into the thoracic cavity with *each* inspiratory effort of the rib cage muscles.

These patterns are not always associated with impending muscle fatigue. Rather, they may be adaptations to high workloads when the respiratory muscle strength is normal.[12] Also, patients with respiratory distress often have tachypnea, along with recruitment of the expiratory muscles. This situation can make it difficult to discern accurately the presence and type of abnormal breathing pattern. The RT must be careful about offering definitive therapeutic suggestions (e.g., absolute need for mechanical ventilation) based solely on his or her perception of an abnormal breathing pattern.

Palpation

Palpation is the art of touching the chest wall to evaluate underlying structure and function. It is used in selected patients to confirm or rule out suspected problems suggested by the history and initial examination findings. Palpation is performed to evaluate vocal fremitus, estimate thoracic expansion, and assess the skin and subcutaneous tissues of the chest.

Vocal and Tactile Fremitus. *Vocal fremitus* refers to vibrations created by the vocal cords during speech. These vibrations are transmitted down the tracheobronchial tree and through the lung to the chest wall. When these vibrations are felt on the chest wall, it is called *tactile fremitus.* Assessing vocal fremitus requires a conscious, cooperative patient.

Increase intensity of vocal and tactile fremitus occurs when the lung becomes consolidated (e.g., filled with inflammatory exudate) as in pneumonia. However, if the consolidated area is not in communication with an open airway, speech cannot be transmitted and fremitus is absent or decreased. In addition, fremitus is reduced in patients who are obese or overly muscular.

Decreased intensity of vocal and tactile fremitus occurs when fluid or air collects in the pleural space (e.g., pleural effusion or pneumothoraces). Similarly, lung tissue density is reduced with hyperinflation (e.g., asthma, emphysema) that decreases transmission of speech vibrations through the lung and thereby reduces fremitus.

Tactile fremitus is assessed by asking the patient to repeat the word "ninety-nine" while the RT systematically palpates the thorax. The palmar aspect of the fingers or the ulnar aspect of the hand can be used for palpation. If one hand is used, it should be moved from one side of the chest to the corresponding area on the other side. The anterior, lateral, and posterior portions of the chest wall are evaluated.

Skin and Subcutaneous Tissues. When the lung ruptures, air frequently leaks out and collects in the subcutaneous tissues of the chest and neck. These fine air bubbles within the subcutaneous tissues produce a crackling sound and sensation when palpated. This condition is referred to as **subcutaneous emphysema**, and the sensation it produces on palpation is called *crepitus.* Crepitus is a classic sign of barotrauma. It can be felt over the chest of a patient who develops this condition as a result of receiving mechanical ventilation with high airway pressures and end-inspiratory volumes. It is also found in patients with blunt or penetrating chest trauma.

Percussion of the Chest

Percussion is the art of tapping on a surface to evaluate the underlying structure. Percussion of the chest wall produces a sound and a palpable vibration useful in evaluating underlying lung tissue. The vibration created by percussion penetrates the lung to a depth of 5 to 7 cm below the chest wall. This assessment technique is not performed routinely on all patients but is reserved for patients with suspected pneumothorax or lung consolidation.

The technique most often used in percussing the chest wall is called *mediate,* or *indirect,* percussion and can be broken down into two steps. First, place the middle finger of the nondominant hand firmly against the patient's chest wall, parallel to the ribs, with the palm and other fingers held off the chest. Second, the tips of middle and index fingers of the dominant hand are then used to strike the finger pressed against the chest. Alternatively, the lateral aspect of the thumb can be used. A quick, sharp blow should be placed near the base of the terminal phalanx. Movement of the hand striking the chest is generated at the wrist, not at the elbow or shoulder.

Percussion Over Lung Fields. Percussion of the lung fields is performed systematically by consecutively testing comparable areas on both sides of the chest. Percussion over the bony structures and over the breasts of female patients has no diagnostic value and should not be performed. Asking patients to raise their arms above their shoulders helps move the scapulae laterally and minimize their interference with percussion on the posterior chest wall.

The sounds generated during chest percussion are evaluated for intensity (loudness). Percussion over normal lung fields produces an easily heard, moderately low-pitched, resonate sound described as *tympanic.* When the percussion note is louder, deeper, and more resonate, it is said to be *hypertympanic.* Percussion may also produce a *damped,* or *dull* noise resembling the sound of a heavily muffled drum. Unilateral problems are easier to detect than bilateral problems because the normal side provides a normal standard for immediate comparison.

Clinical Implications. In modern practice, chest percussion enables rapid bedside assessment of chest abnormalities and may aid in deciding whether to obtain a chest radiograph. Any abnormality that either increases lung tissue density (e.g., pneumonia, tumor, or atelectasis) or increases the density of the pleural space (e.g., pleural effusion, empyema) results in *decreased resonance* or a *dull note* to percussion over the affected area. In contrast, *increased resonance* or a *hyperresonate note* is detected when the lungs are either hyperinflated (e.g., asthma or emphysema) or when the pleural space contains large amounts of air (**pneumothorax**). Percussion of the chest has important limitations. Abnormalities that are small or deep below the surface are not likely to be detected during percussion of the chest.

Auscultation of the Lungs

Auscultation is the process of listening for bodily sounds. Auscultation over the thorax is performed to identify normal and abnormal lung sounds and to evaluate the effects of therapy. Because auscultation can be performed quickly and is noninvasive, it is a particularly useful clinical tool. Auscultation is performed with a stethoscope to enhance sound transmission from the patient's lungs to the examiner's ears. The clinician always must ensure that the room is as quiet as possible whenever performing auscultation.

Stethoscope. A stethoscope has the following four basic parts: (1) a bell, (2) a diaphragm, (3) tubing, and (4) earpieces (Figure 16-5). The bell detects a broad spectrum of sounds and is very useful for listening to low-pitched sounds (e.g., heart sounds). Proper technique for listening to heart sounds is to place the bell lightly against the chest. This avoids stretching the skin, which inadvertently makes auscultating heart sounds more difficult because it filters out low-frequency sounds.

The diaphragm is preferred for auscultation of the lungs because most lung sounds are high frequency. The ideal tubing

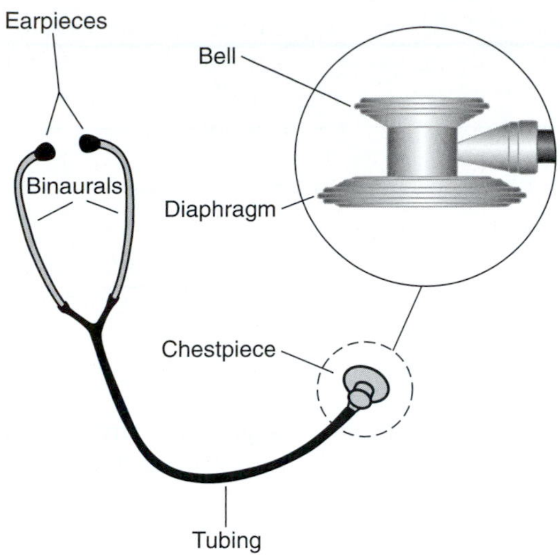

FIGURE 16-5 Acoustic stethoscope.

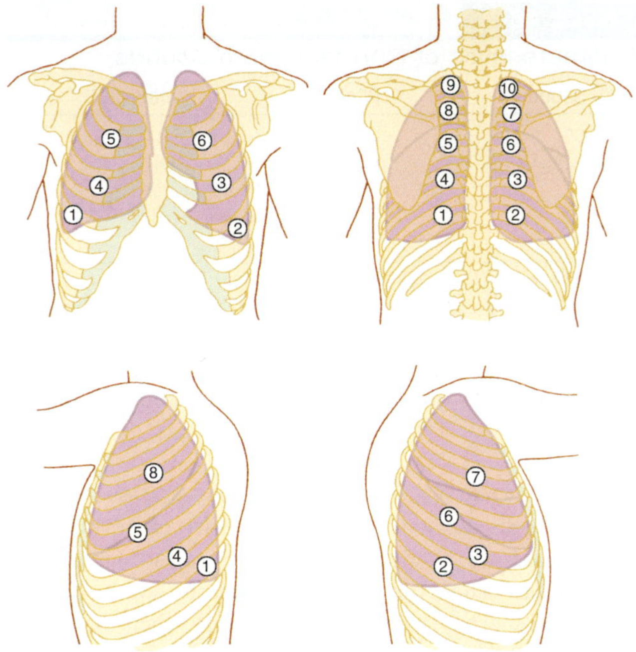

FIGURE 16-6 Sequencing for auscultation technique. (Modified from Wilkins RL, Dexter JR, editors: Respiratory diseases: a case study approach to patient care, ed 3, Philadelphia, 2007, FA Davis.)

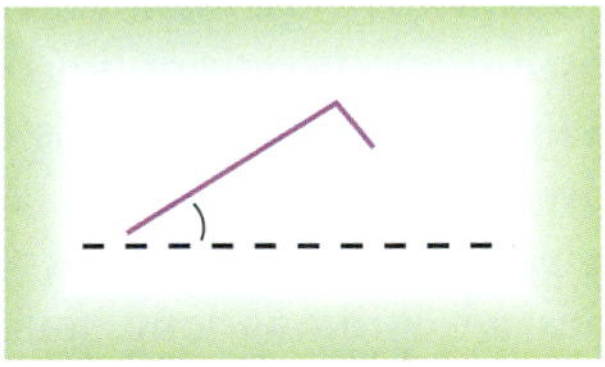

FIGURE 16-7 Diagram of normal breath sound. Upstroke represents inhalation, and downstroke represents exhalation; length of upstroke represents duration; thickness of stroke represents intensity; angle between upstroke and horizontal line represents pitch.

should be thick enough to exclude external noises and approximately 25 to 35 cm (11 to 16 inches) in length. Longer tubing may impair sound transmission.

The stethoscope should be examined regularly for cracks in the diaphragm, wax or dirt in the earpieces, and other defects that may interfere with sound transmission. A hospital-approved disinfectant should be used to clean the stethoscope *after every patient contact* to minimize contamination with microorganisms.[13] Patients who are placed in contact isolation and patients who are in protective isolation because of immunosuppression should have a dedicated stethoscope in the room to prevent cross infection.

Technique. When possible, the patient should be sitting upright in a relaxed position. The patient should be instructed to breathe a little more deeply than normal through an open mouth. Exhalation should be passive. Whenever possible, place the bell or diaphragm directly against the chest wall because clothing may produce distortion. The tubing must not be allowed to rub against any objects because this may produce extraneous sounds, which could be mistaken for adventitious lung sounds (discussed later).

Auscultation of the lungs should be systematic and include all lobes on the anterior, lateral, and posterior chest. Auscultation should begin at the lung bases with comparison of breath sounds side to side, working upward toward the lung apexes (Figure 16-6). It is important to begin at the bases because certain abnormal sounds that occur only in the lower lobes may be altered by several deep breaths. At least one full ventilatory cycle should be evaluated at each stethoscope position. If abnormal sounds are present, the clinician should listen to several breaths to clarify the characteristics.

The clinician should listen for, and distinguish among, the key features of breath sounds. The clinician should identify the pitch (vibration frequency), intensity (loudness), and duration of the inspiratory and expiratory phases. The acoustic characteristics of breath sounds can be illustrated in breath sound diagrams (Figure 16-7). The features of normal breath sounds are described in Table 16-3. One must be familiar with normal breath sounds before one can expect to identify the subtle changes that may signify respiratory disease.

Terminology. The sounds normally heard over the trachea have a loud, tubular quality and are referred to as *tracheal breath sounds*. They are also characterized by an expiratory component of equal length or slightly longer than the inspiratory component. A variation of the tracheal breath sounds can be heard both around the upper half of the sternum and between the scapulae. These are referred to as *bronchovesicular breath sounds* and are slightly lower in pitch and have equal inspiratory and expiratory components compared to tracheal breath sounds.

When auscultating over the lung parenchyma of a healthy individual, soft, muffled sounds are heard. These normal breath sounds, or *vesicular breath sounds*, are lower in pitch and intensity than bronchovesicular breath sounds. Vesicular sounds are heard primarily during inhalation, with an exhalation

TABLE 16-3
Characteristics of Normal Breath Sounds

Breath Sound	Pitch	Intensity	Location	Diagram
Vesicular	Low	Soft	Peripheral lung areas	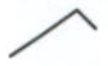
Bronchovesicular	Moderate	Moderate	Around upper part of sternum, between the scapulae	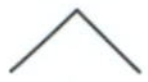
Tracheal	High	Loud	Over the trachea	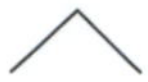

component approximately one-third the duration of inhalation (see Table 16-3).

Lung Sounds in Pulmonary Disease

Respiratory disease may alter the intensity of normal breath sounds heard over the lung fields. Breath sounds are described as *diminished* when the intensity decreases and as *absent* in extreme cases. They are described as *harsh* when the intensity increases. When the expiratory component of harsh breath sounds equals the inspiratory component, they are described as *bronchial breath sounds.*

Adventitious lung sounds are added sounds or vibrations produced by the movement of air through abnormal airways. Adventitious lung sounds are classified as either *discontinuous* or *continuous.* Discontinuous adventitious lung sounds are intermittent, crackling, or bubbling sounds of short duration. Discontinuous adventitious lung sounds are referred to as either **crackles** or **rales** (from the French word for "rattle"), whereas continuous adventitious lung sounds are described with the term **wheezes;** a wheeze is a quasi-musical sound. However, the RT often will encounter the term **rhonchi** (from the Latin word for "wheezing"). It is a term no longer favored, but widely used among older clinicians to describe a low-pitched, continuous sound (vaguely resembling snoring) that is associated with secretions in the larger airways; thus it is synonymous with coarse crackles.[14]

Another continuous type of adventitious lung sound, heard primarily over the larynx and trachea during inhalation, is **stridor.** Stridor is usually a loud, high-pitched sound that sometimes can be heard without a stethoscope. Most common in infants and small children, stridor is a sign of obstruction in the trachea or larynx. Stridor is most often heard during inspiration.

When abnormal lung sounds are heard, their location and specific features should be documented. Abnormal lung sounds may be high-pitched or low-pitched, loud or faint, scattered or diffuse, and inspiratory or expiratory (or both). Faint or low-intensity crackles are often referred to as *fine crackles;* more pronounced or more intense crackles are referred to as *coarse crackles.*

Mechanisms and Significance of Lung Sounds. The exact mechanisms that produce normal and abnormal lung sounds are not fully known. However, there is sufficient agreement to allow a general description.

Normal Breath Sounds. Lung sounds are audible vibrations primarily generated by turbulent airflow in the larger airways. These sounds are altered as they travel through the lung periphery and chest wall. Normal lung tissue acts as a low-pass filter, which means it preferentially passes low-frequency sounds. This filtering effect explains the characteristic differences between tracheal breath sounds, heard directly over the trachea, and vesicular sounds, heard over the lung periphery. Normal vesicular lung sounds essentially are attenuated tracheal breath sounds.

Bronchial Breath Sounds. Bronchial breath sounds are considered abnormal when they are heard over peripheral lung regions. Normal vesicular sounds are replaced with bronchial sounds when lung tissue density increases, and attenuation is reduced. When normal air-filled lung tissue becomes atelectatic or consolidated (e.g., pneumonia), the resulting breath sounds are similar to the sounds normally heard over large upper airways.

Diminished Breath Sounds. Diminished breath sounds occur when the sound intensity at the site of generation (larger airways) is reduced, or when the sound transmission through the lung or chest wall is decreased. Shallow or slow breathing patterns both reduce sound intensity because they create less turbulent flow in the larger airways. Reduced sound transmission also occurs for a variety of other reasons, including (1) when airways are plugged with mucus, (2) the lung tissue is hyperinflated (e.g., COPD, asthma), (3) air or fluid collects in the pleural space (e.g., pneumothorax, hemothorax, pleural effusion), (4) anasarca (generalized body edema), and (5) obesity or when chest muscles are highly developed.

Wheezes and Stridor. Wheezes and stridor represent vibrations of airway wall caused when air flows at a high velocity through a narrowed airway. Airway diameter can be reduced by bronchospasm, mucosal edema, inflammation, tumors, foreign bodies, and pulmonary edema.

This narrowing initially causes an increase in the velocity of airflow, which causes the lateral wall pressure to decrease. This decrease in pressure causes the lateral walls of the narrowed airway to pull closer together, and airflow stops. When airflow stops, the lateral wall pressure increases, and the airway opens back to the previous position. This cycle repeats many times per second and causes the airway walls to vibrate and make a musical type of adventitious lung sound similar to a reed instrument.

RULE OF THUMB

Generally, expiratory wheezes indicate obstruction of intrathoracic airways such as occurs with lung diseases (e.g., bronchitis, asthma). Wheezing may be monophonic (single note) or polyphonic (multiple notes). A monophonic wheeze indicates that a single airway is partially obstructed. Monophonic wheezing may be heard during inhalation and exhalation or during exhalation only. Polyphonic wheezing suggests that many airways are obstructed, such as with asthma, and is heard only during exhalation. Bronchitis and CHF with pulmonary edema also can cause polyphonic wheezing.

It is useful to monitor the pitch and duration of wheezing. Improved expiratory flow is associated with a decrease in the pitch and length of the wheezing. If high-pitched wheezing is present during the entire expiratory time before treatment but becomes lower pitched and occurs only late in exhalation after therapy, the pitch and duration of the wheeze have diminished. This change suggests that the degree of airway obstruction has decreased.

Stridor is a serious adventitious lung sound indicating that the upper airway is compromised. It may occur in patients of any age but most often occurs in children. In children, laryngomalacia is the most common cause of chronic stridor, whereas croup is the most common cause of acute stridor. Generally, inspiratory stridor is consistent with narrowing above the glottis, whereas expiratory stridor indicates narrowing of the lower trachea. In adults, stridor most often occurs from laryngeal or subglottic edema secondary to airway trauma after prolonged intubation.

Crackles. Crackles occur when airflow moves secretions or fluid in the airways. Coarse crackles usually are heard during both inspiration and expiration and often clear when the patient coughs or when the upper airway is suctioned. Crackles also may be heard in patients without excess secretions. These crackles occur when collapsed airways pop open during inspiration. Airway collapse or closure can occur in peripheral bronchioles or in larger, more proximal bronchi.

Larger, more proximal bronchi may close during expiration when there is an abnormal increase in bronchial compliance or when the retractile pressures around the bronchi are low. In this situation, crackles usually occur early in the inspiratory phase and are referred to as *early inspiratory crackles* (Figure 16-8). Early inspiratory crackles may be loud or faint and are not silenced by a cough or a change in position. They frequently occur in patients with COPD (chronic bronchitis, emphysema, or asthma) and usually indicate severe airway obstruction.

Peripheral airways may close during exhalation when the surrounding intrathoracic pressure increases or when surfactant levels are diminished. *Fine, late inspiratory crackles* are produced by the sudden opening of peripheral airways, usually late in the inspiratory phase. They are more common in the dependent lung regions, where the peripheral airways are most prone to collapse during exhalation. They may clear with changes in posture or if the patient performs several deep inspirations. Late inspiratory crackles are most common in patients with respiratory disorders that reduce gas volume of the lung, such as atelectasis, pneumonia, pulmonary edema, and pulmonary fibrosis (Table 16-4).

RULE OF THUMB

Fine, late inspiratory crackles suggest either restrictive lung diseases such as pulmonary fibrosis or the opening of collapsed (atelectatic) alveoli.

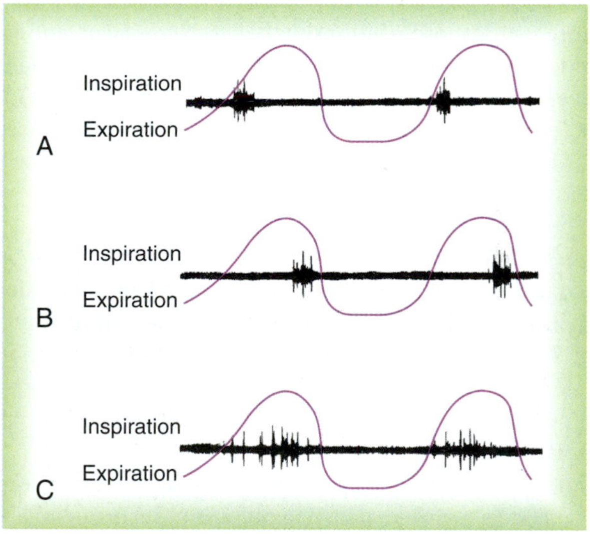

FIGURE 16-8 Timing of inspiratory crackles. **A,** Early inspiratory crackles. **B,** Late inspiratory crackles. **C,** Pan-inspiratory crackles.

TABLE 16-4
Application of Adventitious Lung Sounds

Lung Sound	Possible Mechanism	Characteristics	Causes
Wheezes	Rapid airflow through obstructed airways	High-pitched, usually expiratory	Asthma, congestive heart
Stridor	Rapid airflow through obstructed upper airway	High-pitched, monophonic	Croup, epiglottitis, postextubation laryngeal edema
Coarse crackles	Excess airway secretions moving through airways	Coarse, inspiratory and expiratory	Severe pneumonia, bronchitis
Fine crackles	Sudden opening of peripheral airways	Fine, late inspiratory	Atelectasis, fibrosis, pulmonary edema

Pleural Friction Rub. A pleural friction rub is a creaking or grating sound that occurs when the pleural surfaces become inflamed and rub together during breathing, as in pleurisy. It may be heard only during inhalation but often is identified during both phases of breathing. The rub usually is localized to a certain site on the chest wall. It sounds similar to coarse crackles but is not affected by coughing. The intensity of pleural rubs may increase with deep breathing.

Voice Sounds. Vocal resonance is produced by the same mechanism as vocal fremitus. Normal, air-filled lung tissue filters vocal sounds and reduces the intensity and clarity of spoken words. **Egophony,** or **bronchophony,** is an increased intensity and clarity of vocal resonance produced by enhanced transmission of vocal vibrations through consolidated lung tissue. The patient is instructed to repeat the words "one," "two," "three," or "ninety-nine" while the clinician listens over the chest wall with a stethoscope, comparing one side with the other. When listening over consolidation lung tissue, the words will be transmitted louder, clearer, and with a distinctive *nasal bleating quality*. Alternatively, by having the patient repeatedly pronounce a long A sound, consolidated lung will transmit the sound as an E. This is referred to as *E to A egophony*. Bronchophony often accompanies bronchial breath sounds, a dull percussion note, and increased vocal fremitus.

Cardiac Examination

Because of the close relationship between the heart and lungs, chronic lung diseases often cause cardiac problems. The techniques for physical examination of the chest wall overlying the heart (precordium) include inspection, palpation, and auscultation. Most clinicians examine the precordium at the same time they assess the lungs.

Inspection and Palpation

Inspection and palpation of the precordium help identify normal or abnormal pulsations. Pulsations on the precordium are created by ventricular contraction. Detection of pulsations depends on the force of ventricular contraction and the thickness of the chest wall through which the vibrations travel.

Normally, left ventricular contraction is the most forceful and generates a visible, palpable pulsation during systole. This pulsation is called the *point of maximal impulse* (PMI). To identify the PMI, place the palm of the right hand over the lower left sternal border.

The PMI shifts laterally with left ventricular hypertrophy. Right ventricular hypertrophy produces a systolic **heave** (or thrust) felt near the lower left sternal border. This is a common finding in patients with chronic hypoxemia, pulmonary valvular disease, or primary pulmonary hypertension The PMI may be difficult to locate in patients with severe emphysema, because systolic vibrations are not well transmitted across hyperinflated lungs.

The PMI also may shift with deviations in the mediastinum caused by pneumothorax or lobar collapse. Typically, the PMI shifts *toward* lobar collapse but *away* from a tension pneumothorax. With severe pulmonary hyperinflation the PMI shifts centrally to the epigastric area.

The second left intercostal space near the sternal border is referred to as the *pulmonic area* and is palpated to identify accentuated pulmonary valve closure. Strong vibrations may be felt in this area with the presence of pulmonary hypertension or valvular abnormalities (Figure 16-9). Valvular abnormalities may produce palpable vibrations or **thrills** that often are accompanied by a murmur (see later).

Auscultation of Heart Sounds

Heart sounds are auscultated using either the bell or diaphragm of the stethoscope. Optimal auscultation occurs when the patient leans forward or lies on the left side, as this moves the heart closer to the chest wall.

Normal heart sounds are created by closure of the heart valves (see Chapter 10). The first heart sound (S_1) is produced by closure of the mitral and tricuspid (atrioventricular [AV]) valves during ventricular contraction. When systole ends and the ventricles relax, the pulmonic and aortic (semilunar) valves close, creating the second heart sound (S_2). If either the AV valves or the semilunar valves do not close together, a *pronounced* split heart sound is heard. A third, low-pitched, heart sound (S_3) is heard over the apex of the heart that, in adults, may signify CHF. A fourth heart sound (S_4) occurs later and may be a sign of heart disease. A patient with heart disease who has S_3 and S_4 is said to have a **gallop rhythm.**

Abnormal Heart Sounds

Reduced intensity of heart sounds may result from cardiac or extracardiac abnormalities. Pulmonary hyperinflation, pleural effusion, pneumothorax, and obesity make it difficult to identify S_1 and S_2. Poor ventricular contraction resulting from heart failure or valvular disease also decreases S_1 and S_2. In contrast, an intense S_2 **(loud P2)** occurs in pulmonary hypertension due to forceful closure of the pulmonic valve.

Cardiac **murmurs** are created by (1) a backflow of blood through an incompetent valve, (2) a forward flow of blood through a stenotic ("narrowed") valve, and (3) rapid blood flow through a normal valve (as occurs with heavy exertion). Cardiac murmurs caused by incompetent or stenotic heart valves are classified as systolic or diastolic.

Systolic murmurs from an incompetent AV valve typically produce a high-pitched "whooshing" noise during S_1. In contrast, obstructed blood flow through a stenotic semilunar valve produces a crescendo-decrescendo sound. A *diastolic murmur* occurs with S_2 and is created by the backflow of blood across an incompetent semilunar valve. A *turbulent diastolic murmur* is caused by obstructed blood flow across a stenotic AV valve during diastole.

Abdominal Examination

The abdomen should be inspected and palpated for evidence of distention and tenderness. Abdominal distention and pain impair diaphragmatic movement and may contribute to or cause respiratory insufficiency. Abdominal dysfunction may

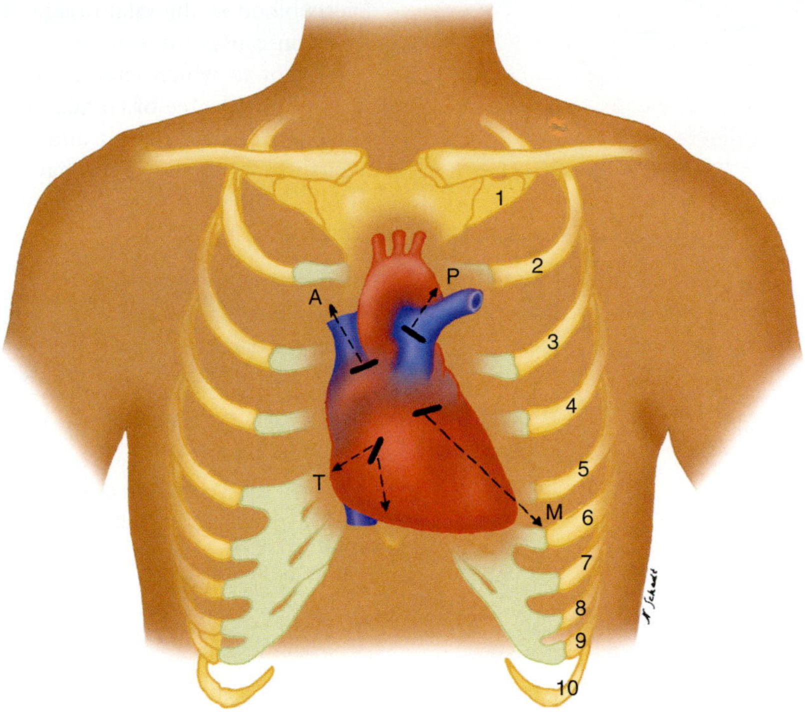

FIGURE 16-9 Anatomic and auscultatory valve area. Location of anatomic valve sites is represented by *solid bars*. *Arrows* designate transmission of valve sounds to their respective auscultatory valve areas. *A,* Aortic valve; *M,* mitral valve; *P,* pulmonic valve; *T,* tricuspid valve.

inhibit deep breathing and coughing and promote atelectasis. Of particular concern is intraabdominal hypertension, which is defined as intraabdominal pressure greater than 12 mm Hg, and is found in between 20% and 30% of critically ill patients.[15] **Abdominal compartment syndrome** occurs when intraabdominal pressures are greater than 20 mm Hg and often requires emergency decompressive surgery. This syndrome causes profound atelectasis and hypoxemia, hypotension, and renal failure.

Intraabdominal hypertension is a common finding in patients with blunt or penetrating abdominal trauma, ruptured aortic aneurysm, bowel infarction, and end-stage liver failure. It is suspected when gross examination of the abdomen reveals very pronounced abdominal distention. Intraabdominal pressure is measured by connecting an intraarterial pressure catheter to the culture port of a Foley urine catheter.

The presence of an enlarged liver (**hepatomegaly**) is a frequent cause of right lower lobe atelectasis and pleural effusion. Hepatomegaly is a common finding in patients with liver disease and patients with cor pulmonale.

Examination of the Extremities

Respiratory disease may cause several abnormalities of the extremities, including digital clubbing, cyanosis, and pedal edema.

Clubbing

Clubbing of the digits is a significant manifestation of cardiopulmonary disease. **Clubbing** is a painless enlargement of the terminal phalanges of the fingers and toes that develops over time. As the process advances, the angle of the fingernail to the nail base increases, and the base of the nail feels "spongy." The profile view of the digits allows easier recognition of clubbing (Figure 16-10), but sponginess of the nail bed is the most important sign. Causes of clubbing include infiltrative or interstitial lung disease, bronchiectasis, various cancers (particularly lung cancer),[16] congenital heart disease, chronic liver disease, and inflammatory bowel disease. COPD alone, even when hypoxemia is present, does not lead to clubbing. Clubbing of the digits in a patient with COPD indicates that something other than obstructive lung disease is occurring.

Cyanosis

Examination of the digits for cyanosis is part of the initial assessment and is done whenever hypoxemia is suspected. Cyanosis is detectable because of the transparency of the fingernails and skin. Cyanosis becomes visible when the amount of unsaturated hemoglobin in the capillary blood exceeds 5 to 6 g/dl; this may be caused by a reduction in arterial or venous O_2 content, or both.

Cyanosis of the digits is referred to as ***peripheral cyanosis*** or *acrocyanosis* and may involve extensive portions of limbs. This condition is mainly the result of poor perfusion, especially in the extremities. When capillary blood flow is poor, the tissues extract more O_2. This reduces the venous O_2 content and therefore increases the amount of reduced hemoglobin. The extremities are usually cool to the touch when peripheral cyanosis is a sign of poor peripheral perfusion. ***Central cyanosis*** on the other hand can be seen in the patient's mucosa or trunk and may

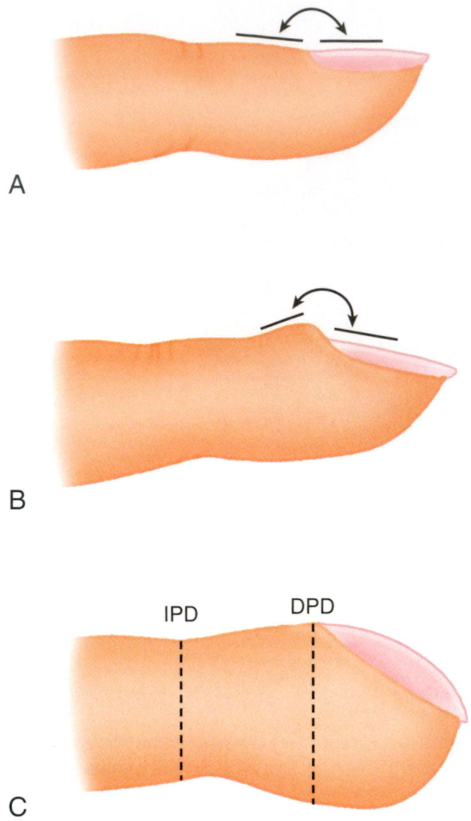

FIGURE 16-10 **A,** Normal digit configuration. **B,** Mild digital clubbing with increased hyponychial angle. **C,** Severe digital clubbing; the depth of the finger at the base of the nail *(DPD)* is greater than the depth of the interphalangeal joint *(IPD)* with clubbing.

signal severe lung disease or when venous blood is shunting as a result of congenital heart disease. However, cyanosis may be masked by room lighting and in people of color, as well as those with severe anemia.

Pedal Edema

See discussions of common cardiopulmonary symptoms.

Capillary Refill

Capillary refill is assessed by pressing briefly and firmly on the patient's fingernail until the nail bed is blanched. When pressure is released, the speed at which the blood flow and color return is noted. When cardiac output is reduced and the digital perfusion is poor, capillary refill is slow, taking several seconds to complete. In healthy individuals with good cardiac output and digital perfusion, capillary refill time is 2 seconds or less. Capillary refill time should be assessed in the context of whether or not the skin is mottled (i.e., blotched skin shade) and skin temperature.

Peripheral Skin Temperature

When systemic perfusion is poor (as in heart failure or shock), there is a compensatory vasoconstriction in the extremities that diverts blood to the vital organs. This reduction in peripheral perfusion causes the extremities to become cool to the touch. The extent to which coolness extends back toward the torso indicates the degree of circulatory failure. In contrast, patients with high cardiac output and peripheral vascular failure (as occurs in septic shock) may have warm, dry skin.

MINI CLINI

Evaluation of Acute-Onset Respiratory Distress

PROBLEM: The RT is called to evaluate a 55-year-old woman with acute respiratory distress and worsening hypoxemia. The patient is 3 days post-admission for right-sided rib fractures. This resulted from falling down a flight of stairs, secondary to alcohol intoxication with brief loss of consciousness. Since admission she had maintained adequate oxygenation with pulse oximetry (SpO_2) of 95% on 3 L/min of nasal O_2. Over the past hour she has become febrile (maximum temperature 39.5° C), tachycardic (heart rate 130 beats/min), and hypotensive (blood pressure 88/50 mm Hg; mean, 63 mm Hg), with new-onset altered mental status. Her SpO_2 is now 87% on 6 L/min nasal O_2 with a respiratory rate of 32 breaths/min. Her medical history is significant for alcoholism and a 30 pack-year smoking history. What can the physical examination and history tell us about the potential source of respiratory distress?

SOLUTION: The signs, symptoms and history suggest bacterial pneumonia possibly from aspiration during her initial loss of consciousness or from a pulmonary contusion. Bacterial pneumonia has an incubation period of 1 to 3 days. The associated high fever, tachycardia, hypotension, and altered mental status also suggest that pneumonia has resulted in sepsis (systemic inflammation). Pulmonary contusion also can result in pneumonia and ARDS (see Chapter 29), with a peak occurrence at approximately 72 hours.[17]

Rib fractures are painful and limit deep breathing and effective coughing, leading to atelectasis and retained secretions that increase the risk for pneumonia. When extensive, rib fractures also cause chest wall instability that limits effective ventilation and heightens the risk for respiratory failure. Both alcoholism and cigarette smoking further increases the susceptibility to pneumonia.[18,19] Also, a history of alcohol abuse may be a contributory factor because the onset of acute alcohol withdrawal typically occurs in this time frame.[20]

The first priority is to increase O_2 therapy to achieve adequate oxygenation ($Sp_{O2} \geq 90\%$) while conducting an examination. Worsening oxygenation, despite doubling O_2 therapy, suggests refractory hypoxemia, which is a hallmark of ARDS. This situation indicates the need for high-concentration O_2 therapy, continuous pulse oximetry and close hemodynamic monitoring.

The RT should be alert for signs suggestive for heightened work of breathing (rapid-shallow breathing, accessory inspiratory muscle use, along with tracheal or intercostal retractions and expiratory muscle recruitment), chest wall instability (paradoxical chest motion), and diminished ventilation (global decrease in breath sound intensity). Breath sounds should be evaluated for evidence suggesting the presence of secretions (coarse, bubbling crackles) or pulmonary edema (fine inspiratory crackles). Another possibility is acute pulmonary embolism, which would become a more prominent consideration if the patient had also suffered pelvic or leg fractures and was immobilized or has redness and swelling of the lower extremities. Although a pneumothorax is unlikely in this situation, the chest should be inspected for signs (e.g., subcutaneous emphysema, JVD, unilateral chest excursion).

Further work-up would include a chest radiograph to confirm the suspicion of pneumonia or chest contusion (and to rule out a pneumothorax), an arterial blood gas to evaluate the severity of hypoxemia and the adequacy of ventilation, and blood samples to evaluate the presence of infection (see Chapter 17). The results of these tests and the patient's response to therapeutic interventions would determine where the patient can be safely and optimally managed.

SUMMARY CHECKLIST

- The interview is used to obtain important diagnostic information and build a rapport between with the patient.
- Dyspnea is the sensation that occurs when breathing effort is excessive relative to the tidal volume achieved and increases with reduced lung compliance and narrowed airways. Breathlessness is the unpleasant sensation associated with a heightened drive to breathe.
- Cough is one of the most common symptoms of lung disease and occurs when the cough receptors in the airways are stimulated by foreign material, mucus, noxious gases, or inflammation.
- Chronic cough is most often caused by upper airway cough syndrome, asthma, chronic bronchitis from cigarette smoking, and gastroesophageal reflux disease.
- The most common cause of hemoptysis (spitting up blood from the lung) is infection.
- Vital signs provide reliable assessment information about the general condition of the patient and the patient's response to therapy.
- Rapid, shallow breathing indicates pathologic changes in the lung consistent with a reduction in the gas volume of the lungs.
- A prolonged expiratory phase suggests that the intrathoracic airways are narrowed.
- Normal breath sounds are generated by turbulent airflow in the larger airways.
- Crackles are generated by the sudden opening of closed airways or by the movement of excessive airway secretions with breathing.
- Wheezes are produced by the rapid vibration of narrow airways as gas passes through at high velocity.
- Cor pulmonale causes JVD, hepatomegaly, a loud P_2, and pedal edema.
- Central cyanosis is a sign of hypoxemia caused by respiratory failure, whereas peripheral cyanosis suggests circulatory failure.

References

1. Terasaki G, Paauw DS: Evaluation and treatment of chronic cough. *Med Clin North Am* 98:391–403, 2014.
2. O'Grady NP, Barie PS, Bartlett JG, et al: Guidelines for evaluation of new fever in critically-ill adult patients: 2008 update from the American College of Critical care medicine and the Infectious Diseases Society of America. *Crit Care Med* 35:1330–1342, 2008.
3. Hayakawa K, Ramasamy B, Chandrasekar PH: Fever of unknown origin: an evidence-based review. *Am J Med Sci* 344:307–316, 2012.
4. Mavros MN, Velmahos GC, Falagas ME: Atelectasis as a cause of postoperative fever: where is the clinical evidence? *Chest* 140:418–424, 2011.
5. Brugha R, Grigg J: Urban air pollution and respiratory infections. *Paediatr Respir Rev* 15:194–199, 2014.
6. Buda AJ, Pinsky MR, Ingels NB, Jr, et al: Effect of intrathoracic pressure on left ventricular performance. *N Engl J Med* 301:453–459, 1979.
7. National High Blood Pressure Education Program: *The 7th report of the Joint National Committee on Prevention, Detection, Evaluation and Treatment of High Blood Pressure*, Besthesda, MD, 2004, National Institutes of Health National Heart, Lung and Blood Institute.
8. Antonelli M, Levy M, Andrews PJD, et al: Hemodynamic monitoring and shock and implications for management. International consensus conference, Paris, France. 27th-28th April 2006. *Intensive Care Med* 33:575–590, 2007.
9. Roussos C, Macklem PT: The respiratory muscles. *N Engl J Med* 307:786–797, 1982.
10. Astiz ME: Pathophysiology and classification of shock states. In Fink MP, Abraham E, Vincent J-L, et al, editors: *Textbook of critical care*, ed 5, Philadelphia, 2005, Saunders, pp 897–904.
11. Kallet RH: Patient-ventilator interactions during acute lung injury and the role of spontaneous breathing. Part 1. Respiratory muscle function in critical illness. *Respir Care* 56:181–189, 2011.
12. Tobin MJ, Perez W, Guenther SM, et al: Does rib cage-abdominal paradox signify respiratory muscle fatigue. *J Appl Physiol* 63:851–860, 1987.
13. Longtin Y, Schneider A, Tschopp C, et al: Contamination of stethoscopes and physician's hands after a physical examination. *Mayo Clin Proc* 89:291–299, 2014.
14. Wilkins RL, Dexter JR, Murphy RLH, et al: Lung sound nomenclature survey. *Chest* 98:886–889, 1990.
15. Atema JJ, vanBuijtenen JM, Lamme B, et al: Clinical studies on intra-abdominal hypertension and abdominal compartment syndrome. *J Trauma Acute Care Surg* 76:234–240, 2013.
16. Rutherford JD: Digital clubbing. *Circulation* 127:1997–1999, 2013.
17. Cohn SM, DuBose JJ: Pulmonary contusion: an update on recent advances in clinical management. *World J Surg* 34:1959–1970, 2010.
18. Kaphalia L, Calhoun WJ: Alcoholic lung injury: metabolic, biochemical and immunological aspects. *Toxicol Lett* 222:171–179, 2013.
19. Huttunen R, Heikkinen T, Syrjanen J: Smoking and outcome of infection. *J Intern Med* 269:258–269, 2011.
20. Awassi D-K, Lebrun G, Fagnan M, et al: Alcohol, nicotine and iatrogenic withdrawals in the ICU. *Crit Care Med* 41:S57–S68, 2013.

Bibliography

Bickley LS: *Bate's guide to physical examination and history taking*, ed 10, Philadelphia, 2008, Lippincott.

Booth S, Dudgeon D: *Dyspnoea in advanced disease: a guide to clinical management*, Oxford, 2006, Oxford University Press.

Bowers AC, Thompson JM: *Clinical manual of health assessment*, ed 4, St Louis, 1992, Mosby.

Gardner WN: The pathophysiology of hyperventilation syndrome. *Chest* 109:516–534, 1996.

Mahler DA, O'Donnell DE: *Dyspnea: mechanisms, measurement and management*, ed 3, Boca Raton, FL, 2014, CRC Press, Taylor & Francis.

Ropper AH, Brown RH: *Adams and Victor's principles of neurology*, ed 8, New York, 2005 McGraw-Hill.

Seidel HM, Ball JW, Dains JE, et al: *Mosby's guide to physical examination*, ed 7, St Louis, 2011, Mosby.

Wilkins RL, Dexter JM, Heuer AJ: *Clinical assessment in respiratory care*, ed 6, St Louis, 2010, Mosby.

Wilkins RL, Hodgkin JE, Lopez B: *Lung sounds: a practical guide*, ed 3, St Louis, 2004, Mosby.

CHAPTER 17

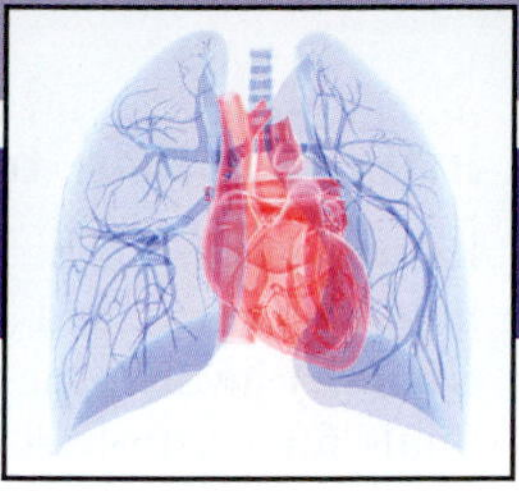

Interpreting Clinical and Laboratory Data

RICHARD H. KALLET

CHAPTER OBJECTIVES

After reading this chapter you will be able to:

- Describe a critical value and its importance in clinical practice.
- Define leukocytosis, leukopenia, anemia, polycythemia, and thrombocytopenia.
- Identify which electrolyte disturbances interfere with normal respiratory function.
- Describe clinical tests used to identify cardiac stress and myocardial infarction.
- Identify the three main tests used to diagnose coagulation disorders.
- Describe how the sputum Gram stain and culture are used to diagnose pulmonary infections.

CHAPTER OUTLINE

KEY TERMS

acid-fast bacterium
anemia
bands
basic chemistry panel
complete blood count
critical test value
erythrocytes
hematology
hematocrit
homeostasis
hyperglycemia
hyperkalemia
hypernatremia
hypoglycemia
hypokalemia
lactate
leukocytes
leukocytosis
leukopenia
neutropenia
polycythemia
reference range
segs
thrombocytes
thrombocytopenia
troponin
troponin I

INTERPRETING CLINICAL LABORATORY TESTS

This chapter discusses common blood tests performed on patients admitted to the hospital. These tests are done to evaluate the general health and baseline status of the patient, identify organ system dysfunction, detect the presence of infection, and determine the effects of therapy. Hence, the respiratory therapist (RT) must be familiar with these tests and their value in helping diagnose respiratory dysfunction.

This chapter also presents a brief review of fundamental physiologic concepts related to these tests, contains comprehensive with reference-range values, and explains the significance of these tests in patient assessment.

Introduction to Laboratory Medicine

Laboratory medicine involves the study of patient tissue and fluid specimens and consists of five disciplines. *Clinical biochemistry* involves the analysis of blood, urine, and other bodily fluids for electrolytes and proteins; **hematology** analyzes the cellular components of blood. *Clinical microbiology* tests blood and other bodily fluids for infectious agents and includes the subspecialties that identify bacteria *(bacteriology)*, viruses *(virology)*, fungi *(mycology)*, and parasites *(parasitology)*. *Immunology* is a closely related discipline focusing on autoimmune and immunodeficiency diseases. Finally, the *anatomic pathology* service assists with diagnosing diseases by analyzing tissue samples.

Reference Range

Laboratory tests help determine a patient's health status and aid medical decisions. Therefore it is important to determine whether a specific test result falls within an expected range of values considered to be "normal." However, the notion of "normal" can be problematic. In the early history of laboratory medicine, determining the normal range for blood chemistry and hematology tests was primitive and not representative of the larger population in terms of age, gender, race, and ethnicity. In addition, the term *normal* is not synonymous with *healthy*. For example, the normal range for cholesterol found in most Americans puts them at risk for cardiovascular disease and therefore cannot be considered healthy.

Beginning in the 1970s,[1] the term *normal ranges* was replaced with more appropriate terms such as *reference ranges, biologic reference intervals*, and *expected value*.[2] This change in terminology acknowledged that what we consider normal must take into account variations related to age, gender, race, and ethnicity, which change over time as the demographic composition of society changes. A **reference range** sets the boundaries for, and expected variability of, any analyte (e.g., electrolyte, blood cell, protein, enzyme) that would likely be encountered in healthy subjects.

Reference ranges differ from laboratory to laboratory for various reasons. These include differences in measurement techniques, the populations of healthy individuals used to establish the reference intervals, and analytic imprecision. Most differences in reference ranges between laboratories are small.[2] Reference ranges and critical values displayed in this chapter serve as representative examples; however, RTs must become familiar with the reference ranges used at their institutions.

Critical Test Value

A **critical test value** is a result *significantly* outside the reference range and represents a pathophysiologic condition. A critical value may be *potentially* life-threatening, and immediate corrective action is often warranted. Critical values are reported in the hospital to alert caregivers, decrease medical errors, and protect patients.

Typically, critical values are communicated by telephone from the clinical laboratory to the unit where the patient is situated. The nurse or RT receiving these results must read back the critical value to the clinical laboratory to ensure accuracy. The nurse or RT then must communicate the critical value in a timely fashion to the physician. The same read-back procedure is used. All communication of critical test values is documented in the medical record.

In this chapter, critical values are listed along with common pathophysiologic states with which they commonly occur. Not all clinical analytes have an associated critical value because sometimes there is no agreement on what constitutes a critical value. Others have only a one-sided value that exists below or above a critical threshold. This is true particularly for substances that do not normally appear in the blood. For example, certain enzymes and proteins are released only after extensive cellular damage following injury (see later section on enzyme tests). Under normal circumstances, these proteins or enzymes may be virtually undetectable in the serum or plasma.

When interpreting derangements for *any* test result, clinicians must consider the *context* of the change. In a patient with chronic renal disease, a serum creatinine of 3.0 mg/dl (approximately twice the upper limit of normal) is not considered urgent. But, in a patient with a bloodstream infection (i.e., sepsis) and hypotension, a sudden increase in serum creatinine to 3.0 mg/dl is considered critical because it indicates acute kidney dysfunction and possibly septic shock.

Complete Blood Count

The **complete blood count** (CBC) describes the number of circulating white blood cells (WBCs), called **leukocytes;** red blood cells (RBCs), called **erythrocytes;** and platelets, called **thrombocytes.** The WBC count is made up of five different types of cells and is reported under the *differential*. RBCs are evaluated for size and hemoglobin (Hb) content. Platelets are evaluated by the number present. Table 17-1 lists the normal CBC results for adults.

An elevated WBC count is termed **leukocytosis** and has multiple causes, including stress, infection, and trauma. The degree of leukocytosis reflects the severity of infection. A significantly elevated WBC count ($>20 \times 10^3$/mcl) suggests the presence of a serious infection and that the patient's immune system is generating a strong response. In contrast, **leukopenia** (or leukocytopenia) is a WBC count below normal that often occurs when the immune system is overwhelmed by infection. Other causes include bone marrow diseases (e.g., leukemia, lymphoma), influenza, systemic lupus erythematosus, tuberculosis, acquired immunodeficiency syndrome (AIDS), and chemotherapy or radiation therapy given to cancer patients.

RULE OF THUMB

Leukocytosis usually represents a vigorous immune response to either infection or trauma.

RULE OF THUMB

Leukocytopenia often signifies that either the immune system has been overwhelmed by infection or there is presence of immunosuppression.

White Blood Cell Count

The WBC differential count determines the number of each type of WBC present in the blood (Table 17-2). Most circulating WBCs are either neutrophils or lymphocytes. Leukocytosis is a significant elevation in the WBC count (>15 × 10^3/mcl) that occurs when either neutrophils or lymphocytes are responding to an abnormality. Basophils, eosinophils, and monocytes make up a small proportion of the circulating WBCs and rarely cause a major increase in the WBC count.

TABLE 17-1

Reference Range Values for Complete Blood Count in an Adult

Test	Reference Range
Red blood cell count	
Men	4.4-5.9 × 10^6/mcl
Women	3.8-5.2 × 10^6/mcl
Hemoglobin	
Men	13.3-17.7 g/dl
Women	11.7-15.7 g/dl
Hematocrit	
Men	40%-52%
Women	35%-47%
White blood cell count	3.9-11.7 × 10^3/mcl
White blood cell differential	
Segmented neutrophils	40%-75%
Bands	0%-6%
Eosinophils	0%-6%
Basophils	0%-1%
Lymphocytes	20%-45%
Monocytes	2%-10%
Platelet count	150-400 × 10^3/mcl

Values for reference ranges and critical test results are from the University of California–San Francisco Moffit-Long Hospital and San Francisco General Hospital.

The WBC count differential is calculated by multiplying the percentage of each WBC subtype by the total WBC count. This prevents misinterpreting the WBC count differential when one cell type changes, causing a *relative change* (percentage) in the other four cell types. For example, if the neutrophil count doubles because of infection, the relative percentage of the other four cells types would decrease, although their absolute number would not change.

The sub-analysis of lymphocytes is important for identifying infection with human immunodeficiency virus (HIV), the causative agent of AIDS. HIV targets and destroys CD4 T lymphocytes. Opportunistic infections such as *Pneumocystis jiroveci* pneumonia generally occur when lymphocytes decrease to less than 200 × 10^6/L, and this information is used in making the diagnosis of AIDS.

Elevation of the absolute value of neutrophils is termed *neutrophilia*. Immature neutrophils are known as **bands** because of the banded shape of the nucleus. Most bands are located in the bone marrow, where they continue to mature. Mature neutrophils are known as **segs** because of the segmented shape of their nucleus. Severe infection causes the bone marrow to release stores of any available neutrophils, and both bands and segs enter the circulating blood volume. When bands and segs are elevated in the CBC, the patient is likely experiencing a more severe bacterial infection.

A reduced number of circulating neutrophils is termed **neutropenia** and is observed in patients with bone marrow disease (e.g., lymphoma, leukemia), autoimmune disorders, HIV infection, and those undergoing chemotherapy or radiation treatment for cancer. Neutropenia increases risk for the developing opportunistic infections.

RULE OF THUMB

Elevation of the WBC count usually is caused by an increase in either neutrophils or lymphocytes in response to infection.

TABLE 17-2

Reference Range Values for White Blood Cell Count Differential and Common Causes for Abnormalities

Cell Type	Relative Value (%)	Absolute Value	Causes for Abnormalities
Neutrophils	40-75	1.8-6.8 × 10^9/L	Increased with bacterial infection and trauma; reduced with bone marrow diseases (critical value <1.0)
Lymphocytes	20-45	1.0-3.4 × 10^9/L	Increased with viral and other infections; reduced with immunodeficiency problems
CD4 T lymphocytes	31-60*	410-1590 × 10^6/L	HIV disease; diagnostic threshold <200
Eosinophils	0-6	0-0.4 × 10^6/L	Increased with allergic reactions and parasitic infections
Basophils	0-1	0-0.1 × 10^6/L	Increased with allergic reactions
Monocytes	2-10	0.2-0.8 × 10^6/L	Increased with invasion of foreign material

Values for reference ranges and critical test results are from the University of California–San Francisco Moffit-Long Hospital and San Francisco General Hospital.

*Percentage of lymphocyte.

RULE OF THUMB

When bands and segs are elevated in the CBC, the patient is likely experiencing a more severe bacterial infection.

Red Blood Cell Count

The primary function of RBCs or erythrocytes is to supply oxygen to the tissues. The RBC count helps determine the ability of the blood to carry O_2. An abnormally low RBC count is referred to as **anemia** and suggests that either bone marrow production of RBCs is inadequate or excessive blood loss has occurred. Regardless, the O_2-carrying capacity of blood is reduced, and the patient is at increased risk for tissue hypoxia. Anemia has different causes: some are related to dietary deficiencies in iron or vitamins (e.g., vitamin B_{12} and folate); others are related to chronic inflammatory diseases, such as Crohn disease, HIV/AIDS, lymphoma, and autoimmune diseases that destroy erythrocytes (hemolytic and aplastic anemia). A hereditary cause is sickle cell anemia, which is common in African-Americans. For most forms of anemia, a blood transfusion may be needed if the RBC count is too low, as discussed later in this chapter.

MINI CLINI

White Blood Cell Count Differential

PROBLEM: A patient admitted to the hospital for acute shortness of breath and fever has a chest radiograph revealing pneumonia. The CBC shows an increased WBC count of 15×10^3/mcl with 75% neutrophils but only 10% lymphocytes. Given that the normal lymphocyte differential is 20% to 45%, does the value of 10% suggest a problem with lymphocyte production by the immune system? What type of pneumonia is probably present in this case?

SOLUTION: The 10% differential for the lymphocytes represents a *relative value*. Because the total WBC count is markedly elevated, the 10% in relative terms represents 1500 lymphocytes in absolute value, which is within normal range. If the total WBC count was reduced to less than normal and the differential showed a lymphocyte count of 10%, an abnormal absolute value would be present and would suggest an immunologic problem. This patient probably has bacterial pneumonia, given the elevated number of neutrophils.

Polycythemia is an abnormally elevated RBC count. It often occurs when the bone marrow is stimulated to produce extra RBCs in response to chronic hypoxemia (secondary polycythemia). Polycythemia counteracts reduced PO_2 by increasing the O_2-carrying capacity of the blood. Patients living at high altitudes and those with chronic lung disease are most likely to experience chronic hypoxia and develop secondary polycythemia.

In addition to the RBC count, the clinical laboratory reports Hb and hematocrit (Hct) levels. Hb is a protein substance with the unique ability to bind with O_2. Each healthy RBC contains 200 million to 300 million molecules of Hb, for an Hb level of 12 to 17 g/dl in a healthy adult. Patients with an inadequate Hb concentration have reduced O_2-carrying capacity. In this condition, the RBCs are smaller than normal *(microcytic anemia)* and lack normal color *(hypochromic anemia)*. The necessity for RBC transfusion depends on the cause of anemia and the patient's overall condition. Transfusions generally are indicated only when the Hb concentration falls to 7.0 g/dl (an Hct of approximately 21%), because this conservative practice actually improves patient outcomes.[3]

The Hct level is the ratio of RBC volume to whole blood. It is determined by spinning a blood sample in a centrifuge to separate the blood cells from the plasma. The proportion of the sample represented by the packed cells is the **hematocrit.** A low Hct occurs with anemia and a high Hct with polycythemia. The Hct also reflects the patient's hydration status. Dehydration causes the Hct to increase (hemoconcentration), whereas overhydration causes it to decrease via hemodilution.

RULE OF THUMB

The recommended threshold for blood transfusion is Hb of 7.0 g/dl or Hct of 21%.

Electrolyte Tests

Basic Concepts for Understanding Electrolyte Balance

Normal cellular function depends on homeostasis of fluids, electrolytes, and acid-base balance. **Homeostasis** is the ability of complex organisms to maintain a *dynamic balance* or *equilibrium* in their internal environments by making constant adjustments. The guiding principle is that the total amount of water, electrolytes, acid, and base gained each day must be balanced by the total amount lost.

Electrolytes are positively or negatively charged ions that influence the functioning of enzymes. The concentration of any electrolyte is determined by the amount of water in which it is suspended. Electrolytes always must be interpreted within the context of fluid balance. Enzymes are proteins that regulate all chemical reactions occurring within cells, such as metabolism and protein synthesis. All cellular functions operate within very narrow parameters of electrolyte concentrations. Disturbances in electrolyte balance disrupt normal cellular functioning.

Two important points must be kept in mind when interpreting blood tests. First, blood samples provide a one-time "snapshot" of processes that are constantly in flux. These "snapshots" provide the clinician with valuable but time-limited insight. Often, the most important information comes from serial measurements, whereby the degree of abnormalities and directional changes can be assessed. Changes over time provide vital information about the severity and progression of disease as well as judging the effectiveness of therapy.

Second, the intravascular blood compartment is remote from the intracellular environment. Serum electrolyte levels provide only a hint of what might be occurring inside the cells of the body. This is because the intracellular fluid compartment represents approximately two-thirds of total body fluid. By comparison, the extracellular fluid compartment represents approximately one-third and the blood plasma is just a small fraction of the extracellular environment. Therefore monitoring blood plasma abnormalities provides important but limited indirect information about the intracellular environment.

Basic Chemistry Panel

The **basic chemistry panel** (BCP) or *basic metabolic panel* includes the predominant electrolytes sodium (Na^+), potassium (K^+), chloride (Cl^-), total carbon dioxide/bicarbonate (CO_2), and glucose. Because the body's electrolyte balance is controlled by the kidneys, excretion of renal-mediated waste products is included: creatinine and blood urea nitrogen. A comprehensive metabolic panel includes electrolytes, such as magnesium (Mg^{++}), phosphorus (PO_4^-), and calcium (Ca^{++}). Each electrolyte plays a crucial role in maintaining normal cellular function. Specific information on the reference range and physiologic significance of each electrolyte and waste product can be found in Table 17-3. Information regarding the terminology used to describe abnormal test values for electrolytes, diseases associated with these disturbances, and sample critical test results are provided in Table 17-4.

There are subtle differences in how electrolytes are reported, and this may cause confusion. The concentration of electrolytes in solution is reported by either the *number of molecules* (millimoles [mmol]) or their associated valence or *electrical charge* (milliequivalents [mEq]). Although customary practice has been to report electrolytes as mEq/L, many laboratories report electrolytes as mmol/L. In an electrolyte solution, milliequivalents are simply millimoles per liter multiplied by the valence. For example, Na^+ possesses a valence of 1, so that the expression as either mmol/L or mEq/L is the same. For Ca^{++} and Mg^{++}, which both possess a valence of 2, then the mEq value is twice the mmol value.

Glucose

Carbohydrate degradation produces serum glucose that is metabolized by cells for energy. Insulin, which comes from the pancreas, is necessary for cells to use glucose circulating in the blood. **Hyperglycemia** is an abnormally elevated blood glucose level most often resulting from either diabetes or severe sepsis. **Hypoglycemia** is an abnormally reduced serum glucose level associated with digestive problems, inadequate dietary intake of carbohydrates, or overtreatment of diabetes with insulin or drug-induced.

TABLE 17-3

Components of Basic Metabolic Panel and Common Electrolyte Tests With Sample Reference Ranges and Physiologic Significance

Test	Reference Range*	Physiologic Importance
Sodium (Na^+)	136-145 mEq/L	Primary extracellular cation; crucial for maintaining fluid balance and nerve impulse conduction
Potassium (K^+)	3.5-5.0 mEq/L	Primary intracellular cation; crucial for maintaining normal heart and kidney function and acid-base balance
Chloride (Cl^-)	98-106 mEq/L	Primary extracellular anion; crucial for maintaining serum osmolarity and acid-base balance
Total carbon dioxide (CO_2)	22-29 mEq/L	Primary metabolic end product of aerobic metabolism; crucial for maintaining acid-base balance
Calcium (Ca)	4.5-5.25 mEq/L	Most abundant mineral in the body; essential for bone strength, muscular contraction, nerve impulse conduction, and coagulation
Ionized calcium (Ca^{++})	2.2-2.7 mEq/L	The approximately 50% of calcium not bound to circulating proteins; represents the biologically active portion
Glucose (Glu)	70-139 mg/dl	Primary cellular energy source
Creatinine (Cr)	0.7-1.3 mg/dl	Waste product from muscle catabolism excreted by the kidneys; one of the key markers of kidney function because it provides a gross estimation of glomerular filtration rate
Blood urea nitrogen (BUN)	8-23 mg/dl	Waste product from metabolism of amino acids; a key marker of kidney function
Magnesium (Mg^{++})	1.7-2.1 mEq/L	Essential for regulation of most biochemical processes; important for normal muscle and neuronal functioning, regulating heart rate and blood pressure, glucose levels, bone strength, and immune function
Phosphorus (PO_4^-)	1.2-2.3 mEq/L	Main intracellular anion (phosphate), exists as PO_4^- in serum; combined with Ca in teeth and bones; serum levels inversely related to serum Ca
Lactate	0.7-2.1 mEq/L	End product of glucose metabolism under anaerobic conditions; clinically significant levels coincide with regional or systemic tissue hypoxia
Osmolarity	275-295 mOsm/kg	Tonicity or ability to attract water molecules; indicates overall ionic concentration in the serum

Values for reference ranges and critical test results are from the University of California–San Francisco Moffit-Long Hospital and San Francisco General Hospital.

*Reference ranges vary among clinical laboratories. See text for explanation.

TABLE 17-4
Sample Critical Test Results Reflecting Abnormalities in Electrolyte and Other Common Laboratory Tests

Test	Sample Critical Test Result*	Common Pathologic Conditions Associated With *Abnormally High Levels*	Common Pathologic Conditions Associated With *Abnormally Low Levels*
Sodium (Na^+)	>155 mEq/L; <125 mEq/L	*Hypernatremia:* Dehydration from excessive water loss or fluid restriction; excessive administration of saline fluids or diuretics (usually ≥180 mmol)	*Hyponatremia:* Overhydration or abnormal secretion of antidiuretic hormone; severe vomiting or diarrhea; congestive heart failure, renal or hepatic failure, Addison disease
Potassium (K^+)	>6.0 mEq/L; <3.0 mEq/L	*Hyperkalemia:* Acute or chronic kidney disease, Addison disease, severe alcoholism, rhabdomyolysis; values ≥6 mmol are life-threatening	*Hypokalemia:* Severe vomiting or diarrhea; chronic renal disease; high-dose beta-agonist therapy
Chloride (Cl^-)	>120 mEq/L; <70 mEq/L	*Hyperchloremia:* Excessive Cl^- administration (usually saline resuscitation during shock); metabolic acidosis, diabetes insipidus	*Hypochloremia:* Severe vomiting or diarrhea; metabolic alkalosis, adrenal insufficiency, severe burns, excessive intravenous dextrose administration
Total carbon dioxide (CO_2)	>40 mEq/L; <15 mEq/L	Ventilatory failure	Metabolic acidosis; hyperventilation syndrome; severe diarrhea
Calcium (Ca)	>13.5 mEq/L; <6.5 mEq/L	*Hypercalcemia:* Hyperparathyroidism, lithium or thiazide diuretic therapy, metastatic cancer, multiple myeloma	*Hypocalcemia:* Hypoparathyroidism, blood transfusions, acute pancreatitis, vitamin D deficiency
Ionized calcium (Ca^{++})	>1.5 mEq/L; <0.8 mEq/L	See above	See above
Glucose (Glu)	>500 mg/dl; <50 mg/dl	*Hyperglycemia:* Diabetes mellitus, severe sepsis	*Hypoglycemia:* Excessive insulin administration, inadequate dietary intake of carbohydrates
Creatinine (Cr)	>10 mg/dl	Acute kidney injury, chronic renal failure	Protein starvation, liver disease
Blood urea nitrogen (BUN)	>100 mg/dl	Acute kidney injury, chronic renal failure, dehydration	Liver disease, malnutrition
Magnesium (Mg^{++})	>3.7 mEq/L; <0.8 mEq/L	*Hypermagnesemia:* Chronic renal failure, Addison disease, diabetic ketoacidosis, dehydration	*Hypomagnesemia:* Cirrhosis, pancreatitis, severe alcoholism, hemodialysis, toxemia of pregnancy, ulcerative colitis
Phosphorus (PO_4^-)	<1.0 mEq/L; >2.5 mEq/L	*Hyperphosphatemia:* Commonly found in patients with renal failure, hepatic failure, bone metastasis, hypocalcemia, hypoparathyroidism	*Hypophosphatemia:* Most often seen in chronic hyperventilation syndrome; also caused by hypercalcemia, hyperparathyroidism, and malnutrition
Lactate	>4 mEq/L		Primarily causes anaerobic metabolism; frequently found in patients with hemorrhagic or septic shock; may also be due to reduced hepatic clearance, dehydration, or trauma
Osmolarity	>320 mOsm/kg; <240 mOsm/kg		

Values for reference ranges and critical test results are from the University of California–San Francisco Moffit-Long Hospital and San Francisco General Hospital.
*Reference ranges and critical test results vary among clinical laboratories. See text for explanation.

Diabetes is diagnosed by measuring fasting blood glucose levels (i.e., a glucose measurement taken after 12 hours without food). A blood glucose level greater than 140 mg/dl on two occasions usually indicates diabetes. Severe hyperglycemia occurring with metabolic acidosis is consistent with *diabetic ketoacidosis* and represents a potentially life-threatening condition if not treated immediately.

In critically ill patients, insulin resistance and severe hyperglycemia (glucose levels >200 mg/dl) are common and are associated with higher incidences of organ failure and mortality. Insulin therapy is used in critically ill surgical and medical patients to control blood sugar. The practice of maintaining tightly controlled glucose levels (80 to 110 mg/dl) in these patients has been controversial. It now appears that the association between hyperglycemia and mortality is limited to critically ill patients who are *not* diabetic at hospital admission, so that less stringent parameters (glucose levels 110 to 150 mg/dl) are probably acceptable.[4]

Anion Gap

As discussed in Chapter 14, metabolic acidosis is caused by either the addition of nonvolatile acids or a primary loss of

HCO_3^-. The anion gap provides a quick method for determining whether a decrease in HCO_3^- is caused by a disruption of normal anion balance or the presence of an abnormal acid anion. A balance normally exists between cations (+ charge) and anions (− charge) in the serum. The normal anion gap occurs because sulfate, phosphate, and organic anions such as lactate are not routinely measured, whereas most cations are measured. The anion gap is calculated by adding the CO_2 and Cl^- values and then subtracting this total from the serum Na^+. The normal anion gap is approximately 8 to 14 mEq/L, and *gap acidosis* usually coincides with an anion gap of 16 mmol/L or greater. However, serum proteins are an important determinant of the anion gap. *Hypoalbuminemia* (decreased serum albumin) is common in critically ill patients and significantly reduces the anion gap. As a rule, for every 1-g reduction in serum albumin below 4 g/dl, the anion gap is corrected upward by 3 mEq/L.

RULE OF THUMB

An anion gap greater than 16 is consistent with the presence of metabolic acidosis.

Lactate

Lactate is the end product of anaerobic glucose metabolism. Blood lactate concentration depends on lactate production in muscle cells and erythrocytes and the rate of lactate metabolism by the liver. Therefore lactic acidosis results either from overproduction of lactate or insufficient metabolism of lactate. Abnormal lactate levels can be found in diverse conditions, such as liver disease, diabetes mellitus, thiamine deficiency, malignancies, and toxic ingestion of ethanol, methanol, or salicylates. However, the most common cause of lactic acidosis is anaerobic metabolism from tissue hypoxia associated with shock. Initial lactate levels greater than 4 mEq/L signifies the inability to rapidly clear high lactate levels and is associated with higher mortality in patients with septic, traumatic, or cardiogenic shock.[5]

RULE OF THUMB

In patients with many forms of shock, a serum lactate level greater than 4 mEq/L is associated with higher mortality.

MINI CLINI

Anion Gap

PROBLEM 1: A patient in the intensive care unit is being treated for shock and acute renal failure. No arterial blood gas (ABG) samples have been drawn yet, but the RT suspects the respiratory system is involved because the patient has been breathing more rapidly over the past 12 hours. The electrolyte panel reveals a serum Na^+ of 146 mEq/L, a total CO_2 of 20 mEq/L, and a serum Cl^- of 100 mEq/L. Does the electrolyte panel suggest any problems, and what should be done if there are any?

SOLUTION: The electrolytes are normal except for a decrease in the serum CO_2. The anion gap is calculated by subtracting the sum of CO_2 and Cl^- from Na^+ (146 − [100 + 20]). In this case, the anion gap is elevated (26 mEq/L) and is consistent with a metabolic acidosis. An ABG analysis is needed to evaluate the acid-base status of the patient further. The patient's rapid breathing probably is related to the metabolic acidosis because hyperventilation decreases CO_2 levels and promotes acid-base compensation.

PROBLEM 2: A patient in the trauma intensive care unit is undergoing large fluid resuscitation with normal saline solution. The patient is in hemorrhagic shock after a motor vehicle accident. An initial ABG measurement reveals a pH of 7.25, PCO_2 of 25 mm Hg, and HCO_3^- of 10.6 with a base deficit of −14.9 mEq/L. The trauma surgeons are debating increasing the amount of normal saline solution infused. They suspect their resuscitation efforts are inadequate, and metabolic acidosis is worsening from continued lactate accumulation. What additional information can be provided by obtaining a BCP to help guide therapy?

SOLUTION: If the BCP reveals Na^+ of 140 mEq/L, Cl^- of 95 mEq/L, and CO_2 of 20 mEq/L (anion gap of 25 mEq/L), the surgeons would be correct in assuming that their resuscitation efforts were inadequate. The anion gap of 25 likely represents a worsening lactic acidosis. However, if the BCP reveals Na^+ of 150 mEq/L, CO_2 of 20 mEq/L, and Cl^- of 122 mEq/L, the anion gap would be normal (8 mEq/L). The metabolic acidosis would be caused by an abnormally high serum Cl^- concentration from excessive normal saline administration. This example represents a common problem in emergency and critical care practice: the overresuscitation of trauma patients from severe shock.

Enzyme Tests

Liver Function Tests

The liver is primarily responsible for converting food into substrates essential for cellular metabolism, protein synthesis, and detoxifying substances in the body. Liver damage is assessed by abnormal increases in the hepatic enzymes *alanine aminotransferase*, *aspartate aminotransferase*, and *alkaline phosphatase*. *Total bilirubin* is produced by the liver from the breakdown of destroyed RBCs. It is a crucial component of the liver panel test because it assesses one of the primary functions of the liver. Protein synthesis, another vital aspect of liver function, is assessed by measuring concentrations of total protein and albumin. Liver disease is characterized by the inability to remove toxins from the bloodstream. One of the primary toxins associated with altered mental function in patients with liver disease is the accumulation of *ammonia*, which forms from the breakdown of proteins.

Pancreatic and Muscle Enzyme Tests

Other diseases also produce abnormal amounts of enzymes in the serum. Patients with pancreatitis have abnormal levels of the pancreatic enzymes *lipase* and *amylase*. *Creatine phosphokinase* (CPK) or *creatinine kinase* is an enzyme found mainly in heart, brain, and skeletal muscle tissue. Patients who have sustained ischemic damage to these tissues have elevated CPK levels. Three types of CPK are associated with each tissue. CPK-1 (CPK-BB) is released primarily from the lungs or brain after injury. Patients with extensive crush injuries involving the skeletal muscles and those with myositis have elevated levels of CPK-3 (CPK-MM). The third type of CPK is associated with cardiac injury and is discussed subsequently.

Lactate dehydrogenase is the enzyme that catalyzes the conversion of pyruvate into lactate. Elevated serum levels of lactate dehydrogenase are associated with tissue breakdown. This breakdown occurs with many conditions, such as rhabdomyolysis (e.g., skeletal muscle breakdown typically from traumatic crush injuries releases myoglobin into the blood), cancer, meningitis, hemolytic anemia, acute pancreatitis, acute myocardial infarction, and HIV disease. Moderate increases in lactate dehydrogenase are associated with myocardial infarction or hemolytic anemia (880 units/L), whereas large increases are seen in extensive cancers, rhabdomyolysis, severe shock, and anoxia (8800 units/L).

TABLE 17-5

Liver Function and Other Enzymatic Tests

Test	Reference Range	Sample Critical Test Result*
Total bilirubin (T Bil)	0.1-1.1 mg/dl	≥15 mg/dl
Alanine aminotransferase (ALT)	7-56 units/L	†
Aspartate aminotransferase (AST)	10-50 units/L	†
Alkaline phosphatase (ALK)	40-125 units/L	†
Total protein (TP)	15-45 mg/dl	†
Albumin (ALB)	3.3-5.2 g/dl	†
Ammonia	18-54 μmol/L	≥500 mcg/dl
Amylase (serum)	20-110 units/L	>330 units/L
Lipase	10-140 units/L	>420 units/L
Creatinine phosphokinase (CPK)	20-220 units/L	>10,000 units/L
Troponin I	0 ng/ml	>0.05 ng/ml
B-type natriuretic peptide	<100 pg/ml	†
Lactate dehydrogenase (LDH)	110-220 units/L	>880 (moderate); >8800 (severe)

Values for reference ranges and critical test results from the University of California–San Francisco Moffit-Long Hospital/San Francisco General Hospital.

*Critical test results vary among clinical laboratories based on instrumentation and calibration procedures. Not all tests have an associated critical result that can be reported.

†No critical value established.

Cardiac Enzyme and Protein Tests

The most common CPK test is CPK-2 (CPK-MB), an enzyme released from the heart after myocardial infarction. Levels notably increase 4 to 6 hours and peak 12 to 24 hours after injury. Serial CPK-2 measurements are monitored in patients with suspected myocardial infarction, cardiac contusion from chest trauma, open heart surgery, or myocarditis. **Troponin** is a complex protein that helps regulate skeletal and cardiac muscle contractility. The protein fragment **troponin I** is associated with cardiac muscle damage. Similar to CPK-2, troponin I levels peak 12 to 16 hours after myocardial infarction. Reference values for these enzyme tests are presented in Table 17-5.

B-type natriuretic peptide (BNP) is secreted by the heart in response to increased cardiac muscle stretch. The BNP test primarily is used to evaluate patients for heart failure, particularly those presenting to the emergency department with dyspnea and pulmonary edema.[6] Values greater than 300 pg/ml indicate mild heart failure, above 600 pg/ml moderate heart failure, and greater than 900 pg/ml severe heart failure. Other conditions such as acute respiratory distress syndrome (ARDS) and severe sepsis also cause increased cardiac muscle stretch, resulting in BNP levels in the range of 300 to 500 pg/ml.[6]

Coagulation Studies

Coagulation is the process by which the blood and vascular tree form clots to stop bleeding and repair damage to the injured blood vessels. In brief, damage to the internal vascular wall (endothelium) exposes the blood to tissue factors (i.e., proteins) that attract and activate platelets, which stimulates clotting. **Thrombocytopenia** (low platelets) and *thrombasthenia* (abnormal platelet functioning) lead to excessive bleeding, whereas *thrombocytosis* (excessive platelets) causes excessive clotting. In addition to direct platelet measurement, the functionality of the entire process of coagulation is measured by the *prothrombin time* (PT) and *partial thromboplastin time* (PTT). These tests assess two different pathways by which fibrin clots are formed.

PT is the time in seconds required by plasma to form a fibrin clot after exposure to tissue factors. It assesses the *extrinsic coagulation pathway* and reflects the function of clotting factors I, II, V, VII, and X. In contrast, PTT primarily assesses the *intrinsic coagulation pathway*. It is used to evaluate abnormalities in blood clotting and monitor the effects of anticoagulation therapy. Abnormalities in PTT are associated with clotting factors I through VI and factors VIII through XII. Clinically, abnormal increases in PT and PTT are found in patients with vitamin K deficiencies and patients receiving anticoagulation therapy such as warfarin or heparin. Increased PT and PTT also occur in patients with *disseminated intravascular coagulation* (DIC) and patients with end-stage liver disease.

Because PT test results (Table 17-6) depend on manufactured animal tissue factors, which have unavoidable variability, PT is accompanied by an additional measurement known as the *international normalized ratio* (INR). The INR expresses PT relative to an established sample value. The reference range for INR is 0.9 to 1.3. INR values of approximately 5.0 indicate a high likelihood for bleeding. Values of 0.5 are associated with a tendency toward increased clotting.

D-dimer is a small protein fragment found in the blood when fibrin clots are dissolving. It belongs to a larger group of substances referred to as *fibrin degradation products*. D-dimer levels are measured to help diagnose deep vein thrombosis,

TABLE 17-6
Coagulation Studies

Test	Reference Range	Critical Test Result
Prothrombin time (PT)	12-15 sec	>30 sec
Partial thromboplastin time (PTT)	25-39 sec	>50 sec
International normalized ratio (INR)	0.8-1.2	>5 sec
Fibrin D-dimer	<200 ng/ml	*
Platelet count	150,000-400,000/mm^3	<25,000/mm^3

Values for reference ranges and critical test results are from the University of California–San Francisco Moffit-Long Hospital and San Francisco General Hospital.
*No critical value established.

pulmonary embolism, or DIC. Unless significant clotting has occurred in the body, the D-dimer test is normal.

Protein C has an integral role in regulating coagulation. In its activated state (activated protein C), it inhibits coagulation and promotes clot degradation. Protein C levels are reduced in patients with severe sepsis and acute respiratory distress syndrome.[7] Low protein C promotes abnormal clot formation and damages blood vessels in the microcirculation throughout the body (DIC). Significant deficiencies in protein C levels (<40% of normal) are associated with increased risk for death in patients with severe sepsis. Protein C levels are sometimes used to assess the severity of inflammation and coagulation disorders in patients with severe sepsis.

Infection Monitoring

Procalcitonin (PCT) is an inactive protein of the hormone calcitonin that is released in response to bacterial infections (particularly sepsis). PCT levels are directly related to the severity of infection. Because PCT does not increase in response to viral infections, it is a unique marker for bacterial infections. PCT levels typically increase within 2 to 4 hours of sepsis with peak levels occurring 24 to 48 hours later. Once infection is controlled with appropriate antibiotic therapy, PCT levels promptly decrease. Therefore measuring PCT increasingly is used to titrate antibiotic therapy. In healthy individuals PCT levels are less than 0.1 ng/ml. A diagnosis of sepsis is confirmed when PCT levels are greater than 0.5 ng/ml and excluded when PCT levels are 0.2 ng/ml or less.[8] Antibiotic therapy often is initiated when PCT levels reach 0.25 to 0.50 ng/ml. Measurements of PCT are repeated every 1 to 2 days to evaluate antibiotic therapy. When PCT decreases by approximately 90% from peak values, antibiotic therapy is usually terminated.

C-reactive protein (CRP) is a plasma protein expressed by the liver in response to infection (particularly sepsis) or trauma. The primary role of CRP is activating the complement system that assists antibodies in destroying bacteria. CRP levels begin to increase 6 to 8 hours after the onset of infection or injury and peak at approximately 36 to 50 hours.[9] Normal CRP levels are approximately 0.8 mg/L with cutoff values of 80 to 100 mg/L indicative of infection and levels of approximately 130 mg/L associated with severe sepsis.

MICROBIOLOGY TESTS

Sputum Gram Stain

Patients suspected of having a serious lung infection require a sputum sample to identify the microorganism causing the infection, thereby facilitating appropriate antibiotic selection. The Gram stain is the first test used in evaluating sputum samples. A laboratory technician smears the sputum sample onto a glass slide, applies a staining solution, and examines it through a microscope.

The Gram stain determines the quality of the sputum sample. Some patients have difficulty producing an adequate sputum sample and may expectorate only saliva into the sputum cup. In such cases, the Gram stain shows few (<25 per low-power field) or no pus cells and numerous epithelial cells, and the sample must be discarded. A sample with numerous pus cells and few epithelial cells is most likely a true lung sample and likely reflects the infection source.

RULE OF THUMB

A legitimate sputum sample has few epithelial cells and many pus cells (leukocytes).

After the sample is verified, the laboratory technician identifies the Gram stain reaction (either positive or negative) and the shape of any bacteria present (rods vs. cocci). For example, *Streptococcus pneumoniae,* a common bacterium associated with pneumonia, is characterized as lancet-shaped, gram-positive diplococci. Although a Gram stain can be helpful in identifying an invading organism so antibiotics can be more quickly started, a definitive diagnosis is made only by culture of the specific organism over several days.

Sputum Culture

If the Gram stain reveals an adequate sample, the technician prepares a portion of the sputum for culture. The sputum sample is placed in a medium permitting growth of the organism. When the organism has matured, it is examined microscopically to determine its exact type and sensitivity to antibiotic therapy. This information allows the physician to initiate appropriate antibiotic therapy. Gram staining and culturing are also applied to samples of blood, pleural fluid, or any other body fluid involved in an infection.

Acid-Fast Testing

Pulmonary tuberculosis is caused by a mycobacterium *(Mycobacterium tuberculosis).* The rapid identification and isolation of patients with suspected tuberculosis infection is an extremely important infection control measure. A rapid and effective method for detecting tuberculosis infection is to perform a Gram stain of a slide containing a sample of sputum followed by an acid wash. A characteristic of all mycobacteria is that after staining, the subsequent acid wash does not weaken the cell wall sufficiently to remove the color dye. This resistance to decolorization classifies the organism as an **acid-fast bacterium.**

Sweat Chloride

Patients with cystic fibrosis have increased levels of Cl^- in their sweat because of an inability to reabsorb it. These patients typically have sweat Cl^- levels greater than 60 mmol/L, whereas values of 40 to 60 mmol/L are considered borderline for cystic fibrosis. Sweat Cl^- levels less than 40 mmol/L are considered unlikely to confirm the diagnosis. Although the sweat electrolyte test is an important tool for diagnosing cystic fibrosis, it must be combined with other tests.

CLINICAL APPLICATION OF LABORATORY DATA

RTs are focused primarily on the pulmonary system and not as much on other organ systems. However, many of the laboratory tests previously discussed in this chapter are relevant to the RT's implementation of various aspects of the plan of care.

Coagulation Disorders

In patients requiring arterial blood gas (ABG) testing or nasotracheal suctioning, the RT must evaluate the clotting characteristics of the blood. For ABG testing, patients with an abnormally low platelet count or an elevated PT and INR need to have the puncture site compressed for a longer time after the arterial sample is obtained to prevent bleeding and hematoma development. Patients with an extremely low platelet count should have an arterial puncture performed (or undergo nasotracheal suctioning) *only* when it is essential because of the extremely high risk for bleeding.

In addition, RTs are intimately involved in assessing patients with suspected pulmonary embolism. Patients with pulmonary embolism present with some of the same symptoms as patients with myocardial infarction (e.g., dyspnea and chest pain), and it is important for the RT to be familiar with tests such as D-dimer, troponin I, CPK-1, and CPK-2, which help make the differential diagnosis.

Electrolyte Disorders

Severe electrolyte disorders have a profound impact on pulmonary function. The primary concern of the RT is the effect of electrolyte disorders on respiratory muscle function. Many electrolyte disorders cause generalized skeletal muscle weakness. This weakness may limit ambulation and increases the risk for patients developing pneumonia and venous thromboembolism that can lead to pulmonary embolism. In a patient with pulmonary disease, respiratory muscle weakness impairs the ability to sustain spontaneous ventilation and the ability to maintain pulmonary hygiene through deep breathing and adequate cough.

Primary electrolyte disorders causing respiratory muscle weakness include low serum levels of Ca^{++}, Mg^{++} and phosphate.[10,11] A patient with hypoglycemia often complains of weakness, so that weaning from a ventilator is unlikely to be successful in the patient with hypoglycemia. In addition, abnormally high serum K^+ levels, or **hyperkalemia** (>8.0 mmol/L), and abnormally low serum K^+, or **hypokalemia** (<2.0 mmol/L), or phosphorus, or hypophosphatemia (<1.0 mg/dl) can lead to respiratory muscle weakness. In addition, severe hyperkalemia (>6.0 mmol/L) increases the likelihood of cardiac arrhythmias. Severe hypocalcemia (<6.5 mmol/L) sometimes leads to laryngeal stridor and dyspnea.

Electrolyte disorders and other toxins in the bloodstream can depress neurologic function. Pulmonary function is profoundly affected because decreased mental functioning may depress respiratory drive, prevent patients from cooperating with therapy, and suppress the ability of patients to protect their airway and clear secretions by depressing the cough mechanism. In severe cases, **hypernatremia** is a major cause of central nervous system depression, which can lead to lethargy, coma, and respiratory arrest.[12] In patients with severe liver disease, elevated ammonia levels also depress neurologic function.

Finally, laboratory tests are used by physicians to assess the overall likelihood of survival of a critically ill patient. For patients with primary pulmonary failure, survival is related to the prevention of secondary multiple organ system failure. As a result, following trends in creatinine, total bilirubin, and platelets is crucial in monitoring the development or progression of renal, hepatic, and hematologic failure.

SUMMARY CHECKLIST

- The three formed elements of the blood are the WBCs (leukocytes), RBCs (erythrocytes), and platelets (thrombocytes).
- Elevation of the WBC count is known as *leukocytosis*. It often occurs with infection, stress, or trauma.
- A reduced WBC count is known as *leukopenia*. It puts the patient at risk for serious infection.
- Abnormal elevation of the RBC count is known as *polycythemia,* and an abnormal reduction in the RBC count is known as *anemia*.
- Anemia reduces the O_2-carrying capacity of the blood and increases the risk for tissue hypoxia. Severe electrolyte abnormalities, including low Ca^{++}, Mg^{++}, and PO_4^-, cause respiratory muscle weakness.
- Weakness from anemia and electrolyte abnormalities can inhibit a patient from participating in their care plan and slow their recovery.
- Severe hyperkalemia (>6 mmol/L) greatly increases the risk for cardiac arrhythmias.
- Troponin I and CPK-MM tests are used to help diagnose myocardial infarction.
- To minimize bleeding risk in arterial punctures and nasotracheal suctioning, extreme caution should be used in patients with thrombocytopenia and elevated PT or INR.
- A sputum Gram stain is useful for determining the quality of the sample and the type of organism present. Samples with many epithelial cells and few pus cells suggest oral and not pulmonary secretions.

References

1. Grasbeck R: The evolution of the reference value concept. *Clin Chem Lab Med* 42:692–697, 2004.
2. Friedberg RC, Soures R, Wagar EA, et al: The origin of reference intervals. *Arch Pathol Lab Med* 131:348–357, 2007.
3. Salpeter SR, Buckley JS, Chatterjee S: Impact of more restrictive transfusion strategies on clinical outcomes: a meta-analysis and systematic review. *Am J Med* 127:124–131, 2014.
4. Abdelmalak BB, Lansang MC: Revisiting tight glycemic control in perioperative and critically ill patients: when one size may not fit all. *J Clin Anesth* 25:499–507, 2013.
5. Andersen LW, Mackenhauer J, Roberts JC, et al: Etiology and therapeutic approach to elevated lactate. *Mayo Clin Proc* 88:1127–1140, 2013.
6. Del Ry S, Cabiati M, Clerico A: Recent advances on natriuretic peptide system: new promising therapeutic targets for the treatment of heart failure. *Pharmacol Res* 76:190–198, 2013.
7. Christiaans SC, Wagener BM, Esmon CT, et al: Protein C and acute inflammation: a clinical and biological perspective. *Am J Physiol Lung Cell Mol Physiol* 305:L455–L466, 2013.
8. Meisner M: Update on procalcitonin measurements. *Ann Lab Med* 34:263–273, 2014.
9. Lelubre C, Anselin S, Boudjeltia KZ, et al: Interpretation of C-reactive protein concentrations in critically ill patients. *BioMed Res Int* 2013:124021, 2013.
10. Gravelyn TR, Brophy N, Siegert C, et al: Hypophosphatemia-associated respiratory muscle weakness and a general inpatient population. *Am J Med* 84:870–876, 1988.
11. Fiaccadori E, Del Canale S, Coffrini E, et al: Muscle and serum magnesium in pulmonary intensive care unit patients. *Crit Care Med* 16:751–760, 1988.
12. Riggs JE: Neurologic manifestations of electrolyte disturbances. *Neurol Clin* 20:227–239, 2002.

Bibliography

Hoffman R, Benz PJ, Shattil SJ, et al: *Hematology basic principles and practice*, ed 4, Philadelphia, 2005, Saunders.

McPherson RA, Pincus MR: *Henry's clinical diagnosis and management by laboratory methods*, ed 21, Philadelphia, 2007, Saunders.

Moffit-Long Hospital; San Francisco General Hospital: *Clinical laboratory reference ranges and critical values.* <http://pathology.ucsf.edu/sfghlab/test/ReferenceRanges.html>.

University of California–San Francisco: *Clinical laboratory reference ranges and critical values.* <http://pathology.ucsf.edu/labmanual/mftlng-mtzn/test/test-index.html>.

University of California–San Francisco: *Clinical laboratory reference ranges and critical values.* <http://pathology.ucsf.edu/labmanual/mftlng-mtzn/test/test-index.html> and <http://pathology.ucsf.edu/sfghlab/test/ReferenceRanges.html>. (Accessed July, 2015.)

University of North Carolina at Chapel Hill: *Conversion factors for clinical laboratory tests between conventional and standardized international units.* <http://www.unc.edu/~rowlett/units/scales/clinical_data.html>. (Accessed July, 2015.)

Wu AHB: *Tietz's Clinical guide to laboratory tests*, ed 4, St Louis, 2006, Saunders.

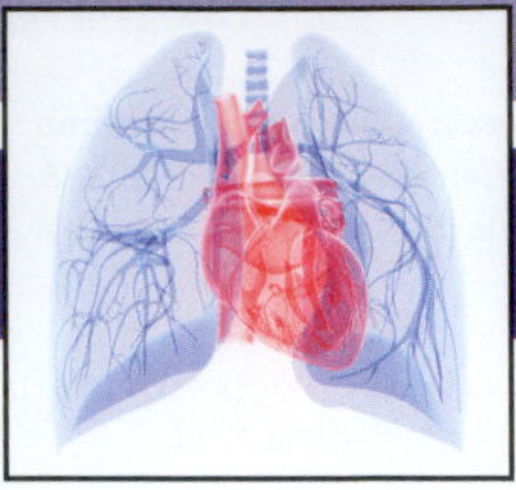

CHAPTER 18

Interpreting the Electrocardiogram

ALBERT J. HEUER

CHAPTER OBJECTIVES

After reading this chapter you will be able to:

- Describe the value and limitations of the electrocardiogram.
- Review the electrocardiogram equipment set-up.
- Describe the electrophysiology of cardiac cells.
- Describe how the cardiac impulse is conducted.
- Recognize various abnormal electrocardiographic recordings and major treatment alternatives.

CHAPTER OUTLINE

KEY TERMS

atrial kick
automaticity
depolarization
ectopic beat
ectopic foci
impulse-conducting system
repolarization

The electrocardiogram (ECG) is an important diagnostic tool that in some settings is obtained by the respiratory therapist (RT). As a result, this can place the RT in a prime position to recognize and respond to life-threatening arrhythmias. This chapter emphasizes the basics of cardiac physiology, lead placement, ECG interpretation, and the identification and key points in the treatment of dysrhythmias. More details of the cardiopulmonary anatomy and emergency cardiovascular life support are presented in Chapters 10 and 37.

An ECG can be done using either a 12-lead system, which provides more diagnostic value than the alternative approach, or a 3-lead system, which is commonly used for telemetry. A 12-lead ECG provides a more complete assessment of the electrical activity of the heart by viewing it from 12 different angles and is the focus of this chapter.

The ECG is a popular evaluation tool because it is inexpensive, noninvasive, and easy to obtain. It is used primarily to help evaluate a patient with signs and/or symptoms of myocardial disease. A physician would order an ECG for most adult patients complaining of certain types of chest pain, shortness of breath, dyspnea with palpitations, weakness, lethargy, or syncope; these are the classic clinical symptoms associated with heart disease. In addition, the ECG is routinely used to detect abnormalities that are occurring or have already occurred, such as a myocardial infarction (MI), the general health status of middle-aged or older patients or for preoperative screening. However, ECGs done at rest have little or no value as a predictor of future heart problems and they cannot directly identify certain abnormalities, such as valvular defects.[1]

MINI CLINI

Acute Chest Pain in the Emergency Room

PROBLEM: A 52-year-old man presents with severe chest pain that radiates to his left shoulder and shortness of breath. The newly graduated resident physician is obtaining a comprehensive history and performing a physical examination; the RT assisting with the evaluation notes that the man is diaphoretic and tachycardic, with pale skin color. After giving an order for O_2, the physician resumes taking the history and performing the physical. What additional tests should the RT recommend be obtained at this time?

SOLUTION: A STAT ECG should be ordered to help differentiate among chest pain associated with an MI or other cardiac abnormality such as angina and other causes such as orthopedic injury. As discussed later in this chapter, T wave inversion and ST segment elevation suggest cardiac ischemia and perhaps an MI, which would warrant immediate treatment.

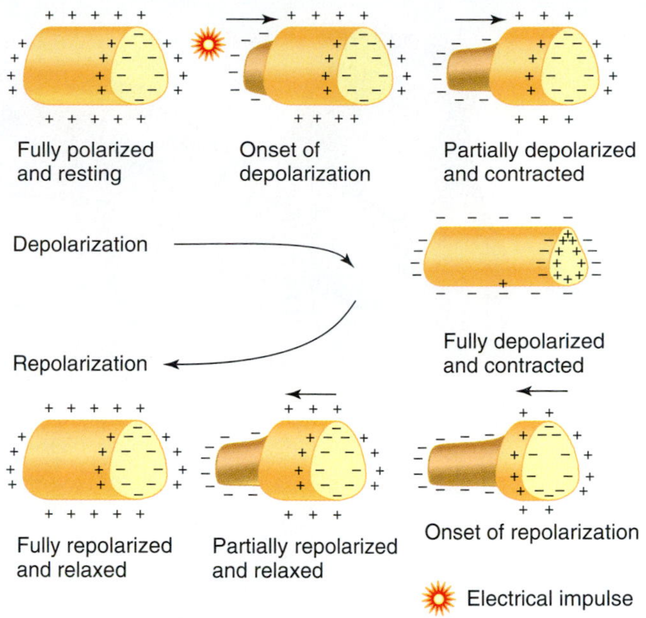

FIGURE 18-1 Depolarization and repolarization of a cardiac cell. (Modified from Wesley K: Huszar's basic dysrhythmias and acute coronary syndromes: interpretation and management, ed 4, St Louis, 2014, Elsevier.)

BASIC PRINCIPLES OF ELECTROPHYSIOLOGY

The muscle cells of the heart normally are stimulated and paced by the electrical activity of the cardiac **impulse-conducting system.** The impulse-conducting system cells have the ability to stimulate the heart without the influence of the nervous system. However, the autonomic nervous system normally plays a major role in controlling heart function.[1]

Cardiac muscle cells normally generate an electrical imbalance across the cell membrane, with a positive charge on the outside and a negative charge on the inside. This is the resting or polarized state in which there is no electrical activity. Stimulation of the "polarized" cells causes an influx of Na^+ into the interior portion of the cell; this is called **depolarization** (Figure 18-1). Depolarization causes the cardiac muscle cells to contract momentarily. Depolarization is immediately followed by **repolarization,** which is a rapid return of the cell to the "polarized" position in which the electrical imbalance across the membrane is reestablished.

The impulse-conducting system has three types of cardiac cells capable of electrical excitation: pacemaker cells (e.g., sinoatrial [SA] node, atrioventricular [AV] node), specialized rapidly conducting tissue (e.g., Purkinje fibers), and atrial and ventricular muscle cells. The ability of these cells to depolarize without stimulation is known as **automaticity.** Each of these cardiac cell groups varies in degree of automaticity.[1-3]

Impulse-Conducting System

The impulse-conducting system is responsible for initiating the heartbeat and controlling the heart rate. It also coordinates the contraction of the heart chambers, which is essential to move blood effectively. A defect in the impulse-conducting system may lead to inadequate cardiac output and decreased tissue perfusion. Normally, the SA node, which is located in the upper portion of the right atrium, has the greatest degree of automaticity and paces the heart (Figure 18-2). Any heartbeat originating outside the SA node is considered an **ectopic beat.**[2] The SA node is innervated by the autonomic nervous system, which allows the sympathetic and parasympathetic nervous systems to influence heart rate. Stimulation of the sympathetic nervous system, such as occurs with the administration of certain medications (e.g., adrenergic bronchodilators), increases the heart rate, whereas activation of the parasympathetic nervous system slows the heart rate by influencing the degree of automaticity within the SA node.

The electrical impulse generated by the SA node travels rapidly across the right atrium, through intraatrial pathways, to the left atrium by way of the Bachmann bundle; this causes a wave of depolarization to occur over the atria, producing atrial contraction. Next, the impulse moves to the AV node, located in the intraventricular septum in the inferior aspect of the right atrium (see Figure 18-2). The AV node is the "backup" pacemaker because it has the second greatest degree of automaticity in the healthy heart. In most cases, if the SA node fails to function properly, the AV node paces ventricular activity at a lower heart rate of 40 to 60 beats/min, which is generally sufficient to maintain adequate cardiac output.[2]

The electrical impulse is temporarily delayed at the AV node to allow the ventricles time to fill with blood. That brief delay also limits the rate of the ventricular stimulation during excessively fast atrial rhythms that, if passed to the ventricles, would lead to inadequate cardiac output.[3,4]

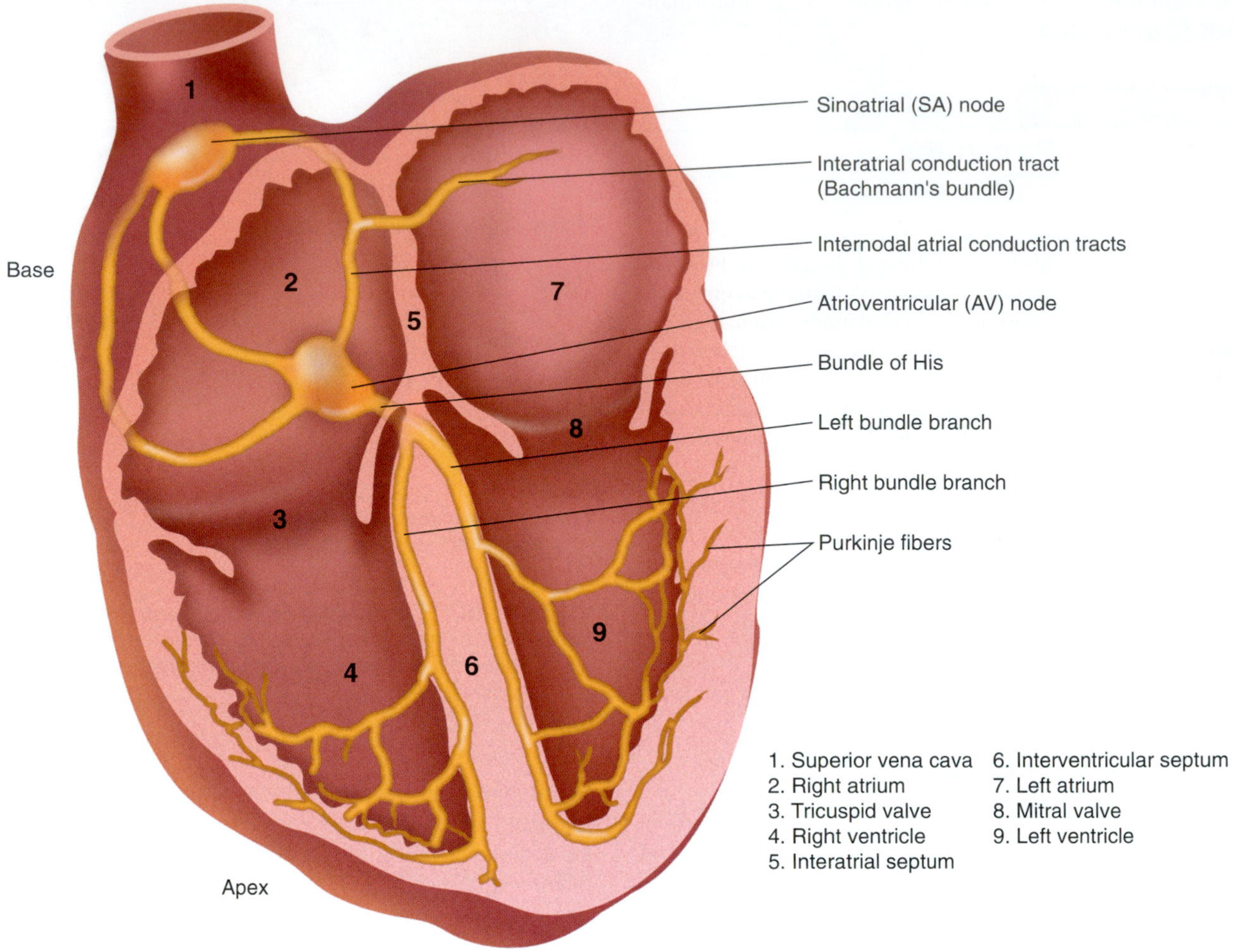

FIGURE 18-2 Anatomy of the impulse-conducting system of the human heart.

The impulse exits the AV node, enters the bundle of His, and rapidly moves to the bundle branches. The bundle branches carry the impulse rapidly into the right and left ventricles. The bundle branches terminate in the Purkinje fibers, which are small, finger-like projections that penetrate the myocardium (see Figure 18-2). These fibers stimulate contraction of the myocardium from the apex of the heart upward toward the base of the heart, causing a coordinated contraction of the ventricles, which normally is effective in moving blood. The impulse travels most rapidly in the Purkinje fibers, which is essential if contraction of the ventricles is to occur in a coordinated fashion. Immediately after depolarization of the ventricles, repolarization occurs in preparation for the next impulse.[3,4]

ELECTROCARDIOGRAM PROCEDURAL SUMMARY

Once the physician orders a 12-lead ECG, the equipment is gathered, which includes the portable ECG unit, lead wires, and electrodes.

The lead wires permit the connection between the ECG unit and the electrodes, which have adhesive permitting temporary attachment to the skin. Generally, the lead wires should be attached to the electrodes before being placed on the skin, to avoid unnecessary pressure to the skin's surface. The lead wires are often marked to help ensure proper placement on the patient's body.

The 12 leads can be subdivided into two groups: 6 extremity (limb) leads and 6 chest (precordial) leads. For the six limb leads, four electrodes are placed on the extremities, one on each wrist and one on each ankle. These leads are bipolar, which permits the measurement of electrical activity in two different directions. Additionally, the ECG unit can vary the orientation of these four electrodes to create six different views. Any electrical activity of the heart that is directed up, down, left, or right is recorded by the limb leads. The limb leads are called leads *I, II, III*, aV_R, aV_L, and aV_F (Table 18-1).

The six chest or precordial leads are called leads V_1, V_2, V_3, V_4, V_5, and V_6. These leads are unipolar, which means that they measure electrical activity in only one direction. These leads are placed in a horizontal plane across the chest, starting with V_1 in the fourth intercostal space to the right of the sternum. The rest of the chest leads are on the left side, starting with V_2, which is placed in the fourth intercostal space just to the left of the

TABLE 18-1
The 12 Leads of an Electrocardiograph and the Myocardial Wall That Each Set Views

Facing Lead*	View
I, aV_L, V_5, V_6	Lateral
II, III, aV_F	Inferior
V_1, V_2	Septal
V_3, V_4	Anterior
	Cells and Function
Pacemaker cells	Specialized cells that have a high degree of automaticity and provide electrical power for the heart
Conducting cells	Cells that conduct the electrical impulse throughout the heart
Myocardial cells	Cells that contract in response to electrical stimuli and pump blood

From Heuer AJ, Scanlan CL: Clinical assessment in respiratory care, ed 7, St Louis, 2013, Elsevier.
*Excludes aV_R, which faces the interior, endocardial surface of the ventricles.

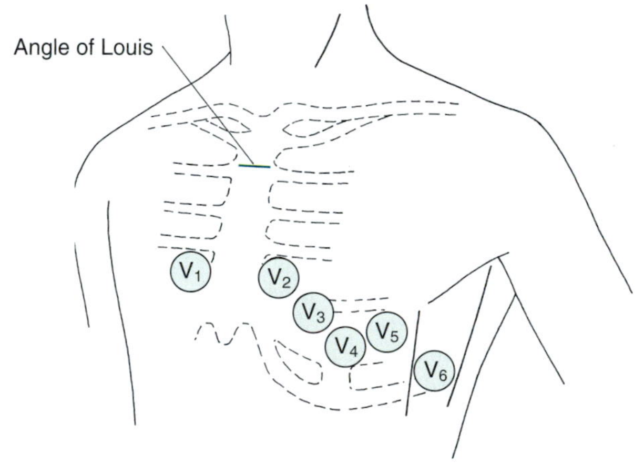

FIGURE 18-3 Proper precordial lead placement. (From Heuer AJ, Scanlan CL: Clinical assessment in respiratory care, ed 7, St Louis, 2013, Elsevier.)

sternum, and ending with V_6, which is placed at the fifth intercostal space at the left midaxillary line (V_6). Figure 18-3 illustrates proper placement of ECG leads. The view from each chest lead provides its own angle of orientation to measure cardiac electrical activity moving anteriorly or posteriorly.[2,4]

After all leads are properly placed and the ECG unit is activated, all 12 leads together provide a comprehensive view of the electrical activity of the heart. Given that an array of conditions, including cardiac ischemia and acute MI can alter electrical conduction through the heart, the ECG has considerable diagnostic value. The balance of this chapter focuses mainly on how electrocardiographic waves are generated, interpreting ECGs, identifying abnormal rhythms, and some treatment considerations.

Basic Electrocardiographic Waves

The wave of depolarization occurring in the atria is seen as the P wave on the ECG (Figure 18-4). The normal P wave is no

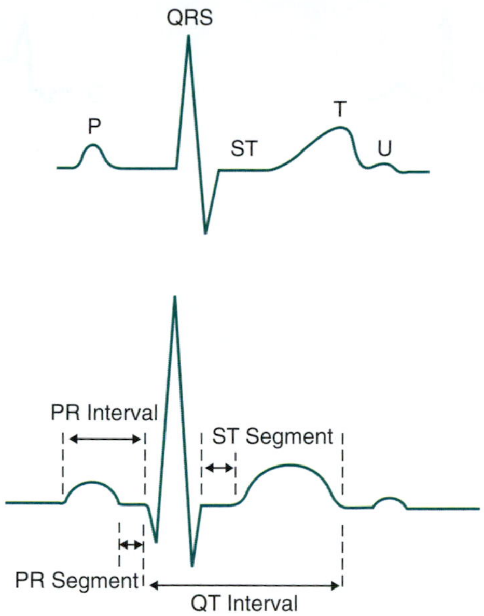

FIGURE 18-4 Normal configuration of electrocardiographic waves, segments, and intervals. (From Heuer AJ, Scanlan CL: Clinical assessment in respiratory care, ed 7, St Louis, 2013, Elsevier.)

more than 2.5 mm high and 3 mm long. Atrial hypertrophy may cause the P wave to enlarge to a larger height and length. Atrial repolarization is not seen on the electrocardiographic tracing because it is obscured by the electrical activity occurring in the ventricles at the same time.

The wave of depolarization occurring over the ventricles is seen as the QRS complex on the electrocardiographic tracing. The QRS complex is normally larger than the P wave because the muscle mass of the ventricles is much greater than that of the atria. The normal QRS complex is not wider than 3 mm (0.12 second) because of the rapid movement of the impulse through the ventricles by the bundle branches and Purkinje fibers. Abnormalities in the ventricular conduction system may lead to irregular QRS complexes that are wider than normal.

The QRS complex usually consists of several distinct waves, each of which has a letter assigned to it as a label. If the first wave of the complex is negative (downward), it is labeled the *Q wave*. The initial positive (upward) deflection is electrocardiographically referred to as the *R wave*, and the next negative deflection after the R wave is labeled the *S wave*. Not all QRS complexes have all three components present, but the waves making up ventricular depolarization are electrocardiographically referred to as the *QRS complex*, regardless of its exact makeup. The wave of repolarization occurring in the ventricles immediately after depolarization is the *T wave* (see Figure 18-4).

Two important segments of the electrocardiographic pattern must be observed and measured. The first is the *PR interval*, which refers to the distance (time) between the start of atrial depolarization and the start of ventricular depolarization. The PR interval represents the time in which the impulse begins in the SA node and travels across the atria to the AV node, where it is held briefly before passing on to the ventricles. Normally,

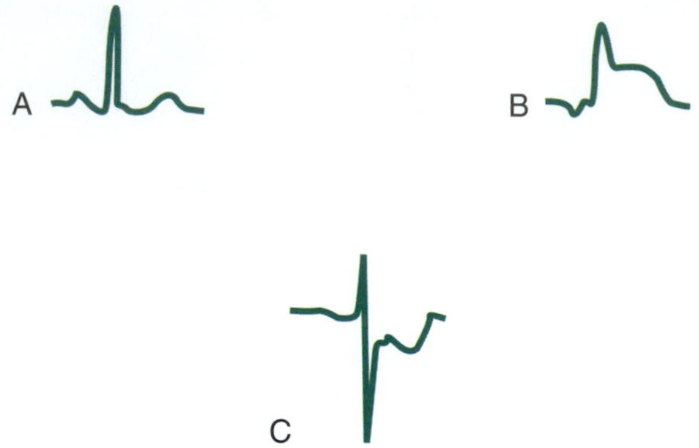

FIGURE 18-5 ST segments. **A,** Normal. **B,** Abnormal elevation. **C,** Abnormal depression. (From Heuer AJ, Scanlan CL: Clinical assessment in respiratory care, ed 7, St Louis, 2013, Elsevier.)

the PR interval represents a period no longer than 0.20 second. PR intervals longer than 0.20 second suggest that the impulse is abnormally delayed at the AV node and a "block" is present, often as a result of a serious defect in the impulse-conducting system.

The next important part of the ECG to evaluate is the *ST segment,* which represents the time from the end of ventricular depolarization to the start of ventricular repolarization. The normal ST segment is isoelectric and is seen as a flat line that is not above or below the neutral baseline. Certain pathologic abnormalities in the myocardium cause the ST segment configuration to become abnormal; this is seen as an elevated or depressed ST segment and is common in cardiac ischemia and MI (Figure 18-5). Because this configuration represents a potentially life-threatening arrhythmia, abnormal ST segments must be identified as soon as possible.[3-5]

RULE OF THUMB

A negative QRS complex in lead I is consistent with right-axis deviation, which is often caused by cor pulmonale.

Electrocardiographic Paper and Measurements

Electrocardiographic paper is made up of gridlike boxes that define time on the horizontal axis and voltage on the vertical axis. Dark lines circumscribe larger boxes that are 5 × 5 mm, and lighter lines define smaller boxes that are 1 × 1 mm (Figure 18-6). Because the paper passes through the electrocardiograph at a set speed of 25 mm/sec, each large box represents 0.20 second, and each small box represents 0.04 second on the horizontal axis. The standard ECG is calibrated so that 1 mV causes an upward deflection of 10 small boxes or 2 large boxes on the vertical axis; this allows measurement of the exact voltage occurring during depolarization of the cardiac muscle fibers.[1,4,6]

Interpreting the Electrocardiogram

The following steps should be followed in interpreting the ECG.

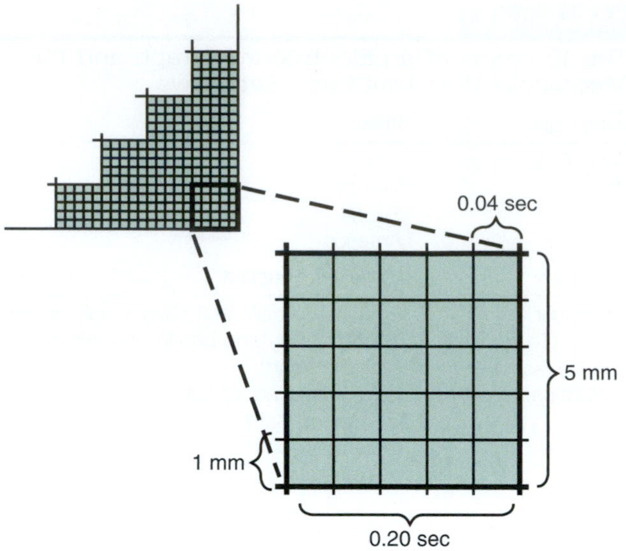

FIGURE 18-6 Gridlike boxes of electrocardiographic paper illustrating the 1 × 1 mm and 5 × 5 mm boxes. (From Heuer AJ, Scanlan CL: Clinical assessment in respiratory care, ed 7, St Louis, 2013, Elsevier.)

MINI CLINI

Weaning Complications

PROBLEM: The clinician is in the intensive care unit (ICU) attending to a 65-year-old woman who is being weaned from the ventilator after 2 weeks of mechanical ventilation. After 15 minutes of T-piece weaning, the patient complains of mild shortness of breath and the bedside ECG shows an increase in heart rate, inverted T waves, and acute elevation of the ST segment. What do the inverted T waves and ST segment elevation indicate? What should be done?

SOLUTION: The inverted T waves and elevated ST segment suggest that the heart is experiencing acute hypoxia, probably caused by the stress of weaning. T wave inversion and ST segment elevation are serious signs indicating that the patient is not tolerating the weaning. She should be put back on full ventilatory support at an elevated FiO_2 and monitored closely. Weaning should not be attempted again until the patient's clinical condition improves significantly. The attending physician should be notified.

Steps to Follow

Step 1. *Identify the atrial and ventricular rates.* Normally, the rate of the atria and ventricles is the same, but rates may differ when a defect in the conduction system is present. The clinician can identify the heart rate by counting the number of QRS complexes (for the ventricular rate) or the number of P waves (for the atrial rate) in 6 seconds (30 large boxes) and multiplying this number by 10. When the rate is regular, the clinician also can count the number of large boxes between two successive complexes and divide this number into 300 to obtain the heart rate.

Step 2. *Measure the PR interval.* This is done by determining the number of small boxes between the start of the P wave and the start of the QRS complex. Normally, this interval is less than 0.20 second (five small boxes) and is consistently the same for each complex. PR intervals that are longer than 0.20 second or vary from one complex to the next indicate an abnormality in the impulse-conducting system.

Step 3. *Evaluate the QRS complex.* Normally, the QRS complex is shorter than 0.12 second. If it is longer, there is an abnormality in the impulse-conducting system within the ventricles, which often leads to a decrease in cardiac output and blood pressure.

Step 4. *Evaluate the T wave.* Normally, the T wave is upright and rounded. Inverted T waves suggest ischemia of the heart muscle, and abnormal configuration of the T wave occurs with electrolyte abnormalities such as hyperkalemia.

Step 5. *Evaluate the ST segment.* The ST segment should be flat or at least no more than 1 mm above or below baseline. As stated earlier, significant elevation or depression of the ST segment indicates serious problems with oxygenation of the myocardium and must be recognized as soon as possible.

Step 6. *Identify the R-R interval.* The R-R interval is identified to assess regularity of the rhythm. The distance, in millimeters or time, is measured between the R waves of several successive QRS complexes. Normally, there is little variance in the R-R interval between QRS complexes, but if the variance between the different R-R intervals exceeds 0.12 second, an abnormal rhythm exists.

Step 7. *Identify the mean QRS axis.* The limb lead exhibiting the largest amount of voltage is identified. If the lead shows a positive QRS complex, the axis is very close to the position on the hexaxial reference circle where that limb lead is labeled. If the QRS complex with the most voltage is negative, the mean axis is moving in the opposite direction from where that lead is labeled on the hexaxial reference circle.[1-3]

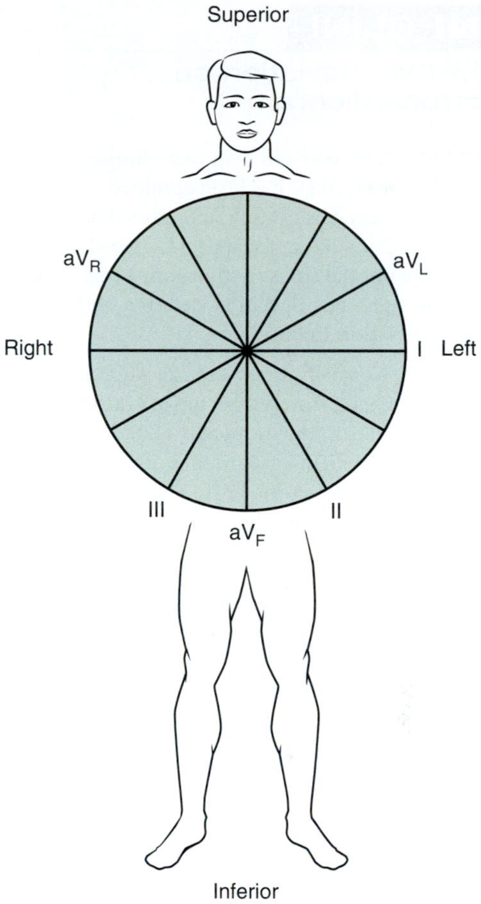

FIGURE 18-7 Hexaxial reference circle used for axis evaluation. (From Heuer AJ, Scanlan CL: Clinical assessment in respiratory care, ed 7, St Louis, 2013, Elsevier.)

Axis Evaluation

A less understood area of ECG interpretation for RTs is the axis evaluation and the identification of related deviations from normal. Axis evaluation is used to determine the general direction of current flow during ventricular depolarization; this is helpful to know when hypertrophy of one of the ventricles is suspected, which would cause the direction of current flow to deviate from normal. Normally, the mean QRS axis (vector) points leftward (patient's left) and downward, between 0 and +90 degrees in the frontal plane (Figure 18-7). The normal position of the QRS axis results from the slight tilt of the heart to the left and from the large muscle mass of the left ventricle compared with the right ventricle.

The mean QRS axis is identified by using the hexaxial reference circle (see Figure 18-7) with the position of each limb lead labeled on the circle. Next, the clinician identifies the limb lead with the most voltage (either positive or negative) from the ECG being evaluated. If the lead with the most voltage is positive (upright), the clinician locates the position of that lead on the hexaxial reference circle. The mean axis must be very close to that position on the circle. If the lead with the most voltage is negative (downward), the mean axis points in the opposite direction from that lead. If the lead with the most voltage is lead II and it is positive, the mean QRS axis must be approximately +60 degrees because this is where lead II is located on the hexaxial reference circle (see Figure 18-7). This is considered a normal axis because it falls between 0 and +90 degrees.[5,6]

In some situations, the most voltage may be equally present in two leads. The mean axis must fall equally between the two leads if they are both upright QRS complexes. If the QRS complexes in leads II and aV_F are equally positive in voltage, the mean axis must be at approximately +75 degrees and is considered normal. This is a common situation. If the mean QRS axis is between +90 degrees and +180 degrees, the patient has right-axis deviation; this is quickly identified by looking at lead I. If lead I is negative, right-axis deviation is present; this is commonly seen in patients with chronic obstructive pulmonary disease with cor pulmonale. Left-axis deviation is present when the mean axis is between +90 degrees and −90 degrees on the hexaxial reference circle. This is common in patients with left ventricular hypertrophy.

MINI CLINI

Right-Axis Deviation on Electrocardiogram

PROBLEM: A 54-year-old man with chronic obstructive pulmonary disease (COPD) has been admitted to the hospital for abdominal surgery. His routine laboratory data are normal, but his heart (cardiac silhouette) appears somewhat enlarged. The ECG shows a normal sinus rhythm with a right-axis deviation. How is the right-axis deviation detected and what does the right-axis deviation suggest?

SOLUTION: Normally, the mean axis (summary of electrical activity) of the heart travels from top to bottom and from right to left. This results in the mean axis of 0 to +90 degrees in the healthy heart. The slight leftward shift of the normal axis results from the angle at which the heart is situated in the chest and the fact that the left ventricle is normally larger than the right one. Right-axis deviation indicates that the electrical activity of the heart has been abnormally shifted to the patient's right side, between +90 degrees and +180 degrees. In this case, right-axis deviation is detected by noting a negative deflection of the QRS in lead I. This is most commonly the result of right ventricle enlargement, such as occurs with cor pulmonale (right heart failure caused by chronic hypoxic lung disease).

Recognizing Arrhythmias

Normal Sinus Rhythm. Recognizing abnormal ECGs results is easier if you have an appreciation for the normal tracing. The normal sinus rhythm begins with an upright P wave that is identical from one complex to the next. The PR interval is consistent throughout the rhythm strip and is 0.12 to 0.20 second. The QRS complexes are identical and no longer than 0.12 second. The ST segment is flat. The R-R interval is regular and does not vary more than 0.12 second between QRS complexes. The heart rate is between 60 and 100 beats/min (Figure 18-8).[2,3]

Sinus Tachycardia. Heart rates exceeding 100 beats/min are abnormal in resting adult patients and are electrocardiographically referred to as *sinus tachycardia* when a P wave is appropriately present before each QRS complex (Figure 18-9). Other than the rate exceeding 100 beats/min, sinus tachycardia does not differ from a normal sinus rhythm. This abnormality is common and can be caused by numerous problems. Most often, sinus tachycardia is caused by anxiety, pain, fever, hypovolemia, or hypoxemia. It also may be a side effect of certain medications, such as adrenergic bronchodilators. Treatment typically involves eliminating the underlying cause.[5,6]

Sinus Bradycardia. A heart rate of less than 60 beats/min that is otherwise normal is electrocardiographically referred to

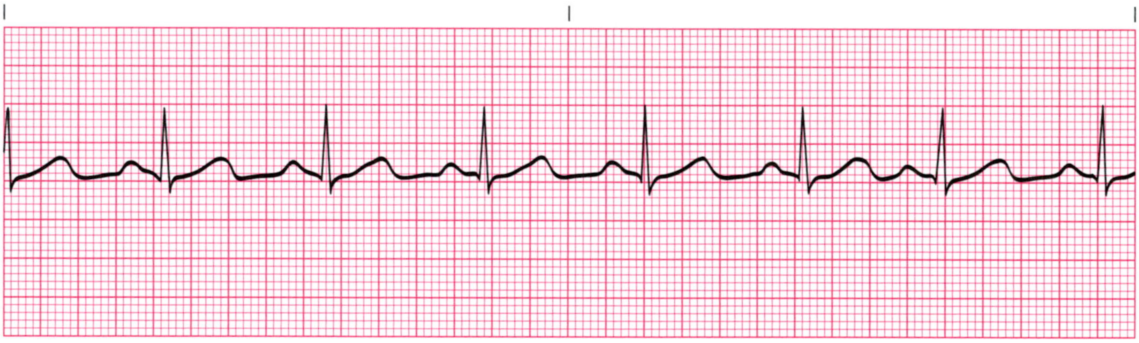

FIGURE 18-8 Electrocardiographic tracing showing a **normal sinus rhythm**. (Modified from Atwood S, Stanton C, Storey Davenport J: Introduction to basic cardiac dysrhythmias, ed 4, St Louis, 2009, Mosby/JEMS.)

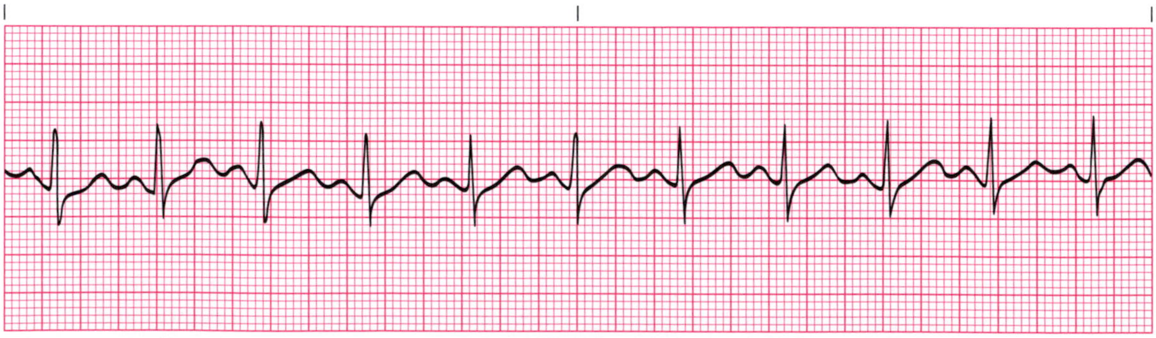

FIGURE 18-9 Electrocardiographic tracing showing **sinus tachycardia**. (Modified from Atwood S, Stanton C, Storey Davenport J: Introduction to basic cardiac dysrhythmias, ed 4, St Louis, 2009, Mosby/JEMS.)

as *sinus bradycardia*. Other than the rate being too slow, sinus bradycardia does not differ from a normal sinus rhythm (Figure 18-10). This abnormal rhythm is not as common as sinus tachycardia, but it represents a significant clinical problem if it causes the patient's blood pressure to decrease significantly or impairs tissue perfusion, causing symptoms such as fatigue, lightheadedness, or syncope. It is most often caused by hypothermia, abnormalities in the SA node, or intense athletic conditioning. Numerous medications, such as atropine, are available to stimulate the heart rate when clinical bradycardic symptoms occur.[5,6]

Sinus Arrhythmia. Sinus arrhythmia is a common arrhythmia and is recognized by the irregular spacing between QRS complexes. The spacing is measured by identifying the intervals between the R waves of successive QRS complexes, which are normally consistent. When the R-R interval varies more than 0.12 second throughout the rhythm strip, sinus arrhythmia is present (Figure 18-11). This arrhythmia may occur with the effects of breathing on the heart or as a side effect of medications such as digoxin. Most cases of sinus arrhythmia are benign and do not need treatment.[5,6]

First-Degree Heart Block. In first-degree heart block, the PR interval is longer than 0.20 second. In addition, there is one P wave before each QRS complex (Figure 18-12). This tracing indicates that the impulse from the SA node is getting through to the ventricles but is abnormally delayed in passing through the AV node or bundle of His. Typically, the QRS complex has

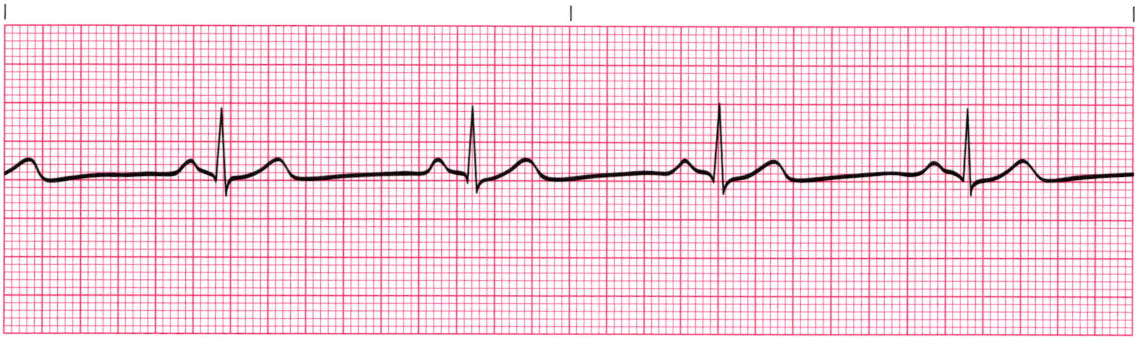

FIGURE 18-10 Electrocardiographic tracing showing **sinus bradycardia** with first-degree heart block. (Modified from Atwood S, Stanton C, Storey Davenport J: Introduction to basic cardiac dysrhythmias, ed 4, St Louis, 2009, Mosby/JEMS.)

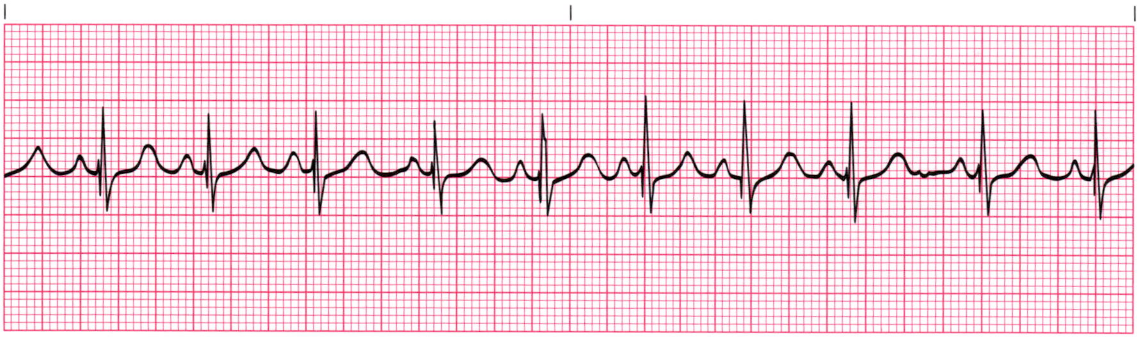

FIGURE 18-11 Electrocardiographic tracing showing **sinus arrhythmia**. (Modified from Atwood S, Stanton C, Storey Davenport J: Introduction to basic cardiac dysrhythmias, ed 4, St Louis, 2009, Mosby/JEMS.)

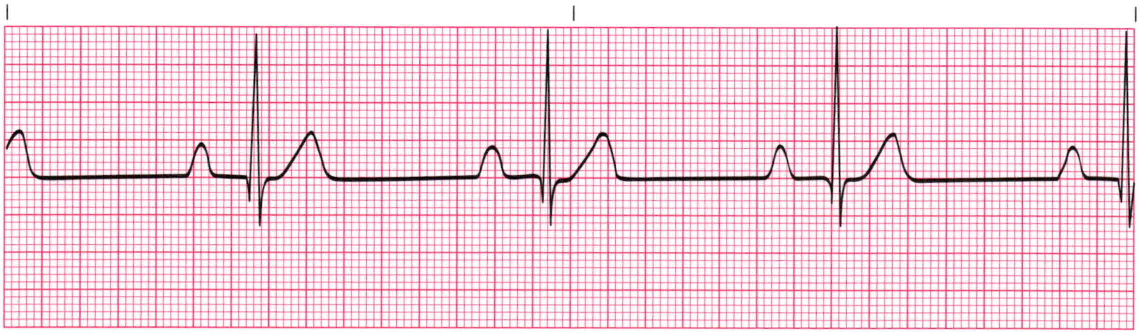

FIGURE 18-12 Electrocardiographic tracing showing **first-degree heart block**. (Modified from Atwood S, Stanton C, Storey Davenport J: Introduction to basic cardiac dysrhythmias, ed 4, St Louis, 2009, Mosby/JEMS.)

a normal configuration, and the R-R intervals are regular. First-degree heart block is common after an MI that damages the AV node, or it may be a complication of certain medications, such as digoxin or beta blockers. Treatment usually is not needed for first-degree heart block if the patient is able to maintain an adequate blood pressure.[6,7]

Second-Degree Heart Block. Second-degree heart block comes in two different types. Type I (Wenckebach or Mobitz type I) block is a relatively benign and often transient arrhythmia. It occurs when an abnormality in the AV junction delays or blocks conduction of some of the impulses through the AV node. It can be recognized by progressive prolongation of the PR interval until one impulse does not pass on to the ventricles at all (seen as a P wave not followed by a QRS complex). The cycle then repeats itself.

Second-degree heart block type II (Mobitz type II) is less common and is more often the result of serious problems such as MI or ischemia. Type II heart block is seen as a series of nonconducted P waves followed by a P wave that is conducted to the ventricles (Figure 18-13). Sometimes the ratio of nonconducted to conducted P waves is fixed at 3:1 or 4:1. The PR interval for the conducted impulses is consistent.[6,7]

Treatment for type I second-degree heart block is not needed because it usually does not impair cardiac output or cause symptoms. Type II second-degree heart block requires treatment in most cases because the resulting reduction in ventricular rate causes a decrease in blood pressure. Medications such as atropine provide a better cardiac output until a pacemaker can be inserted. Because type II block may progress to third-degree heart block without warning, a pacemaker is indicated even if the patient is asymptomatic.[8,9]

Third-Degree Heart Block. Third-degree heart block is the most serious of the different types of heart block. It indicates that the conduction system between the atria and ventricles is completely blocked, and impulses generated in the SA node are not conducted to the ventricles. The atria and ventricles are paced by independent sources. Most commonly, the atria are paced by the SA node, and the ventricles are paced by the AV node. This arrhythmia can be recognized when it is established that there is no relationship between the P waves and the QRS complexes. The P-P intervals are regular and the R-R intervals are regular, but they have no correlation with one another. In addition, the QRS complexes are normal in configuration if the ventricles are paced by the AV node (Figure 18-14). If the ventricles are paced by an ectopic site in the myocardium, the QRS complexes may be abnormally wide. Typically, the ventricular rate is slower than the atrial rate.[6,7]

Third-degree heart block is a serious arrhythmia because it often is caused by MI or drug toxicity (especially digitalis), and it may render the heart unable to meet the normal metabolic demands of the body. In almost all cases, treatment usually includes medication to speed up the ventricles and a temporary external pacemaker until a permanent one can be placed.[8,9]

Atrial Flutter. Atrial flutter is the rapid depolarization of the atria resulting from an ectopic focus that depolarizes at a rate of 250 to 350 times per minute. Typically, only one ectopic

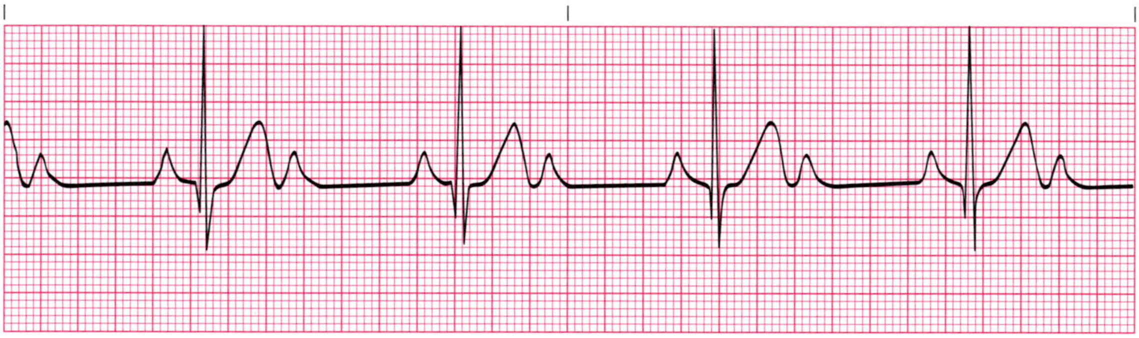

FIGURE 18-13 Electrocardiographic tracing showing **second-degree heart block type II**. (Modified from Atwood S, Stanton C, Storey Davenport J: Introduction to basic cardiac dysrhythmias, ed 4, St Louis, 2009, Mosby/JEMS.)

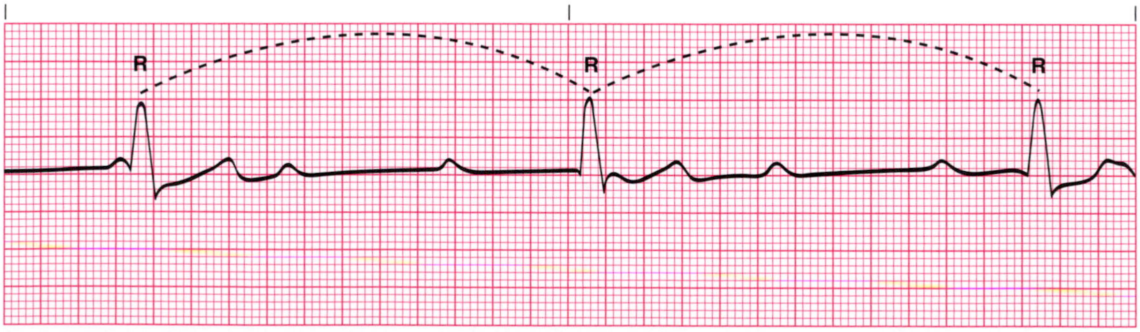

FIGURE 18-14 Electrocardiographic tracing showing **third-degree heart block**. (Modified from Atwood S, Stanton C, Storey Davenport J: Introduction to basic cardiac dysrhythmias, ed 4, St Louis, 2009, Mosby/JEMS.)

focus is causing the arrhythmia, which results in each P wave appearing similar. The result is a characteristic saw-toothed baseline pattern (Figure 18-15). Numerous P waves are present for every QRS complex, and the QRS complexes are normal in configuration. The R-R interval may be regular or it may vary, depending on the ability of the atrial impulse to pass through the AV node.[1,3,4]

Various conditions can produce atrial flutter, including rheumatic heart disease, coronary heart disease, stress, renal failure, and hypoxemia. This arrhythmia is not considered life-threatening, but it may lead to atrial fibrillation if untreated. Treatment usually includes medications such as digoxin, beta blockers, or calcium channel blockers. Once the rate is significantly slowed, cardioversion is attempted to return the heart rhythm back to a normal sinus rhythm.[8,9]

Atrial Fibrillation. Atrial fibrillation is present when the atrial muscle quivers in an irregular pattern that does not result in a coordinated contraction. The baseline electrical activity appears erratic, and no true P waves are seen in atrial fibrillation (Figure 18-16). The AV node determines the ventricular response to the atrial activity by controlling which impulses pass through and which do not. The ventricular rate is often very irregular and results in an abnormal R-R interval.[1,3,4]

The causes of atrial fibrillation are similar to the causes of atrial flutter. However, atrial fibrillation is a more serious arrhythmia because it can lead to a significant reduction in cardiac output resulting from the loss of the **atrial kick** that helps fill the ventricles before systole. The resulting stagnation of blood in the atria can lead to formation of blood clots, which can lead to pulmonary emboli or an embolic stroke. Treatment for atrial fibrillation is similar to the treatment for atrial flutter. However, patients with sustained atrial fibrillation are often treated with anticoagulants or antithrombolytic medications to treat potential blood clot formation, medications to slow the heart rate and cardioversion. [8,9]

RULE OF THUMB

Atrial fibrillation generally results in a reduction in cardiac output due to what is known as a loss of *atrial kick* resulting from a lack of coordination between the atria and ventricles. However, an even bigger problem is the potential for blood clot formation from stagnation of blood in the atria. These blood clots can easily travel to the pulmonary artery, causing a pulmonary embolism, or to the aorta, leading to an embolic stroke. As a result, most patients with atrial fibrillation should receive anticoagulant therapy.

Premature Ventricular Contractions. Premature beats can occur when a portion of the impulse-conducting system or myocardium other than the SA node becomes diseased and triggers depolarization of the surrounding cardiac cells. Sources for the impulse outside the SA node are called **ectopic foci.** Ectopic foci occur when hypoxia, acid-base imbalances, or electrolyte abnormalities are present and cause the cardiac cells in the ventricles to become abnormally excited. PVCs are easy to

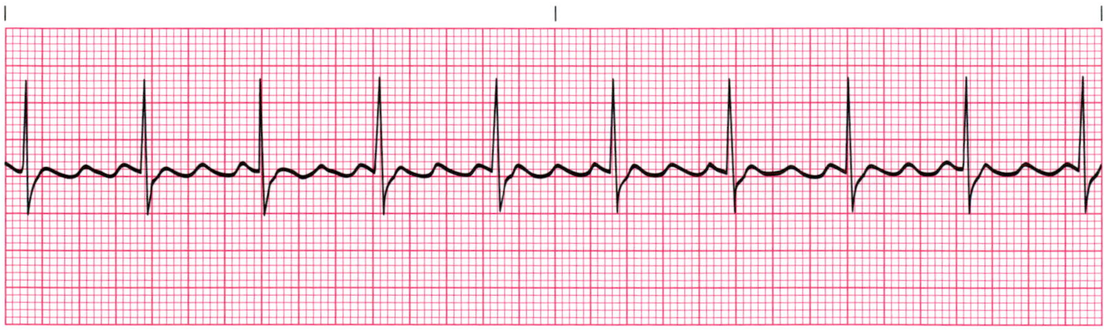

FIGURE 18-15 Electrocardiographic tracing showing **atrial flutter**. (Modified from Atwood S, Stanton C, Storey Davenport J: Introduction to basic cardiac dysrhythmias, ed 4, St Louis, 2009, Mosby/JEMS.)

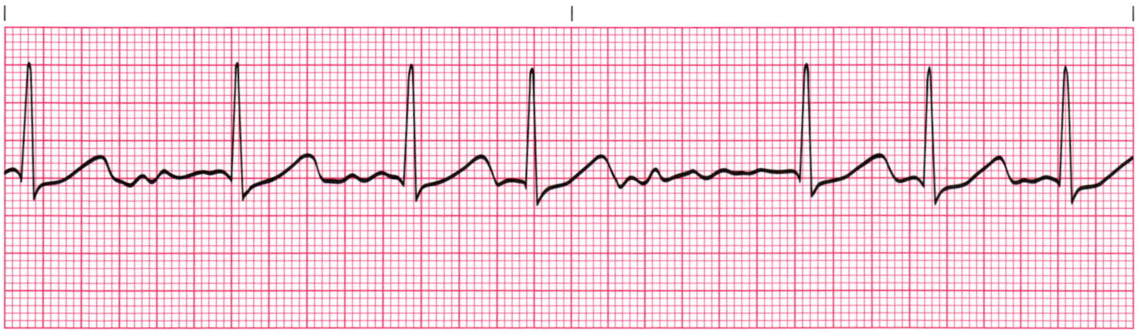

FIGURE 18-16 Electrocardiographic tracing showing **atrial fibrillation**. (Modified from Atwood S, Stanton C, Storey Davenport J: Introduction to basic cardiac dysrhythmias, ed 4, St Louis, 2009, Mosby/JEMS.)

recognize because they cause a unique and bizarre QRS complex that is much wider than normal (Figure 18-17). The QRS complex of a PVC is wider than normal because the ectopic focus is using channels outside the normal conduction system to move the impulse throughout the myocardium. PVCs have no P wave preceding them and may occur as a singular event or, more commonly, as a temporary run of PVCs. They also may occur at every other beat (bigeminy) or every third beat (trigeminy).[1,3,4]

An occasional PVC is not of major concern and may occur as a result of stress, caffeine intake, nicotine use, or electrolyte imbalance. However, frequent PVCs are more serious and most often occur in response to ischemia of the myocardium. They also are commonly seen as a side effect of some medications. Treatment is based on the frequency and cause of the PVCs and is needed when the PVCs are frequent (more than six per minute), paired together, or multifocal (appear differently because they come from more than one ectopic focus) or when they land directly on the T wave *(R on T phenomenon)*. In such cases, treatment must be prompt because the problem may progress rapidly to ventricular tachycardia (VT) and ventricular fibrillation (VF) (see subsequent discussion). Antiarrhythmic medications (e.g., lidocaine) may offer a temporary solution until the underlying cause can be addressed.[8,9]

Ventricular Tachycardia. VT is a run of three or more PVCs. It usually is easy to recognize as a series of wide, bizarre QRS complexes that have no preceding P wave. The ventricular rate is usually 100 to 250 beats/min (Figure 18-18). It is considered sustained VT if it lasts longer than 30 seconds.

Sustained or symptomatic VT is a serious arrhythmia because it indicates that an ectopic focus is rapidly firing from the ventricles, which results from increased automaticity. It suggests a significant pathologic defect in the myocardium and often leads to VF if untreated. MI, coronary artery disease, and hypertensive heart disease are the most common causes.[1,3,4]

Treatment must be prompt and specific and usually consists of cardioversion followed by long-term antiarrhythmic drugs for long-term suppression. Patients at high risk for recurrent VT may have an internal cardioverter-defibrillator (ICD) placed so that if VT occurs it can be treated automatically and promptly. Asymptomatic patients with recurrent nonsustained VT and ventricular ectopic beats may be treated with beta blockers to reduce symptoms of non–life-threatening ventricular arrhythmias. Symptomatic or sustained VT is considered a medical emergency, and the patient must be treated and monitored continuously in the ICU until his or her condition is stabilized.[8-12]

RULE OF THUMB

VT causes the cardiac output to decrease significantly because the ventricles do not have time to fill between contractions. This places the patient in danger of cardiac arrest and death.

Ventricular Fibrillation. VF is the most life-threatening arrhythmia and is defined as erratic quivering of the ventricular muscle mass. It causes the cardiac output to drop to zero; the patient becomes unconscious and represents a true medical

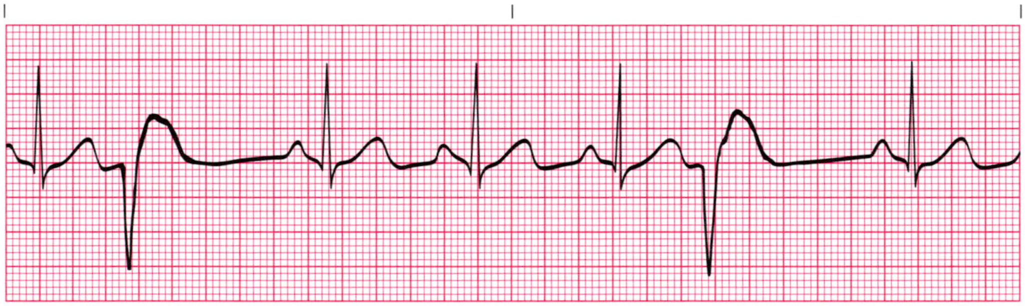

FIGURE 18-17 Electrocardiographic tracing showing **PVCs**. (Modified from Atwood S, Stanton C, Storey Davenport J: Introduction to basic cardiac dysrhythmias, ed 4, St Louis, 2009, Mosby/JEMS.)

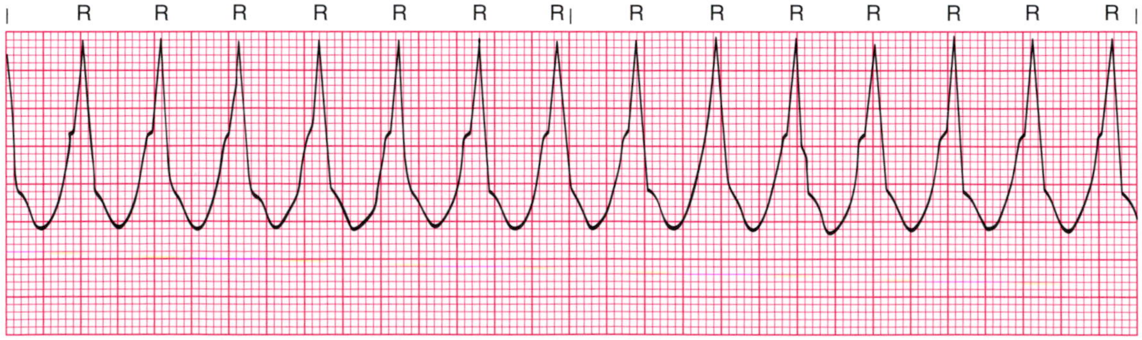

FIGURE 18-18 Electrocardiographic tracing showing **ventricular tachycardia**. (Modified from Atwood S, Stanton C, Storey Davenport J: Introduction to basic cardiac dysrhythmias, ed 4, St Louis, 2009, Mosby/JEMS.)

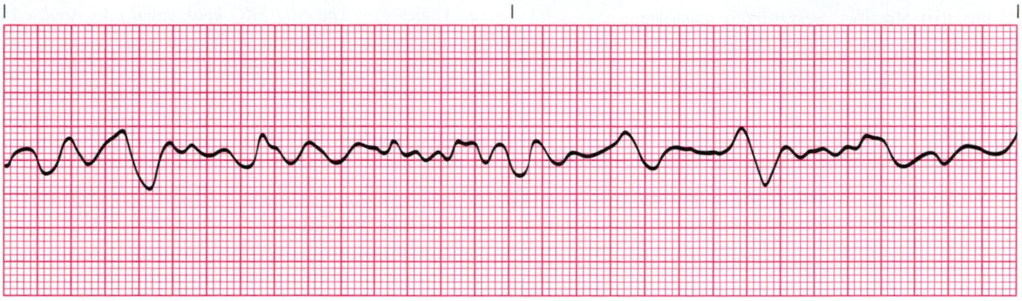

FIGURE 18-19 Electrocardiographic tracing showing **ventricular fibrillation**. (Modified from Atwood S, Stanton C, Storey Davenport J: Introduction to basic cardiac dysrhythmias, ed 4, St Louis, 2009, Mosby/JEMS.)

emergency. The electrocardiographic tracing of VF shows grossly irregular fluctuations with a zigzag pattern (Figure 18-19). This pattern is caused by the same problems associated with VT.

Treatment calls for rapid defibrillation, cardiopulmonary resuscitation, and administration of O_2 and antiarrhythmic medications; treatment of the underlying cause of the ischemia **is also warranted (see Chapter 37).** Survivors of VF usually receive an internal cardioverter-defibrillator.[8-12]

Pulseless Electrical Activity

In addition to the arrhythmias noted throughout this chapter, pulseless electrical activity (PEA) is a serious condition characterized by a disassociation between the electrical and mechanical activity of the heart. In essence, the ECG pattern on the monitor does not generate a pulse. PEA is relatively rare and generally does not occur without a precipitating event, such as a tension pneumothorax, MI, drug overdose, or severe electrolyte or acid-base disturbances.

Treatment involves emergency life support and the immediate reversal of the cause. PEA also illustrates why RTs and other clinicians should never "treat the monitor" and underscores the importance of using ECGs as just one of several clinical indicators in assessing patients.[10-12] The prompt recognition and response to VT, VF, and PEA are discussed in detail in Chapter 37, which covers the broader topic of emergency cardiovascular life support.

MINI CLINI

Pulseless Electrical Activity

PROBLEM: A 68-year-old man with a recent complaint of radiating chest pain is being placed on O_2 therapy with a nasal cannula at 2 L/min. Immediately after being set up on a 12-lead ECG, the patient loses consciousness. The ECG continues to show an apparent sinus bradycardia, but assessment reveals that the patient is pulseless.

SOLUTION: This is an apparent case of PEA, which should be treated as a potentially life-threatening emergency. A "code blue" should be initiated, cardiopulmonary resuscitation should be started immediately, and potential causes, including in this instance MI, should be considered and treated.

SUMMARY CHECKLIST

- The ECG is an inexpensive, noninvasive, and easy way to evaluate patients, but it does not predict future heart problems nor identify all abnormalities (i.e., valvular defects).
- The impulse-conducting system has three types of cardiac muscle cells capable of electrical excitation: pacemaker cells (e.g., SA node, AV node), specialized rapid conducting tissue (e.g., Purkinje fibers), and atrial and ventricular muscle cells. Each of these vary in their degree of automaticity.
- An elevated or depressed ST segment is common in MI and is a potentially life-threatening arrhythmia.
- Axis evaluation is used to determine the general direction of current flow during ventricular depolarization and is helpful in identifying hypertrophy of one of the ventricles.
- Sinus bradycardia is a significant clinical problem only if it causes the patient's blood pressure to decrease significantly or the patient becomes symptomatic.
- Frequent, paired together, multifocal PVCs or the R on T phenomenon with PVCs is serious because it often is due to ischemia of the myocardium and can progress rapidly to ventricular tachycardia and fibrillation.
- Type II second-degree heart block usually causes a significant decrease in cardiac output and may also progress to third-degree heart block. Even if the patient is asymptomatic, treatment calls for medication such as atropine until a pacemaker can be placed.
- Third-degree heart block is the most serious of the different types of heart block often caused by MI or drug toxicity (especially digitalis) and may render the heart unable to meet the normal metabolic demands of the body. Treatment usually includes medication to speed up the ventricles and a pacemaker.
- Atrial fibrillation is a serious arrhythmia that can lead to a significant reduction in cardiac output. In addition, if untreated, over time it can potentially cause an embolic event. Treatment entails medications to control the rate, antithrombolytics or anticoagulants, and potential cardioversion.
- Sustained or symptomatic VT is a serious arrhythmia that often leads to VF if untreated. Prompt treatment usually consists of cardioversion, antiarrhythmic drugs, and transfer to the ICU.

- VF is the most life-threatening arrhythmia, requiring emergent treatment with rapid defibrillation, cardiopulmonary resuscitation, and administration of O_2 and antiarrhythmic medications.
- Always treat the patient, not the rhythm on the ECG monitor. Patients with PEA often have a seemingly productive rhythm on the ECG but are pulseless and require immediate emergency life support.

References

1. Goldberger AL, Goldberger ZD, Shvilkia S: *Clinical electrocardiography: a simplified approach*, ed 8, St Louis, 2012, Elsevier.
2. Conover M: *Understanding electrocardiography*, ed 8, St Louis, 2002, Mosby.
3. Thaler MS: *The only EKG book you'll ever need*, ed 7, Philadelphia, 2012, Lippincott, Williams & Wilkins.
4. Aehlert B: *ECGs made easy*, ed 5, St Louis, 2012, Elsevier.
5. Wesley K: *Huszar's basic dysrhythmias and acute coronary syndromes: interpretation and management*, ed 4, St Louis, 2014, Elsevier.
6. Walraven G: *Basic arrhythmias*, ed 7, Upper Saddle River, NJ, 2010, Prentice Hall.
7. Phalen T, Aehlert B: *The 12-lead ECG in acute coronary syndromes*, ed 2, St. Louis, 2006, Mosby.
8. Barrett D, Gretton M, Quinn T: *Cardiac care: an introduction for healthcare professionals*, Indianapolis, 2006, Wiley.
9. Hazinski MF, Field JM, editors: *2010 guidelines for cardiopulmonary resuscitation and emergency cardiovascular care*, Dallas, 2010, American Heart Association.
10. Darovic GO: *Hemodynamic monitoring: invasive and noninvasive clinical application*, ed 3, Philadelphia, 2002, Saunders.
11. Huff J: *ECG workout exercises in arrhythmia interpretation*, ed 5, Philadelphia, 2005, Lippincott Williams & Wilkins.
12. Heuer AJ, Scanlan CL: *Clinical assessment in respiratory care*, ed 7, St Louis, 2013, Elsevier.

CHAPTER 19

Analysis and Monitoring of Gas Exchange

MICHAEL A. GENTILE, ALBERT J. HEUER, AND RICHARD H. KALLET

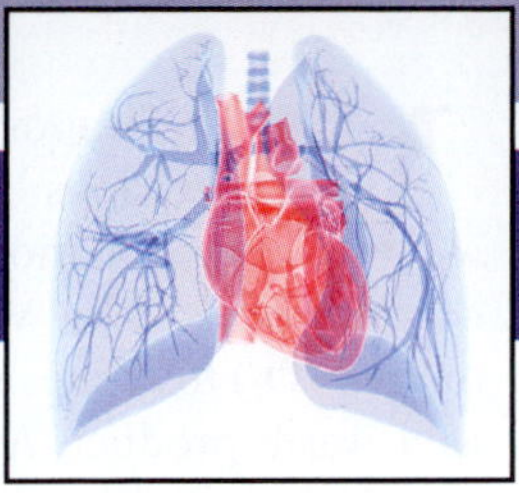

CHAPTER OBJECTIVES

After reading this chapter you will be able to:

- Describe the difference between monitoring and analysis.
- Describe the two types of electrochemical oxygen analyzers.
- Describe calibration and problem-solving techniques for oxygen analyzers.
- State how to obtain, process, and analyze arterial and capillary blood gas samples.
- List the quality control procedures applied to blood gas analysis.
- List the potential advantages of point-of-care testing.
- Describe how to obtain and interpret transcutaneous oxygen and carbon dioxide monitoring.
- Describe the basic principles used by an oximeter to monitor oxygen saturation.
- State how to perform and interpret pulse oximetry.
- Describe how to perform capnometry and interpret capnograms.

CHAPTER OUTLINE

KEY TERMS

analyte
analyzer
arterialized blood
calibration media
capnography
capnometry
collateral circulation
cuvette
electrochemical
invasive
modified Allen test
monitor
needle capping device
noninvasive
optical fluorescence
optode
oximetry
photoplethysmography
point-of-care testing
pre-analytic error
precision
proficiency testing
pulse cooximetry
quality control
random error
spectrophotometry
systematic error
volumetric capnography

Many important and potentially lifesaving clinical decisions are based on a patient's gas-exchange information. Gas exchange takes place inside each of the body's cells, where complex metabolic pathways use oxygen (O_2) to create energy and produce carbon dioxide (CO_2) as a waste product. Although it is possible but clinically not practical to analyze gas exchange at the cellular level, clinical focus normally is on gas exchange between the lungs and blood or between the blood and tissues. Gas exchange between the lungs and blood is usually analyzed by measuring O_2 and CO_2 levels in the arterial blood. Clinicians, including RTs, also can measure CO_2 levels in the expired gas to monitor ventilation. The most common approach to analyzing gas exchange between the blood and tissues is to measure O_2 levels in the mixed venous blood. This chapter focuses on these important parameters related to gas exchange.

ANALYSIS VERSUS MONITORING

Although the term *analysis* is defined broadly as *study* or *interpretation,* analysis conducted in a clinical laboratory has a special meaning, as does the term *monitoring*. In clinical practice, *laboratory analysis* refers to measurements of fluids or tissue that must be removed from the body. Such measurements are made by an **analyzer.** Conversely, monitoring is an ongoing process by which clinicians obtain and evaluate dynamic physiologic processes, usually at the bedside. A **monitor** is a device that provides data to the clinician in real time, usually without removal of samples from the body.

INVASIVE VERSUS NONINVASIVE PROCEDURES

Invasive procedures require insertion of a sensor or collection device into the body, whereas **noninvasive** monitoring gathers data externally.[1] Because laboratory analysis of gas exchange requires blood samples, it is considered invasive. Monitoring can be either invasive or noninvasive. In general, invasive procedures provide more accurate data than noninvasive methods, but carry greater risk.

When both approaches are available, the need for measurement accuracy dictates which is chosen. However, clinicians sometimes combine the approaches—using the invasive approach to establish accurate baseline information and applying the noninvasive method for ongoing monitoring of a patient. After the gradient between the invasive and noninvasive method is established, trending changes by noninvasive methods can be useful in making clinical decisions.

MEASURING FRACTIONAL INSPIRED OXYGEN

Gas-exchange analysis begins with knowledge of the system inputs—the inspired O_2 and CO_2 concentrations. Healthy individuals breathe air that contains a fixed O_2 concentration (21%) and negligible amounts of CO_2 (approximately 0.2%). Hypoxemic patients are routinely given supplemental O_2. In most cases, O_2 analyzers are used to measure the fractional inspired O_2 concentration (FiO_2).

Instrumentation

Although many methods exist for measuring O_2 concentrations, most bedside systems apply electrochemical principles. There are two common types of **electrochemical** O_2 analyzers are the polarographic (Clark) electrode and the galvanic fuel cell. Under ideal conditions of temperature, pressure, and relative humidity, both types are generally accurate to within ± 2% of the actual concentration.[1]

The Clark electrode is similar to electrodes used in blood gas analyzers and transcutaneous monitors, discussed later in this chapter. This system typically consists of a platinum cathode and a silver–silver chloride anode (Figure 19-1). O_2 molecules diffuse through the sensor membrane into the electrolyte, where a polarizing voltage causes electron flow between the anode and cathode. While silver is oxidized at the anode, the flow of electrons reduces O_2 (and water) to hydroxyl ions (OH^-) at the cathode. More O_2 molecules undergoing reduction causes greater electron flow across the poles (current). The resulting current change is proportional to the PO_2, with its value displayed on a galvanometer, calibrated in $\%O_2$. Response times for O_2 analyzers range from 10 to 30 seconds.

Most galvanic fuel cells use a gold anode and a lead cathode. In contrast to the Clark electrode, current flow across these poles is generated by the chemical reaction itself.

The Clark electrode and galvanic cell are suitable for basic FiO_2 monitoring. When greater accuracy or faster response times are needed (e.g., when performing indirect calorimetry), a paramagnetic, zirconium cell, Raman scattering, or mass spectroscopy analyzer should be selected.

Procedure

To obtain accurate results with an O_2 analyzer, the clinician first must calibrate it. Although procedures differ according to the

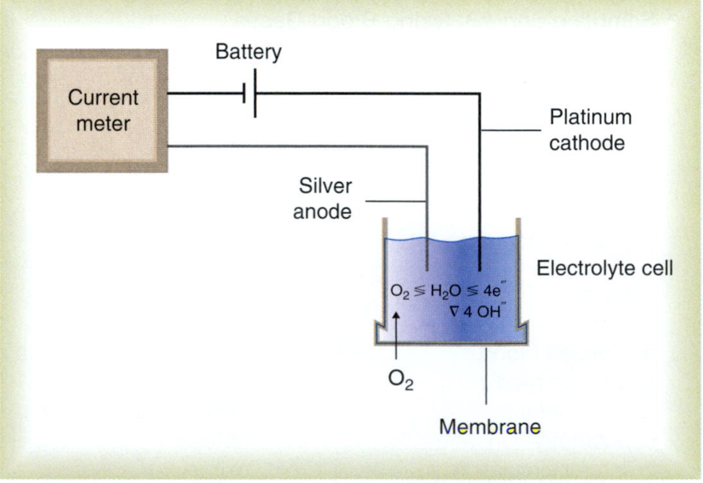

FIGURE 19-1 The basic principle underlying the Clark polarographic analyzer. (Modified from Kacmarek RM, Hess D, Stoller JK, editors: Monitoring in respiratory care, St Louis, 1993, Mosby.)

manufacturer, the basic steps are similar. This requires exposing the sensor to two gases with different O_2 concentrations, usually 100% O_2 and room air (21% O_2). In one common procedure, the sensor is first exposed to 100% O_2. If the analyzer fails to read 100%, the device's *calibration,* or balance control, must be adjusted until it reads 100%. Then the clinician exposes the sensor to room air and confirms a second reading of 21% (±2%). The clinician should use the analyzer to measure a patient's FiO_2 only after confirming both readings.

Problem-Solving and Troubleshooting

Because O_2 analyzers include replaceable components that deteriorate over time (batteries, electrodes, membranes, electrolytes), the best way to avoid problems is through preventive maintenance. This should include both scheduled parts replacement and routine operational testing.

Even with the best preventive maintenance, O_2 analyzers may malfunction. The clinician would know that an analyzer is not working if it fails to calibrate or gives an inconsistent reading during use. Common causes of analyzer malfunction are low batteries, sensor depletion, and electronic failure. Because a low battery condition is common, the first step in troubleshooting is to replace the batteries. If the analyzer still does not calibrate on fresh batteries, the problem is probably a depleted sensor. With most analyzers, a depleted sensor must be replaced. If an analyzer still fails to calibrate after battery and sensor replacement, the most likely problem is an internal failure of its electrical system. In this case, the device should be taken out of service and repaired.

Inaccurate readings also can occur with electrochemical analyzers, resulting from either condensed water vapor or pressure fluctuations. Galvanic cells are particularly sensitive to condensation. To avoid this problem during continuous use in humidified circuits, the clinician should place the analyzer sensor proximal to any humidification device.

Fuel cell and Clark electrode readings also are affected by ambient pressure changes. Under conditions of low pressure (high altitude), these devices read lower than the actual O_2 concentration. Conversely, higher pressures, such as pressures that occur during positive pressure ventilation, cause these devices to read higher than the actual FiO_2. These observations are consistent with the fact that both devices measure the PO_2 but report a percent concentration scale.

RULE OF THUMB

Three common causes of O_2 analyzer malfunction are low batteries, sensor depletion, and electronic failure.

SAMPLING AND ANALYZING BLOOD GASES

In the clinical setting, it is common for the collection of blood specimens (sampling) to be performed separately from their analysis. Each procedure involves different knowledge and skill. For these reasons, these topics are covered separately.

Sampling

Clinicians have been using blood samples to assess gas-exchange parameters for more than 50 years.[2] The definition of *respiratory failure* is based largely on blood gas measurements (i.e., PaO_2, and $PaCO_2$). Depending on the need, blood gas samples can be obtained by percutaneous puncture of a peripheral artery, from an indwelling catheter: arterial, central venous, or pulmonary artery (PA) or by capillary sampling.

Arterial Puncture and Interpretation

Results obtained from sampling arterial blood gas (ABG) are the foundation for the diagnosis and management of oxygenation and acid-base disturbances. ABGs are considered the "gold standard" of gas-exchange analysis, against which all other methods are compared.

Arterial puncture involves drawing blood from a peripheral artery (radial, brachial, femoral, or dorsalis pedis) through a single percutaneous needle puncture (Figure 19-2). The radial artery is the preferred site for arterial blood sampling for the following reasons:

- It is near the surface and relatively easy to palpate and stabilize.
- Effective **collateral circulation** normally exists in the ulnar artery.
- The artery is not near any large veins.

Other sites (brachial, femoral, and dorsalis pedis) are riskier and should be used only by clinicians specifically trained in their use. Likewise, arterial puncture in infants (through either the radial or the temporal artery) requires advanced training. Arterial cannulation sites for indwelling catheters include radial, brachial, femoral, dorsalis pedis, umbilical (in neonates), and axillary arteries. The focus here is on radial artery puncture.

To guide practitioners in providing quality care, the American Association for Respiratory Care (AARC) has published Clinical Practice Guideline: Sampling for Arterial Blood Gas Analysis.[3] Complementary recommendations have been published by the National Committee for Clinical Laboratory Standards.[4] Modified excerpts from the AARC guideline appear in Clinical Practice Guideline 19-1.

Equipment. Box 19-1 lists the equipment needed to perform an arterial puncture. Commercial vendors provide kits containing most of the equipment listed.

Procedure. Box 19-2 outlines the basic procedure for radial artery puncture of adults. Before radial artery puncture is performed, a **modified Allen test** (Figure 19-3) is recommended. The test is normal (indicating adequate collateral circulation) if the palm, fingers, and thumb flush pink within 5 to 10 seconds after pressure on the ulnar artery is released. A normal test result indicates the presence of collateral circulation in the ulnar artery, but may not predict the development of complications after radial artery puncture or cannulation.

The modified Allen test has been a widely used clinical method to assess adequacy of ulnar artery collateral blood flow

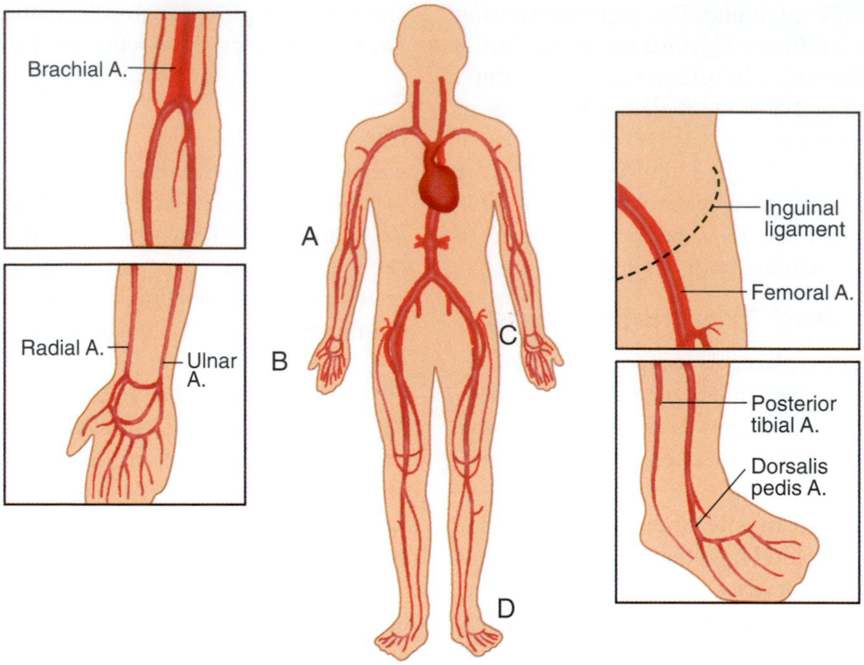

FIGURE 19-2 Arteries *(A.)* used for arterial puncture. **A,** Brachial artery. **B,** Radial artery (with collateral flow through the ulnar arteries). **C,** Femoral artery. **D,** Dorsalis pedis (with collateral flow through the posterior tibial artery). The radial artery is the preferred site.

Box 19-1 Recommended Equipment for Percutaneous Arterial Blood Sampling

- Standard precautions barrier protection (gloves, safety goggles)
- Preheparinized blood gas kit syringe (1 to 3 ml)
- Short-bevel 20- to 22-gauge needle with a clear hub (23- to 25-gauge for children and infants)
- Patient and sample label
- Isopropyl alcohol (70%), povidone-iodine (Betadine) (check patient for iodine sensitivity), or chlorhexidine swabs
- Sterile gauze squares, tape, bandages
- Puncture-resistant container
- Ice slush, depending upon the analyzer. **Note:** For most point-of-care (bedside) analyzers, samples should not be chilled and should be run within 1 to 2 minutes after being obtained.
- Towels
- Sharps container
- Local anesthetic (optional)
- Hypodermic needle (25- or 26-gauge)
- Needle capping device

despite the lack of evidence that it can predict ischemic complications in the setting of complete radial artery occlusion.[5] The criteria for an abnormal test result are not agreed on, and therefore the significance of an abnormal test is unclear. For example, test results (1) may be inaccurate in predicting postcannulation hand ischemia, (2) may vary depending on the clinician performing the test (poor interrater reliability), and (3) are known to yield high incidences of both false normal and abnormal results. In addition, prior radial artery cannulation, severe circulatory insufficiency, wrist or hand burns, or jaundice makes interpreting the results difficult. Despite these limitations, an Allen test may reveal gross circulatory abnormalities and therefore should be performed beforehand and then documented in the patient's medical record.

In patients who have undergone previous radial artery cannulation, the modified Allen test can provide documentation of possible arterial thrombosis and should be used to direct catheter placement. In that circumstance, it is imprudent to ignore totally the utility of the modified Allen test, especially if another arterial site is available for cannulation.[6]

In most cases, a sample volume of 0.5 to 1 ml of blood is adequate. The actual sample volume needed depends on (1) the anticoagulant used, (2) the requirements of the specific analyzer used, and (3) whether other tests will be performed on the sample. It should be noted that point-of-care (bedside) analyzers tend to require less blood (≤0.5 ml) than laboratory analyzers.

The following rules for careful handling of the needle help avoid transmission of blood-borne diseases:

- Never recap a used needle without a safety device.
- Never handle a used needle using both hands.
- Never point a used needle toward any part of the body.
- Never bend, break, or remove used needles from syringes by hand.
- Always dispose of used syringes, needles, and other sharp items in appropriate puncture-resistant sharps containers.

Indications for Blood Gas Sampling. Knowing when to obtain a blood gas sample is just as important as knowing how to perform the procedure. See Clinical Practice Guideline 19-1 for the general indications for ABG sampling. Box 19-3 lists

19-1 Sampling for Arterial Blood Gas Analysis

AARC Clinical Practice Guidelines (Excerpts)*

INDICATIONS

- The need to evaluate ventilation ($PaCO_2$), acid-base balance (pH and $PaCO_2$), oxygenation status (PaO_2 and SaO_2), and oxygen-carrying capacity of blood (PaO_2, HbO_2, total Hb, and dyshemoglobins)
- The need to assess the patient's response to therapy or diagnostic tests (e.g., oxygen or exercise testing)
- The need to monitor the severity and progression of a documented disease process

CONTRAINDICATIONS

- Abnormal results of a modified Allen test (lack of collateral circulation) may be indicative of inadequate blood supply to the hand and suggest the need to select another puncture site.
- Arterial puncture should not be performed through a lesion or distal to a surgical shunt. For example, arterial puncture should not be performed on a patient undergoing dialysis. If there is evidence of infection or peripheral vascular disease involving the selected limb, an alternative site should be selected.
- Because of the need for monitoring the femoral puncture site for an extended period, femoral punctures should not be performed outside the hospital.
- Coagulopathy or medium-dose to high-dose anticoagulation therapy, such as heparin or warfarin (Coumadin), streptokinase, and tissue plasminogen activator (but not aspirin), may be a relative contraindication.

PRECAUTIONS AND POSSIBLE COMPLICATIONS

- Arteriospasm
- Hemorrhage
- Air or clotted blood emboli
- Trauma to the vessel
- Anaphylaxis from local anesthetic
- Arterial occlusion
- Patient or sampler contamination
- Vasovagal response
- Hematoma
- Pain

ASSESSMENT OF NEED

The following assessments are useful for deciding whether arterial blood sampling is needed:

- History and physical indicators, such as positive smoking history, recent onset of difficulty breathing (independent of activity level), or trauma
- Presence of other abnormal diagnostic tests or indices, such as abnormal pulse oximetry reading or chest x-ray examination
- Initiation, change, or discontinuation of therapy (e.g., oxygen therapy or mechanical ventilation)
- Projected enrollment in a pulmonary rehabilitation program

FREQUENCY

The frequency with which sampling is repeated should depend on the clinical status of the patient and the indication for performing the procedure. Because repeated punctures at a single site can cause injury, clinicians should consider either finding alternative sites or using an indwelling catheter.

MONITORING

The following should be monitored as part of arterial blood sampling:

- FiO_2 (analyzed) or prescribed flow
- Patient's respiratory rate
- Proper application of oxygen device
- Patient's temperature
- Mode of ventilatory support and settings
- Appearance of the puncture site (for hematoma) after application of pressure and before dressing

**For the complete guideline, see American Association for Respiratory Care: Clinical practice guideline: sampling for arterial blood gas analysis. Respir Care 37:891, 1992.*

common clinical situations associated with the need for ABG analysis.

Problem-Solving and Troubleshooting. There are two major problem areas associated with arterial puncture. The first problem involves difficulties in getting a good sample. The second problem involves pre-analytic error.

Getting a Good Sample. Problems with getting a good sample include an inaccessible artery, absent pulse, deficient sample return, and alteration of test results caused by the patient's response. If the selected artery cannot be located, another site should be considered. Likewise, if an adequate pulse cannot be palpated at the chosen site, another site should be selected or an acceptable noninvasive approach should be considered as an alternative (e.g., pulse oximetry). Ultrasound guidance may useful in artery identification and sampling success.[7]

If the clinician gets only a small spurt of blood, the needle has probably passed through the artery. In this situation, the needle is slowly withdrawn until a pulsatile flow fills the syringe. The tip of the needle is never redirected without it first being withdrawn to the subcutaneous tissue. If the needle must be withdrawn completely and the clinician does not have an adequate sample, the procedure is repeated with a fresh blood gas kit.

Small sample volumes or the need to apply syringe suction also may indicate that venous blood has been obtained. However,

Box 19-2 Procedure for Radial Artery Puncture

- Check the medical record to (1) confirm the order and indications and (2) determine the patient's primary diagnosis, history (especially bleeding disorders or blood-borne infections), current status, respiratory care orders (especially oxygen therapy or mechanical ventilation), and anticoagulant or thrombolytic therapy.
- Confirm steady-state conditions (20 to 30 minutes after changes).
- Obtain and assemble necessary equipment and supplies.
- Wash hands and don barrier protection (e.g., gloves, eyewear).
- Identify the patient using current patient safety standards.
- Explain the procedure to the patient.
- Position the patient, extending the patient's wrist to approximately 30 degrees.
- Perform a modified Allen test, and confirm collateral circulation.
- Clean site thoroughly with 70% isopropyl alcohol or an equivalent antiseptic.
- Inject a local anesthetic subcutaneously/periarterially, wait 2 minutes for effect (optional).
- Use a preheparinized blood gas kit syringe, or heparinize a syringe and expel the excess (fill dead space only).
- Palpate and secure the artery with one hand.
- Insert the needle, bevel up, through the skin at a 45-degree angle until blood pulsates into the syringe.
- Allow 1 ml of blood to fill syringe (the need to aspirate indicates a venous puncture).
- Apply firm pressure to puncture site with sterile gauze until the bleeding stops.
- Expel any air bubbles from the sample, and cap or plug the syringe.
- Mix the sample by rolling and inverting the syringe.
- Place the sample in a transport container and chilled or not, depending on analyzer manufacturer recommendation. **Note:** For most point-of-care (bedside) analyzers, samples should not be chilled and should be run within 1 to 2 minutes after being obtained.
- Dispose of waste materials and sharps properly.
- Document the procedure and patient status in the medical record and on the specimen label.
- Check the site for hematoma and adequacy of distal circulation.

From Malley WJ: Clinical blood gases: assessment and intervention. St Louis, 2005, Saunders.

Box 19-3 Clinical Indications for Arterial Blood Gas Analysis

- Sudden, unexplained dyspnea
- Cyanosis
- Abnormal breath sounds
- Severe, unexplained tachypnea
- Heavy use of accessory muscles
- Changes in ventilator settings
- Cardiopulmonary resuscitation
- New appearance of diffuse infiltrates in chest radiograph
- Sudden appearance or progression of cardiac arrhythmias
- Acute hypotension
- Acute deterioration in neurologic function

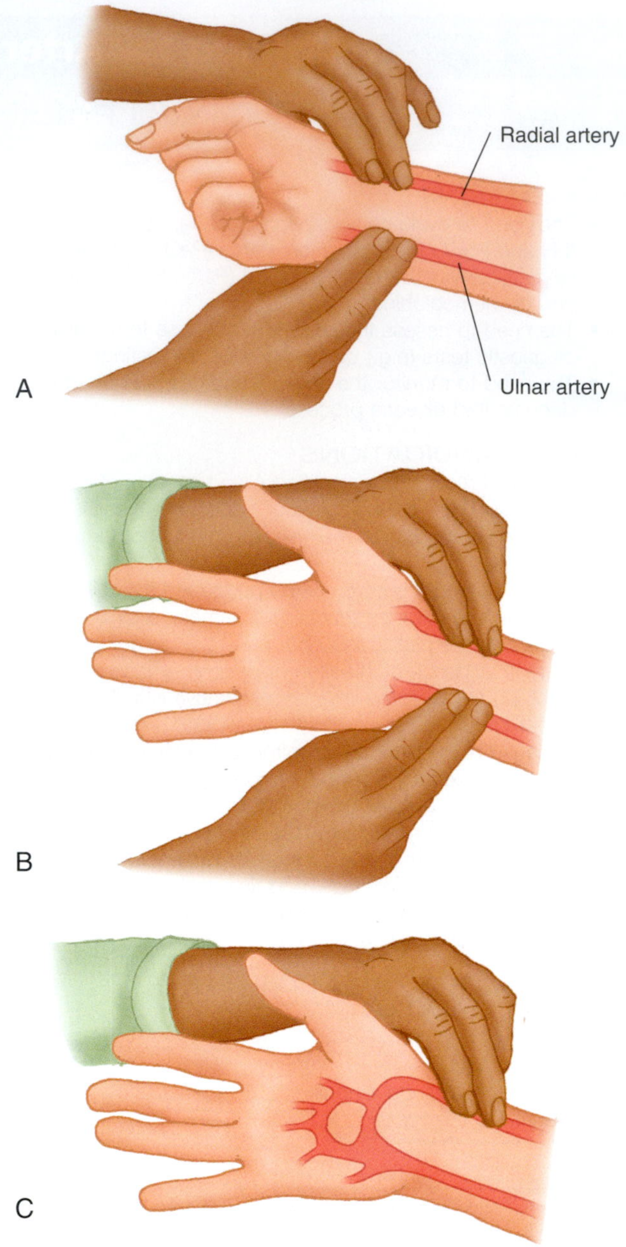

FIGURE 19-3 Modified Allen test. **A,** The hand is clenched into a tight fist, and pressure is applied to the radial and ulnar arteries. **B,** The hand is opened (but not fully extended); the palm and fingers are blanched. **C,** Removal of pressure on the ulnar artery should cause flushing of the entire hand (within 5 to 10 seconds), indicative of adequate collateral circulation or a normal modified Allen test.

when drawing arterial blood from hypotensive patients or when using small needles (<23-gauge), the clinician may need to pull gently on the syringe barrel. If clinicians suspect that pain or anxiety during the procedure may have altered the results (most typically causing hyperventilation, but sometimes breath-holding), they should consider using a local anesthetic for subsequent sampling attempts.

Pre-analytic Error. **Pre-analytic errors** are problems occurring before sample analysis that can alter the accuracy of the blood gas results. Table 19-1 summarizes the most common

TABLE 19-1

Pre-analytic Errors Associated With Arterial Blood

Error	Effect on Parameters	How to Recognize	How to Avoid
Air in sample	↓ PCO_2 ↑ pH ↑ low PO_2 ↓ high PO_2	Visible bubbles or froth Low PCO_2 inconsistent with patient status	Discard frothy samples Fully expel bubbles Mix only after air is expelled Cap syringe quickly
Venous admixture	↑ PCO_2 ↓ pH Can greatly lower PO_2	Failure of syringe to fill by pulsations Patient has no symptoms of hypoxemia	Avoid brachial and femoral sites Do not aspirate sample Use short-bevel needles Avoid artery "overshoot" Cross-check with SpO_2
Excess anticoagulant (dilution)	↓ PCO_2 ↑ pH ↑ low PO_2 ↓ high PO_2	Visible heparin remains in syringe before sampling	Use premade lyophilized (dry) heparin blood gas kits Fill dead space only Collect >2 ml (adults) and >0.6 ml (infants)
Metabolic effects	↑ PCO_2 ↓ pH ↓ PO_2	Excessive time lag since sample collection Values inconsistent with patient status	Analyze within 15 min Place sample in ice slush

errors associated with arterial blood sampling, including recommendations on how to recognize and avoid these problems. Clinicians can avoid most pre-analytic errors by ensuring that the sample is obtained anaerobically (with immediate expulsion of air bubbles), properly anticoagulated, and quickly analyzed.

The traditional method used to avoid pre-analytic errors caused by blood cell metabolism is to chill the sample quickly by placing it in ice.[3] However, some studies suggest that results may be altered if samples are stored in certain types of plastic syringes, especially if placed on ice before being analyzed. In addition, chilled samples can result in potassium transport between blood cells and plasma and can result in erroneous elevation in potassium measured from a blood gas sample. Hence, the best ways to minimize such pre-analytic errors is to use low-diffusability syringes, which minimize the risk for room-air altering the sample, and to analyze the sample as soon as possible after it has been obtained. Furthermore, samples that have been stored for an undetermined time, whether chilled or not, should be discarded.[8,9] Another consideration is that pneumatic tube transport of samples containing small air bubbles can have a noticeable effect on increasing PaO_2.[9] Finally, most point-of-care (bedside), analyzer systems (discussed later in this chapter) require that the sample not be chilled and be analyzed within 1 to 2 minutes after being obtained, depending on the manufacturer.

RULE OF THUMB

Three common methods for avoiding pre-analytic errors in ABG measurements are ensuring that the sample is obtained anaerobically (with immediate expulsion of air bubbles), the sample syringe is properly anticoagulated, and the sample is promptly analyzed.

Interpretation of Arterial Blood Gases. Because gas exchange is a dynamic process, looking at results from a single blood sample is akin to looking at a single frame of streaming video, representing a single point in time rather than an ongoing physiologic process. Blood gas results must be interpreted in light of the patient status at the time the sample was obtained.

Any major change in the patient's condition or therapy disrupts the patient's steady state. However, over time, a new steady state emerges. The time needed to restore steady-state conditions varies with the patient's pulmonary status. Patients with healthy lungs achieve a steady state in only 5 minutes after changes, whereas patients with chronic obstructive pulmonary disease (COPD) may require up to 30 minutes. For example, when FiO_2 is changed, the measured PaO_2 would accurately reflect the patient's gas-exchange status within 5 minutes in healthy individuals but may require up to 30 minutes in patients with COPD.

To document the patient's status, the following need to be recorded: (1) date, time, and site of sampling; (2) results of the modified Allen test, when performed; (3) patient's body temperature, position, activity level, and respiratory rate; and (4) FiO_2 concentration or nasal cannula flow and all applicable ventilatory support settings. Noting such information may prove useful in interpretation of the results.

RULE OF THUMB

To ensure a steady state, waiting up to 30 minutes after any major change in ventilatory support may be necessary before sampling and analyzing the blood gases of a critically ill patient.

In the first step of interpreting results, clinicians must ensure they are looking at the results for the correct patient. The name and patient identification number from the blood gas report must match the patient. Interpretation of the results can be divided into two basic steps: interpretation of the oxygenation status and interpretation of the acid-base status.

TABLE 19-2

Common Sites for Indwelling Vascular Catheters and the Information They Provide

Location	BLOOD COLLECTION		PRESSURE MONITORING	
	Sample	**Reflects**	**Pressure**	**Reflects**
Peripheral, umbilical artery	Arterial blood	Pulmonary gas exchange (O_2 uptake/CO_2 removal)	Systemic arterial pressure	LV afterload, vascular tone, blood volume
Central vein	Venous blood (unmixed)	Not useful for assessing gas exchange; can be used for some other laboratory tests	CVP	Fluid volume, vascular tone, RV preload
Pulmonary artery	Mixed venous blood (balloon deflated)	Gas exchange at tissues (O_2 consumption/ CO_2 production)	PAP, PCWP	RV afterload, vascular tone, blood volume, LV preload

CVP, Central venous pressure; *LV,* left ventricular; *PAP,* pulmonary artery pressure; *PCWP,* pulmonary capillary wedge pressure; *RV,* right ventricular.

The oxygenation status is determined by examining the PaO_2, arterial O_2 saturation (SaO_2), and arterial O_2 content (CaO_2). The PaO_2 represents the partial pressure of O_2 dissolved in the plasma of the arterial blood and is the result of gas exchange between the lung and blood. The PaO_2 is reduced in various settings but most often when lung disease is present. PaO_2 of less than 40 mm Hg is called *severe* hypoxemia, PaO_2 of 40 to 59 mm Hg is called *moderate* hypoxemia, and PaO_2 of 60 mm Hg to the predicted normal is called *mild* hypoxemia.

SaO_2 represents the degree to which the hemoglobin (Hb) is saturated with O_2 (see Chapter 12). Normally, the Hb saturation with O_2 is 95% to 100% with healthy lungs. When the lungs cannot transfer O_2 into the blood at normal levels, the SaO_2 usually decreases in proportion to the degree of lung disease. Blood gas analyzers report a calculated SaO_2. Measurement of SaO_2 by hemoximetry and Hb content is required for accurate determination of CaO_2.

CaO_2 represents the content of O_2 in 100 ml of arterial blood and is a function of the amount of Hb present and the degree to which it is saturated. A normal CaO_2 is 18 to 20 ml of O_2 per 100 ml of arterial blood. A reduced CaO_2 is often the result of low PaO_2 and SaO_2, reduced Hb level, or the presence of dyshemoglobins.

The acid-base status of the patient is determined by evaluating the pH, $PaCO_2$, and plasma bicarbonate (HCO_3^-). The steps for interpreting the acid-base status of the ABG results are described in Chapter 14.

RULE OF THUMB

Mild hypoxemia is defined as a PaO_2 of 60 mm Hg relative to predicted normal, whereas moderate hypoxemia is a PaO_2 between 40 and 59 mm Hg and severe hypoxemia is defined as a PaO_2 less than 40 mm Hg.

Indwelling Catheters (Arterial, and Central Venous Pressure, and Pulmonary Artery Lines)

Indwelling catheters provide ready access for blood sampling and allow continuous monitoring of vascular pressures, without the traumatic risks associated with repetitive percutaneous punctures. However, infection and thrombosis are more likely with indwelling catheters than with intermittent punctures.

The most common route for an indwelling arterial vascular line is the radial artery; less commonly used sites are the dorsalis pedis, brachial, axillary, and femoral arteries. Venous blood gases are obtained from either a central venous catheter or a PA catheter, which can access both the superior vena cava and a main branch of the PA. In neonates, the umbilical artery is cannulated for arterial blood sampling. Table 19-2 summarizes the usefulness of these various sites in providing relevant clinical information. Chapter 51 provides details on the use of these systems for hemodynamic pressure and flow monitoring.

Equipment. Figure 19-4 shows the basic setup used for an indwelling vascular line, in this case, a brachial artery catheter. The catheter connects to a disposable continuous-flush device. This device keeps the line open by providing a continuous low rate of flow (2 to 4 ml/hr) of intravenous (IV) saline solution through the system.

Heparinized saline flush solution may be used with indwelling vascular catheters. However, results of coagulation studies are affected by heparinized flush solution and unnecessary exposure to heparin may increase the risk for heparin-induced thrombocytopenia.[10] Because arterial pressures are much higher than venous pressures, the IV bag supplying these systems must be pressurized, usually by using a hand bulb pump. A strain-gauge pressure transducer connected to the flush device provides an electrical signal to an amplifier or monitor, which displays the corresponding pressure waveform.

Procedure. Access for sampling blood from most intravascular lines is provided by a three-way stopcock (Figure 19-5). Equipment and supplies are the same as specified for arterial puncture, with the addition of a second "waste" syringe. Box 19-4 outlines the proper procedure for taking an arterial blood sample from a three-way stopcock system.

The procedure is slightly different when obtaining mixed venous blood samples from PA catheters because PA catheters have separate sampling and IV infusion ports and a balloon at the tip is used to measure pulmonary capillary wedge pressure. The clinician must ensure that the balloon is deflated and withdraw the sample slowly (e.g., approximately 3 ml/min or 1 ml in 20 seconds). If the clinician fails to deflate the balloon or

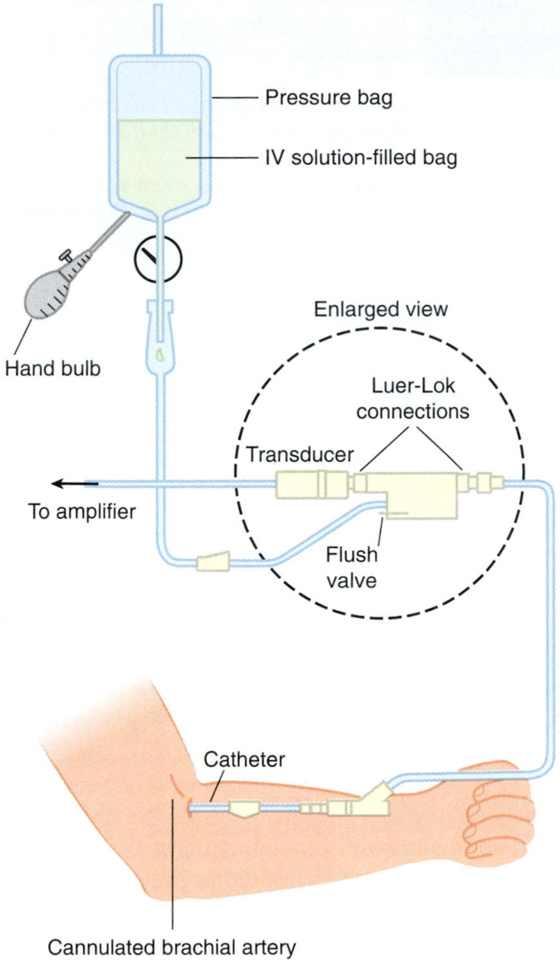

FIGURE 19-4 An indwelling vascular line (brachial artery catheter) used to monitor blood pressure and obtain a blood sample.

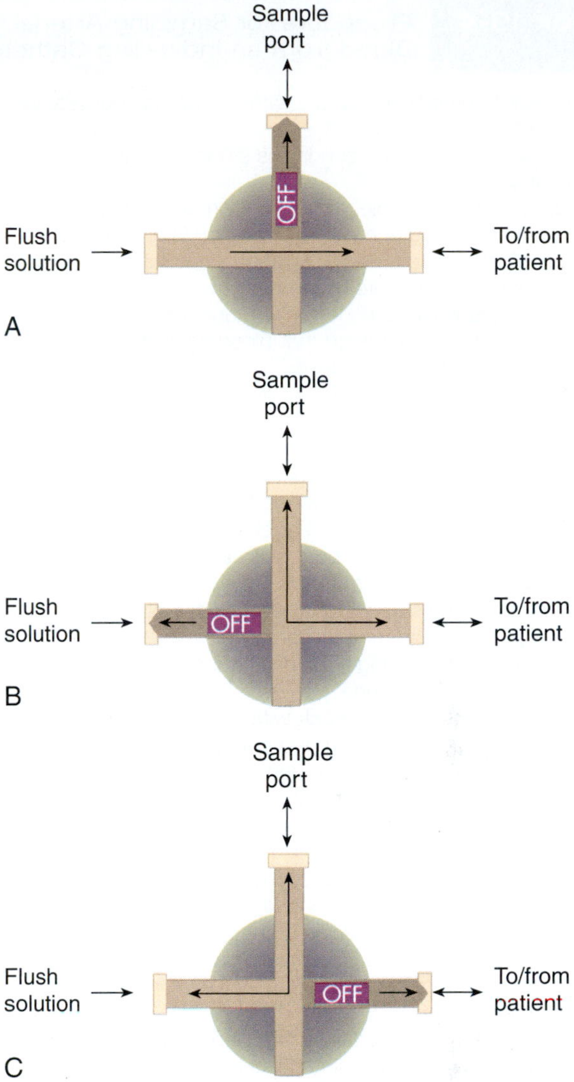

FIGURE 19-5 A three-way stopcock in a vascular line system showing the various positions used. **A,** Normal operating position, with flush solution going to the patient and the sample port closed. **B,** Position to draw a blood sample from the vascular line (closed to flush solution). **C,** Position to flush sample port (closed to patient). In any intermediary position, all ports are closed.

withdraws the sample too quickly, the venous blood may be "contaminated" with blood from the pulmonary capillaries. The result is always a falsely high O_2 level. In addition, close attention must be paid to the infusion rate through the catheter. Rapid flow of IV fluid can dilute the blood sample and affect O_2 content measurements.

Problem-Solving and Troubleshooting. With the exception of venous admixture, the pre-analytic errors that occur when sampling blood from a vascular line are the same as the errors that occur with intermittent puncture, as are the ways to avoid them. For clinicians, the challenge with vascular lines is to maintain their function properly and troubleshoot the many potential problems that can occur. Because these are key components of bedside monitoring skills, they are discussed in the section on hemodynamics in Chapter 51.

Capillary Blood Gases

Capillary blood gas sampling is used as an alternative to direct arterial access in infants and small children. Properly obtained capillary blood from a well-perfused patient can provide clinically useful estimates of arterial pH and PCO_2 levels. However, capillary PO_2 is of little value in estimating arterial oxygenation. Therefore, O_2 saturation by pulse oximetry also must be evaluated when obtaining a capillary blood gas sample. Clinicians must exercise extreme caution when using capillary blood gases to guide clinical decisions. Direct arterial access is still the preferred approach for assessing gas exchange in infants and small children.

Capillary blood values are meaningful only if the sample site is properly warmed. Warming the skin (to approximately 42° C) causes dilation of the underlying blood vessels, which increases capillary flow well above tissue needs. Blood gas values resemble the values in the arterial circulation; this is why a sample obtained from a warmed capillary site is often referred to as **arterialized blood.** It has been shown that capillary blood samples from the earlobe reflect arterial PCO_2 and PO_2 better than samples drawn from a finger stick.[11] The posterior medial or lateral curvature of the heel is the recommended site for

Box 19-4 Procedure for Sampling Arterial Blood from an Indwelling Catheter

- Check the medical record to affirm order (as per arterial puncture).
- Confirm steady-state conditions (20 to 30 minutes after changes).
- Obtain and assemble needed equipment and supplies.
- Wash hands and don barrier protection (e.g., gloves, eyewear).
- Identify the patient using current patient safety standards.
- Explain the procedure to the patient.
- Attach the waste syringe to the stopcock port.
- Position the stopcock so that blood flows into the syringe and the IV bag port is closed.
- Aspirate at least 1 to 2 ml, or five to six times the tubing volume, of fluid or blood.
- Reposition the stopcock handle to close off all ports.
- Disconnect and properly discard waste syringe.
- Attach new heparinized syringe to the sampling port.
- Position the stopcock so that blood flows into the sample syringe and the IV bag port is closed.
- Fill syringe with 1 ml of blood.
- Reposition the stopcock handle to close off the sampling port and open the IV bag port.
- Disconnect the syringe, expel air bubbles from sample, and cap or plug the syringe.
- Flush the line and stopcock with the IV solution.
- Mix the sample by rolling and inverting the syringe.
- Confirm that the stopcock port is open to the IV bag solution and catheter.
- Confirm undampened pulse pressure waveform on the monitor graphic display.
- Place the sample in a transport container (ice slush) if specimen is not to be analyzed within 10 to 30 minutes.
- Dispose of waste materials properly. **Note:** For most point-of-care (bedside) analyzers, samples should not be chilled and should be run within 1 to 2 minutes after being obtained.
- Document the procedure and patient status in the medical record and on the specimen label.

Box 19-5 Procedure for Capillary Blood Sampling

- Check the medical record (as per arterial puncture).
- Confirm steady-state conditions (20 to 30 minutes after changes).
- Obtain and assemble necessary equipment and supplies.
- Wash hands and don barrier protection (e.g., gloves, eyewear).
- Select site (e.g., heel, earlobe, great toe, finger).
- Warm site to 42° C for 10 minutes using a compress, heat lamp, or commercial hot pack.
- Clean skin with an antiseptic solution.
- Puncture the skin (<2.5 mm) with the lancet.
- Wipe away the first drop of blood and observe free flow (do not squeeze).
- Fill the sample tube from the middle of the blood drop until it is completely full (75 to 100 mcl).
- Place the metal flea in the capillary tube, and then seal the tube ends.
- Tape sterile cotton or a bandage over the puncture wound.
- Mix the sample by moving the magnet back and forth along the capillary tube.
- Sample should be immediately chilled or analyzed within 10 to 15 minutes if left at room temperature.
- Dispose of waste materials properly.
- Document the procedure and patient status in the medical record and on the specimen label.

capillary puncture specimens in infants younger than 1 month old to avoid nerve and bone damage.

To guide practitioners in providing quality care, the AARC has published Clinical Practice Guideline: Capillary Blood Gas Sampling for Neonatal and Pediatric Patients.[12] Modified excerpts from the AARC guideline appear in Clinical Practice Guideline 19-2.

Equipment. Equipment needed for capillary blood sampling includes a lancet, preheparinized capillary tubes, small metal stirrer bar (metal flea), a magnet, clay or wax sealant or caps, gauze or cotton balls, bandages, ice, gloves, skin antiseptic, warming pads (42° C), sharps container, and labeling materials.

Procedure. Box 19-5 outlines the basic procedure for capillary blood sampling. The most common site for sampling is the heel, specifically the lateral aspect of the plantar surface.

Problem-Solving and Troubleshooting. Sampling of capillary blood is useful for patient management only if the procedure is performed according to an established quality assurance program. The most common technical errors in capillary sampling are inadequate warming of the capillary bed and squeezing of the puncture site. Squeezing the puncture site may result in venous and lymphatic contamination of the sample.[13] Both errors invalidate the test results. Other pre-analytic errors are essentially the same as the errors described for arterial puncture. Because of the small sample volume (75 to 100 mcl or 0.075 to 0.1 ml) and collection tube size, the clinician must ensure an adequate sample collection while avoiding air contamination and clotting.

Analyzing

The primary **analytes** or parameters of pH, PCO_2, and PO_2 in a blood sample are measured with a blood gas analyzer. Typically, analyzers use these measures to compute several secondary values, such as plasma bicarbonate level, base excess or deficit, and Hb saturation. If actual measurement of total Hb saturation (oxyhemoglobin [HbO_2], methemoglobin [metHb], and carboxyhemoglobin [HbCO]) is required, the sample usually must be analyzed separately using hemoximetry. Some analyzers combine the blood gas and hemoximetry measurements, which may require a larger sample size (usually 100 mcl).

Blood gas analysis and hemoximetry are moderately complex laboratory procedures. Clinicians performing these tests must have documented training and must demonstrate proficiency in performing the procedures, preventive maintenance, troubleshooting, and instrument calibration. In addition, clinicians must be skilled in validating test results using rigorous **quality control** methods that ensure clinical decisions used to determine patient care are based on accurate information.[14]

To guide practitioners in providing quality care, the AARC has published Clinical Practice Guideline: Blood Gas Analysis and Hemoximetry: 2013.[15] Related recommendations have been

19-2 Capillary Blood Gas Sampling for Neonatal and Pediatric Patients

AARC Clinical Practice Guideline (Excerpts)*

INDICATIONS

Capillary blood gas sampling is indicated when:
- ABG analysis is indicated, but arterial access is unavailable
- Noninvasive monitor readings (e.g., $PtcCO_2$: $PETCO_2$, SpO_2) are abnormal
- Assessment of initiation, administration, or change in therapy (e.g., mechanical ventilation) is indicated
- A change in patient status is detected by history or physical assessment
- Monitoring the severity and progression of a documented disease process is desirable

CONTRAINDICATIONS

Capillary punctures should not be performed at or through the following:
- The posterior curvature of the heel (because it can puncture the bone)
- The heel of a patient who has begun walking and has callus development
- The fingers of neonates (because it can cause nerve damage)
- Previous puncture sites
- Inflamed, swollen, or edematous tissues
- Cyanotic or poorly perfused tissues
- Localized areas of infection
- Peripheral arteries

Capillary punctures should not be performed:
- On patients less than 24 hours old (because of poor peripheral perfusion)
- When there is a need for direct analysis of oxygenation
- When there is a need for direct analysis of arterial blood

Relative contraindications include:
- Peripheral vasoconstriction
- Polycythemia (caused by shorter clotting times)
- Hypotension

PRECAUTIONS AND POSSIBLE COMPLICATIONS

- Contamination and infection of the patient, including calcaneus osteomyelitis and cellulitis
- Inappropriate patient management may result from reliance on capillary PO_2 value
- Inadvertent puncture or incision and consequent infection
- Tibial artery laceration (puncture of posterior sample of medial aspect of heel)
- Burns
- Hematoma
- Bruising
- Scarring
- Bleeding

ASSESSMENT OF NEED

Capillary blood gas sampling is an intermittent procedure and should be performed only when a documented need exists and arterial access is unavailable or contraindicated. Documented need exists in response to initiation, administration, or change in therapy and is determined by history and physical assessment or results of noninvasive respiratory monitoring.

MONITORING

The following should be monitored and documented in the medical record as part of the capillary sampling procedure:
- FiO_2 or prescribed oxygen flow
- Appearance of puncture site
- Oxygen modality or ventilator settings
- Complications or adverse reactions to the procedure
- Ease or difficulty of obtaining the sample
- Results of blood gas analysis
- Patient's temperature, respiratory rate, position or level of the foot or finger to obtain a sample of activity, and clinical appearance
- Date, time, and sampling site
- Noninvasive monitoring values (e.g., SpO_2)

**For the complete guideline, see American Association for Respiratory Care: Clinical practice guideline: capillary blood gas sampling for neonatal and pediatric patients. Respir Care 46:506, 2001.*

published by the National Committee for Clinical Laboratory Standards.[9] Modified excerpts from the AARC guideline appear in Clinical Practice Guideline 19-3.

Instrumentation

Many instrumentation companies manufacture laboratory blood gas analyzers. Although available in a range of designs, these devices typically share the following key components:
- Operator interface (e.g., operating controls, display screen, touch screen keypads, software)
- Measuring chamber incorporating the typical three-electrode system
- Calibrating gas tanks
- Reagent containers (buffers used for calibration, rinse solutions)
- Waste container
- Results display, storage, and transmittal system (e.g., screen, printer, disk storage device, network interface)

Measurement of the three primary parameters—pH, PCO_2, and PO_2—is accomplished using three separate electrodes. To measure PO_2, blood gas analyzers use the Clark polarographic electrode (see Figure 19-1).

The pH electrode consists of two electrodes or half cells (Figure 19-6). The measuring half cell contains a silver–silver

19-3 Blood Gas Analysis and Hemoximetry

AARC Clinical Practice Guideline (Excerpts)*

INDICATIONS

- The need to evaluate the adequacy of a patient's ventilatory ($PaCO_2$), oxygenation (PaO_2 and HbO_2), or acid-base balance (pH, $PaCO_2$, HCO_3^-)
- The need to quantify the response to therapeutic intervention (e.g., oxygen therapy, mechanical ventilation) or diagnostic evaluation (e.g., exercise desaturation)
- The need to monitor the severity and progression of disease processes

CONTRAINDICATIONS

Contraindications to pH and blood gas analysis and hemoximetry include:

- An improperly functioning analyzer
- An analyzer for which the performance has not been validated by quality control or proficiency testing procedures
- Any specimen gathered with *known* or suspected preanalytic errors (e.g., aircontamination, improper anticoagulation, improper storage or handling)
- An incomplete requisition that precludes adequate interpretation and documentation of results
- An inadequately labeled specimen lacking the patient's full name or other unique identifier, such as the medical record number, date, and time of sampling

HAZARDS AND POSSIBLE COMPLICATIONS

- Infection of specimen handler from blood (human immunodeficiency virus, hepatitis C, other blood-borne pathogens)
- Inappropriate patient medical treatment based on an improperly analyzed blood specimen, on analysis of an unacceptable specimen, or on incorrect reporting of results

ASSESSMENT OF NEED

Presence of the listed indications in a patient to be tested supports the need for sampling and analysis.

MONITORING

- Monitoring of personnel, sample handling, and analyzer performance to ensure proper handling, analysis, and reporting should be ongoing during the process.
- There must be documented evidence of active review of quality control; proficiency testing; and physician alert, or "panic values" on a level commensurate with the number of tests performed

**For the complete guideline, see American Association for Respiratory Care: Clinical practice guideline: Blood gas analysis and hemoximetry: 2013. Respir Care 58:1694, 2013.*

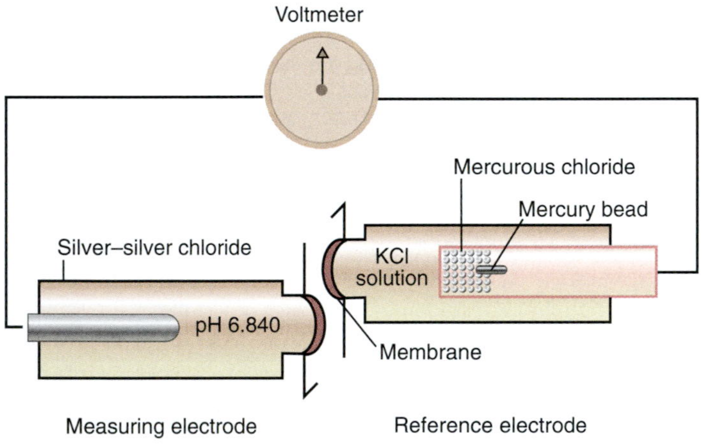

FIGURE 19-6 Blood gas analyzer pH electrode system, consisting of both a measurement and a reference electrode. (Modified from Shapiro BA, Peruzzi WT, Kozelowski-Templin R: Clinical application of blood gases, ed 5, St Louis, 1994, Mosby.)

chloride rod surrounded by a solution of constant pH and enclosed by a pH-sensitive glass membrane. As the sample passes this membrane, the difference in H^+ concentration on either side of the glass changes the potential of the measuring electrode. The reference half cell (mercury–mercurous chloride) produces a constant potential, regardless of sample pH. The difference in potential between the two electrodes is proportional to the H^+ concentration of the sample, which is displayed on a voltmeter calibrated in pH units.

To measure PCO_2, blood gas analyzers use the Severinghaus electrode, which is essentially a pH electrode exposed to an electrolyte solution in equilibrium with the sample through a CO_2-permeable membrane. As CO_2 diffuses through this membrane into the electrolyte solution, it undergoes the following hydration reaction:

$$CO_2 + H_2O \leftrightarrow H_2CO_3 \leftrightarrow H^+ + HCO_3^-$$

The greater the partial pressure of CO_2, the more H^+ that is produced by this reaction and the more the pH of the electrolyte solution changes. The measuring electrode detects the pH change as a change in electrical potential, which is proportional to the PCO_2 of the sample.

Procedure

To provide accurate and clinically useful data, blood gas analysis must be performed as follows:

- On a sample free of pre-analytic errors
- With a properly functioning analyzer (validated by quality control procedures)
- Using a procedure that follows the manufacturer's recommendations

Box 19-6 Basic Procedure for Analyzing a Blood Gas Sample

- Apply standard precautions.
- Confirm that the instrument and its electrodes are operating properly.
- Identify the specimen, and confirm all relevant information provided.
- Note the time at which the sample was obtained (discard sample if >60 minutes has passed).
- Inspect the sample for obvious signs of preanalytic error (e.g., air bubbles, gross dilution, clotting, air exposure).
- Mix the sample (critical for hemoglobin and hematocrit measurements).
- Uncap the syringe, and expel and discard a drop or two of blood from the syringe tip.
- Introduce the sample (manually or by automatic aspiration).
- Confirm the readings.
- Remove the syringe and clear the system.
- Dispose of waste materials properly.
- Transmit the results.
- Contact the responsible clinician if the results warrant.

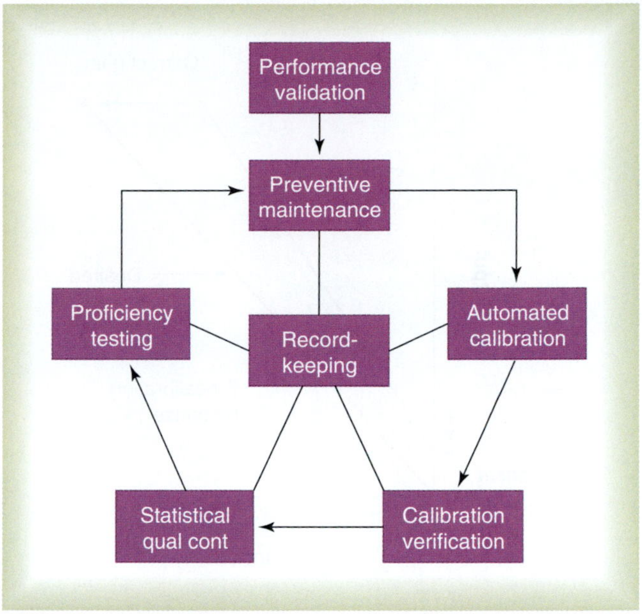

FIGURE 19-7 Blood gas analysis quality control program. (Data from Kozelowski-Templin R: Blood gas analyzers. Respir Care Clin North Am 1:35–46, 1995.)

Prior discussion addressed how to avoid pre-analytic errors. Subsequent discussion focuses on blood gas quality control and key elements involved in the analysis procedure.

Box 19-6 outlines the steps commonly used in most established procedures for laboratory blood gas analysis. One should always refer to the manufacturer's literature for the particular steps to use with a specific analyzer.

Rigorous application of the U.S. Centers for Disease Control and Prevention (CDC) standard precautions is essential. In addition, the Occupational Safety and Health Administration requires personnel to wear personal protective equipment when handling all laboratory specimens. Waste fluids are potentially infectious and should be handled as if they were blood samples. In addition, the National Committee for Clinical Laboratory Standards recommends adding a strong disinfectant, such as 2% glutaraldehyde or a 1:4 solution of sodium hypochlorite, to the waste container of the instrument either during use or before disposal.

Quality Assurance

High-quality patient care depends on consistently accurate blood gas results. Modern laboratory analyzers are often automated, computer-controlled, self-calibrating systems. Likewise, most point-of-care (bedside), analyzer systems are self-calibrating. This sophistication has led to the false assumption that accurate results are "automatic," with clinicians needing only to input the sample properly and record the results. Nothing could be further from the truth. As with all diagnostic laboratory procedures, the accuracy of blood gas testing depends on rigorous quality control.

The Clinical Laboratory Standards Institute (CLSI) established guidelines and standards for blood gas analysis and quality assurance. Government regulatory agencies collaborate to update the Clinical Laboratory Improvement Amendments (CLIA) that establish proficiency testing requirements.[16] Although an in-depth review of laboratory quality control is beyond the scope of this text, all clinicians must understand the key elements.[17]

Figure 19-7 depicts the key components of laboratory quality control. A brief description of each element follows.

Recordkeeping. Meticulous recordkeeping and clearly written, comprehensive policies and procedures are the hallmark of a quality control program. Both statutory law and professional accreditation requirements emphasize this component as the basis for demonstrating and ensuring quality.

Performance Validation. Performance validation is the process of testing a new instrument to confirm accurate measurement. Typically, this process involves using samples with known values to assess both the accuracy (comparing the value from the tested instrument with a known value) and the **precision** (examining the repeatability of results) of the instrument.

Preventive Maintenance and Function Checks. Many blood gas analyzer components (e.g., filters, membranes, electrolyte solution, and single-test and multitest cartridges) have a limited life and deteriorate or fail over time, resulting in faulty analysis. The best way to avoid these problems is to schedule regular preventive maintenance. This should include scheduled parts replacement and routine function tests, as recommended by the manufacturer.

Automated Calibration. Calibration is the only fully automated element of blood gas quality control for laboratory analyzers. Blood gas analyzers regularly calibrate themselves by adjusting the output signal of each electrode when exposed to media having known values. In most units, the media used to calibrate the gas electrodes are precision mixtures of O_2 and CO_2. For the pH electrode, standard pH buffer solutions are

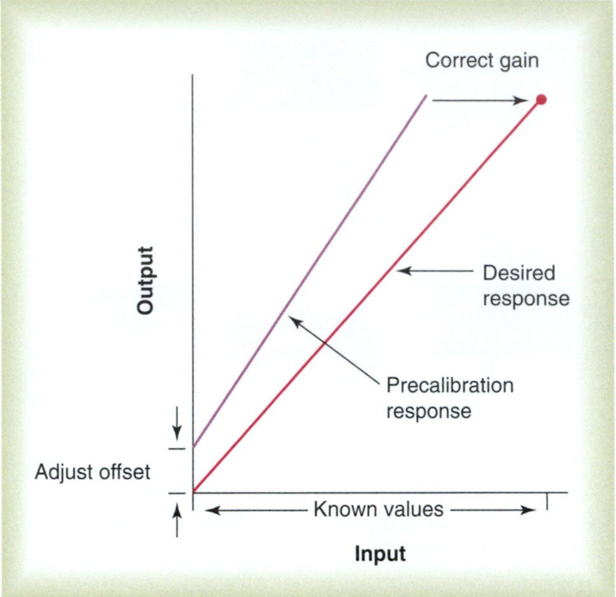

FIGURE 19-8 Two-point calibration procedure. (Modified from Chatburn RL: Fundamentals of metrology: evaluation of instrument error and method agreement. In Kacmarek RM, Hess D, Stoller JK, editors: Monitoring in respiratory care, St Louis, 1993, Mosby.)

used. **Calibration media** must meet the requirements set by nationally recognized standards organizations. Users are responsible for ensuring that calibration media are properly stored and that in-use life and expiration dates are strictly enforced.

Calibration is performed to ensure that the analyzer output is both accurate and linear across the range of measured values. Parameters must be measured with known input values representing at least two points, usually a low and a high value. Figure 19-8 shows a typical two-point calibration procedure. In this example, the instrument's initial precalibration response indicates that the output readings are consistently higher than the actual input, with this positive **bias** worsening at higher levels. Calibration is performed first by adjusting the offset (or balance) of the instrument so that the low output equals the low input (in this case zero). Next, the gain (or slope) of the device is adjusted to ensure that the high output equals the high input. When both offset and gain are adjusted against known inputs, the instrument is properly calibrated and can undergo calibration verification with control samples.

Internal Statistical Quality Control. Internal quality control takes calibration verification a step further by applying statistical and rule-based procedures (Westgard rules)[18,19] to help detect, respond to, and correct instrument error. In one common approach, the results of control media analyses are plotted on a graph and compared with statistically derived limits, usually ± 2 standard deviation (SD) ranges (Figure 19-9). Control results that fall outside these limits indicate analytic error.

There are two categories of analytic error: (1) **random error** and (2) **systematic error.** Random error is observed when sporadic, out-of-range data points occur (see Figure 19-9, point *A*). Random errors are errors of precision or, more precisely, **imprecision.** Conversely, either a trending or an abrupt shift in data points outside the statistical limits (see Figure 19-9, point *B*) is sometimes observed. This phenomenon is called *systematic error* or sometimes *bias.* Bias plus imprecision equals total instrument error, or *inaccuracy.* Table 19-3 outlines the major factors causing these two types of error and suggests some common corrective actions.

TABLE 19-3
Correction of Analytic Errors

Error Type	Common Contributing Factors	Common Corrective Actions
Imprecision (random) errors	Statistical probability Sample contamination Sample mishandling	Rerun control Repeat analysis on different instrument
Bias (systematic) errors	Contaminated buffers Incorrect gas concentrations Incorrect procedures Component failure	Perform function check of suspected problem area Repair or replace failed components

MINI CLINI

Blood Gas Quality Control

PROBLEM: Using control media for calibration verification, the RT responsible for the quality control of a blood gas analyzer in the intensive care unit (ICU) notes that the "high PCO_2" control readings have increased progressively over the last four quality control analyses from 60 ± 1 mm Hg to 66 ± 1 mm Hg. What is the likely cause and what actions should the RT take?

SOLUTION: The observed problem indicates a trending, or systematic, error (bias). If the analyzer solutions and calibrating gases have not been changed during the error period, the likely problem is component failure—probably the PCO_2 electrode. The electrode should be checked, and any faulty components should be replaced.

External Quality Control (Proficiency Testing). The federal government mandated a rigorous program of external quality control for analytic laboratories. CLIA standards were established in 1988. To meet these standards, analytic laboratories must undergo regular proficiency testing designed to evaluate their operating procedures and the competence of their personnel.[20] **Proficiency testing** requires analysis and reporting on externally provided control media with unknown values, usually three times per year, with five samples per test. There are many CLIA-approved proficiency testing providers. A commonly used provider is the College of American Pathologists (CAP) proficiency testing survey. Proficiency testing survey

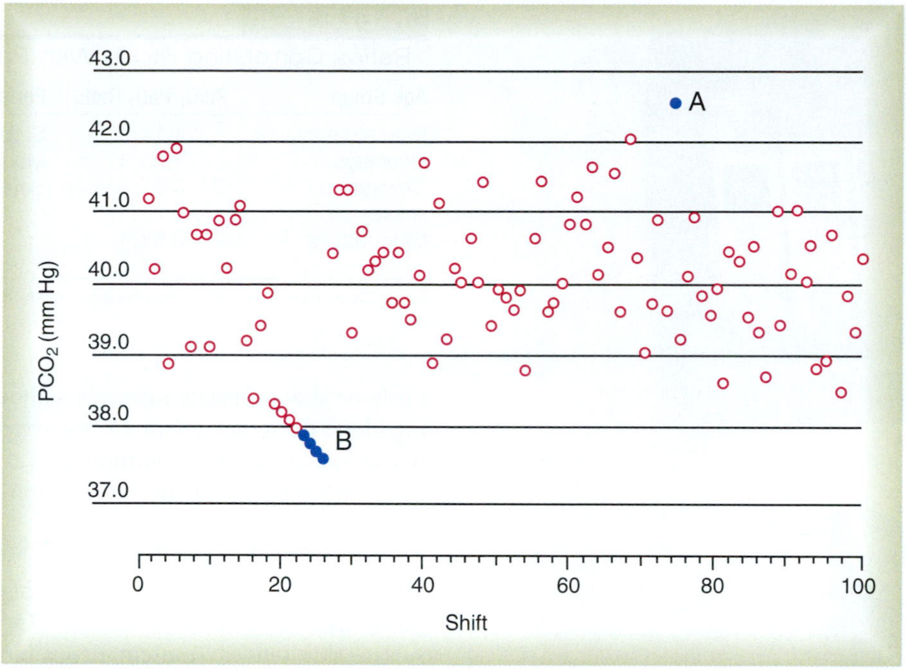

FIGURE 19-9 Schematic representation of a quality control plot for PCO_2. The horizontal axis depicts time. *White circles* represent values within 2 standard deviations of the mean; *blue circles* represent values outside 2 standard deviations of the mean. Point *A* represents a random error; point *B* represents systematic errors. (Modified from Shapiro BA, Peruzzi WT, Kozelowski-Templin R: Clinical application of blood gases, ed 5, St Louis, 1994, Mosby.)

analyses must be performed along with the regular workload by the personnel routinely responsible for testing, following the laboratory's standard testing practices.[21]

Criteria for acceptable performance specify a range around a target value, such as ± 0.04 for pH. A single incidence of unsatisfactory performance requires documentation of remedial action. Multiple or recurring incidences of poor performance can result in severe sanctions, including suspension of Medicare and Medicaid reimbursement or the loss of the laboratory's operating license and accreditation.

Remedial Action. Remedial action is the ongoing process of applying appropriate measures to correct errors identified through the quality assurance cycle. Analytic errors include calibration and internal quality control failures, actual sample errors, and unsatisfactory proficiency test results. A comprehensive quality assurance program also tries to identify and correct both pre-analytic and post-analytic errors, such as clerical misreporting.

Examples of remedial action include procedural changes, staff training and retraining, closer supervision, and more frequent preventive maintenance checks. The remedial action chosen should be appropriate for the identified problem. As with all other components of the process, meticulous documentation is necessary.

Point-of-Care Testing

Point-of-care testing takes blood gas analysis from the specialized laboratory to the patient's bedside.[22] Point-of-care testing reduces turnaround time, which may lead to quicker diagnosis and treatment. Theoretically, cost savings can be accrued by eliminating delays in therapy, decreasing patient length of stay in the hospital and emergency department (ED).[23] Point-of-care testing is used increasingly in the hospital and physician office settings.[24]

Instrumentation. Figure 19-10 shows a typical point-of-care blood gas analyzer (GEM 4000; Instrumentation Laboratory, Bedford, MA). Smaller point-of-care analyzers using similar technology, such as the i-STAT point-of-care system (Abbott Laboratories, Abbott Park, IL), are also gaining popularity. In addition to blood gas analysis, such devices can be used to measure several chemistry and hematology parameters, including serum electrolytes, blood glucose levels, blood urea nitrogen, hematocrit, hemoximetry, lactate, bilirubin, and prothrombin and partial thromboplastin times. It should be noted that unlike conventional analyzers, blood samples for most point-of-care analyzers should not be chilled and should be run within 1 to 2 minutes after being obtained.

These devices are portable, and some can perform 900 tests using a disposable cartridge. They typically include a display screen for accessing menu functions and viewing results. Most devices include a simple keypad or touch screen for data and command entry. Analysis occurs using disposable cartridges or inside a chamber in the body of the unit.

Some devices employ single-use sample cartridges that differ according to the array of tests being performed. Each cartridge contains the necessary calibration solution, a sample handling system, a waste chamber, and miniaturized electrochemical or photochemical sensors. The cartridge system requires no operator oversight because it is self-calibrating and disposable after a single use. After self-calibration and introduction of the sample

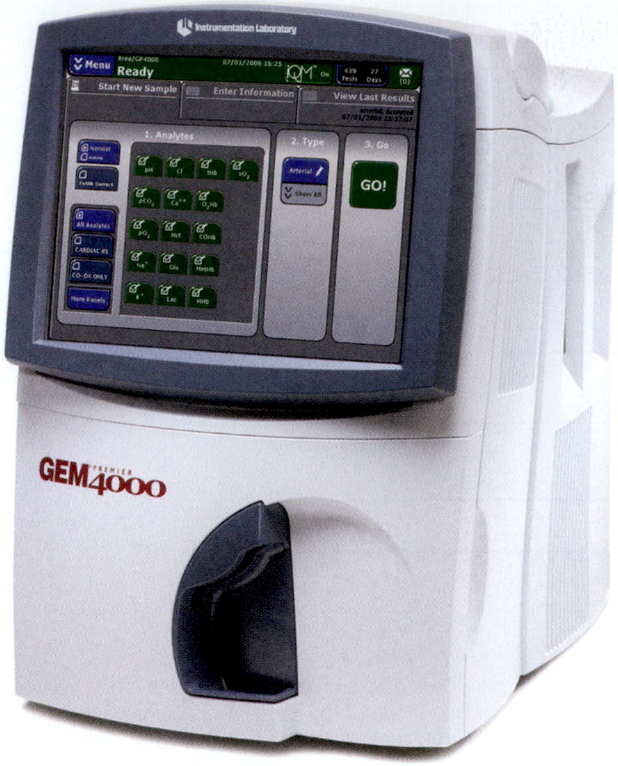

FIGURE 19-10 GEM Premier 4000 critical care analyzer for blood gas, electrolyte, metabolite, and integrated cooximetry testing; the device also performs continuous automated quality assurance. (Courtesy Instrumentation Laboratory, Bedford, MA.)

into the cartridge, the sensors measure the concentration of the analytes and conduct their output signal through conductive contact pads to the analyzer microprocessor. Test results usually are ready within 60 seconds. Waste management involves simple removal and proper disposal of the analysis cartridge.

Other devices use self-contained multiuse cartridge packs that include all testing components, are maintenance-free, and incorporate automated quality control management systems. Multiuse cartridges are typically replaced every 30 days or when testing components are used up.

Clinical Performance. More recent method comparisons indicate that portable point-of-care blood gas analyzers can achieve accuracy and precision levels comparable to those with laboratory-based analyzers.[14,25] Such findings have resulted in the widespread use of these systems.

Clinical laboratories have expanded point-of-care testing solutions to improve operational costs, streamline workflow in the clinical laboratory and critical care setting, and provide blood analysis results more quickly.[26,27] Guidelines for providers who are considering adoption of this new technology have been published in the clinical laboratory literature.[28]

BLOOD GAS MONITORING

A blood gas monitor is a bedside tool (usually dedicated to a single patient) that can provide measurements either continuously or at appropriate intervals without permanently removing blood from the patient. Of the systems which are currently in use, two of the most common ones are transcutaneous blood gas monitoring and tissue oxygen monitoring.

TABLE 19-4
Ratios Correlating $PtcO_2$ With PaO_2

Age Group	$PtcO_2/PaO_2$ Ratio	Perfusion Status	$PtcO_2/PaO_2$
Premature infants	1.14 : 1	Stable	0.79 : 1
Neonates	1.00 : 1	Moderate shock	0.48 : 1
Children	0.84 : 1	Severe shock	0.12 : 1
Adults	0.79 : 1		
Older adults	0.68 : 1		

From Tobin MJ: Respiratory monitoring. JAMA 264:244–251, 1990.

Transcutaneous Blood Gas Monitoring

Transcutaneous blood gas monitoring provides continuous, noninvasive estimates of arterial PO_2 and PCO_2 through a surface skin sensor. Transcutaneous blood gas monitoring has been used for many decades in infants and now is available for use in adults because of advances in technology. As with capillary sampling, the device arterializes the underlying blood by heating the skin. Warming also increases the permeability of the skin to O_2 and CO_2, which enhances diffusion from the capillaries to the sensor, where they are measured as transcutaneous partial pressures ($PtcO_2$ and $PtcCO_2$).

Numerous factors influence the agreement between arterial blood and transcutaneous gas measurements, with O_2 levels being affected most. The two most important factors are age and perfusion status (Table 19-4). With regard to perfusion status, PaO_2 and $PtcO_2$ are similar only in patients with normal cardiac output and fluid balance, because accurate transcutaneous measures require adequate skin perfusion. Peripheral vasoconstriction and impaired capillary flow decrease the $PtcO_2$; common causes include low cardiac output, shock, and dehydration. Some clinicians use $PtcO_2$ not to monitor oxygenation as a surrogate for PaO_2 but to assess blood flow changes during procedures such as vascular surgery and resuscitation. Agreement between $PaCO_2$ and $PtcCO_2$ is better because CO_2 is more diffusible. $PaCO_2$ changes of 5 mm Hg can be monitored or "trended" by transcutaneous blood gas analysis. Based on these factors, $PtcCO_2$ monitoring is a reasonable choice when there is a need for continuous, noninvasive analysis of trends in ventilation and $PaCO_2$. In hemodynamically stable infants and children, PaO_2 can be "correlated" with $PtcO_2$, thus decreasing the need for repeated arterial samples. Because pulse oximetry cannot provide accurate estimates of excessive blood O_2, the transcutaneous monitor may be useful for monitoring hyperoxia in neonates. However, prevention of hyperoxia in premature neonates is more often achieved by maintaining pulse oximetry saturation between 85% and 93%.[29]

Transcutaneous blood gas monitoring of $PtcCO_2$ can be useful in adult patients during deep sedation and mechanical ventilation in the ED, in the ICU, and during surgery.[30-35] $PtcCO_2$

19-4 Transcutaneous Monitoring of Carbon Dioxide and Oxygen: 2012

AARC Clinical Practice Guideline (Excerpts)*

INDICATIONS

- The need to monitor continuously the adequacy of arterial oxygenation or ventilation
- The need to quantify the real-time responses to diagnostic and therapeutic interventions, as evidenced by $PtcO_2$ or $PtcCO_2$ values

CONTRAINDICATIONS

There are no absolute contraindications. In patients with poor skin integrity or adhesive allergy, alternative devices should be considered.

HAZARDS AND POSSIBLE COMPLICATIONS

- False-negative or false-positive results may lead to inappropriate treatment.
- Tissue injury (e.g., erythema, blisters, burns, skin tears) may occur at the measuring site.

ASSESSMENT OF NEED

- When direct measurement of arterial blood is unavailable or not readily accessible, $PtcO_2$ or $PtcCO_2$ measurements may suffice temporarily if the limitations of the data are appreciated.
- Transcutaneous blood gas monitoring is appropriate for continuous and prolonged monitoring (e.g., during mechanical ventilation, continuous positive airway pressure [CPAP], and supplemental oxygen administration).
- $PtcO_2$ values can be used for diagnostic purposes, such as in the assessment of functional shunts or in determining the response to oxygen challenge in the assessment of congenital heart disease.

ASSESSMENT OF OUTCOME

- Results should reflect the patient's clinical condition (i.e., they should validate the basis for ordering the monitoring).
- Results of therapeutic interventions and clinical decisions based on the transcutaneous measurements should be noted in the medical record.

MONITORING

The schedule for patient assessment during transcutaneous monitoring should be integrated into the patient assessment as part of vital signs monitoring. Results should be documented in the patient's medical record and should detail the following conditions:

- Date and time of measurement, transcutaneous reading, patient's position, respiratory rate, and activity level
- Inspired oxygen concentration or supplemental oxygen flow, specifying the type of oxygen delivery device
- Mode of ventilatory support, and ventilator, or CPAP settings
- Electrode placement site, electrode temperature, and time of placement
- Results of simultaneously obtained PaO_2, $PaCO_2$, and pH, when available
- Clinical appearance of the patient and subjective assessment of perfusion, pallor, and skin temperature

**For the complete guideline, see American Association for Respiratory Care: Clinical practice guideline: Transcutaneous monitoring of Carbon Dioxide and Oxygen: 2012s. Respir Care 57:1955, 2012.*

is a more accurate reflection of $PaCO_2$ than both $PETCO_2$ and nasal $ETCO_2$ in intubated and spontaneously breathing adult patients. The use of $PtcCO_2$ in conjunction with pulse oximetry reduces the need for repeated ABG sampling.[36]

To guide practitioners in providing high-quality care, the AARC has published Clinical Practice Guideline: Transcutaneous Blood Monitoring of Carbon Dioxide and Oxygen: 2012.[37] Modified excerpts from the AARC guideline appear in Clinical Practice Guidelines 19-4.

Instrumentation

Figure 19-11 shows a simplified diagram of a transcutaneous blood gas monitor sensor. Included are a heating element and two electrodes, one each for O_2 and CO_2. These electrodes are similar in design to the electrodes found in bench-top analyzers. However, instead of measuring gas tensions in a blood sample, transcutaneous electrodes measure PO_2 and PCO_2 in an

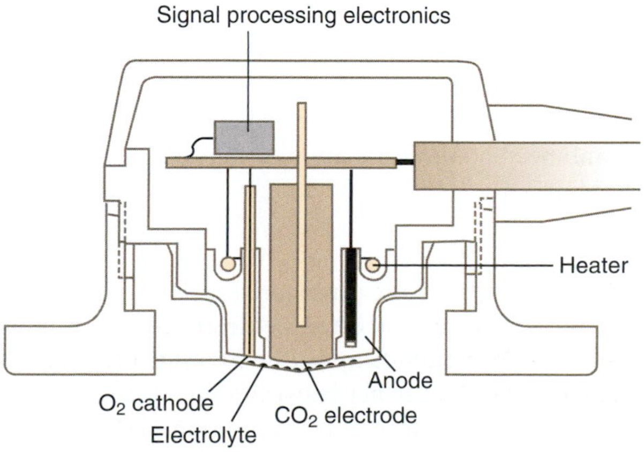

FIGURE 19-11 Schematic diagram of transcutaneous O_2-CO_2 sensor. (Modified from Mahutte CK, Michiels TM, Hassell KT, et al: Evaluation of a single transcutaneous PO_2-PCO_2 sensor in adult patients. Crit Care Med 12:1063–1066, 1984.)

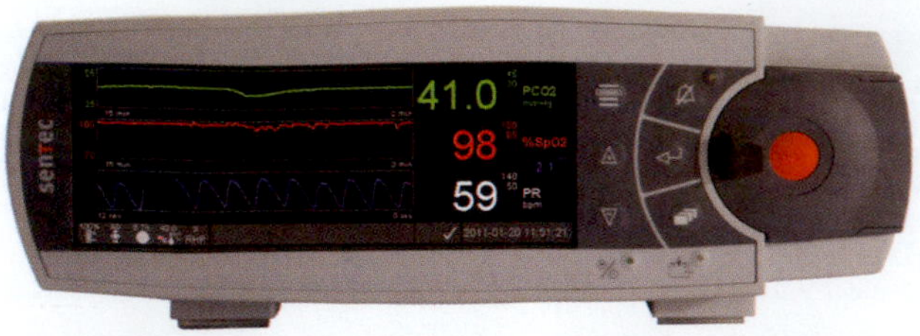

FIGURE 19-12 SenTec Digital Monitoring System, combined $PtcCO_2$ and SpO_2 sensor suitable for neonatal, pediatric, and adult patients. (Courtesy SenTec AG, Therwil, Switzerland.)

Box 19-7 Procedure for Using a Transcutaneous Monitor

- Place the unit at bedside, and provide manufacturer-specified warm-up time.
- Check the membrane to ensure that it is free of bubbles or scratches, and change it if necessary.
- Select the monitoring site by evaluating perfusion, skin thickness, and absence of bones.
- Prepare the sensor with an adhesive ring and electrolyte gel.
- Set the appropriate probe temperature (per the manufacturer's recommendations).
- Prepare the site by removing excess hair and cleaning the skin.
- Securely attach probe to the patient.
- Schedule site change time (2 to 12 hours, depending on patient/device).
- Set the high and low alarms.
- Monitor and document the results per institutional protocol.
- Change site at appropriate intervals.
- Validate the reading against arterial blood gas values.

From Koff PB, Hess D: Transcutaneous oxygen and carbon dioxide measurements. In Kacmarek RM, Hess D, Stoller JK, editors: Monitoring in respiratory care, St Louis, 1993, Mosby.

electrolyte gel between the sensor and the skin. When properly set up, the response time for these electrodes is 20 to 30 seconds, a bit slower than the response time for pulse oximetry.

Figure 19-12 shows a transcutaneous monitor with digital signal processing. A Severinghaus-type $PtcCO_2$ electrode and two-wavelength reflectance SpO_2 are combined into a single sensor. The sensor can be applied to the skin surface in neonates and infants or to the earlobe of pediatric and adult patients for combined noninvasive monitoring of ventilation and oxygenation.

Procedure

Box 19-7 outlines the basic procedure for setting up a transcutaneous blood gas monitor. Once the electrodes are properly set up, the clinician should compare the monitor readings with a concurrent ABG. Consistency between values validates monitor performance under the existing conditions. This validation should be repeated any time the patient's status undergoes a major change. During validation studies of patients with anatomic shunts, the electrode site and arterial sampling site should be on the same "side" of the shunt.

MINI CLINI

Selecting a Monitoring System

PROBLEM: Concerned about retinopathy of prematurity, the RT sets up a noninvasive system to monitor a preterm infant for hyperoxia. What type of system should the RT choose and why?

SOLUTION: Because the infant should be monitored for hyperoxia, a system that provides continuous data would be the best choice. Because hyperoxia is best assessed using PO_2 (as opposed to Hb saturation), the RT needs to use a PO_2 electrode system. A transcutaneous PO_2 electrode system would provide the needed measurement noninvasively.

Problem-Solving and Troubleshooting

Monitoring requires setup and calibration. In terms of technical limitations, transcutaneous blood gas sensors must be calibrated and maintained using methods similar to those described for bench-top analyzers. Improper calibration yields erroneous patient information. Meticulous care of the sensor membranes is also essential for proper maintenance.

Because the sensor is heated, clinicians must take care to avoid thermal injury to the patient's skin. Thermal injury can be avoided by careful monitoring of sensor temperature (the safe upper limit is approximately 42° C) and regularly rotating the sensor site. Proper sensor-electrolyte contact is essential, as is proper application to the skin surface.

When arterial and transcutaneous blood gas values are inconsistent with each other or with the clinical status of the patient, the clinician should explore possible causes before reporting any results. Often, discrepancies can be reduced by switching the monitoring site or recalibrating the instrument. If these steps fail to resolve the inconsistencies, the clinician should recommend an alternative method for assessing gas exchange, such as pulse oximetry or more frequent ABG analysis.

Tissue Oxygen

Tissue O_2 (PtO_2) can be measured by probes inserted directly into organs, tissue, and body fluids. Ease of probe placement and the sensitivity of PtO_2 as an indicator of tissue perfusion make tissue O_2 monitoring attractive for clinical research applications. Clinical indications for measuring PtO_2 include monitoring brain tissue O_2 as an early sign of ischemia, assessing brain blood flow autoregulation, and monitoring the adequacy of brain perfusion in patients with traumatic brain injury.[38] In patients with traumatic brain injury, brain PtO_2 values are between 25 and 30 mm Hg when intracranial pressure and cerebral perfusion are normal. The critical threshold for ischemic brain damage and poor outcome is suspected to be at a brain PtO_2 of approximately 10 to 15 mm Hg.[38]

Instrumentation

Both electrochemical and **optical fluorescence tissue** O_2 probes have been developed for clinical use and research applications.

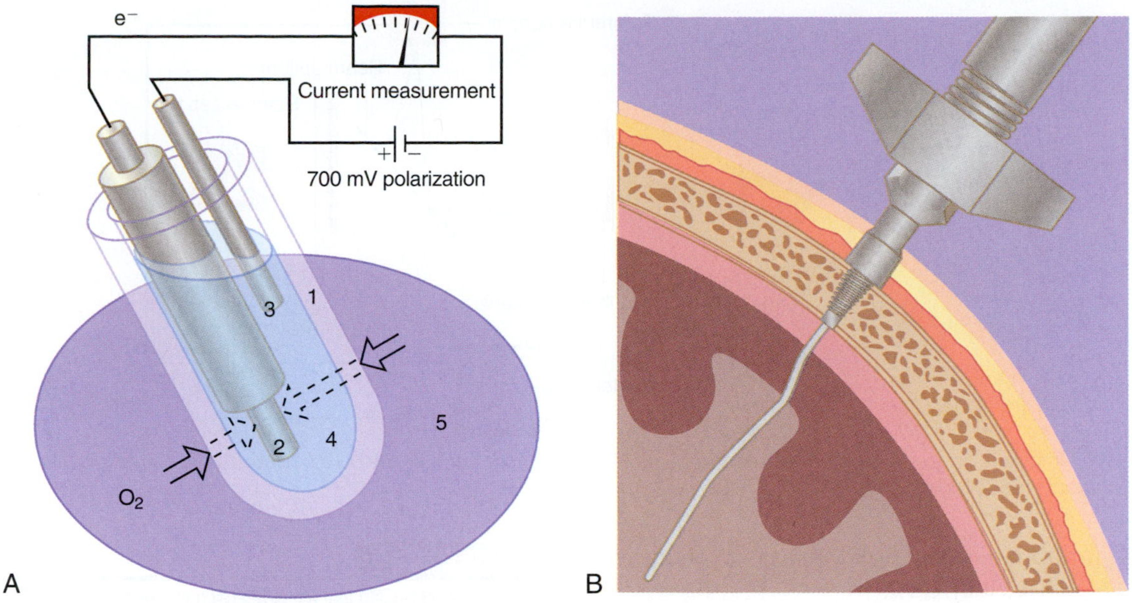

FIGURE 19-13 **A,** Schematic of Clark-type polarographic tissue oxygen probe. Polyethylene membrane *(1)*, gold cathode *(2)*, silver anode *(3)*, electrolyte solution *(4)*, cerebral tissue *(5)*. **B,** Insertion into cerebral tissue. (From Mulvey JM, Dorsch NW, Mudaliar Y, et al: Multimodality monitoring in severe traumatic brain injury: the role of brain tissue oxygenation monitoring. Neurocrit Care 1:391–402, 2004.)

Figure 19-13 shows a Clarke-type polarographic sensor and its insertion into brain tissue through an intracranial bolt. **Optode** probes capable of monitoring tissue pH, CO_2, and O_2 have also been developed.[39]

OXIMETRY

Oximetry is the measurement of blood Hb saturations using **spectrophotometry.** According to the principles of spectrophotometry, every substance has a unique pattern of light absorption, similar to a fingerprint. The pattern of light absorption of a substance varies predictably with the amount present; this is known as the *Lambert-Beer law*. By measuring the light absorbed and transmitted by a substance, scientists can identify its presence and determine its concentration.

The particular pattern of light absorption exhibited by a substance at different wavelengths is called its *absorption spectrum*. As shown in Figure 19-14, each form of Hb (i.e., reduced Hb, HbO_2, HbCO, metHb) has its own unique pattern. By comparing the amount of light transmitted through (or reflected from) a blood sample at two or more specific wavelengths, the relative concentrations of Hb forms can be measured. For example, oxygenated Hb absorbs less red light (600 to 750 nm) and more infrared light (850 to 1000 nm) than deoxygenated or reduced Hb. Comparing a blood sample's light absorption with red and infrared light yields the $\%HbO_2$ and %Hb. When measuring additional forms of Hb, additional (more than two) wavelengths of light must be used.

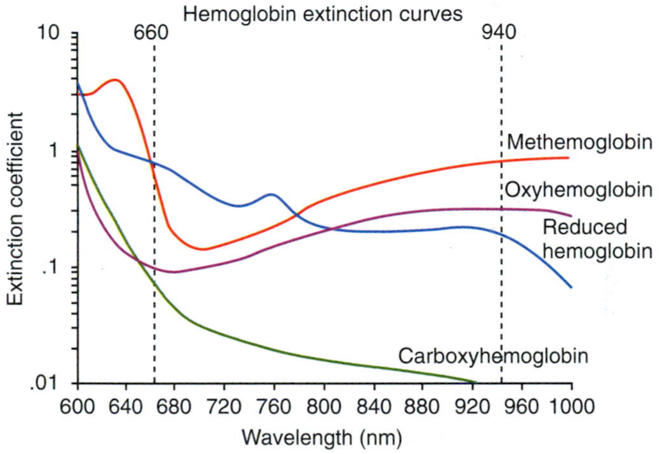

FIGURE 19-14 Principle of spectrophotometric oximetry. Different forms of hemoglobin (e.g., reduced Hb, HbO_2, HbCO, metHb) absorb light differently at different wavelengths. By comparing points of equal absorbance (isobestic points) between pairs of Hb forms (e.g., Hb vs. HbO_2, Hb vs. HbCO), the relative proportion of each can be measured.

Several types of oximetry are used in clinical practice, including hemoximetry (also called *cooximetry*), pulse oximetry, venous oximetry, and tissue oximetry. Hemoximetry is a laboratory analytic procedure requiring invasive sampling of arterial blood. Pulse oximetry is a noninvasive monitoring technique performed at the bedside. Venous oximetry requires invasive monitoring through a fiberoptic catheter placed in the vena cava or PA. Tissue oximetry is a noninvasive method of measuring the saturation of Hb at the tissue level.

Hemoximetry

Hemoximetry (known in some settings as *cooximetry*) is an analytic method of oximetry and is covered in the AARC Clinical Practice Guideline: Blood Gas Analysis and Hemoximetry[15]

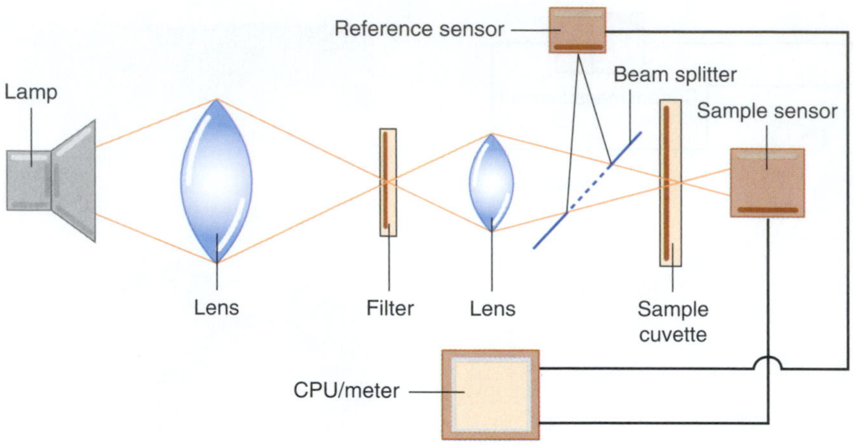

FIGURE 19-15 Simplified diagram showing key components of a laboratory hemoximeter. (Modified from Lane EE: Clinical arterial blood gas analysis, St Louis, 1987, Mosby.)

(see Clinical Practice Guideline 19-3). Related recommendations have been published by CLSI.[9]

Instrumentation

Figure 19-15 is a simplified diagram showing the key components of a laboratory hemoximeter. Light generated by a thallium cathode lamp passes through a series of lenses and filters, yielding the specific wavelengths needed for analysis. A beam splitter divides the light into two portions, directing one through a reference solution and the other through a sample chamber, or **cuvette.** Photodetection sensors measure the amount of light transmitted through these two sources. By comparing the difference in light transmission through the reference and sample solutions, a microprocessor computes the relative amount of Hb present, with its output sent to the calibrated device meter or display. Because a laboratory hemoximeter uses four or more different wavelengths of light, it can simultaneously compute the relative concentrations of multiple forms of Hb, such as reduced Hb, HbO_2, HbCO, and metHb.

Procedure and Quality Assurance

Similar to modern blood gas analyzers, laboratory hemoximeters are highly automated and simple to use. Some devices now combine both technologies into a single instrument. However, the caveats remain the same. Accurate and clinically useful hemoximetry results can be expected only if an error-free sample is assessed on a calibrated analyzer, using the manufacturer's protocol.

Although variations exist among devices, the basic procedure is similar. First, the blood is introduced into the sampling port of the analyzer, usually by either aspiration or injection. Required sample sizes vary from approximately 200 mcl to 40 mcl (microanalysis). Once introduced, erythrocyte Hb is released into the solution by hemolysis. After hemolysis, the sample is transported to the cuvette for analysis. On completion of the analysis, the sampling system (cuvette and tubing) is flushed and cleaned. As with blood gas analysis, operators must follow CDC standard precautions and ensure proper disposal of syringes and waste materials.

TABLE 19-5

Problems Causing Measurement Errors With Hemoximeters

Problem	Potential Error
Incomplete hemolysis	Falsely low total Hb, HbO_2
Sickle cell anemia (caused by incomplete hemolysis)	Falsely low HbO_2
Presence of vascular dyes (e.g., methylene blue)	Falsely low total Hb, HbO_2
High lipid levels (e.g., from parenteral nutrition)	Falsely low total Hb, HbO_2
Presence of high levels of fetal hemoglobin	Falsely high HbCO
Elevated bilirubin levels (>20 mg/dl)	Falsely high total Hb, HbO_2, metHb
Dirty cuvette chamber	Falsely high total Hb, HbO_2

Quality assurance procedures for hemoximetry are essentially the same as the procedures used for blood gas analysis, differing only with regard to the control materials used. In addition, careful cleaning and maintenance of the cuvette chamber is essential because clouding of its walls decreases absorbance and can cause falsely elevated values.[40]

Problem-Solving and Troubleshooting

A major assumption underlying hemoximetry is that the measured changes in light absorbance result only from variations in the relative concentrations of various Hbs. In practice, this assumption does not always hold true. Table 19-5 outlines some of the potential problems and resulting errors that can occur with hemoximetry.

Pulse Oximetry

Pulse oximeters are portable noninvasive monitors that estimate arterial blood oxyhemoglobin saturation levels. So as not to confuse these estimates with actual SaO_2 measures obtained by hemoximetry, the abbreviation SpO_2 is used to refer to pulse oximetry readings. No other device in recent medical history has been so widely and quickly adopted into clinical practice.

19-5 Pulse Oximetry

AARC Clinical Practice Guideline (Excerpts)*

INDICATIONS

- To monitor the adequacy of arterial oxyhemoglobin saturation
- To quantify the response of arterial oxyhemoglobin saturation to therapeutic intervention or to diagnostic procedures, such as bronchoscopy
- To comply with mandated regulations or recommendations by authoritative groups

CONTRAINDICATIONS

The ongoing need for actual measurements of pH, $PaCO_2$, total Hb, and abnormal Hb may be a relative contraindication to pulse oximetry.

PRECAUTIONS

- Device limitations causing false-negative results for hypoxemia or false-positive results for normoxemia or hyperoxemia may lead to inappropriate treatment of patients.
- Factors affecting SpO_2 accuracy include motion artifact, abnormal Hbs, intravascular dyes, low perfusion states, skin pigmentation, and nail polish.

ASSESSMENT OF NEED

- When direct measurement of SaO_2 is unavailable or not readily accessible, a pulse oximetry measurement may temporarily suffice if the limitations of the data are appreciated.
- SpO_2 is appropriate for continuous and prolonged monitoring (e.g., during sleep, exercise, or bronchoscopy).
- SpO_2 may be adequate when assessment of acid-base status or PaO_2 is not required.

ASSESSMENT OF OUTCOME

The following should be used to evaluate the benefits of pulse oximetry:

- SpO_2 results should reflect the patient's clinical condition.
- Documenting the results of therapeutic interventions, and clinical decisions based on the SpO_2 measurements should be noted in the medical record.

FREQUENCY

After initially establishing agreement between SaO_2 and SpO_2, the frequency of SpO_2 monitoring (i.e., continuous vs. spot check) depends on the clinical status of the patient, the indications for performing the procedure, and recommended guidelines. For example, continuous SpO_2 monitoring is indicated throughout a bronchoscopy to detect desaturation, whereas a spot check may suffice for evaluating oxygen therapy in a stable postoperative patient. Direct measurement of SaO_2 is needed whenever SpO_2 does not confirm or verify suspicions about the patient's clinical state.

MONITORING

Continuous pulse oximetry monitoring, should be incorporated into the bedside assessment of a patient's vital signs.

**For the complete guideline, see American Association for Respiratory Care: Clinical practice guideline: sampling for arterial blood gas analysis. Respir Care 37:891, 1992.*

However, its rapid embracement has been accompanied by equally sweeping misconceptions regarding the appropriate applications and technologic limitations.[41] Moreover, the true impact of pulse oximetry on patient outcomes is unknown.[42] To guide practitioners in providing quality care, the AARC has published Clinical Practice Guideline: Pulse Oximetry.[43] Modified excerpts from the AARC guideline appear in Clinical Practice Guideline 19-5.

Instrumentation

The pulse oximeter combines the principle of spectrophotometry, as used by hemoximeters, with **photoplethysmography.** Photoplethysmography uses light to detect the tiny volume changes that occur in living tissue during pulsatile blood flow. However, compared with a hemoximeter, the pulse oximeter usually uses only two wavelengths of light, one red (approximately 660 nm) and one infrared (approximately 940 nm) (see Figure 19-14). In addition, rather than measuring light transmission through a blood sample in a glass cuvette, the pulse oximeter measures transmission through living tissue, such as a finger or earlobe, or reflectance through the skin surface.

Figure 19-16, *A* provides a schematic block diagram of a pulse oximeter, consisting of a transmission sensor, processor, and display unit. The sensor has two sides. From one side, separate red and infrared light-emitting diodes (LEDs) alternately transmit light through the tissue. The transmitted light intensity is measured by a photodetector on the other side. The resulting output signal is filtered and amplified by instrument electronics, with processing and display functions controlled by a microprocessor.

Figure 19-16, *B* shows a schematic of a reflectance pulse oximeter sensor. This type of sensor has only one side, which contains both the LED light sources and the photodetector. The principle of operation is identical to a transmission sensor except that the sensor is placed on the skin surface, usually the forehead, and reflected light from the tissue back to the sensor is used to calculate SpO_2.

Figure 19-17 shows a typical output signal generated by the photodetector (the pulsatile component can be observed on

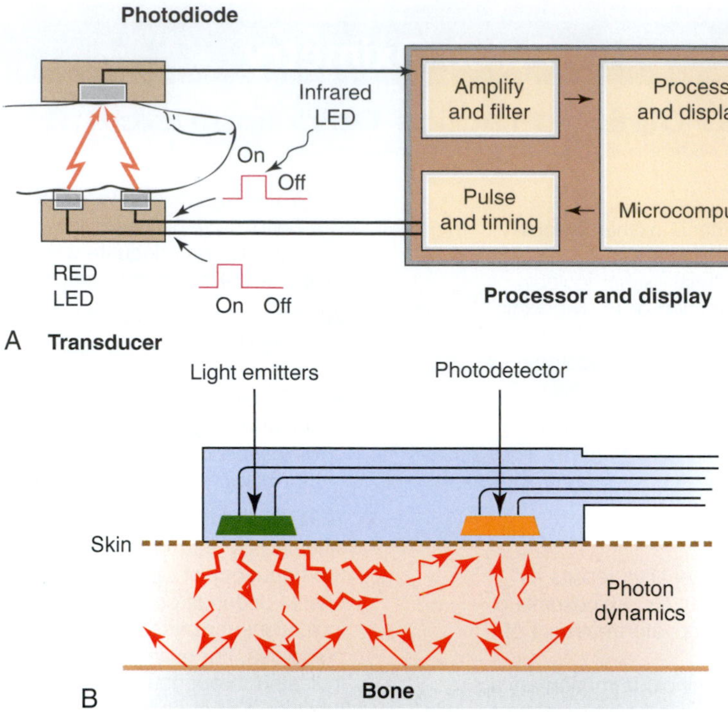

FIGURE 19-16 A, Schematic block diagram of a transmission pulse oximeter sensor and monitor. **B,** Schematic of a reflectance pulse oximeter sensor. *LED,* Light-emitting diode. (**A,** Modified from Gardner R: Pulse oximetry: is it monitoring's "silver bullet"? J Cardiovasc Nurs 1:79–83, 1987; **B,** from Keogh BF, Kopotic RJ: Recent findings in the use of reflectance oximetry: a critical review. Curr Opin Anaesthesiol 18:649–654, 2005.)

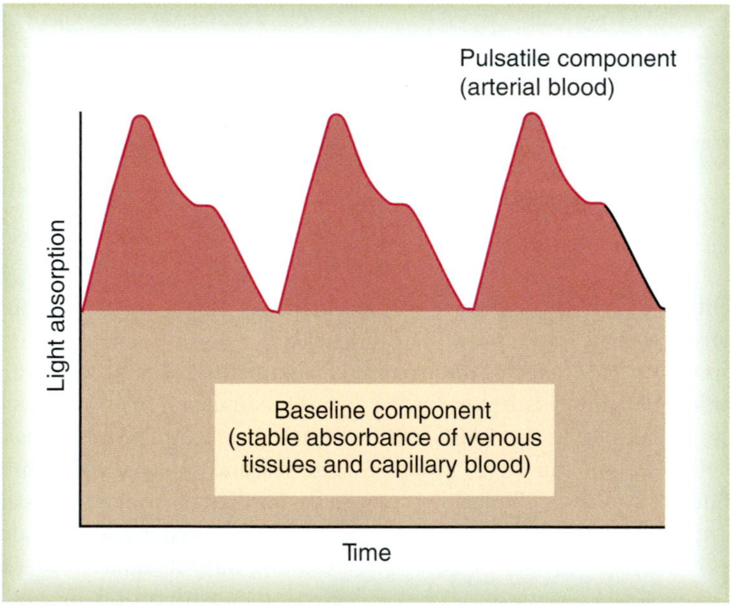

FIGURE 19-17 Output signal generated by pulse oximeter. Saturation is based on the ratio of light absorption between two or more wavelengths during pulsatile and baseline phases.

instruments that have a plethysmographic display). A baseline component represents the stable absorbance of the tissue bed, which mainly represents venous and capillary blood. At the top is the pulsatile component, caused by intermittent arterial flow through the tissues. By comparing light absorbance during the pulsatile phase with the baseline value at each wavelength, a pulse-added measure is obtained. Arterial oxyhemoglobin saturation is computed as the ratio of the pulse-added absorbances at the two different wavelengths.

The accuracy of pulse oximetry readings is usually within ± 3% to 5% of invasive hemoximetry readings.[43,44] Generally, the lower the actual SaO_2, the less accurate and reliable is the SpO_2 measurement. Most clinicians consider pulse oximeter readings unreliable at saturations less than 80%. Instrument response

Box 19-8 Key Points for Performing Pulse Oximetry

- Always follow manufacturer's recommended protocol.
- Never mix sensors among different devices.
- Ensure the sensor is the correct size for the site chosen.
- Ensure the sensor is properly applied (not too tight or loose).
- Before taking or recording a reading, confirm the adequacy and accuracy of the pulse signal.
- When doing spot checks, allow sufficient response time before taking a reading because response times vary greatly.
- For continuous monitoring of adults and children, set the low alarm at 88% to 92%.
- Whenever possible, validate the initial SpO_2 reading against the actual SaO_2.
- Clean multiuse sensors and disinfect the instrument housing between patients.
- Inspect the sensor site frequently throughout the duration of continuous monitoring and change it as needed.
- Never act on SpO_2 readings alone.
- Avoid using pulse oximetry to monitor hyperoxia in neonates.

times vary by manufacturer, sensor location, and the patient's hemodynamic status from 10 seconds to 1 minute or longer.

Procedure

The actual procedure used to measure SpO_2 varies according to the device used, sensor site selected, and whether a spot check or continuous monitoring is required. Box 19-8 lists key points to be considered when performing pulse oximetry.

Given the limits of this technology, meticulous documentation is important. Specifically, all SpO_2 results should be recorded in the patient's medical record. The following details should be documented:

- Date, time of measurement, and reading
- Patient's position, activity level, and location during monitoring
- FiO_2 or O_2 flow and O_2 delivery device
- Probe type and placement site
- Model of device (if more than one device is available for use)
- Results of simultaneously obtained ABGs and hemoximetry (if available)
- Stability of readings (length of observation time and range of fluctuation)
- Patient's clinical appearance, including assessment of perfusion at the measuring site (e.g., cyanosis, skin temperature)
- Agreement between oximeter and actual patient heart rate, as determined by palpation or electrocardiogram

RULE OF THUMB

When using a pulse oximeter to detect hypoxemia in an otherwise healthy adult, never set the low alarm below 92%. Generally, this level ensures that the alarm is activated before true arterial saturation drops below that critical.

MINI CLINI

Troubleshooting Pulse Oximetry

PROBLEM: The RT draws an ABG sample from a conscious and alert patient in a postsurgical unit who also is being monitored with a pulse oximeter, which reads 80% saturation. The patient is breathing 35% O_2 through an air-entrainment mask. The patient's extremities are pink and warm. After running the blood sample through a calibrated ABG analyzer with a hemoximeter, the RT obtains the following values:

PaO_2 = 90 mm Hg
Hb = 12 g/dl
SaO_2 = 98%
metHb = 0.5%
HbCO = 1%

Explain the difference between the pulse oximeter and hemoximeter readings of this patient's blood O_2 levels and what action the RT should take.

SOLUTION: Given that a calibrated hemoximeter provides more accurate results than a pulse oximeter and that the patient exhibits no signs of hypoxemia, it is likely that the pulse oximeter reading is falsely low. Because the total Hb and metHb levels are not grossly abnormal, potential problems include motion artifact, poor sensor placement, and device malfunction. The oximeter and sensor should be rechecked, and, if found to be malfunctioning, they should be replaced.

Problem-Solving and Troubleshooting

Problems with pulse oximetry fall into two categories: (1) inherent technology problems and (2) problems associated with clinical interpretation of the data. Dozens of technical factors may affect the readings, limit the precision, or alter the performance of pulse oximeters. Table 19-6 summarizes the most important of these factors and the types of errors they cause.

Motion artifact probably is the most common source of error and false alarms. Although new technologies promise to reduce motion artifact, relocation of the sensor to the earlobe, toe, or forehead can minimize the problem. Falsely elevated readings can occur with dark skin pigmentation at low saturation levels; this can be compensated for by setting oximeter low alarms 3% to 5% higher in applicable cases.

Early studies on the effects of nail polish found significant differences in lowering SpO_2 readings. More recent studies have found either no effect or small differences that are considered clinically irrelevant; this may be due to improvements in LED light sources.[45,46] The effect of nail polish may be minimized by using a different site or by rotating the sensor so that the light path does not cross the fingernails.

If ambient light interference is creating problems, the sensor can be loosely covered with an opaque towel or cloth. Problems that occur during procedures producing electromagnetic interference (e.g., electrocautery, magnetic resonance imaging) need only be recognized. Careful monitoring of the patient during episodes of false low alarms is essential.

TABLE 19-6

Factors Affecting Accuracy or Precision of Pulse Oximeters

Factor	Potential Error
Presence of HbCO	Falsely high $\%HbO_2$
Presence of high levels of metHb	Falsely low $\%HbO_2$ if SaO_2 >85% Falsely high $\%HbO_2$ if SaO_2 <85%
Presence of fetal hemoglobin	No effect
Anemia (very low hematocrit, <10%)	Falsely low CaO_2 and high $\%HbO_2$
Vascular dyes (e.g., methylene blue)	Falsely low $\%HbO_2$
Elevated bilirubin levels	No effect
Dark skin pigmentation	Falsely high $\%HbO_2$ (3%-5%)
Nail polish (especially black)	Falsely high $\%HbO_2$
Ambient light	Varies (e.g., falsely high $\%HbO_2$ in sunlight); also may cause falsely high pulse reading
Poor perfusion (vasoconstriction)	Inadequate signal; unpredictable results
Motion artifact	Unpredictable, spurious readings
Electrocautery	Falsely low HbO_2
Magnetic resonance imaging	Falsely low HbO_2

RULE OF THUMB

If the pulse oximeter is reading a critically low value (<90%) but the patient appears in no distress, then it is likely that there is an erroneous pulse oximeter reading. In such situations is best to further assess the patient's clinical status and troubleshoot the pulse oximetry equipment setup. If further examination suggests that the patient is stable, it is likely that the problem is the is equipment related and the setup, including the sensor, should be checked.

Regarding problems with interpreting pulse oximetry data, rule number one is to treat the patient, not the monitor. The clinician should never interpret or act on monitoring data without first assessing the patient and verifying proper sensor placement and signal quality. A related problem is simple confusion over the relationship between oxyhemoglobin saturation and PO_2. Many clinicians rely solely on PaO_2 readings to assess oxygenation and do not understand oxyhemoglobin saturation. To these clinicians, an SpO_2 reading of 80% might be confused easily with PaO_2 of 80 mm Hg. The latter measure of partial pressure is normal, whereas a saturation of 80% indicates moderate to severe hypoxemia, equivalent to PaO_2 of approximately 50 mm Hg.

A similar interpretation error (PaO_2 vs. SpO_2) occurs because of the limited accuracy of most pulse oximeters. It is common practice to set the low alarm of a monitoring oximeter to 90%. In theory, this practice makes sense because an SaO_2 reading of 90% normally corresponds to a PO_2 reading of approximately 60 mm Hg (the lower limit of clinically acceptable oxygenation). However, with the accuracy of some oximeters being only ± 4%, an SpO_2 reading of 90% could mean an actual SaO_2 reading of 86%, corresponding to a PO_2 level of 55 mm Hg or less.

At the high end, oximetry data can be even less meaningful. Because of the characteristics of the oxyhemoglobin dissociation curve (see Chapter 12), a patient with an SpO_2 reading of 100% could represent a PaO_2 level between 100 and 600 mm Hg. Therefore pulse oximetry should not be used for monitoring hyperoxia (as is important for neonates).

It is also important to remember that a pulse oximeter does not measure PCO_2. A patient breathing an elevated FiO_2 can have normal SpO_2 readings despite severe hypercarbia. ABG analysis is needed when acute ventilatory failure may be present.

SpO_2 can read falsely high when carbon monoxide poisoning or methemoglobinemia is present. This false reading is due to the fact that the two-wavelength pulse oximeter measures only saturation of the Hb and not specifically saturation with O_2. HbCO and metHb cannot be distinguished from HbO_2 with a pulse oximeter. A falsely high SpO_2 reading occurs when significant HbCO is present. When metHb is elevated, the SpO_2 reading is higher than the actual measured SaO_2. As metHb level increases, SpO_2 decreases and plateaus at approximately 85% when the metHb level reaches 30%.[47]

To address these limitations, pulse oximeters using seven or more wavelengths of light have been developed. Use of multiwavelength pulse oximeters capable of measuring reduced Hb, HbO_2, HbCO, and metHb has been referred to as **pulse cooximetry.** The accuracy of these measurements does not equal that of conventional hemoximetry (cooximetry), but pulse cooximetry may be useful for trend monitoring in some clinical situations (e.g., monitoring therapy for acute carbon monoxide poisoning in the emergency department).[48]

As with transcutaneous monitoring, if pulse oximetry and blood gas values are inconsistent with each other, or the clinical status of the patient, the RT should explore possible causes before reporting, interpreting, or acting on results. Often, discrepancies can be reduced by switching sites or replacing the sensor probe. If these steps fail to resolve the inconsistencies, the RT should document the problem and recommend obtaining an ABG measurement with hemoximetry if indicated.

Venous Oximetry

Continuous central venous (vena cava) and mixed venous (PA) O_2 saturation monitoring ($S\bar{v}O_2$) is performed to assess the balance between O_2 delivery and use as an indirect index of global tissue oxygenation and perfusion. Decreased $S\bar{v}O_2$ is indicative of cardiac failure in patients with myocardial infarction and after cardiovascular surgery, as well as in patients with severe cardiopulmonary disease, including those in septic or cardiogenicshock.[49] Regional and organ-specific $S\bar{v}O_2$ monitoring has been performed via catheters placed in the coronary sinus, hepatic vein, and cranial jugular venous bulb for cerebral perfusion monitoring. Normal values for $S\bar{v}O_2$ range from 60% to 80%.

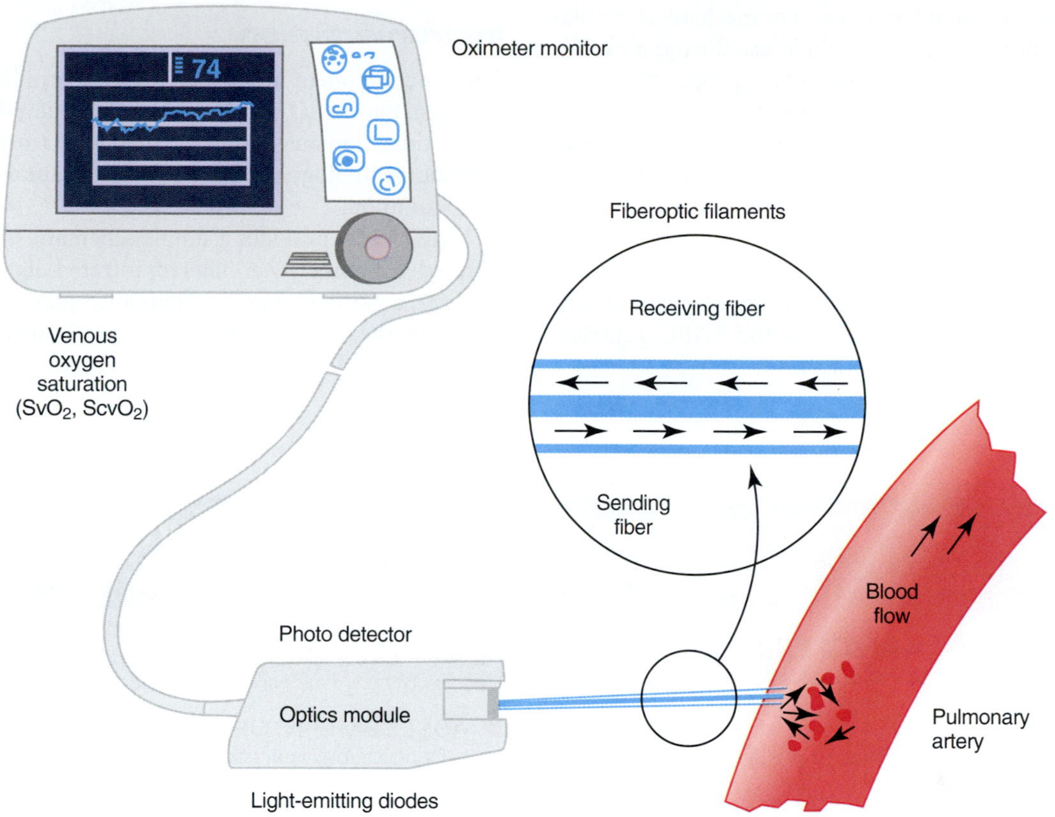

FIGURE 19-18 Diagram of a venous oximetry monitoring system using reflectance oximetry. (Courtesy Edwards Life Science, Irvine, CA.)

Instrumentation

Figure 19-18 shows a diagram of an $S\bar{v}O_2$ monitoring system. Venous oximetry is measured through a fiberoptic catheter by reflectance spectrophotometry. Two or three wavelengths of light are emitted from LEDs through fiberoptic filaments into the venous blood. Some of this light is reflected back and received through another fiberoptic channel, which is read by a photodetector. The amount of light that is absorbed by the venous blood and reflected back is determined by the amount of O_2 that is saturated or bound to Hb. This information is processed by the monitor, updated, and displayed as $S\bar{v}O_2$.

Clinical Usefulness

Continuous $S\bar{v}O_2$ can be monitored through an $S\bar{v}O_2$-equipped PA catheter or venous catheter. Mixed venous oximetry from the PA is an indication of global O_2 use. Central venous oximetry is nearly interchangeable with mixed venous oximetry. Both correlate with mixed venous saturation measured by hemoximetry with an accuracy of $\pm$ 3% to 5%. Accuracy of venous oximetry monitoring depends on several factors, including the frequency of calibration with measured $S\bar{v}O_2$ and Hb, the position of the catheter free floating in the vein, the absence of wall artifact, damage to the fiberoptic filaments, and clot formation at the catheter tip.[50,51]

Tissue Oximetry

Tissue level O_2 saturation (StO_2) assesses the adequacy of circulation and O_2 delivery. Low StO_2 can be used for early detection of tissue hypoperfusion in patients with traumatic injuries.[52] Cerebral StO_2 monitoring also can be used to monitor brain oxygenation and detect cerebral ischemia during neurosurgical or cardiovascular procedures.[53]

Instrumentation

Tissue oximetry is essentially a reflectance oximeter that uses near-infrared spectroscopy to measure StO_2. Multi-wavelengths of light in the near-infrared spectrum transilluminate muscle tissue in the hand or brain through the forehead. Because biologic tissue, including the skull, is relatively transparent in the near-infrared range, the absorbance and reflectance characteristics of HbO_2 and reduced Hb concentrations in the tissue being monitored is used to calculate StO_2. To date, StO_2 monitoring is used primarily for research purposes but may eventually be used for clinical practice.

CAPNOMETRY AND CAPNOGRAPHY

Capnometry is the measurement of CO_2 in respiratory gases. A capnometer is the device that measures CO_2. **Capnography** is the graphic display of CO_2 levels versus time (scalar display) as they change during breathing. **Volumetric capnography** is the graphic displaying of CO_2 versus expired tidal volume that allows for the measurement of physiologic dead-space fraction and volumetric CO_2 excretion.[54]

Although capnography can be applied to any patient, its primary clinical use is for monitoring during either general anesthesia (where it is a standard of care) or mechanical ventilation. Other common indications include use during a cardiopulmonary resuscitation to both identify the proper placement of an artificial airway and to assess the effectiveness in restoring adequate perfusion pressures, which are discussed elsewhere in this text. However, the following section of this chapter focuses mainly on the application of capnography and capnometry during mechanical ventilation. To guide practitioners in providing quality care, the AARC has published Clinical Practice Guideline: Capnography/Capnometry During Mechanical Ventilation: 2011.[55] Modified excerpts from the AARC guideline appear in Clinical Practice Guidelines 19-6.

Instrumentation

The key component in a capnograph is a rapid-responding CO_2 analyzer. Rapid CO_2 analysis can be achieved using infrared absorption, Raman scattering, mass spectroscopy, or photoacoustic technology, with the infrared capnometer being the most common.

Figure 19-19 provides a simple schematic of a double-beam infrared capnometer. A filtered infrared light source passes through a sample chamber. (Because glass absorbs infrared radiation, the chamber "windows" usually are constructed with sodium chloride or sodium bromide.) After the infrared light

19-6 Capnography and Capnometry During Mechanical Ventilation: 2011

AARC Clinical Practice Guideline (Excerpts)*

■ INDICATIONS

There are three broad categories of indications for capnography/capnometry:

- Verification of artificial airway placement (determining that tracheal, rather than esophageal, intubation has been accomplished)
- Assessment of pulmonary circulation and respiratory status
- Improve the matching of $\dot{V}/\dot{Q}$
- Measurement of the volume of CO_2 elimination to assess metabolic rate or alveolar ventilation
- Optimization of mechanical ventilation
- Improve the V_D/V_T ratio
- Continued monitoring of the integrity of the ventilatory circuit, including the artificial airway
- Evaluation of the efficiency of mechanical ventilatory support (by [PaCO2 – $PETCO_2$])

■ CONTRAINDICATIONS

There are no absolute contraindications to capnography in mechanically ventilated patients, provided that the data obtained are evaluated with consideration given to the patient's clinical condition.

■ HAZARDS AND POSSIBLE COMPLICATIONS

- Misunderstanding of the data provided may lead to inappropriate treatment of the patient.
- With mainstream analyzers, too large a sampling window can excessively increase the circuit mechanical dead space.
- The sampling window or the sampling lines can place additional weight on the circuit and increase traction on the patient's artificial airway (primarily a concern in young pediatric patients).
- With sidestream analyzers, the sampling rate may cause auto-triggering of mechanical ventilators.

■ ASSESSMENT OF NEED

- Capnography is a standard of care during general anesthesia. The American Society of Anesthesiologists has suggested that capnography be available for patients with acute ventilatory failure on mechanical ventilatory support.[56] The American College of Emergency Physicians recommends capnography as an adjunctive method to ensure proper endotracheal tube position.[57] The 2010 American Heart Association Guidelines for Cardiopulmonary Resuscitation and Emergency Cardiovascular Care recommend capnography to verify endotracheal tube placement in all age groups.[58]
- Assessing the need for capnography in a specific patient is guided by the clinical situation; in particular both the primary cause and the severity of respiratory failure should be considered.

■ ASSESSMENT OF OUTCOME

Results should reflect the patient's condition. Documentation of results (along with all ventilatory and hemodynamic variables available), therapeutic interventions, and clinical decisions made based on the capnogram should be included in the patient's medical record.

■ MONITORING

During capnography, the following should be considered and monitored:

- *Ventilatory variables:* Tidal volume, respiratory rate, minute ventilation, peak airway pressure, plateau pressure, positive end expiratory pressure, inspiratory/expiratory time ratio, and concentrations of respiratory gas mixture
- *Hemodynamic variables:* Systemic and pulmonary blood pressures, cardiac output, and intrapulmonary shunt

**For the complete guideline, see American Association for Respiratory Care: Clinical Practice Guideline: Capnography/Capnometry During Mechanical Ventilation. Respir Care 56:503, 2011.*

passes through the sample chamber, a lens focuses the remaining, unabsorbed radiation onto an electrical photodetector. Because CO_2 absorbs infrared radiation, the greater the concentration of CO_2 in the sample, the less is the infrared light that arrives at the detector. Variations in the concentration of CO_2 alter the electrical output signal of the detector. This signal is used either to display the CO_2 concentration with LEDs (capnometer) or to generate a real-time graphic display (capnogram).

Capnometers use two different methods to sample the respiratory gases: mainstream sampling and sidestream sampling (Figure 19-20). The mainstream analyzer places an in-line analysis chamber between the patient's airway and the ventilator circuit. The sidestream analyzer uses a sampling tube to pump a small volume of gas continually from the ventilator circuit into the analysis chamber within the device. Box 19-9 lists the

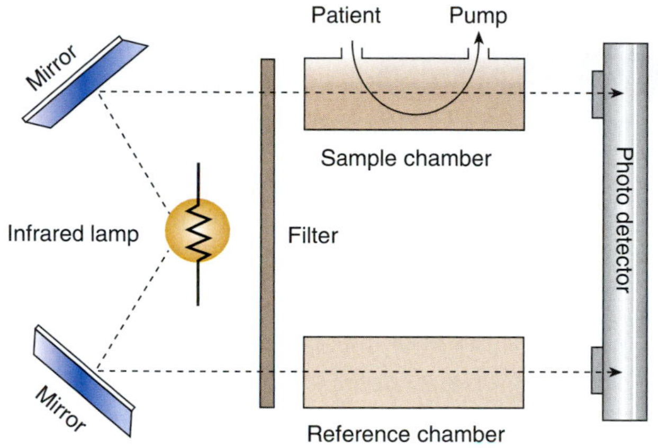

FIGURE 19-19 Schematic representation of infrared capnometer.

Box 19-9 Advantages and Disadvantages of Mainstream and Sidestream Capnometers

MAINSTREAM

Advantages

- Sensor at patient airway
- Fast response (crisp waveform)
- Short lag time (real-time readings)
- No sample flow to reduce tidal volume

Disadvantages

- Secretions and humidity can block sensor window
- Sensor requires heating to prevent condensation
- Requires frequent calibration
- Bulky sensor at patient airway
- Does not measure N_2O
- Difficult to use with nonintubated patients
- Reusable adapters require cleaning and sterilization

SIDESTREAM

Advantages

- No bulky sensors or heaters at airway
- Ability to measure N_2O
- Disposable sample line
- Ability to use with nonintubated patients

Disadvantages

- Secretions block sample tubing
- Trap required to remove water from sample
- Frequent calibration required
- Slow response to CO_2 changes
- Lag time between CO_2 change and measurement
- Sample flow may decrease tidal volume

From Kacmarek RM, Hess D, Stoller J, editors: Monitoring in respiratory care, St Louis, 1993, Mosby.

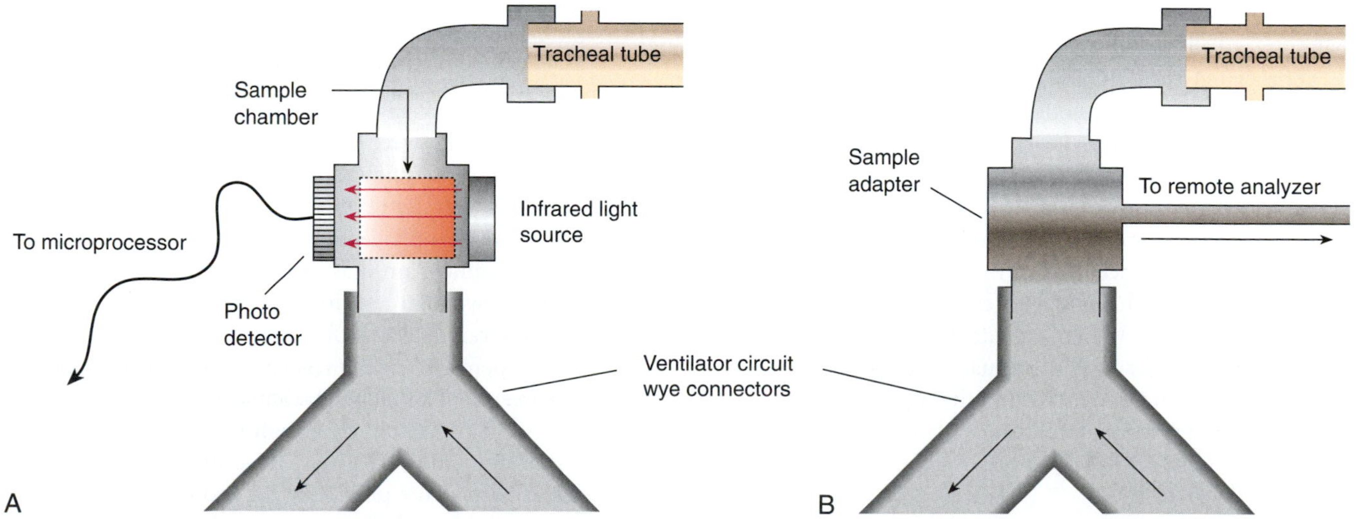

FIGURE 19-20 A, Mainstream CO_2 sampling. The sample chamber, light source, and photodetector are attached to the breathing circuit, with the output signal sent to a microprocessor for analysis and display. **B,** Sidestream CO_2 sampling through an in-line sampling adapter with a small-bore connector. A small sample of expired gas is drawn continuously through the tubing and analyzed inside a remote capnometer.

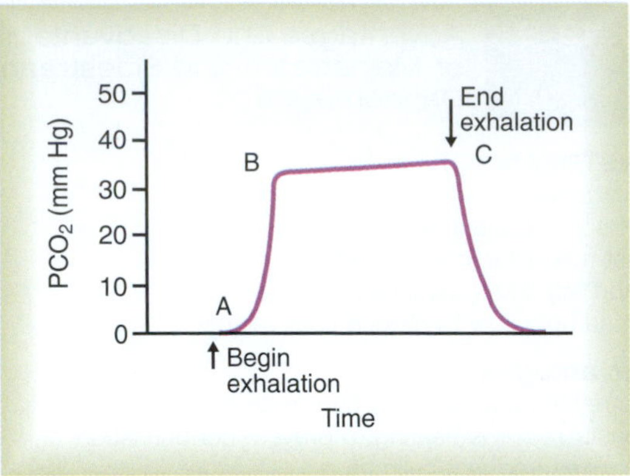

FIGURE 19-21 Normal single-breath capnograph tracing.

TABLE 19-7

Conditions Associated With Changes in $PETCO_2$

Change	High $PETCO_2$	Low $PETCO_2$
Sudden	Sudden increase in cardiac output	Sudden hyperventilation
	Sudden release of a tourniquet	Sudden decrease in cardiac output
	Injection of sodium bicarbonate	Massive pulmonary embolism
		Air embolism
		Disconnection of ventilator
		Obstruction of endotracheal tube
		Leakage in the circuit
Gradual	Hypoventilation	Hyperventilation
	Increase in CO_2 production	Decrease in oxygen consumption
		Decreased pulmonary perfusion

Note: An absent $PETCO_2$ means that a system leak, esophageal intubation, or cardiac arrest has occurred.

advantages and disadvantages of these two approaches. Differences notwithstanding, clinicians should use the method best suited to the patient's needs.

Interpretation

Interpretation of the capnogram can be useful in assessing trends in alveolar ventilation and detecting ventilation/perfusion ratio ($\dot{V}/\dot{Q}$) imbalance caused by either pulmonary disease or cardiovascular disorders. Capnometry also is used to measure physiologic dead space, detect esophageal intubation, assess blood flow during cardiac arrest, and guide setting positive end-expiratory pressure levels. To interpret abnormal events, clinicians first must understand the normal capnogram.

Normal Capnogram

Figure 19-21 shows a typical normal single-breath capnogram. Initially, the expired PCO_2 is 0 mm Hg, indicating exhalation of pure dead space gas from the airways (*A*, phase I). Soon after, alveolar gas begins mixing with dead space gas in the airways, causing a rapid increase in expired PCO_2 (*A* to *B*, phase II). The CO_2 concentration then reaches a plateau indicates exhalation of alveolar gas (*B* to *C*, phase III). Gas sampled at the end of exhalation is called *end-tidal gas,* with its partial pressure of CO_2 abbreviated as $PETCO_2$. In healthy individuals, $PETCO_2$ averages 3 to 5 mm Hg less than $PaCO_2$, or 35 to 43 mm Hg (approximately 5% to 6% CO_2). The sharp downstroke and return to baseline that normally occurs after the end-tidal point indicates inhalation of fresh gas with zero CO_2.

The same phases are also captured during volumetric capnography. The difference is that the area within the V_T-CO_2 curve with each breath is used to calculate the mean expired PCO_2, which in turn is used to calculate physiologic dead-space according to the Bohr-Enghoff equation ($V_D/V_T = [PaCO_2 - PECO_2]/PaCO_2$).[54] The area within the V_T-CO_2 curve (when multiplied by the respiratory rate) calculates CO_2 excretion per minute, which under normal physiologic conditions equals CO_2 production.[54]

Abnormal Capnogram

The first step in assessing the capnogram is to determine the actual $PETCO_2$ and whether it has changed over time. Table 19-7 differentiates between the causes of high and low $PETCO_2$ readings by the suddenness of the change. A $PETCO_2$ of zero usually indicates a system leak, endotracheal tube displacement out of the airway, esophageal intubation, or cardiac arrest.

After the capnogram has been assessed for changes in $PETCO_2$, the waveform and its pattern should be analyzed. A normal capnogram starts with a sharp upstroke, followed by a plateau and then a rapid downstroke. As indicated in Figure 19-22, changes in this normal contour may indicate a $\dot{V}/\dot{Q}$ abnormality. Such patterns, although not diagnostic, can indicate the severity of the $\dot{V}/\dot{Q}$ disturbance and warn of developing problems, such as acute pulmonary emboli.

Waveform changes also may occur with equipment malfunction. Because the normal inspired CO_2 level is zero, the capnogram baseline should also be at zero. An elevated baseline (>0 mm Hg) indicates rebreathing. However, an expired CO_2

MINI CLINI

Interpreting Capnometry Data

PROBLEM: The RT is monitoring an intubated, mechanically ventilated patient in the ICU with a capnograph. She notices the expired CO_2 level suddenly drop to near zero. On auscultation, the patient exhibits good bilateral breath sounds, and all connections between the airway and capnograph are tight. What is the likely problem?

SOLUTION: The most common causes of a zero $PETCO_2$ are extubation and ventilator or monitoring system disconnection. However, a $PETCO_2$ of zero also can occur with shock or cardiac arrest (no CO_2 returns to the lungs for exhalation). The RT should check this patient's cardiovascular status immediately. If the patient's cardiovascular system is functioning within normal limits, the RT should check the position of the endotracheal tube.

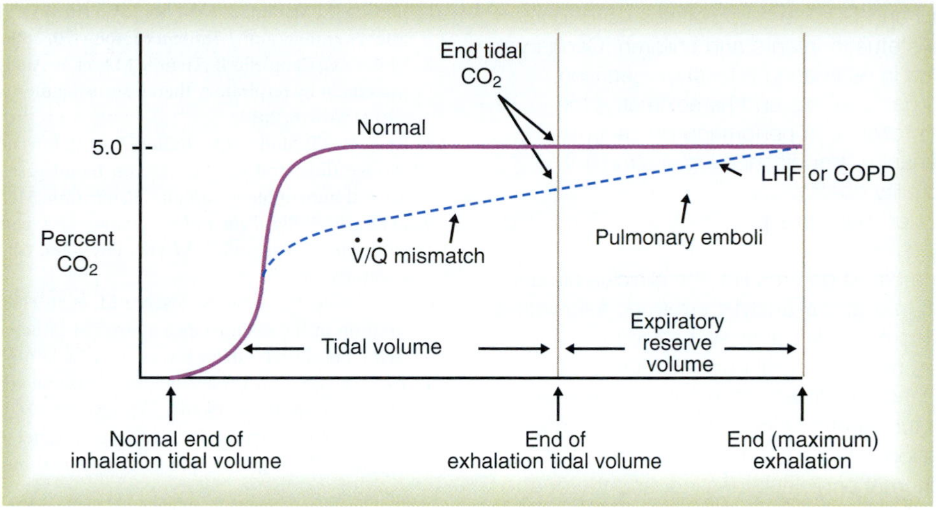

FIGURE 19-22 Normal and abnormal capnogram waveforms. For a healthy individual *(solid line),* the end-tidal CO_2 ($ETCO_2$) at the completion of normal tidal exhalation is equal to end-tidal CO_2 at maximum exhalation. With shock caused by left ventricular heart failure *(LHF)* or chronic obstructive pulmonary disease *(COPD)*, the CO_2 level increases more slowly and does not reach a true end-tidal plateau. The $ETCO_2$ is less than normal at the completion of a normal exhalation (but may increase slightly with a maximum exhalation). Similar findings can be noted with a pulmonary embolus except that the low $ETCO_2$ does not increase with a maximum exhalation. (Modified from Darin J: Capnography. Curr Rev Resp Ther 3:146, 1981; Erickson L, Wollmer P, Olsson CG, et al: Diagnosis of pulmonary embolism based upon alveolar dead space analysis. Chest 96:357–362, 1989; Hatte CJ, Rokseth R: The arterial to end-expiratory carbon dioxide tension gradient in acute pulmonary embolism and other cardiopulmonary diseases. Chest 66:352–357, 1974. In: Pilbeam SP, Cairo JM: Mechanical ventilation, ed 4, St Louis, 2006, Mosby.)

level of zero might indicate patient disconnect. (For more information on the use of capnography during mechanical ventilation, see Chapter 51.)

Procedure

Bedside capnography procedures vary according to the type of equipment used and the manufacturer's recommended protocol. Generally, a capnograph should be calibrated as recommended by its manufacturer, using precision CO_2 mixtures in the clinical range of measurement.

In terms of infection control, nondisposable components that contact the patient's airway or ventilator circuit should undergo high-level disinfection between patients. The monitor should be cleaned as needed, according to the manufacturer's recommendations.

Problem-Solving and Troubleshooting

Monitoring a patient with a capnograph that is properly calibrated and operating according to the manufacturer's specifications presents few major problems. The most significant error is assuming that the end-expired CO_2 levels can substitute for actual $PaCO_2$ measurements. The most common problem is contamination or obstruction of the sampling system or monitor by secretions or condensate.[57] Proper use of water traps and regular changing of sample tubing or chambers can help prevent this problem. Other potential problems include the following:

- False reading caused by the presence of gases with infrared absorption spectra similar to CO_2 (e.g., nitrous oxide)
- Inaccurate readings with high frequencies of breathing (this is more of a problem with sidestream systems)
- Misinterpreting low or absent cardiac output as a disconnect or possible esophageal intubation (all three can result in a $PETCO_2$ of zero)

SUMMARY CHECKLIST

- To measure the inspired O_2 concentration, a properly calibrated electrochemical O_2 analyzer should be used.
- The most common causes of O_2 analyzer malfunction are low batteries, sensor depletion, and electronic failure.
- As the "gold standard" of gas-exchange analysis, ABG results help the clinician assess ventilation, acid-base balance, oxygenation, and the O_2-carrying capacity of blood.
- The radial artery is the preferred site for adult arterial blood sampling. Before radial puncture, a modified Allen test to confirm collateral circulation is performed.
- For critically ill patients, the clinician waits 20 to 30 minutes after a change in treatment before sampling arterial blood.
- Most pre-analytic blood gas errors can be avoided by ensuring that the sample was obtained anaerobically, is properly anticoagulated, and is promptly analyzed.
- Indwelling peripheral artery, central venous, and PA catheters give ready access for blood sampling and allow continuous pressure monitoring but with increased risk for infection and thrombosis.

- Capillary blood pH and PCO_2 are sometimes used to assess acid-base status in infants and children. Capillary PO_2 is of little value in estimating arterial oxygenation.
- To perform blood gas analysis and hemoximetry, the clinician must be proficient in performing procedures, preventive maintenance, troubleshooting, instrument calibration, and quality control.
- A blood gas analyzer measures pH, PCO_2, and PO_2 using three separate electrodes.
- To obtain accurate blood gas results, the clinician ensures that the sample is free of pre-analytic error and follows the manufacturer's recommended analysis protocol.
- Blood gas analysis quality control involves a cycle of performance validation for new instruments, preventive maintenance and function checks, automated calibration, calibration verification with control media, internal statistical quality control, external proficiency testing, and thorough recordkeeping of all processes.
- Portable point-of-care blood gas analyzers can achieve accuracy and precision levels comparable with laboratory-based analyzers.
- Transcutaneous blood gas monitoring provides continuous noninvasive analysis of gas exchange.
- Oximetry is the measurement of blood Hb saturations using spectrophotometry. Hemoximetry is a laboratory procedure that requires an arterial blood sample. Pulse oximetry combines spectrophotometry with photoplethysmography to obtain a noninvasive measure of blood Hb saturations.
- At best, pulse oximetry readings fall within ± 3% to 5% of readings obtained by hemoximetry (cooximetry).
- Technical factors may affect the readings, limit the precision, or alter the performance of pulse oximeters. To interpret test results properly, clinicians must have in-depth knowledge of these factors.
- Capnometry is the measurement of CO_2 in respiratory gases. A capnometer is the device that measures the CO_2. Capnography is the graphic display of CO_2 levels as they change during breathing.
- A capnogram may be used to assess trends in alveolar ventilation, to identify $\dot{V}/\dot{Q}$ imbalance caused by cardiopulmonary disorders, to estimate physiologic dead space, to detect esophageal intubation, and to determine the amount of blood flow during cardiac arrest.

References

1. Epstein CD, Haghenbeck KT: Bedside assessment of tissue oxygen saturation monitoring in critically ill adults: an integrative review of the literature. *Crit Care Res Pract* 19, 2014. doi: 10.1155/2014/709683.
2. Severinghaus JW: The invention and development of blood gas analysis apparatus. *Anesthesiology* 97:253–256, 2002.
3. American Association for Respiratory Care: Clinical practice guideline: sampling for arterial blood gas analysis. *Respir Care* 37:913–917, 1992.
4. Blonshine S: *Procedures for the collection of arterial blood specimens: approved standard, H11-A4*, ed 2, Wayne, PA, 2004, National Committee for Clinical Laboratory Standards.
5. Brzezinski M, Luisetti T, London MJ: Radial artery cannulation: a comprehensive review of recent anatomic and physiologic investigations. *Anesth Analg* 109:1763–1781, 2009.
6. Barone JE, Madlinger RV: Should an Allen test be performed before radial artery cannulation? *J Trauma* 61:468–470, 2006.
7. Miller AG, Cappiello JL, Gentile MA, et al: Analysis of radial artery catheter placement by respiratory therapists using ultrasound guidance. *Respir Care* 59:1813–1816, 2014.
8. Knowles TP, Mullin RA, Hunter JA, et al: Effects of syringe material, sample storage time, and temperature on blood gases and oxygen saturation in arterial human blood samples. *Respir Care* 51:732–736, 2006.
9. D'Orazio P: *Blood gas and pH analysis and related measurements: approved guideline, C46-A2*, ed 2, Wayne, PA, 2009, Clinical Laboratory Standards Institute.
10. Del Cotillo M, Grané N, Llavoré M, et al: Heparinized solution vs. saline solution in the maintenance of arterial catheters: a double blind randomized clinical trial. *Intensive Care Med* 34:339–343, 2008.
11. Zavorsky GS, Cao J, Mayo NE, et al: Arterial versus capillary blood gases: a meta-analysis. *Respir Physiol Neurobiol* 155:268–279, 2007.
12. American Association for Respiratory Care: Clinical practice guideline: capillary blood gas sampling for neonatal and pediatric patients. *Respir Care* 46:506, 2001.
13. Meites S: Skin puncture and blood collecting techniques for infants: update and problems. In Meites S, editor: *Pediatric clinical chemistry*, ed 3, Washington, DC, 1989, American Association for Clinical Chemistry, pp 5–15.
14. De Koninck AS, De Decker K, Van Bocxlaer J, et al: Analytical performance evaluation of four cartridge-type blood gas analyzers. *Clin Chem Lab Med* 50:1083–1091, 2012.
15. American Association for Respiratory Care: Clinical practice guideline: blood gas analysis and hemoximetry—2013. *Respir Care* l58:1694–1703, 2013.
16. Centers for Disease Control and Prevention: <https://www.cms.gov/Regulations-and-Guidance/Guidance/Transmittals/Downloads/R140SOMA.pdf>, (Accessed Sept 15, 2015).
17. Berte L: *Application of a quality management system model for laboratory services: approved guideline, GP26-A3*, ed 3, Wayne, PA, 2004, National Committee for Clinical Laboratory Standards.
18. Westgard JO, Barry PL, Hunt MR, et al: A multi-rule Shewhart medical record for quality control in clinical chemistry. *Clin Chem* 27:493–501, 1981.
19. Westguard SC: <http://www.westgard.com/westgard-rules>, (Accessed December 7, 2014).
20. Centers for Disease Control and Prevention: <http://wwwn. cdc.gov/clia/default.aspx>, (Accessed December 7, 2014).
21. Center for Medicare and Medicine Services: <https://www.cms.gov/CLIA/14_Proficiency_Testing_Providers.asp>, (Accessed December 7, 2014).
22. Pecoraro V, Germagnoli L, Banfi G: Point-of-care testing: where is the evidence? A systematic survey. *Clin Chem Lab Med* 52:313–324, 2014.
23. Singer AJ, Ardise J, Gulla J, et al: Point-of-care testing reduces length of stay in emergency department chest pain patients. *Ann Emerg Med* 45:587–591, 2005.
24. St John A, Price CP: Existing and emerging technologies for point-of-care testing. *Clin Biochem Rev* 35:155–167, 2014.
25. Quinn LM, Hamnett N, Wilkin R, et al: Arterial blood gas analysers: accuracy in determining haemoglobin, glucose and electrolyte concentrations in critically ill adult patients. *Br J Biomed Sci* 70:97–100, 2013.
26. Schimke I: Quality and timeliness in medical laboratory testing. *Anal Bioanal Chem* 393:1499–1504, 2009.
27. Stotler BA, Kratz A: Analytical and clinical performance of the Epoc blood analysis system: experience at a large tertiary academic medical center. *Am J Clin Pathol* 140:715–720, 2013.
28. Jacobs E: *Point-of-care in vitro diagnostic (IVD) testing: approved guideline, POCT4-A2*, Wayne, PA, 2006, Clinical Laboratory Standards Institute.
29. Finer N, Leone T: Oxygen saturation monitoring for the preterm infant: the evidence basis for current practice. *Pediatr Res* 65:375–380, 2009.
30. De Oliveira GS, Jr, Ahmad S, Fitzgerald PC, et al: Detection of hypoventilation during deep sedation in patients undergoing ambulatory gynaecological hysteroscopy: a comparison between transcutaneous and nasal end-tidal carbon dioxide measurements. *Br J Anaesth* 104:774–778, 2010.

31. McVicar J, Eager R: Validation study of a transcutaneous carbon dioxide monitor in patients in the emergency department. *Emerg Med J* 26:344–346, 2009.
32. Rodriguez P, Lellouche F, Aboab J, et al: Transcutaneous arterial carbon dioxide pressure monitoring in critically ill adult patients. *Intensive Care Med* 32:309–312, 2006.
33. Roediger R, Beck-Schimmer B, Theusinger OM, et al: The revised digital transcutaneous PCO_2/SpO_2 ear sensor is a reliable noninvasive monitoring tool in patients after cardiac surgery. *J Cardiothorac Vasc Anesth* 25:243–249, 2011.
34. Chakravarthy M, Narayan S, Govindarajan R, et al: Weaning mechanical ventilation after off-pump coronary artery bypass graft procedures directed by noninvasive gas measurements. *J Cardiothorac Vasc Anesth* 24:451–455, 2010.
35. Xue Q, Wu X, Jin J, et al: Transcutaneous carbon dioxide monitoring accurately predicts arterial carbon dioxide partial pressure in patients undergoing prolonged laparoscopic surgery. *Anesth Analg* 111:417–420, 2010.
36. Hirabayashi M, Fujiwara C, Ohtani N, et al: Transcutaneous PCO_2 monitors are more accurate than end-tidal PCO_2 monitors. *J Anesth* 23:198–202, 2009.
37. American Association for Respiratory Care: Clinical practice guideline: transcutaneous monitoring of carbon dioxide and oxygen: 2012. *Respir Care* 58:1955–1962, 2012.
38. Mulvey JM, Dorsch NW, Mudaliar Y, et al: Multimodality monitoring in severe traumatic brain injury: the role of brain tissue oxygenation monitoring. *Neurocrit Care* 1:391–402, 2004.
39. Mellstrom A, Mansson P, Jonsson K, et al: Measurements of subcutaneous tissue PO_2 reflect oxygen metabolism of the small intestinal mucosa during hemorrhage and resuscitation: an experimental study in pigs. *Eur Surg Res* 42:122–129, 2009.
40. Mathews PJ: Co-oximetry. *Respir Care Clin N Am* 1:47–68, 1995.
41. Moyle JT: Uses and abuses of pulse oximetry. *Arch Dis Child* 74:77–80, 1996.
42. Ochroch EA, Russel MW, Hanson WC, 3rd: The impact of continuous pulse oximetry monitoring on intensive care unit admissions from a postsurgical care floor. *Anesth Analg* 102:868–875, 2006.
43. American Association for Respiratory Care: Clinical practice guideline: pulse oximetry. *Respir Care* 36:1406–1409, 1991.
44. Wahr JA, Tremper KK, Diab M: Pulse oximetry. *Respir Care Clin N Am* 1:77, 1995.
45. Yamamoto LG, Yamamoto JA, Yamamoto JB, et al: Nail polish does not significantly affect pulse oximetry measurements in mildly hypoxic subjects. *Respir Care* 53:1470–1474, 2008.
46. Yont GH, Korhan EA, Dizer B: The effect of nail polish on pulse oximetry readings. *Intensive Crit Care Nurs* 30:111–115, 2014.
47. Barker SJ, Tremper KK, Hyatt J: Effects of methemoglobinemia on pulse oximetry and mixed venous oximetry. *Anesthesiology* 70:112–117, 1989.
48. Feiner JR, Bickler PE: Improved accuracy of methemoglobin detection by pulse CO-oximetry during hypoxia. *Anesth Analg* 111:1160–1167, 2010.
49. Reinhart K, Kuhn HJ, Hartog C, et al: Continuous central venous and pulmonary artery oxygen saturation monitoring in the critically ill. *Intensive Care Med* 30:1572–1578, 2004.
50. Cariou A, Monchi M, Dhainaut JF: Continuous cardiac output and mixed venous oxygen saturation monitoring. *J Crit Care* 13:198–213, 1998.
51. Molnar Z, Umgelter A, Toth I, et al: Continuous monitoring of $ScvO_2$ by a new fibre-optic technology compared with blood gas oximetry in critically ill patients: a multicentre study. *Intensive Care Med* 33:1767–1770, 2007.
52. Santora RJ, Moore FA: Monitoring trauma and intensive care unit resuscitation with tissue hemoglobin oxygen saturation. *Crit Care* 13(Suppl 5): S10, 2009.
53. Prabhakar H, Sandhu K, Bhagat H, et al: Current concepts of optimal cerebral perfusion pressure in traumatic brain injury. *J Anaesthsiol Clin Pharmacol* 30:318–327, 2014.
54. Kallet RH: Measuring dead-space in acute lung injury. *Minerva Anaesthesiol* 78:1297–1305, 2012.
55. American Association for Respiratory Care: Clinical practice guideline: capnography/capnometry during mechanical ventilation: 2011. *Respir Care* 56:503, 2011.
56. American Society of Anesthesiologists: Standards for basic anesthetic monitoring. Committee of Origin: Standards and practice parameters (approved by the ASA House of Delegates, October 21, 1986; amended October 20, 2010 with an effective date of July 1 2011). <https://www.asahq.org/…/Standard>, (Accessed December 24, 2014).
57. Godwin SA, Burton JH, Gerardo CJ, et al: Clinical policy: procedural sedation and analgesia in the emergency department. *Ann Emerg Med* 63:247–277, 2014.
58. Field JM, Hazinski MF, Sayre MR, et al: 2010 American Heart Association guidelines for cardiopulmonary resuscitation and emergency cardiovascular care: executive summary. *Circulation* 122(Suppl 3):S640–S656, 2010.

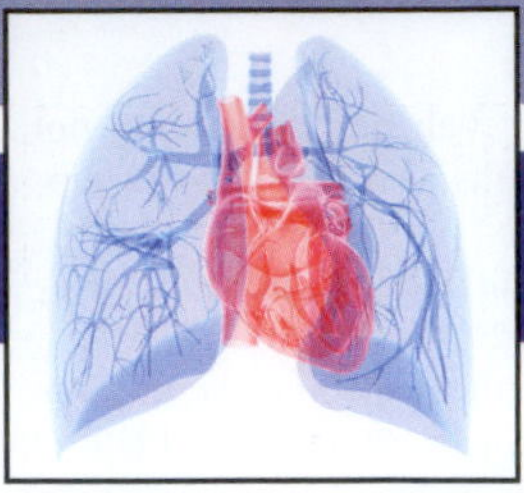

CHAPTER 20

Pulmonary Function Testing

ZAZA COHEN

CHAPTER OBJECTIVES

After reading this chapter you will be able to:

- List the three categories of pulmonary function tests.
- State the primary purposes of pulmonary function testing.
- Describe the pathophysiologic patterns associated with obstructive and restrictive lung disease.
- State what is meant by the term *spirometer,* and list the parameters that can be measured by it.
- List and describe the four general principles that should be considered for pulmonary function tests.
- List and describe the measurements that indicate pulmonary mechanics.
- Describe the purpose and technique for the bronchoprovocation test.
- List and describe the four volumes and four capacities that can be measured with pulmonary function testing.
- Describe the purpose and techniques used to measure diffusing capacity.
- Interpret pulmonary function reports.

CHAPTER OUTLINE

Pulmonary Function Testing
- Purposes
- Pathophysiologic Patterns
- Infection Control
- Equipment

Principles of Measurement and Significance
- Spirometry
- Lung Volumes and Capacities
- Diffusing Capacity

Interpretation of the Pulmonary Function Report

KEY TERMS

compliance
diffusing capacity of the lung
diffusing capacity of the lung for carbon monoxide
diffusing capacity of the lung-to–effective total lung capacity ratio
effective total lung capacity
expiratory reserve volume
forced expiratory flow between 25% and 75% of forced vital capacity ($FEF_{25\%-75\%}$)
forced expiratory flow between 75% and 85% of forced vital capacity ($FEF_{75\%-85\%}$)
forced expiratory flow between 200 ml and 1200 ml of FVC ($FEF_{200-1200}$)
forced expiratory volume in 1 second (FEV_1)
forced expiratory volume in 1 second-to-vital capacity ratio (FEV_1/FVC)
forced expiratory volume in half of a second ($FEV_{0.5}$)
forced vital capacity
functional residual capacity
inspiratory capacity
inspiratory reserve volume
maximal voluntary ventilation
minute ventilation
obstructive pulmonary disease
peak expiratory flow rate
residual volume
restrictive pulmonary disease
thoracic gas volume
tidal volume
total lung capacity
vital capacity

The most important function of the lungs is gas exchange. As mixed venous blood passes through the pulmonary circulation, the lungs add oxygen and remove excess carbon dioxide. The ability of the lungs to perform gas exchange depends on the following four general physiologic functions:

1. The diaphragm and thoracic muscles must be capable of expanding the thorax and lungs to produce a subatmospheric pressure.
2. The airways must be unobstructed to allow gas to flow into the lungs and reach the alveoli.
3. O_2 and CO_2 must be able to diffuse through the alveolar-capillary membrane.
4. The cardiovascular system must circulate blood through the lungs and ventilated alveoli.

Pulmonary function tests can provide valuable information about these important individual processes that support gas exchange. Various measurements are available to aid in the diagnosis and assessment of pulmonary diseases, to determine the need for therapy, and to evaluate the effectiveness of respiratory care. For respiratory therapists (RTs), knowledge of these tests and the ability to interpret the measurements are essential for assessing patients objectively and for planning and implementing effective patient care. The key terms used in this chapter are terms adopted and defined by the pulmonary medical community and should become the standard vocabulary of all RTs.[1]

PULMONARY FUNCTION TESTING

A complete evaluation of the respiratory system includes a patient history, physical examination, radiographic imaging, arterial blood gas analysis, and tests of pulmonary function. Test results become most meaningful when considered in the context of a complete clinical evaluation. Although diagnostic pulmonary function testing is performed in a laboratory setting and usually only on patients in a stable condition, RTs also perform many of these tests at the bedside on patients who are acutely ill or being evaluated for surgical readiness. There are three categories of pulmonary function tests, measuring (1) dynamic flow rates of gases through the airways, (2) lung volumes and capacities, and (3) the ability of the lungs to diffuse gases. A combination of these measurements provides a quantitative picture of lung function. Although pulmonary function tests do not diagnose specific pulmonary diseases, these tests identify the presence and type of pulmonary impairments and the degree of pulmonary disease present. Some basic tests of pulmonary function are often performed at the bedside to provide immediate information about the need for respiratory therapy and its effectiveness.

Purposes

Generally, the primary purposes of pulmonary function testing are to identify pulmonary impairment and quantify the severity of pulmonary impairment if present.[2] Pulmonary function testing has diagnostic and therapeutic roles and helps clinicians answer some general questions about patients with lung disease (Box 20-1).

Box 20-1 Basic Diagnostic and Therapeutic Questions for Clinical Pulmonary Function Testing

DIAGNOSTIC
- Is lung disease present?
- What type of lung impairment is present?
- What is the degree of lung impairment?
    - Is more than one type of lung impairment present?
    - Can multiple lung diseases be separated?

THERAPEUTIC
- Is therapy indicated?
- What treatments are most effective?
- To what degree is the disease reversible?
- Can treatments be evaluated?
- Is rehabilitation feasible?

The indications for pulmonary function testing are as follows[2-5]:

- *To identify and quantify changes in pulmonary function.* The most common purposes of pulmonary function testing are to detect the presence or absence of pulmonary disease, to classify the type of disease as either obstructive, restrictive, or both (mixed), and to quantify the severity of pulmonary impairment as mild, moderate, severe, or very severe. Over time, pulmonary function tests help quantify the progression or the reversibility of the disease.
- *To evaluate need and quantify therapeutic effectiveness.* Pulmonary function tests may aid clinicians in selecting or modifying a specific therapeutic regimen or technique (e.g., bronchodilator medication, airway clearance therapy, rehabilitation exercise protocol). Clinicians and researchers use pulmonary function tests to measure changes in lung function objectively before and after treatment.
- *To perform epidemiologic surveillance for pulmonary disease.* Screening programs may detect pulmonary abnormalities caused by disease or environmental factors in general populations, in people in occupational settings, in smokers, or in other high-risk groups. In addition, researchers have determined what normal pulmonary function is by measuring the pulmonary function of healthy people.
- *To assess patients for risk for postoperative pulmonary complications.* Preoperative testing can identify patients who may have an increased risk for pulmonary complications after surgery. Sometimes the risk for complications can be reduced by preoperative respiratory care, or in some cases, the risk may be significant enough to rule out surgery.
- *To determine pulmonary disability.* Pulmonary function tests can also determine the degree of disability caused by lung diseases, such as occupational asthma or coal workers' pneumoconiosis. Some federal entitlement programs and insurance policies rely on pulmonary function tests to confirm claims for financial compensation.

There are also contraindications to pulmonary function testing.[2,6] Patients with acute, unstable cardiopulmonary problems, such as hemoptysis, pneumothorax, myocardial infarction, pulmonary embolism, and patients with acute chest or abdominal pain should not be tested. Patients who have nausea and who have recently vomited should not be tested because there is a risk of aspiration. Testing for patients who have had recent cataract removal surgery should be delayed because changes in ocular pressure may be harmful to the eye. Pulmonary function testing requires patient effort and cooperation. Patients with dementia or confusion may not achieve optimal or repeatable results. Pulmonary function testing should not be performed if valid and reliable results cannot be predicted. In patients who are acutely ill or who have recently smoked a cigarette, the test validity of measuring the **forced vital capacity** (FVC) may be hindered.

Pathophysiologic Patterns

Pulmonary function testing provides the basis for classifying pulmonary diseases into two major categories, **obstructive pulmonary disease** and **restrictive pulmonary disease**. These two types of lung diseases sometimes occur together as a mixed impairment. Obstructive and restrictive types of lung diseases differ in several important ways. Figure 20-1 shows normal lungs with the pathophysiologic aspects of obstructive lung diseases and restrictive lung diseases, and the differences are summarized in Table 20-1. The primary problem in obstructive pulmonary disease is an increased airway resistance (R_{aw}). R_{aw} is the difference in pressure between the ends of the airways divided by the flow rate of gas moving through the airway, according to the following formula:

$$R_{aw} = \frac{\Delta P}{\dot{V}}$$

There is an inverse relationship between R_{aw} and flow rate $\dot{V}$. If the pressure difference is constant, a reduced flow rate indicates an increase in R_{aw}. Because the radius of the airways normally lessens slightly during expiration, flow rates are usually measured during expiration. According to Poiseuille's law (see Chapter 6), R_{aw} is inversely related to the radius (r) of the airways:

$$R_{aw} = \frac{8\eta l}{r^4}$$

The most important point of this formula is that a small decrease in airway radius (or diameter) leads to exponential increase in the airway resistance. Airway radius can be reduced by excessive contraction of the bronchial and bronchiolar muscles (bronchospasm), excessive secretions in the airways, swelling of the airway mucosa, airway tumors, collapse of the bronchioles, and other causes. By measuring flow rates, pulmonary function tests measure R_{aw}, estimate the size of the airways, and indicate the presence of obstructive disease.

The primary problem in restrictive lung disease is reduced lung compliance, thoracic compliance, or both. **Compliance** is the volume of gas inspired per the amount of inspiratory effort; effort is measured as the amount of pressure created in the lung or in the pleural space when the inspiratory muscles contract. Compliance is calculated according to the following formula:

$$C = \frac{\Delta V}{\Delta P}$$

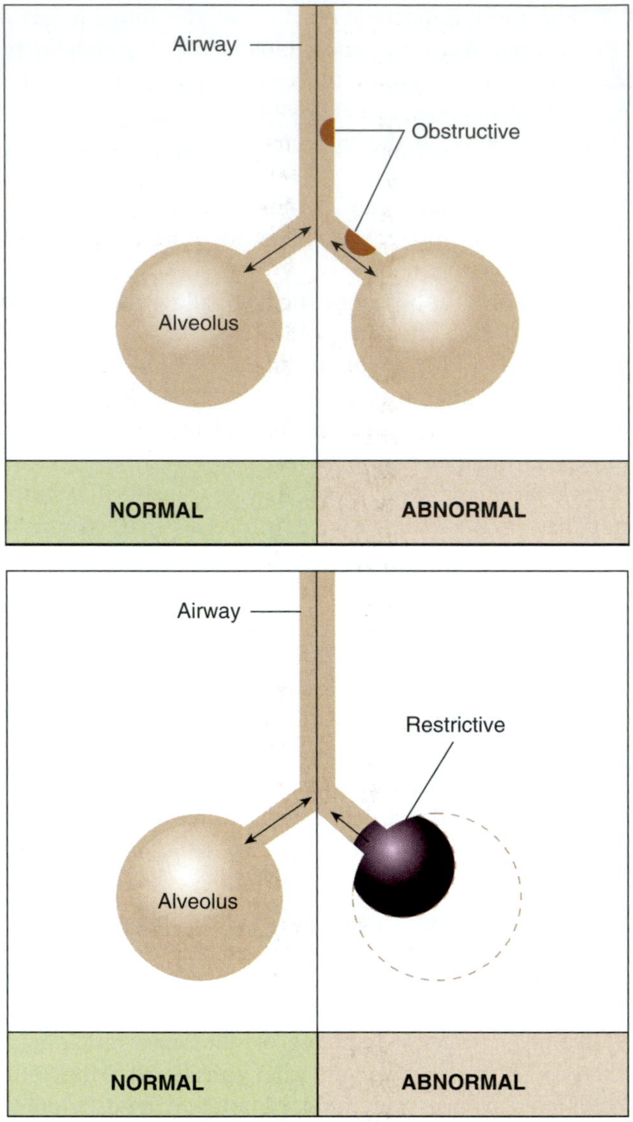

FIGURE 20-1 Pathophysiologic aspects of lung disease.

TABLE 20-1

Comparison of Obstructive and Restrictive Types of Pulmonary Diseases

Characteristic	Obstructive Disease	Restrictive Disease
Anatomy affected	Airways	Lung parenchyma, thoracic pump
Breathing phase difficulty	Expiration	Inspiration
Pathophysiology	Increased airway resistance	Decreased lung or thoracic compliance
Useful measurements	Flow rates	Volumes or capacities

There is a direct relationship between compliance (C) and volume (V). If the pressure difference is constant, a reduced inspiratory volume indicates a reduction in compliance. Reduced lung compliance is usually the result of alveolar inflammation (pneumonia), swelling (pulmonary edema), or scarring (pulmonary fibrosis); a reduced thoracic compliance may be the result of thoracic wall abnormalities, such as kyphoscoliosis, or exogenous pressure exerted on the thoracic cavity, such as ascites or pregnancy. Neuromuscular diseases also can result in reduced lung volumes and restrictive-type pulmonary impairments, mainly by affecting the function of the inspiratory muscles. In these circumstances, lung compliance and thoracic compliance may be normal, but the patient is unable to generate enough sub-atmospheric pressure to take a full, deep breath.

Some obstructive diseases and some restrictive diseases also may affect the ability of the lung to diffuse gases. In some diseases, there is damage to the alveolar-capillary membrane, or less alveolar surface area is accessible for diffusion. Measuring the **diffusing capacity of the lung for carbon monoxide** (DLCO) can identify the destruction of alveolar tissue or the loss of functioning alveolar surface area.

For each measurement of pulmonary function, there is a predicted value and upper and lower limit of normal (ULN, and LLN, respectively). It is expected that most healthy individuals would fall between the values of LLN and ULN. Measurements outside that range often indicates the presence of an abnormality. The severity of pulmonary impairment is based on a comparison of each patient's measurement with the predicted normal value for the patient. Several methods are used for comparison with the normal value. A common method of comparison is to compute a percentage of the predicted normal value according to the following equation:

$$\%\ \text{Predicted} = \frac{\text{Measured value}}{\text{Predicted normal value}} \times 100$$

The percent predicted value can be used to quantify severity of impairment. Typical degrees of severity are listed in Table 20-2.

Infection Control

Pulmonary function testing is generally regarded as a very low-risk procedure. However, there is potential to transmit infective microorganisms to patients and technologists.[2] Transmission can occur by direct or indirect contact. Standard precautions should be applied because of the potential exposure to saliva, mucus, or blood, which can harbor potentially hazardous microorganisms. Patients with oral lesions or active respiratory infections pose the greatest potential hazard, and patients with compromised immune systems are at the greatest risk. Practitioners should wear gloves when handling potentially contaminated mouthpieces, valves, tubing, and equipment surfaces. When performing procedures on patients with potentially infectious airborne diseases, practitioners should wear a personal respirator or a close-fitting surgical mask, especially if the testing induces coughing. Practitioners should always wash their hands between testing patients and after contact with testing equipment. Although it is unnecessary to clean the interior surfaces of the testing instruments routinely between patients,[2] the mouthpiece, nose clips, tubing, and any parts of the instrument that come into direct contact with a patient should be disposed, sterilized, or disinfected between patients. Any equipment surface showing visible condensation from exhaled air should be discarded, disinfected, or sterilized before reuse. When testing instruments are disassembled for cleaning and disinfecting, manufacturer recommendations should be considered and recalibration may be necessary before testing resumes. The routine use of low-resistance, in-line barrier filters is controversial.[2] Filters may be appropriate when internal surfaces of manifolds and valves proximal to mouthpieces are inaccessible or difficult to disassemble for cleaning and disinfecting. Filters provide visible evidence to reassure patients that their protection has been considered.

TABLE 20-2

Severity of Pulmonary Impairments Based on a Percentage of Predicted Normal Values

Degree of Impairment	Obstruction Based on FEV_1 (%)	Gas Exchange Based on DLCO (%)
Normal	80-120	80-120
Mild	70-79	61-79
Moderate	60-69	40-60
Moderately severe	50-59	
Severe	35-49	<40
Very severe	<35	

DLCO, Diffusing capacity of the lung for carbon monoxide.

Equipment

Pulmonary function testing requires measurement of gas volume or flow, and various instruments and measurement principles are used to make these measurements. There are two general types of measuring instruments: instruments that measure gas volume and instruments that measure gas flow. Both types of instruments simultaneously measure time, and both compute various volumes and flow rates used in pulmonary function testing. The term *spirometer* is sometimes used as a generic term for all volume-measuring and flow-measuring devices.

Volume-measuring devices are specifically called *spirometers* and include water-sealed, bellows, and dry rolling seal types. These devices expand as they collect gas volumes. The magnitude of the expansion is the *volume* measured, and the speed of expansion represents the *flow rate.* In the absence of leaks and with low-momentum forces, volume-measuring devices can be extremely accurate for measuring volumes, and with low inertia and friction forces, volume-measuring devices can be extremely accurate when computing flow rates.

Flow-measuring devices are commonly called *pneumotachometers,* although some practitioners reserve this term for only the device originally designed by Fleisch. These devices measure flow using a variety of unique principles. The Fleisch-type pneumotachometer measures the change in pressure as gas flows through it. Known as *thermistors* or *mass flowmeters,* another type of flow-measuring device measures the temperature change created by gas flowing through it. There are also *tubinometers,* which use rotation of a fan or blades similar to a windmill. Detailed descriptions and examples of each type of device are beyond the scope of this chapter.[7]

Regardless of the type of device or the principle of measurement used, several important characteristics are common to all measuring devices. Having an understanding of these common characteristics provides RTs the ability to select and use these devices properly. Every measuring instrument has capacity, accuracy, error, resolution, precision, linearity, and output. The ideal instrument would have unlimited capacity to measure every pulmonary parameter, and it would have perfect accuracy and precision over its entire measurement range. However, in real practice, there are no ideal instruments.

The *capacity* of an instrument refers to the range or limits of how much it can measure. Most instruments are designed with capacities to measure volumes and flow rates of all adults. The *accuracy* of a measuring instrument is how well it measures a known reference value. For volume measurements, standard reference values are provided by a graduated 3.0-L calibration syringe. No measuring instrument is perfect, and there usually is an arithmetic difference between reference values and measured values. This difference is called the *error. Accuracy* and *error* are opposing terms; the greater the accuracy, the smaller is the error. Accuracy and error are commonly expressed as percentages, with their sum always equaling 100%. To determine percent accuracy and percent error, several reference values are measured, and the mean of the measured values is computed and compared with the reference values. *Resolution* is the smallest detectable measurement; instruments with high resolution can measure the smallest volumes, flows, and times. *Precision* is synonymous with reliability (repeatability) of measurements and the opposite of variability. When multiple values are measured for a given test, the standard deviation of these values indicates the extent to which these values vary from the mean, and are therefore an indication of the precision of an instrument. A small standard deviation indicates low variability and high precision. *Linearity* refers to the accuracy of the instrument over its entire range of measurement, or its *capacity.* Some devices may accurately measure large volumes or high flow rates but may be less accurate when measuring small volumes or low flow rates. To determine linearity, accuracy and precision are calculated at different points over the range (capacity) of the device. *Output* includes the specific measurements made or computed by the instrument.

Most volume-measuring and flow-measuring devices measure the FVC and **forced expiratory volume in 1 second (FEV1).** Others calculate various forced expiratory flow (FEF) rates, and some measure tidal volume (V_T) and **minute ventilation** ($\dot{V}_E$). Diagnostic spirometers usually measure and calculate **vital capacity** (VC), FVC, FEV_1, **peak expiratory flow rate** (PEF), and FEF rates. Some measure and calculate **maximal voluntary ventilation** (MVV). Some of these instruments may be a component of a laboratory system providing the volume-measuring or flow-measuring capability for other diagnostic tests of pulmonary function. For example, they may be used with gas analyzers to measure **functional residual capacity** (FRC) and **total lung capacity** (TLC) or the inspiratory VC during *single-breath diffusing capacity (DLCO-SB).* Whether a spirometer or pneumotachometer is used in a diagnostic laboratory, a physician's office, or at the bedside in a hospital, it should meet or exceed the national performance standards for volume-measuring and flow-measuring devices.

In 1978, the American Thoracic Society (ATS) adopted the initial standards for diagnostic spirometers. These standards were most recently updated in 2005 in collaboration with the European Respiratory Society (ERS), are now recognized internationally as the standards for the industry,[2-4] and have been adopted by other medical organizations and government agencies. In clinical practice, RTs should use only devices that meet or exceed current ATS/ERS performance standards. The standards are summarized in Table 20-3. In addition, the spirometer standards also require spirometers to have a thermometer or to produce values corrected for body temperature, ambient pressure, and fully saturated with water vapor (BTPS). For quality control, the standards include verifying volume accuracy at least daily, although best practice in many laboratories is to verify accuracy before each test subject.

Most modern pulmonary function laboratories use computers for data acquisition and reproduction. Computer-assisted testing decreases the time necessary to complete the tests and enhances the effectiveness of pulmonary function testing by increasing accuracy, increasing patient acceptance, and

TABLE 20-3

2005 Spirometer Performance Standards of the American Thoracic Society/European Respiratory Society (ATS/ERS) Task Force

Test	Volume (L)	Flow (L/sec)	Accuracy	Time (sec)	Back Pressure (cm H_2O/L/sec)
VC	0.5-8 L	0-14	≤3% or 0.05 L*	30	
FVC	0.5-8 L	0-14	≤3% or 0.05 L*	15	<1.5%scm H_2O/L/sec at 14 L/sec
FEV_1	0.5-8 L	0-14	≤3% or 0.05 L*	1	<1.5%scm H_2O/L/sec at 14 L/sec
PEF		0-14	≤10% or 0.3 L/sec*		<1.5%scm H_2O/L/sec at 14 L/sec
FEF		±14	≤5% or 0.2 L/sec*		<1.5%scm H_2O/L/sec at 14 L/sec
MVV	250 L/min at 2 L/breath		±10% or 15 L/min*	12-15	<1.5%scm H_2O/L/sec at 14 L/sec

From Miller MR, Hankinson J, Brusasco V, et al: Standardisation of spirometry. Eur Respir J 26:319, 2005.
*Whichever is greater.

monitoring patient performance. Although computer-assisted testing and interpretations of test results are often applied by a computer, pulmonary function testing always requires a trained and competent RT to administer the tests, and computer analysis should not replace human analysis.

PRINCIPLES OF MEASUREMENT AND SIGNIFICANCE

For tests of pulmonary function, these general principles should be considered: test sensitivity and specificity, validity, and reliability.

Sensitivity and specificity address the test's ability to detect disease, or absence of it, respectively. Some tests are extremely *sensitive,* and apparently healthy individuals may have an abnormal test result. However, some tests are not sensitive; individuals must be extremely sick to have an abnormal test result. Most tests of pulmonary function are not *specific* because several different diseases may cause the test result to be abnormal. This limitation of many pulmonary function tests explains why these tests identify a pattern of impairment rather than diagnose specific diseases.

Validity of the test relates to its meaningfulness or the ability to measure what it is intended to measure. When performing pulmonary function testing, strictly following testing procedures, ensuring patient effort and performance, and ensuring equipment accuracy and calibration establish test validity.

Reliability of the test is its consistency. A reliable test produces consistent test results with minimal variability. To be reliable, each test must be performed more than once. Ensuring test validity and reliability is the most important role of the RT. Test results that are invalid or unreliable can lead to misdiagnosis, mistreatment, and poor outcomes.

> **RULE OF THUMB**
>
> Never report test results that are invalid or unreliable.

There are three basic tests of pulmonary function: spirometry, lung volumes, and diffusing capacity. When the purpose of the testing is to identify the presence and the degree of pulmonary impairment and the type of pulmonary disease, all three testing components are required. When the purpose of the testing is more limited, such as to assess postoperative pulmonary risk or to evaluate and quantify therapeutic effectiveness, the scope of measurement also is limited.

General indications, contraindications, and potential complications of pulmonary function testing were briefly discussed at the beginning of this chapter. A complete listing of all indications, contraindications (absolute and relative), hazards, and complications, assessment of need and test quality, techniques and different types of equipment that make the measurements, and quality control measures is outside of the scope of this chapter. They are summarized in the corresponding American Association for Respiratory Care (AARC) Clinical Practice Guidelines and ATS/ERS included in the references for this chapter. Many pulmonary function laboratories also perform arterial blood gas analysis (see Chapter 19), and some laboratories provide more specialized and advanced tests, such as bronchial challenge tests and exercise stress tests.

Spirometry

Spirometry—the measurement of air entering and leaving the lungs—includes measurement of several values of forced airflow and volume during inspiration and expiration. For the most part, the purpose of spirometry is to assess the ability of the lungs to move large volumes of air quickly through the airways to identify airway obstruction. Some measurements are aimed at large intrathoracic airways, some are aimed at small airways, and some assess obstruction throughout the lungs. Measuring flow rates is a surrogate for measuring airways resistance, as discussed earlier in the chapter. To a lesser extent, spirometry can also identify and quantify a restrictive pattern of pulmonary disease. The major values measured during spirometry are discussed below.

Spirometry is an effort-dependent test that requires careful patient instruction, understanding, coordination, and cooperation. Spirometry standards for FVC specify that patients must be instructed in the FVC maneuver, that the appropriate technique be demonstrated, and that enthusiastic coaching occur.[3] When measuring FVC, the RT needs to coach the preceding **inspiratory capacity** (IC) as enthusiastically as the FVC. According to the standards, nose clips are encouraged, but not required and patients may be tested in the sitting or standing position. Although standing usually produces a larger FVC compared with sitting, sitting is considered safer in case of lightheadedness. It is recommended that the position be consistent for repeat testing of the same patient. FVC should be converted to body temperature conditions and reported as liters under BTPS conditions.

Except for PEF rate, all other measurements that originate from FVC come from the "best curve"—these include **forced expiratory flow between 200 ml and 1200 ml of FVC (FEF200-1200); forced expiratory flow between 25% and 75% of FVC ($FEF_{25\%-75\%}$); forced expiratory flow between 75% and 85% of FVC ($FEF_{75\%-85\%}$)**; and instantaneous $FEF_{25\%}$, $FEF_{50\%}$, and $FEF_{75\%}$. The *best test curve* is defined as the trial that meets the acceptability criteria and gives the largest sum of FVC plus FEV_1. The validity and reliability of these other measurements of pulmonary mechanics are based on their origin from a valid and reliable FVC. (See AARC Clinical Practice Guideline 20-1.)

Forced Vital Capacity

FVC is the most commonly performed test of pulmonary mechanics, and many measurements are made while the patient is performing the FVC maneuver (Figure 20-2). Measuring FVC often occurs under baseline or untreated conditions. For baseline testing, patients should temporarily abstain from bronchodilator medications. Short-acting bronchodilators (e.g., beta agonist: albuterol; anticholinergic agent: ipratropium bromide)

20-1 Spirometry

AARC Clinical Practice Guideline (Excerpts)*

INDICATIONS

The indications for spirometry include the need to do the following:

Detect the presence or absence of lung dysfunction suggested by history or physical signs and symptoms or the presence of other abnormal diagnostic tests (e.g., chest radiograph, arterial blood gases).

- Quantify the severity of known lung disease.
- Assess the change in lung function over time or after administration of or change in therapy.
- Assess the potential effects or response to environmental or occupational exposure.
- Assess the risk for surgical procedures known to affect lung function.
- Assess impairment or disability (e.g., for rehabilitation, legal reasons, military).

CONTRAINDICATIONS

Circumstances listed here could affect the reliability of spirometry measurements. In addition, forced expiratory maneuvers may aggravate these conditions, which may make test postponement necessary until the medical condition resolves. The following are some relative contraindications to performing spirometry:

- Hemoptysis of unknown origin (forced expiratory maneuver may aggravate the underlying condition)
- Pneumothorax
- Unstable cardiovascular status (forced expiratory maneuver may worsen angina or cause changes in blood pressure) or recent myocardial infarction or pulmonary embolus
- Thoracic, abdominal, or cerebral aneurysms (danger of rupture resulting from increased thoracic pressure)
- Recent eye surgery (e.g., cataract)
- Presence of an acute disease process that might interfere with test performance (e.g., nausea, vomiting)
- Recent surgery of thorax or abdomen

HAZARDS AND COMPLICATIONS

Although spirometry is a safe procedure, untoward reactions may occur, and the value of the test data should be weighed against potential hazards. The following have been reported anecdotally:

Pneumothorax

- Paroxysmal coughing
- Increased intracranial pressure
- Contraction of nosocomial infections
- Syncope, dizziness, lightheadedness
- O_2 desaturation resulting from interruption of O_2 therapy
- Chest pain
- Bronchospasm

ASSESSMENT OF NEED

Need is assessed by determining that valid indications are present.

ASSESSMENT OF TEST QUALITY

Spirometry performed for the listed indications is valid only if the spirometer functions acceptably and the subject is able to perform the maneuvers in an acceptable and reproducible fashion. All reports should contain a statement about the technician's assessment of test quality and specify which acceptability criteria were not met.

QUALITY CONTROL

Volume verification (i.e., calibration): At least daily before testing, use a calibrated known-volume syringe with a volume of at least 3 L to ascertain that the spirometer reads a known volume accurately. The known volume should be injected or withdrawn at least three times, at flows that vary between 2 L/sec and 12 L/sec (3-L injection times of approximately 1 second, 6 seconds, and between 1 second and 6 seconds). The tolerance limits for an acceptable calibration are ±3% of the known volume. For a 3-L calibration syringe, the acceptable recovered range is 2.91 to 3.09 L. The practitioner is encouraged to exceed this guideline whenever possible (i.e., reduce the tolerance limits to less than ±3%).

- Leak test: Volume-displacement spirometers must be evaluated for leaks daily. One recommendation is that any volume change of more than 10 ml/min while the spirometer is under at least 3 cm H_2O pressure be considered excessive.
- A spirometry procedure manual should be maintained.
- A log that documents daily instrument calibration, problems encountered, corrective action required, and system hardware or software changes should be maintained.
- Computer software for measurement and computer calculations should be checked against manual calculations, if possible. In addition, biologic laboratory standards (i.e., healthy, nonsmoking individuals) can be tested periodically to ensure historic reproducibility, to verify software upgrades, and to evaluate new or replacement spirometers.
- The known-volume syringe should be checked for accuracy at least quarterly using a second known-volume syringe, with the spirometer in the patient-test mode; this validates the calibration and ensures that the patient-test mode operates properly.
- For water-seal spirometers, water level and paper tracing speed should be checked daily. The entire range of volume displacement should be checked quarterly.

QUALITY ASSURANCE

Each laboratory or testing site should develop, establish, and implement quality assurance indicators for equipment calibration and maintenance and patient preparation.

Methods should be devised and implemented to monitor technician performance (with appropriate feedback) while obtaining, recognizing, and documenting acceptability criteria.

MONITORING

The following should be evaluated during the performance of spirometric measurements to ascertain the validity of the results:

- Acceptability of maneuver and reproducibility of FVC and FEV_1
- Level of effort and cooperation by the subject
- Equipment function or malfunction (e.g., calibration)
- The final report should contain a statement about test quality.
- Spirometry results should be subject to ongoing review by a supervisor, with feedback to the technologist.
- Quality assurance or quality improvement programs should be designed to monitor technician competency initially and in an ongoing fashion.

*For the complete guideline, see American Association for Respiratory Care: Clinical practice guideline: spirometry. 1996 update.

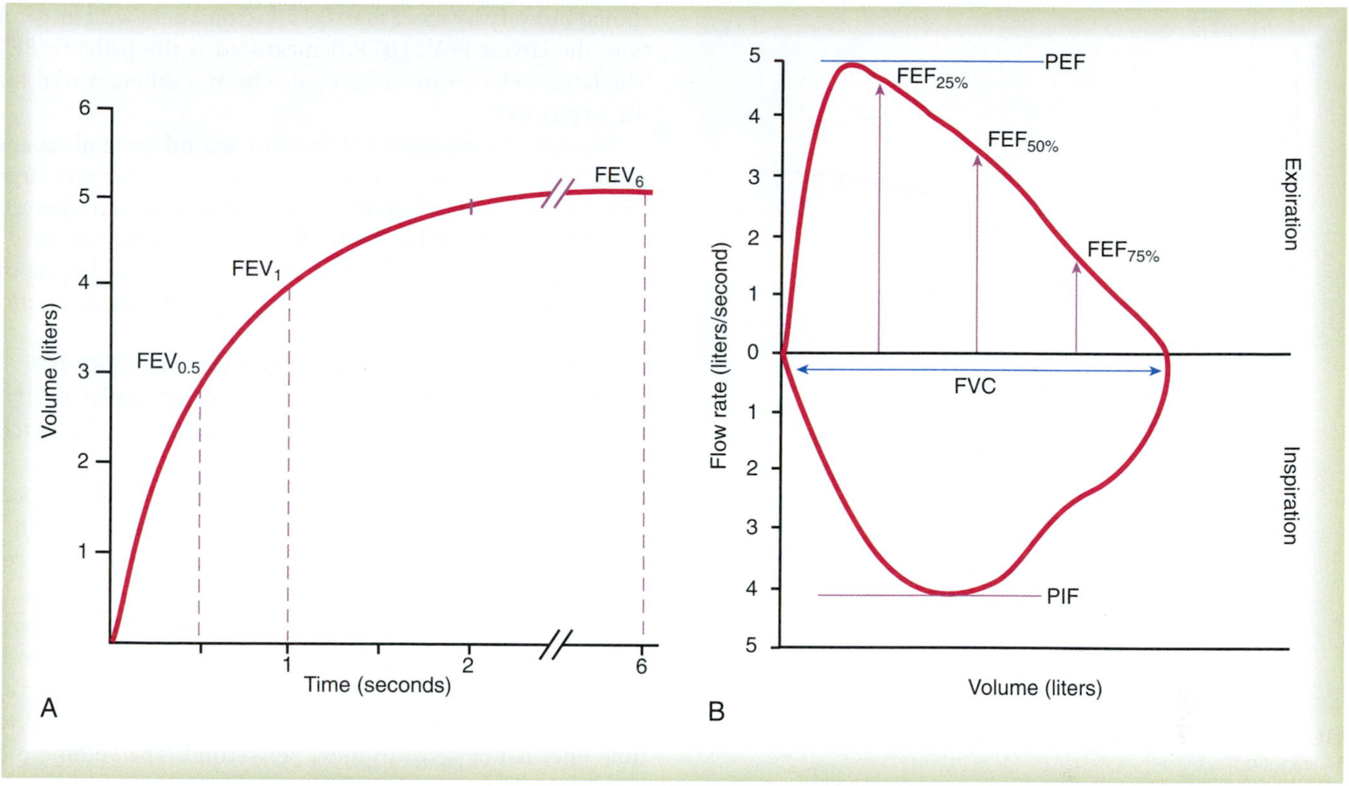

FIGURE 20-2 Forced vital capacity, forced expiratory volumes, and flow rates. **A,** Forced vital capacity on a volume-time graph. **B,** Forced vital capacity on a flow-volume graph. *PEF,* Peak expiratory flow; *PIF,* peak inspiratory flow.

should not be used for 4 hours before baseline spirometry, whereas long-acting beta-agonist bronchodilators and oral therapy with aminophylline should be stopped for 12 hours. When a patient's baseline results show airway obstruction, performing FVC after treatment (e.g., albuterol bronchodilator aerosol or metered dose inhaler) can help determine if the treatment is effective. The FVC maneuver is also performed repeatedly during bronchial provocation testing.

FVC may be measured on a spirometer that reveals volumes or flows, that presents a graph of volume and time or flow and volume, that is mechanical or electronic, and that has a calculator or computer. The forced expiratory VC sometimes is followed by a forced inspiratory VC to produce a complete image of forced breathing called a *flow-volume loop* (see Figure 20-2, *B*).

RULE OF THUMB

If you do not inhale it, you cannot exhale it. So, coach the preceding IC as enthusiastically as the FVC.

To ensure validity, each patient must perform a minimum of three acceptable FVC maneuvers. To ensure reliability, the largest FVC and second largest FVC from the acceptable trials should not vary by more than 0.15 L. To perform an FVC trial, the patient should inhale rapidly and completely to TLC from the resting FRC level. The forced exhalation of an acceptable FVC trial should begin abruptly and without hesitation. A satisfactory start of expiration is defined as an extrapolated volume at the zero time point less than 5% of FVC or 0.15 L, whichever is greater (Figure 20-3). The volume exhaled before the zero time point is called the *extrapolated volume.* To be valid, no more than 5% of the VC or 0.15 L is allowed to be exhaled before the zero time point. An acceptable FVC trial also is smooth, continuous, and complete. A cough, an inspiration, a Valsalva maneuver, a leak, or an obstructed mouthpiece while an FVC maneuver is being performed disqualifies the trial. FVC must be completely exhaled or an exhalation time of at least 6 seconds must occur for adults and children older than 10 years (longer times are commonly needed for patients with airway obstruction). A 3-second exhalation is acceptable for children younger than 10 years old. An end-expiratory plateau must be obvious in the volume-time curve (see Figure 20-3); the objective standard is less than 0.025 L exhaled during the final second of exhalation. Consistent with its definition, the largest acceptable FVC (BTPS) measured from the set of three acceptable trials is the patient's FVC.

Forced Expiratory Volume in 1 Second

During FVC testing, several other measurements are also made. FEV_1 is a measurement of the volume exhaled in the first second of FVC (see Figure 20-2, *A*). To ensure validity of FEV_1, the measurement must originate from a set of three acceptable FVC trials. The first second of forced exhalation begins at the zero time point (see Figure 20-3). To ensure reliability of FEV_1, the largest FEV_1 and second largest FEV_1 from the acceptable trials

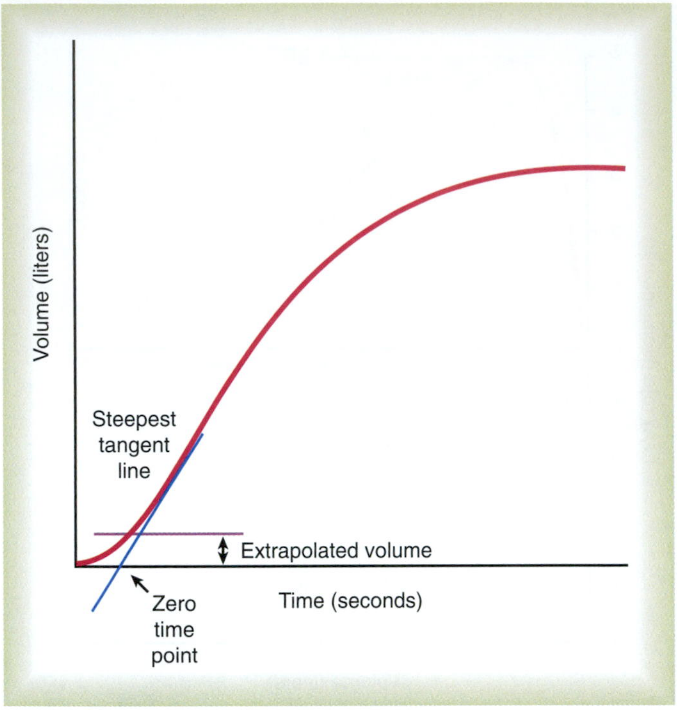

FIGURE 20-3 Extrapolated volume and zero time point determination.

should not vary by more than 0.15 L. Consistent with its definition, the largest FEV_1 (BTPS) measured is the patient's FEV_1. The largest FEV_1 sometimes comes from a different trial than the largest FVC.

The **forced expiratory volume in 1 second-to-vital capacity ratio (FEV1/FVC),** is calculated by dividing the patient's largest FEV_1 by the patient's largest VC and converting it to a percentage (by multiplying by 100). The two values do not have to come from the same trial; the VC should be the largest one measured, even if measured as a slow VC or during inspiration.

Forced Expiratory Flow Between 200 ml and 1200 ml of Forced Vital Capacity and Forced Expiratory Flow Between 25% and 75% of Forced Vital Capacity

$FEF_{200\text{-}1200}$ and $FEF_{25\%\text{-}75\%}$ represent average flow rates that occur during specific intervals of FVC. Both measurements can be made on a volume-time spirogram as the slope of a line connecting the two points in their subscripts. For $FEF_{200\text{-}1200}$, the 200-ml point and the 1200-ml point are identified. A straight line is drawn connecting these points, and the line is extended to intersect two vertical time lines 1 second apart on the graph (Figure 20-4). The volume of air measured between the two time lines is $FEF_{200\text{-}1200}$ in liters per second. The volume measured must be corrected to BTPS.

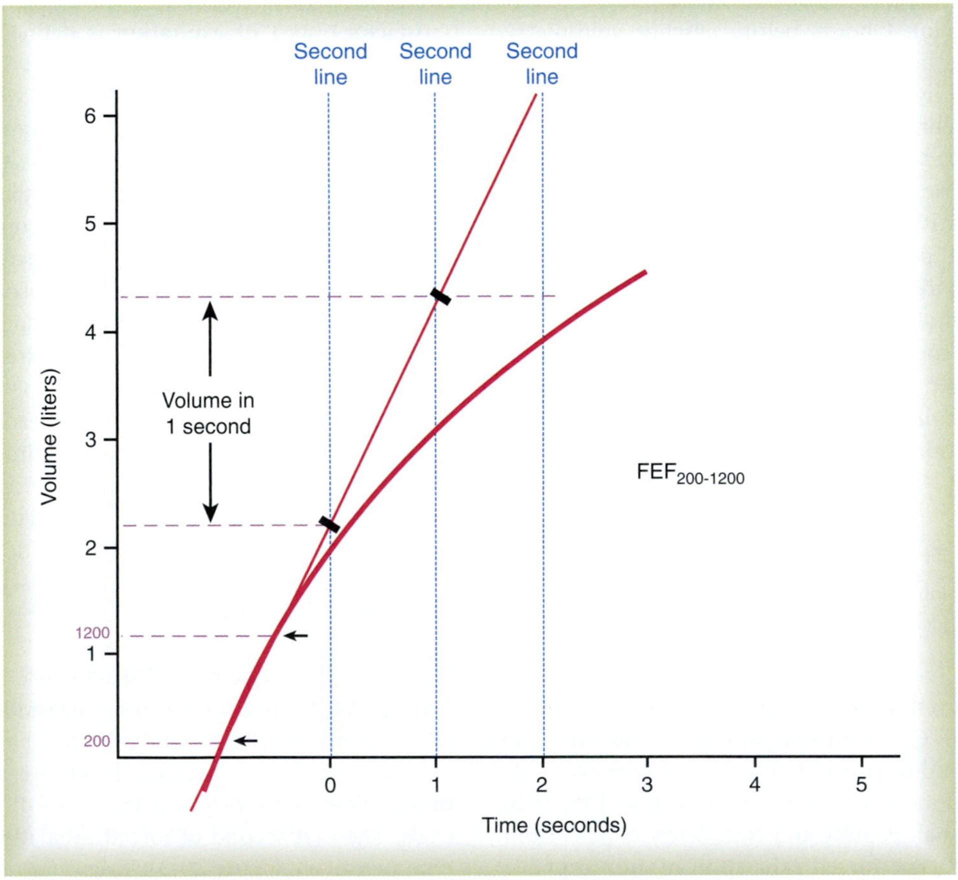

FIGURE 20-4 Forced expiratory flow rate 200 to 1200 ml.

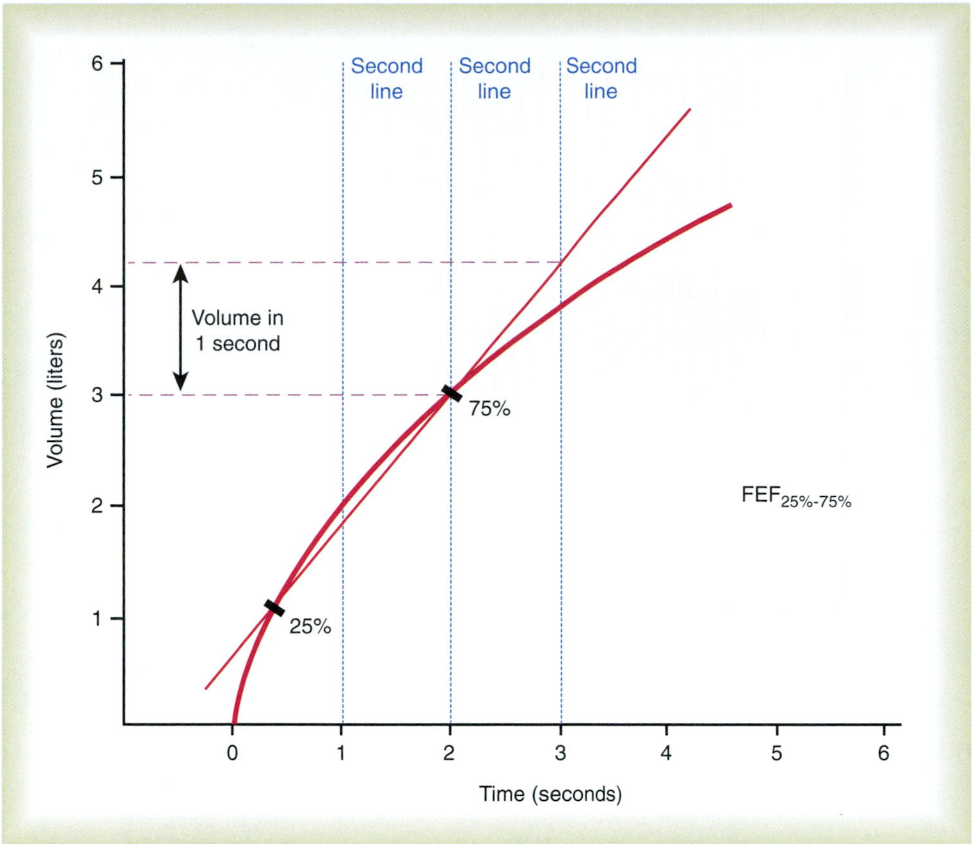

FIGURE 20-5 Forced expiratory flow (FEF) rate 25% to 75% of the forced vital capacity.

$FEF_{25\%-75\%}$ is a measure of the flow during the middle portion of FVC, or the time necessary to exhale the middle 50%. For $FEF_{25\%-75\%}$, the VC of the best curve is multiplied by 25% and 75%, and the points are identified on the tracing. A straight line is drawn connecting these points, and the line is extended to intersect two vertical time lines 1 second apart on the graph. The volume of air measured between the two time lines is $FEF_{25\%-75\%}$ in liters per second. The volume measured must be corrected to BTPS (Figure 20-5).

Peak Expiratory Flow

PEF is difficult to identify on a volume-time graph of FVC. The peak flow is the slope of the tangent to the steepest portion of the FVC curve. PEF is easy to identify on a flow-volume graph as the highest point on the graph (see Figure 20-2, *B*). PEF is sometimes measured independently of FVC with a peak flow meter. These devices are designed to indicate only the greatest expiratory flow rate. The validity of PEF rate is based on a preceding inspiration to TLC and a maximal effort. The FVC principles of ensuring reliability should apply to measurements of PEF rate. The two largest repeated measurements should agree within 5%.

In addition to PEF rate, the other instantaneous flow rates, such as FEF at 25% ($FEF_{25\%}$) of FVC, forced expiratory flow at 50% ($FEF_{50\%}$) of FVC, and forced expiratory flow at 75% ($FEF_{75\%}$) of FVC, during FVC are graphed on a flow-volume curve. When FVC is followed by a forced inspiratory VC, a flow-volume loop is produced (see Figure 20-2, *B*). On the flow-volume loop, the maximal forced inspiratory flow rate at 50% ($FIF_{50\%}$) of VC can be measured and compared with $FEF_{50\%}$.

Maximal Voluntary Ventilation

Another measurement of pulmonary mechanics is maximal voluntary ventilation (MVV). It is another effort-dependent test for which the patient is asked to breathe as deeply and as rapidly as possible for at least 12 seconds. MVV is a test that reflects patient cooperation and effort, the ability of the diaphragm and thoracic muscles to expand the thorax and lungs, and airway patency. Because of the potential for acute hyperventilation and fainting or coughing, the patient should be seated. Measuring systems that incorporate rebreathing may minimize the effects of hyperventilation. After a demonstration of the expected breathing pattern is performed, the patient should be instructed to breathe as rapidly and as deeply as possible for at least 12 seconds. The patient's breathing is measured on a spirogram (Figure 20-6) or electronically for the specific number of seconds (t) and the volume (V) breathed when the MVV is converted to liters per minute. As with all volumes measured on a spirometer, the recorded values should be in BTPS conditions. The validity of MVV depends on the duration of the maneuver, which should be at least 12 seconds; the breathing frequency, which should be at least 90 breaths/min;

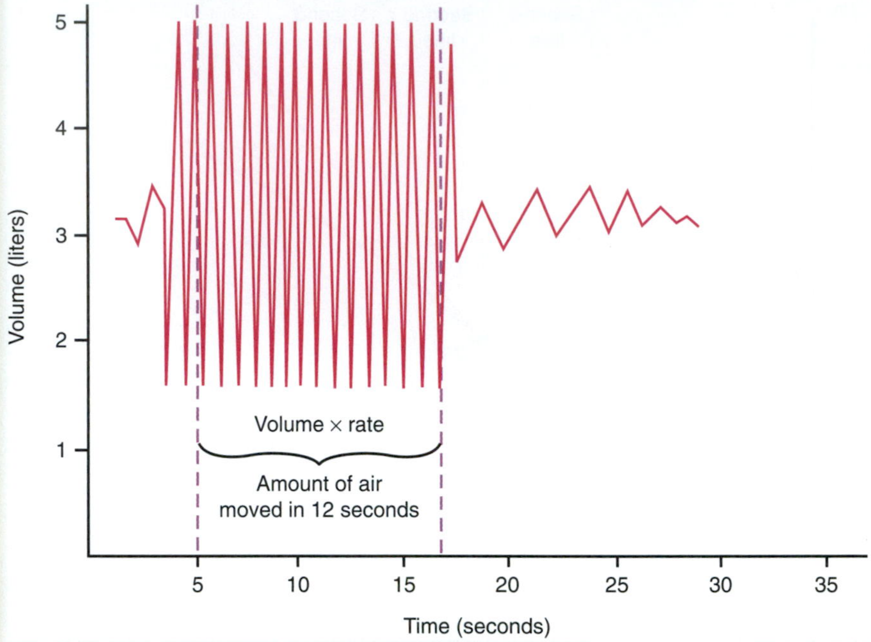

FIGURE 20-6 Maximal voluntary ventilation tracing. Actual ventilations recorded during a 12-second period.

and the average volume, which should be at least 50% of FVC. In addition, measured MVV should be compared to two other values: subject's $FEV_1 \times 40$, and predicted value for MVV. If the measured MVV is less than 80% of either of those values, a repeat test should be performed to ensure accuracy. Reliability is shown when there is less than 20% variability between the two largest trials. The largest MVV (BTPS) should be reported.

Other Values Obtained During Spirometry. During spirometry, a few additional measurements can be obtained, such as V_T, expiratory reserve volume (ERV), and IC. These values are usually interpreted in the context of other lung volumes (see later) and are discussed later in this chapter.

An important caveat during interpretation of spirometry values is the concept of "pseudorestriction." Some patients with obstructive lung disease will not be able to exhale a significant portion of their VC during forced maneuvers, leading to smaller than actual FVC measurement. These patients will have reduced FVC, will have reduced FEV_1, and may actually have normal FEV_1/FVC ratio, suggestive of restrictive physiology, hence the name *pseudorestriction*. In these patients, it is important to give them enough time to fully exhale by making sure that they reach a plateau at the end of FVC maneuver (see Figure 20-3) to allow proper measurement of FVC. Comparing FVC to slow vital capacity (SVC, see later) is another method of looking for obstructive physiology.

Interpretation

The normal values for the spirometric measurements of pulmonary mechanics are based on height, age, gender, and

MINI CLINI

Decreased Forced Vital Capacity and Forced Expiratory Volume in 1 Second: Is It Obstruction or Restriction?

PROBLEM: Both obstructive and restrictive diseases may exhibit decreased FVC and FEV_1. How can the two kinds of patterns be differentiated?

SOLUTION: FVC and FEV_1 are reduced in both obstructive and restrictive diseases for different reasons. With restrictive disease, lung expansion is reduced. If a person can inhale only a small volume, he or she can exhale only a small volume. All lung volumes are smaller than normal, including TLC, FVC, and FEV_1.

With obstructive disease, there is airway obstruction, which slows expiratory flow. FEV_1 is reduced because of the increased airway resistance, which decreases expiratory flow rates. FVC is reduced because airway obstruction in the bronchioles causes air trapping in the lung. If a person cannot exhale all of his or her air because some is trapped in the lungs, the volume the person does exhale is reduced.

To differentiate between obstructive and restrictive patterns of impairment, compare FEV_1 with FVC using the FEV_1/FVC ratio. Only individuals with airway obstruction exhale less than 70% of FVC in the first second. Individuals with restrictive disease or healthy lungs are able to exhale more than 70% of FVC during the first second. Therefore FEV_1/FVC less than 70% is often used as the sign of obstructive lung disease.

TABLE 20-4

Examples of Regression Equations for Predicted Normal Pulmonary Mechanics in White Adults

Parameters	Equations	R^2
Men ≥20 Years Old		
FVC (L)	$0.00018642\ (Ht)^2 + 0.00064\ (A) - 0.000269\ (A)^2 - 0.2033$	0.8668
FEV_6 (L)	$0.00018188\ (Ht)^2 - 0.00842\ (A) - 0.000223\ (A)^2 + 0.1102$	0.8692
FEV_1 (L)	$0.00014098\ (Ht)^2 - 0.01303\ (A) - 0.000172\ (A)^2 + 0.5536$	0.8510
% FEV_1/FVC	$88.066 - 0.2066\ (A)$	0.3448
$FEF_{200\text{-}1200}$ (L/sec)	$0.0429\ (Ht) - 0.047\ (A) + 2.010$	0.440
$FEF_{25\%\text{-}75\%}$ (L/sec)	$0.00010345\ (Ht)^2 - 0.04995\ (A) + 2.7006$	0.5601
PEF (L/sec)	$0.00024962\ (Ht)^2 + 0.08272\ (A) - 0.001301\ (A)^2 + 1.0523$	0.7808
$FEF_{25\%}$ (L/sec)	$0.088\ (Ht) - 0.035\ (A) - 5.618$	
$FEF_{50\%}$ (L/sec)	$0.069\ (Ht) - 0.015\ (A) - 5.4$	
$FEF_{75\%}$ (L/sec)	$0.44\ (Ht) - 0.012\ (A) - 4.143$	
MVV (L/min)	$1.20\ (Ht) - 0.816\ (A) - 37.9$	
Women ≥18 Years Old		
FVC (L)	$0.00014815\ (Ht)^2 + 0.01870\ (A) - 0.000382\ (A)^2 - 0.3560$	0.7344
FEV_6 (L)	$0.00014395\ (Ht)^2 + 0.01317\ (A) - 0.000352\ (A)^2 - 0.1373$	0.7457
FEV_1 (L)	$0.00011496\ (Ht)^2 - 0.00361\ (A) - 0.000204\ (A)^2 + 0.4333$	0.7494
% FEV_1/FVC	$90.809 - 0.2125\ (A)$	0.3955
$FEF_{200\text{-}1200}$ (L/sec)	$0.0570\ (Ht) - 0.036\ (A) - 2.532$	0.530
$FEV_{25\%\text{-}75\%}$ (L/sec)	$0.00006982\ (Ht)^2 - 0.02004\ (A) - 0.000200\ (A)^2 + 2.3670$	0.5005
PEF (L/sec)	$0.00018623\ (Ht)^2 + 0.06929\ (A) - 0.001031\ (A)^2 + 0.9267$	0.5559
$FEF_{25\%}$ (L/sec)	$0.043\ (Ht) - 0.025\ (A) - 0.132$	
$FEF_{50\%}$ (L/sec)	$0.035\ (Ht) - 0.013\ (A) - 0.444$	
$FEF_{75\%}$ (L/sec)	$3.042 - 0.014\ (A)$	
MVV (L/min)	$0.84\ (Ht) - 0.685\ (A) - 4.87$	

A, Age in years; *Ht,* height in centimeters.

ethnicity. Table 20-4 provides common regression equations to predict normal values for the measurements of pulmonary mechanics for individuals of specific height (in centimeters), age (in years), and gender.[8,9] A positive correlation exists between measurements of pulmonary mechanics and height, and a negative correlation exists between measurements of pulmonary mechanics and age for patients older than 20 years. Male values are larger than female values when height and age are equal. The populations that were studied to determine the normal values of pulmonary mechanics were predominantly white. To account for ethnic differences of nonwhites, the predicted normal values for whites commonly are reduced by 12% to 15% when applied to nonwhites. Ethnic-specific equations for special populations, such as African-Americans and Mexican-Americans, have also been developed.[8]

Although traditional textbooks suggest the typical normal VC is 4.80 L, the predicted normal FVC for a 20-year-old, 180-cm man approaches 5.60 L. A reduced FVC may occur with obstructive or restrictive impairments. Figure 20-7 shows FVC from volume-time spirometer tracings for normal, obstructive, and restrictive conditions. The FVC values in both the obstructed and the restricted curves are shown as reduced volumes compared with the normal curve. The primary difference between the curve in the restricted patient compared with the curve in the obstructed patient is the slope of the tracing; obstructive diseases produce flattened slopes and smaller FEV_1.

Figure 20-8 displays the FVC from flow-volume tracings for obstructive and restrictive conditions. The shapes of these tracings are different; obstructive diseases produce lower peaks and lower flow rates at all lung volumes. Forced inspiratory flow rates sometimes are useful for identifying extrathoracic airway obstructions. In moderate and severe obstructive lung diseases, the FVC is reduced if weakened bronchioles collapse and trap air in the lungs, creating an increase in residual volume. Some laboratories compare the volumes of SVC and FVC to identify air trapping. VC is reduced in restrictive lung diseases because the patient's inhaled volume is reduced.

Although FEV_1 is measured as a volume, it is considered a flow rate. The predicted normal FEV_1 for a 20-year-old, 180-cm man approaches 4.70 L. FEV_1 may be reduced with obstructive or restrictive impairments. For patients with airway obstruction, FEV_1 measures the general severity of airway obstruction. For patients with restrictive impairment, FEV_1 may be reduced when the patient's VC is smaller than the predicted FEV_1.

To interpret other flow rates, a generalization may be helpful. Gas exhaled during the early portion of the FVC reflects the resistance in the larger airways, and gas exhaled during the later portion of the FVC reflects the resistance in the smaller airways. As exhalation of FVC proceeds, flow decreases, and the airways reflected in the measurements get smaller. Any flow measured in the first half of the FVC reflects on the bronchi; any flow measured beyond 50% of the VC reflects on the bronchioles.

PEF, $FEF_{200\text{-}1200}$, and $FEF_{25\%}$ occur near the onset of FVC. A reduced PEF rate, $FEF_{200\text{-}1200}$, or $FEF_{25\%}$ may occur as a result of a large airway obstruction and from lack of sufficient effort to inhale maximally and exhale forcibly. $FEF_{25\%\text{-}75\%}$ and $FEF_{50\%}$

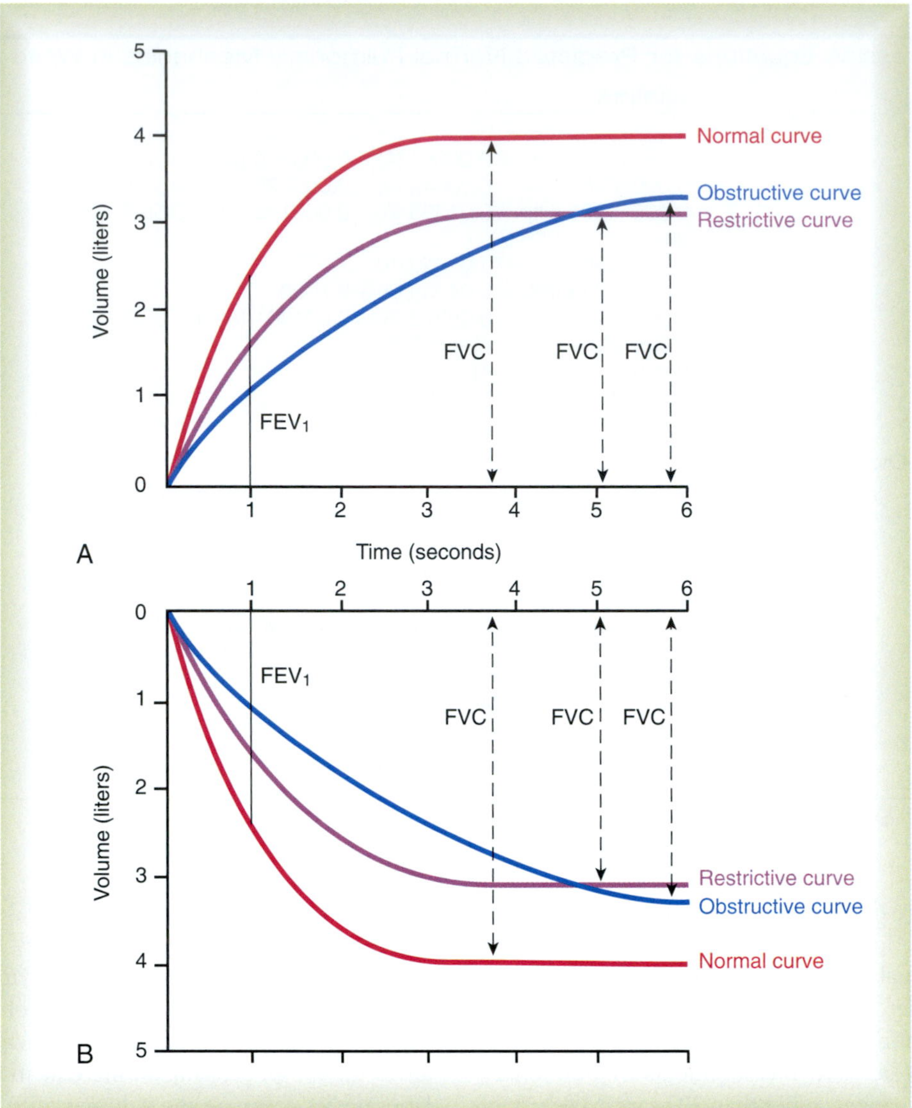

FIGURE 20-7 Forced vital capacity (FVC) curves comparing normal, obstructive, and restrictive disorders. **A,** Curves as they appear on commonly available spirometers with tracings beginning at the bottom left corner. **B,** The same curves as they appear on some spirometers with tracings beginning at upper left corner.

occur in the middle of FVC. Reduced $FEF_{25\%-75\%}$ or $FEF_{50\%}$ may occur because of small airway obstruction and from lack of effort to sustain a maximal exhalation. $FEF_{75\%}$ and $FEF_{75\%-85\%}$ occur late in FVC and reflect on the smallest airways. Experts differ on the significance of these flow rates. A singular reduction in small airway flow may indicate nothing at all or may be an early indicator of obstruction.

The shape of the flow-volume loop and the $FEF_{50\%}/FIF_{50\%}$ ratio provide additional information about upper airway obstruction. Compared with the normal flow-volume loop, a fixed upper airway obstruction produces a curve that appears box-shaped. In Figure 20-9, both expiratory and inspiratory flows are decreased and limited by the solid obstruction; the $FEF_{50\%}/FIF_{50\%}$ ratio remains normal. Variable upper airway obstructions produce two different shapes depending on the site of the obstruction. Because the intraairway pressure during a forced inspiration is less than atmospheric outside the thorax, a variable extrathoracic upper airway obstruction limits inspiratory flow, and the $FEF_{50\%}/FIF_{50\%}$ ratio is greater than 1.0. Because the intraairway pressure during a forced inspiration is greater than atmospheric pressure inside the thorax, a variable intrathoracic upper airway obstruction limits expiratory flow, and the $FEF_{50\%}/FIF_{50\%}$ ratio is less than 1.0.

Similar to other spirometric measurements of pulmonary mechanics, normal values of MVV are based on gender, age, and height. MVV is reduced in patients with moderate and severe airway obstruction. A measured value less than 75% of predicted is significant. The normal for men is approximately 160 to 180 L/min; it is slightly lower in women. In restrictive lung disease, MVV may be normal or only slightly reduced. Respiratory muscle strength is a primary determinant of MVV in patients with interstitial lung disease and an important determinant in patients with chronic obstructive pulmonary disease (COPD). Undernourished patients also may have a reduced MVV.

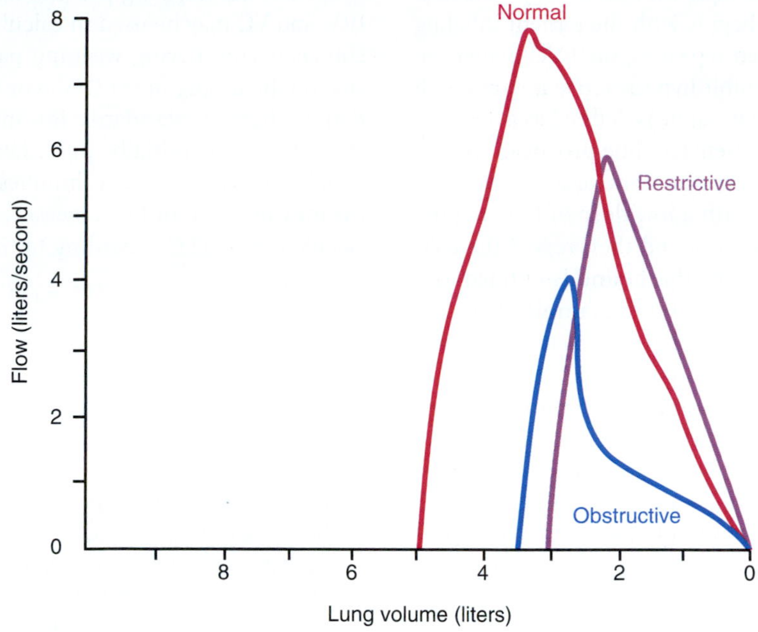

FIGURE 20-8 Maximal expiratory flow volume curves of normal, obstructive, and restrictive patterns.

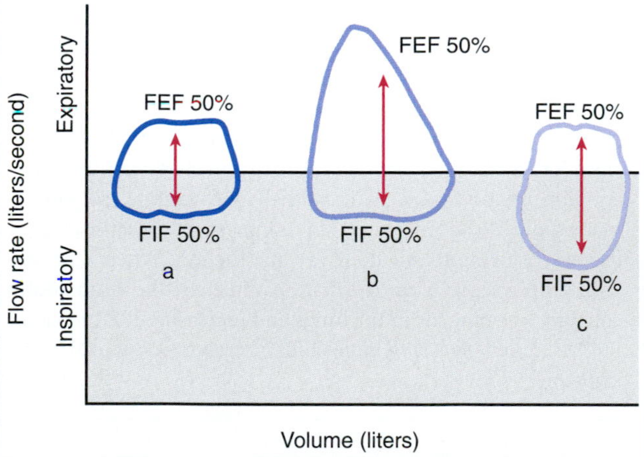

FIGURE 20-9 Flow-volume loops of fixed upper airway obstruction *(a)*, variable extrathoracic upper airway obstruction *(b)*, and variable intrathoracic upper airway obstruction *(c)*. *FEF,* Forced expiratory force; *FIF,* forced inspiratory flow.

RULE OF THUMB

If a person cannot exhale at least 70% of his or her VC in 1 second, it is highly likely the person has an obstructive disorder.

Reversibility

Based on the initial results of baseline spirometry, additional testing of pulmonary mechanics is often desirable. If the baseline test indicates airway obstruction, determining the reversibility of the obstruction is indicated. RTs also use the concept of reversibility when evaluating routine therapy by performing spirometry before and after therapy. In the laboratory, the FVC maneuver is often repeated after the patient has received a bronchodilator administered by small volume nebulizer or metered dose inhaler. This laboratory protocol is commonly known as *spirometry before and after bronchodilator*. Reversibility of the airway obstruction indicates effective therapy. Although improvement in other measurements of pulmonary function is sometimes used, reversibility is defined as a 15% or greater improvement in FEV_1 *and* at least a 200-ml increase in FEV_1. Improvement is determined using the percent change formula:

$$\%\,\text{Improvement} = \frac{\text{PostFEV}_1 - \text{PreFEV}_1}{\text{PreFEV}_1} \times 100$$

Bronchoprovocation

When the patient's history suggests episodic symptoms of hyperreactive airways and airway obstruction, such as seasonal or exercise-induced wheezing, and the results of baseline spirometry are normal, performing a bronchial provocation may be indicated.[10] Bronchial provocation testing uses an agent to stimulate a hyperreactive airway response and to create airway obstruction. Although several types of provocations are possible, such as inhaling histamine or cold air or exercising, provoking a hyperreactive airway response by inhaling methacholine is the most popular technique with the most predictable results. The procedure usually begins with the patient inhaling a normal saline aerosol and then repeating the FVC maneuver. Some very sensitive patients exhibit hyperreactive airways with saline alone; a positive response to saline is defined as a decrease in FEV_1 of 10% or greater. The methacholine provocation protocol systematically exposes the patient to increasing dosages of methacholine. Usually starting with a low dose of 0.03 mg/ml, patients inhale methacholine aerosol and then repeat the FVC maneuver. A *positive response* to methacholine is defined as a decrease in FEV_1 of 20% or greater (another example of percent change). If a positive response does not occur, the methacholine dose is doubled to 0.06 mg/ml, and the FVC maneuver is repeated. The process of "double-dosing" and performing FVC maneuvers continues until there is a positive response or until the full dose, 16 mg/ml, is given. If a positive response occurs, treatment with a fast-acting bronchodilator is indicated, and sometimes administering O_2 is helpful. The final test report should include the concentration of methacholine that caused the 20% decrease in FEV_1 in the form of $PD\%FEV_1$. For example, $PD_{22}FEV_1$ = 4 mg/ml indicates that the provocation dose of 4 mg/ml resulted in a 22% decrease in FEV_1.[10-12]

It should be noted that given the nature and goal of this test to induce bronchospasm, and in many cases do so in patients with a suspicion of preexisting lung disease, certain precautions need to be taken when performing a methacholine challenge. Most notably, it is imperative that an evidence-based protocol be in place to address patients who respond to the test adversely by developing status asthmaticus or other life-threading conditions. In general, the protocol should include the availability of fast-acting bronchodilators, a code/crash cart, and health care professionals who are trained in Advance Cardiac Life Support.

RULE OF THUMB

Normal pulmonary function values are predictably based on the subject's age, height, gender, ethnicity, and sometimes weight. Normal pulmonary function predictably declines with age older than 20 years.

Lung Volumes and Capacities

There are four lung volumes and four lung capacities. A lung capacity consists of two or more lung volumes. The lung volumes are **tidal volume** (V_T), **inspiratory reserve volume** (IRV), **expiratory reserve volume** (ERV), and **residual volume** (RV). The four lung capacities are TLC, IC, FRC, and VC. These volumes and capacities are shown in Figure 20-10. The lung volumes that can be measured directly with a spirometer or pneumotachometer include V_T, IC, IRV, ERV, and VC. Because the RV cannot be exhaled, the RV, FRC, and TLC must be measured using indirect methods.

Knowing TLC is necessary to identify patients with a restrictive pattern of pulmonary impairment. Measuring FRC is necessary to quantify hyperinflation, which may be associated with obstructive impairment. Calculating RV is necessary to gauge any air trapping present. Measurements of V_T, IC, ERV, IRV, and VC may be used in calculations of TLC or be useful to clinicians considering weaning parameters such as the rapid-shallow-breathing index (f/V_T) or inspiration goals of hyperinflation therapy. Standards for measuring lung volumes and capacities were initially published in 2005[4]; these standards focus primarily on the techniques to measure FRC. Following the measurement of FRC, measurements of ERV and VC enable calculation of TLC according to the formulas:

$$TLC = FRC + IC$$

or

$$TLC = (FRC - ERV) + VC$$

MINI CLINI

Why Are Functional Residual Capacity and Residual Volume Increased in Emphysema?

PROBLEM: In the advanced stages of pulmonary emphysema, FRC and RV are increased; in addition, VC is often decreased. Why do these changes occur?

SOLUTION: When the ventilatory muscles relax, the opposing forces of lung recoil and chest wall expansion determine the size of FRC. Emphysema is characterized by a destruction of elastic tissue in the lung, which causes a lower lung recoil force. When lung recoil forces decrease, as in emphysema, chest wall expansion forces predominate and the chest wall expands outward, pulling the lung with it. As the lung stretches to a larger volume, its recoil force increases, and eventually equilibrium is reestablished between the lung and chest wall. This new equilibrium occurs at an increased lung volume, so FRC is increased. RV is increased in emphysema because VC is decreased owing to small airway obstruction. When a person with emphysema tries to exhale completely, the bronchioles collapse, trapping air in the lungs and increasing RV. Increased FRC is called *hyperinflation,* and increased RV is called *air trapping.*

The V_T is measured directly from a spirogram (see Figure 20-10). For the purposes of ensuring test validity and standardization, the patient should be in a sitting or reclining position and wearing a nose clip. It sometimes takes the patient 1 to 2 minutes to be at rest and become accustomed to the nose clip and mouthpiece. The patient breathes through a tight-fitting mouthpiece until a normal, rhythmic breathing pattern is established. Because V_T varies normally from breath to breath, an average V_T is a more reliable measurement. In the laboratory, an average V_T sometimes is measured during 3 minutes of quiet breathing while the spirometer records volumes and graphs volume and time. At the bedside, an average V_T usually is

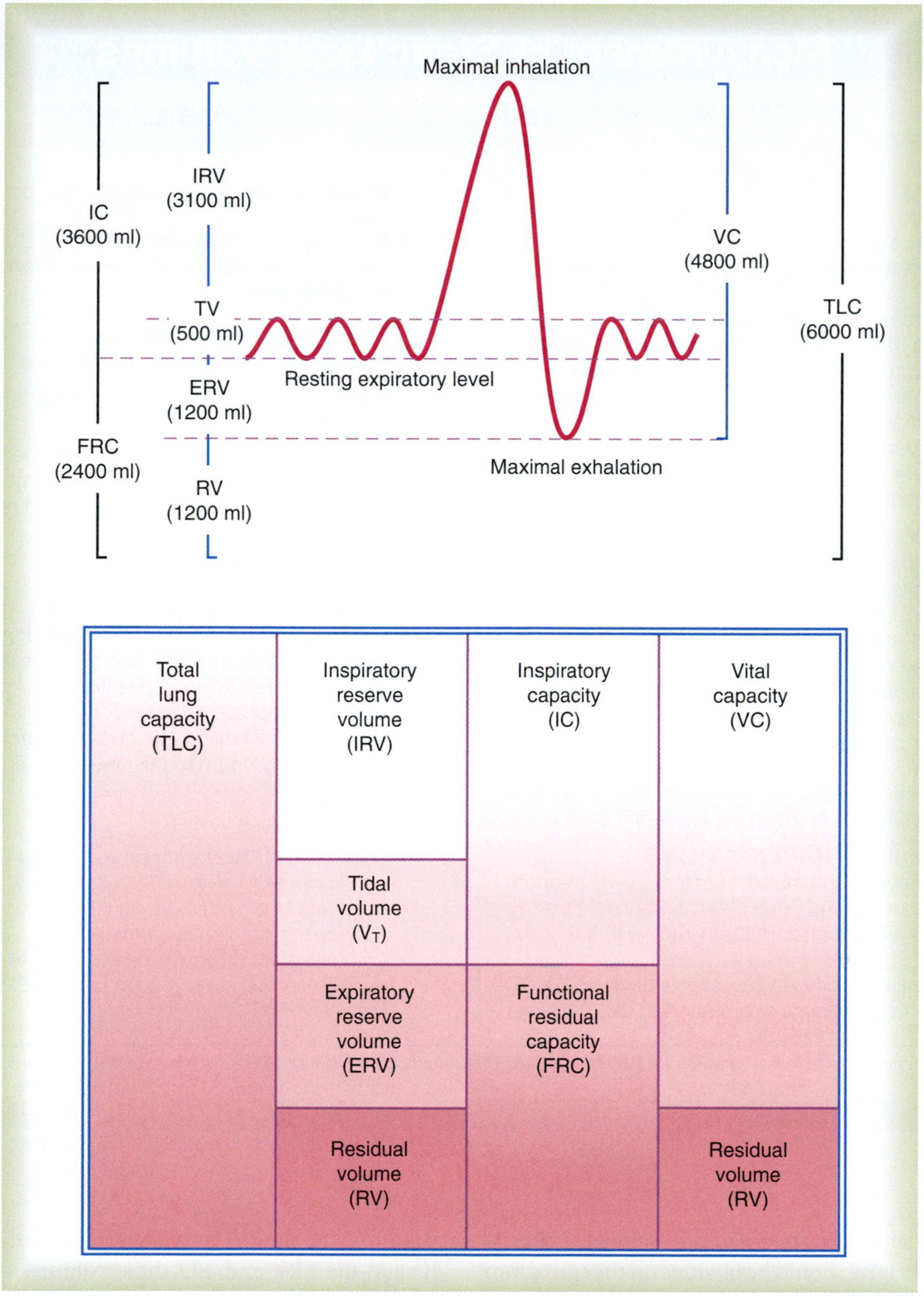

FIGURE 20-10 Lung volumes and capacities. Volumes listed are average normal values for a young, healthy adult man.

measured over 1 minute; the patient breathes normally into a spirometer that stores in memory each volume exhaled for 1 minute and computes an average. An alternative approach is to measure the total volume of air exhaled for 1 minute ($\dot{V}_E$) and divide by the breathing frequency (f) counted during the same period. The following formula can be used to calculate the V_T: $V_T = (\dot{V}_E \div f)$.

The IC is also measured directly from a spirogram. The patient is asked to inhale maximally from the resting FRC at the end of a normal effortless exhalation. To ensure validity, a consistent resting expiratory level should be obvious on the spirogram before inhaling. To ensure reliability, the IC should be measured at least twice, and the two largest measurements should agree within 5%. Because the definition of IC is the maximal volume inhaled, the largest measurement is the patient's IC. (See Clinical Practice Guideline 20-2.)

The ERV is measured directly from the spirogram (see Figure 20-10). The patient is asked to breathe normally for a few breaths and then exhale maximally. The ERV is the volume of air exhaled between the resting expiratory level and the maximal

20-2 Measurement of Static Lung Volumes

AARC Clinical Practice Guideline (Excerpts)*

INDICATIONS

Indications include the need to do the following:

- Diagnose restrictive disease patterns.
- Differentiate between obstructive and restrictive disease patterns.
- Assess response to therapeutic interventions (e.g., transplantation, radiation, chemotherapy, lobectomy).
- Aid in the interpretation of other lung function tests.
- Make preoperative assessments in patients with impaired lung function that would be affected by surgery.
- Evaluate pulmonary disability.
- Quantify the amount of gas trapping by comparing results of different techniques.

CONTRAINDICATIONS

- No apparent absolute contraindications exist; relative contraindications for spirometry include hemoptysis of unknown origin, untreated pneumothorax, unstable cardiovascular status, and thoracic and abdominal or cerebral aneurysms.
- With respect to whole-body plethysmography, factors such as claustrophobia, upper body paralysis, obtrusive body casts, or other conditions that immobilize or prevent the patient from fitting into or gaining access to the "body box" are a concern. In addition, the procedure may necessitate stopping intravenous therapy or supplemental O_2.

HAZARDS AND COMPLICATIONS

- Nosocomial infection contracted from improperly cleaned tubing, mouthpieces, and pneumotachographs.
- Hypoxemia from interruption of O_2 therapy with the body box.
- Depressed ventilatory drive in susceptible subjects (i.e., CO_2 retainers) as a consequence of breathing 100% O_2 during the nitrogen washout; such patients should be carefully observed.
- Hypercapnia and hypoxemia during helium-dilution FRC determinations as a consequence of failure to remove CO_2 or add O_2 adequately.

ASSESSMENT OF NEED

Determine that valid indications are present.

ASSESSMENT OF OUTCOME AND TEST QUALITY

- Outcome and test quality are determined by ascertaining that the desired information has been generated for the specific indication and that validity and reproducibility have been ensured.
- Results are valid if the equipment functions acceptably and the subject is able to perform the maneuvers in an acceptable and reproducible fashion.
- Report of test results should contain a statement by the technician performing the test about test quality (including patient understanding of directions and effort expended) and, if appropriate, which recommendations were not met.
- Equipment calibration and quality control measures specific to measuring lung volumes should be applied and documented.

MONITORING

The following should be monitored during lung-volume determinations:

- Test data of repeated efforts (i.e., reproducibility of results) to ascertain the validity of results
- The patient for any adverse effects of testing (patients on supplemental O_2 may require periods of time to rest on O_2 between trials)

**For the complete guideline, see American Association for Respiratory Care: Clinical practice guideline: static lung volumes: 2001 revisions and updates.*

exhalation level on the spirogram. To ensure validity, a consistent resting expiratory level should be obvious on the spirogram before exhaling maximally. To ensure reliability, the ERV should be measured at least twice and the two largest measurements should agree within 5%. Because the definition of ERV is the maximal volume exhaled, the largest measurement is the patient's ERV.

The VC is the most commonly measured lung volume. There are several methods of measuring the VC. The VC can be measured during inspiration or during a slow prolonged expiration when air trapping is of concern. To measure the VC during inspiration, the patient exhales maximally and then inhales as deeply as possible. The volume of the maximal inspiration is the inspiratory VC. To measure the VC during expiration, the patient inhales maximally and then exhales maximally, taking all the time necessary to exhale completely. The exhaled volume is the slow VC. An alternative method is to measure the IC and the ERV and add these volumes together for a "combined" VC, but this method should be reserved only for patients who cannot otherwise execute the VC. The VC also is measured when it is exhaled forcefully and as rapidly as possible. This technique is called the *FVC*, and it is used to assess pulmonary mechanics under the section spirometry.

Because the RV cannot be exhaled, RV, FRC, and TLC cannot be measured directly with a spirometer or pneumotachometer. There are three indirect techniques to measure these lung volumes: helium dilution, nitrogen washout, and body plethysmography. The He dilution and N washout techniques measure whatever gas is in the lungs at the beginning of the test, if the gas is in contact with unobstructed airways. The body plethysmographic technique measures all the gas in the thorax at the resting expiratory volume. Because the plethysmographic technique measures all gas in the thorax, including gas that is trapped distal to obstructed airways or gas in the pleural space, the lung volume measured by this technique is called the **thoracic gas volume** (TGV) (V_{TG}, or FRC_{Pleth}). In healthy individuals, TGV is identical to FRC measured by both the gas dilution and washout techniques. However, in patients with obstructive lung disease with gas trapping, TGV is often larger than FRC measured by other methods. TGV is also more complex and cumbersome to perform. Therefore, unless specifically requested by a physician, He dilution or N washout methods are routinely used. The latter two allow measurements of either FRC or TLC. Once one of them is measured, the other can be calculated using the previous formulas. For simplicity, we will only describe the maneuvers used to measure FRC below.[13] (See AARC Clinical Practice Guideline 20-2.)

Helium Dilution

The helium dilution technique for measuring lung volumes uses a closed, rebreathing circuit (Figure 20-11).[14-16] This technique is based on the assumptions that the patient has no He in his or her lungs, and that an equilibration of He can occur between the spirometer and the lungs. First, volume (V1) and concentration (C1) of He are measured at the beginning of the test. Next, the valve is turned to connect the patient to the breathing circuit, usually at the resting expiratory level of the FRC. The patient is connected to the He-air mixture, and the concentration of He is diluted slowly by the patient's lung volume. Wearing nose clips, the patient breathes normally in the closed circuit. Exhaled CO_2 is absorbed with soda lime, and O_2 is added at a rate equal to the patient's O_2 consumption. A constant volume is maintained to ensure accurate He concentration measurements. The patient rebreathes the gas in the system until equilibrium of He concentration is established. In healthy patients and patients with a small FRC, equilibration occurs in 2 to 5 minutes. Patients with obstructive lung disease may require 20 minutes to equilibrate because of slow gas mixing in the lungs. The He dilution time or the duration of the test is gives a reasonable indication of the distribution of ventilation.

For FRC to be calculated using the He dilution technique, several observations must be made: V1 and C1 (see earlier discussion), before the patient is connected to the breathing circuit; the final He concentration (C2) after He equilibrium between the spirometer and patient is established, the spirometer temperature, and the time necessary for He equilibration to occur. If there was no absorption of the He across the pulmonary capillaries,

$$V1 \times C1 = V2 \times C2$$

where V2 is the volume of the He at the end of the test. After measuring V1, C1 and C2, V2 is calculated: FRC = V2 − V1 (see Figure 20-11).

Corrections for temperature and He absorption are normally applied. All lung volumes and capacities must be reported under BTPS conditions. Volumes measured by spirometers are at ambient temperature, pressure, and saturated (ATPS) conditions and must be adjusted for the temperature difference between the spirometer and the patient's body temperature. This ATPS to BTPS adjustment can increase volumes 5% to 10%, and the difference is large enough to invalidate the test

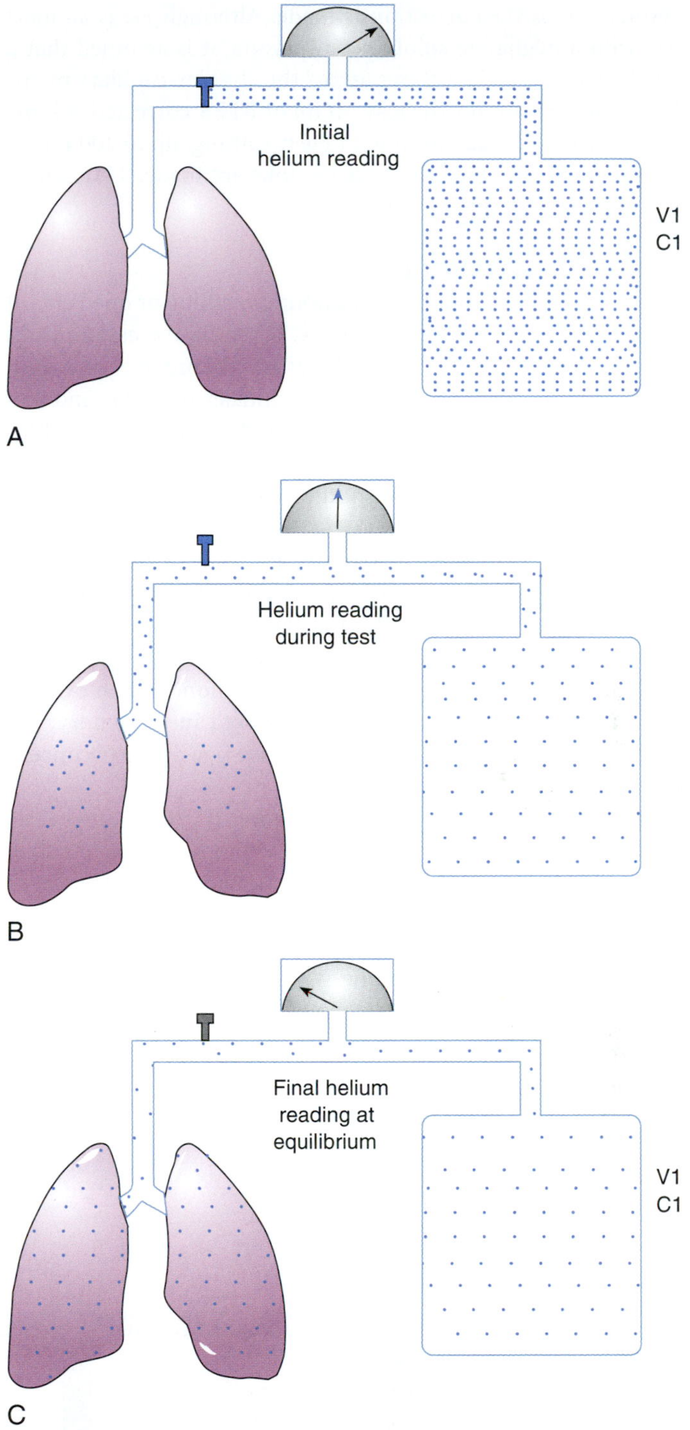

FIGURE 20-11 Helium dilution method for measuring functional residual capacity. **A,** Initial He readings, He volume (V1) and concentration (C1), lung volume is at functional residual capacity. **B,** He reading during test. **C,** Final He concentration reading (C2) at equilibrium. See text for details.

results, unless the correction is made. Although He is an inert gas with a negligible solubility in plasma, it is assumed that a small amount of He diffuses across the alveolar-capillary membrane. To account for the loss, 30 ml of BTPS-corrected volume is subtracted for each minute of He breathing, up to 200 ml for a 7-minute test. Once these corrections are made, TLC can be calculated using spirometry data.

Nitrogen Washout

The nitrogen N technique uses a nonrebreathing or open circuit (Figure 20-12).[15,16] The technique is based on the assumptions that the N concentration in the lungs is 78% and in equilibrium with the atmosphere, that the patient inhales 100% O_2, and that the O_2 replaces all of the N in the lungs. Similar to the He dilution technique, the patient is connected to the system at FRC. The patient's exhaled gas is monitored, and its volume and N percentage are measured.

Generally, two types of circuits are used to measure lung volumes with this technique. In one type of circuit, all of the exhaled gases are collected in a large container, where the volume and concentration of N are measured. In the second type of circuit, the volume and concentration of each exhaled breath are measured separately and stored in a memory; the sum of the volumes and the weighted average of the N concentration are calculated by a computer.

Wearing nose clips, the patient breathes 100% O_2 until nearly all of the N has been washed out of the lungs, leaving less than 1.5% N in the lungs. When the peak exhaled concentration of N is less than 1.5%, the patient exhales completely, and the fractional concentration of alveolar N (F_AN_2) is noted. Similar to the He technique, the time it takes to wash out the N is approximately 2 to 5 minutes in healthy individuals and longer in patients with obstructive lung disease. The test must occur in a leak-proof circuit because the presence of any air increases the measured N percentages and results in grossly elevated measurements of lung volume.

For FRC to be calculated by the N washout technique, several measurements must be made: the total volume of gas exhaled during the test (V_E), the fractional concentration of exhaled N in the total gas volume (F_EN_2), the fractional concentration of N in the alveoli at the end of the test (F_AN_2), and the spirometer temperature. FRC can be calculated with the following equation:

$$FRC = \frac{V_E \times F_EN_2}{0.78 - F_AN_2}$$

The calculated FRC must be adjusted for the temperature difference between the spirometer and the patient's body temperature using the BTPS correction factor. During the test, some N from the plasma and body tissues is usually excreted and exhaled with lung N. For this reason, another correction is needed, using duration of the test and the weight of the patient.

Plethysmography

The plethysmography technique applies Boyle's law and uses measurements of volume and pressure changes to determine lung volume, assuming temperature is constant.[15-17] The plethysmography technique measures the volume of all compressible gas in the thorax, including gas trapped behind airway obstructions or in the pleural space. Gas in the abdomen also may be included in the measurement. The whole-body plethysmograph consists of a sealed chamber in which the patient sits (Figure 20-13). Pressure transducers (electronic manometers) measure pressure at the mouth and in the chamber. An electronically controlled shutter near the mouthpiece allows the airway to be

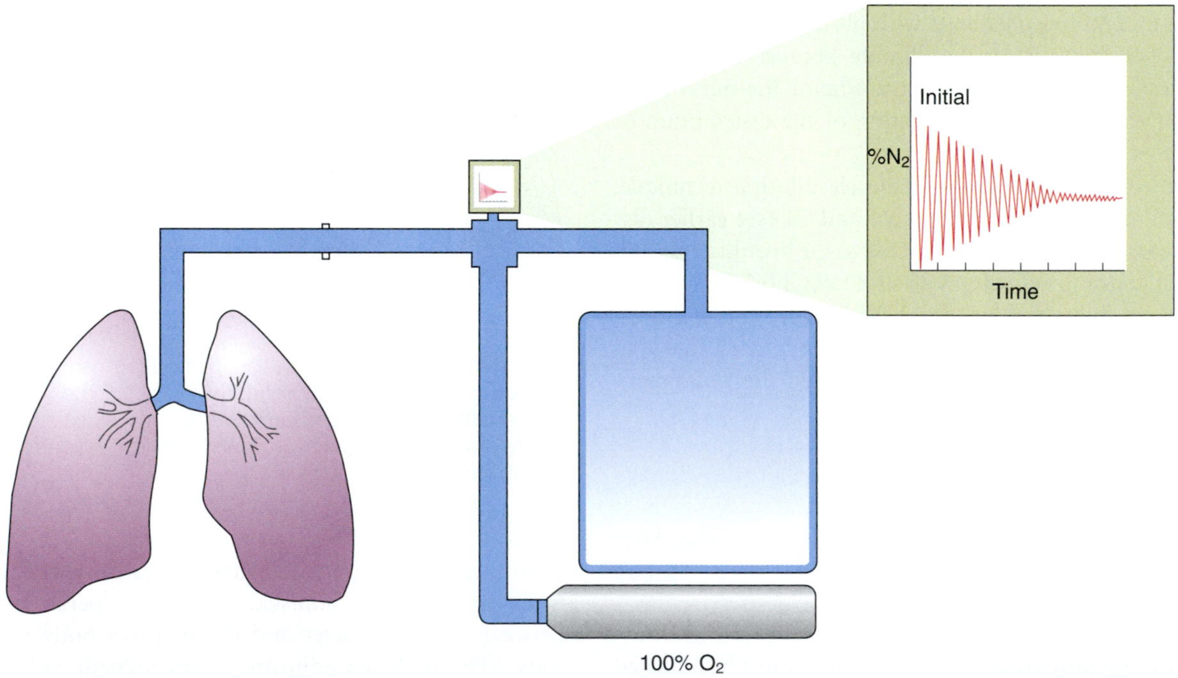

FIGURE 20-12 Nitrogen washout method for measuring functional residual capacity, residual volume, and total lung capacity.

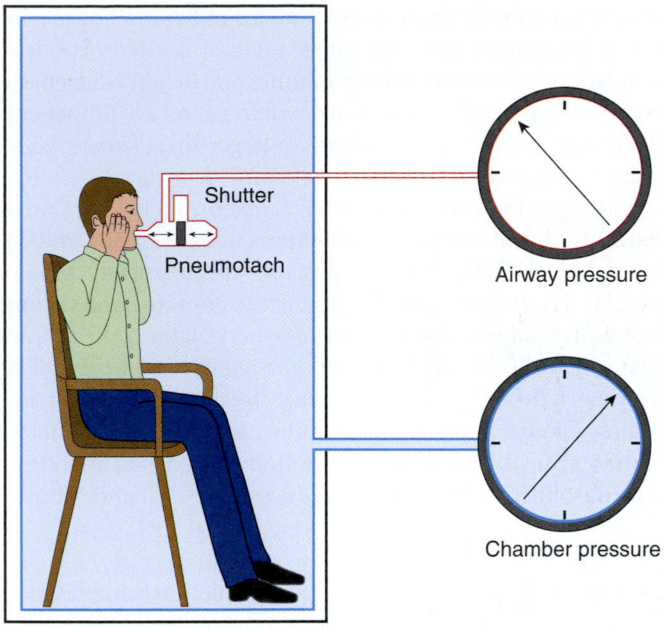

Plethysmograph chamber

$$V(FRC) = P_B \text{ atmospheric} \times \frac{\Delta V}{\Delta P}$$

FIGURE 20-13 Body plethysmography method for measuring lung volumes. *V* is the change in gas volume in the lungs, as sensed by the chamber pressure manometer. *P* is the change in pressure produced by the respiratory efforts of breathing against the shutter, as sensed by the airway pressure manometer.

occluded periodically, measuring airway pressure changes under conditions of no airflow. Without airflow, pressure changes measured at the mouth are pressure changes in the alveoli. According to Boyle's law ($V \times P = k$), when temperature is constant, volume changes in the thorax create volume changes in the chamber, which are reflected by pressure changes in the chamber. When measurement of TGV is being done, the patient sits in the chamber and initially breathes normal tidal volumes through the mouthpiece. When the patient is near FRC, the shutter is closed at end expiration for 2 to 3 seconds. The patient holds his or her cheeks and performs gentle panting at 1 Hz or one pant per second. During panting, changes in airway pressure (ΔP) and changes in chamber volume (ΔV) are measured. Because the panting maneuver occurs with small pressure changes around barometric pressure, the simplified equation used to calculate TGV is:

$$TGV = P_B \times (\Delta V \div \Delta P)$$

where P_B is the barometric pressure in cm H_2O.

A series of three to five panting maneuvers should be performed. After panting, the patient should exhale completely to record ERV and then inhale maximally to record the inspiratory vital capacity.

Because the body plethysmographic method of measuring FRC actually measures TGV, the value obtained for some patients may be larger than values resulting from either the He dilution or N washout techniques. Such a difference occurs whenever there is gas in the thorax that is not in communication with patent airways, as might be the case in patients with pneumothorax, pneumomediastinum, or emphysema. Assuming that TGV actually represents FRC, calculations can be made for TLC and RV, similar to He dilution or N washout methods.

Interpretation

Changes in lung volumes and capacities are generally consistent with the pattern of impairment. TLC, FRC, and RV increase with obstructive lung diseases and decrease with restrictive impairment. Some lung volumes provide valuable diagnostic information. For example, TLC is always reduced in restrictive lung disease, unless obstruction and restriction occur together. When obstruction and restriction occur together, the TLC may be a less sensitive measure of the restrictive impairment. Other volumes and capacities may remain normal with mild obstructive or restrictive disease. The pattern of lung volume changes and the proportion of FRC and RV to TLC are also important.

Normal Values for Lung Volumes. The normal V_T is approximately 500 to 700 ml for an average healthy adult. In the normal population, great variation of tidal volumes and measurements beyond the normal range are not indicative of a disease process. Normal V_T is often observed in both restrictive and obstructive lung diseases. V_T alone is not a valid indicator of the type of lung disease.

The normal IC is approximately 3.6 L, with a significant variation in the normal population. IC may be normal or reduced in restrictive and obstructive lung diseases. A reduction of IC occurs in restrictive lung diseases because the patient's inhaled volume is reduced and there is a reduction in TLC. In mild obstructive lung diseases, IC is usually normal. In moderate and severe obstructive diseases, IC can be reduced because the resting expiratory level of FRC has increased owing to hyperinflation of the lungs. An increase in IC may occur when the patient inhales from below the resting expiratory level when the measurement is performed; athletes and musicians who play wind instruments may have increased inspiratory capacities. RTs use the measurement of IC in clinical protocols to decide between methods of lung expansion therapy (see Chapter 42).

IRV is not commonly measured. Similar to V_T and IC, IRV can be normal in both restrictive and obstructive diseases and is not a useful diagnostic measurement. The normal value for IRV is 3.10 L.

The normal ERV is approximately 1.2 L and represents approximately 20% to 25% of the VC. It can be either normal or reduced in obstructive and restrictive lung diseases. ERV is subtracted from FRC to calculate RV.

The normal value of the VC is 4.8 L and represents approximately 80% of TLC. Normal values for VC can vary significantly depending on age, gender, height, and ethnicity. A reduction of VC occurs in restrictive lung diseases because the patient's inhaled volume is reduced and there is a reduction in TLC. In mild obstructive lung diseases, the slow VC is usually normal if the patient exhales leisurely and has had enough time to exhale completely or if the VC is measured during inspiration. Measurements made from FVC provide valuable data for pulmonary mechanics.

RV, FRC, and TLC are the most important measurements of lung volumes. Age, height, gender, ethnicity, and sometimes weight or body surface area correlate with normal values for these lung volumes.[18] Table 20-5 provides common regression equations to predict the lung volumes for individuals of specific height (in centimeters), age (in years), and gender. A positive correlation exists between lung volumes and height, and a negative correlation exists between lung volumes and age for patients older than 20 years. Male values are larger than female values when height and age are equal.

The typical normal TLC is 6.0 L. The normal RV is approximately 1.2 L and represents approximately 20% of TLC. FRC is approximately 2.4 L, which represents approximately 40% of the TLC. RV and FRC are usually enlarged in acute and chronic obstructive lung diseases because of hyperinflation and air trapping (Figure 20-14). TLC also may be enlarged in COPD. TLC is always reduced in restrictive lung diseases because of a loss of lung volume; RV and FRC are often reduced proportionately. Certain acute disorders, such as pulmonary edema, atelectasis, and consolidation, also cause a reduction of TLC and FRC.

TABLE 20-5

Examples of Regression Equations for Predicting Normal Lung Volumes and Capacities in Adults

Lung Volumes	Equations
Men	
FRC (L)	0.0234 (Ht) + 0.01 (A) − 1.09
RV (L)	0.0131 (Ht) + 0.022 (A) − 1.23
TLC (L)	0.0799 (Ht) − 7.08
FRC/TLC%	43.8 + 0.21 (A)
RV/TLC%	14.0 + 0.39 (A)
Women	
FRC (L)	0.0224 (Ht) + 0.001 (A) − 1.00
RV (L)	0.0181 (Ht) + 0.016 (A) − 2.00
TLC (L)	0.0660 (Ht) − 5.79
FRC/TLC%	45.1 + 0.16 (A)
RV/TLC%	20.0 + 0.34 (A)

From Stocks J, Quanjer PH: Reference values for residual volume, functional residual capacity and total lung capacity. Eur Respir J 8:492–497, 1995.
A, Age in years; *Ht,* height in centimeters.

Diffusing Capacity

The third major category of pulmonary function testing is measuring the ability of the lungs to transfer gases across the alveolar-capillary membrane. As discussed in Chapter 12, the diffusion of gases across a sheet of membrane depends on various factors.

$$V_{gas} = D_L \times (P_1 - P_2)$$

Vgas = Amount of the gas transferred into the lungs
P1 = Partial pressure of the gas in the alveolus
P2 = Partial pressure of the gas in the pulmonary capillary

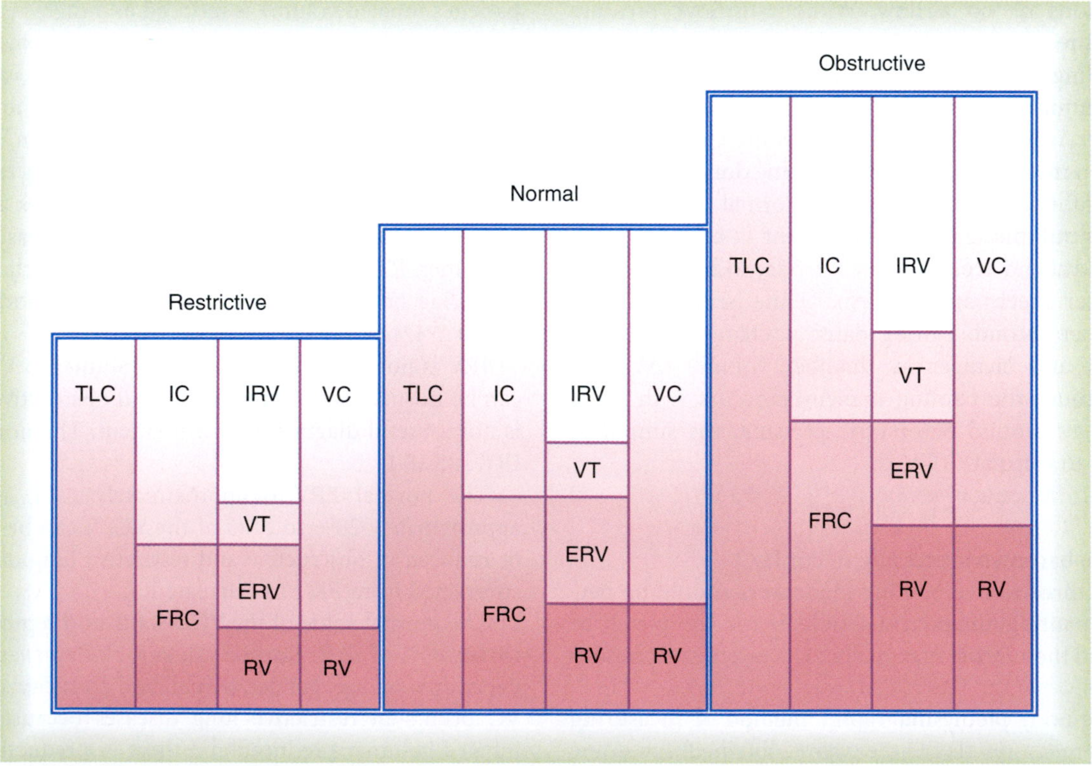

FIGURE 20-14 Changes in lung volumes and capacities with pulmonary disease. *ERV,* Expiratory reserve volume; *FRC,* functional residual capacity; *IC,* inspiratory capacity; *IRV,* inspiratory reserve volume; *TLC,* total lung capacity; *VT,* tidal volume.

Carbon monoxide (CO) is the gas normally used to measure the DL. The **diffusing capacity of the lung for carbon monoxide** (DLCO) is expressed in ml/min/mm Hg under standard temperature and pressure and dry conditions. CO is used as the transfer gas because CO is similar to O_2 in important ways. CO and O_2 have similar molecular weights and solubility coefficients. Similar to O_2, CO also chemically combines with hemoglobin (Hb). CO has a very high affinity for Hb and diffuses rapidly into the pulmonary blood, keeping the *pulmonary capillary partial pressure of CO (P_2 in the formula above)* near zero. Consequently, the formula for the DLCO calculation can be rewritten as follows:

$$DL_{CO} = \frac{\dot{V}_{CO}}{P_ACO}$$

Where $\dot{V}_{CO}$ is the amount of CO taken up by the lungs and P_ACO is the alveolar partial pressure of CO during the test.

Single-Breath Technique

There are several techniques to measure the diffusing capacity of the lung for CO, including steady-state, intrabreath, and rebreathing techniques, but the single-breath method (DLCO-SB) is the most common measurement technique because it is quick and reproducible. Standards for measuring diffusing capacity of the lung were initially published in 1995 and updated in 2005; these standards focus primarily on the DLCO-SB.[5,19] During the single-breath method, the patient exhales completely to RV, rapidly inspires to TLC a volume of air containing small concentration of CO and He, maintains breath holding for 10 seconds, and then exhales at least 1 L rapidly. He is added to the inhaled gas mixture to help with the estimation of effective lung volume, as well as alveolar CO concentration (F_ACO). Note that F_ACO is different from the inhaled CO concentration because dilution by RV and this corrected value should be used in calculation of P_ACO. The dilution of CO is proportional to the dilution of He, and can be calculated using inhaled (F_IHe) and exhaled (F_EHe) He concentrations. A sample of exhaled alveolar gas is collected and analyzed for expired CO (F_ECO). The **effective total lung capacity** (or alveolar volume, V_A) can be similarly calculated using measured VC and inhaled and exhaled He concentrations. The V_A is necessary to calculate $\dot{V}_{CO}$, and it is used in the determination of the diffusing capacity of the lung-to-alveolar volume ratio ($DLCO/V_A$, discussed later). The total time of the test (t) is recorded and used in ultimate calculation of DLCO. To regulate the breath holding period, some measuring systems close the mouthpiece with a timed shutter. The suitable breathing pattern requires patient cooperation and coordination; some patients benefit from a timer as a visual aid.

It is important to note that the rate of CO transfer across the membrane is not uniform throughout the test. When a bolus of CO gas is inhaled, the rate of gas diffusion declines logarithmically with time, meaning that the rate of gas transfer at the beginning of the test (high CO concentration) is much greater than at the end of the test (low CO concentration). The single-breath method (DLCO-SB) is based on the diffusion decay curve described by Forster and colleagues[20] (Figure 20-15). The final formula for DLCO calculation incorporates all measurements used to calculate $\dot{V}_{CO}$ and P_ACO, as well as the correction for nonlinearity of CO transfer.[5]

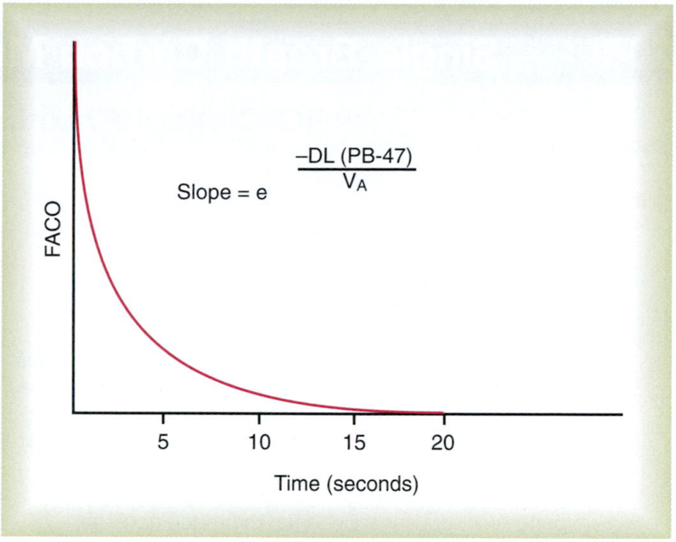

FIGURE 20-15 Concentration of alveolar carbon monoxide after a single breath to total lung capacity.

The reliability of the DLCO is based on repeatability of the test. At least 4 minutes should be allowed between tests to allow an adequate elimination of CO from the lungs. In patients with obstructive airway disease, a longer period (e.g., 10 minutes) may be necessary. The actual DLCO reported should be the mean of two acceptable tests. An acceptable test is defined as one that is reproducible to within 10% or 3 ml of the CO/min/mm Hg value, whichever is greater.[21] (See AARC Clinical Practice Guideline 20-3.)

Interpretation

Normal values for the DLCO using the single-breath technique are based primarily on a patient's age, height, and gender (Table 20-6). A typical normal value for a 20-year-old healthy man is 40 ml/min/mm Hg.[21] Factors known to affect test results should be controlled or standardized; these include body position, activity, PAO_2, Hb and carboxyhemoglobin (COHb) levels, and pulmonary blood volume. To focus the test on diffusion through the alveolar-capillary membrane, the patient should be tested at rest in a seated position, should not breathe supplemental O_2 for 10 minutes before testing, and should not have an abnormal level of COHb before the test. Mathematical corrections can be applied for patients who cannot abstain from O_2. Performing the diffusing capacity on patients who have recently smoked a cigarette or who have been exposed to environmental CO may hinder test validity. Patients should refrain from smoking on the day of the test. All patients undergoing diffusing capacity should have their Hb concentration measured, and a mathematical correction should be applied if it is abnormal. In addition, DLCO measurement may be altered in patients on supplemental O_2, or at high altitude. Provision of formulas that

20-3 Single-Breath Carbon Monoxide Diffusing Capacity

AARC Clinical Practice Guideline (Excerpts)*

INDICATIONS

Tests of diffusing capacity may be indicated in the following situations:

- Evaluation and follow-up of parenchymal lung diseases associated with dusts (e.g., asbestos) or drug reactions (e.g., amiodarone) or related to sarcoidosis.
- Evaluation and follow-up of emphysema and cystic fibrosis.
- Differentiation among chronic bronchitis, emphysema, and asthma in patients with obstructive patterns.
- Evaluation of pulmonary involvement in systemic diseases (e.g., rheumatoid arthritis, lupus erythematosus).
- Evaluation of cardiovascular diseases (e.g., pulmonary hypertension, pulmonary edema, thromboembolism).
- Prediction of arterial desaturation during exercise in chronic obstructive pulmonary disease.
- Evaluation and quantification of disability associated with interstitial lung disease.
- Evaluation of the effects of chemotherapy agents or other drugs known to induce pulmonary dysfunction.
- Evaluation of hemorrhagic disorders.

CONTRAINDICATIONS

The following are relative contraindications to performing a diffusing capacity test:

- Mental confusion or incoordination preventing the subject from adequately performing the maneuver
- A large meal or vigorous exercise immediately before the test.
- Smoking within 24 hours of test administration (may have effect on diffusion capacity of the lung for carbon dioxide [DLCO] independent of carboxyhemoglobin [COHb]).

HAZARDS AND COMPLICATIONS

- Single-breath DLCO requires breath holding at total lung capacity; some patients may perform either a Valsalva (high intrathoracic pressure) or Müller (low intrathoracic pressure) maneuver. Either of these maneuvers can result in alteration of venous return to the heart.
- Transmission of infection is possible via improperly cleaned mouthpieces or from the inadvertent spread of droplet nuclei or body fluids (patient to patient or patient to technologist).

ASSESSMENT OF NEED

The need for DLCO testing exists when any of the aforementioned indications are present.

ASSESSMENT OF TEST QUALITY

Individual test maneuvers and results should be evaluated according to the American Thoracic Society recommendations. In particular, the following recommendations are pertinent:

- The inspiratory volume should exceed 90% of the largest previously measured vital capacity (forced vital capacity [FVC] or vital capacity [VC]).
- Breath hold time should be between 9 and 11 seconds, with a rapid inspiration.
- The washout volume (dead space) should be 0.75 to 1 L, or 0.50 L if the subject's VC is <2 L. If a washout volume other than 0.75 to 1 L is used, it should be noted.
- Two or more acceptable tests should be averaged. The maneuvers should be reproducible to within 10% or 3 ml of CO/min/mm Hg, whichever is greater.
- The subject should have refrained from smoking for 24 hours before the test.
- Corrections for Hb and COHb should be included; correction for tests performed at high altitude is recommended.
- If Hb correction is made, both the corrected and the uncorrected DLCO values should be reported.
- Equipment calibration and quality control measures specific to measuring diffusing capacity should be applied and documented.

MONITORING

- The final report should contain a statement about test quality.
- The final report should contain the DLCO, the corrected DLCO (Hb, COHb, altitude), and the Hb value used for correction. The alveolar volume (VA) and DL/VA (i.e., the ratio of diffusing capacity to the lung volume at which the measurement was made) may be included in the report. These values are helpful for purposes of interpretation.

**For complete guideline, see American Association for Respiratory Care: Clinical practice guideline: single-breath carbon monoxide diffusing capacity.*

are used to obtain the raw DLCO measurement or to correct it for all of these variables is outside of the scope of this chapter and is given in the references.[5]

Some clinicians argue that if the DLCO measurement has to be corrected for variables that have nothing to do with the gas transfer across the membrane, then it must not be the true diffusion that we are measuring with the DLCO. In fact, in European respiratory communities, the DLCO, as we have been describing in this chapter, is called K_{CO}, or transfer factor for CO, to differentiate it from the true diffusion properties of the lung.[5]

The DLCO may be reduced from the predicted normal in patients with obstructive or restrictive lung diseases. With destruction of alveoli in pulmonary emphysema, with small lung volumes, and with fibrosis of alveoli in asbestosis, the DLCO may be less than normal. Pulmonary embolism also may decrease the DLCO. The DLCO may be useful in identifying which patients with obstructive impairment are likely to

TABLE 20-6

Examples of Regression Equations for Predicting Normal Diffusing Capacity in Adults

Parameter	Regression Equations
Men	
DLCO-SB (ml/min/mm Hg)	0.0416 (Ht) – 0.220 (A) – 26.34
DLCO-SB/V_A (ml/min/ mm Hg/L)	6.61 – 0.034 (A)
Women	
DLCO-SB (ml/min/mm Hg)	0.0256 (Ht) – 0.144 (A) – 8.36
DLCO-SB/V_A (ml/min/ mm Hg/L)	7.34 – 0.032 (A)

From Crapo RO, Morris AM: Standardized single breath normal values for carbon monoxide diffusing capacity. Am Rev Respir Dis 123:185, 1981.
A, Age in years; *DLCO-SB,* single-breath diffusing capacity; *Ht,* height in cm.

Box 20-2 Effect of Various Factors on Diffusing Capacity of the Lung for Carbon Monoxide

FACTORS THAT DECREASE DLCO
- Anemia
- Carboxyhemoglobin
- Pulmonary embolism
- Diffuse pulmonary fibrosis
- Pulmonary emphysema

FACTORS THAT INCREASE DLCO
- Polycythemia
- Exercise
- Congestive heart failure

DLCO, Diffusing capacity of the lung for carbon monoxide.

MINI CLINI

Diffusing Capacity of the Lung for Carbon Monoxide in Chronic Obstructive Pulmonary Disease

PROBLEM: A patient has spirometry and lung volumes typical of the obstructive pattern. FEV_1, FEV_1/FVC, and FEFs are significantly reduced, and FRC and TLC are increased. Two common obstructive diseases are chronic bronchitis and pulmonary emphysema. How can pulmonary function data differentiate between these two diseases? The answer is the DLCO.

SOLUTION: Chronic bronchitis involves mostly airways and is characterized by chronic inflammation of the mucosa, hypertrophy of mucous glands, excessive mucus, and possibly bronchospasm, all of which narrow the airways. Pulmonary emphysema primarily involves alveolar structures and is characterized by destruction of alveolar architecture, elastic fibers, and alveolar-capillary membranes. Emphysema decreases gas-exchange surface area. Chronic bronchitis does not involve alveoli and does not change surface area for gas exchange. For these reasons, a decreased diffusion capacity is associated with emphysema rather than with chronic bronchitis. DLCO is a useful way to determine the extent to which emphysema may be present in a patient with COPD.

TABLE 20-7

Pulmonary Function Changes in Advanced Lung Diseases

Measurement	Normal*	Obstructive	Restrictive
V_T	500%smL	N or ↑	N or ↓
IRV	3.10 L	N or ↓	↓
ERV	1.20 L	N or ↓	↓
RV	1.20 L	↑	↓
IC	3.60 L	N or ↓	↓
FRC	2.40 L	↑	↓
TLC	6.00 L	N or ↑	↓
FVC	4.80 L	↓	↓
FEV_1	4.20 L	↓	N or ↓
FEV_1/FVC	>70%	↓	N or ↑
$FEF_{200-1200}$	8.5 L/sec	↓	N
$FEF_{25\%-75\%}$	4.5 L/sec	↓	N
PEF	9.5 L/sec	↓	N
$FEF_{25\%}$	9.0 L/sec	↓	N
$FEF_{50\%}$	6.5 L/sec	↓	N
$FEF_{75\%}$	3.5 L/sec	↓	N
MVV	160 L/min	↓	N or ↓
DLCO	40% mL/min/mm Hg	N or ↓	N or ↓
DLCO/V_A	6.6% mL/min/mm Hg/L	N or ↓	N or ↓

DLCO, Diffusing capacity of the lung for carbon monoxide; *N,* no change.
*Values for 20-year-old, 70-kg man.

experience desaturation during exercise and which may benefit from O_2 therapy. The DLCO may be increased in patients with polycythemia, congestive (left) heart failure (resulting from an increase in pulmonary vascular blood volume), and elevated cardiac output. Variables in health and disease that can alter the DLCO are summarized in Box 20-2.

The **diffusing capacity ratio of the lung-to–effective total lung capacity ratio (DLCO/VA)** differentiates between diffusion abnormalities caused by having a small lung volume compared with diffusion abnormalities caused by alveolar-capillary membrane pathologies. Patients whose only problem is small lungs would have a decreased DLCO, but their DLCO/V_A ratio would be normal. Patients with pulmonary emphysema or fibrosis would have a decreased DLCO and a decreased DLCO/V_A ratio. In contrast, patients with neuromuscular disease will similarly have restrictive lung volumes and reduced DLCO, but DLCO/V_A will likely be normal, because they will likely have normal diffusion.

INTERPRETATION OF THE PULMONARY FUNCTION REPORT

Interpretive strategies for pulmonary function testing abound. Most computer-based pulmonary function testing systems have algorithms in their software programs for computer-assisted interpretations of the pulmonary function report. Table 20-7 summarizes pulmonary function changes that may occur in advanced obstructive and restrictive patterns of lung diseases, and Figure 20-16 presents a simple algorithm to assess pulmonary function test results in clinical practice.[22,23]

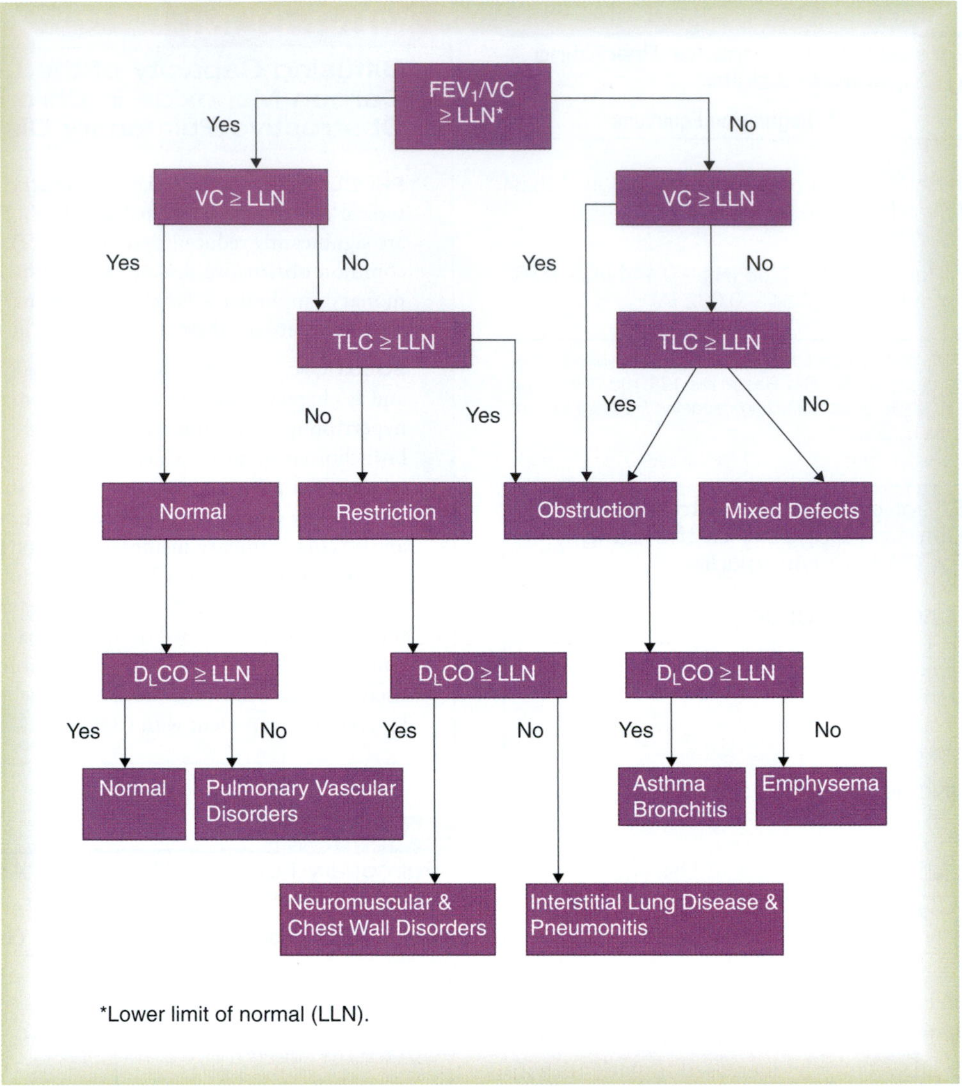

FIGURE 20-16 A simple algorithm to assess pulmonary function test results in clinical practice. *LLN,* Lower limit of normal; *ULN,* upper limit of normal. (From Gardner RM, Crapo RO, Morris AH, et al: Computer guidelines for pulmonary laboratories. Am Rev Respir Dis 134:628, 1986.)

When considering a pulmonary function report, the FEV_1/VC ratio is a good place to start because it provides an initial focus as normal, restrictive, or obstructive impairment. When the FEV_1/FVC is reduced, there is airway obstruction. FEV_1/FVC is normal in healthy individuals and patients with restriction. The LLN for FEV_1/FVC can be determined directly for various populations using regression equations in Table 20-8. However, most clinicians use an arbitrary value of 70%.

The next to consider is TLC. If the TLC is less than the LLN, often defined as less than 80% predicted normal, the patient has a restrictive impairment according to this algorithm. Patients with obstruction will often have normal or elevated TLC. Naturally, some patients may have a mixed obstructive/restrictive pattern. In those patients, TLC may be reduced, normal, or elevated.

Once obstructive/restrictive pattern is ascertained, DLCO will help differentiate between the diseases that do and do not

TABLE 20-8

Examples of Regression Equations for Determining Lower Limit of Normal of Forced Expiratory Volume in 1 Second-to-Vital Capacity Ratio (%FEV_1/FVC) in Adults

Population	Equations	R^2
Men		
White	78.388 – 0.2066 (A)	0.3448
African-American	78.822 – 0.1828 (A)	0.1538
Mexican-American	80.925 – 0.2186 (A)	0.2713
Women		
White	81.015 – 0.2125 (A)	0.3955
African-American	80.978 – 0.2039 (A)	0.2284
Mexican-American	83.044 – 0.2248 (A)	0.3352

From Hankinson JL, Odencratz JR, Fedan KB: Spirometric reference values from a sample of the general U.S. population. Am J Respir Crit Care Med 159:179, 1999.
A, Years.

affect the gas transfer across the alveolar-capillary membrane. If the percent predicted normal DLCO is less than 80%, the patient has a diffusion impairment. Some laboratories also report the DLCO/V_A ratio, which indices the DLCO for lung volume measured during the single-breath test.

According to most recent ATS/ERS guidelines on PFT interpretation, the severity of obstructive *and* restrictive impairment is judged by the patient's FEV_1, and the severity of gas transfer is based on the DLCO.[21] Severity categories, based on percent predicted values, are outlined in Table 20-2. Use of other indices, such as FRC or TLC, to quantify the severity is controversial[23] and will not be discussed here. Although FEV_1 is used to quantify the severity of illness across the disease categories, it is important to note its limitations.[21] FEV_1 is a poor measurement of upper airway obstruction; it may not be suitable comparing different pulmonary conditions, it may not be reliable in the extremes of severity assessment, it has poor correlation with clinical symptoms or progression.

MINI CLINI

Identifying Patterns of Pulmonary Impairment

PROBLEM: Following are three pulmonary function reports that show three distinct examples of pulmonary impairment. Using the algorithm in Figure 20-16, identify the patterns typical of asthma, pulmonary fibrosis, and COPD.

PULMONARY FUNCTION REPORT 1

Pulmonary Measurements	Predicted Normal Value	Measured Baseline Conditions	Percent Predicted
SVC (L)	5.00	3.00	60
FVC (L)	5.00	3.00	60
FEV_1 (L)	4.00	2.80	70
%FEV_1/FVC	80%	94%	—
$FEF_{25\%-75\%}$ (L/sec)	4.00	3.75	94
PEF (L/sec)	8.00	8.25	103
TLC (L)	7.20	3.96	55
FRC (L)	4.10	2.00	49
RV (L)	2.20	1.40	60
DLCO (ml/min/mm Hg)	34.0	15.9	47
DLCO/V_A (ml/min/mm Hg/L)	7.20	3.50	49

SOLUTION REPORT 1: Although FEV_1 is less than 80% of predicted, because the FEV_1/FVC is greater than 70%, there is no apparent airway obstruction. FEV_1 is reduced because FVC is reduced. The patient's measured FVC is less than the predicted FEV_1. Because TLC is less than 80% predicted, the data suggest a restrictive impairment, and because DLCO is less than 80% predicted, there is also a diffusion impairment. The low DLCO/V_A suggests that the diffusion impairment is out of proportion to the lung volume. This finding implies that the impairment to normal diffusion is the result of abnormal lung tissue. Overall, this report shows a mild to moderate restrictive pattern consistent with pulmonary fibrosis.

PULMONARY FUNCTION REPORT 2

Pulmonary Measurements	Predicted Normal Value	Measured Baseline Conditions	Percent Predicted Baseline	Measured After Bronchodilator Treatment	Percent Predicted After Treatment
SVC (L)	5.00	3.50	70	4.25	85
FVC (L)	5.00	3.30	66	4.00	80
FEV_1 (L)	4.00	2.00	50	2.50	62
%FEV_1/FVC	80%	57%	—	62%	—
$FEF_{25\%-75\%}$ (L/sec)	4.00	1.00	25	2.00	50
PEF (L/sec)	8.00	6.00	75	6.50	81
TLC (L)	5.27	5.51	105	5.36	102
FRC (L)	3.11	4.55	146	3.60	116
RV (L)	1.67	2.60	156	2.00	120
DLCO (ml/min/mm Hg)	28.7	25.25	88	—	—
DLCO/V_A (ml/min/mm Hg/L)	5.45	5.17	96	—	—

SOLUTION REPORT 2: The FEV_1/FVC is less than 70%; there is airway obstruction. FEV_1 is 50% of predicted; the obstruction is moderate. Because the $FEF_{25\%-75\%}$ is 25% of predicted, the major site of obstruction is in the bronchioles. After bronchodilator inhalation, FEV_1 improved by 24% (remember to compute percent change), showing effective treatment and partial reversibility of the obstruction. The large FRC and RV show hyperinflation and air trapping, which also improved after bronchodilator therapy. Diffusing capacity is in the normal range, indicating no diffusion impairment and no alveolar problems. Overall, this report shows a moderately severe obstructive pattern with hyperinflation and air trapping responsive to bronchodilators and consistent with acute hyperreactive airways disease, such as asthma.

MINI CLINI

Identifying Patterns of Pulmonary Impairment—cont'd

PULMONARY FUNCTION REPORT 3

Pulmonary Measurements	Predicted Normal Value	Measured Baseline Conditions	Percent Predicted Baseline	Measured After Bronchodilator Treatment	Percent Predicted After Treatment
SVC (L)	5.00	4.00	80	4.25	85
FVC (L)	5.00	3.50	70	4.00	80
FEV_1 (L)	4.00	2.00	50	2.20	55
$\%FEV_1/FVC$	80%	57%	—	55%	—
$FEF_{25\%-75\%}$ (L/sec)	4.00	1.75	50	2.00	50
PEF (L/sec)	8.00	6.00	75	6.50	80
TLC (L)	5.27	5.51	105	5.36	102
FRC (L)	3.11	4.55	146	3.79	122
RV (L)	1.67	2.60	156	2.24	134
DLCO (ml/min/mm Hg)	28.7	14.25	56	—	—
$DLCO/V_A$ (ml/min/mm Hg/L)	5.45	3.17	58%	—	—

SOLUTION REPORT 3: This case is similar to case 2, but there are some important differences. The FEV_1/FVC is less than 70%; there is airway obstruction. FEV_1 is 50% of predicted; the obstruction is moderately severe. After a single bronchodilator treatment, FEV_1 improved by 10% (remember to compute percent change)—not enough to show that bronchodilator therapy was immediately effective. The large FRC and RV show hyperinflation and air trapping, which did improve after bronchodilator therapy. DLCO and $DLCO/V_A$ are reduced, suggesting alveolar involvement. This report shows a moderately severe obstructive pattern with hyperinflation and air trapping not responsive to bronchodilators. There is diffusion impairment and alveolar disease. Overall, this report is consistent with COPD, the combination of chronic bronchitis and pulmonary emphysema.

PULMONARY FUNCTION REPORT 4

Pulmonary Measurements	Predicted Normal Value	Measured Baseline Conditions	Percent Predicted Baseline	Measured After Bronchodilator Treatment	Percent Predicted After Treatment
SVC (L)	5.38	4.84	90		
FVC (L)	5.38	4.92	92	5.16	109
FEV_1 (L)	4.33	2.95	68	3.24	75
$\%FEV_1/FVC$	80%	54%	—	63%	
$FEF_{25\%-75\%}$ (L/sec)	5.23	1.20	23	1.08	21
PEF (L/sec)	9.96	6.32	63	7.53	76
TLC (L)	7.51	6.38	85		
FRC (L)	4.10	3.51	86		
RV (L)	2.10	1.58	75		
DLCO (ml/min/mm Hg)	37.22	29.60	89		
$DLCO/V_A$ (ml/min/mm Hg/L)	4.96	4.06	82		

SOLUTION REPORT 4: This case is similar to Case 3, but there are some important differences. The FEV_1/FVC is less than 70%; there is airway obstruction. FEV_1 is 68% of predicted; the obstruction is mild. After a single bronchodilator treatment, FEV_1 improved by only 9.8% (remember to compute percent change)—not enough to show that the bronchodilator therapy was immediately effective. Lung volumes and diffusing capacity are within the normal range, so there is no hyperinflation, air trapping, or diffusion impairment. This report shows a moderate obstructive pattern not responsive to bronchodilators. Overall, this report is consistent with chronic bronchitis.

PULMONARY FUNCTION REPORT 5

Pulmonary Measurements	Predicted Normal Value	Measured Baseline Conditions	Percent Predicted Baseline
SVC (L)	3.85	1.93	50
FVC (L)	3.85	2.01	52
FEV_1 (L)	3.01	1.66	55
$\%FEV_1/FVC$	78%	86%	—
$FEF_{25\%-75\%}$ (L/sec)	3.40	1.85	55
PEF (L/sec)	6.50	4.55	70
TLC (L)	5.65	3.39	60
FRC (L)	3.01	2.11	70
RV (L)	1.80	1.35	75
DLCO (ml/min/mm Hg)	22.13	13.28	60
$DLCO/V_A$ (ml/min/mm Hg/L)	3.91	3.60	92

SOLUTION REPORT 5: The FEV_1/FVC is greater than 70%, so there is no apparent airway obstruction even though the FEV_1 is less than 80% of predicted. The patient's measured FVC is less than the predicted FEV_1, and FEV_1 is reduced because FVC is reduced. Because TLC is less than 80% predicted, the data suggest a restrictive impairment. Although DLCO is less than 80% predicted, there is no apparent diffusion impairment involving lung tissue because the $DLCO/V_A$ suggests that the diffusion impairment is proportional to the low lung volume. This finding implies that the diffusion impairment is due to the subject having small lungs. Overall, this report shows a moderately severe restrictive pattern consistent with neuromuscular weakness or other extrapulmonary restriction.

SUMMARY CHECKLIST

- Pulmonary function testing includes measurements of airway mechanics, lung volumes and capacities, and the diffusing capacity of the lung.
- The results of pulmonary function testing can aid in the diagnosis of disease and include patterns of obstructive and restrictive impairments.
- Pulmonary function testing provides objective data on which decisions may be made regarding the status of the patient, the selection of appropriate therapy, and the evaluation of therapeutic outcomes.
- There are specific guidelines published by the AARC and other authorities for performance of pulmonary function testing which must be followed by RTs conducting such procedures.
- Patients with obstructive lung disease exhibit reduced expiratory flows and possibly lung hyperinflation, whereas patients with restrictive lung disease exhibit reduced lung volumes and capacities.
- While pulmonary function testing cannot definitively diagnose any disease, when combined with the results of astute patient assessment, such testing can be useful in uncovering and determining the severity of obstructive disorders such as asthma (reversible) and COPD, or restrictive illnesses such as pulmonary fibrosis.

References

1. ACCP-ATS Joint Committee on Pulmonary Nomenclature: Pulmonary terms and symbols: a report. *Chest* 67:583, 1975.
2. Miller MR, Crapo R, Hankinson J, et al: General considerations for lung function testing. *Eur Respir J* 26:153, 2005.
3. Miller MR, Hankinson J, Brusasco V, et al: Standardisation of spirometry. *Eur Respir J* 26:319, 2005.
4. Wanger J, Clausen JL, Coates A, et al: Standardisation of the measurement of lung volumes. *Eur Respir J* 26:511, 2005.
5. MacIntyre N, Crapo R, Viegi G, et al: Standardization of the single breath determination of carbon monoxide uptake in the lung. *Eur Respir J* 26:720, 2005.
6. American Association for Respiratory Care: Clinical practice guideline. Spirometry, 1996 update. *Respir Care* 41:629, 1996.
7. Douce FH: Flow and volume measuring devices. In Branson R, Hess D, Chatburn R, editors: *Respiratory care equipment*, Philadelphia, 1995, Lippincott.
8. Hankinson JL, Odencratz JR, Fedan KB: Spirometric reference values from a sample of the general U.S. population. *Am J Respir Crit Care Med* 159:179, 1999.
9. Crapo RO, Morris AH, Gardner RM: Reference spirometric values using techniques and equipment that meet ATS recommendations. *Am Rev Respir Dis* 123:659, 1981.
10. American Thoracic Society: Guidelines for methacholine and exercise challenge testing. *Am J Respir Crit Care Med* 161:309, 2000.
11. Hathirat S, Renzetti AD, Mitchell M: Measurement of the total lung capacity by helium dilution in a constant volume system. *Am Rev Respir Dis* 102:760, 1970.
12. Dell SD, Bola SS, Foty R, et al: Provocative dose of methacholine causing a 20% drop in FEV1 should be used to interpret methacholine challenge tests with modern nebulizers. *Ann Am Thorac Soc* 12:165, 2015.
13. American Association for Respiratory Care: Clinical practice guideline: static lung volumes: 2001 revisions and updates. *Respir Care* 46:531, 2001.
14. Mottram CD: Lung volumes and gas distribution tests. In *Ruppel's manual of pulmonary function testing*, ed 10, St Louis, 2013, Elsevier.
15. In Hyatt RE, Scanlon PD, Nakamura M, editors: *Static lung volumes. In Interpretation of pulmonary function tests*, ed 4, Philadelphia, 2014, Lippincott, Williams & Wilkins.
16. Dubois AB, Botelho SY, Bedell GN, et al: A rapid plethysmographic method for measuring thoracic gas volume: a comparison with a nitrogen washout method for measuring FRC in normal patients. *J Clin Invest* 35:322, 1956.
17. Stocks J, Quanjer PH: Reference values for residual volume, functional residual capacity and total lung capacity. *Eur Respir J* 8:492, 1995.
18. American Thoracic Society: Single breath carbon monoxide diffusing capacity (transfer factor): recommendations for a standard technique. *Am J Respir Crit Care Med* 152:2185, 1995.
19. Forster RE, Fowler WS, Bates DV, et al: The absorption of carbon monoxide by the lungs during breathholding. *J Clin Invest* 33:1135, 1954.
20. Crapo RO, Morris AM: Standardized single breath normal values for carbon monoxide diffusing capacity. *Am Rev Respir Dis* 123:185, 1981.
21. American Association for Respiratory Care: Clinical practice guideline: single-breath carbon monoxide diffusing capacity, 2099 update. *Respir Care* 44:539, 1999.
22. American Thoracic Society: Lung function testing: selection of reference values and interpretative strategies. *Am Rev Respir Dis* 144:1202, 1991.
23. Pelligrino R, Viegi G, Brusasco V, et al: Interpretive strategies for lung function testing. *Eur Respir J* 26:948, 2005.

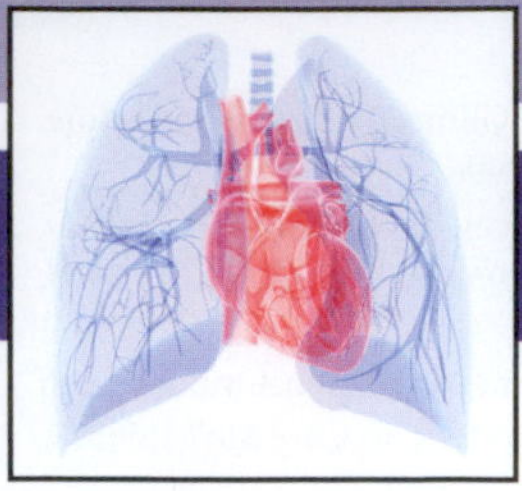

CHAPTER 21

Review of Thoracic Imaging

JOSEPH T. AZOK AND JAMES K. STOLLER

CHAPTER OBJECTIVES

After reading this chapter you will be able to:

- List the four tissue densities seen on a chest radiograph.
- Describe how to evaluate the technical quality of a chest radiograph.
- List the anatomic structures seen on the chest radiograph.
- List the steps used to interpret thoracic imaging studies.
- Understand the value of a computed tomography scan and the use of intravenous contrast.
- Describe the common radiographic abnormalities seen in the pleura, lung parenchyma, and mediastinum.
- Understand the role of ultrasound and magnetic resonance imaging in imaging the chest.

CHAPTER OUTLINE

Overview of the Chest Radiograph
- Approach to Reading a Plain Chest Radiograph
- Chest Radiograph Technique and Quality
- Anatomic Structures Seen on a Chest Radiograph
- Advanced Chest Imaging Techniques

Pleura
- Pleural Effusion (Hydrothorax)
- Pneumothorax

Lung Parenchyma
- Alveolar Disease
- Pulmonary Edema
- Interstitial Disease
- Assessing Lung Volume
- Solitary Pulmonary Nodule

Mediastinum
- Pneumomediastinum
- Catheters, Lines, and Tubes

KEY TERMS

air bronchogram
atelectasis
cephalization
chest radiograph
computed tomography
empyema
hydropneumothorax
infiltrates
interstitial lung disease
Kerley B lines
pleural effusion
pneumomediastinum
pneumothorax
radiograph
radiolucent
radiopaque
roentgenogram
solitary pulmonary nodule

Chest imaging is crucial in the practice of pulmonary and critical care medicine. It is essential that the respiratory therapist (RT) have a solid understanding of chest imaging to accurately assess patients. Various chest imaging techniques exist, including the conventional chest film (more accurately called a **radiograph** or **roentgenogram** after Conrad Wilhelm Roentgen, who first discovered the x-ray), computed tomography (CT) scanning, ultrasound, and magnetic resonance imaging (MRI).

A separate branch of medicine that uses radioactive material to produce images is referred to as *nuclear medicine.* Radioactive material is administered to patients by intravenous (IV) injection, inhalation, or oral ingestion. In the chest, the most commonly performed nuclear medicine studies are called *ventilation-perfusion* ($\dot{V}/\dot{Q}$) *scans* and *positron emission tomography-CT (PET-CT).* $\dot{V}/\dot{Q}$ scans have historically been used to diagnose pulmonary emboli, although chest CT is now the preferred examination for diagnosing pulmonary emboli.[1]

PET-CT combines a nuclear medicine study, the injection of radioactive glucose, with a chest CT and is used to diagnose and stage disease in patients with cancer.

This chapter summarizes important concepts in chest imaging for the RT. The basic elements of chest radiography are addressed first, followed by more advanced techniques such as ultrasound, CT, and MRI. The role of various imaging techniques used to evaluate the different components of the chest (e.g., pleura, mediastinum, lung tissue [lung parenchyma]) will be described, and examples of abnormal findings will be shown.

OVERVIEW OF THE CHEST RADIOGRAPH

A chest radiograph is produced by passing x-rays through the chest to photographic film or a detector. The resulting image is formed as x-rays strike the film or digital screen and darken/expose it. A radiograph is similar to a negative from an old-fashioned black and white film camera. X-rays that pass directly through low-density tissue (e.g., lung) strike the film in greater numbers and cause the resulting shadow to turn darker. X-rays that strike denser tissue (e.g., bone) are absorbed by the tissue to a greater extent and leave the exposed film lighter. The shadows on the radiograph vary in shades of gray based on the density of the tissue through which the x-rays have passed.

Four different tissue densities are visible on a normal **chest radiograph.** The tissue types that generate these densities are *air, fat, soft tissue* (*water density* because soft tissues, similar to muscle, are mainly composed of water), and *bone.* Each tissue type absorbs different proportions of the x-ray beam, which results in a different appearance on the chest radiograph. Air in the lung, stomach, or intestines absorbs very few x-rays and appears virtually black **(radiolucent).** Fat absorbs a small amount of the x-ray beam and is usually seen as a light gray shadow. Soft tissue absorbs a slightly greater amount of the x-ray beam and is usually seen as a medium gray shadow. Bone absorbs a large fraction of the x-ray beam and is seen as a nearly white **(radiopaque)** shadow.

X-ray images have traditionally been recorded on film. Once developed, x-ray films were displayed by placing the film over a viewbox to illuminate the film for the observer. Currently, most radiographs are recorded, displayed, and stored in digital format on a computerized picture archiving and communication system. To record a digital image, an x-ray detector (digital film) replaces the photographic film. A computer takes the data from the x-ray detector and creates the image. The resulting image is displayed on a computer monitor.

Compared with images recorded on traditional film, digital images have advantages for interpreting and retrieving the image. The display of digital images can be manipulated by adjusting the contrast, brightness, and magnification. These adjustments allow findings that would be subtle and difficult to perceive on a traditional photographic film to be seen more easily. Digital images also allow multiple people to view the image simultaneously and in different locations. For example, an RT in a critical care unit, a radiologist in the imaging department, and a critical care physician in another location may collaborate by simultaneously viewing a chest radiograph on a rapidly deteriorating patient. Digital images also can be easily copied and recorded on compact discs so that patients can obtain digital copies of studies to take to their physicians. These technologic advancements facilitate the transmission of patient information as patients move from one hospital to another.

The structures visible on a chest radiograph are seen only when tissue of one density is next to tissue of a different density. The heart is visible as a soft tissue density in the middle of the chest because the lungs, which are primarily air density, normally surround it. If the lungs on either side of the heart fill with water (pulmonary consolidation or pleural effusion), the normal adjacent heart shadow would be invisible on the radiograph. This obscuring of the margin of adjacent structures of the same density is called the *silhouette sign* and can be useful to localize abnormalities within the chest. For example, the right middle lobe is adjacent to the right heart border, so the disappearance of the right heart border on the chest radiograph indicates an airspace opacity (such as pneumonia or atelectasis) in the right middle lobe. Stated simply, a right middle lobe pneumonia or atelectasis would "silhouette" the right heart border (Figure 21-1)

When to obtain a chest radiograph is the decision of the attending physician. However, because the RT is at the bedside, the physician will often welcome the RT's suggestion to obtain a chest x-ray radiograph, such as when a patient in the intensive care unit (ICU) suddenly deteriorates for no apparent reason. The RT needs to be familiar with the common clinical indications for obtaining a chest radiograph (Box 21-1).

Although a chest radiograph is important in evaluating patients with lung disease, it does have limitations. A chest radiograph may appear normal in a patient in respiratory failure; this is common in patients with acute (e.g., pulmonary embolism) or chronic obstructive lung disease (e.g., emphysema that is not apparent on a chest radiograph). In addition, the chest radiograph may lag behind the clinical condition of the patient. This situation is common in pneumonia, with which the patient may present with high fever and cough typical for pneumonia, but an airspace opacity or infiltrate may not appear on a chest film until 12 to 24 hours later. Similarly, the infiltrate on the chest film may persist for days to weeks after the resolution of symptoms.

Approach to Reading a Plain Chest Radiograph

A disciplined approach is required to obtain the maximal information from any diagnostic imaging study. Interpreting the chest radiograph provides an excellent example of this statement. An obvious abnormality such as a 6-cm mass is easily identified, even by the untrained observer. However, more subtle abnormalities, often with equal or even greater diagnostic importance, may go unnoticed if the observer is distracted by a more obvious abnormality. To avoid this pitfall, the observer must develop a step-by-step approach that is applied to interpreting a chest radiograph in a disciplined and consistent

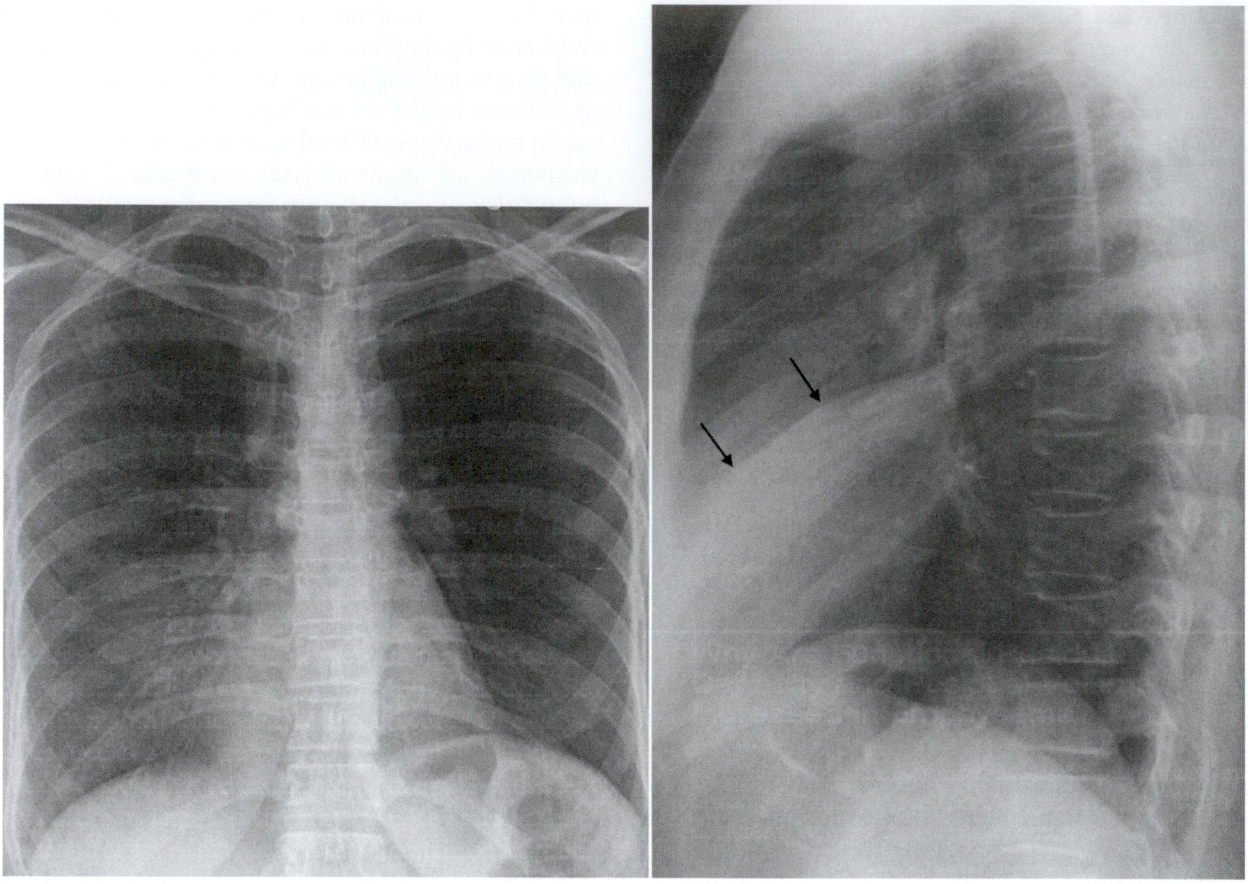

FIGURE 21-1 Posteroanterior view of the chest demonstrates obscuration or silhouetting of the right heart border because of airspace opacity in the right middle lobe. On the lateral view, there is right middle lobe collapse *(arrows)* secondary to an obstructing primary lung neoplasm (adenocarcinoma).

Box 21-1 Clinical Indications for Obtaining a Chest Radiograph

OUTPATIENT
Unexplained dyspnea
Severe persistent cough
Hemoptysis
Fever and sputum production
Acute severe chest pain
Positive tuberculosis skin test

INPATIENT
Placement of endotracheal tube
Placement of pulmonary artery catheter
Placement of central venous pressure catheter
Sudden onset of dyspnea or chest pain
Elevated or changing plateau pressure during mechanical ventilation
Sudden decline in oxygenation

fashion until it becomes routine. The following suggestions are broad guidelines, and each observer must formulate an approach that he or she finds comfortable.

In broad terms, the steps in reviewing a chest film are as follows:

- Confirm the correct patient's name on the radiograph.
- Review the technique and quality of the examination: Is the radiograph well centered (i.e., do the spinous processes project, overlying the trachea on a posteroanterior [PA] film), and is the degree of penetration of the beam adequate, too high (i.e., the lung parenchyma is too dark to see subtle changes), or too low (i.e., the lung parenchyma is too white, causing normal lung markings to appear abnormal)?
- Systematically review the anatomic structures on the chest film to assess their normality or abnormality.

In later sections of this chapter, the following areas will be reviewed: (1) evaluation of the technical quality and adequacy of the film, (2) normal anatomic structures on a chest radiograph, (3) more sophisticated imaging techniques, and (4) major anatomic components seen on the radiograph.

Chest Radiograph Technique and Quality

Several technical factors should be routinely assessed when interpreting a chest radiograph:

1. Is the radiograph appropriately labeled?
2. Is the study performed with PA and lateral views, or is it an anteroposterior (AP) portable examination?

3. Is the entire chest imaged (i.e., are any structures not included)?
4. Was the patient properly positioned?
5. Were the optimal settings for the x-ray beam selected when the film was taken (the term used is *penetration,* which is similar to *exposure* on camera film)?

As the first step, the RT should check the patient's identity and all labels visible on the film. This step helps to avoid the mistake of interpreting a chest radiograph for the wrong patient and establishes which side is which because labels are often placed to indicate the patient's left or right side; such labeling of the side is important in cases in which the patient's chest or abdominal contents are reversed—known as *situs inversus* or *dextrocardia.*

MINI CLINI

Evaluating the Heart Size on a Portable Chest Radiograph

A standard chest radiograph is obtained with the patient standing and facing the film cassette. The x-ray beam first enters the patient's back and then passes through the chest to the film. This standard technique is called the *PA chest radiograph.* The heart is located very close to the film with the standard PA view, and magnification of the heart shadow is minimal.

PROBLEM: In the ICU, patients are generally too ill for a PA chest film to be obtained. The chest film is obtained with the patient lying in bed and the film cassette placed behind the patient. The x-ray beam passes from anterior to posterior, producing an AP portable chest film. In examining an AP portable chest film, how is the appearance of the heart size affected?

DISCUSSION: An AP portable radiograph is obtained with the patient's heart farther from the film, producing a heart shadow that is artificially magnified compared with the shadow produced with a PA chest film; this may give the appearance of an enlarged heart in some cases. The clinician interpreting an AP portable radiograph must keep this in mind to avoid misinterpreting the film as showing that the heart is enlarged heart (cardiomegaly). To illustrate this point, hold a flashlight 3 feet from a wall and turn it on. While holding the flashlight steady, place one hand in the beam. The shadow created by the hand becomes smaller as the hand is moved closer to the wall and farther from the light source (equivalent to a PA film) and bigger as the hand approaches the light source (equivalent to an AP film).

RULE OF THUMB

When evaluating a plain chest radiograph, first assess the technical quality of the chest radiograph—that is, is there rotation or is the patient positioned well? Is the x-ray beam penetration appropriate? Then, use a step-by-step approach to view all the structures on the chest radiograph.

A chest radiograph is taken using one of two techniques: the PA view or the AP view. The views are named for the path of the x-ray beam. In the PA view, the patient puts his or her back to the x-ray source and the chest against the film. The x-ray beam leaves the source, passes through the posterior side of the patient, through the patient, then through the patient's anterior surface, and finally to the film. The PA view is usually performed in the radiology department with equipment that standardizes the distance (typically 6 feet) from the x-ray source to the film and where the x-ray technician can maximize the quality of each film. In addition, as noted, taking the film with the anterior chest closest to the film minimizes magnification of the heart.

The AP film is usually taken with a portable x-ray machine. The AP technique places the x-ray source in front of the patient, with the film behind the patient's back. The source of the x-ray beam is usually much closer to the patient than with a PA film, although the distance varies from patient to patient. The closer x-ray source and the position of the patient both lead to a magnification of the heart shadow. The AP film is usually taken in the ICU because these patients are too ill to travel to the radiology department or to stand for a PA film. Overall, AP portable films are usually of lesser quality than PA films. During the interpretation of the chest radiograph, the RT needs to take into account the view (AP or PA) when evaluating the heart size and subtle findings that may be influenced by film quality and technique.

When a chest radiograph examination is performed, it is sometimes difficult to align the patient properly, and a portion of the chest may not be imaged. Although these problems are more common with portable (AP) examinations, they also may occur with PA and lateral radiographs as well. The RT should ask the following questions: (1) Is the entire chest included on the film? (2) Is the patient well positioned?

Patient rotation can make interpretation more difficult by projecting *midline* structures (e.g., the trachea) to the right or left. The observer can assess for rotation by comparing anterior structures such as the *medial* (toward the middle) ends of the clavicles with a posterior structure such as the spinous processes of the spine. In a perfectly positioned or aligned chest film, the spinous process should be seen midway between the medial ends of the clavicles and in the middle of the tracheal air column (Figure 21-2). Patient rotation makes the mediastinum appear unusually wide and obscures or distorts the appearance of the pulmonary arteries as they emerge from the mediastinum into the lung parenchyma.

The RT also must ensure that the film is adequately penetrated. An improperly penetrated film may conceal important details. A chest radiograph with proper exposure should show the intervertebral disc spaces through the shadow of the heart and should allow the blood vessels in the peripheral regions of the lungs to be visualized. A chest radiograph that is underexposed or underpenetrated (i.e., owing to too-low kilovoltage of the x-ray beam) does not allow visualization of the intervertebral discs through the heart shadow and may make identification of abnormalities in the soft tissue areas such as the mediastinum more difficult. Specifically, an underpenetrated

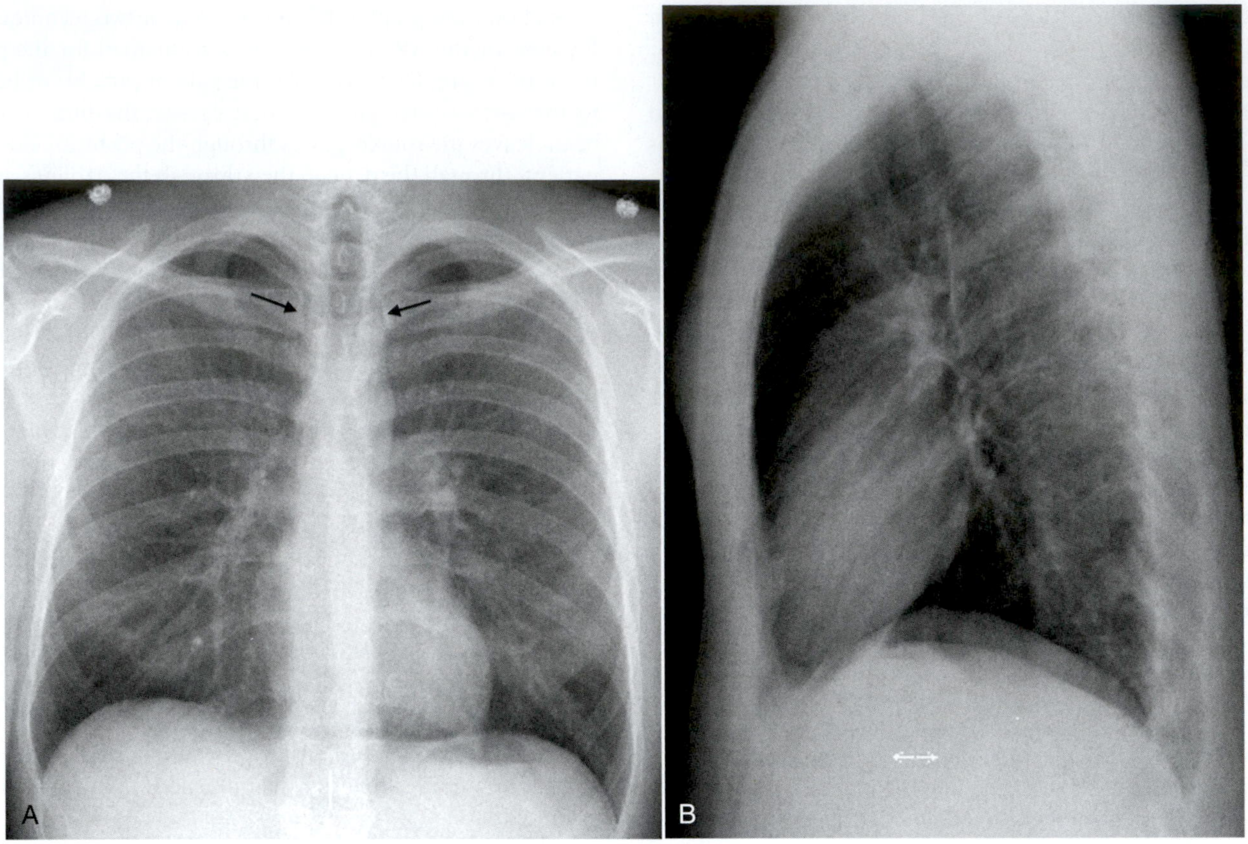

FIGURE 21-2 Normal frontal **(A)** and lateral **(B)** views of the chest radiograph. Note the medial ends of the clavicles *(arrows)* with the spinous process *(arrowhead)* framed between them **(A).**

film may cause the normal branching of the pulmonary arteries in the lung to appear abnormal and be misinterpreted as evidence of interstitial infiltrates. Similarly, an overpenetrated radiograph overexposes the film, leaving the lung parenchyma black and making it difficult to visualize the peripheral blood vessels or abnormalities that may be present (e.g., infiltrates secondary to pneumonia, pulmonary nodules). This overpenetration makes evaluation of the lung parenchyma far more difficult. Adjustment of the contrast and brightness of the chest film on the computer display of a digital image improves the ability to see certain aspects of a chest x-ray with improper penetration. However, adjusting the display cannot completely overcome the loss of important details caused by an improperly penetrated film.

MINI CLINI

Value of Proper Technique on a Chest Radiograph

Careful attention to the technical quality of a chest radiograph is key in both acquiring and interpreting the study. If the settings when the examination is taken are incorrect or if the patient is improperly positioned, this can lead to important changes in the appearance of the chest radiograph that can either hide important details or lead to a misinterpretation.

PROBLEM: A patient presents to the emergency department with chest pain. The initial radiograph obtained demonstrates decreased lung markings (Figure 21-3), which the inexperienced observer may interpret as emphysema or a pneumothorax.

DISCUSSION: The astute observer realizes that the findings on the chest radiograph may be due to overpenetration rather than an abnormality with the lung parenchyma. When radiographs were previously obtained on film, errors in either underpenetration or overpenetration were difficult to overcome. As this study was obtained using a digital detector, inadequate penetration often can be compensated for by changing the contrast or brightness on the digital screen. However, in some instances in which the overpenetration or underpenetration is so severe, changing the contrast and brightness cannot correct the initial error and a repeat study may be necessary. A repeat radiograph (see Figure 21-3) demonstrates normal lung markings without evidence of emphysema or a pneumothorax.

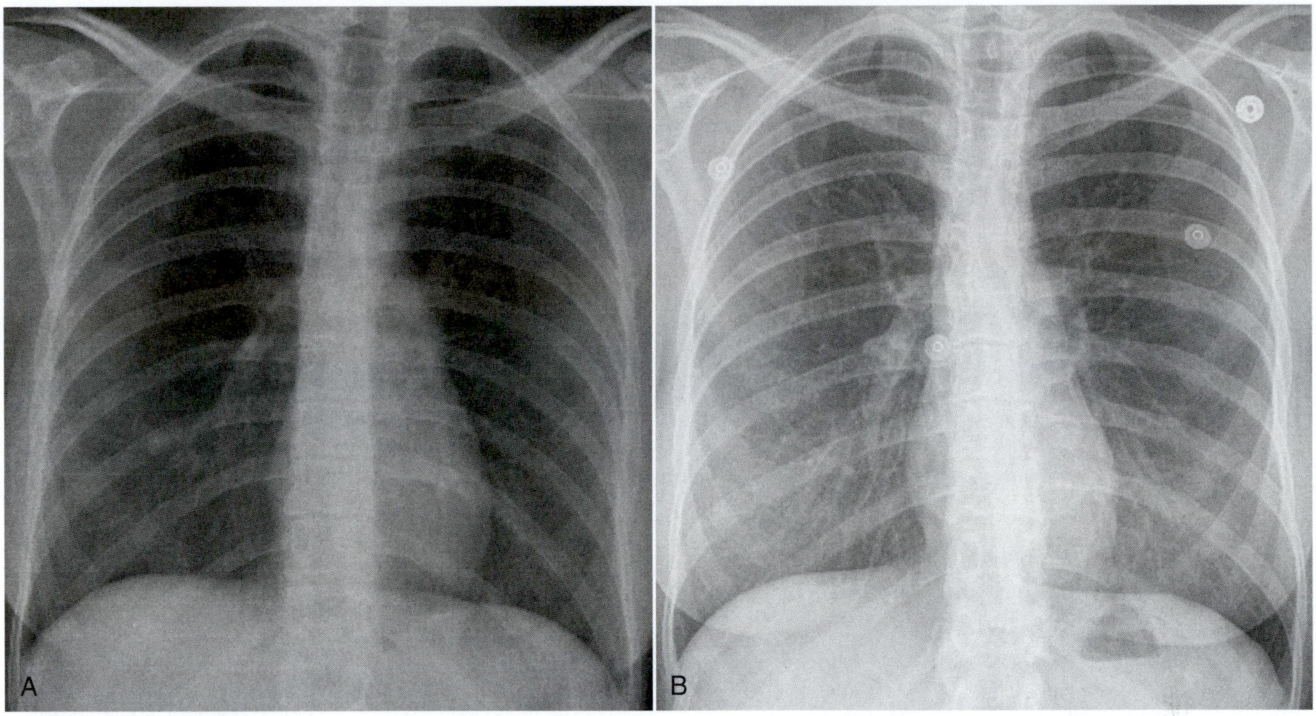

FIGURE 21-3 Radiographs of the chest performed several hours apart. **A,** The chest radiograph is overpenetrated. The lung markings are difficult to visualize which can simulate emphysema or a pneumothorax. **B,** A repeat radiograph performed with adequate penetration demonstrates normal lung markings bilaterally without evidence of emphysema or a pneumothorax.

Anatomic Structures Seen on a Chest Radiograph

After the RT has reviewed the technical aspects of the chest radiograph, it is time to review the anatomic findings on the film. The main structures imaged on a routine chest radiograph are listed next and illustrated in Figure 21-4:

1. Bones (e.g., ribs, clavicles, scapulae, vertebrae)
2. Soft tissues (e.g., tissues of the chest wall, upper abdomen, lymph nodes)
3. Lungs (including the trachea, bronchi, and lung tissue or parenchyma)
4. Pleura (membranous covering of the lung, including the *visceral pleura* [the part attached to the lungs] and the *parietal pleura* [the part lining the inside of the chest wall]; although normally occupied by only a small amount of fluid, the space between the parietal and visceral pleura is called the *pleural space*)
5. Heart, great vessels, and mediastinum (i.e., the tissues between the lungs in the center of the chest, bordered by the sternum anteriorly and the vertebral column posteriorly in the AP dimension and by the thoracic inlet superiorly [where the trachea enters the chest] and the diaphragm inferiorly in the craniocaudal [moving from the head to the feet] direction)
6. Upper abdomen
7. Lower neck

The anatomy seen on the chest radiograph should be reviewed in a thorough, systematic manner. All of the previously listed anatomic structures must be individually assessed. When first interpreting radiographs, it is helpful for the RT to create a list of the anatomic structures that must be assessed and to check off the structures as they are reviewed. With experience, the checklist becomes second nature and automatic.

Assessment of the chest wall should include evaluating for symmetry, rib fractures, or other bone abnormalities. Lung evaluation begins by assessing the lung volumes (size) and density. Any obvious differences in symmetry must be explained. Of the lung parenchyma, 80% to 90% is overlaid with bone in the form of ribs, clavicles, and the thoracic spine. The overlying bone may obscure important lung abnormalities. A lateral view is helpful in clarifying the presence or absence of suspicious lung abnormalities on frontal (PA or AP) projections. The RT must pay specific attention to areas where subtle abnormalities may be hiding; these include the lung apexes (behind the clavicles), the area of lung that projects behind the heart, and the portion of lung that lies deep in the posterior sulcus (the extreme bottom of the lung projecting behind the dome of the diaphragm on the frontal view).

Review of the lung periphery on both frontal and lateral views discloses any pleural abnormalities, such as fluid in the pleural space (e.g., hydrothorax, hemothorax [blood in the pleural space]) and air in the pleural space (pneumothorax). Evaluation of the mediastinum should include assessment of the heart size. On the PA projection, the diameter of the heart shadow (cardiac silhouette) should not exceed one-half the diameter of the chest. An enlarged cardiac silhouette may occur

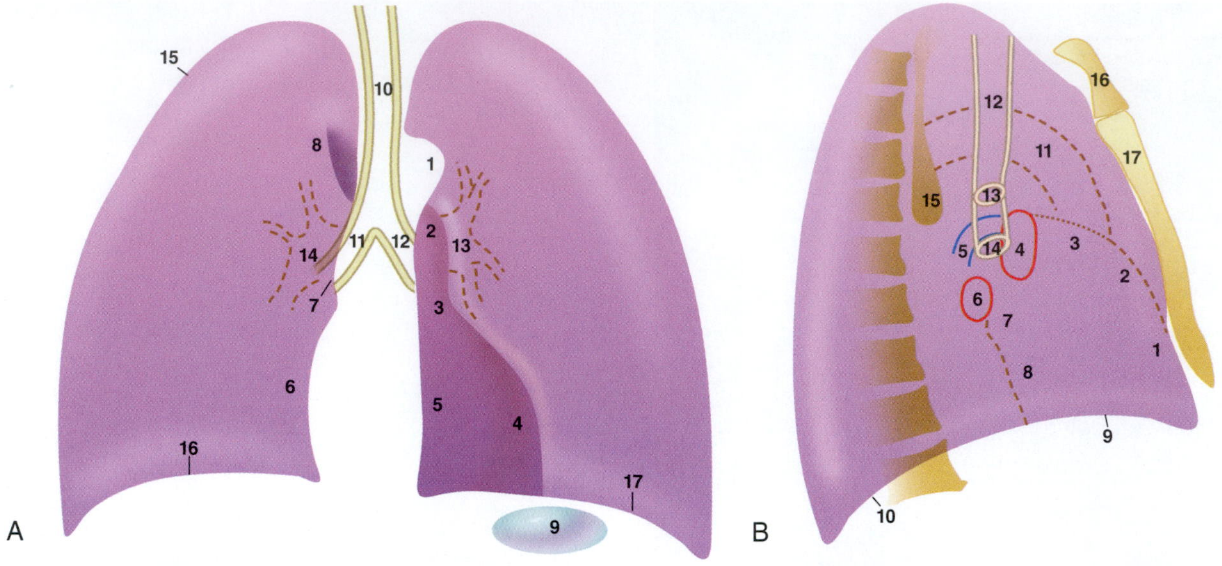

1. Aortic arch
2. Main pulmonary artery
3. Left atrium
4. Left ventricle
5. Descending aorta
6. Right atrium
7. Ascending aorta
8. Superior vena cava
9. Gastric bubble
10. Trachea
11. Right main bronchus
12. Left main bronchus
13. Left pulmonary artery
14. Right pulmonary artery
15. Pleural line
16. Right hemidiaphragm
17. Left hemidiaphragm

1. Right ventricle
2. Pulmonary outflow tract
3. Main pulmonary artery
4. Right pulmonary artery
5. Left pulmonary artery
6. Pulmonary veins
7. Left atrium
8. Left ventricle
9. Right hemidiaphragm
10. Left hemidiaphragm
11. Aortic arch
12. Trachea
13. Right upper lobe bronchus
14. Left upper lobe bronchus
15. Scapulae
16. Manubrium
17. Sternum

FIGURE 21-4 Schematic diagrams of the normal structures seen on a chest radiograph. A, Posteroanterior view. B, Lateral view.

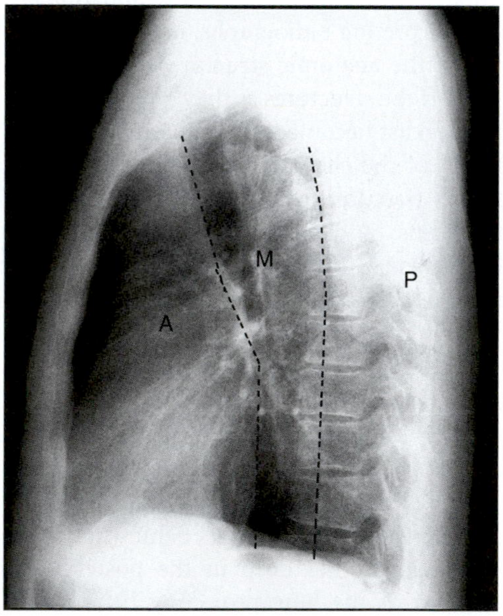

FIGURE 21-5 Lateral view of the chest, indicating the divisions of the mediastinum: anterior *(A)*; middle *(M)*; posterior *(P)*.

with congestive heart failure or with a pericardial effusion (fluid within the space that surrounds the heart encased within the pericardium). The lateral contours of the mediastinum should correspond to normal anatomic structures, as outlined in Figure 21-5.

Advanced Chest Imaging Techniques

Computed Tomography of the Chest

Computed tomography (CT) scanning is an essential and commonly used imaging technique to assess the chest. Advantages include its excellent anatomic detail, wide availability, and short examination time to acquire the images. Structures as small as 1 mm can be visualized, allowing for detailed anatomic depiction of the structures of the chest. Modern CT scanners are fast, with images of the entire chest obtained in less than 10 seconds, allowing for accurate and rapid assessment of critically ill ICU patients in the ICU.

To perform a CT scan, a patient lies on a table called a **gantry.** The gantry is passed through a circular opening in the CT scanner. X-ray sources and detectors surround the opening in the scanner. When the scanning begins, the x-ray source and detectors pass quickly around the patient in a circular motion with the x-ray beam passing through the patient to detectors on the opposite side. The information from the detectors is sent to a computer, which generates a two-dimensional image from the detector data. Each image created by the scan looks like a slice of the patient. Historically, after each CT image was obtained, the patient was advanced in a step-wise fashion until the entire chest was imaged. Modern CT scanners use numerous detectors (typically between 16 and 256) all connected to a highly capable image processing computer. Patients pass rapidly through the CT scanner without stopping for each image. The term *spiral* or *helical* is applied to these more current CT scanners.

TABLE 21-1
Radiation Dose of Common Thoracic Imaging Studies

Study	Radiation Dose (mSv)	Equivalent Normal Background Radiation
Chest radiograph (PA and lateral)	0.1 mSv	10 days
Chest CT (low-dose screen)	1.5 mSv	6 mo
Chest CT (standard dose)	7.0 mSv	2 yr
Coronary CT angiogram	12.0 mSv	4 yr

CT, Computed tomography; *PA,* posteroanterior.

CT scans depict the anatomy in the chest better than the standard chest radiograph but expose the patient to more radiation, which varies depending on the specific CT technique used (Table 21-1). For example, a standard-dose chest CT examination exposes the patient to the equivalent of 70 chest x-rays. Ongoing research and technologic advancements will likely continue to lower the radiation dose of CT scans.

Chest CT provides an excellent view of the chest and allows imaging of portions of the chest that are poorly seen on chest radiographs. Areas such as the mediastinum, the lung apexes and costophrenic sulci of the lungs (the normally sharp shadows where the diaphragm contacts the rib cage laterally), and the pleural surfaces all are easily seen with CT scanning. Chest CT is commonly performed to evaluate lung nodules and masses, the lung parenchyma, great vessels of the chest, the mediastinum, and pleural disease. To evaluate blood vessels and soft tissue structures in close proximity, such as hilar lymph nodes, iodinated contrast can be helpful because contrast makes blood appear denser (radiopaque or white) and allows blood vessels to be distinguished from soft tissue.

Currently, chest CT examinations are generally displayed with a slice thickness of 1 to 5 mm. Each image therefore will include everything within the 1- to 5-mm slice of tissue. Thin slices allow for maximal spatial resolution (i.e., the ability to separate objects that are close together). For example, to evaluate the lung parenchyma in a patient with suspected interstitial lung disease, thin slices, typically 1 mm, are used to evaluate the fine architecture of the lung, referred to as a high-resolution chest CT (HRCT). Thin slices are also helpful in the evaluation of small pulmonary nodules or to evaluate for pulmonary emboli on a pulmonary embolism study. A disadvantage of thin slices is that they have more image noise and there are more images to interpret. For example, pulmonary embolism studies performed with a 1-mm slice thickness generally have approximately 1000 images per study.

Recent evidence suggests that low-dose chest CT scans may be useful in screening high-risk individuals for lung cancer. Specifically, patients who are between the ages 55 and 74, who have smoked more than 30 pack-years, and who are currently smoking or who stopped smoking fewer than 15 years earlier may prolong survival from lung cancer. A large study of greater than 50,000 patients demonstrated that the mortality rate or risk for death from lung cancer was reduced by 20% in patients who underwent screening chest CT compared to a chest radiograph examination.[2] This technique uses a lower peak kilovoltage than standard studies, so the images are grainier than a with standard CT. The benefit is that the radiation dose is approximately one-fifth that of a standard chest CT.

Computed Tomography Angiography

The rapid scanning that can be performed on helical CT scanners has made CT angiography possible. To perform CT angiography, IV contrast dye is injected at a high rate to darken or opacify the vascular structures. A large-bore peripheral IV in an antecubital vein or a peripherally inserted central catheter (PICC) line that can handle a high contrast injection rate is required. CT angiography of the chest has been used for years to identify pulmonary embolism, although advances in technology now allow for visualization of pulmonary emboli in tiny peripheral arteries that were not visible on older models of CT scans (Figure 21-6).[1] Technologic advancements have made possible CT angiography of the coronary arteries, which can serve as an alternative to routine coronary angiography by catheterization in many patients.[3]

Three-Dimensional Reconstruction

The imaging processing capabilities of modern CT scanners allow for reconstruction of the chest in any direction and production of three-dimensional (3-D) representations of some areas of the body (Figure 21-7). These 3-D images can be helpful for surgeons before surgery to visualize how anatomic structures may appear at surgery. The images also can simulate what a physician would see during a bronchoscopy, referred to as *virtual bronchoscopy.*

Magnetic Resonance Imaging of the Chest

MRI has many uses in the chest and is typically used as a problem-solving tool to answer specific clinical questions that cannot be answered by other imaging examinations such as a chest x-ray, chest CT, or ultrasound examination. MRI is generated by placing patients into a strong magnetic field. The physics of MR are complicated and are beyond the scope of this chapter. Briefly, the strong magnetic field aligns nuclei with nonzero spins (nuclei that have an odd number of protons and neutrons), such as hydrogen atoms, with the magnetic field. Because hydrogen atoms are present in high concentration throughout the body, they provide an excellent target for MRI evaluation. Pulses of radio waves are directed at the hydrogen nuclei, resulting in the alignment of hydrogen nuclei to change in orientation with the magnetic field. After the radio signal is stopped, the nuclei flip back to their original alignment and release their own radio waves. MRI uses the radio waves from the realigning nuclei to generate an image.

MRI has advantages over other imaging techniques in the chest that are useful in specific circumstances. MRI does not use x-rays and therefore does not expose patients to ionizing radiation. MRI has superb soft tissue characterization, allowing for detailed analysis of soft tissue masses. The most common uses for MRI in the chest are for imaging the mediastinum, large vessels in the chest (e.g., for pulmonary emboli or

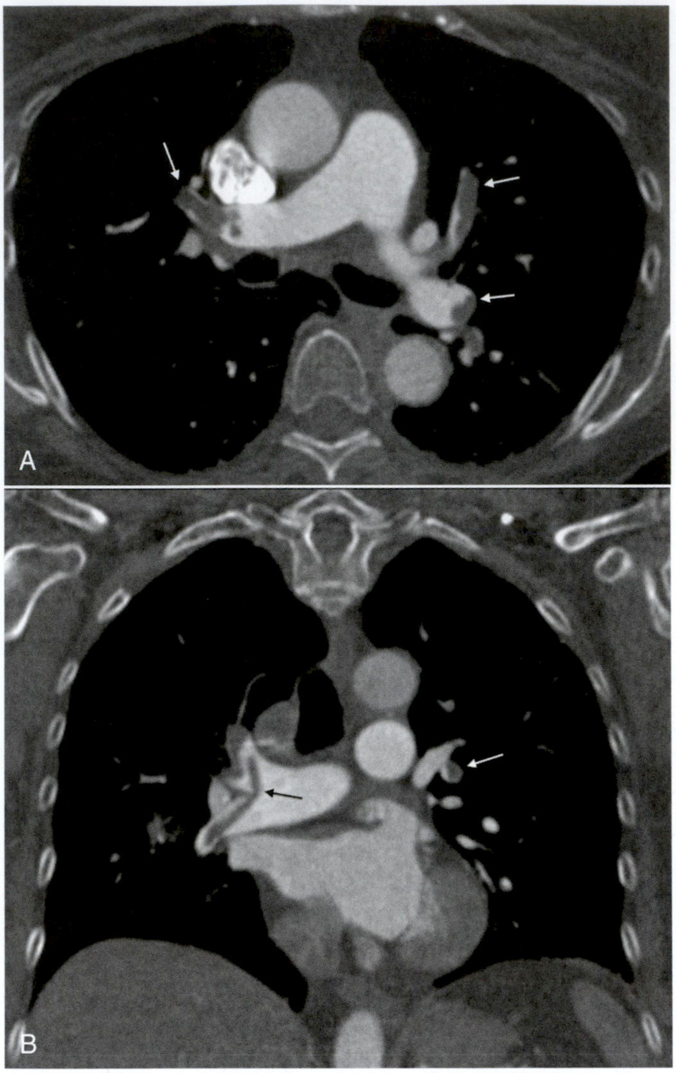

FIGURE 21-6 Computed tomography angiogram of a patient with bilateral acute pulmonary emboli. **A,** The pulmonary emboli are seen as the dark filling defects *(arrows)* outlined by the white contrast-enhanced blood vessels *(arrows)*. Coronally reformatted image **(B)** is helpful to visualize clot entering both the right upper and right lower lobar pulmonary arteries *(arrows)*.

vascular abnormalities), and the heart.[4] The superior soft tissue characterization of MR allows for the confident diagnosis of a benign mediastinal mass (such as a thymoma) and can spare patients surgery to establish a diagnosis.[5] In patients in renal failure in whom there is clinical concern for a pulmonary embolism who cannot receive IV contrast, an MR examination can be performed without contrast to establish a diagnosis. MR has limited uses for imaging the lung parenchyma. For example, in a patient with lung cancer undergoing evaluation for possible resection, MR can determine whether the tumor invades the chest wall by determining if the lesion moves independently of the chest wall during both inspiration and expiration.

However, MRI does have significant limitations when applied to imaging the chest. MRI examinations take longer to acquire (at least 10 minutes and up to 1 hour) than other examinations (such as radiographs or CT), which makes respiratory and cardiac motion more significant obstacles. Imaging of critically ill ICU patients is thus difficult because these patients may be unable to lie in the MR scanner for a long period. The lungs are primarily composed of gas; therefore there is little signal to generate images as is required by MR, making the MRI less useful to evaluate the lung parenchyma.

In addition, the large magnet required for MR examinations makes it generally contraindicated in patients with pacemakers or other significant metal objects in their bodies to undergo MRI. A patient with a small metal object in a crucial place, such as a surgical clip in the brain or eye generally cannot undergo MRI. The powerful magnet will pull metallic objects into the magnet with great force, exposing both patients and health care providers in its path to life-threatening risk. Medical equipment containing metal such as ventilators and gas cylinders also cannot be brought near the MR scanner. Deaths have been reported when metal objects (e.g., oxygen cylinders) have been brought into the magnetic field of the MRI, and RTs must be especially vigilant about this issue. MRI units usually have well-marked warnings and areas beyond which conventional metal objects absolutely must not pass.

Ultrasound

Ultrasound images are created by passing high-frequency sound waves into the body and detecting the sound waves that bounce back (echo) from the tissues of the body. The pattern of the returning sound waves is used to generate an image of the tissue studied. Ultrasound of the chest is excellent for evaluating the heart (echocardiogram) or pleural fluid.[6]

Ultrasound imaging using small portable machines has become common practice in critical care units. Portable ultrasound units allow for the rapid assessment of heart function and volume status and are used to assist in many critical care procedures.[7] Because it can localize excessive pleural fluid which characterizes a pleural effusion, ultrasound can be using in performing a thoracentesis. Ultrasound is also commonly used to guide placement of central venous and arterial catheters. Blood vessels are easily identified using ultrasound. The compressibility of veins is used to differentiate veins from arteries (Figure 21-8). Because the path that the needle is taking is clearly seen on the ultrasound screen, using ultrasound guidance for venous and arterial puncture allows the procedure to be more easily accomplished with less time, risk, and patient discomfort.

The remainder of the chapter outlines commonly encountered abnormalities involving the pleura, lung parenchyma, and mediastinum. The reader is encouraged to fine-tune his or her observational powers for assessing imaging studies because, as noted by Pasteur, "In the field of observation, chance favors the prepared mind."

RULE OF THUMB

Three general steps to assessing a chest film are as follows:

1. Content assurance: Is the entire chest visible on the film?
2. Quality assurance: Is the chest radiograph properly exposed and centered?
3. Disciplined application of a personalized, consistent search pattern

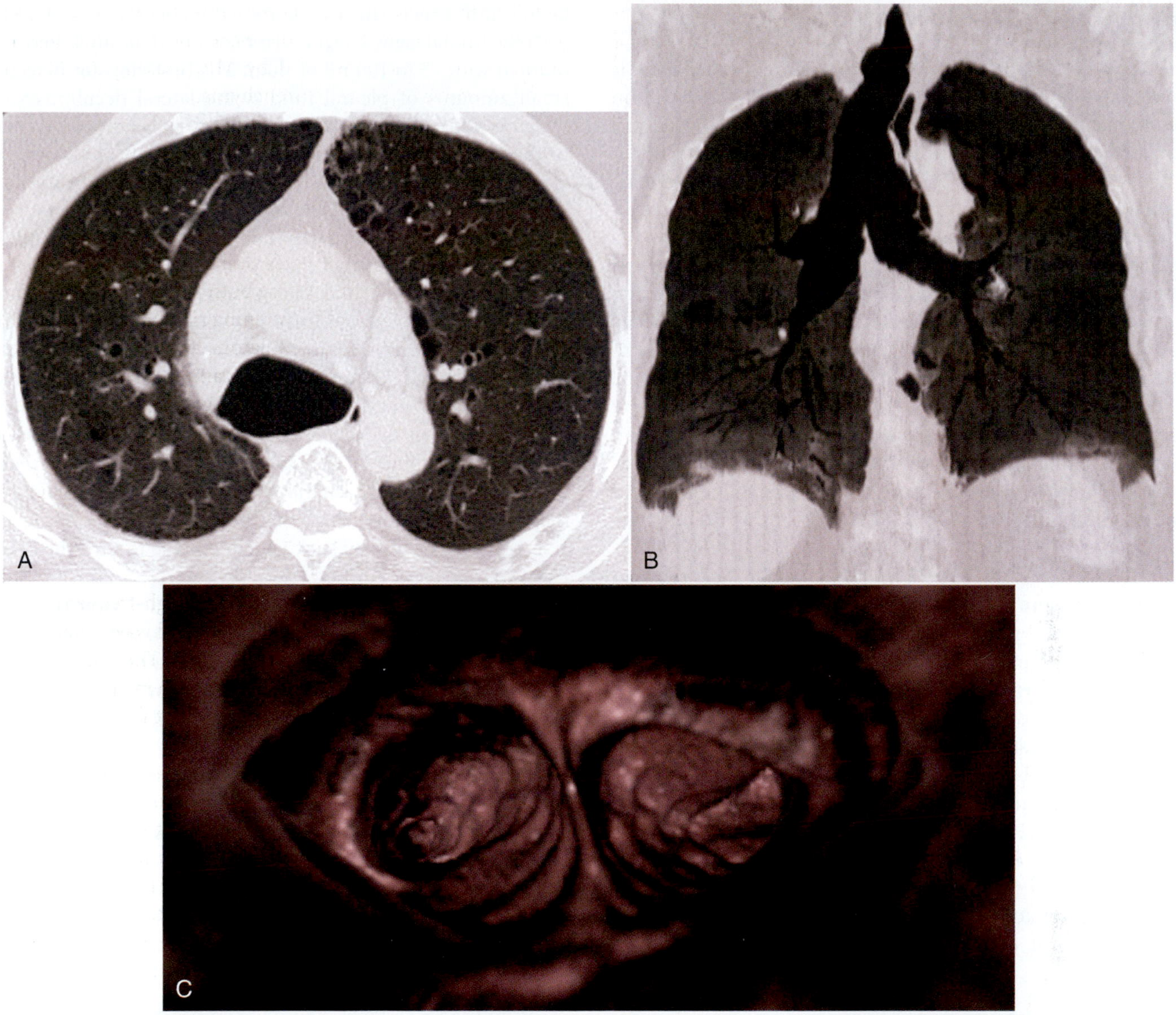

FIGURE 21-7 Use of 2-D and 3-D images for visualization of the trachea. Axial CT **(A)** image demonstrates a massively dilated trachea in a patient with tracheobronchomegaly (Mounier-Kuhn). A coronally reformatted minimum intensity projection (minIP) image **(B)** allows for visualization of the entire trachea and main stem bronchi. A 3-D image **(C)** endoluminal view of the inferior trachea looking downward at the carina with the left and right main stem bronchi located on each side of the carina. The 3-D image, termed *virtual bronchoscopy,* can aid the bronchoscopist in planning a bronchoscopic procedure.

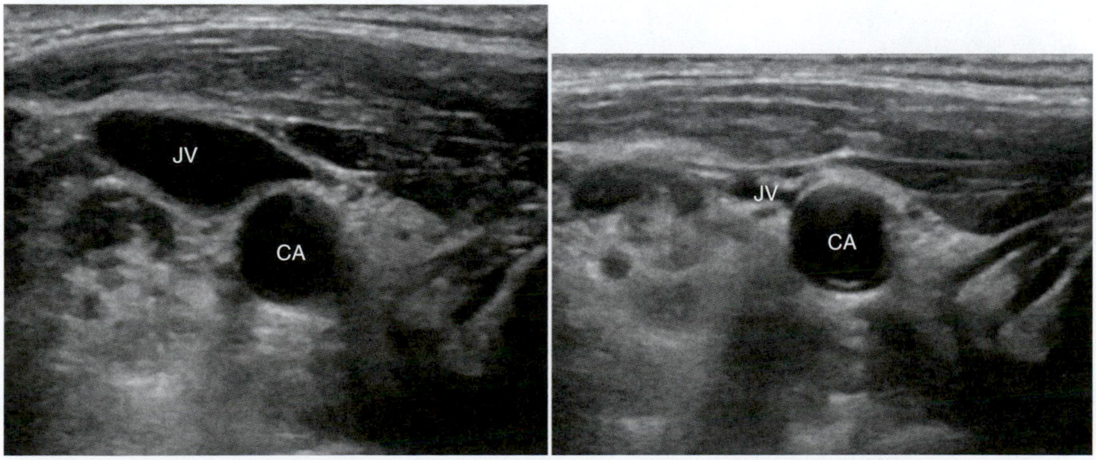

FIGURE 21-8 Two ultrasound images of the right internal jugular vein *(JV)* and right carotid artery *(CA)*. In the first image, the jugular vein is distended; in the second image, the jugular vein is collapsed by gently applying pressure with the ultrasound transducer. The carotid artery did not compress.

PLEURA

The thin membrane surrounding the lung parenchyma is referred to as the *pleura.* The lungs are surrounded by two thin pleural membranes. The outer pleural membrane, known as the *parietal pleura,* adheres to the inside of the chest wall, the upper surface of the diaphragm, and the lateral aspect of the mediastinum. The inner pleural membrane, or *visceral pleura,* closely adheres to the surface of each lung. The visceral pleura extends along the fissures that separate the lobes. The pleural membranes around the lung cannot be seen on a chest radiograph because they blend into the water density of the chest wall, diaphragm, and mediastinum. However, the visceral pleura separating the lobes can be seen if the pleural surface is parallel to the x-ray beam (as with the "minor" or "horizontal" fissure separating the right upper lobe from the right middle lobe on a PA chest x-ray). Although very thin, the visceral pleura separating the lobes is visible because it is contrasted with aerated lung on either side.

Pleural Effusion (Hydrothorax)

A **pleural effusion** refers to the accumulation of excess fluid within the pleural space. In healthy individuals, it is estimated that 1 to 8 ml of pleural fluid is normally present.[8] Normally, the diaphragm forms a dome that curves downward to attach to the chest wall on the lower ribs and thoracic and lumbar vertebra. On a chest radiograph, the arch of the diaphragm and the chest wall meet to form a point called the *costophrenic angle.* The costophrenic angle is seen on both PA and lateral views (see Figure 21-2). If the point of the costophrenic angle is rounded rather than sharp, it usually indicates that a pleural effusion is present (Figure 21-9).[9] For a pleural effusion to cause blunting of the costophrenic angle on the frontal (PA/AP) view, at least 175 to 200 ml of pleural fluid must have accumulated. The lateral film detects smaller pleural effusions than are detected with the frontal view. The posterior costophrenic angle becomes blunted with 75 to 100 ml of fluid. The best view for detecting small amounts of pleural fluid is the lateral decubitus view, which is a frontal view taken as the patient is lying on the side of the suspected effusion; 5 ml of pleural fluid can be detected on a decubitus radiograph.[10] As discussed later, ultrasound is also useful for detecting a pleural effusion.

Sometimes, fluid can accumulate between the lung and the diaphragm and maintain a sharp costophrenic angle, hiding up to 500 ml of fluid.[11] Fluid that accumulates between the lung and the diaphragm is said to be in a *subpulmonic* location. The subpulmonic location is the first place pleural effusions accumulate in an upright patient.[12] The earliest sign of a left-sided pleural effusion on an upright chest radiograph is an increased distance between the inferior margin of the left lung and the stomach gas bubble. With a subpulmonic effusion, there may be an associated slight lateral shift of the point at which the diaphragm dips downward on the frontal chest radiograph (i.e., similar to a hockey stick with the blade toward the lateral chest wall).

If both air and fluid are contained within the same space, the interface between the air and the fluid forms a soft tissue density with a straight, horizontal border that has air density above it. The interface may have a small meniscus on both sides. These straight, level interfaces between air and fluid are called *air-fluid levels.* An air-fluid level in the pleural space indicates a **hydropneumothorax** (Figure 21-10), or both air and fluid in the pleural space.

Occasionally, fluid accumulates in an unusual position, such as within an interlobar fissure (which separates lobes of the lung). Fluid is most commonly seen in the minor fissure, which is between the right middle lobe and the right upper lobe. Fluid within a fissure can be diagnosed on a chest radiograph by a

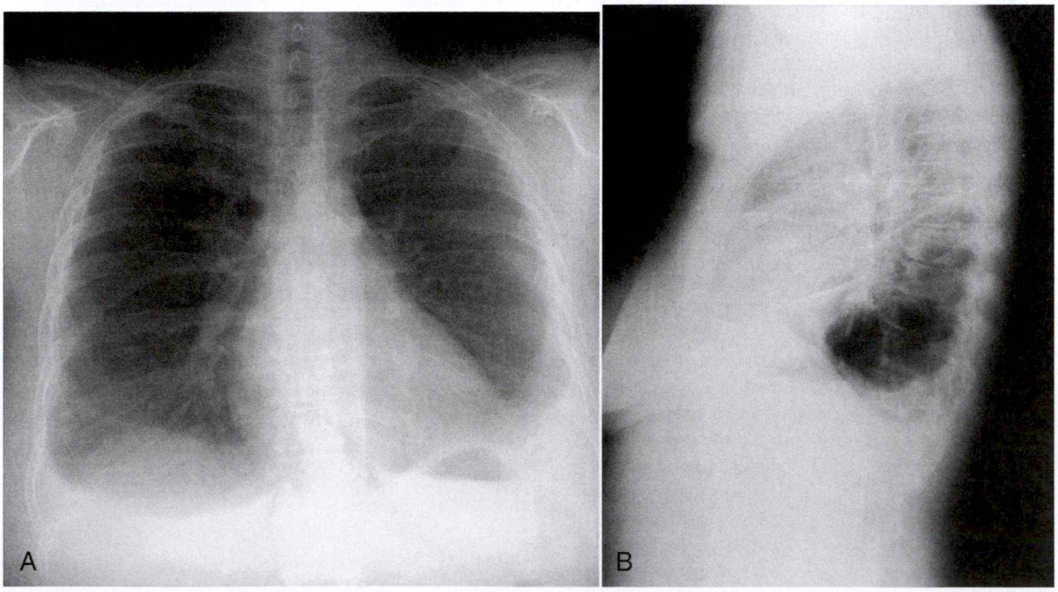

FIGURE 21-9 Pleural effusion. Posteroanterior **(A)** and lateral **(B)** chest films in a 43-year-old patient with long-standing bilateral pleural effusions resulting from rheumatoid arthritis. Note the bilateral meniscus sign is also visualized posteriorly on the lateral view.

characteristic biconvex lenslike, elliptical shape on either the PA or the lateral projection (Figure 21-11).

An increased volume of pleural fluid generally is categorized as either a *transudate* or an *exudate* (see Chapter 27). However, an exudate cannot be distinguished from a transudate on a chest radiograph or chest CT. This distinction requires analyzing a sample of the pleural fluid. *Loculation* of pleural fluid (or trapping so that the fluid does not move freely with changing positions) is more commonly seen in exudative effusions, hemothorax (blood in the pleural space), and empyema (infection of the pleural fluid).

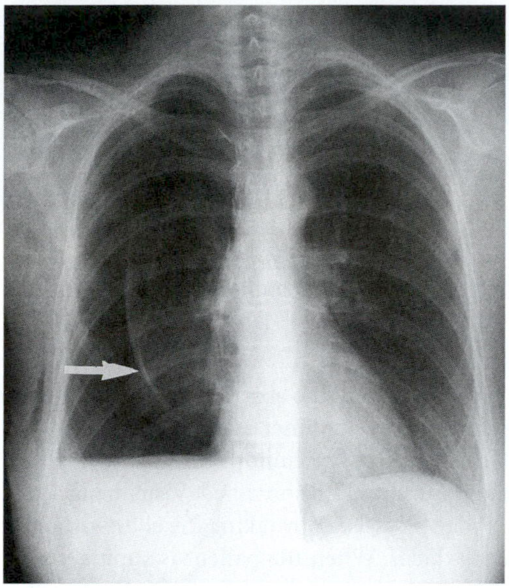

FIGURE 21-10 Hydropneumothorax. Single posteroanterior view of the chest in a patient with a hydropneumothorax. Note the air-fluid level in the pleural space. The arrow points to the visceral pleura (lung border) being compressed by both air and fluid.

Clues as to whether a pleural exudate results from inflammation or from cancer may be present on the chest radiograph. Clues that favor a malignant cause for a pleural effusion include pleural-based nodules, pulmonary nodules, or evidence of prior malignancy, such as surgical absence of the breast in a patient with breast cancer.

Ultrasound for Evaluating Pleural Fluid

Ultrasound reliably detects both small and large pleural effusions (Figure 21-12). It is also very useful in separating pleural

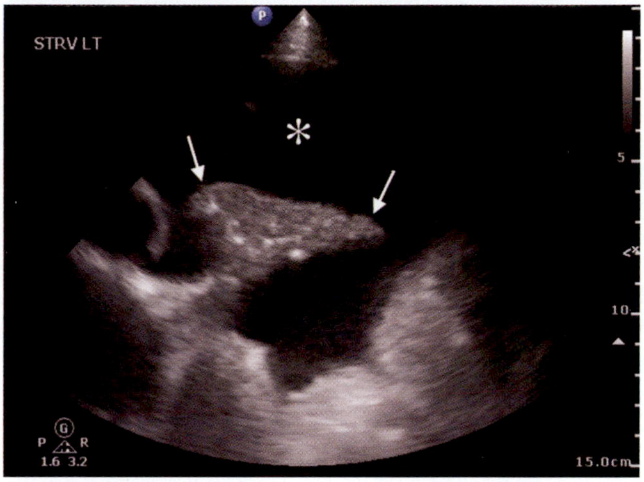

FIGURE 21-12 Pleural effusion. Ultrasound image demonstrates a large pleural effusion (asterisk). Adjacent to the pleural effusion is collapsed lung *(arrows)*.

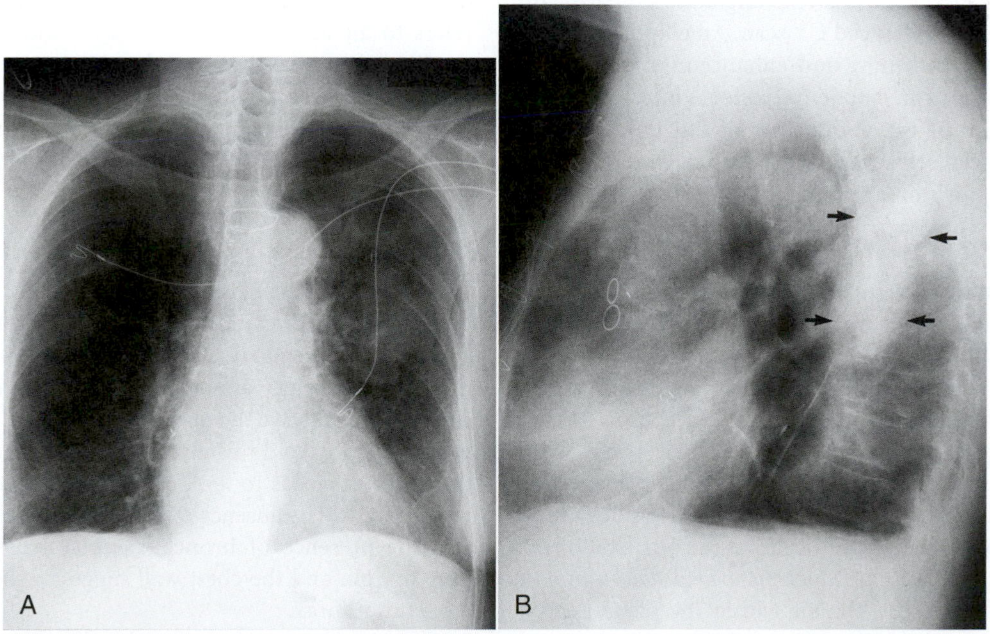

FIGURE 21-11 Intrafissural fluid. Two views of the chest showing fluid accumulating within the superior portion of the major fissure. In the posteroanterior view, the fluid is seen as vague increased density in the left upper lobe. Note the typical elliptic shape of the fluid on the lateral projection *(arrows)*.

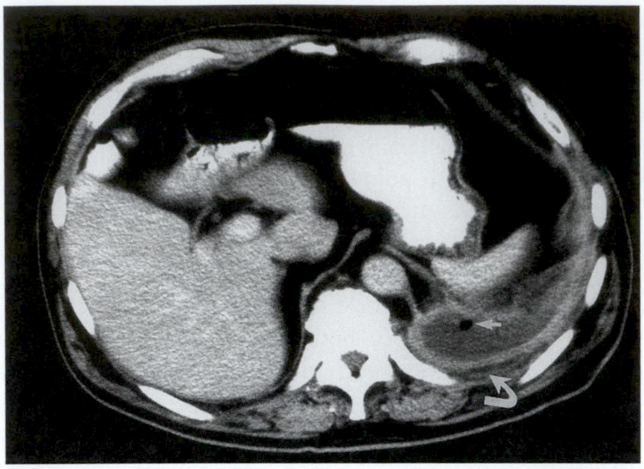

FIGURE 21-13 Empyema. Cross-sectional computed tomography image shows an elliptic pleural fluid collection surrounded by thickened enhancing pleura (split pleural sign). The presence of the gas bubble *(short arrow)* within the fluid and the thickened extrapleural subcostal tissues *(curved arrow)* is strongly suggestive of empyema.

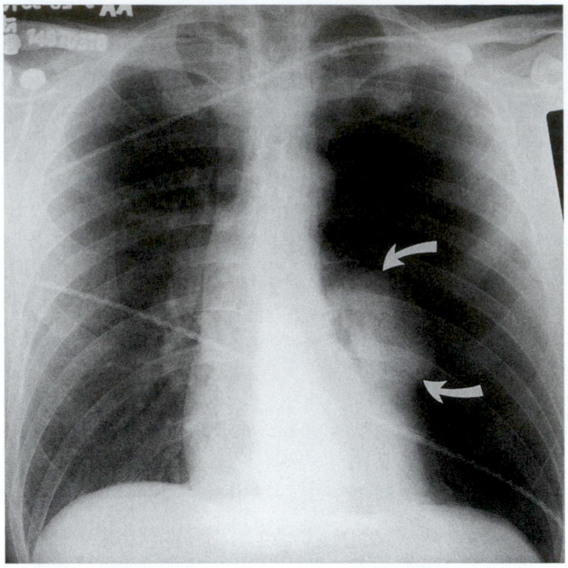

FIGURE 21-14 Pneumothorax. Complete atelectasis of the left lung *(curved arrows)* resulting from a large left pneumothorax.

fluid from solid tissue[13] and readily identifies tissue bands associated with loculated effusions. Ultrasound is also helpful in guiding thoracentesis, in particular, for small or loculated pleural effusions.

Computed Tomography

Pleural fluid can be identified easily on CT scans of the chest. In a supine patient, free fluid accumulates in the most dependent area of the pleura, which is posteriorly. Pleural fluid that does not flow to the posterior thorax is loculated.

The pleural lining is enhanced by contrast media with some forms of pleural disease. Pleural thickening and nodularity are well seen with contrast-enhanced CT scan. An elliptical pleural fluid collection with thickening and enhancement of the surrounding pleura suggests an **empyema,** which is infected pleural fluid.[14] The presence of gas within the pleural fluid without prior surgery or needle insertion (which can introduce air) establishes the diagnosis of empyema (Figure 21-13).

Pneumothorax

The term **pneumothorax** refers to the presence of air within the pleural space. The visceral pleura surrounding the lung becomes visible when air accumulates in the pleural space. A pneumothorax may occur spontaneously because of rupture of a *bleb* (a thin-walled subpleural gas-containing space deep to the pleura—a form of pulmonary air cyst) or may result from trauma or invasive procedures that puncture the pleura, such as transbronchial biopsy or a percutaneous (CT-guided) lung biopsy. Pneumothorax also may occur as a complication of positive pressure ventilation (which is called *barotrauma*). When the patient is upright, the air within the pleural space typically accumulates along the top of the lung (apex) and displaces the lung away from the chest wall. The clinician can detect a pneumothorax by seeing the thin pleural line at the lung margin and noting the absence of lung markings between the lung margin and the inner aspect of the chest wall (Figure 21-14). If a diagnosis of pneumothorax is suspected, an upright chest radiograph should be obtained. Visualizing a small pneumothorax may be assisted by taking the chest radiograph when the patient exhales. When the patient is supine, the air within the pleural space moves to the highest point in the chest, which is the anterior cardiophrenic sulcus.[15] Because air in this region does not create a visible edge between the pleura and the x-ray beam, radiographic clues to the presence of pneumothorax are more subtle in a supine patient.[15] A supine patient with a pneumothorax may have a *deep sulcus sign* (Figure 21-15),[16] which refers to air accumulating anteriorly and outlining the heart border below the dome of the diaphragm. In addition, the upper abdomen on the same side often shows increased lucency. If the diagnosis remains in doubt, a decubitus radiograph or a cross-table lateral radiograph (in which the patient lies face up while the x-ray is directed across the body) can help make the diagnosis of pneumothorax. Ultrasound is an alternative to chest radiograph and has been shown to be highly accurate in the diagnosis of a pneumothorax.[17]

A pneumothorax may be difficult to diagnose if a patient has bullous emphysema. If, after carefully examining the chest film, there is uncertainty about the presence of a pneumothorax, a chest CT can resolve the question. Skin folds can mimic a pneumothorax. To avoid mistaking a skin fold for a pneumothorax, the clinician needs to look carefully at what appears to be the lung margin. The absence of the pleural line at the lung margin and the presence of bronchovascular markings between the lung margin and the chest wall suggest a skin fold rather than a pneumothorax.

Occasionally, air within the pleural space may be under pressure or tension (Figure 21-16); this is called a *tension pneumothorax*. A tension pneumothorax is an emergency that occurs

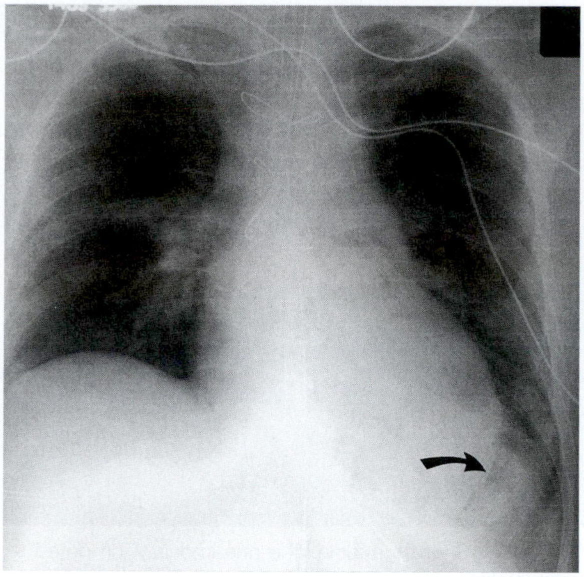

FIGURE 21-15 Deep sulcus sign. Portable supine radiograph in a patient status-post median sternotomy. Note the increased lucency in the left upper quadrant. The highest portion of the thorax in a supine patient is the anterior cardiophrenic sulcus; this accounts for the well-defined low cardiac border *(arrow)* and the adjacent fat pad.

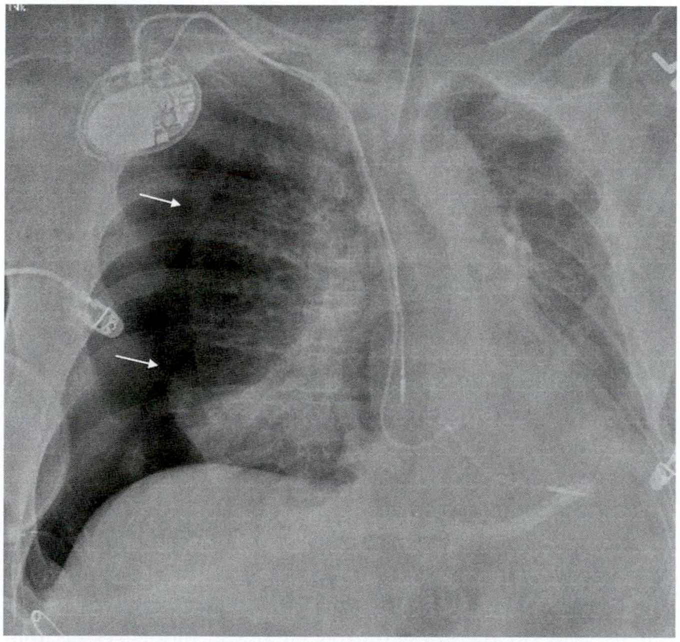

FIGURE 21-16 Tension pneumothorax. Portable chest radiograph after a recent liver transplant. Note the large right pneumothorax displacing the mediastinum to the left and the right hemidiaphragm inferiorly. These findings indicate the presence of a tension pneumothorax on the right requiring immediate chest tube placement.

when the tear in the pleura (which allows air to leave the lung and enter the pleural space) opens on inspiration but closes on expiration. Air continues to accumulate in the pleural space and can compress the heart and adjacent lung. Imaging features of a tension pneumothorax include inferior displacement of the hemidiaphragm on the side of the pneumothorax or mediastinal shift away from the pneumothorax. A tension pneumothorax requires immediate decompression with a chest tube, Heimlich valve, or needle aspiration of the air within the pleural space.

MINI CLINI

Use of the Silhouette Sign

PROBLEM: A patient has an airspace opacity in the lower half of the right lung that is secondary to pneumonia. It is unclear if this abnormality is located in the right middle lobe or in the upper portion of the lower lobe. Is there a way to identify the location of this infiltrate?

DISCUSSION: If the right heart border is visible next to the infiltrate, the pneumonia is located in the lower lobe behind the heart. If the right heart border is invisible, the infiltrate must be located in the right middle lobe next to the right side of the heart. The disappearance of the right heart border in this circumstance is due to the silhouette sign. In this instance, pneumonia is considered a water density, and when two structures of similar density are touching each other in the same plane, the border between the two structures (or the silhouette of the heart border) is not seen. Pneumonia in the upper segments of the lower lobe appears to be next to the heart on the PA chest film but does not obliterate the heart border in such cases because the water density of the pneumonia in the lower lobe is not adjacent to the water density of the heart. In this instance, the heart border or silhouette is seen because the silhouette sign is not present.

LUNG PARENCHYMA

The lung parenchyma is made up of two main components: air sacs (alveoli) and interstitium (the supporting structures of the lung). Lung parenchymal disease involves both components, although one component is usually affected more than the other.

Alveolar Disease

When alveoli are filled with material denser than air, they have a characteristic radiographic appearance regardless of the material that fills them. The type of fluid that fills the alveoli varies depending on the disease process. In the case of pulmonary edema, the alveoli are filled with a watery fluid that contains few cells. With bacterial pneumonia, the alveoli are filled with an exudative fluid containing numerous white blood cells (pus). In the case of pulmonary hemorrhage, the alveoli fill with blood. Both pneumonia and pulmonary hemorrhage can cause identical-appearing patchy, increased density shadows that tend to coalesce over time on the chest radiograph. These shadows are often referred to as *airspace opacities* or ***infiltrates***. Although the term *infiltrate* is commonly used to describe an airspace opacity, caution should be used because some clinicians equate infiltrates with pneumonia whereas others take infiltrates to

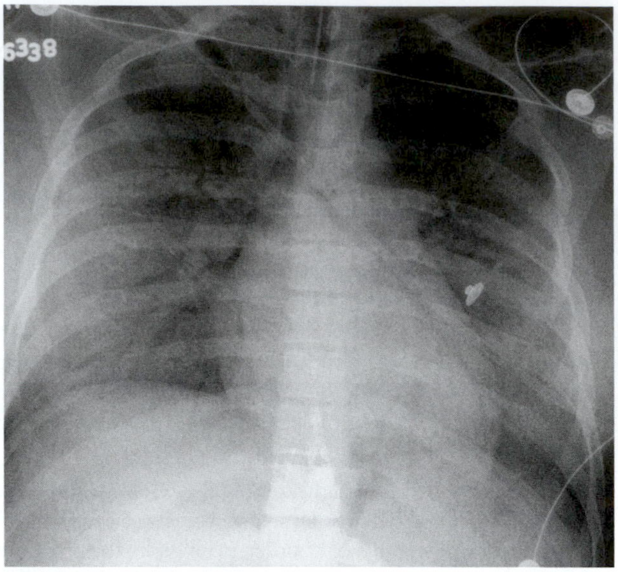

FIGURE 21-17 Air bronchograms. This portable radiograph shows diffuse increased density throughout both lungs highlighted by tubular lucencies. These are air bronchograms. They are visualized because of the alveolar filling that surrounds them. This typical alveolar filling pattern (airspace disease) suggests acute pneumonia, pulmonary hemorrhage, or pulmonary edema.

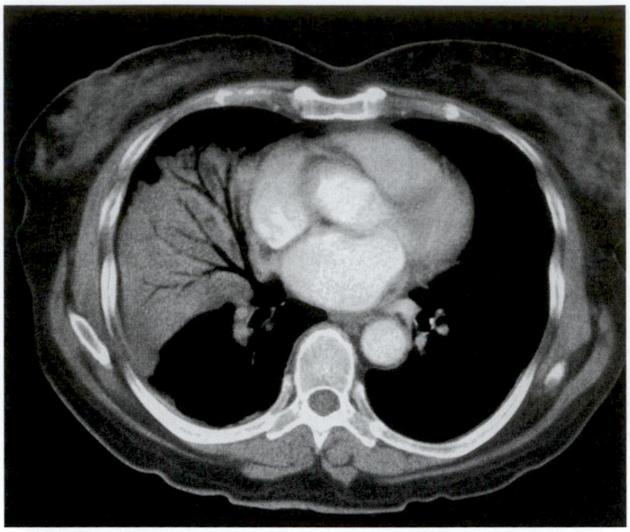

FIGURE 21-18 Right middle lobe pneumonia. Computed tomography slice shows an alveolar filling process in the right middle lobe with tubular air bronchograms running through it. The patient is a 73-year-old woman with right middle lobe pneumonia.

mean a much broader differential diagnosis, including pulmonary edema, pneumonia, and hemorrhage.

The lucent tubular structures that course through dense airspace opacities or infiltrates on both chest radiographs and chest CT images are referred to as **air bronchograms** (Figure 21-17). Normally, patent airways are invisible in the outer two-thirds of the lung on a chest radiograph because of the lack of contrast between air in the airway and air in the lung. However, the increased contrast produced by filling of the surrounding alveoli with fluid makes the airways more visible and causes the air bronchogram sign. Air bronchograms are the hallmark of infiltrates that fill alveoli (so-called *airspace disease*) (Figure 21-18 and Box 21-2).

Box 21-2 Radiographic Features of Alveolar Versus Interstitial Processes

ALVEOLAR (AIRSPACE) DISEASE
Air bronchograms
Fluffy opacities
Rapid coalescence
Acinar nodules
Segmental/lobar distribution

INTERSTITIAL DISEASE
Nodules
Linear/reticular opacities
Septal lines
Cysts
Honeycombing

RULE OF THUMB

Air bronchograms indicate that the imaging abnormality is located in the lung parenchyma and not in the pleural space and suggest that the findings may be secondary to pneumonia.

Pulmonary Edema

Pulmonary edema is one of the most common chest radiographic findings in critically ill patients. Pulmonary edema can be caused by vascular congestion, rupture of the pulmonary capillaries, or a combination of both factors. Edema from vascular congestion can be caused by failure of the left heart (cardiogenic pulmonary edema), renal failure, or fluid overload. Breakdown in the integrity of the lung capillaries also can cause pulmonary edema as in acute respiratory distress syndrome (ARDS; see Chapter 29).

The development of cardiogenic pulmonary edema can be described through a series of changes on the chest film. Before pulmonary edema develops, the pressure in the pulmonary veins increases. The increasing pressure in the pulmonary veins can be seen on the chest film as enlarging blood vessels that extend to the lung apexes. If the blood vessels in the upper lung zones are the same size or larger than the blood vessels in the lower lung zones, the vessels are said to be "cephalized" (Figure 21-19). **Cephalization** of the pulmonary blood flow is often caused by left-sided heart failure.

As fluid builds up from the high venous pressures, thickening of bronchial walls *(peribronchial cuffing)* (see Figure 21-19) and edema in the walls or septa that separate the lung lobules become evident. The thickened septa are most clearly seen as thin lines. Fluid also may accumulate in the lymphatics that drain the lung. Such accumulation within the lymphatics may

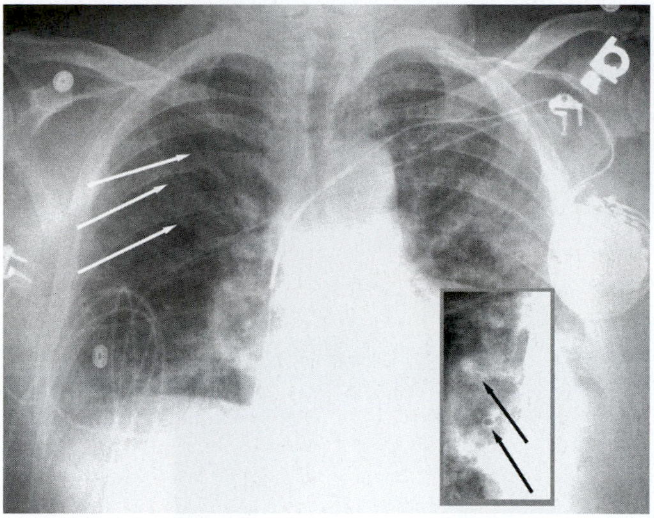

FIGURE 21-19 Moderate pulmonary edema. Cephalization of blood flow is visible *(white arrows)*. The blood vessels to the apex of the lung are enlarged and similar in size to the blood vessels to the base of the lungs. The *inset* displays peribronchial cuffing *(black arrows)*; the *inset* is from the right hilum of the same film but is enhanced to make the peribronchial cuffing easier to see.

appear on the plain radiograph as thin lines against the pleural edge that run perpendicularly away from the pleural edge. These lines are called **Kerley B lines** (Figure 21-20).

RULE OF THUMB

Radiographic signs of cardiac decompensation include the following:

- Cardiac enlargement
- Pleural effusions, usually bilateral
- Redistribution of blood flow to the upper lobes (cephalization of blood flow)
- Poor definition of the central blood vessels (perihilar haze)
- Kerley B lines
- Alveolar filling

Note: These findings are shown in Figure 21-20.

The development of pulmonary edema in the lung is seen first in the hila of the lungs by blurring of the normally distinct walls of the hilar blood vessels; this is followed by blurring and increased haziness caused by the edema progressing outward toward the pleura. The term *bat wing appearance* is applied to the predominance of edema in the hilar regions of both lungs with progressively less edema in the more peripheral areas of the lungs (Figure 21-21).

In addition to the previously mentioned classic signs of pulmonary edema, many patients with long-standing heart failure have enlargement of the heart and pleural effusions. Pleural effusions from heart failure are usually bilateral but if the effusion is visible only on one side, it is more common on the right side than on the left.

The radiographic appearance of ARDS can appear similar to other forms of pulmonary edema. Although they may appear similar, there are some key differences to help distinguish ARDS from pulmonary edema caused by high vascular pressures or congestive heart failure. The edema of ARDS is patchy and bilateral and does not predominate in the central hilar regions. A chest film of a patient with ARDS also lacks cardiomegaly, cephalization, and Kerley B lines, which are often seen in cardiogenic pulmonary edema.

Interstitial Disease

Diseases that primarily involve the interstitium of the lung have a different radiographic appearance than alveolar diseases (see Box 21-2). The interstitium of the lung represents the framework or scaffolding of the lung that supports the vessels and bronchi. The secondary pulmonary lobule is the smallest functional unit of the lung.[18] The *secondary pulmonary lobule* contains alveoli and alveolar ducts built around a central pulmonary arteriole and bronchiole, all surrounded by a thin sheet of fibrous connective tissue called the *intralobular septa*. Intralobular septa are invisible on a normal chest radiograph. Pulmonary edema secondary to poor left-sided heart function causes edema of the intralobular septa. As noted, short thin lines from the edematous intralobluar septa can be seen perpendicular to the pleura (see Figure 21-19); these are Kerley B lines.

Interstitial lung disease (see Chapter 26) refers to a group of diseases that involve the lower respiratory tract. Chest radiographs of patients with interstitial lung disease may have several different appearances, depending on the stage and type of interstitial lung disease (see Box 20-2). A chest radiograph of a patient with interstitial lung disease usually has diffuse, bilateral opacities. The opacities may resemble scattered, poorly defined nodules (nodular); a collection of scattered lines (reticular); or a combination of both lines and nodules (reticulonodular); or *honeycombing*, which is the development of cystic spaces with well-defined walls seen in the periphery of the lung and resembling a bee's honeycomb. Honeycombing is thought to represent irreversible scarring and indicates end-stage lung disease (Figure 21-22). Lung volumes are generally decreased in patients with interstitial lung disease, a key finding that can aid in the diagnosis on a chest radiograph examination.

There are many types of interstitial lung disease. Causes include *infectious* (e.g., viral pneumonia), *occupational* exposures (e.g., to asbestos [asbestosis] or to silica [silicosis]), and *collagen vascular disease* (e.g., rheumatoid arthritis, scleroderma). The two most common interstitial lung diseases, *sarcoidosis* and *idiopathic pulmonary fibrosis,* have no known cause and are said to be idiopathic. Because many different types of interstitial lung diseases have similar appearances on the chest radiograph, the chest film rarely establishes the specific cause of interstitial disease. Clues to specific causes of interstitial lung disease on a plain chest film are reviewed in Table 21-2. HRCT has become an important tool in establishing the specific form of interstitial lung disease that a patient may have. HRCT is particularly helpful in diagnosing idiopathic pulmonary

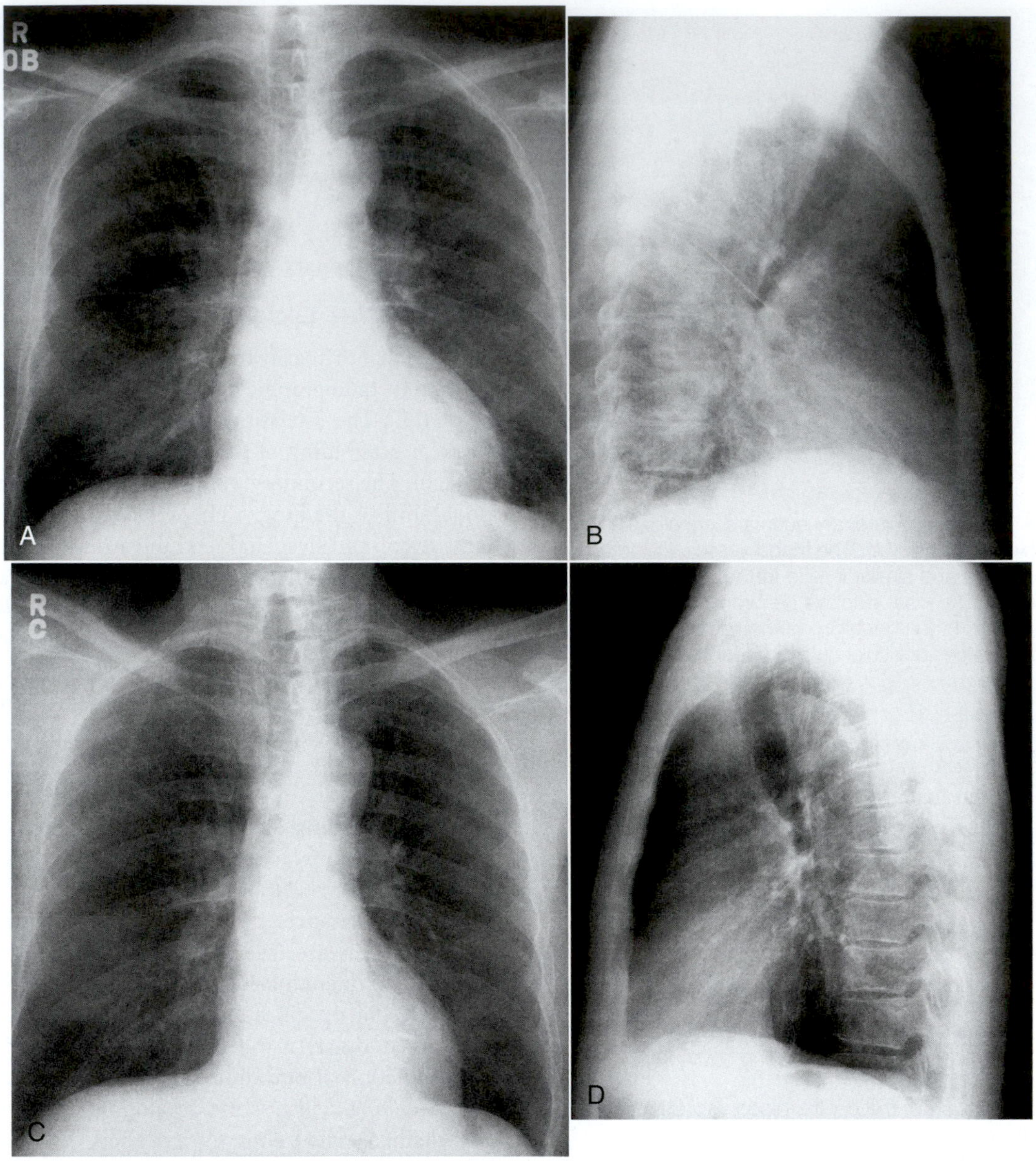

FIGURE 21-20 Posterior **(A)** and lateral **(B)** chest films show an enlarged cardiac silhouette. The lateral lung margins are slightly displaced away from the inner chest wall in both costophrenic angles, which is consistent with bilateral effusions. There is thickening of the fissures on the lateral projection, indicating that the pleural fluid is extending into the interlobar fissures. Numerous Kerley B lines are seen as linear densities extending to the pleural surface in the right lower chest. The definition of the central vessels is suboptimal, indicating interstitial edema. **C** and **D,** The same patient after therapeutic diuresis. Note the decreased heart size, disappearance of Kerley B lines, and improved definition of the central pulmonary vasculature.

fibrosis because of a characteristic pattern with changes in the lower lobes exceeding those in the apexes, a subpleural location, and the presence of honeycombing.[19,20]

Assessing Lung Volume

Volume loss, or *atelectasis,* is a common abnormality on chest radiographs, and the location and extent of volume loss produce characteristic chest radiograph patterns. The degree of atelectasis can be described as subsegmental (involving less than a segment of lung), segmental (involving one or more segments of lung), or lobar (involving one or more lobes of the lung). A specific type of subsegmental atelectasis that has a classic radiographic appearance is called *platelike* or *discoid* ***atelectasis*** (Figure 21-23). Atelectasis commonly occurs after abdominal or thoracic surgery, adjacent to pleural effusions, or after pleural irritation from a rib fracture or pulmonary infarction.

Volume loss involving an entire lobe (lobar atelectasis) is usually caused by central airway obstruction.[21] The collapsed lobe assumes the shape of a wedge with the apex of the wedge at the hilum and the base of the wedge on the pleural surface. This wedge is visible on a PA or lateral x-ray film, depending on which lobe is collapsed (Figure 21-24). The central bronchial obstruction may be caused by cancer, a foreign body, or a mucous plug (Figure 21-25). As shown in Figure 21-26, a bulging convexity to the apex of the wedge indicates a central tumor.

Atelectasis causes changes to the surrounding structures. As lung volume decreases, surrounding tissues collapse in to fill the space of the collapsed lung. The diaphragm becomes elevated on the side of the atelectasis, the mediastinum shifts toward the atelectasis, and poor expansion of the chest causes narrowing of the rib spaces. If the collapsed segment of the lung is in the upper lobe, the hilum is displaced upward, and the minor fissure on the right is displaced upward.

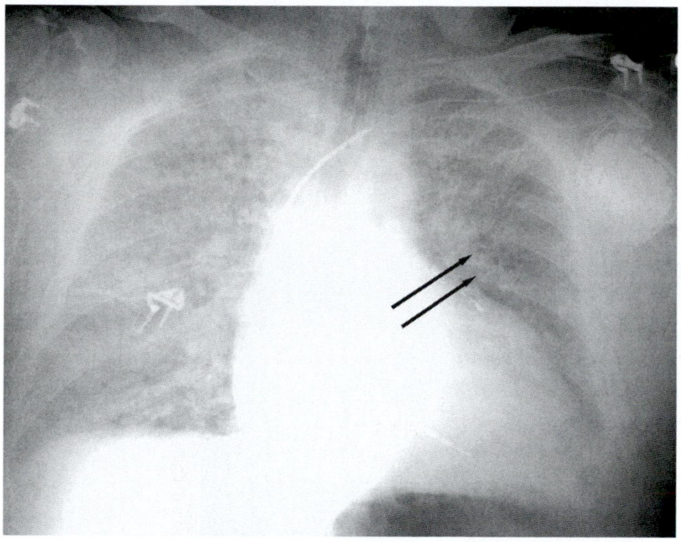

FIGURE 21-21 Severe pulmonary edema. Both lungs are opacified in a bat's wing distribution. The hilar vessels are invisible because of the edema in the lung tissue surrounding these vessels. Peribronchial cuffing is indicated by the *black arrows*.

RULE OF THUMB

Radiographic signs of volume loss include the following:

- Unilateral diaphragmatic elevation
- Mediastinal shift toward the atelectasis
- Narrowing of the space between the ribs
- Hilar displacement toward the atelectasis

See Figures 21-23, 21-24, 21-25, and 21-26.

TABLE 21-2
Clues on Plain Chest Radiograph Indicating the Specific Cause of Interstitial Lung Disease

Clues on Radiograph	Cause of Disease
Pneumothorax	Lymphangioleiomyomatosis, Langerhans cell histiocytosis
Pleural effusion	Rheumatoid arthritis, systemic lupus erythematosus
Dilated esophagus	Scleroderma, CREST syndrome*
Erosive arthropathy (shoulder joints, clavicles)	Rheumatoid arthritis
Mediastinal adenopathy	Sarcoidosis, progressive systemic sclerosis (scleroderma), metastatic cancer
Soft tissue calcification	Dermatomyositis, progressive systemic sclerosis (scleroderma)
Pleural plaque	Asbestosis

*Calcinosis, Raynaud's phenomenon, esophageal dysmotility, sclerodactyly, and telangiectasia.

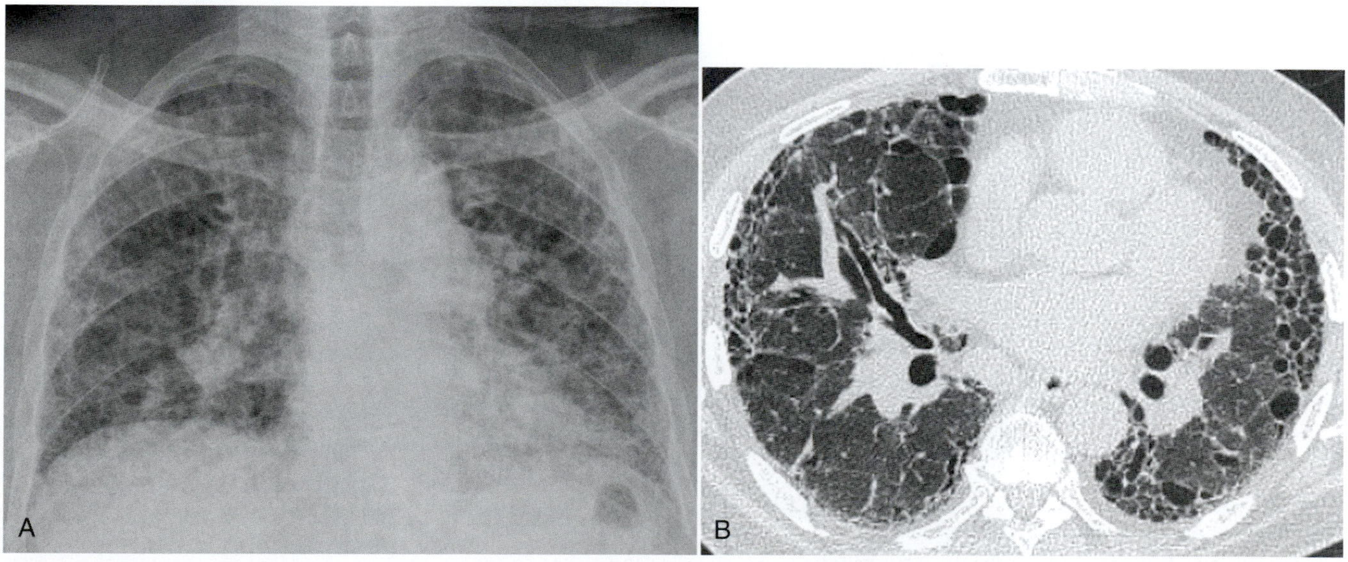

FIGURE 21-22 Posteroanterior view **(A)** of the chest in a patient with shortness of breath. The chest radiograph shows interstitial lung disease. The lung volumes are small. Coarse linear and cystic lucencies represent pulmonary fibrosis. These findings are better visualized on the chest computed tomography image **(B)** where there is bronchiectasis, architectural distortion, and honeycombing. The patient has interstitial pulmonary fibrosis, the most common type of pulmonary fibrosis.

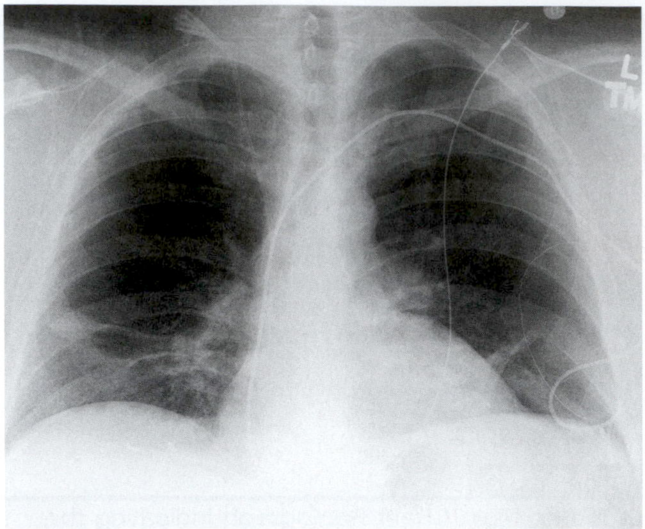

FIGURE 21-23 Plate atelectasis. Posteroanterior chest radiograph shows linear areas of plate atelectasis in both lower lobes.

Assessment of lung volumes on a chest radiograph requires several observations. Rib counting is a popular method to assess lung volume. With a good inspiration, the sixth and sometimes the seventh anterior rib should project above the diaphragm. If more than seven anterior ribs are visible above the diaphragm, *hyperinflation* is present. Obstructive pulmonary disease is classically associated with increased lung volumes (hyperinflation). In patients with chronic obstructive pulmonary disease, there also may be an increase in the AP diameter of the chest, with associated enlargement of the retrosternal and retrocardiac (behind the sternum and the heart, respectively) airspaces and flattening of the hemidiaphragms. These findings all are secondary signs of *pulmonary emphysema*. The only primary signs of emphysema are loss or shifting of pulmonary vessel markings and the appearance of the walls of bullous airspaces (Figure 21-27).

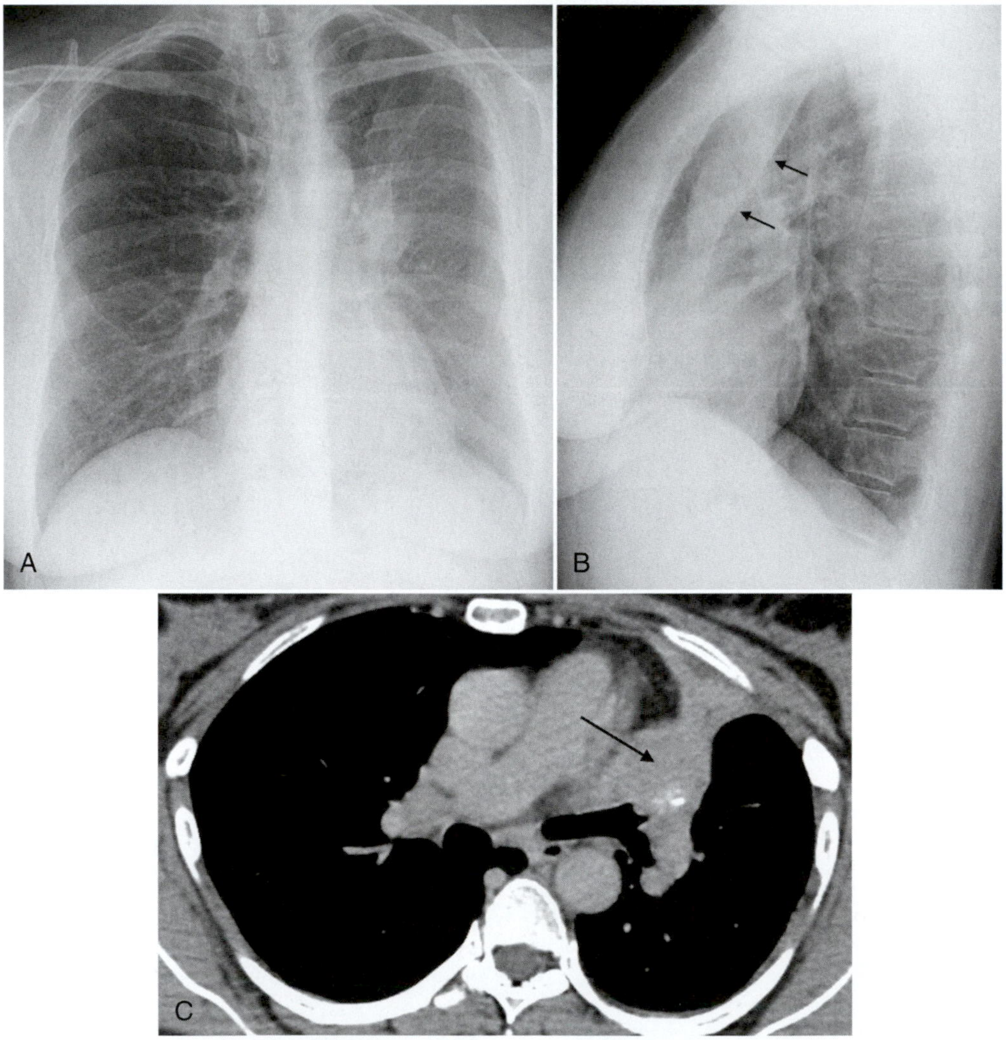

FIGURE 21-24 **A,** Posteroanterior view of the chest shows leftward mediastinal shift, a left hilar mass, and increased density overlying the left chest. **B,** Lateral view shows a wedge of increased density *(arrows)* anteriorly with its apex at the hilum and its base on the pleural surface representing the collapsed left upper lobe. **C,** Computed tomography image shows a partially calcified left hilar mass *(arrow),* with the collapsed left upper lobe distally. Biopsy of the mass revealed carcinoid tumor.

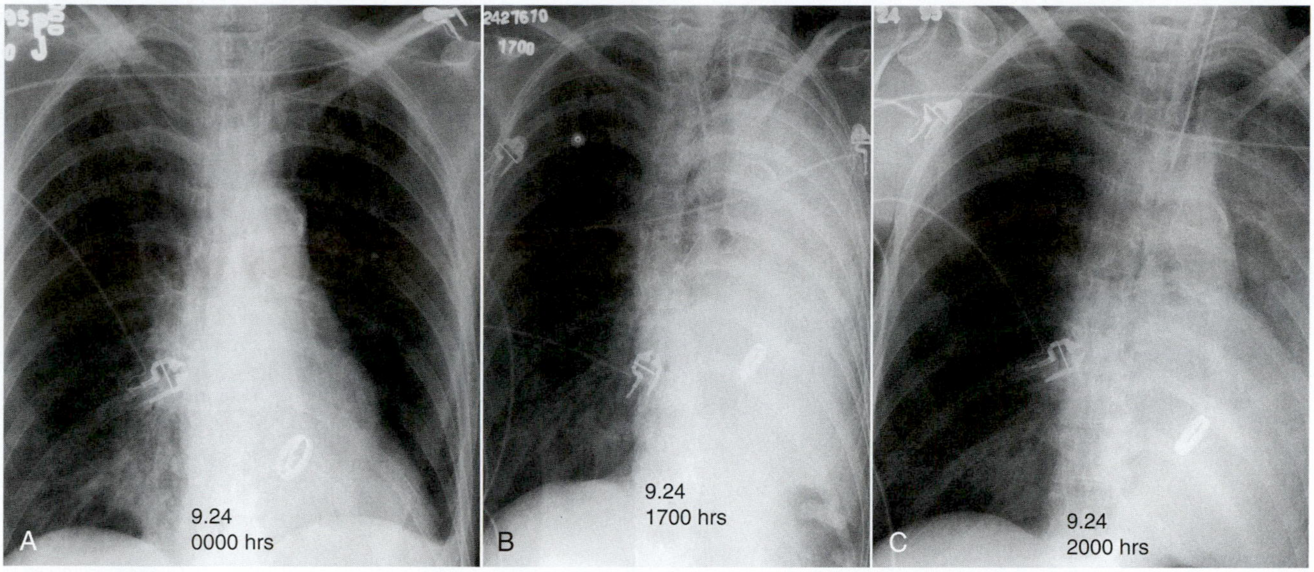

FIGURE 21-25 Three portable chest films obtained within a 20-hour time span. **A,** Good aeration of both lungs. **B,** Film obtained 17 hours later shows complete opacification of the left hemithorax. Bronchoscopy performed after this film revealed a mucous plug in the left main bronchus. It was removed at bronchoscopy. **C,** Partial reexpansion.

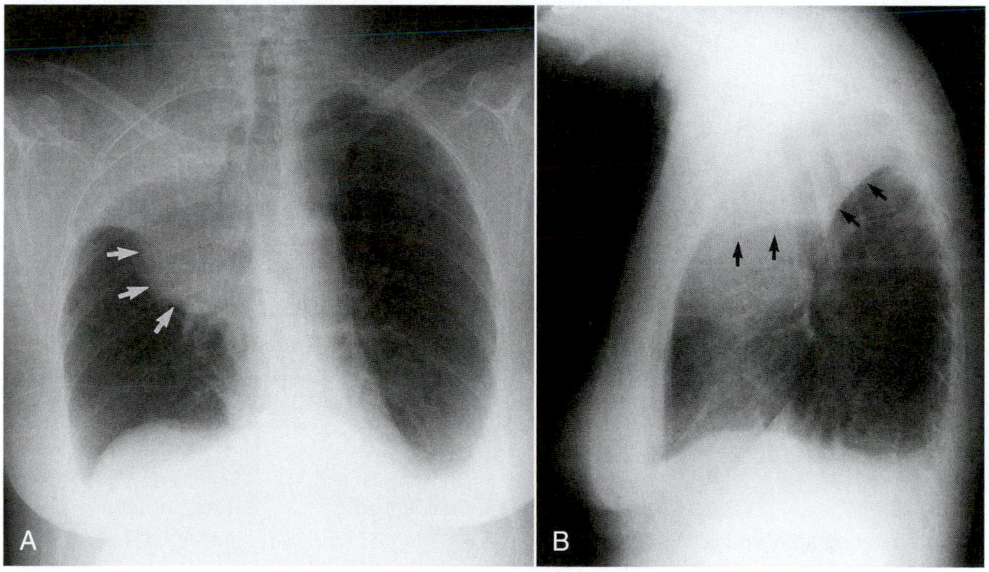

FIGURE 21-26 Posteroanterior **(A)** and lateral **(B)** views of the chest in a patient with right upper lobe collapse. **A,** Note the wedge opacity of the right upper lobe and the inferior bulge *(arrows)* of the minor fissure on the PA film. This bulge indicates the presence of a central mass. **B,** The wedge shape of right upper lobe atelectasis *(arrows)* is well seen on the lateral film.

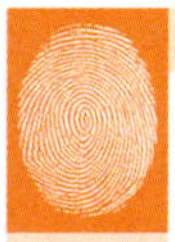

RULE OF THUMB

A good inspiratory effort by the patient is needed to obtain a good-quality chest radiograph examination. Visualization of 6 anterior or 10 posterior ribs above the level of the diaphragm on the PA view indicates a good inspiratory effort by the patient.

Because radiographic signs of emphysema are apparent only with more advanced disease, the chest radiograph is generally considered insensitive for detecting obstructive lung disease. However, CT is far more sensitive and may show evidence of emphysema even when pulmonary function test results are normal.[22] Emphysema is often anatomically described in three patterns depending on which part of the secondary pulmonary lobule is affected. When only the central part of the lobule is affected, the pattern is called *centrilobular* or *centriacinar emphysema*. When the entire lobule is affected, the pattern of emphysema is called *panlobular* or *panacinar*. Finally, when the emphysema is confined to areas near the pleura, the pattern is called *paraseptal emphysema*. Figure 21-28 shows a case of upper lobe paraseptal emphysema, characterized by cystic areas along the pleural surface. A chest CT scan may prove useful to

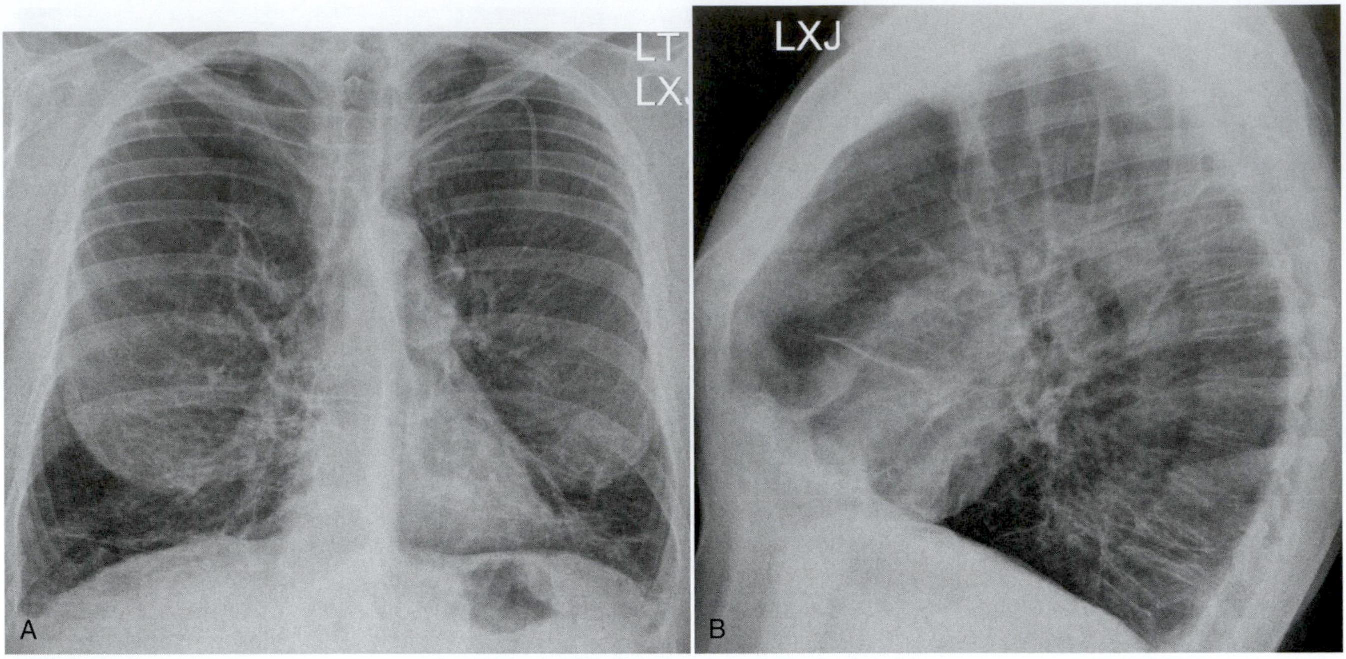

FIGURE 21-27 Posteroanterior **(A)** and lateral **(B)** views of the chest of a patient with bullous emphysema, worse on the right. The lungs are hyperinflated with flattening of the diaphragms, increased retrosternal clear space, and areas in the upper lung zones that are devoid of any vascular markings.

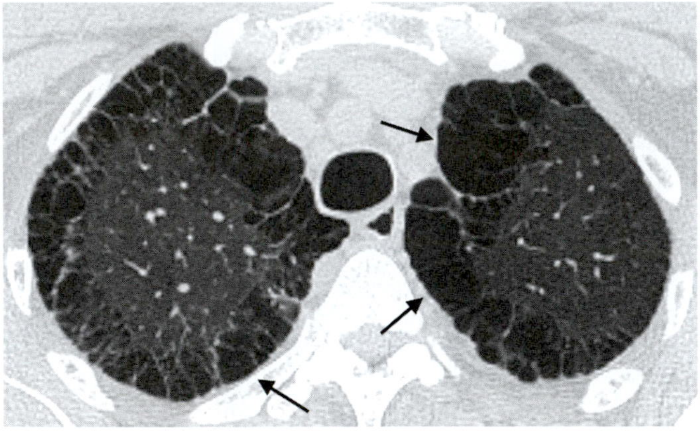

FIGURE 21-28 Computed tomography image through the upper lobes in a patient with pulmonary emphysema. Numerous cystic lucencies are present in both lungs. Note the absence of bronchovascular markings within the lucencies. Most of the emphysematous areas are located in a peripheral distribution *(arrows)* along the pleural surface, representing paraseptal emphysema.

help define which patients may benefit from treatments such as lung volume reduction surgery. Results of the National Emphysema Treatment Trial showed that patients with heterogeneous upper lobe-predominant emphysema (i.e., emphysema that is greater in the apexes of the lung than in the bases) are good candidates for lung volume reduction surgery.[23]

Solitary Pulmonary Nodule

A **solitary pulmonary nodule** (SPN) is a parenchymal opacity smaller than 3 cm in diameter that is surrounded by aerated lung. One or two SPNs are encountered in every 1000 chest radiographs. SPNs are important to identify because they may be caused by lung cancer. The reported prevalence of malignancy in SPN ranges from 3% to 6% in large surveys of the general population. In patients with SPN who have surgical resection, 30% to 60% of the nodules are malignant.[24]

When first encountered, a SPN should be assessed for features listed in Table 21-3 that may help to establish a nonmalignant cause. The goal of imaging SPNs is to avoid resecting benign nodules, while encouraging surgical removal of all potentially curable cancers. The axial anatomic display of CT, along with better density-discriminating powers, makes CT a favored tool for evaluating the SPN. CT provides a detailed

TABLE 21-3

Features Useful in Distinguishing Benign from Malignant Solitary Pulmonary Nodules

Feature	Favoring Malignant Nodule	Favoring Benign Nodule
Patient age	>40 yr old	<40 yr old
Smoking status	Current or former smoker	Lifetime nonsmoker
Size of nodule	>3 cm	<3 cm
Shape of nodule	Lobulated	Spherical
Margins of nodule	Spiculated	Well defined
If cavity	Thick-walled	Thin-walled
Doubling time*	7-465 days	<7 or >465 days
Calcification	Rare, usually eccentric	Central, lamellar, popcorn

*Time necessary for the nodule to double in volume.

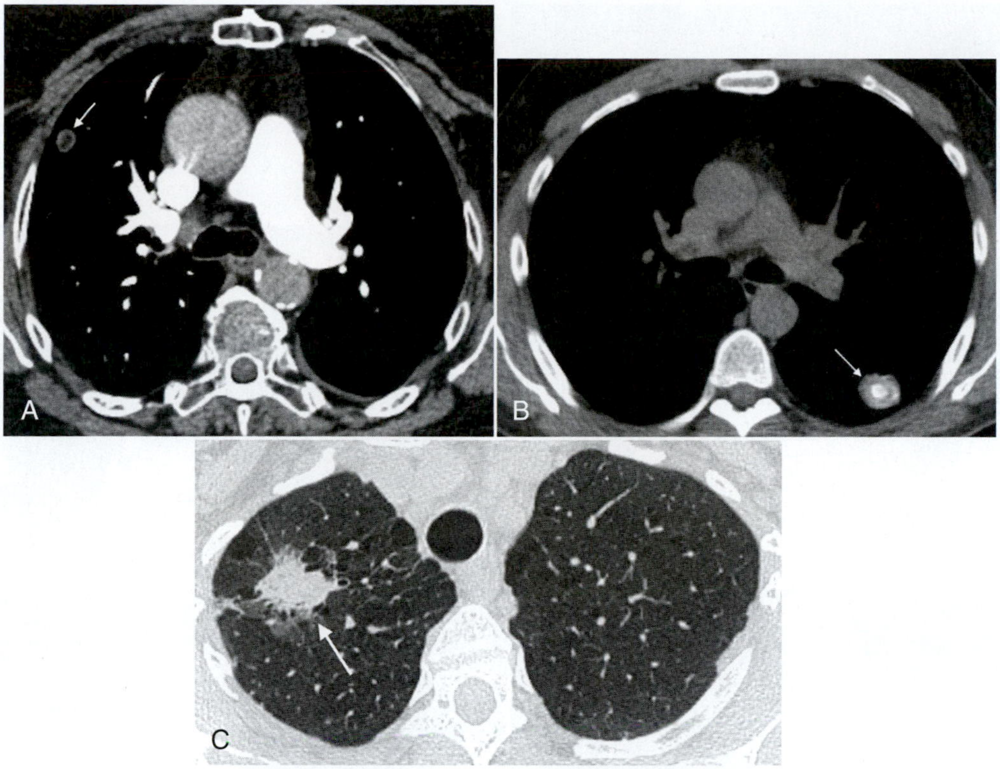

FIGURE 21-29 Computed tomography examples of solitary pulmonary nodules. **A,** Nodular density in the right lung that contains fat. Note the same density within the nodule as the subcutaneous fat. This finding is diagnostic of a pulmonary hamartoma, a benign diagnosis, requiring no further follow-up. **B,** There is central calcification with this pulmonary nodule, a benign form of calcification, and consistent with a granuloma. **C,** The spiculated edge of this nodule *(arrow)* is suggestive of malignancy in this biopsy-proved primary lung adenocarcinoma.

evaluation of the size, shape, border, and density of a nodule. For example, the presence of fat or the pattern of calcification can help to establish that a pulmonary nodule is benign (Figure 21-29).

Central or lamellar (swirls of concentric rings) often result from calcification and strongly suggests a benign cause of an SPN or a granuloma. Eccentric (off-center), speckled, or amorphous calcification may be seen in lung cancer. A smoothly marginated round nodule more often is benign, whereas a lobulated, irregular, or spiculated edge is more likely to be a malignant nodule (see Figure 21-29). PET-CT is often very helpful in evaluating SPNs. Nodules greater than 1 cm in diameter that take up the isotope used in PET-CT studies, fluorodeoxyglucose (FDG), are metabolically active and are more likely to be malignant than nodules without uptake. Unfortunately, FDG uptake by a pulmonary nodule on a PET-CT is not specific for malignancy because infectious or inflammatory nodules (such as nodules caused by fungal infection with *Histoplasmosis*) may also be FDG-avid and "light up." Similarly, slow-growing cancers (such as adenocarcinoma in situ) or small cancers (<1 cm) may not take up FDG or be visible on the PET-CT scan.

MEDIASTINUM

The mediastinum consists of the heart, great vessels, trachea, and other soft tissue structures that lie between the lungs. The mediastinum is divided into three compartments: anterior, middle, and posterior. When a mediastinal abnormality is discovered, determining the precise location of the mediastinum is important to narrow the differential diagnosis. Radiographically, the mediastinal compartments are best defined on a lateral view (see Figure 21-5). A line extending from the diaphragm along the posterior margin of the heart and the anterior margin of the trachea to the neck divides the anterior mediastinum from the middle compartment. A second line traversing the vertebral bodies 1 cm posterior to their anterior margins and extending from the neck to the diaphragm divides the middle from the posterior compartment. Some mediastinal masses are visible on both front and lateral projections, and the specific location within the mediastinum offers the first clue to diagnosis.

Table 21-4 lists the common causes of masses in the three mediastinal compartments. CT is the preferred imaging examination for evaluating most mediastinal masses. Figure 21-30 shows the normal axial anatomic display on contrast-enhanced CT scan at the levels of the great vessels, aortic arch, carina, and cardiac chambers. The CT appearance of an anterior mediastinal mass (thymoma) is shown in Figure 21-31. Figure 21-32 shows a middle mediastinal mass (bronchogenic cyst) on an MRI examination. A large hiatal hernia in the posterior mediastinum can be easily confused with a mass on the frontal chest film but is easily seen on CT in Figure 21-33.

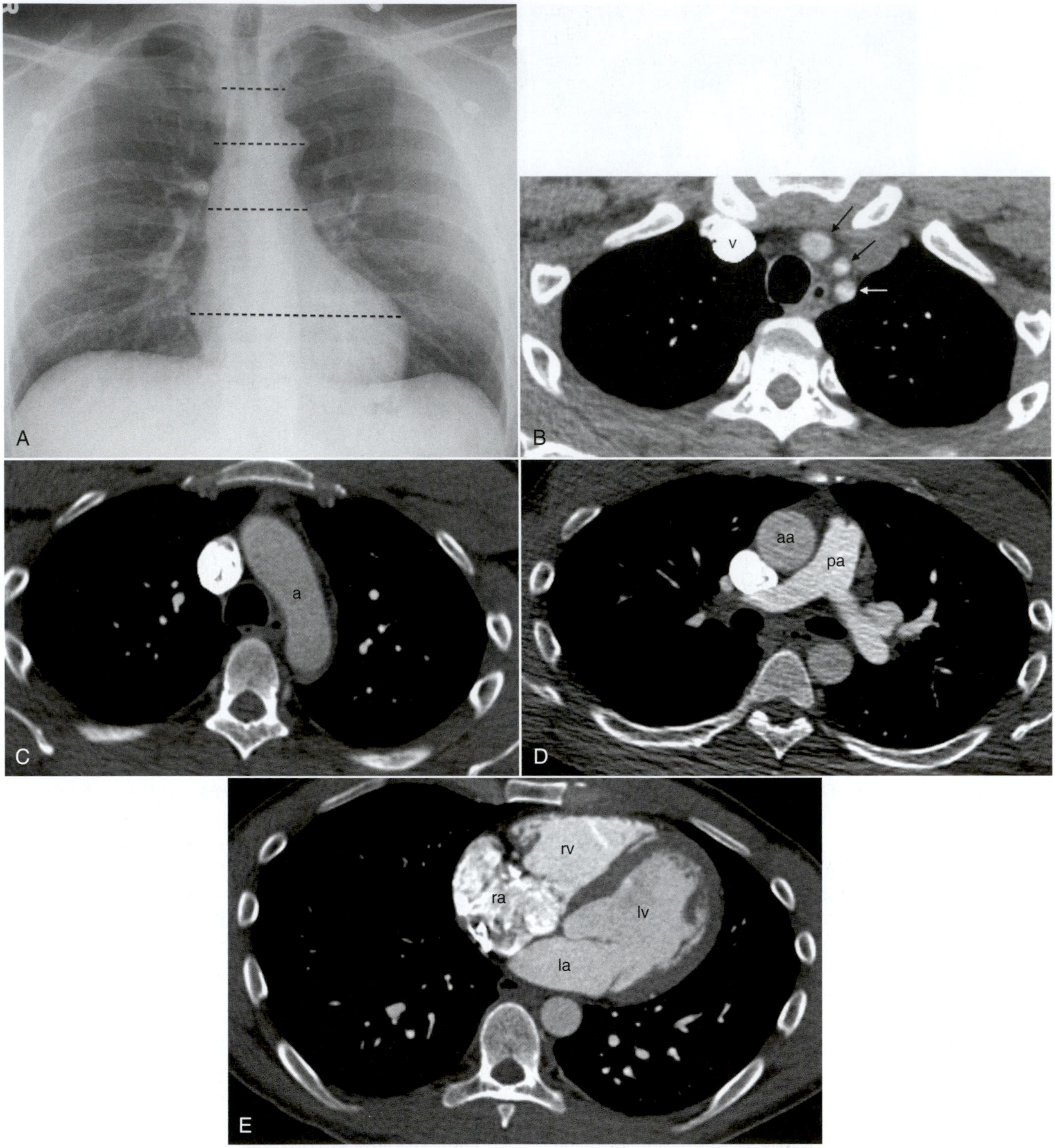

FIGURE 21-30 **A,** Posteroanterior chest radiograph indicating the four levels at which computed tomography scan slices **B** to **E** were obtained. **B,** The most superior image is at the level of the great vessels. Contrast material fills the right brachiocephalic vein *(v)* and the three arch vessels, the right brachiocephalic, left common carotid, and left sublavian arteries. **C,** At this level, the arch of the aorta *(a)* lies on the left side of the airway. The esophagus is seen in front of the vertebral body behind the airway. The opacified superior vena cava lies to the right of the arch anteriorly. **D,** At the level of the pulmonary artery bifurcation, the right pulmonary artery crosses the mediastinum anterior to the right main bronchus. The vena cava lies to the right of the ascending aorta *(aa)*. The descending aorta is seen next to the vertebral body. **E,** At the level of the heart, contrast material is seen filling the right atrium *(ra)* and crossing the atrioventricular (tricuspid) valve into the right ventricle *(rv)*. The thick, muscular left ventricular *(lv)* wall is visualized as it contracts. The left atrium *(la)* is seen anterior to the esophagus.

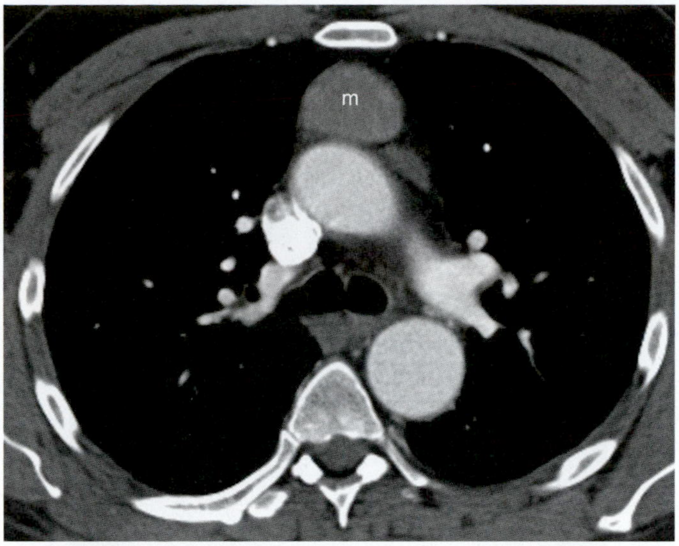

FIGURE 21-31 Anterior mediastinal mass. Computed tomography slice at the level of the aortic arch shows a homogeneous encapsulated anterior mediastinal mass *(m)*. The diagnosis was thymoma.

TABLE 21-4
Mediastinal Abnormalities by Compartment

Anterior Mediastinum	Middle Mediastinum	Posterior Mediastinum
Thyroid or parathyroid mass	Aortic aneurysm (ascending/arch)	Aortic aneurysm (descending)
Thymic lesions	Lymphadenopathy	Neurogenic tumors
Lymphoma	Bronchogenic cyst	Lymphoma
Pericardial cyst/fat pad	Tracheoesophageal masses	Neurenteric cyst
Teratoma	Hiatal hernia	Bochdalek hernia*
Morgagni hernia*		
Ventricular aneurysm		

*Hernia in which the abdominal contents press through a gap in the diaphragm.

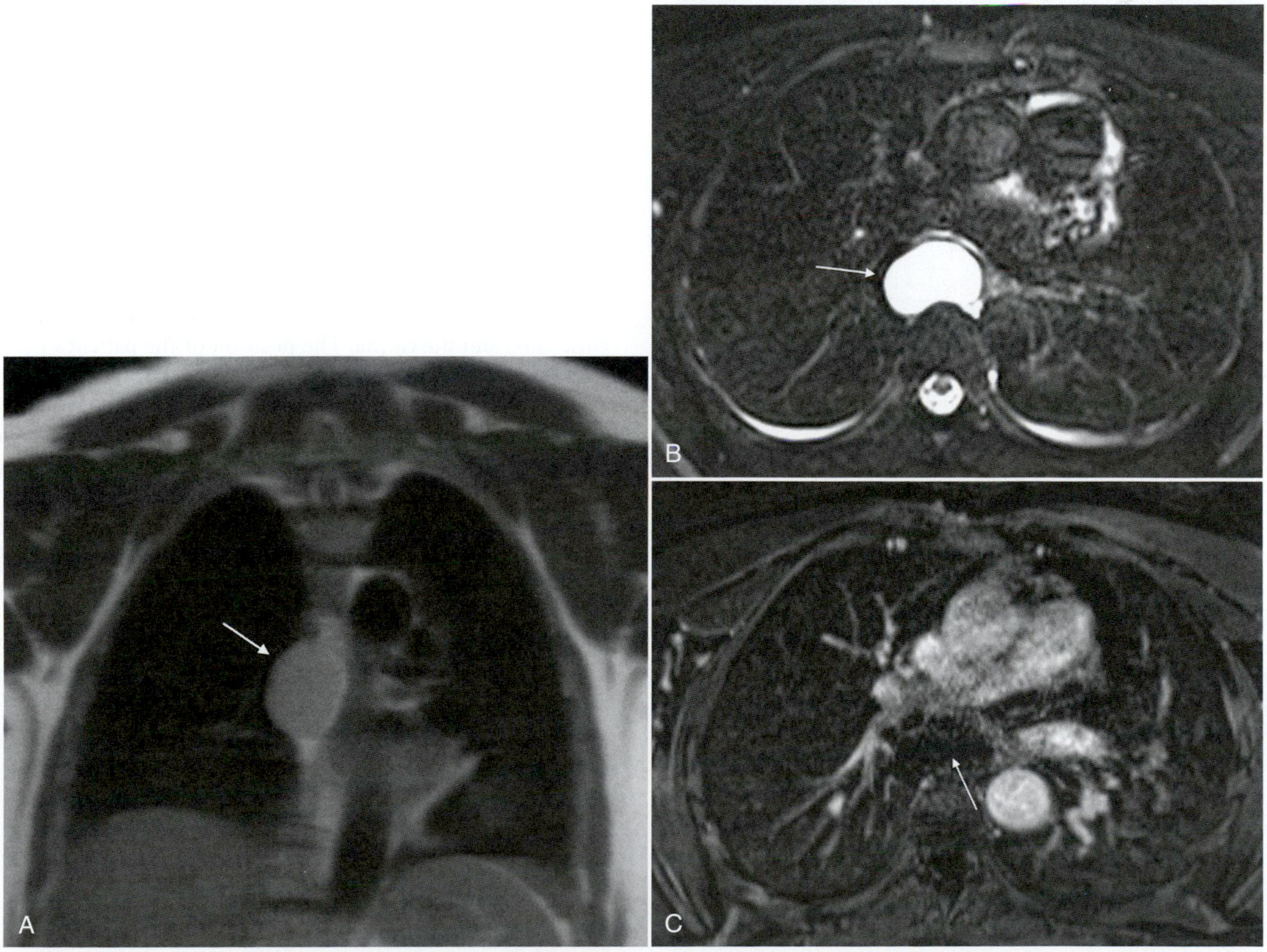

FIGURE 21-32 Middle mediastinal mass. Magnetic resonance images demonstrate a subcarinal mass *(arrows)*. Coronal HASTE **(A)** and axial STIR **(B)** images demonstrate increased T2 signal (appearing gray or white) intensity in this mass, suggestive of a cystic lesion. Substraction VIBE image **(C)** shows no enhancement (the mass is black) confirming no contrast enhancement. The diagnosis is a bronchogenic cyst, a benign lesion.

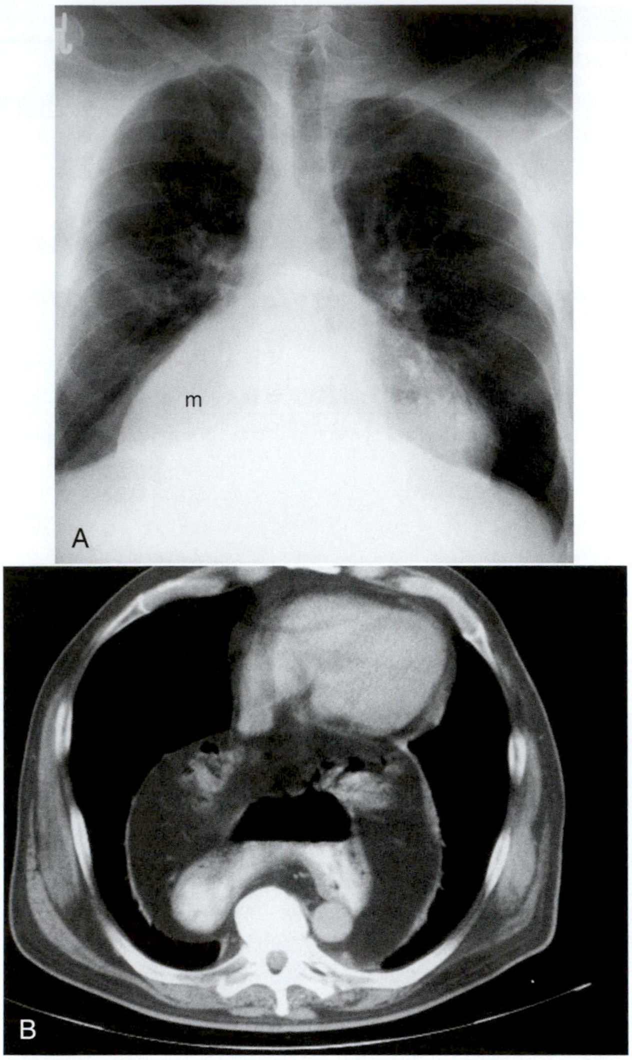

FIGURE 21-33 Posterior mediastinal mass. **A,** Posteroanterior chest film shows a large soft tissue density *(m)* obscuring the right heart border and the right hemidiaphragm. **B,** Computed tomography image at this level shows a large retrocardiac diaphragmatic hernia containing omentum and stomach.

Pneumomediastinum

Pneumomediastinum, a form of barotrauma, may result from movement of air into the mediastinum, as also may be seen in cases of esophageal rupture (Figure 21-34). This condition usually occurs in the distal portion of the esophagus in patients who undergo procedures to stretch or dilate the esophagus. Chest trauma may cause rupture of the trachea or a mainstem bronchus, also allowing movement of air into the mediastinum. Rarely, air dissects down from the soft tissues of the neck after thyroid, parathyroid, or tonsillar surgery. Gas associated with a retrotonsillar abscess may extend inferiorly into the mediastinum through the fascial planes of the neck. Air that accumulates in the retroperitoneum may enter the mediastinum via openings in the diaphragm for the aorta or esophagus.

Catheters, Lines, and Tubes

A common use of a chest radiograph is to evaluate the position of catheters, lines, and tubes after insertion. RTs must be skilled at examining the chest radiograph to determine the position of the endotracheal tube, chest tubes, central and peripheral catheters, and hemodynamic monitoring lines.

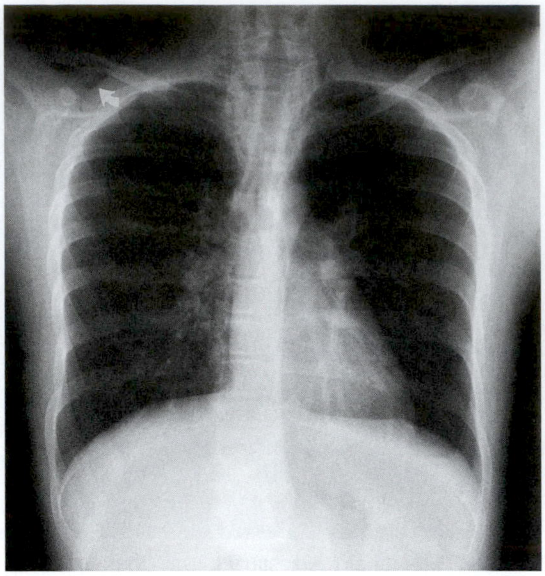

FIGURE 21-34 Pneumomediastinum. Posteroanterior view of the chest of an 11-year-old child with asthma shows linear lucencies (free air) in the mediastinum and extending into the soft tissues of the neck bilaterally. Note the free air around the lateral aspect of the right clavicle *(arrow)*.

Endotracheal Tube

Endotracheal tubes are radiopaque or have an opaque marker indicating the end of the tube. Radiographs are routinely obtained at the bedside after intubation to assess correct tube position. The radiograph shows the distal tip of the endotracheal tube and the carina. The position of the patient's neck is important. The neck position usually is neutral, but the position of the tip of the endotracheal tube can vary with neck position. Specifically, the endotracheal tube position can move appropriately 4 cm toward the main carina as the neck moves from full extension (high position) to full neck flexion (low position), which is one-third the length of the average adult trachea. Though there is some variability in the literature, several studies suggest that when the head and neck are in the neutral position, the endotracheal tube should be positioned in the midtrachea approximately 3 to 7 cm above the carina. Although it may be difficult to see on some chest images, the carina is generally located at the space between T-4 and T-5 in most adults.[25] Placement below the thoracic inlet (usually at C5-6 for adults) ensures that the tube is beyond the vocal cords. (usually at C5-6). Figure 21-35 shows a malpositioned endotracheal tube in the right mainstem bronchus.

RULE OF THUMB

The distal tip of the endotracheal tube should be positioned approximately 3 to 7 cm above the level of the carina in an adult patient.

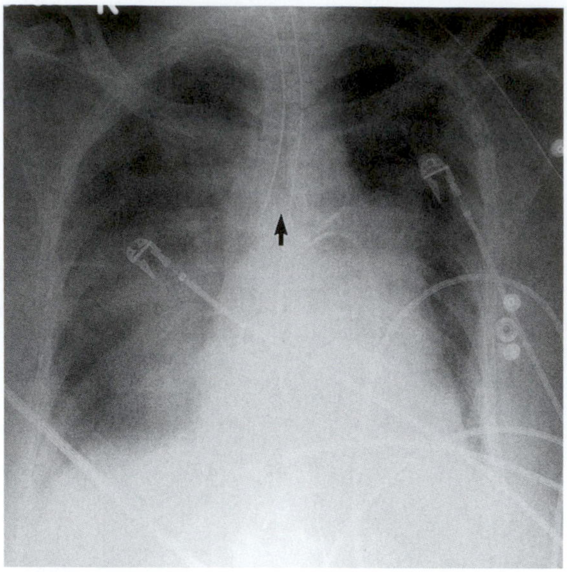

FIGURE 21-35 Portable supine chest film shows malposition of an endotracheal tube in the right main stem bronchus *(arrow)*.

RULE OF THUMB

When the patient flexes his or her neck, the tip of the endotracheal tube moves down (into the lung). When the neck is extended, the endotracheal tube moves up (out of the lung toward the vocal cords). Thus, a well-positioned endotracheal tube is important to prevent migration of the endotracheal tube into a mainstem bronchus (usually the right main stem bronchus) when neck flexion occurs or to prevent accidental extubation when neck extension occurs.

Tracheostomy Tube

Tracheostomy tubes should be two-thirds the diameter of the trachea and should project within the borders of the trachea on the radiograph. The tip should extend beyond half the distance from the stoma to the carina.

Central Line

A central venous catheter is typically placed via either the internal jugular vein or subclavian vein. A chest radiograph should be obtained after placement to assess the position and to exclude a procedural complication (e.g., pneumothorax, hemothorax). Ideally, the tip of the central venous pressure catheter should be in the superior vena cava. This vessel usually forms at the level of the first anterior intercostal space where the brachiocephalic veins come together. The brachiocephalic veins contain valves, and these catheters ideally should be placed central to any valves.

Peripherally Inserted Central Venous Catheter

An alternative to placement of a central venous catheter is a peripherally inserted central venous catheter (PICC), which is placed via a peripheral vein in either the left or right upper extremity. Advantages of a PICC are that it does not have the risk for a pneumothorax as with central venous catheters, it can be used long term (often for several weeks), and it has a lower rate of infection than central venous catheters. The preferred location for a PICC is similar to a central venous catheter, with the tip of the catheter in the superior vena cava.

Pulmonary Artery (Swan-Ganz) Catheter

A Swan-Ganz catheter is used to measure hemodynamic and central pressure variables such as pulmonary artery occlusion pressure (sometimes called the "wedge pressure"). Pulmonary artery catheters are placed at the bedside and ideally should reside in the proximal right or left main pulmonary arteries. They are floated into position using an inflatable balloon on the catheter tip. Because of this floating, they are placed in the right pulmonary artery more than 90% of the time. When measuring the so-called "wedge" or pulmonary artery occlusion pressure, the balloon is inflated, and the catheter moves out into a more peripheral vessel. As soon as the reading is accomplished, the balloon should be deflated, and the catheter should be pulled back to a central location. Persistent peripheral placement (i.e., when the catheter tip is far out in the lung parenchyma) can cause infarction of lung beyond (distal to) the wedged catheter (Figure 21-36) or result in injury to the pulmonary artery such as formation of a pseudoaneurysm or even rupture.

Chest Tube

Chest tubes are small-bore to large-bore tubes placed into the pleural space from outside the chest wall. The most common indications for a chest tube are for a pneumothorax (air in the pleural space) or an empyema (pus in the pleural space), although chest tubes also may be used to drain blood *(hemothorax)* or fluid *(hydrothorax)* or to install a sealant (e.g., the antibiotic doxycycline) to achieve closure of the pleural space, preventing recurrent pneumothorax or hydrothorax. Radiographically, most chest tubes have radiopaque stripes along their axis so they can be seen on the chest radiograph. The chest tube should be within the pleural space; it usually follows the contour of the chest wall or diaphragm on the chest radiograph.

Intraaortic Balloon Pump

The intraaortic balloon pump (IABP) is a counterpulsation device used to improve cardiac output and blood pressure in patients in cardiogenic shock. It is inserted through the femoral artery and advanced into the thoracic aorta. The device is approximately 26 cm long, and a radiopaque tip allows for radiographic verification of position. The balloon inflates during diastole and deflates during systole to enhance perfusion of the coronary arteries and cardiac output. The radiopaque tip should reside just beyond the origin of the left subclavian artery within the proximal descending thoracic aorta. The carina can be used as a landmark with the tip of the IABP approximately 2 cm above the carina.[26] Correct positioning is important as placement too proximal (superiorly) can occlude the branch

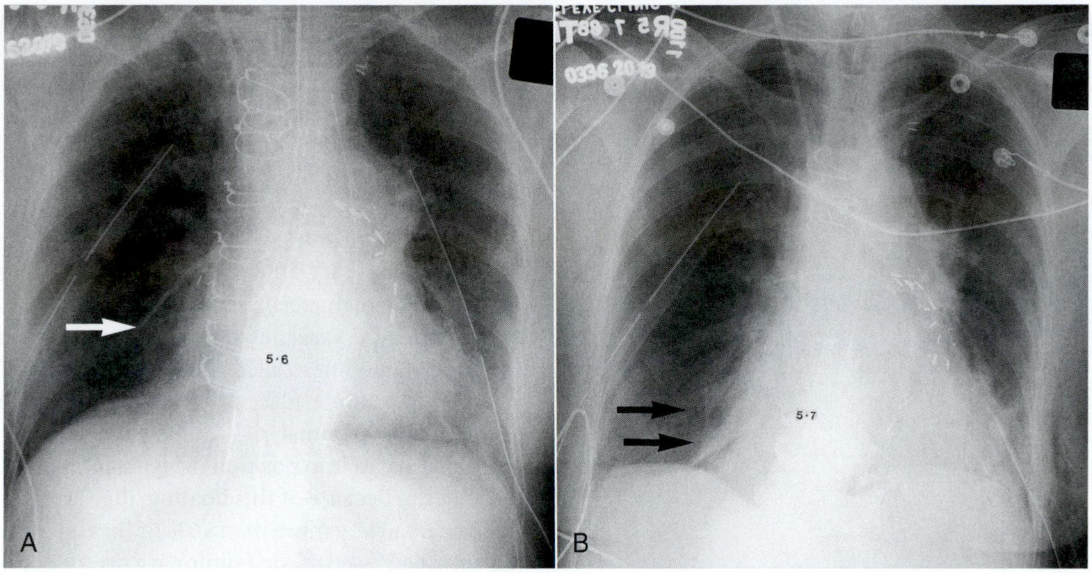

FIGURE 21-36 Two portable supine chest films obtained 30 hours apart. **A,** Wedged Swan-Ganz (pulmonary artery) catheter in the right lower lobe *(arrow)*. **B,** Film obtained after retraction of the catheter shows increased density at the site, reflecting an area of infarction caused by prolonged inadvertent wedging of the catheter *(arrows)*.

aortic vessels to the neck and upper extremities and placement too low (inferiorly) can occlude vessels to the abdominal organs and intestines.

SUMMARY CHECKLIST

- Thoracic imaging is an important tool for evaluating the cause and degree of various pulmonary diseases. Various thoracic imaging techniques are available to assist assessment of patients with lung disease.
- The tissue densities seen on the plain chest radiograph are air, fat, soft tissue (water), and bone.
- The steps in interpreting the chest film include (1) reviewing the technique and quality of the chest film (rotation and penetration) and (2) taking a step-by-step, disciplined approach to reviewing all the anatomic structures seen on the chest film (e.g., bones, soft tissue, heart, lower neck, airways and lungs, pleura, mediastinum, upper abdominal contents).
- The lungs are considered radiolucent and the bones are radiopaque.
- The chest film is useful for detecting pleural diseases such as pleural effusion or pneumothorax.
- Airspace opacities in the lung represent alveolar filling caused by water (pulmonary edema), blood (pulmonary hemorrhage), or pus (pneumonia).
- Air bronchograms are seen when air-filled airways are surrounded by consolidated (infiltrated) lung.
- Radiographic signs of pulmonary edema secondary to heart failure include (1) redistribution of blood flow to the upper lobes, (2) Kerley B lines, and (3) alveolar filling.
- Signs of long-standing heart failure include cardiac enlargement and pleural effusions, which are usually bilateral.
- Signs of volume loss (atelectasis) in the lungs include: (1) unilateral diaphragmatic elevation, (2) mediastinal shift, (3) narrowing of the rib spaces, (4) hilar displacement, and (5) fissure displacement.
- The chest film is useful in identifying the position of catheters and tubes. The tip of the endotracheal tube should be 5 to 7 cm above the carina when the neck is in a neutral position.
- CT has superb anatomic detail compared to chest radiographs but exposes patients to more radiation.
- Ultrasound can be useful in placing central lines, visualizing the presence of pleural fluid (e.g., to help guide thoracentesis), and detecting a pneumothorax.
- MRI is used less commonly for imaging the chest, but has a role in evaluating vascular structures, mediastinal masses, and cardiac structures.

References

1. Schoepf UJ, Costello P: CT angiography for diagnosis of pulmonary embolism: state of the art. *Radiology* 230:329–337, 2004.
2. Aberle DR, Adams AM, Berg CD, et al: Reduced lung-cancer mortality with low-dose computed tomographic screening. *N Engl J Med* 365:395–409, 2011.
3. Bastarrika G, Lee YS, Huda W, et al: CT of coronary artery disease. *Radiology* 253:317–338, 2009.
4. Kluge A, Luboldt W, Bachmann G: Acute pulmonary embolism to the subsegmental level: diagnostic accuracy of three MRI techniques compared with 16-MDCT. *AJR Am J Roentgenol* 187:W7–W14, 2006.
5. Inaoka T, Takahashi K, Mineta M, et al: Thymic hyperplasia and thymus gland tumors: differentiation with chemical shift MR imaging. *Radiology* 243:869–876, 2007.
6. Sachdeva A, Shepherd RW, Lee HJ: Thoracentesis and thoracic ultrasound: state of the art in 2013. *Clin Chest Med* 34:1–9, 2013.
7. Nicolaou S, Talsky A, Khashoggi K, et al: Ultrasound-guided interventional radiology in critical care. *Crit Care Med* 35:S186–S197, 2007.

8. Black LF: The pleural space and pleural fluid. *Mayo Clin Proc* 47:493–506, 1972.
9. Raasch BN, Carsky EW, Lane EJ, et al: Pleural effusion: explanation of some typical appearances. *AJR Am J Roentgenol* 139:899–904, 1982.
10. Moskowitz H, Platt RT, Schachar R, et al: Roentgen visualization of minute pleural effusions: an experimental study to determine the minimum amount of pleural fluid visible on a radiograph. *Radiology* 109:33–35, 1973.
11. Colins JD, Burwell D, Furmanski S, et al: Minimum detectable pleural effusions: a roentgen pathology model. *Radiology* 105:51–53, 1972.
12. Hessen I: Roentgen examination of pleural fluid: a study of the localization of free effusions, the potentialities of diagnosing minimal quantities of fluid and its existence under physiological conditions. *Acta Radiol Suppl* 86:1–80, 1951.
13. Lipscomb DJ, Flower CD, Hadfield JW: Ultrasound of the pleura: an assessment of its clinical value. *Clin Radiol* 32:289–290, 1981.
14. Tocino IM: Pneumothorax in the supine patient: radiographic anatomy. *Radiographics* 5:557–586, 1985.
15. Chiles C, Ravin CE: Radiographic recognition of pneumothorax in the intensive care unit. *Crit Care Med* 14:677–680, 1986.
16. Kong A: The deep sulcus sign. *Radiology* 228:415–416, 2003.
17. Zhang M, Liu ZH, Yang JX, et al: Rapid detection of pneumothorax by ultrasonography in patients with multiple trauma. *Crit Care* 10:R112, 2006.
18. Webb WR: Thin-section CT of the secondary pulmonary lobule: anatomy and the image—the 2004 Fleischner lecture. *Radiology* 239:322–338, 2006.
19. American Thoracic Society: Idiopathic pulmonary fibrosis: diagnosis and treatment. International consensus statement. American Thoracic Society (ATS), and the European Respiratory Society (ERS). *Am J Respir Crit Care Med* 161(2 Pt 1):646–664, 2000.
20. Hobbs S, Lynch D: The idiopathic interstitial pneumonias: an update and review. *Radiol Clin North Am* 52:105–120, 2014.
21. Woodring JH, Reed JC: Types and mechanisms of pulmonary atelectasis. *J Thorac Imaging* 11:92–108, 1996.
22. Gurney JW, Jones KK, Robbins RA, et al: Regional distribution of: emphysema—correlation of high-resolution CT with pulmonary function tests in unselected smokers. *Radiology* 183:457–463, 1992.
23. Fishman A, Martinez F, Naunheim K, et al: A randomized trial comparing lung-volume-reduction surgery with medial therapy for severe emphysema. *N Engl J Med* 348:2059–2273, 2003.
24. Steele JD: The solitary pulmonary nodule: report of a cooperative study of resected asymptomatic solitary pulmonary nodules in males. *J Thorac Cardiovasc Surg* 46:21–39, 1963.
25. Goodman LR, Putman CE: Radiological evaluation of patients receiving assisted ventilation. *JAMA* 245:858–860, 1981.
26. Kim JT, Lee JR, Kim JK, et al: The carina as a useful radiographic landmark for positioning the intraaortic balloon pump. *Anesth Analg* 105:735–738, 2007.

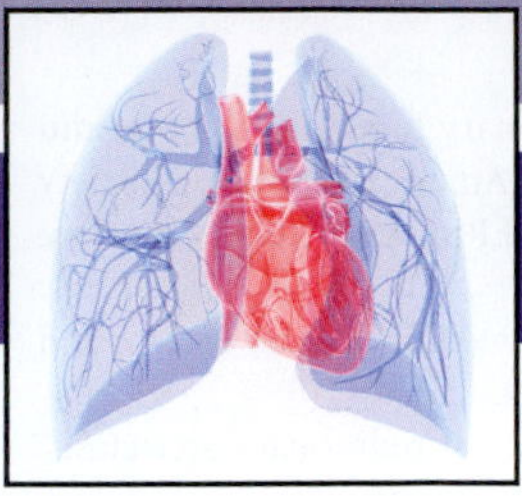

CHAPTER 22

Flexible Bronchoscopy and the Respiratory Therapist

DANAI KHEMASUWAN AND ATUL C. MEHTA

CHAPTER OBJECTIVES

After reading this chapter you will be able to:

- Understand the preprocedure assessment, type of sedation, and patient monitoring during bronchoscopy.
- Understand the indications, contraindications, and complications of various diagnostic and therapeutic bronchoscopic techniques.
- Recognize the difference between each thermal ablation technique.
- Recognize the difference between silicone and metallic stents.
- Identify the emerging bronchoscopic treatment options for patients with steroid-dependent asthma and for patients with severe emphysema.
- Describe the role of the respiratory therapist in assisting with bronchoscopy.
- Identify special considerations for bronchoscopy during mechanical ventilation.

CHAPTER OUTLINE

Flexible Bronchoscopy
- Procedure, Sedation, and Monitoring

Diagnostic Bronchoscopy
- Bronchoalveolar Lavage
- Endobronchial Biopsy
- Transbronchial Biopsy
- Electromagnetic Navigational Bronchoscopy
- Ultrathin Bronchoscopy
- Narrow Band Imaging

Therapeutic Bronchoscopy
- Thermal Ablation of the Endobronchial Lesion
- Cryotherapy
- Brachytherapy
- Endobronchial Stents
- Bronchoscopy in Difficult Intubation

The Role of the Respiratory Therapist in Bronchoscopy

Special Considerations for Bronchoscopy During Mechanical Ventilation

Physiologic and Mechanical Alterations Associated With Flexible Bronchoscopy in Intubated Patients

Emerging Bronchoscopic Interventions

Conclusion

KEY TERMS

airway stents
argon plasma coagulation
brachytherapy
bronchial washings
bronchial brushings
bronchoalveolar lavage
cryotherapy
electromagnetic navigational bronchoscopy
endobronchial biopsy
fiberoptic bundles
laser photocoagulation
Mallampati classification
methemoglobinemia
moderate sedation
narrow band imaging
transbronchial biopsy
transbronchial needle aspiration
ultrathin bronchoscopy

Besides thoracentesis, bronchoscopy is one of the most commonly performed procedures in pulmonary medicine. Bronchoscopy allows physicians to access the inside of the airways for both diagnostic and therapeutic purposes. The procedure can be performed using either a rigid or a flexible instrument. This chapter focuses is mainly on flexible bronchoscopy because it is much more commonly performed than the rigid variation.

The first bronchoscopy was performed by a German laryngologist, Gustav Killian, in the early nineteenth century. He

removed a foreign body via the translaryngeal route with direct bronchoscopy[1] using a rigid esophagoscope. In the United States, Chevalier Jackson is considered to be the pioneer of rigid bronchoscopy. He reported the first bronchoscopic resection of an endobronchial tumor in 1917.[2] Over time, the technology has progressed remarkably. In 1966, the flexible bronchoscope (FB) was introduced by Shigeto Ikeda, a Japanese thoracic surgeon. In 1970, Olympus introduced the first FB for commercial purposes. Since then, the technologic advancements have led to a wide array of minimally invasive endoscopic diagnostic and therapeutic techniques that will be discussed in this chapter.

This chapter will focus on the essential elements of the procedure, including the equipment, indications, contraindications, and variations in the procedures and emerging trends. In addition, the role of the respiratory therapist and special considerations when performing bronchoscopy on patients under specific conditions (e.g., during mechanical ventilation) are also described.

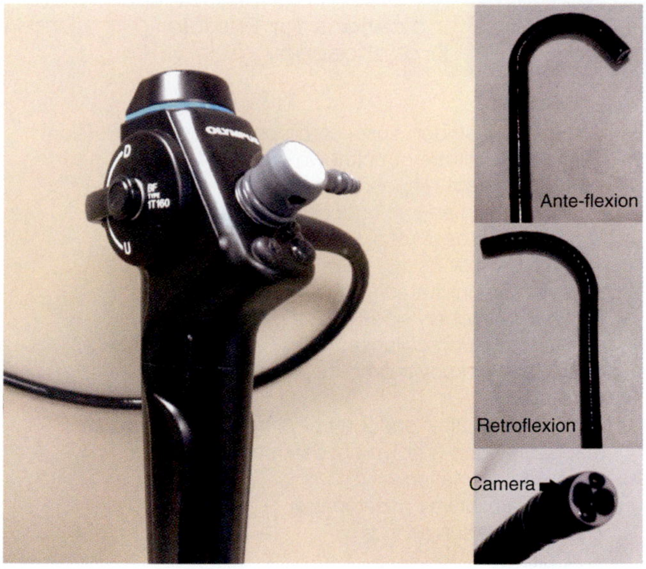

FIGURE 22-1 Flexible bronchoscope. *Left, inset:* Anteflexion *(top),* retroflexion *(middle),* and distal tip *(bottom).*

FLEXIBLE BRONCHOSCOPY

The FB uses **fiberoptic bundles** to illuminate the endobronchial tree. Based on the imaging system, FBs are divided into fiberoptic, video, or hybrid. The fiberoptic bronchoscope carries a second fiberoptic bundle that gathers the images from the distal tip of the instrument, which is visualized through the eye piece. The video bronchoscope uses somewhat different technology which employs a miniaturized charge-coupled devices (CCDs) chip at its distal tip to gather the images from the endobronchial tree and transmit them to the image-processing unit. The hybrid instrument uses a fiberoptic imaging system but also has a CCDs chip to convert the information in a digital format. Most modern FBs use video technology, whereas thinner bronchoscopes are hybrid in nature.

The proximal end of the FB is the controlling unit of the instrument, which helps the operator perform desired maneuvers to control the distal tip of the FB (Figure 22-1). The distal tip of FB can be flexed in two directions up to 180 degree in anteflexion and up to 130 degree in retroflexion positions (see Figure 22-1). In addition to these controls, the operator rotates the instrument on its axis using the wrist. More recently, Olympus also added a feature that allows axial rotation of the instrument without relying on wrist movement (Figure 22-2).

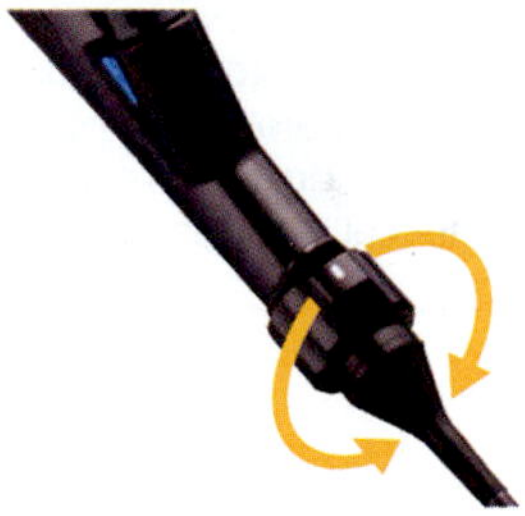
FIGURE 22-2 New Olympus scope with rotating function. (From Olympus. http://www.olympusaustralia.com.au/Document/Detail/328/Advancing-Control-Respiratory.)

Today, flexible bronchoscopy has become a standard procedure because of its diagnostic value, safety, and ease of performance. The procedure can be done in an outpatient setting, under local anesthesia and moderate (or conscious) sedation. The indications for FB have grown over the past years (Box 22-1) and are extensive. Box 22-2 presents the contraindications to performing FB. There are a few absolute contraindications for FB, which include severe hypoxemia, hemodynamics instability, acute bronchospasm, and the inability to obtain informed consent for the procedure.

The discussion as to whether the bronchoscopy is indicated involves the physician and often other members of the bronchoscopy team, including the respiratory therapist. However, in the end, the final decision whether to perform the procedure must be individualized in a conversation between the physician and the patient, based on an open discussion about the risks and benefits of the procedure.

Procedure, Sedation, and Monitoring

FB can be performed on spontaneously breathing patients via the oral or the nasal route and occasionally through a tracheostomy stoma. FB can also be done on patient with artificial airways such as endotracheal or tracheostomy tubes. Most procedures are performed under moderate or deep sedation. When deep sedation is used, the procedure is performed via either a laryngeal mask airway or an endotracheal tube of the appropriate size. Rigid bronchoscopy is performed under deep sedation with muscle relaxation.

The goal of sedation is to improve the patient's comfort during the procedure. In addition to risks for arrhythmias and fluctuations in blood pressure related to the procedure, airway manipulation during bronchoscopy may lead to coughing, hypoxemia, vomiting, bleeding, laryngospasm, and bronchospasm. All of these responses can affect the outcomes of the

Box 22-1 Indications for Flexible Bronchoscopy

- Hemoptysis
- Wheeze and stridor; suspected upper airway obstruction
- Pulmonary infiltrate of unknown cause
  - Infiltrates not responding to conventional treatment
  - Infiltrates in an immunocompromised host
  - Recurrent or unresolved pneumonia
  - Cavitary lesions
  - Interstitial infiltrates
  - New pulmonary nodule
- Unexplained lung collapse
- Suspected or known bronchogenic carcinoma
  - Staging
  - Follow-up after endobronchial treatments
- Mediastinal and hilar lymphadenopathy
- Lung transplantation
  - Evaluate airway anastomosis
  - Rejection surveillance
  - Cultures
- Endotracheal intubation
  - Confirm endotracheal tube position
  - Evaluate tube-related injury
- Evaluation of foreign body aspiration, chemical-related, or burn-related injury to the airway
- Unexplained superior vena cava syndrome
- Unexplained vocal cord paralysis or hoarseness
- Suspected fistulas (e.g., bronchopleural, tracheoesophageal and bronchoesophageal, trachea or bronchoaortic)

Box 22-2 Contraindications to Flexible Bronchoscopy

CONTRAINDICATIONS

Absolute

- Uncorrectable hypoxemia
- Lack of patient cooperation
- Lack of skilled personnel
- Lack of appropriate equipment and facilities
- Unstable angina
- Uncontrolled arrhythmias

Relative

- Unexplained or severe hypercarbia
- Uncontrolled asthma attack
- Lack of patient cooperation
- Uncorrected coagulopathy
- Recent myocardial infarction
- Unstable cervical spine and impaired neck mobility
- Need for large tissue specimen

procedure. Therefore adequate sedation is an important part of the procedure.

There is a wide range in the level of sedation that can be provided, including light sedation (anxiolysis), **moderate (conscious) sedation**, and deep sedation with general anesthesia. Moderate sedation is most commonly used during FB. At this level of sedation, patients can respond to verbal stimuli and demonstrate preserved protective airway reflexes. Several intravenous forms of benzodiazepines and opioids are commonly used during FB. Diazepam, midazolam, lorazepam, morphine sulfate, and fentanyl have been used either as a single agent or in combination based on the availability and physician preference.[3] The combination of a benzodiazepine (like midazolam) and an opioid (like morphine sulfate or fentanyl) has been shown to be safe and effective for sedation during FB.[4]

Several techniques are used to apply local anesthetic agents to the upper and the lower airway. Using approximately 10 mL of 2% viscous lidocaine, "swish and swallow" is a simple and effective method to numb the upper airways. Another common method involves nebulizing 5 mL of 4% lidocaine. The nasal passage is usually anesthetized using 5 mL of 2% lidocaine jelly. In addition, 1% to 2% of lidocaine is instilled directly in to the lower airways through the working channel of the instrument in 2-mL aliquots during the procedure. The drug lidocaine has a very narrow therapeutic range. To help avoid unwanted hazards such as **methemoglobinemia,** the total dose of lidocaine should be limited to 5 to 7 mg/kg in adults (maximum of 400 to 500 mg in a 150-lb adult), during the procedure, with added caution in the elderly and in those with liver or cardiac disease.[5]

MINI CLINIC

Methemoglobinema During Bronchoscopy

PROBLEM: A respiratory therapist (RT) is assisting during a flexible bronchoscopy. The patient had local anesthesia with lidocaine nebulization and benzocaine spray. The patient developed central cyanosis and his oxygen saturation dropped to 85% via pulse oximetry. The procedure was aborted. An arterial blood gas check showed pH, 7.43; PCO_2, 43; and PO_2, 279; with an O_2 saturation of 85%. What condition should an RT consider in this situation?

DISCUSSION: Methemoglobinemia should be suspected. Benzocaine is a common cause of methemoglobinemia during endoscopic procedures. Benzocaine, which is used as a local anesthetic, is a common source of methemoglobinemia during such procedures. Benzocaine causes oxidization of the iron in hemoglobin (Hb) from the ferrous (Fe^{2+}) to the ferric state (Fe^{3+}). Fe^{3+} Hb is unable to carry O_2. The PO_2 is within normal range as shown by the machine measurement of dissolved O_2 in the blood, not in the Hb. Therefore methemoglobinemia causes hypoxemia at the cellular level that is not detected by measuring PO_2 but can be uncovered by co-oximetry to measure methemoglobin directly. In terms of management, a methemoglobin level less than 30% usually resolves spontaneously over 15 to 20 hours after removal of the offending agent and with O_2 administration. Intravenous administration of methylene blue is the management of choice in patients when the methemoglobin levels exceed 30%.

RULE OF THUMB

For patient safety, to help avoid methemoglobinemia, the total dose of lidocaine should not exceed 7 mg/kg of body weight during a routine (<45 min) FB procedure.

The assessment of the upper airway before the procedure helps identify those patients in whom it may be difficult to secure an airway in case of hypoventilation. The **Mallampati classification** is one of the most commonly used methods to identify individuals who may pose difficulty during intubation. The Mallampati score is assessed by having the patient open his or her mount and protrude the tongue as much as possible without phonation (Figure 22-3).

RULE OF THUMB

The Mallampati score should be assessed in every spontaneously breathing patient before flexible bronchoscopy.

Several maneuvers (e.g., chin-lift, jaw-thrust) may become necessary if the patient becomes oversedated during FB. In addition to an unfavorable Mallampati score, comorbidities can also affect the safety and outcome of the procedure. The recommendation from the American Society of Anesthesiologists (ASA) is to categorize patients based on their ASA score, which considers comorbid conditions and their impact on the patient's daily living (Table 22-1).[6]

During the FB procedure, continuous monitoring of oxygenation and hemodynamic stability are important. Pulse oximetry, heart rate, and blood pressure are monitored throughout the procedure. One of the most difficult parameters to monitor during FB is the depth of sedation. Intermittent boluses of sedation may be needed to ensure the adequate depth of sedation during the procedure. However, the depth of sedation must be balanced with the side effects of oversedation during and after the procedure. To monitor the patient, the respiratory therapist or other member of the bronchoscopy team should keep track of the patient's responses to verbal commands or spontaneous movements. Notably, chest movement may continue despite near total obstruction of the airway. To prevent the patient's slipping into deep sedation, the ASA also recommends capnography monitoring while performing FB under moderate sedation.[7]

RULE OF THUMB

Continuous cardiac, blood pressure, and oximetry monitoring must be carried out during bronchoscopy. Capnography is highly recommended.

DIAGNOSTIC BRONCHOSCOPY

A computed tomography (CT) scan of the chest is performed before all elective bronchoscopic procedures being performed for lung cancer diagnosis. The information is very valuable in increasing the diagnostic yield of the procedure among patients suspected to have lung cancer. The scan also may eliminate the need for preforming the procedure in 7% of patients.[8]

Diagnostic bronchoscopy begins with the examination of the upper airways. Proper upper airway examination is crucial to identify lesions involving nasal passages, pharyngeal, and laryngeal structures, including vocal cords. After examination of the

TABLE 22-1
American Society of Anesthesiologists Classification: Comorbid Conditions and Impact on Daily Living

ASA Class	Class Definition
I	A normally healthy patient
II	A patient with mild systemic disease
III	A patient with systemic disease that is not incapacitating
IV	A patient with an incapacitating systemic disease that is a constant threat to life
V	A moribund patient who is not expected to survive for 24 hr with or without operation

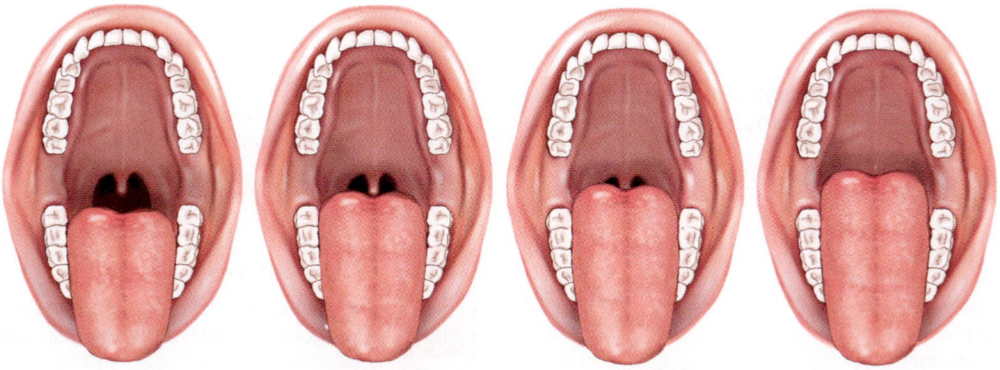

FIGURE 22-3 Mallampati classification.

upper airway structures, the lower airways are examined at least until the fifth- or sixth-generation bronchi. Examining bronchi deeper than this depends on the diameter of the bronchoscope. For diagnostic purposes, besides examining the airways, several different types of specimens can be collected through the working channel of the bronchoscope.

RULE OF THUMB

A CT scan of the chest is generally performed before all elective bronchoscopic procedures done for patients with, or suspected of having, lung cancer.

Bronchoalveolar Lavage

Bronchoalveolar lavage is used to obtain specimens from the alveolar level of the lung. BAL is performed by instilling a small volume (up to 50 mL) of normal saline solution deep into the airways and then suctioning the instilled liquid back. BAL fluid contains both cellular and noncellular components of alveolar lining fluid (Figure 22-4). As a form of "liquid lung" sample, the BAL fluid is thought to represent millions of alveoli as well as respiratory epithelial lining and colonizing organisms. BAL has become a standard diagnostic procedure in patients with pulmonary infiltrates of uncertain cause (Box 22-3). As cellular content, a normal BAL sample includes 95% macrophages; 3% lymphocytes; 1% to 2% neutrophils, eosinophils and basophils; and few epithelial cells. In addition to routine culture and cell count, an estimation of the CD4/CD8 ratio of lymphocytes in the lavage fluid can be helpful in establishing the diagnosis of sarcoidosis and hypersensitivity pneumonitis.

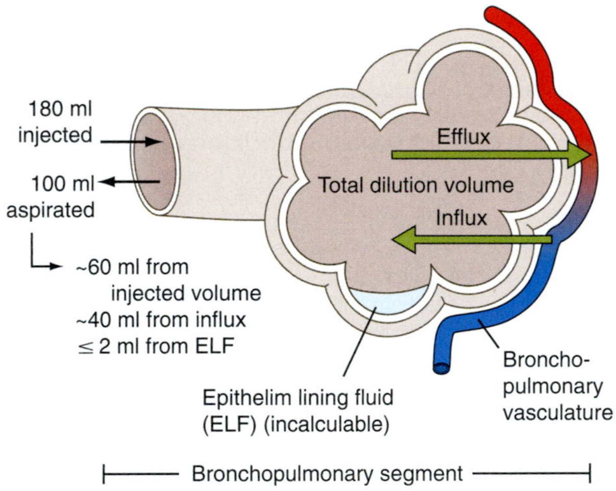

FIGURE 22-4 Schematic presentation of the constituents of the bronchoalveolar lavage.

Box 22-3 Role of Bronchoalveolar Lavage in Diagnosis for Pulmonary Diseases

- Infection (e.g., bacteria, fungus, virus, and mycobacteria)
- Pulmonary hemorrhage
- Malignancy (e.g. solid tumor, lymphoma)
- Eosinophilic lung disease
- Pulmonary alveolar proteinosis
- Langerhans cell histiocytosis
- Lipoid pneumonia
- Diffuse alveolar hemorrhage

Bronchoalveolar Lavage Technique

It is important to avoid suction while inserting the FB through the nasopharynx and central airways, to minimize contamination of the working channel of the bronchoscope with the local organisms.[9–11] The amount of lidocaine used should be minimized both to prevent its bacteriostatic properties from interfering with BAL fluid cultures used to identify infectious organisms and to avoid altering the cellular contents of the lavage fluid. The right middle lobe or the lingua is generally used to perform BAL in patients with diffuse diseases. With the patient in a supine position, gravity helps to augment BAL return from these locations.[9,10] Meanwhile, in localized lung diseases, lavage is performed from the area of the focal abnormality.[10]

To obtain the lavage fluid, the bronchoscope is wedged at the level of fourth- or fifth-generation bronchus. A "good wedge" position means that the bronchoscope is advanced as far as possible while the distal lumen is still visible. In this position, BAL return is maximal. Fluid (20 to 60 mL) is instilled into the appropriate bronchial segment and aspirated back manually for laboratory testing. In general, 15 to 20 mL of BAL volume is enough to conduct common laboratory tests such as microbiologic and cytologic tests.[11]

Several complications are associated with BAL. Hypoxemia is common, and its severity generally depends upon three factors: the volume of fluid administered,[12] the number of segments lavage, and the duration of the procedure. Introduction of 100 mL of lavage fluid can cause O_2 desaturation up to 7%, whereas 200 mL of lavage fluid can drop O_2 saturation up to 15% from the baseline value.[12] O_2 supplementation during BAL may mitigate the degree of O_2 desaturation. However, the volume of lavage fluid and the duration of the procedure are important factors to determine the risk of this complication. Cases of pneumothorax from BAL have also been reported in patients with *Pneumocystis jirovici* pneumonia and during therapeutic BAL for pulmonary alveolar proteinosis (PAP).[13,14]

RULE OF THUMB

BAL should be obtained from the nondependent part of the lung to optimize the fluid return.

RULE OF THUMB

Supplemental O_2 should be administered in all patients undergoing bronchoscopy, to help avoid or minimize hypoxemia.

Mini-BAL is defined as nonbronchoscopic BAL. Mini-BAL is most frequently performed in intubated patients when a catheter is passed through an endotracheal tube into the bronchi until the catheter lodges, after which saline is instilled for the lavage and then withdrawn. The volume of saline instillation is usually 25 mL or less. The return of fluid by aspiration is highly variable. Mini-BAL is a simple procedure for acquiring quantitative lower airway cultures in mechanically ventilated patients.[15] In some settings, RTs perform the procedure. As an example of the impact of mini-BAL, approximately, 46% of mini-BAL cultures are found to contain at least one organism potentially contributing to a suspected episode of ventilator-assisted pneumonia.[16]

Bronchial Washings

Bronchial washings are generally obtained for the cytologic examination for cancer and for microbiologic analysis to diagnose mycobacterial or fungal infections. Unlike BAL, bronchial washings are obtained from the large airways. Bronchial washing is easy to perform, but is not very effective in diagnosing malignancy, successfully diagnosing only 22% to 29% of peripheral lesions[17,18] and is slightly higher for central lesions.[19,20] Bronchial washings are an inexpensive by-product of the bronchoscopy and are routinely obtained in patients suspected to have airway malignancy.[21]

Bronchial Brushings

Bronchial brushings have been used as an adjunct diagnostic test in addition to endobronchial and transbronchial biopsies and transbronchial needle aspiration (TBNA). It involves brushing the surface of the suspicious lesion back and forth 5 to 10 times while rotating the handle. Brushes of various different diameters and bristle strengths are available in the market. Brushing is usually performed under direct visualization or with fluoroscopic guidance to avoid trauma to the bronchial mucosa and pneumothorax, respectively. Brushing establishes a diagnosis in 72% (range 44% to 94%) of patients with central lung cancers and in 45% of patients with peripheral lesions.[22] Bronchial brushing is usually performed after obtaining all the other specimens to avoid bleeding or cellular degradation that may affect the overall interpretation of FB specimens. Once the specimen is collected, the cells are smeared onto a slide and the end of the brush is cut off and placed in a fixative solution for cytologic examination.[23]

Endobronchial Biopsy

Endobronchial biopsy (EBBx) is a technique whereby flexible forceps are used to obtain a tissue sample from a visible endobronchial lesion. It provides specimens for histologic examination. EBBx has been shown to successfully diagnose between 51% and 97% of neoplasms.[24,25] The number of biopsy specimens that should be obtained depends on the diagnosis suspected. In patients suspected to have bronchogenic carcinoma, three biopsy specimens are often able to successfully diagnose almost all such cases.[26] If the specimen is obtained from the surrounding necrotic tissue, the EBBx can fail to contain cancerous cells despite the patient having a malignancy. In such cases, debridement of the necrotic tissue with the forceps or performing a TBNA may improve diagnostic value. Endobronchial biopsy of a highly vascularized lesion may lead to significant bleeding and must be undertaken with caution. The physician may take precautions such as instilling ice cold saline or using the TBNA approach.

Transbronchial Biopsy

Transbronchial biopsy is a technique of obtaining a specimen of the lung parenchyma by using flexible forceps positioned distally through the working channel of the bronchoscope. A fenestrated alligator forceps is most commonly used to obtain the TBBx. Six to ten tissue specimens are obtained, depending on the suspected diagnosis. TBBx can be performed with or without fluoroscopic guidance (Figure 22-5). The latter is a common practice while performing the TBBx in the intensive care unit setting.

The diagnostic value of TBBx varies depending on the underlying lung diseases and the patient population. For infectious diseases, the 88% to 97% of cases of *P. jiroveci* pneumonia[27] and 57% to 79% of cases of *Mycobacterium tuberculosis* have been successfully diagnosed.[28] In lung transplant surveillance, the TBBx can detect a presence of allograft rejection in approximately 70% of the cases.[29] In interstitial lung diseases, the diagnostic value is relatively low compared with the experience in infectious diseases. TBBx can successfully diagnose 40% to 90% of sarcoidosis cases[30] and only 10% to 40% of those with Langerhans cell histiocytosis.[31] In a peripheral pulmonary nodule (PPN), the diagnostic value of TBBx depends upon the size and the location of the nodule. The presence of an airway leading to the nodule as seen on the Computed Tomography scan of the chest is called a "positive bronchus sign" and when combined with TBBx increases successful diagnosis from 31% to 79% for the PPN.[32]

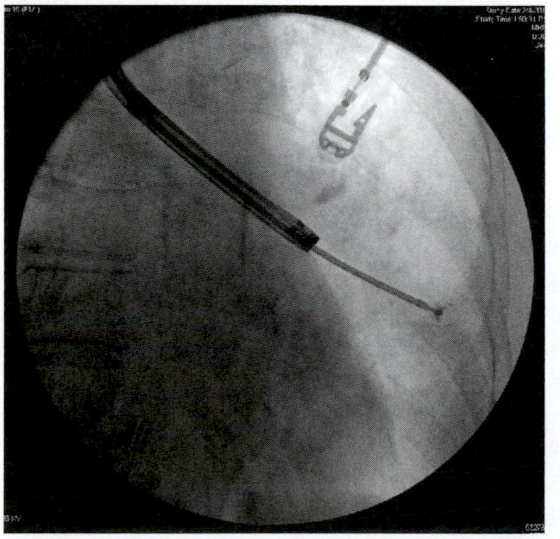

FIGURE 22-5 Transbronchial biopsy under direct visualization with fluoroscopy.

TABLE 22-2

Antithrombotic Therapies and Recommended Interval Between Last Dose and Procedure [Baron]

Agents	Interval from Last Dose Before Procedure
Warfarin	3-5 days; or goal international normalized ratio <1.5
Unfractionated heparin	Intravenous 2-6 hr
Low molecular weight heparin	24 hr; depending on creatinine clearance
Dabigatran	1-2 days with creatinine clearance >50 ml/min 3-5 days with creatinine clearance <50 ml/min
Rivaroxaban	1 day with normal renal function 2-4 days with impaired renal function
Desirudin	2 hr
Clopidogrel, ticlopidine, prasugrel, ticagrelor	5 days
Aspirin and dipyridamole	7-10 days

Data from Baron TH, Kamath PS, McBane RD: Antithrombotic therapy and invasive procedures. N Engl J Med 369:1079–1080, 2013.

The two major complications of TBBx are pneumothorax and bleeding. Adequate sedation and cough suppression are important to reduce the risk for pneumothorax arising from cough-induced barotrauma. Whenever available, fluoroscopy should be used to guide the TBBx, especially in patients with localized lesions. Fluoroscopy is also used to screen for pneumothorax after the TBBx.[33] The risk for developing pneumothorax is three times higher in mechanically ventilated patients compared to that among spontaneously breathing patients.[34,35] To reduce the risk for pneumothorax among the former group, the positive end-expiratory pressure (PEEP) level should be maintained below 5 cm H_2O. Also, the capability of promptly placing a chest tube should be available.

Meanwhile, the incidence of bleeding from TBBx is low (2% to 9%) in the absence of a bleeding tendency or coagulopathies. Risk factors for bleeding after TBBx include renal insufficiency with blood urea nitrogen less than 30 mg/dL and creatinine greater than 3 mg/dL, pulmonary hypertension with a mean pulmonary pressure of greater than 40 mm Hg, thrombocytopenia with platelets less than 50,000/mL and international normalized ratio (INR) greater than 1.5 are considered risk factors for bleeding after TBBx.[36]

TBBx can be safely performed in patients who are receiving aspirin or nonsteroidal inflammatory drugs. However, several antithrombotic and antiplatelet therapies should be withheld for a specific period before TBBx (Table 22-2).[37] In an event of bleeding, wedging the bronchoscope in the involved subsegment helps tamponade, or compress, the bleeding site. Alternatively, 5 to 10 mL of ice cold saline (−4° C) or 2 to 4 mL of either epinephrine or norepinephrine (1:10,000) solution can be instilled through the working channel of the bronchoscope to lessen the bleeding.

MINI CLINIC

Sudden Chest Pain and Clinical Deterioration During Bronchoscopy

PROBLEM: An RT is assisting during a FB on a young female with suspected sarcoidosis. The patient is very anxious and despite an adequate amount of narcotics and anxiolytic agents, continues to cough violently. The physician is performing TBBx under the fluoroscopic guidance from the left lower lobe. In seven attempts, he manages to obtain three pieces of tissue before giving up the procedure. During the last attempt, the patient winced with mild pain. Soon after the last biopsy the patient became tachypnic (respiration rate [RR] 30 breaths/min), with heart rate of 110 beats/min, and SpO_2 dropped to 82% on O_2 6 L/min via nasal cannula. Examination of the chest showed that it was tympanic on percussion with reduced breath sounds on auscultation. What condition should the RT consider in this situation?

DISCUSSION: The RT should consider pneumothorax in this situation and should also consider ruling out a tension pneumothorax. Pneumothorax is a potential complication following a TBBx.[38] The risk is further increased in the situation in which the patient cannot cooperate for the procedure and continues to cough during the biopsy procedure. In this case, fluoroscopic examination can help confirm or rule out the condition. Meanwhile the patient should receive an adequate amount of supplemental O_2, if required via a nonrebreather mask. The RT should be prepared to assist the pulmonologist place either a Heimlich valve or a chest tube, depending on the size of the pneumothorax and the symptoms of the patient. If a tension pneumothorax is suspected, any size needle can be inserted into the pleural space and the air would be expected to rush out as the pressure is relieved.

Transbronchial Needle Aspiration: Conventional and Ultrasound-Guided Procedures

Transbronchial needle aspiration (TBNA) is the technique that allows sampling tissue from the mediastinum or the peripheral lung by inserting needles through the bronchial wall. TBNA can be used to determine the cause of mediastinal lesions and PPNs in a minimally invasive fashion.[39,40]

With the advent of endobronchial ultrasound (EBUS), the accuracy of TBNA has improved dramatically. EBUS is essentially a bronchoscope with a linear ultrasound probe attached at its distal end. EBUS provides real-time ultrasonographic guidance for TBNA of target structures (Figures 22-6 and 22-7). It has recently been found that in patients with potentially operable lung cancer, the diagnostic accuracy of EBUS-TBNA is far superior (98% diagnostic accuracy) to either positron-emission tomography or CT scans of the chest.[41,42] Recently the use of EBUS-TBNA has greatly expanded in the diagnosis and staging of non–small cell lung cancer because of the minimally invasive nature of EBUS-TBNA. Notably, subcarinal lymph

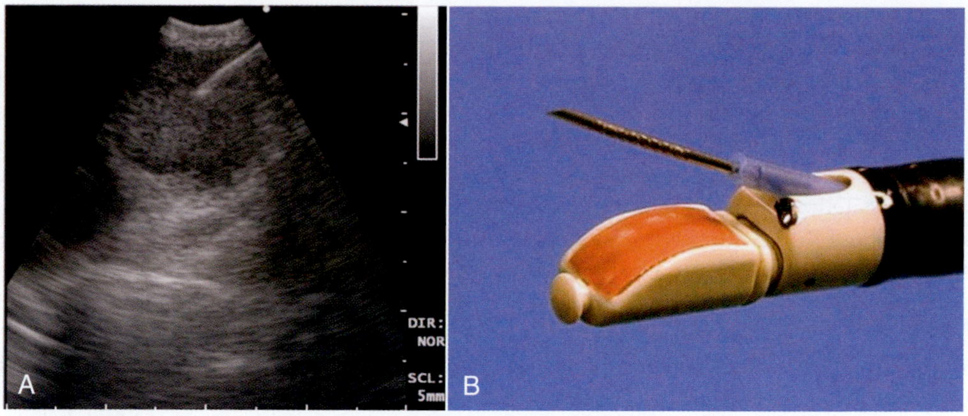

FIGURE 22-6 **A,** The distal tip of the endobronchial ultrasound endoscope with an aspiration needle. **B,** Sonographic image of EBUS-TBNA demonstrating needle inside lymph node. (**B,** From Medford AR: Diagnostic utility of endobronchial ultrasound-guided transbronchial needle aspiration for left paratracheal lesions. *QJM* 105[6]:589–590, 2012.)

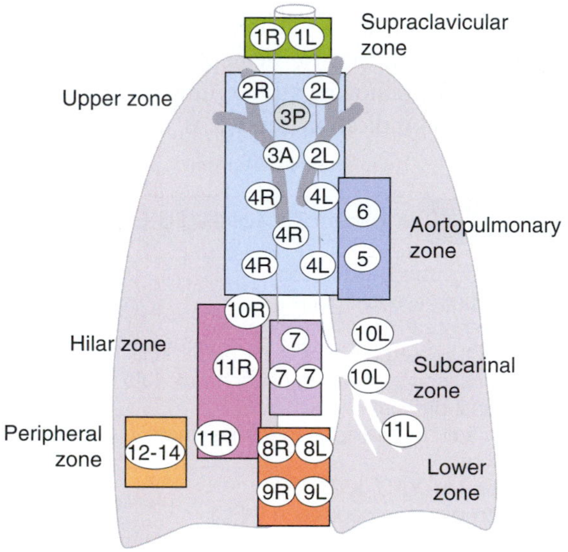

FIGURE 22-7 The International Association for the Study of Lung Cancer (IASLC) lymph node map.

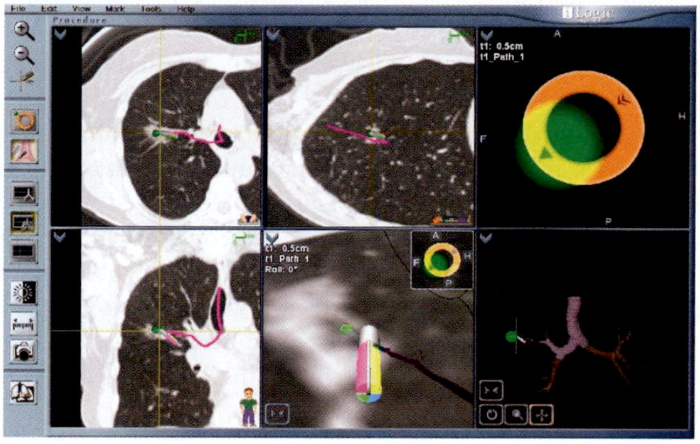

FIGURE 22-8 Electromagnetic navigation monitor. Location of the pulmonary lesion is displayed in three different axis of computed tomography imaging.

nodes can be assessed more accurately with EBUS-TBNA than with conventional mediastinoscopy. Reported complications of EBUS-TBNA include pneumomediastinum, pneumothorax, mediastinitis, bacteremia, and, rarely, death.[43–46]

In the current era, in which genetic profiling of lung cancer is essential to identify biomarkers that significantly influence treatment decisions and responses, EBUS-TBNA can provide adequate tissue for genetic analysis.[47] The utility of EBUS-TBNA also has been investigated for restaging of lung cancer after chemotherapy, and evidence supports it use for this purpose.[48]

Electromagnetic Navigational Bronchoscopy

Recently, an advanced CT imaging technology has been innovatively combined with an electromagnetic navigation system to guide the biopsy of PPNs that lie beyond the reach of standard flexible bronchoscopy. **Electromagnetic navigational bronchoscopy** (ENB), peripheral EBUS, virtual bronchoscopy, ultrathin bronchoscopy, and their combination have significantly increased the diagnostic value of FB for peripheral lesions, with an acceptably low complication rate of bleeding and pneumothorax.[49]

The ENB system uses low-frequency electromagnetic waves transmitted from a magnetic board placed below the patient's chest. As a result, the lesion can be visualized in real time with computer-generated guidance in three dimensions.

ENB is performed in several steps. The first step is planning the procedure by uploading high-quality CT images into the planning software. The software will generate the plan markers from the main carina to the lesion via multiple bronchial subsegments. The next step is aligning the virtual images to the patient's endobronchial anatomy, which is called the *registration* phase. Then, the navigation is conducted by driving the locatable guide probe with its extended working channel (EWC) to the lesion, by following the three dimensional CT images and the "tip view" (Figure 22-8). Once the lesion is reached, the guide probe is removed, leaving the EWC in place. The position of the tip of the EWC may be confirmed by using the radial EBUS probe to determine the location of the lesion (Figure 22-9). Various diagnostic tools such as a needle, brush, or forceps for biopsy can be used through the EWC to obtain a tissue specimen. In terms of diagnostic value, ENB can successfully diagnose almost 75% of peripheral lesions, but pneumothorax occurs in approximately 3.5% of such cases. The combination of radial probe EBUS with ENB can further increase the diagnostic value.[50]

Ultrathin Bronchoscopy

The normal tracheobronchial tree divides approximately 24 times before it reaches the respiratory bronchioles. The external diameter of the adult FB is approximately 5.7 to 6 mm, which allows the physician to reach the fourth- or fifth-order bronchi. The ultrathin bronchoscope is approximately 2.8 mm in external diameter and can reach up to at least the eighth-order bronchi (Figure 22-10). **Ultrathin bronchoscopy** can be helpful in diagnosing PPNs and can be used to inspect peripheral airways or to examine the airway beyond a pathologic airway narrowing.

The major technical challenge of performing ultrathin bronchoscopy is maintaining proper anatomic orientation in the peripheral airways. The instrument is seldom used without a real-time CT guidance, virtual bronchoscopy,[51] or a specially designed peripheral EBUS system. Another drawback of the ultrathin bronchoscope is its narrow working channel (1.7 mm) and miniaturized accessories (1 to 1.2 mm). These limit its diagnostic value because the specimens that can be obtained are very small.

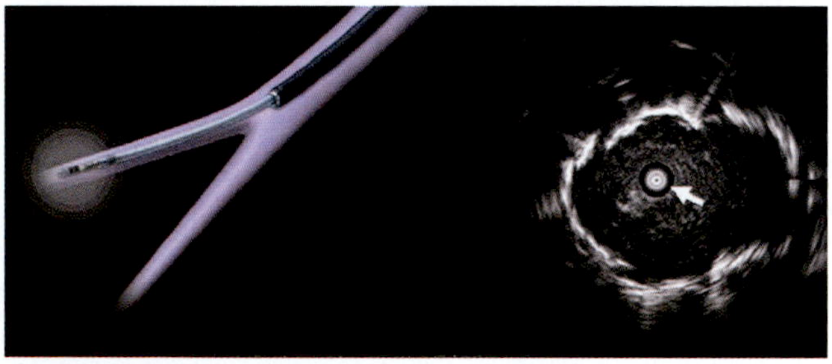

Figure 22-9 Radial probe endobronchial ultrasound *(left)*. A radial probe is surrounded by lesion *(right, arrow)*. (*Left* from http://www.goldcoastrespiratoryandsleep.com.au/gcrsc-services.html.)

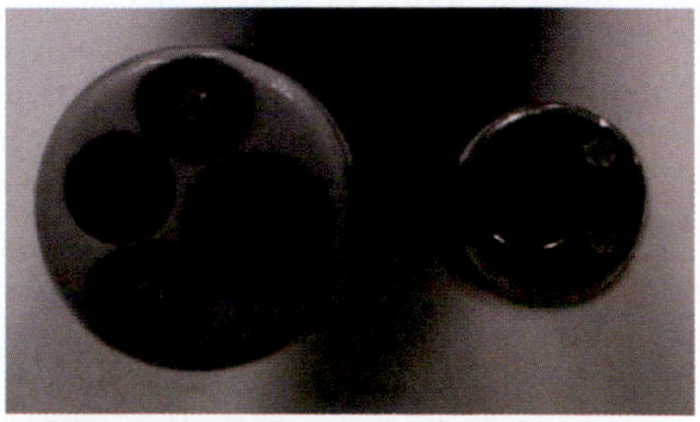

FIGURE 22-10 Comparison of the diameter of the tip of the ultrathin bronchoscope (2.8 mm) *(right)* with that of a standard-size bronchoscope *(left)*.

Narrow Band Imaging

Narrow band imaging is a technique that uses specialized filters to separate wavelengths of white light and selectively emits red, green, and blue bands. The intensification of the blue band detects vessel growth and complex vessel networks in the bronchial mucosa and therefore may be useful to detect early malignant lesions (Figure 22-11). The system involves two narrow band filters, one to detect 415-nm light that is absorbed by the surface level capillaries and a second to detect 540-nm light that is absorbed below the surface layer. This permits visualizing abnormal distribution and dilatation of blood vessels in the mucosa, which can be an early sign of malignancy.[52]

THERAPEUTIC BRONCHOSCOPY

In the past decades, FB has been widely used for therapeutic purposes. Although the role of rigid bronchoscopy (RB) has declined, RB remains an invaluable tool for the control of a compromised airway, massive hemoptysis, and silicone stent placement and for removing asphyxiating foreign bodies (Box 22-4). The major indication for RB is in managing central

Box 22-4 Indications for Rigid Bronchoscopy

- Large foreign body extraction
- Large volume tissue biopsies
- Management of massive hemoptysis
- Silicone or self-expandable stent placement
- Mechanical coring of lesion using beveled tip and sequential mechanical dilation
- Using of adjunct therapies in management of endobronchial obstruction
  - Laser: Nd:YAG, KTP, CO_2
  - Argon plasma coagulation (APC)
  - Electrocautery
  - Cryotherapy
  - Balloon dilation
  - Microdebrider

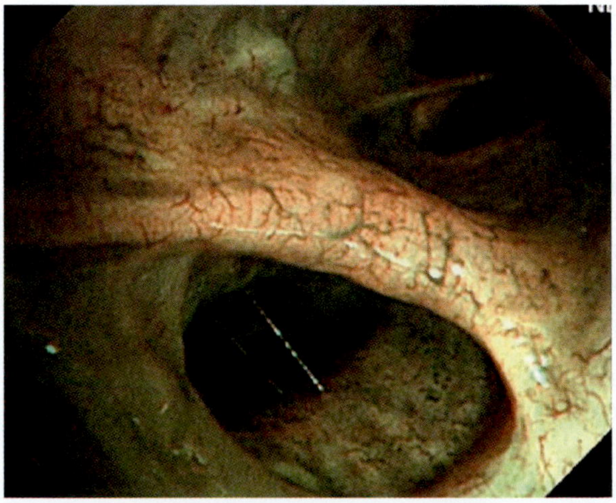

FIGURE 22-11 Narrow band imaging.

airway obstruction. Approximately 30% of patients with lung cancer may present with airway obstruction and its complications, such as hemoptysis, post-obstructive pneumonia, and asphyxia.[53] Reducing the size of a tumor or establishing airway patency with or without stent placement can produce rapid relief of symptoms, improved quality of life, and increased survival.[54] There are very few contraindications to RB. These include the inability to hyperextend the neck and an unstable facial fracture.

Some of the common bronchoscopic therapeutic procedures that are performed through the FB are discussed in the following section.

Thermal Ablation of the Endobronchial Lesion

Newer modalities such as endobronchial electrocautery, **argon plasma coagulation** (APC) or **laser photocoagulation** can be used to coagulate, carbonize, or vaporize lesions that protrude into the airway lumen and obstruct the central airways. These modalities increase the temperature of the tissue by molecular agitation and can be applied either through a flexible or an RB. By applying the appropriate power density, the desired tissue reaction can be achieved.

Application of electrocautery requires use of accessories such as knives, snares, or probes. Argon plasma coagulation is a noncontact technique to apply electric current to the endobronchial lesion. The modalities involved application of an electrically charged argon gas via a special disposable catheter.[55] Presence of a pacemaker or a defibrillator is a relative contraindication for using electrical modalities.[56]

Lasers can produce tissue reaction by thermal, photochemical, or electromagnetic effects. As stated earlier, it is the thermal effect of the laser is mainly use to remove the endobronchial lesion. Most commonly used lasers for this purpose are neodymium:yttrium-aluminum-garnet (Nd-YAG) and neodymium:yttrium-aluminum-perovskite (Ng-YAP) lasers. Lasers produce more précised tissue reaction than the electrosurgery units.[57,58]

The thermal ablation of the endobronchial lesion in properly selected patients produces some relief in close to 90% of patients. Improper use of the thermal modalities can lead to perforation of the airway, vascular structures, or esophagus. In addition, hypoxemia, pneumothorax, bronchopleural and bronchoesophageal fistulas are other reported complications.[57] In the presence of high FiO_2, endobronchial ignition has been reported as a rare complication of such therapies. Refractory hypoxemia (i.e., an O_2 requirement of $FiO_2 > 40\%$) and extrinsic compression of the airway without an endobronchial lesion are contraindications to thermal ablation.

RULE OF THUMB

During the application of "hot therapies" (thermal ablation) such as laser, electrosurgery, or argon plasma coagulation, the FiO_2 always should be maintained below 40% to prevent endobronchial ignition.

Cryotherapy

Cryotherapy is a method of destroying tissue by freezing it. Cryotherapy leads to extracellular ice crystal formation and extraction of intracellular water. In addition, extreme cold induces vasoconstriction, and endothelial injury leading to microthrombus formation and eventually tissue necrosis. The cryoprobe can be used through either a flexible bronchoscope or RB. The cryogen (the agent that causes the freezing) is released from very-high-pressure storage to atmospheric pressure. The sudden drop in the pressure leads to expansion of the cryogen and a drop in its temperature. This effect is also called the *Joule-Thompson effect*. The cryoprobe is placed in contact with the target and the cryogen is released, producing a tissue temperature of −80° C. The temperature increases approximately 10° C per millimeter from the tip. Thus the effective zone is approximately 5 to 8 mm. Multiple cycles of rapid freezing and gradual thawing are applied to cover the entire treatment area. The effects of cryotherapy depend on the sensitivity of the tissue. The cryoresistant structures are fat, cartilage, nerve sheath, and connective tissue, whereas, neoplasms, granulation tissue, skin, mucous membranes, nerves, and endothelium are cryosensitive. The inherent sensitivity of the tissue mainly depends on its water content. Therefore selection of a cryosensitive tumor is essential for a successful outcome with this technique.[59,62]

Cryotherapy has been used as a therapeutic tool for the patients with central airway obstruction. Cyotherapy is ideal for treating stent-related granulation tissue when the stent is made of an inflammable material. It can be used to remove organic foreign bodies, blood clots, and mucus plugs by cryoadhesion; ice crystal formation between the probe and the object that holds them together. In addition, cryotherapy can be used in a high-O_2 requirement. Recently, there is a growing interest in its use for obtaining larger pieces of lung tissue compared to conventional TBBx and EBBx (cryobiopsy) approaches. Further trials are required to prove the safety of this method.

Brachytherapy

The term **brachytherapy** describes a method to deliver short distance radiation therapy. Brachytherapy involves temporary placement of encapsulated radioactive sources within or near the tumor via a bronchoscope. It is used as both an adjuvant to external-beam radiation and a palliative radiation option for lung cancer located near the airways. It also can be used in the management of superficial endobronchial squamous cell carcinoma. In brachytherapy, a catheter is placed adjacent to the lesion and the location is confirmed by fluoroscopy. The catheter is then loaded with the radioactive source, usually radium or iridium, reaching a total dose of 500 to 4000 Gray over a precise duration.[60,61]

The main advantage of brachytherapy is that a higher dose of radiation can be delivered to the tumor cells while minimizing radiation to the normal tissue, thereby reducing complications. Brachytherapy is indicated in patients with inoperable lung cancer or cancer metastatic to the airways.

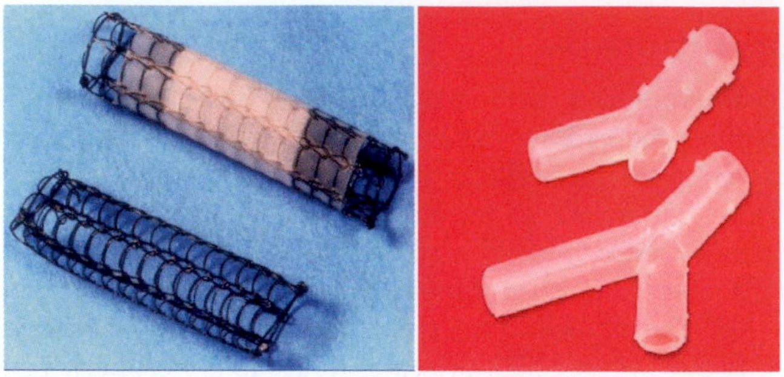

FIGURE 22-12 Self-expanding metallic stents *(left)* and silicone stents *(right)*.

Endobronchial Stents

Stents are the devices designed for internal splinting of the airway lumen. **Airway stents** have been used to help reduce airway obstruction from malignant or benign processes that compress the airway from the outside. Airway stenting can offer immediate relief of acute respiratory distress, can allow successful extubation, and may prolong survival.[62,63] There are two major types of airway stents, metallic and silicone. Self-expanding metallic stents (SEMS) are commercially available in covered and uncovered forms (Figure 22-12). Covered stents are designed primarily to prevent the growth of granulation tissue into the lumen of the stent. Current SEMS are made from nitinol; a nickel-titanium alloy that is well adapted for endobronchial applications. At room temperature, nitinol is extremely elastic. It can tolerate the extreme folding that is required when using a small deployment system but still return to its original shape without compromising its resistance to compression. The advantages of SEMS are ease of deployment, small internal-to-external diameter ratio, better conformity to complex airway shapes, and ventilation across a lobar bronchial orifice (Table 22-3). The indications for SEMS placement include (1) extrinsic compression of central airways; (2) stabilizing airway patency after endoscopic removal of an intrinsic tumor; (3) sealing fistula between the lung and the gastrointestinal tract; and (4) managing of post–lung transplant anastomotic complications. SEMS is rarely used in benign central airway obstruction because there is high-risk for stent-related granulation tissue formation. In 2005 the U.S. Food and Drug Administration issued a medical device safety warning against using self-expanding metallic stents for benign airway obstruction unless all other therapeutic options have been explored.[64]

Silicone stents have two major designs, straight and Y-shape (for disease involving the carina). The stents are either made of transparent silicone (radiolucent) or silicone blended with barium sulfate (to make the stent radiopaque). The silicone stent is usually placed through an RB. The advantages of silicone stents include easy customization, ease of repositioning/removal, minimal granulation tissue overgrowth, and lower cost than metallic stents. The indications for placing a silicone stent are similar to SEMS and include internal splinting for external compression/intraluminal growing cancer, benign strictures, collapsing airways, and tracheoesophageal fistulas. In terms of complications, mucous impaction (3.6%), bacterial colonization, migration (9.5%), and formation of granuloma (7.9%) are most common. After stent placement, the patient should be given a stent alert card with details regarding the type, length/diameter, and location of the stent.

TABLE 22-3

Comparison of Silicone and Metallic Stent Properties

Comparison Factors	Metallic Stents	Silicone Stents
General Considerations		
Deployment	Flexible or rigid bronchoscopy	Rigid bronchoscopy only
Customization	No	Yes
Repositioning	Difficult	Easier
Conforms to complex airway	Yes	No
Internal-to-external diameter	Low	High
Elasticity	Excellent for nitinol	Poor
Mucociliary clearance	Yes for uncovered stents	No
Cost	More	Less
Complications		
Granulation tissue	More	Less
Migration	Less common	Significant
Fracture	Significant	Rare
Infection	More common	Less common
Tracheobronchial fistula formation	Possible	Very rare
Mucus impaction	Uncommon	Common

RULE OF THUMB

SEMS should not be used in benign conditions unless all other therapeutic options have been exhausted.

Bronchoscopy in Difficult Intubation

It may be difficult to establish an artificial airway by conventional means in patients with cervical and oropharyngeal trauma or redundant supraglottic soft tissue. The American Society of Anesthesiologists Task Force on difficult airway recommends alternative techniques to overcome such an airway challenge, including flexible bronchoscopy.[65]

Using an FB can help place an endotracheal tube (ETT) through the mouth or the nose. The ETT is placed over the FB, the vocal cords are visualized, and the ETT is then advanced into the trachea. Using the FB to aid ETT placement also allows for awake intubations with topical anesthesia and is particularly useful in patients with cervical injuries, in which immobilization of the neck is crucial.[66] The bronchoscope also may help identify causes of acute hypoxia and help remove secretions or blood in the airway. The limitations of this approach include operator inexperience and the need for patient cooperation.

THE ROLE OF THE RESPIRATORY THERAPIST IN BRONCHOSCOPY

The respiratory therapist (RT) has a major supportive role in the bronchoscopic procedures. The RT may collaborate with other members of the patient care team to determine if the procedure is indicated. The RT often is responsible for ensuring that all documentation is in place before the procedure and that a preprocedure "time-out" takes place to ensure the correct procedure is being done on the right patient. During preprocedure evaluation, the RT helps recognize the patient's O_2 requirement and anticipates appropriate O_2 supplement during the procedure. The RT also administers inhaled bronchodilators before or during the procedure if the patient exhibits bronchospasm. The FB is usually performed on spontaneously breathing patients via a transoral or transnasal route. The RT assists preparing upper as well as lower airways for the procedure using local anesthetic agents. In mechanically ventilated patients, the RT may help to optimize the length and the size of the endotracheal tube, place a bite-block in place to protect the equipment and adjust ventilator settings before and during the procedure. In addition to monitoring vital signs and O_2 saturation during the procedure, the RT may assist the physician in operating the bronchoscopic accessories, including brush, forceps, needles, laser fibers, cryoprobe, and APC probes. In patients with suspected ventilator-associated pneumonia, the RT may perform mini-BAL, which may guide the escalation and de-escalation of antibiotic therapy. Furthermore, the RT often identifies and can assist in responding to an adverse event associated with FB, such as hypoxemia. These and other aspects of the role of the RT are summarized in Box 22-5.

MINI CLINIC

Bronchoscopy-Induced Hypoxemia

PROBLEM: An RT is assisting during a flexible bronchoscopy on a spontaneously breathing patient that is taking longer than expected because other adjunctive procedures, including BAL. Shortly after instilling the lavage solution into the airway through the bronchoscope, the patient's O_2 saturation drops from 97% to 88% via pulse oximetry, their heart rate increases from 90 to 118 and the patient's skin color changes from pink to pale. What condition that an RT should consider in this situation?

DISCUSSION: Hypoxemia should be suspected in this case. Given that the bronchoscope occupies a significant amount of the anatomic airway during this procedure, additional airway resistance can partially impede ventilation during the procedure. In addition, the BAL solution introduced during into the airway can temporarily interfere with ventilation and gas exchange and hypoxemia can occur. Pausing the procedure and administering a higher FiO_2 or even 100% O_2 will generally alleviate this problem and boost the pulse oximetry to more acceptable levels (mid-90%). Once monitored blood O_2 levels return to normal, the procedure can generally be resumed and the patient's oxygenation and overall clinical status should be monitored for the balance of the procedure and for a period following it.

SPECIAL CONSIDERATIONS FOR BRONCHOSCOPY DURING MECHANICAL VENTILATION

In addition to the role of the RT described earlier, they play an even more important role when this procedure is being performed on patients receiving mechanical ventilation. It is most important to note that FB carries a higher risk when done on patients with reduced cardiopulmonary reserve, particularly

Box 22-5 Role of the Respiratory Therapist in Bronchoscopy

- Preprocedure
  - Help identify potential need for a bronchoscopy such as retained secretions or foreign body removal.
  - Verify, physician's order or protocol; review medical record for contraindications (e.g., excessive clotting times), hazards, and informed consent.
  - Prepare/ensure proper function of equipment, including bronchoscope, light source, TV monitor, video recorder, medications, specimen traps.
  - Outline plan for adequate oxygenation during the procedure.
  - Evaluate patient for bronchospasm and administer aerosolized bronchodilators if required.
  - Assist nursing staff in the application of topical anesthesia to the upper airways (nasal passages, oropharynx, hypopharynx).
  - Identify patient and perform preprocedure "time-out."
  - Mechanically ventilated patients/bedside bronchoscopy
    - Establish adequacy of the length and the diameter of the endotracheal or the tracheostomy tube based on the indication.
    - Ensure a bite-block is in place to avoid equipment damage.
    - Adjust ventilator settings for the safety of the procedure while maintaining proper oxygenation.
- During the procedure
  - Monitor vital parameters during the procedure, including capnography (if available).
  - Help identify and respond to adverse reactions (e.g., hypoxemia or pneumothorax).
  - Administer adequate amount of supplemental oxygen all throughout the procedure by choosing proper appliances (nasal cannula, mask, bilevel positive airway pressure)
  - Provide proper positioning of the patient to maintain patency of the upper airways (jaw-lift etc.).
  - Assist use of endobronchial accessories (bite block, oral airways, nasopharyngeal tube, biopsy forceps, brushes, etc.).
  - Set up instruments for rigid bronchoscopy and silicon stent placement.
  - Attend to emergent situations (pneumothorax, bleeding).
  - Place chest or endotracheal tubes.
- Postprocedure
  - Determine adequate oxygenation and ventilation and respond to adverse reactions.
  - Disinfect and properly store equipment.
  - Document procedure and relevant details.

those requiring mechanical ventilation. In such patients, the RT must ensure the airway is properly secured, verify adequate ventilation and gas exchange, monitor the patient, and quickly communicate the development of any complications to the physician and any other members of the bronchoscopy team.

In mechanically ventilated patients, it is important to consider that the bronchoscope will occupy a greater proportion of the airway than for spontaneously breathing patients. The external diameter of a standard fiberoptic bronchoscope is 5.7 mm, but in some situations a smaller (5 mm or less) or larger (6.4 mm) diameter scope may be used. The narrowest point in the upper airway (and point of maximal resistance) is the cricoid space, the diameter of which averages 14 mm in women and 18 mm in men.[67] Thus, in nonintubated, spontaneously breathing patients, inspiratory and expiratory effort (measured by tracheal pressure) appear minimally affected in most patients (−5 and +3.5 cm H_2O, respectively). However, in intubated, spontaneously breathing patients, the resistance imposed by the bronchoscope may cause tracheal pressures to increase noticeably (−10 and +9 cm H_2O) and may reach clinically unacceptable levels (−20 and +20 cm H_2O) in some patients.[68] Therefore the minimum appropriately sized ETT for a standard 5.7-mm bronchoscope is an 8.0-mm inner diameter.[69]

RULE OF THUMB

The minimal sized endotracheal tube that can be used with a standard 5.7-mm bronchoscope has an 8.0-mm internal diameter.

PHYSIOLOGIC AND MECHANICAL ALTERATIONS ASSOCIATED WITH FLEXIBLE BRONCHOSCOPY IN INTUBATED PATIENTS

Complications associated with flexible bronchoscopy in intubated patients are infrequent (<10%) and usually mild.[70] However, serious complications may occur (Table 22-4). These include the following (along with their reported incidence): transient hypoxemia with SpO_2 less than 90% (8%), tension pneumothorax (14%), bronchial hemorrhage greater than 30 mL (6%), hypotension with mean arterial pressure less than 60 mm Hg (7%), and tachycardia greater than 140 (4%).[70] Pneumothorax is primarily associated with lung biopsy procedures,[71,72] whereas the risk for significant bleeding after biopsy increases when the platelet count is below 50,000/mm^3.[70]

As noted elsewhere in this chapter, some degree of hypoxemia may occur during FB. In those with normal lungs the PaO_2 can decrease by 10 to 30 mm Hg, whereas in critically ill patients, the PaO_2 may be reduced by 60 mm Hg.[70,71] Hypoxemia during FB is partly caused by suctioning through the bronchoscope. This decreases PEEP and functional residual capacity and promotes atelectasis. For example, setting the vacuum at 100 mm Hg through a standard 2-mm suction port can evacuate approximately 7 L/min of gas.[70] The problem is accentuated if tidal volume delivery also is significantly compromised during FB. In fact, frequent suctioning during FB also causes pronounced tidal volume loss.[68] Because FB commonly is used to remove mucus plugs, this problem may be unavoidable. Both the RT and physician performing bronchoscopy need to be mindful of

TABLE 22-4

Physiologic and Mechanical Alterations Associated With Flexible Bronchoscopy in Intubated Patients

System	Effects	Comments/Interventions
Respiratory mechanics	High peak inspiratory pressures and pressure cycling	Obstruction by the bronchoscope causes back-pressure that is not transmitted to the lungs. Use of high inspiratory flow rates/brief inspiratory time will accentuate the problem and may greatly reduce minute ventilation. **Intervention:** *Volume control ventilation:* Use a lower peak flow rate or decreasing ramp pattern and increased inspiratory time. *Pressure control ventilation:* Increase the pressure control level and extend the inspiratory time. *Before bronchoscopy:* Assess minute ventilation demand and blood gases with the physician to determine if the patient might tolerate mild to moderate respiratory acidosis during the anticipated procedure duration. Monitor peak inspiratory pressure.
	Intrinsic PEEP	Increased expiratory resistance can cause a 30% increase in functional residual capacity and may cause high levels of intrinsic PEEP to develop. With an 8-mm endotracheal tube, intrinsic PEEP levels are generally <20 cm H_2O, but have been reported to rise to 35 cm H_2O when bronchoscopy has been attempted with a 7-mm tube. *Consider* removing or reducing PEEP by 50% during the procedure. Monitor blood pressure as a signifier for possible intrinsic PEEP buildup. Either a sustained downward trend or abrupt drop in systolic blood pressure may indicate decreased cardiac output.

TABLE 22-4
Physiologic and Mechanical Alterations Associated With Flexible Bronchoscopy in Intubated Patients—cont'd

System	Effects	Comments/Interventions
	Circuit leak, suctioning, and tidal volume loss	Circuit leaks with substantial loss of tidal volume were a common problem until the creation of specialized bronchoscopy port endotracheal tube adapters. These are commercially available and have largely eliminated the problem. When encountered, the rule of thumb has been to increase the preset tidal volume by 30%-40% to compensate for the leak.[71] Use lower peak inspiratory flow rate and longer inspiratory time. Frequent, prolonged suctioning during FB can greatly reduce tidal volume regardless of ETT size. Monitor: • Expired tidal volume • End-tidal PCO_2 and VCO_2 (CO_2 excretion) if volumetric capnography is available, particularly in those with baseline hypercarbia, acidosis, or hemodynamically unstable.
Gas cxchange	Hypoxemia	Preoxygenate for 15 min on FiO_2 of 1.[71] Ensure adequate sedation before and during FB. Ensure continuous pulse oximetry. *Consider* using recruitment maneuvers to improve functional residual capacity before and (if necessary) after FB in patients with marginal oxygenation. To the extent possible: • Minimize tidal volume loss • Avoid using a brief inspiratory time. • Limit the frequency and duration of suctioning.
	Acute hypercapnia and acidosis	On average, $PaCO_2$ tends to increase by 8 mm Hg during FB.[71] This would decrease arterial pH by only 0.06; and even less in patients with chronic hypercapnia. This mild change in $PaCO_2$ should be interpreted in the context of clinicians adjusting mechanical ventilator settings to attempting to maintain adequate ventilation. Given the relatively brief procedure time for FB, concern over the impact of hypercapnia should be focused on clinically unstable patients. *In at-risk patients:* The procedure time should curtailed. Periodic withdrawal of the bronchoscope to ensure adequate ventilation. Clinicians should determine the limits of what an acute rise in $PaCO_2$ and decrease in pH would be acceptable during the procedure and use clinical equations to estimate the minimum acceptable minute ventilation that must be maintained (see MINI CLINI for details). When FB must be attempted in patients with significant acidosis, consideration should be given to preprocedure buffer therapy with a non–CO_2 generating agent (i.e., THAM) often used for procedures requiring apneic oxygenation.
Hemodynamics	Heart rate and cardiac arrhythmias	Hypoxemia and hypercapnia increase sympathetic tone, which can lead to tachycardia, myocardial ischemia, and arrhythmias may result in hypotension and/or cardiac arrest. Heart rate tends to increase by ~40% during FB.[73] The occurrence of major arrhythmias is 3%-11%. *Reduce the risk for arrhythmias by:* • Preoxygenation with an FiO_2 of 1 • Minimizing procedure time • Periodic withdrawal of the bronchoscope to ensure adequate ventilation Ensure continuous cardiac monitoring.
	Alterations in blood pressure and cardiac output	Mean blood pressure and cardiac output tend to increase during FB by ~30%.[73] Hemodynamic variables tend to return to normal ~15 min after completion of FB.[71]

ETT, Endotracheal tube; *FB,* fiberoptic bronchoscopy; *PEEP,* positive end-expiratory pressure; *THAM,* tris-hydroxymethyl aminomethane.

TABLE 22-5
High-Risk Patients for Flexible Bronchoscopy

Conditions	Considerations
Asthma	Greater tendency for laryngospasm and bronchospasm[72,73]
	Tendency for greater reduction in lung function after FB when lavage or biopsies are done.
	Hypoxemia not uncommon.
	Pretreatment with bronchodilators immediately before FB
	In patients with unstable lung function, consider pretreatment with steroids several days before FB in.
Acute brain injury	Intracranial hypertension is a predominant concern.
	Procedural Goal: intracranial pressure <20 mm Hg with Cerebral Perfusion Pressure ≥70.
	Causes of increased intracranial pressure include sympathetic stimulation from discomfort and hypercapnia, hypoxemia. Build-up of intrinsic PEEP decreases venous return causing cranial venous pooling.
	Procedural sedation and strategies to maintain minute ventilation assume even greater importance.
	Employing continuous drainage when subdural catheters are present should be considered.
	Either curtailing procedure time or frequent periods bronchoscope withdrawal to resume baseline minute ventilation also should be considered.
Acute respiratory distress syndrome (ARDS)	Tendency is for severe hypoxemia and respiratory acidosis, particularly in those with severe ARDS ($PaO_2/FiO_2 < 100$) secondary to low lung volumes and high dead-space ventilation.
	Risk is increased if hemodynamic instability is present (e.g., mean arterial pressure <65 mm Hg and/or high vasopressor requirements).
	Loss of PEEP is particularly problematic.
	Consideration should be given to preprocedure use of recruitment maneuvers to optimize lung volumes and oxygenation and THAM to control acidosis.
Coronary artery disease	Adrenergic discharge during FB in response to undersedation, hypoxemia, and/or acute respiratory acidosis may cause myocardial ischemia, arrhythmias, hypotension are cardiac arrest.
	In nonintubated patients, the need for high doses of topical anesthesia with lidocaine may cause sinus arrest and atrioventricular block.

FB, Fiberoptic bronchoscopy; *THAM*, tris-hydroxymethyl aminomethane.

the frequency and duration of suctioning, along with the total procedure time to limit the potential for severe, prolonged hypoxemia. The risk for significant hypoxemia is elevated in those with acute respiratory distress syndrome (ARDS) and in those insufficiently sedated.[68] Patients undergoing FB should be preoxygenated on FiO_2 of 1 for 15 minutes. Resolution of hypoxemia depends on the presence and severity of underlying pulmonary disease. For example, hypoxemia tends to resolve within 15 minutes after FB in those with normal lungs, whereas hypoxemia may persist for several hours in those with severe lung disease.

RULE OF THUMB

Hypoxemia during FB on mechanically ventilated patients is related to several factors, including loss of lung volume during suctioning, particularly if tidal volume delivery also is compromised. It occurs more frequently in those with ARDS and in those insufficiently sedated.

It is the RT's responsibility to effectively manage the most common of these complications (see Table 22-4). In addition, the RT must anticipate which patients are most likely to suffer significant adverse events during bronchoscopy (Table 22-5). Before the procedure, the members of the bronchoscopy team, including the RT, should assess the patient's condition, discuss which adverse effects most likely will occur, and how they should be managed. This discussion should include the anticipated procedure time, whether the original plan for the procedure should be modified, sedation strategy, hemodynamic management, and ventilator management. A particular emphasis for the RT should be the minimum clinically acceptable level of minute ventilation necessary to complete the procedure. Depending on the procedure goal (e.g., diagnostic, removal of secretions), bronchoscopy tends to last between 7 and 17 minutes.[73,74]

EMERGING BRONCHOSCOPIC INTERVENTIONS

In addition to the interventions described earlier, others are emerging and hold promise for the future. One such intervention is bronchial thermoplasty, which is still considered a novel procedure for patients with bronchial asthma. Also, endobronchial valves and coil placement are being studied in the management of patients with severe emphysema. If shown to be effective, they could represent an alternative to lung volume reduction surgery for severe emphysema.

MINI CLINI

Estimating Minimum Minute Ventilation Requirements During Flexible Bronchoscopy in a Patient With Severe Respiratory Failure

PROBLEM: A patient with ARDS has deteriorating oxygenation associated with a new infiltrate on chest radiograph. Gram-negative bacterial ventilator-associated pneumonia is strongly suspected, and FB is deemed necessary before adjusting antibiotic therapy because the suspected pathogen is likely to be multidrug resistant. The patient has a high minute ventilation demand of 13 L/min to maintain a pH of 7.40 and $PaCO_2$ of 40 mm Hg. The patient has sepsis and currently requires norepinephrine at 12 mcg/min to maintain a mean arterial pressure of 65 mm Hg. The physician decides that during FB, a pH of 7.25 would be tolerable for the estimated procedure time of 10 minutes. The RT is asked if there is a clinical formula to *estimate* what rise in $PaCO_2$ would likely produce the target minimum pH. In addition, the RT is asked to estimate the minimum minute ventilation needed during FB that would likely maintain pH at 7.25.

DISCUSSION: In patients without chronic hypercapnia, an acute rise in $PaCO_2$ of 10 produces a decrease in pH of 0.008.[74] Because tidal volume can be greatly reduced during FB, the RT can reasonably begin with an estimated $PaCO_2$ increase of 20 mm Hg. This would yield an *estimated* drop in pH of 0.16 units (20 × 0.008) and a pH of 7.26 (7.40 − 0.16). The clinical formula for corrected minute ventilation then can be used to estimate the minimum acceptable minute ventilation.[73]

$$VE_{min} = VE_{measured} \times (PaCO_2 \text{ measured} \div PaCO_2 \text{ upper limit})$$
$$VE_{min} = 13\ L/min \times (40 \div 60)$$
$$VE_{min} = 13\ L/min \times 0.67$$
$$VE_{min} = 8.7\ L/min$$

Patients with high minute ventilation demand who require vasopressor support to maintain adequate perfusion may be particularly sensitive to sudden respiratory acidosis. The fact that this patient already requires the highest recommended dose of norepinephrine to maintain an adequate blood pressure is cause for concern about the safety of performing FB. The steps described previously are *only estimates* useful for guiding management during FB and assessing the risk-to-benefit ratio. For example, a preprocedure pH that was substantially lower (e.g., $\leq$7.30) may change the management strategy, including shortening the FB procedure or performing the procedure in steps.

CONCLUSION

Bronchoscopy is a common diagnostic and therapeutic procedure that has reduced the need for procedures such has percutaneous needle aspiration, mediastinoscopy, thoracoscopy, and open lung biopsy. In many settings, RTs play a major role in identifying patients who may benefit from it, setting up the equipment, and assisting with bronchoscopy procedure and patient monitoring.

SUMMARY CHECKLIST

- FB has been used for most diagnostic and therapeutic indications in patients with pulmonary diseases. The goal of sedation is to improve the patient's comfort during the procedure. Continuous monitoring of oxygenation and hemodynamic stability are important during the procedure.
- BAL, biopsy, and TBNA are the most commonly used diagnostic procedures in FB. BAL obtains samples from the alveoli. Needle aspiration has a role in sampling mediastinal lymph nodes to diagnose lung cancer, sarcoidosis, and some infectious processes. Biopsy has value in the diagnosis of infiltrative pulmonary diseases.
- Various thermal ablation techniques have been used along with FB as treatments. The most important point is to ensure a low FiO_2 environment before the use of any thermal ablative therapy.
- Airway stenting has been used to maintain airway patency after dilation of any obstructed major airways. It is important to recognize the difference between silicone and metallic stents.
- Bronchial thermoplasty is a novel bronchoscopic technique for patients with steroid-dependent asthma. Also, endobronchial valves and coil placement are being studied in the management of patients with severe emphysema as a minimally invasive lung volume reduction therapy.
- The RT plays a vital role in assisting before, during, and after bronchoscopy. There are many aspects to this role, but they include ensuring appropriate documentation (e.g., physician's order), preparing the patient and the equipment, patient monitoring, and responding to adverse events.
- There are special considerations the RT and other members of the bronchoscopy team must consider when performing this procedure on mechanically ventilated patients, who are more susceptible to adverse events. These considerations include ensuring adequate ventilation and gas exchange before, during, and after the procedure.

References

1. Becker HD: Bronchoscopy: the past, the present, and the future. *Clin Chest Med* 31:1–18, 2010.
2. Jackson C: Endothelioma of the right bronchus removed by peroral bronchoscopy. *Am J Med Sci* 153:371–375, 1917.
3. Maltais F, Laberge F, Laviolette M: A randomized, double-blind, placebo-controlled study of lorazepam as premedication for bronchoscopy. *Chest* 109:1195–1198, 1996.
4. Stolz D, Chhajed PN, Leuppi JD, et al: Cough suppression during flexible bronchoscopy using combined sedation with midazolam and hydrocodone: a randomized, double blind, placebo controlled trial. *Thorax* 59:773–776, 2004.
5. British Thoracic Society: Guidelines on diagnostic bronchoscopy. *Thorax* 56(Suppl 1):i1–i21, 2001.
6. Wolters U, Wolf T, Stützer H, et al: ASA classification and perioperative variables as predictors of postoperative outcome. *Br J Anaesth* 77:217–222, 1996.
7. Abdelmalak B, Wang J, Mehta A: Capnography monitoring in procedural sedation for bronchoscopy. *J Bronchology Interv Pulmonol* 21:188–191, 2014.

8. Boiselle PM: Computed tomography screening for lung cancer. *JAMA* 309:1163–1170, 2013.
9. Costabel U, Guzman J: Bronchoalveolar lavage in interstitial lung disease (review). *Curr Opin Pulm Med* 7:255–261, 2001.
10. Helmers RA, Hunninghake GW: Bronchoalveolar lavage and opportunistic pulmonary infections. *Mayo Clin Proc* 62:630–631, 1987.
11. American Thoracic Society: Clinical role of bronchoalveolar lavage in adults with pulmonary disease. *Am Rev Respir Dis* 142:481–486, 1990.
12. Pirozynski M, Sliwinski P, Zielinski J: Effect of different volumes of BAL fluid on arterial oxygen saturation. *Eur Respir J* 1:943–947, 1988.
13. Krueger JJ, Sayre VA, Karetzky MS: Bronchoalveolar lavage induced pneumothorax. *Chest* 94:440–441, 1988.
14. Prakash UB, Barham SS, Carpenter HA, et al: Pulmonary alveolar phospholipoproteinosis: experience with 34 cases and a review. *Mayo Clin Proc* 62: 499–518, 1987.
15. Kollef MH, Bock KR, Richards RD, et al: The safety and diagnostic accuracy of minibronchoalveolar lavage in patients with suspected ventilator-associated pneumonia. *Ann Intern Med* 122:743–748, 1995.
16. Kollef MH, Ward S: The influence of mini-BAL cultures on patient outcomes: implications for the antibiotic management of ventilator-associated pneumonia. *Chest* 113:412–420, 1998.
17. Trisolini R, Cancellieri A, Tinelli C, et al: Performance characteristics and predictors of yield from transbronchial needle aspiration in the diagnosis of peripheral pulmonary lesions. *Respirology* 16:1144–1149, 2011.
18. Rhee CK, Kang HH, Kang JY, et al: Diagnostic yield of flexible bronchoscopy without fluoroscopic guidance in evaluating peripheral lung lesions. *J Bronchology Interv Pulmonol* 17:317–322, 2010.
19. Reichenberger F, Weber J, Tamm M, et al: The value of transbronchial needle aspiration in the diagnosis of peripheral pulmonary lesions. *Chest* 116:704–708, 1999.
20. Baaklini WA, Reinoso MA, Gorin AB, et al: Diagnostic yield of fiberoptic bronchoscopy in evaluating solitary pulmonary nodules. *Chest* 117:1049–1054, 2000.
21. Mak VH, Johnston ID, Hetzel MR, et al: Value of washings and brushings at fibreoptic bronchoscopy in the diagnosis of lung cancer. *Thorax* 45:373–376, 1990.
22. Mazzone P, Jain P, Arroliga AC, et al: Bronchoscopy and needle biopsy techniques for diagnosis and staging of lung cancer. *Clin Chest Med* 23:137–158, 2002.
23. Mehta AC, Ahmad M, Nunez C, et al: Newer procedures using the fiberoptic bronchoscope in the diagnosis of lung cancer. *Cleve Clin J Med* 54:195–203, 1987.
24. Buccheri G, Barberis P, Delfino MS: Diagnostic, morphologic, and histopathologic correlates in bronchogenic carcinoma: a review of 1,045 bronchoscopic examinations. *Chest* 99:809–814, 1991.
25. Dasgupta A, Jain P, Minai OA, et al: Utility of transbronchial needle aspiration in the diagnosis of endobronchial lesions. *Chest* 115:1237–1241, 1999.
26. Rivera MP, Mehta AC, Wahidi MM: Establishing the diagnosis of lung cancer: diagnosis and management of lung cancer, ed 3: American College of Chest Physicians evidence-based clinical practice guidelines. *Chest* 143 (5 Suppl):e142S–e165S, 2013.
27. Saldana MJ, Mones JM: Pulmonary pathology in AIDS: atypical *Pneumocystis carinii* infection and lymphoid interstitial pneumonia. *Thorax* 49(Suppl):S46–S55, 1994.
28. Venkateshiah S, Mehta AC: Role of flexible bronchoscopy in the diagnosis of pulmonary tuberculosis in immunocompetent individuals. *J Bronchol* 10:300–308, 2003.
29. Trulock EP, Ettinger NA, Brunt EM, et al: The role of transbronchial lung biopsy in the treatment of lung transplant recipients: an analysis of 200 consecutive procedures. *Chest* 102:1049–1054, 1992.
30. American Thoracic Society: Statement on sarcoidosis. *Am J Respir Crit Care Med* 160:736–755, 1999.
31. Green MB, Allen JN: Cough, dyspnea and reticulonodular opacities in a 58-year-old smoker. *Chest* 132:700–703, 1999.
32. Ernst A, Anantham D: Bronchus sign on CT scan rediscovered. *Chest* 138:1290–1292, 2010.
33. Simpson FG, Arnold AG, Purvis A, et al: Postal survey of bronchoscopic practice by physicians in the United Kingdom. *Thorax* 41:311–317, 1986.
34. Papin TA, Grum CM, Weg JG: Transbronchial biopsy during mechanical ventilation. *Chest* 89:168–170, 1986.
35. O'Brien JD, Ettinger NA, Shevlin D, et al: Safety and yield of transbronchial biopsy in mechanically ventilated patients. *Crit Care Med* 25:440–446, 1997.
36. Wahidi MM, Rocha AT, Hollingsworth JW, et al: Contraindications and safety of transbronchial lung biopsy via flexible bronchoscopy: a survey of pulmonologists and review of the literature. *Respiration* 72:285–295, 2005.
37. Baron TH, Kamath PS, McBane RD: Antithrombotic therapy and invasive procedures. *N Engl J Med* 369:1079–1080, 2013.
38. Cordasco EM, Jr, Mehta AC, Ahmad M: Bronchoscopically induced bleeding: a summary of nine years' Cleveland Clinic experience and review of the literature. *Chest* 100:1141–1147, 1991.
39. Toloza EM, Harpole L, Detterbeck F, et al: Invasive staging of non-small cell lung cancer: a review of the current evidence. *Chest* 123(1 Suppl):157S–166S, 2003.
40. Schreiber G, McCrory DC: Performance characteristics of different modalities for diagnosis of suspected lung cancer: summary of published evidence. *Chest* 123(1 Suppl):115S–128S, 2003.
41. Yasufuku K, Nakajima T, Motoori K, et al: Comparison of endobronchial ultrasound, positron emission tomography, and CT for lymph node staging of lung cancer. *Chest* 130:710–718, 2006.
42. Gu P, Zhao YZ, Jiang LY, et al: Endobronchial ultrasound-guided transbronchial needle aspiration for staging of lung cancer: a systematic review and meta-analysis. *Eur J Cancer* 45:1389–1936, 2009.
43. Huang CT, Chen CY, Ho CC, et al: A rare constellation of empyema, lung abscess, and mediastinal abscess as a complication of endobronchial ultrasound-guided transbronchial needle aspiration. *Eur J Cardiothorac Surg* 40:264–265, 2011.
44. Steinfort DP, Johnson DF, Irving LB: Incidence of bacteraemia following endobronchial ultrasound-guided transbronchial needle aspiration. *Eur Respir J* 36:28–32, 2010.
45. Almeida FA: Bronchoscopy and endobronchial ultrasound for diagnosis and staging of lung cancer. *Cleve Clin J Med* 79(Suppl 1):eS11–eS16, 2012.
46. Al-Qadi MO, Maldonado F: Focal tracheal stenosis due to intramural hematoma following endobronchial ultrasound-guided transbronchial needle aspiration. *J Bronchology Interv Pulmonol* 21:274–276, 2014.
47. Folch E, Yamaguchi N, VanderLaan PA, et al: Adequacy of lymph node transbronchial needle aspirates using convex probe endobronchial ultrasound for multiple tumor genotyping techniques in non-small-cell lung cancer. *J Thorac Oncol* 8:1438–1444, 2013.
48. Nasir BS, Bryant AS, Minnich DJ, et al: The efficacy of restaging endobronchial ultrasound in patients with non-small cell lung cancer after preoperative therapy. *Ann Thorac Surg* 98:1008–1012, 2014.
49. Gildea TR, Mazzone PJ, Karnak D, et al: Electromagnetic navigation diagnostic bronchoscopy: a prospective study. *Am J Respir Crit Care Med* 174: 982–989, 2006.
50. Eberhardt R, Anantham D, Ernst A, et al: Multimodality bronchoscopic diagnosis of peripheral lung lesions: a randomized controlled trial. *Am J Respir Crit Care Med* 176:36–41, 2007.
51. Asano F, Shinagawa N, Ishida T, et al: Virtual bronchoscopic navigation combined with ultrathin bronchoscopy: a randomized clinical trial. *Am J Respir Crit Care Med* 188:327–333, 2013.
52. Herth FJ, Eberhardt R, Ananthan D, et al: Narrow-band imaging bronchoscopy increases the specificity of bronchoscopic early lung cancer detection. *J Thorac Oncol* 4:1060–1065, 2009.
53. Lee P, Mehta AC: Management of obstruction airway lesions in patients with lung cancer. *PCCU Chest* 18:5, 2004.
54. Lee P, Kupeli E, Mehta AC: Therapeutic bronchoscopy in lung cancer: laser therapy, electrocautery, brachytherapy, stents, and photodynamic therapy. *Clin Chest Med* 23:241–256, 2002.
55. Seijo LM, Sterman DH: Interventional pulmonary. *N Engl J Med* 344:740–749, 2001.
56. Bolliger CT, Sutedja TG, Strausz J, et al: Therapeutic bronchoscopy with immediate effect: laser, electrocautery, argon plasma coagulation and stents. *Eur Respir J* 27:1258–1271, 2006.

57. Diaz-Jimenez JB, Rodriguez AN: Laser bronchoscopy for malignant disease. In Beams JF, Mathur PN, Mehta AC, editors: *Interventional pulmonary medicine: lung biology in health and disease*, Leflant C (executive editor), New York, 2004, Marcel Dekker, pp 80–125.
58. Colt H: Laser bronchoscopy for benign disease. In Beams JF, Mathur PN, Mehta AC, editors: *Interventional pulmonary medicine: lung biology in health and disease*, Leflant C (executive editor), New York, 2004, Marcel Dekker, pp 127–155.
59. Vergnon JM, Mathur PN: Cryotherapy for endobronchial disorders. In Bolliner CT, Mathur PN, editors: *Progress in respiratory research, vol 30. Interventional bronchology*, Basel, 2000, S Karger, pp 133–145.
60. Sheski FD, Mathur PN: Cryotherapy, electrocautery, and brachytherapy. *Clin Chest Med* 20:123–138, 1999.
61. Brenner B, Kramer MR, Katz A, et al: High dose rate brachytherapy for nonmalignant airway obstruction: new treatment option. *Chest* 124:1605–1610, 2003.
62. Dumon JF, Cavalier S, Diaz-Jimenez JP, et al: Seven experience with the Dumon prosthesis. *J Bronchol* 31:6–10, 1996.
63. Rafanan AL, Mehta AC: Stenting of the tracheobronchial tree. *Radiol Clin North Am* 38:395–408, 2000.
64. U.S. Food and Drug Administration: Medical devices: safety alert. <http://www.fda.gov/MedicalDevices/Safety/AlertsandNotices/PublicHealthNotifications/ucm062115.htm>, Accessed July 4, 2013.
65. Practice Guidelines for Management of the Difficult Airway: An updated report by the American Society of Anesthesiologists task force on management of the difficult airway. *Anesthesiology* 118:251–270, 2013.
66. Ovassapian A: The flexible bronchoscope: a tool for the anesthesiologist. *Clin Chest Med* 22:281–299, 2001.
67. Randestad A, Lindholm C-E, Fabian P: Dimensions of the cricoid cartilage and the trachea. *Laryngoscope* 110:1957–1961, 2000.
68. Lindholm C-E, Ollman B, Snyder JV, et al: Cardiorespiratory effects of flexible fiberoptic bronchoscopy in critically ill patients. *Chest* 74:362–368, 1978.
69. Jolliet PH, Chevrolet JC: Bronchoscope in the intensive care unit. *Intensive Care Med* 18:160–169, 1992.
70. Raoof S, Mehrishi S, Prakash UB: Role of bronchoscopy in modern medical intensive care unit. *Clin Chest Med* 22:1–26, 2001.
71. Agarwal R, Khan A, Aggarwal AN, et al: Bronchoscopic lung biopsy using noninvasive ventilatory support: case series and review of literature of NIV-assisted bronchoscopy. *Respir Care* 57:1927–1936, 2012.
72. Clarkson K, Power CK, O'Connell F, et al: A comparative evaluation of propofol and midazolam as sedative agents in fiberoptic bronchoscopy. *Chest* 104:1029–1031, 1993.
73. Kallet RH, Liu K, Tang J: Management of acidosis in acute respiratory distress syndrome. *Respir Care Clin N Am* 9:437–456, 2003.
74. Wexler HR, Lok P: A simple formula for adjusting arterial carbon dioxide tension. *Can Anaesth Soc J* 28:370–372, 1981.

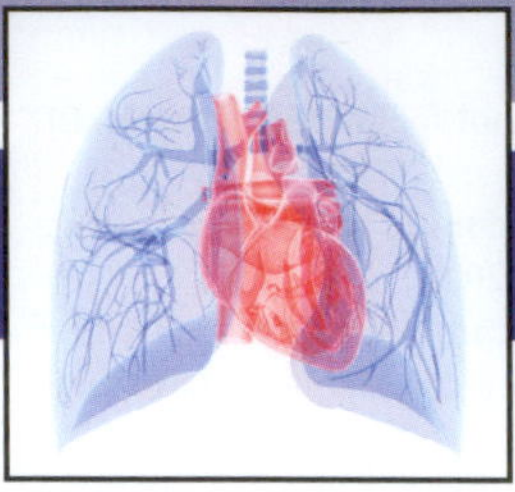

CHAPTER 23

Nutrition Assessment

JAMI E. BALTZ

CHAPTER OBJECTIVES

After reading this chapter you will be able to:

- Describe how a comprehensive nutrition assessment is conducted.
- Calculate and interpret body mass index.
- Distinguish between two forms of protein-energy malnutrition.
- List the biochemical indicators of nutrition status.
- Describe the clinical manifestations of malnourishment.
- Describe how to obtain and evaluate a nutrition history.
- Estimate daily resting energy expenditure.
- List the indications, contraindications, hazards, and limitations of indirect calorimetry.
- Describe how to prepare a patient for indirect calorimetry.
- Interpret the results of indirect calorimetry.
- Adjust resting energy expenditure values to reflect the actual patient energy needs.
- Describe the effects of malnutrition on the respiratory system.
- Describe how to identify patients at high risk for malnutrition.
- State when enteral nutrition and parenteral nutrition are needed.
- Identify and minimize common respiratory complications of enteral feedings.
- List specific nutrition guidelines for specific pulmonary diseases.
- Explain how common pulmonary medications affect nutrition.

CHAPTER OUTLINE

Nutrition Assessment
- Food-Related and Nutrition-Related History
- Anthropometrics
- Biochemical Indicators
- Other Tests and Procedures
- Pulmonary Function
- Nutrition-Focused Physical Findings

Outcomes of Nutrition Assessment

Macronutrients and Energy Requirements
- Estimating Energy Requirements
- Indirect Calorimetry
- Alternative Resting Energy Expenditure Measures

General Aspects of Nutrition Support
- Meeting Overall Energy Needs
- Respiratory Consequences of Malnutrition
- Providing the Appropriate Combination of Substrates

Routes of Administration

Nutrition Support in Specific Circumstances
- General Guidelines for Critically Ill Patients
- Systemic Inflammatory Response Syndrome
- Mechanical Ventilation
- Chronic Obstructive Pulmonary Disease
- Asthma
- Cystic Fibrosis

KEY TERMS

anergy
anthropometrics
azotemia
basal metabolic rate
body mass index
cachexic
indirect calorimetry
kwashiorkor
marasmus
normometabolic
protein-energy malnutrition
resting energy expenditure

Nutrition is vital to life, health, and well-being. Second to the provision of oxygen is the provision of nutrients to sustain the function, growth, maintenance, and repair of the body. A human deprived of O_2 for minutes can no longer function. Similarly, a human deprived of food for days to weeks can no longer function.

Adequate nutrition is essential for health. The relationship between nutrition and respiratory status is reciprocal. A balanced supply of nutrients is needed for proper respiratory function; O_2 is required for adenosine triphosphate synthesis and muscle function, including the respiratory muscles. Poor or inadequate nutrient intake disrupts energy use and impairs normal organ function. Conversely, disease can impair nutrient intake or alter metabolism, causing malnutrition.

Traumatized tissue requires the provision of nutrients for healing. To achieve healthy living requires daily, consistent attention to providing essential nutrients. Patients with respiratory disease are particularly challenged because it is difficult to breathe and swallow at the same time. This chapter focuses on nutrition assessment—determining the nutrient needs of individuals.

NUTRITION ASSESSMENT

Nutrition assessment is the process of collecting and evaluating data to determine the nutrition status of an individual. Typically, a registered dietitian gathers data to compare various social, pharmaceutical, environmental, physical, and medical factors to evaluate the nutrient needs of an individual. The purpose of nutrition assessment is to develop a *nutrition care plan* that ensures continual adequate nutrition for health.

Data are obtained from numerous sources for nutrition assessment. Interviewing the individual or the caregiver to determine past and current eating practices is most helpful. Reviewing the patient's medical record provides additional information regarding pertinent social, pharmaceutical, environmental, and medical issues. Information gathered for a nutrition assessment is grouped into five domains: (1) food/nutrition-related history, (2) anthropometric measurements, (3) biochemical data and tests/procedures, (4) nutrition-focused physical findings and (5) client history (Box 23-1).[1]

Box 23-1 Components of a Comprehensive Nutrition Assessment

MEDICAL CHART
- History and physical examination
- Present diseases
- Current medications
- Activity level
- Physical assessment
- Social history

ANTHROPOMETRICS
- Usual weight and height
- History of weight loss
- Actual versus ideal body weight
- Body mass index
- Body composition (triceps skin fold, arm muscle area)

PHYSICAL ASSESSMENT
- Signs of weight loss (cachexia)
- Edema that may mask weight loss
- Hair, skin, mouth, and tongue

CLINICAL LABORATORY TESTS
- Visceral proteins
- C-reactive protein
- Creatinine-height index
- Immune-related tests
- Nitrogen balance

DIETARY HISTORY
- Usual food intake
- Food likes and dislikes
- Appetite

TOTAL CALORIC REQUIREMENTS
- Resting energy expenditure predictive equations
- Indirect calorimetry

ACCESS TO FOOD
- Income
- Education
- Mobility
- Mechanical impediments

Food-Related and Nutrition-Related History

Past dietary practices are identified to determine the pattern of food intake. Numerous means are available to determine food consumed by an individual. A registered dietitian may use a 24-hour recall or a usual daily intake recall, a food diary or food record, or a food frequency questionnaire. The 24-hour recall and the usual daily intake recall depends on past information in which the patient states the foods and amount consumed in an average day. This technique is easily incorporated into a clinical setting. Food frequency questionnaires incorporate information on the frequency and amount of the specific foods consumed and can help identify eating patterns. Patients are asked to write down daily everything they have eaten. The patient may record food intake over an extended time, most frequently, a 3-day or 7-day period.

Evaluation of Nutrition History

The information from a diet history may be evaluated for nutrient intake using MyPlate, a nutrient analysis handbook, or a nutrient analysis software package.

MyPlate. The U.S. Department of Agriculture and the U.S. Department of Health and Human Services recommend balanced nutrition for U.S. citizens.[2] The clinician or patient can go to http://www.choosemyplate.gov and compare diet history information to estimate the adequacy of the patient's diet.[3]

Nutrient Analysis Handbook. A handbook listing the nutrient content of specific foods may be used to calculate manually the adequacy of a 24-hour recall. This is a tedious and time-consuming task.

Nutrient Analysis Software. Computer programs can determine total calories, percent of calories of macronutrients (protein, carbohydrate, and fat), and units of micronutrients and fiber. The patient's individual foods and serving size are entered into a computer file to determine quickly the nutrient content of a diet history.

Anthropometrics

Anthropometrics refers to body measurements; the most frequently used are height and weight. Skin fold thicknesses, arm muscle measurements, waist and hip measurements, head circumference, and wrist diameter are useful body composition measurements when assessing nutrition status.

Height and Weight

A measured height and weight is preferred, but the clinician may ask the patient or caregiver for the height and weight. When recording this data note the date and whether the height and weight were stated or measured.

Body Mass Index. Body mass index (BMI) expresses the relationship between weight and height and is used to classify patients as underweight, healthy weight, overweight, obese, or morbidly obese. The formula for calculating BMI in kilograms and meters is:

$$BMI = \frac{\text{Actual body weight (kg)}}{\text{height}^2\ (\text{m}^2)}$$

And when using pounds and inches is:

$$BMI = \frac{\text{Actual body weight (lb)} \times 703}{\text{height}^2\ (\text{in}^2)}$$

An Internet calculator for BMI is available at: http://www.cdc.gov/bmi.

RULE OF THUMB

BMI categories for adults and children (male and female, age 2 to 20 years) are as follows[4,5]:

	Adult (BMI)	Children (BMI for Age)
Underweight	<18.5	<10th percentile
Healthy weight	18.5-24.9	10th-85th percentiles
Excessive weight	25.0-29.9	85th-95th percentiles
Obesity	>30	>95th percentile
Morbid obesity	>35	>99th percentile

Overweight and Obesity. Simply defined, overweight and obesity occur over time with the consumption of too many calories or too little expenditure of calories through activity or exercise or both overconsumption and underexpenditure. Other contributory factors include rare diseases, genetic predisposition, and loss of mobility through trauma or disease. Regardless, too many calories are ingested for the amount of energy (calories) expended.

Kwashiorkor and Marasmus. Undernutrition classifications include kwashiorkor and marasmus. Typically seen in children 6 to 18 months of age residing in impoverished areas of the world, **marasmus** results from a prolonged, extreme lack of calories and protein associated with food shortage, early weaning, or infrequent feeding of infants.[6] "Matchstick" arms and obvious lack of muscle and fat characterize a child or adult with marasmus. Table 23-1 compares the two forms of protein energy malnutrition (PEM). **Kwashiorkor** results from a more sudden lack of protein and calories, as in a first-born infant weaned suddenly on the arrival of a new sibling, when a diet of nutrient-rich breast milk is traded for a nutrient-poor, cereal-based diet.[6] The protruding belly and edematous face and limbs characteristic of kwashiorkor result from decreased plasma proteins needed to maintain fluid balance and transport fat out of the liver.

TABLE 23-1
Comparison of Two Primary Forms of Protein-Energy Malnutrition

Parameter	Starvation (Marasmus)	Hypercatabolism (Kwashiorkor)
Cause	Inadequate energy intake	Response to injury or infection
Examples	Cancer, pulmonary emphysema	Sepsis, burns
Body habitus	Thin, wasted, cachexic	May be normal, edematous
Rate of malnutrition	Slow	Rapid
Metabolic rate	↓	↑
Fuel	Glucose/fat	Mixed
Catabolism	↓	↑
Gluconeogenesis	↑	Markedly ↑
Glucagon	↑	Markedly ↑
Insulin	↓	↑
Ketogenesis	↑	Slightly ↑
Catecholamines	Unchanged	↑
Cortisol	Unchanged	↑
Growth hormone	Increased	↑
Visceral proteins	Normal	Decreased ↓
Cytokines	Variable	Increased
Immune function	Normal	Impaired
Clinical course	Adequate responsiveness to short-term stress	Infections, poor wound healing, decubitus ulcers, skin breakdown
Mortality	Low unless related to underlying disease	High

Body Composition

Other anthropometric measurements useful in nutrition assessment evaluate body weight variations in individuals. Someone with similar height may differ in the proportion of lean body mass, fat mass, and skeletal size. Common measurements are *arm muscle area* (index for muscle), *skin folds* (measures of fat), and waist-to-hip ratios. More sophisticated imaging technologies such as bioelectric impedance analysis or dual-energy x-ray absorptiometry scans determine body fat, body mass, ratio of intracellular water to extracellular water, and bone density. These methods are generally expensive and time-consuming and are not clinically relevant but may be used in research.

Skin Fold. Skin-fold thickness measures subcutaneous fat with the assumption that it compromises 50% of total body fat. Usually, the triceps and subscapular skin folds are the most useful for evaluation.[7] Skin-fold thickness measurements have limited clinical application in the acute care setting because of proper equipment and examiner technique.

Arm Muscle Area. The triceps skin-fold measurement with the midarm circumference is used to calculates arm muscle area (AMA). The AMA indicates muscle stores available for protein synthesis or energy needs. AMA changes over time may signify protein or caloric deprivation and is useful as a predictor of mortality.[8]

Waist Circumference. An alternative to BMI, waist circumference, can be a more accurate predictor of excess body fat and risks associated with obesity.[9,10] According to the U.S. Department of Health and Human Services, the following individuals are at increased risk for developing chronic diseases:

- Women with a waist circumference of more than 35 inches
- Men with a waist circumference of more than 40 inches

The World Health Organization has recommended lower thresholds for waist circumference for Asian populations.[11] Therefore those at increased risk for developing chronic disease include:

- Asian women with a waist circumference of more than 31 inches
- Asian men with a waist circumference of more than 35 inches

Biochemical Indicators

Particularly significant laboratory values used in assessing nutrition status include serum proteins. PEM may be reflected in low values for albumin, transthyretin (prealbumin), and retinol-binding protein. Blood levels of these markers indicate the level of protein synthesis and yield information on overall nutrition status. However, inadequate intake may not be the cause of low values; certain disease states, level of hydration, liver and kidney function, pregnancy, infection, and medical therapies may alter laboratory values for each of the circulating proteins.[12] Diagnosing a nutritional disorder cannot be done based on a single laboratory value but should be used with other assessment data to determine the nutritional status of the patient. The majority of laboratory values used in nutritional assessments lack sensitivity and specificity for malnutrition.[13]

Albumin

Albumin is the largest constituent protein in plasma. Because its half-life is only 14 to 21 days, its usefulness for monitoring the effectiveness of nutrition in the critical care setting is limited.[14] Albumin often reflects the metabolic response to and severity of disease, injury, or infection and can be a useful prognostic indicator. Albumin synthesis is affected by both nutrition and inflammation. Proinflammatory states diminish albumin production, and the combination of inflammation and hypoalbuminemia is linked with increased morbidity, mortality, and longer hospitalization.[15]

Transthyretin and Retinol-Binding Protein

Transthyretin, or *prealbumin,* has a half-life of 2 to 3 days, and retinol-binding protein has a half-life of 12 hours. Each of these proteins responds to nutrition changes more quickly than either albumin. However, numerous metabolic states, diseases, therapies, and infections influence the laboratory values.[16]

Levels of each protein are influenced by many factors other than nutrition status. Because these conditions are so common among critically ill patients, visceral protein markers are of limited usefulness for assessing nutrition deficiency. *Nonetheless, plasma proteins are useful in assessing illness severity and the risk for future malnutrition.*[16] Inflammatory metabolism causes a 25% decrease in the synthesis of these visceral proteins; causing lean body mass depletion and anorexia. Therefore it is important to evaluate their values with biomarkers of inflammation where there is a reverse relationship.

RULE OF THUMB

Nutritional disorders cannot be made from a single laboratory value because, by themselves, they are not sufficiently sensitive or specific to diagnose malnutrition. Instead, laboratory test results are used with other data as part of a holistic assessment of a patient's nutritional status.

RULE OF THUMB

Increased metabolism associated with inflammation causes a 25% decrease in protein synthesis resulting in loss of lean body mass.

In proinflammatory states the combination of inflammation and hypoalbuminemia is linked with increased morbidity, mortality, and longer hospitalization.

Biomarkers of Inflammation

Inflammation adversely affects a patient's nutritional status by both increasing catabolism and causing albumin leakage out of the vascular compartment. Inflammation triggers a chemical cascade that causes loss of appetite or anorexia, thereby decreasing dietary protein intake and further catabolism.[13]

The most commonly used clinical biomarker of inflammation is C-reactive protein (CRP), which increases with infection and inflammation while the production of albumin and prealbumin decreases.[17] Increased levels of C-reactive protein during stress, illness, and trauma have been linked to increased nutrition risk.[18] Other common biomarkers of inflammation include white cell count and erythrocyte sedimentation rate (ESR).[19]

Other Tests and Procedures

Creatinine-Height Index

Because the rate of creatinine formation in skeletal muscle is constant, the amount of creatinine excreted in the urine every 24 hours reflects skeletal muscle mass. Predicted values are based on gender and height, with reference values of approximately 18 mg/kg body weight per day for women and approximately 23 mg/kg body weight per day for men.[7] Factors that influence creatinine excretion and complicate its interpretation include age, diet, exercise, stress, trauma, fever, and sepsis.[17]

Nitrogen Balance (Protein Catabolism)

Approximately 16% of protein is nitrogen, and nitrogen is a major by-product of protein catabolism. Therefore measuring nitrogen balance is an important aspect of nutritional assessment. The urinary excretion rate of nitrogen is used to assess protein adequacy. Nitrogen balance is calculated as follows:

$$\text{Nitrogen balance} = \text{Nitrogen intake} - \text{Nitrogen losses}$$

$$\text{Nitrogen intake} = \frac{\text{Protein intake}}{6.25}$$

$$\text{Nitrogen losses} = \text{UUN excretion in grams} + \text{3-5 g (for insensible losses)}$$

The dietary protein conversion factor is 6.25 g of nitrogen per 1 g of protein. The amount of nitrogen excretion in the urine is typically measured as the 24-hour urinary urea nitrogen. Between 3 g/day and 5 g/day is added to the 24-hour urinary urea nitrogen to estimate the average daily unmeasured nitrogen lost through other sources (skin and gastrointestinal [GI] sloughing, hair loss, sweat, feces). Theoretically, increasing exogenous protein, reduces endogenous protein loss. However, the accuracy of 24-hour urine collection is limited by alterations in renal or liver function, large insensible losses (burns, high-output fistulas, wounds, or ostomies), and inflammatory conditions.[20]

TABLE 23-2
Physical Signs of Malnutrition

	Normal	Abnormal
Demeanor	Alert, responsive Positive outlook	Lethargic Negative attitude
Weight	Reasonable for build	Underweight Overweight, obese
Hair	Glossy, full, firmly rooted Uniform color	Dull, sparse; easily, painlessly plucked
Eyes	Bright, clear, shiny	Pale conjunctiva Redness, dryness
Lips	Smooth	Chapped, red, swollen
Tongue	Deep red Slightly rough One longitudinal furrow	Bright red, purple Swollen or shrunken Several longitudinal furrows
Teeth	Bright, painless	Caries, painful, mottled, or missing
Gums	Pink, firm	Spongy, bleeding, receding
Skin	Clear, smooth, firm, slightly moist	Rashes, swelling Light or dark spots Dry, cracked
Nails	Pink, firm	Spoon-shaped or ridged Spongy bases
Mobility	Erect posture Good muscle tone Walks without pain or difficulty	Muscle wasting Skeletal deformities Loss of balance

From Lutz C, Przytulski K: Nutrition and diet therapy, ed 5, Jackson Community College; Jackson, MS, 2011, FA Davis.

Immune Status

Impaired immunity (**anergy**) is common in malnutrition, especially the kwashiorkor type. Two laboratory values, white blood cell count and percentage of lymphocytes, are indices of compromised immunity. The result is often a reduction in the total lymphocyte count. Many nonnutrition variables, including disease states and drugs, influence these laboratory values, so their usefulness in assessing nutrition status is questioned.[21]

Pulmonary Function

Pulmonary function test results may change with malnutrition. Respiratory muscle weakness reduces both maximal inspiratory and expiratory pressures and reduced vital capacity. These limitations in turn reduce the ability to maintain sufficient lung volumes to prevent atelectasis and produce an effective cough to clear secretions. Diminished strength and endurance of respiratory muscles increases the susceptibility to respiratory muscle fatigue and the inability to maintain effective spontaneous breathing. The negative effects of malnutrition on both respiratory muscle function and immunologic function increase the risk for respiratory infections and pneumonia.[22]

Nutrition-Focused Physical Findings

The physical signs of malnutrition often appear first in specific tissues where high cell turnover occurs[23] (e.g., hair, eyes, lips, mouth and gums, skin and nails), so incorporating the appearance of these features into the physical examination can alert the clinician to signs of nutrient deficiencies (see Table 23-2 for physical signs of nutrition status). In addition to malnutrition, other causes of these abnormalities include medical therapies, anemia, allergies, sunburn, medications, poor hygiene practices, aging, or various pathologic processes.[24] Patients with persistent malnutrition often appear very thin. When the bony structures of the chest are conspicuously visible, a patient is said to be **cachexic.** Special attention should be given to fluid retention because this can mask weight loss.[25] Other physical findings such as skeletal muscle depletion can be clinical indicators of inflammation or signs of systemic inflammatory response.

OUTCOMES OF NUTRITION ASSESSMENT

With nutrition intervention, patients improve their nutrient intake and reduce mortality and morbidity. Improved nutrition status increases the patient's tolerance of therapeutic regimens in the treatment of disease and decreases recovery time. The resulting economic benefits are multifaceted and include shorter and less frequent hospital stays, reduced need for medication or medical care or extended care, and increased years of productivity.[26]

MACRONUTRIENTS AND ENERGY REQUIREMENTS

The nutrition assessment determines a nutrition care plan for the patient. Calorie or energy needs are fundamental to these recommendations. Several means are available to determine calorie needs. These include calculating total calories using a mathematical formula or predictive equation.

Macronutrients supply the energy requirements of the body. The three macronutrients are *protein, carbohydrate,* and *fat.* Each contributes to calorie intake with 4, 4, and 9 calories (kcal) per gram. Alcohol is the only other calorie source, with approximately 7 kcal/g. Box 23-2 outlines the factors influencing energy and macronutrient needs.

Estimating Energy Requirements

An individual's energy requirement represents the ratio of energy intake to energy expenditure relative to body weight, activity level, and stressors. The classic measure of energy expenditure is the **basal metabolic rate (BMR)**. Obtained after 10 hours of fasting, the BMR measures the number of calories (kcal) expended at rest per square meter of body surface per hour (kcal/m^2/hr). BMR varies by body size, age, and sex. Caloric needs for energy expenditure increase beyond the BMR based on activity level, stage of growth (pregnancy, lactation), and extent of injury.

In clinical practice, interest is focused on a patient's *daily* energy requirements (kilocalories per day). Multiple methods are available for estimating daily energy needs. The "quick method," based on a 1997 equation provided by the American College of Chest Physicians, estimates daily energy needs based on a simple body weight factor of 20 to 35 kcal/kg.[27] Alternatively, predictive equations (Box 23-3) such as the classic *Harris-Benedict equation* estimate daily **resting energy expenditure (REE)**.

Several other predictive equations focus on specific patient populations and medical conditions. Additional data such as injury-stress, activity, medications received, and obesity have been added to improve accuracy. The *Mifflin-St. Jeor equation* is the most reliable in both nonobese and obese ill patients.[28] Other equations, such as the *Ireton-Jones* and *Penn State equations* are used specifically in intubated patients to account for temperature and ventilation parameters. Although the predicted REE averages approximately 10% higher than the BMR, predictive equations may still tend to overestimate or underestimate actual energy need.[29]

Box 23-2 Factors Influencing Energy and Macronutrient Needs

ENERGY NEEDS
- Height and weight
- Activity level
- Growth state: Infants through teens, pregnancy, and lactation
- Presence of infection or fever
- Surgery
- Trauma and fractures
- Presence of infection or inflammation

PROTEIN NEEDS
- State of growth
- Surgery, trauma, fractures, and infection
- Renal (kidney) function
- Liver function
- Corticosteroid administration

FAT NEEDS
- Total energy needs
- Hyperlipidemia, and diabetes mellitus
- Liver, gallbladder, and pancreatic disorders
- Cardiovascular disease

Box 23-3 Predictive Equations

HARRIS-BENEDICT EQUATIONS

Men: Resting metabolic rate (RMR) = 66.47 + 13.75(W) + 5(H) – 6.76 (A)

Women: RMR = 655.1 + 9.56 (W) + 1.7 (H) – 4.7 (A)

Equation uses weight (W) in kilograms (kg), height (H) in centimeters (cm), and age (A) in years.

IRETON-JONES ENERGY EQUATIONS (IJEE) 1992

Spontaneously breathing IJEE
(s) = 629 – 11 (A) + 25 (W) – 609 (O)

Ventilator dependent IJEE
(v) = 1925 – 10 (A) + 5 (W) + 281 (S) + 292 (T) + 851 (B)

Equations uses age (A) in years, body weight (W) in kilograms, sex (S, male = 1, female = 0), diagnosis of trauma (T, present = 1, absent = 0), diagnosis of burn (B, present = 1, absent = 0), obesity more than 30% above initial body weight from 1959 Metropolitan Life Insurance tables or body mass index (BMI) more than 27 kg/m^2 (present = 1, absent = 0).

MIFFLIN-ST. JEOR EQUATIONS

Men: RMR = (9.99 × weight) + (6.25 × height) – (4.92 × age) + 5

Women: RMR = (9.99 × weight) + (6.25 × height) – (4.92 × age) – 161

Equations use weight in kilograms and height in centimeters.

PENN STATE EQUATIONS (PSU)
Also known as *PSU 2010* (Modified Penn State Equation)

$$RMR = Mifflin\,(0.71) + \dot{V}_E\,(64) + T_{max}\,(85) - 3085$$

Used for patients with BMI over 30 and older than 60 years old. Validated in 2010 by the ADA Evidence Analysis Library (EAL).

PSU 2003b (Penn State Equation)

$$RMR = Mifflin\,(0.96) + \dot{V}_E\,(31) + T_{max}\,(167) - 6212$$

Used for patient of any age with BMI below 30 or patients who are younger than 60 years with BMI over 30. This equation was validated in 2009 by the EAL and is also referred to as the Penn State equation.

PSU 2003a (Penn State 2003a)

Invalidated in 2007 and 2009 by EAL

$$RMR = HBE\,(0.85) + \dot{V}_E\,(33) + T_{max}\,(175) - 6433$$

(Use actual weight in all patients.)

From Academy of Nutrition and Dietetics. Evidence analysis library, 2014. Available http://www.andeal.org. Accessed September 2014.

To overcome the limitations of estimating formulas, energy needs can be measured using O_2 consumption and carbon dioxide production. From these data, an actual REE can be quickly computed. Indirect calorimetry is described in more detail later.

Energy needs vary according to activity level and state of health. Energy needs of sick patients can be significantly greater than predicted normal values. Energy needs for obese individuals are less because adipose tissue uses less energy than muscle. Energy needs should be reevaluated and adjusted whenever weight changes more than 10 lb.

RULE OF THUMB

To estimate the energy needs of an average adult in kilocalories per day, identify the goal and multiply the individual's actual body weight in kilograms times the factor listed as follows[27]:

Goal	Energy Needs (kcal/kg)
Weight maintenance	25-30
Weight gain	30-35
Weight loss	20-25

Indirect Calorimetry

Indirect calorimetry is the estimation of energy expenditure by measurement of O_2 consumption and CO_2 production. Data obtained can be used to assess a patient's metabolic state, to determine nutrition needs, or to assess response to nutritional therapy.[30] To guide practitioners in using indirect calorimetry, the American Association for Respiratory Care (AARC) has published the Clinical Practice Guideline: Metabolic Measurement Using Indirect Calorimetry During Mechanical Ventilation. Excerpts appear in Clinical Practice Guideline 23-1.[31]

In regard to the indications for indirect calorimetry, the determination of energy and protein needs by an empiric formula is sufficient for most patients. However, the use of indirect calorimetry improves nutritional care and reduces complications associated with underfeeding and overfeeding.[30] Specific clinical conditions supporting the need for indirect calorimetry as a tool in nutrition assessment are listed in Box 23-4.[30]

Box 23-4 Clinical Situations in Which Indirect Calorimetry May Be Indicated

- Patients with morbid obesity
- Patients who are difficult to wean from ventilatory support
- Patients for whom weight estimates are unclear
- Patients with severe malnutrition
- Patients with high level of stress
- Patients at the extremes of weight or age
- Patients failing to respond to nutrition support

Equipment and Technique

Good calorimetry results require extensive preparation. Box 23-5 outlines the key preparatory steps to be taken before testing.[32] Indirect calorimetry can be performed with a Douglas bag, a Tissot spirometer, and CO_2 and O_2 gas analyzers. The patient's expired gas is collected in the Douglas bag, where it is sampled for O_2 and CO_2 concentrations; the Tissot spirometer measures expired volume. Commercially available metabolic carts are much easier to use. These automated systems either use a mixing chamber or perform breath-by-breath analysis. The breath-by-breath method provides real-time data, which may aid in ensuring optimal measurement conditions, particularly in mechanically ventilated patients.[33]

Figure 23-1 shows the basic configuration for open-circuit indirect calorimetry during mechanical ventilation using a metabolic cart with mixing chamber. Gas sampled from the inspiratory limb of the ventilator circuit is assessed for fractional inspired oxygen (FiO_2) using a paramagnetic or zirconium oxide O_2 analyzer. Volume exhaled by the patient is measured using a flow transducer. The patient's exhaled gas enters a mixing chamber, from which a sample is drawn to measure fractional expired carbon dioxide ($FeCO_2$) by infrared analysis and fractional expired oxygen (FeO_2). Exhaled gas is returned to the ventilator after volume and gas concentration measurements. After all measurements are obtained, O_2 consumption, CO_2 production, and *respiratory quotient (RQ)* are computed using the equations shown in Box 23-6. *All measurements must be corrected to standard temperature and pressure and dry conditions (STPD) before computation.*[31] The values are used in the abbreviated Weir equation to determine REE:

$$REE = [(O_2 \times 3.9) + (CO_2 \times 1.1)] \times 1.44$$

Box 23-5 Preparation for Indirect Calorimetry

30 HOURS BEFORE TEST

- 24-Hour urine urea nitrogen collection (with sufficient time to receive result) if determination of carbohydrate, fat, and protein use desired

10 HOURS BEFORE TEST

- Patient fasting if measuring energy requirements; if feeding is continued, results will reflect the patient's energy expenditure in response to feeding (may be spuriously high if patient is being overfed)

4 HOURS BEFORE TEST

- Patient resting and avoiding physical activity, physical therapy, dressing changes

2 HOURS BEFORE TEST

- Endotracheal tube suctioned for the last time before test; further ventilator changes or suctioning avoided

1 HOUR BEFORE TEST

- Supine position, complete rest; analgesic or sedative administered if needed

23-1 Metabolic Measurement Using Indirect Calorimetry During Mechanical Ventilation

AARC Clinical Practice Guideline (Excerpts)*

INDICATIONS

Metabolic measurements may be indicated:

- In patients with known nutrition deficits or derangements
- When patients fail attempts at weaning from mechanical ventilation to measure the O_2 cost of breathing in mechanically ventilated patients
- When the need exists to assess the $\dot{V}/\dot{Q}_2$ to evaluate the hemodynamic support of mechanically ventilated patients

CONTRAINDICATIONS

When a specific indication is present, there are no contraindications to performing a metabolic measurement using indirect calorimetry, unless short-term disconnection of ventilatory support for connection of measurement lines results in hypoxemia, bradycardia, or other adverse effects.

HAZARDS AND COMPLICATIONS

Performing metabolic measurements using an indirect calorimeter is a safe, noninvasive procedure with few hazards or complications. Under certain circumstances and with particular equipment, the following hazards or complications may be seen:

- Closed-circuit calorimeters may cause a reduction in alveolar ventilation secondary to increased compressible volume of the breathing circuit.
- Closed-circuit calorimeters may decrease the trigger sensitivity of the ventilator and result in increased patient work of breathing.
- Short-term disconnection of the patient from the ventilator for connection of the indirect calorimetry apparatus may result in hypoxemia, bradycardia, and patient discomfort.
- Inappropriate calibration or system setup may result in erroneous results causing incorrect patient management.

ASSESSMENT OF NEED

Metabolic measurements should be performed only on the order of a physician after review of indications (see earlier) and objectives.

ASSESSMENT OF TEST QUALITY

Test quality can be evaluated by determining whether:

- Respiratory quotient is consistent with the patient's nutrition intake.
- Respiratory quotient is in the normal physiologic range (0.67 to 1.3).
- Variability of the measurements of $\dot{V}O_2$ and $\dot{V}CO_2$ should be 5% or less for a 5-minute data collection.
- The measurement is of sufficient length to account for variability in $\dot{V}O_2$ and $\dot{V}CO_2$ if these conditions are not met.
- Outcome may be assessed by comparing the measurement results with the patient's condition and nutrition intake. Outcome also may be assessed by observation of the patient before and during the measurement to determine if the patient is at steady state.

MONITORING

The following should be evaluated during the metabolic measurement to ascertain the validity of the results:

- Clinical observation of the resting state
- Patient comfort and movement during testing
- Values in concert with the clinical situation
- Equipment function
- Results within the specifications of test quality (see earlier)
- FiO_2 stability

Measurement data should include a statement of test quality and list the current nutrition support, ventilator settings, FiO_2 stability, and vital signs.

For the complete guidelines, see American Association of Respiratory Care: Clinical practice guideline. Respir Care 49:1073, 2004. http://www.rcjournal.com/contents/09.04/09.04.1073.pdf. Accessed June 1, 2014.

Box 23-6 Equations Used to Calculate $\dot{V}O_2$ and $\dot{V}CO_2$ Using the Gas-Exchange Method

$$\dot{V}O_2 = \dot{V}_E \times (3\,FiO_2 4) - (\dot{V}_E \times FeO_2)$$
$$\dot{V}CO_2 = \dot{V}_E \times FeCO_2$$
$$RQ = \dot{V}CO_2/\dot{V}O_2$$

Indirect calorimetry is more difficult to perform on spontaneously breathing patients, especially patients breathing supplemental O_2. Although a mouthpiece with nose clips or a mask can be used to collect expired gas, these items tend to alter the patient's steady state and invalidate results.[33] Instead, most clinicians recommend using a plastic canopy that covers the patient's head. Expired gases are cleared from the canopy by a preset flow of air; expired gas concentrations are sampled and corrected for the air dilution.

Because standard modes of O_2 therapy do not deliver a consistent FiO_2 to spontaneously breathing patients, special delivery systems must be used. To overcome this problem, the clinician can substitute a precise O_2 mixture for the gas used to clear the canopy. Alternatively, a large gas reservoir (e.g., a Douglas bag) can be placed between an O_2 flow source and the subject[33] to ensure a stable FiO_2 throughout the test procedure.

Problems and Limitations

Indirect calorimetry is a technically complex procedure requiring rigorous attention to both instrument and procedure quality

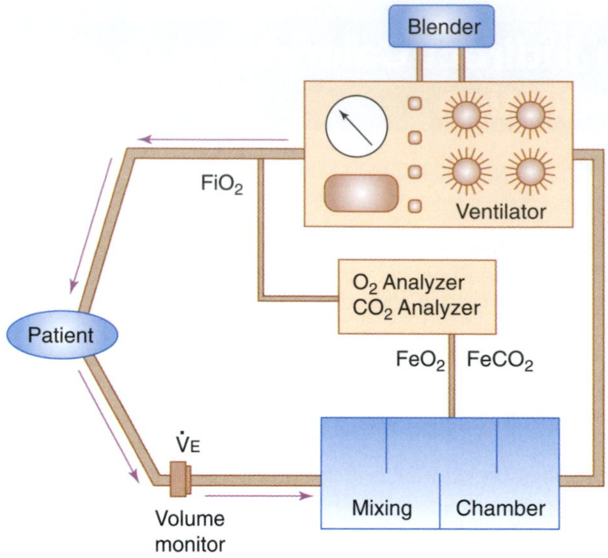

FIGURE 23-1 Open-circuit indirect calorimetry in a mechanically ventilated patient. Inspiratory gas is sampled for determination of FiO_2, volume is measured in the expiratory limb of the ventilator circuit, and mixed exhaled gas is drawn from the mixing chamber for analysis of FeO_2 and $FeCO_2$. *Arrows* indicate direction of gas flow. (Modified from Witte MK: Metabolic measurements during mechanical ventilation in the pediatric intensive care unit. Respir Care Clin N Am 2:573, 1996.)

control. Regarding instrumentation, small errors in measurements can result in large errors in calculated O_2, CO_2, and therefore energy expenditure. For this reason, the calorimeter's gas analyzers and volume measurement device must be properly calibrated before each patient use. Gas analyzers should be accurate to the hundredth percent and linear over the clinical range of O_2 concentrations.[32]

Regarding procedure quality control, it is essential that measurements be made during steady-state conditions. Although proper patient preparation (see Box 23-5) is helpful in this regard, steady-state conditions can be confirmed only during the test procedure itself. A common standard for ensuring steady-state conditions is five consecutive 1-minute averages with a variability of 5% or less.[33]

Perhaps the most significant problem in performing indirect calorimetry on mechanically ventilated patients is the presence of leaks (circuit, tracheal tube cuff, chest tubes).[31] Because any leak invalidates test results, no procedure should begin until a leak-free patient-ventilator-calorimeter system is confirmed. Other sources of error during open-circuit indirect calorimetry of mechanically ventilated patients are listed in Box 23-7.[31]

Interpretation and Use of Results

Results obtained from indirect calorimetry are used to assess metabolic status and plan nutrition support. Energy expenditure varies during illness and injury (Figure 23-2),[34] which occurs in three phases: the stress response, the catabolic phase and the anabolic phase. Because of the changing metabolic rate, it is important to reassess metabolic needs when there is a change in clinical status. Indirect calorimetry is an important tool because it can demonstrate these changes in energy expenditure. Energy expenditure can vary on a daily basis by 15% to 30%.[33]

In regard to assessing metabolic status, the first step is to compare the REE obtained by calorimetry with the REE predicted by predictive equations. If the calorimetry REE is within 10% of the predicted value, the patient is considered **normometabolic.** Measured REEs greater than 10% above predicted values indicate a hypermetabolic state, whereas values less than 90% of predicted indicate hypometabolism.

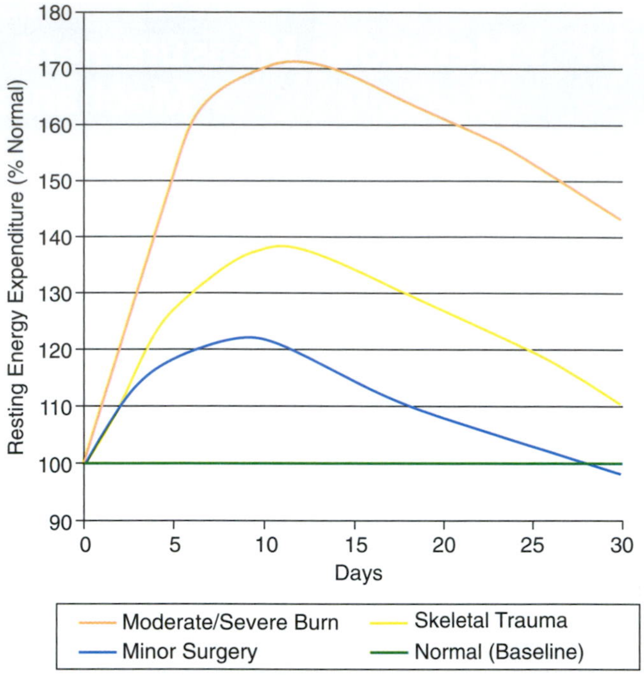

FIGURE 23-2 Resting energy expenditure variation during illness and injury.

Box 23-7 Sources of Error During Open-Circuit Indirect Calorimetry of Mechanically Ventilated Patients

- Instability of FiO_2 because of changes in source gas pressure or ventilator or blender variability
- Delivery of high FiO_2 levels (>0.60)
- Inability to separate inspired and expired gases because of bias flow from flow-triggering systems, intermittent mandatory ventilation systems, or specific ventilator characteristics
- Presence of anesthetic gases or gases other than O_2, CO_2, and nitrogen in the ventilation system
- Presence of water vapor resulting in sensor malfunction
- Inappropriate calibration
- Adverse effect on functions of some ventilators (triggering, expiratory resistance, pressure measurement)
- Total circuit flow exceeding internal calorimeter flow (if using dilutional principle)
- Concurrent peritoneal dialysis or hemodialysis

TABLE 23-3

Traditional Interpretation and Use of the Respiratory Quotient

Value	Interpretation	General Nutrition Strategy
>1.00	Overfeeding	Decrease total kilocalories
0.9-1.00	Carbohydrate oxidation	Decrease carbohydrates or increase lipids
0.8-0.9	Fat, protein, and carbohydrate oxidation	Target range for mixed substrate
0.7-0.8	Fat and protein oxidation Starvation	Increase total kilocalories

Note: Acute hyperventilation or acute metabolic acidosis increases the respiratory quotient (RQ) and can lead to misinterpretation. Metabolism of ketones or ethyl alcohol decreases RQ to less than 0.7.

The second step in metabolic assessment is to interpret the RQ. The RQ is the ratio of moles of CO_2 expired to moles of O_2 consumed. Traditionally, the RQ has been used to determine substrate use, where carbohydrates have an RQ of 1.0, protein has an RQ of 0.82, and fat has an RQ of 0.7. Table 23-3 outlines the basic significance of the RQ relative to substrate use and traditional nutrition strategies.[33] RQ has been shown to have low sensitivity and reduced specificity in critically ill patients.[35,36] This finding limits the RQ as an indicator for substrate use and should be used only as a measure of test validity. If the RQ is outside its physiologic range of 0.67 to 1.3, this should alert the clinician to assess the validity of the study.

RULE OF THUMB

RQ	0.67 to 1.3	Ideal range for test validity

Alternative Resting Energy Expenditure Measures

In patients with pulmonary artery catheters, REE can be measured using a modification of the Fick equation[37]:

$$\text{REE (kcal/day)} = \text{Cardiac output} \times \text{Hemoglobin} \times (\text{SaO}_2 - \text{S}\bar{\text{v}}\text{O}_2) \times 95.18$$

In a patient with cardiac output of 4.2 L, hemoglobin of 11 g/dl, SaO_2 of 89%, and SVO_2 of 69%, the REE would be computed as follows:

$$\text{REE} = 4.2 \times 11 \times (0.89 - 0.69) \times 95.18$$
$$\text{REE} = 4.2 \times 11 \times (0.20) \times 95.18$$
$$\text{REE} = 879 \text{ kcal/day}$$

MINI CLINI

Comparison of Resting Energy Expenditure from Predictive Equations and Indirect Calorimetry

PROBLEM: A 57-year-old male construction worker fell three stories and after being intubated and mechanical ventilation initiated was admitted to the intensive care unit for multiple orthopedic injuries, several rib fractures, and a pulmonary contusion. On hospital day 2, after the patient was stabilized, a nasogastric feeding tube was placed and a nutrition consult was requested for enteral nutrition recommendations. Anthropometrics: Height: 5 ft, 9 inches; measured body weight: 127.3 kg; BMI: 43.8 kg/m^2.

The dietitian used and compared the follow predictive equations to determine the patient's energy expenditure:

Predictive Equation:	kcal/day
Harris-Benedict × 1.3-1.6*	2269-2792
Mifflin-St. Joer × 1.3	2718
Ireton-Jones	3081
Penn State	2137

*Factor to correct for stress and/or activity levels.

The initial goal recommended by the dietitian for the tube feeding would provide 2280 calories. An indirect calorimetry study was also requested by the dietitian because the patient is a perfect candidate for the indirect calorimetry because of his BMI and clinical status.

The indirect calorimetry study was conducted on a weekly basis and the results were as follows:

Hospital Day	Measured Metabolic Rate (kcal/day)	RQ
3	1980	1.1
10	3150	0.83
17	2700	0.85

Interpret the results and compare to the predictive equations. Based on the results, suggest what changes would be made.

DISCUSSION: The following conclusions can be made based on retrospective data review. Overall, the predictive equations estimations vary widely. Initially the Penn State equation was the most accurate equation compared to the indirect calorimetry study results. The RQ is within physiologic range of 0.67 to 1.3, suggesting a valid study; however, it further indicates the patient is possibly being overfed. As a result the tube feed goal was adjusted to provide 1980 calories to match the patient's current metabolic phase. However, as the patient moved into the catabolic phase, if the patient continued to receive 2280 calories as initially recommended by the dietitian (or the adjusted level of 1980 calories) and subsequent indirect calorimetry was not done on day 10, resulting in a tube feed increase to 3150 calories, the patient would be significantly underfed. Finally, entering into the anabolic phase, the patient's energy expenditure begins to decrease, as shown by the indirect calorimetry on day 17. As a result, the tube feed regimen should be further adjusted (decreased) to match the measured metabolic rate.

Modified from Wooley JA, Frankenfield D: Energy. In: Mueller CM, Merritt RJ, McClave S, et al, editors: The ASPEN adult nutrition support core curriculum, ed 2, Silver Spring, MD, 2012, American Society for Parenteral and Enteral Nutrition.

RULE OF THUMB

Although predictive equations are highly useful tools in calculating a patient's energy expenditure needs, they do not always replace the need for performing indirect calorimetry, which is generally more accurate and provides additional information, including calculation of the RQ.

GENERAL ASPECTS OF NUTRITION SUPPORT

The primary goal of nutrition support is the maintenance or restoration of lean body (skeletal muscle) mass. This goal is accomplished by (1) meeting the patient's overall energy needs and (2) providing the appropriate combination of substrates to do so. The route of administration used to provide the support is also important.

Meeting Overall Energy Needs

When the patient's REE is derived, it needs to be adjusted to account for variations in activity and stress levels. If using a predictive equation, such as the Harris-Benedict or Mifflin-St. Joer equations, the predicted REE should be corrected for stress, activity levels, or both.[20] When the REE is derived from the Penn State equations or indirect calorimetry, a stress or activity factor should not be used.

Insufficient Energy Consumed

Malnutrition from undernutrition results from insufficient energy (calorie) intake over time. This insufficient intake leads to a state of impaired metabolism in which the intake of essential nutrients falls short of the body's needs. Certain factors may place a patient at risk for malnutrition (Box 23-8).

Protein-Energy Malnutrition

Protein-energy malnutrition (PEM) has adverse effects on respiratory musculature and the immune response.[24] PEM may be either primary or secondary. Primary PEM results from inadequate intake of calories, protein, or both and is typically seen only in developing countries.[20]

Secondary PEM is due to underlying illness. Illness may cause (1) decreased caloric or protein intake (e.g., anorexia, dysphagia), (2) increased nutrient losses (e.g., malabsorption or diarrhea), and (3) increased nutrient demands (e.g., injury or infection).[38]

RULE OF THUMB

Fifty percent of hospitalized patients present with secondary PEM.

When PEM is due to inadequate nutrient intake or excessive loss, the body responds by decreasing its metabolic rate, ventilatory drive, thyroid function, and adrenergic activity.[38] As calorie intake decreases, energy for metabolic processes is initially supplied by converting liver glycogen stores into glucose *(gluconeogenesis)*. However, liver reserves of glycogen are adequate for less than 1 day at rest and only a few hours during exercise.[14] Thereafter endogenous fat stores are mobilized in the form of free fatty acids *(ketogenesis)*. When fat stores are depleted, nutrient needs must be met by catabolizing skeletal muscle protein. This type of PEM usually manifests as a gradual wasting process, as seen in patients with chronic diseases such as cancer and emphysema. The primary clinical sign is progressive weight loss.

When PEM results from increased nutrient demand, metabolism, thyroid function, and adrenergic activity all increase. Visceral protein levels tend to decrease early in the course of illness and are associated with impaired immunity.[37] This type of PEM typically occurs with acute catabolic disease, such as in sepsis, burns, or trauma. The two types of PEM are often referred to as *marasmus* and *kwashiorkor,*[6,20] as previously described (see Table 23-1).

Box 23-8 Patients at High Risk for Malnutrition

- Underweight (BMI <18.5) or recent loss of 10% or greater of usual body weight
- Poor intake: Anorexia, food avoidance (e.g., psychiatric condition), nothing allowed by mouth (NPO) status for greater than 5 to 7 days
- Protracted nutrient losses: Malabsorption, enteric fistulas, draining abscesses or wounds, or renal dialysis
- Hypermetabolic states: Sepsis, protracted fever, extensive trauma, or burns
- Chronic use of alcohol or drugs with antinutrient or catabolic properties: Steroids, antimetabolites (e.g., methotrexate), immunosuppressants, antitumor agents
- Impoverishment, isolation, advanced age, limited mobility

Micronutrient Malnutrition

The same problems causing PEM can produce deficiencies in micronutrients. Deficiencies of nutrients that are stored only in small amounts (e.g., water-soluble vitamins) or lost through external secretions (e.g., zinc in diarrhea, fluid or burn exudate) are quite common.[20] Although the causes and results of micronutrient deficiencies are beyond the scope of this chapter, a few of the most common problems are described.

Signs of scurvy (vitamin C deficiency) may be observed in chronically ill patients and patients with alcoholism hospitalized for acute illnesses. Low folic acid blood levels are common whenever illness, alcoholism, or poverty is present. Alcoholism is also associated with thiamin deficiency. Zinc deficiencies impair immunity, clotting, and slow wound healing. Magnesium deficiencies can result in cardiovascular, neurologic, and electrolyte abnormalities (hypocalcemia, hypokalemia) and decreased respiratory muscle strength. Hypophosphatemia is seen frequently with cachexia or alcoholism, especially in patients receiving intravenous glucose or taking antacids. Severe

Box 23-9 Respiratory Consequences of Malnutrition

RESPIRATORY MUSCLE DYSFUNCTION
- Loss of diaphragmatic mass and contractility
- Loss of accessory muscle mass and contractility

EFFECT ON CONTROL OF VENTILATION
- Decreased hypoxic and hypercapnic response

INCREASED INCIDENCE OF RESPIRATORY INFECTIONS
- Decreased lung clearance mechanisms
- Decreased secretory immunoglobulin A
- Increased bacterial colonization

CHANGES IN LUNG PARENCHYMAL STRUCTURE
- Unopposed enzymatic digestion
- Reduced production of surfactant

hypophosphatemia can result in decreased muscle strength and contractility and acute cardiopulmonary failure.

Respiratory Consequences of Malnutrition

Malnutrition affects all organ systems. In addition, malnutrition seems to interact with disease processes to increase the morbidity and mortality of respiratory, cardiac, and renal failure.[39] Specific effects of malnutrition on the respiratory system are listed in Box 23-9.[40]

Approximately one-third of all patients with acute respiratory failure have malnutrition. In these patients, the underlying diseases (e.g., sepsis, burns, trauma) increase energy expenditure and promote skeletal muscle catabolism. These patients are prone to hypercapnia and can be difficult to wean from mechanical ventilation. Malnourished patients who require mechanical ventilation also have higher mortality rates than patients with normal nutrition status.[41]

Malnutrition also plays a role in chronic obstructive pulmonary disease (COPD). The combined effect of increased energy expenditure (because of high work of breathing) and inadequate caloric intake contributes to a marasmus-type malnutrition. The resulting progressive muscle weakness and dyspnea can limit caloric intake further, as can several profound psychosocial factors. Box 23-10 summarizes factors contributing to malnutrition in patients with COPD.[42] The RT may notice signs that could lead to malnutrition in patients for whom they provide care (Box 23-11).

Providing the Appropriate Combination of Substrates

After estimating energy requirements, the physician or registered dietitian determines the appropriate combination of macronutrients (protein, carbohydrate, fat) needed.

Protein

Amino acids or proteins are essential to maintaining or restoring lean body mass. Because illness usually increases protein catabolism and protein requirements, the Recommended Dietary Allowance (RDA) of 0.8 g/kg/day is generally insufficient for sick patients. Based on the assessment of the protein catabolism rate, protein intake may need to be doubled or tripled above the RDA (1.5 to 2.5 g/kg/day).[43] Ideally, approximately

Box 23-10 Underlying Causes of Malnutrition in Patients With Chronic Obstructive Pulmonary Disease

INCREASED ENERGY EXPENDITURE
- Increased caloric cost of breathing
- Increased systemic inflammation
- Thermogenic effect of medications (e.g., bronchodilators)

INADEQUATE CALORIC INTAKE
- Dyspnea while eating
- Chewing and swallowing difficulties
- Early satiety
- Taste alterations from medications, nasal cannulas, or a tracheostomy
- Suppressed appetite from medications (e.g., theophylline)

PSYCHOSOCIAL FACTORS
- Depression
- Poverty
- Difficulty shopping
- Tire easily when preparing food

Box 23-11 Nutrition Status Changes Observable by Respiratory Therapists

- Mechanics of breathing can be affected by cachexia, obesity, pregnancy.
- Increased coughing effort may indicate poor nutrition.
- Viscosity of sputum, jugular venous pressure, ascites, and edema suggest fluid imbalance.
- Lung crackles relate to fluid overload or oncotic pressure changes (loss of blood protein).
- Wheezing may be associated with food intolerances, alcohol, or aspirated food particles.
- Late inspiratory crackles of atelectasis may result from decreased surfactant production from malnutrition.
- S_3 heart sounds of congestive heart failure may indicate fluid imbalance.
- S_4 heart sounds may be associated with severe anemia.
- Pulmonary function measures may be related to:
  FVC or FEV_1 decrease: Severe malnutrition
  FVC: Excess fat weight
  PEP and PIP decrease: Poor nutrition
  Lung compliance: Fluid and serum albumin changes acutely or chronic malnutrition
- Arterial blood gas values may be related to:
  $PaCO_2$ increases: Excess glucose, inadequate ventilation from lack of muscle energy
  O_2 saturation, O_2 content, hemoglobin: Nutrition status
- Meal acceptance may be related to visible equipment—suction bottles, sputum specimens.
- Lack of O_2 may increase difficulty of eating—ensure availability of O_2 via cannula if needed.

FEV_1, Forced expiratory volume in 1 second; *FVC,* forced vital capacity; *PEP,* positive expiratory pressure; *PIP,* peak inspiratory pressure.

20% of a patient's estimated caloric needs should be provided by protein. Higher percentages of protein may be needed in patients who are cachexic, have severe infections, or are otherwise critically ill. However, whenever high protein intake is administered, the patient should be monitored for progressive **azotemia** (blood urea nitrogen >100 mg/dl).[14]

Too much protein is harmful, especially for patients with limited pulmonary reserves. Excess protein can increase O_2 consumption, REE, minute ventilation, and central ventilatory drive.[43] In addition, overzealous protein feeding may lead to symptoms such as dyspnea.

Carbohydrate

Carbohydrates are the main source of fuel for the body. Adequate amounts of carbohydrates and fat help prevent protein catabolism. Glucose (dextrose) is the most commonly administered intravenous carbohydrate. Total calories per day from carbohydrates can range from 45% to 65%. In an average-sized patient, daily glucose provision is generally estimated at 200 g/day.[44]

For patients with pulmonary disease or patients requiring mechanical ventilation, high carbohydrate loads were initially blamed for increased CO_2 production and the RQ, resulting in increased ventilatory demand, O_2 consumption, and work of breathing.[45] More recent evidence indicates that this problem is probably more closely related to total calorie load (overfeeding) than to the proportion of carbohydrate in the diet.[46,47] Therefore overfeeding should be carefully avoided in patients with pulmonary disease and patients requiring mechanical ventilation.

Fat

The remaining calories (20% to 30%) should be provided from fat.[48] A minimum of 2% to 4% is needed to prevent essential fatty acid deficiency. Fat intakes greater than 50% of energy needs are associated with fever, impaired immune function, liver dysfunction, and hypotension.[14]

The initiation of nutrition support is determined by the patient's nutrition status and the estimated length of time the patient will be unable to consume a diet by mouth to meet nutrition needs. To ensure satisfactory nutrition and metabolic response, early enteral nutrition begun within 24 to 48 hours provides significant benefits to critically ill patients, including reduced infectious complications and lengths of stay.[49]

> **RULE OF THUMB**
>
> Begin enteral nutrition within 24 to 48 hours of intubation

ROUTES OF ADMINISTRATION

The two primary routes for supplying nutrients to patients are *enteral* (oral and tube feeding) and *parenteral* (peripheral or central venous alimentation). Box 23-12 provides guidelines for initiating nutrition support as recommended by the American Society for Parenteral and Enteral Nutrition.[49-51]

Box 23-12 Guidelines for Initiation of Nutrition Support

CLINICAL SETTINGS IN WHICH ENTERAL NUTRITION SHOULD BE PART OF ROUTINE CARE

- Protein-calorie malnutrition (>10% loss of usual weight) with inadequate oral intake of nutrients for previous 5 to 7 days
- Normal nutritional status with less than 50% of required nutrient intake orally for previous 7 to 10 days
- Severe dysphagia
- Moderate to severe pancreatitis (bowel rest anticipated beyond 5 to 7 days)
- Burns of greater than 15% total BSA in infants and children and greater than 25% total BSA in older children and adults
- Massive small bowel resection in combination with administration of total parenteral nutrition
- Low output (<500 ml/day) enterocutaneous fistulas

CLINICAL SETTINGS IN WHICH PARENTERAL NUTRITION SHOULD BE PART OF ROUTINE CARE

- Patients with inability to absorb nutrients by the GI tract
- Severe malnutrition in the face of a nonfunctional GI tract (within 1 to 3 days)
- Severely catabolic patients with or without malnutrition when the GI tract is not usable within 7 to 10 days

From Mueller CM, Merritt RJ, McClave S, et al, editors: The ASPEN adult nutrition support core curriculum, ed 2, Silver Spring, MD, 2012, American Society for Parenteral and Enteral Nutrition.
BSA, Body surface area; *GI,* gastrointestinal.

Enteral Feeding

Enteral feedings are the route of choice: "If the gut works, use it." The enteral route is safer and cheaper than the parenteral route. Enteral feeding stimulates gut hormones, subjects nutrients to the absorptive and metabolic controls of the intestinal tract and liver, and produces less hyperglycemia (providing for better immune function) than the parenteral route. In addition, the buffering capacity of enteral feeding can improve resistance against stress ulcers.[52] Finally, enteral feeding maintains a more normal intestinal mucosa than the parenteral route (the intestinal mucosa may undergo atrophy during parenteral nutrition).[53]

Enteral Tube Routes. There are six primary routes for enteral tube feeding: (1) nasogastric, (2) nasoduodenal, (3) nasojejunal, (4) gastrostomy, (5) jejunostomy, and (6) esophagotomy. Site selection depends on GI function, respiratory status, surgical state, and anticipated length of time the patient will be receiving tube feeding.

Gastric feedings are indicated if there are no physiologic factors affecting GI function (e.g., gastroparesis, delayed gastric emptying, or obstruction or upper GI tract surgery). Small bowel (duodenum and jejunum) feedings are indicated if the upper GI tract cannot be used. Intestinal feeding tube placement is recommended to minimize aspiration risk because it is believed to decrease the risk for gastric distention and gastroesophageal reflux; however, this remains controversial.[54]

Nasogastric and *nasoenteric* tubes are indicated for short-term enteral therapy (<30 days). The tubes are placed at the bedside and generally have a large internal diameter, which helps deliver viscous feedings and medications. *Nasoduodenal* and *nasojejunal* tubes are placed through the nose past the pylorus.

Long-term feeding tubes can be placed endoscopically and surgically. Percutaneous endoscopic placement of a feeding tube can be done to establish gastric (percutaneous endoscopic gastrostomy) or intestinal (percutaneous endoscopic jejunostomy) access. This method is preferred to surgical placement because of reduced costs associated with operating room time and the need for anesthesia.[55] Surgical laparotomy is indicated if endoscopy is contraindicated.

Tube Feeding Administration. There are three basic methods of tube feeding administration: bolus, intermittent, and continuous drip. *Bolus* feedings involve the rapid infusion of 250 to 500 ml of feeding several times daily. Feedings are provided by a syringe into the feeding tube port. There is an increased risk for aspiration associated with bolus feedings because of the rapid infusion of formula into the stomach. Nausea, vomiting, abdominal pain, and distention can develop in conjunction with this feeding route. This feeding method can be used only with gastric tubes and is primarily applied to patients who are stable and patients receiving enteral nutrition support at home.

Intermittent feedings are also administered several times per day, but are infused over at least 30-minutes. Feedings can be given only into the gastric cavity. Intermittent feedings are associated with the same problems as bolus feedings.

Continuous drip infusion provides a constant, steady flow of formula at a predetermined rate for a set period, generally 12 to 24 hours per day. Drip regulators, roll clamps, or pumps are used to control rates. Because the small bowel lacks storage capacity, feedings delivered beyond the pylorus must be provided by the continuous drip method. This method is preferred for critically ill patients because it is associated with reductions in gastric residual volume, abdominal distention, gastroesophageal reflux, and pulmonary aspiration.[56]

Trophic feeding is the practice of feeding minimal amounts (10 to 30 ml/hr) of enteral nutrition with the primary goal to maintain GI function and integrity. Studies in mechanically ventilated patients with respiratory failure or ARDS show that trophic feedings resulted in fewer episodes of GI intolerance but resulted in similar clinical outcomes compared to early advancement to full enteral feedings.[57]

Enteral Formula Selection. Selection of an enteral formula depends on the patient's medical and surgical state, GI function, energy and nutrient needs, and route of administration. There are eight broad categories of enteral formulas: oral supplements, blenderized, whole-protein lactose-free, fiber containing, nutrient-dense, elemental, disease-specific, and modular. Table 23-4 describes the indications for the various enteral formulas and lists examples of commercial preparations.

Complications of Enteral Therapy. Complications associated with enteral nutrition are categorized as GI, mechanical, or metabolic. These may be avoided by careful selection of formulas, proper administration, and consistent patient monitoring.

Pulmonary aspiration is of particular concern in a critically ill patient with respiratory disease. Aspiration can occur because of one or more of the following factors: if the patient is lying flat, has a depressed gag reflux or vocal cord dysfunction, has delayed gastric emptying, or has improper tube placement. The incidence of pulmonary aspiration varies depending on the patient population and technique used to identify aspiration in the tube-fed patient. The three following practices are proved to minimize aspiration risk[51]: (1) raise the head of the bed at

TABLE 23-4
Enteral Product Reference Guide

Category	Indications	Examples
Oral supplements	Given with an oral diet to increase calorie and protein intake	Boost,* Ensure,† Carnation Breakfast Essentials
Standard/Polymeric	Made with intact nutrients. May vary in concentration (1.0-2.0 kcal/ml) and fiber content	Osmolite,† Jevity,† Promotel HN,† Nutren,† Isosource,† Fibersource,* Replete*
Blenderized	Made from natural foods and usually lower in sucrose and corn syrup than other formulas; beneficial if intolerance to synthetic formulas exists	Compleat,* Compleat Pediatric*
Elemental and semi-elemental	Impaired gastrointestinal function with impaired ability to digest or absorb intact nutrients	Peptamen,† Peptamen 1.5,† Tolerex,† Vivonex,† Vital,* Vital 1.5,* Vital HN*
Disease specific	Liver disease; renal disease; pulmonary disease; glucose intolerance; immune-enhancing; critically ill obese	Nutrihe*; Nepro,* NovaSource Renal,† Suplena,* Renalcal†; Pulmocare,* Oxepa,* Nutren Pulmonary†; Diabetisource AC,† Glucerna,* Glytrol†; Impact,† Pivot*; Peptamen Bariatric† Vital High Protein†*
Modular	Need to modify a single nutrient (carbohydrate, protein, fat)	Beneprotein,* Benecalorie,† Promod,* Glutasolve,† Arginaid,†, MCT oil†

*Nestle Health Sciences.
†Abbott Nutrition.

least 30 degrees, (2) use of bowel motility agents such as metoclopramide, and (3) using postpyloric feeding with the continuous drip method in patients at risk for gastric atony or gastroesophageal reflux. Tube placement always should be verified by x-ray examination before feeding. Pulmonary aspiration has not been proved to be a result of high gastric residual volumes.[58]

Aggressive suctioning of oropharyngeal secretions can help prevent aspiration. The greatest risk is in patients with endotracheal tubes. Endotracheal tubes increase aspiration risk because they alter sensation, impair glottic closure, increase secretion volume, and act as "wicks" to allow secretions to enter the airway.[59] The use of special endotracheal tubes that provide continuous, low-level suctioning of subglottic secretions reduce the microaspiration common in tube-fed patients.[60] The use of blue dye to detect aspiration is no longer a standard practice because of numerous problems, including a U.S. Food and Drug Administration Public Health Advisory issued in 2003. Blue discoloration of body parts and fluids followed by refractory hypotension, metabolic acidosis, and death were reported in some patients receiving blue food dye.[61]

Parenteral Nutrition Support

When it is impossible to provide nutrition support through the GI tract, intravenous or parenteral nutrition support may be needed. Parenteral nutrition support is administered through a peripheral or central vein. Ideally, the vascular access line should be restricted to nutrition use and maintained as a sterile route. Because the volume and concentration of nutrients given through a small vein are limited, peripheral parenteral nutrition is considered only for short-term support. Mechanical, infectious, and metabolic complications have been reported in patients fed parenterally.[62]

NUTRITION SUPPORT IN SPECIFIC CIRCUMSTANCES

Details on the appropriate nutrition support provided to all the various types of patients seen by RTs are beyond the scope of this chapter. This section emphasizes key points related to nutrition support and management of the most common conditions encountered by practitioners.

General Guidelines for Critically Ill Patients

The general goal of nutrition support in critically ill patients is to provide the energy and protein necessary to meet metabolic demands and to preserve lean body mass. Nutritional support is also an important therapy in critical illness because it attenuates the metabolic response to stress, prevents oxidative cellular injury, and modulates the immune response. Nutritional modulation of the stress response includes early enteral nutrition, appropriate macronutrient and micronutrient delivery, and meticulous glycemic control.[57]

Table 23-5 outlines the general guidelines recommended to achieve these goals.[49]

TABLE 23-5
General Nutrition Guidelines for Chronically Critically Ill Patients

Category	Guideline
Route of delivery	Enteral nutrition is preferred when the gut is functional. Start 24-48 hr after resuscitation. If gut is not functional, consider starting parenteral nutrition. If enteral nutrition cannot provide goal within 7-10 days, consider starting parenteral nutrition.
Energy need	Indirect calorimety should be used when available for estimation of energy goal. Target is 65% of goal within the first week. Hypocaloric feeding recommended for obese (11-14 kcal/kg).
Protein	Provide supplemental protein to achieve 1.2-2.0 g/kg/day; 2.0-2.5 g/kg/day for obese.
Glycemic control	An intensive insulin therapy protocol should be in place Goal: 110-150 mg/dl
Micronutrients	Adequate vitamins and minerals such as vitamins A, B_6, C, E; potassium; magnesium; zinc; iron; selenium; phosphate
Fluid	Approximately 1 ml/kcal
Specialized nutrients	Glutamine (may improve nitrogen stores), arginine (may improve immune system in surgical patients), and omega-3 fatty acids (may reduce inflammatory processes in ARDS/ALI)

Compiled from: McClave SA, Martindale RG, Vanek VW, et al, Society of Critical Care Medicine (SCCM) and American Society for Parenteral and Enteral Nutrition: Guidelines for the provision and assessment of nutrition support therapy in the adult critically ill patient. JPEN J Parenter Enteral Nutr 33:277, 2009.
ALI, Acute lung injury; *ARDS,* acute respiratory distress syndrome.

Systemic Inflammatory Response Syndrome

The *systemic inflammatory response syndrome (SIRS)* underlies many critical illnesses, including *sepsis* and *acute respiratory distress syndrome (ARDS)*. Metabolism in systemic inflammatory response syndrome is characterized by increased total caloric requirements, hyperglycemia, triglyceride intolerance, increased net protein catabolism, and increased macronutrient and micronutrient requirements.[39]

Micronutrient requirements also are increased in SIRS. Because of the potential high losses of potassium, zinc, magnesium, calcium, and phosphorus, serum levels of these minerals need to be closely monitored and maintained within the normal range.[39]

Mechanical Ventilation

Adequate nutrition support is crucial for ventilator-dependent patients. During acute illness, proper nutrition helps prevent the loss of lean body mass. After the resolution of the acute phase of illness, good nutrition helps the muscles regain strength and improves the likelihood of successful weaning.[20]

For most patients requiring ventilatory support, following the guidelines provided in Table 23-5 is generally sufficient. As always, care must be taken to avoid overfeeding and the increased ventilatory demands that follow. Patients with COPD present a special situation, in terms of both nutrition needs and ventilatory support. More details regarding these patients are provided in the next section.

Nutrition support alone is insufficient to ensure weaning of ventilator-dependent patients. For these patients, appropriate nutrition may need to be combined with a tailored exercise program designed to strengthen and retrain muscles. Methods used to wean ventilator-dependent patients are discussed in detail in Chapter 52.

Chronic Obstructive Pulmonary Disease

Malnutrition is common in patients with COPD and can occur in 30% to 60% of inpatients and 10% to 45% of outpatients.[63] Progressive weight loss from malnutrition is common in patients with COPD and appears to have two causes: prolonged periods of insufficient caloric intake coupled with increased nutritional needs resulting from increased metabolism demand associated with chronic disease. Both malnutrition and low body weight seem to be factors associated with a poor prognosis.[64]

The degree of weight loss generally correlates with deterioration of pulmonary function values. COPD can create a cycle in which respiratory dysfunction promotes weight loss and weight loss further hinders respiratory function.[40] Figure 23-3 illustrates the cycle.

Factors contributing to poor intake include fatigue, shortness of breath, frequent coughing, early fullness because of pressure on the abdominal cavity, increased dyspnea during eating, side effects from medications (nausea, vomiting, diarrhea, dry mouth, taste changes), and depression. The increased metabolic rate is due to the added effort to breathe and frequent

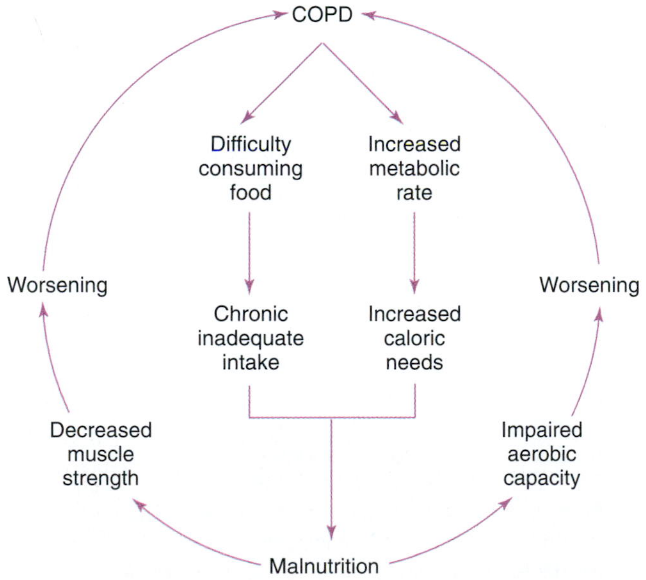

FIGURE 23-3 The vicious cycle of respiratory impairment and malnutrition in chronic obstructive pulmonary disease.

respiratory infections, both of which increase calorie and fluid needs.

The goal is to increase nutrient intake carefully without overfeeding. Cachexic patients with COPD should be refed cautiously.[65] Functional capacity and the patient's overall health status may improve with an anabolic stimulus, such as exercise, along with nutrition supplementation.[66]

In patients with COPD, satisfactory conventional macronutrient allocations are 15% to 20% as protein, 50% to 60% as carbohydrates, and 20% to 30% as fat. Specialized nutrition formulation consisting of high fat and, reduced carbohydrate have been marketed for patients with COPD; however, there is little evidence to support its use.[63,67] As previously stated, setting an appropriate total calorie load is more important than fine-tuning the ratio of carbohydrates to fat.

Given the positive link between dietary intake and knowledge of diet and health, good patient education is crucial. Patients should be taught to select easy-to-consume, calorically dense foods. Emphasis should be placed on small, frequent feedings, and encourage use of high-calorie, high-protein nutrition supplements. Other considerations in providing nutrition support to patients with COPD are listed in Box 23-13.[68-70]

When patients with COPD are hospitalized for ventilatory failure, the clinical outcome is affected by nutrition support. Patients who receive adequate nutrition support are more readily weaned from mechanical ventilation than patients with diets deficient in protein and energy.

MINI CLINI

Methods to Increase Nutrient Intake in Chronic Obstructive Pulmonary Disease

PROBLEM: An 82-year-old woman with known history of COPD has been hospitalized for several days and treated with multiple inhalers and nebulizers. She lost 12 pounds in the last month. She presents with muscle wasting, sparse hair, dry and cracked lips and skin. She reports decrease in oral intake because of shortness of breath and decreased appetite satiety. The dietitian receives a nutrition consult to evaluate the patient's nutrition status and provides nutrition counseling to prevent further weight loss.

List sample foods and potential strategies the dietitian reviewed with the patient that the RT can reinforce with the patient.

- Dried fruits, nuts, Popsicles, milkshakes
- Whole milk or skim milk powder added to milk, soup, gravies
- Nutrition supplements
- Puddings, custards, yogurt, ice cream
- Cream soups
- Add butter or oil or cheese to vegetables, soups, mashed potatoes, and rice
- Casseroles and egg dishes with sauces and gravies
- Peanut butter or other nut butters, spread on bananas, celery, crackers, apple slices, breads

Box 23-13 Nutrition Support for Patients With Pulmonary Disease

- Perform a complete nutrition assessment.
- Evaluate energy needs and provide an appropriate amount (do not overfeed or underfeed).
- Ensure protein balance.
- Monitor fluids and electrolytes, especially phosphorus.
- Evaluate vitamin and mineral status as indicated.

Asthma

Because breathing and eating are mutually exclusive, feeding should generally be avoided during severe asthma attacks. However, nutrient-dense, small meals high in quality protein, calories, vitamins, and minerals are recommended during prolonged, mild asthma attacks. Foods identified as allergens (most often milk, eggs, seafood, and fish) should be avoided. Fluid intake should be generous, unless contraindicated. Saturated fats may aggravate the airway, whereas omega-3 fatty acids may be beneficial; these are available in walnuts and flaxseed if the patient is allergic to fish.[68]

Cystic Fibrosis

Exocrine gland dysfunction associated with cystic fibrosis causes chronic lung disease with recurrent infections. The same disturbance causes pancreatic insufficiency. Metabolic problems in patients with cystic fibrosis are similar to metabolic problems in patients with COPD, with reduced intake and increased metabolic needs. However, the associated pancreatic insufficiency with cystic fibrosis also causes malabsorption of all nutrients, especially fat. The administration of pancreatic enzyme supplements with meals enhances absorption but requires trial and error and intense education on how to balance the amount of food and the intake of enzymes. In addition, the time spent in various treatment programs reduces the ability to consume small frequent feedings.

The goals of nutrition management in cystic fibrosis are to (1) maximize nutrition intake through calorically dense foods, (2) balance intake with pancreatic enzymes to maximize absorption, and (3) provide a nutrition plan that meets the patient's changing clinical and psychosocial status.[68] Use of calorically dense foods and nutrition supplements consumed throughout the day has proved helpful in achieving weight gain.[68] Because of the malabsorption of micronutrients, vitamin and mineral supplementation is encouraged, especially of fat-soluble vitamins.[68] Helping patients with cystic fibrosis achieve optimal nutritional health may minimize the decline in pulmonary function and improve their quality of life.[71]

SUMMARY CHECKLIST

- Nutrition assessment is the basis for developing a nutrition care plan.
- The components of a nutrition assessment include dietary history, anthropometry, biochemical indicators, nutrition-focused physical assessment, and client history.
- BMI is a comparison of weight to height used to determine underweight, healthy weight, overweight, obesity, or morbid obesity.
- Classifications of undernutrition, called *protein-energy malnutrition,* include kwashiorkor, marasmus, and a combination of the two (lack of circulating protein, starvation, and a mixture of the two).
- Laboratory values of albumin, transferrin, transthyretin, and retinal-binding protein may indicate malnutrition. CRP may be elevated during acute illness, indicating an inflammatory response and causing low values of serum proteins.
- The creatinine-height index reflects skeletal muscle mass.
- Nitrogen balance compares protein intake to nitrogen excretion in the urine.
- Observable signs in hair, eyes, lips, mouth and gums, skin, and nails may indicate malnutrition.
- Resting energy expenditure (REE) may be determined by the predictive equations or indirect calorimetry.
- Estimation of total caloric need involves multiplying the REE by a factor that accounts for activity and stressors.
- Indirect calorimetry involves measurement of whole-body $\dot{V}O_2$, $\dot{V}CO_2$, and respiratory quotient (RQ); results are used to assess a patient's metabolic state, determine nutrition needs, or assess response to nutrition therapy.
- RQ greater than 1.00 indicates overfeeding and the need to decrease total calories; RQ between the ranges of 0.67 to 1.3 should be used as an indicator of test validity.
- Malnutrition is a state of impaired metabolism in which the intake of essential nutrients is less than the body's needs; marasmus is malnutrition associated with inadequate nutrient intake (starvation), and kwashiorkor is the hypercatabolic form.
- Malnutrition can affect the respiratory system by causing loss of respiratory muscle mass and contractility, decreased ventilatory drive, impaired immune response, and alterations in lung parenchymal structure.
- Approximately one-third of all patients with acute respiratory failure have malnutrition, mainly the hypercatabolic form; these patients are prone to hypercapnia, can be difficult to wean from ventilatory support, and have higher mortality rates than patients with a normal nutrition status.
- In chronic lung disease, the combined effect of increased energy expenditure (secondary to increased work of breathing) and inadequate caloric intake contributes to a marasmus-type malnutrition.
- The primary goal of nutrition support is to maintain or restore lean body (skeletal muscle) mass by (1) meeting the overall energy needs of the patient and (2) providing the appropriate combination of macronutrients (protein, carbohydrate, and fat) and micronutrients (vitamins and minerals). Nutrition support also attenuates the metabolic response to stress, prevents oxidative cellular injury, and modulates the immune response.
- For most patients, a balance of 20% of daily calorie needs from protein, 50% to 60% from simple carbohydrate, and 20% to 30% from fat is adequate.
- Nutrients can be supplied enterally (oral and tube feeding) or parenterally (peripheral or central venous alimentation); the enteral route should be used whenever possible.

- The likelihood of aspiration during tube feedings can be minimized by raising the head of the bed at least 30 degrees, use of motility agents, and delivering the feeding beyond the pylorus using the continuous drip method.
- Nutrition support should be individualized according to patient needs and condition or disease process; accepted guidelines for SIRS, COPD, mechanical ventilation, asthma, and cystic fibrosis should be followed.

References

1. Academy of Nutrition and Dietetics: *International dietetic and nutrition terminology (IDNT) reference manual*, ed 4, Chicago, 2013, The Academy.
2. U.S. Department of Agriculture and U.S. Department of Health and Human Services: *Nutrition and your health: dietary guidelines for Americans*, Washington, DC, 2010, U.S. Government Printing Office.
3. U.S. Department of Agriculture: *MyPlate*. <http://www.choosemyplate.gov>, Accessed June 3, 2014.
4. U.S. Department of Agriculture, U.S. Department of Health and Human Services: *Nutrition and your health: dietary guidelines for Americans*, Washington, DC, 2005, U.S. Government Printing Office.
5. Centers for Disease Control and Prevention, National Center for Health Statistics: *Growth charts*. <http://www.cdc.gov/growthcharts>, Accessed June 3, 2014.
6. Shils ME, Shike M, Ross AC, et al, editors: *Modern nutrition in health and disease*, ed 10, Philadelphia, 2006, Lippincott Williams & Wilkins.
7. Lee RD, Neiman DC: *Nutritional assessment*, ed 4, Boston, 2007, McGraw-Hill.
8. Soler-Cataluna JJ, Sanchez-Sanchez L, Martinez-Garcia MA, et al: Mid-arm muscle area is a better predictor of mortality than body mass index in COPD. *Chest* 128:2108–2115, 2005.
9. Janssen I, Katzmarzyk PT, Ross R: Waist circumference and not body mass index explains obesity-related health risk. *Am J Clin Nutr* 79:379–384, 2004.
10. Snijder MG, van Dam RM, Visser M, et al: What aspects of body fat are particularly hazardous and how do we measure them? *Int J Epidemiol* 35:83–92, 2006.
11. Ness-Ambramof R, Apovian CM: Waist circumference measurement in clinical practice. *Nutr Clin Pract* 23:397–404, 2008.
12. Forse RA, Shizgal HM: Serum albumin and nutritional status. *JPEN J Parenter Enteral Nutr* 4:450–454, 1980.
13. Jensen GL: Inflammation as the key interface of the medical and nutrition universe a provocative examination of the future of clinical nutrition and medicine. *JPEN J Parenter Enteral Nutr* 30:453–463, 2006.
14. Whitney EN, Rolges SR: *Understanding nutrition*, ed 13, Belmont, CA, 2012, Wadsworth.
15. Don BR, Kaysen G: Serum albumin: relationship to inflammation and nutrition. *Semin Dial* 17:432–437, 2004.
16. Bloch AS, Maillet J, Howell WH, et al, editors: *Issues and choices in clinical nutrition practice*, Philadelphia, 2007, Lippincott Williams & Wilkins.
17. Lelubre C, Anselin S, Boudjeltia KZ, et al: Interpretation of C-reactive protein concentrations in critically ill patients. *Bio Med Res Int* 124021, 2013.
18. Deodhar SD: C-reactive protein: the best laboratory indicator available for monitoring disease activity. *Cleve Clin J Med* 56:126–130, 1989.
19. Lowe GD: Circulating inflammatory markers and risks of cardiovascular and non-cardiovascular disease. *J Thromb Haemost* 3:1618–1627, 2005.
20. Gropper SS, Smith JL, Groff JL: *Advanced nutrition and human metabolism*, ed 5, Belmont CA, 2009, Wadsworth, Cengage Learning.
21. Kuzuya M, Kanda S, Koike T, et al: Lack of correlation between total lymphocyte count and nutritional status in the elderly. *Clin Nutr* 24:427–432, 2005.
22. Sopena N, Heras E, Casas I, et al: Risk factors for hospital acquired pneumonia outside the intensive care unit: a case-control study. *Am J Infect Control* 42:38–42, 2014.
23. Jensen GL, Hsiao PY, Wheeler D: Adult nutrition assessment tutorial. *JPEN J Parenter Enteral Nutr* 36:267–274, 2012.
24. Lutz C, Przytulski K: *Nutrition and diet therapy*, ed 5, Jackson Community College; Jackson MS, 2011, FA Davis.
25. White JV, Guenter P, Jensen G, et al; Academy of Nutrition and Dietetics and American Society for Parenteral and Enteral Nutrition: Consensus statement: characteristics recommended for the identification and documentation of adult malnutrition (undernutrition). *JPEN J Parenter Enteral Nutr* 36:275–283, 2012.
26. Barker LA, Gout BS, Crowe TC: Hospital malnutrition: prevalence, identification and impact on patients and the healthcare system. *Int J Environ Res Public Health* 8:514–527, 2011.
27. Cerra FB, Benitez MR, Blackburn GL, et al: Applied nutrition in ICU patients: a consensus statement of the American College of Chest Physicians. *Chest* 111:769–778, 1997.
28. Academy of Nutrition and Dietetics. *Evidence analysis library*, 2014. <http://www.andeal.org>, Accessed September, 2014.
29. Frankenfield D, Hise M, Malone A, et al: Prediction of resting metabolic rate in critically ill adult patients: results of a systematic review of the evidence. *J Am Diet Assoc* 107:1552–1561, 2007.
30. Wooley JA, Frankenfield D: Energy. In Mueller CM, Merritt RJ, McClave S, et al, editors: *The ASPEN adult nutrition support core curriculum*, ed 2, Silver Spring, MD, 2012, American Society for Parenteral and Enteral Nutrition.
31. American Association of Respiratory Care: Clinical practice guideline: metabolic measurement using indirect calorimetry during mechanical ventilation. *Respir Care* 49:1073–1076, 2004.
32. Branson RD: The measurement of energy expenditure: instrumentation, practical considerations and clinical application. *Resp Care* 35:640–659, 1990.
33. McArthur C: Indirect calorimetry. *Respir Care Clin North Am* 3:291–304, 1997.
34. Long CL, Schaffel N, Geiger JW, et al: Metabolic response to injury and illness: estimation of energy and protein needs from indirect calorimetry and nitrogen balance. *JPEN J Parenter Enteral Nutr* 3:452–456, 1979.
35. McClave SA, Lowen CC, Kleber MJ, et al: Clinical use of the respiratory quotient obtained from indirect calorimetry. *JPEN J Parenter Enteral Nutr* 27:21–26, 2003.
36. Haugen HA, Chan LN, Li F: Indirect calorimetry: a practical guide for clinicians. *Nutr Clin Pract* 22:377–388, 2007.
37. Mehta NM, Smallwood CD, Joosten KF, et al: Accuracy of a simplified equation for energy expenditure based on bedside volumetric carbon dioxide elimination measurement: a two-center study. *Clin Nutr* 2014. (in press).
38. Hoffer LJ, Bistrian BR: Why critically ill patients are protein deprived. *JPEN J Parenter Enteral Nutr* 37:300–309, 2013.
39. Miller K, Kiraly L, Martindale RG: Critical care sepsis. In Mueller CM, Merritt RJ, McClave S, et al, editors: *The ASPEN adult nutrition support core curriculum*, ed 2, Silver Spring, MD, 2012, American Society for Parenteral and Enteral Nutrition.
40. Mechanick JI, Brett EM: Nutrition and the chronically critically ill patient. *Curr Opin Clin Nutr Metab Care* 8:33–39, 2005.
41. Bergman EA, Buergel NS: Diseases of the respiratory system. In Nelms M, Sucher K, Long S, editors: *Nutrition therapy and pathophysiology*, Belmont, CA, 2007, Thomson.
42. Baltz JE: Nutrition assessment. In Egan DF, Kacmarek RM, Stoller JK, et al, editors: *Egan's fundamentals of respiratory care*, ed 10, St Louis, 2013, Mosby.
43. Young LS, Kearns LR, Schoefel SL, et al: Protein. In Mueller CM, Merritt RJ, McClave S, et al, editors: *The ASPEN adult nutrition support core curriculum*, ed 2, Silver Spring, MD, 2012, American Society for Parenteral and Enteral Nutrition.
44. Ling PR, McCowen KC: Carbohydrates. In Mueller CM, Merritt RJ, McClave S, et al, editors: *The ASPEN adult nutrition support core curriculum*, ed 2, Silver Spring, MD, 2012, American Society for Parenteral and Enteral Nutrition.
45. Shikora SA, Benotti PN: Nutritional support of the mechanically ventilated patient. *Respir Care Clin North Am* 3:69–90, 1997.

46. Baker JP, Detsky AS, Stewart S, et al: Randomized trial of total parenteral nutrition in crucially ill patients: metabolic effects of varying glucose-lipid ratios as the energy source. *Gastroenterology* 87:53–59, 1984.
47. Talpers SS, Romberger DJ, Bunce SB, et al: Nutritionally associated increased carbon dioxide production: excess total calories versus high proportion of carbohydrate calories. *Chest* 102:551–555, 1992.
48. Institute of Medicine of the National Academies: *Dietary reference intakes for energy, carbohydrate, fiber, fat, fatty acids, cholesterol, protein, and amino acids*, Washington, DC, 2005, National Academy Press.
49. McClave SA, Martindale RG, Vanek VW, et al; Society of Critical Care Medicine, American Society for Parenteral and Enteral Nutrition: Guidelines for the provision and assessment of nutrition support therapy in the adult critically ill patient. *JPEN J Parenter Enteral Nutr* 33:277–282, 2009.
50. American Society for Parenteral and Enteral Nutrition: Standards of practice for nutrition support dietitians. *Nutr Clin Pract* 22:558–586, 2007.
51. Mueller CM, Merritt RJ, McClave S, et al, editors: *The ASPEN adult nutrition support core curriculum*, ed 2, Silver Spring, MD, 2012, American Society for Parenteral and Enteral Nutrition.
52. Hurt RT, Frazier TH, McClave SA, et al: Stress prophylaxis in intensive care unit patients and the role of enteral nutrition. *J Parenter Enteral Nutr* 36:721–731, 2012.
53. Mahan LK, Escott-Stump S, editors: *Krause's food, nutrition, and diet therapy*, ed 11, Philadelphia, 2004, Saunders.
54. Zhang Z, Xu X, Ding J, et al: Comparison of postpyloric tube feeding and gastric tube feeding in intensive care unit patients: a meta-analysis. *Nutr Clin Pract* 28371–28380, 2013.
55. Fang JC, Bankhead R, Kinikini M: Enteral access devices. In Mueller CM, Merritt RJ, McClave S, et al, editors: *The ASPEN adult nutrition support core curriculum*, ed 2, Silver Spring, MD, 2012, American Society for Parenteral and Enteral Nutrition.
56. Rolanelli RH, Bankhead R, Boullata J, editors: *Clinical nutrition enteral and tube feeding*, ed 4, Philadelphia, 2000, Saunders.
57. Rice TW, Wheeler AP, Thompson BT, et al: Initial trophic vs full enteral feeding in patients with acute lung injury: the EDEN randomized trial. *JAMA* 307:795–803, 2012.
58. McClave SA, Lukan JK, Stefater JA, et al: Poor validity of residual volumes as a marker for risk for aspiration in critically ill patients. *Crit Care Med* 33:324–330, 2005.
59. Elpern EH: Pulmonary aspiration in hospitalized adults. *Nutr Clin Pract* 12:5–13, 1997.
60. Muscedere J, Rewa O, Mckechnie K, et al: Subglottic secretion drainage for prevention of ventilator-associated pneumonia: a systematic review and meta-analysis. *Crit Care Med* 39:1985–1991, 2011.
61. U.S. Food and Drug Administration. *FDA Public Health Advisory September 29, 2003: reports of blue discoloration and death in patients receiving enteral feedings tinted with dye*, FD&C Blue No. 1.
62. Kumpf VJ, Gervasio J: Complications of parenteral nutrition. In Mueller CM, Merritt RJ, McClave S, et al, editors: *The ASPEN adult nutrition support core curriculum*, ed 2, Silver Spring, MD, 2012, American Society for Parenteral and Enteral Nutrition.
63. Turner KL: Pulmonary failure. In Mueller CM, Merritt RJ, McClave S, et al, editors: *The ASPEN adult nutrition support core curriculum*, ed 2, Silver Spring, MD, 2012, American Society for Parenteral and Enteral Nutrition.
64. Collins PF, Elia M, Stratton RJ: Nutritional support and functional capacity in chronic obstructive pulmonary disease: a systematic review and meta-analysis. *Respirology* 18:616–629, 2013.
65. Mehanna HM, Moledina J, Tracis J: Refeeding syndrome: what it is, and how to prevent it and treat it. *BMJ* 336:1495–1498, 2008.
66. Mallampalli A: Nutritional management of the patient with chronic obstructive pulmonary disease. *Nutr Clin Pract* 19:550–556, 2004.
67. Akrabawi SS, Mobarhan S, Stoltz RR, et al: Gastric emptying, pulmonary function, gas exchange, and respiratory quotient after feeding a moderate versus high fat enteral formula meal in chronic obstructive pulmonary disease patients. *Nutrition* 12:260–265, 1996.
68. Escott-Stump S: *Nutrition and diagnosis-related care*, ed 7, Philadelphia, 2012, Lippincott Williams & Wilkins.
69. Pronsky ZM: *Food medication interactions*, ed 14, Birchrunville, PA, 2006, Food-Medication Interactions.
70. Physicians' desk reference. <http://www.pdr.net>, Accessed September 19, 2014.
71. McPhail GL, Acton JD, Fenchel MC, et al: Improvements in lung function outcomes in children with cystic fibrosis are associated with better nutrition fewer chronic pseudomona aeruginosa infections, and dornase alfa use. *J Pediatr* 153:752–757, 2008.

SECTION IV

REVIEW OF CARDIOPULMONARY DISEASE

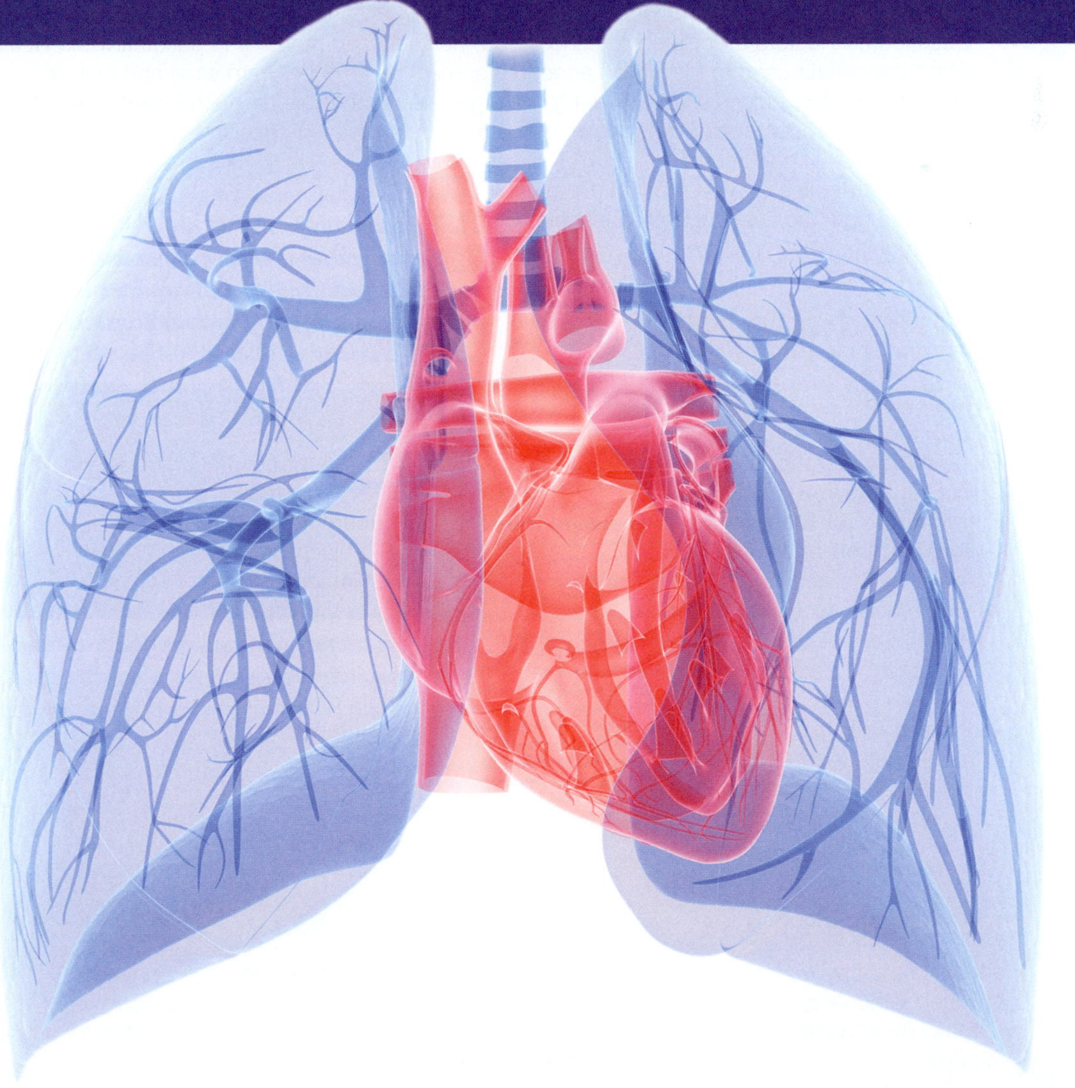

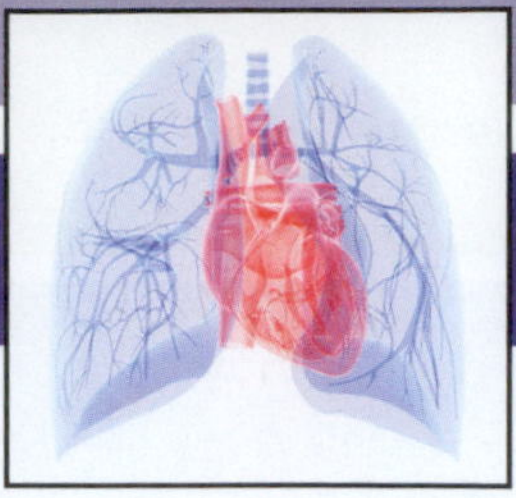

CHAPTER 24

Pulmonary Infections

SARAH A. LONGWORTH, STEVEN K. SCHMITT, AND DAVID L. LONGWORTH

CHAPTER OBJECTIVES

After reading this chapter you will be able to:

- State the incidence and economic impact of pneumonia in the United States.
- Discuss the current classification scheme for pneumonia and be able to define hospital-acquired pneumonia, health care–associated pneumonia, and ventilator-associated pneumonia.
- Recognize the pathophysiology and common causes of lower respiratory tract infections in specific clinical settings.
- List the common microbiologic organisms responsible for community-acquired and nosocomial pneumonias.
- Describe the clinical and radiographic findings seen in patients with pneumonia.
- Describe risk factors associated with increased morbidity and mortality in patients with pneumonia.
- State the criteria used to identify an adequate sputum sample for Gram stain and culture.
- Describe the techniques used to identify the organism responsible for nosocomial pneumonia.
- List the latest recommendations regarding empiric and pathogen-specific antibiotic regimens used to treat various types of pneumonia.
- Discuss strategies to prevent pneumonia.
- Describe how the respiratory therapist aids in diagnosis and management of patients with suspected pneumonia.

CHAPTER OUTLINE

Classification
Pathogenesis
Microbiology
Clinical Manifestations
Chest Radiograph
Risk Factors for Mortality and Assessing the Need for Hospitalization
Diagnostic Studies
- Community-Acquired Pneumonia
- Health Care–Associated Pneumonia, Hospital-Acquired Pneumonia, and Ventilator-Associated Pneumonia

Antibiotic Therapy
- Community-Acquired Pneumonia
- Health Care–Associated Pneumonia, Hospital-Acquired Pneumonia, and Ventilator-Associated Pneumonia

Prevention
- Community-Acquired Pneumonia
- Health Care–Associated Pneumonia, Hospital-Acquired Pneumonia, and Ventilator-Associated Pneumonia

Tuberculosis
- Epidemiology
- Pathophysiology
- Diagnosis
- Precautions
- Treatment

Role of the Respiratory Therapist in Pulmonary Infections

KEY TERMS

antibiotic therapy
atypical pathogens
community-acquired pneumonia
fomites
health care–associated pneumonia
hospital-acquired pneumonia
lower respiratory tract infection
nosocomial pneumonia
pneumonia
tuberculosis
ventilator-associated pneumonia

Infection involving the lungs is termed **pneumonia** or **lower respiratory tract infection** (LRTI) and is a common clinical problem in the practice of respiratory care. Today, pneumonia remains a major cause of morbidity and mortality in the United States and worldwide. Each year, 5 million people die from pneumonia worldwide. Five million cases of pneumonia occur annually in the United States, of which approximately 1.1 million require hospitalization at a projected yearly cost of more than $20 billion.[1] Pneumonia is the ninth leading cause of death in the United States and the leading cause of infection-related mortality.[2]

CLASSIFICATION

Pneumonia can be classified based on the clinical setting in which it occurs (Table 24-1). This classification is useful because it predicts the likely microbial causes and guides empiric antimicrobial therapy while a definitive microbiologic diagnosis is awaited. (The term *empiric therapy* refers to treatment that is initiated based on the most likely cause of infection when the specific causative organism is still unknown.)

TABLE 24-1

Classifications and Possible Causes of Pneumonia

Classification	Likely Organisms
Community-Acquired: Acute	
Typical	*Streptococcus pneumoniae*
	Haemophilus influenzae
	Moraxella catarrhalis
	Staphylococcus aureus
Atypical	*Legionella pneumophila*
	Chlamydophila pneumoniae
	Mycoplasma pneumoniae
	Viruses
	Coxiella burnetii
Community-acquired: Chronic	*Mycobacterium tuberculosis*
	Histoplasma capsulatum
	Blastomycosis dermatitidis
	Coccidioides immitis
Health care-associated	Mixed aerobic and anaerobic mouth flora
	S. aureus
	Enteric gram-negative bacilli
	Influenza
	Mycobacterium tuberculosis
Immunocompromised host	*Pneumocystis jiroveci*
	Cytomegalovirus
	Aspergillus species
	Cryptococcus neoformans
	Reactivation tuberculosis or histoplasmosis
Nosocomial	
Aspiration	Mixed aerobes and anaerobes, gram-negative bacilli
Health care-associated	*S. aureus*
Ventilator-associated	*Pseudomonas aeruginosa*
	Acinetobacter species
	Enterobacter species
	Klebsiella species
	Stenotrophomonas maltophilia
	S. aureus

Community-acquired pneumonia (CAP) can be divided into two types—acute and chronic—based on its clinical presentation. *Acute* pneumonia presents with sudden onset over a few hours to several days. The clinical presentation may be typical or atypical, depending on the pathogen. The onset of *chronic* pneumonia is more insidious, often with gradually escalating symptoms over days, weeks, or months.

Pneumonia acquired in health care settings is often caused by microorganisms different from those that cause CAP. Previously termed **nosocomial pneumonia**, this clinical entity has been further classified as **health care–associated pneumonia** (HCAP), **hospital-acquired pneumonia** (HAP), and **ventilator-associated pneumonia** (VAP).[3] HCAP is defined as pneumonia occurring in any patient hospitalized for 2 or more days in the past 90 days in an acute-care setting or who in the past 30 days has resided in a long-term care or nursing facility; attended a hospital or hemodialysis clinic; or received intravenous antibiotics, chemotherapy, or wound care. HAP is defined as an LRTI that develops in hospitalized patients more than 48 hours after admission and excludes community-acquired infections that are incubating at the time of admission. VAP is defined as an LRTI that develops more than 48 to 72 hours after endotracheal intubation.

HAP is a common clinical problem and represents the second most common nosocomial infection in the United States, accounting for 15% to 22% of all such infections.[4-6] Current estimates suggest that more than 150,000 individuals develop HAP each year. HAP increases hospital length of stay 7 to 9 days at an average incremental per-patient cost of $40,000. In selected populations, such as patients in the intensive care unit (ICU) and bone marrow transplant recipients, the crude mortality rate from HAP may approach 30% to 70%, with attributable mortality of 33% to 50%. Certain microorganisms, such as *Pseudomonas aeruginosa* and *Acinetobacter* species, are associated with higher rates of mortality.[7]

PATHOGENESIS

Six pathogenetic mechanisms may contribute to the development of pneumonia (Table 24-2). Knowledge of these mechanisms is important to both the understanding of the various disease processes and the formulation of effective strategies within the hospital to minimize nosocomial spread. Inhalation of infectious particles is a common route of inoculation; this method of acquiring an infection occurs with pulmonary tuberculosis and justifies the policy of respiratory isolation for patients with suspected or proved tuberculosis who are coughing.

Aspiration of oropharyngeal secretions is the second mechanism that may contribute to the development of LRTI. Healthy individuals may aspirate periodically, especially during sleep. Aspiration of even a small volume of oropharyngeal secretions, which can be colonized with potential pathogens such as *Streptococcus pneumoniae* and *Haemophilus influenzae,*

TABLE 24-2
Pathogenetic Mechanisms Responsible for the Development of Pneumonia

Mechanism of Disease	Examples of Specific Infections
Inhalation of aerosolized infectious particles	Tuberculosis Histoplasmosis Cryptococcosis Blastomycosis Coccidioidomycosis Q fever Legionellosis
Aspiration of organisms colonizing the oropharynx	Community-acquired bacterial pneumonia Aspiration pneumonia Hospital-acquired pneumonia Ventilator-associated pneumonia
Direct inoculation of organisms into the lower airway	Hospital-acquired pneumonia Ventilator-associated pneumonia
Spread of infection to the lungs from adjacent structures	Mixed anaerobic and aerobic pneumonia from subdiaphragmatic abscess Amebic pneumonia from rupture of amebic liver abscess into the lung
Spread of infection to the lung through the blood	*Staphylococcus aureus* pneumonia arising from right-sided bacterial endocarditis Parasitic pneumonia: Strongyloidiasis, ascariasis, hookworm
Reactivation of latent infection, usually resulting from immunosuppression	*Pneumocystis jiroveci* pneumonia Reactivation tuberculosis Cytomegalovirus

may contribute to development of CAP. Certain patient populations are at risk for large-volume aspiration, such as patients with impaired gag reflexes from narcotic use, alcohol intoxication, or prior stroke. Aspiration also may occur after a seizure, cardiac arrest, or syncope.

Aspiration seems to be the major mechanism responsible for the development of some types of mixed aerobic and anaerobic, gram-negative, and staphylococcal HAPs. In intubated patients, chronic aspiration of colonized secretions through a tracheal cuff has been linked to the subsequent occurrence of pneumonia,[4] which led to the development of strategies to prevent HAP, such as continuous suctioning of subglottic secretions in mechanically ventilated patients and elevation of the head of the bed.[8,9]

Direct inoculation of microorganisms into the lower airway is a less common cause of pneumonia. In mechanically ventilated patients who undergo frequent suctioning of lower airway secretions, passage of a suction catheter through the oropharynx may result in inoculation of colonizing organisms into the trachea and subsequent development of VAP.

Contiguous spread of microorganisms to the lungs or pleural space from adjacent areas of infection, such as subdiaphragmatic or liver abscesses, is an infrequent cause of pneumonia. This may occur in patients with pyogenic or amebic liver abscesses involving the dome of the liver in whom rupture of the abscess through the diaphragm leads to the development of pulmonary infection or empyema.

Hematogenous dissemination is the spread of infection through the bloodstream from a remote site; it is an uncommon cause of pneumonia. It may occur in the setting of right-sided bacterial endocarditis, in which fragments of an infected heart valve break off and embolize through the pulmonary arteries to the lungs, producing either pneumonia or septic pulmonary infarcts. Certain parasitic pneumonias, including strongyloidiasis, ascariasis, and hookworm, arise through hematogenous dissemination. In such cases, migrating parasite larvae travel to the lungs through the bloodstream from remote sites of infection, such as the skin or the gastrointestinal (GI) tract.

Pneumonia may develop when a latent infection, acquired earlier in life, is reactivated. This may occur for no apparent reason, as in the case of reactivation pulmonary tuberculosis. However, reactivation is usually attributable to the development of cellular immunodeficiency, as is the case with *Pneumocystis jiroveci* (previously called *Pneumocystis carinii*) pneumonia. In developed countries, most healthy individuals have acquired *P. jiroveci* by age 3 years and show serologic evidence of prior infection. The organism remains dormant in the lung but may reactivate later in life and produce pneumonia in individuals with compromised cell-mediated immunity, such as patients with human immunodeficiency virus (HIV) infection or recipients of long-term immunosuppressive therapy. Cytomegalovirus pneumonia is another example of a latent infection that can reactivate during chronic immunosuppression, especially in solid organ and bone marrow transplant recipients. Immunosuppressive drugs used to modify inflammatory diseases, such as tumor necrosis factor (TNF) inhibitors, have been associated with the development of pulmonary and extrapulmonary tuberculosis.[10]

MICROBIOLOGY

The microbiology of CAP and nosocomial pneumonia has been studied extensively. Knowledge of which organisms are most commonly associated with pneumonia in different settings is essential because the microbial differential diagnosis guides the diagnostic evaluation and the selection of empiric antimicrobial therapy.

In most studies, *S. pneumoniae,* also called *pneumococcus,* is the most commonly identified cause of CAP, accounting for 20% to 75% of cases (Table 24-3). Various other organisms have been implicated with varying frequencies. *H. influenzae, Staphylococcus aureus,* and gram-negative bacilli each account for 3% to 10% of isolates in many reports.[11] Notably, the incidence of *H. influenzae* pneumonia has decreased dramatically since the introduction of the type B *H. influenzae* (also known as *Hib*) vaccine in the 1980s. *Legionella* species, *Chlamydophila pneumoniae,* and *Mycoplasma pneumoniae* together account for 10% to 20% of cases. These latter organisms, called **atypical pathogens**, vary in frequency in more recent reports, depending on the age of the patient population, the season of the year, and

TABLE 24-3

Frequency of Pathogens in Community-Acquired Pneumonia

Cause	Cases (%)
Streptococcus pneumoniae	20-75
Aspiration	6-10
Chlamydophila pneumoniae	4-11
Haemophilus influenzae	3-10
Gram-negative bacilli	3-10
Staphylococcus aureus	3-5
Legionella species	2-8
Viruses	2-16
Moraxella catarrhalis	1-3
Mycoplasma pneumoniae	1-24
Pneumocystis jiroveci	0-13
Mycobacterium tuberculosis	0-5
No diagnosis	25-50

geographic locale. Legionellosis and *C. pneumoniae,* in particular, exhibit significant geographic variation in incidence.

RULE OF THUMB

S. pneumoniae remains the most common cause of CAP.

Many studies examining the epidemiology and microbiology of CAP are potentially biased because they focus on patients requiring hospitalization. In patients with less severe illnesses not requiring hospitalization, more recent studies suggest that *M. pneumoniae* and *C. pneumoniae* account for 38% of cases and may be more common than typical bacterial pathogens such as pneumococcus and *H. influenzae.*[12] In patients who are ill enough to require admission to the ICU, *Legionella* species, gram-negative bacilli, and pneumococcus are disproportionately more common.[13] A virulent strain of methicillin-resistant *S. aureus* (MRSA) has emerged as a cause of severe necrotizing CAP.[14]

In urban settings that have a high incidence of endemic HIV infection, *P. jiroveci* may be an occasional cause of CAP.[15] Viruses such as influenza, respiratory syncytial virus, parainfluenza, and adenovirus can cause CAP, especially in patients with milder illnesses not requiring hospitalization, and are encountered in the late fall and winter months. A worldwide pandemic of H1N1 influenza during 2009 to 2010 and ongoing sporadic cases of transmission of H5N1 influenza from birds to humans have led to heightened international awareness of influenza epidemiology, pathogenesis, and prevention.[16]

Mixed aerobic and anaerobic aspiration pneumonia may account for 10% of cases. This cause of pneumonia is an important consideration for nursing home residents and for individuals with impaired gag reflexes or recent loss of consciousness.

The outbreak in 2000 to 2001 of inhalation anthrax in the United States adds another microbial differential diagnostic consideration in patients with fulminant community-acquired LRTI.[17] To date, inhalation anthrax remains a rare disease. Several new coronaviruses have emerged as important pathogens within the past decade. *Severe acute respiratory syndrome* (SARS) emerged out of Asia and spread globally in 2002 to 2003. Fortunately, no cases have been identified since 2004.[18] More recently, *Middle East respiratory syndrome* (MERS) has arisen as a global health concern. First described in Saudia Arabia in 2012, the virus is found within the Arabian peninsula and causes a severe respiratory illness with a 30% mortality rate. The first cases imported to the United States were confirmed in 2014, both in travelers from Saudia Arabia.[19] Albeit rare in the United States, both viruses also should be considered in the appropriate clinical and epidemiologic setting. In addition, enterovirus D68 is an emerging cause of pneumonia in children.[20]

In most published series, no microbiologic diagnosis is established in 50% of patients. This is attributable to many factors, including:

- Inability of many patients to produce sputum
- Acquisition of sputum specimen after antibiotics have been started
- Failure to perform numerous serologic studies routinely in all patients
- The fact that many organisms (e.g., viruses and anaerobic bacteria) were not routinely sought
- Failure, until more recently, to recognize pneumonia pathogens, such as *C. pneumoniae* and some viral agents.

The common microbial agents producing HCAP, HAP, and VAP are summarized in Table 24-1 and include gram-negative bacilli, *S. aureus, Legionella* species, and rarely viruses such as influenza or respiratory syncytial virus. The last-mentioned viruses are considerations only during the winter months, when they are endemic in the community and may enter the hospital via health care workers, visitors, or patients with incubating or active infections.

The relative frequencies and antimicrobial susceptibilities of these respective bacteria may vary considerably from one institution to another. Knowledge of which nosocomial isolates are most common within one's own institution and community, along with their drug-sensitivity profiles, has important implications with regard to selecting **antibiotic therapy**, formulating infection control policies, investigating potential outbreaks, and selecting antimicrobial agents for the hospital formulary. For example, patients developing severe VAP in ICUs with a high prevalence of carbapenem resistance among gram-negative organisms such as *Klebsiella pneumoniae* and *Acinetobacter baumannii* may warrant empiric antimicrobial therapy for these organisms pending culture information. Similarly, nosocomial legionellosis occurs with variable frequency at different institutions, such that empiric therapy in critically ill patients with nosocomial LRTI may or may not require coverage of this pathogen.

Nosocomial pathogens capable of producing HAP can be transmitted directly from one patient to another, as in the case for tuberculosis. However, transmission from health care workers (including respiratory therapists [RTs]), contaminated equipment, or **fomites** (objects capable of transmitting infection through physical contact with them) is more common, especially for gram-negative bacilli, *S. aureus,* and viruses. The RT has an important role to play in preventing the transmission and development of nosocomial pneumonia.

MINI CLINI

Distinguishing Between Different Types of Nosocomial Pneumonia

PROBLEM: A 52-year-old man with a history of severe low back pain is admitted to the hospital with a GI bleed in the setting of excessive NSAID use. He has not seen a doctor in 5 years. His presenting symptoms include epigastric abdominal pain, black stools, and dizziness with standing. Admission hemoglobin is 5.2 g/dl and white blood count (WBC) count is 6.2×10^9. He is transfused red blood cells (RBCs) and undergoes upper GI endoscopy, which reveals a large bleeding duodenal ulcer. Three days into his admission, the patient develops a fever to 40.2°C, shortness of breath, and cough. Laboratory testing reveals a WBC count of 16.8×10^9. Chest radiography reveals a patchy infiltrate in the right lower lobe. What type of pneumonia does this patient have? How might this infection have developed?

DISCUSSION: The patient has HAP, because he did not have any evidence of pneumonia at the time of admission and developed his infection more than 48 hours into his hospital stay. He may have developed pneumonia secondary to inhalation of infectious particles via exposure to patients or health care providers working with a respiratory illness. More likely, he aspirated oropharyngeal or gastric secretions during his upper endoscopy procedure or during a vomiting episode. Empiric antimicrobial coverage should target mixed aerobic and anaerobic mouth flora, *S.aureus,* enteric gram-negative bacilli, and potentially influenza, depending on the season.

CLINICAL MANIFESTATIONS

Patients with CAP typically have fever and respiratory symptoms, such as cough, sputum production, pleuritic chest pain, and dyspnea. Not all of these symptoms are present all the time, especially in elderly patients in whom the presentation may be subtle. Other problems, such as hoarseness, sore throat, headache, and diarrhea, may accompany certain pathogens. Fever, cough, and sputum production may occur in other illnesses such as acute bronchitis or exacerbations of chronic bronchitis.

In the past, clinicians often distinguished between typical and atypical clinical syndromes as a means of predicting the most likely microbial causes. A typical presentation consisted of the sudden onset of high fever, shaking, chills, and cough with purulent sputum. Such a presentation was considered more common with bacterial pathogens such as pneumococcus and *H. influenzae.* An atypical presentation was an illness characterized by the gradual onset of fever, headache, constitutional symptoms, diarrhea, and cough, often with minimal sputum production. Cough was often a relatively minor symptom at the outset, and the illness was initially dominated by nonrespiratory symptoms. Such a presentation was thought to be more common with pathogens such as *M. pneumoniae, C. pneumoniae, Legionella* species, and viruses. More recent studies have shown that considerable overlap exists in the clinical presentations of pneumonia with typical and atypical pathogens.[21] The occurrence of concomitant diarrhea, previously considered indicative of legionellosis, is now known to be common in pneumococcal and mycoplasmal pneumonia.

Despite the limitations in predicting the microbial diagnosis based on the clinical presentation, clinicians use certain historical clues and physical findings at the bedside to determine the likely cause of pneumonia in patients presenting from the community. In patients presenting with high fever, teeth-chattering chills, pleuritic pain, and a cough producing rust-colored sputum, pneumococcal pneumonia is the most likely diagnosis. Patients with pneumonia accompanied by foul-smelling breath, an absent gag reflex, or recent loss of consciousness are most likely to have a mixed aerobic and anaerobic infection as a consequence of aspiration. CAP accompanied by hoarseness suggests *C. pneumoniae.* Pneumonia in a patient with a history of splenectomy suggests infection with an encapsulated pathogen such as pneumococcus or *H. influenzae.* Pneumonia occurring after resolution of a flulike illness raises concern for *S. aureus.* Epidemics of pneumonia occurring within households or closed communities, such as dormitories or military barracks, suggest pathogens such as *M. pneumoniae* or *C. pneumoniae.* Pneumonia accompanied by splenomegaly suggests psittacosis (caused by *Chlamydophila psittaci* and associated with bird exposure) or Q fever (caused by *Coxiella burnetii* and associated with exposure to farm animals). Bullous myringitis and erythema multiforme are associated with *Mycoplasma* infection. Relative bradycardia (defined as a heart rate <100 beats/min) in the presence of fever and in the absence of preexisting cardiac conduction system disease or beta-blocker therapy may suggest infection with an atypical pathogen. Pneumonia accompanied by conjunctivitis suggests adenovirus infection.

The clinical presentation of CAP in elderly patients warrants special mention because it may be subtle. Older individuals with pneumonia may not have a fever or cough and may simply present with shortness of breath, confusion, worsening congestive heart failure (CHF), or failure to thrive.

Inhalation anthrax is a rare disease, but warrants mention because of the small epidemic believed to have been an act of bioterrorism.[17] This outbreak affected mainly postal workers who were exposed to mail containing anthrax spores. Most patients presented with a febrile flulike illness of several days' duration accompanied by dry cough and shortness of breath. Some patients went on to develop septic shock, meningitis, and disseminated intravascular coagulation over several days, culminating in death.

Because of a lack of prior host immunity or unique viral virulence factors, patients infected with pandemic influenza strains may have unusually severe presentations. During the 2009 to 2010 pandemic of H1N1 influenza, clinical presentations varied from mild upper respiratory syndromes to fulminant pneumonias with acute respiratory distress syndrome (ARDS) and shock.[16] SARS manifests with high fever and myalgia for 3 to 7 days followed by nonproductive cough and progressive hypoxemia with progression to mechanical ventilation in 20%.[18] MERS presents similarly, with an added history of travel to or close contact with a symptomatic person who has traveled to the Arabian peninsula within 14 days of symptom onset.[19]

HCAP, HAP, and VAP usually manifest with new onset of fever in hospitalized or institutionalized patients. Nonintubated patients may have a recent history of vomiting, seizure, or syncope, during which aspiration of oropharyngeal or gastric secretions may have occurred. In intubated patients, VAP traditionally manifests with new onset of fever, leukocytosis, purulent endotracheal secretions, and a new pulmonary infiltrate. The diagnosis of HCAP, HAP, or VAP can be extremely difficult to make in patients with preexisting abnormalities on the chest radiograph, such as CHF or ARDS. In mechanically ventilated patients, purulent tracheobronchitis may be accompanied by fever, and in patients with preexisting abnormalities on chest radiograph, the distinction between bronchitis and pneumonia can be especially difficult.

CHEST RADIOGRAPH

In patients with a compatible clinical syndrome, the diagnosis of CAP is established by the presence of a new pulmonary infiltrate on the chest radiograph. Not all healthy outpatients with suspected pneumonia require a chest radiograph, and physicians may choose not to obtain a chest radiograph and treat empirically for CAP in individuals with mild illnesses who are at low risk for morbidity or mortality.

Also, a normal chest radiograph does not exclude the diagnosis of pneumonia. The chest radiograph may be normal in patients with early infection, dehydration, or *P. jiroveci* infection. The pattern of radiographic abnormality is not diagnostic of the causative agent, although specific radiographic findings should suggest specific microbial differential diagnoses (Table 24-4).

Consolidation involving an entire lobe is called *lobar consolidation* (Figure 24-1), whereas *bronchopneumonia* refers to the presence of a patchy infiltrate surrounding one or more bronchi, without opacification of an entire lobe. Both radiographic patterns suggest the presence of a bacterial pathogen. Pleural effusions are common in patients with bacterial pneumonia and uncommon in patients with viral, *P. jiroveci, C. pneumoniae,* or fungal pneumonia. Pleural effusions are seen in approximately 10% of patients with *M. pneumoniae* and *Legionella pneumophila* pneumonia and occur occasionally in patients with reactivation pulmonary tuberculosis. Interstitial infiltrates (Figure 24-2), especially if diffuse, suggest viral disease, *P. jiroveci,* or miliary tuberculosis in patients with CAP. Cavitary infiltrates (Figure 24-3) are seen in reactivation pulmonary tuberculosis; fungal pneumonias, such as histoplasmosis, blastomycosis, and aspergilosis; nocardiosis; pyogenic lung abscess; and, rarely, *P. jiroveci* pneumonia. Patients with severe staphylococcal or gram-negative pneumonias may develop small cavities called *pneumatoceles.* Legionellosis should be considered in sicker

TABLE 24-4
Radiographic Patterns Produced by Pathogens in Community-Acquired Pneumonia

Pattern	Pathogens
Lobar consolidation	Bacterial
Bronchopneumonia	Bacterial
Pleural effusion	Bacterial Inhalation anthrax
Interstitial infiltrates	Viruses *Pneumocytis jiroveci*
Cavities	Mycobacteria Fungi *Nocardia* species *Staphylococcus aureus* Gram-negative bacilli Polymicrobial aerobic and anaerobic lung abscess *P. jiroveci* (rare)
Mediastinal widening without infiltrates	Inhalation anthrax
Rapidly progressive multilobar	*Legionella* species *Streptococcus pneumoniae* Endobronchial tuberculosis

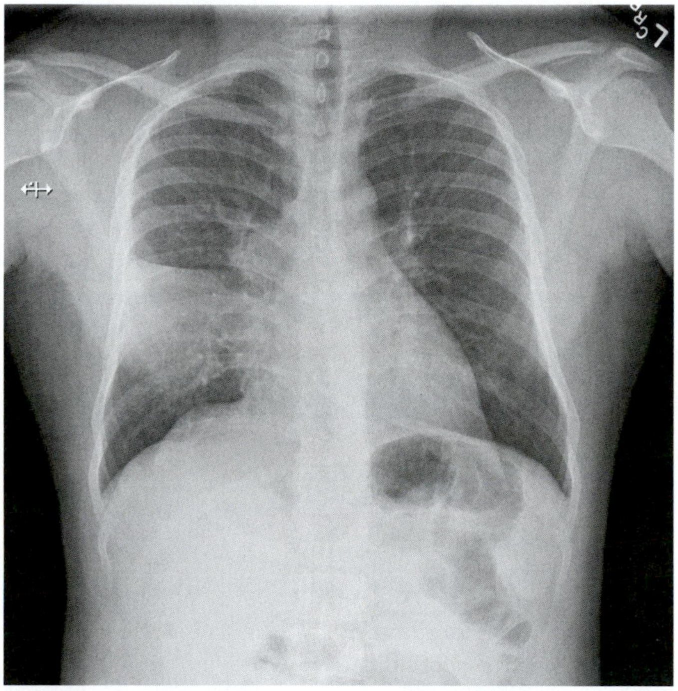

FIGURE 24-1 Lobar pneumonia caused by *Streptococcus pneumoniae.* A 36-year-old previously healthy woman presents with abrupt onset of fevers and shaking chills, cough productive of yellow sputum, and right-sided pleuritic chest pain. Chest radiograph reveals lobar consolidation. Sputum culture yields *S. pneumoniae.*

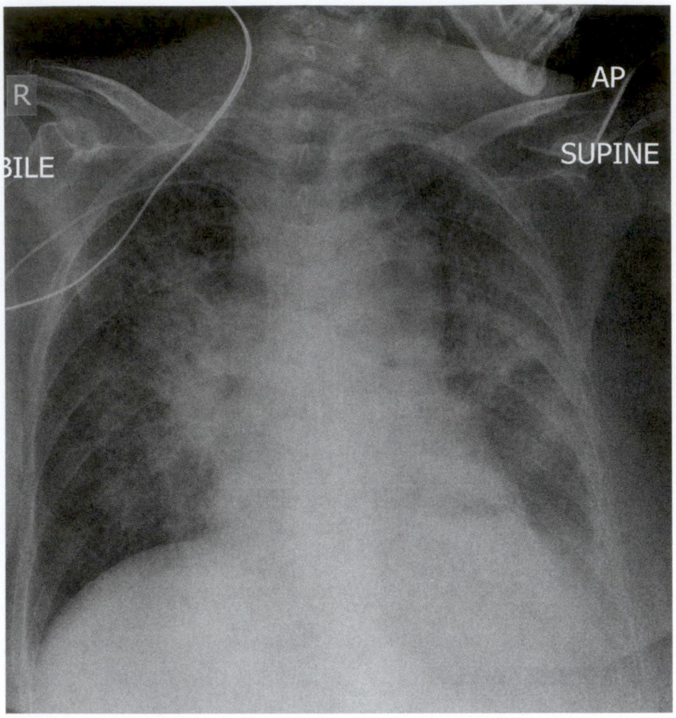

FIGURE 24-2 *Pneumocystis jiorveci* pneumonia (PCP). A 23-year-old male intravenous drug user presents with 2 weeks of dyspnea on exertion, nonproductive cough, and fevers to 40.4° C. The chest radiograph shows an interstitial infiltrate. Human immunodeficiency virus antibody test is positive, serum beta-D glucan level is elevated, and bronchoalveolar lavage toluidine blue O stain is positive for *P. jiroveci.* The interstitial infiltrate in a "bat-wing" distribution is classic for PCP pneumonia.

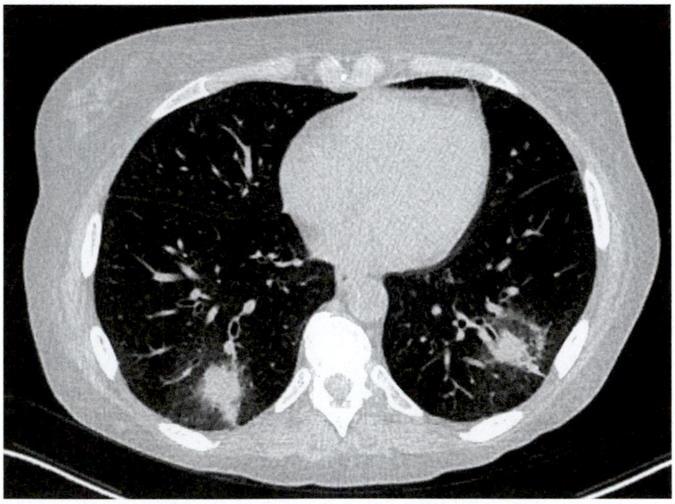

FIGURE 24-3 Cavitary nodular pneumonia caused by *Aspergillus*. A 34-year-old woman undergoing induction chemotherapy for newly diagnosed acute myeloid leukemia presents with persistent neutropenic fevers and cough productive of scant hemoptysis. Sputum cultures are negative, but serum galactomannan antigen is markedly elevated, highly suggestive of *Aspergillus* infection. Computed tomography reveals multicentric cavitary nodules, some of which have a halo of ground glass opacity surrounding them, findings that are classic for invasive pulmonary aspergillosis.

patients with pneumonia of a single lobe, which quickly spreads to involve multiple lobes over 24 to 48 hours.

The chest radiograph may be helpful in diagnosing HCAP or HAP in nonintubated patients with a suspected aspiration event and a prevously normal chest film. In such cases, development of a new infiltrate may confirm the clinical suspicion of aspiration pneumonia. The chest radiograph is often less helpful in the diagnosis of VAP because mechanically ventilated patients often have other reasons for radiographic abnormalities, such as ARDS, CHF, pulmonary thromboembolism, alveolar hemorrhage, or atelectasis. In these patients, the accurate diagnosis of a new nosocomial LRTI can be difficult. *Clinical diagnosis,* defined as the presence of fever, purulent respiratory secretions, new leukocytosis, and a new pulmonary infiltrate, is sensitive but not specific for the diagnosis of VAP. Other strategies to diagnose VAP more accurately have been investigated.

RISK FACTORS FOR MORTALITY AND ASSESSING THE NEED FOR HOSPITALIZATION

Many cases of CAP can be managed successfully on an outpatient basis. The challenge for the clinician is to identify individuals at higher risk of morbidity and mortality for whom hospitalization is indicated. Over the past 20 years, numerous studies have analyzed risk factors for mortality in patients with CAP.[21-23] Risk factors predicting a high risk for death are summarized in Box 24-1.

Fine and associates[23] performed a meta-analysis of 127 cohorts of patients with CAP to examine risk factors for death. The overall mortality for the 33,148 patients in these cohorts was 13.7%. Eleven prognostic variables were significantly associated with mortality, including male sex, absence of pleuritic chest pain, hypothermia, systolic hypotension, tachypnea, diabetes mellitus, cancer, neurologic disease, bacteremia, leukopenia, and multilobar infiltrates on chest radiograph. Mortality varied according to the infecting agent and was highest for *P. aeruginosa* (61.1%), *Klebsiella* species (35.7%), *Escherichia coli* (35.3%), and *S. aureus* (31.8%). Mortality rates for more common pathogens were lower but still substantial: *Legionella* species (14.7%), *S. pneumoniae* (12.3%), *C. pneumoniae* (9.8%), and *M. pneumoniae* (1.4%).

Because some variables are unknown at the time a patient seeks treatment for pneumonia, such as the causative agent and whether bacteremia is present, more recent studies have sought to assess the risk for fatal outcome by using clinical and laboratory data that are readily available at the time of the initial evaluation. Based on an analysis of the 30-day mortality in more than 40,000 patients, Fine and associates[24] proposed a prediction rule to identify low-risk and high-risk patients with CAP. Their algorithm uses the demographic, clinical, and laboratory data available at presentation to stratify the risk for death and the criteria for hospitalization in outpatient groups. Points are assigned for the presence of numerous variables, and cumulative point scores are used to stratify patients into one of five different risk groups with predictable mortality rates

Box 24-1 Risk Factors for Mortality in Community-Acquired Pneumonia from Multiple Studies

I. Patient variables
  A. Age >50 years
  B. Male sex
  C. Comorbid illnesses
    1. Cerebrovascular disease
    2. Cancer
    3. Congestive heart failure
    4. Renal disease
    5. Liver disease
    6. Immunosuppression
    7. Alcoholism
    8. Diabetes mellitus
    9. Chronic lung disease
II. Clinical parameters at presentation
  A. Altered mentation
  B. Systolic hypotension <90 mm Hg
  C. Tachypnea >30 breaths/min
  D. Hypothermia (temperature <35° C)
  E. Fever (temperature >40° C)
  F. Pulse rate >125 beats/min
  G. Extrapulmonary site of infection
III. Laboratory and radiographic findings at presentation
  A. Arterial pH <7.35
  B. Blood urea nitrogen >30 mg/dl
  C. Serum sodium <130 mmol/L
  D. Glucose >250 mg/dl
  E. Hematocrit <30%
  F. Hypoxia (PaO_2 <60 mm Hg) or hypercarbia (PCO_2 > 50 mm Hg) on room air
  G. White blood cell count <4 × 10^9/L, >30 × 10^9/L, or an absolute neutrophil count <1 × 10^9
  H. Multilobar infiltrate
  I. Bacteremia
  J. Pleural effusion
  K. High-risk cause
    1. Gram-negative bacilli
    2. *Staphylococcus aureus*
    3. Postobstructive pneumonia
    4. Aspiration

From Fine MJ, Smith MA, Carson CA, et al: Prognosis and outcomes of patients with community-acquired pneumonia: a meta-analysis. JAMA 275:134–141, 1996.

(Tables 24-5 and 24-6). In this model, which has been validated in large prospective cohorts of patients, the patients at the lowest risk for death fall into groups I and II. In most instances, these patients may be treated successfully as outpatients, unless they are hypoxemic, vomiting and unable to take oral antibiotics, noncompliant, or immunocompromised. Patients in group I are patients younger than 50 years of age without comorbid illnesses and abnormal physical findings at presentation (see Box 24-1 and Table 24-5). This group of patients has a 0.1% risk for death.

Because of the complexity of the pneumonia severity index, many practitioners prefer a simpler stratification system, CURB-65. Risk criteria in this system include confusion, blood urea nitrogen greater than 20 mg/dl, respiratory rate greater than 30 breaths/min, systolic blood pressure less than 90 mm Hg or diastolic blood pressure less than 60 mm Hg, and age older than 65 years. Based on their data analysis, the authors recommend that patients with one or two risk criteria should be treated as outpatients, patients with two criteria treated on general hospital wards, and patients with three or more criteria admitted to the ICU.[25]

TABLE 24-5 Scoring System for Stratifying Risk of 30-Day Mortality in Adults With Community-Acquired Pneumonia

Variable	Points Assigned
Age	
Men	Age (yr)
Women	Age (yr) – 10
Nursing home resident	+10
Comorbid illnesses	
Cancer	+30
Liver disease	+20
Kidney disease	+10
Cerebrovascular disease	+10
Congestive heart failure	+10
Physical findings	
Altered mentation	+20
Tachypnea >30 breaths/min	+20
Systolic hypotension <90 mm Hg	+20
Temperature <35° C or >40° C	+15
Heart rate >125 beats/min	+10
Laboratory and radiographic findings	
Acidemia (arterial pH <7.35)	+30
Azotemia (blood urea nitrogen >30 mg/dl)	+20
Hyponatremia (sodium <130 mmol/L)	+20
Hypoxia (PaO_2 <60 mm Hg)	+10
Hyperglycemia (glucose >250 mg/dl)	+10
Anemia (hematocrit <30%)	+10
Pleural effusion	+10

Modified from Fine MJ, Auble TE, Yealy DM, et al: A prediction rule to identify low-risk patients with community-acquired pneumonia. N Engl J Med 336:243–250, 1997.

NOTE: Plus sign (+) denotes adding points; minus sign (–) denotes subtracting points (e.g., for women, points assigned equal age in years – 10).

TABLE 24-6 Risk Class Mortality Rates Using Prediction Model Cumulative Point Scores in Patients With Community-Acquired Pneumonia

Risk Class (Cumulative Point Score)	Mortality Rate (%)
I	0.1
II (≤70)	0.6
III (71-90)	2.8
IV (91-130)	8.2
V (>130)	29.2

Modified from Fine MJ, Auble TE, Yealy DM, et al: A prediction rule to identify low-risk patients with community-acquired pneumonia. N Engl J Med 336:243–250, 1997.

NOTE: Patients in risk class I are <50 years old and lack existing illness or physical findings listed in Table 19-5. Points are assigned to patients in risk classes II and higher.

Many studies have examined risk factors for the development of HAP and VAP, which in broad terms can be divided into (1) factors that interfere with host defense and (2) factors that encourage exposure to large numbers of bacteria.[7] Examples of factors that interfere with host defense include the following:

- Underlying illnesses such as diabetes mellitus, malignancy, chronic heart and lung disease, and renal failure
- Critical illnesses such as sepsis syndrome and ARDS
- Therapeutic interventions such as endotracheal intubation, tracheostomy, and administration of medications such as sedatives and corticosteroids

Factors that promote exposure of the lung to pathogenic microorganisms include the following:

- Use of endotracheal or nasogastric tubes
- Contaminated ventilator equipment or water supplies
- Prior antibiotic therapy
- Neutralization of gastric pH

Although many studies have emphasized the substantial mortality rate (20% to 50%) for patients who develop HAP or VAP, few studies have examined the specific risk factors associated with mortality in hospital-acquired LRTI. For nonventilated patients, risk factors for mortality include bilateral infiltrates, respiratory failure, and infection with high-risk organisms.[26,27] In mechanically ventilated patients, factors associated with fatal outcome include the following[27,28]:

- Infection with high-risk organisms such as *P. aeruginosa*, *Acinetobacter* species, and *Stenotrophomonas maltophilia*
- Multisystem organ failure
- Nonsurgical diagnosis
- Therapy with antacids or histamine-2 (H_2)-receptor antagonists
- Transfer from another hospital or ward
- Renal failure
- Prolonged mechanical ventilation
- Coma or shock
- Inappropriate antibiotic therapy
- Hospitalization in a noncardiac ICU

MINI CLINI

Estimating Risk from Pneumonia

PROBLEM: The RT is called to the emergency department to perform an arterial blood gas analysis on a 70-year-old woman who has been sent from a nursing home with confusion and shortness of breath. Her history is notable for end-stage renal disease caused by hypertension and a recent stroke, which has resulted in left-sided hemiplegia. The emergency physician ordered a chest x-ray examination, which revealed a right lower lobe infiltrate and a right pleural effusion.

On physical examination, the patient is somnolent. Her vital signs are temperature, 35° C; blood pressure, 85/50 mm Hg; and heart rate, 130 beats/min. Additional findings include the following:

- Absent gag reflex
- Right basilar rales (crackles) and left hemiplegia
- Peripheral white blood cell (WBC) count, 3000 cells/mm^3
- Blood urea nitrogen, 100 mg/dl
- Hematocrit, 31%
- Blood glucose, 110 mg/dl
- Serum sodium, 144 mmol/L

The RT collects the arterial blood gas on room air, which shows a pH of 7.30; PaO_2, 58 mm Hg; and PCO_2, 25 mm Hg. Should the patient be admitted to the hospital, or should she be sent back to the nursing home? What is her risk for 30-day mortality?

DISCUSSION: This patient is at substantial risk for dying from pneumonia and should be admitted to the hospital. The Fine prediction rule[24] may be used as follows to estimate the risk for 30-day mortality (see Tables 24-5 and 24-6):

Variable	Points
Age 70 yr	+70
Sex female	−10
Nursing home resident	+10
Cerebrovascular disease	+10
Renal disease	+10
Altered mentation	+20
Systolic hypotension	+20
Hypothermia	+15
Tachycardia	+10
Acidemia	+30
Renal failure	+20
Hypoxemia, with PaO_2 <60 mm Hg	+10
Pleural effusion	+10
Total	*225*

Her cumulative point score is 225, she belongs in risk class V, and her estimated risk for mortality is 29.2% (see Table 24-6). She should be admitted to the hospital for treatment.

DIAGNOSTIC STUDIES

Community-Acquired Pneumonia

Many patients with CAP who are treated as outpatients never have a microbiologic diagnosis established. Many are treated based on the history and examination findings, with or without a chest radiograph to confirm the presence of an infiltrate. Patients who are sick enough to warrant hospitalization or consideration of hospitalization should undergo appropriate studies to stratify risk for mortality and establish a microbiologic diagnosis (Box 24-2). Complete blood count, blood glucose, serum sodium, and blood urea nitrogen are all necessary to derive a point score for estimating mortality risk. An arterial blood gas analysis is used to detect the presence of hypoxemia and acidemia, which indicate more serious illness.

The value of Gram stain and culture of expectorated sputum has been debated for years.[29] Many patients lack a productive cough, making collection of an adequate specimen difficult. Prior antibiotic therapy reduces the yield from both tests. Only 50% of patients with bacteremic pneumococcal pneumonia have a positive sputum culture.[30] Nevertheless, the finding of a predominant organism on Gram stain in an appropriately collected specimen can be very helpful in selecting appropriate

Box 24-2 Recommended Tests for Adults With Community-Acquired Pneumonia Warranting Consideration of Hospitalization

- Chest radiograph
- Complete blood count
- Blood chemistries
  - Glucose
  - Serum sodium
  - Blood urea nitrogen
- Arterial blood gas
- Sputum Gram stain and culture
- Additional sputum studies as clinically indicated
  - Acid-fast stains and culture for mycobacteria
  - Potassium hydroxide examination and fungal culture
  - Stain for *Pneumocystis jiroveci*
  - Direct fluorescent antibody stain for *Legionella* species
- Blood cultures
- Pleural fluid analysis if sizable effusion is present
  - Cell count with differential
  - Glucose, protein, and lactate dehydrogenase
  - pH
  - Gram stain and routine aerobic and anaerobic culture
  - Acid-fast stain and culture for mycobacteria
- Additional other studies as clinically indicated
  - *Legionella* urinary antigen
  - Pneumococcal urinary antigen
  - Acute and convalescent sera for *Mycoplasma pneumoniae, Legionella* species, and *Chlamydophila pneumoniae*
  - Fungal serologies
  - HIV test for individuals 15 to 65 years old or for individuals engaging in high-risk behavior

antibiotic therapy.[31] A routine sputum culture must be interpreted within the context of the sputum Gram stain. Specimens contaminated with oropharyngeal epithelial cells are unsatisfactory for analysis and specimens lacking neutrophils from nonneutropenic patients are unlikely to be helpful.

RULE OF THUMB

A routine sputum culture can be interpreted only within the context of the sputum Gram stain.

The RT has an important role in collecting an appropriate specimen of expectorated sputum. Patients should be advised to rid the mouth of contaminating saliva by rinsing with water or by spitting and then to expectorate a specimen from deep within the tracheobronchial tree into a collection container. Prompt transportation to the laboratory is essential and improves the diagnostic yield from culture.[12] Most microbiology laboratories screen the adequacy of the specimen by cytologic examination. A satisfactory specimen contains more than 25 leukocytes and fewer than 10 squamous epithelial cells per high-power field.[32] In routine sputum culture, the isolation of bacteria such as *S. pneumoniae* and *H. influenzae* must be interpreted within the context of the Gram stain because these organisms can colonize the oropharynx, and their presence in culture may not signify true LRTI. The culture isolation of other organisms, such as *Mycobacterium tuberculosis, Histoplasma capsulatum, Blastomyces dermatitidis, Coccidioides immitis,* and *Legionella* species is diagnostic of disease because these organisms almost never colonize the respiratory tract.

RULE OF THUMB

The presence of *Candida* species on sputum smear or culture is almost never clinically significant.

Other stains and cultures of expectorated sputum should be obtained as dictated by the clinical circumstance, when management would be changed, or for purposes of tracking unusual or resistant organisms in an institution or population. In patients with suspected tuberculosis, the finding of acid-fact bacilli in stained sputum specimens often prompts initiation of antituberculous therapy because culture isolation of *M. tuberculosis* may take 6 weeks. A direct fluorescence antibody stain of sputum for *Legionella* species may reveal the organism in 25% to 80% of individuals with Legionnaire's disease, and cultures are positive in 50% to 70%.[33] Toluidine blue O stains of sputum may disclose the organism in 80% of patients with *P. jiroveci* pneumonia. Potassium hydroxide preparations of sputum show fungi in only a few patients with histoplasmosis, blastomycosis, or coccidioidomycosis but are very helpful if positive.

Blood cultures should be obtained in hospitalized patients with CAP and may be helpful in establishing the diagnosis in patients with typical bacterial pathogens. Blood cultures are positive in approximately 30% of patients with pneumococcal pneumonia and in 70% of patients with *H. influenzae* pneumonia.[34] Blood cultures are not helpful in patients with legionellosis, *M. pneumoniae, C. pneumoniae, P. jiroveci,* or viral infections. Collection of blood cultures within 24 hours of hospitalization in elderly patients with pneumonia has been associated with improved survival.[35]

Parapneumonic pleural effusions are common and occur in 30% to 50% of patients with CAP.[11] Thoracentesis is indicated for patients with large pleural effusions and patients with smaller effusions who fail to respond to therapy or for whom the microbiologic diagnosis is not established. Pleural fluid should be tested for cell count, glucose, protein, pH, lactate dehydrogenase, Gram and acid-fast bacilli stains, and routine (aerobic and anaerobic) and mycobacterial cultures. Effusions with a fluid pH less than 7.20, a positive Gram stain or culture, or fluid that appear grossly purulent on inspection require tube thoracostomy for drainage.[36]

Other studies may be helpful in establishing a microbiologic diagnosis in the appropriate clinical setting. *L. pneumophila* serogroup 1 accounts for 80% of cases of Legionnaire's disease.[37] The urinary antigen test for *L. pneumophila* serogroup 1 is a sensitive and rapid test and usually becomes positive within 3 days of illness onset, but the test has limitations. First is its inability to detect the non–serogroup 1 *L. pneumophila* and non–*L. pneumophila* species that account for 20% of cases of Legionnaire's disease. Second, it can be negative if patients present very early in the disease course, potentially misleading clinicians with a negative result and requiring repeat testing if clinical suspicion remains high. Third, the test may remain positive for 1 year, obviating the ability to distinguish new from remote infection in patients with a recent history of pneumonia.

Serologic tests for immunoglobulin M (IgM) and IgG antibodies to *M. pneumoniae, Legionella* species, or *C. pneumoniae* are rarely helpful during the initial stages of pneumonia, but convalescent titers 3 to 4 weeks later may permit a retrospective microbiologic diagnosis by showing a fourfold increase in IgG titer or the development of IgM antibody against a specific pathogen. Acute sera should be analyzed in patients who are critically ill with pneumonia and for whom the microbiologic diagnosis is unavailable. Fungal serologic findings are occasionally helpful in supporting the diagnosis of blastomycosis, histoplasmosis, or coccidioidomycosis, pending culture isolation of the organism.

Fungal antigen assays are increasingly being used in settings in which there is a high clinical suspicion for invasive fungal infection. Invasive aspergillosis is is an important cause of pneumonia in immunocompromised hosts, particularly in those with prolonged neutropenia. Galactomannan is a polysaccharide that is a major constituent of *Aspergillus* cell walls. A large meta-analysis revealed that galactomannan antigen assays have a sensitivity of 71% and specificity of 89% for *Aspergillus* infection.[38] However, the sensitivity of the test is decreased by concomitant administration of antifungal therapy and false-positive results can occur in patients receiving the antibiotic combination piperacillin-tazobactam in infections with other fungi that share cross-reacting antigens (*Fusarium* and *Penicillium* species, *H. capsulatum*) and in patients with chemotherapy-induced mucositis or transplant-associated graft-versus-host disease (in whom bacteria with cross-reactive antigens translocate across the intestinal mucosal wall). Similarly, 1,3-beta-D-glucan is a cell wall component of many fungi, and levels of this molecule are elevated in many types of invasive fungal infection, including those with *Aspergillus, P. jiroveci, H. capsulatum*, and *C. immitis*. Beta-D glucan assays have a sensitivity of 77% and specificity of 85% for invasive fungal infection.[39] Like the galactomannan assay, there are some drawbacks to this test. First, the assay cannot distinguish between infections from various fungal pathogens. False-positive results can occur in patients receiving intravenous immunoglobulin or albumin infusions, in patients undergoing hemodialysis or receiving intravenous infusions that use cellulose filters, in patients with glucan-containing gauze packing of serosal surfaces, and patients who are bacteremic with certain organisms, including *Pseudomonas aeruginosa.*[39]

Because pneumococcal and *H. influenzae* pneumonia occur with higher frequency in patients with HIV infection than in the average population, an HIV test is recommended for patients ages 15 to 65 with CAP. HIV testing is also recommended for other individuals who engage in behaviors that put them at risk for HIV infection.

Molecular techniques, such as DNA probes and polymerase chain reaction (PCR), used for detecting specific organisms such as *M. pneumoniae* or *M. tuberculosis* or for confirming the identity of culture isolates, are being developed and used in some larger centers. Rapid diagnostic testing of nasopharyngeal specimens for viral pathogens such as influenza, parainfluenza, and respiratory syncytial virus may be helpful in diagnosing CAP because of these organisms in patients with compatible clinical presentations.

MINI CLINI

Importance of Clinical Setting for Determining the Cause of Pneumonia

PROBLEM: The RT is caring for a 32-year-old man admitted to the hospital 24 hours earlier with fever, shaking chills, and a new left lower lobe infiltrate. His WBC count on admission was 3500 cells/mm^3, with 96% neutrophils and 4% lymphocytes. A sputum Gram stain disclosed many polymorphonuclear leukocytes and lancet-shaped, gram-positive diplococci. Blood cultures have grown *S. pneumoniae* at 24 hours. He remains febrile 24 hours into therapy with penicillin G. While checking pulse oximetry, the RT notes that the patient is emaciated and that multiple needle tracks are present in each antecubital fossa. He tells the RT that he uses intravenous heroin. What other tests are indicated?

DISCUSSION: This patient, who is an intravenous drug user, has bacteremic pneumococcal pneumonia. These findings, along with the presence of cachexia and leukopenia with lymphopenia, should suggest the possibility of underlying HIV infection. An HIV test is indicated and should be performed after the patient's consent is obtained.

Both pneumococcal and *H. influenzae* pneumonia occur with higher frequency in HIV-infected individuals than in the general population. Occasionally, an HIV-infected patient has his or her first contact with the health care system as a result of one of these infections. New guidelines recommend that all average-risk individuals ages 15 to 65 undergo testing for HIV once in their lives and persons at higher risk for HIV infection undergo more frequent testing.[40]

Flexible bronchoscopy is usually reserved for severe cases of CAP, for immunocompromised individuals in whom opportunistic pathogens must be excluded, or for cases in which *P. jiroveci* infection is suspected. The yield from flexible bronchoscopy is higher if performed before starting antibiotic therapy in patients with bacterial pneumonia. Open lung biopsy is rarely indicated for patients with CAP.

Health Care–Associated Pneumonia, Hospital-Acquired Pneumonia, and Ventilator-Associated Pneumonia

The accurate diagnosis of nosocomial pneumonia is challenging and has been the subject of intense investigation over the

Box 24-3 Techniques for Diagnosing Nosocomial Pneumonia

- Clinical diagnosis
- Direct visualization of the airway by bronchoscopy
- Quantitative cultures of:
  - Endotracheal aspirates
  - Protected brush–bronchoscopy specimens
  - Nonbronchoscopic distally protected specimens
  - Conventional or protected BAL specimens, plus microscopic examination of recovered cells
  - PSB and BAL specimens, plus microscopic examination of BAL fluid cells
- RT-directed mini-BAL
- Transthoracic fine-needle aspiration

BAL, Bronchoalveolar lavage; *PSB,* protected specimen brush; *RT,* respiratory therapist.

past three decades. Numerous techniques have been extensively evaluated (Box 24-3); however, none is absolutely sensitive and specific.[41,42] *Clinical diagnosis* has been defined as the development of a new infiltrate on chest radiograph in the setting of fever, purulent tracheal secretions, and leukocytosis in a hospitalized patient. Clinical diagnosis lacks specificity because many other causes of pulmonary infiltrates exist in hospitalized patients, especially in patients on mechanical ventilation.[43] In addition, the upper airway commonly is colonized with nosocomial gram-negative bacilli and staphylococci, even in the absence of pneumonia. The qualitative culture isolation of these organisms from tracheal secretions correlates poorly with the presence or absence of pneumonia.

Direct visualization of the lower airway by bronchoscopy in ventilated patients is sometimes helpful to support the diagnosis of VAP. In one study, the presence of distal, purulent secretions, persistence of secretions surging from distal bronchi during exhalation, and a decrease in the PaO_2/FiO_2 ratio of less than 50 were independently associated with the presence of pneumonia. The presence of two of three of these factors had a sensitivity of 78% in the diagnosing nosocomial pneumonia; these factors were absent 89% of the time when there was no pneumonia (89% specific).[44]

Because the specificity of qualitative sputum cultures has been unreliable, several studies have examined the role of quantitative cultures of endotracheal aspirates using various breakpoints ranging from 10^3 to 10^7 *colony-forming units (CFUs)* per milliliter of respiratory secretions. Results with this technique have been best using a breakpoint of 10^6 CFU/ml, but sensitivities have been only 68% to 82%, with specificities of 84% to 96% with this test.[45,46]

The protected specimen brush (PSB) was developed in the 1970s and uses a special double-catheter brush system to minimize contamination by upper airway flora. Specimens obtained with this technique are cultured quantitatively. Numerous studies have validated the sensitivity of PSB in diagnosing nosocomial pneumonia.[47,48] However, PSB may be less useful in cases in which antibiotics have already been started, in cases of early infection, and in cases in which the wrong lobe is sampled.[41]

Nonbronchoscopic techniques using telescoping protected catheters have also been developed to obtain specimens for quantitative culture from the lower airway. In most studies, sensitivity has been comparable to bronchoscopic techniques, but results have disagreed in 20% of cases.[41]

Bronchoalveolar lavage (BAL), in which a lung segment is lavaged with sterile saline through the bronchoscope and recovered fluid is quantitatively cultured, has been studied extensively as a tool for diagnosing nosocomial pneumonia (see Chapter 24). Some studies have supported the usefulness of this technique, and others have questioned its specificity because of upper airway contamination.[47,48] BAL has proved useful for obtaining alveolar cells for microscopic analysis; several studies have suggested that the presence of intracellular bacteria in 3% to 5% of BAL cells distinguishes patients with nosocomial pneumonia from patients without pneumonia.[47,48] In one study, the combination of PSB cultures and microscopic examination of BAL cells for intracellular bacteria was 100% sensitive and 96% specific in identifying patients with nosocomial pneumonia.[47]

Mini-BAL performed by RTs also has been advocated for diagnosing VAP. In one study, results obtained using this technique were comparable with results obtained by bronchoscopy using PSB.[49] Some centers use this technique as the primary method of sampling respiratory secretions in suspected nosocomial pneumonia. Transthoracic ultrathin needle aspiration of the lung in nonventilated patients with nosocomial pneumonia also has been studied and in one report was found to have a sensitivity of 60%, a specificity of 100%, and a positive predictive value of 100%.[50]

Accurately diagnosing HAP, HCAP, and VAP remains a challenge for the physician and the RT. None of the available diagnostic techniques is 100% sensitive or specific; all are limited in the populations at greatest risk for getting nosocomial pneumonia—mechanically ventilated patients and patients receiving prior antibiotic therapy.

ANTIBIOTIC THERAPY

Community-Acquired Pneumonia

The selection of antibiotic therapy for patients with CAP should be guided by several considerations, including the age of the patient, severity of the illness, presence of risk factors for specific organisms, and results of initial diagnostic studies. Pathogen-specific therapy should be used when clinical circumstances and initial evaluation strongly suggest the microbiologic diagnosis or when cultures or other studies confirm the cause. In many instances, initial studies fail to establish a diagnosis, and empiric therapy must be started. Major classes of antibiotics used to treat pneumonia are listed in Table 24-7. Consensus guidelines for therapy have been published by the American Thoracic Society (ATS) and the Infectious Diseases Society of America (IDSA) (Table 24-8).[51-53] Therapy initiated within 4 hours of hospital admission has been associated with improved survival.[35]

For hospitalized patients who are not critically ill and who are admitted to the ward, an empiric regimen of a respiratory fluoroquinolone alone or an advanced macrolide plus a beta-lactam (cefotaxime, ceftriaxone, or ampicillin) is recommended (see Table 24-8). For critically ill patients requiring admission to the ICU, the IDSA and ATS recommend as empiric therapy a beta-lactam (cefotaxime, ceftriaxone, or ampicillin-sulbactam) plus either an advanced macrolide or a respiratory fluoroquinolone for legionella coverage. Certain pathogens require specific consideration in the ICU setting. If *Pseudomonas* is a concern, recommended regimens include two drugs with antipseudomonal coverage: an antipseudomonal beta-lactam (piperacillin-tazobactam, cefepime, imipenem, or meropenem) and ciprofloxacin or levofloxacin; an antipseudomonal beta-lactam, an aminoglycoside, and azithromycin; or an antipseudomonal beta-lactam, an aminoglycoside, and a respiratory fluoroquinolone (see Table 24-8). When MRSA is a concern, addition of vancomycin or linezolid is recommended.

When a microbiologic diagnosis is established, the antimicrobial regimen should be tailored to the isolated pathogen. Pathogen-specific treatment recommendations from the IDSA and ATS are summarized in Table 24-9. For isolates of *S. pneumoniae* susceptible to penicillin, penicillin remains the preferred agent. Many strains of *H. influenzae* produce beta-lactamase, making them resistant to penicillin. Second- or third-generation cephalosporins and amoxicillin/clavulanate are the agents of choice. Legionellosis should be treated with a macrolide or with a fluoroquinolone alone. Pneumonia caused by *M. pneumoniae* and *C. pneumoniae* should be treated with a macrolide or doxycycline. Trimethoprim-sulfamethoxazole (TMP-SMX) is the drug of choice for *P. jiroveci* pneumonia. However, 50% of HIV-infected patients may develop fever or a rash while taking this medication. For patients with mild to moderate disease, atovaquone, clindamycin, and primaquine, or trimethoprim and dapsone, are treatment alternatives; pentamidine is indicated for severe infection in patients unable to tolerate TMP-SMX. Treatment for staphylococcal or gram-negative pneumonias is dictated by the antibiotic susceptibility profiles of the offending organism. For patients with staphylococcal pneumonia, vancomycin is preferred, pending antibiotic susceptibility results. If the isolate is methicillin-susceptible, a semisynthetic penicillin, such as oxacillin or nafcillin, should be used because these antibiotics kill the bacteria more effectively than vancomycin; in seriously ill patients, rifampin or an aminoglycoside may be added. A detailed discussion regarding the treatment of fungal and viral pneumonias is beyond the scope of this chapter.

The duration of therapy of CAP is guided by the specific pathogen and the patient's clinical course. Recommendations

TABLE 24-7

Major Classes of Antibiotics Used in the Treatment of Pneumonia

Antibiotic Class	Representative Drugs
Penicillins	Penicillin G, ampicillin
Ureidopenicillins	Ticarcillin, piperacillin, mezlocillin
Semisynthetic penicillins	Oxacillin, nafcillin
First-generation cephalosporins	Cefazolin
Second-generation cephalosporins	Cefuroxime
Third-generation cephalosporins	Cefotaxime, ceftriaxone, ceftizoxime
Antipseudomonal cephalosporins	Ceftazidime, cefepime
Carbapenems	Imipenem, meropenem, ertapenem
Monobactams	Aztreonam
Beta-lactam/beta-lactamase inhibitor combinations	Ticarcillin/clavulanate, piperacillin/tazobactam, ampicillin/sulbactam
Quinolones	Ciprofloxacin, levofloxacin, moxifloxacin, gemifloxacin
Macrolides	Erythromycin, clarithromycin, azithromycin
Tetracyclines	Doxycycline
Glycopeptides	Vancomycin
Oxazolidinones	Linezolid

TABLE 24-8

Empiric Regimens for Treatment of Hospitalized Adults With Community-Acquired Pneumonia

Patient Group	Likely Pathogens	Empiric Regimens
Hospitalized on ward	*Streptococcus pneumoniae, Haemophilus influenzae, Chlamydophila pneumoniae, Staphylococcus aureus, Mycoplasma pneumoniae,* anaerobes, viruses	Respiratory fluoroquinolone (levofloxacin, moxifloxacin, gemifloxacin) alone or beta-lactam (cefotaxime, ceftriaxone, ampicillin, ertapenem) and macrolide
Critically ill, ICU	*S. pneumoniae, Legionella* species, *S. aureus,* gram-negative bacilli, *M. pneumoniae, C. pneumoniae*	If *Pseudomonas aeruginosa* unlikely: Beta-lactam (cefotaxime, ceftriaxone, ampicillin-sulbactam) plus either azithromycin or a respiratory fluoroquinolone If *P. aeruginosa* possible: IV antipseudomonal beta-lactam (piperacillin-tazobactam, cefepime, imipenem, meropenem) plus fluoroquinolone (ciprofloxacin or levofloxacin) or IV antipseudomonal beta-lactam plus aminoglycoside plus either IV macrolide or fluoroquinolone

Modified from Mandell MA, Wunderink RG, Anzueto A, et al: Infectious Disease Society of America/American Thoracic Society consensus guidelines on the management of community-acquired pneumonia in adults. Clin Infect Dis 44:S27–S72, 2007.
IV, Intravenous; *PO*, by mouth.

TABLE 24-9

Pathogen-Specific Treatment Recommendations for Adults With Community-Acquired Pneumonia: Infectious Disease Society of America Guidelines

Pathogen	Recommended Regimen
Streptococcus pneumoniae	
Penicillin susceptible	Penicillin G or amoxicillin
Penicillin resistant	Ceftriaxone, cefotaxime, fluoroquinolone, or vancomycin
Haemophilus influenzae	Second- or third-generation cephalosporin, azithromycin, or TMP-SMX
Legionella species	Macrolide ± rifampin or fluoroquinolone alone
Mycoplasma pneumoniae	Macrolide or doxycycline
Chlamydophila pneumoniae	Macrolide or doxycycline
Staphylococcus aureus	
Methicillin susceptible	Semisynthetic penicillin ± rifampin or gentamicin
Methicillin resistant	Vancomycin or linezolid
Enterobacteriaceae	Third-generation cephalosporin ± aminoglycoside or carbapenem
Pseudomonas aeruginosa	Aminoglycoside + antipseudomonal beta-lactam or carbapenem
Influenza with suspected secondary pneumococcal or staphylococcal infection	Neuraminidase inhibitor (oseltamivir or zanamivir) and vancomycin or linezolid

From Mandell MA, Wunderink RG, Anzueto A, et al: Infectious Disease Society of America/American Thoracic Society consensus guidelines on the management of community-acquired pneumonia in adults. Clin Infect Dis 44:S27–S72, 2007.
TMP-SMX, Trimethoprim-sulfamethoxazole.

have evolved from the traditional 14 days to a minimum of 5 days of therapy with clinical stability. Exceptions include Legionnaire's disease or staphylococcal pneumonia, for which a minimum of 2 weeks of therapy is recommended. Older individuals and patients with comorbidities also may require longer courses of treatment. When fever has resolved and patients begin to improve clinically, oral therapy may be used to complete the treatment program. Failure of the patient's temperature to normalize within 4 or 5 days suggests a missed pathogen, a metastatic or closed-space infection (e.g., empyema), drug fever, or the presence of an obstructing endobronchial lesion. Empyema should be treated with tube thoracostomy. Abnormal findings on physical examination may persist beyond 1 week in 20% to 40% of patients, despite clinical improvement. By 1 month, radiographic resolution occurs in 90% of individuals younger than 50 years.[54] After 1 month, radiographic abnormalities may persist in 70% of cases involving older individuals or in patients with significant underlying illnesses.[54]

RULE OF THUMB

Empyema should be ruled out in patients with CAP and a large pleural effusion who fail to respond to therapy. In cases of CAP, patients often get better before the chest radiograph shows any improvement.

MINI CLINI

Evaluating Persisting Fever in Pneumonia

PROBLEM: The RT is caring for a 68-year-old man admitted 1 week ago with bacteremic *H. influenzae* pneumonia. His admitting chest radiograph showed right lower lobe consolidation and a large right pleural effusion. He has a history of chronic obstructive pulmonary disease (COPD) and reports a 100 pack-year smoking history. He was treated initially with erythromycin and ceftizoxime until his blood cultures became positive. The organism was susceptible to ceftizoxime, which was continued as monotherapy (i.e., treatment with one antibiotic drug). Despite treatment, the patient has remained persistently febrile (39° C) and his chest radiograph has not shown improvement. Why is he not responding to therapy?

DISCUSSION: Patients with CAP who have comorbid illnesses such as alcoholism or COPD may recover more slowly than healthy individuals despite appropriate therapy. Nevertheless, persistent fever 7 days into optimal treatment should prompt several considerations.

The two most likely concerns for this patient are (1) an undrained empyema and (2) an obstructing endobronchial malignancy, given his substantial smoking history. Other less likely considerations are drug fever; a new nosocomial infection; a missed pathogen that is not responsive to ceftizoxime, contributing to his pneumonia; or a deep venous thrombosis resulting from bed rest.

The next step should be to repeat the history and physical examination. If these do not reveal a cause of the persistent fever, a thoracentesis should be performed to exclude empyema. If thoracentesis findings are negative, further investigation looking for an endobronchial-obstructing lesion should be considered.

Health Care–Associated Pneumonia, Hospital-Acquired Pneumonia, and Ventilator-Associated Pneumonia

Empiric and definitive therapy of nosocomial pneumonia is determined by institution-specific data regarding the most common organisms and their antibiotic-susceptibility profiles and by patient-specific risk factors. Although general guidelines have been published,[3] the importance of local data cannot be overemphasized because there is great variation across regions and across health care facilities regarding the prevalence and susceptibility profiles of specific pathogens.

Generally, in-hospital aspiration should be treated with a regimen that provides coverage against anaerobes and gram-negative bacilli, such as a beta-lactam/beta-lactamase inhibitor combination or clindamycin with a third-generation cephalosporin. Although vancomycin has been the traditional drug of choice for MRSA pneumonia, evolving data suggest that linezolid may be better than vancomycin. In a randomized controlled trial of vancomycin versus linezolid for treatment of MRSA pneumonia, clinical resolution of pneumonia occurred more frequently in patients treated with linezolid, but there was no difference in 60-day mortality between the two groups.[55] For VAP, empiric coverage may be targeted at organisms known to colonize the patient's oropharynx or pathogens that are present in the ICU. Patients with *P. aeruginosa* pneumonia usually are treated with two agents, such as a ureidopenicillin or antipseudomonal cephalosporin together with an aminoglycoside or fluoroquinolone. Other gram-negative pneumonias generally are treated with a single agent, except in cases involving critically ill patients, for whom a second drug is sometimes added. If nosocomial legionellosis is present within an institution, a macrolide may be added to the empiric regimen.

Similar to CAP, the duration of therapy for cases of nosocomial pneumonia is dictated by the clinical course. A study comparing 8 days versus 15 days of therapy in patients with VAP found that short-course therapy was associated with comparable outcomes to long-course therapy, although the rate of relapse was slightly higher in patients with *Pseudomonas* or *Acinetobacter* infections.[56] More prolonged courses of therapy may be required in patients who are slow to respond but are associated with a greater risk for new colonization with other organisms. Failure of the patient to improve should prompt the following considerations: the presence of an occult empyema; an unrecognized pathogen; a new, unrelated nosocomial infection; or other noninfectious causes of fever common in the ICU, such as deep venous thrombosis, drug fever, occult pancreatitis, or acalculous cholecystitis (gallbladder inflammation without gallstones).

The RT has an important role in diagnosing and managing patients with CAP and nosocomial pneumonia. Helping patients clear infected secretions aids clinical improvement and maintaining adequate oxygenation is essential. The usefulness of chest physiotherapy in the treatment of pneumonia is still unproved but some patients seem to benefit from it.

PREVENTION

Community-Acquired Pneumonia

Preventive strategies for CAP have focused on immunizing high-risk individuals against influenza and *S. pneumoniae.* Influenza is a risk factor for subsequent development of CAP during the fall and winter months. In 2010, the Advisory Committee on Immunization Practices (ACIP) expanded its recommendation for influenza vaccination to include all individuals older than 6 months.[57] Immunization is particularly important for individuals older than 60 years (because it reduces the incidence of illness for this age group by half[58]) and for those with chronic lung or heart disease in whom the morbidity of influenza may be substantial. Recent studies suggest that widespread immunization of healthy working adults is cost-effective because the number of sick days taken and the number of visits to a physician are reduced.[59] Health care workers, including RTs, should be immunized annually to prevent transmission of influenza to patients.

Currently available pneumococcal vaccines provide protection against the 23 serotypes of *S. pneumoniae,* which cause 85% to 90% of invasive pneumococcal infections in the United States. Vaccination is indicated for all individuals older than 65 years and for individuals older than 2 years who have functional or anatomic asplenia (i.e., lack a spleen). Vaccination is also indicated in patients with chronic illnesses such as CHF, chronic lung disease, or chronic liver disease; alcoholism; cerebrospinal fluid leaks; or conditions characterized by impaired immunity.[60] Routine pneumococcal vaccination of all health care workers is not currently recommended; health care workers who possess one of the specific indications for vaccination outlined previously should be immunized.

Immunity against *Bordetella pertussis* fades over time, leading to transmission from older adults to other adults and infants. Because secondary bacterial pneumonia occurs in a significant number of cases of pertussis, the ACIP has recommended that the tetanus-diphtheria-acellular pertussis (Tdap) vaccine replace the tetanus-diphtheria (Td) vaccine in the adult immunization schedule.[61]

Health Care–Associated Pneumonia, Hospital-Acquired Pneumonia, and Ventilator-Associated Pneumonia

Preventing nosocomial pneumonia has been intensely studied over the past 30 years. Table 24-10 summarizes currently available strategies and their relative efficacy. No preventive strategy is uniformly effective. Many institutions now employ a "ventilator bundle" including several of these measures.

Handwashing is an important but frequently overlooked measure that can reduce transmission of nosocomial bacteria from one patient to another. Handwashing is especially important for RTs who may be caring for several ventilated patients in the ICU. Failure to wash the hands between patient contacts may result in transmission of respiratory pathogens from one patient to another. Handwashing is important even if gloves are worn. Gloves should be changed between patient contacts because they also can become contaminated with and transmit bacteria.

TABLE 24-10
Strategies for Prevention of Nosocomial Pneumonia

Strategy	Efficacy
Handwashing	Probably effective
Isolation of patients with resistant organisms	Probably effective
Infection control and surveillance	Probably effective
Enteral feeding, rather than total parenteral nutrition	Possibly effective
Semierect position	Possibly effective
Sucralfate for bleeding prophylaxis	Possibly effective
Careful handling of respiratory therapy equipment	Possibly effective
Subglottic secretion aspiration	Possibly effective
Selective digestive decontamination	Unproved efficacy
Topical tracheobronchial antibiotics	Unproved efficacy

Infection control surveillance to detect outbreaks of nosocomial pneumonia with specific pathogens and to monitor antibiotic resistance patterns is important. Isolation and caring for infected patients in the same place can limit the scope and duration of outbreaks, especially in ICUs.

In patients requiring nutrition support, the use of enteral feeding via jejunostomy has been associated with a lower risk for nosocomial pneumonia than the use of total parenteral nutrition.[62] In addition, patients who are fed enterally (i.e., using the gut to feed) have a lower incidence of pneumonia if kept semierect rather than recumbent.[8]

Two studies suggest that GI bleeding prophylaxis with sucralfate is associated with a lower risk for pneumonia compared with antacid or H_2-blockers.[63,64] Careful handling of respiratory therapy equipment may reduce the risk for LRTI in ventilated patients. Condensate within the tubing may be colonized with bacteria and should be drained away from the patient because passage of this material into the airway may encourage colonization with nosocomial pathogens. One study found that continuous subglottic aspiration of secretions was effective in reducing the incidence of nosocomial pneumonia in intubated patients.[65] Many studies have failed to show that selective digestive decontamination is effective to prevent nosocomial pneumonia; this is a strategy that uses topical antibiotics in the oropharynx and GI tract along with a brief course of systemic therapy. A meta-analysis suggested that topical oral decontamination may reduce the incidence of VAP but not mortality, duration of mechanical ventilation, or length of ICU stay.[66]

Prevention of nosocomial pneumonia remains a challenge to the RT. Careful attention to basic infection control practices, such as frequent handwashing, using new gloves with each patient contact, and careful handling of respiratory care equipment, is important in preventing nosocomial pneumonia.

TUBERCULOSIS

Tuberculosis, caused by *M. tuberculosis,* can sometimes mimic CAP and poses special management challenges for the RT. Knowledge of the epidemiology, clinical manifestations, diagnosis, infection control management, and treatment of patients with suspected or proved tuberculosis is essential.

Epidemiology

The epidemiology of tuberculosis in the United States has changed over the past 25 years. After the introduction of effective drugs to treat tuberculosis in the 1950s, the incidence of tuberculosis steadily declined. Tuberculosis increasingly became a disease affecting elderly patients, and most cases represented reactivation of old latent disease. With the emergence of the acquired immunodeficiency syndrome (AIDS) epidemic in the early 1980s, there was a resurgence of tuberculosis in the United States and worldwide. This resurgence began in 1985 and peaked in 1992. Since 1992, the incidence of tuberculosis has declined. This resurgence of tuberculosis was accompanied by dramatic shifts in the patients at risk and the clinical manifestations of the disease. Multidrug-resistant tuberculosis, defined as resistance of *M. tuberculosis* to both isoniazid and rifampin, emerged as a major public health problem in some populations and areas. Compared with frequency of the era before AIDS, tuberculosis now more often occurs in younger individuals with HIV infection, especially inner-city minority populations with a history of injection drug use. Foreign-born nationals residing in the United States have accounted for half of cases reported annually in recent years.

Tuberculosis has increasingly become a disease affecting individuals of lower socioeconomic status in whom homelessness or crowded living conditions, poor access to health care, and unemployment have contributed to the persistence of the disease.[67] Other risk factors include the presence of hematologic malignancies, head and neck cancer, celiac disease (a bowel disease characterized by poor absorption), and the receipt of medications such as corticosteroids and TNF-alpha antagonists.[67-70]

Pathophysiology

Tuberculosis is acquired by inhaling airborne droplets containing the responsible microorganism, *M. tuberculosis,* and the lungs are the major site of infection. Microorganism-laden droplets are deposited in the terminal airways and cause a host immune response. Most exposed individuals successfully contain the infection and remain asymptomatic, although they remain at risk for reactivation of infection later in life, especially if they become immunosuppressed.

Patients with tuberculosis can present with pulmonary or extrapulmonary manifestations. The major syndromes of pulmonary tuberculosis include primary, reactivation, and endobronchial tuberculosis and tuberculoma.

Primary Tuberculosis

Symptomatic primary tuberculosis occurs in a few individuals shortly after exposure. Primary tuberculous pneumonia is a more common clinical presentation in children and in HIV-infected individuals compared with non–HIV-infected adults. Fever is the most common symptom and occurs in 70% of patients; it persists for 14 to 21 days on average.[71] Chest pain occurs in approximately 25%; cough is even less common. The chest radiograph shows hilar lymphadenopathy in 65%, pleural effusion in 33%, and an infiltrate in approximately 25%. Diagnosis may be difficult given the infrequency of cough and a pulmonary infiltrate.

Reactivation and Endobronchial Tuberculosis

Reactivation tuberculosis develops months to years after initial infection and may occur spontaneously or in the setting of immunosuppression. In individuals without HIV infection, reactivation disease accounts for 90% of cases of tuberculosis. The most common symptoms include fever, cough, night sweats, and weight loss. Sputum production increases as the infection progresses and is occasionally accompanied by hemoptysis, which is seldom massive. Older patients may present with a more indolent illness in which fever and night sweats are absent. Physical examination is often unrevealing in patients with reactivation tuberculosis. Chest radiograph shows apicoposterior upper lobe disease in 80% to 90% of patients, and cavities are present in 20% to 40%.

Endobronchial tuberculosis involves the airways and may be seen in both primary and reactivation tuberculosis. In primary tuberculosis, hilar nodal enlargement may impinge on the bronchi, resulting in compression and ultimately ulceration. In patients with reactivation disease, endobronchial involvement may occur as a result of direct extension from the parenchyma or pooling of secretions from upper lobe cavities in the dependent distal airways. Symptoms of endobronchial tuberculosis include a barking cough in two-thirds of patients, sputum production, wheezing, and hemoptysis. On physical examination, wheezing is common. The chest radiograph most often shows an upper lobe cavitary infiltrate with an ipsilateral (i.e., on the same side) lower lobe infiltrate. Extensive endobronchial disease may produce bronchiectasis.

Tuberculomas

Tuberculomas are rounded solitary mass lesions and may occur in primary or reactivation tuberculosis. They are often asymptomatic and may mimic malignancy. Tuberculoma is in the differential diagnosis of solitary pulmonary nodule and may be difficult to diagnose without biopsy or excision because expectorated sputum in patients with tuberculoma rarely shows *M. tuberculosis* on smear or culture.

Complications

Complications of pulmonary tuberculosis include tuberculous empyema, bronchiectasis, extensive pulmonary parenchymal destruction, spontaneous pneumothorax, and massive hemoptysis from rupture of a Rasmussen aneurysm in the wall of a cavity.

Extrapulmonary Tuberculosis

Extrapulmonary tuberculosis is defined as spread of *M. tuberculosis* infection beyond the lung and may involve virtually any organ. The central nervous system, musculoskeletal system, genitourinary tract, and lymph nodes (scrofula) are the most common sites of extrapulmonary tuberculosis. HIV-infected patients who acquire tuberculosis often present with unique clinical manifestations compared with non–HIV-infected patients. HIV-infected patients may develop rapidly progressive primary infection and present with both pulmonary and extrapulmonary disease. In patients with advanced AIDS, tuberculosis may manifest as disseminated disease with involvement of multiple organs, including lymph nodes, bone marrow, liver, and spleen. Symptoms in this setting include high fevers, sweats, and progressive weight loss. Findings on examination may include fever, wasting, and hepatosplenomegaly. Laboratory testing may show pancytopenia (decreased cell counts in WBCs, RBCs, and platelets) and advanced immunodeficiency. Imaging studies often show mediastinal and abdominal lymphadenopathy and hepatosplenomegaly.

Diagnosis

The history is important in diagnosing and managing patients with suspected tuberculosis. In addition to eliciting the patient's symptoms, the clinician should inquire about any history of tuberculosis, the presence of risk factors for acquiring tuberculosis and/or HIV infection, any history of travel, and potential contacts with individuals with known or suspected tuberculosis. In patients with a history of tuberculosis, outside medical records, including drug susceptibility results of prior isolates, should be obtained. If the patient has been previously treated, the drugs chosen, duration of treatment, and adherence to therapy should be evaluated. Risk factors for drug-resistant tuberculosis should be sought, which include prior treatment for tuberculosis, exposure to individuals with known drug-resistant disease, exposure to individuals with active tuberculosis who have been previously treated, travel to parts of the world with a high prevalence of drug resistance, or exposure to individuals with active tuberculosis from those areas.

The gold standard for diagnosing tuberculosis from pulmonary and extrapulmonary sites is culture isolation of the organism on solid or liquid media. The major disadvantage of culture is that *M. tuberculosis* may take 4 to 6 weeks to grow, thereby delaying diagnosis. Acid-fast staining of expectorated sputum, bronchoscopic specimens, and other body fluids or tissues may be used in patients with suspected pulmonary or extrapulmonary disease. In patients with pulmonary tuberculosis, it is estimated that 10^4 organisms/ml is required for the smear to be positive. Acid-fast smears of both sputum and other body sites are less sensitive than culture for detecting disease. The presence of acid-fast bacilli on a smear is not synonymous with a diagnosis of *M. tuberculosis* because nontuberculous mycobacteria (NTM) can produce pulmonary and extrapulmonary disease in selected populations. More rapid diagnostic techniques for identifying *M. tuberculosis* in clinical specimens and for confirming the identity of the organism in culture are being developed and are available in some centers. These techniques include nucleic acid amplification, nucleic acid probes, PCR genomic analysis, and molecular tests for chromosomal mutations associated with drug resistance.

A 5 tuberculin unit purified protein derivative (5 TU PPD) skin test or interferon-gamma release assay (IGRA) may be performed in individuals with suspected tuberculosis. Both tests evaluate for cell-mediated immunity to tuberculosis in individuals with prior exposure to the organism. A PPD consists of intradermal injection of tuberculin material, which stimulates a delayed-type hypersensitivity response mediated by T cells and causes skin induration within 48 to 72 hours. False-positive results can occur in patients with prior bacille Calmette-Guérin (BCG) vaccination or infection with NTM species. IGRAs are blood tests that measure T-cell release of the cytokine interferon-gamma after stimulation by antigens unique to *M. tuberculosis.* IGRAs are unaffected by BCG vaccination status and most NTM infections (except *Mycobacterium marinum* and *Mycobacterium kansasii*) and require only a single patient encounter, all of which are advantages over the PPD.[72] Both tests become positive

3 to 8 weeks after acquisition of infection. A positive skin test or IGRA supports the diagnosis in the appropriate clinical setting, but a negative result does not exclude the diagnosis. Patients with HIV infection, other causes of immunodeficiency, advanced age, or other comorbidities may be anergic and unable to mount either a positive skin test or IGRA result.[72,73]

Precautions

Patients hospitalized with suspected or proved active pulmonary tuberculosis should be placed in respiratory isolation in private negative pressure airflow rooms because they pose a risk for transmitting infection to others by coughing up aerosolized droplets containing *M. tuberculosis*. Individuals entering the patient's room should wear fit-tested National Institute for Occupational Safety and Health–approved N-95 or higher masks or respirators. A surgical mask should be placed on a patient with suspected or proved active pulmonary tuberculosis during transport outside the negative pressure room.

Treatment

Treatment recommendations for tuberculosis have been published by the ATS, U.S. Centers for Disease Control and Prevention (CDC), and the IDSA.[74] The goals of therapy are to cure the patient and prevent transmission of *M. tuberculosis* to others. Treatment must address clinical and social issues and should be customized to the patient's circumstance. At the outset, daily observed therapy (DOT) should be part of the treatment program; this consists of observing the patient taking the antituberculous medications. Treatment programs that use comprehensive case management and DOT have a higher rate of successful completion of therapy than other treatment strategies. Social service support, housing assistance, and treatment for substance abuse may be required for selected individuals with tuberculosis and should be part of the treatment plan. Patients with tuberculosis must be promptly reported to the local department of public health so that contact tracing can be performed. This includes identification, if possible, of the index case from whom the patient has contracted the infection and identification of close personal contacts to whom the patient may have transmitted *M. tuberculosis*.

Isoniazid, rifampin, pyrazinamide, and ethambutol are first-line antituberculous medications. Pending antimicrobial susceptibility results, treatment with four drugs at the outset is recommended. In patients with drug-susceptible pulmonary tuberculosis, many 6- to 9-month treatment regimens have been shown to be effective as outlined in guidelines by the ATS, CDC, and IDSA.[74] Patients with multidrug-resistant tuberculosis require more prolonged courses of therapy with multidrug regimens.

ROLE OF THE RESPIRATORY THERAPIST IN PULMONARY INFECTIONS

The RT plays a key role in managing patients with pulmonary infections, including helping to diagnose and treat the illnesses. Diagnostically, RTs participate in the collection of sputum by expectoration or assisting physicians during bronchoscopy. In some settings, RTs may perform mini-BAL.

RTs often administer chest physiotherapy when indicated, as in patients with bronchiectasis and cystic fibrosis. They also may be involved in counseling patients in other clearance techniques, such as autogenic drainage and positive expiratory pressure (PEP) therapy. RTs also play key roles in modeling optimal infection control and prevention practices (e.g., handwashing, implementing and complying with respiratory precautions, vaccination) and in advising patients about preventive interventions, such as influenza, pneumococcal, and Tdap vaccines.

SUMMARY CHECKLIST

- CAP and nosocomial pneumonia are common and important clinical problems with significant morbidity and mortality.
- *S. pneumoniae* remains the most common cause of CAP. Gram-negative bacilli and *S. aureus* are the most common causes of nosocomial pneumonia, but their relative incidence and antimicrobial susceptibility profiles may vary across institutions.
- The mortality risk can be quantified at presentation for most patients with CAP, which helps in determining the need for hospitalization.
- Routine sputum cultures for patients with CAP must be interpreted within the context of the sputum Gram stain, which provides valuable information regarding the adequacy of the specimen and the predominance of potential pathogens.
- The accurate diagnosis of nosocomial pneumonia remains a challenge; none of the diagnostic methods currently available is completely reliable.
- Guidelines exist for the treatment of CAP and nosocomial pneumonia. When possible, pathogen-specific antibiotic therapy should be used.
- Immunizing high-risk individuals against influenza and *S. pneumoniae* is the major strategy in preventing CAP.
- Strategies for preventing nosocomial pneumonia are not uniformly effective.
- Pulmonary tuberculosis may mimic CAP; the recognition and appropriate isolation, diagnostic evaluation, and management of individuals with possible pulmonary tuberculosis are essential.
- The RT can help prevent nosocomial pneumonia by careful attention to basic infection control procedures such as handwashing.

References

1. Centers for Disease Control and Prevention: Pneumonia statistics. <http://www.cdc.gov/nchs/fastats/pneumonia.htm>, Accessed July, 2014.
2. Heron M: Deaths: leading causes for 2010. *Natl Vital Stat Rep* 62:1–97, 2013.
3. American Thoracic Society: Guidelines for the management of adults with hospital-acquired, ventilator-associated, and healthcare-associated pneumonia. *Am J Respir Crit Care Med* 171:388–416, 2005.

4. Craven DE, Steger KA, Barber TW: Preventing nosocomial pneumonia: state of the art and perspectives for the 1990s. *Am J Med* 91:44S–53S, 1991.
5. Wiblin RT, Wenzel RP: Hospital-acquired pneumonia. *Curr Clin Top Infect Dis* 16:194–214, 1996.
6. Magill SS, Edwards JR, Bamberg W, et al: Multistate point-prevalence survey of health care associated infections. *N Engl J Med* 370:1198–1208, 2014.
7. Bassin A, Niederman MS: New approaches to prevention and treatment of nosocomial pneumonia. *Semin Thorac Cardiovasc Surg* 7:70–77, 1995.
8. Torres A, Serra-Batlles J, Ros E, et al: Pulmonary aspiration of gastric contents in patients receiving mechanical ventilation: the effect of body position. *Ann Intern Med* 116:540–543, 1992.
9. Valles J, Artigas A, Rello J, et al: Continuous aspiration of subglottic secretions in preventing ventilator-associated pneumonia. *Ann Intern Med* 122: 179–186, 1995.
10. Wallis RS, Broder MS, Wong JY, et al: Granulomatous infectious diseases associated with tumor necrosis factor antagonists. *Clin Infect Dis* 38:1261–1265, 2004.
11. Bartlett JG, Mundy LM: Community-acquired pneumonia. *N Engl J Med* 333:1618–1624, 1995.
12. Marrie TJ, Peeling RW, Fine MJ, et al: Ambulatory patients with community-acquired pneumonia: the frequency of atypical agents and clinical course. *Am J Med* 101:508–515, 1996.
13. Rello J, Bodi M, Mariscal M, et al: Microbiological testing and outcomes in patients with severe community-acquired pneumonia. *Chest* 123:174–180, 2003.
14. Kollef MH, Micek ST: Methicillin-resistant *Staphylococcus aureus:* a new community-acquired pathogen? *Curr Opin Infect Dis* 19:161–168, 2006.
15. Mundy LM, Auwaerter PG, Oldach D, et al: Community-acquired pneumonia: impact of immune status. *Am J Respir Crit Care Med* 152:1309–1315, 1995.
16. World Health Organization: Clinical management of human infection with avian influenza A (H5N1) virus. <http://www.who.int/csr/disease/avian_influenza/guidelines/Clinical Management07.pdf>, August 2007 Accessed June 2015.
17. Bush LM, Abrams BH, Beall A, et al: Index case of fatal inhalational anthrax due to bioterrorism in the United States. *N Engl J Med* 345:1607–1610, 2001.
18. Christian MD, Poutanen SM, Loutfy MR, et al: Severe acute respiratory syndrome. *Clin Infect Dis* 38:1420–1427, 2004.
19. Bialek SR, Allen D, Alvarado-Ramy F, et al: First confirmed cases of Middle East respiratory syndrome coronavirus (MERS-CoV) infection in the United States: updated information on the epidemiology of MERS-CoV infection, and guidance for the public, clinicians, and public health authorities—May 2014. *MMWR Morb Mortal Wkly Rep* 63:431–436, 2014.
20. Centers for Disease Control and Prevention: Enterovirus D68 in the United States: 2014. <http://www.cdc.gov>, Accessed September 27, 2014.
21. Fang GD, Fine M, Orloff J, et al: New and emerging etiologies for community-acquired pneumonia with implications for therapy: a prospective multicenter study of 359 cases. *Medicine* 69:307–316, 1990.
22. Fine MJ, Smith DN, Singer DE: Hospitalization decision in patients with community-acquired pneumonia: a prospective cohort study. *Am J Med* 89:713–721, 1990.
23. Fine MJ, Smith MA, Carson CA, et al: Prognosis and outcomes of patients with community-acquired pneumonia: a meta-analysis. *JAMA* 275:134–141, 1996.
24. Fine MJ, Auble TE, Yealy DM, et al: A prediction rule to identify low-risk patients with community-acquired pneumonia. *N Engl J Med* 336:243–250, 1997.
25. Lim WS, van der Erden MM, Laing R, et al: Defining community acquired pneumonia severity on presentation to hospital: an international derivation and validation study. *Thorax* 58:377–382, 2003.
26. Torres A, Aznar R, Gatell JM, et al: Incidence, risk, and prognosis factors of nosocomial pneumonia in mechanically ventilated patients. *Am Rev Respir Dis* 142:523–528, 1990.
27. Craven DE, Steger KA: Epidemiology of nosocomial pneumonia: new perspectives on an old disease. *Chest* 108:1S–16S, 1995.
28. Kollef MH, Silver P, Murphy DM, et al: The effect of late-onset ventilator-associated pneumonia in determining patient mortality. *Chest* 108:1655–1662, 1995.
29. Rein MF, Gwaltney JM, Jr, O'Brien WM, et al: Accuracy of Gram's stain in identifying pneumococci in sputum. *JAMA* 239:2671–2673, 1978.
30. Barrett-Connor E: The nonvalue of sputum culture in the diagnosis of pneumococcal pneumonia. *Am Rev Respir Dis* 103:845–848, 1971.
31. Gleckman R, DeVita J, Hibert D, et al: Sputum Gram's stain assessment in community-acquired bacteremic pneumonia. *J Clin Microbiol* 26:846–849, 1988.
32. Murray PR, Washington JA: Microscopic and bacteriologic analysis of expectorated sputum. *Mayo Clin Proc* 50:339–344, 1975.
33. Nguyen ML, Yu VL: *Legionella* infection. *Clin Chest Med* 12:257–268, 1991.
34. Farley MM, Stephens DS, Harvey RC, et al: Invasive *Haemophilus influenzae* disease in adults. *Ann Intern Med* 116:806–812, 1992.
35. Houck PM, Bratzler DW, Nsa W, et al: Timing of antibiotic administration and outcomes for Medicare patients hospitalized with pneumonia. *Arch Intern Med* 164:637–644, 2004.
36. Colice GL, Curtis A, Deslauriers J, et al: Medical and surgical treatment of parapneumonic effusions: an evidence-based guideline. *Chest* 118:1158–1171, 2000.
37. Kohler RB: Antigen detection for the rapid diagnosis of mycoplasma and *Legionella* pneumonia. *Diagn Microbiol Infect Dis* 4:47S–59S, 1986.
38. Pfeiffer CD, Fine JP, Safdar N: Diagnosis of invasive Aspergillosis using a galactomannan assay: a meta-analysis. *Clin Infect Dis* 42:1417–1427, 2006.
39. Karageorgopoulos DE, Vouloumanou EK, Ntziora F, et al: β-D-glucan assay for the diagnosis of invasive fungal infections: a meta-analysis. *Clin Infect Dis* 52:750–770, 2011.
40. Moyer VA: Screening for HIV: U.S. Preventive Services Task Force recommendation statement. *Ann Intern Med* 159:51–60, 2013.
41. Chastre J, Fagon JY, Trouillet JL: Diagnosis and treatment of nosocomial pneumonia in patients in intensive care units. *Clin Infect Dis* 21(Suppl 3): S226–S237, 1995.
42. Garrard CS, A'Court CD: The diagnosis of pneumonia in the critically ill. *Chest* 108(Suppl 2):17S–25S, 1995.
43. Fagon JY, Chastre J, Hance AJ, et al: Evaluation of clinical judgment in the identification and treatment of nosocomial pneumonia in ventilated patients. *Chest* 103:547–553, 1993.
44. Timsit JF, Misset B, Azoulay E, et al: Usefulness of airway visualization in the diagnosis of nosocomial pneumonia in ventilated patients. *Chest* 110: 172–179, 1996.
45. Marquette CH, Georges H, Wallet F, et al: Diagnostic efficacy of endotracheal aspirates with quantitative bacterial cultures in intubated patients with suspected pneumonia. *Am Rev Respir Dis* 148:138–144, 1993.
46. Jourdain B, Novara A, Joly-Guillou ML, et al: Role of quantitative cultures of endotracheal aspirates in the diagnosis of nosocomial pneumonia. *Am J Respir Crit Care Med* 152:241–246, 1995.
47. Chastre J, Fagon JY, Soler P, et al: Quantification of BAL cells containing intracellular bacteria rapidly identifies ventilated patients with nosocomial pneumonia. *Chest* 95:S190–S192, 1989.
48. Chastre J, Fagon JY, Soler P, et al: Diagnosis of nosocomial bacterial pneumonia in intubated patients undergoing ventilation: comparison of the usefulness of bronchoalveolar lavage and the protected specimen brush. *Am J Med* 85:499–506, 1988.
49. Kollef MH, Bock KR, Richards RD, et al: The safety and diagnostic accuracy of minibronchoalveolar lavage in patients with suspected ventilator-associated pneumonia. *Ann Intern Med* 122:743–748, 1995.
50. Dorca J, Manresa F, Esteban L, et al: Efficacy, safety, and therapeutic relevance of transthoracic aspiration with ultrathin needle in non-ventilated nosocomial pneumonia. *Am J Respir Crit Care Med* 151:1491–1496, 1995.
51. Mandell MA, Wunderink RG, Anzueto A, et al: Infectious Disease Society of America/American Thoracic Society consensus guidelines on the management of community-acquired pneumonia in adults. *Clin Infect Dis* 44: S27–S72, 2007.
52. Bartlett JG, Dowell SF, Mandell LA, et al: Practice guidelines for the management of community-acquired pneumonia in adults. *Clin Infect Dis* 31: 347–382, 2000.

53. Mandell LA, Bartlett JG, Dowell SF, et al: Update of practice guidelines for the management of community-acquired pneumonia in immunocompetent adults. *Clin Infect Dis* 37:1405–1433, 2003.
54. Mittl RL, Jr, Schwab RJ, Duchin JS, et al: Radiographic resolution of community-acquired pneumonia. *Am J Respir Crit Care Med* 149:630–635, 1994.
55. Wunderink RG, Niederman MS, Kollef MH, et al: Linezolid in methicillin-resistant *Staphylococcus aureus* nosocomial pneumonia: a randomized, controlled study. *Clin Infect Dis* 54:621–629, 2012.
56. Chastre J, Wolff M, Fagon JY, et al: Comparison of 8 vs 15 days of antibiotic therapy for ventilator-associated pneumonia in adults: a randomized trial. *JAMA* 290:2588–2598, 2003.
57. Centers for Disease Control and Prevention: Prevention and control of influenza with vaccines: recommendations of the Advisory Committee on Immunization Practices (ACIP), 2010. *MMWR Recomm Rep* 59(RR-8):1–59, 2010.
58. Govaert TM, Thijs CT, Masurel N, et al: The efficacy of influenza vaccination in elderly individuals: a randomized double-blind placebo-controlled trial. *JAMA* 272:1661–1665, 1994.
59. Nichol KL, Lind A, Margolis KL, et al: The effectiveness of vaccination against influenza in healthy, working adults. *N Engl J Med* 333:889–893, 1995.
60. Centers for Disease Control and Prevention: Prevention of pneumococcal disease: recommendations of the Advisory Committee on Immunization Practices (ACIP). *MMWR CDC Surveill Summ* 46(RR-8):1–24, 1997.
61. Centers for Disease Control and Prevention: Updated recommendations for the use of tetanus toxoid, reduced diphtheria toxoid and acellular pertussis (Tdap) vaccine from the Advisory Committee on Immunization Practices (ACIP): 2010. *MMWR* 60:13–15, 2011.
62. Moore FA, Moore EE, Jones TN, et al: TEN versus TPN following major abdominal trauma: reduced septic mortality. *J Trauma* 29:916–922, 1989.
63. Tryba M: Sucralfate versus antacids or H_2-antagonists for stress ulcer prophylaxis: a meta-analysis on efficacy and pneumonia rate. *Crit Care Med* 19:942–949, 1991.
64. Cook DJ, Laine LA, Guyatt GH, et al: Nosocomial pneumonia and the role of gastric pH: a meta-analysis. *Chest* 100:7–13, 1991.
65. Valles J, Artigas A, Rello J, et al: Continuous aspiration of subglottic secretions in preventing ventilator-associated pneumonia. *Ann Intern Med* 122: 179–186, 1995.
66. Chan EY, Ruest A, O'Meade M, et al: Oral decontamination for prevention of pneumonia in mechanically ventilated adults: systematic review and meta-analysis. *BMJ* 334:889, 2007.
67. Centers for Disease Control and Prevention: Trends in tuberculosis: United States, 2005. *MMWR Morb Mortal Wkly Rep* 55:305–308, 2006.
68. Kamboj M, Sepkowitz KA: The risk of tuberculosis in patients with cancer. *Clin Infect Dis* 42:1592–1595, 2006.
69. Jick SS, Lieberman ES, Rahman MU, et al: Glucocorticoid use, other associated factors, and the risk of tuberculosis. *Arthritis Rheum* 55:19–26, 2006.
70. Ludvigsson JF, Wahlstrom J, Grunewald J, et al: Coeliac disease and risk of tuberculosis: a population based cohort study. *Thorax* 62:23–28, 2007.
71. Poulson A: Some clinical features of tuberculosis. 2. Initial fever. 3. Erythema nodosum. 4. Tuberculosis of lungs and pleura in primary infection. *Acta Tuberc Scand* 33:37–92, 1951.
72. Mazurek GH, Jereb J, Vernon A, et al: Updated guidelines for using interferon gamma release assays to detect *Mycobacterium tuberculosis* infection: United States, 2010. *MMWR Recomm Rep* 59(RR-5):1–25, 2010.
73. Pai M, Denkinger CM, Kik SV, et al: Gamma interferon release assays for detection of *Mycobacterium tuberculosis* infection. *Clin Microbiol Rev* 27:3–20, 2014.
74. Blumberg HM, Burman WJ, Chaisson RE, et al: ATS/CDC/IDSA: treatment of tuberculosis. *Am J Respir Crit Care Med* 167:603–662, 2003.

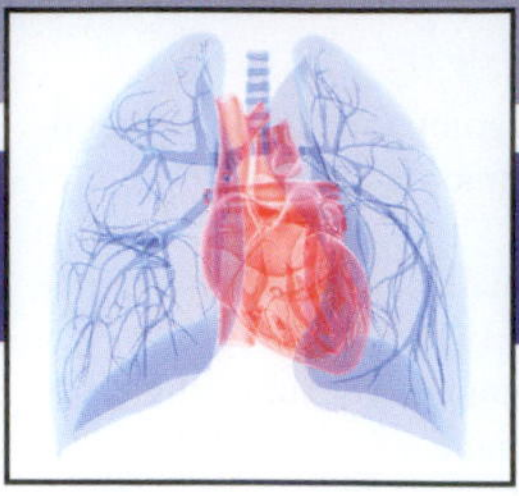

CHAPTER 25

Obstructive Lung Disease: Chronic Obstructive Pulmonary Disease, Asthma, and Related Diseases

ENRIQUE DIAZ-GUZMAN AND JAMES K. STOLLER

CHAPTER OBJECTIVES

After reading this chapter you will be able to:

- State definitions of chronic obstructive pulmonary disease (COPD), asthma, and bronchiectasis.
- Understand the major risk factors associated with COPD.
- Identify the common signs and symptoms associated with COPD.
- Describe a treatment plan for a patient with stable COPD and for a patient with an acute exacerbation of COPD.
- State the typical clinical presentation of a patient with asthma.
- Identify the treatment currently available for a patient with acute asthma.
- Describe the treatment currently available for patients with bronchiectasis.

CHAPTER OUTLINE

Chronic Obstructive Pulmonary Disease
- Overview and Definitions
- Epidemiology
- Risk Factors and Pathophysiology
- Clinical Signs and Symptoms
- Management
- Establishing the Diagnosis
- Optimizing Lung Function
- Maximizing Functional Status
- Preventing Progression of Chronic Obstructive Pulmonary Disease and Enhancing Survival
- Additional Therapies

Asthma
- Definition
- Incidence
- Etiology and Pathogenesis
- Clinical Presentation and Diagnosis
- Management
- Objective Measurement and Monitoring
- Pharmacotherapy
- Emergency Department and Hospital Management
- Bronchial Thermoplasty
- Immunotherapy
- Environmental Control
- Patient Education
- Special Considerations in Asthma Management

Bronchiectasis
- Clinical Presentation
- Evaluation
- Management

Role of the Respiratory Therapist in Obstructive Lung Disease

KEY TERMS

acute exacerbation of COPD
airway hyperresponsiveness
airway inflammation
airway obstruction
asthma
bronchiectasis
bronchodilator
bronchospasm
chronic bronchitis
cystic fibrosis
emphysema
noninvasive ventilation
supplemental oxygen

The category of obstructive lung diseases is broad and includes chronic obstructive pulmonary disease (COPD) and **asthma** as the most common diseases and **bronchiectasis** and **cystic fibrosis** as less common forms. Airflow obstruction also may be a feature of other lung diseases such as sarcoidosis, lymphangioleiomyomatosis, and congestive heart failure. This chapter reviews the major obstructive lung diseases, emphasizing their defining features, epidemiology, pathophysiology, clinical signs and symptoms, prognosis, and management. Cystic fibrosis is discussed in Chapter 34.

CHRONIC OBSTRUCTIVE PULMONARY DISEASE

Overview and Definitions

The term *chronic obstructive pulmonary disease (COPD)*, or sometimes *chronic obstructive lung disease (COLD)*, refers to a disease state characterized by the presence of incompletely reversible airflow obstruction. Current guidelines by the American Thoracic Society (ATS) and the Global Initiative for Chronic Obstructive Lung Disease (GOLD) guidelines recommend the use of the term *COPD* to encompass both chronic bronchitis and emphysema. The ATS guidelines statement regarding COPD defines this entity as follows[1]:

> *Chronic obstructive pulmonary disease (COPD) is a preventable and treatable disease state characterized by airflow limitation that is not fully reversible. The airflow limitation is usually progressive and is associated with an abnormal inflammatory response of the lungs to noxious particles or gases, primarily caused by cigarette smoking. Although COPD affects the lungs, it also produces significant systemic consequences.*

Similarly, the GOLD guidelines define COPD as follows[2]:

> *A disease state characterized by persistent airflow limitation that is usually progressive, and is associated with an enhanced inflammatory response in the airways and the lung to noxious particles or gases. Exacerbations and comorbidities contribute to the overall severity in individual patients.*

The spectrum of COPD is shown in Figure 25-1, which presents a nonproportional Venn diagram representing the major components of COPD—chronic bronchitis and emphysema. Although asthma is no longer conventionally considered to be part of the spectrum of COPD, the diagram shows that there is overlap between asthma and COPD. In actual practice, it may not be possible to distinguish between individuals with a history of asthma but with incompletely reversible airflow obstruction and individuals with COPD.

The two major diseases that make up COPD—emphysema and chronic bronchitis—are defined in different ways. **Emphysema** is defined in anatomic terms as a condition characterized by abnormal, permanent enlargement of the airspaces beyond the terminal bronchiole, accompanied by destruction of the walls of the airspaces without fibrosis. **Chronic bronchitis** is defined in clinical terms as a condition in which chronic productive cough is present for at least 3 months per year for at least 2 consecutive years. The definition specifies further that other causes of chronic cough (e.g., gastroesophageal reflux, asthma, and postnasal drip) have been excluded. Figure 25-1 shows considerable overlap between chronic bronchitis and emphysema and some overlap with asthma—that is, when airflow obstruction is incompletely reversible. Figure 25-1 also shows that chronic bronchitis and emphysema can occur without airflow obstruction, although the clinical significance of these diseases usually comes from obstruction to airflow.

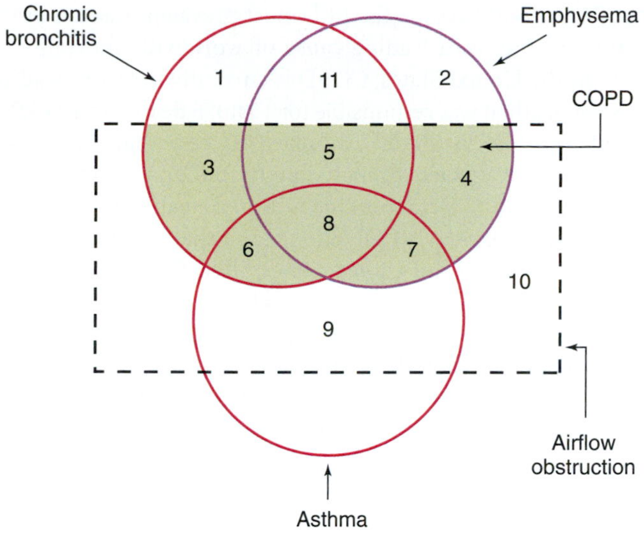

FIGURE 25-1 Schema of chronic obstructive pulmonary disease (COPD). This nonproportional Venn diagram shows subsets of patients with chronic bronchitis, emphysema, and asthma. The subsets constituting COPD are *shaded.* Subset areas are not proportional to actual relative subset sizes. Asthma is by definition associated with reversible airflow obstruction, although in variant asthma special maneuvers may be necessary to make the obstruction evident. Patients with asthma whose airflow obstruction is completely reversible *(subset 9)* are not considered to have COPD. Because in many cases it is virtually impossible to differentiate patients with asthma whose airflow obstruction does not remit completely from patients with chronic bronchitis and emphysema who have partially reversible airflow obstruction with airway hyperreactivity, patients with unremitting asthma are classified as having COPD (*subsets 6, 7,* and *8*). Chronic bronchitis and emphysema with airflow obstruction usually occur together *(subset 5),* and some patients may have asthma associated with these two disorders *(subset 8).* Individuals with asthma who are exposed to chronic irritation, as from cigarette smoke, may develop a chronic, productive cough, a feature of chronic bronchitis *(subset 6).* Such patients are often referred to as having *asthmatic bronchitis* or the *asthmatic form of COPD.* Individuals with chronic bronchitis or emphysema without airflow obstruction (*subsets 1, 2,* and *11*) are not classified as having COPD. Patients with airway obstruction caused by diseases with a known cause or specific pathologic process, such as cystic fibrosis or obliterative bronchiolitis *(subset 10)*, are not included in this definition.

Epidemiology

COPD is one of the most frequent causes of morbidity and mortality worldwide.[3] The World Health Organization predicts that COPD will become the fifth most prevalent disease in the world and the third leading cause of worldwide mortality by 2030. In the United States, COPD is currently the third leading cause of death; it was responsible for 134,676 deaths and 715,000 hospitalizations in 2010.[4] Estimates suggest that 24 million Americans are affected, though only 15 million U.S. adults have been diagnosed.[4-6] Data from the National Health and Nutrition Examination Survey (NHANES) suggest that among adults 25 to 75 years old in the United States, mild COPD (defined as forced expiratory volume in 1 second [FEV_1]/forced vital capacity [FVC] < 70%, and FEV_1 > 80% predicted) occurs in 6.9% and moderate COPD (defined as FEV_1/FVC < 79% and $FEV_1 \leq$ 80% predicted) occurs in 6.6%.[3] COPD prevalence increases with aging, with a five-fold increased risk for adults older than 65 years compared with adults younger than 40 years, and some studies estimate a prevalence of 20% to 30% in adults older than 70 years.[7]

The growing health burden from COPD is caused in part by the aging of the population but mainly by the continued use of tobacco. The socioeconomic burden of COPD is also substantial. In 2010, COPD caused 715,000 hospitalizations (which accounted for 1.9% of all hospitalizations in the United States), and, in 2010, COPD resulted in a total health expenditure of $49.9 billion.[4] In this regard, COPD is a problem that is a frequent challenge for the respiratory clinician.

Risk Factors and Pathophysiology

Although many risk factors exist for COPD (Box 25-1), the two most common are *cigarette smoking* (which has been estimated to account for 80% to 90% of all COPD-related deaths) and *alpha-1 antitrypsin (AAT) deficiency*.[8] Evidence linking cigarette smoking to the development of COPD is strong and includes the following:

- Symptoms of COPD (e.g., chronic cough and phlegm production) are more common in smokers than in nonsmokers.
- Impaired lung function with evidence of an obstructive pattern of lung dysfunction is more common in smokers than in nonsmokers.
- Pathologic changes of airflow obstruction and chronic bronchitis are evident in the lungs of smokers.
- So-called *susceptible smokers,* who represent approximately 15% of all cigarette smokers, experience more rapid rates of decline of lung function than nonsmokers.

Information from the Lung Health Study (Figure 25-2) highlighted the accelerated rate of decrease of FEV_1 in smokers compared with former smokers who have achieved sustained quitting.[9,10] Overall, the strength of evidence implicating cigarette smoking as a cause of COPD has allowed the U.S. Surgeon General to conclude, "Cigarette smoking is the major cause of chronic obstructive lung disease in the United States for both men and women. The contribution of cigarette smoking to chronic obstructive lung disease morbidity and mortality far outweighs all other factors."[11]

As the second well-recognized cause of emphysema, AAT deficiency, sometimes called *genetic emphysema* or *alpha-1 antiprotease deficiency,* is a condition that features a reduced amount of the protein alpha-1 antitrypsin (AAT), which may result in the early onset of emphysema and which is inherited as a so-called *autosomal codominant condition*. AAT deficiency

Box 25-1 Causes of Chronic Obstructive Pulmonary Disease*

COMMON CAUSES
- Cigarette smoking
- Alpha-1 antitrypsin (AAT) deficiency
- Outdoor air pollution
- Long-standing asthma
- Biomass and occupational exposure (e.g., chronic exposure to wood smoke with poorly ventilated indoor cooking)

LESS COMMON CAUSES
- Hypocomplementemic urticarial vasculitis
- Intravenous methylphenidate (Ritalin) abuse
- Ehlers-Danlos syndrome
- Marfan syndrome
- Cutix laxa
- Menke syndrome
- Salla disease†
- Alpha-1 antichymotrypsin deficiency†
- Human immunodeficiency virus infection (emphysema-like illness)

*Multiple causes (e.g., cigarette smoking and alpha-1 antitrypsin deficiency) may coexist in a single patient.
†Putative cause; firm evidence is unavailable.

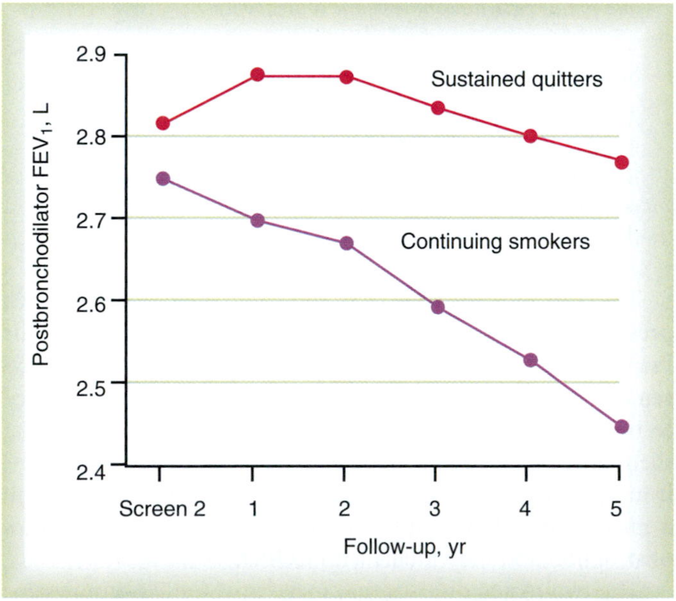

FIGURE 25-2 Mean postbronchodilator FEV_1 for participants in the smoking intervention and placebo groups who were sustained quitters *(red circles)* and continuing smokers *(purple circles)*. The two curves diverge sharply after baseline. (From Anthonisen SR, Connett JE, Kiley JP, et al: Effects of smoking intervention and the use of an anticholinergic bronchodilator on the rate of decline of FEV_1: the Lung Health Study. JAMA 272:1497–1504, 1994.)

accounts for 2% to 3% of all cases of COPD and affects 100,000 Americans but is underrecognized by health care providers. In one 1995 survey, the mean interval between the first onset of pulmonary symptoms and initial diagnosis of AAT deficiency was 7.2 years, and 43% of individuals with severe deficiency of AAT reported seeing at least three physicians before the diagnosis of AAT deficiency was first made.[12] More recent studies suggest that underrecognition of AAT deficiency persists and that the diagnostic delay interval has not decreased significantly.[12-15]

Identifying individuals with AAT deficiency is simple, often requiring only a blood test of the serum AAT level. Respiratory therapists (RTs) can contribute importantly to detecting individuals with AAT deficiency (e.g., by suggesting or offering testing when airflow obstruction is diagnosed in the pulmonary function laboratory by an RT performing the test and by making patients aware of available free, home-based testing kits) (see http://www.alpha-1foundation.org). Several observations suggest the importance of detection: (1) first-degree relatives (e.g., siblings, parents, and children) also may be affected but unaware of their risk; (2) early detection allows appropriate monitoring and therapy, including the very important step of smoking cessation; and (3) for individuals with established emphysema, consideration can be given to available specific therapy, called *intravenous augmentation therapy* (which is the administration of purified AAT intravenously to individuals with severe deficiency of AAT). The risk for developing emphysema for individuals with AAT deficiency increases as the serum AAT level decreases to less than 11 μmol/L, or less than approximately 57 mg/dl using a testing technique called *nephelometry;* these levels in serum define the so-called *protective threshold value,* which is the serum level below which the risk for emphysema is felt to increase. Cigarette smoking markedly accelerates the rate of emphysema progression in individuals with AAT deficiency.[14]

Study of AAT deficiency has helped formulate the protease-antiprotease hypothesis of emphysema.[14,16] In this explanatory model (Figure 25-3), lung elastin, a major structural protein that supports the alveolar walls of the lung, is normally protected by AAT, a protein that defends the lung against tissue destruction by neutrophil elastase. Neutrophil elastase is a protein contained within a category of white blood cells called *neutrophils* that is released when neutrophils are attracted to the lung during inflammation or infection. Under normal circumstances of an adequate amount of AAT, neutrophil elastase is counteracted so as not to digest lung elastin. However, in the face of a severe deficiency of AAT (i.e., when serum levels decrease below the "protective threshold" serum value of 11 μmol/L, or 57 mg/dl), neutrophil elastase may go unchecked, causing breakdown of elastin and of alveolar walls. This protease-antiprotease model explains the pathogenesis of emphysema in AAT deficiency, but evidence suggesting its role in COPD in individuals with normal amounts of AAT is conflicting. Also, other enzymes that break down proteins (e.g., matrix metalloproteinases) are thought to contribute to the destruction of alveolar walls that produces emphysema.[17]

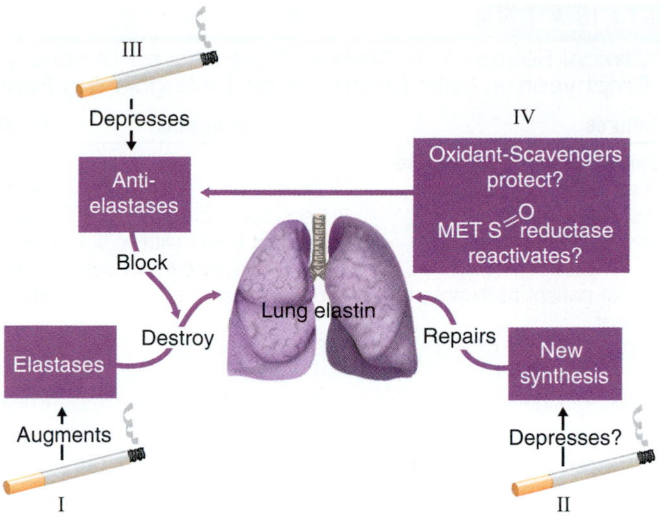

FIGURE 25-3 Proposed biochemical links between cigarette smoking and the pathogenesis of emphysema. *(I)* Smoking recruits monocytes, macrophages, and (through macrophage chemotactic factors) polymorphonuclear neutrophils to the lung, elevating the connective tissue "burden" of elastolytic serine and metalloproteases. *(III)* At the same time, oxidants in smoke plus oxidants produced by smoke-stimulated lung phagocytes (and oxidizing products of chemical interactions between these two) inactivate bronchial mucus proteinase inhibitor and alpha-1 antitrypsin (AAT), the latter representing the major antielastase "shield" of the respiratory units. *(II)* Other, unidentified water-soluble, gas-phase components of cigarette smoke (cyanide, copper chelators) inhibit lysyl oxidase–catalyzed oxidative deamination of epsilon-amino groups in tropoelastin and block formation of desmosine and presumably other cross-links during elastin synthesis, decreasing connective tissue repair. *(IV)* Antioxidants (ceruloplasmin, methionine-sulfoxide-reductase) may protect or reactivate elastase inhibitors, and other unidentified factors may modulate the chemical lesions induced in the lung by smoking to influence the risk for developing COPD. (Modified from Janoff A, Carp H, Laurent P, et al: The role of oxidative processes in emphysema. Am Rev Respir Dis 127[Suppl]:S31, 1983.)

COPD may occur without active cigarette smoking or AAT deficiency (see Box 25-1).[18,19] Factors such as passive smoking, air pollution, occupational exposure, and airway hyperresponsiveness may contribute to airflow obstruction that is not reversible.

The mechanisms of airflow obstruction in COPD include inflammation and obstruction of small airways (<2 mm in diameter); loss of elasticity, which keeps small airways open when elastin is destroyed in emphysema; and active **bronchospasm.** Although traditionally considered to be characteristic of asthma, some reversibility of airflow obstruction has been observed in up to two-thirds of patients with COPD when tested multiple times with inhaled bronchodilators.[20]

Clinical Signs and Symptoms

Common symptoms of COPD include cough, phlegm production, wheezing, and shortness of breath, typically on exertion. Dyspnea is often slow but progressive in onset and occurs later in the course of the disease, characteristically in the late sixth or seventh decade of life. One notable exception is AAT

TABLE 25-1

Clinical Features of Chronic Obstructive Pulmonary Disease: Distinctions Between Chronic Bronchitis and Emphysema, With Emphasis on Distinguishing Features of Alpha-1 Antitrypsin Deficiency

Features	Chronic Bronchitis	Emphysema	Severe Alpha-1 Antitrypsin Deficiency
Symptoms and Signs			
Chronic cough, phlegm	Common	Less common	Less common, but may be present
Dyspnea on exertion	Less common	Common	Common
Cor pulmonale	Present (often with multiple exacerbations)	Present (but often in end-stage emphysema)	Present (but often in end-stage emphysema)
Age of patient at symptom onset	6th-7th decade	6th-7th decade	4th-5th decade (although late onset is possible)
Family history of COPD	Possible but not characteristic	Possible but not characteristic	Common in parents, children, and siblings
History of cigarette smoking	Present, often heavy	Present, often heavy	May be present, but COPD can occur in the absence of smoking
Physiologic Function			
Airflow (FEV_1, FEV_1/FVC)	Decreased	Decreased	Decreased
Lung volumes, residual volume	Normal	Increased, suggesting air trapping	Increased
Gas exchange, diffusion PaO_2	Often decreased	Often preserved until advanced stage	Often preserved until advanced stage
$PaCO_2$	May be increased	Often preserved until advanced disease, then elevated	Often preserved until advanced disease, then elevated
Diffusion capacity	Often normal	Decreased	Decreased
Static lung compliance	Normal	Increased	Increased
Chest radiograph	"Dirty lungs" with peribronchial cuffing, suggesting thickened bronchial walls	Hyperinflation, with evidence of emphysema; greater at lung apex than at lung base	Hyperinflation, with evidence of emphysema; frequently greater at lung base than at lung apex (basilar hyperlucency)

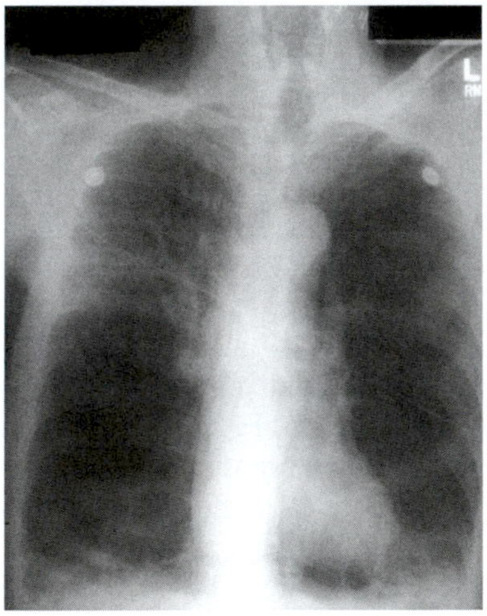

FIGURE 25-4 Posteroanterior plain chest radiograph in a patient with severe deficiency of alpha-1 antitrypsin and emphysema. Note that the emphysematous changes (hyperlucency) are more pronounced at the lung bases than at the apexes.

deficiency, in which dyspnea characteristically begins sooner (mean age approximately 45 years).[8]

Table 25-1 reviews the characteristic features of emphysema and chronic bronchitis and emphasizes traits that should suggest the possibility of AAT deficiency, including early onset of emphysema, emphysema in a nonsmoker, a family history of emphysema, or emphysema with a chest x-ray (Figure 25-4) or computed tomography (CT) (Figure 25-5), in which emphysematous changes are more pronounced at the lung bases than at the apexes (so-called *basilar hyperlucency*). Suspicion of AAT deficiency should lead to a simple blood test by which the serum level can be established.[8,14]

Physical examination of the chest early on in a patient with COPD may reveal wheezing or diminished breath sounds. Later, signs of hyperinflation may be evident—that is, increased anteroposterior diameter of the chest (sometimes called a *barrel chest*), diaphragm flattening, and dimpling inward of the chest wall at the level of the diaphragm on inspiration (called the *Hoover sign*). Other late signs of COPD include use of accessory muscles of respiration (e.g., sternocleidomastoid), edema from cor pulmonale, mental status changes caused by hypoxemia or hypercapnia (especially in acute exacerbations of chronic, severe disease), or asterixis (i.e., involuntary flapping of the hands when held in an extended position, as in "stopping traffic").

RULE OF THUMB

In patients with COPD, $PaCO_2$ is usually preserved until airflow obstruction is severe (i.e., $FEV_1 < 1$ L), when $PaCO_2$ may increase.

RULE OF THUMB

Digital clubbing is not caused by COPD alone, even if hypoxemia is present. Clubbing in a patient with COPD warrants consideration of another cause (e.g., bronchogenic cancer, bronchiectasis).

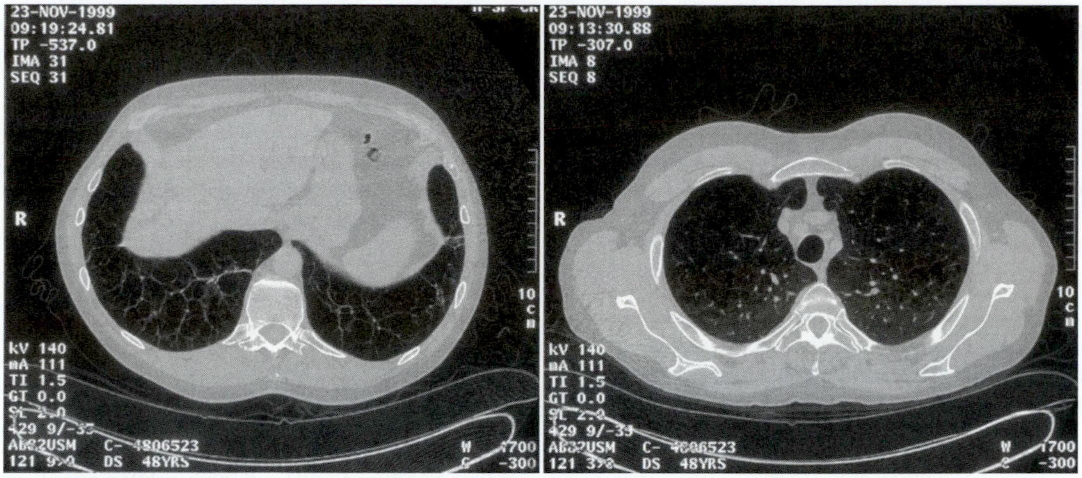

FIGURE 25-5 Computed tomography chest image from an individual with severe deficiency of alpha-1 antitrypsin. Note the changes of emphysema *(arrows)* are more pronounced in the lung bases **(B)** than in the lung apexes **(A).**

RULE OF THUMB

When COPD occurs in a nonsmoker, a young person, an individual with a family history of liver or lung disease, or an individual with emphysematous changes more pronounced at the lung bases than apexes on a chest radiograph (see Figure 25-4) or chest CT (see Figure 25-5), AAT deficiency should be suspected. Guidelines suggest that *all* adult, symptomatic patients with COPD should be tested for AAT deficiency.

Management

In managing patients with chronic, stable COPD, the following goals must guide the clinician[1,2]:

- Establish the diagnosis of COPD.
- Optimize lung function.
- Maximize the patient's ability to perform daily activities.
- Simplify the medical treatment program as much as possible.
- Avoid exacerbations of COPD.
- Prolong survival.

In managing an **acute exacerbation of COPD,** additional considerations are to reestablish the patient to baseline status as quickly and with as little morbidity and mortality as possible.[21,22] Each of the treatments that are discussed in this section is considered in regard to these goals, recognizing differences in management between patients with chronic, stable COPD versus an acute exacerbation of COPD. In patients with COPD, $PaCO_2$ usually is generally preserved until airflow obstruction is severe ($FEV_1 < 1$ L), when the $PaCO_2$ level may increase.

Establishing the Diagnosis

Although a spectrum of diseases can give rise to obstructive lung disease, including some unusual entities such as chronic eosinophilic pneumonia, bronchiectasis, and allergic bronchopulmonary aspergillosis, the major challenge facing the clinician who encounters a patient with airflow obstruction is to distinguish COPD (i.e., emphysema or chronic bronchitis or both) from asthma. Distinguishing asthma from COPD may be very difficult in practice; features that tend to favor COPD include chronic daily phlegm production, which establishes the diagnosis of chronic bronchitis; diminished vascular shadows on the chest radiograph (called *hyperlucency*); and a decreased diffusing capacity. The diagnosis of asthma is favored if the diminished FEV_1 obtained on spirometry returns to normal after **bronchodilator** treatment.

After the diagnosis of COPD is established, another issue is for the clinician to consider whether the patient has an underlying predisposition to COPD, such as AAT deficiency or other cause listed in Box 25-1.[18,19] Underlying causes are present in fewer than 5% of patients with COPD, with AAT deficiency being the most common (2% to 3% of all patients with COPD).

Optimizing Lung Function

Stable Chronic Obstructive Pulmonary Disease

Although airflow obstruction from emphysema itself is irreversible, most (up to two-thirds) patients with stable COPD exhibit a reversible component of airflow obstruction, defined as a 12% and 200-ml increase in post-bronchodilator FEV_1 or FVC or both. For this reason, as shown in an algorithm developed by GOLD (Figure 25-6),[2,22,25,26] bronchodilator therapy is recommended for patients with COPD.

Bronchodilators produce smooth muscle relaxation resulting in improved airflow obstruction, improved symptoms and exercise tolerance, and decrease in the frequency and severity of exacerbations, but they do not enhance survival. The results of the Lung Health Study,[9] which compared the effects of inhaled ipratropium bromide (two puffs four times daily) with placebo in patients with mild, stable COPD, showed that regular,

MINI CLINI

Determining the Severity of Chronic Obstructive Pulmonary Disease

PROBLEM: You are asked to see a new patient in clinic who was recently discharged from the hospital with a COPD exacerbation. The patient describes being hospitalized at least twice per year because of lung problems and complains of severe dyspnea when walking up a hill. Spirometry revealed an FEV_1 of 40% predicted. How do you characterize the severity of COPD in this patient?

DISCUSSION: In 2001 GOLD created a classification system based on the severity of airflow obstruction.[2] According to this staging system, severity of COPD was graded based on the degree of airflow obstruction into one of the following four stages:

Stage	Description
I	Patients with $FEV_1/FVC < 70\%$ and $FEV_1 > 80\%$ predicted
II	Patients with $FEV_1/FVC < 70\%$ and FEV_1 50%-79% predicted
III	Patients with $FEV_1/FVC < 70\%$ and FEV_1 30%-49% predicted
IV	Patients with $FEV_1/FVC < 70\%$ and $FEV_1 < 30\%$ or $FEV_1 <$ 50% predicted plus chronic respiratory failure

The GOLD guidelines were revised in 2011 to include symptoms and exacerbation history, and now COPD severity is graded (A to D) as follows:

A = Low risk, low symptom burden
- Low symptom burden (mMRC of 0 to 1 OR CAT score < 10) AND
- FEV_1 of 50% or greater (old GOLD 1 to 2) AND low exacerbation rate (0 to 1/year)

B = Low risk, higher symptom burden
- Higher symptom burden (mMRC of 2 or more OR CAT of 10 or more) AND
- FEV_1 of 50% or greater (old GOLD 1 to 2) AND low exacerbation rate (0 to 1/year)

C = High risk, low symptom burden
- Low symptom burden (mMRC of 0 to 1 OR CAT score < 10) AND
- $FEV_1 < 50\%$ (old GOLD 3 to 4) AND/OR high exacerbation rate (2 or more/year)

D = High risk, higher symptom burden
- Higher symptom burden (mMRC of 2 or more OR CAT of 10 or more) AND
- $FEV_1 < 50\%$ (old GOLD 3 to 4) AND/OR high exacerbation rate (2 or more/year)

The new classification categorizes patients first by symptom burden and then adds degree of airflow obstruction and exacerbation history to refine risk. This system uses two different scales to define symptom burden, the modified Medical Research Council questionnaire (mMRC)[23] and the COPD assessment test (CAT).[24] Based on severity of airflow obstruction, high symptom burden, and history of exacerbations, this patient is classified as GOLD D, indicating severe COPD with high risk for complications.

mMRC

1. Dyspnea with strenuous exercise
2. Dyspnea when hurrying on the level or walking up a slight hill
3. Walks slower than most people on the level, stops after a mile or so, or stops after 15 minutes of walking at own pace
4. Stops for breath after walking 100 yards or after a few minutes of level ground
5. Too breathless to leave the house, or breathless when undressing

CAT

Cough (none to all the time): Total 0 to 5
Phlegm (mucus) in my chest: Total 0 to 5 (none to severe)
Chest tightness: Total 0 to 5 (none to severe)
Dyspnea walking flight of stairs: Total 0 to 5 (none to severe)
Limitation for home activities: Total 0 to 5 (none to severe)
Confident leaving home despite lung condition: Total 0 to 5 (very confident to nonconfident)
Sleep quality: Total 0 to 5 (sound sleep to no sleep because of lung condition)
Energy: Total 0 to 5 (full energy to none)

long-term use of ipratropium did not change the rate of decline of lung function but offered a one-time, small increase in FEV_1.

Both anticholinergic and adrenergic (beta agonist) bronchodilators can improve airflow in patients with COPD, although some clinicians favor an inhaled anticholinergic medication (e.g., ipratropium bromide or tiotropium[25,26]) as first-line therapy (see Figure 25-6). More recent concerns about the possible adverse cardiovascular effects of anticholinergic therapy in patients with COPD[27,28] have been dismissed by the results of a multicenter trial (Understanding Potential Long-Term Impacts on Function with Tiotropium [UPLIFT]), which found a significantly lower rate of cardiac adverse events and cardiovascular death in patients who received tiotropium.[27]

The GOLD guidelines[2] recommend the use of short-acting beta-adrenergic agents (≤6 hours) for symptomatic management of all patients with COPD. Also, the use of a long-acting beta agonist (e.g., salmeterol) or a long-acting anticholinergic drug (e.g., tiotropium) can lessen the frequency of acute exacerbations of COPD.[26]

Other treatment options to optimize lung function include administering corticosteroids and, as a second-line option, methylxanthines. Systemic corticosteroids can produce significant improvements in airflow in a few (6% to 29%) patients with stable COPD.[29,30] To assess whether airflow obstruction is completely reversible (i.e., the patient has asthma) and whether a patient with COPD is responsive to steroids, a brief course of corticosteroids (20 to 40 mg/day of prednisone or equivalent for 5 to 8 days) is sometimes recommended. Patients with a significant clinical response often are treated with long-term inhaled corticosteroids or, rarely, with the smallest necessary dose of systemic corticosteroids, recognizing that long-term systemic steroid therapy has risks.[31] Also, results of several major clinical trials (e.g., Lung Health Study II, Euroscop, Inhaled Steroids in Obstructive Lung Disease [ISOLDE] study,

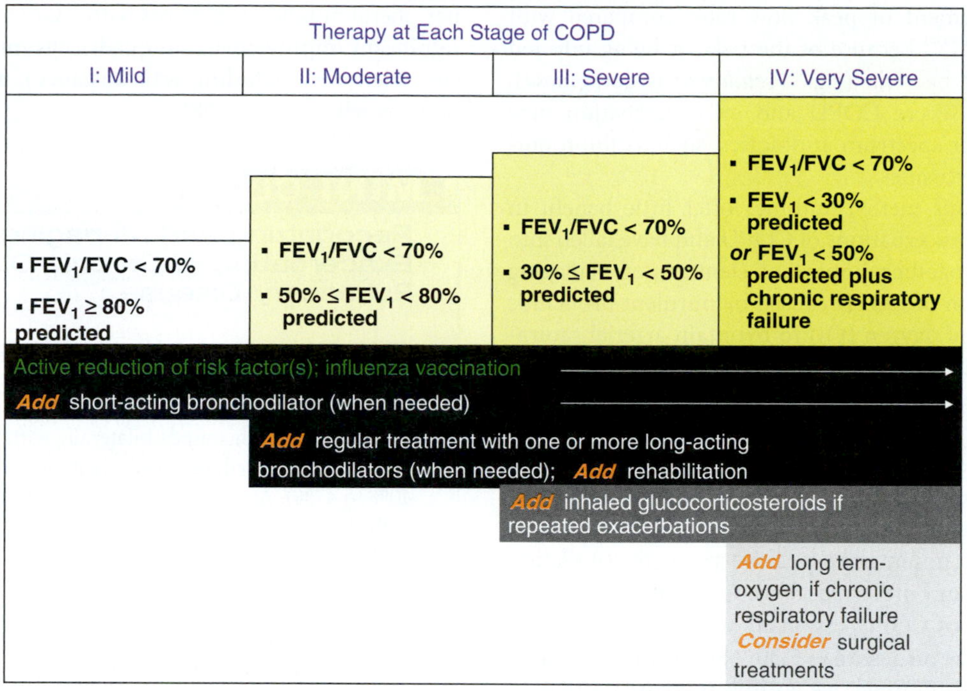

FIGURE 25-6 Initial Pharmacologic Management of COPD. (From The Global Strategy for the Diagnosis, Management and Prevention of COPD. Global Initiative for Chronic Obstructive Lung Disease [GOLD], 2014. http://www.goldcopd.com. Accessed July 29, 2015.)

and Copenhagen City Study, but not another trial, Towards a Revolution in COPD Health [TORCH] study) agree that inhaled corticosteroids do not change the rate of decline of FEV_1 in patients with COPD, although their use is associated with a decreased frequency of acute exacerbations.[32-34]

Studies of combined salmeterol and fluticasone versus placebo in patients with COPD suggest that adding an inhaled corticosteroid (fluticasone) to the long-acting beta agonist (salmeterol) can improve FEV_1 and reduce the frequency of acute exacerbations of COPD but does not improve survival.[32,33] The finding of a higher rate of pneumonia in inhaled corticosteroid users is concerning. Overall, the GOLD guidelines[2] recommend use of inhaled corticosteroids in patients with FEV_1 less than 50% and history of recurrent exacerbations (three episodes in the last 3 years), whereas the ATS/European Respiratory Society (ERS) guidelines recommend use of inhaled corticosteroids in patients with FEV_1 less than 50% who have required use of oral corticosteroids or oral antibiotics at least once within the last year.[3]

Treatment with methylxanthines offers little additional bronchodilation in patients using inhaled bronchodilators and generally is reserved for patients with debilitating symptoms from stable COPD despite optimal inhaled bronchodilator therapy. Controlled trials show lessened dyspnea in methylxanthine recipients despite a lack of measurable increases in airflow.[35] Side effects of methylxanthines include anxiety, jitteriness (tremulousness), nausea, cardiac arrhythmias, and seizures. To minimize the chance of toxicity, current recommendations suggest maintaining serum theophylline levels at 8 to 10 mcg/ml.

Acute Exacerbation of Chronic Obstructive Pulmonary Disease

Strategies for improving lung function during acute exacerbations of COPD generally include inhaled bronchodilators (especially beta-2 agonists), antibiotics, and systemic corticosteroids. Because of their rapid onset of action and efficacy, short-acting beta-2 agonists are first-line therapy for patients with COPD exacerbation. Inhaled beta-2 agonists are frequently administered through a nebulizer, although metered dose inhaler devices may have equal efficacy if administered appropriately.[2] A common practice is to administer 2.5 mg of albuterol by nebulizer every 1 to 4 hours as needed. Higher doses of albuterol (i.e., 5 mg) do not produce further improvement in pulmonary function and may cause cardiac side effects.[36] Similarly, continuous nebulization of short-acting beta-2 agonists in patients with COPD exacerbation is not recommended.

In addition to inhaled bronchodilator therapy, short-term systemic corticosteroids are recommended to reduce inflammation and improve lung function. An early randomized, controlled trial of intravenous methylprednisolone for patients with acute exacerbations showed accelerated improvement in FEV_1 within 72 hours.[37] Larger, more recent trials have confirmed the benefits of systemic corticosteroids in acute exacerbations and have shown that short-term oral courses (i.e., approximately 2 weeks) are as effective as longer courses (i.e., 8 weeks) with fewer adverse steroid effects.[38] For patients with acute exacerbations characterized by purulent phlegm, oral antibiotics (e.g., trimethoprim-sulfamethoxazole, amoxicillin, or doxycycline) administered for 7 to 10 days have produced accelerated improvement of peak flow rates compared with placebo recipients.[21,39,40] Because of the risk for being infected with more virulent bacteria (e.g., *Pseudomonas aeruginosa*), patients who have severe COPD and an exacerbation may benefit from broader spectrum antibiotics, such as fluoroquinolones or aminoglycosides.

Finally, intravenous methylxanthines offer little benefit in the setting of acute exacerbations of COPD and have fallen into disfavor.[41,42] Taken together, important elements of managing an acute exacerbation of COPD caused by purulent bronchitis include supplemental oxygen (O_2) to maintain arterial saturation at greater than 90%, inhaled bronchodilators, oral antibiotics, and a brief course of systemic corticosteroids.[21]

For patients with hypercapnia and acute respiratory acidemia, the clinician also must decide whether to provide ventilatory assistance. Although intubation and mechanical ventilation historically have been the preferred approach, more recent studies suggest that noninvasive positive pressure ventilation can be an effective and preferred alternative for patients with acute exacerbations of COPD, especially with severe exacerbations characterized by pH less than 7.30.[43] Specifically, based on studies that show that noninvasive positive pressure ventilation can shorten intensive care unit (ICU) stay and avoid the need for intubation, the American Association for Respiratory Care consensus conference and guidelines on noninvasive ventilation from other official societies have endorsed use of noninvasive ventilation for such patients (unless a contraindication to noninvasive ventilation is present).[44,45] Criteria defining candidacy for **noninvasive ventilation** include acute respiratory acidosis (without frank respiratory arrest), hemodynamic stability, ability to tolerate the interface needed for noninvasive ventilation, and ability to protect the airway. Relative contraindications include craniofacial trauma or burns, copious secretions, or massive obesity.[4]

Maximizing Functional Status

In symptomatic patients with stable COPD, maximizing their ability to perform activities of daily living is a priority. Pharmacologic treatments to maximize functional status include administration of bronchodilators to enhance lung function as much as possible and consideration of methylxanthine therapy, based on data that such drugs can lessen dyspnea and improve functional status ratings even though airflow is not increased.[3]

Comprehensive pulmonary rehabilitation is another important treatment for patients with COPD that has the goal of improving patients' ability to function.[46] Pulmonary rehabilitation is a multidisciplinary intervention that consists of lower and upper extremity exercise conditioning, breathing retraining, education, and psychosocial support. Randomized, controlled trials show that although pulmonary rehabilitation does not improve lung function or survival, pulmonary rehabilitation results in decreased dyspnea perception, improved health-related quality of life, fewer days of hospitalization, and decreased health care usage.[47,48]

Finally, transcutaneous neuromuscular electrical stimulation is a newer therapy that has been successfully used to stimulate peripheral muscles in patients with COPD. Studies have shown significant improvements in quadriceps muscle function, exercise tolerance (including walk distance), and health status in patients with severe COPD.[49]

MINI CLINI

Recognizing and Managing an Acute Exacerbation of Chronic Obstructive Pulmonary Disease

PROBLEM: A 70-year-old man with long-standing COPD is admitted to the hospital with an acute exacerbation. On physical examination, he is not dehydrated and examination shows diminished breath sounds bilaterally without wheezing. Pertinent laboratory values show a hematocrit of 54% (normal is 40% to 47%). An arterial blood gas (ABG) analysis performed with the patient on room air showed the following:

PaO_2 = 47 mm Hg
PCO_2 = 67 mm Hg
pH = 7.30
HCO_3^- = 34 mEq/L

How do you describe his current status, what do his current laboratory values suggest about his long-term gas exchange status, and what treatment should be considered?

SOLUTION: The patient has an acute exacerbation of COPD. The acidemia (pH 7.30) on his ABG analysis suggests an acute increase in PCO_2 superimposed on chronic hypercapnia, which is suggested by the elevated serum bicarbonate (HCO_3^-), indicating renal compensation for chronic respiratory acidosis. Although his current hypoxemia may be due to worsened gas exchange accompanying the current flare-up of COPD, his elevated hematocrit, in the absence of dehydration, suggests chronic hypoxemia and secondary erythrocytosis. The goal of therapy is to restore his gas exchange to baseline and to avoid invasive or high-risk interventions, while optimizing survival.

To achieve these goals, treatment would consist of aggressive use of bronchodilators, intravenous corticosteroids, supplemental O_2, and antibiotics (if there is evidence of acute lung infection, either bronchitis or pneumonia). In view of the patient's acute chronic respiratory acidemia, ventilatory support should be implemented. As indicated by several randomized, controlled trials, noninvasive positive pressure ventilation is an effective alternative to intubation.

Preventing Progression of Chronic Obstructive Pulmonary Disease and Enhancing Survival

Cigarette smoking is widely recognized as the major risk factor for accelerating airflow obstruction in smokers who are "susceptible." For these individuals, smoking cessation can generally slow the rate of decline of FEV_1 and restore the rate of lung decline to that seen in healthy, age-matched nonsmokers.

Follow-up data from the Lung Health Study[9] confirm that a comprehensive smoking cessation program (including instruction, group counseling, and nicotine replacement therapy) can achieve sustained smoking cessation in 22% of participants and that the rate of annual FEV_1 decline in these sustained nonsmokers was significantly less than it was for continuing smokers, even over 11 years of follow-up.[10] Participation in aggressive smoking cessation can enhance survival rates in patients with COPD.[10]

Critical elements in achieving successful smoking cessation include identifying "teachable moments" (i.e., during episodes of illness in which smoking can be identified as a contributing factor[50]), identifying the role of smoking in adverse health outcomes, negotiating a "quit date," and providing frequent follow-up reminders from health care providers.[51] A helpful strategy during counseling is to use the five *A*s of smoking cessation[2]:

*A*sk if they are smoking
*A*dvise to quit
*A*ssess willingness to quit
*A*ssist by providing a plan
*A*rrange a follow-up

In this regard, the RT, who sees the patient frequently, has a special responsibility to provide frequent, constructive reminders about the advisability of smoking cessation.[52]

Among available treatments for COPD, **supplemental oxygen** is important because, similar to smoking cessation and lung volume reduction surgery in selected individuals (see later discussion), it can prolong survival.[53-56] Box 25-2 reviews the indications for supplemental O_2, and Figure 25-7 shows the results of the American Nocturnal Oxygen Therapy Trial[53] and the British Medical Research Council trial of domiciliary O_2 (1980 to 1981).[54,55] Survival was improved when eligible patients used supplemental O_2 for as close to 24 hours as possible; survival improved less for patients using O_2 only 15 hours per day. No survival benefit was observed when O_2 was used during sleeping hours only. Patients should be assessed for supplemental O_2 use only after receiving optimal bronchodilator therapy because one-third of potential O_2 candidates can experience sufficient improvement with aggressive bronchodilation to avoid the need for long-term supplemental O_2. Also, patients prescribed to receive supplemental O_2 during acute exacerbations should be reassessed several months later to determine whether they continue to need supplemental O_2.[57] RTs can play a key role in ensuring compliance with this recommendation and optimizing O_2 therapy.[57,58]

Finally, preventive strategies such as annual influenza and pneumococcal vaccinations are recommended for all patients with chronic debilitating conditions such as COPD.[59] Specific indications for pneumococcal vaccination are presented in Box 25-3. Recent recommendations for those age 65 or older also include a 13-valent pneumococcal vaccine in addition to the existing 23-valent pneumococcal vaccine.

Other measures to prevent exacerbations of COPD include use of long-acting anticholinergic agents (e.g., tiotropium, aclidinium, umeclidinium), inhaled corticosteroids, especially in combination with long-acting beta agonists, macrolide antibiotics (e.g., erythromycin and azithromycin),[60] phosphodiesterase-4 inhibition with roflumilast,[61] and antioxidants such as oral N-acetylcysteine.[62]

Box 25-2 Indications for Long-Term Oxygen Therapy

I. Continuous O_2
   A. Resting $PaO_2 \leq 55$ mm Hg
   B. Resting PaO_2 56 to 59 mm Hg or SaO_2 89% in the presence of any of the following:
      1. Dependent edema, suggesting congestive heart failure
      2. P pulmonale on the electrocardiogram (P wave > 3 mm in standard lead II, III, or aV_F)
      3. Erythrocytosis (hematocrit > 56%)
         a. Reimbursable only with additional documentation justifying O_2 prescription and a summary of more conservative therapy that has failed
II. Noncontinuous O_2
   A. O_2 flow rate and number of hours per day must be specified
      1. During exercise: $PaO_2 \leq 55$ mm Hg or $SaO_2 \leq 88\%$ with a low level of exertion
      2. During sleep: $PaO_2 \leq 55$ mm Hg or $SaO_2 \leq 88\%$ with associated complications, such as pulmonary hypertension, daytime somnolence, or cardiac arrhythmias

From Tarpy SP, Celli BR: Long-term oxygen therapy. N Engl J Med 333:710–714, 1995.

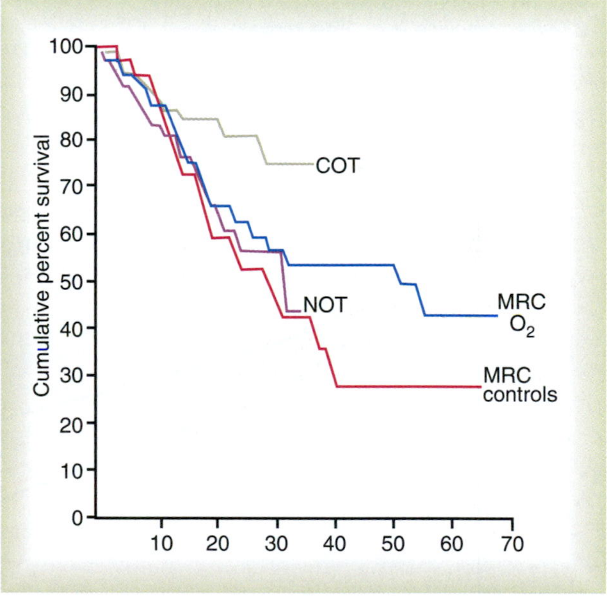

FIGURE 25-7 Cumulative percent survival of patients in the Nocturnal Oxygen Therapy Trial (NOTT) and Medical Research Council (MRC) controlled trials of long-term domiciliary O_2 therapy for men older than 70 years. MRC control subjects *(red line)* received no O_2. NOTT subjects *(purple line)* received O_2 for 12 hours in the 24-hour day, including the sleeping hours. MRC O_2 subjects *(blue line)* received O_2 for 15 hours in the 24-hour day, including the sleeping hours, and continuous O_2 therapy (COT) subjects *(green line)* received O_2 for 24 hours in the 24-hour day (on average, 19 hours). (Modified from Flenley DC: Long-term oxygen therapy. Chest 87:99–193, 1985.)

Box 25-3 Indications for Pneumococcal Vaccine Administration

Vaccination is recommended for the following adults:

- Adults age 65 years and older and adults of all ages with long-term illnesses that are associated with a high risk for contracting pneumococcal disease, including heart or lung diseases, diabetes, alcoholism, cirrhosis, or cerebrospinal fluid leaks
- Adults with diseases or conditions that lower the body's resistance to infections, including abnormal function of the spleen or removed spleen, Hodgkin disease, lymphoma, multiple myeloma, kidney failure, nephrotic syndrome, or organ transplantation, and adults who are taking drugs that lower the body's resistance to infections
- Adults with human immunodeficiency virus infection and acquired immunodeficiency syndrome (HIV/AIDS), with or without symptoms

Revaccination should be considered for the following groups:

- Individuals at the highest risk for fatal pneumococcal infection, such as individuals with abnormal function or removal of the spleen, who received the original pneumococcal vaccination (from 1979 to 1983) or who received the current vaccine (1983 to present) 6 or years or longer ago
- Individuals shown to lose protection rapidly (e.g., individuals with nephrotic syndrome, kidney failure, or transplants), who received the current vaccine 6 years or longer ago
- Children 10 years old or younger with nephrotic syndrome, abnormal function or removal of the spleen, or sickle cell anemia, who received the vaccine 3 to 5 years ago
- Adults age ≥65 should receive the 13-valent pneumococcal vaccine (Prevnar) followed 6-12 months later by the 23-valent vaccine (e.g., Pneumovax)

Additional Therapies

Additional therapies for individuals with end-stage COPD include lung transplantation[63] and lung volume reduction surgery (LVRS),[64-66] in which small portions of emphysematous lung are removed to reduce hyperinflation and improve lung mechanics of the remaining tissue. COPD is the most common current indication for lung transplantation. Lung transplantation is a consideration for patients with severe airflow obstruction (i.e., FEV_1 < 20% predicted and a Body-mass index, Obstruction, Dyspnea, and Exercise [BODE] index > 7 who are younger than 70 years old, and who are psychologically suitable and motivated). Double lung transplantation is preferred; nevertheless, because the supply of donor lungs to transplant is less than the number of patients needing lung transplantation, single-lung transplantation is also frequently performed. Although lung transplantation may be associated with significantly improved quality of life and functional status, major risks include rejection (manifested as bronchiolitis obliterans and progressive, debilitating airflow obstruction), infection with unusual opportunistic organisms, and death from these and other complications. The 5-year actuarial survival rate after lung transplantation in patients with COPD is approximately 54%[63] (Figure 25-8).

LVRS has regained popularity after initial experiences were reported in 1957.[64] Results of randomized controlled trials of LVRS, including the large National Emphysema Treatment

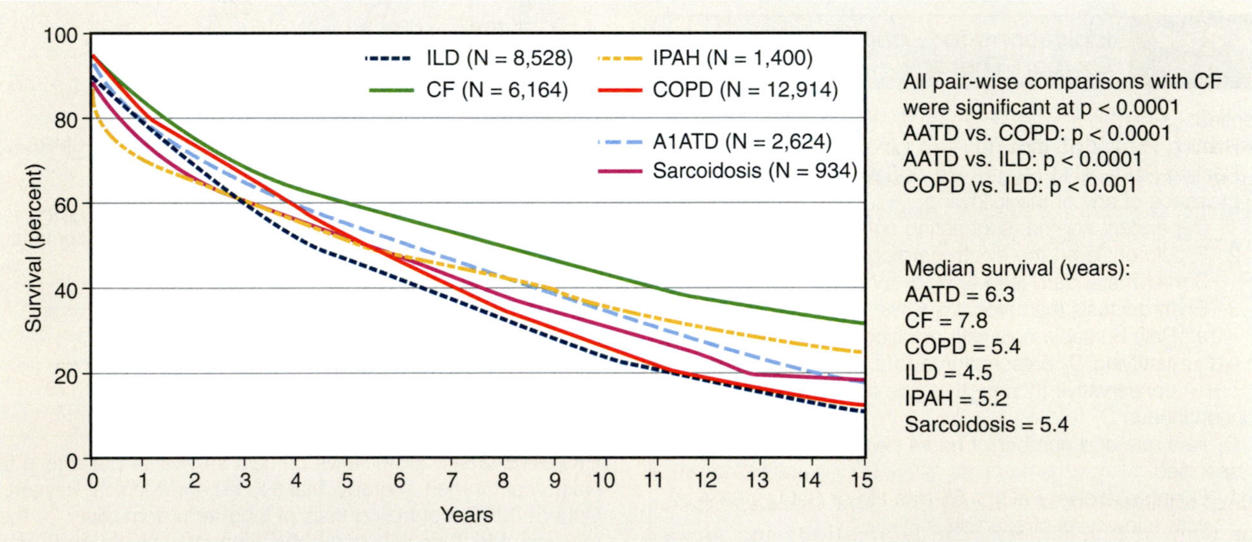

FIGURE 25-8 Adult recipient Kaplan-Meier survival by diagnosis (transplants: January 1990 to June 2011). The overall survival rate of patients with alpha-1 antitrypsin (AAT) deficiency is significantly higher than the survival rate of patients with chronic obstructive pulmonary disease (COPD) and interstitial lung disease (ILD), which includes idiopathic pulmonary fibrosis (IPF). Similarly, the overall survival rate of patients with COPD is higher than the survival rate of patients with idiopathic pulmonary fibrosis. *AATD,* alpha-1 antitrypsin deficiency associated COPD; *COPD,* non-AATD associated COPD; *CF,* cystic fibrosis; IPAH, idiopathic pulmonary arterial hypertension. (From Yusen RD, Christie JD, Edwards LB, et al: 30th official adult lung and heart-lung transplant report, 2013 in the Registry of the International Society for Heart and Lung Transplantation. http://www.ishlt.org. Accessed September 17, 2014.)

Trial, indicate that in selected subsets of patients with COPD (i.e., patients with heterogeneous emphysema that is upper lobe–predominant and who have low exercise capacity after pulmonary rehabilitation), LVRS can prolong survival, improve quality of life, and increase exercise capacity.[65,66] LVRS should not be considered in individuals with very severe COPD (i.e., characterized by FEV_1 <20% predicted with either a homogeneous pattern of emphysema or a diffusing capacity <20% predicted), because the mortality rate of LVRS is higher in such individuals than in medically treated patients.[67]

Given the positive results associated with LVRS in selected patients with COPD, nonsurgical bronchoscopic techniques have been developed in an attempt to reduce costs and expand treatment options for patients with high operative risk.[68] With the use of the bronchoscope, deployment of unidirectional endobronchial valves or coils into the airways results in collapse of the targeted lung parenchyma. Other techniques that have been studied include application of biodegradable gel to induce lung collapse or application of bronchial stents to create fenestrations and allow gas escape from hyperinflated areas of the lung. None of the aforementioned devices is currently approved by the U.S. Food and Drug Administration (FDA) for treatment of emphysema in the United States.[69]

Finally, for patients with AAT deficiency and established COPD, so-called *intravenous augmentation* with a purified preparation of AAT from human blood donors is recommended.[14] The best available evidence[70,71] suggests that for individuals with severe AAT deficiency and moderate degrees of airflow obstruction (i.e., FEV_1 35% to 60% predicted), weekly augmentation therapy may be associated with a slower rate of decline of lung function, a slower rate of loss of lung density on chest CT, and improved survival. Difficulties with intravenous augmentation therapy include the substantial expense (approximately $100,000 per year); the inconvenience of frequent intravenous infusions for life; and the infusion itself, which poses a theoretical risk for transmitting a blood-borne infection. Despite these drawbacks, the facts that augmentation therapy can slow the rate of FEV_1 decline, can possibly slow the rate of CT lung density loss, and is currently the only specific therapy for AAT deficiency have led to its endorsement in official guidelines from the ATS, the ERS, and the Canadian Thoracic Society.[14,72]

ASTHMA

Definition

Asthma is a clinical syndrome characterized by **airway obstruction,** which is partially or completely reversible either spontaneously or with treatment; **airway inflammation;** and **airway hyperresponsiveness** (AHR) to various stimuli.[73-75] Past definitions of asthma emphasized AHR and reversible obstruction; however, newer and more accurate definitions of asthma focus on asthma as a primary inflammatory disease of the airways, with clinical manifestations of increased airway hyperreactivity and airflow obstruction caused by the inflammation.

Incidence

Asthma is a chronic illness that has been increasing in prevalence in the United States since 1980. The number of people with asthma in the United States grew from 20 million in 2001 to 25 million in 2010 (8% of the U.S. population). According to data from the National Health Interview Survey performed by the Centers for Disease Control and Prevention in 2012, 18.7 million adults and 6.8 million children (9.3% of American children) reported having asthma. Asthma accounted for 1.8 million emergency room visits, or 25% of all emergency room visits. Asthma also accounted for 14.2 million outpatient visits, 439,000 hospitalizations, and, approximately 3400 deaths in 2010. Asthma costs in the United States grew from approximately $53 billion in 2002 to about $56 billion in 2007.[76,77]

Etiology and Pathogenesis

In the genetically susceptible host, allergens, respiratory infections, certain occupational and environmental exposures, and many unknown hosts or environmental stimuli can produce the full spectrum of asthma, with persistent airway inflammation, bronchial hyperreactivity, and subsequent airflow obstruction. When inflammation and bronchial hyperreactivity are present, asthma can be triggered by additional factors, including exercise; inhalation of cold, dry air; hyperventilation; cigarette smoke; physical or emotional stress; inhalation of irritants; and pharmacologic agents, such as methacholine and histamine.[78-80]

When a patient with asthma inhales an allergen to which he or she is sensitized, the antigen cross-links to specific immunoglobulin E (IgE) molecules attached to the surface of mast cells in the bronchial mucosa and submucosa. The mast cells degranulate rapidly (within 30 minutes), releasing multiple mediators including leukotrienes (previously known as *slow-reacting substance of anaphylaxis* [SRS-A]), histamine, prostaglandins, platelet-activating factor, and other mediators. These mediators lead to smooth muscle contraction, vascular congestion, and leakage resulting in airflow obstruction, which can be assessed clinically as a decline in FEV_1 or *peak expiratory flow rate* (PEFR) (Figures 25-9 and 10). This is the *early (acute) asthmatic response*, which is an immediate hypersensitivity reaction that usually subsides in approximately 30 to 60 minutes. In approximately 50% of asthmatic patients, however, airflow obstruction recurs in 3 to 8 hours.[80] This *late asthmatic response* is usually more severe and lasts longer than the early asthmatic response (see Figure 25-10).[81] The late asthmatic response is characterized by increasing influx and activation of inflammatory cells such as mast cells, eosinophils, and lymphocytes.[81,82]

Clinical Presentation and Diagnosis

The diagnosis of asthma requires a two-pronged approach of clinical assessment supported by laboratory evaluation. Because no single measurement can absolutely establish the diagnosis, and physical examination can be entirely normal between episodes, the history plays a key role in suggesting, and later establishing, the diagnosis of asthma. The classic symptoms of asthma are episodic wheezing, shortness of breath, chest

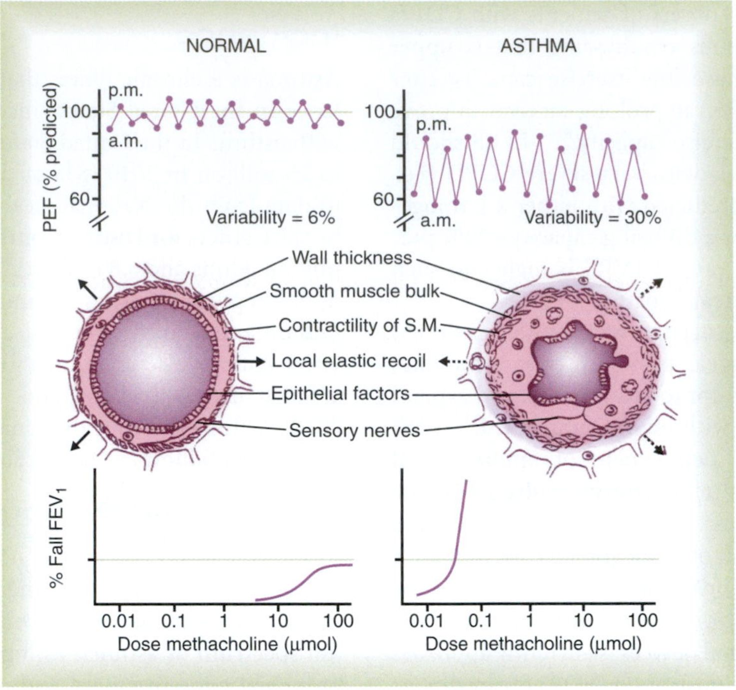

FIGURE 25-9 Inflammation in asthma. Cross sections of an airway from a healthy individual and a patient with asthma are shown. Multiple cells and multiple mediators are involved in asthma. Inflammatory cells, such as mast cells, eosinophils, lymphocytes, and macrophages, release a variety of chemical mediators, such as histamine, prostaglandins, and leukotrienes. These mediators result in increased wall thickness, airway smooth muscle hypertrophy and constriction, epithelial sloughing, mucus hypersecretion, mucosal edema, and stimulation of nerve endings. *Top,* Daily variability in peak airflow measurements. The normal increase in smooth muscle tone in the early morning, which causes airway narrowing in healthy individuals, is more exaggerated in asthmatics. *Bottom,* Dose-response curves to methacholine. (Modified from Woolcock AJ: Asthma. In: Murray JF, Nadel JA, editors: Textbook of respiratory medicine, Philadelphia, 1994, Saunders.)

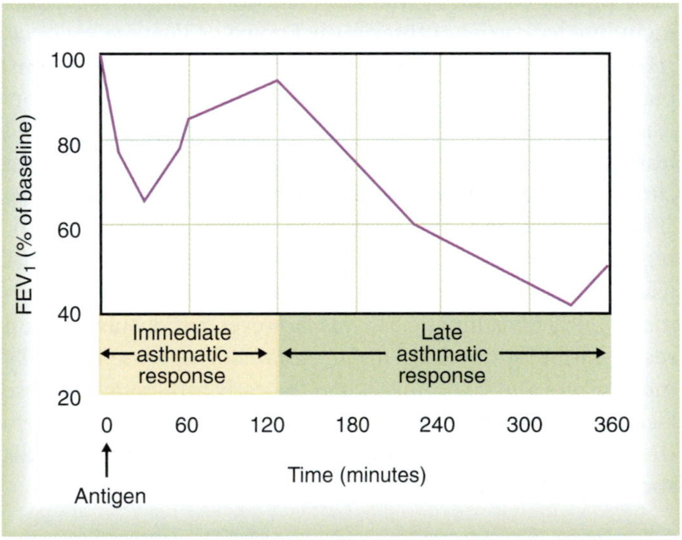

FIGURE 25-10 Early and late asthmatic responses. When a person with asthma is exposed to an allergen to which he or she is sensitized, the challenge results in a biphasic decline in respiratory function. An early asthmatic response occurs within minutes and usually subsides within 2 hours. In approximately half of asthmatic patients, a late asthmatic response occurs within 3 to 8 hours and may last for 24 hours or longer. (Modified from Wiedemann HP, Kavuru MS: Diagnosis and management of asthma, Caddo, OK, 1994, Professional Communications.)

tightness, and cough. The absence of wheezing does not exclude asthma, and sometimes a cough can be the only manifestation (cough-variant asthma). Not all wheezing is due to asthma, however. Obstruction of the upper airway by tumors, laryngospasm, aspirated foreign objects, tracheal stenosis, or functional laryngospasm (vocal cord dysfunction) can mimic the wheezing of asthma.

Confirmation of the diagnosis of asthma requires demonstration of reversible airflow obstruction. Pulmonary function tests may be normal in asymptomatic patients with asthma, but more commonly they reveal some degree of airway obstruction manifested by decreased FEV_1 and FEV_1/FVC ratio. By convention, improvement in the FEV_1 by at least 12% and 200 ml after administration of a bronchodilator is considered evidence of reversibility. Spontaneous variation in self-recorded PEFR by 15% or more also can provide evidence of reversibility of airway obstruction. Elevated values of exhaled nitric oxide also can be used to support the diagnosis of asthma when eosinophilic inflammation is present.[83]

Patients with asthma evaluated in a symptom-free period may have a normal chest x-ray examination and normal pulmonary function tests. Under these circumstances, provocative testing can be used to induce airway obstruction. Bronchoprovocation is a well-established method to detect and quantify

MINI CLINI

Recognizing Severity of Asthma

PROBLEM: A 20-year-old woman with a diagnosis of asthma is seen in the outpatient clinic for increased dyspnea with exertion requiring daily use of short-acting bronchodilators. The patient complains of difficulty attending classes in college and wakes up a couple of times a week feeling short of breath. She describes two visits to the emergency department in the last 12 months because of asthma, requiring use of corticosteroids for a short period. Physical examination shows normal breath sounds bilaterally without wheezing. Spirometry shows FEV_1 of 78% percent predicted with FEV_1/FVC of 75%. How do you describe the severity of her asthma?

SOLUTION: Classification of asthma severity is based on a combination of symptoms, medication requirements, and lung function. Although this patient has a spirometry consistent with mild airflow obstruction, her asthma is classified as moderately persistent because of the presence of daily symptoms, daily use of short-acting bronchodilators, frequent nighttime awakenings, limitation with normal activities, and history of exacerbations (see the following table).

Components of Severity		Classification of Asthma Severity (Youths ≤12 Years of Age and Adults)			
			Persistent		
		Intermittent	Mild	Moderate	Severe
Impairment FEV_1/FVC:	Symptoms	≤2 days/wk	>2 days/wk but not daily	Daily	Throughout the day
18-19 yr, 85%	Nighttime awakenings	≤2 ×/mo	3-4 ×/mo	>1 ×/wk but not nightly	Often 7 ×/wk
20-39 yr, 80% 40-59 yr, 75% 60-80 yr, 60%	Short-acting beta-2 agonist use for symptom control (not prevention of exercise-induced bronchospasm)	≤2 days/wk	>2 days/wk but not >1 time/day	Daily	Several times per day
	Interference with normal activity	None	Minor limitation	Some limitation	Extremely limited
	Lung function	Normal FEV_1 between exacerbations FEV_1 > 80% predicted FEV_1/FVC normal	FEV_1 ≥ 80% predicted FEV_1/FVC normal	FEV_1 ≥ 60% but < 80% predicted FEV_1/FVC reduced > 5%	FEV_1 ≥ 60% predicted FEV_1/FVC reduced > 5%
Risk	Exacerbations requiring oral systemic corticosteroids	0-1/yr	≥ 2/yr		
		Consider severity and interval since last exacerbation. Frequency and severity may fluctuate over time for patients in any severity category. Relative annual risk for exacerbations may be related to FEV_1.			

AHR. Pharmacologic agents, including acetylcholine, methacholine, histamine, cysteinyl leukotrienes, and prostaglandins, and physical stimuli such as exercise and isocapnic hyperventilation with cold, dry air have been used to detect, quantify, and characterize nonspecific AHR in asthma.

The most commonly used stimulus for bronchoprovocation is methacholine. The generally accepted criterion for hyperresponsiveness is a decrease in FEV_1 by 20% or more below the baseline value after inhalation of methacholine.

The methacholine provocation test has few false-negative results (<5%), but a false-positive result may be found in 7% to 8% of the average population and patients with other obstructive lung diseases. Elevated IgE levels and eosinophilia may be present in patients with asthma, but their presence is not specific and their absence does not exclude asthma, making them less useful for the diagnosis.[73-75] Although ABG analysis is not helpful or necessary in diagnosing asthma, it can be helpful in assessing the severity of an acute asthma attack.

A patient experiencing an acute asthma attack usually has a low $PaCO_2$ as a result of hyperventilation. A normal $PaCO_2$ in such a situation is concerning because it indicates a severe attack and impending respiratory failure.

Management

The goal of asthma management is to maintain a high quality of life for the patient, uninterrupted by asthma symptoms, side effects from medications, or limitations on the job or during exercise. This goal can be accomplished by preventing acute exacerbations, with their potential mortality and morbidity, or by returning the patient to a stable baseline when exacerbations occur. Asthma management relies on the following four important components recommended by the National Asthma Education Program (NAEP) expert panel[73]:

1. Objective measurements and monitoring of lung function
2. Pharmacologic therapy
3. Environmental control
4. Patient education

Table 25-2 outlines the stepwise approach currently recommended for long-term management of asthma. This approach provides a framework for adjusting the dose of medication

TABLE 25-2

Stepwise Approach to Long-Term Management of Asthma Based on Severity

Severity*	Clinical Features Before Treatment†	PEFR or FEV_1	Long-Term Preventive Medications	Quick Relief Medications
Step 4				
Severe persistent	Continuous symptoms	≤60% predicted	Inhaled corticosteroids ≥800-2000 mcg/day	Inhaled beta-2 agonist as needed for symptoms
Red zone	Frequent exacerbations Nocturnal symptoms Symptoms limit activity	>30% variability	Long-acting bronchodilator‡ Oral corticosteroids	
Step 3				
Moderate persistent	Daily symptoms	>60%-<80% predicted	Inhaled corticosteroids ≥800-2000 mcg/day	Inhaled beta-2 agonist as needed for symptoms, not to exceed 3-4 times per day
Yellow zone	Exacerbations affect activity and sleep Nocturnal symptoms more than once per week Daily use of short-acting beta-2 agonist	>30% variability	Long-acting bronchodilator,‡ especially for nocturnal symptoms	
Step 2				
Mild persistent	Symptoms at least once per week but <1 time per day	≥80% predicted	Inhaled corticosteroid, 200-500 mg/day	Inhaled beta-2 agonist as needed for symptoms, not to exceed 3-4 times per day
Yellow zone	Exacerbations may affect activity or sleep Nocturnal symptoms more than twice per month	20%-30% variability	Long-acting bronchodilator‡ for nocturnal symptoms	
Step 1				
Intermittent	Intermittent symptoms less than once per week	≥80% predicted	None needed	Inhaled beta-2 agonist needed for symptoms but less than once per week
Green zone	Nocturnal symptoms not more than twice per month Asymptomatic with normal lung function between exacerbations	<20% variability		Inhaled beta-2 agonist or cromolyn before exercise or exposure to allergen

Modified from: Global Initiative for Asthma: Asthma management and prevention: a practical guide for public health officials and health care professionals, NIH publication no. 96-3659A, Bethesda, MD, 1995, National Institutes of Health, National Heart, Lung, and Blood Institute, and World Health Organization.
**Step-down:* Review treatment every 3 to 6 months. If control is sustained for at least 3 months, consider a gradual stepwise reduction in treatment. *Step-up:* If control is not achieved, consider step-up, but first review patient medication technique, compliance, and environmental control.
†The presence of one of the features of severity is sufficient to place a patient in that category.
‡Long-acting beta-2 agonist or sustained-release theophylline.

based on the severity of asthma in any patient at a particular time. This approach also takes into consideration the fact that asthma is a chronic and dynamic disease, which needs optimum control. Control of asthma is defined as minimal to no chronic diurnal or nocturnal symptoms, infrequent exacerbations, minimal to no need for beta-2 agonists, no limitation to exercise activity, PEFR or FEV_1 greater than 80% predicted with less than 20% diurnal variation, and minimal to no adverse effects of medication.[73-75]

Objective Measurement and Monitoring

Objective measurement of lung function is particularly important in asthma because subjective measures, such as patient reports of the degree of dyspnea and physical examination findings, often do not correlate with the variability and severity of airflow obstruction. It is recommended that spirometry be performed as part of the initial assessment of all patients being evaluated for asthma and periodically thereafter as needed.

Either spirometry or PEFR measurement can be used to assess response to therapy in the outpatient setting, emergency department, or hospital. NAEP guidelines also recommend that home PEFR measurement be used for patients with moderate to severe asthma.

When patients learn how to take PEFR measurements at home, the clinician is better able to recommend effective treatment. Daily monitoring of PEFR helps detect early stages of airway obstruction. All PEFR measurements are compared with the patient's personal best value, which can be established during a 2- to 3-week asymptomatic period when the patient is being treated optimally.[73-75]

MINI CLINI

Diagnosis of Wheezing

PROBLEM: You are asked to see a patient with a history of wheezing. The patient notes that the wheezing has been continuous, has been present for several months, and has been unresponsive to bronchodilator medications, including systemic corticosteroids and various inhaled bronchodilators.

SOLUTION: The patient has either refractory asthma or a condition mimicking asthma. The aphorism "all that wheezes is not asthma" applies here, and the clinician should suspect alternative diagnoses. Features that are atypical for asthma in this patient are the continuous nature of the wheezing and its complete refractoriness to medication. With this in mind, consideration of other "wheezy" disorders should include abnormalities of the upper airway. Specifically, tracheal stenosis or fixed upper airway obstruction (e.g., caused by tracheal tumors) could account for the patient's symptoms. Another condition that mimics asthma is vocal cord dysfunction. Characteristically, vocal cord dysfunction causes stridor with convergence of the vocal cords on inspiration (a paradoxical response). However, vocal cord dysfunction also can cause expiratory wheezing, with closure of the vocal cords on expiration. Further assessment of this patient might include a flow-volume loop or a flexible bronchoscopic examination of the upper airway, observing both the vocal cords and the trachea to the level of the main stem bronchi.

To help patients understand home PEFR monitoring, a zonal system corresponding to the traffic light system may be helpful (see Table 25-2). A PEFR measurement of 80% to 100% of the personal best is considered to be in the *green zone*. No asthma symptoms are present, and maintenance medications can be continued or tapered. A PEFR in the 60% to 80% range of the personal best is in the *yellow zone* and may indicate an acute exacerbation and requires a temporary step-up in treatment. A PEFR less than 60% of the personal best is in the *red zone* and signals a medical alert, requiring immediate medical attention if the patient does not return to the yellow zone or green zone with bronchodilator use.[75]

Pharmacotherapy

Pharmacotherapy for asthma reflects the basic understanding that asthma is a chronic inflammatory airway disease that requires long-term antiinflammatory therapy for adequate control.[73-82] Antiinflammatory agents such as corticosteroids suppress the primary disease process and its resultant airway hyperreactivity. Bronchodilators, such as beta-2–adrenergic agonists, anticholinergics, and theophylline, relieve asthma symptoms. Because asthma is a disease of the airways, inhalation therapy is preferred to oral or other systemic therapy. Inhaled therapy using metered dose inhalers or dry powder inhalers allows high concentration of the medication to be delivered directly to the airways, resulting in fewer systemic side effects. Spacer devices can be used to improve delivery of inhaled medication, but training and coordination are still required for patients using metered dose inhalers. Table 25-3 lists commonly used medications in the treatment of asthma.

Corticosteroids

Corticosteroids are the most effective medication currently available for the treatment of asthma. Although their mode of action is still unclear, corticosteroids probably act on various components of the inflammatory response in asthma.[84] Inhaled corticosteroids are effective locally, and regular use suppresses inflammation in the airways, decreases bronchial hyperreactivity and airflow obstruction, and reduces the symptoms of and mortality from asthma. Long-term, high-dose inhaled corticosteroids have far fewer side effects than oral corticosteroids. Side effects such as oropharyngeal candidiasis and dysphonia are controllable with spacer use and by rinsing the mouth after each treatment. Patients should be informed of other side effects of chronic inhaled corticosteroid use such as skin bruising and increased risks for glaucoma and cataracts.

Oral corticosteroids are effective for treating asthma, but the potential for devastating side effects during long-term use restricts their use to patients not responding to other forms of asthma therapy. Short-term, high-dose (0.5 to 1 mg/kg/day) oral corticosteroid therapy during exacerbation reduces the severity and duration, decreases the need for emergency department visits and hospitalization, and reduces mortality.[84]

Leukotriene Inhibitors

Leukotrienes are mediators of inflammation and bronchoconstriction and are thought to play a role in the pathogenesis of asthma. Three leukotriene antagonists are currently available for the treatment of asthma. Montelukast (Singulair; Merck, Whitehouse Station, NJ) and zafirlukast (Accolate; Astra Zeneca, London, UK) are leukotriene receptor antagonists, and zileuton (Zyflo; Abbott Laboratories, Chicago, IL) is a leukotriene synthesis inhibitor. These agents all are modestly effective for maintenance of mild to moderate asthma, but their exact role in asthma therapy remains to be determined. Inhaled steroids remain the preferred antiinflammatory drugs for treating asthma.[84,85]

Beta-2-Adrenergic Agonists

Inhaled beta-2–adrenergic agents are the most rapid and effective bronchodilators for treating asthma. They are the drugs of choice for all types of acute bronchospasm, and they provide protection from all bronchoconstrictor challenges when given prophylactically. However, they do not prevent the late asthmatic response. Beta-2 agonists are the drugs of choice for exercise-induced asthma. They exert their action by attaching to beta receptors on the cell to produce smooth muscle relaxation and by blocking mediator release from mast cells.

The effectiveness of beta-2 agonists as bronchodilators is not disputed, and they are the drug of choice for acute emergency management of asthma. However, there is concern that they may worsen asthma control if used regularly and that excessive

TABLE 25-3
Medications Commonly Used in the Treatment of Asthma or Chronic Obstructive Pulmonary Disease

Medication	Trade Names	Available Preparations	Usual Dosage	Comment
Inhaled Corticosteroids (Single Medication)				
Beclomethasone	Beclovent, QVAR	MDI 42 mcg/puff, 200 puffs/canister	2 puffs tid-qid, maximum 20 puffs/day	
Flunisolide	Aerobid	MDI 250 mg/puff, 100 puffs/canister	2 puffs bid, maximum 8 puffs/day	
Fluticasone	Flovent	MDI 44, 110, 220 mcg/puff	88-880 mcg/day	
Mometasone	Asmanex	DPI 220 mcg/spray	1-2 sprays daily-bid, maximum 4 puffs/day	
Budesonide	Pulmicort	DPI 90, 180 mcg/puff	360-720 mcg/day	
Inhaled Corticosteroids (Combined Medication)				
Fluticasone and salmeterol	Advair	DPI 100 mcg fluticasone/50 mcg salmeterol/puff, 250 mcg/50 mcg, 500 mcg/50 mcg/puff MDI HFA 45 mcg/21 mcg/puff, 115 mcg/21 mcg/puff, and 230 mcg/21 mcg/puff	400-2000 mcg/day (corticosteroid dose)	
Budesonide and formoterol	Symbicort	160 mcg budesonide/4.5 mcg formoterol/puff and 80 mcg/4.5 mcg/puff	160-640 mcg/day (corticosteroid dose)	
Fluticasone and vilanterol	Breo Ellipta	DPI 100 mcg fluticasone/25 mcg vilanterol/puff	100 mcg/day (corticosteroid dose)	Only approved for patients with COPD.
Systemic Corticosteroids				
Prednisone	Many	Tablets 1, 5, 20, 50 mg	5-50 mg/day	
Methylprednisolone	Medrol	Tablets 2, 4, 8, 16, 24, 32 mg	4-48 mg/day	
	Solu-Medrol	IV 40, 125, 500, 1000 mg	1-2 mg/kg q4-6h	
Hydrocortisone	Solu-Cortef	IV 100, 250, 500, 1000 mg	4 mg/kg q4-6h	
Beta-2 Agonists				
Albuterol	Proventil	MDI 90 mcg/puff, 200 puffs/canister	2-4 puffs q4-6h, maximum 20 puffs/day	
	Ventolin	Solution for nebulizer 0.083% and 0.5%	2.5-10 mg q6-8h	
		Tablets 2, 4 mg	2-4 mg q6-8h	
	Volmax	Sustained-release tablets 4, 8 mg	4-8 mg q12h	
Metaproterenol	Alupent	MDI 650 mcg/puff, 200 puffs/canister	2-3 puffs q3-4h, maximum 12 puffs/day	
	Metaprel	Solution 0.5%	2.5-10 mg q4-6h	
		Tablets 10, 20 mg	10 mg q6-8h	
Pirbuterol	Maxair	MDI 200 mcg/puff, 300 puffs/canister	1-2 puffs q4-6h, maximum 12 puffs/day	
Terbutaline	Breathaire	MDI 200 mcg/puff, 300 puffs/canister 1-2 puffs q4-6h		
	Bricanyl	Tablets 2.5, 5 mg	2.5-5 mg tid, maximum 15 mg/day	
		Solution 1 mg/ml	0.25 mg subcutaneously q15-30min	
Long-Acting Beta Agonists				
Salmeterol	Serevent	MDI 50 mcg/puff	2 puffs q12h	
Formoterol	Foradil	DPI 12 mcg/capsule	1 capsule inhaled q12h	
Indacaterol	Arcapta	DPI 75 mcg/capsule	75 mcg/day	Not indicated in patients with asthma.
Arformoterol	Brovana	Solution 15 mcg/ml	15 mcg inhaled bid	
Anticholinergics (Single Medication)				
Ipratropium bromide	Atrovent	MDI 18 mcg/puff, 200 puffs/canister Solution for nebulizer 0.02% 0.5 mg/2.5 ml vial, 0.5 mg qid	2-4 puffs q6h	
Tiotropium	Spiriva	DPI 18 mcg/capsule	1 capsule inhaled/day	
Aclinidium	Tudorza	DPI 400 mcg/actuation	800 mcg/day	M_2/M_3 muscarinic antagonist. Only approved for COPD.

TABLE 25-3
Medications Commonly Used in the Treatment of Asthma or Chronic Obstructive Pulmonary Disease—cont'd

Medication	Trade Names	Available Preparations	Usual Dosage	Comment
Anticholinergics (Combined Medication)				
Umeclidinium and vilanterol	Anoro Ellipta	DPI 62.5 mcg umeclidinium/25 mcg vilanterol/puff	62.5 mcg of umeclidinium/day	Umeclidinium is a muscarinic antagonist. Vilanterol is a long-acting bronchodilator. Not approved for patients with asthma.
Methylxanthines				
Aminophylline		IV	Load 5-6 mg/kg, maintenance 0.5-0.9 mg/kg/hr	
		Tablets or capsules		
Theophylline	Theo-Dur		300-1200 mg/day divided q6-8h for immediate and q12-24h for sustained	
	Slo-bid			
	Theovent Uniphyl (immediate or sustained release)			
Leukotriene Inhibitors				
Zafirlukast	Accolate	Tablets 20 mg	20 mg bid	
Zileuton	Zyflo	Tablets 600 mg	600 mg qid	
Montelukast	Singulair	Tablets 10 mg	10 mg daily	
Other				
Roflumilast	Daliresp	Tablets 500 mcg	500 mcg/day	PDE-4 inhibitor. Primary use prevention of COPD exacerbations, not indicated for acute bronchospasm or asthma.
Azithromycin	Zithromax	Tablets 250 mg, 500 mg	250 mg/day	Macrolide antibiotic associated with reduction in number of COPD exacerbations.*
N-Acetylcysteine (NAC)	Mucomyst	Tablets 300 mg, 600 mg	1200 mg/day	High dose NAC is associated with decrease in exacerbation frequency in patients COPD.†
Omalizumab	Xolair	150 mg / 5 mL	150-375 mg subcutaneously every month	Anti-IgE therapy only approved for patients with moderate to severe asthma.

*Albert RK, Connett J, Bailey WC, et al: Azithromycin for prevention of exacerbations of COPD. N Engl J Med 365:689–698, 2011.
†Zheng JP, Wen FQ, Bai CX, et al: Twice daily N-acetylcysteine 600 mg for exacerbations of chronic obstructive pulmonary disease (PANTHEON): a randomised, double-blind placebo-controlled trial. Lancet Respir Med: 2:187–194, 2014.
COPD, Chronic obstructive pulmonary; *DPI,* dry powder inhaler; *HFA,* hydrofluoroalkane; *IgE,* immunoglobulin E; *MDI,* metered dose inhaler.

use may increase the risk for death from asthma, which makes the role of beta-2 agonists alone in long-term maintenance therapy questionable. It is clear that excessive beta-2 agonist use by asthmatics indicates an increased risk for death from asthma and indicates the need for more effective antiinflammatory therapy. Furthermore, because use of long-acting beta-2-agonosists in asthmatics has been associated with increased mortality, such agents should not be used in asthmatics but rather in combination with an anti-inflammatory drug such as an inhaled corticosteroid medication. Treatment with conventional doses of the short-acting beta-2 agonists available in the United States is felt to be safe for asthmatic patients.[82,84,86] The NAEP guidelines recommend that inhaled beta-2 agonists be used as needed. If a patient needs more than 3 or 4 puffs per day of a beta-2 agonist, additional antiinflammatory therapy should be considered.[84]

Longer acting (12 to 24 hours) beta-2 agonists, such as salmeterol and formoterol, are available in the United States. Their mechanism of action is different from that of the shorter acting beta-2 agonists discussed earlier. Long-acting beta-2 agonists have use in treating nocturnal asthma but again, should not be used alone in managing asthma.[73-75,86-88]

Inhaled corticosteroids remain the first choice of therapy in asthma.

Methylxanthines

The role of theophylline and similar drugs in the treatment of acute asthma is controversial. The NAEP expert panel did not recommend using theophylline routinely in the emergency treatment of asthma but did recommend its use orally or intravenously for patients admitted to the hospital for an acute asthma attack. Sustained-release theophylline drugs added to long-term asthma management therapy may be helpful in controlling nocturnal asthma symptoms because they maintain therapeutic plasma concentrations overnight. They also are helpful in soothing the symptoms of patients with labile asthma. However, the efficacy of theophylline is limited by its side effects of nausea, vomiting, headache, insomnia, seizures, and cardiac arrhythmias. Toxicity increases with blood levels greater than 15 mcg/ml, but levels of 8 to 10 mcg/ml are adequate for long-term therapy and are associated with fewer side effects.

Several factors affect the plasma levels of theophylline by increasing or decreasing hepatic metabolism of the drug. Conditions that tend to increase plasma concentrations include acute viral infections, cardiac failure, hepatic disease, and concomitant use of certain medications such as erythromycin or cimetidine. In these cases, the maintenance dose should be halved and the theophylline blood levels should be monitored. Conditions that tend to decrease plasma levels of theophylline include cigarette smoking and use of medications that increase hepatic clearance, such as phenobarbital.[73-75]

Anticholinergics

Inhaled anticholinergic agents, such as ipratropium bromide, are effective dilators of airway smooth muscles. Ipratropium produces bronchodilation by reduction of intrinsic vagal tone and blocking vagal reflex bronchospasm. However, ipratropium does not stabilize mast cells or prevent mediator release and is a less potent bronchodilator than beta-2 agonists. Ipratropium has few side effects, is safe because it is poorly absorbed, adds a bronchodilator effect to beta-2 agonists, and is useful for treating cough-variant asthma. Ipratropium also can be used in treating acute asthma when first-line bronchodilators are ineffective. The long-acting anticholinergic agent tiotropium has been shown to enhance asthma control (e.g., improved peak expiratory flow, increased FEV_1, and improved symptoms) when added to an inhaled corticosteroid compared with doubling the inhaled steroid dose.[89]

Anti–Immunoglobulin E Therapy

IgE plays a key role in the pathogenesis of asthma, and many asthmatic patients have elevated levels of IgE.[90] Corticosteroids do not inhibit synthesis of IgE by activated lymphocytes. Omalizumab, an antibody that binds IgE and blocks its biologic effects, has been approved by the FDA for patients with a history of allergy and with moderate to severe asthma that is poorly controlled with inhaled corticosteroids.[91] Studies have shown that treatment with omalizumab results in a reduction in the dose of inhaled glucocorticoids required to control symptoms and a reduction in the number of asthma exacerbation episodes.[92] For this reason, the NAEP asthma guidelines recommended that omalizumab should be considered as adjunctive therapy for patients with severe persistent asthma.[73]

Emergency Department and Hospital Management

Emergency management of acute asthma should include early and frequent administration of aerosolized beta-2 agonists and therapy with systemic corticosteroids. Frequent assessment for response with PEFR should be performed. The NAEP guidelines recommend that only selective beta-2 agonists (i.e., albuterol, levalbuterol, pirbuterol) should be used in high doses to avoid cardiotoxicity.[73]

Hospital and ICU care for patients with asthma should be aggressive. The goal is to decrease mortality and morbidity and to return the patient to preadmission stability and function as quickly as possible. Management includes O_2 supplementation, periodic administration of high doses of aerosolized beta-2 agonists (limited only by tachycardia or tremor), high-dose parenteral corticosteroids (>0.5 to 1 mg/kg/day), and antibiotics if there is evidence of infection. Sedatives and hypnotics should be avoided. Symptoms, PEFR, and ABGs should be monitored.

Patients with severe asthma and respiratory failure (hypoxemia, hypercapnia, increased work of breathing) need ventilatory support and present special challenges. Mortality rates for these patients can reach 22%, and complications are common, especially barotrauma. These complications can be minimized by limiting peak inspiratory pressure to less than 50 cm H_2O and by the use of small tidal volumes, allowing "permissive hypercapnia" if necessary. When asthma control is achieved, hospital discharge criteria include not needing supplemental O_2; having a PaO_2 greater than 60 mm Hg and a stable PEFR or FEV_1, with values close to the patient's best or greater than 70% of predicted; feeling that asthma symptoms are returning to preadmission levels and are not occurring at night; and 12- to 24-hour stability on discharge medications.[73-75]

RULE OF THUMB

In a patient presenting with an acute asthma attack, $PaCO_2$ is usually low because of hyperventilation. A normal $PaCO_2$ in this situation indicates a severe attack and impending respiratory failure.

Bronchial Thermoplasty

Bronchial thermoplasty is an approved addition to treatment options for adults whose asthma remains uncontrolled despite use of inhaled steroids and long-acting beta agonists.[93] Bronchial thermoplasty is a procedure in which a probe is introduced into the central airways through a bronchoscope and heat is applied (through radiofrequency waves) to airways of 3 to 10 mm diameter with the goal to reduce the airway smooth muscle mass, reducing the ability of the airways to constrict. Studies have shown that bronchial thermoplasty improves asthma-specific quality of life and reduces the number of severe

MINI CLINI

Assessing the Severity of an Acute Asthma Attack

PROBLEM: You have just obtained an ABG analysis on a patient who sought treatment at the emergency department for an acute attack of asthma. How would the ABG analysis help you assess the severity of the attack?

SOLUTION: In the early stages of an asthma attack, the ABG analysis shows a low $PaCO_2$ caused by hyperventilation. As the asthma attack progresses, and the FEV_1 decreases to less than 25% of predicted, the $PaCO_2$ returns to normal. When the FEV_1 decreases to less than 15% of predicted, carbon dioxide retention begins to occur. Changes in the pH reflect changes in the $PaCO_2$ level. The following table summarizes the ABG abnormalities based on the severity of an asthma attack:

Asthma Severity	Stage	PaO_2	$PaCO_2$	pH
Mild	I	Normal	Decreased	Increased
Moderate	II	Decreased	Decreased	Increased
Severe	III	Decreased	Normal	Normal
Very severe (respiratory failure)	IV	Decreased	Increased	Decreased

asthma exacerbation episodes and emergency department visits.[94,95] Moreover, there are now data suggesting that these effects are long-lasting (approximately 5 years) with regard to both asthma control (based on maintained reduction in severe exacerbations and emergency department visits for respiratory symptoms) and safety.[96] Although bronchial thermoplasty is a promising treatment for patients with asthma that is difficult to control, some controversy remains and more studies are needed before it can be recommended to all patients with poorly controlled asthma.[97]

Immunotherapy

Immunotherapy is based on the theoretical rationale that part of the immunologic response to an administered allergen is the production of IgG-specific antibody to the allergen injected. This newly generated IgG does not affix to most cells but can react with the allergen diffusing into the tissues and "neutralize" it. Although immunotherapy is acceptable in the treatment of allergic rhinitis, its use in the treatment of asthma is not standardized and remains controversial. However, a meta-analysis of 88 randomized controlled trials of injection allergen immunotherapy for asthma reported that immunotherapy is effective, with evidence of significant reductions in asthma medications and symptoms and a reduction in the degree of bronchial hyperreactivity.[98]

Environmental Control

The association between asthma and allergy has long been recognized. Among patients with asthma, 75% to 85% are reported to have positive immediate skin test reaction to common inhalant allergens. A thorough history is essential to diagnosing whether a patient's asthma has an allergic component and determining the relationship between exposure to an allergen and the occurrence of symptoms. Skin tests are more helpful for excluding an allergen as a cause of asthma symptoms because clinical sensitivity to an aeroallergen is rare in the absence of a positive skin test, whereas many positive skin tests do not have clinical relevance.

To prevent allergic reactions in patients with asthma, environmental control measures to reduce exposure to indoor and outdoor allergens and irritants are essential. Patients should be advised to avoid outdoor antigens, primarily ragweed, grass, pollens, and molds. Exposure to outdoor allergens is best reduced by staying indoors with the windows closed, in an air-conditioned environment, particularly during the midday and afternoon, when pollen and some mold counts are highest. Patients who are allergic to indoor allergens, primarily house-dust components and indoor molds, should take steps to eliminate these allergens from the home environment (e.g., single-room air purifier). All warm-blooded pets, including small rodents and birds, should be removed from the house because they produce dander, urine, and saliva that can cause allergic reactions. House-dust mites depend on atmospheric moisture and human dander for survival. Essential house-dust mite control measures include encasing mattresses and pillows in airtight covers, washing the bedding in water of 130° F weekly, avoiding sleeping on upholstered furniture, and removing carpets that are laid on concrete.

Additional helpful control measures include reducing the indoor humidity to less than 50%, removing carpets from the bedroom, and using chemical agents to kill mites. Indoor air-cleaning devices, especially high-efficiency particulate air/aerosol filters, may be useful, but they cannot substitute for controlling the allergen source. Humidifiers are potentially harmful because they can harbor and aerosolize mold spores, and the increased humidity they generate may encourage production of both mold and house-dust mites.[73-75]

Patient Education

With close back-up by the informed physician, respiratory therapist, or nurse, much of the day-to-day responsibility for managing asthma falls on the patient and the patient's family. Patient education is a powerful motivational tool, helping patients attain the skills and gain the confidence to control their asthma. Patient education involves helping patients understand asthma and learning and practicing the skills necessary to manage it. Patient education includes providing information; developing a partnership with the patient; involving the patient in decision-making; and demonstrating and observing asthma management practices such as the proper use of inhalers, nebulizers, and peak flowmeters.[86]

Special Considerations in Asthma Management

Exercise-Induced Asthma

Exercise-induced asthma is common in asthmatics, especially after participation in outdoor activities in cold weather. The causes of exercise-induced asthma are not fully understood, but heat loss from the airways seems to be one of the causes.[81] Treatment consists of prophylactic inhalation of a beta-2 agonist.[99,100] Leukotriene inhibitors also may have a role in treatment of exercise-induced asthma.[73,74]

Occupational Asthma

An estimated 2% to 5% of all asthma episodes may be caused by exposure to a specific sensitizing agent in the workplace. Occupational asthma is the most common form of occupational lung disease in many industrialized countries. In an attempt to distinguish occupational from preexisting asthma, occupational asthma is defined as a disease characterized by a variable airflow limitation or AHR secondary to causes and conditions attributable to a particular working environment and not to stimuli encountered outside the workplace. Toluene diisocyanate is the most common cause of occupational asthma and is the best studied. Other causes of occupational asthma are listed in Table 25-4.

Generally, the treatment of occupational asthma is identical to treatment of other types of asthma. However, early diagnosis is important and in environmental control, in particular, cessation of exposure is key. Complete elimination of exposure is usually necessary because once sensitization has occurred, bronchoconstriction can be triggered by minimal subsequent exposure.[74,81]

Cough-Variant Asthma

Coughing may be the only complaint of patients with asthma. In such patients, the cough may be relieved by a bronchodilator or by avoiding inhaled allergens. If bronchospasm is not present at the time of examination and spirometry is normal (which is often the case), the diagnosis can be confirmed by showing reversible airway obstruction by a methacholine challenge test or suggested by elevated levels of exhaled NO.[83] Ipratropium bromide may be particularly helpful in the treatment of cough-variant asthma. Otherwise, the treatment is the same as for other types of asthma.

TABLE 25-4
Occupational Causes of Asthma

Occupation or Industry	Agent
Laboratory animal workers, veterinarians	Animals (dander, urine protein)
Food processing	Shellfish, egg proteins, pancreatic enzymes
Dairy farming	Storage mites
Poultry farming	Poultry mites, droppings, feathers
Detergent manufacturing	*Bacillus subtilis* enzymes
Baking	Flour
Sawmill workers, carpentry	Wood dust (western red cedar, oak, mahogany, zebrawood, redwood)
Nursing	Psyllium
Refining	Platinum salts
Plating	Nickel salts
Stainless steel welding	Chromium salts
Cosmetology	Persulfate
Refinery workers	Vanadium
Rubber processing	Formaldehyde, ethylenediamine
Plastics industry	Toluene diisocyanate, trimellitic anhydride

Nocturnal Asthma

Nocturnal asthma is a characteristic problem in poorly controlled asthma and is reported by more than two-thirds of patients who receive treatment that is less than ideal. It probably is due to the known physiologic decrease in the airway tone during sleep, which has been attributed to variation in catecholamine and cortisol secretion. Aspiration of gastric acid also may play a role in some patients with increased symptoms at night.

After ensuring adequate antiinflammatory therapy, medications for nocturnal asthma should be focused toward the night and especially the early morning hours, when the airway tone is lowest. Sustained-release theophylline and long-acting beta-2 agonists such as salmeterol are particularly helpful for controlling nocturnal asthma symptoms.[73] Addition of a proton pump inhibitor medication such as esomeprazole has not been shown to enhance asthma control.[101]

Aspirin Sensitivity

At least 5% of adults with asthma experience severe and even fatal exacerbation of asthma after taking aspirin or other nonsteroidal antiinflammatory drugs (NSAIDs). Many of these patients have nasal polyps, although the relationship is not causal. The presumed mechanism is the inhibition of the cyclooxygenase pathway by aspirin and NSAIDs, with subsequent shunting of all arachidonic acid into the 5-lipoxygenase pathway, causing overproduction of bronchoconstrictor leukotrienes. Individuals with asthma should avoid aspirin and NSAIDs and instead use alternatives such as acetaminophen (e.g., Tylenol). Patients should be informed that many over-the-counter medications contain aspirin and should be avoided as well.[73,81]

Gastroesophageal Reflux

The relationship between asthma and gastroesophageal reflux is controversial, although gastroesophageal reflux is nearly three times more prevalent in patients with asthma than in persons without asthma. Presumably, acid reflux into the esophagus causes vagal stimulation, resulting in a reflex increase in bronchial tone in patients with asthma. However, addition of a proton pump inhibitor to an asthma regimen has not been shown to enhance asthma control significantly.[101]

Asthma During Pregnancy

During pregnancy, one-third of patients have worse control of their asthma, one-third have better control of asthma, and one-third have asthma that is unchanged. The potential threat of adverse effects from asthma medications is far outweighed by the danger of uncontrolled asthma to the fetus and mother. Poorly controlled asthma during pregnancy can cause increased perinatal mortality, increased prematurity, and low birth weight.

Theophyllines, beta-2 agonists, or inhaled or oral corticosteroids can be used during pregnancy without significant risk for fetal abnormalities.[102]

Sinusitis

Acute sinusitis and chronic sinusitis have been related to exacerbations and poor control of asthma by causing postnasal drip and interfering with nasal patency. A limited CT scan of the sinuses should be obtained for patients with uncontrolled asthma. If sinusitis is present, therapy with antibiotics for 2 to 3 weeks, nasal decongestants, and nasal corticosteroid inhalers may help improve asthma control.[73,81]

Surgery

Patients with asthma are predisposed to respiratory complications after surgery, including respiratory arrest during induction of anesthesia, hypoxemia and possible hypercapnia, impaired effectiveness of cough, atelectasis, and respiratory infection. The likelihood of these complications depends on the severity of the patient's airway hyperreactivity, the degree of airflow obstruction, and the amount of excess airway secretions at the time of surgery. Optimizing the patient's lung function before surgery, including the administration of perioperative corticosteroids, is an important strategy for minimizing perioperative complications.[73,81]

BRONCHIECTASIS

Clinical Presentation

Bronchiectasis refers to the abnormal, irreversible dilation of the bronchi caused by destructive and inflammatory changes in the airway walls. Bronchiectasis has the following three major anatomic patterns[103]:

1. *Cylindrical bronchiectasis:* Airway wall is regularly and uniformly dilated
2. *Varicose bronchiectasis:* Irregular pattern, with alternating areas of constriction and dilation
3. *Cystic bronchiectasis:* Progressive, distal enlargement of the airways, resulting in saclike dilations

Bronchiectasis is thought to result from damage to the bronchial wall by chronic inflammation. Predisposing conditions are listed in Box 25-4.

Box 25-4 Causes of Bronchiectasis

LOCAL BRONCHIECTASIS

- Foreign body
- Benign airway tumor (e.g., adenoma)
- Bronchial compression by surrounding lymph nodes (e.g., middle lobe syndrome)

DIFFUSE BRONCHIECTASIS

- Cystic fibrosis
- Ciliary dyskinesia disorders (e.g., Kartagener syndrome, Young syndrome)
- Hypogammaglobulinemia
- Alpha-1 antitrypsin deficiency
- Allergic bronchopulmonary aspergillosis
- Rheumatoid arthritis
- Serious childhood lung infection (e.g., from whooping cough, measles, or influenza)

Evaluation

The hallmark of bronchiectasis is the chronic production of large quantities of purulent sputum. Dyspnea is variable and depends on the extent of involvement and the underlying disease. Hemoptysis occurs frequently and is usually mild, but severe hemoptysis can be seen. Radiographic studies confirm the diagnosis by showing airway dilation. A chest radiograph may show cystic spaces and tram tracks (thin parallel lines representing the airway walls). CT is the diagnostic standard; the diagnosis of bronchiectasis is established when the diameter of the bronchus exceeds the diameter of the adjacent pulmonary artery branch.[104] Because reversible airway changes consistent with bronchiectasis can follow pneumonia, CT should be deferred for 6 to 8 weeks after pneumonia resolves. Only then can a diagnosis of bronchiectasis be made.

Management

Antibiotics and bronchopulmonary hygiene are the mainstays of bronchiectasis management. Antibiotics can be given as needed or following a regularly scheduled regimen. Sputum cultures may be helpful in guiding antibiotic choice. Inhaled aminoglycosides may be a useful option for patients with chronic colonization by *P. aeruginosa*. Additionally, inhaled fluoroquinolones (ciprofloxacin) are currently being evaluated in patients with cystic fibrosis and noncystic fibrosis bronchiectasis.[105] Infection by *P. aeruginosa* in patients with bronchiectasis is a marker of severity but is not linked to accelerated decline in pulmonary function.[106] Secretions can be cleared by chest physiotherapy with postural drainage, cough maneuvers, and humidification. Inhaled bronchodilators may be helpful in some patients because accompanying airflow obstruction is common.[103] Inhaled hyperosmolar substances may be helpful in clearing secretion in patients with bronchiectasis. A Cochrane review concluded that dry powder mannitol improves tracheobronchial clearance in patients with bronchiectasis, patients with cystic fibrosis, those with asthma, and normal individuals.[107] Hypertonic saline has been studied to a limited extent in bronchiectasis and may be helpful. In cases that are complicated by massive hemoptysis, embolization of the bleeding bronchial artery may be helpful. Surgical resection should be reserved for patients with localized disease who develop massive hemoptysis or who are severely symptomatic despite appropriate medical therapy.[108-110]

ROLE OF THE RESPIRATORY THERAPIST IN OBSTRUCTIVE LUNG DISEASE

RTs play key roles in all aspects of managing patients with obstructive lung diseases; they are involved in diagnosis, acute treatment, and follow-up and monitoring. In diagnosing obstructive lung diseases, RTs often perform the lung function testing that indicates the presence of airflow obstruction that is essential for diagnosis. Because of their close involvement with patients, RTs also play important roles in recognizing clinical features that may prompt physicians' appreciation of COPD variants, such as the presence of copious secretions, hemoptysis, or both that might lead to suspicion of bronchiectasis or the early onset or familial clustering of COPD that might prompt suspicion of AAT deficiency.[111] In the current environment of value-based care in which all health care providers must function at the "top of their license," RTs are increasingly at the front line of diagnosis and may be the first health care provider that patients see in evaluation for dyspnea.[112]

In acute management, hospital-based RTs often administer medications and therapies to patients with acute exacerbations of asthma or COPD. Examples include the delivery of bronchodilators in small-volume nebulizers, administration of chest physiotherapy in the management of bronchiectasis, and setup of supplemental O_2. For patients with severe exacerbations, ICU management of arterial lines, blood gases, and mechanical ventilation (with both noninvasive and conventional mechanical ventilation) usually involves RTs in key management roles. In managing patients with bronchiectasis, RTs are pivotal in administering chest physiotherapy and instructing in the use of flutter valves and percussive vests that may be critical parts of acute management.

Finally, in longitudinal follow-up of patients with obstructive lung diseases, RTs are involved in counseling (e.g., smoking cessation, medication management), administering pulmonary rehabilitation programs, and certifying and recertifying long-term O_2 therapy. RTs working in home care may conduct home visits to patients and set up and adjust equipment in the home. This description of activities of the RT in care of the patient with obstructive lung disease suggests that RTs are indispensable caregivers for patients with asthma, COPD, and bronchiectasis and that the care of patients with obstructive lung diseases constitutes a major component of RTs' activities.

SUMMARY CHECKLIST

- The spectrum of obstructive lung diseases includes chronic obstructive lung disease (consisting of emphysema and chronic bronchitis), asthma, and bronchiectasis. Airflow obstruction may be a feature of other lung diseases as well, such as sarcoidosis, lymphangioleiomyomatosis, and congestive heart failure.
- Chronic obstructive lung disease features persistent airflow obstruction despite therapy.
- Classically, asthma causes airway obstruction that is fully reversible with therapy and features symptoms such as episodic wheezing, shortness of breath, chest tightness, and cough.
- Bronchiectasis features permanent dilation of bronchi or bronchioles on chest imaging (often chest CT) and may result from various causes (e.g., childhood lung infection, cystic fibrosis, hypogammaglobulinemia, etc.).
- Major risk factors for COPD include cigarette smoking, chronic exposure to noxious fumes (e.g., cooking with biomass fuels in enclosed spaces), and genetic factors, the best characterized of which is AAT deficiency.
- The most common symptom of patients with COPD is dyspnea. Cough, chronic phlegm production, and wheezing also may be present.
- Goals in treating COPD are to improve airflow, maximize the patient's functional status, avoid exacerbations, and prolong the patient's survival as possible.
- Important treatments for COPD include inhaled bronchodilators, inhaled corticosteroids, supplemental O_2 when indicated, pulmonary rehabilitation, and preventive vaccinations (e.g., against influenza and pneumococcus). Lung transplantation and lung volume reduction surgery are also available for specific subsets of patients with advanced disease.
- The goal of stable asthma management is to maintain a high quality of life for the patient, uninterrupted by asthma symptoms, side effects from medications, or limitations on the job or during exercise. This goal can be accomplished by objective measurements and monitoring lung function, pharmacologic therapy, environmental control, and patient education.
- The goals of emergency management of acute asthma are to decrease mortality and morbidity and to return the patient to preadmission stability and function as quickly as possible. These goals are accomplished by O_2 supplementation and frequent administration of high doses of aerosolized beta-2 agonists, high-dose parenteral corticosteroids, and antibiotics if there is evidence of infection.
- The hallmark of bronchiectasis is the chronic production of large quantities of purulent sputum. Dyspnea is variable and depends on the extent of involvement and the underlying disease. Antibiotics and bronchopulmonary hygiene are important treatments.

References

1. American Thoracic Society: COPD guidelines. <http://www.thoracic.org/COPD>, (Accessed September 30, 2014.)
2. The Global Initiative for Chronic Obstructive Lung Disease (GOLD): <http://www.goldcopd.com>, (Accessed May 16, 2014.)
3. World Health Organization: Burden of COPD. <http://www.who.int>, (Accessed May 16, 2014.)
4. American Lung Association: Trends in COPD morbidity and mortality. <http://www.lung.org>, (Accessed May 16, 2014.)
5. Centers for Disease Control and Prevention: Chronic obstructive pulmonary disease among adults: United States, 2011. *MMWR Morb Mortal Wkly Rep* 61:938–943, 2012.
6. Mannino DM, Homa DM, Akinbami LJ, et al: Chronic obstructive pulmonary disease surveillance: United States, 1971–2000. *MMWR Morb Mortal Wkly Rep* 51:1–16, 2002.
7. Hardie JA, Vollmer WM, Buist AS, et al: Respiratory symptoms and obstructive pulmonary disease in a population aged over 70 years. *Respir Med* 99:186–195, 2005.
8. Stoller JK, Aboussouan LS: Alpha-1 antitrypsin deficiency. *Lancet* 365: 2225–2236, 2005.
9. Anthonisen SR, Connett JE, Kiley JP, et al: Effects of smoking intervention and the use of an anticholinergic bronchodilator on the rate of decline of FEV_1: the Lung Health Study. *JAMA* 272:1497–1504, 1994.

10. Anthonisen NR, Skeans MA, Wise RA, et al: Lung Health Study Research Group: the effects of a smoking cessation intervention on 14.5-year mortality: a randomized clinical trial. *Ann Intern Med* 142:233–239, 2005.
11. U.S. Department of Health and Human Services: *The health consequences of smoking: chronic obstructive lung disease: a report of the Surgeon General*, No. (PHS) 84-50205, Rockville, MD, 1984, U.S. Department of Health and Human Services, Public Health Service, Office on Smoking and Health.
12. Stoller JK, Smith P, Yang P, et al: Physical and social impact of alpha-1 antitrypsin deficiency: results of a survey. *Cleve Clin J Med* 61:461–467, 1994.
13. Stoller JK, Sandhaus RA, Turino G, et al: Delay in diagnosis of alpha-1 antitrypsin deficiency: a continuing problem. *Chest* 128:1989–1994, 2005.
14. American Thoracic Society/European Respiratory Society: Standards for the diagnosis and management of patients with alpha-1 antitrypsin deficiency. *Am J Respir Crit Care Med* 168:816–900, 2003.
15. Gruelich T, Ottaviani S, Bals RC, et al: Alpha-1 antitrypsin deficiency: diagnostic testing and disease awareness in Germany and Italy. *Respir Med* 107:1400–1408, 2013.
16. Gadek JE, Fells GA, Zimmerman RL, et al: Antielastases of the human alveolar structures: implications for the protease-antiprotease therapy of emphysema. *J Clin Invest* 68:889–898, 1981.
17. Stockley RA, Mannino D, Barnes PJ: Burden and pathogenesis of chronic obstructive pulmonary disease. *Proc Am Thorac Soc* 6:524–526, 2009.
18. Eisner MD, Anthonisen N, Coultas D, et al: Committee on Nonsmoking COPD, Environmental and Occupational Health Assembly. An official American Thoracic Society public policy statement: novel risk factors and the global burden of chronic obstructive pulmonary disease. *Am J Respir Crit Care Med* 182:693–718, 2010.
19. Stoller JK, Aboussouan LS: Other causes of emphysema. In Albert RK, Spiro S, Jett J, editors: *Principles of respiratory medicine*, St. Louis, 1999, Mosby-Year Book.
20. Anthonisen NR, Wright EC, IPPB Trial Group: Response to inhaled bronchodilators in COPD. *Chest* 91:36S–39S, 1987.
21. Stoller JK: Clinical practice: acute exacerbations of chronic obstructive pulmonary disease. *N Engl J Med* 346:988–994, 2002.
22. Sutherland ER, Cherniack RM: Management of chronic obstructive pulmonary disease. *N Engl J Med* 350:2689–2697, 2004.
23. Stenton C: The MRC breathlessness scale. *Occup Med (Lond)* 58:226–227, 2008.
24. Jones PW, Harding G, Berry P, et al: Development and first validation of the COPD Assessment Test. *Eur Respir J* 34:648–654, 2009.
25. Barr RG, Bourbeau J, Camargo CA, et al: Inhaled tiotropium for stable chronic obstructive pulmonary disease. *Cochrane Database Syst Rev* (2):CD002876, 2005.
26. Niewoehner DE, Rice K, Cote C, et al: Prevention of exacerbations of chronic obstructive pulmonary disease with tiotropium, a once-daily inhaled anticholinergic bronchodilator: a randomized trial. *Ann Intern Med* 143:317–326, 2005.
27. Celli B, Decramer M, Kesten S, et al: Mortality in the 4-year trial of tiotropium (UPLIFT) in patients with chronic obstructive pulmonary disease. *Am J Respir Crit Care Med* 180:948–955, 2009.
28. Singh S, Loke YK, Furberg CD: Inhaled anticholinergics and risk of major adverse cardiovascular events in patients with chronic obstructive pulmonary disease: a systematic review and meta-analysis. *JAMA* 300:1439–1450, 2008.
29. Callahan D, Dittus R, Katz B: Oral corticosteroid therapy for patients with stable chronic obstructive pulmonary disease: a meta-analysis. *Ann Intern Med* 114:216–223, 1991.
30. Sin DD, McAlister FA, Man SF, et al: Contemporary management of chronic obstructive pulmonary disease: scientific review. *JAMA* 290:2301–2312, 2003.
31. McEvoy CE, Niewohener DE: Adverse effects of corticosteroid therapy for COPD: a critical review. *Chest* 111:732–743, 1997.
32. Calverley PM, Anderson JA, Celli B, et al: TORCH investigators: salmeterol and fluticasone propionate and survival in chronic obstructive pulmonary disease. *N Engl J Med* 356:775–789, 2007.
33. Kardos P, Wencker M, Glaab T, et al: Impact of salmeterol/fluticasone propionate versus salmeterol on exacerbations in severe chronic obstructive pulmonary disease. *Am J Respir Crit Care Med* 175:144–149, 2007.
34. Celli BR, MacNee W: Standards for the diagnosis and treatment of patients with COPD: a summary of the ATS/ERS position paper. *Eur Respir J* 23:932–946, 2004.
35. Mahler D, Matthay RA, Snyder PE, et al: Sustained-release theophylline reduces dyspnea in nonreversible obstructive airway disease. *Am Rev Respir Dis* 131:22–25, 1985.
36. Nair S, Thomas E, Pearson SB, et al: A randomized controlled trial to assess the optimal dose and effect of nebulized albuterol in acute exacerbations of COPD. *Chest* 128:48–54, 2005.
37. Albert R, Martin T, Lewis S: Controlled clinical trial of methylprednisolone in patients with chronic bronchitis and acute respiratory insufficiency. *Ann Intern Med* 92:753–758, 1980.
38. Niewoehner DE, Erbland ML, Deupree RH, et al: Effect of systemic glucocorticoids on exacerbations of chronic obstructive pulmonary disease. *N Engl J Med* 340:1941–1947, 1999.
39. Saint S, Bent S, Vittinghoff E, et al: Antibiotics in chronic obstructive pulmonary disease exacerbations: a meta-analysis. *JAMA* 273:957–960, 1995.
40. Anthonisen NR, Manfreda J, Warren CPW, et al: Antibiotic therapy in exacerbations of chronic obstructive pulmonary disease. *Ann Intern Med* 106:196–204, 1987.
41. Rice KL, Leatherman JW, Duane PG, et al: Aminophylline for acute exacerbations of chronic obstructive pulmonary disease: a controlled trial. *Ann Intern Med* 107:305–309, 1987.
42. Duffy N, Walker P, Diamantea F, et al: Intravenous aminophylline in patients admitted to hospital with non-acidotic exacerbations of chronic obstructive pulmonary disease: a prospective randomized controlled trial. *Thorax* 60:713–717, 2005.
43. Keenan SP, Sinuff T, Cook DJ, et al: Which patients with acute exacerbation of chronic obstructive pulmonary disease benefit from noninvasive positive-pressure ventilation? A systematic review of the literature. *Ann Intern Med* 138:861–870, 2003.
44. Bach JR, Brougher P, Hess DR, et al: Consensus statement: non-invasive positive pressure ventilation. *Respir Care* 42:365–369, 1997.
45. International Consensus Conferences in Intensive Care Medicine: Noninvasive positive pressure ventilation in acute respiratory failure. *Am J Respir Crit Care Med* 163:283–291, 2001.
46. Troosters T, Janssens W, Decramer M: Pulmonary rehabilitation. In Barnes PJ, Drazen JM, Rennard SI, et al, editors: *Asthma and COPD: basic mechanisms and clinical management*, ed 2, Waltham, MA, 2009, Academic Press.
47. Ries AL, Kaplan RM, Limberg TM, et al: Effects of pulmonary rehabilitation on physiological and psychosocial outcomes in patients with chronic obstructive pulmonary disease. *Ann Intern Med* 122:823–832, 1995.
48. Celli BR: Is pulmonary rehabilitation an effective treatment for chronic obstructive pulmonary disease? *Am J Respir Crit Care Med* 155:781–783, 1997.
49. Sillen MJ, Speksnijder CM, Eterman RM, et al: Effects of neuromuscular electrical stimulation of muscles of ambulation in patients with chronic heart failure or COPD: a systematic review of the English-language literature. *Chest* 136:44–61, 2009.
50. Shi Y, Warner DO: Surgery as a teachable moment for smoking cessation. *Anesthesiology* 112:102–107, 2010.
51. Kottke TE, Battista RN, DeFriese GH, et al: Attributes of successful cessation interventions in medical practice: a meta-analysis of 39 controlled trials. *JAMA* 259:2882–2889, 1988.
52. Marlow S, Stoller JK: Smoking cessation. *Respir Care* 48:1238–1256, 2003.
53. Nocturnal Oxygen Therapy Trial Group: Continuous or nocturnal oxygen therapy in hypoxemic chronic obstructive lung disease: a clinical trial. *Ann Intern Med* 93:391–398, 1980.
54. British Medical Research Council Working Party: Long-term domiciliary oxygen therapy in chronic hypoxic cor pulmonale complicating chronic bronchitis and emphysema. *Lancet* 1:681–685, 1981.
55. Flenley DC: Long-term oxygen therapy. *Chest* 87:99–103, 1985.

56. Stoller JK, Panos R, Krachman S, et al: Oxygen therapy for patients with COPD: evidence for current therapy and the Long-term Oxygen Treatment Trial (LOTT). *Chest* 138:179–187, 2010.
57. Guyatt GH, Nomoyama M, Lachetti C, et al: A randomized trial of strategies for assessing the eligibility for long-term domiciliary oxygen therapy. *Am J Respir Crit Care Med* 172:573–580, 2005.
58. Chaney JC, Jones K, Grathwohl K, et al: Implementation of an oxygen therapy clinic to manage users of long-term oxygen therapy. *Chest* 122: 1661–1667, 2002.
59. Gardner P, Schaffner W: Immunization of adults. *N Engl J Med* 328:1252–1258, 1993.
60. Albert RK, Connett J, Bailey WC, et al: Azithromycin for prevention of exacerbations of COPD. *N Engl J Med* 365:689–698, 2011.
61. Calverley PM, Rabe KF, Goehring UM, et al: Roflumilast in symptomatic chronic obstructive pulmonary disease: two randomised clinical trials. *Lancet* 374:685–694, 2009.
62. Zheng JP, Wen FQ, Bai CX, et al: Twice daily N-acetylcysteine 600 mg for exacerbations of chronic obstructive pulmonary disease (PANTHEON): a randomised, double-blind placebo-controlled trial. *Lancet Respir Med* 2:187–194, 2014.
63. International Society for Heart and Lung Transplantation: <http://www.ishlt.org>, (Accessed September 27, 2014.)
64. Brantigan OC, Mueller E: Surgical treatment of pulmonary emphysema. *Am Surg* 23:789, 1957.
65. National Emphysema Treatment Trial: Randomized trial comparing lung-volume-reduction surgery with medical therapy for severe emphysema. *N Engl J Med* 348:2059–2073, 2003.
66. Naunheim KS, Wood DE, Mohsenifar Z, et al: National Emphysema Treatment Trial Research Group: long term follow-up of patients receiving lung-volume-reduction surgery versus medical therapy for severe emphysema. *Ann Thorac Surg* 82:431–443, 2006.
67. National Emphysema Treatment Trial Research Group: Patients at high risk of death after lung-volume-reduction surgery. *N Engl J Med* 345:1075–1083, 2001.
68. Sciurba FC, Ernst A, Herth FJ, et al: VENT Study Research Group: A randomized study of endobronchial valves for advanced emphysema. *N Engl J Med* 363:1233–1244, 2010.
69. Berger RL, DeCamp MM, Criner GJ, et al: Lung volume reduction therapies for advanced emphysema: an update. *Chest* 138:407–417, 2010.
70. Dirksen A, Dijkman JH, Madsen F, et al: A randomized clinical trial of alpha1-antitrypsin augmentation therapy. *Am J Respir Crit Care Med* 160:1468–1472, 1999.
71. Dirksen A, Piitulainen E, Parr DG, et al: Exploring the role of CT densitometry: a randomised study of augmentation therapy in alpha1-antitrypsin deficiency. *Eur Respir J* 33:1345–1353, 2009.
72. Abboud RT, Ford GT, Chapman KR: Standards Committee of the Canadian Thoracic Society: Alpha1-antitrypsin deficiency: a position statement of the Canadian Thoracic Society. *Can Respir J* 8:81–88, 2001.
73. National Asthma Education and Prevention Program: *Expert Panel Report III: guidelines for the diagnosis and management of asthma*, NIH Publication No. 07-4051, Bethesda, MD, 2007, National Institutes of Health, National Heart, Lung, and Blood Institute.
74. National Heart, Lung, and Blood Institute: *International consensus report on diagnosis and treatment of asthma*, No. 92-3091, Bethesda, MD, 1992, U.S. Department of Health and Human Services, National Institutes of Health.
75. Asthma Management and Prevention/Global Initiative for Asthma: *A practical guide for public health officials and healthcare professionals*, No. 96-3659A, Bethesda, MD, 1995, U.S. Department of Health and Human Services, National Institutes of Health.
76. Blackwell DL, Lucas JW, Clarke TC: Summary health statistics for U.S. adults: national health interview survey, 2012. *Vital Health Stat* 10:1–161, 2014.
77. Akinbami LJ, Moorman JE, Bailey C, et al: Trends in asthma prevalence, health care use and mortality in the United States 2001-2010. U.S. Department of Health and Human Services. *NCHS Data Brief* 94:2012.
78. McFadden ER, Jr, Gilbert IA: Asthma. *N Engl J Med* 327:1928–1937, 1992.
79. Barnes PJ: A new approach to the treatment of asthma. *N Engl J Med* 321:1517–1527, 1989.
80. Wiedemann HP, Kavuru MS: *Diagnosis and management of asthma*, Caddo, OK, 1994, Professional Communications.
81. Woolcock AJ: Asthma. In Murray JF, Nadel JA, editors: *Textbook of respiratory medicine*, Philadelphia, 2005, Saunders.
82. Fanta CH: Asthma. *N Engl J Med* 360:1002–1014, 2009.
83. Dweik RA, Boggs PB, Erzurum SC, et al: An official ATS clinical practice guideline: interpretation of exhaled nitric oxide levels (FENO) for clinical applications. *Am J Respir Crit Care Med* 184:602–615, 2011.
84. Barnes PJ: Inhaled corticosteroids for asthma. *N Engl J Med* 332:868–875, 1995.
85. Zafirlukast for asthma. *Med Lett Drugs Ther* 38:111–112, 1996.
86. Kavuru MS, Pien L, Litwin D, et al: Asthma: current controversies and emerging therapies. *Cleve Clin J Med* 62:293–304, 1995.
87. Salpeter SR, Buckley NS, Ormiston TM, et al: Meta-analysis: effect of long-acting β-agonists on severe asthma exacerbations and asthma-related deaths. *Ann Intern Med* 144:904–912, 2006.
88. U.S. Food and Drug Administration, Center for Drug Evaluation and Research: Advair Diskus, Advair HFA, Brovana, Foradil, Serevent Diskus, and Symbicort information (long acting beta agonists. <http://www.fda.gov/cder/drug/infopage/LABA/default.htm>, (Accessed December 28, 2010.)
89. Peters SP, Kunselman SJ, Icitovic N, et al: Tiotropium bromide step-up therapy for adults with uncontrolled asthma. *N Engl J Med* 363:1715–1726, 2010.
90. Burrows B, Martinez FD, Halonen M, et al: Association of asthma with serum IgE levels and skin-test reactivity to allergens. *N Engl J Med* 320: 271–277, 1989.
91. Omalizumab (Xolair): an anti-IgE antibody for asthma. *Med Lett Drugs Ther* 45:67–68, 2003.
92. Busse W, Corren J, Lanier BQ, et al: Omalizumab, anti-IgE recombinant humanized monoclonal antibody, for the treatment of severe allergic asthma. *J Allergy Clin Immunol* 108:184–190, 2001.
93. Wahidi MM, Kraft M: Bronchial thermoplasty for severe asthma. *Am J Respir Crit Care Med* 185:709–714, 2012.
94. Cox G, Thomson NC, Rubin AS, et al: AIR Trial Study Group: asthma control during the year after bronchial thermoplasty. *N Engl J Med* 356: 1327–1337, 2007.
95. Castro M, Rubin AS, Laviolette M, et al: AIR2 Trial Study Group: effectiveness and safety of bronchial thermoplasty in the treatment of severe asthma: a multicenter, randomized, double-blind, sham-controlled clinical trial. *Am J Respir Crit Care Med* 181:116–124, 2010.
96. Wechsler ME, Laviolette M, Rubin AS, et al: Bronchial thermoplasty: long-term safety and effectiveness in patients with severe persistent asthma. *J Allergy Clin Immunol* 132:1295–1302, 2013.
97. Torrego A, Solà I, Munoz AM, et al: Bronchial thermoplasty for moderate or severe persistent asthma in adults. *Cochrane Database Syst Rev* (3): CD009919, 2014.
98. Abrahamson MJ, Puy RM, Weiner JM: Injection allergen immunotherapy for asthma. *Cochrane Database Syst Rev* 8:6–114, 2010.
99. Bonini M, Di Mambro C, Calderon MA, et al: Beta$_2$-agonists for exercise-induced asthma. *Cochrane Database Syst Rev* (10):CD003564, 2013.
100. Spooner CH, Saunders LD, Rowe BH: Nedocromil sodium for preventing exercise-induced bronchoconstriction. *Cochrane Database Syst Rev* (1): CD001183, 2002.
101. Kiljander TO, Junghard O, Beckman O, et al: Effect of esomeprazole 40 mg once or twice daily on asthma: a randomized, placebo-controlled study. *Am J Respir Crit Care Med* 181:1042–1048, 2010.
102. National Asthma Education Program Report of the Working Group on Asthma and Pregnancy: *Management of asthma during pregnancy*, No. 93-3279A, Bethesda, MD, 1993, U.S. Department of Health and Human Services, National Institutes of Health.
103. Barker AF: Bronchiectasis. *N Engl J Med* 346:1383–1393, 2002.
104. Stanford W, Galvin JR: The diagnosis of bronchiectasis. *Clin Chest Med* 9:691–699, 1988.

105. Stass H, Weimann B, Nagelschmitz J, et al: Tolerability and pharmacokinetic properties of ciprofloxacin dry powder for inhalation in patients with cystic fibrosis: a phase I, randomized, dose-escalation study. *Clin Ther* 35:1571–1581, 2013.
106. Davies G, Wells AU, Doffman S, et al: The effect of *Pseudomonas aeruginosa* on pulmonary function in patients with bronchiectasis. *Eur Respir J* 28:974–979, 2006.
107. Wills P, Greenstone M: Inhaled hyperosmolar agents for bronchiectasis. *Cochrane Database Syst Rev* (2):CD002996, 2006.
108. Dweik RA, Stoller JK: Role of bronchoscopy in massive hemoptysis. *Clin Chest Med* 20:89–105, 1999.
109. Fujimoto T, Hillejan L, Stamatis G: Current strategy for surgical management of bronchiectasis. *Ann Thorac Surg* 72:1711–1715, 2001.
110. Mal H, Rullon I, Mellot F, et al: Immediate and long-term results of bronchial artery embolization for life-threatening hemoptysis. *Chest* 115:996–1001, 1999.
111. Rahaghi FF, Sandhaus RA, Strange C, et al: The prevalence of alpha-1 antitrypsin deficiency among patients found to have airflow obstruction. *COPD* 9:352–358, 2012.
112. Porter ME: What is value in health care? *N Engl J Med* 363:2477–2481, 2010.

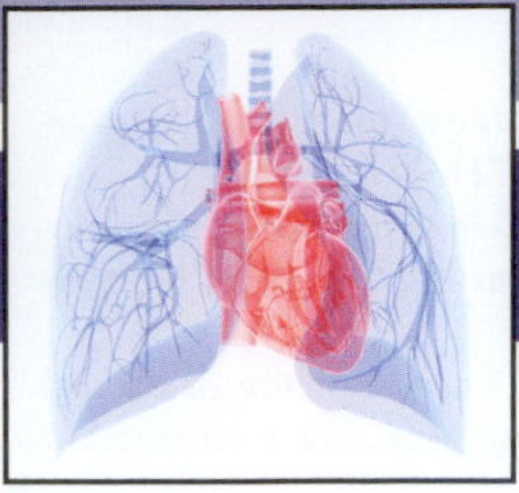

CHAPTER 26

Interstitial Lung Disease

JEFFREY T. CHAPMAN AND JASON BORDELON

CHAPTER OBJECTIVES

After reading this chapter you will be able to:

- Organize and distinguish among the interstitial lung diseases (ILDs).
- Interpret symptoms, examination signs, and pulmonary function test results in ILD.
- List causes, exposures, or pathologic characteristics associated with selected ILDs.
- Describe how to manage ILD in general and how some specific ILDs can be treated.

CHAPTER OUTLINE

KEY TERMS

asbestosis
connective tissue disease
corticosteroids
hypersensitivity pneumonitis
idiopathic pulmonary fibrosis
interstitial lung disease
lymphangioleiomyomatosis
occupational interstitial lung disease
organizing pneumonia
pulmonary Langerhans cell histiocytosis
sarcoidosis
silicosis

Interstitial lung disease (ILD) refers to a broad category of lung diseases rather than a specific disease process.[1,2] This category includes various illnesses affecting the lung parenchyma with many different causes, treatments, and prognoses. These disease processes are grouped together because of similarities in their clinical presentations, appearance on plain chest radiography, and physiologic features.

With over 100 separate disorders, it is essential to group ILDs based on cause, disease associations, or pathologic processes. An organizational scheme is presented in Figure 26-1. In evaluating patients with an ILD, diseases with known causes or associations, such as diseases related to specific exposures, diseases associated with systemic conditions, and diseases with a known genetic basis must be considered first. Most patients are classified with an ILD of unknown cause, the so-called *idiopathic interstitial diseases*. Their disorder is classified by pathologic pattern. These groups are divided into specific disease entities. Using this organizational scheme to guide a careful and complete history, one is able to understand the disease processes and work efficiently toward an accurate diagnosis and treatment.

As the name ILD implies, the histologic abnormalities that characterize ILD involve the pulmonary interstitium to a greater extent than the alveolar spaces or airways, although exceptions exist. Figure 26-2 illustrates the components of the normal pulmonary parenchyma. The interstitium is the area between the capillaries and the alveolar space. As Figure 26-2 shows, in the

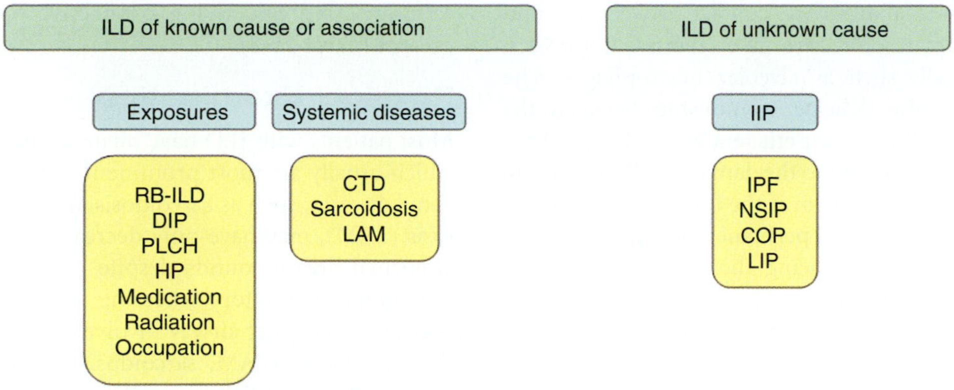

FIGURE 26-1 Current organization of interstitial lung disease (ILD). *COP,* Cryptogenic organizing pneumonia; *CTD,* connective tissue disease; *IBD,* inflammatory bowel disease; *IPF,* idiopathic pulmonary fibrosis; *LAM,* lymphangioleiomyomatosis; *LIP,* lymphocytic interstitial pneumonia; *NSIP,* nonspecific interstitial pneumonitis; *PAP,* pulmonary alveolar proteinosis; *PLCH,* pulmonary Langerhans cell histiocytosis.

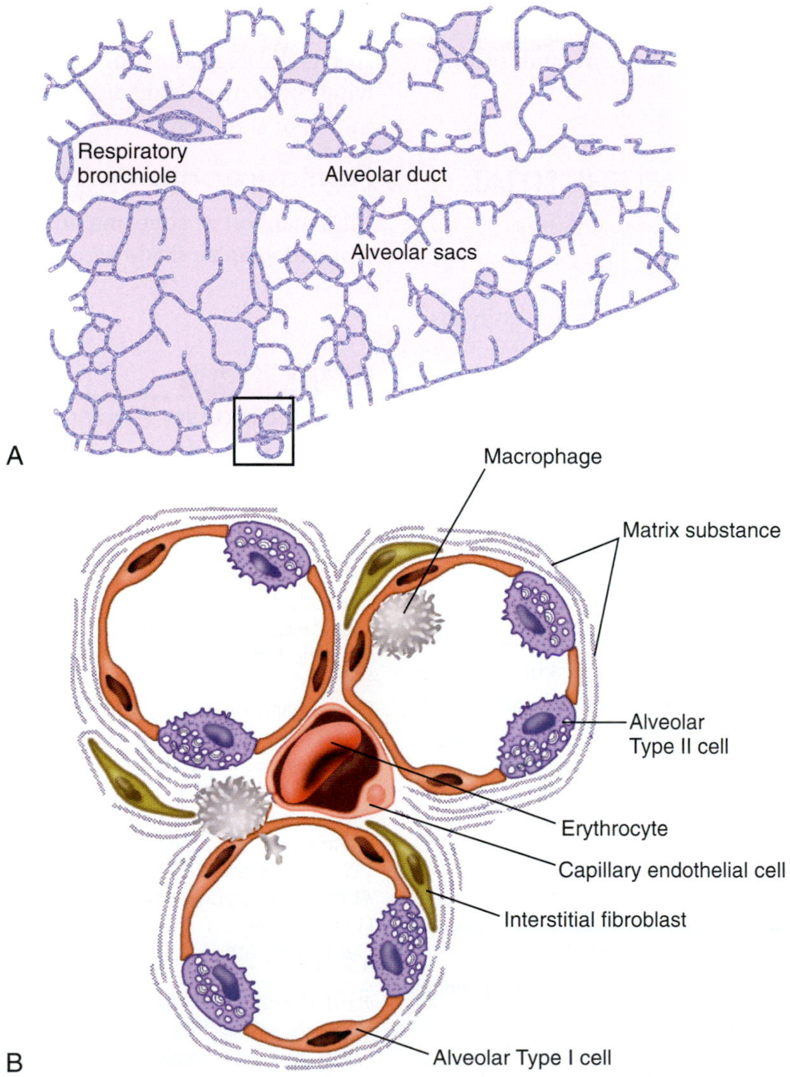

FIGURE 26-2 A, Diagram of the pulmonary parenchyma shows the respiratory bronchiole, alveolar duct, and alveolar sacs. **B,** The constituents of the interstitial space, including type I and type II alveolar epithelial cells, a capillary with vascular endothelial cells and erythrocytes in transit, resident macrophages, interstitial fibroblasts, and matrix substance.

normal state, this space allows close contact between gas and capillaries with minimal connective tissue matrix, fibroblasts, and inflammatory cells such as alveolar macrophages. The interstitium supports the delicate relationship between the alveoli and capillaries, allowing for efficient gas exchange. After an injury, the lung must respond to the damage and repair itself. If the exposure or injury persists or if the injury repair process is imperfect, the lung may be permanently damaged with increased interstitial tissue replacing the normal capillaries, alveoli, and healthy interstitium.

These pathologic abnormalities can lead to profound impairment in lung physiology and function. Gas exchange is impaired secondary to $\dot{V}/\dot{Q}$ mismatching, shunt, and decreased diffusion across the abnormal interstitium. The work of breathing in patients with interstitial lung disease (ILD) can be markedly increased because of decreased lung compliance. Together, these physiologic impairments lead to the exercise intolerance seen in all ILDs. If the injury that causes the ILD or the abnormal repair from injury is not halted, progressive tissue damage can occur, leading to worsening physiologic impairment and possibly death.

CHARACTERISTICS OF INTERSTITIAL LUNG DISEASE

Clinical Signs and Symptoms

Many ILDs have similar clinical features and are not easily distinguished based on history or examination. Symptoms are generally limited to the respiratory tract. However, extrapulmonary symptoms should not be ignored because they may point to an ILD associated with a systemic diagnosis. Exertional breathlessness (dyspnea) and a nonproductive cough are the most common reasons that patients with ILD seek medical attention. Other respiratory symptoms, such as sputum production, hemoptysis, pneumothorax, or wheezing, can occur and may suggest specific diseases (Table 26-1). If the patient also has prominent extrapulmonary symptoms, such as myalgia, arthralgia, sclerodactyly (tightening of the skin over the fingers), gastroesophageal reflux, or Raynaud phenomenon (discoloration of the digits, often initially with a white color because of spasm of the arteries that supply the digits), ILD resulting from underlying **connective tissue disease** may be present (Table 26-2).

Physical Examination

Most patients with ILD have bilateral fine inspiratory crackles, which usually are most prominent at the lung bases. However, some diseases, such as sarcoidosis and lymphangioleiomyomatosis (LAM), may have only decreased breath sounds without abnormal breath sounds despite a markedly abnormal chest radiograph. Expiratory wheezing is uncommon, and its presence suggests either airway involvement as part of the primary disease process (LAM, sarcoidosis, respiratory bronchiolitis–associated interstitial lung disease [RB-ILD], desquamative interstitial pneumonitis [DIP], pulmonary Langerhans cell histiocytosis [PLCH]) or concomitant airways disease, such as emphysema or asthma. Signs of pulmonary arterial hypertension with right ventricular dysfunction, such as lower extremity edema or jugular venous distention, may occur late in the course of any ILD and are not helpful in the diagnosis of a specific ILD. Examination also may show features of an underlying connective tissue disease, including synovitis, joint deformities, or skin rash.

Radiographic Features

ILDs manifest as abnormal lung parenchyma that casts abnormal radiographic shadows. For most ILDs, the chest radiograph

TABLE 26-1
Unusual Pulmonary Findings and Likely Diagnosis

Pulmonary Findings	Disease	Frequency
Hemoptysis	LAM	Rare
Chyloptysis (coughing up chyle)	LAM	Rare
Pneumothorax	LAM, BHD	Common
Wheeze	Sarcoidosis, LAM	Common
Chylous pleural effusion	LAM	Common
Exudative pleural effusion	RA	Common

BHD, Birt-Hogg-Dubé syndrome; *RA,* rheumatoid arthritis.

TABLE 26-2
Extrapulmonary Findings and Likely Diagnosis

Extrapulmonary Findings	Disease	Frequency
Raynaud phenomenon	All CTD	Common
Arthralgia	All CTD	Common
Myalgia	Polymyositis	Common
Large muscle weakness	Polymyositis	Common
Sclerodactyly	Scleroderma	Common
Rheumatoid skin nodules	RA	Rare
Fingertip fissures	Antisynthetase syndrome	Common
Dorsal hand rash	Dermatomyositis	Common
Facial rash	Dermatomyositis	Common
Exudative pleural effusion	RA	Common
Shawl distribution skin nodules	TSC	Common
"Pencil eraser" facial skin nodules	BHD	Common
Central nervous system benign cortical tuber	TSC	Common
Abdominal angiomyolipoma	LAM	Common
Renal cancer	BHD	Common
Cardiomyopathy	Sarcoidosis, polymyositis	Rare
Cardiac conduction block	Sarcoidosis	Rare
Violaceous facial skin nodules	Sarcoidosis	Common
Subcutaneous nodules	Sarcoidosis	Common
Cranial neuropathy	Sarcoidosis	Rare
Small fiber neuropathy	Sarcoidosis	Rare

BHD, Birt-Hogg-Dubé syndrome; *CTD,* connective tissue disease; *LAM,* lymphangioleiomyomatosis; *RA,* rheumatoid arthritis; *TSC,* tuberous sclerosis complex.

reveals reduced lung volumes with bilateral reticular or reticulonodular opacities. However, the chest radiograph has limited value because the three-dimensional abnormalities are summed into a two-dimensional image with loss of spatial information. High-resolution cross-sectional imaging via computed tomography (CT) provides detailed images representing pulmonary pathology.[3] High-resolution CT images allow noninvasive evaluation of ILDs and are a key element in making a confident diagnosis and managing ILD.[4]

Plain chest radiographs and high-resolution CT images of usual interstitial pneumonitis (UIP) show the typical fibrotic injury pattern. The chest radiograph (Figure 26-3, *A*) and high-resolution CT image (see Figure 26-3, *B*) in UIP typically reveal a bilateral, patchy, peripheral (subpleural), and basilar-predominant disease with reticulonodular infiltrates, often with honeycomb, cystic change. Honeycomb change refers to a pattern of scarring that looks like a bee's honeycomb, most characteristically at the lung bases in UIP. The lung architecture is distorted in patients with moderate or severe disease burden, with reduced lung volume and traction bronchiectasis, especially at the lung bases. Reticulogranular (ground-glass) abnormalities, increased attenuation of the lung tissue without distortion of the underlying blood vessels or bronchi, are absent or minimal in idiopathic pulmonary fibrosis (IPF). Pleural disease, air trapping, micronodules, and significant lymphadenopathy are not seen, although two-thirds of patients with UIP (also known as *IPF*) can have mild mediastinal adenopathy.[5]

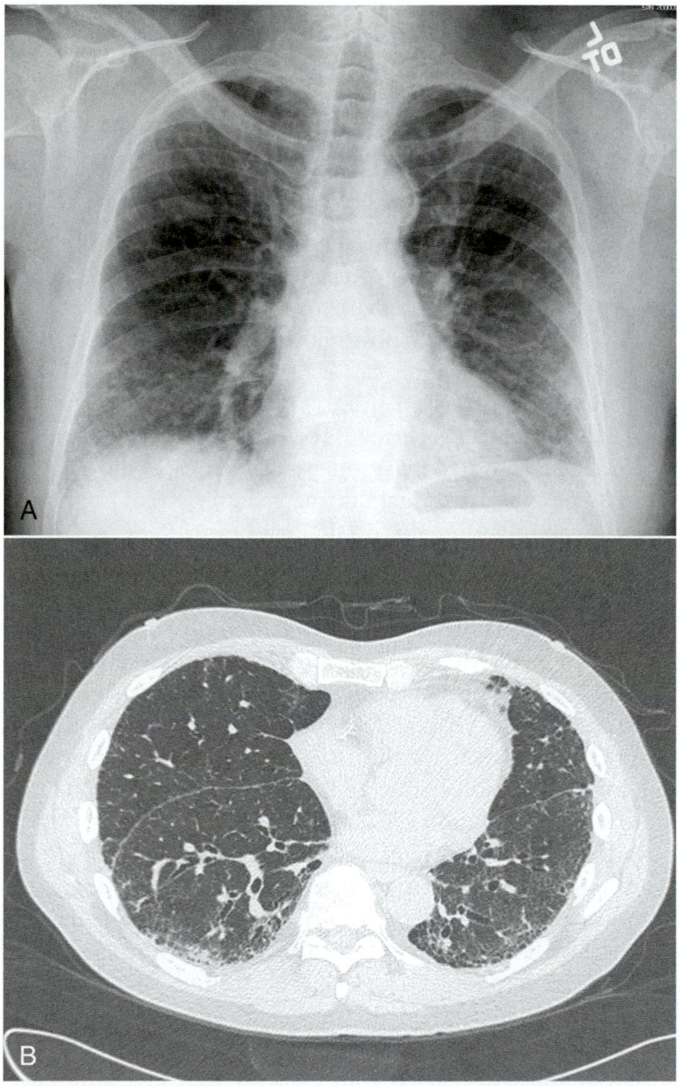

FIGURE 26-3 A, Posteroanterior chest radiograph showing the characteristic features of idiopathic pulmonary fibrosis, a common interstitial lung disease. Notice the bilateral lower zone reticulonodular infiltrates and the loss of lung volume in the lower lobes. **B,** Chest computed tomography image shows the peripheral nature of the fibrosis.

As the burden of disease increases, the chest radiograph may reveal multiple, tiny cysts in the most markedly involved regions. This cystic pattern, called *honeycombing,* reflects end-stage fibrosis and is a feature of many end-stage ILDs. These fibrotic cysts represent irreversible destruction of normal alveoli; therapies are aimed at preserving the remaining normal parenchyma and reducing symptoms.

RULE OF THUMB

In patients with spontaneous pneumothorax and interstitial infiltrates, LAM or PLCH should be considered.

In contrast to UIP, cellular nonspecific interstitial pneumonitis (NSIP) is a pattern of injury dominated by inflammation and has imaging findings distinct from those with UIP. Reticulogranular (ground-glass) attenuation predominates and is found centrally and peripherally in the middle and lower lung zones. If the inflammation can be reduced, these abnormalities may improve. A mixed pattern of injury with fibrotic nonspecific UIP also can be seen and is suggested by ground-glass attenuation in the presence of fibrotic changes. Ground-glass attenuation refers to a pattern of patchy infiltrates, with a fine texture like that of ground glass.

RULE OF THUMB

Calcification along the pleura on a chest radiograph suggests previous exposure to asbestos. Although such calcified areas (called *plaques*) do not cause symptoms or physiologic abnormality, they can provide a clue that the cause of ILD is asbestos exposure.

Physiologic Features

Similar to the radiographic findings, specific ILDs can vary considerably regarding the degree of physiologic abnormalities that occur. However, a restrictive physiologic impairment is the most common finding.[6] With this restrictive pattern, both forced expiratory volume in 1 second (FEV_1) and forced vital capacity (FVC) are diminished, and the FEV_1/FVC ratio is preserved or even above normal. Lung volumes are reduced, as is the diffusing capacity of the lung for carbon monoxide (DLCO).

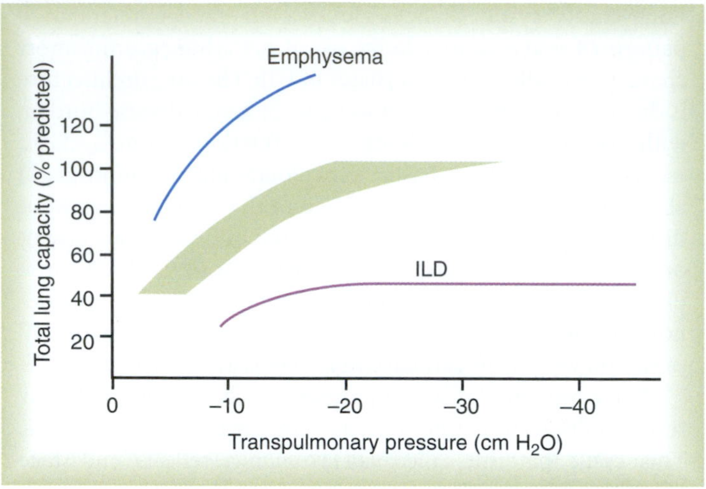

FIGURE 26-4 Static pressure-volume curve. The compliance characteristics of the lung are illustrated with a plot of lung volume against the corresponding transthoracic pressure measured during static (i.e., no flow) conditions. The *shaded area* represents the range of values expected with a normally compliant lung. The line labeled *ILD* represents an example of a patient with interstitial lung disease (ILD). At any particular lung volume, the transthoracic pressure is greater than expected. For comparison, the line labeled *Emphysema* shows the compliance characteristics of patients with emphysema.

This reduction in diffusing capacity reflects a pathologic disturbance of the alveolar-capillary interface, reflecting the abnormality in the interstitium of the lung.

Although not commonly evaluated under usual clinical circumstances, the compliance characteristics of the lungs can be evaluated with an esophageal balloon to measure intrathoracic pressure at various lung volumes. In almost all ILDs, the lungs have reduced compliance and require above normal transpleural pressures to ventilate (Figure 26-4). This lack of compliance results in small lung volumes and increased work of breathing.

Less frequently, a pattern of physiologic obstruction may be seen. This obstruction can be the result of the primary disease process (e.g., LAM, PLCH, or sarcoidosis in some patients) or concomitant emphysema or asthma.[7] If ILD develops in a patient with significant emphysema, the opposing physiologic effects of the two disease processes (i.e., restriction for the ILD and obstruction from the emphysema) may result in deceptively normal spirometry and lung volume measurements and apparently normally compliant lungs. For example, emphysema might cause lung volumes to increase whereas the restriction would be reflected by decreased lung volumes. The net effect of both processes in the same patient could be a normal lung volume. However, because both emphysema and ILD result in impaired gas exchange, DLCO is significantly decreased.

RULE OF THUMB

Among smokers with IPF, normal spirometry and lung volumes with reduced DLCO suggest the presence of coexisting emphysema.

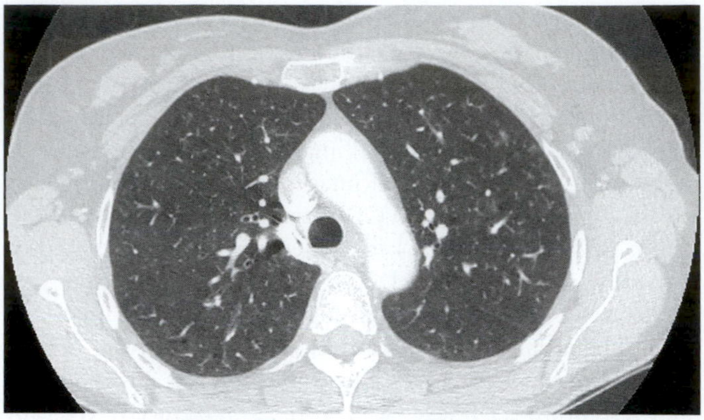

FIGURE 26-5 Respiratory bronchiolitis–associated interstitial lung disease (RB-ILD). There are numerous indistinct centrilobular nodules. Air trapping can be seen in RB-ILD but is not present in this case.

SELECTED SPECIFIC TYPES OF INTERSTITIAL LUNG DISEASE AND THERAPIES

Exposure-Related Disease

Tobacco-Associated Lung Disease

Although the association of first-hand tobacco smoke and obstructive lung disease is common and well known, tobacco smoke is also an avoidable cause of ILD. Although the association is rarer than with obstructive lung disease, first-hand tobacco smoke inhalation can lead to three types of ILD in susceptible individuals: RB-ILD, DIP, and PLCH. The first two disorders are related. Each disease consists of increased numbers of polyclonal activated macrophages. The diseases differ by the location of these overly abundant cells. In RB-ILD, macrophages accumulate in the respiratory bronchioles leading to bronchiolar remodeling and fibrosis of adjacent alveoli. As expected for a disease with combined airway and alveolar injury, pulmonary function testing reveals mixed restriction and obstruction with frequent air trapping. High-resolution CT images show this mixed pathologic location with indistinct centrilobular nodules (Figure 26-5). In DIP, the increased macrophages fill the alveoli, manifesting as restrictive impairment on pulmonary function testing and diffuse ground-glass attenuation on high-resolution CT imaging (Figure 26-6).

Pulmonary Langerhans cell histiocytosis (PLCH) is the third interstitial manifestation of tobacco smoke. Increased numbers of polyclonal macrophages play a prominent role. However, in PLCH, they are accompanied by fibroblasts and eosinophils in nodules concentrated around small airways. These nodules are star-shaped (or stellate) and destroy adjacent lung tissue, leading to the classic high-resolution CT image of stellate nodules associated with cysts, as seen in Figure 26-7. Although adult smoking-associated PLCH is pathologically similar to childhood Langerhans cell histiocytosis, the adult form does not involve bone and has not proved to respond to chemotherapy as the childhood form does. The relationship of these two disorders has yet to be defined.

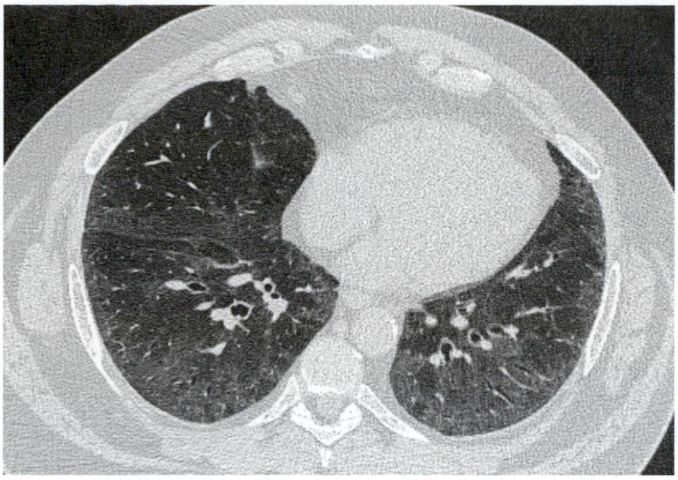

FIGURE 26-6 Desquamative interstitial pneumonitis. Note the diffuse ground-glass attenuation.

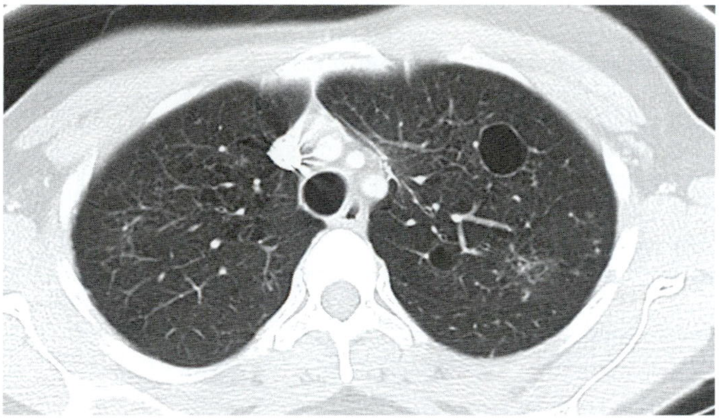

FIGURE 26-7 Pulmonary Langerhans cell histiocytosis. Note the left upper lobe cysts and indistinct stellate-shaped nodule around an airway, which will become a cyst.

In each of these three diseases, the primary treatment is stopping smoking completely. With abstinence from smoking, most patients either minimally improve or remain stable,[8] but a few progressively worsen, sometimes to the point of needing lung transplantation. Active treatment with prednisone or other immunosuppressive medications is discouraged because few, if any, patients improve and the medications have significant side effects.[9]

Drug-Related and Radiation-Related Disease

Many drugs have been associated with pulmonary complications of various types, including interstitial inflammation and fibrosis, bronchospasm, pulmonary edema, and pleural effusions. Drugs from many different therapeutic classes can cause ILD, most commonly chemotherapeutic agents, antibiotics, antiarrhythmic drugs, and immunosuppressive agents (Box 26-1). There are no distinct physiologic, radiographic, or pathologic patterns of drug-induced ILD, and the diagnosis is usually made when a patient is exposed to a medication known to result in lung disease, the timing of the exposure is appropriate for the development of the disease, and other causes of ILD have been excluded. Treatment is avoidance of further exposure and systemic corticosteroids in markedly impaired or declining patients. In the specific instance of ILD related to exposure to the chemotherapeutic agent bleomycin, bleomycin injury is accentuated by exposure to increased fractional inspired oxygen (FiO_2), even months after last drug exposure. Thus, supplemental oxygen (O_2) should be used only if absolutely necessary patients with bleomycin-induced ILD.[10]

Box 26-1 Drugs Associated With the Development of Interstitial Lung Disease

ANTIBIOTICS
- Nitrofurantoin
- Sulfasalazine

ANTIINFLAMMATORY AGENTS
- Leflunomide
- Methotrexate
- Etanercept
- Infliximab

CARDIOVASCULAR AGENTS
- Amiodarone
- Tocainide

CHEMOTHERAPEUTIC AGENTS
- Bleomycin
- Mitomycin C
- Busulfan
- Cyclophosphamide
- Chlorambucil
- Melphalan
- Methotrexate
- Etoposide
- Vinblastine
- Imatinib

DRUGS USED IN AN ILLEGAL WAY
- Heroin
- Methadone
- Talc as an intravenous drug contaminant

Exposure to therapeutic radiation used to treat cancer may result in ILD. Patients presenting within 6 months of radiation therapy generally have ground-glass abnormalities thought to represent acute inflammation. The ground-glass abnormalities can occur in both radiation-exposed tissue and unexposed tissue. Short-term systemic corticosteroid treatment can improve lung function. In contrast, radiographic abnormalities that develop more than 6 months after therapy typically appear as densely fibrotic tissue within the radiation port. On CT scan, a straight line indicating the margin of radiation is frequently evident, as seen in Figure 26-8. These patients do not improve with corticosteroid therapy, and treatment is supportive.

Hypersensitivity Pneumonitis

Hypersensitivity pneumonitis (HP) is a cell-mediated immune reaction to inhaled antigens in susceptible persons.[11] Patients

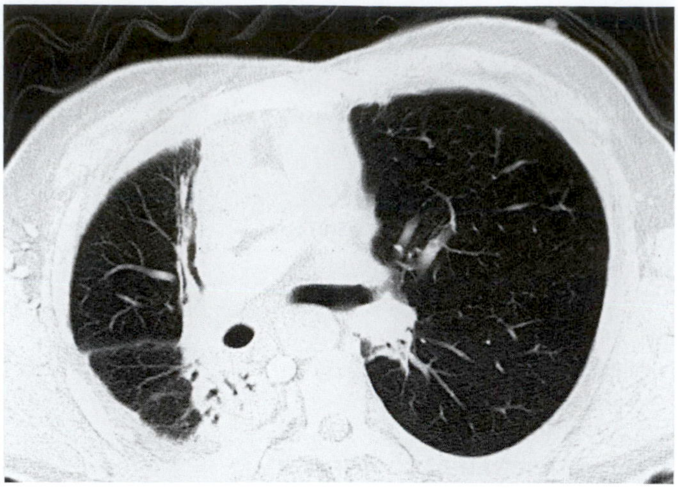

FIGURE 26-8 High-resolution computed tomography slice shows dense fibrosis with a nonanatomic straight line boundary.

must be sensitized by an initial exposure, with subsequent reexposure leading to either an acute or chronic development of HP. Patients with acute HP present to medical attention with a history of a few days of shortness of breath, chest pain, fever, chills, malaise, and a cough that may be productive of purulent sputum. Patients who are chronically exposed to low levels of inhaled antigens may develop subtle interstitial inflammatory reactions in the lung that do not result in noticeable symptoms for months to years and can present with severe, impairing disease, which can be very difficult to distinguish from IPF.

Common organic antigens known to cause HP include bacteria and fungi, which may be found in moldy hay (farmer's lung) or in the home environment, in particular, in association with central humidification systems (humidifier lung), indoor hot tubs, and animal proteins (e.g., bird breeder's lung). Inorganic antigens from vaporized paints and plastics also can lead to HP. Numerous established antigens are listed in Table 26-3 along with the typical source of exposure and the associated syndrome.

Because the causal relationship between exposure and lung disease may not be obvious, a careful systematic occupational, environmental, and avocational history is crucial in evaluating patients with ILD. Elements that strongly suggest a diagnosis of HP are exposure to an appropriate antigen and the correct timing of symptom onset to the exposure. Blood samples may be obtained to determine whether there has been an antibody response to certain antigens associated with HP (serum precipitins). However, the presence of such antibodies is insufficient to establish the diagnosis of HP because many individuals develop antibodies in the absence of disease. Likewise, the absence of detectable antibodies does not rule out the diagnosis of HP because the culprit may be an antigen that is not included in the blood test panel that is analyzed.[12]

Specific therapies for HP are strict antigen avoidance and immunosuppression with corticosteroids in patients with symptomatic or physiologically impairing disease. In acute HP,

TABLE 26-3

Causes of Hypersensitivity Pneumonitis

Antigen	Exposure	Syndrome
Bacteria		
Thermophilic Bacteria		
Saccharopolyspora rectivirgula	Moldy hay	Farmer's lung
Thermoactinomyces vulgaris	Moldy sugarcane	Bagassosis
Thermoactinomyces sacchari	Mushroom compost	Mushroom worker's lung
Thermoactinomyces candidus	Heated water reservoirs	Humidifier lung Air conditioner lung
Nonthermophilic Bacteria		
Bacillus subtilis, Bacillus cereus	Water, detergent	Humidifier lung Washing powder lung
Fungi		
Aspergillus species	Moldy hay	Farmer's lung
Aspergillus clavatus	Barley	Malt worker's lung
Penicillium casei, Penicillium roqueforti	Cheese	Cheese washer's lung
Alternaria species	Wood pulp	Woodworker's lung
Merulius lacrymans	Rotten wood	Dry rot lung
Penicillium frequentans	Cork dust	Suberosis
Aureobasidium pullulans	Water	Humidifier lung
Cladosporium species	Hot tub mists	Hot tub HP*
Trichosporon cutaneum	Damp wood and mats	Japanese summer-type HP*
Animal Proteins		
Avian proteins	Bird droppings, feathers	Bird-breeder's lung
Urine, serum, pelts	Rats, gerbils	Animal handler's lung
Chemicals		
Isocyanates, trimellitic anhydride	Paints, resins, plastics	Chemical worker's lung
Copper sulfate	Bordeaux mixture	Vineyard sprayer's lung
Phthalic anhydride	Heated epoxy resin	Epoxy resin lung

corticosteroids seem to hasten recovery but do not improve ultimate lung function.[13] In chronic HP, patients with fibrosis on CT scan have a shorter survival and the benefits of long-term immunosuppression is unknown.[14]

Occupational Disease

The three most common types of **occupational interstitial lung disease** are **asbestosis,** chronic **silicosis,** and coal workers' pneumoconiosis. Awareness of the associated risk and reduction in exposure has greatly reduced the incidence of these diseases in developed countries. However, they remain common in developing countries and among emigrants from these countries.

Predictable clinical and radiographic abnormalities occur in susceptible patients who have been exposed to asbestos.[15] These abnormalities include pleural changes (plaques, fibrosis, effusions, atelectasis, and mesothelioma) and parenchymal scarring and lung cancer. Asbestos exposure alone increases the risk for lung cancer only minimally (1.5 to 3.0 times). However, asbestos exposure and cigarette smoking act synergistically to increase greatly the risk for cancer. Asbestos exposure also may result in benign asbestos pleural effusions or an entity known as *rounded atelectasis*. Benign asbestos pleural effusions may be asymptomatic or may be associated with acute chest pain, fever, and dyspnea. Benign asbestos pleural effusions usually resolve on their own, but may recur. Treatment is drainage to reduce symptoms. Rounded atelectasis typically manifests as a pleural-based parenchymal mass that may be mistaken for carcinoma. The characteristic CT features, such as local volume loss, pleural thickening, and the "comet tail" appearance of bronchi and vessels curving into the lesion, help distinguish rounded atelectasis from carcinoma.

The term *asbestos-related pulmonary disease* encompasses all of these entities, whereas *asbestosis* is reserved for patients who have evidence of parenchymal fibrosis. Most patients with asbestosis have had considerable airborne asbestos exposure many years before the lung disease becomes apparent. Exposure frequently is associated with occupations such as shipbuilding or insulation work. Patients report very slowly progressive dyspnea on exertion[16] and have crackles on lung examination. Physiologic testing shows restrictive impairment with a reduced DLCO. The chest radiograph reveals bilateral lower zone reticulonodular infiltrates similar to infiltrates seen in IPF. With an appropriate exposure history, the presence of radiographic pleural plaques or rounded atelectasis indicates asbestos as the likely cause of ILD, although neither history nor radiographic findings is required for establishing the diagnosis. Surgical lung biopsy with asbestos body determination can establish a definitive diagnosis, but this is infrequently performed owing to the age and debility of these patients. No medical therapy has been shown to improve or decrease progression of asbestosis. Severe impairment typically occurs 30 to 40 years after exposure, making almost all patients ineligible for lung transplantation because of advanced age. Management of asbestosis is supportive.

Chronic silicosis results from chronic exposure to inhaled silica particles. Occupations that commonly involve exposure to silica include mining, tunneling, sandblasting, and foundry work. The chest radiograph commonly shows upper lung zone–predominant abnormalities characterized by multiple small nodular opacities in the central lung tissue. These nodules (simple silicosis) are asymptomatic and may never progress or cause symptoms. However, in susceptible individuals, the nodules coalesce into large midlung zone masses known as *progressive massive fibrosis*. Some patients with abnormal chest radiographs report few, if any, symptoms and may have normal lung examination and pulmonary function testing. Many patients are impaired and have mixed restrictive and obstructive impairment with reduced diffusion capacity. The physiologic impairment may remain stable or, if progressive, massive fibrosis occurs, may progress even without continued exposure. Symptoms are typically exertional dyspnea and variable mucus production.

It is important to recognize the association of silicosis with lung cancer and active tuberculosis.[17] Patients with silicosis are at increased risk for lung cancer, and the risk is increased when combined with exposure to tobacco smoke, diesel exhaust, or radon gas. Patients with silicosis develop active tuberculosis 2 to 30 times more frequently than co-workers without silicosis. This association is especially important in societies with a high incidence of human immunodeficiency virus infection, which markedly increases the risk for silicosis-associated active tuberculosis.

Coal workers' pneumoconiosis develops as the result of chronic inhalation of coal dust. In the past, it was assumed that silica dust was responsible for the pulmonary disease seen among coal miners because the clinical and radiographic features are quite similar to those of chronic silicosis. However, it is now recognized that coal workers' pneumoconiosis and silicosis are the result of different exposures. Simple coal workers' pneumoconiosis, characterized by multiple small nodular opacities on the chest radiograph, is asymptomatic. Cough and shortness of breath do not develop unless the disease progresses to progressive massive fibrosis similar to that seen in silicosis.

There are no proved therapies for either silicosis or coal workers' pneumoconiosis other than eliminating future exposure. In patients with significant obstructive impairment or mucus production, inhaled bronchodilators and **corticosteroids** may relieve some symptoms. Exacerbations can be frequent and are treated with antibiotics and systemic corticosteroids.

Associated Systemic Disease

Connective Tissue Disease

ILD is a well-known complication of various connective tissue diseases.[18] The most commonly implicated disorders are scleroderma, rheumatoid arthritis, Sjögren syndrome, polymyositis/dermatomyositis, and systemic lupus erythematosus.

In any of these disorders, pulmonary involvement may remain undetected until significant impairment is present, because these patients may be inactive owing to the underlying connective tissue disease. In addition, there is generally poor correlation between the severity of the pulmonary and nonpulmonary manifestations of these diseases. In some instances, the lung disease may overshadow or may occur earlier than the other symptoms of the underlying disease. When symptoms develop, dyspnea and cough are common. On chest examination, crackles, wheezing, or a pleural rub may be heard because of the varied patterns of lung involvement in these disorders. The physiologic features are usually restrictive with decreased DLCO but may be obstructive depending on the anatomic location of the disease, especially with Sjögren syndrome (because the collections of lymphocytes that define this disease are most frequent in the bronchioles).

High-resolution CT findings are variable and range from normal lung architecture to ground-glass abnormalities to reticular and fibrotic changes.[19] The pathologic pattern of injury with these diseases is equally diverse and correlates with the high-resolution CT findings. Inflammatory injury patterns are most commonly seen, such as NSIP and organizing pneumonia. The NSIP inflammatory injury pattern appears as ground-glass abnormalities on high-resolution CT scan, whereas organizing pneumonia is shown by patchy consolidated lung with air bronchograms. Both of these pathologic patterns can improve with aggressive immunosuppression. At the other end of the pathologic response spectrum is fibrotic injury, which manifests as UIP and shows reticular fibrotic opacities and honeycomb cystic changes on high-resolution CT scan. These abnormalities typically do not improve with immunosuppression, although long-term controlled studies are lacking.

Specific treatment of connective tissue disease–associated ILD must be individualized. Patients with evidence of extrapulmonary inflammation, an inflammatory pathologic pattern such as NSIP or organizing pneumonia on high-resolution CT or biopsy, or rapidly progressive symptoms, are usually treated with prolonged immunosuppressive agents such as cyclophosphamide, azathioprine, mycophenolate, or tacrolimus.[20,21]

More recent studies have begun to provide evidence-based therapy for these diverse patients. The Scleroderma Lung Study showed that 1 year of oral cyclophosphamide modestly improved lung function compared with modest decline in the control group.[20] However, after 1 year off immunosuppressive therapy, the patients treated with cyclophosphamide worsened and were indistinguishable from the untreated patients in the control group.[22] Many clinicians hypothesize that to preserve any lung function gained by cyclophosphamide, continued immunosuppression may be necessary, and mycophenolate is most often used.

Polymyositis-associated ILD is being increasingly recognized as a common disease entity. Patients usually present with "mechanic's hands" consisting of thickened skin and painful fingertip fissures, and 50% have Jo-1 antibodies on antinuclear antibody testing. Lung pathologic results typically show fibrotic NSIP or organizing pneumonia. As would be expected with these inflammatory patterns of injury, patients usually benefit from immunosuppression. Classic treatment is with cyclophosphamide, but tacrolimus and rituximab are emerging as salvage agents.

Sarcoidosis

Sarcoidosis is an idiopathic multisystem inflammatory disorder that commonly involves the lung.[23] It is the most common ILD in the United States. The tissue inflammation that occurs in sarcoidosis has a characteristic pattern in which the inflammatory cells collect in microscopic nodules called *granulomas*. In contrast to IPF, sarcoidosis is more common among young adults than among older adults. Sarcoidosis often follows a benign course of inflammation without symptoms or long-term consequences that spontaneously remits.

The most common manifestation of sarcoidosis is asymptomatic hilar adenopathy. Less frequently, the chest radiograph shows parenchymal opacities in the midlung zone that may be nodular, reticulonodular, or alveolar. When symptoms occur, cough, chest pain, dyspnea, and wheezing are most common. Pulmonary physiology may be normal, restrictive, obstructive, or mixed, all with reduced DLCO. Obstructive impairment may be related to endobronchial granulomatous inflammation or scarring.[24]

Corticosteroids are commonly used in the management of sarcoidosis, but treatment usually is reserved for patients with marked symptoms or physiologic impairment attributable to the disease.[25] Although corticosteroids almost always reduce active sarcoid inflammation, long-term side effects should limit the duration of steroid treatment. For patients requiring long-term immunosuppression, alternative immunosuppressive agents such as methotrexate, azathioprine, leflunomide, or tumor necrosis factor-alpha inhibitors such as infliximab should be used.[26] Involvement of other organs that may require corticosteroid therapy include cardiac involvement, uveitis, and peripheral or central nervous system involvement with cranial nerve abnormalities. Disease activity is difficult to detect in many patients. Serum angiotensin-converting enzyme levels and gallium scans are not well correlated with disease activity, and their routine use is discouraged.[27]

Lymphangioleiomyomatosis

Lymphangioleiomyomatosis (LAM) is a rare disorder of abnormal smooth muscle tissue proliferating around small airways and leading to severe obstruction and destruction of alveoli with resultant thin-walled cyst formation.[28] All patients are women, although both men and women with tuberous sclerosis complex can develop lung pathologic findings identical to those of LAM that is called *tuberous sclerosis complex LAM*. This peculiar pathologic process is caused by abnormalities in the *TSC-2* gene.[29]

Dyspnea on exertion and an obstructive ventilatory impairment with reduced DLCO is almost always present, except in very early disease. Disease progression is quite variable; some women having steadily worsening lung function during midlife, whereas some elderly women experience extremely slow decline over many years. Risk factors for worsening lung function include a significant bronchodilator response and possibly pregnancy. Other important disease manifestations include pneumothorax from a ruptured subpleural cyst. Unilateral or, less commonly, bilateral chylothorax is seen in about one-third of patients. This results from lymphatic obstruction by abnormal smooth muscle tissue. Treatment with a low-fat diet or blocking gut fat absorption is usually ineffective, and pleurodesis is required. Pleurodesis does not preclude subsequent lung transplantation.

Treatment is with inhaled bronchodilators and inhaled corticosteroids. Younger patients may ultimately require lung transplantation. Ongoing studies with rapamycin, which blocks the abnormal *TSC-2* gene and inhibits LAM cell proliferation, show promise for the first disease-specific therapy for an ILD.

Interstitial Lung Disease of Unknown Cause

Idiopathic Interstitial Pneumonias

Despite a careful history, physical examination, and high-resolution CT scan, most patients are not found to have an exposure or systemic illness as a cause of ILD. These patients have a disorder isolated to the lung termed *idiopathic interstitial pneumonia (IIP)*. Prognosis and potential therapies are completely dependent on the type of pathologic pattern of IIP.

Idiopathic Pulmonary Fibrosis. **Idiopathic pulmonary fibrosis** (IPF) is the most common IIP and is a progressive fibrotic disease isolated to the lung.[30] Although the precise cause of IPF is unknown, studies have demonstrated that susceptible individuals have lung injury from diverse causes, such as metal dust, farming dust, tobacco smoke, subclinical gastric aspiration, and mechanical stress from abnormal surfactant proteins that lead to abnormal lung healing and progressive fibrosis.[31] Most patients are older than 60 years, and IPF is extremely unusual in persons younger than 40 years. Patients present with chronic cough and exertional dyspnea, and high-resolution CT suggests a fibrotic process.

The diagnosis of IPF is made by noting a lack of exposure or systemic disease known to cause ILD and determining UIP as the pathologic pattern of injury. The diagnosis of UIP is made when high-resolution CT shows bilateral and basilar-predominant peripheral reticular fibrosis and honeycomb cystic change with absence of significant ground-glass abnormalities, micronodules, and air trapping. Without these classic findings, a surgical lung biopsy is needed for diagnosis.[32,33] Patients who do not have IPF can have UIP on surgical lung biopsy (e.g., connective tissue disease), so this pattern of injury and repair is not unique to IPF.

Most patients die as a result of progressive fibrotic lung disease within 4 years of diagnosis. Data show that approximately half of patients die with gradually progressive disease over several years.[34] The other half experience stable lung function or minimal decline for months to years and then have sudden worsening over a few weeks or months, leading to death.[35] Baseline parameters that predict an increased risk for death include severity of dyspnea, severity of restrictive physiologic defect, reduced DLCO, presence of pulmonary arterial hypertension, degree of fibrosis on high-resolution CT, and SaO_2 desaturation on exertion.[36] Serial parameters that predict poor survival include worsening dyspnea, FVC, and DLCO.

Specific treatment for IPF is emerging after decades of IPF trials showing no benefit with aggressive immunosuppression,[37-39] interferon gamma,[40] etanercept,[41] bosentan, macitentan, ambrisentan, sildenafil,[42] imatinib,[43] warfarin, *N*-acetylcysteine,[44] and azathioprine in combination with both oral corticosteroids and *N*-acetylcysteine.[45] Pirfenidone and nintedanib, both molecules with multiple antifibrotic properties, have recently been shown to slow disease progression in selected patients with IPF. Perfenidone has been approved for use in Japan, Canada, and in several European countries at this writing,[46,47] and both perfenidone and nintendanib were approved for use in the United States by the U.S. Food and Drug Administration on October 15, 2014.

Studies have demonstrated concomitant pulmonary arterial hypertension in IPF leading to worse exercise intolerance and increased mortality.[48,49] Significant pulmonary arterial hypertension is suggested in patients with markedly impaired diffusion capacity but relatively preserved FVC. Medications that benefit pulmonary arterial hypertension such as bosentan and sildenafil generally have not proved beneficial for IPF either with or without pulmonary arterial hypertension.[50,51]

Nonspecific Interstitial Pneumonia. NSIP is an IIP with diffuse inflammation seen on surgical lung biopsy.[52] Patients are on average 7 to 10 years younger than patients with IPF, but considerable overlap exists. The degree of accompanying interstitial fibrosis is variable among patients. The most common presentation of NSIP is fibrotic NSIP. This type involves fibrosis and inflammation. Cellular NSIP is less common. Patients present with chronic or subacute cough and dyspnea. High-resolution CT shows predominant ground-glass abnormalities in cellular NSIP and both ground-glass abnormalities and fibrotic changes in fibrotic NSIP. Given that there is significant clinical and radiographic overlap between fibrotic NSIP and IPF, surgical lung biopsy is frequently required to distinguish these two entities, such as when elements of classic UIP are not present on high-resolution CT images.

The prognosis is much better for NSIP than IPF, with most patients surviving 7 to 10 years. Immunosuppression with oral corticosteroids and cytotoxic immunosuppressive agents is the primary therapy. Type and duration of therapy are guided by disease activity and degree of inflammation on biopsy and ground-glass abnormalities on high-resolution CT. Pathologic NSIP is found frequently as an IIP and is the most common pattern of injury seen in connective tissue disease–associated ILD. Owing to this frequent association, many authors consider NSIP a connective tissue disease isolated to the lung.[53,54]

Organizing Pneumonia. **Organizing pneumonia** (OP) is the revised term for *bronchiolitis obliterans organizing pneumonia*. The term *cryptogenic organizing pneumonia* is used when this pattern of injury occurs as an IIP, and it is termed *organizing pneumonia* when found in the setting of connective tissue disease. Patients with organizing pneumonia are typically younger than patients with IPF and present with acute or subacute dyspnea and cough. Approximately one-third describe a preceding viral illness. However, no other risk factors are known. High-resolution CT shows alveolar filling with air bronchograms mimicking acute pneumonia, and the patient with classic organizing pneumonia presents after having failed to improve despite several courses of antibiotics. Diagnosis usually requires surgical lung biopsy, especially if the clinical and radiographic features are uncertain because small areas of organizing pneumonia can be seen in various inflammatory and fibrotic disorders on transbronchial lung biopsy. Surgical lung biopsy specimens show young fibroblasts within the alveoli that are presumably recovering from an injury. The alveolar basement membrane is intact, allowing for significant recovery if the inflammation or injury can be suppressed.

Most patients improve with oral corticosteroids (0.5 to 1 mg/kg for 6 to 12 weeks). However, many patients have recurrence after corticosteroid withdrawal and require long-term immunosuppression with cytotoxic immunosuppressive agents. A few patients develop progressive fibrosis despite aggressive immunosuppression and may be candidates for lung transplantation.

Lymphocytic Interstitial Pneumonia

Lymphocytic interstitial pneumonia is a rare disorder of polyclonal lymphocyte aggregates that accumulate diffusely in the interstitium.[55] The diagnosis almost always requires surgical lung biopsy. Patients are typically younger than patients with IPF and present with subacute dyspnea and cough. Pulmonary function testing may show a mixed picture, and high-resolution CT typically shows diffuse ground-glass attenuation with variable amounts of fibrosis. Most patients respond well to oral corticosteroids, with a few requiring long-term immunosuppression. Lymphocytic interstitial pneumonia is frequently associated with connective tissue diseases, especially Sjögren syndrome, and with immunodeficiency, and these possibilities should be investigated in all patients with lymphocytic interstitial pneumonia.

MINI CLINI

Clinical Deterioration in a Patient With Interstitial Lung Disease

PROBLEM: A 50-year-old man with fibrotic NSIP is being treated with oral corticosteroids and cyclophosphamide. After 6 months of therapy, he begins to report progressive breathlessness. Why is this occurring?

SOLUTION: Many ILDs follow a gradually progressive course to end-stage disease and death. The available treatments may result in temporary improvement or retard progression of the disease. These treatments seldom are curative, however. Progressive symptoms (exertional dyspnea or cough) in a patient being treated for ILD often, although not always, indicates disease progression.

The following possibilities must be considered and separated from progression of the disease:

1. *Superimposed infection:* Immunosuppressive agents used in the management of some ILDs increase the risk for infection in the lung and elsewhere. Common bacteria or uncommon opportunistic infections may be responsible. Pneumonia may be difficult to detect radiographically because of preexisting radiographic abnormalities, and bronchoscopy with bronchoalveolar lavage and transbronchial lung biopsy may be needed.
2. *Drug reaction:* Almost all medications used to treat ILD have been reported to be capable of causing an adverse pulmonary reaction. Some medications, such as methotrexate, have been described to result in pulmonary reactions in 5% to 10% of users. An adverse drug reaction should be considered in all patients with ILD who are being actively treated, particularly if there is a clear temporal relationship between starting the medication and the new or progressive respiratory symptoms.
3. *Steroid-related muscle weakness.* This is a less common complication of corticosteroid therapy and can cause exercise intolerance indistinguishable from progression of the underlying lung disease. Steroid-related muscle weakness (steroid myopathy) is difficult to diagnose because the weakness can result in worsening of the underlying restrictive physiologic defect. When proximal muscle weakness occurs in combination with progressive respiratory symptoms, the possibility of steroid myopathy should be considered. A greater than 20% drop in the FVC in the supine position compared with the sitting position suggests neuromuscular dysfunction.
4. *Pulmonary embolism:* Inactivity as a result of disease-related physiologic impairment and right ventricular dysfunction may be a risk factor for thromboembolic disease. A sudden decline in respiratory status, sometimes associated with pleuritic chest pain, should raise the possibility of acute pulmonary embolism.
5. *Lung carcinoma:* Patients with pulmonary fibrosis have an increased risk for lung cancer, and the development of lung cancer can contribute to clinical decline.
6. *Atherosclerotic vascular disease:* Many patients with ILD have independent risk factors for atherosclerotic vascular disease. They may have unrelated cardiac disease, such as coronary artery disease, left ventricular dysfunction, or valvular disease, which can be mistaken for a worsening of the pulmonary process.

Each of the possible explanations for the patient's breathlessness should be considered before ascribing it to progression of the ILD.

NONSPECIFIC THERAPIES

Oxygen Therapy

Because hypoxemia is common in ILD, supplemental O_2 therapy is frequently prescribed, although it has not been studied as extensively as in chronic obstructive pulmonary disease (COPD). Patients with ILD should have arterial O_2 saturation determined at rest and especially during exertion because many patients with only mild disease desaturate with exertion despite normal saturation at rest. Although studies are limited, supplemental O_2 delivered via nasal cannula can prevent resting hypoxemia and allow greater exertion before desaturation. These benefits may improve quality of life and potentially ward off development of pulmonary arterial hypertension, although further studies are needed.

We favor continuous rather than pulsed delivery of O_2 in patients with ILD because the desaturation with activity seen in most patients is not corrected with pulse therapy, and pulse units vary greatly in the amount of O_2 delivered.[56] For most patients, liquid O_2 is the best source to provide adequate flow rates. In motivated patients, transtracheal delivery of supplemental O_2 increases the efficiency of delivery and improves cosmetic appearance. However, patients must be chosen carefully because of the need for frequent care and risk for mucus drying, tracheal blockage by dried secretions, and rare bleeding.

MINI CLINI

Tobacco Use and Interstitial Lung Disease

PROBLEM: A 30-year-old woman has ILD and is a current smoker. She is concerned that quitting on her own is too difficult and comments that tobacco use is associated with emphysema, not with scarring. Should she be encouraged to quit smoking? Why or why not?

SOLUTION: Yes! Although the association between tobacco use and COPD is well known, the relationship with ILD is less well-appreciated. Smoking is a risk factor for the development of IPF but not the sole cause. However, the IIPs of DIP, RB-ILD, and PLCH have a strong association with cigarette smoking.

Approximately 90% of patients with DIP and RB-ILD are current or former tobacco smokers. More than 90% of patients with PLCH smoke, often quite heavily. As with other toxic exposures, complete avoidance of all smoke is important for these patients. In RB-ILD and PLCH, physiologic stabilization and occasionally even improvement can occur after stopping smoking. In DIP, the benefits of smoking cessation are unclear.

In addition to having concerns about these specific disease considerations, patients with ILD of any type cannot afford to risk the development of additional, smoking-related cardiorespiratory impairment. The patient should be strongly encouraged to stop smoking.

Pulmonary Rehabilitation and Exercise Therapy

Pulmonary rehabilitation, a very important part of treating obstructive lung disease, also has proved beneficial in the management of ILD. Pulmonary rehabilitation is important in building aerobic fitness, maintaining physical activity, and improving quality of life. When pulmonary rehabilitation is stopped, the benefits decrease over a few months.[57] We encourage all of our patients to enroll in outpatient pulmonary rehabilitation and to continue maintenance rehabilitation.

Vaccinations and Infection Avoidance

Because patients with ILD have increased consequences of respiratory infections, patients with ILD should receive a pneumococcal vaccine per U.S. Centers for Disease Control and Prevention guidelines and a yearly influenza virus vaccine. Additionally, we recommend that patients practice good hand hygiene (frequent handwashing). We do not recommend use of masks or special antibacterial products. Patients treated with prednisone in doses greater than 15 mg daily or with a steroid-sparing immunosuppressant should receive *Pneumocystis* prophylaxis (e.g., with oral trimethoprim-sulfamethoxazole, inhaled pentamidine, etc.).

Transplantation

The only therapy shown to prolong life in patients with end-stage, particularly fibrotic, ILD is lung transplantation.[58] Transplantation has been performed successfully in the management of most ILDs. A recommendation for lung transplantation must consider the significant risk for mortality at 1 year (10% to 25%) and 5 years (50% to 60%). Many patients with ILD are older than the upper age limit of "physiologic" age 65. Additionally, comorbidities such as gastroesophageal reflux disease, which is common in many ILDs, preclude lung transplantation because of the increased risk for chronic rejection and death.

Summary

The entities grouped as ILDs are a diverse group of illnesses of varied cause, treatment, and prognosis. These diseases generally manifest as chronic, progressive dyspnea on exertion and cough. Findings on examination are often limited to the chest in the form of fine, inspiratory crackles. The most common finding on chest radiograph is diffuse reticular or reticulonodular infiltrates with reduced lung volumes. Pulmonary function testing usually reveals restrictive physiology and decreased diffusion capacity; however, other patterns can be seen. Therapy depends on the underlying disease and may consist of immunosuppressive drugs and the avoidance of disease-inducing exposures.

ROLE OF THE RESPIRATORY THERAPIST

- The respiratory therapist (RT) sees patients with ILD in one of two settings. RTs assess and treat outpatients in several manners. In the role of pulmonary function technician, the RT assesses disease burden and serial changes in lung function. At the initial evaluation, the RT needs to provide accurate spirometry, lung volume, and DLCO, along with 6-minute walk distance and saturation, because these measures have important prognostic value. At subsequent visits, serial changes in these parameters are important to assess a patient's response to therapy or disease progression. Besides having important prognostic values, changes in lung function over time help determine whether to continue therapy or refer eligible patients for lung transplantation.
- RTs determine supplemental O_2 requirements at rest and with exertion and recommend the appropriate delivery amount, mode, and source of O_2. Also, RTs typically perform outpatient pulmonary rehabilitation, which can benefit many patients with ILD. RTs also may administer inhaled pentamidine, which is used to prevent *Pneumocystis jirovecii* infection in patients receiving immunosuppressive drugs for an ILD.
- The needs of patients with ILD change when admitted to the hospital. The RT plays a crucial role in assessing supplemental O_2 needs and delivering O_2 by the proper mode (nasal cannula, face mask, high-flow O_2 with nonrebreathing face mask, or intubation and mechanical ventilation). If obstructive impairment is suspected, the RT can recommend and deliver the appropriate bronchodilators or inhaled corticosteroids. Owing to the tenuous nature of these patients, careful monitoring by the RT of patients with ILD is required to prevent hypoxemia and its acute complications.

SUMMARY CHECKLIST

- ILDs are a diverse group of illnesses that can be organized into groups based on related causes.
- These diseases generally cause chronic, progressive dyspnea on exertion and cough.
- Findings on examination are often limited to the chest in the form of fine, inspiratory crackles.
- The most common chest radiograph finding is diffuse reticular or reticulonodular infiltrates with reduced lung volumes.
- Pulmonary function testing usually reveals restrictive physiology and decreased diffusion capacity; however, other patterns can be seen.
- Causes of the ILDs are diverse but are most frequently from exposure (tobacco, hypersensitivity pneumonitis antigens, silica, asbestos), autoimmune dysfunction (sarcoidosis, connective tissue disease associated), and abnormal injury healing (IPF).
- Nonspecific treatment may be considered in all ILD patients (e.g., supplemental O_2, pulmonary rehabilitation), but specific ILD treatment depends on the underlying disease and may consist of immunosuppressive drugs and avoidance of disease-inducing exposures.

References

1. Raghu G, Brown KK: Interstitial lung disease: clinical evaluation and keys to an accurate diagnosis. *Clin Chest Med* 25:409–419, 2004.
2. King TE, Jr: Clinical advances in the diagnosis and therapy of the interstitial lung diseases. *Am J Respir Crit Care Med* 172:268–279, 2005.
3. Elliot TL, Lynch DA, Newell JD, Jr, et al: High-resolution computed tomography features of non-specific interstitial pneumonia and usual interstitial pneumonia. *J Comput Assist Tomogr* 29:339–345, 2005.
4. Hunninghake GW, Lynch DA, Galvin JR, et al: Radiologic findings are strongly associated with a pathologic diagnosis of usual interstitial pneumonia. *Chest* 124:1215–1223, 2003.
5. Souza CA, Muller NL, Lee KS, et al: Idiopathic interstitial pneumonias: prevalence of mediastinal lymph node enlargement in 206 patients. *AJR Am J Roentgenol* 186:995–999, 2006.
6. Chetta A, Marangio E, Olivieri D: Pulmonary function testing in interstitial lung diseases. *Respiration* 71:209–213, 2004.
7. Cottin V, Nunes H, Brillet PY, et al: Combined pulmonary fibrosis and emphysema: a distinct underrecognised entity. *Eur Respir J* 26:586–593, 2005.
8. Ryu JH, Myers JL, Capizzi SA, et al: Desquamative interstitial pneumonia and respiratory bronchiolitis-associated interstitial lung disease. *Chest* 127:178–184, 2005.
9. Portnoy J, Veraldi KL, Schwarz MI, et al: Respiratory bronchiolitis-interstitial lung disease: long-term outcome. *Chest* 131:664–671, 2007.
10. Goldiner PL, Carlon GC, Cvitkovic E, et al: Factors influencing postoperative morbidity and mortality in patients treated with bleomycin. *Br Med J* 1:1664–1667, 1978.
11. Selman M: Hypersensitivity pneumonitis: a multifaceted deceiving disorder. *Clin Chest Med* 25:531–547, 2004.
12. Lacasse Y, Selman M, Costabel U, et al: Clinical diagnosis of hypersensitivity pneumonitis. *Am J Respir Crit Care Med* 168:952–958, 2003.
13. Monkare S: Influence of corticosteroid treatment on the course of farmer's lung. *Eur J Respir Dis* 64:283–293, 1983.
14. Vourlekis JS, Schwarz MI, Cherniack RM, et al: The effect of pulmonary fibrosis on survival in patients with hypersensitivity pneumonitis. *Am J Med* 116:662–668, 2004.
15. American Thoracic Society: Diagnosis and initial management of nonmalignant diseases related to asbestos. *Am J Respir Crit Care Med* 170:691–715, 2004.
16. Schwartz DA, Davis CS, Merchant JA, et al: Longitudinal changes in lung function among asbestos-exposed workers. *Am J Respir Crit Care Med* 150:1243–1249, 1994.
17. Ross MH, Murray J: Occupational respiratory disease in mining. *Occup Med (Lond)* 54:304–310, 2004.
18. Strange C, Highland KB: Interstitial lung disease in the patient who has connective tissue disease. *Clin Chest Med* 25:549–559, 2004.
19. Tanaka N, Newell JD, Brown KK, et al: Collagen vascular disease-related lung disease: high-resolution computed tomography findings based on the pathologic classification. *J Comput Assist Tomogr* 28:351–360, 2004.
20. Tashkin DP, Elashoff R, Clements PJ, et al: Cyclophosphamide versus placebo in scleroderma lung disease. *N Engl J Med* 354:2655–2666, 2006.
21. Swigris JJ, Olson AL, Fischer A, et al: Mycophenolate mofetil is safe, well tolerated, and preserves lung function in patients with connective tissue disease-related interstitial lung disease. *Chest* 130:30–36, 2006.
22. Tashkin DP, Elashoff R, Clements PJ, et al: Effects of 1-year treatment with cyclophosphamide on outcomes at 2 years in scleroderma lung disease. *Am J Respir Crit Care Med* 176:1026–1034, 2007.
23. Baughman RP: Pulmonary sarcoidosis. *Clin Chest Med* 25:521–530, 2004.
24. Shorr AF, Torrington KG, Hnatiuk OW: Endobronchial involvement and airway hyperreactivity in patients with sarcoidosis. *Chest* 120:881–886, 2001.
25. Paramothayan NS, Lasserson TJ, Jones PW: Corticosteroids for pulmonary sarcoidosis. *Cochrane Database Syst Rev* (2):CD001114, 2005.
26. Rossman MD, Newman LS, Baughman RP, et al: A double-blinded, randomized, placebo-controlled trial of infliximab in subjects with active pulmonary sarcoidosis. *Sarcoidosis Vasc Diffuse Lung Dis* 23:201–208, 2006.
27. Keir G, Wells AU: Assessing pulmonary disease and response to therapy: which test? *Semin Respir Crit Care Med* 31:409–418, 2010.
28. Ryu JH, Moss J, Beck GJ, et al: The NHLBI lymphangioleiomyomatosis registry: characteristics of 230 patients at enrollment. *Am J Respir Crit Care Med* 173:105–111, 2006.
29. McCormack FX: Lymphangioleiomyomatosis: a clinical update. *Chest* 133:507–516, 2008.
30. Raghu G, Weycker D, Edelsberg J, et al: Incidence and prevalence of idiopathic pulmonary fibrosis. *Am J Respir Crit Care Med* 174:810–816, 2006.
31. Renzoni E, Srihari V, Sestini P: Pathogenesis of idiopathic pulmonary fibrosis: review of recent findings. *F1000Prime Rep* 6:69, 2014.
32. Raghu G, Mageto YN, Lockhart D, et al: The accuracy of the clinical diagnosis of new-onset idiopathic pulmonary fibrosis and other interstitial lung disease: a prospective study. *Chest* 116:1168–1174, 1999.
33. Hunninghake GW, Zimmerman MB, Schwartz DA, et al: Utility of a lung biopsy for the diagnosis of idiopathic pulmonary fibrosis. *Am J Respir Crit Care Med* 164:193–196, 2001.
34. Martinez FJ, Safrin S, Weycker D, et al: The clinical course of patients with idiopathic pulmonary fibrosis. *Ann Intern Med* 142:963–967, 2005.
35. Collard HR, Moore BB, Flaherty KR, et al: Acute exacerbations of idiopathic pulmonary fibrosis. *Am J Respir Crit Care Med* 176:636–643, 2007.
36. Collard HR, King TE, Jr, Bartelson BB, et al: Changes in clinical and physiologic variables predict survival in idiopathic pulmonary fibrosis. *Am J Respir Crit Care Med* 168:538–542, 2003.
37. Richeldi L, Davies HR, Ferrara G, et al: Corticosteroids for idiopathic pulmonary fibrosis. *Cochrane Database Syst Rev* (3):CD002880, 2003.
38. Davies HR, Richeldi L, Walters EH: Immunomodulatory agents for idiopathic pulmonary fibrosis. *Cochrane Database Syst Rev* (3):CD003134, 2003.
39. Collard HR, Ryu JH, Douglas WW, et al: Combined corticosteroid and cyclophosphamide therapy does not alter survival in idiopathic pulmonary fibrosis. *Chest* 125:2169–2174, 2004.
40. King TE, Jr, Albera C, Bradford WZ, et al: Effect of interferon gamma-1b on survival in patients with idiopathic pulmonary fibrosis (INSPIRE): a multicentre, randomised, placebo-controlled trial. *Lancet* 374:222–228, 2009.

41. Raghu G, Brown KK, Costabel U, et al: Treatment of idiopathic pulmonary fibrosis with etanercept: an exploratory, placebo-controlled trial. *Am J Respir Crit Care Med* 178:948–955, 2008.
42. Idiopathic Pulmonary Fibrosis Clinical Research Network, Zisman DA, Schwarz M, et al: A controlled trial of sildenafil in advanced idiopathic pulmonary fibrosis. *N Engl J Med* 363:620–628, 2010.
43. Daniels CE, Lasky JA, Limper AH, et al: Imatinib treatment for idiopathic pulmonary fibrosis: randomized placebo-controlled trial results. *Am J Respir Crit Care Med* 181:604–610, 2010.
44. Idiopathic Pulmonary Fibrosis Clinical Research Network, Martinez FJ, de Andrade JA, et al: Randomized trial of acetylcysteine in idiopathic pulmonary fibrosis. *N Engl J Med* 370:2093–3101, 2014.
45. Idiopathic Pulmonary Fibrosis Clinical Research Network, Raghu G, Anstrom KJ, et al: Prednisone, azathioprine, and N-acetylcysteine for pulmonary fibrosis. *N Engl J Med* 366:1968–1977, 2012.
46. King TE, Jr, Bradford WZ, Castro-Bernardini S, et al: A phase 3 trial of pirfenidone in patients with idiopathic pulmonary fibrosis. *N Engl J Med* 370:2083–2092, 2014.
47. Richeldi L, du Bois RM, Raghu G, et al: Efficacy and safety of nintedanib in idiopathic pulmonary fibrosis. *N Engl J Med* 2014 370:2071–2082, 2014.
48. Nadrous HF, Pellikka PA, Krowka MJ, et al: Pulmonary hypertension in patients with idiopathic pulmonary fibrosis. *Chest* 128:2393–2399, 2005.
49. Lettieri CJ, Nathan SD, Barnett SD, et al: Prevalence and outcomes of pulmonary arterial hypertension in advanced idiopathic pulmonary fibrosis. *Chest* 129:746–752, 2006.
50. King TE, Brown KK, Raghu G, et al: BUILD-3: a randomized, controlled trial of bosentan in idiopathic pulmonary fibrosis. *Am J Respir Crit Care Med* 184:92–99, 2011.
51. Corte TJ, Keir GJ, Dimopoulos K, et al: Bosentan in pulmonary hypertension associated with fibrotic idiopathic interstitial pneumonia. *Am J Respir Crit Care Med* 190:208–217, 2014.
52. Martinez FJ: Idiopathic interstitial pneumonias: usual interstitial pneumonia versus non-specific interstitial pneumonia. *Proc Am Thorac Soc* 3:81–95, 2006.
53. Fischer A, West SG, Swigris JJ, et al: Connective tissue disease-associated interstitial lung disease: a call for clarification. *Chest* 138:251–256, 2010.
54. Kinder BW, Collard HR, Koth L, et al: Idiopathic non-specific interstitial pneumonia: lung manifestation of undifferentiated connective tissue disease? *Am J Respir Crit Care Med* 176:691–697, 2007.
55. Cha SI, Fessler MB, Cool CD, et al: Lymphoid interstitial pneumonia: clinical features, associations and prognosis. *Eur Respir J* 28:364–369, 2006.
56. Palwai A, Skowronski M, Coreno A, et al: Critical comparisons of the clinical performance of oxygen-conserving devices. *Am J Respir Crit Care Med* 181:1061–1071, 2010.
57. Holland AE, Hill CJ, Conron M, et al: Short term improvement in exercise capacity and symptoms following exercise training in interstitial lung disease. *Thorax* 63:549–554, 2008.
58. Orens JB, Estenne M, Arcasoy S, et al: International guidelines for the selection of lung transplant candidates: 2006 update—a consensus report from the Pulmonary Scientific Council of the International Society for Heart and Lung Transplantation. *J Heart Lung Transplant* 25:745–755, 2006.

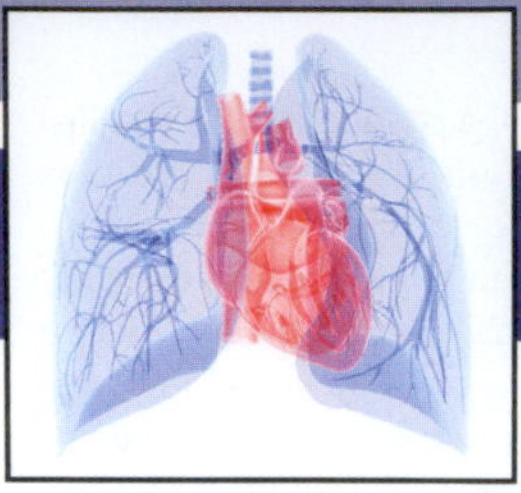

CHAPTER 27

Pleural Diseases

CHARLIE STRANGE

CHAPTER OBJECTIVES

After reading this chapter you will be able to:

- Describe the anatomy and function of the visceral and parietal pleura.
- Describe how pleural effusions occur and the difference between transudative and exudative effusions.
- Identify common causes of transudative and exudative pleural effusions.
- Write definitions of chylothorax, hemothorax, and pneumothorax.
- Describe the impact of moderate to large pleural effusions on lung function.
- State the role of the chest radiograph in recognizing pleural effusions.
- State the purpose of thoracentesis and the potential complications.
- Identify the definitions of spontaneous, secondary, and tension pneumothorax.
- Describe the diagnosis and treatment of pneumothorax.

CHAPTER OUTLINE

KEY TERMS

alveolopleural fistula
bronchopleural fistula
chyle
chylothorax
empyema
exudative pleural effusion
hemothorax
parietal pleura
pleural effusion
pleurisy
pleurodesis
pneumothorax
primary spontaneous pneumothorax
reexpansion pulmonary edema
secondary spontaneous pneumothorax
stomata
tension pneumothorax
thoracentesis
transudative pleural effusion
visceral pleura

A spectrum of pleural diseases affects respiratory function. An understanding of pleural anatomy, physiology, and pathology is essential to delivering effective respiratory care. This chapter focuses on the two major diseases that occur in the pleural space: pleural effusion and pneumothorax.

THE PLEURAL SPACE

Each lung is covered by a thin membrane called the **visceral pleura** that adheres closely to the underlying lung (Figure 27-1). The visceral pleura dips into the fissures of the lung, allowing the surgeon easy access between the lung lobes and allowing pleural fluid to travel freely between the lobes while remaining in the pleural space.

The ribs and connective tissue of the chest wall are covered on the inner surface by a similar membrane called the **parietal pleura.** The parietal pleura can be thought of as a sac that covers not only the rib surface (costal pleura) but also the diaphragm (diaphragmatic pleura) and the mediastinum (mediastinal pleura).

The blood vessels and airways that enter the lung connect to the mediastinum at the lung hilum. It is at this juncture that the visceral pleura meet the mediastinal parietal pleura to form a single, continuous pleural membrane (Figure 27-2).

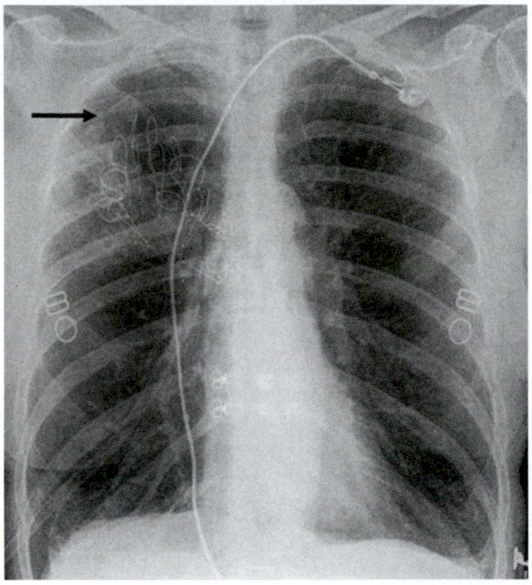

FIGURE 27-1 The presence of a pneumothorax is diagnosed by identification of a pleural line *(arrow)*, in this case after bronchoscopic placement of lung volume reduction coils. A hydropneumothorax requires identification of both a pleural line *(arrow)* and the air-fluid interface of pleural fluid that causes a straight line in the chest. A high-quality monitor is needed to optimally detect the pleura.

Because the lung usually is completely inflated, it might be thought that the pleural membranes always touch. However, freeze-fracture imaging has demonstrated that there is a space between the visceral and parietal pleura that averages 10 to 20 mm in width and is filled with pleural fluid. This thin film of fluid allows the lung to slide over the ribs and a gliding movement that takes little energy and produces little friction.

The average person has approximately 8 ml of pleural fluid per hemithorax.[1] It is estimated that this pleural fluid has a total protein concentration similar to that of interstitial fluid elsewhere in the body: between 1.3 and 1.4 g/dl.[2]

In humans, the pleural spaces surrounding each lung are completely independent, being separated by the mediastinum. This is not the case in all other mammals. The slaughter of the American buffalo could occur with a single spear or rifle shot because the pleural spaces of the buffalo lung are connected. Consequently, air in the pleural space collapses both lungs. A similar situation can occur in any patient who has undergone median sternotomy, during which both pleural spaces were entered. Common operations resulting in this condition are lung volume reduction surgery and bilateral lung transplantation.

The pleural space is under negative pressure except during forced expiration. The intact thoracic rib cage provides elastic recoil pressure outward, whereas the intrinsic recoil pressure of the lung is inward toward the lung hilum. The diaphragm further decreases the intrapleural pressure below atmospheric pressure to allow inspiration to occur. In an upright person, the pressure is more negative at the top of the lung than at the bottom of the lung because of the weight of the lung and the effects of gravity. The net effect of the negatively pressurized pleural space is that fluid moves into the pleural space from adjacent sites when a communication is present. A patient with

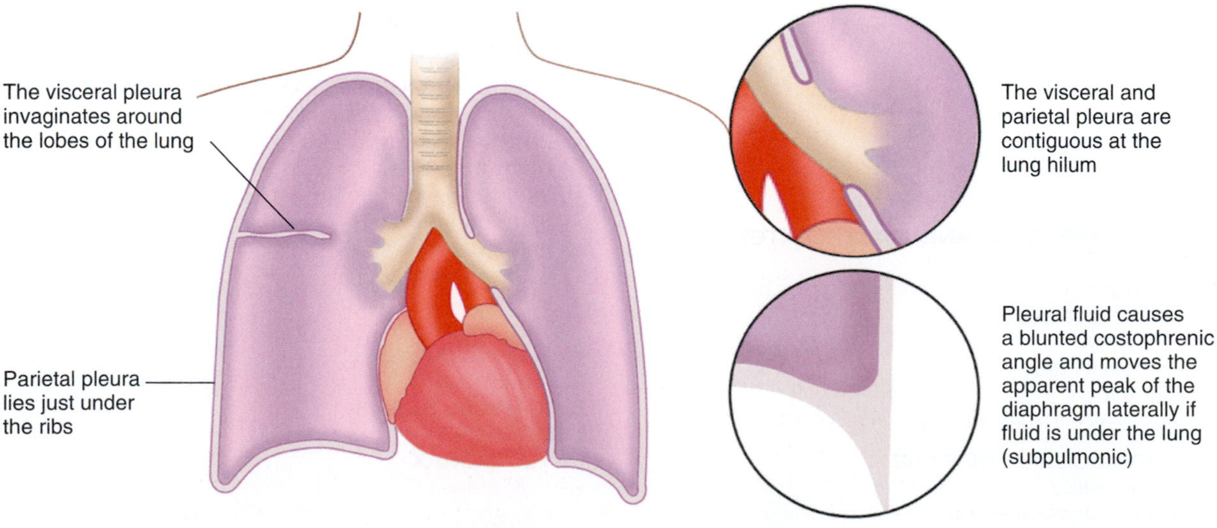

FIGURE 27-2 Anatomy of the pleura.

ascitic fluid and a hole in the diaphragm usually pulls fluid into the pleural space.

PLEURAL EFFUSIONS

Any abnormal amount of pleural fluid in the pleural space is called **pleural effusion.** The many causes of pleural effusion are categorized according to the factor that causes it and the content of the fluid.[3]

Pleural fluid enters the pleural space across both the visceral and the parietal pleura, particularly when the interstitial pressure within either the lung or the chest wall is increased. The main route for pleural fluid removal is small holes within the parietal pleura called **stomata** that are large enough to allow a red blood cell to enter and be cleared from the pleural space. The parietal pleural stomata connect with intercostal lymphatic vessels under the ribs that drain posteriorly into the mediastinum. In the mediastinum, these lymphatic vessels enter lymph nodes before draining into the thoracic duct, a large lymphatic channel within the chest, which empties into the left subclavian vein. Abnormalities of increased pleural fluid production or blockade of drainage can cause pleural fluid to accumulate.

Transudative Effusions

Any pleural effusion that forms when the pleural space is intact is called a **transudative pleural effusion.** A pleural fluid total protein concentration less than 50% of the serum total protein level and lactate dehydrogenase (LDH) values in the pleural fluid less than 60% of the serum value indicate the presence of a transudative pleural effusion. In the absence of serum values, an absolute pleural fluid LDH level less than two-thirds normal for serum suggests the presence of a transudate. These numbers were derived from large patient series in which pleural fluid and serum protein concentrations were measured while the cause of the effusion was being determined and corrected.[4]

The classification system listed in Box 27-1 is not perfect, and refinements continue to be proposed. For practical purposes, these numbers help narrow the possible causes of pleural fluid formation.

Transudative pleural effusions form when hydrostatic and oncotic pressures are abnormal[5] (Figure 27-3). The list of diseases that cause transudative pleural effusions is short. Therefore these diseases remain relatively easy to diagnose.

Box 27-1 Causes of Pleural Effusion

TRANSUDATIVE PLEURAL EFFUSION
- Congestive heart failure
- Cirrhosis
- Nephrotic syndrome
- Hypoalbuminemia
- Lymphatic obstruction
- Peritoneal dialysis
- Atelectasis
- Central venous catheter in pleural space
- Urinothorax

EXUDATIVE PLEURAL EFFUSION NEOPLASTIC DISEASE
- Carcinoma
- Lymphoma
- Mesothelioma

INFECTIOUS DISEASE
- Bacterial infection
- Tuberculosis
- Fungal infection
- Paragonimiasis
- Viral pleurisy

PULMONARY EMBOLISM AND GASTROINTESTINAL DISEASE
- Pancreatic disease
- Intraabdominal abscess
- Splenic infarction
- Esophageal perforation
- Abdominal surgery
- Endoscopic variceal sclerotherapy

COLLAGEN VASCULAR DISEASE
- Rheumatoid pleurisy
- Systemic lupus erythematosus
- Drug-induced lupus
- Immunoblastic lymphadenopathy
- Sjögren's syndrome
- Familial Mediterranean fever
- Churg-Strauss syndrome
- Granulomatosis with polyangiitis (formerly called *Wegener granulomatosis*)

DRUG-INDUCED PLEURAL DISEASE
- Nitrofurantoin
- Minoxidil
- Dantrolene
- Methysergide
- Bromocriptine
- Amiodarone
- Procarbazine, bleomycin, mitomycin
- Methotrexate

MISCELLANEOUS DISEASES AND CONDITIONS
- Benign asbestos pleural effusion
- Postcardiac injury syndrome (Dressler syndrome)
- Meigs syndrome
- Yellow nail syndrome
- Sarcoidosis
- Pericardial disease
- Fetal pleural effusion
- Uremic pleural effusion
- Trapped lung
- Radiation pleurisy
- Amyloidosis

ELECTRICAL BURNS
HEMOTHORAX
CHYLOTHORAX

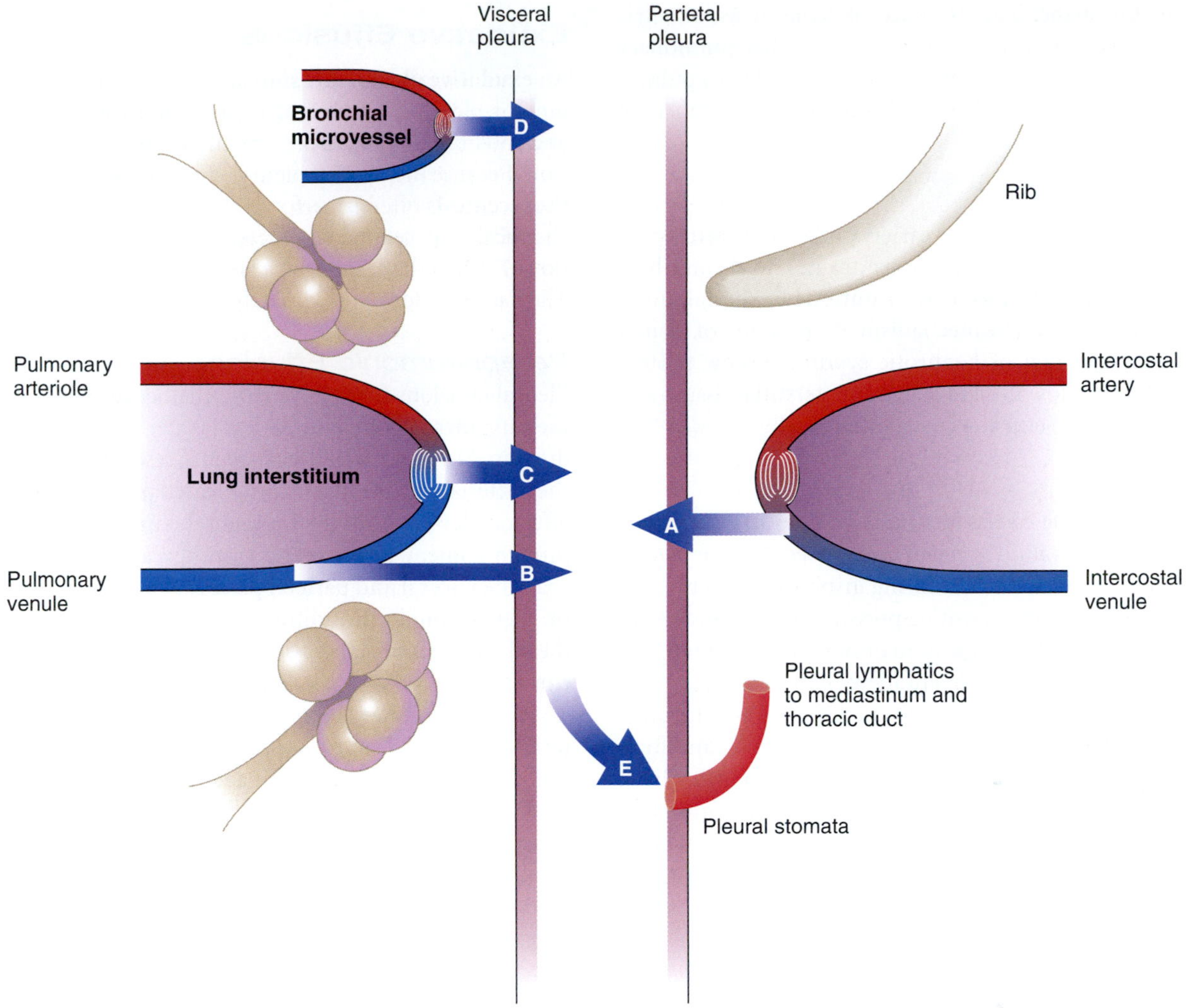

FIGURE 27-3 Pleural fluid formation requires both excess fluid formation and decreased elimination. In diseases such as pulmonary arterial hypertension, in which right-sided heart pressure is increased and systemic veins, such as the intercostal veins *(A)*, are pressurized, pleural fluid does not form because pleural fluid formation is not increased and lymphatic drainage remains intact. However, when left ventricular failure causes pulmonary venule pressure *(B)* to increase, the addition of interstitial lung water overwhelms the drainage and produces a transudative pleural effusion. Injury to the capillaries *(C)*, as in pneumonia or acute respiratory distress syndrome, causes fluid to leak into the lung interstitium and pleural space at increased rates. Under these conditions, fibrin can occlude the pleural lymphatic vessels *(E)* and cause fluid to accumulate. The bronchial microvessels *(D)* supply the pleura with blood and likely participate to some extent in production of pleural fluid.

Congestive Heart Failure

Elevation of pressure in the left atrium and pulmonary veins is the hallmark defining feature of *congestive heart failure* (CHF). Elevation of pulmonary venous pressure increases the amount of interstitial fluid in the lung. In severe cases, flooding of the alveoli causes pulmonary edema, but in less severe cases, interstitial lung water increases and decompresses into the pleural space. Because systemic venous pressure also is elevated, there is limited capability to remove pleural fluid through the intercostal veins. Therefore pleural fluid must be predominantly removed by the lymphatic vessels. Pleural effusions result when the capacity of pleural lymphatic drainage is overcome.[6]

CHF is the most common cause of pleural effusions in clinical practice. The effusions can be massive, filling the entire hemithorax and compressing the lung. More commonly, they are small and bilateral. The effusions are rarely drained because outcome is heavily influenced by successful management of the underlying CHF, which also clears the effusions.[7]

Nephrotic Syndrome

In *nephrotic syndrome* (also known as *nephrosis*), the kidneys leak more than 3 g of protein per day into the urine. Because patients become protein depleted, there is insufficient oncotic pressure within the blood to hold appropriate amounts of fluid within the blood vessels. These patients become edematous, and fluid leaks into the lung interstitium and pleural space. Pleural effusions are common but usually are small.

Patients with nephrosis are at increased risk for deep venous thrombosis and pulmonary embolism. In nephrosis, protein S, which keeps blood from clotting, becomes deficient from leaking into the urine. The presence of large or asymmetric pleural effusions should raise the possibility that pulmonary emboli have occurred. Pleural effusions associated with pulmonary emboli usually are exudates and contain large numbers of red blood cells.

Hypoalbuminemia

Hypoalbuminemia is caused by a variety of debilitating diseases, such as acquired immunodeficiency syndrome and chronic liver disease. Pleural effusions rarely form until the serum albumin level is less than 1.8 g/dl. The mechanism of formation of pleural fluid is identical to that of nephrotic syndrome. Low protein levels in the blood allow fluid to leak into interstitial tissues and the pleural space. The effusions usually are small.

Liver Disease

End-stage liver disease causes transudative fluid to accumulate in the abdomen. This fluid is called *ascites.* Because the pleural space is under negative pressure during inspiration and because ascitic fluid often is under positive pressure, any small hole in the diaphragm can result in movement of ascitic fluid into the pleural space to form *hepatic hydrothorax.*

All ascitic fluid can end up in the chest because of the pressure gradient, and true ascites can be absent. This condition often is quite difficult to manage except with methods that limit ascites formation, such as sodium restriction and diuretics. Excessive pleural fluid is present in approximately 6% of patients with ascites, and 70% of these fluid collections are on the right side.[8]

Atelectasis

When segments of the lung collapse, intrapleural pressure becomes more negative and can produce small effusions. With relief of bronchial obstruction and postoperative pain, these effusions may go away.

Lymphatic Obstruction

Lymphatic obstruction within the mediastinum causes poor pleural fluid removal from the pleural space, although the pleural space is otherwise normal. The most common condition that causes this abnormality is cancer that metastasizes to the mediastinum. This condition should be differentiated from a true malignant pleural effusion, defined as cancer cells within the pleural space.

Rare Causes

There are other rare causes of transudative pleural effusions. Urinothorax occurs after rupture of the ureter causing a urine leak into the retroperitoneal space that refluxes into the chest. The pleural fluid has a low pH. A central venous line that is inappropriately placed into the pleural space can put large amounts of transudative fluid into the pleural space before this abnormality is recognized. The level of glucose in the pleural fluid can be very elevated, depending on the infusion. Peritoneal dialysate can migrate into the pleural cavity in patients undergoing continuous ambulatory peritoneal dialysis.

Exudative Effusions

An **exudative pleural effusion** is caused by inflammation in the lung or pleura. This type of pleural effusion has more protein and inflammatory cells present than does a transudative effusion. Because therapy for pleural effusion depends on the cause, **thoracentesis** often is performed to determine the specific biochemical and cellular characteristics of the pleural effusion. Box 27-1 lists the common causes of exudative pleural effusion. They account for approximately 70% of all pleural effusions.

Parapneumonic Effusion

Pleural effusions form in pneumonia because inflammation in the lung increases interstitial lung water and pleural fluid production. Most effusions are small and resolve with resolution of the bacterial pneumonia.[9] Complicated parapneumonic pleural effusion develops when the pleural fluid has a high enough protein content to clot. The clotting causes fibrin strands to span the visceral and parietal pleura. The net result is collection of pleural fluid into different pockets called *loculi* within the pleural cavity. These often cannot be drained by a single chest tube.

Progression to **empyema** is marked by the presence of bacteria within the pleural space, seen as pus or bacteria on Gram stain. Empyemas require drainage. Whether complicated parapneumonic effusions require drainage remains controversial, although most physicians perform drainage because some of these effusions can progress to empyema.[10]

Parapneumonic effusions are common causes of persistent fever among intensive care unit (ICU) patients with pneumonia. Sampling by thoracentesis is commonly performed to exclude empyema. Pleural fluid drainage can improve ventilation and dyspnea if the volume of fluid removed is large.[11]

Viral Pleurisy

Viral lung infections (**pleurisy**) can cause pleural inflammation, small pleural effusions, and pain. The effusions may be so small they may be overlooked on a routine chest radiograph, and even when they can be seen, the effusions often are too small to sample. Pleural pain, which is called *pleurodynia,* and which can be the result of many other pleural processes, often is difficult to manage. The typical patient with pleurodynia has shallow respirations; deeper breaths are limited by pain. The subsequent atelectasis can cause oxygenation difficulty caused by shunting.

Tuberculous Pleurisy

In many parts of the world, any lymphocyte-predominant exudative effusion is considered tuberculosis until proved otherwise. Tuberculous pleural effusions occur when a caseous granuloma in the lung ruptures through the visceral pleural surface causing an exudative inflammatory effusion. Experiments in which purified protein derivative (PPD) is placed into the pleural space of animals have shown that such effusions result from the body's immune reaction to tuberculin proteins.

Although these patients need respiratory isolation, only 25% of them have sputum that subsequently grows *Mycobacterium tuberculosis.* The PPD skin test result is negative in 30% of patients when they come to medical attention but turns positive in 6 to 8 weeks in almost everyone.[12]

Malignant

Malignant disease is the most common cause of large unilateral pleural effusions among persons older than 60 years. Common cancers that form malignant pleural effusions include lung cancer and breast cancer, although any cancer can metastasize to the pleural surface. The effusions usually are lymphocyte predominant; malignant cells are found during cytologic examination of the pleural fluid.

Some malignant pleural effusions, such as those from lymphoma, respond to therapy for the malignant disease. However, most patients with symptomatic malignant pleural effusions need primary therapy with pleurodesis. **Pleurodesis** occurs when the visceral and parietal pleural membranes are fused by talc, other chemicals, or surgery to obliterate the pleural space.

Postoperative Effusion

A variety of operations involving the chest or upper abdomen produce pleural fluid.[13] Effusions after cardiac surgery usually are predominant on the left side and tend to be bloody. These effusions are particularly prevalent after a cutdown of the internal mammary artery for coronary artery bypass.

Small transudative pleural effusions are common when there is any atelectasis in the lung. Upper abdominal operations cause inflammation of the diaphragm. The resulting effusion has been termed a *sympathetic* effusion. Lung surgery in which the lung is unable to fill the thoracic cavity leaves a space under negative pressure, which fills with inflammatory pleural fluid. When the lung is unable to fill the space because of small postoperative size or visceral pleural fibrosis, the resulting pleural effusion can never be completely drained because of the "trapped lung."

Chylothorax

The thoracic duct is a lymphatic channel that runs from the abdomen through the mediastinum to enter the left subclavian vein. Disruption of the thoracic duct anywhere along its course can cause leakage of **chyle** into the mediastinum, which then may rupture into the pleural space and cause a **chylothorax.** The most common causes of rupture are malignancy (50%), surgery (20%), and trauma (5%).[14] The thoracic duct courses through the right side of the mediastinum in the lower thoracic cavity before crossing to the left side of the mediastinum at the level of T4 to T6. Rupture below this level causes right-sided pleural effusion, whereas rupture above this level causes left-sided pleural effusion.

In a patient who has eaten recently, the effusions are milky white as a result of the presence of chylomicrons (microscopic fat particles) absorbed by abdominal lymphatic vessels. In a fasting patient, these effusions usually are yellow. They may be bloody. A pleural fluid triglyceride concentration greater than 110 mg/dl confirms the diagnosis.[15] Computed tomography (CT) should be performed to evaluate the cause of the chylothorax.

Hemothorax

Hemothorax is the presence of blood in the pleural space. Hemothorax is arbitrarily defined as a pleural fluid hematocrit more than 50% of the serum value. Small amounts of blood in otherwise clear fluid can turn the fluid red, so measurement of the pleural fluid hematocrit is necessary to make this diagnosis.

Although hemothorax is seen most commonly after blunt or penetrating chest trauma, a number of medical conditions can give rise to blood in the pleural space. These should be considered in the absence of trauma. Any vein or artery in the thorax can bleed into the pleural space. A chest tube usually is inserted to monitor the rate of bleeding and determine whether the source is arterial or venous.[16]

Connective Tissue Diseases

Pleural effusions are found in a variety of connective tissue diseases, although the effusions usually are small. Effusions caused by inflammation of small blood vessels are the most common chest manifestation of systemic lupus erythematosus (SLE). Pleural effusions often accompany pericardial effusions in SLE and disappear with corticosteroid therapy.

Rheumatoid arthritis produces a characteristic effusion with a very low glucose content and low pH. These effusions can cause visceral pleural fibrosis and a trapped lung.

Uremic Effusion

Uremic pleurisy occurs under the same conditions as uremic pericarditis. The typical patient is undergoing dialysis that is inadequate in duration or frequency. Although the cause of pleural and pericardial inflammation in kidney failure remains unknown, the inflammatory process can take weeks to resolve.

Miscellaneous Causes

Discussion of the other causes of exudative effusions is beyond the scope of this chapter. Nevertheless, thoracentesis that yields findings compatible with any of those in the systemic diseases listed in Box 27-1 can narrow the differential diagnosis.

Physiologic Importance

Mechanics of Ventilation

Pleural effusions cause lung atelectasis because the capacity of the thorax is limited and fluid collapses the lung. Spirometry shows restriction. Studies correlating the volume of pleural fluid removed with improvement in forced vital capacity (FVC) show much variability from patient to patient.

Dyspnea is common with small pleural effusions, even when lung mechanics are relatively preserved. The mechanisms remain unknown but likely involve activation of stretch receptors or irritant receptors within the airways or nonadrenergic, noncholinergic C fibers in the chest wall or diaphragm. The net result is that dyspnea relief is variable after pleural fluid removal. Some patients have symptomatic relief after removal of small

RULE OF THUMB

The patient's vital capacity improves by approximately one-third of the pleural fluid volume removed. The remainder of the pleural fluid volume causes diaphragmatic compression and chest wall expansion. Some patients have a delay of 24 to 48 hours before the improvement can be seen as atelectasis resolves. Lack of any improvement suggests that lung consolidation or endobronchial obstruction is present. Improvement is less when the underlying disease is acute respiratory distress syndrome (ARDS).

pleural fluid volumes. Others can actually have more dyspnea if the fluid is removed in situations such as trapped lung, in which neural activation may increase with fluid withdrawal.

In rare instances, the pleurae thicken with a disease process sufficient to cause fibrothorax. Technically, fibrothorax is any process that causes fibrosis of the thoracic cage that affects pulmonary function. Fibrothorax can be caused by skin (e.g., fibrothorax that occurs, rarely, in scleroderma), soft tissue, bone (e.g., myositis ossificans, a disease in which muscles calcify), or pleura. The causes of pleural thickening significant enough to produce restriction include severe asbestos pleurisy, rheumatoid pleurisy, complicated trauma, cancer, and empyema. Treatment of fibrothorax from a pleural cause requires surgery, which is rarely performed because it is a very difficult operation.

Hypoxemia

Most patients with a pleural effusion have an increased alveolar-arterial (A-a) gradient resulting from the pathologic changes in the lung that are causing the effusion. Oxygenation can worsen after thoracentesis because changes in ventilation/perfusion ($\dot{V}/\dot{Q}$) matching are not instantaneous. Recovery to baseline PO_2 and subsequent improvement usually occurs a short time after thoracentesis.[16]

Diagnostic Tests

Chest Radiography

The chest radiograph is the most common method of detecting a pleural effusion. It is important that, if possible, the chest radiograph be obtained with the patient in an upright position to show a pleural fluid meniscus at the costophrenic angles. Many ICUs have rules that all radiographs are taken with patients sitting upright to optimize the value of the test. When the same patient undergoes radiography in the supine position, the effusion is distributed throughout the posterior part of the chest. The chest radiograph shows a generalized haze, which interferes with the detection of pulmonary infiltrates and quantifies the amount of fluid in the pleural effusion.

Lateral decubitus chest radiographs are performed by having patients lie on their side with the radiograph taken across the bed or table. This technique can show an effusion as small as 5 ml. This technique is used less often than other tests.

Ultrasonography and Computed Tomography

Pleural fluid and loculi can be detected easily with ultrasonography of the chest. The sensitivity of ultrasonography for pleural effusions is high, although ultrasonography is an operator-dependent study. Small portable ultrasound machines with high diagnostic accuracy have become available to localize the presence and location of pleural effusions. Most physicians use them routinely to optimize thoracentesis success.

CT scanning of the chest is the most sensitive study for identifying a pleural effusion. A contrast-enhanced scan is needed to delineate the pleural membrane and differentiate peripheral lung consolidation from pleural fluid. In addition to showing the size and location of a pleural effusion, the chest CT scan often gives information about the underlying lung parenchyma and the primary process causing the effusion.

Thoracentesis

In thoracentesis, pleural fluid is sampled percutaneously by means of inserting a needle into the pleural space (Figure 27-4). Administering an adequate local anesthetic ensures a painless procedure if care is taken to place lidocaine at the skin insertion site, along the periosteum of the involved rib, and at the parietal pleura, which is richly innervated with sensory nerve fibers. Diagnostic sampling of pleural fluid for cell counts, cultures, chemistries, and cytologic examination usually can be performed with a single syringe and a small needle. Samples for pleural pH should be kept from contact with room air. Pleural fluid drainage with lung reexpansion involves placing a larger catheter into the pleural space.

Thoracentesis involves the following three major risks: (1) intercostal artery laceration, (2) infection, and (3) pneumothorax.[17] Both an artery and a vein course under every rib, and the vessels become increasingly serpiginous with aging. Ensuring needle passage just over the rib margin makes bleeding during thoracentesis rare.

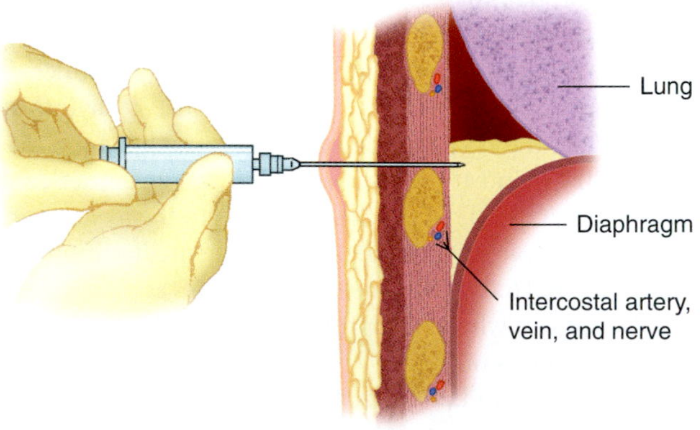

FIGURE 27-4 The technique of thoracentesis involves passage of a needle just superior to the rib. If the needle is placed too low on the chest, the diaphragm or organs below the diaphragm can be punctured. Diagnostic thoracentesis can be performed with small amounts of pleural fluid.

Because infection can be introduced into the pleural space, a totally sterile procedure is necessary. In some situations, the risk for infection is so high that thoracentesis rarely should be performed. When a lung is surgically removed, the space fills with sterile fluid. An infection introduced into this space usually necessitates open surgical drainage. Any trapped lung also carries a high risk for empyema because of the inability of the visceral and parietal pleura to meet and contain any infectious process. Needle puncture remains one of the most common causes of pneumothorax (see discussion of pneumothorax later in this chapter).

RULE OF THUMB

Chest tubes are usually removed when the volume of pleural fluid that comes out is less than 50 ml/24 hr. Chest tubes should not be kinked, to optimize pleural space drainage. Higher volumes suggest that the primary process has not been treated adequately. Daily monitoring of pleural fluid volume requires that the pleural fluid drainage system not be tipped over. Volumes should be recorded in the medical chart and marks made on the pleural drainage system to help determine the best time for chest tube removal.

Chest Thoracotomy Tubes

Chest tubes currently are manufactured in a variety of sizes and shapes, from 7F to 40F catheters. Catheter choice is frequently a matter of physician preference. Larger tubes are less likely to become obstructed and are capable of high airflow rates. Smaller tubes are easier to place over guidewire systems and cause less pain.

Intercostal placement is designed for the skin and soft tissue to approximate the tube and prevent air from entering the pleural space from the outside. The chest tube is then connected to a water-sealed chamber, which usually is contained within a commercially marketed three-bottle system that also regulates pleural pressure and is used to measure pleural fluid volume (Figure 27-5).

Thoracoscopy

The video-assisted thoracoscope is ideally designed for diagnostic and therapeutic work in the pleural space. Diagnostic thoracoscopy often is performed in a medical procedure room using local anesthesia and conscious sedation. The procedure involves placing the thoracoscope through an intercostal incision to visualize the lung surfaces, drain pleural fluid, perform biopsy under direct visualization, and perform pleurodesis if needed.

Pleurodesis

Pleurodesis is the process of fusing the parietal and visceral pleura with a fibrotic reaction that prevents further pleural fluid formation or seals the pleural space. Methods to produce pleurodesis include surgical abrasion and the application of intrapleural chemicals such as doxycycline, minocycline, and talc. Talc has been applied as a powder suspended in sterile saline solution and injected through the chest tube (talc slurry) or dusted through a thoracoscope (talc insufflation). The success rate of talc pleurodesis, approximately 90%, is higher than that of all alternatives except surgical abrasion.[18,19] Pleurodesis is used most commonly in managing symptomatic pleural effusions caused by cancer.

Although pleurodesis of benign effusions, such as those occurring with CHF, nephrotic syndrome, and idiopathic

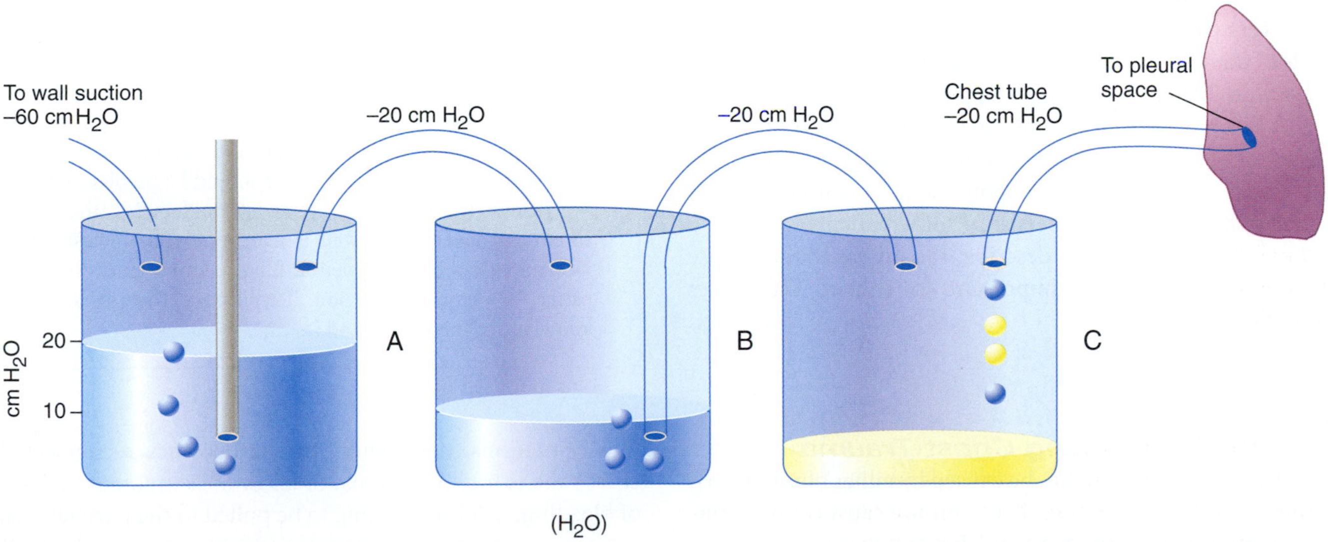

FIGURE 27-5 The standard three-bottle system is the basis for all commercial chest tube drainage systems. Pleural fluid and pleural air enter compartment **C,** which serves as a fluid collection trap so that the water-seal fluid volume will not rise (compartment **B**) and create resistance to air escaping the chest. Air cannot be inspired into the chest because of the water in compartment **B.** Open entrainment of room air through a submerged tube in compartment **A** buffers the amount of wall suction applied (–60 cm H_2O) to the height of the water column to standardize the pressure (–20 cm H_2O) transmitted to the chest.

chylothorax, has been performed successfully, the procedure is discouraged for pleural effusions that are not malignant. Most pleural effusions are best managed by controlling the underlying condition.[20]

Pleuroperitoneal Shunt and Indwelling Catheter

In refractory pleural effusions that cannot be treated adequately with pleurodesis, a small pump (PleurX, CareFusion, San Diego, CA) can be placed subcutaneously and tubes placed in the pleural and peritoneal spaces. The pleuroperitoneal connection has a one-way valve and a pumping mechanism to allow the patient to expel pleural fluid from the negatively pressurized chest to the positively pressurized peritoneum. The pleuroperitoneal shunt is placed as a last resort for refractory pleural effusions for which there is no other treatment.

More commonly, an indwelling catheter is placed into the pleural space and tunneled under the skin to prevent infections. This catheter then exits the skin and has an adapter that hangs outside of the body. The patient or family member then connects this catheter to vacuum bottles that fill with pleural fluid. Pleural fluid can be removed at home for recurrent effusions. If the pleural space is kept dry, a pleurodesis often results and the catheter can then be removed.[21]

PNEUMOTHORAX

Pneumothorax is air in the pleural space. Although air can enter the pleural space from outside the body, as occurs in sucking chest wounds, most cases of pneumothorax occur when disruption of the visceral pleura allows air from the lung to enter the pleural space. Pneumothorax is discussed according to the causative (etiologic) factor because traumatic pneumothorax is managed differently from spontaneous pneumothorax.

Chest pain, which is typically sharp and abrupt, occurs in nearly every patient with pneumothorax. Palpation of the chest wall does not worsen the pain, although respiratory efforts may be difficult. Dyspnea occurs in approximately two-thirds of patients when decreases in vital capacity and PO_2, probably as a result of airway closure at low lung volumes, cause $\dot{V}/\dot{Q}$ defects and shunting. When a spontaneous pneumothorax is evacuated, hypoxemia may persist in some patients.

The following sections describe the diseases that cause pneumothorax and the important treatment differences among them.

> **MINI CLINI**
>
> **Indwelling Catheter Care**
>
> **PROBLEM:** A patient with a malignant pleural effusion has an indwelling PleurX catheter placed during his hospitalization and is now ready for hospital discharge. The nurse on the ward asks you to assist with discharge planning of the patient with this device.
>
> **SOLUTION:** The care of an indwelling catheter at home requires the involvement of a dedicated caregiver who needs to be taught about proper catheter care, timing and technique of drainage, and vacuum bottle inventory. There is often one individual in a hospital that is most knowledgeable to provide this teaching. Often, this person is a respiratory therapist. Note that the brand name of PleurX is unique to the first company that advanced this technology and other catheter systems are available.
>
> Teaching is facilitated by online resources from the catheter manufacturer that provide reading materials for home use. However, there is no substitute for hands-on training. If a PleurX catheter arrives on the hospital ward, dedicated time for teaching home care is best done a few days before hospital discharge. This allows the home care provider to have a better comfort level and causes fewer questions after the patient returns to home.
>
> One major risk is infection. The risk for infection is sometimes worse than with other wounds because many of these patients have cancer and may be immune suppressed by chemotherapy or radiation. Infection can occur at the skin surface or by introducing an infection at the vacuum bottle adapter. The skin wound should be kept with a clean dressing, and signs of colored discharge or redness should prompt medical evaluation. A suture is left in place for some time after placement, and a suture abscess should prompt medical evaluation. To prevent introducing bacteria inside the catheter, the adapter should be cleaned before vacuum bottle attachment.
>
> The number of vacuum bottles needed and the timing of drainage is determined by the volume of pleural fluid on previous drainage days. The goal of the catheter is to keep the pleural space dry enough to allow a natural pleurodesis by growth of cancer cells between the parietal and visceral pleura. The other goal is dyspnea relief. Vacuum bottle inventory and access is determined by local resources but should be preplanned.
>
> Ultimately, the management of a PleurX catheter and whether it can be removed is a medical team decision best informed by a diary of pleural fluid volume removal and the patient's medical condition. Respiratory therapists should know about this device and its care.

Traumatic

Blunt and Penetrating Chest Trauma

Traumatic pneumothorax can be caused by either blunt or penetrating wounds of the thorax. The common causes of penetrating wounds include gunshots and knife punctures. In many cases, penetrating trauma to the chest can be managed conservatively with a chest tube. The clear indications for entering the chest surgically are uncontrolled bleeding from intercostal or pulmonary arteries and injury to the heart or great vessels. In these situations, the pneumothorax becomes secondary. The chest tube is multifunctional to allow measurement of the rate of bleeding, to allow the lung to be pulled to the parietal pleural surface to compress or tamponade bleeding, and to allow maximum ventilation.

In blunt trauma to the chest, pneumothorax can be the result of a rib fracture that enters the lung parenchyma and allows air to leak into the pleural space. For this type of injury, a chest tube is placed and the rib fractures need no specific therapy. A more common injury is alveolar rupture, which breaks through the pleural membrane.

Two special injuries that produce pneumothorax are tracheal fracture and esophageal rupture. Tracheal fracture results from severe deceleration injury and often occurs along with fractures of the anterior aspect of the first through third ribs. In this case, urgent bronchoscopy is appropriate because tracheal fracture must be corrected surgically. Esophageal rupture produces an air fluid level in the pleural space. Pleural fluid amylase level is elevated from a salivary source.

Large-caliber chest tubes are placed for trauma-related pneumothoraces to allow exit of blood and blood clots, which can be difficult to remove through small-bore catheters. Air leaks from an injured lung can be large. When bleeding is a major component of pleural injury, two chest tubes are used: a posterior chest tube to drain blood that is gravity-dependent and an anterior and apical chest tube to drain air that moves to the lung apex in the absence of pleural disease.

Iatrogenic

Iatrogenic pneumothorax is the most common type of traumatic pneumothorax. Common causes are punctures of the lung from needle aspiration lung biopsy, thoracentesis, and central venous catheter placement. Unusual causes, such as feeding tube placement into the pleural space, also have been recorded. Because the pleural rupture is typically small in the absence of parenchymal lung disease, these lung punctures usually resolve within 24 hours and can be observed without chest tubes as long as serial radiographs are obtained.

Neonatal

In radiographic series, spontaneous pneumothorax occurs in 1% to 2% of all infants soon after birth.[22] The cause of pneumothorax is likely high transpulmonary pressure during birth coupled with transient bronchial blockade caused by meconium, mucus, or aspiration of blood that can produce transpulmonary pressure gradients as high as 100 cm H_2O.

Recognizing pneumothorax is difficult because breath sounds are transmitted widely through the chest of the neonate. A shift of the heart sounds away from the side of the pneumothorax may provide a clue. Transillumination of the chest with a high-intensity light is used in some centers. Almost all neonates with pneumothorax need a chest tube.

Spontaneous

Spontaneous pneumothorax is defined as any pneumothorax caused by the escape of air into the pleural space without an obvious cause. Spontaneous pneumothoraces are of two types: (1) **primary spontaneous pneumothorax,** in which there is no underlying lung disease, and (2) **secondary spontaneous pneumothorax,** in which lung disease is present.

Primary

Primary spontaneous pneumothorax occurs without underlying lung disease. In a way, this term is a misnomer because high-resolution CT scans have shown the presence of small subpleural blebs in more than 80% of patients.[23]

Primary spontaneous pneumothorax usually occurs in patients in their late teenage years or early 20s. Patients often are tall and slender, and the lungs and pleural membrane may not have grown at the same pace; the result is airspace enlargement and a thin pleural membrane.

Results of some studies suggest that cigarette smoking is a risk factor in more than 90% of cases of primary spontaneous pneumothorax.[24] The smoking history is typically short, and smoking cessation is recommended.

Secondary

Secondary spontaneous pneumothorax occurs in patients with underlying lung disease. In most cases, the underlying lung disease is chronic obstructive pulmonary disease with some component of emphysema. Pneumothorax also can occur with asthma and cystic fibrosis, usually during an exacerbation of disease.

Interstitial lung diseases in which lung volumes are spared, such as sarcoidosis, bronchiolitis obliterans with organizing pneumonia, Langerhans cell histiocytosis, and lymphangioleiomyomatosis, have a higher incidence than do diseases without any component of obstruction.

Depending on the extent of parenchymal lung disease, pneumothorax in this population can be devastating. A Veterans Affairs cooperative study included 185 patients with secondary spontaneous pneumothorax and monitored them for 5 years.[25] Although only 3 patients died of pneumothorax, the mortality rate was 43%.[1] Severe underlying lung disease caused most of these deaths. This finding suggested that most pneumothoraces occur in patients with severe lung dysfunction. The degree of dyspnea is disproportionate to the size of pneumothorax in this group of patients because pulmonary reserve is already diminished. Pneumothorax usually should be evacuated and not simply watched in this patient cohort.

Catamenial Pneumothorax

Catamenial pneumothorax occurs in association with menstruation and usually is recurrent and right-sided. The reason for the right-sided predominance is unclear. Many patients have endometriosis on the pleural surface, although it may be impossible to see because of hormonal involution during menses. Once the diagnosis is considered, catamenial pneumothorax is not difficult to manage in that most patients do not have a recurrence when ovulation is suppressed.

Complications

Tension Pneumothorax

Tension pneumothorax occurs when air in the pleural space exceeds atmospheric pressure. The radiographic appearance includes mediastinal shift to the contralateral side, diaphragmatic depression, and expansion of the ribs. The lung does not necessarily collapse completely if it is involved with a disease process such as ARDS.

MINI CLINI

Subcutaneous Emphysema

PROBLEM: A patient with ARDS experiences subcutaneous emphysema. How does the clinician determine where the air leak is occurring? Is a pneumothorax always present?

SOLUTION: Subcutaneous emphysema occurs when air enters the soft tissues. Although physical examination reveals subcutaneous bubbles, the patient's family needs to be reassured that the condition is rarely, if ever, physiologically significant. What is important to recognize, however, is that alveolar disruption has occurred, most commonly as the result of barotrauma.

Barotrauma disrupts alveoli and allows air to enter the interstitium of the lung. Rupture of the visceral pleura allows air to produce a pneumothorax, or the air can travel along the low-resistance tissue planes of the bronchovascular bundles and through the hilum of the lung to enter the mediastinum. From the mediastinum, air has easy access to the retroperitoneal space, including the scrotum and the neck. The presence of subcutaneous air does not necessarily mean that pneumothorax has occurred, although the risk factors for its development are present.

Air under pressure in the pleural space can enter the subcutaneous tissues through the intercostal incision made for chest tube placement. Subcutaneous air often is seen on a chest radiograph after chest tube placement, but the air rarely spreads unless the chest tube is occluded.

In the absence of pneumothorax, there is no way to determine which lung is causing subcutaneous emphysema. For any deterioration in gas exchange, radiographs should be repeated. Because air in the mediastinum can displace the mediastinal parietal pleura, it can be difficult to tell without chest CT whether a small pneumothorax is present. Because patients often are too unstable to be moved, a chest tube sometimes is placed because the potential benefits are greater than the risks.

Not all patients with radiographic tension have the physiologic changes commonly associated with tension pneumothorax. However, almost all pneumothoraces that occur during mechanical ventilation enlarge if not drained.

As pressure in the thorax increases and mediastinal shift places torsion on the inferior vena cava, venous return to the right side of the heart decreases. Cardiac output decreases, and hypotension with tachycardia results. Hypoxemia occurs as the lung continues to compress because of intrapulmonary shunting through the collapsed lung.

The respiratory therapist can make the diagnosis of tension pneumothorax. Treatment is emergency decompression of the chest. This procedure usually is done with an 18-gauge intravenous (e.g., Jelco, Smiths Medical, Dublin, OH) catheter inserted just over the second rib on the anterior aspect of the chest in the midclavicular line. Catheter placement should elicit a rush of air through the catheter, and this sign confirms the diagnosis. The blood pressure should recover rapidly, although resolution of hypoxemia depends on complete lung reexpansion and can be delayed. The soft intravenous catheter can be left in place while a more conventional chest tube is inserted.

RULE OF THUMB

Tension pneumothorax is a clinical diagnosis made at the bedside in more than 50% of cases. The clinical signs are diminished breath sounds, hyperresonance to percussion, tachycardia, and hypotension.

In one case series of 74 patients with tension pneumothorax, a clinical diagnosis was made for 45 patients; the associated mortality rate was 7%. In the other cases, the diagnosis was delayed from the onset of clinical signs by 30 minutes to 8 hours, resulting in a 31% mortality rate.[26]

Respiratory therapists are in the perfect position to make a timely diagnosis because ventilator alarms give early warnings.

Reexpansion Pulmonary Edema

Reexpansion pulmonary edema occurs in a lung that has been rapidly reinflated from low lung volumes, particularly when the pneumothorax has been long-standing or when the pressure gradient across the lung has become high, as might occur when there is endobronchial obstruction from cancer, mucus, or blood.

For many years, it was believed that alveolar edema occurs because intraalveolar pressure becomes negative and pulls fluid from the vasculature. However, the lung fluid has high protein content, a finding that suggests blood vessels have been injured as well.

One of the proposed mechanisms of vascular injury is a phenomenon of reperfusion injury caused by reactive oxygen (O_2) species. Support for this hypothesis has come from experimental studies that have shown administration of antioxidants before reexpansion decreases the amount of reexpansion pulmonary edema.

Regardless of the cause, lung reexpansion in nonemergency situations should proceed slowly and transpulmonary pressure should not become excessive. Most physicians who insert a chest tube for a large pneumothorax first place it to water seal without suction. If the lung is not completely inflated on the subsequent chest radiograph, the chest tube is placed to suction. Reexpansion pulmonary edema also occurs after drainage of pleural effusions. As a rule, thoracentesis should be limited to approximately 1000 ml, unless pleural pressures are monitored and not allowed to fall below −20 cm H_2O.

Diagnosis

The diagnosis of pneumothorax is established with chest radiography or ultrasound. The diagnosis requires a high-quality film to visualize a visceral pleural line. In the ICU, as many as 30% of cases of pneumothorax may be missed on a chest radiograph in retrospect. Impediments to diagnosis include a low-quality radiograph or using a computer monitor, supine position of the patient, concomitant presence of mediastinal air, and subpulmonic or mediastinal position of the pneumothorax. Diagnosis is enhanced with additional upright radiographs or decubitus views.

The size of a pneumothorax is difficult to assess with a chest radiograph because a two-dimensional picture is being taken of a three-dimensional thorax. Size can be estimated with volume equations and can be confirmed with CT if needed.

RULE OF THUMB

The size of a pneumothorax on a chest radiograph can be estimated with the knowledge that the volume of the lung and thorax is proportional to the cube of their diameters.

For example, on a chest radiograph, the chest measures 8 cm from the spine to the lateral chest wall. A pneumothorax is measured 2 cm from the chest wall.

$$\text{Volume of the lung} = (6\text{ cm})^3 \approx 216\text{ cm}^3$$
$$\text{Volume of the hemithorax} = (8\text{ cm})^3 = 512\text{ cm}^3$$
$$\text{Lung size} = 216/512 = 42\%$$
$$\text{Pneumothorax size} \approx 58\%$$

The equation shows the large volume of lung that a pneumothorax can displace despite a "small" distance from the lung to the chest wall. Use of the equation is not as accurate as chest CT because many pneumothoraces collapse asymmetrically.

The diagnosis of pneumothorax by ultrasound occurs when the normal finding of lung sliding is lost. Ultrasound is not capable of judging the size of the pneumothorax because air in the pleural space does not transmit sound waves and the lung is not seen.

Therapy

Oxygen

O_2 should be administered to all patients who have a pneumothorax. Most of the air in a pneumothorax is nitrogen (N) because O_2 is readily absorbed. If an air leak is continuing, supplemental O_2 rather than N leaks into the pleural space. After an air leak has been stopped, administering O_2 decreases the blood and tissue partial pressure of N surrounding the pleural space. Pneumothorax resolution is normally 1.25% of the air per day. O_2 speeds recovery by increasing the gradient of N from the pleural space to the pleural tissues.

Observation

A 2001 consensus conference recommended observing patients in stable condition with primary spontaneous pneumothorax and also some patients with small secondary spontaneous pneumothorax before recurrence prevention is administered.[27] A small iatrogenic pneumothorax also should be managed with observation. Primary spontaneous pneumothorax often is observed for 4 hours in the emergency department (ED) before discharge to home follow-up care as long as the pneumothorax is not found to enlarge on serial chest radiographs. Discharged patients should have ready access to emergency care facilities and should be advised to return if they experience any worsened dyspnea or pain.

Patients with secondary spontaneous pneumothorax should be admitted to the hospital. During observation, it is important to record the respiratory rate and any signs of deteriorating respiratory function. A decrease in the patient's O_2 saturation can be an early warning of pneumothorax enlargement. Any deterioration indicates that the pneumothorax must be drained.

Simple Aspiration

Simple aspiration can be used in the ED when pneumothorax is first detected. A small catheter is placed into the pleural space, and air is sequentially evacuated with a three-way stopcock until no more air can be removed. If more than 4 L of air is aspirated and no resistance to further aspiration is felt, a chest tube is needed for continuing pleural air leak.

The goal of aspiration is to reexpand the lung. Many patients have a pneumothorax from air leak that subsequently heals between the time of onset and the time treatment is sought in the ED. Patients with primary spontaneous pneumothorax who undergo simple aspiration for lung reexpansion and who have a stable chest radiograph 4 hours after aspiration can go home without hospital admission.

Chest Tubes

Chest thoracostomy tubes (chest tubes) come in a variety of sizes, from 7F to 40F, and can be connected to a variety of one-way devices (e.g., Heimlich valves) that prevent entry of air into the pleural space from the outside environment. Regardless of chest tube size and the presence of a Heimlich valve or water seal, the effectiveness of chest tube placement for pneumothorax resolution depends more on lung surface healing than on the device used.

Small Bore. One simple device is a small-bore 7F catheter with a one-way valve apparatus (Heimlich valve) that prevents air movement back into the chest. Small-bore catheters can be placed with a small skin incision followed by either a guidewire and dilator technique or a trocar to get through the parietal pleura.

All chest tubes used to drain pneumothorax should be directed to the apex of the lung. Small-bore catheters can be placed in the second intercostal space anteriorly in the midclavicular line or laterally in the chest from the fifth through the seventh intercostal space.

It is difficult to determine whether a Heimlich valve has an ongoing leak unless it is placed to seal under water. This procedure can be done in the ED by placing the Heimlich valve into a cup of water or by placing it in line with a water-seal chamber to see whether an air leak is continuing after lung expansion.

Large Bore. Large-bore chest tubes usually are connected to a commercial equivalent of a three-bottle system to collect any pleural fluid present, determine whether an air leak is ongoing, and measure intrapleural pressure (Figure 27-6). Inserting large-bore catheters is done with local anesthetic and blunt dissection of soft tissue down to the parietal pleura.

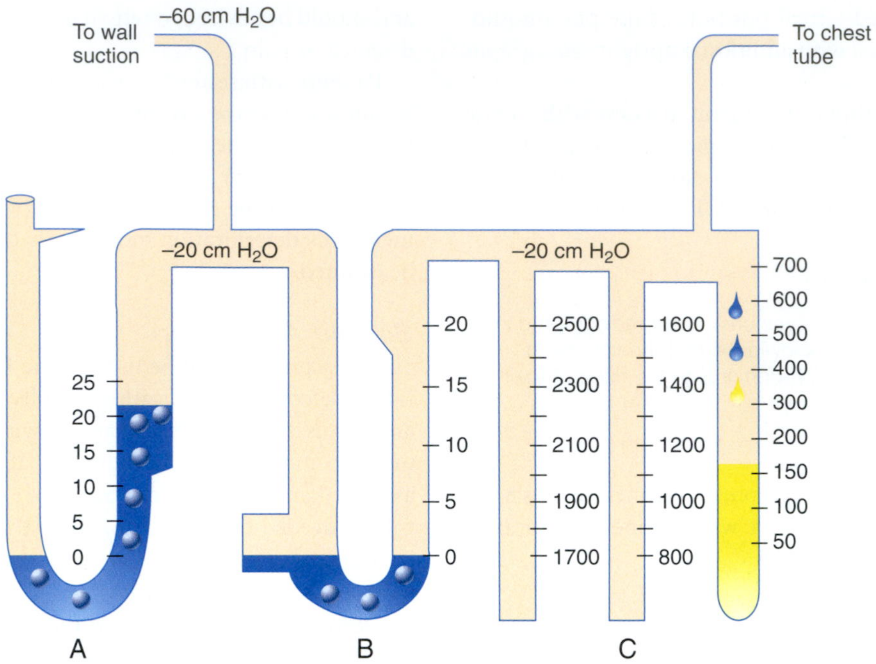

FIGURE 27-6 The Pleur-evac chest tube collection system collects fluid in compartment *C* so that it will not spill into the water-seal compartment *(B)*. A patent chest tube should cause respiratory variation to be seen on the scale adjacent to compartment *B*, which measures intrapleural pressure. Compartment *B* also is the place to see bubbles if an air leak is present. The water level in compartment *A* controls intrapleural pressure and should be adjusted daily.

Dissection should be wide enough to allow insertion of a finger into the pleural space to ensure that no adhesions are holding the lung close to the insertion site and to allow unobstructed entrance of the tube into the pleural space, where it can be directed to the position of choice.

Chest tubes are secured with sutures. The insertion distance should be recorded and be checked on subsequent days to ensure that the chest tube does not migrate outward. Should the most proximal hole in the tube emerge from the skin, air will enter the tube and it will appear as if the lung is persistently leaking.

Another problem of apparent chest tube leak can occur when the insertion wound is large enough to allow air entry into the pleural space. This usually is accompanied by a sucking sound at the entrance, which can be occluded with petroleum gauze.

A chest radiograph is routinely obtained, although unless a lateral radiograph also is obtained, confirming the precise placement of the tube is often difficult. In addition, many chest tubes end up in the major fissure, where their function may be suboptimal.

Chest tube removal remains a highly variable practice. Removal of a chest tube as soon as an air leak visually ceases is associated with a 25% rate of recurrence of pneumothorax. The recurrence rate is near zero when chest tubes are removed 48 hours after the air leak no longer is seen in the water-seal chamber.[28] A common practice of clamping the chest tube, with chest radiographs before and after a 4-hour observation period, can be accompanied by the return of pneumothorax. If symptoms develop during chest tube clamping, the clamp should be removed immediately and the presence of air leak assessed.

Bronchopleural Fistula

Two terms are used for continuing air leaks from the lung through a chest tube. A **bronchopleural fistula** (BPF) is a large air leak that classically was described after surgery in which the airway was cut. Because some surgeons insist that BPF be reserved for this situation, the term **alveolopleural fistula** has been recently used for large air leaks that come from the lung tissue and that do not heal rapidly. Many patients with persistent air leaks are receiving mechanical ventilation, and positive airway pressures contribute to perpetuating the pleural air.

Because persistent air leaks can leak large quantities of air, more than one chest tube may be used to approximate the lung to the chest wall. This maneuver results in tamponade of the site of the air leak and allows pleural healing to occur.

Therapy for BPF involves meticulous monitoring of tidal volume, airway pressures, and positive end-expiratory pressure (PEEP); avoidance of auto-PEEP; and consideration of bronchoscopic closure or thoracoscopic surgery.[29]

Pleurodesis

Patients who have had one pneumothorax are more likely than the general population to have a second. The recurrence rate is greater than 30% among patients with primary spontaneous pneumothorax and approximately 40% among patients with secondary spontaneous pneumothorax. These high recurrence rates indicate that preventing a recurrent pneumothorax should be a priority, particularly for patients in whom pneumothorax may be life-threatening. Preventing recurrence involves production of adhesions between the parietal and the visceral pleurae in the involved area and is termed *pleurodesis*.

The most noninvasive approaches to pleurodesis involve chemical sclerosis of the pleural space through the chest tube once the pleural air leak has stopped. The two most common preparations used for pleurodesis currently in the United States include 500 mg of doxycycline or 5 g of talc mixed into a 50-ml syringe of sterile saline solution. The agent is injected through the chest tube into the pleural space. Then the chest tube is clamped for 2 hours before drainage is allowed.

More invasive methods have included thoracoscopy with pleural poudrage (blowing talc onto the pleural surface under direct visualization), pleural abrasion through a thoracoscope, and thoracotomy with pleurectomy (removing the pleural surface to ensure lung adhesion). Recent recommendations are for pleurodesis to occur after the first secondary spontaneous pneumothorax with thoracoscopic bullae stapling and talc poudrage.[27]

MINI CLINI

Alveolopleural Fistula

PROBLEM: Pneumothorax develops in a patient undergoing ventilation for pneumonia. A 20F chest tube is placed and the lung fails to reexpand, although a large amount of air is passing through the water-seal chamber. The patient's minute ventilation is 20 L/min to keep gas exchange stable. What is the problem?

SOLUTION: The problem is an alveolopleural fistula caused by a large hole in the pleura that is difficult to manage. The lung surface of patients with underlying emphysema can contain large bullae that do not heal readily once ruptured. Large pleural holes also can develop in patients with necrotizing pneumonia and those who have undergone surgery on the lung.

The Fanning equation tells us that humidified airflow through a chest tube is proportional to the chest tube radius to the fifth power. Therefore the chest tube radius is the most important determinant of maximal airflow. Airflow through large air leaks has been measured as high as 16 L/min, a volume impossible to remove through a chest tube smaller than 24F, regardless of the amount of pressure applied.

This patient should receive a second, larger chest tube. The seal of the chest tube at the skin surface should be inspected to ensure that no air is entering the body from the outside. The position of both chest tubes should be confirmed either by x-ray examination or by hand to ensure the tubes are in the pleural space. Once the lung is expanded, the minute ventilation should decrease because effective alveolar ventilation will be improved.

Flow through stopcocks and chest tube collection devices is governed by the same considerations as chest tube size. The manufacturer of the chest tube collection device in your hospital will have the resistance figures necessary to ensure that 16 L/min of airflow can be accommodated.

Because the diseases that produce pneumothorax often involve both lungs, patients may experience sequential events in opposite lungs. In this situation, median sternotomy with bilateral abrasion or pleurectomy can be performed, particularly for patients at considerable risk for developing a pneumothorax, such as divers and aviators.

MINI CLINI

Measuring a Pleural Air Leak

PROBLEM: Pneumothorax develops in a patient with ARDS, and a chest tube is placed to reexpand the lung. Before the pneumothorax developed, the patient was ventilated easily at a rate of 16 breaths/min, which delivered a tidal volume (V_T) of 500 ml, and was exhaling 450 ml (a small difference caused by endotracheal cuff leak and tubing compliance). Since the pneumothorax developed, the patient needs a rate of 30 breaths at the same V_T to keep the $PaCO_2$ level the same. Exhaled V_T is 300 ml. What is the approximate size of this patient's air leak? What ventilation options are appropriate?

SOLUTION: Although research laboratories can measure airflow through a chest tube precisely with a pneumotachometer, clinical care can be provided by estimating the pleural air leak.

The following simple calculations suggest that the excess difference in returned V_T (450 to 300 ml or 150 ml) is due to air passing through the BPF:

30 breaths/min (150 ml differential = 4.5 L of pleural ventilation)

One other problem is that large amounts of carbon dioxide (CO_2) (up to 20%) may be removed through the chest tube.[30] Removal of CO_2 is beneficial because it allows lower V_T and respiratory rates for any given PCO_2. However, as the BPF closes, CO_2 will no longer be eliminated through the chest tube but only through the endotracheal tube, necessitating higher minute ventilation to maintain CO_2 clearance. This need for higher minute ventilation might falsely suggest that ARDS is worsening, when in reality the BPF is closing.

Nevertheless, when the air leak is measured with every ventilatory change, the mode of ventilation that minimizes air leak is the one most likely to allow pleural healing. Breath-by-breath analysis shows the difference between delivered V_T and exhaled V_T and approximates the volume of the pleural leak.

PEEP can be a major cause of large air leaks and should be turned off unless necessary for maintaining PO_2. Because there is no such thing as a true plateau pressure when air is exiting a BPF, V_T should be adjusted to produce the lowest peak airway pressure that can sustain ventilation and oxygenation. Position the patient so that the lung with the air leak is down (i.e., in the bed).[31]

Auto-PEEP can be impossible to measure if the fistula is large and decompressing the airways. Therefore, long expiratory times are preferred. Trials of pressure-controlled and high-frequency jet ventilation are appropriate. In a practical sense, these adjustments are the same ones made to prevent barotrauma in the first place and are limited by the severity of lung injury, which requires more support than would optimally close the air leak.

MINI CLINI

Management of a Bronchopleural Fistula

PROBLEM: A 40-year-old trauma patient with ARDS cannot be ventilated because of a large (16 L/min) BPF located entirely in the left lung. If surgery is not possible, what ventilatory options would be appropriate?

SOLUTION: Two ventilatory interventions have been attempted for large BPFs. The first is placement of a double-lumen endotracheal tube, which can carry most ventilation and PEEP on the right lung while underventilating the lung with the fistula to aid in its closure.[32] Long-term double-lumen ventilation is difficult because of tenuous tube position, the need for continuous paralysis, difficulty with secretion clearance, and high airway resistance through the small endotracheal tube lumens.

The second intervention is applying positive pressure to the chest tube. This back pressure increases resistance across the BPF and allows the remainder of the lung to better ventilate. One simple way to add chest tube resistance is to connect a PEEP valve to the expiratory port of the water-seal chamber.[33] PEEP usually is placed at the same level as the ventilator PEEP. Inspiratory pressures exceed PEEP, and air flows through the chest tube. However, as expiratory pressures equilibrate, PEEP can be held within the lung, allowing the beneficial effects on oxygenation.

Pressurizing the chest tube entails synchronous closure of the chest tube during inspiration[34] and requires specialized equipment that must be set up under controlled conditions. When used in combination with an in-line PEEP valve, BPF flow can be slowed during both inspiration and expiration.

These techniques usually increase the volume of intrapleural air. The net effect on oxygenation requires careful bedside observation because hypoxemia can worsen with any degree of lung collapse. Tension pneumothorax can occur so the patient must be monitored closely.

ROLE OF THE RESPIRATORY THERAPIST IN PLEURAL DISEASES

The respiratory therapist (RT) may play an important role in both the diagnosis and management of pleural disease. Diagnostically, the therapist's careful palpation and auscultation of the chest may show the dullness and decreased breath sounds that may prompt suspicion of a pleural effusion and lead the physician to order the imaging studies to confirm the presence of a pleural effusion. The RT who is managing the ventilator is often in the earliest position to appreciate a pneumothorax because the patient's ventilatory function would change when a pneumothorax develops. Furthermore, the RT may be called on to assist in performing a thoracentesis or placing a chest tube. Therapeutically, the RT may be called on to assist in setting up the fluid collection chamber after the chest tube is placed or in performing a talc pleurodesis. This broad spectrum of potential roles for the RT makes knowledge of the diagnosis and management of pleural disease essential for the capable RT.

SUMMARY CHECKLIST

- Pleural effusions form when excess pleural fluid is produced by the lung or chest wall in sufficient quantities to overcome the resorptive capacity of the pleural lymphatic vessels.
- Pleural fluid analysis is the key to understanding the specific cause of any pleural effusion.
- Transudates have a pleural fluid total protein level less than 0.5 and an LDH level less than 0.6 of the respective serum values. Common causes of a transudative effusion include CHF, nephrosis, and cirrhosis.
- Pleural fluid drainage returns approximately one-third of the lung volume as measured by FVC. The other two-thirds of fluid drainage allow the diaphragm to rise and the chest wall to normalize.
- Pneumothorax size is underestimated with a one-dimensional view of the chest. Measurement accuracy requires a three-dimensional perspective.
- The risk factors for pneumothorax and pneumomediastinum are the same. Air ruptures a pleural membrane in pneumothorax, and air passes through the lung hilum in pneumomediastinum.
- O_2 therapy speeds resolution of all pneumothoraces by improving N absorption.
- Chest tube flow depends on tube size, stopcock size, and collection system resistance.
- Breath-by-breath measurement of an air leak can be approximated by the difference between inspired and expired volumes (in the absence of endotracheal cuff leaks).
- The mode of ventilation that produces the least fistula airflow is the most likely to produce healing.
- Methods to decrease BPF airflow include lowering *tidal volume,* lowering respiratory rate, lowering PEEP, and avoiding auto-PEEP. In more severe cases, positioning the affected lung down, double-lumen tube ventilation, adding PEEP valves to the chest tube, inspiratory chest tube occlusion, or thoracic surgery should be considered.

References

1. Noppen M, De Waele M, Li R, et al: Volume and cellular content of normal pleural fluid in humans examined by pleural lavage. *Am J Respir Crit Care Med* 162:1023–1026, 2000.
2. Light RW: *Pleural diseases*, ed 2, Philadelphia, 1990, Lea & Febiger.
3. Sahn SA: The diagnostic value of pleural fluid analysis. *Semin Respir Crit Care Med* 16:269–278, 1995.
4. Light RW, Macgregor MI, Luchsinger PC, et al: Pleural effusions: the diagnostic separation of transudates and exudates. *Ann Intern Med* 77:507–513, 1972.
5. Staub NC, Wiener-Kronish JP, Albertine JP: Transport through the pleura: physiology of normal liquid and solute exchange in the pleural space. In Chrétien J, Bignon J, Hirsch A, editors: *The pleura in health and disease*, New York, 1985, Marcel Dekker.
6. Wiener-Kronish JP, Matthay MA, Callen PW, et al: Relationship of pleural effusions to pulmonary hemodynamics in patients with congestive heart failure. *Am Rev Respir Dis* 132:1253–1256, 1985.
7. Peterman TA, Brothers SK: Pleural effusions in congestive heart failure and in pericardial disease. *N Engl J Med* 309:313, 1983.

8. Lieberman FL, Hidemura R, Peters RL, et al: Pathogenesis and treatment of hydrothorax complicating cirrhosis with ascites. *Ann Intern Med* 64:341–351, 1966.
9. Lieberman FL, Hidemura R, Peters RL, et al: Parapneumonic effusions. *Am J Med* 69:507–511, 1980.
10. Colice GL, Curtis A, Deslauriers J, et al: Medical and surgical treatment of parapneumonic effusions: an evidence-based guideline. *Chest* 118:1158–1171, 2000.
11. Razazi K, Thille AW, Carteaux G, et al: Effects of pleural effusion drainage on oxygenation, respiratory mechanics, and hemodynamics in mechanically ventilated patients. *Ann Am Thorac Soc* 11:1018–1024, 2014.
12. Berger HW, Mejia E: Tuberculous pleurisy. *Chest* 63:88–92, 1973.
13. Light RW, George RB: Incidence and significance of pleural effusion after abdominal surgery. *Chest* 69:621–625, 1976.
14. Sahn SA: State of the art: the pleura. *Am Rev Respir Dis* 138:184–234, 1988.
15. Seriff NS, Cohen ML, Samuel P, et al: Chylothorax: diagnosis by lipoprotein electrophoresis of serum and pleural fluid. *Thorax* 32:98–100, 1977.
16. Strange C: Hemothorax. *Semin Respir Crit Care Med* 16:324, 1995.
17. Collins TR, Sahn SA: Thoracocentesis: clinical value, complications, technical problems, and patient experience. *Chest* 91:817–822, 1987.
18. Walker-Renard PB, Vaughan LM, Sahn SA: Chemical pleurodesis for malignant pleural effusions. *Ann Intern Med* 120:56–64, 1994.
19. Kennedy L, Sahn SA: Talc pleurodesis for the treatment of pneumothorax and pleural effusion. *Chest* 106:1215–1222, 1994.
20. Sudduth CD, Sahn SA: Pleurodesis for nonmalignant pleural effusions: recommandations. *Chest* 102:1855–1860, 1992.
21. Bhatnagar R, Maskell NA: Indwelling pleural catheters. *Respiration* 88:74–85, 2014.
22. Chernick V, Reed MH: Pneumothorax and chylothorax in the neonatal period. *J Pediatr* 76:624–632, 1970.
23. Bense L, Lewander R, Eklund G, et al: Nonsmoking, non-alpha 1-antitrypsin deficiency-induced emphysema in nonsmokers with healed spontaneous pneumothorax, identified by computed tomography of the lungs. *Chest* 103:433–438, 1993.
24. Bense L, Eklund G, Wiman LG: Smoking and the increased risk of contracting spontaneous pneumothorax. *Chest* 92:1009–1012, 1987.
25. Light RW, O'Hara VS, Moritz TE, et al: Intrapleural tetracycline for the prevention of recurrent spontaneous pneumothorax: results of a Department of Veterans Affairs cooperative study. *JAMA* 264:2224–2230, 1990.
26. Steier M, Ching N, Roberts EB, et al: Pneumothorax complicating continuous ventilatory support. *J Thorac Cardiovasc Surg* 67:17–23, 1979.
27. Baumann MH, Strange C, Heffner JE, et al: Management of spontaneous pneumothorax: an American College of Chest Physicians Delphi consensus statement. *Chest* 119:590–602, 2001.
28. Sharma TN, Agnihotri SP, Jain NK, et al: Intercostal tube thoracostomy in pneumothorax. *Indian J Chest Dis Allied Sci* 30:32–35, 1988.
29. Baumann MH, Sahn SA: Medical management and therapy of bronchopleural fistulas in the mechanically ventilated patient. *Chest* 97:721–738, 1990.
30. Bishop MJ, Benson MS, Pierson DJ: Carbon dioxide excretion via bronchopleural fistulas in adult respiratory distress syndrome. *Chest* 91:400–402, 1987.
31. Lau KY: Postural management of bronchopleural fistula. *Chest* 94:1122, 1988.
32. Dodds CP, Hillman KM: Management of massive air leak with asynchronous independent lung ventilation. *Intensive Care Med* 8:287–290, 1982.
33. Weksler N, Ovadia L: The challenge of bilateral bronchopleural fistula. *Chest* 95:938–939, 1989.
34. Gallagher TJ, Smith RA, Kirby RR, et al: Intermittent inspiratory chest tube occlusion to limit bronchopleural cutaneous airleaks. *Crit Care Med* 4:328–382, 1976.

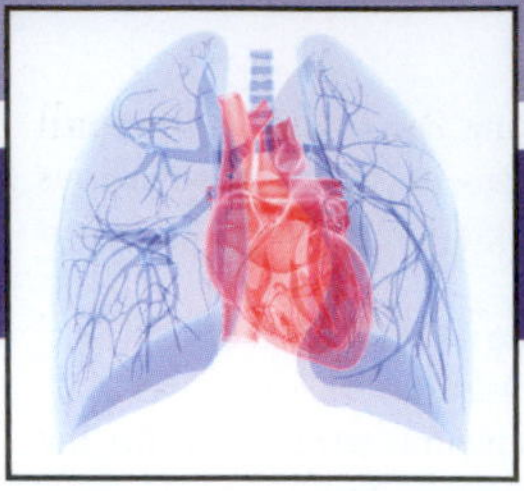

CHAPTER 28

Pulmonary Vascular Disease

ADRIANO R. TONELLI AND RAED A. DWEIK

CHAPTER OBJECTIVES

After reading this chapter you will be able to:
- State how many patients develop venous thromboembolism each year.
- Describe how and where thromboemboli originate.
- Describe how pulmonary emboli alter lung and cardiac function.
- Identify the clinical features and electrocardiographic, chest radiograph, and arterial blood gas findings associated with pulmonary embolism.
- Describe how pulmonary embolism is diagnosed and managed.
- Describe the hemodynamic findings associated with pulmonary hypertension.
- Describe the possible mechanisms believed to be responsible for pulmonary arterial hypertension (PAH).
- State who is at risk for the development of PAH.
- Identify the clinical features associated with PAH.
- Describe the treatment used to care for patients with PAH.
- Describe the pathogenesis and management of PH associated with chronic obstructive pulmonary disease.

CHAPTER OUTLINE

KEY TERMS

deep venous thrombosis
pulmonary embolism
pulmonary arterial hypertension
pulmonary hypertension
venous thromboembolism

The vessels of the lung can be affected by many conditions, including clots and narrowing of the pulmonary arteries, conditions referred as **pulmonary embolism** (PE) and **pulmonary hypertension** (PH). PE occurs when a fragment of the thrombus in the venous system travels to the lung and pulmonary circulation. The thrombus usually originates in the deep veins of the lower extremities and therefore is called **deep venous thrombosis** (DVT). DVT and PE are grouped in the category named *venous thromboembolism* (VTE). *Pulmonary hypertension* is a term that defines an increase in the pressure in the pulmonary arteries that could result from a large number of conditions that affect the lung vessels, lung parenchyma, and/or the heart.

This chapter reviews disorders associated with the pulmonary vasculature. It predominantly focuses on venous thromboembolic disease and **pulmonary arterial hypertension** (PAH). PAH is a particular subgroup of patients with PH who have progressive narrowing of the pulmonary arteries that, if left untreated, leads to right heart failure (cor pulmonale) and death.[1]

VENOUS THROMBOEMBOLIC DISEASE

Venous thromboembolism (VTE) is a major national health problem with an estimated prevalence of 117 cases per 100,000 persons (i.e., DVT at 48 cases per 100,000 and PE at 69 cases per 100,000) and an incidence of 200,000 to 300,000 new cases per year in the United States.[2] VTE is treatable but requires prompt diagnosis and treatment to avert serious consequences, because one-third of deaths from PE occur within 1 hour of the onset of symptoms. In more than 70% of patients who die of PE, the diagnosis is not suspected.[3] In fact, the frequency of recognizable emboli in routine autopsies of adult patients varies from 1.5% to almost 30%.[4-6] In a population-based study of PE as a cause of death in New Mexico, only 34% of 812 documented cases of PE were diagnosed before death.[5] Similarly, another study[7] showed that only 28% of cases of massive or submassive PE were diagnosed before death, a finding that emphasizes the high rate of underrecognition of this disease.

Patients with undiagnosed PE have a higher mortality rate (approximately 30%[8]) compared to those in whom the condition was recognized and treated (mortality rate <8% with generally favorable long-term outcome).[9] A high index of suspicion to detect the disease is essential, particularly in patients at risk for VTE, such as those with multiple injuries, immobilization, bed rest, or intravascular catheters and the elderly (Table 28-1). Because clinical findings of VTE are frequently misleading,[10] objective tests are needed to confirm or exclude the diagnosis.

Pathogenesis

PE is a frequent complication of DVT[11]; however, the actual source of PE is found in only half of patients[7]. PE usually arises from detached portions of venous thrombi that form in deep veins of the lower extremities or pelvis (86%). A small percentage of PE arises from the right-sided heart cavities (3.15%) or from the superior vena cava (3%).[7]

Venous thrombosis can be due to heritable and/or acquired conditions, and in more than 80%, a risk factor can be identified. Conditions that favor thrombus formation include blood *stasis,* the presence of hypercoagulable states, and vessel wall abnormalities (factors known as the *Virchow triad*). Causes of blood stagnation include local pressure, venous obstruction, immobilization, congestive heart failure, shock and dehydration, varicose veins, and enlargement of the right heart chambers. Several conditions increase the intravascular coagulability of the blood and predispose to VTE disease[12] (Box 28-1). The most frequent causes of an inherited hypercoagulable state are the factor V Leiden mutation and prothrombin gene mutation, which together account for 50% to 60 % of cases.[13] Meanwhile, the major acquired conditions associated with an hypercoagulable state are recent major surgery, trauma, immobilization, antiphospholipid antibodies, malignancy, myeloproliferative disorders, pregnancy, and use of oral contraceptives.[14] Vessel wall abnormalities are found most often in patients who have sustained trauma or have undergone major surgery.

In general, more than one risk factor is responsible for VTE.[15] In the postoperative period, diminished blood flow favors the deposition of platelets and fibrin in the venous valve cups. Associated trauma and toxins can worsen endothelial damage and promote the release of mediators that encourage further adhesion, aggregation, and degranulation of platelets, which results in activation of the coagulation cascade and clot production.

TABLE 28-1
Frequency of Venous Thrombosis in Various Hospitalized Patient Groups

Group	Frequency (%)
Orthopedic (e.g., fractured hip)	54-67
Urologic (e.g., prostatectomy)	25
Surgical patients older than 40 yr	28
Gynecologic surgery	18
Cardiovascular surgery (e.g., acute myocardial infarction)	39
Obstetrics	3

From Arroliga AC, Matthay MA, Matthay RA: Pulmonary thromboembolism and other pulmonary vascular diseases. In George RB, editor: Chest medicine: essentials of pulmonary and critical care medicine, ed 3, Baltimore, 1995, Williams & Wilkins.

Box 28-1 Conditions Predisposing to Venous Thrombosis and Pulmonary Thromboembolism

- Advanced age
- Postoperative status
- Previous venous thrombosis
- Trauma
- Oral contraceptive use
- Pregnancy
- Prolonged bed rest
- Long periods of travel
- Diagnosis of cancer
- Obesity
- Cerebrovascular accidents
- Thrombocytosis
- Erythrocytosis
- Hyperhomocysteinemia
- Mutation in gene coding for factor V (factor V Leiden)
- Mutation of prothrombin gene
- Antiphospholipid antibody
- Antithrombin deficiency
- Proteins C and S deficiency
- Abnormalities of fibrinogen
- Deficiency of plasminogen
- Sickle cell anemia
- Myeloproliferative disorder
- Paroxysmal nocturnal hemoglobinuria
- Heparin-induced thrombocytopenia

Modified from Arroliga AC, Matthay MA, Matthay RA: Pulmonary thromboembolism and other pulmonary vascular diseases. In George RB, editor: Chest medicine: essentials of pulmonary and critical care medicine, ed 3, Baltimore, 1995, Williams & Wilkins.

Pathology

PE is more frequently observed in the lower lobes and more commonly in the right rather than in the left lung, a phenomenon related to the pulmonary flow distribution that tends to favor the right side and the lower lobes.[4] Embolism to the pulmonary arteries produces pulmonary hemorrhage in the poorly perfused or infarcted lung in fewer than 10% of cases. Infarction secondary to thromboembolism is less common in the lung than in other tissues because the lung has two blood supplies, namely the pulmonary arterial and the bronchial circulations. At a capillary level, extensive connections exist between the pulmonary and bronchial circulations that prevent serious damage to lung tissue that is deprived of its pulmonary artery supply.[4] Cardiovascular diseases may affect bronchial circulation, which may lead to lung tissue necrosis when emboli occur. Pulmonary infarction is associated with thromboembolic obstruction of a medium-sized pulmonary artery and generally occurs at the lung bases, where it usually manifests as a wedge-shaped opacity on chest images. Microscopic examination of the lung in pulmonary infarction shows necrosis of alveolar walls, alveoli filled with red blood cells, and a mild inflammatory response in the periphery.[4]

RULE OF THUMB

PE is a complication of venous thrombosis. Patients with clots in the proximal venous system of the lower extremities and in the upper extremities are at high risk for developing PE.

Pathophysiology

The sudden obstruction of a pulmonary arterial branch causes a decrease or total cessation of blood flow to the distal area of the lung. This interruption of blood flow can cause respiratory and hemodynamic alterations.[16] The obstruction of the pulmonary artery by a clot increases the alveolar dead space (in which areas of the lung parenchyma are ventilated but not perfused), causes bronchoconstriction, and decreases the production of alveolar surfactant. As a compensatory mechanism, the body increases the total ventilation ($\dot{V}$), which in turn contributes to the sensation of dyspnea that accompanies PE and results in hypocapnia. Further ventilation/perfusion ($\dot{V}/\dot{Q}$) mismatching may be caused by bronchoconstriction from hypocapnia, regional hypoxia, and the production of serotonin and histamine.[17]

Not all patients with PE have significant arterial hypoxemia, but the presence of a widened alveolar-arterial oxygen tension gradient and reduced arterial O_2 tension (PaO_2) are common.[18] Hypoxemia develops because of $\dot{V}/\dot{Q}$ mismatch, intrapulmonary shunt, and in some cases shock. Shock is caused by a large obstruction of the pulmonary vasculature or by numerous small emboli in the presence of cardiopulmonary disease. In this case, cardiac output decreases, peripheral O_2 extraction increases and the O_2 saturation of the venous blood markedly falls. In patients with elevated right heart pressures, an intracardiac right-to-left shunt may develop through a patent foramen ovale (present in one-third of the population).[16,17] Moreover, the depletion of pulmonary surfactant as a result of embolic occlusion can lead to atelectasis and intrapulmonary shunt, which also cause hypoxemia.[16]

The main consequence of PE is the increased resistance to blood flow caused by obstruction of the pulmonary arterial bed. The hemodynamic impact is determined by the extent of the pulmonary circulation involved (cross-sectional area), the underlying cardiopulmonary reserve, and the neurohumoral response to the embolism. PH occurs when approximately 50% or more of the pulmonary vascular bed has been occluded[16,17] and is made worse by pulmonary vasoconstriction resulting from hypoxemia and the release of vasoactive mediators such as serotonin and thromboxane A_2.[19,20] When PH occurs, the right ventricle must work harder to maintain the same flow given the higher pressure. This added strain results in dilation and dysfunction of the right ventricle. When the mean pulmonary arterial pressure increases to greater than 40 mm Hg during an acute first PE, the right ventricle fails and hemodynamic collapse and death occur.[21] Therefore a massive PE should be suspected any time there is unexplained hypotension accompanied by an elevated central venous pressure (jugular vein distention).[22] Death from massive PE is the result of cardiovascular collapse rather than of respiratory failure. Even massive emboli are likely to resolve within weeks, particularly in young individuals. Although the usual course of PE is to resolve rapidly (because the body dissolves the embolism with endogenous fibrinolytic agents), permanent residual emboli do occur.[23] Overall, fewer than 10% of patients have lung perfusion defects after 6 weeks and approximately 4% of patients with acute PE may develop long-standing PH.

Clinical Features

A high index of suspicion for VTE is crucial to make the diagnosis. Unfortunately, no specific signs or symptoms indicate the presence of VTE and a significant proportion of patients are asymptomatic (32%).[3,24] The physical findings of DVT in the lower extremities include erythema and warm skin in one-third of patients and swelling and tenderness in three-fourths of patients. In addition to the lack of sensitivity, the physical examination is not specific for diagnosing DVT. For instance, patients who have swelling above and below the knee, fever, and a history of immobility and cancer, the likelihood of finding DVT on a venogram is only 42%.[25]

The most frequent symptoms in patients with PE are dyspnea, followed by pleuritic chest pain (sharp pain predominantly during inhalation) and cough (Table 28-2).[26] The onset of dyspnea is usually rapid, within seconds (46%) or minutes (26%) of the PE.[26] Hemoptysis occurs in 13% to 20% of patients. The combination of dyspnea of sudden onset, fainting, and acute chest pain should raise suspicion of PE. In one study, this combination of symptoms was present in 96% of patients with confirmed PE compared with 59% of patients in whom PE was suspected but not confirmed.[27] In some patients, dyspnea lasts

TABLE 28-2

Clinical Characteristics in Patients With Pulmonary Embolism and No Cardiopulmonary Disease

Symptoms	Frequency (%)
Dyspnea at rest or with exercise	73
Pleuritic pain	44
Calf or thigh pain	44
Cough	34
Orthopnea	28
Wheezing	21
Signs	**Frequency (%)**
Tachypnea	54
Tachycardia	24
Rales	18
Decrease breath sounds	17
Loud P2	15
Jugular venous distension	14

From Stein PD, Beemath A, Matta F, et al. Clinical characteristics of patients with acute pulmonary embolism: data from PIOPED II. Am J Med 120:871–879, 2007.

only a few minutes, and this episode may be wrongly dismissed as being trivial.[16,18,27,28] There are no characteristic physical findings of PE. The most frequent physical findings include tachypnea, rales on chest examination, and tachycardia. These signs, like dyspnea, may be short-lived. Other common physical findings include an accentuated pulmonary component of the second heart sound (loud P_2) consistent with PH. Fever may be present in as many as 54% of patients.[18,27,28] Similar to what occurs in the diagnosis of DVT, fewer than 35% of patients in whom PE is clinically suspected actually have it.[3]

Because the clinical features lack specificity and treatment is anticoagulation (which carries risk for bleeding over time), confirming or excluding the diagnosis with appropriate testing is necessary, rather than committing the patients to long-term anticoagulation on the basis of clinical suspicion alone. At the same time, unless there is a contraindication (e.g., recent bleeding, head trauma, etc.), anticoagulation is begun when the diagnosis of PE is first suspected and continued until it is ruled out by tests. The rationale for this approach is based on the high mortality rate soon after the occurrence of PE.

Chest Radiograph

The chest radiograph cannot confirm or exclude the presence of PE but is helpful to rule out other potentially life-threatening conditions, such as pneumothorax or pneumonia, which can manifest in a similar way. In patients with dyspnea, a normal chest radiograph may be a clue to the presence of PE; however, the plain chest radiograph is abnormal in more than 80% of the patients who present with dyspnea.[29] Some of the abnormalities include enlargement of the right descending pulmonary artery (66%), elevation of the diaphragm (61%), cardiomegaly (55%), and a small pleural effusion (50%). Patchy radiographic opacities or round nodular lesions predominantly appearing next to the pleural surface are present in patients who have infarction or atelectasis. Other less common findings include the *Westermark sign,* in which there is pulmonary hyperlucency caused by a marked reduction in blood flow and the *Hampton hump,* a pleural-based opacity in the costophrenic angle that represents alveolar hemorrhage from a pulmonary infarction. These signs may be present in only 25% to 30% of patients with PE.[27,29,30]

Electrocardiogram

The electrocardiogram (ECG) is helpful to rule out other diagnoses, such as acute myocardial infarction and pericarditis. The ECG is frequently abnormal in patients with PE (87% of the time), but the ECG abnormalities are nonspecific in most cases (70% to 75%); tachycardia and ST-segment depression are most common.[27] Abnormalities such as depression of the ST segment and T-wave inversion in V_1 and V_2 may be present. An $S_1Q_3T_3$ pattern (S wave in lead D_I and Q wave with negative T wave in D_{III}) is associated with massive PE and is present in 19% of such patients.[25]

Arterial Blood Gases

Most patients with acute PE have hypoxemia and hypocapnia,[27] but many patients (15% to 25%) have a Pao_2 greater than 80 mm Hg.[18] Although a widened alveolar-arterial O_2 gradient is frequently present, a normal alveolar-arterial O_2 gradient may occur in approximately 20% of patients with angiographically documented PE.[18,27] Thus the ABGs can never establish the diagnosis of PE.

In intubated patients or those with chronic obstructive lung disease (COPD), a decrease in PaO_2 and an increase in $PaCO_2$ can accompany PE and should prompt suspicion. Massive PE with hypotension and respiratory collapse can result in hypercapnia and respiratory acidosis. Overall, the value of arterial blood gas (ABG) values in PE is to document hypoxemia, direct O_2 supplementation, or demonstrate hypercapnia in patients with limited cardiopulmonary reserve.

Diagnostic Modalities

The diagnosis of VTE disease relies on the diagnosis of DVT or PE. Importantly, the absence of one condition does not exclude the other.

By-Products of Thrombin and Plasmin

Clot formation is always associated with thrombin generation. Measurement of cross-linked fibrin split products (D-dimers) has been found sensitive for the diagnosis of acute VTE. D-dimer results have been particularly useful in the emergency department and outpatient area for the evaluation of patients with suspected DVT[31] and PE.[32] The D-dimer test has good sensitivity and negative predictive value but poor specificity and positive predictive value. The specificity of the test is only 39%, but a value less than the recommended cutoff for current quantitative enzyme-linked immunosorbent assay (ELISA) has been shown to rule out VTM in 98% of patients.[31-33] The negative predictive value of a negative D-dimer result with low pretest probability for DVT or PE is greater than 99%.[32,33]

Although there are several laboratory methods to measure D-dimer levels, tests using ELISAs are the most widely used and best-performing among the D-dimer assays regarding the sensitivity and negative likelihood ratio. For excluding PE or DVT, a negative result on quantitative rapid ELISA is as diagnostically useful as a normal lung scan or negative duplex ultrasonography finding. The D-dimer ELISA can be used to exclude PE in outpatients with a low to moderate suspicion without the need for further costly testing. In-patients, however, should undergo an imaging study as the initial test for PE because most will already have elevated D-dimer levels as a result of comorbid conditions.[32]

Testing for Lower-Extremity Deep Venous Thromboembolism

To evaluate the clinical pretest probability of DVT, the Wells score is frequently used. This score is calculated using the following clinical parameters: presence of cancer, immobilization, localized tenderness, swelling, edema, previous DVT, collateral superficial veins, and absence of an alternative diagnosis.[34] In cases in which there is a moderate to high pretest probability, several modalities could be used for diagnosing DVT, such as compression ultrasonography (most commonly used), impedance plethysmography (a noninvasive method that measures venous outflow by changes in impedance, which in turn estimates blood volume after rapid deflation of a cuff), and venography (involves the injection of contrast dye into a foot vein to allow venous visualization by x-rays). In patients with low pretest probability of DVT and a negative D-dimer, further testing may not be necessary.[31,35-37]

Compression ultrasonography has proved to be sensitive and specific for diagnosing symptomatic proximal DVT. This test is noninvasive, portable, and accurate and is the modality of choice for the diagnosing DVT. Compression ultrasonography combines B-mode scanning with a tightly focused pulse Doppler beam directed at the vessels of interest. DVT is diagnosed with the findings of venous noncompressibility, an echogenic filling defect, absence of Doppler flow, free-floating thrombus in the vein, and venous distention.[38] The most reliable sign of DVT is lack of compressibility of the vein, although a free-floating thrombus has the highest embolic potential (Figure 28-1). The sensitivity and specificity of compression ultrasound in symptomatic patients vary between 95% and 100% for detecting a proximal lower-extremity thrombus.[38,39]

Testing for Pulmonary Embolism

Noninvasive tests for the diagnosis of PE include the $\dot{V}/\dot{Q}$ scan and computed tomography angiography (CTA) scan of the chest. Either of these tests, depending on the resources available, may be the initial diagnostic examination if the presence of acute PE is clinically suspected.[40] Echocardiography can suggest the diagnosis (right ventricle dilation, dysfunction, or thrombus) and can provide prognostic information.[41] In certain cases when these noninvasive tests are nondiagnostic, pulmonary angiography may be needed to confirm or exclude the diagnosis of PE.

$\dot{V}/\dot{Q}$ scanning involves the inhalation of a radiolabeled gas (usually xenon-133 or technetium-99 m) and the intravenous injection of macroaggregated albumin tagged with a gamma-emitting radioisotope (^{99m}Tc-labeled macroaggregated albumin). The distribution of lung ventilation ($\dot{V}$) and lung perfusion ($\dot{Q}$) is studied, and areas of mismatch in which $\dot{Q}$ is less than $\dot{V}$ are sought. The presence of mismatches most often indicates embolic occlusion of the blood vessel, although other

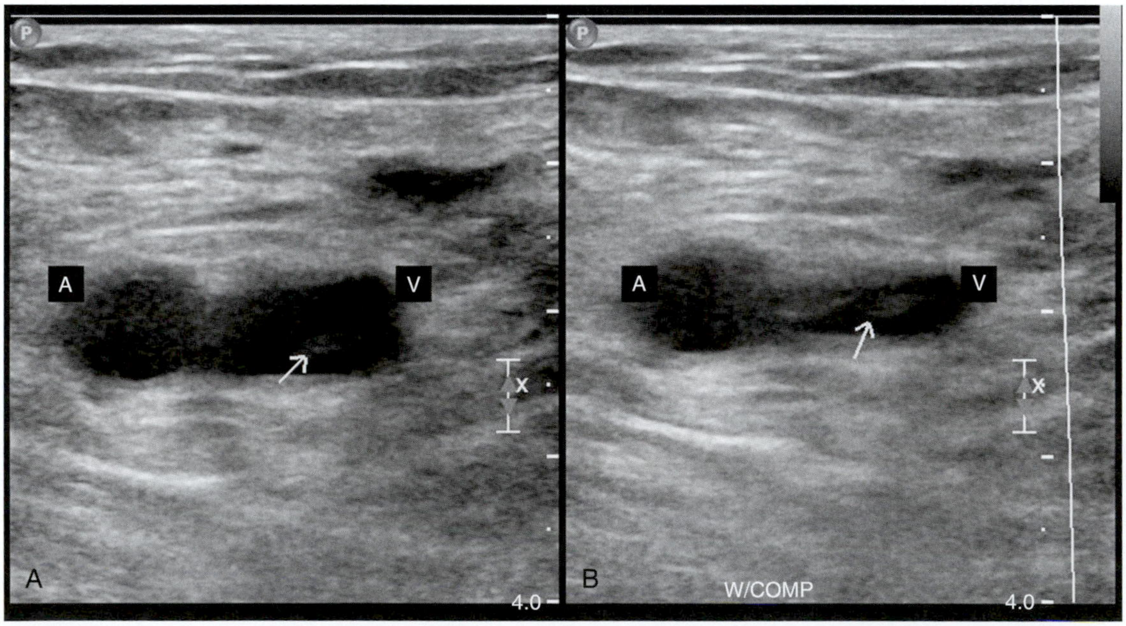

FIGURE 28-1 Deep vein thrombosis diagnosed by ultrasonography. **A,** An intraluminal thrombus is visible in the right common femoral vein *(arrow)*. **B** Incomplete collapse of the femoral vein secondary to the presence of a clot. *A,* Femoral artey; *V,* femoral vein.

rare causes exist, such as extrinsic compression of the vessel by a mass, intraluminal obstruction by angiosarcoma, or obliteration of a vessel by vasculitis. The addition of a ventilation scan increases the specificity of the perfusion scan.[42] In general, with the presence of a parenchymal abnormality, the $\dot{V}$ defect coincides with the $\dot{Q}$ defect, and matched abnormalities are found. Normal results of a $\dot{V}/\dot{Q}$ scan exclude the presence of a clinically significant PE in the context of a low clinical probability of PE.[43] Abnormal $\dot{V}/\dot{Q}$ scan results can be classified as high probability, intermediate (or indeterminate) probability, and low probability for PE, according to the size of the defect and the degree of mismatch between the $\dot{V}$ and $\dot{Q}$.[42] Diagnostic accuracy is greatest when $\dot{V}/\dot{Q}$ scan results are combined with clinical probability[44] (Table 28-3). The presence of concomitant cardiopulmonary disease (e.g., chronic obstructive pulmonary disease), even if severe, does not diminish the diagnostic usefulness of $\dot{V}/\dot{Q}$ scans in the diagnosis of acute PE.[45-47]

Spiral (helical) CTA has been used extensively in the diagnostic evaluation of PE and has become the principal diagnostic imaging modality to evaluate suspected PE (Figure 28-2).[48,49] The reported sensitivity of CTA ranges from 53% to 100%, and the specificity ranges from 81% to 100%.[49] The variability is due to the experience of the radiologists and image quality.[50] Studies indicate that CTA scanning detects large PEs involving main and lobar emboli. However, this test is generally unable to detect smaller PEs. One potential advantage of helical CTA is its ability to identify alternative diagnoses in cases in which PE is not present (e.g., pneumonia, pleural disease, etc.). Multicenter trials suggest that helical CT scanning is safe to use for ruling out PE, at least in patients with a low or intermediate clinical probability of embolism. The Prospective Investigation of Pulmonary Embolism Diagnosis (PIOPED) II trial evaluated the accuracy of multidetector CTA alone and combined with venous-phase imaging (CTA-CTV) for the diagnosis of acute PE. Excluding inconclusive studies (6%), the sensitivity of CTA was 83% and the specificity was 96%. The sensitivity of CTA-CTV for PE was 90%, and specificity was 95%. The predictive value of either CTA or CTA-CTV was high with a concordant clinical assessment, but additional testing was necessary when the clinical probability is inconsistent with the imaging results.[49,51] Several algorithms for diagnosing PE are available, but no approach has proved to be the best.[52-55] Figure 28-3 summarizes the diagnostic approach to pulmonary embolus using CTA.

For the patients who do not receive a definitive diagnosis on the basis of the results of noninvasive studies, *pulmonary angiography* is the test of choice. Pulmonary angiographic signs of acute PE include filling defects and cutoff of the pulmonary arteries. Other angiographic signs include absent, decreased, or delayed filling of pulmonary arteries; delayed venous emptying; pruning; and abnormal tapering. None of these findings is as specific as filling defects, particularly in the presence of other cardiopulmonary diseases. Table 28-4 presents the probability of finding PE with angiography on the basis of results of $\dot{V}/\dot{Q}$ scan and clinical probability.[56] A definite diagnosis can be established with noninvasive diagnostic tools in two-thirds of cases.[57]

Because of the history of surgery on the right hip, DVT and PE are the most likely diagnoses. The next examinations are duplex ultrasonography of the lower extremities followed by a $\dot{V}/\dot{Q}$ radionuclide study or a CTA scan of the chest. DVT should be sought in patients diagnosed with PE, to investigate the origin of the thrombus and assess prognosis, because individuals with PE and coexisting DVT are at increased risk for death.[58] The presence of a "normal" PaO_2 of 85 mm Hg in this patient

TABLE 28-3

Revised Prospective Investigation of Pulmonary Embolism Diagnosis Ventilation/Perfusion Scan Interpretation Criteria

High probability	Two or more large (>75% of a segment) segmental $\dot{Q}$ defects without corresponding $\dot{V}$ or abnormalities on chest radiograph
	One large segment $\dot{Q}$ defect and two or more moderate (25%-75% of a segment) segmental $\dot{Q}$ defects without corresponding $\dot{V}$ or abnormalities on chest radiograph
	Four or more moderate segmental $\dot{Q}$ defects without corresponding $\dot{V}$ or abnormalities on chest radiograph
Intermediate probability	One moderate or up to two large segmental $\dot{Q}$ defects without corresponding $\dot{V}$ defect or abnormalities on chest radiograph
	Corresponding $\dot{V}/\dot{Q}$ defects and parenchymal opacity in lower lung zone on chest radiograph
	Corresponding $\dot{V}/\dot{Q}$ defects and small pleural effusion
	Single moderate matched $\dot{V}/\dot{Q}$ defects with normal findings on chest radiograph
	Findings difficult to categorize as normal, low, or high probability
Low probability	Multiple matched $\dot{V}/\dot{Q}$ defects, regardless of size, with normal findings on chest radiograph
	Corresponding $\dot{V}/\dot{Q}$ defects and parenchymal opacity in upper or middle lung zone on chest radiograph
	Corresponding $\dot{V}/\dot{Q}$ defects and large pleural effusion
	Any $\dot{Q}$ defects with substantially larger abnormality on chest radiograph
	Defects surrounded by normally perfused lung (stripe sign)
	Single of multiple small (<25% of a segment) segmental $\dot{Q}$ defects with a normal chest radiograph
	Nonsegmental $\dot{Q}$ defects (cardiomegaly, aortic impression, enlarged hila)
Normal	No $\dot{Q}$ defects; $\dot{Q}$ outlines the shape of the lung on chest radiograph

Modified from Worsley DF, Alavi A, Palevsky JH: Role of radionuclide imaging in patients with suspected pulmonary embolism. Radiol Clin North Am 31:849, 1993.

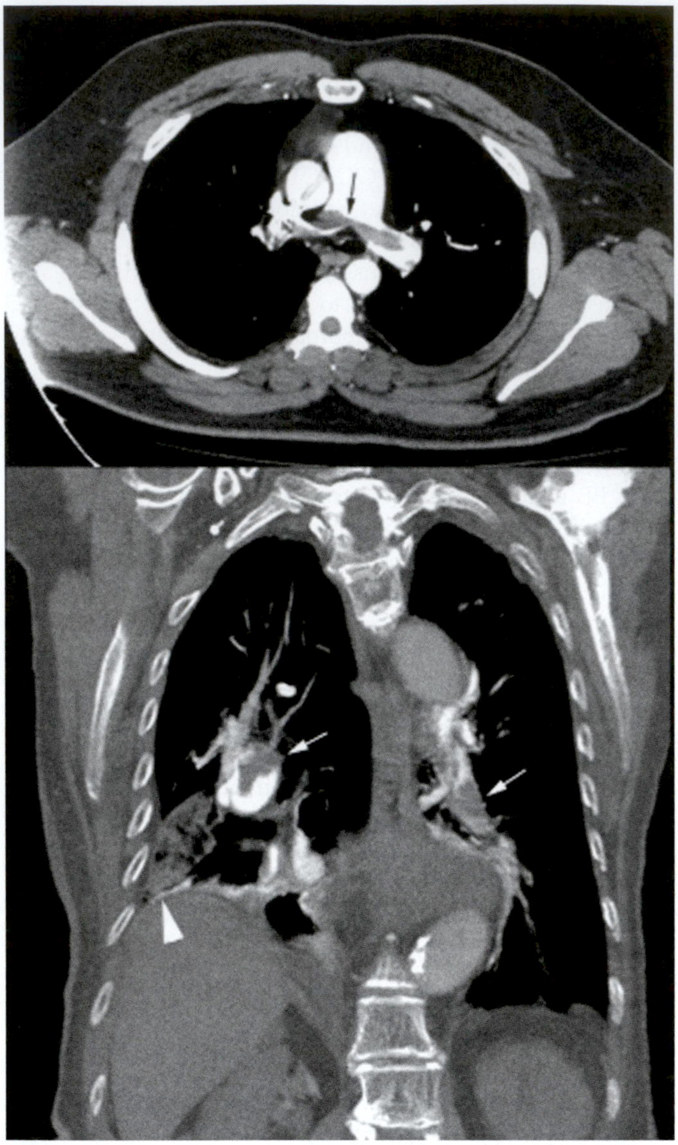

FIGURE 28-2 Pulmonary embolism diagnosed by computed tomography angiography. Axial (at the level of the pulmonary artery bifurcation, *upper panel*) and coronal cuts (just anterior to the thoracic spine, *lower panel*) showing the presence of pulmonary embolism involving the right and left pulmonary arteries, also known as *saddle embolism (arrows).* On the coronal cut, there is a wedge-shaped area in the right lower lobe that represents lung infarction *(arrow head).*

TABLE 28-4

Likelihood of Identifying Pulmonary Embolism on Pulmonary Angiogram on the Basis of Results of Ventilation/Perfusion Lung Scan and Clinical Probability

Scan Interpretation	High Clinical Probability (%)	Intermediate Clinical Probability (%)	Low Clinical Probability (%)
High probability	96	88	56
Intermediate probability	66	28	16
Low probability	40	16	4
Near normal/normal	0	6	2

From Arroliga AC, Matthay MA, Matthay RA: Pulmonary thromboembolism and other pulmonary vascular diseases. In George RB, editor: Chest medicine: essentials of pulmonary and critical care medicine, ed 3, Baltimore, 1995, Williams & Wilkins.

MINI CLINI

Respiratory Distress After Hip Replacement

PROBLEM: You are asked to evaluate a 65-year-old man who has undergone right hip replacement. On the third day after surgery, the patient experienced dyspnea and pleuritic chest pain in the right hemithorax. On physical examination, his heart rate is 120 beats/min; respiratory rate, 25 breaths/min; and blood pressure, 120/85 mm Hg. The lungs are clear, and the heart examination does not show any gallops or murmurs. ABG measurements on room air show a pH of 7.49; $PaCO_2$, 30 mm Hg; and PO_2, 85 mm Hg. The chest radiograph is unremarkable. What is your differential diagnosis, and how should you treat this patient?

DISCUSSION: The differential diagnosis is extensive and should include an ischemic cardiac event such as myocardial infarction, as well as bacterial pneumonia. The type of chest pain is not typical of myocardial infarction. An ECG may be of value because in patients with myocardial infarction, elevation of the ST segments is prominent in the acute phase. Other laboratory data include elevation of the creatinine kinase and troponin levels, although these tests may become abnormal after several hours. The normal chest radiograph decreases the likelihood of the presence of pneumonia.

may be misleading. The wide alveolar-arterial gradient probably is caused by the presence of a pulmonary embolus. The patient should be anticoagulated.

Treatment

Prophylaxis

Prophylactic therapy reduces the risk for VTE in patients at risk. The frequency of proximal DVT varies from 2% to 4% among general surgical patients undergoing minor surgery to 40% to 80% among patients at the highest risk, such as those who have undergone hip or knee surgery.[59] Patients at moderate to high risk include those with acute spinal cord injury, myocardial infarction, ischemic stroke, or other medical conditions such as heart failure and pneumonia.[59] Patients admitted to medical intensive care units are another group at risk for DVT; indeed, DVT has been detected in 33% of these patients.[60] Unfortunately, compliance in the use of prophylaxis is variable.[59]

Pharmacologic choices for prophylaxis include low-dose subcutaneous heparin, low-molecular-weight heparin (LMWH; enoxaparin and dalteparin) and the factor Xa inhibitor (fondaparinux).[61-63] Mechanical measures to reduce venous stasis include early ambulation, wearing elastic stockings,

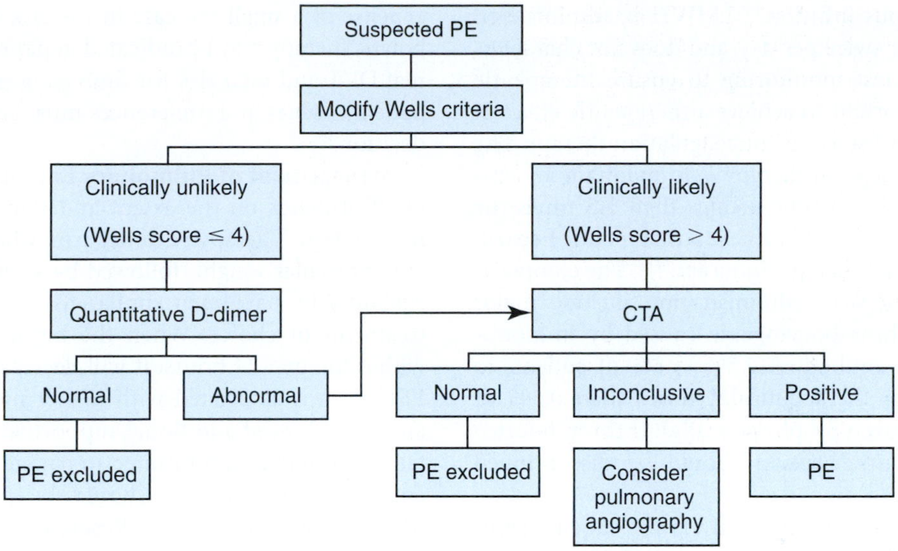

FIGURE 28-3 Strategy for diagnosis of pulmonary embolism using D-dimer and computed tomography angiography (CTA). Diagnosis is based on clinical suspicion (using the Wells modified criteria) and the results of CTA scan. The modified Wells criteria include the following: clinical symptoms of deep venous thrombosis (DVT) (3 points), other diagnoses less likely than pulmonary embolism (PE) (3 points), heart rate greater than 100 beats/min (1.5 points), immobilization 3 days or longer, surgery in the previous 4 weeks (1.5 points), previous DVT/PE (1.5 points), hemoptysis (1 point), or malignancy (1 point). (Modified from van Belle A, Buller HR, Huisman MV, et al. Effectiveness of managing suspected pulmonary embolism using an algorithm combining clinical probability, D-dimer testing, and computed tomography. JAMA 295:172–179, 2006.)

TABLE 28-5

Thromboembolism Risk and Recommended Thromboprophylaxis in Hospitalized Patients

Risk		DVT Risk Without Prophylaxis (%)	Suggested Option
Low	1. Minor surgery in mobile patient 2. Medical patients fully mobile	<10	1. No specific prophylaxis 2. Early and aggressive ambulation
Moderate	1. For general and abdominal-pelvic surgery 2. Medical patients, bed rest or sick 3. High bleeding risk	10-40	1. LMWH, unfractionated heparin, or fondaparinux 2. LMWH, unfractionated heparin or fondaparinux 3. Mechanical prophylaxis
High	1. Hip or knee arthroplasty, major trauma, hip fracture, and spinal cord injury 2. High bleeding risk	40-80	1. LMWH, fondaparinux, apixiban, dabigatran, rivaroxaban, unfractionated heparin, warfarin (Coumadin) (INR 2-3) for a minimum of 10-14 days 2. Mechanical prophylaxis

Modified from Guyatt GH, Akl EA, Crowther M, et al: Executive summary: Antithrombotic therapy and prevention of thrombosis, 9th ed: American College of Chest Physicians evidence-based clinical practice guidelines. Chest 141(2 Suppl):7S–47S, 2012.
INR, International normalized ratio; *LMWH,* low molecular weight heparin. unfractionated.
Note: Mechanical prophylaxis includes graduated compression stockings or intermittent pneumatic compression. Recommendations suggest thromboprophylaxis in acutely ill hospitalized patients until they regain mobility.

pneumatic calf compression, and electrical stimulation of calf muscles. Mechanical methods are reserved for patients with contraindications to anticoagulant thromboprophylaxis.[64] Current prophylactic strategies for DVT and PE are summarized in Table 28-5. Most hospitalized patients who are immobile need prophylaxis for VTE.

RULE OF THUMB

Most hospitalized patients who are immobile need prophylaxis for VTE.

Management of Venous Thromboembolism: Anticoagulation

Management of Deep Venous Thrombosis. Unfractionated heparin is the time-honored drug treatment, but LMWH (e.g., enoxaparin, etc.) is widely used and has been endorsed in guidelines as first-line therapy.[65] Heparin has an immediate action and is relatively safe. Heparin is an indirect thrombin inhibitor that forms a complex with antithrombin, potentiating the cofactor potency to inactivate thrombin, factor Xa, and, to a lesser extent, factors XIIa, XIa, and IXa. Heparin does not lyse existing clots but prevents formation and propagation of new clots. Unfractionated heparin should is administered as a bolus followed by a continuous infusion.[59] LMWH is administered subcutaneously, once or twice per day, and does not characteristically require blood test monitoring to ensure therapeutic benefit.[65] It is very important to achieve a therapeutic effect in the first 24 to 48 hours of starting anticoagulation therapy. The goal of unfractionated heparin therapy is to maintain an activated partial thromboplastin time greater than 1.5 times the control value.[66] The fastest way to achieve a therapeutic heparin effect is to follow an established normogram.[66-68] The complications of intravenous heparin administration include major bleeding (3.8%) and thrombocytopenia caused by immunoglobulin G antiheparin antibodies (2.5% to 3% of patients to whom heparin is given therapeutically, fewer than 0.5% of patients to whom it is given prophylactically). If thrombocytopenia or bleeding occurs, heparin should be discontinued promptly.

LMWH, once or twice per day given via the subcutaneous route, is the suggested therapy for proximal DVT if no contraindication exists.[69] This agent has been shown to be as effective and as safe as intravenous heparin therapy but less expensive. At the same time, in selected patients, LMWH can be administered at home in an efficacious and safe way that can potentially decrease the number of days of hospital admission for acute DVT.[66] The patients chosen for outpatient therapy should be in stable condition, should have a low risk for bleeding, and should not have renal insufficiency.

Several oral anticoagulants are approved by the U.S. Food and Drug Administration (FDA) for the treatment of VTE disease. These include vitamin K antagonists (warfarin) and the newer factor Xa (rivaroxaban,[70,71] apixaban,[72] and direct thrombin inhibitors (dabigatran[73]—unlabeled use). Warfarin should not be started before initiating heparin[69] because it also decreases production of proteins C and S, therefore causing a relative hypercoagulable state in the first 24 hours as a result of the depletion of these proteins. Factor Xa and direct thrombin inhibitors are fixed-dose oral treatments that do not require laboratory monitoring and reach their peak efficacy within 1 to 4 hours after ingestion, obviating the need for prolonged bridging. They have no readily available antidotes for bleeding events. These novel agents have similar efficacy as conventional anticoagulants for hemodynamically stable patients with VTE disease. Patients with the first episode of DVT generally need treatment with oral anticoagulants for at least 3 to 6 months.[66,74,75] Patients who need therapy for more than 6 months include those with idiopathic VTE, cancer, and/or recurrent DVTs.[66,76]

The role of thrombolytic therapy with streptokinase, urokinase, or tissue plasminogen activator is not well defined in the management of acute DVT. The administration of early thrombolytic therapy decreases the pain and the incidence of postthrombotic syndrome (characterized by persistent pain, swelling, skin discoloration, or venous ulceration), but the risks and benefits of this particular therapy are not well established.[66] A systematic review of the efficacy and the safety of the use of thrombolysis in the management of lower extremity DVT showed that this treatment increased the patency of the veins and reduced the incidence of postthrombotic syndrome at the expense of a small increase in the risk for bleeding.[77] Thrombolytic therapy may be indicated in patients with massive proximal DVT and high risk for limb gangrene.[69] Knowledge of the patient's values and preferences must be used to guide the best decision.[78]

Management of Pulmonary Embolism. The management of PE depends on the extent and status of the cardiopulmonary system. Therapy with heparin, whether unfractionated or low molecular weight, followed by warfarin (or newer anticoagulants) in a regimen similar to that for acute DVT is the treatment of choice. When the heparin effect is therapeutic within the first 24 hours, it will decrease the risk for recurrent PE, which is associated with higher mortality.[79] Patients with an acute PE need additional supportive measures. Supplemental O_2 should be administered to patients who have hypoxemia, and adequate analgesia should be prescribed for patients who have pain and anxiety. Resuscitation with fluids and vasopressor agents is necessary for patients who develop hypotension and shock. In the care of patients with severe hypoxemia, acute right heart failure,[80] or shock, thrombolytic therapy may be considered for lysis of the emboli. Persistent hypotension secondary to massive PE is the most commonly accepted indication for thrombolytic therapy; however, no major trial has conclusively demonstrated a mortality benefit of this intervention.[69,81,82]

Other options in the care of a patient with confirmed massive PE, in whom thrombolysis is either contraindicated or unsuccessful, include pulmonary embolectomy, catheter tip embolectomy (physical removal of the embolism), and catheter tip fragmentation. Because of associated risks, these techniques should be used in centers with appropriate experience.[40] For patients in whom anticoagulation is contraindicated (e.g., because of bleeding risk), placement of a filter into the inferior vena cava to prevent embolism of clot to the pulmonary arteries is a treatment option. Another reason for placing an inferior vena caval filter is that a recurrent embolism has occurred despite adequate anticoagulation or that the patient has experienced multiple past emboli and is considered not able to tolerate another PE. Filter placement reduces the risk for PE in the period immediately after insertion but is associated over the longer term with a higher incidence of recurrent DVT.

Prognosis

Factors associated with increased risk for death include right ventricular dysfunction,[41] right ventricular thrombus,[83] coexisting DVT,[58] higher serum brain natriuretic peptide (which is associated with right ventricular dysfunction)[84] and troponin levels (marker of myocardial injury),[85] low serum sodium (reflects neurohormonal activation),[86] and elevated lactic acid.[87] The prognostic model Simplified Pulmonary Embolism Severity Index (sPESI)[88] assigns a high risk for dying to those patients with any of the following factors: age older than 80, history of cancer, chronic cardiopulmonary disease, pulse 110/min or greater, systolic blood pressure less than 100 mm Hg, and arterial O_2 saturation less than 90%. Those with low risk (without risk factors) have a 30-day mortality of 1%; meanwhile, those with high risk (at least one risk factor) have a 30-day mortality of 10.9%.[88]

If left untreated, PE has an overall mortality of 30%.[89] Early death is due to shock and/or a secondary embolic event. Long-term mortality is related to predisposing comorbidities and recurrent PE. Although the mortality from PE has decreased in recent years,[89] the death rate for the first episode of PE among hospitalized patients may be as high as 17.4% at 3 months.[90] Recurrent PE carries a much higher mortality rate, because only a quarter of patients will survive 3 months.[91]

PULMONARY HYPERTENSION

PH is defined by an elevation in mean pulmonary arterial pressure 25 mm Hg or greater at rest. PH is grouped in five categories, a classification that was updated in 2013 by the 5th World Symposium on Pulmonary Hypertension in Nice, France (Box 28-2).[92,93] The importance of the clinical system, besides allowing a better understanding of pathophysiology, is to give a framework for understanding important branch-points in the management and treatment of different conditions known to cause PH. The first category, PAH, is characterized by an elevation in pulmonary arterial pressure associated with high pulmonary vascular resistance (≥3 Wood units) and normal left ventricular filling pressures (pulmonary artery occlusion pressure ≤15 mm Hg).[94] PAH may be associated with several conditions, including collagen vascular disease, congenital heart disease, cirrhosis of the liver, human immunodeficiency virus (HIV) infection, and drugs and toxins (diet pills or anorexigens).[92,93] In patients in whom no underlying cause of PH can be identified, the disease is referred to as *idiopathic pulmonary arterial hypertension* (IPAH), previously known as *primary pulmonary hypertension* (PPH).[95-98]

PH also can develop as a consequence of PE, and this entity is known as *chronic thromboembolic PH*.[99] In addition, PH can be associated to heart or lung diseases or may result from a variety of other conditions grouped in PH with unclear or multifactorial mechanisms. PH resulting from lung diseases is further divided into several groups: PH associated with COPD, interstitial lung disease, other diseases with mixed obstructive and restrictive patterns, sleep breathing disorders, alveolar hypoventilation, chronic exposure to high altitude, and developmental abnormalities. A rare type of PH, pulmonary venoocclusive disease, is characterized by narrowing of the small pulmonary venules. Although challenging, recognizing pulmonary venoocclusive disease is important given that the response to PAH-specific treatment in this disease is limited and lung transplantation is frequently needed. These patients commonly develop pulmonary edema when treated with PH-specific therapies.

Box 28-2 Simplified Clinical Classification of Pulmonary Hypertension (Nice, 2013)

1. Pulmonary arterial hypertension
2. Pulmonary hypertension owing to left heart disease
3. Pulmonary hypertension owing to lung diseases and/or hypoxia
4. Chronic thromboembolic pulmonary hypertension
5. Pulmonary hypertension with unclear multifactorial mechanisms

Modified from Simonneau G, Gatzoulis MA, Adatia I, et al: Updated clinical classification of pulmonary hypertension. J Am Coll Cardiol 62(25 Suppl):D34–D41, 2013.

Pathogenesis

The initial event of PAH is probably an insult to the pulmonary endothelium (the cells that line the blood vessel) in patients with certain genetic predisposition.[100-102] This damage to the endothelium alters the balance between vasoconstrictive mediators (e.g., thromboxane and endothelin I) and vasodilators such as nitric oxide and prostacyclin, resulting in vasoconstriction. Vasoconstriction might not be the primary event, but it is an important component in the pathogenesis of PAH.[103-105] In addition to vasoconstriction, there is inflammation, thrombosis, cell proliferation, apoptosis and fibrosis, all of which can lead to pulmonary vascular remodeling and irreversible PAH.[106] Recent research suggests the presence of other potential pathways that contribute to PAH, including downregulation of potassium channels,[107] increased matrix metalloproteinases,[108] decreased vasoactive intestinal peptide,[109] disruption and progressive loss of endothelial caveolin-1 with enhanced expression in smooth muscle cells,[110] elevated serotonin,[111] and transforming growth factor-beta,[112] among others.[113] Potential new biomarkers and lines of therapies could result from these discoveries.[95-98,103-105,114]

Epidemiology and Clinical Findings

The true prevalence of PH is unknown. The prevalence of idiopathic and heritable PAH is estimated to be 5 to 15 cases per million adults.[115,116] Overall, PH affects all age groups as well as both genders. Idiopathic PAH is more common among women than among men, with a ratio of 3:1. Approximately 7% of all cases are heritable. Idiopathic PAH can occur at any age, although it is more common from ages 20 to 50 years.

On average, the diagnosis of PAH is delayed for 2 years after the onset of symptoms.[117] The condition frequently is misdiagnosed as asthma, anxiety, or depression because it is characterized by the onset of vague respiratory symptoms and hyperventilation. The most common initial symptom is dyspnea (60% of patients). Other common symptoms include chest pain (50% of patients), probably secondary to underperfusion of the right ventricle or stretching of the large pulmonary arteries, and syncope (passing out) (8% of patients) because of insufficient cardiac output, predominantly with activities. Less frequent symptoms include cough, hemoptysis, hoarseness, and Raynaud's phenomenon (blanching of the fingers on exposure to cold) in approximately 10% of patients.

Physical findings associated with PAH include a loud second heart sound and a right-sided third or fourth heart sound. Other common signs are a palpable right ventricular heave and both pulmonary ejection and pulmonary tricuspid regurgitation murmurs. Signs of right ventricular failure are common. Cyanosis often is present as a result of low cardiac output or the presence of an intracardiac right-to-left shunt in patients with a patent foramen ovale or advanced stages of congenital heart diseases. Clubbing does not occur in PAH. The chest radiographic findings include enlargement of the main and hilar pulmonary arteries, "pruning" (or narrowing) of the peripheral arteries, enlargement of the right ventricle and atrium, and pleural effusion, although the chest radiograph may remain normal in 6% of patients.

Diagnosis

Before the diagnosis of PAH can be made, other underlying diseases associated with PAH must be excluded. Tests commonly ordered to establish the precise cause of PH include blood testing, ECG, pulmonary function testing, echocardiogram, $\dot{V}/\dot{Q}$ scan, CTA, and pulmonary artery catheterization.

Laboratory tests include a complete blood cell count, comprehensive metabolic panel, HIV test, rheumatologic panel, and liver function tests. These tests help identify conditions associated with PAH, such as systemic sclerosis, systemic lupus erythematosus, and mixed connective tissue diseases. Schistosomiasis, a parasitic disease and the most common cause of PH worldwide, must be ruled out in the appropriate setting. Electrocardiographic findings usually include right-axis deviation, right ventricular hypertrophy, and strain.[118] Pulmonary function tests are useful to rule out the presence of significant restrictive or obstructive airway disease. The most common abnormality on pulmonary function testing in patients with PAH is a low carbon monoxide diffusing capacity (DLCO), associated with relatively normal pulmonary mechanics.

The echocardiogram may show dilation of the right ventricle and right atrium, dysfunction of the right ventricle, and tricuspid regurgitation (Figure 28-4). One important noninvasive test for PAH is the $\dot{V}/\dot{Q}$ scan lung scan, which helps rule out the possibility of chronic thromboembolic PH, a mimic of PAH that has a different treatment, that is, possible thromboendarterectomy. In patients with PAH, the perfusion scan may be normal or show only patchy subsegmental defects. In patients with chronic thromboembolic PH, the $\dot{V}/\dot{Q}$ scan shows segmental defects; in these cases, confirmation of chronic thromboembolic PH requires pulmonary angiography. High-resolution CT is helpful to rule out associated causes such as interstitial lung disease, emphysema, or their co-occurrence.

Right heart catheterization is required to confirm the diagnosis and determine the degree of hemodynamic impairment, presence of vasoreactivity, and prognosis of patients with PAH (Figure 28-5). Patients with severe degrees of PH defined hemodynamically as high right atrial pressure and pulmonary vascular resistance, as well as low cardiac output, have a worse prognosis.[12,95-98]

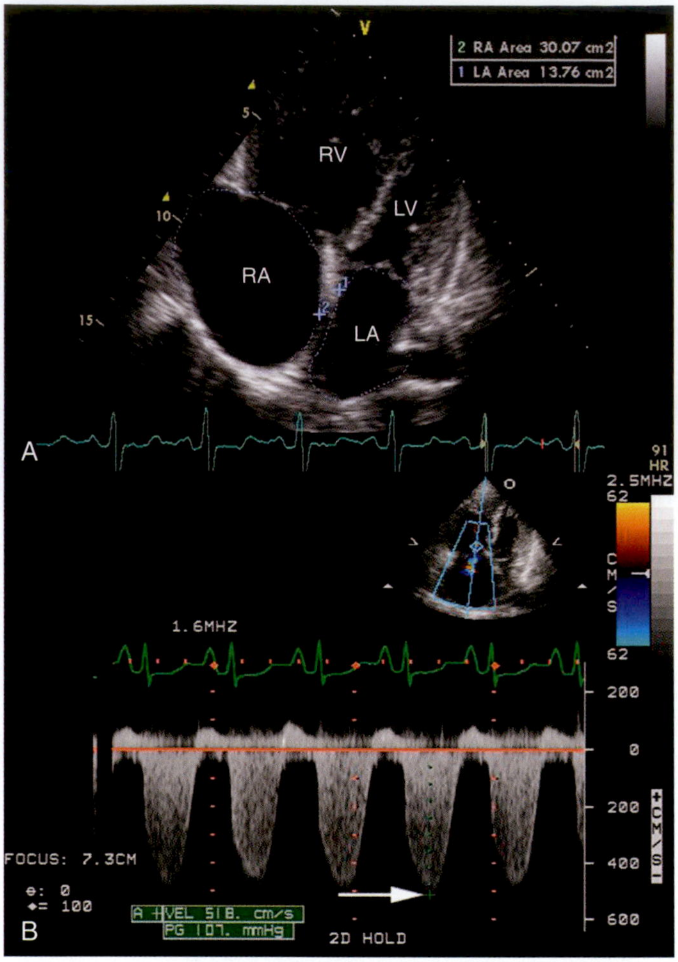

FIGURE 28-4 Echocardiography in pulmonary hypertension. Apical four-chamber view of the heart, revealing enlarged right atrium and ventricle compressing the left cardiac chambers **(A).** Doppler echocardiography showing tricuspid insufficiency jet *(arrow)* used to estimate the right ventricular systolic pressure, in this case 107 mm Hg. *LA,* Left atrium; *LV,* left ventricle; *RA,* right atrium; *RV,* right ventricle.

Management

PAH can be life-threatening and carries a poor prognosis. Without therapy, only 33% of patients are alive 5 years after the onset of the disorder. During the past two decades, treatment has improved considerably.[119-124] Current treatment options include using calcium channel blockers, prostanoids, endothelin receptor antagonists, and phosphodiesterase-5 inhibitors.

General Measures

Oral anticoagulation is recommended for patients with IPAH unless there is a contraindication to anticoagulation.[125,126] The recommended target international normalized ratio (INR) is 2 to 3. The role of anticoagulation in other forms of PAH is less clear and possibly not beneficial.[125] Supplemental O_2 should be used to maintain O_2 saturation greater than 90%, especially because hypoxemia is a major cause of pulmonary vasoconstriction. This is of particular importance in air travel or when staying at places with altitudes above 1000 m. Diuretics are indicated for right ventricular volume overload, and digoxin might be indicated for patients with refractory right ventricular

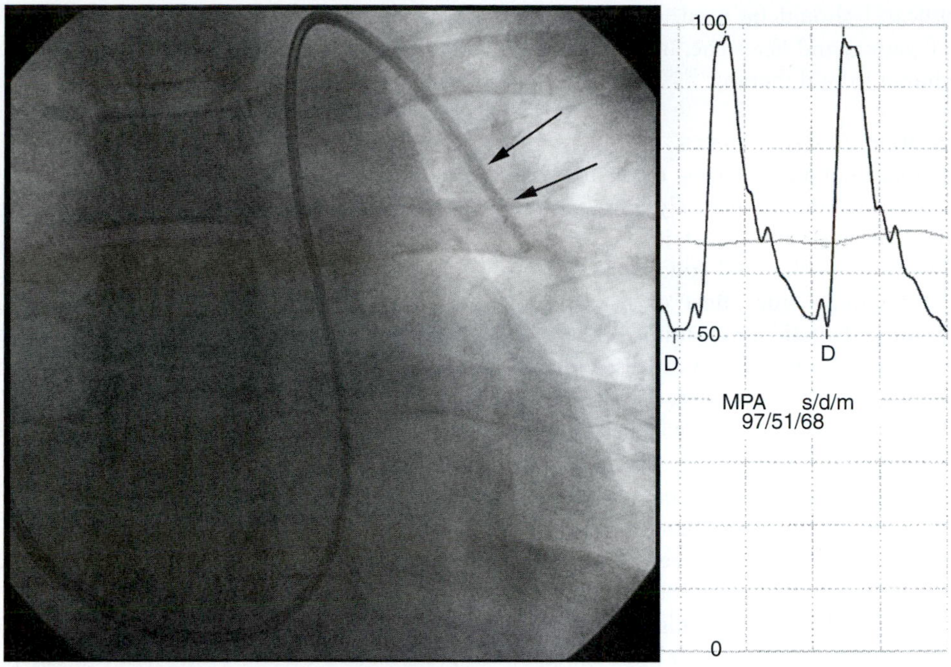

FIGURE 28-5 Right heart catheterization in pulmonary hypertension. On the *left panel* a pulmonary artery catheter is observed in the left pulmonary artery *(arrows)*. On the *right panel* the corresponding pulmonary artery pressure tracing is shown, confirming the diagnosis of pulmonary hypertension. In this case the pulmonary artery, systolic, diastolic, and mean pressures were 97, 51, and 68 mm Hg, respectively.

failure and for rate control in atrial flutter or fibrillation.[123,124] Pregnancy is generally contraindicated in women with PH.

Calcium Channel Blockers

Patients with IPAH who respond to vasodilators in the short term have improved survival with long-term use of calcium channel blockers. Thus these agents should be considered only in IPAH patients who have significant and definite response to a short-acting vasodilator such as NO (others include intravenous epoprostenol or adenosine). Unfortunately, only a small fraction of IPAH patients qualify for and benefit from long-term therapy with oral calcium channel blockers.[123,124] Patients with other causes of PAH usually have negative acute vasodilator testing or, even if the testing was positive, they would not respond to long-term calcium channel blockers.[127]

NO is the preferred agent for pulmonary vasodilator testing because its half-life is very short, it does not affect cardiac output, and it enhances $\dot{V}/\dot{Q}$ matching.[127] NO is usually administered by mask at 10 to 40 parts per million for 2 to 5 minutes.[127] Protocols for using NO vary by institution. We use 40 ppm of NO delivered on room air (or the percentage of O_2 need to keep a pulse oximetry saturation ≥90%) for 5 minutes; others use 40 ppm of NO combined with 100% O_2.

Prostanoids

Several prostanoids are currently available for treating patients with severe PAH, including epoprostenol, treprostinil, and iloprost. Epoprostenol delivered via continuous intravenous infusion improves exercise capacity, hemodynamic variables, and survival in PAH patients.[128] Epoprostenol is unstable at room temperature and needs continuous intravenous infusion because of the short half-life of the drug. Common side effects include headache, flushing, jaw pain, diarrhea, nausea, skin rash, and musculoskeletal pain. Catheter-related complications include infection, sometimes serious (e.g., bacteremia), and thrombosis. By changing the buffer, a thermostable epoprostenol was developed and has been approved for clinical use by the FDA.

Another prostanoid, treprostinil, is a stable prostacyclin analogue with a longer half-life, allowing for subcutaneous,[129] intravenous,[130] inhaled,[131] or oral delivery. In addition to side effects seen with epoprostenol, patients receiving treprostinil subcutaneously may also experience pain at the infusion site. Inhaled teprostinil is administered by using the Tyvaso Inhalation System (ultrasonic, pulsed-delivery device; United Therapeutics, Research Triangle, NC). It is initially dosed at 3 inhalations, 4 times per day. If this dose is tolerated, it may be increased up to 9 inhalations, 4 times per day. Oral treprostinil has been approved by the FDA for the treatment of PAH. This mode of delivery is associated with gastrointestinal side effects and requires a slow titration. Iloprost is a stable prostacyclin analogue that can be delivered by inhalation and is an effective therapy for PAH.[132] Because of the relatively short duration of action of inhaled iloprost, it needs to be taken as 1 or 2 inhalations, 6 to 9 times per day. For its administration, the I-neb AAD System (Phillips Healthcare, Andover, MD) or Prodose AAD

System (Phillips Healthcare) should be used. Common side effects include cough, flushing, and headache. Inhaled iloprost may be useful as an adjunct to oral therapy.[119,120,123,124]

Endothelin-Receptor Antagonists

Endothelin antagonists represent another class of medications available for treating PAH. Bosentan, an orally administered nonselective endothelin-1 receptor antagonist, improves walking distance, hemodynamic variables, and functional class in patients with PAH.[133] The main side effect of bosentan is an asymptomatic increase in hepatic aminotransferase levels, which necessitates monitoring liver function at least monthly in all patients receiving bosentan. Ambrisentan, a selective type A endothelin-1 receptor antagonist, is also beneficial in patients with PAH. Its main side effect is peripheral edema.[134,135] Macitentan also has been approved by the FDA for treatment of PAH patients.[136] Macitentan blocks both endothelin type A and B receptors. Ambrisentan and macitentan are once-daily medications that do not need monthly hepatic aminotransferase determinations. All endothelin receptor antagonists are potent teratogens, and very careful contraception must be observed by patients receiving these medications.

Phosphodiesterase-5 Inhibitors

Sildenafil, a phosphodiesterase type 5 (PDE5) inhibitor, reduces pulmonary arterial pressure and is effective in treating PH.[121] By inhibiting PDE5, sildenafil stabilizes cyclic guanosine monophosphate (cGMP; the second messenger of NO), allowing a more sustained effect of endogenous NO, which is an indirect but effective and practical way of using the NO-cGMP pathway. Tadalafil, a long-acting PDE5 inhibitor, also improves outcomes in PAH and has some differences in acute effects when compared to sildenafil.[137,138] These medications are usually well tolerated; rarely, patients can have vision or hearing loss, priapism, and hypotension.

Soluble Guanylate Cyclase Stimulators

Riociguat has also been approved by the FDA for the treatment of PAH[139] and for patients with chronic thromboembolic PH who are not candidates for pulmonary thromboendarterectomy (i.e., surgery to remove clots from the pulmonary artery) or in whom the PH persists or recurs after thromboendarterectomy surgery.[140] This medication is associated with embryo-fetal toxicity; therefore patients need to follow strict recommendations to avoid pregnancy.

Surgical Therapy

Atrial Septostomy. The role of balloon atrial septostomy in treating patients with PAH is uncertain. Septostomy might be of benefit in the setting of severe disease with recurrent syncope and/or right heart failure despite maximal medical therapy. The procedure also can be used as a palliative bridge to lung transplantation. The rationale for its use is that the controlled creation of an atrial septal defect would allow right-to-left shunting, leading to increased systemic output and systemic O_2 transport despite the accompanying fall in systemic arterial O_2 saturation. The shunt at the atrial level would also allow decompression of the right atrium and right ventricle, alleviating signs and symptoms of right heart failure. Balloon atrial septostomy is a high-risk procedure and should be performed only in experienced centers to reduce the procedural risks.[123]

Lung Transplantation. Single or double lung transplantation has been used successfully in the treatment of patients with PAH. Patients who undergo lung transplantation have an immediate decrease in pulmonary artery pressure at the time of surgery and rapid improvement in right heart function despite severe preoperative cor pulmonale.[123] This option is reserved for special cases not responsive to medical treatment who have indicators of poor prognosis (syncope, refractory right heart failure, function class III/IV, or severe hypoxemia).[141] Perioperative mortality for transplantation is higher in PAH, but after the immediate postoperative period, some patients have an excellent response with dramatic improvements in symptoms and quality of life.[142] Although lung transplantation is an alternative for treating patients with PAH, the disadvantages of transplantation are the need for lifelong immunosuppression and the morbidity and mortality, which increase over time. The survival rate 3 years after lung transplantation is approximately 60%. Unfortunately, by the time PAH patients are considered for transplantation, they are usually poor candidates for transplantation because of the multiple organ system failures that may accompany PAH.

> **RULE OF THUMB**
>
> In patients with shortness of breath who have an unremarkable physical examination, the presence of a low DLCO and normal pulmonary mechanics suggests a pulmonary vascular cause (e.g., PH) as a cause of the shortness of breath.

Pulmonary Hypertension in Chronic Lung Disease

PH is a frequent complication of COPD (see Chapter 25). Approximately 50% of elderly patients with COPD have PH with significant reduction in survival and quality of life. The PH associated with COPD is multifactorial. Alveolar hypoxia, because of its potent pulmonary vasoconstrictive effect, is probably the most important factor contributing to PH in patients with COPD. Sustained alveolar hypoxia causes pulmonary vasoconstriction and eventually medial hypertrophy, fibrosis of the intima, and narrowing of the lumen of the pulmonary blood vessels. Other factors include the loss of vascular surface caused by destruction of lung parenchyma, compression of the vascular bed as a result of hyperinflation, hyperviscosity of the blood as a result of polycythemia, and left ventricular diastolic dysfunction. The presence of PH in patients with COPD correlates with the severity of the disease. Patients with severe hypoxemia (PaO_2 <55 mm Hg) may have more elevated pulmonary artery pressures, although the mean pulmonary artery pressure resulting from COPD alone rarely exceeds 35 to

40 mm Hg.[143-146] Patients with mean pulmonary artery pressure higher than 35 to 40 mm Hg have a poor prognosis.[147]

MINI CLINI

Dyspnea and Near-Syncope

PROBLEM: A 35-year-old woman has shortness of breath. She had an episode of near-syncope approximately 6 months ago; a diagnostic evaluation was done, and the results were negative. The physical examination shows a loud second heart sound. A chest radiograph shows questionable cardiomegaly. The forced vital capacity and forced expiratory volume in 1 second are normal, but the DLCO is only 40% of the predicted value. What is the cause of the dyspnea and the low DLCO?

DISCUSSION: This patient could have PH of unknown cause, that is, IPAH. She has physical findings consistent with high pressure in the right side of the heart (a loud second heart sound), and she has symptoms that are common in this disorder, such as dyspnea and near-syncope or syncope. The differential diagnosis is broad, but a low DLCO in the presence of normal lung mechanics could indicate an abnormality of the pulmonary vasculature.

An echocardiogram is usually the first test of choice to assess for the presence of PH. If the echocardiogram is consistent with the diagnosis, pulmonary artery (also known as *right heart*) catheterization is needed to confirm the diagnosis, determine the severity, and exclude left heart disease. For the diagnosis of IPAH, other underlying diseases that can be associated with PAH must be excluded. A $\dot{V}/\dot{Q}$ scan and/or pulmonary angiogram can exclude chronic thromboembolic disease, a CT scan of the chest and pulmonary function tests can help determine the presence of parenchymal lung disease, and blood serologic tests can be used to evaluate for connective tissue disease. A 6-minute walk test may help in determining the functional capacity of the patient and assess her response to treatment. Several treatment options are currently available for patients with PH. The best option depends on the underlying cause of the PH and the severity of the disease.

O_2 therapy is the main treatment that improves survival among patients with COPD and PH, although smoking cessation and lung volume reduction (in selected individuals) may also offer survival benefits in patients with COPD. Vasodilator agents used for PAH are sometimes used in these patients, but the results of large clinical trials are not yet available.[145,147,148]

ROLE OF THE RESPIRATORY THERAPIST IN PULMONARY VASCULAR DISEASE

Respiratory therapists (RTs) can play a key role in diagnosing and managing individuals with pulmonary vascular disease. Diagnostically, the astute RT may help diagnose VTE and PH by recognizing the signs and symptoms of DVT/PE and PH (e.g., acute onset of dyspnea, pleuritic pain, pedal edema). Communication with the managing physician to point out these findings and suggest a workup may prove lifesaving.

Therapists also may play an important role in both preventing and managing pulmonary vascular disease. Ensuring patients' compliance with vascular compression stockings can help prevent PE. Therapists may also be members of teams that care for patients with PH, as in administering NO during pulmonary vasodilator challenge and managing inhaled therapies that are used to treat PAH (e.g., inhaled iloprost and treprostinil).

SUMMARY CHECKLIST

- VTE (DVT and PE) is an important cause of morbidity and mortality among hospitalized patients.
- Early recognition and treatment are essential and can be lifesaving. One-third of the deaths caused by PE occur within 1 hour of the symptom onset. The mortality rate in the group of patients with PE that goes undiagnosed is 30%; if the venous thrombosis is recognized and managed, the mortality rate is less than 8%.
- The point of origin of PE is DVT of the lower extremities or pelvis in 86% of cases.
- Most of the time, the clinical presentation of PE and DVT is nonspecific. A high index of suspicion is important to make the diagnosis in patients at risk.
- Prophylactic therapy reduces the risk for VTE in patients at risk, but, unfortunately, prophylactic therapy is underused.
- Pharmacologic choices for prophylaxis include low-dose subcutaneous heparin, warfarin, LMWH, and dextran. Mechanical measures include early ambulation, wearing elastic stockings, pneumatic calf compression, and electric stimulation of calf muscles.
- Management of VTE includes anticoagulation therapy (heparin and warfarin).
- IPAH is a rare disease that mainly affects young adults. In IPAH, damage to the endothelium of the pulmonary artery alters the balance between vasoconstrictors and vasodilators, favoring vasoconstriction. Thrombosis and cellular proliferation are contributors to PH.
- Management of IPAH includes anticoagulation and the administration of vasodilators (calcium channel blockers, prostanoids, endothelin receptor antagonists, PDE5 inhibitors, and soluble guanylate cyclase stimulators). Lung transplantation is an option for refractory cases.

References

1. Tonelli AR, Arelli V, Minai OA, et al: Causes and circumstances of death in pulmonary arterial hypertension. *Am J Respir Crit Care Med* 188:365–369, 2013.
2. Silverstein MD, Heit JA, Mohr DN, et al: Trends in the incidence of deep vein thrombosis and pulmonary embolism: a 25-year population-based study. *Arch Intern Med* 158:585–593, 1998.
3. Rosenow EC, 3rd: Venous and pulmonary thromboembolism: an algorithmic approach to diagnosis and management. *Mayo Clin Proc* 70:45–49, 1995.
4. Wagenvoort CA: Pathology of pulmonary thromboembolism. *Chest* 107(1 Suppl):10S–17S, 1995.
5. Sperry KL, Key CR, Anderson RE: Toward a population-based assessment of death due to pulmonary embolism in New Mexico. *Hum Pathol* 21:159–165, 1990.

6. Sandler DA, Martin JF: Autopsy proven pulmonary embolism in hospital patients: are we detecting enough deep vein thrombosis? *J R Soc Med* 82: 203–205, 1989.
7. Morpurgo M, Schmid C: The spectrum of pulmonary embolism: clinicopathologic correlations. *Chest* 107(1 Suppl):18S–20S, 1995.
8. Dalen JE, Alpert JS: Natural history of pulmonary embolism. *Prog Cardiovasc Dis* 17:259–270, 1975.
9. Carson JL, Kelley MA, Duff A, et al: The clinical course of pulmonary embolism. *N Engl J Med* 326:1240–1245, 1992.
10. Dalen JE: When can treatment be withheld in patients with suspected pulmonary embolism? *Arch Intern Med* 153:1415–1418, 1993.
11. Girard P, Decousus M, Laporte S, et al: Diagnosis of pulmonary embolism in patients with proximal deep vein thrombosis: specificity of symptoms and perfusion defects at baseline and during anticoagulant therapy. *Am J Respir Crit Care Med* 164:1033–1037, 2001.
12. Arroliga AC, Matthay M, Matthay R: Pulmonary thromboembolism and other pulmonary vascular diseases. In George RB, editor: *Chest medicine: essentials of pulmonary and critical care medicine*, ed 4, Philadelphia, 2000, Lippincott Williams & Wilkins.
13. Crowther MA, Kelton JG: Congenital thrombophilic states associated with venous thrombosis: a qualitative overview and proposed classification system. *Ann Intern Med* 138:128–134, 2003.
14. Goldhaber SZ: Risk factors for venous thromboembolism. *J Am Coll Cardiol* 56:1–7, 2010.
15. Haemostasis and Thrombosis Task Force, British Committee for Standards in Haematology: Investigation and management of heritable thrombophilia. *Br J Haematol* 114:512–528, 2001.
16. Riedel M: Acute pulmonary embolism. I. Pathophysiology, clinical presentation, and diagnosis. *Heart* 85:229–240, 2001.
17. Elliott CG: Pulmonary physiology during pulmonary embolism. *Chest* 101(4 Suppl):163S–171S, 1992.
18. Stein PD, Terrin ML, Hales CA, et al: Clinical, laboratory, roentgenographic, and electrocardiographic findings in patients with acute pulmonary embolism and no pre-existing cardiac or pulmonary disease. *Chest* 100:598–603, 1991.
19. Egermayer P, Town GI, Peacock AJ: Role of serotonin in the pathogenesis of acute and chronic pulmonary hypertension. *Thorax* 54:161–168, 1999.
20. Smulders YM: Pathophysiology and treatment of haemodynamic instability in acute pulmonary embolism: the pivotal role of pulmonary vasoconstriction. *Cardiovasc Res* 48:23–33, 2000.
21. Benotti JR, Dalen JE: The natural history of pulmonary embolism. *Clin Chest Med* 5:403–410, 1984.
22. Kucher N, Goldhaber SZ: Management of massive pulmonary embolism. *Circulation* 112:e28–e32, 2005.
23. Thomas D, Stein M, Tanabe G, et al: Mechanism of bronchoconstriction produced by thromboemboli in dogs. *Am J Physiol* 206:1207–1212, 1964.
24. Stein PD, Matta F, Musani MH, et al: Silent pulmonary embolism in patients with deep venous thrombosis: a systematic review. *Am J Med* 123:426–431, 2010.
25. Landefeld CS, McGuire E, Cohen AM: Clinical findings associated with acute proximal deep vein thrombosis: a basis for quantifying clinical judgment. *Am J Med* 88:382–388, 1990.
26. Stein PD, Beemath A, Matta F, et al: Clinical characteristics of patients with acute pulmonary embolism: data from PIOPED II. *Am J Med* 120:871–879, 2007.
27. Miniati M, Prediletto R, Formichi B, et al: Accuracy of clinical assessment in the diagnosis of pulmonary embolism. *Am J Respir Crit Care Med* 159: 864–871, 1999.
28. Manganelli D, Palla A, Donnamaria V, et al: Clinical features of pulmonary embolism: doubts and certainties. *Chest* 107(1 Suppl):25S–32S, 1995.
29. Worsley DF, Alavi A, Aronchick JM, et al: Chest radiographic findings in patients with acute pulmonary embolism: observations from the PIOPED Study. *Radiology* 189:133–136, 1993.
30. Algin O, Gokalp G, Topal U: Signs in chest imaging. *Diagn Interv Radiol* 17:18–29, 2011.
31. Wells PS, Anderson DR, Rodger M, et al: Evaluation of D-dimer in the diagnosis of suspected deep-vein thrombosis. *N Engl J Med* 349:1227–1235, 2003.
32. Stein PD, Hull RD, Patel KC, et al: D-dimer for the exclusion of acute venous thrombosis and pulmonary embolism: a systematic review. *Ann Intern Med* 140:589–602, 2004.
33. Kearon C, Ginsberg JS, Douketis J, et al: A randomized trial of diagnostic strategies after normal proximal vein ultrasonography for suspected deep venous thrombosis: D-dimer testing compared with repeated ultrasonography. *Ann Intern Med* 142:490–496, 2005.
34. Tamariz LJ, Eng J, Segal JB, et al: Usefulness of clinical prediction rules for the diagnosis of venous thromboembolism: a systematic review. *Am J Med* 117:676–684, 2004.
35. Carrier M, Le Gal G, Bates SM, et al: D-dimer testing is useful to exclude deep vein thrombosis in elderly outpatients. *J Thromb Haemost* 6:1072–1076, 2008.
36. Stender MT, Frokjaer JB, Hagedorn Nielsen TS, et al: Combined use of clinical pre-test probability and D-dimer test in the diagnosis of preoperative deep venous thrombosis in colorectal cancer patients. *Thromb Haemost* 99:396–400, 2008.
37. Qaseem A, Snow V, Barry P, et al: Current diagnosis of venous thromboembolism in primary care: a clinical practice guideline from the American Academy of Family Physicians and the American College of Physicians. *Ann Fam Med* 5:57–62, 2007.
38. Cronan JJ: Venous thromboembolic disease: the role of US. *Radiology* 186:619–630, 1993.
39. Lensing AW, Prandoni P, Brandjes D, et al: Detection of deep-vein thrombosis by real-time B-mode ultrasonography. *N Engl J Med* 320:342–345, 1989.
40. ACCP Consensus Committee on Pulmonary Embolism: American College of Chest Physicians. Opinions regarding the diagnosis and management of venous thromboembolic disease. *Chest* 113:499–504, 1998.
41. ten Wolde M, Sohne M, Quak E, et al: Prognostic value of echocardiographically assessed right ventricular dysfunction in patients with pulmonary embolism. *Arch Intern Med* 164:1685–1689, 2004.
42. Worsley DF, Alavi A, Palevsky HI: Role of radionuclide imaging in patients with suspected pulmonary embolism. *Radiol Clin North Am* 31:849–858, 1993.
43. van Beek EJ, Kuyer PM, Schenk BE, et al: A normal perfusion lung scan in patients with clinically suspected pulmonary embolism. Frequency and clinical validity. *Chest* 108:170–173, 1995.
44. Wren C, Rowland E, Burn J, et al: Familial ventricular tachycardia: a report of four families. *Br Heart J* 63:169–174, 1990.
45. Stein PD, Coleman RE, Gottschalk A, et al: Diagnostic utility of ventilation/perfusion lung scans in acute pulmonary embolism is not diminished by pre-existing cardiac or pulmonary disease. *Chest* 100:604–606, 1991.
46. Henry JW, Stein PD, Gottschalk A, et al: Scintigraphic lung scans and clinical assessment in critically ill patients with suspected acute pulmonary embolism. *Chest* 109:462–466, 1996.
47. Hartmann IJ, Hagen PJ, Melissant CF, et al: Diagnosing acute pulmonary embolism: effect of chronic obstructive pulmonary disease on the performance of D-dimer testing, ventilation/perfusion scintigraphy, spiral computed tomographic angiography, and conventional angiography. ANTELOPE Study Group: advances in new technologies evaluating the localization of pulmonary embolism. *Am J Respir Crit Care Med* 162:2232–2237, 2000.
48. Perrier A, Nendaz MR, Sarasin FP, et al: Cost-effectiveness analysis of diagnostic strategies for suspected pulmonary embolism including helical computed tomography. *Am J Respir Crit Care Med* 167:39–44, 2003.
49. Perrier A, Roy PM, Sanchez O, et al: Multidetector-row computed tomography in suspected pulmonary embolism. *N Engl J Med* 352:1760–1768, 2005.
50. Rathbun SW, Raskob GE, Whitsett TL: Sensitivity and specificity of helical computed tomography in the diagnosis of pulmonary embolism: a systematic review. *Ann Intern Med* 132:227–232, 2000.
51. Stein PD, Fowler SE, Goodman LR, et al: Multidetector computed tomography for acute pulmonary embolism. *N Engl J Med* 354:2317–2327, 2006.

52. Wells PS, Ginsberg JS, Anderson DR, et al: Use of a clinical model for safe management of patients with suspected pulmonary embolism. *Ann Intern Med* 129:997–1005, 1998.
53. van Belle A, Buller HR, Huisman MV, et al: Effectiveness of managing suspected pulmonary embolism using an algorithm combining clinical probability, D-dimer testing, and computed tomography. *JAMA* 295:172–179, 2006.
54. Wells PS, Anderson DR, Rodger M, et al: Excluding pulmonary embolism at the bedside without diagnostic imaging: management of patients with suspected pulmonary embolism presenting to the emergency department by using a simple clinical model and d-dimer. *Ann Intern Med* 135:98–107, 2001.
55. Anderson DR, Kahn SR, Rodger MA, et al: Computed tomographic pulmonary angiography vs ventilation-perfusion lung scanning in patients with suspected pulmonary embolism: a randomized controlled trial. *JAMA* 298:2743–2753, 2007.
56. PIOPED Investigators: Value of the ventilation/perfusion scan in acute pulmonary embolism: results of the Prospective Investigation of Pulmonary Embolism Diagnosis (PIOPED). *JAMA* 263:2753–2759, 1990.
57. Stein PD, Woodard PK, Weg JG, et al: Diagnostic pathways in acute pulmonary embolism: recommendations of the PIOPED II investigators. *Am J Med* 119:1048–1055, 2006.
58. Jimenez D, Aujesky D, Diaz G, et al: Prognostic significance of deep vein thrombosis in patients presenting with acute symptomatic pulmonary embolism. *Am J Respir Crit Care Med* 181:983–991, 2010.
59. Geerts WH, Heit JA, Clagett GP, et al: Prevention of venous thromboembolism. *Chest* 119(1 Suppl):132S–175S, 2001.
60. Hirsch DR, Ingenito EP, Goldhaber SZ: Prevalence of deep venous thrombosis among patients in medical intensive care. *JAMA* 274:335–337, 1995.
61. Alikhan R, Cohen AT: Heparin for the prevention of venous thromboembolism in general medical patients (excluding stroke and myocardial infarction). *Cochrane Database Syst Rev* (3):CD003747, 2009.
62. King CS, Holley AB, Jackson JL, et al: Twice vs three times daily heparin dosing for thromboembolism prophylaxis in the general medical population: a metaanalysis. *Chest* 131:507–516, 2007.
63. Cohen AT, Davidson BL, Gallus AS, et al: Efficacy and safety of fondaparinux for the prevention of venous thromboembolism in older acute medical patients: randomised placebo controlled trial. *BMJ* 332:325–329, 2006.
64. Geerts WH, Bergqvist D, Pineo GF, et al: Prevention of venous thromboembolism: American College of Chest Physicians evidence-based clinical practice guidelines (8th edition). *Chest* 133(6 Suppl):381S–453S, 2008.
65. Snow V, Qaseem A, Barry P, et al: Management of venous thromboembolism: a clinical practice guideline from the American College of Physicians and the American Academy of Family Physicians. *Ann Intern Med* 146: 204–210, 2007.
66. Hyers TM, Agnelli G, Hull RD, et al: Antithrombotic therapy for venous thromboembolic disease. *Chest* 119(1 Suppl):176S–193S, 2001.
67. Raschke RA, Reilly BM, Guidry JR, et al: The weight-based heparin dosing nomogram compared with a "standard care" nomogram: a randomized controlled trial. *Ann Intern Med* 119:874–881, 1993.
68. Raschke RA, Gollihare B, Peirce JC: The effectiveness of implementing the weight-based heparin nomogram as a practice guideline. *Arch Intern Med* 156:1645–1649, 1996.
69. Kearon C, Kahn SR, Agnelli G, et al: Antithrombotic therapy for venous thromboembolic disease: American College of Chest Physicians evidence-based clinical practice guidelines (8th edition). *Chest* 133(6 Suppl):454S–545S, 2008.
70. Bauersachs R, Berkowitz SD, Brenner B, et al: Oral rivaroxaban for symptomatic venous thromboembolism. *N Engl J Med* 363:2499–2510, 2010.
71. Buller HR, Prins MH, Lensin AW, et al: Oral rivaroxaban for the treatment of symptomatic pulmonary embolism. *N Engl J Med* 366:1287–1297, 2012.
72. Agnelli G, Buller HR, Cohen A, et al: Oral apixaban for the treatment of acute venous thromboembolism. *N Engl J Med* 369:799–808, 2013.
73. Schulman S, Kearon C, Kakkar AK, et al: Dabigatran versus warfarin in the treatment of acute venous thromboembolism. *N Engl J Med* 361:2342–2352, 2009.
74. Pinede L, Ninet J, Duhaut P, et al: Comparison of 3 and 6 months of oral anticoagulant therapy after a first episode of proximal deep vein thrombosis or pulmonary embolism and comparison of 6 and 12 weeks of therapy after isolated calf deep vein thrombosis. *Circulation* 103:2453–2460, 2001.
75. Schulman S, Rhedin AS, Lindmarker P, et al: A comparison of six weeks with six months of oral anticoagulant therapy after a first episode of venous thromboembolism. Duration of Anticoagulation Trial Study Group. *N Engl J Med* 332:1661–1665, 1995.
76. Boutitie F, Pinede L, Schulman S, et al: Influence of preceding length of anticoagulant treatment and initial presentation of venous thromboembolism on risk of recurrence after stopping treatment: analysis of individual participants' data from seven trials. *BMJ* 342:d3036, 2011.
77. Watson L, Broderick C, Armon MP: Thrombolysis for acute deep vein thrombosis. *Cochrane Database Syst Rev* 1:002783, 2014.
78. O'Meara JJ, 3rd, McNutt RA, Evans AT, et al: A decision analysis of streptokinase plus heparin as compared with heparin alone for deep-vein thrombosis. *N Engl J Med* 330:1864–1869, 1994.
79. Hull RD, Raskob GE, Brant RF, et al: Relation between the time to achieve the lower limit of the APTT therapeutic range and recurrent venous thromboembolism during heparin treatment for deep vein thrombosis. *Arch Intern Med* 157:2562–2568, 1997.
80. Meyer G, Vicaut E, Danays T, et al: Fibrinolysis for patients with intermediate-risk pulmonary embolism. *N Engl J Med* 370:1402–1411, 2014.
81. Kearon C, Akl EA, Comerota AJ, et al: Antithrombotic therapy for VTE disease: antithrombotic therapy and prevention of thrombosis, 9th ed: American College of Chest Physicians Evidence-Based Clinical Practice Guidelines. *Chest* 141(2 Suppl):e419S–e494S, 2012.
82. Wan S, Quinlan DJ, Agnelli G, et al: Thrombolysis compared with heparin for the initial treatment of pulmonary embolism: a meta-analysis of the randomized controlled trials. *Circulation* 110:744–749, 2004.
83. Torbicki A, Galie N, Covezzoli A, et al: Right heart thrombi in pulmonary embolism: results from the International Cooperative Pulmonary Embolism Registry. *J Am Coll Cardiol* 41:2245–2251, 2003.
84. Cavallazzi R, Nair A, Vasu T, et al: Natriuretic peptides in acute pulmonary embolism: a systematic review. *Intensive Care Med* 34:2147–2156, 2008.
85. Becattini C, Vedovati MC, Agnelli G: Prognostic value of troponins in acute pulmonary embolism: a meta-analysis. *Circulation* 116:427–433, 2007.
86. Scherz N, Labarere J, Mean M, et al: Prognostic importance of hyponatremia in patients with acute pulmonary embolism. *Am J Respir Crit Care Med* 182:1178–1183, 2010.
87. Vanni S, Viviani G, Baioni M, et al: Prognostic value of plasma lactate levels among patients with acute pulmonary embolism: the thromboembolism lactate outcome study. *Ann Emerg Med* 61:330–338, 2013.
88. Jimenez D, Aujesky D, Moores L, et al: Simplification of the pulmonary embolism severity index for prognostication in patients with acute symptomatic pulmonary embolism. *Arch Intern Med* 170:1383–1389, 2010.
89. Horlander KT, Mannino DM, Leeper KV: Pulmonary embolism mortality in the United States, 1979–1998: an analysis using multiple-cause mortality data. *Arch Intern Med* 163:1711–1717, 2003.
90. Goldhaber SZ, Visani L, De Rosa M: Acute pulmonary embolism: clinical outcomes in the International Cooperative Pulmonary Embolism Registry (ICOPER). *Lancet* 353:1386–1389, 1999.
91. Nijkeuter M, Sohne M, Tick LW, et al: The natural course of hemodynamically stable pulmonary embolism: clinical outcome and risk factors in a large prospective cohort study. *Chest* 131:517–523, 2007.
92. Simonneau G, Gatzoulis MA, Adatia I, et al: Updated clinical classification of pulmonary hypertension. *J Am Coll Cardiol* 62(25 Suppl):D34–D41, 2013.
93. Simonneau G, Robbins IM, Beghetti M, et al: Updated clinical classification of pulmonary hypertension. *J Am Coll Cardiol* 54(1 Suppl):S43–S54, 2009.
94. Hoeper MM, Bogaard HJ, Condliffe R, et al: Definitions and diagnosis of pulmonary hypertension. *J Am Coll Cardiol* 62(25 Suppl):D42–D50, 2013.

95. Farber HW, Loscalzo J: Pulmonary arterial hypertension. *N Engl J Med* 351:1655–1665, 2004.
96. Ghamra ZW, Dweik RA: Primary pulmonary hypertension: an overview of epidemiology and pathogenesis. *Cleve Clin J Med* 70(Suppl 1):S2–S8, 2003.
97. Fishman AP: Primary pulmonary arterial hypertension: a look back. *J Am Coll Cardiol* 43(12 Suppl S):2S–4S, 2004.
98. Arroliga AC, Dweik RA, Kaneko FJ, et al: Primary pulmonary hypertension: update on pathogenesis and novel therapies. *Cleve Clin J Med* 67:175–190, 2000.
99. Kline JA, Steuerwald MT, Marchick MR, et al: Prospective evaluation of right ventricular function and functional status 6 months after acute submassive pulmonary embolism: frequency of persistent or subsequent elevation in estimated pulmonary artery pressure. *Chest* 136:1202–1210, 2009.
100. Deng Z, Morse JH, Slager SL, et al: Familial primary pulmonary hypertension (gene *PPH1*) is caused by mutations in the bone morphogenetic protein receptor-II gene. *Am J Hum Genet* 67:737–744, 2000.
101. Harrison RE, Flanagan JA, Sankelo M, et al: Molecular and functional analysis identifies ALK-1 as the predominant cause of pulmonary hypertension related to hereditary haemorrhagic telangiectasia. *J Med Genet* 40:865–871, 2003.
102. Eddahibi S, Humbert M, Fadel E, et al: Serotonin transporter overexpression is responsible for pulmonary artery smooth muscle hyperplasia in primary pulmonary hypertension. *J Clin Invest* 108:1141–1150, 2001.
103. Christman BW, McPherson CD, Newman JH, et al: An imbalance between the excretion of thromboxane and prostacyclin metabolites in pulmonary hypertension. *N Engl J Med* 327:70–75, 1992.
104. Giaid A, Yanagisawa M, Langleben D, et al: Expression of endothelin-1 in the lungs of patients with pulmonary hypertension. *N Engl J Med* 328: 1732–1739, 1993.
105. Kaneko FT, Arroliga AC, Dweik RA, et al: Biochemical reaction products of nitric oxide as quantitative markers of primary pulmonary hypertension. *Am J Respir Crit Care Med* 158:917–923, 1998.
106. Rabinovitch M: Pulmonary hypertension: pathophysiology as a basis for clinical decision making. *J Heart Lung Transplant* 18:1041–1053, 1999.
107. Newman JH, Fanburg BL, Archer SL, et al: Pulmonary arterial hypertension: future directions: report of a National Heart, Lung and Blood Institute/Office of Rare Diseases workshop. *Circulation* 109:2947–2952, 2004.
108. Lepetit H, Eddahibi S, Fadel E, et al: Smooth muscle cell matrix metalloproteinases in idiopathic pulmonary arterial hypertension. *Eur Respir J* 25:834–842, 2005.
109. Petkov V, Mosgoeller W, Ziesche R, et al: Vasoactive intestinal peptide as a new drug for treatment of primary pulmonary hypertension. *J Clin Invest* 111:1339–1346, 2003.
110. Mathew R: Pathogenesis of pulmonary hypertension: a case for caveolin-1 and cell membrane integrity. *Am J Physiol Heart Circ Physiol* 306:H15–H25, 2014.
111. Guignabert C, Izikki M, Tu LI, et al: Transgenic mice overexpressing the 5-hydroxytryptamine transporter gene in smooth muscle develop pulmonary hypertension. *Circ Res* 98:1323–1330, 2006.
112. Zaiman AL, Podowski M, Medicherla S, et al: Role of the TGF-beta/Alk5 signaling pathway in monocrotaline-induced pulmonary hypertension. *Am J Respir Crit Care Med* 177:896–905, 2008.
113. Morrell NW, Adnot S, Archer SL, et al: Cellular and molecular basis of pulmonary arterial hypertension. *J Am Coll Cardiol* 54(1 Suppl):S20–S31, 2009.
114. Erzurum S, Rounds SI, Stevens T, et al: Strategic plan for lung vascular research: an NHLBI-ORDR Workshop Report. *Am J Respir Crit Care Med* 182:1554–1562, 2010.
115. Humbert M, Sitbon O, Chaouat A, et al: Pulmonary arterial hypertension in France: results from a national registry. *Am J Respir Crit Care Med* 173:1023–1030, 2006.
116. Ling Y, Johnson MK, Kiely DG, et al: Changing demographics, epidemiology, and survival of incident pulmonary arterial hypertension: results from the pulmonary hypertension registry of the United Kingdom and Ireland. *Am J Respir Crit Care Med* 186:790–796, 2012.
117. Brown LM, Chen H, Halpern S, et al: Delay in recognition of pulmonary arterial hypertension: factors identified from the REVEAL Registry. *Chest* 140:19–26, 2011.
118. Tonelli AR, Baumgartner M, Alkukhun L, et al: Electrocardiography at diagnosis and close to the time of death in pulmonary arterial hypertension. *Ann Noninvasive Electrocardiol* 19:258–265, 2014.
119. Kuhn KP, Byrne DW, Arbogast PG, et al: Outcome in 91 consecutive patients with pulmonary arterial hypertension receiving epoprostenol. *Am J Respir Crit Care Med* 167:580–586, 2003.
120. McLaughlin VV, Gaine SP, Barst RJ, et al: Efficacy and safety of treprostinil: an epoprostenol analog for primary pulmonary hypertension. *J Cardiovasc Pharmacol* 41:293–299, 2003.
121. Galie N, Ghofrani HA, Torbicki A, et al: Sildenafil citrate therapy for pulmonary arterial hypertension. *N Engl J Med* 353:2148–2157, 2005.
122. Channick RN, Simonneau G, Sitbon O, et al: Effects of the dual endothelin-receptor antagonist bosentan in patients with pulmonary hypertension: a randomised placebo-controlled study. *Lancet* 358:1119–1123, 2001.
123. Rubin LJ, Badesch DB: Evaluation and management of the patient with pulmonary arterial hypertension. *Ann Intern Med* 143:282–292, 2005.
124. Humbert M, Sitbon O, Simonneau G: Treatment of pulmonary arterial hypertension. *N Engl J Med* 351:1425–1436, 2004.
125. Olsson KM, Delcroix M, Ghofrani HA, et al: Anticoagulation and survival in pulmonary arterial hypertension: results from the Comparative, Prospective Registry of Newly Initiated Therapies for Pulmonary Hypertension (COMPERA). *Circulation* 129:57–65, 2014.
126. Johnson SR, Mehta S, Granton JT: Anticoagulation in pulmonary arterial hypertension: a qualitative systematic review. *Eur Respir J* 28:999–1004, 2006.
127. Tonelli AR, Alnuaimat H, Mubarak K: Pulmonary vasodilator testing and use of calcium channel blockers in pulmonary arterial hypertension. *Respir Med* 104:481–496, 2010.
128. Barst RJ, Rubin LJ, Long WA, et al: A comparison of continuous intravenous epoprostenol (prostacyclin) with conventional therapy for primary pulmonary hypertension. The Primary Pulmonary Hypertension Study Group. *N Engl J Med* 334:296–302, 1996.
129. Simonneau G, Barst RJ, Galie N, et al: Continuous subcutaneous infusion of treprostinil, a prostacyclin analogue, in patients with pulmonary arterial hypertension: a double-blind, randomized, placebo-controlled trial. *Am J Respir Crit Care Med* 165:800–804, 2002.
130. Tapson VF, Gomberg-Maitland M, McLaughlin VV, et al: Safety and efficacy of IV treprostinil for pulmonary arterial hypertension: a prospective, multicenter, open-label, 12-week trial. *Chest* 129:683–688, 2006.
131. Channick RN, Olschewski H, Seeger W, et al: Safety and efficacy of inhaled treprostinil as add-on therapy to bosentan in pulmonary arterial hypertension. *J Am Coll Cardiol* 48:1433–1437, 2006.
132. Olschewski H, Simonneau G, Galie N, et al: Inhaled iloprost for severe pulmonary hypertension. *N Engl J Med* 347:322–329, 2002.
133. Rubin LJ, Badesch DB, Barst RJ, et al: Bosentan therapy for pulmonary arterial hypertension. *N Engl J Med* 346:896–903, 2002.
134. Galie N, Olschewski H, Oudiz RJ, et al: Ambrisentan for the treatment of pulmonary arterial hypertension: results of the ambrisentan in pulmonary arterial hypertension, randomized, double-blind, placebo-controlled, multicenter, efficacy (ARIES) study 1 and 2. *Circulation* 117:3010–3019, 2008.
135. Oudiz RJ, Galie N, Olschewski H, et al: Long-term ambrisentan therapy for the treatment of pulmonary arterial hypertension. *J Am Coll Cardiol* 54:1971–1981, 2009.
136. Pulido T, Adzerikho I, Channick RN, et al: Macitentan and morbidity and mortality in pulmonary arterial hypertension. *N Engl J Med* 369:809–818, 2013.
137. Galie N, Brundage BH, Ghofrani HA, et al: Tadalafil therapy for pulmonary arterial hypertension. *Circulation* 119:2894–2903, 2009.
138. Ghofrani HA, Voswinckel R, Reichenberger F, et al: Differences in hemodynamic and oxygenation responses to three different phosphodiesterase-5

inhibitors in patients with pulmonary arterial hypertension: a randomized prospective study. *J Am Coll Cardiol* 44:1488–1496, 2004.
139. Ghofrani HA, Galie N, Grimminger F, et al: Riociguat for the treatment of pulmonary arterial hypertension. *N Engl J Med* 369:330–340, 2013.
140. Ghofrani HA, D'Armini AM, Grimminger F, et al: Riociguat for the treatment of chronic thromboembolic pulmonary hypertension. *N Engl J Med* 369:319–329, 2013.
141. Klepetko W, Mayer E, Sandoval J, et al: Interventional and surgical modalities of treatment for pulmonary arterial hypertension. *J Am Coll Cardiol* 43(12 Suppl S):73S–80S, 2004.
142. Trulock EP: Lung and heart-lung transplantation: overview of results. *Semin Respir Crit Care Med* 22:479–488, 2001.
143. Matthay RA, Arroliga AC, Wiedemann HP, et al: Right ventricular function at rest and during exercise in chronic obstructive pulmonary disease. *Chest* 101(5 Suppl):255S–262S, 1992.
144. Weitzenblum E, Kessler R, Oswald M, et al: Medical treatment of pulmonary hypertension in chronic lung disease. *Eur Respir J* 7:148–152, 1994.
145. Higenbottam T: Pulmonary hypertension and chronic obstructive pulmonary disease: a case for treatment. *Proc Am Thorac Soc* 2:12–19, 2005.
146. American Thoracic Society: Standards for the diagnosis and care of patients with chronic obstructive pulmonary disease. *Am J Respir Crit Care Med* 152(5 Pt 2):S77–S121, 1995.
147. Weitzenblum E, Chaouat A, Canuet M, et al: Pulmonary hypertension in chronic obstructive pulmonary disease and interstitial lung diseases. *Semin Respir Crit Care Med* 30:458–470, 2009.
148. Guyatt GH, Akl EA, Crowther M, et al: Executive summary: Antithrombotic therapy and prevention of thrombosis, 9th ed: American College of Chest Physicians evidence-based clinical practice guidelines. *Chest* 141(2 Suppl):7S–47S, 2012.

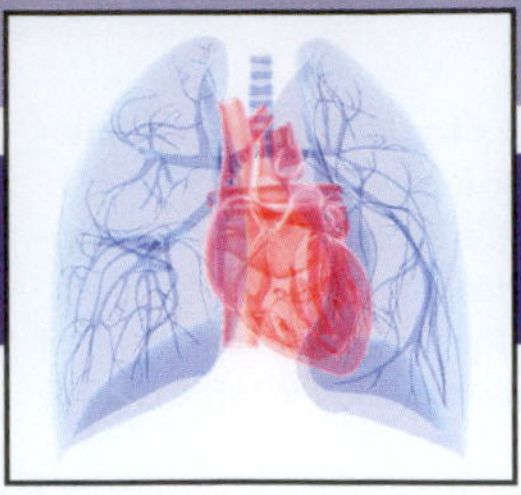

CHAPTER 29

Acute Respiratory Distress Syndrome

MATTHEW C. EXLINE, EDUARDO MIRELES-CABODEVILA, AND R. DUNCAN HITE

CHAPTER OBJECTIVES

After reading this chapter you will be able to:

- Diagnose patients with acute respiratory distress syndrome (ARDS) using currently recommended criteria (Berlin criteria).
- Differentiate normal lung function that prevents pulmonary edema versus common disease mechanisms that lead to pulmonary edema, including nonhydrostatic edema (e.g., ARDS) and hydrostatic pulmonary edema (e.g., congestive heart failure).
- Describe the effect pulmonary edema has on lung function, including gas exchange and lung compliance.
- Identify the histopathologic findings associated with the exudative phase and the fibroproliferative phase of ARDS.
- Describe the common risk factors associated with the onset of ARDS.
- Quantify the impact of ARDS on individual patients (e.g., mortality and morbidity), hospitals, and health care systems.
- State the approaches to managing ARDS, including therapies that directly target improving lung function and care designed to support and protect other vital organs.
- Describe how ventilator settings (e.g., mode, tidal volume, positive end expiratory pressure, inspiratory flow rate) should be adjusted for patients with ARDS.
- Describe how mechanical ventilation can cause lung injury and how ventilator-induced lung injury can be avoided.
- Describe the use of innovative and alternative strategies for assisting ventilation in ARDS, including modes of mechanical ventilation, prone positioning, neuromuscular blockade (paralytics), extracorporeal support, and other interventions.
- Describe the current status of evidence to support the use of pharmacologic therapies (e.g., nitric oxide, surfactant, corticosteroids) in treating patients with ARDS.

CHAPTER OUTLINE

KEY TERMS

acute hypoxemic respiratory failure
acute lung injury
acute respiratory distress syndrome
airway pressure release ventilation
barotrauma
congestive heart failure
conservative fluid management
extracorporeal carbon dioxide removal
extracorporeal membrane oxygenation
high-frequency oscillatory ventilation
hydrostatic pulmonary edema
inspiratory-to-expiratory ratio
nonhydrostatic pulmonary edema
lung protective ventilation
multiple organ dysfunction syndrome
positive end-expiratory pressure
prone positioning
pulmonary edema
ventilator–induced lung injury
volutrauma

Acute hypoxemic respiratory failure (AHRF) may develop in many clinical settings and is a common reason for admission to the intensive care unit (ICU). There are a wide variety of causes for AHRF, including infection (e.g., bacterial or viral pneumonia), pulmonary embolus, airway obstruction (e.g., tumor, mucous plug), and more. Two common causes of AHRF are the abnormal leakage of fluid from inside the vascular space (i.e., alveolar capillary) into the alveoli, which is commonly referred to as pulmonary edema. This chapter will focus on understanding the diseases that cause pulmonary edema formation by highlighting one common source of pulmonary edema known as the **acute respiratory distress syndrome** (ARDS).[1] In addition, the chapter will explore the clinical syndrome of ARDS, including current management strategies, and the vital role of the respiratory therapist (RT) in helping manage ARDS.

PHYSIOLOGY OF PULMONARY EDEMA

Liquid and Solute Transport in the Lungs

In addition to maintaining gas exchange and lung perfusion, as detailed in other chapters, a key component of normal lung function is to maintain a net flux of fluid through the lung parenchyma without causing lung edema or alveolar consolidation. For maximal gas exchange, the entire cardiac output must pass through the extensive capillary network that surrounds the total surface area of the alveolar airspaces. As a feature of the anatomy of the alveolus, the walls of the alveolus are separated from the capillary walls by the very thin lung interstitium (Figure 29-1). This close approximation of the alveolus to the

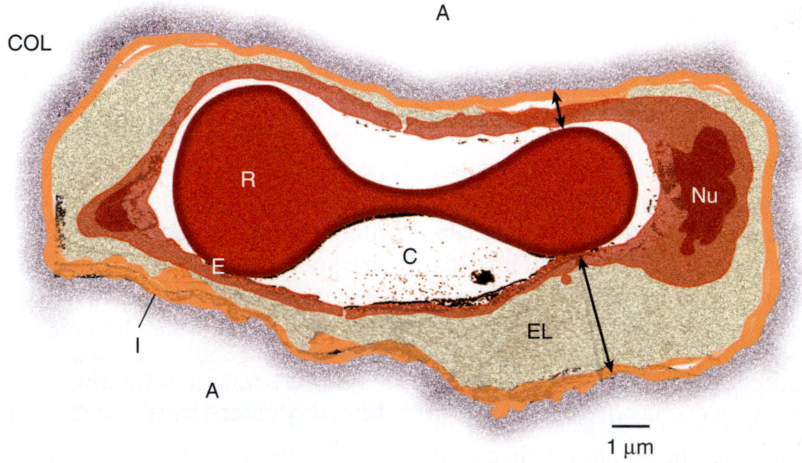

FIGURE 29-1 Cross section of an alveolar wall shows the path for O_2 and CO_2 diffusion. The thin side of the alveolar wall barrier *(short double arrow)* consists of type I epithelium *(I)*, interstitium formed by the fused basal laminae of the epithelial and endothelial cells, capillary endothelium *(E)*, plasma in the alveolar capillary *(C)*, and the cytoplasm of the red blood cell (RBC) *(R)*. The thick side of the gas-exchange barrier *(long double arrow)* has an accumulation of elastin *(EL)*, collagen *(COL)*, and matrix that separates the alveolar epithelium from the alveolar capillary endothelium. As long as the RBCs are flowing, O_2 and CO_2 diffusion probably occur across both sides of the air-blood barrier. *A*, Alveolus; *Nu*, nucleus of the capillary endothelial cell. (Human lung surgical specimen, transmission electron photomicrograph.)

capillary walls minimizes the distance for gases (i.e., O_2 and carbon dioxide [CO_2]) to diffuse between the airspace and blood. However, this small barrier also serves as a conduit for leakage of fluid out of the lumen of the capillary into the lung interstitium and alveolar airspace. Under normal conditions, the vascular and lung compartments work synergistically to maintain a physiologic amount of fluid leakage. Under normal circumstances, the alveoli contain air and are without fluid. In pathologic disease states involving either the capillaries or the alveoli, the rate of leakage of fluid into the lung can exceed the lung's capacity to clear the fluid (i.e., through the lymphatic drainage of the lung), thereby leading to excessive fluid accumulation in the airspace (called *pulmonary edema*) and abnormal lung function and gas exchange.

On average, the entire blood volume of the body circulates through the lungs in 1 minute or less. This incredible feat is achieved through an ingenious design that begins at the outflow tract of the right ventricle and passes through the thick-walled branches of the pulmonary artery, which successively divide into bronchial and bronchiolar branches. Beyond the terminal bronchioles, the pulmonary vasculature divides further to form a fine capillary meshwork that surrounds the alveoli. The large surface area of the capillary network provides for a low–hydrostatic pressure (5 to 12 mm Hg), high-volume system wherein large volumes of blood come into immediate contact with alveolar gases. At the capillary level, the vessel walls are composed solely of endothelial cells bound to basal lamina.

The interstitial space of the lung is separated into two compartments: (1) the alveolar side, which is the space between the capillaries and epithelial lining of the alveolus, and (2) the nonalveolar side. The alveolar interstitium is composed of several structural proteins (collagens and elastin) and proteoglycans, which form a relatively stiff, noncompliant basement membrane between the membranes of the vascular endothelium and the alveolar epithelium. All combined, this structure is very thin (<0.5 μm) and facilitates gas exchange (see Figure 29-1). In contrast, the interstitium on the nonalveolar side of the capillaries is composed of collagen, elastin proteins, and mucopolysaccharides in a hyaluronic acid gel that is more compliant and serves to interconnect membranes of the airway epithelium, vascular endothelium, and fibroblasts.

Under normal conditions, the physical properties of the interstitium allow absorption of water by these tissues with no leakage of fluid into the alveoli and no impact on pulmonary gas exchange. This interstitial fluid content leads to an interstitial pressure that keeps fluid in the interstitial space, thereby serving as a hydrostatic pressure that is similar to but opposes the hydrostatic pressure in the vascular space. Overall, the interstitium, particularly the nonalveolar component, is highly compliant and able to accommodate relatively large increases in fluid volume in the interstitium without significant change in interstitial hydrostatic pressure or leakage of fluid into the alveolar airspace.

The alveolar capillaries contain pores (pumps and channels) that selectively permit the leakage of protein and allow movement of electrolytes and nutrients between the intravascular space and the interstitium of the lungs.[2] The net exchange of fluids between the intravascular space (i.e., within the capillaries) and the interstitium of the lungs is determined by the combined influences of hydrostatic and osmotic forces within the blood and interstitium. Osmotic forces reflect the effects of dissolved proteins to retain fluid within the interstitial space. Under normal conditions, the capillary hydrostatic force and interstitial osmotic force influencing the movement of fluid out of the bloodstream into the interstitium are slightly greater than the capillary osmotic force and interstitial hydrostatic forces opposing this movement. This balance is governed by the Starling forces. As a result of the normal balance of these forces, a small fraction of the cardiac output (approximately 0.01%) normally filters from the capillaries into the interstitial space of the lungs.[3] This filtration process plays a role in the immune defenses of the lung and is a major determinant of total lung fluid content.

The lung protects itself from excessive fluid accumulation by several mechanisms. The lung *lymphatic drainage system* is the primary system for removing filtered fluid and protein from the lungs. Fluid and solutes enter the lymphatic drainage channels from small lymphatic capillaries located around the respiratory bronchioles. This process is assisted by the presence of a modest pressure gradient within the lungs. Higher pressure near the dense alveolar interstitium forces fluid away from the alveolar surface toward the lower pressured nonalveolar interstitium and terminal lymphatic vessels. Drainage is enhanced further by intrathoracic pressure alterations that occur with respiration, and retrograde (backward) flow is prevented by the presence of one-way lymphatic valves. Ultimately, lymphatic fluid drains out of the lung into the superior vena cava through the thoracic duct.[4]

When the rate of fluid leakage into the interstitium exceeds the capacity for drainage through the pulmonary lymphatic vessels, backup mechanisms exist for storing additional fluid and protecting against alveolar flooding. Loose connective tissue surrounding the bronchioles and bronchi is capable of storing twice the normal fluid content of the lungs.[4] Also, fluid can fill the interlobular septal spaces or cuffs; when this happens, the fluid-filled septal spaces can be seen on a chest radiograph as linear interstitial infiltrates (known as *Kerley lines*) at the lung periphery (Figure 29-2). As total lung fluid accumulates, the capacity of the gel-like matrix in the nonalveolar lung interstitium to accommodate fluid is maximized. Once this capacity is maximized and the rate of fluid accumulation exceeds the rate of lymphatic drainage, fluid will start to accumulate within the alveoli; the alveoli then become flooded.

Hydrostatic Versus Nonhydrostatic Edema

Despite these extensive protective mechanisms to protect the alveolus from excess fluid leakage, common disease states can result in fluid flux that exceeds the lung's capacity to remove or store the fluid. Under such circumstances, small increases in lung fluid content produce large increases in interstitial hydrostatic pressure, accumulation of intraalveolar fluid, and the

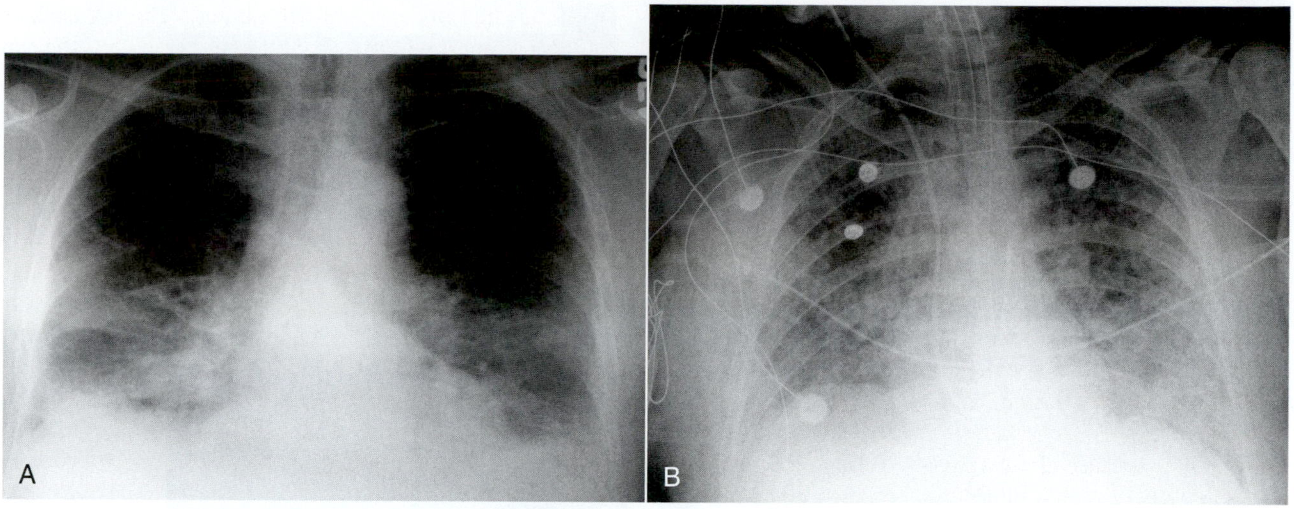

FIGURE 29-2 Chest radiographs show typical radiographic features of congestive heart failure (CHF) and acute respiratory distress syndrome (ARDS). **A,** CHF is characterized by cardiomegaly, interstitial infiltrates, bilateral perihilar and basilar alveolar infiltrates, and bilateral pleural effusions, which cause blunting of the costophrenic angles. **B,** ARDS is commonly associated with normal cardiac size, diffuse peripheral alveolar infiltrates, and minimal or absent pleural effusions.

clinical entity called **pulmonary edema.** The diseases that cause pulmonary edema are typically categorized as either hydrostatic or nonhydrostatic edema. To clarify the distinction between hydrostatic and nonhydrostatic edema, a simple analogy is to consider the intravascular hydrostatic force within the capillary as a body of water and the alveolar barrier as an impermeable dam with pumps that help regulate the water levels behind the dam (Figure 29-3). Hydrostatic pulmonary edema occurs when the pressure or volume of water exceeds the capacity of the dam's pumps to maintain the water levels. Water then floods the land below the dam (the alveolus in this metaphor). Nonhydrostatic pulmonary edema occurs when the dam is cracked or damaged and the water leaks through it onto the land below the dam. It should also be noted that the type or color of water is different in nonhydrostatic edema because the cracks in the dam permit leakage of more sediment (equivalent of protein and cells in patients with ARDS).

Box 29-1 Common Causes of Hydrostatic Pulmonary Edema

CARDIAC
- Left ventricular failure
  - Systolic (e.g., myocardial infarction, myocarditis)
  - Diastolic (e.g., left ventricular hypertrophy)
- Valvular heart disease (e.g., aortic, mitral)

VOLUME OVERLOAD
- Excessive fluid administration
- Renal failure
- Hepatic failure
- Hypoalbuminemia (e.g., malnutrition)

Hydrostatic Pulmonary Edema

Hydrostatic pulmonary edema is often also called *cardiogenic pulmonary edema* because of its close association with abnormalities in intravascular hydrostatic pressures that cause edema. Whereas increased hydrostatic pressures in the pulmonary arteries lead to pulmonary arterial hypertension and problems with right heart failure, increased hydrostatic pressures in the pulmonary veins lead to increased hydrostatic pressures in the alveolar capillaries that increase fluid leakage out of the capillary. In most patients, elevation of pulmonary venous pressures are caused by increased pressures in left-sided heart pressures (left atrial or left ventricular end-diastolic pressure), which are key characteristics of left-sided congestive heart failure, both diastolic and systolic (Box 29-1). The elevated hydrostatic pressures within the capillary ultimately lead to elevated interstitial fluid pressure and alveolar flooding through leakage of fluid from the respiratory epithelium.[5] In the setting of increased hydrostatic pressure, the endothelial and epithelial barriers remain intact and impermeable to large proteins and molecules. As a result, the fluid that accumulates within the alveoli, when measured from bronchoalveolar lavage (BAL) fluid samples, has characteristics identical to those of interstitial fluid, that is, with low protein levels similar to those of transudative fluid collections sampled from the pleural and peritoneal spaces in the same disease states.[4]

Nonhydrostatic Pulmonary Edema

Nonhydrostatic pulmonary edema, also called *noncardiogenic pulmonary edema*, results from injury to the vascular endothelium and/or alveolar epithelium. This injury creates a loss of integrity in the barrier between the vascular and alveolar spaces (like cracks in a dam; see Figure 29-3). In contrast to hydrostatic pulmonary edema, nonhydrostatic pulmonary edema is associated with increased total lung water despite normal microvascular hydrostatic pressure. Although many seemingly unrelated

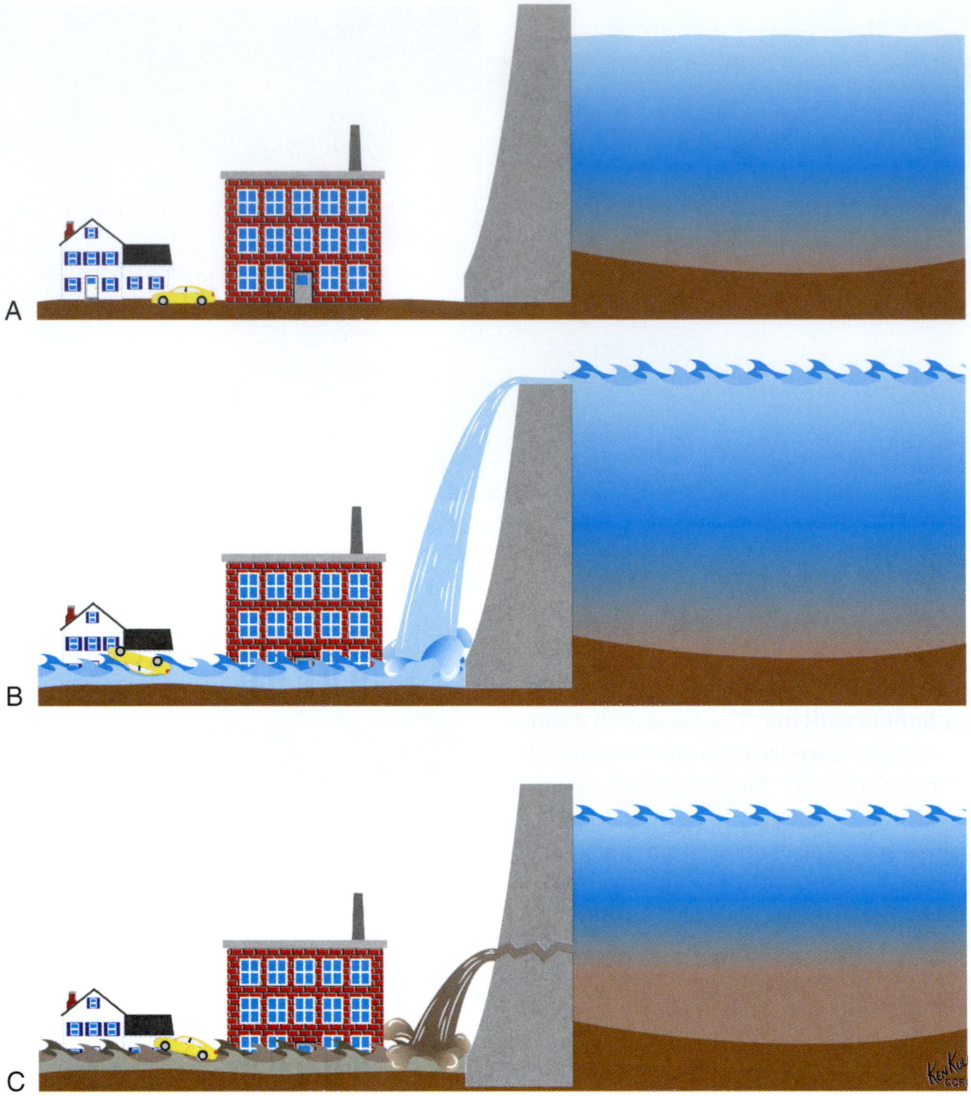

FIGURE 29-3 The intact dam **(A)** represents the normal condition in which oncotic and hydrostatic forces (Starling forces) are balanced, keeping the town dry (where the town represents the alveolar space). In **B,** the dam remains intact but the water level has risen, overwhelming the dam (i.e., exceeding the forces that resist alveolar flooding) and flooding the town representing the alveoli. This condition resembles hydrostatic pulmonary edema. In **C,** a crack in the dam (simulating the alveolar-capillary interface) allows water through the dam, flooding the town. Note that the water flooding the town is darker because it contains more sediment and mud from the lake. The condition in **C** simulates the damage to the alveolar-capillary interface that accompanies inflammation in acute respiratory distress syndrome, causing nonhydrostatic pulmonary edema. The muddier water flooding the town (representing the alveolar space) in **C** than in **B** represents the more proteinaceous, inflammatory nature of the fluid that floods the alveoli in nonhydrostatic pulmonary edema.

risk factors for ARDS have been identified, all causes of ARDS feature disruption of endothelial and epithelial barriers and typically occur under conditions associated with widespread microvascular injury to the lungs. Vascular endothelial injury in the lungs causes increased microvascular permeability and allows fluid to pass from the capillaries into the interstitial space. As protein-rich fluid enters the pulmonary interstitium from the vasculature, the osmotic gradient between the capillary and the lung approaches zero and no longer opposes the hydrostatic forces that favor fluid movement from the capillary into the lung. This process is likely facilitated both by damage to the normally impermeable alveolar epithelial barrier, which is a key feature of ARDS,[6] and by impaired alveolar fluid clearance in ARDS.[7]

Many acute illnesses can lead to the development of ARDS (Box 29-2), but a common mechanism was proposed by Weiland and colleagues.[8] Regardless of the cause, ARDS is typically associated with an influx of polymorphonuclear neutrophils (PMNs), which release inflammatory by-products, such as proteases, phospholipases, and oxygen radicals into the lung.[2,9] These inflammatory by-products degrade the endothelial and epithelial barriers and recruit additional PMNs to continue the

Box 29-2 Clinical Features of Congestive Heart Failure and Acute Respiratory Distress Syndrome

FEATURES COMMON TO BOTH CONGESTIVE HEART FAILURE AND ACUTE RESPIRATORY DISTRESS SYNDROME

- Symptoms of anxiety, dyspnea, tachypnea
- Decreased compliance and reduced lung volumes
- Hypoxemia (mild to severe), often requiring ventilator assistance
- Chest radiograph shows diffuse alveolar and interstitial infiltrates

FEATURES FAVORING CONGESTIVE HEART FAILURE

- Clinical history suggestive of CHF (see Box 29-1)
- Symmetric pulmonary infiltrates, cardiomegaly, or pleural effusions on chest radiograph (see Figure 29-2)
- Elevated pulmonary artery catheter wedge pressure (18 to 30 mm Hg)
- Bronchoalveolar lavage fluid: Low protein and minimally increased cellularity
- Prompt (<12 to 24 hours) and lasting response to diuretics and CHF therapy

FEATURES FAVORING ACUTE RESPIRATORY DISTRESS SYNDROME

- Clinical history of a risk factor for ARDS (see Box 29-3)
- Asymmetric, peripheral infiltrates on chest radiograph (see Figure 29-3)
- Bronchoalveolar lavage fluid: Very high protein level and marked cellular influx
- Transient improvement with CHF therapy, but uncommon to significantly improve during initial 12 to 36 hours

CHF, congestive heart failure.

inflammatory cascade. In contrast to hydrostatic pulmonary edema, the fluid that accumulates in ARDS, when sampled using BAL, typically demonstrates very high levels of protein, neutrophils, and total cells (Figure 29-4).[1]

Although PMNs play a central role in the development of ARDS, multiple pathways lead to the inflammatory cascade in the lung and subsequent loss of alveolar membrane integrity. Other chemical insults (e.g., gastric aspiration), inhalational injury (e.g., of noxious gas such as chlorine), or immunologic pathways (e.g., tumor necrosis factor [TNF] or interleukin-8 [IL8]) all contribute to the hemodynamic and inflammatory events characteristic of ARDS.[10] Sepsis, one of the most common causes of ARDS, features activation of many of these inflammatory pathways. The relative contributions and exact roles of these proinflammatory mediators in the pathogenesis of ARDS are not known.[1,11] Attempts to control the inflammatory response in sepsis and ARDS by blocking specific mediators (e.g., steroids and antibodies to TNF and IL-1) unfortunately have not proved beneficial and are not currently used.

It is important to note that acute illnesses associated with the development of ARDS also can lead to widespread systemic organ injury (e.g., renal failure, encephalopathy), which is caused by similar inflammatory pathways leading to injury and fluid leak in those organs.[12,13] This syndrome of diffuse organ impairment is frequently referred to as the **multiple organ dysfunction syndrome** (MODS). ARDS is the pulmonary manifestation of MODS, and MODS is a common cause of death in ICUs. In contrast to ARDS, illnesses that lead to hydrostatic pulmonary edema typically do not cause MODS.

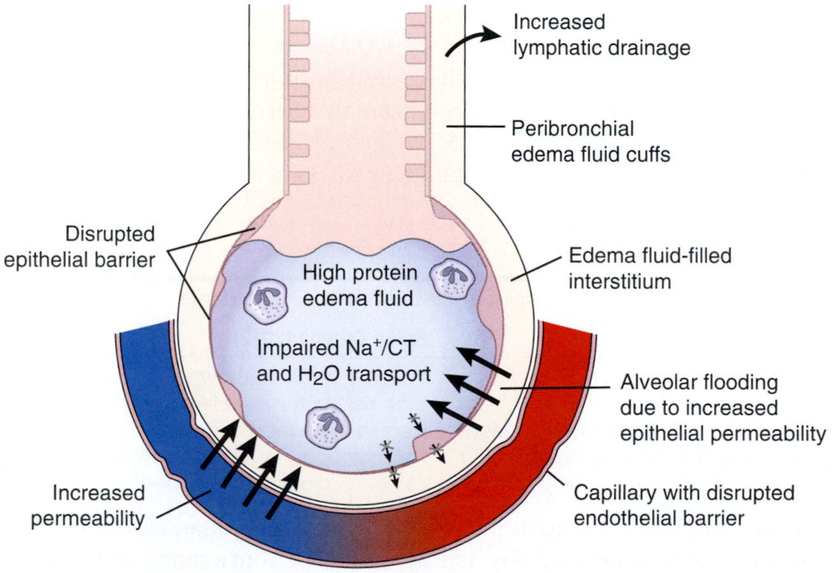

FIGURE 29-4 In this cartoon, the anatomy of the normal alveolus is on the left side of the figure including the alveolar epithelium (type I and type II cells), pulmonary capillary with its endothelium, surfactant layer, and alveolar macrophages. In the normal alveolus, little or no excess fluid is present. The right side of the picture represents the changes associated with acute respiratory distress syndrome, including injury and leak of the capillary endothelium and alveolar epithelium, damage and depletion of surfactant, influx of inflammatory cells (neutrophils) and cytokines, and leak of fluid with high protein levels. (Modified with permission from Matthay MA, Zimmerman GA: Acute lung injury and the acute respiratory distress syndrome: four decades of inquiry into pathogenesis and rational management. Am J Respir Cell Mol Biol 33:319–327, 2005.)

Gas Exchange and Lung Mechanics in Pulmonary Edema

Hydrostatic pulmonary edema and ARDS are both associated with restrictive physiology, reduced lung compliance, and refractory hypoxemia, which are largely the result of the accumulation of interstitial and alveolar fluid. In addition, impaired gas exchange that results from pulmonary edema is complicated further by an increase in the work of breathing. The increased work of breathing is caused by dramatic reductions in lung compliance that in turn result from alveolar collapse and interstitial fluid accumulation. This scenario commonly causes acute respiratory failure and the need for ventilatory assistance (invasive or noninvasive). In most cases, the severity of lung dysfunction and hypoxemia is worse and more prolonged in ARDS compared to the hydrostatic pulmonary edema of **congestive heart failure** (CHF). The inflammatory nature of the intraalveolar fluid in ARDS also impairs surfactant synthesis, secretion, and function. The resulting surfactant abnormalities further impair pulmonary gas exchange (i.e., related to atelectasis and impaired compliance). The negative effects of alveolar consolidation and atelectasis on pulmonary gas exchange are further worsened by a loss of the normal vascular response to alveolar hypoxemia. Normally, pulmonary arteries in areas of alveolar hypoxia will constrict as a physiologic response to preserve ventilation/perfusion ($\dot{V}/\dot{Q}$) matching. However, in ARDS, this normal vasoconstrictive response is impaired. Because the body is unable to shunt blood away from the diseased alveoli, these nonaerated alveoli receive excessive blood flow, which contributes to severe $\dot{V}/\dot{Q}$ mismatching and an intrapulmonary right-to-left shunting of blood flow, which causes hypoxemia.

In summary, pulmonary edema may arise from acute illnesses associated with increased pulmonary venous pressure (hydrostatic pulmonary edema or CHF) or may result from conditions associated with acute injury to the lung, in which the normal barriers to fluid movement within the lungs are disrupted, as in the nonhydrostatic pulmonary edema of ARDS. Although CHF and ARDS are distinct disease processes that require different management strategies, differentiating these two forms of pulmonary edema in patients is frequently challenging because signs and symptoms of both are often very similar. The remainder of this chapter will focus on the distinct characteristics and management approaches for ARDS. In so doing, the reader should gain further ability to understand which characteristics and management approaches are both similar and distinct to CHF.

DEFINITION AND DIAGNOSIS

Early in the 20th century, the clinical problem of respiratory distress shortly after birth was identified in premature infants. By the 1950s, the mechanism for the respiratory distress syndrome (RDS) of neonates was identified as a primary deficiency of pulmonary surfactant caused by birth at a stage of gestation (typically ≤32 weeks) before fetal lung maturation.[14] The first formal report of RDS in adults was published in the late 1960s, and the entity of adult respiratory distress syndrome (ARDS) was created.[15] Over the next 25 years, extensive research was focused on this highly lethal condition (i.e., initially with an associated mortality rate of 60% to 70%), but outcomes did not improve significantly during this period.[16] Progress was challenged by a lack of consensus in the definition of the syndrome and by variation in approaches to clinical management.[17] A key component of the challenge of defining ARDS is the close similarity to other disease entities, including CHF, pneumonia, and lung contusion. In the absence of a key distinguishing feature that easily separates ARDS from these other common disease conditions; the definition of ARDS must include several features, which in combination form a syndrome.

In response to these challenges, a consensus definition for acute (no longer called *adult*) respiratory distress syndrome (ARDS) was created in 1994 with input from key thought leaders from both Europe and the United States and is commonly referred to as the American-European Consensus Conference (AECC) definition (Table 29-1).[17] Because the syndrome of ARDS in children (older than newborns) is not significantly

TABLE 29-1

Recommended Definitions for the Acute Respiratory Distress Syndrome

	AECC Criteria (1994)	Berlin Criteria (2012)
Timing of onset	Acute onset (no definition)	Within 1 week of known risk factor (trigger)
Risk factor	Not included	If no risk factor identified, hydrostatic edema must be formally excluded
Exclusion of hydrostatic edema	Right heart catheterization with wedge pressure ≤18 mm Hg *or* no clinical evidence of left atrial hypertension	Requirement for wedge pressure measurement removed. Clinical vignettes using history, clinical signs/symptoms, and echocardiography provided
Hypoxemia	ALI: P/F ratio ≤300 ARDS: P/F ≤200 (regardless of PEEP level)	Three categories of ARDS (no ALI): *Mild:* P/F ratio = 201-300 *Moderate:* P/F = 101-200 *Severe:* P/F ≤100 (must have PEEP or CPAP ≥5 cm H_2O)
Chest imaging	Bilateral infiltrates seen on frontal chest radiograph (no specific criteria)	Bilateral infiltrates not explained by effusions, collapse, or nodules

Modified from Acute Respiratory Distress Syndrome Task Force; Ranieri VM, Rubenfeld GD, Thompson BT, et al: Acute respiratory distress syndrome: the Berlin definition. JAMA 307:2526–2533, 2012.

different from that in adults, the AECC definition discontinued using the term *adult* in favor of *acute* for the syndrome's title. The AECC definition includes five central components: (1) reduced lung compliance, (2) hypoxemia (ratio of PaO_2/FiO_2 [P/F] <200), (3) bilateral infiltrates on chest radiograph, (4) an acute illness associated with the development of ARDS that can trigger the onset of ARDS, and (5) no evidence of CHF (based on measurements from a pulmonary artery catheter or other means to estimate elevated pressures on the left side of the heart). The AECC definition includes a condition known as **acute lung injury** (ALI) which shares all characteristics of ARDS except hypoxemia that is less severe (i.e., P/F ratio of <300 compared to <200 to qualify as ARDS). Since 1994, The AECC definition has served as the gold standard for identifying and enrolling patients with ARDS into clinical trials. The combination of this consistent definition and enhanced collaboration between investigators around the world has led to dramatic discoveries and marked improvements in the outcomes of patients.

In 2012, the AECC definition of ARDS was updated by a new international consensus group that met in Berlin, Germany in 2011. These updates were made in response to limitations of the AECC that had been identified over the ensuing two decades. This new definition is commonly referred to as the Berlin definition or Berlin criteria (see Table 29-1).[18] The key new features of the Berlin definition include the following:

1. Replacement of the distinction between ALI and ARDS with three categories of ARDS severity (mild, moderate, and severe) based on ranges of P/F ratio and levels of **positive end expiratory pressure** (PEEP)
2. Inclusion of noninvasive techniques to estimate left heart pressures, including echocardiography
3. Enhanced specificity for interpretation of chest radiographs when trying to determine the presence of bilateral infiltrates or opacities
4. Enhanced specificity regarding the timeframe referred to as "acute" (i.e., occurring within 1 week of the triggering condition)

With the introduction of the Berlin definition, it is anticipated that use of the term *acute lung injury* will diminish because it has become clear that ALI and ARDS are not distinct conditions and only represent differences in severity of the same condition. Although no major clinical trials have yet been completed using the Berlin definition, it is expected that the Berlin definition will become the basis for future trials and for communication among clinicians caring for patients with ARDS.

Distinguishing Acute Respiratory Distress Syndrome from Nonhydrostatic Pulmonary Edema in Clinical Practice

Despite the strength of these definitions for ARDS and nonhydrostatic pulmonary edema, differentiating ARDS from **hydrostatic pulmonary edema** (CHF) based on the AECC or Berlin definition can remain challenging, even for experienced clinicians. In Box 29-2, clinical features that are common to both CHF and ARDS and those that can distinguish each are outlined. CHF is more common than ARDS and should be considered whenever the history or physical examination findings suggest one of the causes of CHF listed in Box 29-3. A clinical history of infection, recent trauma, or risk factors for aspiration may be present in either patient group, but the presence of these risk factors (triggers) favors a diagnosis of ARDS. To underscore the difficulty in distinguishing the cause of pulmonary edema, many patients with ARDS are older and have preexisting illnesses that also place them at risk for CHF.

It is difficult to distinguish between CHF and ARDS based on the radiographic findings alone. Both CHF and ARDS are characterized by diffuse alveolar infiltrates that especially occur in dependent lung zones (see Box 29-2). CHF is more often associated with cardiomegaly, perihilar infiltrates, and pleural effusions, whereas ARDS is more often associated with the presence

RULE OF THUMB

The severity of hypoxemia can be measured in many ways with the most complex method, known as the *alveolar-arterial (A-a) gradient*. Calculation of the A-a gradient is cumbersome; therefore many clinicians choose to use methods that are simple and quick and that provide useful estimates for trending the response of a patient to therapy. The P/F ratio is calculated using the PaO_2 obtained from an arterial blood gas (ABG) analysis and the fraction of inspired oxygen (FiO_2) at the time the ABG value was obtained. When calculating P/F ratios, it is important to remember the difference between a fraction and a percent. In other words, a patient who is receiving 40% supplemental O_2 has a FiO_2 of 0.40 (not 40). As an example, the P/F ratio of a patient on 50% O_2 whose PaO_2 is 100 mm Hg calculates to be 200. Assuming the patient met the other points of the Berlin criteria to have ARDS, the P/F ratio would indicate the patient has moderate ARDS.

Box 29-3 Risk Factors for Acute Lung Injury and Acute Respiratory Distress Syndrome

DIRECT INJURY
- Pneumonia (viral, bacterial, fungal)
- Gastric aspiration
- Toxic inhalation (phosgene, cocaine, smoke, high concentration of oxygen)
- Near drowning
- Lung contusion

INDIRECT INJURY
- Sepsis and prolonged shock
- Burn injury (chemical or heat-induced)
- Multiple trauma
- Transfusions (transfusion-related acute lung injury [TRALI])
- Pancreatitis
- Gynecologic causes (abruptio placentae, amniotic embolism, eclampsia)
- Drug effect (e.g., *trans*-retinoic acid for acute leukemia)
- Sickle cell crisis

of peripheral alveolar infiltrates, air bronchograms, sparing of the costophrenic angles, and normal cardiac size. However, cardiac size and pleural effusions may be difficult to interpret on portable chest x-ray studies with patients lying supine in the ICU. Consequently, differentiating between CHF and ARDS on the basis of the chest radiograph is often difficult.

Pulmonary edema of any cause is associated with impaired gas exchange and abnormal lung mechanics. Both CHF and early ARDS (especially in the exudative phase; see below later discussion) are associated with interstitial and alveolar accumulation of fluid. As a result of $\dot{V}/\dot{Q}$ mismatching and shunt accompanying this fluid accumulation, arterial hypoxemia develops. Because of associated reduced lung compliance and increased ventilator rates, patients with interstitial and alveolar edema of any cause use a higher fraction (25% to 50%) of their total metabolic output to support their increased work of breathing.

Intuitively, invasive measurement of hemodynamic variables using a pulmonary artery (Swan-Ganz) catheter would seem to offer a definitive way to differentiate hydrostatic and nonhydrostatic edema. However, in practice, the measurement of the cardiac output or pulmonary arterial pressure either invasively or noninvasively has not been shown to be essential for diagnosis of ARDS or beneficial in the daily management of ARDS patients.[19] The increasing availability and accuracy of noninvasive assessment of cardiac function by means of echocardiography, when combined with other physical examination features (capillary refill and mottling), can provide reliable information that can effectively guide clinical decision making.[20]

A potential method of separating CHF from ARDS is based on differences in the characteristics of the edema fluid. As previously discussed, ARDS is associated with inflammatory injury to the pulmonary microvasculature, which allows the influx of inflammatory cells and proteinaceous fluid into the interstitium and alveolar spaces. The inflammatory nature of this exudative fluid is reflected by the presence of large quantities of inflammatory cells (predominantly neutrophils) in BAL fluid (BALF). The BALF findings also can provide diagnostic insights regarding respiratory infections that may be present, and potentially the primary source for ARDS. In contrast, the alveolar edema fluid in CHF is typically noninflammatory, and the protein content is much lower than the protein content of normal BALF.[21] Despite its potential value, performing BAL and analyzing BALF is not currently a standard clinical practice in managing patients with acute respiratory failure caused by pulmonary edema.

MINI CLINI

A careful history and evaluation of the overall clinical presentation often are the most useful means by which CHF and ARDS can be initially differentiated in a patient who has refractory hypoxemia and bilateral infiltrates on the chest radiograph. For example, a patient presents to the emergency department with complaints of increased cough and shortness of breath and a low-grade fever (38.2° C). His medical history includes a long history of systolic congestive heart failure (ejection fraction of 20% to 25% on recent echocardiogram). On examination, he has rales noted in both bases, engorged neck veins, bilateral lower extremity edema and bilateral infiltrates with cardiomegaly on chest radiograph. His P/F ratio on ABG analysis and 50% FiO_2 are 175. His white blood cell count is within normal range, and he has no other signs of systemic inflammatory response syndrome (SIRS) or other organ failure (e.g., renal, hepatic, central nervous system). Based on this manifesting information, the patient is more likely to have CHF as a cause of his pulmonary edema than ARDS, despite his fever and a P/F less than 200. Low-grade fever can be commonly seen in exacerbations of CHF. It would be typical for this patient to improve quickly with diuretic therapy and other measures to lower afterload.

Histopathologic Findings

During the early years of understanding RDS and ARDS, pathologists were critically important in helping characterize and understand the primary abnormalities in the lung tissue by examining lung biopsies and autopsies.[14] Although biopsy of the lung can provide specific information that can reliably distinguish ARDS from nonhydrostatic forms of pulmonary edema, lung biopsy is typically not required for managing patients with ARDS. The changes in the lung tissue in ARDS are typically separated into two phases based on the overall duration of the disease process: (1) the exudative phase (1 to 7 days) and (2) the fibroproliferative phase (3 days to weeks).

The exudative phase is characterized by diffuse damage to alveoli and blood vessels and the influx of proteinaceous fluid and inflammatory cells into the interstitium and alveolar spaces. Also, many of the alveolar spaces are filled with *hyaline membranes,* which are composed of cellular debris and condensed plasma proteins (Figure 29-5). As a result of these characteristic changes, an early name for ARDS was hyaline membrane disease. Pathologically, there is destruction of the alveolar wall, which includes type I pneumocytes (the predominant structure cells lining the alveoli) and type II pneumocytes (which make and secrete surfactant).[22,23] The pathologic findings of ARDS also include cellular injury to the lining (endothelium) of the pulmonary capillaries. When the primary condition that triggered the onset of ARDS is quickly identified and treated, the exudative phase is typically short, lasting only a few days and is fully reversible, leaving no significant chronic signs of injury to the lung.

After the cause of lung injury is established and the initiating events are controlled, a process of lung repair begins. On pathologic examination, this appears as an overabundance of alveolar type II pneumocytes and infiltration or proliferation by fibroblasts within the alveolar basement membrane and intraalveolar spaces. Fibroblasts drive intraalveolar and interstitial fibrosis.[23] The extent of fibrosis determines the degree of pulmonary disability in patients who survive ARDS. The exact mechanisms controlling lung remodeling in ARDS are not well established but very likely involve by-products of inflammatory cells (e.g., proteases, antiproteases, IL-6) and

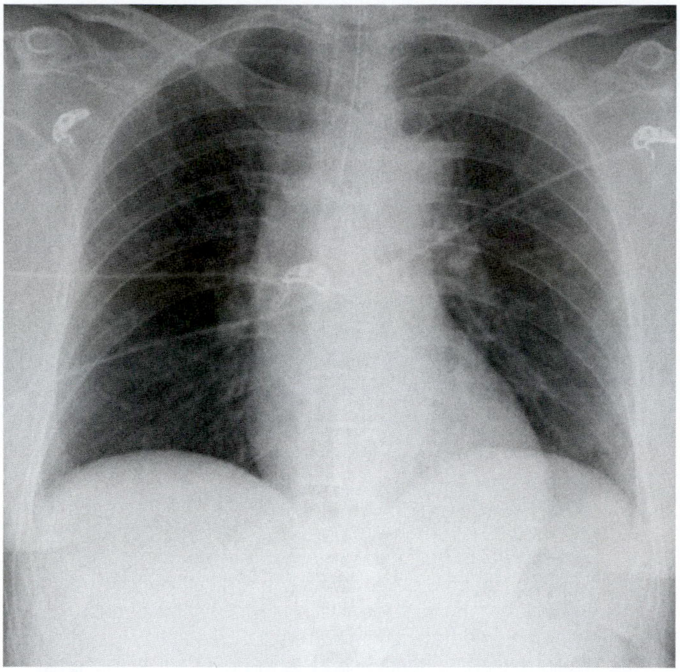

FIGURE 29-5 Light microscopic image of an alveolus in acute respiratory distress syndrome (ARDS) with injury to the alveolar epithelium, interstitial edema, and the development of hyaline membranes *(arrow)*. Hyaline membranes form as the coalescence of cells and serum proteins, particularly clotting factors. These membranes were an early hallmark of findings in premature newborns with RDS and led many to refer to RDS as hyaline membrane disease. (Modified with permission from Tomashefski JF, Jr: Pulmonary pathology of adult respiratory distress syndrome. Clin Chest Med 11;593–619, 1990.)

various growth factors (transforming growth factor [TGF]-alpha, TGF-beta).[24,25] However, the remodeling process after ARDS is quite variable. Typically, patients have nearly complete normalization of lung compliance and oxygenation 6 to 12 months after the illness, with a persistent slight impairment of the diffusing capacity. However, in a small percentage (5% to 10%) of patients the architecture of the lung does not fully return to normal and patients can experience chronic respiratory disability related to irreversible pulmonary fibrosis and obliteration of the pulmonary vasculature. The extent of recovery depends on the severity and duration of the initial trigger that led to ARDS and the influence of potential secondary forms of injury that may develop over the patient's complete hospital course. Secondary forms of lung injury include nosocomial infection, O_2 toxicity, and forms of **ventilator-induced lung injury** (VILI), which will be reviewed in detail in the following section.

KEY FEATURES

Risk Factors (Triggers) and Host Susceptibility

Whether using the AECC or the Berlin definition for ARDS, an essential component of ARDS is that the patient must have an associated illness that stimulates an acute inflammatory response that leads to lung injury. These acute illnesses are typically referred to as risk factors or triggers for ARDS. It has been proposed that the risk factors for ARDS should be categorized into problems that lead to either direct injury or indirect injury to the lung (see Box 29-3).[17] In this concept, direct injury occurs as the result of triggers that begin in the lung (e.g., pneumonia and aspiration) and create an acute inflammatory reaction within the lung that ultimately leads to the alveolar injury characteristic of ARDS. Conversely, indirect injury is caused by acute illnesses that trigger an acute inflammatory reaction that begins outside of the lung (e.g., pyelonephritis or massive hemorrhage) and spreads to the lung by the SIRS, thereby leading to the alveolar injury of ARDS. Some studies have suggested that the response of patients to treatment in ARDS may differ depending on whether the initial injury is direct versus indirect. However, thus far, this distinction has not proved to predict response to treatment or other important clinical outcomes.[26] This lack of distinction is most likely explained by the fact that all risk factors share the ability to initiate SIRS, which when severe enough, leads to ARDS.

It is important to recognize that only a minority of patients with risk factors for ARDS ultimately develop the full clinical syndrome. The key factors that determine which patients will develop ARDS are the severity and duration of the risk factor, and variables that lead some patients to be more susceptible. In all patients with ARDS, sepsis is the most common risk factor, but even among all patients with sepsis; fewer than 20% will develop ARDS. As the severity of sepsis increases to include severe sepsis and/or septic shock, the likelihood of ARDS developing increases dramatically and can exceed 50%. Among direct insults that lead to ARDS, pneumonia is the most common. Pneumonia caused by influenza infection is believed to carry an especially high risk for developing ARDS and a higher severity of ARDS once it develops.[27] Similarly, patients who are likely to have recurrent problems with a known risk factor, such as aspiration, are more likely to develop ARDS after multiple aspirations than after a single aspiration. Transfusion-related acute lung injury (TRALI), which occurs particularly after transfusions of platelets or plasma (less likely from packed red blood cells) from female donors, has become an increasingly recognized trigger for ARDS, but only carries a risk of less than 5%. The risk of TRALI increases with the number of transfusions.[28] Furthermore, patients can have more than one risk factor for ARDS, which also increases the risk for developing ARDS.[29] As for the susceptibility of the host to develop ARDS after any risk factor, important variables are increased age (i.e., age >50 years), prior liver disease, alcoholism, and genetic polymorphisms related to inflammatory mediators (e.g., IL-1, TNF, and surfactant).[30] Evidence suggests that cigarette smoking may also increase susceptibility to ARDS.[31]

Epidemiology and Outcomes

The exact incidence of ARDS (including ALI) varies depending on the population, but most recent estimates in the United

States suggest that each year there are 75 to 90 cases per population of 100,000, which represents almost 200,000 cases for the entire country.[32] ARDS may account for up to 16% of mechanically ventilated patients on admission to the ICU in big tertiary care centers.[33] Although there are more common conditions that require ICU care and mechanical ventilation, the high severity of illness associated with ARDS creates a substantial burden on providers and the health care system. Recent estimates indicate that ARDS patients in the ICU use over 2 million days in the ICU and almost 4 million days in the hospital, with total costs measured in billions of dollars. These burdens address the impact of the illness only on society and health care system. As for the impact on the individual patients with ARDS, the associated mortality and morbidity is even more substantial.

The early mortality rates associated with ARDS between the late 1960s and the early 1990s were very high, that is, 60% to 80%. Given our ability to maintain respiratory function in ARDS using mechanical ventilation, only a small minority (10% to 15%) of patients with ARDS die from respiratory failure. The most common cause of death in patients with ARDS relates to the original risk factor that triggered ARDS and from the MODS that develops in patients whose original risk factor is more severe or prolonged. Fortunately, the mortality rate over the past 20- to 25 years has declined dramatically, with most recent mortality rates typically reported between 20% to 40% and some experience as low as 20%.[34-36] The reasons for this improved survival is likely multifactorial and include advances in supportive care, early detection, effective management of comorbid diseases such as nosocomial infection, and the broad application of approaches to mechanical ventilation that limit VILI.

Beyond a risk for death, many important morbidities affect survivors of ARDS, including a long period on mechanical ventilation, time in the ICU and hospital, and slow recovery of lung function. Lessening these morbidities has increasingly become the primary target for recent, large ARDS clinical trials. In the early 1990s, patients with ARDS required an average of more than 21 days on mechanical ventilation, whereas more recent clinical trials have reported that most patients require mechanical ventilation for less than 10 days.[37] As the duration of the time spent on mechanical ventilation has declined, so has the number of days in the ICU and hospital. However, the recent increasing use of long-term acute care facilities has made these comparisons with early experience more complicated. Recovery of lung function as assessed by pulmonary function tests such as spirometry, diffusion capacity (DLCO), and 6 minute walk test (6MWT) demonstrates that ARDS survivors typically recover more than 80% of lung function over 3 to 12 months.[38] The rate of recovery depends on several variables, including ARDS severity, the original risk factor, patient age, and more. Recovery of vital capacity, expiratory volume, and total lung capacity typically occur earliest, whereas recovery of DLCO and 6MWT is more prolonged. This difference is likely explained by the slower pace of recovery for the vascular (capillary) component of the lung after ARDS.

In addition to outcomes primarily linked with lung function, morbidities are associated with the other aspects of ICU care that are needed in managing ARDS patients (e.g., sedation, delirium, and immobility) that have long-term impact on other organ function, such as muscle strength and cognition.[38] Using a variety of techniques to assess muscular and cognitive function, survivors of ARDS consistently demonstrate prolonged impairments in both for at least 6 to 12 months; however, in some patients the changes may never reverse. Consequently, increasing attention and urgency has been placed on identifying and using supportive care strategies to minimize these morbidities and accelerate recovery.

RULE OF THUMB

Although ARDS was once considered a diagnosis that carried a high likelihood for death (≥70%), current rates of survival in patients with ARDS are much higher, with far more than 50% surviving. As a result of our ability to provide mechanical ventilation that does not cause harm, very few patients with ARDS die from respiratory failure. Consequently, short-term periods of hypoxemia in patients with ARDS do not significantly increase the likelihood for death. Patients with more severe disease (more hypoxemia) that persists do have higher mortality rates. Most patients who die from mechanical ventilation die from the disease that triggered the ARDS. Accurate early diagnosis and treatment of the risk factor is a key factor to increase the patient's chance for survival. For the RT, this means that patients with severe hypoxemia may need to undergo diagnostic tests that require transportation to radiology (e.g., CT scans) or that might disrupt their ventilation (e.g., bronchoscopy). Until the triggering risk factor has been clearly established, these risks must generally be taken.

THERAPEUTIC APPROACH

Once the diagnosis of ARDS is made, one of the most important steps for managing and determining the outcome of patients with ARDS is to establish the triggering risk factor. Identifying and controlling the cause of ARDS is an important step to stop progression of the lung injury. After diagnosis, the care focuses on preventing further injury (lung and other organs) and supporting the body while it recovers. This section presents an overview of the current approach to supportive care (ventilator and overall), rescue interventions, and potential therapies for ARDS (Box 29-4). Furthermore, Table 29-2 provides a summary of the recommendations regarding specific interventions that are reviewed and that are currently considered and used by clinicians.

As previously mentioned, efforts to improve outcomes in ARDS up until and through much of the 1990s were largely unsuccessful.[16] A key factor contributing to the lack of success was the large variation in research and management approaches across investigators and institutions. The results of early efforts

Box 29-4 Key Points in the Care of Patients With Acute Respiratory Distress Syndrome

1. Diagnose ARDS (use screening and current Berlin definition):
   a. Diagnose the cause of ARDS
   b. Treat the cause of ARDS
2. Organ support: Key points in ARDS
   a. Minimize delirium
      i. Treat anxiety and pain
      ii. Promote patient awareness, ability to interact, and orientation
   b. Support lung function
      i. Maintain effective gas exchange
      ii. Balance the benefits of PEEP in oxygenation and recruitment with the increased intrathoracic pressure and its potential negative impact on hemodynamics
   c. Fluid balance
      i. Once patient has achieved hemodynamic stability, initiate protocolized conservative fluid management
      ii. Maintain perfusion pressures
3. Prevent further lung injury:
   a. Avoid barotrauma and volutrauma (to avoid further lung injury)
      i. Set V_T according to height
      ii. Keep tidal volume as low as possible, ideally 4 to 6 ml/kg ideal body weight
      iii. Keep plateau pressure below 30 cm H_2O
      iv. Tolerate hypercapnia
   b. Avoid O_2 toxicity (avoid biotrauma)
      i. Titrate FiO_2 and PEEP to a SpO_2 of 88% to 95%
   c. Avoid aspiration (to avoid pneumonia)
      ii. Keep head of bed elevated at 30 degrees
      iii. Subglottic suctioning
   d. Liberate from mechanical ventilation as soon as possible
      i. Daily assessment of spontaneous breathing
      ii. Minimize sedation (give sedation holidays), use a protocol for sedation
      iii. Encourage mobility and alertness

PEEP, positive end expiratory pressure.

were often conflicting, which made interpretation and application of study findings to patients very difficult. In response to this challenge, the National Institutes of Health launched a multicenter network of investigators and institutions to specifically collaborate on clinical treatment strategies for ARDS, a group that has since been known as the *ARDS Network* (ARDSNet).[39] Not by coincidence, the launch of ARDSNet was in 1994 at the same time that the AECC ARDS definition was created. Several landmark clinical trials by ARDSNet have demonstrated improvements in patient outcomes, including increased survival. The ARDSNet remains active, has been renamed the *Prevention and Early Treatment of Acute Lung Injury* (PETAL) Network, and is now expanding its focus to include ARDS prevention.[40] Similar networks of ARDS investigators have successfully formed outside the United States, including in Canada, France, Australia, and New Zealand, and have provided important contributions.

Mechanical Ventilation and Other Respiratory Supportive Care

Mechanical ventilation is the cornerstone of supportive care for patients with ARDS. In general, the three goals of mechanical ventilation are safety, comfort, and liberation from mechanical ventilation. Safety encompasses two main clinical objectives: ensuring gas exchange and preventing further lung injury caused by mechanical ventilation or ventilator-induced lung injury (VILI). Comfort focuses on ensuring synchrony with the ventilator and balancing the work of breathing distribution. Keeping in mind these goals and clinical objectives of ventilation, one can see that some are more important at different stages of ARDS. In the early exudative phase of ARDS, the main goal is to ensure gas exchange and prevent further lung injury. As the disease process resolves and the patient-ventilator interaction and awareness is more important, comfort and liberation become the main goals. This does not mean that each goal is

TABLE 29-2
Summary of Current Treatment Strategies in Acute Respiratory Distress Syndrome

Treatment	LEVEL OF RECOMMENDATION		
	Recommended	Not Recommended	Alternative/Rescue Therapy
Lung protective (low tidal volume—6 ml/kg ideal body weight) ventilation	X (all patients)		
Conservative fluid management	X (all patients)		
Prone positioning (with or without neuromuscular blockade)	X (P/F < 150)		
Inhaled vasodilators		X	
Beta-2 agonists		X	
Supplemental nutrition		X	
Corticosteroids			X
Surfactant replacement therapy		X	
Inverse-ratio ventilation		X	
Airway pressure release ventilation			X
High-frequency ventilation			X
Extracorporeal support			X

mutually exclusive, but it does help explain choices about which mode of ventilation to apply to a given patient at a given time.

Setting Tidal Volume

Although mechanical ventilation provides lifesaving support to patients with ARDS and other forms of acute respiratory failure, mechanical ventilation can be dangerous and can cause further lung injury, which is often referred to as ventilator-induced lung injury (VILI). Although there are multiple forms of VILI, the most important and well-established forms of VILI are volutrauma and barotrauma. **Barotrauma** is the rupture of alveolar structures that results in gross leak of air outside of the lung parenchyma into adjacent tissue spaces (e.g., pleura and mediastinum). Pneumothorax and pneumomediastinum are the common clinical manifestations of barotrauma, and although not certain, these complications are thought to be most closely related to excess airway pressures on mechanical ventilation. **Volutrauma** is similarly a form of injury to the alveolar structure but that does not lead to a macroscopic rupture of the wall with clinically recognizable leak of air, but instead leads to an overstretching and subsequent microscopic cellular injury to the alveolar and capillary walls, causing them to become leaky. This cellular injury then becomes the trigger for an inflammatory cascade that may cause further nonhydrostatic pulmonary edema. A critically important point for every RT is that the volutrauma related to mechanical ventilation must be included on the list of potential risk factors and triggers for ARDS. The strategy of using V_Ts that avoid volutrauma is commonly referred to as low tidal volume ventilation (LTVV) or **lung protective ventilation** (LPV).

The first highly successful trial completed by the ARDSNet in 2000 using LPV demonstrated a 22% reduction in mortality in patients with ARDS managed with a "low stretch" or low V_T approach. The study compared a strategy of low V_T (of 6 ml/kg ideal body weight [IBW]) versus a larger V_T of 12 ml/kg IBW. Until this trial, the standard of practice for mechanical ventilation for several decades had been to use a V_T of 12 to 15 ml/kg.[41] The results of this trial showing a significant survival benefit associated with low V_T transformed the standards for care of patients with ARDS and is considered one of the most important reasons for the dramatic improvements in mortality and morbidity associated with ARDS over the past 10 to 15 years. More recent trials of mechanical ventilation in patients without ARDS have suggested that VILI may happen in many more patients than just those with ARDS and that LPV may be a preferred approach for choosing a V_T in other clinical settings (e.g., chronic obstructive pulmonary disease [COPD], etc.). These trials include even patients requiring only brief exposures to mechanical ventilation during elective abdominal surgical procedures.[42]

To deliver LPV to patients effectively, two important points must be understood. First, the target of 6 ml/kg (range 4 to 7 ml/kg) is based on a patient's IBW not the actual weight. During growth and maturation of the lung parenchyma during childhood and early adult life, the length/height of the patient will be the variable that most determines the size and capacity of the lungs. Gender also plays a small role, with males having slightly larger lung capacity than females of similar height. Changes in weight associated with obesity, edema, or loss of an extremity from amputation do not affect the IBW. Also, surgical removal of a lung (pneumonectomy) or portion of a lung (lobectomy) should be considered, with a relative reduction in target V_T based on the percent of total lung that has been removed. There are many sources online and in print providing calculators or tables to assist bedside providers with a patient's IBW once the patient's height has been measured.

MINI CLINI

Tidal Volume

V_T in mechanical ventilation should be kept within a safe range to prevent volutrauma or VILI. The recommended size of V_T is 6 ml/kg of IBW (not actual body weight). IBW is determined by knowing a patient's gender, weight, and height, and tables with formulas for calculating IBW are readily available. It is important for the RT to accurately calculate each patient's IBW when starting mechanical ventilation and throughout the patient's course of mechanical ventilation.

For example, a 50-year-old male who is 6 feet and 0 inches tall and weighs 224 lb (100 kg) has an ideal body weight of only 70 to 75 kg. Using his IBW and the V_T target of 6 ml/kg, the ventilator should be set for a V_T of 420 to 450 ml. If his actual body weight were incorrectly used, a V_T of 600 ml would have been selected and would be too large and could lead to VILI and increased mortality. The RT should also consider whether the patient has any history of surgical lung resection. For example, if the same patient had undergone a left-sided pneumonectomy, leaving only the right lung for function, the selected V_T should be reduced by approximately 50% to 200 to 250 ml.

The second point is that the use of a lower V_T in LPV often will result in worsened gas exchange, with patients demonstrating worsening oxygenation and ventilation, including lower P/F ratios and higher levels of $PaCO_2$. These seemingly adverse effects of LPV on ABGs often create confusion and concern for families and care providers, including RTs. However, these changes are not associated with worse overall patient outcomes (e.g., as measured by mortality or time on mechanical ventilation). Quite the contrary, by keeping a V_T lower, the patient's outcomes will be dramatically improved.

Selecting the Mode of Mechanical Ventilation

For decades, the discussion of which mode of mechanical ventilation is best for ARDS has caused vigorous debate with many strong and divergent opinions. In practice, the clinician may use any mode of mechanical ventilation to deliver the recommended V_T. At this time, there is no definitive evidence that one mode is better than the other in delivering LPV. To simplify this issue, the mode of ventilation should principally serve the goals of safety (i.e., ensuring and limiting the inhaled V_T) while also ensuring minute ventilation/gas exchange. More complete details outlining mechanical ventilation and the available associated modes are provided in Chapter 45.

The mode that most directly achieves the goal of controlling V_T is volume control, which includes continuous mandatory ventilation (also known as *volume control* or *assist/control*). In this traditional mode, which is still present on most ventilators, the clinician sets the V_T (6 ml/kg of IBW) and the ventilator delivers the target V_T on every breath, whether patient-initiated or not. However, there are several potential shortcomings to this mode, of which the most important are patient-ventilator dysynchrony, requiring heavier patient sedation, and double triggering, in which the patient's actual inspiratory time exceeds the set inspiratory time on the ventilator, thereby triggering a second mechanical breath during the same inspiratory cycle and causing delivery of a V_T twice the targeted size. In response to this limitation, many ventilator manufacturers have refined their volume control modes to use other targeting schemes. For example, on the Maquet Servo-I (Rastatt, Germany), volume control has a dual targeting scheme, which turns into a pressure-controlled breath when the patient initiates a sufficient inspiration. On the Drager Evita XL (Lubeck, Germany), when the autoflow feature is activated, volume control converts to a pressure control mode with an adaptive targeting scheme.[43,44]

In pressure control modes, the V_T depends on the set inspiratory pressure above PEEP, inspiratory time, patient effort, airway resistance, and lung compliance. In practice, this means that to consistently achieve the target V_T, the set inspiratory pressure and inspiratory time need to be adjusted manually or automatically by the ventilator. The same variation in patient respiratory effort that creates challenges for volume control modes also creates problems in these modes by limiting the ability to maintain targeted V_T and minute ventilation and less ability to prevent excessive V_T, which can lead to VILI. In response to this challenge, some newer ventilators include technologic features that may improve the ability to maintain LPV, including adaptive or intelligent targeting schemes[45] in which the inspiratory pressure is automatically adjusted to achieve a target V_T. Whether these technologic advances lead to advantages that provide improved clinical care for patients remains unproved currently.

In the volume control and pressure control modes, variation in patient effort is a challenge. This challenge can be addressed with sedation, analgesia, and/or neuromuscular blockade to blunt patient respiratory effort. However, the adverse effects of these pharmacologic interventions must be considered (discussed further later) and are increasingly recognized as affecting the long-term outcome of ARDS survivors.

Positive End Expiratory Pressure

The use of PEEP in patients with ARDS was first reported in 1967,[15] and by the mid-1970s, the effects of PEEP on lung compliance, oxygenation, and cardiac output (Figure 29-6) had been well characterized.[46] Of interest, since that time, even after much debate and research, there is no standardized method to set PEEP in ARDS.[47-49]

The rationale for using PEEP requires understanding the pressure-volume (P-V) curve of the lung. The P-V relationship can be established for a given patient by measuring lung volume during step increases in airway pressure. The classic P-V curve has an S, or sigmoid, shape (Figure 29-7). The initial limb has large changes in pressure for each step increase in volume, the middle limb has the "best" change in pressure per volume, and the final limb again has large pressure changes for each step increase in volume. From the resulting curve, we can obtain a

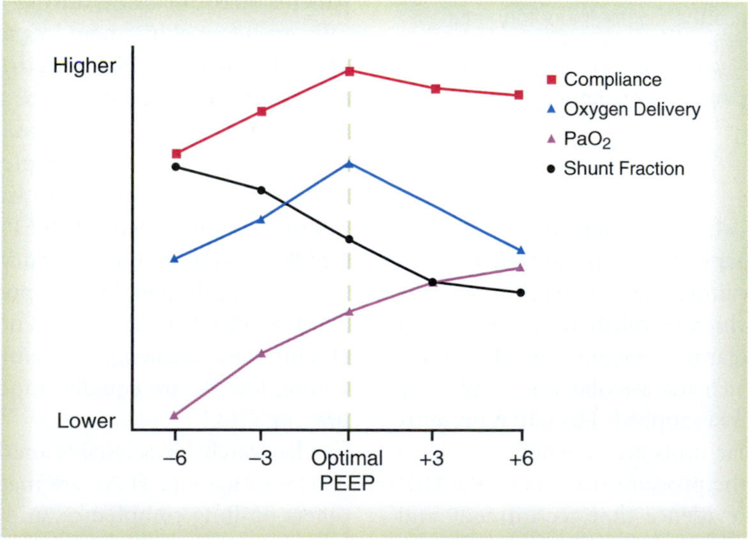

FIGURE 29-6 Determination of optimal PEEP from simultaneous measurements of hemodynamic (DO_2), gas exchange (shunt fraction and arterial oxygenation [PaO_2]), and physiologic values. Optimal PEEP does not correspond to PEEP associated with optimal pulmonary gas exchange. When adjusting PEEP, the clinician should consider its effects on systemic DO_2 and lung compliance such that systemic organ injury and lung injury are minimized.

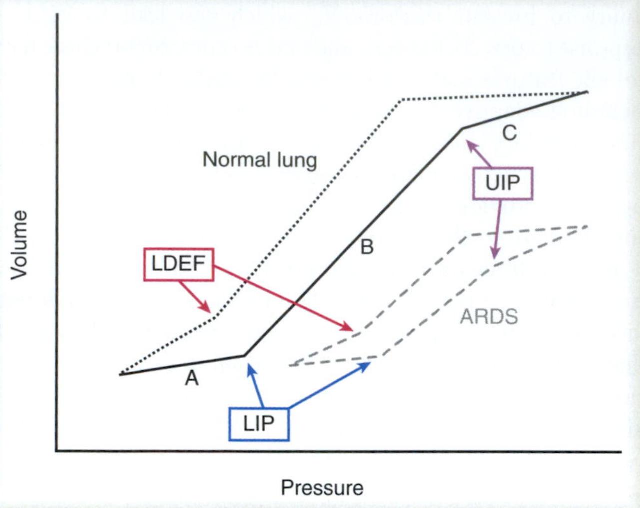

FIGURE 29-7 Typical pressure-volume relationships during normal conditions and during acute respiratory distress syndrome (ARDS). At low lung volume, inspiratory pressure increases faster than lung volume *(line A)* owing to high alveolar surface tension. As alveoli open, surface tension decreases, and the pressure required to increase lung volume further decreases *(line B)*. The lower inflection point *(LIP)* occurs between *lines A* and *B* and represents the volume above which most alveolar units are open. The upper inflection point *(UIP)* occurs at near-maximal lung volume and corresponds to the point at which further increases in pressure result in minimal increases in lung volume *(line C)*. Pressure applied above the *UIP* is associated with alveolar distention. During the expiratory phase of the respiratory cycle *(dotted line)*, the lower deflection point *(LDEF)* is the point below which lung volumes slowly decrease (alveolar units collapse). During ARDS *(gray dashed curve)*, pressure-volume relationships change such that higher pressure is needed to maintain alveolar patency, and alveolar distention occurs at lower V_T levels. Near-maximal lung volumes are typically achieved at an inspiratory pressure of approximately 35 cm H_2O in normal conditions and during *ARDS*. Attempts to increase inspiratory pressure to more than 35 cm H_2O provide little additional ventilation and substantially increase the risk for injury to the lungs. During *ARDS*, the *LIP* often occurs at a pressure of 5 to 15 cm H_2O. PEEP at levels greater than *LIP* may prevent end-expiratory alveolar collapse and reduce lung injury secondary to alveolar shear stress.

lower inflection point (LIP), which is where the initial and middle limbs meet, and an upper inflection point (UIP), which is where the middle and upper limbs meet. The LIP represents the point in the P-V curve at which recruitment (i.e., opening) of a significant number of alveolar units begins. The LIP is typically the same point below which the alveolar units will close (atelectasis) if no airway pressure is applied. The UIP represents the point beyond which alveolar units are generally unable to expand or distend further, so the pressure rises above the UIP. Imaging studies have shown evidence that recruitment and overdistention occurs throughout the P-V curve, which may be interpreted as showing that there is no absolute point at which safety can be guaranteed.[50] From the physiologic standpoint, PEEP increases the functional residual capacity (residual volume + expiratory reserve volume) and decreases the amount of unaerated lung (atelectasis), leading to improved gas exchange and lung compliance.

RULE OF THUMB

Changes in physiologic markers (oxygenation, compliance) take time after changing the level of PEEP. When decreasing PEEP, the changes in physiology becomes evident early, usually within 5 minutes. On the other hand, when increasing PEEP, the changes in physiology make take at least 60 minutes to become fully evident and may continue to change with time.[51]

During mechanical ventilation, the goal is to maintain the PEEP above the LIP to avoid repeated cycles of alveolar collapse and recruitment (also known as *cyclic recruitment* or *atelectrauma*) and keep the V_T below the UIP to avoid cyclic overdistention. Although creating P-V curves on patients receiving mechanical ventilation can be done so that the LIP and UIP can be actually quantified, measuring P-V curves is both technically challenging (requiring patient to be heavily sedated and off PEEP) and time-consuming. Because the actual LIP and UIP are not typically measured and available to the providers, titration of PEEP is typically performed using best estimates from the more commonly available pressure and volume data collected daily during mechanical ventilation. Thus identifying the level of PEEP that allows the patient to remain within the middle limb of the P-V curve during daily practice in the ICU can be challenging.

In ARDS, the challenge to estimate the P-V relationships to determine the "optimal" or "best" PEEP settings is even greater. The P-V curves are flatter and more deviated to the right (Figure 29-6), which creates a smaller window for the settings to maximize benefits while avoiding overdistention. Furthermore, these patients' need for PEEP during mechanical ventilation is typically greater, making them less tolerant to a formal assessment of the P-V curve (which requires a brief period with PEEP set to 0 cm H_2O). It must also be noted that in ARDS, the P-V relationships are highly dynamic and depend on the patient's overall condition. For example, administering or removing additional fluids can result in worsening or improvement that can require adjustment of PEEP to maintain the patient in the middle portion of the P-V curve. Finally, the use of PEEP is further complicated by the potential adverse hemodynamic effect of PEEP to decrease venous return to the right heart. Despite these challenges, careful titration of PEEP and maintaining low V_T are equally important components of LPV to prevent VILI.[52]

The search for a reliable method to accurately set PEEP in ARDS is ongoing. There are methods focused on oxygenation, others on lung compliance, and still others using CT imaging to determine best PEEP.[53] In a recent study, a comparison of methods based on lung mechanics versus using a table based on oxygenation (like the one used in the ARDSNet trials) favored the table approach.[53] Overall, trials assessing different levels of PEEP in ARDS do not demonstrate a difference in mortality; however, higher levels of PEEP in more severe disease (P/F ratio <150) may lead to decreased mortality and less use of rescue strategies.[49,54] Taking all of this into account, it is reasonable to use a table to set the PEEP (see http://www.ARDSNet.org) and FiO_2 and in severe ARDS a higher PEEP may be better.

MINI CLINI

Avoiding Ventilator-Induced Lung Injury

PROBLEM: How can VILI be minimized in patients with ARDS through adjustments of PEEP and V_T?

DISCUSSION: Alveolar shear stress occurs when alveoli collapse during expiration and are reopened as the next V_T is delivered. Patients with ARDS are prone to developing this form of lung injury because surface tension increases as a result of impaired surfactant synthesis and function and decreased lung compliance. Alveolar collapse at end-expiration (the LIP of the P-V curve) can be avoided with PEEP, which reduces alveolar shear stress by preventing the cyclic opening and closing of the alveoli during each ventilatory cycle. Because partially patent alveoli require less pressure to inflate than collapsed alveoli, PEEP also improves lung compliance. Improved compliance is reflected by an increase in the slope of the P-V curve (see Figure 29-7).

The clinician can gauge the effects of PEEP on the basis of calculated changes in lung compliance (see Figure 29-6). In the clinical setting, changes in lung compliance are estimated from the compliance of the entire respiratory system, which includes the combined influences of lung compliance, chest wall compliance, and abdominal pressure:

$$\text{Compliance of the respiratory system} = \text{Tidal volume}/-(\text{Plateau pressure} - \text{Total PEEP})$$

As PEEP increases, risk also increases for alveolar overdistention and volutrauma. This is identified as a decrease of compliance as the PEEP increases. Just as alveolar collapse during end-expiration is associated with decreased lung compliance; alveolar overinflation during end-inspiration is reflected by decreasing compliance and corresponds to the UIP of the P-V curve (see Figure 29-7).

RULE OF THUMB

In most patients with ARDS, PEEP levels below 20 cm H_2O are generally preferred. Levels of PEEP greater than 20 cm H_2O should *not* be routinely used unless the benefits of higher levels of PEEP are supported by objective end points, such as improved lung compliance (see Figure 29-6) or optimal alveolar recruitment (see Figure 29-7).

Respiratory Rate and Inspiratory Time

ARDS is associated with alveolar consolidation and $\dot{V}/\dot{Q}$ mismatching, causing increased physiologic shunt and dead space ventilation. Also, critically ill patients typically have elevated rates of metabolism rates and CO_2 production, explaining why patients with ARDS require much higher minute ventilation to maintain $PaCO_2$ in the normal range. The challenge is that we use low V_Ts to prevent lung injury in ARDS, resulting in the need to increase the ventilator rate to achieve adequate $PaCO_2$ levels. In conventional practice and most large ARDS trials, the respiratory frequency is kept below 35 breaths/min. The concern with faster ventilator rates is that these faster rates will cause auto-PEEP and impaired perfusion.[55-57] Thus, in managing patients with ARDS, the clinician must resist the urge to correct the $PaCO_2$ value to normal. Instead, in the absence of a contraindication to hypercapnia (e.g., elevated intracranial pressure), we allow hypercapnia ("permissive hypercapnia") with a goal to maintain the arterial pH at no less than 7.15 to 7.20. Even when $PaCO_2$ rises to a point during which pH may become dangerously low (e.g., <pH 7.15), the absolute need to keep the V_T at 6 ml/kg IBW remains. In this circumstance, the pH can be corrected by other means, for example, either through normal physiologic retention of bicarbonate by the kidneys over time, pharmacologic supplementation (intravenous or oral) of bicarbonate, or, in rare instances, use of extracorporeal removal of CO_2.[58] Animal models and human studies have confirmed the safety of controlled hypoventilation or "permissive hypercapnia."[59]

In conventional modes of mechanical ventilation, the respiratory cycle is characterized by an **inspiratory-to-expiratory ratio** (I/E) exceeding 1:2 (i.e., the time for expiration is at least two times that of the time for inspiration). Patients with obstructive lung diseases (COPD and asthma), typically benefit from I/E rates with even longer expiratory times (i.e., I/E ratios of 1:3 to 1:4) to allow full lung emptying. However, in patients with ARDS, the impact of pulmonary and interstitial edema is to create a stiffer lung, which characteristically does not require as much time for exhalation. As a result, using I/E ratios of 1:1 are generally recommended in managing patients with ARDS. An I/E ratio of 1:1 can be achieved by using slower inspiratory flow rates, which also can help minimize airway pressures during inspiration (i.e., lower the peak inspiratory pressure). More extreme reductions in inspiratory time (i.e., I/E ratios = 1.5:1 to 2:1), a technique known as *inverse-ratio ventilation (IRV),* also have also been used in ARDS, but inverting the I/E ratio is generally not recommended and is considered an alternative ventilatory approach.

RULE OF THUMB

Administering high levels of supplemental O_2 can cause lung injury as a result of O_2 toxicity. O_2 toxicity is considered to be time-dependent and dose-dependent; that is, the longer the exposure and the higher the FiO_2, the worse the injury will be. The RT must continuously titrate the FiO_2 and PEEP to keep the target SpO_2 in the range of 88% to 95%.

Nonventilatory Supportive Care

Supportive care in the ICU, including patients with ARDS, focuses on maintaining function of key organs and minimizing the complications associated with critical illnesses and spending several days in an ICU. These points of management do not directly treat the primary risk factor that triggered ARDS, but are nonetheless critically important to optimize patient outcomes both during and after their time in the ICU. Supportive care measures apply to many (if not most) patients on mechanical ventilation in the ICU and can be very general (e.g., prophylaxis against deep vein thrombosis, gastric acid suppression, and prevention of nosocomial infections), but many first have been tested and most are well proved for patients with ARDS (e.g., LPV). Ventilatory support of the lungs with mechanical ventilation is a key component, but it is not the only supportive measure that has benefit on lung function (e.g., conservative fluid management). This section will briefly review a few key aspects of supportive care related to both the lungs and other key organs.

Conservative Fluid Management. In managing the critically ill patient, blood pressure, cardiac output, and oxygenation must be preserved to ensure perfusion of vital organs (e.g., kidney, brain). Fluids are given both intravenously and orally to critically ill patients to preserve perfusion and hydration. The amount of fluids taken in by critically ill patients invariably exceeds the amount of fluids that the patient loses, and patients often gain approximately 1 L of fluid per day. Such fluid retention was widely accepted in ARDS management until the ARDSNet Fluids and Catheters Treatment Trial (FACTT), which was completed in 2006 and changed the approach to fluid management in ARDS. In this study, a new, protocol-driven **conservative fluid management** strategy was compared to a so-called *liberal strategy* that was typical of standard practice before the beginning of the study. The two strategies (conservative vs. liberal) were applied for the first 7 days of ARDS treatment in patients who were no longer in shock. The key finding of the FACTT study was that a conservative strategy led to improved gas exchange (oxygenation), shorter duration of mechanical ventilation and ICU length of stay for survivors, and no increased frequency of other organ failures, including renal failure.[60]

In practice, once patients with ARDS are hemodynamically stable (i.e., not needing fluid boluses or vasopressors to maintain blood pressure for at least 12 hours), a conservative fluid management should begin. This approach includes reducing all unnecessary maintenance fluids and aggressively giving diuretics to reduce total body fluid, while closely monitoring for negative effects of diuresis on tissue perfusion and responding promptly to electrolyte changes caused by diuretics (e.g., hypokalemia, hypernatremia, and alkalosis). Using a conservative fluid approach, the total amount of nonhydrostatic pulmonary edema can be more actively and promptly reduced than with a liberal approach, in which normal alveolar processes are expected to slowly clear alveolar flooding. At the bedside, a common clue that diuresis may be appropriate is the presence of significant edema in the patient's face, hands and feet and/or persistent evidence of pulmonary edema and pleural effusions on the chest radiograph.

MINI CLINI

Managing Hydrostatic Pressure in Patients With Acute Respiratory Distress Syndrome

PROBLEM: Critically ill patients requiring mechanical ventilation for acute respiratory failure often receive large volumes of fluid in the form of intravenous medications, maintenance fluids, and nutrition (enteral or parenteral). Excessive or nonessential fluid administration should be avoided in patients with ARDS because they have "leaky capillaries" and are remarkably sensitive to changes in pulmonary vascular hydrostatic pressure. How can iatrogenic pulmonary edema be avoided in these patients so they can be liberated from mechanical ventilator sooner?

DISCUSSION: Noninvasive estimates of total body water, such as daily weights and total fluid intake and output measurements, are helpful tools but often are not accurate. The inaccuracy of noninvasive estimates of total body fluid content are tolerable as long as the patient's overall clinical status is improving and the patient is hemodynamically stable (i.e., with acceptable blood pressure and tissue perfusion). The use of a protocol to guide fluid management leads to faster liberation of mechanical ventilation. In the conservative fluid management strategy used in the FACTT trial,[60] the approach combined clinical and invasive monitoring to guide fluid therapy. While patients are in shock (requiring fluid boluses and/or vasopressors to maintain a mean arterial pressure ≥60 mm Hg), fluid conservative management is not attempted. Once patients are no longer in shock for 12 hours (a much shorter timeframe than previously considered safe), the protocol uses clinical signs of effective circulation (capillary refill), urine output, and central venous pressure (CVP) measured by a central venous catheter to determine when diuretics should be given. These parameters are reassessed every 4 hours, and diuretic therapy is given when patients meet the appropriate criteria. The target level for CVP was less than 4 mm Hg, which is the range for CVP under normal conditions. The use of the conservative fluid protocol (compared to liberal or usual fluid management) caused patients to have significantly reduced fluid accumulation during their ICU course and to be liberated from mechanical ventilation an average of 2 or 3 days sooner.

Sedation and Analgesia

Over the past 10 to 15 years, the approach to managing sedation and analgesia in critically ill patients has changed dramatically. Protocolized sedation and scheduled daily interruptions of sedation (awakenings) lead to shorter times on mechanical ventilation and decreased length of ICU stay.[61,62] Furthermore, evidence from survivors of ARDS has demonstrated that many experience persistent problems with memory and cognition and that these changes relate to the types of sedation that patients receive during their care in the ICU. In particular, using benzodiazepines (e.g., lorazepam or midazolam) seems to carry the greatest risk for these adverse neurocognitive effects. One of the earliest neurocognitive warning signs in the ICU is the development of ICU-associated *delirium*, which can be caused by several common environmental challenges in the ICU, including lack of sleep, noise, use of restraints, and immobility. The use of benzodiazepines also has been strongly linked to the development and progression of delirium in the ICU.

Given these concerns related to the acute and long-term adverse effects of ICU sedation, current strategies for sedation aim to minimize the exposure to all sedatives, in particular benzodiazepines.[63] Preferred agents to treat patient agitation (including ventilator dyssynchrony) are analgesic (e.g., narcotics) and antipsychotic drugs, which are more likely to directly address delirium. This recent emphasis on reducing the level of sedation for patients on mechanical ventilation poses a challenge for the RT, who along with the nursing staff, must manage patients who are more awake and who breathe spontaneously while receiving lung protective ventilation. We can no longer assume that a heavy sedation to optimize a patient's synchrony with mechanical ventilation is the best and safest approach for the patient. An approach that balances the short-term risks of mechanical ventilation with the longer term risks of sedation is recommended, and the goals of care should be discussed daily among all caregivers to ensure success.

Nutrition

Malnutrition in the ICU leads to poor outcomes, but so does overfeeding. Further, the type of alimentation may affect how the body reacts to disease. Although the literature on nutritional management of patients with ARDS is rather scant, two recent studies deserve comment. The ARDSNet EDEN trial studied whether using trophic feeds (a small amount of enteral nutrition just to keep the gut working) was better than full enteral nutrition for the first 6 days of care of patients with ARDS. The results of the study showed no benefit for the full nutritional approach either during the ICU stay or 1 year later.[64]

Although an early small trial suggested benefit from supplementing nutrition with omega-3 fatty acids, another recent ARDSNet trial, the OMEGA trial,[65] in which omega-3 fatty acids, along with γ-linolenic acid and antioxidants (given to help modulate the inflammatory response in ARDS), were compared to placebo. Again, no differences were observed between the treatment and placebo groups. A recent meta-analysis of seven trials examining omega-3 fatty acids also found no effect from nutritional supplements in patients with ARDS.[66] Currently, there is no specific recommendation regarding nutrition in patients with ARDS. Guidelines recommend the same nutritional management as for any critically ill patient.

Mobility

It has long been recognized that the prolonged period patients spend lying in bed on mechanical ventilation has an adverse effect on the mass and function of muscles for patients in the ICU, including those with ARDS.[67,68] As mentioned previously, profound weakness is a commonly reported symptom in ARDS survivors, and can persist for 6 to 12 months or more. This adverse consequence of ICU care is related to both drugs (e.g., steroids, neuromuscular blocking paralytic agents) and just the simple lack of mobility (immobility). Mobilizing a small, select group of patients receiving mechanical ventilation in ICUs has been done for decades, but this has been typically limited to patients after tracheostomy, after several weeks of immobility. Over the past decade, numerous clinical trials from the United States and Europe have demonstrated that early mobilization of patients on mechanical ventilation, including ARDS patients with severe hypoxemia, is both highly beneficial and safe. In these studies, early mobilization typically refers to allowing capable patients to sit on the side of the bed, stand, and/or walk within 48 to 72 hours of ARDS onset, even while they are still endotracheally intubated. The benefits of early mobility include reducing the length of time ARDS survivors spend in the ICU and hospital and accelerating the recovery and return to their baseline functional status after hospital discharge, including return to work. This important element of supportive care has not yet become the standard of care in many ICUs because of apprehension by caregivers (physicians, nurses, and RTs) about the safety of mobilizing critically ill patients. Also, the costs associated with increased commitment of physical therapists and RTs to the ICU have often been considered prohibitive. However, when all costs of patient care (ICU, hospital, and posthospital discharge) are considered, the cost of mobilizing patients is no higher or is actually reduced.[69]

Adjunctive Strategies to Improve Lung Function

Prone Positioning

In view of the heterogeneous distribution of lung injury in patients with ARDS, it has been proposed that changing the position of the patient could result in improved $\dot{V}/\dot{Q}$ matching within the lungs. In this regard, it is known that alveolar consolidation in ARDS tends to be most pronounced in the dependent lung zones (posterior regions when patient is lying supine), where blood flow is greatest.[70] These observations led investigators to experiment with positioning the patient so that aerated lung fields (nondependent lung zones) become dependent by positioning of the patient in the prone position (i.e., placing chest and face down). So-called *proning* the patient recalls the old adage to "put the good lung down."

The mechanisms by which **prone positioning** improves oxygenation is the subject of debate. Some proposed mechanisms include improved matching of ventilation with perfusion, increased functional residual capacity, increased cardiac output, more effective drainage of upper and lower airway secretions, and improved diaphragmatic excursion. Investigations using animal models of ARDS have shown that ventilation in the supine position causes compressive forces on the dorsal airspaces, resulting in derecruitment of lung units. This phenomenon is reversed by ventilation in the prone position.[71,72]

In 1977, Douglas and colleagues[73] were the first to describe improved oxygenation with prone positioning of patients with

ARDS. However, because of concerns over the logistics and safety of proning patients, prone ventilation strategy remained unpopular. This concern prevailed even in the face of studies that had demonstrated a beneficial effect of prone ventilation.[74] Recently, a large multicenter, randomized clinical trial demonstrated that using prone positioning for more than 16 hours per day improved survival when started within the first 36 hours of onset of mechanical ventilation[75] for patients with moderate to severe hypoxemia (P/F ratio <150 mm Hg). These new studies have again demonstrated the advantages of prone ventilation, including improved oxygenation and improved long-term survival over supine ventilation without the need for expensive pharmacologic interventions or new ventilator modalities. Despite these advantages, prone positioning of patients with ARDS requires an experienced and committed staff (nursing and RT) and may require special equipment to facilitate turning, especially for obese patients. Some patients may not tolerate prone ventilation or may have a relative contraindication to proning, such as open surgical wounds or late trimester pregnancy. However, as more centers gain comfort with the logistics of rotating patients, prone position ventilation has emerged as one of the first-line adjunctive therapies available to assist in oxygenating the patient with severe ARDS and is considered by many to now be the standard of care for patients with sustained severe ARDS (P/F ratio <150 for more than 12 to 24 hours on stable ventilator settings).

Neuromuscular Blockade

Neuromuscular blocking paralytic agents have been used for decades to enhance compliance with mechanical ventilation in patients with ARDS, especially when the ventilatory mode has involved low-volume ventilation or inverse-ratio ventilation. Furthermore, with severe dyspnea and/or ventilator dyssynchrony, a substantial portion of the patient's arterial O_2 content can be consumed by accessory respiratory muscles. Therefore, in patients who continue to remain hypoxemic despite maximal ventilator settings and adequate sedation, a trial of neuromuscular blockade is usually warranted.

Although earlier studies showed improved oxygenation with neuromuscular blockade for the first 48 hours, they did not address whether neuromuscular blockade conferred any survival advantage. A multicenter randomized trial considered 90-day in-hospital mortality as the outcome measure after treatment with a bolus of the paralytic drug cisatracurium followed by a 48-hour infusion. The cisatracurium group showed improved adjusted 90-day survival, more days off the ventilator, and a lower incidence of barotrauma complications. In a post hoc analysis of the study, the benefit of neuromuscular blockade was most evident in patients with more severe disease as defined by a P/F ratio less than 120. Although problems with muscle weakness related to neuromuscular blocker use were thought to be more likely in the intervention group, no such effect was seen, perhaps related to the short duration of paralysis in the study.[76] Despite the promising nature of these results, many clinicians remain concerned about the adverse neuromuscular effects of neuromuscular blockers in ARDS, particularly in patients with only mild to moderate ARDS who are oxygenating adequately on conventional ventilation.

Inhaled Vasodilators

The potential role of inhaled vasodilators in ARDS is based on the idea that vasodilators that enter via the airways (as compared to intravenously) are preferentially distributed to well-ventilated portions of the lung, where the vasodilator can cause local vasodilation. In this way, well-ventilated areas of the lung receive a greater portion of the total pulmonary blood flow, which results in improved oxygenation by reducing $\dot{V}/\dot{Q}$ mismatch (Figure 29-8).

Nitric oxide (NO) and prostacyclin are naturally occurring potent vasodilators that play a critical role regulating blood flow within the normal lungs. NO is soluble in liquids and gases and diffuses readily through various tissues. When NO diffuses from the alveolus into the capillary, it is bound by hemoglobin. As a result, the vasodilatory effects of NO are short-lived (few minutes) and are localized to the area of tissue where the NO is released.

Prostacylin is a prostaglandin byproduct of arachadonic acid metabolism and several analogues have been pharmacologically developed (e.g., epoprostenol [Flolan]) and revolutionized the treatment of pulmonary hypertension over the past 20 years.[77] Although not gaseous, epoprostenol and other prostacyclin analogues can be nebulized and provide a similar effect as inhaled NO.

When given clinically, the beneficial effects of NO can be achieved at low concentrations of inhaled NO (5 to 10 ppm) and are typically not improved with higher doses. Because of its profound effects on pulmonary hemodynamics, discontinuing inhaled NO or other pulmonary vasodilators may be associated with severe rebound pulmonary vasoconstriction and

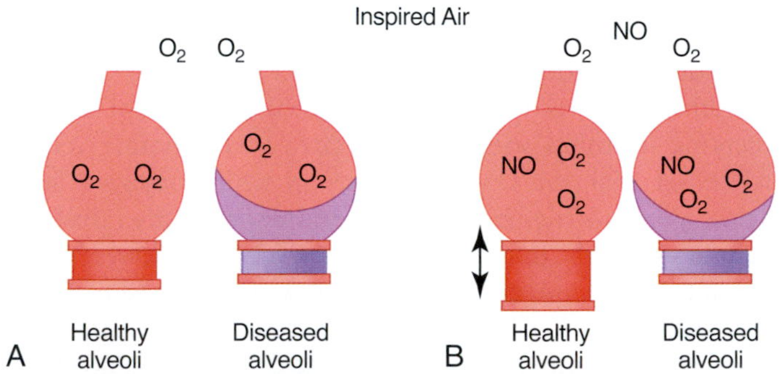

FIGURE 29-8 The damage of acute lung injury and acute respiratory distress syndrome is heterogeneous. **A,** Despite autoregulatory changes that favor vasodilation of well-oxygenated alveoli, perfusion goes to both the healthy, unaffected alveoli and the diseased alveoli that are unable to oxygenate blood. This results in $\dot{V}/\dot{Q}$ mismatch or a shuntlike state resulting in deoxygenated blood returning from the lung and hypoxemia. **B,** The addition of inhaled NO to the inspired gas results in vasodilation of the capillaries adjacent to healthy alveoli promoting increased blood flow to the "good" alveoli and diminishing the percentage of blood going to diseased alveoli, resulting in improved $\dot{V}/\dot{Q}$ match and improved oxygenation.

hypoxemia. A large multicenter randomized trial involving more than 300 patients reported that NO at a dose of 5 ppm provided a short-term benefit in oxygenation, but was ineffective in altering mortality or duration of ventilator support.[78] No large clinical trials of nebulized prostacyclin analogues have been completed in ARDS, but the current consensus is that the results of those trials would likely resemble those for inhaled NO.

Beyond the lack of proved outcome benefit for pulmonary vasodilators, other adverse consequences that should be considered include potential toxicities and cost. There are breakdown products of NO that are potentially toxic, including reactive free radicals (e.g., peroxynitrite and methemoglobin). As a result, use of inhaled NO during mechanical ventilation must involve close monitoring and special exhaust systems to prevent exposure of health care personnel. The cost of NO and its patented delivery system (INOmax, Ikaria, Perryville, IL) is substantial, causing many institutions to limit its use until new evidence supporting a more significant improvement in patient outcomes is available. Nebulized epoprostenol serves as a less expensive alternative to NO at many centers.[79]

The apparent discrepancy in the effects of inhaled vasodilators—with improvements on oxygenation without a favorable effect on survival or time on mechanical ventilation—further emphasizes that enhancing oxygenation alone is insufficient to establish the efficacy of a treatment.[78,80] In the case of pulmonary vasodilators, oxygenation has improved but the patient's overall chances for survival and time on mechanical ventilation have not changed while being exposed to potential risks and unnecessary costs. Given these limitations and adverse consequences, use of inhaled vasodilators should be limited to patients with refractory, severe ARDS (P/F < 80) to prevent the need for and/or use as a bridge to more invasive adjunctive therapies (e.g., extracorporeal support). If inhaled vasodilators are started, clinicians should reassess the need for continuing their use within 24 hours of starting, and daily thereafter.

MINI CLINI

In the management of a patient with ARDS, oxygenation (PaO_2 or SpO_2) is a readily available measure that often attracts the attention of bedside providers. In an attempt to improve oxygenation, providers are often faced with decisions as to whether they should increase V_T or PEEP, change ventilator mode, or use additional therapies such as pulmonary vasodilators (e.g., inhaled NO). In all instances, the severity of the patient's hypoxemia is typically not closely linked with likelihood of survival, so that these changes or additions are not likely to positively affect the patient. Increasing V_T or PEEP can have very harmful effects by increasing VILI, and inhaled vasodilators add to the cost and complexity of the patient's care. These maneuvers should be reserved for patients with persistent and severe hypoxemia and should not be pursued without close consultation with the patient's intensivist.

Corticosteroids

Although most patients who survive ARDS have minimal residual pulmonary impairment, a small but significant number of patients require prolonged mechanical ventilatory support because of abundant fibroproliferation in the lung during recovery from ARDS. The high mortality rate among these patients seems to relate to the extent and severity of pulmonary fibrosis.[81] High-dose corticosteroids have been used to manage uncomplicated pulmonary fibrosis following ARDS. In small studies from single institutions,[82] patients treated with corticosteroids for ARDS-related pulmonary fibrosis have demonstrated improved gas exchange and low mortality (24%). In a larger, multicenter ARDSNet trial, corticosteroids were used for patients with late fibroproliferative ARDS (>7 days' duration) and did not demonstrate a survival benefit.[83] Importantly, patients given steroids after 14 days from ARDS onset experienced a higher mortality rate than control patients. Currently, the routine use of corticosteroids for the treatment of established ARDS cannot be recommended and should be avoided after 14 days from ARDS onset.[84]

Use of steroids in the earliest stages of ARDS has been evaluated, but they have not yet proved to provide a significant outcome benefit. It should be noted that many patients who meet the syndrome definition of ARDS can have other pulmonary disease processes that mimic ARDS (e.g., alveolar hemorrhage, interstitial lung disease, organizing pneumonia). Many of these conditions can respond to steroid therapy. In patients in whom the triggering risk factor cannot be easily identified and/or the course of illness is atypical or prolonged, clinicians often will consider these conditions and perform an open lung biopsy before starting steroid therapy. Potential adverse consequences of high-dose steroid therapy are numerous, including hyperglycemia, altered mental status, and muscular weakness. Thus routine use of systemic steroids in patients with ARDS is not advised at this time.

Beta-2 Agonists

In addition to their effects as bronchodilators, high doses of beta-2 agonists (e.g., albuterol, salbutamol) have been shown to accelerate clearance of alveolar edema by the epithelium of the alveolar wall.[85] Although beta-2 agonists are often used in patients with ARDS, their therapeutic benefits were not formally studied in ARDS until recently. Two recently completed trials in both the United States (ARDSNet) and Europe did not demonstrate a clinically significant benefit in patients with ARDS when using either aerosolized albuterol or intravenous salbutamol.[86,87] Demonstrated effects of beta-2 agonists have included reduced lung water using a surrogate measurement and improved lung function (lower plateau pressures), but no change in oxygenation (i.e., P/F ratio) has been observed.[86] In the ARDSNet trial, which is the largest to date, the trial was terminated early because of potential concern for increased mortality in the patients receiving beta-2 agonists, although the difference did not achieve statistical significance.[87] At this time, beta-2 agonist therapy cannot be recommended for use in ARDS.

Exogenous Surfactant Administration

Surfactant dysfunction and deficiency is a well-established component of RDS in premature infants as well as in children and adults with ARDS. Surfactant abnormalities contribute to the development of ARDS by promoting instability of the alveolar units (airway shear trauma, atelectasis, and right-to-left shunt) and by allowing inflammatory injury to alveoli to continue unchecked. Delivery of exogenous surfactants via direct intratracheal administration has become a cornerstone of therapy in RDS since the early 1990s.[88,89] Multiple surfactant preparations are commercially available, including natural surfactants (harvested from lungs of animals used in the meat industry) and synthetic surfactants, which are created artificially.[90]

Unfortunately, the pathogenesis of surfactant deficiency in the ARDS of children and adults is more challenging. The depletion of surfactant in premature newborns is related to the lack of lung maturation and surfactant production. In contrast, the surfactant depletion of ARDS is caused by inflammation of the alveolus and subsequent degradation of the endogenous surfactant (i.e., that normally produced by the patient's lungs). Numerous clinical trials have demonstrated improvement in oxygenation with intratracheal surfactant administration, including both natural and synthetic preparations.[91,92] However, the improvements in gas exchange have typically proven to be short-lived (24 to 72 hours) and have not demonstrated significant impact on clinical outcomes such as mortality or duration of mechanical ventilation in survivors.[34,93] These negative results in ARDS (in contrast to clear benefit in neonatal RDS) are thought to largely be explained by the degradation of the exogenously administered surfactant via the same inflammatory mechanisms that depleted the patient's native surfactant. Future studies of surfactant therapy are likely to include a combined approach that includes specific (e.g., monoclonal antibodies) or nonspecific (e.g., steroids) antiinflammatory agents. Despite the strong scientific rationale that surfactant replacement therapy may still prove beneficial for ARDS in the future, its cost is substantial and it is not considered a part of current ARDS management.

Alternative and Rescue Ventilation Strategies

In addition to the LPV approach of mechanical ventilation in ARDS (discussed previously), other ventilatory strategies are available and may prove beneficial in selected patients, but are less well-studied. These alternative approaches should be considered for patients who have failed LPV and the other components of "routine care." As such, these therapies are often considered primarily in patients with refractory severe ARDS and are often referred to as "rescue" or "salvage" therapies. In research trials and at some medical centers, the threshold for using such rescue approaches is defined by markers of unsafe ventilation, such as high plateau pressures (i.e., >30 cm H_2O) or high O_2 requirements (e.g., FiO_2 > 60%). Because the level of evidence regarding these alternative modes of ventilation is lower, variation in practice is greater and the choice of which ventilator strategy to use depends on the patient's clinical condition, the hospital's expertise (especially among intensivists, RTs, and nurses), and the availability of the necessary equipment.

Inverse-Ratio Ventilation

Inverse-ratio ventilation (IRV) is a form of pressure control (most often) or volume control ventilation with either a continuous mandatory or intermittent mandatory breath scheme. In conventional modes of mechanical ventilation, the respiratory cycle is characterized by I/E ratios exceeding 1:2; that is, the amount of time in the respiratory cycle in which expiration occurs is at least twice as long as the time for inspiration. During IRV, the inspiratory time on the ventilator is prolonged so that the I/E ratio is reversed (i.e., inspiratory time now exceeds expiratory time) and the I/E ratio characteristically ranges between 2:1 and 4:1. The clinical goal of IRV is to elevate the mean airway pressure to recruit alveolar units through prolongation of the inspiratory phase, hopefully improving oxygenation. The increase in mean airway pressure primarily results from incomplete lung emptying during a shortened exhalation time, causing air trapping and the development of additional PEEP, referred to as either *auto-PEEP* or *intrinsic PEEP.* Initial reports using IRV suggested significant improvement in oxygenation in patients with ARDS,[94] but subsequent studies that controlled for the level of PEEP did not demonstrate an advantage.[95] The IRV approach can lead to increased patient discomfort and ventilator dysynchrony, which often requires more sedation or even paralysis. As a result, use of IRV has declined significantly in recent years.

Airway Pressure Release Ventilation

Airway pressure release ventilation (APRV) was described by Stock and colleagues[96] in 1987 as a mode to allow unrestricted spontaneous breathing (e.g., IMV) in the setting of lung injury. The mode is a form of pressure control intermittent mandatory ventilation with IRV (the I/E ratio may exceed 4:1). The clinical aim of APRV is to increase the mean airway pressure to allow recruitment of alveoli while allowing the patient to spontaneously breathe. Ventilator manufacturers vary in how they implement APRV, but this mode generally features two levels of PEEP: a high PEEP (also named P_{high}), often set to approximately 25 to 30 cm H_2O, and a low PEEP (also known as P_{low}) that is usually set to zero. In APRV, patients can spontaneously breathe, which should make APRV more comfortable than traditional IRV. After a period at the high PEEP level, there are brief, approximately 0.5-second, decreases in airway pressure to the low PEEP level, allowing volume release and generating a mandatory V_T. Owing to the prolonged inspiratory times, APRV is associated with an increase in mean airway pressure and intrinsic PEEP. Indeed the literature demonstrates increases in oxygenation when APRV is used; however, the clinician is cautioned in using APRV because of technical issues with its application (e.g., no protocol has been tested and proved) and because there is a risk for injuriously large V_T and transpulmonary pressures.[97] Regarding the use of APRV as a routine mode for management of ARDS, the evidence so far is not conclusive, with no large randomized control trial comparing APRV to conventional ventilation.[98] However, some centers use APRV routinely.[99] In terms of using APRV as a rescue therapy, there is scant literature; the H1NI influenza pandemic generated as few case reports.[100] Taken together, we suggest that APRV remains as an alternative to manage patients with severe hypoxemia when conventional ventilation has failed and the clinician must exercise caution based on the concerns mentioned previously.

High-Frequency Ventilation

High-frequency ventilation (HFV) was initially devised as a method to minimize the hemodynamic effects of conventional mechanical ventilation (i.e., the large inflating pressures and volumes).[101] It soon became evident that HFV had theoretical advantages for managing ARDS. HFV is different from any of the conventional modes of ventilation because it uses a rapidly moving piston to create movement of air through a circuit. The device allows setting a mean airway pressure over which oscillations happen. V_Ts generated by HFV are very small (i.e., characteristically smaller than the patient's dead space), and higher mean airway pressures are provided to maintain alveolar patency, thereby theoretically preventing VILI. HFV has been successfully used in ventilating neonates with RDS and has been used both as routine therapy and rescue therapy.[102,103] Use of HFV in ARDS has been the subject of considerable debate as available trials have shown widely differing results.

To date, four randomized control trials have assessed the use of HFV versus conventional ventilation for the routine care of patients with severe ARDS. The first two of these trials[104,105] were conducted before later studies proved the benefits of using lower V_Ts in ARDS; both of these studies showed that using HFV was feasible and could support gas exchange without hemodynamic compromise.[106] Until the H1N1 influenza pandemic of 2009, few centers in the world used HFV routinely because no protocol had been proved, few devices were available (i.e., only a single device was available in the United States), and their use required specific training. With the H1N1 influenza outbreak in 2009 and the frequent development of ARDS among affected patients, a resurgence of interest in HFV occurred. After this renewed interest, two additional trials—OSCILLATE[107] (which assessed the efficacy of HFV; i.e., under conditions of ideal use, can HFV provide benefit?) and OSCAR[108] (testing effectiveness; i.e., how does HFV work under conditions of usual care?)—evaluated the routine use of HFV versus conventional lung protective ventilation in managing patients with early ARDS.—The OSCILLATE trial showed an increased mortality rate in patients treated with HFV and had to be stopped early.[107] In contrast, the OSCAR trial showed no difference between HFV and conventional modes of mechanical ventilation in treating ARDS.[108] At the current time, we do not recommend HFV in routine ARDS management, and, when being considered, its use should be reserved to referral centers with established experience.

Regarding the use of HFV as a rescue strategy for patients with severe hypoxemia from ARDS, there is less definitive information but a larger clinical experience. Anecdotal evidence, as well as published case series, suggests that HFV can have a role as a rescue strategy.[109,110] For example, in the CESAR trial[111] using HFV as part of a protocol prevented the need for extracorporeal membrane oxygenation in patients with severe ARDS. Thus, in some centers, **high-frequency oscillatory ventilation** is used as a rescue therapy for patients with severe ARDS.[112] The RT must remember that patients on HFV will be exposed to high mean airway pressures and also to high levels of PEEP, which may reduce cardiac output and overall O_2 delivery despite elevated arterial oxygenation.

Extracorporeal Support

Extracorporeal membrane oxygenation (ECMO) was first introduced in 1972 as a form of respiratory support for patients with severe AHRF. ECMO involves establishing a circuit for diverting a large proportion of the cardiac output through an artificial gas-exchange device, or "artificial lung," to facilitate the exchange of CO_2 and O_2. There are two types of ECMO, which differ according to which vessels are cannulated for the circuit: venoarterial and venovenous ECMO. In the case of a venoarterial circuit, both gas exchange and hemodynamic support can be offered through the ECMO circuit. However, venoarterial ECMO carries the risk associated with having a large indwelling arterial catheter in the patient (e.g., clots, bleeding, accidental withdrawal of the catheter). For pure respiratory failure, a venovenous circuit allows for gas exchange without hemodynamic support and can now be offered through a single venous cannula with fewer potential risks than venoarterial ECMO.

After an initial flurry of interest during the 1970s, a clinical trial comparing ECMO to conventional mechanical ventilation in ARDS showed no survival benefit with ECMO and enthusiasm subsided.[113] However, with continued improvements in equipment and delivery methods along with anecdotal cases with favorable results, more recent studies have been performed and suggest improved outcomes including survival[114] and less severe disability at 6 months.[111] These promising results and the experience gained during the 2009 H1N1 influenza pandemic led many institutions to use ECMO as rescue therapy for patients with ARDS who cannot be managed with conventional ventilatory modes.[114] The role of ECMO in the routine management in ARDS remains an area of intense debate and conflicting opinions. Overall, we consider ECMO to be a reasonable alternative to conventional ventilation strategies when the ARDS patient experiences refractory hypoxemia despite conventional management.[115] Unfortunately, this debate may never be fully resolved, because a rigorous randomized trial for patients with severe disease will require that the control group not be offered the therapy, which many clinicians and families are unwilling to support.

Similar to ECMO, **extracorporeal carbon dioxide removal** ($ECCO_2R$) entails the use of artificial membranes to supplement the gas-exchange deficiencies of damaged lungs. $ECCO_2R$ has a venovenous circuit that diverts a fraction of the cardiac output (approximately 20%) through a membrane lung. $ECCO_2R$ is primarily designed to remove CO_2 and does not directly influence oxygenation though oxygenation is indirectly facilitated through the removal of CO_2, which would otherwise compete with O_2 exchange within the alveoli. By this mechanism, $ECCO_2R$ allows the clinician to maintain the same level of oxygenation at lower ventilatory rates and reduce the risk for lung injury related to mechanical ventilation. A small clinical trial (with 40 adults) compared $ECCO_2R$ with conventional mechanical ventilation and found improved gas exchange, lower peak airway pressure, lower ventilatory rates, and reduced thoracic volumes (i.e., less overinflation of the lungs).[116] However, there was no survival benefit with $ECCO_2R$ at 30 days in that trial.[117]

Not all patients are good candidates for extracorporeal support, especially those with multisystem organ failure as opposed to primary respiratory failure. In considering ECMO or $ECCO_2R$, we favor early assessment and avoiding barotrauma and lung injury induced by prior prolonged mechanical ventilation. In conclusion, severely hypoxemic patients who do not respond to conventional ventilation, with or without some of the adjunctive therapies discussed previously, should be considered for early referral to centers that specialize in ECMO use.

THE ROLE OF THE RESPIRATORY THERAPIST IN ACUTE RESPIRATORY DISTRESS SYNDROME

The RT is essential as the expert in mechanical ventilation and respiratory support for the ICU team. Patients with ARDS represent some of the most challenging patients to manage on mechanical ventilation and require the greatest experience and expertise. The pivotal roles that RTs play in caring for patients with ARDS include ventilator setup, monitoring and frequent adjustments, equipment checks, drawing ABGs, placing arterial lines or performing hemodynamic assessments, and monitoring pulse oximetry and/or exhaled CO_2 monitors.

In treating patients with ARDS, RTs are essential members of the ICU team. In multiple randomized trials, RT-driven ventilator management protocols have outperformed usual care protocols in management of ARDS, including using the most advanced techniques (e.g., ECMO) and achieving liberation from the ventilator.[61,118] The assistance of RTs in ventilator management—offering advice concerning ventilatory strategies, reinforcing the value of low stretch approaches to all members of the team, and performing key technical tasks—is invaluable.

More specific to the management of patients with ARDS, the RT must learn and consistently apply the following key general aspects of supportive care:

1. ARDS is a diffuse injury of the lungs, but is not homogenous. Despite the presence of widespread pulmonary injury on radiographs and altered gas exchange in ARDS, there are areas of the lung with near-normal mechanical characteristics.
2. Better oxygenation (in terms of PaO_2 or SpO_2) is not always linked to better survival. This is an essential concept, because at the bedside we sometimes confuse improvement in oxygenation with success.
3. Mechanical ventilation can lead to VILI, which when not addressed can worsen ARDS and increase mortality secondary to MODS. The RT must always remember that it is the volume, not the pressure, that causes VILI.[119]
4. Initiation and maintenance of LPV, including $V_T = 6$ ml/kg of IBW and sufficient PEEP to exceed the lower inflection point, should become the priority and focus of daily care. The RT should take an active role in making sure that an accurate estimate of the patient's height has been obtained so an accurate IBW can be calculated.
5. Modes of mechanical ventilation that emphasize control of the V_T should be preferred. Although many modes are capable of maintaining V_T and no single mode has been proved to be superior, respiratory therapists should become familiar with how to manage each mode in a manner that prioritizes control of the V_T. Unnecessary transitions to multiple modes of mechanical ventilation in patients with ARDS are typically not helpful and further complicate interpretation of the patient's response to therapy.[120-122]
6. Inspiratory time can be prolonged in ARDS patients to target I/E ratios as low as 1 : 1. Hypercapnia can and should be tolerated (permissive hypercapnia) as long as pH remains above 7.15 to 7.20.
7. Adjunctive therapies, including prone positioning and neuromuscular blockade, may benefit respiratory function and be warranted in patients with severe ARDS.
8. Other nonrespiratory measures of supportive care are now proved to improve the outcomes of patients with ARDS, and RTs should be familiar with these approaches and should support and encourage their consistent application to all ARDS patients.
9. Pharmacologic therapies (e.g., inhaled NO, surfactant) are available and can enhance oxygenation in patients with ARDS but are expensive and do not change patient outcomes. Their routine use in ARDS is not recommended, and should be discouraged.
10. A small percent of patients with ARDS will develop refractory, severe hypoxemia in which the conventional approaches fail. Alternative or "rescue" therapies are as yet unproved but are available at large referral centers. Transfer of patients with refractory hypoxemia should be considered early in the course of disease within the initial 24 to 72 hours.

SUMMARY CHECKLIST

- Pulmonary edema from both hydrostatic (e.g., CHF) and nonhydrostatic (e.g., ARDS) causes may give rise to acute respiratory failure and are often difficult to differentiate on initial clinical evaluation.
- Pulmonary edema leads to bilateral alveolar infiltrates on the chest radiograph, restriction in lung volumes, and significant decline in gas exchange, particularly oxygenation.

- The pathologic findings of ARDS are characterized early by acute alveolar inflammation and injury with neutrophils and cytokines, which can rapidly reverse. In severe and/or persistent ARDS, a fibrotic phase can develop and can lead to a more prolonged course of recovery.
- The clinical definition and diagnosis of ARDS is based on the presence of a syndrome of characteristics that include abnormalities on the chest radiograph, hypoxemia, and a known risk factor or trigger that generates acute inflammation. There are well-established consensus definitions for ARDS that should be used by all caregivers.
- Although ARDS is a common critical illness with high associated mortality and morbidity, recent improvements in the care of patients with ARDS have substantially improved the likelihood of survival and have reduced recovery time for survivors.
- Although the physical examination and chest radiograph frequently do not provide sufficient information to distinguish CHF from ARDS, the clinical history and noninvasive methods to evaluate cardiac function (e.g., echocardiography) often provide key insights that can assist with accurately differentiating the cause of pulmonary edema. Alternative diagnostic techniques such as bronchoscopy or pulmonary artery catheterization can be helpful but are typically not required.
- The management of ARDS focuses on identification and treatment of the triggering risk factor and comprehensive supportive care of vital organs, particularly optimization of gas exchange and avoidance of VILI.
- Currently recommended ventilatory strategies for patients with ARDS are designed to minimize VILI using LPV that emphasizes low V_TS and sufficient levels of PEEP. Multiple modes of mechanical ventilation can be used to achieve LPV, but providers must prioritize avoiding VILI and be willing to tolerate reduced gas exchange, including lower oxygenation and higher $PaCO_2$.
- Adjunctive strategies beyond mechanical ventilation, such as prone positioning and neuromuscular blockade, have recently demonstrated benefit in patients with severe ARDS.
- Other nonventilatory supportive care measures (e.g., conservative fluid management, reduced sedation, early mobility) have been shown to improve outcomes in ARDS and should be encouraged and supported by RTs when possible.
- Alternative ventilation strategies, such as APRV, HFV, and ECMO still lack definitive proof of efficacy, but are available for patients who fail conventional LPV as suggested by severe, refractory hypoxemia. Using these rescue strategies should be considered early in the disease course, because their potential benefits lessen with more prolonged disease.

References

1. Ware LB, Matthay MA: The acute respiratory distress syndrome. *N Engl J Med* 342:1334–1349, 2000.
2. Matthay MA, Zimmerman GA: Acute lung injury and the acute respiratory distress syndrome: four decades of inquiry into pathogenesis and rational management. *Am J Respir Cell Mol Biol* 33:319–327, 2005.
3. West JB: *Respiratory physiology: the essentials*, ed 9, Baltimore, MD, 2012, Lippincott Williams & Wilkins.
4. Flick M, Matthay M: *Pulmonary edema and acute lung injury*, Philadelphia, 1994, WB Saunders.
5. Conhaim RL: Airway level at which edema liquid enters the air space of isolated dog lungs. *J Appl Physiol* 67:2234–2242, 1989.
6. Pugin J, Verghese G, Widmer MC, et al: The alveolar space is the site of intense inflammatory and profibrotic reactions in the early phase of acute respiratory distress syndrome. *Crit Care Med* 27:304–312, 1999.
7. Ware LB, Matthay MA: Alveolar fluid clearance is impaired in the majority of patients with acute lung injury and the acute respiratory distress syndrome. *Am J Respir Crit Care Med* 163:1376–1383, 2001.
8. Weiland JE, Davis WB, Holter JF, et al: Lung neutrophils in the adult respiratory distress syndrome: clinical and pathophysiologic significance. *Am Rev Respir Dis* 133:218–225, 1986.
9. Seeds MC, Grier BL, Suckling BN, et al: Secretory phospholipase A2-mediated depletion of phosphatidylglycerol in early acute respiratory distress syndrome. *Am J Med Sci* 343:446–451, 2012.
10. Marsh CB, Wewers MD: The pathogenesis of sepsis: factors that modulate the response to gram-negative bacterial infection. *Clin Chest Med* 17:183–197, 1996.
11. Parsons PE: Mediators and mechanisms of acute lung injury. *Clin Chest Med* 21:467–476, 2000.
12. Crouser ED, Julian MW, Weisbrode SE, et al: Acid aspiration results in ileal injury without altering ileal $V(O_2)$-$D(O_2)$ relationships. *Am J Respir Crit Care Med* 153:1965–1971, 1996.
13. St John RC, Mizer LA, Kindt GC, et al: Acid aspiration-induced acute lung injury causes leukocyte-dependent systemic organ injury. *J Appl Physiol* 74:1994–2003, 1993.
14. Wrobel S, Clements JA: Bubbles, babies and biology: the story of surfactant. Second breath: a medical mystery solved. *FASEB J* 18:1624e, 2004.
15. Ashbaugh DG, Bigelow DB, Petty TL, et al: Acute respiratory distress in adults. *Lancet* 2:319–323, 1967.
16. Hudson LD, Steinberg KP: Epidemiology of acute lung injury and ARDS. *Chest* 116:74S–82S, 1999.
17. Bernard GR, Artigas A, Brigham KL, et al; American-European Consensus Conference on ARDS: Definitions, mechanisms, relevant outcomes, and clinical trial coordination. *Am J Respir Crit Care Med* 149:818–824, 1994.
18. Force ADT, Ranieri VM, Rubenfeld GD, et al: Acute respiratory distress syndrome: the Berlin Definition. *JAMA* 307:2526–2533, 2012.
19. National Heart, Lung, and Blood Institute Acute Respiratory Distress Syndrome Clinical Trials Network, Wheeler AP, Bernard GR, Thompson BT, et al: Pulmonary-artery versus central venous catheter to guide treatment of acute lung injury. *N Engl J Med* 354:2213–2224, 2006.
20. National Heart, Lung, and Blood Institute Acute Respiratory Distress Syndrome Clinical Trials Network, Wheeler AP, Bernard GR, Thompson BT, et al: Comparison of two fluid-management strategies in acute lung injury. *N Engl J Med* 354:2564–2575, 2006.
21. Idell S, Cohen AB: Bronchoalveolar lavage in patients with the adult respiratory distress syndrome. *Clin Chest Med* 6:459–471, 1985.
22. Matthay MA, Robriquet L, Fang X: Alveolar epithelium: role in lung fluid balance and acute lung injury. *Proc Am Thorac Soc* 2:206–213, 2005.
23. Tomashefski JF, Jr: Pulmonary pathology of acute respiratory distress syndrome. *Clin Chest Med* 21:435–466, 2000.
24. Fahy RJ, Lichtenberger F, McKeegan CB, et al: The acute respiratory distress syndrome: a role for transforming growth factor-beta 1. *Am J Respir Cell Mol Biol* 28:499–503, 2003.
25. Marinelli WA, Henke CA, Harmon KR, et al: Mechanisms of alveolar fibrosis after acute lung injury. *Clin Chest Med* 11:657–672, 1990.
26. Rubenfeld GD, Herridge MS: Epidemiology and outcomes of acute lung injury. *Chest* 131:554–562, 2007.
27. Riscili BP, Anderson TB, Prescott HC, et al: An assessment of H1N1 influenza-associated acute respiratory distress syndrome severity after adjustment for treatment characteristics. *PLoS ONE* 6:e18166, 2011.
28. Fowler AA, Hamman RF, Good JT, et al: Adult respiratory distress syndrome: risk with common predispositions. *Ann Intern Med* 98:593–597, 1983.

29. Sloane PJ, Gee MH, Gottlieb JE, et al: A multicenter registry of patients with acute respiratory distress syndrome: physiology and outcome. *Am Rev Respir Dis* 146:419–426, 1992.
30. Meyer NJ, Garcia JG: Wading into the genomic pool to unravel acute lung injury genetics. *Proc Am Thorac Soc* 4:69–76, 2007.
31. Iribarren C, Jacobs DR, Jr, Sidney S, et al: Cigarette smoking, alcohol consumption, and risk of ARDS: a 15-year cohort study in a managed care setting. *Chest* 117:163–168, 2000.
32. Rubenfeld GD, Caldwell E, Peabody E, et al: Incidence and outcomes of acute lung injury. *N Engl J Med* 353:1685–1693, 2005.
33. Brun-Buisson C, Minelli C, Bertolini G, et al: Epidemiology and outcome of acute lung injury in European intensive care units: results from the ALIVE study. *Intensive Care Med* 30:51–61, 2004.
34. Spragg RG, Lewis JF, Walmrath HD, et al: Effect of recombinant surfactant protein C-based surfactant on the acute respiratory distress syndrome. *N Engl J Med* 351:884–892, 2004.
35. Sheu CC, Gong MN, Zhai R, et al: Clinical characteristics and outcomes of sepsis-related vs non-sepsis-related ARDS. *Chest* 138:559–567, 2010.
36. Milberg JA, Davis DR, Steinberg KP, et al: Improved survival of patients with acute respiratory distress syndrome (ARDS): 1983-1993. *JAMA* 273: 306–309, 1995.
37. National Heart, Lung, and Blood Institute ARDS Clinical Trials Network, Truwit JD, Bernard GR, Steingrub J, et al: Rosuvastatin for sepsis-associated acute respiratory distress syndrome. *N Engl J Med* 370:2191–2200, 2014.
38. Herridge MS, Tansey CM, Matté A, et al: Functional disability 5 years after acute respiratory distress syndrome. *N Engl J Med* 364:1293–1304, 2011.
39. National Heart, Lung, and Blood Institute, National Institutes of Health: <http://www.ARDSNet.org>, (Accessed September 12, 2015).
40. PETAL Network: Prevention and treatment of acute lung injury. <http://www.petalnet.org>, (Accessed September 12, 2015).
41. Acute Respiratory Distress Syndrome Network: Ventilation with lower tidal volumes as compared with traditional tidal volumes for acute lung injury and the acute respiratory distress syndrome. *N Engl J Med* 342:1301–1308, 2000.
42. Futier E, Constantin J-M, Paugam-Burtz C, et al: A trial of intraoperative low-tidal-volume ventilation in abdominal surgery. *N Engl J Med* 369:428–437, 2013.
43. Mireles-Cabodevila E, Chatburn RL: Work of breathing in adaptive pressure control continuous mandatory ventilation. *Respir Care* 54:1467–1472, 2009.
44. Volsko TA, Hoffman J, Conger A, et al: The effect of targeting scheme on tidal volume delivery during volume control mechanical ventilation. *Respir Care* 57:1297–1304, 2012.
45. Chatburn RL, Mireles-Cabodevila E: Closed-loop control of mechanical ventilation: description and classification of targeting schemes. *Respir Care* 56:85–102, 2011.
46. Suter PM, Fairley B, Isenberg MD: Optimum end-expiratory airway pressure in patients with acute pulmonary failure. *N Engl J Med* 292:284–289, 1975.
47. PROVE Network Investigators for the Clinical Trial Network of the European Society of Anaesthesiology, Hemmes SN, Gama de Abreu M, Pelosi P, et al: High versus low positive end-expiratory pressure during general anaesthesia for open abdominal surgery (PROVHILO trial): a multicentre randomised controlled trial. *Lancet* 384:495–503, 2014.
48. Brower RG, Lanken PN, MacIntyre N, et al: Higher versus lower positive end-expiratory pressures in patients with the acute respiratory distress syndrome. *N Engl J Med* 351:327–336, 2004.
49. Santa Cruz R, Rojas JI, Nervi R, et al: High versus low positive end-expiratory pressure (PEEP) levels for mechanically ventilated adult patients with acute lung injury and acute respiratory distress syndrome. *Cochrane Database Syst Rev* (6):CD009098, 2013.
50. Crotti S, Mascheroni D, Caironi P, et al: Recruitment and derecruitment during acute respiratory failure: a clinical study. *Am J Respir Crit Care Med* 164:131–140, 2001.
51. Chiumello D, Coppola S, Froio S, et al: Time to reach a new steady state after changes of positive end expiratory pressure. *Intensive Care Med* 39:1377–1385, 2013.
52. Gattinoni L, Protti A, Caironi P, et al: Ventilator-induced lung injury: the anatomical and physiological framework. *Crit Care Med* 38:S539–S548, 2010.
53. Chiumello D, Cressoni M, Carlesso E, et al: Bedside selection of positive end-expiratory pressure in mild, moderate, and severe acute respiratory distress syndrome. *Crit Care Med* 42:252–264, 2014.
54. Briel M, Meade M, Mercat A, et al: Higher vs lower positive end-expiratory pressure in patients with acute lung injury and acute respiratory distress syndrome: systematic review and meta-analysis. *JAMA* 303:865–873, 2010.
55. Richard JC, Brochard L, Breton L, et al: Influence of respiratory rate on gas trapping during low volume ventilation of patients with acute lung injury. *Intensive Care Med* 28:1078–1083, 2002.
56. Vieillard-Baron A, Jardin F: The issue of dynamic hyperinflation in acute respiratory distress syndrome patients. *Eur Respir J Suppl* 42:43s–47s, 2003.
57. Vieillard-Baron A, Prin S, Augarde R, et al: Increasing respiratory rate to improve CO_2 clearance during mechanical ventilation is not a panacea in acute respiratory failure. *Crit Care Med* 30:1407–1412, 2002.
58. O'Croinin D, Ni Chonghaile M, Higgins B, et al: Bench-to-bedside review: permissive hypercapnia. *Crit Care* 9:51–59, 2005.
59. Kregenow DA, Rubenfeld GD, Hudson LD, et al: Hypercapnic acidosis and mortality in acute lung injury. *Crit Care Med* 34:1–7, 2006.
60. Wiedemann HP, Wheeler AP, Bernard GR, et al: Comparison of two fluid-management strategies in acute lung injury. *N Engl J Med* 354:2564–2575, 2006.
61. Girard TD, Kress JP, Fuchs BD, et al: Efficacy and safety of a paired sedation and ventilator weaning protocol for mechanically ventilated patients in intensive care (Awakening and Breathing Controlled trial): a randomised controlled trial. *Lancet* 371:126–134, 2008.
62. Kress JP, Pohlman AS, O'Connor MF, et al: Daily interruption of sedative infusions in critically ill patients undergoing mechanical ventilation. *N Engl J Med* 342:1471–1477, 2000.
63. Barr J, Fraser GL, Puntillo K, et al: Clinical practice guidelines for the management of pain, agitation, and delirium in adult patients in the intensive care unit. *Crit Care Med* 41:263–306, 2013.
64. Needham DM, Dinglas VD, Bienvenu OJ, et al: One year outcomes in patients with acute lung injury randomised to initial trophic or full enteral feeding: prospective follow-up of EDEN randomised trial. *BMJ* 346:f1532, 2013.
65. Rice TW, Wheeler AP, Thompson BT, et al: Enteral omega-3 fatty acid, gamma-linolenic acid, and antioxidant supplementation in acute lung injury. *JAMA* 306:1574–1581, 2011.
66. Zhu DJ, Zhang Y, Li S, et al: Enteral omega-3 fatty acid supplementation in adult patients with acute respiratory distress syndrome: a systematic review of randomized controlled trials with meta-analysis and trial sequential analysis. *Intensive Care Med* 40:504–512, 2014.
67. Morris PE, Goad A, Thompson C, et al: Early intensive care unit mobility therapy in the treatment of acute respiratory failure. *Crit Care Med* 36: 2238–2243, 2008.
68. Schweickert WD, Pohlman MC, Pohlman AS, et al: Early physical and occupational therapy in mechanically ventilated, critically ill patients: a randomised controlled trial. *Lancet* 373:1874–1882, 2009.
69. Morris PE: Moving our critically ill patients: mobility barriers and benefits. *Crit Care Clin* 23:1–20, 2007.
70. Boonyapisit K, Katirji B: Multifocal motor neuropathy presenting with respiratory failure. *Muscle Nerve* 23:1887–1890, 2000.
71. Gattinoni L, Tognoni G, Pesenti A, et al: Effect of prone positioning on the survival of patients with acute respiratory failure. *N Engl J Med* 345: 568–573, 2001.
72. Mutoh T, Guest RJ, Lamm WJ, et al: Prone position alters the effect of volume overload on regional pleural pressures and improves hypoxemia in pigs in vivo. *Am Rev Respir Dis* 146:300–306, 1992.
73. Douglas WW, Rehder K, Beynen FM, et al: Improved oxygenation in patients with acute respiratory failure: the prone position. *Am Rev Respir Dis* 115:559–566, 1977.
74. Sud S, Friedrich JO, Taccone P, et al: Prone ventilation reduces mortality in patients with acute respiratory failure and severe hypoxemia: systematic review and meta-analysis. *Intensive Care Med* 36:585–599, 2010.

75. Guerin C, Reignier J, Richard JC, et al: Prone positioning in severe acute respiratory distress syndrome. *N Engl J Med* 368:2159–2168, 2013.
76. Papazian L, Forel JM, Gacouin A, et al: Neuromuscular blockers in early acute respiratory distress syndrome. *N Engl J Med* 363:1107–1116, 2010.
77. Corris P, Degano B: Severe pulmonary arterial hypertension: treatment options and the bridge to transplantation. *Eur Respir Rev* 23:488–497, 2014.
78. Taylor RW, Zimmerman JL, Dellinger RP, et al: Low-dose inhaled nitric oxide in patients with acute lung injury: a randomized controlled trial. *JAMA* 291:1603–1609, 2004.
79. van Heerden PV, Barden A, Michalopoulos N, et al: Dose-response to inhaled aerosolized prostacyclin for hypoxemia due to ARDS. *Chest* 117:819–827, 2000.
80. Adhikari NK, Dellinger RP, Lundin S, et al: Inhaled nitric oxide does not reduce mortality in patients with acute respiratory distress syndrome regardless of severity: systematic review and meta-analysis. *Crit Care Med* 42:404–412, 2014.
81. Martin C, Papazian L, Payan MJ, et al: Pulmonary fibrosis correlates with outcome in adult respiratory distress syndrome: a study in mechanically ventilated patients. *Chest* 107:196–200, 1995.
82. Meduri GU, Chinn AJ, Leeper KV, et al: Corticosteroid rescue treatment of progressive fibroproliferation in late ARDS: patterns of response and predictors of outcome. *Chest* 105:1516–1527, 1994.
83. Meduri GU, Headley AS, Golden E, et al: Effect of prolonged methylprednisolone therapy in unresolving acute respiratory distress syndrome: a randomized controlled trial. *JAMA* 280:159–165, 1998.
84. Steinberg KP, Hudson LD, Goodman RB, et al: Efficacy and safety of corticosteroids for persistent acute respiratory distress syndrome. *N Engl J Med* 354:1671–1684, 2006.
85. Frank JA, Wang Y, Osorio O, et al: Beta-adrenergic agonist therapy accelerates the resolution of hydrostatic pulmonary edema in sheep and rats. *J Appl Physiol* 89:1255–1265, 2000.
86. Perkins GD, McAuley DF, Thickett DR, et al: The beta-agonist lung injury trial (BALTI): a randomized placebo-controlled clinical trial. *Am J Respir Crit Care Med* 173:281–287, 2006.
87. National Heart, Lung, and Blood Institute Acute Respiratory Distress Syndrome Clinical Trials Network, Matthay MA, Brower AG, Carson S, et al: Randomized, placebo-controlled clinical trial of an aerosolized beta(2)-agonist for treatment of acute lung injury. *Am J Respir Crit Care Med* 184:561–568, 2011.
88. Fujiwara T, Konishi M, Chida S, et al: Surfactant replacement therapy with a single postventilatory dose of a reconstituted bovine surfactant in preterm neonates with respiratory distress syndrome: final analysis of a multicenter, double-blind, randomized trial and comparison with similar trials. The Surfactant-TA Study Group. *Pediatrics* 86:753–764, 1990.
89. Jobe AH: Pulmonary surfactant therapy. *N Engl J Med* 328:861–868, 1993.
90. Ramanthan RK, Kamholz K, Fujii A: Is there a difference in surfactant treatment of respiratory distress syndrome in premature neonates? A review. *J Pulmon Respir Med* S13, 2013.
91. Gregory TJ, Steinberg KP, Spragg R, et al: Bovine surfactant therapy for patients with acute respiratory distress syndrome. *Am J Respir Crit Care Med* 155:1309–1315, 1997.
92. Walmrath D, Grimminger F, Pappert D, et al: Bronchoscopic administration of bovine natural surfactant in ARDS and septic shock: impact on gas exchange and haemodynamics. *Eur Respir J* 19:805–810, 2002.
93. Kesecioglu J, Beale R, Stewart TE, et al: Exogenous natural surfactant for treatment of acute lung injury and the acute respiratory distress syndrome. *Am J Respir Crit Care Med* 180:989–994, 2009.
94. Tharratt RS, Allen RP, Albertson TE: Pressure controlled inverse ratio ventilation in severe adult respiratory failure. *Chest* 94:755–762, 1988.
95. Mercat A, Graini L, Teboul JL, et al: Cardiorespiratory effects of pressure-controlled ventilation with and without inverse ratio in the adult respiratory distress syndrome. *Chest* 104:871–875, 1993.
96. Stock MC, Downs JB, Frolicher DA: Airway pressure release ventilation. *Crit Care Med* 15:462–466, 1987.
97. Sasidhar M, Chatburn RL: Tidal volume variability during airway pressure release ventilation: case summary and theoretical analysis. *Respir Care* 57:1325–1333, 2012.
98. Varpula T, Valta P, Niemi R, et al: Airway pressure release ventilation as a primary ventilatory mode in acute respiratory distress syndrome. *Acta Anaesthesiol Scand* 48:722–731, 2004.
99. Gonzalez M, Arroliga AC, Frutos-Vivar F, et al: Airway pressure release ventilation versus assist-control ventilation: a comparative propensity score and international cohort study. *Intensive Care Med* 36:817–827, 2010.
100. Sundar KM, Thaut P, Nielsen DB, et al: Clinical course of ICU patients with severe pandemic 2009 influenza A (H1N1) pneumonia: single center experience with proning and pressure release ventilation. *J Intensive Care Med* 27:184–190, 2012.
101. Lunkenhe PP, Dickhut HH, Keller H, et al: Application of transtracheal pressure oscillations as a modification of diffusion respiration. *Br J Anaesth* 44:627, 1972.
102. Cools F, Askie LM, Offringa M, et al: Elective high-frequency oscillatory versus conventional ventilation in preterm infants: a systematic review and meta-analysis of individual patients' data. *Lancet* 375:2082–2091, 2010.
103. Zivanovic S, Peacock J, Alcazar-Paris M, et al: Late outcomes of a randomized trial of high-frequency oscillation in neonates. *N Engl J Med* 370:112–130, 2014.
104. Derdak S, Mehta S, Stewart TE, et al: High-frequency oscillatory ventilation for acute respiratory distress syndrome in adults: a randomized, controlled trial. *Am J Respir Crit Care Med* 166:801–808, 2002.
105. Bollen CW, van Well GT, Sherry T, et al: High frequency oscillatory ventilation compared with conventional mechanical ventilation in adult respiratory distress syndrome: a randomized controlled trial [ISRCTN24242669]. *Crit Care* 9:R430–R439, 2005.
106. Sud S, Sud M, Friedrich JO, et al: High frequency oscillation in patients with acute lung injury and acute respiratory distress syndrome (ARDS): systematic review and meta-analysis. *BMJ* 340:c2327, 2010.
107. Ferguson ND, Cook DJ, Guyatt GH: et: High-frequency oscillation in early acute respiratory distress syndrome. *N Engl J Med* 368:795–805, 2013.
108. Young D, Lamb SE, Shah S, et al: High-frequency oscillation for acute respiratory distress syndrome. *N Engl J Med* 368:806–813, 2013.
109. Fort P, Farmer C, Westerman J, et al: High-frequency oscillatory ventilation for adult respiratory distress syndrome: a pilot study. *Crit Care Med* 25:937–947, 1997.
110. Gluck E, Heard S, Patel C, et al: Use of ultrahigh frequency ventilation in patients with ARDS: a preliminary report. *Chest* 103:1413–1420, 1993.
111. Peek GJ, Elbourne D, Mugford M, et al: Randomised controlled trial and parallel economic evaluation of conventional ventilatory support versus extracorporeal membrane oxygenation for severe adult respiratory failure (CESAR). *Health Technol Assess* 14:1–46, 2012.
112. Pipeling MR, Fan E: Therapies for refractory hypoxemia in acute respiratory distress syndrome. *JAMA* 304:2521–2527, 2010.
113. Zapol WM, Snider MT, Schneider RC: Extracorporeal membrane oxygenation for acute respiratory failure. *Anesthesiology* 46:272–285, 1977.
114. Australia, New Zealand Extracorporeal Membrane Oxygenation Influenza I, Davies A, Jones D, Beca J, et al: Extracorporeal membrane oxygenation for 2009 influenza A(H1N1) acute respiratory distress syndrome. *JAMA* 302:1888–1895, 2009.
115. Park PK, Dalton HJ, Bartlett RH: Point: efficacy of extracorporeal membrane oxygenation in 2009 influenza A (H1N1)—sufficient evidence? *Chest* 138:776–778, 2010.
116. Brunet F, Mira JP, Belghith M, et al: Extracorporeal carbon dioxide removal technique improves oxygenation without causing overinflation. *Am J Respir Crit Care Med* 149:1557–1562, 1994.
117. Freed DH, Henzler D, White CW, et al: Extracorporeal lung support for patients who had severe respiratory failure secondary to influenza A (H1N1) 2009 infection in Canada. *Can J Anaesth* 57:240–247, 2010.
118. Morris AH, Wallace CJ, Menlove RL, et al: Randomized clinical trial of pressure-controlled inverse ratio ventilation and extracorporeal CO_2 removal for adult respiratory distress syndrome. *Am J Respir Crit Care Med* 149:295–305, 1994.

119. Dreyfuss D, Soler P, Basset G, et al: High inflation pressure pulmonary edema: respective effects of high airway pressure, high tidal volume, and positive end-expiratory pressure. *Am Rev Respir Dis* 137:1159–1164, 1988.
120. Esteban A, Alia I, Gordo F, et al: Spanish Lung Failure Collaborative Group: Prospective randomized trial comparing pressure-controlled ventilation and volume-controlled ventilation in ARDS. *Chest* 117:1690–1696, 2000.
121. Lessard MR, Guerot E, Lorino H, et al: Effects of pressure-controlled with different I:E ratios versus volume-controlled ventilation on respiratory mechanics, gas exchange, and hemodynamics in patients with adult respiratory distress syndrome. *Anesthesiology* 80:983–991, 1994.
122. Meade MO, Cook DJ, Guyatt GH, et al: Ventilation strategy using low tidal volumes, recruitment maneuvers, and high positive end-expiratory pressure for acute lung injury and acute respiratory distress syndrome: a randomized controlled trial. *JAMA* 299:637–645, 2008.

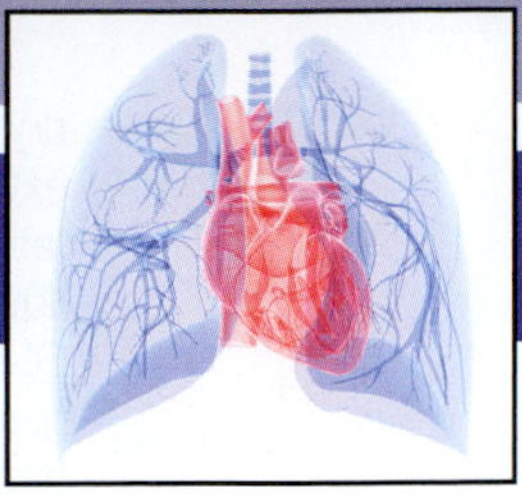

CHAPTER 30

Respiratory Management of Trauma, Obesity, Near Drowning, and Burns

LORENZO BERRA

CHAPTER OBJECTIVES

After reading this chapter you will be able to:

- Discuss the clinical presentation and the differences in approach to the assessment of patients with life-threatening trauma, pulmonary and body surface burns, obesity, and near drowning.
- Discuss the specific pathophysiology that would guide the application of respiratory care to the management of patients with life-threatening trauma, pulmonary and body surface burns, obesity, and near drowning.
- List the factors affecting gas exchange in each of these patient types.
- Discuss indications for oxygen therapy, noninvasive ventilation, and invasive mechanical ventilation.
- Describe concerns associated with the application of mechanical ventilation to patients with life-threatening trauma, pulmonary and body surface burns, obesity, and near drowning.
- Discuss the application of lung protective ventilation to patients with life-threatening trauma, pulmonary and body surface burns, obesity, and near drowning.
- Discuss the use of positive end expiratory pressure, lung recruitment maneuvers, and prone positioning in patients with life-threatening trauma, pulmonary and body surface burns, obesity, and near drowning.
- Discuss the process of ventilator discontinuation in patients with life-threatening trauma, pulmonary and body surface burns, obesity, and near drowning.

CHAPTER OUTLINE

Life-Threatening Trauma
- Epidemiology
- Clinical Assessment and Specific Pathophysiologic Concerns
- Respiratory Management

Obesity
- Epidemiology
- Specific Pathophysiologic Concerns
- Clinical Assessment
- Respiratory Management

Near Drowning
- Epidemiology
- Specific Pathophysiologic Concerns
- Respiratory Management
- Airway Clearance Therapy
- Mechanical Ventilation
- Positioning

Burns
- Epidemiology
- Clinical Assessment
- Pathophysiology of Burn Patients
- Specific Concerns
- Respiratory Management

KEY TERMS

% total body surface area
blunt trauma
carbon monoxide poisoning
cold shock cardiac-respiratory reflexes
cyanide toxicity
cyanocobalamin
cytochrome oxidase
decremental PEEP trial

dry drowning
exudates
fasciotomy
fluvial or brackish water
Glasgow Coma Scale
glomerular filtration rate
hydrophilic drugs
lipophilic drugs
morbid obesity
obesity hypoventilation syndrome
obstructive sleep apnea
penetrating trauma
pulmonary contusion
recruitment maneuvers
severe obesity
super obesity
tension pneumothorax
thiosulfate
thoracic flap (flail chest)
transudates
wet drowning

LIFE-THREATENING TRAUMA

Epidemiology

Trauma is the third overall cause of death in the United States and the primary cause of death for Americans between 1 and 44 years of age.[1] Each year, trauma accounts for 41 million admissions to emergency departments (EDs) and 2 million hospital admissions. Each year, more than 190,000 Americans lose their lives to trauma. But what exactly is trauma? In the most basic sense, trauma is an injury to the body that threatens life and limb integrity. The injury is caused by a physical agent (a force, heat, radiations, etc.) acting on one or more regions of the human body. As a result, trauma patients can have vastly different presentations and clinical manifestations and can require different levels of care. Not every trauma that involves the thorax requires intensive care and respiratory support, just as some traumas that do not involve the chest might require intensive care and respiratory support (e.g., in the setting of transfusion-related acute lung injury or head trauma). Additionally, patients who suffer from trauma and require invasive mechanical ventilation (for trauma that directly involves the thorax, because of the need for an artificial airway, or as a result of massive transfusion) are at higher risk for ventilator-associated pneumonia (VAP), thus complicating these patients' clinical courses. Among patients admitted to the intensive care unit (ICU) after trauma, it has been shown that the presence of traumatic brain injury (TBI) and a poor **Glasgow Coma Scale** score (GCS, Table 30-1) (GCS < 8) on admission are the main determinants of patient outcome, measured as post-ICU disability and quality of life.[2] Neurologic damage appears to be pivotal in determining patient mortality and disability; therefore the respiratory therapist must pay special attention to maintaining adequate oxygenation without compromising perfusion and hemodynamics. Because of the heterogeneous presentation of trauma, there is no overarching rule of thumb regarding patient respiratory management, and the respiratory therapist plays a key role in identifying life-threatening problems and tailoring the support of respiratory function.

Clinical Assessment and Specific Pathophysiologic Concerns

During the first evaluation of a trauma patient, the respiratory therapist, together with the medical team, should focus on the airway and breathing. If blunt injury is present, cervical spine injury always should be suspected and immobilization of the cervical spine must be instituted immediately.[3]

Assessment of a victim of major trauma should start with a GCS evaluation. If a patient is fully awake, responsive (GCS = 15), and able to maintain a patent airway, close respiratory and neurologic monitoring should be instituted until the medical team completes surveillance. If a patient's GCS range is between 14 and 9, the respiratory therapist should pay extra attention to the status of the patient because the clinical condition might quickly deteriorate, requiring endotracheal intubation and invasive ventilation. A GCS lower than 8 always mandates securing the airway by endotracheal intubation and further diagnostic evaluation.

RULE OF THUMB

Trauma victims with TBI and a GCS scores of less than 8 require endotracheal intubation and generally have poorer postinjury quality of life and greater disability.

TABLE 30-1
Glasgow Coma Score

Response	Score
Best Eye Response (E)	
Spontaneously	4
To speech	3
To pain	2
No response	1
Best Verbal Response (V)	
Oriented to time, place, and person	5
Confused	4
Inappropriate words	3
Incomprehensible sounds	2
No response	1
Best Motor Response (M)	
Obeys commands	6
Moves to localized pain	5
Flexion withdrawal from pain	4
Abnormal flexion (decorticate)	3
Abnormal extension (decerebrate)	2
No response	1
Total Score	**15**
Change in Mental Status	
Close monitoring is required.	14-9
Comatose. Securing the airway is required.	≤8
Totally unresponsive	3

Head, Neck, and Upper Airway Injuries

The presence of external injuries to the head should raise the suspicion of TBI. These patients are at risk for rapid neurologic deterioration as a result of an array of alterations in mental status, ranging from confusion to seizures to coma. The respiratory function of these patients can be compromised by upper airway obstruction because of loss of muscular tone or, as with seizures, to excessive muscular tone that requires immediate sedation, paralysis, and endotracheal intubation. Endotracheal intubation might be challenging because of the mandatory immobilization of the cervical spine (Figure 30-1). Management of the upper airways is complicated by anatomic alterations of the rhino-oropharynx caused by the traumatic injury. Severe maxillofacial injuries or destructive trauma of the upper airway prompts tracheal access for definitive airway management.[4] The presence of blood, gastric contents, oral secretions, and foreign material complicate artificial airway placement and management.

Lower Respiratory Injuries

Chest trauma is usually classified either as **penetrating trauma** (i.e., high force applied to a small surface area of the body, such as with a gunshot) or **blunt trauma** (i.e., high force applied over a larger body surface, such as the case of a head-on-end motor vehicle accident).[5] However, most chest injuries do not fall into one of these two categories but instead represent a mix of the two. Depending on the depth of the penetrating lesions, patients can present different clinical features. A lesion that breaches the chest wall violating the pleural space without injuring the lung causes a decoupling of the chest wall/lung relationship. During spontaneous breathing the chest wall tends to expand while the lung tends to collapse. This results in a physiologically negative pleural pressure. When the pleural space is exposed to atmospheric pressure, as in the case of a penetrating trauma injury, the negative pleural pressure causes air to enter the pleural space. At this point the chest wall expands and the lung collapses, resulting in a pneumothorax. If the penetrating injury violates both the pleural space and the lung, air can enter the pleural cavity from both the chest wall and the lung. Patients with this particular injury are at high risk for developing a **tension pneumothorax**. A tension pneumothorax develops when the pleural lesion acts as a one-way valve allowing the entrance of air into the pleural space and progressively trapping air in the expanding pleural cavity. With every breath, the volume of air increases in the pleural cavity. As volume increases, pressure increases, resulting in a force directed toward the opposite pleural cavity. The high unilateral pressure causes a shift of mediastinal structures, resulting in distortion and eventual collapse of the main vascular structures, specifically the vena cava. This phenomenon leads to rapid hemodynamic deterioration that, if unrecognized, results in cardiovascular collapse and death. Penetrating traumas may involve one or more bronchial structures.

Bronchial injuries cause large volumes of air to rapidly enter the pleural cavity as well as the mediastinum, depending on the location of the injury.[6] The presence of bronchial injury should be suspected when, after the placement of a chest tube for pleural drainage, large amounts of air continue to exit the chest tube in a synchronized pattern with positive pressure ventilation. Tracheal lesions can be life-threatening and require prompt surgical evaluation and appropriate airway management. The chosen artificial airway should be capable of bypassing the tracheal lesion to provide adequate pressurization and mechanical ventilation to both lungs. Mechanical ventilation through a tracheal disruption leads to pneumomediastinum, hemodynamic instability, and mediastinal infection.

Esophageal rupture may result in a communicating lesion with the respiratory tract or with the mediastinum. In the first case, the main clinical features are gas leakage during mechanical ventilation and aspiration of gastric material, which can result in chemical pneumonia or full-blown acute respiratory distress syndrome (ARDS). It is vital to recognize and treat these lesions as soon as possible.[7]

Blunt trauma is the other main mechanism that can cause physical injury to the human body. The main sign that a significant blunt trauma has affected the thoracic region is the presence of rib fractures.[8] Rib fractures can be unifocal (one point of fracture per rib) or multifocal (two or more points of fracture in a single rib). This difference is fundamental in understanding the effects of rib fractures on respiratory function. Unifocal fractures can be either nondisplaced or displaced. Nondisplaced rib fractures do not usually require particular attention if the number of fractured ribs is low. However, multiple fractured ribs can be extremely painful and impair proper inspiration, leading to shallow breathing and fatigue. These patients benefit from pain medication and, eventually, pneumatic stabilization of the chest wall through CPAP.[9]

RULE OF THUMB

The presence of bronchial injury should be suspected when, after the placement of a chest tube for pleural drainage, large amounts of air continue to exit the chest tube in a synchronized pattern with positive pressure ventilation.

Displaced rib fractures are even more painful, and sharp bone edges can cause pneumothorax through laceration of the visceral pleura. Pain control and pneumatic stabilization are encouraged. These patients should be routinely monitored because they can develop internal pleural bleeding, especially in the setting of anticoagulant therapy. The presence of blood in the pleural cavity (hemothorax) requires pleural drainage and close monitoring of the bleeding (total amount of blood lost and presence of active bleeding). Surgical evaluation is mandatory. Multifocal fractures of one or more ribs create a **thoracic flap (flail chest)** that is extremely painful and impairs normal respiratory mechanics. During inspiration, when pleural pressure becomes negative, the free flap will be pushed inward, whereas during exhalation, when pleural pressure is positive, it will be pushed outward. This causes extreme pain because the edges of the ribs will be subjected to continuous friction. Based

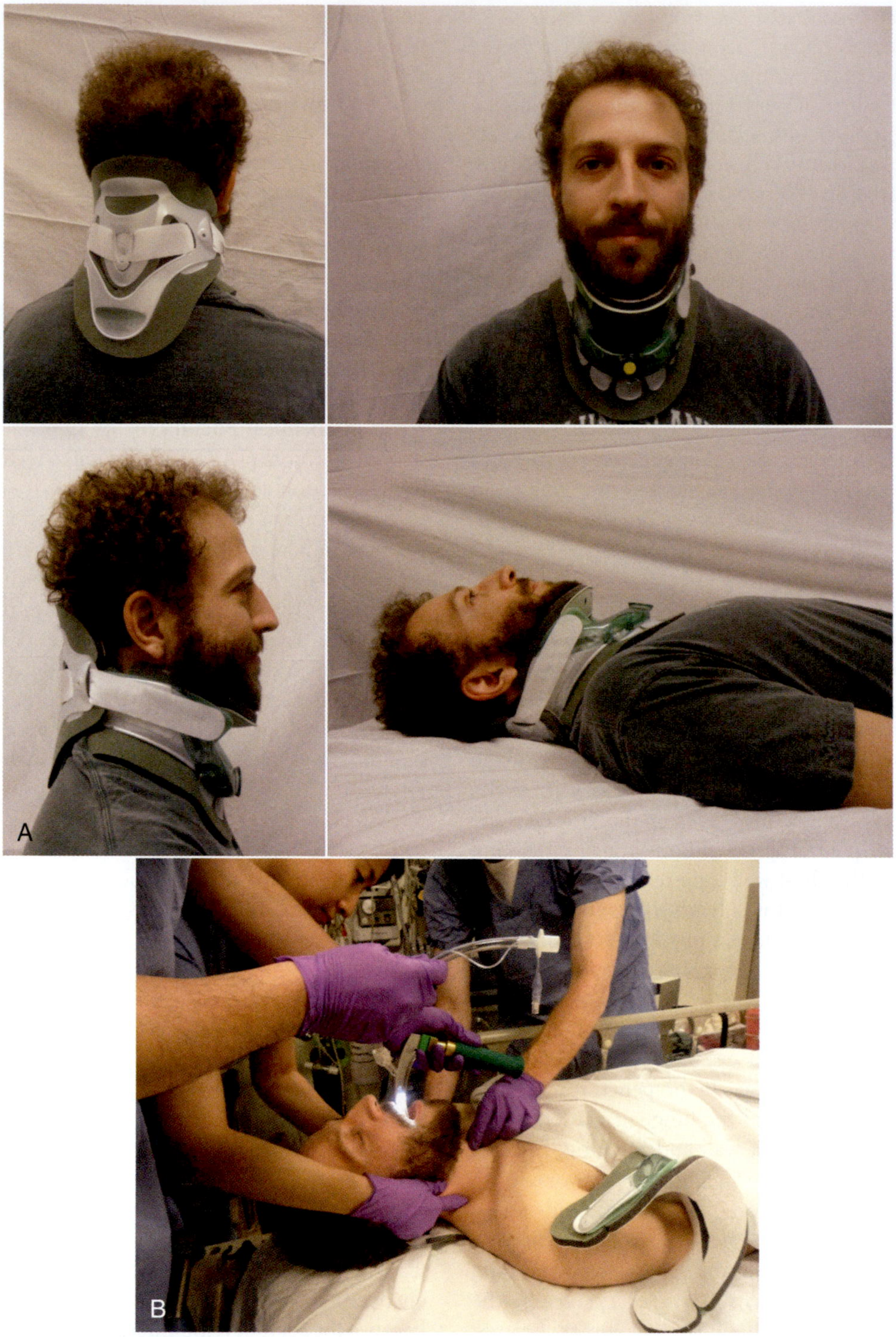

FIGURE 30-1 **A,** In trauma cervical stabilization is generally obtained by a rigid collar that encircles the neck and supports the chin and the back of the head. The goal of cervical collars is to restrict a certain motion in flexion and extension, while supporting the chin and the occiput. When rigid cervical collar are applied venous outflow at the neck should always be maintained, to avoid increased intracranial pressure. **B,** During intubation, it is tolerated to undo the anterior part of the cervical collar while an assistant maintains in-line stabilization with the occiput held firmly in neutral position (hands are placed along the side of the head with fingertips on the mastoid holding the occiput down). When possible, another assistant applies cricoid pressure. This orientation might limit visualization of the vocal cords for the operator; however, reduction of atlantooccipital motion should be the priority. Awake or asleep fiberoptic intubation or newer airway management instrumentation should be planed before intubation of a patient with unstable cervical spine.

on the extent of the lesion, flail chest can impair normal ventilation. The current therapeutic approach is based on pain management and continuous positive airway pressure (CPAP). Needless to say, the presence of flail chest is associated with a high risk for pneumohemothorax.

Blunt trauma also can cause **pulmonary contusions**. This injury is characterized by acute inflammation and exudation of plasma and blood components into the alveolar space. Even though these lesions resolve spontaneously, they are at high risk for bacterial or viral infection, leading to pneumonia.[10] These inflammatory processes are usually located in the regions of the lung that were subject to the traumatic force.

The application of a traumatic blunt force on the abdomen causes a rapid increase of intraabdominal pressure. This could lead to diaphragmatic rupture. A rupture of the diaphragm impairs normal respiratory function and represents a medical and surgical emergency. If positive pressure ventilation is not applied, the negative intrathoracic pressure during inspiration literally sucks visceral organs into the pleura, causing massive lung collapse, acute bowel obstruction, and possibly splanchnic ischemia.

RULE OF THUMB

All patients with chest trauma, regardless of whether the injury is penetrating or blunt, require careful assessment for pneumothorax, airway injuries, disruption of thoracic vessels, and chest contusion leading to ARDS.

Special Considerations in Patients With Chest Trauma

All bedridden patients are at increased risk for atelectasis secondary to decreased tidal volume and residual volume. Mucus clearance is impaired by inadequate mobilization and excessive or inadequate pain control. Secretion retention might aggravate atelectasis by creating thick mucus plugs in the distal bronchial tree. This phenomenon exposes the bedridden patient to hospital-acquired pneumonia. Secretion retention is a major issue in patients with chest trauma. The pain associated with the trauma (i.e., rib fractures) further impairs the cough reflex. In addition, direct chest trauma might be complicated by lung contusion. The presence of edema and blood in the lung parenchyma represents a perfect growth medium for pathogenic bacteria. The role of the respiratory therapist is crucial in the prevention of potentially life-threatening respiratory complications. There are four interventions on which the respiratory therapist should focus (Box 30-1):

1. *Mobilization.* The patient should be assisted in changing positions periodically to help with mucus drainage and prevention of atelectasis. If tolerated, patient should be helped to move out of bed and to spend some time in a chair.[11]
2. *Humidification of the airways.* Regardless of mechanical ventilation, bedridden patients should receive optimal humidification of the airways to prevent the accumulation of dry secretions.

Box 30-1 Basic Respiratory Interventions in the Bedridden Trauma Patients

- Mobilization
- Humidification
- Pain control
- Incentive spirometry
- Noninvasive continuous positive airway pressure and bilevel positive airway pressure

3. *Pain control.* Control of pain in the trauma patient is one of the most challenging tasks of the critical care team. Inadequate pain control generally results in minimal chest expansion as a reflex response to minimize pain associated with breathing. Excessive use of pain medications (i.e., opioids) also will decrease chest expansion and cough reflex because of sedative effects. Both scenarios exacerbates the pathophysiologic sequence of events described earlier, leading to pneumonia.[12]
4. *Incentive spirometry and noninvasive ventilation (NIV).* Patients should be encouraged as soon as possible to take advantage of incentive spirometry. Incentive spirometry consists of regular breathing exercises performed with the aid of a dedicated device. Regular exercise has shown this prevents formation of atelectasis and reduces secretion retention. The use of such devices requires the full collaboration and dedication of the patient. Secretions clearance can be aided by gentle external chest percussion (i.e., chest physiotherapy), avoiding sites of injury, if tolerated. Should these interventions fail, the respiratory therapist should consider the use of intermittent NIV (CPAP or bilevel positive airway pressure) to reexpand the residual volume and assist tidal ventilation. Recruitment maneuvers should be carefully performed in patients with chest trauma. The presence of silent lesions could cause hypertensive pneumothorax under elevated airways pressures.[13]

Respiratory Management

Every trauma patient represents a case by itself, and the respiratory management of trauma patients should focus on the mechanism of chest injury. Supplemental oxygen is generally administered immediately after the trauma to prevent secondary hypoxic injury. However, any sign of pending respiratory failure should prompt endotracheal intubation and initiation of mechanical ventilation (Box 30-2). Upper airway disruption might require emergent tracheostomy. Advanced airways management such as a double-lumen endotracheal tube (ETT) may be required for injury of the trachea or for selective lung ventilation for bronchial injuries. Injury to the lung parenchyma always should be suspected after major trauma. Extensive lung injury frequently evolves into traumatic ARDS requiring protective lung ventilation strategies (see Chapters 29 and 52). In addition, trauma patients are at higher risk for developing lung injury resulting from the large volume of blood components that these patients may require (i.e., transfusion-related lung injury and/or transfusion-associated circulatory overload).

Box 30-2 Mechanical Ventilation of the Trauma Patient

- Mode: Pressure or volume ventilation
- Tidal volume: 6 to 8 ml/kg predicted body weight
- Inspiratory time 0.6 to 1.0 second
- Plateau pressure: Less than 28 cm H_2O
- Driving pressure of 15 cm H_2O or less
- Rate only limited by the development of auto-PEEP
- Minute volume to maintain normal $PaCO_2$
- PEEP 5 to 10 cm H_2O
- FiO_2 set to maintain target PaO_2
- If ARDS, manage as any other ARDS patient

Bronchoscopy plays a major role in the respiratory care of trauma patients. It first allows removal of foreign bodies and drainage of blood clots and provides an excellent method for removal of tenacious mucus plugs. Moreover, it is the gold standard for diagnosis of proximal and distal major airway lesions and is capable of providing a first-line treatment. Trauma patients are at high risk for VAP, and preventive clinical bundles should be applied as soon as possible (see Chapter 24). Recent reports outlined beneficial effects of these bundles (i.e., decreased sedation, early mobilization, and improved secretion clearance) compared to early tracheostomy for patients requiring prolonged mechanical ventilation. However, it is still difficult to predict the time for weaning from mechanical ventilation. A number of factors play a role in liberation from mechanical ventilation, such as neurologic status, muscular strength, adequate pain management, proper healing of major injury, and hemodynamic instability.

OBESITY

Epidemiology

Obesity is defined by an excess of weight in relation to a person's height. It is mainly measured through the body mass index (BMI), which is the ratio of an individual's weight (kg) divided by the square of the individual's height (m):

$$BMI = (weight)/(height)^2 = kg/m^2$$

A normal BMI range for a healthy individual is between 20 and 25 kg/m^2, and a BMI over 30 kg/m^2 is defined as obesity. Among the different excesses of BMI, a BMI greater than 40 kg/m^2 is defined as **severe obesity**, a BMI greater than 45 kg/m^2 is defined as **morbid obesity**, and a BMI greater than 50 kg/m^2 is defined as **super obesity**. In the last decade, the prevalence of obesity progressively has increased in the U.S. population, reaching a plateau of almost a third of the total population. There are differences in obesity prevalence among different ethnic groups, with non-Hispanic Asians having a lower prevalence compared to non-Hispanic whites, non-Hispanic African Americans, and Hispanic groups. Obesity is connected to a plethora of adverse health conditions and imposes considerable burdens on the U.S. health care system.

MINI CLINI

Trauma: Recognizing Common Life-Threatening Acute Respiratory Complications in Trauma Patients

PROBLEM: A water-skier was sent by medical flight to the hospital after collision with a boat following a 30-feet acrobatic jump. The unknown young man was intubated with a 7.0-mm ETT at the scene for hypoxemia and GCS 6 with no lower limb movements. Vital signs at admission in the ED were heart rate 40 beats/min, blood pressure 80/40 mm Hg, O_2 saturation 99%, and body temperature 35° C. He weighs 160 lb and is 6 ft tall. The ventilator settings are as follows: volume-controlled ventilation mode, tidal volume (V_T) 500 ml, respiratory rate 14 breaths/min, and positive end expiratory pressure (PEEP) 5 cm H_2O. During central line placement, the RT notices that the peak airway pressure increased from 18 cm H_2O to 35 cm H_2O, activating the high pressure alarm, and SaO_2 declined rapidly from 99% to 90%. What are the next steps the RT should take?

SOLUTIONS:
1. Immediately inform the medical team regarding the alarming acute increased peak pressure and decreased SaO_2.
2. Verify that the ETT did not migrate into the right main stem bronchus during neck positioning for central line placement by confirming tube positioning.
3. Pass a suctioning catheter to verify absence of ETT kinking or occlusion resulting from secretions or blood.
4. Visually inspect that the inspiratory and expiratory ventilator circuit is not kinked and that the water trap is not filled.
5. Auscultate breath sounds on all lung fields and inspect tracheal deviation or asymmetry in chest movements during ventilation. Tension pneumothorax should be suspected when breath sounds are absent on the affected part of the thorax and the trachea deviates away from the affected side. The thorax may also be hyperresonant with jugular venous distention. Increased intrathoracic pressure might cause hypotensive and hypoxemia. If not recognized, tension pneumothorax leads to cardiovascular collapse and death.
6. Immediate chest radiograph and arterial blood gas (ABG) analysis should be requested to confirm hypoxemia and rule out acute changes (i.e., pneumothorax, acute pleural effusion, hemothorax, bronchial mucus plug causing large lobar or entire lung collapse).
7. Until a pneumothorax is ruled out, V_T should be decreased and respiratory rate increased ideally by use of a manual ventilator. This is to ensure that limited pressure is applied to minimize the volume of gas extending the possible pneumothorax.
8. Regardless of the final diagnosis, the respiratory therapist has a key role in the care of the trauma patient in the acute settings. Common tasks of the RT are titration of the ventilator after acute changes in the patient's condition, travel to a computed tomography (CT) scan or other emergent hospital location (i.e., operating room or ICU), and assistance with procedures such as bronchoscopy, chest tube placements, or intracranial pressure monitoring.

Obesity is associated with increased morbidity and mortality in the context of both acute and chronic medical problems, including diabetes mellitus and related complications, hypertension, dyslipidemia, cardiovascular disease, gallstones, cholecystitis, and certain forms of cancer. Although there is now a considerable amount of data available on the impact of obesity on ICU outcomes, there are still contradictory conclusions concerning the nature of this impact, possibly because obese ICU patients on average are younger and are affected with less severe diseases compared to nonobese ICU patients; however, obese ICU patients require the same level of intensive care.

Among people with a BMI within the range of severe obesity, the distribution of adipose tissue plays a major role in determining the risks for chronic diseases. Current guidelines concerned with the clinical care of the obese recommend measurement of waist circumference in people with a BMI greater than 25 kg/m^2 and propose that waist circumferences of 102 cm in men and 88 cm in women define abdominal adiposity. Most studies examining the association between fat distribution and mortality have shown that abdominal adiposity is an important predictor of mortality. In particular, waist circumference has been associated with mortality even in people with a normal BMI, indicating that BMI might be of limited use in assessing the severity of a person's obesity and that fat tissue distribution plays a major role in the pathophysiology of obesity.[14]

RULE OF THUMB

Patients who are obese have a greater likelihood of mortality in the ICU if their waist circumstance is greater 102 cm in men and 88 cm in women.

Specific Pathophysiologic Concerns

Adipose tissue is a potent source of proinflammatory molecules that induce a chronic inflammatory state mimicking critical illness and diminishing immune and metabolic reserves (Box 30-3). Moreover, an increased BMI requires additional cardiovascular, respiratory, and metabolic work, further diminishing an individual's physiologic reserves.[15]

Obesity is a risk factor for cardiovascular disease independent of diabetes mellitus and hypertension. The mechanism of obesity-related cardiovascular disease involves an increase in both preload and afterload. Adipose tissue is perfused on average by 3 ml of blood per each 100 g of tissue. The resulting expansion of blood volume increases venous return (preload), cardiac output, and cardiac work. Afterload is increased by secretion of steroids and catecholamines and through the renin-angiotensin endocrine axis. Myocardial hypertrophy and diastolic dysfunction are the results of these alterations, eventually leading to heart failure, arrhythmias, or sudden cardiac arrest. Myocardial hypertrophy and the consequently reduced heart-wall compliance, as well as reduced heart chamber volumes, are responsible for poor tolerance of intravenous fluids in these patients. Additionally, the presence of diabetes mellitus and hypertension in this setting exponentially increases the risk for myocardial infarction. Moreover, the presence of diabetes mellitus increases the risk for a silent myocardial infarction being present at the time of admission or happening as a complication of critical illness. This risk is especially pertinent to the extreme range of obese patients, whose physical activity is very limited and who may not manifest symptoms of myocardial ischemia or show signs of congestive heart failure before ICU admission.

Box 30-3 Physiologic Concerns Associated With Obesity

- Cardiovascular disease
- Venous thrombosis and pulmonary embolism
- Chronic renal failure
- Obstructive sleep apnea
- Obesity hypoventilation syndrome
- Reduced lung volumes
- Expiratory flow resistance
- Air-trapping and auto-PEEP

The presence of a proinflammatory/procoagulatory state induced by adipose tissue and associated with a sedentary lifestyle and venous stasis puts these patients at high risk for venous thrombosis and pulmonary embolism. The increased cardiac output of obese patients is responsible for an increased glomerular filtration rate in patients whose obesity-related complications have not yet compromised kidney function. However, diabetes mellitus and hypertension can be responsible for chronic kidney failure. Thus an evaluation of kidney function is mandatory in this patient population. Abnormal glomerular filtration and excess adipose tissue alter the clearance and the volume distribution of most drugs that are administered to obese patents.

Dosing of **lipophilic drugs** should be based on the actual body weight of the patient, whereas for **hydrophilic drugs** dosage is best determined using the ideal body weight (IBW) or predicted body weight (PBW) of the patient and corrected for higher renal clearance if an abnormally high **glomerular filtration rate** is present. Because of altered clearance, distribution, and accumulation of drugs, obese patients are particularly prone to underdosage and overdosage of hypnotic medications. Because most of these drugs are lipophilic, allowing them to cross the blood-brain barrier, the accumulation of drugs in excess adipose tissue can occur and result in a slowed release into the bloodstream. Frequent spontaneous awakening trials are necessary to assess the accumulation of drugs in the adipose tissue and to determine the ability of the patient to promptly recover from sedation to avoid delaying liberation from mechanical ventilation.[16]

RULE OF THUMB

Over two-thirds of obese patients have sleep apnea. All obese patients on admission should be evaluated for sleep apnea if not already being treated for it.

More than two-thirds of obese people have **obstructive sleep apnea** (OSA). However, the factors that lead to a higher incidence of OSA in obese patients are still poorly understood. It has been argued that obesity can act in different ways on the respiratory system, that it narrows the upper airway, causes upper airway collapsibility, and disrupts the normal physiologic respiratory drive. Specifically, it has been shown that obesity is associated with the deposition of peripharyngeal fat, which may increase pharyngeal collapsibility. In addition to this, it has been shown that the proinflammatory state associated with obesity alters the pharyngeal-patency control mechanisms, resulting in additional airway occlusion. Neuromuscular control of pharyngeal patency is of the utmost importance in these patients. Any increase in a proinflammatory state or loss of active neuromuscular control (e.g., because of a neurologic condition or sedation) further aggravates upper airway occlusion.

Lung volumes progressively decrease as BMI increases. Total lung capacity and residual volume decrease linearly as BMI increases, while functional residual capacity is exponentially reduced at higher BMI values, especially in patients with a central fat distribution (high waist circumference). Furthermore, forced vital capacity, forced expiratory volume in 1 second, maximum voluntary ventilation and forced mid-expiratory flow are significantly reduced in obese persons, with airway closure occurring during tidal breathing in the extreme range of obesity. Low functional residual capacity increases the risk for expiratory flow limitation and airway closure. This is thought to be due to an increase in pleural pressure caused by the transmission of the gravitational weight of the abdomen. The weight of the abdomen displaces the diaphragm in a cephalad position, causing passive atelectasis in the most gravity-dependent regions of the lung. The collapsed lung tissue exerts less elastic recoil on adjacent structures, particularly on the smaller airways, reducing their diameter. The increase in pleural pressure further aggravates airway collapse. The ensuing expiratory flow limitation can lead to incomplete exhalation with air trapping, resulting in dynamic hyperinflation. Dynamic hyperinflation (auto-PEEP) is one of the most common sources of increased work of breathing and patient-ventilator asynchrony in mechanically ventilated patients.

Trapped end-expiratory gas causes auto-PEEP. This trapping of gas behind collapsed airways acts as a recoil pressure that needs to be released at the beginning of inspiration before the generation of a V_T, resulting in wasted work of breathing.[17,18] It has been observed that the sitting position can increase functional residual capacity, reverse expiratory flow limitation, improve respiratory mechanics and gas exchange, and lower the PEEP required to restore functional residual capacity to a normal physiologic level—another indication of the pathophysiologic role of abdominal weight in obesity.[19] The presence of expiratory flow limitation and atelectasis in the dependent zones of the lung is pivotal in the development of ventilation/perfusion ($\dot{V}/\dot{Q}$) mismatch and hypoxemia. To supplement the increased rates of O_2 consumption and carbon dioxide (CO_2) production in the setting of impaired gas exchange, obese patients increase their respiratory drive and minute ventilation, maintaining adequate alveolar ventilation at the expense of higher dead space ventilation. However, the most severely obese patients acquire a reduced chemosensitivity, impairing their ventilatory response to hypoxemia and hypercapnia (**obesity hypoventilation syndrome** [OHS]). These patients tend to slowly progress to hypoventilation with hypercapnic respiratory failure. It has been shown that noninvasive nocturnal ventilation is effective in restoring a more normal physiologic chemosensitivity and compensatory respiratory drive.[20]

RULE OF THUMB

The majority of patients with severe obesity develop flow limitation, air trapping, and auto-PEEP, especially when ventilated in the supine position.

Clinical Assessment

Given an unstable respiratory/cardiovascular equilibrium, obese patients are particularly prone to acute respiratory failure in the setting of disease. Particular attention must be paid to gas exchange and signs of increased work of breathing (labored breathing, high respiratory rates, use of accessory muscles), because any deterioration in their clinical status can quickly precipitate respiratory failure requiring mechanical ventilation.

BMI, body fat distribution, and history of snoring, sleepiness, and headaches should be determined or collected on admission. The degree of self-mobilization and physical daily activity should be investigated, and the risk for deep venous thrombosis or pulmonary embolism should be assessed. A plan for airway management and intubation should be discussed before the onset of respiratory failure, especially if the patient shows signs of a particularly difficult airway for intubation. The past use of, and settings for, home nocturnal CPAP or NIV should be investigated, and their continued use should be encouraged. In the presence of a history suggestive of OSA/OHS, intermittent/nocturnal noninvasive bilevel positive airway pressure/CPAP should be started regardless of the patient's respiratory status.

Respiratory Management

See Box 30-4.

Box 30-4 Respiratory Management of Obesity

- Oxygen therapy for management of hypoxemia
- Inhalational bronchodilators for management of asthma symptoms
- Noninvasive CPAP for management of sleep apnea
- NIV for obesity hypoventilation syndrome and hypercarbic respiratory failure
- Invasive mechanical ventilation for management of hypoxemic and hypercarbic respiratory unresponsive to NIV

CPAP, Continuous positive expiratory pressure; *NIV,* noninvasive ventilation.

Oxygen Therapy

Hypoxemia is the most common gas-exchange abnormality in obese patients. It can be mild and easily corrected by O_2 supplementation, or it can be severe enough to require mechanical ventilation. However, a mild, progressive hypoxemia should prompt close monitoring of gas exchange, work of breathing, and mental status, because it might be a sign of impending respiratory failure. A sudden onset of hypoxemic respiratory failure should raise the suspicion for pulmonary embolism. If the patient's response to O_2 supplementation is inadequate but the patient has sufficient mental status, NIV should be initiated.

Aerosolized Pharmacology

Obese patients have a higher incidence and severity of asthma, and they frequently require inhalation therapy. For a detailed discussion, see Chapter 35.

Noninvasive Ventilation

NIV should be attempted when the patient's neurologic status is sufficient but O_2 therapy alone is ineffective at correcting hypoxemia or when hypercapnia complicates the respiratory failure. By the time NIV is attempted, a plan for airway management and intubation already should have been made. NIV should be instituted immediately in the setting of hypercapnic respiratory failure. If qualified staff is available, noninvasive mechanical ventilation can be set up and begun in EDs or respiratory wards. An alert and cooperative mental status, proper mask-fitting, ability to clear secretions, and relative hemodynamic stability are essential factors that contribute to the success of NIV. Pressure-support ventilation with adequate PEEP is the preferred mode of ventilation. Vital signs, level of consciousness, respiratory pattern, oxygenation, delivered V_T, gas exchange, and circuit leaks should be frequently assessed to guarantee proper ventilatory therapy.[21]

Approach to Noninvasive Ventilation

The approach to noninvasive ventilation is as follows.

1. Explain the indications of NIV and the possible outcomes (requirement of intubation or prolonged use of NIV) to the patient. Explain to the patient that he or she is not allowed to drink or eat anything by mouth until able to avoid the risk for aspiration during NIV.
2. Perform an ABG analysis to assess baseline gas exchange.
3. Fit the mask appropriately. If more than one model is available, quickly check with the patient which one is most comfortable.
4. Suggested initial settings are 10 cm H_2O of pressure support and 10 cm H_2O of PEEP.
5. Monitor vital signs, gas exchange, respiratory rate, V_T, and comfort of the patient.
6. Gradually increase PEEP in 2–cm H_2O increments to improve airway patency and oxygenation ($SpO_2 > 90\%$). Check hemodynamics carefully.
7. Gradually increase pressure support in 2–cm H_2O increments to improve V_T (until 6 to 8 ml/kg of IBW), reduce the respiratory rate (<25 breaths/min), reduce ventilatory distress, and improve CO_2 clearance.
8. Check gas exchange at 60 minutes. If noticeable improvement has been observed and there is no clinical deterioration, NIV can be continued. If NIV did not improve oxygenation or hypercapnia, the patient should be intubated and mechanically ventilated.

> **RULE OF THUMB**
>
> If the first hour of NIV does not at least partially correct the patient's clinical presentation, hypoxemia, and hypercarbia, endotracheal intubation should be immediately considered.

Invasive Mechanical Ventilation

Intubation. Airway management in obese patients can be challenging because of the anatomic and physiologic alterations described earlier that make this population prone to airway obstruction and severe hypoxemia. BMI is a predictor of mask ventilation difficulties because of reduced upper airway space, difficulty fitting the mask, increased pressure required for V_T generation, and reduced diaphragmatic excursion. Intubation is difficult as well; however, BMI is not an effective predictor of intubation difficulty, but neck circumference above 40 cm is associated with difficult intubation. There is no common agreement on which approach to intubation should be used in obese patients. A possible strategy is awake intubation through the use of fiberoptics, although this technique requires coordination, proper anesthesia of the upper airways, and complete collaboration of the patient, with this final factor being particularly important for success, although particularly difficult in the critically ill obese patient. The advent of video-laryngoscopy has significantly reduced the amount of difficulty clinicians face in airway management, and the use of a video-laryngoscope should be strongly considered in any intubation plan for the critically ill obese patient. A kit for rapid airway access should be present at the bedside or within reach until the airway is secured. Regardless of the device or technique adopted—which should be based on patient evaluation and personal expertise—optimal positioning is mandatory to increase the chance of securing the airways. The "ramped position" consists of elevating the upper body and head of the patient to align the sternum and ear horizontally. This positioning technique results in a significantly improved laryngoscopic view. In addition, the elevated head of bed positioning typical of the ramped position improves respiratory mechanics and lung volumes during preoxygenation, increasing the time to desaturation. The use of CPAP during preoxygenation can additionally increase the nonhypoxemic apnea time by 50%.

Tidal Volume, Minute Volume, and Respiratory Rate. Pressure control ventilation or volume control ventilation can be equally effectively used to mechanically ventilate the obese patient (Box 30-5). However, regardless of mode of ventilation, V_T settings *must not be calculated* based on actual body weight,

Box 30-5 Mechanical Ventilation of the Obese Patient

- Mode: Pressure or volume ventilation
- Tidal volume: Average 6 ml/kg PBW, range 4 to 8 ml/kg PBW
- Inspiratory time 0.6 to 1.0 second
- Plateau pressure: Less than 28 cm H_2O, unless TPP measured then TPP less than 20 cm H_2O
- Driving pressure equal to or less than 15 cm H_2O
- Rate only limited by the development of auto-PEEP
- Minute volume generally 10 L/min or greater
- Lung recruitment maneuver with decremental PEEP trial to set PEEP
- FiO_2 set to maintain target PaO_2
- Position head of the bed to 30 degrees or greater elevation
- Noninvasive ventilation for 24 to 48 hours after extubation

PBW, predicted body weight; *TTP*, transpulmonary pressure.

but on PBW or IBW, because an increased BMI does not reflect increased lung size. The best current evidence and practice stresses the importance of lung protective ventilation with a V_T target of 6 ml/kg PBW (range, 4 to 8 ml/kg PBW) in all critically ill patients. There are different equations and formulas to calculate the predicted or IBW, and there could be significant differences in the calculations. The most widely recommended formulas are listed below. These are the formulas used by the NIH/NHLBI ARDS Network in their landmark study:

$$PBW_{MEN} = 50.0 + 0.905^{*}([\text{Height in cm}] - 152.4)$$
$$PBW_{WOMEN} = 45.5 + 0.905^{*}([\text{Height in cm}] - 152.4)$$

Minute ventilation and respiratory rate should be adjusted to ensure an adequate clearance of CO_2. Because of the increased metabolic rate, minute ventilation is commonly greater than 10 L/min. In assisted partial ventilatory support, respiratory rate and volumes should be carefully monitored, especially in the setting of OHS, as central desensitization to CO_2 might result in depressed respiratory drive in the setting of normal oxygenation. It is reasonable in this context to have a lower oxygenation target (SpO_2 88% to 92%).

RULE OF THUMB

V_T in obese patients always should be determined based on PBW, *not* actual body weight because lung size is not based on weight, it is based on height and gender.

Lung Recruitment. It has been demonstrated in intraoperative settings that **recruitment maneuvers** in obese, mechanically ventilated patients are effective at improving respiratory system compliance and oxygenation without affecting hemodynamics. This effect is due to the reversal of atelectasis that forms during induction and persists without adequate levels of PEEP during mechanical ventilation. It is advisable to perform a recruitment maneuver whenever PEEP is increased or after temporary PEEP discontinuation (e.g., disconnection of the patient from the ventilator circuit in the setting of high PEEP).[22] A recruitment maneuver during volume or pressure control ventilation can be performed as follows:

1. Assess hemodynamic stability of the patient.
2. Switch to pressure control ventilation with the following settings:
   Pressure control: +15 cm H_2O
   PEEP: +10 cm H_2O
   Respiratory rate: 10 breaths/min
   I/E ratio: 1 : 1
3. If patient is stable, after 30 seconds increase PEEP by 5 cm H_2O (PEEP: +15 cm H_2O).
4. Check oxygenation and hemodynamics.
5. If patient is stable, after 30 seconds increase PEEP by 5 cm H_2O (PEEP: +20 cm H_2O).
6. Check oxygenation and hemodynamics.
7. If patient is stable, after 30 seconds increase PEEP by 5 cm H_2O (PEEP: +25 cm H_2O).
8. Check oxygenation and hemodynamics.
9. Switch to volume control and perform a **decremental PEEP trial**. Set ventilator setting similar to that before recruitment maneuvers (RM) but keep PEEP at 25 cm H_2O and FiO_2 at 1.0. Measure total respiratory system compliance (Crs) after 3 to 5 minutes.
10. Decrease PEEP to 21 cm H_2O after 3 to 5 minutes and measure Crs.
11. Decrease PEEP to 19 cm H_2O after 3 to 5 minutes and measure Crs.
12. Decrease PEEP to 17 cm H_2O after 3 to 5 minutes and measure Crs.
13. Continue this process until the best Crs PEEP can be identified.
14. Recruit the lung again and then set PEEP at the best Crs PEEP plus 2 cm H_2O.
15. Decrease the FiO_2 to the lowest level maintaining PaO_2 in the target range.

This approach to setting PEEP works well in morbidly obese patients and results in improved lung mechanics compared to the routine use of 8 to 12 cm H_2O PEEP in these patients. In patients with less severe obesity PEEP in the range of 10 to 15 cm H_2O generally stabilizes the lung and avoids atelectasis.[23]

Positioning. It has been shown that elevation of the head of the bed is effective at improving respiratory system compliance and oxygenation, reducing expiratory flow limitation, and reducing PEEP requirements for optimal ventilation in obese patients. This phenomenon is related to the gravitational effects of the abdomen on the diaphragm. When obese patients lie in the supine position, the abdominal content pushes against the diaphragm and displaces it in a cranial direction, resulting in increased pleural pressure and passive atelectasis in the dependent zones of the lung (see the section on pathophysiology). The adoption of a sitting position changes the vector of the gravitational forces of the abdomen, partially releasing the diaphragm from abdominal pressure. Changes in bed position in morbidly obese patients (e.g., from sitting to supine, and back to sitting) should be followed by a recruitment maneuver in order to reexpand the regions of the lungs that collapsed during the transient increase in pleural pressure. In general, unless contraindicated, obese patients should be managed with the head of the bed elevated above 30 degrees.

RULE OF THUMB

FiO_2 and pressure support level should always be weaned before PEEP level is decreased. When FiO_2 is approximately 0.40 and pressure support is 10 cm H_2O or less, PEEP can be decreased.

Ventilator Discontinuation. One of the most challenging aspects of ventilatory management of obese patients is liberation from mechanical ventilation. Expiratory flow limitation, low respiratory system compliance, atelectasis, and impaired neurologic respiratory drive play an important role in determining increased work of breathing in morbidly obese patients. As critical illness resolves, catabolic muscular wasting and post–critical illness muscular weakness aggravate the patient's respiratory condition. There is still no consensus or scientific data on what might be the best approach for ventilatory weaning in these patients. Requiring a longer time on mechanical ventilation and more prone to fail liberation from mechanical ventilation, these patients more often require tracheostomy and transfer to long-term respiratory care facilities. However, it has been shown that morbidly obese patients who undergo tracheostomy have a higher morbidity and mortality and are more prone to tracheostomy-related complications. As the beneficial effects of PEEP and positioning in this population become more clear, especially in partially reversing the phenomena that lead to increased work of breathing, it is advisable that PEEP should be carefully reduced only after the FiO_2 has stabilized at approximately 0.40. In addition, it is preferable to gradually reduce the level of pressure support while keeping the PEEP level stable, and eventually test a careful reduction of PEEP down to 8 to 10 cm H_2O, if feasible. It would be best to extubate these patients while they are on PEEP and start noninvasive CPAP or bilevel positive airway pressure immediately after extubation. Noninvasive mechanical ventilation then can be gradually adjusted and weaned in the following 48 to 72 hours.

MINI CLINI

Obesity: The Role of Postoperative Noninvasive Ventilation

PROBLEM: A 550-lb patient is recovering in the postoperative care unit after a laparoscopic cholecystectomy. The procedure was uneventful. The nurse called you because the SpO_2 decreased from 95% to 88% over the past hour despite a nonrebreather facemask at 12 L/min. You see the patient; she is calm, resting in no pain, and breathing regularly at 8 breaths/min. Other vital signs are heart rate 66 beats/min, blood pressure 128/70 mm Hg and body temperature 36.5° C. After reviewing the nursing notes, you notice that patient required 4 mg of midazolam before surgery for anxiety, 4 mg of hydromorphone during surgery, and additionally 10 mg of morphine in the recovery room.

SOLUTIONS: Inform the medical/surgical team of the increased hypoxemia in this high-risk obese postsurgical patient. Suggest the medical/surgical team perform an ABG analysis to confirm hypoxemia and determine PCO_2 to rule out pharmacologic narcosis and request a chest radiograph to rule out postoperative atelectasis. In agreement with the medical/surgical team, this patient should receive NIV and be monitored for 24 hours by telemetry.

In this patient, NIV instead of CPAP is required because not only is there most likely marked atelectasis but this patient's ventilatory drive has been depressed by sedatives and narcotics, requiring ventilatory support. NIV may be required for only 24 hours, but considering the size of the patient and the likelihood that the patient has sleep apnea, the use of CPAP during sleep should be considered on an ongoing basis and the patient evaluated for sleep apnea once recovered from the acute episode.

NEAR DROWNING

Epidemiology

Drowning is one of the major causes of accidental pediatric death and is more common in low-income and middle-income countries. In adults, drowning is generally associated with alcohol and drug abuse. From 2005 to 2009 in the United States, there were approximately 4000 deaths resulting from drowning, of which almost 1000 were children younger than 14 years of age. It has been calculated that for each drowning casualty there are at least five times as many near-drowning–related admissions to EDs, of which half require hospitalization.

The essential feature of drowning and the primary cause of death is asphyxia leading to cardiopulmonary collapse. Permanent injuries include a spectrum of brain damage, starting with minor memory problems, to severe learning disabilities, including a permanent vegetative state.[24-26]

Specific Pathophysiologic Concerns

The pathophysiologic mechanisms of drowning comprise the following two reflexes:

1. Inhalation of fluid causes irritation and cough response, resulting in fluid being either swallowed or inhaled. Laryngospasm with closure of the glottis prevents aspiration of large amounts of fluid in the lungs (**"dry drowning"**), diverting these fluids to the stomach. Generally, the laryngospasm lessens with unconsciousness, leading to **"wet drowning"**—the aspiration of fluid, which is a more common occurrence.
2. **Cold shock cardiac-respiratory reflexes** occur with sudden immersion in water cooler than 25° C. The breathing pattern is characterized by gasping followed by hyperventilation and

shallow breathing at almost total lung capacity. At lower water temperatures, sudden peripheral vasoconstriction can acutely increase systemic vascular resistance, leading to sudden cardiovascular collapse if the heart is unable to overcome the acute increase in preload and afterload.[27]

During "wet drowning," specific respiratory and blood chemistry dysfunction depend on whether fresh or seawater has been inhaled.

1. Inhalation of fresh water.[28]
    a. *Inhalation of fresh water and its effects on the respiratory system.* Inhalation of fresh water rapidly depletes alveolar surfactant, leading to $\dot{V}/\dot{Q}$ mismatch. Inhaled water is quickly absorbed into the vascular system from the alveolar space by osmosis, causing alveolar collapse and worsening shunt and hypoxia. Additionally, in the setting of inhaled fresh water, acute neurogenic pulmonary edema secondary to cerebral hypoxia has been shown to worsen alveolar flooding. However, if hypoxia is reversed, normal pulmonary function can be quickly restored.
    b. *The effects of inhalation of fresh water on other organs.* If a large volume of fresh water is inhaled, it is rapidly absorbed into the circulation, leading to electrolyte imbalance. Hyponatremia can lead to seizures, especially in pediatric patients. Additionally, diluted plasma causes water to rapidly enter into erythrocytes by osmosis, causing hemolysis. The resulting hyperkalemia and hyponatremia can cause ventricular fibrillation, and the liberation of hemoglobin into the plasma can precipitate acute renal failure.
2. Inhalation of salt water.[29]
    a. *Inhalation of salt water and its effects on the respiratory system.* Seawater has a three-fold higher osmolarity than blood. Hypertonic fluid inhalation therefore causes water to move from the circulation into the lungs. In experimental studies in animals, inhaled seawater accounted for less than 50% of the volume of water retrieved from the lungs at autopsy. In contrast with the inhalation of fresh water, this phenomenon explains the sustained edema and prolonged shunt after the inhalation of salt water. Additionally, salt water causes direct damage to the alveolar-capillary membrane, enhancing lung injury.
    b. *The effects of inhalation of salt water on other organs.* If a large volume of salt water is inhaled, the rapid loss of circulating volume into the alveolar space across the injured alveolar capillary membrane may cause hemoconcentration, hypernatremia, and hypoalbuminemia. This phenomenon, if not recognized and rapidly reversed, leads to vascular collapse and hypovolemic shock.

Despite the pathophysiologic differences and the obvious circumstantial differences between drowning in salt water versus fresh water, at autopsy a definitive diagnosis cannot be made.[30-32]

Respiratory Management

Immediate management of patients who present with drowning or near-drowning events must follow the classic airway-breathing-circulation approach, and cardiopulmonary resuscitation should be started immediately, if needed (Box 30-6). If possible, prone positioning of the patient is preferable, because it allows optimal clearance of water from the tracheobronchial tree, especially in the case of salt water drowning. Temperature monitoring and active body temperature control should be initiated as soon as possible because submersion and inhalation of water drastically reduces body temperature.

Box 30-6 Respiratory Management of Near Drowning

- Basic cardiopulmonary
- Airway clearance
    - Bronchoscopy
    - Lavage
    - Prone positioning
- Mechanical ventilation as in all ARDS patients

RULE OF THUMB

Near-drowning victims almost always develop ARDS and should be managed from a mechanical ventilation perspective like any other ARDS patient.

Airway Clearance Therapy

The aspiration of foreign matter occurs relatively commonly in drowning or near-drowning events, particularly events involving drowning in shallow water. The most common aspirated material is sand, mud, or dirt. This can be easily recognized if solid material is found in the upper airways or in the stomach. It has been reported that a CT scan can show distinct hyperdense "sand bronchograms" in cases of sand aspiration. The inhalation of foreign material in the setting of drowning or near drowning is particularly harmful, because the material is usually solid, is nonsoluble, has a high density, and tends to consolidate and clog distal airways. This further worsens the onset of ARDS that follows drowning by enhancing the inflammatory response and by mechanically sealing the airways. Upper airway clearance should be performed as soon as possible. Foreign material in the distal airways can be washed after intubation through repeated bronchoscopy and bronchoalveolar lavages.[33,34]

Mechanical Ventilation

Almost every patients who experiences drowning or near-drowning events will develop ARDS. Ventilatory management of these patients should follow ARDS ventilation guidelines as outlined in Chapter 27 and 48 (Box 30-7). Frequently, these patients develop bronchospasm as a result of the irritant effects of water in the airways. Laryngospasm and persistent upper airway closure are usually resolved on the administration of paralysis at intubation, but severe bronchospasm might persist, requiring antibronchospasm inhalatory or intravenous therapy (see Chapter 35). Drowning in **fluvial or brackish water** or

Box 30-7 Mechanical Ventilation of the Near-Drowning Patient

- Mode: Pressure or volume ventilation
- Tidal volume: Average 6 to 8 ml/kg PBW
- Inspiratory time 0.6 to 1.0 sec
- Plateau pressure: less than 28 cm H_2O
- Driving pressure equal to or less than 15 cm H_2O
- Rate only limited by the development of auto-PEEP
- Minute volume to maintain $PaCO_2$
- PEEP 5 to 10 cm H_2O
- FiO_2 set to maintain target PaO_2
- Prone position
- If ARDS, manage as normal for ARDS patients

seawater is usually complicated by pneumonia caused by opportunistic pathogens inhaled at the moment of drowning. However, these bacteria usually do not show antibiotic resistance and prompt antibiotic prophylaxis should be able to prevent pneumonia.

Positioning

Whenever feasible, prone positioning is preferable immediately after cardiovascular stabilization, especially in the case of brackish water or saltwater drowning, in which the osmotic activity of the inhaled salt causes continuous refilling of the lungs with water. The prone position allows clearance of salt-containing fluids from the lungs and might prove useful in the setting of severe ARDS.

RULE OF THUMB

Once stabilized, salt-water near-drowning victims generally benefit from prone positioning, which allows better clearance of inhaled fluids from the lungs.

BURNS

Epidemiology

In the United States, each year approximately 450,000 people receive medical treatment for burn injuries; of these patients, 40,000 are hospitalized. Over 60% of the estimated U.S. acute hospitalizations related to burn injury were admitted to 127 burn centers. Each year 3400 patients die as a result of burn and smoke inhalation. In a selected case series from 2003 to 2012 the reason for admission was 43% fire, 34% scald, 9% contact, 4% electrical, 3% chemical, and 7% other burn injuries.[35] The main feature characterizing the natural history of serious burns is burn shock. Burn shock can lead to death within the first hours after injury. The most important cause of mortality, among those who survive burn shock is wound sepsis (Box 30-8). After recovery from the acute inflammatory phase, postburn deformities delay full functional recovery. Improved survival has been associated with early resuscitation, prevention of postburn sepsis, aggressive surgical treatment, improved perioperative care, and the development of multidisciplinary treatment teams. The first phase of the care of patients with serious burn injury is challenging in both respiratory care and hemodynamic management. Intensivists and respiratory therapists during the initial management period must work cooperatively in the management of these critically ill patients.[36]

Box 30-8 Survival in Burn Patients

Survival in burn patients has been associated with:

- Early fluid resuscitation
- Prevention of post burn sepsis
- Aggressive surgical treatment
- Improved perioperative care
- Development of multidisciplinary teams

MINI CLINI

Near Drowning: Recognizing Life-Threatening Acute Respiratory Complications

PROBLEM: An unresponsive 3-year-old boy is brought into the ED by his parents after he was rescued from their swimming pool. The parents were hosting a midsummer barbecue when they heard screaming kids and found their son face-down in the swimming pool. Vital signs at admission to the ED were heart rate 40 beats/min, blood pressure 50/20 mm Hg, $SatO_2$ 88%, and body temperature 33° C. What are the next steps and how should the RT respond?

SOLUTIONS: This is an emergency, and the team should be prepared for impending cardiac arrest because of near drowning. Advance Cardiac Life Support (ACLS) should be started right away without delay. While the medical team supports the circulation, the RT should be prepared for emergent and possibly difficult intubation because of aspiration, oral/pharyngeal/tracheobronchial fluids, and edema. A few pediatric ETT sizes, a pediatric intubation kit, and a difficult airway cart with an emergent tracheostomy kit should be at the bedside.

Wall suctioning should be readily available, and a pediatric fiberoptic bronchoscope for deep suctioning and/or foreign body retrieval should be at the bedside.

In summary, a pediatric near drowning should be treated as an emergency with standard pediatric ACLS. However, immediately after recovery, the RT should focus on pulmonary toilette by body positioning, suctioning, and titration of the ventilator in anticipation of impending respiratory complications; refractory hypoxemia; and ARDS.

Clinical Assessment

During the clinical assessment of burn patients the airway is the first priority. Burn patients always should be considered trauma patients; airways evaluation and management should follow what is described in the previous section on airways management of the trauma patient. Airways of burn patients should be monitored closely because exposure to hot gases, flames, and toxic gases causes airways obstruction as a result of acute edema. Early intubation in these patients is essential, and early initiation of mechanical ventilation is required. Signs for early intubation include gradual but progressive compromise of respiratory mechanics and gas exchange and the presence of facial burns or any direct or indirect evidence of upper airways involvement.

Respiratory assessment of burn patients should focus on the following[37]:

1. Extension (**total body surface area**, [TBSA]) and depth of external burns
2. Degree of involvement of lung tissue
3. Inhalation of toxic gases (carbon monoxide and cyanide)

The surface area of external burns can be easily quantified by the rule of nines, which estimates the total amount of the body surface area involved by the burns (%TBSA). The evaluation of external burns with the rule of nines is crucial to the medical team to guide fluid management during the first hours of treatment (Table 30-2). An adult patient of approximately 80 kg and with burns of 50% of TBSA would require 16 L of fluids in the first 24 hours, of which 8 L is given within the first 8 hours (1 L/hr of fluid infusion). It is imperative for the RT to know the rate of fluid resuscitation and the hemodynamic response during the first critical hours after major burn. The severity of the burn depth is classified based on the anatomic planes progressively involved in the injury (Table 30-3). A first-degree burn is a superficial injury that involves only the epidermis. The second-degree involves the dermis. Third-degree injury is characterized by the destruction of both the epidermis and dermis above the fascia. Fourth-degree involves the muscles and the bones. Surgical intervention with debridement and grafting should be considered starting from second-degree burns.

Extensive chest-wall burns commonly lead to worsening gas exchange and work of breathing. The accumulation of edema in the chest wall and upper abdomen lowers chest wall compliance. The deterioration of respiratory mechanics can be so severe to require early **fasciotomy**.

Lung injury frequently results from inhalation of hot gases and smoke. ARDS is the typical presentation of heat-related lung injury. Fluid overload and systemic inflammatory response usually complicates the respiratory status and respiratory management of burn patients. Direct visualization of the tracheobronchial tree by fiberoptic bronchoscopy can be extremely helpful in revealing mucosal alterations and disruptions characterized by inflammation, erythema, carbonaceous debris, and ulcerations.

Carbon monoxide poisoning and **cyanide toxicity** are common findings in patients who have fire-related burns. The respiratory therapist should be aware that CO and cyanide poisoning do not cause cyanosis. SaO_2 in blood should be measured by ABG analyses because most SpO_2 sensors are unable to distinguish SO_2Hb from methemoglobin (MetHb) and carboxyhemoglobin (COHb). This phenomenon results in false 100 SpO_2 readings even when the patient is lethally hypoxemic. In the absence of blood gas analyses, a cooximeter can measure concentration of MetHb and COHb. CO has an affinity for hemoglobin a hundred times greater than that for O_2, and this can shift the oxyhemoglobin dissociation curve to the left. Patients become symptomatic when COHb levels are higher than 15%; levels greater than 50% are lethal. In these patients, 100% O_2 should be administered as soon as possible because it reduces the half-life of COHb to 40 to 60 minutes. When feasible, hyperbaric O_2 should be considered to prevent serious neurologic sequelae.[38,39] Inhalation of cyanide-containing gas during combustion of nitrogenous materials is characterized by

TABLE 30-2

Quantification of Total Burn Surface Area by the Rule of Nines

Anatomic Structure	% TBSA
Adult	
Head, anterior	4.5
Head, posterior	4.5
Torso, anterior	18
Torso, posterior	18
Leg, anterior, each	9
Leg, posterior, each	9
Arm, anterior, each	4.5
Arm, posterior, each	4.5
Genitalia/perineum	1
Child	
Head, anterior	9
Head, posterior	9
Torso, anterior	18
Torso, posterior	18
Leg, anterior, each	6.75
Leg, posterior, each	6.75
Arm, anterior, each	4.5
Arm, posterior, each	4.5
Genitalia/perineum	1
Infant	
Head and neck	20
Torso, anterior	16
Torso, posterior	16
Leg, each	16
Arm, each	8
Genitalia/perineum	1

TBSA, Total burn surface area.

TABLE 30-3

Severity of Burn Depth

Degree of Burn	Depth of Injury	Level of Pain
First degree	Superficial, only involving the epidermis	Tender and sore
Second degree	Involves the dermis	Very painful
Third degree	Destruction of the epidermis and dermis above the fascia	Very little to no pain
Fourth degree	Full-thickness burns involving the fascia, muscles, and bones	Painless

Box 30-9 Early Clinical Features of Carbon Monoxide and Cyanide Poisoning

- Anxiety
- Tachycardia
- Arrhythmias
- Tachypnoea
- Hypertension followed by:
  - Headache
  - Confusion
- Dyspnea
- Hypotention
- Bradycardia followed by:
  - Neurologic system symptoms (seizures, reduced consciousness)
  - Respiratory failure with pulmonary edema
  - Coma
  - Death

the presence of an adequate O_2 delivery and metabolic acidosis with anion gap. Cyanide compounds work by interfering with mitochondrial O_2 usage, blocking the final step of the oxidative phosphorylation cascade. The O_2 use impairment, despite a normal O_2 delivery, is confirmed by a high mixed venous O_2 saturation. Concentration of cyanide higher than 20 parts per million (ppm) is considered dangerous, and 100 ppm is lethal. **Thiosulfate** and **cyanocobalamin** are administered as soon as possible to reduce the half-life of this toxic compound. For both CO and cyanide poisoning, early clinical features are anxiety, tachycardia and/or arrhythmia, tachypnea, and hypertension, followed by headache, confusion, dyspnea, hypotension, and bradycardia leading to neurologic symptoms, such as seizures and reduced consciousness, respiratory failure with pulmonary edema, coma, and death (Box 30-9).[40]

RULE OF THUMB

CO and cyanide poisoning do not cause cyanosis. SaO_2 in blood should be measured by ABG analyses, because most SpO_2 sensors are unable to distinguish SO_2Hb from MetHb and COHb. This phenomenon results in false normal SpO_2 readings (100%) even when the patient is lethally hypoxemic.

Pathophysiology of Burn Patients

Burn injury can cause extensive tissue destruction, leading to a vast inflammatory process, which starts with the release of inflammatory cytokines. To simplify, there is a local burn effect at the site of the burn and a systemic effect mediated by inflammatory mediators that are released. However, these two effects are interlinked and difficult to separate from each other.

It is generally better to divide burn patients according to the systemic response over time: a severe systemic response that lasts up to the first 48 hours followed by a late response starting at 48 hours, and ending at approximately 72 hours after the burn accident.[37]

1. Commonly, if TBSA exceeds 25%, a systemic inflammatory process becomes evident and fluids from the intravascular space enter the extravascular space and develop a generalized edema. Edema expands quickly within the first hours after the injury. If patients are not sufficiently hydrated, this fluid shift rapidly leads into an impairment of local and systemic perfusion with tissue and organ damage causing ischemia, metabolic acidosis, and mixed venous desaturation, as a result of hypovolemic and distributive shock. The hematocrit gradually increases secondary to hemoconcentration. At the same time, the massive systemic inflammation commonly leads to cardiovascular instability followed by myocardial depression if not treated.
2. The first few hours after injury are characterized by a hyperdynamic state with high metabolic requirements with elevated CO_2 production and O_2 consumption. Massive vasodilation increases pulmonary shunt fraction, worsening hypoxemia that can develop into full pulmonary edema. However, this phase is short-lived and progresses to a catabolic state. At this stage, patients are at high risk for developing infections, with pneumonia being the most common.
3. The effects of the inhalation injury on the tracheobronchial tree and the lungs lead to edema, bronchospasm, and buildup of secretions. Different degrees of ARDS usually follow lung burn injury. When the burn circumferentially surrounds the chest, a mechanical constriction can develop worsening chest and respiratory system compliance.

Specific Concerns

Burn-injured patients with an inhalation injury have a significantly increased risk for morbidity and mortality. Inhalation injury can complicate 20% of burn patients, and these patients often present with facial burns. Patients presenting with facial burns, burnt nasal hairs, soot in the oral and nasal pharynx, and any signs of upper airway burns should be immediately intubated because of the probability of serious airway obstruction developing over time is nearly 100%. At admission it is difficult to identify characteristic radiographic features of inhalation injury. The effects become evident over time only when secondary complications such as inflammation, infection, or atelectasis develop. For this reason, the respiratory status and the airway patency of burn victims should be continuously monitored for the high risk for developing airway obstruction if an artificial airway is not already in place. Securing the airways as soon as possible should be the priority before catastrophic, irreversible airways obstruction occurs. One of the challenges in the respiratory care for severely injured burn patients is the clearance of copious and tenacious secretions. Secretions are accumulating throughout the tracheobronchial tree as a result of increased mucus secretion, buildup of toxic debris and necrotic cells, and peribronchial inflammatory **exudates** and **transudates**. In addition, mucociliary transport is severely impaired by disrupted tracheal-bronchial epithelium causing small airways plugs, worsening alveolar collapse, and predisposing to pulmonary infections. Optimization of airway humidification, careful endotracheal tube suctioning, and bronchoscope toilette are milestones of daily respiratory care of these particular vulnerable patients.[41-43]

RULE OF THUMB

Burn-injured patients with an inhalation injury have a significantly increased risk for morbidity and mortality.

Respiratory Management

Respiratory care of burn patients is complex. Hemodynamics, fluid resuscitation, %TBSA involvement and related injuries, time from the injury, and upper and lower respiratory conditions are some of the key elements that the RT needs to know while caring for these patients.

Oxygen Therapy

The SaO_2 of burn patients has to be monitored continuously. Until proved otherwise, all victims rescued from a fire should be treated with O_2 for suspected cyanide and CO poisoning. In the presence of cyanide and CO poisoning and to monitor response to treatment, noninvasive portable cooximetry or ABG analysis allows measurements of SaO_2, COHb, and MetHb levels. Cyanide poisoning is treated pharmacologically. The RT should monitor continuously the level of MetHb in the blood, especially if cyanide is treated with nitrite donors. Methylene blue should be administered if levels of MetHb become symptomatic. CO poisoning treatment is focused on dislodging CO from the hemoglobin. High concentration of inspired O_2 via nonrebreathing mask is mandatory in these patients, because O_2 shortens the half-life of CO. When available, a hyperbaric chamber is used in the treatment of the most severely CO poisoned burn patients; CO is quickly dissociated from hemoglobin and **cytochrome oxidase**. Hyperbaric O_2 at three times atmospheric pressure reduces the half-life of CO to approximately 3 minutes, compared to 80 minutes for regular 100% O_2 via nonrebreather mask. It also may reduce the brain (and other organs) tissue ischemia by increasing O_2 transport in plasma to the brain.[44,45]

RULE OF THUMB

Patients presenting with facial burns, burnt nasal hairs, soot in the oral and nasal pharynx, and any signs of upper airway burns should be immediately intubated because the probability of serious airway obstruction developing over time is nearly 100%.

Early Endotracheal Intubation

In these patients early endotracheal intubation is generally recommended for four reasons: (1) Protection of the airways from the risk for occlusion secondary to mucosal and interstitial edema, (2) the need for extensive pulmonary toilette by multiple bronchoscopies, (3) delivery of high fraction of inspired O_2 during CO poisoning, and (4) initiation of early lung protected ventilation in patients at high risk for developing ARDS.

Fiberoptic Bronchoscopy

Fiberoptic bronchoscopy is often used in these patients for diagnostic and treatment purposes. Bronchoscopy is used in acute settings for clearance of foreign bodies from the airways, disrupted mucosa, and mucous debris that might precipitate hypoxemia by alveolar obstruction, collapse, and atelectasis. The copious and tenacious secretions and necrotic tissue often require multiple fiberoptic bronchoscopies over time. Clearance of the tracheobronchial tree has three purposes: (1) Improving ventilation while avoiding $\dot{V}/\dot{Q}$ mismatch, (2) preventing bacterial overgrowth within the bloody-necrotic secretions and pneumonia, and (3) enhancing nebulized drug delivery that is commonly used in these patients (e.g., bronchodilators, antioxidants, and pulmonary vasodilator). Other use of bronchoscopy in these patients includes inspection of injury and monitoring over time of major lesions and distal bronchoalveolar lavage for a microbiologic sample if pneumonia is clinically suspected.[46]

RULE OF THUMB

Hyperbaric O_2 at three times atmospheric pressure reduces the half-life of CO to approximately 3 minutes, compared to 80 minutes for regular 100% O_2 via nonrebreather mask.

Active Humidification

Active humidification with heated humidifiers supplied by heated wire circuit should be used when possible. The aim of using continuous heated well-humidified ventilation is avoidance of mucus plugs in the distal airways and endotracheal tube while preventing body temperature loss.

Mechanical Ventilation

Mechanical ventilation should be titrated according to the underlying major respiratory condition of the patient (i.e., upper airway edema, lower airway injury, intoxication, ARDS, or pulmonary edema). In addition, the respiratory therapist should be prepared to change ventilation management according to the rapid cardiovascular and respiratory changes of the patient's clinical course during hospitalization. A typical early pulmonary scenario is a combination of pulmonary edema resulting from the high rate of fluid infusion and distal atelectasis secondary to secretions and mucus accumulation. Often ARDS develops, complicating the multifactorial respiratory failure and worsening lung compliance and hypoxemia. An early protective lung ventilation approach with low V_T and high PEEP is especially advantageous in these patients. Neuromuscular-blocking drugs are often beneficial to optimize low V_T ventilation (Box 30-10). In refractory hypoxemia, prone positioning and the use of inhaled pulmonary vasodilators might be considered an adjunct to respiratory treatment when

Box 30-10 Mechanical Ventilation of Patients With Smoke Inhalation and Pulmonary Burns

- Mode: Pressure or volume ventilation
- Tidal volume: 4 to 8 ml/kg PBW
- Inspiratory time 0.6 to 1.0 sec
- Plateau pressure: less than 28 cm H_2O unless chest wall compliance decreased
- If compliance decreased, plateau pressure can exceed 28 cm H_2O
- Measure end inspiratory transpulmonary pressure to determine acceptable plateau pressure, \
- Driving pressure equal to or less than 15 cm H_2O
- Rate only limited by the development of auto-PEEP
- Minute volume to maintain normal $PaCO_2$
- PEEP 5 to 10 cm H_2O, unless ARDS
- FIO_2 1.0 initially because of concern for CO poisoning
- If ARDS, manage as any other ARDS patient

feasible. The use of venovenous extracorporeal membrane oxygenation remains highly controversial in patients with extensive burn because of the risk for exsanguination. Early tracheostomy is often advocated because it improves secretion management by cough and suctioning, patient recovery by weaning from anesthetic medications, and wound care by patient collaboration.[47,48]

SUMMARY CHECKLIST

- In trauma patients, careful assessment for injuries of the head, neck, upper airway, and chest should occur immediately on presentation.
- Obese patient are at significant risk for cardiovascular disease. In addition, lung volumes are generally decreased, with atelectasis and airflow limitation that can result in air trapping and auto-PEEP. High levels of PEEP are frequently required.
- Near-drowning victims frequently have aspirated foreign material and present with significant pulmonary edema and electrolyte imbalances.
- Patients with smoke inhalation and pulmonary burns require careful assessment of their airways. Any clinical signs of upper airway injury generally require immediate intubation and mechanical ventilation.
- Chest trauma frequently results in injuries that cause disruption of major vessels and the development of tension hemothorax or pneumothorax.
- All obese patients should be assessed for sleep apnea and obesity hypoventilation syndrome.
- Fresh water drowning frequently results in hyponatremia, hemolysis, hyperkalemia, and ventricular fibrillation. Salt water drowning frequently results in marked pulmonary edema, hemoconcentration, hypernatremia, and hypoalbuminemia.
- Respiratory assessment of burn patients should focus on percent of TBSA, degree of tissue involvement, and inhalation of toxic gases.

MINI CLINI

Burn: Recognizing Hypoxemia in Patients After a Fire and Titrating Ventilation

PROBLEM: A 55-year-old firefighter presents at the hospital with 60% TBSA second- and third-degree burns after the successful rescue of an entire family from their burning house. The patient is 6 feet, 2 inches and 240 lb. During transport to the hospital he was intubated with an 8.0-mm ETT for increased shortness of breath and changes in mental status. Breath sounds are audible bilaterally. Ventilator settings are pressure support ventilation 15, PEEP 5 cm H_2O, and FiO_2 0.5. The patient's vital signs are heart rate 110 beats/min, blood pressure 90/50 mm Hg, respiratory rate 30 breaths/min, and SpO_2 98%. Endotracheal suctioning shows moderate dark/black secretions. The medical team started fluid resuscitation at a rate of 1 L/hr of normal saline. An arterial line was placed in his right radial artery, and the medical team has been struggling for the past half hour in the emergency room to place a central line. His SpO_2 has declined to 92%, but the other vital signs are unchanged. What should the RT do?

SOLUTIONS: Immediately confirm ETT positioning by auscultation of bilateral breath sounds and suggest a chest radiograph to the medical team if it was not requested already. Confirm by ETT suctioning the dark/black secretions in the airways, which imply a severe inhalation burn and cyanide poisoning.

Obtain a blood gas sample as soon as possible to rule out CO poisoning and evaluate metabolic acidosis. It is imperative to perform a blood gas analysis as soon as possible in any burn patient with a TBSA greater than 25% admitted to the ED even when SaO_2 is 99% to 100%. It might be a falsely high reading because of MetHb and COHb. The blood gas analysis should include PaO_2, MetHb, COHb, $PaCO_2$, pH, anion gap, lactate, and base excess. If available, noninvasive continuous monitoring for MetHb and COHb should be applied to trend MetHb and COHb values and evaluate response to treatment.

This is a critically ill patient with extensive and severe burns (TBSA 60%, second- and third-degree burn) and inhalation injury with an ongoing massive fluid resuscitation requirement. Ventilator settings should be titrated according to the clinical scenario; however, the following should be recommended: (1) increase FiO_2 up to 100% until the presence of CO and cyanide poisoning has been ruled out; (2) increase minute volume ventilation, avoiding increased V_T and mean airway pressure, to minimize effects of metabolic acidosis; (3) titrate PEEP by performing best PEEP trial. This patient most likely will develop pulmonary edema secondary to inflammation and fluid resuscitation and ARDS secondary to inhalation injury.

- Generally, gas-exchange abnormalities in trauma victims are a result of disruption of the chest wall and pulmonary contusion.
- Generally, gas-exchange abnormalities in obesity are a result of low lung volumes and the development of atelectasis.
- Generally, gas-exchange abnormalities in near drowning are a result of fluid shifts and the activation of inflammatory mediators.
- Generally, gas-exchange abnormalities in burns are a result of burns to the lung parenchyma and inhalation of foreign materials and toxic gases, specifically CO and cyanide.
- O_2 therapy is immediately indicated in the management of near drowning and pulmonary burns. Obese patients and trauma victims require O_2 therapy based on the severity of the patient's clinical presentation.
- Noninvasive ventilation is primarily indicated in the management of patients with sleep apnea, patients with OHS, and trauma patients with unstable chest walls.
- Invasive mechanical ventilation can be indicated in all four settings based on the severity of the injury.
- The primary concern during mechanical ventilation to trauma patients is the presence of a tension pneumothorax and hemodynamic instability.
- The primary concern with the application of mechanical ventilation to obese patients is the appropriate selection of V_T (based on PBW) and the appropriate application of PEEP.
- Near-drowning victims and pulmonary burn patients frequently and rapidly develop ARDS.
- In all four categories of patients, lung protective mechanical ventilation should be used from the onset of mechanical ventilation.
- PEEP and lung recruitment maneuvers should be applied to the markedly obese patient and any patient who develops ARDS. Prone positioning should be considered early in near-drowning patients and any patient with refractory hypoxemia unresponsive to the lung recruitment maneuvers and the setting of PEEP by decremental trial.
- Spontaneous breathing trials are the primary approach to weaning from ventilatory support for all of these patients.

References

1. Centers for Disease and Control and Prevention. <http://www.cdc.gov/injury/overview/leading_cod.html>. Accessed April 17, 2015.
2. Brain Trauma Foundation, American Association of Neurological Surgeons, Joint Section on Neurotrauma and Critical Care: Glasgow Coma Scale score. *J Neurotrauma* 17:563–571, 2000.
3. Theodore N, Hadley MN, Aarabi B, et al: Prehospital cervical spinal immobilization after trauma. *Neurosurgery* 72(Suppl 2):22–34, 2012.
4. Kellman RM, Losquadro WD: Comprehensive airway management of patients with maxillofacial trauma. *Craniomaxillofac Trauma Reconstr* 1:39–47, 2008.
5. American Association for the Surgery of Trauma. A resource for trauma care professional. <http://www.aast.org/library/traumatools/injuryscoringscales.aspx>. Accessed April 17, 2015.
6. Lawrence DA, Branson B, Oliva I, et al: The wonderful world of the windpipe: a review of central airway anatomy and pathology. *Can Assoc Radiol J* 66:30–43, 2015.
7. Nirula R: Esophageal perforation. *Surg Clin North Am* 94:35–41, 2014.
8. Vana PG, Neubauer DC, Luchette FA: Contemporary management of flail chest. *Am Surg* 80:527–535, 2014.
9. Karcz MK, Papadakos PJ: Noninvasive ventilation in trauma. *World J Crit Care Med* 4:47–54, 2015.
10. Cohn SM, Dubose JJ: Pulmonary contusion: an update on recent advances in clinical management. *World J Surg* 34:1959–1970, 2010.
11. Branson RD: The scientific basis for postoperative respiratory care. *Respir Care* 58:1974–1984, 2013.
12. Carrier FM, Turgeon AF, Nicole PC, et al: Effect of epidural analgesia in patients with traumatic rib fractures: a systematic review and meta-analysis of randomized controlled trials. *Can J Anaesth* 56:230–242, 2009.
13. Beckers SK, Brokmann JC, Rossaint R: Airway and ventilator management in trauma patients. *Curr Opin Crit Care* 20:626–631, 2014.
14. Ogden CL, Carroll MD, Kit BK, et al: Prevalence of childhood and adult obesity in the United States, 2011–2012. *JAMA* 311:806–814, 2014.
15. Kress JP, Pohlman AS, Alverdy J, et al: The impact of morbid obesity on oxygen cost of breathing (VO2RESP) at rest. *Am J Respir Crit Care Med* 160:883–886, 1999.
16. Anzueto A, Frutos-Vivar F, Esteban A, et al: Ventila Group: Influence of body mass index on outcome of the mechanically ventilated patients. *Thorax* 66:66–73, 2011.
17. Jones RL, Nzekwu MM: The effects of body mass index on lung volumes. *Chest* 130:827–833, 2006.
18. Behazin N, Jones SB, Cohen RI, et al: Respiratory restriction and elevated pleural and esophageal pressures in morbid obesity. *J Appl Physiol* 108:2012–2018, 2010.
19. Lemyze M, Mallat J, Duhamel A, et al: Effects of sitting position and applied positive end-expiratory pressure on respiratory mechanics of critically ill obese patients receiving mechanical ventilation. *Crit Care Med* 41:2592–2599, 2013.
20. Valenza F, Vagginelli F, Tiby A, et al: Effects of the beach chair position, positive end-expiratory pressure, and pneumoperitoneum on respiratory function in morbidly obese patients during anesthesia and paralysis. *Anesthesiology* 107:723–732, 2007.
21. Manzano F, Fernández-Mondéjar E, Colmenero M, et al: Positive-end expiratory pressure reduces incidence of ventilator-associated pneumonia in nonhypoxemic patients. *Crit Care Med* 36:2225–2231, 2008.
22. Reinius H, Jonsson L, Gustafsson S, et al: Prevention of atelectasis in morbidly obese patients during general anesthesia and paralysis: a computerized tomography study. *Anesthesiology* 111:979–987, 2009.
23. Pirrone M, Mietto C, Chipman D, et al: Tailored ventilation in morbid obese patients. *Crit Care Med* 42:A1523, 2014.
24. Centers for Disease Control and Prevention, National Center for Injury Prevention and Control. Web-based Injury Statistics Query and Reporting System (WISQARS). <http://www.cdc.gov/injury/wisqars>. Accessed April 17, 2015.
25. Hyder AA, Borse NN, Blum L, et al: Childhood drowning in low- and middle-income countries: urgent need for intervention trials. *J Paediatr Child Health* 44:221–227, 2008.
26. Mtaweh H, Kochanek PM, Carcillo JA, et al: Patterns of multiorgan dysfunction after pediatric drowning. *Resuscitation* 19:90–96, 2015.
27. Datta A, Tipton M: Respiratory responses to cold water immersion: neural pathways, interactions, and clinical consequences awake and asleep. *J Appl Physiol* 100:2057–2064, 2006.
28. Rumbak MJ: The etiology of pulmonary edema in fresh water near drowning. *Am J Emerg Med* 14:176–179, 1996.
29. Modell JH, Calderwood HW, Ruiz BC, et al: Effects of ventilatory patterns on arterial oxygenation after near-drowning in sea water. *Anesthesiology* 40:376–384, 1974.
30. Golden FS, Tipton MJ, Scott RC: Immersion, near-drowning and drowning. *Br J Anaesth* 79:214–225, 1997.
31. DiMaio D, Vincent JM: *Forensic Pathology*, ed 2, New York, 2001, Taylor & Francis.

32. Laosee OC, Gilchrist J, Rudd R: Drowning 2005–2009. *MMWR* 61:344–347, 2012.
33. Kapur N, Slater A, McEniery J, et al: Therapeutic bronchoscopy in a child with sand aspiration and respiratory failure from near drowning: case report and literature review. *Pediatr Pulmonol* 44:1043–1047, 2009.
34. Metcalf KB, Michaels AJ, Edlich RF, et al: Extracorporeal membrane oxygenation can provide cardiopulmonary support during bronchoscopic clearance of airways after sand aspiration. *J Emerg Med* 45:380–383, 2013.
35. Burn Incidence and Treatment in the United States. 2013 fact sheet. <http://ameriburn.org>. Accessed April 17, 2015.
36. Sheridan R: Burns. *Crit Care Med* 30:S500–S514, 2002.
37. Bittner EA, Shank E, Woodson L, et al: Acute and perioperative care of the burn-injured patient. *Anesthesiology* 122:448–464, 2015.
38. Wu PE, Juurlink DN: Carbon monoxide poisoning. *CMAJ* 186:611–617, 2014.
39. Hampson NB, Piantadosi CA, Thom SR, et al: Practice recommendations in the diagnosis, management, and prevention of carbon monoxide poisoning. *Am J Respir Crit Care Med* 186:1095–1101, 2012.
40. Baud FJ, Barriot P, Toffis V, et al: Elevated blood cyanide concentrations in victims of smoke inhalation. *N Engl J Med* 325:1761–1766, 1991.
41. Wise B, Levine Z: Inhalation injury. *Can Fam Physician* 61:47–49, 2015.
42. Rehberg S, Maybauer MO, Enkhbaatar P, et al: Pathophysiology, management and treatment of smoke inhalation injury. *Expert Rev Respir Med* 3:283–297, 2009.
43. Weiss SM, Lakshminarayan S: Acute inhalation injury. *Clin Chest Med* 15:103–116, 1994.
44. Weaver LK: Hyperbaric oxygen therapy for carbon monoxide poisoning. *Undersea Hyperb Med* 41:339–354, 2014.
45. Buckley NA, Juurlink DN, Isbister G, et al: Hyperbaric oxygen for carbon monoxide poisoning. *Cochrane Database Syst Rev* (4):002041, 2011.
46. Valdez TA, Desai U, Ruhl C, et al: Early laryngeal inhalation injury and its correlation with late sequelae. *Laryngoscope* 116:283–287, 2006.
47. Sen S, Heather J, Palmieri T, et al: Tracheostomy in pediatric burn patients. *Burns* 41:248–251, 2015.
48. Dunham CM, Cutrona AF, Gruber BS, et al: Early tracheostomy in severe traumatic brain injury: evidence for decreased mechanical ventilation and increased hospital mortality. *Int J Burns Trauma* 4:14–24, 2014.

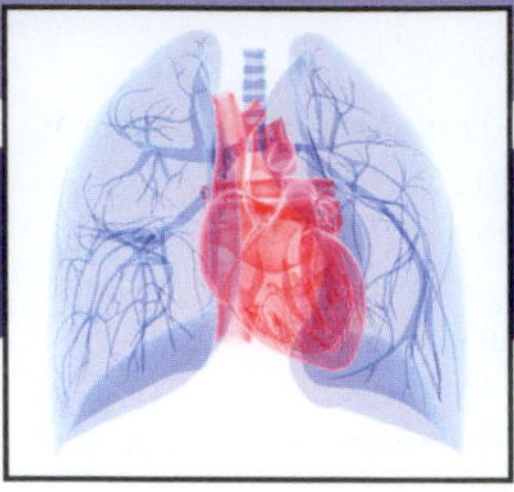

CHAPTER 31

Lung Cancer

PETER J. MAZZONE AND HILARY PETERSEN

CHAPTER OBJECTIVES

After reading this chapter you will be able to:

- Describe the epidemiology of lung cancer in the United States, particularly current trends.
- Identify risk factors for lung cancer.
- State the classification of lung cancer types and the cellular features of the four common types of lung cancer.
- Describe our current understanding of the pathophysiology of lung cancer.
- Identify the clinical features of the common types of lung cancer.
- Describe the diagnostic approach to lung cancer.
- State the importance of proper staging for lung cancer.
- Describe the treatment and outcomes for the common types of lung cancer by stage.
- State the role of the respiratory therapist in managing patients with lung cancer.

CHAPTER OUTLINE

Epidemiology
  New Cases
  Deaths
Classification
Pathophysiology
Clinical Features
Diagnosis
Staging
Preoperative Evaluation for Lung Resection Surgery
Screening
Treatment and Outcomes
  Non–Small Cell Lung Cancer
  Small Cell Lung Cancer
Future Scenario
Role of the Respiratory Therapist in Managing Patients With Lung Cancer

KEY TERMS

adenocarcinoma
chemotherapy
computed tomography
flexible bronchoscopy
large cell carcinoma
magnetic resonance imaging
mass
nodule
non–small cell carcinoma
Pancoast syndrome
paraneoplastic syndrome
positron emission tomography
radiotherapy
screening
small cell carcinoma
squamous cell carcinoma
staging system
surgical resection
tumor, node, metastasis (TNM) staging
transbronchial needle aspiration
transthoracic needle biopsy

Lung cancer is a major public health problem. In the United States, approximately 28% of cancer deaths are due to lung cancer.[1] Most of these deaths could be avoided if people did not smoke tobacco-related products. Worldwide tobacco consumption has not been declining, however, suggesting lung cancer will remain an epidemic for years to come. Advances in early detection and treatment have been slow, but steady. The overall prognosis remains poor, with just over one in eight lung cancer patients still living 5 years after diagnosis. This chapter provides an overview of lung cancer for the respiratory therapist (RT).

EPIDEMIOLOGY

New Cases

In 2014 an estimated 224,210 new cases of lung cancer were diagnosed in the United States.[1] Lung cancer is the second most frequently diagnosed cancer in men and women. The incidence of lung cancer peaked in men in 1984 and has since been declining. In women, however, the incidence increased during the 1990s, with a leveling off toward the end of the decade. These trends parallel the smoking patterns of men and women.[1] The World Health Organization estimates that there are 2 million cases of lung cancer worldwide each year.

Deaths

Lung cancer is the number one cause of cancer-related death in men and women; it surpassed colon cancer in the early 1950s in men and breast cancer in the late 1980s in women. There are more deaths from lung cancer than breast, colon, and prostate cancer combined. Mortality rates in men declined significantly in the 1990s, whereas a slow increase occurred in women. These rates parallel the smoking patterns of men and women (Figures 31-1). In 2014 in the United States, an estimated 159,260 deaths were due to lung cancer. In men, lung cancer is the leading cause of cancer-related deaths from age 40 years to end of life. In women, lung cancer surpasses breast cancer in the age group of 60 and older.[1]

Tobacco-Related Products

Direct exposure to tobacco has occurred in 85% to 90% of individuals with lung cancer. Many tobacco-related carcinogens have been identified. The age at which smoking began, the number of cigarettes smoked per day, and the duration of smoking all influence the likelihood of developing lung cancer. Also, the intensity of smoking, the depth of inhalation, and the composition of the cigarette influence the risk. All types (see later) of lung cancer are associated with smoking. The strongest associations are with two of the cell types: *small cell* and *squamous cell carcinoma.* The risk for developing lung cancer decreases over time after smoking cessation, although it never reaches that of a lifelong nonsmoker.

There is evidence that *nicotine,* a chemical in tobacco, is highly addictive.[2] Approximately one-fifth of all adults in the United States smoke cigarettes. Progress had been made in the fight against cigarette use; in the decades from 1970 to 1990, the percentage of women who smoked declined from 33% to 25% and the rate of smoking among men decreased from 43% to 28%. The annual decline that had occurred since the early 1970s began to slow through the 1990s despite mounting evidence associating smoking with disease and death.[3] In addition, a decrease in smoking has not been observed among adults 18 to 24 years old. Cigarette smoking among young people remains a major public health concern. Of young adults (18 to 24 years), 33% have been reported to be current users of tobacco,[4] and 3000 teenagers begin smoking each day.[5] Approximately 13% of middle school children and 28% of high school students use tobacco products. In the context that a person who has not started smoking as a teenager is unlikely ever to become a

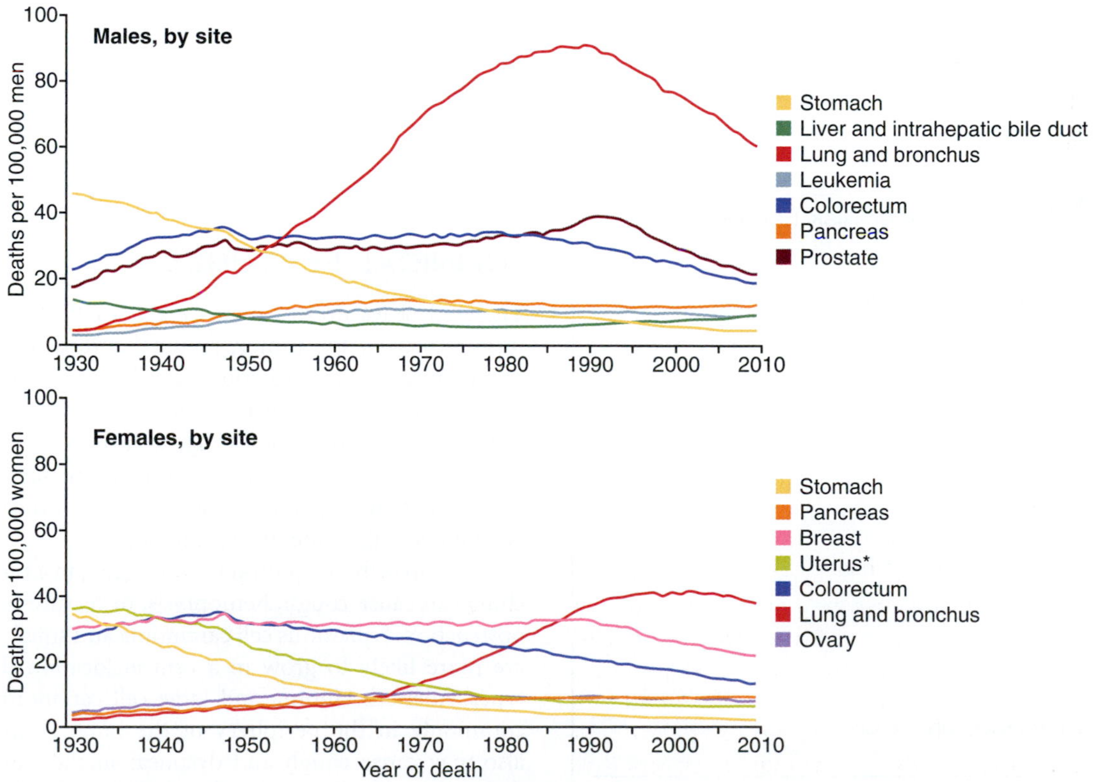

FIGURE 31-1 Death rate from lung cancer by gender from 1930 to 2010. (Modified from Siegel R, Ma J, Zou Z, et al: Cancer statistics, 2014. *CA Cancer J Clin* 64:9–29, 2014.)

smoker, the tobacco industry has focused on young people and developing countries as the primary sources of new customers.[6,7]

Other forms of exposure to tobacco-related products also pose risk for promoting lung cancer. Cigar smoking, which has increased considerably over the past several years, is known to be an independent risk factor for developing lung cancer.[8]

Exposure to *sidestream smoke,* or *passive smoking,* also may lead to an increased risk for lung cancer. The risk is generally much lower than active smoking but varies with the intensity of exposure.[7] It has been estimated that 3000 to 5000 deaths in the United States and 21,400 deaths worldwide from lung cancer occur each year because of second-hand smoke exposure.[9]

Occupational Agents and Other Risks

Many other risk factors have been identified (Box 31-1). Occupational agents are known to act as lung cancer carcinogens. Arsenic, asbestos, and chromium confer the highest risk. This risk is increased when there is concomitant exposure to tobacco products. Indoor radon exposure is also a risk factor for developing lung cancer. Radon is a naturally occurring gas produced by the breakdown of uranium ore or other rocks such as shale and granite. Indoor radon exposure generally comes from the soil underneath homes and buildings.[10] Particulates in the atmosphere (i.e., pollution) also can increase the risk for lung diseases including lung cancer.

Family members of people who develop lung cancer have an increased risk.[11–13] Women seem to have a higher baseline risk for developing lung cancer and a greater susceptibility to the effects of smoking. Differences in the metabolism of tobacco-related carcinogens and their metabolites, an effect of hormone differences, or both are thought to account for the increased susceptibility.[14] Dietary factors also can modify risks. Higher consumption of fruits and vegetables is associated with a reduced lung cancer risk, and increased dietary fat intake may lead to a higher risk.[15,16] Supplementation with vitamin A, vitamin E, or beta-carotene has not positively influenced risk.[15] The presence of chronic obstructive pulmonary disease (COPD) is an independent risk factor.[17,18]

Box 31-1 Lung Cancer Risk Factors

Tobacco smoke exposure
- Active (mainstream)—cigarette, cigar
- Passive (sidestream)

Occupational and environmental exposures
- Arsenic
- Asbestos
- Chromium
- Beryllium
- Bis(chloromethyl)ether
- Cadmium
- Nickel
- Polycyclic aromatic hydrocarbons
- Radon
- Vinyl chloride

Genetic predisposition
Gender
Dietary factors
Chronic obstructive pulmonary disease
Air pollution

Courtesy The Cleveland Clinic, Cleveland, OH.

CLASSIFICATION

Lung cancers are divided into two major groups—**small cell carcinoma** and **non–small cell carcinoma**—based on pathologic features that are visible under light microscopy. The evaluation and management of a patient are guided by the type and stage (see later) of lung cancer. The non–small cell cancer category consists of **adenocarcinoma, squamous cell carcinoma, large cell carcinoma,** and variants (Figure 31-2). Table 31-1 presents the pathologic and epidemiologic features of the four most common types of lung cancer.

PATHOPHYSIOLOGY

The pathophysiology of lung cancer development is complex and incompletely understood. Damage to genetic material in lung cells is the result of exposure to chemical carcinogens such as the carcinogens contained in tobacco smoke.[18] People who develop lung cancer may have a genetic predisposition to the effects of these carcinogens. The genes influenced in the pathogenesis of lung cancer produce proteins involved in cell growth and differentiation, cell cycle processes, *apoptosis* (programmed cell death), *angiogenesis* (production of new blood vessels), tumor progression, and immune regulation. If enough of these pathways have been affected, the uncontrolled growth of cells that defines cancer occurs. By understanding the mechanisms that lead to genetic damage and the impact of that damage, novel means of risk stratification, prevention, early detection, and therapy should be able to be developed.

CLINICAL FEATURES

The clinical features of lung cancer result from the effects of local growth of the tumor, regional spread through the lymphatic system, hematogenous (blood-borne) distant metastatic spread, and remote effects from tumor products or immune cross reaction with tumor antigens (Box 31-2). Some manifestations occur more commonly with a particular cell type. Only 15% of patients with a diagnosis of lung cancer do *not* have symptoms at the time of presentation.

Local growth in a central location (e.g., in a main stem bronchus) can cause cough, hemoptysis, or features of large airway obstruction. Squamous cell carcinoma and small cell carcinoma are more likely to grow in a central location than other cell types. Adenocarcinoma and large cell carcinoma occur more commonly in the periphery of the lung. Peripheral growths also may cause cough and dyspnea; smaller tumors may not cause any symptoms. If the pleura or chest wall is involved, pain may occur.

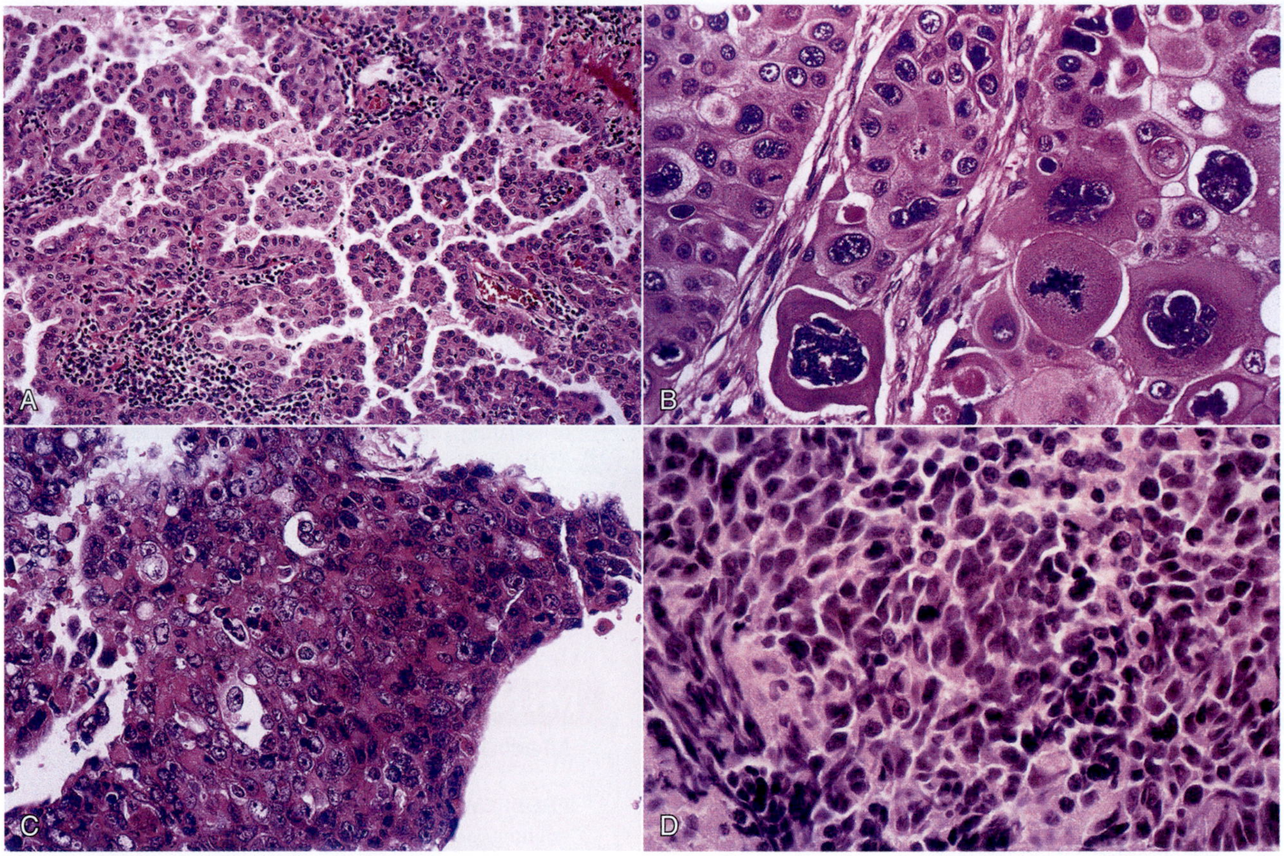

FIGURE 31-2 Lung cancer histology. **A,** Adenocarcinoma, characterized by heterogeneous differentiation in the same tumor. **B,** Squamous cell carcinoma, characterized by the presence of cytokeratin differentiation with keratinization and intercellular bridges. **C,** Large cell carcinoma, characterized by sheets and nest with extensive necrosis, large nuclei with prominent nucleoli, and lack of definitive evidence of squamous or glandular differentiation. **D,** Small cell carcinoma, characterized by round to fusiform nuclei, nuclear molding, faint or absent nucleoli, and scant cytoplasm. (Courtesy The Cleveland Clinic, Cleveland, Ohio.)

TABLE 31-1

Classification of Most Common Types of Lung Cancer

Category	Cell Type	Pathologic Features (Light Microscopy)	Epidemiology
Non–small cell carcinoma	Adenocarcinoma	Formation of glandular structures; heterogeneous differentiation	Accounts for >40% of lung cancers in North America; increasing frequency in women
	Squamous cell carcinoma	Cytokeratin and intercellular bridges	Second most frequent type of lung cancer in United States
	Large cell carcinoma	Sheets and nests of cells, necrosis, lack of squamous cell or glandular features	Less common than adenocarcinoma or squamous cell carcinoma
Small cell carcinoma	Small cell carcinoma	Round to fusiform nuclei; faint to absent nucleoli; scant cytoplasm	Accounts for 13% of lung cancers

Regional spread may lead to esophageal compression *(dysphagia),* recurrent laryngeal nerve paralysis (hoarseness), phrenic nerve paralysis with an elevated hemidiaphragm (dyspnea), and sympathetic nerve paralysis leading to Horner syndrome (ptosis [droopy eyelid], miosis [small pupils], anhidrosis [lack of facial sweating], and enophthalmos [sunken eye]). Growth at the very top of the lung may lead to a **Pancoast syndrome,** with shoulder pain radiating in an ulnar distribution as a result of involvement of the brachial plexus. The superior vena cava can become obstructed, resulting in swelling of the face, neck, and upper chest, plethora (swollen facial veins causing a ruddy complexion), and dilation of superficial veins over these areas. This is called the *superior vena cava syndrome.* Lung cancer can grow to involve the heart and pericardium. Lymphatic obstruction and spread can lead to dyspnea, hypoxemia, and pleural effusions.

Box 31-2 Lung Cancer Manifestations

Local growth
- Cough
- Dyspnea
- Hemoptysis
- Pain

Regional growth
- Dysphagia
- Dyspnea
- Hoarseness
- Horner syndrome
- Hypoxia
- Pancoast syndrome

Pericardial and pleural effusions
- Superior vena cava syndrome

Metastatic disease
- Headache
- Hepatomegaly
- Mental status change
- Pain
- Papilledema
- Seizures
- Skin or soft tissue mass
- Syncope
- Weakness

Paraneoplastic
- Cutaneous or skeletal
  - Acanthosis nigricans
  - Clubbing
  - Dermatomyositis
  - Hypertrophic osteoarthropathy
- Endocrine
  - Cushing syndrome
  - Humoral hypercalcemia
  - Syndrome of inappropriate antidiuretic hormone
  - Tumor necrosis factor (cachexia)
- Hematologic
  - Anemia or polycythemia
  - Disseminated intravascular coagulation
  - Eosinophilia
  - Granulocytosis
  - Thrombophlebitis
- Neurologic
  - Cancer-associated retinopathy
  - Encephalomyelitis
  - Lambert-Eaton syndrome
  - Neuropathies
  - Cerebellar degeneration
- Renal
  - Glomerulonephritis
  - Nephrotic syndrome

Courtesy The Cleveland Clinic, Cleveland, OH.

Distant metastatic disease can affect most organs; the brain, bones, liver, and adrenal glands are most commonly involved. Neurologic symptoms such as headaches, vision changes, and seizures may suggest brain metastases. Back pain and changes in strength or sensation in an extremity may indicate spinal cord compression. Bone pain could indicate bone metastases. Laboratory abnormalities may point to bone marrow or liver involvement. Imaging may detect adrenal involvement.

MINI CLINI

Pancoast Tumor

PROBLEM: A 65-year-old man who has smoked two packs of cigarettes per day for the past 40 years has had drooping of the left eyelid for the past 3 weeks. A chest radiograph reveals a mass in the apex of the left lung. Is there a link between the drooping of the eyelid and the lung mass?

DISCUSSION: Lung tumors involving the apex of the lung (superior sulcus tumors) are also known as *Pancoast tumors*. If they involve the cervical sympathetic nerves in the neck, these tumors result in Horner syndrome. This syndrome is characterized by ptosis (drooping of the eyelid), anhidrosis (absence of sweating), and miosis (constricted pupil) on the same side as the tumor. Other manifestations of Pancoast tumor include pain and weakness in the upper extremity (owing to involvement of the brachial plexus), rib destruction, and destruction of vertebral bodies. Treatment depends on local and distant spread of the tumor.

MINI CLINI

Mediastinal Adenopathy

PROBLEM: A 60-year-old man has been found to have small cell lung cancer on the basis of results of bronchoscopic biopsy findings. Computed tomography (CT) scan of the chest shows extensive mediastinal adenopathy. The patient has been admitted to the oncology floor for chemotherapy. You are called to assess him because he cannot lie down owing to shortness of breath (orthopnea). When you arrive, the patient is sitting on the edge of the bed. You notice that his face and neck are swollen. He also has dilated veins over the face, neck, chest, and arms. How do you explain these findings?

DISCUSSION: This patient has superior vena cava obstruction caused by compression by the mediastinal tumor. The swelling of the face, neck, and arms is caused by impairment of the venous drainage from the upper body (the superior vena cava distribution). The dilated chest and arm veins are collateral vessels (or alternative pathway vessels) that compensate for the superior vena cava obstruction. Superior vena cava obstruction can be caused by various benign or malignant conditions that involve the mediastinum or the right upper lung. Treatment usually is therapy for the underlying problem.

When symptoms develop that are the result of the presence of cancer but are not related to the growth or spread of the cancer, these symptoms constitute a **paraneoplastic syndrome.** Paraneoplastic syndromes can result from the effects of proteins produced by the tumor that circulate through the body to have their effects on distant organs or result from the immune response of the body to a tumor antigen that is similar to antigens in other parts of the body, causing immune injury to the distant organ. Paraneoplastic syndromes may occur before the primary tumor appears and be the first sign of disease or an indication of tumor recurrence. Examples of tumor secretion include the production of excess glucocorticoids (ectopic Cushing syndrome), parathyroid hormone (hypercalcemia of malignancy), and antidiuretic hormone (syndrome of inappropriate antidiuretic hormone [SIADH]). Immune cross-reactivity leads to paraneoplastic neurologic syndromes that can affect all parts of the neurologic system, resulting in emotional lability (limbic encephalitis), loss of balance (cerebellar degeneration), or proximal muscle weakness of the arms and legs with autonomic dysfunction (Lambert-Eaton myasthenic syndrome). Other paraneoplastic syndromes include skeletal and connective tissue syndromes (digital clubbing, hypertrophic pulmonary osteoarthropathy), coagulation and hematologic disorders, cutaneous and renal manifestations, and systemic symptoms (anorexia, cachexia, and weight loss).[19]

MINI CLINI

Paraneoplastic Syndrome

PROBLEM: A 55-year-old man is brought to the emergency department by family members because of confusion and progressive generalized weakness. Examination in the emergency department shows the patient is dehydrated, lethargic, and confused. Chest radiograph reveals a cavitary lesion in the right upper lobe. Results of arterial blood gas analysis are normal. Results of chemical analysis urgently performed with the blood gas analysis reveal a sodium level of 150 mEq/L (normal 135 to 145 mEq/L) and a calcium level of 17 mg/dL (normal 9 to 10.5 mg/dL). How is the lung mass related to this patient's presentation and biochemical abnormalities?

DISCUSSION: This patient's confusion and weakness are due to hypercalcemia, which is a paraneoplastic presentation of lung cancer, especially squamous cell carcinoma (the cavitating mass on the chest radiograph). Paraneoplastic syndromes are systemic manifestations of lung cancer that are not caused by metastasis. Most paraneoplastic syndromes are associated with small cell lung cancer. However, hypercalcemia is more common with squamous cell carcinoma and is caused by secretion by the tumor of parathyroid hormone–related peptide. Treatment consists of hydration, diuresis, and use of medications that can reduce the levels of calcium.

DIAGNOSIS

Approximately 85% of patients with lung cancer present with one or more of the previously described symptoms. In the remainder, lung cancer is detected by radiographic evaluation performed for an unrelated problem. This proportion may change in the future as **computed tomography** (CT) screening programs become widespread. Most patients have a chest radiograph and CT scan of the chest performed in their initial evaluation. These studies show a small spot (<3 cm in diameter) termed a **nodule** in the lungs or a larger spot (>3 cm in diameter) termed a **mass.** Other findings on imaging include enlarged lymph nodes in the hila (where the bronchi and central blood vessels emerge from the mediastinum into the lung) or mediastinum or a pleural effusion. An individual patient's clinical and radiographic presentation dictates further evaluation.

The symptoms of lung cancer are nonspecific. There are many reasons that someone could have a cough or be short of breath. Similarly, an abnormality such as a lung nodule can be present on chest imaging for various reasons. Certain clinical and radiographic features make it more likely that the presentation represents lung cancer. The older the patient is and the more he or she has smoked over time, the more likely the chest finding is lung cancer. Also, individuals with prior cancers are more likely to have lung cancer. Hemoptysis increases concern about cancer.

Radiographic features are also used to determine the probability of cancer. The larger the lung abnormality, the more likely it is to be cancer. When the abnormality has reached the size of a mass (3 cm), it needs to be considered a cancer until proved otherwise. The rate of growth of the lesion is also helpful. If a nodule grows rapidly (doubles in size in <1 month) or grows very slowly or not at all over a couple of years, it is unlikely to be due to cancer. If the nodule appears to be heavily calcified on imaging, it has likely been present for quite some time and is unlikely to represent cancer. If the abnormality has an irregular border, is lobulated, or is spiculated, it is more likely to be a cancer than if the border is smooth and rounded. Finally, if the lesion is cavitary, the thickness of the wall of the cavity can suggest cancer. A wall thickness of 14 mm or greater is likely to represent a cancer.[20]

RULE OF THUMB

A solid solitary pulmonary nodule that has not grown in 24 months is unlikely to be malignant.

MINI CLINI

No Response to Antibiotics

PROBLEM: A 55-year-old woman who does not smoke has a 3-month history of dyspnea on exertion, weight loss, and cough productive of copious amounts of clear, frothy sputum. She has no fever or chills. She has been treated for 2 weeks for "double pneumonia" without relief of the symptoms. Examination reveals finger clubbing and decreased air entry in both lung bases with dullness to percussion. A chest radiograph shows bilateral alveolar infiltrates. What should be done next?

DISCUSSION: The patient has a variant of adenocarcinoma of the lung. Cough productive of copious amounts of clear, frothy sputum is characteristic of this type of lung cancer. The radiographic appearance may be indistinguishable from that of pneumonia, especially when there is sputum production. The absence of fever, the chronic presence of infiltrates, and the lack of response to antibiotic therapy should raise suspicion for this type of lung cancer. Bronchoscopy with transbronchial biopsy would be a reasonable next step to confirm the diagnosis.

After the clinical and standard imaging features are reviewed, a probability of malignancy can be determined. If the probability is very high, the potential cancer does not seem to have spread, and the individual is fit, proceeding directly to surgery would be reasonable. If the previously mentioned features suggest a very low probability of malignancy, the clinician and patient might choose to follow along with serial chest imaging over time to assess for further growth. When the probability falls between these extremes, adjunctive imaging and invasive procedures can be used to help alter the probability. The most commonly used additional imaging technique is **positron emission tomography** (PET) with fluorodeoxyglucose (FDG-PET). Because malignant cells are metabolically very active, they take up the glucose analogue more avidly than nonmalignant cells. The attached radioactive tracer becomes trapped in the cells, allowing it to be imaged. When this test is used to help predict the presence of lung cancer, it has a sensitivity of 97% and a specificity of 78%. PET imaging can produce false-positive results in other metabolically active conditions such as infections. It can be falsely negative if the lesion is too small (<10 mm) or if the tumor is slow growing and not very metabolically active (e.g., some adenocarcinomas, carcinoid tumor).[21]

Ultimately, tissue is obtained to confirm the diagnosis of lung cancer. **Flexible bronchoscopy** and **transthoracic needle biopsy** are invasive, nonsurgical approaches used to obtain tissue. If these procedures fail or are deemed unnecessary, a surgical approach is used.

Flexible bronchoscopy is a procedure in which a long, thin, flexible camera is passed through a patient's nostril or mouth into the lungs. The camera can be extended into the branches of the lung as far as the branches are large enough to admit it. The camera has a small channel through which very thin biopsy instruments can be passed out deeper into the lung to take samples from concerning areas. Flexible bronchoscopy has a high diagnostic yield for lesions that are endoscopically visible within the larger airways. Samples are collected by washing saline over the lesion, sending a small brush through the camera to collect cells on its bristles, and taking biopsy samples with a forceps or needle.

Addition of needle aspiration to the conventional sampling techniques (washing, brushing, and forceps biopsy) improves the yield. The diagnostic yield from lesions in the periphery of the lung, beyond where the camera is able to see, is lower. Conventional sampling techniques and peripheral **transbronchial needle aspiration** complement each other. Factors that influence the diagnostic yield of flexible bronchoscopy for peripheral lesions include the size of the lesion, its location, and the presence of a "bronchus sign" on CT (an airway leading directly into the lesion). Smaller, more peripheral lesions, without a visible bronchus within or leading directly to them, are unlikely to be diagnosed by flexible bronchoscopy.[22] More recent technologic advances, such as multiplanar imaging, electromagnetic navigation of the bronchoscopy instruments, and peripheral endobronchial ultrasound, have been able to improve the yield of flexible bronchoscopy for these small peripheral lesions.[23] Not infrequently, the hilar or mediastinal lymph nodes are enlarged as a result of spread of the tumor. Diagnosis and staging can be accomplished during bronchoscopy with endobronchial ultrasound to guide biopsies of these lymph nodes.[24,25]

Transthoracic needle biopsy, using fluoroscopic or CT guidance, also can be used to obtain tissue. With this procedure, an aspirating needle is passed through the skin into the lung lesion under the guidance of chest imaging. The positive predictive value of this procedure is high, the negative predictive value is modest, and the rate of establishing a specific benign diagnosis is low. Smaller nodules in central locations have lower diagnostic rates. A higher rate of pneumothorax occurs with transthoracic needle biopsy.[24] The choice of which procedure to use is guided by the size and location of the lesion and by the local expertise with each technique.

STAGING

A major factor that determines the prognosis of lung cancer and guides the selection of appropriate treatment is the extent to which the cancer has spread in the lungs and throughout the body. The extent of cancer spread is termed the *stage* of the cancer. Non–small cell lung cancer is staged using the **TNM staging** system (*T* for extent of primary tumor, *N* for regional lymph node involvement, and *M* for metastases).

The T component of the **staging system** is divided into T1 through T4 lesions, as follows:

- A *T1 tumor* is a small tumor confined to the lung. It must be less than 3 cm in diameter and be surrounded by lung or visceral pleura and cannot extend into a main bronchus. T1a tumors are less than 2 cm in diameter, and T1b tumors are 2 to 3 cm.
- A *T2 tumor* is between 3 cm and 7 cm in diameter or any size tumor that invades the visceral pleura, or extends into the main bronchus, but remains greater than 2 cm from the main carina. It may cause segmental or lobar atelectasis.
- A *T3 tumor* is locally advanced or invasive up to but not including the major intrathoracic structures. It can be any size, and it may involve the chest wall, diaphragm, mediastinal pleura, parietal pericardium, or main bronchus within 2 cm of the main carina (but not involving the main carina). It may cause atelectasis of an entire lung. There may be separate tumor nodules in the same lobe as the primary tumor. A tumor larger than 7 cm in diameter is considered T3 even if unaccompanied by local invasion.
- A *T4 tumor* is a tumor of any size that has invaded one of the major intrathoracic structures, such as the mediastinum, heart, great vessels, trachea, esophagus, vertebral body, or main carina. The tumor is also classified T4 if there are tumor nodules in a different ipsilateral lobe of the lung.

The N component of the staging system is determined by which lymph nodes, if any, are involved with tumor, as follows:

- *N0 spread* does not involve any lymph nodes.
- *N1 spread* indicates the presence of cancer in nodes within the ipsilateral lung (the same side as the tumor).
- *N2 spread* signifies cancer in nodes in the mediastinum ipsilateral to the primary tumor.

TABLE 31-2
TNM Staging for Lung Cancer

Stage	
IA	T1a,bN0M0
IB	T2aN0M0
IIA	T1a,bN1M0, T2aN1M0, T2bN0M0
IIB	T2bN1M0, T3N0M0
IIIA	T3N1M0, T(1-3)N2M0, T4N0-1
IIIB	T4N2M0, T(1-4)N3M0
IV	T(any)N(any)M1a,b

- *N3 spread* signifies cancer in *contralateral* ("opposite side") mediastinal or hilar nodes, *ipsilateral* or contralateral scalene, or supraclavicular nodes.[25–27]

The M part of the staging system represents the absence *(M0)* or presence *(M1)* of metastases outside of the chest. *M1a* refers to metastasis of separate tumor nodules in the contralateral lung or the presence of a malignant pleural or pericardial effusion. *M1b* refers to distant metastatic spread, such as liver, bone, or brain lesions.

The most recent revision[26] to this staging system occurred in 2009 (Table 31-2 and Figure 31-3). The stages are labeled from stage IA to stage IV based on the combination of T, N, and M features.

For patients with small cell lung cancer, the TNM staging system was previously thought to be less useful. Instead, small cell lung cancer has been staged as limited or extensive disease. *Limited stage* disease is present when the tumor is confined to a hemithorax (including ipsilateral mediastinal and supraclavicular lymph nodes) and can be contained within a radiotherapy port. *Extensive stage* disease is present when the tumor extends beyond these boundaries. The recent lung cancer staging revision recognized a benefit to applying the TNM staging system used for non–small cell cancer to small cell cancer as well.[26-29]

The proper use of testing to stage a patient with lung cancer is addressed in a more recent set of guidelines.[27] The history and physical examination are important in guiding testing. The extent of spread is best evaluated using CT of the chest extending to the upper abdomen to include the liver and adrenal glands; this should be ordered in all patients. **Magnetic resonance imaging** (MRI) has not proved to be more accurate except in the setting of a Pancoast tumor. Evidence shows that integrated PET/CT scanning has better test characteristics for staging lymph node and distant disease involvement than other types of imaging (Figure 31-4).[30-32]

Because noninvasive tests can have false-positive results, tissue confirmation is necessary. Bronchoscopy with transbronchial needle aspiration is useful to stage the mediastinum. The addition of endobronchial and endoscopic ultrasound has increased the yield of nonsurgical mediastinal staging.[26,33] If such staging is negative, mediastinoscopy, mediastinotomy, or thoracoscopy can confirm the nodal status. Despite the advances in imaging technology and sampling techniques, definitive staging with **surgical resection** and mediastinal dissection remains the gold standard in a patient with resectable disease. The assigned clinical stage (determined by the previously listed testing, including mediastinoscopy) can be lower than the pathologic staging (assigned after surgery).

The evaluation of metastatic disease also takes into consideration the history, physical examination, laboratory results (electrolytes, calcium, alkaline phosphatase, liver profile, and creatinine), and pathologic examination results.

Per guidelines, a head CT or MRI scan should be performed if symptoms or signs of metastatic disease are present or when evaluating what appears to be stage IIIA through IV disease. Although there is no proved survival benefit from CT versus MRI, many clinicians prefer to use MRI of the brain because it has greater sensitivity to detect metastatic disease.[30,34] The rest of the body is assessed by PET imaging, as was the mediastinum. PET imaging is recommended for all patients.

Along with evaluating the anatomic extent of disease, a patient's performance status is important in determining his or her prognosis and ability to tolerate any proposed treatment. The two most commonly used scales of performance status are the *Zubrod scale* and the *Karnofsky scale*. Although their definitions differ, the general principles of the two scales are the same, with ratings based on activity level, independence in daily activities, and severity of symptoms.

RULE OF THUMB

Staging for lung cancer is complex and should involve a multidisciplinary team. Stage I cancers are small tumors. Stage II cancers involve hilar nearby lymph nodes or larger tumors. When mediastinal nodes are positive, the patient is at least stage III. When a malignant pleural effusion or distant sites such as the brain or bones are involved, the patient is stage IV.

PREOPERATIVE EVALUATION FOR LUNG RESECTION SURGERY

To determine if a patient would tolerate lung resection surgery, patients go through testing of their pulmonary, cardiovascular, and overall health. Reports of activity tolerance, pulmonary function testing, and exercise testing are used to assess the risk. The amount of risk is weighed against the benefit of having a traditional lung resection surgery (a lobectomy—one lobe removed, or pneumonectomy—a lung removed) versus a sublobar resection or nonsurgical treatment. Traditional resection is the best chance for cure and reduces local recurrence. As would be expected, a pneumonectomy requires better preoperative lung function than a lobectomy. When a lobe is removed, patients generally have a 10% to 15% drop in lung function. With a pneumonectomy, 30% to 35% is lost.

Cardiac conditions requiring medications, or an inability to climb two flights of stairs, should prompt a cardiac evaluation. The **thoracic revised cardiac risk index** can be used to identify

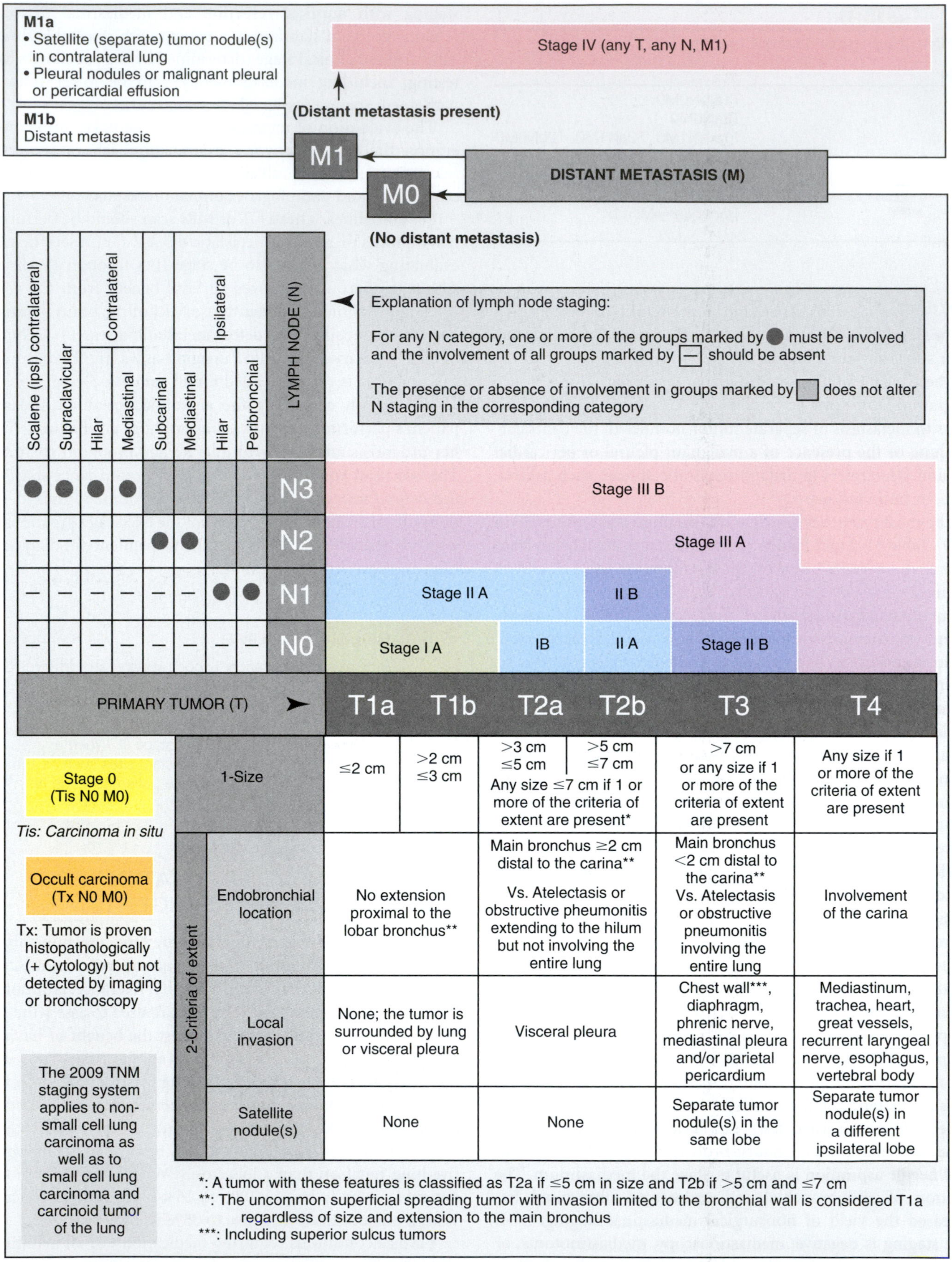

FIGURE 31-3 Reference chart for TNM staging of lung cancer. (Modified from Lababede O, Meziane P, Rice T: Seventh edition of the cancer staging manual and stage grouping of lung cancer: quick reference chart and diagrams. *Chest* 139:183–189, 2011.)

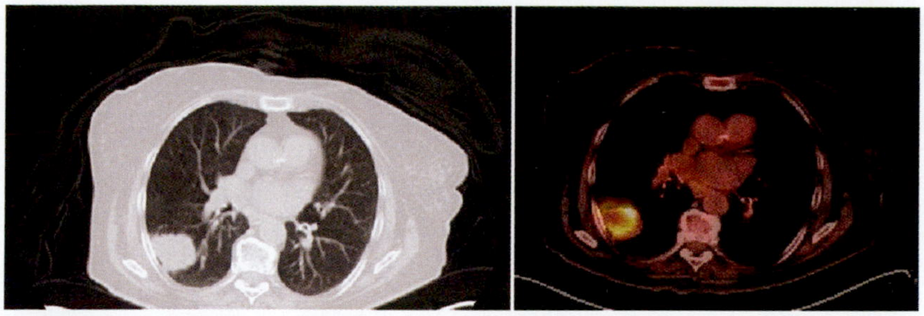

FIGURE 31-4 Positron emission tomography image of right lower lobe 4.7cm lung mass. Standardized uptake valve (SUV) of 10. Corresponding computed tomography chest imaging of right lower lobe 4.7-cm lung mass. (Courtesy Cleveland Clinic, Cleveland, OH.)

Box 31-3 To Calculate Percent Predicted Postoperative Values

The segment method

PPO FEV1 = preoperative FEV1 × (1 − number of resected segments/19)

19 representing the total number of segments in both lungs:
- Right upper lung: 3
- Right middle lung: 2
- Right lower lung: 5
- Left upper lung: 5
- Left lower lung: 4

patients at risk for cardiac complications. Those with any combination of the following conditions (i.e., score ≥ 2) should have noninvasive cardiac stress testing or a cardiology consultation: previous ischemic heart disease, stroke or transient ischemic attack, creatinine > 2 mg/dL or planned pneumonectomy. Similarly, those with a cardiac condition requiring medication, or with a newly suspected cardiac condition, and those unable to climb two flights of stairs should be considered for noninvasive cardiac stress testing or a cardiology consultation.

The evidence shows that the volume exhaled during the first second of a forced expiratory maneuver (FEV_1) (see Chapter 20) and diffusing capacity for carbon monoxide (DLCO) are the most frequently used pulmonary function tests and the best predictors for postoperative complications, including death. Traditional preoperative cutoff values have been replaced by percent predicted postoperative (PPO) values as starting points. PPO values of FEV_1 and DLCO can be calculated by multiplying the percent predicted *pre*operative value by the fraction of the total number of lung segments that will remain postoperatively. This is the segment method (Box 31-3). Alternatively, quantitative perfusion imaging can be used to guide the calculation. If the PPO FEV_1 and DLCO are greater than 60%, the patient is considered at low risk for lung resection. If PPO values fall between 30% to 60%, an exercise test should be performed. The stair climb test, shuttle walk, and 6 minute walk tests can be used. For patients with PPO values below 30%, inadequate low technology exercise testing results, or when measured values and predictions seem discordant with an individual's reported activity tolerance, a formal cardiopulmonary exercise test should be performed (Figure 31-5). If the peak oxygen uptake is greater than 20 mL/kg/min (or 75% predicted), the patient is considered at low risk for any resection. If the peak O_2 uptake is less than 10 mL/kg/min (35% predicted), the patient is considered at high risk and conventional surgery should not be performed. Patients with a maximum O_2 consumption value between these two limits are at moderate risk and should be considered on a case-by-case basis.[33]

RULE OF THUMB

Patients with an FEV_1 greater than 80% predicted value or 2 L can safely undergo surgical resection for lung cancer, even if pneumonectomy is needed.

SCREENING

Given the poor prognosis for advanced-stage lung cancer and the high proportion of patients who present in an advanced stage, there has been great interest in **screening** for lung cancer. The earliest efforts at radiographic screening involved the analysis of mass chest radiograph screenings from the population of an individual city. Subsequently in the 1970s, there were large efforts to use chest radiograph, sputum, or a combination of the two as screening tools. Finally, a large randomized trial of chest radiography as a screening did not show any benefit. Thus screening with chest radiography is not recommended.[36-38]

Given the disappointing overall results from studies of chest radiograph as a screening technique, efforts have centered on the use of low-dose CT imaging as a screening tool.[37,38]

One trial, the National Lung Screening Trial, reported a 20% reduction in lung cancer–specific mortality in patients with very high risk for developing lung cancer. This finding has changed the clinical discussion regarding lung cancer screening. The U.S. Preventive Services Task Force gave low-dose CT chest screening a grade B recommendation for high-risk individuals (age 55 to 80 and at least 30 pack-years of current smoking [pack years = the number of packs per day × years smoked], or at least 30 pack-years of former smoking and quit within 15 years). The evidence shows that CT lung screening is most effective when patient selection adheres closely to the

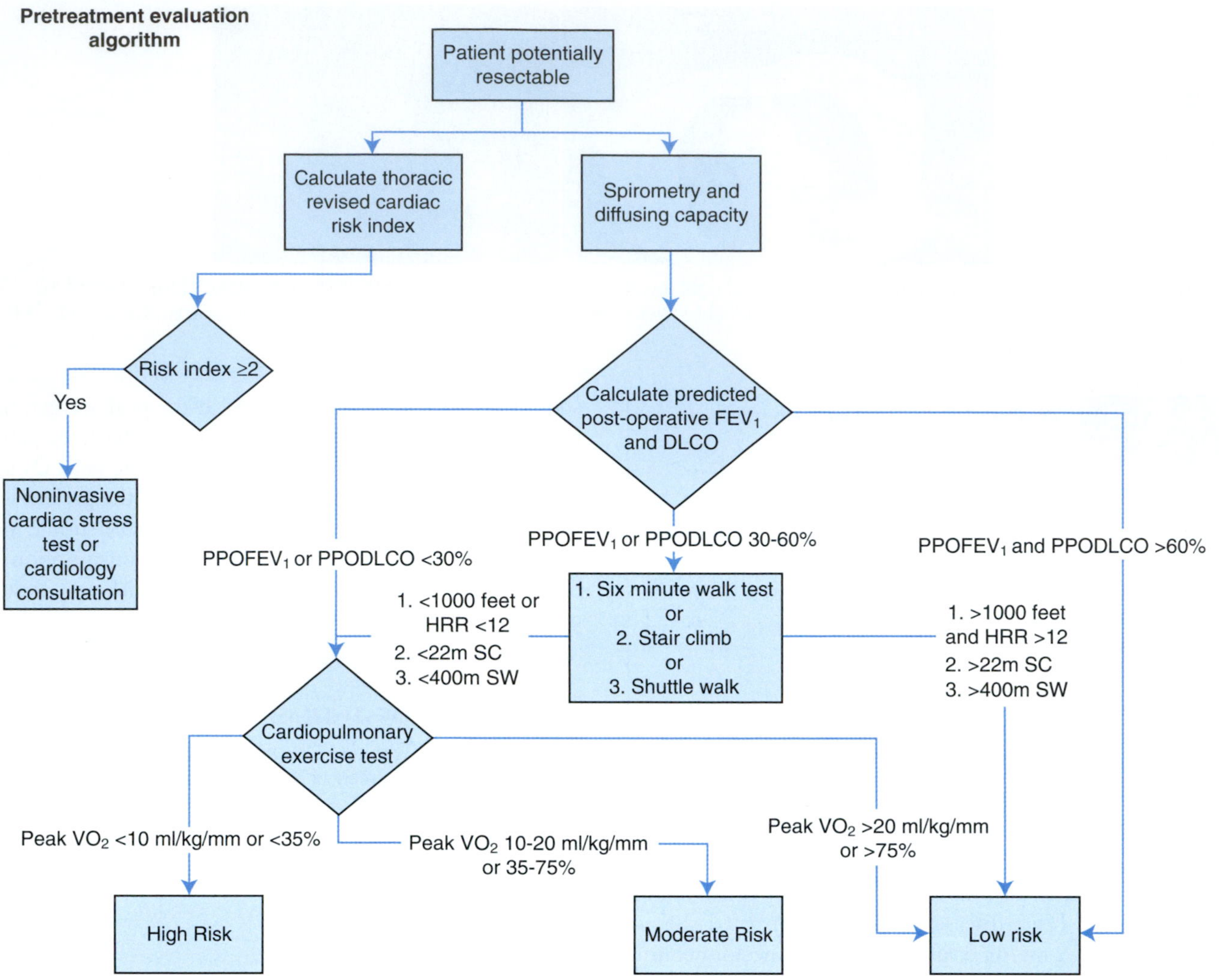

FIGURE 31-5 Algorithm for patients considered for lung resection surgery. **Note 1:** The algorithm represents an assessment of risk for traditional resection (lobectomy, pneumonectomy). One must consider the benefits of traditional resection over alternative therapies (sublobar resection, ablative therapies), the relative risks of the therapeutic choices and the patient's values when selecting treatment. **Note 2:** The 6-minute walk is included in this algorithm but is not part of other guidelines due to relatively small literature support. It is a more practical and available low-technology exercise study than the recommended tests and we have substantial experience with this test, leading us to include it in our algorithm. **Note 3:** Potential modifiers of risk include smoking cessation, adequate treatment of comorbid pulmonary conditions, preresection or postresection pulmonary rehabilitation, and the surgical approach (VATS versus thoracotomy). Each of these should be considered when assessing risk. **Note 4:** For lobectomy, the segment method or quantitative perfusion scan can be used to calculate predicted postoperative values. For pneumonectomy, the quantitative perfusion scan should be used. **Note 5:** Management of cardiac disease per American College of Cardiology/American Heart Association guidelines. *PPO,* Predicted postoperative values; *FEV_1*, forced expiratory volume in 1 second; *DLCO,* diffusion capacity for carbon monoxide; *PPO,* predicted post-operative; *HRR,* heart rate recovery; *SC,* stair climb; *SW,* shuttle walk; *VO_2*, oxygen consumption; ml/kg/min, milliliters per kilogram per minute.

criteria described earlier and when the CT is performed in a setting where expertise in lung cancer and lung nodules is available.[39–41]

TREATMENT AND OUTCOMES

Although the RT would not be administering the treatments for lung cancer, and the therapies change with advances over time, a brief discussion to familiarize the RT with the approach to treatment and the types of available therapy is important.

Non–Small Cell Lung Cancer

Three types of treatment are used to treat non–small cell lung cancer: surgical resection, **radiotherapy,** and **chemotherapy** (Box 31-4). The first two treatments provide local control of the cancer, and the last is used to treat systemic disease. Which therapy or combination of therapies is recommended depends on the stage of the cancer, the patient's ability to tolerate treatment, and the type of cancer (or its histology). Molecular changes within the tumor are beginning to influence treatment choices as well.

MINI CLINI

Lung Cancer Screening

PROBLEM: A 68-year-old man presents to the clinic with the concern of developing lung cancer in the future. He currently smokes one pack of cigarettes per day and has smoked for 45 years. He does not cough or feel shortness of breath. He has a history of high blood pressure and high cholesterol. He is otherwise in his regular state of health. Should this man have lung cancer screening?

DISCUSSION: Based on the evidence, he meets criteria to have a low-dose CT chest to screen for lung cancer. He does not have any symptoms that also make screening appropriate. A vitally important part of the conversation with this patient should be tobacco cessation. Quitting smoking at any age reduces the risk for lung cancer and other health problems.

TABLE 31-3

Non–Small Cell Lung Cancer: 5-Year Survival by Stage

Stage	Clinical Stage (%)	Pathologic Stage (%)
IA	50	73
IB	43	58
IIA	36	46
IIB	25	36
IIIA	19	24
IIIB	7	9
IV	2	13

Modified from Goldstraw P, Crowley J, Chansky K, et al; International Association for the Study of Lung Cancer International Staging Committee; IASLC Lung Cancer Staging Project: Proposals for the revision of the TNM stage groupings in the forthcoming (seventh) edition of the TNM classification of malignant tumors. *J Thorac Oncol* 2:706–714, 2007.

Box 31-4 Options for Treatment of Lung Cancer

NON–SMALL CELL

Stages IA, IB, IIA, IIB

- Surgical resection standard of care if patient deemed able to tolerate resection
- Sublobar resection if patient is unable to tolerate larger resection
- Radiotherapy, particularly stereotactic body radiotherapy in N0 disease, if patient is unable to tolerate or chooses not to undergo resection
- Adjuvant radiotherapy possibly of use if incomplete resection has occurred
- Adjuvant chemotherapy in patient with stage II disease who can tolerate it; consider in stage IB

Stage IIIA

- Concurrent chemoradiotherapy using platinum-based regimen if performance status is reasonable
- Induction chemoradiotherapy followed by resection and adjuvant chemotherapy in selected patients, ideally as part of a study protocol

Stage IIIB

- Concurrent chemoradiotherapy using platinum-based regimen if performance status is reasonable
- Induction chemoradiotherapy followed by resection in highly selected patients, only as part of a study protocol

Stage IV

- Platinum-based chemotherapy regimen in patients with adequate performance status
- Targeted therapies (EGFR, VEGF, and ALK inhibitors) in appropriate subgroups

SMALL CELL

Limited Stage

- Combination chemotherapy with concurrent hyperfractionated radiotherapy if performance status is adequate
- Prophylactic cranial radiation for patients with complete response to chemoradiotherapy

Extensive Stage

- Combination chemotherapy if performance status is adequate

Courtesy The Cleveland Clinic, Cleveland, OH.
ALK, Anaplastic lymphoma kinase; *EGFR,* epithelial growth factor receptor; *VEGF,* vascular endothelial growth factor.

Early Stage Non–Small Cell Carcinoma

Surgical resection offers the best chance of cure for early stage non–small cell lung cancer (stages I and II) (Table 31-3). Survival after resection in pathologic stage IA approaches 70% at 5 years; in pathologic stage IB, 5-year survival is closer to 55%. The surgery of choice is a *lobectomy,* in which the entire lobe of the lung containing the cancer is removed. If the tumor is very central, a pneumonectomy may be required. Sublobar resections, such as *segmentectomy,* or *wedge resection,* can be performed in patients with modest lung function to spare as much lung tissue as possible. In most patients, sublobar resection leads to a slightly lower survival rate and a higher rate of local recurrence of cancer.[42,43] In the smallest cancers and in patients who are older than 70 years, a sublobar resection may be as effective as a lobectomy.[44] Recurrence usually involves distant metastases.

Survival after resection in pathologic stage IIA is 50% to 55% at 5 years and in pathologic stage IIB is approximately 40% (see Table 31-3). Sublobar resections are not typically an option in stage II cancers. Most recurrences involve distant metastases.

Radiotherapy has been used with curative intent in early-stage non–small cell lung cancer in patients who cannot tolerate surgery or in patients who elect not to undergo surgery. The 5-year survival rate in stage I and II disease approaches 15% with standard radiotherapy alone. There is a high rate of local recurrence, and most deaths are due to lung cancer. Stereotactic body radiotherapy is a novel radiation therapy technique in which multiple convergent beams of radiation are precisely targeted on the tumor. This targeting allows very high doses of radiation to be delivered to the tumor while sparing the normal lung tissue. Rates of local control and survival are impressive in selected groups reported in many case series, approaching the rates of lung resection.[45] Lung resection and stereotactic body radiotherapy have not been compared head to head. Lung resection remains the standard of care in patients able to tolerate it. *Adjuvant* ("applied after initial treatment") radiotherapy in patients who have undergone surgical resection may improve local control but does not improve survival (with the possible exception of patients who have undergone incomplete resection).

Adjuvant platinum-based chemotherapy leads to a significant survival benefit in selected patients with completely resected stage II lung cancers.[46] The potential benefit of adjuvant chemotherapy in patients with stage IB disease is debated.

Locally and Regionally Advanced Non–Small Cell Carcinoma

Locally advanced tumors (T3) frequently can be completely resected, although central T3 tumors are less resectable than tumors involving the chest wall. The survival in patients with T3 tumors and chest wall involvement without lymph node involvement approximates the survival of other patients with stage IIB disease. The best results occur when complete resection is possible. With nodal involvement at any level, survival decreases dramatically and the tumor is classified in a higher stage. T3 involvement of the mediastinum or main stem bronchus portends a poorer prognosis, with 5-year survival rates less than 30%.

When a Pancoast tumor is present, chemoradiotherapy followed by surgical resection (lobectomy ± chest wall resection) is performed if possible. The invasion of local structures (rib, vertebral body, subclavian artery, or sympathetic chain) is a poor prognostic sign. Two-thirds of patients have a recurrence, and two-thirds of these recurrences are local.

The approach to N2 (stage IIIA, mediastinal lymph node involvement) disease varies among institutions. Patients without radiographic evidence of N2 disease but who are found at surgery to have N2 disease do better than patients with preoperative evidence of N2 disease. Adjuvant chemotherapy should be offered to this group. Generally, the more advanced the node involvement (number, extension, or location), the poorer the prognosis. Induction with chemotherapy with or without radiotherapy leads to objective responses in most patients. Patients who have bulky nodes or who require a pneumonectomy are less likely to benefit from resection after induction therapy. At the present time, concurrent chemoradiotherapy should be considered the standard of care, with resection included in specialized centers, often in the setting of a study. Survival rates are 5% to 13% at 5 years. With advances in each of the modes of therapy, treatment will evolve over time.[47–49]

T4 disease without advanced nodal status (stage IIIB) may be considered for surgical treatment in only a few settings. T4 disease involving the main carina may be considered for resection at centers with expertise. The role of induction therapy in this setting has not yet been defined. Disease at the N3 level (stage IIIB) is generally considered nonsurgical.[50,51]

Metastatic Non–Small Cell Carcinoma

In stage IV lung cancer, platinum-based chemotherapy regimens have been shown to improve survival and enhance quality of life. They are also cost-effective. This treatment is most appropriate for individuals with a good performance status. Resection of an isolated brain metastasis in patients with a good performance status can improve survival. Standard chemotherapy typically involves two agents administered in cycles, each approximately 3 weeks apart, for a total of four to six cycles. The addition of a third agent or additional cycles has traditionally added risk without benefit. More recently, agents with improved tolerance have been shown to benefit patients who have shown a good response to treatment when administered as maintenance treatment, until progression is noted.[52]

Standard chemotherapy targets all growing cells, not just cancer cells (hence the common side effects seen). Targeted therapies have been developed where the mechanism of action is more specific to the cancer cell. In lung cancer, inhibitors of epidermal growth factor receptors (EGFRs), vascular endothelial growth factor (VEGF), and anaplastic lymphoma kinase (ALK) translocations have been studied. EGFR and ALK inhibitors have been most successful in patients with EGFR-activating mutations and ALK translocations in their cancer tissue. The patients most likely to have EGFR mutations include female never-smokers with adenocarcinoma, in particular, patients of Asian origin. This subgroup has been found to have an improved survival overall, which is improved further by the use of an EGFR inhibitor. The VEGF receptor inhibitor has been shown to improve survival when added to standard chemotherapy in patients with nonsquamous cell histology. These treatments can be continued until progression is noted. Other promising agents in late-phase development include immune system stimulators.[53,54]

Small Cell Lung Cancer

Treatment of small cell lung cancer is based on its staging (see Box 31-4). In limited-stage disease, combination chemotherapy with concurrent hyperfractionated radiotherapy is recommended. The drug etoposide and a platinum agent are standard. Prophylactic brain radiation is generally recommended for patients who have a complete response to chemoradiotherapy. Surgery is limited to cases in which the diagnosis is in doubt or in rare cases that manifest as a single lung nodule. In patients with extensive-stage disease, combination chemotherapy improves the quality of life and median survival. A poor performance status and an elevated lactate dehydrogenase level portend a poor prognosis.[55]

RULE OF THUMB

Surgery is the treatment of choice for early-stage non–small cell lung cancer. Chemotherapy is the modality of choice for advanced non–small cell lung cancer. Chemotherapy with or without radiation therapy is used to treat small cell lung cancer.

Palliation of symptoms related to lung cancer is an important aspect of overall management. The judicious use of analgesic agents for pain, antiemetics for nausea, and antidepressants can improve quality of life. Radiotherapy can be used to palliate bone pain related to metastatic disease, hemoptysis, or symptoms of airway obstruction. Invasive bronchoscopic procedures (e.g., laser ablation, electrocautery, stent placement) may be palliative in patients with airway obstruction. Evidence shows that in patients with end-stage non–small cell lung cancer early integration of palliative care has an increased median survival when compared to standard aggressive treatment.[56]

FUTURE SCENARIO

The prospect of major advances in the prevention, detection, and treatment of lung cancer is strong. An attainable vision for 2034 could be as follows: Primary prevention campaigns have successfully minimized the number of individuals who are smoking, legislation has passed broadly to prevent exposure to tobacco smoke in public places, progress has been made in occupational exposure avoidance, and successful measures have been enacted to clean the air. Individuals are now identified who have changes in lung cells that suggest lung cancer could develop and are being treated with medication to prevent it from developing. Individuals at risk for developing lung cancer are part of a screening program that detects early-stage lung cancer with a test that is inexpensive and acceptable to all. Technology has improved diagnostic abilities by making imaging more specific and biopsies more accurate. Noninvasive diagnostics have expanded with advances in blood and breath testing. In addition to tumor appearance, researchers are identifying characteristics of tumor biology that allow more selection in choosing treatments. The best form of local control for a given tumor (resection, radiation) is known, and means have been developed to minimize the effect of these interventions on the quality of life. Novel agents have been developed that can reach and kill tumor cells while avoiding injury to healthy tissue. As evidence of successes, lung cancer is no longer the leading cause of cancer-related mortality in the United States.

ROLE OF THE RESPIRATORY THERAPIST IN MANAGING PATIENTS WITH LUNG CANCER

RTs perform many important roles in the evaluation and management of patients with lung cancer. Many patients in the care of the RT are smokers, and the RT has the opportunity to educate these individuals on the dangers of smoking and on the means available to help them quit. Because many of these patients also have smoking-related lung disorders (e.g., COPD), RTs can offer guidance on the proper use of inhaled medications, the use of supplemental O_2, and the role of pulmonary rehabilitation before and after treatment. Also, many RTs assist with diagnostic tests such as bronchoscopy and the measurement of pulmonary function. Finally, in the context that the RT may spend substantial time with the patient with lung cancer, the RT may be an important source of psychologic support and help. Taken together, these various diagnostic and treatment roles establish that the RT plays a crucial role in helping to manage patients with lung cancer.

MINI CLINI

Evaluating Surgical Risk

PROBLEM: A 62-year-old man with a long history of smoking has a chronic, productive cough. A chest CT obtained because of a recent episode of hemoptysis reveals a lung mass in the right upper lobe. Results of transbronchial biopsy suggest the presence of large cell carcinoma. There is no evidence of metastasis. As part of the patient's evaluation for surgery, he has the following spirometry and diffusing capacity results:

Forced vital capacity (FVC) 4.2 L (80% of predicted value)
FEV_1 1.6 L (60% of predicted value)
FEV_1/FVC 0.4
DLCO 15.5 (60% of predicted)

Can he undergo surgery?

DISCUSSION: Assessment of lung reserve is an important step in the preoperative evaluation of patients with lung cancer being considered for surgical resection. After calculating his PPO values with the segment method ($60 \times [1 - 3/19]$), he is found to have a PPO FEV_1 and PPO DLCO of 50%. This patient, similar to most patients with lung cancer, has PPO values between 30% and 60% because of underlying COPD. He needs further evaluation with exercise testing such as a stair climb or shuttle walk test to better assess his risk. Furthermore, he needs treatment optimization for his COPD. If the patient's lung function remains at moderate risk after these steps, a cardiopulmonary exercise test may help to clarify his risk.

SUMMARY CHECKLIST

- Approximately 224,210 cases of bronchogenic carcinoma were newly diagnosed in the United States in 2014, making bronchogenic carcinoma a major health hazard. It is the leading cause of cancer-related mortality in the United States.
- Approximately 85% of all cases of bronchogenic carcinoma are linked to smoking.
- The major histopathologic types of bronchogenic carcinoma include adenocarcinoma, squamous cell carcinoma, small cell carcinoma, and large cell carcinoma. Adenocarcinoma is the most common type, representing more than 40% of all cases.
- The clinical manifestations of bronchogenic carcinoma result from local growth of the tumor, regional spread, metastases to extrathoracic and intrathoracic organs, and paraneoplastic syndromes.
- The staging system most commonly used for non–small cell bronchogenic carcinoma is based on status of the primary tumor (T), local and regional lymph node involvement (N), and the presence of metastasis (M). The TNM classification groups patients in stages or categories that correlate with survival. Small cell lung cancer is classified in two stages, limited and extensive, although the TNM system can be used as well.
- The most commonly used treatments for patients with non–small cell lung cancer are surgical resection, radiation therapy, and chemotherapy. Treatment of most patients

with small cell carcinoma includes chemotherapy, with radiation therapy added if a limited stage disease.

- The most effective way to prevent lung cancer is to prevent smoking.

References

1. Siegel R, Ma J, Zou Z, et al: Cancer statistics, 2014. *CA Cancer J Clin* 64:9–29, 2014.
2. Fontham ET, Correa P, Reynolds P, et al: Environmental tobacco smoke and lung cancer in nonsmoking women: a multi-center study. *JAMA* 271:1752–1759, 1994.
3. Bartecchi CE, MacKenzie TD: Schrien RW: The human cost of tobacco use. *N Engl J Med* 330:907–912, 1994.
4. Rigotti NA, Lee JE, Wechsler H: U.S. college students' use of tobacco products: results of a national survey. *JAMA* 284:699–705, 2000.
5. Kessler DA: Nicotine addiction in young people. *N Engl J Med* 333:186–189, 1995.
6. Marshall L, Schooley M, Ryan H, et al: Youth tobacco surveillance: US, 2001–2002. *MMWR Surveill Summ* 55:1–56, 2006.
7. Iribarren C, Tekawa IS, Sidney S, et al: Effect of cigar smoking on the risk of cardiovascular disease, chronic obstructive pulmonary disease, and cancer in men. *N Engl J Med* 340:1773–1780, 1999.
8. Vineis P, Airoldi L, Veglia F, et al: Environmental tobacco smoke and risk of respiratory cancer and chronic obstructive pulmonary disease in former smokers and never smokers in the EPIC prospective study. *BMJ* 330:277–281, 2005.
9. Oberg M, Jaakkola MS, Woodward A, et al: Worldwide burden of disease from exposure to second hand smoke: a retrospective analysis of data from 193 countries. *Lancet* 377:139–146, 2011.
10. Choi H, Mazzone P: Radon and lung cancer: assessing and mitigating the risk. *Cleve Clin J Med* 81:567–575, 2014.
11. Cote ML, Kardia SLR, Wenzlaff AS, et al: Risk of lung cancer among white and black relatives of individuals with early-onset lung cancer. *JAMA* 293:3036–3042, 2005.
12. Nitadori J, Inoue M, Iwasaki M, et al: Association between lung cancer incidence and family history of lung cancer: data from a large-scale population-based cohort study, the JPHC study. *Chest* 130:968–975, 2006.
13. Dresler CM, Fratelli C, Babb J, et al: Gender differences in genetic susceptibility for lung cancer. *Lung Cancer* 30:153–160, 2000.
14. Schabath MD, Hernandez LM, Wu X, et al: Dietary phytoestrogens and lung cancer risk. *JAMA* 294:1493–1504, 2005.
15. Brennan P, Hsu C, Moullan N, et al: Effect of cruciferous vegetables on lung cancer in patients stratified by genetic status: a mendelian randomization approach. *Lancet* 366:1558–1560, 2005.
16. Virtamo J, Pietinen P, Huttunen JK, et al: ATBC Study Group: Incidence of cancer and mortality following alpha-tocopherol and beta-carotene supplementation: a postintervention follow-up. *JAMA* 290:476–485, 2003.
17. Mannino DM, Aguayo SM, Petty TL, et al: Low lung function and incident lung cancer in the United States: data from the first National Health and Nutrition Examination Survey follow-up. *Arch Intern Med* 163:1475–1480, 2003.
18. Alberg A, Brock M, Ford JG, et al: Epidemiology of lung cancer: diagnosis and management of lung cancer, ed 3, American College of Chest Physicians evidence-based clinical practice guidelines. *Chest* 143(5 Suppl):e1S–e29S, 2013.
19. Gerber RB, Mazzone PJ, Arroliga AC: Paraneoplastic syndromes associated with bronchogenic carcinoma. *Clin Chest Med* 23:257–264, 2002.
20. Mazzone P, Stoller JK: The pulmonologist's perspective regarding the solitary pulmonary nodule. *Semin Thorac Cardiovasc Surg* 14:250–260, 2002.
21. Gould MK, Maclean CC, Kuschner WG, et al: Accuracy of positron emission tomography for diagnosis of pulmonary nodules and mass lesions: a meta-analysis. *JAMA* 285:914–924, 2001.
22. Mazzone PJ, Jain P, Arroliga AC, et al: Bronchoscopy and needle biopsy techniques for the diagnosis and staging of lung cancer. *Clin Chest Med* 23:137–158, 2002.
23. Ha D, Choi H, Almeida FA, et al: Histologic and molecular characterization of lung cancer with tissue obtained by electromagnetic navigation bronchoscopy. *J Bronchology Interv Pulmonol* 20:10–15, 2013.
24. Wallace MB, Pascaul JM, Raimondo M, et al: Minimally invasive endoscopic staging of lung cancer. *JAMA* 299:540–546, 2008.
25. Detterbeck FC, Boffa DJ, Tanour LT: The new lung cancer staging system. *Chest* 126:260–271, 2009.
26. Lababede O, Meziane M, Rice T: Seventh edition of the cancer staging manual and stage grouping of lung cancer: quick reference chart and diagrams. *Chest* 139:183–189, 2011.
27. Silvestri GA, Gonzalez AV, Jantz MA, et al: Methods for staging non-small cell lung cancer staging methods for NSCLC: diagnosis and management of lung cancer, ed 3: American College of Chest Physicians evidence-based clinical practice guidelines. *Chest* 143(5 Suppl):e211S–e250S, 2013.
28. Lardinois D, Weder W, Hany TF, et al: Staging of non-small-cell lung cancer with integrated positron-emission tomography and computed tomography. *N Engl J Med* 348:2500–2507, 2003.
29. Annema JT, Versteegh MI, Veselic M, et al: Endoscopic ultrasound-guided fine-needle aspiration in the diagnosis and staging of lung cancer and its impact on surgical staging. *J Clin Oncol* 23:8357–8361, 2005.
30. Yokoi K, Kamiya N, Matsuguma H, et al: Detection of brain metastasis in potentially operable non-small cell lung cancer: a comparison of CT and MRI. *Chest* 114:714–719, 1999.
31. Pieterman RM, van Putten JW, Meuzelaar JJ, et al: Preoperative staging of non-small-cell lung cancer with positron-emission tomography. *N Engl J Med* 343:254–261, 2000.
32. Mazzone PJ, Arroliga AC: Lung cancer: preoperative pulmonary evaluation of the lung resection candidate. *Am J Med* 118:578–583, 2005.
33. Brunelli A, Kim AW, Berger KI, et al: Physiologic evaluation of the patient with lung cancer being considered for resectional surgery: diagnosis and management of lung cancer. *Chest* 143(5 Suppl):e166S–e190S, 2013.
34. Manser RL, Irving LB, Byrnes G, et al: Screening for lung cancer: a systematic review and meta-analysis of controlled trials. *Thorax* 58:784–789, 2003.
35. Henschke CI, Naidich DP, Yankelevitz DF, et al: Early Lung Cancer Action Project: initial findings on repeat screening. *Cancer* 92:153–159, 2001.
36. Swensen SJ, Jett JR, Hartman TE, et al: CT screening for lung cancer: five-year prospective experience. *Radiology* 235:259–265, 2005.
37. Mahadevia PJ, Fleisher LA, Frick KD, et al: Lung cancer screening with helical computed tomography in older adult smokers: a decision and cost-effectiveness analysis. *JAMA* 289:313–322, 2003.
38. International Early Lung Cancer Action Program Investigators, Henschke CI, Yankelevitz DF, et al: Survival of patients with stage I lung cancer detected on CT screening. *N Engl J Med* 355:1763–1771, 2006.
39. National Lung Cancer Screening Research Team, Aberle DR, Berg CD, et al: The National Lung Cancer Screening Trial: overview and study design. *Radiology* 258:243–253, 2011.
40. Mazzone P: Lung cancer screening: examining the issues. *Cleve Clin J Med* 79(electronic Suppl 1):eS1–eS16, 2012.
41. Hocking W, Hu P, Oken M, et al: Lung cancer screening in the randomized prostate, lung, colorectal, and ovarian (PLCO) cancer screening trial. *J Natl Cancer Inst* 102:722–731, 2010.
42. Ginsberg RJ, Rubenstein LV: Randomized trial of lobectomy versus limited resection for T1N0 non-small cell lung cancer. Lung Cancer Study Group. *Ann Thorac Surg* 60:615–622, 1995.
43. Landreneau RJ, Sugarbaker DJ, Mack MJ, et al: Wedge resection versus lobectomy for stage I (T1N0M0) non-small-cell lung cancer. *J Thorac Cardiovasc Surg* 113:691–700, 1997.
44. Okada M, Nishio W, Sakamoto T, et al: Effect of tumor size on prognosis in patients with non-small cell lung cancer: the role of segmentectomy as a type of lesser resection. *J Thorac Cardiovasc Surg* 129:87–93, 2005.
45. Timmerman R, Paulus R, Galvin J, et al: Stereotactic body radiation therapy for inoperable early stage lung cancer. *JAMA* 303:1070–1076, 2010.
46. Arriagada R, Bergman B, Dunant A, et al: International Adjuvant Lung Cancer Trial Collaborative Group: Cisplatin-based adjuvant chemotherapy

in patients with completely resected non-small-cell lung cancer. *N Engl J Med* 350:351–360, 2004.

47. Spira A, Ettinger DS: Multidisciplinary management of lung cancer. *N Engl J Med* 350:379–392, 2004.
48. Georgoulias V, Papadakis E, Alexopoulos A, et al: Platinum-based and non-platinum-based chemotherapy in advanced non-small-cell lung cancer: a randomised multicentre trial. *Lancet* 357:1478–1484, 2001.
49. Albain KS, Swann RS, Rusch VW, et al: Radiotherapy plus chemotherapy with or without surgical resection for stage III non-small-cell lung cancer: a phase III randomised controlled trial. *Lancet* 374:379–386, 2009.
50. van Meerbeeck JP, Kramer GW, Van Schil PE, et al: Randomized controlled trial of resection versus radiotherapy after induction chemotherapy in stage IIIA-N2 non- small-cell lung cancer. *J Natl Cancer Inst* 99:442–450, 2007.
51. Azzoli CG, Baker S, Jr, Temin S, et al: American Society of Clinical Oncology Clinical Practice Guideline update on chemotherapy for stage IV non-small-cell lung cancer. *J Clin Oncol* 27:6251–6266, 2009.
52. Sharma SV, Bell DW, Settleman J, et al: Epidermal growth factor receptor mutations in lung cancer. *Nat Rev Cancer* 7:169–181, 2007.
53. Silvestri GA, Rivera P: Targeted therapy for the treatment of advanced non-small cell lung cancer: a review of the epidermal growth factor receptor antagonists. *Chest* 128:3975–3984, 2005.
54. Kwak EL, Bang Y, Camidge R, et al: Anaplastic lymphoma kinase inhibition in non-small cell lung cancer. *N Engl J Med* 363:1693–1703, 2010.
55. Jackman DM, Johnson BE: Small-cell lung cancer. *Lancet* 366:1385–1396, 2005.
56. Kelley AU, Meier AS: Palliative care-a shifting paradigm. *N Engl J Med* 363:781–782, 2010.

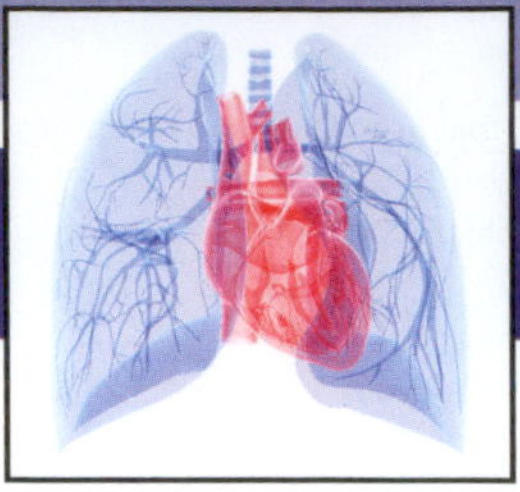

CHAPTER 32

Neuromuscular and Other Diseases of the Chest Wall

RENDELL W. ASHTON

CHAPTER OBJECTIVES

After reading this chapter you will be able to:

- Identify pulmonary function test results typically seen in patients with neuromuscular disease.
- List the potential respiratory complications associated with neuromuscular disease.
- Identify the clinical signs and symptoms associated with respiratory muscle weakness.
- Describe techniques for monitoring patients with respiratory muscle weakness.
- Describe general respiratory care management of patients with respiratory muscle weakness.
- Describe the clinical findings and treatment for each of the following neuromuscular disorders: Duchenne muscular dystrophy, myotonic dystrophy, polymyositis, myasthenia gravis, Lambert-Eaton syndrome, Guillain-Barré syndrome, unilateral diaphragmatic paralysis, amyotrophic lateral sclerosis, critical illness myopathy and polyneuropathy, spinal cord injury, stroke, traumatic brain injury, kyphoscoliosis, and flail chest.
- Understand the role of the RT in caring for patients with neuromuscular and chest wall diseases.

CHAPTER OUTLINE

General Principles Related to Neuromuscular Weakness of the Ventilatory Muscles
- Pathophysiology and Pulmonary Function Testing
- Clinical Signs and Symptoms
- Monitoring and Assessing Patients With Muscle Weakness for Respiratory Insufficiency

Management of Respiratory Muscle Weakness

Specific Neuromuscular Diseases
- Disorders of the Muscle (Myopathic Disease)
- Disorders of the Neuromuscular Junction
- Disorders of the Nerves
- Disorders of the Spinal Cord
- Disorders of the Brain

Disorders of the Thoracic Cage
- Kyphoscoliosis
- Flail Chest
- Ankylosing Spondylitis

The Role of Respiratory Therapists in Caring for Patients With Neuromuscular Weakness and Other Diseases of the Chest Wall

KEY TERMS

amyotrophic lateral sclerosis
ankylosing spondylitis
apneustic breathing
ataxic breathing
Becker muscular dystrophy
central neurogenic hyperventilation
Cheyne-Stokes respirations
critical illness myopathy
critical illness polyneuropathy
dermatomyositis
Duchenne muscular dystrophy
flail chest
gasping
Guillain-Barré syndrome
inclusion body myositis
kyphoscoliosis
Lambert-Eaton syndrome
Lou Gehrig disease
myasthenia gravis
myopathy
myositis
myotonic dystrophy
neuropathy
Ondine curse
paradoxical motion
periodic breathing
polymyositis
stroke
traumatic brain injury

Neuromuscular diseases are the group of conditions that affect the strength and ability of muscles to function. In addition to the lungs, which provide an interface between inhaled air and circulating blood, the respiratory system includes the *thoracic cage,* which forms the structure of the ventilatory pump, and the *muscles of respiration,* whose action on the thoracic cage produces movement of air into and out of the lungs. Diseases that affect the brain, nerves, muscles, or thoracic cage can lead to respiratory failure or hypoxemia even if the lungs are normal.

Understanding the interactions between these components is essential to understanding how their dysfunction leads to disease. The neuromuscular components of the respiratory system are shown in Figure 32-1. Maintenance of normal ventilation depends on intact, functional components of the neuromuscular system, which contribute to breathing in three main ways: (1) regulation of respiratory drive and rate, (2) control of the mechanics of ventilation, and (3) cough and other airway protection. The pulmonary consequences of neuromuscular disease include the following:

1. Dysregulation of respiratory drive or rate
   - Hyperventilation
   - Hypoventilation
   - Central apnea
   - Other pathologic breathing patterns (listed in Table 32-4)
2. Loss of strength or control of the mechanics of breathing
   - Respiratory failure as a result of excessive work of breathing
   - Atelectasis leading to hypoxemia
   - Secondary effects of chronic hypoxemia (e.g., pulmonary hypertension, cor pulmonale)
3. Loss of strength or control of the muscles responsible for airway protection and cough
   - Aspiration
   - Obstructive apnea
   - Mucous plugging
   - Pneumonia

Some systemic diseases that affect the neuromuscular system also cause interstitial lung disease, which can lead to considerable respiratory dysfunction (see Chapter 26). Respiratory failure, often associated with pulmonary infection, is a frequent cause of death in patients with neuromuscular disorders.

A thorough understanding of the physiology of ventilation and chest wall mechanics (see Chapters 11 and 19) is needed to understand how abnormalities of the upper airway, chest wall, diaphragm, and abdominal muscles cause disease. This chapter reviews major disorders of the neuromuscular and skeletal systems that affect breathing. Disorders are grouped according to which functional unit of the neuromuscular system is affected, focusing on pulmonary manifestations of these disease processes (Table 32-1).

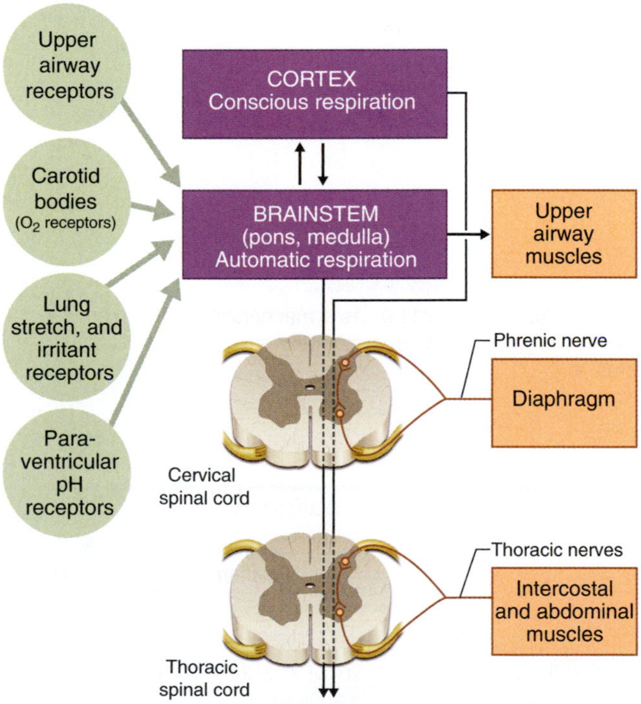

FIGURE 32-1 The neuromuscular components of the respiratory system include elements of the cortex (which allow conscious alteration of breathing) and motor centers (which maintain upper airway tone). Brainstem structures receive input from peripheral oxygen, pH, and stretch receptors and generate automatic respiration. Efferent nerves carry central nervous impulses to the muscles of respiration through the phrenic and spinal nerves, which drive the muscles of respiration.

GENERAL PRINCIPLES RELATED TO NEUROMUSCULAR WEAKNESS OF THE VENTILATORY MUSCLES

This section describes the evaluation and testing of patients with suspected neuromuscular weakness of the respiratory muscles, regardless of the disease causing the weakness.

TABLE 32-1

Locations at Which Several Neuromuscular Diseases Affect the Respiratory System

Location	Disease
Cerebral cortex, brainstem (including the respiratory center) and upper motor neurons	Stroke, traumatic brain injury
Spinal cord	Trauma, transverse myelitis, multiple sclerosis
Anterior horn cells (lower motor neurons)	ALS, spinal muscular atrophy, poliomyelitis, and postpoliomyelitis
Peripheral nerves	Guillain-Barré syndrome, critical illness polyneuropathy, Lyme disease
Neuromuscular junction	Myasthenia gravis, Lambert-Eaton syndrome, botulism
Muscle	Duchenne muscular dystrophy, polymyositis, acid maltase deficiency
Interstitial lung disease*	Polymyositis, dermatomyositis, tuberous sclerosis, neurofibromatosis

*A category of systemic diseases that can affect neuromuscular function as well as lung function.

Pathophysiology and Pulmonary Function Testing

Weakness of the respiratory muscles leads to the inability to generate or maintain normal respiratory pressures. Pulmonary function testing in patients with neuromuscular weakness typically reveals a restrictive ventilatory defect even if the lungs are normal. Vital capacity (VC), forced expiratory volume in 1 second (FEV_1), and total lung capacity (TLC) are decreased. Functional residual capacity is normal or decreased. Residual volume (RV) may be increased, especially as weakness becomes more severe. Diffusing capacity corrected for alveolar volume is usually normal or near-normal but can be decreased.[1] Comparison of spirometric results obtained with the patient in seated and supine positions can be useful in showing that orthopnea is caused by neuromuscular weakness. A decrease in VC or FEV_1 of 20% or more when a patient moves from the seated to the supine position suggests diaphragmatic weakness (Table 32-2 and Figure 32-2). The inability to generate normal respiratory pressures is reflected in a decreased maximal inspiratory pressure (PImax), which is generally specific for diaphragm weakness. Expiratory muscle weakness is characterized by a decreased maximal expiratory pressure (PEmax) and is not specific to any single muscle group.[2]

Arterial blood gases (Pmax) in the setting of a rapid, shallow breathing pattern may show a decreased $PaCO_2$, although progressive inspiratory muscle weakness leads to hypoventilation and hypercapnia. Hypoxemia can occur in patients unable to take deep breaths and may be caused by microatelectasis, which leads to ventilation/perfusion ($\dot{V}/\dot{Q}$) mismatching within the lung and a resulting decrease in PaO_2 (Figure 32-3). Chronic hypoxemia in this situation may be protective against acute respiratory muscle failure. Some studies suggest that when hypoxemia is chronic, it may increase diaphragm muscle endurance.[3] Hypoventilation that occurs with progressive neuromuscular disease may be a protective mechanism that avoids acute respiratory muscle fatigue. However, when hypoxemia is acute, it potentiates respiratory muscle fatigue, hastening respiratory failure.[4]

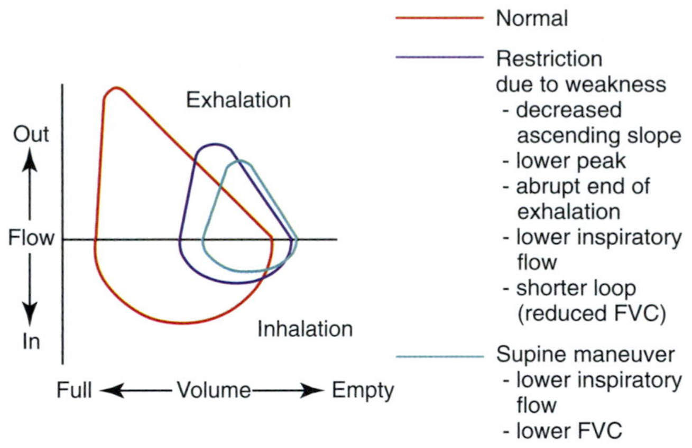

FIGURE 32-2 Normal flow-volume loop compared with loops from a patient with neuromuscular weakness, showing characteristic ventilatory restriction, which worsens when the patient is placed in the supine position. *FVC,* Forced vital capacity.

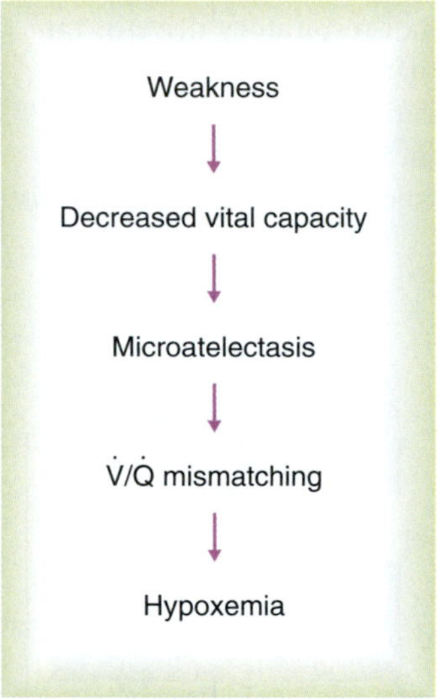

FIGURE 32-3 Atelectasis as a mechanism of hypoxemia in patients with respiratory muscle weakness. $\dot{V}/\dot{Q}$, Ventilation/perfusion.

TABLE 32-2

Pulmonary Function Testing Results from a Patient With Profound Diaphragm Weakness

	Predicted Value	Lower Limit of Normal	Sitting Position	% of Predicted	Supine Position	% Change from Sitting
FVC	4.42	3.55	1.85	42	0.89	–52
FEV_1	3.36	2.62	1.51	45	0.68	–55
FEV_1/FVC	75.88	66.20	81.75	108	75.76	–7
TLC	6.53	4.92	4.21	64		
RV	2.10	1.34	2.39	114		
DLCO	24.93	16.67	17.16	69		
DLCO/VA	3.88	2.38	5.57	144		
PImax	110.58	75.02	18.46	17		
PEmax	207.29	140.04	26.52	13		

DLCO, Diffusing capacity for carbon dioxide; *DLCO/VA, DLCO* divided by alveolar volume; *FEV_1,* forced expiratory volume in 1 second; *FVC,* forced vital capacity; *PEmax,* decreased maximum expiratory pressure; *PImax,* decreased maximal inspiratory pressure; *RV,* residual volume; *TLC,* total lung capacity.

RULE OF THUMB

Neuromuscular weakness of the respiratory muscles may be present before any substantial decrease in VC or FEV_1 is noticed. Values of PEmax may be decreased by 50% or more before any decrease in VC or FEV_1 is noticed.

Clinical Signs and Symptoms

In the early stages of neuromuscular disease, patients with respiratory muscle weakness initially report exertional dyspnea and fatigue. As the disease process progresses, patients may complain of orthopnea or symptoms of cor pulmonale (remodeling of the right ventricle, usually in response to pulmonary hypertension, which causes symptoms of dyspnea, fatigue, anorexia, chest pain, and syncope). These symptoms occur because the muscles involved with respiration can no longer generate or maintain normal ventilation. The response to hypoxemia and respiratory drive is preserved in most patients with neuromuscular weakness.[5] This drive is assessed by a measurement of the negative airway pressure generated during 100 msec of airway occlusion, the so-called *airway occlusion pressure,* abbreviated P0.1, which indicates respiratory effort and intact pathways from the respiratory center in the brainstem to the muscles of respiration. Because these patients often do not have the strength to take deep breaths, they maintain minute ventilation by increasing respiratory rate and adopting a rapid, shallow breathing pattern, which uses less respiratory muscle strength but provides less efficient ventilation. Patients with poor inspiratory muscle function (especially diaphragm weakness) may have marked orthopnea and prefer to sleep in a seated position. They also may experience a decline in voice volume, power, or quality. Muscle weakness can progress to the point at which adequate ventilation is no longer maintained and hypercapnia occurs.

RULE OF THUMB

When a patient complains of immediate shortness of breath on lying down, especially if one side is worse than the other, the problem is diaphragm weakness until proved otherwise.

Monitoring and Assessing Patients With Muscle Weakness for Respiratory Insufficiency

If respiratory muscle weakness progresses and cannot be stopped, the eventual result is respiratory failure. The onset of respiratory failure is acute or chronic depending on the time course of the disease process and the circumstances of the patient. When this progression toward respiratory failure is noted, careful follow-up and monitoring of symptoms and pulmonary function are necessary to assess the need for mechanical ventilation.

MINI CLINI

Consider Neuromuscular Weakness When a Patient Complains of Dyspnea

PROBLEM: A 27-year-old woman was referred to the pulmonary clinic for persistent shortness of breath for 2 months, along with a sore throat and a hoarse voice. The symptoms had begun with a viral syndrome including sore throat, myalgias, and fever, progressing to cough and chest discomfort. All symptoms except her shortness of breath and hoarseness had resolved. She complained of being particularly short of breath while lying down and not being able to lie down on her left side at all because she felt she could not breathe in that position. She also described running out of breath in the middle of sentences and of her voice having a hoarse, "airy" quality. She had been evaluated previously, including a normal chest radiography and spirometry, and had been told her dyspnea was due to anxiety. No other diagnosis was made. What clues in her history might suggest a pulmonary disease, and what additional testing could help identify it?

DISCUSSION: This patient had already been evaluated and had been told that her dyspnea was psychologic because her chest radiography and standard pulmonary function testing were normal. Spirometry was within the normal range of values, but when repeated in the supine position, FVC decreased by 41%. Lung volumes were normal except for a slight elevation of residual volume. Diffusing capacity also was normal. A fluoroscopic sniff test, in which her diaphragms were visualized in real time as she performed a simple sniff maneuver, showed paradoxical motion of the right hemidiaphragm. She was diagnosed with neuralgic amyotrophy, a rare neuromuscular condition affecting the phrenic nerve, which is often triggered by a viral syndrome and which usually improves gradually with time.

The important clue that led to the diagnosis of neuromuscular weakness was her complaint of orthopnea, especially the inability to breathe comfortably lying on one specific side. When one diaphragm is weak or paralyzed, a patient often cannot breathe when lying on the opposite side because this prevents the good side from compensating for the weak side. When the details of her history were recognized as classic symptoms of diaphragm weakness, testing to establish the diagnosis was straightforward.

PROBLEM: What physical findings may suggest respiratory distress in a patient with diaphragmatic weakness?

DISCUSSION: Patients whose diaphragmatic strength is inadequate to meet their ventilatory needs may use *accessory* muscles of inspiration. The sternocleidomastoid, intercostal, and scalene muscles all may be activated in the setting of respiratory distress. Use of these muscles in the setting of a weak or paralyzed diaphragm can lead to cephalad movement of the diaphragm during inspiration that is accompanied by paradoxical inward movement of the abdomen during inspiration (which is called *paradoxical breathing*). The presence of these signs in this patient should prompt evaluation of ventilatory adequacy and the need for ventilatory support.

Monitoring the ventilatory function of a patient with neuromuscular weakness can involve repeated measurement of inspiratory pressure, VC, and ABG values. Depending on the condition, the need for mechanical support can be signaled by reaching either a critical value on testing or an overall clinical condition that does not allow unassisted ventilation to continue. Additional measurements that may indicate early respiratory insufficiency, at least in amyotrophic lateral sclerosis, include maximal sniff nasal inspiratory force[2] and nocturnal oximetry.[6]

At least two caveats to this general approach should be mentioned. First, patients with myasthenia gravis having an acute myasthenic crisis may have normal test results within minutes of acute ventilatory failure because of the nature of the disorder.[7] Second, the need to protect the upper airway from secretions and aspiration may not be clearly reflected in results of pulmonary function tests, which evaluate only the mechanical function of the ventilatory pump.

Neuromuscular weakness may not manifest uniformly in all muscle groups. Ventilation may be only moderately reduced in patients with gross oropharyngeal dysfunction leading to aspiration. Patients with ventilatory weakness can have a high risk for acute respiratory failure if upper respiratory tract infection or pneumonia develops. In these patients, inability to clear secretions can increase the work of breathing; the results are muscle fatigue, hypoventilation, and acute respiratory failure.

Patients with significant weakness of the respiratory muscles can have a high risk for respiratory failure when any additional process increases the work of breathing. Pulmonary edema, pneumonia, and mucous plugging are examples of clinical conditions that can precipitate respiratory failure rapidly in patients with significant neuromuscular weakness. Although the underlying disease may not have progressed to the point that these patients need continual or routine ventilatory support at their baseline function, that support may be critical in the setting of acute, exacerbating illness.

Nocturnal oximetry or formal sleep testing with polysomnography may be suggested in some clinical settings when patients have cor pulmonale, sleep disturbance, or excessive daytime somnolence that is otherwise unexplained.

MINI CLINI

Assessment of a Patient With Neuromuscular Weakness

PROBLEM: A 50-year-old man with ALS is admitted to the hospital because of right lower lobe pneumonia. The patient is moderately hypoxemic, with PO_2 of 68 mm Hg on room air. ALS was diagnosed 3 years previously, and he has had progressive worsening of dyspnea since then. These symptoms first occurred with mild exertion and then with supine position, which the patient has noticed in the last 1 or 2 months. A recent measurement of VC at the physician's office was 35 ml/kg. The patient has recent noticed difficulty with swallowing and frequent coughing at meals. What features in the patient's history may be relevant with regard to management?

DISCUSSION: This patient has a disease that is associated with respiratory compromise, which progresses slowly in most cases, in contrast to the acute case described here. All patients with ALS ultimately have respiratory insufficiency. The earliest symptom of neuromuscular weakness in the respiratory muscles is exertional dyspnea, which this patient has had for some time. A more significant finding is orthopnea, which is highly suggestive of diaphragmatic weakness. Patients with significant diaphragmatic weakness prefer an upright position, which allows the abdominal contents to shift toward the feet and allows unimpeded diaphragmatic descent. Although the patient may not have had a critically low VC recently, this value is low. Additional loading of already compromised ventilatory machinery can lead to fatigue and frank respiratory failure. It is important to recognize that the underlying neuromuscular weakness coupled with pneumonia may predispose this patient to respiratory fatigue and subsequent respiratory failure. The history of feeding difficulty may suggest that the pneumonia is related to aspiration. The location of pneumonia in the lower lobe also favors the diagnosis if the aspiration occurred when the patient was seated upright.

MANAGEMENT OF RESPIRATORY MUSCLE WEAKNESS

Respiratory insufficiency and failure to clear secretions are the major consequences of inspiratory and expiratory muscle weakness. Treatment of these patients involves consideration of mechanical ventilation via face mask or other noninvasive interfaces or via tracheostomy. Although often overlooked, therapies to augment secretion clearance and assist with cough are important in these patients (see Chapters 42 and 43). Used together, these interventions can decrease hospitalizations for respiratory complications in patients with neuromuscular disease.[8] These measures also may be useful in delaying or preventing the need for intubation or tracheostomy, although severe bulbar muscle weakness may limit a patient's ability to avoid invasive ventilatory support.[9] In addition to these interventions, general rehabilitation focusing on aerobic conditioning, muscle strengthening, and respiratory muscle training often can delay the need for ventilatory support and improve the overall quality of life for patients with muscle weakness.[10]

Noninvasive ventilation is being used increasingly for short-term and intermittent ventilatory support of patients with neuromuscular disease.[11] Acute deterioration, such as during pneumonia, and surgical procedures such as gastrostomy tube insertion are situations in which noninvasive ventilation is safe and effective if used carefully.[9,12] If a patient needs long-term ventilatory support on an intermittent basis, such as at night only, noninvasive ventilation may be appropriate.[13] Decisions to begin mechanical ventilation in some patients with neuromuscular weakness have varied greatly among physicians[14] and may be motivated by many different patient factors.[15] No uniform guidelines exist for the use of long-term mechanical ventilation for patients with neuromuscular weakness. However, it is considered a standard option for patients who have reached the point of respiratory failure. Starting a patient on long-term mechanical ventilation requires careful planning and consideration of various issues related to respiratory care in alternative settings. These issues have been addressed in consensus statements[16,17] and are discussed in Chapter 56.

Diaphragm pacing in patients with spinal cord injury has been described using direct stimulation of an intact phrenic nerve to contract the diaphragm and produce negative intrathoracic pressure and inspiration.[18] This technique usually requires a thoracotomy, with its associated risks and high cost, and carries some risk for phrenic nerve injury. These objections have led to the development of an alternative system for diaphragm pacing using direct pacing of the diaphragm muscle by laparoscopically implanted electrodes.[19] When the electrodes can be placed in the diaphragm muscle at an electrophysiologically mapped *motor point,* the result is often elimination of the need for mechanical ventilation in patients with spinal cord injury and delay in the need to start mechanical ventilation in patients with ALS and other progressive neuromuscular diseases.[20]

MINI CLINI

Care of a Patient With Neuromuscular Weakness

PROBLEM: A 45-year-old man has myotonic dystrophy. He has progressive dyspnea that has increased, particularly in the last year. PCO_2 determined from ABG analysis is 55 mm Hg. VC is 45% of the predicted value. The patient has no underlying lung disease. Cough is decreased, but the patient maintains adequate control of secretions. The patient sleeps in a seated to semirecumbent position. What interventions are indicated for this patient?

DISCUSSION: The patient has a disease that can result in respiratory insufficiency. VC is decreased, and arterial carbon dioxide levels are increased. These factors are consistent with hypoventilation secondary to neuromuscular weakness. The patient has dyspnea on exertion and orthopnea. All these factors suggest that mechanical ventilation should be considered.

Noninvasive positive pressure ventilation (NIPPV) may be a reasonable first choice in the care of this patient. The patient's mental status and bulbar function are intact. He has no significant problems with secretions. (Important factors for successful application of NIPPV are discussed in Chapter 49.) Use of a nasal mask with a biphasic positive airway pressure unit may be instituted and titrated to patient tolerance. (Most pressure or volume-cycled ventilators can be used to deliver NIPPV and invasive ventilation.) A time-cycled backup rate can be set on some ventilators to facilitate ventilation of patients who may inadequately trigger the ventilator. If the ability to clear secretions becomes compromised, cough augmentation strategies should be implemented. As long as bulbar function—swallowing and secretion management—are maintained, noninvasive ventilation is a reasonable choice for ventilatory support.

RULE OF THUMB

Patients with neuromuscular weakness who require noninvasive ventilation generally prefer a low expiratory pressure (2 to 3 cm H_2O) with a significantly higher inspiratory pressure (7 to 15 cm H_2O).

SPECIFIC NEUROMUSCULAR DISEASES

Disorders of the Muscle (Myopathic Disease)

Primary muscle disease can decrease the ability of a normal neural impulse to generate effective muscle contraction. Some commonly recognized myopathies include Duchenne muscular dystrophy, myotonic dystrophy, and polymyositis. Box 32-1 presents a more complete list of myopathic diseases associated with ventilatory dysfunction.

Duchenne Muscular Dystrophy and Becker Muscular Dystrophy

Duchenne muscular dystrophy (DMD) is a genetic muscle-wasting disorder caused by mutations in the dystrophin gene.[21] Because it is an X-linked recessive disorder, it affects mostly males. The diagnosis is made when a dystrophin mutation is

Box 32-1 Myopathic Diseases With Associated Respiratory Dysfunction

MUSCULAR DYSTROPHIES
- Duchenne muscular dystrophy
- Becker muscular dystrophy
- Myotonic dystrophy
- Facioscapulohumeral muscular dystrophy
- Limb-girdle dystrophy
- Oculopharyngeal dystrophy

MYOPATHIES
- Congenital myopathies
- Nemaline rod myopathy
- Centronuclear myopathy
- Metabolic myopathies
- Acid maltase deficiency
- Mitochondrial myopathies (Kearns-Sayre syndrome)
- Inflammatory myopathies
- Polymyositis
- Dermatomyositis
- Hypothyroid-related and hyperthyroid-related myopathies
- Endocrine myopathies
- Steroid-induced myopathies (including critical illness myopathy)
- Miscellaneous myopathies
- Electrolyte disorders (e.g., hypophosphatemia, hypokalemia)
- Rhabdomyolysis
- Periodic paralysis
- Postneuromuscular blockade myopathy

found in DNA from circulating white blood cells or when dystrophin is found to be absent or abnormal in biopsied muscle tissue.

DMD manifests early in life with proximal muscle weakness that leads to a waddling gait, exaggerated lumbar curvature (lordosis), and frequent falls. Most affected children need a wheelchair by 12 years of age. Death generally occurs by 20 years of age, usually as a result of declining respiratory muscle strength and subsequent infection. **Becker muscular dystrophy**, a milder form of DMD, also is associated with the dystrophin gene and manifests later in life.

Other systemic effects of DMD include scarring of the left ventricle and decreased bowel motility (intestinal pseudoobstruction). The progressive decline in respiratory function in patients with DMD parallels limb weakness and typically manifests at the time of wheelchair dependence. Respiratory failure is primarily due to loss of muscle strength and features a lower PImax at all lung volumes than is present in healthy persons.

Progressive scoliosis is associated with DMD and can contribute further to respiratory insufficiency. Many patients undergo spine fusion surgery, and often the procedure allows greater comfort and ease in maintaining an upright posture. Although no randomized trials have proved any benefit of surgery on pulmonary function,[22] it appears that the rate of respiratory decline is slower after fusion surgery.[23]

Obstructive sleep apnea is present in a significant proportion of patients with DMD, prompting some experts to recommend formal polysomnography in patients with symptoms of obstructive sleep apnea or at the time of becoming wheelchair-bound.[24] Instituting positive pressure ventilation (PPV) is a decision most patients face at some point in the disease. The point at which to begin different methods of ventilatory support depends on both test results and clinical condition. Nocturnal PPV is usually indicated when FVC reaches 30% of predicted with signs of hypoventilation.[25,26] It can be started in response to oxygen (O_2) desaturation during sleep, which is common in patients with increased disability and scoliosis.

Nocturnal ventilation usually improves daytime ventilatory function in patients with DMD,[27] presumably through prevention of respiratory muscle fatigue. Despite this improvement, studies of early "prophylactic" PPV for patients with DMD have shown that early PPV failed to delay the need for invasive ventilatory support.[28] Long-term inspiratory muscle training using resistive loading has been shown to improve PImax in patients with DMD and VC of at least 27%,[29] theoretically delaying the need for ventilatory support. Although there are concerns that pulmonary rehabilitation might produce deleterious effects through overloading weak respiratory muscles, such concerns have not been confirmed in studies in Becker muscular dystrophy.[30]

Myotonic Dystrophy

Myotonic dystrophy is the most common form of muscular dystrophy in adults, with an estimated frequency of 1 in 8000 persons.[31] *Myotonia,* or delayed muscle relaxation, is the hallmark of this neuromuscular disorder but does not clearly target respiratory muscles or directly cause respiratory insufficiency.[32] This autosomal dominant disorder causes progressive muscle weakness, abnormalities of the cardiac conduction system, endocrine dysfunction, and cataracts. There are two main types of myotonic dystrophy, both caused by an expansion of a repeated DNA sequence on chromosome 19.[33]

Respiratory dysfunction in myotonic dystrophy is common, usually occurring late in the course of disease, and can include respiratory muscle weakness, obstructive sleep apnea, central sleep apnea, and bulbar muscle dysfunction leading to aspiration. Sleep-related disorders are particularly common, even at an early age.[34]

Patients with myotonic dystrophy can be very sensitive to anesthesia and respiratory depressants. Both respiratory failure and prolonged neuromuscular blockade have been reported in patients with myotonic dystrophy given usual doses of these agents. For this reason, prolonged perioperative monitoring after surgery is important.[35,36]

Nocturnal ventilation by nasal mask often is effective for these patients and should be considered if the patient has declining SaO_2 or hypercapnia. If patients develop central hypoventilation, they may require tracheostomy and mechanical ventilation. Because cough is often weak, cough assistive devices and techniques may play an important role to clear secretions.

Polymyositis

Polymyositis, **dermatomyositis**, and **inclusion body myositis** are inflammatory myopathies of unknown cause. Respiratory compromise is rare in inclusion body myositis but can be seen in both polymyositis and dermatomyositis. Clinical respiratory muscle weakness is uncommon but can lead to respiratory weakness or failure within weeks to months in the setting of rapidly progressing disease. Diagnosis of these diseases is based on clinical findings of myalgia, elevated muscle enzyme levels (creatine phosphokinase or aldolase), and compatible electromyographic or muscle biopsy results. Diagnostic criteria may apply to any inflammatory **myopathy**, and specific findings or antibody identification may be needed to differentiate the various diseases (Table 32-3).[37,38]

Ventilatory insufficiency and failure caused by these inflammatory myopathies are unusual but tend to parallel the development of limb muscle weakness when they occur. In rare instances, diaphragmatic function is decreased disproportionately to the degree of limb weakness.[39]

Corticosteroids are important in the initial management of polymyositis and dermatomyositis, although other immunosuppressive and cytotoxic regimens are used to limit long-term steroid exposure; 35% to 40% of patients with inflammatory myopathy have interstitial lung disease associated with their myopathy. This lung disease appears as diffuse interstitial infiltrates that may be caused by various lung processes, but the most common (56%) is nonspecific interstitial pneumonia.[40] Various antisynthetase antibodies (e.g., the Jo-1 antibody) have been identified that are associated with polymyositis and dermatomyositis,[41-43] although the role of these antibodies in these

TABLE 32-3

Diagnostic Criteria for Inflammatory Myopathies

Criterion	Polymyositis	Dermatomyositis	Inclusion Body Myositis
Symmetric proximal muscle weakness on physical examination	Yes	Yes	May be asymmetric and more distal weakness
Elevation of serum muscle enzymes (creatine kinase, aldolase, glutamate oxaloacetate, pyruvate transaminases, and lactate dehydrogenase)	Yes	Yes	Yes, lower levels than in polymyositis or dermatomyositis
Electromyographic triad of (1) short, small polyphasic potentials, (2) fibrillations, (3) high-frequency repetitive discharges	Yes	Yes	Yes
Muscle biopsy showing mononuclear inflammation, phagocytosis, necrosis, degeneration, and regeneration	Yes	Yes	Yes, may have fatty infiltration
Skin findings: Gottron sign and papules; heliotrope rash	No	Common	No
Anti–Jo-1 antibody (or other antisynthetase antibodies)	30%-50%, may indicate antisynthetase syndrome		No
Interstitial lung disease	86% in patients with antisynthetase syndrome		No

MINI CLINI

Care of an Intensive Care Unit Patient to Minimize the Risk for Critical Care Myopathy

PROBLEM: A 60-year-old man is in the ICU with respiratory failure secondary to severe influenza pneumonia. He has developed acute respiratory distress syndrome (ARDS), and gas exchange is severely impaired, with a PaO_2/FiO_2 ratio of 90. He is requiring relatively high positive end expiratory pressure (PEEP) and FiO_2 to maintain adequate SaO_2. He has been hypotensive because of septic shock from his influenza and required pressors via a central line immediately after admission to the unit and intubation for the initiation of mechanical ventilation. He also has diabetes. Along with the immediate needs for stabilization, resuscitation, and supportive care, the ICU team needs to consider what impact their therapeutic choices now will have on his risk for developing critical illness myopathy.

DISCUSSION: Patients like this are commonly seen in high-acuity ICUs, in which patients with severe ARDS and sepsis are frequently found. He has a number of risk factors for critical care myopathy, some of which may be avoidable and others may not. As the critical care team provides supportive care for him, they need to consider how each risk factor could be avoided or minimized, as followed:

- *Corticosteroids:* So far he has not required corticosteroids, but they are sometimes used for refractory hypotension in septic shock. The sepsis guidelines are somewhat ambiguous about the use of corticosteroids in this setting, because the evidence for their usefulness is mixed. In this case, if the blood pressure can be maintained without them, it would eliminate one risk factor for critical care myopathy.
- *Paralytic agents:* In severe ARDS, patients are sometimes paralyzed to improve oxygenation and ventilator synchrony. There is evidence that paralysis for the first 48 hours may improve survival in such patients. If paralytics are used, they should be discontinued as soon as they are no longer needed, certainly by the 48-hour mark, thus minimizing another risk factor.
- *Hyperglycemia:* As a diabetic who is critically ill, this patient may experience wide fluctuations in his blood glucose level. ICU protocols usually aim to maintain the glucose level at about 150 mg/dl, and if this can be done, it will minimize an additional risk factor. Because corticosteroids would likely raise the blood glucose level, this is another reason to avoid them in this patient.
- *Systemic inflammatory response syndrome (SIRS):* Because this patient has septic shock, by definition he has SIRS. Once a patient has SIRS, the only option for the ICU team is to treat the underlying infection if possible and support the patient through the septic period. This risk factor is not modifiable directly, but treating the influenza appropriately should minimize the duration and severity of SIRS.

diseases is unclear. Pulmonary vasculitis can occur with polymyositis and dermatomyositis and can lead to O_2 exchange abnormalities and pulmonary hypertension.

Critical Illness Myopathy

Critical illness myopathy is a heterogeneous entity that occurs commonly in intensive care units (ICUs) in which patients develop flaccid weakness of proximal muscles. Although this condition does not specifically target the diaphragm muscle, these patients are often very difficult to wean from mechanical ventilation. Risk factors for developing this myopathy include use of corticosteroids (likely dose-dependent); use of paralytic agents; hyperglycemia; hyperthyroidism; and possibly systemic inflammatory response syndrome, with or without sepsis.[44] Weakness improves on its own in most cases but may take weeks or months to resolve, often incompletely. There is no specific therapy, and prevention by avoiding the risk factors as much as possible is the best approach.[45]

Disorders of the Neuromuscular Junction

Disorders of the neuromuscular junction decrease conduction of nervous system impulses to the peripheral muscles, resulting in muscle weakness. Different clinical syndromes are caused by defects in different molecules or components of the neuromuscular junction, which is represented schematically in Figure 32-4, which compares a normal neuromuscular junction with an abnormal junction in myasthenia gravis. Disorders of the neuromuscular junction include the following:

1. Myasthenia gravis
2. Lambert-Eaton syndrome
3. Poisoning (organophosphate, tetanus, botulism)

Myasthenia Gravis

Myasthenia gravis (MG) is characterized by intermittent muscular weakness, which worsens on repetitive stimulation and improves with administration of anticholinesterase medications, such as edrophonium (Tensilon) or neostigmine. Most cases of MG arise from production of antibodies directed against the acetylcholine receptor (ACh-R). The antibodies inactivate the ACh-R and block transmission of electrical impulses from the nerve to the muscle.[46]

Approximately 20% of patients with MG do not exhibit such antibodies but may have antibodies to alternative targets, such as muscle-specific kinase.[47] Abnormalities of the thymus gland are common in MG. Approximately 10% of patients with MG have a neoplastic growth within the thymus called *thymoma,* which can be malignant but usually is not. Patients without thymoma typically have some degree of thymic hyperplasia. Congenital or fetal myasthenic syndromes are caused by either autoantibodies or inherited defects in the ACh-R.

MG typically occurs earlier in life in women and later in men. As the population has aged, more patients are diagnosed with MG later in life, and now there are more men affected than women.[48] This disorder may be associated with other autoimmune diseases, such as thyroid disease, diabetes, rheumatoid arthritis, ulcerative colitis, sarcoidosis, and pernicious anemia.

MG is characterized by progressive loss of muscular function, which may affect only the eye muscles (ocular myasthenia) or may be more widespread. The initial symptom is diplopia (double vision) or ptosis (a drooping eyelid) in more than 65% of patients (Figure 32-5).[49] The patient typically reports weakness of the affected muscles that may vary through the day or progress, especially with repetitive use. The diagnosis of MG is supported by the detection of anti–ACh-R antibodies in the blood, a characteristic fading of nerve impulses with repeated nerve stimulation testing during electromyography, and improvement of strength or symptoms in response to an anticholinesterase inhibitor drug (edrophonium) (Figure 32-6).

The pulmonary complications of MG depend on the magnitude and location of the affected muscle groups and tend to occur in patients most severely disabled with the disease. Upper airway obstruction, exertional dyspnea, and overt ventilatory failure all are reported in MG. Pulmonary function testing of MG patients who have respiratory muscle weakness shows decreased TLC, VC, PImax, and PEmax, similar to other

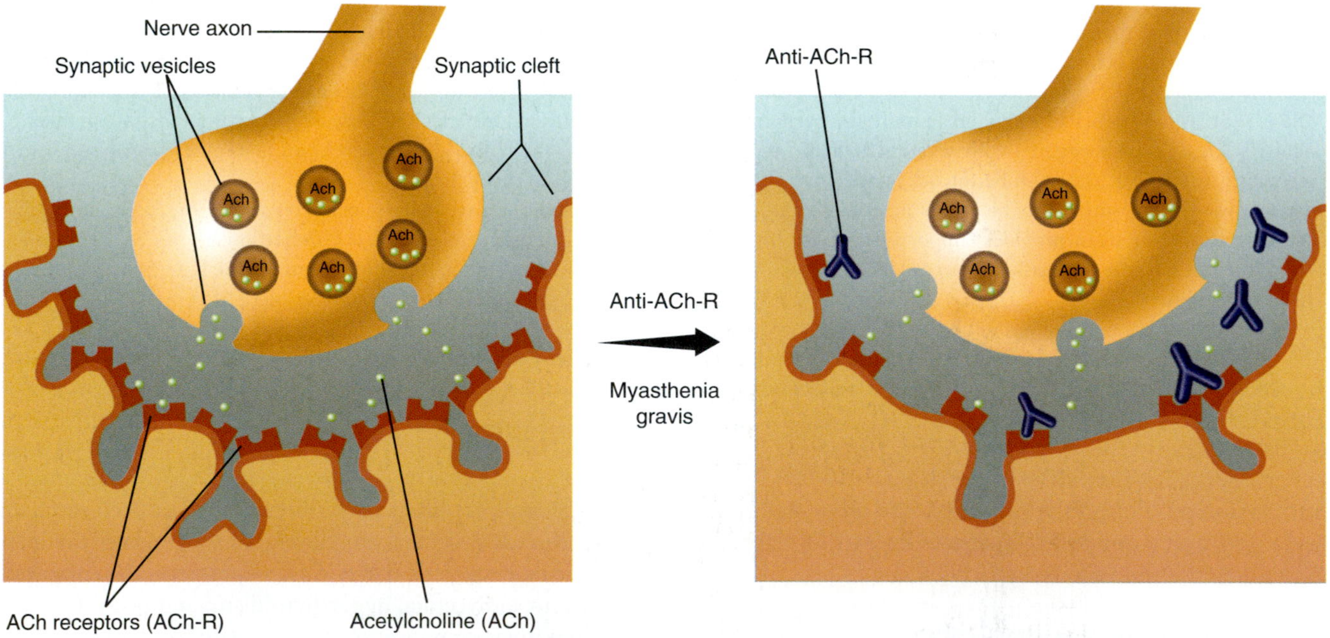

FIGURE 32-4 The neuromuscular junction with acetylcholine *(ACh)* stored in presynaptic vesicles. ACh is released by exocytosis into the synaptic cleft in response to a presynaptic nerve impulse. ACh binds to its cognate *ACh-R* on the postsynaptic membrane. This process depolarizes the nerve, propagates the impulse, and causes muscle contraction. Binding of anti–ACh-R antibodies to ACh-R mediates autoimmune destruction of the receptors. This process leads to abnormal muscle activation and the weakness that occurs in patients with myasthenia gravis.

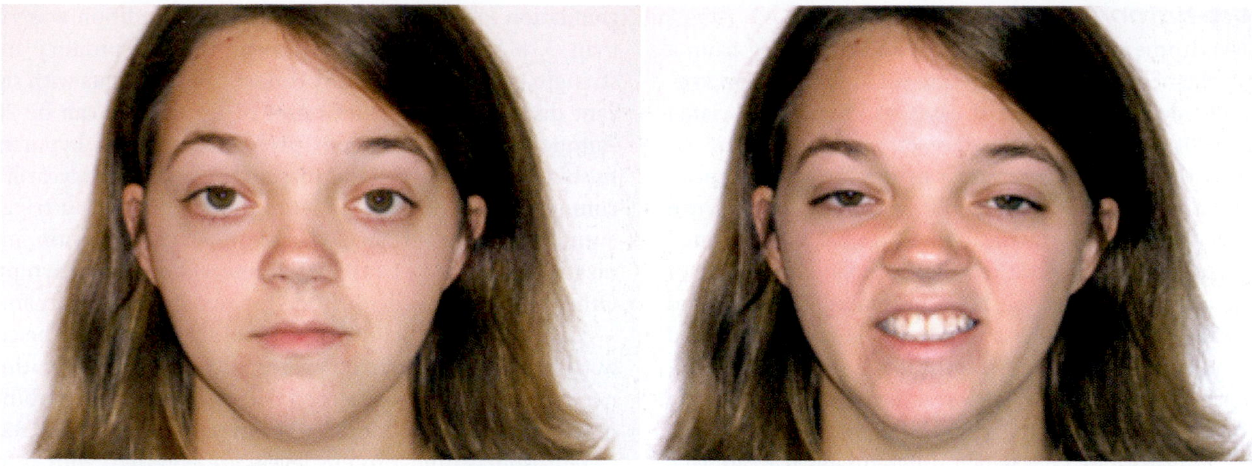

FIGURE 32-5 Features of ocular and facial weakness in a patient with myasthenia gravis. At rest *(left),* there is slight bilateral lid ptosis, which is partially compensated by asymmetric contraction of the frontalis muscle, raising the right eyebrow. During attempted smile *(right),* there is contraction of the medial portion of the upper lip and horizontal contraction of the corners of the mouth without the natural upward curling, producing a "sneer." (From Sanders DB, Howard JF: Disorders of neuromuscular transmission. In: Bradley, editor: Neurology in clinical practice, ed 5, Philadelphia, 2008, Butterworth Heinemann.)

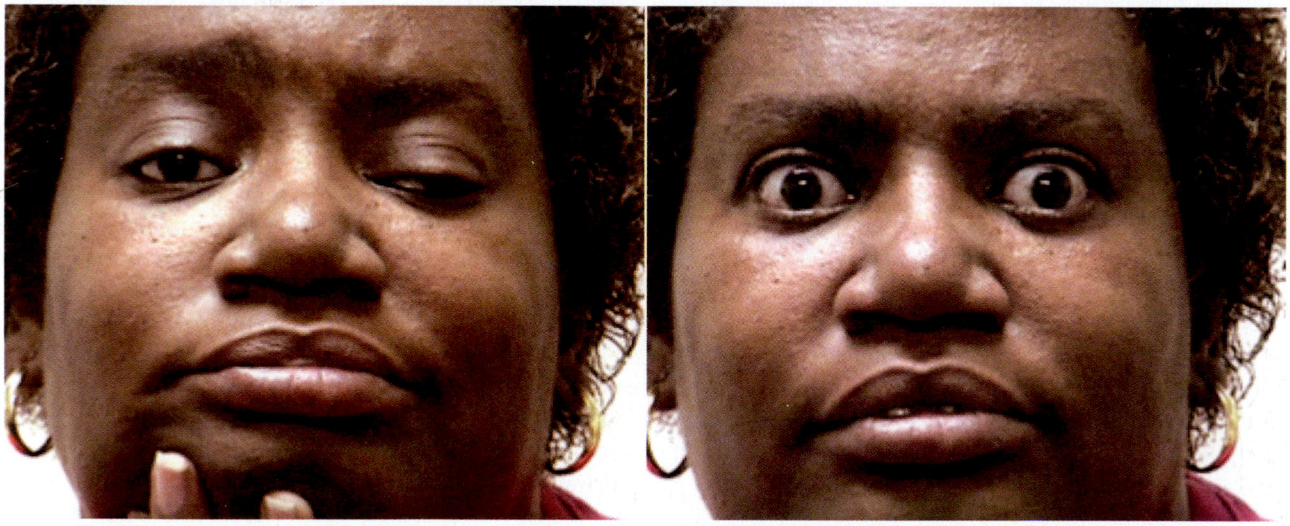

FIGURE 32-6 Clinical effect of edrophonium on a patient with myasthenia gravis. Before testing *(left),* the patient has ptosis of the left eyelid and lateral deviation of the left eye, and she must support her jaw. At 5 seconds after injection of 0.1 mg of edrophonium *(right)*, ptosis and lateral deviation are resolved, and her jaw no longer requires support. (From Sanders DB, Massey JM: Clinical features of myasthenia gravis. In: Engel AG, editor: Neuromuscular junction disorders, New York, 2008, Elsevier.)

neuromuscular disorders, with PImax and PEmax being more sensitive markers of early respiratory muscle weakness.[50]

Myasthenic crisis is an acute event in MG and is characterized either by respiratory failure or inability to maintain a patent airway. Myasthenic crisis can occur acutely in response to worsening of disease, intercurrent infection, or surgery or when excess anticholinesterase inhibitors have been given. Endotracheal intubation and mechanical ventilation are required immediately and may be prolonged.[51]

Treatment of MG is generally effective, although it is largely empiric because clinical trials are rare. Long-term management includes thymectomy[52] and administration of anticholinesterase medications (edrophonium, neostigmine, pyridostigmine) with or without corticosteroids or other immunosuppressants such as azathioprine or cyclosporine.[49] For patients in acute myasthenic crisis, who often have respiratory failure requiring mechanical ventilation, circulating antibodies can be removed by plasmapheresis, which results in clinical improvement[53,54] usually after five or six treatments and has been used to facilitate weaning from mechanical ventilation in the care of these patients.[55] Intravenous immunoglobulin G (IgG) has been used and can improve muscle strength and hasten recovery from respiratory failure. Neither plasmapheresis nor intravenous IgG is generally used for long-term management of MG. The effect of both treatments is temporary but may last several months.[49] Clinical trials comparing these treatments have shown a slight advantage with plasmapheresis but also a higher complication rate.[56,57]

Lambert-Eaton Syndrome

Another syndrome of neuromuscular weakness arising from a disorder at the neuromuscular junction is **Lambert-Eaton syndrome** (LES). More than 50% of cases of LES are associated with cancer. Of these cancer-related cases, greater than 80% are associated with small cell carcinoma of the lung.[58] The mean age at presentation is approximately 60 years, although LES can occur in all age groups. Autoantibodies against voltage-gated calcium channels at the nerve terminals impair the release of acetylcholine and can lead to both muscular weakness and autonomic insufficiency.[59] These autoantibodies can be detected in a patient's serum, which confirms the diagnosis.[58,60] The clinical diagnosis of LES is supported by results of nerve conduction studies. Increasing muscle strength with repetitive stimuli is a characteristic feature of LES, which differentiates it from MG, which is characterized by progressive fatigue of muscular contraction with repetitive stimulation.

Patients with LES usually present with tiredness or weakness of proximal muscle groups out of proportion to findings on clinical examination. Although patients are subject to respiratory complications because of their increased sensitivity to the effects of anesthesia, respiratory failure is rare. The clinical course of LES tends to be one of relative stability with less fluctuation than MG. Management of LES includes treatment of the underlying malignancy when present. If no malignancy is found, surveillance for lung cancer is recommended every 6 months, and LES is managed symptomatically with immunosuppressive medication or acetylcholinesterase inhibitors.[58,60]

Disorders of the Nerves

The peripheral nerves may be affected by toxic agents, inflammatory processes, vascular disorders, malignant diseases, and metabolic or nutritional imbalances. Hundreds of conditions have been associated with neuropathies leading to respiratory muscle dysfunction. Representative conditions are listed in Box 32-2.

Guillain-Barré Syndrome

Guillain-Barré syndrome (GBS) is acute inflammatory demyelinating polyneuropathy and is the most common peripheral **neuropathy** causing respiratory insufficiency. GBS is characterized by paralysis and hyporeflexia with or without sensory symptoms. GBS is typically a self-limited disease, but overall mortality ranges from 3% to 10%.[61] Before modern mechanical ventilation techniques, mortality in this condition was greater than 33%.[62] Most patients recover their respiratory muscle strength completely, but the proportion of patients with significant disability 1 year after onset of the disease can be 20%.[63] Autonomic nervous system problems, such as hypotension, flushing, bronchorrhea, dermatographia, and bradycardia, are common. Two-thirds of patients with GBS report a triggering event, such as respiratory or gastrointestinal infection, immunization, or surgery, 1 to 4 weeks before the onset of symptoms. Other reported triggers include pregnancy and malignancy.[62]

GBS is a demyelinating process widely believed to be caused by autoantibodies directed against the myelin constituting the nerve sheath. The diagnosis of GBS is based on a combination of clinical, laboratory, and electrophysiologic data (Box 32-3).[64] Cerebrospinal fluid protein levels are elevated, with minimal cellularity after approximately 1 week of illness. Nerve conduction studies show slowing of conduction with preserved amplitude, which is typical of demyelination. Approximately one-third of all patients with GBS have respiratory muscle compromise. Although the diaphragm is typically affected later in the course of GBS, cases of respiratory failure in the absence of substantial peripheral weakness have been reported. The need for mechanical ventilatory support for patients with GBS increases with age.[62]

Treatment strategies that have improved outcome in GBS include intravenous IV infusions and plasmapheresis. These treatments are equally effective in hastening recovery of muscle strength. The benefit is greatest when treatment is started within 2 weeks of symptom onset. There is no additional benefit of combining the two therapies. Corticosteroids have no beneficial role in GBS.[65]

Patients with dyspnea, orthopnea, or impaired ability to maintain a patent airway should receive spirometry every 4 to 6 hours for documentation of function and assessment of the need for endotracheal intubation. Patients with poor upper airway control, weak cough, or large amounts of secretions should be considered for endotracheal intubation even though their VC is greater than 20 ml/kg. The increased work of breathing imposed by mucous plugging or atelectasis can hasten

Box 32-2 Causes of Phrenic Nerve Dysfunction Leading to Respiratory Dysfunction

- Cardiac surgery (cold cardioplegia to arrest the heart can cause "frostbitten" phrenic nerves; ischemic injury to nerves also can complicate cardiac surgery)
- Diabetes
- Trauma
- Thoracic aneurysm

Box 32-3 Diagnostic Criteria for Guillain-Barré Syndrome

REQUIRED FOR DIAGNOSIS
- Progressive weakness of both legs and arms
- Areflexia

SUPPORTIVE OF DIAGNOSIS
- Symptoms progress over days to weeks
- Symmetry of weakness
- Cranial nerve involvement (facial palsies)
- Improvement begins 2 to 4 weeks after progression stops
- Absence of fever at onset of symptoms
- Pain
- Laboratory features not suggestive of alternative diagnosis
- Cerebrospinal fluid with high protein, low cell count
- Nerve conduction slowing or block with normal amplitude

decompensation. A small subgroup may need mechanical ventilation for 1 year or more. Weaning of patients with GBS from mechanical ventilation is predicted by VC greater than 18 ml/kg,[66] transdiaphragmatic pressure greater than 31 cm H_2O, or a PImax stronger than −30 cm H_2O.[67]

RULE OF THUMB

Patients with GBS whose VC becomes less than 20 ml/kg or declines more than 30% from baseline or whose PImax is less negative than −30 cm H_2O and PEmax is less than 40 cm H_2O are at risk for respiratory failure and may need ventilatory support. Patients who meet the criteria of this "20-30-40 rule" should be observed in an ICU.[66,67]

RULE OF THUMB

Patients with GBS should be intubated for mechanical ventilatory support when VC decreases to 12 to 15 ml/kg or sooner if they have bulbar dysfunction with difficulty managing oral secretions or when PaO_2 values are less than 70 mm Hg while breathing room air.[62] As with all patients requiring intubation, as soon as it is clear that intubation will exceed 2 weeks' duration, a tracheostomy should be considered.[68]

Phrenic Nerve Damage and Diaphragmatic Paralysis

Each hemidiaphragm is supplied by its own phrenic nerve. The phrenic nerves emerge from the spinal cord at level C3-5 and descend through the mediastinum along the great vessels of the chest and pericardium. Damage to or interruption of either phrenic nerve leads to paralysis of the ipsilateral hemidiaphragm. Bilateral interruption is seen in high spinal cord injury and causes complete diaphragmatic paralysis. Unilateral diaphragmatic paralysis can be seen in various disease processes. Reversible unilateral diaphragmatic paralysis is a rare complication of acute pneumonia, but it can occur in 10% of patients who undergo cardiac surgery with cardiopulmonary bypass, usually secondary to cold cardioplegia or traction on the nerve during surgery or ischemic nerve injury.[69]

Patients with unilateral diaphragmatic paralysis may have a 15% to 20% reduction in VC and TLC in the upright position and a further reduction while supine. If they have no other diseases, patients with unilateral diaphragmatic paralysis may have no symptoms. Athletes, musicians, and others who use their lungs more fully are more likely to notice the decreased ventilatory capacity caused by unilateral diaphragm weakness. Diaphragmatic paralysis is diagnosed most often with chest radiography. The paralyzed side retains its contour but is displaced upward (Figure 32-7, *A*). At fluoroscopy, the paralyzed hemidiaphragm paradoxically rises into the thorax during a sudden forceful inspiration (sniff test). This paradoxical motion damps the effect of the normal diaphragm on the opposite side.

For patients with unilateral diaphragm paralysis, surgical plication of the weak side can move the diaphragm downward to a more normal position (see Figure 32-7, *B*), minimize paradoxical motion, and improve overall lung function.[70,71] Historically, results of diaphragm plication procedures have been disappointing, but newer laparoscopic techniques are more promising.[72,73] Appropriate patient selection is crucial to avoid operating on patients whose diaphragms would recover their strength in time and patients whose weakness is due to primary neuromuscular disorders, which would not be improved by plication.

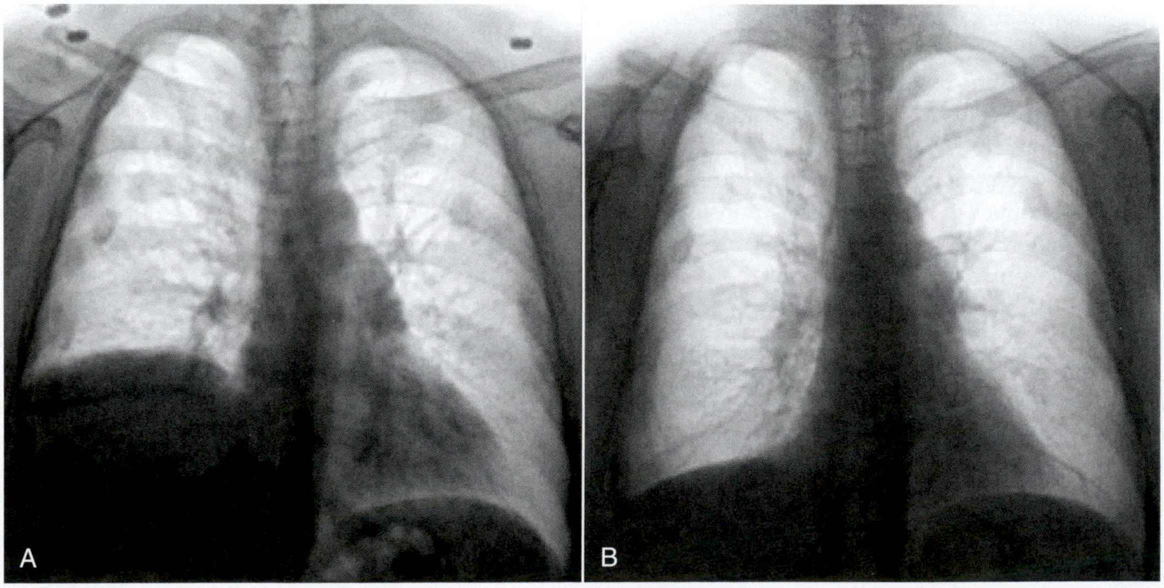

FIGURE 32-7 **A,** Chest radiograph showing elevation of a right hemidiaphragm. **B,** Chest radiograph in the same patient 1 year after laparoscopic diaphragm plication. (From Groth SS, Andrade RS: Diaphragm plication for eventration or paralysis: a review of the literature. Ann Thorac Surg 89:S2146–S2150, 2010.)

RULE OF THUMB

Diaphragm weakness resulting from phrenic nerve injury (not transection) often improves very slowly, sometimes over years, so plication should be delayed until serial testing shows that no further improvement is occurring, usually at least 1 to 2 years from the onset of weakness.

Critical Illness Polyneuropathy

In contrast to critical illness myopathy, discussed previously, **critical illness polyneuropathy** is associated almost entirely with severe sepsis in the ICU. Patients develop muscle weakness and atrophy, loss of deep tendon reflexes, and loss of peripheral sensation to pinprick and touch. Cranial nerve function is usually spared. The mechanism of nerve damage is unknown but, similar to other complications of sepsis, may be related to ischemia caused by thrombosis or underperfusion of the microcirculation, or both, in this case of the affected nerves.[45]

Effects of critical illness polyneuropathy may persist for years, or permanently, but often improve with time and rehabilitation. As in critical illness myopathy, there is no specific treatment; optimal management of the patient's severe sepsis following protocols to restore adequate circulation and limit the length of organ system failure is probably beneficial.

Disorders of the Spinal Cord

Upper motor neurons arise from cell bodies in the motor areas of the brain and terminate at the anterior horn cells in the spinal cord, which constitute the lower motor neurons because it is axons from these cells that extend out of the central nervous system to the skeletal muscles. Disorders in this group (e.g., ALS) can affect specific parts of this chain or nonspecifically disrupt these tracts (e.g., spinal cord injury). Other examples of lesions in this anatomic location include transverse myelitis, syringomyelia, poliomyelitis, and spinal cord tumors.

Amyotrophic Lateral Sclerosis

Amyotrophic lateral sclerosis, or **Lou Gehrig disease**, is a neuromuscular disease characterized by progressive degeneration of both upper and lower motor neurons; early in the disease, degeneration of either upper or lower motor neurons may predominate. Approximately 5% to 10% of cases are familial; others are sporadic. The male-to-female ratio for ALS is approximately 1.2 : 1, and the peak incidence is between 65 and 75 years old, although cases have been reported in patients younger than 30 years old. The prognosis of ALS is poor, with a mean survival from diagnosis of 3 years. By 5 years, 80% of patients have died and 90% have died by 10 years.[74] Medical treatment of ALS is disappointing. There is no cure, and therapies to halt or slow progression of the disease are few and ineffective. One approved therapy for ALS is riluzole, an antiglutamate agent. Randomized trials have shown modest improvements in median survival of 4.2 months.[75] The high cost of the medication makes it hard to get for many patients, especially in light of the modest benefits that are usually seen.

Muscle weakness from ALS usually begins in a localized muscle group and spreads out geographically from there. It most often begins in the arms but may originate in the bulbar muscles (i.e., muscles supplied by nerves in the upper spinal cord, such as the nerves controlling swallowing and speaking) 25% of the time. In 1% to 2% of cases, ALS manifests initially as isolated respiratory muscle dysfunction in an otherwise relatively intact patient. Respiratory involvement eventually occurs in all patients with ALS, and pulmonary complications are the most frequent cause of death. Muscle weakness is associated with fasciculations, or involuntary quivering of the affected muscles. If muscle fasciculation does not develop in a patient with presumed ALS soon after weakness, another diagnosis should be considered.[76]

Inspiratory muscle decline, measured by FVC, tends to be linear with time in any one patient, although the rate of decline may be different between patients. As respiratory muscle strength gradually declines, acute respiratory decompensation may occur in the setting of respiratory infection or aspiration. ALS patients may have respiratory difficulty for various disease-related reasons, not all of which are direct results of respiratory muscle weakness. Nocturnal hypoxemia and hypoventilation can lead to disrupted sleep, frequent arousal, daytime headaches, and somnolence.

Monitoring FVC, PImax, and PEmax or maximal sniff nasal inspiratory force is helpful in these patients and can provide important information regarding the ability to clear secretions and maintain gas exchange. Ineffective cough can lead to atelectasis, pneumonia, worsening gas exchange, and hypoxemia.

RULE OF THUMB

Effective cough typically requires a PEmax greater than 40 cm H_2O to compress airways and generate sufficient flow velocities within the tracheobronchial tree to clear obstructing secretions or aspirated material.

Preventing respiratory complications and assessing the need for ventilatory assistance are central in caring for patients with advancing ALS. Helpful treatments include (1) modification of food consistency or placement of feeding tubes in patients with marked bulbar dysfunction, (2) clearing of secretions with assisted cough techniques or postural drainage, and (3) ventilatory assistance with positive or negative pressure devices. Noninvasive techniques are a reasonable option for many patients and have been shown to slow the rate of pulmonary decline, improve symptoms, and prolong survival.[77] When these techniques no longer suffice, many patients with ALS choose not to receive invasive mechanical ventilation and opt for palliative management at that point. However, many patients do desire invasive ventilatory support, and up to 90% of such patients report satisfaction with their decision and would choose tracheostomy and ventilation again in the same situation.[78] Although overall survival with ALS is poor, prolonged survival of ventilated patients has been reported.

RULE OF THUMB

The timing and type of ventilatory intervention (noninvasive or invasive) in the care of patients with ALS are the subject of much discussion. General guidelines for considering ventilatory assistance[79] include VC less than 50% predicted, orthopnea, maximal sniff nasal inspiratory force more negative than −40 cm H_2O, and abnormal nocturnal oximetry.

MINI CLINI

Respiratory Care of a Patient With Amyotrophic Lateral Sclerosis

PROBLEM: A 57-year-old practicing attorney with a diagnosis of ALS for 2 years has a tracheostomy for nocturnal mechanical ventilation. He is still able to function and practice law in a specialized wheelchair and wants to maintain his independence and professional practice as long as possible. What measures can be offered to help him maintain his respiratory function, avoid exacerbations that could lead to acute respiratory failure, and preserve his quality of life?

DISCUSSION: Respiratory muscle failure can be influenced by many factors in addition to the primary neuromuscular disease. These additional factors can be significant contributors to a patient's quality of life or progressive decline in function, and they provide additional therapeutic targets for care providers trying to maintain a patient's function and comfort.

Reduced lung compliance secondary to atelectasis or retained secretions can greatly increase the work of breathing for weakened muscles and worsen gas exchange. Maneuvers to recruit collapsed alveoli and augment his cough to clear secretions can counteract these factors. These maneuvers include chest physiotherapy and mechanical insufflation and exsufflation devices. Increased secretion production is another factor in many patients' illness, which can be managed with medications such as atropine or amitriptyline. In some cases, salivary glands are treated with low-dose radiation. Patients with bulbar dysfunction may lose additional respiratory muscle strength as a result of poor nutrition; placement of a percutaneous endoscopic gastrostomy tube for nutrition may avoid this as eating becomes more difficult. Keeping these additional aspects in mind allows a care provider to address them along with the primary weakness, and it is this care in many cases that prolongs a patient's ability to breathe independently and function as he or she would like.[80]

RULE OF THUMB

ALS is a complex and devastating disease and often requires a multidisciplinary approach, with input and active participation from numerous clinical specialties, including pulmonary, neurology, critical care, gastroenterology, palliative medicine, physical therapy, occupational therapy, social work, home nursing, psychiatry, and spiritual care.

RULE OF THUMB

Patients with ALS typically need psychologic support because of the progressive, incurable nature of their disease. Care providers must address issues such as depression, social and family support and education, and end-of-life planning. Because end-of-life discussions with patients can be uncomfortable for care providers, many avoid them and assume someone else will address this difficult topic, but that is a disservice to patients who need to understand and confront issues of eventual respiratory failure and death from their disease.

Spinal Cord Trauma

Approximately 12,000 new spinal cord injuries occur in the United States each year, and 55% involve the cervical spine. The causes are varied, but the most common causes are motor vehicle accidents, falls, violence, and sports. Many patients with a spine injury have other injuries associated with their trauma, including 25% to 50% with traumatic head injury.[81] Of spinal cord injuries, 5% to 10% cause quadriplegia. Complete cord injury is associated with absent motor and sensory function below the level of injury, and the patient's condition rarely improves. Patients with incomplete injury have residual function and tend to improve to varying degrees.

The respiratory manifestations of spinal cord injury depend on the level of injury and extent of damage. Cervical cord injuries can be functionally divided into two classes: high cervical cord lesions (C1-2) and middle to low cervical cord lesions (C3-8). The diaphragm receives innervation from nerve roots exiting the spinal cord at levels C3-5. Complete injury above this level results in total respiratory muscle paralysis and death, unless urgent intubation and ventilation are performed. Injury to the cord at C3-5 can severely reduce respiratory strength, as manifested by reductions in PEmax, PImax, FVC, and FEV_1, consistent with a restrictive ventilatory defect. Patients adopt a rapid, shallow breathing pattern and use accessory inspiratory muscles (scalene and sternocleidomastoid muscles) unless these muscles are also affected. *Abdominal paradox* (inward movement of the abdomen while the thorax expands) is the hallmark of significant bilateral diaphragmatic weakness. Despite the serious nature of injury between C3 and C5, 80% of intubated patients with this lesion can ultimately be liberated from mechanical ventilation. The muscles of expiration receive neural input from spinal levels T1-L1 and are predominantly affected by middle to low cervical cord lesions. This condition manifests as a marked reduction in PEmax compared with PImax and a diminished or absent effective cough.

The differential weakness of respective muscle groups in patients with neuromuscular weakness affects ventilatory capacity in the supine and seated positions. Patients with predominantly diaphragmatic weakness have orthopnea and are most comfortable in the upright seated position. The upright seated position favors gravity-assisted descent of the diaphragm, which is less affected by the abdominal contents that shift caudally (toward the bottom of the patient's spine) in the seated patient.

Recumbent patients with bilateral diaphragmatic weakness accompanying spinal cord injury may display paradoxical breathing, or abdominal paradox. Observation of the chest and abdomen of patients reveals paradoxic inward movement of the abdomen during inspiration. Conversely, patients with expiratory muscle weakness similar to that produced by low cervical cord injury prefer the supine position, in which the tendency of the abdominal contents to move toward the head assists expiration in the absence of marked expiratory muscle tone. These physiologic principles form the basis for the use of "rocking beds" and pneumatic belt devices as ventilatory adjuncts in the care of patients with significant respiratory muscle weakness.

MINI CLINI

Respiratory Dysfunction in Spinal Cord Injury

PROBLEM: A young man who is otherwise healthy falls from a ladder and transects the spinal cord at the level of C6. Which muscles of the respiratory system will be affected, and what will be the effect?

DISCUSSION: Transection of the spinal cord at the level of the sixth cervical vertebra paralyzes any muscle group that receives its innervation from nerve roots that exit the spinal vertebral canal below C6. A review of the innervation of the major muscles of inspiration and expiration is important:

Upper airway, tongue, palate: Cranial nerves IX, X, XI, and XII
C3-5: Diaphragm
C4-8: Shoulder girdle muscle (scalenes)
T1-12: Intercostal muscles
T7-L1: Abdominal muscles

The upper airway, tongue, shoulder girdle muscles, and diaphragm should be intact in this patient's injury. Maintenance of intrathoracic volume depends partly on continuous activation of intercostal muscles, which stabilize and expand the thoracic cage. With these muscles paralyzed, expiratory reserve volume decreases and normal activation of the diaphragm results in a tendency toward inward excursion of the chest wall and loss of effective volume. Forceful exhalation and the development of cough depend on activation of abdominal and intercostal muscle groups, both of which are paralyzed in this injury. Although he has an intact diaphragm, this patient has a poor cough, which is a predisposing factor for atelectasis, pooling of secretions, and pneumonia. Successful management of spinal cord injury at this level includes aggressive postural drainage and percussion (when the injury has been stabilized) and possibly assisted cough in the respiratory care regimen.

Disorders of the Brain

Traumatic brain injury (TBI), stroke, hemorrhage, and infection can lead to abnormality of respiration through various mechanisms. The motor cortex contains voluntary centers for control of the upper airway and pharynx (see Chapter 15). The pons and medulla, located in the brainstem, contain (1) chemoreceptors for automatic control of ventilation in response to increasing pH and hypercapnia and (2) centers that generate and modify patterns of automatic ventilation in response to visceral and chemical afferent information (see Figure 32-1). Both stroke and TBI can lead to disordered patterns of breathing, which are listed in Table 32-4,[82-84] and abnormalities in the lungs themselves, such as neurogenic pulmonary edema. This section describes the clinical entities of stroke and TBI and their effects on the respiratory system.

Stroke

Stroke is a clinical syndrome produced by acute interruption of the normal blood flow to an area of the brain. The result is persistent dysfunction related to the affected structures. Stroke can be thrombotic (related to local formation of a clot), embolic (related to a clot traveling from a remote place in the body), or hemorrhagic. The effect of a stroke on respiration depends on which of the control elements of ventilation are damaged.

Strokes in the cerebral cortex can produce decreased chest wall and diaphragmatic movement. Infarction in this area usually does not lead to significant alteration of ventilation. However, the patient may have significant impairment of speech and movement, including impairment of muscles that affect upper airway tone and control secretions. Swallowing is frequently a problem, leading to aspiration or poor nutrition. Chronic changes in pharyngeal muscle tone can lead to obstructive sleep apnea. Rarely, localized strokes lead to profound alterations of the respiratory system. These alterations often result from strokes in the midbrain and brainstem or from subarachnoid hemorrhage. They often resolve or improve after the acute timeframe of the stroke (Table 32-4).

Therapy for stroke has evolved considerably. Previous therapy for thrombotic stroke was largely supportive. At the present time, early use of thrombolytic therapy to dissolve the clot and restore circulation and function has been shown to improve function and survival, particularly if the thrombolytic agent is given less than 3 hours after the onset of symptoms.[85,86] More recent trials also have shown benefit in a more restricted patient population when thrombolytic therapy was given in the 3- to 4.5-hour time frame.[87,88] Physical therapy and occupational therapy continue to be important components for optimizing function in the setting of residual deficit after stroke. Patients with substantial impairment of speech and swallowing may be at risk for aspiration pneumonia. As in many catastrophic illnesses, stroke presents a complex set of problems, and patients do best when managed using a multidisciplinary approach in a center with high volumes of similar patients and well-developed expertise.[85,86]

Traumatic Brain Injury

Traumatic brain injury (TBI) is a general term referring to numerous focal or diffuse lesions of the brain resulting from blunt or penetrating force. In some patients, direct trauma to the respiratory centers in the brain may cause the same

TABLE 32-4
Abnormal Respiratory Patterns Associated With Stroke

Pattern	Definition
Cheyne-Stokes respiration	Common abnormal pattern characterized by crescendo-decrescendo breathing force and tidal volume; it is not specific for stroke and is more commonly the result of cardiopulmonary disease
Periodic breathing	Similar to Cheyne-Stokes but with complete central apneas in between periods of crescendo-decrescendo breathing; it is seen in 25% of acute strokes, especially in patients with subarachnoid hemorrhage
Gasping	Very short inspiration, often involving contraction of accessory muscles, with long expiratory phase; it often heralds impending respiratory failure
Ataxic breathing	Irregularly irregular respiratory rate and tidal volumes; it nearly always means a medullary stroke or lesion; it is not the sign of a poor prognosis
Apneustic breathing	Very long inspiratory phase (several seconds), then brief, rapid exhalation followed by a respiratory pause; it is usually associated with bulbar dysfunction with difficulty protecting airway from secretions, so usually requires intubation, and may be difficult to wean from ventilator
Central neurogenic hyperventilation	Rapid deep breaths resulting in hypocapnia; other causes of hyperventilation must be ruled out, but if so, this pattern signifies a poor prognosis
Apnea	Unusual in strokes except in brain death; prognosis is generally poor
Ondine curse	Apnea during sleep with normal respiration while awake; it is treated with mechanical ventilation during sleep only; some patients improve and no longer need ventilatory support

Data from North JB, Jennett S: Abnormal breathing patterns associated with acute brain damage. Arch Neurol 31:338-344, 1974; Lee MC, Klassen AC, Resch JA: Respiratory pattern disturbances in ischemic cerebral vascular disease. Stroke 5:612-616, 1974; Frank JI: Abnormal breathing patterns. In: Hanley DC, Einhaupl KM, Bleck TP, et al, editors: Neurocritical care, Heidelberg, 1994, Springer-Verlag.

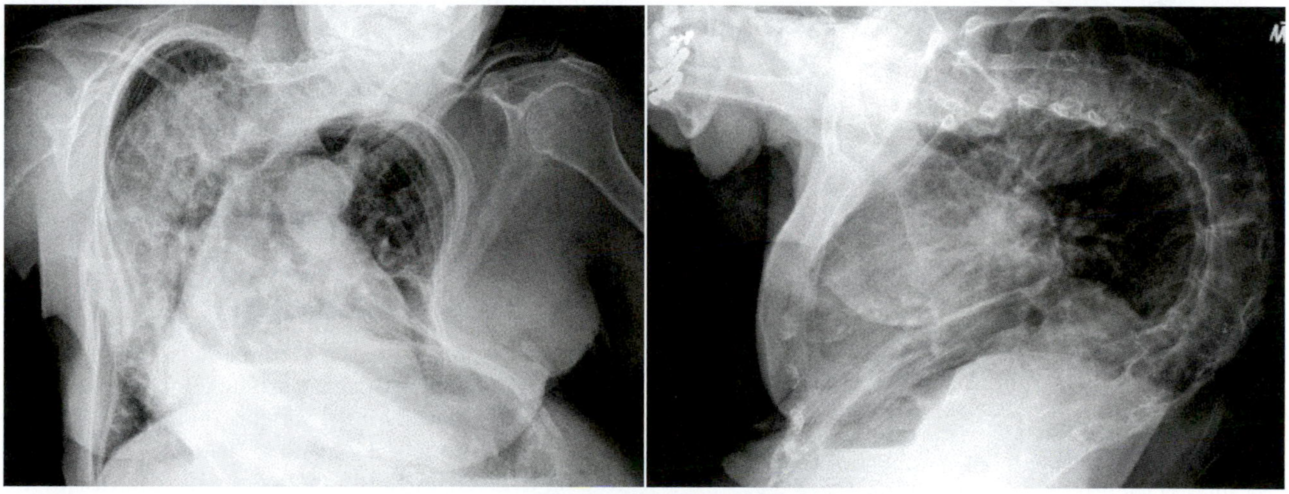

FIGURE 32-8 Frontal and lateral chest radiograph views of the same patient, showing severe scoliosis and kyphosis.

abnormalities of ventilation as strokes (mentioned previously); TBI also can lead to secondary effects on the respiratory system, such as neurogenic pulmonary edema and hypersecretion of mucus, leading to hypoxemia and respiratory insufficiency through mechanisms other than muscular weakness. There may be other injuries in patients with TBI that affect the respiratory system, such as spinal cord injury or rib fractures, or there may be factors that helped lead to the injury, which may independently affect breathing, such as intoxication or underlying illness.

DISORDERS OF THE THORACIC CAGE

The thoracic cage contains the lungs and supports the muscles of respiration. Normal ventilatory mechanics depend on a compliant thoracic cage with free excursion throughout the respiratory cycle.

Kyphoscoliosis

Kyphosis is posterior angulation of the thoracic cage. *Scoliosis* is lateral curvature of the spine (Figure 32-8). These two deformities often occur together (called **kyphoscoliosis**) as a result of the compensatory effects of the spine in response to the primary lateral curve in scoliosis.

Scoliosis is typically noticed during childhood and progresses during adolescence, although idiopathic adult kyphoscoliosis has been reported. The degree of scoliosis is measured by the *Cobb angle*, which is determined by the intersection of lines drawn between the upper and lower limbs of the primary curve in scoliosis (Figure 32-9). Severe kyphoscoliosis (Cobb

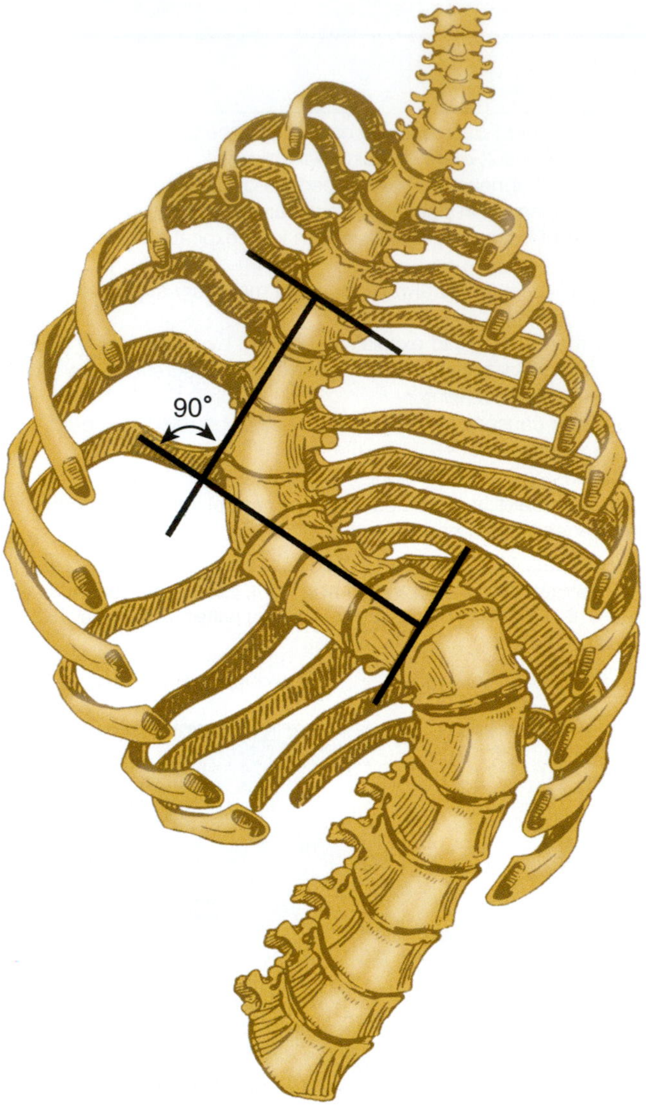

FIGURE 32-9 Scoliosis is lateral curvature of the spine. The degree of scoliosis is measured by the Cobb angle, which is determined by the intersection of lines drawn between the upper and lower limbs of the primary curve in scoliosis. Respiratory insufficiency rarely occurs until the Cobb angle exceeds 90 to 100 degrees. (Modified from Fishman AP: Acute respiratory failure. In Fishman AP, editor: Pulmonary disease, New York, 1992, McGraw-Hill, p 2300.)

angle > 90 to 100 degrees) can lead to hypoventilation, hypercapnia, and, if untreated, complications of pulmonary hypertension. However, the degree of pulmonary dysfunction cannot be predicted from the Cobb angle alone.[89,90] Respiratory dysfunction is probably multifactorial in most patients. Compliance of the chest wall and lung is decreased in patients with significant kyphoscoliosis. The result is a restrictive ventilatory defect with decreased TLC and VC in pulmonary function testing. Maximal transdiaphragmatic pressure also is decreased, a sign of impaired diaphragmatic function in the pathogenesis of respiratory dysfunction in severe kyphoscoliosis.

Anterior or posterior spinal fixation can stabilize kyphoscoliosis and restore the thoracic curvature to a condition close to normal. Fixation prevents complications resulting from progressive curvature, loss of compliance, and subsequent ventilatory dysfunction. Few options are available to restore pulmonary function to older patients with established kyphoscoliosis. Surgery to correct the deformity can be undertaken, but this treatment generally does not improve pulmonary function.[91] Better long-term results are seen when surgery or brace therapy to correct the angulation is undertaken in adolescence.[92]

Both noninvasive and invasive ventilation are used in some patients with severe kyphoscoliosis, with improvement in blood gas values, respiratory muscle strength, symptoms of dyspnea,[93] and exercise capacity.[94] Both negative pressure[95] and positive pressure[96] ventilation have been used to stabilize respiratory function in patients with severe kyphoscoliosis.

Flail Chest

Flail chest is defined in different ways but occurs as a result of multiple rib fractures that cause a portion of the chest wall to become free-floating. The destabilized segment of the thoracic cage exhibits **paradoxical motion** during the respiratory cycle, bowing out with expiration and collapsing inward during a spontaneous breath. The movement is associated with a decreased pressure gradient to drive inspiration and expiration and can result in respiratory failure. Flail chest frequently is accompanied by other pulmonary injuries as a result of the mechanism of injury and the force required to fracture multiple ribs. Pulmonary contusion, hemothorax, and pneumothorax are frequently associated with flail chest and often necessitate urgent or emergency treatment in the trauma patient.[97] Flail chest is managed by controlling pain and by PPV until the fractured ribs heal.

Ankylosing Spondylitis

Ankylosing spondylitis is a rheumatologic disease that affects the spine and thoracic cage. Chronic joint inflammation ultimately leads to fusion of the vertebral bodies and the costovertebral joints (sometimes called a "bamboo spine"), typically leading to severe kyphosis and a dramatic decrease in thoracic cage compliance. Because diaphragmatic movement is retained, TLC and VC are only slightly reduced. The most severe respiratory consequence is parenchymal lung disease, which occurs in approximately 10% of patients with ankylosing spondylitis in the form of apical fibrocystic changes that can decrease gas exchange and often provide a location for infection, especially fungal infection.[98]

THE ROLE OF RESPIRATORY THERAPISTS IN CARING FOR PATIENTS WITH NEUROMUSCULAR WEAKNESS AND OTHER DISEASES OF THE CHEST WALL

Many of the diseases discussed in this chapter are chronic, progressive conditions that evolve into respiratory failure over time. Optimal management depends on the degree, rate, and specific manifestations of the disease process, and there is considerable variability. Physicians, nurses, and respiratory therapists (RTs) caring for these patients must be familiar with the course and symptoms of this progression, so they can provide appropriate diagnostic testing and therapy at the right time.

RTs with expertise in caring for these patients can be essential to their care. Many patients require close monitoring of their respiratory symptoms and function, and these results must be reliable and consistent, because decisions such as when to begin a new supportive therapy may rely heavily on them. Maneuvers such as spirometry and maximal respiratory pressures, as well as the use of respiratory devices such as noninvasive ventilation and cough assist technology require explanation, education, reinforcement, and troubleshooting. Without this kind of supervision and support, many patients will use their devices improperly or not at all, which will be of no benefit to them and may lead to the inaccurate conclusion that the therapies have failed.

Neuromuscular diseases also carry with them the burdens common to many chronic and progressive diseases, including depression and other psychological burdens. Respiratory therapists involved in the care of these patients can provide longitudinal support, including encouragement to not give up on therapies that may be effective and perspective when there are still additional measures that can be added to improve the patient's quality of life. The more familiar an RT is with specific disease entities as well as the diagnostic and therapeutic options, the better they can help patients understand and cope with their chronic diseases.

SUMMARY CHECKLIST

- The components of the neuromuscular system that affect respiration include the brain (especially respiratory centers in the brainstem), the nerves (the phrenic nerve supplying the diaphragm, the intercostal nerves supplying many of the other respiratory muscles, and the bulbar muscles coordinating the throat), the neuromuscular junction, and the muscles of inspiration, expiration, and upper airway control.
- Respiratory muscle weakness or ventilatory failure is often the most important clinical dysfunction for many patients with neuromuscular diseases.
- Other effects of neuromuscular disease on the respiratory system include hyperventilation or hypoventilation, sleep apnea, aspiration, atelectasis, pulmonary hypertension, and cor pulmonale.
- Signs and symptoms that may indicate weakness of the respiratory muscles include exertional dyspnea, orthopnea, decreased volume of voice, weak or ineffective cough, accessory muscle use, and paradoxical breathing pattern (abdominal paradox).
- Pulmonary function abnormalities in patients with inspiratory muscle weakness typically include decreases in PImax, TLC, VC, and FEV_1. Residual volume can be increased. There often is an abnormally large decrease in FVC and FEV_1 (30% to 50%) when patients repeat testing in the supine position, compared to the seated position. Diffusing capacity corrected for alveolar volume typically is normal.
- Common neuromuscular disorders that cause respiratory compromise include ALS, myotonic dystrophy, spinal cord injury, GBS, Duchenne muscular dystrophy, and MG.
- Cervical spine injury above the C3 level results in complete paralysis of the respiratory muscles and necessitates emergency mechanical ventilation. Cervical spine injury below C5 leads to weakness of the expiratory muscles with decreased ability to cough and clear secretions.
- Unilateral diaphragmatic paralysis resulting from phrenic nerve damage usually is asymptomatic and is associated with minor reductions in respiratory function in an otherwise healthy patient.
- Scoliosis is abnormal lateral curvature of the spine. Respiratory insufficiency can occur if the curve is severe.
- Flail chest typically results from trauma to the chest. Multiple fractures of adjacent ribs produce a free-floating segment of the thoracic cage, which displays paradoxical excursion during the respiratory cycle. Flail chest often is associated with serious damage to the lungs, heart, or great vessels. Respiratory insufficiency in patients with flail chest can occur through numerous mechanisms.

References

1. American Thoracic Society/European Respiratory Society: ATS/ERS statement on respiratory muscle testing. *Am J Respir Crit Care Med* 166:518–624, 2002.
2. Cabrera Serrano M, Rabinstein AA: Usefulness of pulmonary function tests and blood gases in acute neuromuscular respiratory failure. *Eur J Neurol* 19:452–456, 2012.
3. McMorrow C, Fredsted A, Carberry J, et al: Chronic hypoxia increases rat diaphragm muscle endurance and Na^+-K^+ ATPase pump content. *Eur Respir J* 37:1474–1481, 2010.
4. Verges S, Bachasson D, Wuyam B: Effect of acute hypoxia on respiratory muscle fatigue in healthy humans. *Respir Res* 11:109, 2010.
5. Begin R, Bureau MA, Lupien L, et al: Control of breathing in Duchenne's muscular dystrophy. *Am J Med* 69:227–234, 1980.
6. Elman LB, Siderowf AD, McCluskey LF: Nocturnal oximetry: utility in the respiratory management of amyotrophic lateral sclerosis. *Am J Phys Med Rehabil* 82:866–870, 2003.
7. Yavagal DR, Mayer SA: Respiratory complications of rapidly progressive neuromuscular syndromes: Guillain-Barré syndrome and myasthenia gravis. *Semin Respir Crit Care Med* 23:221–229, 2002.
8. Tzeng AC, Bach JR: Prevention of pulmonary morbidity for patients with neuromuscular disease. *Chest* 118:1390–1396, 2000.
9. Servera E, Sancho J, Zafra MJ, et al: Alternatives to endotracheal intubation for patients with neuromuscular diseases. *Am J Phys Med Rehabil* 84:851–857, 2005.
10. Aboussouan LS: Mechanisms of exercise limitation and pulmonary rehabilitation for patients with neuromuscular disease. *Chron Respir Dis* 6:231–249, 2009.
11. Vianello A, Bevilacqua M, Arcaro G, et al: Non-invasive ventilatory approach to treatment of acute respiratory failure in neuromuscular disorders: a comparison with endotracheal intubation. *Intensive Care Med* 26:384–390, 2000.
12. Boitano LJ, Jordan T, Benditt JO: Noninvasive ventilation allows gastrostomy tube placement in patients with advanced ALS. *Neurology* 56:413–415, 2001.

13. Robert D, Argaud L: Clinical review: long-term noninvasive ventilation. *Crit Care* 11:210, 2007.
14. Melo J, Homma A, Iturriaga E, et al: Pulmonary evaluation and prevalence of non-invasive ventilation in patients with amyotrophic lateral sclerosis: a multicenter survey and proposal of a pulmonary protocol. *J Neurol Sci* 169:114–117, 1999.
15. Laub M, Berg S, Midgren B: Symptoms, clinical and physiological finding motivating home mechanical ventilation in patients with neuromuscular diseases. *J Rehabil Med* 38:250–254, 2006.
16. Make BJ, Hill NS, Goldberg AI, et al: Mechanical ventilation beyond the intensive care unit: report of a consensus conference of the American College of Chest Physicians. *Chest* 113(Suppl):289S–344S, 1998.
17. MacIntyre NR, Epstein SK, Carson S, et al: Management of patients requiring prolonged mechanical ventilation: report of a NAMDRC consensus conference. *Chest* 128:3937–3954, 2005.
18. Elefteriades JA, Quin JA, Hogan JF, et al: Long-term follow-up of pacing of the conditioned diaphragm in quadriplegia. *Pacing Clin Electrophysiol* 25:897–906, 2002.
19. DiMarco AF, Onders RP, Ignagni A, et al: Phrenic nerve pacing via intramuscular diaphragm electrodes in tetraplegic subjects. *Chest* 127:671–678, 2005.
20. Onders RP, Elmo M, Kaplan C, et al: Extended use of diaphragm pacing in patients with unilateral or bilateral diaphragm dysfunction: a new therapeutic option. *Surgery* 156:776–786, 2014.
21. Hoffman E, Brown R, Kunkel L: Dystrophin: the product of the Duchenne muscular dystrophy locus. *Cell* 51:919–928, 1987.
22. Cheuk DK, Wong V, Wraige E, et al: Surgery for scoliosis in Duchenne muscular dystrophy. *Cochrane Database Syst Rev* 24:005375, 2007.
23. Velasco MV, Colin AA, Zurakowski D, et al: Posterior spinal fusion for scoliosis in Duchenne muscular dystrophy diminishes the rate of respiratory decline. *Spine (Phila)* 32:459–465, 2007.
24. Suresh S, Wales P, Harris M, et al: Sleep-related breathing disorder in Duchenne muscular dystrophy: disease spectrum in the paediatric population. *J Paediatr Child Health* 41:500–503, 2005.
25. Bushby K, Finkel R, Birnkrant DJ, et al; Care Considerations Working Group: Diagnosis and management of Duchenne muscular dystrophy. II. Implementation of multidisciplinary care. *Lancet Neurol* 9:177–189, 2010.
26. Birnkrant DJ, Bushby KM, Amin RS, et al: The respiratory management of patients with Duchenne muscular dystrophy: a DMD care considerations working group specialty article. *Pediatr Pulmonol* 45:739–748, 2010.
27. Mohr C, Hill N: Long-term follow-up of nocturnal ventilatory assistance in patients with respiratory failure due to Duchenne-type muscular dystrophy. *Chest* 97:91–96, 1990.
28. Raphael JC, Chevret S, Chastang C, et al: Randomized trial of preventive nasal ventilation in Duchenne muscular dystrophy: French Multicentre Cooperative Group on Home Mechanical Ventilation Assistance in Duchenne de Boulogne Muscular Dystrophy. *Lancet* 343:1600–1604, 1994.
29. Kessler W, Wanke T, Winkler G, et al: 2 Years experience with inspiratory muscle training in patients with neuromuscular disorders. *Chest* 120:765–769, 2001.
30. Sveen ML, Jeppesen TD, Hauerslev S, et al: Endurance training improves fitness and strength in patients with Becker muscular dystrophy. *Brain* 131:2824–2831, 2008.
31. Harper P: *Myotonic dystrophy: major problems in neurology* (vol 21). Philadelphia, 1989, Saunders.
32. Rimmer K, Golar SD, Lee MA, et al: Myotonia of the respiratory muscles in myotonic dystrophy. *Am Rev Respir Dis* 148:1018–1022, 1993.
33. Pizzuti A, Friedman D, Caskey C: The myotonic dystrophy gene. *Arch Neurol* 50:1173–1179, 1993.
34. Culebras A: Sleep and neuromuscular disorders. *Neurol Clin* 23:1209–1223, 2005.
35. Mathieu J, Allard P, Gobeil G, et al: Anesthetic and surgical complications in 219 cases of myotonic dystrophy. *Neurology* 49:1646–1650, 1997.
36. Gupta N, Saxena K, Kumar PA, et al: Myotonic dystrophy: an anaesthetic dilemma. *Indian J Anaesth* 53:688–691, 2009.
37. Dimachkie MM, Barohn RJ, Amato AA: Idiopathic inflammatory myopathies. *Neurol Clin* 32:595–628, 2014.
38. Tansley S, Gunawardena H: The evolving spectrum of polymyositis and dermatomyositis: moving towards clinicoserological syndromes—a critical review. *Clin Rev Allergy Immunol* 47:264–273, 2014.
39. Blumbergs P, Byrne E, Kakulas B: Polymyositis presenting with respiratory failure. *J Neurol Sci* 65:221–229, 1984.
40. Connors GR, Christopher-Stine L, Oddis CV, et al: Interstitial lung disease associated with the idiopathic inflammatory myopathies: what progress has been made in the past 35 years? *Chest* 138:1464–1474, 2010.
41. Hallowell RW, Danoff SK: Interstitial lung disease associated with the idiopathic inflammatory myopathies and the antisynthetase syndrome: recent advances. *Curr Opin Rheumatol* 26:684–689, 2014.
42. Targoff IN: Myositis specific autoantibodies. *Curr Rheumatol Rep* 8:196–203, 2006.
43. Mahler M, Miller FW, Fritzler MJ: Idiopathic inflammatory myopathies and the anti-synthetase syndrome: a comprehensive review. *Autoimmun Rev* 13:367–671, 2014.
44. Zhou C, Wu L, Ni F, et al: Critical illness polyneuropathy and myopathy: a systematic review. *Neural Regen Res* 9:101–110, 2014.
45. Osias J, Manno E: Neuromuscular complications of critical illness. *Crit Care Clin* 30:785–794, 2014.
46. Gilhus NE: Myasthenia and the neuromuscular junction. *Curr Opin Neurol* 25:523–529, 2012.
47. Hoch W, McConville J, Helms S, et al: Auto-antibodies to the receptor tyrosine kinase MuSK in patients with myasthenia gravis without acetylcholine receptor antibodies. *Nat Med* 7:365–368, 2001.
48. Phillips LH: The epidemiology of myasthenia gravis. *Semin Neurol* 24:17–20, 2004.
49. Sanders DB, Howard JF: Disorders of neuromuscular transmission. In Bradley WG, Davoff RB, Fenichel GM, et al, editors: *Neurology in clinical practice*, ed 5, Philadelphia, 2008, Butterworth Heinemann.
50. Prigent H, Orlikowski D, Letilly N, et al: Vital capacity versus maximal inspiratory pressure in patients with Guillain-Barré syndrome and myasthenia gravis. *Neurocrit Care* 17:236–239, 2012.
51. Gracey D, Divertie M, Howard FJ: Mechanical ventilation for respiratory failure in myasthenia gravis: two year experience with 22 patients. *Mayo Clin Proc* 58:597–602, 1983.
52. Gronseth GS, Barohn RJ: Practice parameter: thymectomy for autoimmune myasthenia gravis (an evidence-based review). *Neurology* 55:5–15, 2000.
53. Norris FH, Jr, Denys EH, Mielke CH, Jr: Plasmapheresis (plasma exchange) in neurologic disorders. *Clin Neuropharmacol* 5:93–114, 1982.
54. Batocchi AP, Evoli A, Di Schino C, et al: Therapeutic apheresis in myasthenia gravis. *Ther Apher* 4:275–279, 2000.
55. Gracey DR, Howard FM, Jr, Divertie MB: Plasmapheresis in the treatment of ventilator-dependent myasthenia gravis patients: report of four cases. *Chest* 85:739–743, 1984.
56. Gajdos P, Chevret S, Clair B, et al: Clinical trial of plasma exchange and high-dose intravenous immunoglobulin in myasthenia gravis. Myasthenia Gravis Clinical Study Group. *Ann Neurol* 41:789–796, 1997.
57. Qureshi AI, Choudhry MA, Akbar MS, et al: Plasma exchange versus intravenous immunoglobulin treatment in myasthenic crisis. *Neurology* 52:629–632, 1999.
58. Gilhus NE: Lambert-Eaton myasthenic syndrome: pathogenesis, diagnosis, and therapy. *Autoimmune Dis* 2011:973808, 2011.
59. Lennon VA, Lambert EH: Autoantibodies bind solubilized calcium channel-omega-conotoxin complexes from small cell carcinoma: a diagnostic aid for Lambert-Eaton myasthenic syndrome. *Mayo Clin Proc* 64:1498–1504, 1989.
60. Mareska M, Gutmann L: Lambert-Eaton myasthenic syndrome. *Semin Neurol* 24:149–153, 2004.
61. van Doorn PA: Diagnosis, treatment and prognosis of Guillain-Barré syndrome (GBS). *Presse Med* 42(6 Pt 2):2193–2201, 2013.
62. Harati Y, Bosch EP: Disorders of peripheral nerves. In Bradley WG, Davoff RB, Fenichel GM, et al, editors: *Neurology in clinical practice*, ed 5, Philadelphia, 2008, Butterworth Heinemann.
63. Winer J, Hughes R, Osmond C: A prospective study of acute idiopathic neuropathy. I. Clinical features and their prognostic value. *J Neurol Neurosurg Psychiatry* 51:605–612, 1988.

64. van den Berg B, Walgaard C, Drenthen J, et al: Guillain-Barré syndrome: pathogenesis, diagnosis, treatment and prognosis. *Nat Rev Neurol* 10:469–482, 2014.
65. Lehmann HC, Hartung HP, Hetzel GR, et al: Plasma exchange in neuroimmunological disorders. II. Treatment of neuromuscular disorders. *Arch Neurol* 63:1066–1071, 2006.
66. Chevrolet JC, Deleamont P: Repeated vital capacity measurements as predictive parameters for mechanical ventilation need and weaning success in Guillain-Barré syndrome. *Am Rev Respir Dis* 144:814–818, 1991.
67. Lawn ND, Fletcher DD, Henderson RD, et al: Anticipating mechanical ventilation in Guillain-Barré syndrome. *Arch Neurol* 58:893–898, 2001.
68. Marsh M, Gillespie D, Baumgartner A: Timing of tracheostomy in critically ill patients. *Chest* 96:190–193, 1989.
69. Canbaz S, Turgut N, Halici U, et al: Electrophysiological evaluation of phrenic nerve injury during cardiac surgery: a prospective, controlled, clinical study. *BMC Surg* 4:2, 2004.
70. Groth SS, Andrade RS: Diaphragm plication for eventration or paralysis: a review of the literature. *Ann Thorac Surg* 89:S2146–S2150, 2010.
71. Celik S, Celik M, Aydemir B, et al: Long-term results of diaphragmatic plication in adults with unilateral diaphragm paralysis. *J Cardiothorac Surg* 15:111, 2010.
72. Groth SS, Rueth NM, Kast T, et al: Laparoscopic diaphragmatic plication for diaphragmatic paralysis and eventration: an objective evaluation of short-term and midterm results. *J Thorac Cardiovasc Surg* 139:1452–1456, 2010.
73. Hu J, Wu Y, Wang J, et al: Thoracoscopic and laparoscopic plication of the hemidiaphragm is effective in the management of diaphragmatic eventration. *Pediatr Surg Int* 30:19–24, 2014.
74. Murray B: Natural history and prognosis in amyotrophic lateral sclerosis. In Mitsumoto H, Przedborski S, Gordon PH, editors: *Amyotrophic lateral sclerosis*, New York, 2006, Taylor & Francis Group, pp 227–255.
75. Traynor BJ, Alexander M, Corr B, et al: An outcome study of riluzole in amyotrophic lateral sclerosis: a population based study in Ireland, 1996–2000. *J Neurol* 250:473–479, 2003.
76. Murray B, Mitsumoto H: Disorders of upper and lower motor neurons. In Bradley WG, Davoff RB, Fenichel GM, et al, editors: *Neurology in clinical practice*, ed 5, Philadelphia, 2008, Butterworth Heinemann.
77. Aboussouan LS, Khan SU, Arroliga AC, et al: Effect of noninvasive positive-pressure ventilation on pulmonary function, respiratory muscle strength and arterial blood gases in amyotrophic lateral sclerosis. *Muscle Nerve* 24:403–409, 2001.
78. Moss AH, Casey P: Home ventilation for amyotrophic lateral sclerosis patients: outcomes, costs and patient, family and physician attitudes. *Neurology* 43:438–443, 1993.
79. Miller RG, Jackson CE, Kasarskis EJ, et al: Practice parameter update: the care of the patient with amyotrophic lateral sclerosis: drug, nutritional, and respiratory therapies (an evidence-based review). Report of the Quality Standards Subcommittee of the American Academy of Neurology. *Neurology* 73:1218–1226, 2009.
80. Hardiman O: Management of respiratory symptoms in ALS. *J Neurol* 258:359–365, 2011.
81. Gala VC, Vovadzis JM, Kim DH, et al: Trauma of the nervous system: spinal cord trauma. In Bradley WG, Davoff RB, Fenichel GM, et al, editors: *Neurology in clinical practice*, ed 5, Philadelphia, 2008, Butterworth Heinemann.
82. North JB, Jennett S: Abnormal breathing patterns associated with acute brain damage. *Arch Neurol* 31:338–344, 1974.
83. Lee MC, Klassen AC, Resch JA: Respiratory pattern disturbances in ischemic cerebral vascular disease. *Stroke* 5:612–616, 1974.
84. Frank JI: Abnormal breathing patterns. In Hanley DC, Einhaupl KM, Bleck TP, et al, editors: *Neurocritical care*, Heidelberg, 1994, Springer-Verlag.
85. Jauch EC, Saver JL, Adams HP, Jr, et al; for the American Heart Association Stroke Council; Council on Cardiovascular Nursing; Council on Peripheral Vascular Disease; Council on Clinical Cardiology: Guidelines for the early management of patients with acute ischemic stroke: a guideline for healthcare professionals from the American Heart Association/American Stroke Association. *Stroke* 44:870–947, 2013.
86. Maldonado NJ, Kazmi SO, Suarez JI: Update in the management of acute ischemic stroke. *Crit Care Clin* 30:673–697, 2014.
87. Hacke W, Kaste M, Bluhmki E, et al: ECASS Investigators: Thrombolysis with alteplase 3 to 4.5 hours after acute ischemic stroke. *N Engl J Med* 359:1317–1329, 2008.
88. Bluhmki E, Chamorro A, Davalos A, et al: Stroke treatment with alteplase given 3.0–4.5 h after onset of acute ischaemic stroke (ECASS III): additional outcomes and subgroup analysis of a randomised controlled trial. *Lancet Neurol* 8:1095–1102, 2009.
89. Upadhyay SS, Mullaji AB, Luk KD, et al: Evaluation of deformities and pulmonary function in adolescent idiopathic thoracic scoliosis. *Eur Spine J* 4:274–279, 1995.
90. Kearon C, Viviani GR, Kirkley A, et al: Factors determining pulmonary function in adolescent idiopathic thoracic scoliosis. *Am Rev Respir Dis* 148:288–294, 1993.
91. Wong CA, Cole AA, Watson L, et al: Pulmonary function before and after anterior spinal surgery in adult idiopathic scoliosis. *Thorax* 51:534–536, 1996.
92. Pehrsson K, Danielsson A, Nachemson A: Pulmonary function in adolescent idiopathic scoliosis: a 25 year follow up after surgery or start of brace treatment. *Thorax* 56:388–393, 2001.
93. Gonzalez C, Ferris G, Diaz J, et al: Kyphoscoliotic ventilatory insufficiency: effects of long-term intermittent positive-pressure ventilation. *Chest* 124:857–862, 2003.
94. Fuschillo S, De Felice A, Gaudiosi C, et al: Nocturnal mechanical ventilation improves exercise capacity in kyphoscoliotic patients with respiratory impairment. *Monaldi Arch Chest Dis* 59:281–286, 2003.
95. Jackson M, Kinnear W, King M, et al: The effects of five years of nocturnal cuirass-assisted ventilation in chest wall disease. *Eur Respir J* 6:630–635, 1993.
96. Hoeppner V, Cockcroft DW, Dosman JA, et al: Nighttime ventilation improves respiratory failure in secondary kyphoscoliosis. *Am Rev Respir Dis* 129:240–243, 1984.
97. Ciraulo D, Elliott D, Mitchell KA, et al: Flail chest as a marker for significant injuries. *J Am Coll Surg* 178:466–470, 1994.
98. Kanathur N, Lee-Chiong T: Pulmonary manifestations of ankylosing spondylitis. *Clin Chest Med* 31:547–554, 2010.

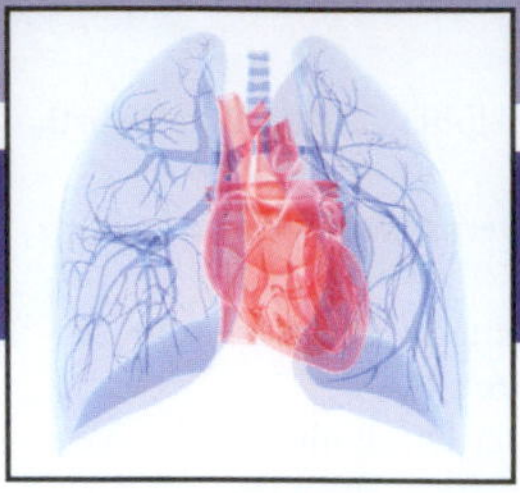

CHAPTER 33

Disorders of Sleep

EUHAN JOHN LEE AND PATRICK J. STROLLO, JR.

CHAPTER OBJECTIVES

After reading this chapter you will be able to:

- Define obstructive sleep apnea (OSA).
- Identify why airway closure occurs only during sleep.
- State the long-term consequences of uncontrolled OSA.
- State how a diagnosis of OSA is made.
- Identify what groups of patients are at particular risk for OSA.
- State the treatments available for patients with OSA.
- Describe how continuous positive airway pressure (CPAP) works.
- Identify problems associated with CPAP.
- Determine when bilevel pressure is useful in the treatment of OSA.
- Define "auto-titrating" CPAP.
- Identify the surgical alternatives for patients with severe OSA.

CHAPTER OUTLINE

KEY TERMS

bilevel positive airway pressure	excessive daytime sleepiness	sleep-disordered breathing
central sleep apnea	obesity hypoventilation	uvulopalatopharyngoplasty
continuous positive airway pressure	obstructive sleep apnea	upper airway stimulation

Obstructive sleep apnea (OSA) syndrome is a common clinical problem that is underdiagnosed.[1] It is estimated that approximately 2% to 4% of adults have OSA.[2] This prevalence is equivalent to those of asthma and diabetes in the general population. The spectrum of disease ranges from sleep disruption related to increased airway resistance to profound daytime sleepiness in conjunction with severe oxyhemoglobin desaturation, pulmonary hypertension, and right heart failure. The common feature in all variants of OSA syndrome is sleep disruption secondary to increased ventilatory effort that results in increased daytime sleepiness (or hypersomnolence) (Figure 33-1).[3] Treatment decreases morbidity and mortality.

Sleep apnea is defined as repeated episodes of complete cessation of airflow for 10 seconds or longer. The events can be obstructive (caused by upper airway closure) or central (caused by lack of ventilatory effort). Primary central nervous system lesions, stroke, congestive heart failure, and high-altitude

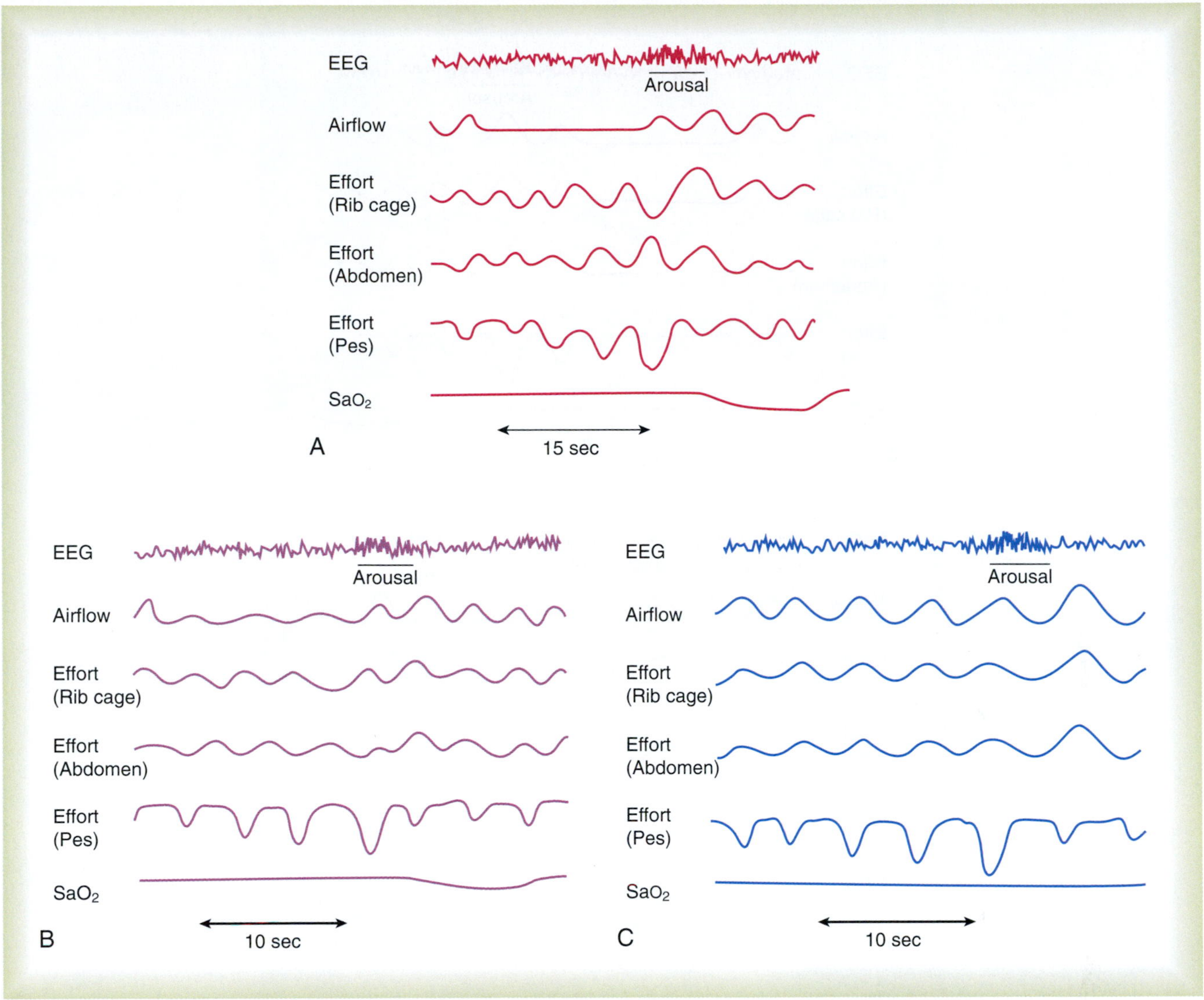

FIGURE 33-1 Spectrum of sleep-related upper airway obstruction. **A,** Obstructive sleep apnea. These events are defined as cessation of airflow for 10 seconds or longer. Paradoxical movement of the rib cage and abdomen in response to the closed airway occurs. Ventilatory effort, measured with an esophageal pressure balloon, usually increases until a threshold is reached that triggers a brief arousal seen on the electroencephalogram *(EEG),* and airway opening occurs. Oxyhemoglobin desaturation usually accompanies the event. **B,** Obstructive hypopnea. These events have been defined as a reduction of airflow by 30% to 50% for 10 seconds or longer. Paradoxical movement of the rib cage and abdomen in response to the narrowed airway occurs. Ventilatory effort, measured with an esophageal pressure balloon, usually increases until a threshold is reached that triggers a brief arousal seen on the EEG, and complete airway opening occurs. Oxyhemoglobin desaturation usually accompanies the event and usually is of a lesser degree than occurs with apnea. **C,** Respiratory effort–related arousals. These events are characterized by no discernible reduction in airflow. Subtle paradoxical movement of the rib cage and abdomen in response to narrowing of the airway may occur. As in apnea and hypopnea, ventilatory effort, measured with an esophageal pressure balloon, usually increases until a threshold is reached that triggers a brief arousal seen on the EEG, and complete airway opening occurs. By definition, no oxyhemoglobin desaturation is associated with the event.

hypoxemia can diminish respiratory control and cause central apnea events.[3] **Central sleep apnea** (CSA) is not as common as OSA. Only 10% to 15% of patients with sleep-disordered breathing are classified as having CSA.[4] Mixed sleep apnea has an initial central component followed by an obstructive component (Figure 33-2).

Hypopnea is a significant decrease in breathing without complete cessation of airflow.[5] Hypopnea is defined as a 30% decrease in airflow in conjunction with 4% oxygen (O_2) desaturation.[6] Most investigators agree that physiologically significant hypopnea is associated with a decrease in O_2 saturation (SaO_2) and/or arousal from sleep.[7]

Respiratory therapists (RTs) are likely to encounter both OSA and CSA when treating patients. OSA is the most commonly encountered type of sleep apnea and is underdiagnosed by health professionals; therefore the focus of this chapter is on the pathophysiology and management of the variants of OSA.

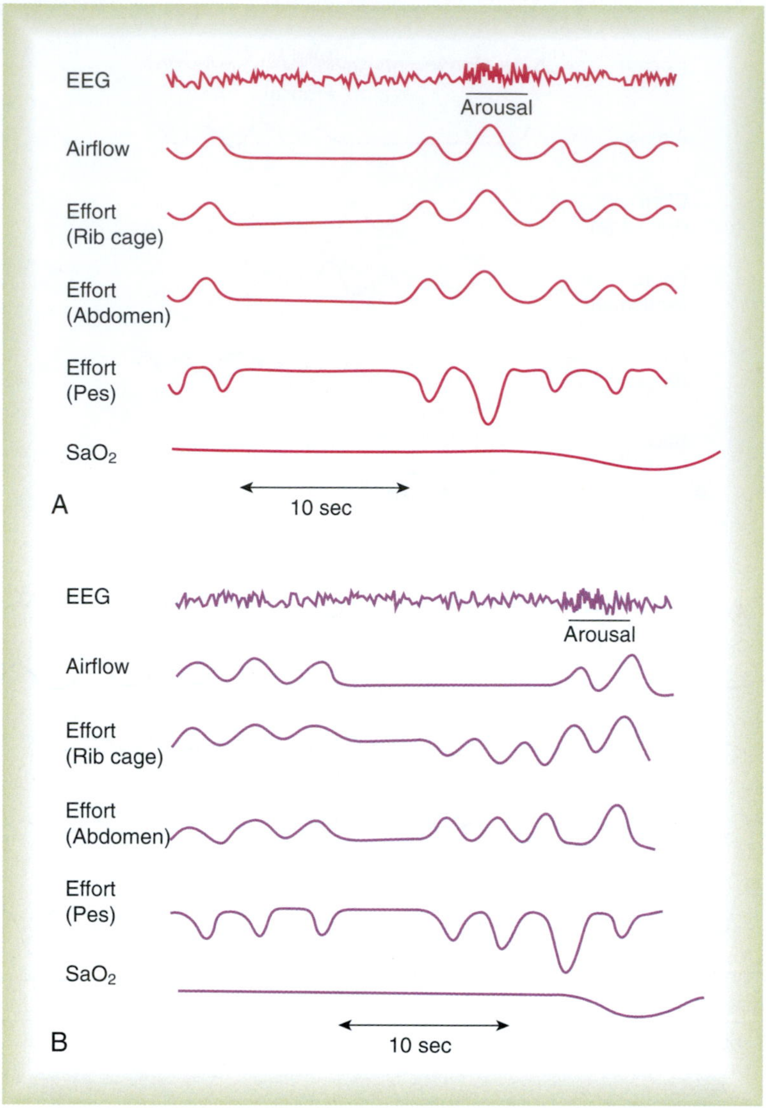

FIGURE 33-2 Central sleep apnea (CSA) and mixed sleep apnea. **A,** CSA. These events are defined as cessation of airflow for 10 seconds or longer. Compared with the events of obstructive sleep apnea (OSA), no movement of the rib cage or abdomen is present and the airway remains open. During an apneic event, there is a lack of ventilatory effort, measured with an esophageal pressure balloon. A brief arousal on the electroencephalogram *(EEG)* is associated with a maximal ventilatory effort that usually follows the episode of apnea. Oxyhemoglobin desaturation may be associated with the event. **B,** Mixed sleep apnea. These events have characteristics of both CSA and OSA. They are 10 seconds or longer in duration, and the central portion precedes the obstructive component. As with other sleep-related upper airway obstructive events, termination of the event is characterized by a maximal ventilatory effort and is associated with brief arousal on the EEG. Mixed sleep apnea usually is associated with oxyhemoglobin desaturation.

PATHOPHYSIOLOGY

Obstructive Sleep Apnea

The primary cause of OSA is a small or unstable pharyngeal airway. This condition can be caused by soft tissue factors, such as upper body obesity or tonsillar hypertrophy (rare in adults), and skeletal factors, such as a small or recessed chin.[8] During the waking state, pharyngeal patency is maintained by increased activity of the upper airway dilator muscles. Sleep onset is associated with a decrease in the activity of these muscles. The result is airway narrowing or closure of airways that are at risk.[9] In an unstable upper airway, narrowing and closure during sleep frequently involves multiple sites.[10]

Partial or complete closure of the upper airway during sleep is associated with a number of serious neurobehavioral, metabolic, and cardiopulmonary consequences (Box 33-1). Compared with the general population, patients with untreated OSA have an increased risk for systemic and pulmonary hypertension, stroke, nocturnal arrhythmia, heart failure, and myocardial infarction.[11,12] The repetitive cycle of upper airway closure and opening during sleep is believed to have effects on the autonomic nervous system—specifically, an increase in sympathetic tone.[13] These effects are caused in part by recurrent

Box 33-1 Adverse Consequences of Obstructive Sleep Apnea

CARDIOPULMONARY
- Nocturnal arrhythmia
- Diurnal hypertension
- Pulmonary hypertension
- Right or left ventricular failure
- Myocardial infarction
- Stroke

NEUROBEHAVIORAL
- Excessive daytime sleepiness
- Diminished quality of life
- Adverse personality change
- Motor vehicle accidents

METABOLIC
- Insulin resistance
- Altered lipid metabolism

episodes of hypoxemia and hypercapnia that are due to airway closure and hypoventilation that can occur throughout the night in patients with OSA. The arousals and microarousals during sleep also play an important role in the increase in sympathetic tone.[13] Over time, increased sympathetic tone may result in systemic hypertension and modest pulmonary hypertension.[14] Patients with OSA may develop right ventricular hypertrophy and right heart failure if they are not treated.[15,16]

Obesity, especially of the upper body, has been found to correlate positively with the presence of OSA. In most instances, patients with OSA are obese with a large amount of peripharyngeal adipose tissue along with adipose tissue in the neck.[17] A body mass index greater than 28 (>120% of ideal body weight normalized for height) should alert the practitioner to the possibility of OSA, particularly if the patient has excessive daytime sleepiness.[2]

Patients who are of normal body weight can be predisposed to OSA if they have an abnormal craniofacial configuration. Men may grow a beard to disguise such a craniofacial abnormality. If the chin is recessed (retrognathic) or small (micrognathic), the upper airway space may be narrow, and the risk for airway closure during sleep increases.[2, 8, 14] Patients with a deviated nasal septum or trauma to the nasal passages may be predisposed to upper airway closure during sleep as a result of the increased resistive load to the upper airway. An isolated nasal abnormality is an unusual cause of OSA.

OSA also can have a genetic predisposition.[18] There have been reports of families in which obesity alone does not explain the increased prevalence of OSA.[19] It has been postulated that craniofacial abnormalities and defects in ventilatory control explain the increased frequency of OSA in these families.

Central Sleep Apnea

Although a detailed discussion of the pathophysiology of CSA is beyond the scope of this chapter, several concepts are important to RTs. In contrast to OSA, which represents a spectrum of the same disease, CSA is a heterogeneous group of disorders. Patients have a ventilatory pattern known as *periodic breathing,* in which there is a waxing and waning of respiratory drive, which is reflected clinically as an increase and then a decrease in respiratory rate and tidal volume (V_T). Cheyne-Stokes respiration, which often occurs in patients with congestive heart failure or stroke, is a severe type of periodic breathing characterized by a crescendo-decrescendo pattern of hyperpnea alternating with apnea. After apnea occurs, there may be an increase in central ventilatory drive and an increase in V_T.[3]

Overlap Syndrome

Some patients with chronic obstructive pulmonary disease (COPD) have coexisting OSA. This combination is referred to as *overlap syndrome.*[20] Patients are usually obese and have a history of smoking. They have moderate to severe nocturnal oxyhemoglobin desaturation secondary to both OSA and COPD. The worst desaturation values occur during rapid eye movement (REM) sleep and are related to the loss of accessory muscle use encountered in this physiologic state. Patients with overlap syndrome tend to have a worse prognosis and more severe blood gas abnormalities than patients with the same degree of OSA but without COPD.[20] they may arrive in the intensive care unit with a "COPD exacerbation" and decompensated right heart failure. Undiagnosed OSA complicates the course at night with arousals, increased dyspnea, and O_2 desaturation values resistant to supplemental O_2.[20]

Hypoventilation Syndromes

In addition to OSA and CSA, chronic hypoventilation syndromes are increasingly being recognized.[21, 22] Patients with neuromuscular disorders such as amyotrophic lateral sclerosis (ALS) or muscular dystrophy, obesity hypoventilation syndrome, and spinal cord injury with diaphragm dysfunction may have underlying restrictive lung physiology. These patients may benefit from early detection of sleep-related hypoventilation. Treatment with nocturnal noninvasive ventilation may result in improved breathing during sleep, as well as better daytime energy and quality of life.[21, 22] Alternative therapies such as placement of a diaphragm pacer also may benefit a select subset of these patients.[23]

CLINICAL FEATURES

Patients with sleep apnea are more commonly men (three times greater frequency than among women), are older than 40 years, and have hypertension (Box 33-2). Most patients with sleep apnea report habitual snoring that has become progressively worse.[2, 24] Sensations of nocturnal choking, gasping, or resuscitative snorting are frequently reported. If a bed partner observes periods of apnea, the diagnosis of OSA is highly likely.

The presence of **excessive daytime sleepiness** (EDS) may be underestimated because OSA manifests in a subacute manner. As a result, patients with OSA may report symptoms of fatigue alone. These patients also frequently report nocturnal reflux, nocturia, chronic nasal congestion, morning headaches, and symptoms of depression.

Box 33-2 Common Clinical Features of Obstructive Sleep Apnea

- Male
- Age greater than 40 years
- Upper body obesity (neck >16.5 inches)
- Habitual snoring
- Fatigue or daytime sleepiness
- Diurnal hypertension

Patients with OSA have arousals from sleep and sleep fragmentation, which can lead to fatigue, EDS, and irritability.[25] Patients who have an increased frequency of awakenings and microarousal have more daytime sleepiness and greater difficulty with daytime functioning than the general population.[26] Patients with OSA may have neuropsychologic deficits and impaired vigilance.[27] Compared with the general population, untreated OSA patients are at increased risk for motor vehicle accidents because of EDS.[28-30]

The physical examination of most patients reveals evidence of obesity, particularly in the upper body. Upper body obesity can be quantitated with neck size. A neck circumference of 42 cm (16.5 inches) in men increases the likelihood of the diagnosis of sleep apnea.[14] Examination of the oropharynx frequently reveals a long soft palate. Although tonsillar hypertrophy is common in children with sleep apnea, it is seldom found in adults. Large palatine tonsils may increase the risk for airway closure during sleep. A retrognathic or micrognathic mandible can narrow the pharyngeal airway, placing a patient of normal weight at risk for airway closure during sleep.[8]

The cardiovascular examination may reveal evidence of pulmonary hypertension or right heart failure (lower extremity edema).[31,32] These findings are determined primarily by the hypoxic burden experienced by the patient. Pulmonary hypertension or right heart failure is more commonly encountered in patients with concomitant daytime hypoxemia. Patients with OSA and COPD or severe obesity (body mass index > 40) appear to be at particular risk for this complication.[33] Recurrent moderate to severe oxyhemoglobin desaturation secondary to OSA can be associated with an increased incidence of cardiac arrhythmias.[34,35] Repeated nocturnal desaturation also can cause secondary polycythemia.[14,36]

OSA and poor sleep quality are also associated with the metabolic syndrome independent of obesity.[37,38] The metabolic syndrome includes three of the following: waist circumference 102 cm or greater in men or 88 cm or greater in women, hypertension, impaired glucose tolerance, insulin resistance, and elevated triglycerides.[39,40] These interactions also can increase a patient's cardiac risks and are associated with increased morbidity and mortality from cardiovascular disease.[12,41]

In the acute care setting, patients who present with previously undiagnosed OSA can pose a particular challenge for diagnosis and management.[42-44] A high clinical suspicion for OSA in hospitalized patients is necessary because untreated or unrecognized OSA can complicate recovery from acute illness, trauma, heart failure, and recent surgery.[45-52] Patients with known OSA are frequently not placed on continuous positive airway pressure (CPAP) while in the hospital or may require a temporary adjustment in pressure settings.[53] Patients who are unstable for testing in a sleep laboratory can undergo portable bedside testing or empiric treatment with positive pressure if the diagnosis cannot be confirmed.[54] Outpatient follow-up with confirmatory sleep evaluation is important for long-term treatment and compliance.

RULE OF THUMB

Untreated OSA can cause daytime hypoxemia. The diagnosis of OSA should be considered when the degree of hypoxemia is out of proportion to the defect on pulmonary spirometry. When the arterial partial pressure of O_2 is less than 60 mm Hg but the FEV_1 is greater than 30% of predicted, COPD alone is inadequate to explain the hypoxemia and coexisting OSA should be considered. OSA in this setting is frequently associated with pulmonary hypertension and evidence of right heart failure on physical examination. Hypoxemia, pulmonary hypertension, and right heart failure can be substantially improved with management of OSA. If the patient adheres to therapy, the need for supplemental O_2 may be reduced or eliminated.

SCREENING QUESTIONNAIRES

An initial history and physical examination may be inadequate for identifying OSA. Several screening questionnaires have been developed to aid in rapidly identifying individuals with OSA. In general, screening questionnaires have good sensitivity but limited specificity for diagnosis of OSA. The Berlin Questionnaire, the American Society for Anesthesiology (ASA) screening questionnaire, and the Sleep Apnea Clinical Score (SACS) have been validated for use as screening for OSA.[48-50] The STOP-BANG has been used commonly because of simplicity and ease of use, particularly in patients undergoing elective surgery[50] (Box 33-3). However useful and suggestive these questionnaires may be, a diagnostic sleep study remains the gold standard for diagnosing OSA.

LABORATORY TESTING

When sleep apnea is suspected, an overnight polysomnogram (PSG) should be obtained to confirm the clinical diagnosis. A full-night PSG in the sleep laboratory monitored by a sleep technologist is considered the standard method for diagnosing OSA.

In a laboratory sleep study, several physiologic signals are recorded to determine whether airway closure occurs during sleep and to what extent the events disturb sleep continuity and cardiopulmonary function. An electroencephalogram (EEG), electrooculogram (EOG), and chin electromyogram (EMG) are obtained for assessment of sleep stage and documentation of sleep disruption secondary to sleep-related breathing disturbance. Airflow (measured at the nose and mouth), ventilatory

Box 33-3 STOP-BANG Questionnaire to Screen for Obstructive Sleep Apnea

***S**nore:*	Do you snore loudly (louder than talking or loud enough to be heard through closed doors)?
***T**ired:*	Do you often feel tired, fatigued, or sleepy during the daytime?
***O**bserved:*	Has anyone observed you stop breathing during sleep?
***P**ressure:*	Do you have or are you being treated for high blood pressure?
***B**MI:*	Greater than 35 kg/m^2?
***A**ge:*	Age older 50 years?
***N**eck:*	Neck circumference greater than 40 cm?
***G**ender:*	Gender male?

One point assigned for each positive question.
Total score less than three = low probability for OSA.
Total score three or greater = high probability for OSA.
Total score five or greater = high probability of moderate to severe OSA.

From Chung F, Subramanyam R, Liao P, et al: High STOP-BANG score indicates a high probability of obstructive sleep apnoea. Br J Anaesth 108:768–775, 2012.

Box 33-4 Key Features of Sleep Studies to Be Analyzed and Reported for Obstructive Sleep Apnea

- Apnea-hypopnea index
- Arousal index
- Sleep stage distribution
- Frequency of oxyhemoglobin desaturations
- Mean oxyhemoglobin saturation
- Nadir of oxyhemoglobin saturation

effort (using inductive plethysmography or piezoelectric belts), cardiac rhythm (with a modified lead II electrocardiogram [ECG]), and SaO_2 (measured with pulse oximetry) are included in the standard testing montage.

In obstructive apnea or hypopnea, airflow is absent or decreased in the presence of continued ventilatory effort. Asynchronous (paradoxical) movement of the abdomen and rib cage can be observed. O_2 desaturation may or may not occur. The degree of the O_2 desaturation depends on the length of the apneic event or the patient's baseline saturation (see Figure 33-1). Respiratory effort–related arousals are characterized by increased respiratory effort, leading to arousal from sleep that does not meet the criterion of an apneic or a hypopneic event (see Figure 33-1).[55,56]

Measuring devices that are adequate for assessing hypopnea also are adequate for assessing apnea; however, devices used for measuring apnea cannot always detect hypopnea. The diagnosis of hypopnea may be affected by the measurement technique used. In 1999, an American Academy of Sleep Medicine (AASM) task force conducted an evidence-based review of measurement techniques for detection of hypopnea.[57] The scoring system was as follows: *A,* good to excellent agreement with a reference standard (face mask pneumotachygraph); *B,* limited data, but good theoretical framework and clinical experience suggest the method is valid; *C,* no data, weak theoretical framework or clinical experience; and *D,* research or clinical experience suggests the method is invalid.

The measuring techniques were scored as follows: nasal pressure, B; respiratory inductance plethysmography (RIP) with sum of chest and abdominal signals, B; dual-channel RIP, C; single-channel RIP, C; piezoelectricity sensors, strain gauges, and thoracic impedance, D; breathing measurement signal with a desaturation or arousal, B; expired carbon dioxide (CO_2), D; and thermal sensors, D. A face mask pneumotachygraph allows the greatest precision in measuring airflow, but it is poorly tolerated. Nasal pressure is a reliable way to detect hypopnea and is well tolerated by patients undergoing a diagnostic PSG.[5,57]

After the sleep study is completed, the sleep technologist scores it. The number of apneas and hypopneas per hour of sleep are reported as an apnea-hypopnea index (AHI) or respiratory disturbance index (RDI). The AASM has operationally defined the severity of OSA as follows: mild, AHI 5 to 15; moderate, AHI 15 to 30; and severe, AHI greater than 30. AHI less than 5 is considered within the normal range for adults. The number of arousals per hour (arousal index), percentage of each sleep stage, frequency of SaO_2, mean SaO_2, and nadir of SaO_2 also are reported (Box 33-4).

RULE OF THUMB

Intermittent checks of SaO_2 cannot reliably exclude sleep-related desaturation secondary to OSA. Placing the oximetry probe on the patient frequently awakens the patient. In addition, isolated readings may not allow sampling of all sleep stages, especially rapid eye movement (REM) sleep, during which sleep-disordered breathing and nocturnal desaturation tend to be prominent. Continuous overnight oximetry is a better assessment of the degree of oxyhemoglobin desaturation with sleep.

Abbreviated (portable) cardiopulmonary testing has been used to confirm a diagnosis of OSA. These studies do not record the electrophysiologic signals (EEG, EOG, and EMG) required to stage and score sleep. The portable studies vary in the type and number of cardiopulmonary values recorded. Controversy exists whether portable systems are sufficient to diagnose OSA. Many variables, such as airflow, ventilatory effort, sleep stage, and SaO_2 values, may be less precise or may not be measured at all with these devices. Currently, portable monitoring for the diagnosis of OSA is acceptable in patients with high pretest probability but without significant comorbidities that may affect the accuracy of testing.[58] A growing body of evidence supports the use of portable testing for additional patient populations, including patients undergoing elective surgery and patients admitted to the hospital with acute heart failure or stroke.[59]

Excerpts of American Association for Respiratory Care (AARC) Clinical Practice Guidelines for a PSG are provided in Clinical Practice Guideline 33-1.

TREATMENT

Management of OSA should be individualized but generally can be classified into three options: behavioral, medical, and surgical interventions.[60] Behavioral therapy should be pursued in the care of all patients. Medical and surgical therapy must be tailored to the individual patient. The likelihood of acceptance and adherence to the prescribed therapeutic intervention must be considered. The goals of treatment are to normalize SaO_2 and ventilation; eliminate apnea, hypopnea, and snoring; and improve sleep architecture and continuity (Box 33-5).

Behavioral Interventions and Risk Counseling

Patients must be informed of the risks of uncontrolled sleep apnea. Several behavioral interventions can be beneficial,

33-1 Polysomnography

AARC Clinical Practice Guideline (Excerpts)*

INDICATIONS

Polysomnography may be indicated in patients with:

- COPD whose awake PaO_2 is greater than 55 mm Hg but whose illness is complicated by pulmonary hypertension, right heart failure, polycythemia, or excessive daytime sleepiness
- Restrictive ventilatory impairment secondary to chest wall and neuromuscular disturbances whose illness is complicated by chronic hypoventilation, polycythemia, pulmonary hypertension, disturbed sleep, morning headaches, or daytime somnolence or fatigue
- Disturbances in respiratory control whose awake $PaCO_2$ is greater than 45 mm Hg or whose illness is complicated by pulmonary hypertension, polycythemia, disturbed sleep, morning headaches, or daytime somnolence or fatigue
- Nocturnal cyclic bradyarrhythmia or tachyarrhythmia, nocturnal abnormalities of atrioventricular conduction, or ventricular ectopy that seems to increase in frequency during sleep
- Excessive daytime sleepiness or insomnia
- Snoring associated with observed apneas or excessive daytime sleepiness or both
- Other symptoms of sleep-disordered breathing as described in *The International Classification of Sleep Disorders, Diagnostic and Coding Manual*

CONTRAINDICATIONS

There are no absolute contraindications to polysomnography when indications are clearly established. However, risk-to-benefit ratios should be assessed if transferring medically unstable inpatients.

PRECAUTIONS AND COMPLICATIONS

- Skin irritation may occur as a result of the adhesive used to attach electrodes to the patient.
- At the conclusion of the study, adhesive remover is used to dissolve adhesive on the patient's skin. Adhesive removers (e.g., acetone) should be used only in well-ventilated areas.
- The integrity of the electrical isolation of polysomnographic equipment must be certified by engineering or biomedical personnel qualified to make such assessment.
- The adhesive used to attach EEG electrodes should not be used to attach electrodes near the patient's eyes and should always be used in well-ventilated areas.
- Because of the high flammability of adhesives and acetone, these substances should be used with caution, especially in patients who require supplemental O_2.
- Adhesives should be used with caution in patients with reactive airways disease and in small infants.
- Patients with parasomnias or seizures may be at risk for injury related to movements during sleep.
- Institution-specific policies and guidelines describing personnel responsibilities and appropriate responses should be developed.

ASSESSMENT OF NEED

Polysomnography is indicated for patients suspected to have sleep-related respiratory disturbances described in *The International Classification of Sleep Disorders, Diagnostic and Coding Manual*.

ASSESSMENT OF TEST QUALITY

- Polysomnography should either confirm or eliminate a sleep-related diagnosis.
- Documentation of findings, suggested therapeutic intervention, and other clinical decisions resulting from polysomnography should be noted in the patient's chart.
- Each laboratory should implement a quality assurance program that addresses equipment calibration and maintenance, patient preparation and monitoring, scoring methodology, and intertechnician scoring variances.

MONITORING

- Patient variables to be monitored include EEG, EOG, EMG, ECG, respiratory effort, nasal or oral airflow, SpO_2, body position, and limb movement; intervention should occur if the physiologic signals are lost.
- Infrared or low-light video cameras and recording equipment should permit visualization of the patient by the technician throughout the procedure.
- The technician should intervene if an acute change in physiologic status occurs and communicate that change to appropriate medical personnel.

**For complete guidelines, see AARC-APT (American Association for Respiratory Care-Association of Polysomnography Technologists) clinical practice guideline. Polysomnography. Respir Care 40:1336–1343, 1995.*

Box 33-5 Goals of Treating Obstructive Sleep Apnea

- Eliminate apnea, hypopnea, and snoring
- Normalize SaO_2 and ventilation
- Improve sleep architecture and continuity

including weight loss in obese patients; avoiding alcohol, sedatives, and hypnotics; and avoiding sleep deprivation. Although weight loss clearly influences the severity of sleep apnea, it is frequently difficult to accomplish. Involving the patient with a dietitian or nutritionist can be helpful. Alcohol decreases the arousal threshold and so can increase the duration of apnea. Alcohol also reduces upper airway muscle tone, causing the airway to be more compliant and more prone to complete or partial closure.[61] For these reasons, alcohol should be avoided by patients believed to have sleep apnea. Sedatives and hypnotics can decrease the stability of the upper airway and suppress certain stages of sleep.[62]

Positional Therapy

When a sleep study indicates that apnea and snoring occur only in the supine position, instruction on sleeping in the lateral position or head of bed elevation can be beneficial.[63,64] Use of the "tennis ball" technique, in which a ball is sewn onto the back of the patient's sleeping garment, or other positional devices that discourage the patient from rolling into the supine position can be effective in treating positional OSA.[65] However, the long-term effects of positional therapy are unknown. Positional therapy is generally recommended for milder cases of positional OSA.

Medical Interventions

Positive Pressure Therapy

Continuous Positive Airway Pressure Therapy. Continuous positive airway pressure (CPAP) therapy was introduced for management of OSA in 1981.[66] CPAP has become the first-line medical therapy for OSA. Many studies have documented the effectiveness of CPAP in decreasing the morbidity and mortality associated with OSA.[9,11,67,68] For most patients, obstruction of the upper airway is abolished by CPAP pressures between 7.5 cm H_2O and 12.5 cm H_2O.[69] The level of CPAP required for optimal management of OSA is best determined with a titration performed in the sleep laboratory.[68] Attempts to use an algorithm or a prediction equation as a replacement for in-laboratory titration have not been uniformly successful.[70]

CPAP therapy has been shown to decrease daytime sleepiness and improve neurocognitive testing, vigilance scores, insulin sensitivity, and lipid profiles. CPAP decreases the incidence of pulmonary hypertension and right heart failure and decreases the number of ventilation-related arousals and nocturnal cardiac events. Reductions in daytime hypoxemia and hypercapnia also have been attributed to CPAP therapy.[69,71-75]

CPAP therapy primarily works by splinting the upper airway open, increasing the intraluminal pressure of the upper airway

MINI CLINI

Nocturnal Angina in an Obese Middle-Aged Man

HISTORY: A 45-year-old, morbidly obese nonsmoker is admitted to the coronary care unit after awakening at 4 AM with chest pain typical of angina pectoris. The pain has resolved by the time he reaches the emergency department. The patient is unsure of the duration of the pain before he called for his wife, who sleeps in a separate bedroom because of his very loud habitual snoring. The patient reports exertional shortness of breath but no chest pain before this event. He states that he frequently gets "indigestion" that sometimes is worse at night, but that this pain was different.

MEDICATIONS:

- Captopril, 25 mg by mouth twice per day
- Furosemide (Lasix), 20 mg by mouth every day
- Cimetidine (Tagamet), 300 mg by mouth at bedtime

MEDICAL HISTORY:

- Hypertension and gastroesophageal reflux
- No significant cardiac disease
- Cardiac catheterization 1 year ago showed normal left ventricular function and minimal coronary artery occlusion

PHYSICAL EXAMINATION:

- *Vital signs:* Blood pressure 160/98 mm Hg, heart rate 100 beats/min, temperature 98.6° F (37° C), respiration 18 breaths/min
- *General:* Mildly diaphoretic obese white man
- *Neck:* 52 cm (20.5 inches) in circumference
- *Lungs:* Clear breath sounds bilaterally
- *Heart:* Regular rate and rhythm
- *Abdomen:* Obese; soft, normal bowel sounds
- *Extremities:* 4-mm pretibial pitting edema

LABORATORY DATA:

- *Room air arterial blood gases (ABGs):* pH 7.36, PCO_2 37 mm Hg, PO_2 62 mm Hg, SaO_2 92%
- *Chest radiograph:* Pulmonary congestion, otherwise normal
- *ECG:* Sinus tachycardia without acute changes

PROBLEM: Why did this patient experience angina during sleep?

DISCUSSION: Serial cardiac enzyme values show no myocardial infarction. A stress test result is negative, but a submaximal effort is obtained. The patient's weight precludes an adenosine thallium stress test. A repeat cardiac catheterization shows no change in the minimal coronary artery occlusion reported previously. The pulmonary consultant called to evaluate the patient's shortness of breath recommends a nocturnal PSG to rule out sleep apnea. The sleep study result is positive for severe sleep apnea (AHI 110; lowest SaO_2 70% on the oximeter during REM sleep). A CPAP titration test is performed. The patient is discharged home on CPAP 17.5 cm H_2O via a nasal mask. He returns to the pulmonary clinic 1 month after discharge. He reported no further episodes of nocturnal angina. Reflux and shortness of breath have been relieved. The patient has lost 10 lb (4.5 kg) without dieting. Lower extremity edema is markedly relieved. A download of data from his CPAP machine shows excellent compliance with usage on 85% of nights, as well as good response to therapy with an average estimated AHI 3.5.

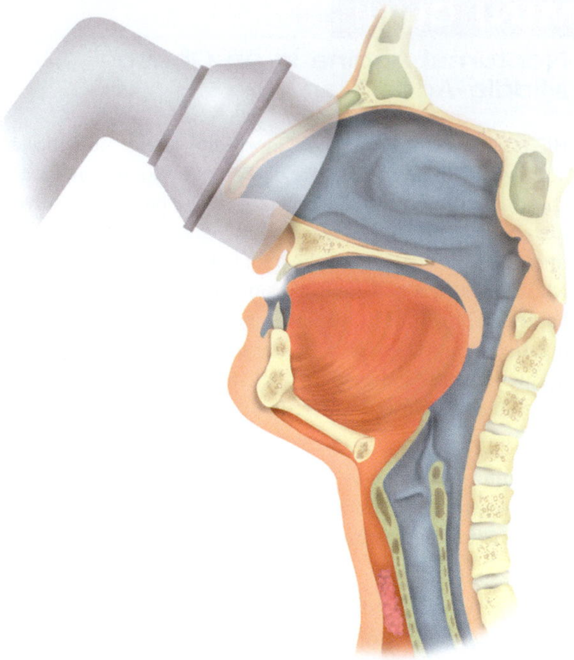

FIGURE 33-3 Nasal continuous positive airway pressure (CPAP). Positive airway pressure is applied with a nasal mask. The soft palate falls against the base of the tongue so that the upper airway is pneumatically splinted open.

above a critical transmural pressure of the pharynx and hypopharynx that is associated with airway closure. The soft palate is effectively moved anteriorly up against the tongue, "pressurizing" the upper airway (Figure 33-3).[76] CPAP allows the upper airway to be splinted open whether there is a single site (uncommon) or multiple sites (more common) of airway narrowing or closure. Investigators have found that when nasal CPAP is applied, EMG activity of the upper airway dilator muscles is decreased.[77]

To be successful, CPAP titration should eliminate all apneic episodes and reduce the number of hypopneic episodes for preventing arterial O_2 desaturation. Paradoxical thoracoabdominal movement and snoring should be eliminated.[78] For improvement of sleep continuity, respiration-related EEG arousals and microarousals must be abolished. There is no evidence to support the misconception that a higher level of CPAP always is necessary in patients with severe sleep apnea. There is variability in the CPAP requirement to treat OSA effectively. Some patients with relatively mild elevation of the AHI need higher levels of CPAP than patients with a substantially higher AHI.[79]

Patients who report EDS without an increase in AHI may have repetitive 2- to 3-second transient EEG arousals during episodes of snoring. These short arousals occur during episodes of increased upper airway resistance, and although not associated with any significant arterial O_2 desaturation, they may cause EDS and fatigue.[80,81] This pattern is known as *upper airway resistance syndrome,* generally occurs in younger patients, and is characterized by respiratory effort–related arousals (see Figure 33-1). With the emergence of upper airway resistance syndrome as a clinical entity, some researchers have suggested that CPAP titrations may be suboptimal without measurement of esophageal pressure.[79,82,83] Many sleep laboratories do not measure esophageal pressure. In addition, many patients refuse this type of monitoring because of perceived or real discomfort.

The contour of the inspiratory flow signal, when measured by a pressure transducer, correlates with ventilatory effort as reflected by esophageal pressure.[55] When esophageal pressure is not used, nasal pressure can be useful to facilitate CPAP titrations.[83] It has been hypothesized that during CPAP titration, there is a period during the transition to deeper stages of sleep when there is flow limitation and increased intrathoracic pressure without EEG arousals.[63] It has been suggested that if this condition is not corrected, patients may have incomplete and suboptimal titrations. The clinical significance of flow limitation without EEG arousals is currently uncertain.

Despite numerous studies documenting the efficacy of CPAP in treating patients in the sleep laboratory, many patients have difficulty adhering to CPAP therapy. Approximately 80% of patients accept CPAP initially, although long-term objective compliance is frequently lower. *Objective compliance*—defined as use of the machine for more than 4 hours per night for more than 70% of observed nights—has been measured to be 46%.[84,85] Data can be downloaded from CPAP machines that reveal patient compliance, average usage per night, average estimated AHI, presence of air leak, and other parameters.

The severity of AHI does not always correlate with compliance, and the benefit perceived by the patient is a better predictor. Research indicates that patients who are subjectively sleepy and have an AHI of 30 or greater are likely to accept and comply with CPAP therapy.[94] Clinic follow-up with objective compliance monitoring is essential. Compliance 1 month after the initiation of therapy is reported to be a good predictor of CPAP use at 3 months.

It is unclear whether higher levels of CPAP cause a decrease in compliance. Some patients report that breathing against a continuous pressure is uncomfortable. Discomfort with the interface and the device also may reduce acceptance and compliance.[87-89] Since introducing CPAP, various interfaces have been designed to improve comfort and have a favorable impact on compliance. Nasal pillows or prongs, nasal masks with comfort flaps or bubbles, oronasal masks, and full-face masks are available.[90-94] No studies have been conducted to directly compare efficacy, subjective patient comfort, or objective patient compliance with these interfaces.[90] In clinical practice, some patients tolerate one interface better than another. Technician bias may affect the choice of an interface, and this may have a positive or negative impact.

Bilevel Pressure Therapy. Another form of positive pressure therapy is **bilevel positive airway pressure (bilevel PAP).** Bilevel PAP therapy was developed to take advantage of the fact that some patients may have different pressure requirements between inspiration and expiration.[89] It was hypothesized that because a patient may have a lower expiratory pressure

MINI CLINI

Young Man Hospitalized for Observation After a Single-Vehicle Accident in the Midafternoon

HISTORY: A 27-year-old nonsmoker is admitted to the coronary care unit for monitoring so that the diagnosis of cardiac contusion can be ruled out. The patient has been involved in a single-vehicle automobile accident. The accident occurred at 3:30 PM on a clear day. The patient felt drowsy immediately before the event. He became conscious after hitting the guardrail. The patient's chest hit the steering wheel. The patient reports anterior chest wall pain and denies having angina or feeling faint.

MEDICATIONS:
- None

MEDICAL HISTORY:
- Negative

PHYSICAL EXAMINATION:
- *Vital signs:* Blood pressure 140/88 mm Hg, heart rate 100 beats/min, temperature 98.6° F (37° C), respirations 16 breaths/min
- *General:* Well-developed, well-nourished white man
- *Head, eyes, ears, nose throat:* Elongated soft palate, mild crowding of tonsillar pillars, retrognathic chin
- *Neck:* 40 cm (16 inches) in circumference
- *Chest:* Contusion on anterior portion of the chest
- *Lungs:* Clear breath sounds bilaterally
- *Heart:* Regular rate and rhythm
- *Abdomen:* Soft with normal bowel sounds
- *Extremities:* No clubbing, cyanosis, or edema
- *Skin:* Multiple small lacerations

LABORATORY DATA:
- *Chest radiograph:* No cardiomegaly, mass, infiltrate, or effusion
- *ECG:* Sinus tachycardia
- *Creatine kinase:* 350 international/L (no myocardial bond fraction)

PROBLEM: What caused the patient to fall asleep at the wheel?

DISCUSSION: The patient is found to have bradycardia during sleep on the night of admission. These episodes appear to be associated with snoring and oxyhemoglobin desaturation on O_2 at 2 L/min through a nasal cannula. The cardiology consultant recommends a diagnostic nocturnal PSG to rule out sleep apnea. The study shows severe sleep apnea (AHI 85 with a low SaO_2 of 60%). A CPAP titration study reveals that the patient requires 10 cm H_2O of CPAP via nasal pillows. At follow-up 1 month later, the patient states he no longer experiences the fatigue he had previously. In retrospect, the patient believes that before treatment with CPAP, he was quite sleepy during the day. Despite this improvement, he wants to explore other treatment options. A surgical consultation is obtained.

RULE OF THUMB

Retrognathia can be the cause of OSA in young patients who are at or close to ideal body weight. CPAP therapy is highly effective for these patients, but upper airway reconstruction (phases I and II surgery) can be curative.

requirement to splint the airway open, patient acceptance and compliance would be favorably affected. Bilevel units operate on household electricity and are similar in size and appearance to conventional CPAP units. There is a difference in cost, however, with bilevel devices generally more expensive than CPAP devices.

Although patient acceptance may be slightly better with bilevel PAP, published data have shown no difference in compliance between conventional CPAP and bilevel PAP in patients who have not previously received CPAP therapy.[95] However, bilevel PAP may be better tolerated by the subgroup of patients who need higher CPAP settings or who are uncomfortable exhaling against a continuous pressure.

In contrast to conventional CPAP, bilevel PAP is titrated by increasing inspiratory positive airway pressure and expiratory positive airway pressure separately in response to apnea, hypopnea, and desaturation. The specific titration algorithm may vary from laboratory to laboratory. Generally, inspiratory positive airway pressure and expiratory positive airway pressure are titrated upward together (as CPAP) until apnea is eliminated. Inspiratory positive airway pressure is then increased independently to eliminate hypopnea, snoring, and arousals.

Autotitrating Devices. A new generation of self-titrating CPAP devices has been developed to address issues of patient compliance, patient comfort, and variability of the CPAP requirement throughout the night.[96-99] These devices are referred to as *auto-CPAP, intelligent CPAP,* or *smart CPAP*. These devices use a computer algorithm for adjusting the level of CPAP in response to dynamic changes in airflow or vibration caused by snoring or both. Abnormal function manifests as snoring, hypopnea, and apnea. The average overnight pressure required to treat OSA effectively may be decreased, which may have a favorable impact on interface-related leaks. It is unknown whether these devices are capable of eliminating the need for standard CPAP titration in a sleep laboratory. Self-titrating devices may help facilitate therapeutic CPAP titrations by technologists in the sleep laboratory but cannot replace proper diagnostic testing.[54] Further studies are needed to determine whether self-titrating CPAP devices provide any improvement over conventional CPAP units in the areas of compliance and EDS, particularly in patients who have not previously received CPAP therapy. More advanced auto-titrating devices can be used for CSA and hypoventilation syndromes.

Side Effects and Troubleshooting Strategies. Side effects of positive pressure therapy are related to the interface and to the pressure prescribed. These effects include feelings of claustrophobia, nasal congestion, rhinorrhea, skin irritation, and

MINI CLINI

Middle-Aged Woman With Pulmonary Hypertension

HISTORY: A 59-year-old former smoker is admitted to the hospital for right and left heart catheterization. A previous ECG showed pulmonary hypertension. The patient denies having angina or exertional chest discomfort. She admits to dyspnea on exertion that has been increasing over the past few months and to a chronic nonproductive cough. She denies taking "diet pills."

MEDICATIONS:

- Nifedipine, 10 mg by mouth three times per day
- Furosemide (Lasix), 20 mg by mouth daily
- Potassium chloride, 20 mEq by mouth twice per day

MEDICAL HISTORY:

- Hypertension and allergic rhinitis
- No cardiac disease

PHYSICAL EXAMINATION:

- *Vital signs:* Blood pressure 140/88 mm Hg, heart rate 90 beats/min, temperature 98.6° F (37° C), respirations 12 breaths/min
- *General:* Obese white woman in no acute distress
- Neck: 40 cm (16 inches) in circumference
- Lungs: Clear breath sounds bilaterally
- *Heart:* Regular rate and rhythm, increased second heart sound (P_2)
- *Abdomen:* Obese; soft, normal bowel sounds
- *Extremities:* 2-mm pretibial pitting edema

LABORATORY DATA:

- *Chest radiograph:* Mildly enlarged heart, no mass, infiltrate, or effusion
- *ECG:* Normal sinus rhythm with P pulmonale
- *Left heart catheterization:* No significant coronary artery disease, normal left ventricular function
- *Right heart catheterization:* Pulmonary hypertension (75/25 mm Hg), pulmonary artery wedge pressure 23 mm Hg
- *Room air ABGs:* pH 7.45, PCO_2 41 mm Hg, PO_2 54 mm Hg, SaO_2 84%
- *Spirometry:* Forced vital capacity (FVC) 1.69 L (55% of predicted value), FEV_1 1.27 L (55% of predicted value), FEV_1/FVC 75, forced expiratory flow midexpiratory phase ($FEF_{25\%-75\%}$) 0.96 L/sec (37% of predicted value); no significant improvement with single-dose bronchodilator

PROBLEM: What is the cause of the pulmonary hypertension?

DISCUSSION: The pulmonary service is consulted for evaluation for pulmonary hypertension in association with abnormal spirometric results. Results of bilateral lower extremity Doppler examinations and a ventilation/perfusion scan are normal. Because of a history of snoring, an overnight portable cardiopulmonary sleep study is performed. The study reveals evidence of snoring, nonpositional apnea and hypopnea, and desaturation to less than 60% on the oximeter for most of the monitoring period. Results of a PSG performed in the sleep laboratory verify the presence of moderate to severe OSA with AHI 28, which responds well to the application of CPAP titrated to 12 cm H_2O. Follow-up examinations show the dyspnea is relieved and that ABG values have improved. The patient no longer needs portable liquid O_2 to maintain SaO_2 greater than 90% at rest or with exercise.

It is likely this patient has pulmonary hypertension that is due to OSA, as opposed to idiopathic pulmonary artery hypertension, which generally affects younger women. Chronic thromboembolic disease should be excluded, as it was in this case. Chronic right heart failure secondary to sleep apnea can be improved with proper treatment.

nasal dryness (Figure 33-4). Claustrophobia and skin irritation can be managed by changing the interface to one that is more easily tolerated by the patient. Nasal congestion, rhinorrhea, skin irritation, and nasal dryness can be managed by using combinations of topical nasal steroids, antihistamines, nasal saline sprays, and lotions. A humidifier can be used in-line with the machine. Heated humidification has been shown to improve compliance.[100] If the patient has a sensation of too much pressure in the nose, adding a system equipped with a ramp may be beneficial.[62] The ramp allows a gradual increase in pressure over 5 to 45 minutes. The ramp time is empirically determined by the prescribing physician. There is no objective evidence that a ramp feature improves patient acceptance or compliance.[84]

Pressure leaks are another problem that RTs may encounter. Most interfaces use the nose. Some patients tend to breathe partially or mainly through the mouth. The addition of a chin strap may not resolve the problem. Changing the interface to an oronasal mask may be required for effective "pressurization" of the upper airway in these patients.[90] Mask and equipment availability varies depending on the home care company or medical facility, which can affect patient accommodation and long-term adherence to therapy

Oral Appliances

Oral appliances are devices that enlarge the airway by moving the mandible forward or by keeping the tongue in an anterior position (Figure 33-5). Patients who have mild sleep apnea and are unwilling to use CPAP may benefit from these devices. Oral appliances are worn only during sleep and come in various forms. The appliances are custom-fitted by dentists and are generally well tolerated by patients. They are overall less effective than CPAP therapy and are regarded as a second-line intervention, particularly for severe OSA.[101,102] The role of oral appliance therapy in the acute care setting, such as patients hospitalized for acute heart failure or after elective surgery, is unclear.

Medications

Medications have proved ineffective for most patients with sleep apnea. Benzodiazepines and other sedative-hypnotics

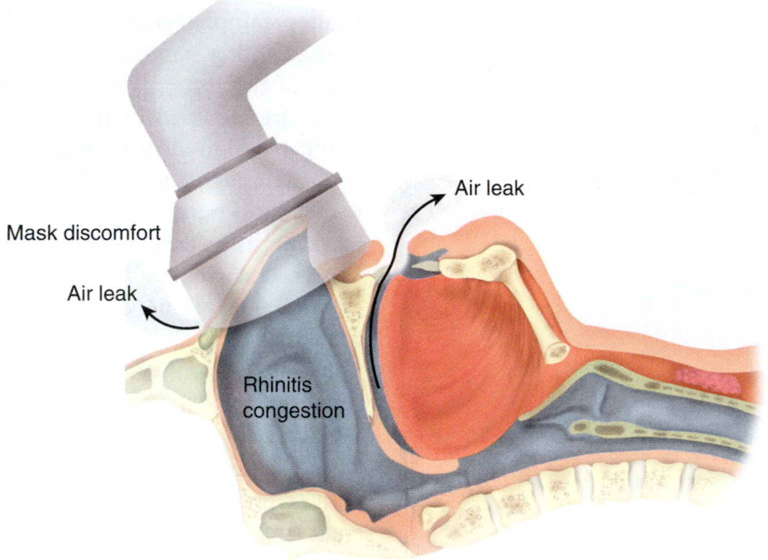

FIGURE 33-4 Positive airway pressure problems. Various problems can be encountered with continuous positive airway pressure.

MINI CLINI

Worsening Right-Sided Heart Failure in a Patient With Chronic Obstructive Pulmonary Disease Who Is Using Oxygen

HISTORY: A 50-year-old former smoker previously found to have severe COPD, with FEV_1 of 0.9 L (30% of predicted value), is admitted to the hospital for evaluation and management of worsening shortness of breath and persistent bilateral leg swelling. He has been using O_2 at 2 L/min 24 hours per day for the last 3 months. A chronic productive cough of clear sputum has been unchanged. He denies having chest pain.

MEDICATIONS:

- Ipratropium bromide by metered dose inhaler, 2 puffs four times per day
- O_2, 2 L/min 24 hours per day
- Hydrochlorothiazide, 50 mg by mouth daily
- Theophylline, 300 mg by mouth twice per day

MEDICAL HISTORY:

- Hypertension and chronic bronchitis
- No cardiac disease

PHYSICAL EXAMINATION:

- *Vital signs:* Blood pressure 150/90 mm Hg, heart rate 100 beats/min, temperature 98.6° F (37° C), respirations 18 breaths/min
- *General:* Obese white man who appears short of breath
- *Neck:* 46 cm (18 in) in circumference
- *Lungs:* Decreased breath sounds bilaterally
- *Heart:* Faint sounds but regular rate and rhythm
- *Abdomen:* Obese; soft, normal bowel sounds
- *Extremities:* "Dusky" lower extremities with 4 mm pitting edema to the knees

LABORATORY DATA:

- *Theophylline level:* 12 mcg/ml
- *ABGs:* pH 7.36, PCO_2 44 mm Hg, PO_2 56 mm Hg, SaO_2 89% (on 2 L/min O_2)
- *Chest radiograph:* "Pulmonary congestion"; otherwise normal
- *ECG:* Sinus tachycardia without acute changes
- *Echocardiogram:* "Technically limited" but reported to be without segmental wall abnormalities or to show normal left ventricular function
- *Bilateral lower extremity Doppler examination:* Negative for deep venous thrombosis

PROBLEM: What could be the cause of this patient's continued signs of right heart failure?

DISCUSSION: The patient has overlap syndrome (COPD and OSA). He has been appropriately treated for COPD (bronchodilators and O_2) but has not been treated for OSA. His physician never asked and the patient never volunteered a history of nightly loud snoring with observed apnea and daytime fatigue. Subsequent evaluation with a nocturnal PSG reveals severe nocturnal desaturation to 40% on the oximeter despite treatment with O_2 at 2 L/min. A CPAP titration study is performed. The patient is discharged with CPAP set at 15 cm H_2O via a nasal mask. He returns to the outpatient clinic 3 months later and reports "feeling great." He reports that the shortness of breath has decreased and that he has much more energy during the day. Physical examination shows trace pedal edema. ABG studies on 2 L/min of O_2 reveal pH 7.40, PCO_2 40 mm Hg, PO_2 75 mm Hg, and SaO_2 93%.

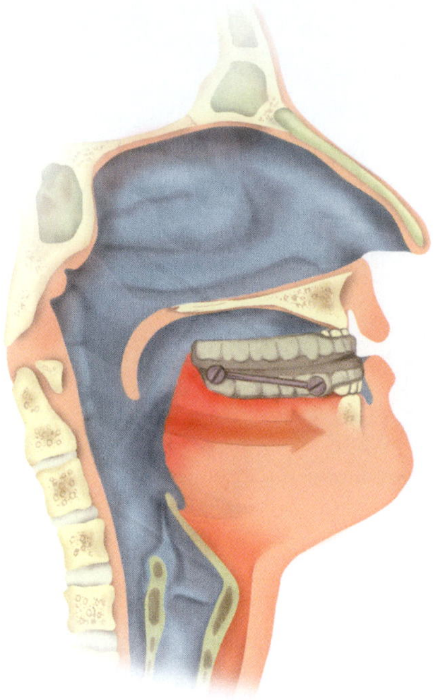

FIGURE 33-5 Oral appliance. The oral appliance covers the teeth of the upper and lower jaws and is adjusted to move the mandible (lower jaw) forward mechanically to open the airway.

Box 33-6 Surgical Alternatives for Obstructive Sleep Apnea

- Bypass of the upper airway
- Tracheostomy
- Reconstruction of the upper airway
- Nasal surgery
- Palatal surgery
- Maxillofacial surgery

should be avoided because they can potentiate upper airway collapse. The antidepressants protriptyline and fluoxetine have been used to manage mild sleep apnea but are ineffective in most patients.[14] O_2 therapy is useful for patients with oxyhemoglobin desaturation who refuse positive pressure therapy. O_2 therapy can improve nocturnal desaturation but has no significant effect on ventilatory arousals and daytime sleepiness.[103] O_2 therapy should be used with caution by patients with concomitant severe COPD, who may retain CO_2.

Surgical Interventions

Surgical alternatives can be divided into two broad categories: procedures that bypass the upper airway and procedures that reconstruct the upper airway (Box 33-6). Before the advent of CPAP therapy, tracheostomy was the primary therapy for severe OSA. Because of the psychosocial and medical morbidity associated with the procedure, use of tracheostomy today is limited to managing severe OSA when all other therapies have been exhausted.[104,105]

Palatal Surgery

Uvulopalatopharyngoplasty (UPPP) is palatal surgery performed with a standard "cold knife" technique or a laser. Portions of the soft palate, the uvula, and additional redundant tissue are removed in these procedures. The success rate of UPPP is reported to be less than 50% overall.[106] The site of the physiologic obstruction cannot be predicted correctly with preoperative imaging. Laser-assisted UPPP has been marketed as an outpatient procedure; however, substantial efficacy in managing OSA has not been documented. UPPP cannot be recommended for the management of OSA at the present time.[107,108]

Maxillofacial Surgery

Maxillofacial surgery shows more promise for patients with OSA (Figure 33-6). Phase I surgical procedures combine UPPP with genioglossal advancement. Patients are identified preoperatively with a combination of radiologic imaging and direct visualization of the upper airway. It is beneficial to have these patients use CPAP therapy perioperatively to reduce the chronic upper airway swelling and edema present before surgery and to reduce postoperative airway edema.[109] When phase I surgery is unsuccessful, phase II surgery involves advancement of the maxilla and the mandible.[110] These surgical procedures are performed at only a few specialized centers. A coordinated effort by a dedicated team of otolaryngologists, oral surgeons, and sleep specialists is essential. Regardless of the surgical option chosen, a postoperative PSG should be obtained to document improvement objectively.[111]

Additional Therapies

Newer treatment options for OSA are being developed and tested, including nasal resistance devices, negative pressure appliances, and implantable **upper airway stimulators**.[112,113] Long-term benefits have yet to be established, but initial results have been promising.

RULE OF THUMB

Sleep symptoms may present early in patients with neuromuscular disease. Treatment with noninvasive ventilation during sleep may improve daytime symptoms.

ROLE OF THE RESPIRATORY THERAPIST IN DISORDERS OF SLEEP

RTs play a vital role in diagnosing and treating OSA. As part of the multidisciplinary team, RTs prepare patients for the overnight PSG and obtain key information relating to their sleep history. During the study, RTs assess for **sleep-disordered breathing** and apply and titrate positive pressure. They are also involved with education, which is important in assisting with the patient's understanding and compliance with positive

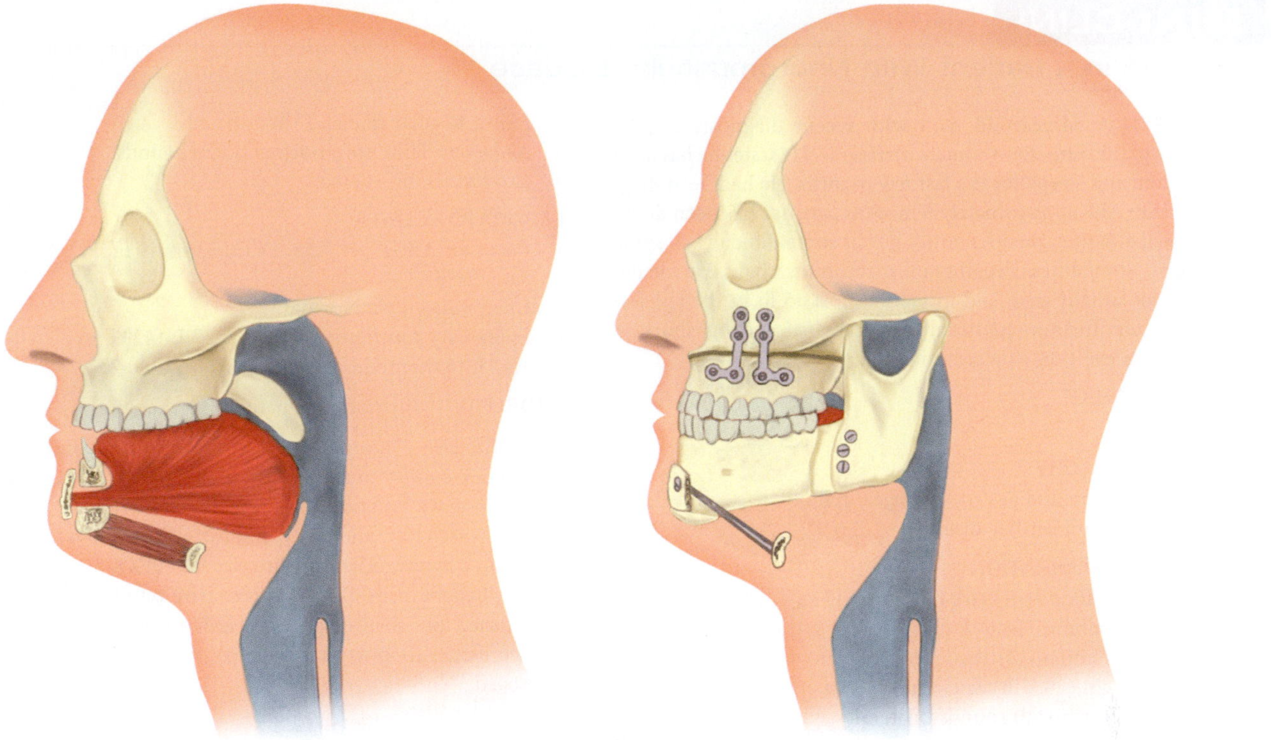

FIGURE 33-6 Phase I and phase II upper airway reconstruction. **A,** Phase I surgery. Lateral cutaway view of the skull shows tongue (genioglossal) and hyoid bone advancement in conjunction with uvulopalatopharyngoplasty. **B,** Phase II surgery. Lateral cutaway view of the skull shows advancement of the maxilla (upper jaw) and mandible (lower jaw) in a patient who has undergone a phase I procedure.

MINI CLINI

Young Woman With Mental Status Changes After Orthopedic Surgery

HISTORY: A 37-year-old obese smoker is admitted to the hospital after elective surgical repair of a biceps tendon and ulnar collateral ligament. She initially sustained the injury after a fall when riding a bicycle. After outpatient orthopedic evaluation and preoperative cardiac clearance, an elective repair of the tendon and ligament was scheduled. She was intubated electively for the procedure, and her operative course was unremarkable. Postoperatively, she was extubated and noted to be slightly lethargic but easily arousable and in pain while in postoperative recovery. On transfer to the floor, she became increasingly lethargic and hypoxemic despite the addition of up to 6 L/min of supplemental O_2 via nasal cannula. An emergency code is called. She is transferred to a step-down bed and further testing is performed.

MEDICATIONS AT HOME:

- None

MEDICAL HISTORY:

- Hypertension, not on medications

PHYSICAL EXAMINATION:

- *Vital signs:* Blood pressure 158/74 mm Hg, heart rate 68 beats/min, temperature 98.6° F (38.6° C), respirations 12 breaths/min
- *General:* Obese woman, lethargic and arousable
- *Neck:* 46 cm (18 in) in circumference
- *Lungs:* Diminished breath sounds bilaterally
- *Heart:* Faint sounds but regular rate and rhythm
- *Abdomen:* Obese; soft, normal bowel sounds
- *Extremities:* Right arm wound intact with bandages in place, pulses equal

LABORATORY DATA:

- *ABGs on 6 L/min O_2 via nasal cannula:* pH 7.11, PCO_2 109 mm Hg, PO_2 110 mm Hg, SaO_2 87%
- *Chest x-ray:* No mass, infiltrate, or effusion
- *ECG:* Normal sinus rhythm
- *CT scan of the head without contrast agent:* No mass, hemorrhage, or midline shift
- *CT scan of the chest with contrast agent:* No evidence of pulmonary embolism or parenchymal abnormality
- *EEG:* No seizure activity

PROBLEM: How should this patient be managed?

DISCUSSION: The patient requires bilevel noninvasive ventilator support intermittently for the next several days. After her workup reveals nothing remarkable, a pulmonary and sleep consultation is obtained. Review of the medical records reveals the patient has been receiving hydromorphone (Dilaudid) frequently for pain control. After stopping opioid medication, the patient's mental status gradually returns to baseline. Repeat ABGs on room air show pH 7.39, PCO_2 62 mm Hg, PO_2 110 mm Hg, and SaO_2 93%. A diagnostic nocturnal PSG is performed, which reveals severe OSA with AHI of 55 and low SaO_2 of 72% and evidence of chronic **obesity hypoventilation.** Positive pressure titration is performed successfully with average volume assisted pressure support with goal V_T of 8 ml/kg. The patient is discharged home with a follow-up appointment in the sleep clinic.

MINI CLINI

Fatigue in a Patient With Neuromuscular Disease

HISTORY: A 54-year-old man with recent diagnosis of ALS presents to the outpatient clinic with fatigue. He states he has been more tired and sleepy for the last few months. He had been diagnosed with ALS approximately 6 months ago, but has been doing fairly well at home. He does notice he has some difficulty sleeping at night, sometimes sleeping in a reclining chair. He denies snoring or weight gain, and in fact has lost 15 lb in the last few months. On further questioning, he reports feeling short of breath with exertion or when lying flat.

MEDICATIONS:

- None

MEDICAL HISTORY:

- Hypertension and gastroesophageal reflux
- No significant cardiac disease

PHYSICAL EXAMINATION:

- *Vital signs:* Blood pressure 135/70 mm Hg, heart rate 80 beats/min, temperature 98.6° F (37° C), respiration 16 breaths/min
- *General:* Thin, no distress, pleasant man
- *Neck:* 52 cm (20.5 in) in circumference
- *Lungs:* Clear breath sounds bilaterally
- *Heart:* Regular rate and rhythm
- *Abdomen:* Thin; soft, normal bowel sounds
- *Extremities:* no edema

LABORATORY DATA:

- *Room air ABGs:* pH 7.38, PCO_2 52 mm Hg, PO_2 88 mm Hg, SaO_2 94%
- *Chest radiograph:* Normal
- *Pulmonary function tests:* FVC 1.52 L (42% predicted), FEV_1 1.41 L (53% predicted), FEV_1/FVC ratio 0.73

PROBLEM: Why does this patient have fatigue?

DISCUSSION: The patient's symptoms are concerning for respiratory compromise because of his neuromuscular disease. His pulmonary function tests reveal restrictive lung physiology, with decreased FVC and FEV_1 on spirometry. He also has evidence for chronic hypoventilation with elevated PCO_2 on ABG analysis. He may benefit from starting noninvasive ventilation. The patient was started on positive pressure therapy with average volume assist pressure support and his sleep quality and daytime energy improved.

pressure therapy. Some RTs pursue special certification in Sleep Technology.

RTs may see patients with sleep disorder–related symptoms in the course of their clinical practice and can encourage diagnostic testing by discussion with the patient or the managing physician or both. In the acute care setting, RTs and nursing staff are in a unique position to observe directly evidence of abnormal breathing during sleep or other clinical clues that may prompt further clinical action.

Therapeutically, RTs may see patients in their home and help manage the CPAP or bilevel PAP machines, interfaces, and supplemental O_2. In the context of rehabilitation or bariatric surgery, RTs may help care for patients recovering from surgery or participating in rehabilitation programs for weight loss or improvement in cardiopulmonary function. The role of the RT may be key in serving as the bridge between physician and patient to enable education, identify obstacles to therapy, and improve overall compliance. In all these ways, RTs play an invaluable role as members of the sleep medicine team.

SUMMARY CHECKLIST

- There are three types of sleep apnea: OSA, CSA, and mixed sleep apnea; OSA is the most common.
- OSA is common, underdiagnosed, and controllable.
- The major risk factor for airway narrowing or closure during sleep is a small or unstable upper airway.
- The shift in the physiologic state from wakefulness to sleep and the consequent decrease in muscle tone result in partial or complete airway closure of the upper airway in patients with OSA.
- The long-term harmful effects of OSA include poor daytime functioning, impaired metabolic function, and increased risk for cardiovascular morbidity and mortality.
- Risk factors for OSA include male sex, age greater than 40 years, upper body obesity (neck size >16.5 in), habitual snoring, and diurnal hypertension.
- PSG is the most accurate way to make the diagnosis of OSA. The PSG measures several physiologic variables and allows for the staging of sleep and measurement of airflow, ventilatory effort, ECG, and SaO_2.
- First-line medical therapy for OSA is CPAP. This modality is almost always effective in the laboratory, although long-term adherence with CPAP therapy may be suboptimal.
- Bilevel PAP therapy may be useful in salvaging selected patients who have difficulty accepting or complying with CPAP.
- The role of auto-titrating positive airway pressure devices (auto-CPAP or auto–bilevel PAP) in managing OSA remains to be defined.
- Oral appliances can be effective, in particular, in patients with mild to moderate OSA.
- Surgical therapy may be an option for a select group of patients who have undergone an extensive preoperative analysis of the upper airway and do not accept or comply poorly with medical therapy. Optimal management of OSA, regardless of the modality, requires patient education, continued monitoring, and reassessment.

References

1. Kapur V, Strohl KP, Redline S, et al: Underdiagnosis of sleep apnea syndrome in U.S. communities. *Sleep Breath* 6:49–54, 2002.
2. Young T, Peppard PE, Gottlieb DJ: Epidemiology of obstructive sleep apnea: a population health perspective. *Am J Respir Crit Care Med* 165:1217–1239, 2002.
3. White DP: Pathogenesis of obstructive and central sleep apnea. *Am J Respir Crit Care Med* 172:1363–1370, 2005.
4. Bradley TD, Phillipson EA: Central sleep apnea. *Clin Chest Med* 13:493–505, 1992.
5. Iber C: *The AASM manual for the scoring of sleep and associated events: rules, terminology and technical specifications*, Westchester, IL, 2007, American Academy of Sleep Medicine.
6. Meoli AL, Casey KR, Clark RW, et al: Hypopnea in sleep-disordered breathing in adults. *Sleep* 24:469–470, 2001.
7. Moser NJ, Phillips BA, Berry DT, et al: What is hypopnea, anyway? *Chest* 105:426–428, 1994.
8. Schellenberg JB, Maislin G, Schwab RJ, et al: Physical findings and the risk for obstructive sleep apnea: the importance of oropharyngeal structures. *Am J Respir Crit Care Med* 162:740–748, 2000.
9. Ayas NT, FitzGerald JM, Fleetham JA, et al: Cost-effectiveness of continuous positive airway pressure therapy for moderate to severe obstructive sleep apnea/hypopnea. *Arch Intern Med* 166:977–984, 2006.
10. Morrison DL, Launois SH, Isono S, et al: Pharyngeal narrowing and closing pressures in patients with obstructive sleep apnea. *Am Rev Respir Dis* 148:606–611, 1993.
11. Marin JM, Carrizo SJ, Vicente E, et al: Long-term cardiovascular outcomes in men with obstructive sleep apnoea-hypopnoea with or without treatment with continuous positive airway pressure: an observational study. *Lancet* 365:1046–1053, 2005.
12. Shahar E, Whitney CW, Redline S, et al: Sleep-disordered breathing and cardiovascular disease: cross-sectional results of the Sleep Heart Health Study. *Am J Respir Crit Care Med* 163:19–25, 2001.
13. Shamsuzzaman AS, Gersh BJ, Somers VK: Obstructive sleep apnea: implications for cardiac and vascular disease. *JAMA* 290:1906–1914, 2003.
14. Strollo PJ, Jr, Rogers RM: Obstructive sleep apnea. *N Engl J Med* 334:99–104, 1996.
15. Guidry UC, Mendes LA, Evans JC, et al: Echocardiographic features of the right heart in sleep-disordered breathing: the Framingham Heart Study. *Am J Respir Crit Care Med* 164:933–938, 2001.
16. Shivalkar B, Van de Heyning C, Kerremans M, et al: Obstructive sleep apnea syndrome: more insights on structural and functional cardiac alterations, and the effects of treatment with continuous positive airway pressure. *J Am Coll Cardiol* 47:1433–1439, 2006.
17. Schwab RJ, Gupta KB, Gefter WB, et al: Upper airway and soft tissue anatomy in normal subjects and patients with sleep-disordered breathing: significance of the lateral pharyngeal walls. *Am J Respir Crit Care Med* 152:1673–1689, 1995.
18. Palmer LJ, Buxbaum SG, Larkin E, et al: A whole-genome scan for obstructive sleep apnea and obesity. *Am J Hum Genet* 72:340–350, 2003.
19. Mathur R, Douglas NJ: Family studies in patients with the sleep apnea-hypopnea syndrome. *Ann Intern Med* 122:174–178, 1995.
20. Gay PC: Chronic obstructive pulmonary disease and sleep. *Respir Care* 49:39–51, 2004.
21. Balachandran JS, Masa JF, Mokhlesi B: Obesity hypoventilation syndrome: epidemiology and diagnosis. *Sleep Med Clin* 9:341–347, 2014.
22. Deak MC, Kirsch DB: Sleep-disordered breathing in neurologic conditions. *Clin Chest Med* 35:547–556, 2014.
23. Pinto S, Carvalho MD: Breathing new life into treatment advances for respiratory failure in amyotrophic lateral sclerosis patients. *Neurodegener Dis Manag* 4:83–102, 2014.
24. Malhotra A, White DP: Obstructive sleep apnoea. *Lancet* 360:237–245, 2002.
25. Seneviratne U, Puvanendran K: Excessive daytime sleepiness in obstructive sleep apnea: prevalence, severity, and predictors. *Sleep Med* 5:339–343, 2004.
26. Gottlieb DJ, Whitney CW, Bonekat WH, et al: Relation of sleepiness to respiratory disturbance index: the Sleep Heart Health Study. *Am J Respir Crit Care Med* 159:502–507, 1999.
27. Adams N, Strauss M, Schluchter M, et al: Relation of measures of sleep-disordered breathing to neuropsychological functioning. *Am J Respir Crit Care Med* 163:1626–1631, 2001.
28. George CF, George CFP: Sleep. 5: driving and automobile crashes in patients with obstructive sleep apnoea/hypopnoea syndrome. *Thorax* 59:804–807, 2004.
29. Hartenbaum N, Collop N, Rosen IM, et al: Sleep apnea and commercial motor vehicle operators: statement from the joint task force of the American College of Chest Physicians, the American College of Occupational and Environmental Medicine, and the National Sleep Foundation. *Chest* 130:902–905, 2006.
30. Teran-Santos J, Jimenez-Gomez A, Cordero-Guevara J: The association between sleep apnea and the risk of traffic accidents. Cooperative Group Burgos-Santander. *N Engl J Med* 340:847–851, 1999.
31. Blankfield RP, Hudgel DW, Tapolyai AA, et al: Bilateral leg edema, obesity, pulmonary hypertension, and obstructive sleep apnea. *Arch Intern Med* 160:2357–2362, 2000. [erratum in Arch Intern Med 2000;160:2650].
32. Badesch DB, Raskob GE, Elliott CG, et al: Pulmonary arterial hypertension: baseline characteristics from the REVEAL Registry. *Chest* 137:376–387, 2010.
33. Kessler R, Chaouat A, Schinkewitch P, et al: The obesity-hypoventilation syndrome revisited: a prospective study of 34 consecutive cases. *Chest* 120:369–376, 2001.
34. Mehra R, Benjamin EJ, Shahar E, et al: Association of nocturnal arrhythmias with sleep-disordered breathing: the Sleep Heart Health Study. *Am J Respir Crit Care Med* 173:910–916, 2006.
35. Monahan K, Storfer-Isser A, Mehra R, et al: Triggering of nocturnal arrhythmias by sleep-disordered breathing events. *J Am Coll Cardiol* 54:1797–1804, 2009.
36. Yamashiro Y, Kryger M: Why should sleep apnea be diagnosed and treated? *Clin Pulm Med* 1:250, 1994.
37. Coughlin SR, Mawdsley L, Mugarza JA, et al: Obstructive sleep apnoea is independently associated with an increased prevalence of metabolic syndrome. *Eur Heart J* 25:735–741, 2004.
38. Troxel WM, Buysse DJ, Matthews KA, et al: Sleep symptoms predict the development of the metabolic syndrome. *Sleep* 33:1633–1640, 2010.
39. Reaven GM: Banting Lecture 1988. Role of insulin resistance in human disease. *Nutrition* 13:65, 1997.
40. Punjabi NM, Beamer BA: Alterations in glucose disposal in sleep-disordered breathing. *Am J Respir Crit Care Med* 179:235–240, 2009.
41. Gottlieb DJ, Yenokyan G, Newman AB, et al: Prospective study of obstructive sleep apnea and incident coronary heart disease and heart failure: the Sleep Heart Health Study. *Circulation* 122:352–360, 2010.
42. Gay PC: Sleep and sleep-disordered breathing in the hospitalized patient. *Respir Care* 55:1240–1254, 2010.
43. Gross JB, Bachenberg KL, Benumof JL, et al: Practice guidelines for the perioperative management of patients with obstructive sleep apnea: a report by the American Society of Anesthesiologists Task Force on Perioperative Management of patients with obstructive sleep apnea. *Anesthesiology* 104:1081–1093, 2006.
44. Meoli AL, Rosen CL, Kristo D, et al: Upper airway management of the adult patient with obstructive sleep apnea in the perioperative period: avoiding complications. *Sleep* 26:1060–1065, 2003.
45. Khayat RN, Jarjoura D, Patt B, et al: In-hospital testing for sleep-disordered breathing in hospitalized patients with decompensated heart failure: report of prevalence and patient characteristics. *J Card Fail* 15:739–746, 2009.
46. Memtsoudis S, Liu SS, Ma Y, et al: Perioperative pulmonary outcomes in patients with sleep apnea after noncardiac surgery. *Anesth Analg* 112:113–121, 2011.
47. Weingarten TN, Flores AS, McKenzie JA, et al: Obstructive sleep apnoea and perioperative complications in bariatric patients. *Br J Anaesth* 106:131–139, 2011.
48. Rowley JA, Aboussouan LS, Badr MS: The use of clinical prediction formulas in the evaluation of obstructive sleep apnea. *Sleep* 23:929–938, 2000.

49. Chung F, Yegneswaran B, Liao P, et al: Validation of the Berlin questionnaire and American Society of Anesthesiologists checklist as screening tool for obstructive sleep apnea in surgical patients. *Anesthesiology* 108:822–830, 2008.
50. Abrishami A, Khajehdehi A, Chung F: A systematic review of screening questionnaires for obstructive sleep apnea. *Can J Anaesth* 57:423–438, 2010.
51. Chung F, Subramanyam R, Liao P, et al: High STOP-BANG score indicates a high probability of obstructive sleep apnoea. *Br J Anaesth* 108:768–775, 2012.
52. Adesanya AO, Lee W, Greilich NB, et al: Perioperative management of obstructive sleep apnea. *Chest* 138:1489–1498, 2010.
53. Spurr KF, Graven MA, Gilbert RW: Prevalence of unspecified sleep apnea and the use of continuous positive airway pressure in hospitalized patients, 2004 National Hospital Discharge Survey. *Sleep Breath* 12:229–234, 2008.
54. Morgenthaler TI, Aurora RN, Brown T, et al: Practice parameters for the use of autotitrating continuous positive airway pressure devices for titrating pressures and treating adult patients with obstructive sleep apnea syndrome: an update for 2007. An American Academy of Sleep Medicine report. *Sleep* 31:141–147, 2008.
55. Condos R, Norman RG, Krishnasamy I, et al: Flow limitation as a noninvasive assessment of residual upper-airway resistance during continuous positive airway pressure therapy of obstructive sleep apnea. *Am J Respir Crit Care Med* 150:475–480, 1994.
56. Cracowski C, Pepin JL, Wuyam B, et al: Characterization of obstructive nonapneic respiratory events in moderate sleep apnea syndrome. *Am J Respir Crit Care Med* 164:944–948, 2001.
57. American Academy of Sleep Medicine Task Force: Sleep-related breathing disorders in adults: recommendations for syndrome definition and measurement techniques in clinical research. *Sleep* 22:667–689, 1999.
58. Collop NA, Anderson WM, Boehlecke B, et al: Clinical guidelines for the use of unattended portable monitors in the diagnosis of obstructive sleep apnea in adult patients. Portable Monitoring Task Force of the American Academy of Sleep Medicine. *J Clin Sleep Med* 3:737–747, 2007.
59. Qaseem A, Dallas P, Owens DK, et al: Diagnosis of obstructive sleep apnea in adults: a clinical practice guideline from the American College of Physicians. *Ann Intern Med* 161:210–220, 2014.
60. Epstein LJ, Kristo D, Strollo PJ, Jr, et al: Clinical guideline for the evaluation, management and long-term care of obstructive sleep apnea in adults. *J Clin Sleep Med* 5:263–276, 2009.
61. Herzog M, Riemann R, Herzog M, et al: Alcohol ingestion influences the nocturnal cardio-respiratory activity in snoring and non-snoring males. *Eur Arch Otorhinolaryngol* 261:459–462, 2004.
62. Guilleminault C, Guilleminault C: Benzodiazepines, breathing, and sleep. *Am J Med* 88:25S–28S, 1990.
63. Skinner MA, Kingshott RN, Jones DR, et al: Elevated posture for the management of obstructive sleep apnea. *Sleep Breath* 8:193–200, 2004.
64. Mador MJ, Kufel TJ, Magalang UJ, et al: Prevalence of positional sleep apnea in patients undergoing polysomnography. *Chest* 128:2130–2137, 2005.
65. Permut I, Diaz-Abad M, Chatila W, et al: Comparison of positional therapy to CPAP in patients with positional obstructive sleep apnea. *J Clin Sleep Med* 6:238–243, 2010.
66. Sullivan CE, Issa FG, Berthon-Jones M, et al: Reversal of obstructive sleep apnoea by continuous positive airway pressure applied through the nares. *Lancet* 1:862–865, 1981.
67. Kushida CA, Littner MR, Hirshkowitz M, et al: Practice parameters for the use of continuous and bilevel positive airway pressure devices to treat adult patients with sleep-related breathing disorders. *Sleep* 29:375–380, 2006.
68. Kushida CA, Chediak A, Berry RB, et al: Clinical guidelines for the manual titration of positive airway pressure in patients with obstructive sleep apnea. *J Clin Sleep Med* 4:157–171, 2008.
69. Hoffstein V, Viner S, Mateika S, et al: Treatment of obstructive sleep apnea with nasal continuous positive airway pressure: patient compliance, perception of benefits, and side effects. *Am Rev Respir Dis* 145:841–845, 1992.
70. Miljeteig H, Hoffstein V: Determinants of continuous positive airway pressure level for treatment of obstructive sleep apnea. *Am Rev Respir Dis* 147:1526–1530, 1993.
71. Engleman HM, Martin SE, Deary IJ, et al: Effect of continuous positive airway pressure treatment on daytime function in sleep apnoea/hypopnoea syndrome. *Lancet* 343:572–575, 1994.
72. Sforza E, Lugaresi E: Daytime sleepiness and nasal continuous positive airway pressure therapy in obstructive sleep apnea syndrome patients: effects of chronic treatment and 1-night therapy withdrawal. *Sleep* 18:195–201, 1995.
73. Montplaisir J, Bedard MA, Richer F, et al: Neurobehavioral manifestations in obstructive sleep apnea syndrome before and after treatment with continuous positive airway pressure. *Sleep* 15:S17–S19, 1992.
74. Lamphere J, Roehrs T, Wittig R, et al: Recovery of alertness after CPAP in apnea. *Chest* 96:1364–1367, 1989.
75. Leech JA, Onal E, Lopata M: Nasal CPAP continues to improve sleep-disordered breathing and daytime oxygenation over long-term follow-up of occlusive sleep apnea syndrome. *Chest* 102:1651–1655, 1992.
76. Strollo PJ, Sanders MH, Striller RA: Continuous and bilevel positive airway pressure therapy in sleep disordered breathing. *Oral Maxillofac Surg Clin N Am* 7:221, 1995.
77. Strohl KP, Redline S: Nasal CPAP therapy, upper airway muscle activation, and obstructive sleep apnea. *Am Rev Respir Dis* 134:555–558, 1986.
78. Grunstein RR: Sleep-related breathing disorders. V. Nasal continuous positive airway pressure treatment for obstructive sleep apnoea. *Thorax* 50: 1106–1113, 1995.
79. Sforza E, Krieger J, Bacon W, et al: Determinants of effective continuous positive airway pressure in obstructive sleep apnea: role of respiratory effort. *Am J Respir Crit Care Med* 151:1852–1856, 1995.
80. Guilleminault C, Stoohs R, Clerk A, et al: From obstructive sleep apnea syndrome to upper airway resistance syndrome: consistency of daytime sleepiness. *Sleep* 15:S13–S16, 1992.
81. Guilleminault C, Stoohs R, Clerk A, et al: A cause of excessive daytime sleepiness: the upper airway resistance syndrome. *Chest* 104:781–787, 1993.
82. Guilleminault C, Stoohs R, Duncan S: Snoring. I. Daytime sleepiness in regular heavy snorers. *Chest* 99:40–48, 1991.
83. Montserrat JM, Ballester E, Olivi H, et al: Time-course of stepwise CPAP titration: behavior of respiratory and neurological variables. *Am J Respir Crit Care Med* 152:1854–1859, 1995.
84. Zozula R, Rosen R: Compliance with continuous positive airway pressure therapy: assessing and improving treatment outcomes. *Curr Opin Pulm Med* 7:391–398, 2001.
85. Sin DD, Mayers I, Man GC, et al: Long-term compliance rates to continuous positive airway pressure in obstructive sleep apnea: a population-based study. *Chest* 121:430–435, 2002.
86. McArdle N, Devereux G, Heidarnejad H, et al: Long-term use of CPAP therapy for sleep apnea/hypopnea syndrome. *Am J Respir Crit Care Med* 159:1108–1114, 1999.
87. Sanders MH, Gruendl CA, Rogers RM: Patient compliance with nasal CPAP therapy for sleep apnea. *Chest* 90:330–333, 1986.
88. Kribbs NB, Pack AI, Kline LR, et al: Objective measurement of patterns of nasal CPAP use by patients with obstructive sleep apnea. *Am Rev Respir Dis* 147:887–895, 1993.
89. Sanders MH, Kern N: Obstructive sleep apnea treated by independently adjusted inspiratory and expiratory positive airway pressures via nasal mask: physiologic and clinical implications. *Chest* 98:317–324, 1990.
90. Sanders MH, Kern NB, Stiller RA, et al: CPAP therapy via oronasal mask for obstructive sleep apnea. *Chest* 106:774–779, 1994.
91. Prosise GL, Berry RB: Oral-nasal continuous positive airway pressure as a treatment for obstructive sleep apnea. *Chest* 106:180–186, 1994.
92. Criner GJ, Travaline JM, Brennan KJ, et al: Efficacy of a new full face mask for noninvasive positive pressure ventilation. *Chest* 106:1109–1115, 1994.
93. Mayer LS, Kerby GR, Whitman RA: Evaluation of a new nasal device for administration of continuous positive airway pressure for treatment of obstructive sleep apnea. *Am Rev Respir Dis* 139:A114, 1989.
94. Harris C, Daniels B, Herold D, et al: Comparison of cannula and mask systems for administration of nasal continuous positive airway pressure for treatment of obstructive sleep apnea. *Sleep Res* 19:233, 1990.

95. Reeves-Hoche MK, Hudgel DW, Meck R, et al: Continuous versus bilevel positive airway pressure for obstructive sleep apnea. *Am J Respir Crit Care Med* 151:443–449, 1995.
96. Littner M, Hirshkowitz M, Davila D, et al: Practice parameters for the use of auto-titrating continuous positive airway pressure devices for titrating pressures and treating adult patients with obstructive sleep apnea syndrome. An American Academy of Sleep Medicine report. *Sleep* 25:143–147, 2002.
97. d'Ortho MP: Auto-titrating continuous positive airway pressure for treating adult patients with sleep apnea syndrome. *Curr Opin Pulm Med* 10:495–499, 2004.
98. Berry RB, Parish JM, Hartse KM, et al: The use of auto-titrating continuous positive airway pressure for treatment of adult obstructive sleep apnea. An American Academy of Sleep Medicine review. *Sleep* 25:148–173, 2002.
99. Ayas NT, Patel SR, Malhotra A, et al: Auto-titrating versus standard continuous positive airway pressure for the treatment of obstructive sleep apnea: results of a meta-analysis. *Sleep* 27:249–253, 2004.
100. Rakotonanahary D, Pelletier-Fleury N, Gagnadoux F, et al: Predictive factors for the need for additional humidification during nasal continuous positive airway pressure therapy. *Chest* 119:460–465, 2001.
101. Kushida CA, Morgenthaler TI, Littner MR, et al: Practice parameters for the treatment of snoring and obstructive sleep apnea with oral appliances: an update for 2005. *Sleep* 29:240–243, 2006.
102. Ferguson KA, Cartwright R, Rogers R, et al: Oral appliances for snoring and obstructive sleep apnea: a review. *Sleep* 29:244–262, 2006.
103. Fletcher EC, Munafo DA: Role of nocturnal oxygen therapy in obstructive sleep apnea: when should it be used? *Chest* 98:1497–1504, 1990.
104. Guilleminault C, Simmons FB, Motta J, et al: Obstructive sleep apnea syndrome and tracheostomy: long-term follow-up experience. *Arch Intern Med* 141:985–988, 1981.
105. Conway WA, Victor LD, Magilligan DJ, Jr, et al: Adverse effects of tracheostomy for sleep apnea. *JAMA* 246:347–350, 1981.
106. Sher AE, Schechtman KB, Piccirillo JF: The efficacy of surgical modifications of the upper airway in adults with obstructive sleep apnea syndrome. *Sleep* 19:156–177, 1996.
107. Sundaram S, Bridgman SA, Lim J, et al: Surgery for obstructive sleep apnoea. *Cochrane Database Syst Rev* (4):001004, 2005.
108. Littner M, Kushida CA, Hartse K, et al: Practice parameters for the use of laser-assisted uvulopalatoplasty: an update for 2000. *Sleep* 24:603–619, 2001.
109. Johnson NT, Chinn J: Uvulopalatopharyngoplasty and inferior sagittal mandibular osteotomy with genioglossus advancement for treatment of obstructive sleep apnea. *Chest* 105:278–283, 1994.
110. Dattilo DJ, Drooger SA: Outcome assessment of patients undergoing maxillofacial procedures for the treatment of sleep apnea: comparison of subjective and objective results. *J Oral Maxillofac Surg* 62:164–168, 2004.
111. Kushida CA, Littner MR, Morgenthaler T, et al: Practice parameters for the indications for polysomnography and related procedures: an update for 2005. *Sleep* 28:499–521, 2005.
112. White DP: New therapies for obstructive sleep apnea. *Semin Respir Crit Care Med* 35:621–628, 2014.
113. Strollo PJ, Jr, Soose RJ, Maurer JT, et al: STAR Trial Group: Upper-airway stimulation for obstructive sleep apnea. *N Engl J Med* 370:139–149, 2014.

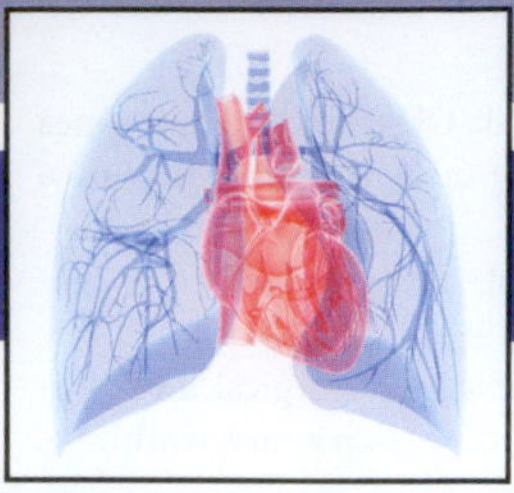

CHAPTER 34

Neonatal and Pediatric Respiratory Disorders

DOUGLAS D. DEMING AND KIMBERLY N. OTSUKA

CHAPTER OBJECTIVES

After reading this chapter you will be able to:

- Discuss the clinical findings, radiographic abnormalities, and treatment of patients with respiratory distress syndrome.
- Describe the clinical manifestations and treatment of patients with transient tachypnea of the newborn.
- Describe the pathophysiology, presentation, and treatment of meconium aspiration syndrome.
- Identify the clinical signs and symptoms associated with bronchopulmonary dysplasia and the approaches used to manage these infants.
- State the cause and treatment of apnea of prematurity.
- Describe the pathophysiology, diagnosis, and treatment of persistent pulmonary hypertension of the newborn.
- Discuss the pathophysiology, diagnosis, and treatment of congenital diaphragmatic hernia.
- Identify the anatomic defects associated with tetralogy of Fallot.
- Describe the clinical presentation of a ventricular septal defect.
- Describe types and associated conditions for abdominal wall defects.
- Define the epidemiologic factors associated with increased risk for sudden infant death syndrome.
- Identify the respiratory problems associated with gastroesophageal reflux disease.
- State the clinical findings commonly observed in patients with bronchiolitis.
- Describe the clinical features and treatment of children with epiglottitis.
- Describe the clinical manifestations and treatment of cystic fibrosis.

CHAPTER OUTLINE

Neonatal Respiratory Disorders
- Lung Parenchymal Disease
- Control of Breathing
- Pulmonary Vascular Disease
- Congenital Abnormalities Affecting Respiration
- Congenital Heart Disease
- Hypertension of the Newborn

Neonatal Resuscitation

Pediatric Respiratory Disorders
- Sudden Infant Death Syndrome
- Gastroesophageal Reflux Disease
- Bronchiolitis
- Croup
- Epiglottitis
- Cystic Fibrosis

Role of the Respiratory Therapist in Neonatal and Pediatric Respiratory Disorders

KEY TERMS

apnea of prematurity
bronchiolitis
bronchopulmonary dysplasia
croup
cystic fibrosis
ductus arteriosus
epiglottitis
gastroesophageal reflux disease
meconium aspiration syndrome
nasal flaring
persistent pulmonary hypertension of the newborn
respiratory distress syndrome
sudden infant death syndrome
tetralogy of Fallot
transient tachypnea of the newborn
transposition of the great arteries

Many perinatal disorders affect the respiratory system. Some disorders are developmental abnormalities of the heart, lungs, or airways; some are caused by prematurity; some are caused by problems during labor and delivery; and some are caused by treatments. Common disorders in the neonatal period with which respiratory therapists (RTs) should be familiar are respiratory distress syndrome, transient tachypnea of the newborn, meconium aspiration syndrome, apnea of prematurity, bronchopulmonary dysplasia, persistent pulmonary hypertension of the newborn, and congenital cardiopulmonary abnormalities.

NEONATAL RESPIRATORY DISORDERS

Lung Parenchymal Disease

Respiratory Distress Syndrome

Background. Neonatal **respiratory distress syndrome** (RDS) affects approximately 40,000 infants each year in the United States.[1] Although the death rate has decreased dramatically over the past 4 decades, many infants still die or have chronic effects of the syndrome. RDS, also known as *hyaline membrane disease,* is a disease of prematurity. The incidence increases with decreasing gestational age. The major factors in the pathophysiology of RDS are qualitative surfactant deficiency, decreased alveolar surface area, increased small airways compliance, and presence of a **ductus arteriosus**.

> **RULE OF THUMB**
> The incidence of RDS increases with decreasing gestational age.

Surfactant production depends on both the relative maturity of the lung and the adequacy of fetal perfusion. Maternal factors that impair fetal blood flow, such as abruptio placentae and maternal diabetes, also may lead to RDS.

Pathophysiology. In preterm infants, adequate amounts of surfactant are present in the lung; however, the surfactant is trapped inside type II cells. In infants with RDS, type II cells do not release adequate amounts of surfactant. The surfactant that is released is incompletely formed, so it does not make tubular myelin and does not decrease alveolar surface tension. Because the surfactant molecule in the alveolus is structurally abnormal, the type II cells and alveolar macrophages have more rapid uptake for recycling. Thus, there is a qualitative deficiency of alveolar surfactant.

Figure 34-1 outlines the pathophysiologic events associated with RDS. A qualitative decrease in surfactant increases alveolar surface tension forces, which causes alveoli to become unstable and collapse and leads to atelectasis and increased work of breathing. At the same time, the increased surface tension draws fluid from the pulmonary capillaries into the alveoli. In combination, these factors impair oxygen (O_2) exchange and cause severe hypoxemia. The severe hypoxemia and acidosis increase

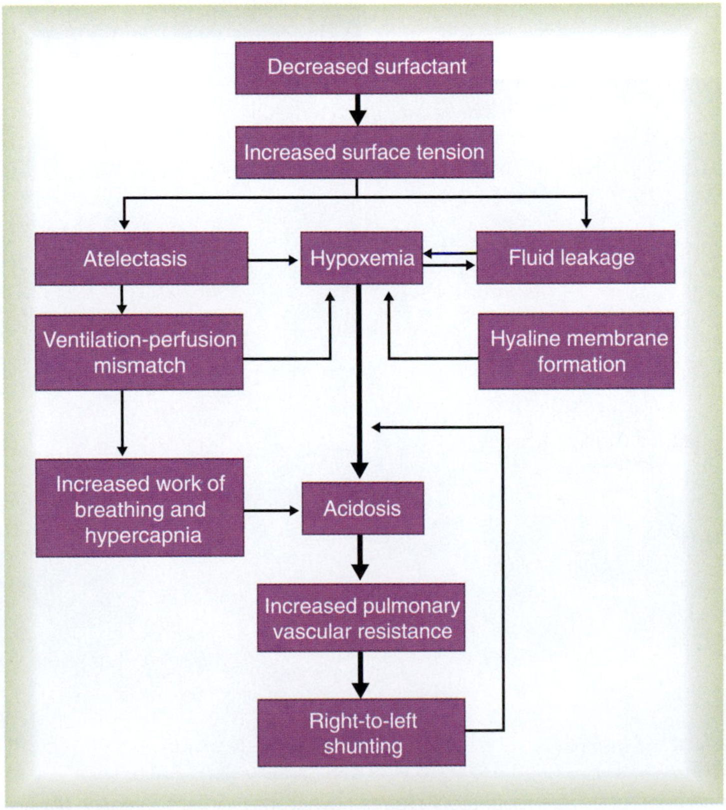

FIGURE 34-1 Pathophysiology of respiratory distress syndrome.

pulmonary vascular resistance (PVR). As pulmonary arterial pressure increases, extrapulmonary right-to-left shunting increases, and hypoxemia worsens. Hypoxemia and acidosis also impair further surfactant production. Steroids given before birth (antenatally) have been shown to mature surfactant function in the fetus, decrease the severity of RDS, and improve outcomes.[2,3]

Clinical Manifestations. The first signs of respiratory distress in infants with RDS normally appear soon after birth. Tachypnea usually occurs first. After tachypnea, worsening retractions, paradoxical breathing, and audible grunting are observed. **Nasal flaring** also may be seen. Chest auscultation often reveals fine inspiratory crackles. Cyanosis may or may not be present. If central cyanosis is observed, it is likely that the infant has severe hypoxemia. Certain other conditions, such as systemic hypotension, hypothermia, and poor perfusion, can mimic this aspect of RDS.

A definitive diagnosis of RDS usually is made with chest radiography (Figure 34-2). Diffuse, hazy, reticulogranular densities with the presence of air bronchograms with low lung volumes are typical of RDS. The reticulogranular pattern is caused by aeration of respiratory bronchioles and collapse of the alveoli. Air bronchograms appear as aerated, dark, major bronchi surrounded by the collapsed or consolidated lung tissue.

Treatment. *Continuous positive airway pressure (CPAP)* and *positive end expiratory pressure (PEEP)* are the traditional support modes used to manage RDS. Surfactant replacement therapy and *high-frequency ventilation (HFV)* have been added to these traditional approaches.[1-8] Unless the infant's condition is severe, a trial of nasal CPAP is indicated (4 to 6 cm H_2O).[4-6,8-13] Because of the hazards of endotracheal tubes (ETTs), nasal prongs are preferred. If the infant's clinical condition deteriorates rapidly, a more aggressive approach is required. Endotracheal intubation should be performed under controlled conditions as an elective procedure. Mechanical ventilation with PEEP should be initiated if oxygenation does not improve with CPAP or if the patient is apneic or acidotic. There is significant interest in an approach comprising intubation, delivery of surfactant, extubation, and then nasal CPAP.[14,15] However, more research is needed to understand the risks and benefits of this approach.

The aim of mechanical ventilation for RDS is to prevent lung collapse and maintain alveolar inflation. In severe RDS, collapse of alveoli with every breath necessitates very high reinflation pressure. To prevent the need for this high reinflation pressure, use of end-tidal pressure is necessary.

Because of the relationship between arterial partial pressure of carbon dioxide ($PaCO_2$) and functional residual capacity (FRC), $PaCO_2$ is lowest when PEEP is used to optimize FRC.

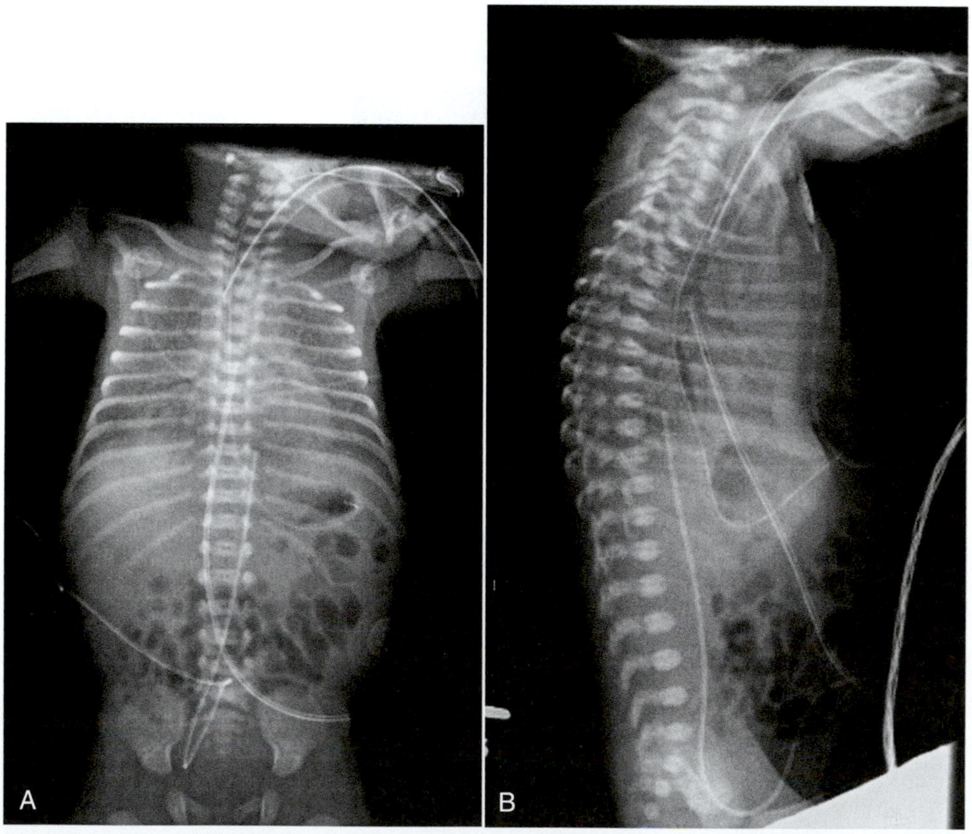

FIGURE 34-2 Radiopaque appearance of severe respiratory distress syndrome. Anteroposterior **(A)** and lateral **(B)** radiographs show diffuse hazy appearance with low lung volumes and air bronchograms that extend into the periphery.

TABLE 34-1

Surfactant Dosing

Dosing Information	Beractant (Survanta)	Calfactant (Infasurf)	Poractant Alfa (Curosurf)	Lucinactant (Surfaxin)
Dose mg/kg of birth weight	100	100	100-200	20
Dose: mL/kg birth weight	4	3	1.25-2.5	5.8
Administration	¼ dose quickly in each of four positions	½ dose slowly supine then rotated	Whole or ½ dose supine	Dose in each of four positions
Dosing interval	Every 6 hr or more often	Every 12 hr or more often	Every 12 hr or more often	Up to 4 doses in 48 hr, minimum of 6-hr interval

The time constant of the lungs in RDS is short, so the lung empties very quickly with each ventilator cycle. If alveolar ventilation is inadequate, either peak inspiratory pressure or rate should be increased. For minimizing the possibility of volutrauma, the peak inspiratory pressure should be kept less than 30 cm H_2O for larger premature infants, and even lower peak inspiratory pressure is indicated for more immature infants.

Four surfactant preparations are currently available in the United States for managing neonatal RDS: beractant (Survanta; Abbott Laboratories, North Chicago, IL), calfactant (Infasurf; ONY, Amherst, NY), poractant alfa (Curosurf; Chiesi, Cheadle, United Kingdom), and lucinactant (Surfaxin, Discovery Labs, Warrington, PA).[4,5,7,8,16-26]

Beractant and calfactant are natural bovine surfactant extracts. Poractant alfa is a natural porcine surfactant extract. Lucinactant is a completely synthetic surfactant. Each of three natural surfactants has surfactant proteins B and C as part of the formulation. The synthetic surfactant uses an amino acid sequence that acts like surfactant protein. Surfactant proteins are important for decreasing alveolar surface tension. All of these preparations are liquid suspensions that are instilled directly into the trachea. The current standard of care is to deliver replacement surfactant to all infants with RDS. There are investigations of an aerosol delivery system that would not require intubation for the synthetic surfactant. Currently, there is no evidence to support the use of a particular brand of surfactant over another.

Surfactant replacement therapy also is used as both a rescue treatment (in infants who already have RDS) and a prophylactic therapy (in the care of infants delivered prematurely).[4,7-9,27] Some centers use prophylactic surfactant replacement therapy in the care of all very small infants (<1500 g). Therapies aimed at decreasing pulmonary edema, improving cardiac output, and weaning from O_2 and high ventilator pressures are essential in the successful treatment of infants receiving surfactant. Recent evidence supports the use of noninvasive ventilatory support (e.g., bubble CPAP) to support even the smallest of infants.[13,28-30]

RULE OF THUMB

FRC is best supported by positive end-expiratory pressure (CPAP or PEEP).

All surfactants are delivered by ETT. Animal studies suggest that surfactant is rapidly distributed throughout the lung.[6] Each specific surfactant has different dosing volumes and intervals (Table 34-1). The surfactant product insert describes the positioning of the infant for surfactant delivery. Basically, the infant is positioned with different sections of the lung dependent so that the surfactant enters that section of the lung with gravity flow. If the infant is very sick and cannot be repositioned, surfactant can be administered with the infant in the supine position.

MINI CLINI

Respiratory Distress Syndrome

PROBLEM: A woman is about to deliver at 26 weeks of gestational age. What should the RT have available for resuscitation of the infant?

DISCUSSION: An infant at 26 weeks of gestational age is most likely going to have RDS—ranging from mild to severe disease. The RT should have equipment, supplies, and drugs necessary to support the infant. Many infants require mask-bag ventilation. It is crucial that the RT be acutely attuned to using the lowest pressures necessary to move the chest. It is very easy to injure the lung with high V_T. Most authorities recommend the use of a T-piece resuscitator that delivers manual breaths at fixed pressures, decreasing the risk for traumatic injury from high V_T.[31]

Some infants have severe disease that requires intubation and immediate administration of surfactant. Some infants have only mild disease. These less sick infants may require only nasal CPAP. For infants who have intermediate disease, at some centers clinicians intubate the infant, administer surfactant, and then extubate the infant back to nasal CPAP.[14,15,28,32]

Transient Tachypnea of the Newborn

Background. Transient tachypnea of the newborn (TTN), often called *type II RDS,* is probably the most common respiratory disorder of newborns.[33-36] The cause of TTN is unclear, but it is most likely related to delayed clearance of fetal lung liquid.[36-42] During most births, approximately two-thirds of this fluid is expelled by thoracic squeeze in the birth canal; the rest is reabsorbed through the lymphatic vessels during initial breathing. These mechanisms are impaired in infants born by cesarean section or infants with incomplete development of the lymphatic vessels (preterm or small-for-gestational-age infants). The residual lung fluid causes an increase in airway resistance and an overall decrease in lung compliance. Because compliance is low, the infant must generate more negative pleural pressure to breathe. This process can result in hyperinflation of some areas and air trapping in others. Most infants with TTN are born at term without any specific predisposing factors in common. Mothers of neonates who have TTN tend to have longer labor intervals and a higher incidence of failure to progress in labor, which leads to cesarean delivery. In many cases, however, maternal history and labor and delivery are normal.

Clinical Manifestations. During the first few hours of life, infants with TTN breathe rapidly. Alveolar ventilation, as measured by arterial pH and $PaCO_2$, usually is normal. The chest radiographic findings, which may initially be indistinguishable from pneumonia, are hyperinflation, which is secondary to air trapping, and perihilar streaking. The perihilar streaking probably represents lymphatic engorgement. Pleural effusions may be evident in the costophrenic angles and interlobar fissures.

Treatment. Infants with TTN usually respond readily to a low FiO_2 by infant O_2 hood or nasal cannula. Infants requiring a higher FiO_2 may benefit from CPAP. Because the retention of lung fluid may be gravity-dependent, frequent changes in the infant's position may help speed lung fluid clearance. Because TTN and neonatal pneumonia have similar clinical signs, intravenous administration of antibiotics should be considered for at least 3 days after appropriate culture samples are obtained. Mechanical ventilation is rarely needed, and, when it is, this probably indicates a complication. Clearing of the lungs evident on a chest radiograph and with clinical improvement usually occurs within 24 to 48 hours. A few infants with TTN eventually have persistent pulmonary hypertension.

Meconium Aspiration Syndrome

Background. Meconium aspiration syndrome is a disease of term and near-term infants. It involves aspiration of meconium into the central airways of the lung. It usually is associated with perinatal depression and asphyxia.

Pathophysiology. Amniotic fluid consists mainly of fetal lung fluid, fetal urine, and transudate from the uterine wall. *Meconium,* the contents of the fetal intestine, occasionally is expelled from the fetus into the surrounding amniotic fluid. Meconium consists of mucopolysaccharides, cholesterol, bile acids and salts, intestinal enzymes, and other substances. Meconium normally is not passed until after delivery.[43] Infants who have marked perinatal depression or perinatal asphyxia may pass meconium in utero. The pathophysiologic control mechanisms for the passage of meconium in utero are not completely understood. It is widely accepted that infants can have meconium aspiration in utero. Amniotic fluid stained with meconium is found in approximately 12% of all births.[43] Meconium-stained amniotic fluid is rare among infants younger than 37 weeks of gestational age. The clinical syndrome develops in 2 of every 1000 infants. Of infants with inhaled meconium, 95% clear their lungs spontaneously.[30] Amniotic fluid infusion into the uterus before the delivery of infants with meconium-stained fluid has been shown to improve neonatal outcomes.[44,45]

For many years, the aspirated meconium itself was considered the primary cause of MAS. More recent evidence suggests that the real causative agent is fetal asphyxia that precedes aspiration. Fetal asphyxia causes pulmonary vasospasm and hyperreactivity of the vasculature, which lead to persistent pulmonary hypertension.[46-48]

MAS involves three primary problems: pulmonary obstruction, lung tissue damage, and pulmonary hypertension.[46] Obstruction occurs because of plugging of the airways with particulate meconium. This obstruction often is of the ball-valve type, which allows gas entry but prevents gas exit. Ball-valve obstruction causes air trapping and can lead to volutrauma (Figure 34-3). The lung tissue injury caused by MAS is chemical pneumonitis. Additionally, there are various chemical effects, inflammatory responses, cytokine and chemokine activations, complement activation, and phospholipase A_2 activation.[45,46,49-54] Persistent pulmonary hypertension with intracardiac and extracardiac right-to-left shunting frequently complicates MAS.[46]

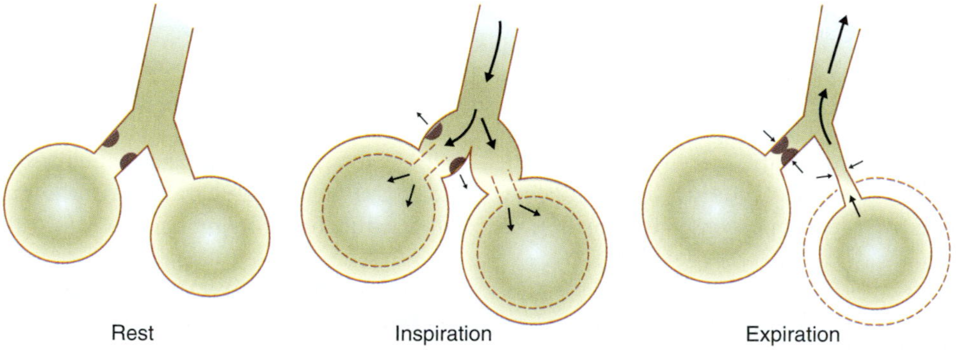

FIGURE 34-3 Ball-valve effect. At rest, the airway lumen is partially obstructed. With inspiration, negative intrathoracic pressure opens the airway and relieves obstruction. Gas enters and expands the alveoli. With expiration, intrathoracic pressure changes to positive force, which narrows the airway and causes total occlusion. Gas cannot be expelled and is trapped within the alveoli. (Modified from Koff PB, Eitzman DV, Neu J: Neonatal and pediatric care, ed 2, St Louis, 1993, Mosby.)

Clinical Manifestations. Before birth, thick meconium, fetal tachycardia, and absent fetal cardiac accelerations during labor are evidence that the fetus is at high risk for MAS.[55] After delivery, if the infant has a low umbilical artery pH, an Apgar score less than 5, and meconium aspirated from the trachea, intensive care and close observation for MAS are warranted. Infants with MAS typically have gasping respirations, tachypnea, grunting, and retractions. The chest radiograph usually shows irregular pulmonary densities, which represent areas of atelectasis, and hyperlucent areas, which represent hyperinflation secondary to air trapping (Figure 34-4). Arterial blood gases (ABGs) typically show hypoxemia with mixed respiratory and metabolic acidosis. In the most severe cases, there is right-to-left shunting and persistent pulmonary hypertension.[43]

Treatment. It is no longer recommended that vigorous infants with meconium-stained fluid be intubated and suctioned.[44,50,56-60] However, it is important that an ETT be inserted immediately in severely depressed infants with thick meconium, and suction should be applied directly to the ETT.[58] The ETT is removed and inspected for meconium. If meconium is present, the procedure is repeated with a new ETT until no further meconium is aspirated or until two to four aspirations have been performed. The ETT should be left in place, and mechanical ventilation should be started. For prevention of hypoxemia, a flow of warmed 100% O_2 should be blown across the infant's face during the aspiration efforts. No evidence suggests an improved outcome because of endotracheal suctioning in the care of infants who have meconium and are vigorous and would not otherwise require intubation.[56,60] There is evidence that tracheal lavage with dilute surfactant improves the clinical course and outcome of infants with MAS.[51,61,62]

If the infant's condition worsens, CPAP or mechanical ventilation may be indicated. CPAP is indicated if the primary problem is hypoxemia. By distending the small airways, CPAP can sometimes overcome the ball-valve obstruction and improve both oxygenation and ventilation. If respiratory acidosis is severe or clinical assessment indicates excessive work in breathing, mechanical ventilation should be started. Figure 34-3 shows the ball-valve effect. At rest, the airway lumen is partially obstructed. With inspiration, negative intrathoracic pressure opens the airway and relieves the obstruction. Gas enters and expands the alveoli. With expiration, intrathoracic pressure changes to a positive force, which narrows the airway and causes total occlusion. Gas cannot be expelled and is trapped within the alveoli. It is difficult to provide ventilation to infants with severe MAS. These infants often retain CO_2 and need increased ventilator support. Because of high airway resistance, the lungs have a long time constant. High ventilator rates and pressures increase the risk for air trapping and volutrauma.

Evidence suggests that both HFV and synchronous intermittent mechanical ventilation decrease the risk for air leak.[63,64] Various studies have shown improvement in MAS with the use of HFV and surfactant.[51,54,61,65-67] Nitric oxide (NO) has become a major adjunct in the management of persistent pulmonary hypertension.[47-49,68] Corticosteroids have not yet been shown to improve outcomes for infants with MAS.[69] High mean airway pressures may worsen pulmonary hypertension and aggravate right-to-left cardiac shunting.[55]

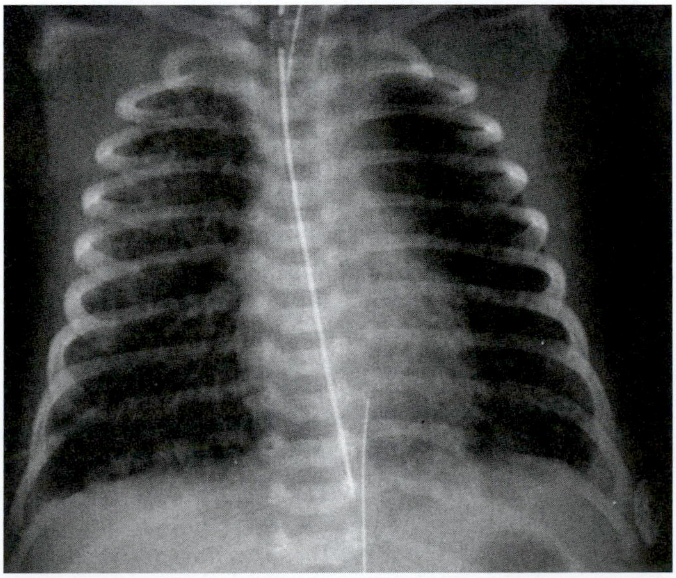

FIGURE 34-4 Radiograph of a patient with meconium aspiration syndrome. Anteroposterior radiograph shows diffuse patchy areas of atelectasis and emphysema.

MINI CLINI

Meconium Aspiration Syndrome

PROBLEM: The RT is called to the delivery room to attend the delivery of a term infant with meconium-stained amniotic fluid. What should the RT have available for the resuscitation of this infant?

DISCUSSION: The RT should have the standard resuscitation equipment available. Current recommendations for resuscitating a newborn with meconium staining do not include immediate intubation and tracheal suctioning for a vigorous infant. If the infant is depressed and not breathing, the infant should be resuscitated similar to any other depressed and apneic infant, which includes intubation. However, there is no evidence for whether the depressed infant would benefit from intubation and tracheal suctioning.[57,58,70]

Bronchopulmonary Dysplasia

Background. Infants, especially preterm infants, with severe respiratory failure in the first few weeks of life may develop a chronic pulmonary condition called **bronchopulmonary dysplasia** (BPD). BPD is a complex disease that is poorly defined.[71-75] Historical definitions have included radiographic patterns and the requirement for supplemental O_2 at fixed time points in the infant's life. Immaturity, genetics, malnutrition, O_2 toxicity, and mechanical ventilation all have been suspected to cause BPD.[56,73,76-79]

Pathophysiology. The development of BPD is complex and involves many pathways. The initiating factors are related to *atelectrauma* (lung collapse) and *volutrauma* (large tidal volume [V_T]). Factors such as hyperoxia and hypoxia, mechanical forces, vascular maldevelopment, inflammation, nutrition, and genetics contribute to the abnormal development of the lung and lead to BPD.[77,78,80-86] *Atelectrauma* is a term coined to describe loss of alveolar volume that is both a result and a cause of lung injury. *Volutrauma* is the term used to describe local overinflation (and stretch) of airways and alveoli. Atelectrauma leads to derecuitment (e.g., areas of alveolar collapse) of the lung. Volutrauma leads to damage to airways, pulmonary capillary endothelium, alveolar and airway epithelium, and basement membranes. The combination of atelectrauma and volutrauma synergistically increases lung injury.[87]

Both atelectrauma and volutrauma cause a need for increased supplemental O_2 concentrations. This use of supplemental O_2 leads to overproduction of superoxide, hydrogen peroxide, and perhydroxyl radicals. Preterm infants are particularly susceptible to O_2 radicals because the antioxidant systems develop in the last trimester of pregnancy. Prolonged hyperoxia begins a sequence of lung injury that leads to inflammation, diffuse alveolar damage, pulmonary dysfunction, and death.

The response of the lungs to the combination of trauma and O_2 toxicity is the production and release of soluble mediators. These mediators probably are released from granulocytes residing in the lung. The release of these mediators can injure the alveolar-capillary barrier and cause an inflammatory response.[71,79] A "new" BPD is being described that shows decreased alveolarization rather than the prominent airway damage of the "old" BPD.[77-88] This change in the pathologic characteristics of BPD is thought to be related to improvements in ventilator management, the use of surfactant, and processes that interrupt alveolar development (e.g., postnatal steroid therapy).[74,89,90]

Clinical Manifestations. BPD has various clinical manifestations. Some very immature infants may start with little or no O_2 requirement and little or no mechanical ventilation requirement. Progressive respiratory distress develops at approximately 2 to 3 weeks of life, and then the infant needs O_2 and mechanical ventilation. Other immature infants may begin with pneumonia or sepsis and need very high levels of O_2 and mechanical ventilation. In either of these scenarios, progressive vascular leakage and areas of atelectasis and emphysema develop in the lungs, and progressive pulmonary damage occurs. The chest radiograph in severe disease shows areas of atelectasis, emphysema, and fibrosis diffusely intermixed throughout the lung (Figure 34-5).[77,78] ABG measurements reveal varying degrees of hypoxemia and hypercapnia secondary to airway obstruction, air trapping, pulmonary fibrosis, and atelectasis. There is a marked increase in airway resistance with an overall decrease in lung compliance.

Treatment. The best management of BPD is prevention. Prevention of atelectrauma and volutrauma begins in the delivery room. Establishment of an optimal FRC without overstretching the lung requires careful attention to detail in providing end-tidal pressure and avoiding large V_T. Surfactant should be delivered early in the course of treatment.

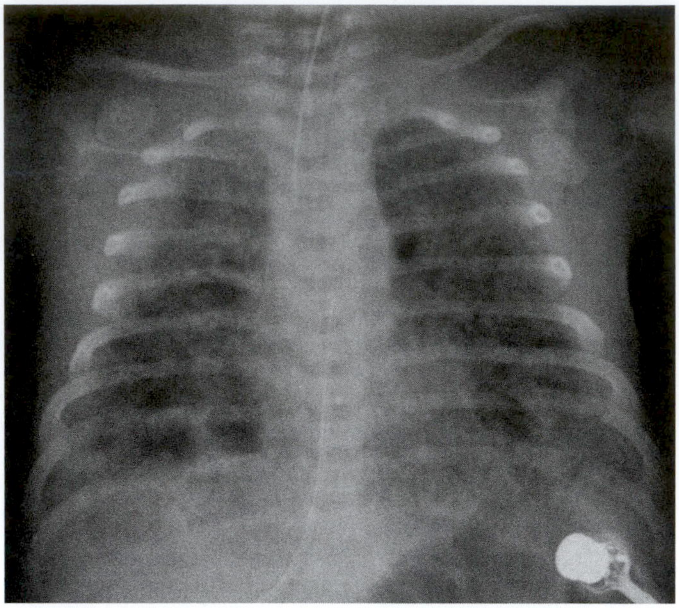

FIGURE 34-5 Radiograph of a patient with bronchopulmonary disease (BPD). Anteroposterior radiograph shows areas of scarring, atelectasis, emphysema, and cysts. This film is consistent with severe BPD.

Treatment of infants with BPD involves steps to minimize additional lung damage and prevent pulmonary hypertension and cor pulmonale. Infants with severe disease may be dependent on supplemental O_2 or mechanical ventilation for months and have symptoms of airway obstruction for years. Therapy usually is supportive throughout the course of the disease. An infant with BPD is given respiratory support as needed. Supplemental O_2 can help decrease the pulmonary hypertension that is common with BPD.[80]

Multiple treatments have been suggested for infants with BPD.[73,76,84,90-92] Diuretics are given as needed to decrease pulmonary edema; antibiotics are given to manage existing pulmonary infection.[93-95] Chest physical therapy may help mobilize secretions and prevent further atelectasis. Bronchodilator therapy may help decrease airway resistance.[93] Steroid therapy with dexamethasone can produce substantial short-term improvement in lung function, often allowing rapid weaning from ventilatory support. However, steroid therapy has little effect on long-term outcome such as mortality and duration of O_2 therapy.[96] Steroid therapy also has been implicated in decreased alveolarization and increased developmental delay.[92] Although steroids are still given in clinical practice, they should be used cautiously and only after the risks have been thoroughly explained to the parents. The use of NO to prevent or improve BPD is controversial.[97,98]

Control of Breathing

Apnea of Prematurity

Background. Apnea of prematurity is a common, controllable disorder among premature infants. It usually resolves over time.[99-103] Premature infants frequently have periodic respiration, which comprises sequential short apneic episodes of 5 to 10 seconds followed by 10 to 15 seconds of rapid respiration. Apneic spells are abnormal if (1) they last longer than 15 seconds or (2) they are associated with cyanosis, pallor, hypotonia, or bradycardia.

If no effort to breathe occurs during a spell, the apnea is called *central* apnea. If breathing efforts occur, but obstruction prevents airflow, the apnea is termed *obstructive*. Mixed apnea is a combination of the central and obstructive types that starts as obstructive apnea and then develops into central apnea.[99,100,104,105]

Cause. Premature infants have immature control of respiratory drive in response to O_2 and carbon dioxide (CO_2). In mature animals, an increase in alveolar $PaCO_2$ elicits an increase in V_T and respiratory rate. A decrease in FiO_2 below room air also triggers an increase in V_T. Conversely, in premature animals, an increase in $PaCO_2$ temporarily increases V_T but does not increase respiratory rate. A decrease in FiO_2 below room air decreases V_T and respiratory rate. This effect can lead to apnea in a premature infant. Several factors in addition to prematurity can cause apnea in infants. Table 34-2 summarizes the potential causes, associated signs, and diagnostic indicators.[99,105-107]

Treatment. Infants with apnea need continuous monitoring of heart and respiratory rates. Continuous noninvasive monitoring of oxygenation by transcutaneous electrode or pulse oximetry is recommended. Most apneic incidents can be quickly ended with gentle mechanical stimulation, such as picking the infant up, flicking the sole of the foot, or rubbing the skin.[106,108] If the cause of apnea is not prematurity, treatment must be directed at resolving the underlying condition. Table 34-3 outlines current treatment strategies for infants with apnea.[86,109] Apnea secondary to prematurity responds well to methylxanthines, especially theophylline and caffeine.[110-112] These agents stimulate the central nervous system and increase the infant's responsiveness to CO_2. For infants with apnea that does not respond to treatment with theophylline, doxapram can be used.[113-115] However, doxapram is delivered by continuous infusion and has multiple toxicities.

The "Back to Sleep" program initiated by the American Academy of Pediatrics has significantly decreased the incidence of SIDS.[116] It is thought that when a newborn, which has a relatively heavy head and weak neck muscles, manages to position its face into a soft surface (e.g., mattress, pillow, bunting, etc.) it will develop increased CO_2 retention and become apneic. Unlike older infants, newborns will not have a response to awaken and move, they become apneic, then become bradycardic, then have cardiopulmonary arrest.[100-116]

CPAP also can be used to manage infant apnea.[117] Although the mechanism of action is not established, CPAP probably increases FRC and improves arterial partial pressure of oxygen (PaO_2) and $PaCO_2$. CPAP may stimulate vagal receptors in the lung, increasing the output of the brainstem respiratory centers. Severe or recurrent apnea that is unresponsive to these interventions may necessitate mechanical ventilatory support.

As the respiratory control mechanisms mature, apnea of prematurity normally resolves without intervention. Apneic spells begin to disappear by weeks 37 to 44 of postmenstrual age with no apparent long-term effects. Infants who have apnea of prematurity are not at higher risk for **sudden infant death syndrome** (SIDS) than other infants.

Apnea monitoring can allow infants who are otherwise ready for discharge but still having occasional episodes of apnea to go home.[103,109,118] However, the presence of a home apnea monitor

TABLE 34-2

Evaluation of an Infant With Apnea

Possible Cause	Associated Signs	Investigation
Infection	Lethargy, respiratory distress, temperature instability	Complete blood count, sepsis evaluation
Metabolic disorder	Poor feeding, lethargy, jitteriness	Glucose, calcium, electrolyte levels
Impaired oxygenation	Respiratory distress, tachypnea, cyanosis	O_2 monitoring, arterial blood gases, chest radiograph
Maternal drugs	Maternal history, hypotonia, central nervous system depression	Magnesium level, urine drug screen
Intracranial lesion	Abnormal neurologic findings, seizures	Cranial ultrasonography
Environmental	Lethargy	Monitor temperature (infant and environment)
Gastroesophageal reflux	Feeding difficulty	Specific observation, radiographic barium swallow examination

From Stark AR: Disorders of respiratory control in infants. Respir Care 36:673, 1991.

TABLE 34-3

Treatment Strategies for Infants With Apnea

Treatment	Rationale
Manage underlying cause if identified	Removes precipitating factor
Tactile stimulation	Increases respiratory drive by sensory stimulation
CPAP	Reduces mixed and obstructive apnea by splinting the upper airway
Theophylline or caffeine	Increases respiratory center output and CO_2 response, enhances diaphragm strength, adenosine antagonist
Doxapram	Stimulates respiratory center and peripheral chemoreceptors
Transfusion	Decreases hypoxic depression by increasing O_2-carrying capacity
Mechanical ventilation	Provides support when respiratory effort is inadequate

From Stark AR: Disorders of respiratory control in infants. Respir Care 36:673, 1991.
CPAP, Continuous positive airway pressure.

is a significant inconvenience to the family. Home monitors lack the sophisticated filtering systems of hospital monitors, and they have very frequent false alarms.[118] Also, there is no evidence that apnea monitors prevent SIDS.

Pulmonary Vascular Disease

Persistent Pulmonary Hypertension of the Newborn

Background. **Persistent pulmonary hypertension of the newborn** (PPHN) is a complex syndrome with many causes.[119-132] The common denominator in PPHN is a return to fetal circulatory pathways, usually because of elevated PVR. This condition results in further right-to-left shunting, severe hypoxemia, and metabolic and respiratory acidosis.

Pathophysiology. In the uterus, the fetus does not use the lungs as a gas-exchange organ. PVR is high, and systemic vascular resistance (SVR) is low. This condition produces a PVR/SVR ratio greater than 1. A fetus has two anatomic shunts that are not present in older infants, children, or adults: the foramen ovale and ductus arteriosus. With a PVR/SVR ratio greater than 1 and the anatomic shunts, blood flow bypasses the lung either at the atrial level (foramen ovale) or at the pulmonary artery (ductus arteriosus). Intrauterine total pulmonary blood flow and systemic arterial O_2 saturation (SaO_2) are low.

In the transition to extrauterine life, PVR decreases owing to gas filling the lungs and increasing PaO_2 in the pulmonary venous circulation. SVR increases with the removal of the placenta from the circulation, and this makes the PVR/SVR ratio less than 1. If PVR does not decrease to allow the PVR/SVR ratio to become less than 1, the infant has PPHN.

The three fundamental types of PPHN are vascular spasm, increased muscle wall thickness, and decreased cross-sectional area of pulmonary vessels.[123] Vascular spasm is an acute event that can be triggered by many different conditions, including hypoxemia, hypoglycemia, hypotension, and pain. Increased muscle wall thickness is a chronic condition that develops in utero in response to several different causative factors, including chronic fetal hypoxia, increased pulmonary blood flow (e.g., intrauterine closure of the ductus arteriosus), and pulmonary venous obstruction (e.g., total anomalous pulmonary venous return with obstructed below-diaphragm return). Decreased cross-sectional area is related to hypoplasia of the lungs and occurs with congenital diaphragmatic hernia, Potter sequence (absent kidneys), and oligohydramnios syndromes (decreased amniotic fluid).

Clinical Manifestations. PPHN should be suspected when an infant has rapidly changing O_2 saturation (SaO_2) without changes in FiO_2 or has hypoxemia out of proportion to the lung disease detected with chest radiography or $PaCO_2$ measurement. In infants with a significant shunt through the ductus arteriosus, there usually is a substantial gradient (>5%) between preductal and postductal O_2 saturation. This gradient can be found easily if two pulse oximeters are placed on the infant, one on the right arm and the other on either leg.

Treatment. Initial therapy for PPHN is removal of the underlying cause, such as administration of O_2 for hypoxemia, surfactant for RDS, glucose for hypoglycemia, and inotropic agents for low cardiac output and systemic hypotension. If correction of the underlying problem does not correct hypoxemia, the infant needs intubation and mechanical ventilation. Because pain and anxiety may contribute to PPHN, the infant may need sedation and, frequently, paralysis. If these measures do not improve oxygenation, the next step is HFV. This mode of ventilation allows a higher FRC without a large V_T. Inhaled NO is considered the next intervention.[68,133-136] If all of these modalities fail to improve oxygenation, the infant may be a candidate for extracorporeal membrane oxygenation (ECMO).[137-139] Also, types 3 and 5 phosphodiesterase inhibitors are being used in infants and children with refractory pulmonary hypertension.[140-143] Even with all of these treatments, PPHN remains a complex disease with high morbidity and mortality.

MINI CLINI

PROBLEM: The RT is called to the bedside of a term infant who has mild respiratory distress, is receiving nasal cannula O_2 of 1 L/min, has an FIO_2 of 1.0, and has a SpO_2 of 75%. Shortly after birth, the infant's chest radiograph revealed a normal size heart and clear, slightly hyperlucent lung fields with no infiltrates. The bedside nurse describes that she has just finished taking the infant's vital signs and changing its diaper. Before her touching the infant, the infant's saturation was 96%. What is this infant's problem? What should the RT do?

DISCUSSION: This infant is exhibiting signs of persistent pulmonary hypertension. The immediate interventions potentially could include increasing the O_2 flow, lowering the lights in the room, decreasing the activity and ambient noise in the room, swaddling the infant, and minimizing the physical contact with the infant. All of these interventions are aimed at getting the infant into a quiet, calm environment and allowing the infant to relax.

Additionally, the RT and nurse should contact the physician who is caring for this infant and alert him or her to the possibility of persistent pulmonary hypertension. Potential additional therapies could include sedation, intubation, mechanical ventilation, and inhaled NO.

Congenital Abnormalities Affecting Respiration

Congenital abnormalities that affect respiration can be divided into several groups: airway diseases, lung malformations, chest wall abnormalities, abdominal wall abnormalities, and diseases of neuromuscular control.

Airway Diseases

Airway abnormalities have three fundamental mechanisms: internal obstruction, external obstruction, and disruption. Internal obstruction includes common problems, such as laryngomalacia, that cause obstructive apnea. Less common problems caused by internal obstruction are tracheomalacia, laryngeal webs, tracheal stenosis, and hemangiomas. All of these diseases usually manifest as a combination of inspiratory stridor, gas trapping, expiratory wheezing, and accessory respiratory muscle activity.

External compression can be caused by hemangiomas, neck or thoracic masses, and vascular rings. These lesions are far less common than diseases caused by internal obstruction, but they are not rare. The symptoms are similar to those of internal obstruction. Neck masses usually are obvious at visual inspection. Intrathoracic masses and vascular rings must be suspected on the basis of the clinical manifestations: noise during the respiratory cycle that worsens with exertion. The infant may have difficulty with swallowing.

Airway disruptions usually are related to tracheoesophageal fistula (TEF) in a newborn. This malformation usually is associated with esophageal atresia. There are five types of TEF: esophageal atresia with a proximal fistula, esophageal atresia with a distal fistula, esophageal atresia with both a proximal and a distal fistula, esophageal atresia without either fistula, and an intact esophagus with a so-called *H fistula*.[144] The most common of these malformations is esophageal atresia with a distal fistula, which accounts for 85% to 90% of all TEFs. The least common is the H fistula. All of these malformations manifest as difficulty swallowing, bubbling and frothing at the mouth, and choking, particularly during attempts at feeding. These anomalies can occur in isolation or as part of an association of defects. The most common is the VATER or VACTERL association of vertebral anomalies, imperforate anus, TEF, and renal or radial anomalies. In VACTERL, cardiac anomalies are added, and renal and limb anomalies replace renal or radial anomalies in the acronym. These associated anomalies must be sought in any infant with TEF. TEF is managed with surgical ligation of the fistula (tying it closed) and reconnection of the interrupted esophagus.[145] Most infants with TEF have a good outcome; however, some infants have severe malformations that can cause chronic problems. Infants with TEF usually need only supportive respiratory care. They usually do not have lung disease. However, some infants need HFV because the air leak through the fistula can become larger than the airflow to the alveoli.

Lung Malformations

There is a broad spectrum of rare lung malformations that occur in the newborn period.[106-108] These lesions are thought to be part of a continual spectrum of diseases that originate as defects in lung segmentation. The most common is congenital pulmonary adenomatoid malformation (CPAM); this was previously known as *cystic adenomatoid malformation of the lung*. CPAM is classified into five types on the basis of the type and size of the cyst.[146,147] The disease may affect entire lobes of the lung. The affected parts of the lung do not exchange gas and can become infected. The usual treatment is surgical removal of the affected lobe. There is also the potential for malignant transformation.

Some affected fetuses can develop hydrops in utero. Most infants with CPAM have symptoms of lung volume loss. As the mass expands, the normal surrounding lung is compressed. Some CPAMs resolve spontaneously. A few infants have severe cardiorespiratory compromise and need respiratory support and emergency surgery. However, better results are seen when surgery can be performed electively.

Other, less common lung malformations include pulmonary sequestration and lobar emphysema. Both of these diseases involve maldevelopment of lobes of the lung. Sequestration is a primitive, frequently cystic, lung lobe that is not in communication with the tracheobronchial tree and frequently receives no pulmonary vascular blood flow.

Lobar emphysema is an airway malformation that causes gas trapping in a lobe of the lung. These malformations manifest as space-occupying masses within the thorax. They usually are treated by surgical removal.

Congenital Diaphragmatic Hernia

Congenital diaphragmatic hernia is a severe disease that usually manifests in newborns as severe respiratory distress.[148-150] The pathophysiologic mechanism is a complex combination of lung hypoplasia, including decreased alveolar count and decreased pulmonary vasculature, pulmonary hypertension, and unusual anatomy of the inferior vena cava.[148-150] This disorder varies between asymptomatic (rare) and severe life-threatening disease (frequent). There are two types of hernia: Bochdalek hernia (lateral and posterior defect, usually on the left) and Morgagni hernia (medial and anterior, may be on either side). Hernias that occur in the right hemidiaphragm may be less severe because the liver can block the defect and decrease the volume of abdominal contents that can enter the thorax.[150]

Some authors speculate that the diaphragmatic hernia complex is a developmental field defect and not just a simple cascade of events related to a hole in the diaphragm. This theory is partly based on long-term outcomes of survivors with diaphragmatic hernias. These survivors frequently have severe scoliosis in the direction of the diaphragm defect. They also frequently have severe esophageal reflux disease.

Most cases of congenital diaphragmatic hernia can be diagnosed in utero with ultrasonography. Physical examination may yield the following findings: scaphoid abdomen (because the abdominal contents are in the thorax), decreased breath sounds, displaced heart sounds (because the heart is pushed away from the hernia), and severe cyanosis (from lung hypoplasia and pulmonary hypertension). The diagnosis is established with chest radiography.

The general treatment of infants with congenital diaphragmatic hernia involves neonatologists and pediatric surgeons. Initial treatment is insertion of an ETT, paralysis, and mechanical ventilation. A large sump tube is placed in the stomach and connected to continuous suction. These therapies allow adequate ventilation and oxygenation and prevent gas insufflation of the intestine. Most centers delay surgical repair for several days to allow the natural decrease in PVR. On day 7 to 10 of life, a surgeon closes the defect. This scenario occurs only for infants with easily correctable pulmonary hypertension. Infants with severe pulmonary hypertension may need HFV and ECMO. At some centers, the diaphragm is repaired during ECMO. Most centers try to wean the infant from ECMO and then perform the repair. Despite all these advanced therapies, the mortality for this disease is high.[151] Survival depends on many complex variables (e.g., liver herniation into the thorax, fetal head-to-lung ratio, initial PaO_2, and $PaCO_2$).[149,151]

Abdominal Wall Abnormalities

Because all newborns are primarily abdominal breathers, the abdominal wall is an intrinsic part of the respiratory system. Large defects in the abdominal wall can cause severe respiratory compromise.[152-154] One of the most common of these defects is omphalocele. An omphalocele is an abdominal wall defect that involves the insertion of the umbilical cord. The umbilical cord goes into the omphalocele. The bowel of an infant with an omphalocele is usually covered by a membrane that looks like the surface of the umbilical cord. Occasionally, the omphalocele membrane ruptures and exposes the bowel of the infant. Omphaloceles must be distinguished from gastroschisis. Gastroschisis is an abdominal wall defect that is completely separate from the insertion of the umbilical cord. The bowel of an infant with a gastroschisis is not covered by a membrane and is outside of the abdomen. Because the bowel has been out of the abdomen, the abdominal cavity is small. There are two methods of repairing gastroschisis. If the abdominal cavity is of sufficient size and the amount of bowel outside is small, a primary closure is done in which all of the bowel is returned to the abdominal cavity and the small defect is closed. However, if the abdominal cavity is too small or the amount of bowel is too large, the surgeons will place the bowel into a Silastic chimney (or silo). The open end is inserted into the defect and the closed end is suspended from the bed. Over the next several days, gravity and the gradual stretching of the abdominal wall will allow the bowel to come back into the abdomen.

Usually only large omphaloceles cause respiratory distress. When they are greater than 10 cm in diameter, these defects can cause severe respiratory distress and frequently require prolonged mechanical ventilation. Infants with gastroschisis usually have normal lungs. However, if they need to be have a silo placed, this is like a water column (the height of bowel in the silo) applying pressure against the diaphragm. These infants will need an end-tidal pressure to support FRC.

Neuromuscular Control

Many diseases of poor neuromuscular control affect newborns,[155-159] including spinal muscular atrophy, congenital myasthenia gravis, and myotonic dystrophy. These diseases frequently require respiratory support in the newborn and pediatric periods. The morbidity and mortality of these diseases are extremely variable. New technologies may allow noninvasive respiratory support of some patients.[158,160,161] Some diseases can be quite severe in the newborn period and be relieved with age. It is important to make an accurate diagnosis to be able to estimate prognosis and provide genetic counseling. Many of these diseases are inherited with known inheritance patterns.

MINI CLINI

Delivery of an Infant With an Abdominal Wall Defect

PROBLEM: The RT is called to the delivery room to assist in the delivery of a term infant with an abdominal wall defect. What should the RT consider for assisting this infant?

DISCUSSION: There are many types of abdominal wall defects. The two most common are gastroschisis and omphalocele. These anomalies can be differentiated by whether the insertion of the umbilical cord into the abdomen is involved in the defect. In a gastroschisis, the umbilical cord inserts directly into the abdomen and is separate from the defect. In an omphalocele, the umbilical cord inserts directly into the defect. Although there is usually a membrane covering the bowel in an omphalocele, if the membrane has ruptured, the only means of distinguishing an omphalocele is by the umbilical cord insertion.

Most infants with these abdominal wall defects are term. Most do not have significant lung disease. An abdominal wall defect increases the intraabdominal pressure. It pushes the diaphragm up into the thorax, decreasing FRC. The RT should be aware that these patients will need support of their FRC. Typically, if the FRC can be supported with CPAP or PEEP, the infant will not need high rates or a high V_T to achieve adequate gas exchange.

Congenital Heart Disease

A full discussion of congenital heart disease is beyond the scope of this chapter. However, basic knowledge of the common defects is essential to good practice in pediatric and neonatal respiratory care. Congenital heart diseases usually are divided into two large categories: cyanotic and acyanotic heart disease.[162,163] Cyanotic heart diseases are diseases in which blood shunts from right to left, bypassing the lungs, and is deoxygenated. Acyanotic heart diseases are diseases in which blood shunts from left to right, causing congestive heart failure. Figure 34-6 compares normal cardiac anatomy with the features of the five most common congenital defects.

Cyanotic Heart Diseases

The two most common cyanotic heart diseases are tetralogy of Fallot and transposition of the great arteries.

Tetralogy of Fallot. **Tetralogy of Fallot** is a defect that includes (1) obstruction of right ventricular outflow (pulmonary stenosis), (2) ventricular septal defect (a hole between the right and left ventricles), (3) dextroposition of the aorta, and (4) right ventricular hypertrophy. Tetralogy of Fallot varies between mild disease, which is initially diagnosed in early childhood, and severe disease, which is diagnosed in the newborn period.[163-165] The mild form of the disease manifests as a heart murmur, intermittent severe cyanotic spells, a history of the infant squatting or entering a knee-chest position, or a combination of these features. The severe form of the disease manifests as a heart murmur and severe continuous cyanosis. Most

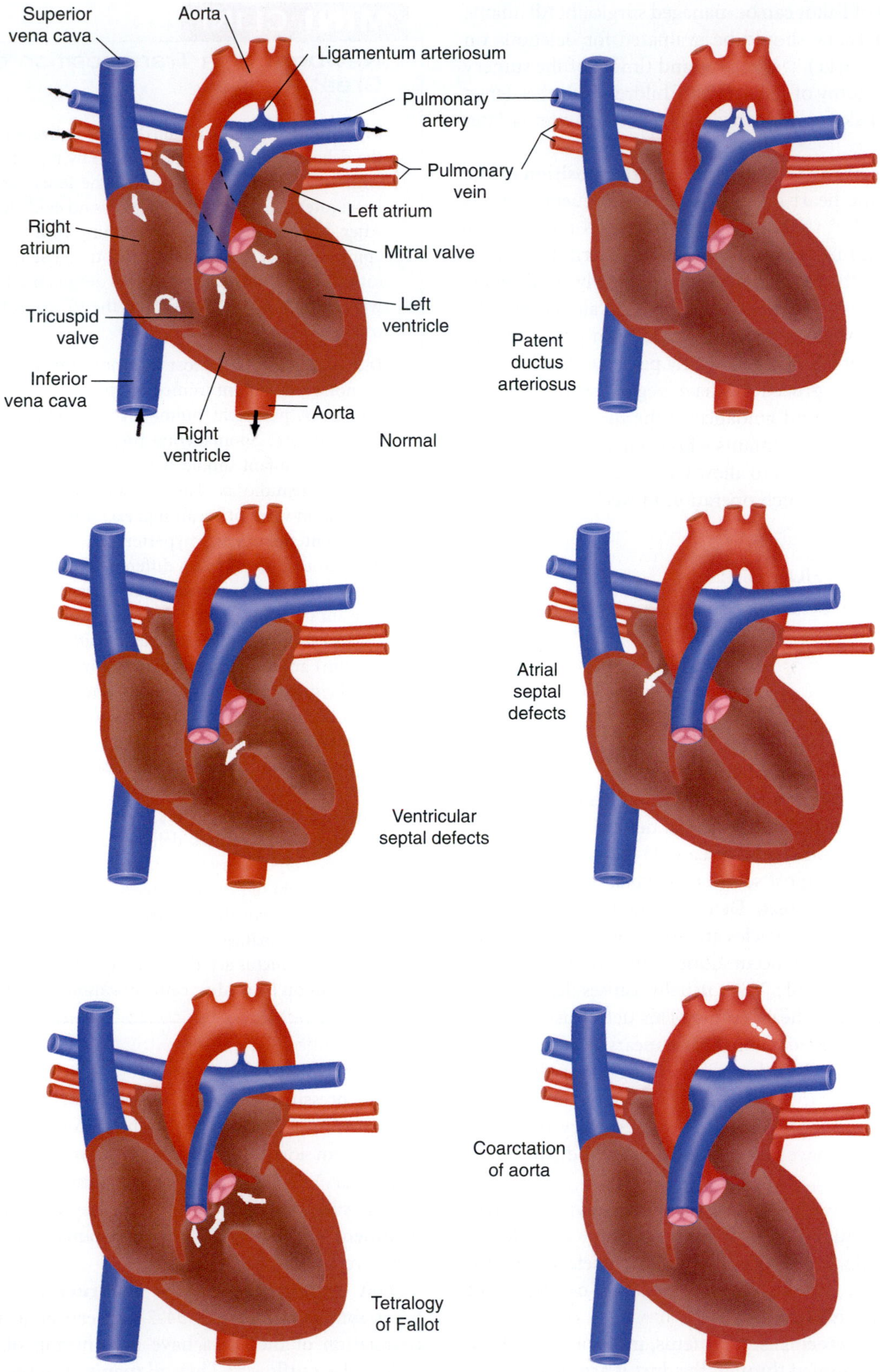

FIGURE 34-6 Normal flow of blood through the heart and some congenital defects that cause abnormal flow. (Modified from Jacob S, Francone C, Lossow WJ: Structure and function in man, ed 5, Philadelphia, 1982, Saunders.)

types of tetralogy of Fallot can be managed surgically. All infants with tetralogy of Fallot should be evaluated for deletions on chromosome 22 (22q11).[166] The type and timing of the surgery depend on the anatomy of the defects. Children with this defect are at increased risk for sudden death from arrhythmia later in life.

Transposition of the Great Arteries. **Transposition of the great arteries** is the heart disease that most frequently causes severe cyanosis.[162,163,167,168] It usually manifests as moderate to severe cyanosis immediately after birth. A murmur may be present. Infants with this abnormality frequently need emergency atrial septostomy (cutting a hole in the wall between the two atria). This procedure historically has been performed in heart catheterization laboratories. Many pediatric cardiologists who perform invasive procedures have begun performing this procedure with ultrasound guidance in the neonatal intensive care unit. The condition of infants who need atrial septostomy usually stabilizes. The goal is to allow PVR to decrease and then to perform the arterial switch operation in week 2 or 3 of life.

RULE OF THUMB

An infant with profound cyanosis at birth most likely has cyanotic heart disease or PPHN.

MINI CLINI

Newborn With Transposition of the Great Arteries

PROBLEM: The RT is called to the delivery room to assist in the delivery of an infant to be born by repeat cesarean section without rupture of membranes. The fetus has had reassuring heart rate patterns in utero. There is no evidence of meconium. After delivery, the infant is breathing comfortably but fails to "pink up" (i.e., the infant is cyanotic). The transcutaneous O_2 saturation stabilizes in the low 70s despite mask-bag ventilation with an FiO_2 of 1. What should the RT consider as the source of this problem?

DISCUSSION: The most common reasons for a significantly cyanotic term infant immediately after delivery include pneumothorax, persistent pulmonary hypertension, and cyanotic heart disease. Spontaneous pneumothorax occasionally can occur. The infant should have decreased breath sounds in the affected hemithorax. These infants usually have a significant increase in work of breathing; excluding pneumothorax leaves persistent pulmonary hypertension and cyanotic congenital heart disease as the main differential diagnoses. The two most likely cyanotic congenital heart diseases to manifest with significant cyanosis immediately after birth are transposition of the great arteries (particularly with an intact ventricular septum) and tetralogy of Fallot (particularly with pulmonary atresia instead of pulmonary stenosis). An echocardiogram must be done as soon as possible to distinguish between these three possibilities.

Infants with cyanotic heart diseases are cyanotic. Some of these infants have saturations in the low 80s. Some of them have saturations in the 40s to 50s. Attempts to improve oxygenation with increased delivery of O_2 would be unsuccessful. Increased O_2 delivery would lead to problems with O_2 toxicity. Improvement in systemic oxygenation occurs only by developing a left-to-right shunt in the central circulation. Acutely, this shunt can be managed with administration of prostaglandin to reopen the ductus arteriosus. Long-term management requires intervention by cardiac catheterization or surgery.

Hypertension of the Newborn

Acyanotic Heart Diseases

Some of the most common and most severe congenital heart diseases are acyanotic. Ventricular septal defect is probably the most common congenital heart disease. Hypoplastic left heart syndrome is one of the most severe congenital heart diseases.

Ventricular Septal Defect. Defects along the septum separating the right and left ventricles are quite common. Ventricular septal defect (VSD) can occur alone or in combination with other anomalies. A simple VSD usually causes left-to-right shunting and congestive heart failure. This defect usually does not appear immediately after birth. It appears at 6 to 8 weeks of age, when the PVR has decreased enough that the shunt becomes large.

Historically, closure of VSDs has required surgery. In the last few years many VSDs have been able to be closed during heart catheterization.[169-173]

Atrial Septal Defect. The most common type of atrial septal defect is a small, slitlike opening that persists after closure of the foramen ovale.[174] An isolated atrial septal defect is of little clinical importance. As with VSDs, some ASDs can be closed during heart catheterization.[171,175-178]

Patent Ductus Arteriosus. In a fetus, most of the pulmonary blood flow is shunted through the ductus arteriosus to the aorta. Closure of the ductus normally occurs 5 to 7 days after birth of a term infant. Patent ductus arteriosus usually is a disease of immature, preterm infants. Factors altering pressure gradients or affecting smooth muscle contraction can cause the ductus not to close or to reopen after it has closed. Depending on the pressure gradients established, shunting through an open ductus may be either right to left (pulmonary pressure greater than aortic) or left to right (aortic pressure greater than pulmonary). Treatment is either pharmacologic (indomethacin) or surgical (ligation). In recent years, the best timing of treatment and the treatment mechanism have become quite controversial.[179,180]

Left Ventricular Outflow Obstructions. Hypoplastic left heart syndrome (Figure 34-7), interrupted aortic arch, and coarctation of the aorta have in common obstruction of left ventricular outflow.[181] They all manifest in the newborn period with symptoms of acute heart failure. Systemic blood flow depends on patency of the ductus arteriosus. When the ductus spontaneously closes (usually at 5 to 7 days of age), severe congestive heart failure develops. The symptoms range from moderate respiratory distress to complete cardiovascular collapse.

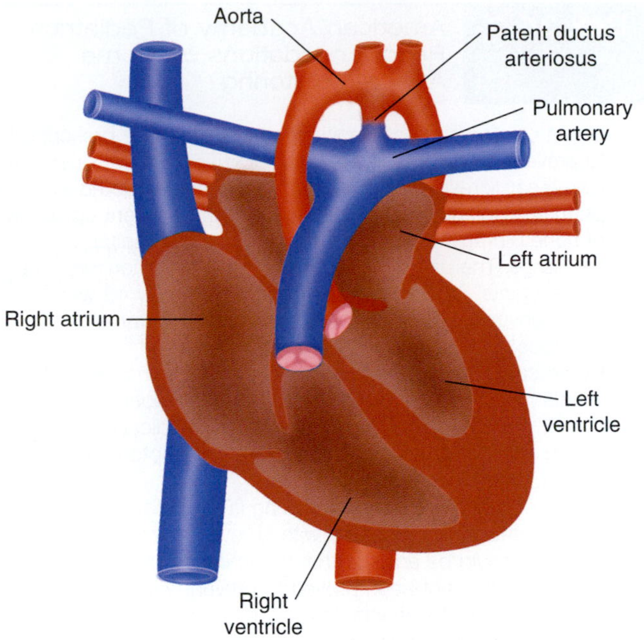

FIGURE 34-7 Hypoplastic left heart syndrome.

Box 34-1 Factors Associated With Increased Frequency of Sudden Infant Death Syndrome

MATERNAL CHARACTERISTICS
- Younger than 20 years
- Poor
- African American, Native American, or Alaskan Native
- Previous fetal loss
- Cigarette smoking
- Narcotic abuse
- Illness during pregnancy
- Inadequate prenatal care

INFANT CHARACTERISTICS AT BIRTH
- Male gender
- Premature birth
- Small for gestational age
- Low Apgar score
- Resuscitation with O_2 and ventilation at birth
- Second or third in birth order or of a multiple birth
- Sibling death from SIDS

From Koff PB, Eitzman DV, Neu J: Neonatal and pediatric respiratory care, ed 2, St Louis, 1993, Mosby.

Initial treatment is intravenous administration of prostaglandin E_1. Most infants with these defects need support with mechanical ventilation. These infants do not have lung disease. The pressures and rates used should be set appropriately.

There are standard surgical repairs for both interrupted aortic arch and coarctation of the aorta. Hypoplastic left heart syndrome has several accepted treatments, including a palliative surgical procedure (Norwood) and transplantation.[181-184] Neither the Norwood procedure nor transplantation is ideal, and each option has significant associated problems. The decision must be made in consultation with the family.

NEONATAL RESUSCITATION

Resuscitation of the newborn is a subset of resuscitation techniques. Most infant resuscitations occur in the delivery room. Although these resuscitations can range from minimal intervention to full resuscitation, more than 90% of them can be successfully dealt with by stimulation, ensuring the presence of an airway, and providing breathing support.[185-188] RTs are very important members of any resuscitation team. Their expertise in establishing and supporting an airway and initiating respiratory support is essential. It is beyond the scope of this chapter to delineate the guidelines of neonatal resuscitation. The reader should refer to the neonatal resuscitation guidelines published by the American Academy of Pediatrics (AAP).[185-188]

PEDIATRIC RESPIRATORY DISORDERS

Compared with the common cardiopulmonary diseases in the neonatal period, the pulmonary conditions that occur among older infants and children commonly result from airway obstruction caused by bacterial or viral infections. Other entities discussed in this section include asthma, SIDS, gastroesophageal reflux disease, and cystic fibrosis.

Sudden Infant Death Syndrome

SIDS is the leading cause of death (40%) among infants younger than 1 year in the United States. Approximately 7000 infants die of SIDS each year in the United States.[99,102,189,190] A presumptive diagnosis is based on the conditions of death in which a previously healthy infant dies unexpectedly, usually during sleep. Autopsy shows that many infants who die of SIDS have evidence of repeated episodes of hypoxemia or ischemia. Factors associated with increased frequency of SIDS are presented in Box 34-1. If the infant is found and resuscitation is successful, the diagnosis would be apparent.

Cause

The cause of SIDS is unknown. Apnea of prematurity is not a predisposing factor, and there is no evidence that immaturity of the respiratory centers is a cause. Although infants in families in which two or more SIDS deaths have occurred are at slightly higher risk, there is no evidence of a genetic link. The best knowledge of SIDS comes from population or epidemiologic studies and is summarized in Box 34-2. An infant who dies of SIDS typically is a preterm African-American boy born to a poor mother younger than 20 years of age who received inadequate prenatal care. Infants 1 to 3 months old are most susceptible, and death is most likely to occur at night during the winter. The risk for SIDS also is high among infants who previously experienced an apparent life-threatening event. Such an event occurs when an infant becomes apneic, cyanotic, or limp enough to frighten the parent or caregiver. The prone sleeping position has been strongly associated with increased risk for SIDS. It is difficult to differentiate death from SIDS and death

Box 34-2 Infant Characteristics Near the Time of Death From Sudden Infant Death Syndrome

- Age younger than 6 months (peak between 1 month and 3 months)
- Winter season
- Asleep at night
- Mild illness in week before death
- History of apparent life-threatening event
- Prone sleep position
- Mother smokes cigarettes

from intentional suffocation. The possibility of intentional suffocation must be investigated but with great sensitivity.[109,191,192]

Prevention

Because of the unknown causation and unexpected occurrence, there is no therapy for SIDS. Prevention is the goal. Successful prevention requires that infants at high risk be identified through a history of risk factors and documented monitoring or event recording. After identification that an infant is at risk, the family is trained in apnea monitoring and cardiopulmonary resuscitation. The AAP recommends placing infants in either the supine or the side-lying position for the first 6 months of life and reducing soft objects in the infant's sleeping environment.[109,191-193] To define the need and appropriate approach for home monitoring of infants, the AAP has developed a policy statement on infantile apnea and home monitoring.[109,191] The AAP recommendations for the need for and use of home monitoring are summarized in Box 34-3.

Box 34-3 American Academy of Pediatrics Recommendations on Home Apnea Monitoring

1. Home cardiorespiratory monitoring should not be prescribed to prevent SIDS.
2. Home cardiorespiratory monitoring may be warranted for premature infants who are at high risk for recurrent episodes of apnea, bradycardia, and hypoxemia after hospital discharge. The use of home cardiorespiratory monitoring in these infants should be limited to approximately 43 weeks postmenstrual age or after the cessation of extreme episodes, whichever comes last.
3. Home cardiorespiratory monitoring may be warranted for infants who are technology-dependent (tracheostomy, CPAP), have unstable airways, have rare medical conditions affecting regulation of breathing, or have symptomatic chronic lung disease.
4. If home cardiorespiratory monitoring is prescribed, the monitor should be equipped with an event recorder.
5. Parents should be advised that home cardiorespiratory monitoring has not been proved to prevent sudden unexpected deaths in infants.
6. Pediatricians should continue to promote proved practices that decrease the risk for SIDS, including supine sleep position, safe sleeping environments, and elimination of prenatal and postnatal exposure to tobacco smoke.

From Committee on Fetus and Newborn: American Academy of Pediatrics: Apnea, sudden infant death syndrome, and home monitoring. Pediatrics 111(4 Pt 1):914–917, 2003.

Gastroesophageal Reflux Disease

Gastroesophageal reflux disease (GERD) is the regurgitation of stomach contents into the esophagus and is common in childhood. Some causes of GERD are not pathologic. There is general agreement that there are important interactions between GERD and various disorders of the respiratory system.[194] Respiratory problems caused by gastroesophageal reflux include reactive airways disease, wheezing, aspiration pneumonia, laryngospasm, stridor, chronic cough, choking spells, and apnea.[194-198] GERD should be considered when an infant has faced a sudden life-threatening event and when an older child has unexplained chronic head and neck problems. GERD can be diagnosed with esophageal pH testing, upper gastrointestinal contrast studies, and gastric scintiscan. When GERD has been diagnosed, medical therapy can begin.[199-205] Occasional cases that do not respond to medical management may require surgical intervention.

Bronchiolitis

Bronchiolitis is an acute infection of the lower respiratory tract, usually caused by respiratory syncytial virus (RSV). Nearly 1 in 10 infants younger than 2 years of age acquires a bronchiolitis infection. The outcome is generally good, although approximately 1% of infants hospitalized for bronchiolitis die of respiratory failure. Infants most prone to respiratory failure as a consequence of bronchiolitis are very young and immunodeficient and have a comorbidity, such as congenital heart disease, BPD, CF, or childhood asthma.[206-210]

Clinical Manifestations

The clinical manifestations of bronchiolitis are inflammation and obstruction of the small bronchi and bronchioles. Bronchiolitis commonly occurs soon after a viral upper respiratory tract infection. The infant may have a slight fever with an intermittent cough. After a few days, signs of respiratory distress develop, particularly dyspnea and tachypnea. Progressive inflammation and narrowing of the airways cause inspiratory and expiratory wheezing and increase airway resistance. A chest radiograph shows signs of hyperinflation with areas of consolidation. The diagnosis of RSV infection can be established by immunofluorescent assay the same day and assists in the implementation of a treatment plan.

Prophylaxis. In recent years, passive immunization for RSV has become available.[208,210-216] Initially, passive immunization was recommended only for preterm infants with BPD. However, passive immunization is now recommended for high-risk infants younger than 2 years of age who require medical therapy for chronic lung disease, infants born at less than 32 weeks of gestational age, and infants with congenital heart disease who have cardiovascular compromise (Box 34-4).[216]

Box 34-4 American Academy of Pediatrics Recommendations for Respiratory Syncytial Virus Prophylaxis

INDICATIONS FOR RSV PROPHYLAXIS

- Preterm infants without CLD or congenital heart disease
    - Preterm infants born before 29 weeks, 0 days gestation who are younger than 12 months at the start of the RSV season
    - Not recommended for the 2 year of life
- Preterm infants with CLD
    - Infants with CLD of prematurity defined as gestational age <32 weeks, 0 days and requiring FiO_2 >21% oxygen for at least the first 28 days after birth
    - Second year of life recommendation only for those infants who continue requiring medical support during the 6-month period before the start of the second RSV season
- Infants with hemodynamically significant CHD
    - Acyanotic heart disease requiring medications to control congestive heart failure and will require cardiac surgical procedures in infants with moderate to severe pulmonary hypertension
    - Cyanotic heart defects in the first year of life
    - Infants after surgical procedures that involve cardiopulmonary bypass
        - These infants may need a postoperative dose.
    - Infants younger 2 years of age undergoing cardiac transplantation
- Children with anatomic pulmonary abnormalities or neuromuscular disorder
- Immunocompromised children
    - Children younger than 24 months of age with severe immunocompromise
- Children with Down syndrome
    - Routine us is not recommended unless they have qualifying heart disease, CLD, airway clearance issues, or prematurity
- Children with cystic fibrosis
    - Routine use not recommended unless other indications are present
    - Infants with CF and CLD or nutritional compromise in the first year of life
    - Infants with CF and severe lung disease requiring hospitalization, or abnormalities on chest radiograph/computed tomography, or weight for length less than 10%
- Alaska Native and American Indian Infants

CF, Cystic fibrosis; *CLD,* chronic lung disease; *RSV,* respiratory syncytial virus.

Treatment. Treatment of a patient with bronchiolitis varies with the severity of the infection and the clinical signs and symptoms. Many patients can be treated at home with humidification and oral decongestants. Patients with more severe symptoms (apnea) and comorbidity usually are hospitalized, and treatment is directed at relieving the airway obstruction and associated hypoxemia. Hospitalized children frequently are treated with systemic hydration and O_2 via nasal cannula, high-flow nasal cannula, hood, croup tent, or nasal cannula and assisted with airway clearance.[208,212,215,217-220] Antibiotics may be administered to control secondary bacterial infections. If bronchiolitis progresses to acute respiratory failure, mechanical ventilation is required. Because of the obstructive nature of this disorder, low respiratory rates and long expiratory times may be needed to prevent air trapping. Heliox has been used for severe airways disease requiring mechanical ventilation.[219] Vigorous bronchial hygiene, occasionally including tracheobronchial aspiration, usually is needed to maintain a patent airway (Box 34-5).

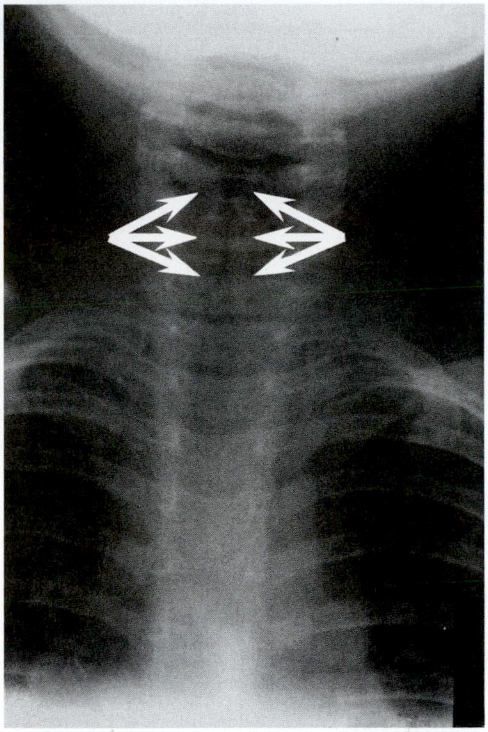

FIGURE 34-8 Anteroposterior chest radiograph of a patient with croup. Subglottic narrowing typical of croup is evident *(arrows).*

Croup

Croup is a viral disorder of the upper airway that normally results in subglottic swelling and obstruction. Termed *laryngotracheobronchitis,* viral croup is usually caused by the parainfluenza virus and is the most common form of airway obstruction in children 6 months to 6 years old. RSV and influenza virus are less common as causative agents. Bacterial superinfection with *Staphylococcus aureus,* group A *Streptococcus pyogenes,* or *Haemophilus influenzae* may worsen croup.

Clinical Manifestations

Symptoms become evident after 2 or 3 days of nasal congestion, fever, and coughing. A child typically has slow, progressive inspiratory and expiratory stridor and a barking cough. As the disease progresses, dyspnea, cyanosis, exhaustion, and agitation occur. A radiograph of the upper airway is helpful in confirming the diagnosis and ruling out epiglottitis but is usually not needed in most cases of croup. Classic croup is seen on an anteroposterior radiograph as characteristic subglottic narrowing of the trachea, called the *steeple sign* (Figure 34-8).

Box 34-5 American Academy of Pediatrics Recommendations for Diagnosis and Management of Bronchiolitis

DIAGNOSIS

1a Diagnosis and severity should be made on the basis of history and physical examination. Routine laboratory and radiologic studies are not needed.
1b Assess for history of risk factors in patients younger than 12 weeks of age.
Prematurity
Underlying cardiopulmonary disease
Immunodeficiency

TREATMENT

2a Bronchodilators should not be routinely used.
2b A carefully monitored trial of α-adrenergic or β-adrenergic is an option. Inhaled bronchodilators should be continued only if there is a documented positive clinical response.
3 Corticosteroids should not be used routinely.
4 Ribavirin should not be used routinely.
5 Antibacterial medications should be used only with specific indications of the coexistence of a bacterial infection.
6a Assess hydration and the ability to take oral fluids.
6b Chest physiotherapy should not be used routinely.
Supplemental oxygen is indicated if oxyhemoglobin saturation (SpO_2) falls persistently below 90%.
7a Supplemental O_2 should be discontinued if SpO_2 is ≥90% and the infant is feeding well and has minimal respiratory distress.
7b As the child's clinical course improves, continuous measurement of SpO_2 is not routinely needed.
7c Infants with a known history of hemodynamically significant heart or lung disease and premature infants require close O_2 monitoring as the O_2 is being weaned.

PROPHYLAXIS

8a Palivizumab prophylaxis should be done according to the new AAP Guidelines (Box 34-4).
9a Hand decontamination is the most important step in preventing nosocomial spread of RSV.
Hands should be decontaminated before and after direct contact with the patient and after contact with inanimate objects in the direct vicinity of the patient.
9b Alcohol-based rubs are preferred for hand decontamination.
9c Educate personnel and family members on hand sanitation.
10a Infants should not be exposed to passive smoking.
10b Breastfeeding is recommended to decrease a child's risk for developing a lower respiratory tract disease.
11 Inquire about the use of complementary and alternative medicines.

- Infants with chronic lung disease
  - Infants born at younger than 32 weeks of gestational age
  - Infants born at 32 to 35 weeks to gestational age who are at high risk for severe infection and younger than 90 days of age
- If two or more of following risks are present
  - Child care attendance
  - School-age siblings
  - Exposure to environmental air pollutants
  - Congenital abnormalities of the airways
  - Severe neuromuscular disease
- Infants with hemodynamically significant congenital heart disease (cyanotic and acyanotic)
- Following cardiopulmonary bypass

American Academy of Pediatrics Subcommittee on Diagnosis and Management of Bronchiolitis: Diagnosis and management of bronchiolitis. Pediatrics 118:1774–1193, 2006.

Treatment

The evaluation and treatment of a child with croup must focus on the degree of respiratory distress and associated clinical findings. If stridor is mild or occurs only on exertion and cyanosis is not present, hospitalization is generally not required and the child is treated at home. If there is stridor at rest (accompanied by harsh breath sounds, suprasternal retractions, and cyanosis with breathing of room air), hospitalization is indicated. The traditional treatment of a child with mild to moderate croup has involved cool mist therapy with or without supplemental O_2. However, there is no evidence that this practice is beneficial.[221] Corticosteroids and epinephrine have been shown to have the greatest benefit for decreasing the length and severity of respiratory symptoms associated with viral croup.[222-225] The addition of budesonide has been shown to reduce the severity of symptoms in mild to moderate cases of croup.[222-225] Progressive worsening of the clinical signs despite treatment indicates the need for intubation and mechanical ventilation. Heliox has been used for infants and children with severe disease. There is some evidence to show short-term benefit; however, long-term benefit has not yet been shown.[226]

Epiglottitis

Epiglottitis is an acute and often life-threatening infection of the upper airway that causes severe obstruction secondary to supraglottic swelling. Evidence suggests that the incidence of epiglottitis is decreasing among children and increasing in adults,[227] probably because of the use of vaccines. The most common cause is *H. influenzae* type B infection. Other organisms that are increasingly found to be causes of acute epiglottitis include group A *S. pneumoniae, S. aureus, Klebsiella pneumoniae, Haemophilus parainfluenzae,* and beta-hemolytic streptococci (groups A, B, C, and F).[228]

Clinical Manifestations

A child with epiglottitis usually has a high fever, sore throat, stridor, and labored breathing.[228-233] The patient does not have a croupy bark but instead has a muffled voice. Older children may report a sore throat and difficulty swallowing. Difficulty swallowing may cause drooling. Lateral radiographs of the neck (Figure 34-9) show the epiglottis is markedly thickened and flattened (thumb sign) and the aryepiglottic folds are swollen; the vallecula may not be visualized. Visual examination of the

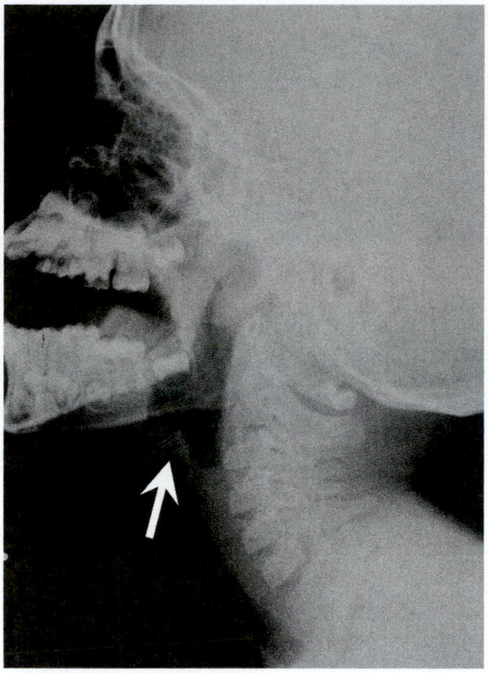

FIGURE 34-9 Lateral radiograph of the neck of a patient with epiglottitis. The thumb sign is prominent *(arrow)*.

upper airway is dangerous in these children and always should be performed in a controlled setting by personnel expert in emergency intubation. Inadvertent traction of the tongue can cause further and immediate swelling of the epiglottis and abrupt and total upper airway obstruction. Children with suspected epiglottitis should be accompanied by personnel expert in emergency intubation during any transport for diagnostic procedures.

MINI CLINI

Extubation

PROBLEM: A 3-year-old child underwent emergency intubation 5 days earlier for epiglottitis. The physician asks the RT to evaluate the patient for extubation. What would the RT evaluate before making the decision to extubate? What equipment would the RT want to have at the bedside during extubation?

DISCUSSION: Clinical examination of vital signs (e.g., body temperature), breath sounds, sensorium, and degree of airway leak should be considered. Equipment for rapid reintubation must be at the bedside, including racemic epinephrine for aerosolization.

Extubation of any patient should take into consideration the pathophysiologic condition that led to intubation. In this case, the RT should look for evidence that the infection is resolving and that the upper airway is no longer inflamed. A lack of fever for at least 12 hours and visual inspection of the throat that reveals minimal inflammation would be most helpful. After extubation, close monitoring must be performed for evidence of airway compromise. Cool mist may be helpful to minimize inflammation after extubation.

Treatment

Children with epiglottitis need elective intubation under general anesthesia in the operating room. Tracheostomy may be needed if the patient's condition warrants it; however, this procedure is rarely used. There should be no attempt to lie the child down or attempts to intubate until the child is sedated. Premature attempts at intubation can precipitate acute airway obstruction and respiratory arrest. After an airway is secured, a sample for bacterial culture should be obtained and antibiotic therapy should be started. Corticosteroids may decrease the swelling.[228,229,231,233] Children with an ETT should be sedated and restrained to prevent inadvertent extubation. Extubation should not be attempted until an upper airway leak is readily detected.

Cystic Fibrosis

Cystic fibrosis (CF) is one of the most common life-limiting autosomal recessive diseases, occurring in approximately 1 in every 3500 newborns in the United States.[234] It affects approximately 30,000 persons in the United States and 70,000 persons worldwide.[234] The incidence varies by race and ethnicity affecting approximately 1:3200 whites, 1:9500 Hispanics, 1:15,000 African Americans, and 1:31,000 in Asian Americans.[235] CF is caused by mutations in the gene that encodes a multifunctional protein called the *CF transmembrane conductance regulator (CFTR)*.[236] One of the main functions of this protein is to serve as an apical chloride channel in airway, intestinal, and exocrine cells.[237] The movement of chloride ions and regulation of sodium ions is important to the proper regulation of the water content of secretions.[238] The dehydrated viscous secretions that result from the *CFTR* abnormality lead to organ dysfunction resulting in the clinical manifestations of the disease.[238] There are over 1900 known *CFTR* mutations,[239] which are grouped into six classes that result in varying levels of *CFTR* production and dysfunction.[237] The variety of *CFTR* mutations explains some of the variability in the severity of the clinical manifestations of the disease.

RULE OF THUMB

Both parents must be carriers of the mutated CF gene *(CFTR)* for a child to be born with CF. If both parents have a deleterious *CFTR* mutation, the chance that CF will develop in their offspring is 1 in 4.

Clinical Manifestations

Patients with CF primarily experience abnormalities in the respiratory, digestive, and reproductive tracts.[240] Complications of lung disease are the leading cause of death in patients with CF.[241] The decreased airway surface liquid secondary to *CFTR* dysfunction leads to impaired mucus clearance, resulting in inflammation and infection of the airways[238] that causes a patient to have a chronic productive cough. Chronic airway infections can occur early in life, most frequently with *S. aureus, H. influenzae*, or *Pseudomonas aeruginosa*.[234] Certain organisms, including *P. aeruginosa*, methicillin resistant *S. aureus*, and *Burkholderia cepacia*, have been associated with greater declines in lung function.[242-244] There are infection control guidelines to reduce the risk for acquiring pathogens that can be detrimental to the health of patients with CF.[245] As the disease progresses, the cycle of inflammation, infection, and lung damage results in lung hyperinflation and bronchiectasis.[237] Patients with end-stage CF lung disease have severe debility from respiratory failure and may develop pulmonary hypertension and cor pulmonale.[241]

Approximately 85% of patients with CF have exocrine pancreatic insufficiency.[234] *CFTR* dysfunction in the pancreas dramatically reduces the amount of digestive enzymes, leading to malabsorption of fats and proteins and less so for carbohydrates.[246] Malabsorption results in bulky, greasy, foul-smelling stools, fat-soluble vitamin deficiencies, and poor weight gain with failure to thrive. Some newborns present with a condition called *meconium ileus* secondary to bowel obstruction of thick and hardened meconium that sometimes results in intestinal perforation.[247] Rectal prolapse also can occur as a result of malabsorption and elimination of bulky stools.[248] Patients with pancreatic sufficiency can have recurrent bouts of pancreatitis.[249] Liver disease can result in prolonged obstructive jaundice in the newborn period.[250] Some children and adults have progressive liver disease leading to cirrhosis and portal hypertension.[251]

Males with CF have obstructive azospermia as a result of congenital absence of the vas deferens.[252] Males and females with CF often have pubertal delays.[253] Females also have reduced fertility.[254]

As children with CF age, the risk for diabetes increases, and by adulthood the majority of patients have abnormal glucose tolerance testing.[234]

The electrolyte composition of sweat in CF patients is abnormal because of the higher content of salt.[255] Increased salt losses in the sweat may lead to the initial presentation of some CF patients with hyponatremic hypochloremic metabolic alkalosis.[256] The sweat chloride test used for the diagnosis of CF is based on the abnormal concentration of chloride in the sweat of patients with the disease.[257]

Diagnosis

Since 2010, screening for CF in newborns indicating persistent hypertrypsinogenemia is performed in all 50 states and the District of Columbia.[234] The diagnosis is confirmed by a sweat chloride test performed at an accredited CF center. The skin is stimulated to produce sweat (pilocarpine iontophoresis), and a sweat chloride level greater than 60 mEq/L confirms the diagnosis of CF.[258] The diagnosis in some infants is challenging because they have two *CFTR* mutations, but a normal sweat chloride (<30 mEq/L in infants younger than 6 months).[258]

The diagnosis of CF in patients not identified by newborn screening can be made by performing a sweat test in children or adults with signs or symptoms suggestive of CF, including recurrent sinus or lung infections, bronchiectasis, nasal polyps, digital clubbing, malabsorption, failure to gain weight as expected, recurrent pancreatitis, salt-losing syndromes, and male infertility resulting from obstructive azoospermia, or if they have a sibling with CF.[258] Having two sweat chloride test results greater than 60 mEq/L confirms the diagnosis.[258]

Pancreatic insufficiency is most often diagnosed with a stool fecal elastase testing.[259]

Monitoring

CF patients should be managed at an accredited CF center.[234] The CF Foundation recommends that newborns with CF are seen soon after a positive newborn screen result and then at least on a monthly basis until 6 months of age, then every 2 months until age 1 year, and every 2 to 3 months thereafter.[259] It is recommended that older children and adults are seen quarterly at a minimum. Because CF lung disease is progressive, patients are closely monitored by symptom assessment, physical examinations, sputum cultures to monitor airway flora, and objective measurements with spirometry and chest radiography.[234] The nutritional status of each patient is also monitored very closely, including their growth, body mass index, protein stores, and fat-soluble vitamin levels.

Treatment

Multiple therapies are used to maintain a patient's lung health. Airway clearance has been a mainstay of therapy in CF.[260] There are many options for airway clearance, including percussion and postural drainage, positive expiratory pressure, autogenic drainage, autocycle of breathing technique, oscillatory positive expiratory pressure, and high-frequency chest compression.[260] Airway clearance therapies have been shown to increase sputum production, improve exercise tolerance, and decrease the rate of lung function decline.[260] In general, no specific airway clearance technique is superior to another; therefore airway clearance must be tailored to the individual patient.[260]

As a result of the cellular debris from chronic infection and inflammation, there is free DNA in the airways that contributes to the viscosity of secretions. To treat this, inhaled recombinant deoxyribonuclease (DNase) is used to degrade the viscous DNA.[261] The routine daily use of inhaled DNase has been shown to improve pulmonary function and reduce exacerbations in patients with CF.[261,262] Inhaled DNase is recommended for daily use in patients 6 years of age and older.[263] Nebulized 7% hypertonic saline is thought to improve mucociliary clearance and has been shown to improve lung function and reduce exacerbations.[264] Nebulized 7% hypertonic saline is currently recommended for twice-daily use in patients 6 years and older.[263] High doses of the antiinflammatory drug ibuprofen, when used at doses resulting in appropriate levels, reduce the progression of CF lung disease and is recommended for use in children 6 to 17 years of age with a forced expiratory volume in 1 second greater than 60% predicted.[263] The regular use of azithromycin, possibly through its antiinflammatory and antimicrobial properties, helps preserve lung function and decreases the frequency of pulmonary exacerbations. Azithromycin is recommended in patients 6 years and older.[263] Patients taking azithromycin should be monitored for the acquisition of nontuberculous mycobacteria, at which time their azithromycin monotherapy should be discontinued.[263]

The lungs of CF patients are chronically colonized with bacteria. One of the most common organism is *P. aeruginosa,*[234] which has been associated with more rapid decline in lung function and decreased survival.[242] Inhaled antibiotics directed against this organism are recommended for eradiation and chronic suppression. Currently two inhaled antibiotics—inhaled tobramycin and inhaled aztreonam—are available for use.[263,265,266]

More recently developed therapies are aimed at correcting the underlying *CFTR* defect or potentiating its function.[237] In 2012, ivacaftor, a potentiator that activates defective *CFTR,* was approved for use in the United States in patients with a specific variant of CF—the G551D *CFTR* mutation. In 2014 the approval for use of ivacaftor was expanded to some other gating *CFTR* mutations. Ivacaftor has been shown to improve lung function and significantly reduce pulmonary exacerbations.[267] Ivacaftor also was observed to significantly decrease the sweat chloride concentration.

Lung transplantation is an option for patients with advanced severe CF lung disease.

The malabsorption secondary to deficiency of pancreatic enzymes is managed with pancreatic enzyme supplementation and vitamin supplementation.[240] Some patients also require oral calorie supplements to assist with their nutritional needs.

Prognosis

When CF was first described in 1938, children lived approximately 6 months.[268] As a result of improvements in CF care and advances in therapies, survival has significantly improved.[234] In 2002 the median age of survival was 31.3 years, and 10 years later in 2012, the median survival of patients with CF rose to 41.1 years.[234] In the near future, the number of adults will outnumber the children with CF.[234]

ROLE OF THE RESPIRATORY THERAPIST IN NEONATAL AND PEDIATRIC RESPIRATORY DISORDERS

As with any clinical situation, the role of the RT in the special environment of neonatal and pediatric care is to use his or her expertise and knowledge to improve patient outcome. Because there are significant differences in the diseases, pathophysiologies, and function of respiratory support equipment between adult and pediatric patients, the RT must be thoroughly familiar with all aspects of pediatric care. The old adage "children are not little adults" is true. Equally, newborns are not little children. Each of these age groups has unique characteristics that require specialized knowledge and experience. The RT is an important part of a team that is dedicated to the health and well-being of these fragile patients.

Also, the RT has an important role in providing education and emotional support, not only of the pediatric patient but also of the families and caregivers. Frequently, the RT is at the bedside of patients when the parents or caregivers are present. The RT is invaluable in helping patients and parents understand the respiratory goals of each individual patient.

SUMMARY CHECKLIST

- The incidence of RDS increases with decreasing gestational age.
- A qualitative decrease in surfactant increases alveolar surface tension forces in RDS patients. This process causes alveoli to become unstable and collapse and leads to atelectasis and increased work of breathing.
- The definitive diagnosis of RDS usually is made with chest radiography. Diffuse, hazy, reticulogranular densities with the presence of air bronchograms and low lung volumes are typical of RDS.
- TTN, often referred to as type II RDS, is probably the most common respiratory disorder of the newborn. The cause of TTN is unclear but is most likely related to delayed clearance of fetal lung liquid. Infants with TTN usually respond readily to low FiO_2 by O_2 hood or nasal cannula. Infants who need higher FiO_2 levels may benefit from CPAP.
- MAS is a disease of term and near-term infants. It involves aspiration of meconium into the central airways of the lung. This disorder usually is associated with perinatal depression and asphyxia.
- The best management of BPD is prevention. Prevention of atelectrauma and volutrauma begins in the delivery room.
- PPHN should be suspected when an infant has rapidly changing SaO_2 without changes in FiO_2 or has hypoxemia out of proportion to the lung disease detected on the chest radiograph or on the basis of $PaCO_2$.
- Congenital diaphragmatic hernia is a severe disease that usually manifests as severe respiratory distress in the newborn period. The pathophysiologic mechanism is a complex combination of lung hypoplasia, including decreased alveolar count and decreased pulmonary vasculature; pulmonary hypertension; and unusual anatomy of the inferior vena cava.
- The cause of SIDS is unknown. Apnea of prematurity is not a predisposing factor, and there is no evidence that immaturity of the respiratory centers is a cause.
- Bronchiolitis is an acute infection of the lower respiratory tract usually caused by RSV.
- Croup is a viral disorder of the upper airway that normally results in subglottic swelling and obstruction. Termed *laryngotracheobronchitis,* viral croup is caused by the parainfluenza virus and is the most common form of airway obstruction in children 6 months to 6 years old.
- Epiglottitis is an acute, often life-threatening infection of the upper airway that causes severe obstruction secondary to supraglottic swelling. Evidence suggests that the incidence of epiglottitis is decreasing among children,

probably because of the use of vaccines. A child with epiglottitis usually has a high fever, sore throat, stridor, and labored breathing.

- CF is the most common lethal genetic disorder among whites. It is inherited as an autosomal recessive trait that affects approximately 30,000 people in the United States. Treatment of CF lung disease requires aggressive efforts to control pulmonary infections and clear pulmonary secretions. RTs often play a key role in treating patients with CF.

References

1. Kamath BD, Macguire ER, McClure EM, et al: Neonatal mortality from respiratory distress syndrome: lessons for low-resource countries. *Pediatrics* 127:1139–1146, 2011.
2. Eriksson L, Haglund B, Ewald U, et al: Short and long-term effects of antenatal corticosteroids assessed in a cohort of 7,827 children born preterm. *Acta Obstet Gynecol Scand* 88:933–938, 2009.
3. Gyamfi-Bannerman C, Gilbert S, Landon MB, et al: Effect of antenatal corticosteroids on respiratory morbidity in singletons after late-preterm birth. *Obstet Gynecol* 119:555–559, 2012.
4. Bahadue FL, Soll R: Early versus delayed selective surfactant treatment for neonatal respiratory distress syndrome. *Cochrane Database Syst Rev* (11): 001456, 2012.
5. Curley AE, Halliday HL: The present status of exogenous surfactant for the newborn. *Early Hum Dev* 61:67–83, 2001.
6. Davis JM, Russ GA, Metlay L, et al: Short-term distribution kinetics of intratracheally administered exogenous lung surfactant. *Pediatr Res* 31: 445–450, 1992.
7. Lopez E, Gascoin G, Flamant C, et al: Exogenous surfactant therapy in 2013: what is next? Who, when and how should we treat newborn infants in the future? *BMC Pediatr* 13:165, 2013.
8. Rojas-Reyes MX, Morley CJ, Soll R: Prophylactic versus selective use of surfactant in preventing morbidity and mortality in preterm infants. *Cochrane Database Syst Rev* (3):000510, 2012.
9. Kugelman A, Durand M: A comprehensive approach to the prevention of bronchopulmonary dysplasia. *Pediatr Pulmonol* 46:1153–1165, 2011.
10. Ramanathan R, Sekar KC, Rasmussen M, et al: Nasal intermittent positive pressure ventilation after surfactant treatment for respiratory distress syndrome in preterm infants <30 weeks' gestation: a randomized, controlled trial. *J Perinatol* 32:336–343, 2012.
11. Sweet D, Bevilacqua G, Carnielli V, et al: European consensus guidelines on the management of neonatal respiratory distress syndrome. *J Perinat Med* 35:175–186, 2007.
12. Sekar KC, Corff KE: To tube or not to tube babies with respiratory distress syndrome. *J Perinatol* 29(Suppl 2):S68–S72, 2009.
13. Verder H, Bohlin K, Kamper J, et al: Nasal CPAP and surfactant for treatment of respiratory distress syndrome and prevention of bronchopulmonary dysplasia. *Acta Paediatr* 98:1400–1408, 2009.
14. Dani C, Berti E, Barp J: Risk factors for INSURE failure in preterm infants. *Minerva Pediatr* 62(3 Suppl 1):19–20, 2010.
15. Dani C, Corsini I, Bertini G, et al: The INSURE method in preterm infants of less than 30 weeks' gestation. *J Matern Fetal Neonatal Med* 23:1024–1029, 2010.
16. Donn SM: Lucinactant: a novel synthetic surfactant for the treatment of respiratory distress syndrome. *Expert Opin Investig Drugs* 14:329–334, 2005.
17. Donn SM, Sinha SK: Aerosolized lucinactant: a potential alternative to intratracheal surfactant replacement therapy. *Expert Opin Pharmacother* 9:475–478, 2008.
18. Jordan BK, Donn SM: Lucinactant for the prevention of respiratory distress syndrome in premature infants. *Expert Rev Clin Pharmacol* 6:115–121, 2013.
19. Moen MD, Perry CM, Wellington K: Lucinactant: in neonatal respiratory distress syndrome. *Treat Respir Med* 4:139–145, discussion 46–47, 2005.
20. Seger N, Soll R: Animal derived surfactant extract for treatment of respiratory distress syndrome. *Cochrane Database Syst Rev* (2):007836, 2009.
21. Soll R, Ozek E: Multiple versus single doses of exogenous surfactant for the prevention or treatment of neonatal respiratory distress syndrome. *Cochrane Database Syst Rev* (1):000141, 2009.
22. Soll RF: Synthetic surfactant for respiratory distress syndrome in preterm infants. *Cochrane Database Syst Rev* (2):001149, 2000.
23. Soll RF: Prophylactic synthetic surfactant for preventing morbidity and mortality in preterm infants. *Cochrane Database Syst Rev* (2):001079, 2000.
24. Soll RF: Prophylactic natural surfactant extract for preventing morbidity and mortality in preterm infants. *Cochrane Database Syst Rev* (2):000511, 2000.
25. Soll RF: Natural surfactant extract versus synthetic surfactant for neonatal respiratory distress syndrome. *Cochrane Database Syst Rev* (2):000144, 2000.
26. Soll RF: Multiple versus single dose natural surfactant extract for severe neonatal respiratory distress syndrome. *Cochrane Database Syst Rev* (2): 000141, 2000.
27. Speer CP: Neonatal respiratory distress syndrome: an inflammatory disease? *Neonatology* 99:316–319, 2011.
28. Yagui AC, Vale LA, Haddad LB, et al: Bubble CPAP versus CPAP with variable flow in newborns with respiratory distress: a randomized controlled trial. *J Pediatr* 87:499–504, 2011.
29. Narendran V, Donovan EF, Hoath SB, et al: Early bubble CPAP and outcomes in ELBW preterm infants. *J Perinatol* 23:195–199, 2003.
30. Kawaza K, Machen HE, Brown J, et al: Efficacy of a low-cost bubble CPAP system in treatment of respiratory distress in a neonatal ward in Malawi. *PLoS ONE* 9:e86327, 2014.
31. Hartung JC, Dold SK, Thio M, et al: Time to adjust to changes in ventilation settings varies significantly between different T-piece resuscitators, self-inflating bags, and manometer equipped self-inflating bags. *Am J Perinatol* 31:505–512, 2014.
32. Tagare A, Kadam S, Vaidya U, et al: Bubble CPAP versus ventilator CPAP in preterm neonates with early onset respiratory distress: a randomized controlled trial. *J Trop Pediatr* 59:113–119, 2013.
33. Jain L: Morbidity and mortality in late-preterm infants: more than just transient tachypnea! *J Pediatr* 151:445–446, 2007.
34. Jain L: Respiratory morbidity in late-preterm infants: prevention is better than cure! *Am J Perinatol* 25:75–78, 2008.
35. Jain L, Dudell GG: Respiratory transition in infants delivered by cesarean section. *Semin Perinatol* 30:296–304, 2006.
36. Jain L, Eaton DC: Physiology of fetal lung fluid clearance and the effect of labor. *Semin Perinatol* 30:34–43, 2006.
37. Eaton DC, Chen J, Ramosevac S, et al: Regulation of Na+ channels in lung alveolar type II epithelial cells. *Proc Am Thorac Soc* 1:10–16, 2004.
38. Eaton DC, Helms MN, Koval M, et al: The contribution of epithelial sodium channels to alveolar function in health and disease. *Annu Rev Physiol* 71:403–423, 2009.
39. Eaton DC, Malik B, Bao HF, et al: Regulation of epithelial sodium channel trafficking by ubiquitination. *Proc Am Thorac Soc* 7:54–64, 2010.
40. Jain L: Alveolar fluid clearance in developing lungs and its role in neonatal transition. *Clin Perinatol* 26:585–599, 1999.
41. Jain L, Eaton DC: Alveolar fluid transport: a changing paradigm. *Am J Physiol Lung Cell Mol Physiol* 290:L646–L648, 2006.
42. Johnson MD, Bao HF, Helms MN, et al: Functional ion channels in pulmonary alveolar type I cells support a role for type I cells in lung ion transport. *Proc Natl Acad Sci U S A* 103:4964–4969, 2006.
43. Katz VL, Bowes WA, Jr: Meconium aspiration syndrome: reflections on a murky subject. *Am J Obstet Gynecol* 166(1 Pt 1):171–183, 1992.
44. de Beaufort AJ: Early human development at the perinatal interface: meconium stained amniotic fluid (MSAF) and meconium aspiration syndrome (MAS). *Early Hum Dev* 85:605, 2009.
45. Hofmeyr GJ, Xu H: Amnioinfusion for meconium-stained liquor in labour. *Cochrane Database Syst Rev* (1):000014, 2010.

46. Ivanov VA, Gewolb IH, Uhal BD: A new look at the pathogenesis of the meconium aspiration syndrome: a role for fetal pancreatic proteolytic enzymes in epithelial cell detachment. *Pediatr Res* 68:221–224, 2010.
47. Storme L, Aubry E, Rakza T, et al: Pathophysiology of persistent pulmonary hypertension of the newborn: impact of the perinatal environment. *Arch Cardiovasc Dis* 16:169–177, 2013.
48. Teng RJ, Wu TJ: Persistent pulmonary hypertension of the newborn. *J Formos Med Assoc* 112:177–184, 2013.
49. Gadzinowski J, Kowalska K, Vidyasagar D: Treatment of MAS with PPHN using combined therapy: SLL, bolus surfactant and iNO. *J Perinatol* 28(Suppl 3):S56–S66, 2008.
50. Hahn S, Choi HJ, Soll R, et al: Lung lavage for meconium aspiration syndrome in newborn infants. *Cochrane Database Syst Rev* (4):003486, 2013.
51. Jeng MJ, Soong WJ, Lee YS: Effective lavage volume of diluted surfactant improves the outcome of meconium aspiration syndrome in newborn piglets. *Pediatr Res* 66:107–112, 2009.
52. Kaapa P, Soukka H: Phospholipase A2 in meconium-induced lung injury. *J Perinatol* 28(Suppl 3):S120–S122, 2008.
53. Mokra D, Calkovska A: How to overcome surfactant dysfunction in meconium aspiration syndrome? *Respir Physiol Neurobiol* 187:58–63, 2013.
54. Mokra D, Mokry J, Tonhajzerova I: Anti-inflammatory treatment of meconium aspiration syndrome: benefits and risks. *Respir Physiol Neurobiol* 187:52–57, 2013.
55. Rossi EM, Philipson EH, Williams TG, et al: Meconium aspiration syndrome: intrapartum and neonatal attributes. *Am J Obstet Gynecol* 161:1106–1110, 1989.
56. Halliday HL: Endotracheal intubation at birth for preventing morbidity and mortality in vigorous, meconium-stained infants born at term. *Cochrane Database Syst Rev* (1):000500, 2001.
57. Vain NE, Szyld EG, Prudent LM: Evidence based practice and the prevention and management of meconium aspiration syndrome. *Eur J Pediatr* 164:789, author reply 90, 2005.
58. Vain NE, Szyld EG, Prudent LM, et al: What (not) to do at and after delivery? Prevention and management of meconium aspiration syndrome. *Early Hum Dev* 85:621–626, 2009.
59. Vain NE, Szyld EG, Prudent LM, et al: Oropharyngeal and nasopharyngeal suctioning of meconium-stained neonates before delivery of their shoulders: multicentre, randomised controlled trial. *Lancet* 364:597–602, 2004.
60. van Ierland Y, de Boer M, de Beaufort AJ: Meconium-stained amniotic fluid: discharge vigorous newborns. *Arch Dis Child* 95:F69–F71, 2010.
61. Dargaville PA: Innovation in surfactant therapy. I. Surfactant lavage and surfactant administration by fluid bolus using minimally invasive techniques. *Neonatology* 101:326–336, 2012.
62. Halliday HL, Speer CP, Robertson B: Treatment of severe meconium aspiration syndrome with porcine surfactant. Collaborative Surfactant Study Group. *Eur J Pediatr* 155:1047–1051, 1996.
63. Jeng MJ, Lee YS, Tsao PC, et al: Neonatal air leak syndrome and the role of high-frequency ventilation in its prevention. *J Chin Med Assoc* 75:551–559, 2012.
64. Greenough A, Dimitriou G, Prendergast M: et a1: Synchronized mechanical ventilation for respiratory support in newborn infants. *Cochrane Database Syst Rev* (1):000456, 2008.
65. Mokra D, Drgova A, Kopincova J, et al: Anti-inflammatory treatment in dysfunction of pulmonary surfactant in meconium-induced acute lung injury. *Adv Exp Med Biol* 756:189–196, 2013.
66. Soll RF, Dargaville P: Surfactant for meconium aspiration syndrome in full term infants. *Cochrane Database Syst Rev* (2):002054, 2000.
67. Wang PW, Jeng MJ, Wang LS, et al: Surfactant lavage decreases systemic interleukin-1 beta production in meconium aspiration syndrome. *Pediatr Int* 52:432–437, 2010.
68. Finer NN, Barrington KJ: Nitric oxide for respiratory failure in infants born at or near term. *Cochrane Database Syst Rev* (4):000399, 2006.
69. Ward M, Sinn J: Steroid therapy for meconium aspiration syndrome in newborn infants. *Cochrane Database Syst Rev* (4):003485, 2003.
70. Wiswell TE: Delivery room management of the meconium-stained newborn. *J Perinatol* 28(Suppl 3):S19–S26, 2008.
71. Bancalari E: Bronchopulmonary dysplasia: old problem, new presentation. *J Pediatr* 82:2–3, 2006.
72. Bancalari E, Claure N: Definitions and diagnostic criteria for bronchopulmonary dysplasia. *Semin Perinatol* 30:164–170, 2006.
73. Bancalari E, Gerhardt T: Bronchopulmonary dysplasia. *Pediatr Clin North Am* 33:1–23, 1986.
74. Merritt TA, Deming DD, Boynton BR: The "new" bronchopulmonary dysplasia: challenges and commentary. *Semin Fetal Neonatal Med* 14:345–357, 2009.
75. Northway WH, Jr, Rosan RC, Porter DY: Pulmonary disease following respiratory therapy of hyaline-membrane disease: bronchopulmonary dysplasia. *N Engl J Med* 276:357–368, 1967.
76. Bancalari E: Caffeine reduces the rate of bronchopulmonary dysplasia in very low birth weight infants. *J Pediatr* 149:727–728, 2006.
77. Coalson JJ: Pathology of new bronchopulmonary dysplasia. *Semin Neonatol* 8:73–81, 2003.
78. Coalson JJ: Pathology of bronchopulmonary dysplasia. *Semin Perinatol* 30:179–184, 2006.
79. Nickerson BG: Bronchopulmonary dysplasia: chronic pulmonary disease following neonatal respiratory failure. *Chest* 87:528–535, 1985.
80. Ambalavanan N, Carlo WA: Ventilatory strategies in the prevention and management of bronchopulmonary dysplasia. *Semin Perinatol* 30:192–199, 2006.
81. Bhandari A, Bhandari V: Bronchopulmonary dysplasia: an update. *Indian J Pediatr* 74:73–77, 2007.
82. Bhandari V, Gruen JR: The genetics of bronchopulmonary dysplasia. *Semin Perinatol* 30:185–191, 2006.
83. Biniwale MA, Ehrenkranz RA: The role of nutrition in the prevention and management of bronchopulmonary dysplasia. *Semin Perinatol* 30:200–208, 2006.
84. Blanchard PW, Brown TM, Coates AL: Pharmacotherapy in bronchopulmonary dysplasia. *Clin Perinatol* 14:881–910, 1987.
85. Chess PR, D'Angio CT, Pryhuber GS, et al: Pathogenesis of bronchopulmonary dysplasia. *Semin Perinatol* 30:171–178, 2006.
86. Frank L, Sosenko IR: Undernutrition as a major contributing factor in the pathogenesis of bronchopulmonary dysplasia. *Am Rev Respir Dis* 138:725–729, 1988.
87. Bjorklund LJ, Ingimarsson J, Curstedt T, et al: Manual ventilation with a few large breaths at birth compromises the therapeutic effect of subsequent surfactant replacement in immature lambs. *Pediatr Res* 42:348–355, 1997.
88. Nakanishi H, Sugiura T, Streisand JB, et al: TGF-beta-neutralizing antibodies improve pulmonary alveologenesis and vasculogenesis in the injured newborn lung. *Am J Physiol Lung Cell Mol Physiol* 293:L151–L161, 2007.
89. Stenmark KR, Abman SH: Lung vascular development: implications for the pathogenesis of bronchopulmonary dysplasia. *Annu Rev Physiol* 67:623–661, 2005.
90. Stenmark KR, Balasubramaniam V: Angiogenic therapy for bronchopulmonary dysplasia: rationale and promise. *Circulation* 112:2383–2385, 2005.
91. Baveja R, Christou H: Pharmacological strategies in the prevention and management of bronchopulmonary dysplasia. *Semin Perinatol* 30:209–218, 2006.
92. Grier DG, Halliday HL: Corticosteroids in the prevention and management of bronchopulmonary dysplasia. *Semin Neonatol* 8:83–91, 2003.
93. Ghanta S, Leeman KT, Christou H: An update on pharmacologic approaches to bronchopulmonary dysplasia. *Semin Perinatol* 37:115–123, 2013.
94. Oh W: Fluid and electrolyte management of very low birth weight infants. *Pediatr Neonatol* 53:329–333, 2012.
95. Tin W, Wiswell TE: Adjunctive therapies in chronic lung disease: examining the evidence. *Semin Fetal Neonatal Med* 13:44–52, 2008.
96. Harkavy KL, Scanlon JW, Chowdhry PK, et al: Dexamethasone therapy for chronic lung disease in ventilator- and oxygen-dependent infants: a controlled trial. *J Pediatr* 115:979–983, 1989.
97. Soll RF: Inhaled nitric oxide in the neonate. *J Perinatol* 29(Suppl 2):S63–S67, 2009.
98. Soll RF: Inhaled nitric oxide for respiratory failure in preterm infants. *Neonatology* 102:251–253, 2012.

99. Abu-Shaweesh JM, Martin RJ: Neonatal apnea: what's new? *Pediatr Pulmonol* 43:937–944, 2008.
100. Hunt CE: Ontogeny of autonomic regulation in late preterm infants born at 34-37 weeks postmenstrual age. *Semin Perinatol* 30:73–76, 2006.
101. Hunt CE, Corwin MJ, Lister G, et al: Precursors of cardiorespiratory events in infants detected by home memory monitor. *Pediatr Pulmonol* 43:87–98, 2008.
102. Hunt CE, Hauck FR: Sudden infant death syndrome. *CMAJ* 174:1861–1869, 2006.
103. Silvestri JM, Weese-Mayer DE, Hunt CE: Home monitoring during infancy: what is normal? *Paediatr Respir Rev* 3:10–17, 2003.
104. Elder DE, Campbell AJ, Galletly D: Current definitions for neonatal apnoea: are they evidence based? *J Paediatr Child Health* 49:E388–E396, 2013.
105. Martin RJ, Wilson CG: Apnea of prematurity. *Compr Physiol* 2:2923–2931, 2012.
106. Di Fiore JM, Martin RJ: Gauda EB: Apnea of prematurity: perfect storm. *Respir Physiol Neurobiol* 189:213–222, 2013.
107. Mayer CA, Ao J, Di Fiore JM, et al: Impaired hypoxic ventilatory response following neonatal sustained and subsequent chronic intermittent hypoxia in rats. *Respir Physiol Neurobiol* 187:167–175, 2013.
108. Henderson-Smart DJ, Osborn DA: Kinesthetic stimulation for preventing apnea in preterm infants. *Cochrane Database Syst Rev* (2):000373, 2000.
109. Committee on Fetus and Newborn, American Academy of Pediatrics: Apnea, sudden infant death syndrome, and home monitoring. *Pediatrics* 111(4 Pt 1):914–917, 2003.
110. Abu Jawdeh EG, O'Riordan M, Limrungsikul A, et al: Methylxanthine use for apnea of prematurity among an international cohort of neonatologists. *J Neonatal Perinatal Med* 6:251–256, 2013.
111. Henderson-Smart DJ, Davis PG: Prophylactic methylxanthine for extubation in preterm infants. *Cochrane Database Syst Rev* (2):000139, 2000.
112. Schoen K, Yu T, Stockmann C, et al: Use of methylxanthine therapies for the treatment and prevention of apnea of prematurity. *Paediatr Drugs* 16:169–177, 2014.
113. Henderson-Smart D, Steer P: Doxapram treatment for apnea in preterm infants. *Cochrane Database Syst Rev* (4):000074, 2004.
114. Henderson-Smart DJ, Davis PG: Prophylactic doxapram for the prevention of morbidity and mortality in preterm infants undergoing endotracheal extubation. *Cochrane Database Syst Rev* (3):001966, 2000.
115. Henderson-Smart DJ, Steer P: Doxapram versus methylxanthine for apnea in preterm infants. *Cochrane Database Syst Rev* (2):000075, 2000.
116. Hunt CE, Lesko SM, Vezina RM, et al: Infant sleep position and associated health outcomes. *Arch Pediatr Adolesc Med* 157:469–474, 2003.
117. Henderson-Smart DJ, Subramanian P, Davis PG: Continuous positive airway pressure versus theophylline for apnea in preterm infants. *Cochrane Database Syst Rev* (2):001072, 2000.
118. Silvestri JM: Indications for home apnea monitoring (or not). *Clin Perinatol* 36:87–99, 2009.
119. Abman SH, Wolfe RR, Accurso FJ, et al: Pulmonary vascular response to oxygen in infants with severe bronchopulmonary dysplasia. *Pediatrics* 75:80–84, 1985.
120. Berkelhamer SK, Mestan KK, Steinhorn RH: Pulmonary hypertension in bronchopulmonary dysplasia. *Semin Perinatol* 37:124–131, 2013.
121. Dudell GG, Jain L: Hypoxic respiratory failure in the late preterm infant. *Clin Perinatol* 33:803–830, abstract viii–ix, 2006.
122. Dukarm RC, Steinhorn RH, Morin FC, 3rd: The normal pulmonary vascular transition at birth. *Clin Perinatol* 23:711–726, 1996.
123. Gao Y, Raj JU: Regulation of the pulmonary circulation in the fetus and newborn. *Physiol Rev* 90:1291–1335, 2010.
124. Ivy DD, Abman SH, Barst RJ, et al: Pediatric pulmonary hypertension. *J Am Coll Cardiol* 62(25 Suppl):D117–D126, 2013.
125. Lakshminrusimha S, Steinhorn RH: Pulmonary vascular biology during neonatal transition. *Clin Perinatol* 26:601–619, 1999.
126. Lakshminrusimha S, Steinhorn RH, Wedgwood S, et al: Pulmonary hemodynamics and vascular reactivity in asphyxiated term lambs resuscitated with 21 and 100% oxygen. *J Appl Physiol (1985)* 111:1441–1447, 2011.
127. Lakshminrusimha S, Swartz DD, Gugino SF, et al: Oxygen concentration and pulmonary hemodynamics in newborn lambs with pulmonary hypertension. *Pediatr Res* 66:539–544, 2009.
128. Porta NF, Steinhorn RH: Pulmonary vasodilator therapy in the NICU: inhaled nitric oxide, sildenafil, and other pulmonary vasodilating agents. *Clin Perinatol* 39:149–164, 2012.
129. Steinhorn RH: Persistent pulmonary hypertension of the newborn. *Acta Anaesthesiol Scand Suppl* 111:135–140, 1997.
130. Steinhorn RH: Neonatal pulmonary hypertension. *Pediatr Crit Care Med* 11(2 Suppl):S79–S84, 2010.
131. Steinhorn RH: Diagnosis and treatment of pulmonary hypertension in infancy. *Early Hum Dev* 89:865–874, 2013.
132. Wedgwood S, Steinhorn RH: Role of reactive oxygen species in neonatal pulmonary vascular disease. *Antioxid Redox Signal* 21:1926–1942, 2014.
133. Ball MK, Steinhorn RH: Inhaled nitric oxide for preterm infants: a Marksman's approach. *J Pediatr* 161:379–380, 2012.
134. Golombek SG: The use of inhaled nitric oxide in newborn medicine. *Heart Dis* 2:342–347, 2000.
135. Steinhorn RH, Porta NF: Use of inhaled nitric oxide in the preterm infant. *Curr Opin Pediatr* 19:137–141, 2007.
136. Steinhorn RH, Shaul PW, deRegnier RA, et al: Inhaled nitric oxide and bronchopulmonary dysplasia. *Pediatrics* 128:e255–e256, author reply e6–e7, 2011.
137. Farrow KN, Fliman P, Steinhorn RH: The diseases treated with ECMO: focus on PPHN. *Semin Perinatol* 29:8–14, 2005.
138. Keller RL, Steinhorn RH: Extracorporeal membrane oxygenation in resource-limited countries. *Pediatr Crit Care Med* 14:900–902, 2013.
139. Steinhorn RH, Green TP: Use of extracorporeal membrane oxygenation in the treatment of respiratory syncytial virus bronchiolitis: the national experience, 1983 to 1988. *J Pediatr* 116:338–342, 1990.
140. Dukarm RC, Russell JA, Morin FC, 3rd, et al: The cGMP-specific phosphodiesterase inhibitor E4021 dilates the pulmonary circulation. *Am J Respir Crit Care Med* 160:858–865, 1999.
141. Dukarm RC, Steinhorn RH, Russell JA, et al: Selective type 5 phosphodiesterase inhibition alters pulmonary hemodynamics and lung liquid production in near-term fetal lambs. *J Appl Physiol (1985)* 99:2331–2336, 2005.
142. Farrow KN, Lakshminrusimha S, Czech L, et al: SOD and inhaled nitric oxide normalize phosphodiesterase 5 expression and activity in neonatal lambs with persistent pulmonary hypertension. *Am J Physiol Lung Cell Mol Physiol* 299:L109–L116, 2010.
143. Farrow KN, Steinhorn RH: Phosphodiesterases: emerging therapeutic targets for neonatal pulmonary hypertension. *Handb Exp Pharmacol* 204:251–277, 2011.
144. El-Gohary Y, Gittes GK, Tovar JA: Congenital anomalies of the esophagus. *Semin Pediatr Surg* 19:186–193, 2010.
145. Holland AJ, Fitzgerald DA: Oesophageal atresia and tracheo-oesophageal fistula: current management strategies and complications. *Paediatr Respir Rev* 11:100–106, quiz 6–7, 2010.
146. Gupta K, Sundaram V, Das A, et al: Extralobar sequestration associated with congenital pulmonary airway malformation (CPAM), type I: an autopsy report. *Fetal Pediatr Pathol* 30:167–172, 2011.
147. Pizzi M, Fassan M, Ludwig K, et al: Congenital pulmonary airway malformation (CPAM) [congenital cystic adenomatoid malformation] associated with tracheoesophageal fistula and agenesis of the corpus callosum. *Fetal Pediatr Pathol* 31:169–175, 2012.
148. Cullen ML, Klein MD, Philippart AI: Congenital diaphragmatic hernia. *Surg Clin North Am* 65:1115–1138, 1985.
149. de Buys Roessingh AS, Dinh-Xuan AT: Congenital diaphragmatic hernia: current status and review of the literature. *Eur J Pediatr* 168:393–406, 2009.
150. Keijzer R, Puri P: Congenital diaphragmatic hernia. *Semin Pediatr Surg* 19:180–185, 2010.
151. Hoffman SB, Massaro AN, Gingalewski C, et al: Predictors of survival in congenital diaphragmatic hernia patients requiring extracorporeal membrane oxygenation: CNMC 15-year experience. *J Perinatol* 30:546–552, 2010.

152. Islam S: Clinical care outcomes in abdominal wall defects. *Curr Opin Pediatr* 20:305–310, 2008.
153. Morgan RD, Hanna L, Lakhoo K: Management of giant omphalocele: a case series. *Eur J Pediatr Surg* 23:254–256, 2013.
154. Islam S: Advances in surgery for abdominal wall defects: gastroschisis and omphalocele. *Clin Perinatol* 39:375–386, 2012.
155. Danov Z, Schroth MK: Respiratory management of pediatric patients with neuromuscular disease. *Pediatr Ann* 39:769–776, 2010.
156. Panitch HB: Respiratory issues in the management of children with neuromuscular disease. *Respir Care* 51:885–893, discussion 94–95, 2006.
157. Panitch HB: The pathophysiology of respiratory impairment in pediatric neuromuscular diseases. *Pediatrics* 123(Suppl 4):S215–S218, 2009.
158. Schroth MK: Special considerations in the respiratory management of spinal muscular atrophy. *Pediatrics* 123(Suppl 4):S245–S249, 2009.
159. Wang CH, Finkel RS, Bertini ES, et al: Consensus statement for standard of care in spinal muscular atrophy. *J Child Neurol* 22:1027–1049, 2007.
160. Benditt JO: Initiating noninvasive management of respiratory insufficiency in neuromuscular disease. *Pediatrics* 1239(Suppl 4):S236–S238, 2009.
161. Kennedy JD, Martin AJ: Chronic respiratory failure and neuromuscular disease. *Pediatr Clin North Am* 56(1):261–273, xii, 2009.
162. Dob DP, Naguib MA, Gatzoulis MA: A functional understanding of moderate to complex congenital heart disease and the impact of pregnancy. I. the transposition complexes. *Int J Obstet Anesth* 19:298–305, 2010.
163. Naguib MA, Dob DP, Gatzoulis MA: A functional understanding of moderate to complex congenital heart disease and the impact of pregnancy. II. Tetralogy of Fallot, Eisenmenger's syndrome and the Fontan operation. *Int J Obstet Anesth* 19:306–312, 2010.
164. Duro RP, Moura C, Leite-Moreira A: Anatomophysiologic basis of tetralogy of Fallot and its clinical implications. *Rev Port Cardiol* 29:591–630, 2010.
165. Starr JP: Tetralogy of Fallot: yesterday and today. *World J Surg* 34:658–668, 2010.
166. Momma K: Cardiovascular anomalies associated with chromosome 22q11.2 deletion syndrome. *Am J Cardiol* 105:1617–1624, 2010.
167. Martins P, Castela E: Transposition of the great arteries. *Orphanet J Rare Dis* 3:27, 2008.
168. Skinner J, Hornung T, Rumball E: Transposition of the great arteries: from fetus to adult. *Heart* 94:1227–1235, 2008.
169. Butera G, Chessa M, Carminati M: Percutaneous closure of ventricular septal defects. *Cardiol Young* 17:243–253, 2007.
170. Butera G, Chessa M, Carminati M: Percutaneous closure of ventricular septal defects: state of the art. *J Cardiovasc Med* 8:39–45, 2007.
171. Butera G, Romagnoli E, Saliba Z, et al: Percutaneous closure of multiple defects of the atrial septum: procedural results and long-term follow-up. *Catheter Cardiovasc Interv* 76:121–128, 2010.
172. Sykes JA, Verma R, Peshkovsky C, et al: Early repair of large infant ventricular septal defect despite respiratory syncytial virus-induced respiratory failure with postrepair chylous pericardial effusion requiring pleuropericardial window: a case report and review of the literature. *Pediatr Emerg Care* 28:1072–1077, 2012.
173. Wilson W, Osten M, Benson L, et al: Evolving trends in interventional cardiology: endovascular options for congenital disease in adults. *Can J Cardiol* 30:75–86, 2014.
174. Geva T, Martins JD, Wald RM: Atrial septal defects. *Lancet* 383:1921–1932, 2014.
175. Butera G, Biondi-Zoccai G, Sangiorgi G, et al: Percutaneous versus surgical closure of secundum atrial septal defects: a systematic review and meta-analysis of currently available clinical evidence. *EuroIntervention* 7:377–385, 2011.
176. Butera G, Romagnoli E, Sangiorgi G, et al: Patent foramen ovale percutaneous closure: the no-implant approach. *Expert Rev Med Devices* 5:317–321, 2008.
177. Chessa M, Medda M, Moharram A, et al: Simultaneous percutaneous atrial septal defect closure and percutaneous coronary intervention. *Anatol J Cardiol* 7:51–53, 2007.
178. Scacciatella P, Butera G, Meynet I, et al: Percutaneous closure of patent foramen ovale in patients with anatomical and clinical high-risk characteristics: long-term efficacy and safety. *J Interv Cardiol* 24:477–484, 2011.
179. Benitz WE: Treatment of persistent patent ductus arteriosus in preterm infants: time to accept the null hypothesis? *J Perinatol* 30:241–252, 2010.
180. Laughon M, Bose C, Benitz WE: Patent ductus arteriosus management: what are the next steps? *J Pediatr* 157:355–357, 2010.
181. Barron DJ, Kilby MD, Davies B, et al: Hypoplastic left heart syndrome. *Lancet* 374:551–564, 2009.
182. Bacha E: Re: Results of orthotopic heart transplantation for failed palliation of hypoplastic left heart. *Eur J Cardiothorac Surg* 43:604, 2013.
183. Bacha EA: Individualized approach in the management of patients with hypoplastic left heart syndrome (HLHS). *Semin Thorac Cardiovasc Surg Pediatr Card Surg Annu* 16:3–6, 2013.
184. Harada Y: Current status of the hybrid approach for the treatment of hypoplastic left heart syndrome. *Gen Thorac Cardiovasc Surg* 62:334–341, 2014.
185. Kattwinkel J, Perlman JM, Aziz K, et al: Part 15: neonatal resuscitation—2010 American Heart Association guidelines for cardiopulmonary resuscitation and emergency cardiovascular care. *Circulation* 122(18 Suppl 3): S909–S919, 2010.
186. Kattwinkel J, Perlman JM, Aziz K, et al: Neonatal resuscitation: 2010 American Heart Association guidelines for cardiopulmonary resuscitation and emergency cardiovascular care. *Pediatrics* 126:e1400–e1413, 2010.
187. Kleinman ME, Chameides L, Schexnayder SM, et al: Part 14: pediatric advanced life support—2010 American Heart Association guidelines for cardiopulmonary resuscitation and emergency cardiovascular care. *Circulation* 122(18 Suppl 3):S876–S908, 2010.
188. American Academy of Pediatrics, American Heart Association: *Neonatal resuscitation*, ed 6, Elk Grove Village, IL, 2011, American Academy of Pediatrics, American Heart Association, p 329.
189. Hunt CE: Sudden infant death syndrome and other causes of infant mortality: diagnosis, mechanisms, and risk for recurrence in siblings. *Am J Respir Crit Care Med* 164:346–357, 2001.
190. Jobe AH, Tibboel D: Update in pediatric lung disease 2013. *Am J Respir Crit Care Med* 189:1031–1036, 2014.
191. American Academy of Pediatrics Task Force on Sudden Infant Death Syndrome: Syndrome TFoSID: the changing concept of sudden infant death syndrome—diagnostic coding shifts, controversies regarding the sleeping environment, and new variables to consider in reducing risk. *Pediatrics* 116:1245–1255, 2005.
192. Hall KL, Zalman B: Evaluation and management of apparent life-threatening events in children. *Am Fam Physician* 71:2301–2308, 2005.
193. Grazel R, Phalen AG, Polomano RC: Implementation of the American Academy of Pediatrics recommendations to reduce sudden infant death syndrome risk in neonatal intensive care units: an evaluation of nursing knowledge and practice. *Adv Neonatal Care* 10:332–342, 2010.
194. Tolia V, Vandenplas Y: Systematic review: the extra-oesophageal symptoms of gastro-oesophageal reflux disease in children. *Aliment Pharmacol Ther* 29:258–272, 2009.
195. Abu Jawdeh EG, Martin RJ: Neonatal apnea and gastroesophageal reflux (GER): is there a problem? *Early Hum Dev* 89(Suppl 1):S14–S16, 2013.
196. Roden DF, Altman KW: Causes of dysphagia among different age groups: a systematic review of the literature. *Otolaryngol Clin North Am* 46:965–987, 2013.
197. Rosen R: Gastroesophageal reflux in infants: more than just a phenomenon. *JAMA Pediatr* 168:83–89, 2014.
198. Thakkar K, Boatright RO, Gilger MA, et al: Gastroesophageal reflux and asthma in children: a systematic review. *Pediatrics* 125:e925–e930, 2010.
199. Chung EY, Yardley J: Are there risks associated with empiric acid suppression treatment of infants and children suspected of having gastroesophageal reflux disease? *Hosp Pediatr* 3:16–23, 2012.
200. Corvaglia L, Martini S, Aceti A, et al: Nonpharmacological management of gastroesophageal reflux in preterm infants. *BioMed Res Int* 2013:141967, 2013.
201. Horvath A, Dziechciarz P, Szajewska H: The effect of thickened-feed interventions on gastroesophageal reflux in infants: systematic review and

meta-analysis of randomized, controlled trials. *Pediatrics* 122:e1268–e1277, 2008.
202. Shakhnovich V, Ward RM, Kearns GL: Failure of proton pump inhibitors to treat GERD in neonates and infants: a question of drug, diagnosis, or design. *Clin Pharmacol Ther* 92:388–392, 2012.
203. Tjon JA, Pe M, Soscia J, et al: Efficacy and safety of proton pump inhibitors in the management of pediatric gastroesophageal reflux disease. *Pharmacotherapy* 33:956–971, 2013.
204. Vandenplas Y: Management of paediatric GERD. *Nat Rev Gastroenterol Hepatol* 11:147–157, 2014.
205. Ward RM, Kearns GL: Proton pump inhibitors in pediatrics : mechanism of action, pharmacokinetics, pharmacogenetics, and pharmacodynamics. *Paediatr Drugs* 15:119–131, 2013.
206. Cox DW, Le Souef PN: Rhinovirus and the developing lung. *Paediatr Respir Rev* 15:268–274, 2014.
207. Del Vecchio A, Ferrara T, Maglione M, et al: New perspectives in respiratory syncytial virus infection. *J Matern Fetal Neonatal Med* 26(Suppl 2): 55–59, 2013.
208. Rodriguez R, Ramilo O: Respiratory syncytial virus: how, why and what to do. *J Infect* 68:S115–S118, 2014.
209. Wainwright C: Acute viral bronchiolitis in children: a very common condition with few therapeutic options. *Paediatr Respir Rev* 11:39–45, quiz, 2010.
210. Zorc JJ, Hall CB: Bronchiolitis: recent evidence on diagnosis and management. *Pediatrics* 125:342–349, 2010.
211. Fitzgerald DA: Preventing RSV bronchiolitis in vulnerable infants: the role of palivizumab. *Paediatr Respir Rev* 10:143–147, 2009.
212. Mitchell I: Treatment of RSV bronchiolitis: drugs, antibiotics. *Paediatr Respir Rev* 10(Suppl 1):14–15, 2009.
213. Murray J, Saxena S, Sharland M: Preventing severe respiratory syncytial virus disease: passive, active immunisation and new antivirals. *Arch Dis Child* 99:469–473, 2014.
214. Robinson KA, Odelola OA, Saldanha IJ: Palivizumab for prophylaxis against respiratory syncytial virus infection in children with cystic fibrosis. *Cochrane Database Syst Rev* (5):007743, 2014.
215. Turner TL, Kopp BT, Paul G, et al: Respiratory syncytial virus: current and emerging treatment options. *Clinicoecon Outcomes Res* 6:217–225, 2014.
216. American Academy of Pediatrics Committee on Infectious D, American Academy of Pediatrics Bronchiolitis Guidelines C: Updated guidance for palivizumab prophylaxis among infants and young children at increased risk of hospitalization for respiratory syncytial virus infection. *Pediatrics* 134:415–420, 2014.
217. Beggs S, Wong ZH, Kaul S, et al: High-flow nasal cannula therapy for infants with bronchiolitis. *Cochrane Database Syst Rev* (1):009609, 2014.
218. Fernandes RM, Bialy LM, Vandermeer B, et al: Glucocorticoids for acute viral bronchiolitis in infants and young children. *Cochrane Database Syst Rev* (10):004878, 2010.
219. Liet JM, Ducruet T, Gupta V, et al: Heliox inhalation therapy for bronchiolitis in infants. *Cochrane Database Syst Rev* (4):006915, 2010.
220. Ralston S, Comick A, Nichols E, et al: Effectiveness of quality improvement in hospitalization for bronchiolitis: a systematic review. *Pediatrics* 134:571–581, 2014.
221. Moore M, Little P: Humidified air inhalation for treating croup: a systematic review and meta-analysis. *Fam Pract* 24:295–301, 2007.
222. Bjornson C, Russell K, Vandermeer B, et al: Nebulized epinephrine for croup in children. *Cochrane Database Syst Rev* (10):006619, 2013.
223. Bjornson CL, Johnson DW: Croup. *Lancet* 371:329–339, 2008.
224. Bjornson CL, Johnson DW: Croup in children. *CMAJ* 185:1317–1323, 2013.
225. Cherry JD: Clinical practice: croup. *N Engl J Med* 358:384–391, 2008.
226. Moraa I, Sturman N, McGuire T, et al: Heliox for croup in children. *Cochrane Database Syst Rev* (12):006822, 2013.
227. Berger G, Landau T, Berger S, et al: The rising incidence of adult acute epiglottitis and epiglottic abscess. *Am J Otolaryngol* 24:374–383, 2003.
228. Sobol SE, Zapata S: Epiglottitis and croup. *Otolaryngol Clin North Am* 41:551–566, ix, 2008.
229. Alcaide ML, Bisno AL: Pharyngitis and epiglottitis. *Infect Dis Clin North Am* 21:449–469, 2007.
230. Bowman M, Vanderford V: Acute epiglottitis. *Radiol Technol* 72:275–278, 2001.
231. Katori H, Tsukuda M: Acute epiglottitis: analysis of factors associated with airway intervention. *J Laryngol Otol* 119:967–972, 2005.
232. Loftis L: Acute infectious upper airway obstructions in children. *Semin Pediatr Infect Dis* 17:5–10, 2006.
233. Rotta AT: Wiryawan B: Respiratory emergencies in children. *Respir Care* 48:248–258, discussion 58–60, 2003.
234. Cystic Fibrosis Foundation: *Patient Registry 2012 annual data report*, Bethesda, MD, 2013, Cystic Fibrosis Foundation.
235. Hamosh A, FitzSimmons SC, Macek M, Jr, et al: Comparison of the clinical manifestations of cystic fibrosis in black and white patients. *J Pediatr* 132:255–259, 1998.
236. Anderson MP, Gregory RJ, Thompson S, et al: Demonstration that CFTR is a chloride channel by alteration of its anion selectivity. *Science* 253:202–205, 1991.
237. Boyle MP, Boeck KD: A new era in the treatment of cystic fibrosis: correction of the underlying CFTR defect. *Lancet Respir Med* 1:158–163, 2013.
238. Boucher RC: Cystic fibrosis: a disease of vulnerability to airway surface dehydration. *Trends Mol Med* 13:231–240, 2007.
239. Cystic Fibrosis Mutation Database. <http://www.genet.sickkids.on.ca/cftr/StatisticsPage.html>, (Accessed 15 October 2007.)
240. Paranjape SM, Mogayzel PJ, Jr: Cystic fibrosis. *Pediatr Rev* 35:194–205, 2014.
241. Kerem E, Reisman J, Corey M, et al: Prediction of mortality in patients with cystic fibrosis. *N Engl J Med* 326:1187–1191, 1992.
242. Emerson J, Rosenfeld M, McNamara S, et al: *Pseudomonas aeruginosa* and other predictors of mortality and morbidity in young children with cystic fibrosis. *Pediatr Pulmonol* 34:91–100, 2002.
243. Courtney JM, Dunbar KEA, McDowell A, et al: Clinical outcome of *Burkholderia cepacia* complex infection in cystic fibrosis adults. *J Cyst Fibros* 3:93–98, 2004.
244. Ren CL, Morgan WJ, Konstan MW, et al: Presence of methicillin resistant *Staphylococcus aureus* in respiratory cultures from cystic fibrosis patients is associated with lower lung function. *Pediatr Pulmonol* 42:513–518, 2007.
245. Saiman L, Siegel JD, LiPuma JJ, et al: Infection prevention and control guideline for cystic fibrosis: 2013 update. *Infect Control Hosp Epidemiol* 35(Suppl 1):S1–S67, 2014.
246. Lapey A, Kattwinkel J, Di Sant'Agnese PA, et al: Steatorrhea and azotorrhea and their relation to growth and nutrition in adolescents and young adults with cystic fibrosis. *J Pediatr* 84:328–334, 1974.
247. FitzSimmons SC: The changing epidemiology of cystic fibrosis. *Curr Probl Pediatr* 24:171–179, 1994.
248. Kulczycki LL, Shwachman H: Studies in cystic fibrosis of the pancreas: occurrence of rectal prolapse. *N Engl J Med* 259:409–412, 1958.
249. Atlas AB, Orenstein SR, Orenstein DM: Pancreatitis in young children with cystic fibrosis. *J Pediatr* 120:756–759, 1992.
250. Valman HB, France NE, Wallis PG: Prolonged neonatal jaundice in cystic fibrosis. *Arch Dis Child* 46:805–809, 1971.
251. Scott-Jupp R, Lama M, Tanner MS: Prevalence of liver disease in cystic fibrosis. *Arch Dis Child* 66:698–701, 1992.
252. Kaplan E, Shwachman H, Perlmutter AD, et al: Reproductive failure in males with cystic fibrosis. *N Engl J Med* 279:65–69, 1968.
253. Johannesson M, Gottlieb C, Hjelte L: Delayed puberty in girls with cystic fibrosis despite good clinical status. *Pediatrics* 99:29–34, 1997.
254. Ahmad A, Ahmed A, Patrizio P: Cystic fibrosis and fertility. *Curr Opin Obstet Gynecol* 25:167–172, 2012.
255. Quinton PM, Bijman J: Higher bioelectric potentials due to decreased chloride absorption in the sweat glands of patients with cystic fibrosis. *N Engl J Med* 308:1185–1189, 1983.
256. Arvanitakis SN, Lobeck CC: Metabolic alkalosis and salt depletion in cystic fibrosis. *J Pediatr* 82:535–536, 1973.
257. Gibson LE, Cooke RE: A test for concentration of electrolytes in sweat in cystic fibrosis of the pancreas utilizing pilocarpine by iontophoresis. *Pediatrics* 23:545–549, 1959.

258. Farrell PM, Rosenstein BJ, White TB, et al: Guidelines for diagnosis of cystic fibrosis in newborns through older adults: Cystic Fibrosis Foundation consensus report. *J Pediatr* 153:S4–S14, 2008.
259. Borowitz D, Robinson KA, Rosenfeld M, et al: Cystic Fibrosis Foundation evidence-based guidelines for management of infants with cystic fibrosis. *J Pediatr* 155(6 Suppl):S73–S93, 2009.
260. Flume PA, Robinson KA, O'Sullivan BP, et al: Cystic fibrosis pulmonary guidelines: airway clearance therapies. *Respir Care* 54:522–537, 2009.
261. Fuchs HJ, Borowitz DS, Christiansen DH, et al: Effect of aerosolized recombinant human DNase on exacerbations of respiratory symptoms and on pulmonary function in patients with cystic fibrosis. The Pulmozyme Study Group. *N Engl J Med* 331:637–642, 1994.
262. Furuya ME, Lezana-Fernandez JL, Vargas MH, et al: Efficacy of human recombinant DNase in pediatric patients with cystic fibrosis. *Arch Med Res* 32:30–34, 2001. 2001/04/03.
263. Mogayzel PJ, Jr, Naureckas ET, Robinson KA, et al: Cystic fibrosis pulmonary guidelines: chronic medications for maintenance of lung health. *Am J Respir Crit Care Med* 187:680–689, 2013.
264. Elkins MR, Robinson M, Rose BR, et al: A controlled trial of long-term inhaled hypertonic saline in patients with cystic fibrosis. *N Engl J Med* 354:229–240, 2006.
265. Ramsey BW, Pepe MS, Quan JM, et al: Intermittent administration of inhaled tobramycin in patients with cystic fibrosis. Cystic Fibrosis Inhaled Tobramycin Study Group. *N Engl J Med* 340:23–30, 1999.
266. McCoy KS, Quittner AL, Oermann CM, et al: Inhaled aztreonam lysine for chronic airway *Pseudomonas aeruginosa* in cystic fibrosis. *Am J Respir Crit Care Med* 178:921–928, 2008.
267. Yu H, Burton B, Huang CJ, et al: Ivacaftor potentiation of multiple CFTR channels with gating mutations. *J Cyst Fibros* 11:237–245, 2012.
268. Davis PB: Cystic fibrosis since 1938. *Am J Respir Crit Care Med* 173:475–482, 2006.

SECTION V

BASIC THERAPEUTICS

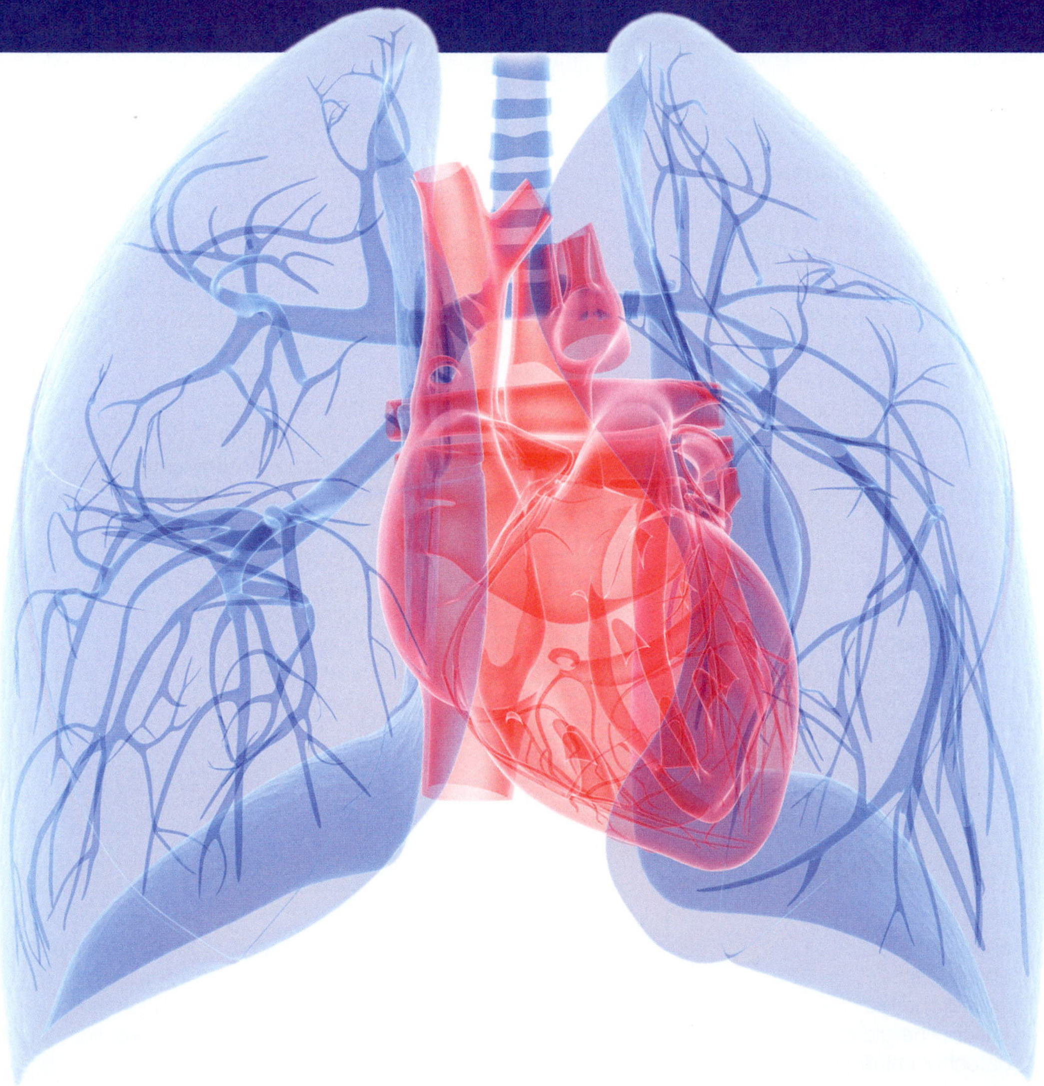

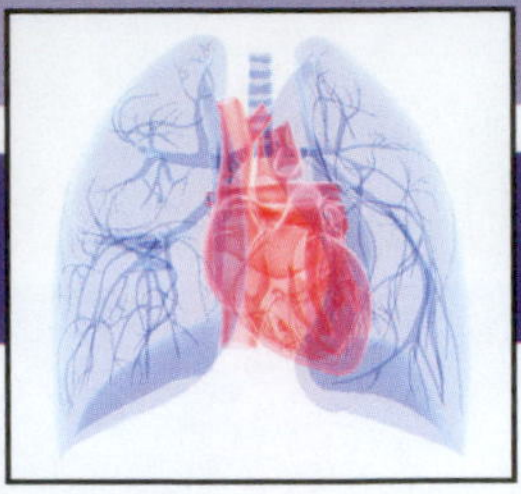

CHAPTER 35

Airway Pharmacology

DOUGLAS S. GARDENHIRE

CHAPTER OBJECTIVES

After reading this chapter you will be able to:

- Analyze three phases that constitute the course of drug action from dose to effect.
- Describe classes of drugs that are delivered via the aerosol route.
- Compare mode of action, indications, and adverse effects that characterize each major class of aerosolized drug.
- Compare available aerosol formulations, brand names, and dosages for each specific drug class.
- Select the appropriate drug class for a specific patient or clinical situation.
- Assess the outcomes for each class of aerosol drug therapy.

CHAPTER OUTLINE

Principles of Pharmacology
- Drug Administration Phase
- Pharmacokinetic Phase
- Pharmacodynamic Phase
- Airway Receptors and Neural Control of the Lung

Adrenergic Bronchodilators
- Indications for Use
- Mode of Action and Effects
- Adrenergic Bronchodilator Agents
- Adverse Effects
- Assessment of Bronchodilator Therapy

Anticholinergic Bronchodilators
- Indications for Use
- Mode of Action
- Adverse Effects
- Assessment

Mucus-Controlling Agents
- *N*-Acetyl Cysteine
- Dornase Alfa
- Other Mucoactive Agents
- Assessment of Mucoactive Drug Therapy

Inhaled Corticosteroids
- Indications and Purposes
- Mode of Action
- Adverse Effects
- Special Considerations
- Assessment of Drug Therapy

Nonsteroidal Antiasthma Drugs
- Indication for Use
- Mode of Action
- Adverse Effects
- Assessment of Drug Therapy

Aerosolized Antiinfective Agents
- Pentamidine Isethionate
- Ribavirin
- Inhaled Tobramycin
- Inhaled Aztreonam
- Colistimethate Sodium
- Inhaled Zanamivir

Inhaled Pulmonary Vasodilators
- Nitric Oxide
- Iloprost
- Treprostinil

KEY TERMS

adrenergic
agonists
antagonists
antiadrenergic
anticholinergic
catecholamine
cholinergic
drug signaling
L/T ratio
leukotriene
muscarinic
neutropenia
pharmacodynamic phase
pharmacokinetic phase
prodrug
tachyphylaxis
vasopressor

The primary focus of respiratory care pharmacology is the delivery of inhaled aerosols to the respiratory tract for the diagnosis and treatment of pulmonary diseases. Although other drug classes are used in respiratory care, discussion in this chapter is limited to bronchoactive inhaled aerosols. Other drug classes are discussed in pharmacology texts.[1,2]

PRINCIPLES OF PHARMACOLOGY

The course of drug action from dose to effect comprises three phases: *drug administration, pharmacokinetic,* and *pharmacodynamic phases.* These three phases of drug action can be applied to drug treatment of the respiratory tract with inhaled agents.

Drug Administration Phase

The drug administration phase describes the method by which a drug dose is made available to the body. Administering drugs directly to the respiratory tract uses the inhalation route, and the dose form is an aerosol of liquid solutions, suspensions, or dry powders. The most commonly used devices to administer orally or nasally inhaled aerosols are the metered dose inhaler (MDI), the soft-mist inhaler Respimat, the small volume nebulizer (SVN), and the dry powder inhaler (DPI). Reservoir devices, including holding chambers with one-way inspiratory valves and simple, nonvalved spacer devices, are often added to MDIs to reduce the need for complex hand-breathing coordination and to reduce oropharyngeal impaction of the aerosol drug (see Chapter 39).

The advantages of treatment of the respiratory tract with inhaled aerosols are as follows:

- Aerosol doses are usually smaller than doses for systemic administration.
- Onset of drug action is rapid.
- Delivery is targeted to the organ requiring treatment.
- Systemic side effects are often fewer and less severe.

Disadvantages of the delivery of inhaled aerosols in treating respiratory disease include the number of variables affecting the delivered dose and lack of adequate knowledge of device performance and use among patients and caregivers.[3]

Pharmacokinetic Phase

The **pharmacokinetic phase** of drug action describes the time course and disposition of a drug in the body based on its absorption, distribution, metabolism, and elimination. Inhaled aerosols are intended for local effects in the airway. Undesired systemic effects result from absorption and distribution throughout the body.

An inhaled aerosol distributes to the lung by inhalation and the stomach through swallowing of drug that deposits in the oropharynx. The therapeutic effect of the aerosol drug is caused by the portion in the airway, whereas systemic effects are due to absorption of the drug from the airway and gastrointestinal (GI) tract. The ideal aerosol would distribute only to the airway, with none reaching the stomach. The ratio of lung availability to total systemic availability (**L/T ratio**) quantifies the efficiency of aerosol delivery to the lung:

$$\text{L/T ratio} = \text{Lung availability}/(\text{Lung} + \text{GI availability})$$

This concept, proposed by Borgström[4] and elaborated by Thorsson,[5] is illustrated in Figure 35-1, showing delivery of albuterol by inhalation using an MDI and a DPI.

Pharmacodynamic Phase

The **pharmacodynamic phase** describes the mechanisms of drug action by which a drug molecule causes its effects in the body. Drug effects are caused by the combination of a drug with a matching receptor. **Drug signaling** mechanisms include the following:

Signaling Mechanism	Example
Mediation by G protein (guanine nucleotide)–linked receptors	Beta-adrenergic agonists, antimuscarinic agents
Attachment to intracellular receptors by lipid-soluble drugs	Corticosteroids

The mechanisms of drug action are briefly described for each class of bronchoactive drug.

Airway Receptors and Neural Control of the Lung

Pharmacologic control of the airway is mediated by receptors found on airway smooth muscle, secretory cells, bronchial epithelium, and pulmonary and bronchial blood vessels. There are *sympathetic (adrenergic)* and *parasympathetic (cholinergic)* receptors in the lung. The terminology for drugs acting on these receptors is based on the usual neurotransmitter that acts on the receptor. The usual neurotransmitter in the sympathetic system is norepinephrine, which is similar to epinephrine. The usual neurotransmitter in the parasympathetic system is acetylcholine. The receptors responding to these neurotransmitters are termed *adrenergic* and *cholinergic.* **Agonists** (stimulating agents) and **antagonists** (blocking agents) that act on these receptors are given the following classifications:

- **Adrenergic** (adrenomimetic): Drug that stimulates a receptor responding to norepinephrine or epinephrine
- **Antiadrenergic:** Drug that blocks a receptor for norepinephrine or epinephrine
- **Cholinergic** (cholinomimetic): Drug that stimulates a receptor for acetylcholine
- **Anticholinergic:** Drug that blocks a receptor for acetylcholine
- **Muscarinic:** Drug that stimulates acetylcholine receptors specifically at parasympathetic nerve–ending sites

Because cholinergic receptors exist at autonomic ganglia and at the myoneural junction in skeletal muscle, the terms *muscarinic* and *antimuscarinic* distinguish cholinergic agents whose action is limited to parasympathetic sites. Neostigmine is a cholinergic (indirect-acting) drug that increases receptor stimulation at both the myoneural junction and the parasympathetic sites. By contrast, atropine is an antimuscarinic agent that blocks the action of acetylcholine only at the parasympathetic sites. Table 35-1 summarizes receptors and their effects for the cardiopulmonary system. A more detailed description of the

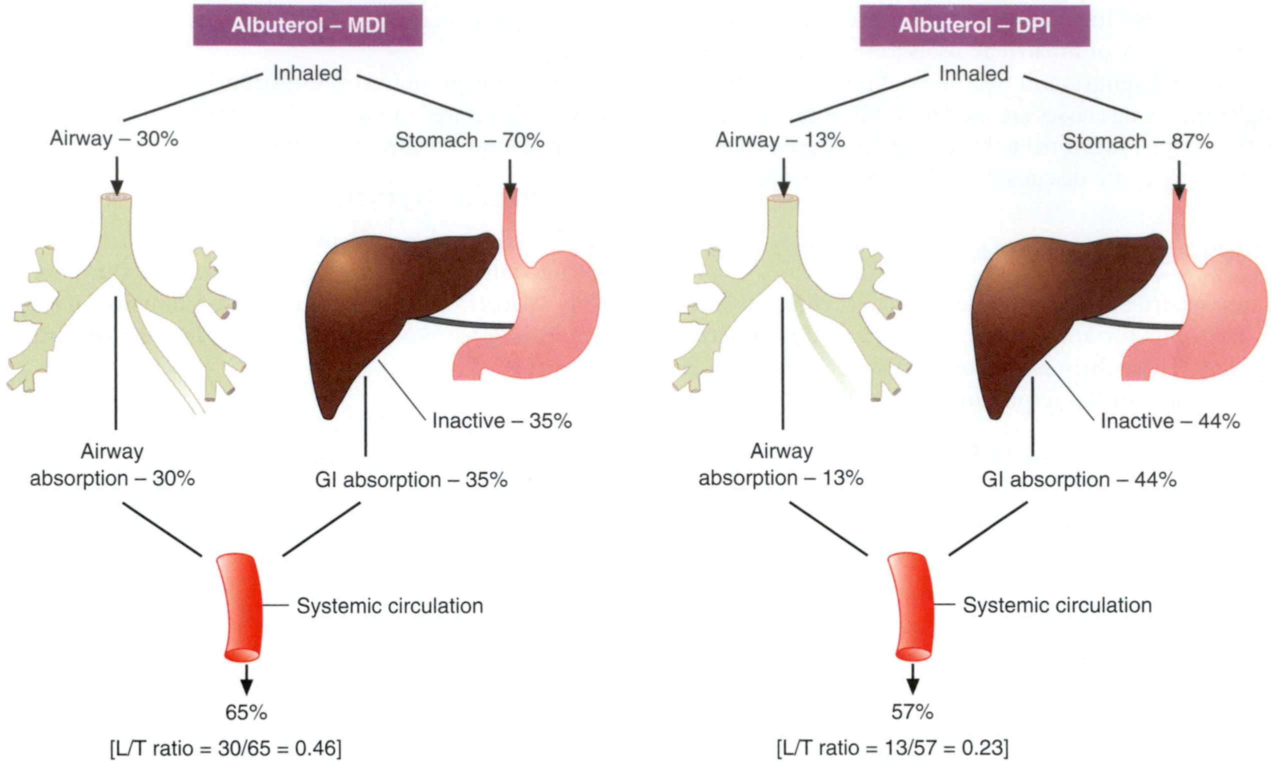

FIGURE 35-1 Comparison of efficiency of aerosol delivery with MDI and DPI using the L/T availability ratio. *L/T,* Ratio of lung availability to total systemic availability. (From Gardenhire DS: Rau's respiratory care pharmacology, ed 9, St. Louis, 2016, Elsevier.)

TABLE 35-1
Airway Receptors and Their Effects in the Cardiopulmonary System*

Location	Receptor	Effect
Heart	Beta-1-adrenergic	Increased rate, force
	M_2-cholinergic	Decreased rate
Bronchiolar smooth muscle	Beta-2-adrenergic	Bronchodilation
	M_3-cholinergic	Bronchoconstriction
Pulmonary blood vessels	Alpha-1-adrenergic	Vasoconstriction
	Beta-2-adrenergic	Vasodilation
	M_3-cholinergic	Vasodilation
Bronchial blood vessels	Alpha-1-adrenergic	Vasoconstriction
	Beta-2-adrenergic	Vasodilation
Submucosal glands	Alpha-1-adrenergic	Increased fluid, mucin
	Beta-2-adrenergic	Increased fluid, mucin
	M_3-cholinergic	Exocytosis, secretion

M_2, M_3, Subtypes of muscarinic *(M)* cholinergic receptors.
*Adrenergic and muscarinic cholinergic receptor subtypes are indicated.

autonomic nervous system and receptor subtypes is provided by Katzung and colleagues.[2]

ADRENERGIC BRONCHODILATORS

Adrenergic bronchodilators represent the largest group of drugs among the aerosolized agents used for oral inhalation. Table 35-2 lists bronchodilators in this group, with their aerosol formulations, selected brand names, and dosages.

Indications for Use

The general indication for use of an adrenergic bronchodilator is the presence of reversible airflow obstruction. The most common use of these agents clinically is to improve flow rates in asthma (including exercise-induced asthma), acute and chronic bronchitis, emphysema, bronchiectasis, cystic fibrosis (CF), and other obstructive airway states.

Indication for Short-Acting Agents

Short-acting beta-2 agonists (SABAs), such as albuterol and levalbuterol, are indicated for relief of acute reversible airflow obstruction in asthma or other obstructive airway diseases. Short-acting agents are termed *rescue agents* in the 2007 National Asthma Education and Prevention Program Expert Panel III (NAEPP EPR III) guidelines.[6]

Indication for Long-Acting Agents

Long-acting beta agonists (LABAs), such as salmeterol, formoterol, arformoterol, indacaterol, and olodaterol are indicated for maintenance bronchodilation and control of bronchospasm and nocturnal symptoms in asthma or other obstructive diseases, such as chronic obstructive pulmonary disease (COPD). NAEPP EPR III guidelines consider LABAs a *controller;* its slower time to peak effect makes it a poor rescue drug. In

TABLE 35-2
Adrenergic Bronchodilator Agents Available in the United States

Drug	Brand Name	Receptor Preference	Adult Dosage	Time Course (Onset, Peak, Duration)
Ultra-Short-Acting Adrenergic Bronchodilator Agents				
Racemic epinephrine	Asthmanefrin*	Alpha, beta	SVN: 2.25% solution, 0.25-0.5 ml (5.63-11.25 mg) 4 times daily	*Onset:* 3-5 min *Peak:* 5-20 min *Duration:* 0.5-2 hr
Short-Acting Adrenergic Bronchodilator Agents				
Metaproterenol	Alupent	Beta-2	SVN: 0.4%, 0.6% solution, tid, qid Tab: 10 mg and 20 mg, tid, qid Syrup: 10 mg per 5 ml	*Onset:* 1-5 min *Peak:* 60 min *Duration:* 2-6 hr
Albuterol	Proventil HFA999, Ventolin HFA, ProAir HFA, AccuNeb, VoSpire ER	Beta-2	SVN: 0.5% solution, 0.5 ml (2.5 mg), 0.63 mg, 1.25 mg and 2.5 mg unit dose, tid, qid MDI: 90 µg/puff, 2 puffs tid, qid Tab: 2 mg, 4 mg, and 8 mg, bid, tid, qid Syrup: 2 mg/5 ml, 1-2 tsp tid, qid	*Onset:* 15 min *Peak:* 30-60 min *Duration:* 5-12 hr
Levalbuterol	Xopenex, Xopenex HFA	Beta-2	SVN: 0.31 mg/3 ml 3 times daily, 0.63 mg/3 ml 3 times daily, or 1.25 mg/3 ml 3 times daily, concentrate 1.25 mg/0.5 ml, 3 times daily MDI: 45 µg/puff, 2 puffs every 4-6 hr	*Onset:* 15 min *Peak:* 30-60 min *Duration:* 5-8 hr
Long-Acting Adrenergic Bronchodilator Agents				
Salmeterol	Serevent Diskus	Beta-2	DPI: 50 µg/blister twice daily	*Onset:* 20 min *Peak:* 3-5 hr *Duration:* 12 hr
Formoterol	Perforomist, Foradil	Beta-2	SVN: 20 µg/2 ml unit dose, bid DPI: 12 µg/inhalation, bid	*Onset:* 15 min *Peak:* 30-60 min *Duration:* 12 hr
Arformoterol	Brovana	Beta-2	SVN: 15 µg/2 ml unit dose, twice daily	*Onset:* 15 min *Peak:* 30-60 min *Duration:* 12 hr
Indacaterol	Arcapta Neohaler	Beta-2	DPI: 75 µg/inhalation, once daily	*Onset:* 5 min *Peak:* 30 min *Duration:* 24 hr
Olodaterol	Stiverdi Respimat	Beta-2	SMI: 2.5 µg/actuation, 2 actuations daily	*Onset:* 15 min *Peak:* 30-60 min *Duration:* 12 hr

DPI, Dry powder inhaler; *MDI,* metered dose inhaler; *SMI,* soft mist inhaler; *SVN,* small volume nebulizer.
*Available over-the-counter.

asthma, a long-acting bronchodilator is usually combined with antiinflammatory medication for control of airway inflammation and bronchospasm. Although some LABAs have a rapid onset and peak effect similar or better than that of albuterol, its prolonged activity makes it a better maintenance drug compared with an acute reliever or rescue agent.

Indication for Racemic Epinephrine

Racemic epinephrine is often used by inhaled aerosol or direct lung instillation for its strong vasoconstricting effect to reduce airway swelling after extubation or during epiglottitis, croup, or to control airway bleeding during endoscopy.

Mode of Action and Effects

Adrenergic bronchodilators can stimulate one or more of the following receptors, with the effects described:

- *Alpha-receptor stimulation:* Causes vasoconstriction and a **vasopressor** effect (increased blood pressure)
- *Beta-1-receptor stimulation:* Causes increased heart rate and myocardial contractility
- *Beta-2-receptor stimulation:* Relaxes bronchial smooth muscle, stimulates mucociliary activity, and has some inhibitory action on inflammatory mediator release

Bronchodilation, through stimulation of beta-2 receptors, is the desired therapeutic effect. Both alpha-adrenergic and beta-adrenergic receptors are G protein–linked receptors. Figure 35-2 illustrates the mode of action for relaxation of airway smooth muscle when a beta-2 receptor is stimulated. The nature of the beta receptor and its activity is presented in more detail by Chung and colleagues.[7]

Adrenergic Bronchodilator Agents

Adrenergic bronchodilator agents represent the evolution of a drug class. Although all of these agents are adrenergic agonists, the differences among individual agents are due to their receptor preference (alpha-adrenergic, beta-1-adrenergic,

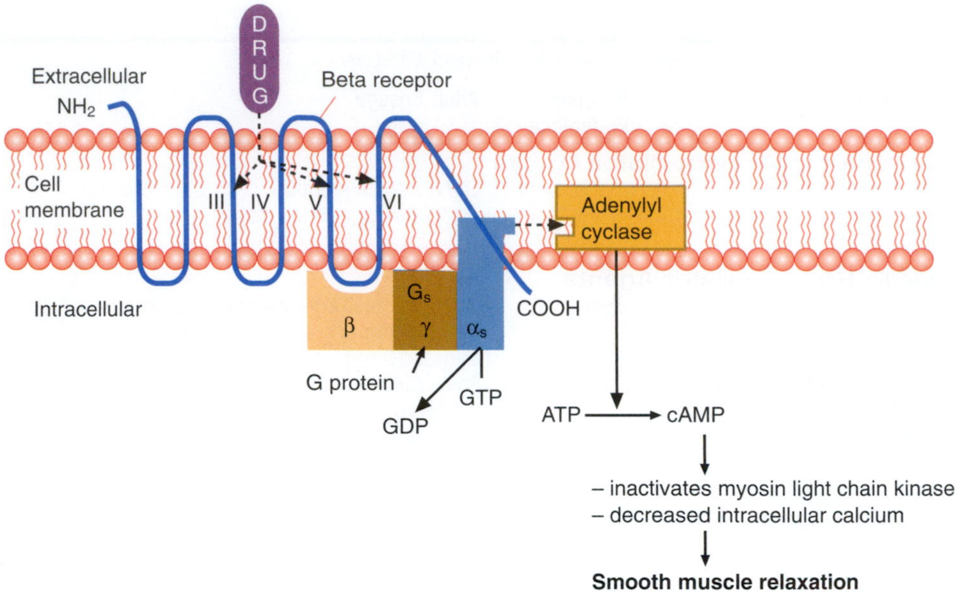

FIGURE 35-2 Mode of action by which a beta agonist stimulates the G protein–linked beta receptor to cause smooth muscle relaxation. Adrenergic agonists, such as albuterol or epinephrine, attach to beta receptors, which are polypeptide chains traversing the cell membrane seven times. This causes activation of the stimulatory G protein, designated G_S, linked to the receptor. When stimulated, the receptor undergoes a conformational change, and the alpha subunit of the G protein attaches to adenyl cyclase. Activation of adenyl cyclase by the G_S protein causes an increased synthesis of the second messenger, cyclic adenosine monophosphate (cAMP). This ultimately causes smooth muscle relaxation and bronchodilation. *ATP,* Adenosine triphosphate; *COOH,* carboxy terminus; *GDP,* guanosine diphosphate; *GTP,* guanosine triphosphate. (From Gardenhire DS: Rau's respiratory care pharmacology, ed 9, St. Louis, 2016, Elsevier.)

beta-2-adrenergic) and their different pharmacokinetics, as listed in Table 35-2. These differences determine the clinical application of individual agents. The adrenergic bronchodilators form three subgroups.

Ultra-Short-Acting Catecholamines

The older agent racemic epinephrine is a **catecholamine.** This agent lacks beta-2 specificity. As a result, cardiac effects, especially tachycardia and increased blood pressure, are common. Catecholamines are metabolized by the enzyme catechol *O*-methyltransferase, which causes a short duration of action. Because of a strong alpha-1 activity and vasoconstricting effect, racemic epinephrine is used to reduce swelling in the nose (nasal decongestant) and larynx (croup, epiglottitis) and to control bleeding during bronchoscopic biopsy.

Short-Acting Noncatecholamine Agents

Because of their short duration of action and lack of beta-2 specificity, catecholamines were replaced with longer acting, beta-2-specific agents, including metaproterenol, albuterol, and levalbuterol. Because their duration of action averages 4 to 6 hours, these drugs are better bronchodilating agents than catecholamines and can be taken on a four-times-daily schedule. However, their modest duration of action results in loss of bronchodilating effect overnight.

Single-Isomer Beta Agonists. Levalbuterol is approved as a single-isomer beta-2-selective agonist. Previous inhaled formulations of adrenergic bronchodilators all were synthetic racemic mixtures, containing both the (*R*)-isomer and the (*S*)-isomer in equal amounts. Levalbuterol is the pure (*R*)-isomer of racemic albuterol. Both stereoisomers of albuterol are shown in Figure 35-3 with the single-isomer (*R*-isomer) form of levalbuterol. Although the (*S*)-isomer is physiologically inactive on adrenergic receptors, there is evidence that the (*S*)-isomer is not completely inactive. Box 35-1 lists some of the physiologic effects of (*S*)-albuterol noted in the literature.[8-14] The effects antagonize the bronchodilating effects of the (*R*)-isomer and promote bronchoconstriction. In addition, the (*S*)-isomer is more slowly metabolized than the (*R*)-isomer.

Box 35-1 Effects and Characteristics of (*S*)-Isomer of Albuterol

- Increases intracellular calcium concentration in vitro[8]
- Activity is blocked by the anticholinergic atropine[8]
- Does not produce pulmonary or extrapulmonary beta-2–mediated effects[9]
- Enhances experimental airway responsiveness in vitro[10]
- Increases contractile response of bronchial tissue to histamine or leukotriene C_4 in vitro[11]
- Enhances eosinophil superoxide production with interleukin-5 stimulation[12]
- Slower metabolism than *(R)*-albuterol in vivo[13]
- Preferential retention in the lung when inhaled by MDI (in vivo)[14]

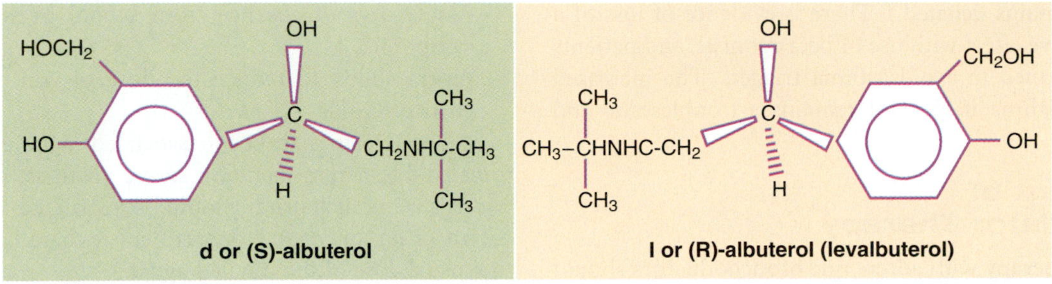

FIGURE 35-3 *(R)*- and *(S)*-isomers of racemic albuterol. Levalbuterol is the single, *(R)*-isomer form of racemic albuterol and contains no *(S)*-isomer.

Levalbuterol is available in many strengths and formulas that can be found in Table 35-2. Side effects of tremor and heart rate changes were less with the single-isomer formulation.[15] The 1.25-mg dose showed a higher peak effect on forced expiratory volume in 1 second (FEV_1) with an 8-hour duration compared with racemic albuterol. Side effects with this dose were equivalent to the side effects seen with racemic albuterol. An equivalent clinical response was seen with one-fourth of the racemic dose (0.63 mg) using the pure isomer, although the racemic mixture contains 1.25 mg of the *(R)*-isomer (half of the total 2.5-mg dose).

Long-Acting Adrenergic Bronchodilators

The release of salmeterol offered the first LABA in the United States. In contrast to previous agents, the duration of action of salmeterol is approximately 12 hours. The pharmacokinetics of salmeterol makes it suitable for maintenance therapy, in particular, with nocturnal asthma. However, it should not be used for relief of acute airflow obstruction or bronchospasm because its onset is longer than 20 minutes, with a peak effect occurring by 3 to 5 hours. Although this agent is a beta-2 agonist, its exact mode of action differs from previous beta-2 agonists, allowing persistent receptor stimulation over a prolonged period of hours.

Formoterol has a duration of effect of approximately 12 hours, but in contrast to salmeterol, the onset of action and peak effect of formoterol are rapid and similar to those of albuterol.[16] Formoterol should not be used as a rescue inhaler. As with salmeterol, the extensive side chain or tail makes formoterol more lipophilic than shorter acting bronchodilators and is the basis for its longer duration of effect.

Arformoterol, the single *(R)*-isomer of formoterol is available as a 2-ml unit dose vial inhalation solution delivering 15 mcg per dose. The recommended dosage is 1 unit dose twice daily. Arformoterol is indicated for the maintenance of bronchospasm in COPD, including chronic bronchitis and emphysema.

Indacaterol (Arcapta Neohaler) a novel once-daily therapy, LABA has been used mainly to treat asthma; however, in the United States it is indicated only in the treatment of COPD. Indacaterol is similar to formoterol, with a quick onset; however, it is even faster—with onset at approximately 5 minutes and a duration of 24 hours.[17] Indacaterol is also being studied in combination with tiotropium bromide with successful preliminary outcomes.[1]

Olodaterol is an ultra-long-acting beta agonist for once-daily treatment of COPD. Olodaterol has a quick onset similar to that of formoterol and indacaterol, with a change in FEV_1 at approximately 5 minutes.[18] Currently, olodaterol is not approved for asthma; however, it has been shown to be effective as monotherapy and in combination with tiotropium.[19]

Vilanterol is an ultra-long-acting beta agonist that is available in fixed combinations with fluticasone (Breo Ellipta) and umeclidinium (Anoro Ellipta). Vilanterol in not available as monotherapy, but has been studied with effective results in COPD.[20]

Adverse Effects

Older adrenergic agents, such as isoproterenol, commonly caused tachycardia, palpitations, and an "adrenaline effect" of shakiness and nervousness. Newer, more beta-2-selective agents are safer and typically cause tremor as the main side effect. Other common side effects with the inhaled agents include headache, insomnia, and nervousness. Patients should be reassured that some tolerance to these effects does occur. Potential adverse effects with use of adrenergic bronchodilators include the following:

- Dizziness
- Hypokalemia
- Loss of bronchoprotection
- Nausea
- Tolerance (**tachyphylaxis**)
- Worsening ventilation/perfusion ($\dot{V}/\dot{Q}$) ratio (decrease in PaO_2/SpO_2)

Inhalation results in fewer and less severe side effects than oral administration. Although tolerance develops to the bronchodilating effect, this is not a contraindication to use of the drugs, and relaxation of airway smooth muscle still occurs. Desaturation resulting from mismatching of $\dot{V}/\dot{Q}$ with inhalation of the aerosol is not clinically significant and reverses quickly. The implication of beta-2-adrenergic agonists in deaths from asthma—termed the *asthma paradox* or the *beta agonist controversy*—remains debated.[21] There is evidence of loss of a bronchoprotective effect with use of beta agonists, and patients should be cautioned to avoid asthma triggers. The increased prevalence of asthma in general remains a troublesome and unresolved issue.

Assessment of Bronchodilator Therapy

Assessment of therapy with adrenergic bronchodilators should be based on the indication for the aerosol agent (presence of reversible airflow obstruction owing to primary bronchospasm or other obstruction secondary to an inflammatory response or secretions, either acute or chronic). Basic vital signs (respiratory rate and pattern, pulse, breath sounds) should be assessed before and after treatment, especially for initial drug use, and the patient's subjective reaction (complaints of breathing difficulty). Patients should be instructed in the correct use of the aerosol device, with verification of correct use. Finally, the patient's subjective reaction to the treatment should be monitored for any change in breathing effort. This assessment applies to all subsequent drug groups by aerosol and is not repeated for each class. The following specific actions are suggested to evaluate patient response to this class of drugs:

- Monitor flow rates using bedside peak flowmeters, portable spirometry, or laboratory reports of pulmonary function before and after bronchodilator studies to assess reversibility of airflow obstruction.
- Assess arterial blood gases (ABGs) or pulse oximetry saturation, as needed, for acute states with asthma or COPD to monitor changes in gas exchange.
- Beta agonists increase blood glucose and decrease K^+ if using high doses, such as with continuous nebulization or emergency department treatments.
- In the long term, monitor pulmonary function studies of lung volumes, capacities, and flows.
- Instruct asthmatic patients in the use and interpretation of disposable peak flowmeters to assess severity of asthmatic episodes and provide an action plan for treatment modification.
- Emphasize in patient education that beta agonists do not treat underlying inflammation and do not prevent progression of asthma and that additional antiinflammatory treatment or more aggressive medical therapy may be needed if there is a poor response to the rescue beta agonist.
- Instruct and then verify correct use of aerosol delivery device (SVN, MDI, reservoir, Respimat, DPI).
- Instruct patients in use, assembly, and cleaning of aerosol inhalation devices.

The following actions are suggested to evaluate patient response to long-acting beta agonists:

- Assess ongoing lung function, including predose FEV_1 over time and variability in peak expiratory flows.
- Assess amount of rescue beta agonist use and nocturnal symptoms.
- Assess number of exacerbations, unscheduled clinic visits, and hospitalizations.
- Assess days of absence from school or work because of symptoms.
- Assess ability to reduce the dose of concomitant inhaled corticosteroids.

Note: Death has been associated with excessive use of inhaled adrenergic agents in severe acute asthma crises. Individuals using such drugs should be instructed to contact a physician or an emergency department if there is no response to the usual dose of the inhaled agent.

Because of the ongoing safety concerns of long-acting beta-2 agonists, the U.S. Food and Drug Administration (FDA) is requiring changes on how long-acting beta-2 agonists are used in the treatment of asthma. The FDA suggests that if a LABA is used, it should be done in conjunction with a corticosteroid. Once the asthma episode has improved, the LABA should be discontinued. If a child needs a LABA it is preferred that a combination product (with a corticosteroid) be used to increase adherence.

MINI CLINI

Assessing Beta-Agonist Side Effects

PROBLEM: The respiratory therapist (RT) has administered an aerosol treatment of albuterol using an MDI with a holding chamber to a 67-year-old patient with newly diagnosed COPD who was admitted for an acute exacerbation and shortness of breath. When the RT returns for the second treatment that day, the patient informs the RT that he began to feel very shaky and nervous, beginning about 30 minutes after the previous treatment. He also noticed a tremor when he held his water cup and took a drink. His pulse during the earlier treatment was 84 beats/min. Clinical assessment shows that he is coherent, has good color, is not diaphoretic, and is in no respiratory distress. His respiratory rate is 16 breaths/min and regular, and his pulse is 82 beats/min and regular. Auscultation reveals mild wheezing and scattered rhonchi, with little change from earlier breath sounds. A mild tremor is apparent when he holds his hand out. On questioning, he states that he is now feeling better, and the "shakiness" has subsided a bit.

DISCUSSION: This patient's situation exemplifies a common reaction to inhaled adrenergic bronchodilators. Although albuterol is beta-2 preferential, it is still an epinephrine-like drug and can produce side effects secondary to sympathetic stimulation. The description of the symptoms is suggestive of common adrenergic side effects (tremor, shakiness). The timing of the symptoms coincides with the pharmacokinetics of albuterol (peak effect in 30 to 60 minutes). As presented in the case description, it is important to rule out other complications. The physical examination shows no changes from the earlier treatment in his vital signs.

It is important to caution patients about "normal" expected side effects and to reassure them that the side effects decrease with tolerance to the medication. In addition, the RT needs to be alert to the possibility that patients may have deteriorated or changed their respiratory status.

RULE OF THUMB

Choosing an Aerosol Agent

An aerosol agent to treat the respiratory tract is chosen based on the indication for the agent or class of drugs and a corresponding presence of the indication in the patient.

- *Example:* Adrenergic bronchodilator. The indication is presence of reversible airflow obstruction. The patient shows a 20% improvement in FEV_1 on spirometry with use of inhaled albuterol. Choose an adrenergic bronchodilator.
- *Example:* Inhaled corticosteroid. The indication is mild, moderate, or persistent asthma. The patient with asthma reports a need to use a beta-agonist inhaler more than a few days each week and complains of waking up at night with shortness of breath. Choose an inhaled corticosteroid.

ANTICHOLINERGIC BRONCHODILATORS

A second method of producing airway relaxation is through blockade of cholinergic-induced bronchoconstriction. An important difference between beta agonists and anticholinergic bronchodilators is the active stimulatory action of the former versus the passive blockade of the latter. A cholinergic blocking agent is effective only if bronchoconstriction exists secondary to cholinergic activity.

Indications for Use

Table 35-3 lists the dosage, forms, and pharmacokinetics of anticholinergic bronchodilators available in the United States. Generally, anticholinergic agents have been found to be as effective as beta agonists in airflow improvement in COPD but less so in asthma. A nasal formulation of ipratropium is also available for relief of allergic and nonallergic perennial rhinitis, including the common cold.

Indication for Anticholinergic Bronchodilators

Anticholinergic agents are indicated as bronchodilators for maintenance treatment in COPD, including chronic bronchitis and emphysema.

Indication for Combined Anticholinergic and Beta-Agonist Bronchodilators

A combination anticholinergic and beta agonist, such as ipratropium bromide and albuterol (Combivent Respimat; DuoNeb), is indicated for use in patients with COPD receiving regular treatment who require additional bronchodilation for relief of airflow obstruction. Ipratropium bromide is also commonly used in severe asthma in addition to beta agonists, especially in acute bronchoconstriction that does not respond well to beta agonist therapy.

Mode of Action

Anticholinergic or antimuscarinic agents act as a competitive antagonist for acetylcholine at muscarinic receptors on airway

TABLE 35-3

Inhaled Anticholinergic Bronchodilator Agents*

Drug	Brand Name	Adult Dosage	Time Course (Onset, Peak, Duration)
Ipratropium bromide	Atrovent HFA	HFA MDI: 17 µg/puff, 2 puffs 4 times daily SVN: 0.02% solution (0.2 mg/ml), 500 µg 3-4 times daily Nasal spray: 21 µg or 40 µg, 2 sprays per nostril 2-4 times daily (dosage varies)	*Onset:* 15 min *Peak:* 1-2 hr *Duration:* 6 hr
Ipratropium bromide and albuterol	Combivent Respimat DuoNeb	SMI: Ipratropium 20 µg/puff and albuterol 100 µg/puff, 1 inhalation qid SVN: Ipratropium 0.5 mg and albuterol 2.5 mg	*Onset:* 15 min *Peak:* 1-2 hr *Duration:* 6 hr
Aclidinium Bromide	Tudorza Pressair	DPI: 400 µg/inhalation, 1 inhalation bid	*Onset:* 10 min *Peak:* 2 hr *Duration:* 12 hr
Tiotropium bromide	Spiriva	DPI: 18 µg/inhalation, 1 inhalation daily (1 capsule)	*Onset:* 30 min *Peak:* 3 hr *Duration:* 24 hr
Umeclidinium bromide	Incruse Ellipta	DPI: 62.5 µg/inhalation, 1 inhalation daily	*Onset:* 5-15 min *Peak:* 1-3 hr *Duration:* 24 hr
Umeclidinium bromide and vilanterol	Anoro Ellipta	DPI: Umeclidinium 62.5 µg/inhalation and vilanterol 25 µg/inhalation, 1 inhalation daily	*Onset:* 5-15 min *Peak:* 1-3 hr *Duration:* 24 hr

DPI, Dry powder inhaler; *HFA,* hydrofluoroalkane; *MDI,* metered dose inhaler; *SMI,* soft mist inhaler; *SVN,* small volume nebulizer.
*A holding chamber is recommended with MDI administration to prevent accidental eye exposure.

smooth muscle. Part of the airflow obstruction in COPD may be due to vagally mediated, reflex cholinergic stimulation. Airway irritation and inflammation stimulate afferent sensory C-fibers in the airway, which synapse with efferent vagal (cholinergic) fibers to the airway and mucous glands. The muscarinic receptor subtype on smooth muscle and submucosal mucous glands is the M_3 receptor, which is a G protein–linked receptor. The effect of acetylcholine, the usual neurotransmitter, on the muscarinic (M_3) receptors on airway smooth muscle is bronchoconstriction. The M_1 receptor at the ganglionic junction enhances cholinergic nerve transmission. The M_2 receptor is an autoreceptor inhibiting further release of acetylcholine so that blockade can increase acetylcholine release and may offset the bronchodilating effect of antimuscarinics.[22]

All anticholinergic agents have affinity for M_1, M_2, and M_3 receptors; however, the main difference is how slowly they dissociate from the receptor. Ipratropium dissociates much faster; therefore it does not have as long duration. Aclidinium, tiotropium, and umeclidinium dissociate from the M_3 receptor much slower, allowing for a much longer duration.[1] The site of action of anticholinergic agents in reversing cholinergic-induced airflow obstruction is shown in Figure 35-4.

Adverse Effects

Side effects of inhaled anticholinergics usually include the local topical effect of dry mouth, pupillary dilation, lens paralysis, increased intraocular pressure, increased heart rate, urinary retention, and altered mental state. Box 35-2 details the side effects of anticholinergics.

The actual amount of drug delivered should be considered; for example, the nebulizer dose of ipratropium is more than 10 times greater than the MDI dose (500 mcg vs. 34 mcg). If a patient receives approximately 10% of the SVN volume in the lung, a much larger dose is given with an SVN than with an MDI. Although ipratropium is not contraindicated in patients with prostatic hypertrophy, urinary retention, or glaucoma, the drug should be used with caution and adequate evaluation for possible systemic side effects in these patients. The eyes must be protected from drug exposure with aerosol use owing to accidental spraying from an MDI or with nebulizer-mask delivery. There is less chance for eye exposure with the MDI formulation than the SVN solution; a holding chamber is recommended with MDI use.

Box 35-2 Side Effects Seen With Anticholinergic Aerosol Agents*

SVN, MDI, AND DPI (COMMON)
- Cough, dry mouth

MDI (OCCASIONAL)
- Nervousness, irritation, dizziness, headache, palpitation, rash

SVN AND DPI
- Pharyngitis, dyspnea, flulike symptoms, bronchitis, upper respiratory tract infections, nausea, occasional bronchoconstriction, eye pain, urinary retention

Precautions: Use with caution in patients with narrow-angle glaucoma, prostatic hypertrophy, bladder neck obstruction, constipation, bowel obstruction, or tachycardia.

DPI, Dry powder inhaler; *MDI,* metered dose inhaler; *SVN,* small volume nebulizer.

*Side effects were reported in a small percentage (1% to 5%) of patients.

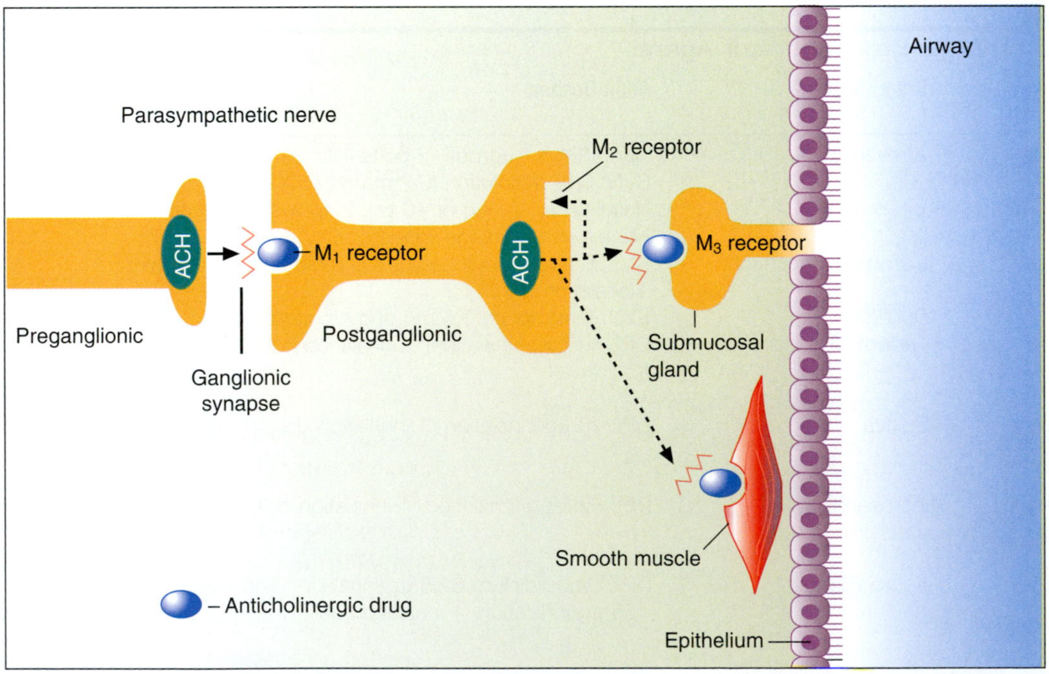

FIGURE 35-4 Mode of action of anticholinergic agents in blocking muscarinic receptors in the airway to inhibit cholinergic-induced bronchoconstriction. *ACH,* Acetylcholine. (From Gardenhire DS: Rau's respiratory care pharmacology, ed 9, St. Louis, 2016, Elsevier.)

TABLE 35-4
Mucoactive Agents Available for Aerosol Administration

Drug	Brand Name	Adult Dosage	Use
N-Acetylcysteine 10% N-Acetylcysteine 20%	Mucomyst	SVN: 3-5 ml	Efficacy has not been demonstrated for any lung disease
Dornase alfa	Pulmozyme	SVN: 2.5 mg/ampule, 1 ampule daily*	CF
Aqueous water, saline		SVN: 3-5 ml, as ordered	Sputum induction
Hyperosmolar 7% saline		SVN: 4 ml	Airway clearance
Hyperosmolar 3% saline		SVN: 4 ml	Infantile bronchiolitis
Mannitol	Bronchitol†	DPI: 400 mg, bid	Airway clearance in CF

CF, Cystic fibrosis; *DPI,* dry power inhaler; *SVN,* small volume nebulizer.
*Nebulizer system recommended (see package insert).
†Orphan designation only.

Assessment

The assessment of bronchodilator therapy with an anticholinergic agent is the same as assessment for adrenergic agents. In addition, preexisting conditions of narrow-angle glaucoma, prostatic hypertrophy, or urinary retention warrant caution with continued evaluation.

MUCUS-CONTROLLING AGENTS

The two agents approved in the United States for oral inhalation with an effect on mucus are *N*-acetyl cysteine (NAC) and dornase alfa. Both agents are mucolytic, although their modes of action differ. Table 35-4 lists these agents, their formulations, dosages, and bland aqueous aerosols. A review by Rubin[23] provides additional detail.

N-Acetyl Cysteine

NAC is the *N*-acetyl derivative of the amino acid L-cysteine and is given by either nebulization or direct tracheal instillation.

Indications for Use

NAC is indicated to reduce accumulation of airway secretions, with concomitant improvement in pulmonary function and gas exchange and prevention of recurrent respiratory infection and airway damage. Diseases of excessive viscous mucous secretions and poor airway clearance include COPD, acute tracheobronchitis, and bronchiectasis. NAC also is used to treat or prevent liver damage that can occur when a patient takes an overdose of acetaminophen.[24] Despite excellent in vitro mucolytic activity and a long history of use, no data clearly demonstrate that oral or aerosolized NAC is effective therapy for treating any lung disease.[25] This situation may be partially due to NAC selectively depolymerizing the essential mucin polymer structure and leaving the pathologic polymers of DNA and F-actin intact in respiratory secretions.[26]

Mode of Action

NAC acts as a classic mucolytic to reduce the viscosity of mucus by substituting its own sulfhydryl group for the disulfide group in mucus, breaking a portion of the bond forming the gel structure.[26] When NAC comes into physical contact with mucus it begins to reduce viscosity and mucolytic activity increases with a higher pH of 7.0 to 9.0.

MINI CLINI

Calculating Drug Doses

PROBLEM: The dose of ipratropium bromide (Atrovent) released from the valve of the MDI is 17 mcg. With a usual dose of two actuations, this would release 34 mcg total. The SVN solution is a vial of 2.5 ml of a 0.02% strength concentration, all of which is placed in the nebulizer. Does the nebulizer dose contain the same amount of drug as the two actuations from the MDI?

DISCUSSION: The amount of drug in milligrams or micrograms can be calculated for the nebulizer solution, using the following formula for percentage strength:

$$\%\,(\text{as decimal}) = \frac{\text{Drug solute (in g)}}{\text{Total solution (in ml)}}$$

$$0.0002 = \frac{x\text{ g}}{2.5\text{ ml}}$$

$$x\text{ g} = 0.0002 \times 2.5\text{ ml} = 0.0005\text{ g}$$

Converting 0.0005 g to milligrams gives 0.5 mg, or 500 mcg. Two actuations of the MDI release 34 mcg, whereas the dose contained in the SVN is 500 mcg (or >10 times more). The lower dose MDI is the reason that additional actuations of four or six are needed if a patient does not obtain relief. The SVN solution also may provide relief by giving a higher dose of the drug.

Side Effects

Several side effects to NAC have led to less use in patients with hypersecretory states. The drug is irritating to the airway and can produce bronchospasm, especially in subjects with asthma and hyperreactive airways. The general effect of airway irritation is counterproductive to reduction of mucus hypersecretion. To reduce the occurrence of bronchospasm, use of the 10% solution, which is less hypertonic than the 20% solution, is recommended. Pretreatment with an adrenergic bronchodilator, allowing adequate time for production of a bronchodilatory effect, can prevent or reduce airway resistance with NAC.

Other side effects that can occur include the following:

- Airway obstruction secondary to rapid liquefaction of secretions
- Disagreeable odor secondary to hydrogen sulfide
- Incompatibility with certain antibiotics (sodium ampicillin, amphotericin B, erythromycin, tetracyclines, and aminoglycosides) if mixed in solution
- Increased concentration and toxicity of nebulizer solution toward end of treatment. It is recommended to dilute with equal volume of sterile water to reduce concentration that may lead to airway irritation
- Nausea and rhinorrhea
- Stomatitis
- Reactivity of acetylcysteine with rubber, copper, iron, and cork

Dornase Alfa

Dornase alfa (Pulmozyme) is a genetically engineered clone of the natural human pancreatic DNase enzyme, which can digest extracellular DNA material. It is a peptide mucolytic and can reduce extracellular DNA and F-actin polymers. It is occasionally referred to as *rhDNase* (recombinant human DNase). It is designated as an orphan drug. Administration and dosage are given in Table 35-4.

Indication for Use

Dornase alfa is indicated in the management of CF to reduce the frequency of respiratory infections requiring parenteral antibiotics and to improve pulmonary function of these patients.[27]

Mode of Action

Dornase alfa is a proteolytic enzyme that can break down the DNA material from neutrophils found in purulent secretions (Figure 35-5). This agent is more effective than acetylcysteine in reducing the viscosity of infected sputum in CF.[28]

Side Effects

In contrast to its predecessor, pancreatic dornase (Dornavac), a natural enzyme obtained from animal preparations, dornase alfa has not been shown to produce antibodies that might cause allergic reactions, including bronchospasm. Common side effects associated with the drug include pharyngitis and voice alteration, laryngitis, rash, chest pain, and conjunctivitis. Other effects are less common but are reported as various respiratory symptoms (cough, dyspnea, pneumothorax, hemoptysis, rhinitis, sinusitis), flu syndrome, GI obstruction, hypoxia, malaise, and weight loss. Contraindications to the drug include hypersensitivity to dornase, Chinese hamster ovary (CHO) cell products, or other components of the drug preparation.

Other Mucoactive Agents

Bland aerosols of water, including distilled water and normotonic, hypertonic, and hypotonic saline, have traditionally been nebulized to improve mobilization of secretions in respiratory disease states. The mucous gel layer is relatively resistant to the addition or removal of water after it is formed. Bland aerosols have been found to increase secretion clearance and sputum production and cause productive coughing.[29] The effect is probably a vagally mediated reflex production of cough and mucus secretion. Bland aerosols are more properly considered expectorants rather than mucolytic agents. Clinicians must be alert to the possibility of bronchospasm with nonisotonic solutions, in particular, in patients with hyperreactive airways.

Inhaled mannitol administered by DPI (Bronchitol) has been approved outside the United States. Studies have shown Bronchitol to be safe and well tolerated in treating patients with CF or bronchiectasis. However, because some children with CF experience bronchial hyperreactivity with inhaled mannitol,[30] it is important to pretreat with a short-acting bronchodilator before use.

Sodium bicarbonate has been aerosolized and directly instilled into the airway in intubated patients to reduce the

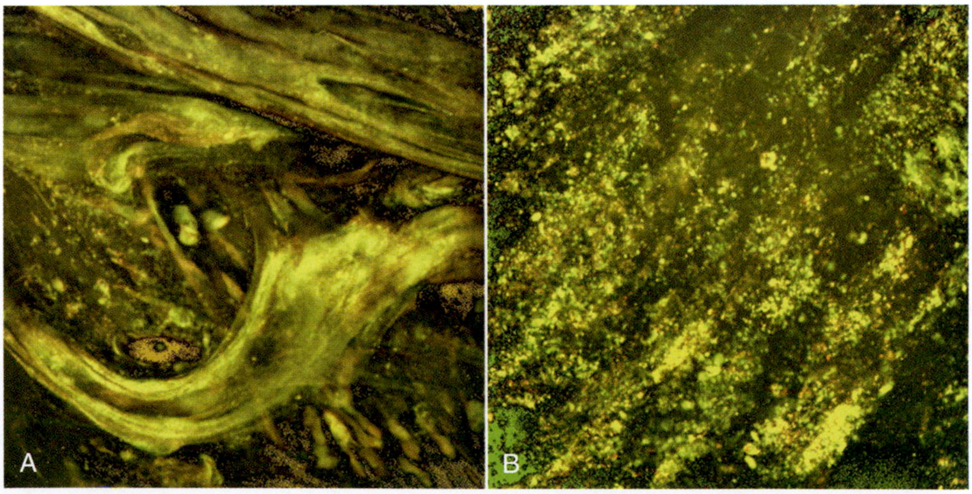

FIGURE 35-5 Illustration of the mode of action of dornase alfa in reducing DNA polymers in cystic fibrosis (CF) sputum. Confocal micrograph showing CF sputum stained (with YOYO-1) for DNA before **(A)** and after **(B)** treatment with dornase alfa in vitro. The long DNA polymers are degraded after dornase treatment. (From Gardenhire DS: Rau's respiratory care pharmacology, ed 9, St. Louis, 2016, Elsevier.)

viscosity of airway secretions. This agent is not approved for such use. The reduction in secretion viscosity is thought to be caused by the increase in topical airway pH, with degradation of bonding in the mucin polysaccharide.

Expectorants are mucoactive but stimulate the production and clearance of airway secretions rather than cause mucolysis. Examples of such agents include guaifenesin (also known as *glyceryl guaiacolate*), iodinated glycerol, and saturated solution of potassium iodide (SSKI). Guaifenesin is found in many over-the-counter cough and cold products.

Assessment of Mucoactive Drug Therapy

Assessment of drug therapy for respiratory secretions is difficult. FEV_1 is relatively insensitive to changes in mucociliary clearance. The rate of change in lung function over time is a better marker. In addition, during maintenance therapy, the volume of sputum expectorated varies from day to day and does not reflect effective therapy. The following assessments should be performed.

Before Treatment

- Assess the patient's adequacy of cough and level of consciousness to determine need for treatment with mechanical suctioning or adjunct bronchial hygiene (postural drainage or percussion, positive expiratory pressure therapy) to clear the airway or if treatment is contraindicated.

During Treatment and Short Term

- Teach and then verify correct use of aerosol nebulization system, including cleaning.
- Assess therapy based on indication for drug.
- Monitor changes in FEV_1.
- Assess the patient's breathing pattern and rate.
- Assess the patient's breathing effort or pattern.
- Discontinue therapy if the patient experiences adverse reactions.

Long Term

- Discontinue therapy if the patient experiences adverse reactions.
- Monitor number and severity of respiratory tract infections and need for antibiotic therapy, emergency visits, and hospitalizations.
- Monitor pulmonary function for improvement or slowing in the rate of deterioration.

General Contraindications

Mucoactive therapy should be used with caution in patients with severely compromised vital capacity and expiratory flow, such as in the presence of end-stage pulmonary disease or neuromuscular disorders. Generally, if FEV_1 is less than 25% of predicted, it becomes difficult to mobilize and expectorate secretions. Theoretically, with profound airflow compromise, secretion clearance could decline.

Gastroesophageal reflux and inability of the patient to protect the airway are risk factors for postural drainage that should be considered if postural drainage is necessary with mucoactive therapy. Mucoactive agents should be discontinued if there is evidence of clinical deterioration. Patients with acute bronchitis or exacerbation of chronic disease (CF, COPD) may be less responsive to mucoactive therapy, possibly secondary to infection and muscular weakness, which can reduce airflow-dependent mechanisms further.

INHALED CORTICOSTEROIDS

Corticosteroids are endogenous hormones produced in the adrenal cortex that regulate basic metabolic functions in the body and exert an antiinflammatory effect.[30] The use of aerosolized corticosteroids is reviewed in this section. All corticosteroids used to treat asthma and COPD are glucocorticoids.

Indications and Purposes

The two general formulations of aerosolized glucocorticoids are orally inhaled and intranasal aerosol preparations. Orally inhaled preparations are listed in Table 35-5. The primary use of orally inhaled corticosteroids is for antiinflammatory maintenance therapy of persistent asthma[6] and severe COPD.[31] The use of intranasal steroids is for control of seasonal allergic or nonallergic rhinitis. Most agents in Table 35-5 are available as intranasal preparations, with the exception of the combination drugs.

Mode of Action

Glucocorticoids are lipid-soluble drugs that act on intracellular receptors. The complex action of steroids is illustrated in Figure 35-6.[32-34] It is important for patients to understand that inhalation of an aerosolized steroid does not provide immediate relief as with an adrenergic bronchodilator. However, daily compliance with the inhaled medication is essential to controlling the inflammation of asthma. Oral corticosteroids may be needed initially to clear the airway or as "burst" therapy to control asthma exacerbations.

Adverse Effects

The type and severity of side effects seen with inhaled aerosolized corticosteroids are much less than with systemic use, as with other classes of aerosolized drugs. Box 35-3 lists systemic and local effects that can occur with inhaled steroids. The systemic effect of adrenal suppression is not usually seen with inhaled doses less than 800 mcg/day in adults or less than 400 mcg/day in children. Use of a reservoir device should be routine with inhaled steroids to prevent the swallowed portion adding to the systemic effect and to prevent the local effects of oral candidiasis and dysphonia. Allen and colleagues[35] published a comprehensive review of inhaled steroids.

Special Considerations

The modes of action of all inhaled glucocorticoids are the same with one exception. Ciclesonide, a **prodrug,** is given as an

TABLE 35-5

Corticosteroids and Combination Products Available by Aerosol for Oral Inhalation*

Drug	Brand Name	Formulation and Dosage
Beclomethasone dipropionate	QVAR	MDI: 40 and 80 μg/puff Adults and children ≥12 yr: 40-80 μg twice daily[†] or 40-160 μg twice daily[‡] Children ≥5 yr: 40-80 μg twice daily
Ciclesonide	Alvesco	MDI: 80 μg/puff and 160 μg/puff Adults and children ≥12 yr: 80-160 μg twice daily[†] or 80-320 μg twice daily[‡]
Flunisolide hemihydrate	AeroSpan	MDI: 80 μg/puff Adults and children ≥12 yr: 2 puffs twice daily, adults no more than 4 puffs daily[§] Children 6-11 yr: 1 puff daily, no more than 2 puffs daily
Fluticasone propionate	Flovent HFA	MDI: 44, 110, and 220 μg/puff Adults and children ≥12 yr: 88 μg twice daily,[†] 88-220 μg twice daily,[‡] or 880 μg twice daily[§] Children 4-11 yr: 88 μg twice daily[¶]
	Flovent Diskus	DPI: 50, 100, and 250 μg Adults and children ≥12 yr: 100 μg twice daily,[†] 100-250 μg twice daily,[‡] 1000 μg twice daily[§] Children 4-11 yr: 50 μg twice daily
Fluticasone furoate	Arnuity Ellipta	DPI: 100 μg/actuation and 200 μg/actuation Adults and children ≥12 yr: 100 μg or 200 μg, once daily
Budesonide	Pulmicort Flexhaler	DPI: 90 μg/actuation and 180 μg/actuation Adults and children ≥12 yr: 180-360 μg bid,[†] 180-360 μg bid,[‡] 360-720 μg bid[§] Children ≥6 yr: 180-360 μg bid
	Pulmicort Respules	SVN: 0.25 mg/2 ml, 0.5 mg/2 ml, 1 mg/2 ml Children 1-8 yr: 0.5-mg total dose given once daily or twice daily in divided doses[†,‡] 1 mg given as 0.5 mg twice daily or once daily[§]
Mometasone furoate	Asmanex Twisthaler	DPI: 110 μg/actuation; or 220 μg actuation Adults and children ≥12 yr: 220-440 μg daily,[†] 220-440 μg daily,[‡] 440-880 μg daily[§]; children 4-11 yr: 110-220 μg daily
	Asmanex HFA	MDI: 100 μg/actuation; or 200 μg actuation Adults and children ≥12 yr: 100-200 μg bid
Fluticasone propionate/ salmeterol	Advair Diskus	DPI: 100 μg fluticasone/50 μg salmeterol, 250 μg fluticasone/50 μg salmeterol, or 500 μg fluticasone/50 μg salmeterol Adults and children ≥12 yr: 100 μg fluticasone/50 μg salmeterol, 1 inhalation twice daily, ~12 hr apart (starting dose if not currently taking inhaled corticosteroids) Maximal recommended dose 500 μg fluticasone/50 μg salmeterol twice daily Children ≥4 yr: 100 μg fluticasone/50 μg salmeterol, 1 inhalation twice daily, ~12 hr apart (for patients who are symptomatic while taking an inhaled corticosteroid)[§]
	Advair HFA	MDI: 45 μg fluticasone/21 μg salmeterol, 115 μg fluticasone/21 μg salmeterol, or 230 μg fluticasone/21 μg salmeterol[§] Adults and children ≥12 yr: 2 inhalations twice daily, ~12 hr apart
Budesonide/formoterol fumarate HFA	Symbicort	MDI: 80 μg budesonide/4.5 μg formoterol and 160 μg budesonide/4.5 μg formoterol twice daily Adults and children ≥12 yr: 320 μg budesonide/9 μg formoterol; or 160 μg budesonide/9 μg formoterol twice daily
Mometasone furoate/ formoterol fumarate HFA	Dulera	MDI: 100 μg mometasone/5 μg formoterol and 200 μg mometasone/5 μg formoterol Adults and children ≥12 yr: If previously on medium dose of corticosteroids, ≤400 μg mometasone/20 μg formoterol daily; if previously on high dose of corticosteroid, ≤800 μg mometasone/20 μg formoterol daily
Fluticasone furoate/vilanterol	Breo Ellipta	DPI: 100 μg fluticasone/25 μg vilanterol Adults: 100 μg fluticasone/25 μg vilanterol daily

HFA, Hydrofluoroalkane.
*Individual agents are discussed in the text. Detailed information about each agent should be obtained from the manufacturer's drug insert.
[†]Recommended starting dose if taking only bronchodilators.
[‡]Recommended starting dose if previously taking inhaled corticosteroids.
[§]Recommended starting dose if previously taking oral corticosteroids.
[¶]This dose should be used regardless of previous therapy.

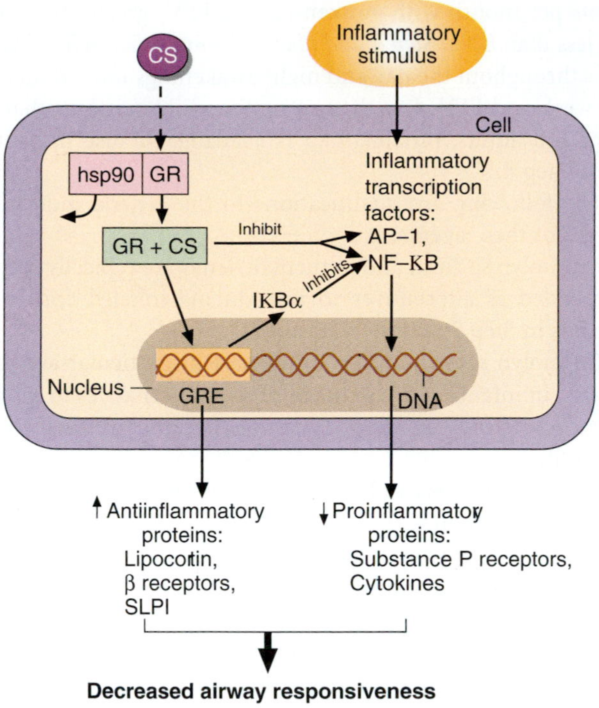

FIGURE 35-6 Mode of action by which corticosteroids modify cell response to inhibit inflammatory response in the airway. Corticosteroids *(CS)* diffuse into the cell and bind to a glucocorticoid receptor *(GR)*. When the steroid binds to the GR, a protein, heatshock protein 90 (hsp 90), dissociates from the GR, and the steroid-GR complex moves into the cell nucleus. The drug-receptor complex binds to glucocorticoid response elements *(GRE)* of the nuclear DNA to upregulate transcription of antiinflammatory substances such as lipocortin, a protein that inhibits the generation of the arachidonic acid cascade by phospholipase A_2. There is evidence that steroids also upregulate inhibitors of factors in the cell, such as nuclear factor-κB (NF-κB), which can cause transcription of inflammatory substances. There may be direct inhibition of factors such as NF-κB to limit the inflammatory process further. *AP-1,* Activator protein-1; *iκBα,* inhibitor of nuclear factor-κBα; *SLPI,* secretory leukocyte protease inhibitor. (From Gardenhire DS: Rau's respiratory care pharmacology, ed 9, St. Louis, 2016, Elsevier.)

Box 35-3 Potential Hazards and Side Effects of Aerosolized Corticosteroids

SYSTEMIC
- Adrenal insufficiency*,†
- Extrapulmonary allergy*
- Acute asthma*
- HPA suppression (minimal, dose dependent)
- Growth retardation†
- Osteoporosis†

LOCAL (TOPICAL)
- Oropharyngeal fungal infections
- Dysphonia
- Cough, bronchoconstriction
- Incorrect use of MDI

*Following substitution for systemic corticosteroid therapy.
†Effect with inhaled corticosteroids alone is unclear.
HPA, Hypothalamo-pituitary-adrenocortical.

inactive compound and is converted to an active metabolite, desisobutyryl ciclesonide, by intracellular enzymes. Ciclesonide is available as an intranasal formulation (Omnaris and Zetonna) and a pressurized MDI (Alvesco).

Assessment of Drug Therapy

The basic actions to evaluate an aerosol drug treatment should be followed (see section on Assessment of Bronchodilator Therapy). As with other drug therapy, the indications for this class of drug should be present. The NAEPP and Global Initiative on Obstructive Lung Disease (GOLD) COPD guidelines are recommended for guidance.[6,31] In addition, with inhaled corticosteroids, the following actions are suggested:

- Verify that the patient understands that a corticosteroid is a controller agent and is different from a rescue bronchodilator; assess the patient's understanding of the need for consistent use of an inhaled corticosteroid (compliance).
- Instruct the patient in the use of a peak flowmeter to monitor baseline peak expiratory flow (PEF) and changes. Verify that there is a specific action plan, based on symptoms and PEF results. The patient should understand when to contact a physician with deterioration in PEF or exacerbation of symptoms.

Long Term

- Assess severity of symptoms (coughing, wheezing, nocturnal awakenings, symptoms during exertion; use of rescue bronchodilator; number of exacerbations; missed work or school days; and pulmonary function) and modify level or dosage as recommended by NAEPP and GOLD guidelines.[6,31]
- Assess for the presence of side effects with inhaled steroid therapy (oral thrush, hoarseness or voice changes, cough or wheezing with MDI use); use a reservoir (preferably a holding chamber) with MDI use, and verify correct technique.

NONSTEROIDAL ANTIASTHMA DRUGS

Nonsteroidal antiinflammatory drugs constitute a growing class of drugs in the treatment of asthma. These include mast cell stabilizers (cromolyn sodium); antileukotrienes, also termed **leukotriene** modifiers (zafirlukast, zileuton, montelukast); and monoclonal antibodies or antiimmunoglobulin E (IgE) agents (omalizumab). Antileukotrienes are administered orally, and the monoclonal antibody agent omalizumab is given parenterally, but these are included as bronchoactive drugs. Table 35-6 lists pharmaceutical details for each agent.

Indication for Use

The general indication for clinical use of nonsteroidal antiasthma agents is prophylactic management (control) of persistent asthma (Step 2 or greater asthma, using the classification in the NAEPP guidelines[6]). *Step 2 asthma* is defined as more than 2 days per week with but not daily symptoms and more than 2 nights per month with awakenings and FEV_1 of 80% or greater. *Step 3 asthma* is defined as daily symptoms and 3 to 4

MINI CLINI

Patient Education

PROBLEM: A 24-year-old patient with asthma has complained of waking up at night and being short of breath. She also reports feeling tight in her chest and needs to use her albuterol inhaler 5 to 6 days per week to get relief. She is not currently on other inhaled medications. Her allergist prescribes an inhaled MDI corticosteroid and salmeterol to be taken on a daily basis. What instructions should she be given in using these agents by inhalation?

DISCUSSION: The key points with corticosteroid inhalation should be reviewed. These are small doses and safe to take. However, it is important to take the prescribed corticosteroid dose regularly every day if the drug is to have an antiinflammatory effect in the lung. She should also use a reservoir device with the MDI. Rinsing her mouth with water after a treatment can reduce further the chance of oral candidiasis or dysphonia. With salmeterol, she should be instructed to follow her prescribed dose, which is usually two inhalations, twice daily. Because of its pharmacokinetics, salmeterol is considered a long-term controller and not a quick reliever. It is not helpful in relieving bronchospasm if she experiences acute difficulty in breathing. For acute respiratory problems, she should have a quick-acting adrenergic agent such as albuterol or levalbuterol. If she experiences wheezing or chest tightness, one or two actuations of one of these agents would help. Salmeterol should be taken at the regularly prescribed time, usually every 12 hours.

nights per month with awakening and FEV_1 greater than 60% but less than 80%. *Step 4 and above asthma* is defined as symptoms throughout the day and night awakenings more than once per week and FEV_1 less than 60%. For children older than 12 years and adults, omalizumab is available for use in asthma above Step 4.[36]

The following are qualifications to the general indications for use of these agents:

- Cromolyn sodium and antileukotrienes are typically recommended as alternatives to introducing inhaled corticosteroids in Step 2 and Step 3 asthma.
- Cromolyn sodium and montelukast in particular are often used in infants and young children as alternatives to inhaled corticosteroids in Step 2 asthma because of their safety profiles.
- Antileukotrienes can be useful in combination with inhaled steroids to reduce the dose of the steroid and are listed as alternatives in Step 2 through Step 4 asthma.
- The monoclonal antibody omalizumab is available for consideration in the appropriate population.[37]

All of the nonsteroidal antiasthma drugs described in this chapter are controllers, not relievers, and are used in asthma requiring antiinflammatory drug therapy (Box 35-4).

Mode of Action

Cromolyn sodium acts by inhibiting the degranulation of mast cells in response to allergic and nonallergic stimuli. This inhibition prevents release of histamine and other mediators of

TABLE 35-6

Nonsteroidal Antiasthma Medications*

Generic Drug	Brand Name	Formulation and Dosage
Mast Cell Stabilizer		
Cromolyn sodium		SVN: 20 mg/ampule or 20 mg/2 ml Adults and children ≥2 yr: 20 mg inhaled 4 times daily Spray†: 40 mg/ml (4%) (5.2 mg per actuation) Adults and children ≥32 yr: 1 spray each nostril, 3-6 times daily every 4-6 hr
	Gastrocrom	Oral concentrate: 100 mg/5 ml Adults and children ≥13 yr: 2 ampules 4 times daily, 30 min before meals and at bedtime Children 2-12 yr: 1 ampule 4 time daily, 30 min before meals and at bedtime
Antileukotrienes		
Zafirlukast	Accolate	Tablets: 10 and 20 mg Adults and children ≥12 yr: 20 mg twice daily, without food Children 5-11 yr: 10 mg twice daily
Montelukast	Singulair	Tablets: 10 mg and 4-mg and 5-mg cherry-flavored chewable; 4-mg packet of granules Adults and children ≥15 yr: One 10-mg tablet daily Children 6-14 yr: One 5-mg chewable tablet daily Children 2-5 yr: One 4-mg chewable tablet or one 4-mg packet of granules daily 6-23 mo: One 4-mg packet of granules daily
Zileuton	Zyflo; Zyflo CR	Tablets: 600 mg Adults and children ≥12 yr: One 600-mg tablet 4 times per day; CR, 2 tablets twice daily, within 1 hr of morning and evening meals
Monoclonal Antibody		
Omalizumab	Xolair	Adults and children ≥12 yr: subcutaneous injection every 4 wk; dose dependent on weight and serum IgE level

*Detailed prescribing information should be obtained from the manufacturer's package insert.
†Available over-the-counter.

inflammation. These mediators cause bronchospasm and trigger an increasing cascade of further mediator release and inflammatory cell activity in the airway.[38]

Zafirlukast and montelukast act as leukotriene receptor antagonists and are selective competitive antagonists of leukotriene receptors LTD_4 and LTE_4. Leukotrienes such as LTC_4, LTD_4, and LTE_4 (previously known as *SRS-A*) stimulate leukotriene receptors termed $CysLT_1$ to cause bronchoconstriction, mucus secretion, vascular permeability, and plasma exudation into the airway. The mode of action is shown in Figure 35-7. The drug inhibits asthma reactions induced by exercise, cold air, allergens, and aspirin.[39]

Zileuton inhibits the 5-lipoxygenase enzyme that catalyzes the formation of leukotrienes from arachidonic acid (see Figure 35-7).[40] Omalizumab is a recombinant DNA–derived humanized antibody that binds to IgE. The agent inhibits the attachment of IgE to mast cells and basophils, reducing the release of chemical mediators of the allergic response.[41]

Box 35-4 Bronchoactive Agents Distinguished as Controllers or Relievers in Treating Asthma

LONG-TERM CONTROL
- Inhaled corticosteroids
- Cromolyn sodium
- Long-acting beta-2 agonists
  - Inhaled: Salmeterol, formoterol
  - Oral: Sustained-release albuterol
- Leukotriene modifiers
- Systemic corticosteroids
- Methylxanthines (theophylline)

QUICK RELIEF
- Short-acting inhaled beta-2 agonists: Albuterol, levalbuterol
- Anticholinergic (antimuscarinic): Ipratropium
- Systemic corticosteroids (oral burst therapy, IV)

From National Asthma Education and Prevention Program, National Heart, Lung and Blood Institute, National Institutes of Health: Expert Panel Report 3: Guidelines for the diagnosis and management of asthma, NIH Publication No. 08-4051. Bethesda, MD, 2007, National Institutes of Health.

Adverse Effects

A potential adverse effect with any nonsteroidal antiasthma drug is inappropriate use. These agents are not bronchodilators and offer no benefit for acute airway obstruction in asthma.

Table 35-7 summarizes information and comparative features of the three antileukotriene agents, including drug interactions, common side effects, and contraindications. The most

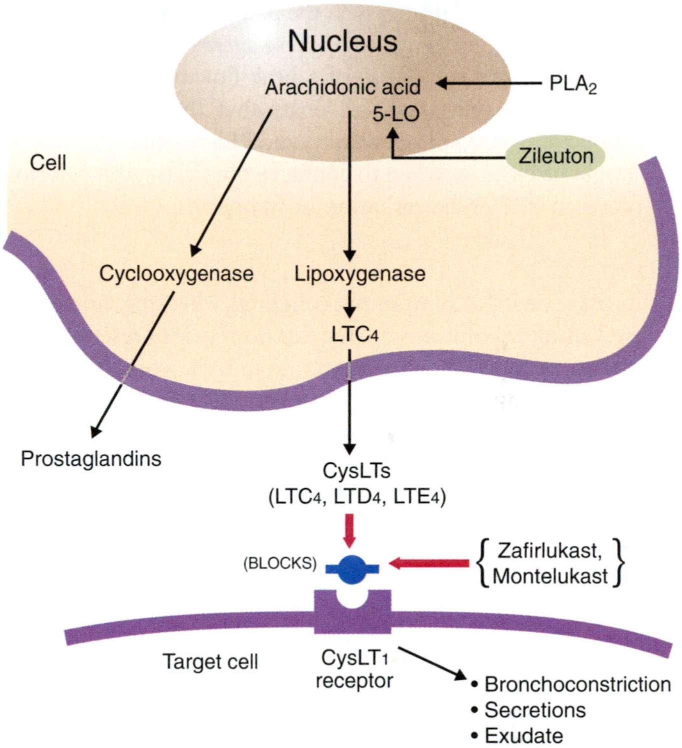

FIGURE 35-7 Modes and sites of action for leukotriene modifiers zileuton, zafirlukast, and montelukast. Zileuton inhibits the 5-LO enzyme, whereas zafirlukast and montelukast block the leukotriene receptor ($CysLT_1$). *LT,* Leukotriene; *PLA,* phospholipase A.

TABLE 35-7 Summary of Comparative Features of Three Available Antileukotriene Agents

Features	Zileuton	Zafirlukast	Montelukast
Brand name	Zyflo; Zyflo CR	Accolate	Singulair
Action	5-LO inhibitor	$CysLT_1$ receptor block	$CysLT_1$ receptor block
Age range	≥12 yr	≥5 yr	≥6 mo
Dosage	600-mg tab, qid; CR: 2 600-mg tab bid; 1 hr within morning and evening meal	Adult: 20-mg tab bid Children 5-11 yr: 10-mg tab bid	Adult: 10-mg tab q evening 6-14 yr: 5-mg tab q evening 2-5 yr: 4-mg tab q evening 6-23 mo: 4-mg oral granules q evening
Administration	Can be taken with food	1 hr before or 2 hr after meal	Taken with or without food
Drug interaction	Yes (theophylline, warfarin, propranolol)	Yes (warfarin, theophylline, aspirin)	No
Side effects (common)	Headache, dyspepsia, unspecified pain, liver enzyme elevations	Headache, infection, nausea, possible liver enzyme changes	Headache, influenza, abdominal pain
Contraindications	Active liver disease or elevated liver enzyme levels, hypersensitivity to components	Hypersensitivity to components	Hypersensitivity to components

common adverse reactions seen with omalizumab include injection site reaction, viral infections, respiratory tract infections, headache, sinusitis, and pharyngitis.

Assessment of Drug Therapy

The basic actions to evaluate an aerosol drug treatment should be followed (see section on Assessment of Bronchodilator Therapy). As with other drug therapy, the indication for this class of drug should be present.

- Verify that the patient understands that nonsteroidal antiasthma agents are controller drugs and their difference from rescue bronchodilators; assess the patient's understanding of the need for consistent use of these agents (compliance).
- Instruct the patient in use of a peak flowmeter to monitor baseline PEF and changes. Verify that there is a specific action plan, based on symptoms and PEF results. The patient should be clear on when to contact a physician with deterioration in PEF or exacerbation of symptoms.

Long Term

- Assess severity of symptoms (coughing, wheezing, nocturnal awakenings, symptoms during exertion); use of rescue medication; number of exacerbations; missed work or school days; pulmonary function), and modify level of asthma therapy (up or down, as described in the NAEPP EPR III guidelines for step therapy).
- Assess for the presence of side effects with nonsteroidal antiasthma agents; refer to the particular agent and its side effects (listed previously).

AEROSOLIZED ANTIINFECTIVE AGENTS

Multiple aerosolized antiinfective agents are available. Some agents may be used less often than others in respiratory therapy. The antiinfective agents pentamidine, ribavirin, inhaled tobramycin, inhaled aztreonam, and zanamivir are briefly outlined here. Drug formulations and dosages are given in Table 35-8.

Pentamidine Isethionate

Pentamidine isethionate (NebuPent) is an antiprotozoal agent that has been used in the treatment of opportunistic pneumonia caused by *Pneumocystis jiroveci,* which is the causative agent of *Pneumocystis* pneumonia (PCP). PCP is seen in immunocompromised patients, especially patients with AIDS.

Indication for Use

General recommendations for prophylaxis of PCP were published by the U.S. Centers for Disease Control and Prevention (CDC) for HIV-positive children[42] and adults.[43] In the 2013 CDC recommendations, oral trimethoprim-sulfamethoxazole (TMP-SMX) was preferred for prophylaxis of PCP as long as adverse side effects from TMP-SMX were absent or acceptable.[43] Aerosolized pentamidine is recommended as an alternative therapy for prophylaxis of PCP if TMP-SMX cannot be tolerated.

Adverse Effects

Possible side effects with aerosolized pentamidine include cough, bronchial irritation, bronchospasm, wheezing, shortness of breath, fatigue, bad or metallic taste, pharyngitis, conjunctivitis, rash, and chest pain. Systemic effects also have been noted with inhaled pentamidine, including decreased appetite, dizziness, rash, nausea, night sweats, chills, spontaneous pneumothoraces, **neutropenia**, pancreatitis, renal insufficiency, and hypoglycemia. Extrapulmonary infection with *P. jiroveci* can occur with prophylactic inhaled pentamidine.

Assessment

When administering aerosolized pentamidine, isolation, an environmental containment system (e.g., a booth or negative pressure room), and personnel barrier protection should be provided. Patients should be screened for tuberculosis. The drug is given using a nebulizer system with one-way valves and scavenging expiratory filters (e.g., Respirgard); this reduces environmental contamination. Nebulizer systems capable of

TABLE 35-8
Inhaled Antiinfective Agents*

Drug	Brand Name	Formulation and Dosage	Clinical Use
Pentamidine isethionate	NebuPent	300 mg powder in 6 ml sterile water; 300 mg once every 4 wk	PCP prophylaxis
Ribavirin	Virazole	6 g powder in 300 ml sterile water (20 mg/ml solution); given every 12-18 hr/day for 3-7 days by SPAG nebulizer	RSV
Tobramycin	TOBI	300-mg/5-ml ampule; adults and children ≥6 years: 300 mg bid, 28 days on/28 days off drug	*Pseudomonas aeruginosa* infection in CF
Tobramycin	Bethkis	300-mg/4-ml ampule; adults and children ≥6 years: 300 mg bid, 28 days on/28 days off drug	*P. aeruginosa* infection in CF
Aztreonam	Cayston	75 mg/1 ml; adults and children ≥7 yr: 75 mg tid, 28 days on/28 days off drug	*P. aeruginosa* infection in CF
Zanamivir	Relenza	DPI: 5 mg/inhalation; adults ≥5 years: 2 inhalations (one 5-mg blister per inhalation) bid, 12 hr apart for 5 days	Influenza

CF, Cystic fibrosis; *RSV,* respiratory syncytial virus; *PAP, Pneumocystis jiroveci* pneumonia; *SPAG,* small particle aerosol generator.
*Details on use and administration should be obtained from manufacturer's drug insert material before use.

producing a mass median diameter of 1 to 2 μm for peripheral lung deposition may reduce coughing. The patient should be monitored for onset of any of the previously described adverse reactions. In addition, the following actions are recommended:

- If coughing and bronchospasm are present, provide a short-acting beta agonist or an anticholinergic bronchodilator such as ipratropium with inhaled pentamidine.
- Monitor for occurrence rate of PCP and rate of long-term hospitalizations.
- Monitor for presence of side effects (shortness of breath, possible pneumothorax, conjunctivitis, rash, neutropenia, dysglycemia) or appearance of extrapulmonary *P. jiroveci* infection.
- Evaluate need for prior use of a bronchodilator if symptoms of bronchospasm or coughing occur after inhalation of pentamidine.

Long Term. Over the long term, monitor the efficacy of pentamidine prophylaxis in preventing episodes of PCP.

Ribavirin

Ribavirin (Virazole) is an antiviral agent used in the treatment of severe lower respiratory tract infections caused by respiratory syncytial virus (RSV). RSV is a common seasonal respiratory infection in infants and young children that is usually self-limiting. Recommendations for use of the drug were published in a statement by the American Academy of Pediatrics.[44] Generally, the drug is not recommended for routine RSV infection, but it may be considered for life-threatening infections.

Administration of the aerosol requires use of a special large-reservoir nebulizer called a *small particle aerosol generator (SPAG)*. The mode of action of ribavirin is similar to that of the drug guanosine, a natural nucleoside. Substitution of ribavirin for the natural nucleoside interrupts the viral replication process in the host cell.

Adverse Effects

Skin rash, eyelid erythema, and conjunctivitis have been noted with aerosol administration. Important equipment-related effects during mechanical ventilation include endotracheal tube occlusion and occlusion of ventilator expiratory valves or sensors. Deterioration of pulmonary function can occur. Patients or practitioners who are pregnant should not have exposure to ribavirin.

Assessment

- Monitor signs of improvement in RSV infection severity, including vital signs, respiratory pattern and work of breathing, level of FiO_2 needed, level of ventilatory support, ABGs, body temperature, and other indicators of pulmonary gas exchange.
- Monitor the patient for evidence of side effects, such as deterioration in lung function, bronchospasm, occlusion of endotracheal tube, cardiovascular instability, skin irritation from the aerosol drug, and equipment malfunction related to drug residue.

Inhaled Tobramycin

Patients with CF have chronic respiratory infection with *Pseudomonas aeruginosa* and other microorganisms. Such chronic infection causes recurrent acute respiratory infections and deterioration of lung function. With the exception of the quinoline derivatives such as ciprofloxacin, antibiotics such as the aminoglycosides (e.g., tobramycin), which are effective against *Pseudomonas* organisms, have poor lung bioavailability when taken orally. Consequently, these antibiotics must be given either intravenously or by inhalation. The aminoglycoside tobramycin has been approved for inhaled administration (TOBI) and is intended to manage chronic infection with *P. aeruginosa* in patients with CF. Goals of therapy are to treat or prevent early colonization with *P. aeruginosa* and maintain present lung function or reduce the rate of deterioration. The emergence of bacterial resistance has not been seen in clinical trials with inhaled tobramycin.[45]

Adverse Effects

Side effects with parenteral aminoglycosides include possible auditory and vestibular damage with potential for deafness and nephrotoxicity. Other possible effects are listed in Box 35-5. Risk for more serious side effects with tobramycin, whether by inhaled or parenteral routes, increases with the use of other aminoglycosides, in the presence of poor renal function and dehydration, with preexisting neuromuscular impairment, or with use of other ototoxic drugs.

The following precautions are suggested with use of inhaled tobramycin:

- Inhaled tobramycin should be used with caution in patients with preexisting renal, auditory, vestibular, or neuromuscular dysfunction.
- Tobramycin solution should not be mixed with beta-lactam antibiotics (penicillins, cephalosporins) because of admixture incompatibility, and mixing with other drugs in general is discouraged.
- Nebulization of antibiotics during hospitalization should be performed under conditions of containment, as previously described for pentamidine and ribavirin, to prevent

Box 35-5 Side Effects With Aminoglycosides and Tobramycin

PARENTERAL ADMINISTRATION

- Ototoxicity (auditory and vestibular)
- Nephrotoxicity
- Neuromuscular blockade
- Hypomagnesemia
- Cross-allergenicity
- Fetal harm (deafness)

INHALED NEBULIZED TOBRAMYCIN

- Voice alteration
- Tinnitus
- Nonsignificant increase in bacterial resistance

environmental saturation and development of resistant organisms in the hospital.

- Aminoglycosides can cause fetal harm if administered to pregnant women; exposure to ambient aerosol drug should be avoided by women who are pregnant or trying to become pregnant.
- Local airway irritation resulting in cough and bronchospasm with decreased ventilatory flow rates is possible with inhaled antibiotics and seems to be related to the osmolality of the solution.[46,47] Peak flow rates and chest auscultation should be used before and after treatments to evaluate airway changes. Pretreatment with a beta agonist may be needed.
- Allergic reactions in the patient, staff, or family should be considered if exposure to the aerosolized drug is not controlled. The use of a nebulizing system with a scavenging filter, one-way valves, and thumb control could reduce ambient contamination with the drug, as previously described.

In clinical trials, inhaled tobramycin was administered using the PARI LC Plus nebulizer with a DeVilbiss Pulmo-Aide compressor. Studies have reported that not all nebulizer-compressor systems perform adequately with antibiotic solutions, and higher flow rates of 10 to 12 L/min may be needed with nebulizers.[48,49]

Assessment

- Verify that the patient understands that nebulized tobramycin should be given after other CF therapies, including other inhaled drugs.
- Check whether the patient has renal, auditory, vestibular, or neuromuscular problems or is taking other aminoglycosides or ototoxic drugs. Consider whether tobramycin should be used for the patient based on severity of preexisting or concomitant risk factors.
- Monitor lung function to note improvement in FEV_1.
- Assess rate of hospitalization before and after institution of inhaled tobramycin.
- Assess need for intravenous antipseudomonal therapy.
- Assess improvement in weight.
- Monitor for occurrence of side effects, such as tinnitus or voice alteration; have the patient rinse and expectorate after aerosol treatments.
- Evaluate for changes in hearing or renal function during use of inhaled tobramycin.

Inhaled Aztreonam

Aztreonam was approved in December 1986 by the FDA as a monobactam, a synthetic bactericidal antibiotic; it is given as an intravenous solution. Inhaled aztreonam (Cayston) was approved in 2010 to improve pulmonary symptoms in patients with CF colonized with *P. aeruginosa.*[50] Inhaled aztreonam is not indicated for patients younger than 7 years old or patients with *Burkholderia cepacia* infection. This agent has been studied only in patients with FEV_1 greater than 25% or less than 75% of predicted. The agent is delivered by itself using the Altera Nebulizer System.

Adverse Effects

Inhaled aztreonam can cause bronchospasm and decrease FEV_1. All patients should be screened for baseline pulmonary function results and treated with a bronchodilator before administering inhaled aztreonam.

Patients have been reported to experience severe allergic reactions with injectable aztreonam. Careful observation is warranted when first using inhaled aztreonam because it could cause an allergic reaction.

The use of antibiotics in the absence of infection may lead to the development of drug-resistant bacteria. Inhaled aztreonam should not be used in patients with CF not infected with *P. aeruginosa.*

Colistimethate Sodium

Colistimethate sodium (colistin) is an antibiotic used to treat sensitive strains of gram-negative bacilli, particularly *P. aeruginosa.* Colistimethate sodium is available as an inhaled formulation in Europe as Promixin; this agent is not approved by the FDA for inhalation. However, nebulization of the parenteral formulation is commonly used in patients with CF. Falagas and colleagues[51] published a review of intravenous and aerosolized colistimethate sodium.

Adverse Effects

Side effects seen with parenteral administration include neurotoxic events and nephrotoxicity. Because colistimethate sodium is mainly eliminated by the renal system, renal insufficiency should be considered. Neurotoxic events associated with colistimethate sodium include dizziness, confusion, muscle weakness, and possible neuromuscular blockade, leading to respiratory arrest. When using aerosolized colistimethate sodium, the most common complication seen is bronchospasm. Pretreatment with a beta agonist can decrease the potential for this complication.

Inhaled Zanamivir

Zanamivir is an inhaled powder aerosol (DPI). Despite the availability of zanamivir and the oral antiinfluenza agent oseltamivir (Tamiflu), prophylactic vaccination against influenza is still recommended, especially in high-risk individuals with cardiovascular or pulmonary disease. Zanamivir and oseltamivir represent a new class of antiviral agents termed *neuraminidase inhibitors.*

Indication for Use

Inhaled zanamivir is indicated for the treatment of uncomplicated acute illness caused by influenza virus in adults and children 5 years or older who have been symptomatic for no longer than 2 days. The agents have an off-label use for treatment and prophylaxis of H1N1 influenza A.

Mode of Action

The influenza virus attaches to respiratory tract cells by binding of viral surface hemagglutinin to the cell's surface molecule of sialic acid (Figure 35-8). The viral particle also has an enzyme,

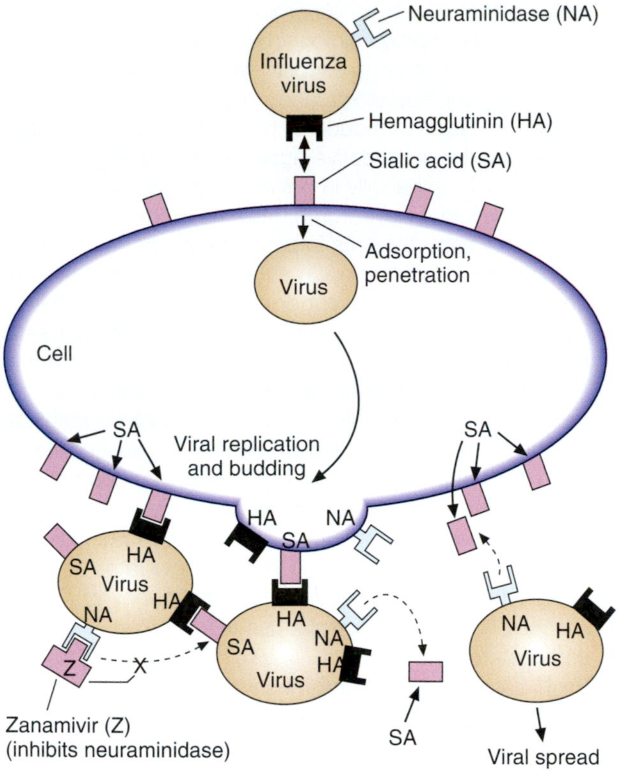

FIGURE 35-8 Mode of action by which inhaled zanamivir exerts an antiviral effect on influenza virus. Zanamivir is a sialic acid analogue and binds to neuraminidase, the enzyme responsible for cleaving sialic acid and preventing viral binding to sialic acid. This causes viral aggregation, with binding of viral particles to each other and to the host cell, preventing viral spread. *HA,* Hemagglutinin; *NA,* neuraminidase; *SA,* sialic acid. (From Gardenhire DS: Rau's respiratory care pharmacology, ed 9, St. Louis, 2016, Elsevier.)

neuraminidase, on its surface. When replicated viral particles are released from the host cell after infection, the viral neuraminidase cleaves the sialic acid on both the host cell surface and other viral particle surfaces so that mature virus can be released and spread. Without neuraminidase, influenza virus would clump together and to the host cell, preventing spread. Zanamivir and oseltamivir combine with the surface neuraminidase, preventing its action and the spread of viral particles.

Adverse Effects

Several adverse effects can occur with inhaled zanamivir:

- Bronchospasm and deterioration in lung function, especially in patients with COPD or asthma
- Possible undertreatment of bacterial infection masquerading as a viral infection or a secondary bacterial infection in the presence of influenza
- Allergic reactions, as may occur with any drug
- Adverse reactions, such as diarrhea, nausea, vomiting, bronchitis, cough, sinusitis, dizziness, and headaches

Because of the effect on lung function in patients with respiratory disease and reports of adverse reactions, revised labeling for the drug carries a warning that zanamivir is not generally recommended for patients with underlying airways disease.[52] However, other studies have determined that high-risk patients such as patients with asthma and COPD were not affected by the use of zanamivir.[53]

Clinical Efficacy

In studies of clinical efficacy, the use of zanamivir resulted in shortening of the median time to alleviation of symptoms by 1 day. In subjects who began treatment within 30 hours of illness, the median time to alleviation of symptoms was reduced by approximately 3 days.[54] Zanamivir is not approved for prophylaxis of influenza, although some data suggest a preventive effect in patients exposed to influenza virus.[53] Cost-versus-efficacy issues revolve around the modest reduction in symptoms and inability to confirm the presence of influenza quickly, easily, and inexpensively as the basis for the drug treatment.

Assessment

- Assess improvement in influenza symptoms, including fever reduction, less myalgia and headache, reduced coughing and sore throat, and less systemic fatigue.
- Monitor for airway irritation and symptoms of bronchospasm, especially during initial use of the dry powder aerosol. Provide a short-acting beta agonist if needed or if the patient is at risk for airway reactivity (COPD, asthma).

INHALED PULMONARY VASODILATORS

The use of nitric oxide gas to treat neonates with persistent pulmonary hypertension is approved by the FDA and is discussed in detail in Chapters 41 and 53. In addition to this medical gas, inhaled medications are being tested and used to treat pulmonary hypertension. Several such agents are being studied, including epoprostenol (Flolan) and alprostadil (Prostin VR Pediatric); however, only two, iloprost, and treprostinil, are approved by the FDA for widespread use. Siobal[55] published a review of aerosolized prostacyclins and nitric oxide (NO).

Nitric Oxide

Indications for Use

As described in more detail in Chapters 41 and 53, NO (INOmax) is indicated in the treatment of neonates (>34 weeks of gestational age) with hypoxic respiratory failure.[56] The patient should have evidence of pulmonary hypertension in which NO would improve oxygenation and decrease the need for extracorporeal membrane oxygenation. Off-label uses include reducing pulmonary artery pressure in the neonate, pediatric patient, and adult.[57] NO is frequently used in cardiac surgical patients who present with perioperative pulmonary hypertension although this indication is considered off label.

Mode of Action

NO is produced by cells in the body. It relaxes vascular smooth muscle by binding to the heme group of cytosolic guanylate cyclase, activating guanylate cyclase, and increasing cyclic guanosine monophosphate. When inhaled, NO produces pulmonary vasodilation, reducing pulmonary artery pressure and improving $\dot{V}/\dot{Q}$ mismatching.

Adverse Effects

NO is contraindicated in neonates with dependent right-to-left shunts. Precautions include methemoglobinemia and NO_2 formation. The most common adverse events are hypotension and withdrawal.[58]

Iloprost

Indications for Use

Iloprost (Ventavis) inhalation is indicated for the treatment of pulmonary hypertension.[59] Iloprost inhalation is administered with the I-neb nebulizer.

Mode of Action

Iloprost is a synthetic analogue of prostacyclin (PGI_2). This agent dilates pulmonary arterial vascular beds and affects platelet aggregation. It is unknown whether platelet aggregation plays a role in the treatment of pulmonary hypertension.

Adverse Effects

Syncope and pulmonary edema may occur secondary to the vasodilatory properties of iloprost. During the 12-week clinical trial, headache and increased cough were the most noted adverse reactions.

Treprostinil

Indication for Use

Treprostinil (Tyvaso) is indicated for the treatment of pulmonary arterial hypertension to increase walking distance in patients with New York Heart Association class III symptoms.[60] It is administered using the Tyvaso Inhalation System, which is an ultrasonic, pulsed-delivery device.

Mode of Action

Treprostinil is a prostacyclin analogue that causes vasodilation of the pulmonary and systemic arterial vascular beds and inhibits platelet aggregation. Treprostinil is available in a 2.9-mL ampule, which contains 1.74 mg of treprostinil (0.6 mg/mL). It is provided as an aerosol in the Tyvaso Inhalation System.

Adverse Effects

Treprostinil has not been studied in patients with underlying lung disease (e.g., asthma, COPD). Treprostinil may cause bronchospasm. This agent should not be mixed with any other agents.

SUMMARY CHECKLIST

- Orally inhaled aerosol drug classes include beta-agonist bronchodilators, anticholinergic (antimuscarinic) bronchodilators, mucolytics, corticosteroids, nonsteroidal antiasthma drugs, antiinfective agents, and anti–pulmonary hypertensive agents.
- Beta-agonist and anticholinergic bronchodilators are used to reverse or improve airflow obstruction; mucolytics are used to reduce mucus viscosity and improve mucociliary clearance; corticosteroids and nonsteroidal antiasthma agents are used to reduce or prevent airway inflammation in asthma; the antiinfective agent pentamidine is used to treat PCP, especially in patients with acquired immunodeficiency syndrome; ribavirin is used to treat respiratory syncytial virus infection in at-risk infants and children; inhaled tobramycin and aztreonam are used in patients with CF to prevent or manage gram-negative *Pseudomonas* infections; and inhaled zanamivir is used to treat acute influenza.
- All aerosol treatments are assessed immediately by monitoring respiratory vital signs, which include respiratory rate and pattern, pulse, breath sounds on auscultation, general patient appearance (e.g., color, diaphoresis), and patient report of subjective reaction (e.g., chest tightness). Additional assessment should be related to the indication for the drug (e.g., monitoring of peak flow rates or bedside spirometry with bronchodilator use; frequency of exacerbation or beta agonist use with inhaled corticosteroids in asthma).
- Each class of aerosol drug has its own mode of action. Practitioners should be familiar with how agents they administer work. Common side effects with each class of drug include tremor and shakiness with beta agonists, dry mouth with anticholinergic agents, bronchial irritation with acetylcysteine, dysphonia and voice changes with dornase alfa, and oral fungal infections with corticosteroids.
- Agents used in asthma that provide quick relief include short-acting beta agonists (albuterol, levalbuterol, metaproterenol) and anticholinergic bronchodilators. Agents that provide long-term control include long-acting beta agonists (salmeterol, formoterol, arformoterol, indacaterol, olodaterol); inhaled corticosteroids; and nonsteroidal antiasthma drugs (cromolyn, montelukast, and other leukotriene antagonists). Systemic corticosteroids are used for both quick relief (intravenously) and long-term control (orally).
- Newer inhaled medications within a class known as *aerosolized prostacyclins* are being introduced to help treat pulmonary hypertension. Several agents are being studied, including epoprostenol (Flolan) and alprostadil (Prostin VR Pediatric); however, only treprostinil (Tyvaso) and iloprost (Ventavis) are being used on a widespread basis.

References

1. Gardenhire DS: *Rau's respiratory care pharmacology*, ed 9, St. Louis, 2016, Elsevier.
2. Katzung BG, Masters SB, Trevor AJ: *Basic and clinical pharmacology*, ed 12, New York, 2012, McGraw-Hill.
3. Rau JL: The inhalation of drugs: advantages and problems. *Respir Care* 50:367–382, 2005.
4. Borgström L: A possible new approach of comparing different inhalers and inhaled substances. *J Aerosol Med* 4:A13, 1991.

5. Thorsson L: Influence of inhaler systems on systemic availability, with focus on inhaled corticosteroids. *J Aerosol Med* 8(Suppl 3):S29–S36, 1995.
6. National Asthma Education and Prevention Program: *National Heart, Lung and Blood Institute, National Institutes of Health: Expert Panel Report 3: Guidelines for the diagnosis and management of asthma, NIH Publication No. 08-4051*, Bethesda, MD, 2007, NIH.
7. Chung LP, Waterer G, Thompson PJ: Pharmacogenetics of β_2 adrenergic receptor gene polymorphisms, long-acting β-agonists and asthma. *Clin Exp Allergy* 41:312–326, 2011.
8. Mitra S, Ugur M, Ugur O, et al: (S)-Albuterol increases intracellular free calcium by muscarinic receptor activation and a phospholipase C-dependent mechanism in airway smooth muscle. *Mol Pharmacol* 53:347–354, 1998.
9. Lipworth BJ, Clark DJ, Koch P, et al: Pharmacokinetics and extrapulmonary β_2 adrenoceptor activity of nebulised racemic salbutamol and its R- and S-isomers in healthy volunteers. *Thorax* 52:849, 1997.
10. Johansson FJ, Rydberg I, Aberg G, et al: Effects of albuterol enantiomers on in vitro bronchial reactivity. *Clin Rev Allergy Immunol* 14:57–64, 1996.
11. Templeton AG, Chapman ID, Chilvers ER, et al: Effects of S-salbutamol on human isolated bronchus. *Pulm Pharmacol Ther* 11:1–6, 1998.
12. Volcheck GW, Gleich GJ, Kita H: Pro- and anti-inflammatory effects of β-adrenergic agonists on eosinophil response to IL-5. *J Allergy Clin Immunol* 101:S35, 1998.
13. Schmekel B, Rydberg I, Norlander B, et al: Stereoselective pharmacokinetics of S-salbutamol after administration of the racemate in healthy volunteers. *Eur Respir J* 13:1230–1235, 1999.
14. Dhand R, Goode M, Reid R, et al: Preferential pulmonary retention of (S)-albuterol after inhalation of racemic albuterol. *Am J Respir Crit Care Med* 160:1136–1141, 1999.
15. Nelson HS, Bensch G, Pleskow WW, et al: Improved bronchodilation with levalbuterol compared with racemic albuterol in patients with asthma. *J Allergy Clin Immunol* 102:943–952, 1998.
16. Sears MR, Ottosson A, Radner F, et al: Long-acting β-agonists: a review of formoterol safety data from asthma clinical trials. *Eur Respir J* 33:21–32, 2009.
17. Cazzola M, Bardaro F, Stirpe E: The role of indacaterol for chronic obstructive pulmonary disease (COPD). *J Thorac Dis* 5:559–566, 2013.
18. van Noord JA, Smeets JJ, Drenth BM, et al: 24-hour bronchodilation following a single dose of the novel β2-agonist olodaterol in COPD. *Pulm Pharmacol Ther* 24:666–672, 2011.
19. Smit M, Zuidhof AB, Bos SIT, et al: Bronchoprotection by olodaterol is synergistically enhanced by tiotropium in a guinea pig model of allergic asthma. *J Pharmacol Exp Ther* 348:303–310, 2013.
20. Hanania NA, Feldman G, Zachgo W, et al: The efficacy and safety of the novel long-acting β2 agonist vilanterol in COPD patients: a randomized placebo-controlled trial. *Chest* 142:119–127, 2012.
21. Hall IP: The β-agonist controversy revisited. *Lancet* 363:183–184, 2004.
22. Barr RG, Bourbeau J, Camargo CA, Jr, et al: Tiotropium for stable chronic obstructive pulmonary disease: a meta-analysis. *Thorax* 61:854–862, 2006.
23. Rubin BK: The pharmacologic approach to airway clearance: mucoactive agents. *Paediatr Respir Rev* 7:S215–S219, 2006.
24. Macy AM: Preventing hepatotoxicity in acetaminophen overdose. *Am J Nurs* 79:301–303, 1979.
25. Decramer M, Rutten-van Molken M, Dekhuijzen PN, et al: Effects of N-acetylcysteine on outcomes in chronic obstructive pulmonary disease (Bronchitis Randomized on NAC Cost-Utility Study, BRONCUS): a randomised placebo-controlled trial. *Lancet* 365:1552–1560, 2005.
26. King M, Rubin BK: Mucus-controlling agents: past and present. *Respir Care Clin N Am* 5:575–594, 1999.
27. Consensus Conference: Practical applications of Pulmozyme. *Pediatr Pulmonol* 17:404–408, 1994.
28. Shak S, Capon DJ, Hellmiss R, et al: Recombinant human DNase I reduces the viscosity of cystic fibrosis sputum. *Proc Natl Acad Sci U S A* 87:9188–9192, 1990.
29. Robinson M, Regnis JA, Bailey DL, et al: Effect of hypertonic saline, amiloride, and cough on mucociliary clearance in patients with cystic fibrosis. *Am J Respir Crit Care Med* 153:1503–1509, 1996.
30. Minasian C, Wallis C, Metcalfe C, et al: Bronchial provocation testing with dry powder mannitol in children with cystic fibrosis. *Pediatr Pulmonol* 43:1078–1084, 2008.
31. Global Initiative for Asthma (GINA): *Global strategy for asthma management and prevention*. National Heart, Lung, and Blood Institute (Bethesda, MD) and World Health Organization (Geneva, Switzerland), Available at: <http://www.ginasthma.org/local/uploads/files/GINA_Report_2014_Jun11.pdf>. Accessed December, 2014.
32. Baraniuk JN: Molecular actions of glucocorticoids: an introduction. *J Allergy Clin Immunol* 97:141–142, 1996.
33. Anderson GP: Interactions between corticosteroids and β-adrenergic agonists in asthma disease induction, progression, and exacerbation. *Am J Respir Crit Care Med* 161:S188–S196, 2000.
34. Barnes PJ: Inhaled glucocorticoids for asthma. *N Engl J Med* 332:868–875, 1995.
35. Allen DB, Bielory L, Derendorf H, et al: Inhaled corticosteroids, past lessons and future issues. *J Allergy Clin Immunol* 112(Suppl 3):S1–S40, 2003.
36. Ayres JG, Higgins B, Chilvers ER, et al: Efficacy and tolerability of anti-immunoglobulin E therapy with omalizumab in patients with poorly controlled (moderate-to-severe) allergic asthma. *Allergy* 59:701–708, 2004.
37. Lanier BQ, Corren J, Lumry W, et al: Omalizumab is effective in the long-term control of severe allergic asthma. *Ann Allergy Asthma Immunol* 91: 154–159, 2003.
38. Holgate ST: Inhaled sodium cromoglycate. *Respir Med* 90:387–390, 1996.
39. Bisgaard H: Role of leukotrienes in asthma pathophysiology. *Pediatr Pulmonol* 30:166–176, 2000.
40. Drazen JM, Israel E, O'Byrne PM: Treatment of asthma with drugs modifying the leukotriene pathway. *N Engl J Med* 340:197–206, 1999.
41. Holgate ST, Djukanovic R, Casale T, et al: Anti-immunoglobulin E treatment with omalizumab in allergic diseases: an update on anti-inflammatory activity and clinical efficacy. *Clin Exp Allergy* 35:408–416, 2005.
42. Mofenson LM, Brady MT, Danner SP, et al: Guidelines for the prevention and treatment of opportunistic infections among HIV-exposed and HIV-infected children: recommendations from CDC, the National Institutes of Health, the HIV Medicine Association of the Infectious Diseases Society of America, the Pediatric Infectious Diseases Society, and the American Academy of Pediatrics. *MMWR Recomm Rep* 58(RR-11):1–166, 2009.
43. Kaplan JE, Benson C, Holmes KH, et al: Guidelines for prevention and treatment of opportunistic infections in HIV-infected adults and adolescents: recommendations from CDC, the National Institutes of Health, and the HIV Medicine Association of the Infectious Diseases Society of America. *MMWR Recomm Rep* 58(RR-4):1–198, 2009.
44. American Academy of Pediatrics, Committee on Infectious Diseases: Respiratory syncytial virus. In Pickering LK, editor: *Red Book: 2009 report of the Committee on Infectious Diseases*, ed 28, Elk Grove Village, IL, 2009, American Academy of Pediatrics.
45. Ramsey BW, Pepe MS, Quan JM, et al: Intermittent administration of inhaled tobramycin in patients with cystic fibrosis. *N Engl J Med* 340:23–30, 1999.
46. Littlewood JM, Smye SW, Cunliffe H: Aerosol antibiotic treatment in cystic fibrosis. *Arch Dis Child* 68:788–792, 1993.
47. Dally MB, Kurrle S, Breslin AB: Ventilatory effects of aerosol gentamicin. *Thorax* 33:54–56, 1978.
48. Hurley PK, Smye SW, Cunliffe H: Assessment of antibiotic aerosol generation using commercial jet nebulizers. *J Aerosol Med* 7:217–228, 1994.
49. Newman SP, Pellow PG, Clay MM, et al: Evaluation of jet nebulizers for use with gentamicin solution. *Thorax* 40:671–676, 1985.
50. Anderson P: Emerging therapies in cystic fibrosis. *Ther Adv Respir Dis* 4:177–185, 2010.
51. Falagas ME, Kasiakou SK, Tsiodras S, et al: The use of intravenous and aerosolized polymyxins for the treatment of infections in critically ill patients: a review of the recent literature. *Clin Med Res* 4:138–146, 2006.
52. U.S. Food and Drug Administration: Revised labeling for zanamivir. *JAMA* 284:1234, 2000.
53. Gubareva LV, Kaiser L, Hayden FG: Influenza virus neuraminidase inhibitors. *Lancet* 355:827–835, 2000.

54. Hayden FG, Gubareva LV, Monto AS, et al: Inhaled zanamivir for the prevention of influenza in families. *N Engl J Med* 343:1282–1289, 2000.
55. Siobal M: Aerosolized prostacyclins. *Respir Care* 49:640–652, 2004.
56. Taylor RW, Zimmerman JL, Dellinger RP, et al: Inhaled Nitric Oxide in ARDS Study Group: Low dose inhaled nitric oxide in patients with acute lung injury. *JAMA* 291:1603–1609, 2004.
57. Palevsky HI: Treatment of pulmonary hypertension. In Leff AR, editor: *Pulmonary and critical care pharmacology and therapeutics*, New York, 2000, McGraw-Hill.
58. Martin WJ, Rehm S: Toxic injury of the lung parenchyma. In Leff AR, editor: *Pulmonary and critical care pharmacology and therapeutics*, New York, 2000, McGraw-Hill.
59. Olschewski H, Simonneau G, Galie N, et al: Aerosolized Iloprost Randomized Study Group: Inhaled iloprost for severe pulmonary hypertension. *N Engl J Med* 347:322–329, 2002.
60. Channick RN, Olschewski H, Seeger W, et al: Safety and efficacy of inhaled treprostinil as add-on therapy to bosentan in pulmonary arterial hypertension. *J Am Coll Cardiol* 48:1433–1437, 2006.

CHAPTER 36

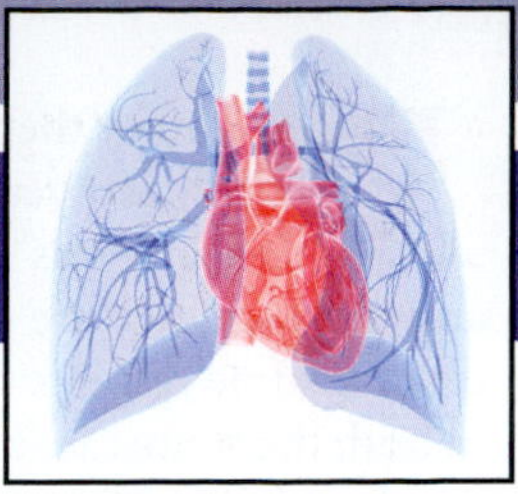

Airway Management

NEILA ALTOBELLI

CHAPTER OBJECTIVES

After reading this chapter you will be able to:

- Describe how to perform endotracheal and nasotracheal suctioning safely.
- Describe how to obtain sputum samples properly.
- Assess the need for and select an artificial airway.
- Identify the complications and hazards associated with insertion of artificial airways.
- Describe how to perform orotracheal and nasotracheal intubation of an adult.
- Assess and confirm proper endotracheal tube placement.
- Describe the rationale and the methods for performing a tracheotomy.
- Identify the types of damage that artificial airways can cause.
- Describe how to maintain and troubleshoot artificial airways properly.
- Describe techniques for measuring and adjusting tracheal tube cuff pressures.
- Identify when and how to extubate or decannulate a patient.
- Describe how to use alternative airway devices.
- Describe how to assist a physician in setting up and performing bronchoscopy.

CHAPTER OUTLINE

KEY TERMS

bronchoscopy
decannulation
endotracheal tubes
extubation
fenestrated
intubation
laryngectomy
obturator
pharyngeal airways
radiopaque
stenosis
suctioning
tracheoesophageal fistula
tracheoinnominate artery fistula
tracheomalacia
tracheostomy
tracheostomy tubes
tracheotomy

Respiratory therapists (RTs) are an important part of the health care team who aim to optimize patient ventilation and gas exchange. Because adequate ventilation and gas exchange are impossible without a patent airway, RTs often assume responsibility for airway management of patients in both the acute care and the post–acute care settings. RTs must develop skills in three broad areas of airway care. First, the RT must be proficient in airway clearance techniques, including methods designed to ensure the patency of the patient's natural or artificial airway. Second, the RT must be able to insert and maintain artificial airways designed to support patients whose own natural airways are inadequate. Third, the RT must be able to assist physicians in performing special procedures related to airway management. This chapter explores each of these areas.

SUCTIONING

Airway obstruction can be caused by retained secretions, foreign bodies, and structural changes such as edema, tumors, or trauma. Retained secretions increase airway resistance and the work of breathing and can cause hypoxemia, hypercapnia, atelectasis, and infection. Difficulty in clearing secretions may be due to the thickness or amount of the secretions or to the patient's inability to generate an effective cough.

RTs can remove retained secretions or other semi-liquid fluids from the airways by suctioning. **Suctioning** is the application of negative pressure (vacuum) to the airways through a collecting tube (flexible catheter or suction tip). Removal of foreign bodies, secretions, or tissue masses beyond the main stem bronchi requires bronchoscopy, which is generally performed by a physician; however, an increasing number of centers have trained RTs to perform therapeutic bronchoscopy. RTs often assist physicians in performing bronchoscopy, which is discussed at the end of the chapter.

Suctioning can be performed by way of either the upper airway (oropharynx) or the lower airway (trachea and bronchi). Secretions or fluids also can be removed from the oropharynx by using a rigid tonsillar or Yankauer suction tip (Figure 36-1). Access to the lower airway is by introduction of a flexible suction catheter (Figure 36-2) through the nose (nasotracheal suctioning) or artificial airway (endotracheal suctioning). Tracheal suctioning through the mouth should be avoided because it causes gagging.

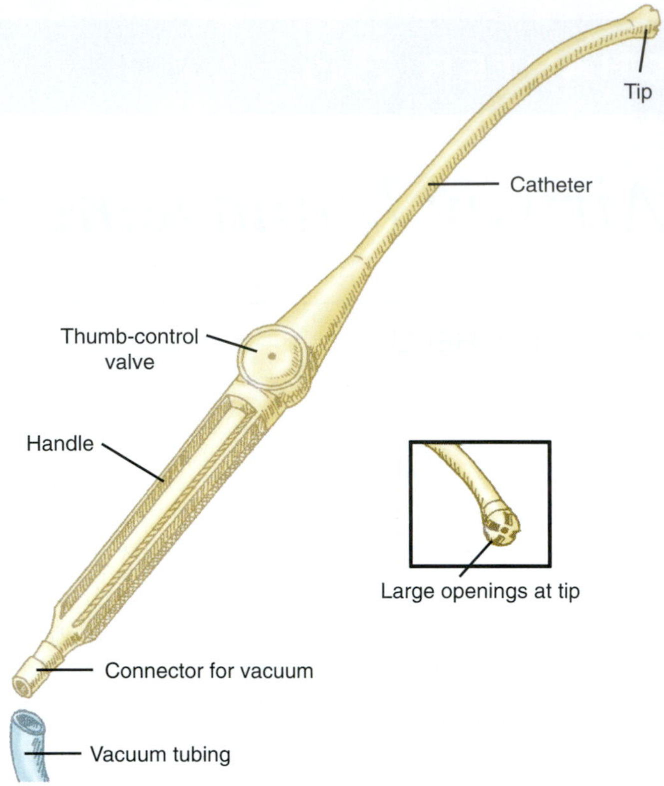

FIGURE 36-1 Rigid tonsillar, or Yankauer, suction tip. (Modified from Sills JR: The comprehensive respiratory therapist exam review, entry and advanced levels, ed 5, St. Louis, 2010, Mosby.)

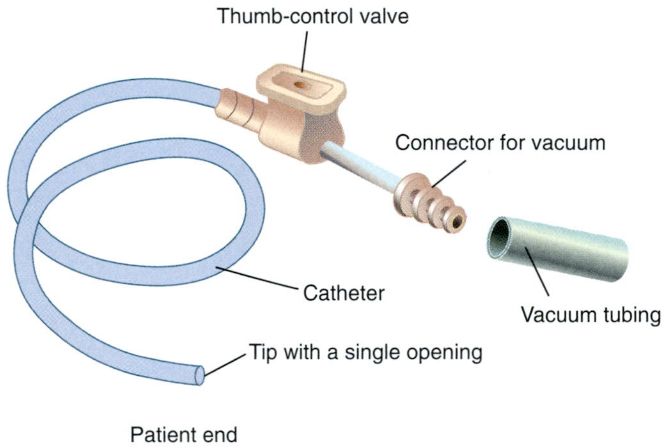

FIGURE 36-2 Flexible suction catheter for lower airway suctioning.

Endotracheal Suctioning

Clinical Practice Guideline

To guide practitioners in safe and effective application of this procedure, the American Association for Respiratory Care (AARC) has developed a clinical practice guideline on endotracheal suctioning of mechanically ventilated patients with artificial airways. Excerpts from the AARC guideline, including indications, contraindications, hazards and complications, assessment of need, assessment of outcome, and monitoring, appear in Clinical Practice Guideline 36-1.[1]

Equipment and Procedure

The procedure described here is for endotracheal suctioning of adults or children. Nasotracheal suctioning is described separately later in this chapter. There are two techniques for endotracheal suctioning: open and closed. The open, sterile technique requires disconnecting the patient from the ventilator. The closed technique uses a sterile, closed, in-line suction catheter that is attached to the ventilator circuit so that the suction

36-1 Endotracheal Suctioning of Mechanically Ventilated Patients With Artificial Airways

AARC Clinical Practice Guideline (Excerpts)*

INDICATIONS

- Need to maintain patency and integrity of the artificial airway
- Need to remove accumulated pulmonary secretions as evidenced by one of the following:
  - Sawtooth pattern on the flow-volume loop on the monitor screen of the ventilator or the presence of coarse crackles over the trachea—both are strong indicators of retained pulmonary secretions
  - Increased peak inspiratory pressure on volume-control ventilation or decreased tidal volume on pressure control ventilation
  - Deterioration of O_2 saturation or blood gas values
  - Visible secretions in the airway
  - Inability of patient to generate an effective cough
  - Acute respiratory distress
    - Suspected aspiration of gastric or upper airway secretions
- Need to obtain a sputum specimen to rule out or identify pneumonia or other pulmonary infection or for sputum cytology

CONTRAINDICATIONS

Endotracheal suctioning is a necessary procedure for patients with artificial airways. Most contraindications are relative to the patient's risk for developing adverse reactions or worsening clinical condition as a result of the procedure. When indicated, there is no absolute contraindication to endotracheal suctioning because the decision to withhold suctioning to avoid possible adverse reaction may be lethal.

HAZARDS AND COMPLICATIONS

- Decrease in dynamic lung compliance and functional residual capacity
- Atelectasis
- Hypoxia or hypoxemia
- Tissue trauma to the tracheal or bronchial mucosa
- Bronchoconstriction or bronchospasm
- Increased microbial colonization of lower airway
- Changes in cerebral blood flow and increased intracranial pressure
- Hypertension
- Hypotension
- Cardiac dysrhythmias

Routine use of normal saline instillation may be associated with the following adverse events:

- Excessive coughing
- Decreased O_2 saturation
- Bronchospasm
- Dislodgment of the bacterial biofilm that colonizes the endotracheal tube into the lower airway
- Pain, anxiety, dyspnea
- Tachycardia
- Increased intracranial pressure

ASSESSMENT OF NEED

Qualified personnel should assess the need for endotracheal suctioning as a routine part of a patient and ventilator system assessment as detailed under Indications.

ASSESSMENT OF OUTCOME

- Improvement in appearance of ventilator graphics and breath sounds
- Decreased peak inspiratory pressure with narrowing of peak inspiratory pressure to plateau pressure difference; decreased airway resistance or increased dynamic compliance; increased tidal volume delivery during pressure-limited ventilation
- Improvement in arterial blood gas values or saturation as reflected by pulse oximetry (SpO_2)
- Removal of pulmonary secretions

MONITORING

The following should be monitored before, during, and after the procedure:

- Breath sounds
- O_2 saturation
- Skin color
- Pulse oximeter
- Respiratory rate and pattern
- Hemodynamic parameters
- Pulse rate
- Blood pressure, if indicated and available
- Electrocardiogram, if indicated and available
- Sputum characteristics—color, volume, consistency, odor
- Cough characteristics
- Intracranial pressure, if indicated and available
- Ventilator parameters
- Peak inspiratory pressure and plateau pressure
- Tidal volume
- Pressure, flow, and volume graphics, if available
- FiO_2

**For complete guidelines, see American Association for Respiratory Care: Clinical practice guideline: endotracheal suctioning of mechanically ventilated patients with artificial airways. Respir Care 55:758, 2010.*

catheter can be advanced into the patient's endotracheal airway without disconnecting the patient from the ventilator.

There are also two methods of suctioning based on how deep the suction catheter is inserted in the artificial airway: deep suctioning and shallow suctioning. Deep suctioning is when the catheter is inserted until resistance is met and then withdrawn approximately 1 cm before applying suction. Shallow suctioning is when the catheter is advanced to a predetermined depth, which is usually the length of the airway plus the adapter.[2] Using shallow suctioning rather than deep suctioning is recommended in infants and children.[3]

Step 1: Assess Patient for Indications.

Generally, a patient should never be suctioned according to a preset schedule. Although very thick secretions may not move with airflow and may not create any adventitious sounds, the patient should be assessed for clinical indicators, such as rhonchi heard on auscultation, which suggest the need for suctioning (see Clinical Practice Guideline 36-1).

Step 2: Assemble and Check Equipment.

The equipment needed for endotracheal suctioning is listed in Box 36-1. The suction catheter, gloves, and cup are often prepackaged together in disposable sterile kits for use during the open suctioning technique. The AARC Clinical Practice Guideline suggests the closed suctioning technique to avoid disconnecting the patient from the ventilator, which interrupts ventilation and exposes the patient to infection risk. Suction pressure should always be checked by occluding the end of the suction tubing before attaching the suction catheter. The suction pressure should be set at the lowest effective level. Negative pressures of 80 to 100 mm Hg in neonates and less than 150 mm Hg in adults are generally recommended.[4]

Suction catheters are available in various designs, most with side ports to minimize mucosal damage. Most suction catheters for adult general purposes are 22 inches long (sufficient to reach the main stem bronchi) and sized in French units (external circumference). A curved-tip catheter, or catheter coudé, is available to help direct access to the left main stem bronchus. The size of the catheter may be more important than its design. A catheter that is too large can obstruct part or all of the airway by occupying too much of its opening. Too large a suction catheter combined with negative pressure quickly evacuates lung volume and can cause atelectasis and hypoxemia. To avoid this problem, the diameter of the catheter should be less than 50% of the internal diameter of the artificial airway in adults.[5,6] In infants and small children, the diameter of the suction catheter should be less than 70% of the internal diameter of the artificial airway.[7]

Box 36-1 Equipment Needed for Suctioning

- Vacuum source
- Calibrated, adjustable regulator
- Collection bottle and connecting tubing
- Disposable gloves: sterile (open suction) or clean (closed suction)
- Sterile suction catheter
- Sterile water and cup (open suction), if needed to clear catheter
- Goggles, mask, and other appropriate equipment for standard precautions
- Oxygen (O_2) source with a calibrated flowmeter (open suction) or ventilator (closed suction)
- Pulse oximeter
- Manual resuscitation bag equipped with O_2-enrichment device for emergency backup use
- Stethoscope

OPTIONAL EQUIPMENT

- Electrocardiograph
- Sterile sputum trap for culture specimen

RULE OF THUMB

To estimate quickly the proper size of suction catheter to use with a given tracheal tube, first multiply the tube's inner diameter by 2. Then use the next smallest size catheter.

Example: 6-mm endotracheal tube: $2 \times 6 = 12$; next smallest catheter is 10F

Example: 8-mm endotracheal tube: $2 \times 8 = 16$; next smallest catheter is 14F

An in-line suction catheter can be used for patients receiving ventilatory support (Figure 36-3). These systems are incorporated directly into the ventilator circuit and used repeatedly. Because this system allows suctioning without disconnecting the patient from the ventilator, it is recommended for suctioning patients who require high fractional inspired oxygen (FiO_2) and positive end-expiratory pressure (PEEP), who are at risk for lung derecruitment, and for neonates.[8-10] In addition, cross contamination is less likely with such systems. The use of in-line suction catheters has been shown to be cost-effective because they need to be changed only if soiled or malfunctioning and not on a daily basis.[11] However, in-line suction catheters have not been shown either to increase or to decrease the risk for ventilator-associated pneumonia (VAP).[12] The extra weight an in-line catheter adds to a ventilator circuit may increase tension on the endotracheal tube (ETT), so care should be taken to support the ventilator tubing appropriately.

Basic indications for the use of closed suction catheters are listed in Box 36-2.[13] Routine instillation of sterile normal saline to aid secretion removal before suctioning is not recommended because there is insufficient evidence that this practice is beneficial, and it may increase infection risk (see Hazards and Complications in Clinical Practice Guideline 36-1). If the secretions are extremely tenacious, instillation of acetylcysteine or sodium bicarbonate (2%) may be more effective than normal saline; this generally requires a physician's order. The use of these medications is discussed in more detail in Chapter 35.

After connecting the catheter to the suction source, the level of suction pressure should be checked by closing the

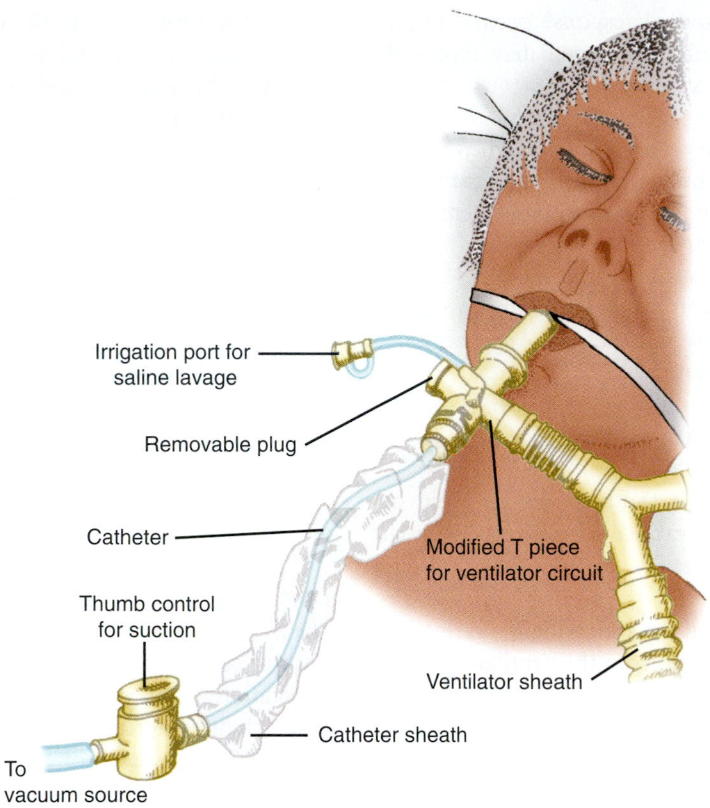

FIGURE 36-3 In-line, closed-system multiuse suction catheter. (Modified from Sills JR: The comprehensive respiratory therapist exam review, entry and advanced levels, ed 5, St. Louis, 2010, Mosby.)

Box 36-2 Indications for Use of Closed Suctioning Technique

Mechanically ventilated patients, especially neonates and patients with:
- Positive end expiratory pressure ≥10 cm H_2O
- Mean airway pressure ≥20 cm H_2O
- Inspiratory time ≥1.5 seconds
- FiO_2 ≥0.60
- Frequent suctioning (≥6 times/day)
- Hemodynamic instability associated with ventilator disconnection
- Respiratory infections requiring airborne or droplet precautions (see Chapter 4)
- Inhaled agents that cannot be interrupted by ventilator disconnection (e.g., nitric oxide, helium/oxygen mixture)

catheter thumb port and aspirating some sterile water or saline from the basin. If no vacuum is generated, it is necessary to check for leaks in the tubing, at the collection container, or at the suction regulator. In addition, if the collecting bottle is full, the float-valve closes and prevents vacuum transmission.

RULE OF THUMB

Set suction pressure 120 to150 mm Hg for adults, 100 to 120 mm Hg for children, and 80 to 100 mm Hg for infants.

Step 3: Assess Patient for Hyperoxygenation.

Before suctioning, delivery of 100% oxygen (O_2) for 30 to 60 seconds to pediatric and adult patients is suggested, especially to patients who are at risk for hypoxemia. Also, the O_2 concentration should be increased by 10% in neonates before suctioning[14]; this may be done by increasing the set FiO_2 or activating the temporary 100% setting on microprocessor ventilators. Manual ventilation is not recommended because it is sometimes difficult to deliver 100% O_2 this way and high pressure potentially causing lung injury can inadvertently be applied.[15] However, if there is no other alternative to hyperoxygenate the patient, PEEP should be maintained by adding a PEEP valve to the manual resuscitator during manual ventilation with 100% O_2.

Step 4: Insert Catheter.

To prevent tracheal mucosal trauma, especially in infants, the shallow suction method should be used, advancing the catheter just to the end of the artificial airway as recommended in the AARC guidelines.

Step 5: Apply Suction and Clear Catheter.

Suction is applied while withdrawing the catheter. Total suction time should be kept to less than 15 seconds.[16,17] After removing the catheter, it should be cleared using a sterile cup filled with sterile water or saline. The closed suction catheter has an adapter for saline vials to be placed in line with the device. The catheter is cleared by squeezing the saline vial and applying suction at the same time. Caution must be used to ensure saline is being drawn into the catheter and not down the airway. If any untoward response occurs during suctioning, the catheter should be immediately removed, and the patient should be oxygenated.

Step 6: Reoxygenate Patient.

The patient should be hyperoxygenated by the same method used in Step 3 for at least 1 minute. Routine hyperventilation is not recommended. If there are indications of derecruitment, lung recruitment maneuvers may be used.

Step 7: Monitor Patient and Assess Outcomes.

Steps 3 through 7 are repeated as needed until improvement is seen or an adverse response is observed. Any necessary corrective steps should be taken.

Minimizing Complications and Adverse Responses

Careful adherence to procedure is the best way to avoid or minimize complications of endotracheal suctioning. Potential complications are as follows:

- Hypoxemia
  - Minimized by preoxygenating the patient, preferably without disconnecting patient from the ventilator.[18]
  - Minimized by using closed suction technique, especially in neonates and adults requiring high FiO_2 or PEEP, or both or at risk for lung derecruitment.
- Cardiac dysrhythmias
  - Bradycardia may occur secondary to vagal nerve stimulation.
  - Tachycardia may occur as a result of agitation and/or hypoxemia.
  - If either occurs, stop suctioning, administer O_2 and ventilation, and notify the nurse and physician.
- Hypotension or hypertension
  - May occur as a result of cardiac dysrhythmia, hypoxemia, anxiety, stress, pain, or coughing.
  - If either occurs, stop suctioning, administer O_2 and ventilation, and notify the nurse and physician.
- Atelectasis (collapse of alveoli)/lung derecruitment
  - Limit amount of negative suction pressure used (see Rule of Thumb).
  - Keep duration of suctioning less than 15 seconds.
  - Use appropriate-size catheter (see Rule of Thumb).
  - Avoid disconnection from ventilator by using closed suction technique, especially in neonates and adults who require high FiO_2 or PEEP.
- Mucosal trauma
  - Limit amount of negative suction pressure used (see Rule of Thumb).
  - Use shallow suctioning method.
- Increased intracranial pressure (ICP)
  - Usually transient and returns to baseline within 1 minute.
  - For patients who already have increased ICP, administer aerosolized topical anesthetic (lidocaine) 15 minutes before suction to minimize cough, discomfort, and increased ICP.[19]
- Bacterial colonization of lower airway
  - Use sterile technique during open suctioning.
  - Do not routinely instill normal saline; only instill normal saline to help mobilize very thick secretions.
  - Use closed suction technique to avoid disconnection from ventilator.

RULE OF THUMB

To minimize hypoxemia and lung derecruitment when suctioning a mechanically ventilated patient, preoxygenate and suction the artificial airway with a closed-system in-line catheter to avoid disconnecting the patient from the ventilator.

Nasotracheal Suctioning

Nasotracheal suctioning is indicated for patients who have retained secretions but do not have an artificial airway.

Clinical Practice Guideline

The AARC has published a clinical practice guideline on nasotracheal suctioning to guide practitioners in safe and effective application of this procedure. Excerpts from the AARC guideline, including indications, contraindications, hazards and complications, assessment of need, assessment of outcome, and monitoring, appear in Clinical Practice Guideline 36-2.[20]

Equipment and Procedure

The equipment and procedure for nasotracheal suctioning are similar to the equipment and procedure for endotracheal suctioning. Only the key differences are highlighted here. In addition to the equipment and supplies used for endotracheal suctioning (see Box 36-1), sterile water-soluble lubricating jelly is needed to aid catheter passage through the nose. Use of a nasopharyngeal airway should be considered to help reduce mucosal trauma in the nose of patients who require repeated, long-term nasotracheal suctioning.

The key aspect of the nasotracheal suctioning procedure is catheter insertion. After lubricating the catheter, the RT inserts it gently through the nostril, directing it toward the septum and floor of the nasal cavity, without applying negative pressure. The catheter is gently twisted if any resistance in the nose is felt. If twisting does not help, the catheter is withdrawn and inserted through the other nostril.

As the catheter enters the lower pharynx, the patient should assume a "sniffing" position (Figure 36-4). This position helps align the opening of the larynx with the lower pharynx, making catheter passage through the larynx more likely. The catheter is continually advanced until the patient coughs or a resistance is felt.

Minimizing Complications and Adverse Responses

Complications of nasotracheal suctioning are as follows:

- Gagging and/or regurgitation
  - To minimize this risk, avoid suctioning soon after a meal or tube feeding; coordinate with nurse.

36-2 Nasotracheal Suctioning

AARC Clinical Practice Guideline (Excerpts)*

INDICATIONS

- Need to maintain a patent airway and remove saliva, pulmonary secretions, blood, vomitus, or foreign material from the trachea in the presence of inability to clear secretions when audible or visible evidence of secretions in the large or central airways that persist despite patient's best cough effort, as evidenced by one or more of the following:
  - Visible secretions in airway
  - Chest auscultation of coarse, gurgling breath sounds, rhonchi, or diminished breath sounds
  - Feeling of secretions in the chest (increased tactile fremitus)
  - Suspected aspiration of gastric or upper airway secretions
  - Clinically apparent increased work of breathing
  - Deterioration of arterial blood gas values suggesting hypoxemia or hypercarbia
  - Chest radiographic evidence of retained secretions resulting in atelectasis or consolidation
  - Restlessness
- Stimulate cough or for unrelieved coughing
- Obtain a sputum sample for microbiologic or cytologic analysis

CONTRAINDICATIONS

Listed contraindications are relative unless noted to be absolute.

- Occluded nasal passages
- Nasal bleeding
- Epiglottitis or croup—absolute
- Acute head, facial, or neck injury
- Coagulopathy or bleeding disorder
- Laryngospasm
- Irritable airway
- Upper respiratory tract infection
- Tracheal surgery
- Gastric surgery with high anastomosis
- Myocardial infarction
- Bronchospasm

HAZARDS AND COMPLICATIONS

- Mechanical trauma
- Laceration of nasal turbinates
- Perforation of pharynx
- Nasal irritation or bleeding
- Tracheitis
- Mucosal hemorrhage
- Edema of uvula
- Hypoxia or hypoxemia
- Cardiac dysrhythmias or arrest
- Bradycardia
- Increased blood pressure
- Hypotension
- Respiratory arrest
- Uncontrolled coughing
- Gagging or vomiting
- Laryngospasm
- Bronchoconstriction or bronchospasm
- Discomfort and pain
- Nosocomial infection
- Atelectasis
- Misdirection of the catheter
- Increased intracranial pressure
- Intraventricular hemorrhage
- Exacerbation of cerebral edema
- Pneumothorax

ASSESSMENT OF NEED

Personnel should perform a baseline assessment for indications of respiratory distress and the need, as recognized by the previously listed presenting indications. This assessment should include but not be limited to the following:

- Auscultation of the chest
- Monitoring of heart rate
- Assessment of respiratory rate
- Assessment of cardiac rhythm
- Assessment of O_2 saturation
- Assessment of skin color and perfusion
- Assessment of effectiveness of cough

Prepare the patient for the procedure by providing an appropriate explanation along with adequate sedation and pain relief as needed.

ASSESSMENT OF OUTCOME

Assess the patient after suction for the following:

- Improved breath sounds
- Removal of secretions
- Improved blood gas data or pulse oximetry
- Decreased work of breathing (decreased respiratory rate or dyspnea)

MONITORING

The following should be monitored before, during, and after the procedure:

- Breath sounds
- Skin color
- Breathing pattern and rate
- Pulse rate, dysrhythmia, electrocardiogram if available
- Color, consistency, and volume of secretions
- Presence of bleeding or evidence of physical trauma
- Subjective response, including pain
- Oxygenation (pulse oximeter)
- Intracranial pressure, if equipment is available
- Arterial blood pressure, if available
- Laryngospasm

For complete guidelines, see American Association for Respiratory Care: Clinical practice guideline: nasotracheal suctioning—2004 revision and update. Respir Care 49:1080, 2004.

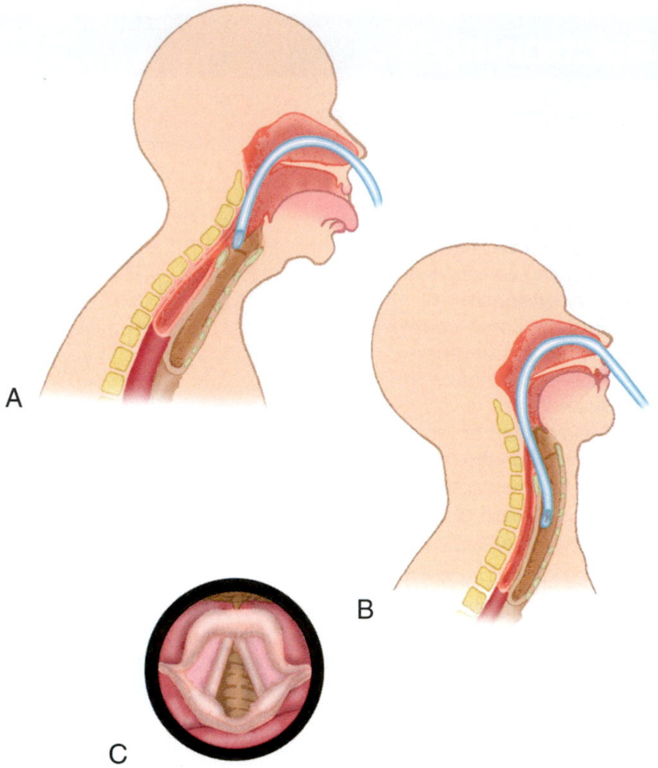

FIGURE 36-4 Nasotracheal suctioning technique. **A,** Optimal position of the head to insert catheter into the trachea. The neck is flexed, and the head is extended. The tongue is protruded (and held by a 4 × 4 gauze pad). **B,** After catheter has advanced into the trachea, the tongue is released, and the patient's head is allowed to assume a comfortable position. **C,** View of vocal cords from above. The cords are most widely separated during inspiration. (Modified from Sanderson RG: The cardiac patient: a comprehensive approach, Philadelphia, 1972, Saunders.)

- If this occurs, reposition patient and suction oropharynx if necessary.

- Airway trauma (bleeding)
  - To avoid, before suctioning, assess patient for any bleeding disorder (check platelet count and/or bleeding studies and anticoagulation medications) before suctioning.
  - To minimize, do not use excessive force when advancing catheter.
  - To minimize, lubricate catheter.
  - To minimize, use nasopharyngeal airway to protect nasal mucosa.
- Contamination of the lungs
  - Immunosuppressed patients are especially at risk.
  - To avoid, use sterile technique and gentle insertion of catheter.
- Bronchospasm or laryngospasm
  - These incidents may be stimulated by the catheter in the lower airway.
  - Patients with hyperactive airway disease are especially at risk.
  - If these occur, stop suctioning and administer aerosolized bronchodilator if needed.

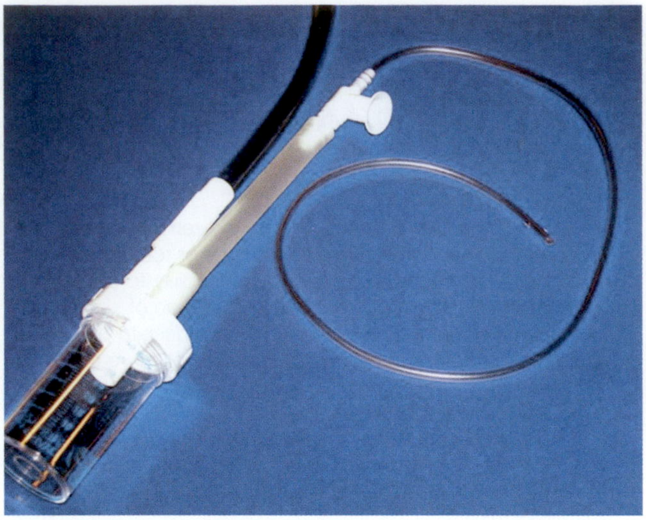

FIGURE 36-5 Specimen container placement between the suction catheter and wall suction source.

Sputum Sampling

Sputum samples are often collected to identify organisms infecting the airway. To obtain the samples, the suctioning procedures described previously should be followed. In addition to the usual equipment, a sterile specimen container is needed. This device consists of a plastic tube or cup with flexible tubing on one end to attach to the suction catheter. The other outlet is a stiff plastic nozzle that connects to the suction tubing from the wall vacuum unit (Figure 36-5).

It is important to maintain sterile technique when touching the connection points on the trap. If a closed suction system is being used, a new catheter should be placed just before suctioning the patient for the sample. When an adequate sample is obtained, the container is removed from the suction catheter and suction tubing. The flexible tubing on the container is attached to the open nozzle; this creates a closed container. The container should be labeled according to hospital or facility policy. The suctioning procedure is completed as previously described.

ESTABLISHING AN ARTIFICIAL AIRWAY

Clinical Practice Guideline

An artificial airway is required when the patient's natural airway can no longer perform its proper functions. To guide practitioners in the identification, assessment, and treatment of patients requiring artificial airways, the AARC has developed a clinical practice guideline on management of airway emergencies. Excerpts from the AARC guideline, including indications; contraindications; precautions, hazards, and possible complications; assessment of need and outcome; and monitoring, appear in Clinical Practice Guideline 36-3.[21]

36-3 Management of Airway Emergencies

AARC Clinical Practice Guideline (Excerpts)*

INDICATIONS

In general, conditions requiring management of the airway are impending or actual (1) airway compromise, (2) respiratory failure, and (3) need to protect the airway. Specific conditions include but are not limited to the following:

- Airway emergency before endotracheal intubation
- Obstruction of the artificial airway
- Apnea
- Acute traumatic coma
- Penetrating neck trauma
- Cardiopulmonary arrest and unstable dysrhythmias
- Severe bronchospasm
- Severe allergic reactions with cardiopulmonary compromise
- Pulmonary edema
- Sedative/narcotic drug effect
- Foreign body obstruction
- Choanal atresia in neonates
- Aspiration
- Risk for aspiration
- Severe laryngospasm
- Self-extubation

Conditions requiring emergency tracheal intubation include but are not limited to:

- Persistent apnea
- Traumatic upper airway obstruction
- Accidental extubation of a patient unable to maintain adequate spontaneous ventilation
- Obstructive angioedema
- Massive uncontrolled upper airway bleeding
- Infection-related upper airway obstruction (partial or complete)
  - Epiglottitis in children or adults
  - Acute uvular edema
  - Tonsillopharyngitis or retropharyngeal abscess
  - Suppurative parotitis
- Coma with potential for increased intracranial pressure
- Neonatal- or pediatric-specific conditions
  - Perinatal asphyxia
  - Severe adenotonsillar hypertrophy
  - Severe laryngomalacia
  - Bacterial tracheitis
  - Neonatal epignathus
  - Obstruction from abnormal laryngeal closure owing to arytenoid masses
  - Mediastinal tumors
  - Congenital diaphragmatic hernia
  - Presence of thick or particulate meconium in amniotic fluid
  - Absence of airway protective reflexes
  - Cardiopulmonary arrest
  - Massive hemoptysis

A patient in whom airway control is not possible by other methods may require surgical placement of an airway (needle or surgical cricothyrotomy).

Conditions in which endotracheal intubation may be impossible and in which alternative techniques may be used include but are not limited to the following:

- Restriction of endotracheal intubation by policy or statute
- Difficult or failed intubation in the presence of risk factors associated with difficult tracheal intubations such as:
  - Short neck or bull neck
  - Protruding maxillary incisors
  - Receding mandible
  - Reduced mobility of atlantooccipital joint
  - Temporomandibular ankylosis
  - Congenital oropharyngeal wall stenosis
  - Anterior osteophytes of the cervical vertebrae, associated with diffuse idiopathic skeletal hyperostosis
  - Large substernal or cancerous goiters
  - Treacher Collins syndrome
  - Morquio-Brailsford syndrome
  - Endolaryngeal tumors
  - When endotracheal intubation is not immediately possible

CONTRAINDICATIONS

Aggressive airway management (intubation or establishment of a surgical airway) may be contraindicated when the patient's desire not to be resuscitated has been clearly expressed and documented in the patient's medical record or other valid legal document.

PRECAUTIONS, HAZARDS, AND COMPLICATIONS

Possible hazards or complications related to the major facets of management of airway emergencies include the following:

- Failure to establish a patent airway
- Failure to intubate the trachea
- Failure to recognize intubation of esophagus
- Upper airway trauma, laryngeal, and esophageal damage
- Aspiration
- Cervical spine trauma
- Unrecognized bronchial intubation
- Eye injury
- Vocal cord paralysis
- Problems with endotracheal tubes
  - Cuff perforation
  - Cuff herniation
  - Pilot-tube-valve incompetence
  - Tube kinking during biting
  - Inadvertent extubation
  - Tube occlusion
  - Bronchospasm
  - Laryngospasm
  - Dental accidents
  - Dysrhythmias
  - Hypotension and bradycardia secondary to vagal stimulation
  - Hypertension and tachycardia
  - Inappropriate tube size
  - Bleeding
  - Mouth ulceration
- Nasal intubation specific
  - Nasal damage, including epistaxis
  - Tube kinking in pharynx
  - Sinusitis and otitis media

Continued

AARC Clinical Practice Guideline (Excerpts)*

- Tongue ulceration
- Tracheal damage, including tracheoesophageal fistula, tracheal innominate fistula, tracheal stenosis, and tracheomalacia
- Pneumonia
- Laryngeal damage with consequent laryngeal stenosis, laryngeal ulcer, granuloma, polyps, synechiae

- Surgical cricothyrotomy or tracheostomy specific
  - Stomal stenosis
  - Innominate erosion
- Needle cricothyrotomy specific
  - Bleeding at insertion site with hematoma formation
  - Subcutaneous and mediastinal emphysema
  - Esophageal perforation
  - Emergency ventilation
  - Inadequate O_2 delivery
  - Hypoventilation or hyperventilation
  - Gastric insufflation or rupture
  - Barotrauma
  - Hypotension owing to reduced venous return secondary to high mean intrathoracic pressure
  - Vomiting and aspiration
  - Prolonged interruption of ventilation for intubation
  - Failure to establish adequate functional residual capacity in a newborn
  - Movement of unstable cervical spine (more than by any commonly used method of endotracheal intubation)
  - Failure to exhale owing to upper airway obstruction during percutaneous transtracheal ventilation

ASSESSMENT OF NEED

The need for airway management is dictated by the clinical condition of the patient. Careful observation, implementation of basic airway management techniques, and laboratory and clinical data should help determine the need for more aggressive measures. Specific conditions requiring intervention include the following:

- Inability to protect airway adequately (e.g., coma, lack of gag reflex, inability to cough) with or without other signs of respiratory distress.
- Partially obstructed airway. Signs of a partially obstructed upper airway include ineffective patient efforts to ventilate, paradoxical respiration, stridor, use of accessory muscles, patient pointing to neck, choking motions, cyanosis, and distress. Signs of lower airway obstruction may include the above-mentioned signs and wheezing.
- Complete airway obstruction. Respiratory efforts with no breath sounds or suggestion of air movement are indicative of complete obstruction.
- Apnea. No respiratory efforts are seen; may be associated with cardiac arrest.
- Hypoxemia, hypercarbia, or acidemia seen on arterial blood gas analysis, oximetry, or exhaled gas analysis.
- Respiratory distress. Elevated respiratory rate, high or low ventilatory volumes, and signs of sympathetic nervous system hyperactivity may be associated with respiratory distress.

ASSESSMENT OF PROCESS AND OUTCOME

Timely intervention to maintain the patient's airway can improve outcomes. Under rare circumstances, maintenance of an airway by nonsurgical means may be impossible. Despite optimal airway maintenance, outcomes are affected by patient-specific factors. Lack of appropriate equipment and personnel may adversely affect outcomes. Monitoring and recording can help improve emergency airway management. Some aspects (e.g., frequency of complications of tracheal intubations or time to establishment of a definitive airway) are easy to quantify and can help improve hospital-wide systems. The patient's condition after the emergency should be evaluated from this perspective.

MONITORING

Clinical Signs

Continuous patient observation and repeated clinical assessment by a trained observer provide optimal monitoring of the airway. Special consideration should be given to the following:

- Level of consciousness
- Presence and character of breath sounds
- Ease of ventilation
- Symmetry and amount of chest movement
- Skin color and character (temperature and presence or absence of diaphoresis)
- Presence of upper airway sounds (crowing, snoring, stridor)
- Presence of excessive secretions, blood, vomitus, or foreign objects in the airway
- Presence of epigastric sounds
- Presence of retractions
- Presence of nasal flaring

Physiologic Variables

Repeated assessment of physiologic data by trained professionals supplements clinical assessment in managing patients with airway difficulties. Monitoring devices should be available, accessible, functional, and periodically evaluated for function. These data include but are not limited to:

- Ventilatory frequency, tidal volume, and airway pressure
- Presence of CO_2 in exhaled gas
- Heart rate and rhythm
- Pulse oximetry
- Arterial blood gas values
- Chest radiograph

Endotracheal Tube Position

Regardless of the method of ventilation used, the most important consideration is detection of esophageal intubation.

- Tracheal intubation is suggested but may not be confirmed by:
  - Bilateral breath sounds over the chest
  - Symmetric chest movement
  - Absence of ventilation sounds over the epigastrium
  - Presence of condensate inside the tube, corresponding with exhalation
  - Visualization of the tip of the tube passing through the vocal cords
  - Esophageal detector devices may be useful in differentiating esophageal from tracheal intubation
- Tracheal intubation is confirmed by detection of CO_2 in the exhaled gas, although cases of transient CO_2 excretion from the stomach have been reported.
- Tracheal intubation is confirmed by endoscopic visualization of the carina or tracheal rings through the tube.
- Position of the endotracheal tube (i.e., depth of insertion) should be appropriate on chest radiograph.

AIRWAY MANAGEMENT PROCESS

A properly managed airway may improve patient outcome. Continuous evaluation of the process identifies components needing improvement. These include response time, equipment function, equipment availability, practitioner performance, complication rate, and patient survival and functional status.

**For complete guidelines, see American Association for Respiratory Care: Clinical practice guideline: management of airway emergencies. Respir Care 40:749, 1995.*

Routes

Artificial airways are inserted for various reasons and involve varying degrees of invasion into the upper airway. **Pharyngeal airways** extend only into the pharynx. Artificial airways that are placed through the mouth or nose into the trachea are called **endotracheal tubes (ETTs).** The process of placing an artificial airway into the trachea is referred to as **intubation.** When the ETT is passed through the nose first, the procedure is referred to as *nasotracheal intubation*. When the tube is passed through the mouth on its way into the trachea, the procedure is called *orotracheal intubation*.

Pharyngeal Airways

Pharyngeal airways prevent airway obstruction by keeping the tongue pulled forward and away from the posterior pharynx. This type of obstruction is common in an unconscious patient as a result of a loss of muscle tone.

A *nasopharyngeal airway* (Figure 36-6) is most often placed in a patient who requires frequent nasotracheal suctioning. Although it does not ensure entry into the trachea, it minimizes damage to the nasal mucosa that can be caused by the suction catheter. A nasopharyngeal airway also may be placed in a patient who was recently extubated after facial surgery. The nasopharyngeal airway helps maintain the patency of the upper airway despite swelling.

Oropharyngeal airways (see Figure 36-6) are inserted into the mouth over the tongue. Use of oropharyngeal airways should be restricted to unconscious patients to avoid gagging and regurgitation. These airways maintain a patent airway when the tongue would otherwise obstruct the oropharynx. The airway also can be used as a bite block for patients with oral tubes.

Pharyngeal airways are used mainly in emergency life support. Further details on their use, insertion techniques, and size selection are provided in Chapter 37.

Tracheal Airways

Tracheal airways extend beyond the pharynx into the trachea. The two basic types of tracheal airways are *endotracheal (translaryngeal) tubes* and *tracheostomy tubes*. ETTs are inserted through either the mouth or the nose (orotracheal or nasotracheal), through the larynx, and into the trachea. **Tracheostomy tubes** (TTs) are inserted through a surgically created opening in the neck directly into the trachea. Table 36-1 summarizes the advantages and disadvantages of each of these three approaches.

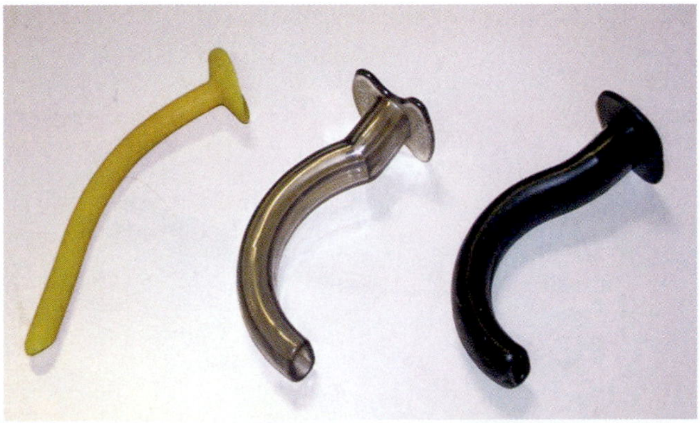

FIGURE 36-6 Pharyngeal airways. **A,** Nasopharyngeal airway. **B** and **C,** Oropharyngeal airways.

Airway Tubes

Endotracheal Tubes

ETTs are semi-rigid tubes most often composed of polyvinyl chloride or related plastic polymers.[22] Figure 36-7 shows a typical ETT, its key components, and a stylet used for insertion. The proximal end of the tube is attached to a standard adapter with a 15-mm external diameter. The curved body of the tube usually has length markings, indicating the distance (in centimeters) from the beveled tube tip. In addition to the beveled opening at the tip, there is a side port, or "Murphy eye," that ensures gas flow if the main port should become obstructed. The angle of the bevel minimizes mucosal trauma during insertion. The tube cuff is permanently bonded to the tube body. Inflation of the cuff seals off the lower airway, either for protection from gross aspiration or to provide positive pressure ventilation. A small filling tube leads from the cuff to a pilot balloon, used to monitor cuff status and pressure when the tube is in place. Finally, a valve with a standard connector for a syringe allows inflation and deflation of the cuff. Although not shown in Figure 36-7, included with most modern ETTs is a **radiopaque** indicator that is embedded in the distal end of the tube body. This indicator allows for easy identification of tube position on the radiograph.

Specialized Endotracheal Tubes. Some standard ETTs have been modified for specific uses, including special ventilation methods, lung pathologic conditions, and surgical procedures. Some more common tubes, including double-lumen

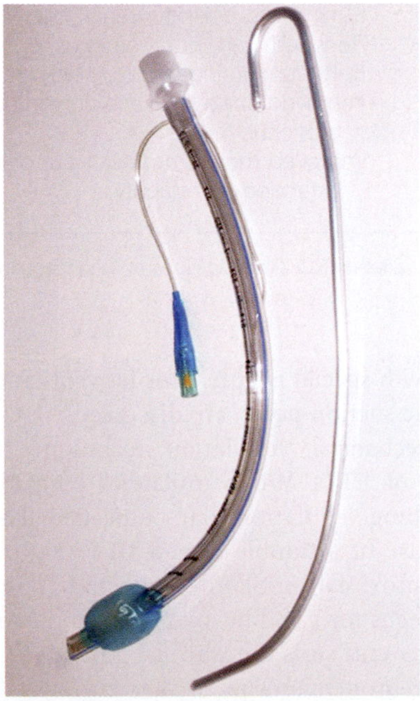

FIGURE 36-7 Typical endotracheal tube and stylet.

TABLE 36-1
Advantages and Disadvantages of Tracheal Airway Routes

Route	Advantages	Disadvantages
Oral intubation	Insertion is faster, easier, less traumatic, and more comfortable Larger tube is tolerated Easier suctioning Less airflow resistance Decreased work of breathing Easier passage of bronchoscope Reduced risk for tube kinking Avoidance of nasal and paranasal complications, including epistaxis and sinusitis	Esthetically displeasing, especially long term Greater risk for self-extubation or inadvertent extubation Greater risk for main stem intubation Risk of tube occlusion by biting or trismus Risk of injury to lips, teeth, tongue, palate, and oral soft tissues May require additional use of oral airway Great risk for retching, vomiting, and aspiration Pain and discomfort, especially with inadequate preparation
Nasal intubation	Less retching and gagging Greater comfort in long-term use Less salivation Improved ability to swallow oral secretions Improved communication Improved mouth care and oral hygiene Avoidance of occlusion by biting or trismus Easier nursing care Avoidance of oral route complications Less posterior laryngeal ulceration Better tube anchoring, less chance of inadvertent extubation Reduced risk for main stem intubation Some patients can swallow liquids, providing a means of nutritional support Blind nasal intubation does not require muscle relaxants or sedatives May avert "crash" oral intubation	Nasal and paranasal complications, including epistaxis, sinusitis, otitis More difficult to perform Spontaneous breathing required for blind nasal intubation Smaller tube is necessary Greater suctioning difficulty Increased airflow resistance Increased work of breathing Difficulty passing bronchoscope Smaller risk for transient bacteremia
Tracheotomy	Avoidance of laryngeal and upper airway complications of translaryngeal intubation Greater comfort Aids feeding, oral care, suctioning, speech Psychologic benefit (improved motivation) Easier passage of fiberoptic bronchoscope Easier reinsertion Esthetically less objectionable Facilitation of weaning from ventilator Elimination of risk for main stem intubation Reduced work of breathing Better anchoring (reduced risk for decannulation) Improved ability to place curve-tipped suction catheter in left bronchus Improved mobility (transfer out of intensive care unit to ward or extended-care facility)	Greater expense Requirement for use of operating room in most cases Need for general anesthesia in most cases Permanent scar More severe complications Greater mortality rate Delayed decannulation Increased frequency of aspiration Greater bacterial colonization rate Persistent open stoma after decannulation, reducing cough efficiency

From Stauffer JL, Silvestri RC: Complications and consequences of endotracheal intubation and tracheostomy. Respir Care 27:417, 1982.

tubes, tubes with special adapters for jet ventilation, and tubes with subglottic suction ports, are discussed.[23]

Special mechanical ventilation techniques may require unique types of ETTs. When unilateral lung disease occurs, independent lung ventilation may be needed. This ventilation requires the use of a double-lumen ETT (Figure 36-8). This tube has two proximal ventilator connectors (15-mm adapter), two inner lumens for gas flow, two cuffs, and two distal openings. The larger cuff seals the tracheal lumen and allows gas to flow into one bronchus. The smaller cuff seals the opposite bronchial lumen (Figure 36-9).

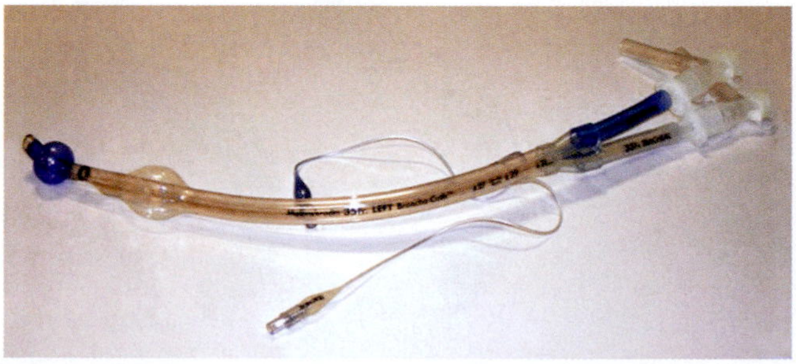

FIGURE 36-8 Double-lumen endotracheal tube for independent lung ventilation.

There are important points to consider when using double-lumen ETTs. These tubes are stiffer and bulkier to insert than standard tubes and must be rotated during insertion to align with the proper bronchus. Fiberoptic bronchoscopy should be performed to ensure proper placement. The resistance to flow through each tube is increased because each lumen is smaller than the same-size single-lumen tubes.

High-frequency jet ventilation uses a special ETT adapter (Figure 36-10). This adapter replaces the standard ETT adapter. There is a jet port for the injection of high-flow pulses from the jet ventilator and a 15-mm connection for conventional ventilation. A pressure monitoring tube also is available for monitoring airway pressures.

A specialized ETT with an attached subglottic suction port has been designed to allow for removal of secretions that often accumulate above the cuff (Figure 36-11). A separate channel in the wall of the tube attaches to a wall suction source. The suction source is run continuously at negative pressures of 20 to 30 cm H_2O. The aspirated material is collected in a small container, which is emptied on a regular basis. Every 4 hours, a small amount of air should be injected into the suction port to ensure the port and tubing are not clogged. Use of this tube has been reported to decrease the incidence of VAP.[24,25]

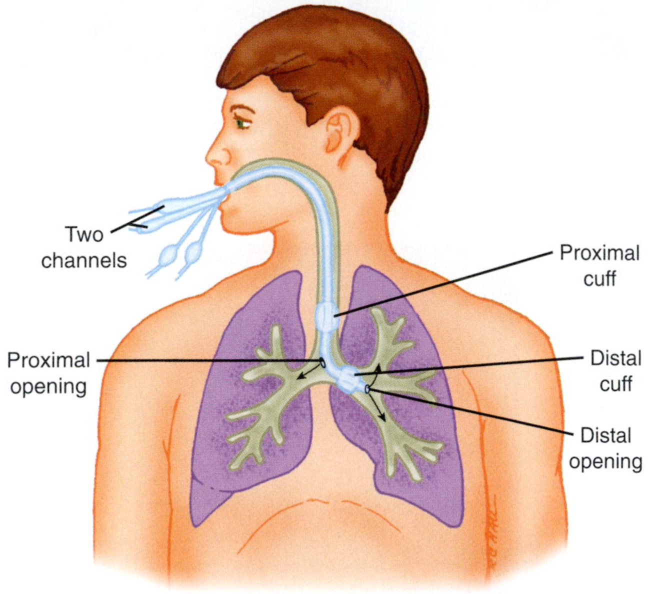

FIGURE 36-9 Correct positioning of double-lumen endotracheal tube.

Tracheostomy Tubes

Tracheostomy tubes are generally made from polyvinyl chloride or silicone, although some are still made from metal.

Figure 36-12 shows a typical tracheostomy tube and its key components. The outer cannula forms the primary structural unit of the tube, to which the cuff and a flange are attached. The flange prevents tube slippage into the trachea and provides the means to secure the tube to the neck. There are single-cannula and double-cannula tracheostomy tubes. The double-cannula tube has a removable inner cannula with a standard 15-mm adapter. It is normally kept in place within the outer cannula. To prevent accidental removal, the inner cannula can be locked in place at the proximal end of the outer cannula. The inner cannula may be disposable or nondisposable. If the tube becomes occluded with very thick secretions or blood clots, the inner cannula can be easily removed and cleaned or replaced to establish a patent airway. This prevents the necessity of emergently changing the entire tracheostomy tube in this situation.

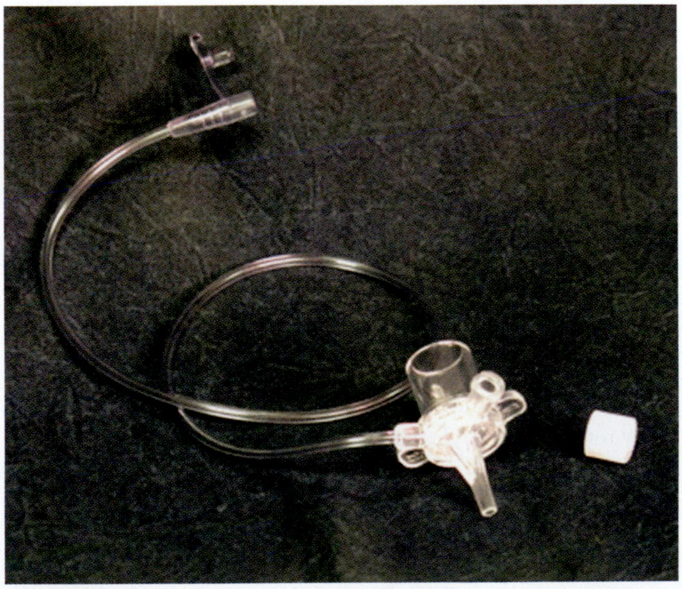
FIGURE 36-10 Endotracheal tube adapter for jet ventilation. LifePort Adapter. (Courtesy Bunnell Incorporated, Salt Lake City, Utah.)

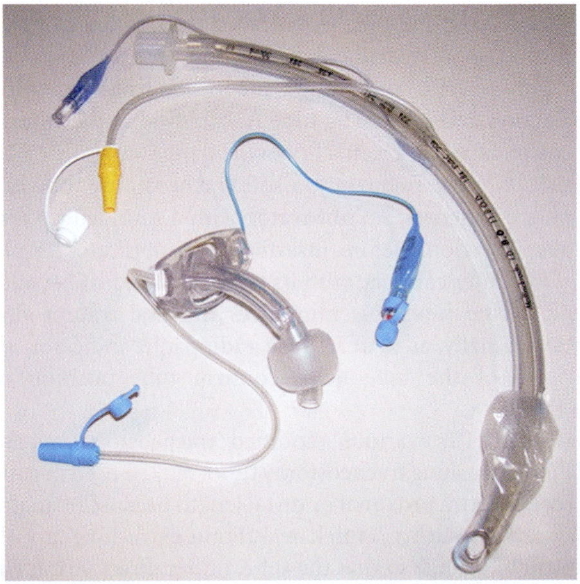
FIGURE 36-11 Endotracheal and tracheostomy tubes with subglottic suction ports.

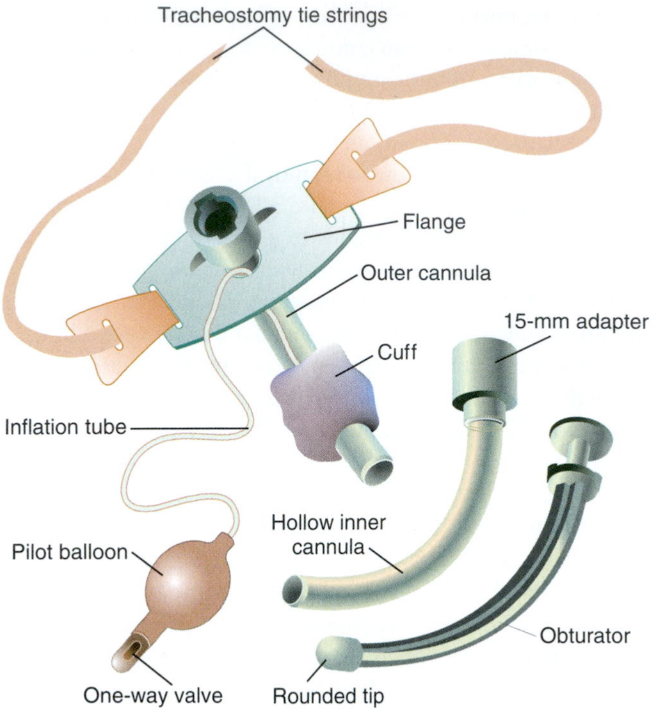

FIGURE 36-12 Parts of a tracheostomy tube.

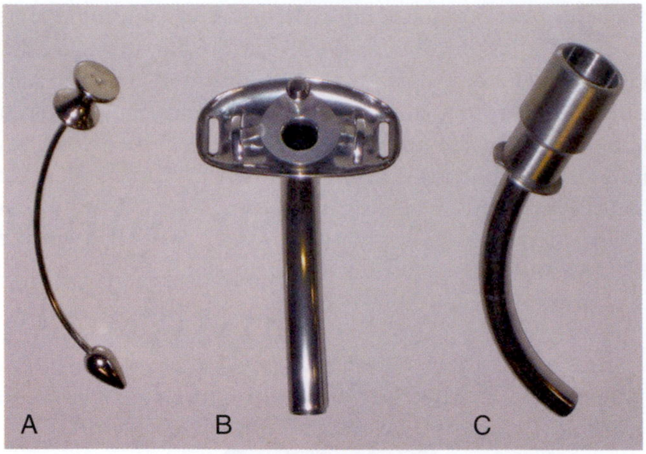

FIGURE 36-13 Jackson tracheostomy tube made from stainless steel. It has no cuff and no 15-mm adapter. **A,** Obturator. **B,** Outer cannula. **C,** Inner cannula.

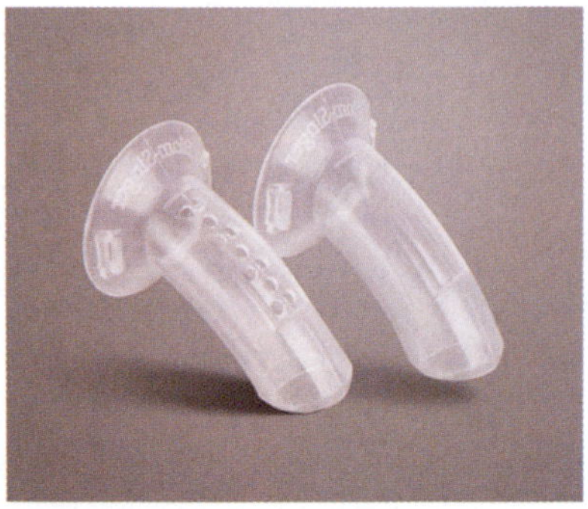

FIGURE 36-14 Laryngectomy tubes.

Double cannula tubes are especially recommended for patients who are going home with a tracheostomy tube or in situations in which the humidity delivered to the airway is less than optimal. However, the inner cannula in some tracheostomy tubes can decrease the inner diameter of the tube, causing some patients to have difficulty breathing through the tube because of the increased airway resistance. In other double-cannula tubes the outer diameter is larger than the outer diameter of the same-size single cannula tube. This can decrease the room around the tube with the cuff deflated so that a patient may not be able to breathe around it with a speaking valve or cap on the tube. In this case the tube would need to be changed to a one with a smaller outer diameter.[26]

As with an ETT, an inflation tube leads from the cuff to a pilot balloon and valve. The tube is stabilized at the stoma site with cotton tape, which attaches to the flange and is tied around the neck or, more frequently, a soft tracheostomy tube holder with Velcro fasteners. An **obturator** with a rounded tip is used for tube insertion. Before insertion, the obturator is placed within the outer cannula, with its tip extending just beyond the far end of the tube; this minimizes mucosal trauma during insertion. Finally, as with ETTs, a radiopaque indicator in the distal end of the tube helps confirm tube position on a radiograph.

As with ETTs, various modified tracheostomy tubes are available. Extra-long tracheostomy tubes may be used in patients who require extra proximal or distal length because of anatomic considerations, such as a thick neck. Some extra-long tubes have an adjustable flange so that the tube, under direct vision with a bronchoscope, can be placed past an abnormality in the trachea, such as a tumor or tracheal stenosis.

The metal Jackson tracheostomy tube is made of stainless steel with an inner and outer cannula (Figure 36-13). There is no cuff at the distal end or 15-mm adapter at the proximal end. This tracheostomy tube is generally used in patients with a long-term need for an airway but who do not require a seal to protect the airway from aspiration or to facilitate positive pressure ventilation. If the patient requires manual ventilation, a 15-mm adapter should be inserted into the proximal opening. If the patient requires a sealed airway, the tube needs to be changed to the standard cuffed tube described earlier. A laryngectomy tube is a shorter tube without a cuff inserted into the stoma after a laryngectomy. The tube keeps the stoma open until it heals. There are several different types, some with a flange that can be secured with a fastener around the patient's neck and some without a flange (low profile). The tube may be easily removed to be cleaned and then reinserted (Figure 36-14).

Procedures

Orotracheal Intubation

Orotracheal intubation is the preferred route for establishing an emergency tracheal airway because the oral passage is the quickest and easiest route in most cases. Orotracheal intubation can be safely performed by an appropriately trained physician, RT, nurse, or paramedic.[27] Typically, this training involves manikin practice and application on anesthetized patients under the guidance of an anesthesiologist or other appropriately skilled individual. The basic steps in orotracheal intubation are described here.[28] Proficiency in this technique can be developed only with extensive training and experience.

Step 1: Assemble and Check Equipment.

Box 36-3 lists the equipment necessary for intubation. All suction equipment is assembled, and the vacuum pressure is checked before intubation because vomitus or secretions may obscure the pharynx or glottis. The appropriate-size laryngoscope blade (see Box 36-3) is attached to its handle, and the light source is checked for secure attachment and brightness. If the light does not function, the bulb first should be checked to see if it is tight. If the scope still does not light, the batteries should be checked or the bulb should be replaced.

An appropriate-size tube should be selected, and other tubes should be available that are at least one size larger and one size smaller. Table 36-2 lists recommended orotracheal tube sizes according to patient weight or age. ETTs are sized by their internal diameter (in millimeters). Tube lengths given in Table 36-2 are averages after insertion, confirmed placement, and fixation (teeth to tube tip).

RULE OF THUMB

Generally, a woman is intubated with a No. 7 or No. 7.5 orotracheal tube and a man is intubated with a No. 8.0 or No. 8.5 orotracheal tube.

After selecting the correct size of tube, the RT inflates the tube cuff and checks for leaks. The RT must be sure to deflate the cuff before insertion. To ease insertion, the outer surface of the tube should be lubricated with a water-soluble gel. Finally, many clinicians insert a stylet into the tube to add rigidity and maintain shape during insertion. The tip of the stylet must never extend beyond the ETT tip.

Step 2: Position Patient.

To visualize the glottis and insert the tube, the RT aligns the patient's mouth, pharynx, and larynx. This alignment is achieved by combining moderate cervical flexion with extension of the atlantooccipital joint. Placement of one or more rolled towels under the patient's shoulders helps. Next the RT flexes the patient's neck and tilts the head backward with his or her hand, placing the patient into the sniff position (Figure 36-15).

Box 36-3 Equipment Needed for Endotracheal Intubation

- Oxygen flowmeter and tubing
- Suction apparatus
- Flexible sterile suction catheters
- Sterile gloves for endotracheal suctioning
- Yankauer (tonsillar) tip suction
- Manual resuscitation bag and mask
- Colorimetric carbon dioxide detector
- Oropharyngeal airways
- Laryngoscope (two) with assorted blades (size 2 or 3 for adults, size 1 or 2 for children, size 0 or 1 for infants)
- Endotracheal tubes (three appropriate sizes)
- Tongue depressor
- Stylet
- Stethoscope
- Tape or endotracheal tube holder
- 10- or 12-ml syringe
- Water-soluble lubricating gel
- Magill forceps
- Local anesthetic (spray)
- Towels (for positioning)
- CDC barrier precautions (gloves, gowns, masks, goggles, or face shields)

CDC, U.S. Centers for Disease Control and Prevention.

TABLE 36-2 Guideline for Infant, Pediatric, and Adult Oral Endotracheal Tube Sizes

Age	Tube Size (mm Internal Diameter)	Distance (in cm) from Incisors (Lip in Infants) to Tip of Tube
Infant, <1 kg	2.5	6.5-8
Infant, 1-2 kg	3.0	7-8
Infant, 2-3 kg	3.5	8-9
Infant, 4 kg	3.5-4.0	9-10
6 mo	3.5-4.0	10-11
18 mo	3.5-4.5	11-13
3 yr	4.5-5.0	12-14
5 yr	4.5-5.0	13-15
6 yr	5.5-6.0	14-16
8 yr	6.0-6.5	15-17
12 yr	6.0-7.0	17-19
16 yr/small women	6.5-7.0	18-20
Women (average)	7.5-8.0	19-21
Men	8.0-9.0	21-23

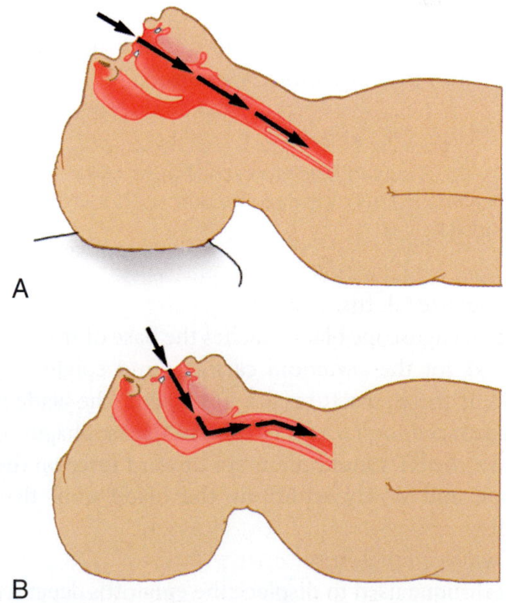

FIGURE 36-15 **A,** Correct head position before intubation. **B,** Incorrect head position before intubation.

MINI CLINI

Indications for Artificial Airway Management

PROBLEM: A woman is admitted to the emergency department after sustaining chest trauma during a motor vehicle accident. The patient is unconscious, cyanotic, and tachypneic and has blood in the mouth and pharynx. Breath sounds are diminished on both sides. The physician requests that the RT immediately perform orotracheal intubation. Why?

DISCUSSION: This patient exhibits several indications for insertion of an artificial airway. First, being unconscious, the patient is probably unable to protect her lower airway adequately. With blood in the mouth and pharynx, there should be increased concern for protecting her lungs from aspiration. The blood also may indicate partial airway obstruction; the breath sounds, cyanosis, and respiratory distress contribute to that conclusion. Finally, the cyanosis and chest trauma indicate potential hypoxemic respiratory failure, which may require positive pressure ventilatory support via a cuffed ETT.

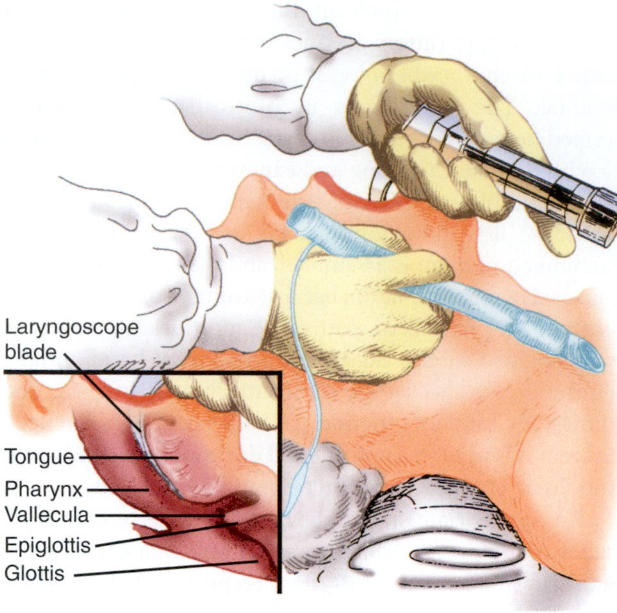

FIGURE 36-16 To achieve orotracheal intubation, the respiratory therapist holds the laryngoscope in the left hand, introduces the blade into the right side of mouth, and displaces the tongue to the left. (Modified from Ellis PD, Billings DM: Cardiopulmonary resuscitation: procedures for basic and advanced life support, St. Louis, 1980, Mosby.)

Step 3: Preoxygenate and Ventilate Patient.

A patient in need of intubation is often apneic or in respiratory distress. Providing ventilation and oxygenation by manual resuscitator bag and mask with 100% O_2 before intubation helps ensure the patient tolerates the intubation procedure. No more than 30 seconds should be devoted to any intubation attempt. If intubation fails, immediate ventilation and oxygenation of the patient for 3 to 5 minutes before the next attempt should occur.

Step 4: Insert Laryngoscope.

The RT should use the left hand to hold the laryngoscope and the right hand to open the mouth (Figure 36-16). The laryngoscope is inserted into the right side of the mouth and moved toward the center, displacing the tongue to the left. The tip of the blade is advanced along the curve of the tongue until the epiglottis is visualized.

RULE OF THUMB

A No. 3 curved Macintosh or straight Miller laryngoscope blade is commonly used to intubate adults.

Step 5: Visualize Glottis.

As the laryngoscope blade reaches the base of the tongue, the RT looks for the arytenoid cartilage and epiglottis (Figure 36-17). If these structures are not visible, the blade is probably advanced too far and may be in the esophagus. If this is the case, the RT should maintain upward force on the laryngoscope and slowly withdraw the blade until the larynx is seen.

Step 6: Displace Epiglottis.

The technique used to displace the epiglottis depends on the type of blade chosen (Figure 36-18). With the curved or MacIntosh blade, the epiglottis is displaced indirectly by advancing the tip of the blade into the vallecula (at the base of the tongue), and the laryngoscope is lifted up and forward (see Figure 36-18, *A*). With the straight or Miller blade, the epiglottis is displaced directly by advancing the tip of the blade over its posterior surface and the laryngoscope is lifted up and forward (see Figure 36-18, *B*).

One should avoid levering the laryngoscope against the teeth while lifting the tip of the blade because this can damage the teeth and gums. This problem can be avoided by keeping the wrist fixed and moving the handle of the laryngoscope in the direction it is pointing when visualizing the epiglottis.

Step 7: Insert Tube.

When the epiglottis is displaced and the glottis is visualized, the tube is inserted from the right side of the mouth and advanced without obscuring the glottic opening (Figure 36-19). When the tube tip is seen passing through the glottis, it is advanced until the cuff has passed the vocal cords. When the tube is in place, the RT stabilizes it with the right hand and uses the left hand to remove the laryngoscope and stylet. The cuff is inflated to seal the airway, and ventilation and oxygenation are immediately provided.

Step 8: Assess Tube Position.

Ideally, the tip of an ETT should be positioned in the trachea about 3 to 6 cm above the carina.[29] One or more of several bedside methods can be used to assess positioning of the ETT before stabilization (Box 36-4). With the exception of fiberoptic laryngoscopy or bronchoscopy and videolaryngoscopy, none of these methods can absolutely confirm proper tube placement.

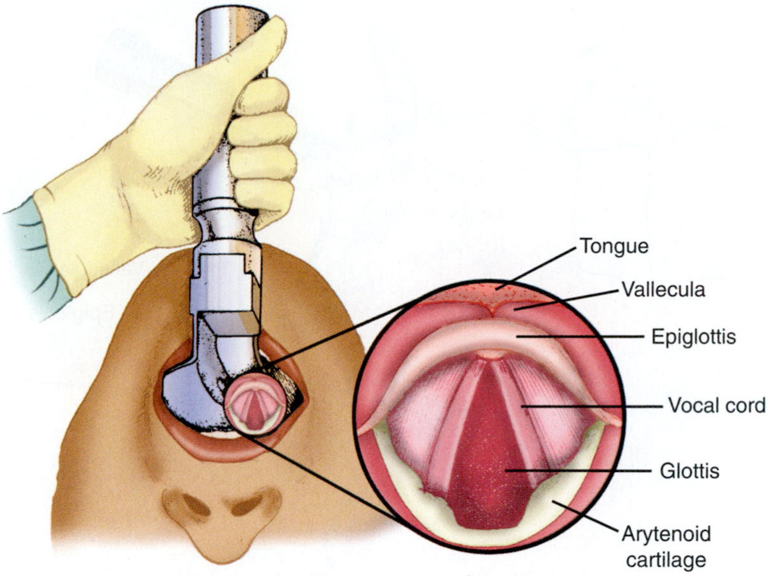

FIGURE 36-17 Visualization of vocal cords is achieved with a laryngoscope. (Modified from Ellis PD, Billings DM: Cardiopulmonary resuscitation: procedures for basic and advanced life support, St. Louis, 1980, Mosby.)

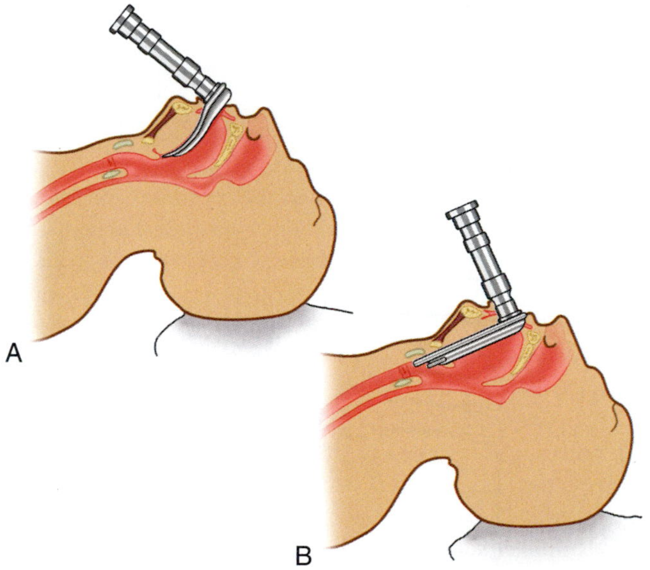

FIGURE 36-18 Placement of curved **(A)** versus straight **(B)** laryngoscope blade.

Box 36-4 Bedside Methods to Assess Endotracheal Tube Position

- Auscultation of chest and abdomen
- Observation of chest movement
- Tube length (centimeters to teeth)
- Esophageal detection device
- Light wand
- Capnometry
- Colorimetry
- Fiberoptic laryngoscopy or bronchoscopy
- Videolaryngoscopy

After tube passage and cuff inflation, the RT listens for equal and bilateral breath sounds as the patient is being ventilated. Air movement or gurgling sounds over the epigastrium indicate possible esophageal intubation. In addition, the chest wall is observed for adequate and equal chest expansion. These movements, combined with good breath sounds, are reinforcing. The combination of decreased breath sounds and decreased chest wall movement on the left side may indicate right main stem intubation. Right main stem intubation is corrected by slowly withdrawing the tube while listening for the return of left-side breath sounds. Other conditions may cause decreased breath sounds in the left lung (e.g., atelectasis, pleural effusion).

The depth of tube insertion (length from teeth to tip) is useful to help determine tube position. As indicated in Table 36-2, the average length from the teeth (incisors) to the tip of a properly positioned oral ETT in men is 21 to 23 cm. For women, this distance is approximately 2 cm less. Tube length alone cannot confirm proper placement; a tube with the 23-cm mark positioned at the teeth could just as well be in the esophagus as in the trachea.

An esophageal detection device may be used to determine whether the tube is in the esophagus or trachea.[30] This device is more commonly used outside the hospital setting. The original device consists of a squeeze-bulb aspirator attached to a standard 15-mm adapter. After a negative pressure (−80 to −90 mm Hg) is created by squeezing the bulb, the adapter is attached to the positioned ETT. If the tube is placed correctly, the bulb quickly reexpands on release because the tracheal lumen is held open by cartilaginous rings. If the tube is in the esophagus, it does not reinflate because the more pliable esophagus collapses around the tip of the ETT and prevents the bulb from reinflating. Instead of a squeeze-bulb, a large syringe with a 15-mm adapter can be used. If

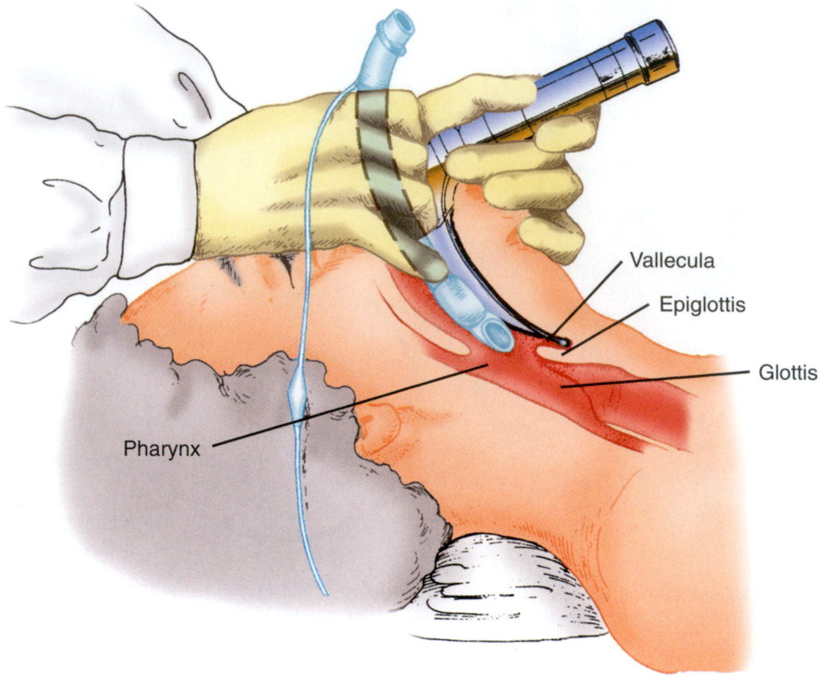

FIGURE 36-19 Insertion of endotracheal tube. (Modified from Ellis PD, Billings DM: Cardiopulmonary resuscitation: procedures for basic and advanced life support, St. Louis, 1980, Mosby.)

the ETT is in the esophagus, strong resistance is noticed when aspirating air (the barrel tends to recoil if released); if the tube is in the trachea, aspirating air into the syringe is easy. In patients with copious secretions, the esophageal detection device may become occluded and not reexpand. The esophageal detection device is not recommended for detecting esophageal intubation in children younger than 1 year.[30]

A light wand is a flexible stylet with a lighted bulb at the tip. If a light wand is used during intubation, as the stylet and ETT pass into the larynx, a characteristic glow is seen under the skin, just above the thyroid cartilage.[31] This glow is not as bright or focused if the tube is in the esophagus.

Esophageal intubation can be assessed using exhaled carbon dioxide (CO_2) analysis (capnometry). Because inspired air contains only approximately 0.04% CO_2 and end-tidal gas contains approximately 5% CO_2, placement of an ETT in the respiratory tract causes CO_2 levels to increase abruptly during expiration. This increase is evident on a capnographic display (Figure 36-20). If the tube is in the esophagus, CO_2 levels remain near zero.[32]

Colorimetric CO_2 analysis is an inexpensive alternative to capnometry. Functioning similar to pH paper, a colorimetric system has an indicator that changes color when exposed to different CO_2 levels.[33] Figure 36-21 shows a disposable colorimetric system designed specifically to confirm tube placement during intubation. Colorimetric devices are portable and disposable and are commonly used in hospitals.

Both devices are effective in detecting most esophageal intubations. However, in patients with cardiac arrest, expired CO_2 levels may be near zero because of poor pulmonary

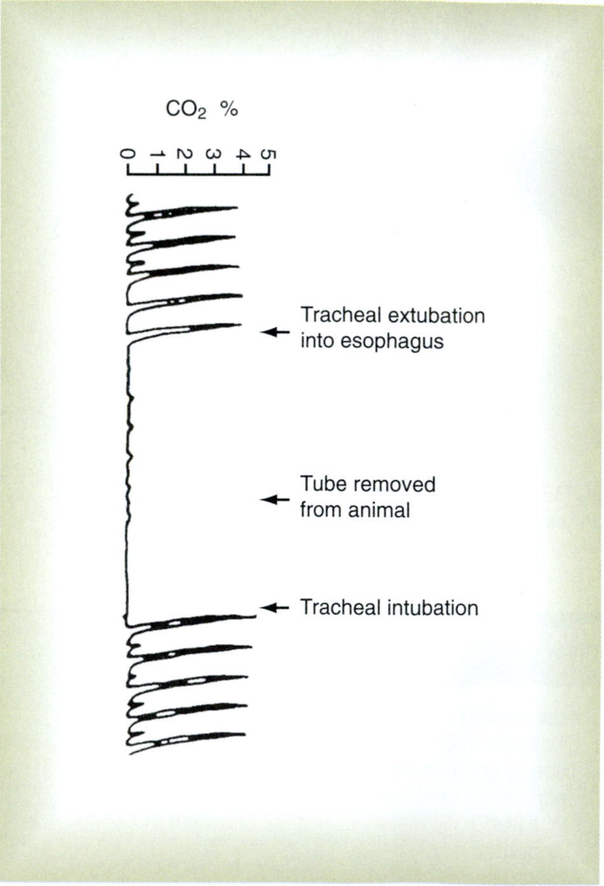

FIGURE 36-20 Capnogram tracing showing changes in expired percent carbon dioxide with proper and improper placement of endotracheal tube in test animals.

blood flow, yielding a false-negative result.[31-33] Generally, expired CO_2 levels increase with the return of spontaneous circulation. CO_2 analysis is an unreliable indicator of main stem bronchial intubation.

RULE OF THUMB

Generally, an orotracheal tube initially should be inserted to the 21- to 23-cm mark at the teeth in men and to the 19- to 21-cm mark at the teeth in women and adjusted based on the results of the patient assessment (bilateral breath sounds) and chest radiograph findings after intubation.

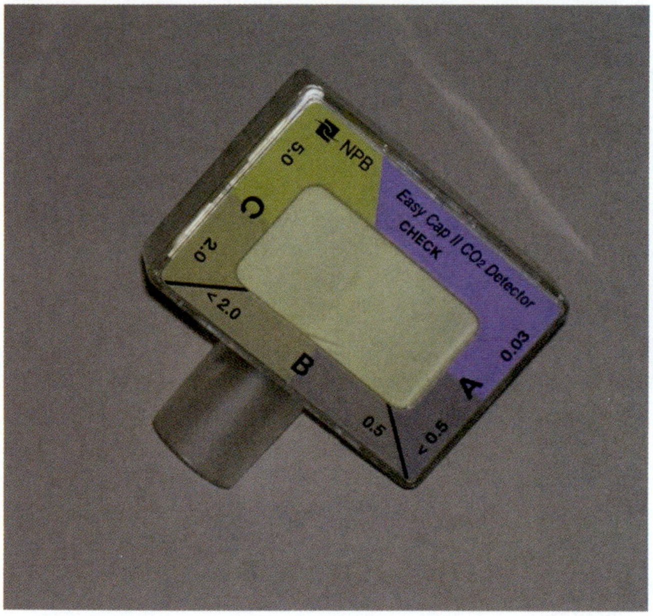

FIGURE 36-21 Disposable colorimetric carbon dioxide detector for confirming tracheal intubation. (Used by permission from Nellcor Puritan Bennett LLC, Boulder, Colorado, doing business as Covidien.)

Proper tube placement in the trachea can be confirmed without a chest radiograph by using a fiberoptic laryngoscope or bronchoscope[34] (Figure 36-22). After ensuring patient reoxygenation, a fiberoptic bronchoscope can be inserted directly into the ETT. Visualization of the carina distal to the tip of the ETT ensures proper placement in the trachea. More precise placement is possible by moving the bronchoscope from the tube tip to the carina, while measuring this distance. Also, a videolaryngoscope can be used to ensure proper placement of the ETT, especially in anticipated difficult intubations. It provides a better view of the airway, especially when there is limited mobility of the patient's neck or mouth. Also, other clinicians can see the airway and help if needed.[35]

MINI CLINI

Capnometry and Endotracheal Tube Placement

PROBLEM: At a code blue in the emergency department, a patient is intubated by the RT. A capnometer is attached to the ETT to confirm placement in the trachea. The end-expired CO_2 reads 0% as the patient is ventilated with a manual resuscitator. At this time, no one is performing cardiac compressions. Should the RT conclude that the ETT is not in the trachea?

DISCUSSION: No. If the patient is in cardiac arrest, no blood is perfusing the alveoli and no CO_2 is entering the alveoli. The result is an end-tidal CO_2 of 0%. When cardiac compressions begin (and they should begin immediately in confirmed cardiac arrest) and if compressions are effective, one should see an increase in end-tidal CO_2 as blood begins to perfuse the alveoli and CO_2 diffuses the blood.

There are other simple ways to assess ETT placement in the trachea, such as bilateral breath sounds on auscultation and chest excursions.[36] However, an increase in end-tidal CO_2 is a sure indication that the endotracheal tube is in the lungs because the only source of CO_2 is in the alveoli.

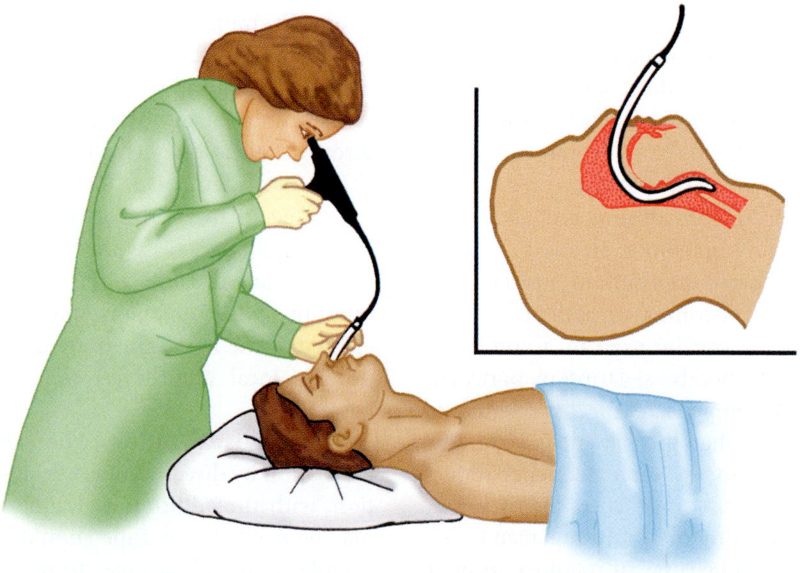

FIGURE 36-22 Fiberoptic laryngoscopy used to confirm endotracheal tube placement.

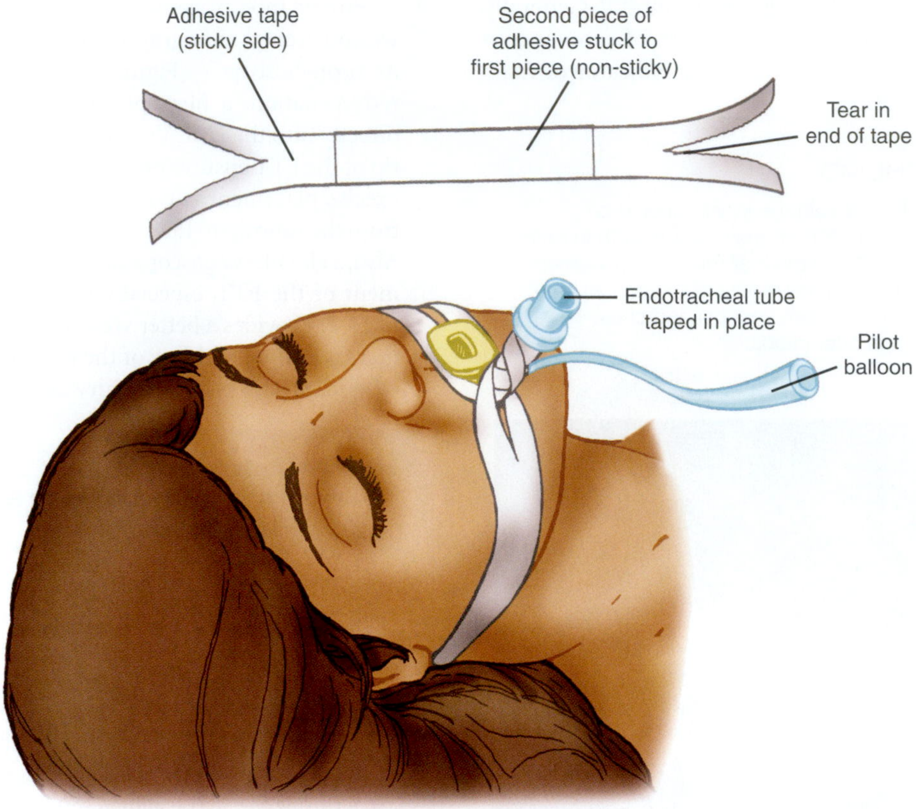

FIGURE 36-23 Securing the endotracheal tube.

Step 9: Stabilize Tube and Confirm Placement.

The tube should not be secured until correct placement has been assessed by using one or more of the previously mentioned methods. After assessing placement and while holding the tube in position, the RT secures the tube to the skin above the lip and on the cheeks using tape or an ETT holder. A bite block, oropharyngeal airway, or similar device may be needed to prevent the patient from biting down on the tube (Figure 36-23). After the tube is stabilized, a chest radiograph should be taken to confirm its position.

The most common complication of emergency airway management is tissue trauma. The most serious complications are acute hypoxemia, hypercapnia, bradycardia, and cardiac arrest.[37,38] These problems can be minimized by using proper technique, providing the patient with adequate ventilation and oxygenation (before, during, and after), and strictly adhering to intubation time limits. In addition, sedation and anesthesia can reduce complications and facilitate intubation in a semicomatose or combative patient.[27] Muscle relaxing or paralyzing agents can be used in a combative patient who cannot be controlled by sedation. A paralyzed patient has no ability to compensate for hypoxemia or hypercapnia. It is imperative that the patient can be adequately ventilated by bag and mask. Rapid-sequence induction is used with the administration of a sedative-hypnotic medication and a muscle relaxing or paralyzing agent.

Difficult intubations occur because of inability to open the patient's mouth, inability to position the patient, or unusual airway anatomy. Special intubation equipment (e.g., laryngoscope blades, videolaryngoscopy, or specialized stylets) or alternative techniques can be employed.[27,36] Additional details of these techniques are beyond the scope of this chapter.

Nasotracheal Intubation

Although nasotracheal intubation is more difficult than orotracheal intubation, it is the route of choice in certain clinical situations. Examples include intubation of patients when the oral route is unavailable, such as patients with maxillofacial injuries or undergoing oral surgery.

Nasotracheal intubation is performed either blindly or by direct visualization.[37] The direct visualization approach requires either a standard or a fiberoptic laryngoscope. For the blind technique to work, the patient must be breathing spontaneously. Equipment assembly, patient positioning, and preoxygenation are essentially the same as with oral intubation. A mixture of 0.25% phenylephrine and 3% lidocaine may be applied to the nasal mucosa with a long cotton-tipped swab to provide local anesthesia and vasoconstriction of the nasal passage.

Direct Visualization. The equipment needed for nasal intubation by direct visualization is the same as for oral intubation, with the addition of Magill forceps. A smaller ETT also may be needed. The tube should be prelubricated with water-soluble gel to aid passage. To insert the tube, the bevel is positioned toward the septum and advanced along the floor of the

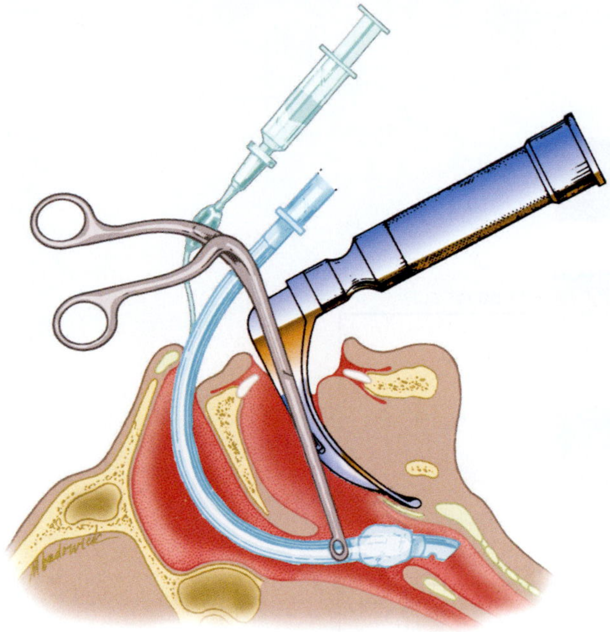

FIGURE 36-24 Nasal intubation using Magill forceps. (Modified from Finucane BT, Santora AH: Principles of airway management, Philadelphia, 1988, FA Davis.)

nasal cavity (inferiorly). When the tip of the tube is in the patient's oropharynx, the RT opens the patient's mouth, inserts the laryngoscope (with the left hand), and visualizes the glottis. The RT uses the Magill forceps with the right hand to grasp the tube just above the cuff and direct it between the vocal cords (Figure 36-24). To help advance the tube past the vocal cords, the neck may need to be flexed. Confirmation of position and stabilization follows, as with the oral route.

Alternatively, a fiberoptic bronchoscope or laryngoscope can be used to guide tube passage.[34] With the bronchoscopic method, the distal end of the scope is passed through the ETT and directly into the trachea. When placement is ensured, the RT slides the ETT down over the scope into proper position. The procedure is similar with a fiberoptic laryngoscope. However, because directional control of the scope is limited, the RT may have to reposition the patient's head and neck to help guide the tube.

Blind Passage. For blind nasal intubation, the patient is placed in either the supine or the sitting position. As with direct visualization, the tube is inserted through the nose. As the tube approaches the larynx, one can listen through the tube for air movement. The breath sounds become louder and more tubular when the tube passes through the larynx. Successful passage of the tube through the larynx usually is indicated by a harsh cough, followed by vocal silence. If the sounds disappear, the tube is moving toward the esophagus. A malpositioned tube can be corrected by manipulating the tube and repositioning the patient's head and neck. Confirmation of tube placement and stabilization should follow. As previously indicated, a light wand can help ensure proper tracheal placement during blind nasotracheal intubation.

Box 36-5 Factors to Consider in Switching from Endotracheal Tube to Tracheostomy

- Projected time the patient will need an artificial airway
- Patient's tolerance of endotracheal tube
- Patient's overall condition (including nutritional, cardiovascular, and infection status)
- Patient's ability to tolerate a surgical procedure
- Relative risks of continued endotracheal intubation versus tracheostomy

Tracheotomy

Tracheotomy is the procedure of establishing access to the trachea via a neck incision. The opening created by this procedure is called a **tracheostomy.** Tracheotomy may be performed as a regular surgical procedure or by a percutaneous dilation procedure.

Tracheotomy is the preferred, primary route for overcoming upper airway obstruction or trauma and for patients with poor airway protective reflexes. Another indication for tracheotomy is the continuing need for an artificial airway after a prolonged period of oral or nasal intubation. The patient should be assessed daily for the continued need for intubation. If the patient still needs an artificial airway after approximately 7 to 14 days, a tracheostomy is commonly considered. The benefits of a tracheostomy versus oral or nasal intubation are elimination of vocal cord injury, increased patient comfort, less need for deep sedation, easier removal of secretions, decreased work of breathing, and potentially shorter weaning time.[38] The decision when to switch from an ETT to a tracheostomy tube should be individualized. Pertinent factors that should be considered in making this decision are summarized in Box 36-5. Figure 36-25 is a decision-making algorithm useful for timing tracheotomy in critically ill patients.

Procedure. Tracheotomy should be performed as an elective procedure by a skilled physician or surgeon after the patient's airway is stabilized. Mortality and morbidity are greater when the procedure is performed on an emergency basis. The RT may be asked to assist in tracheotomy, especially if performed at the bedside. For this reason, we briefly describe both the traditional surgical procedure and the percutaneous dilation method.[38]

A local anesthetic is used, and the patient is mildly sedated if conditions permit. If an ETT is in place, it should not be removed until just before the insertion of the tracheostomy tube. Keeping the ETT in place this way ensures a patent airway and provides additional stability to the trachea during the procedure.

In traditional surgical tracheotomy, the surgeon makes an incision in the neck over the second or third tracheal ring. After the skin and subcutaneous tissue have been incised, the surgeon divides the superficial muscles and locates the underlying thyroid gland. The surgeon divides and ligates the thyroid isthmus, which overlies the second and third tracheal rings. The surgeon then enters the trachea through either a horizontal incision between rings or a vertical incision through the second

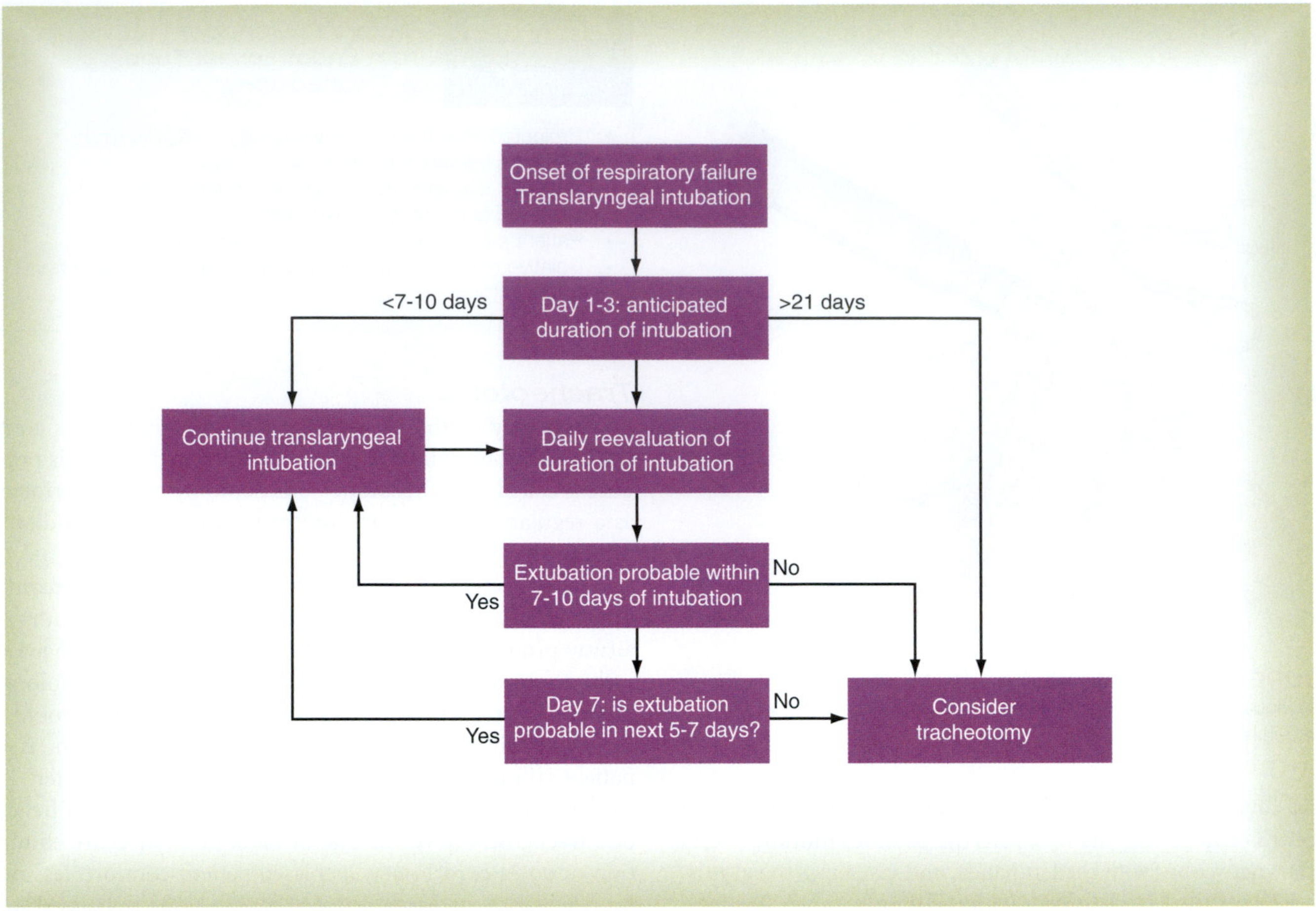

FIGURE 36-25 Approach to timing tracheotomy in patients intubated and mechanically ventilated for respiratory failure. (From Heffner JE: Timing of tracheostomy in ventilator-dependent patients. Clin Chest Med 12:611, 1991.)

and third rings. As little cartilage as possible should be removed to promote better closure after extubation.

In percutaneous dilation tracheotomy, the initial steps to prepare the patient are similar to the steps in the traditional tracheotomy procedure. After dissection to the anterior tracheal wall, the ETT is retracted to keep the tip of the tube inside the larynx. A bronchoscope can be used to reassess placement for the ETT for the duration of the procedure. A large leak around the ETT may develop, requiring adjustment of mechanical ventilation. If the patient is unable to tolerate the large leak, and adjustments to ventilatory support cannot compensate for the leak, a surgical procedure may be indicated for that patient.

The physician inserts a needle and sheath into the trachea between the cricoid and first tracheal ring or between the first and second rings. The physician then inserts a guidewire through the sheath, the sheath is removed, and a dilator is passed over the guidewire. Increasingly larger dilators are introduced until the stoma is large enough for a standard tracheostomy tube. The physician slips the tracheostomy tube over the last dilator used. An alternative to the use of multiple dilators is to use a single dilator with increasing diameter from the proximal to the distal end.

The procedure may be performed under direct vision with a bronchoscope passed through the ETT or a laryngeal mask airway (LMA). Compared with the traditional surgical procedure, a percutaneous dilation tracheotomy is rapid, with fewer complications from the surgical site, and has a better cosmetic appearance after decannulation. Contraindications for percutaneous tracheotomy are listed in Box 36-6.

Insertion of the tube, inflation of the cuff, and securing the tube follow both methods. Tracheostomy tube ties should be secure enough to prevent movement of the tube but not so tight as to cause skin ulceration. The role of the RT in the procedure may include managing the ETT, making ventilator changes as needed, assisting with the bronchoscope, and monitoring the patient. Advantages and disadvantages of percutaneous and open surgical tracheotomy are listed in Table 36-3.

Generally, the tube size is correct if it occupies two-thirds to three-quarters of the internal tracheal diameter. Tracheostomy tubes come in various sizes, lengths, and shapes depending on the manufacturer. The size marked on the flange usually indicates the internal diameter, but some tracheostomy tubes with inner cannulas use Jackson sizing. Table 36-4 lists the sizes, internal diameter, external diameter, and length of commonly used brands and styles of adult tracheostomy tubes. Table 36-5 provides guidelines for selecting a tracheostomy tube according to a patient's age. Within an age category, the exact size of tube chosen depends on the patient's height, weight, and airway

Box 36-6 Contraindications for Percutaneous Dilation Tracheostomy

ABSOLUTE

- Need for emergent surgical airway

RELATIVE

- Children younger than 12 years of age
- Poor landmarks secondary to body habitus, abnormal anatomy, or occluding thyroid mass
- Positive end expiratory pressure less than 15 cm H_2O
- Coagulopathy
- Pulsating blood vessel over tracheotomy site
- Limited ability to extend cervical spine
- History of difficult intubation
- Infection, burn, or malignancy at tracheotomy site

From Park S, Goldenberg D: Percutaneous tracheotomy: Griggs technique. Op Tech Otolaryngol 18:95, 2007.

TABLE 36-3 Comparison of Percutaneous and Open Surgical Tracheotomy

Procedure	Advantages	Disadvantages
Percutaneous tracheotomy	May be done in intensive care unit	Not done in children younger than 12 yr
	Sedation and local anesthetic given	
	Stoma usually stabilizes in 5 days	May be difficult to insert because of calcified cartilaginous rings
Open surgical tracheotomy	Done in patients with poor landmarks because of abnormal anatomy or body habitus	Usually done in operating room
	May be done emergently	General anesthesia given
	Done in children younger than 12 yr	Stoma usually takes longer to stabilize (7 to 10 days)

TABLE 36-4 Comparison of Commonly Used Brands of Adult Tracheostomy Tubes

PORTEX FLEX DIC: SIZED BY ID; ALSO AVAILABLE CUFFLESS OR FENESTRATED

ID (mm)	OD (mm)	Length (mm)*
6.0	8.2	64
7.0	9.6	70
8.0	10.9	74

SHILEY SCT: SIZED BY ID; ALSO AVAILABLE CUFFLESS

ID (mm)	OD (mm)	Length (mm)*
6.0	8.3	67
7.0	9.6	80
8.0	10.9	89

SHILEY DOUBLE CANNULA (LPC, DC, CFS, CFN, FEN, PERC) WITH DISPOSABLE OR NONDISPOSABLE INNER CANNULA: SIZED BY JACKSON SCALE; ALSO AVAILABLE CUFFLESS OR FENESTRATED

Size (Jackson)	ID (mm)	OD (mm)	Length (mm)
4	5.0	9.4	65
6	6.4	10.8	76 (PERC 74)
8	7.6	12.2	81 (PERC 79)

JACKSON DOUBLE CANNULA STAINLESS STEEL TUBE; AVAILABLE CUFFLESS ONLY; AVAILABLE FENESTRATED

Size (Jackson)	ID (mm)	OD (mm)	Length (mm)
4	5.3	8.0	62
6	7.2	10.0	69
8	9.2	12.0	69

EXTRA LENGTH TUBES: SHILEY TRACHEOSOFT XLT PROXIMAL OR DISTAL EXTENSION WITH DIC: SIZED BY ID

ID (mm)	OD (mm)	Length (mm)
6.0	11	95
7.0	12.3	100
8.0	13.3	105

BIVONA MID-RANGE AIRE-CUF EXTRA LENGTH FIXED OR ADJUSTABLE NECK FLANGE: SIZED BY ID

ID (mm)	OD (mm)	Length (mm)
6.0	8.7	100 (adjustable 110)
7.0	10.0	110 (adjustable 120)
8.0	11.0	120 (adjustable 130)

BIVONA TTS: SIZED BY ID; CUFF INFLATED WITH STERILE WATER NOT AIR

ID (mm)	OD (mm)	Length (mm)
6.0	8.7	70
7.0	10.0	80
8.0	11.0	88

DIC, Disposable inner cannula; *ID*, inner diameter; *OD*, outer diameter; *SCT*, single cannula tracheostomy.
*The main difference between these tubes is the length.

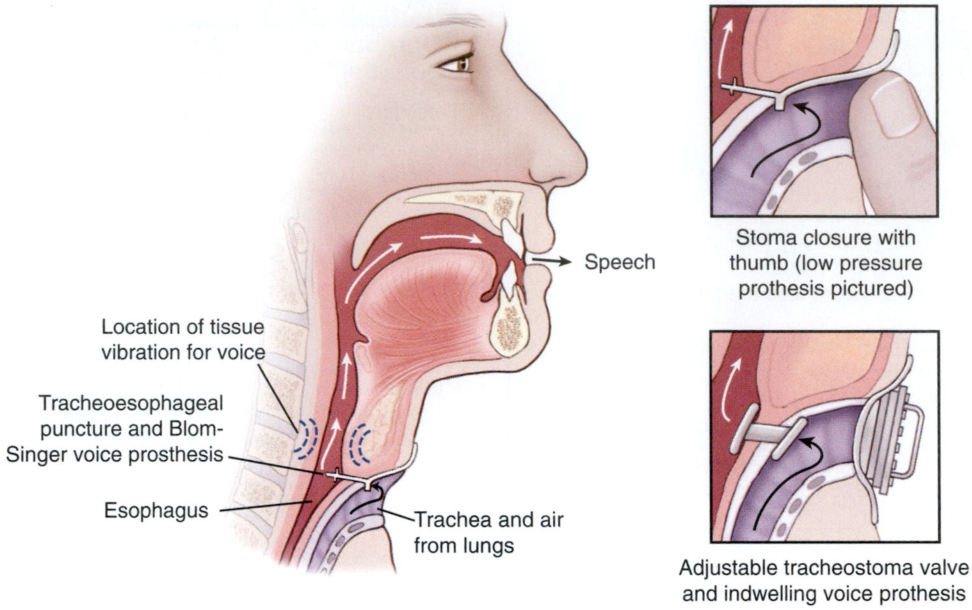

FIGURE 36-26 Laryngectomy with tracheoesophageal voice prosthesis (TEP). (Courtesy INHEALTH technologies: Blom-Singer voice restoration systems.)

TABLE 36-5

Guideline for Infant, Pediatric, and Adult Tracheostomy Tube Sizes

Age/Weight*	ID (mm)
Premature <2 kg	2.5 cuffless neonatal
Infant	3.0-3.5 cuffless neonatal
6-18 mo	3.5-4.0 neonatal or pediatric
18 mo to 4-5 yr	4.0-4.5 pediatric
4-5 yr to 10 yr	4.5-6.0 pediatric
10-14 yr	5.0-6.5 pediatric or adult
14 years to adult	6.0-9.0 adult

Note: The difference between the same size (ID) neonatal and pediatric tube or pediatric and adult tube is the length; that is, the adult tube is longer than the pediatric tube, and the pediatric tube is longer than the neonatal tube.
ID, Inner diameter.
*Typical pediatric size = (16 + age)/4 or (age/4) + 4.

anatomy. To choose a tracheostomy tube that fits a patient properly, it is important to consider not only the internal and external diameter of the tube but also the length and shape of the tube.

Laryngectomy

Total **laryngectomy,** removal of the larynx (voice box), is usually done to treat laryngeal cancer. It also may be done to treat severe trauma, such as from a gunshot wound to the neck or damage to the larynx from radiation (radiation necrosis). Besides removing the larynx the surgeon creates a hole in the neck (stoma) and attaches the trachea to the stoma. The patient will now breathe through this permanent stoma. A laryngectomy tube may be inserted into the stoma to keep it open while it heals.

The surgeon may also do a tracheoesophageal puncture (TEP), which is a small opening between the posterior wall of the trachea and esophagus. The surgeon will insert a small device (prosthesis) that has a one-way valve. This prosthesis allows the patient to speak when the patient occludes the stoma during exhalation once the patient has been trained by a speech and language pathologist (Figure 36-26). Some patients with TEP use their thumb, and others use an attached tracheostoma adjustable valve to occlude the stoma during exhalation to be able to speak. Another way a laryngectomy patient can speak is by holding an electrolarynx against the throat. This is a battery-operated device that creates vibrations that are transmitted through the pharynx and mouth to produce a voice.[39]

The risks associated with this surgery are hematoma, wound infection, fistulas, stomal stenosis (narrowing), leaking around tracheoesophageal prosthesis, difficulty swallowing and eating, and problems speaking.

Sometimes the surgeon will perform only a partial laryngectomy to remove the cancer. A tracheotomy is also done and a tracheostomy tube is inserted while the surgical site is allowed to heal. There is still communication between the pharynx and trachea, so the patient should eventually be able to breathe using the normal upper airway and may even be able to speak once the tracheostomy tube is removed by the surgeon.[40]

It is important to know whether a patient has had a total or partial laryngectomy, in case the patient accidentally loses the artificial airway and requires manual ventilation. In the case of a total laryngectomy the RT would apply bag-mask ventilation over the stoma, ideally using a small pediatric mask that would fit more closely over the stoma than an adult mask. In a partial laryngectomy the RT would cover the stoma with a gauze pad and apply bag-mask ventilation over the nose and mouth with the standard adult mask because there is still communication between the trachea and upper airway.

AIRWAY TRAUMA ASSOCIATED WITH TRACHEAL TUBES

Artificial airways do not conform exactly to patient anatomy, which may result in pressure on soft tissues that can result in ischemia and ulceration.[41] In addition, artificial airways tend to shift position as the patient's head and neck move or as the tube is manipulated. This shifting can result in friction-like injuries. Occasional reaction to the materials composing the tube also may cause problems.

Depending on the type of tube, damage to the patient's airway can occur anywhere from the nose down into the lower trachea. Because tracheostomy tubes do not pass through the larynx, structural injury resulting from these airways is limited to tracheal sites. Laryngeal dysfunction may occur secondary to a lack of stimulation from airflow or restricted movement secondary to equipment.[14]

Because injury often cannot be assessed while an artificial airway is in place, the patient's airway should always be evaluated carefully after extubation. Techniques commonly used to diagnose airway damage include physical examination, air tomography, fluoroscopy, laryngoscopy, bronchoscopy, magnetic resonance imaging, and pulmonary function studies.[42]

Laryngeal Lesions

The most common laryngeal injuries associated with endotracheal intubation are glottic edema, vocal cord inflammation, laryngeal or vocal cord ulcerations, and vocal cord polyps or granulomas. Less common and more serious injuries are vocal cord paralysis and laryngeal stenosis.[29,41]

Glottic edema and vocal cord inflammation are transient changes that occur as a result of pressure from the ETT or trauma during intubation.[41] The primary concern with glottic edema and vocal cord inflammation occurs after extubation. Because swelling can worsen over 24 hours after extubation, patients should be evaluated periodically for delayed development of glottic edema.

The primary symptoms of glottic edema and vocal cord inflammation are hoarseness and stridor. Hoarseness occurs in most extubated patients and usually resolves quickly. Stridor is a more serious symptom than hoarseness, indicating a significant decrease in diameter of the airway. Stridor is often treated with epinephrine (2.25% racemic solution or levoepinephrine 1:1000) via aerosol.[41] The treatment goal is to reduce glottic or airway edema by mucosal vasoconstriction. A steroid also may be added to the aerosol to reduce inflammation further. Both of these techniques are more commonly used in children than in adults.

To reduce laryngeal edema in patients who have had prolonged intubation or patients who have failed prior extubation because of glottic edema, intravenous steroids may be given 24 hours before extubation.[41] If stridor continues and is unresponsive to treatment, structural changes that narrow the airway should be suspected.

Laryngeal and vocal cord ulcerations may cause hoarseness soon after extubation. Symptoms usually resolve spontaneously, and no treatment is indicated. Vocal cord polyps and granulomas develop more slowly, taking weeks or months to form.[24] Symptoms include difficulty in swallowing, hoarseness, and stridor. If symptoms are severe or persistent, the polyps or granulomas may have to be removed surgically.

Vocal cord paralysis is likely in extubated patients with hoarseness and stridor that does not resolve with treatment or time. In some patients, symptoms may resolve within 24 hours, and full movement of the vocal cords can return over several days. If the obstructive symptoms continue, tracheotomy may be indicated.

Laryngeal **stenosis** occurs when the normal tissue of the larynx is replaced by scar tissue, which causes stricture and decreased mobility. The symptoms of laryngeal stenosis are similar to symptoms of vocal cord paralysis—stridor and hoarseness. Because laryngeal stenosis does not resolve spontaneously, surgical correction is usually required. Some patients require a permanent tracheostomy.

Tracheal Lesions

Although laryngeal lesions occur only with oral or nasal ETTs, tracheal lesions can occur with any tracheal airway. These tracheal lesions include granulomas, **tracheomalacia,** and tracheal stenosis.[1,24,43] Less common, but more serious complications are tracheoesophageal and tracheoinnominate artery fistulas.

Tracheomalacia and tracheal stenosis can occur either separately or together. *Tracheomalacia* is the softening of the cartilaginous rings, which causes collapse of the trachea during inspiration and expiration. *Tracheal stenosis* is a narrowing of the lumen of the trachea, which can occur as fibrotic scarring, causes the airway to narrow. In patients with ETTs, this type of damage most often occurs at the cuff site. In patients with tracheostomy tubes, stenosis may occur at the cuff, tube tip, or stoma sites; the stoma site is the most common. Stenosis at the stoma site is associated with too large a stoma, infection of the stoma, movement of the tube, frequent tube changes, and advanced age.[44]

Signs of possible tracheal damage before extubation include difficulty in sealing the trachea with the cuff and evidence of tracheal dilation on chest radiograph.[41] Signs and symptoms of postextubation problems include difficulty with expectoration, dyspnea, and stridor. Although these findings may appear acutely, they may develop over several months and may not be present until the radius is reduced by 50% to 75%. Dyspnea at rest may not be seen until the diameter of the trachea is less than 5 mm. Symptoms are often incorrectly attributed to the development of asthma or chronic lung disease.[24]

Tomography, fluoroscopy, and pulmonary function studies (especially flow-volume loops) may be helpful in quantifying the severity of the damage. Flow-volume loops are also helpful in distinguishing between tracheomalacia and tracheal stenosis. Tracheomalacia appears as a variable obstruction with different inspiratory and expiratory patterns. Tracheal stenosis appears as a fixed obstructive pattern, with flattening of both the inspiratory and the expiratory limbs of the flow-volume loop (Figure 36-27).

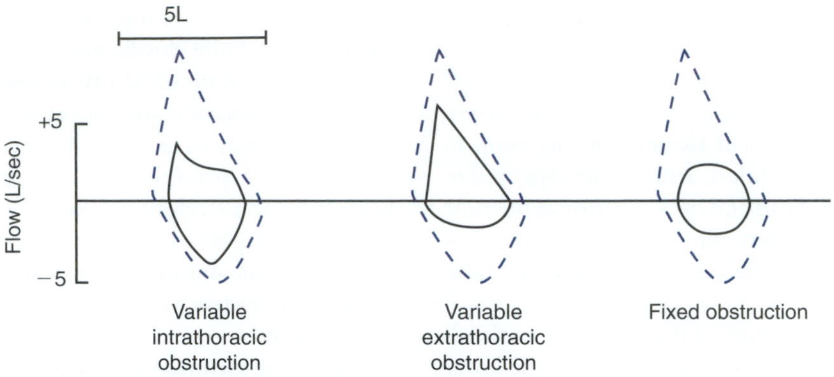

FIGURE 36-27 Patterns of pulmonary dysfunction revealed by flow-volume loops. *Dashed lines* are normal values for comparison. Tracheomalacia is typically seen as a variable obstruction, whereas stenosis most often manifests with a fixed obstruction pattern. (Modified from Mottram C: Ruppel's manual of pulmonary function testing, ed 10, Mosby, 2013, St. Louis.)

Treatment depends on the severity of the lesion, especially the length and circumference of the damage.[42] Laser therapy may be useful if the lesion is small. Resection and end-to-end anastomosis may be indicated when the damage involves fewer than three tracheal rings. More involved damage may require staged repair. Stents may be placed to maintain the patency of the airway.

A **tracheoesophageal fistula** is a direct communication between the trachea and the esophagus. Tracheoesophageal fistula is a rare complication of both tracheotomy and endotracheal intubation. If it occurs soon after a tracheotomy, incorrect surgical technique may be the cause. Later development is related to sepsis, malnutrition, tracheal erosion from the cuff and tube, and esophageal erosion from nasogastric tubes.[41] The diagnosis can be made based on a history of recurrent aspiration and abdominal distention as air is forced into the esophagus during positive pressure ventilation. Diagnosis is also made by direct endoscopic examination of the trachea and esophagus. Treatment involves surgical closure of the defect.

A **tracheoinnominate artery fistula** can occur when a tracheostomy tube causes tissue erosion through the innominate artery. The result is massive hemorrhage and, in most cases, death. Tracheoinnominate artery fistula is a rare complication, probably caused by improper low positioning of the stoma or excessive movement of the tube.[42] Pulsation of the tracheostomy tube may be the only clue before actual hemorrhage. When hemorrhage begins, hyperinflation of the cuff may slow the bleeding, but the patient still needs surgical intervention.[42] Even with proper corrective action, only 25% of patients who develop this serious complication survive.

Prevention

Several actions can minimize the trauma caused by tracheal airways. Many studies suggest that tube movement is a primary cause of injury.[41,42] Several methods can be used to limit tube movement. Sedation can help keep patients comfortable and decrease the likelihood of self-extubation. Nasotracheal tubes are easier to stabilize and may move less than orotracheal tubes. Swivel adapters can be used to minimize tube traction whenever respiratory therapy equipment is attached to patients with tracheostomies. If a patient with a tracheostomy requires O_2 therapy, tracheostomy collars are preferred to T-tubes or Briggs adapters.

Selection of the correct airway size is also important. Once in place, endotracheal and tracheostomy tubes should not be changed unless necessary. To minimize vocal cord closure around ETTs, patients should be discouraged from unnecessary coughing or efforts to talk. Tracheal wall injury from the endotracheal or tracheostomy tube cuff can be reduced by maintaining pressures of 20 to 30 cm H_2O.[13,43] If the airway is in place solely for suctioning or to bypass an obstruction, a cuff may not be needed.

Infected secretions have been implicated in the development of tracheitis and mucosal destruction, and infection of the tracheotomy stoma has been linked to tracheal stenosis.[42] Sterile techniques should be used when cleaning or suctioning tracheostomy tubes. Good tracheostomy care, including aseptic cleaning of the stoma with sterile normal saline or half-strength hydrogen peroxide, should be carried out routinely, and soiled tracheostomy dressings should be changed as needed. If there is significant drainage from the stoma, it is better to use a foam dressing, which will absorb the drainage away from the skin, rather than a standard gauze dressing, which when wet will keep the skin moist. (See discussion of tracheostomy care procedure later in the chapter.) When sutures are used to secure the trach tube flange to the patient's neck it can be very difficult to properly clean around the stoma. So if sutures are present, it is recommended to remove them as soon as possible, ideally by day 7 after the tracheostomy was performed. If there are any signs of pressure injury from the trach flange, place a hydrocolloid dressing under the flange. Sometimes because of a patient's neck anatomy, changing the tracheostomy tube to another type with a different style of flange as soon as it is safe to do so may also prevent further skin injury.

RULE OF THUMB

In adults, tracheal tube cuff pressure should be maintained at 20 to 30 cm H_2O to minimize tracheal mucosal injury and aspiration of oral secretions.

AIRWAY MAINTENANCE

The RT must attend to several aspects of airway maintenance when a tracheal airway is in place. Critical responsibilities in this area include (1) securing the tube and maintaining its proper placement, (2) providing for patient communication, (3) ensuring adequate humidification, (4) minimizing the possibility of infection, (5) aiding in secretion clearance, (6) providing appropriate cuff care, and (7) troubleshooting airway-related problems.

Securing the Airway and Confirming Placement

The most common way to secure ETTs is with tape. The tape is secured to one side of the face and then wound around the tube and airway once or twice before the end is secured to the skin again (see Figure 36-23). Silk tape is adequate if the period of intubation is short, such as during surgery; however, silk tape is easily loosened by oral secretions. Cloth tape seems to be better for longer use and may adhere better if the skin is prepared with a nonirritating medical liquid adhesive. Instead of using tape to secure the tube, practitioners can choose among several commercial ETT or stabilizers. Case reports indicate that use of these stabilizers can result in less skin damage, tube movement, and self-extubations than with traditional taping. However, of and by themselves, these stabilizing devices cannot prevent airway or skin trauma. So the skin around the mouth or nose should be checked regularly. If there is evidence of skin irritation, the tube should be moved to the other side of the mouth or the other nares and then resecured.

A tracheostomy tube can be secured by threading cloth ties through the tube flange and tying them together on the side of the patient's neck. Alternatively, a commercial tracheostomy tube holder made of soft foam with Velcro attachments threaded through the tube flange can be used. This soft tracheostomy tube holder is easier to change and does not cause skin ulceration as often as cloth ties. Whichever tube holder is used, skin damage can be minimized by keeping the ties loose enough to slip one finger underneath easily.

Proper placement of an endotracheal or tracheostomy tube normally is confirmed by radiograph. The tube tip should be approximately 3 to 6 cm above the carina in adults, or between the second and fourth tracheal rings.[29,44] Keeping the tube position in this range minimizes the chance of the tube moving down into the main stem bronchi or up into the larynx. Even so, the ETT position changes with movement of the head and neck (Figure 36-28).[45] Flexion of the neck moves the tube toward the carina, whereas extension pulls the tube toward the larynx.[46,47] When reviewing a radiograph for tube placement, the clinician should also check the position of the head and neck. If the tube is malpositioned, the old tape should be removed and the tube repositioned, using the centimeter markings as a guide. This maneuver usually requires two people to prevent extubation.

As an alternative to using chest films to confirm tube placement, a practitioner trained in fiberoptic laryngoscopy or bronchoscopy may confirm the position of the tube visually.[48] With this method, the fiberoptic scope is inserted into the tube, and the carina is directly visualized. By moving the scope from the tube tip to the carina and measuring the distance of bronchoscopy displacement, the exact distance of insertion can be determined.

Providing for Patient Communication

One of the most frustrating aspects of caring for a patient with a tracheal tube is his or her inability to talk. Phonation requires moving vocal cords, resulting in airflow between them. ETTs prevent vocal cord movement and airflow through the cords. Standard tracheostomy tubes allow vocal cord movement but prevent airflow. Without the ability to speak, the patient cannot easily inform the health care providers of changes in symptoms or make basic requests. This situation may lead to agitation and stress in the patient. If that agitation is treated with sedatives, a patient on a ventilator may wean more slowly.[47]

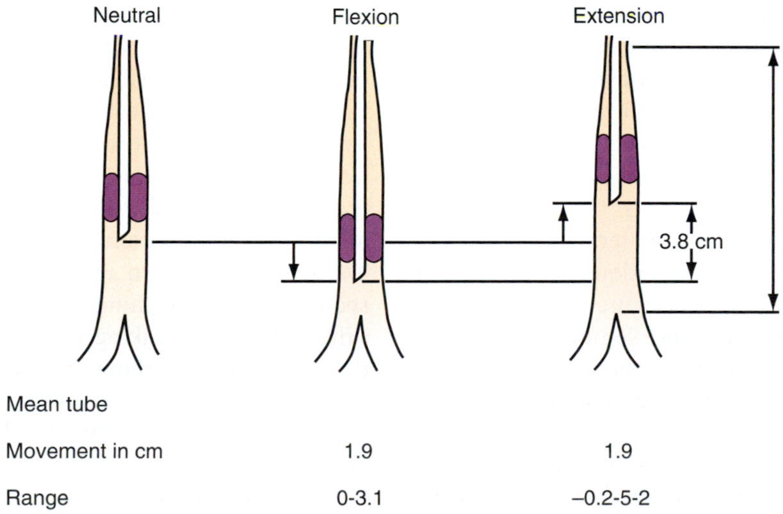

FIGURE 36-28 Effect of neck flexion and extension on endotracheal tube position. (Modified from Conrardy PA, Goodman L, Lainge F, et al: Alteration of endotracheal tube position: flexion and extension of the neck. Crit Care Med 4:8, 1976.)

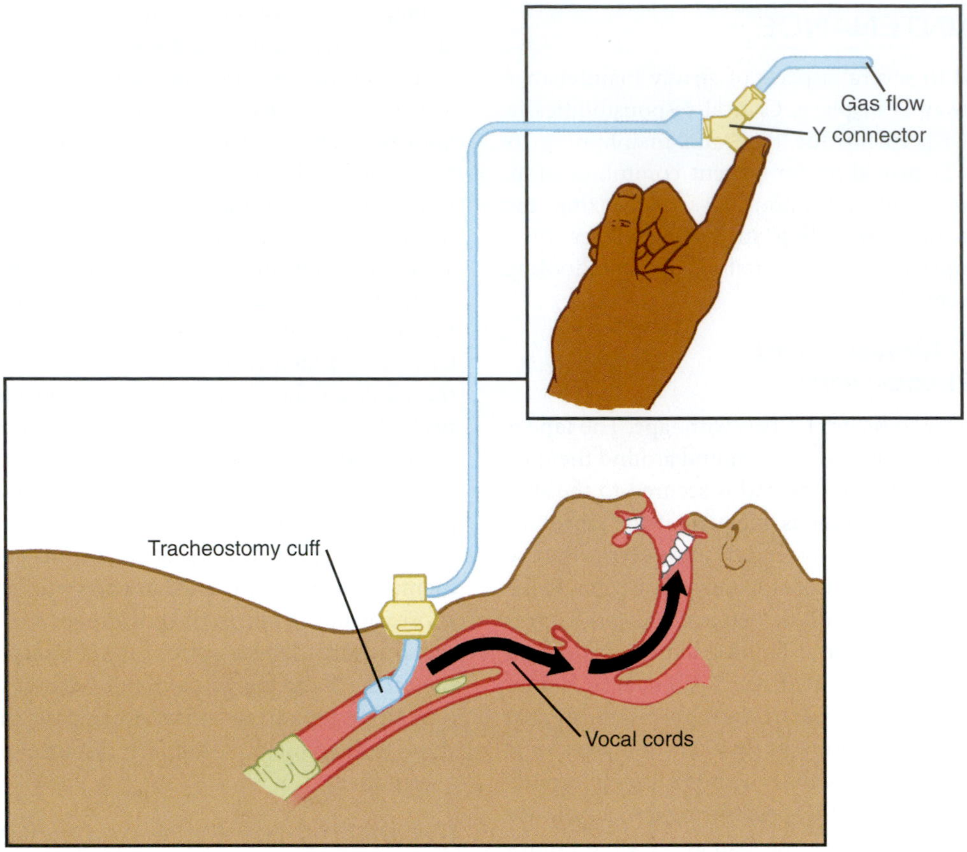

FIGURE 36-29 "Talking" tracheostomy tube.

An experienced practitioner may use lip reading, but this technique is very difficult in patients with orotracheal tubes. Alternatively, an alert patient may write messages on paper or some other writing surface. For many patients, however, restricted hand movement because of restraints or vascular catheters makes writing impossible. Some critically ill patients simply cannot hold up their heads. A better solution is a letter, phrase, or picture board.[47] These devices allow patients to communicate by simple pointing. Large and simple drawings are particularly important for patients who cannot see print clearly. Some patients may choose to use special electronic devices to communicate, especially patients who have a tracheostomy tube because of the need for chronic mechanical ventilation. Speech language pathologists often work with these patients to figure out which device will work best so an individual patient can communicate.

For conscious patients with a long-term tracheostomy who are ventilator-dependent, communication can be enhanced with a "talking" tracheostomy tube (Figure 36-29).[28] These special airways provide a separate inlet for compressed gas, which escapes above the tube, allowing phonation. There are some problems associated with these tubes, however. The continuous gas flow through a new tracheostomy may cause air leaks. High flow rates may cause mucosal drying and irritation. Finally, secretions may occlude the speaking gas outlets. Although not life-threatening, these problems can be frustrating for both the patient and the practitioner.

Another tracheostomy tube, the Blom fenestrated tracheostomy tube, has a special speech cannula that allows ventilator-dependent patients to speak with the cuff fully inflated. With the speech cannula inserted during inhalation the flap valve opens and the flexible bubble valve expands, blocking the fenestrations. During exhalation the flap valve closes and the bubble valve collapses, which allows air to pass through the fenestrations so the patient can speak.[28] (Figure 36-30)

An alternative to a speaking tracheostomy tube is to place a one-way valve (speaking valve) on the external opening of the tracheostomy tube.[28] With this device in place and the tracheostomy tube cuff deflated, the patient inhales around and through the tube and exhales only around the tube through the larynx. Speech is coordinated with exhalation through the larynx. A patient who is a good candidate for a speaking valve is one who is medically stable, is able to communicate, and has a low risk for aspiration. Several types of speaking valves are available, as shown in Figure 36-31. They can be used with spontaneously breathing or ventilator-dependent patients. When using the speaking valve, the cuff on the tube must be deflated to allow airflow around the tube. This deflation of the cuff causes a leak on inspiration and a decrease in tidal volume (V_T) delivery during mechanical ventilation. However, an increase in the set V_T on the ventilator during initial trials of the valve should compensate for this.

During the initial placement of the speaking valve, the patient's ability to exhale around the tracheostomy tube should

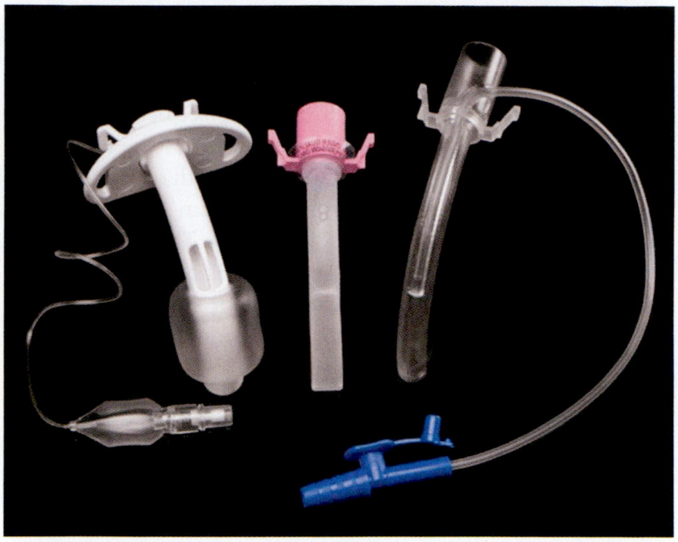

FIGURE 36-30 Blom fenestrated trach tube with speech cannula.

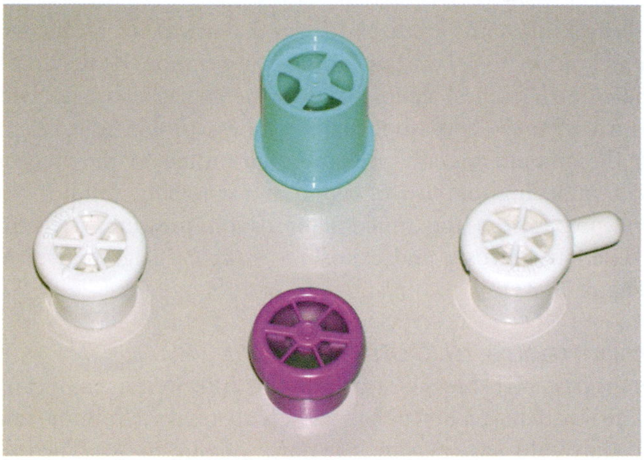

FIGURE 36-31 Speaking valves.

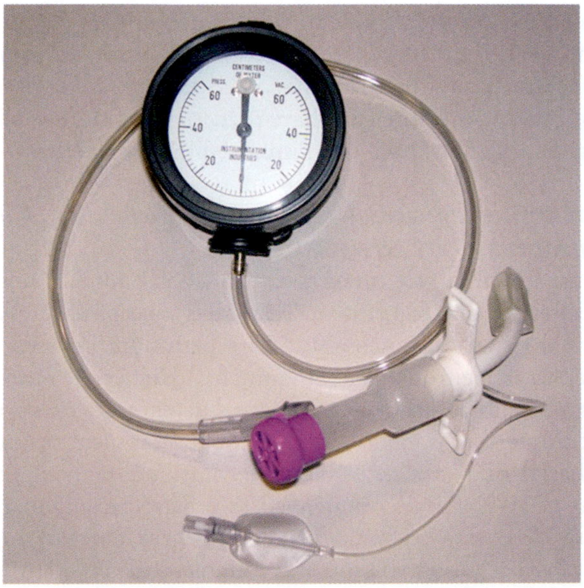

FIGURE 36-32 Setup to measure transtracheal pressures with speaking valve on tracheostomy tube.

be assessed by measuring the tracheal pressure during exhalation with the valve in place as shown in Figure 36-32. If the tracheal pressure is greater than 5 cm H_2O, it may indicate that there is increased resistance during exhalation. The most common causes of this problem are the size of the tracheostomy tube relative to the size of the trachea, tube position, inadequate cuff deflation, or an upper airway abnormality.[28] The tube may need to be changed to a smaller size, to a cuffless tube, or to a tube with a tight-to-shaft cuff. The speaking valve then can be placed and the tracheal pressure measured again. If an upper airway abnormality is suspected, an otolaryngologist should be consulted. A speech-language pathologist may be consulted to assist in the assessment of the patient's risk for aspiration and tolerance of the speaking valve.

Assessment of heart rate, respiratory rate, and saturation should follow initial placement of the valve for all patients. In addition to facilitating communication, other benefits of airflow over the upper airway include better function of the vocal cords, better sense of smell, and fewer secretion problems. Improved swallowing function and less aspiration have been reported with the speaking valve.[48,49]

RULE OF THUMB

The tracheostomy tube cuff must be deflated before a speaking valve is placed on the tracheostomy tube.

Ensuring Adequate Humidification

Although tracheal tubes provide an artificial airway to conduct gas to and from the lungs, they do not function as well as natural airways. Specifically, artificial tracheal airways bypass the normal humidification, filtration, and heating functions of the upper airway. The decreased humidity in the inspired air can cause secretions to thicken. Cool air also can decrease ciliary function. These conditions may impair mucociliary clearance and cause retention of secretions. If a patient is intubated to help clear secretions, failure to provide adequate humidification only worsens the problem. In the worst case, thick secretions can obstruct a tracheal tube and cause asphyxiation.

Either a heated humidifier or a large-volume jet nebulizer should be used to deliver heated humidity to nonventilated patients with a tracheostomy. However, some patients may have increased airway resistance or bronchospasm from the aerosol produced by a large-volume jet nebulizer. A heat and moisture exchanger may be used to provide humidity to patients who do not require O_2 and do not have thick secretions. For ventilated patients, a heated humidifier or heat and moisture exchanger can be used. These devices can provide saturated gas to the airway at temperatures between 32° C and 35° C.[50] The selection of a humidification device ultimately should be based on patient needs and assessment of the airway and include the volume and thickness of secretions and the history of mucous plugging or tube occlusions. More details are provided in the AARC Clinical Practice Guideline for humidification during mechanical ventilation, which is included in Chapter 38.[51]

Minimizing Nosocomial Infections

Patients with tracheal airways are very susceptible to bacterial colonization and infection of the lower respiratory tract. The presence of infection is suggested by changes in the patient's sputum (color, consistency, or amount), breath sounds (wheezes, crackles, or rhonchi), or chest radiograph (infiltrates or atelectasis).[52] Additional changes associated with bacterial infection include fever, increased heart rate, and leukocytosis.

There are several reasons why tracheal tubes increase the incidence of pulmonary infection (Box 36-7).[52,53] To guard against infection, the clinician first should avoid introducing organisms into the airway. The clinician does this by (1) adhering to sterile technique during suctioning, (2) ensuring that only aseptically clean or sterile respiratory equipment is used for each patient, and (3) consistently performing hand hygiene between patient contacts (see Chapter 4).[54]

In addition, efforts should be made to prevent retention of secretions. Suctioning, chest physiotherapy, and adequate humidification are useful to this end. Closed suction systems may be preferred to open suction systems in the prevention of infection.[54] Routinely cleaning or changing the inner cannula on tracheostomy tubes also may help minimize bacterial contamination and infection. Techniques to decrease the consequences of pharyngeal aspiration include (1) use of medications for stress ulcer prophylaxis, such as sucralfate, that maintain normal gastric pH; (2) positioning of patients with the head of the bed elevated 30 degrees or more to decrease reflux; and (3) continuous aspiration of subglottic secretions.[55]

Facilitating Secretion Clearance

The most common cause of airway obstruction in critically ill patients is retained secretions. To remove retained secretions, blood, or other semiliquid fluids from the large airways, the patient is suctioned as described previously in this chapter. Suctioning involves application of negative pressure to the large airways through a catheter. This method may be used alone or in combination with noninvasive techniques described in Chapter 43.

One noninvasive technique is the mechanical insufflator-exsufflator (Cough Assist, J. H. Emerson, Cambridge, MA). It has been shown to facilitate secretion clearance in patients with an ineffective cough, especially secondary to neuromuscular disease, such as amyotrophic lateral sclerosis and muscular dystrophy.[56,57] These patients have decreased vital capacities and expiratory flows. During inspiration, the mechanical insufflator-exsufflator delivers positive pressure usually set between 30 and 40 cm H_2O for 1 to 3 seconds to inflate the lungs. During expiration, it delivers negative pressure usually set between 30 and 40 cm H_2O for 2 to 3 seconds, which increases the expiratory flow rates mobilizing secretions upward into the larger airways.

The mechanical insufflator-exsufflator can be used with a face mask, mouthpiece, or artificial airway. The patient's oropharynx may need to be suctioned after using the mechanical insufflator-exsufflator with a face mask or mouthpiece if the patient is unable to expectorate the secretions. A patient with a tracheostomy tube may require suctioning to clear the tube of secretions after using the mechanical insufflator-exsufflator. The mechanical insufflator-exsufflator may also be used to improve secretion clearance in patients with chronic obstructive pulmonary disease (COPD) and in pediatric patients, but the evidence is unclear as to how beneficial it is in these patients.[58]

Box 36-7 Why Tracheal Airways Increase the Incidence of Pulmonary Infection

- Bypassed upper airway filtration
- Increased aspiration of pharyngeal secretions
- Contaminated equipment or solutions
- Impaired mucociliary clearance in trachea
- Increased mucosal damage owing to tube or suctioning
- Ineffective clearance via cough

Providing Cuff Care

Tracheal tube cuffs are used to seal the airway for mechanical ventilation or to prevent or minimize aspiration. As previously mentioned, tracheal stenosis and tracheomalacia are associated with cuff use. The pathogenesis of these problems is related to the amount of cuff pressure transmitted to the tracheal wall, impeding the flow of blood and lymphatic fluid. If cuff pressure exceeds the mucosal perfusion pressure, ischemia, ulceration, necrosis, and exposure of the cartilage may result (Figure 36-33).

Importance of Cuff Pressure

In the past, high-pressure tracheal tube cuffs were a major cause of airway damage. Since the 1970s, high-residual-volume, low-pressure cuffs have become the norm (Figure 36-34). The fully inflated diameter of these cuffs is greater than the diameter of the trachea. This means that the cuff does not have to be fully inflated to seal the airway, and less internal cuff pressure is needed. When properly used, these cuffs transmit less pressure to the tracheal wall than the older high-pressure designs. Although low-pressure cuffs have reduced the incidence of tracheal damage, they have not eliminated the problem entirely.

Cuff Inflation and Measuring and Adjusting Cuff Pressure

Key aspects of airway care are cuff inflation and cuff pressure measurement and adjustment. The goal is to keep cuff pressures below the tracheal mucosal capillary perfusion pressure, estimated to range from 20 to 30 mm Hg.[43] Higher pressure cuts off mucosal blood flow and causes tissue damage. However, if the cuff pressure is too low, it does not prevent silent aspiration of pharyngeal secretions, which can contribute to the development of VAP. It is recommended to inflate the cuff to 20 to 30 cm H_2O, which should prevent tracheal mucosal injury. Minimal occluding volume and minimal leak inflation techniques are no longer recommended because they increase the risk for silent aspiration.[43]

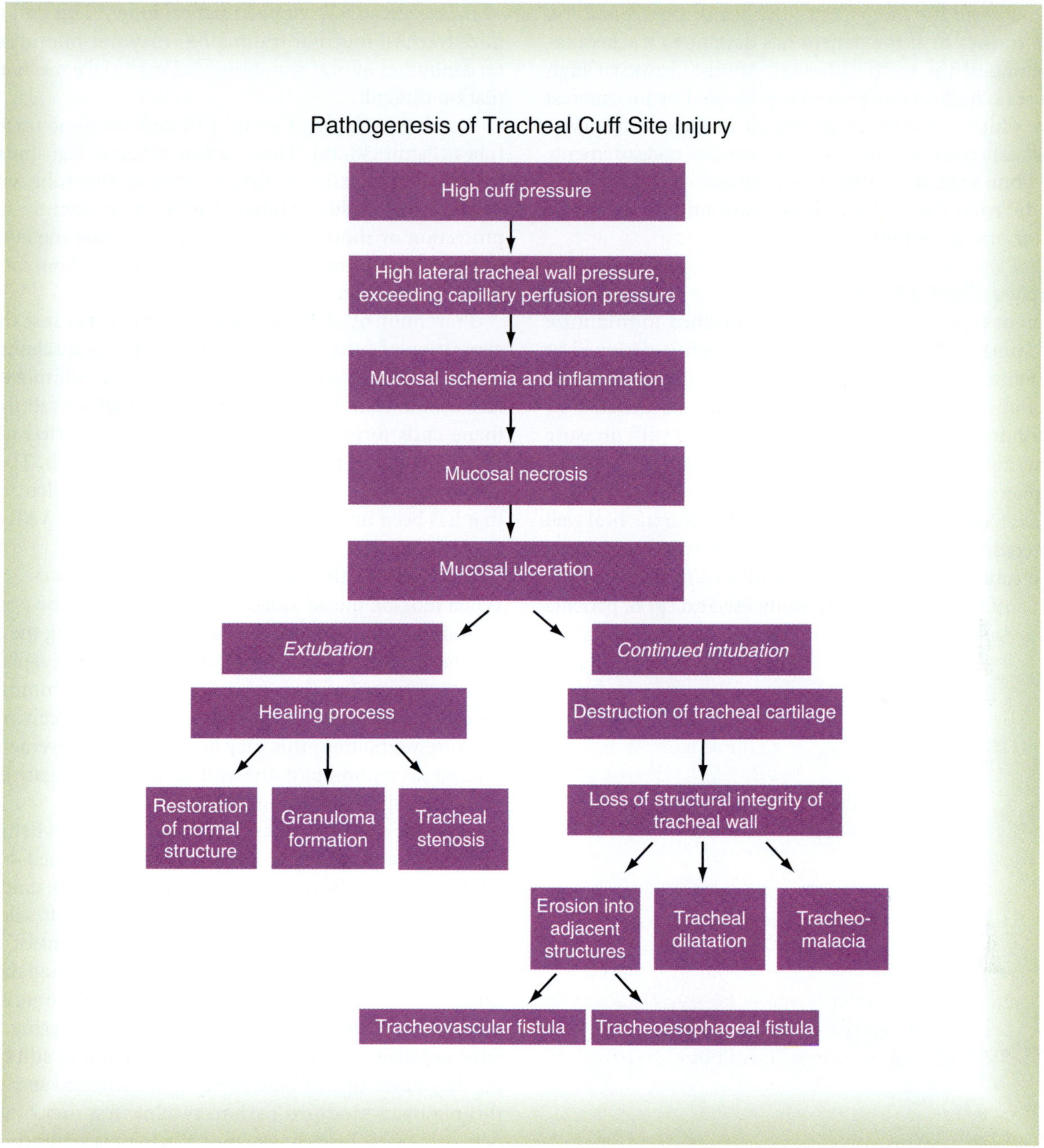

FIGURE 36-33 Tracheal injury may occur secondary to trauma from the cuff. (Modified from Stauffer JL: Complications of endotracheal intubation and tracheostomy. Respir Care 44:828, 1999.)

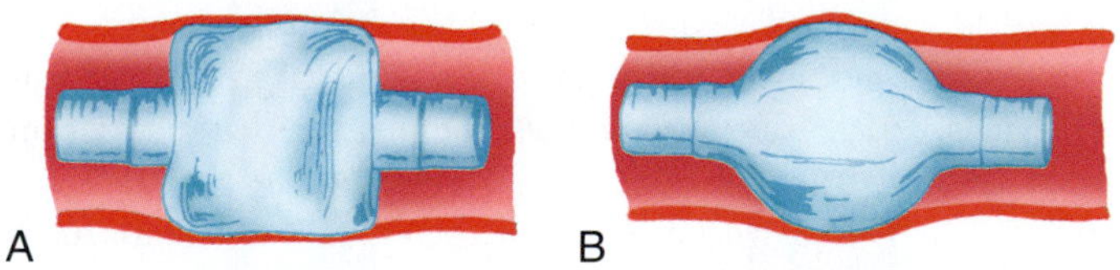

FIGURE 36-34 Comparison of shapes of high-residual-volume, low-pressure cuff **(A)** and low-residual-volume, high-pressure cuff **(B).** (Modified from McPherson SP: Respiratory therapy equipment, ed 4, St. Louis, 1989, Mosby.)

Cuff pressure can be measured with various devices designed for this purpose. These devices have the ability to measure the pressure and allow air to be added or withdrawn from the cuff. There are two key considerations when making these adjustments. First, most manometers are calibrated in centimeters of water, with the "acceptable range" of pressure 20 to 30 cm H_2O.[42] Second, attaching the measurement system to the pilot tube evacuates some volume from the cuff (and decreases its pressure). For this reason, the clinician should always adjust the pressure to the desired level and never just measure it.

High cuff pressures may be caused by the need to overinflate the cuff to seal the airway. This problem is common if the tube chosen is too small for the patient's trachea or positioned too high in the trachea or if the patient has developed tracheomalacia (softening of the tracheal tissue). Another cause of high cuff pressures is high airway pressures generated by mechanical ventilation, which may require adding air to the cuff to maintain an adequate tracheal seal. Intracuff pressure measurements should be done regularly to maintain the cuff pressure in the safe range to avoid tracheal wall injury and minimize risk for aspiration of oral secretions.

Alternative Cuff Designs

Some different types of cuffs have been designed to minimize mucosal trauma.[24] The foam cuff is one, which is designed to seal the trachea with atmospheric pressure in the cuff (Figure 36-35). Before insertion, the foam cuff must be deflated by actively withdrawing air from the cuff with a cuff pressure device or syringe. When in position, the pilot tube is opened to the atmosphere, and the foam is allowed to expand against the tracheal wall. Expansion of the cuff stops when the tracheal wall is encountered. If too much air leak and volume loss occur around the tube, the pilot tube can be placed in line with the ETT. Foam cuff tubes are not commonly used except in patients who have already developed tracheal injury. This cuff can minimize tracheal mucosal trauma but may not minimize the risk for aspiration of oral secretions and may make mechanical ventilation difficult.

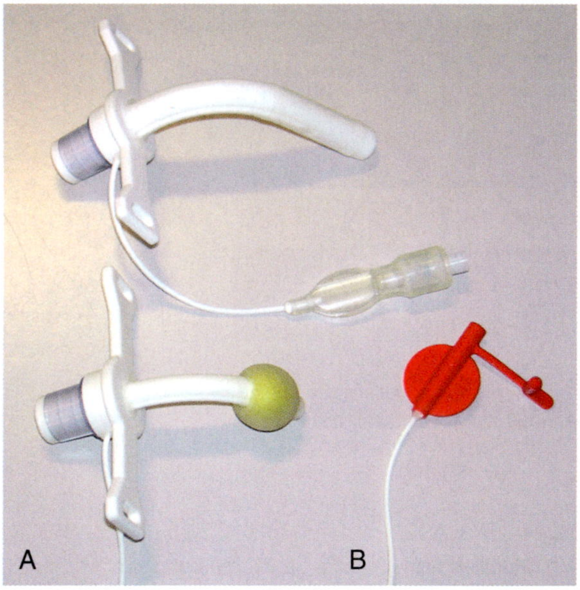

FIGURE 36-35 Tracheostomy tubes (TTs) with different types of cuffs. **A,** TTS cuff. **B,** Self-inflating foam cuff.

Another cuff design is the TTS cuff on some tracheostomy tubes (Figure 36-36). This is a low-volume, high-pressure cuff designed to maximize airflow around the tube when it is deflated. It should be inflated only intermittently for airway protection or short-term ventilation. Because the cuff is made of a porous silicone material, it can be inflated only with sterile water and not air.

Prevention of silent aspiration is difficult because the current generation of cuffs when inflated properly create channels along the cuff in which secretions from above the cuff move by capillary action. Newer tubes with longer length ultrathin polyurethane cuffs form a cylinder shape or an inverted pear shape when inflated so that they do not form channels. These newer cuff designs and material seem to minimize silent aspiration that has been implicated in the development of VAP.[59]

Minimizing Likelihood of Aspiration

When judging the adequacy of a tracheal seal, the potential for aspiration should be taken into account. Keeping the cuff pressure between 20 and 30 cm H_2O helps minimize aspiration and injury. Also, aspiration is reported to be more common in spontaneously breathing patients than in patients receiving positive pressure ventilation; this may be due to the movement of pharyngeal secretions past the cuff during the negative pressure phase of a spontaneous inspiration.

A simple swallowing test can help determine whether aspiration is occurring. These tests can be performed by various clinicians, including speech therapists, nurses, and RTs. To perform this test, blue food coloring is added to the patient's feedings or the patient swallows a small amount of blue food coloring in water. The patient's trachea is suctioned through the artificial airway. If blue-tinged secretions are obtained when performing suctioning, some aspiration is occurring. However, false-negative results can occur; the patient may still be aspirating despite no sign of blue coloring in suctioned secretions. For this reason, a modified barium swallow test may be needed to determine conclusively whether a patient is aspirating.[60]

If aspiration is confirmed, efforts must be made to minimize the aspiration. Ideally, the patient should be switched to a tube that continually aspirates subglottic secretions (see the previous

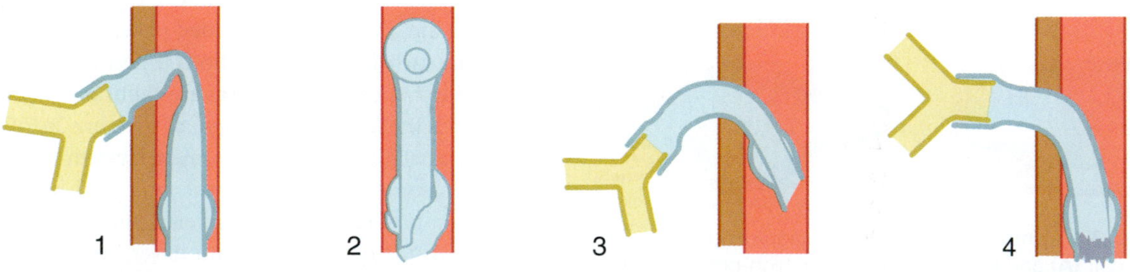

FIGURE 36-36 Causes of tube obstruction. (See text for details.) (Modified from Sykes MK, McNichol MW, Campbell EJM: Respiratory failure, Philadelphia, 1969, FA Davis.)

Box 36-8 Equipment for Tracheostomy Care

- Personal protective equipment: Goggles and mask or face shield
- Sterile gloves
- Suction equipment
- Resuscitation bag
- Oxygen
- Tracheostomy care kit (basin and brush)
  - Spare inner cannula
  - Disposable inner cannula (if appropriate)
  - Hydrogen peroxide and sterile water
  - Cotton-tipped applicators
  - Precut gauze pad or precut foam dressing (to absorb excessive drainage)
  - New tracheostomy tube tie or Velcro tracheostomy tube (TT) holder
  - Another TT of the same size as backup
  - Additional equipment needed if changing TT
  - New TT with component parts and another tube one size smaller
  - Water-soluble lubricant
  - 10- or 12-ml syringe

section on Specialized Endotracheal Tubes). If it is impossible to make this switch, oropharyngeal suctioning (above the tube cuff) should be performed as needed. To decrease the possibility of aspiration with feedings, the head of the bed should be elevated 30 degrees or more when possible.[55] Also, the feeding tube can be inserted into the duodenum, with its position confirmed by radiograph. The use of slightly higher cuff pressure during and after feedings may minimize aspiration.

Care of Tracheostomy and Tube

Tracheostomy tubes require daily care to clean the site and change the tie or holder securing the tube. The tubes also may be removed and replaced for routine cleaning or in an emergency, such as obstruction of the tube. The procedures for tracheostomy care and changing a tracheostomy tube are described in the following section.[61-63]

Tracheostomy Care

Step 1: Assemble and Check Equipment.

Box 36-8 lists the equipment needed for routine tracheostomy care. The equipment needed is for cleaning through the tube, around the tube, and the tube itself. Personal protective equipment (face shield or mask and goggles) for the clinician is needed because the stimulation of the trachea may result in coughing and expectorated secretions. Use of suction equipment to remove secretions from the tube before the procedure can decrease the possibility of secretions contaminating the environment. O_2 and a manual resuscitator are needed for the suctioning procedure and in case any problems such as desaturation occur. To clean around the tube, hydrogen peroxide (diluted to half-strength with sterile water or saline), sterile water, cotton-tipped applicators, and tracheostomy sponges are needed along with a new tie or tracheostomy tube holder to secure the tube. A tracheostomy tube kit includes a basin and brush to clean the inner cannula of the tube. Alternatively, a disposable inner cannula may be used. The function of the manual resuscitator, O_2 flow, and suction control must be checked before starting.

Step 2: Explain Procedure to Patient.

Explain the procedure and confirm the patient understands what will be done.

Step 3: Suction Patient.

The procedures previously described for endotracheal suctioning are appropriate for this situation. A tracheostomy tube is much shorter than an ETT. The catheter is inserted just to the end of the tracheostomy tube to avoid causing mucosal injury to the carina.

Step 4: Clean Inner Cannula (If Present and Nondisposable).

The inner cannula is removed and placed in the basin. If appropriate, such as in the case of a ventilator-dependent patient, the spare inner cannula is inserted. Patients with certain types of tracheostomy tubes (Portex) can be mechanically ventilated without an inner cannula in place. If the patient is not mechanically ventilated, the O_2 therapy device is reapplied as necessary. Sterile water and hydrogen peroxide are added to the basin, and the cannula is left to soak. The brush is used to remove any dried secretions from the inner lumen or the outside of the cannula. The cannula is rinsed with sterile water and allowed to air dry on sterile gauze.

Step 5: Clean and Examine Stoma Site.

The dressing (if present) is removed and disposed. Applicators that have been dipped in sterile normal saline or half-strength hydrogen peroxide are used to clean around the stoma site. After cleaning liquid, a skin barrier should be applied to protect the skin from moisture. A clean dressing, if needed to absorb drainage, is placed under the flange of the tube. Either precut gauze or an absorbent foam dressing, especially if there is excessive drainage around stoma, should be used. If the stoma site appears red or swollen, has pus around it, or is emitting a foul smell, the physician and nurse should be notified.

Step 6: Change Tie or Holder.

The clinician cuts the old tie or loosens the Velcro holder. One hand is kept on the flange of the tracheostomy tube to keep it secure. The old tie or holder is removed and discarded. The clinician replaces the tie or holder, keeping one finger-width of space between the neck and tie or holder.

Step 7: Replace Clean Inner Cannula (If Present).

If the inner cannula is marked disposable and is not to be reused, a new one is inserted.

Step 8: Reassess Patient.

The clinician checks for adequate breath sounds, checks vital signs and oxygenation, and confirms no adverse effects.

RULE OF THUMB

An extra tracheostomy tube of the same size and another, one size smaller, should be kept readily available in or near the patient's room in case of an accidental decannulation.

Changing a Tracheostomy Tube

A tracheostomy tube may need to be replaced according to schedule in the case of long-term mechanical ventilation; if the current tube develops a problem, such as a mucous plug or damage to the cuff; or if a different size or type of tube is needed.[63] If a tube needs to be replaced before the stoma heals (7 to 10 days), it is best done by a physician. Intubation equipment should also be available. Because a single cannula tube has no inner cannula to remove for cleaning, it may need to be replaced periodically.

Step 1: Assemble and Prepare Equipment.

In addition to the equipment described previously, the new tube, an extra tube one size smaller, and water-soluble lubricant are necessary.

Step 2: Explain Procedure to Patient.

Step 3: Prepare Equipment.

Sterile technique must always be maintained for the distal portion of the cannula, which goes into the trachea. The inner cannula is removed and placed on a sterile surface. The obturator is inserted. The tie or tracheostomy tube holder is attached to one side of the flange of the tube. The clinician inflates the cuff, checks for leaks, and deflates the cuff. Lubricant is applied to the distal portion of the cannula.

Step 4: Prepare Patient.

The patient should be placed with the neck extended so that the tracheal stoma is accessible. The patient is suctioned and hyperoxygenated.

Step 5: Remove Old Tube.

The tie is cut, or the Velcro tracheostomy tube holder is opened. The cuff is deflated. The clinician removes the tube by following the curve of the tube. The clinician grasps the outer portion of the tracheostomy tube with one hand and rotates the wrist toward the chest. The stoma is inspected for any bleeding or other problems, such as granuloma or ulceration.

Step 6: Insert New Tube and Assess Patient.

The new tube is picked up by the proximal portion. The surface that enters the trachea should not be touched. The tip of the obturator is inserted into the stoma, and the tube is advanced following the curve of the tube. While holding the flange of the tube against the neck, the clinician immediately removes the obturator. The clinician assesses for airflow through the tube. Coughing may reflect pressure on the outside of the trachea. The patient is assessed for proper tube placement and tolerance of the procedure. If extreme difficulty is encountered inserting the new tube, insertion of the "stand-by" tube, which is one size smaller, is attempted.

Step 7: Secure Tube.

While still holding onto the flange, the clinician secures the tracheostomy tube tie or holder without overtightening. The inner cannula, if present, is inserted. The clinician reassesses for airflow and reapplies the O_2 therapy device or ventilator.

Step 8: Reassess Patient.

Suctioning may be required again. The clinician checks vital signs and O_2 saturation (SaO_2) and assesses the patient's overall tolerance of the procedure.

Troubleshooting Airway Emergencies

The areas discussed so far are routine aspects of airway care. Three emergency situations that may occur are tube obstruction, cuff leaks, and accidental extubation. Clinical signs frequently encountered under these circumstances include various degrees of respiratory distress; changes in breath sounds; air movement through the mouth; or, if the patient is mechanically ventilated, changes in pressures.

Decreased breath sounds are a common finding in airway emergencies. The RT must try to identify specific indications of decreased breath sounds, such as the inability to pass a suction catheter (obstruction, occluded tube) or airflow around the tube (leaking cuff). Replacement airways, a manual resuscitator, mask, and gauze pads (for patients with tracheostomies) should be kept at the bedside.

Tube Obstruction

Obstruction of the tube is one of the most common causes of airway emergencies. Tube obstruction can be caused by (1) the kinking of the tube or the patient biting on the tube, (2) herniation of the cuff over the tube tip,[64] (3) obstruction of the tube orifice against the tracheal wall,[67] and (4) mucous plugging (see Figure 36-36).

Different clinical signs are present depending on whether the tube obstruction is partial or complete.[39,65] A spontaneously breathing patient with partial airway obstruction exhibits decreased breath sounds and decreased airflow through the tube. If the patient is receiving volume-controlled ventilation, peak inspiratory pressures increase, often causing the high-pressure alarm to sound; during pressure-controlled ventilation, delivered V_Ts decrease. With complete tube obstruction, the patient exhibits severe distress, no breath sounds are heard, and there is no gas flow through the tube.

If the tube is kinked or positioned against the tracheal wall, the obstruction can be reversed by moving the patient's head and neck or repositioning the tube.[39] If this action does not relieve the obstruction, a herniated cuff may be blocking the airway. Deflating the cuff relieves the obstruction in such cases. If these steps fail to overcome the obstruction, the clinician can try to pass a suction catheter through the tube. The distance the catheter inserts before stopping helps determine the site of obstruction. If the catheter does not travel much beyond the tube tip and insertion does not cause coughing, the likely problem is a herniated cuff or a mucous plug. In the case of mucous plugging, the clinician can attempt to remove the plug by suctioning the tube before considering more drastic action. Although instillation of sterile normal saline into the tube is not routinely needed during suctioning, it may facilitate mobilizing the mucous plug so that it can be more easily removed by suctioning. Also, a mucus shaving device may be used to clear thick, dried secretions from the inner lumen of the ETT. This device has a balloon at the end of the catheter. Once the catheter is inserted into the ETT, the balloon is inflated. When the catheter is withdrawn, the balloon scrapes the thick, dried mucus from the inside of the tube[66] (Figure 36-37).

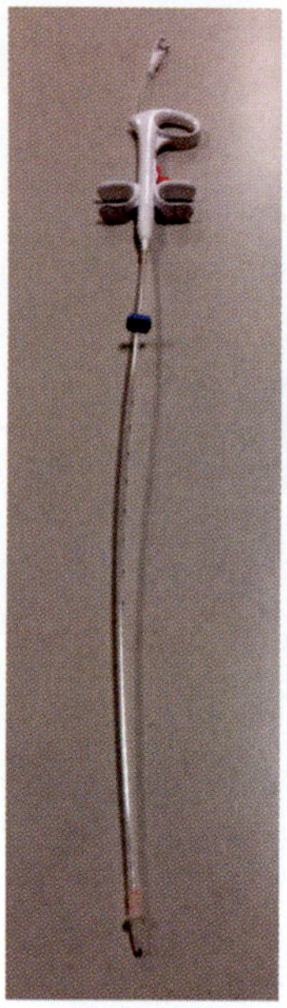

FIGURE 36-37 Mucus shaving device.

When the patient has a tracheostomy tube with an inner cannula, it should be removed and checked to see if the plug is lodged in the tube. O_2 should be provided to the patient through the outer cannula, or the inner cannula should be replaced with a spare one to facilitate manual ventilation.

If the obstruction cannot be cleared by using these techniques, the airway should be removed and replaced. In patients who have undergone recent tracheotomy (4 or 5 days earlier), the stoma may not be well established and may close when the tube is removed. If suture ties were left in place by the surgeon, they can be used to pull open the stoma.

After the obstructed airway is removed, the clinician should immediately try to restore adequate ventilation and oxygenation. For a patient with a tracheotomy stoma, the stoma may need to be covered with a gauze pad and the patient may need to be manually ventilated with a mask. Airway reinsertion by a properly trained RT or physician should be undertaken only after adequate ventilation and oxygenation are restored.

Cuff Leaks

A leak in the cuff, pilot tube, or one-way valve is a problem mostly for patients receiving mechanical ventilation. This leak causes a system leak, with a resultant loss of delivered volume or decreased inspiratory pressure or both.

A small cuff leak can be detected by noting decreasing cuff pressures over time. A large leak, such as occurs with a ruptured cuff, generally has a more rapid onset. Breath sounds are decreased, but a spontaneously breathing patient has air movement through the tube. With positive pressure breaths, airflow often is felt at the mouth. Under such circumstances, the RT should try to reinflate the cuff while checking the pilot tube and valve for leaks.[13] If the pilot tube or valve is leaking, the tube needs to be changed as soon as possible. However, a pilot valve (pilot balloon) repair kit, which permits the insertion of a replacement valve into the pilot tubing, can offer a safe and effective alternative until a replacement tube can be inserted.

A ruptured cuff requires extubation and reintubation emergently if the patient is being mechanically ventilated. This procedure can be done via the standard reintubation procedure or by using an ETT exchanger, which is a semirigid guide over which the damaged tube can be removed and the new tube promptly inserted. An ETT exchanger should be used only by an individual trained in its use, and all necessary intubation equipment and personnel should be available to perform a standard intubation if problems occur. An ETT that is positioned too high in the trachea and near the glottic opening can mimic a cuff leak. Before presuming a cuff leak, the RT should check the tube depth by noting the markings, and if the tube appears shallow, the RT should attempt to advance the tube slightly and reassess the leak. A leak around a tracheal tube can occur from a tube or cuff problem. Figure 36-38 is a diagram of the process to investigate the source of a leak around a tube.[13]

MINI CLINI

Airway Cuff Problems

PROBLEM: The RT is called to assist with a 220-lb, 6-ft, 2-inch male patient who is intubated with a 7-mm ETT and receiving positive pressure ventilation. The patient's nurse reports to the RT that over the last week it has been increasingly difficult to get a good seal with the tube cuff and that she has had to add "more and more air" to prevent gross leakage. When asked if the cuff pressures have been monitored, she says no. What is the likely problem and solution?

DISCUSSION: "Low-pressure" cuffs can exert high pressure at high inflation volumes. The need for high volumes to get a good seal usually indicates that the ETT or tracheostomy tube is too small for the patient. This large man probably should have been intubated with at least an 8-mm tube. In addition, because cuff pressures were not monitored, it is possible that tracheal damage has already occurred. The fact that the nurse reports having to add "more and more air" to get a seal suggests tracheomalacia, which could be confirmed by radiographic or bronchoscopic examination.

Tracheomalacia can cause a vicious cycle in which high pressure causes more tracheal dilation, which requires higher pressures to seal the cuff, and so on. If tracheomalacia is confirmed, and the patient still needs an artificial airway, the smaller tube should be replaced with a larger one that allows a good seal at acceptable cuff pressures. It also may be necessary to reposition the tube so that the cuff is not proximal to the original site of damage.

Accidental Extubation

Partial displacement of an airway out of the trachea can be detected by noting decreased breath sounds, decreased airflow through the tube, and the ability to pass a catheter to its full length without meeting an obstruction or eliciting a cough.

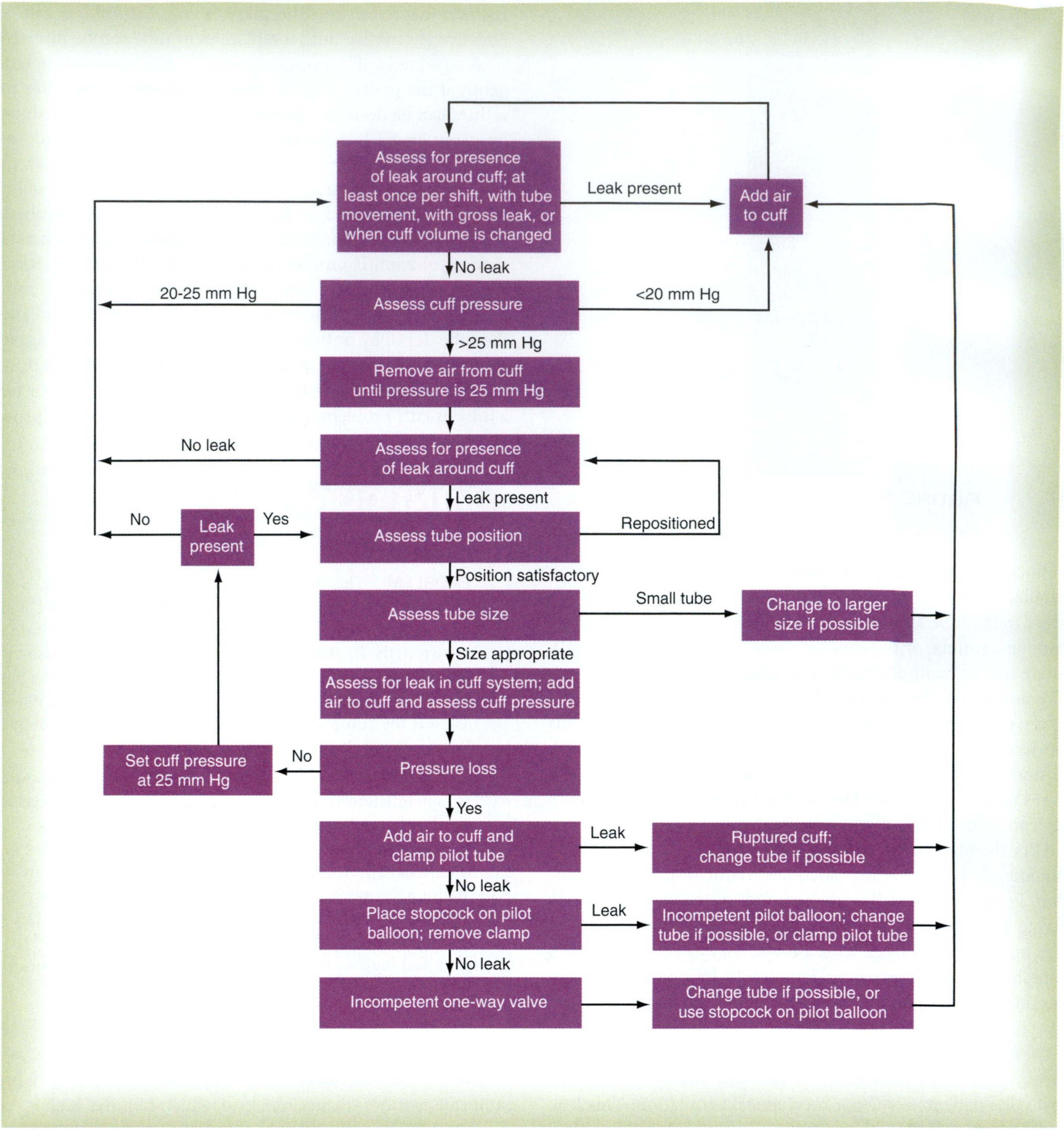

FIGURE 36-38 Algorithm for solving leaking cuff problems. (From Hess D: Managing the artificial airway. Respir Care 44:759, 1999.)

With positive pressure ventilation, airflow through the mouth or into the stomach may be heard and a decrease in delivered volumes or pressures occurs. In these cases, the tube should be completely removed and ventilatory support should be provided by manual resuscitator and mask as needed until the patient can be reintubated or the tracheostomy tube reinserted. To monitor trends and optimize quality outcomes associated with unplanned extubations, hospitals often require certain details of such incidents to be recorded.

EXTUBATION OR DECANNULATION

For most patients, tracheal intubation is a temporary measure. The artificial airway should be removed when it is no longer needed. The process of removing an artificial tracheal airway is called **extubation** (ETT) or **decannulation** (tracheostomy tube). Although most patients eventually undergo extubation, a few need to maintain a permanent artificial route, usually by tracheostomy. Permanent tracheostomies are common among patients with surgically treated throat or laryngeal cancer and patients requiring long-term positive pressure ventilation. Advances in noninvasive mechanical ventilation have reduced the need for permanent tracheostomies in the latter group.

Assessing Patient Readiness for Extubation

A patient is ready to be extubated when the original need for the artificial airway no longer exists. Because artificial airways are inserted for many different reasons, several different criteria to establish readiness for extubation need to be considered.[67] Some basic assessments include the ability of the patient to protect the airway by the presence of a gag reflex, the ability to manage secretions based on cough strength, the quantity and thickness of secretions, and the patency of the upper airway.

MINI CLINI

Extubation Assessment

PROBLEM: A physician informs the RT that a patient recently removed from a ventilator is maintaining adequate oxygenation and ventilation via spontaneous breathing through an oral ETT. She requests that the RT evaluate the patient for extubation. What would the RT assess and why?

DISCUSSION: Because the patient is maintaining adequate oxygenation and ventilation off the ventilator, two key criteria for extubation have already been met. Further assessment is needed to determine (1) the risk for upper airway obstruction after extubation, (2) the level of protection against aspiration, and (3) the ability of the patient to clear secretions after extubation. First, the RT should perform a leak test to assess for upper airway edema. Second, the RT should determine the patient's level of consciousness and neuromuscular function by assessing the gag reflex or having the patient try to raise and hold his or her head off the bed. Third, the RT should determine the patient's ability to cough, using either subjective assessment (on suctioning) or measurement of maximum expiratory pressure or peak cough flow. Extubation should be recommended only if all three areas yield positive results.

The decision to remove the airway may not be the same as the decision to discontinue mechanical ventilation. The ventilator and airway may be removed simultaneously in the case of patients with normal lungs intubated for surgery. If a patient was intubated because of respiratory failure and has improved, but the upper airway problems remain (e.g., no gag reflex), the ventilator may be discontinued before extubation.

The cuff-leak test is designed to help predict the occurrence of glottic edema or stridor after extubation.[68,69] The clinician totally deflates the tube cuff and assesses the leak around the tube during positive pressure ventilation in a volume-controlled mode. The percent of the cuff leak should be approximately 15% or greater, as determined by the difference between the measured expiratory V_T with the cuff inflated and then deflated.[68] If the exhaled volume is 500 ml with the cuff inflated and 400 ml with the cuff deflated, the difference is 100 ml. The percent cuff leak is 20% (100 ml divided by 500 ml), which suggests that there is no significant upper airway edema or obstruction. However, some data suggest that this test may not always be predictive of the presence of upper airway obstruction or edema.[70] This test may be most useful in patients who are at greatest risk for postextubation stridor, such as children, women, and patients intubated for more than 6 days.[71] Some patients who fail the test or who have questionable results may still be extubated, but they must be closely monitored with the appropriate personnel and equipment available to reestablish the airway if needed.

Clinical Practice Guideline

To guide practitioners in safe and effective application of this procedure, the AARC has developed a clinical practice guideline on removal of the ETT. Excerpts from the AARC guideline, including indications, contraindications, hazards and complications, assessment of need, assessment of outcome, and monitoring, appear in Clinical Practice Guideline 36-4.[67]

Procedures

Because RTs play a key role in extubation and decannulation and the techniques differ, the procedures for removing orotracheal or nasotracheal (extubation) and tracheostomy tubes (decannulation) are reviewed separately.

Orotracheal or Nasotracheal Tubes

The procedure for orotracheal or nasotracheal extubation is as follows.

Step 1: Assemble Needed Equipment.
Needed equipment includes suctioning apparatus; two age-appropriate suction kits with sterile suction catheters and gloves; tonsillar suction tip (Yankauer); 10-ml or 12-ml syringe; O_2 and aerosol therapy equipment; manual resuscitator and mask; aerosol nebulizer with racemic epinephrine and normal saline (if ordered); and intubation equipment (laryngoscope blades, handle, ETTs, stylets, water-soluble lubricant, syringe to inflate cuff, tape or holder to secure tube).

Step 2: Suction Endotracheal Tube and Pharynx to Above Cuff.
Suctioning before extubation helps prevent aspiration of secretions after cuff deflation. After use, the first suction kit should be discarded, and another should be prepared for use, or a rigid tonsillar (Yankauer) suction tip should be prepared to suction the oropharynx.

Step 3: Oxygenate Patient Well After Suctioning.
Extubation is a stressful procedure that can cause hypoxemia and unwanted cardiovascular side effects. To help avoid these problems, 100% O_2 should be administered for 1 to 2 minutes.

Step 4: Deflate Cuff.
The 10- or 12-ml syringe is attached to the pilot tubing. All the air is withdrawn from the cuff while applying positive pressure to direct any pooled secretions above the cuff up into the oropharynx, where they can immediately be

36-4 Removal of the Endotracheal Tube

AARC Clinical Practice Guideline (Excerpts)*

ENVIRONMENT

The endotracheal tube should be removed in an environment in which the patient can be physiologically monitored and in which emergency equipment and appropriately trained health care providers with airway management skills are immediately available.

INDICATIONS

- The airway control afforded by the endotracheal tube is deemed to be no longer necessary for the continued care of the patient.
- Subjective or objective determination of improvement of the underlying condition impairing pulmonary function or gas-exchange capacity, or both, is made before extubation. To maximize the likelihood for successful extubation, the patient should be capable of maintaining a patent airway and generating adequate spontaneous ventilation. Generally, the patient needs to possess adequate central inspiratory drive, respiratory muscle strength, cough strength to clear secretions, laryngeal function, nutritional status, and clearance of sedative and neuromuscular blocking effects.
- Occasionally, acute airway obstruction of the artificial airway caused by mucus or mechanical deformation mandates immediate removal of the artificial airway. Reintubation or other appropriate techniques for reestablishing the airway (i.e., surgical airway management) must be used to maintain effective gas exchange.
- Patients in whom an explicit declaration of the futility of further medical care is documented may have the endotracheal tube removed despite failure to meet the previously listed indications.

CONTRAINDICATIONS

There are no absolute contraindications to extubation. However, some patients may require one or more of the following to maintain acceptable gas exchange after extubation: Noninvasive ventilation, continuous positive airway pressure (CPAP), high inspired O_2 fraction, or reintubation. Airway protective reflexes may be depressed immediately after as well as for some time after extubation. Measures to prevent aspiration should be considered.

HAZARDS AND COMPLICATIONS

- Hypoxemia after extubation may result from but is not limited to
  - Failure to deliver adequate FiO_2 through the natural upper airway
  - Acute upper airway obstruction secondary to laryngospasm
  - Development of postobstruction pulmonary edema
  - Bronchospasm
  - Development of atelectasis, or lung collapse
  - Pulmonary aspiration
  - Hypoventilation
- Hypercapnia after extubation may be caused by but is not limited to
  - Upper airway obstruction resulting from edema of the trachea, vocal cords, or larynx
  - Respiratory muscle weakness
  - Excessive work of breathing
  - Bronchospasm
- Death may occur when medical futility is the reason for removing the endotracheal tube.

ASSESSMENT OF EXTUBATION READINESS

The endotracheal tube should be removed as soon as the patient no longer requires an artificial airway. Patients should show some evidence for the reversal of the underlying cause of respiratory failure and should be capable of maintaining adequate spontaneous ventilation and gas exchange. The determination of extubation readiness may be individualized using the following guidelines:

- Patients with an artificial airway to facilitate treatment of respiratory failure should be considered for extubation when they have met established extubation readiness criteria; examples of these criteria include but are not limited to:
  - The capacity to maintain adequate arterial partial pressure of O_2 (PaO_2/FiO_2 ratio >150 to 200) on inspired O_2 fractions provided with simple O_2 devices ($FiO_2 \le 0.4$ to 0.5) and with low levels of PEEP (≤5 to 8 cm H_2O)
  - The capacity to maintain appropriate pH (pH ≥ 7.25) and arterial partial pressure of CO_2 during spontaneous ventilation
  - Successful completion of 30- to 120-minute spontaneous breathing trial performed with a low level of CPAP (e.g., 5 cm H_2O) or low level of pressure support (e.g., 5 to 7 cm H_2O) showing adequate respiratory pattern and gas exchange, hemodynamic stability, and subjective comfort
  - In adults, respiratory rate less than 35 breaths/min during spontaneous breathing; in infants and children, acceptable respiratory rate decreases inversely with age and can be measured with good repeatability with a stethoscope
  - Adequate respiratory muscle strength
  - Maximum negative inspiratory pressure greater than −30 cm H_2O, although current clinical practice may accept greater than −20 cm H_2O
  - Vital capacity greater than 10 ml/kg ideal body weight or in neonates greater than 150 ml/m^2
  - Pressure measured across the diaphragm during spontaneous ventilation less than 15% of maximum
  - In adults, spontaneous exhaled minute ventilation less than 10 L/min
  - In adults, a rapid shallow breathing index (ratio of respiratory rate to tidal volume of ≤105); in infants and children, variables standardized by age or weight prove more useful
  - Thoracic compliance greater than 25 ml/cm H_2O
  - Work of breathing less than 0.8 J/L
  - O_2 cost of breathing less than 15% total, especially for patients with chronic respiratory insufficiency requiring long-term mechanical ventilation
  - Ratio of dead space to tidal volume (V_D/V_T) less than 0.6; in children, V_D/V_T of 0.5 or less equates to 96% successful extubation, 0.51 to 0.64 equates to 60% successful extubation, 0.65 equates to 20% successful extubation.
  - Airway occlusion pressure at 0.1 second (P0.1) less than 6 cm H_2O and when normalized for maximal inspiratory

36-4 Removal of the Endotracheal Tube—cont'd

AARC Clinical Practice Guideline (Excerpts)*

pressure (MIP), as indicated by P0.1/MIP (107 to 109) (this measurement is primarily a research tool)
- Maximum voluntary ventilation more than twice the resting minute ventilation
- In preterm infants, minute ventilation testing versus standard clinical evaluation resulted in shorter time to extubation.
- Peak expiratory flow of 60 L/min or greater after three cough attempts measured with an in-line spirometer.
- Time to recovery of minute ventilation to pre–spontaneous breathing trial baseline levels
- Sustained maximal inspiratory pressures greater than 57.5 pressure time units predicted extubation outcome.
- In neonates, total respiratory compliance (derived from V_T/PIP – PEEP) of 0.9 ml/cm H_2O or less was associated with extubation failure, whereas a value of 1.3 ml/cm H_2O or greater was associated with extubation success.
- Preterm infants extubated directly from low-rate ventilation without a trial of endotracheal tube CPAP showed a trend toward increased chance of successful extubation.
- Integrated indices of measured vital capacity (threshold value 635 ml), respiratory frequency-to-tidal volume ratio (threshold value 88 breaths/min/L), and maximal expiratory pressure (threshold value 28 cm H_2O)

- In addition to treatment of respiratory failure, artificial airways are sometimes placed for airway protection. Resolution of the need for airway protection may be assessed by but is not limited to
  - Appropriate level of consciousness
  - Adequate airway protective reflexes
  - Reduced cough strength (grade 0 to 2) measured by the white card test and increased secretion burden predicted unsuccessful extubation
  - Easily managed secretions
- In addition to resolution of the processes requiring the insertion of an artificial airway, issues that should be considered in all patients before extubation include the following:
  - No immediate need for reintubation
  - Known risk factors for extubation failure
  - Patient features of high risk for extubation failure include admission to medical intensive care unit, age older than 70 years or younger than 24 months, higher severity of illness on weaning, hemoglobin less than 10 mg/dl, use of continuous intravenous sedation, longer duration of mechanical ventilation, presence of a syndromic or chronic medical condition, known medical or surgical airway condition, frequent pulmonary toilet, and loss of airway protective reflexes.
  - Risk factors for a known history of a difficult airway include syndromic or congenital conditions associated with cervical instability (i.e., Klippel-Feil syndrome or trisomy 21); limited physical access to the airway (i.e., halo vest or anatomic hindrances); and multiple failed direct laryngoscopy attempts by an experienced laryngoscopist or a failed laryngoscopy attempt followed by tracheal intubation using fiberoptic bronchoscopy or a nasal light wand or requiring placement of a laryngeal mask airway.
  - In the pediatric patients undergoing cardiothoracic surgery, presence of one or more of these variables increases the likelihood of failed extubation: age younger than 6 months, history of prematurity, congestive heart failure, and pulmonary hypertension.
  - For pediatric patients, validated bedside measures of respiratory function identifying low risk (<10%) and high risk (>25%) threshold values of extubation failure may be useful in generating discussion but do not apply to individual risk.
  - Presence of upper airway obstruction or laryngeal edema as detected by diminished gas leak around the endotracheal tube with positive pressure breaths
  - Percent cuff leak or the difference between expiratory tidal volume measured with the cuff inflated and then deflated in a volume-controlled mode of 15.5% or greater; this test was found not to be predictive in a study of patients undergoing cardiothoracic surgery.
  - Air leak may be an age-dependent predictor of postextubation stridor in children. An air leak greater than 20 cm H_2O was predictive of postextubation stridor in children 7 years old or older but was not predictive in children younger than 7 years.
  - Air leak test has been predictive of postextubation stridor or extubation failure for children with upper airway pathology, including trauma patients, patients with croup, and patients after tracheal surgery.
  - Evidence of stable, adequate hemodynamic function
  - Evidence of stable nonrespiratory functions
  - Electrolyte values within normal range
  - Evidence of malnutrition decreasing respiratory muscle function and ventilatory drive
  - Anesthesia literature indicates the patient must have no intake of food or liquid by mouth for a time before airway manipulation; continuation of transpyloric feedings during an extubation procedure is controversial.
- Prophylactic medication before extubation to avoid or reduce the severity of postextubation complications
  - Consider use of lidocaine to prevent cough or laryngospasm in patients at risk
  - Prophylactic administration of steroids may be helpful to prevent reintubation rates in high-risk neonates but not in children.
  - Prophylactic administration of steroids may help reduce the incidence of postextubation stridor in children but not in neonates or adults.
  - Prophylactic administration of steroids for patients with laryngotracheobronchitis (croup) correlates with reduced rates of reintubation.
  - Caffeine citrate reduced the risk for apnea for infants but did not reduce the risk for extubation failure.
  - Methylxanthine treatment stimulates breathing and reduces the rate of apnea for neonates with poor respiratory drive, especially low-birth-weight infants.

ASSESSMENT OF OUTCOME

- Removal of the endotracheal tube should be followed by adequate spontaneous ventilation through the natural airway, adequate oxygenation, and no need for reintubation.

Continued

36-4 Removal of the Endotracheal Tube—cont'd

AARC Clinical Practice Guideline (Excerpts)*

- Clinical outcome may be assessed by physical examination, auscultation, invasive and noninvasive measurements of gas exchange, and chest radiography.
- When a patient experiences an unplanned self-extubation and does not require reintubation, this suggests that planned extubation should have been considered earlier.
- Some patients may require support after extubation or intervention to maintain adequate gas exchange independent of controlled mechanical ventilation.

Noninvasive Respiratory Support

- Nasal continuous positive airway pressure (CPAP) is used in infants.
- Routine use of noninvasive positive pressure ventilation in adults is not supported.
- In patients with chronic obstructive pulmonary disease, CPAP of 5 cm H_2O and pressure support ventilation of 15 cm H_2O have improved pulmonary gas exchange, decreased intrapulmonary shunt fraction, and reduced patient work of breathing.

Postextubation Medical Therapy

- Aerosolized levoepinephrine is as effective as aerosolized racemic epinephrine in the treatment of postextubation laryngeal edema in children.
- Heliox may alleviate symptoms of partial airway obstruction and resultant stridor, improve patient comfort, decrease work of breathing, and prevent reintubation.

Diagnostic Therapy

- For patients with postextubation complications such as stridor or obstruction, fiberoptic bronchoscopy may provide direct airway inspection and therapeutic interventions (secretion clearance, instillation of drugs, removal of aspirated foreign objects).

**For complete guidelines, see American Association for Respiratory Care: Clinical practice guideline: removal of the endotracheal tube—2007 revision and update. Respir Care 52:81, 2007.*

suctioned with the tonsillar suction tip. The RT should listen for an audible leak around the tube. If no audible leak is present, the RT should reinflate the cuff and discuss with the physician how to proceed.

Step 5: Remove Tube.

The tape or holder that is securing the tube is removed. The technique used to remove the tube should help avoid aspiration of pharyngeal secretions and maximally abduct the vocal cords. Clinicians use one of two different techniques to accomplish these goals. In the first method, a large breath is given with the manual resuscitator, and the tube is removed at peak inspiration (when the vocal cords are maximally abducted). In the second method, the patient coughs and the tube is pulled during the expulsive expiratory phase. This technique also results in maximal abduction of the vocal cords.

Step 6: Apply Appropriate Oxygen and Humidity Therapy.

Patients who have been receiving mechanical ventilation may still require O_2 therapy, usually at a higher FiO_2. Other patients may require some O_2 because this is a stressful procedure. If humidity or aerosol therapy is indicated, most clinicians suggest a cool mist immediately after extubation.

Step 7: Assess or Reassess Patient.

After extubation, auscultation is performed to check for good air movement. Stridor or decreased air movement after extubation indicates upper airway problems. Next, the patient's respiratory rate, breathing pattern, heart rate, blood pressure, and SaO_2 are checked. Mild hypertension and tachycardia immediately after extubation are common and resolve spontaneously in most cases. The patient should be monitored for nosebleed after nasotracheal extubation. The patient is encouraged to cough, with assistance as needed. Because laryngeal edema may worsen with time and stridor may develop, racemic epinephrine for nebulization should be available. Arterial blood gas (ABG) values should be sampled and analyzed as needed.

The most common problems that occur after extubation are hoarseness, sore throat, and cough.[41] These problems are benign and improve with time. A rare but serious complication associated with extubation is laryngospasm. Postextubation laryngospasm is usually a transient event, lasting several seconds. If laryngospasm occurs, oxygenation can be maintained with a high FiO_2 and the application of positive pressure. If laryngospasm persists, a neuromuscular blocking agent may need to be given, which necessitates manual ventilation or reintubation.

Because the vocal cords have had limited function during the intubation period, they may not close fully as needed when the airway has been removed. To avoid aspiration, oral feedings, especially liquids, should be withheld for 24 hours after extubation. Patients may aspirate liquids even with an intact gag reflex.[48]

Extubation failure, defined as the sudden need for reinsertion of the airway because of airway problems, often occurs within 8 hours of extubation. Aspiration and edema are the most common problems. If the patient also is mechanically ventilated, reintubation may be required for work of breathing issues unrelated to the airway.

Tracheostomy Tube Removal (Decannulation)

Decannulation refers to removal of the tracheostomy tube. Several approaches exist to remove tracheostomy tubes. Patients who received a tracheostomy as a result of upper airway obstruction that has been resolved may have their tube removed in one step. Patients who have been on mechanical ventilation for an extended time may have problems with muscle weakness, problems adjusting to the increase in anatomic dead space, and upper airway problems with secretions and glottic closure. For these patients, a weaning process is used rather than abrupt removal of the tube. Weaning is accomplished by using fenestrated tubes, progressively smaller tubes, or tracheostomy buttons.[70]

Before decannulation, a comprehensive patient assessment is required. The patient should have sufficient muscle strength (peak expiratory pressure > 40 cm H_2O) to generate an effective cough. Ideally, there should be no active pulmonary infection, and the volume and thickness of secretions should be acceptable. Patency of the upper airway can be assessed via bronchoscopy.[71] An adequate swallow must be present to decrease the risk for aspiration. After removal of the tube, the stoma closes on its own in a few days. After cleaning around the stoma, a sterile occlusive dressing should be applied over the stoma until it closes. The particular decannulation technique used depends on the patient's needs and the experience and preferences of the attending physician.

Fenestrated Tracheostomy Tubes

A **fenestrated** tracheostomy tube is a double cannulated tube that has an opening in the posterior wall of the outer cannula above the cuff (Figure 36-39). Removal of the inner cannula opens the fenestration, allowing air to pass into the upper airway. Capping or placing a speaking valve on the proximal opening of the tube's outer cannula, accompanied by deflation of the cuff, allows for assessment of upper airway function. Removal of the cap or speaking valve allows access for suctioning. If mechanical ventilation is needed, the inner cannula can be reinserted and the cuff can be reinflated.

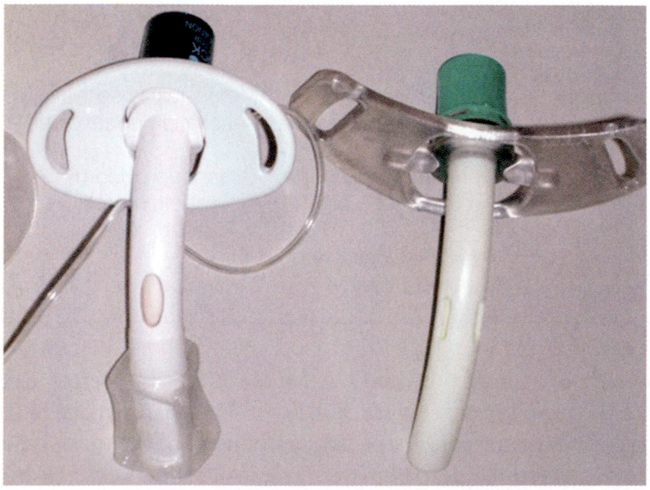

FIGURE 36-39 Fenestrated tracheostomy tubes.

One problem associated with this type of tracheostomy tube is malposition of the fenestration, such as between the skin and stoma or against the posterior wall of the larynx.[43] Customizing the fenestration or trying a fenestrated tube of a different size or by a different manufacturer can help avoid this problem. Proper placement can be confirmed by using fiberoptic bronchoscopy.

Case reports have shown granular tissue formation in some patients using a fenestrated tracheostomy tube. Granular tissue tends to form on the posterior tracheal wall, above the tube fenestration. This granular tissue may occlude the fenestration, cause bleeding (especially with tube changes), or result in airway obstruction on decannulation. Given the location of this granular tissue, these problems may be due to poor positioning of the fenestration within the airway.

Progressively Smaller Tubes

A second airway weaning technique is to use progressively smaller tracheostomy tubes. Similar to fenestrated tubes, this approach maintains the airway, but it allows for increasing use of the upper airway. This technique is also indicated in patients whose airway is too small for the available fenestrated tubes. The use of progressively smaller tubes may also allow for better healing of the stoma.

The problem with these techniques is the continued presence of a tube within the lumen of the airway.[70] The presence of the tube (cuffed or uncuffed) increases airway resistance. In patients with preexisting obstructive disorders, this added airway resistance may be too much to bear, resulting in failed decannulation. These tubes also can impair coughing by preventing full compression of the inspired thoracic volume. The last factor to consider when using smaller tubes is the fit of the tube within the trachea. Smaller tubes not only have a smaller diameter but also a different length; this may result in the curve of the tube impacting the posterior tracheal wall.

Tracheal Buttons

The tracheal button also may be used to maintain a tracheal stoma.[43] In contrast to the fenestrated tube, the tracheal button fits through the skin to just inside the anterior wall of the trachea (Figure 36-40), which avoids the problem of added resistance. Because the tracheal button has no cuff, its use is limited to relieving airway obstruction and aiding the removal of secretions. When the inner cannula is removed, the clinician can suction through the outer cannula. However, when the inner cannula is removed, the clinician needs to hold the outer cannula in place to prevent it from being coughed out during suctioning.

Assessment After Tracheostomy Decannulation

After tracheostomy decannulation, the patient should be assessed for vocal cord responses.[71] Vocal cord abnormalities can result in either aspiration or acute airway obstruction.

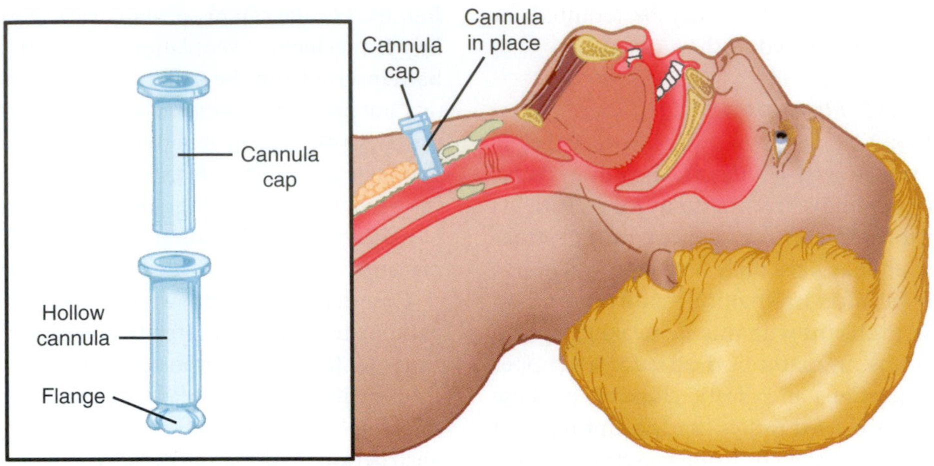

FIGURE 36-40 Tracheostomy button.

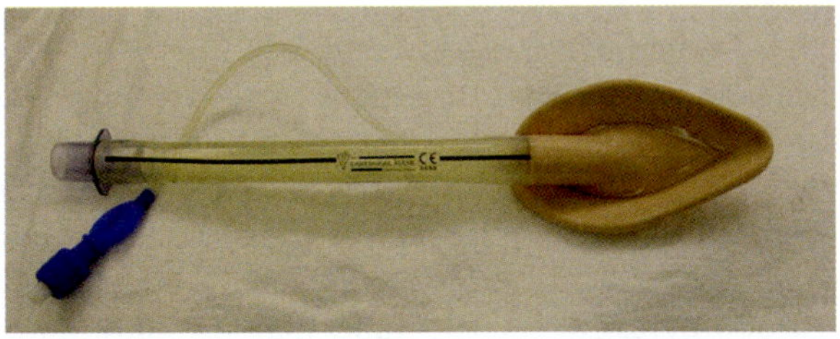

FIGURE 36-41 Largneal mask airway (LMA). (From Gartsman G: Shoulder arthroscopy, ed 2, Philadelphia, 2009, Saunders.)

Symptoms such as stridor, retractions, and inability to feel airflow through the upper airway indicate upper airway obstruction. A replacement tracheostomy tube and suctioning equipment should be available in case the patient develops any of these symptoms of obstruction.

ALTERNATIVE AIRWAY DEVICES

Placement of an ETT is a complex skill and is not always accomplished easily, even in experienced hands. Emergency medical services personnel are not always in the best situation to intubate. A patient's particular anatomy may make intubation difficult. Several alternative devices and techniques can be used in such circumstances. An algorithm for difficult intubations created by the American Society of Anesthesiologists provides extensive options.[72] Video-assisted laryngoscopy or intubating over a fiberoptic bronchoscope are alternative approaches during a difficult intubation. Two devices, the *LMA* and the *double-lumen airway* (Combitube), are referred to as *nonintermediate airways*. They can be used to ventilate a patient, but an ETT or tracheostomy tube may be needed eventually. These two devices may be inserted by respiratory care practitioners and are discussed subsequently. The advantages and disadvantages of each device are summarized in Table 36-6.

Laryngeal Mask Airway

The algorithm for management of a difficult airway has been modified to show the various uses of the LMA. The LMA consists of a short tube and a small mask that is inserted deep into the oropharynx (Figure 36-41).[72,73] The open surface of the mask faces the laryngeal opening, and the tip of the mask is just above the esophageal sphincter. The short tube has a 15-mm adapter that can be connected to a manual resuscitator bag. A

TABLE 36-6

Advantages and Disadvantages of Alternatives to Endotracheal Intubation for Maintaining Upper Airway Patency

Device	Advantages	Disadvantages
Oral and nasal airways	Little training required	Does not guarantee airway patency
	No special equipment necessary	May worsen obstruction
	Inexpensive	Poorly tolerated by awake patient
	Can be quickly placed	Does not prevent aspiration
		Short-term use
		Does not facilitate positive pressure ventilation
Double-lumen airway (Combitube) placement	Less skill than bag-valve-mask or intubation	Difficulty distinguishing tracheal versus esophageal insertion
	No special equipment necessary	Short-term use
	Protection against aspiration	Aspiration during removal
	Facilitates positive pressure ventilation	Cannot suction in esophageal position
		Only one size (adult)
		Potential for esophageal injury
Laryngeal mask airway (LMA)	Easy to insert	Short-term use
	No special equipment necessary	Aspiration not avoided
	Can intubate without removing LMA	Cannot provide high ventilation pressures if needed
	Avoids laryngeal and tracheal trauma	

small tube is used to inflate a cuff when the device is in place. LMAs range in size from size 5 for adults to size 1 for infants.

Compared with bag and mask ventilation, a greater amount of ventilation is directed to the lungs by the LMA. The ease and speed of insertion offer an advantage over intubation when the intubator is inexperienced, the patient cannot be positioned for intubation, or the intubation is difficult.

The insertion of the LMA does not require any equipment (Figure 36-42).[73] Before insertion, the posterior surface of the mask must be lubricated and the cuff must be fully deflated. The index finger is used to guide insertion of the mask along the palate and down into the oropharynx. When the cuff is in place, it is inflated to a maximum of 60 cm H_2O. Inflation causes the mask to rise slightly out of the mouth.

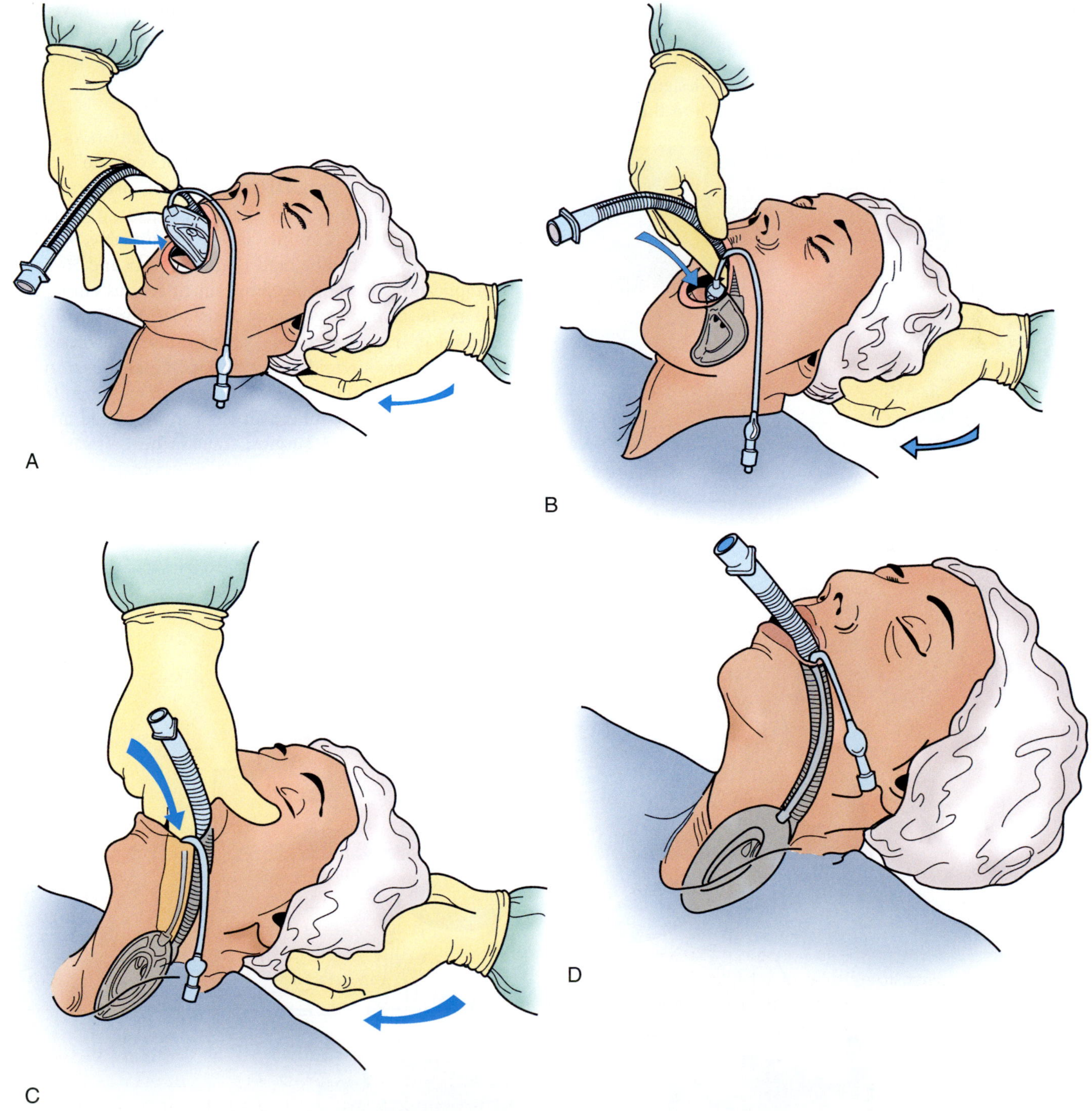

FIGURE 36-42 Insertion of largneal mask airway. (Modified from Cairo JM, Pilbeam SP: Mosby's respiratory care equipment, ed 8, St. Louis, 2010, Mosby.)

Use of the LMA has two major limitations.[73] First, it cannot be used in a conscious or semicomatose patient because of stimulation of the gag reflex. Second, if ventilating pressures greater than 20 cm H_2O are needed, gastric distention may occur. This device does not protect against aspiration should regurgitation occur.

The classic LMA can be used to facilitate intubation because the opening faces the glottis. However, because of the small size of the ventilating tube on the mask, a small ETT is needed. A specially designed LMA with a small handle facilitates intubation (Figure 36-43).

Double-Lumen Airway

The double-lumen airway (Combitube) is designed to be inserted blindly through the oropharynx and into the trachea or the esophagus (Figure 36-44).[73] Its external design is similar to that of a double-lumen ETT with two external openings, two 15-mm adapters, two lumens, and two cuffs. One cuff seals the oropharynx. The second seals the trachea or the esophagus.

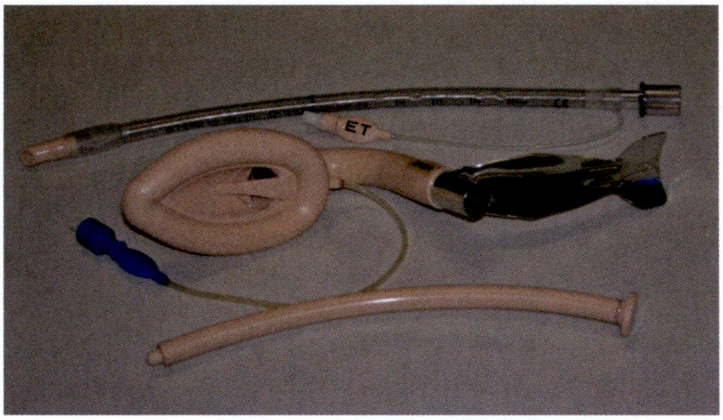

FIGURE 36-43 Intubating laryngeal mask airway.

If the tube is placed into the esophagus and the cuffs are inflated, ventilation is accomplished by air passing through a series of holes in the area of the hypopharynx and into the trachea. The pharyngeal cuff prevents air from leaving through the mouth. The distal cuff in the esophagus helps decrease regurgitation. If the tube is placed in the trachea, it functions like an ETT. To assess placement, the RT can manually ventilate through the external adapters and determine which gives the best breath sounds.

Surgical Emergency Airways

Despite various alternatives to establish ventilation, occasionally the problem of "cannot intubate/cannot ventilate" occurs.[27] In these situations, a surgical transtracheal airway must be established. Cricothyroidotomy and percutaneous transtracheal ventilation are options. Commercial kits are available, or a series of available supplies can be used (Figures 36-45 and 36-46).[74]

Complications include bleeding, subcutaneous emphysema secondary to inspiratory airway resistance through a small lumen, and air trapping secondary to expiratory flow resistance. Nevertheless, cricothyroidotomy and percutaneous transtracheal ventilation are the preferred routes over emergent tracheotomy until a more definitive airway can be placed after the emergency has passed. A surgical transtracheal airway should be accomplished in 48 to 72 hours.[39,74]

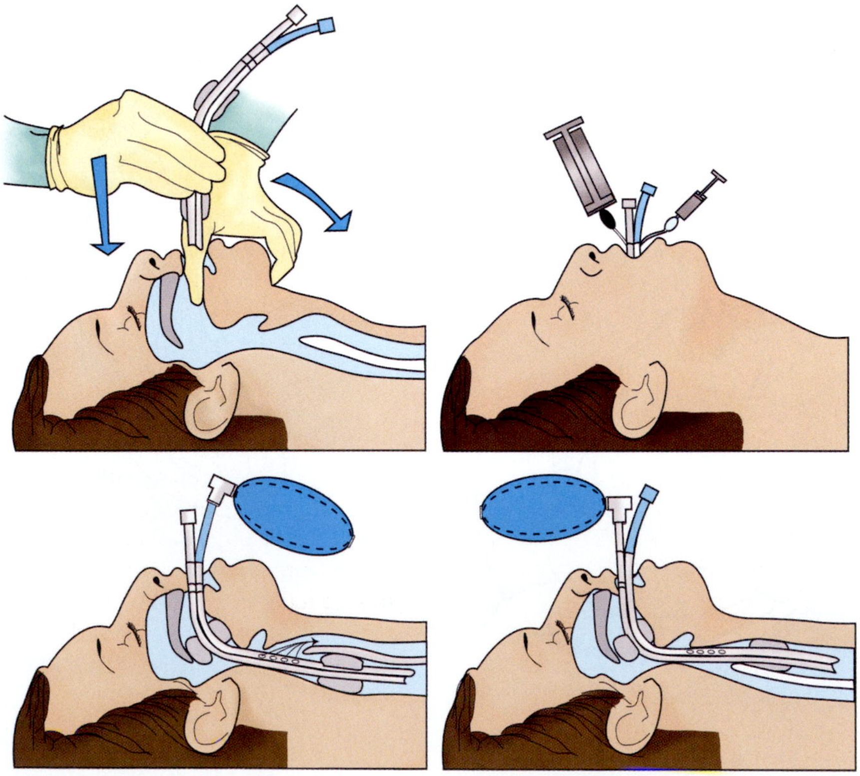

FIGURE 36-44 Insertion of a double-lumen airway (Combitube). (Modified from Cairo JM, Pilbeam SP: Mosby's respiratory care equipment, ed 8, St. Louis, 2010, Mosby.)

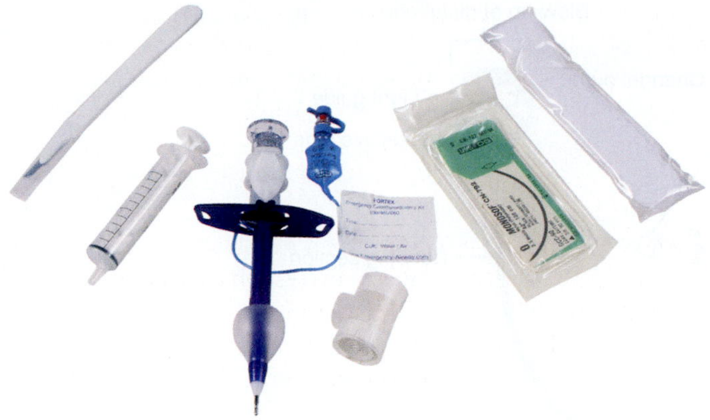

FIGURE 36-45 Commercially available cricothyroidotomy kit. (Courtesy Smith's Medical International, Kent, United Kingdom.)

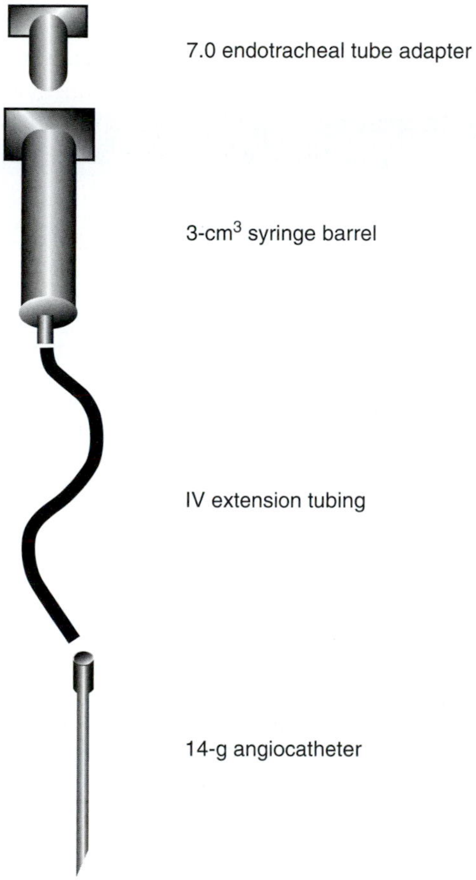

FIGURE 36-46 Percutaneous tracheal ventilation supplies. (Modified from Rodrick MB, Deutschman CS: Emergent airway management: indications and methods in the face of confounding conditions. Crit Care Clin 16:396, 2000.)

BRONCHOSCOPY

Bronchoscopy is the general term used to describe the insertion of a visualization instrument (endoscope) into the bronchi. The purposes of bronchoscopy are to inspect the airway, remove objects from the airway, collect samples from the airway, and place devices into the airway.[34] Two different bronchoscopic techniques are in use: rigid tube bronchoscopy and flexible bronchoscopy. Although RTs most often assist in flexible fiberoptic bronchoscopy, they should understand the differences between these two approaches.

Rigid Tube Bronchoscopy

A *rigid bronchoscope* is an open metal tube with a distal light source and a port for attaching O_2 or ventilating equipment. A rigid bronchoscope is used most often by otorhinolaryngologists or thoracic surgeons. The tube is passed through the mouth, down into the trachea, and as far as the bronchi. A telescoping tube with mirrors is used to advance to and view segmental bronchi. Suctioning is accomplished via a metal tube passed through the bronchoscope. The large internal diameter of this suction tube allows for aspiration of thick inspissated secretions and large mucous plugs. Grasping forceps passed through the device allow removal of foreign bodies and biopsies of airway tumors.

Rigid bronchoscopy has several disadvantages. First, it is very uncomfortable for conscious patients. It usually requires the assistance of an anesthesiologist and the use of an operating room. Last, and most important, rigid bronchoscopy cannot access the smaller airways.

Flexible Fiberoptic Bronchoscopy

Flexible fiberoptic bronchoscopy has gained popularity over the years as a result of both its versatility and its ability to access very small airways. A typical fiberoptic bronchoscope has a light transmission channel, a visualizing channel, and a multipurpose open channel (Figure 36-47). The open channel can be used for aspiration, tissue sampling, or O_2 administration. After insertion, the physician can direct the tip of the scope via the control section to the location desired. This type of bronchoscope is most often used by the pulmonologist, often with the assistance of the RT.[75]

To guide practitioners in assisting physicians performing this procedure, the AARC has developed and published a clinical practice guideline on fiberoptic bronchoscopy assisting. Excerpts from the AARC guideline, including indications, contraindications, precautions and possible complications, assessment of need, assessment of outcome, and monitoring, appear in Clinical Practice Guideline 36-5.[76]

Fiberoptic Bronchoscopy Procedure

Key factors in planning and conducting fiberoptic bronchoscopy include premedication, equipment preparation, airway preparation, and monitoring.[76,77] To reduce the risk for aspiration secondary to gagging and loss of airway reflexes, the patient should refrain from food or drink for at least 8 hours before the start of the procedure. In addition, if the intravenous route is not already available, vascular access should be obtained before the start of the procedure.

Premedication

Bronchoscopy is an uncomfortable procedure. To decrease anxiety, the patient should be premedicated 30 to 45 minutes

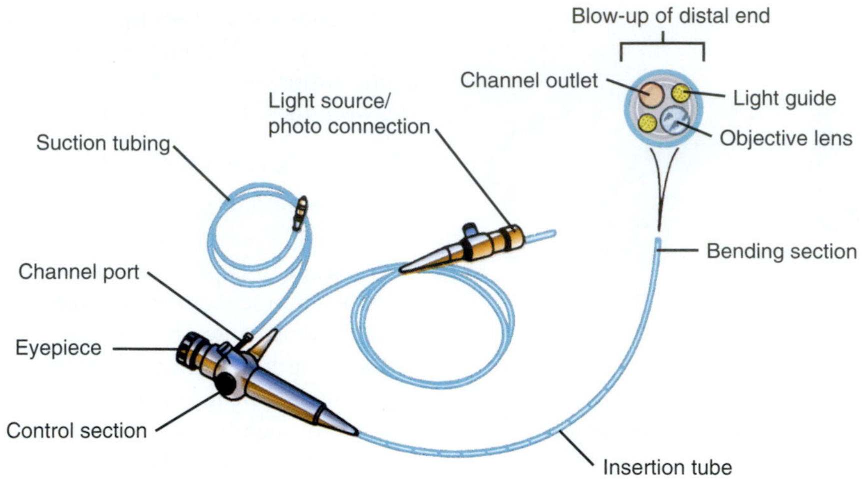

FIGURE 36-47 Flexible fiberoptic bronchoscope.

36-5 Bronchoscopy Assisting

AARC Clinical Practice Guideline (Excerpts)*

INDICATIONS

- Presence of lesions of unknown cause on the chest radiograph or need to evaluate recurrent pneumonia, persistent atelectasis, or pulmonary infiltrates
- Need to assess patency or mechanical properties of the upper airway
- Need to investigate hemoptysis, unexplained cough, wheeze, or stridor
- Suspicious or positive sputum cytology results
- Suspicion that secretions or mucous plugs are causing atelectasis
- Need to obtain lower respiratory tract secretions, cell washings, and biopsy specimens for cytologic, histologic, and microbiologic evaluation
- Need to determine location and extent of injury from toxic inhalation or aspiration
- Need to evaluate problems associated with endotracheal or tracheostomy tubes (tracheal damage, airway obstruction, or tube placement)
- Need for aid in performing difficult intubations or percutaneous tracheostomies
- Suspicion that secretions or mucous plugs are responsible for lobar or segmental atelectasis
- Need to remove abnormal endobronchial tissue or foreign material by forceps, basket, or laser
- Need to retrieve a foreign body (although rigid bronchoscopy is preferred under most circumstances)
- Therapeutic management of endobronchial toilet in ventilator-associated pneumonia
- Selective intubation of a main stem bronchus
- Need to place or assess airway stent function
- Need for airway balloon dilation in treatment of tracheobronchial stenosis

CONTRAINDICATIONS

Flexible bronchoscopy should be performed only when the relative benefits outweigh the risks. Absolute contraindications include the following:

- Absence of consent from the patient or his or her representative unless a medical emergency exists and patient is not competent to give permission
- Absence of an experienced bronchoscopist to perform or supervise closely and directly the procedure
- Lack of adequate facilities and personnel to care for emergencies such as cardiopulmonary arrest, pneumothorax, or bleeding
- Inability to oxygenate the patient adequately during the procedure
- Danger of a serious complication from bronchoscopy is especially great in patients with the following disorders, and these conditions are usually considered absolute contraindications unless the risk-benefit assessment warrants the procedure:
  - Coagulopathy or bleeding diathesis that cannot be corrected
  - Severe refractory hypoxemia
  - Unstable hemodynamic status including dysrhythmias

Relative contraindications (or conditions involving increased risk), according to the American Thoracic Society guidelines for fiberoptic bronchoscopy in adults, include the following:

- Lack of patient cooperation
- Recent (within 6 weeks) myocardial infarction or unstable angina
- Partial tracheal obstruction
- Moderate to severe hypoxemia or any degree of hypercarbia

36-5 Bronchoscopy Assisting—cont'd

AARC Clinical Practice Guideline (Excerpts)*

- Uremia and pulmonary hypertension (possible serious hemorrhage after biopsy)
- Lung abscess (danger of flooding airway with purulent material)
- Obstruction of superior vena cava (possibility of bleeding and laryngeal edema)
- Debility and malnutrition
- Disorders requiring laser therapy, biopsy of lesions obstructing large airways, or multiple transbronchial lung biopsies
- Known or suspected pregnancy (safety concern of possible radiation exposure)
- Safety of bronchoscopic procedures in asthmatic patients is a concern, but the presence of asthma does not preclude use of these procedures
- Patients with recent head injury are susceptible to increased intracranial pressures
- Inability to sedate (including time constraints of oral ingestion of solids or liquids)

HAZARDS AND COMPLICATIONS

- Adverse effects of medication used before and during bronchoscopic procedure
- Hypoxemia
- Hypercarbia
- Bronchospasm
- Hypotension
- Laryngospasm, bradycardia, or other vagally mediated phenomena
- Mechanical complications such as epistaxis, pneumothorax, and hemoptysis
- Increased airway resistance
- Cross-contamination of specimens or bronchoscopes
- Nausea, vomiting
- Fever and chills
- Cardiac dysrhythmias
- Death
- Infection hazard for health care workers or other patients

ASSESSMENT OF NEED

Need is determined by bronchoscopist assessment of the patient and treatment plan in addition to the presence of clinical indications and the absence of contraindications, as described previously.

ASSESSMENT OF OUTCOME

Patient outcome is determined by clinical, physiologic, and pathologic assessment. Procedural outcome is determined by the accomplishment of the procedural goals as indicated and by appropriate quality assessment indicators.

MONITORING

The following should be monitored continuously before, during, and after bronchoscopy, until the patient returns to presedation level of consciousness.

Patient

- Level of consciousness
- Medications administered, dosage, route, and time of delivery
- Subjective response to procedure (e.g., pain, discomfort, dyspnea)
- Blood pressure, breath sounds, heart rate, rhythm, and changes in cardiac status
- SpO_2, FiO_2, and end-tidal CO_2
- Tidal volume, peak inspiratory pressure, adequacy of inspiratory flow, and other ventilator parameters if patient is mechanically ventilated
- Lavage volumes (delivered and retrieved)
- Monitor and document site of biopsies and washings; record which laboratory tests were requested on each sample
- Periodic follow-up monitoring of patient condition after the procedure is advisable for 24 to 48 hours for inpatients. Outpatients should be instructed to contact the bronchoscopist regarding fever, chest pain or discomfort, dyspnea, wheezing, hemoptysis, or any new findings manifesting after procedure has been completed. Oral instructions should be reinforced by written instructions that include names and phone numbers of persons to be contacted in emergency.
- Chest radiograph 1 hour after transbronchial biopsy to exclude pneumothorax

Technical Devices

- Bronchoscope integrity (fiberoptic or channel damage, passage of leak test)
- Strict adherence to the manufacturer's and institutional recommended procedures for cleaning, disinfection, and sterilization of the devices and integrity of disinfection or sterilization packaging
- Smooth, unhampered operation of biopsy devices (forceps, needles, brushes)

Recordkeeping

- Quality assessment indicators determined appropriate by the institution's quality assessment committee
- Documentation of patient and device monitoring
- Identification of bronchoscope used for each patient
- Annual assessment of the institutional or departmental bronchoscopy procedure, including (1) evaluation of the adequacy of bronchoscopic specimens; (2) review of infection control procedures and compliance with current guidelines for semicritical patient care objects; (3) synopsis of complications; (d) control washings to ensure that infection control and disinfection and sterilization procedures are adequate, and that cross contamination of specimens does not occur; and (e) annual review of the bronchoscopy service and all of the previously listed records with physician bronchoscopists

before the procedure. The patient should be calm but alert enough to follow commands, such as taking a deep breath. Conscious sedation is normally performed for this procedure.

Another goal of premedication is to dry the patient's airway. A dry airway promotes anesthetic deposition, aids visibility, and can reduce procedure time. An anticholinergic agent, such as atropine, may be given before the procedure. Atropine also may help decrease vagal responses (e.g., bradycardia and hypotension) that can occur during bronchoscopy.

Narcotic analgesics such as morphine or fentanyl also may be given. In addition to reducing pain, these agents help diminish laryngeal reflexes. However, narcotics should be withheld until procedures requiring patient cooperation are completed. Caution must be exercised to avoid respiratory depression. Naloxone (Narcan) must be available in the event of respiratory depression.

Additional narcotics and sedatives (e.g., propofol) may be needed for patient comfort and should be available. The need for antiarrhythmics, resuscitative drugs, narcotic antagonists, and intravenous fluids is harder to predict. Advance preparation results in a more efficient and rapid response.

Equipment Preparation

The RT is often responsible for preparing the equipment needed for bronchoscopy. Box 36-9 lists needed equipment. Special procedure rooms are often used for bronchoscopy and usually have most of the ancillary equipment already in place. All equipment must be thoroughly checked for function, tight connections, and integrity. This check is especially important for small parts and connectors, which can be aspirated if they loosen and disconnect.

Airway Preparation

The goals of airway preparation are to prevent bleeding, decrease cough and gagging, and decrease pain. Topical vasoconstrictors such as pseudoephedrine or dilute epinephrine (usually 1 : 10,000) may be used to prevent or treat bleeding.

Airway anesthesia is achieved by topical anesthetics or nerve block. Topical anesthetics are more common. The particular anesthetic and route of administration vary depending on experience and locale. Lidocaine (1%, 2%, or 4%) is often used. Lidocaine is commonly delivered via an atomizer to the nose, via mouthwash to the oropharynx, and via nebulizer or instillation through the bronchoscope to the lower airways. The RT will usually administer the lidocaine by nebulizer. The use of lidocaine by nebulizer before bronchoscopy may limit the need for lidocaine instillations into the lower airways and can make the procedure less unpleasant for the patient. Superior laryngeal nerve block provides anesthesia in the upper larynx, but it does not affect the vocal cords. Transtracheal block through the cricoid membrane anesthetizes both the vocal cords and the trachea.

Monitoring

The RT has an active role in monitoring the patient and should communicate any changes to the physician. Oxygenation should

Box 36-9 Equipment Needed for Bronchoscopy

EQUIPMENT FOR BRONCHOSCOPIST AND ASSISTANT
- Masks and goggles
- Gloves (sterile for bronchoscopist)
- Gown

BRONCHOSCOPIC DEVICES
- Appropriate size bronchoscope, as determined by bronchoscopist
- Bronchoscopic light source
- Bronchoscope adapter for endotracheal tube (ETT)
- Cytology brushes, flexible forceps, transbronchial aspiration needles, retrieval baskets, as determined by the bronchoscopist
- Syringes for medication delivery, normal saline lavage, and needle aspiration
- Sterile normal saline
- Specimen collection devices and fixatives as determined by institutional policies
- Bite block
- Sterile gauze pads for cleaning tip of bronchoscope, as needed
- Water-soluble lubricant
- Venous access equipment
- In case intubation is required
  - ETTs (various sizes, laryngoscope, laryngeal mask airway, thoracostomy set/tray)
  - Appropriate procedure documentation paperwork, including laboratory requisitions

FOR PATIENT SUPPORT AND MONITORING
- Pulse oximeter
- Oxygen and related delivery equipment
- Electrocardiographic monitoring equipment
- Sphygmomanometer
- Suction system with suction supplies for mouth and scope
- Resuscitation equipment, in case needed

MEDICATIONS*
- Topical anesthetics: Lidocaine 1%, 2%, 4%; lidocaine 3% with phenylephrine (for nares)
- Sedatives: Codeine, midazolam, morphine, diazepam, fentanyl, propofol
- Benzodiazepine antagonist (flumazenil), narcotic antagonist (naloxone)
- Anticholinergic agent (atropine, glycopyrrolate) to reduce secretions and minimize vasovagal reflexes
- Sterile nonbacteriostatic 0.9% sodium chloride solution for bronchial washings or lavage
- Dilute epinephrine (usually 1 : 10,000) for bleeding control
- Inhaled beta agonist (albuterol, levalbuterol)
- Nasal decongestants (pseudoephedrine)
- Water-soluble lubricant or combined lubricant and anesthetic (viscous lidocaine)
- Mucolytics or mucokinetics (10% or 20% acetylcysteine, 7.5% sodium bicarbonate, rhDNAse)
- Emergency and resuscitation drugs as deemed appropriate

From American Association for Respiratory Care: Clinical practice guideline: bronchoscopy assisting—2007 revision and update. Respir Care 52:74, 2007.

*Depend on institutional policy and bronchoscopist preference. Aerosolized, atomized, or instilled drugs may be administered by an appropriately trained respiratory therapist. Intravenous medications must be administered by a physician or nurse.

be monitored continuously via pulse oximetry. If desaturation occurs, FiO_2 is increased with an O_2 therapy device. Alternatively, the procedure can be temporarily halted, and O_2 can be given through the scope's open channel. The latter technique has the advantage of defogging the scope.

The respiratory rate and depth are also observed. Decreases in rate or depth may indicate oversedation. Continuous electrocardiogram and periodic blood pressure monitoring also should be routine. Arrhythmias and changes in blood pressure that occur are usually due to hypoxemia, vagal stimulation, pain, or anxiety. Prompt recognition of a problem and appropriate response aid recovery.

Assisting With the Procedure

The physician inserts the bronchoscope into the airway and guides it by directing the tip with the thumb lever. While monitoring the patient, the RT may also assist the physician by supplying syringes filled with anesthetic, vasoconstrictor, mucolytic agents, or lavage solutions. Forceps or brushes are often inserted into the bronchoscope by the RT. The physician guides these devices to the desired area. In addition, sputum or tissue samples obtained by the physician may be collected by the RT and prepared for laboratory analysis. When the goals of the procedure have been achieved, the bronchoscope is removed, and the patient's recovery period begins.

Recovery

Hypoxemia that occurs during the procedure may persist after completion. O_2 therapy should be maintained for up to 4 hours. Adequate oxygenation, via pulse oximetry, should be confirmed before therapy is discontinued.

The risk for aspiration persists as long as the airway is anesthetized. Patients should remain in a sitting position and refrain from eating or drinking until sensation returns. Patients are assessed for the development of stridor or wheezes. The physician is notified, and appropriate aerosol therapy with nebulized racemic epinephrine or bronchodilators is given in such cases.

Complications

The complications of bronchoscopy are similar to the complications associated with suctioning. However, the greater patient discomfort, longer duration, and the extent of airway penetration make bronchoscopy a more hazardous and complex procedure.

Hypoxemia is most severe in patients with underlying lung disease. To minimize this problem, all patients should receive O_2 before and during the procedure. When the nasal route is used to insert the bronchoscope, O_2 can be administered by a nasal catheter (in the opposite naris) or by a mask adapted to allow passage of the bronchoscope.

Hemodynamic changes (heart rate, blood pressure, and cardiac output) vary and may be related to differences in techniques or medications. Bronchospasm also has been reported and is most severe in patients with asthma. Premedication with albuterol and ipratropium bromide may help relieve this problem; the use of sedatives or narcotic analgesics, which do not release histamine, would also be helpful. Meperidine (Demerol) and fentanyl are better for patients with asthma.[34]

In patients with artificial airways, placing a bronchoscope through an ETT or tracheostomy tube may decrease the radius by 50%. If the patient is on a ventilator, peak inspiratory pressure may increase, or V_Ts may decrease. Inadvertent PEEP also may increase. An RT should be present during the procedure to adjust the ventilator and monitor SaO_2 and exhaled volumes.

SUMMARY CHECKLIST

- Retained secretions or other semiliquid fluids are removed from the large airways via suctioning. Removal of foreign bodies or tissue masses beyond the main stem bronchi requires bronchoscopy.
- To avoid or minimize the complications of suctioning, the RT needs to (1) preoxygenate, (2) limit negative pressure and suction time, and (3) use sterile technique.
- The primary indications for an artificial tracheal airway are (1) to relieve airway obstruction, (2) to facilitate secretion removal, (3) to protect against aspiration, and (4) to provide positive pressure ventilation.
- There are two basic types of tracheal airways: endotracheal (translaryngeal) tubes and tracheostomy tubes.
- Orotracheal intubation is the preferred route for establishing an emergency tracheal airway.
- Before intubation, adequate ventilation and 100% O_2 by manual resuscitator and mask should be provided.
- No more than 30 seconds should be devoted to any intubation attempt.
- There are many ways to assess ETT position; only laryngoscopy or bronchoscopy can confirm correct positioning.
- Serious complications of emergency airway management include acute hypoxemia, hypercapnia, bradycardia, and cardiac arrest.
- Nasotracheal intubation is the preferred route for intubation of patients with maxillofacial injuries.
- The primary indication for tracheotomy is the continuing need for an artificial airway after a prolonged period of oral or nasal intubation; the decision when to switch from ETT to tracheostomy tube should be individualized.
- The most common laryngeal injuries associated with endotracheal intubation are glottic edema, vocal cord inflammation, laryngeal or vocal cord ulcerations, and vocal cord polyps or granulomas.
- Although laryngeal lesions occur only with oral or nasal ETTs, tracheal lesions can occur with any tracheal airway. The most common tracheal lesions are granulomas, tracheomalacia, and tracheal stenosis.
- To minimize or prevent trauma secondary to tracheal airways, the RT needs to (1) select the correct size of airway, (2) avoid tube movement or traction, (3) limit cuff pressures, and (4) use sterile techniques.
- To minimize the risk for infection, the RT needs to (1) use closed suction devices, (2) use passive humidification, (3) monitor cuff pressure carefully, (4) use subglottic suction, and (5) keep the head of the bed elevated.

- ETT obstruction can be caused by (1) kinking of or biting on the tube, (2) herniation of the cuff over the tube tip, (3) obstruction of the tube orifice against the tracheal wall, and (4) mucous plugging.
- If a tracheal airway appears to be completely obstructed, the RT needs to perform the following steps in order until the obstruction is relieved: (1) Reposition the patient's head and neck, (2) deflate the tube cuff, (3) try passing a suction catheter, (4) try removing the inner cannula of the tracheostomy tube, (5) remove the airway and provide bag-valve-mask ventilation and oxygenation.
- A patient is ready for extubation if the patient (1) can maintain adequate spontaneous oxygenation and ventilation, (2) is at minimal risk for upper airway obstruction, (3) has adequate airway protective reflexes, and (4) can adequately clear secretions.
- Tracheostomy decannulation can be accomplished by using fenestrated tubes, progressively smaller tubes, or tracheostomy buttons.
- An LMA or a double-lumen airway (Combitube) can be used in a difficult intubation.
- Cricothyroidotomy is performed when a patient cannot be intubated or ventilated.
- Key factors in planning and conducting fiberoptic bronchoscopy include premedication, equipment preparation, airway preparation, and monitoring.

References

1. American Association for Respiratory Care: Clinical practice guideline: endotracheal suctioning of mechanically ventilated patients with artificial airways. *Respir Care* 55:758, 2010.
2. Koeppel R: Endotracheal tube suctioning in the newborn: a review of the literature. *Newborn Infant Nurs Rev* 6:94, 2006.
3. Spence K, Gillies D, Waterworth L: Deep versus shallow suction of endotracheal tubes in ventilated neonates and young infants. *Cochrane Database Syst Rev* (3):CD003309, 2004.
4. Plevak D, Ward J: Airway management. In Burton G, Hodgkin J, editors: *Respiratory care: a guideline to clinical practice*, New York, 1997, Lippincott Williams & Wilkins.
5. Tiffin NH, Keim MR, Trewen TC: The effects of variations in flow through an insufflating catheter and endotracheal tube and suction catheter size on test lung pressures. *Respir Care* 35:889, 1990.
6. Vanner R, Bick E: Tracheal pressures during open suctioning. *Anaesthesia* 63:313, 2008.
7. Singh NC, Kissoon N, Frewen T, et al: Physiological responses to endotracheal and oral suctioning in pediatric patients: the influence of endotracheal tube sizes and suction pressures. *Clin Intensive Care* 2:345, 1991.
8. Maggiore S, Lellouche F, Pigeot J, et al: Prevention of endotracheal suctioning-induced alveolar derecruitment in acute lung injury. *Am J Respir Crit Care Med* 1:1215, 2003.
9. Kalyn A, Blatz S, Feuerstake S, et al: Closed suctioning of intubated neonates maintains better physiologic stability: a randomized trial. *J Perinatol* 23:218, 2003.
10. Caramez M, Schettino G, Suchodolski K, et al: The impact of endotracheal suctioning on gas exchange and hemodynamics during lung-protective ventilation in acute respiratory distress syndrome. *Respir Care* 51:497, 2006.
11. Stoller J, Orens D, Fotica C, et al: Weekly versus daily changes of in-line suction catheters: impact on rates of ventilator-associated pneumonia and associated costs. *Respir Care* 48:494, 2003.
12. Topeli A, Harmanci A, Cetinkaya Y, et al: Comparison of the effect of closed versus open endotracheal suction systems on the development of ventilator-associated pneumonia. *J Hosp Infect* 58:14, 2004.
13. Hess DR: Managing the artificial airway. *Respir Care* 44:759, 1999.
14. Pritchard MA, Flenady V, Woodgate P: Systematic review of the role of pre-oxygenation for tracheal suctioning in ventilated newborn infants. *J Paediatr Child Health* 39:163, 2003.
15. Barnes TA, McGarry WP: Evaluation of ten disposable manual resuscitators. *Respir Care* 35:960, 1990.
16. Woodgate PG, Flenady V: Tracheal suctioning without disconnection in intubated ventilated neonates. *Cochrane Database Syst Rev* (2):CD003065, 2001.
17. Pedersen C, Rosendahl-Nielsen M, Hjermind J, et al: Endotracheal suctioning of the adult intubated patient: what is the evidence? *Intensive Crit Care Nurs* 25:21, 2009.
18. Morrow BM, Argent AC: A comprehensive review of pediatric endotracheal suctioning: effects, indications, and clinical practice. *Pediatr Crit Care Med* 9:465, 2008.
19. Oh H, Seo W: A meta-analysis of the effects of various interventions in preventing endotracheal suction-induced hypoxemia. *J Clin Nurs* 12:912, 2003.
20. American Association for Respiratory Care: Clinical practice guideline: nasotracheal suctioning—2004 revision and update. *Respir Care* 49:1080, 2004.
21. American Association for Respiratory Care: Clinical practice guideline: management of airway emergencies. *Respir Care* 40:749, 1995.
22. ANSI/AAMI/ISO 5361: Anaesthetic and respiratory equipment: tracheal tubes and connectors, 2012.
23. Jaeger JM, Durbin CG: Special purpose endotracheal tubes. *Respir Care* 44:661, 1999.
24. Diaz E, Rodriquez A, Rello J: Ventilator-associated pneumonia: issues related to the artificial airway. *Respir Care* 50:900, 2005.
25. Deem S, Treggiari M: New endotracheal tubes designed to prevent ventilator-associated pneumonia: do they make a difference? *Respir Care* 55:1046, 2010.
26. Hess DR, Altobelli NP: Tracheostomy tubes. *Respir Care* 59:956, 2014.
27. Gudzenko V, Bittner E, Schmidt U: Emergency airway management. *Respir Care* 55:1026, 2010.
28. Levitan R, Ochroch EA: Airway management and direct laryngoscopy: a review and update. *Crit Care Clin* 16:373, 2000.
29. Reed D, Clinton J: Proper depth of placement of nasotracheal tubes in adults prior to radiographic confirmation. *Acad Emerg Med* 4:1111, 1997.
30. American Heart Association: 2010 American Heart Association Guidelines for Cardiopulmonary Resuscitation and Emergency Cardiovascular Care. *Circulation* 122:S729, 2010.
31. Salem MR: Verification of endotracheal tube position. *Anesthesiol Clin N Am* 19:813, 2001.
32. Li J: Capnography alone is imperfect for endotracheal tube placement confirmation during emergency intubation. *J Emerg Med* 20:223, 2001.
33. Hogg K, Teece S: Colourimetric CO_2 detector compared with capnography for confirming ET tube placement. *Emerg Med J* 20:265, 2003.
34. Leibler JM, Markin CJ: Fiberoptic bronchoscopy for diagnosis and treatment. *Crit Care Clin* 16:83, 2000.
35. Hurford WE: Video revolution: a new view of laryngoscopy. *Respir Care* 55:1036, 2010.
36. Jaber S, Amraoui J, Lefrant JY, et al: Clinical practice and risk factors for immediate complications of endotracheal intubation in the intensive care unit: a prospective, multiple-center study. *Crit Care Med* 34:2355, 2006.
37. Hurford WE: Nasotracheal intubation. *Respir Care* 44:643, 1999.
38. Durbin CG: Tracheostomy: why, when, and how? *Respir Care* 55:1056, 2010.
39. Rassekh CH, Haughey BH: Total laryngectomy and larynpharyngectomy. In Feber T, editor: *Otolaryngology: head and neck surgery*, ed 5, St. Louis, 2010, Mosby.
40. Zeitels SM, Wain JC, et al: Aortic homograft reconstruction of partial laryngectomy defects: a new technique. *Ann Otol Laryngol* 121:301, 2012.

41. Stauffer JL: Complications of endotracheal intubation and tracheostomy. *Respir Care* 44:828, 1999.
42. Epstein SK: Late complications of tracheostomy. *Respir Care* 50:542, 2005.
43. Hess DR: Tracheostomy tubes and related appliances. *Respir Care* 50:495, 2005.
44. Lotano R, Gerber D, Aseron C, et al: Utility of postintubation chest radiographs in the intensive care unit. *Crit Care* 4:50, 2000.
45. Olufolab AJ, Charlto GA, Sparg PM: Effect of head posture on tracheal tube position in children. *Anesthesia* 59:1069, 2004.
46. Reyes G, Ramilo J, Horowitz I, et al: Use of an optical fiber scope to confirm endotracheal tube placement in pediatric patients. *Crit Care Med* 24:175, 2001.
47. Williams ML: An algorithm for selecting a communication technique with intubated patients. *Dimens Crit Care Nurs* 11:222, 1992.
48. Prigent H, Lejaille M, et al: Effect of a tracheostomy speaking valve on breathing-swallowing interaction. *Intensive Care Med* 38:85, 2012.
49. Shikani AH, Dietrich-Burns K: Comparison of speech parameters and olfaction using different tracheotomy speaking valves. *Int Forum Allergy Rhinol* 2:348, 2012.
50. Branson RD: Humidification for patients with artificial airways. *Respir Care* 44:630, 1999.
51. American Association for Respiratory Care: Clinical practice guideline: humidification during mechanical ventilation. *Respir Care* 37:887, 1992.
52. Levine SA, Neederman MS: The impact of tracheal intubation on host defenses and risks for nosocomial pneumonia. *Clin Chest Med* 12:523, 1991.
53. Safdar N, Crinch CJ, Maki DG: The pathogenesis of ventilator-associated pneumonia: its relevance to developing effective strategies for prevention. *Respir Care* 50:725, 2005.
54. Hess DR, Kallstrom T, Mottram CD, et al: Care of the ventilator circuit and its relation to ventilator-associated pneumonia. *Respir Care* 48:869, 2003.
55. Hijazi M, Al-Ansari M: Therapy for ventilator associated pneumonia: what works and what doesn't. *Respir Care Clin N Am* 10:341, 2004.
56. Boitano LJ: Management of airway clearance in neuromuscular disease. *Respir Care* 51:913, 2006.
57. Panitch HB: Respiratory issues in the management of children with neuromuscular disease. *Respir Care* 51:885, 2006.
58. Homnick DN: Mechanical insufflation-exsufflation for airway mucus clearance. *Respir Care* 52:1296, 2007.
59. Pitts R, Fisher D, Sulemanji D, et al: Variables affecting leakage past endotracheal tube cuffs: a bench study. *Intensive Care Med* 36:2066, 2010.
60. Kacmarek R, Dimas S, Mack C: Airway care. In *The essentials of respiratory care*, St. Louis, 2005, Mosby.
61. Dennis-Rouse MD, Davidson JE: An evidence-based evaluation of tracheostomy care practices. *Crit Care Nurs Q* 31:150, 2008.
62. Dhand R, Johnson J: Care of chronic tracheostomy. *Respir Care* 51:984, 2006.
63. White AC, Kher S, O'Connor HH: When to change a tracheostomy tube. *Respir Care* 55:1069, 2010.
64. Saini S, Taxak S, Singh MR: Tracheostomy tube obstruction caused by an overinflated cuff. *Otolaryngol Head Neck Surg* 122:768, 2000.
65. Schmidt U, Hess D, et al: Tracheostomy tube malposition in patients admitted to a respiratory acute care unit following prolonged ventilation. *Chest* 134:288, 2008.
66. Berra L, Coppadoro A, et al: A clinical assessment of the mucus shaver, a device to keep the endotracheal tube free from secretions. *Crit Care Med* 40:119, 2012.
67. American Association for Respiratory Care: Clinical practice guideline: removal of the endotracheal tube—2007 revision and update. *Respir Care* 52:81, 2007.
68. Kriner EJ, Shafazand S, Coilice GL: The endotracheal tube cuff-leak test as a predictor of postextubation stridor: a prospective study. *Respir Care* 50:1632, 2005.
69. Deem S: Limited value of the cuff leak test. *Respir Care* 50:1627, 2005.
70. Christopher KL: Tracheostomy decannulation. *Respir Care* 50:538, 2005.
71. O'Connor H, White A: Tracheostomy decannulation. *Respir Care* 55:1076, 2010.
72. Apfelbaum JL, Task Force on Management of the Difficult Airway: Practice guidelines for management of the difficult airway: an updated report by the American Society of Anesthesiologists Task Force on Management of the Difficult Airway. *Anesthesiology* 118:251, 2013.
73. Foley LJ, Ochroch EA: Bridges to establish an emergency airway and alternate intubating techniques. *Crit Care Clin* 16:429, 2000.
74. Roderick MB, Duetschman CS: Emergent airway management: indications and methods in the face of confounding conditions. *Crit Care Med* 16:389, 2000.
75. Treanor S, Benitez WD, Raffin TA: Respiratory therapists as fiberoptic bronchoscopy assistants. *Respir Care* 30:321, 1985.
76. American Association for Respiratory Care: Clinical practice guideline: bronchoscopy assisting—2007 revision and update. *Respir Care* 52:74, 2007.
77. Ernst A, Silvestri GA, Johnstone D: Interventional pulmonary procedures: guidelines from the American College of Chest Physicians. *Chest* 123:1693, 2003.

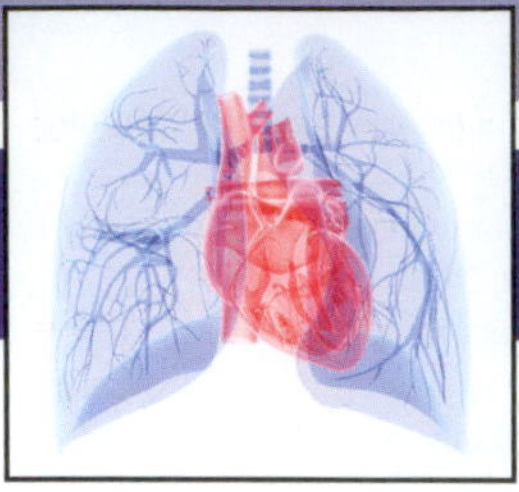

CHAPTER 37

Emergency Cardiovascular Life Support

THOMAS A. BARNES

CHAPTER OBJECTIVES

After reading this chapter you will be able to:

- List the causes of sudden cardiac arrest (SCA).
- List the signs of SCA, heart attack, and foreign body airway obstruction.
- Describe how to perform cardiopulmonary resuscitation (CPR) on adults, children, and infants.
- Describe how to perform defibrillation with automated external defibrillators and manual defibrillators.
- State how to administer synchronized cardioversion.
- Describe how to evaluate quality and effectiveness of CPR.
- List the complications that can occur as a result of resuscitation of SCA.
- State when not to initiate CPR.
- Describe how to apply key adjunct equipment during Advanced Cardiac Life Support (ACLS).
- State common drugs and drug routes used during ACLS.
- Describe how to monitor patients before cardiac arrest, during CPR, and after cardiac arrest.

CHAPTER OUTLINE

Causes and Prevention of Sudden Death
Basic Life Support
- Determining Unresponsiveness
- Restoring Circulation
- Restoring the Airway
- Restoring Ventilation
- One-Rescuer Versus Two-Rescuer Adult Cardiopulmonary Resuscitation
- Automated External Defibrillation
- Evaluating Effectiveness of Cardiopulmonary Resuscitation
- Hazards and Complications
- Contraindications to Cardiopulmonary Resuscitation
- Treating Foreign Body Airway Obstruction

Advanced Cardiovascular Life Support
- Support for Oxygenation
- Airway Management
- Ventilation
- Bag-Mask Devices
- Restoring Cardiac Function
- Monitoring Provider Team Performance During Advanced Cardiac Life Support
- Patient Care After Resuscitation
- Respiratory Management
- Cardiovascular Management

KEY TERMS

abdominal thrust
Advanced Cardiovascular Life Support
automated external defibrillators
basic life support
cardiopulmonary resuscitation
cardioversion
defibrillation
gastric inflation
synchronized cardioversion

Respiratory therapists (RTs) play a vital role in emergency cardiovascular life support. In hospitals, RTs serve as key members of the medical emergency teams, also known as *rapid response teams.* In addition to managing the airway, RTs often provide ventilatory and circulatory support; drug and electrical therapy; and monitoring immediately before, during, and after a cardiac arrest.

In the community, RTs also may be certified **cardiopulmonary resuscitation** (CPR) instructors, extending their knowledge to laypeople through organizations such as the American Heart Association (AHA) and the American Red Cross. Mastery of an extensive knowledge base and the development of various, sometimes difficult, manual skills are required for teaching and performing CPR. The practitioner is encouraged to obtain further competencies by completion of formal courses in CPR, **Advanced Cardiovascular Life Support** (ACLS), pediatric advanced life support, and neonatal resuscitation program.

CAUSES AND PREVENTION OF SUDDEN DEATH

Sudden cardiac arrest (SCA) is a leading cause of death among adults over the age of 40 in the United States and many parts of the world.[1] In the United States, approximately 500,000 people per year experience SCA and receive an attempted resuscitation.[1] Pulseless ventricular rhythms are the first manifestation of 23% of emergency medical services (EMS)-treated out-of-hospital cardiac arrests.[2] Successful resuscitation depends on immediate CPR and delivery of a shock before pulseless ventricular rhythms deteriorate into asystole. In cases of SCA related to asphyxia secondary to trauma, drug overdose, or upper airway obstruction, CPR with chest compressions and ventilation before the shock is critical.

BASIC LIFE SUPPORT

The goal of **basic life support** (BLS) is to restore ventilation and circulation to victims of airway obstruction and respiratory or cardiac arrest. These skills can be used by a single practitioner to restore ventilation and circulation until the victim is revived or until ACLS equipment and personnel are available. The steps for administering BLS by a single health care practitioner are as follows:

1. Check for lack of movement or response and no normal breathing or only gasping.
2. Activate the emergency response system (get automated external defibrillator [AED] if close to your location).
3. If no AED is available, start chest compressions and rescue breathing for adult cardiac arrest (use cycles of 30 compressions to 2 ventilations).
4. Open airway and check breathing.
5. If person is not breathing, give 2 breaths that produce chest rise.
6. Immediately resume chest compressions (push hard and deep with a minimum depth of 2 inches [5 cm] and a minimum rate of 100 to 120/min. Do not exceed 120/min compressions because depth of compression and release of pressure during chest compression will be affected).
7. AED arrives with response team.

Steps 3 through 6 are referred to as the *CABDs* of resuscitation—*c*irculation, *a*irway, *b*reathing, and *d*efibrillation. Table 37-1 summarizes the CABDs of CPR for adults, children (1 year old to puberty), and infants (younger than 1 year old).

Determining Unresponsiveness

BLS begins with immediate recognition of SCA and activation of the emergency response system, based on assessment of unresponsiveness, not moving, and no normal breathing (only gasping).

Whatever the location, the victim's level of consciousness should be assessed quickly by checking for signs of life (e.g., movement and normal breathing). The rescuer should call for help and activate the EMS system if the patient is not moving or breathing or only gasping. Outside the hospital, someone may need to call 911 or the emergency number for the local EMS system. Within the hospital, specific protocols exist for "calling a code." All RTs must be familiar with the protocols of their institution for handling these emergency situations.

Restoring Circulation

Determining Pulselessness

For ease of training, the lay rescuer should be taught to assume that a cardiac arrest is present if the unresponsive victim is not breathing or gasping and not take time to check for a pulse. Health care workers also may take too long for a pulse check and have difficulty determining if a pulse is present. For this reason, health care rescuers should proceed immediately with chest compressions if no pulse is found within 10 seconds.

RULE OF THUMB

Assessment of the pulse of an unresponsive patient by health care providers should be limited to 10 seconds to avoid delaying chest compressions. Pulse checks are difficult to accomplish with any fidelity. Pulse and rhythm checks should not be done after a shock until five cycles of CPR have been completed. Pulse checks should not be done by lay rescuers.[3]

Pulselessness is evaluated by palpating a major artery. In adults and children older than 1 year, the carotid artery in the neck or femoral artery should be palpated. To locate the carotid artery, the rescuer should maintain the head-tilt with one hand while sliding the fingers of the other hand into the groove created by the trachea and the large neck muscles (Figure 37-1). The carotid artery area must be palpated gently to avoid compressing the artery or pushing on the carotid sinus. Because the pulse may be slow, weak, or irregular, the artery may need to be assessed for approximately 10 seconds for the presence or absence of a pulse to be confirmed.

For infants, the brachial artery is preferred for assessing pulselessness. To palpate the brachial artery, the rescuer must

TABLE 37-1

Steps for Cardiopulmonary Resuscitation in Adults, Children, and Infants

Procedure	Adult	Child	Infant
Compressions			
Where to check pulse (limit pulse check to <10 sec)	Carotid artery	Carotid or femoral artery	Brachial artery
Hand placement	Heel of one hand on sternum in center of chest, between nipples. Second hand on top of first with hands overlapped and parallel.	Lower half of sternum with heel of one hand or with two hands (for larger children). Do not compress over xiphoid.	Sternum with two fingers placed just below nipple line in center of chest
Compression-to-ventilation ratio	One or two rescuers 30:2	One rescuer 30:2; two rescuers 15:2	One rescuer 30:2; two rescuers 15:2 Newly born or newborn 3:1
Cycles of compression-to-ventilation	5	5	5
Depth of compressions (push in hard and fast, allow chest to recoil fully)	Minimum of 2 in (50 mm)	At least one-third anteroposterior diameter of chest or 2 inches (50 mm)	At least one-third anteroposterior diameter of chest or 1½ inch (4 cm).
Compression rate	Minimum of 100/min (do not exceed 120/min)	100/min	100/min
Breathing			
Obstructive procedure	*Responsive:* If mild, allow victim to clear the airway by coughing. If severe, repeat abdominal thrusts until foreign body is expelled, or the choking victim becomes unresponsive. Consider chest thrusts if abdominal thrusts are ineffective, if rescuer is unable to encircle victim's abdomen, or if victim is in the late stages of pregnancy. *Unresponsive:* Carefully move victim to the ground, immediately activate EMS system, and begin CPR, compressions first, then look into the mouth before giving breaths. If a foreign body is seen, it should be removed. Follow ventilation with chest compressions.	Same as for adult	*Responsive:* If mild, allow infant to clear the airway by coughing. If infant is unable to make a sound (severe obstruction), deliver five back blows (slaps) followed by chest thrusts repeatedly until object is expelled or infant becomes unresponsive. Abdominal thrusts should not be done on infants because they may damage the largely unprotected liver. *Unresponsive:* Activate EMS system and begin CPR, 30 chest compressions first, then look into the mouth before giving breaths. If a foreign body is seen, it should be removed. Follow ventilations with cycles of 30 chest compressions and 2 ventilations.
Rescue Breathing			
Palpable pulse, but no spontaneous breaths or inadequate breathing	10-12/min, 1 breath every 5-6 sec	12-20/min, 1 breath every 3-5 sec, if palpable pulse ≥60/min	20/min, 1 breath every 3 sec, if palpable pulse ≥60/min

grasp the infant's arm with his or her thumb outward, slide his or her fingers down toward the antecubital fossa, and press gently to feel for a pulse. The femoral artery also can be palpated, which may be done for an adult, a child, or an infant.

In hospital critical care settings, bedside monitoring equipment may provide supporting or confirming information regarding the respiratory or circulatory status of a patient. However, information obtained from these devices should never be a substitute for careful clinical assessment.

If the patient has a pulse but is not breathing, ventilation must be started immediately, at the appropriate rate of 8 to 10 breaths/min (every 6 to 8 seconds). If no pulse is palpable, external chest compressions must be interposed with ventilatory support. Deliver cycles of 30 compressions and 2 ventilations until an advanced airway is placed; then deliver uninterrupted chest compressions with asynchronous ventilations at a rate every 6 to 8 seconds (8 to 10/min) (see Table 37-1).

Providing Chest Compressions

Adequate circulation can be restored in a pulseless victim using external chest compressions. The rescuer manually compresses the lower half of the sternum (for an adult patient) at a minimum rate of 100 compressions/min without exceeding 120/min. The duty cycle for downstroke and upstroke (release) is 1:1 downstroke-to-upstroke ratio. It is very important to

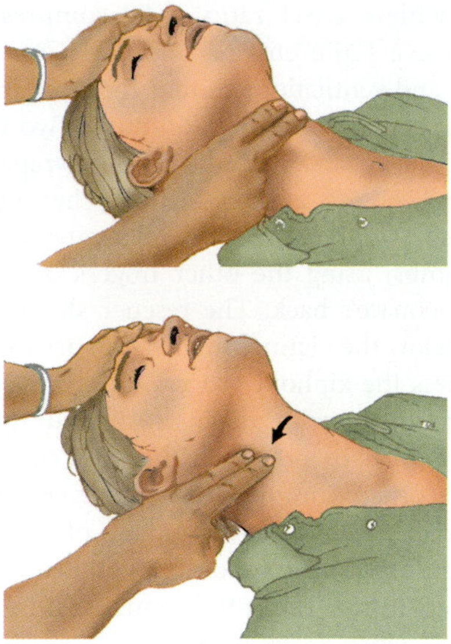

FIGURE 37-1 Determining pulselessness.

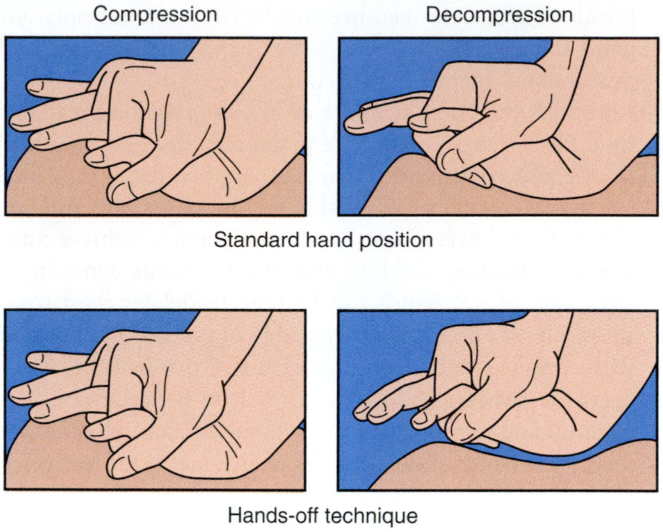

FIGURE 37-3 Techniques for hand position.

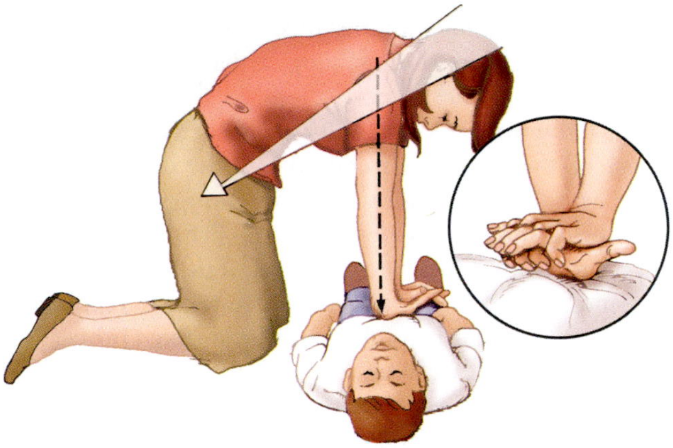

FIGURE 37-2 Position of practitioner for external cardiac compression. Note interlocked fingers to prevent pressure on rib cage.

have a complete upstroke so as not to increase intrathoracic pressure during the diastolic phase. The best way to ensure that the upstroke is complete is for the rescuer to take his or her hand slightly off the chest between compressions.[4,5] Cardiac output produced by external chest compressions is approximately one-fourth of normal cardiac output, with arterial systolic blood pressures between 60 and 80 mm Hg. Blood flow during chest compression probably results from changes in the intrathoracic pressure.

Adults. The procedure for providing chest compressions to adults is as follows (Figures 37-2 and 37-3):

1. Place the victim in a supine position on a firm surface because chest compressions are more effective when the victim is on a firm surface.
2. Choose a position close to the patient's upper chest so that the weight of your upper body can be used for compression. If the patient is on a bed or stretcher, stand next to it with the patient close to that side. If the bed is high or you are short, you may need to lower the bed, stand on a stool or chair, or kneel on the bed next to the victim. If the patient is on the ground, kneel at his or her side.
3. Identify the lower half of the victim's sternum, in the center of the chest between the nipples, place the heel of your hand on the sternum with your other hand on top, and lock your elbows.[6]
4. Perform compression with the weight of your body exerting force on your outstretched arms, elbows held straight. Your shoulders should be positioned above the patient so that the thrust of each compression goes straight down onto the sternum, using your upper body weight and the hip joints as a fulcrum (see Figure 37-2). It is acceptable to let your hands leave the victim's chest ever so slightly to ensure a complete upstroke (see Figure 37-3).
5. Compress the sternum 2 inches (5 cm) at a minimum rate of 100 compressions/min; however, do not exceed a rate of 120/min. The compression phase of the cycle should be equal in duration to the upstroke phase.
6. If CPR must be interrupted for transportation or advanced life-support measures, resume chest compressions as quickly as possible. Compressions should not cease for more than 5 seconds (30 seconds if the victim is being intubated).

Children. Children who have reached puberty should receive chest compressions as outlined for adults. The procedure for younger children (1 year old to puberty) is as follows:

1. Place the victim in the supine position on a firm surface. Small children may require additional support under the upper body; this is particularly true when chest compressions are given with mouth-to-mouth ventilation because extension of the neck raises the shoulders. The head should be no higher than the body.
2. As with an adult, identify the lower half of the sternum. Because the liver and spleen of younger children lie higher in the abdominal cavity, take special care to ensure proper

positioning as described previously. However, use only one hand to compress. Use the other hand to maintain head position and maintain an airway.

3. Compress the chest at a rate of at least 100 compressions/min. Push with enough force to depress the chest one-third of the anteroposterior diameter, approximately 1½ inch (4 cm) in infants or at least 2 inches (5 cm) in children. Generally, the heel of one hand is sufficient to achieve compression. Because children and rescuer hands come in all sizes, one or two hands can be used to deliver chest compressions to ensure that adequate compression depth and with complete release occur. The use of two hands to compress the chest of children will result in better release (less leaning) and less fatigue.[6,7] As with adults, compression and relaxation times should be equal in length and delivered smoothly.

Infants. The procedure for infants (1 year of age or younger) is as follows (Figure 37-4):

1. Use the lower half of the sternum for compression in an infant. Proper placement is determined by imagining a line across the chest connecting the nipples. Place your index finger along this line on the sternum. Then place your middle and ring fingers next to the index finger. Raise your index finger and perform compressions with the middle and ring fingers. Use the other hand to maintain the infant's head position and airway.
2. Compress the sternum approximately 1.5 inch (4 cm) at a rate of at least 100 compressions/min. Compression and upstroke phases should be equal in length and delivered smoothly. Your fingers should remain on the chest at all times.

Neonates. Chest compressions are indicated if the neonate's heart rate decreases to less than 60/min despite adequate ventilation with supplemental oxygen (O_2) for 30 seconds.[8] Before starting chest compressions, the rescuer should ensure that the neonate is being ventilated optimally.[8] Neonatal chest compressions are delivered on the lower third of the sternum to a depth of approximately one-third of the anteroposterior diameter of the chest to achieve a 3:1 ratio of 90 compressions and 30 breaths to achieve 120 events per minute.[8] Coordinated chest compressions and ventilations should continue until the spontaneous heart rate is greater than 60/min.[8] Two methods have been described. The first method uses a "wraparound" technique (Figure 37-5). To use this method, the rescuer encircles the neonate's chest with both hands and compresses the sternum with two thumbs, using the other fingers of both hands to support the neonate's back. The rescuer should position the thumbs just below the victim's intermammary line, taking care not to compress the xiphoid process. Compression should be performed smoothly, with downstroke and upstroke times approximately equal. In all infants, the chest should be allowed to expand fully after a compression. After every third compression, the neonate should receive a breath of 100% O_2, coordinated with compressions to avoid simultaneous delivery. The second method, the two-finger technique (see Figure 37-4), may have advantages when access to the umbilicus is required.

Chest Compressions Under Special Circumstances

The following unique circumstances require modification of the normal procedures for applying cardiac compressions: near drowning and electrical shock.

Near Drowning. Use the A-B-C approach instead of C-A-B because of the hypoxemia caused by near drowning. When cardiac arrest occurs as a result of drowning, the victim must be moved as quickly as possible to a firm surface. Cardiac compressions are difficult to perform while a victim is in the water and may be ineffective. Mouth-to-mouth ventilation in shallow water may be helpful when administered properly. Stabilization of the cervical spine is unnecessary unless circumstances leading to the incident indicate that trauma is likely. Manual cervical spine and spine immobilization equipment

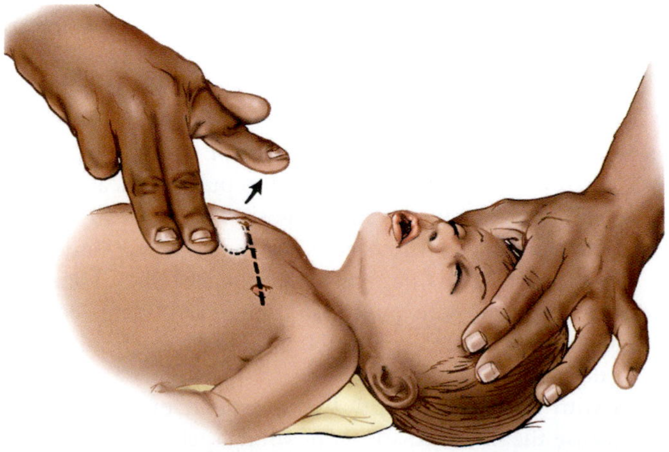

FIGURE 37-4 Position for chest compression in infants.

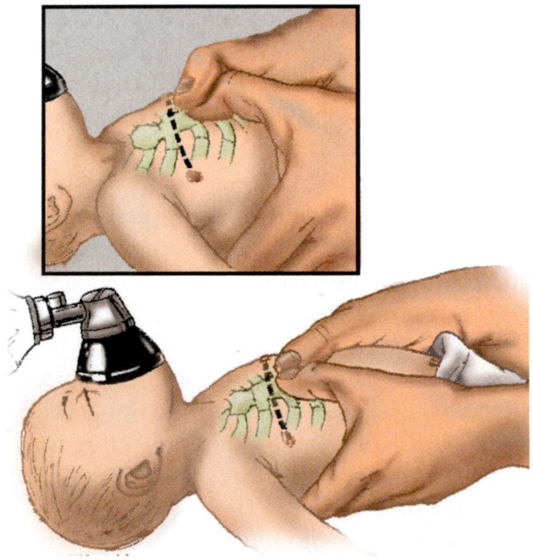

FIGURE 37-5 Neonatal chest compression using the wraparound technique.

may restrict adequate opening of the airway and may delay the delivery of adequate ventilation.

Electrical Shock. Electrical shock can cause either cardiac or respiratory arrest. Cardiac arrest is caused by ventricular fibrillation (VF). Respiratory arrest may occur secondary to paralysis of ventilatory muscles. Initially, the victim must be removed from contact with the source of electricity and evaluated. The rescuers must pay special attention to their own safety. A victim who is still connected to an electrical source must not be touched. The power must be turned off. If cardiac arrest has occurred, airway control, CPR, and attempts at defibrillation should be administered immediately.

Restoring the Airway

After calling for help and activating the EMS system, the lay rescuer providing "hands only" CPR should not use a passive airway such as hyperextending the neck. There is insufficient evidence indicating that a passive airway improves ventilation while administering chest compressions.[3]

The health care provider after activating the emergency response system and sending someone for an automatic external defibrillator should deliver 30 chest compressions and use the head-tilt/chin-lift or jaw-thrust maneuver to open the airway (Figures 37-6 and 37-7). The victim should be quickly inspected for any neck or facial trauma. If spinal cord trauma is suspected, the neck must be carefully positioned in a neutral in-line position and procedures requiring hyperextension must be modified. In addition, when a victim is found lying on his or her side or stomach, he or she should be moved to a supine position before airway procedures are begun. Manual in-line spinal motion restriction should be employed when moving the patient. The rescuer must ensure that the victim is positioned on a hard, flat surface.

One of two procedures can be used. (1) The head-tilt/chin-lift method is the primary procedure recommended when spinal trauma is not suspected. (2) The jaw thrust is used mainly by trained clinicians when spinal neck injuries are suspected. Health care providers should use the head-tilt/chin-lift procedure if the jaw-thrust maneuver does not open the airway.[4] After the airway is cleared and opened, the rescuer must immediately deliver 2 breaths.

Restoring Ventilation

Breathlessness exists if no chest movement or normal breath sounds are present or only gasping is present. This evaluation should take no longer than 3 to 5 seconds to complete. Delivery of chest compressions should always precede attempts to ventilate the patient using a ratio of 30 compressions to 2 breaths.

Providing Artificial Ventilation

During respiratory arrest, the victim must be provided with O_2 within 4 to 6 minutes, or biologic death follows. The lay rescuer can restore O_2 supply to the victim's lungs by exhaling into the victim's mouth, nose, or tracheal stoma. These procedures can be used for any victim, with appropriate modification for the patient's age. Health care providers should be able to provide bag-mask ventilation with 100% O_2.

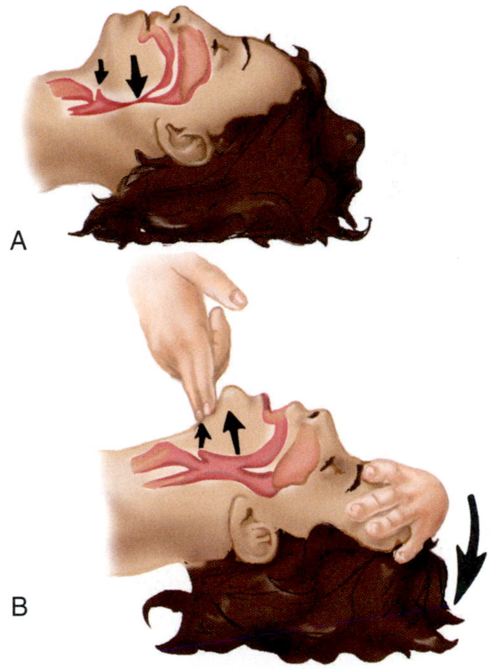

FIGURE 37-6 Opening the airway. **A,** Airway obstruction produced by tongue and epiglottis. **B,** Relief by head-tilt/chin-lift method.

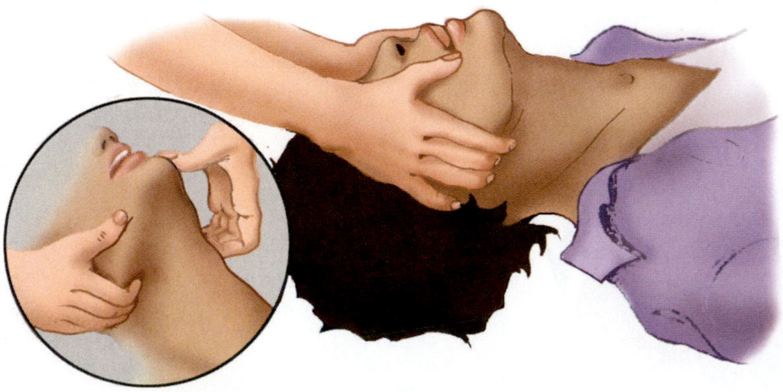

FIGURE 37-7 Jaw-thrust maneuver.

Mouth-to-Mouth Ventilation. **Untrained lay rescuers should be encouraged to deliver hands-only (chest compression only) CPR** (i.e., continuous chest compression over the middle of the chest). Trained rescuers can restore adequate oxygenation through mouth-to-mouth ventilation. To do this, the rescuer should take a normal breath (500 to 600 mL) and exhale directly into the victim's mouth over 1 second to produce visible chest rise. Exhaled air provides approximately 16% O_2, which is sufficient to achieve an arterial O_2 tension (PaO_2) of 50 to 60 mm Hg. A tidal volume (V_T) of 500 mL should be delivered when chest compressions are being administered. Children require proportionally smaller volumes.

During resuscitation of a victim of cardiac arrest, 2 breaths should be given over a period of 1 second each. Excessive volumes (>500 mL) or an inspiratory rate that is too fast (>10 breaths/min) must be avoided because this can push air into the stomach, causing **gastric inflation** and increase intrathoracic pressure. Increased intrathoracic pressure can decrease coronary and cerebral perfusion. Visible chest rise should be used to gauge the V_T needed in children and adults.

Adults. Thirty chest compressions should be delivered to unresponsive victims with apnea or abnormal breathing (gasping) before attempting mouth-to-mouth breathing. The exception would be a hypoxic event such as a near-drowning victim. The procedure for mouth-to-mouth ventilation of adults with spontaneous circulation (i.e., strong palpable pulses) is as follows (Figure 37-8).

1. Place the person on his or her back on a hard, flat surface.
2. Kneel at the person's side, and open and clear the airway as previously described. Pinch the person's nose with your thumb and index finger close to the nares to prevent air from escaping during ventilation.
3. Take a normal breath and deliver 500 mL over 1 second, while making a seal over the person's mouth and watching for chest rise. A good seal over the person's mouth is essential. If a good seal cannot be obtained using this method, attempt mouth-to-nose ventilation.
4. Remove your mouth from the person's mouth, and allow him or her to exhale passively. Provide a second breath after exhalation is complete.
5. After successfully delivering 2 breaths, immediately assess the circulatory status (take <10 seconds to accomplish).
6. Should the initial attempt to ventilate fail, reposition the person's head and repeat the effort. If a second attempt at ventilation fails, the person may have foreign body airway obstruction (FBAO), and the procedures for handling such situations described elsewhere in this chapter should be followed.
7. Assuming mouth-to-mouth ventilation is successful and the person remains apneic, continue the effort at a rate of 1 breath every 5 to 6 seconds to maintain the minimal adult rate of 10 to 12 breaths/min.[3]

Infants and Children. Airway opening maneuvers for children and infants are similar to maneuvers for adults, with several key differences. Anatomic differences in the infant's airway make it especially susceptible to occlusion by the tongue. The infant's head should be extended only slightly, or it should be tilted back gently into a neutral position when the head-tilt/chin-lift maneuver is used. The procedure for children and infants is as follows:

1. If the child is an infant (younger than 1 year), create an airtight seal by placing your mouth over the infant's nose and mouth (Figure 37-9).
2. If the patient is a child between 1 year old and puberty, ventilate the child's lungs using the same technique as would be used for an adult (see Figure 37-8).
3. Provide an initial breath (over 1 second) sufficient to cause a visible rise in the chest. In infants, small puffs of air from the rescuer's cheeks are usually sufficient to achieve adequate ventilation.
4. Remove your mouth, and allow the child to exhale passively. Provide a second breath after this deflation pause.
5. After successfully delivering 2 breaths, immediately assess the pulse (<5 seconds). Provide chest compressions if the pulse is less than 60/min despite adequate oxygenation and ventilation.
6. If the initial attempt to ventilate fails, reposition the child's head and repeat the effort. A child's head may need to be

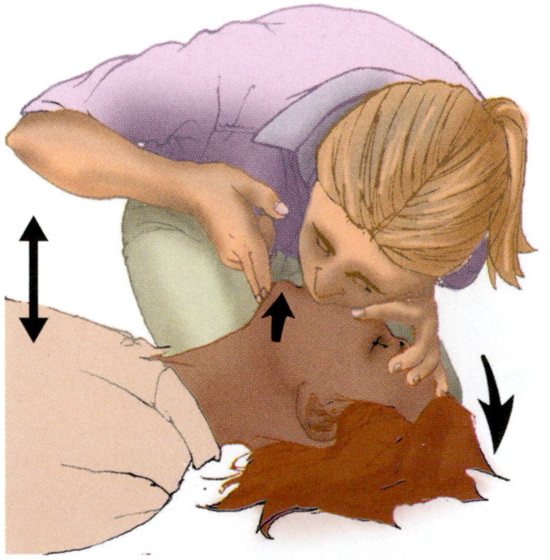

FIGURE 37-8 Adult mouth-to-mouth ventilation.

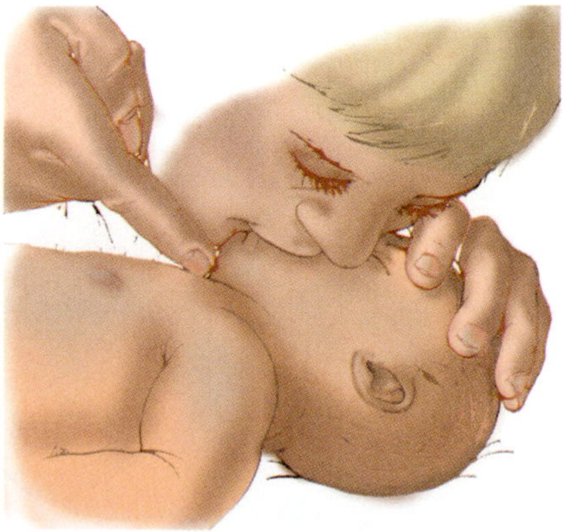

FIGURE 37-9 Mouth-to-mouth and nose seal for infants.

moved through a wide range of positions to secure an open airway. Hyperextension of a child's neck can cause obstruction and should be avoided. If a second attempt at ventilation fails, the victim may have FBAO, and the appropriate procedures outlined elsewhere in this chapter should be followed.

7. Assuming mouth-to-mouth ventilation is successful and the child remains apneic, continue to provide 1 breath every 3 to 5 seconds to maintain a rate of 12 to 20 breaths/min. Recheck pulse every 2 minutes.

Mouth-to-Nose Ventilation. Mouth-to-mouth ventilation cannot be performed in some situations; these include trismus (involuntary contraction of the jaw muscles, also known as *lockjaw*) and traumatic jaw or mouth injury. Also, sometimes it is difficult to maintain a tight seal with the lips using the mouth-to-mouth method. In these situations, mouth-to-nose ventilation should be used. The procedure is as follows (Figure 37-10):

1. Place the person in a supine position.
2. Use the head-tilt/chin-lift maneuver to establish the airway, taking care to close the mouth completely.
3. Inhale normally and exhale into the person's nose. Greater force may need to be applied than would be used with mouth-to-mouth ventilation because the nasal passageways are smaller.
4. Remove your mouth from the person's nose to allow the person to exhale passively. If the person does not exhale through the nose (because of nasopharyngeal obstruction from the soft palate), open the mouth or separate his or her lips to facilitate exhalation.
5. After successfully delivering 2 slow breaths, immediately assess the circulatory status (limit pulse check to <10 seconds).
6. If the person remains apneic, maintain ventilation at the rate appropriate for his or her age.

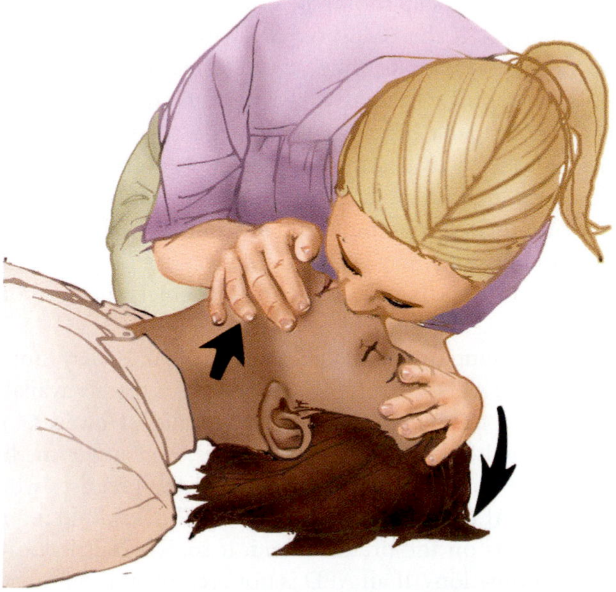

FIGURE 37-10 Mouth-to-nose ventilation.

Mouth-to-Stoma Ventilation. Patients with tracheostomies or laryngectomies can be ventilated directly through the stoma or tube. These patients can be identified by an obvious stoma or a tracheostomy or laryngectomy tube in place. Some patients wear a medical alert tag or bracelet indicating that a stoma is present. The procedure for mouth-to-stoma ventilation is as follows:

1. Place the person on his or her back with the neck in vertical alignment. Usually, the neck does not need to be extended and the nose or mouth does not need to be sealed because oropharyngeal structures are bypassed by the stoma.
2. Ensure that the stoma is clear of any obstructing matter and breathe directly into the stoma (or tube). If the person has a cuffed tracheostomy tube in place, inflate the cuff to prevent air from escaping around the tube. If the tube is uncuffed, the mouth and nose may need to be sealed off with your hand or a tight-fitting face mask. A pediatric face mask may be used to create an adequate peristomal seal for bag-mask ventilation to persons with stomas without artificial airways.
3. After delivering 2 breaths, immediately assess the circulatory status.
4. If the person remains apneic, maintain ventilation at the rate appropriate for his or her age.

One-Rescuer Versus Two-Rescuer Adult Cardiopulmonary Resuscitation

Outside the hospital, one-rescuer CPR is common. In such cases, the rescuer must assess the victim, call for help, and begin CPR without assistance from others. The rescuer must remain calm and remember the steps of one-rescuer CPR. The technique for performing chest compressions, opening the airway, and giving mouth-to-mouth breaths is the same, regardless of the number of rescuers.

When performing CPR alone, the lay rescuer must remember to give only compressions for adults, children, and infants until an AED arrives. When two rescuers are available, the second rescuer ventilates and evaluates the effectiveness of CPR. The other rescuer administers cardiac compressions. To facilitate movement, each rescuer should assume the appropriate rescue position on opposite sides of the victim. For an adult and child, the compression-to-ventilation ratio is the same as for a single rescuer (30:2) and the timing for compressions is "one and two and three and four and five" (a minimum rate of 100 times/min). In infants, two rescuers should use a compression-to-ventilation ratio of 3:1 with 90 compressions and 30 breaths delivered per minute (120 events/min). Each breath is delivered over a half-second with exhalation occurring on the next compression.

RULE OF THUMB

Lay rescuers should be taught to do a minimum of 100 compressions/min (do not exceed 120/min) until the AED arrives for all age groups because it is easier to remember. Emphasis should be placed on teaching lay rescuers to "push hard and fast" on the sternum.

RULE OF THUMB

Health care providers should use a 30:2 compression-to-ventilation ratio on adults and children. However, when two health care providers work together to resuscitate a child or infant the compression-to-ventilation ratio should be 15:2.[9]

When two health care providers resuscitate a patient, the individual providing compressions briefly pauses after 30 compressions so that the other person can administer two ventilations. The cycle is repeated without interruption of compressions to check for signs of circulation or response until an AED arrives or until the hospital code team take over CPR. Health care providers should limit interruptions in chest compressions to no longer than 10 seconds except for interventions such as insertion of an advanced airway or defibrillation.

To provide rest for the individual delivering cardiac compressions, the rescuers should change positions every five cycles (approximately 2 minutes). The individual doing cardiac compressions calls for the change, saying "we will change next time" in sequence with compressions. The switch should be accomplished in less than 5 seconds. The cycle continues with the two rescuers in their new positions. Alternatively, to avoid fatigue, teams of three health care providers can be assigned to do chest compression, switching every five cycles of 30:2 compression-to-ventilation ratio. The goal is to push "hard and fast" at a minimum rate of 100/min (do not exceed 120/min) without fatigue diminishing that goal.

RULE OF THUMB

The person doing chest compressions should be changed every 2 minutes. Doing chest compressions is tiring, and fatigue occurs within a few minutes, leading to a compression rate less than 100 compressions/min, shallow chest compressions (<50 mm), and incomplete chest recoil.[4]

Rescue attempts continue until advanced life support is available, the rescuers note spontaneous pulse and breathing, or a physician pronounces the victim dead. A cardiopulmonary emergency is a crisis for the victim and his or her family, and appropriate support and intervention should be provided all individuals affected. Victims who survive CPR should be transported quickly to tertiary care facilities, ideally only after advanced life support is instituted.

Automated External Defibrillation

Early Defibrillation

Since 1990 the AHA has recommended adding a fourth step to the treatment of cardiac arrest. This step involves early **defibrillation** after CPR has been initiated. The rationale is as follows:

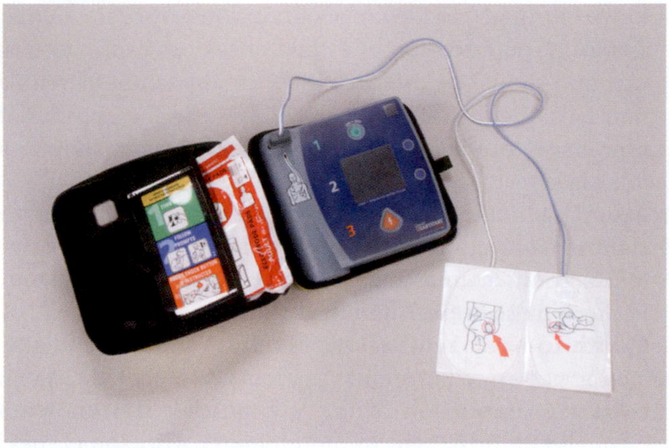

FIGURE 37-11 Automated external defibrillator with pads attached. (From Chapleau W: Emergency first responder, making the difference, revised ed 2, St. Louis, 2011, St. Louis, Mosby JEMS.)

1. The most common initial rhythm in witnessed sudden cardiac arrest is VF.
2. The treatment for VF is electrical defibrillation.
3. The probability of successful defibrillation diminishes rapidly over time.
4. VF tends to convert to asystole within a few minutes.

Studies have shown that survival rates are highest when immediate bystander CPR is provided and defibrillation occurs within 5 minutes after SCA.[10,11]

The AHA recommendation is that **automated external defibrillators** (AEDs) be made available to individuals expected to respond to emergencies, such as police, security personnel, ski patrol personnel, flight attendants, and first-aid volunteers (Figure 37-11). Early defibrillation has already proved effective in saving lives of people who otherwise may not have been successfully resuscitated.[10,11] After appropriate training and implementation of the *CABs,* this step is inserted as the letter *D,* for defibrillation. This step should be initiated within 2 minutes of beginning CPR. If the EMS provider witnesses the collapse or for in-hospital situations, the rescuer should use the defibrillator as soon as it is available. When more than one health care provider is available, one should provide chest compressions while the other activates the emergency response system and retrieves the defibrillator. In an adult drowning victim or a victim of FBAO who becomes unconscious, a health care provider working alone may give about five cycles (approximately 2 minutes) of CPR before activating the emergency response system.[3]

Personnel employed at high-acuity hospitals may not be equipped with AEDs because access to ACLS is readily available, usually within minutes of the code being called. However, low-acuity hospitals, skilled nursing facilities, and other medical facilities that do not have a code team on the premises would benefit from AEDs. RTs working at such facilities should inquire whether one is on the premises and, if so, where it is located and how it functions. If an AED is not present, a recommendation should be made to the administration of the facility to purchase one. The AHA recommends that an AED be available wherever CPR is likely to be performed.

VF cardiac arrest is less common in children than adults and accounts for 5% to 15% of pediatric and adolescent arrests.[12] The AHA recommends use of an AED for children older than 1 year who are in cardiac arrest and encourages the use of a pediatric dose-attenuator system if one is available. If such a system is unavailable, a standard AED is recommended. The standard doses recommended by the AHA for manual defibrillation of children are 2 J/kg for the first attempt and 4 J/kg for the subsequent attempt, increasing the dose in additional subsequent attempts not to exceed 10 J/kg.[13] Research has shown that lower energy (120 to 200 J) biphasic waveform shocks have equivalent or higher success in terminating VF than three stacked monophasic waveform shocks delivering escalating energy of 200 J, 300 J, and 360 J.[14,15] AEDs should be deployed in locations where there is a high incidence of witnessed SCA, such as airports, casinos, and sports facilities.

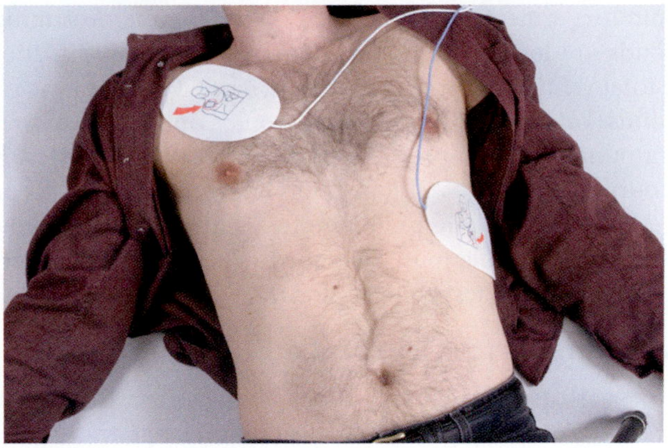

FIGURE 37-12 Positioning of rescuer and placement of pads when using automated external defibrillator. (From Chapleau W: Emergency first responder, making the difference, revised ed 2, St. Louis, 2011, St. Louis, Mosby JEMS.)

Automated External Defibrillators

AEDs function in a semiautomatic fashion; the device only recommends that a shock be delivered, rather than initiating one automatically. Adhesive electrodes from the AED are attached to the patient. When all of the equipment is hooked up, the "Analyze" button should be pressed to begin. A rhythm recognition program analyzes the patient's rhythm. If it detects ventricular tachycardia (VT) or VF, it advises the rescuer through voice and visual prompts that a shock should be delivered. If a shock is indicated, the rescuer should "Clear" the patient and press the "Shock" button. After pressing the shock button, the rescuer should deliver five cycles of CPR beginning with chest compressions using a compressions-to-ventilations ratio of 30 : 2.

The rescuer should not delay chest compressions by stopping to recheck the rhythm or pulse. The rhythm is checked by the AED after five cycles (approximately 2 minutes) of CPR have been completed. The rescuers should be prepared to initiate another five cycles of CPR immediately after a second shock has been delivered. The rescuer administering chest compressions should be changed every 2 minutes. The rescuer providing 2 minutes of chest compressions should be prepared to deliver a shock as soon as he or she removes hands from the victim's chest. The second rescuer should be in position to start chest compressions as soon as the shock is delivered. If no shock is advised by the AED, the AED voice prompt should instruct the rescuer to resume CPR immediately, starting with chest compressions. If the message reads "No shock indicated," CPR should be performed for 1 to 2 minutes and then the rhythm analysis should be repeated. A 1- to 2-minute period of CPR after a no-shock prompt from the AED delivers O_2 and metabolic substrates to the myocardium, increasing the probability that a perfusing rhythm will occur. The rescuer should not be concerned that chest compressions might trigger the return of VF in the presence of a postshock organized rhythm.[16] Figure 37-12 demonstrates how the AED is attached to the victim.

RULE OF THUMB

Patients in VF or pulseless VT cardiac arrest should receive only one shock followed immediately by five cycles of CPR before the next shock is delivered. Time should not be taken to check for a pulse or ventilate the patient before delivering the second shock if needed. Biphasic AEDs have a 90% conversion rate of VF on the first shock, so it is unlikely there will be a need for a second shock. However, chest compressions immediately after the first shock increase O_2 delivery and increase the chance of VF conversion to a normal rhythm.[13]

Evaluating Effectiveness of Cardiopulmonary Resuscitation

CPR providers need to judge continuously both the effectiveness of CPR and the victim's response. Ventilation can be evaluated by observing visible rise and fall of the victim's chest during mouth-to-mouth resuscitation. Air that is escaping can be heard and felt during exhalation. A consensus statement from the AHA on the quality of CPR reached the following conclusions on five quality metrics of CPR performance.[17]

1. Minimize the frequency and duration of interruptions in chest compressions.
2. Compress the adult chest at a rate of 100 to 120 compressions/min.
3. Ensure chest compression depth of 50 mm or greater ($\geq$2 inches) in adults and at least one-third the anteroposterior dimension of the chest in infants and children.
4. Allow the chest to recoil completely after each compression, that is, no residual leaning.
5. Avoid excessive ventilation: rate less than 12 breaths/min (minimal chest rise).

The time to deliver 30 compressions is 18 seconds or less if the compression rate is at least 100 compressions/min. It takes a rescuer 4 seconds to deliver 2 breaths with a 1-second inspiratory time and a 1-second expiratory time. Assuming 2 seconds are lost switching from compressions to ventilations, the total ventilation time is 6 seconds. The CPR cycle time is 24 seconds or less; 2.5 cycles/min would optimally deliver a minimum of 75 compressions and five breaths. The AHA has encouraged the use of CPR prompts after studies showed compression and ventilation rates are frequently too fast or slow.[17] Every effort possible must be made to decrease the number of interruptions in chest compressions.

Hazards and Complications

The most common complications that occur with CPR are worsening of existing neck or spine injuries, gastric inflation and vomiting, trauma to internal structures during chest compressions, and problems associated with the removal of foreign objects to clear an obstructed airway.

Neck and Spine Injuries

Health care providers can aggravate neck or spinal injuries by inappropriately moving the victim's head. However, only approximately 2% to 5% of victims with blunt trauma have a spinal injury. Spinal injury risk is greatest if the victim has craniofacial injury or a Glasgow Coma Scale score of less than 8.[18] The victim should be carefully assessed for head, neck, or spinal injuries. If this type of injury is apparent, the head should be carefully supported, and side-to-side motion must be avoided. In such situations, using the jaw thrust maneuver rather than the head-tilt/chin-lift method to open the airway is recommended by the AHA.[3] If jaw thrust is unsuccessful in establishing an airway, the rescuer should try a slight head-tilt.[3]

Gastric Inflation

During prolonged mouth-to-mouth ventilation, air enters the esophagus and stomach. Some gastric inflation is not unusual, particularly in children, and occurs in approximately 17% of cases.[19,20] Severe gastric inflation puts pressure on the diaphragm, restricting lung expansion. Gastric inflation also can increase vagal tone and cause reflex bradycardia and hypotension.

> **RULE OF THUMB**
>
> The best way to avoid gastric inflation during bag-mask ventilation is to deliver breaths with low to moderate flow (<30 L/min) over 1 second.[21] V_T size should be only large enough to cause visible chest rise. The health care provider should not ventilate and compress the chest simultaneously with a bag-mask device.

However, most important is the fact that severe gastric inflation prompts regurgitation. Because an unconscious patient lacks normal upper airway reflexes, regurgitated stomach contents can be aspirated easily into the lungs. Aspiration of stomach contents into the lungs may cause death by making ventilation virtually impossible or lead to severe lung injury such as aspiration pneumonia that may cause death days or weeks later.

Vomiting

Vomiting is another complication associated with **abdominal thrusts,** and it is impossible to avoid in some victims. Vomiting itself is a minor problem. The hazard is the aspiration of vomitus into the lung. Aspiration can be prevented only by using advanced airway devices such as an endotracheal tube, laryngeal mask airway, or esophageal-tracheal double-lumen airway (Combitube, Medtronic, Minneapolis, MN).

Internal Trauma

External cardiac compression is hazardous, and every attempt should be made to minimize trauma by using the correct technique. Complications associated with chest compression include rare incidents of gastric perforation, laceration of the liver, pneumothorax, hemothorax, cardiac tamponade, and soft tissue emphysema. More common complications are contusion of the lung and fractured ribs or sternum.[22,23] These complications most often are linked to improper hand position. Placement of the hands too far to either the left or the right can cause fractured ribs or lacerated lung. Incorrect placement on the left can injure the heart. Placing the hands too high on the sternum can fracture the sternum; placing the hands too low can cause a fractured xiphoid process or a lacerated liver. Correct identification of landmarks and proper hand placement minimize the likelihood of these complications.

Foreign Body Airway Obstruction

Manual removal of FBAO from the upper airway also can be hazardous because of the possibility of forcing the object deeper into the airway or traumatizing the airway. This hazard can be minimized by attempting to remove an FBAO only when the provider can see solid material obstructing the airway in an unresponsive patient and using extreme care in removing it.[3]

Contraindications to Cardiopulmonary Resuscitation

A pulseless, apneic patient dies within 4 to 6 minutes without intervention. Fear of further harm should never influence the decision to begin CPR. CPR is contraindicated only when the patient is obviously biologically dead (as noted by such findings as rigor mortis). In the hospital, CPR is contraindicated when a valid "do-not-resuscitate" order is in effect or when a properly executed living will (advance directive) specifically requests that CPR not be initiated.

Health Concerns and Cardiopulmonary Resuscitation

The actual risk for disease transmission during mouth-to-mouth ventilation is very small. However, the reluctance to initiate CPR poses a clear threat to the effectiveness of early intervention in life-threatening emergencies, which affects the public as a whole. A bystander should provide hands-only (chest compression only) CPR, with an emphasis on "push hard and fast," or follow the directions of the emergency medical dispatcher.[4]

RULE OF THUMB

Rescuers of adult VF cardiac arrest should provide chest compressions at a rate of at least 100 compressions/min, with an emphasis on "push hard and fast." Periodic gasps and chest recoil in adult cardiac arrest may provide some ventilation if the airway is open. Most children and infants with cardiac arrest require both prompt ventilations and chest compressions.

Health care providers with a duty to provide CPR should follow the guidelines established by the U.S. Centers for Disease Control and Prevention (CDC) and the Occupational Safety and Health Administration. These recommendations include the use of latex gloves, masks, and goggles. Mechanical barrier aids to ventilation (e.g., masks, filters, valves, bag-mask) also have been suggested to allay fear and protect the rescuer. However, these devices require training to be used properly.

Equipment contaminated with blood or other body fluids during a resuscitation effort always should be discarded in appropriate receptacles or thoroughly cleaned and disinfected according to hospital protocols.

Treating Foreign Body Airway Obstruction

Early recognition of FBAO is critical. Foreign bodies may cause partial or complete obstruction. Partial obstruction may allow nearly adequate air exchange, in which case the patient remains conscious and coughing. As long as air exchange is present, the patient should be reassured and allowed to clear his or her own airway by coughing. If partial obstruction persists, or air exchange worsens, the EMS system should be activated. Poor air exchange exists when the patient has a weak or ineffective cough, increased inspiratory difficulty, or cyanosis.

With a completely obstructed airway, the patient commonly clutches at his or her throat. This is known as the *universal distress signal for foreign body obstruction.* A person with a complete obstruction cannot talk, cough, or breathe and is in dire need of emergency intervention using abdominal thrusts, chest thrusts, back blows, or a combination of two or more maneuvers.

Several procedures can be used to obtain a clear passageway if attempts to open a victim's airway are unsuccessful or if a foreign body is observed but cannot be removed from the mouth or pharynx. For adults and children, the procedure for health care providers for clearing a foreign body is the *abdominal thrust.* The rescuer should attempt back blows first for infants with an obstructed airway; if these are unsuccessful, the rescuer should try chest thrusts. *Chest thrusts* may be used in place of abdominal thrusts on women in advanced stages of pregnancy and on markedly obese individuals. Both abdominal thrusts and chest thrusts normally are followed by a visual check and manual removal of any observed obstructing foreign material.

Abdominal Thrusts (Heimlich Maneuver)

Forceful thrusts applied to the epigastrium can dislodge an obstruction caused by a food bolus, vomitus, or other foreign body. Quick thrusts to the abdomen rapidly displace the diaphragm upward, increasing intrathoracic pressure and creating expulsive expiratory airflow. As with a normal cough, this expulsive airflow may be sufficient to expel the foreign body from the airway. The procedure for performing abdominal thrusts on adults and children is as follows (Figure 37-13). If the victim is sitting or standing, stand behind the victim and wrap your arms around his or her waist. Make a fist with one hand, and place the thumb side midline on the abdomen slightly above the navel and well below the tip of the xiphoid process (see Figure 37-13). Grasp the fist with the other hand and deliver a quick upward and inward thrust. Each thrust should be a separate and distinct movement. Repeat the process until the obstruction is removed or the victim loses consciousness.

If an adult victim with FBAO becomes unresponsive, the rescuer should move the patient to the ground, activate the EMS system, and begin CPR. Each time the mouth is opened during cycles of compressions and ventilation, the rescuer should look into the victim's mouth for FBAO and remove it; this should be done without increasing the time to deliver 2 breaths (approximately 6 seconds). The routine use of blind finger sweeps to remove FBAO in adults, children, and infants is not recommended by the AHA.[3,8]

A conscious victim who is alone can attempt to dislodge the foreign body with self-administered abdominal thrusts, performed by pressing his or her fist into the abdomen or pushing the abdomen against a firm surface such as a counter top, sink, chair back, railing, or tabletop.

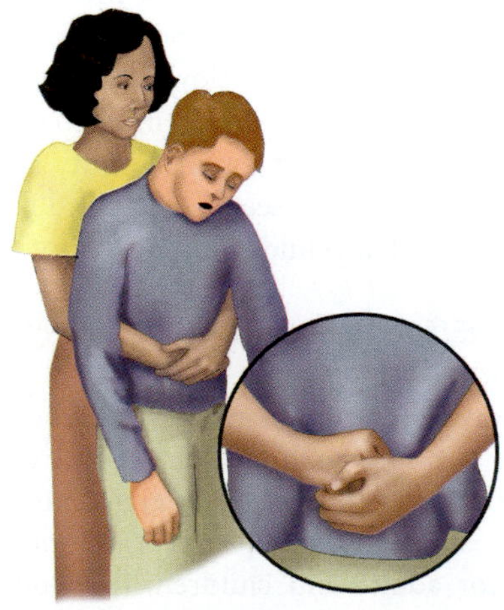

FIGURE 37-13 Abdominal thrusts, adult victim standing. (From Chapleau W: Emergency First Responder, Making the Difference, Revised 2nd edition, 2011, St. Louis, Mosby JEMS.)

Internal Organ Damage. The major hazard associated with abdominal thrusts that are performed when an individual has choked and lost consciousness is possible damage to internal organs, such as laceration or rupture of abdominal or thoracic viscera.[24] The body of clinical data regarding choking is largely retrospective and anecdotal. Abdominal thrusts have been recommended for relief of FBAO in adults and children since 1975, based mostly on early anecdotal case reports. Abdominal thrusts are recommended by the AHA and several other resuscitation councils for use for *unresponsive* adult and child (but not infant) victims. Abdominal thrusts are not recommended for infants younger than 1 year of age because of their relatively unprotected abdomens and large livers. Rational conjecture and common practices suggest that back blows may loosen obstruction so that subsequent abdominal or chest thrusts may relieve obstruction. The risk for internal organ damage from abdominal thrusts in a conscious patient can be minimized by the rescuer placing his or her arms and fist below the victim's xiphoid process and the lower margin of the ribs.

Back Blows and Chest Thrusts

Because an abdominal maneuver can easily cause abdominal injury when applied to infants, a combination of back blows and chest thrusts should be used to clear foreign bodies from the upper airway. Back blows alone may create sufficient force to dislodge trapped objects, but if this is ineffective, the back blows should be followed with five chest thrusts. The rescuer should continue inspecting the airway until the airway is restored. This procedure is as follows:

1. Back blows can be administered to infants more efficiently if the child is held straddled over one arm with the head lower than the body (Figure 37-14).
2. Use the flat portion of your hand to deliver gently, but quickly, five back blows between the shoulder blades.
2. If the back blows do not clear the infant's airway, turn the infant over and institute a series of five chest thrusts (see Figure 37-14). Similar to abdominal thrust, chest thrust creates a rapid increase in intrathoracic pressure, aiding expulsion of the foreign body. Chest thrusts for infants are performed in the same manner and at the same location as cardiac compressions but at a slower rate.
3. Try to clear the airway between attempts to expel the foreign body. First, visually inspect the oral cavity and remove any foreign matter that can be seen. Deep blind finger sweeps of the mouth of an infant, child, or adult are not recommended.

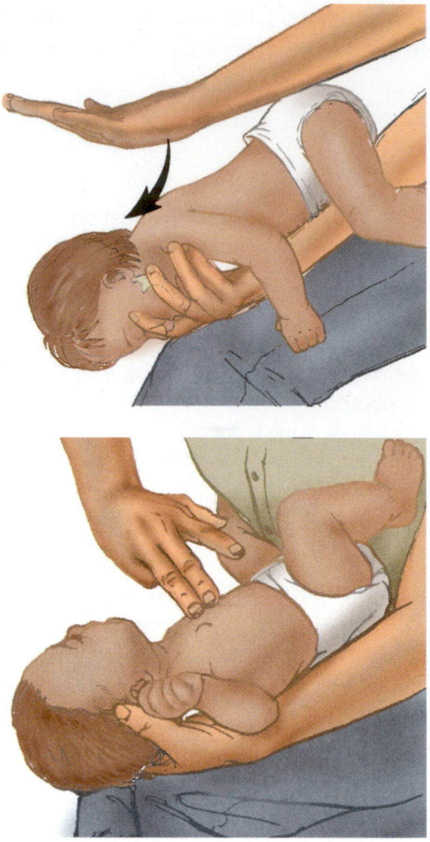

FIGURE 37-14 Use of back blows and chest thrusts to clear foreign bodies from infant airway.

Evaluating Effectiveness of Foreign Body Removal

After each airway restoration maneuver, the rescuer must determine whether the foreign body has been expelled and the obstructed airway cleared. If the foreign body has not been dislodged, the appropriate sequence (abdominal thrusts or chest thrusts for adults and children, back blows and chest thrusts for infants) should be repeated until successful. Successful removal of an obstructing body is indicated by the following:

- Confirmed expulsion of foreign body
- Clear breathing and ability to speak
- Return of consciousness
- Return of normal color

If successive attempts to clear the airway fail, more aggressive techniques are indicated, if available. These include direct laryngoscopy and foreign body removal with Magill forceps, transtracheal catheterization, cricothyrotomy, and tracheotomy. These methods require specially trained health care professionals and equipment, and they are aptly categorized as advanced life-support techniques. Transtracheal catheterization and cricothyrotomy are discussed later in this chapter, and laryngoscopy, bronchoscopy, and tracheotomy are described in Chapter 36.

ADVANCED CARDIOVASCULAR LIFE SUPPORT

ACLS extends BLS capabilities by providing additional measures beyond immediate ventilatory and circulatory assistance. These measures include using accessory equipment to support ventilation and oxygenation, monitoring the electrocardiogram (ECG), establishing an intravenous (IV) route for drug administration, and applying selected pharmacologic agents and electrical therapies (Figure 37-15). The AHA claims that "the

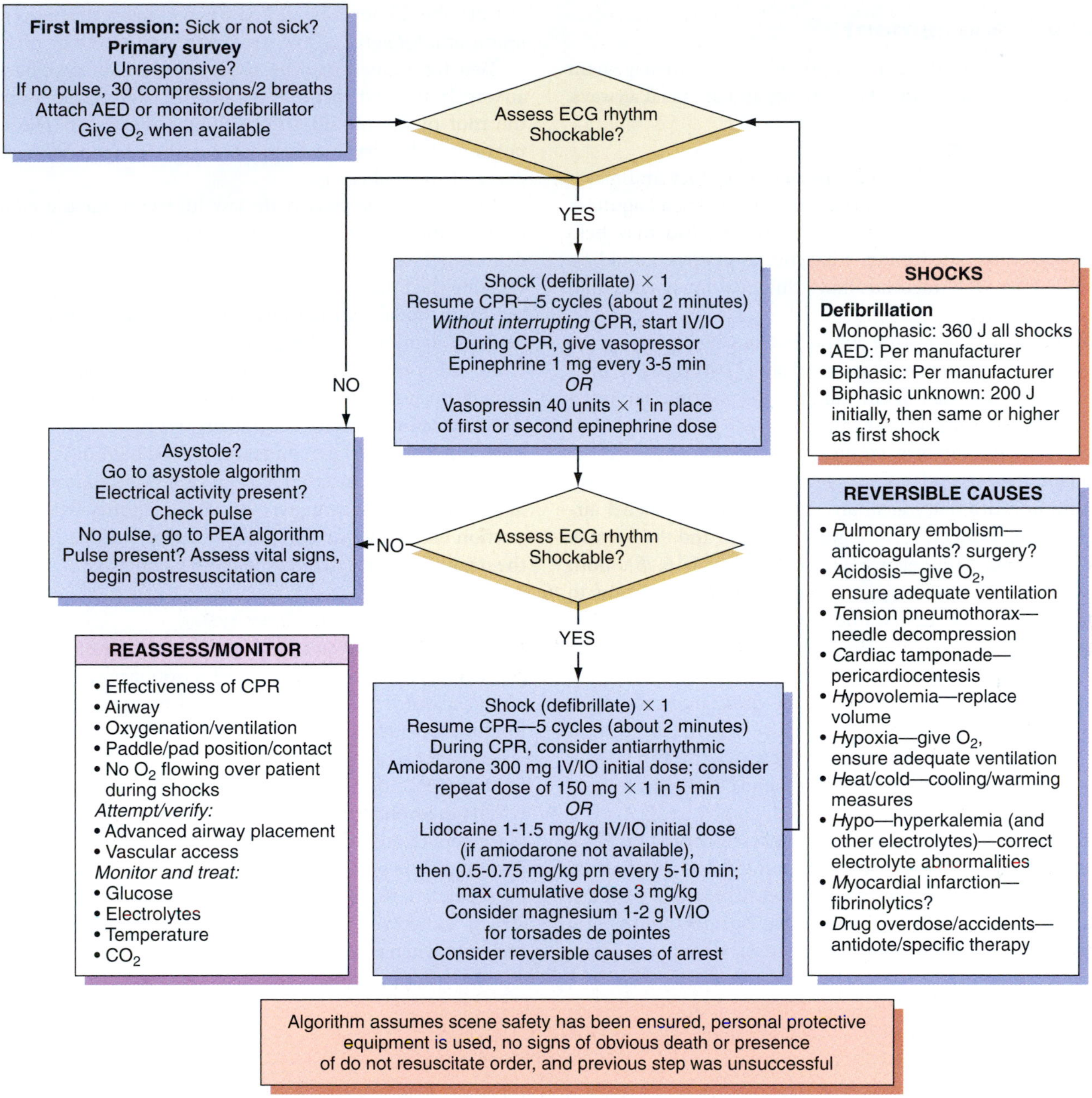

FIGURE 37-15 Pulseless VT/VF algorithm. (From Aehlert B: ACLS study guide, ed 4, St. Louis, 2012, Mosby.)

foundation of ACLS is good BLS care, beginning with prompt high-quality bystander CPR and, for pulseless ventricular rhythms, attempted defibrillation within minutes of collapse."[25]

During ACLS in the hospital, the RT assumes primary responsibility for supporting oxygenation, establishing and maintaining the airway, and providing ventilation. RTs must demonstrate high levels of proficiency in these advanced life-support skills and other ACLS skills that may be assigned by the resuscitation team leader.

Support for Oxygenation

Although expired air ventilation provides an acceptable level of oxygenation, low cardiac output, pulmonary shunting, and abnormalities during CPR lead to hypoxia. Hypoxia results in anaerobic metabolism and metabolic acidosis. Metabolic acidosis impedes the action of certain drugs and can diminish the effectiveness of electrical therapies. For these reasons, the highest possible concentration of O_2 should be administered as soon as possible to adults and children. Concerns about O_2 toxicity are not valid during this period of resuscitation. Less than 100% O_2 may be used during neonatal resuscitation at birth.

During ACLS, supplemental O_2 is normally given through accessory devices designed to support ventilation. The ability of these devices to provide high fractional inspired O_2 (F_IO_2) is a key factor in judging their performance.

Airway Management

Accessory equipment designed to provide airway management during ACLS includes a variety of masks and artificial airways.

Pharyngeal Airways

Pharyngeal airways can help restore airway patency and maintain adequate ventilation, in particular, when using a bag-mask device. A properly placed pharyngeal airway also may help provide access for suctioning. Pharyngeal airways should be used only after BLS methods have successfully opened and cleared the airway.

Pharyngeal airways restore airway patency by separating the tongue from the posterior pharyngeal wall. Two types of pharyngeal airways are used in clinical practice: the oropharyngeal airway and the nasopharyngeal airway.

Oropharyngeal airways come in many different sizes to fit adults, children, and infants. Figure 37-16 shows the two most common oropharyngeal airway designs: the Guedel airway (Flexicare, Irvine, CA; see Figure 37-16, *A*) and the Berman airway (Medline, Mundelein, IL; see Figure 37-16, *B*). Both types have an external flange, a curved body that conforms to the shape of the oral cavity, and one or more channels. The Guedel airway has a single center channel, whereas the Berman airway uses two parallel side channels.

To choose the correct size airway, the clinician should place the devices on the side of the patient's face with the flange even with the patient's mouth. The correct size airway measures from the corner of the patient's mouth to the angle of the jaw following the natural curve of the airway.

Because insertion of an oropharyngeal airway can provoke a gag reflex, vomiting, or laryngeal spasm, these devices generally are contraindicated for conscious or semiconscious patients. They also are contraindicated when there is trauma to the oral cavity or the mandibular or maxillary areas of the skull. These airways should never be placed when either a space-occupying lesion or a foreign body obstructs the oral cavity or pharynx.

Two techniques may be used to insert an oropharyngeal airway. In the first method, the tongue is displaced away from the roof of the mouth with a tongue depressor. The curved portion of the airway is slipped over the tongue, following the curve of the oral cavity.

In the second approach, the jaw-lift technique is used to help displace the tongue. The oropharyngeal airway is rotated 180 degrees before insertion. In this manner, the airway itself helps separate the tongue from the posterior wall of the pharynx. As the tip of the airway reaches the hard palate, it is rotated 180 degrees, aligning it in the pharynx.

In either approach, incorrect placement can displace the tongue, pushing it farther back into the pharynx and worsening the obstruction. Oropharyngeal airways must be inserted carefully and by trained personnel only. As shown in Figure 37-16, *C,* when properly inserted, the tip of an oropharyngeal airway lies at the base of the tongue above the epiglottis, with the flange portion extending outside the teeth. Only in this position can the device properly maintain airway patency.

Nasopharyngeal Airways

Nasopharyngeal airways are inserted through the nose instead of the mouth. A properly inserted nasopharyngeal airway provides a passageway from the external nares to the base of the tongue. As with the oropharyngeal airway, the nasopharyngeal airway helps restore airway patency by separating the tongue from the posterior pharyngeal wall.

The nasopharyngeal airway generally is indicated when placement of an oropharyngeal airway is impossible. The nasopharyngeal airway also is used when the jaws of a victim cannot be separated, as may occur with seizures. A nasopharyngeal airway should not be used when there is trauma to the nasal region or when space-occupying lesions or foreign objects block

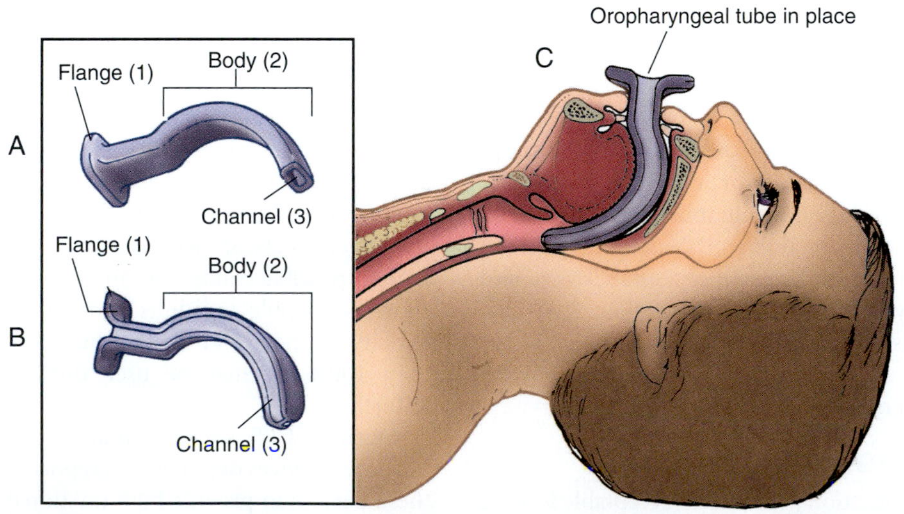

FIGURE 37-16 Oropharyngeal airways. **A,** Guedel airway. **B,** Berman airway. **C,** Airway in place.

the nasal passages. Because the nasal passageway in children and infants is small, the use of nasal airways is generally limited to adults.

Most nasal airways are made from either rubber or plastic polymers and sized by external diameter according to the French scale, with 26F to 32F being the usual range for adults. Anatomically, the length of the airway is more critical than the diameter. The appropriate length can be estimated by measuring the distance from the patient's earlobe to the tip of the nose.

To insert a nasopharyngeal airway, the victim's head is tilted slightly backward. The airway is lubricated with a water-soluble agent to ease insertion, and it is positioned perpendicular to the frontal plane of the victim's face. The airway is advanced slowly through the inferior meatus of either the right or the left nasal cavity, with the bevel edge facing the septum. If an obstruction is felt during insertion, gentle twisting may facilitate placement. If the resistance continues, the most likely cause is a deviated nasal septum. In this case, attempt to insert the airway through the other naris or try a smaller diameter tube.

After the airway is inserted, try to visualize and confirm its correct position quickly, using a tongue depressor if necessary. When properly positioned, a nasopharyngeal airway is usually stabilized by its own flange.

Masks

A mask that fits the patient is a useful tool for the application of artificial ventilation by appropriately trained rescuers. An ideal mask should be made of transparent material, be capable of sealing tightly against the face, provide an inlet for supplemental O_2, and have a standard 22-mm port for connection to a bag-mask device. The mask should be available in various sizes to accommodate adults, children, and infants. Infant masks often have a 15-mm male connector instead of a 22-mm port. The use of masks to support ventilation presumes that the airway can be maintained by conventional BLS techniques. Which mask should be used in a given situation depends on careful assessment of the status of the victim and an in-depth knowledge of the capabilities and limitations of the equipment at hand.

Endotracheal Intubation

An advanced airway allows the rescuer to achieve one or more of the following goals:

1. Deliver ventilations that are not synchronous with chest compressions
2. Restore airway patency
3. Maintain adequate ventilation
4. Isolate and protect the airway from aspiration
5. Provide access for clearance of secretions

Endotracheal intubation is the preferred method for securing the airway during CPR. When positioned properly, an endotracheal tube can maintain a patent airway, prevent aspiration of stomach contents, permit suctioning of the trachea and main stem bronchi, facilitate ventilation and oxygenation, and provide a route for drug administration.

Attempts to intubate the trachea must never interfere with providing adequate ventilation and oxygenation by other means. Only highly trained personnel should perform endotracheal intubation, and each attempt ideally should not exceed 10 seconds because chest compressions will not be possible during the procedure. Continuous waveform capnography is recommended by the AHA Guidelines in addition to physical assessment as the initial method for confirming and monitoring correct placement of an endotracheal tube.[25] When capnometry is not available, auscultation and direct visualization should be used to confirm tracheal position of the endotracheal tube. Adequate ventilation and oxygenation must be provided between attempts. Figure 37-17 shows a cuffed orotracheal tube properly positioned in the trachea. It is being used with a manual bag-mask device to provide ventilation and oxygenation. Adequate ventilation and oxygenation can be provided with 10 to 12 breaths/min.

RTs should be trained in endotracheal intubation techniques, as applied in both emergency life support and mechanical ventilation situations. Details about the necessary equipment,

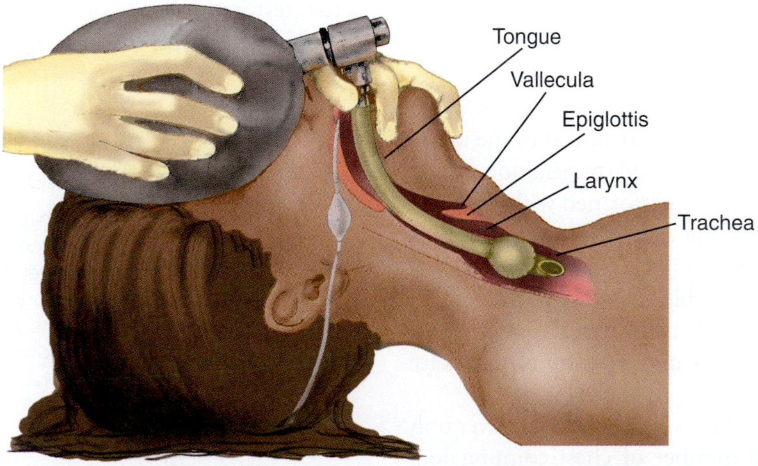

FIGURE 37-17 Orotracheal tube in place, being used with a bag-valve resuscitator.

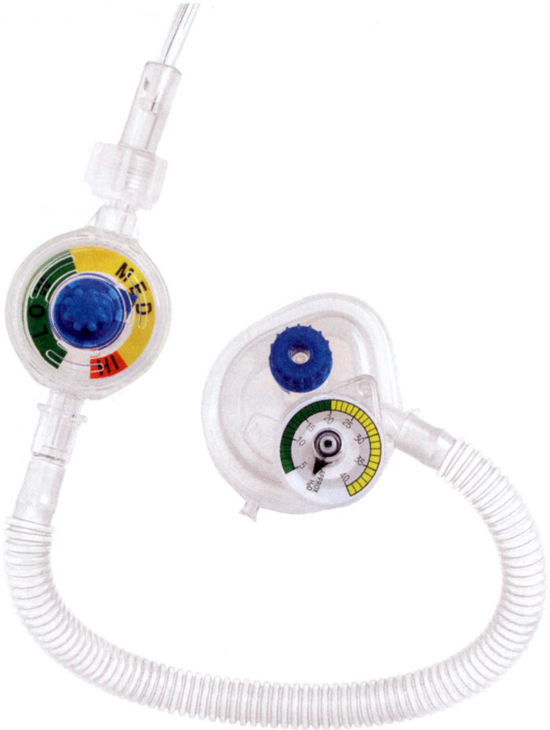

FIGURE 37-18 T-tube resuscitator used to ventilate newly born neonates. (Courtesy Mercury Medical, Clearwater, FL.)

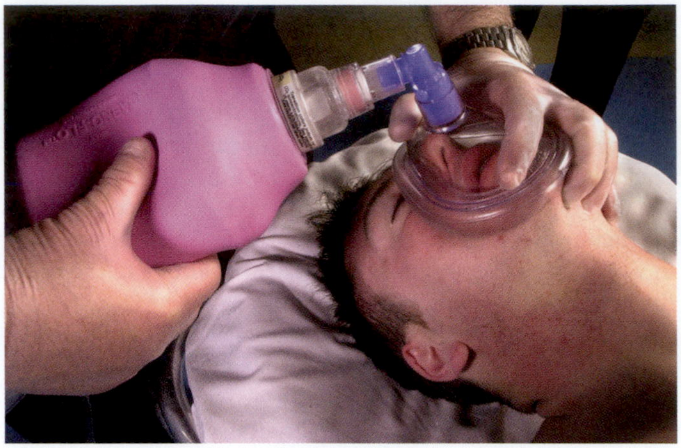

FIGURE 37-19 Ventilation using a bag-mask device and head-tilt/chin-lift method to open the airway. (From Henry MC, Stapleton ER: EMT prehospital care, revised ed 4, St. Louis, 2009, Mosby.)

procedures, and short-term and long-term complications of endotracheal intubation are provided in Chapter 36.

Ventilation

Accessory equipment used to support ventilation in advanced life support includes manual and O_2-powered resuscitators. Manual resuscitators, also called *bag-mask devices,* are available for adults, children, and infants. Conversely, O_2-powered resuscitators are strictly limited to adult application and are not discussed in this chapter. T-tube devices have been used successfully to ventilate and oxygenate neonates at birth (Figure 37-18).

Bag-Mask Devices

One-way valves on bag-mask devices should be simple, dependable, and jam-free. All health care professionals responding to a cardiac arrest call should be familiar and skilled in the use of such a device for support of ventilation and oxygenation. Application of the bag-mask device is best performed with the practitioner positioned at the head of the victim, using the head-tilt maneuver to maintain the airway (Figure 37-19). The rescuer delivers V_T adequate to produce visible chest rise (6 to 7 mL/kg predicted body weight or 400 to 500 mL) over 1 second. Using this smaller V_T decreases airway pressure and minimizes risk for gastric inflation.

It is important to deliver the 2 breaths during CPR over only 3 seconds so that the optimal number of chest compressions per minute can be delivered (75 compressions/min, rate of delivery 100 to 120 compressions/min). The ratio of 30 compressions to 2 ventilations allows for only 5 breaths to be delivered per minute. All 5 breaths should be delivered with no more than visible chest rise.[17] After an advanced airway replaces the face mask, the ventilatory rate should be 8 to 10 breaths/min during CPR. Slower rates of 6 to 8 breaths/min might be needed for patients with chronic obstructive pulmonary disease (COPD) to prevent air trapping and the development of auto–positive end expiratory pressure (PEEP). Ventilatory rates greater than 12 breaths/min are not recommended during CPR because they lead to increased intrathoracic pressure, impeding venous return to the heart during chest compressions,[26] and hyperventilation.

The rescuer delivers each breath over 1 second and should not attempt to synchronize ventilations with the chest compressions. Nonsynchronized delivery of ventilation and compressions allows the number of chest compressions delivered per minute to increase from 75 to 100 (33% increase) and breaths delivered per minute increase from 5 to 10 (100% increase). After restoration of a perfusing rhythm, the ventilation rate should be 10 to 12 breaths/min delivered over 1 second.

RULE OF THUMB

Rescuers should not hyperventilate victims of cardiac arrest. Once an advanced airway is placed, ventilations should be delivered over 1 second at a rate of 8 to 10 breaths/min (every 6 to 8 seconds). Do not attempt to synchronize ventilations with chest compressions. Ventilation for patients with a perfusing rhythm should be at a rate of 10 to 12 breaths/min (1 breath every 5 to 6 seconds). Patients with COPD may need ventilation rates of 6 to 8 breaths/min to prevent auto-PEEP.

Bag-mask devices combine a mask with a self-inflating bag and a nonrebreathing valve mechanism. These devices may be used to ventilate patients by applying the mask over the patient's mouth and nose or by attaching the self-inflating bag directly to an endotracheal tube or other advanced airways. All devices are capable of providing ventilation with air or with supplemental O_2. Bag-mask devices can provide 100% O_2 when properly applied. Although initially designed as adjuncts for emergency life support, they are used extensively in other respiratory care settings, particularly in the areas of airway management and continuous mechanical ventilation.

Design

Figure 37-20 is a schematic of a typical bag-mask device, showing gas movement and valve action during both the inhalation-compression and exhalation-relaxation phases. The key components shown in this schematic are the nonrebreathing valve *(left)*, the bag itself, the O_2 inlet and bag inlet valve *(to the right of the bag)*, and the O_2 reservoir tube *(far right)*.

During exhalation (see Figure 37-20, *A*), gas flows out from the patient's lungs through the nonrebreathing valve into the atmosphere. At the same time (while the bag expands), the intake valve opens and 100% O_2 flows into the bag from both the reservoir and the O_2 inlet.

During the inhalation phase (see Figure 37-20, *B*), the bag is compressed manually, causing bag pressure to increase. This increase in bag pressure simultaneously closes the inlet valve and opens the nonrebreathing valve, forcing gas into the patient. While the bag inlet valve is closed, O_2 coming in through the O_2 inlet goes into the reservoir tube, where it is stored for the next breath.

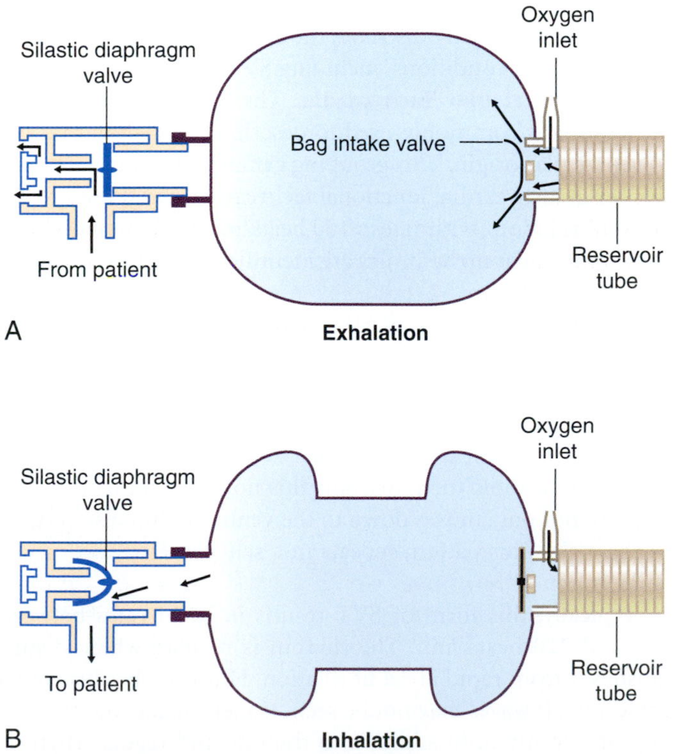

FIGURE 37-20 Components of bag-mask device.

Use

To use a bag-mask device, the health care provider is positioned at the head of the patient's bed. Ideally, an oral airway is inserted, and the head-tilt method is used to keep the airway open (assuming there are no neck injuries). While using one hand to keep the patient's head extended and the mask tightly sealed to the patient's face, the health care provider uses the other hand to compress the bag (see Figure 37-19).

In addition to providing adequate ventilation, bag-mask devices can provide high FiO_2. Theoretically, all such devices on the market can deliver 100% O_2; however, the actual FiO_2 provided at the bedside depends on several factors, including O_2 input flow, reservoir volume, delivered volume and rate, and bag refill time. As a guideline to achieve the highest possible FiO_2 with a bag-mask device, the following always should be done:

1. Use an O_2 reservoir of adequate size.
2. Set the O_2 input flow at 10 to 15 L/min.
3. Deliver appropriate V_T for a 1-second period (when using a mask).
4. Ensure the longest possible bag refill time.

Hazards and Troubleshooting

Bag-mask devices are simple and safe advanced life-support devices. However, several major hazards are associated with their use. The first and most common problem is unrecognized equipment failure. Knowledge of how such devices operate can help clinicians understand the operational testing of and troubleshooting for these devices. Gastric inflation is another common hazard encountered when using a bag-valve device with a face mask. Gastric inflation can be minimized by providing low to moderate inspiratory flows (<30 L/min).[23] For an adult, a full 1 second should be used to deliver V_T of 500 mL.

Barotrauma has long been recognized as a potential hazard of bag-mask device use. However, with the full-bag volume of adult-size devices (generally ≤2000 mL), the potential for barotrauma is small if the nonrebreathing valve is working properly and a bronchial intubation has not occurred. The average mask leak with bag-mask devices ranges from 20% to 40% of stroke volume and substantially reduces the risk for barotrauma, especially if no more than visible chest rise is used to determine adequate V_T. Some pediatric bag-mask devices have bag volumes of more than 500 mL, and rescuers may cause barotrauma to small children or infants if they do not adjust stroke volume by squeezing the bag so that only half to one-third of the volume is delivered to the mask.

Hyperventilation during resuscitation of a cardiac arrest victim markedly decreases coronary perfusion pressure and survival rates.[26] Overzealous ventilation with high rates (>12 breaths/min) during resuscitation of cardiac arrest increases intrathoracic pressure, impedes venous return, decreases cardiac output, decreases coronary artery perfusion pressure, increases gastric inflation, and provides more ventilation than is needed.

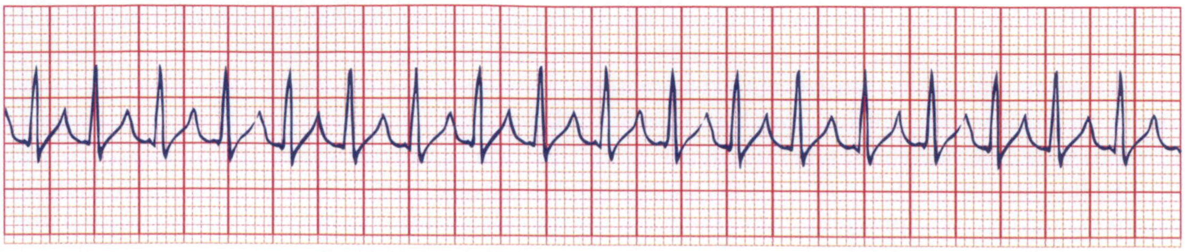

FIGURE 37-21 Supraventricular tachycardia, lead II.

MINI CLINI

Ventilation During Cardiopulmonary Resuscitation

PROBLEM: A student is observing a code blue in progress in the intensive care unit. The patient has had a cardiac arrest, and CPR is being administered. The student notices that the RT is ventilating the patient's lungs with a bag-valve device through an endotracheal tube at a considerably higher rate and minute ventilation than would normally be established on a mechanical ventilator for a patient of this size. Is this increased minute ventilation needed?

SOLUTION: No, it is not. The ventilation rate should be 8 to 10 breaths/min, and V_T should be limited to achieve no more than a visible chest rise to avoid excessive ventilation.[17] Ventilation rates greater than 12 breaths/min and large V_T (>6 to 7mL/kg) increase intrathoracic pressure and impede venous return to the heart during chest compressions.[26] During CPR, hyperventilation reduces cardiac output and decreases coronary and cerebral perfusion. Increases in central venous pressure, as a result of increased intrathoracic pressure, can decrease cerebral blood flow. Increased airway pressures and auto-PEEP generated by hyperventilation should be avoided. The AHA guidelines for CPR and emergency cardiovascular care state that "routine hyperventilation during and after cardiac arrest is detrimental and it is considered a Class III procedure" (i.e., the risk is greater than the benefit).[3,17] Ventilation with V_T of 400 to 500 mL at rates of 1 breath every 6 to 8 seconds is all that is needed to maintain a normocarbic level during CPR.

Restoring Cardiac Function

Perfusion support techniques, such as chest compressions, can restore circulation only temporarily. ACLS must go beyond simple perfusion support to identify, remove, or relieve the underlying cause of cardiac failure; this is done by combining ECG monitoring with pharmacologic and electrical therapies.

Electrocardiogram Monitoring

Because most cases of cardiac arrest are caused by arrhythmias, ECG monitoring should be started as soon as the necessary equipment and personnel arrive. Monitoring may be done with either standard electrocardiographic equipment or the quick-look paddles now available on most defibrillators.

Given their important role in ACLS, RTs must be skilled in recognizing arrhythmias. Although an RT may be able to quickly interpret gross arrhythmias appearing on electrocardiographic monitors at the bedside, these skills develop only after much practice with actual rhythm strips. Chapter 18 presents a review of ECG interpretation. The reader should focus on the following arrhythmias:

- VT
- VF
- Sinus tachycardia
- Sinus bradycardia
- Sinus arrest
- Premature atrial contractions
- SVT—a classification of arrhythmias, including but not limited to sinus tachycardia, atrial flutter, and atrial fibrillation
- Atrioventricular blocks—first degree, second degree types I and II, and third degree
- Premature ventricular contractions
- Pulseless electrical activity (PEA)
- Systole

This section briefly discusses the arrhythmias closely associated with CPR conditions, including SVT, VT, VF, and PEA.

Supraventricular Tachycardia. The term *supraventricular tachycardia* is commonly used to describe any tachycardia not of ventricular origin. This grouping can include sinus tachycardia, atrial tachycardia, junctional tachycardia, atrial flutter, and atrial fibrillation (with rates >100 beats/min). These individual supraventricular arrhythmias are identified by ECG and treated accordingly (Figure 37-21).

A more specific form of SVT involves rapid impulse formation caused by a reentry mechanism that develops in the atria or atrioventricular junction. Normally, a single impulse from the sinoatrial node traverses the atria and continues down into the ventricles, causing depolarization and contraction. In reentry, an ectopic focus disrupts this normal conduction. The impulse not only moves down to the ventricles but also returns to the atria. This pattern repeats in a self-perpetuating, or circular, manner.

Typically, this form of SVT results in heart rates between 160 and 220 beats/min. The rhythm is regular, which distinguishes it from rapid atrial fibrillation. However, because of its rapid rate, P waves may not be seen. If identifiable, the P waves appear abnormal. In addition to the rate and regular rhythm, SVT is characterized by a normal QRS complex. At very high

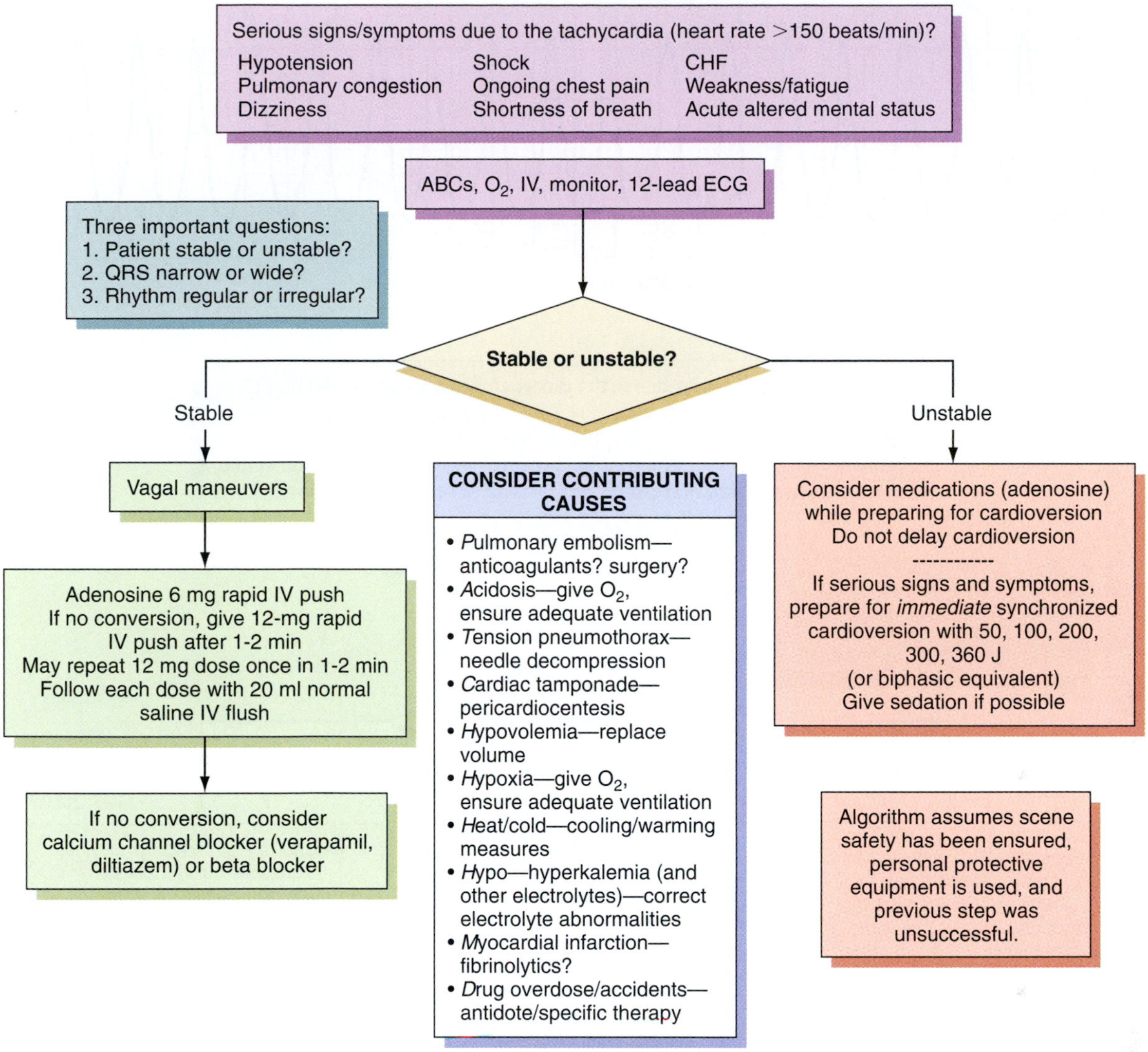

FIGURE 37-22 Narrow-complex QRS tachycardia. (From Aehlert B: ACLS study guide, ed 4, St. Louis, 2012, Mosby.)

rates, the ventricles may not have enough time to fill completely. Incomplete ventricular filling can result in decreased cardiac output, congestive heart failure, and tissue hypoxia. SVT may deteriorate to VT if it is not recognized and treated in a timely manner.

The treatment of SVT varies according to the clinical situation (Figure 37-22). If a patient with SVT is ill or unstable, the treatment of choice is immediate synchronized electrical cardioversion, as described elsewhere in this chapter. If the patient is stable, other interventions are tried before cardioversion is considered. The most common nonelectrical treatment for SVT is vagal stimulation by carotid artery massage or Valsalva maneuver. If these attempts are ineffective and the patient remains stable, drugs such as adenosine, diltiazem, verapamil, or beta blockers (as a second-line agent) may halt SVT. These drugs work primarily on the nodal tissue by slowing ventricular response to atrial arrhythmias, or they block the reentry SVT that travels through the atrioventricular node.[25]

Ventricular Tachycardia. VT occurs when one or more irritable foci within the ventricle discharge at rapid rates, creating the appearance of a prolonged chain of premature ventricular contractions. Rates typically range from 140 to 220 beats/min and usually are regular (Figure 37-23). Although VT may come and go in brief episodes, or *paroxysms,* it is always a sign of a serious underlying pathologic condition and should be treated immediately. In stable patients, VT is managed with amiodarone, procainamide, and/or sotalol.[25] Procainamide and sotalol should be avoided in patients with prolonged QT.[25] For patients with sustained VT who exhibit hypotension, ischemic chest pain, shortness of breath, decreased consciousness, or signs of pulmonary edema, immediate **synchronized cardioversion** is indicated (Figure 37-24). Patients with sustained VT in full cardiac arrest are treated similarly to patients with VF.

Ventricular Fibrillation. VF is a rapid, sustained, and uncontrolled depolarization of the ventricles. During VF, the ECG is characterized by irregular, widened, and poorly defined

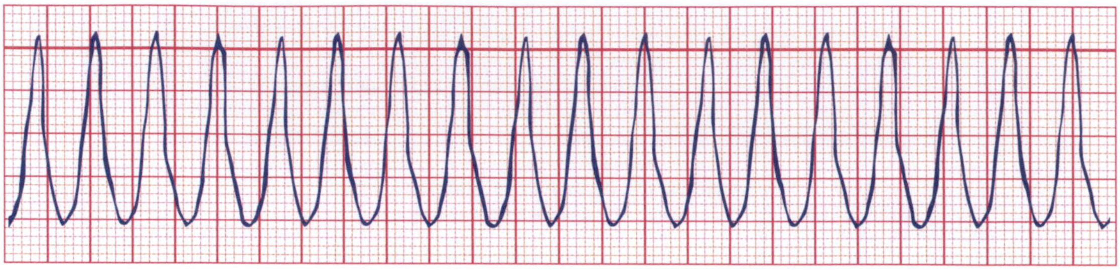

FIGURE 37-23 Ventricular tachycardia, lead II.

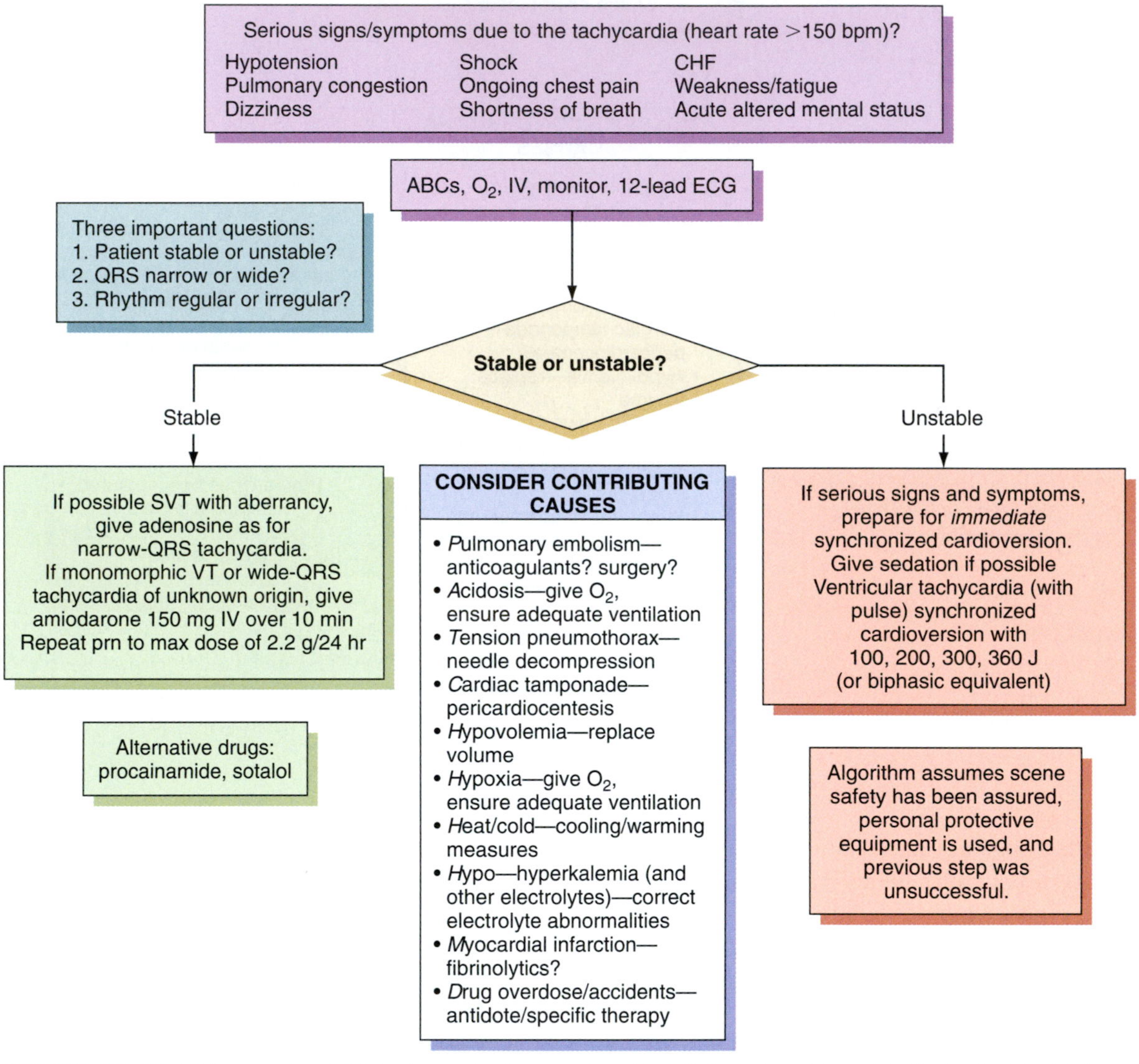

FIGURE 37-24 Wide-complex QRS tachycardia. (From Aehlert B: ACLS study guide, ed 4, St. Louis, 2012, Mosby.)

QRS complexes, known as *coarse* VF (Figure 37-25, *A*). These complexes widen farther and lose amplitude, resembling a coarse asystole, which now is defined as *fine* VF (see Figure 37-25, *B*). Rather than exhibiting coordinated contractions, the ventricles quiver in a totally disorganized manner. Cardiac output during VF is zero. The rapid decrease in cardiac output produces acute cerebral hypoxia, often manifested by seizures. VF is uniformly fatal if not corrected immediately.

Many conditions cause VF. The most common causes include hypoxia, hypovolemia, acidosis, hypokalemia and hyperkalemia, hypothermia, toxins, cardiac tamponade, tension pneumothorax, pulmonary thrombosis, and coronary thrombosis.[25] Regardless of the cause, VF constitutes a true emergency. Patient survival depends on immediate provision of ACLS, especially electrical defibrillation. Early defibrillation is the major determinant of survival in cardiac arrest caused by VF.

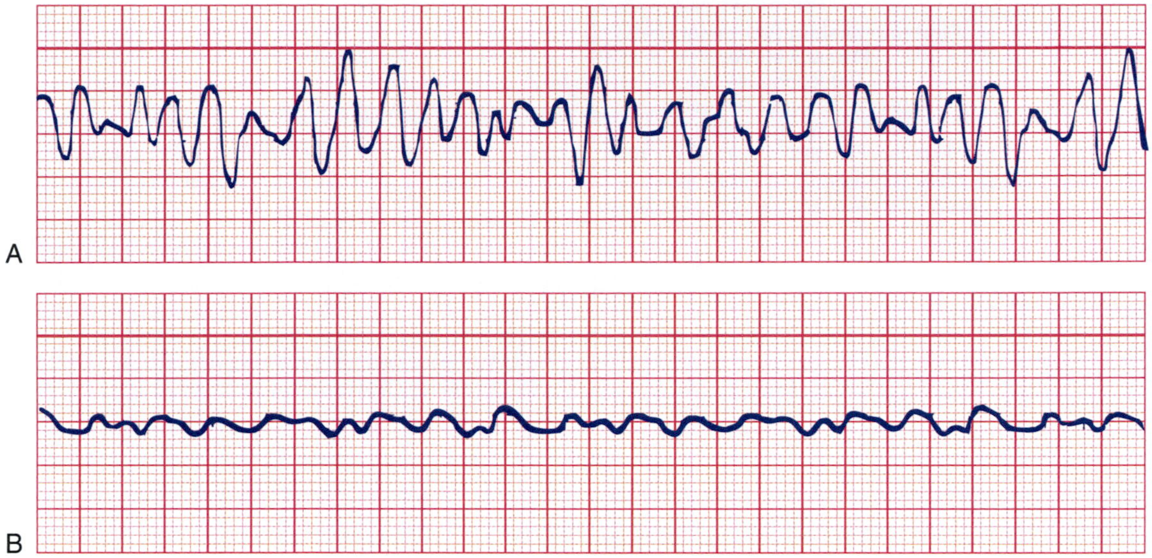

FIGURE 37-25 Ventricular fibrillation (VF). **A,** Coarse VF. **B,** Fine VF, lead II.

Pulseless Electrical Activity. PEA that is not shockable can result from several reversible causes (Figure 37-26). The immediate primary treatment is uninterrupted CPR for approximately 2 minutes with vasopressor given simultaneously. The best secondary approach is to identify and treat reversible causes (e.g., for hypovolemia, replace volume; for tension pneumothorax, needle decompression). In asystole or slow PEA, vasopressin administration should be considered (see Figure 37-26).[25]

Pharmacologic Intervention

Although the full range of drug use in ACLS is beyond the scope of this chapter, RTs must have a general knowledge of both the various drug categories and the specific agents used in emergency situations.[27] Table 37-2 summarizes the major drug categories and primary agents currently used in ACLS.

Routes of Administration. Unless a central vein is already cannulated, the ideal route for drug administration in emergency situations is a peripheral IV line. IV drugs should be given by rapid bolus injection, followed by a 20-mL bolus of IV fluid and elevation of the extremity.

Selected drugs, such as epinephrine, vasopressin, lidocaine, and atropine, also may be given through intraosseous access when IV access is not readily available.[28]

The intraosseous route always is an option, especially in small children or infants.[29] Chapter 35 provides information about pharmacologic agents often used in ACLS.

Electrical Therapy

The following three general types of electrical therapy are used in emergency cardiac care: (1) unsynchronized countershock, or defibrillation; (2) synchronized countershock, or cardioversion; and (3) electrical pacing.

Unsynchronized Countershock (Defibrillation). When an electrical shock of appropriate strength is applied to the myocardium, all myocardial fibers simultaneously depolarize. Theoretically, when all cells depolarize, the cells that spontaneously fire at the fastest rate should be able to regain control and pace the heart. Normally, the sinus node spontaneously depolarizes most rapidly. After electrical shock, the sinus node should discharge first and capture all parts of the myocardium as the depolarization wave travels through the still, silent heart.

MINI CLINI

Route of Drug Administration During Advanced Cardiovascular Life Support

PROBLEM: An RT working in a small, rural hospital is called to the emergency department, where a patient is in cardiac arrest. The RT is able to intubate and ventilate the patient, using a bag-valve device with 100% O_2.

Nurses are performing cardiac compressions and attempting unsuccessfully to start a peripheral IV line. The ECG monitor reveals a fine VF pattern. Electrical defibrillation is unsuccessful on the first attempt, and five cycles of 30 compressions to 2 ventilations are in progress. Immediate administration of epinephrine without interrupting CPR is indicated before or after the next shock. Attempts to secure an IV line continue to be unsuccessful. What action is appropriate at this time?

SOLUTION: Because of its strong inotropic and alpha-adrenergic effects, epinephrine should be the first drug during resuscitation of cardiac arrest and it should be administered as soon as possible. Drugs given via a peripheral vein require 1 to 2 minutes to reach the central circulation. Epinephrine can convert fine VF to coarse VF and improves the chance for successful electrical defibrillation. In this case, because IV routes are unavailable, epinephrine should be administered using the intraosseous route, which can be quickly established with minimal complications by providers with varied levels of training.[25,28,29]

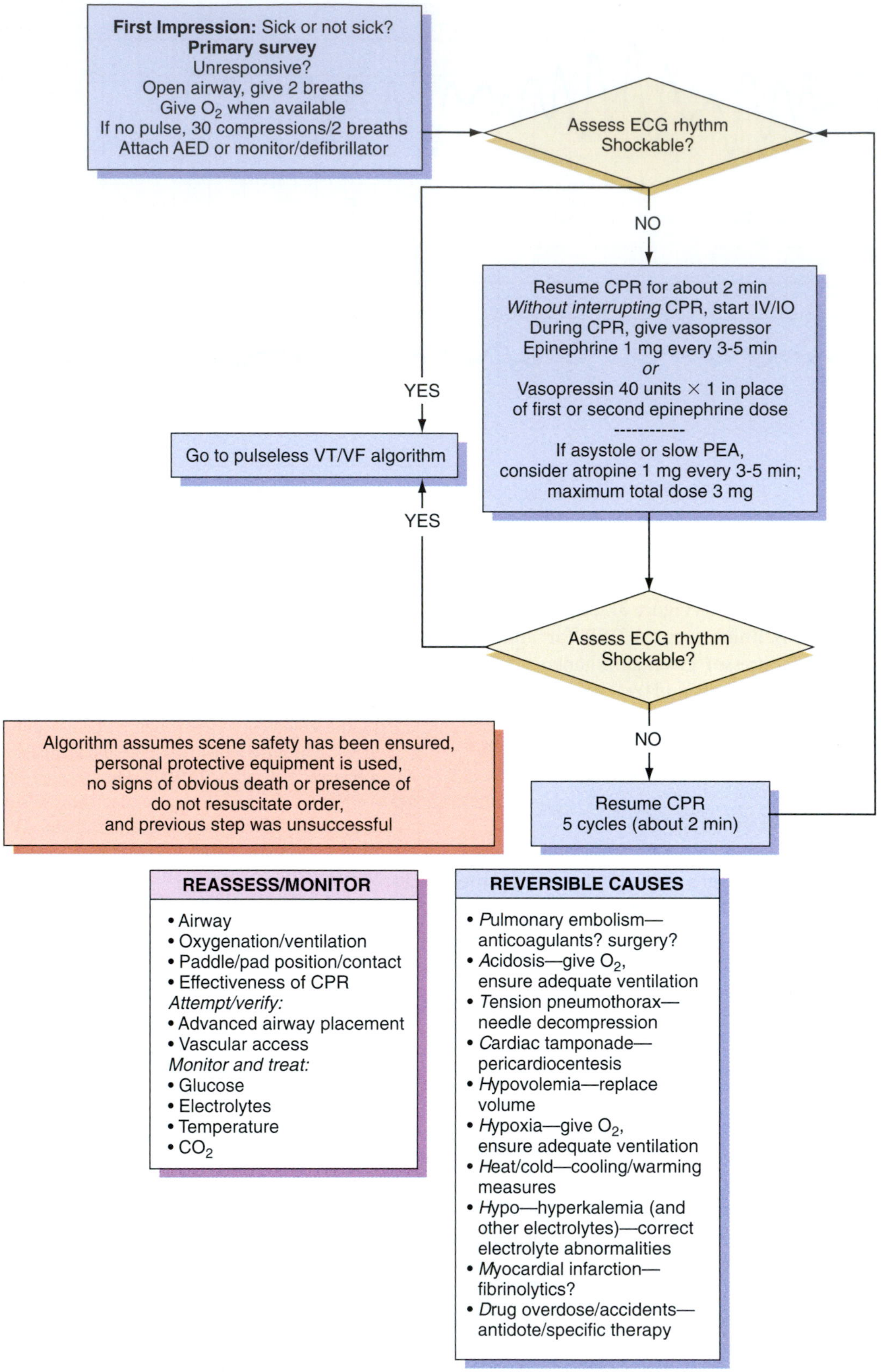

FIGURE 37-26 Asystole or pulseless electrical activity algorithm. (From Aehlert B: ACLS study guide, ed 4, St. Louis, 2012, Mosby.)

TABLE 37-2

Drugs Used in Advanced Cardiovascular Life Support

Drug	Indications	Contraindications	Route	Dosage[26]	Pharmacologic Effects
Adenosine	PSVT	Use with caution if patient has asthma; may precipitate atrial fibrillation; poison-induced or drug-induced tachycardia; second-degree or third-degree heart block	IV bolus	6 mg IV for 1-2 sec followed by 20-mL saline bolus; repeat twice with 12 mg in 1-2 min if needed	Decrease in AV node conduction
Amiodarone	Stable regular narrow-complex tachycardia to control rapid ventricular rate secondary to accessory pathway conduction in preexcited atrial arrhythmias	Prolonged QT interval	IV; IO	150 mg IV over 10 min; may repeat every 10 min to maximum of 2.2 g in 24 hr	Multichannel blocker (calcium, potassium); inhibited alpha- and beta-adrenergic responses
Atropine sulfate	Acute symptomatic bradycardia	Sinus, atrial, and ventricular tachycardia; hypothermic bradycardia; infranodal (type II) AV block; new third-degree with wide QRS complexes	IV bolus; IO	0.5-1 mg IV repeated every 3-5 min to total dose of 3 mg	Increased heart rate; increased force of atrial contractions
Dopamine	Hypotension with signs and symptoms of shock; second-line drug for symptomatic bradycardia	Use with caution in cardiogenic shock with accompanying CHF	IV infusion	2-20 mcg/kg/min	Increased renal and splenic flow at low doses (1-5 mcg/kg/min); beta-adrenergic effects at moderate doses (5-10 mcg/kg/min); alpha-adrenergic effects at high doses (>10 mcg/kg/min)
Epinephrine	Cardiac arrest; VF; pulseless tachycardia; asystole; PEA; symptomatic bradycardia; severe hypotension; anaphylaxis; severe allergic reaction	VT and frequent PVCs	IV bolus; IO; endotracheal* use only if IV or IO cannot be established; IV infusion	1 mg every 3-5 min in cardiac arrest, up to 0.2 mg/kg; 2-10 mcg/min infusion, titrate to patient response	Increased heart rate; increased force of contractions; vasoconstriction; increased coronary perfusion pressure; increased myocardial irritability; increased myocardial O_2 consumption
Isoproterenol	Alternative when a bradyarrhythmia is unresponsive to or inappropriate for treatment with atropine, or as a temporizing measure while awaiting the availability of a pacemaker. Refractory torsades de pointes unresponsive to magnesium sulfate	Cardiac arrest; VT; frequent PVCs	IV infusion	2-10 mcg/min, titrate to adequate heart rate	Increased heart rate; increased force of contractions; vasodilation

Continued

TABLE 37-2
Drugs Used in Advanced Cardiovascular Life Support—cont'd

Drug	Indications	Contraindications	Route	Dosage[26]	Pharmacologic Effects
Lidocaine	Second-line antiarrythmic therapy for monomorphic VT. Alternative to procainamide, sotalol, and amiodarone in cardiac arrest from VF/VT	Signs of lidocaine toxicity; prophylactic use in acute MI	IV bolus; IV infusion; IO; endotracheal[†]	1-1.5 mg/kg bolus every 5-10 min up to 3 mg/kg	Increased electrical stimulation threshold; depressed ventricular electrical activity
Magnesium sulfate	Cardiac arrest only if torsades de pointes or hypomagnesemia is present; life-threatening arrhythmias caused by digitalis toxicity	Routine administration in hospitalized patients with acute MI; use with caution in renal failure	IV infusion; IO infusion	Cardiac arrest: 1-2 g (2-4 mL of 50% solution) diluted in 10 mL of 5% dextrose in water over 20 min	Hypomagnesemia hinders replenishment of intracellular potassium
Procainamide	Stable monomorphic VT with normal QT interval and preserved left ventricular function; treatment of PSVT uncontrolled by adenosine and vagal maneuvers if blood pressure is stable; stable wide-complex tachycardia of unknown origin; AF with Wolff-Parkinson-White syndrome	Heart block, asystole, PEA, proarrhythmic especially in setting of acute MI, hypokalemia, or hypomagnesemia; avoid with in patients with CHF and prolonged QT interval	IV bolus; IV infusion	20 mg/min, 50 mg/min in urgent situations up to maximum dose of 17 mg/kg;	Sodium and potassium channel blocker
Propranolol	Suspected MI and unstable angina; SVTs	Bronchospastic disease; severe bradycardia; hypotension; second-degree or third-degree heart block; cocaine-induced acute coronary syndrome	IV	Total dose: 0.1 mg/kg by slow IV push, divided into 3 equal doses at 2- to 3-min intervals. Do not exceed 1 mg/min, repeat in 2 min to a total dose of 0.1 mg/kg if required	Reduce heart rate; decreased stroke volume; decreased myocardial O_2 consumption; increased LVEDP
Vasopressin	Alternative pressor to epinephrine in treatment of adult shock-refractory VF; alternative to epinephrine in asystole and PEA, hemodynamic support in vasodilatory shock	Responsive patients with coronary artery disease	IV bolus; IO bolus; if IV or IO access cannot be established, vasopressin or epinephrine may be administered via endotracheal tube	40-unit push may replace either first or second dose of epinephrine	Potent peripheral vasoconstrictor

TABLE 37-2
Drugs Used in Advanced Cardiovascular Life Support—cont'd

Drug	Indications	Contraindications	Route	Dosage[26]	Pharmacologic Effects
Verapamil, diltiazem	Alternative drug (after adenosine or vagal maneuvers) to terminate PSVT with narrow QRS complex, adequate blood pressure, and preserved left ventricular function; control ventricular rate in patients with atrial fibrillation or atrial flutter	Wide-complex QRS tachycardias of uncertain origin, Wolff-Parkinson-White syndrome and AF, sick sinus syndrome, second-degree or third-degree block without pacemaker, concurrent IV administration with IV beta blockers	IV bolus	*First dose:* Verapamil: 2.5- to 5-mg IV bolus over 2 min (over 3 min in older patients) *Second dose:* 5-10 mg, if needed, every 15-30 min; maximum dose 20 mg *Alternative:* 5-mg bolus every 15 to 30 min to a total dose of 20 to 30 g *Diltiazem:* initial dose 15 to 20 mg (0.25 mg/kg) IV over 2 min; an additional 20 to 25 mg (0.35 mg/kg) IV in 15 min if needed; 5-15 mg/hr IV titrated maintenance infusion titrated AF heart rate (if given for rate control)	Decreased sinoatrial node automaticity; slowed AV node conduction

AF, Atrial fibrillation; *AV,* atrioventricular; *CHF,* congestive heart failure; *IO,* intraosseous; *LVEDP,* left ventricular end-diastolic pressure; *MI,* myocardial infarction; *PSVT,* paroxysmal supraventricular tachycardia; *PEA,* pulseless electrical activity; *PVC,* premature ventricular contraction; *SVT,* supraventricular tachycardia; *VF,* ventricular fibrillation; *VT,* ventricular tachycardia.

*Endotracheal tube dosage is usually double IV dosage.

†Dose of lidocaine via an endotracheal tube is 2.0 to 2.5 times the normal IV dose diluted in 10 mL of normal saline or sterile water to be used only when IV and IO access is unavailable.

Defibrillation is an unsynchronized shock used to depolarize the myocardial fibers simultaneously. It is the definitive treatment for both VF and pulseless VT. If one of these arrhythmias is present, and the proper equipment and trained personnel are available, defibrillation of the patient should be performed immediately.

If a biphasic defibrillator is available, the AHA recommends an initial energy level of 120 to 200 J for defibrillation of adults and 2 to 4 J/kg for defibrillation of children and infants.[13] For children older than 1 year, if a shockable rhythm persists after five cycles of CPR, the rescuer should give one shock (4 J/kg) and resume compressions immediately. Use a 360-J shock for monophasic defibrillators for the first and subsequent shocks for adults.[13] If VF recurs, the previously successful energy level should be used for subsequent shocks and compressions should be resumed immediately.

Electrode paddle size and placement are important in ensuring that the full energy of the countershock is applied. For adults, paddles should be 8 to 12 cm in diameter to decrease resistance; adult paddles are adequate size for children older than 1 year. Normally, one paddle is placed below the clavicle and just to the right of the upper portion of the sternum, with the other positioned on the midaxillary line to the left of the left nipple. Alternatively, one paddle may be placed on the left precardium, with the other positioned posteriorly under the patient, behind the heart. Paddles should be prepared with conducting gel and applied with firm pressure (approximately 25 lb).

Synchronized Countershock (Cardioversion). **Cardioversion** is similar to defibrillation, with two major exceptions. First, the countershock is synchronized with the heart's electrical activity (the R wave). Synchronization is necessary because electrical stimulation during the refractory phase (part of the T wave) can cause VF or VT. Second, the energy used during cardioversion usually is less than the energy applied during defibrillation.

Cardioversion is considered when a patient with an organized arrhythmia producing a high ventricular rate exhibits signs or symptoms of cardiac decompensation. These so-called *tachyarrhythmias* include SVT, atrial flutter, atrial fibrillation, and monomorphic VT with pulses. Cardioversion is ineffective for treatment of junctional tachycardia or multifocal atrial tachycardia.[13]

If the arrhythmia is not causing serious signs or symptoms, drug therapy is used first. However, if the patient is hypotensive, exhibits signs of decreased consciousness or pulmonary congestion, or complains of chest pain, cardioversion is indicated.

Electrical Pacing. Another application of electrical therapy uses intermittently timed, low-energy discharges to replace or supplement the natural pacemaker of the heart. There are two primary types of electrical pacing. First, the electrical discharge can be delivered from an external power pack through wires inserted into the patient's chest wall (transcutaneous, or transthoracic, pacing). Alternatively, wire electrodes may be floated through the large veins and implanted directly inside the heart (transvenous pacing). Because it can be started quickly, transcutaneous pacing is the method used most often in emergency cardiac care.

Pacemaker therapy is used to treat sinus bradycardias that produce serious signs and symptoms and that do not respond to atropine (Figure 37-27). Electrical pacing also is used to manage second-degree type II and third-degree heart block.

Because defibrillation can cause damage to permanent pacemakers, care should be taken not to place the electrode paddles near these devices. After a patient with a permanent pacemaker undergoes either cardioversion or defibrillation, the device should be checked for proper functioning. Pacing is not recommended by the AHA for patients in asystolic cardiac arrest because it is ineffective and may delay or interrupt the delivery of chest compressions.[13]

Monitoring Provider Team Performance During Advanced Cardiac Life Support

1. Five main components of high-performance CPR have been identified by an AHA consensus statement for inside and outside the hospital.[17] Minimize interruptions in chest compressions to less than 20% of the time chest compressions are performed during cardiac arrest.

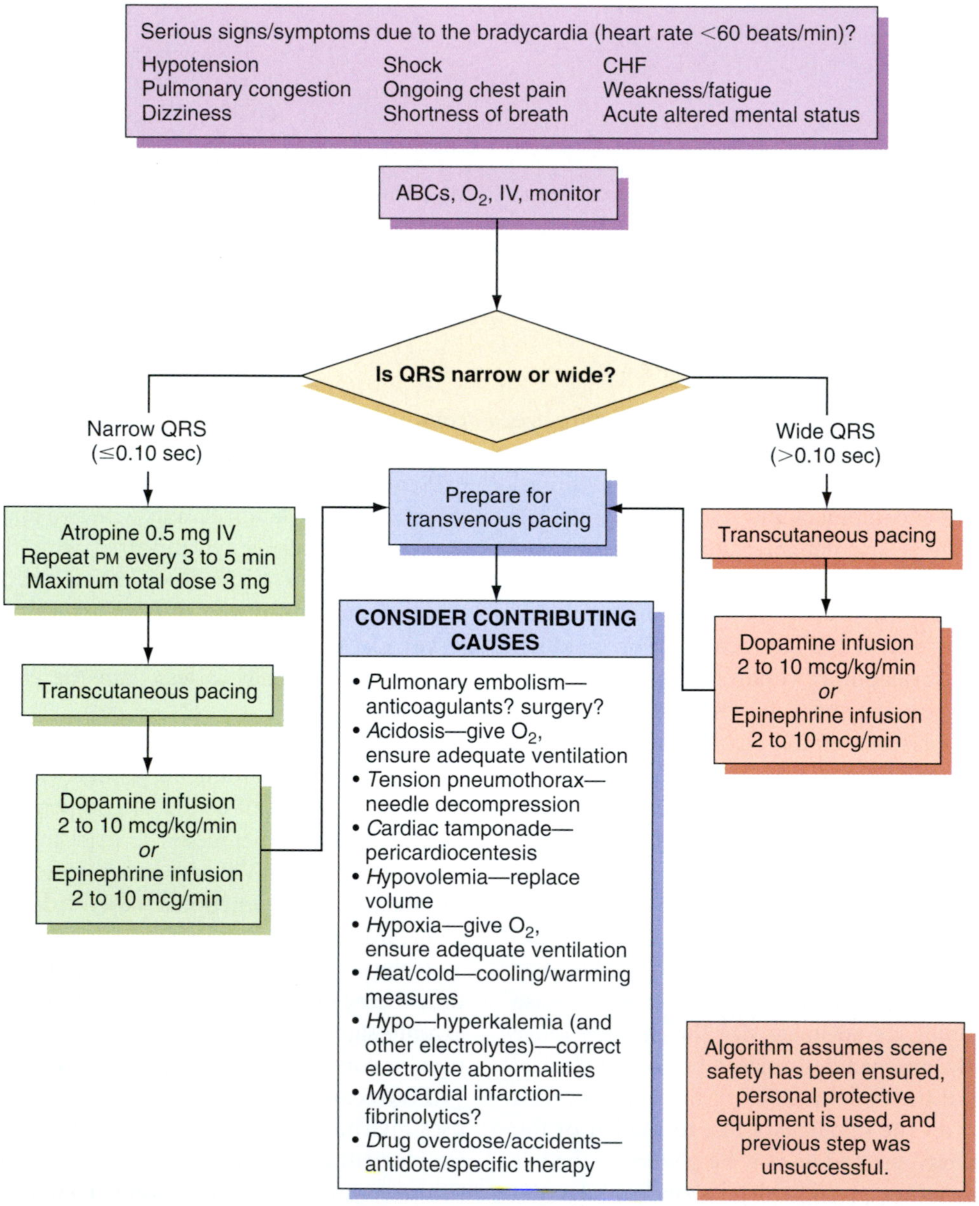

FIGURE 37-27 Symptomatic bradycardia algorithm. (From Aehlert B: ACLS study guide, ed 4, St. Louis, 2012, Mosby.)

2. Maintain a chest compression rate of 100 to 120/min.
3. Chest compression depth should be 50 mm (2 inches) or greater in adults and at least one-third of the anterior to posterior chest diameter in children and infants.
4. Allow the chest to recoil completely during chest compressions (i.e., no residual leaning).
5. Avoid excessive ventilation by keeping the rate to less than 12/min and use a rate of 8 to 10 with an advanced airway.

MINI CLINI

Cardiopulmonary Resuscitation Quality Control

PROBLEM: The RT is part of a code team resuscitating a patient in VF cardiac arrest. The RT notices several quality control issues. Another therapist is providing bag-mask ventilation with breaths that are too large and delivered with a fast inspiratory flow and rate. Another member of the team is administering chest compressions at rate of 80 compressions/min and appears to be tiring. A house-staff member has failed to place an endotracheal tube on the first attempt and is preparing for a second attempt. What steps can the RT take to improve the quality of CPR?

SOLUTION: The RT providing ventilations should be asked to deliver breaths that are large enough only to create visible chest rise and to deliver them over 1 second at a rate of 10 to 12/min. The RT should say silently "one-one thousand" to estimate a 1-second delivery time. The team member doing chest compression should be asked to push "hard and fast" at a rate of 100 to 120 compressions/min at a depth greater than 50 mm and allow complete chest recoil. The hands of the person doing chest compressions should be lifted slightly off the chest on each upstroke to ensure complete chest recoil. Interruptions in chest compressions should be held to less than 20% of CPR time and should not be interrupted by a second attempt to place an advanced airway (endotracheal tube, laryngeal mask airway, double-lumen airway [Combitube]) until five cycles (approximately 2 minutes) of CPR have been completed using a 30 : 2 compression-to-ventilation ratio. Postponing the second intubation attempt assumes that the victim can be ventilated with a bag-mask device. The team members doing chest compressions should be rotated every 2 minutes to prevent fatigue from affecting performance. One cycle of CPR takes approximately 24 seconds with 30 compressions delivered in 18 seconds and 2 breaths delivered in 6 seconds (1 second for inspiration and 1 second for exhalation × 2, with 2 seconds lost to transitioning between compressions and ventilation). Perfect CPR would result in 75 compressions and five breaths being delivered each minute. Code team members should not stop CPR to check the rhythm or a pulse immediately after shock delivery. After the shock, they should immediately administer five cycles of uninterrupted CPR beginning with chest compressions and should check the rhythm and pulse after about 2 minutes.

The ECG is the most common and one of the most useful types of monitoring used during ACLS. The ECG provides the basis for selecting various drug and electrical therapies during CPR and helps indicate patient response to these interventions. However, an acceptable ECG rhythm does not mean that cardiac output is adequate. Other indices of perfusion, such as pulse, blood pressure, and skin temperature, are needed to confirm adequate cardiac output.

Patient Care After Resuscitation

After cardiac arrest, a patient may exhibit an optimal response, in which case the patient regains consciousness, is responsive, and breathes spontaneously. More often, however, the patient requires support of one or more organ systems. Acidemia associated with cardiac arrest usually improves when normal ventilation and perfusion are restored.

If the patient is conscious and breathing spontaneously after resuscitation, supplemental O_2, maintenance of an IV infusion, and continuous cardiac and hemodynamic monitoring may be all that is necessary. A 12-lead ECG, chest x-ray, arterial blood gas (ABG) analysis, and clinical chemistry profile should be performed as soon as possible. Providers of care after cardiac arrest should do the following: "(1) control body temperature to optimize survival and neurologic recovery; (2) identify and treat acute coronary syndromes; (3) optimize mechanical ventilation to minimize lung injury; (4) reduce the risk for multiorgan injury and support organ function if required; (5) objectively assess prognosis for recovery; and (6) assist survivors with rehabilitation services when required."[30] The patient should be closely supervised in an intensive care or coronary care unit, especially during the first 24 hours after a cardiac arrest.

Only in this setting can underlying organ system insufficiency or failure be properly identified and managed. The organs most likely to exhibit failure after resuscitation are the lung, heart, and vasculature, and kidneys. Central nervous system failure is an ominous sign and generally indicates a failed resuscitation attempt.

Respiratory Management

If the patient remains apneic or exhibits irregular breathing after resuscitation, mechanical ventilation is instituted through a properly positioned endotracheal tube, with an initial O_2 concentration of 100%. ABGs, preferably obtained through an arterial line, are analyzed as needed until the oxygenation and acid-base status of the patient stabilize. ABG analysis also helps differentiate between pulmonary and nonpulmonary (or cardiac) causes of hypoxemia and tissue hypoxia. Mechanical ventilation is adjusted to maintain a normal $PaCO_2$ level. Hyperventilation is detrimental and should be avoided. Higher ventilatory rates and larger V_T may cause hyperventilation. This hyperventilation may generate increased airway pressures and auto-PEEP, leading to an increase in cerebral venous and intracranial pressures and a decrease in coronary artery and cerebral arterial pressures.[31] Cerebral blood flow may decrease, causing increased brain ischemia, if hyperventilation results in increased intrathoracic pressure. For details of the selection and use of mechanical ventilators and appropriate patient monitoring procedures, see Chapters 44 to 49, 51, and 52.

Cardiovascular Management

The 12-lead ECG, chest radiograph, clinical chemistry profile, cardiac enzyme results, and current and past drug histories should be reviewed. Invasive hemodynamic monitoring may be needed to monitor blood pressure and cardiac output. This monitoring provides needed data on the adequacy of vascular volumes, left ventricular performance, and overall tissue perfusion. Based on these data, judgments can be made regarding the need for fluid therapy and the selection and use of appropriate drugs.

SUMMARY CHECKLIST

- The most common cause of sudden death in adults is coronary artery disease; accidents are the most common cause of death in young people.
- The fundamental steps of basic CPR of health care providers for a witnessed cardiac arrest are as follows:
  1. Confirm unresponsiveness.
  2. Call for help and activate the EMS system.
  3. Check for a pulse (<10 seconds).
  4. Perform 30 cardiac compressions.
  5. Give two 1-second breaths to produce visible chest rise.
  6. Initiate automated external defibrillation immediately (perform defibrillation as soon as possible).
- Five cycles of 30 compressions to 2 ventilations CPR for adults should be given between attempts at defibrillation using only one shock followed immediately by chest compressions.
- Evaluating the effectiveness of CPR is important and requires rescuers to watch for visible chest rise and fall with ventilation and to push hard and fast when delivering chest compression.
- Complications of CPR include worsening of potential neck injuries, gastric inflation and vomiting, and internal trauma during chest compressions. Correct technique minimizes the risk for such complications.
- The RT is most often called on to establish an airway and ventilation with elevated FiO_2 during ACLS of hospitalized patients. Most often, knowledge and skill with bag-valve devices and oropharyngeal airways are required. Special care should be taken not to hyperventilate the patient during or after cardiac arrest.
- Common pharmacologic agents used during ACLS include atropine for bradycardia, epinephrine and amiodarone or lidocaine for ventricular arrhythmias, and epinephrine or vasopressin for cardiac arrest and hypotension.
- The RT is often involved in care after cardiac arrest of a victim who responds favorably to CPR. In the postresuscitative phase, the RT may need to maintain normal ventilation and oxygenation and assist the physician and nurses in monitoring the patient's condition.

References

1. Berdowski J, Berg RA, Tijssen JG, et al: Global incidences of out-of-hospital cardiac arrest and survival rates: systematic review of 67 prospective studies. *Resuscitation* 81:1479–1487, 2010.
2. Go AS, Mozzafferian D, Roger VL, et al: American Heart Association Statistics Committee and Stroke Statistics Subcommittee: Heart disease and stroke statistics: 2014 update. *Circulation* 129:e28–e292, 2014.
3. Berg RA, Hemphill R, Abella BS, et al: Part 5: Adult basic life support: 2010 American Heart Association guidelines for cardiopulmonary resuscitation and emergency cardiovascular care. *Circulation* 122(Suppl 3):S685–S705, 2010.
4. Aufderheide TP, Pirallo RG, Yannopoulos D, et al: Incomplete chest wall decompression: a clinical evaluation of CPR performance by trained laypersons and an assessment of alternative manual chest compression-decompression techniques. *Resuscitation* 71:341–351, 2006.
5. Yannopoulos D, McKnite S, Aufderheide TP, et al: Effects of incomplete chest wall decompression during cardiopulmonary resuscitation on coronary and cerebral perfusion pressures in a porcine model of cardiac arrest. *Resuscitation* 64:363–372, 2005.
6. Sutton RM, Maltese MR, Niles D, et al: Quantitative analysis of chest compression interruptions during in-hospital resuscitation of older children and adolescents. *Resuscitation* 80:1259–1263, 2009.
7. Niles D, Nyseather J, Sutton R, et al: Leaning is common during in-hospital pediatric CPR, and decreased with automated corrective feedback. *Resuscitation* 80:553–557, 2009.
8. Kattwinkel J, Perlman JM, Aziz K, et al: Part 15: Neonatal resuscitation 2010 American Heart Association guidelines for cardiopulmonary resuscitation and emergency cardiovascular care. *Circulation* 122(Suppl 3):S909–S919, 2010.
9. Berg MD, Sayre MR, Chameides L, et al: Part 13: Pediatric basic life support: 2010 American Heart Association guidelines for cardiopulmonary resuscitation and emergency cardiovascular care. *Circulation* 122(Suppl 3):S862–S875, 2010.
10. White RD, Bunch TJ, Hankins DG: Evolution of a community-wide early defibrillation program experience over 13 years using police/fire personnel and paramedics as responders. *Resuscitation* 65:279–283, 2005.
11. Sasson C, Rogers MA, Dahl J, et al: Predictors of survival from out-of-hospital cardiac arrest: a systematic review and metaanalysis. *Circ Cardiovasc Qual Outcomes* 3:63–81, 2010.
12. Atkins DL, Everson-Stewart S, Sears GK, et al: Epidemiology and outcomes from out-of-hospital cardiac arrest in children: the Resuscitation Outcomes Consortium Epistry-Cardiac Arrest. *Circulation* 119:1484–1491, 2009.
13. Link MS, Atkins DL, Passman RS, et al: Part 6: Electrical therapies: automated external defibrillators, defibrillation, cardioversion, and pacing—2010 American Heart Association Guidelines for Cardiopulmonary Resuscitation and Emergency Cardiovascular Care. *Circulation* 122(Suppl 3):S706–S719, 2010.
14. Tang W, Weil MH, Sun S, et al: A comparison of biphasic and monophasic waveform defibrillation after prolonged ventricular fibrillation. *Chest* 120: 948–954, 2001.
15. Stiell IG, Walker RG, Nesbitt LP, et al: BIPHASIC Trial: a randomized comparison of fixed lower versus escalating higher energy levels for defibrillation in out-of-hospital cardiac arrest. *Circulation* 115:1511–1517, 2007.
16. Hess EP, White RD: Ventricular fibrillation is not provoked by chest compression during post-shock organized rhythms in out-of-hospital cardiac arrest. *Resuscitation* 66:7–11, 2005.
17. Meaney PA, Bobrow BJ, et al, CPR Quality Summit Investigators, the American Heart Association Emergency Cardiovascular Care Committee, and the Council on Cardiopulmonary, Critical Care, Perioperative and Resuscitation: Cardiopulmonary resuscitation quality: improving cardiac resuscitation outcomes both inside and outside the hospital—a consensus statement from the American Heart Association. *Circulation* 128:417–435, 2013.
18. Austin N, Krishnamoorthy V, Dagal A: Airway management in cervical spine injury. *Int J Crit Illn Inj Sci* 4:50–56, 2014.
19. Gabrielli A, Layon AJ, Wenzel V, et al: Alternative ventilation strategies in cardiopulmonary resuscitation. *Curr Opin Crit Care* 8:199–211, 2002.
20. Berg MD, Idris AH, Berg RA: Severe ventilatory compromise due to gastric distention during pediatric cardiopulmonary resuscitation. *Resuscitation* 36:71–73, 1998.

21. Barnes TA, Catino ME, Burns EC, et al: Comparison of an oxygen-powered flow-limited resuscitator to manual ventilation with an adult 1,000 mL self-inflating bag. *Respir Care* 50:1445–1450, 2005.
22. Choi SJ, Kim HS, Kim EY, et al: Thoraco-abdominal CT examinations for evaluating cause of cardiac arrest and complications of chest compression in resuscitated patients. *Emerg Radiol* 21:485–490, 2014.
23. Buschmann CT, Tsokos M: Frequent and rare complications of resuscitation attempt. *Intensive Care Med* 35:397–404, 2009.
24. Fearing NM, Harrison P: Complications of the heimlich maneuver: case report and literature review. *J Trauma* 53:978–979, 2002.
25. Neumar RW, Otto CW, Link MS, et al: Part 8: Adult advanced cardiovascular life support: 2010 American Heart Association guidelines for cardiopulmonary resuscitation and emergency cardiovascular care. *Circulation* 122:S729–S767, 2010.
26. Aufderheide TP, Sigurdsson G, Pirrallo RG, et al: Hyperventilation-induced hypotension during cardiopulmonary resuscitation. *Circulation* 109:1960–1965, 2004.
27. Barnes TA, Gale DD, Kacmarek RM, et al: Competencies needed by graduate respiratory therapists in 2015 and beyond. *Respir Care* 55:601–615, 2010.
28. Horton MA, Beamer C: Powered intraosseous insertion provides safe and effective vascular access for pediatric emergency patients. *Pediatr Emerg Care* 24:347–350, 2008.
29. Kleinman ME, Chameides L, Schexnayder SM, et al: Part 14: Pediatric advanced life support: 2010 American Heart Association guidelines for cardiopulmonary resuscitation and emergency cardiovascular care. *Circulation* 122(Suppl 3):S876–S908, 2010.
30. Peberdy MA, Callaway CW, Neumar RW, et al: Part 9: post–cardiac arrest care: 2010 American Heart Association guidelines for cardiopulmonary resuscitation and emergency cardiovascular care. *Circulation* 122(Suppl 3): S768–S786, 2010.
31. Herff H, Paal P, von Goedecke A, et al: Influence of ventilation strategies on survival in severe controlled hemorrhagic shock. *Crit Care Med* 36: 2613–2620, 2008.

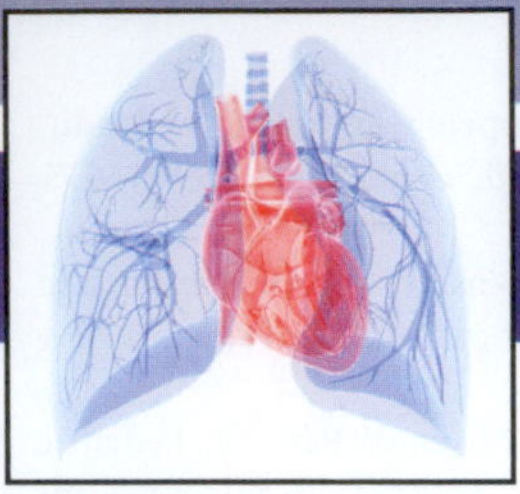

CHAPTER 38

Humidity and Bland Aerosol Therapy

JAMES B. FINK AND ARZU ARI

CHAPTER OBJECTIVES

After reading this chapter you will be able to:

- Describe how airway heat and moisture exchange normally occurs.
- State the effect dry gases have on the respiratory tract.
- State when to humidify and warm inspired gas.
- Describe how various types of humidifiers work.
- Describe how to enhance humidifier performance.
- State how to select and use humidifier heating and feed systems safely.
- Identify the indications, contraindications, and hazards that pertain to humidification during mechanical ventilation.
- Describe how to monitor patients receiving humidity therapy.
- Describe how to identify and resolve common problems with humidification systems.
- State when to apply bland aerosol therapy.
- Describe how large-volume aerosol generators work.
- Identify the delivery systems used for bland aerosol therapy.
- Describe how to identify and resolve common problems with aerosol delivery systems.
- Describe how to perform sputum induction.
- State how to select the appropriate therapy to condition a patient's inspired gas.

CHAPTER OUTLINE

KEY TERMS

American Society for Testing and Materials
baffling
body humidity
heat and moisture exchangers
humidifier
hydrophobic
hygrometer
hygroscopic
hypothermia
inspissated
International Organization for Standardization
isothermic saturation boundary
nebulizer
piezoelectric crystal
servo-controlled heating system
ultrasonic nebulizer

Vapors and mists have been used for millenia to treat respiratory disease. Modern respiratory care still uses these treatments at the bedside, in the form of water vapor (humidity) and bland water aerosols. Concepts of absolute and relative humidity are essential for understanding humidity therapy and are covered in Chapter 6. This chapter reviews the principles, methods, equipment, and procedures for using these concepts appropriately.

HUMIDITY THERAPY

Humidity therapy involves adding water vapor and (sometimes) heat to the inspired gas. To understand the need for humidity therapy, clinicians must understand the normal control of heat and moisture exchange.

Physiologic Control of Heat and Moisture Exchange

Heat and moisture exchange is a primary function of the upper respiratory tract, mainly the nose.[1] The nose heats and humidifies gas on inspiration and cools and reclaims water from gas that is exhaled. The nasal mucosal lining is kept moist by secretions from mucous glands, goblet cells, transudation of fluid through cell walls, and condensation of exhaled humidity. The nasal mucosa is very vascular, actively regulating temperature changes in the nose and serving as an active element in promoting effective heat transfer. Similarly, the mucosa lining the sinuses, trachea, and bronchi aid in heating and humidifying inspired gases.

During inspiration through the nose, the tortuous path of gas through the turbinates increases contact between the inspired air and the mucosa. As the inspired air enters the nose, it warms *(convection)* and picks up water vapor from the moist mucosal lining *(evaporation)*, cooling the mucosal surface.

During exhalation, the expired gas transfers heat back to the cooler tracheal and nasal mucosa by convection. As the saturated gas cools, it holds less water vapor. Condensation occurs on the mucosal surfaces during exhalation, and water is reabsorbed by the mucus *(rehydration)*. In cold environments, the formation of condensate may exceed the ability of the mucus to reabsorb water (resulting in a "runny nose").

The mouth is less effective at heat and moisture exchange than the nose because of the low ratio of gas volume to moist and warm surface area and the less vascular squamous epithelium lining the oropharynx and hypopharynx. When a person inhales through the mouth at normal room temperature, pharyngeal temperatures are approximately 3° C less than when the person breathes through the nose, with 20% less relative humidity. During exhalation, the relative humidity of expired gas varies little between mouth breathing and nose breathing, but the mouth is much less efficient in reclaiming heat and water.[2]

As inspired gas moves into the lungs, it achieves BTPS conditions (i.e., body temperature, 37° C; barometric pressure; saturated with water vapor [100% relative humidity at 37° C]) (Figure 38-1). This point, normally approximately 5 cm below the carina, is called the **isothermic saturation boundary** (ISB).[3]

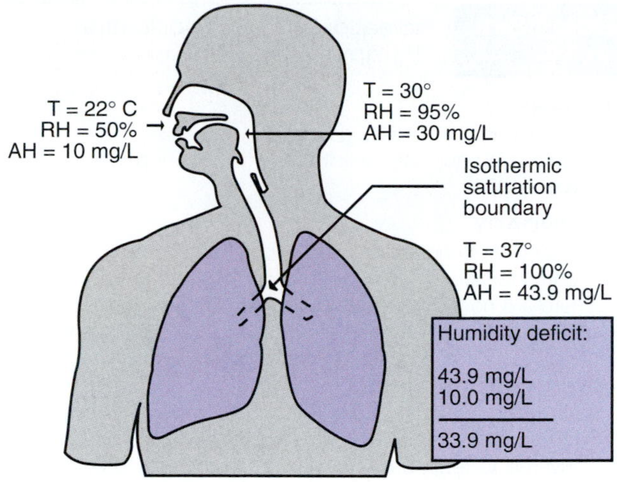

FIGURE 38-1 As a person breathes typical ambient air, the upper airway adds 20 mg/L of water vapor and the lower airway adds 13.9 mg/L. If all of that humidity were exhaled, this would represent a 33.9 mg/L humidity deficit. *AH,* Absolute humidity; *RH,* relative humidity; *T,* temperature. (From Fink J: Humidity and aerosol therapy. In Cairo J, Pilbeam S, editors: Mosby's respiratory equipment, ed 8, St. Louis, 2010, Mosby.)

Above the ISB, temperature and humidity decrease during inspiration and increase during exhalation. Below the ISB, temperature and relative humidity remain constant (BTPS).

Numerous factors can shift the ISB deeper into the lungs. The ISB shifts distally when a person breathes through the mouth rather than the nose; when the person breathes cold, dry air; when the upper airway is bypassed (breathing through an artificial tracheal airway); or when the minute ventilation is higher than normal. When this shift of ISB occurs, additional surfaces of the airway are recruited to meet the heat and humidity requirements of the lung. This recruitment of airways that do not typically provide this level of heat and humidity can have a negative impact on epithelial integrity. These shifts of the ISB can compromise the body's normal heat and moisture exchange mechanisms, and humidity therapy is indicated.

Indications for Humidification and Warming of Inspired Gases

The primary goal of humidification is to maintain normal physiologic conditions in the lower airways. Proper levels of heat and humidity help ensure normal function of the mucociliary transport system. Humidity therapy is also used to treat abnormal conditions. Box 38-1 summarizes the indications and contraindications for humidity therapy.

Administration of dry medical gases at flows greater than 4 L/min to the upper airway causes immediate heat and water loss and, if prolonged, causes structural damage to the epithelium. As the airway is exposed to relatively cold, dry air, ciliary motility is reduced, airways become more irritable, mucus production increases, and pulmonary secretions become **inspissated** (thickened owing to dehydration).

As listed in Box 38-2, the hazard of breathing dry gas is even greater when the normal heat and water exchange capabilities

Box 38-1 Indications for Humidification Therapy

PRIMARY
- Humidifying dry medical gases
- Overcoming humidity deficit created when upper airway is bypassed

SECONDARY
- Treating bronchospasm caused by cold air
- Contraindications for humidification therapy

There are no contraindications to providing physiologic conditioning of inspired gas during mechanical ventilation. However, a heat and moisture exchanger (HME) is contraindicated for patients:
- With thick, copious, or bloody secretions
- With an expired tidal volume (V_T) less than 70% of the delivered V_T (e.g., patients with large bronchopleural fistulas or incompetent or absent endotracheal tube cuffs)
- With body temperature less than 32° C
- With high spontaneous minute volumes (>10 L/min)
- Receiving noninvasive ventilation with large mask leaks, because the patient does not exhale enough V_T to replenish heat and moisture to adequately condition the inspired gas. Also, the resistance and dead space of the HME may negate the effects of the noninvasive positive pressure and add additional work of breathing.
- Receiving lung protective ventilation strategies such as in acute respiratory distress syndrome (additional dead space of HME may increase the ventilation requirement and $PaCO_2$).
- Receiving in-line aerosol drug treatments (a standard HME must be removed from the patient circuit during treatments. An HME designed for aerosol delivery must be switched to the aerosol bypass mode)

Box 38-2 Hazards and Complications for Humidification Therapy

Hazards and complications associated with the use of heated humidifier (HH) and HME devices during mechanical ventilation include the following:
- Potential electrical shock (HH)
- Potential for burns to caregivers from hot metal (HH)
  - Hypothermia (HME or inadequately set HH)
  - Hyperthermia (HH)
  - Thermal injury (HH)
- Underhydration and mucous impaction (HME or HH)
  - Hypoventilation and/or alveolar gas trapping resulting from mucus plugging of airways (HME or HH)
  - Hypoventilation secondary to hypercapnia caused by the increase in dead space (HME)
  - Increased work of breathing (HME)
  - Possible hypoventilation resulting from hypercapnia caused by the increase in dead space (HME)
  - Inadvertent overfilling or pooled condensate resulting in unintentional tracheal lavage (HH)
  - High flow rates during disconnect may aerosolize contaminated condensate (HH)
  - Elevated airway pressures caused by condensation (HH)
  - Ineffective low-pressure alarm during disconnection (HME)
  - Patient-ventilator dyssynchrony and improper ventilator function caused by condensation in the circuit (HH)
  - Airway burns or tubing meltdown if heated wire circuits are covered or incompatible with humidifier (HH)

of the upper airway are lost or bypassed, as occurs with endotracheal intubation. Breathing dry gas through an endotracheal tube (ETT) can cause damage to tracheal epithelium within minutes. However, as long as the inspired humidity is at least 60% of BTPS conditions, no injury occurs in normal lungs.[4,5] Prolonged breathing of improperly conditioned gases through a tracheal airway can result in **hypothermia** (reduced body temperature), inspissation of airway secretions, mucociliary dysfunction, destruction of airway epithelium, and atelectasis.[6] Box 38-3 summarizes the signs and symptoms associated with breathing cold, dry gases. A reduction of 20 mg/L below BTPS (44 mg/L) is less than 60% relative humidity at BTPS.

The amount of heat and humidity that a patient needs depends on the site of gas delivery (e.g., nose or mouth, hypopharynx, trachea). Table 38-1 summarizes the recommended levels based on standards.[7]

Warmed, humidified gases are used to prevent or treat various abnormal conditions. For treatment of hypothermia, heating and humidifying the inspired gas is one of several techniques used to raise core temperatures back to normal.[8,9] Heated humidification is used to prevent intraoperative hypothermia.[10] Of possibly greater clinical significance, warming and humidifying the inspired gas can help alleviate bronchospasm in patients who develop airway narrowing after exercise or when they breathe cold air. Although the cause of this condition is not known for certain, the primary stimulus is probably a combination of airway cooling and drying, which leads to hypertonicity of airway lining fluid and the release of chemical mediators.[11] The incidence of cold air–induced bronchospasm can be reduced by wearing a scarf over the nose and mouth in cold weather; the scarf becomes a crude passive heat and moisture exchanger.

TABLE 38-1 Recommended Heat and Humidity Levels

Delivery Site	Temperature Range (° C)	Relative Humidity (%)	Absolute Humidity (mg/L)
Nose/mouth	20-22	50	10
Hypopharynx	29-32	95	28-34
Trachea	32-35	100	36-40

From Chatburn R, Primiano F: A rational basis for humidity therapy. Respir Care 32:249, 1987.

Box 38-3 Clinical Signs and Symptoms of Inadequate Airway Humidification

- Atelectasis
- Dry, nonproductive cough
- Increased airway resistance
- Increased incidence of infection
- Increased work of breathing
- Patient complaint of substernal pain and airway dryness
- Thick, dehydrated secretions

The delivery of cool humidified gas is used to treat upper airway inflammation resulting from croup, epiglottitis, and postextubation edema. This technique is used most often in conjunction with bland aerosol delivery (see the section on Bland Aerosol Delivery).

Equipment

A **humidifier** is a device that adds molecular water to gas. This process occurs by evaporation of water from a surface (see Chapter 6), whether the water is in a reservoir, a wick, or a sphere of water in suspension (aerosol).

Physical Principles Governing Humidifier Function

The following four variables or principles affect the quality of performance of a humidifier: (1) temperature, (2) surface area, (3) time of contact, and (4) thermal mass. These factors are exploited to various degrees in the design of humidification devices (Box 38-4).

Temperature. Temperature is an important factor affecting humidifier performance. The greater the temperature of a gas, the more water vapor it can hold (increased capacity). As gas expansion and evaporation cool water in unheated humidifiers to 10° C below ambient temperature, the humidifiers become less efficient.

Figure 38-2 shows this concept, where, owing to evaporative cooling, the unheated humidifier on the left is operating at 10° C. Although the humidifier fully saturates the gas, the low operating temperature limits total water vapor capacity to approximately 9.4 mg/L water vapor, equivalent to approximately 21% of **body humidity.** Simply heating the humidifier to 40° C (Figure 38-2, right) increases its output to 51 mg/L, which is sufficient to meet BTPS conditions.

Surface Area. The greater the area of contact between water and gas, the more opportunity there is for evaporation to occur. Passover humidifiers pass gas over a large surface area of water. More space-efficient ways to increase the ratio of water to gas surface area include bubble diffusion, aerosol, and wick technologies.

Bubble-diffusion directs a stream of gas underwater, where it is broken up into small bubbles. As the gas bubbles rise to the surface, evaporation increases the water vapor content within the bubble. The smaller the bubble, the greater is the ratio of water to air surface area.

Box 38-4 Physical Principles Governing Humidifier Function

Temperature: The higher the temperature of a gas, the more water vapor it can hold (increased capacity) or vice versa.
Surface area: The greater the surface area of contact between water and gas, the more opportunity there is for evaporation to occur.
Contact time: The longer a gas remains in contact with water, the greater is the opportunity for evaporation to occur.
Thermal mass: The greater the mass of water or the core element of a humidifier, the greater is its capacity to hold and transfer heat.

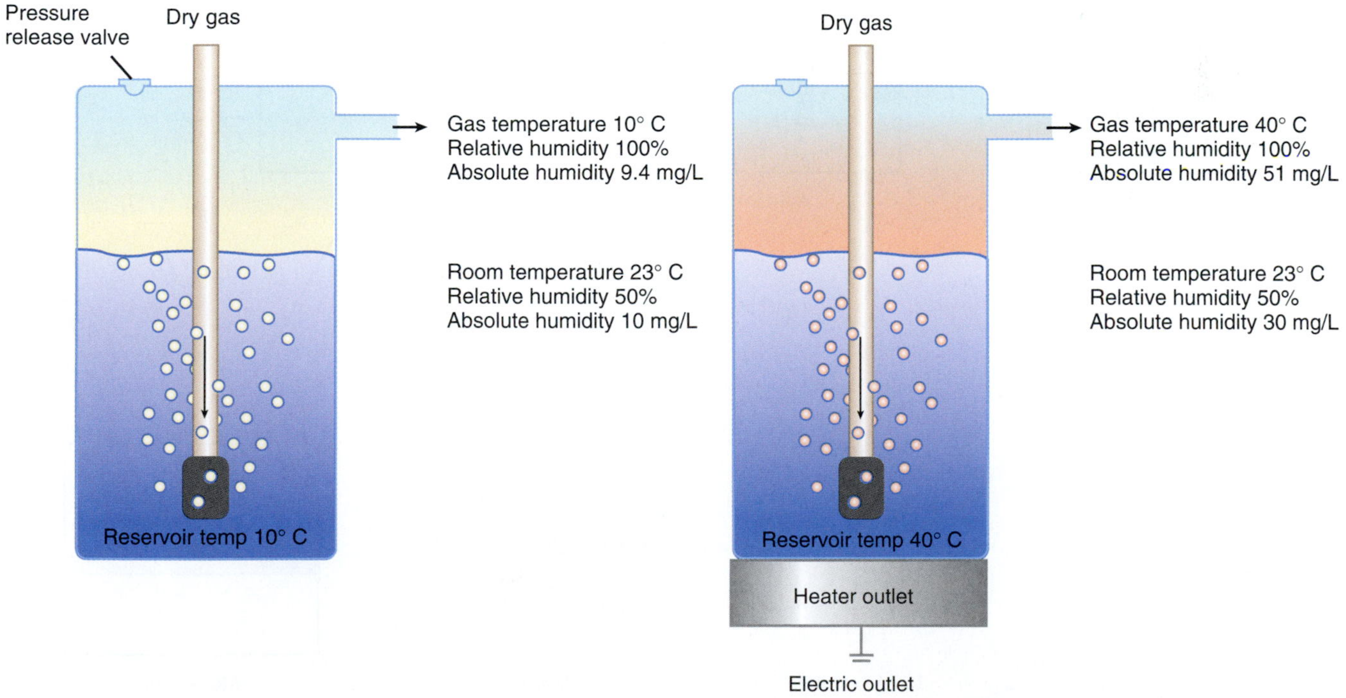

FIGURE 38-2 Effects of reservoir temperature on humidity output with unheated *(left)* and heated *(right)* bubble-type humidifiers. (Modified from Fink J, Cohen N: Humidity and aerosols. In Eubank D, Bone R, editors: Principles and applications of cardiorespiratory care equipment, St. Louis, 1994, Mosby.)

An alternative to dispersing gas bubbles in water is spraying water particles (aerosol) into the gas. The higher the aerosol density (number of particles per volume of gas), the greater is the gas to water surface area available for evaporation.

Wicks use porous water-absorbent materials to draw water (similar to a sponge) into its fine honeycombed structure by means of capillary action. The surfaces of the wick increase the area of contact between the water and gas, which aids evaporation.

Contact Time. The longer a gas remains in contact with water, the greater the opportunity is for evaporation to occur. For bubble humidifiers, contact time depends on the depth of the water column; the deeper the column, the greater is the time of contact as the bubbles rise to the surface. In passover and wick-type humidifiers, the flow rate of gas through the humidifier is inversely related to contact time, with high flow rates reducing the time available for evaporation to occur. Aerosols suspended in a gas stream have extended contact time (and opportunity for evaporation) as the aerosol and gas travel to the patient.

Thermal Mass. The greater the amount of water in a humidifier, the greater is the thermal mass. Increased thermal mass equates to increased capacity to hold and transfer heat to therapeutic gases. Larger reservoir humidifiers can provide more consistent heat and humidification with a broader range of gas flow.

Types of Humidifiers

Humidifiers are either *active* (actively adding heat or water or both to the device-patient interface) or *passive* (recycling exhaled heat and humidity from the patient). Active humidifiers typically include (1) bubble humidifiers, (2) passover humidifiers, (3) nebulizers of bland aerosols, and (4) vaporizers. Passive humidifiers refer to typical **heat and moisture exchangers** (HMEs). Specifications covering the design and performance requirements for medical humidifiers are established by the **American Society for Testing and Materials** (ASTM).[12]

Active Humidifiers

Bubble. A bubble humidifier breaks (diffuses) an underwater gas stream into small bubbles (Figure 38-3). Use of a foam or mesh diffuser produces smaller bubbles than an open lumen, allowing greater surface area for gas/water interaction. Unheated bubble humidifiers are commonly used with oxygen (O_2) delivery systems (see Chapter 41) to raise the water vapor content of the gas to ambient levels.

As indicated in Table 38-2, unheated bubble humidifiers can provide absolute humidity levels between approximately 15 mg/L and 20 mg/L.[13,14] At room temperature, 10 mg/L absolute humidity corresponds to approximately 80% relative humidity but only approximately 25% body humidity (see Chapter 6). As gas flow increases, the reservoir cools and contact time is reduced, limiting effectiveness at flow rates greater than 10 L/min. Heating the reservoirs can increase humidity content,

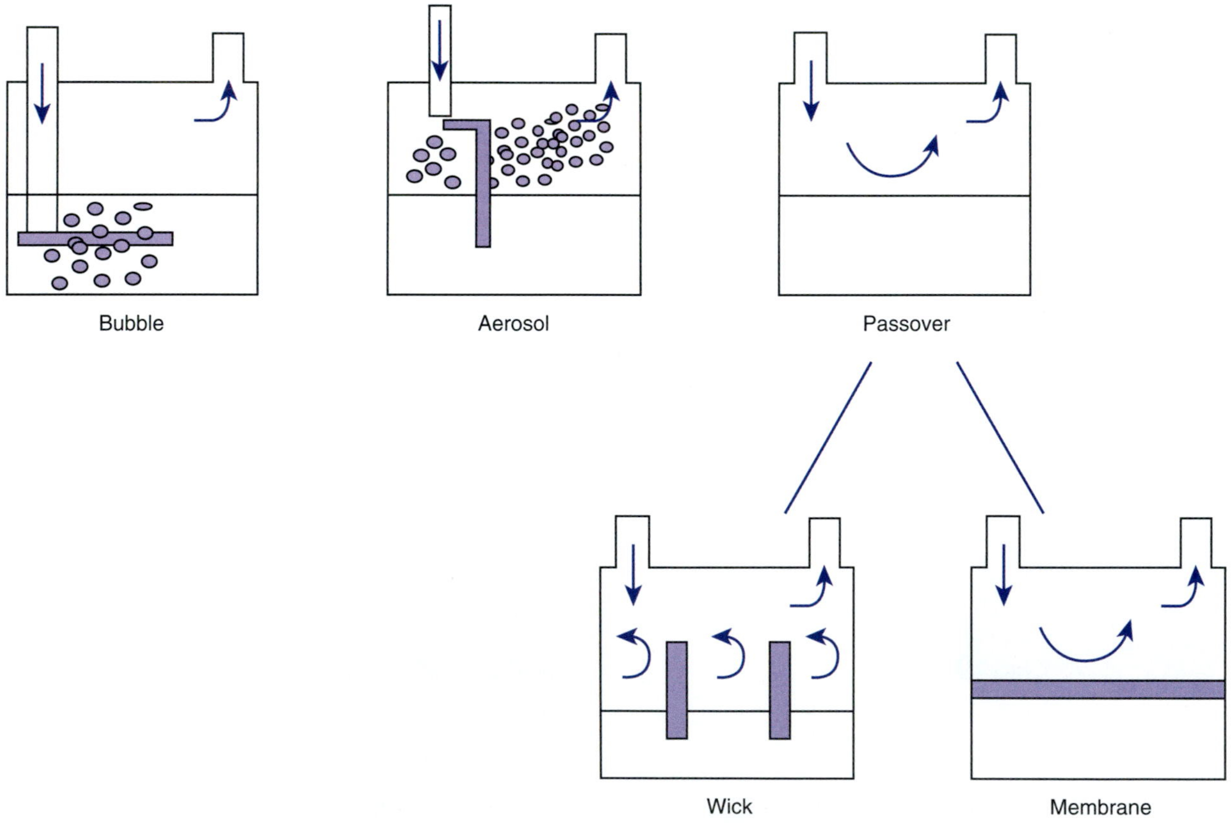

FIGURE 38-3 Primary types of active humidifiers. Gas passes through the water (bubble), around drops of water (aerosol) or over the surface of water (Passover), a saturated material (wick) or a semipermeable membrane (membrane). (From Fink J: Humidity and aerosol therapy. In Cairo J, Pilbeam S, editors: Mosby's respiratory equipment, ed 8, St. Louis, 2010, Mosby.)

TABLE 38-2

Absolute Humidity (mg/L) Provided by Unheated Bubble Humidifiers

L/min	Aquapak 301 (Hudson RCI, Dunham, NC)	Traveral 500 (Baxter-Travenol, Deerfield, IL)
2	17.6	20.4
4	17.7	19.5
6	16.9	16.2
8	14.9	15.7

Modified from Darin J, Broadwell J, MacDonell R: An evaluation of water-vapor output from four brands of unheated, prefilled bubble humidifiers. Respir Care 27:41, 1982.

but this is not recommended because cooling produces condensate that obstructs small-bore delivery tubing.

To warn of flow-path obstruction and prevent bursting of the humidifier bottle, bubble humidifiers incorporate a simple pressure-relief valve, or *pop-off*. The pop-off is commonly a gravity or spring-loaded valve that releases pressures greater than 2 psi. Humidifier pop-offs should provide both an audible and a visible alarm and resume normal position when pressures return to normal.[12] The pop-off can be used to test an O_2 delivery system for leaks by obstructing delivery tubing at or near the patient interface. If the pop-off sounds, the system is leak-free; failure of the pop-off to sound may indicate a leak (or a faulty pop-off valve).

As gas flow increases, bubble humidifiers can produce aerosols. Although invisible to the naked eye, these water droplet suspensions can transmit pathogenic bacteria from the humidifier reservoir to the patient.[15] Because any device that generates an aerosol poses a high risk for spreading infection, strict infection control procedures must be followed when using these systems (see Chapter 4).

Passover. Passover humidifiers direct gas over a surface containing water. There are three common types of passover humidifiers: (1) simple reservoir type, (2) wick type, and (3) membrane type (see Figure 38-3).

The simple reservoir device directs gas over the surface of a volume of water (or fluid). The surface for gas-fluid interface is limited. Typically used with heated fluids with invasive mechanical ventilation, room temperature fluids may be used with noninvasive ventilatory support (nasal continuous positive airway pressure or bilevel ventilation).

A wick humidifier uses an absorbent material to increase the surface area for dry air to interface with heated water. Typically, a wick is placed upright with the gravity-dependent end in a heated water reservoir. Heating elements might be below or surrounding the wick. Capillary action draws water up from the reservoir and keeps the wick saturated. As dry gas enters the chamber, it flows around the wick, quickly picking up heat and moisture and leaving the chamber saturated with water vapor. No bubbling occurs, so no aerosol is produced.

A membrane-type humidifier separates the water from the gas stream by means of a **hydrophobic** membrane (Figure 38-4). Water vapor molecules can easily pass through this membrane, but liquid water (and pathogens) cannot. As with a wick humidifier, bubbling does not occur. If a membrane-type humidifier were to be inspected while it was in use, no liquid water would be seen in the humidifier chamber.

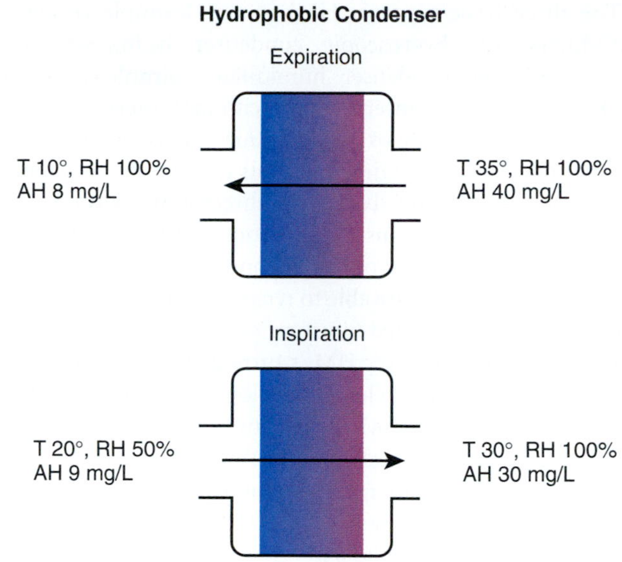

FIGURE 38-4 Process of humidification with a hydrophobic condenser humidifier. *AH,* Absolute humidity; *RH,* relative humidity; *T,* temperature.

Compared with bubble humidifiers, passover humidifiers offer several advantages.[15,16] First, in contrast to bubble devices, passover humidifiers can maintain saturation at high flow rates. Second, they add little or no flow resistance to spontaneous breathing circuits. Third, they do not generate any aerosols, and they pose a minimal risk for spreading infection.

Vaporizer Humidifiers. Simple vaporizers heat water to the point of expansion as a gas. Simple room vaporizers have been used in ambulatory settings for years as room humidifiers. A capillary force vaporizer is a thin-film, high-surface-area boiler that combines capillary force and phase transition to impart pressure onto an expanding gas (water vapor) and ejects it into the gas stream.

Heat and Moisture Exchangers. An HME is a passive humidifier, also described as an "artificial nose." Similar to the nose, an HME captures exhaled heat and moisture and returns up to 70% of the heat and humidify to the patient during the next inspiration. In contrast to the nose, with its rich vasculature and endothelium, most HMEs do not actively add heat or water to the system.[6]

Traditionally, use of HMEs has been limited to providing humidification to patients receiving ventilatory support via endotracheal or tracheostomy tubes. More recently, HMEs have been used successfully in meeting the short-term humidification needs of spontaneously breathing patients with tracheostomy tubes.[17-22] Reports of increased incidence of blocked tracheal tubes associated with long duration of HME use in the intensive care unit,[23] are in contrast with evidence supporting long-term use of HMEs for spontaneously breathing patients.[24]

The three basic types of HMEs are (1) simple condenser humidifiers, (2) hygroscopic condenser humidifiers, and (3) hydrophobic condenser humidifiers. Simple condenser HMEs contain a condenser element with high thermal conductivity, usually consisting of metallic gauze, corrugated metal, or parallel metal tubes. Inspired air cools the condenser element, and expired water vapor condenses directly on its surface and rewarms it. On the next inspiration, cool, dry air is warmed and humidified as its passes over the condenser element. Simple condenser humidifiers are able to recapture only approximately 50% of a patient's exhaled moisture.

Hygroscopic condenser HMEs provide higher efficiency by (1) using a condensing element of low thermal conductivity (e.g., paper, wool, or foam) and (2) impregnating this material with a hygroscopic salt (calcium or lithium chloride). By using an element with low thermal conductivity, hygroscopic condenser HMEs can retain more heat than simple condenser systems while hygroscopic salt helps capture extra moisture from the exhaled gas. The lower water vapor pressure in the inspired gas liberates water molecules directly from the hygroscopic salt, without cooling. Figure 38-5 depicts the overall process of humidification with a hygroscopic condenser humidifier, showing the changes in temperature and the relative and absolute humidity occurring during the cycle of breathing. As shown, these devices typically achieve approximately 70% efficiency (40 mg/L exhaled, 27 mg/L returned).

Hydrophobic condenser HMEs use a water-repellent element with a large surface area and low thermal conductivity (see Figure 38-4). During exhalation, the condenser temperature increases to approximately 25° C because of conduction and the latent heat of condensation. On inspiration, cool gas and evaporation reduce the condenser temperature down to 10° C. This large temperature change results in the conservation of more water to be used in humidifying the next breath. The efficiency of these devices is comparable to that of hygroscopic condenser HMEs (approximately 70%). However, some hydrophobic HMEs that provide bacterial filtration may reduce the risk for pneumonia but be unsuitable for patients with limited respiratory reserve or who are prone to airway blockage because they may increase artificial airway occlusion.[25,26] HMEs that deliver at least 30 mg H_2O/L should be used because they are associated with a lower incidence of ETT occlusion.[18]

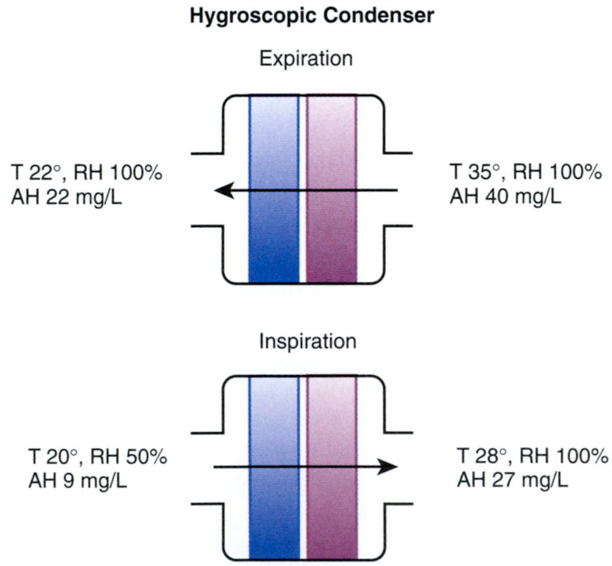

FIGURE 38-5 Process of humidification with a hygroscopic condenser humidifier. *AH*, Absolute humidity; *RH*, relative humidity; *T*, temperature.

Design and performance standards for HMEs are set by the **International Organization for Standardization** (ISO).[27] The ideal HME should operate at 70% efficiency or better (providing at least 30 mg/L water vapor); use standard connections; have a low compliance; and add minimal weight, dead space, and flow resistance to a breathing circuit.[28] HME performance varies from brand to brand and may differ from manufacturers' specifications.[29] Insufficient heat and humidification can occur with some HMEs causing complications.[30,31] Table 38-3 compares performance of several commercially available HMEs

TABLE 38-3

Comparison of 25 Heat and Moisture Exchangers

Device	Manufacturer	Measured AH (mg H_2O/L)	AH/ml of Dead Space	Measured Resistance at 60 L/min cm H_2O
Hygrovent	Peters	31.9 ± 0.6	0.34	1.8
Hygrobac	Mallinckrodt	31.7 ± 0.7	0.33	2.1
Hygrovent S	Peters	31.7 ± 0.5	0.58	2.8
Hygrobac S	Mallinckrodt	31.2 ± 0.2	0.69	2.3
9000/100	Allégiance	31.2 ± 1.4	0.35	2.7
Servo Humidifier 172	Siemens	30.9 ± 0.3	0.56	NA
Humid Vent Filter	Hudson	30.8 ± 0.3	0.88	2.3
Hygroster	Mallinckrodt	30.7 ± 0.6	0.32	2.3
Humid Vent 2	Hudson	29.7 ± 0.4	1.03	NA
Servo Humidifier 162	Siemens	29.7 ± 0.8	0.78	NA
Humid Vent 2S	Hudson	29.2 ± 0.4	1.01	NA
9040/01	Allégiance	28.6 ± 1.1	0.61	2.4
9000/01	Allégiance	28.5 ± 0.8	0.32	3.9
BB100E	Pall	27.2 ± 0.7	0.32	1.4
BB100	Pall	26.8 ± 0.5	0.30	2.0
Stérivent	Mallinckrodt	23.8 ± 0.9	0.26	1.9
Iso Gard Hepa Light	Hudson	23.6 ± 0.3	0.47	2.4
Stérivent S	Mallinckrodt	22.2 ± 0.2	0.36	1.7
BB25	Pall	19.6 ± 1.4	0.56	2.6
BB2000AP	Pall	18.9 ± 0.4	0.54	3.1
Stérivent Mini	Mallinckrodt	16.6 ± 1.0	0.47	2.2
4444/66	Allégiance	16.4 ± 0.6	0.35	3.4
4000/01	Allégiance	15.1 ± 0.9	0.40	2.2
Barrierbac S	Mallinckrodt	13.2 ± 0.2	0.38	2.1

Modified from Lellouche F, Taille S, Lefrancois F, et al: Humidification performance of 48 passive airway humidifiers: comparison with manufacturer data. Chest 135:276, 2009.
AH, Absolute humidity; *NA*, not available.

according to their moisture output, flow resistance, and dead space.[29]

As shown in Table 38-3, the moisture output of HMEs tends to decrease at high volumes and rates of breathing. In addition, high inspiratory flows and high FiO_2 levels can decrease HME efficiency.[28] Flow resistance through the HME also is important. When an HME is dry, resistance across most devices is minimal. However, because of water absorption, HME flow resistance increases after several hours of use.[32] For some patients, the increased resistance imposed by the HME may not be well tolerated, particularly if the underlying lung disease already causes increased work of breathing. An increase in work of breathing through the HME may lead to elevated airway pressures and possible disconnect.[33]

Because HMEs eliminate the problem of breathing circuit condensation, many clinicians consider these devices (especially hydrophobic filter HMEs) to be helpful in preventing nosocomial infections and ventilator-associated pneumonia (VAP).[34] Compared with active humidification systems, HMEs reduce bacterial colonization of ventilator circuits.[35] However, circuit colonization plays a minor role in the development of nosocomial infections, provided that usual maintenance precautions are applied.[36] Although there is no evidence of an overall difference between HMEs and heated humidifiers in preventing mortality and other complications in patients who are mechanically ventilated,[26] and previous research indicates no difference in incidence of ventilator-associated infections, with HMEs and heated humidifiers.[26,29,30,35,37-39] The position of the HME relative to the patient's airway can affect its ability both to heat and to humidify inhaled gas. Secretions can foul HMEs attached directly to the airway. The use of devices such as closed suction catheters and airway monitor ports requires placement of the HME closer to the ventilator. Previous research tested performance of HMEs placed directly at the airway, 10 cm away from ETT and proximal to the ventilator circuit.[40] It was reported that HME performance was best at the airway (Figure 38-6).[40]

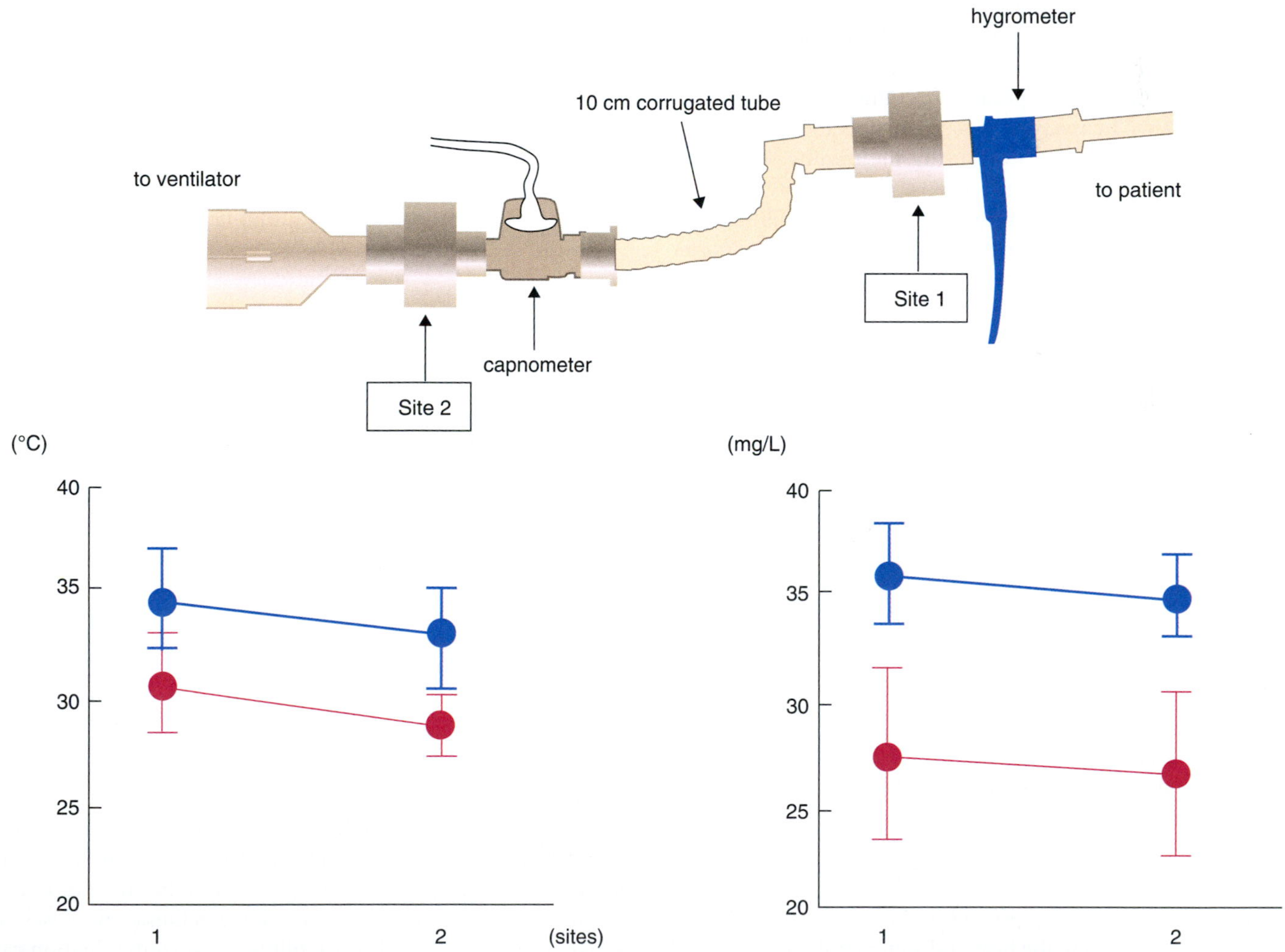

FIGURE 38-6 Placement of heat and moisture exchangers (HMEs) (Hygrobac S [Mallinckrodt-Dar, Mirandola, Italy, *blue circle*] or Thermovent HEPA [Smiths Medical International, Kent, U.K., *red circle*]) at the airway *(site 1)* or proximal to the ventilator circuit *(site 2)*. Temperature mean ± SD (TEMP; *left*) and absolute humidity were significantly higher with both HMEs. $P < .05$ placed at *site 1* compared with *site 2*. (Modified from Inui D, Oto J, Nishimura M: Effect of heat and moisture exchanger [HME] positioning on inspiratory gas humidification. BMC Pulm Med 6:19, 2006.)

Clinicians should select HMEs that perform adequately when placed at the intended position. Although use of HMEs has been associated with thickened and increased volume of secretions in some patients, the incidence of ETT occlusion when HMEs are used is equivalent to that with heated humidifiers.[38,41]

HMEs are not recommended for use with infants and small children for several reasons. First, HMEs add 30 to 90 ml of mechanical dead space, exceeding the tidal volume of the infant. In addition, infants are commonly ventilated through uncuffed ETTs, which allow exhaled gas to leak around the tube and bypass the HME reducing recovered heat and humidity.

Active Heat and Moisture Exchangers. Active HMEs add humidity or heat or both to inspired gas by chemical or electrical means.[42] The Humid-Heat (Louis Gibeck AB, Upplands Väsby, Sweden) consists of a supply unit with a microprocessor, water pump, and humidification device, which is placed between the Y-piece and the ETT. The humidification device is based on a hygroscopic HME, which absorbs the expired heat and moisture and releases it into the inspired gas. External heat and water are added to the patient side of the HME, so the inspired gas should reach 100% humidity at 37° C (44 mg H_2O/L air). The external water is delivered to the humidification device via a pump onto a wick and evaporated into the inspired air by an electrical heater. The microprocessor controls the water pump and the heater by an algorithm using the minute ventilation (which is fed into the microprocessor) and the airway temperature measured by a sensor mounted in the flex-tube on the patient side of the humidification device. The HME Booster (King Systems, Noblesville, IN) has a T-piece containing an electrically heated element that was designed for use as an adjunct to a passive HME. The heating element heats water so that water vapor passes into the airway between the artificial airway and ETT, via a Gore-Tex membrane and aluminum. Using a gravity feedbag via a flow regulator that limits flow to 10 mL/hr, water is fed to the heater, which operates at 110° C and adds 3 to 5.5 mg/L of humidity and 3° C to 4° C to inspired gas compared with the HME alone. The Humid-Booster was designed for patients with minute volumes of 4 to 20 L, and it is not appropriate for use with pediatric patients or infants. Active HMEs add weight and complexity at the patient airway.

> **RULE OF THUMB**
>
> HMEs should be replaced if secretions have contaminated the filter and/or if flow resistance has increased causing an increase in the work of breathing.

Heated Humidifiers

Heat improves the water output of humidifiers. Heated humidifiers are used to increase the heat and water content of inspired gas for patients with bypassed upper airways and patients receiving noninvasive mechanical ventilatory support.[6] Humidifier heating systems generally have a controller that regulates the power to the heating element by monitoring the heating element, which matches a preset or adjustable temperature. They also may use a thermistor placed at the outlet of the humidifier, with a heater set to control output temperature. Servo-controlled heating systems monitor the temperature at the humidifier's outlet and at the patient's airway using a thermistor probe. The controller adjusts the heater power to reach the desired airway temperature and incorporates alarms and an alarm-activated heater shutdown function.

An electrical heating element provides the needed energy. Five types of heating elements are common: (1) a hotplate element at the base of the humidifier; (2) a wraparound type that surrounds the humidifier chamber; (3) a yolk, or collar, element that sits between the water reservoir and the gas outlet; (4) an immersion-type heater, with the element placed in the water reservoir; (5) a heated wire in the inspiratory limb warming a saturated wick or hollow fiber; and (6) a thin-film, high surface area broiler.

Humidifier heating systems have a controller that regulates the element's electrical power. In the simplest systems, the controller monitors the heating element, varying the delivered current to match either a preset or an adjustable temperature. In these systems, the temperature of the patient's airway has no effect on the controller. Conversely, a **servo-controlled heating system** monitors temperature at or near the patient's airway using a thermistor probe. The controller adjusts heater power to achieve the desired airway temperature. Systems usually have alarms and alarm-activated heater shutdown. Box 38-5 outlines key features of modern heated humidification systems.

> **RULE OF THUMB**
>
> Place heated humidifier thermistor probes in the inspiratory limb of a ventilator circuit far enough from the patient Y adaptor to ensure that warm exhaled gas does not fool the controller system. Never place a thermistor probe in an isolette or a radiant warmer, where the probe is warmed externally and the humidifier is fooled into shutting down, reducing the humidity available to the patient.

Reservoir and Feed Systems

Heated humidifiers operating continuously in breathing circuits can evaporate more than 1 L of water per day. An ideal reservoir or feed system should be safe, dependable, easy to set up, and use allowing continuity of therapy, even when the reservoir is being replenished.

Manual Systems. Simple large-reservoir systems are manually refilled (with sterile or distilled water). If a manual system is used, momentary interruption of humidifier operation and mechanical ventilation is required for refilling. Because the system must be "opened" for refilling, cross contamination can occur. Water levels in manually filled systems are constantly changing, and changes in the humidifier fill volume alter the gas compression factor and the delivered volume during mechanical ventilation.

Box 38-5 Key Features for Heated Humidification Systems

- Gas temperature delivered to the patient should not be greater than 40° C. When temperatures greater than 40° C are reached, audible and visual alarms should indicate an overly high temperature condition and interrupt power to the heater.
- Audible and visual alarms should indicate when remote temperature sensors are disconnected, absent, or defective, and power to the heater should be interrupted to prevent overheating.
- Temperature overshoot should be minimized. Overshoot can occur when servo-controlled units warm up without flow through the circuit, when the temperature probe is not inserted in the circuit (or becomes dislodged), or when flow changes during normal operation. Non–servo-controlled units can overshoot when temperature controls are set too high or when gas flow is abruptly reduced.
- Indicators for delivered gas temperature should be accurate to ± 3° C of the indicated value.
- Humidifier temperature output should not vary more than 2° C from the set value (proximal to the patient).
- Warmup time should not exceed 15 minutes.
- The water level should be readily visible in either the humidifier or the remote reservoir.
- Humidifiers should be able to withstand ventilation pressures greater than 100 cm H_2O.
- Internal compliance should be low and stable so that changes in the water level do not significantly alter the delivered tidal volume.
- The exposed surface of a humidifier should not be too hot to touch during operation. Readily accessible surfaces should not be greater than 37.5° C. A warning label is needed for hotter surfaces.
- Operator, or feed, systems must not be able to overfill the humidifier to the point that water can block gas flow through the humidifier or ventilator circuit. Humidifiers should not be damaged by spilled fluids.
- Electromagnetic interference from other devices should not affect humidifier performance. The unit should not be damaged by 95 to 135 Volts.
- Fuses or circuit breakers should be clearly labeled and easily reset or replaced. The unit should have adequate overcurrent protection to prevent ventilator shutdown or loss of power to other equipment on the same branch circuit because of internal equipment failures.
- It should be impossible to assemble the unit in a way that would be hazardous to the patient. The direction of gas flow should be indicated on interchangeable components, for which proper direction is essential.
- The humidifier should be assembled and filled in a manner that minimizes the introduction of infectious materials or foreign objects.
- Service and operation manuals should be provided with the humidifier and should cover all aspects of its use and service.

Modified from Emergency Care Research Institute: Heated humidifiers, Health Devices. 1987. http://www.fda.gov/oc/po/firmrecalls/Vapotherm2000i_01_06.html. Accessed March 2, 2011.

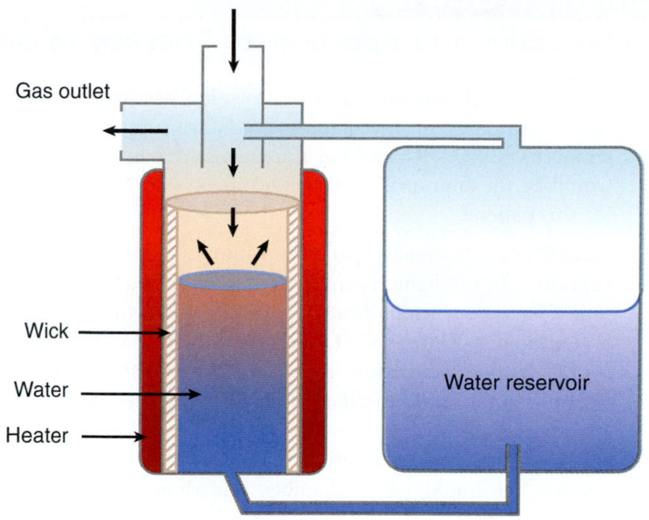

FIGURE 38-7 Schematic of the Concha-Column wick-type humidifier with level-compensated reservoir feed system (Hudson RCI, Temecula, CA). (Modified from Fink J, Cohen N: Humidity and aerosols. In Eubank D, Bone R, editors: Principles and applications of cardiorespiratory care equipment, St. Louis, 1994, Mosby.)

A small inlet that can be attached to a gravity-fed intravenous bag and line allows refilling without interruption of ventilation. Such systems still require constant checking and manual replenishment by opening the line valve or clamp. If not checked regularly, the reservoir in these systems can go dry, placing the patient at considerable risk.

Automatic Systems. Automatic feed systems avoid the need for constant checking and manual refilling of humidifiers. The simplest type of automatic feed system is the level-compensated reservoir (Figure 38-7). In these systems, an external reservoir is aligned horizontally with the humidifier, maintaining relatively consistent water levels between the reservoir and the humidifier chamber.

With flotation-type systems, a float rises and falls with the water level. As the water level falls below a preset value, the float opens the feed valve; as the water rises back to the set fill level, the float closes the feed valve. Alternatively, optical sensors can be used to sense water level, driving a solenoid valve to allow refilling of the humidifier reservoir.

RULES OF THUMB

Humidification of inspired gas is mandatory in mechanically ventilated patients with ETT or tracheostomy tube. During noninvasive ventilation, active humidification is suggested to improve comfort.

Setting Humidification Levels

The American National Standards Institute (ANSI) recommends *minimum* levels of humidity for intubated patients (>30 mg/L). However, optimum humidity targets the temperature and humidity for normal conditions at the point that the

MINI CLINI

Selecting the Appropriate Therapy to Condition a Patient's Inspired Gas

PROBLEM: A survivor of near drowning has just been intubated and placed on mechanical ventilatory support. Her body temperature is 31° C, and her minute ventilation is high. What would be the appropriate humidification system to recommend for this patient?

SOLUTION: Normally, patients without pulmonary disease supported by mechanical ventilation can be started with an HME, unless its use is contraindicated. Using an HME with this patient is contraindicated because (1) she is hypothermic and (2) she has a high minute ventilation. Based on this assessment, the best choice is a heated humidifier, preferably with servo-controlled airway temperature.

Membrane-type humidifiers require no flow control system because the liquid water chamber underlying the membrane cannot overfill and they require only an open gravity feed system. Two examples are the Vapotherm (Vapotherm, Stevensville, MD) membrane cartridge system and the Hummax II (Metran Medical Instruments, Saitama, Japan), which uses a heated wire to warm the polyethylene microporous hollow fiber placed in the inspiratory circuit.

A capillary force vaporizer is driven by software that controls a heater element and water flow. The 19-mm diameter disc can deliver 2.2 mg of water vapor/min at 37° C. Data from prototypes suggest temperature control from 33° C to 41° C for flows 2 to 40 L/min (Figure 38-8).[43]

A gas temperature above 41° C may lead to a potential thermal injury to the patient; over-temperature alarms protect the patient from thermal injury.[6]

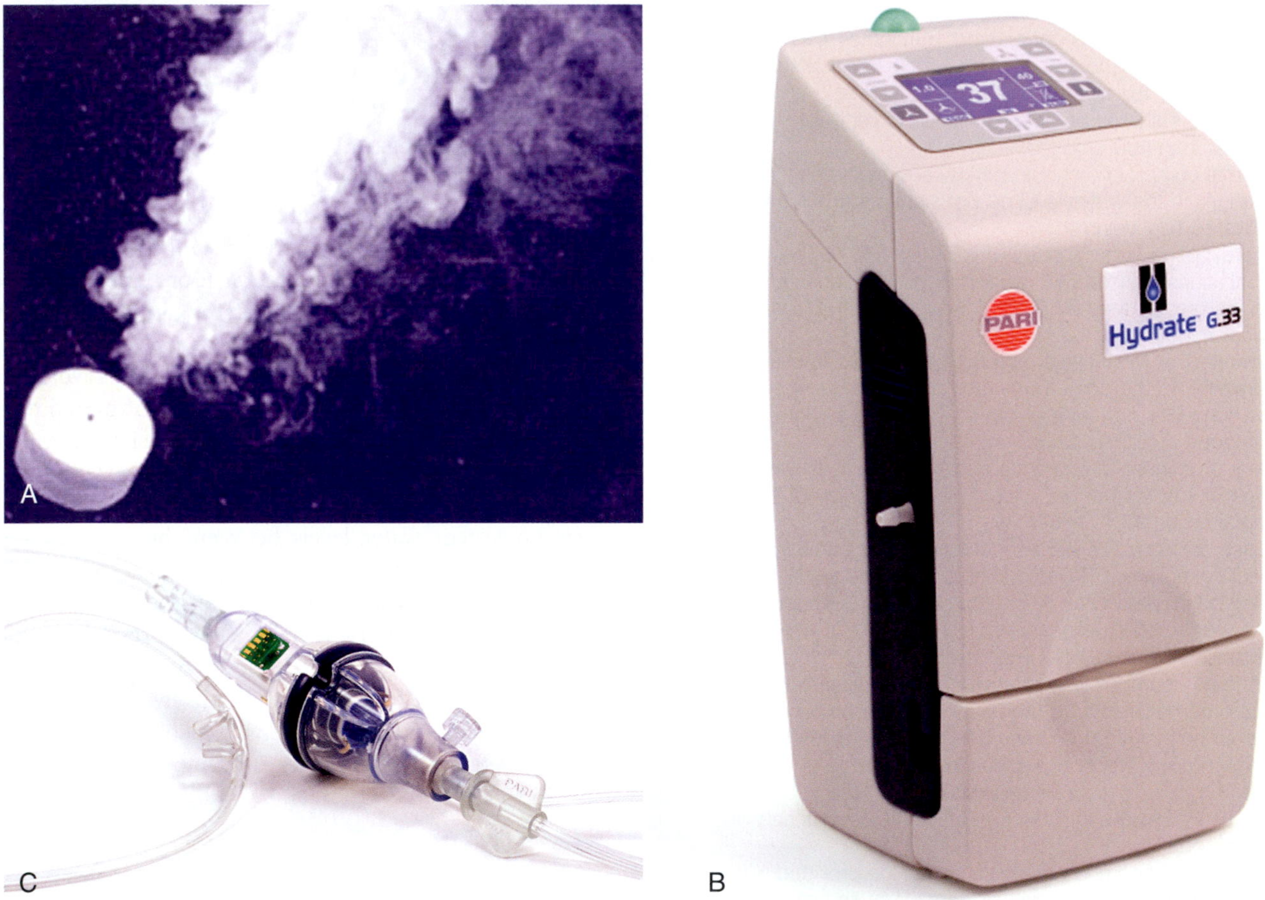

FIGURE 38-8 The capillary force vaporizer (CFV) is a thin-film, high-surface-area boiler that combines capillary force and phase transition. **A,** Inducing phase transition in a capillary environment, the CFV imparts pressure onto the expanding gas and ejects it. **B,** The CFV is incorporated to provide controlled heated humidity in the Hydrate (Pari, Midlothian, VA). **C,** Temperature probe. (Courtesy Pari.)

gas is entering the airway. For example, the humidity of air entering the carina is typically 37 to 40 mg/L. When humidifiers run too cold (<32° C), humidity can be reduced to the point of increased airway plugging. Not all active heated humidifiers perform the same under all conditions.[40] Previous research emphasized the need to set humidifiers to maintain airway temperatures between 35° C and 37° C.[44]

Controversy exists regarding the appropriate temperature and humidity of inspired gas delivered to mechanically ventilated patients with artificial airways. The current AARC Clinical

Practice Guideline recommends 33° C, within 2° C, with a minimum of 30 mg/L of water vapor. (see Clinical Practice Guideline 38-1). In a comprehensive review, Williams[45] suggested that inspired humidity be maintained at an optimal level, 37° C with 100% relative humidity and 44 mg/L, to minimize mucosal dysfunction. Theoretically, optimal humidity offers improved mucociliary clearance. The benefits of this strategy are theory based but have yet to be shown conclusively in the clinical setting. Further controlled studies are needed to support better the need for optimal humidity.

38-1 Humidification During Invasive and Noninvasive Mechanical Ventilation

AARC Clinical Practice Guideline (Excerpts)*

INDICATIONS

Humidification of inspired gas during mechanical ventilation is mandatory when an endotracheal or a tracheostomy tube is present. Humidification of inspired gas during mechanical ventilation is mandatory when an endotracheal or tracheostomy tube is present but optional with noninvasive ventilation.

CONTRAINDICATIONS

There are no contraindications to providing physiologic conditioning of inspired gas during mechanical ventilation. However, a heat and moisture exchanger (HME) is contraindicated in the following circumstances:

- For patients with thick, copious, or bloody secretions
- For patients with an expired tidal volume less than 70% of the delivered tidal volume (e.g., patients with large bronchoneural fistulas or incompetent or absent endotracheal tube cuffs)
- For patients whose body temperature is less than 32° C
- For patients with high spontaneous minute volumes (>10 L/min)
- For patients receiving in-line aerosol drug treatments (an HME must be removed from the patient circuit during treatments)

HAZARDS AND COMPLICATIONS

Hazards and complications associated with the use of heated humidifier (HH) and HME devices during mechanical ventilation include the following:

- High flow rates during disconnect may aerosolize contaminated condensate (HH)
- Underhydration and mucous impaction (HME or HH)
- Increased work of breathing (HME or HH)
- Hypoventilation caused by increased dead space (HME)
- Elevated airway pressures caused by condensation (HH)
- Ineffective low-pressure alarm during disconnection (HME)
- Patient-ventilator dyssynchrony and improper ventilator function caused by condensation in the circuit (HH)
- Hypoventilation or gas trapping caused by mucous plugging (HME or HH)
- Hypothermia (HME or HH)
- Potential for burns to caregivers from hot metal (HH)
- Potential electrical shock (HH)
- Airway burns or tubing meltdown if heated wire circuits are covered or incompatible with humidifier (HH)
- Possible increased resistive work of breathing caused by mucous plugging (HME or HH)
- Inadvertent overfilling resulting in unintended tracheal lavage (HH)
- Inadvertent tracheal lavage from pooled condensate in circuit (HH)

ASSESSMENT OF NEED

- Either an HME or an HH can be used to condition inspired gases:
- HMEs are better suited for short-term use (≤96 hours) and during transport.
- HHs should be used for patients requiring long-term mechanical ventilation (>96 hours) or for patients for whom HME use is contraindicated.

ASSESSMENT OF OUTCOME

Humidification is assumed to be appropriate if, on regular, careful inspection, the patient exhibits none of the listed hazards or complications.

MONITORING

The humidifier should be inspected during the patient-ventilator system check, and condensate should be removed from the circuit as needed. HMEs should be inspected and replaced if secretions have contaminated the insert or filter. The following should be recorded during equipment inspection:

- During routine use on an intubated patient, an HH should be set to deliver inspired gas at 33° C ± 2° C and should provide a minimum of 30 mg/L of water vapor.
- Inspired gas temperature should be monitored at or near the patient's airway opening (HH).
- Specific temperatures may vary with the patient's condition; airway temperature should never exceed 37° C.
- For heated wire circuits used with infants, the probe must be placed outside the incubator or away from the radiant warmer.
- The high-temperature alarm should be set no higher than 37° C, and the low setting should not be less than 30° C.
- The water level and function of automatic feed system (if applicable) should be monitored.
- Quantity, consistency, and other characteristics of secretions should be noted and recorded. When using an HME, if secretions become copious or appear increasingly tenacious, an HH should replace the HME.

*For the complete guideline, see Restrepo RD, Walsh BK: Humidification during invasive and noninvasive mechanical ventilation: 2012. Respir Care 57:782–788, 2012.

Problem Solving and Troubleshooting

Common problems with humidification systems include condensation, avoiding cross contamination, and ensuring proper conditioning of the inspired gas.

Condensation

In standard heated humidifier systems, saturated gas cools as it leaves the point of humidification and passes through the delivery tubing en route to the patient. As gas cools, water vapor capacity decreases, resulting in condensation or "rain out." Factors influencing the amount of condensation include (1) the temperature difference across the system (humidifier to airway); (2) the ambient temperature; (3) the gas flow; (4) the set airway temperature; and (5) the length, diameter, and thermal mass of the breathing circuit.

Figure 38-9 illustrates the condensation process. Because cooling occurs as gas transits the circuit, the humidifier is set to a higher temperature (50° C) than desired at the airway. At 50° C, saturated gas has an absolute humidity level of 84 mg/L of water. As cooling occurs along the tubing, the capacity of the gas to hold water vapor decreases as temperature decreases to 37° C, and holds only 44 mg/L of water vapor. Although BTPS conditions have been achieved, 40 mg/L, half the total output of the humidifier (84 mg/L − 44 mg/L = 40 mg/L), condenses in the inspiratory limb of the circuit.

This condensation poses risks to patients and caregivers and can waste a lot of water. Condensation can disrupt or occlude gas flow through the circuit, potentially altering ventilator function. Because condensate can enter the patient airway and be aspirated, circuits must be positioned to drain condensate away from the patient and checked often, with condensate drained from breathing circuits frequently.

Patients contaminate ventilator circuits within hours, with condensate colonized with bacteria posing an infection risk.[46] Health care personnel should treat all breathing circuit condensate as infectious waste. See Chapters 4 and 46 for more detail on control procedures used with breathing circuits, including the American Association for Respiratory Care (AARC) Clinical Practice Guideline on changing ventilator circuits (see Clinical Practice Guideline 4-1).

RULES OF THUMB

Always treat breathing circuit condensate as infectious waste. Use standard precautions, including wearing gloves and goggles. Always drain the tubing away from the patient's airway into an infectious waste container, and dispose of the waste according to the policies and procedures of the institution.

A common method to minimize problems with condensate is to place water traps at low points in the circuit (both the inspiratory and the expiratory limbs of ventilator circuits) to collect condensate and reduce the likelihood of gas flow obstruction. Water traps should have little effect on circuit compliance, allow emptying without disrupting ventilation, and not be prone to leakage.

Nebulizers, with medication reservoirs positioned below the ventilator circuit, can act as a "water trap," collecting contaminated condensate. This creates a risk that contaminated aerosols can be generated and pathogens delivered to deep into the lung. To minimize this risk, nebulizers should be placed in a superior position so that any condensate travels downstream from the nebulizer. In addition, these nebulizers should be rinsed and air dried, washed, and sterilized or disposed of and replaced between treatments.

One way to avoid condensation problems is to prevent condensation from forming. Because the decrease in temperature

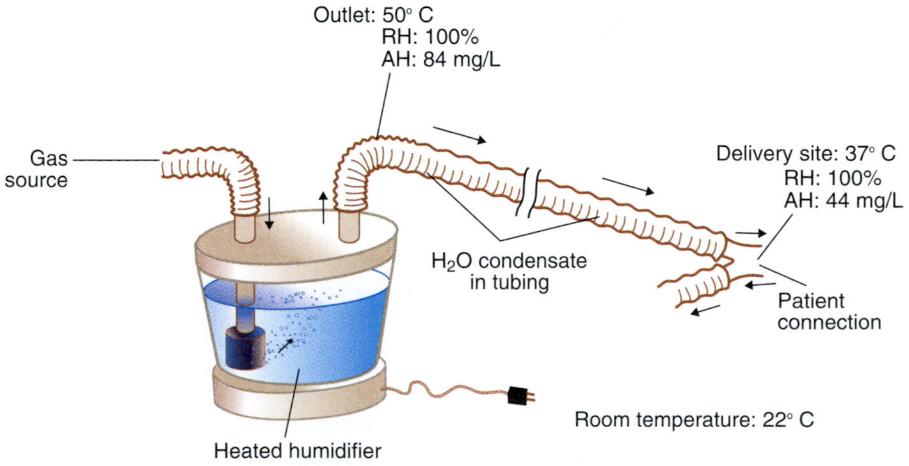

FIGURE 38-9 Gases leaving a standard heated humidifier are cooled en route to the patient. Although the gas remains saturated (100% relative humidity *[RH]*), cooling reduces its water vapor capacity, and condensation forms. Almost half of the original water (500 ml/day) is lost to condensation. The temperature at the patient connection (37° C) shown here is for illustrative purposes only. Heated humidifiers should be set to deliver inspired gas at 35° C ± 2° C. *AH,* Absolute humidity.

in gas traveling from the humidifier to the airway causes condensation, maintaining heat in the circuit can prevent formation of condensate. Several methods, such as insulation or increasing the thermal mass of the circuit, can reduce circuit cooling by keeping the circuit at a constant temperature. The most common approach uses wire heating elements inserted into the ventilator circuit.

Most heated wire circuits use dual controllers with two temperature sensors: one monitoring the temperature of gas leaving the humidifier and the other placed at or near the patient's airway[47-50] (Figure 38-10). The controller regulates the temperature difference between humidifier output and patient airway. When heated wire circuits are used, the humidifier heats gas to a lower temperature (32° C to 40° C) than with conventional circuits (45° C to 50° C). Reduction in condensate in the tubing results in less water use, reduced need for drainage, and less infection risk for patients and health care workers.

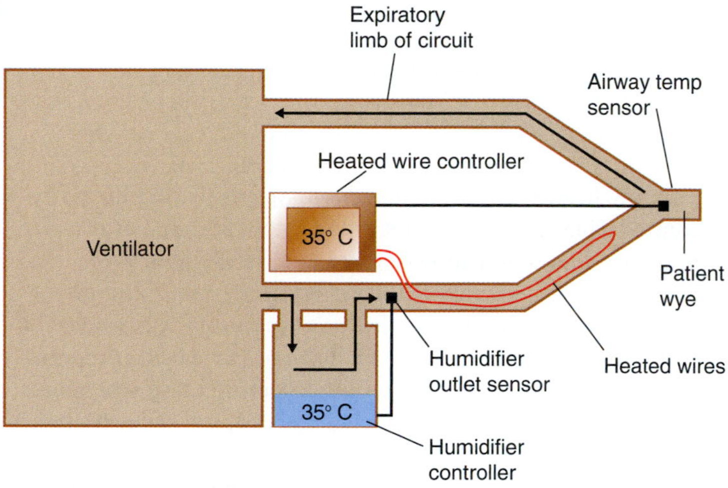

FIGURE 38-10 Heated wire humidifier system. The dual sensor system keeps the temperature constant throughout the inspiratory limb of the ventilator circuit, minimizing condensation. Cooling of exhaled gas in the expiratory limb can cause condensation unless it also is heated.

RULES OF THUMB

Heated humidifiers should be set to deliver an inspired gas temperature of 34° C or greater but less than 41° C at the inspiratory limb near the Y adaptor during invasive mechanical ventilation. Gas temperatures in patients receiving noninvasive ventilation should be selected based on patient comfort, tolerance, adherence, and underlying pulmonary condition.

Unwanted levels of condensate can still occur with heated wires. Absorptive material in the inspiratory limb of the ventilator circuit acts as a wick warmed by the heated wire system (Fisher & Paykel Healthcare, Irvine, CA).

Use of heated wire circuits in neonates is complicated by the use of incubators and radiant warmers. Incubators provide a warm environment surrounding the infant and radiant warmers use radiant energy to warm objects that intercept radiant light. In both cases, a temperature probe placed in the heated environment would affect humidifier performance, resulting in reduced humidity received by the patient. Figure 38-11 shows the impact of temperature probe placement, in or out of the incubator, on absolute humidity delivered to the neonate. Consequently, temperature probes always should be placed outside of the radiant field or incubator (Figure 38-12).

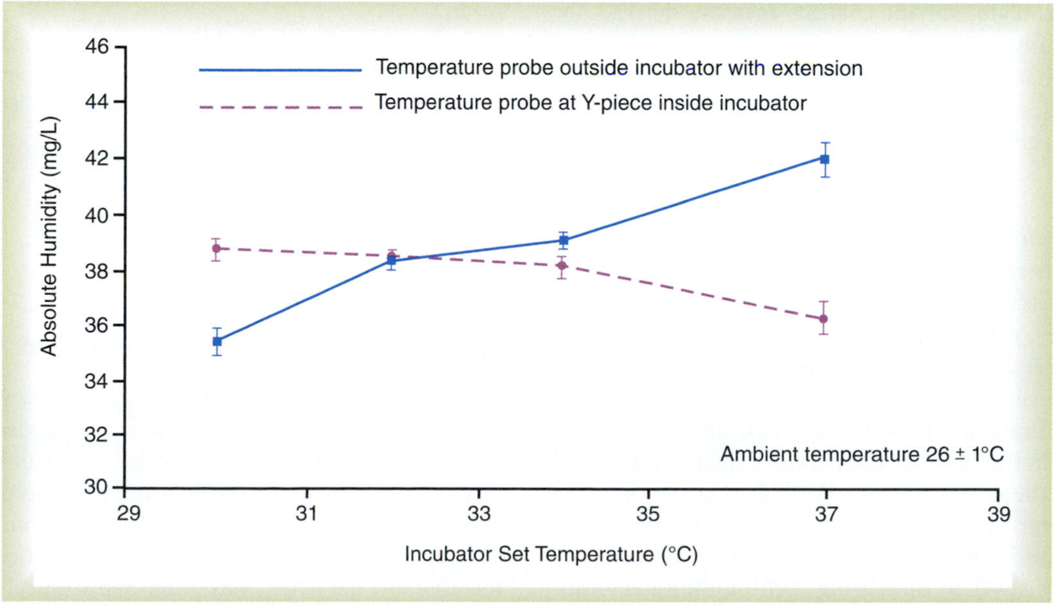

FIGURE 38-11 Humidity achieved at the Y-piece of a neonatal humidification system when used inside an incubator *(dotted line)* and outside or under an incubator *(solid line).*

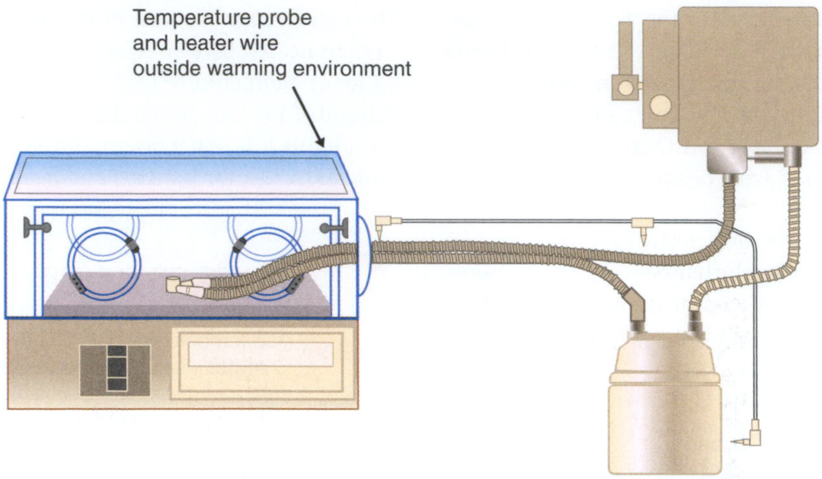

FIGURE 38-12 Neonatal breathing circuit configuration used with an incubator, with the temperature probe placed outside of the warming environment and an unheated portion of the inspiratory circuit delivering the gases to the Y-piece.

Cross Contamination

Aerosol and condensate from ventilator circuits are known sources of bacterial colonization.[46] However, advances in both circuit and humidifier technology have reduced the risk for nosocomial infection when these systems are used. Wick-type or membrane-type passover humidifiers prevent formation of bacteria-carrying aerosols. Heated wire circuits reduce production and pooling of condensate within the circuit. In addition, the high reservoir temperatures in humidifiers are bactericidal.[51] In ventilator circuits using wick-type humidifiers with heated wire systems, circuit contamination usually occurs from the patient to the circuit, rather than vice versa.

For decades, the traditional way to minimize the risk for circuit-related nosocomial infection in critically ill patients receiving ventilatory support was to change the ventilator tubing and its attached components daily.[52] It is now known that frequent ventilator circuit changes increase the risk for nosocomial pneumonia.[45] There is minimal risk for VAP with weekly circuit changes and there may be no need to change circuits at all unless visibly soiled.[35,36,53,54] In addition, substantial cost savings can accrue with decreased frequency of circuit changes.

Proper Conditioning of Inspired Gas

All respiratory therapists (RTs) are trained to measure patient inspired FiO_2 levels regularly and, in ventilatory care, to monitor selected pressures, volumes, and flows. However, few clinicians take the steps needed to ensure proper conditioning of the inspired gas received by patients.

The most accurate and reliable way to ensure that patients are receiving gas at the expected temperature and humidity level is to measure these parameters. Portable battery-operated digital **hygrometer**-thermometer systems are available for less than $300 and are invaluable in ensuring proper conditioning of the inspired gas. When measuring high-humidity environments, hygrometers become saturated and nonresponsive over time and so should be used for spot checks only.

Many heated wire humidification systems have a humidity control. This control does not reflect either absolute or relative humidity but only the temperature differential between the humidifier and the airway sensor. If the heated wires are set warmer than the humidifier, less relative humidity is delivered to the patient. To ensure that the inspired gas is being properly conditioned, clinicians always should adjust the temperature differential to the point at which a few drops of condensation form near the patient connection, or "wye." Lacking direct measurement of humidity, observation of this minimal condensate is the most reliable indicator that the gas is fully saturated at the specified temperature. If condensate cannot be seen, there is no way of knowing the level of relative humidity without direct measurement—it could be anywhere between 99% and 0%. HME performance can be evaluated in a similar manner.[55]

RULES OF THUMB

You can estimate whether an HME is performing well at the bedside by visually confirming condensation in the flex tube between the airway and HME. Lack of condensate may be a clue that humidification is inadequate and that alternative systems may be appropriate for use with the patient.

BLAND AEROSOL THERAPY

Humidity is simply water in the gas phase, whereas a bland aerosol consists of liquid particles suspended in a gas (see Chapter 39 for details on aerosol physics). Bland aerosol therapy involves the delivery of sterile water or hypotonic, isotonic, or hypertonic saline aerosols. Bland aerosol administration may be accompanied by O_2 therapy. To guide practitioners in applying this therapy, the AARC has published Clinical Practice Guideline: Bland Aerosol Administration; excerpts appear in Clinical Practice Guideline 38-2.[56]

38-2 Bland Aerosol Administration

AARC Clinical Practice Guideline (Excerpts)

INDICATIONS
- Presence of upper airway edema—cool, bland aerosol
- Laryngotracheobronchitis
- Subglottic edema
- Postextubation edema
- Postoperative management of the upper airway
- Presence of a bypassed upper airway
- Need for sputum specimens or mobilization of secretions

CONTRAINDICATIONS
- Bronchoconstriction
- History of airway hyperresponsiveness

HAZARDS AND COMPLICATIONS
- Wheezing or bronchospasm
- Bronchoconstriction when artificial airway is used
- Infection
- Overhydration
- Patient discomfort
- Caregiver exposure to airborne contagions produced during coughing or sputum induction
- Edema of the airway wall
- Edema associated with decreased compliance and gas exchange and with increased airway resistance
- Sputum induction by hypertonic saline inhalation can cause bronchoconstriction in patients with chronic obstructive pulmonary disease, asthma, cystic fibrosis, or other pulmonary diseases.

ASSESSMENT OF NEED

The presence of one or more of the following may be an indication for administration of a water or isotonic or hypotonic saline aerosol:
- Stridor
- Brassy, crouplike cough
- Hoarseness after extubation
- Diagnosis of laryngotracheobronchitis or croup
- History of upper airway irritation and increased work of breathing (e.g., smoke inhalation)
- Patient discomfort associated with airway instrumentation or insult
- Bypassed upper airway
- Need for sputum induction (e.g., *Pneumocystis* pneumonia or tuberculosis) is an indication for administration of hypertonic saline aerosol.

ASSESSMENT OF OUTCOME

With administration of water or hypotonic or isotonic saline, the desired outcome is one or more of the following:
- Decreased work of breathing
- Improved vital signs
- Decreased stridor
- Decreased dyspnea
- Improved arterial blood gas values
- Improved O_2 saturation, as indicated by pulse oximetry
- With administration of hypertonic saline, the desired outcome is a sputum sample that is adequate for analysis.

MONITORING

The extent of patient monitoring should be determined based on the stability and severity of the patient's condition:
- Patient subjective response—pain, discomfort, dyspnea, restlessness
- Heart rate and rhythm, blood pressure
- Respiratory rate, pattern, mechanics; accessory muscle use
- Sputum production—quantity, color, consistency, odor
- Skin color
- Breath sounds
- Pulse oximetry (if hypoxemia is suspected)
- Spirometry equipment (if adverse reaction is a concern)

From Kallstrom T, American Association for Respiratory Care: Clinical practice guideline: bland aerosol administration, 2003 revision and update. Respir Care 5:529–533, 2003.

Equipment

The equipment needed for bland aerosol therapy includes an aerosol generator and a delivery system. Devices used to generate bland aerosols include large-volume jet nebulizers and **ultrasonic nebulizers** (USNs). Delivery systems include various direct airway appliances and enclosures (mist tents).

Aerosol Generators

Large-Volume Jet Nebulizers. A large-volume jet nebulizer is the most common device used to generate bland aerosols. As depicted in Figure 38-13, these devices are pneumatically powered, attaching directly to a flowmeter and compressed gas source. Liquid particle aerosols are generated by passing gas at a high velocity through a small "jet" orifice. The resulting low pressure at the jet draws fluid from the reservoir up to the top of a siphon tube, where it is sheared off and shattered into liquid particles. The large, unstable particles fall out of suspension or impact on the internal surfaces of the device, including the fluid surface **(baffling).** The remaining small particles leave the nebulizer through the outlet port, carried in the gas stream. A variable air-entrainment port allows air mixing to increase flow rates and to alter FiO_2 levels (see Chapter 41).

Similar to humidifiers, if heat is required, a hot plate, wrap-around, yolk collar, or immersion element can be added. These devices rarely have sophisticated servo-controlled systems to control delivery temperature. They may not shut down when the reservoir empties, resulting in the delivery of hot, dry gas to the patient. Failure of the heating element also can cause a loss of heating capacity, without warning to the clinician.

Depending on the design, input flow, and air-entrainment setting, the total water output of unheated large-volume jet

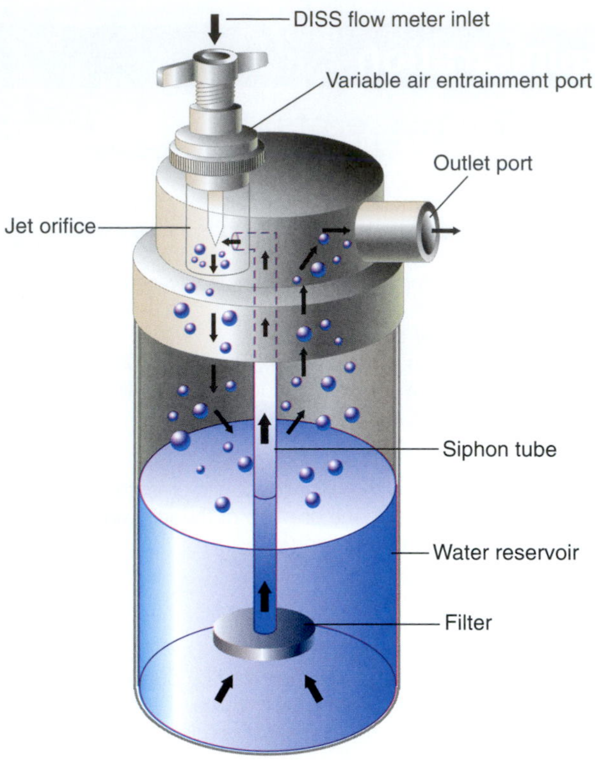

FIGURE 38-13 All-purpose large-volume jet nebulizer.

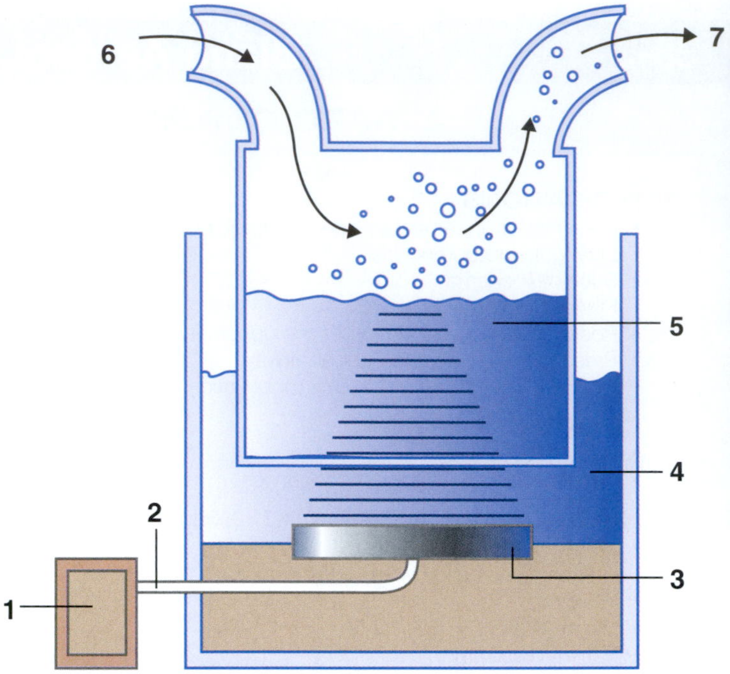

FIGURE 38-14 Functional schematic of a typical large-volume ultrasonic nebulizer. *1,* Radiofrequency generator; *2,* shielded cable; *3,* piezoelectric crystal transducer; *4,* water-filled couplant reservoir; *5,* solution chamber; *6,* chamber inlet; and *7,* chamber outlet. (Modified from Barnes TA: Core textbook for respiratory care practice, ed 2, St. Louis, 1994, Mosby.)

nebulizers varies between 26 mg H_2O/L and 35 mg H_2O/L. When heated, output increases to between 33 mg H_2O/L and 55 mg H_2O/L, mainly because of increased vapor capacity.[56,57] Larger versions of these devices (with 2-L to 3-L reservoirs) are used to deliver bland aerosols into mist tents. These enclosure systems can generate flow rates greater than 20 L/min, with water outputs of 5 ml/min (300 ml/hr). Because heat buildup in enclosures is a problem, these systems are always run unheated.

Ultrasonic Nebulizers. A USN is an electrically powered device that uses a **piezoelectric crystal** to generate aerosol. This crystal transducer converts radiowaves into high-frequency mechanical vibrations (sound). These vibrations are transmitted to a liquid surface, where the intense mechanical energy creates a cavitation in the liquid, forming a standing wave, or "geyser," that sheds aerosol droplets. Figure 38-14 provides a schematic of a large volume USN. Output from a radiofrequency generator is transmitted over a shielded cable to the piezoelectric crystal. Vibrational energy is transmitted either indirectly through a water-filled couplant reservoir or directly to a solution chamber. Gas entering the chamber inlet picks up the aerosol particles and exits through the chamber outlet.

The properties of the ultrasonic signal determine the characteristics of the aerosol generated by these nebulizers. The frequency at which the crystal vibrates, preset by the manufacturer, determines aerosol particle size. Particle size is inversely proportional to signal frequency. A USN operating at a frequency of 2.25 MHz may produce an aerosol with a mass median aerodynamic diameter (MMAD) of approximately 2.5 μm, whereas another nebulizer operating at 1.25 MHz produces an aerosol with MMAD between 4 and 6 μm. Signal amplitude directly affects the amount of aerosol produced; the greater the amplitude, the greater is the volume of aerosol output. In contrast to frequency, signal amplitude may be adjusted by the clinician.

Particle size and aerosol density delivered to the patient also are affected by the source and flow of gas through the aerosol-generating chamber. Some large-volume USNs have built-in fans that direct room air through the solution chamber conducting the aerosol to the patient. The airflow may be adjusted by changing the fan speed or use of a simple damper valve. Alternatively, compressed anhydrous gases can be delivered to the chamber inlet through a flowmeter. For precise control over delivered O_2 concentrations, clinicians can attach a flowmeter with an O_2 blender or air-entrainment system to the chamber inlet.

The flow and amplitude settings interact to determine aerosol density (mg/L) and total water output (ml/min). Amplitude affects water output. At a given amplitude setting, the greater the flow through the chamber, the less the density of the aerosol. Conversely, low flows result in aerosols of higher density. Total aerosol output (ml/min) is greatest when both flow and amplitude are set at the maximum. Using these settings, some units can achieve total water outputs of 7 ml/min.

Particle size, aerosol density, and output are also affected by the relative humidity of the carrier gas (see Chapter 39). In contrast to jet nebulizers, the temperature of the solution placed in a USN increases up to 10° C during use. Although this increase in temperature affects water vapor capacity, its impact on aerosol output is minimal.

RULES OF THUMB

To produce a high-density aerosol using a USN (useful for sputum induction), set the amplitude high and the flow rate low. To maximize aerosol delivery per minute (when trying to help mobilize secretions), set the flow rate to match and slightly exceed patient inspiratory flow rate, and set the amplitude at the maximum.

Although USNs have some unique capabilities, in most cases of bland aerosol administration, their relative advantages over jet nebulizers are outweighed by their high cost and erratic reliability. Exceptions include the use of a USN for sputum induction, where the high output (1 to 5 ml/min) and aerosol density seem to yield higher quantity and quality of sputum specimens for analysis, although at some cost in increased airway reactivity.[58] Although a major manufacturer of USNs (DeVilbiss) discontinued their product line, other companies in both the United States and Europe still manufacture units for clinical use.

Commercially available USNs (usually marketed as "cool" mist devices) have found a place in the home, being used as room humidifiers. As with any nebulizer, the reservoirs of these devices can easily become contaminated, resulting in airborne transmission of pathogens. Care should be taken to ensure that these units are cleaned according to the manufacturer's recommendations and that water is discarded from the reservoir periodically between cleanings. In the absence of a manufacturer's recommendation, these units should undergo appropriate disinfection at least every 6 days.[59] Generally, passover and wick-type humidifiers present less risk than the USN as a room humidifier.

Airway Appliances

Airway appliances used to deliver bland aerosol therapy include the aerosol mask, face tent, T-tube, and tracheostomy mask (Figure 38-15). The aerosol mask and face tent are used for patients with intact upper airways. The T-tube is used for patients who are orally or nasally intubated or who have a tracheostomy. The tracheostomy mask is used only for patients who have a tracheostomy. In all cases, large-bore tubing is required to minimize flow resistance and prevent occlusion by condensate.

For short-term therapy to patients with intact upper airways, the aerosol mask is the device of choice. However, some patients cannot tolerate masks and may do better with a face tent. No data support preferential use of an open aerosol mask versus a face tent.

Although the T-tube is the most common application for tracheostomy patients, unless moderate to high FiO_2 levels are needed, a tracheostomy mask is a better choice. In contrast to

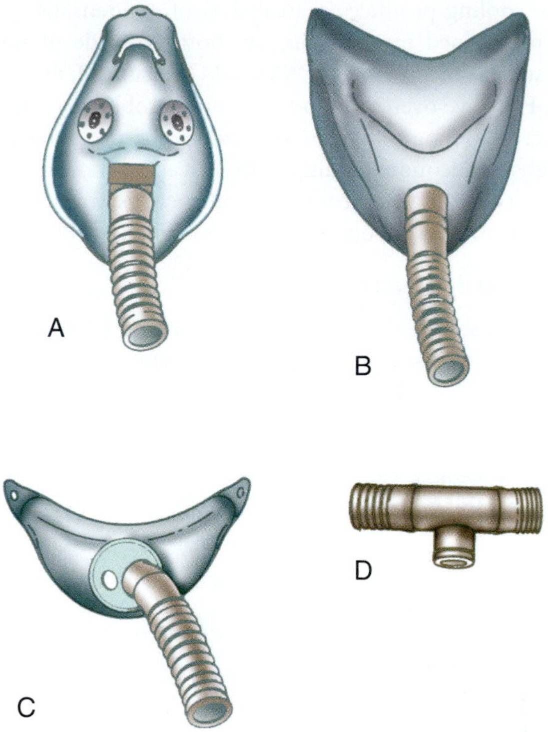

FIGURE 38-15 Airway appliances used to deliver bland aerosol therapy. *A*, Aerosol mask. *B*, Face tent. *C*, Tracheostomy mask. *D*, T-tube.

T-tubes, tracheostomy masks exert no traction on the airway and they allow secretions and condensate to escape from the airway, reducing airway resistance.

Enclosures (Mist Tents and Hoods)

Infants and small children may not readily tolerate direct airway appliances such as masks, so enclosures such as mist tents and aerosol hoods are used to deliver bland aerosol therapy to these patients. More recent studies have shown that aerosol hoods can provide aerosol delivery with similar efficiency to a properly fitted aerosol mask in infants, with less discomfort for the patient.[60]

Mist tents were used for more than 40 years mainly to treat croup and thus called *croup tents*. The cool aerosol provided through these enclosures promotes vasoconstriction, decreases edema, and reduces airway obstruction.

Any body enclosure poses two problems: carbon dioxide (CO_2) buildup and heat retention. CO_2 buildup can be reduced by providing sufficiently high gas flow rates. These high flows of fresh gas circulate continually through the enclosure and "wash out" CO_2 while helping maintain desired O_2 concentrations. Heat retention may be handled with high fresh gas flows to prevent heat buildup or use of a separate cooling device such as a simple ice compartment to cool the aerosol. The Ohmeda Ohio Pediatric Aerosol Tent (Ohmeda Ohio, Gurnee, IL) and other similar units use electrically powered refrigeration units to cool the circulating air.

The cooling produces a great deal of condensation, which must be drained into a collection bottle outside of the tent. Units such as the Mistogen CAM-3M (Mercury Medical, Clearwater, FL) have overcome some of these problems with a thermoelectric cooling system, in which an electrical current passing through a semiconductor augments heat absorption and release. As warm air is taken from the tent, heat is transferred and released in the room, and cool air is returned to the tent.

Sputum Induction

As a diagnostic procedure, sputum induction (Box 38-6) warrants separate attention from other modes of bland aerosol therapy. Sputum induction is a useful, cost-effective, and safe method for diagnosing tuberculosis, pneumocystis pneumonia (caused by *Pneumocystis jiroveci* [formerly *Pneumocystis carinii*]), and lung cancer.[61,62]

Sputum induction involves short-term application of high-density hypertonic saline (3% to 10%) aerosols to the airway to assist in mobilizing pulmonary secretions for evacuation and recovery. These high-density aerosols are often made using ultrasonic nebulization. Box 38-7 outlines a procedure for sputum induction using a 3% saline solution.[63]

To ensure a good sputum sample, every effort must be made to separate saliva from true respiratory tract secretions.[62] Some protocols have patients brush their teeth and tongue surface thoroughly and rinse their mouths before sputum induction. Although the distinction between saliva and sputum can be made in the diagnostic laboratory, care during the collection procedure reduces the need for repeat inductions.

Box 38-6 Sputum-Induction Procedure

- Gather the necessary equipment: Ultrasonic nebulizer, aerosol mask, large-bore tubing, specimen container, 3% sterile saline, and stethoscope.
- Check the chart for order or protocol, diagnosis, history, and other pertinent information.
- Wash your hands and follow applicable standard, airborne, and tuberculosis precautions.
- Introduce yourself and identify your department, verify the patient's identity, and explain the procedure and verify that the patient understands it.
- Have the patient assume an upright, seated position if possible.
- Have the patient rinse his or her mouth with water, blow his or her nose, and clear any excess saliva.
- Perform pretreatment assessment, including vital signs, muscle tone, ability to cough, and auscultation.
- Assemble the nebulizer; fill the couplant chamber with tap water; plug the unit into a grounded electrical outlet; and attach the delivery tubing and mask.
- Aseptically fill the medication chamber of the nebulizer with 3% sterile saline.
- Turn the unit on and adjust the output control to achieve adequate flow and high density.
- Place the mask comfortably on the patient's face, and instruct the patient to take slow, deep breaths, with occasional inspiratory hold as tolerated.
- Periodically reassess the patient's condition (including breath sounds) throughout the application.
- Modify the technique and reinstruct the patient as needed, based on his or her response.
- Terminate the treatment after 15 to 30 minutes, if significant adverse reactions occur, or when sputum specimen has been obtained.
- Encourage the patient to cough and expectorate sputum into specimen cup; observe for volume, color, consistency, odor, and presence or absence of blood.
- Label the specimen container with patient identification and required information, and deliver to the appropriate personnel.
- Chart the therapy according to departmental and institutional protocol.
- Notify the appropriate personnel of any adverse reactions or other concerns.

Modified from Butler TJ: Laboratory exercises for competency in respiratory care, ed 2, Philadelphia, 2009, FA Davis.

Problem Solving and Troubleshooting

The most common problems with bland aerosol delivery systems are cross contamination and infection, environmental safety, inadequate mist production, overhydration, bronchospasm, and noise.

Box 38-7 Monitoring

The humidifier should be inspected during the patient-ventilator system check, and condensate should be removed from the circuit as needed. HMEs should be inspected and replaced if secretions have contaminated the insert or filter. The following should be recorded during equipment inspection:

- *Humidifier settings*: During routine use on an intubated patient, a heated humidifier (HH) should be set to deliver inspired gas at 34° C or greater but less than 41° C at the Y adaptor in the circuit and should provide a minimum of 33 mg/L of water vapor.
- *Inspired gas temperature*: Inspired gas temperature should be monitored at or near the patient's airway opening (HH).
- *Location of probe:* For heated wire circuits used with infants, the probe must be placed outside the incubator or away from the radiant warmer.
- *Temperature:* High-temperature alarm should be set no higher than 41° C, and the low-temperature alarm should be set no lower than 2° C below the desired temperature at the circuit Y piece.
- *Water level and feed system:* Water level and function of automatic feed system (if applicable) should be monitored.
- *Quantity and consistency of secretions:* Quantity, consistency, and other characteristics of secretions should be noted and recorded. When using an HME, if secretions become copious or appear increasingly tenacious, an HH should replace the HME.
- *Airway obstruction:* The presence of copious secretions increases the resistance of airflow through the HME. This even may increase peak pressures and induce changes of the flow waveforms consistent with those observed with airway obstruction. If these changes persist after changing the HME because of copious secretions, an HH should be used instead.

Cross Contamination

Rigorous adherence to the infection control guidelines detailed in Chapter 4, especially guidelines covering solutions and equipment processing, should help minimize the cross contamination and infection risks involved in using these systems. In addition, the water should be changed regularly and the couplant compartments and nebulizer chambers of USNs should be disinfected or replaced regularly.

Environmental Exposure

Environmental safety issues from secondhand and exhaled aerosol arise mainly when aerosol therapy is prescribed for immunosuppressed patients or for patients with tuberculosis. A survey suggested that RTs may be at increased risk for developing asthma-like symptoms, attributed partly to secondhand exposure to aerosols such as ribavirin or albuterol.[64] To minimize problems in this area, all clinicians should strictly follow U.S. Centers for Disease Control and Prevention standards and airborne precautions, including precautions specified for control of exposure to tuberculosis (see Chapter 4). Additional methods for dealing with environmental control of drug aerosols are described in Chapter 39.

Inadequate Aerosol Output

Inadequate mist production is a common problem with all nebulizer systems. With pneumatically powered jet nebulizers, poor mist production can be caused by inadequate input flow of driving gas, siphon tube obstruction, or jet orifice misalignment. With the exception of inadequate driving gas flow, these problems require unit repair or replacement. If a USN is not functioning properly, the electrical power supply (cord, plug, and fuse or circuit breakers) should be checked first. The clinician next should check to confirm that (1) carrier gas is flowing through the device and (2) the amplitude, or output, control is set above minimum. If there is still no visible mist output, the clinician should inspect the couplant chamber to confirm proper fill level and the absence of any visible dirt or debris. Finally, the clinician must ensure that the couplant chamber solution meets the manufacturer's specifications (most units do not function properly with distilled water).

Overhydration

Overhydration is a problem with continuous use of heated jet nebulizers and USNs. With USNs capable of such extraordinarily high water outputs, they should never be used for continuous therapy. The risk for overhydration is highest for infants, small children, and patients with preexisting fluid or electrolyte imbalances. Even if used only to meet BTPS conditions, bland aerosol therapy effectively eliminates insensible water loss through the lungs and should be equated to a daily water gain (approximately 200 ml/day for an average adult). In addition to overhydration of the patient, inspissated pulmonary secretions can swell after high-density aerosol therapy, worsening airway obstruction. Careful patient selection and monitoring can prevent most potential problems with overhydration. Box 38-6 Lists variables that should be recorded during inspection and monitoring of humidification devices.

Bronchospasm

Bland water aerosols are irritating and can cause bronchospasm in some patients. Ultrasonic nebulization of distilled water is used in some pulmonary function laboratories to provoke bronchospasm and to assess bronchial hyperactivity.[63] Always carefully review the patient's history and diagnosis before administering any bland aerosol, especially a hypotonic water solution. As indicated in the AARC practice guideline (see Clinical Practice Guideline 38-2), patients receiving continuous bland aerosol therapy should be initially monitored carefully (including breath sounds and subjective response) and reevaluated every 8 hours or with any change in clinical condition.[56] If bronchospasm occurs during therapy, treatment must be stopped immediately, O_2 provided, and appropriate bronchodilator therapy initiated as soon as possible. If the physician still requests bland aerosol therapy, pretreatment with a bronchodilator may be needed. Isotonic solutions (0.9% saline) may be better tolerated by these patients than water.

A problem unique to large-volume, air-entrainment jet nebulizers is the noise they generate, especially at high flows. The American Academy of Pediatrics recommends that sound levels remain less than 58 dB to avoid hearing loss for infants being cared for in incubators and O_2 hoods. Because many commercial nebulizers exceed this noise level when in operation, careful selection of equipment is necessary. However, the best way to avoid this problem and minimize infection risks further is to use heated passover humidification instead of nebulization.

SELECTING THE APPROPRIATE THERAPY

Figure 38-16 provides a basic algorithm for selecting or recommending the appropriate therapy to condition a patient's inspired gas. Key considerations include (1) gas flow, (2) presence or absence of an artificial tracheal airway, (3) character of the pulmonary secretions, (4) need for and expected duration of mechanical ventilation, and (5) contraindications to using an HME.

Regarding delivery of O_2 to the upper airway, the American College of Chest Physicians advises against using a bubble humidifier at flow O_2 rates of 4 L/min or less.[65] For the occasional patient who complains of nasal dryness or irritation when receiving low-flow O_2, a humidifier should be added to the delivery system. Conversely, the relative inefficiency of unheated bubble humidifiers means that the clinician may need to consider heated humidification for patients receiving long-term O_2 at high flow rates (>10 L/min without air entrainment).

HMEs provide an inexpensive alternative to heated humidifiers when used for ventilation of patients who do not have complex humidification needs. However, passive HMEs may not provide sufficient heat or humidification for long-term management of certain patients. When an HME is to be used, it should be selected based on individual patient need and

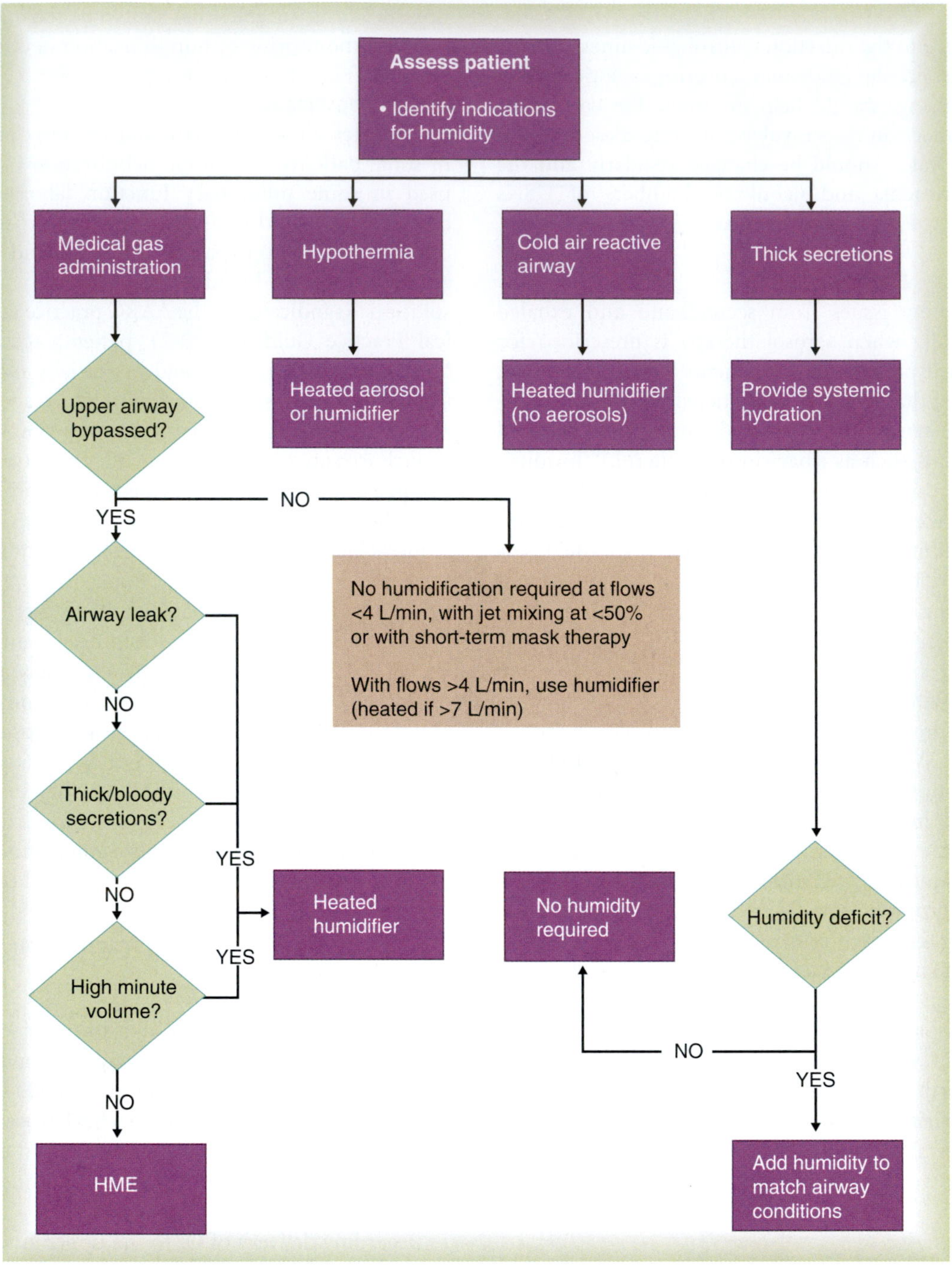

FIGURE 38-16 Selection algorithm for humidity and bland aerosol therapy. *HME,* Heat and moisture exchanger.

ventilatory pattern and the unit's performance, efficiency, and size. All patients using HMEs should be reevaluated regularly to confirm the appropriateness of continued use.

RULES OF THUMB

HMEs are better suited for short-term use and during transport, and heated humidifiers should be used for patients requiring long-term mechanical ventilation (>96 hours) or for patients for whom HME use is contraindicated.

MINI CLINI

Cost-Effectiveness of Humidification Systems

PROBLEM: There is a lot of controversy over which is more cost-effective—heated water humidifiers or HMEs. How can the cost of passover humidifiers, with standard circuit and heated wire circuits, be compared with the cost of HMEs?

SOLUTION: First, determine the frequency of circuit setup and component changes for each type of humidification system. Second, determine supplies and time required to set up the system and operate the system on a daily basis.

The following table compares illustrative costs associated with three humidification strategies in terms of circuit setup costs, water usage, and labor for a typical patient requiring 12 days of mechanical ventilation at a large, comprehensive acute care hospital. Labor costs were calculated as the time required to perform setup or maintenance multiplied by the average salary. This example assumes no circuit changes for a patient over 14 days and that the HME is changed daily.

Components of Circuit Setup and Operating Costs	Heated Humidifier With Standard Circuit	Heated Humidifier With Heated Wire Circuit	Heat Moisture Exchanger
Vent circuit	$3.00	$11.00	$3.00
Humidifier/water feed system	$12.00	$12.00	—
HME filter	—	—	$5.00
Setup cost (labor)	$18.00	$23.00	$8.00
Daily cost (labor)	$11.00	$1.50	$5.00
Total costs (5 days)	$62.00	$29.00	$28.00
Total costs (12 days)	$139.00	$39.50	$63.00

In this example, the standard circuit costs less than the heated wire circuit but has twice the daily water usage, with an additional labor cost of $9.50 per day for adding and removing water from the system. The HME has the lowest setup cost, but after ventilator day 5, total costs of daily filter replacement exceed the cost associated with operation of the heated wire circuit. However, most modern ventilator humidification systems require the purchase of their prepackaged water. This can markedly increase the cost of both unheated and heated wire circuits. Although different component costs may shift the analysis, in general there is not a significant cost difference associated with the use of HME, unheated wire, and heated wire systems. The decision to use each is generally based on the clinical needs of the patient.

SUMMARY CHECKLIST

- Conditioning of inhaled and exhaled gas is accomplished primarily by the nose and upper airway. Bypassing the upper airway without providing similar levels of heat and humidity to inhaled gas can cause damage to the respiratory tract.
- Gases delivered to the nose and mouth should be conditioned to 20° C to 22° C with 10 mg/L water vapor (50% relative humidity).
- When being delivered to the trachea, gases should be warmed and humidified to 32° C to 40° C with 36 to 40 mg/L water vapor (>90% relative humidity).
- A humidifier is a device that adds invisible molecular water to gas.
- A nebulizer generates and disperses liquid particles in a gas stream.
- Water vapor cannot carry pathogens, but aerosols and condensate can carry pathogens.
- Temperature is the most important factor affecting humidifier output. The higher the temperature, the greater is the water vapor content of the delivered gas.
- Bubble humidifiers, passover humidifiers, wick humidifiers, and HMEs are the major types of humidifiers. Active humidifiers incorporate heating devices and reservoir and feed systems.
- At high flow rates, some bubble humidifiers can produce microaerosol particles, which can carry infectious bacteria.
- Most HMEs are passive, capturing both heat and moisture from expired gas and returning it to the patient, at approximately 70% efficiency. HMEs are not recommended for use with infants because of the increased mechanical dead space and use of uncuffed ETTs, which allow some exhaled gas to bypass the HME.
- Common problems with humidification systems include condensation, cross contamination, and ensuring proper conditioning of the inspired gas.
- Breathing circuit condensate must always be treated as infectious waste.
- Bland aerosol therapy with sterile water or saline is used to (1) treat upper airway edema, (2) overcome heat and humidity deficits in patients with tracheal airways, and (3) help obtain sputum specimens.
- Large-volume jet nebulizers and USNs are used to generate bland aerosols. Delivery systems include various direct airway appliances and mist tents.
- Common problems with bland aerosol therapy are cross contamination and infection, environmental safety, inadequate mist production, overhydration, bronchospasm, and noise.

References

1. Kapadia F, Shelley M: Normal mechanisms of humidification. *Probl Respir Care* 4:395–402, 1991.
2. Primiano F, Montague F, Saidel G: Measurement system for water vapor and temperature dynamics. *J Appl Physiol* 56:1679–1685, 1984.
3. Shelley M, Lloyd G, Park G: A review of the mechanisms and the methods of humidification of inspired gas. *Intensive Care Med* 14:1–9, 1988.
4. Chalon J, Loew D, Malbranche J: Effects of dry air and subsequent humidification on tracheobronchial ciliated epithelium. *Anesthesiology* 37:338–343, 1972.
5. Marfatia S, Donahoe P, Henderson W: Effect of dry and humidified gases on the respiratory epithelium in rabbits. *J Pediatr Surg* 10:583–592, 1975.
6. Restrepo RD, Walsh BK: Humidification during invasive and noninvasive mechanical ventilation: 2012. *Respir Care* 57:782–788, 2012.
7. Chatburn R, Primiano F: A rational basis for humidity therapy. *Respir Care* 32:249–254, 1987.
8. Anderson S, Herbring B, Widman B: Accidental profound hypothermia. *Br J Anaesth* 42:653–655, 1970.
9. Weinberg A: Hypothermia. *Ann Emerg Med* 22:370–377, 1993.
10. Chen T: The effect of heated humidifier in the prevention of intra-operative hypothermia. *Acta Anaesthesiol Sin* 32:27–30, 1994.
11. Giesbrecht G, Younes M: Exercise and cold-induced asthma. *Can J Appl Physiol* 20:300–314, 1995.
12. American Society for Testing and Materials (ASTM): *Standard specification for humidifiers for medical use (F1690)*, Conshohocken, PA, 1996, ASTM.
13. Gray H: Humidifiers. *Probl Respir Care* 4:423–429, 1991.
14. Darin J, Broadwell J, MacDonell R: An evaluation of water-vapor output from four brands of unheated, prefilled bubble humidifiers. *Respir Care* 27:41–50, 1982.
15. Rhame F, Streifel A, McComb C: Bubbling humidifiers produce microaerosols which can carry bacteria. *Infect Control* 7:403–407, 1986.

16. Fink JB, Ari A: Humidity and aerosol therapy. In *Mosby's respiratory care equipment*, St. Louis, 2013, Mosby.
17. Chiumello D, Pelosi P, Park G, et al: In vitro and in vivo evaluation of a new active heat moisture exchanger. *Crit Care* 8:R281–R288, 2004.
18. Lemmens H, Brock-Utne J: Heat and moisture exchange devices: are they doing what they are supposed to do? *Anesth Analg* 98:382–385, 2004.
19. Thomachot L, Boisson C, Arnaud S, et al: Changing heat and moisture exchangers after 96 hours rather than after 24 hours: a clinical and microbiological evaluation. *Crit Care Med* 28:714–720, 2000.
20. Thomachot L, Leone M, Razzouk K, et al: Randomized clinical trial of extended use of a hydrophobic condenser humidifier: 1 vs. 7 days. *Crit Care Med* 30:232–237, 2002.
21. Boyer A, Thiery G, Lasry S, et al: Long-term mechanical ventilation with hygroscopic heat and moisture exchangers used for 48 hours: a prospective clinical, hygrometric, and bacteriologic study. *Crit Care Med* 31:823–829, 2003.
22. Rathgeber J: Devices used to humidify respired gases. *Respir Care Clin N Am* 12:165–182, 2006.
23. Kapadia F: Changing patterns of airway accidents in intubated ICU patients. *Intensive Care Med* 27:296–300, 2001.
24. Bien S, Okla S, van As-Brooks CJ, et al: The effect of a heat and moisture exchanger (Provox HME) on pulmonary protection after total laryngectomy: a randomized controlled study. *Eur Arch Otorhinolaryngol* 267:429–435, 2010.
25. Hedley R, Allt-Graham J: A comparison of the filtration properties of heat and moisture exchangers. *Anaesthesia* 47:414–420, 1992.
26. Kelly M, Gillies D, Todd DA, et al: Heated humidification versus heat and moisture exchangers for ventilated adults and children. *Cochrane Database Syst Rev* (4):004711, 2010.
27. International Organization for Standardization: *Heat and moisture exchangers for use in humidifying respired gases in humans (ISO 9360)*, Geneva, 1992, International Organization for Standardization.
28. Shelly M: Inspired gas conditioning. *Respir Care* 37:1070–1080, 1992.
29. Lellouche F, Taille S, Lefrancois F, et al: Humidification performance of 48 passive airway humidifiers: comparison with manufacturer data. *Chest* 135: 276–286, 2009.
30. Siempos II, Vardakas KZ, Kopterides P, et al: Impact of passive humidification on clinical outcomes of mechanically ventilated patients: a meta-analysis of randomized controlled trials. *Crit Care Med* 35:2843–2851, 2007.
31. Parmar V: Heat and moisture exchanger: importance of humidification in anaesthesia and ventilatory breathing system. *J Indian Med Assoc* 106:533–535, 537, 2008.
32. Branson R, Davis K: Evaluation of 21 passive humidifiers according to the ISO 9360 standard: moisture output, deadspace, and flow resistance. *Respir Care* 41:736–743, 1996.
33. Ikuta Y, Fujita M, Miyazaki N, et al: Increased airway resistance in the prone position associated with heat and moisture exchangers with integral bacterial/viral filters. *J Anesth* 21:291–292, 2007.
34. Kola A, Eckmanns T, Gastmeier P: Efficacy of heat and moisture exchangers in preventing ventilator-associated pneumonia: meta-analysis of randomized controlled trials. *Intensive Care Med* 31:5–11, 2005.
35. Ricard JD, Boyer A, Dreyfuss D: The effect of humidification on the incidence of ventilator-associated pneumonia. *Respir Care* 12:263–273, 2006.
36. Dreyfuss D: Mechanical ventilation with heated humidifiers or heat and moisture exchangers: effect on patient colonization and incidence of nosocomial pneumonia. *Am J Respir Crit Care Med* 151:986–992, 1995.
37. Lacherade JC, Auburtin M, Cerf C, et al: Impact of humidification systems on ventilator-associated pneumonia: a randomized multicenter trial. *Am J Respir Crit Care Med* 172:1276–1282, 2005.
38. Jean-Claude L: Impact of humidification systems on ventilator-associated pneumonia. *Am J Respir Crit Care Med* 17:1276–1282, 2005.
39. Lorente L, Lecuona M, Jimenez A, et al: Ventilator-associated pneumonia using a heated humidifier or a heat and moisture exchanger: a randomized controlled trial [ISRCTN88724583]. *Crit Care* 10:R116, 2006.
40. Inui D, Oto J, Nishimura M: Effect of heat and moisture exchanger (HME) positioning on inspiratory gas humidification. <http://www.biomedcentral.com/1471-2466/6/19>, 2007, (Accessed September 28, 2015.)
41. Solomita M, Palmer LB, Daroowalla F, et al: Humidification and secretion volume in mechanically ventilated patients. *Respir Care* 54:1329–1335, 2009.
42. Larsson A, Gustafsson A, Svanborg L: A new device for 100 per cent humidification of inspired air. *Crit Care Med* 4:54–60, 2000.
43. Tiffin N, Weinstein L, Sunstein D: The performance of a novel humidification device for mechanical ventilation. European Respiratory Society 16th Annual Congress; 2006; Munich, Germany.
44. Nishida T: Performance of heated humidifiers with a heated wire according to ventilatory settings. *J Aerosol Med* 14:43–51, 2001.
45. Williams R: Relationship between the humidity and temperature of inspired gas and the function of the airway mucosa. *Crit Care Med* 24:1920–1929, 1996.
46. Craven D, Goularte T, Make B: Contaminated condensate in mechanical ventilator circuits: a risk factor for nosocomial pneumonia. *Am Rev Respir Dis* 129:625–628, 1984.
47. Davies MW, Dunster KR, Cartwright DW: Inspired gas temperature in ventilated neonates. *Pediatr Pulmonol* 38:50–54, 2004.
48. Chiumello D, Chierichetti M, Tallarini F, et al: Effect of a heated humidifier during continuous positive airway pressure delivered by a helmet. *Crit Care* 12:R55, 2008.
49. Lellouche F, Maggiore SM, Lyazidi A, et al: Water content of delivered gases during non-invasive ventilation in healthy subjects. *Intensive Care Med* 35:987–995, 2009.
50. Prat G, Renault A, Tonnelier JM, et al: Influence of the humidification device during acute respiratory distress syndrome. *Intensive Care Med* 2912: 2211–2215, 2003.
51. Gilmour I, Boyle M, Streifel A: Humidifiers kill bacteria. *Anesthesiology* 75:498, 1991.
52. Craven D: Risk factors for pneumonia and fatality in patients receiving continuous mechanical ventilation. *Am Rev Respir Dis* 33:792–796, 1986.
53. Kollef M: Mechanical ventilation with or without 7-day circuit changes: a randomized controlled study. *Ann Intern Med* 123:168–174, 1995.
54. Fink J: Extending ventilator circuit change interval beyond two days reduces the likelihood of ventilator associated pneumonia (VAP). *Chest* 113:405–411, 1998.
55. Beydon L: Correlation between simple clinical parameters and the in vitro humidification characteristics of filter heat and moisture exchangers. *Chest* 112:739–744, 1997.
56. Kallstrom T, American Association for Respiratory Care: Clinical practice guideline: bland aerosol administration, 2003 revision and update. *Respir Care* 5:529–533, 2003.
57. Hill T, Sorbello J: Humidity outputs of large-reservoir nebulizers. *Respir Care* 32:225–260, 1987.
58. Loh L, Eg K, Puspanathan P, et al: A comparison of sputum induction methods: ultrasonic vs compressed-air nebulizer and hypertonic vs isotonic saline inhalation. *Asian Pac J Allergy Immunol* 1:11–17, 2004.
59. Chatburn R, Lough M, Klinger J: An in-hospital evaluation of the sonic mist ultrasonic room humidifier. *Respir Care* 29:893–899, 1984.
60. Kugelman A, Amirav I, Mor F, et al: Hood versus mask nebulization in infants with evolving bronchopulmonary dysplasia in the neonatal intensive care unit. *J Perinatol* 26:31–36, 2006.
61. Anderson C, Inhaber N, Menzies D: Comparison of sputum induction with fiberoptic bronchoscopy in the diagnosis of tuberculosis. *Am J Respir Crit Care Med* 152:1570–1574, 1995.
62. Godwin C, Brown D, Masur H: Sputum induction: a quick and sensitive technique for diagnosing *Pneumocystis carinii* pneumonia in immunosuppressed patients. *Respir Care* 36:33–39, 1991.
63. Gershman N: Comparison of two methods of collecting induced sputum in asthmatic subjects. *Eur Respir J* 9:2448–2453, 1996.
64. Dimich-Ward H, Wymer ML, Chan-Yeung M: Respiratory health survey of respiratory therapists. *Chest* 126:1048–1053, 2004.
65. American College of Chest Physicians, National Heart, Lung and Blood Institute: National Conference on Oxygen Therapy. *Respir Care* 29:922–935, 1984.

CHAPTER 39

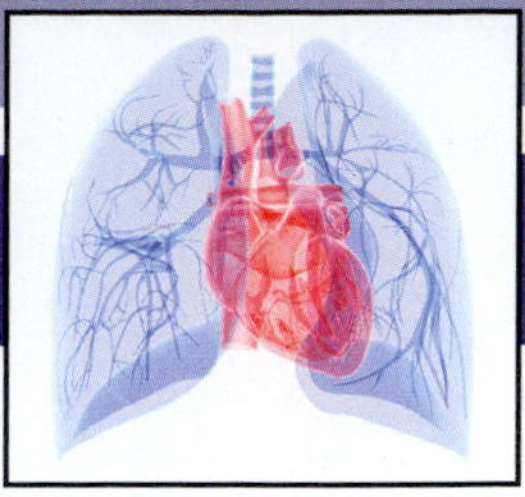

Aerosol Drug Therapy

JAMES B. FINK AND ARZU ARI

CHAPTER OBJECTIVES

After reading this chapter you will be able to:

- Define the term *aerosol*.
- Describe how particle size, motion, and airway characteristics affect aerosol deposition.
- Describe how aerosols are generated.
- List the hazards associated with aerosol drug therapy.
- Describe how to select the best aerosol drug delivery system for a patient.
- Describe how to initiate and modify aerosol drug therapy.
- State the information patients need to know to self-administer drug aerosol therapy properly.
- Describe how to assess patient response to bronchodilator therapy at the point of care.
- Describe how to apply aerosol therapy in special circumstances.
- Describe how to protect patients and caregivers from exposure to aerosolized drugs.

CHAPTER OUTLINE

KEY TERMS

aerosol
aerosol output
aging
atomizer
baffle
breath-actuated nebulizer
breath-enhanced nebulizer
chlorofluorocarbons (CFCs)
deposition
emitted dose
fine-particle fraction
geometric standard deviation (GSD)
heterodisperse
hydrofluoroalkane (HFA)
hygroscopic
inertial impaction
inhaled mass
mass median aerodynamic diameter (MMAD)
monodisperse
nebulizer
propellant
residual drug volume
respirable mass
scintigraphy
sedimentation
therapeutic index
volume median diameter (VMD)

An **aerosol** is a suspension of solid or liquid particles in gas. Aerosols occur in nature as pollens, spores, dust, smoke, smog, fog, and mist.[1] The upper airway and respiratory tract filter out larger particles to protect the lungs from invasion by these aerosols. In the clinical setting, medical aerosols are generated with **atomizers**, **nebulizers**, and inhalers. Aerosols can be used to deliver bland water solutions to the respiratory tract (see Chapter 38) or to administer drugs to the lungs, throat, or nose for local and systemic effect. This chapter focuses on the principles of medical aerosol drug therapy.

The aim of aerosol therapy is to deliver a therapeutic dose of the selected agent (drug) to the desired site of action (nose, throat, airways, or deep lung). The indication for any specific aerosol is based on the need for the specific drug.[1] Administration of drugs by aerosol offers higher local drug concentrations in the lung with lower systemic levels compared with other forms of administration. Improved therapeutic action with fewer systemic side effects provides a higher **therapeutic index**.[2]

CHARACTERISTICS OF THERAPEUTIC AEROSOLS

Effective use of medical aerosols requires an understanding of the characteristics of aerosols and their effect on drug delivery to the desired site of action. Key concepts include aerosol output, particle size, deposition, and changes in the aerosol over time (*aging*).

Aerosol Output

Aerosol output is the mass of fluid or drug produced by an aerosol generator. Output is described as the mass of drug or liquid emitted (leaving) from the aerosol generator. For nebulizers the output rate is the mass of aerosol generated per unit of time. Output varies greatly among different nebulizers and inhalers. For drug delivery systems, **emitted dose** describes the mass of drug leaving the mouthpiece of a nebulizer or inhaler as aerosol.

Aerosol output can be measured by collecting the aerosol that leaves the nebulizer on filters and measuring either their weight (gravimetric analysis) or quantity of drug (assay). Gravimetric measurements of aerosols are easier but less reliable than drug assay techniques because weight changes with water evaporation while drug mass does not. A drug assay provides the most reliable measure of aerosol output.

A large proportion of particles that leave a nebulizer may never reach the lungs. The ability of aerosols to travel through the air, enter the airways, and become deposited in the lungs is based on numerous variables ranging from particle size to breathing pattern. Understanding and skillful manipulation of these variables can greatly improve pulmonary delivery of aerosols.

Particle Size

Aerosol particle size depends on the substance for nebulization, the method used to generate the aerosol, and the environmental conditions surrounding the particle.[3] It is impossible to determine visually whether a nebulizer is producing an optimal particle size. The unaided human eye cannot see particles less than 50 to 100 μm in diameter (equivalent to a small grain of sand). The only reliable way to determine the characteristics of an aerosol suspension is laboratory measurement. The two most common laboratory methods used to measure medical aerosol particle size distribution are cascade impaction and laser diffraction. *Cascade impactors* are designed to collect aerosols of different size ranges on a series of stages or plates. The mass of aerosol deposited on each plate is quantified by drug assay, and a distribution of drug mass across particle sizes is calculated. In *laser diffraction,* a computer is used to estimate the range and frequency of droplet volumes crossing the laser beam.

Because medical aerosols contain particles of many different sizes (**heterodisperse**), the average particle size is expressed with a measure of central tendency, such as **mass median aerodynamic diameter (MMAD)** for cascade impaction or **volume median diameter (VMD)** for laser diffraction. These measurement techniques of the same aerosol may report different sizes, so it is important to know which measurement is used. The MMAD and VMD both describe the particle diameter in micrometers (μm). In an aerosol distribution with a specific MMAD, 50% of the particles are smaller and have less mass, and 50% are larger and have greater mass.

The **geometric standard deviation (GSD)** describes the variability of particle sizes in an aerosol distribution set at 1 standard deviation above or below the median (15.8% and 84.13%). Most aerosols found in nature and used in respiratory care are composed of particles of different sizes, described as heterodisperse. The greater the GSD, the wider the range of particle sizes, and the more heterodisperse the aerosol. Aerosols consisting of particles of similar size (GSD ≤1.2) are referred to as **monodisperse**. Nebulizers that produce monodisperse aerosols are used mainly in laboratory research and in nonmedical industries.

Deposition

When aerosol particles leave suspension in gas, they deposit on (attach to) a surface. Only a portion of the aerosol generated and emitted from a nebulizer (emitted dose) may be inhaled (inhaled dose). A fraction of the inhaled dose is deposited in the lungs (respirable dose). **Inhaled mass** is the amount of drug inhaled. The proportion of the drug mass in particles that are small enough **(fine-particle fraction)** to reach the lower respiratory tract is the **respirable mass.** Not all aerosol particles delivered to the lung are retained, or deposited. A small percentage (1% to 5%) of inhaled drug may be exhaled. Whether aerosol particles that are inhaled into the lung are deposited in the respiratory tract depends on the size, shape, and motion of the particles and on the physical characteristics of the airways and breathing pattern. Key mechanisms of aerosol **deposition** include inertial impaction, gravimetric sedimentation, and brownian diffusion.[1,3]

Inertial Impaction

Inertial impaction occurs when suspended particles in motion collide with and are deposited on a surface; this is the primary deposition mechanism for particles larger than 5 μm. The greater the mass and velocity of a moving object, the greater its inertia, and the greater the tendency of that object to continue moving along its set path (Figure 39-1). When a particle of sufficient (large) mass is moving in a gas stream and that stream changes direction, the particle tends to remain on its initial path and collide with the airway surface.

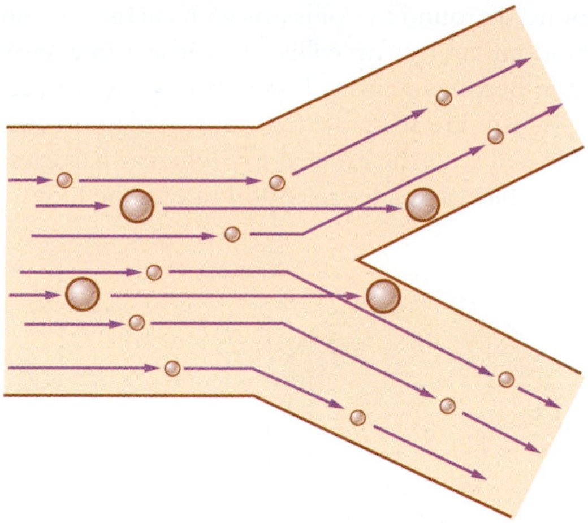

FIGURE 39-1 Inertial impaction of large particles, the masses of which tend to maintain their motion in straight lines. As airway direction changes, the particles are deposited on nearby walls. Smaller particles are carried around corners by the airstream and fall out less readily.

Because inertia involves both mass and velocity, the higher the flow of a gas stream, the greater the tendency for particles to impact and be deposited in the airways. Turbulent flow patterns, obstructed or tortuous pathways, and inspiratory flow rates greater than 30 L/min are associated with increased inertial impaction. Turbulent flow and convoluted passageways in the nose cause most particles larger than 10 μm to impact and become deposited. This process produces an effective filter that protects the lower airway from particulates such as dust and pollen. However, particles 5 to 10 μm tend to become deposited in the oropharynx and hypopharynx, especially with the turbulence created by the transition of air as it passes around the tongue and into the larynx.

Sedimentation

Sedimentation occurs when aerosol particles settle out of suspension and are deposited owing to gravity. The greater the mass of the particle, the faster it settles (Figure 39-2). During normal breathing, sedimentation is the primary mechanism for deposition of particles 1 to 5 μm. Sedimentation occurs mostly in the central airways and increases with time, affecting particles 1 μm in diameter. Breath holding after inhalation of an aerosol increases the residence time for the particles in the lung and enhances distribution across the lungs and sedimentation. A 10-second breath hold can increase aerosol deposition 10% and increase the ratio of aerosol deposited in lung parenchyma to central airway by fourfold.[4]

Diffusion

Brownian diffusion is the primary mechanism for deposition of small particles (<3 μm), mainly in the respiratory region where bulk gas flow ceases and most aerosol particles reach the alveoli by diffusion. These aerosol particles have very low mass and are easily bounced around by collisions with carrier gas molecules. These random molecular collisions cause some particles to contact and become deposited on surrounding surfaces. Particles 1 to 0.5 μm are so stable that most remain in suspension and are cleared with the exhaled gas, whereas particles smaller than 0.5 μm have a greater retention rate in the lungs.

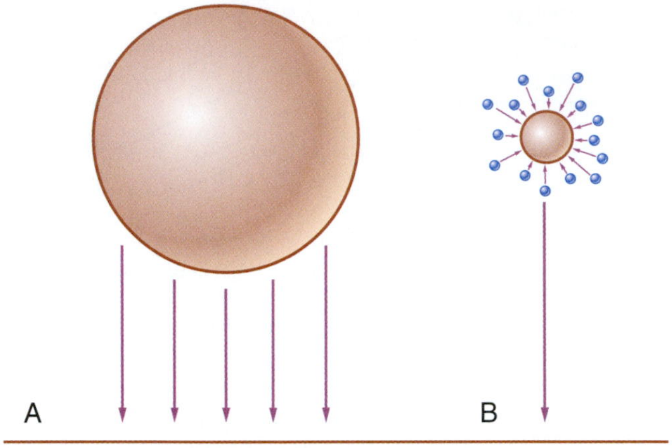

FIGURE 39-2 Effect of mass on particle size. Large particles **(A)** are more susceptible to the force of gravity than smaller particles **(B),** which are more affected by the bombardment of molecules deposited by diffusion.

Figure 39-3 summarizes the relationships between particle size and aerosol deposition in the respiratory tract. The depth of penetration and deposition of a particle in the respiratory tract tend to vary with size and tidal volume (V_T).[5] With this knowledge, it may be possible to target aerosol deposition to specific areas of the lung by using the proper particle size and breathing pattern.

RULE OF THUMB

The site of deposition in the respiratory tract varies with the size of the particle. Use of nebulizers that produce particles in a specific size range improves the targeting of aerosols for deposition to a desired site in the respiratory tract, as follows:

Desired Location	Recommended MMAD
Upper airway: nose, larynx, trachea	5 to >50 μm
Lower airways	2 to 5 μm
Parenchyma: alveolar region	1 to 3 μm
Parenchyma	<0.1 μm

Aging

Aerosols are dynamic suspensions. Individual particles constantly grow, shrink, coalesce, and fall out of suspension. The

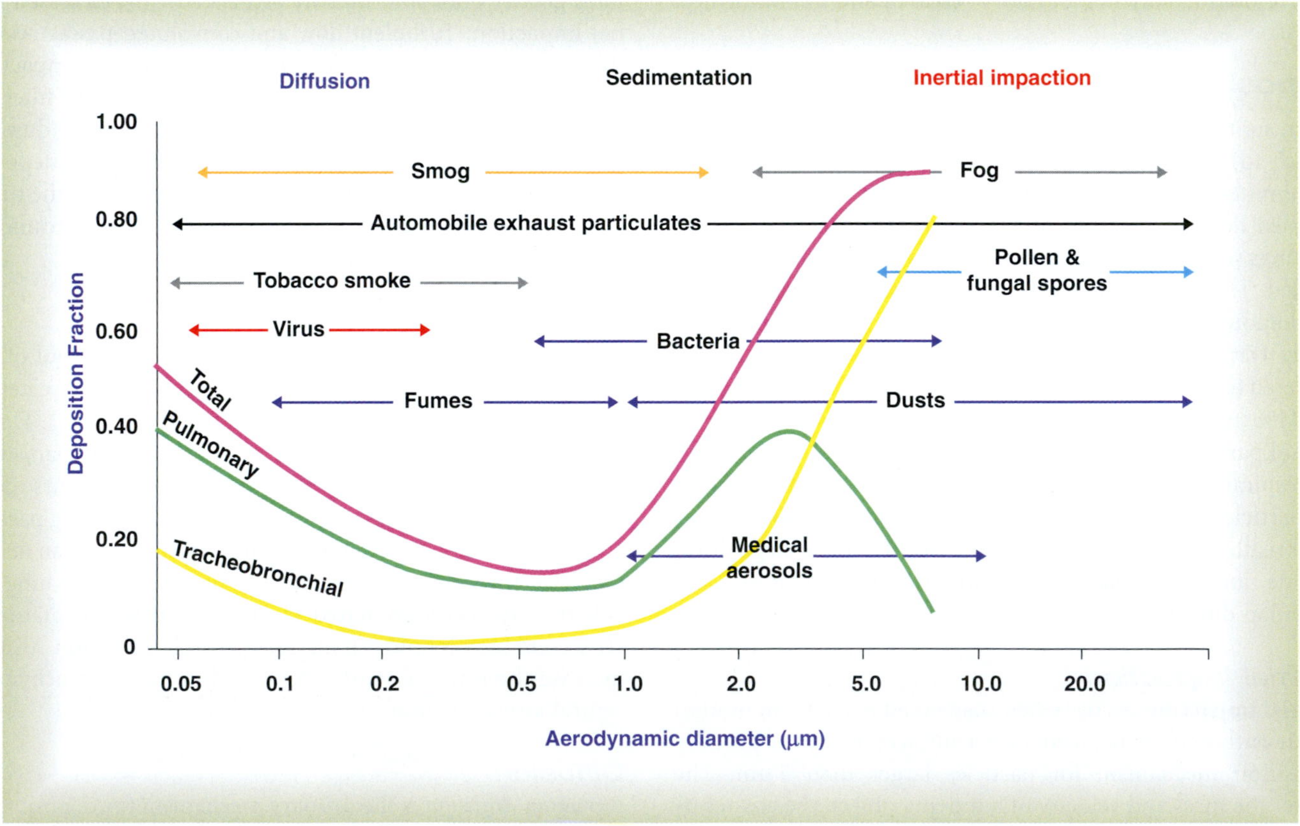

FIGURE 39-3 Range of particle size for common aerosols in the environment and the influence of inertial impactions, sedimentation, and diffusion. (Modified from Yu CP, Nicolaides P, Soong TT, et al: Effect of random airway sizes on aerosol deposition. Am Ind Hyg Assoc J 40:999, 1979.)

process by which an aerosol suspension changes over time is called **aging**. How an aerosol ages depends on the composition of the aerosol, the initial size of its particles, the time in suspension, and the ambient conditions to which it is exposed.

Aerosol particles can change size as a result of either evaporation or **hygroscopic** water absorption. The relative rate of particle size change is inversely proportional to the size of a particle, so small particles grow or shrink faster than large particles. Small water-based particles shrink when exposed to relatively dry gas. Aerosols of water-soluble materials, especially salts, tend to be hygroscopic, absorbing water and growing when introduced into a high-humidity environment.[5]

Particle size is not the only determinant of deposition. Inspiratory flow rate, flow pattern, respiratory rate, inhaled volume, ratio of inspiratory time to expiratory time (I : E ratio), and breath holding all influence where a particle of any specific size is deposited. The presence of airway obstruction is one of the greatest factors influencing aerosol deposition. It has been shown that total pulmonary deposition is greater in smokers and patients with obstructive airway disease than in healthy persons (Figure 39-4). Similarly, when inspiratory flow rates are constant, the deposition fraction of monodisperse aerosols increases with increased V_T, length of inspiration, and particle size (Figure 39-5).

These dynamic variables make it difficult to predict exactly what occurs to aerosol particles when they enter a gas stream and are inhaled. For this reason, prediction of actual aerosol deposition for an individual patient is difficult.

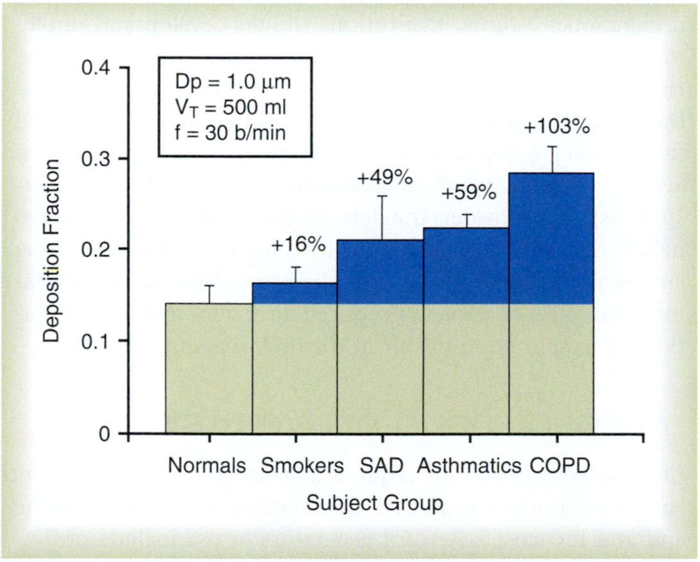

FIGURE 39-4 Total lung deposition of a fine aerosol of particles 1 µm in diameter in healthy adults and in subjects with obstructive airway disease. Numbers over the bar indicate the percentage increase above normal value. *COPD,* Patients with chronic obstructive pulmonary disease; *Dp,* particle diameter; *SAD,* smoker with symptoms of small airways disease; *f,* respiratory rate; *V_T,* tidal volume. (Modified from Kim CS: Methods of calculating lung delivery and deposition of aerosol particles. Respir Care 45:695, 2000.)

Quantifying Aerosol Delivery

As mentioned in the preceding sections, many characteristics of aerosols can account for the variances in quantity of aerosolized medication delivered to the patient. Although the precise amount of drug delivered to the patient's airways can be difficult to determine, it can be measured in terms of the patient's clinical response to aerosol drug therapy, including the desired therapeutic effects and any unwanted adverse effects. The amount of aerosol deposited to a patient's airways can be quantified using specialized equipment and tests.

One approach used to quantify aerosol deposition (in vivo) involves **scintigraphy**, in which a drug is "tagged" with a radioactive substance (e.g., technetium), aerosolized, and inhaled. A scanner (similar to scanners used in nuclear medicine) measures the distribution and intensity of radiation across the device and the patient's head and thorax. The result is a radiation map of aerosol deposition in the upper airway, the lungs (central and peripheral airways), and the stomach. This information is used to calculate the percentage of drug retained by the device and delivered to various areas in the patient.[6]

A less direct approach relates the systemic pharmocokinetic profile of a drug delivered by aerosol to an assay of the drug in a patient's blood or urine over time. This method does not estimate actual lung delivery, but it provides insight into systemic drug levels achieved after aerosol administration. Care must be taken to differentiate drug absorbed through the lungs from drug absorbed through the gastrointestinal tract. Simple laboratory, or in vitro, models, which simulate a range of V_T values, inspiratory flow rates, I : E ratios, and respiratory rates, have been useful in predicting inhaled mass of drug and relative performance of nebulizers.[7]

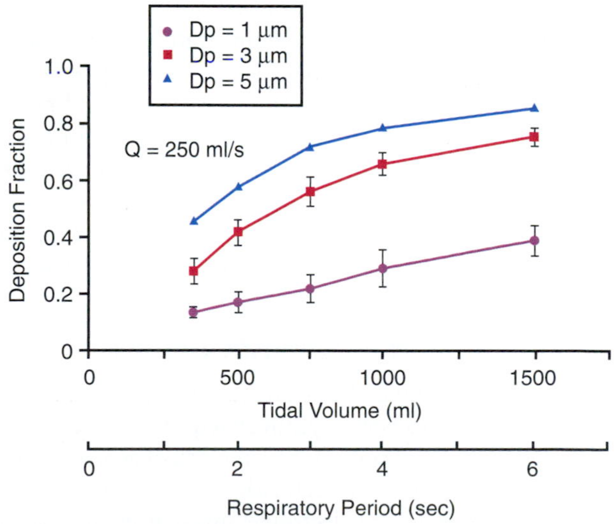

FIGURE 39-5 Total lung deposition versus V_T and respiratory time at a fixed flow: respiratory flow (Q) = 250 ml/sec. *Dp,* Particle diameter. (Modified from Kim CS: Methods of calculating lung delivery and deposition of aerosol particles. Respir Care 45:695, 2000.)

HAZARDS OF AEROSOL THERAPY

The primary hazard of aerosol drug therapy is an adverse reaction to the medication being administered (see Chapter 35). Other hazards to the patient include infection, airway reactivity, systemic effects of bland aerosols, drug concentration, and eye irritation. Care providers and bystanders risk these hazards as a result of exposure to secondhand aerosol drugs.

Infection

Aerosol generators can contribute to nosocomial infections by spreading bacteria by the airborne route.[8] The most common sources of bacteria are patient secretions, contaminated solutions (i.e., multiple-dose drug vials), and caregivers' hands. Offending organisms are primarily gram-negative bacilli, in particular, *Pseudomonas aeruginosa* and *Legionella pneumophila* (the cause of the highly virulent legionnaires' disease).[9]

Various procedures can help reduce contamination and infection associated with respiratory care equipment. Guidelines from the U.S. Centers for Disease Control and Prevention (CDC) state that nebulizers should be sterilized between patients, frequently replaced with disinfected or sterile units, or rinsed with sterile water (not tap water) and air dried every 24 hours (see Chapter 4). In addition, some recommend one nebulizer for one treatment. The cystic fibrosis foundation recommends that standard small volume nebulizers should be discarded after each treatment to prevent infection in cystic fibrosis patients.

Airway Reactivity

Cold air and high-density aerosols can cause reactive bronchospasm and increased airway resistance, especially in patients with preexisting respiratory disease.[10] Medications such as acetylcysteine, antibiotics, steroids, cromolyn sodium, ribavirin, and distilled water have been associated with increased airway resistance and wheezing during aerosol therapy. Administration of bronchodilators before or with administration of these agents may reduce the risk or duration of increased airway resistance.

The risk of inducing bronchospasm always should be considered when aerosols are administered. Monitoring for reactive bronchospasm should include auscultation for adventitious breath sounds; observation of the patient's breathing pattern and overall appearance before and after therapy; and, most essential, communicating with the patient during therapy to determine the perceived work of breathing.

Pulmonary and Systemic Effects

Pulmonary and systemic effects are associated with the site of delivery and the drug being administered. Preliminary assessment should balance the need versus the risk of aerosol therapy, especially among patients at high risk, such as infants, patients who are prone to fluid and electrolyte imbalances, and patients with atelectasis or pulmonary edema. For patients unable to clear their own secretions, suctioning or other airway clearance techniques may be indicated as an adjunct to aerosol therapy. Care must be taken to ensure that patients are capable of clearing secretions when the secretions are mobilized by aerosol therapy. Appropriate airway clearance techniques should accompany any aerosol therapy designed to help mobilize secretions (see Chapter 43).

Drug Concentration

During nebulization, the evaporation, heating, baffling, and recycling of drug solutions undergoing jet or ultrasonic nebulization increase solute concentrations.[11] This process can expose the patient to increasingly higher concentrations of the drug over the course of therapy and result in a larger concentration of drug remaining in the nebulizer at the end of therapy. This increase in concentration usually is time-dependent; the greatest effect occurs when nebulization of medications occurs over extended periods, as in continuous aerosol drug delivery.

Eye Irritation

Aerosol administration via a face mask may deposit drug in the eyes and cause eye irritation. In very rare cases, anticholinergic medications (see Chapter 35) have been suspected to worsen preexisting eye conditions, such as forms of glaucoma. Caution should be exercised when a face mask is used during aerosol drug therapy. In addition, special mask designs that have been shown to reduce drug deposition in the eyes or mouthpieces should be considered for at-risk patients.[12,13]

Secondhand Exposure to Aerosol Drugs

Workplace exposure to aerosols may be detectable in the plasma of bystanders and health care providers. Repeated secondhand exposure to bronchodilators is associated with increased risk of occupational asthma. Institutions should develop and implement an occupational health and safety policy to minimize the risk of secondhand aerosol exposure for care providers and bystanders.[14-16] Implementation of an occupational health and safety policy could include using systems that introduce less aerosol to the atmosphere (pressurized metered dose inhalers [pMDIs], dry powder inhalers [DPIs], and breath-actuated nebulizers), filtering exhalation to contain aerosol, and using environmental controls. Unless filters are placed in the expiratory limb, 40% of aerosols produced during mechanical ventilation are exhausted to the air of the intensive care unit.[17]

AEROSOL DRUG DELIVERY SYSTEMS

Effective aerosol therapy requires a device that quickly delivers sufficient drug to the desired site of action with minimal waste and at a low cost.[18] Aerosol generators in use include pMDIs with or without spacers or VHCs, DPIs, small and large volume (jet) nebulizers, hand-bulb atomizers (including nasal spray pumps), ultrasonic nebulizers (USNs), and vibrating mesh (VM) nebulizers as well as numerous emerging technologies.[2]

Pressurized Metered Dose Inhalers

The pMDI is the most commonly prescribed method of aerosol delivery in the United States. The pMDI is portable, compact, and easy to use and provides multidose convenience. A uniform dose of drug is dispensed within a fraction of a second after actuation and is reproducible throughout the canister life. The pMDI and actuator are designed for the specific drug formulation and dose volume to be delivered. The pMDI is used to administer bronchodilators, anticholinergics, and steroids. More formulations of these drugs are available for use by pMDIs than for use with nebulizers. When properly used, pMDIs are at least as effective as other nebulizers for drug delivery. For this reason, pMDIs often are the preferred method for delivering bronchodilators to spontaneously breathing patients and patients who are intubated and undergoing mechanical ventilation.[19,20]

Although pMDIs have a relatively easy-to-use design, patients commonly misuse them during therapy. Most pMDIs are "press and breathe," but there is increasing presence of a variation known as *breath-actuated pMDIs*. The basic components of pMDI are similar regardless of type, manufacturer, or active ingredient; commonly used pMDIs are shown in Figure 39-6.

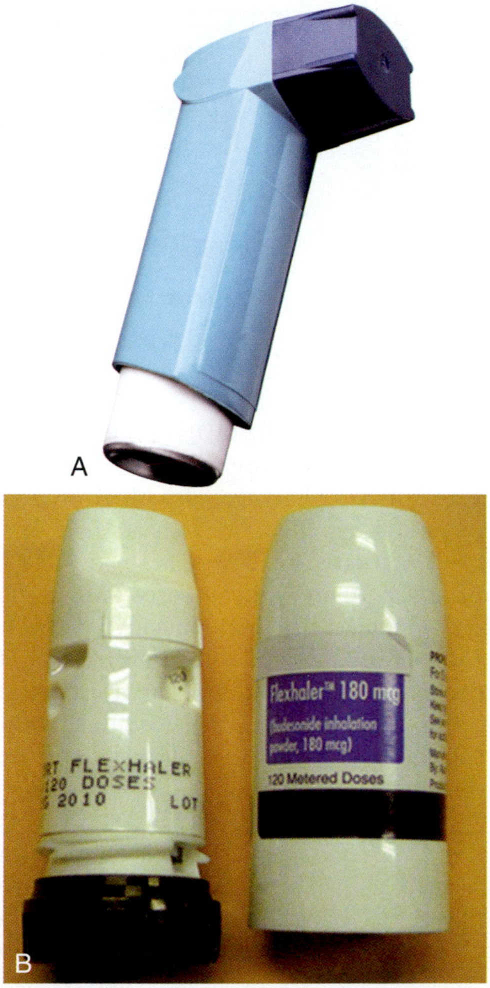

FIGURE 39-6 Examples of commonly used pMDIs. **A,** Albuterol inhaler **B,** The ASMANEX TWISTHALER. (**A,** Courtesy Hemera, Thinkstock. **B,** Reproduced with permission of Schering Corporation, subsidiary of Merck & Co. All rights reserved. ASMANEX and TWISTHALER are registered trademarks of Schering Corporation.)

The pMDI appears to be a simple device, but it represents sophisticated technology and engineering. A pMDI is a pressurized canister that contains the prescribed drug (a micronized powder or aqueous solution) in a volatile **propellant** combined with a surfactant and dispersing agent (Figure 39-7). When the canister is inverted (nozzle down) and placed in its actuator, or "boot," the volatile suspension fills a metering chamber that controls the amount of drug delivered. Pressing down on the canister aligns a hole in the metering valve with the metering chamber. The high propellant vapor pressure quickly forces the metered dose out through this hole and through the actuator nozzle.

Aerosol production takes approximately 20 msec. As the liquid suspension is forced out of the pMDI, it forms a plume, within which the propellants vaporize. Initially, the velocity of this plume is high (approximately 15 m/sec). However, within 0.1 second, the plume velocity decreases to less than half its maximum as the plume moves away from the actuator nozzle. At the same time, propellant evaporation causes the initially large particles (35 μm) generated at the actuator orifice to decrease rapidly in size.

The output volume of pMDIs ranges from 30 to 100 mcl. Approximately 60% to 80% by weight of this spray consists of the propellant, with only approximately 1% being active drug (50 mcg to 5 mg, depending on the drug formulation). For a

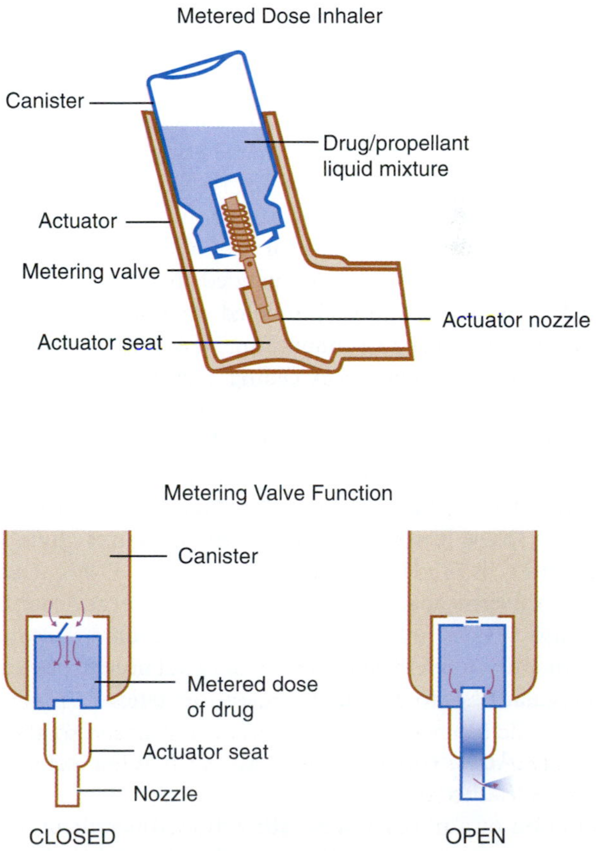

FIGURE 39-7 Components of a pMDI, including function of the metering valve. (From Gardenhire DS: Rau's respiratory care pharmacology, ed 8, St. Louis, 2012, Mosby.)

chlorofluorocarbon (CFC) pMDI used in a standard actuator, loss of drug in the valve stem housing and on the actuator mouthpiece amounts to 10% to 15% of the nominal dose from the metering valve.

From their inception in the mid-1950s to the beginning of the twenty-first century, **chlorofluorocarbons (CFCs)** such as Freon were the propellants used in pMDIs. Manufacture of CFCs for most applications has now been prohibited because of the effect of these compounds on global warming, with a period of transition provided for pMDIs. A consortium of eight pharmaceutical companies developed **hydrofluoroalkane (HFA)**-134a to be more environment-friendly and possibly clinically safer than CFCs.[21] Redesign of key components of the pMDI has resulted in improved performance.[22]

In addition to the propellant, pMDIs use dispersal agents to improve drug delivery by keeping the drug in suspension. The most common dispersal agents are surfactants, such as soy lecithin, sorbitan trioleate, and oleic acid. These agents help keep the drug suspended in the propellant and lubricate the valve mechanism but may also cause adverse responses (coughing or wheezing) in some patients.

Every pMDI should be primed by shaking and actuating the device to atmosphere one to four times (see label for the specific device) before initial use and after storage. Without priming, the initial dose actuated from a new pMDI canister contains less active substance than subsequent actuations.[23] This "loss of dose" from a pMDI occurs when drug particles rise to the top of the canister over time ("cream"). A reduction in emitted dose with the first actuation commonly occurs with a pMDI after storage, particularly with the valve pointed in the downward position. Loss of prime is related to valve design and occurs when propellant leaks out of the metering chamber during periods of nonuse (e.g., 4 hours). The result is reduced pressure and drug released with the next actuation.[23] Improved designs of metering valves developed for use with HFA propellants reduce these losses. It is recommended that a single dose be wasted before the next dose is inhaled when a CFC pMDI has not been used for 4 to 6 hours. An HFA pMDI requires no wasting of dose for periods exceeding 2 days.

New Pressurized Metered Dose Inhaler Technologies

Aerospan™. The Aerospan™ (Meda Pharmaceuticals, Somerset, New Jersey) was developed to deliver flunisolide hemhydrate as an HFA formulation (Figure 39-8). It has a built-in valveless spacer that improves hand-breath coordination. Also, it does not have a built-in dose counter. According to the manufacturer, the Aerospan™ does not need to be cleaned on a regular basis to maintain proper orientation.

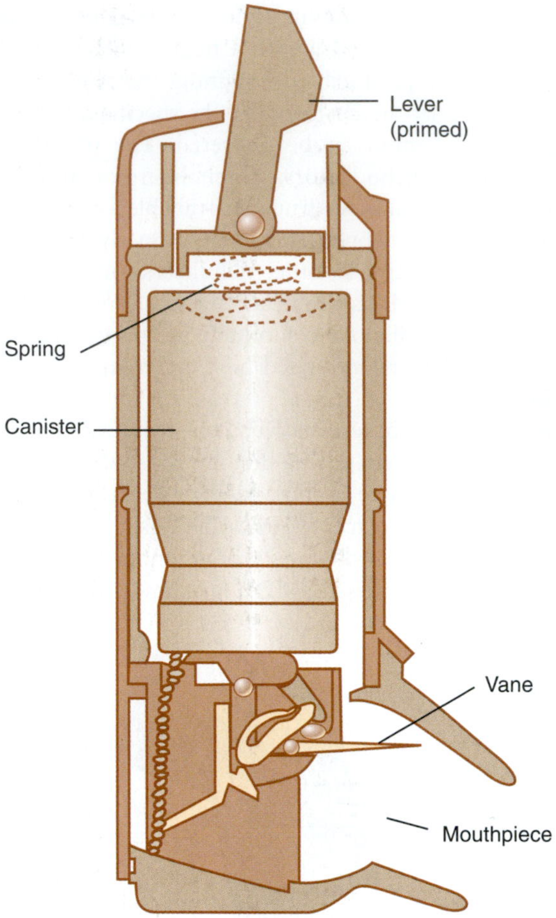

FIGURE 39-8 New pressurized metered dose inhaler (pMDI) technologies.

Breath-Actuated Pressurized Metered Dose Inhaler

A variation of a pMDI is a **breath-actuated nebulizer**, which incorporates a trigger that is activated during inhalation. The trigger theoretically reduces the need for the patient or caregiver to coordinate pMDI actuation with inhalation.[24] Evaluation of the efficacy of breath-actuated pMDIs in children younger than 6 years is limited, and their use should be restricted to older children and adults. Oropharyngeal deposition of steroids using these devices is still very high.

New Breath-Actuated pMDIs

Tempo Inhaler. A new generation of pMDIs such as the Tempo (MAP Pharmaceuticals, Mountain View, CA) have been designed to be breath actuated with lower force of the plume exiting the mouthpiece, reducing oropharyngeal deposition and increasing lung dose. It is used for the treatment of migraines and is seeking approval from the U.S. Food and Drug Administration (FDA).

RULE OF THUMB

- A pMDI has a press-and-breath design; a breath-actuated pMDI incorporates a trigger that is activated with inspiration.
- Before initial use and after storage, every pMDI should be primed by shaking and actuating the device to atmosphere one to four times, depending on the label.

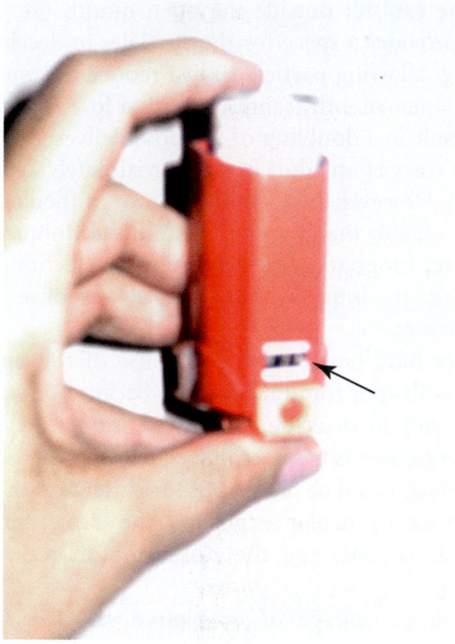

FIGURE 39-9 Dose counters may be mounted on the top of a pMDI canister integrated in the actuator boot.

MINI CLINI

Using Universal Pressurized Metered Dose Inhaler Actuator or Boot

PROBLEM: The association of CFCs with degradation of the earth's atmosphere and the ozone layer has resulted in an international treaty banning use of these compounds. As HFAs become the propellants of choice, a problem arises. If the CFC and HFA drug formulations are bioequivalent, can these compounds be used with the same (universal) pMDI actuator, or boot?

Discussion: In the case of HFA-based albuterol (e.g., Proventil HFA), the operating pressure and stem orifice differ from those used for the CFC formulation. The result is different plume geometries. When HFA albuterol is used in a universal adapter designed for CFC albuterol, the MMAD and GSD are greatly increased. The result is that significantly less drug is available to the patient. When possible, accessory devices that are used in the manufacturer's boot with the pMDI should be selected. If these devices are unavailable, the universal adapter device that is available should be evaluated to determine how much additional dose may be required to provide an equivalent dose through a third-party adapter.

Dose Counters

A serious limitation of pMDIs is the lack of a "counter" to indicate the number of doses remaining in the canister. After the number of label doses has been administered, the pMDI may seem to give another 20 to 60 doses, which may deliver little or no medications as the doses "tail-off." The *tail-off effect* refers to variability in the amount of drug dispensed toward the end of the life of the canister. The result of tail-off is swings from normal to almost no dose emitted from one breath to the next with no reliable indicator to the user. Without a dose counter, there is no viable method to determine remaining drug in a pMDI other than manually keeping a log of every dose taken. The FDA is requiring all new pMDIs to have counter technology to track pMDI actuations remaining. Third-party dose counters may be added to older pMDI models but may not have the accuracy of built-in technology (Figure 39-9).

Factors Affecting Pressurized Metered Dose Inhaler Performance and Drug Delivery

Temperature. Low temperature (<10° C) decreases the output of CFC pMDIs. Patients with cold air–induced bronchospasm who keep their pMDIs in outer coat pockets when outside in cold winter weather may receive only a small percentage of drug compared with that administered with the same pMDI at 25° C. This problem has been less serious with the newer HFA pMDIs.[23]

Nozzle Size and Cleanliness. Aerosol drug delivery is influenced by nozzle size and cleanliness. Nozzle size is pMDI-specific. As debris builds up on the nozzle or actuator orifice, the emitted dose is reduced.[24] Manufacturer recommendations should be followed for cleaning. pMDI canisters should never be placed under water.

Priming. Priming is defined as shaking the device and releasing one or more sprays into the air when the pMDI is new or has not been used for awhile. It is done to mix the drug and the propellant, which can separate in the canister over time. Priming is required to provide an adequate dose, according to the manufacturer's guidelines.

Timing of Actuation Intervals. Manufacturers recommend 30 seconds to 1 minute between actuations. When propellants are released, the device cools, changing aerosol output. The pause allows the device to return to room temperature and recover normal output. However, previous research[25] showed that pMDI output is similar at 15-second intervals. Very rapid actuation of multiple puffs per breath reduces inhaled drug per puff.

Aerosol Delivery Characteristics

Although pMDIs can produce particles in the respirable range (MMAD 2 to 6 μm),[23] the initial velocity and dispersion of the aerosol plume generate larger particles that decrease in size as they leave the pMDI, resulting in approximately 80% of the dose leaving the actuator to impact and become deposited in the oropharynx. A significant proportion of this oropharyngeal deposition is swallowed and may be a factor in systemic absorption of some drugs. Pulmonary deposition ranges from 10% to 20% in adults and larger children (less in infants).[26] The exact amount of drug delivered to an individual patient is unpredictable because of high variability between patients and because pMDI drug administration is technique-dependent.

Box 39-1 Optimal Technique for Use of a Pressurized Metered Dose Inhaler

1. Warm the pMDI canister to hand or body temperature, and shake it vigorously.
2. Before first use of a new pMDI and when the pMDI has not been used for several days, prime the pMDI by pointing it into the air (away from people) and actuating a couple of times.
3. Assemble the apparatus and uncap the mouthpiece, ensuring there are no loose objects in the device.
4. Open-mouth technique: Open your mouth wide, keeping tongue down. Hold the pMDI with the canister oriented downward and the outlet aimed at your mouth. Position the pMDI approximately 4 cm (two fingerbreadths) away from your mouth.
5. Closed-mouth technique: Place mouthpiece between lips, with tongue out of the path of the outlet.
6. Breathe out normally.
7. As you slowly begin to breathe in (<0.5 L/sec), actuate the pMDI.
8. Continue inspiration to total lung capacity.
9. Hold your breath for up to 10 seconds. Then relax and breathe normally.
10. Wait 1 minute between puffs.
11. Disassemble the apparatus, and recap the mouthpiece.

Technique

The successful administration of aerosol drugs by pMDI is highly technique-dependent. Two-thirds of patients and health care professionals who teach pMDI use do not perform the procedure properly.[27] Box 39-1 outlines the recommended steps for self-administering a bronchodilator by pMDI. Patient instruction should last 10 to 30 minutes and should include demonstration, practice, and confirmation of patient performance (demonstration pMDIs with placebo are available from manufacturers for this purpose). Repeated instruction improves performance; repeat instruction is done most appropriately with follow-up clinic or home visits. Demonstration and return demonstration must occur several times for best patient adherence to device use.

For best effect, the pMDI should be actuated once at the beginning of inspiration. Common hand-breath coordination problems include actuating the pMDI before or after the breath. Some patients, especially infants, young children, elderly adults, and patients in acute distress, may be unable to coordinate actuation of the pMDI with inspiration. Some patients exhibit a "cold Freon effect," which occurs when the cold aerosol plume reaches the back of the mouth and the patient stops inhaling. All of these problems reduce aerosol delivery to the lung to the point that the patient does not benefit from the medication, but they can be corrected entirely or in part by use of the proper pMDI accessory device.

Most pMDI labels call for placing the mouthpiece between the lips. However, positioning the outlet of the pMDI approximately 4 cm (two fingerbreadths) in front of the mouth improves lung deposition by decreasing oropharyngeal impaction.[28] Holding the canister outside the open mouth (at two fingerbreadths) provides a space for the particles to decelerate while evaporating, allowing particle size to reduce to respirable size. Use of the open-mouth technique with a low inspiratory flow rate can result in a doubling of the dose delivered to the lower respiratory tract of an adult from approximately 7% to 10% to 14% to 20%. However, this technique is more difficult for patients to perform reliably than the closed-mouth technique. Although it may reduce oropharyngeal deposition, the technique has not been shown to improve the clinical response to pMDI bronchodilators.

Concerns have been raised about use of the open-mouth technique with ipratropium bromide because poor coordination can result in drug being sprayed into the eyes. Use of anticholinergic agents has been associated with increased ocular pressure, which could be dangerous for patients with glaucoma. For avoidance of ocular exposure, the drug manufacturer recommends patients use the closed-mouth technique with ipratropium.

The high percentage of oropharyngeal drug deposition with use of steroid pMDIs can increase the incidence of oral yeast infection (thrush) and changes in the voice (dysphonia). Rinsing the mouth after steroid use can help avoid this problem, but most pMDI steroid aerosol impaction occurs deep in the hypopharynx, which cannot be easily rinsed with gargling. For this reason, steroid pMDIs should not be used alone but always in combination with a spacer or valved holding chamber. See Box 39-2 for instructions for determining dosage left in the pMDI.

Pressurized Metered Dose Inhaler Accessory Devices

Various pMDI accessory devices have been developed to overcome the two primary limitations of these systems: hand-breath coordination problems and high oropharyngeal deposition. Accessory devices include spacers, and valved holding chambers.

Spacers and Valved Holding Chambers. Spacers and valved holding chambers (VHCs) are designed to reduce both oropharyngeal deposition and the need for hand-breath coordination. A spacer is a simple valveless extension device that adds distance between the pMDI outlet and the patient's mouth. This distance allows the aerosol plume to expand and the propellants to evaporate before the medication reaches the oropharynx. Larger particles leaving the pMDI tend to impact on the spacer walls. In combination, this phenomenon reduces oropharyngeal impaction and increases pulmonary deposition. VHCs incorporate one or more valves that prevent aerosol in the chamber from being cleared on exhalation. This allows patients with a small V_T to empty the aerosol from the chamber over two or more successive breaths. Generally, holding chambers provide less oropharyngeal deposition, higher respirable drug dosages, and better protection from poor hand-breath coordination than simple spacers. VHCs protect the patient from poor hand-breath coordination, with exhaled gas venting to the atmosphere, allowing aerosol to remain in the chamber

Box 39-2 Determining Dose Left in Pressurized Metered Dose Inhaler

Tracking the number of actuations (puffs) remaining in a pMDI can be done with or without dose counters (see Figure 39-9).

WITH DOSE COUNTERS

The user should[29]:

1. Determine how many puffs of drug the pMDI has when full.
2. Learn to read the counter display because each dose counter has a different way of displaying doses left in the canister.
3. Check the counter display to track the pMDI actuations remaining in the canister.
4. Reorder the pMDI when there are a few days of drug remaining.
5. Dispose of the pMDI properly, after the last dose is dispensed.

WITHOUT DOSE COUNTERS

The user should[29]:

1. Read the label to determine how many puffs of drug the pMDI has when full.
2. Calculate how long the pMDI will last by dividing the total number of puffs in the pMDI by the total puffs used per day. If the pMDI is used more often than planned, it will run out sooner.
3. Identify the date that the medication will run out, and mark it on the canister or on a calendar.
4. For drugs that are prescribed to be taken as needed, track the number of puffs of drug administered on a daily log sheet and subtract them from the remaining puffs to determine the amount of medication left in the pMDI.
5. Keep the daily log sheet in a convenient place, such as taped to the bathroom mirror.
6. Refill the pMDI prescription when there are a few days of use remaining in the pMDI.
7. Dispose of the pMDI properly when the last dose is dispensed.

available to be inhaled with the next breath. VHCs allow infants, small children, and adults who cannot control their breathing pattern to be treated effectively with pMDIs.

Types of Accessory Devices. Basic concepts for spacer devices include (1) small volume adapters, (2) open tube designs, (3) bag reservoirs, and (4) valved holding chambers (Figure 39-10). More than a dozen different devices with volumes ranging from 15 to 750 ml have been developed over the past 30 years. Despite differences in design, all spacers add distance between the pMDI and the mouth, reducing the initial forward velocity of the pMDI droplets, which occurs with partial evaporation of propellant in the time the aerosol traverses the length of the spacer. The reduction in initial forward velocity decreases the number of nonrespirable particles reaching the airway. The same drug used with different accessory devices may produce differences in MMAD, GSD, and fine-particle fraction. The quantity of respirable drug available at the spacer or valved holding chamber depends on spacer volume and design and formulation. The placement of a valve between the pMDI, the chamber, and the mouthpiece works like a baffle reducing the size of particles inhaled. A simple tube spacer may reduce oral deposition by 90%, whereas a valved holding chamber can reduce oral deposition by 99%.

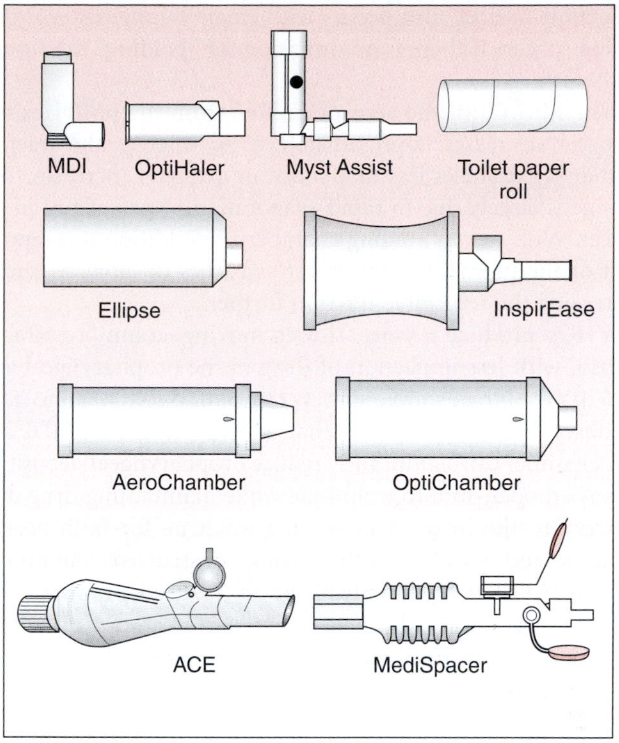

FIGURE 39-10 pMDI and accessory devices consisting of spacer and holding chambers. All of the accessory devices reduce oropharyngeal deposition. Small volume spacers (e.g., Optihaler [Philips Respironics, Murrysville, PA] and Myst Assist [Philips Respironics, Murrysville, PA]) offer no additional advantage, but large volume spacers (e.g., toilet paper roll and Ellipse [Ellipse Technologies, Irving, CA]) improve inhaled aerosol with delay between actuation and inspiration. Only the bag (e.g., Inspirease [Schering Plough, Kenilworth, NJ]) and valved holding chambers (VHCs) (e.g., Aerochamber [Invicare, Elyria, OH], Optichamber [Philips Respironics, Murrysville, PA], Ace [Smiths Medical, Kent, UK], and Medispacer [Cardinal Health, Dublin, OH]) protect the patient from blowing the dose away when the pMDI is actuated during expiration. (Modified from Wilkes W, Fink J, Dhand R: Selecting an accessory device with a metered-dose inhaler: variable influence of accessory devices on fine particle dose, throat deposition, and drug delivery with asynchronous actuation from a metered dose inhaler. J Aerosol Med 14:351, 2001.)

It is increasingly common practice to provide asthmatic patients an accessory device to use with the pMDI and to teach them how to use the pMDI with and without the accessory device. Patients are instructed to use the device with the pMDI whenever they feel short of breath. Many of these patients find that they get much better relief from the pMDI with an accessory device than with the pMDI alone.

Proper use of a simple open-tube spacer still requires some hand-breath coordination because a momentary delay between triggering and inhaling the discharged spray results in a substantial loss of drug and reduced lung delivery. Exhalation into a simple spacer after pMDI actuation clears the aerosol from the device and wastes most of the dose to the atmosphere. This reduction in dose also occurs with small volume reverse-flow design spacers if there is no provision for "holding" the aerosol in the device.[29]

The MMAD of the aerosol emitted from the pMDI exiting a spacer decreases approximately 25%, whereas the fraction containing particles less than 5 µm in diameter increases. This change is largely due to rapid evaporation of propellant in the spacer. With valved holding chambers, in addition to evaporation of the plume, the valves act as baffles of larger particles, increasing the respirable fraction further.

VHCs produce a finer, slower moving, more "respirable" aerosol with less impaction of drug in the oropharyngeal area (1% of dose) than simple spacers (10%) or a pMDI alone (80% of dose). Research suggests that a properly used pMDI and aerochamber can significantly reduce oropharyngeal deposition versus an open-mouth technique while maintaining drug dose delivery to the lungs. This finding was true for both healthy subjects and patients with chronic obstructive pulmonary disease (COPD).[30] The advantage of reduced oropharyngeal deposition is fewer side effects from steroid aerosols. Multiple actuations of one or more drugs into a spacer reduce both the total dose and the respirable dose of drug available for inhalation. The extent of these losses may vary for different drugs and spacer designs.[23]

VHCs with masks are available for use in the care of infants, children, and adults. These units allow effective administration of aerosol from a pMDI to patients who are unable to use a mouthpiece device (because of their size, age, coordination, or mentation). VHCs are helpful in administration of pMDI steroids because deposition of the drug in the mouth is largely eliminated, and systemic side effects can be minimized.

Even with a VHC, respirable particles containing drug settle out and become deposited within the device, causing a whitish buildup on the inner chamber walls. This residual drug poses no risk to the patient but should be be rinsed out periodically. Plastic spacers decrease drug output due to the presence of an electrostatic charge. With these devices, a buildup of material can be seen on the walls of the chamber. As more material builds up on the wall of the chamber, the charge is dissipated, and more drug is inhaled by the patient. Washing the chamber with water (without soap) causes the electrostatic charge to be reestablished, making the device less effective for the next few puffs, until the static charge in the chamber (which attracts small particles) is again reduced.[32] Optimal technique is outlined in Box 39-3.

Use of conductive metal or nonelectrostatic plastic chambers or washing the plastic chamber periodically with deionizing detergent (liquid dishwashing soap) can overcome the loss of fine-particle mass owing to electrostatic charge and increase the inhaled mass from 20% to 50% of the emitted dose of the pMDI, even in children (Figure 39-11).[31] The effect of washing the chamber with conventional dishwashing soap reduces this static charge for up to 30 days. All manufacturers recommend that VHCs and spacers should be cleaned regularly, typically monthly using dilute liquid dishwashing soap, with or without rinsing, and allowing them to air dry.

Box 39-3 Optimal Technique for Use of a Metered Dose Inhaler With a Valved Holding Chamber

1. Warm the pMDI to hand or body temperature.
2. Assemble the apparatus, ensuring there are no objects or coins in the chamber that could be aspirated or obstruct outflow.
3. Hold the canister vertically, and shake it vigorously. Prime if necessary.
4. Place the pMDI in the holding chamber inlet, position chamber outlet in the mouth (or place the mask over nose and mouth), and encourage the patient to breathe through the mouth. Visually inspect for proper valve function.
5. With normal breathing, actuate the pMDI once and have the patient breathe through the device for three to seven breaths (three breaths for adults and seven breaths for infants).*
6. Allow 30 to 60 seconds between actuations.

*For a cooperative patient, synchronizing actuation at the beginning of larger breaths with breath holding may be encouraged. However, this maneuver has not been shown to increase clinical response to inhaled bronchodilators.

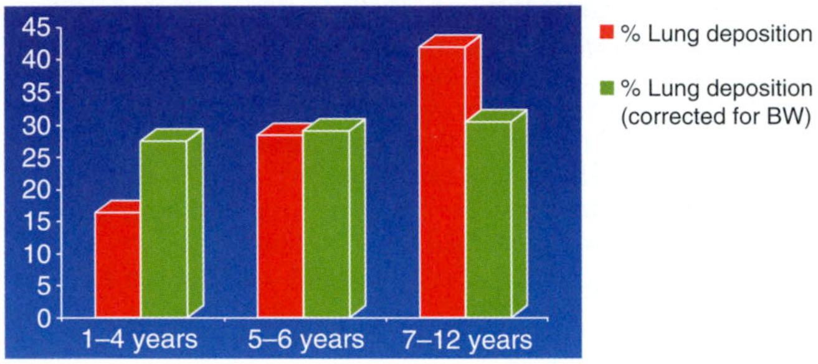

FIGURE 39-11 Although the percentage of drug deposited in the lung varies with age *(red bars)*, the percentage of lung deposition corrected for body weights is consistent across age groups. (Modified from Wildhaber JH, Janssens HM, Piérart F, et al: High percentage lung delivery in children from detergent-treated spacers. Pediatr Pulmonol 29:389-393, 2000.)

The addition of a one-way valve to convert an open tube into a reservoir for the aerosol, the incorporation of the actuator in the pMDI, the shape of the device, flow of air through the device, edge effects, masks, and manufacturing materials all affect aerosol characteristics. The inhalation valve, which is used to contain the aerosol, also acts as a baffle to reduce oropharyngeal deposition. This valve must be able to withstand the initial pressure from the pMDI when the device is triggered to retain aerosol and have sufficiently low resistance to open readily when the user inhales, in particular, when the user is a child or an infant. Exhalation valves in a face mask attached to a spacer device must also provide low resistance. Issues of spacer volume, V_T, frequency of breathing, and mechanical dead space between the spacer and mouth are of particular concern when these devices are used by children.[32] There are twofold to threefold differences in the amount of drug available at the mouth when different spacers are used to treat infants. Clinicians should

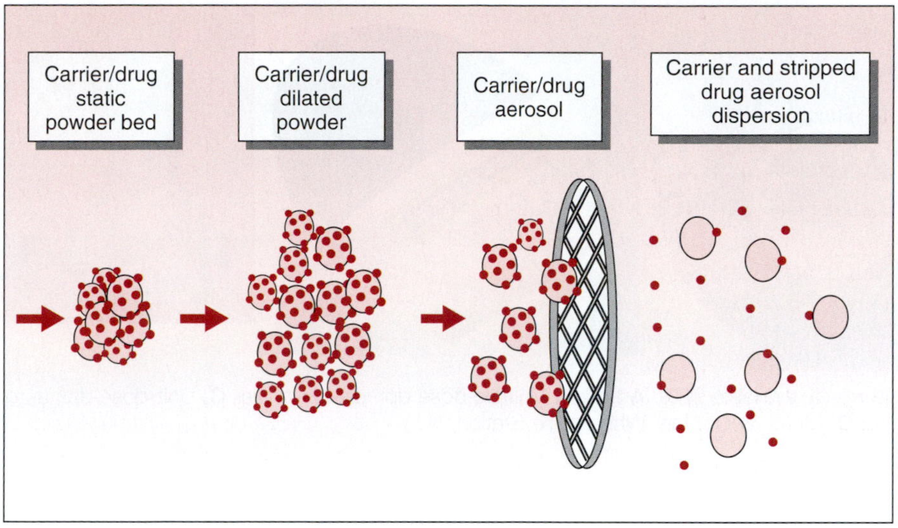

FIGURE 39-12 Aerosolization of dry powder. (Modified from Dhand R, Fink J: Dry powder inhalers. Respir Care 44:940, 1999.)

determine the delivery efficiencies of spacer devices before using the device in a particular population.

Accessory devices are used with either the manufacturer-designed boot that comes with the pMDI or with a "universal adapter" that triggers the pMDI canister. Different formulations of pMDI drugs operate at different pressures and have a different-sized orifice in the boot that is specifically designed by the manufacturer for use exclusively with that pMDI. The output characteristics of a pMDI change when an adapter with a different-sized orifice is used. With HFA pMDIs, the diameter of the actuator orifice is smaller, and the spray is predictably finer. When the HFA pMDI is used in an actuator designed for use with CFC pMDIs, output is reduced. When these HFA formulations are used with any particular spacer, it is important to know how comparable the available dose and particle size distribution are to the dose and particle size from an existing CFC pMDI.[23]

Cost

Many hospitals are moving away from the use of HFA pMDIs because of the high cost of these devices. Regardless of drug delivered, these devices cost between $200 to $300 dollars compared to pennies a dose for the same drug in a preparation to be used in a nebulizer. The use of these less expensive preparations with a vibrating mesh nebulizer (see later discussion) has now become the norm in many hospitals because of cost.

Dry Powder Inhalers

A DPI is typically a breath-actuated dosing system. With a DPI, the patient creates the aerosol by drawing air though a dose of finely milled drug powder with sufficient force to disperse and suspend the powder in the air. DPIs are inexpensive, do not need propellants, and do not require the hand-breath coordination needed for pMDIs. However, dispersion of the powder into respirable particles depends on the creation of turbulent flow in the inhaler. Turbulent flow is a function of the ability of the patient to inhale the powder with a sufficiently high inspiratory flow rate (Figure 39-12). In terms of both lung deposition and drug response, DPIs are as effective as pMDIs.[33]

Equipment Design and Function

Most passive dry powder–dispensing systems require the use of a carrier substance (lactose or glucose) mixed into the drug to enable the drug powder to deaggregate more readily and flow out of the device. Reactions to lactose or glucose seem to be fewer than reactions to the surfactants and propellants used in pMDIs, even though the amount of these substances is substantially greater than the amount of the drug and can represent 98% or more of the weight per inhaled dose in some formulations.

As shown in Figure 39-13, *A*, *B*, and *C*, there are numerous DPIs on the market, which can be divided into three categories based on the design of their dose containers: (1) unit-dose DPI, (2) multiple unit-dose DPI, and (3) multiple dose drug reservoir DPI.

Unit-dose DPIs, such as the Aerolizer (Schering-Plough, Kenilworth, NJ) and the HandiHaler (Boehringer Ingleheim, Ingelheim am Rhein, Germany), dispense individual doses of drug from punctured gelatin capsules. Multiple unit-dose DPIs (Diskhaler; GlaxoSmithKline, Philadelphia) contain a case of four or eight individual blister packets of medication on a disk inserted into the inhaler. Multiple dose DPIs include the Twisthaler (Schering-Plough), Flexhaler (AstraZeneka, London), and the Diskus (GlaxoSmithKline). The Twisthaler and Flexhaler have a multidose reservoir powder system preloaded with a quantity of pure drug sufficient for dispensing 120 doses of medication, and the Diskus incorporates a tape system that contains up to 60 sealed single doses (Figure 39-14).

The particle size of the dry powder particles of drug ranges from 1 to 3 μm. However, the size of the lactose or glucose particles can range from approximately 20 to 65 μm, so most of the carrier (≤80%) is deposited in the oropharynx.

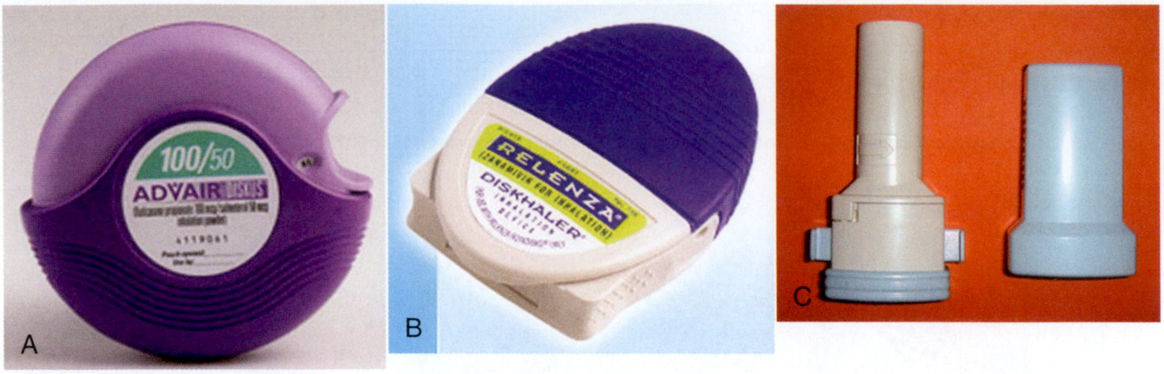

FIGURE 39-13 Some currently available DPIs: **A** and **B,** Multiple-dose dpi: diskus inhaler **C,** Unit-dose dpi: aerolizer. (**A,** GlaxoSmithKline, used with permission. **B** and **C,** Merck & Co. Inc. Whitehouse Station, NJ.)

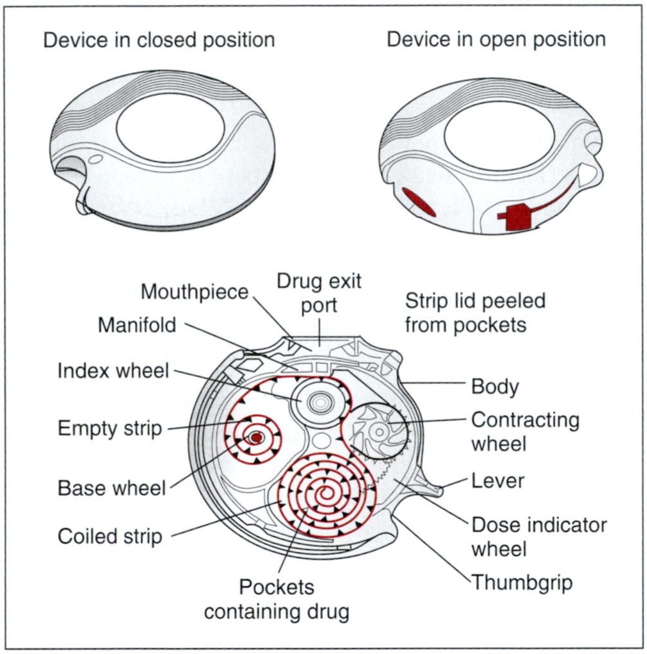

FIGURE 39-14 Diskus DPI (Glaxo Wellcome, Research Triangle Park, NC). The doses are contained in 60 sealed pockets along an aluminum-foil strip that is advanced by the lever. As the drug pocket reaches the mouthpiece, the cover is peeled away, making the drug available for inhalation. A dose counter indicates the number of doses remaining in the device. (Modified from Dhand R, Fink J: Dry powder inhalers. Respir Care 44:940, 1999.)

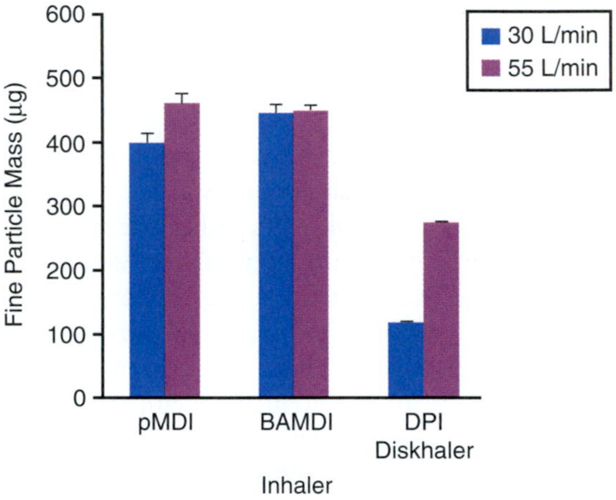

FIGURE 39-15 Fine particle mass delivered from a 1000-mg dose (± standard deviation) as a function of flow. *BAMDI,* Breath-actuated pMDI (Autohaler); *DPI,* dry powder inhaler (Diskhaler); *pMDI,* pressurized metered dose inhaler. (Modified from Smith KJ, Chan HK, Brown KF: Influence of flow rate on aerosol particle size distributions from pressurized and breath-actuated inhalers. J Aerosol Med 11:231, 1998.)

Factors Affecting Dry Powder Inhaler Performance and Drug Delivery

Intrinsic Resistance and Inspiratory Flow Rate. Optimal performance for each DPI design occurs at a specific inspiratory flow rate. The fine-particle fraction of respirable drug from existing DPIs ranges from 10% to 60% of the nominal dose. The amount varies with inspiratory flow and device design. The higher the resistance or the greater the flow requirement of a DPI device, the more difficult it is for a compromised or young patient to generate inspiratory flow sufficient to obtain the maximum dose of drug from the device.

Exposure to Humidity and Moisture. The emitted dose of DPI decreases in a humid environment, likely because of powder clumping. The longer the exposure and the greater the level of absolute humidity, the lower the dose emitted. New DPIs with multiple unit-doses minimize the effects of moisture on the powder as long as individual doses are inhaled as soon as the seal is broken.

Patient's Inspiratory Flow Ability. High peak inspiratory flow rates (>60 L/min) are required to dispense the drug powder from most current DPI designs and result in a pharyngeal dose comparable to the dose received from a typical pMDI without an add-on device. If a patient does not inhale at the optimal inspiratory flow rate for a particular device, delivery to the lung decreases as the dose of drug dispensed decreases and the particle size of the powder aerosol increases (Figure 39-15).[33]

Passive, or patient-driven, DPIs rely on the patient's inspiratory effort to dispense the dose. The result is differences in lung delivery and clinical response. Active or powered DPI devices, which deaggregate the powder before inhalation, are independent of patient effort. Active DPIs use an energy source to deaggregate the powder and suspend the powder into an aerosol, allowing the dose to be suspended independent of patient inspiratory flow rates.

Technique. Proper technique is essential to derive the maximum benefit from a DPI. Box 39-4 outlines the basic steps for ensuring optimal drug delivery. The most critical factor in using a passive DPI is the need for high inspiratory flow. Patients must generate an inspiratory flow rate of at least 40 to 60 L/min to produce a respirable powder aerosol. Because infants, small children (<5 years old) (Figure 39-16), and patients who are unable to follow instructions cannot develop inspiratory flows this high, these patients cannot use DPIs. Because patients with severe airway obstruction may be unable to achieve the required flow, they should not use DPIs during acute bronchospasm.

Exhalation into a DPI before inspiration can result in loss of drug delivery to the lung. Some DPIs also require assembly, which can be cumbersome or difficult for some patients, especially in an emergency. It is important that patients receive demonstrations with their inhalers and have the opportunity to assemble and use the DPI (return demonstration) before self-administration. Although the DPI may require cleaning in accordance with the product label, the device should never be submerged in water. Moisture in the device dramatically reduces available dose. Table 39-1 provides methods to determine the dose of the different types of DPI.

Box 39-4 Optimal Technique for Use of a Dry Powder Inhaler

1. Assemble the apparatus.
2. Load dose, keeping device upright.
3. Exhale slowly to functional residual capacity.
4. Seal lips around the mouthpiece.
5. Inhale deeply and forcefully (>60 L/min). A breath hold should be encouraged but is not essential.
6. Repeat the process until dose is completed.
7. Monitor adverse reactions.
8. Assess beneficial effects.

Modified from Pedersen S: How to use a Rotahaler. Arch Dis Child 61:11, 1986; and Hansen OR, Pedersen S: Optimal inhalation technique with terbutaline. Turbuhaler Eur Respir J 2:637, 1989.

New Dry Powder Inhaler Technologies

Easyhaler®. The Easyhaler® (Orion Corporation, Espoo, Finland) is approved for marketing in Europe for delivery of beclomethasone, albuterol, formoterol, and budesonide. The device is similar to the pMDI in terms of its shape and operation. However, it is a DPI and has a dose counter which gives a red signal when 20 doses are left in the device.

Ellipta®. The Ellipta® (GlaxoSmithKline, Research Triangle Park, NC) is a disposable multidose DPI in which the drug is stored in double-foil blister strips. The device has a 3-step technique (open-inhale-close) and provides auditory feedback with the opening of the inhaler that results in loading the dose and an advancement in the dose counter. When a patient does not inhale the dose from the Ellipta®, the drug is dumped internally to prevent overdosing. The Ellipta® has three categories that provide different drugs or drug combinations: (1) Incruse™

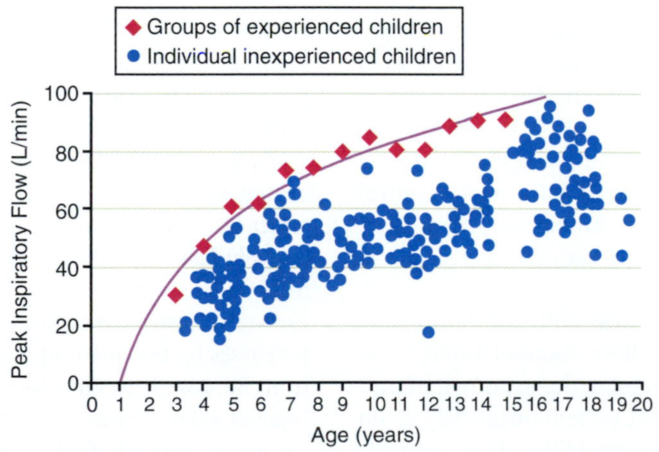

FIGURE 39-16 Peak inspiratory flows in individual inexperienced children (Pedersen et al, 1990) and groups of experienced children (Agertoft et al, 1995). (Modified from Pedersen S: Delivery options for inhaled therapy in children over the age of 6 years. J Aerosol Med 10[Suppl 1]:S41, 1997.)

TABLE 39-1

Determining Doses Left in the Dry Powder Inhaler

		Drug Container	Doses	Type Indicator	Meaning of Dose Indicator
Unit-Dose DPI	Aerolizer or HandiHaler	Single capsule	1	None	Check capsule to ensure full dose was inhaled. Repeat to empty capsule
Multiple Unit-Dose DPI	Diskhaler	Dose blisters	4 or 8	None	Inspect visually to confirm use of all blisters
	Diskus	Blister strip	60	Red numbers	Red numbers indicate that ≤5 doses are left in DPI
Multiple Dose DPI	Flexhaler	Reservoir	60 or 120	"0"	Marked in intervals of 10 doses; "0" indicates empty
	Twisthaler	Reservoir	30	"01"	"01" indicates last dose

Ellipta® delivers umeclidinium, a long-acting muscarinic antagonist that is used in the treatment of COPD, (2) Breo™ Ellipta® has a combination of fluticasone furoate and vilanterol (long-acting β2-agonist), and (3) Anoro™ Ellipta® includes a combination of umeclidinium and vilanterol.

Podhaler™. As a single-dose reusable DPI, the Podhaler™ (Novartis Pharmaceutical Corporation, San Carlos, CA) delivers TOBI for the treatment of chronic infection in patients with cystic fibrosis. The device produces light porous particles with improved flow and dispersion characteristics by using the PulmoSphereTM technology that has less interparticle cohesive forces. When using the Podhaler, a patient opens the mouthpiece, inserts the capsule in the device, and then inhales. The manufacturer suggests disposing of the device after 7 days of use.

Taifun™. The TaifunTM is a reservoir based multidose DPI in which drug within the reservoir is protected from moisture. It is a user friendly device with a dose counter that is used to deliver salbutamol, fentanyl, formoterol, and budesonide in Europe. Although the TaifunTM has reproducible and uniform metered doses, more research is needed about patient acceptance, preference, safety, and clinical efficacy of the device.

Tudorza™ Pressair™. The Tudorza™ Pressair™ (Forest Laboratories, St Louis, MO) is a multidose DPI that delivers aclidinium bromide, a long-acting anticholinergic. The device has a dose counter that decreases by 10 doses and shows a red mark with a "0" sign when it is empty. It also has a lockout system at the end of the dose. The Tudorza™ Pressair™ provides both visual feedback and auditory feedback during therapy. The visual feedback displays red color in the control window with incorrect technique and shows green color when the patient inhales the dose completely with the correct use of the device.

Spiromax®. As a multidose passive DPI, the Spiromax® (Teva Pharmaceuticals) is used to deliver albuterol, fluticasone/salmeterol, and budesonide/formoterol in the treatment of pulmonary diseases in Europe. When the patient opens the cap on the mouthpiece, the dose is loaded to the DPI and then is ready for the patient to inhale the medication.

Staccato®. The Staccato® (Alexza Pharmaceuticals) uses a thermal aerosol technology that has three components including a heating substrate, a thin film of pure drug, and a channel where aerosol forms. It is a small, portable, breath-actuated device that does not require any type of special breathing technique. Therefore, unlike other DPIs, the Staccato is insensitive to patient inhalation rates. The device generates aerosols by heating a thin film of drug to form pure drug vapor. When the patient inhales, the vapor cools and condenses into 1- to 3-μm-diameter particles. Thus, pure drug can be delivered to the alveoli without extensive thermal degradation and with the optimal range of particle diameter, promoting very fast systemic drug absorption. The Staccato has been approved in the United States for delivery of loxapine.

Nebulizers

Nebulizers generate aerosols from solutions and suspensions. The three categories of nebulizers include (1) pneumatic jet nebulizers, (2) USNs, and (3) vibrating mesh (VM) nebulizers. Nebulizers are also described in terms of their reservoir size. Small volume nebulizers (SVNs) most commonly used for medical aerosol therapy hold 5 to 20 ml of medication. Large volume nebulizers, also known as *jet nebulizers,* hold up to 200 ml and may be used for either bland aerosol therapy (see Chapter 38) or continuous drug administration.

Pneumatic (Jet) Nebulizers

Gas-powered jet nebulizers (Figure 39-17, *A*) have been in clinical use for longer than 100 years. Most modern jet nebulizers are powered by high-pressure air or oxygen (O_2) provided by a portable compressor, compressed gas cylinder, or 50-psi wall outlet.

Factors Affecting Nebulizer Performance. Nebulizer design, gas pressure, gas density, and medication characteristics affect SVN performance (Box 39-5).

Nebulizer Design. As shown in Figure 39-17, *B,* a typical SVN is powered by a high-pressure stream of gas directed through a restricted orifice (the jet). The gas stream leaving the jet passes by the opening of a capillary tube immersed in solution. Because it produces low lateral pressure at the outlet, the high jet velocity draws the liquid up the capillary tube and into the gas stream, where it is sheared into filaments of liquid that break up into droplets. This primary spray produces a heterodisperse aerosol with droplets ranging from 0.1 to 500 μm.[34]

This spray is directed against one or more baffles. A **baffle** is a surface on which large particles impact and fall out of suspension, whereas smaller particles remain in suspension, reducing

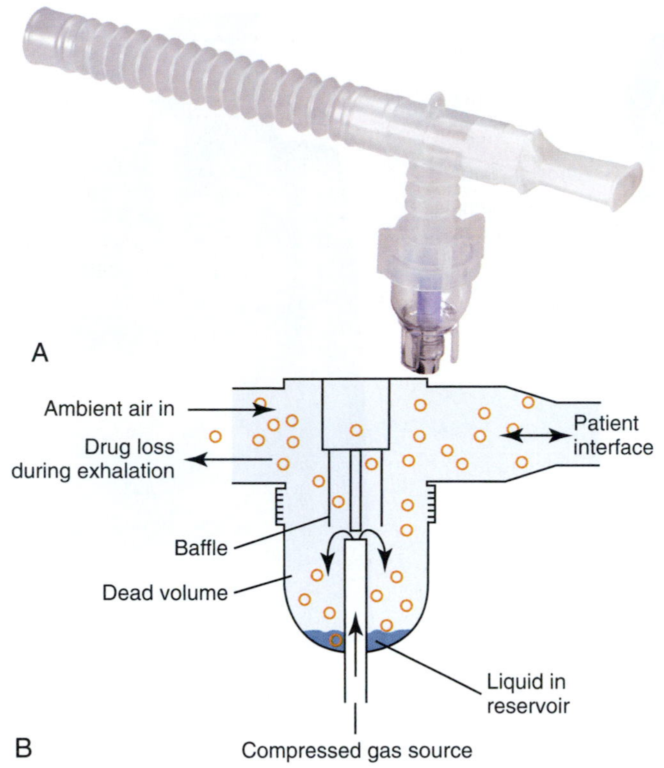

FIGURE 39-17 A, Small volume jet nebulizer with tube reservoir for liquid drug delivery. **B,** Schematic of a small volume jet nebulizer. (**A,** DeVilbiss Healthcare, Somerset PA. **B,** From Gardenhire, D: Rau's Respiratory Care Pharmacology, ed 8, St. Louis, 2012, Mosby.)

Box 39-5 Factors Affecting Performance of Small Volume Nebulizers

NEBULIZER DESIGN
- Baffles
- Fill volume
- Residual drug volume
- Nebulizer position
- Continuous vs. intermittent nebulization
- Reservoirs and extensions
- Vents, valves, and gas entrainment
- Tolerances in manufacturing within lots

GAS SOURCE: WALL, CYLINDER, COMPRESSOR
- Pressure
- Flow through nebulizer
- Gas density
- Humidity
- Temperature

CHARACTERISTICS OF DRUG FORMULATION
- Viscosity
- Surface tension
- Homogeneity

the size of particles remaining in the aerosol. In many designs, droplets that impact baffles in the SVN return to the medication reservoir for nebulization again.

Baffles are key elements in nebulizers; well-designed baffling systems decrease both the MMAD (size) and the GSD (range of sizes) of the generated aerosol. Atomizers operate with the same basic principles as nebulizers without baffling and produce aerosols with larger MMAD and GSD. **Residual drug volume**, or dead volume, is the medication that remains in the SVN after the device stops generating aerosol and "runs dry."[35] The residual volume of a 3-ml dose can range from 0.5 to more than 2.2 ml, which can be more than two-thirds of the total dose. The greater the residual drug volume, the more drug that is unavailable as aerosol, and the less efficient the delivery system. Residual volume also depends on the position of the SVN. Some SVNs stop producing aerosol when tilted 30 degrees from vertical. Increasing the fill volume allows a greater proportion of active medication to be nebulized. In a nebulizer with a residual volume of 1.5 ml, a fill of 3 ml would leave only 50% of the nebulizer volume (nominal dose) available for nebulization. In contrast, a fill of 5 ml would make 3.5 ml, or more than 70% of the medication, available to be inhaled. The unit-dose volumes of drugs were based on clinical response of patients using nebulizers with substantial residual drug volumes. Although increasing dose volume may increase available dose, it should be considered off-label administration, and there is no significant difference in clinical response with varying diluent volumes and flow rates.

Flow. Droplet size and nebulization time are inversely proportional to gas flow through the jet. The higher the flow of gas to the nebulizer, the smaller the particle size generated, and the shorter is the time required for nebulization of the full dose. Nebulizers that produce smaller particle sizes by use of baffles, such as one-way valves, may reduce total drug output per minute compared with the same nebulizer without baffling and require more time or nominal dose to deliver a standard dose of medication to the lungs.

Gas Source (Hospital Versus Home). Gas pressure and flow through the nebulizer affect particle size distribution and output. Within operating limits, the higher the pressure or flow, the smaller the particle size, the greater the output, and the shorter the treatment time. A nebulizer that produces an MMAD of 2.5 μm when driven by a gas source of 50 psi at 6 to 10 L/min may produce an MMAD of more than 5 μm when operated on a home compressor (or ventilator) developing 10 psi. Too low a gas pressure or flow can result in negligible nebulizer output. Consequently, nebulizers used for home care should be matched to the compressor according to data supplied by the manufacturer. Thus, the combination of specific equipment improves efficient nebulization of the desired medications prescribed for the patient.

Other concerns in the use of disposable nebulizers with compressors at home involve possible degradation of performance of the plastic device over multiple uses. One study showed that repeated use of nebulizers did not alter MMAD or output as long as the nebulizer was cleaned properly. Failure to clean the nebulizer properly caused degradation of performance because of clogging of the jet orifice, reducing the output flow, and buildup of electrostatic charge in the device.

Density. Gas density affects both aerosol generation and delivery to the lungs. The lower the density of the carrier gas,

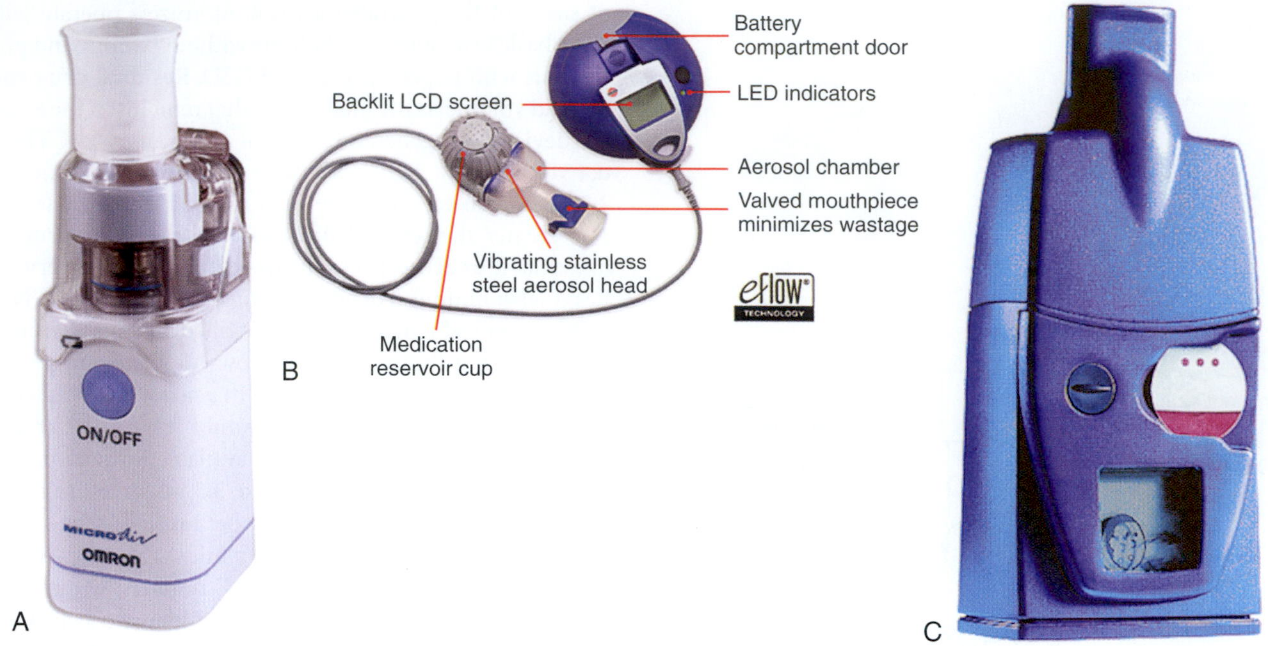

FIGURE 39-18 Variety of available aerosol devices. **A** and **C,** Passive mesh. **B,** Active vibrating mesh. (**A** and **C,** Courtesy Omron Healthcare, Inc. Bannockburn, IL. **B,** Courtesy PARI Respiratory Equipment, Inc., Midlothian, VA.)

the less aerosol impaction as gas passes through the airways, and the greater the deposition of aerosol in the lungs.[36] However, when heliox is used to drive a jet nebulizer at standard flow rates, aerosol output is substantially less than with air or O_2, and aerosol particles are considerably smaller. When driving a nebulizer with heliox, twofold to threefold greater flow is required to produce a comparable aerosol output. Heliox concentrations of 40% or greater have been shown to improve aerosol deposition.[37]

Humidity and Temperature. Humidity and temperature can affect particle size and the concentration of drug remaining in the nebulizer. Evaporation of water and adiabatic expansion of gas can reduce the temperature of the aerosol to 10° C less than ambient temperature. This cooling may increase solution viscosity and reduce the nebulizer output, while decreasing particle MMAD.[38] Aerosol particles entrained into a warm and fully saturated gas stream increase in size. These particles also can coalesce (stick together), increasing the MMAD further and, in the case of a DPI, can severely compromise the output of respirable particles. How much these particles enlarge depends primarily on the tonicity of the solution. Aerosols generated from isotonic solutions probably maintain their size as they enter the respiratory tract. Hypertonic solutions tend to enlarge, whereas evaporation can cause hypotonic droplets to evaporate and shrink.

Characteristics of Drug Formulation. The viscosity and density of a drug formulation affect both output and particle size. Some drugs, such as antibiotics, are so viscous that they cannot be used effectively for nebulization in some standard SVNs. Also, in some suspensions, some aerosolized particles contain no active drug, whereas other particles, generally larger, carry the active medication.

Small Volume Nebulizers

Four categories of jet SVNs include (1) continuous nebulizer with simple reservoir, (2) continuous nebulizer with collection reservoir bag, (3) breath-enhanced nebulizer, and (4) breath-actuated nebulizer (Figure 39-18, *A*, *B*, and *C*). The most commonly used SVN is the constant output design. Aerosol is generated continuously, with 30% to 60% of the nominal dose being trapped as residual volume in the nebulizer, and more than 60% of the emitted dose is wasted to the atmosphere. Continuous nebulization wastes medication because the aerosol is produced throughout the respiratory cycle and is largely lost to the atmosphere, as shown in Figure 39-19. Patients with an I : E ratio of 40 : 60 (or 1 : 1.5) lose 60% of the aerosol generated to the atmosphere. If 50% of the total dose is emitted from the nebulizer, and 50% of that aerosol is in the respiratory range and 40% of that is inhaled by the patient, less than 10% deposition is commonly measured in adults receiving continuous nebulizer therapy. In neonates and infants, given the small minute volumes and small airways with increased impaction and reduced sedimentation, deposition can be only 0.5%.

Aerosolized medication can also be conserved with reservoirs.[39] A reservoir on the expiratory limb of the nebulizer conserves drug aerosol.

Small Volume Nebulizer With a Reservoir. Many types of disposable SVNs are packaged with a 6-inch (15-cm) piece of aerosol tubing to be used as a reservoir (Figure 39-17, *A*). This may increase inhaled dose by 5% to 10% or increase the inhaled dose from 10% to approximately 11% with the reservoir tube.

Continuous Small Volume Nebulizer With Collection Bag. Bag reservoirs hold the aerosol generated during exhalation and allow the small particles to remain in suspension for inhalation with the next breath, while larger particles rain out.

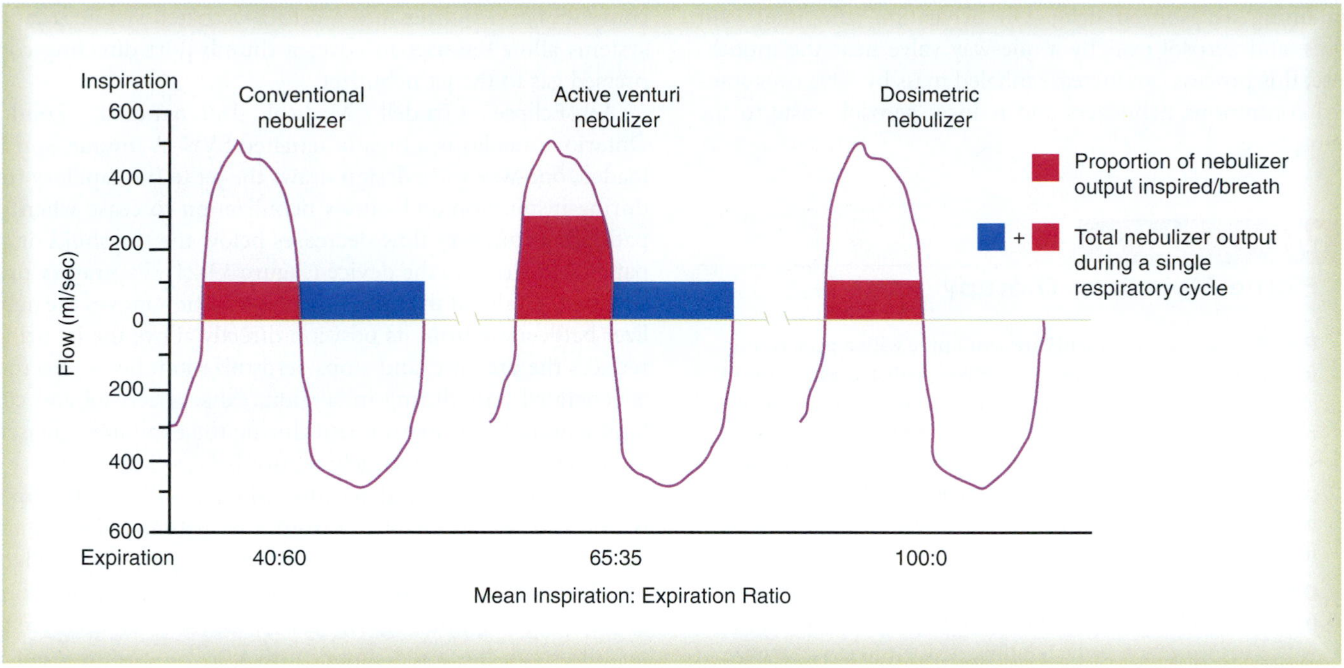

FIGURE 39-19 Proportions of nebulizer output inhaled with continuous standard jet nebulizer, vented nebulizer, and dosimetric (breath-actuated) nebulizer. (Modified from Nikander K: Drug delivery systems. Aerosol Med 7[Suppl 1]:S19, 1994.)

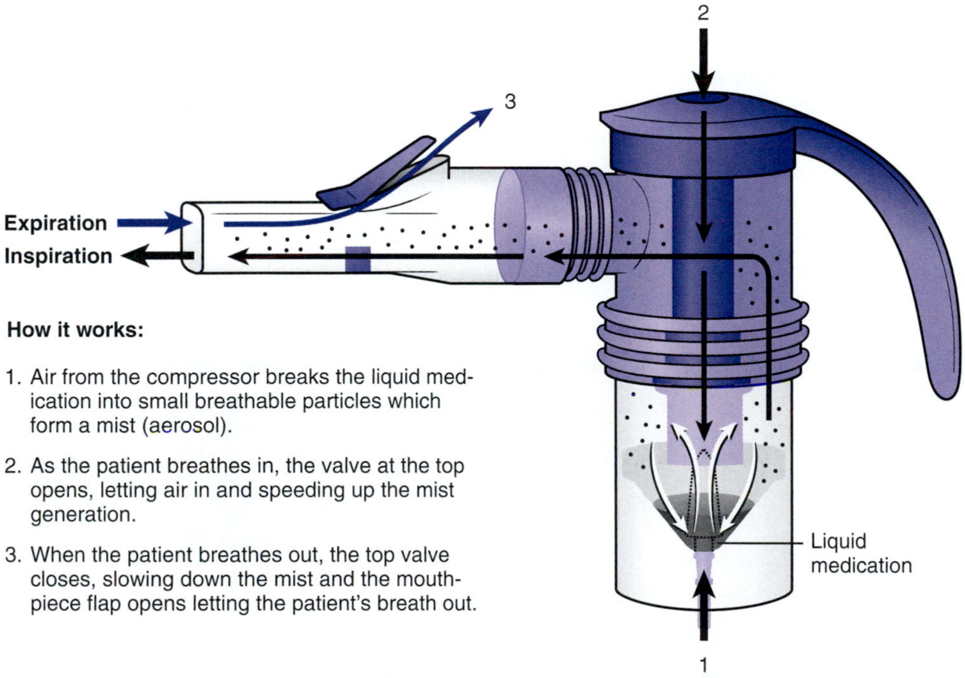

FIGURE 39-20 Operating principles of the Sprint (Pari, Midlothian, VA) breath-enhanced nebulizer. (From Cairo JM, Pilbeam SP: Mosby's respiratory care equipment, ed 8, St. Louis, 2009, Mosby.)

These additions have been attributed with a 30% to 50% increase in inhaled dose.[39] A collection bag is attached on the expiratory side of the nebulizer "T," which collects aerosol leaving the SVN when the patient is not actively inhaling. Some of the aerosol in the bag is inhaled with the next inspiration, increasing total dose efficiency.

Breath-Enhanced Nebulizers. Breath-enhanced nebulizers generate aerosol continuously, using a system of vents and one-way valves to minimize aerosol waste.[40] In the Pari LC Sprint (Pari, Midlothian, VA) breath-enhanced nebulizer (Figure 39-20), an inspiratory vent allows the patient to draw in air through the nebulization chamber generating and containing aerosolized drug. On exhalation, the inlet vent closes, and aerosol exits by a one-way valve near the mouthpiece; this process can increase inhaled mass by 50% over standard continuous nebulizers and reduces aerosol waste to the atmosphere.

MINI CLINI

Home Nebulizer Therapy

PROBLEM: Many patients are sent home with a prescription for home nebulizer therapy prescribed with the intention of giving the patient the same quality of aerosol therapy he or she received in the hospital. However, the patient often is given the same type of nebulizer used in the hospital because it is inexpensive. These nebulizers provide an aerosol that is too large for optimal deposition in the lungs. What should be done instead?

DISCUSSION: Home nebulizers designed for use with compressors should be matched to ensure an MMAD of 1 to 5 μm with the medication being administered. Nebulizer manufacturers such as Pari and Medic-Aid offer matched nebulizer-compressor systems for home use. Although these devices cost a little more, they are more likely to meet therapeutic objectives.

Breath-Actuated Nebulizers. Breath-actuated nebulizers synchronize aerosol generation with inspiration, reducing waste of aerosol during exhalation and increasing inhaled dose up to threefold more than continuous and breath-enhanced nebulizers. Dosimeters, used in pulmonary function laboratories, sense inspiration and pulse airflow to the jet orifice and transform a conventional nebulizer into a breath-actuated system. Manual systems allow the user to cover a thumb port directing compressed gas to the jet nebulizer.

AeroEclipse (Trudell Medical International, London, Ontario, Canada) is a breath-actuated SVN. A unique, spring-loaded, one-way valve design draws the jet to the capillary tube during inspiration and causes nebulization to cease when the patient's inspiratory flow decreases below the threshold or the patient exhales into the device (Figure 39-21). Expiratory pressure on the valve at the initiation of exhalation moves the nebulizer baffle away from its position directly above the jet orifice, reduces the pressure, and stops aerosolization. Because aerosol is generated only during inhalation, exhaled aerosol and contamination of the environment during the expiratory phase of the breathing cycle are largely reduced.

It can be difficult to determine when a nebulizer treatment is complete. Aerosol delivery from a jet nebulizer ceased after the onset of inconsistent nebulization (sputtering) (Figure 39-22).[41] Aerosol output declined by one-half within 20 seconds of the onset of sputtering. The concentration of albuterol in the nebulizer cup increased significantly when the aerosol output declined, and further weight loss in the nebulizer was caused primarily by evaporation. Most consider aerosolization past the point of initial nebulizer sputter ineffective.

Table 39-2 summarizes some of these key factors for many commercially available SVNs.[42] Numerous SVNs are on the market, and they vary widely in design and performance. SVNs of the same design and lot number can exhibit variable performance, even to the point that some nebulizers of the same model number do not work at all.[43] Managers and clinicians always must evaluate SVNs carefully before purchasing or using them. Manufacturers should provide data on the performance of their nebulizers under common use conditions.

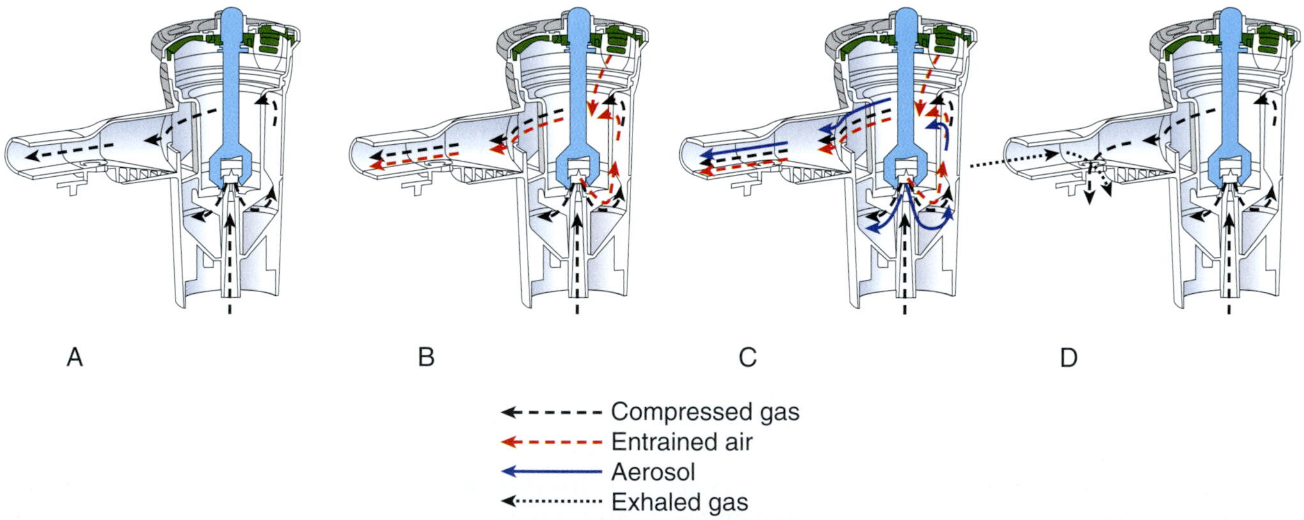

FIGURE 39-21 Breath-actuated pneumatic nebulizer (AeroEclipse BANII) flow path diagram. **A,** Before inhalation, actuator is up, and compressed gas freely circulates with no aerosol produced. **B,** Patient inhales, and actuator starts to move down. **C,** Negative pressure pulls the diaphragm down (with actuator moved down sealing around the nozzle cover), producing aerosol. **D,** Patient exhales through valve in mouthpiece; as pressure increases, the diaphragm and actuator move up, stopping aerosol production. (Courtesy Trudell Medical International, London, Ontario, Canada.)

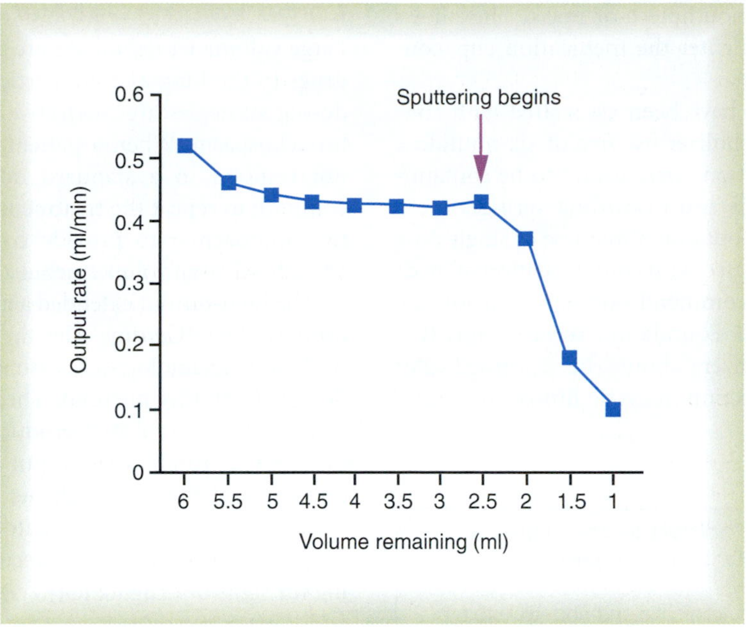

FIGURE 39-22 Output rate for jet nebulizers is substantially reduced as the nebulizer begins to sputter. The decrease in output rate correlates with reduced drug output. This finding supports a recommendation to end treatment when sputtering begins. (Modified from Malone RA, Hollie MC, Glynn-Barnhart A, et al: Optimal duration of nebulized albuterol therapy. Chest 104:1114, 1993.)

TABLE 39-2
Comparison of Different Nebulizers

	Jet	Ultrasonic	Vibrating Mesh
Features			
Power source	Compressed gas or electrical mains	Electrical mains	Batteries or electrical mains
Portability	Restricted	Restricted	Portable
Treatment time	Long	Intermediate	Short
Output rate	Low	Higher	Highest
Residual volume	0.8-2.0 ml	Variable but low	≤0.2 ml
Environmental Contamination			
Continuous use	High	High	High
Breath-activated	Low	Low	Low
Performance variability	High	Intermediate	Low
Formulation Characteristics			
Temperature	Decreases*	Increases†	Minimum change
Concentration	Increases	Variable	Minimum change
Suspensions	Low efficiency	Poor efficiency	Variable efficiency
Denaturation	Possible‡	Probable‡	Possible‡
Cleaning	Required, after single use	Required, after multiple use	Required after single use
Cost	Very low	High	High

Modified from Dolovich MB, Dhand R: Aerosol drug delivery: developments in device design and clinical use. Lancet 377:1032, 2011.
*For jet nebulizers, the temperature of the reservoir fluid decreases about 15° C during nebulization because of evaporation.
†For ultrasonic nebulizers, vibration of the reservoir fluid causes a temperature increase during aerosol generation, which can be 10° C to 15° C.
‡Denaturation of DNA occurs with all the nebulizers.

Technique. Box 39-6 outlines the optimal technique for using an SVN for aerosol drug delivery. Use of an SVN is less technique-dependent and device-dependent than use of a pMDI or DPI delivery system. Slow inspiratory flow optimizes SVN aerosol deposition. However, deep breathing and breath holding during SVN therapy do little to enhance deposition over normal tidal breathing.[44] Because the nose is an efficient filter of particles larger than 5 μm, many clinicians prefer not to use a mask for SVN therapy. As long as the patient is mouth breathing, there is little difference in clinical response between therapy given by mouthpiece and therapy given by mask. The selection of delivery method (mask or mouthpiece) should be based on patient ability, preference, and comfort.

Infection Control Issues. The CDC recommends that nebulizers be cleaned and disinfected, rinsed with sterile water, or air dried between uses. Jet SVNs have reservoirs that are open to and positioned below the mouthpiece or mask. This allows secretions from the patient to enter the medication cup, contaminating medication.

Multidose drug containers have been associated with contamination. After 7 days of nebulizer use five of six multidose containers of medication solutions were found to be contaminated.[45] Refrigerating solutions and discarding syringes every 24 hours eliminated bacterial contamination. Use of single dose ampoules have not been associated with contamination of medications. In addition, some recommend one nebulizer for one treatment. The Cystic Fibrosis Foundation recommends that standard small volume nebulizers should be discarded after each treatment to prevent infection in cyctic fibrosis patients.

Box 39-6 Optimal Technique for Using a Small Volume Nebulizer

1. Assess the patient for need (clinical signs and symptoms, breath sounds, peak flow, $\%FEV_1$).
2. Select mask or mouthpiece delivery (nose clips may be needed with mouthpiece).
3. Use conserving system (thumb port, breath actuator or reservoir) if indicated.
4. Place drug in the nebulizer. If using a multidose vial, add saline to approved dose volume (per drug label).
5. Set gas flow to nebulizer at 6 to 10 L/min (per manufacturer label).
6. Coach patient to breathe slowly through the mouth at normal V_T.
7. Continue treatment until nebulizer begins to sputter.
8. Rinse the nebulizer with sterile water and air dry, or discard, between treatments.
9. Monitor patient for adverse response.
10. Assess outcome (change in peak flow, $\%FEV_1$).

Large Volume Jet Nebulizers

Large volume jet nebulizers are also used to deliver aerosolized drugs to the lung and are particularly useful when traditional dosing strategies are ineffective in the management of severe bronchospasm. When a patient with airway obstruction does not respond to a standard dosage of bronchodilator, it is common to repeat the treatment every 15 minutes. An alternative approach is to provide continuous nebulization with a specialized large volume nebulizer.

The high-output extended aerosol respiratory therapy nebulizers HEART (Cardinal Health, Dublin, OH) and HOPE (B & B Medical Technologies, Carlsbad, CA) are examples of devices designed for this purpose. These nebulizers have a reservoir greater than 200 ml that produces an aerosol with an MMAD of 2.2 to 3.5 μm. Actual output and particle size vary with the pressure and flow at which the nebulizer operates. A concern with continuous bronchodilator therapy (CBT) is increased drug concentration. Patients receiving CBT need close monitoring for signs of drug toxicity (e.g., tachycardia and tremor). An additional strategy is to use an intravenous infusion pump to drip premixed bronchodilator solution into a standard SVN. Although this is an equipment-intensive approach, this technique can provide dosing equivalent to therapy performed every 15 minutes.[46]

Another special-purpose large volume nebulizer is a *small particle aerosol generator (SPAG)* (Figure 39-23). The SPAG was developed in the 1940s to study pathogen aerosols, and subsequently manufactured by ICN Pharmaceuticals specifically for administration of ribavirin (Virazole) to infants with respiratory syncytial virus infection. The device is unique in clinical respiratory care practice. It incorporates a drying chamber with its own flow control to produce a stable aerosol. The SPAG reduces medical gas source from the normal 50 *pounds per square inch gauge (psig)* line pressure to 26 psig with an

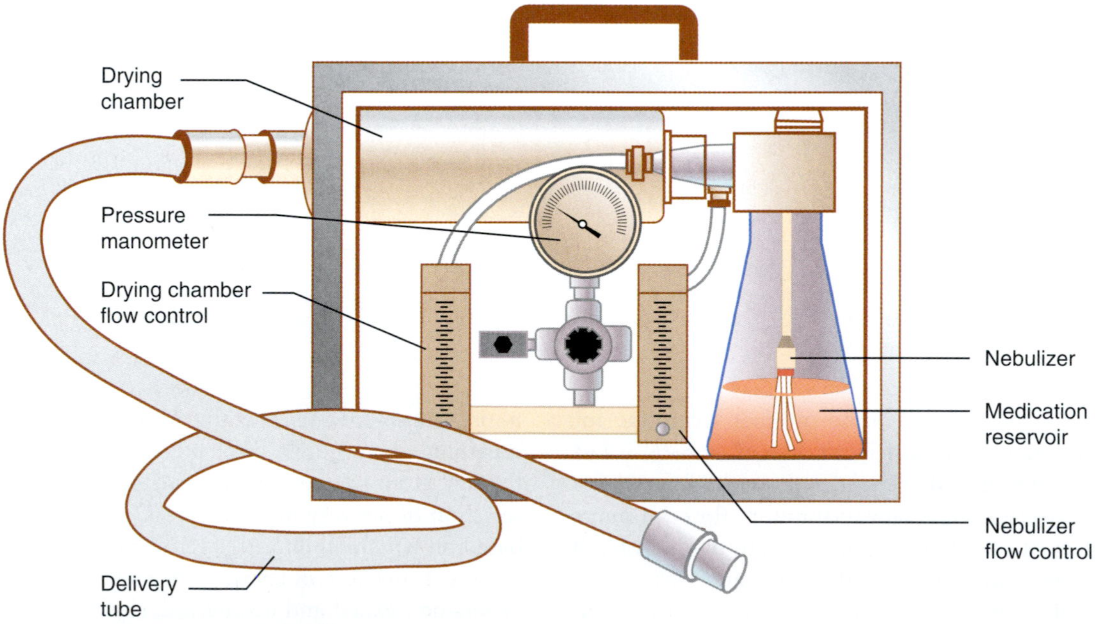

FIGURE 39-23 Small particle aerosol generator (SPAG).

adjustable regulator. The regulator is connected to two flowmeters that separately control flow to the nebulizer and flow through the drying chamber. The nebulizer is located within the glass medication reservoir, the fluid surface and wall of which serve as primary baffles. As it leaves the medication reservoir, the aerosol enters a long, cylindrical drying chamber. Here the second (separate) flow of dry gas is added, reducing particle size by evaporation, creating a monodisperse aerosol with an MMAD of 1.2 to 1.4 μm. Nebulizer flow should be maintained at approximately 7 L/min with total flow from both flowmeters not less than 15 L/min. The latest model operates consistently even with back pressure and can be used with masks, hoods, tents, or ventilator circuits.

Two specific problems are associated with SPAG use to deliver ribavirin. The first is caregiver exposure to the drug aerosol. Approaches to limit caregiver exposure are discussed later (see the section on Controlling Environmental Contamination). The other problem occurs only when the SPAG is used to deliver ribavirin through a mechanical ventilator circuit. Drug precipitation can jam breathing valves or occlude the ventilator circuit. This problem can be overcome by (1) placing a one-way valve between the SPAG and the circuit and (2) filtering out the excess aerosol particles before they reach the exhalation valve, and changing filters frequently to avoid increasing expiratory resistance.[44]

Hand-Bulb Atomizers and Spray Pumps

Hand-bulb atomizers and nasal spray pumps are used to administer sympathomimetic, anticholinergic, antiinflammatory, and anesthetic aerosols to the upper airway, including nasal passages, pharynx, and larynx (see also Chapter 35). These agents are used to manage upper airway inflammation and rhinitis, to provide local anesthesia, and to achieve systemic effects.

Because the spray pump generates relatively low pressure and does not have baffles, it produces an aerosol with large particle size (high MMAD and GSD), ideal for upper airway deposition. (Nasopharyngeal deposition is greatest for particles 5 to 40 μm.) Deposition with the hand-bulb atomizer applied to the nose occurs mostly in the anterior nasal passages with clearance to the nasopharynx. The 100-mcl puffs appear to deposit more medication than 50-mcl puffs, and deposition to a greater surface area occurs with a 35-degree spray angle than with a 60-degree angle.

Ultrasonic Nebulizers

The USN uses a piezoelectric crystal to generate an aerosol. The crystal transducer converts an electrical signal into high-frequency (1.2- to 2.4-MHz) acoustic vibrations. These vibrations are focused in the liquid above the transducer, where they disrupt the surface and create oscillation waves (Figure 39-24). If the frequency of the signal is high enough and its amplitude strong enough, the oscillation waves form a standing wave that generates a geyser of droplets that break free as fine aerosol particles.

USNs are capable of higher aerosol outputs (0.2 to >1.0 ml/min) and higher aerosol densities than conventional jet nebulizers. Output is determined by the amplitude setting (sometimes user-selected). The greater the signal amplitude, the greater the nebulizer output. Particle size is inversely proportional to the frequency of vibrations. Frequency is device-specific and is not user-adjustable. For example, the DeVilbiss (Somerset, PA) Portasonic nebulizer operating at a frequency of 2.25 MHz produces particles with an MMAD of 2.5 μm, whereas the DeVilbiss Pulmosonic nebulizer operating at 1.25 MHz produces particles in the 4- to 6-μm range. Particle size and aerosol density also depend on the source and flow of gas conducting the aerosol to the patient.

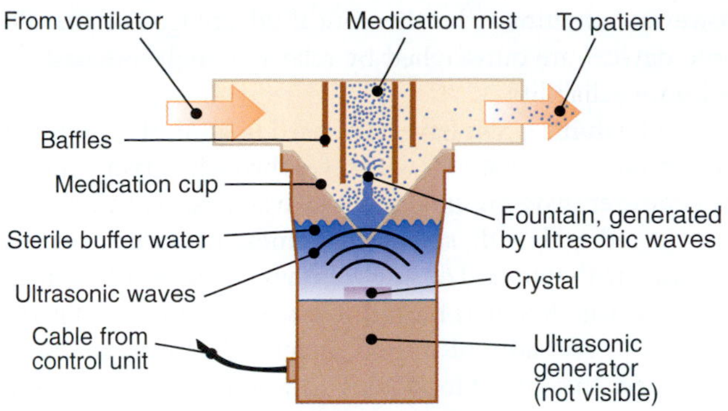

FIGURE 39-24 Small volume USN designed for use with mechanical ventilation. A vibrating piezoceramic crystal generates ultrasonic waves that pass through couplant (sterile buffer water) and the medication cup to generate a fountain (or standing wave) of medication that produces aerosol particles. (Courtesy Siemens, Tarrytown, New York.)

Large Volume Ultrasonic Nebulizers. Large volume USNs (used mainly for bland aerosol therapy or sputum induction) incorporate air blowers to carry the mist to the patient (Chapter 38). Low flow through the USN is associated with higher mist density. In contrast to jet nebulizers, the temperature of the solution placed in a USN increases during use. As the temperature increases, the drug concentration increases, and proteins can be denatured.

Small Volume Ultrasonic Nebulizers. Many small volume USNs have been marketed for aerosol drug delivery (see Figure 39-24). In contrast to the larger units, some of these systems do not use a couplant compartment; the medication is placed directly into the manifold on top of the transducer. The transducer is connected by a cable to a power source, often battery-powered to increase portability. These devices have no blower; the patient's inspiratory flow draws the aerosol from the nebulizer into the lung.

Small volume USNs administer a wide variety of formulations ranging from bronchodilators to antiinflammatory agents and antibiotics.[47] Suspensions such as budesonide may not nebulize well with USNs, because large suspension aerosol particles that are larger than the aerosol particles remain in the medication cup. Use of a small volume USN may increase available respirable mass for designs with less residual drug volume than SVNs; this may reduce the need for a large quantity of diluent to ensure delivery of the drugs. The contained portable power source adds a great deal of convenience in mobility.

However, sometimes the theoretical advantages of the ultrasonic devices are outweighed by relatively high purchase costs and poor reliability.

Small volume USNs have been used to administer undiluted bronchodilators to patients with severe bronchospasm.[47] Because the nebulizers have minimal residual drug volume, the treatment time is reduced with smaller volumes; however, it may be increased with standard dosing volumes. Some ventilator manufacturers (e.g., Maquet, Rastatt, Germany) have promoted the use of USNs for administration of aerosols during mechanical ventilation. In contrast to SVNs, USNs do not add extra gas flow to the ventilator circuit during use. This feature reduces the need to change and reset ventilator and alarm settings during aerosol administration.[48]

Vibrating Mesh Nebulizers

Two types of VM nebulizers, active and passive, are available commercially.[49] Active VM nebulizers use a dome-shaped aperture plate, containing more than 1000 funnel-shaped apertures. The dome is attached to a plate that is also connected to a piezoceramic element surrounding the aperture plate. Electrical energy applied to the piezoceramic element vibrates the aperture plate at a frequency of approximately 130 kHz (or one-tenth that of a USN), moving the aperture plate up and down by approximately 1 μm, creating an electronic micropump. The plate actively pumps the liquid through the apertures, where it is broken into fine droplets. The exit velocity of the aerosol is low (<4 m/sec), and the particle size can range from 3 to 4 μm (MMAD), varying with the exit diameter of the apertures (Figure 39-25, *A* and *B*). Examples of an active VM nebulizer include the Aeroneb Go, Pro, and Solo nebulizers (Aerogen, Inc, Galway, Ireland) and the eFlow nebulizers (Pari, Midlothian, VA). An active VM nebulizer can nebulize single drops of 15 mcl of formulations containing small and large molecules, suspensions, microsuspensions, and liposomes.

Passive VM nebulizers use a mesh separated from an ultrasonic horn by the liquid solution for nebulization. A piezoelectric transducer vibrates the ultrasonic horn, which pushes fluid through the mesh. Passive VM nebulizers include the NEU-22 (Omron, Kyoto, Japan) and the I-Neb (Philips Respironics, Murraysville, PA).

The residual drug volumes with either type of VM nebulizer range from 0.1 to 0.4 ml, in contrast to other types of liquid aerosol generators with residual drug volumes of 0.8 to 1.5 ml. Because a greater percentage of standard unit doses is emitted as aerosol, care should be exercised when transitioning to these devices to ensure that the higher dose does not create adverse effects.

New-Generation Nebulizers

Low-velocity (soft mist) aerosol, smaller particle size distribution, and systems that minimize residual volume of medication left in the nebulizer substantially improve aerosol device efficiency. Along with improved performance, some "smart" nebulizers have the capability to monitor patient compliance and aid in managing the patient's treatment schedule.

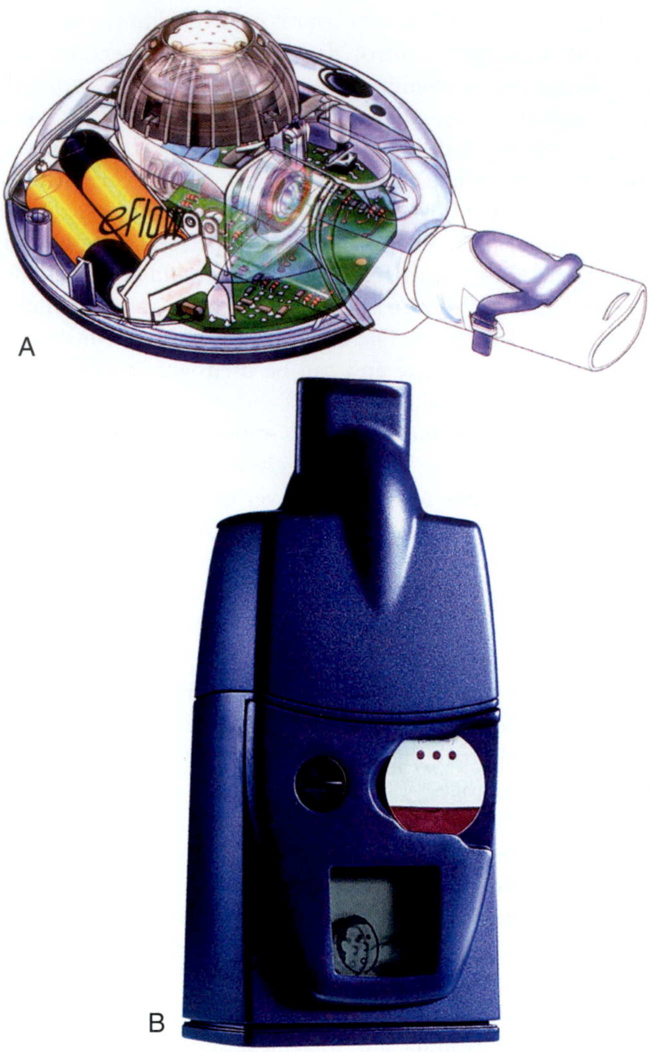

FIGURE 39-25 VM nebulizers use two basic configurations. Active VM nebulizer **(A)** has an aperture plate with funnel-shaped holes vibrated by a piezoelectric transducer surrounding the aperture plate found in the Aeroneb Solo (Aerogen, Galway, Ireland) and eFlow (Pari, Midlothian, VA; **A**). Passive VM nebulizer **(B)** uses an ultrasonic horn to push fluid through a stationary mesh found in the NEU-22 (Omron; **B**) and iNeb (Phillips/Respironics, Murrysville, PA).

With pulmonary deposition increased from the old standard of approximately 10% to more than 60% of the nominal dose, these recent device improvements may be accompanied by greater systemic side effects, unless the delivered dose is reduced. The key is to be able to target an effective delivered dose to the lungs.

New Nebulizer Designs for Liquids. New nebulizer designs are available for delivery of liquids.[50,51]

AERx. The AERx (Aradigm Corp, Hayward, CA) uses a drug solution in a unit-dose, sterile, preservative-free blister pack containing 25 to 50 mcl of fluid. The drug is extruded under pressure through a nozzle containing many small, precision-drilled holes that produce a fine, respirable spray on inhalation. The aerosolization nozzle is part of the disposable blister and is not reused. The dose from a single blister is metered in approximately 1.5 seconds. The emitted dose is more than 70% of the dose contained in the blister with an inspiratory flow rate range of 30 to 85 L/min. The AERx is being tested for use with numerous drugs in liquid form for both topical and systemic therapy. It has built-in electronic monitoring capabilities for measuring *inspiratory flow rate* during dosing and for triggering and dispensing the dose at the appropriate inspiratory flow rate for optimal delivery. The dose administered is logged to provide a record of treatments and an indication of patient compliance with therapy.

Fox. The Fox inhalation system (Vectura Group, Wilshire, UK) is an active vibrating mesh nebulizer with a flow- and volume-controlled inhalation system that increases intrapulmonary deposition. The device targets aerosol deposition in the peripheral and central airways by controlling the time of aerosol release during therapy. While releasing the aerosol at the beginning of inspiration leads to peripheral deposition, the release of aerosols in the middle of inhalation results in aerosol deposition in central airways. The Fox inhalation system is approved for delivery of different medications in Europe but not available in the United States.

Tyvaso®. The Tyvaso® Optineb is a pulsed ultrasonic nebulizer that is used for delivery of treprostinil. Device preparation requires assembly of different parts of the device including dome, inhalation piece, filters, and mouthpiece. A couplant chamber is filled with water between the piezo and the medication cup. A daily dose is placed in the medication cup and patients are instructed to take a set number of breaths per treatment, at set intervals during the day, with the device cleaned at the end of the day. The Optineb provides auditory and visual feedback on the patient's inhalation technique. Also, if a patient stops inhalations during therapy, the device shows the remaining breaths in the numerical display that are needed to complete the treatment.

Respimat. The Respimat soft mist inhaler (Boehringer, Ingelheim am Rhein, Germany) is a small hand-held inhaler that uses mechanical energy to create an aerosol from liquid solutions to produce a low-velocity spray (10 mm/sec) that delivers a unit dose of drug in a single actuation. To operate the device, patients twist the body of the device to load an internal spring, place the mouthpiece of the Respimat between the lips, and press a button to release the drug through a uniblock to create the aerosol, which is released over 1.1 to 1.4 seconds, depending on the formulation configuration. The Respimat requires hand-breath coordination on the part of the patient, as does a pMDI, but because of the longer aerosolization time, it seems more likely that the patient will get a greater percent of emitted dose despite coordination issues. Because of the small particle size and low-velocity spray, pulmonary deposition of 40% is independent of inspiratory flows with oral deposition (40%) half the oral deposition with most pMDIs and DPIs (80%). The Respimat is currently available with several drugs in Europe and with tiotropium in the United States.[52]

Smart Nebulizers. The I-Neb (Phillips Respironics, Murrysville, PA) is a breath-actuated passive VM nebulizer with *adaptive aerosol delivery* that monitors pressure changes and inspiratory time for the patient's first three consecutive breaths (Figure 39-26).[53] Drug is then aerosolized over 50% of the inspiratory maneuver during the fourth and all subsequent breaths. *Targeted inhalation mode* guides the patient to take serially longer inspirations to achieve optimal inhalation duration, reducing the time for administration. When the prescribed emitted dose has been aerosolized, the system provides an audible signal indicating the treatment should be stopped and the remaining medication discarded. Built-in electronics monitor patient treatment schedules and delivered doses with the goal to improve compliance with therapy. The I-Neb has been released for delivery of prostacyclin.

The Akita (Activaero, Gemuenden/Wohra, Germany) allows controlled inhalation of aerosol produced by either a jet or VM nebulizer. The Akita controls inspiratory flow to keep it slow (12 to 15 L/min), reducing impaction loss of aerosols in the upper airways. Patient pulmonary function is stored on a smart card programmed to tell the device when to generate aerosol during inspiration. Aerosol generated early targets distal airways, whereas aerosol generated later in the breath targets larger, more central airways.[54] Smart nebulizers can track the actual time, duration, and dose administered for each treatment and provide logs of use that can be downloaded for the medical or research record.

Advantages and Disadvantages of Aerosol Systems

Knowledge of the advantages and disadvantages of various aerosol drug delivery systems is crucial for proper selection and application. Table 39-3 compares pMDI, DPI, SVN, and USN delivery systems.

Special Medication Delivery Issues for Infants and Children

Children and infants have a smaller airway diameter than adults. In addition, their breathing rate is faster, and nose breathing filters out large particles and deposits more medication in the upper airway. Also, mouthpiece administration often cannot be used before 3 years of age. Patient cooperation and ability vary with age and developmental ability. Finally, infants and small children have lower minute volumes than adults and so inhale a smaller proportion of the output of continuous nebulizers than adults.[6]

Normal tidal breathing is the most effective method for administering aerosols to an infant. Mouth breathing enhances medication delivery to the airways of adults, but there is little evidence to show that this is true for infants, who are preferential nose breathers up to 1 year of age. Crying greatly reduces lower airway deposition of aerosol medication; therefore, aerosols should not be administered to a crying child (Figure 39-27).

For infants and children who can tolerate a mask, a medication nebulizer can be fitted to an appropriately sized aerosol mask. There is no difference in clinical response between mouthpiece and close-fitting mask treatment, so patient tolerance, compliance, and preference should guide selection of the

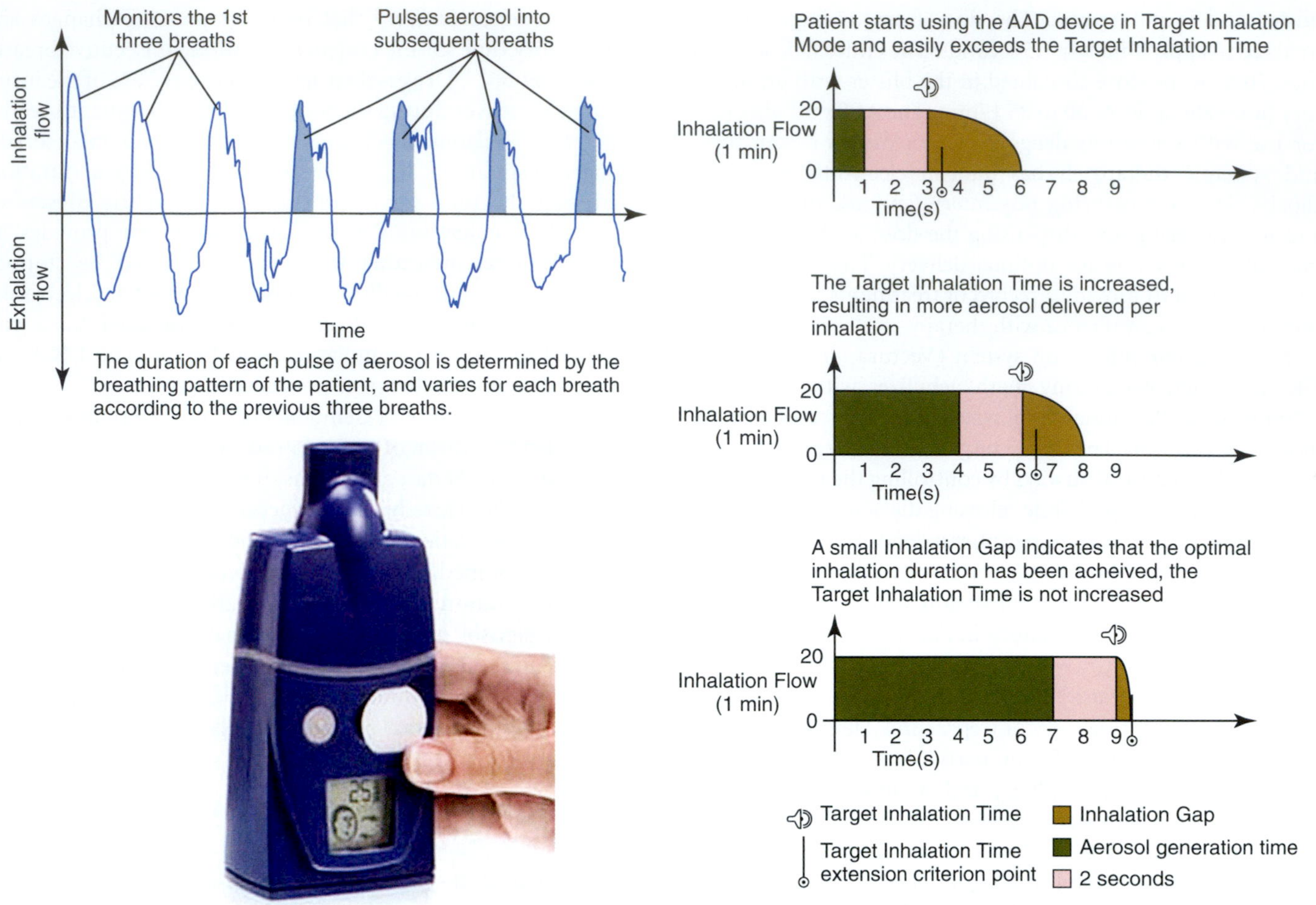

FIGURE 39-26 The iNeb *(bottom left)* is a smart nebulizer with adaptive aerosol delivery (AAD) and targeted inhalation mode (TIM). AAD delivers a precise preset dose with variation between patients. A microprocessor tracks the patient's breathing pattern on a running average of the previous three breaths, generating aerosol for 50% of the predicted inspiration *(upper left)*. TIM progressively guides the patient to take longer inspirations, increasing to achieve optimal inhalation duration *(right)*.

device. There is evidence that the aerosol available to the patient is substantially less when a loosely fitting mask (>1-cm leak) is used rather than a snug mask or mouthpiece with either a nebulizer or a pMDI with a holding chamber.[54,55] If a patient cannot tolerate mask treatment (e.g., will not wear a close-fitting mask without agitation), a commonly used strategy is the "blow-by" technique, in which the practitioner directs the aerosol from the nebulizer toward the patient's nose and mouth from a distance of several inches from the face. Studies suggest a greatly reduced inhaled dose with blow-by. Rather than "blow-by," it may be more efficient to take the time to condition the infant or child to tolerate the mask without crying or to deliver medication with a close-fitting mask when the patient is asleep.[56]

A pediatric mask with an integrated pacifier uses the infant's pull on the pacifier to hold the mask in place with improved face-mask seal which may reduce agitation and crying associated with standard masks (Soothermask InspiRx Inc, Somerset, NJ). Given the cognitive and functional limitations of very young patients, not all delivery devices are suitable for these patients. To help guide clinicians, the accompanying Rule of Thumb outlines age-specific guidelines for using aerosol devices in pediatric and neonatal patients.

RULE OF THUMB

Guidelines for Use of Aerosol Devices in the Care of Infants and Children

Device	Age Group
SVN	Neonate to all ages
Valved chamber with mask	Neonate/infant/toddler
Valved chamber with mouthpiece	>3 years
pMDI alone	>4 years
Breath-actuated Neb	>4 years
DPI	≥4 years

Spontaneous breathing in all patient populations results in greater deposition of aerosol from an SVN than occurs with positive pressure breaths (e.g., intermittent positive pressure ventilation [IPPB]). IPPB reduces aerosol deposition more than 30% compared with spontaneously inhaled aerosols.[57]

TABLE 39-3

Advantages and Disadvantages of Aerosol Drug Delivery Systems

Advantages	Disadvantages
pMDI	
Convenient	Patient coordination required
Inexpensive	Patient activation required
Portable	High percentage of pharyngeal deposition
No drug preparation required	Risk of abuse
Difficult to contaminate	Difficult to deliver high doses
	Not all medications are available
	Most units still use ozone-depleting CFCs
	Expensive
pMDI With Accessory Device	
Less patient coordination required	More complex for some patients
Less pharyngeal deposition	More expensive than MDI alone
No drug preparation required	Less portable than MDI alone
	Not all medications available
DPI	
Less patient coordination required	Requires high inspiratory flow
Breath-activated	Most units are single dose
Breath hold not required	Risk of pharyngeal deposition
Can provide accurate dose counts	Not all medications are available
No CFCs	Difficult to deliver high doses
	Expensive
SVN	
Inexpensive	Wasteful
Less patient coordination required	Drug preparation required
High doses possible (even continuous)	Contamination possible if device not cleaned carefully
No CFC release	Not all medications available
	Pressurized gas source required
	Long treatment times
USN	
Moderate residual volume	Expensive
Quiet	Prone to electrical or mechanical breakdown
Smaller residual drug volume than SVN	Not all medications available
Aerosol accumulates during exhalation	Drug preparation required
VM Nebulizer	
Low residual volume	Expensive
Quiet	Not all medications available
Does not require gas or propellant	Drug preparation required
Flow-independent delivery	
Shorter treatment times	

Modified from Hess D: Aerosol delivery. Respir Care Clin N Am 1:235, 1995.

Selecting an Aerosol Drug Delivery System

pMDIs, DPIs, and nebulizers all work with comparable clinical results, as long as they are prescribed for the appropriate patients and are used properly.[58-60] Consequently, clinicians need to know the strengths and limitations of each type of device, match the device to each patient, and ensure that the patient or caregiver is trained to use the device properly.[51] Figure 39-28 is an algorithm that provides guidance regarding device selection.

Box 39-7 Factors Associated With Reduced Aerosol Drug Deposition in the Lung

- Mechanical ventilation
- Artificial airways
- Reduced airway caliber (e.g., infants and children)
- Severe airway obstruction
- High gas flows
- Low minute volumes
- Poor patient compliance or technique
- Limitation of specific delivery device

Regardless of the device used, the clinician must be aware of the limitations of aerosol drug therapy. First, depending on the device and patient, 10% or less of drug emitted from an aerosol device may be deposited in the lungs (Figure 39-29). As indicated in Box 39-7, additional reductions in lung deposition can occur in many clinical situations that sometimes necessitate the use of higher dosages. Clinical efficacy varies according to both patient technique and device design. For these reasons, the best approach to aerosol drug therapy is to use an assessment-based protocol that emphasizes individually tailored therapy modified according to patient response.

ASSESSMENT-BASED BRONCHODILATOR THERAPY PROTOCOLS

Although the choice of delivery system affects how well an aerosolized drug works, it is ultimately the patient's response that determines the therapeutic outcome. Because patients vary markedly in response to the dose and route of drug administration, it makes sense to tailor aerosol drug therapy to each patient. This approach is best determined with an assessment-based protocol.

Sample Protocol

Figure 39-30 is an algorithm of a bronchodilator therapy protocol for acutely ill adults or children admitted to an emergency department.[61] The protocol relies heavily on bedside assessment of the severity of airway obstruction based on the patient's response to varying drug dosages.

According to the algorithm, a patient with acute airway obstruction (wheezing, cough, dyspnea, and peak expiratory flow rate [PEFR] <60% of predicted value) would receive up to three SVN treatments with a standard dose of albuterol, repeated at 20-minute intervals, or 4 puffs of pMDI albuterol with a holding chamber (up to 12 puffs). Each treatment is followed by a dose-response assessment to determine the "best" dose. Once determined, this best dose, with the pMDI or SVN, is repeated 1 hour later, then every 4 hours as needed, supplemented with patient education. If use of the SVN or pMDI with

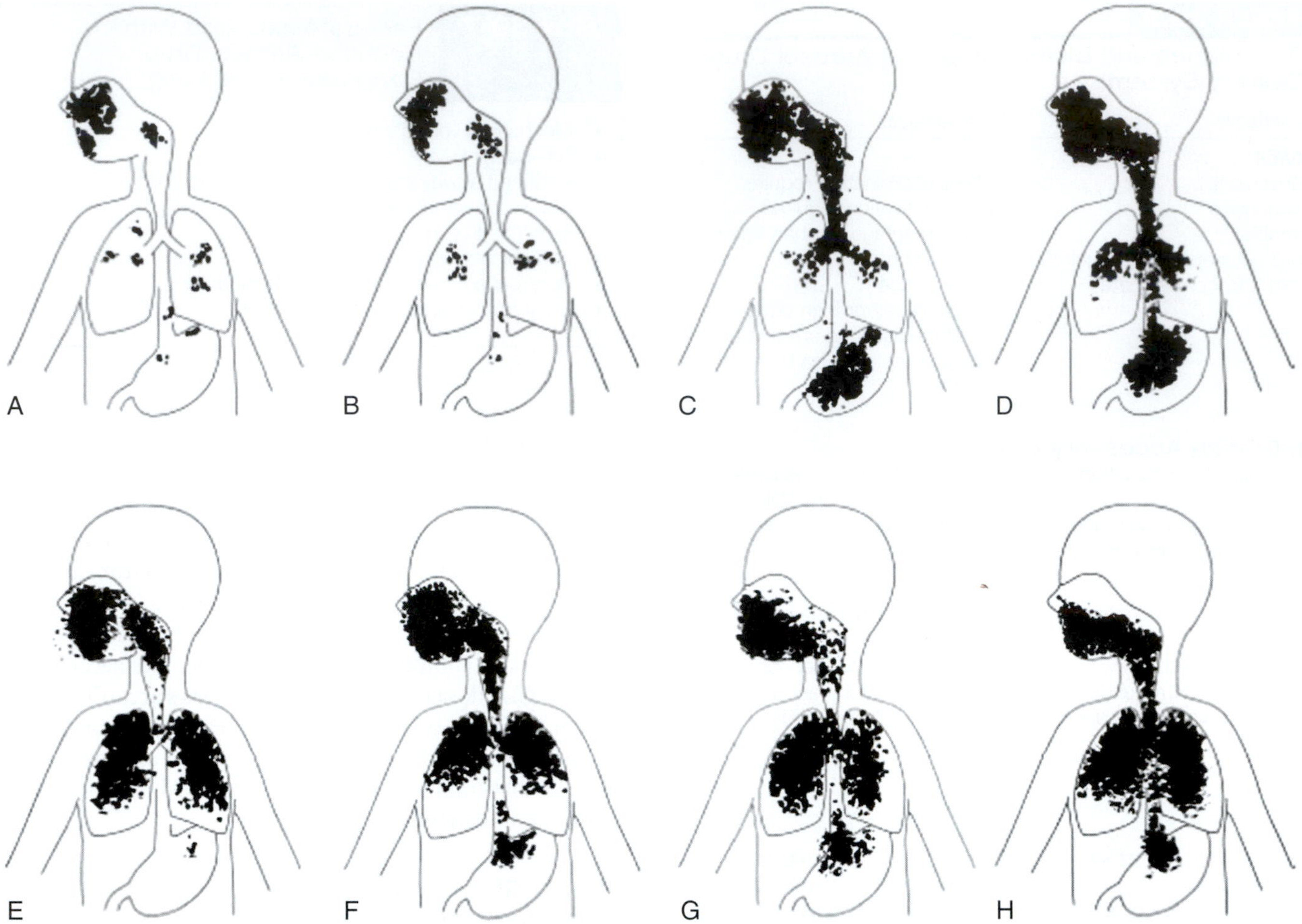

FIGURE 39-27 Drug deposition of radiolabeled albuterol in a young child **(A)** inhaling with a pMDI/space through a non-tightly fitted facemask; **(B)** inhaling with a nebulizer through a non-tightly fitted facemask; **(C)** inhaling with a pMDI/spacer through a tightly fitted facemask, screaming during inhalation; **(E, F)** inhaling with a pMDI/spacer through a tightly fitted facemask, quietly inhaling; and **(G, H)** inhaling from a nebulizer through a tightly fitted facemask, quietly inhaling. (Redrawn from Erzinger, S, Schueepp, KG, Brooks-Wildhaber, J, et al: Facemasks and aerosol delivery in vivo. J Aerosol Med 2007;20(Suppl 1.):S78–S84.)

holding chamber fails to relieve the symptoms, CBT with 15 mg/hr albuterol is generally started.

Assessing Patient Response

Careful, ongoing patient assessment is key to an effective bronchodilator therapy protocol.

Use and Limitations of Peak Flow Monitoring

Because the peak flow measurement is effort-dependent and volume-dependent, evaluation of patient performance is subjective, and there are no good acceptability criteria. In addition, agreement between conventional spirometry values, such as forced vital capacity (FVC) and FEV_1, and bedside PEFR values are poor for individual patients. Although peak flow measurement can be used at the bedside to assess treatment effectiveness and to monitor trends, conventional spirometry remains the standard for determining bronchodilator response.

Some peak flowmeters are more accurate and reliable than others. Even different units of the same model may give variable results. For this reason, when monitoring trends, the same unit should be used for a given patient and the patient's range be reestablished if a different flowmeter is used.

Other Components of Patient Assessment

Tests of expiratory airflow for assessing patient response to therapy are commonly used, but not all patients can perform these maneuvers. Other components of patient assessment useful in evaluating bronchodilator therapy include patient interviewing and observation, measurement of vital signs, auscultation, blood gas analysis, and oximetry.

When possible, the patient should be interviewed to determine the pertinent respiratory history and current level of dyspnea. A validated dyspnea rating scale may be useful for this purpose. Initial determination of patient age and level of consciousness is helpful in selecting both delivery device and starting drug dosage. Observing the patient for signs of increased work of breathing (e.g., tachypnea, accessory muscle use) provides a baseline for assessing status as therapy progresses. Restlessness, diaphoresis, and tachycardia also may indicate severity

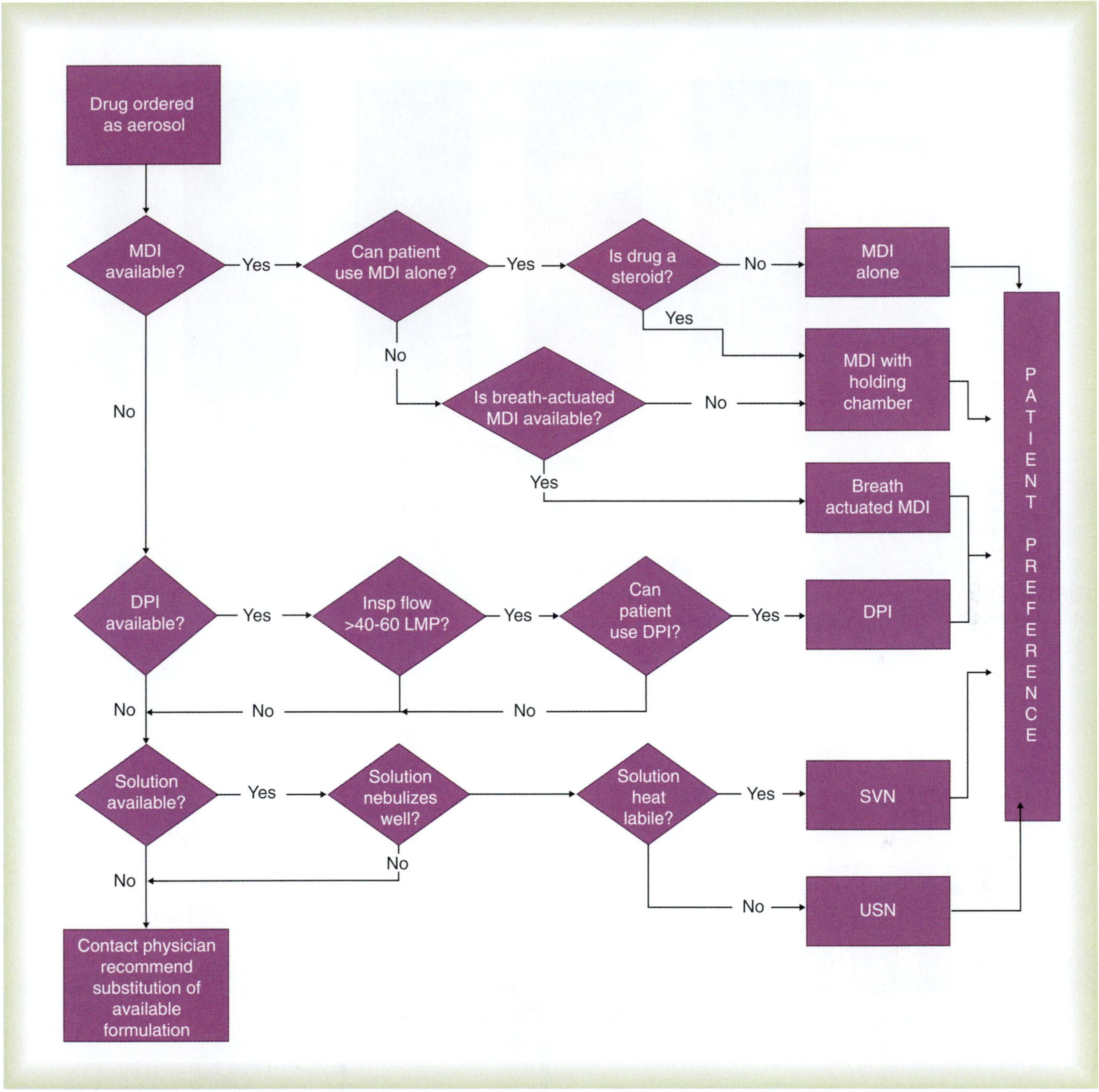

FIGURE 39-28 Selecting an aerosol drug delivery system. When the need is established for aerosol drug delivery, the formulations available for the prescribed medication should be determined. If a pMDI is available, it is the first choice for cost and convenience. The patient's ability to coordinate actuation with inspiration and the need to reduce oropharyngeal deposition (e.g., steroids) determine need for a holding chamber or a breath-actuated unit. Nebulizers are the first choice when the formulation is available only as a solution. When the ordered medication is unavailable for inhalation use, the RT should recommend a substitution to the ordering physician.

of airway obstruction but must not be confused with bronchodilator overdose.

Increased cough has been associated with the onset of asthma. The frequency, severity, and effectiveness of cough should be assessed before and after therapy.

In terms of breath sounds, a decrease in wheezing accompanied by an overall decrease in the intensity of breath sounds indicates worsening airway obstruction or patient fatigue. Improvement is indicated when wheezing decreases and the overall intensity of breath sounds increases.

All patients with acute airway obstruction should be monitored for oxygenation status with pulse oximetry. This value can be used in conjunction with observational assessment to titrate the level of inspired O_2 given to the patient (see Chapter 38).

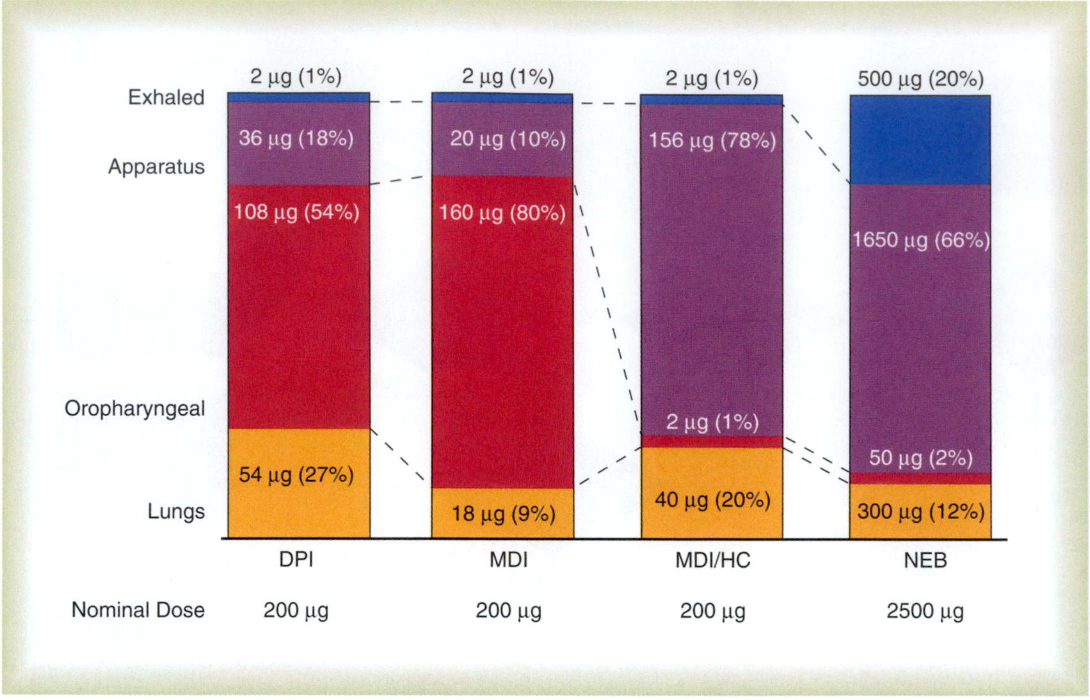

FIGURE 39-29 Distribution of albuterol via nebulizer, pMDI, pMDI with a holding chamber, and DPI. (Modified from Fink J: Metered-dose inhalers, dry powder inhalers and transitions. Respir Care 45:623, 2000.)

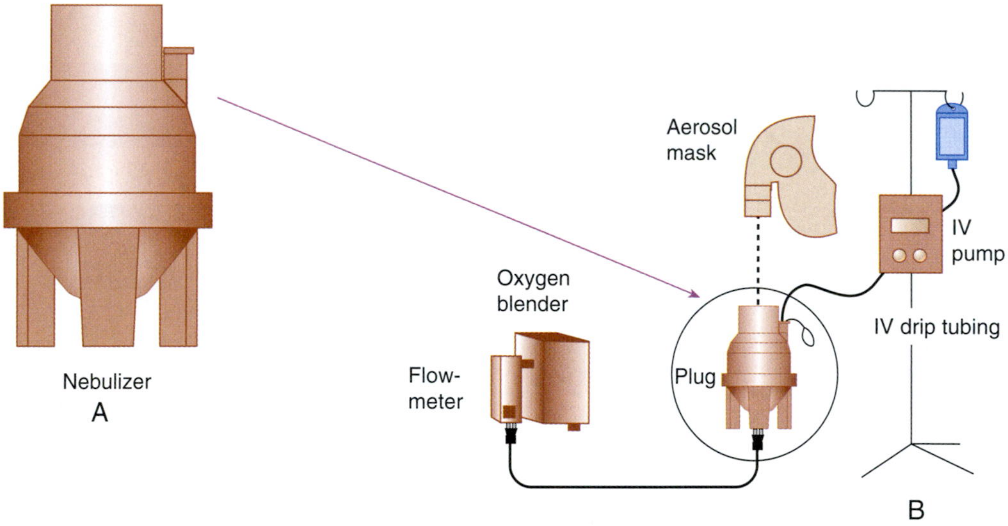

FIGURE 39-30 Algorithm underlying a bronchodilator therapy protocol for acutely ill adults or children admitted to an emergency department. *PEFR,* Peak expiratory flow rate; *VS,* vital signs.

Arterial blood gases are not essential for determining patient response to bronchodilator therapy but may be needed for patients in severe distress to assess for hypercapnic respiratory failure.

Dose-Response Assessment

Poor patient response to bronchodilator therapy often occurs because an inadequate amount of drug reaches the airway. To determine the "best" dose for patients with moderate obstruction, the respiratory therapist should conduct a dose-response titration.

A simple albuterol dose-response titration involves giving an initial 4 puffs (90 mcg/puff) at 1-minute intervals through a pMDI with a holding chamber. After 5 minutes, if airway obstruction is not relieved, the RT gives 1 puff per minute until symptoms are relieved, heart rate increases by more than

Box 39-8 Frequency of Assessment of Bronchodilator Therapy

FOR PATIENT WITH AN ACUTE DISORDER WHO IS IN UNSTABLE CONDITION

- Whenever possible, perform a full assessment and obtain a pretreatment baseline.
- Assess and document all appropriate variables before and after each treatment (breath sounds, vital signs, side effects during therapy, and PEFR or FEV_1).
- The frequency with which physical examination and PEFR or FEV_1 are repeated should be based on the acuteness of the disorder and the severity of the patient's condition.
- SpO_2 should be monitored continuously, if possible.
- Assessment should continue as dosages are changed to optimize patient response (e.g., if an asthmatic patient achieves 70% to 90% of predicted or "personal best" or becomes symptom-free).

FOR STABLE PATIENT

- In the hospital, PEFR should be measured initially before and after each bronchodilator administration. Thereafter, twice-daily determinations may be adequate.
- In the home, PEFR ideally should be measured three or four times a day: on rising, at noon, between 4 PM and 7 PM, and at bedtime.
- For a stable COPD patient at home, measuring PEFR twice a day may be adequate.
- Patients with asthma should adjust the frequency of PEFR measurement according to the severity of symptoms.
- PEFR levels before and after bronchodilator use, medication dose, date and time, and dyspnea score should be documented.
- The patient should be reevaluated periodically for response to therapy.

20 beats/min, tremors increase, or 12 puffs are delivered. The best dose is the dose that provides maximum relief of symptoms and the highest PEFR without side effects.

Frequency of Patient Assessment

How frequently patients should undergo assessment for bronchodilator therapy depends primarily on the acuity of the condition. An unstable patient in acute distress should undergo closer and more frequent scrutiny than a patient in stable condition. Box 39-8 provides guidance regarding the frequency of assessment according to acuity.

Patient Education

The desired outcome of all bronchodilator protocols is restoration of normal airflow and cessation of therapy. For patients who need ongoing maintenance therapy after the acute phase of illness, the goal should be effective self-administration. An effective program of aerosol drug self-administration depends on thorough patient education.

The patient's ability to understand the therapy and its goals significantly affects the therapeutic efficacy of any treatment. Whenever possible, patients should be taught to understand the basic administration techniques, to keep track of dosing requirements, to recognize undesirable side effects, and to understand the options and actions required to reduce or eliminate these effects. In addition, patients should be able to demonstrate good technique regarding the use of each aerosol device that they are expected to use in self-care. Practitioner demonstration followed by repeated patient return demonstration is a must and should be done frequently, with each office or clinic visit.

SPECIAL CONSIDERATIONS

Aerosol Therapy for Treatment of Pulmonary Arterial Hypertension

Epoprostenol (Veletri®, Actelion Pharmaceuticals US, Inc, South San Francisco, CA), epoprostenol sodium (Flolan®, GlaxoSmithKline, Research Triangle Park, NC), iloprost (Ventavis®, Actelion Pharmaceuticals US Inc, South San Francisco, CA), and treprostinil (Tyvaso) are inhaled prostacyclins used for treatment of pulmonary arterial hypertension. Whereas epoprostenol administration is associated with positive effects on symptoms, hemodynamics, exercise capacity, disease progression and survival,[62-64] it has not been approved for inhalation, and due to its short half-life of 30 to 90 seconds, requires continuous nebulization. In contrast, iloprost and treprostinil are approved for inhalation with a half-life of 60 to 90 minutes, allowing more convenient dosing to ambulatory patients.

Acute Care and Off-Label Use

Every drug approved for inhalation to date has been designed for and tested in populations of ambulatory patients with moderate disease. As patients with lung disease become acutely and critically ill, the approved label doses, frequency of administration, and devices may not be practical or effective, especially for treatment of patients requiring ventilatory support. In such cases, clinicians may explore and consider nonstandard methods (doses, frequency, and devices) for administration of approved inhaled drugs to patients in the acute care environment, known as *off-label use*. Another type of off-label use involves drugs that have not been approved for inhalation, ranging from heparin to certain antibiotics. Although physicians may order such drugs via inhalation, the risk to the patient and institution is greater when the administration of such drugs via inhalation has not been thoroughly studied. All forms of off-label use should be avoided when approved and viable alternatives exist. Likewise, off-label administration should always be backed by appropriate departmental or institutional policies and procedures.

Continuous Nebulization for Refractory Bronchospasm

Patients in the emergency department with severe exacerbation of asthma or acute bronchospasm often have been taking standard doses of their bronchodilators for 24 to 36 hours before admission without response. Giving nebulizer treatments with standard bronchodilator doses and repeating the treatments until the symptoms are relieved can require hours of staff time. Administering higher doses of albuterol in short time frames can be accomplished by nebulization of undiluted albuterol (8 to 20 breaths) or by protocol titration with a pMDI and holding chamber (up to 12 puffs). If these strategies fail to provide relief, CBT with albuterol nebulization doses ranging from 5 to 20 mg/hr have proved safe and effective for adult and pediatric patients (Figure 39-31).

Figure 39-32 is a treatment algorithm for high-dose therapy and CBT for pediatric patients with status asthmaticus who are unable to perform peak flow maneuvers.[65] Candidates for this protocol are children who, despite frequent beta agonist treatments, remain in extremis with bronchospasm, dyspnea, cough, chest tightness, and diminished breath sounds.

According to this protocol, children older than 6 years with tachypnea, hypoxemia, increased work of breathing, and restlessness who do not respond to standard therapy are given CBT

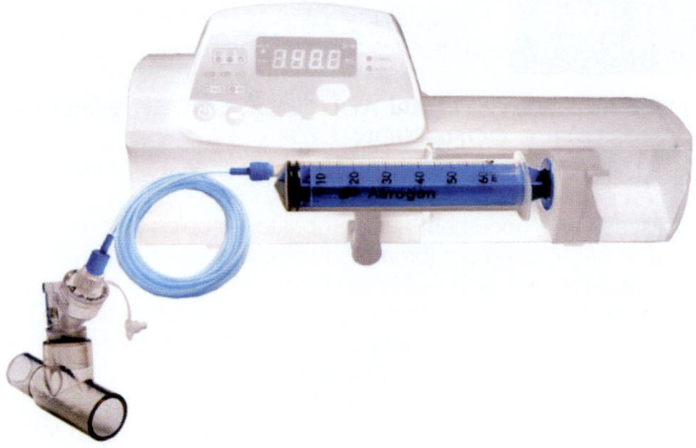

FIGURE 39-31 Continuous line from a syringe pump attached to a nebulizer.

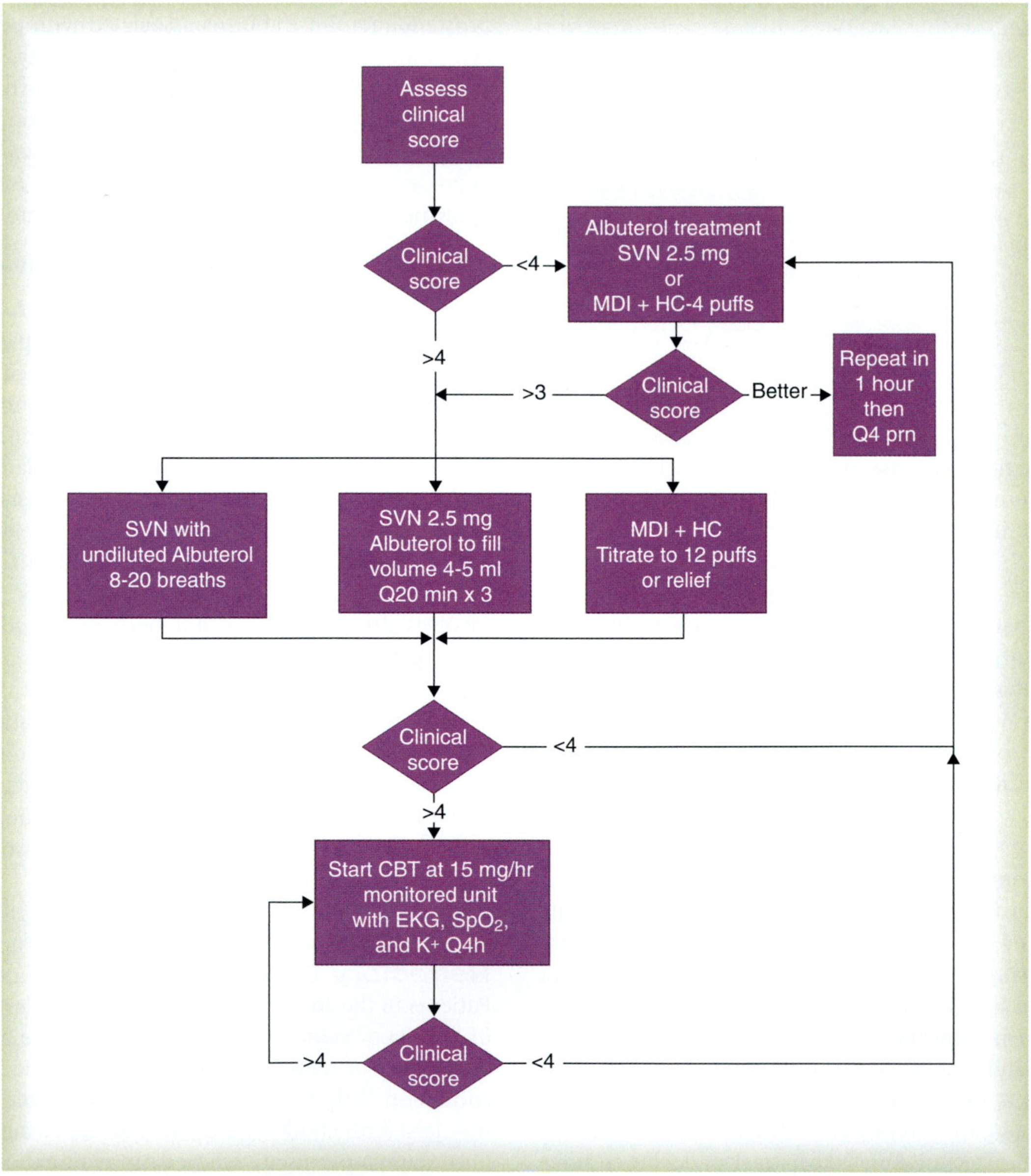

FIGURE 39-32 Algorithm for CBT for patients younger than 5 years with pediatric asthma in extremis.

TABLE 39-4

Pediatric Asthma Score

Indicator	SCORE 0	1	2
PaO_2	>70 mm Hg (air)	<70 mm Hg (air)	<70 mm Hg (40% O_2)
SpO_2	>94% (air)	<94% (air)	<94% (40% O_2)
Cyanosis	No	Yes	Yes
Breath sounds	Equal	Unequal	Absent
Wheezing	None	Moderate	Marked
Accessory muscle use	None	Moderate	Marked
Level of consciousness	Alert	Agitated or depressed	Comatose

Modified from Volpe J: Therapist-driven protocols for pediatric patients. Respir Care Clin N Am 2:117, 1996.

with a large volume nebulizer or SVN at a dose rate of 15 mg/hr (see the accompanying Mini Clini "CBT Dosage Computations" for dosage computations). A standardized asthma score is used to evaluate children younger than 6 years for the severity of the condition (Table 39-4). Patients with an asthma score of 4 or higher are given CBT.

After CBT is started, the patient is carefully assessed every 30 minutes for the first 2 hours and thereafter every hour. A positive response is indicated by an increase in PEFR of at least 10% after the first hour of therapy. The goal is at least 50% of the predicted value. For small children, improved oxygenation (oxygen saturation by pulse oximeter [SpO_2] >92% on room air) with evidence of decreased work of breathing indicates a favorable response. Once the patient "opens up," intermittent SVN administration is resumed, or a pMDI dose-response assessment is conducted.

The patient has responded poorly to CBT if any of the indicators listed in Table 39-4 worsens. The patient must be observed for adverse drug responses, including worsening tachycardia, palpitations, and vomiting. In these situations, the attending physician must be contacted immediately.

As an alternative to large volume drug nebulizers, some protocols are based on high-dose pMDI therapy (12 to 24 puffs per hour).[66] To provide an extra margin of safety, some clinicians recommend that patients receiving CBT undergo continuous electrocardiogram monitoring and measurement of serum potassium level every 4 hours.

Aerosol Administration to Mechanically Ventilated Patients

Since the advent of modern mechanical ventilation, clinicians have administered aerosols to patients with the sickest of lungs. Four primary forms of aerosol generator are used to deliver aerosols during mechanical ventilation: SVN, USN, VM nebulizer, and pMDI with third-party adapter. Table 39-5 summarizes the factors affecting aerosol drug delivery to mechanically ventilated patients. Techniques to optimize delivery to patients receiving ventilatory support are described.[67]

TABLE 39-5

Factors Affecting Aerosol Drug Delivery During Mechanical Ventilation

Category	Factor
Ventilator-related	Mode of ventilation
	V_T
	Respiratory rate
	Duty cycle
	Inspiratory waveform
	Breath-triggering mechanism
Circuit-related	Size of endotracheal tube
	Type of humidifier
	Relative humidity
	Density and viscosity of inhaled gas
Device-related MDI	Type of spacer or adapter used
	Position of spacer in circuit
	Timing of MDI actuation
SVN	Type of nebulizer used
	Fill volume
	Gas flow
	Cycling: inspiration vs. continuous
	Duration of nebulization
	Position in circuit
Patient-related	Severity of airway obstruction
	Mechanism of airway obstruction
	Presence of dynamic hyperinflation
	Spontaneous ventilation
	Disease process
Drug-related	Dose
	Aerosol particle size
	Targeted site for delivery
	Duration of action

MINI CLINI

Continuous Bronchodilator Therapy Dosage Computations

PROBLEM: Dosages for CBT are ordered in milligrams per hour, and delivery depends on both drug concentration and nebulizer output. Compute the volume of 1 : 200 (0.5%) albuterol and the volume of diluent (normal saline solution) needed to provide 4 hours of CBT with 15 mg/hr of albuterol in a nebulizer with an output of 25 ml/hr.

DISCUSSION: *Step 1:* Compute the volume of albuterol given per hour (mg/hr × ml/mg).

$$15.0\ \text{mg/hr} \times 0.2\ \text{ml/mg} = 3.0\ \text{ml/hr albuterol}$$

Step 2: Compute the volume of albuterol for the treatment period (hours × ml/hr).

$$4\ \text{hours} \times 3.0\ \text{ml/hr} = 12\ \text{ml/4 hr albuterol}$$

Step 3: Compute the volume of nebulization solution (ml/hr nebulizer output × hours).

$$25\ \text{ml/hr} \times 4\ \text{hours} = 100\ \text{ml}$$

Step 4: Compute the volume of diluent required.

$$100\ \text{ml} - 12\ \text{ml} = 88\ \text{ml normal saline solution}$$

To prepare this dosage, mix 12 ml of 0.5% albuterol with 88 ml of normal saline solution, for a total nebulizer solution volume of 100 ml. In this example, residual volume of the nebulizer decreases total treatment time and dose.

Regarding doses, the amount of drug required to achieve the same therapeutic end point is substantially similar for medications delivered by pMDI to intubated patients (8%) and patients who are not intubated (8% to 10%). In stable patients with COPD receiving ventilatory support, 4 puffs of albuterol via pMDI with chamber and 2.5 mg via SVN were shown to produce maximum bronchodilation with effects lasting for 4 hours. However, some differences in response were noted that may have been due to the level of airway obstruction and the techniques used for assessing response.

Techniques for assessing the response to a bronchodilator in intubated patients undergoing mechanical ventilation differ from techniques used in the care of spontaneously breathing patients because expiration is passive during mechanical ventilation, and forced expiratory values (PEFR, FVC, FEV_1) cannot normally be obtained. Additional techniques can be used for mechanically ventilated patients because (1) a change in the differences between peak and plateau pressures (volume ventilation with constant flow, the most reliable indicator of a change in airway resistance during continuous mechanical ventilation) can be measured, (2) automatic positive end expiratory pressure levels may decrease in response to bronchodilators (see Chapter 44), and (3) breath-to-breath variations make measurements more reliable when the patient is not actively breathing with the ventilator.[68]

Techniques for aerosol administration vary by type of aerosol generator and device used. The optimal technique for drug delivery to mechanically ventilated patients with each type of aerosol generator is described in Box 39-9.

Box 39-9 Optimal Technique for Aerosolized Drug Delivery to Mechanically Ventilated Patients

1. Review order, identify the patient, gather equipment, and assess the need for bronchodilators.
2. Clear the airways as needed, by suctioning the patient as needed.
3. If using a circuit with heat and moisture exchanger (HME), remove HME from between the aerosol generator and the patient.
4. If using heated humidifier, do not turn off or disconnect before or during treatment.
5. Assemble equipment (tubing, nebulizer, circuit adapter).
6. Fill the nebulizer with recommended volume and medication per physician order and label.
7. Place adapter in the inspiratory limb, 6 inches from the "wye," and connect aerosol generator.
8. Turn off or minimize bias flow during treatment.
9. Connect the nebulizer to a gas or power source, as appropriate.

10a. For jet nebulizer (including SVN): Use gas source on ventilator to synchronize nebulization with inspiration, if available; otherwise, set gas flow 6 to 10 L/min as recommended on nebulizer label, and adjust ventilator volume or pressure limit and alarms to compensate for added flow and volume.
10b. For USN and VM nebulizer: Attach power source and cable from controller.
10c. For pMDI: Shake canister and connect to spacer or adapter; actuate at beginning of inspiration.

11. Observe aerosol cloud for adequate aerosol generation during nebulization.
12. After appropriate dose is administered, remove aerosol generator from the ventilator circuit.
13. Reconnect HME, as appropriate.
14. Return ventilator settings and alarms to previous values.
15. Ensure there is no leak in the ventilator circuit.
16. Rinse the nebulizer with sterile or distilled water, shake off excess water, and allow to air dry.
17. Store aerosol device in a clean, dry place.
18. Monitor heart rate, SpO_2, blood pressure, and patient-ventilator synchronization.
19. Monitor the patient for adverse response.
20. Assess the airway, and suction as needed; document findings.

Use of a Small Volume Nebulizer During Mechanical Ventilation

The aerosol administered by SVN to intubated patients receiving mechanical ventilation tends to be deposited mainly in the tubing of the ventilator circuit and expiratory filter. Under normal conditions with heated humidification and standard jet nebulizers, pulmonary deposition ranges from 1.5% to 3.0%.[68,69] When nebulizer output, humidity level, V_T, flow, and I : E ratio are optimized, deposition can increase to 15%.

There are several disadvantages with SVN use during mechanical ventilation. Although in vitro models showed 40% higher aerosol delivery with an unheated, unhumidified circuit compared with heated humidity, these effects have not been shown in patients, whereas the risks associated with administering cold and dry gas through an endotracheal tube include drying of secretions, bronchospasm, and airway obstruction. A heat and moisture exchanger should be considered a barrier to aerosol administration and should always be removed if placed between the nebulizer and the patient airway. When available with the specific ventilator being used, breath actuation can increase aerosol delivery by 30%, but it may extend administration time by more than threefold. Introducing additional flow into the ventilator circuit may change parameters of flow and delivered volumes and require changes to alarm settings during and after nebulization. The smaller the patient, the greater the impact of added flow into the ventilator circuit, where 6 L/min of additional gas flow can more than double V_T and inspiratory pressure, placing the patient at risk. Risk is high for not changing ventilator parameters and not returning parameters to pretreatment levels after administration. There is also a tendency for condensate and secretions to drain into the nebulizer reservoir, contaminating medication being delivered to the lungs.

Use of a Vibrating Mesh Nebulizer During Mechanical Ventilation

Aerosol administration by a VM nebulizer has been estimated to deliver greater than 10% deposition in adults and infants without the addition of gas into the ventilator circuit. The low residual drug volume and small particle size are associated with higher efficiency. Similar to the USN, the VM nebulizer does not add gas flow into the ventilator circuit, so ventilator

MINI CLINI

Never Emptying Nebulizer

PROBLEM: Jet nebulizers and USNs are commonly used to administer aerosol to patients during mechanical ventilation. Commonly, a nebulizer is filled with a standard unit dose of 3 ml of medication at the beginning of the aerosol treatment, and the RT finds as much or more fluid in the medication reservoir 20 to 30 minutes later. The additional fluid is usually condensate (often contaminated from patient secretions), which drains from the inspiratory limb into the gravity-dependent reservoir of the nebulizer. Even heated wire circuits may have condensate. Although pathogens in a dry circuit have minimal chance of contaminating the patient's airway, aerosolizing the pathogens provides a vehicle for infectious material to enter the airway and the lung parenchyma.

SOLUTION: The nebulizer should be positioned so that the upper end of the reservoir is superior to (higher than) the ventilator tubing attached to both ends of the nebulizer. This position allows the condensate and secretions to drain away from the nebulizer. Alternatively, nebulizers with physical barriers between the ventilator circuit tubing and the medication reservoir can be used. These options include use of a pMDI with spacer or a VM nebulizer.

parameters and alarms do not need to be adjusted before, during, or after nebulization. In contrast to jet SVNs and USNs, the medication reservoir of the VM nebulizer is above the circuit and separated from the ventilator tubing by the mesh, reducing the risk of retrograde contamination of medication in the reservoir from the ventilator circuit. Because of the nature of the mesh, the reservoir can be opened and medication can be added to the nebulizer without creating a perceptible leak during ventilation.

Use of a Pressurized Metered Dose Inhaler During Mechanical Ventilation

Results of in vitro studies show that effective aerosol delivery by pMDIs during mechanical ventilation can range from 2% to 30%. Direct pMDI actuation by simple elbow adapters typically results in the least pulmonary deposition, with most of the aerosol impacting in either the ventilator circuit or the tracheal airway. Higher aerosol delivery percentages occur only when an actuator or spacer is placed in-line in the ventilator circuit. These spacers allow an aerosol "plume" to develop before the bulk of the particles impact on the surface of the circuit or endotracheal tube. The result is a more stable aerosol mass that can penetrate beyond the artificial airway and be deposited mainly in the lung. This situation leads to a better clinical response at lower doses.[49]

Aerosol Generator Placement

Placement of aerosol generators in the ventilator circuit can have a substantial impact on the available lung dose of drug. During adult ventilation without bias flow, placement of aerosol generators 18 to 24 inches from the patient in the inspiratory limb increases inhaled dose for jet nebulizers, where continuous gas flow acts to charge the inspiratory limb of the ventilator circuit with aerosol. In contrast, pMDI, USN, and VM nebulizer devices are more efficient when placed close to the patient at the circuit wye.[70,71] With continuous or bias flow through the adult and pediatric ventilator circuit, the delivery is reduced as flow increases, whereas placement of a VM or USN nebulizer near the ventilator increases delivery (Figure 39-33).[71,72]

Placement During Noninvasive Ventilation

Noninvasive ventilation may be administered with standard and bilevel ventilators. Bilevel ventilators often use a flow turbine, with a fixed leak in the circuit that permits excess flow to vent to atmosphere. Placement of the aerosol generator between the leak and the patient's airway seems to provide the highest aerosol delivery efficiency.[73,74] A VM nebulizer delivers a greater inhaled dose than an SVN during noninvasive ventilation, presumably because of the lower residual drug volume and lower total flow in the circuit.[75]

Placement During High-Flow Nasal Cannula

Delivery of aerosol via a high-flow nasal cannula (HFNC) with infant, pediatric, and adult cannulas, is markedly limited.[76] Figure 39-34 shows the setup with HFNC, including the location of the VM nebulizer. However, placement of the VM nebulizer prior to the humidifier increases aerosol deposition with HFNC.[77] In addition to the location of the nebulizer with HFNC, the inhaled dose seems to vary based on cannula size, respiratory pattern, and O_2 flow. Heliox (80 : 20) appears to improve aerosol delivery at higher flow rates with these setups.[77] The administration of aerosolized medications via HFNC is less efficient than removing the cannula during administration.[78] When delivering aerosolized medications by mask, the benefit of increased aerosol delivery must be weighed against the risk of desaturation when nasal prongs are removed.

Placement During Intrapulmonary Percussive Ventilation

Intrapulmonary percussive ventilation provides high-frequency oscillation of the airway while administering aerosol particles. During intrapulmonary percussive ventilation, the aerosol generator should be placed in the circuit as close to the patient's airway as practical. A comparison study found the MMAD was smaller with intrapulmonary percussive ventilation than with the jet (0.2 μm vs. 1.89 μm), and the fine-particle fraction was lower (16.2% vs. 67.5%). However, lung dose was similar (2.49% with intrapulmonary percussive ventilation vs. 4.2% with the jet nebulizer). It was concluded that intrapulmonary percussive ventilation was too variable and too unpredictable to recommend for drug delivery to the lung.[79]

Placement During High-Frequency Oscillatory Ventilation

When used in conjunction with high-frequency oscillatory ventilation, administration of albuterol sulfate via a VM nebulizer

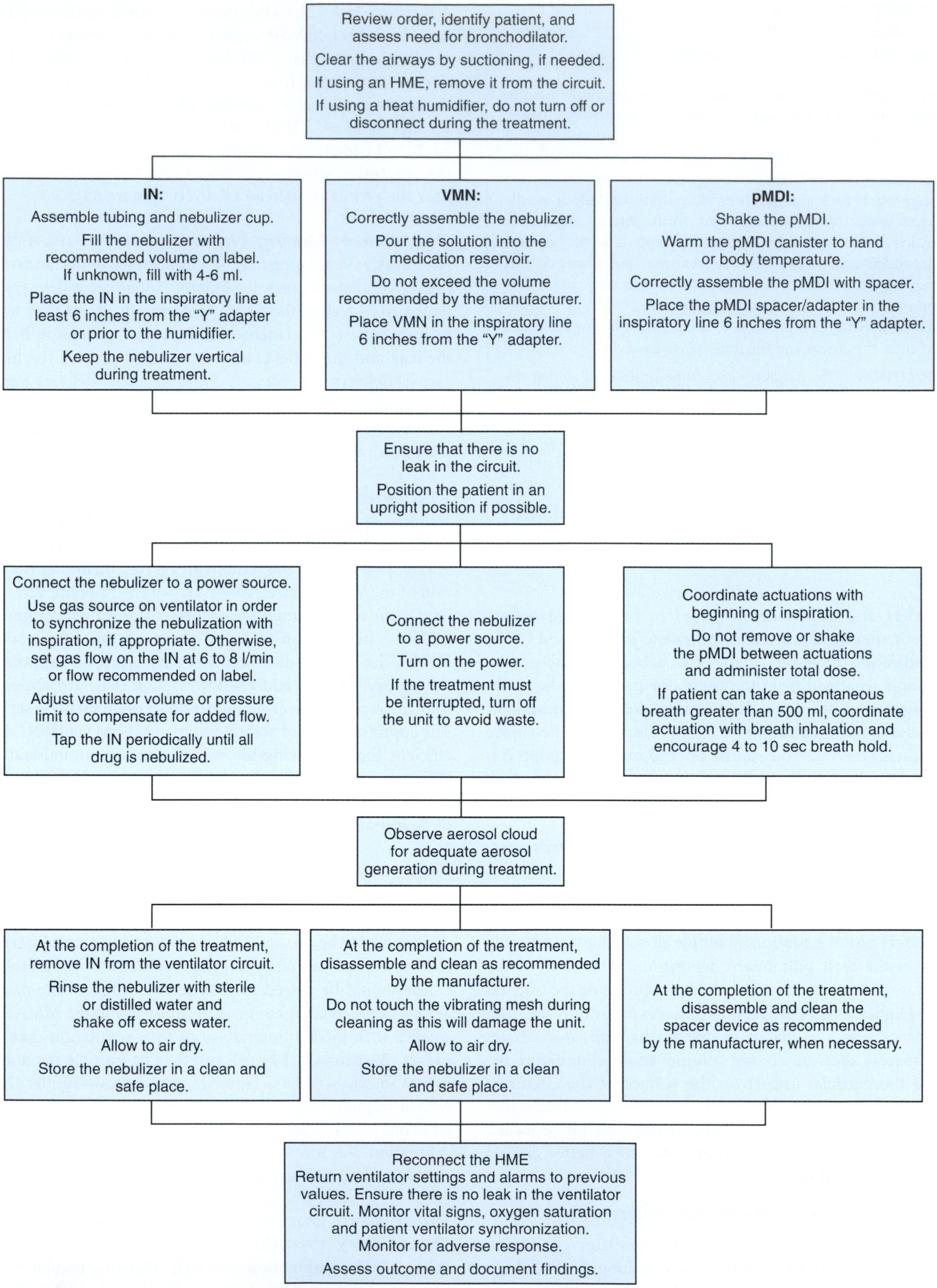

FIGURE 39-33 Frequency of assessment according to acuity. (From Ari A, Fink TB: Factors affecting bronchodilator delivery in mechanically ventilated adults. Nurs Crit Care 15:192, 2010.)

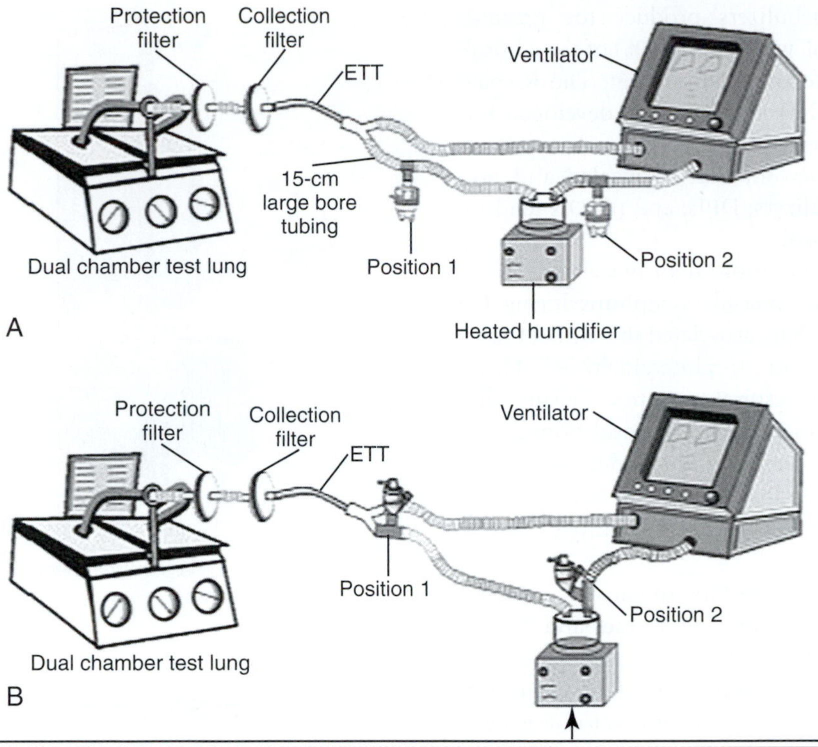

	Percent of nominal or emitted dose (mean ± SD %)							
	Adult lung model				Pediatric lung model			
	Position 1		Position 2		Position 1		Position 2	
	Bias flow 2 L/min	Bias flow 5 L/min	Bias flow 2 L/min	Bias flow 5 L/min	Bias flow 2 L/min	Bias flow 5 L/min	Bias flow 2 L/min	Bias flow 5 L/min
Jet nebulizer	4.7 ± 0.1*	4.0 ± 0.1*	5.2 ± 0.2*	4.7 ± 0.4*	4.2 ± 0.2*	3.8 ± 0.3*	5.2 ± 0.3*	4.1 ± 0.4*
Vibrating-mesh nubulizer	13.4 ± 1.1	9.7 ± 0.6	23.8 ± 1.0	21.4 ± 0.4	11.4 ± 0.7	8.4 ± 0.2	13.6 ± 1.3	10.6 ± 0.3

*Significant difference between jet nebulizer and vibrating-mesh nebulizer (p< 05).

FIGURE 39-34 Placement of SVN and VM nebulizer aerosol generators in two positions in the ventilator circuit with 2 L/min and 5 L/min of bias flow results in different deposition efficiency.

placed between the ventilator circuit and the patient airway has been reported to deliver greater than 10% of dose to both infants and adults.[80,81] A pMDI with adapter placed immediately proximal to the endotracheal tube achieved similar results in adult patients ventilated via high-frequency oscillatory ventilation.[82]

CONTROLLING ENVIRONMENTAL CONTAMINATION

Drugs for nebulization that escape from the nebulizer into the atmosphere or are exhaled by the patient can be inhaled by anyone in the vicinity of the treatment. The risk imposed by this environmental exposure is clear and is associated with a range of drugs and patients with infectious disease. Pentamidine and ribavirin were associated with health risks to health care providers even when used in conjunction with filters on exhalation ports of nebulizers, containment and scavenger systems, and *high-efficiency particulate air (HEPA)* filter hoods and ventilation systems (Figure 39-35).

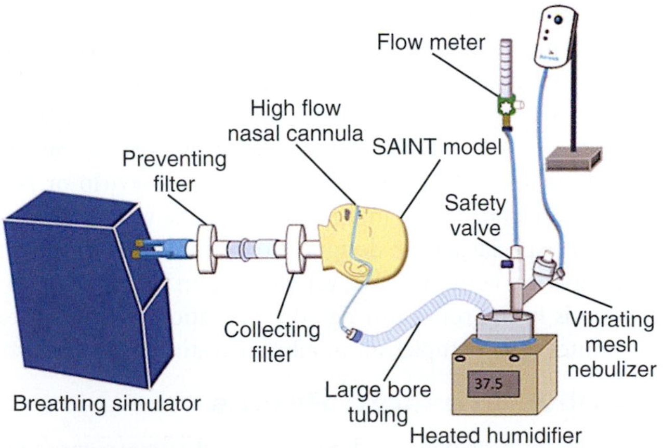

FIGURE 39-35 In vitro model. (From Bhashyam AR, Wolf MT, Marcinkowski AL, et al: Aerosol delivery through nasal cannulas: an in vitro study. J Aerosol Med Pulm Drug Deliv 21:181, 2008.)

Continuous pneumatic nebulizers produce the greatest amount of secondhand aerosol, with most (60%) of the aerosol produced passing directly into the environment. The Respirgard II (Vital Signs, Totowa, NJ) nebulizer was developed for administration of pentamidine, adding one-way valves and an expiratory filter to contain aerosol that is exhaled and not inhaled. Breath-actuated nebulizers, DPIs, and pMDIs tend to generate less secondhand aerosol.

A survey found that RTs were more than twice as likely as physical therapists to develop asthma-like symptoms during the course of their careers. The authors associated this with administration of ribavirin and exposure to gluteraldehyde.[16] There have been anecdotal reports of respiratory care clinicians who have developed a sensitivity to secondhand aerosol from bronchodilators. Further research is required to understand more thoroughly the hazards of secondhand exposure to aerosols in the clinical setting. Most nebulizer therapy currently delivered does not include filtering systems.

Patients with infectious and resistant organisms, such as tuberculosis, severe acute respiratory syndrome, and H1N1 virus, require respiratory isolation, and caregivers require protection. RTs have a duty to take appropriate steps to protect themselves and their patients. In these cases, the aerosols generated by the patient from coughing, speaking, or laughing can transmit disease. These aerosols can travel substantial distances between rooms and even floors in institutions. Although exposure to secondhand aerosol generated by a nebulizer is undesirable, it poses less risk than the infected aerosols produced by mucosa of patients.[83] In essence, it is unlikely that any medical aerosol that is inhaled by the patient would be contaminated. Nonetheless, during the severe acute respiratory syndrome outbreak, some centers outlawed use of medical aerosols to reduce exposure. Efforts should be taken to reduce transmission of both nebulizer aerosols and patient-generated aerosols to the environment.

Various techniques are available for protecting patients and caregivers from environmental exposure during aerosol drug therapy. The greatest occupational risk for RTs has been associated with the administration of ribavirin and pentamidine. Conjunctivitis, headaches, bronchospasm, shortness of breath, and rashes have been reported among individuals administering these drugs.[84] Patients given aerosolized ribavirin or pentamidine must be treated in a private negative room, booth, or tent or at a special station designed to minimize environmental contamination with the caregiver wearing an N95 mask during all periods in the room during administration and at for least 10 minutes after completion of administration of the aerosol.

Negative Pressure Rooms

When ribavirin or pentamidine is given, the treatment is provided in a private room. The room should be equipped for negative pressure ventilation with adequate air exchanges (at least six per hour) to clear the room of residual aerosols before the next treatment. HEPA filters should be used to filter room or tent exhaust, or the aerosol should be scavenged to the outside.

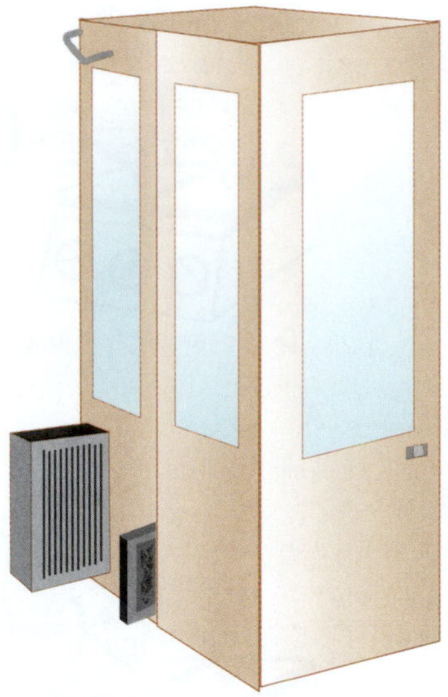

FIGURE 39-36 Emerson treatment booth provides containment of aerosol during therapy.

Booths and Stations

Booths or stations should be used for sputum induction and aerosolized medication treatments given in any area where more than one patient is treated. The area should be designed to provide adequate airflow to draw aerosol and droplet nuclei from the patient into an appropriate filtration system or an exhaust system directly to the outside. Booths and stations should be adequately cleaned between patients.

A variety of booths and specially designed stations are available for delivery of pentamidine or ribavirin. The Emerson containment booth (Figure 39-36) is an example of a system that completely isolates the patient during aerosol administration. The AeroStar Aerosol Protection Cart (Respiratory Safety Systems, San Diego, CA) is a portable patient isolation station for administration of hazardous aerosolized medication. It has been used during sputum induction and for pentamidine treatment. The patient compartment is collapsible with a swing-out counter and three polycarbonate walls. Captured aerosols are removed with a HEPA filter. A prefilter is used to retain larger dust particles and to prevent early loading of the more expensive HEPA filter.

Filters and nebulizers used in treatments with pentamidine and ribavirin should be treated as hazardous wastes and disposed of accordingly. Goggles, gloves, and gowns should be used as splatter shields and to reduce exposure to medication residues and body substances. Staff members should be screened for adverse effects of exposure to the aerosol medication. The risks and safety procedures should be reviewed regularly.

In addition to the risks associated with administration of aerosol medication, risk of tuberculosis transmission has become a great concern because of an increase in case numbers and the development of multidrug-resistant strains of the organism. Tuberculosis is transmitted in the form of droplet nuclei (0.3 to 0.6 μm) that carry tuberculosis bacilli. Patients with known or suspected tuberculosis need private rooms with negative pressure ventilation that exhausts to the outside. If environmental isolation is impossible or the health care worker must enter the patient's room, personal protective equipment should be used.

Personal Protective Equipment

Personal protective equipment is recommended when caring for any patient with a disease that can be spread by the airborne route.[85] The greatest risk is communication of tuberculosis or chickenpox. Although environmental controls should be instituted in the care of these patients, standard and airborne precautions should also be implemented. Various masks and respirators have been recommended for use when caring for a patient with tuberculosis or other respiration-transmitted diseases. Traditional surgical masks, particulate respirators, disposable and reusable HEPA filters, and powered air-purifying respirators (PAPR) have been used. No data are available for determining the most effective and most clinically useful device to protect health care workers and others, although the U.S. Occupational Safety and Health Administration requires specific levels of protection (HEPA filters and powered air-purifying respirators). Guidelines from the World Health Organization recommend surgical masks for all patient care with the exception of N95 masks for aerosol-generating procedures such as sputum induction. Evidence from laboratory studies of potential airborne spread of influenza from contagious patients indicates that guidelines related to the current 1-m respiratory zone may need to be extended to a larger respiratory zone and include eye protection.[86]

SUMMARY CHECKLIST

- An aerosol is a suspension of solid or liquid particles in gas. In the clinical setting, therapeutic aerosols are made with atomizers or nebulizers.
- The general aim of aerosol drug therapy is delivery of a therapeutic dose of the selected agent to the desired site of action.
- Where aerosol particles are deposited in the respiratory tract depends on their size, shape, and motion and on the physical characteristics of the airways. Key mechanisms causing aerosol deposition include inertial impaction, sedimentation, and brownian diffusion.
- For targeting aerosols for delivery to the upper airway (nose, larynx, trachea), particles in the 5- to 20-μm MMAD range are used; for the lower airways, 2- to 5-μm particles are used; and for the lung parenchyma (alveolar region), 1- to 3-μm particles are used.
- The primary hazard of aerosol drug therapy is an adverse reaction to the medication being administered. Other hazards include infection, airway reactivity, systemic effects of bland aerosols, and drug reconcentration.
- Drug aerosol delivery systems include pMDIs, DPIs, SVNs, large volume jet nebulizers, hand-bulb atomizers (nasal spray pumps), USNs, and VM nebulizers.
- MDIs are the preferred method for maintenance delivery of bronchodilators and steroids to spontaneously breathing patients. The effectiveness of this therapy is highly technique-dependent.
- Accessory devices, spacers, and holding chambers are used with pMDIs to reduce oropharyngeal deposition of a drug and to overcome problems with poor hand-breath coordination.
- Effective use of DPIs does not require hand-breath coordination, but it does require high inspiratory flows. Some patients in stable condition prefer DPI delivery systems.
- Compared with pMDI and DPI delivery systems, use of an SVN is less technique-dependent and is more commonly used in acute care.
- Large volume drug nebulizers can be used to provide continuous aerosol delivery when traditional dosing strategies are ineffective in controlling severe bronchospasm.
- Small volume USNs can be used to administer bronchodilators, antiinflammatory agents, and antibiotics.
- Because patients vary greatly in their response to a particular drug dose and route of administration, aerosol drug therapy should be tailored to each patient with an assessment-based protocol.
- Careful, ongoing patient assessment is the key to an effective bronchodilator therapy protocol. Components of the assessment include a patient interview, observation, expiratory airflow tests, vital sign measurements, auscultation, blood gas analysis, and oximetry.
- Protocols for CBT have proved safe and effective in the management of refractory bronchospasm in both adults and children.
- Many factors affect the efficiency of aerosol drug delivery during mechanical ventilation. Proper selection of aerosol generator type, position in the circuit, dose, and accessory equipment is needed to optimize deposition and achieve the desired clinical outcome.
- Various techniques are available to protect patients and caregivers from environmental exposure during aerosol drug therapy.

References

1. Dolovich MA, MacIntyre NR, Anderson PJ, et al: Consensus statement: aerosols and delivery devices. American Association for Respiratory Care. *Respir Care* 45(6):589–596, 2000.
2. Dolovich M: Aerosols and aerosol drug delivery systems. In Adkinson N, Busse W, Bochner B, et al, editors: *Middleton's allergy: principles and practice*, ed 7, Philadelphia, 2009, Mosby, Elsevier, pp 679–700.
3. O'Callaghan C, Barry PW: The science of nebulised drug delivery. *Thorax* 52(Suppl 2):S31–S44, 1997.
4. Newhouse M, Dolovich M: Aerosol therapy in children. In Chermick V, Mellins R, editors: *Basic mechanisms of pediatric respiratory disease: cellular and integrative*, Toronto, 1991, BC Decker.
5. Lange C, Finlay W: Overcoming the adverse effect of humidity in aerosol delivery via pressurized metered-dose inhalers during mechanical ventilation. *Am J Respir Crit Care Med* 161:1614–1618, 2000.
6. Dolovich M, Labiris NR: Imaging drug delivery and drug responses in the lung. *Proc Am Thorac Soc* 1:329, 2004.

7. Dolovich M: Assessing nebulizer performance. *Respir Care* 47:1290, 2002.
8. Pierce A, Sanford J, Thomas G: Long-term evaluation of inhalation therapy equipment and the occurrence of necrotizing pneumonia. *N Engl J Med* 282:528, 1970.
9. Hamill R, Houston E, Georghiou P: An outbreak of *Burkholderia cepacia* respiratory tract colonization and infection associated with nebulized albuterol therapy. *Ann Intern Med* 122:762, 1995.
10. Wojnarowski C: Comparison of bronchial challenge with ultrasonic nebulized distilled water and hypertonic saline in children with mild-to-moderate asthma. *Eur Respir J* 9:1896, 1996.
11. Glick R: Drug reconcentration in aerosol generators. *Inhal Ther* 15:179, 1970.
12. Smaldone GC, Sangwan S, Shah A: Facemask design, facial deposition, and delivered dose of nebulized aerosols. *J Aerosol Med* 20(Suppl 1):S66–S75, discussion S75-67, 2007.
13. Geller DE: Clinical side effects during aerosol therapy: cutaneous and ocular effects. *J Aerosol Med* 20(Suppl 1):S100–S108, discussion S109, 2007.
14. Jakobsson B, Onnered A, Hjelte L, et al: Low bacterial contamination of nebulizers in home treatment of cystic fibrosis patients. *J Hosp Infect* 28:347–351, 1997.
15. Carnathan B, Martin B, Colice G: Second hand (S)-albuterol: RT exposure risk following racemic albuterol. *Respir Care* 46:1084, 2001.
16. Dimich-Ward H, Wymer ML, Chan-Yeung M: Respiratory health survey of respiratory therapists. *Chest* 126(4):1048–1053, 2004.
17. Ari A, Fink J, Harwood R, et al: Secondhand aerosol exposure during mechanical ventilation with and without expiratory filters: an in-vitro study. *Respir Care* 55(11):1566, 2010.
18. The Nebuliser Project Group of the British Thoracic Society Standards of Care Committee: Current best practice for nebuliser treatment. *Thorax* 52(Suppl 2):S4, 1997.
19. Fink J, Ari A: Aerosol therapy in intubated patients. *Expert Opin Drug Deliv* 10(8):1077–1093, 2013.
20. Ari A, Fink JB, Dhand R: Inhalation therapy in patients receiving mechanical ventilation: an update. *J Aerosol Med Pulm Drug Deliv* 25(6):319–332, 2012.
21. Leach CL: Safety assessment of the HFA propellant and the new inhaler. *Eur Respir Rev* 7:41, 1997.
22. Leach CL: The CFC to HFA transition and its impact on pulmonary drug development. *Respir Care* 50(9):1201–1208, 2005.
23. Fink J: Metered-dose inhalers, dry powder inhalers and transitions. *Respir Care* 45:623–635, 2000.
24. Slader CA, Reddel IH, Bosnic-Anticevich SZ: Lack of awareness of need to clean CFC-free metered-dose inhalers. *J Asthma* 41(3):367–373, 2004.
25. Fink JB, Dhand R, Grychowski J, et al: Reconciling in vitro and in vivo measurements of aerosol delivery from a metered-dose inhaler during mechanical ventilation and defining efficiency-enhancing factors. *Am J Respir Crit Care Med* 159(1):63–68, 1999.
26. Newman S: Aerosol generators and delivery systems. *Respir Care* 36(9):939–951, 1991.
27. Fink JB, Rubin BK: Problems with inhaler use: a call for improved clinician and patient education. *Respir Care* 50(10):1360–1374, 2005.
28. Chhabra SK: A comparison of "closed" and "open" mouth techniques of inhalation of a salbutamol metered-dose inhaler. *J Asthma* 31(2):123–125, 1994.
29. Wilkes W, Fink J, Dhand R: Selecting an accessory device with a metered-dose inhaler: variable influence of accessory devices on fine particle dose, throat deposition, and drug delivery with asynchronous actuation from a metered-dose inhaler. *J Aerosol Med* 14:351, 2001.
30. Dolovich M, Ruffin R, Corr D: Clinical evaluation of a simple demand inhalation MDI aerosol delivery device. *Chest* 84:36, 1983.
31. Wildhaber JH, Janssens HM, Pierart F, et al: High-percentage lung delivery in children from detergent-treated spacers. *Pediatr Pulmonol* 29(5):389–393, 2000.
32. Rubin B, Fink J: Optimizing aerosol delivery by pressurized metered-dose inhalers. *Respir Care* 50:1191, 2005.
33. Dhand R, Fink J: Dry powder inhalers. *Respir Care* 44:940, 1999.
34. Nerbrink O, Dahlback M, Hansson H: Why do medical nebulizers differ in their output and particle characteristics? *J Aerosol Med* 7:259, 1994.
35. Hess D, Fisher D, Williams P, et al: Medication nebulizer performance. Effects of diluent volume, nebulizer flow, and nebulizer brand. *Chest* 110(2):498–505, 1996.
36. Goode ML, Fink JB, Dhand R, et al: Improvement in aerosol delivery with helium-oxygen mixtures during mechanical ventilation. *Am J Respir Crit Care Med* 163(1):109–114, 2001.
37. Hess DR, Fink JB, Venkataraman ST, et al: The history and physics of heliox. *Respir Care* 51(6):608–612, 2006.
38. Phipps P, Gonda I: Droplets produced by medical nebulizers. Some factors affecting their size and solute concentration. *Chest* 97(6):1327–1332, 1990.
39. Thomas S, Lanford J, George R: Improving the efficiency of drug administration with jet nebulisers. *Lancet* 1:126, 1988.
40. Rau JL, Ari A, Restrepo RD: Performance comparison of nebulizer designs: constant-output, breath-enhanced, and dosimetric. *Respir Care* 49(2):174–179, 2004.
41. Malone RA, Hollie MC, Glynn-Barnhart A, et al: Optimal duration of nebulized albuterol therapy. *Chest* 104(4):1114–1118, 1993.
42. Kendrick A, Smith E, Wilson R: Selecting and using nebulizer equipment. *Thorax* 52:92–101, 1997.
43. Alvine GF, Rodgers P, Fitzsimmons KM, et al: Disposable jet nebulizers. How reliable are they? *Chest* 101(2):316–319, 1992.
44. Kacmarek R, Kratohvil J: Evaluation of a double-enclosure double-vacuum unit scavenging system for ribavirin administration. *Respir Care* 37:37, 1992.
45. Oie S, Kamiya A: Bacterial contamination of aerosol solutions containing antibiotics. *Microbios* 82:109, 1995.
46. Colacone A, Wolkove N, Stern E: Continuous nebulization of albuterol (salbutamol) in acute asthma. *Chest* 97:693, 1990.
47. Phillips G, Millard F: The therapeutic use of ultrasonic nebulizers in acute asthma. *Respir Med* 88:387–389, 1994.
48. Thomas SH, O'Doherty MJ, Page CJ, et al: Delivery of ultrasonic nebulized aerosols to a lung model during mechanical ventilation. *Am Rev Respir Dis* 148(4):872–877, 1993.
49. Dhand R: Nebulizers that use a vibrating mesh or plate with multiple apertures to generate aerosol. *Respir Care* 47(12):1406–1416, discussion 1416-1408, 2002.
50. Dolovich M, Fink J: Aerosols and devices. *Respir Care Clin N Am* 7:131, 2001.
51. Dolovich MB, Dhand R: Aerosol drug delivery: developments in device design and clinical use. *Lancet* 377(9770):1032–1045, 2010.
52. Henriet AC, Marchand-Adam S, Mankikian J, et al: [Respimat(R), first Soft Mist inhaler: new perspectives in the management of COPD]. *Rev Mal Respir* 27(10):1141–1149, 2010.
53. Denyer J, Nikander K, Smith N: Adaptive aerosol delivery (AAD) technology. *Expert Opin Drug Deliv* 1:165, 2004.
54. Erzinger S, Schueepp KG, Brooks-Wildhaber J, et al: Facemasks and aerosol delivery in vivo. *J Aerosol Med* 20(Suppl 1):S78–S83, discussion S83-74, 2007.
55. Rubin B, Fink J: Aerosol therapy for children. *Respir Care Clin N Am* 7(2):100–108, 2001.
56. Janssens H, Tiddens H: Aerosol therapy: the special needs of young children. *Paediatr Respir Rev* 7:S83–S85, 2006.
57. Dolovich MB, Killian D, Wolff RK, et al: Pulmonary aerosol deposition in chronic bronchitis: intermittent positive pressure breathing versus quiet breathing. *Am Rev Respir Dis* 115(3):397–402, 1977.
58. Dolovich MB, Ahrens RC, Hess DR, et al: Device selection and outcomes of aerosol therapy: evidence-based guidelines: American College of Chest Physicians/American College of Asthma, Allergy, and Immunology. *Chest* 127(1):335–371, 2005.
59. Ari A, Restrepo RD: Aerosol delivery device selection for spontaneously breathing patients: 2012. *Respir Care* 57(4):613–626, 2012.
60. Ari A, Fink J: Guidelines to aerosol devices in infants, children and adults: which to choose, why and how to achieve effective aerosol therapy? *Expert Rev Respir Med* 5(4):561–572, 2011.

61. Volpe J: Therapist-driven protocols for pediatric patients. *Respir Care Clin N Am* 2:117, 1996.
62. Barst RJ, Rubin LJ, Long WA, et al: A comparison of continuous intravenous epoprostenol (prostacyclin) with conventional therapy for primary pulmonary hypertension. *N Engl J Med* 334(5):296–301, 1996.
63. Badagliacca R, Pezzuto B, Poscia R, et al: Prognostic factors in severe pulmonary hypertension patients who need parenteral prostanoid therapy: the impact of late referral. *J Heart Lung Transplant* 31(4):364–372, 2012.
64. Vachiery JL: Prostacyclins in pulmonary arterial hypertension: the need for earlier therapy. *Adv Ther* 28(4):251–269, 2011.
65. Papo MC, Frank J, Thompson AE: A prospective, randomized study of continuous versus intermittent nebulized albuterol for severe status asthmaticus in children. *Crit Care Med* 21(10):1479–1486, 1993.
66. Fink J, Dhand R: Bronchodilator resuscitation in the emergency department, part 2: dosing. *Respir Care* 45(5):497, 2000.
67. Dhand R, Guntur VP: How best to deliver aerosol medications to mechanically ventilated patients. *Clin Chest Med* 29(2):277–296, vi, 2008.
68. Duarte AG, Fink JB, Dhand R: Inhalation therapy during mechanical ventilation. *Respir Care Clin N Am* 7(2):233–260, 2001.
69. Ari A, Fink JB: Factors affecting bronchodilator delivery in mechanically ventilated adults. *Nurs Crit Care* 15(4):192–203, 2010.
70. Ari A, Areabi H, Fink JB: Evaluation of position of aerosol device in two different ventilator circuits during mechanical ventilation. *Respir Care* 55(7):837–844, 2010.
71. Berlinski A, Willis JR: Albuterol delivery by 4 different nebulizers placed in 4 different positions in a pediatric ventilator in vitro model. *Respir Care* 58(7):1124–1133, 2013.
72. Ari A, Atalay OT, Harwood R, et al: Influence of nebulizer type, position, and bias flow on aerosol drug delivery in simulated pediatric and adult lung models during mechanical ventilation. *Respir Care* 55(7):845–851, 2010.
73. Hess DR: The mask for noninvasive ventilation: principles of design and effects on aerosol delivery. *J Aerosol Med* 20(Suppl 1):S85–S98, discussion S98-89, 2007.
74. White CC, Crotwell DN, Shen S, et al: Bronchodilator delivery during simulated pediatric noninvasive ventilation. *Respir Care* 58(9):1459–1466, 2013.
75. Abdelrahim ME, Plant P, Chrystyn H: In-vitro characterisation of the nebulised dose during non-invasive ventilation. *J Pharm Pharmacol* 62(8):966–972, 2010.
76. Bhashyam AR, Wolf MT, Marcinkowski AL, et al: Aerosol delivery through nasal cannulas: an in vitro study. *J Aerosol Med Pulm Drug Deliv* 21(2):181–188, 2008.
77. Sunbul F, Fink J, Harwood R, et al: Comparison of HFNC, bubble CPAP and SiPAP on aerosol delivery in premature babies: an in-vitro study. *Pediatr Pulmonol* 2015. (Accepted).
78. Alalwan M, Ari A, Fink J, et al: Delivery of albuterol by pressurized metered-dose inhaler and jet nebulizer via mask with high flow nasal cannula in place reduces aerosol delivery. *Respir Care* 57(10):1702, 2012.
79. Reychler G: Comparison of lung deposition in two types of nebulization: intrapulmonary percussive ventilation vs jet nebulization. *Chest* 125:502, 2004.
80. Demers B, Gilley D, Fink J: *Nebulizer position impacts aerosol deposition during high frequency oscillatory ventilation (HFOV)*, San Diego, 2005, American Thoracic Society (ATS) International Conference.
81. Siobal M, Ari A, Fink J: Aerosol lung deposition using a vibrating mesh nebulizer during high frequency oscillatory ventilation in the adult lung model. *Respir Care* 55(11):1565, 2010.
82. Alzahrani W, Harwood R, Fink J, et al: Comparison of albuterol delivery during high frequency oscillatory ventilation and conventional mechanical ventilation of a simulated adult. *Respir Care* 55(11):1576, 2010.
83. Lindsley WG, Blachere FM, Thewlis RE, et al: Measurements of airborne influenza virus in aerosol particles from human coughs. *PLoS ONE* 5(11):e15100, 2010.
84. Harrison R: Reproductive risk assessment with occupational exposure to ribavirin aerosol. *Pediatr Infect Dis J* 9(Suppl):S1025, 1990.
85. Garner J: Guideline for isolation precautions in hospitals. *Infect Control Hosp Epidemiol* 17:53, 1996.
86. Gralton J, McLaws ML: Protecting healthcare workers from pandemic influenza: N95 or surgical masks? *Crit Care Med* 38(2):657–667, 2010.

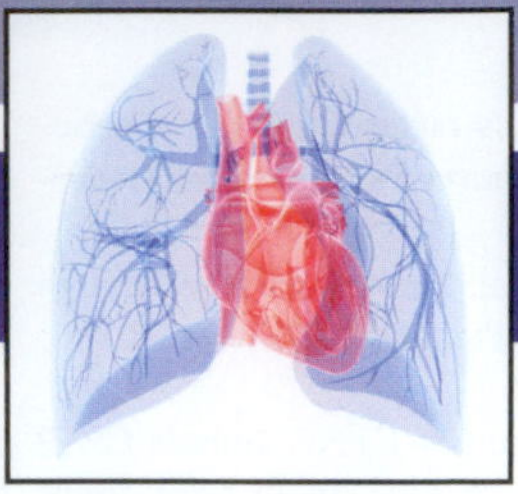

CHAPTER 40

Storage and Delivery of Medical Gases

DAVID L. VINES

CHAPTER OBJECTIVES

After reading this chapter you will be able to:

- Describe how medical gases and gas mixtures are produced.
- Discuss the clinical applications for medical gases and gas mixtures.
- Distinguish between gaseous and liquid storage methods.
- Calculate the duration of remaining contents of a compressed oxygen cylinder.
- Calculate the duration of remaining contents of a liquid oxygen cylinder.
- Describe how to store, transport, and use compressed gas cylinders properly.
- Distinguish between gas supply systems.
- Describe what to do if a bulk oxygen supply system fails.
- Differentiate among safety systems that apply to various equipment connections.
- Select the appropriate devices to regulate gas pressure or control flow in various clinical settings.
- Describe how to assemble, check for proper function, and identify malfunctions in gas delivery equipment.
- Identify and correct common malfunctions of gas delivery equipment.

CHAPTER OUTLINE

KEY TERMS

American standard safety system
Bourdon gauge
cryogenic
diameter-index safety system
downstream
filling density
flammable
flowmeter
fractional distillation
heliox
manifold
nonflammable
oxidizing
pin-index safety system
psig
reducing valve
regulator
Thorpe tube
upstream
zone valves

The hospital "oxygen service" is the origin from which the current technology-laden field of respiratory care evolved. Although respiratory therapists (RTs) have assumed many more challenging duties, ensuring the safe and uninterrupted supply of medical gases remains a key responsibility.

There are many commercially produced gases, but only a few are used medically (Table 40-1). Medical gases are classified as laboratory gases, therapeutic gases, or anesthetic gases. *Laboratory gases* are used for equipment calibration and diagnostic testing. *Therapeutic gases* are used to relieve symptoms and improve oxygenation of patients with hypoxemia. *Anesthetic*

TABLE 40-1
Physical Characteristics of Medical Gases

Gas	Chemical Symbol	Color	Taste	Odor	Can Support Life	Flammability
Laboratory Gases						
Nitrogen	N	Colorless	Tasteless	Odorless	No	Nonflammable
Helium	He	Colorless	Tasteless	Odorless	No	Nonflammable
Carbon dioxide	CO_2	Colorless	Slightly acidic	Odorless	No	Nonflammable
Therapeutic Gases						
Air	AIR	Colorless	Tasteless	Odorless	Yes	Supports combustion
Oxygen	O_2	Colorless	Tasteless	Odorless	Yes	Supports combustion
Helium/oxygen (heliox)	He/O_2	Colorless	Tasteless	Odorless	Yes	Supports combustion
Carbon dioxide/oxygen	CO_2/O_2	Colorless	Slightly acidic	Odorless	No	Supports combustion
Nitric oxide	NO	Colorless	Tasteless	Metallic	No	Supports combustion
Anesthetic Gas						
Nitrous oxide	N_2O	Colorless	Slightly sweet	Slightly sweet	No	Supports combustion

gases are combined with oxygen (O_2) to provide anesthesia during surgery. It is important for RTs to be familiar with all aspects of gases used in the clinical setting, especially the chemical symbols, physical characteristics, ability to support life, and fire risk. In regard to fire risk, medical compressed gases are classified as either **nonflammable** (do not burn), nonflammable but supportive of combustion (also termed **oxidizing**), or **flammable** (burns readily, potentially explosive).[1] Of the gases listed in Table 40-1, the focus of this chapter is on the therapeutic gases.

CHARACTERISTICS OF MEDICAL GASES

Oxygen

Characteristics

O_2 is a colorless, odorless, transparent, and tasteless gas.[1] It exists naturally as free molecular O_2 and as a component of a host of chemical compounds. At *standard temperature, pressure, and dry (STPD),* O_2 has a density of 1.429 g/L, being slightly heavier than air (1.29 g/L). O_2 is not very soluble in water. At room temperature and 1 atm pressure, only 3.3 ml of O_2 dissolves in 100 ml of water.

O_2 is nonflammable, but it greatly accelerates combustion. Burning speed increases with either (1) an increase in O_2 percentage at a fixed total pressure or (2) an increase in total pressure of O_2 at a constant gas concentration. Both O_2 concentration and partial pressure influence the rate of burning.[1,2]

Production

O_2 is produced through one of several methods. Chemical methods for producing small quantities of O_2 include *electrolysis of water* and *decomposition of sodium chlorate* ($NaClO_3$). Most large quantities of medical O_2 are produced by fractional distillation of atmospheric air.[1] Small quantities of concentrated O_2 are produced by physical separation of O_2 from air.

Fractional Distillation. **Fractional distillation** is the most common and least expensive method for producing O_2. The process involves several related steps. First, atmospheric air is filtered to remove pollutants, water, and carbon dioxide (CO_2). The purified air is liquefied by compression and cooled by rapid expansion *(Joule-Thompson effect).*

The resulting mixture of liquid O_2 and nitrogen (N, N_2) is heated slowly in a distillation tower. N_2, with its boiling point of 195.8° C (320.5° F), escapes first, followed by the trace gases of argon, krypton, and xenon. The remaining liquid O_2 is transferred to specially insulated **cryogenic** (low-temperature) storage cylinders. An alternative procedure is to convert O_2 directly to gas for storage in high-pressure metal cylinders. These methods produce O_2 that is approximately 99.5% pure. The remaining 0.5% is mostly N_2 and trace argon. U.S. Food and Drug Administration (FDA) standards require an O_2 purity of at least 99.0%.[3]

Physical Separation. Two methods are used to separate O_2 from air.[4] The first method entails use of molecular "sieves" composed of inorganic sodium aluminum silicate pellets. These pellets absorb N_2, "trace" gases, and water vapor from the air, providing a concentrated mixture of more than 90% O_2 for patient use. The second method entails use of a vacuum to pull ambient air through a semipermeable plastic membrane. The membrane allows O_2 and water vapor to pass through at a faster rate than N_2 from ambient air. This system can produce an O_2 mixture of approximately 40%. These devices, called *oxygen concentrators,* are used primarily for supplying low-flow O_2 in the home care setting. For this reason, details about the principles of operation and appropriate use are discussed in Chapter 56.

Air

Atmospheric air is a colorless, odorless, naturally occurring gas mixture that consists of 20.95% O_2, 78.1% N_2, and approximately 1% "trace" gases, mainly argon. At STPD, the density of air is 1.29 g/L, which is used as the standard for measuring specific gravity of other gases. O_2 and N_2 can be mixed to produce a gas with an O_2 concentration equivalent to that of air. Medical-grade air usually is produced by filtering and compressing atmospheric air.[1,5]

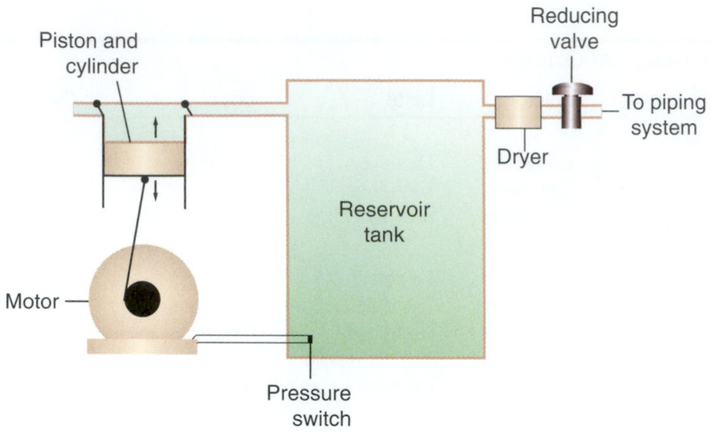

FIGURE 40-1 Large medical air compressor. The compressor sends gas to the reservoir at higher than line pressure. When the preset pressure level is reached, the pressure switch shuts off the compressor. Gas leaves the reservoir and passes through the dryer to remove moisture, and the reducing valve reduces gas to the desired line pressure. When reservoir pressure has decreased to near line pressure, the pressure switch turns the compressor back on. (Modified from McPherson SP, Spearman CB: Respiratory therapy equipment, ed 5, St Louis, 1995, Mosby.)

Figure 40-1 shows a typical large medical *air compressor system*. In these systems, an electric motor is used to power a piston in a compression cylinder. On its downstroke, the piston draws air through a filter system with an inlet valve. On its upstroke, the piston compresses the air in the cylinder (closing the inlet valve) and delivers it through an outlet valve to a reservoir tank. Air from the reservoir tank is reduced to the desired working pressure by a pressure-reducing valve before being delivered to the piping system.

For medical gas use, air must be dry and free of oil or particulate contamination.[5] The most common method used for drying air is cooling to produce condensation. For avoidance of oil or particulate contamination, medical air compressors have air inlet filters and polytetrafluoroethylene (Teflon) piston rings as opposed to oil lubrication. Large medical air compressors must provide high flow (at least 100 L/min) at the standard working pressure of 50 *pounds per square inch gauge* (**psig**) for all equipment in use. The psig is the pressure read on the gauge. It reads the pressure above atmosphere pressure. See Chapter 6 for more information on this concept.

Smaller compressors (Figure 40-2) are available for bedside or home use. These compressors have a diaphragm or turbine that compresses the air and generally do not have a reservoir. This design limits the pressure and flow capabilities of these devices. For this reason, small compressors must never be used to power equipment that needs unrestricted flow at 50 psig, such as pneumatically powered ventilators (see Chapter 45). However, small diaphragm or turbine compressors are ideal for powering devices such as small-volume medication nebulizers (see Chapter 39).

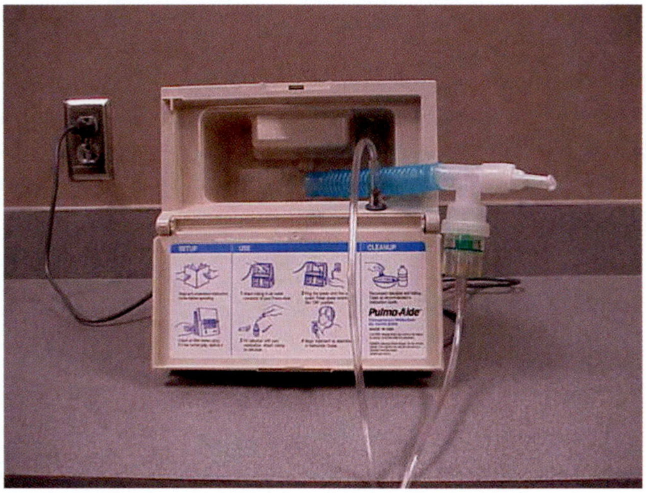

FIGURE 40-2 Small portable compressor used with a hand-held nebulizer to aerosolize medication.

Carbon Dioxide

At STPD, CO_2 is a colorless and odorless gas with a specific gravity of 1.52 (approximately 1.5 times heavier than air).[1] CO_2 does not support combustion or maintain animal life. For medical use, CO_2 usually is produced by heating limestone in contact with water. The gas is recovered from this process and liquefied by compression and cooling. The FDA purity standard for CO_2 is 99%.[3]

Mixtures of O_2 and 5% to 10% CO_2 are occasionally used for therapeutic purposes, as noted in Chapter 41. Therapeutic uses include the management of singultus (hiccups), prevention of the complete washout of CO_2 during cardiopulmonary bypass, and regulation of pulmonary vascular pressures in some congenital heart disorders. However, CO_2 mixtures are more commonly used for the calibration of blood gas analyzers (see Chapter 19) and for diagnostic purposes in the clinical laboratory.

Helium

Helium (He) is second only to hydrogen as the lightest of all gases; it has a density at STPD of 0.1785 g/L. He is odorless, tasteless, nonflammable, and chemically and physiologically inert. It is a good conductor of heat, sound, and electricity but is poorly soluble in water. Although He is present in small quantities in the atmosphere, it is commercially produced from natural gas through liquefaction to purity standards of at least 99%.[1,3]

He cannot support life, so breathing 100% He would cause suffocation and death. For therapeutic use, He must always be mixed with at least 20% O_2. **Heliox** (a gas mixture of O_2 and He) may be used clinically to manage severe cases of airway obstruction. Its low density decreases the work of breathing by making gas flow more laminar. He is discussed in more detail in Chapter 41.

RULE OF THUMB

He must always be combined with at least 20% O_2. The higher the concentration of O_2 used in a heliox mixture, the less likely it is that heliox would be beneficial. Heliox mixtures of less than 60% He are rarely used clinically.

Nitric Oxide

Nitric oxide (NO) is a colorless, nonflammable, toxic gas that supports combustion. It is produced by oxidation of ammonia at high temperatures in the presence of a catalyst. In combination with air, NO forms brown fumes of nitrogen dioxide (NO_2). Together, NO and NO_2 are strong respiratory irritants that can cause chemical pneumonitis and a fatal form of pulmonary edema. Exposure to high concentrations of NO alone can cause methemoglobinemia (see Chapter 41). High levels of methemoglobin can cause tissue hypoxia.

As discussed in Chapter 41, NO is approved by the FDA for use in the treatment of term and near-term infants for hypoxic respiratory failure. The American Academy of Pediatrics (AAP) published a policy statement recommending the use of NO in the care of term and near-term infants when mechanical ventilation is failing because of hypoxic respiratory failure. The AAP suggests that NO be used before extracorporeal membrane oxygenation.[6] A systemic review from the Cochrane database supports the recommendation that inhaled NO at 20 ppm may be beneficial in term and near-term infants who do not have a diaphragmatic hernia (see Chapter 34).[7] The use of inhaled NO in the treatment of premature neonates with hypoxic respiratory failure does not improve outcomes and may increase the risk for intracranial hemorrhage.[8]

Nitrous Oxide

Nitrous oxide (N_2O) is a colorless gas with a slightly sweet odor and taste that is used clinically as an anesthetic agent. Similar to O_2, N_2O can support combustion. However, N_2O cannot support life and causes death if inhaled in pure form. For this reason, inhaled N_2O must always be mixed with at least 20% O_2. N_2O is produced by thermal decomposition of ammonium nitrate.[1]

The use of N_2O as an anesthetic agent is based on its central nervous system depressant effect. However, only dangerously high levels of N_2O provide true anesthesia. N_2O/O_2 mixtures are almost always used in combination with other anesthetic agents.

Long-term human exposure to N_2O has been associated with a form of neuropathy. In addition, epidemiologic studies have linked chronic N_2O exposure with an increased risk for fetal disorders and spontaneous abortion.[1] On the basis of this knowledge, the National Institute for Occupational Safety and Health (a division of the Occupational Safety and Health Administration) set an upper exposure limit for hospital operating rooms of 25 ppm N_2O.[1]

STORAGE OF MEDICAL GASES

Medical gases are stored either in portable high-pressure cylinders or in large bulk reservoirs. Bulk reservoirs require a separate distribution system to deliver the gas to the patient.

Gas Cylinders

The containers used to store and ship compressed or liquid medical gases are high-pressure cylinders. The design, manufacture, transport, and use of these cylinders are carefully controlled by both industrial standards and federal regulations. Gas cylinders are made of seamless steel and are classified by the U.S. Department of Transportation (DOT) according to their fabrication method. DOT type 3A cylinders are made from carbon steel, and DOT type 3AA containers are manufactured with a steel alloy tempered for higher strength.[1]

Markings and Identification

Medical gas cylinders are marked with metal stamping on the shoulders that supplies specific information (Figure 40-3).[1,9] Although the exact location and order of these markings vary, the practitioner should be able to identify several key items of information.

The letters *DOT* or *ICC* (Interstate Commerce Commission) are followed by the cylinder classification (*3A* or *3AA*) and the normal filling pressure in pounds per square inch (psi). Below this information usually is the letter size of the cylinder (*E, G,* and so on) followed by the cylinder serial number. A third line provides a mark of ownership, often followed by the manufacturer's stamp or a mark identifying the inspecting authority. An abbreviation indicating the method of cylinder manufacturer is usually on the opposite side of the cylinder. Also in this area is information about the original safety test and dates of all subsequent tests.

Safety tests are conducted on each cylinder every 5 or 10 years, as specified in DOT regulations.[1,9] During these tests, cylinders are pressurized to five thirds of their service pressure. While the cylinder is under pressure, technicians measure cylinder leakage, expansion, and wall stress. The notation *EE* followed by a number indicates the elastic expansion of the cylinder in cubic centimeters under the test conditions. An asterisk (*) next to the test date indicates DOT approval for 10-year testing. A plus sign (+) means the cylinder is approved

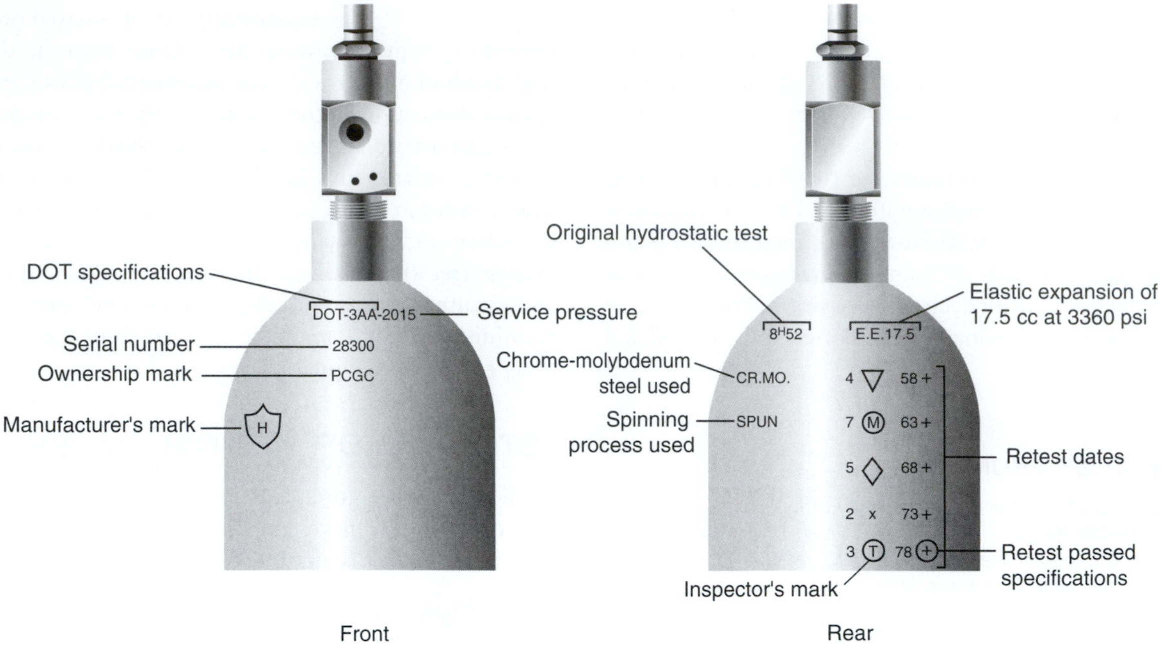

FIGURE 40-3 Typical markings of cylinders containing medical gases. Front and back views are for illustration purposes only; exact location and order of markings vary. *DOT,* Department of Transportation.

TABLE 40-2

Color Codes for Medical Gas Cylinders

Gas	United States	Canada
O_2	Green	White*
CO_2	Gray	Gray
N_2O	Blue	Blue
Cyclopropane	Orange	Orange
He	Brown	Brown
C_2H_4	Red	Red
CO_2-O_2	Gray/green	Gray/white
He-O_2	Brown/green	Brown/white
N_2	Black	Black
Air	Yellow*	Black/white
N_2-O_2	Black/green	Pink

*Vacuum systems historically are identified as white in the United States and yellow in Canada. For this reason, the Compressed Gas Association recommends that white not be used for any cylinders in the United States and that yellow not be used in Canada.
C_2H_4, Ethylene.

for filling to 10% greater than its service pressure. An approved cylinder with a service pressure of 2015 psi can be filled to approximately 2200 psi. After hydrostatic testing, cylinders are subjected to internal inspection and cleaning.

In addition to these permanent marks, all cylinders are color-coded and labeled for identification of their contents.[1,10] Table 40-2 lists the color codes for medical gases as adopted by the Bureau of Standards of the U.S. Department of Commerce.[10,11] For comparison, the color codes adopted by the Canadian Standards Association also are included. Color codes are not standardized internationally. For this reason, cylinder color should be used only as a guide. As with any drug agent, the cylinder contents always must be identified through careful inspection of the label. It has been reported that gas mixtures such as heliox can become unmixed.[12] To be absolutely sure about the O_2 concentration provided by a cylinder, the user must analyze the gas before administering it (see Chapter 19).

Cylinder Sizes and Contents

Letter designations are used for different sizes of cylinders (Figure 40-4). Sizes E through AA are referred to as "small cylinders" and are used most often for transporting patients and anesthetic gases. These small cylinders are easily identified because of their unique valves and connecting mechanisms. Small cylinders have a post valve and yoke connector. Large cylinders (F through H and K) have a threaded valve outlet (Figure 40-5).

Cylinder Safety Relief Valves

In a closed cylinder, any increase in gas temperature increases gas pressure. Should the temperature increase too much (as in a fire), the high gas pressure could rupture and explode the cylinder. To prevent this type of accident, all cylinders have high-pressure relief valves. These relief valves are of three basic designs: frangible disk, fusible plug, and spring-loaded. The *frangible metal disk* ruptures at a specific pressure. The *fusible plug* melts at a specific temperature. The *spring-loaded valve* opens and vents gas at a set high pressure. In each case, the activated valve vents gas from the cylinder and prevents pressure from becoming too high.

Most small cylinders have a fusible plug relief valve. Most large cylinders have a spring-loaded relief valve. These safety relief valves are always located in the cylinder valve stems.

Filling (Charging) Cylinders

How a cylinder is filled depends on whether its contents will be gaseous or liquid. Some gases stored in liquid form can remain at room temperature, but others must be maintained in a cryogenic (low-temperature) state.

Compressed Gases. A gas cylinder normally is filled to its service pressure (the pressure stamped on the shoulder) at 21.1° C (70° F). However, approved cylinders can be filled to 10% greater than service pressure.

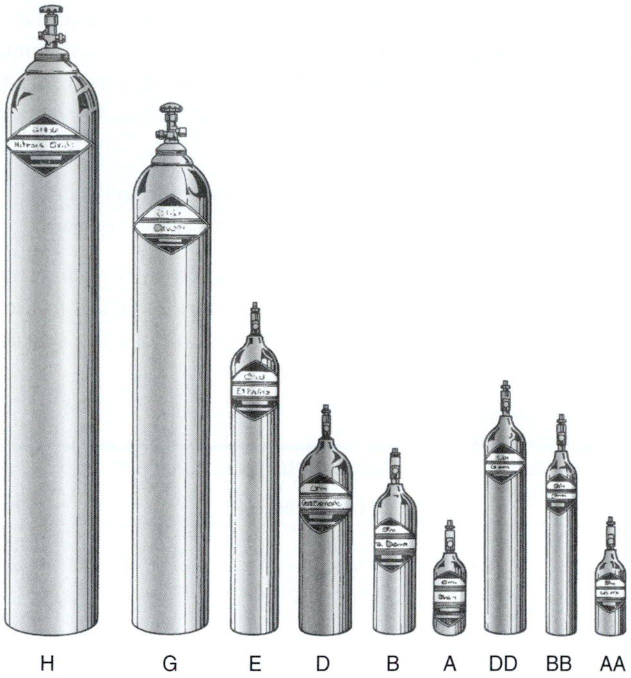

FIGURE 40-4 Cylinder sizes are identified by letter designations.

Liquefied Gases. Gases with critical temperatures greater than room temperature can be stored as liquids at room temperature (see Chapter 6). These gases include CO_2 and N_2O. Rather than being filled to filling pressure, cylinders of these gases are filled according to a specified filling density. The **filling density** is the ratio between the weight of liquid gas put into the cylinder and the weight of water the cylinder could contain if full. The filling density for CO_2 is 68%. This system allows the manufacturer to fill a cylinder with liquid CO_2 up to 68% of the weight of water that a full cylinder could hold. The filling density of N_2O is 55%.

Cylinder pressures for gases stored in the liquid phase are much lower than for gases stored in the gas phase. Because the liquid does not fill the entire volume of a cylinder, the space above the liquid surface contains gas in equilibrium with the liquid. The pressure in a liquid-filled cylinder equals the pressure of the vapor at any given temperature.

Pressure in a cylinder depends on the state of its contents. In a gas-filled cylinder, the pressure represents the force required to compress the gas into its smaller volume. In contrast, the pressure in a liquid-filled cylinder is the vapor pressure needed to keep the gas liquefied at the current temperature.

Measuring Cylinder Contents

Because of the previously described differences in the physical state of matter of compressed and liquid gases, different methods are needed to measure the contents of the cylinder.

Compressed Gas Cylinders. For gas-filled cylinders, the volume of gas in the cylinder is directly proportional to its pressure at a constant temperature. If a cylinder is full at 2200 psig, it will be half full when the pressure decreases to 1100 psig. To know how much gas is contained in a compressed gas cylinder, one needs only to measure its pressure.

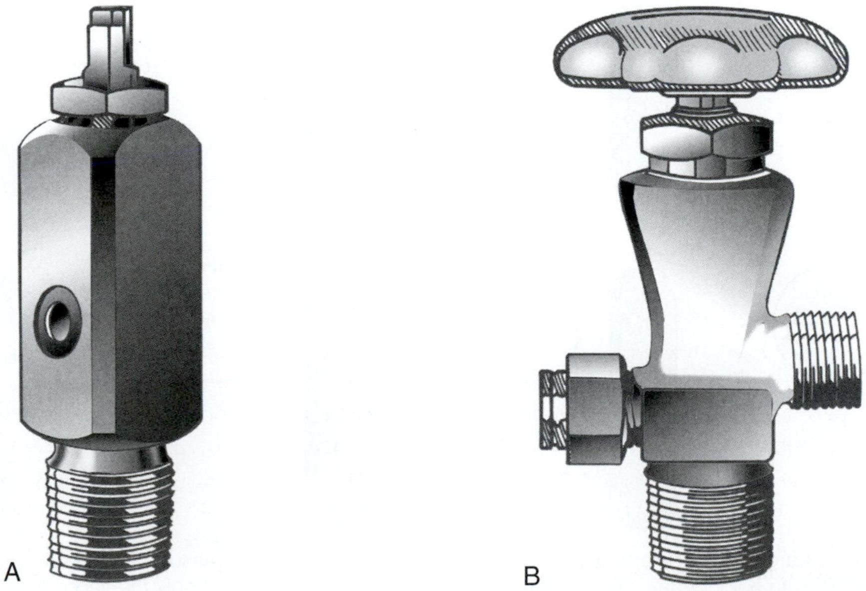

FIGURE 40-5 A, Post valve for yoke connector used with small cylinders (E through AA). **B,** Large, threaded valve outlet used with large cylinders (H/K, G, and M).

Liquid Gas Cylinders. In a liquid gas cylinder or container, the measured pressure is the vapor pressure above the liquid. This pressure bears no relationship to the amount of liquid remaining in the cylinder. As long as some liquid remains (and the temperature remains constant), the vapor pressure and the gauge pressure remain constant. When all the liquid is gone and the cylinder contains only gas, the pressure decreases in proportion to a reduction in volume. Monitoring the gauge pressure of liquid gas cylinders is useful only after all the liquid vaporizes. Weighing a liquid-filled cylinder is the only accurate method for determining the contents.

Figure 40-6 compares the behavior of compressed gas and liquid gas cylinders during use. The vapor pressure of liquid gas cylinders varies with the temperature of the contents. The pressure in an N_2O cylinder at 21.1° C (70° F) is 745 psig; at 15.6° C (60° F), the pressure decreases to 660 psig. As the temperature increases toward the critical point, more liquid vaporizes, and the cylinder pressure increases. If a cylinder of N_2O warms to 36.4° C (97.5° F) (its critical temperature), all the contents convert to gas. Only at this temperature and higher does the cylinder gauge pressure accurately reflect cylinder contents.

Estimating Duration of Cylinder Gas Flow

When a cylinder of therapeutic gas is used, it often is necessary to predict how long the contents will last at a given flow. The duration of flow of a cylinder can be estimated if the following are known: (1) the gas flow, (2) the cylinder size, and (3) the cylinder pressure at the start of therapy. For a given flow, the more gas a cylinder holds, the longer it lasts. The higher the gas flow, the shorter the cylinder emptying time. The duration of flow from a cylinder is directly proportional to the contents and inversely proportional to flow, as expressed in the following formula:

$$\text{Duration of flow} = \frac{\text{Contents}}{\text{Flow}}$$

The units commonly used in the United States for measurement of these quantities are not the same. Cylinder contents are generally specified in cubic feet or gallons, whereas gas flow normally is measured in liters. Table 40-3 provides the factors needed to convert these units.

Rather than memorizing various cylinder contents and constantly converting metric and English units, the user can quickly calculate duration of flow by using *cylinder factors.* Cylinder factors are derived for each common gas and cylinder size with the following formula:

$$\text{Cylinder factor (L/psig)} = \frac{\text{Cubic feet (full cylinder)} \times 28.3}{\text{Pressure (full cylinder) in psig}}$$

In the numerator of the previous equation, the English-metric conversion constant (28.3) is used to convert cubic feet to liters. Dividing the resulting volume by the pressure in a full cylinder

TABLE 40-3
Gas Volume Conversion Factors

Liters	Cubic Feet	Gallons
28.316	1	7.481
1	0.03531	0.2642
3.785	0.1337	1

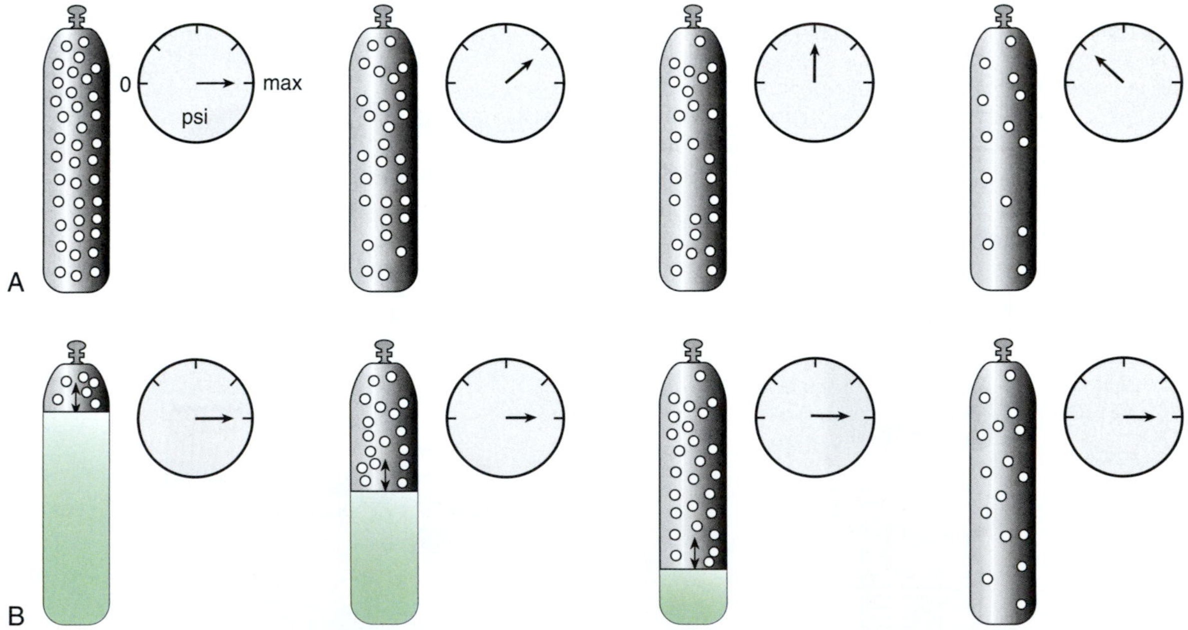

FIGURE 40-6 The content of a gas-filled cylinder **(A)** is directly proportional to the gas pressure. A pressure decrease of 50% indicates a loss of 50% of the contained gas. In a liquid-gas cylinder **(B),** gauge pressure is a measure of only the vapor pressure of gas in equilibrium with the liquid phase. This value remains constant at a given temperature as long as liquid is present. Only when all the liquid has vaporized, as the cylinder nears depletion, does the gauge pressure decrease proportionately to the terminal volume of remaining gas.

TABLE 40-4

Factors for Calculation of Cylinder Duration of Flow (Minutes)

Gas	CYLINDER SIZE			
	D	E	G	H and K
O_2, O_2/N_2, air	0.16	0.28	2.41	3.14
O_2/CO_2	0.20	0.35	2.94	3.84
He/O_2	0.14	0.23	1.93	2.50

yields the cylinder factor. The derived factor represents the volume of gas leaving a given cylinder for every 1-psig decrease in pressure. Table 40-4 provides cylinder factors for the therapeutic medical gases and common cylinder sizes.

When the factor for a given gas and cylinder is known, calculating the duration of flow is a simple matter of applying the following equation:

$$\text{Duration of flow (min)} = \frac{\text{Pressure (psig)} \times \text{Cylinder factor}}{\text{Flow (L/min)}}$$

A margin of safety must be allowed in estimation of cylinder duration of flow. This principle is especially important if the RT cannot be present during use and must return with a full cylinder. Some clinicians return 30 to 40 minutes before the calculated time; others compute duration of flow to a level of 300 to 500 psig rather than 0 psig (empty). Assuming the calculations are correct and there is no change in flow, both methods ensure an uninterrupted supply. The accompanying Rule of Thumb presents a shortcut for estimating cylinder duration of flow.

RULE OF THUMB

A full E O_2 cylinder running at 10 L/min lasts approximately 60 minutes (1 hour). A full H/K cylinder lasts at least 10 times longer (>10 hours). Use these two simple rules to estimate flow duration. For example, a half-full E O_2 cylinder running at 10 L/min lasts approximately 30 minutes, whereas a full H cylinder running at 5 L/min lasts more than 20 hours.

MINI CLINIC

Computing Cylinder Duration of Flow

PROBLEM: The RT needs to determine how long a G cylinder of O_2 with a gauge pressure of 800 psi set to deliver 8 L/min will last until empty.

SOLUTION: *Step 1:* Determine the cylinder factor for an O_2 G cylinder (see Table 40-4), which in this case is 2.41.

Step 2: Apply the duration of flow equation:

$$\text{Duration of flow (min)} = \frac{\text{Pressure (psig)} \times \text{Cylinder factor}}{\text{Flow (L/min)}}$$

$$\text{Duration of flow (min)} = \frac{800 \times 2.41}{8} = 241 \text{ minutes}$$

(approximately 4 hours)

Estimating Duration of Liquid Oxygen Cylinder Gas Flow

The only accurate method for determining the volume of gas in a liquid-filled cylinder is by weight. Because 1 L of liquid O_2 weighs 2.5 lb and produces 860 L of O_2 in its gaseous state, the amount of gas in a liquid O_2 cylinder can be calculated with the following formula:

$$\text{Amount of gas in cylinder} = \frac{\text{Liquid } O_2 \text{ weight (lb)} \times 860}{2.5 \text{ lb/L}}$$

After the amount of O_2 remaining in the cylinder is determined, the duration of the gas in minutes can be calculated with the following formula:

$$\text{Duration of gas (min)} = \frac{\text{Amount of gas in cylinder (L)}}{\text{Flow (L/min)}}$$

As with gaseous O_2 cylinders, a wide margin of safety is needed for estimation of cylinder duration. This margin of safety varies with the size of the portable O_2 unit or large storage container.

MINI CLINIC

Computing the Duration of a Liquid Oxygen Container

PROBLEM: The RT needs to estimate how long Mrs. Jones' portable liquid O_2 container will last if it contains 3 lb of liquid O_2 that supplies an O_2 delivery device running at 2 L/min.

SOLUTION: *Step 1:* Determine the amount of O_2 in the cylinder.

$$\text{Amount of gas in cylinder} = \frac{\text{Liquid } O_2 \text{ weight (lb)} \times 860}{2.5 \text{ lb/L}}$$

$$= \frac{3 \times 860}{2.5}$$

$$= 1032 \text{ L}$$

Step 2: Calculate the duration of the gas in the container.

$$\text{Duration of gas} = \frac{\text{Amount of gas in the cylinder (L)}}{\text{Flow (L/min)}}$$

$$= \frac{1032 \text{ L}}{2} = \frac{516 \text{ minutes}}{60 \text{ (min/hr)}}$$

$$= 8 \text{ hours } 36 \text{ minutes}$$

Gas Cylinder Safety

The following guidelines for cylinder safety are from the recommendations of the National Fire Protection Agency (NFPA)[2] and the Compressed Gas Association (CGA).[1,11] For ease of use, these safety guidelines are divided into cylinder storage, transport, and use.

Cylinder Storage. The following guidelines apply to cylinder storage:

- Store gas cylinders in racks or chain cylinders to the wall to prevent them from falling or becoming damaged.

- Store cylinders away from any combustible material.
- Store gas cylinders away from sources of heat. Keep the cylinder temperature less than 125° F (<51.7° C).
- Store flammable gases separately from gases that support combustion, such as air, O_2, and N_2O.
- If a cylinder is not in use, keep the protective cylinder cap in place.
- Do not store air compressors and gas cylinders together. A fire involving one or the other can damage both gas delivery systems.
- Contain and store cylinder supply systems in an enclosure constructed of a material with at least a 1-hour fire resistive rating that is well ventilated and well drained.
- Segregate full and empty cylinders; store them separately if possible.
- Place on each door or gate of the enclosure a sign that cautions the presence of an oxidizing gas and alerts against smoking. This sign must be readable from a distance of at least 5 ft (1.5 m).
- Store liquid O_2 containers in a cool, well-ventilated area because of the venting of small amounts of O_2 from these low-pressure containers. The venting of O_2 prevents these containers from overpressurizing because liquid O_2 is continuously converting to gaseous O_2.

Cylinder Transport. The following guidelines apply to cylinder transport:

- Use cylinder carts with a securing mechanism for transportation of cylinders.
- Keep the protective cylinder caps in place during transportation of cylinders.
- Protect gas cylinders from striking other cylinders or objects to avoid damaging the safety devices, valve stems, or the cylinder itself.
- Avoid dropping, dragging, or rolling cylinders in transport.
- Do not transport cylinders for use that are not appropriately labeled.

Cylinder Use. The following guidelines apply to cylinder use:

- Secure gas cylinders at the patient's bedside in a way that prevents them from falling. Secure cylinders to the wall with a chain, bind or chain them to a suitable cart, or support the cylinder with a stand.
- Do not use flammable materials, especially oil or grease, on regulators, cylinders, fittings, or valves. This restriction includes oily hands, rags, and gloves.
- Open the cylinder valve slightly to remove dust and dirt before attaching the regulator. When slightly opening the valve, ensure no one is in front of the valve. "Crack" the cylinder before bringing it to the patient's bedside.
- Never use cylinder valves or regulators that need repair.
- Do not alter or deface cylinder markings or color.
- Never place cylinders near sources of heat.
- Never secure cylinders to movable objects unless the object has an apparatus that can contain the cylinder safely.
- Ensure that the connection between the regulator and the cylinder valve is an **American standard safety system** (ASSS) for H and G cylinders and a **pin-index safety system** (PISS) for E cylinders.
- When O_2 is in use, post a "No Smoking" sign unless signs in the entrances are posted that prohibit smoking in the facility.

Bulk Oxygen

Large acute care facilities use large volumes of O_2 every day. To meet these needs, a centralized bulk storage and delivery system is required. By definition, bulk O_2 storage systems hold at least 20,000 ft^3 of gas, including the onsite unconnected reserves.[2] Bulk O_2 may be stored in either gaseous or liquid form, but liquid storage is most common. When needed, the O_2 flows from this central source throughout the facility through a piping system with outlets conveniently located.

A bulk O_2 system has several advantages over portable cylinders. Although initially expensive to construct, bulk O_2 systems are far less expensive over the long term. Bulk O_2 systems are less prone to interruption. These systems eliminate the inconvenience and hazard of transporting and storing numerous cylinders. Bulk O_2 systems regulate delivery pressures centrally, eliminating the need for separate pressure-reducing valves at each outlet. These systems also operate at low pressures, making them much safer than high-pressure cylinders.

Safety standards for bulk O_2 systems are set by the NFPA and are subject to further control by local fire and building codes.[2]

Gas Supply Systems

The three types of centrally located gas supply systems are an alternating supply system or cylinder **manifold** system, a cylinder supply system with reserve supply, and a bulk gas system with a reserve.[2] The *alternating supply* or *cylinder manifold system* consists of large (normally H or K size) cylinders of compressed O_2 banked together in series (Figure 40-7). This alternating supply system has two sides: a primary bank and a reserve bank. When the pressure in the primary bank decreases to a set level, a control valve automatically switches over to the reserve bank. When this occurs, the primary bank is taken offline, and the empty cylinders are replaced with full ones. The replenished primary bank becomes the reserve bank. Some large alternating supply systems are permanently fixed and are refilled on site by a supply truck. These cylinder manifold systems have pressure-reducing valves for regulation of delivered pressure and normally have low-pressure alarms. These alarms sound when reserve switchover occurs, and they warn of impending depletion or malfunction. Cylinder manifolds or alternating supply systems are used to supply O_2 from a central location in small facilities or to supply specialty gases, such as N_2O, to operating rooms (Figure 40-8).

A *cylinder supply system with a reserve* consists of a primary supply, a secondary supply, and a reserve supply. When the primary gas supply is depleted by the demand, this supply system automatically switches to the secondary supply. Master signal panels indicate that the changeover has occurred. This supply system operates in a manner similar to the alternating system except that this system has a reserve supply if primary

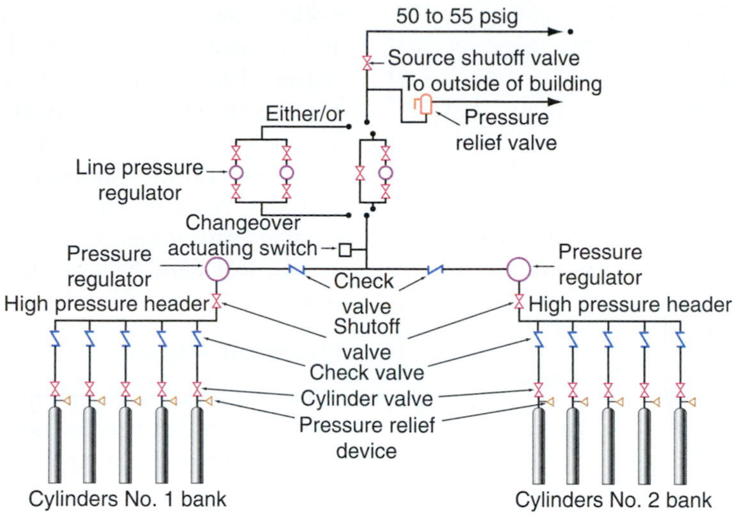

FIGURE 40-7 Gas cylinder manifold system. The alternating supply system is composed of primary and reserve banks, which alternate to charge the piping system. (Modified from Standard for nonflammable medical gas systems, NFPA No. 56F. Copyright 1973, National Fire Protection Association, Boston, MA.)

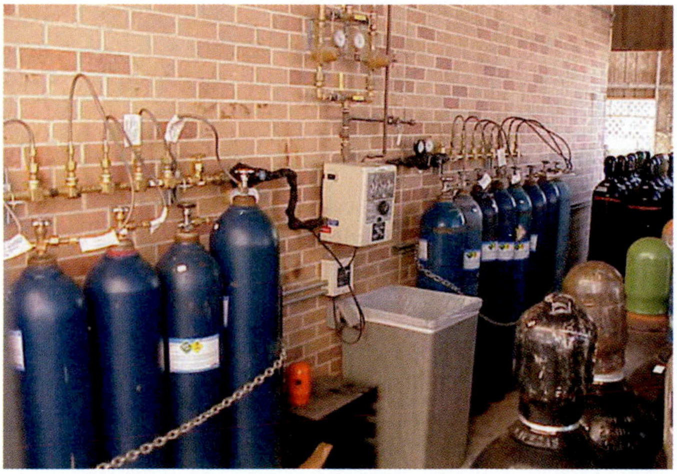

FIGURE 40-8 Alternating supply system of N_2O.

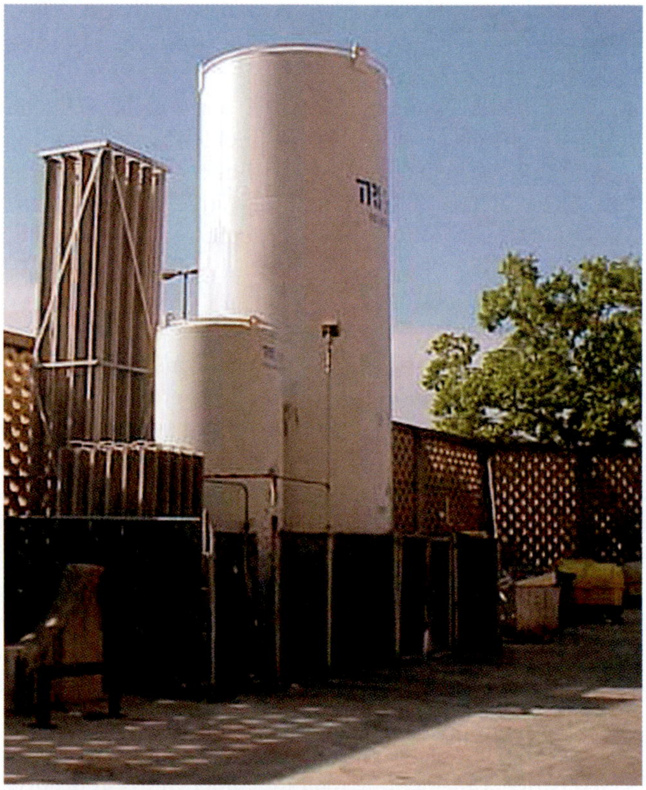

FIGURE 40-9 Large stand tank and reserve tank of liquid O_2 represents a typical bulk gas system with a reserve.

and secondary supplies become depleted. Liquid containers may be used as the primary and secondary gas sources, but the reserve supply usually is high-pressure gas cylinders. Gas cylinders are used as the reserve supply because low-pressure liquid containers lose approximately 3% of the supply per day.[2]

For economy, safety, and convenience, most large health care facilities use a *liquid bulk O_2 system*. A small volume of liquid O_2 provides a very large amount of gaseous O_2 and minimizes space requirements. However, along with this advantage comes a major problem. O_2 has a critical temperature well below room temperature (−118.6° C [−181.4° F]).[1] Liquid O_2 must continually be stored below this temperature, or it reverts to its gaseous state.

To stay in liquid form, O_2 is stored in large stand tanks (Figure 40-9) at relatively low pressure (<250 psig). These stand tanks are similar to giant thermos bottles, consisting of inner and outer steel shells separated by an insulated vacuum chamber (Figure 40-10). Because it eliminates heat conduction, the vacuum keeps the liquid O_2 below its critical temperature without refrigeration. When it flows through vaporizer coils exposed to ambient temperature, the liquid O_2 quickly converts back to a gas. With the O_2 in its gaseous form, the pressure is decreased to the standard working pressure of 50 psi by a

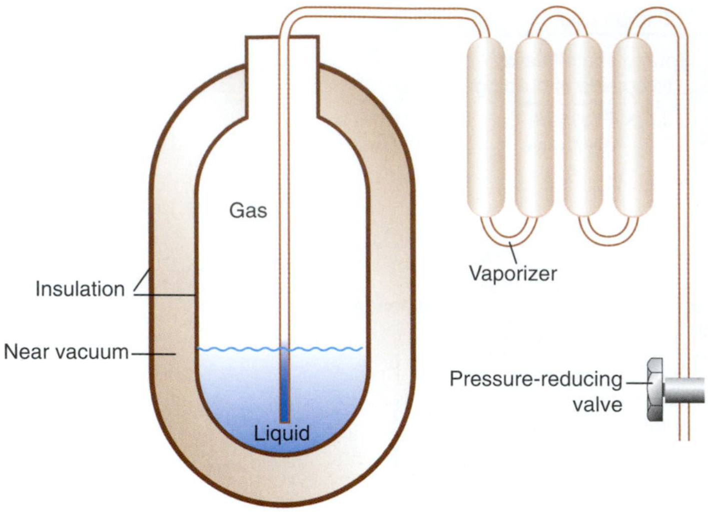

FIGURE 40-10 Liquid-O_2 stand tank (fixed station). (Modified from Cairo JM, Pilbeam SP: Mosby's respiratory care equipment, ed 8, St Louis, 2010, Mosby.)

pressure-reducing valve. A safety vent allows vaporized liquid O_2 to escape if warming causes cylinder pressure to increase above a set limit.

Smaller liquid cylinders are used for home O_2 supply. These cylinders come in several sizes and hold between ⅔ ft^3 and 1½ ft^3 of liquid O_2. Small liquid O_2 cylinders are refilled onsite by means of transfer of liquid O_2 from a large cylinder. Chapter 56 describes the use of these small liquid O_2 cylinders in the home.

Bulk Oxygen Safety Precautions

The NFPA sets standards for the design, construction, placement, and use of bulk O_2 systems.[2] A key provision in these standards is the requirement for a reserve or backup gas supply to equal the average daily gas usage of the hospital. To meet this requirement, most large facilities have a second, smaller liquid stand tank. Smaller facilities may use a cylinder gas manifold as the backup.

Failure of bulk O_2 supply systems has been reported with resultant major problems.[13-16] Failure of a bulk O_2 supply can be life-threatening to any patient receiving O_2 or gas-powered ventilatory support. For this reason, the respiratory care staff must be prepared. Adherence to an established protocol is a quick way to identify and prioritize all affected patients. When affected patients are identified, staff members move appropriate backup equipment to the bedside (e.g., portable cylinders, bag-valve-mask resuscitators). Trained personnel bypass the failed system and provide needed patient support, while engineers determine the cause of the failure and correct it.

DISTRIBUTION AND REGULATION OF MEDICAL GASES

Before it can be administered to a patient, a medical gas must be delivered to the bedside and the pressure reduced to a workable level. This is the primary function of gas distribution and regulation systems. Modern hospital gas distribution systems deliver bulk O_2 and compressed air to patient rooms and special care areas through an elaborate piping network. This network may include a vacuum source and, for surgical areas, N_2O. Patient transport still requires the use of portable cylinders. Whether delivery occurs by central bulk supply or cylinder, patient safety is always the primary aim. For this reason, RTs must be proficient in the use of both delivery systems.

Central Piping Systems

Structural standards for piping systems are established by the NFPA and are described in more detail elsewhere.[2] Figure 40-11 shows a simple central piping gas system. The gas pressure in a central piping system normally is reduced to the standard working pressure of 50 psi at the bulk storage location. A main alarm warns of decreases in pressure or interruptions in flow from the source. **Zone valves** (Figure 40-12) throughout the system can be closed for system maintenance or in case of fire. Wall or station outlets at the delivery sites allow connection of various types of equipment to the gas distribution system. Because most delivery outlets include O_2, air, vacuum, and possibly N_2O, special safety connectors are used to help prevent accidental misconnections.

Safety Indexed Connector Systems

One of the greatest risks in medical gas therapy is giving the wrong gas to a patient. Carefully reading the cylinder or outlet labels is the best way to avoid these accidents. However, human error does occur. For this reason, the industry has developed indexed safety systems for gas delivery and regulation equipment. These safety systems make misconnection between pieces of equipment nearly impossible. For example, an indexed safety system normally prevents connecting a cylinder of N_2O to an O_2 delivery system. Three basic indexed safety systems are used in the delivery and regulation of medical gases: (1) the American National Standard/Compressed Gas Association Standard for Compressed Gas Cylinder Valve Outlet and Inlet Connections, or the ASSS; (2) the **diameter-index safety system** (DISS); and (3) the pin index safety system (PISS).[17,18]

American Standard Safety System

Adopted in the United States and Canada, the ASSS provides standards for threaded high-pressure connections between large compressed gas cylinders (sizes F through H/K) and their attachments.[17] Specifications exist for more than 60 gases and gas mixtures. Figure 40-13 shows a typical ASSS connection between a threaded cylinder outlet and a pressure-reducing valve nipple. Use of the ASSS standards makes misconnections difficult because the size (bore) of the cylinder outlet and its threading differ based on the type of gas in the cylinder.

Because there are only 26 connections for the 62 listed gases and mixtures, each gas may not have a unique connection. Some gases have identical connections. Catalogues of cylinder equipment show the connection specifications for each type of

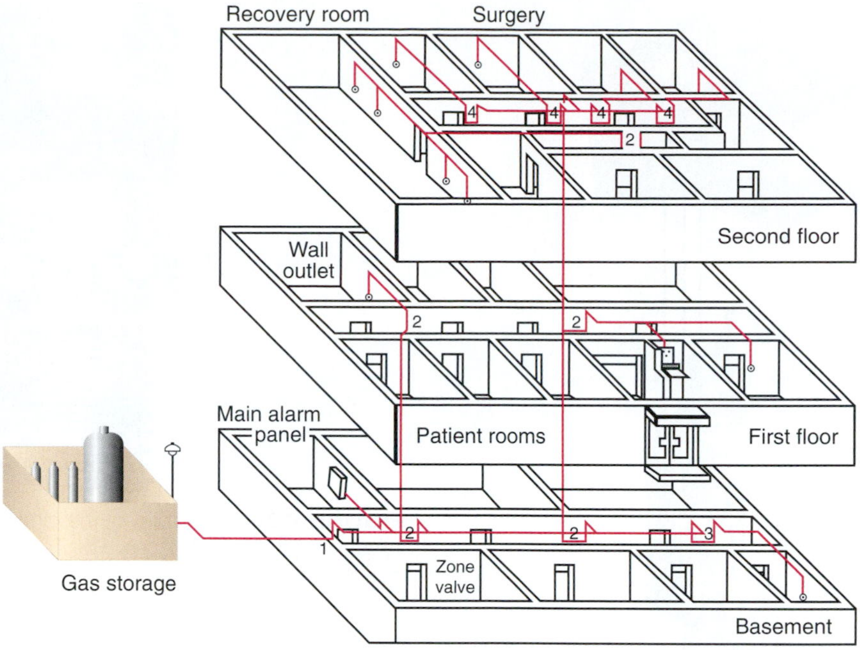

FIGURE 40-11 A hospital piping system. Numbers indicate zone valves.

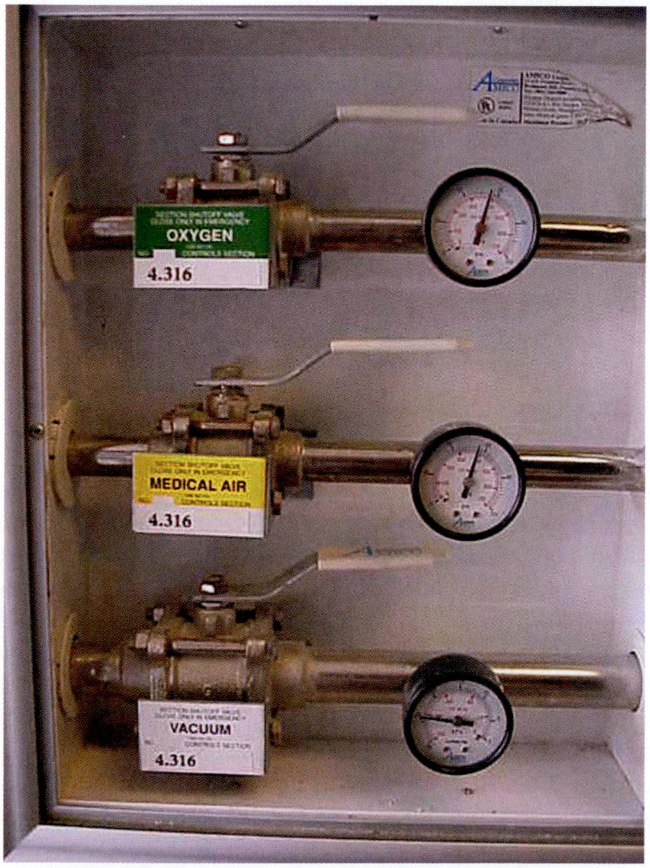

FIGURE 40-12 O_2, air, and vacuum zone valves.

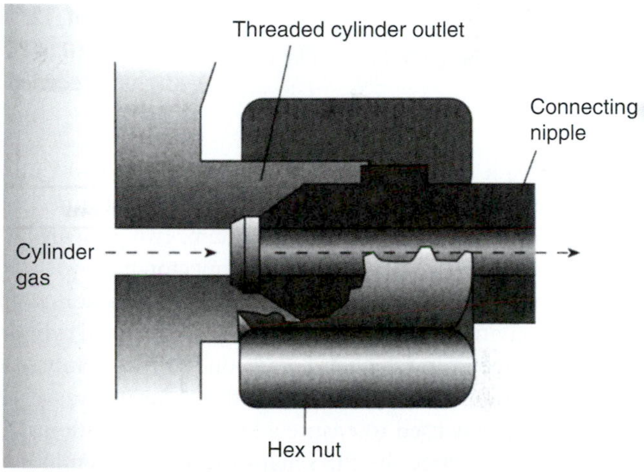

FIGURE 40-13 Typical American standard supply system connection used to attach a reducing valve to a large high-pressure cylinder. A hexagonal nut is held on the nipple of the reducing valve by a circular collar. The connection is made by (1) aligning the reducing valve nipple with the conical cylinder valve outlet and (2) tightening the reducing valve hex nut onto the threaded cylinder outlet. Different threading and cylinder outlet sizes make accidental misconnections difficult.

cylinder and gas. A typical description for a large cylinder of O_2 is as follows: CGA-540 0.903-14NGO-RH-Ext. The connection for the threaded outlet of this cylinder is listed by the CGA as connection number 540. The outlet has a thread diameter (bore) of 0.903 inch; there are 14 threads per inch; and the threads are right-handed (RH) and external (Ext). It generally is necessary to use only one or two outlet connections because most of the gases that are used by RTs are grouped within a few connector sizes. However, practitioners should be familiar with the classification scheme in general because expanding instrumentation and scope of services may bring RTs in contact with other gases and gas systems.

Pin-Index Safety System

Pin indexing is part of the ASSS but applies only to the valve outlets of small cylinders, up to and including size E. These

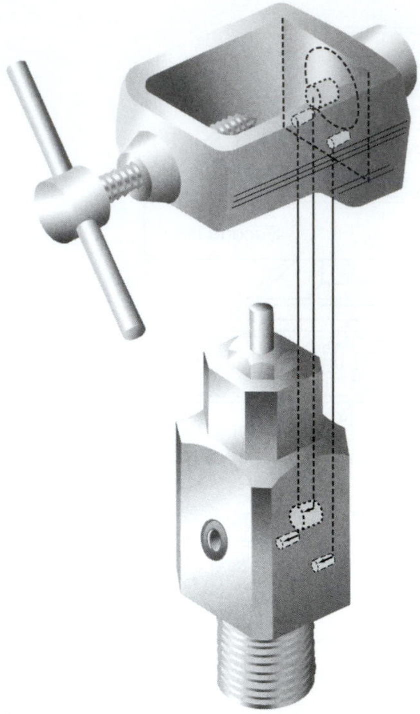

FIGURE 40-14 Yoke connector showing regulator inlet and pin-indexed safety system (for cylinders size AA to E).

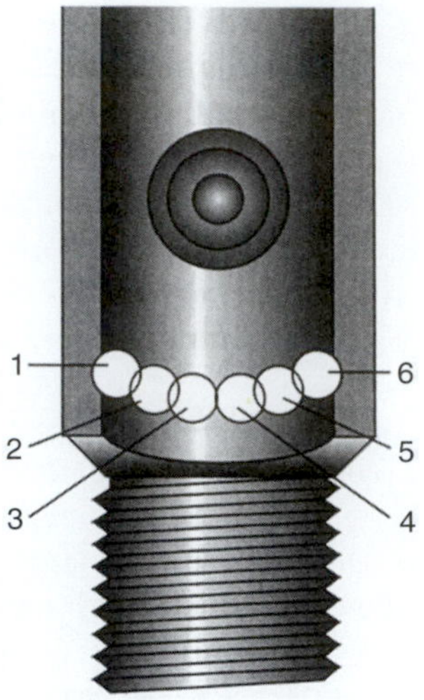

FIGURE 40-15 Location of the pin-index holes in the cylinder valve face for different gases. See Table 40-5 for pin-index hole locations for various gases.

cylinders have a yoke type of connection. Figure 40-14 illustrates the general structure of the pin-indexed yoke connection. The upper yoke fits over the lower valve stem. Two pins, projecting from the inner surface of the yoke connector, mate with two pinholes bored into the valve stem. Proper pin position aligns the small receiving nipple of the yoke with the recessed cylinder valve outlet. Tightening the hand screw on the yoke firmly seats the receiving nipple into the valve outlet. A nylon washer or bushing typically is used to ensure a leak-free connection.

Similar to the ASSS, the PISS helps prevent accidental misconnections between pieces of equipment. The exact positions of pins and pinholes vary for each gas. Unless the pins and holes align perfectly, the yoke nipple cannot seat in the recessed valve outlet. Six holes and pin positions constitute the total system. Because overlapping holes cannot be used, there are 10 possible pin combinations. Figure 40-15 is a diagram of the location of all six possible holes and their index numbers. Table 40-5 lists the gases included in the PISS system, including their index positions.

Diameter-Index Safety System

The ASSS and the PISS provide standards for high-pressure connections between cylinders and equipment; the DISS was established to prevent accidental interchange of low-pressure (<200 psig) medical gas connectors.[18] RTs typically find DISS connections (1) at the outlets of pressure-reducing valves attached to cylinders; (2) at the station outlets of central piping systems; and (3) at the inlets of blenders, flowmeters, ventilators, and other pneumatic equipment.

TABLE 40-5

Pin-Index Hole Positions*

Gas	Pin Positions
O_2	2-5
O_2/CO_2 (CO_2 not >7%)	2-6
He/O_2 (He not >80%)	2-4
C_2H_4	1-3
N_2O	3-5
C_3H_6	3-6
He/O_2 (He > 80%)	4-6
O_2/CO_2 (CO_2 > 7%)	1-6
Air	1-5

*See Figure 40-15.
C_2H_4, Ethylene; *C_3H_6*, cyclopropane.

As shown in Figure 40-16, the DISS connection consists of an externally threaded body and a mated nipple with a nut. As the two parts are joined, the shoulders of the nipple and the bores of the body mate, with the union held together by a hand-tightened hex nut. Indexing is achieved by varying the dimensions of the borings and shoulders. There are 11 indexed DISS connections and 1 connection for O_2, for a total of 12.[18] The standard threaded O_2 connector (0.5625 inch in diameter and 18 threads per inch) preceded adoption of this safety system. Nonetheless, it has been assigned a DISS number of 1240.

Although O_2 and air are generally used from a central outlet, it may be necessary to administer other gases that have different DISS connections. To avoid stocking a large variety of pressure regulators, flowmeters, and connectors for special gas use, adapters can be used to convert various DISS connections so they can be used for different purposes. Using adapters to bypass a safety system carries the increased risk for misconnection. For this reason, RTs should exercise extreme caution

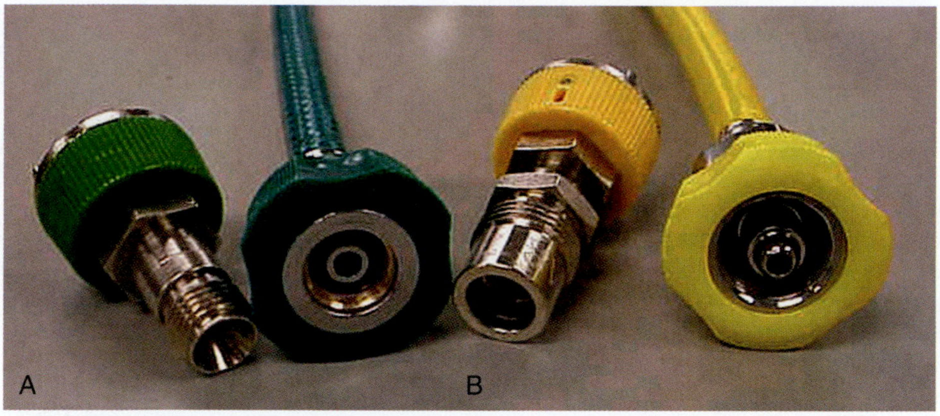

FIGURE 40-16 O_2 **(A)** and air **(B)** diameter index safety system (DISS) connections. The two shoulders of the nipple allow the nipple to unite only with a body that has corresponding borings. If the match is incorrect, the nut does not engage the body threads. The difference in the shoulders and bore between the O_2 **(A)** and air **(B)** DISS connections is evident.

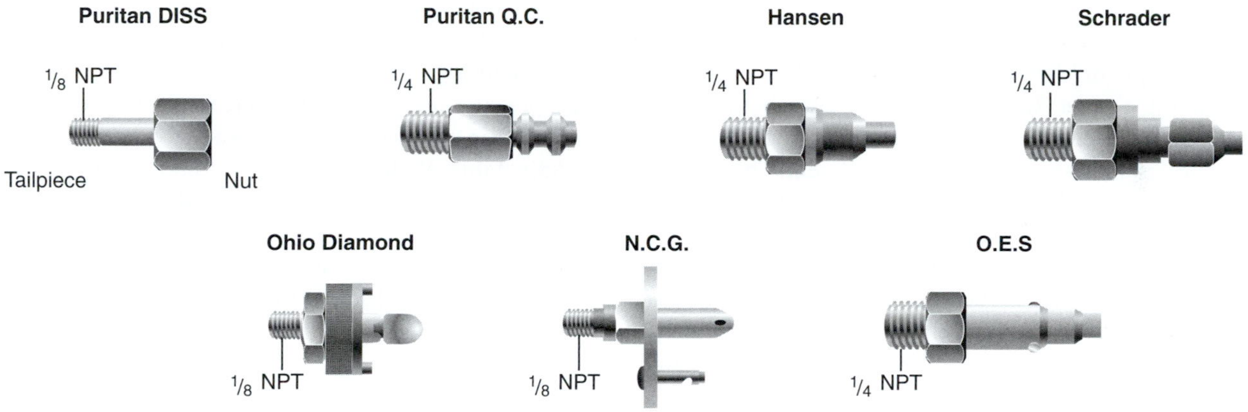

FIGURE 40-17 Common brands of quick connects. *NPT,* National pipe thread taper. (Courtesy Nellcor Puritan Bennett, Pleasanton, CA.)

when adapting equipment connections. Misconnections have occurred, with negative patient consequences.[13,19]

Quick-Connect Systems

Station outlets at the patient's bedside allow quick access to a bulk supply of O_2 and air or a vacuum source. Station outlets have DISS connections or quick-connect systems that are gas-specific or vacuum-specific. Various manufacturers have designed specially shaped connectors for each gas (Figure 40-17). Because each connector has a distinct shape, it does not fit into an outlet for another gas and each manufacturer has its own unique design. For this reason, connectors from different manufacturers are not interchangeable. As long as a facility is standardized for a single quick-connect system, this incompatibility is seldom a problem.

A variety of safety systems help prevent inadvertent misconnections between medical delivery systems and equipment. Figure 40-18 summarizes the use of and relationships between the ASSS, PISS, and DISS systems as applied to cylinder gases. Proficiency in the proper use of these systems is a basic skill of RTs.

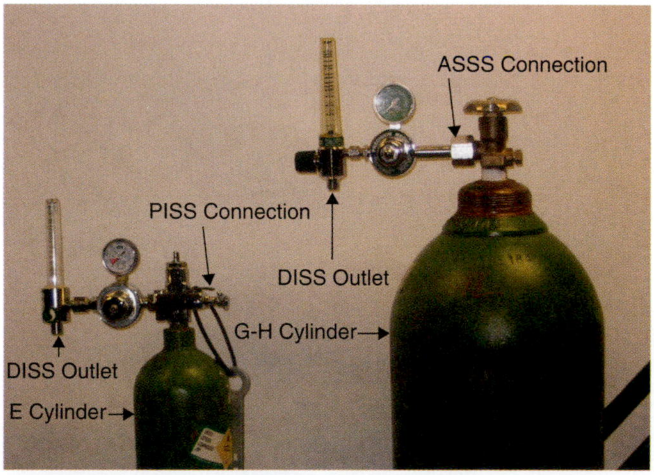

FIGURE 40-18 Comparison of safety systems used for compressed gases. The diameter-index safety system (DISS) connections are for low-pressure outlets (<200 psig). The American standard safety system (ASSS) provides for high-pressure connections with large cylinders. A variation of the ASSS entails a yoke and pin system (PISS) for connecting to small cylinders (AA through E).

Regulating Gas Pressure and Flow

Whatever the source of medical gas, for safe administration to a patient, the pressure and flow must be regulated. If the goal is solely a reduction in gas pressure, a **reducing valve** is used. For control of gas flow to a patient, a **flowmeter** is used. If control of both pressure and flow is needed, a regulator is used.

Cylinder gases such as O_2 and air exert a pressure that is much too high for use with respiratory care equipment. For use at the bedside, these high pressures must be reduced to a lower "working" level. In the United States, this working pressure is 50 psig. For bulk delivery systems with individual station outlets, built-in reducing valves decrease the delivered pressure to 50 psig. This standard pressure can be directly applied to power devices such as ventilators (see Chapter 45). However, if the goal is to control gas delivery to a patient for O_2 therapy or nebulized medication (see Chapters 39 and 41), a flowmeter also must be used.

High-Pressure Reducing Valves

The two basic types of high-pressure reducing valves are single-stage and multiple-stage. Reducing valves are available as preset or adjustable. Although all of these valves function on the same principle, the design, features, and use are different. This section differentiates preset reducing valves and adjustable reducing valves and discusses multiple-stage reducing valves.

Preset Reducing Valve. Figure 40-19 shows the basic design of a high-pressure preset reducing valve. High-pressure gas (2200 psig for O_2) enters through the valve *(A)*, with the inlet pressure displayed on the pressure gauge *(B)*. The body of the valve is divided into a high-pressure chamber *(C)* and an ambient-pressure chamber *(D)* by a flexible diaphragm *(E)*. Attached to the diaphragm in the ambient-pressure chamber is a spring *(F)*, which is fixed to the other side of the chamber. Also attached to the diaphragm, but in the high-pressure chamber, is a valve stem *(G)* that sits on the high-pressure inlet *(H)*. Gas flows through the valve inlet *(H)* into the high-pressure chamber and on to the gas outlet *(I)*. The pressure chamber is supplied with a safety vent *(L)* preset to 200 psig to release pressure in the event of malfunction.

The spring tension is calibrated to give when the pressure on the diaphragm exceeds 50 psig. When this happens, the valve stem is pushed forward and closes the high-pressure inlet, preventing further entry of gas into the reducing valve. However, as long as gas is allowed to escape from the pressure chamber through the outlet *(I)*, the inlet valve remains open and allows gas flow. The regulator maintains a balance between outlet flow and inlet pressure. Automatic adjustment of the diaphragm-spring combination keeps the pressure in the high-pressure chamber at a near-constant 50 psig—hence the name *preset*. Preset reducing valves are normally used in conjunction with high-pressure gas cylinders to decrease the pressure to the standard 50 psig used with most respiratory care equipment.

Adjustable Reducing Valve. Although most respiratory care equipment works at the standard 50 psig, some devices need variable pressures. To provide variable outlet pressures from a high-pressure gas source, an adjustable reducing valve is needed. Figure 40-20 shows the basic design of a high-pressure

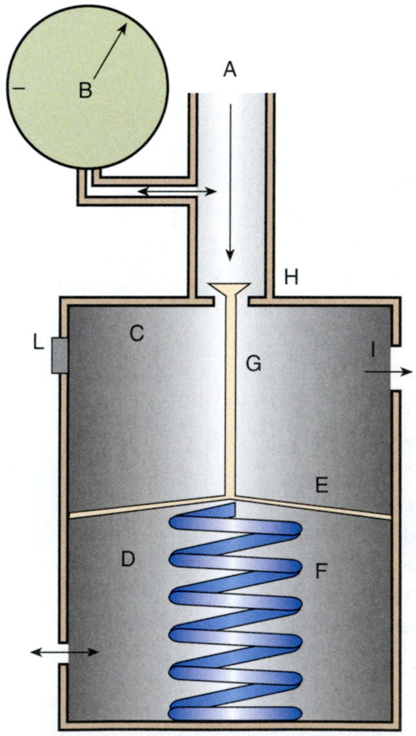

FIGURE 40-19 Preset high-pressure reducing valve.

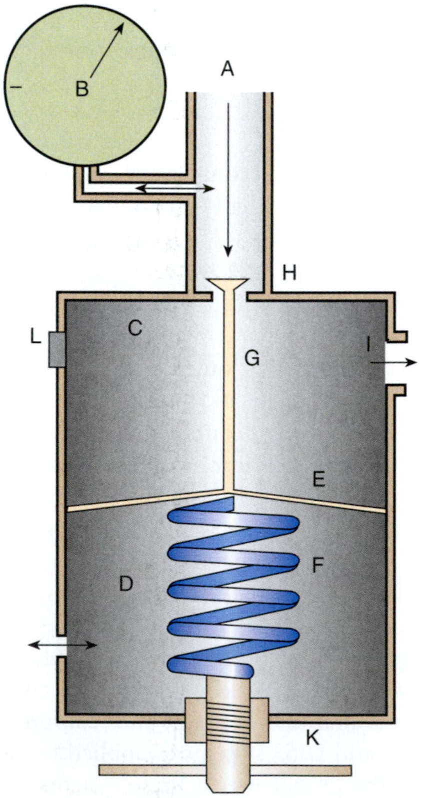

FIGURE 40-20 Adjustable high-pressure reducing valve.

adjustable reducing valve. As with the preset design, the inlet valve *(H)* remains open until the gas pressure exceeds the spring tension, displacing the diaphragm and blocking further gas entry. However, whereas the preset reducing valve provides a fixed pressure, the adjustable reducing valve allows a change in outlet pressure. Outlet pressure can be changed with a threaded hand control *(K)* attached to the end of the diaphragm spring. Changing the tension on the valve spring varies pressure over a wide range, usually between 0 psig and 100 psig.

The adjustable reducing valve commonly is used in combination with a Bourdon-type flow gauge (discussed later). The combination of a flowmeter with a reducing valve is called a **regulator.**

Multiple-Stage Reducing Valve. As the name suggests, a *multiple-stage reducing valve* reduces pressure in two or more steps. Multiple-stage reducing valves can be either preset or adjustable and can be combined with a flowmeter device as a true regulator. Two-stage reducing valves are used occasionally, and three-stage units are rarely needed. A two-stage reducing valve functions as two single-stage reducing valves working in series. Gas enters the first stage, where the pressure is reduced to an intermediate level (usually 200 to 700 psig). Gas then enters the second stage, where the pressure is decreased to working level (usually 50 psig). Because each pressure chamber has one safety relief vent, the user usually can determine the number of stages in a reducing valve by noting the number of relief vents present. Because they reduce pressure in multiple steps, these valves provide more precise and smooth flow control. However, they are larger and more expensive than single-stage reducing valves. For this reason, a multiple-stage reducing valve should be considered only if minimal fluctuations in pressure or flow are critical factors, as in research activities. For routine hospital work, single-stage reducing valves are satisfactory.

Proper Use of High-Pressure Reducing Valves. When a cylinder attached to a high-pressure reducing valve is open, gas undergoes rapid decompression followed by rapid recompression. Because the recompression is adiabatic (see Chapter 6), the gas temperature quickly increases. These rapid pressure and temperature changes may cause failure of the reducing valve. Rapid temperature changes can ignite combustible materials; this risk is increased in the presence of 100% O_2. Box 40-1 provides guidelines for minimizing the risk associated with setting up O_2 cylinders with a high-pressure reducing valve or regulator.[1]

Box 40-1 Safe Procedure for Setup of an Oxygen Cylinder and Reducing Valve or Regulator

1. Secure the cylinder according to the CGA guidelines. Verify the contents from the label that matches the color code and valve indexing.
2. Remove the protective cap or wrap, and inspect the cylinder valve to ensure that it is free of dirt, debris, and oil.
3. Warn any persons present that the cylinder valve is about to be "cracked" and that it will make some noise. Turn the cylinder valve away from persons present, stand to the side, and quickly open and close the valve. This removes any dust or small debris from the cylinder valve outlet.
4. Inspect the valve or regulator inlet for debris, dirt, and oil. Check the device label, and confirm that it is intended for high-pressure service and for use with the gas to be administered. O_2-reducing valves and regulators should have a label stating: *Oxygen: Use No Oil.*
5. After the valve or regulator inlet is confirmed to be free of contaminants, securely tighten (but do not force) the device onto the cylinder outlet. When making connections to the cylinder, use appropriate wrenches that are free of oil and grease. Never use pipe wrenches. Use only cylinder valve connections that conform to the ASSS and the PISS. Low-pressure connections must comply with the DISS or be noninterchangeable, low-pressure quick connects. Never connect fixed or adjustable orifices or metering devices directly to a cylinder without a pressure-reducing valve.
6. Confirm that the regulator or reducing valve is in the *off* or *closed* position, and slowly open the cylinder valve to pressurize the attached reducing valve or regulator. After pressurization has occurred, open the cylinder valve completely and turn it back one-fourth to one-half turn (this maneuver prevents a condition known as "valve freeze," in which the valve cannot be turned).

ASSS, American standard safety system; *CGA,* Compressed Gas Association; *DISS,* diameter-index safety system; *PISS,* pin-index safety system.

Low-Pressure Gas Flowmeters

As with drugs, giving a medical gas to a patient requires knowledge of the dosage being delivered. Physicians often prescribe O_2 dosage as a flow, in liters per minute. In addition, certain gas-mixing equipment requires accurate knowledge of input flows, sometimes involving two or more gases. Flowmeters allow the rate of gas flow to a patient to be set and controlled. When the gas source is a high-pressure gas cylinder, a regulator (reducing valve plus flowmeter) is required. However, when the source is a bulk central supply system, the pressure has already been reduced to 50 psig by the time it reaches the outlet stations; this eliminates the need for pressure reduction and requires only a flowmeter.

Three categories of flowmeters are used in respiratory care: the flow restrictor, the **Bourdon gauge,** and the **Thorpe tube.** The Thorpe tube has two different designs: pressure compensated or not pressure compensated (uncompensated). Although uncompensated Thorpe tubes are rare, they may still be used at some institutions. For this reason, the principles underlying each of the four types of flow metering devices are compared and contrasted.

Flow Restrictor. The flow restrictor is the simplest and least expensive flowmeter device. As shown in Figure 40-21, a flow restrictor consists solely of a fixed orifice calibrated to deliver a specific flow at a constant pressure (50 psig). The operation of the flow restrictor is based on the principle of flow resistance, as described in Chapter 6. Specifically, the flow of gas through a tube can be quantified with the following equation:

$$R = \frac{P_1 - P_2}{\dot{V}}$$

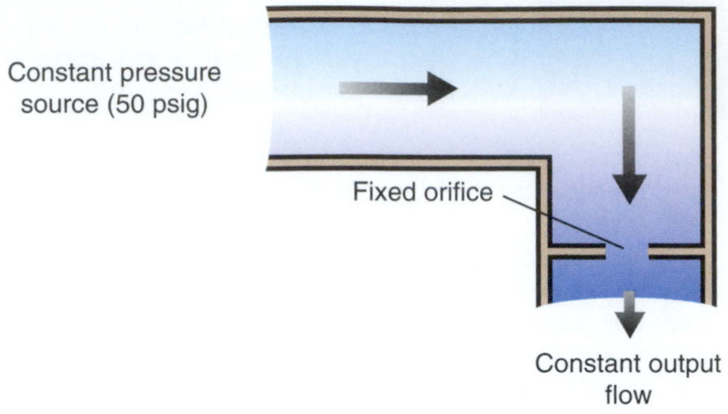

FIGURE 40-21 Flow restrictor.

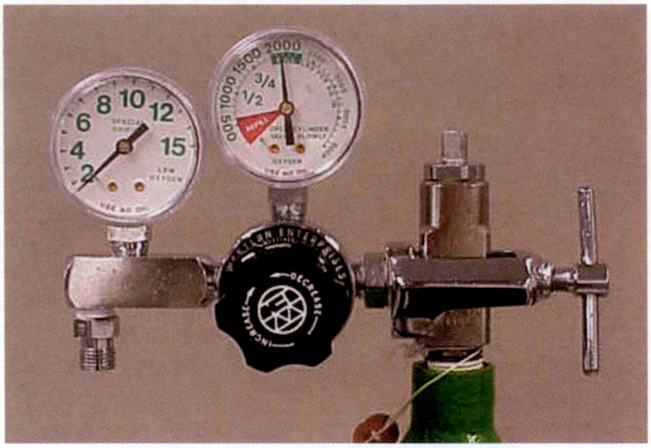

FIGURE 40-22 Bourdon gauge regulator.

MINI CLINIC

Leaky Connections

PROBLEM: Following standard procedure, the RT attaches a pressure-reducing valve to an O_2 cylinder. When the RT opens the cylinder valve, gas leaking at or near the connection can be heard.

SOLUTION: A leak usually indicates that the connection between the pressure-reducing valve and the cylinder outlet is not tight. If the cylinder outlet is a standard ASSS threaded connector, the connection is either cross-threaded or not properly seated and tightened. To solve this problem, the RT closes the cylinder valve and removes and reattaches the pressure-reducing valve, taking care to thread the connection properly and to tighten with a wrench. If the cylinder outlet is a pin-indexed connector, the RT closes the cylinder valve and removes the pressure-reducing valve. The RT checks to ensure that the nylon washer is present, in good condition, and properly fitted. The RT then reattaches the pressure-reducing valve, taking care to seat the connection properly and to hand tighten. If the leak continues after these corrective actions, it is likely that the pressure-reducing valve is malfunctioning and should be replaced.

TABLE 40-6

Advantages and Disadvantages of Flow Restrictors

Advantages	Disadvantages
Low-cost, simple, reliable (no moving parts)	Different versions required for different flows
Cannot be set to incorrect flow	Accuracy varies with changes in source and downstream pressures
Can be used in any position (gravity-independent)	Cannot be used with high-resistance equipment

Rearranging the equation to solve for flow *(V)* yields the following:

$$V = \frac{P_1 - P_2}{R}$$

where *V* is the volumetric flow per unit time, P_1 is the pressure at the **upstream** point (point 1), P_2 is the pressure at the **downstream** point (point 2), and *R* is the total resistance to gas flow.

By design, a flow restrictor requires a source of constant pressure (usually 50 psig). As long as the source pressure remains fixed, $P_1 - P_2$ should stay constant. With a fixed-size orifice, the flow resistance *(R)* also remains constant. The rate of gas flow through a flow restrictor can be increased by increasing P_1 (upstream pressure) or by selecting a larger orifice size. Both fixed and adjustable orifice flow restrictors are used clinically. Commercially produced flow restrictors are calibrated at 50 psig. Table 40-6 summarizes the advantages and disadvantages of flow restrictors.

Bourdon Gauge. A Bourdon gauge (Figure 40-22) is a flowmeter device that is always used in combination with an adjustable pressure-reducing valve. Similar to the flow restrictor, the Bourdon gauge uses a fixed orifice. In contrast to the flow restrictor, the Bourdon gauge operates under variable pressures, as adjusted with the pressure-reducing valve. The Bourdon gauge is a fixed-orifice, variable-pressure flowmeter, so increasing the upstream pressure increases gas flow out of the device unless downstream pressure also increases.

As shown in Figure 40-23, a Bourdon gauge has a calibrated fixed orifice *(A)*, which creates outflow resistance. The gauge itself is attached with a connector *(B)* located proximal to the orifice. Inside the gauge is a curved, hollow, closed tube *(C)* that responds to pressure changes by changing shape. The force of gas pressure tends to straighten the tube, causing its distal end to move. This motion is transmitted to a gear assembly and indicator needle *(D)*. Although it changes based on pressure, the numbered scale is calibrated to read the needle movement in units of flow (liters per minute).

As with the flow restrictor with a fixed orifice, the output flow of the Bourdon gauge is proportional to the driving pressure. However, the Bourdon gauge provides a continuous range of flow, which the user adjusts by altering the driving pressure.

Although the gauge actually measures pressure changes, it displays the corresponding flow.

As with a flow restrictor, gravity does not affect a Bourdon gauge. The Bourdon gauge is the best choice when a flowmeter cannot be maintained in an upright position. This situation is common when a patient is being transported with a portable O_2 source. In these instances, keeping the E cylinder upright is seldom easy, and movement of both the O_2 supply and the patient is common. Combined with its continuous range of flows, this feature makes the Bourdon gauge the metering device of choice for patient transport.

The main disadvantage of the Bourdon gauge is its inaccuracy when pressure distal to the orifice (downstream pressures) changes. Specifically, if downstream pressure increases (as when high-resistance equipment is used), the pressure difference across the orifice and actual output flow decrease. However, the Bourdon gauge flow reading depends on upstream pressure, which stays constant. In this situation, the gauge reading is falsely higher than the actual delivered flow. Because it measures upstream pressure, the gauge registers flow even when the outlet is completely blocked (Figure 40-24). A user who needs accurate flow when using a device that creates high resistance should not select a Bourdon gauge. A compensated Thorpe tube should be used instead.

Integrated O_2 cylinders (Figure 40-25), including the Grab 'n Go System (Praxair, Danbury, CT), have combined the O_2 cylinder with a pressure regulator and an adjustable flow restrictor to meter O_2 flow. These portable O_2 systems eliminate the need for separate O_2 tanks, Bourdon gauge regulators, and O_2 keys or wrenches (needed to turn on standard E-cylinders). These integrated systems virtually eliminate problems and delays associated with incorrectly mounted regulators. The practitioner simply selects the flow on the flow-adjusting knob and connects the O_2 tubing to the system connection and the patient.

Thorpe Tube. The Thorpe tube flowmeter (Figure 40-26) is always attached to a 50-psig source, either a preset pressure-reducing valve or a bedside station outlet. Compared with the flow restrictor and the Bourdon gauge, the Thorpe tube functions as a variable-orifice, constant-pressure flowmeter, so

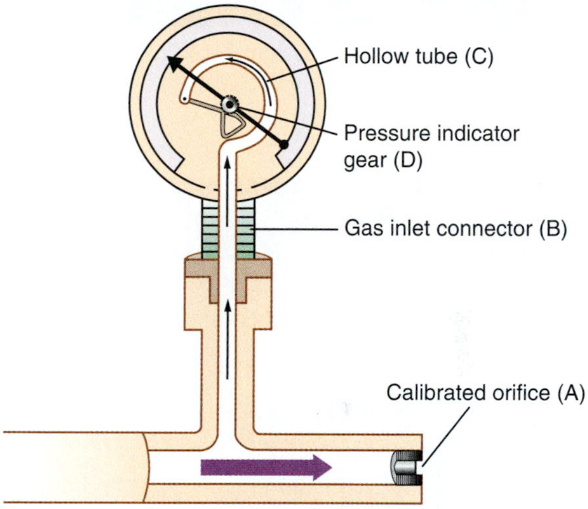

FIGURE 40-23 Components of a Bourdon pressure gauge. See text for more information.

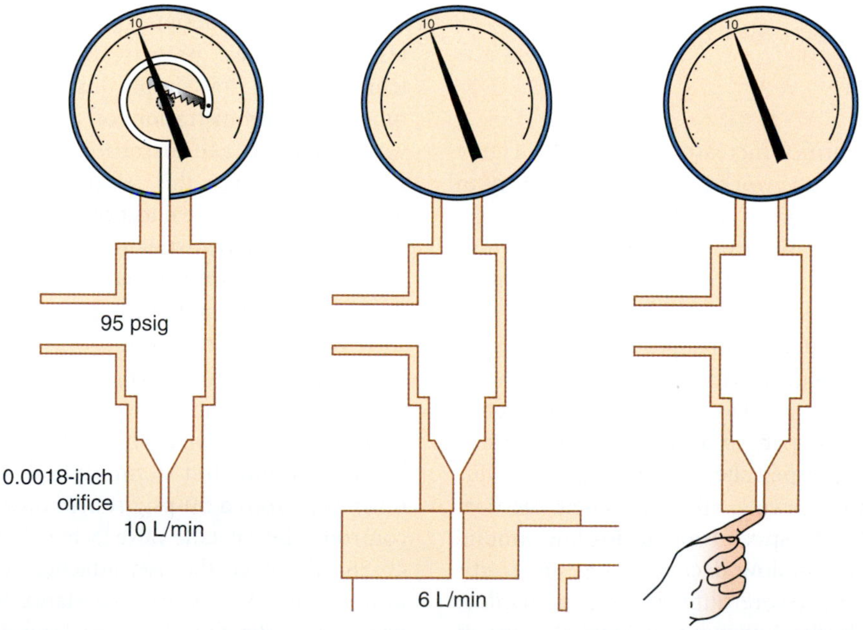

FIGURE 40-24 Bourdon performance when downstream pressures increase as a result of high-resistance equipment or blockage. *Left,* Normal state with fixed orifice and no downstream resistance results in an accurate flow reading. *Center,* High-resistance nebulizer increases downstream pressure, or back pressure. The result is a falsely high reading (10 L/min vs. actual flow of 6 L/min). *Right,* Complete blockage (zero flow) results in flow reading on gauge.

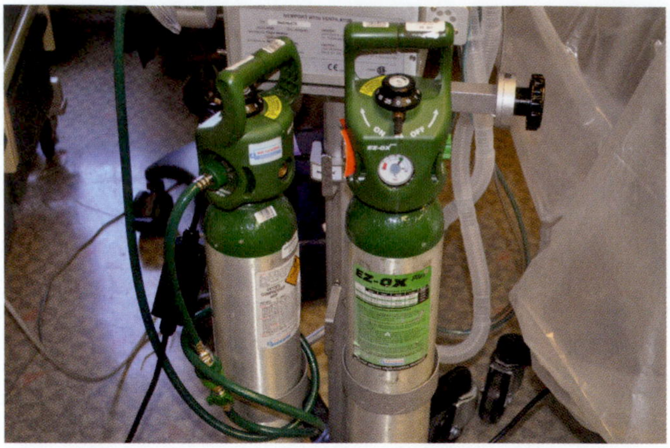

FIGURE 40-25 Grab 'n Go System (Praxair, Danbury, Connecticut).

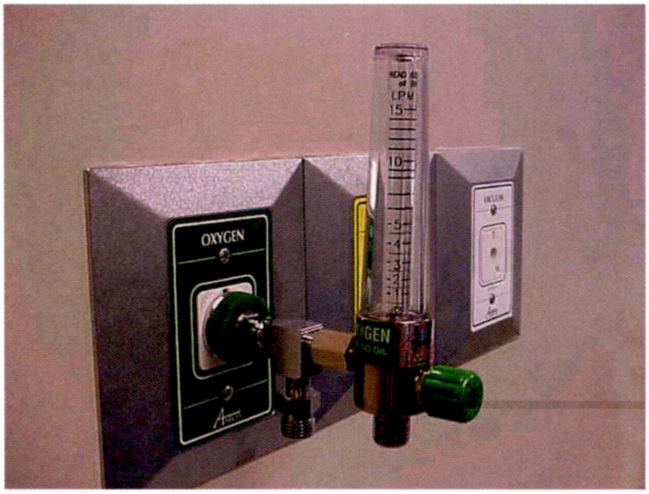

FIGURE 40-26 Thorpe tube flowmeter.

increasing the size of the orifice increases the gas flow. Figure 40-27 shows how a Thorpe tube works. The key component in this device is a tapered transparent tube that contains a float. The diameter of the tube increases from bottom to top. Gas flow suspends the float against the force of gravity. To read the flow, one simply compares the float position with an adjacent calibrated scale, normally calibrated in liters per minute.

Although the Bourdon gauge measures pressure, the Thorpe tube is used to measure true flow. Flow measurement involves the complex interaction of gravity and fluid dynamics. When gas begins to flow into a Thorpe tube, the initial pressure difference lifts the float. As the needle valve is opened, the float rises in the widening tube, the space available for flow around it increases, and resistance to flow decreases. The float ultimately stabilizes when the pressure difference across the float (an upward force) equals the opposing downward force of gravity.

As the needle valve of the flowmeter is opened, the increase in flow initially disrupts this balance, causing an increase in the pressure difference across the float. With the upward pressure difference greater than the downward force of gravity, the float rises. However, as the float rises, the available "orifice" increases in diameter. Flow resistance around the float decreases, and the pressure difference again equilibrates with gravity. The float position stabilizes at a higher level, proportionate to the greater flow around it.

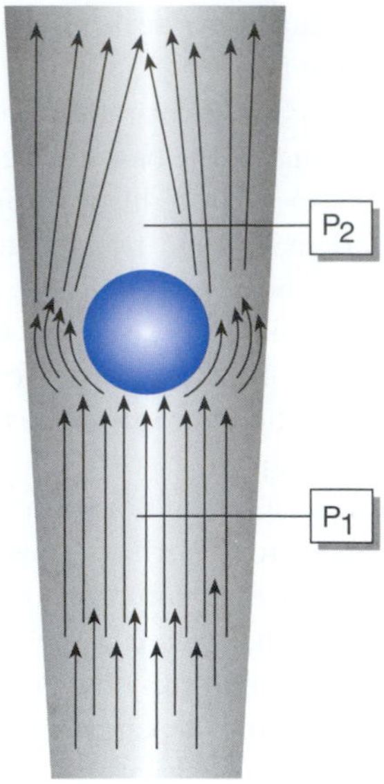

FIGURE 40-27 The position of the float in a Thorpe tube flowmeter is based on a balance between the force of gravity and the pressure difference ($P_2 - P_1$) across it, as determined by the variable-sized orifice between the float and the tube wall.

Thorpe tubes come in two basic designs: pressure compensated and pressure uncompensated. The term *pressure compensation* refers to a design that prevents changes in downstream resistance, or back pressure, from affecting meter accuracy. All manufacturers now supply only pressure-compensated Thorpe tubes for administration of a medical gas. However, some ventilators and anesthesia machines still use uncompensated Thorpe tubes. For this reason, clinicians using these devices must understand the effect of back pressure on the accuracy of these devices. Downstream resistance increases when the user connects a flowmeter to certain types of equipment. Almost all therapy gas equipment produces some flow restriction. Devices such as jet nebulizers produce very high downstream resistance. Depending on their design, Thorpe tube flowmeters respond to resistance in one of two ways.

The *uncompensated* Thorpe tube flowmeter is calibrated in liters per minute but at atmospheric pressure (without restriction). Gas from a 50-psig source flows into the meter at a rate controlled by a needle valve located before the flow tube (Figure 40-28, *A*). When the user attaches flow-restricting equipment to the meter, downstream resistance increases, which increases pressure in the flow tube. As long as this pressure does not exceed 50 psig, gas continues to flow through the tube. However, the added downstream resistance increases the pressure in the flow tube above atmospheric pressure. At this higher pressure,

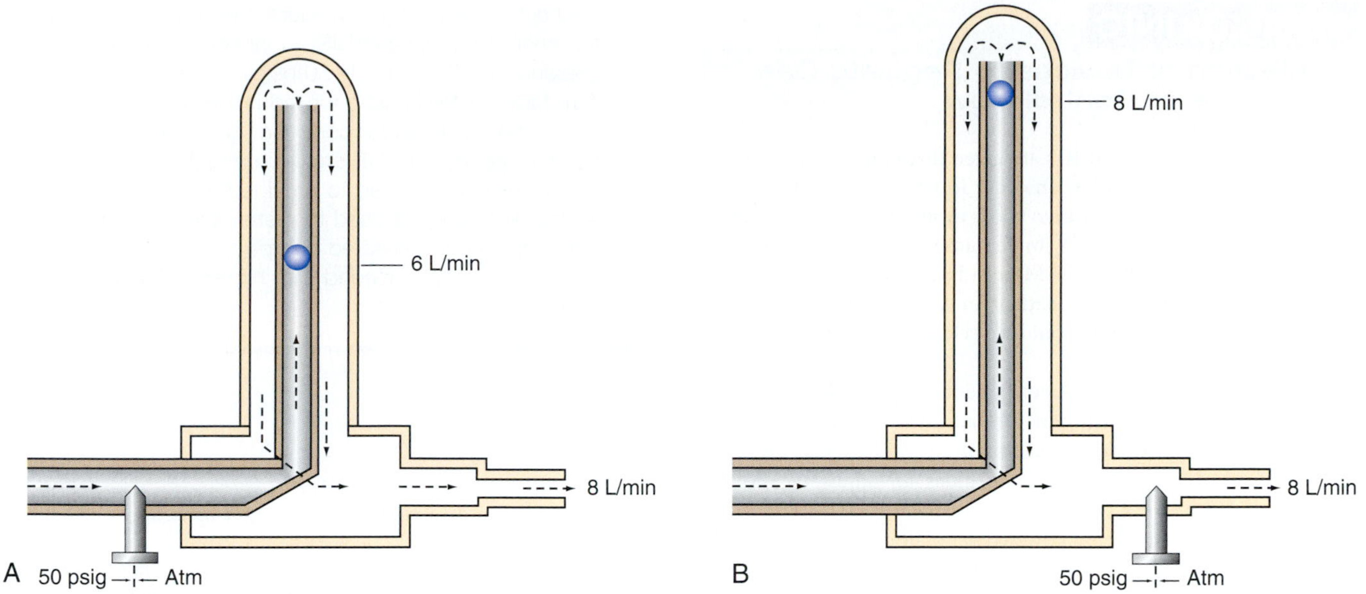

FIGURE 40-28 Comparison of pressure-uncompensated **(A)** and pressure-compensated **(B)** Thorpe tube flowmeters. In the pressure-uncompensated flowmeter, the flow-control valve is proximal to the meter, and the gauge records less than the actual output. In the pressure-compensated flowmeter, location of the valve distal to the meter correlates the gauge reading with the output.

a greater amount of gas flows through a given restriction than at atmospheric pressure so that the float at a given height on the scale indicates more gas flow through the tube than is actually occurring. Under these conditions, an uncompensated Thorpe tube falsely shows a flow lower than that actually delivered to the patient.[4]

In contrast, the scale of the compensated Thorpe tube flowmeter is calibrated at 50 psig instead of at atmospheric pressure. Its flow control needle valve is placed after (distal to) the flow tube (see Figure 40-28, *B*). The entire meter operates at constant 50-psig pressure. Knowing that the compensated Thorpe tube operates at 50 psig helps identify it. When a compensated Thorpe tube is connected to a 50-psig gas source with the needle valve closed, the float "jumps" and then returns to zero as the Thorpe tube is pressurized. Because the entire meter operates at constant pressure, an increase in downstream resistance increases pressure distal to the needle valve only. As long as the downstream pressure does not exceed 50 psig (in which case flow ceases), the position of the float accurately reflects actual outlet flow. For this reason, the pressure-compensated Thorpe tube is the preferred instrument in most clinical situations.

The only factor limiting the use of a pressure-compensated Thorpe tube is gravity. Because it is accurate only in an upright position, a Thorpe tube is not the ideal choice for patient transport. In these cases, the gravity-independent Bourdon gauge is a satisfactory alternative. Figure 40-29 summarizes the effects of downstream resistance, or back pressure, on the Bourdon gauge and pressure-compensated and uncompensated Thorpe tube flow metering devices.

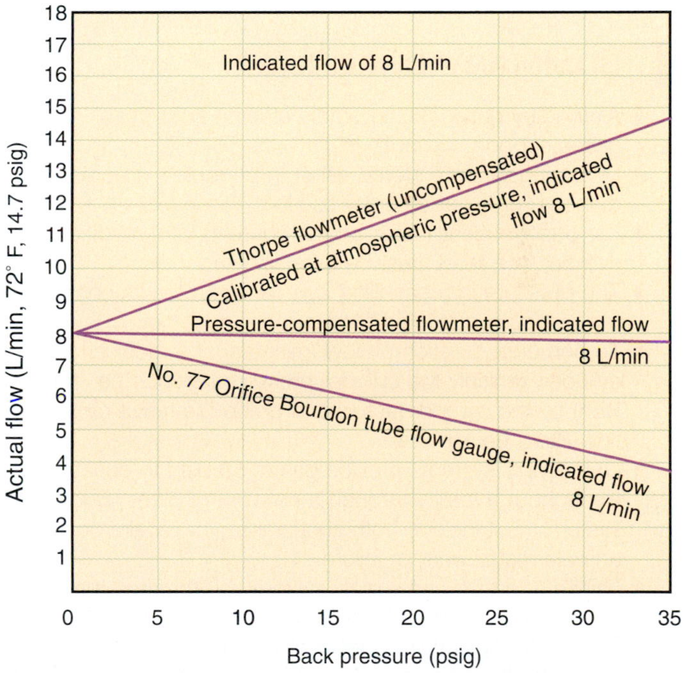

FIGURE 40-29 Comparative accuracy of flowmeter devices against increasing downstream pressure (back pressure). With the pressure-compensated Thorpe tube, indicated flow equals actual flow, regardless of downstream pressure. With the uncompensated Thorpe tube, indicated flow is progressively lower than actual flow as downstream pressure increases. With the Bourdon gauge, indicated flow is progressively higher than actual flow as downstream pressure increases. (Modified from McPherson SP, Spearman CB: Respiratory therapy equipment, ed 5, St Louis, 1995, Mosby. Modified from Puritan-Bennett Corp, Los Angeles, California.)

MINI CLINIC

Selection of Devices to Regulate Gas Pressure or Control Flow

PROBLEM: Three staff RTs are given three separate requests to set up O_2. (1) Mark has an order to transport Ms. Patel to radiology with O_2. (2) Carmen needs to set up a pneumatically powered ventilator with O_2 in the ambulatory clinic (where there are no O_2 outlets). (3) Monica has to set up O_2 therapy with a jet nebulizer for a patient in the intensive care unit (ICU). What equipment should RT select?

SOLUTIONS:

1. Because he has to transport a patient using O_2, Mark should select an E cylinder with an adjustable regulator that includes a Bourdon gauge (unaffected by gravity) or an integrated O_2 cylinder that includes an adjustable flow restrictor.
2. Because pneumatically powered ventilators require 50 psig and no central outlets are available, Carmen needs a preset (50 psig) reducing valve and a large G or H size O_2 cylinder.
3. Because all modern ICUs have central wall outlets for O_2, Monica need only select a flowmeter with the appropriate quick connect. A compensated Thorpe tube is required for metering flow through high-resistance equipment such as jet nebulizers.

SUMMARY CHECKLIST

- All therapy gases must contain at least 20% O_2; all such gases support combustion.
- Medical gases are stored either in portable high-pressure cylinders or in large centralized bulk reservoirs.
- For positive identification of the contents of a medical gas cylinder, the label must be carefully read.
- The pressure in a gas-filled cylinder indicates its contents; the pressure in a liquid-filled cylinder does not.
- To compute duration of flow (minutes) of a medical gas cylinder, multiply the cylinder pressure (pounds per square inch) by the cylinder factor, and divide the result by the set flow (liters per minute).
- Gas supply systems provide gas at 50 psig to outlets throughout a facility through a network of pipes. Such a system must include both zone valves for repairs or fire and alarms to warn of failure.
- Failure of a bulk gas supply system can threaten the lives of patients receiving O_2 therapy or being supported with pneumatically powered devices. A protocol must exist to deal with this emergency.
- Indexed safety systems help prevent misconnections between equipment. The ASSS provides high-pressure connections with large cylinders; the PISS does the same for small cylinders; and DISS connections are for low-pressure outlets, typically 50 psig.
- A reducing valve is used for reduction of gas pressure. A flowmeter is used for control of gas flow. A regulator is used for control of both pressure and flow.
- A flow restrictor is used to provide fixed low flows of O_2. A Bourdon gauge is used to meter flow during patient transport. A compensated Thorpe tube is used when accurate flows are needed with high-resistance equipment.

References

1. Compressed Gas Association: *Handbook of compressed gas*, ed 4, Boston, 1999, Kluwer Academic.
2. National Fire Protection Association 99: *Health care facilities code*, 2015 ed, Quincy, MA, 2014, National Fire Protection Association.
3. *United States Pharmacopeia/National Formulary*, Rockville, MD, 2000, United States Pharmacopeial Convention.
4. Cairo JM: *Mosby's respiratory care equipment*, ed 9, St Louis, 2013, Mosby.
5. Compressed Gas Association: *Compressed air for human respiration (CGA G-7)/ANSI Z86.1)*, Arlington, VA, 2014, Compressed Gas Association.
6. American Academy of Pediatrics: Policy statement: use of inhaled nitric oxide. *Pediatrics* 106:344, 2000. (Reaffirmed December 2009, *Pediatrics* 125:e98, April 2010).
7. Finer NN, Barrington KJ: Nitric oxide for respiratory failure in infants born at or near term. *Cochrane Database Syst Rev* (4):00399, 2008.
8. Barrington KJ, Finer NN: Inhaled nitric oxide for respiratory failure in preterm infants. *Cochrane Database Syst Rev* (12):000509, 2010.
9. United States Department of Transportation: Qualification, maintenance and use of cylinders, 180.213. Requalification markings (revised June 12, 2010), Washington, DC.
10. Compressed Gas Association: *Standard color marking of compressed gas containers for medical use (CGA C-9)*, Arlington, VA, 2013, Compressed Gas Association.
11. Compressed Gas Association: *Characteristics and safe handling of medical gases (P-2)*, Arlington, VA, 2013, Compressed Gas Association.
12. Cylinders with unmixed helium/oxygen. *Health Devices* 19:146, 1990.
13. Bernstein DB, Rosenberg AD: Intraoperative hypoxia from nitrogen tanks with oxygen fittings. *Anesth Analg* 84:225–227, 1997.
14. Stoller JK, Stefanak M, Orens D, et al: The hospital oxygen supply: an "O2K" problem. *Respir Care* 5:300–305, 2000.
15. Schumacher SD, Brockwell RC, Andrews J, et al: Bulk liquid oxygen supply failure. *Anesthesiology* 100:186, 2004.
16. Deleris LA, Yeo GL, Seiver A, et al: Engineering risk analysis of a hospital oxygen supply system. *Med Decis Making* 26:162–172, 2006.
17. Compressed Gas Association: *Compressed gas cylinder valve outlet and inlet connections (ANSI/CGA V-1)*, Arlington, VA, 2013, Compressed Gas Association.
18. Compressed Gas Association: *Diameter index safety systems (CGA V-5)*, Arlington, VA, 2008, Compressed Gas Association.
19. Mismating of precision brand medical gas fittings. *Health Devices* 19:333, 1990.

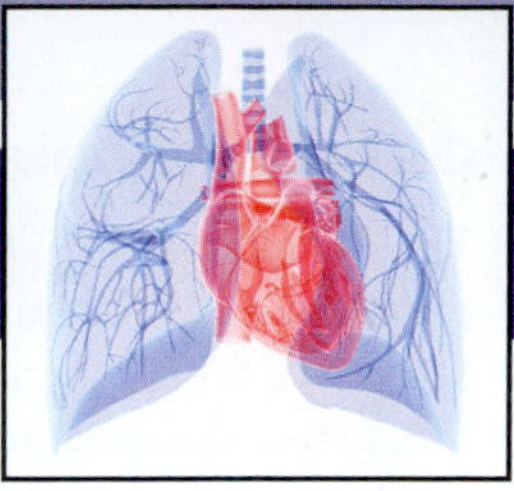

CHAPTER 41

Medical Gas Therapy

ALBERT J. HEUER

CHAPTER OBJECTIVES

After reading this chapter you will be able to:

- Describe when oxygen (O_2) therapy is needed.
- Assess the need for O_2 therapy.
- Describe what precautions and complications are associated with O_2 therapy.
- Select an O_2 delivery system appropriate for the respiratory care plan.
- Describe how to administer O_2 to adults, children, and infants.
- Describe how to identify and correct malfunctions of O_2 delivery systems.
- Assess and monitor a patient's response to O_2 therapy.
- Describe how and when to modify or recommend modification of O_2 therapy.
- Describe how to implement protocol-based O_2 therapy.
- Identify the indications, complications, and hazards of hyperbaric O_2 therapy.
- Identify when and how to administer specialty therapeutic gases.

CHAPTER OUTLINE

Oxygen Therapy
- General Goals and Clinical Objectives
- Clinical Practice Guideline
- Assessing the Need for Oxygen Therapy
- Precautions and Hazards of Supplemental Oxygen
- Oxygen Delivery Systems: Design and Performance
- Selecting a Delivery Approach
- Protocol-Based Oxygen Therapy

Hyperbaric Oxygen Therapy
- Physiologic Effects
- Methods of Administration
- Indications
- Complications and Hazards
- Troubleshooting

Other Medical Gas Therapies
- Nitric Oxide Therapy
- Helium-Oxygen Therapy
- Carbon Dioxide–Oxygen (Carbogen) Therapy

KEY TERMS

atmospheric pressure absolute (ATA)
bronchopneumonia
bronchopulmonary dysplasia
croup
exudative
heliox therapy
high-flow system
high-flow nasal cannula (HFNC)
hyperbaric oxygen (HBO) therapy
low-flow system
neovascularization
neutral thermal environment (NTE)
nitric oxide (NO)
reservoir system
retinopathy of prematurity (ROP)

Gas therapy is the most common mode of respiratory care. Most medical gases are drugs. As with any drug, in consultation with the physician, respiratory therapists (RTs) recommend a dosage and delivery method for medical gases, initiate therapy, monitor the response, and alter therapy accordingly in relation to the patient care plan.

OXYGEN THERAPY

There is general agreement among clinicians about the proper use of O_2 therapy.[1-4] However, as the primary member of the health care team responsible for O_2 administration, the RT must be well versed in all aspects of its use in clinical practice.

General Goals and Clinical Objectives

The overall goal of O_2 therapy is to maintain adequate tissue oxygenation, while minimizing cardiopulmonary work. Clinical objectives for O_2 therapy are the following:

- Correct documented or suspected acute hypoxemia
- Decrease symptoms associated with chronic hypoxemia
- Decrease the workload hypoxemia imposes on the cardiopulmonary system

Correcting Hypoxemia

O_2 therapy corrects hypoxemia by increasing alveolar and blood levels of O_2. Correction of hypoxemia is the most tangible objective of O_2 therapy and the easiest to measure and document.

Decreasing Symptoms of Hypoxemia

In addition to relieving hypoxemia, O_2 therapy can help relieve the symptoms associated with certain lung disorders, including dyspnea.[5] O_2 therapy also may improve mental function among patients with chronic hypoxemia.[6]

Minimizing Cardiopulmonary Workload

The cardiopulmonary system compensates for hypoxemia by increasing ventilation and cardiac output. In cases of acute hypoxemia, supplemental O_2 can decrease demands on both the heart and the lungs. Patients with hypoxemia breathing air can achieve acceptable arterial oxygenation only by increasing ventilation. Increased ventilatory demand increases the work of breathing. In these cases, O_2 therapy can reduce both the high ventilatory demand and the work of breathing.

Patients with arterial hypoxemia can maintain acceptable tissue oxygenation only by increasing cardiac output. Because O_2 therapy increases blood O_2 content, the heart does not have to pump as much blood per minute to meet tissue demands. This reduced workload is particularly important when the heart is already stressed by disease or injury, as in myocardial infarction, sepsis, or trauma.

Hypoxemia causes pulmonary vasoconstriction and pulmonary hypertension. Pulmonary vasoconstriction and hypertension increase workload on the right side of the heart. For patients with chronic hypoxemia, this increased workload over the long-term can lead to right ventricular failure (cor pulmonale). O_2 therapy can reverse pulmonary vasoconstriction and decrease right ventricular workload.[7]

Clinical Practice Guideline

To guide practitioners in safe and effective patient care, the American Association for Respiratory Care (AARC) has developed and published clinical practice guidelines for O_2 therapy. Excerpts from the AARC guideline on O_2 therapy in acute care hospitals appear in Clinical Practice Guideline 41-1.[2] Additional AARC guidelines for O_2 therapy in the home or an extended care facility[3] and for selection of O_2 delivery devices for neonatal and pediatric patients[4] are provided in Chapters 53 and 56.

Assessing the Need for Oxygen Therapy

There are three basic ways to determine whether a patient needs O_2 therapy. The first is the use of laboratory measures to document hypoxemia. Second, a patient's need for O_2 therapy can be based on the specific clinical problem or condition. Third, hypoxemia has many manifestations, such as tachypnea, tachycardia, cyanosis, and distressed overall appearance, and therefore bedside assessment can identify such a need.

Laboratory measures for documenting hypoxemia include hemoglobin saturation and partial pressure of oxygen (PO_2), as determined by either invasive or noninvasive means (see Chapter 19). Threshold criteria defining hypoxemia with these measures are described in the AARC clinical practice guideline (see Clinical Practice Guideline 41-1).[2]

O_2 therapy is needed for patients with disorders associated with hypoxemia. Examples are postoperative patients; patients with carbon monoxide or cyanide poisoning, shock, trauma, or acute myocardial infarction; and some premature infants.[1,2,8]

Careful bedside physical assessment can disclose a patient's need for O_2 therapy. Table 41-1 summarizes the common respiratory, cardiovascular, and neurologic signs used in the detection of hypoxia. This information can be combined with more quantitative measures such as arterial blood gas results to confirm the need for supplemental O_2.

Precautions and Hazards of Supplemental Oxygen

Excerpts from the relevant AARC clinical practice guidelines (see Clinical Practice Guideline 41-1) outline the major precautions and hazards associated with administration of supplemental O_2.[2] Five of these hazards are common enough to warrant additional discussion.

TABLE 41-1
Clinical Signs of Hypoxia

Finding	Mild to Moderate	Severe
Respiratory	Tachypnea Dyspnea Paleness	Tachypnea Dyspnea Cyanosis
Cardiovascular	Tachycardia	Tachycardia, eventual bradycardia, arrhythmia
	Mild hypertension, peripheral vasoconstriction	Hypertension and eventual hypotension
Neurologic	Restlessness Disorientation Headaches Lassitude	Somnolence Confusion Distressed appearance Blurred vision Tunnel vision Loss of coordination Impaired judgment Slow reaction time Manic-depressive activity Coma

41-1 Oxygen Therapy

AARC Clinical Practice Guideline (Excerpts)

INDICATIONS
- Documented hypoxemia as evidenced by
  - PaO_2 less than 60 mm Hg or SaO_2 less than 90% in subjects breathing room air
  - PaO_2 or SaO_2 below desirable range for a specific clinical situation
- Acute care situations in which hypoxemia is suspected
- Severe trauma
- Acute myocardial infarction
- Short-term therapy or surgical intervention (e.g., postanesthesia recovery)

CONTRAINDICATIONS
- With a few exceptions, no specific contraindications to O_2 therapy exist when indications are present.
- Certain delivery devices are contraindicated, such as nasal cannulas and nasopharyngeal catheters in pediatric and neonatal patients with nasal obstruction.

PRECAUTIONS AND/OR POSSIBLE COMPLICATIONS
- PaO_2 greater than or equal to 60 mm Hg; ventilator depression may occur rarely in spontaneously breathing patients with elevated $PaCO_2$
- With FiO_2 greater than 0.5, absorption atelectasis, O_2 toxicity, or depression of ciliary or leukocyte function may occur
- In premature infants, PaO_2 greater than 80 mm Hg may contribute to retinopathy of prematurity
- In infants with certain congenital heart lesions such as hypoplastic left heart syndrome, high PaO_2 can compromise the balance between pulmonary and systemic blood flow
- In infants, O_2 flow directed at the face may stimulate an alteration in respiratory pattern
- Increased FiO_2 can worsen lung injury in patients with paraquat poisoning or patients receiving bleomycin
- During laser bronchoscopy or tracheostomy, minimal FiO_2 should be used to avoid intratracheal ignition
- Fire hazard increased in the presence of high FiO_2
- Bacterial contamination can occur when nebulizers or humidifiers are used

ASSESSMENT OF NEED
Need is determined by measurement of inadequate PaO_2 or SaO_2, or both, by invasive or noninvasive methods and the presence of clinical indicators.

ASSESSMENT OF OUTCOME
Outcome is determined by clinical and physiologic assessment to establish adequacy of patient response to therapy.

MONITORING
Patient
- Clinical assessment including but not limited to cardiac, pulmonary, and neurologic status
- Assessment of physiologic parameters (PaO_2, SaO_2, SpO_2) in any patient treated with O_2 (consider need or indication to adjust FiO_2 for increased levels of activity and exercise) in conjunction with the initiation of therapy or
  - Within 12 hours of initiation with FiO_2 less than 0.40
  - Within 8 hours with FiO_2 of 0.40 or greater (including postanesthesia recovery)
  - Within 72 hours in acute myocardial infarction
  - Within 2 hours for any patient with principal diagnosis of COPD
  - Within 1 hour for the neonate
- Appropriate O_2 therapy use protocol is suggested as a method to decrease waste and to realize increased cost savings

Equipment
- All O_2 delivery systems should be checked at least once per day
- More frequent checks by calibrated analyzer are necessary in systems
  - Susceptible to variation in FiO_2 (e.g., hood, high-flow blending systems)
  - Applied to patients with artificial airways
  - Delivering a heated gas mixture
  - Applied to patients who are clinically unstable or who require FiO_2 greater than 0.50
  - Equipment supplying supplemental O_2 to newborn or premature infants

For complete guidelines, see American Association for Respiratory Care: Clinical practice guideline: selection of an oxygen delivery device for neonatal and pediatric patients, Respir Care 47:707, 2002; and American Association for Respiratory Care: Clinical practice guideline: oxygen therapy for adults in the acute care facility, Respir Care 47:717, 2002.

Oxygen Toxicity
O_2 toxicity primarily affects the lungs and the central nervous system (CNS).[9-11] Two primary factors determine the harmful effects of O_2: PO_2 and exposure time (Figure 41-1). The higher the PO_2 and the longer the exposure, the greater the likelihood of damage. Effects on the CNS, including tremors, twitching, and convulsions, tend to occur only when a patient is breathing O_2 at pressures greater than 1 atm (hyperbaric pressure). Pulmonary effects can also occur with enriched O_2 environments at normal atmospheric pressures.

Table 41-2 summarizes the physiologic response to breathing 100% O_2 at sea level. A patient exposed to a high PO_2 for a prolonged period has signs similar to **bronchopneumonia.** Patchy infiltrates appear on chest radiographs and usually are most prominent in the lower lung fields.

Exposure to high PO_2 first damages the capillary endothelium. Interstitial edema follows and thickens the alveolar-capillary membrane. If the process continues, type I alveolar cells are destroyed, and type II cells proliferate. An **exudative** phase follows, resulting from alveolar fluid buildup, which leads

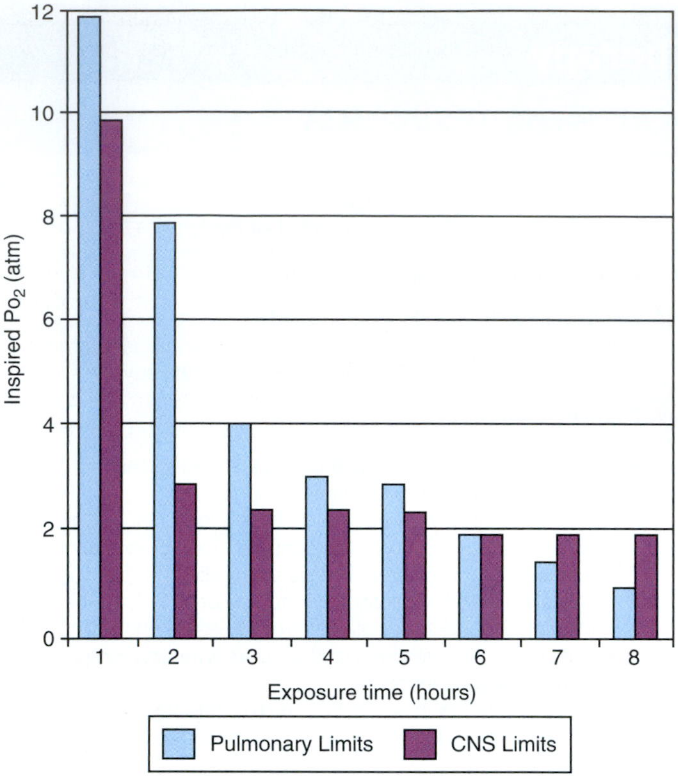

FIGURE 41-1 Relationship between PO_2 and exposure time causing O_2 toxicity.

TABLE 41-2

Physiologic Responses of Healthy Individuals to Exposure to 100% Inspired Oxygen

Exposure Time (hr)	Physiologic Response
0-12	Normal pulmonary function Tracheobronchitis Substernal chest pain
12-24	Decreasing vital capacity
25-30	Decreasing lung compliance Increasing $P(A\text{-}a)O_2$ Decreasing exercise PO_2
30-72	Decreasing diffusing capacity

to a low ventilation/perfusion ratio, physiologic shunting, and hypoxemia. In the end stages, hyaline membranes form in the alveolar region, and pulmonary fibrosis and hypertension develop.

As the lung injury worsens, blood oxygenation deteriorates. If this progressive hypoxemia is managed with additional O_2, the toxic effects worsen (Figure 41-2). However, if the patient can be kept alive while fractional inspired oxygen concentration (FiO_2) is decreased, the pulmonary damage sometimes resolves.

The toxicity of O_2 is caused by overproduction of O_2 free radicals. O_2 free radicals are by-products of cellular metabolism. If unchecked, these radicals can severely damage or kill cells.[9]

In the presence of high PO_2, free radicals can overwhelm the body's normal antioxidant system and cause cell damage. Cell

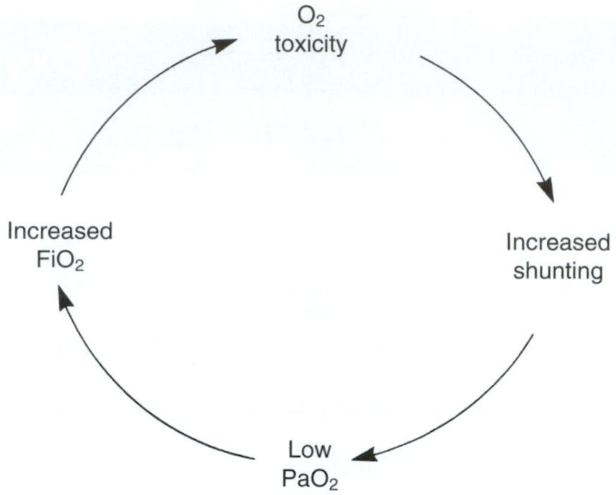

FIGURE 41-2 The vicious circle that can occur in managing hypoxemia with high FiO_2. High FiO_2 can be toxic to the lung parenchyma and cause further physiologic shunting. Increased shunting worsens the hypoxemia, necessitating higher FiO_2. (Modified from Flenley DC: Long-term oxygen therapy—state of the art. Respir Care 28:876, 1983.)

damage provokes an immune response and causes tissue infiltration by neutrophils and macrophages. These scavenger cells release inflammatory mediators that worsen the initial injury. At the same time, local neutrophils and platelets may release more free radicals, which continue the process.

Exactly how much O_2 is safe is the subject of debate (see the following Rule of Thumb). Results of most studies indicate that adults can breathe up to 50% for extended periods without major lung damage.[12] Rather than applying strict cutoffs, the goal always should be to use the lowest possible FiO_2 to achieve adequate tissue oxygenation.[13]

RULE OF THUMB

Avoiding Oxygen Toxicity

Limit patient exposure to 100% O_2 to less than 24 hours whenever possible. High FiO_2 is acceptable if the concentration can be decreased to 70% within 2 days and 50% or less in 5 days.

Because the growing lung may be more sensitive to O_2, more caution is needed with infants. High PO_2 also is associated with retinopathy of prematurity (ROP) and **bronchopulmonary dysplasia** in infants.

Regardless of approach, supplemental O_2 never should be withheld from hypoxic patients. Although the toxic effects of high O_2 concentrations can be serious, it is not FiO_2 but rather PO_2 that results in such harmful effects. If a patient needs a high FiO_2 to maintain adequate tissue O_2, the patient should receive it.

Depression of Ventilation

When breathing moderate to high O_2 concentrations, a very small percentage of patients with COPD and chronic hypercapnia may ventilate less.[14] Decreases in ventilation of nearly 20% have been observed in these patients with accompanying elevations in arterial partial pressure of carbon dioxide ($PaCO_2$) of

20 to 23 mm Hg.[15] However, this hypoventilation is not typical of patients with COPD and appropriate management of hypoxemia with supplemental O_2 should never be avoided in them.

The primary reason some patients with COPD hypoventilate when given O_2 is most likely suppression of the hypoxic drive. In these patients, the normal response to high partial pressure of carbon dioxide (PCO_2) is blunted, the primary stimulus to breathe being lack of O_2 as sensed by the peripheral chemoreceptors. The increase in the blood O_2 level in these patients suppresses peripheral chemoreceptors, depresses ventilatory drive, and elevates the PCO_2.[16,17] High blood O_2 levels may disrupt the normal ventilation/perfusion balance and cause an increase in dead space-to-tidal volume ratio (V_D/V_T) and in $PaCO_2$.[18]

Retinopathy of Prematurity

Retinopathy of prematurity (ROP), also called *retrolental fibroplasia,* is an abnormal eye condition that occurs in some premature or low-birth-weight infants who receive supplemental O_2. An excessive blood O_2 level causes retinal vasoconstriction, which leads to necrosis of the blood vessels. In response, new vessels form and increase in number. Hemorrhage of these delicate new vessels causes scarring behind the retina. Scarring often leads to retinal detachment and blindness.[19] ROP most often affects neonates up to approximately 1 month of age, by which time the retinal arteries have sufficiently matured. Excessive O_2 is not the only factor associated with ROP; other factors associated with ROP include hypercapnia, hypocapnia, intraventricular hemorrhage, infection, lactic acidosis, anemia, hypocalcemia, and hypothermia.

Because premature infants often need supplemental O_2, the risk of ROP poses a serious management problem. The American Academy of Pediatrics recommends keeping arterial PO_2 in an infant less than 80 mm Hg as the best way to minimize the risk of ROP.[8]

Absorption Atelectasis

FiO_2 greater than 0.50 presents a significant risk of absorption atelectasis.[20] Nitrogen normally is the most plentiful gas in both the alveoli and the blood. Breathing high levels of O_2 quickly depletes body nitrogen levels. As blood nitrogen levels decrease, the total pressure of venous gases rapidly decreases. Under these conditions, gases that exist at atmospheric pressure within any body cavity rapidly diffuse into the venous blood. This principle is used for removing trapped air from body cavities. Giving patients high levels of O_2 can help clear trapped air from the abdomen or thorax.

This same phenomenon can cause lung collapse, especially if the alveolar region becomes obstructed (Figure 41-3). Under these conditions, O_2 rapidly diffuses into the blood (see Figure 41-3, *A*). With no source for repletion, the total gas pressure in the alveolus progressively decreases until the alveolus collapses. Because collapsed alveoli are perfused but not ventilated, absorption atelectasis increases the physiologic shunt and worsens blood oxygenation.[20]

The likelihood of absorption atelectasis is greatest when present with other risk factors associated with low tidal volumes such as sedation, surgical pain, or CNS dysfunction. In these cases, poorly ventilated alveoli may become unstable when they lose O_2 faster than it can be replaced. The result is a more

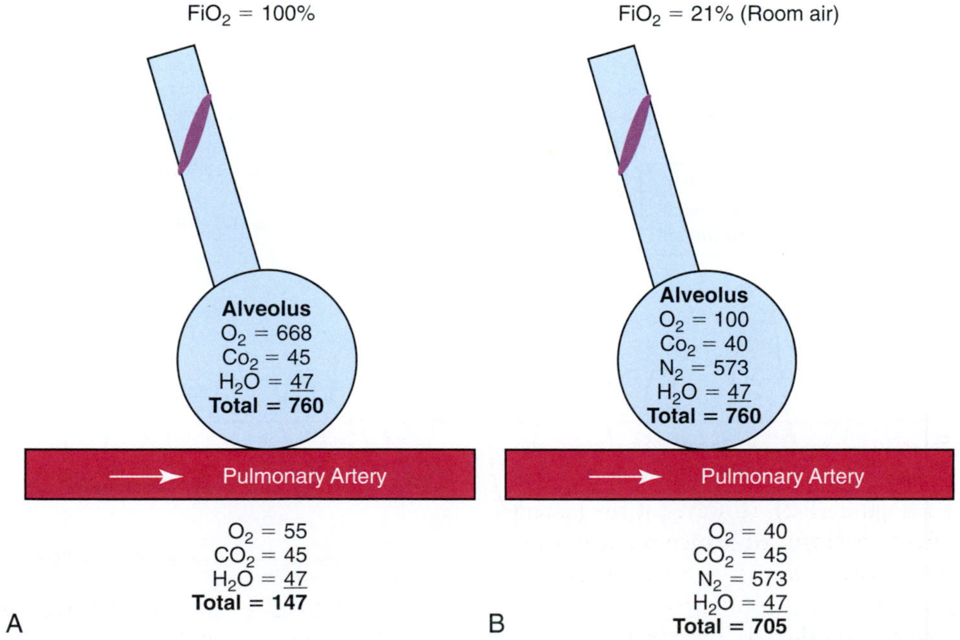

FIGURE 41-3 The development of atelectasis beyond blocked airways when breathing of 100% O_2 **(A)** and room air **(B).** In each case, the sum of the gas pressures in mixed venous blood (pulmonary artery) is less than in the alveoli. The pressure gradient is much greater when breathing 100% O_2 **(A),** causing more rapid diffusion from the alveoli. *Note:* The gas pressures in the room air alveolus will change slightly over time, but the total will remain close to 760 mm Hg.

gradual shrinking of the alveoli that may lead to complete collapse, even when the patient is not breathing supplemental O_2 (see Figure 41-3, *B*).

Fire Hazard

Despite numerous preventive measures, fires involving enriched O_2 environments continue to occur in health care facilities. Fires seem to pose the greatest risk in operating rooms and in association with selected respiratory procedures. During surgery and procedures such as tracheotomies, electronic scalpels and similar devices are often used while the patient is receiving supplemental O_2. To complicate matters, even higher O_2 concentrations may exist under surgical drapes.[21] Other situations associated with increased fire risk involve home care patients smoking while receiving low-flow O_2 and the use of aluminum O_2 regulators. Additionally, hyperbaric oxygen (HBO) therapy or therapy at increased atmospheric pressures (discussed later in this chapter) often involves the administration of supplemental O_2 and greatly increases fire risk.

Some simple strategies can be used to reduce the fire risk in health care facilities. Effectively managing the fire triangle of O_2, heat, and fuel is key. An essential component is always using the lowest effective FiO_2 for a given clinical situation. In addition, using scavenging systems to minimize O_2 buildup beneath sterile drapes during surgery or while performing tracheostomies can help reduce fire risk. Educating clinicians, patients, and caregivers on safe O_2 use is also important. Additionally, fire prevention protocols for HBO therapy should be strictly followed.[21]

Oxygen Delivery Systems: Design and Performance

Proper device selection requires in-depth knowledge of both the general performance characteristics of these systems and the individual capabilities.[22] O_2 delivery devices traditionally are categorized by design. Three basic designs exist: **low-flow systems, reservoir systems**, and **high-flow systems.** Enclosures are commonly identified as a fourth category. The design categories share functional characteristics, capabilities, and limitations.

Although design plays an important role in the selection of these devices, clinical performance ultimately determines how the device is used. The user judges the performance of an O_2 delivery system by answering two key questions: (1) How much O_2 can the system deliver (FiO_2 or FiO_2 range)? (2) Does the delivered FiO_2 remain fixed or vary under changing patient demands?[22]

Regarding the FiO_2 range, O_2 systems can be broadly divided into systems designed to deliver a low (<35%), moderate (35% to 60%), or high (>60%) O_2 concentration. Some designs can deliver O_2 across the full range of concentrations (21% to 100%).

Whether a device delivers a fixed or variable FiO_2 depends on how much of the patient's inspired gas it supplies. If the system provides all of the patient's inspired gas, FiO_2 remains stable. If the device provides only some of the inspired gas, the patient must draw the remainder from the surrounding air. In this case, the more the patient breathes, the more air dilutes the delivered O_2, and FiO_2 is lower. If the patient breathes less with this type of device, less air dilutes the O_2, and FiO_2 increases. A system that supplies only a portion of the inspired gas always provides a variable FiO_2.[23] FiO_2 supplied with such systems can vary widely from minute to minute and even from breath to breath.

Figure 41-4 shows these concepts as applied to low-flow, reservoir, and high-flow systems. With the low-flow system (see Figure 41-4, *A*) the patient's inspiratory flow often exceeds the flow delivered by the device; the result is air dilution *(shaded*

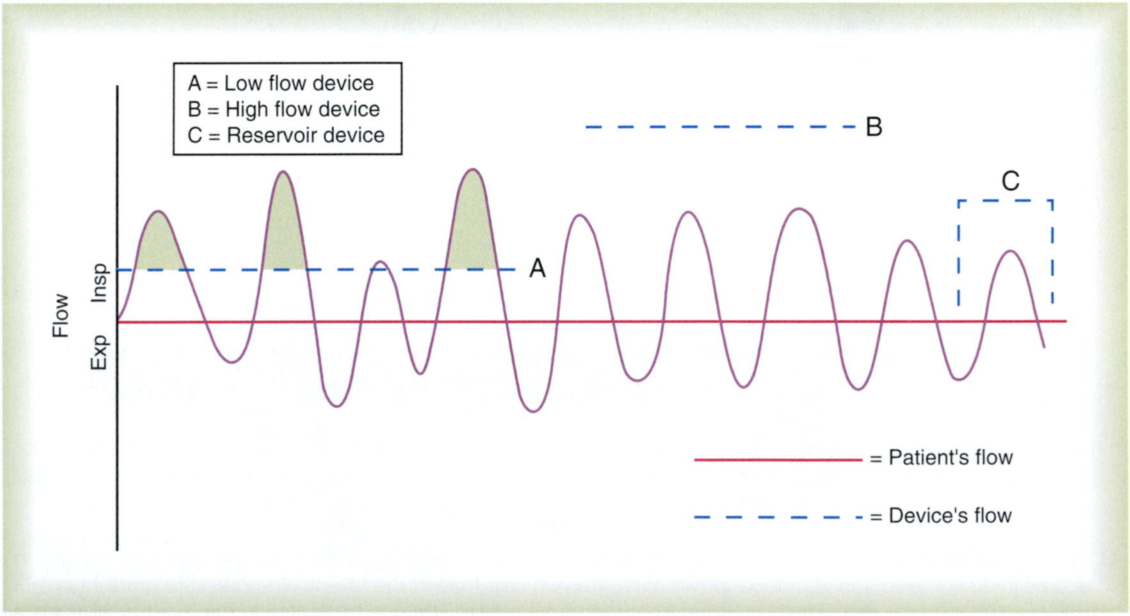

FIGURE 41-4 Differences between O_2 delivery systems. *A,* Low-flow device. *B,* High-flow device. *C,* Reservoir device.

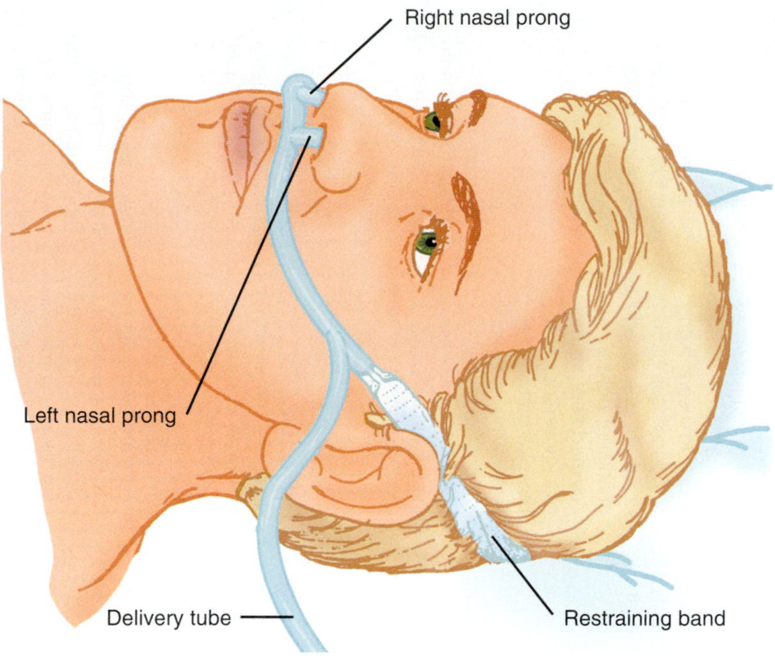

FIGURE 41-5 Nasal cannula.

areas). The greater the patient's inspiratory flow, the more air is breathed, and FiO_2 is lower. The high-flow system (see Figure 41-4, *B*) always exceeds the patient's flow and provides a fixed FiO_2. A fixed FiO_2 can be achieved with a reservoir system (see Figure 41-4, *C*), which stores a reserve volume (flow × time) that equals or exceeds the patient's tidal volume. For a reservoir system to provide a fixed FiO_2, the reservoir volume must always exceed the patient's tidal volume, and there cannot be any air leaks in the system. Table 41-3 outlines the general specifications for the common O_2 therapy systems in current use.

Low-Flow Systems

Typical low-flow systems provide supplemental O_2 directly to the airway at a flow of 8 L/min or less. Because the inspiratory flow of a healthy adult exceeds 8 L/min, the O_2 provided by a low-flow device is always diluted with air; the result is a low and variable FiO_2. Low-flow O_2 delivery systems include nasal cannula, nasal catheter, and transtracheal catheter.

Nasal Cannula. A nasal cannula is a disposable plastic device consisting of two tips or prongs approximately 1 cm long that are connected to several feet of small-bore O_2 supply tubing (Figure 41-5). The user inserts the prongs directly into the vestibule of the nose while attaching the supply tubing either directly to a flowmeter or to a bubble humidifier. In most cases, a humidifier is used only when the input flow is greater than 4 L/min.[2] However, flows greater than 6 to 8 L/min can cause patient discomfort.[22] Cannulas should not be used in newborns and infants if their nasal passages are obstructed, and flows generally should be limited to 2 L/min unless a specialized high-flow cannula system, discussed later in this chapter, is being used.[2] Table 41-3 lists the FiO_2 range, FiO_2 stability, advantages, disadvantages, and best use of a nasal cannula.

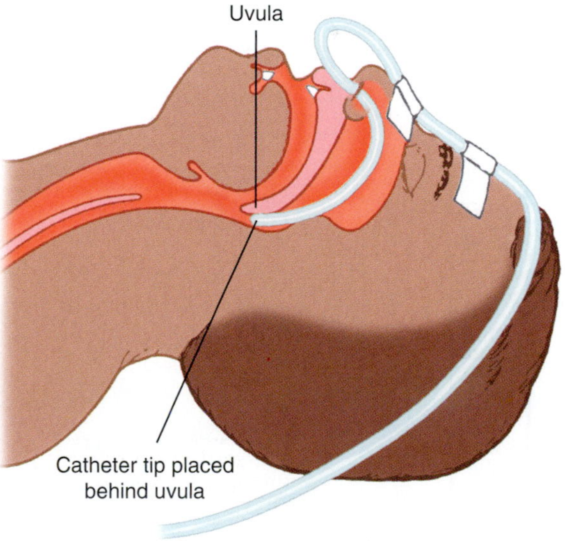

FIGURE 41-6 Placement of nasal catheter in the nasopharynx.

Nasal Catheter. The use of nasal catheters is generally limited to short-term O_2 administration during specialized procedures such as a bronchoscopy. A nasal catheter is a soft plastic tube with several small holes at the tip that is inserted by gently advancing it along the floor of either nasal passage and visualizing it just behind and above the uvula (Figure 41-6). Once in position, the catheter is taped to the bridge of the nose. If direct visualization is impossible, the catheter may be blindly inserted to a depth equal to the distance from the nose to the earlobe.

When placed too deep, the catheter can provoke gagging or swallowing of gas, which increases the likelihood of aspiration. In general, a nasal catheter should be replaced with a new one

TABLE 41-3
Overview of Oxygen Therapy Systems

Category	Device	Flow	FiO_2 Range	FiO_2 Stability	Advantages	Disadvantages	Best Use
Low flow	Nasal cannula	¼-6 L/min (adults) ≤2 L/min (infants)	22%-40%	Variable	Use on adults, children, infants; easy to use; disposable; low cost; well tolerated	Unstable, easily dislodged; high flow uncomfortable; can cause dryness, bleeding; polyps; deviated septum and mouth breathing may reduce FiO_2	Patient in stable condition who needs low FiO_2; home care patient who needs long-term therapy, low to moderate FiO_2 while eating
	Nasal catheter	¼-5 L/min	22%-45%	Variable	Use on adults, children, infants; good stability; disposable; low cost	Difficult to insert; high flow increases back pressure; needs regular changing; polyps, deviated septum may block insertion; may provoke gagging, air swallowing, aspiration	Procedures in which cannula is difficult to use (bronchoscopy); long-term care of infants
	Transtracheal catheter	¼-4 L/min	22%-35%	Variable	Lower O_2 use and cost; eliminates nasal and skin irritation; improved compliance; increased exercise tolerance; increased mobility; enhanced image	High cost; surgical complications; infection; mucous plugging; lost tract	Home care or ambulatory patients who need increased mobility or do not accept nasal O_2
	Reservoir cannula	¼-4 L/min	22%-35%	Variable	Lower O_2 use and cost; increased mobility; less discomfort because of lower flow	Unattractive, cumbersome; poor compliance; must be regularly replaced; breathing pattern affects performance	Home care or ambulatory patients who need increased mobility
	Simple mask	5-10 L/min	35%-50%	Variable	Use on adults, children, infants; quick, easy to apply; disposable; inexpensive	Uncomfortable; must be removed for eating; prevents radiant heat loss; blocks vomitus in unconscious patients	Emergencies; short-term therapy requiring moderate FiO_2; mouth breathing patients requiring moderate FiO_2
	Partial rebreathing mask	Minimum of 10 L/min (prevent bag collapse on inspiration)	40%-70%	Variable	Same as simple mask; moderate to high FiO_2	Same as simple mask; potential suffocation hazard	Emergencies; short-term therapy requiring moderate to high FiO_2
	Nonrebreathing mask	Minimum of 10 L/min (prevent bag collapse on inspiration)	60%-80%	Variable	Same as simple mask; high FiO_2	Same as simple mask; potential suffocation hazard	Emergencies; short-term therapy requiring high FiO_2
	Nonrebreathing circuit (closed)	>3 × V_E (prevent bag collapse on inspiration)	21%-100%	Fixed	Full range of FiO_2	Potential suffocation hazard; requires 50 psi air/O_2; blender failure common	Patients who need precise FiO_2 at any level (21%-100%)

High flow	AEM	Varies; should provide output flow >60 L/min	24%-50%	Fixed	Easy to apply; disposable, inexpensive; stable, precise FiO_2	Limited to adult use; uncomfortable, noisy; must be removed for eating; FiO_2 >0.40 not ensured; FiO_2 varies with back pressure	Patients in unstable condition who need precise low FiO_2
	Air-entrainment nebulizer	10-15 L/min input; should provide output flow of at least 60 L/min	28%-100%	Fixed	Provides temperature control and extra humidification	FiO_2 <0.28 or >0.40 not ensured; FiO_2 varies with back pressure; high infection risk	Patients with artificial airways who need low to moderate FiO_2
	Blending system (open)	Should provide output flow of at least 60 L/min	21%-100%	Fixed	Full range of FiO_2	Requires 50 psi air/O_2; blender failure or inaccuracy common	Patients with high VE who need high FiO_2
	High-flow nasal cannula system	Up to 50 L/min, or more (depending on system)	35%-90%	Generally fixed, depending on system, input flow, and patient breathing pattern	Wide range of FiO_2 and relative/absolute humidity; use on adults, children, infants	FiO_2 is often ensured but depends on system, input flow, and patient breathing pattern; infection risk	Patients of all ages with high or variable VE who need supplemental O_2, positive pressure and humidity
Enclosure	Oxyhood	≥7 L/min	21%-100%	Fixed	Full range of FiO_2	Difficult to clean, disinfect	Infants who need supplemental O_2
	Isolette	8-15 L/min	40%-50%	Variable	Provides temperature control	Expensive, cumbersome, unstable FiO_2 (leaks); difficult to clean, disinfect; limits patient mobility; fire hazard	Infants who need supplemental O_2 and precise thermal regulation
	Tent	12-15 L/min	40%-50%	Variable	Provides concurrent aerosol therapy	Expensive, cumbersome, unstable FiO_2 (leaks); requires cooling; difficult to clean, disinfect; limits patient mobility; fire hazard	Toddlers or small children who need low to moderate FiO_2 and aerosol

VE, Minute volume.

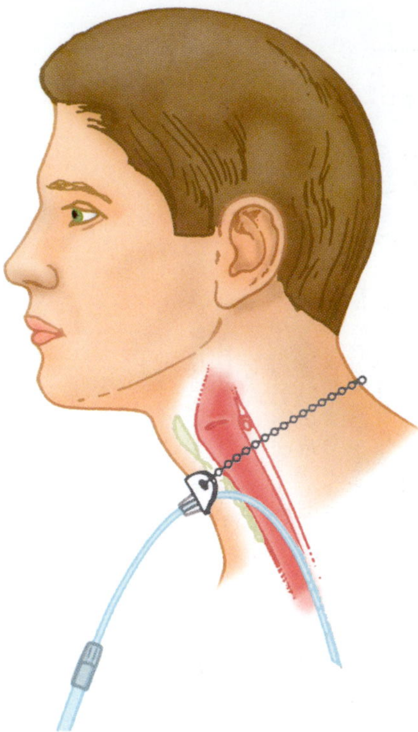

FIGURE 41-7 Transtracheal O_2 catheter.

(placed in the opposite naris) at least every 8 hours. Nasal catheters are inappropriate for neonatal patients. As a result of these notable limitations, nasal catheters are rarely used today.[4]

Transtracheal Catheter. A transtracheal O_2 catheter is a thin polytetrafluoroethylene (Teflon) catheter inserted into the trachea between the second and third tracheal rings (Figure 41-7), secured by a chain necklace. Standard tubing connected directly to a flowmeter provides the O_2 source flow.[24, 25] Because flow is so low, no humidifier is needed.

Because the transtracheal catheter resides directly in the trachea, O_2 builds up both there and in the upper airway during expiration. This process effectively expands the anatomic reservoir and increases the FiO_2 at any given flow. Compared with a nasal cannula, a transtracheal catheter needs about half of the O_2 flow to achieve a given arterial partial pressure of oxygen (PaO_2).[25] This reduced flow can be of great economic and practical benefit to patients needing continuous long-term O_2 therapy because it can greatly increase the duration of flow of portable O_2 systems. Transtracheal O_2 therapy can pose problems and risks, however, and these devices have not received widespread acceptance. Chapter 56 provides some additional details on maintaining transtracheal O_2 set-ups. Table 41-3 lists the FiO_2 range, FiO_2 stability, advantages, disadvantages, and best use of a transtracheal catheter.

Performance Characteristics of Low-Flow Systems

Low-flow nasal systems provide O_2 concentrations ranging from 22% at 1 L/min to 60% at 15 L/min.[2,3,22] The range of 22% to 45% cited in Table 41-3 is based on 8 L/min as the upper limit of comfortable flow. These wide FiO_2 ranges occur because the O_2 concentration delivered by a low-flow system varies with the amount of air dilution. The amount of air dilution depends on several patient and equipment variables. Table 41-4 summarizes these key variables and how they affect FiO_2 provided by low-flow systems.

Simple formulas exist for estimating FiO_2 provided by low-flow systems (see the accompanying Rule of Thumb). Given the large number of variables affecting FiO_2, however, the RT can never know precisely how much O_2 a patient is receiving with these systems. Without knowing the patient's exact FiO_2, the RT must rely on assessing the actual response to O_2 therapy.

TABLE 41-4
Variables Affecting FiO_2 of Low-Flow Oxygen Systems

Increases FiO_2	Decreases FiO_2
Higher O_2 input	Lower O_2 input
Mouth-closed breathing*	Mouth-open breathing*
Low inspiratory flow	High inspiratory flow
Low tidal volume	High tidal volume
Slow rate of breathing	Fast rate of breathing
Small minute ventilation	Large minute ventilation
Long inspiratory time	Short inspiratory time
High I:E ratio	Low I:E ratio

I:E, Inspiratory/expiratory.
*Cannula only.

RULE OF THUMB

Estimating FiO_2 Provided by Low-Flow Systems

For patients with a normal rate and depth of breathing, each 1 L/min of nasal O_2 increases FiO_2 approximately 4%. For example, a patient using a nasal cannula at 4 L/min has an estimated FiO_2 of approximately 37% (21 + 16).

Troubleshooting Low-Flow Systems

Common problems with low-flow O_2 delivery systems include inaccurate flow, system leaks and obstructions, device displacement, and skin irritation. The problem of inaccurate flow is greatest when low-flow flowmeters (≤3 L/min) are used. Given the trend toward assessment of outcome of O_2 therapy (with either blood gases or pulse oximetry), ensuring the absolute accuracy of O_2 input flow generally is not essential. Nonetheless, similar to all respiratory care equipment, flowmeters should be subjected to regular preventive maintenance and testing for accuracy. Equipment that fails preventive maintenance standards should be removed from service and repaired or replaced. Table 41-5 provides guidance on troubleshooting the most common clinical problems with nasal cannulas.

TABLE 41-5
Troubleshooting Common Problems With a Nasal Oxygen Cannula

Problem or Clue	Cause	Solution
No gas flow can be felt coming from the cannula	Flowmeter not on	Adjust flowmeter
	System leak	Check connections
Humidifier pop-off is sounding	Obstruction distal to humidifier	Find and correct the obstruction
	Flow is set too high	Use alternative device
	Obstructed naris	Use alternative device
Patient reports soreness over lip or ears	Irritation or inflammation caused by appliance straps	Loosen straps
		Place cotton balls at pressure points
		Use a different device
Mouth breathing	Habitual mouth breathing, blocked nasal passages	Switch to simple mask or venturi mask

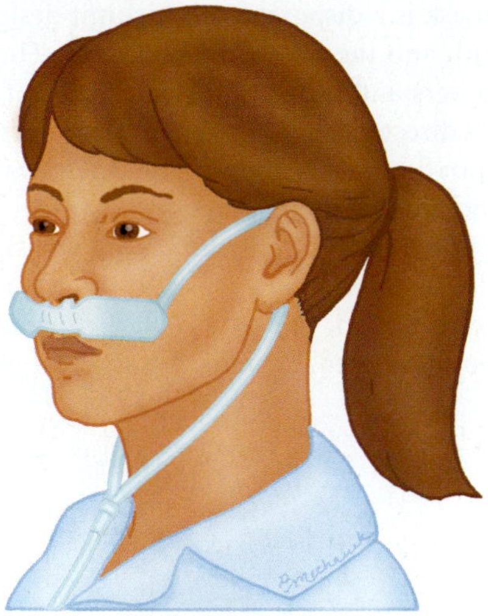

FIGURE 41-8 Reservoir cannula.

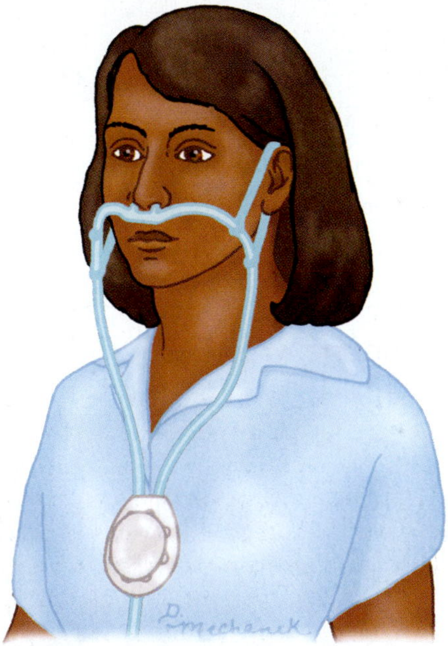

FIGURE 41-9 Pendant reservoir cannula.

Reservoir Systems

Reservoir systems incorporate a mechanism for gathering and storing O_2 between patient breaths. Patients draw on this reserve supply whenever inspiratory flow exceeds O_2 flow into the device. Because air dilution is reduced, reservoir devices generally provide higher FiO_2 than low-flow systems. Reservoir devices can decrease O_2 use by providing FiO_2 comparable with nonreservoir systems but at lower flow. Reservoir systems currently in use include reservoir cannulas, masks, and nonrebreathing circuits. In principle, enclosure systems, such as tents and hoods, operate as reservoirs surrounding the head or body.

Reservoir Cannula. Reservoir cannulas are designed to conserve O_2 and are an alternative to the pulse-dose or demand-flow O_2 systems described in Chapter 56. There are two types of reservoir cannula: nasal reservoir and pendant reservoir. Table 41-3 lists the FiO_2 range, FiO_2 stability, advantages, disadvantages, and best use of a reservoir cannula.

A nasal reservoir cannula operates by storing approximately 20 ml of O_2 in a small membrane reservoir during exhalation (Figure 41-8). The patient draws on this stored O_2 during early inspiration. The amount of O_2 available increases with each breath and decreases the flow needed for a given FiO_2. Although the device is comfortable to wear, many patients object to its appearance and may not always comply with prescribed therapy.

The pendant reservoir system helps overcome esthetic concerns by hiding the reservoir under the patient's clothing on the anterior chest wall (Figure 41-9). Although the device is less visible, the extra weight of the pendant can cause ear and facial discomfort.

At low flow, reservoir cannulas can reduce O_2 use 50% to 75%. A patient at rest who needs 2 L/min through a standard cannula to achieve an arterial oxygen saturation (SaO_2) greater than 90% may need only 0.5 L/min through a reservoir cannula to achieve the same blood oxygenation.[26] Although flow savings is predictable, factors such as nasal anatomy and breathing pattern can affect the performance of the device. For these devices to function properly at low flow, patients must exhale through the nose (this reopens or resets the reservoir membrane). In addition, exhalation through pursed lips may impair performance, especially during exercise. For these reasons, prescribed flow settings should be individually determined by clinical assessment, including SaO_2 monitoring.[26]

The low flow at which the reservoir cannula operates makes humidification unnecessary. Excess moisture can hinder proper action of the reservoir membrane.[26] Even regular use can cause membrane wear. For this reason, patients should replace the reservoir cannula approximately every 3 weeks.

Reservoir Masks. Masks are the most commonly used reservoir systems. There are three types of reservoir masks: (1) simple mask, (2) partial rebreathing mask, and (3) nonrebreathing mask. Table 41-3 lists the FiO_2 range, FiO_2 stability, advantages, disadvantages, and best use of each of these devices.

A simple mask is a disposable plastic unit designed to cover both the mouth and the nose (Figure 41-10). The body of the mask itself gathers and stores O_2 between patient breaths. The patient exhales directly through open holes or ports in the mask body. If O_2 input flow ceases, the patient can draw in air through these holes and around the mask edge.

The input flow range for an adult simple mask is 5 to 10 L/min. Generally, if flow greater than 10 L/min is needed for satisfactory oxygenation, use of a device capable of a higher FiO_2 should be considered. At a flow less than 5 L/min, the mask volume acts as dead space and causes carbon dioxide (CO_2) rebreathing.[27]

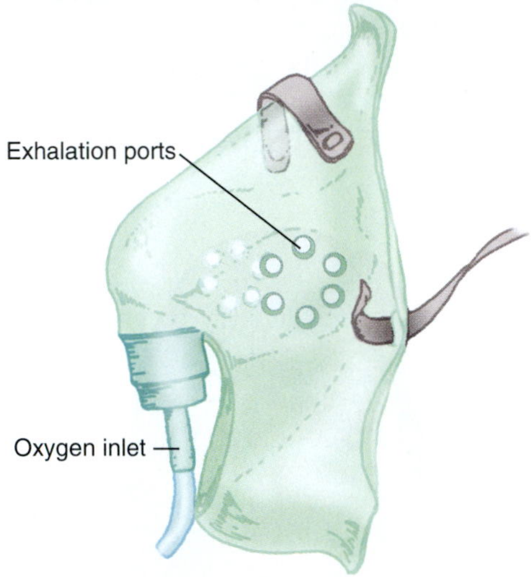

FIGURE 41-10 Simple O_2 mask.

Because air dilution easily occurs during inspiration through its ports and around its body, a simple mask provides a variable FiO_2. How much FiO_2 varies depends on the O_2 input flow, the mask volume, the extent of air leakage, and the patient's breathing pattern.[28]

As shown in Figure 41-11, a partial rebreathing mask and a nonrebreathing mask have a similar design. Each has a 1-L flexible reservoir bag attached to the O_2 inlet. Because the bag increases the reservoir volume, both masks provide higher FiO_2 capabilities than a simple mask. The key difference between these designs is the use of valves. A partial rebreathing mask has no valves (see Figure 41-11, *A*). During inspiration, source O_2 flows into the mask and passes directly to the patient. During exhalation, source O_2 enters the bag. However, because no valves separate the mask and the bag, some of the patient's exhaled gas also enters the bag (approximately the first third). Because it comes from the anatomic dead space, the early portion of exhaled gas contains mostly O_2 and little CO_2. As the bag fills with both O_2 and dead space gas, the last two-thirds of exhalation (high in CO_2) escapes out the exhalation ports of the mask. As long as the O_2 input flow keeps the bag from collapsing more than about one-third during inhalation, CO_2 rebreathing is negligible.

Although it can provide a higher FiO_2 than a simple mask (see Table 41-3), a standard disposable partial rebreathing mask is subject to considerable air dilution. The result is delivery of a moderate but variable FiO_2 dependent on the same factors as with a simple mask.

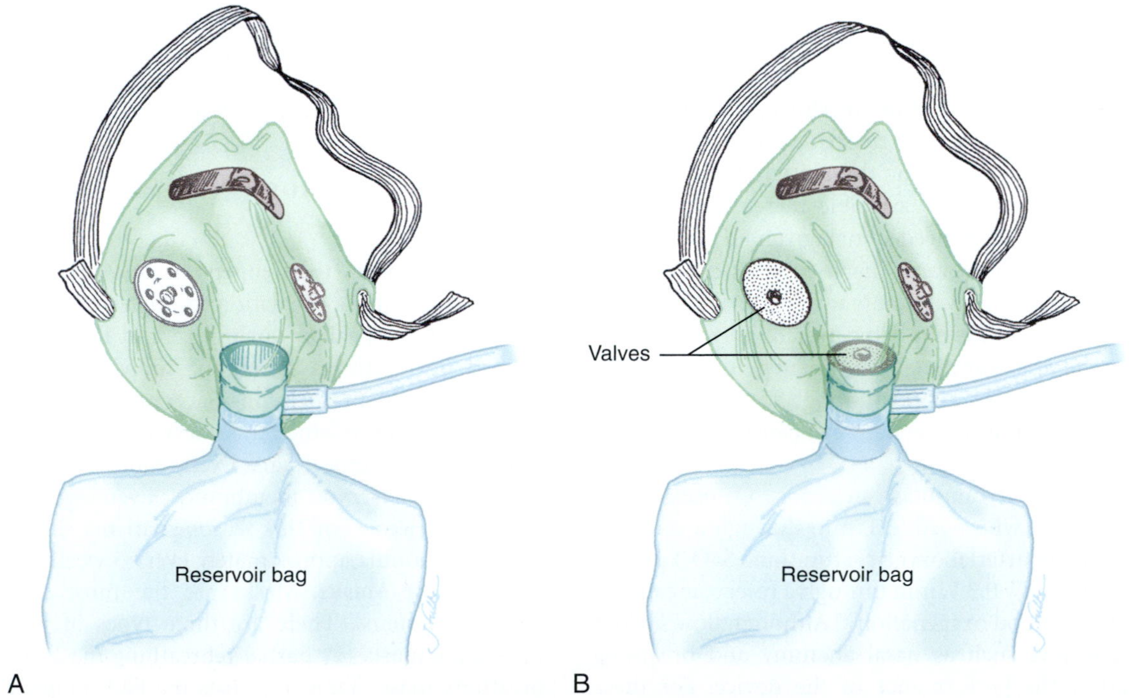

FIGURE 41-11 **A,** Partial rebreathing mask. **B,** Nonrebreathing mask.

A nonrebreathing mask, which is much more commonly used than a partial rebreathing mask, prevents rebreathing with one-way valves (see Figure 41-11, *B*). An inspiratory valve sits on top of the bag, and expiratory valves cover the exhalation ports on the mask body. During inspiration, slight negative mask pressure closes the expiratory valves, preventing air dilution. At the same time, the inspiratory valve on top of the bag opens, providing O_2 to the patient. During exhalation, valve action reverses the direction of flow. Slight positive pressure closes the inspiratory valve, which prevents exhaled gas from entering the bag. Concurrently, the one-way expiratory valves open and divert exhaled gas out to the atmosphere.

Because it is a closed system, a leak-free nonrebreathing mask with competent valves and enough flow to prevent more than one-third bag collapse during inspiration can deliver 100% source gas. As indicated in Table 41-3, however, modern disposable nonrebreathing masks normally do not provide much more than approximately 70% O_2.[22]

Large air leaks which occur both around the mask body and through the open (nonvalved) exhalation port can pose a problem. This open exhalation port is a common safety feature designed to allow air breathing if the O_2 source fails, but can result in air dilution (leakage) and a variable FiO_2 whenever inspiratory flow or volume are high.

Nonrebreathing Reservoir Circuit. A nonrebreathing circuit operates with the same design principles as a nonrebreathing mask. Although the nonrebreathing circuit requires an elaborate combination of equipment and supplies, it can be more versatile than a nonrebreathing mask because it provides a full range of FiO_2 (21% to 100%) and can be used for both intubated and nonintubated patients.[22] As shown in Figure 41-12, a typical nonrebreathing circuit incorporates a blending system to premix air and O_2. The gas mixture is warmed and humidified, ideally with a servo-controlled heated humidifier. Gas flows through large-bore tubing into an inspiratory volume reservoir, which includes a fail-safe inlet valve. The patient breathes through a closed airway appliance, in this case, a mask with one-way valves. A valved T-tube also can be used in the care of a patient with an endotracheal or a tracheostomy tube.

Troubleshooting Reservoir Systems. Common problems with reservoir masks include device displacement, system leaks and obstructions, improper flow adjustment, and skin irritation. Table 41-6 provides guidance on troubleshooting the most common clinical problems with reservoir masks.

High-Flow Systems

High-flow systems supply a given O_2 concentration at a flow equaling or exceeding the patient's peak inspiratory flow. An air-entrainment or a blending system is used. As long as the delivered flow exceeds the patient's flow, both systems can ensure a fixed FiO_2. The accompanying Rule of Thumb can help determine which devices truly qualify as high-flow systems.

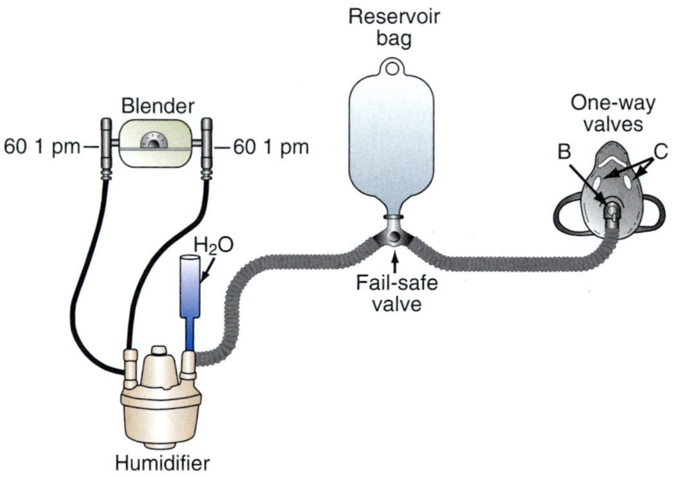

FIGURE 41-12 Nonrebreathing reservoir circuit with a valved face mask. Reservoir bag in combination with high-flow (0 to 100 L/min) flowmeters ensures delivery of set FiO_2. (Modified from Foust GN, Potter WA, Wilons MD, et al: Shortcomings of using two jet nebulizers in tandem with an aerosol face mask for optimal oxygen therapy, Chest 99:1346, 1991.)

TABLE 41-6
Troubleshooting Common Problems With Reservoir Masks

Problem or Clue	Cause	Solution
Patient constantly removes mask	Claustrophobia	Use alternative device
	Confusion	Restrain patient
No gas flow can be detected	Flowmeter not on	Adjust flowmeter
	System leak	Check connections
Humidifier pop-off is sounding	Obstruction distal to humidifier	Find and correct obstruction
	High input flow	Omit humidifier if therapy is short-term
	Jammed inspiratory valve	Fix or replace valve
Reservoir bag collapses when the patient inhales	Flow is inadequate	Increase flow
Reservoir bag remains inflated throughout inhalation	Large mask leak	Correct leak
	Inspiratory valve jammed or reversed	Repair or replace mask
Erythema develops over face or ears	Irritation or inflammation owing to appliance or straps	Reposition mask or straps
		Place cotton balls over ear pressure points
		Provide skin care

RULE OF THUMB

High-Flow Devices

To qualify as a high-flow device, a system should provide at least 60 L/min total flow. This flow criterion is based on the fact that the average adult peak inspiratory flow during tidal ventilation is approximately three times the minute volume. Because 20 L/min is close to the upper limit of sustainable minute volume for an ill person, a flow of 3 × 20, or 60 L/min, should suffice in most situations. In a few rare circumstances, flow must reach or exceed 100 L/min.

Principles of Gas Mixing. All high-flow systems mix air and O_2 to achieve a given FiO_2. These gases are mixed with air-entrainment devices or blending systems. Computations involving mixtures of air and O_2 are based on a modified form of the dilution equation for solutions:

$$V_F C_F = V_1 C_1 + V_2 C_2$$

In this equation, V_1 and V_2 are the volumes of the two gases being mixed; C_1 and C_2, the O_2 concentration in these two volumes; and V_F and C_F, the final volume and concentration of the resulting mixture.

Box 41-1 shows how to apply variations of this equation to compute (1) the final concentration of a mixture of air and O_2, (2) the air-to-O_2 ratio needed to obtain a given FiO_2, (3) the total output flow from an air-entrainment device, and (4) the amount of O_2 that must be added to a volume of air to obtain a given FiO_2. Clinical examples of these computations are provided in the accompanying Mini Clini boxes.

Box 41-1 Equations for Computing Oxygen Percentage, Ratio, and Flow

To compute the O_2 percentage of a mixture of air and O_2:

$$\%O_2 = \frac{(\text{Airflow} \times 21) + (O_2 \text{ flow} \times 100)}{\text{Total flow}} \quad \textbf{(Eq. 41-1)}$$

1. To compute the air-to-O_2 ratio needed to obtain a given O_2 percentage:

$$\frac{\text{Liters air}}{\text{Liters } O_2} = \frac{(100 - \%O_2)}{(\%O_2 - 21)} \quad \textbf{(Eq. 41-2)}$$

2. To compute the total output flow from an air-entrainment device (given the O_2 input):
   a. Compute the air-to-O_2 ratio (see Equation 41-2).
   b. Add the air-to-O_2 ratio parts.
   c. Multiply the sum of the ratio parts by the O_2 input flow.
3. To compute the flow of O_2 and air needed to obtain a given O_2 percentage at a given total flow:
   a. Compute the O_2 flow:

$$O_2 \text{ flow} = \frac{\text{Total flow} \times (O_2\% - 21)}{79} \quad \textbf{(Eq. 41-3)}$$

   b. Compute the airflow:

$$\text{Airflow} = \text{Total flow} - O_2 \text{ flow}$$

MINI CLINI

Conflicting Assessment Information

PROBLEM: A disoriented postoperative male patient breathing room air exhibits tachypnea, tachycardia, and mild cyanosis of the mucous membranes. Using a pulse oximeter, the RT measures the patient's oxyhemoglobin saturation as 90%. What should the RT recommend to the patient's surgeon?

Discussion: This is a classic example of how monitoring data and results of bedside assessment can conflict. Both the patient's condition and the observed clinical signs indicate hypoxemia, but the pulse oximeter indicates adequate oxygenation. In situations such as this, it is always better to err on the side of the patient and recommend O_2 therapy—treat the patient, not the monitor. This concept is particularly important in the use of monitoring technologies known to have limited accuracy, such as pulse oximetry (see Chapter 19).

MINI CLINI

Determining FiO_2 of an Air-Oxygen Mixture

PROBLEM: An air-entrainment device mixes at a fixed ratio of three volumes of air to each volume of O_2 (3:1 ratio). What is the resulting FiO_2?

Solution: Substituting air, O_2, and total (air + O_2) volumes into Equation 41-1:

$$\%O_2 = \frac{(\text{Airflow} \times 21) + (O_2 \text{ flow} \times 100)}{\text{Total flow}}$$

$$\%O_2 = \frac{(3 \times 21) + (1 \times 100)}{3 + 1}$$

$$\%O_2 = 41$$

An air-entrainment device that mixes three volumes of air with one volume of O_2 provides a gas mixture with FiO_2 of approximately 0.40.

Air-Entrainment Systems. Air-entrainment systems direct a high-pressure O_2 source through a small nozzle or jet surrounded by air-entrainment ports (Figure 41-13). The amount of air entrained at these ports varies directly with the size of the port and the velocity of O_2 at the jet. The larger the intake ports and the higher the gas velocity at the jet, the more air is entrained.

Because they dilute source O_2 with air, entrainment devices always provide less than 100% O_2. The more air they entrain, the higher the total output flow, but the delivered FiO_2 is lower. High flow is possible only when low O_2 concentration is delivered. For these reasons, air-entrainment devices function as true high-flow systems only at low FiO_2. If the flow output from an air-entrainment device decreases to less than a patient's inspiratory flow, air dilution occurs, and FiO_2 becomes variable.

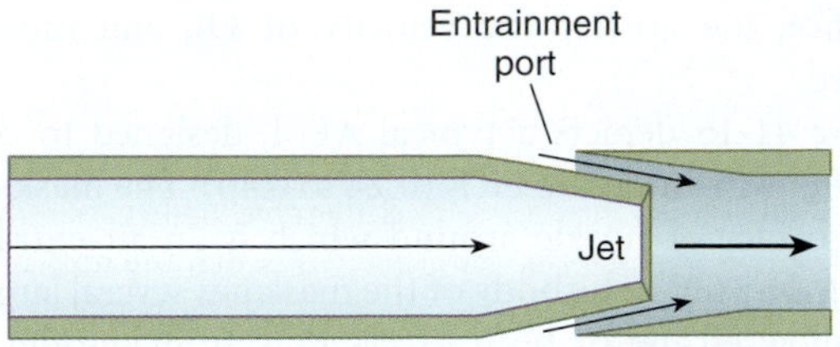

FIGURE 41-13 Basic components of an air-entrainment system. Pressurized gas passes through a nozzle or jet, beyond which are air-entrainment ports. Shear forces at the jet orifice entrain air into the primary gas stream, diluting the O_2 and increasing the total flow output of the device.

MINI CLINI

Computing Total Flow Output of an Air-Entrainment Device

PROBLEM: A patient is receiving O_2 through an air-entrainment device set to deliver 50% O_2. The input O_2 flow is set to 15 L/min. What is the total output flow of this system?

Solution: Step 1: Compute the air-to-O_2 ratio by substituting 50 for the %O_2 in Equation 41-2:

$$\frac{\text{Liters air}}{\text{Liters O}_2} = \frac{(100 - \%\text{O}_2)}{(\%\text{O}_2 - 21)}$$

$$\frac{\text{Liters air}}{\text{Liters O}_2} = \frac{(100 - 50)}{(50 - 21)}$$

$$\frac{\text{Liters air}}{\text{Liters O}_2} = \frac{50}{29}$$

$$\frac{\text{Liters air}}{\text{Liters O}_2} = \frac{1.7}{1}$$

Step 2: Add the air-to-O_2 ratio parts:

$$1.7 + 1 = 2.7$$

Step 3: Multiply the sum of the ratio parts times the O_2 input flow:

$$2.7 \times 15\ \text{L/min} = 41\ \text{L/min}$$

An air-entrainment device set to deliver 50% O_2 that has an input flow of 15 L/min provides a total output flow of approximately 41 L/min.

FiO_2 provided by air-entrainment devices depends on two key variables: the air-to-O_2 ratio and the amount of flow resistance downstream from the mixing site. Changing the input flow of an air-entrainment device alters the total output flow but has little effect on delivered FiO_2. Generally, FiO_2 remains within 1% to 2% of that specified by the manufacturer, regardless of input flow.[29]

The size of the jet and entrainment ports of a device determines the air-to-O_2 ratio and the delivered FiO_2. The accompanying Mini Clini entitled Determining FiO_2 of an Air-Oxygen Mixture shows how to compute the FiO_2 provided by an air-entrainment system if the air-to-O_2 ratio is known.

A more common clinical problem arises when the total output flow from an air-entrainment system must be determined. As described in the previous Rule of Thumb, the total flow output of a system determines whether it truly performs as a high-flow device. The accompanying Mini Clini entitled Computing Total Flow Output of an Air-Entrainment Device shows how to determine the total output flow of an air-entrainment system.

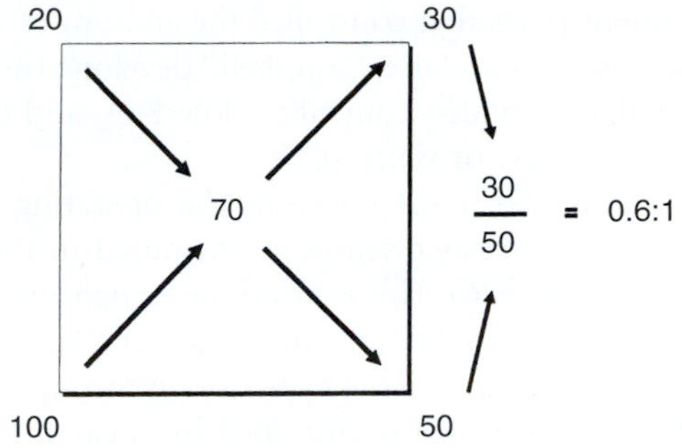

FIGURE 41-14 The magic box used to estimate air-to-O_2 ratio.

Rather than using Equation 41-2 in Box 41-1 to compute air-to-O_2 ratio, many RTs derive quick estimates by using a simple mathematical aid called the ***magic box*** (Figure 41-14). To use the magic box, one draws a square and places 20 in the top left corner and 100 in the bottom left corner. One places the desired O_2 percentage in the center of the box (as in the case illustrated in Figure 41-14, 70%). One subtracts diagonally from lower left to the upper right (disregard the sign). One subtracts diagonally again from upper left to lower right (disregard the sign). The resulting numerator (30) is the value for air, and the denominator (50) is the value for O_2.

By convention, the air-to-O_2 ratio is expressed with the denominator (liters of O_2) set to 1. To reduce any ratio to a ratio of x:1, divide both the numerator and the denominator by the denominator. In the magic box example (also see Figure 41-14):

$$\frac{30}{50} = \frac{30/50}{50/50} = \frac{0.61}{1}$$

The magic box can be used only for estimation of air-to-O_2 ratio. For absolute accuracy, Equation 41-2 in Box 41-1 always should be used. Based on Equation 41-2, Table 41-7 lists the approximate air-to-O_2 ratios for several common O_2 percentages.

The other major factor determining the O_2 concentration provided by an air-entrainment device is downstream flow resistance. In the presence of flow resistance distal to the jet, the volume of air entrained always decreases. With less air being entrained, total flow output decreases, and the delivered O_2 concentration increases. More detail on this phenomenon is provided later in this chapter.[29]

The two most common O_2 delivery systems in which air entrainment is used are the air-entrainment mask (AEM) and the air-entrainment nebulizer.

Air-Entrainment (Venturi) Mask. The use of an O_2 mask with controlled FiO_2 by means of air entrainment was first reported in 1941 by Barach and Eckman.[30] The system provided relatively high FiO_2 (>40%) through the use of adjustable air-entrainment ports that controlled the amount of air mixed with O_2. Almost 20 years later, Campbell[31] developed an entrainment mask that provided controlled, low FiO_2 and called the device a *venturi mask* or *venti-mask*.

As the name *venti-mask* suggests, the operating principle behind these devices has often been attributed to the Venturi principle (see Chapter 6). This assumption is incorrect.[32] Rather than having an actual Venturi tube that entrains air, these devices have a simple restricted orifice or jet through which O_2 flows at high velocity. Air is entrained by shear forces at the boundary of jet flow, not by low lateral pressures. The smaller the orifice, the greater the velocity of O_2, and more air is entrained.

Figure 41-15 depicts a typical AEM, designed to deliver a range of low to moderate FiO_2 (0.24 to 0.40). The mask consists of a jet orifice or nozzle around which is an air-entrainment port *(top drawing)*. The body of the mask has several large ports, which allow escape of both excess flow from the device and exhaled gas from the patient. In this design, FiO_2 is regulated by selection and changing of the jet adapter. The smallest jet provides the highest O_2 velocity, the most air entrainment, and the lowest FiO_2 (0.24). The largest jet provides the lowest O_2 velocity, the least air entrainment, and the highest FiO_2 (0.40). Other AEM designs may vary both jet and entrainment port size to provide an even broader range up to 50% FiO_2. The aerosol entrainment collar fits over the air-entrainment ports (see later).

For controlled FiO_2 at flow high enough to prevent air dilution, the total output flow of an AEM must exceed the patient's peak inspiratory flow.[29] With an entrainment ratio exceeding 5:1, an AEM set to deliver less than 35% O_2 has little trouble meeting or exceeding the 60 L/min high-flow criterion (see previous Rule of Thumb). At settings greater than 35%, total AEM flow decreases significantly, and FiO_2 becomes variable. For example, when set to deliver 50% O_2, some AEMs provide 0.39 FiO_2.[32-34]

Air-Entrainment Nebulizer. Pneumatically powered air-entrainment nebulizers have most of the features of AEMs but have added capabilities, including additional humidification and temperature control. Humidification is achieved through

TABLE 41-7

Approximate Air-to-Oxygen Ratios for Common Oxygen Concentrations*

Percentage O_2	Approximate Air-to-O_2 Ratio	Total Ratio Parts
100	0:1	1
80	0.3:1	1.3
70	0.6:1	1.6
60	1:1	2
50	1.7:1	2.7
45	2:1	3
40	3:1	4
35	5:1	6
30	8:1	9
29	10:1	11
24	25:1	26

*Total output flow (air + O_2) in L/min can be calculated by multiplying the total ratio parts by the O_2 input flow (L/min).

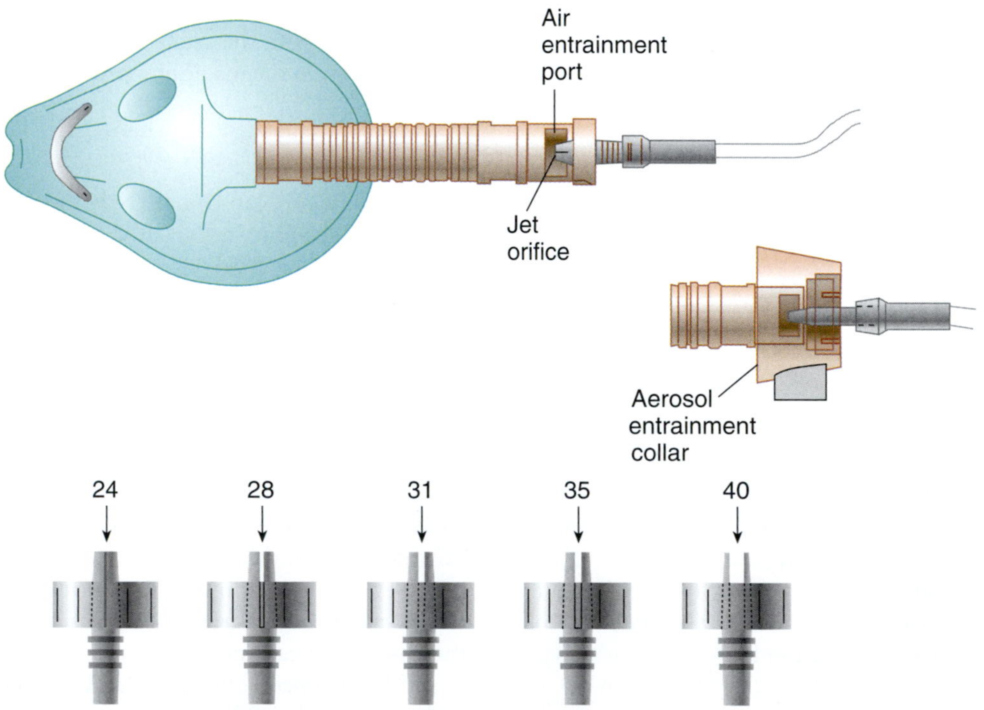

FIGURE 41-15 Typical AEM. FiO_2 is regulated by changing a jet adapter. The aerosol collar allows high humidity or aerosol entrainment from an air source. (Modified from Kacmarek RM: In-hospital O_2 therapy. In Kacmarek RM, Stoller J, editors: Current respiratory care, Toronto, 1988, BC Decker.)

production of aerosol at the nebulizer jet. Temperature control is provided by an optional heating element. In combination, these added features allow delivery of particulate water (in excess of needs for body temperature and pressure, saturated) to the airways. These devices are also widely known as *jet nebulizers* or *large volume nebulizers.*

Because of added humidification and heat control, air-entrainment nebulizers have been the traditional device of choice for delivering O_2 to patients with artificial tracheal airways. O_2 typically is delivered with a T tube or a tracheostomy mask. An alternative is to use an aerosol mask or a face tent to deliver an O_2 mixture via aerosol to patients with intact upper airways (Figure 41-16).[35]

AEMs can vary both jet and entrainment port size to obtain a given FiO_2; however, gas-powered nebulizers have a fixed orifice. Air-to-O_2 ratios can be altered only by varying entrainment port size. Disposable nebulizers usually have a continuous range of settings from 28% to 100%.[22]

Similar to AEMs, air-entrainment nebulizers perform as fixed-performance devices only when output flow meets or exceeds the patient's inspiratory demand. In contrast to AEMs, air-entrainment nebulizers do not allow easy increases in nebulizer output flow by means of an increase in O_2 input. With most nebulizer systems, the extremely small size of the jet needed for aerosol production limits the maximum O_2 input flow to 12 to 15 L/min at 50 psig. For example, the total output flow of an air-entrainment nebulizer set to deliver 40% O_2 ranges from 48 to 60 L/min. Although this amount may be adequate for most patients, it is insufficient for patients with very high inspiratory flow or minute volume.[35]

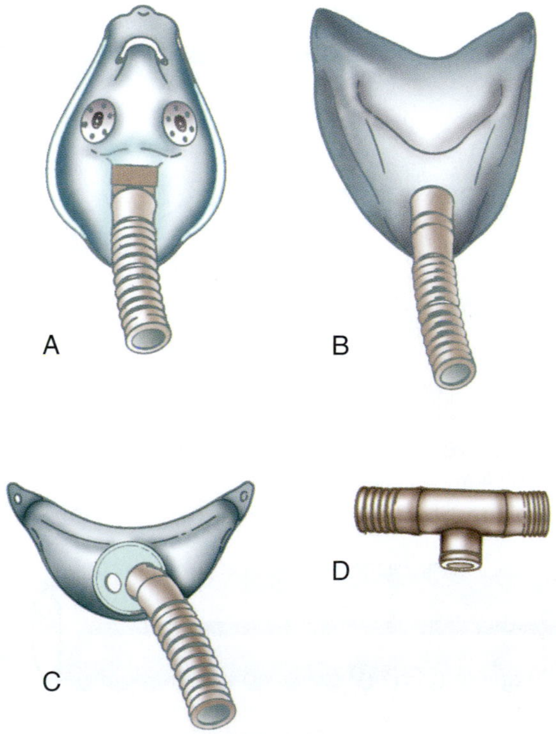

FIGURE 41-16 Devices for delivery of O_2 mixtures with aerosol. **A,** Aerosol mask. **B,** Face tent. **C,** Tracheostomy collar. **D,** T tube. (Modified from Kacmarek RM: In-hospital O_2 therapy. In Kacmarek RM, Stoller J, editors: Current respiratory care, Toronto, 1988, BC Decker.)

The actual FiO_2 received by patients may be affected by the choice of airway appliance. The FiO_2 delivered by face tent is consistently less than the set nebulizer concentration, especially at higher levels.[36]

Air-entrainment nebulizers should be treated as fixed-performance devices only when set to deliver low O_2 concentration (≤35%).[33] When a nebulizer is used to deliver a higher concentration of O_2, the output flow is insufficient to meet patient needs. There are two ways to assess whether the flow of an air-entrainment nebulizer meets the patient's needs. The first method is simple visual inspection. With this approach (generally used only with a T tube), the RT sets up the device to deliver the highest possible flow at the prescribed FiO_2 and observes the mist output at the expiratory side of the T tube. As long as mist can be seen escaping throughout inspiration, flow is adequate and the delivered FiO_2 is ensured.

The second way to assess the adequacy of nebulizer flow is to compare it with the patient's peak inspiratory flow. A patient's peak inspiratory flow during tidal breathing is at least three times minute volume. As long as the nebulizer flow exceeds this value, the delivered FiO_2 is ensured. If the patient's peak flow exceeds that provided by the nebulizer, the device functions as a low-flow system with variable FiO_2 (see the accompanying Mini Clini for an example).[35]

MINI CLINI

Computing Minimum Flow Needs

PROBLEM: A physician orders 40% O_2 through an air-entrainment nebulizer to a patient with a tidal volume of 0.6 L and a respiratory rate of 33 breaths/min. If maximum nebulizer input flow is 12 L/min, will the patient receive 40% O_2? If not, what total flow is needed to meet this patient's needs?

Solution: 1. Estimate the patient's inspiratory flow:

$$\text{Peak inspiratory flow} = \text{VE} \times 3 = (0.6 \times 33) \times 3 = 59.4\ \text{L/min}$$

2. Compute the total flow of the nebulizer:

$$\text{Sum of ratio parts}(3:1) \times \text{Input flow}(12\ \text{L/min}) = 48\ \text{L/min}$$

3. Compare value 1 with value 2 (patient with nebulizer):

$$59.4\ \text{L/min}(\text{patient}) > 48\ \text{L/min}(\text{nebulizer})$$

Under these conditions, the patient does not receive 40% O_2. To deliver a stable 40% O_2 concentration, the total flow would have to be at least 59.4 L/min.

Troubleshooting Air-Entrainment Systems. The major problem with air-entrainment systems is ensuring that the set FiO_2 actually is delivered to the patient. Problems usually do not occur when the devices are used to deliver low FiO_2 (<0.35). However, the design of these devices makes it difficult to provide even moderate FiO_2 at the high flow needed to ensure a set

O_2 concentration. The performance of all air-entrainment devices is affected by downstream resistance. The result can be inaccurate FiO_2 that makes delivery of a low O_2 concentration difficult with air-entrainment nebulizers.

Providing Moderate to High FiO_2 at High Flow. AEMs and air-entrainment nebulizers differ in ratio settings and input and output flow capabilities. Most AEMs can be set to deliver no more than 50% O_2. When set according to the manufacturer's specifications to provide much more than 35% O_2, AEMs simply do not generate enough flow to ensure the set FiO_2. The solution is to boost the total output flow. With AEMs, total output flow can be boosted with a simple increase in input flow. For a 35% AEM (5:1 ratio) with an input flow of 8 L/min, the total output flow is 48 L/min. This flow is insufficient to ensure 35% O_2 delivery to all patients. Simply increasing the input flow to 12 L/min boosts the output flow of the AEM by 50%, to 72 L/min. The new high flow ensures delivery of the set O_2 concentration to essentially all patients.

This solution is impossible with most air-entrainment nebulizers. Because the small jets in many of these devices limit O_2 flow to 12 to 15 L/min, the input flow cannot be increased beyond these levels. A few nebulizer models, such as the Thera-Mist Barrel Nebulizer (Smiths Medical, London, England), supposedly can provide moderately high output flows of 54 L/min at FiO_2 80%. However, most air-entrainment nebulizers cannot because of the total flow-to-FiO_2 tradeoff. The five alternatives for boosting the FiO_2 capabilities in these situations are presented in Box 41-2.

The simplest approach to achieving higher FiO_2 with these devices is to add a 50- to 150-ml aerosol tubing reservoir to the expiratory side of the T tube (Figure 41-17). Given its simplicity, adding an open volume reservoir to the expiratory side of T tubes is standard procedure in most clinical settings. This approach can be used only in the treatment of intubated patients. Even then, the small reservoir size limits the ability of this system to ensure stable FiO_2, especially greater than 40%, and larger reservoirs can cause rebreathing.

Rather than a simple open reservoir, a closed reservoir or nonrebreathing system similar to that shown in Figure 41-12 can be used. These systems combine an inspiratory volume reservoir (usually a compliant 3- to 5-L anesthesia bag) with a one-way expiratory valve. Whenever patient flow exceeds nebulizer flow, the expiratory valve closes, and the patient draws additional gas from the reservoir. Although they can ensure delivery of the set O_2 concentration, these systems pose considerable hazards. If source flow stops for any reason, the patient can suffocate. For this reason, these systems must be equipped with an emergency inlet valve that allows room air breathing in the event of source gas failure.

The third approach to higher FiO_2 with air-entrainment nebulizers is to connect two or more devices together with a "wye" adapter (Figure 41-18).[22] Although a single air-entrainment nebulizer set at 60% (1:1 ratio) with a maximum input flow of 15 L/min has a total output flow of only 30 L/min, connecting two of these devices together doubles the total output flow to 60 L/min (the minimum needed for a high-flow device). This approach works well only for delivery of a concentration of 60% or less to patients with a minute volume less than 10 L/min.[35,36]

A fourth method for boosting FiO_2 provided by air-entrainment nebulizers is to set the device to a lower

Box 41-2 Increasing FiO_2 Capabilities of Air-Entrainment Nebulizers

- Add open reservoir to expiratory side of T tube
- Provide inspiratory reservoir with one-way expiratory valve
- Connect two or more nebulizers together in parallel
- Set nebulizer to low concentration; bleed-in O_2; analyze and adjust
- Use a commercial dual-flow system

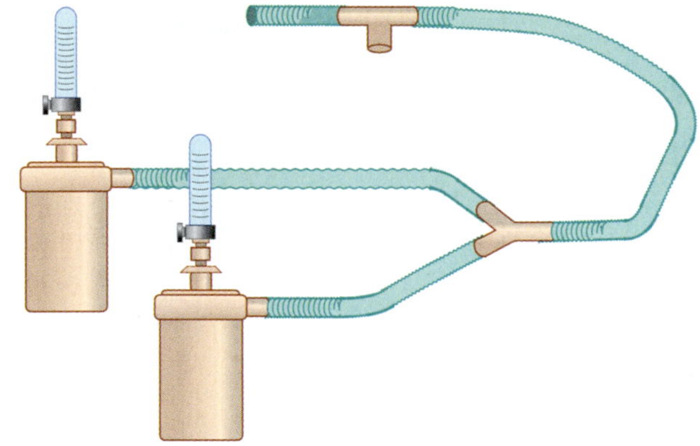

FIGURE 41-18 Use of two nebulizers in parallel to provide high FiO_2 at high flow.

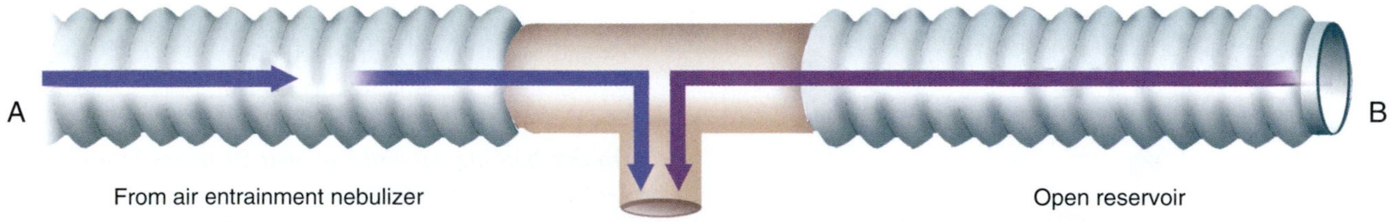

FIGURE 41-17 Use of an open volume reservoir to enhance delivered O_2 concentration with a T tube. From 50 to 150 ml of aerosol tubing is connected to the expiratory side of the T tube. **A,** When the patient inhales, gas at the set FiO_2 is drawn first through the inspiratory side of the circuit. **B,** If the patient's flow exceeds nebulizer flow, gas is drawn from the reservoir side. After the reservoir volume is fully tapped, room air is entrained, and FiO_2 decreases.

concentration than that prescribed (to generate high flow) while bleeding supplemental O_2 into the delivery tubing. This method increases both FiO_2 and total output flow. To achieve a specific FiO_2 the delivered concentration should be analyzed and the supplemental O_2 input flow adjusted until the desired concentration is achieved.

Commercial dual-flow systems entail a similar approach. One flow source powers the jet, while another flow source provides supplemental O_2. The Misty Ox (Vital Signs, Totowa, New Jersey) gas injection nebulizer is an example. This system is not an air-entrainment system because it does not depend on entrainment ports to increase total flow or O_2 concentration to the patient. Rather, it uses two flowmeters: one that operates the jet and one that feeds into the side of the jet manifold. The Misty Ox system can provide FiO_2 of 0.96 at a flow of 42 L/min and offers O_2 concentrations ranging from 0.21 to nearly 1.00.[35]

Problems With Downstream Flow Resistance. Any increase in flow resistance downstream from (distal to) the point of air entrainment alters the performance of all air-entrainment systems. Increased downstream flow resistance causes back pressure. The back pressure decreases both the volume of entrained air and the total flow output of these devices. With less air entrained, the delivered O_2 concentration increases; however, because total flow output also decreases, the effect on FiO_2 varies. High downstream flow resistance usually turns air-entrainment systems from high-flow (fixed) O_2 delivery systems into low-flow (variable) O_2 delivery systems incapable of delivering a precise and constant FiO_2.[29]

This problem explains why it is extremely difficult to deliver less than 28% to 30% O_2 with an air-entrainment nebulizer. The 5 to 6 ft (1.5 to 1.8 m) of aerosol tubing normally used with these devices produces enough flow resistance to decrease air entrainment and prevent a lower FiO_2.

A similar situation can occur when the entrainment ports of an air-entrainment device become obstructed (most common with AEMs). Delivered O_2 concentration increases, but total output flow decreases. The net effect usually is a variable FiO_2. The accompanying Mini Clini is an example of the effect of increased downstream flow resistance on the performance of an air-entrainment device.

High-Flow Nasal Cannula. A variation of the standard nasal cannula discussed earlier in this chapter is a **high-flow nasal cannula (HFNC)**. Various systems are available, including the Vapotherm Precision Flow System (Vapotherm, Exeter, New Hampshire), which can deliver both FiO_2 and relative humidity greater than 90% by using heated, humidified O_2 flows up to 40 L/min. HFNC units offered by other manufacturers such as Fisher and Paykel's Optiflow (Irvine, California) featured in Figure 41-19, have been shown to provide even higher flows of 50 L/min, as well as a maximum FiO_2 of more than 90%. These devices feature a variety of proprietary designs that facilitate the separate control of flow and humidified supplemental oxygen. The ability to maintain a consistent FiO_2 under varying patient breathing patterns makes these devices suitable for a great many patients. As a result, these systems have been shown to successfully treat moderate hypoxemia through a combination of the three main features: (1) delivery of a high FiO_2, (2) meeting or exceeding the patient's minute ventilation and therefore acting as a fixed oxygen delivery device, and (3) generating a distending positive airway pressure. Furthermore, the heated-humidity feature enables these systems to deliver highly humidified oxygen, thus preventing the drying effects that some high-flow devices have on the mucosa. This point and the less confining design of these devices generally mean that they are more comfortable and better tolerated by many patients than are alternative oxygen delivery devices. As a result, such devices have become a popular substitute for both traditional high-flow oxygen devices and continuous positive airway pressure setups for infants with disorders including bronchiolitis and bronchopulmonary dysplasia. Furthermore, HFNC devices are rapidly

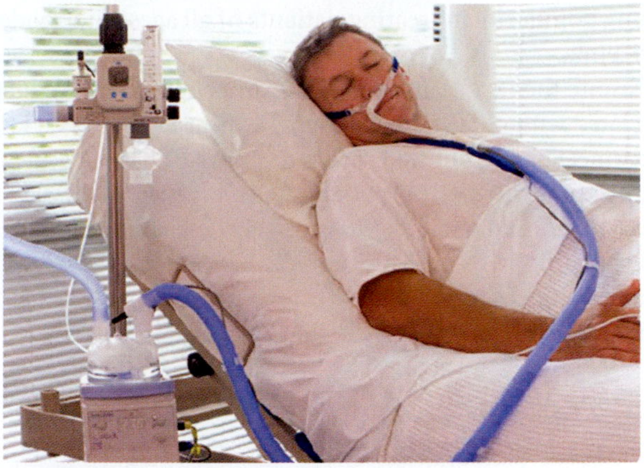

FIGURE 41-19 High-flow nasal cannula set-up (Courtesy of Fisher & Paykel Healthcare, Inc., Irvine, California.)

MINI CLINI

Effect of Downstream Flow Resistance on Performance of an Air-Entrainment Device

PROBLEM: A tracheostomy patient is receiving O_2 therapy through a T tube attached to an air-entrainment nebulizer set at 35% O_2 with an input flow of 10 L/min. Over the past 30 minutes, the patient's SpO_2 has decreased from 93% to 88%. When assessing the patient, the RT finds that the large-bore delivery tubing of the nebulizer is partially obstructed with condensate and that aerosol mist at the T tube is not visible throughout inspiration. What is the likely problem, and what is the best solution?

Solution: The likely problem is a decrease in FiO_2 owing to the increased downstream resistance caused by the condensate. At 10 L/min input flow, the device was probably delivering approximately 60 L/min of 35% O_2 before the tubing became obstructed. Because aerosol mist is not visible at the T tube throughout inspiration, it is clear that the total output flow is no longer sufficient and that the patient is now diluting the delivered O_2 with room air. Draining the tubing solves this problem.

gaining popularity in treating patients of all ages with moderate hypoxemia.

Despite the fact that some earlier infection control concerns associated with older HFNC designs appear to have been largely overcome, a few limitations seem to persist. These include contraindications for use on patients with blocked nasal passages, problems from the inability to precisely determine and monitor the level of positive pressure actually applied to the airway, and in rare instances, nasal skin erosions, mainly in neonates and infants, from an improperly fitting cannula.[37]

MINI CLINI

Indications for High-Flow Nasal Oxygen

PROBLEM: A recently extubated patient experiencing moderate hypoxemia is having trouble tolerating a 50% venturi mask due to claustrophobia and airway dryness. When switched to a nasal cannula, his SpO_2 drops to 88%. The physician wants the patient SpO_2 to remain at 92% or higher and asks the RT what options are available for delivering moderate oxygen concentrations to this patient while maximizing patient comfort.

Solution: A high-flow nasal oxygen setup is able to provide a moderate to high and consistent FiO_2 through varying patient breathing patterns. In addition, features including a less-confining design and delivery of a highly humidified gas tend to make them better tolerated than many other oxygen delivery systems. Hence, in this instance, the RT should recommend a high-flow nasal oxygen setup.

Blending Systems. When air-entrainment devices cannot provide a high enough O_2 concentration or flow, use of a gas blending system should be considered. With a blending system, separate pressurized air and O_2 sources are input, and the gases are mixed either manually or with a precision valve (blender). This system allows precise control over both FiO_2 and total flow output. Most blending systems can provide flow much greater than 60 L/min, qualifying them as true fixed-performance delivery devices. For adults, gas is delivered from the blender either through an open system, such as an aerosol mask or T tube, or with a closed nonrebreathing system. For many patients requiring high FiO_2 and breathing spontaneously, this is the ideal setup, provided that the gas is humidified. The use of high-flow blended systems with heated humidity, as opposed to a heated aerosol, are very well tolerated by most patients, including patients with tracheostomies.

Mixing Gases Manually. When gases are mixed manually, separate air and O_2 flowmeters must be adjusted for the desired FiO_2 and flow (see the accompanying Mini Clini). For adults, this approach requires calibrated high-flow flowmeters (at least 60 L/min) and monitoring of delivered FiO_2.

Oxygen Blenders. Rather than manually mixing air and O_2, the RT more often uses an O_2 blender. Figure 41-20 shows the major components of a typical O_2 blender. Air and O_2 enter the blender and pass through dual pressure regulators that exactly match the two pressures. Gas flows to a precision proportioning valve. Because the two gas pressures at this point are equal, varying the size of the air and O_2 inlets provides precise control over the relative concentration.

An alarm system gives an audible warning when either source gas fails or the pressure decreases below a specified value.

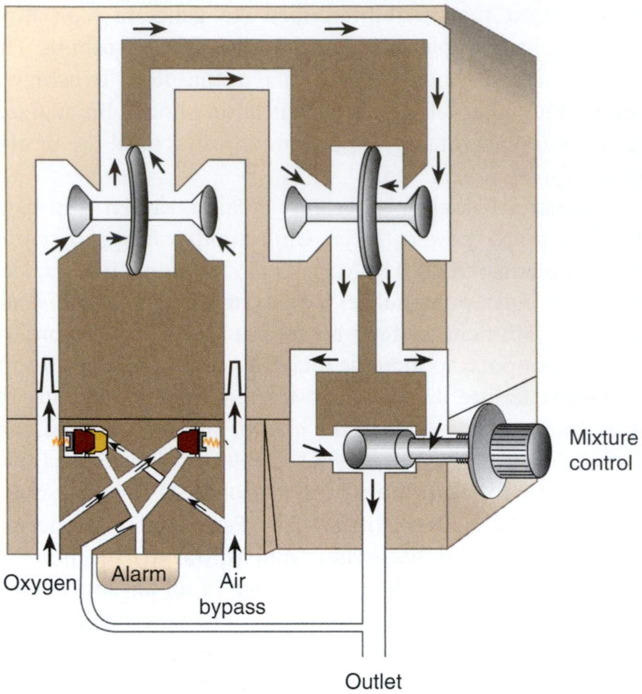

FIGURE 41-20 O_2 blending device. (Modified from McPherson SP: Respiratory therapy equipment, ed 3, St. Louis, 1985, Mosby.)

MINI CLINI

Manually Mixing Air and Oxygen to Achieve Specified Concentration at a Given Flow

PROBLEM: To mix air and O_2 manually to provide a patient with 50% O_2 at a total flow of 60 L/min, what O_2 and airflow would the RT set?

Solution: 1. Use Equation 41-3 to compute the O_2 flow:

$$O_2 \text{ flow} = \frac{\text{Total flow} \times (O_2\% - 21)}{79}$$

$$O_2 \text{ flow} = \frac{60 \times (50 - 21)}{79}$$

$$O_2 \text{ flow} = 22 \text{ L/min}$$

2. Compute the airflow:

$$\text{Airflow} = \text{Total flow} - O_2 \text{ flow}$$

$$\text{Airflow} = 60 - 22$$

$$\text{Airflow} = 38 \text{ L/min}$$

To provide a patient with 50% O_2 at a total flow of 60 L/min, blend 22 L of O_2 with 38 L of air.

Box 41-3 **Procedure for Confirming Operation of an Oxygen Blender**

1. Confirm that inlet pressures of air and O_2 are within manufacturer's specifications.
2. Test low air and O_2 alarms by disconnecting each source; also confirm safety bypass or crossover system.
3. Analyze O_2 concentration at 100%, 21%, and specified FiO_2.

The alarm system usually has a crossover or bypass feature whereby failure of one gas source causes the blender system to switch to the other. If the air source fails when delivering 60% O_2, the alarm sounds, and the blender switches over to delivery of 100% O_2.

Although they allow ideal control over both FiO_2 and flow, blenders are especially prone to inaccuracy and failure.[38,39] Hence, an operational check of any blender should be conducted before using it on a patient (Box 41-3). FiO_2 should be checked and confirmed with a calibrated O_2 analyzer at least once per shift.[2] When a blender is used in the care of a neonate, an O_2 analyzer should be kept in-line at all times. In the use of a nonrebreathing or closed delivery system, (1) all breathing valves should be inspected and tested before application to a patient, and (2) a fail-safe inspiratory valve should be included in the delivery system.

Enclosures. The concept of enclosing a patient in a controlled-O_2 atmosphere is among the oldest approaches to O_2 therapy. Entire rooms once were used for this purpose. With today's simpler airway devices, enclosures are generally used only in the care of infants and children. The primary types of O_2 enclosures used for infants and children are tents, incubators, and hoods.

Oxygen Tents. O_2 tents previously were the most common method of O_2 therapy in the treatment of both adults and children. Use of O_2 tents in both adults and children is rare at the present time. However, when they are used, it is common for tents to be air-conditioned or cooled with ice to provide a comfortable temperature within a plastic sheet canopy (Figure 41-21).

The main problem with tents is that frequent opening and closing of the canopy cause wide swings in O_2 concentration. Constant leakage makes a high FiO_2 impossible. In large tents, O_2 input flow of 12 to 15 L/min can provide only 40% to 50% O_2 levels. Comparable FiO_2 can be achieved in smaller pediatric or **croup** tents with flow of 8 to 10 L/min.

Hoods. An O_2 hood, also known as an *oxyhood,* is often the best method for administration of controlled O_2 therapy to infants. As shown in Figure 41-22, an O_2 hood covers only the head, leaving the infant's body free for nursing care. O_2 is delivered to the hood through either a heated air-entrainment nebulizer or a blending system with a heated humidifier. A minimum flow of 7 L/min should be set to prevent accumulation of CO_2.[40] Depending on the size of the hood, flow of 10 to 15 L/min may be needed to maintain a stable high O_2 concentration. Higher flow generally is not needed and may produce a harmful noise level and additional stress on neonatal patients.[41]

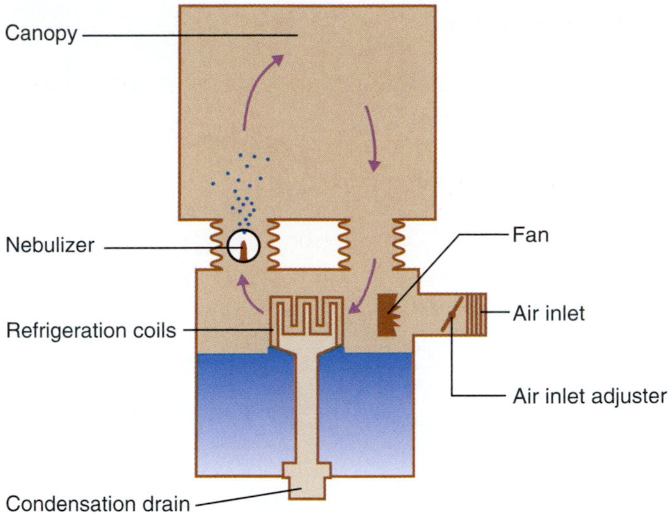

FIGURE 41-21 O_2 tent incorporating refrigeration coils for cooling. (Modified from Cairo JM: Mosby's respiratory care equipment, ed 9, St. Louis, 2014, Mosby.)

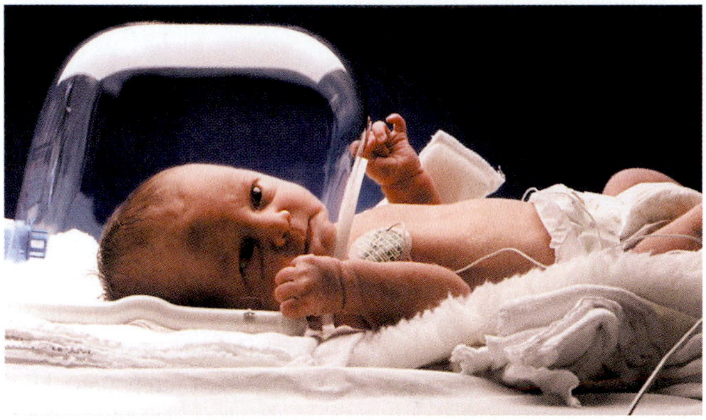

FIGURE 41-22 Infant O_2 hood. (Courtesy Utah Medical Products, Inc, Midvale, Utah.)

In the care of premature infants, it is especially important to ensure that the gas mixture is properly warmed and humidified and not directed toward the patient's face or head. Low temperatures or convection cooling produced by high flow over the head can cause heat loss and cold stress. In premature infants, cold stress can increase O_2 consumption and cause apnea.[42]

The temperature of gases provided to an infant in an O_2 hood should be precisely set to maintain a **neutral thermal environment (NTE)**. The NTE temperature varies according to an infant's age and weight. The NTE temperature for newborns weighing less than 1200 g is 95° F (35° C). For older infants weighing 2500 g or more, the NTE is lower, approximately 86° F (30° C).[42]

Incubators. Incubators, also known by the trade name Isolette (Dräger Medical AG & Co, Lübeck, Germany) are polymethyl methacrylate (Plexiglas) enclosures that combine servo-controlled convection heating with supplemental O_2 (Figure 41-23). When it is needed, supplemental humidity usually is provided with an external heated humidifier or nebulizer.

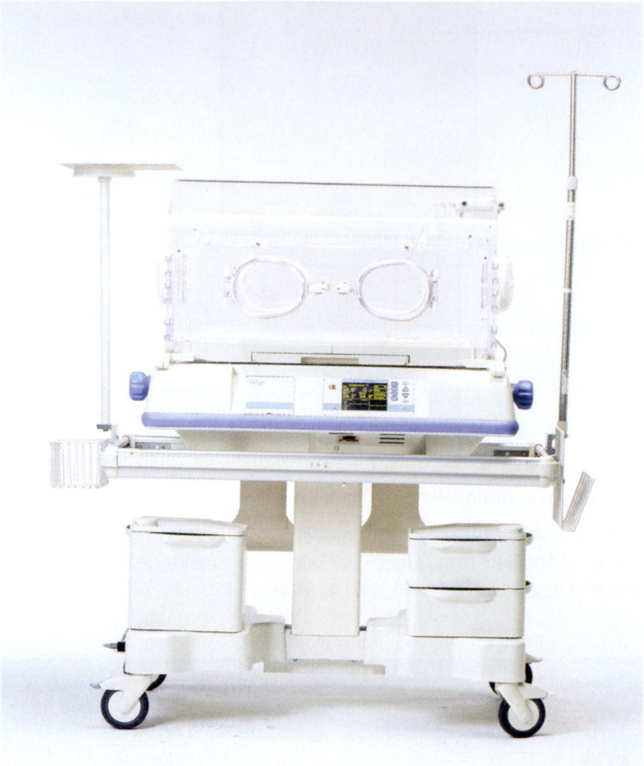

FIGURE 41-23 Infant isolette. (Courtesy Dräger Medical AG & Co, Lübeck, Germany.)

Supplemental O_2 can be administered with a direct connection between the incubator and a flowmeter that has a heated humidifier. In some units, a filtered air-entrainment device limits the delivered concentration to approximately 0.40. However, leaks and frequent opening of the isolette dilute the O_2 levels to much less than 40%. Blockage of the inlet filter can cause less air entrainment and a higher O_2 concentration.[42]

Given the highly variable O_2 concentration provided by these devices, the best way to control O_2 delivery to infants in an isolette is with an oxyhood. The oxyhood is placed over the infant's head inside the isolette. The O_2 concentration and gas temperature within the oxyhood, not in the isolette, must be assessed. It is ideal to monitor isolette or oxyhood O_2 concentration continuously (see later).[2,4]

Because hoods allow better FiO_2 control, and because servo-controlled radiant heating warmers are generally more convenient, Plexiglas isolettes are not as popular as they used to be. However, these devices are still the best choice for providing O_2 to infants in stable condition with a NTE.[42]

Other Oxygen Delivery Devices

Bag-Mask Devices. Bag-mask devices use a self-inflating bag and nonrebreathing valve features to provide up to 100% O_2. Bag-mask devices are often used in emergency life support and in critical care and are more completely discussed in Chapter 37.

Demand-Flow and Pulse-Dose Systems. Demand-flow or pulse-dose systems use a flow sensor and valve to synchronize gas delivery with inspiration. These devices can substantially extend duration of flow of a liquid or gaseous O_2 tank and are popular in alternative settings, as described in Chapter 56.

Box 41-4 Patient Factors in Selecting Oxygen Therapy Equipment

- Severity and cause of hypoxemia
- Patient age group (infant, child, adult)
- Degree of consciousness and alertness
- Presence or absence of tracheal airway
- Stability of minute ventilation
- Mouth breathing vs. nose breathing patient

Selecting a Delivery Approach

The RT is often involved in the initial selection of an appropriate delivery system. This generally involves making recommendations—on the basis of sound patient assessment—to initiate, change or discontinue the treatment regimen (see later section on Protocol-Based Oxygen Therapy).

The three *Ps*—*purpose, patient,* and *performance*—are used in the initial selection or recommendation of a change in O_2 delivery system. The goal is to match the performance characteristics of the equipment to both the objectives of therapy (purpose) and the patient's special needs.

Purpose

The general purpose or objective of all O_2 therapy is to increase FiO_2 sufficiently to correct arterial hypoxemia. Other objectives, including decreasing hypoxic symptoms and minimizing increased cardiopulmonary work, follow from this primary purpose.

Patient

Key patient considerations in selecting O_2 therapy equipment for use in acute care are summarized in Box 41-4. Knowledge of these factors helps guide the RT in selecting the appropriate equipment. For example, a simple mask at 5 to 6 L/min is probably more suitable than a nasal cannula at 4 L/min for a mouth breathing, mildly hypoxemic patient. An infant with moderate hypoxia and a normal airway usually needs an O_2 enclosure (hood or enclosed incubator).

Performance

O_2 systems vary according to actual FiO_2 delivered and stability of FiO_2 under changing patient demands. Generally, the more critically ill the patient, the greater the need for a stable, high FiO_2. Less acutely ill patients generally need a lower, less exact FiO_2. Table 41-8 lists guidelines for selecting an O_2 delivery system on the basis of the level and stability of the FiO_2 needed.

General Goals and Patient Categories

On the basis of overall consideration of the three *Ps*, general goals can be set for several patient categories. In emergencies in which tissue hypoxia is suspected, patients should be given the

TABLE 41-8

Selection of an Oxygen Delivery System Based on Desired FiO_2 Level and Stability

Desired FiO_2 Level	DESIRED FiO_2 STABILITY	
	Fixed	Variable
Low (<35%)	AEM Air-entrainment nebulizer Blending system Isolette, incubator (infant)	Nasal cannula Nasal catheter Transtracheal catheter
Moderate (35%-60%)	Air-entrainment nebulizer Blending system Oxyhood (infant)	Simple mask Air-entrainment nebulizer Tent (child)
High (>60%)	Blending system Oxyhood (infant) High-flow nasal cannula	Partial rebreather Nonrebreather

highest FiO_2 possible—ideally 100%. This level can be achieved with a true high-flow or a closed reservoir system. The goal is the highest possible blood O_2 content. Clinical examples include respiratory or cardiac arrest, severe trauma, shock, carbon monoxide poisoning, and cyanide poisoning. Carbon monoxide and cyanide poisoning may necessitate HBO therapy (see later).

A critically ill adult patient with moderate to severe hypoxemia needs either a reservoir or a high-flow system capable of at least 60% O_2. Thereafter, changes in FiO_2 (and device) should be based on results of assessment of physiologic values. The goal is a PaO_2 greater than 60 mm Hg or oxyhemoglobin saturation greater than 90%.

In the care of adult patients in more stable condition but who are acutely ill with mild to moderate hypoxemia, a system capable of low to moderate O_2 concentration can be used. In these cases, stability of FiO_2 is not critical. Applicable devices include a nasal cannula at moderate flow or a simple mask. Common examples include patients in the immediately postoperative phase and patients recovering from acute myocardial infarction.

Adult patients with chronic lung disease and accompanying acute-on-chronic hypoxemia present a special case. In the care of these patients, the goal is to ensure adequate arterial oxygenation without depressing ventilation. Adequate oxygenation of these patients generally means SaO_2 of 85% to 92% with PaO_2 of 50 to 70 mm Hg.[31,43] These values usually are achieved with either low-flow nasal O_2 or a low-concentration (24% to 28%) AEM. The less stable the patient's condition, the greater the need for a high-flow AEM.[22]

Because of size, discomfort, and appearance, AEMs are less well tolerated than nasal cannulas for long-term therapy. In contrast to a cannula, an AEM must be removed for eating and drinking. Because even a short break in O_2 therapy can cause a rapid decrease in PaO_2 in some patients, these patients should be taught to switch to a nasal cannula whenever they must remove the mask.[22]

Lastly, it is sometimes necessary to modify O_2 delivery systems to facilitate patient transport. An example is a spontaneously breathing patient with a tracheostomy tube receiving a moderate FiO_2 via a blended system or an air-entrainment nebulizer connected to a tracheostomy mask. Given the impracticalities of transporting a patient on an air-entrainment nebulizer, it may be more suitable to connect a venturi adapter temporarily to provide the appropriate FiO_2 to the tracheostomy mask during the transport, and then reconnect them back to the original aerosol set-up immediately after the transport.

Box 41-5 Physiologic Effects of Hyperbaric Oxygen Therapy

- Bubble reduction (Boyle's law)
- Hyperoxygenation of blood and tissue (Henry's law)
- Vasoconstriction
- Enhanced host immune function
- Neovascularization

Protocol-Based Oxygen Therapy

O_2 therapy is ideally suited for a protocol. Bedside assessment of oxygenation by RTs and other clinicians has progressed to where it is more cost-effective and clinically appropriate to use a protocol rather than obtaining a new physician order for each change in FiO_2. An order for "O_2 therapy via protocol" permits O_2 therapy to be initiated, modified, or discontinued by the RT, provided that an assessment reveals that the patient meets previously approved clinical criteria. A well-designed O_2 protocol ensures the patient (1) undergoes initial assessment, (2) is evaluated for protocol criteria, (3) receives a treatment plan that is modified according to need, and (4) stops receiving therapy as soon as it is no longer needed.[44]

Figure 41-24 shows the decision algorithm underlying an O_2 therapy titration protocol developed at the Cleveland Clinic Foundation. In the algorithm, a pulse oximetry saturation (SpO_2) of 92% is the point at which therapy is to be initiated. The patient is assessed each shift for the need of supplemental O_2, which is adjusted depending on need. When the SpO_2 is consistently 92% or greater on room air, therapy is discontinued.

HYPERBARIC OXYGEN THERAPY

Hyperbaric oxygen (HBO) therapy is the therapeutic use of O_2 at pressures greater than 1 atm.[45-47] Pressures during HBO therapy usually are expressed in multiples of **atmospheric pressure absolute (ATA)**: 1 ATA equals 760 mm Hg (101.32 kPa). Most HBO therapy is conducted at pressures between 2 ATA and 3 ATA, although other pressures may be used, often based on U.S. Navy diving treatment tables.[46-48]

Physiologic Effects

The known physiologic effects of HBO therapy are summarized in Box 41-5.[45] These effects are mainly due to either high pressure or high O_2 tension in body fluids and tissues. In conditions

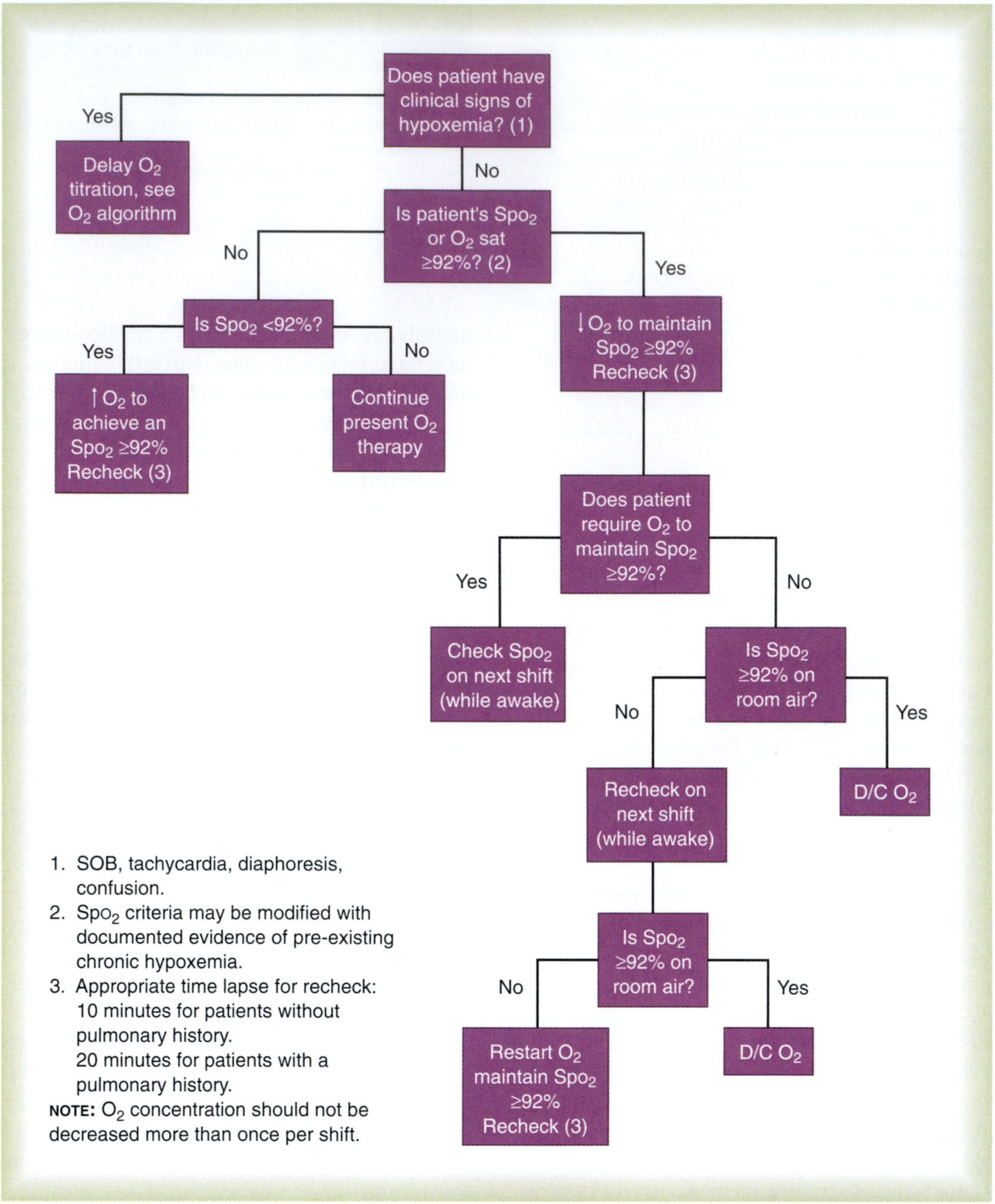

FIGURE 41-24 Protocol for titration of O_2 therapy. (Courtesy the Respiratory Therapy Section, Cleveland Clinic Foundation, Cleveland, Ohio.)

such as air embolism and decompression sickness, Boyle's law dictates that high pressure exerts a physical effect on air or nitrogen bubbles trapped in the blood or tissues, reducing their size, and minimizing potential harm. Because pressure is crucial in these cases, HBO treatments may be conducted at 6 ATA or more.[46,48]

The second beneficial effect of HBO is hyperoxia. When a patient is breathing room air, only a small amount of O_2 dissolves in the plasma (approximately 0.3 ml/dl). At 3 ATA, plasma contains nearly 7 ml/dl dissolved O_2, a level exceeding average resting tissue uptake.[46]

O_2 supply to the tissues affects the immune system, wound healing, and vascular tone. A tissue PO_2 of at least 30 mm Hg is necessary for normal cellular function. Damaged and infected tissues often have a lower PO_2. Increasing O_2 supply to these tissues can help restore both white blood cell function and antimicrobial activity.

Hyperoxia affects the cardiovascular system. HBO therapy causes generalized vasoconstriction and a small decrease in cardiac output. Although these changes may decrease blood flow to a region, this effect is more than offset by the increase in O_2 content. In conditions such as burns, cerebral edema, and crush injuries, vasoconstriction may be helpful because it reduces edema and tissue swelling while maintaining tissue oxygenation.

Hyperoxia also helps form new capillary beds, a process called **neovascularization.** Although the exact mechanism is unknown, neovascularization is an essential component of tissue repair, especially in radiation-induced injuries.[46,47]

Study results suggest that HBO may be useful in many other conditions, including the management of stroke, wound healing, and treating stubborn soft tissue infections. Because HBO has emerged as a highly effective therapy for various conditions, its use in recent years has expanded.[49,50]

Methods of Administration

HBO is administered in either a multiplace or a monoplace chamber. A multiplace chamber is a large tank capable of holding a dozen or more people (Figure 41-25, *A*). Because patients are directly cared for by medical staff inside the tank, multiplace chambers have air locks that allow entry and exit without altering the pressure. The multiplace chamber is generally filled with air. If indicated, only the patient breathes supplemental O_2 (through a mask or another device). Because they can achieve pressures of 6 ATA or more, multiplace chambers are ideal for the management of decompression sickness and air embolism.[46-48]

A typical monoplace chamber consists of a transparent Plexiglas cylinder large enough only for a single patient (see Figure 41-25, *B*). During therapy, the cylinder O_2 concentration is kept at 100%. The patient need not wear a mask. Because of the high O_2 concentration, most electronic equipment cannot be used in a monoplace chamber. In addition, many ventilators do not function properly under the high atmospheric pressures. However, monitoring systems and ventilators can be adapted to allow treatment of a critically ill patient with hyperbaric pressure. Additionally, artificial airways suited to function properly under hyperbaric conditions should be used.[45]

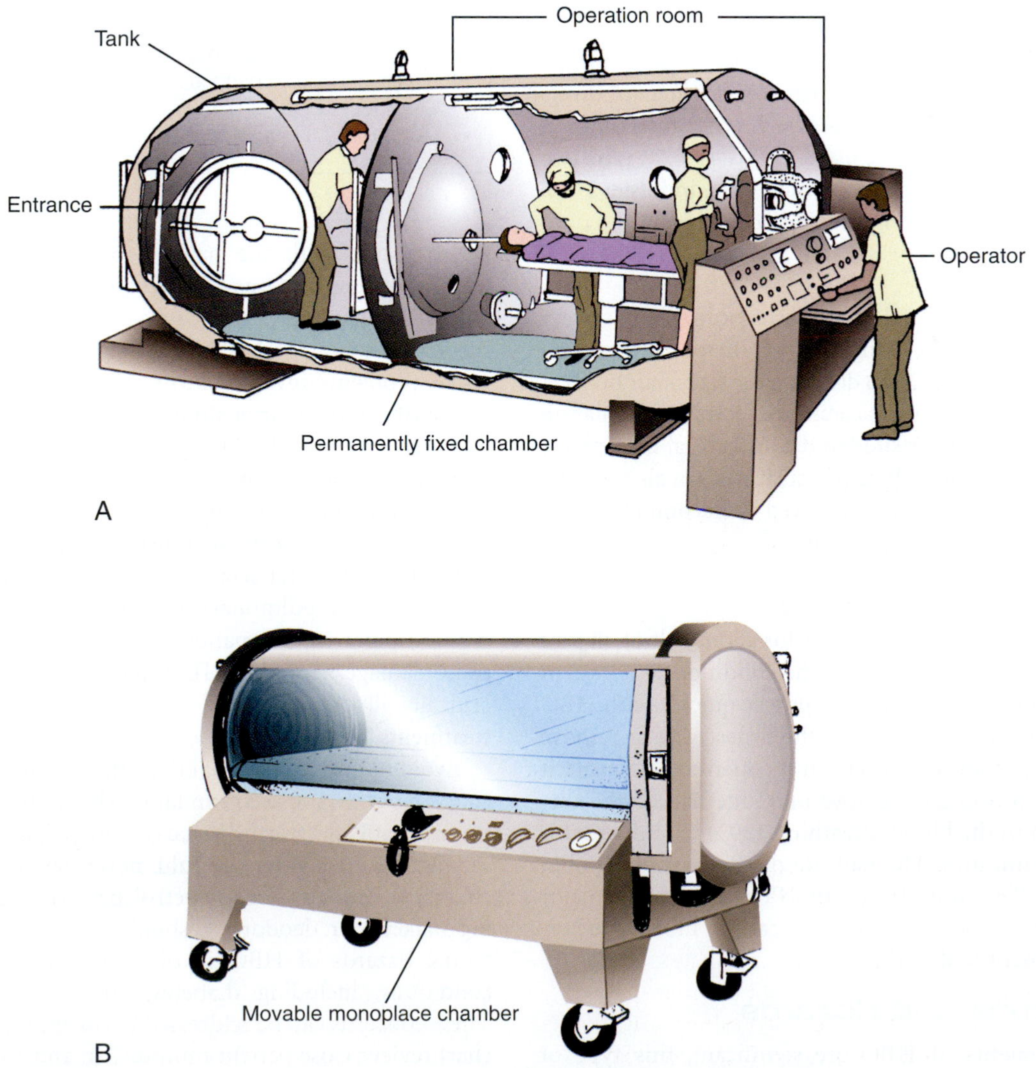

FIGURE 41-25 A, Fixed hyperbaric chamber. **B,** Monoplace chamber.

Box 41-6 Indications for Hyperbaric Oxygen Therapy

ACUTE CONDITIONS
- Decompression sickness
- Air or gas embolism
- Carbon monoxide and cyanide poisoning
- Acute traumatic ischemia (compartment syndrome, crush injury)
- Acute peripheral arterial insufficiency
- Intracranial abscesses
- Crush injuries and suturing of severed limbs
- Clostridial gangrene
- Necrotizing soft tissue infection
- Ischemic skin graft or flap

CHRONIC CONDITIONS
- Diabetic wounds of the lower extremities and other nonhealing wounds
- Refractory osteomyelitis
- Actinomycosis (chronic systemic abscesses)
- Radiation necrosis (HBO as an adjunct to conventional treatment)

Box 41-7 Criteria for Hyperbaric Oxygen Therapy for Acute Carbon Monoxide Poisoning

- History of unconsciousness
- Presence of neuropsychiatric abnormality
- Presence of cardiac instability or cardiac ischemia
- Carboxyhemoglobin level 25% (lower levels for children and pregnant women)

Box 41-8 Major Complications of Hyperbaric Oxygen Therapy

BAROTRAUMA
- Ear or sinus trauma
- Tympanic membrane rupture
- Alveolar overdistention and pneumothorax
- Gas embolism

OXYGEN TOXICITY
- CNS toxic reaction
- Pulmonary toxic reaction

OTHER
- Fire
- Sudden decompression
- Reversible visual changes
- Claustrophobia
- Decreased cardiac output

Indications

HBO has long been accepted as the primary treatment of divers with decompression sickness. Several other of the most common indications for HBO therapy are listed in Box 41-6.[45,47] The two most common acute conditions for which RTs administer HBO are air embolism and carbon monoxide poisoning.[45,48,51]

Air Embolism

Air embolism is a complication that can occur with certain cardiovascular procedures, lung biopsy, hemodialysis, and central line placement. HBO can decrease the size of air bubbles which may otherwise reach the cerebral or cardiac circulation and can cause symptoms or sudden death. Typical therapy for air embolism involves immediate pressurization in air to 6 ATA for 15 to 30 minutes. This step is followed by decompression to 2.8 ATA with prolonged O_2 treatment.[46-48]

Carbon Monoxide Poisoning

Carbon monoxide poisoning accounts for about half of all poisoning deaths in the United States. The condition of a patient with carbon monoxide poisoning improves quickly with HBO treatment because this treatment is the fastest way to remove carbon monoxide from the blood.[51] If a patient breathes air, it takes more than 5 hours to remove only one half of the carboxyhemoglobin in the blood. Breathing 100% O_2 reduces this “half-life” to 80 minutes. The half-life of carboxyhemoglobin under HBO at 3 ATA is only 23 minutes. Box 41-7 lists the major criteria for selecting patients with acute carbon monoxide poisoning for treatment with HBO.[51]

Complications and Hazards

Although the benefits of HBO are significant, this type of therapy also has significant risks. As a result, the benefits should be compared with the hazards before therapy is initiated. Common complications of HBO are listed in Box 41-8.[46] These complications are generally caused by high pressure, O_2 toxicity, fire, or worsening of certain existing conditions. The most frequent problems involve barotrauma to closed body cavities, such as the middle ear or sinuses. Pneumothorax and air embolism also are possible during HBO treatment but are rare in patients with normal lungs.

O_2 at high pressure can rarely be neurotoxic. Early signs of impending CNS toxicity include twitching, sweating, pallor, and restlessness, and later seizures and convulsions.[47]

In terms of pulmonary O_2 toxicity, HBO treatments do not normally expose patients to high PO_2 long enough to cause damage. However, HBO may have an additive effect on critically ill patients who receive high FiO_2 between HBO treatments.[46,47]

Avoiding fire and sudden decompression are primary safety concerns. Only 100% cotton fabric should be used to avoid fire from a static electrical discharge. Other ignition sources such as matches or lighters should never be brought into HBO chambers, and alcohol- or petroleum-based products, including makeup or deodorant, should never be used. Other potential hazards of HBO involve the aggravation of existing conditions, including diabetes, epilepsy, and hypertension. These concerns can be addressed by an appropriate history and chart review, close patient monitoring, and appropriate adjustment of therapy.

There are numerous relative contraindications for HBO, many of which relate to the potential complications and hazards noted earlier. Relative contraindications include inner ear infections and seizure disorders. Absolute contradictions include an untreated pneumothorax and congenital heart defects resulting in dependency on a patent ductus arteriosus for survival.[47]

Troubleshooting

Although fire hazards restrict the use of certain electronic equipment, some state-of-the-art monitors and ventilators with solid-state circuitry can be used within the chamber. This equipment allows intensive care of critically ill patients.[45]

In regard to ventilator use, reductions in delivered tidal volume should be expected and corrected. Additionally, tracheostomy or endotracheal tubes with foam or fluid-filled cuffs should generally be used to preserve cuff integrity under pressure. If not accounted for, reduced tidal volumes and leaks can lead to respiratory hypercapnia and acidosis. Hypercapnia can result in respiratory acidosis and can worsen CNS toxicity owing to cerebral vasodilation.[47] Generally, pressure-regulating and flow-regulating equipment used in a hyperbaric chamber must be specifically designed for operation or equipment appropriately modified to function properly in such conditions.

OTHER MEDICAL GAS THERAPIES

O_2 is not the only medical gas administered by RTs. The potent pulmonary vasodilator **nitric oxide (NO)**, and helium-O_2 mixtures are also among other medical gases administered by RTs.

Nitric Oxide Therapy

Mode of Action

NO gas is a colorless, odorless, highly diffusible, and lipid-soluble free radical that oxidizes quickly to nitrogen dioxide (NO_2) in the presence of O_2. NO is normally produced in small amounts within the human body and activates guanylate cyclase, which catalyzes the production of cyclic guanosine 3′,5′-monophosphate (cGMP). The end result is that increased cGMP levels cause vascular smooth muscle relaxation.[52] The therapeutic benefit of inhaled NO stems from improved blood flow to ventilated alveoli. The result is a reduction in intrapulmonary shunting, improvement in arterial oxygenation, and a decrease in pulmonary vascular resistance and pulmonary arterial pressure.

Indications

Inhaled NO has been approved by the U.S. Food and Drug Administration (FDA) for use in conjunction with mechanical ventilation, in treating term and near-term (>34 weeks) neonates with hypoxic (type I) respiratory failure with associated pulmonary hypertension. As a result of the clinical benefits of reduced pulmonary vascular resistance, improved oxygenation, and less need for a highly invasive method for increasing tissue oxygenation known as *extracorporeal membrane oxygenation,* inhaled NO is a mainstay therapy for near-term neonates with this type of respiratory failure.[53]

In adults, studies have shown that inhaled NO has been effective in treating pulmonary hypertension associated with acute respiratory distress syndrome (ARDS). However, these benefits seem to be short-lived, and no significant improvement in clinical outcomes, including ventilator days and mortality, have been shown to date. However, inhaled nitric oxide is frequently used for the management of patients with acute or chronic pulmonary hypertension as a result of pulmonary or cardiac disease and as a diagnostic tool for assessing pulmonary vascular responsiveness prior to heart transplantation or other cardiac surgical procedures. But because of the high cost of nitric oxide, and the lower cost of alternative drug therapies, including inhaled epoprostenol sodium (Flolan) and similar medications (discussed in Chapter 35), most try to avoid the use of nitric oxide. Inhaled NO in adults has not been approved by the FDA. Irrespective, the potential indications for inhaled NO are listed in Box 41-9.[53,54]

Dosing

The amount of NO needed to improve oxygenation or decrease pulmonary vascular pressure in neonates or adults is relatively low. The therapeutic range of NO is 2 to 20 ppm, and an initial dose of 20 ppm is commonly used. Treatment should be continued until underlying oxygenation desaturation has resolved. For many patients, dosages often can be reduced to less than 20 ppm at the end of 4 hours of initial treatment, as tolerated. At these levels, NO has minimal toxicity.[52-54]

Toxicity and Adverse Effects

Most of the toxic effects of NO are caused by its chemical by-products, especially NO_2. NO_2 is produced spontaneously whenever NO is exposed to O_2. NO_2 is more toxic than NO. Levels greater than 10 ppm can cause cell damage, hemorrhage, pulmonary edema, and death. The U.S. Occupational Safety and Health Administration has set the safety limit for NO_2 exposure at 5 ppm. Properly set up NO delivery systems safely and easily achieve this limit.[55]

Other harmful chemical by-products produced in reaction with NO include methemoglobin and peroxynitrite (produced when NO reacts with superoxide). Although it can occur with NO administration, methemoglobinemia probably is not a large problem considering the doses commonly used and the

Box 41-9 Potential Uses for Inhaled Nitric Oxide

- ARDS
- Persistent pulmonary hypertension of the newborn
- Primary pulmonary hypertension
- Pulmonary hypertension after cardiac surgery
- Cardiac transplantation
- Acute pulmonary embolism
- COPD
- Congenital diaphragmatic hernia
- Sickle cell disease
- Testing pulmonary vascular responsiveness

Box 41-10	Adverse Effects Associated With Nitric Oxide Therapy

- Poor or paradoxical response
- Methemoglobinemia
- Increased left ventricular filling pressure
- Complications of certain cardiac anomalies (coarctation of the aorta)
- Rebound hypoxemia, pulmonary hypertension

Box 41-11	Features of Ideal Nitric Oxide Delivery System

- Dependability and safety
- Delivery of a precise and stable dose of NO
- Limited production of nitrogen dioxide
- Accurate monitoring of NO and nitrogen dioxide levels
- Maintenance of adequate patient ventilation

required monitoring systems discussed later in this section. Peroxynitrite can cause severe cell damage; however, there is no hard evidence supporting its toxic effects during NO administration.

Potential adverse effects associated with NO therapy are listed in Box 41-10.[55] A poor or paradoxical response to NO has been observed in some patients. Of patients with ARDS, 40% do not have initial improvement in oxygenation with NO therapy, and some patients have experienced more severe hypoxemia (probably because of a worsening ventilation/perfusion imbalance when no shunt was present). NO inhibits platelet agglutination; however, no significant increase in bleeding time has been reported in NO trials with human subjects. Because it can quickly reduce right ventricular afterload, NO may increase left ventricular filling pressure in some patients. In the presence of congestive heart failure, this effect could cause or worsen pulmonary edema. Concerns involving increased left heart pressures also account for inhaled NO being contraindicated for neonates with certain cardiac and vascular anomalies such as coarctation of the aorta.[53] In certain patients, the withdrawal of NO has resulted in development of hypoxemia and pulmonary hypertension, perhaps worse than they were before therapy was started. This phenomenon is known as a *rebound effect*. This rebound effect occurs because the administration of nitric oxide depresses the body's normal production of NO. When NO is finally discontinued, FiO_2 frequently needs to be initially increased then slowly reduced to baseline.[52]

Although NO has been used safely with other drugs and treatments such as dopamine, steroids, surfactant, and high-frequency ventilation, the interaction of NO with other medications is still being studied. One investigational area may involve the study of patients receiving both inhaled NO and other NO-related compounds such as nitroglycerin and the possible development of methemoglobinemia or systemic hypotension.[54]

Methods of Administration

NO is administered to mechanically ventilated patients through a system with the capability for operator-determined concentration of NO in the breathing gas, a constant concentration throughout the breathing cycle, and a concentration that does not cause generation of excessive inhaled NO_2. Features of an ideal NO delivery system are listed in Box 41-11.

The INOmax® DS_{IR}® Plus (Delivery System-Infrared) (Ikaria, Hampton, New Jersey) shown in Figure 41-26 provides these features.[54,56] The INOmax DS_{IR} Plus delivers INOmax (nitric oxide) for inhalation into the inspiratory limb of the patient's breathing circuit in a manner that provides a constant dose of NO, as preset by the clinician, throughout inspiration. This configuration tracks the ventilator flow waveforms and delivers

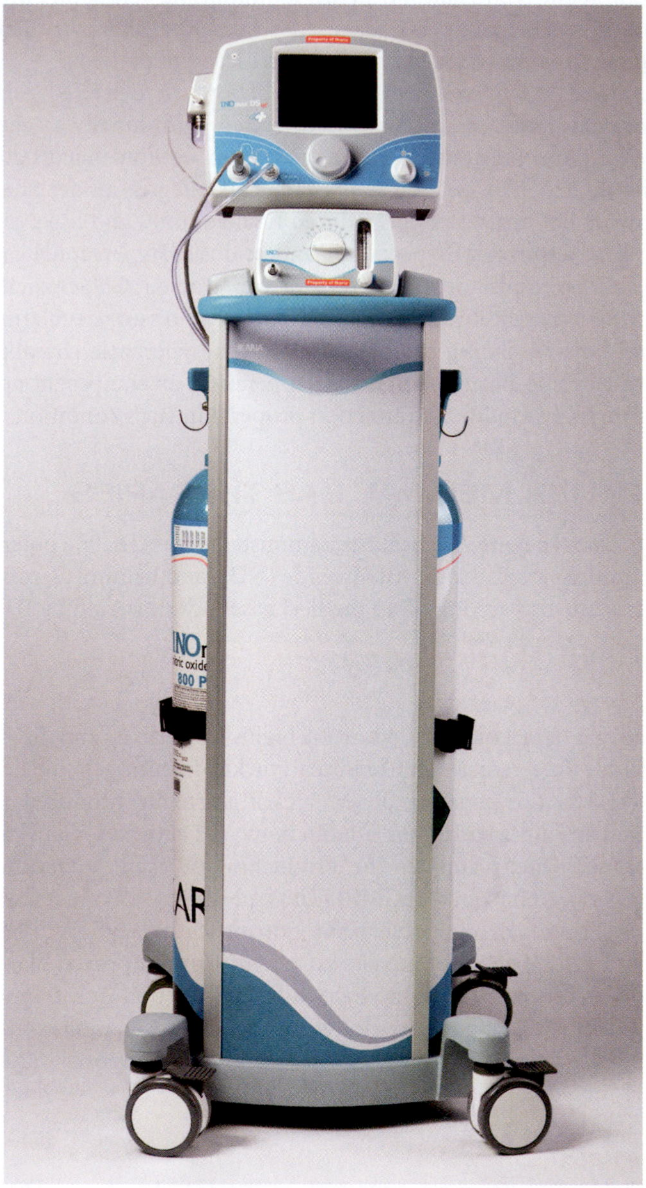

FIGURE 41-26 INOmax DS Plus (Delivery System-Plus) delivery system for administration of NO to mechanically ventilated patients. (Courtesy Ikaria, Hampton, New Jersey.)

a synchronized and proportional dose of NO through the injector module into the ventilator circuit. A monitoring system continuously displays inspired FiO_2, NO_2, and NO. The INOmax DS_{IR} Plus employs several alarm systems to alert clinicians, including alarms for high and low NO and FiO_2 and high NO_2. Other alarms notify clinicians when the source gas (INOmax) pressure is low, or if there is a monitoring failure. The device also informs clinicians when high calibrations for the monitoring system are due; low calibrations are performed automatically by the device without requiring user intervention.[57]

The delivery system entails the use of cylinder mixtures of NO containing up to 800 ppm of NO with the balance being nitrogen. This high concentration of NO is diluted by gases in the ventilator circuit before delivery to the patient. Because adding NO to the circuit decreases the FiO_2 (up to 10 percent at 80 ppm), O_2 concentration must be continuously monitored downstream from the titration site.

The INOmax DS_{IR} Plus can also be interfaced with several specialty ventilators including high-frequency oscillators, jet ventilators, and anesthesia machines. Inhaled NO has also been used with noninvasive ventilation. Other special considerations apply, and resources such as ventilator procedure manuals and department policy and procedures should be reviewed to help ensure proper setup and patient safety.[56]

The administration of inhaled NO to spontaneously breathing patients is also possible. The INOmax DS_{IR} Plus has been validated with high- and low-flow nasal cannula systems and some nasal CPAP systems.[56]

Withdrawing Therapy

Care must be taken when NO therapy is withdrawn to prevent the rebound effect. First, the NO level should be reduced to the lowest effective dose (ideally ≤5 ppm). Second, the patient's condition should be hemodynamically stable, and the patient should be able to maintain adequate oxygenation while breathing a moderate FiO_2 (≤0.4) on low levels of positive end expiratory pressure. Third, the patient should be hyperoxygenated (FiO_2 0.6 to 0.7) just before discontinuation of NO inhalation. Close monitoring of patients and use of these measures usually avoid an increase in pulmonary artery pressure and hypoxemia with withdrawal of nitric oxide.[53]

Helium-Oxygen Therapy

Indications

The value of helium as a therapeutic gas is based solely on its low density. As detailed in Chapter 6, when flow is turbulent, driving pressure varies with the square of the flow. Because flow in the large airways is mainly turbulent, breathing a low-density gas mixture can decrease the driving pressure needed to move gas in and out of this area. With less pressure needed to move gas through the large airways, the patient's work of breathing decreases. However, this effect is limited to large airway obstruction (flow in the small airways is not turbulent).

Helium-O_2 has been used for more than 70 years as an adjunct tool in the management of large airway obstruction.[58] **Heliox therapy** has been shown to be effective in treating acute obstructive disorders.[59,60] Either alone or combined with other therapies such as bronchodilators, helium-O_2 therapy has been shown to decrease the respiratory rate, the level of dyspnea, and the need for intubation and mechanical ventilation in patients with reversible obstructive disorders.[61] Specifically, heliox therapy has yielded promising results in the management of acute upper airway obstruction of varying origin,[62] postextubation stridor in pediatric trauma patients,[63] acute severe asthma, and croup.[64]

Guidelines for Use

Because it is inert and unable to support life, helium always must be mixed with at least 20% O_2. The most common combination is 80% helium and 20% O_2. From the standpoint of its ability to oxygenate, this mixture is comparable to air, but helium is used in place of nitrogen. Although air has a density of 1.293 g/L, the density of an 80% helium mixture is 0.429 g/L. For a comparable flow through constricted large airways, this low-density mixture can dramatically decrease the work of breathing.

Most commonly, premixed, commercial heliox cylinders are used at the bedside. These premixed cylinders are commonly available in an 80:20 or a 70:30 combination. The 70% helium and 30% O_2 mixture has a density of 0.554 g/L and can provide additional O_2 for the management of the hypoxemia that can occur with large airway obstruction. Other combinations such as 60:40 and 65:35 mixtures are being examined and show promising results.[61,65]

The low-density benefit of heliox is the same attribute that presents challenges in selecting a delivery device. Because helium is highly diffusible, administration through low-flow systems such as a nasal cannula tends not to deliver sufficient concentrations to treat obstructive disorders in adults. However, heliox administered via cannulas with an adequate seal at the nares has shown to be effective in some infants.[66] Irrespective, heliox should generally be delivered to most spontaneously breathing patients via a tight-fitting nonrebreathing mask with a fully functional valved exhalation port. The delivery system should be high flow, sufficient to meet or exceed the patient's minute ventilation requirements. Closed systems with demand valves and reservoirs or the use of demand regulators has proved to be suitable for delivering heliox to patients with artificial airways. Ideally, an O_2 analyzer should be used to confirm the FiO_2 of the heliox mixture output flowing to the patient and all such patients should be closely monitored, including with a pulse oximetry.[67]

Helium mixtures can be given through a cuffed tracheal airway with a positive pressure ventilator. However, the performance of ventilators in delivering heliox tends to vary significantly by model, and only some of them have received FDA clearance for such use. Consequently, RTs should ensure that an appropriate ventilator is being used to administer heliox, determine if a conversion factor is needed to adjust settings, and ensure that the patient is monitored closely while such an approach is being used.[68] Pressure measurements on mechanical ventilators are always accurate during the use of heliox but volume measurements can be grossly inaccurate if the ventilator is not calibrated to a heliox mixture.

Blenders have also been used to administer heliox. When a blender is used, the 80:20 heliox is generally attached to the air inlet, and an O_2 analyzer is placed downstream. However, because the accuracy of blenders tends to vary, the system's FiO_2 readings should first be tested, and the difference between the set and actual FiO_2 should be known.

Heliox has also been combined with bronchodilator therapy to treat acute obstructive disorders such as status asthmaticus. Heliox improves aerosol deposition mainly because of a reduction in turbulence and less impaction and medication loss. Because of the low density of heliox, when a nebulizer is driven by heliox, the liter flow must be increased from the customary 6 L/min to 10 to 12 L/min to achieve the same volume of aerosol generated per unit of time.

When heliox is given alone or as part of nebulization, the RT should realize that a typical hospital O_2 flowmeter is inaccurate because of the lower density of helium. Flowmeters calibrated for helium should be used to ensure accurate delivery. However, correction factors are available for O_2 flowmeters. The correction for an 80:20 helium-O_2 mixture is 1.8; this means that for every 10 L/min indicated flow, 10 × 1.8, or 18 L/min, of the 80:20 mixture actually leaves the flowmeter. For delivery of a specific flow from an 80:20 helium-O_2 source, the RT sets the flowmeter to the desired flow divided by 1.8. If a flow of 9 L/min of an 80:20 helium-O_2 mixture is needed, the RT sets the flowmeter to 9/1.8, or 5 L/min. Factors for any other mixture can be calculated if needed. The factor for a 70:30 helium-O_2 mixture is 1.6.

In addition to special flow considerations, the RT should use an O_2 analyzer to monitor heliox (actually O_2) concentrations continuously between the source of the mixture and the patient. The basis for this recommendation is that the gas is either helium or O_2, and if the FiO_2 is known, assuming there are no leaks, the remaining gas is helium. This monitoring helps ensure that the patient is receiving the therapeutic benefits of a less dense gas while maintaining the appropriate FiO_2.

Troubleshooting and Hazards

The low density of helium mixtures makes them poor vehicles for aerosol transport. High-density bland water aerosols are difficult to deliver with helium mixtures. The low density of helium mixtures also makes coughing less effective. If the patient can develop an effective cough, this problem can be rectified by means of washing out the helium before coughing.

The most common side effect of helium is a benign one. When a patient is breathing a helium mixture, the spoken word is badly distorted at a pitch so high as to make it almost unintelligible. This effect is caused by the passage of a low-density gas through the vocal cords on exhalation.

A more serious problem is hypoxemia associated with breathing helium mixtures.[66,69] Although this problem may have been caused by using too low an O_2 concentration (20%), there is another possibility. Very rarely, some commercial helium-O_2 cylinders stored for long periods of time have been found to contain these gases in an unmixed, or separated, state. The only way to avoid this potential hazard is to analyze the O_2 concentration coming from the cylinder before administering the gas.

As clinical applications for heliox have expanded, other hazards have emerged. One potential problem is volume-induced lung injury when heliox is administered via a mechanical ventilator. This risk can be addressed by using only ventilators approved by the FDA for heliox administration. In addition, the lower density of helium-O_2 mixtures may result in greater variability in medication delivery to the airways. Careful patient monitoring during such therapy can help minimize this concern. Another rare but possible problem is hypothermia to infants receiving heliox via an oxyhood. This risk results from the high thermal conductivity of helium and can be avoided by warming and humidifying the heliox gas.[66]

Carbon Dioxide–Oxygen (Carbogen) Therapy

Although rarely used, CO_2-O_2 mixtures (carbogen) have been employed to treat hiccups, carbon monoxide poisoning, and some neonates with congenital cardiac anomalies, and to prevent complete washout of CO_2 during cardiopulmonary bypass and extracorporeal gas exchange. More recently, it has been investigated as a treatment for hearing loss and seizures. However, the application of carbogen in clinical settings has been quite limited given the potential adverse effects of hypoxemia, premature ventricular contractions, hypertension, and muscle twitching.[70]

Carbogen is supplied in compressed gas cylinders as either 5%:95% or 7%:93% CO_2-O_2 mixtures. It can be administered to patients with a snug-fitting nonrebreathing mask, with a flow sufficient to prevent the reservoir from collapsing during inhalation. Because of the potential adverse effects, patients receiving carbogen should be monitored closely, especially at 7%:93% mixtures. If any significant adverse effects are noted, the therapy should be stopped.[70]

SUMMARY CHECKLIST

- O_2 therapy is used to (1) correct acute hypoxemia, (2) decrease the symptoms of chronic hypoxemia, and (3) decrease cardiopulmonary workload.
- The need for supplemental O_2 can be assessed with laboratory measures, clinical history, and bedside patient evaluation.
- In the care of adults, children, and infants older than 28 days, O_2 therapy is indicated if PaO_2 is less than 60 mm Hg or SaO_2 is less than 90%.
- Exposure to 100% O_2 for more than 24 hours should be avoided whenever possible; high FiO_2 is acceptable if the concentration can be decreased to 0.70 within 2 days and to 0.50 or less in 5 days.
- Concern that O_2 therapy can cause hypoventilation should never preclude administration of O_2 to a patient in need. Prevention of hypoxia always is the first priority.

- If an O_2 delivery system provides all of a patient's inspired gas, FiO_2 remains stable. If the device provides only part of the inspired gas, air dilutes the O_2, and FiO_2 can vary.
- O_2 provided with low-flow devices such as a nasal cannula always is diluted with air; the result is a low and variable FiO_2.
- Reservoir devices can provide higher FiO_2 than low-flow systems or can be used to conserve O_2.
- To avoid rebreathing, a flow of at least 5 L/min should be used with O_2 masks; for reservoir masks with bags, the flow must be sufficient to prevent bag collapse.
- A nonrebreathing reservoir circuit can provide a full range of FiO_2 (21% to 100%) at any needed flow to both intubated and nonintubated patients.
- High-flow systems supply a given O_2 concentration at a flow of at least 60 L/min.
- A high-flow nasal cannula can be useful in treating moderate hypoxemia, especially for patients who don't tolerate oxygen masks and need supplemental humidity.
- Because entrainment devices dilute source O_2 with air, they always provide less than 100% O_2. The more air entrained, the higher the total flow, but the delivered FiO_2 is lower.
- Air-entrainment nebulizers should be treated as fixed-performance devices only when set to deliver low O_2 concentration (≤35%).
- One way to achieve high FiO_2 with air-entrainment nebulizers is to connect two or more devices together in parallel.
- Back pressure decreases both the volume of entrained air and the total flow output of air-entrainment devices.
- A blending system allows precise control over FiO_2 and total flow output; most blending systems qualify as true fixed-performance delivery devices.
- An operational check of an O_2 blender should always be conducted before the device is used.
- O_2 therapy enclosures are used mainly in the care of children and infants. Problems include limited and highly variable FiO_2 and temperature control.
- The three Ps—purpose, patient, and performance of the device—should be considered in the selection or recommendation of an O_2 delivery system.
- In HBO therapy, O_2 is administered at a pressure greater than 1 atm for management of conditions such as air embolism and carbon monoxide poisoning.
- Inhaled NO improves blood flow to ventilated alveoli, reduces intrapulmonary shunting, improves arterial oxygenation, and decreases pulmonary vascular resistance and pulmonary arterial pressure.
- Heliox mixtures are used to reduce the work of breathing in large airways obstruction. The low density of heliox makes standard O_2 flowmeters inaccurate and provides inaccurate volume and flow measurement on ventilators not calibrated for its use.
- Carbogen is used in the management of some neonates with congenital heart disease, to treat hiccups and to prevent complete washout of CO_2 during cardiopulmonary bypass or extracorporeal gas exchange.

References

1. Fulmer JF, Snider GL: American College of Chest Physicians/National Heart, Lung and Blood Institute National Conference on Oxygen Therapy. *Chest* 86:224, 1984.
2. American Association for Respiratory Care: Clinical practice guideline: oxygen therapy for adults in the acute care facility. *Respir Care* 47:717, 2002.
3. American Association for Respiratory Care: Clinical practice guideline: oxygen therapy in the home or extended care facility—2007 revision and update. *Respir Care* 52:1063, 2007.
4. American Association for Respiratory Care: Clinical practice guideline: selection of an oxygen delivery device for neonatal and pediatric patients. *Respir Care* 47:707, 2002.
5. Stoller JK, Panos RJ, Krachman S, et al: Oxygen therapy for patients with COPD: current evidence and the long-term oxygen treatment trial. *Chest* 138:179, 2010.
6. Li J, Huang Y, Fei GH: The evaluation of cognitive impairment and relevant factors in patients with chronic obstructive pulmonary disease. *Respiration* 85:98, 2013.
7. Orr R, Smith LJ, Cuttica NJ: Pulmonary hypertension in advanced chronic obstructive pulmonary disease. *Curr Opin Pulm Med* 18:138, 2012.
8. Saugstad OD, Aune D: Optimal oxygenation of extremely low birth weight infants: a meta-analysis and systematic review of the oxygen saturation target studies. *Neonatology* 105:55, 2014.
9. Thomson L, Paton J: Oxygen toxicity. *Paediatr Respir Rev* 15:120, 2014.
10. Auten RL, Davis JM: Oxygen toxicity and reactive oxygen species: the devil is in the details. *Pediatr Res* 66:121, 2009.
11. Sola A: Oxygen in neonatal anesthesia: friend or foe? *Curr Opin Anaesthesiol* 21:332, 2008.
12. Eastwood GM, Peck L, Young H, et al: Oxygen administration and monitoring for ward adult patients in a teaching hospital. *Intern Med J* 16:332, 2010.
13. Moradkhan R, Sinoway LI: Revisiting the role of oxygen therapy in cardiac patients. *J Am Coll Cardiol* 56:1013, 2010.
14. Austin MA, Wills KE, Blizzard L, et al: Effect of high flow oxygen on mortality in chronic obstructive pulmonary disease patients in prehospital setting: randomized controlled trial. *BMJ* 341:5462, 2010.
15. Pilcher J, Cameron L, Braithwaite I, et al: Comparative audit of oxygen use in the prehospital setting, in acute COPD exacerbation, over 5 years. *Emerg Med* 10:1136, 2013.
16. Make B, Krachman S, Panos RJ, et al: Oxygen therapy in advanced COPD: in whom does it work? *Semin Respir Crit Care Med* 31:334, 2010.
17. Lima DF, Dela Coleta K, Tanni SE, et al: Potentially modifiable predictors of mortality in patients treated with long-term oxygen therapy. *Respir Med* 105:470, 2011.
18. Wick JY: Long-term oxygen therapy: battling breathlessness. *Consult Pharm* 27:826, 2012.
19. Chen ML, Guo L, Smith LE, et al: High or low oxygen saturation and severe retinopathy of prematurity: a meta-analysis. *Pediatrics* 125:e1483, 2010.
20. O'Brien J: Absorption atelectasis: incidence and clinical implications. *AANA J* 81:205, 2013.
21. Yardley IE: Surgical fires, a clear and present danger. *Surgeon* 8:87, 2010.
22. Lee GJ, Lee SW, Oh YM, et al: A pilot study comparing two oxygen delivery methods for patients' comfort and administration of oxygen. *Respir Care* 59:1191, 2013.
23. Ayhan H, Iyigun E, Tastan S, et al: Comparison of two different oxygen delivery methods in early postoperative period: randomized trial. *J Adv Nurs* 65:1237, 2009.
24. Udoji TN, Berkowitz DM, Bechara RI, et al: The use of transtracheal oxygen therapy in the management of severe hepatopulmonary syndrome after liver transplant. *Transplant Proc* 45:3316, 2013.
25. Lenfant F, Pean D, Brisard L, et al: Oxygen delivery during transtracheal oxygenation: a comparison of two manual devices. *Anesth Analg* 111:922, 2010.
26. Marti S, Pajares V, Morante F, et al: Are oxygen –conserving devices effective for correcting exercise hypoxemia? *Respir Care* 58:1606, 2013.

27. Slessarev M, Somogyi R, Preiss D, et al: Efficiency of oxygen administration: sequential gas delivery versus "flow into cone" methods. *Crit Care Med* 34: 829, 2006.
28. Lee GJ, Oh YM, Oh SK, et al: Synchronization of oxygen delivery with breathing pattern for enhanced comfort: a bench study. *Respir Care* 58:498, 2013.
29. Hui DS, Chow BK, Chu LC, et al: Exhaled air and aerosolized droplet dispersion during application of a jet nebulizer. *Chest* 135:648, 2009.
30. Barach AL, Eckman M: A physiologically controlled oxygen mask apparatus. *Anesthesiology* 2:421, 1941.
31. Soto-Ruiz KM, Peacock WF, Varon J: The men and history behind the Venturi mask. *Resuscitation* 82:244, 2011.
32. Maggiore SM, Idone FA, Vaschetto R, et al: Nasal high-flow vs venturi mask oxygen therapy after extubation: effects on oxygenation, comfort and clinical outcome. *Am J Respir Crit Care Med* 190:282, 2014.
33. Redding JS, McAfee DD, Parham AM: Oxygen concentrations received from commonly used delivery systems. *South Med J* 71:169, 1978.
34. Woolner DF, Larkin J: An analysis of the performance of a variable Venturi-type oxygen mask. *Anaesth Intensive Care* 8:44, 1980.
35. Cairo JM: *Respiratory care equipment*, ed 9, St. Louis, 2014, Mosby.
36. Caille V, Ehrmann S, Boissinot E, et al: Influence of jet nebulization and oxygen delivery on the fraction of inspired oxygen: an experimental model. *J Aerosol Med Pulm Drug Del* 22:255, 2009.
37. Parke RL, Eccleston ML, McGuinness SP: The effects of flow on pressure during high-flow oxygen therapy. *Respir Care* 56:1151, 2011.
38. Karmann U, Roth F: Prevention of accidents associated with air-oxygen mixers. *Anaesthesia* 37:680, 1982.
39. Inaccurate O_2 concentrations from oxygen-air proportioners. *Health Devices* 18:366, 1989.
40. Walsh BK, Brooks TM, Grenier BM: Oxygen therapy in the neonatal environment. *Respir Care* 54:1193, 2009.
41. Kapadis VS, Chalak LF, Sparks JE, et al: Resuscitation of preterm with limited versus high oxygen strategy. *Pediatrics* 132:1488, 2013.
42. Hummler H, Fuchs H, Schmid M: Automated adjustments of inspired fraction of oxygen to avoid hypoxemia and hyperoxemia in neonates—a systematic review on clinical studies. *Klin Padiatr* 226:204, 2014.
43. Bettoncelli G, Blasi F, Brusasco V: The clinical and integrated management of COPD. *Sarcoidosis Vasc Diffuse Lung Dis* 12:31, 2014.
44. Stoller JK: Implementing change in respiratory care. *Respir Care* 55:749, 2010.
45. Camporesi EM, Bosco G: Mechanisms of action of hyperbaric oxygen therapy. *Undersea Hyperb Med* 41:247, 2014.
46. Bullock MR: Hyperbaric oxygen therapy. *J Neurosurg* 112:1078, 2010.
47. Savage S: New medical therapy: hyperbarics. *Tenn Med* 103:39, 2010.
48. Moon RE: Hyperbaric oxygen treatment for air or gas embolism. *Undersea Hyperb Med* 41:159, 2014.
49. Rollins MD, Gibson JJ, Hunt TK, et al: Wound oxygen levels during hyperbaric oxygen treatment in healing wounds. *Undersea Hyperb Med* 33:17, 2006.
50. Feldman J, Renda N, Markovits GH, et al: Treatment of carbon monoxide poisoning with hyperbaric oxygen and therapeutic hypothermia. *Undersea Hyperb Med* 40:71, 2013.
51. Clower JH, Hampson NB, Iqbal S, et al: Recipients of hyperbaric oxygen treatment for carbon monoxide poisoning and exposure circumstances. *Am J Emerg Med* 30:846, 2012.
52. Khan MF, Azfar MF, Khurshid SM: The role of inhaled nitric oxide beyond ARDS. *Indian J Crit Care Med* 18:392, 2014.
53. Gadhia MM, Cutter GR, Abman SH: Effects of early inhaled nitric oxide therapy and vitamin A supplementation on the risk for bronchopulmonary dysplasia in premature newborns with respiratory failure. *J Pediatr* 164:744, 2014.
54. Center for Drug Evaluation and Research: *NO labeling (revised)*, Washington, DC, 2010, U.S. Food and Drug Administration.
55. *INOmax (nitric oxide) for inhalation package insert (revised)*, Ikaria, Hampton, 2013, New Jersey.
56. Sosenko IR, Bancalari E: NO for preterm infants at risk for bronchopulmonary dysplasia. *Lancet* 376:308, 2010.
57. Lundberg JO, Weitzberg E: Extrapulmonary effects of nitric oxide inhalation therapy: time to consider new dosing regimes? *Crit Care* 12:406, 2008.
58. Hess DR, Fink JB, Venkataraman ST, et al: The history and physics of heliox. *Respir Care* 51:608, 2006.
59. Moraa I, Sturman N, McGuire T, et al: Heliox for croup in children. *Cochrane Datbase Syst Rev* 7:12, 2013.
60. Hess DR: Heliox and noninvasive positive-pressure ventilation: a role for heliox in exacerbations of chronic obstructive pulmonary disease? *Respir Care* 51:640, 2006.
61. El-Khatib MF, Jamaleddine G, Kanj N, et al: Effect of heliox- and air-driven nebulized bronchodilator therapy on lung function in patients with asthma. *Lung* 192:377, 2014.
62. Frazier MD, Cheifetz IM: The role of heliox in paediatric respiratory diseases. *Paediatr Respir Rev* 11:46, 2010.
63. Berkenbosch JW, Grueber RE, Graff GR, et al: Patterns of helium-oxygen (heliox) usage in the critical care environment. *J Intensive Care Med* 19:335, 2004.
64. Kline-Krammes S, Reed C, Giuliano JS, Jr, et al: Heliox in children with croup: a strategy to hasten improvement. *Air Med J* 31:131, 2012.
65. Bathke P, Gallagher T: Respiratory problems in accident and emergency—the role of helium-oxygen mixtures. *Anaesthesia* 64:576, 2009.
66. Ari A, Harwood R, Sheard M, et al: In vitro comparison of heliox and oxygen in aerosol delivery using pediatric high flow nasal cannula. *Pediatr Pulmonol* 46:795, 2011.
67. Roche-Campo F, Vignaux L, Galia F, et al: Delivery of helium–oxygen mixture during spontaneous breathing: evaluation of three high-concentration face masks. *Intensive Care Med* 37:1787, 2011.
68. Hurford WE, Cheifetz IM: Respiratory controversies in the critical care setting: should heliox be used for mechanically ventilated patients? *Respir Care* 52:582, 2007.
69. Cylinders with unmixed helium/oxygen. *Health Devices* 19:146, 1990.
70. Hare HV, Germuska M, Kelly ME, et al: Comparison of CO_2 in air versus Carbogen for the measurement of cerebrovascular reactivity with magnetic resonance imaging. *J Cereb Blood Flow Metab* 33:1799, 2013.

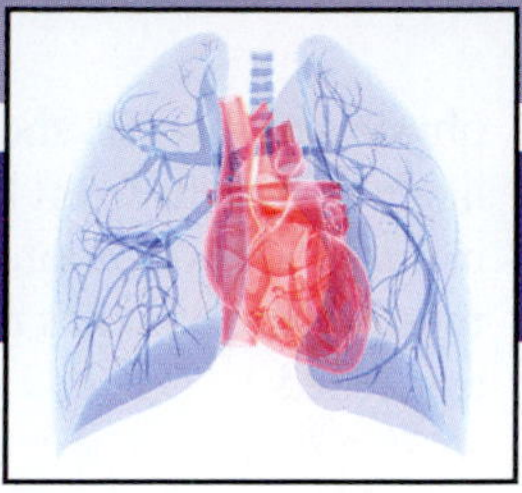

CHAPTER 42

Lung Expansion Therapy

DANIEL F. FISHER

CHAPTER OBJECTIVES

After reading this chapter you will be able to:

- Describe the various causes of atelectasis.
- Identify which patients need lung expansion therapy.
- Define the clinical findings seen in atelectasis.
- Describe how lung expansion therapy works.
- List the indications, hazards, and complications associated with the various modes of lung expansion therapy.
- Describe the primary responsibilities of the respiratory therapist in planning, implementing, and evaluating lung expansion therapy.

CHAPTER OUTLINE

Causes and Types of Atelectasis
 Factors Associated With Causing Atelectasis
Clinical Signs of Atelectasis
Lung Expansion Therapy
 Incentive Spirometry
 Noninvasive Ventilation
 Intermittent Positive Airway Pressure Breathing
 Other Therapies
 Positive Airway Pressure Therapy
Selecting an Approach
 Early Mobilization of the ICU Patient

KEY TERMS

atelectasis
compression atelectasis
continuous positive airway pressure (CPAP)
deep breathing/directed cough
gas absorption atelectasis
incentive spirometry (IS)
intermittent positive airway pressure breathing (IPPB)
lobar atelectasis
noninvasive ventilation (NIV)
positive expiratory pressure (PEP)

Pulmonary complications are common serious problems seen in patients who have undergone thoracic or abdominal surgery.[1,2] Such complications include **atelectasis** (alveolar collapse), pneumonia, and acute respiratory failure. These respiratory problems can be minimized or avoided if proper respiratory care is implemented during the perioperative period. The most common form of therapy used in high-risk patients is lung expansion therapy.

Lung expansion therapy encompasses a variety of respiratory care procedures designed to prevent or correct atelectasis. The most common modalities include **deep breathing/directed cough, incentive spirometry (IS), continuous positive airway pressure (CPAP), positive expiratory pressure (PEP), intermittent positive airway pressure breathing (IPPB)**, and early patient mobilization. The common purpose that all of these techniques share is improving pulmonary function by maximizing alveolar recruitment and optimizing airway clearance.

Various lung expansion therapies can be effective in preventing or correcting atelectasis in selected patients.[1] There is no one specific method to apply in a given situation because no advantage of any one method has been established. In fact, evidence suggests that patient preference is as important as the chosen therapy.[3] The most efficient use of resources is a primary concern with any plan to apply lung expansion therapy.

All of the following therapies share a common goal, to increase functional residual capacity (FRC). In other words, all of these supplemental techniques are designed to simulate a deep breath or sigh. In consultation with the prescribing physician, the RT should assist in identifying patients most likely to benefit from lung expansion therapy, recommend and initiate the appropriate and most efficient therapeutic approach, monitor the patient's response, and alter the treatment regimen as needed.

CAUSES AND TYPES OF ATELECTASIS

Although atelectasis can occur from a large variety of problems, this chapter focuses on the two primary types associated with postoperative or bedridden patients who are breathing spontaneously without mechanical assistance: (1) gas absorption atelectasis and (2) compression atelectasis. **Gas absorption atelectasis** can occur either when there is a complete interruption of ventilation to a section of the lung or when there is a significant shift in ventilation/perfusion ($\dot{V}/\dot{Q}$). Gas distal to an obstruction is absorbed by blood passing through the pulmonary capillaries, which eventually causes partial collapse of the nonventilated alveoli. When ventilation is compromised in a larger airway or bronchus, **lobar atelectasis** can develop.

Compression atelectasis occurs when the transthoracic pressure (the pressure difference between the body surface and the alveoli) exceeds the transalveolar pressure (the pressure difference between the alveoli and pleural space).[2,4,5] Compression atelectasis is primarily caused by mechanisms that increase this pressure gradient. This situation is common with general anesthesia, with the use of sedatives and bed rest, and when deep breathing is painful, as when broken ribs are present or surgery has been performed on the upper abdominal region. Weakening or impairment of the diaphragm can also contribute to compression atelectasis. Compression atelectasis also results from fluid overload. It is a common cause of atelectasis in hospitalized patients. It may occur in combination with gas absorption atelectasis in a patient with excessive airway secretions who breathes with small tidal volumes for a prolonged period.

Factors Associated With Causing Atelectasis

Patients who have difficulty taking deep breaths without assistance include those with significant obesity, patients with neuromuscular disorders, patients under heavy sedation, and patients who have undergone upper abdominal or thoracic surgery. Diaphragmatic position and function is the major contributor to the onset of atelectasis. In an anesthetized patient, there is a cephalad (toward the head) shift of the diaphragm. For patients who are supine and breathing spontaneously, the lower, dependent portion of the diaphragm performs the most movement. The opposite occurs in patients who are paralyzed—the upper portion of the diaphragm is involved in movement.[4,5] Patients undergoing lower abdominal surgery are at relatively less risk for developing atelectasis than patients undergoing upper abdominal or thoracic surgery. Neuromuscular injury patients are prone to respiratory complications, the most common of which is atelectasis. Atelectasis can occur in any patient who cannot or does not take deep breaths periodically and in patients who are restricted to bed rest for any reason.[6] Atelectasis is one of the leading causes of hypoxemia after abdominal surgery and may account for 24% of deaths within 6 days of surgery.[7] It is good clinical practice to consider atelectasis during assessment of postoperative patients.

Impairment of the function of pulmonary surfactant can also have an impact on the development of atelectasis. Surfactants decrease the surface tension of the walls of the alveoli. When there is deterioration of the function of this vital protein, the relative increase in surface tension can cause alveoli to collapse.[5]

Most postoperative patients also have problems coughing effectively because of their reduced ability to take deep breaths. An ineffective cough impairs normal clearance mechanisms and increases the likelihood of retained secretions, which could lead to the development of absorption atelectasis and pneumonia in a patient with excessive mucus production. Patients with a history of lung disease that causes increased mucus production (e.g., chronic bronchitis) are most prone to develop complications in the postoperative period. Similarly, a significant history of cigarette smoking should alert the RT to the high risk for respiratory complications with surgery. Such patients must be identified in the preoperative period and considered strong candidates for airway clearance and lung expansion therapy. Elective surgery for these patients may need to be postponed in some cases until such therapies can be included in the treatment plan. Lung expansion therapy in the postoperative period may help improve clearance of secretions by improving the effectiveness of coughing and secretion removal.

RULE OF THUMB

The closer the incision is to the diaphragm, the greater the risk for postoperative atelectasis. Patients with a history of inadequate nutritional intake, as shown by an albumin level less than 3.2 mg/dl, have an increased risk for pulmonary complications in the postoperative period. This increased risk is most likely due to inadequate strength of the inspiratory muscles to maintain a normal VC.

Laproscopic surgery uses a fiberoptic bundle with small incisions to perform the procedure. Use of this technique has gained widespread acceptance in gastrointestinal procedures because of shortened recovery time, less pain for the patient, and smaller incisions. All of this also lessens the opportunities for development of postoperative pulmonary complications.[8,9] Some studies have shown there is a slightly higher cost both monetarily and in personel time for laparoscopic procedures when compared with open incisions. The benefit of this procedure is the shortened recovery time and fewer complications.[8]

CLINICAL SIGNS OF ATELECTASIS

RTs must be able to recognize the clinical signs of atelectasis in patients so that appropriate therapy can be implemented in a

MINI CLINI

Risk Factors for Atelectasis

PROBLEM: The RT is called to evaluate a 47-year-old obese man admitted to the hospital for upper abdominal surgery. He has a 60 pack-year smoking history and is scheduled for surgery tomorrow morning. Examination reveals bilateral inspiratory and expiratory coarse crackles and expiratory wheezes. He is alert and oriented with normal vital signs. His past medical history is positive for diabetes and kidney stones. What factors are present that predispose this patient for postoperative atelectasis, and what treatment plan should the RT recommend?

Discussion: Several important risk factors are present in this patient. The three most important are positive smoking history, obesity, and the site of surgery (upper abdomen). The findings of adventitious lung sounds and positive smoking history are very suggestive of a current pulmonary problem that would probably require bronchial hygiene and bronchodilators before surgery. Delaying the surgery may be necessary if significant secretion retention is present. Postoperatively, this high-risk patient would need careful monitoring for risks of atelectasis.

timely fashion. The patient's medical history often provides the first clue in identifying atelectasis. Recent upper abdominal or thoracic surgery in any patient should suggest possible atelectasis. A history of chronic lung disease or cigarette smoking or both provides additional evidence that the patient is prone to respiratory complications after major surgery or prolonged bed rest.

The physical signs of atelectasis may be absent or very subtle if the patient has minimal atelectasis. When the atelectasis involves a more significant portion of the lungs, the patient's respiratory rate increases proportionally. Fine, late-inspiratory crackles may be heard over the affected lung region. These crackles are produced by the sudden opening of distal airways with deep breathing. Bronchial-type breath sounds may be present as the lung becomes more consolidated with atelectasis. Diminished breath sounds are common when excessive secretions block the airways and prevent transmission of breath sounds. Tachycardia may be present if atelectasis leads to significant hypoxemia.

RULE OF THUMB

There is a direct relationship between the spontaneous respiratory rate and the degree of atelectasis present. Typically, as atelectasis progresses, respiratory rate increases proportionally.

The chest radiograph is often used to confirm the presence of atelectasis. The atelectatic region of the lung has increased opacity. Evidence of volume loss is present in patients with significant atelectasis. Direct signs of volume loss on the chest film include displacement of the interlobar fissures, crowding of the pulmonary vessels, and air bronchograms. Indirect signs include elevation of the diaphragm; shift of the trachea, heart, or mediastinum; pulmonary opacification; narrowing of the space between the ribs; and compensatory hyperexpansion of the surrounding lung.

LUNG EXPANSION THERAPY

All modes of lung expansion therapy increase lung volume by increasing the transpulmonary pressure (P_{TP}) gradient. As detailed elsewhere in this text (Chapters 46 and 51), P_{TP} gradient represents the difference between the alveolar pressure (P_{alv}) and the pleural pressure (P_{pl}):

$$P_{TP} = P_{alv} - P_{pl}$$

With all else being constant, the greater the P_{TP} gradient, the more that the alveoli expand.

As depicted in Figure 42-1, the P_{TP} gradient can be increased by either (1) decreasing the surrounding P_{pl} (see Figure 42-1, *A*) or (2) increasing the P_{alv} (see Figure 42-1, *B*). A spontaneous deep inspiration increases the P_{TP} gradient by decreasing the P_{pl}. The application of positive pressure to the lungs increases the P_{TP} gradient by increasing the pressure inside the lung (P_{alv}).

All lung expansion therapies use one of these two approaches. IS enhances lung expansion via a spontaneous and sustained decrease in P_{pl}. Positive airway pressure techniques increase P_{alv} in an effort to expand the lung. Positive pressure lung expansion therapies may apply pressure during inspiration only (as in IPPB), during expiration only (as in PEP and flutter valves), or during both inspiration and expiration (CPAP). Although all of these approaches are used in lung expansion therapy, the methods that decrease P_{pl} (e.g., IS) have more of a physiologic effect than the methods that increase P_{alv} and often are most effective. IS and other patient-directed therapies require an alert, cooperative patient who is capable of taking a deep breath.

The goal of any lung expansion therapy should be to implement a plan that provides an effective strategy in the most efficient manner. Staff time and equipment are the two major issues related to efficiency. For a patient with minimal risk of postoperative atelectasis, deep breathing exercises, frequent repositioning, and early ambulation are usually effective and can be done with minimal coaching and time from clinicians

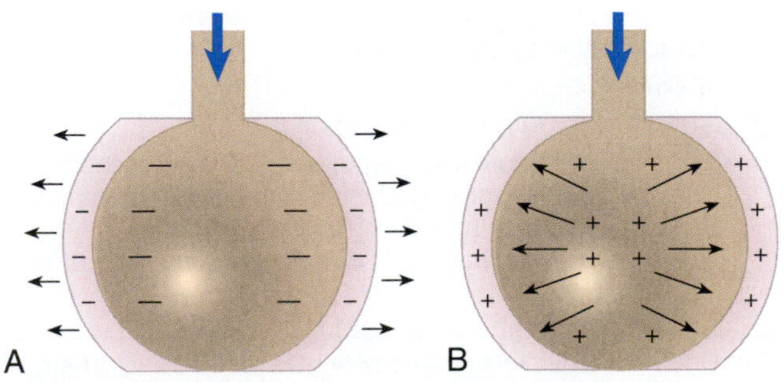

FIGURE 42-1 Transpulmonary pressure gradients with spontaneous inspiration **(A)** and positive pressure inspiration **(B)**.

and without equipment.[5] For a patient at high risk for atelectasis (e.g., a patient undergoing upper abdominal surgery), IS is usually instituted. The additional staff time and equipment are justified in this high-risk group. Positive pressure therapy requires significantly more staff time and equipment and is reserved for high-risk patients who cannot perform IS techniques.

Incentive Spirometry

The purpose of IS is to coach the patient to take a sustained maximal inspiratory (SMI) effort resulting in a decrease in P_{pl} and maintaining the patency of airways at risk for closure. Because of its simplicity, IS has been the mainstay of lung expansion therapy for many years. IS devices are designed to mimic natural sighing by encouraging patients to take slow, deep breaths simulating a yawn or sigh. IS can be performed using devices that provide visual cues to patients when the desired inspiratory flow or volume has been achieved. Incentive spirometry was first described in 1972, which led to the development of a visual feedback device in 1973.[10]

The desired volume and number of repetitions to be performed are initially set by the RT or other qualified caregiver. The inspired volume goal is set on the basis of predicted values or observation of initial performance. The true benefit from IS is best achieved by repeated use and proper technique.[11] The American Association for Respiratory Care (AARC) has developed and published a clinical practice guideline on IS; excerpts from this guideline appear in Clinical Practice Guideline 42-1.

42-1 Incentive Spirometry

AARC Clinical Practice Guideline (Excerpts)*

INDICATIONS

- Presence of conditions predisposing to the development of pulmonary atelectasis (upper abdominal surgery, thoracic surgery, surgery in patients with COPD)
- Presence of pulmonary atelectasis
- Presence of restrictive lung defect associated with quadriplegia or dysfunctional diaphragm

CONTRAINDICATIONS

- Patient cannot be instructed or supervised to ensure appropriate use of device
- Patient cooperation is absent, or patient is unable to understand or demonstrate proper use of device
- Patient is unable to deep breathe effectively (e.g., with VC <10 ml/kg or IC <⅓ predicted)
- Presence of an open tracheal stoma is not a contraindication but requires adaptation of the spirometer

HAZARDS AND COMPLICATIONS

- Ineffective unless closely supervised or performed as ordered
- Inappropriate as sole treatment for major lung collapse or consolidation
- Hyperventilation
- Barotrauma (emphysematous lungs)
- Discomfort secondary to inadequate pain control
- Hypoxia owing to break in mask O_2 therapy
- Exacerbation of bronchospasm
- Fatigue

ASSESSMENT OF NEED

- Surgical procedure involving upper abdomen or thorax
- Conditions predisposing to atelectasis, including immobility, poor pain control, and abdominal binders
- Presence of neuromuscular disease involving respiratory musculature

ASSESSMENT OF OUTCOME

- Absence of or improvement in signs of atelectasis
- Decreased respiratory rate
- Resolution of fever
- Normal pulse rate
- Absence of crackles or presence of or improvement in previously absent or diminished breath sounds
- Normal chest radiograph
- Improved PaO_2 and decreased alveolar-arterial O_2 tension gradient
- Increased VC and peak expiratory flows
- Return of FRC or VC to preoperative values, in absence of lung resection
- Improved inspiratory muscle performance (e.g., attainment of preoperative flow and volume levels, increased FVC)

MONITORING

Direct supervision of every patient performance is unnecessary after the patient has demonstrated mastery of technique; however, preoperative instruction, volume goals, and feedback are essential to optimal performance.

- Observation of patient performance and use
- Frequency of sessions
- Number of breaths per session
- Inspiratory volume or flow goals achieved and 3- to 5-second breath hold maintained
- Effort and motivation
- Periodic observation of patient compliance with technique, with additional instruction as necessary
- Device within reach of patient and patient encouraged to perform independently
- New and increasing inspiratory volumes established each day
- Vital signs

**For complete guidelines, see American Association for Respiratory Care: Clinical practice guidelines: incentive spirometry. Respir Care 56:1600, 2011.*

Physiologic Basis

An SMI is functionally equivalent to performing a functional residual capacity (FRC) to inspiratory capacity (IC) maneuver, followed by a breath hold. Figure 42-2 compares the alveolar and P_{pl} changes occurring during a normal spontaneous breath and an SMI during IS.

During the inspiratory phase of spontaneous breathing, the decrease in P_{pl} caused by expansion of the thorax is transmitted to the alveoli. With P_{alv} now negative, a pressure gradient is created between the airway opening and the alveoli. This transrespiratory pressure gradient causes gas to flow from the airway into the alveoli. Within certain limits, the greater the transrespiratory pressure gradient, the more that lung expansion occurs.

Indications

Indications for IS are listed in Box 42-1. The primary indication for IS is to treat existing atelectasis. IS may also be used as a preventive measure when conditions exist that make the development of atelectasis likely.[7]

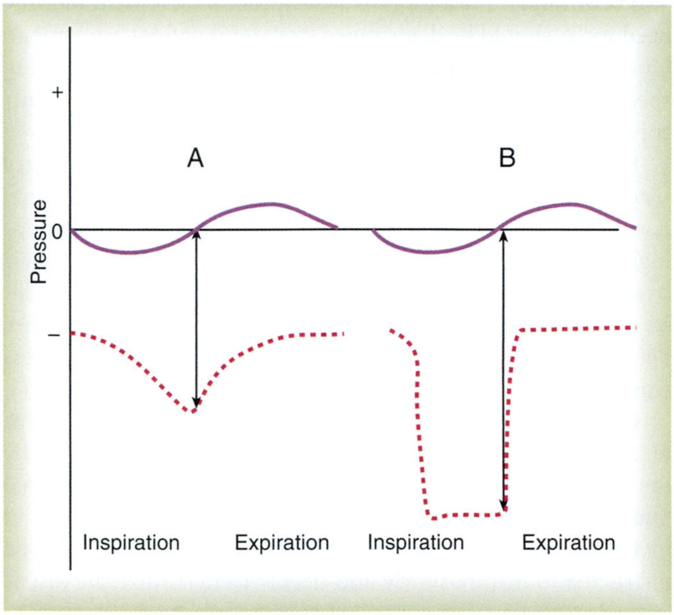

FIGURE 42-2 Alveolar *(solid lines)* and pleural *(dotted lines)* pressure changes during spontaneous breathing *(A)* and SMI *(B)*. Note the difference in P_{TP} gradients *(double arrows)*.

Box 42-1 Indications for Incentive Spirometry

- Presence of pulmonary atelectasis
- Presence of conditions predisposing to atelectasis
  - Upper abdominal surgery
  - Thoracic surgery
  - Surgery in patients with COPD
- Presence of a restrictive lung defect associated with quadriplegia or dysfunctional diaphragm

Contraindications

IS is a simple and relatively safe modality. For this reason, contraindications are few (Box 42-2).

Hazards and Complications

Given its normal physiologic basis, IS presents few major hazards and complications; those that can occur are listed in Box 42-3. Acute respiratory alkalosis is the most common problem and occurs when the patient performs IS too rapidly, or if the prescribed frequency of therapy is mismatched.[12] Dizziness and numbness around the mouth are the most frequently reported symptoms associated with respiratory alkalosis. This can be easily corrected with careful instruction and monitoring of the patient. Discomfort with deep inspiratory efforts secondary to pain is usually the result of inadequate pain control in a postoperative patient. Appropriate pain control prior to and during therapy is important.

Equipment

The equipment needed for SMI is typically simple, portable, and inexpensive. Although advances in technology have produced more complex devices, there is no evidence that these devices produce any better outcomes than their lower cost, disposable counterparts.

IS devices can generally be categorized as volume-oriented or flow-oriented. True volume-oriented devices measure and visually indicate the volume achieved during an SMI. The most popular true volume-oriented IS devices employ a bellows that rises according to the inhaled volume. When the patient reaches a target inspiratory volume, a controlled leak in the device allows the patient to sustain the inspiratory effort for a short period (usually 5 to 10 seconds). Because the bellows types of IS devices are bulky and large, smaller devices that indirectly indicate volume based on flow through a fixed orifice have been

Box 42-2 Contraindications for Incentive Spirometry

- Patient cannot be instructed or supervised to ensure appropriate use of device
- Patient cooperation is absent, or patient is unable to understand or demonstrate proper use of device
- Patients unable to deep breathe effectively (VC <10 ml/kg *or* IC <⅓ predicted)

Box 42-3 Hazards and Complications of Incentive Spirometry

- Hyperventilation and respiratory alkalosis
- Discomfort secondary to inadequate pain control
- Pulmonary barotrauma
- Exacerbation of bronchospasm
- Fatigue

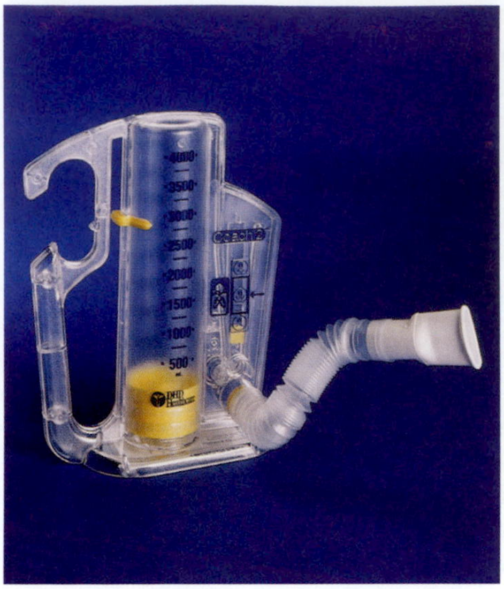

FIGURE 42-3 Volumetric incentive spirometer. (Courtesy DHE Healthcare, Canastota, NY.)

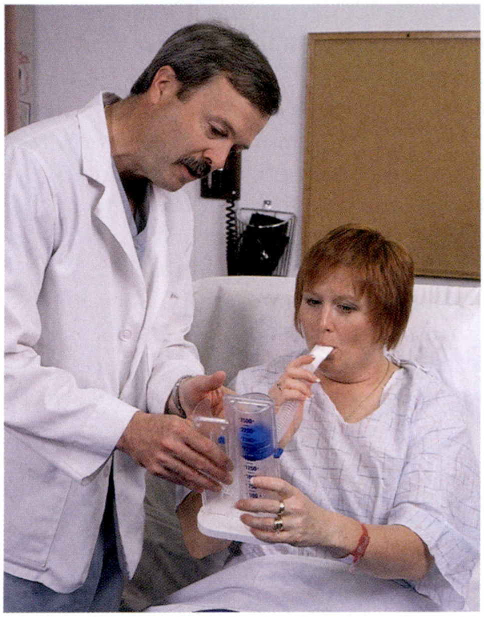

FIGURE 42-4 Flow-oriented incentive spirometer. (From DeWit, S: Fundamental concepts and skills for nursing, ed 2, St Louis, 2004, Saunders.)

developed. These devices sacrifice accurate measurement of the inhaled volume to achieve portability and smaller size (Figure 42-3).

Flow-oriented devices measure and visually indicate the degree of inspiratory flow (Figure 42-4). This flow can be equated with volume by assessing the duration of inspiration or time (flow × time = volume). Both flow-oriented and volume-oriented devices attempt to encourage the same goal for the patient: a sustained maximal inspiratory effort to prevent or correct atelectasis. There is no benefit of one type of IS over the other.

Box 42-4 Potential Outcomes of Incentive Spirometry

- Absence of or improvement in signs of atelectasis
- Decreased respiratory rate
- Normal pulse rate
- Resolution of abnormal breath sounds
- Normal or improved chest radiograph
- Improved PaO_2 and decreased $PaCO_2$
- Increased SpO_2
- Increased VC and peak expiratory flows
- Restoration of preoperative FRC or VC
- Improved inspiratory muscle performance and cough
- Attainment of preoperative flow and volume levels
- Increased FVC

Administration

The successful application of IS involves three phases: planning, implementation, and follow-up. Because many of the components of this process are similar to those previously described, we highlight only the key points and differences in approach.

Preliminary Planning. During preliminary planning, the need for IS should be determined by careful patient assessment. Once the need is established, planning should focus on selecting specific therapeutic outcomes. Box 42-4 lists potential outcomes that can be considered for patients receiving IS.

Patients scheduled for upper abdominal or thoracic surgery should be screened before undergoing the surgical procedure. Assessment conducted at this point helps to identify patients at high risk for complications and allows determination of their baseline lung volumes and capacities. This approach provides an opportunity to orient high-risk patients to the procedure before undergoing surgery, increasing the likelihood of success when IS is provided after surgery.

Implementation. Successful IS requires effective patient teaching. The RT should set an initial goal that is attainable by the patient yet requires a moderate effort. Setting an initial goal that is too low for the patient results in little incentive and an ineffective maneuver, at least initially. The patient should be instructed to inspire slowly and deeply to maximize the distribution of ventilation.

The RT should observe the patient perform the initial inspiratory maneuvers and ensure the patient uses correct technique. Correct technique calls for diaphragmatic breathing at slow to moderate inspiratory flows. Demonstration is probably the most effective way to assist patient understanding and cooperation. Both the operation of the device and the proper breathing technique can be explained easily when the RT uses himself or herself as an example, and much trial and error can be avoided.

Many patients have difficulty with the slow inspiration followed by the breath hold. Nonetheless, patients should be encouraged to try not to breathe in too fast or slowly and to attempt a brief breath hold.

A normal exhalation should follow the breath hold, and the patient should be given the opportunity to rest as long as needed before the next SMI maneuver. Some patients in the early postoperative stage may need to rest for 30 seconds to 1 minute between maneuvers. This rest period helps avoid a common tendency by some patients to repeat the maneuver at rapid rates, causing respiratory alkalosis. The goal is not rapid, partial lung inflation but intermittent, maximal inspiration.

The exact number of sustained maximal inspirations needed to reverse or prevent atelectasis is not known and probably varies according to the patient's clinical status. However, because healthy individuals average about 6 sighs per hour, an IS regimen should probably aim to ensure a minimum of 5 to 10 SMI maneuvers each hour.[12]

Follow-up. Assessing the patient's performance is vital to ensuring achievement of goals. To do so, the RT should make return visits to monitor treatment sessions until the correct technique and appropriate effort are achieved. Suggested monitoring activities for IS are outlined in Box 42-5.

After the patient has demonstrated mastery of technique, IS may be performed with minimal supervision. For patients with a neuromuscular disease or spinal injury, the use of a mechanical cough device (in-exsufflator) may provide a similar therapeutic objective. There is a lack of supporting data that IS has an effect of preventing or reversing pulmonary complications in post cardiac surgery patients, or those patients who have recently had upper abdominal surgery.[10,13] This is not implying that the therapy does not work, but strengthens the need to have more robust studies to evaluate this modality.

Noninvasive Ventilation

Noninvasive ventilation (NIV) provides breathing support to patients with inadequate ability to ventilate. NIV has been documented to have beneficial effects for patients who may need periodic, short-term support or patients who are experiencing exacerbations of pulmonary disease. NIV offers some benefits over traditional, invasive ventilation owing to lower infection risk and reduced need for sedation because of the absence of an artificial airway. NIV is discussed in detail elsewhere (Chapter 49). In addition, variations of NIV, including IPPB and PEP therapy, can be potentially valuable lung expansion tools and are discussed in the following sections.

Box 42-5 Monitoring Patients Receiving Incentive Spirometry

Observe patient performance and use:
- Frequency of sessions
- Number of breaths per session
- Volume and flow goals achieved
- Breath hold maintained
- Effort and motivation
- Periodic observation of patient compliance, with additional instruction as needed
- Device within reach of patient and patient encouraged to perform independently
- New and increasing inspiratory volumes established each day
- Vital signs and breath sounds

Intermittent Positive Airway Pressure Breathing

Physiologic Basis

IPPB is a specialized form of NIV used for relatively short treatment periods (approximately 15 minutes per treatment). The intent of IPPB, unlike NIV, is not to provide full ventilatory support but to provide machine-assisted deep breaths assisting the patient to deep breathe and stimulate a cough. This section discusses the use of IPPB as a modality for the treatment of atelectasis.

IPPB has historically consisted of providing an aerosol under positive pressure, augmenting the patient's own inspiratory efforts and thus resulting in a larger tidal volume (V_T) than could be spontaneously generated. The effectiveness of IPPB as an enhancement for aerosol delivery has been shown to be incorrect. In fact, IPPB does not improve aerosol deposition at all.[3] The AARC CPG for IPPB even recommends a 10-fold increase in medication dosage when compared with other aerosol delivery methods.[14] Lung volumes are increased in IPPB because $P_{alv} > P_{pl}$. Depending on the mechanical properties of the lung, P_{pl} may exceed atmospheric pressure during a portion of inspiration. As with spontaneous breathing, the recoil force of the lung, stored as potential energy during the positive pressure breath, causes a passive exhalation. As gas flows from the alveoli out to the airway opening, P_{alv} decreases to atmospheric level, while P_{pl} is restored to its normal subatmospheric range (Figure 42-5). The AARC has developed and published a clinical practice guideline for IPPB; excerpts from this guideline appear in Clinical Practice Guideline 42-2.

Indications

Although IPPB is not an effective aerosol delivery system, periodic sessions of positive pressure ventilation provided noninvasively can be useful in the treatment of pulmonary complications

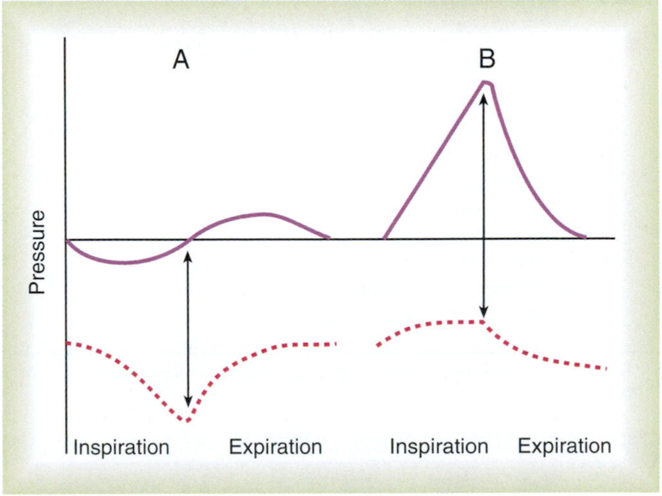

FIGURE 42-5 Alveolar *(solid lines)* and pleural *(dotted lines)* pressure changes during spontaneous breathing *(A)* and IPPB *(B)*. Note the difference in P_{TP} gradients *(double arrows)*.

42-2 Intermittent Positive Pressure Breathing

AARC Clinical Practice Guideline (Excerpts)*

INDICATIONS

- Need to improve lung expansion
- Presence of clinically significant pulmonary atelectasis when other forms of therapy (e.g., IS) have been unsuccessful or the patient cannot cooperate
- Inability to clear secretions adequately because of pathology that severely limits the ability to ventilate or cough effectively and failure to respond to other modes of treatment
- Need for short-term noninvasive ventilatory support for hypercapnic patients (as an alternative to intubation and continuous ventilatory support)
- Need to deliver aerosol medication
- Although some authors oppose the use of IPPB in the treatment of severe bronchospasm (e.g., acute asthma), we recommend a careful, closely supervised trial of IPPB when treatment using other techniques (metered dose inhaler [MDI] or nebulizer) has been unsuccessful
- IPPB may be used to deliver aerosol medications to patients with ventilatory muscle weakness or fatigue or chronic conditions in which intermittent noninvasive ventilatory support is indicated.

CONTRAINDICATIONS

Although no absolute contraindications to use of IPPB therapy (except tension pneumothorax) have been reported, a patient with any of the following should be carefully evaluated before a decision is made to initiate IPPB therapy:

- ICP >15 mm Hg
- Hemodynamic instability
- Recent facial, oral, or skull surgery
- Tracheoesophageal fistula
- Recent esophageal surgery
- Active hemoptysis
- Nausea
- Air swallowing
- Active, untreated tuberculosis
- Radiographic evidence of bleb
- Singultus (hiccups)

HAZARDS AND COMPLICATIONS

- Increased airway resistance
- Barotrauma, pneumothorax
- Nosocomial infection
- Hyperventilation or hypocapnia
- Hemoptysis
- Hyperoxia when O_2 is the gas source
- Gastric distention
- Secretion impaction (inadequate humidity)
- Psychological dependence
- Impedance of venous return
- Exacerbation of hypoxemia
- Hypoventilation
- Increased $\dot{V}/\dot{Q}$ mismatch
- Air trapping, auto-PEEP, overdistended alveoli

ASSESSMENT OF NEED

- Presence of clinically significant atelectasis
- Reduced timed volumes or VC (e.g., FEV_1 <65% predicted, FVC <70% predicted, maximum voluntary ventilation <50% predicted, or VC <10 ml/kg) precluding an effective cough
- Neuromuscular or skeletal disorders associated with decrease in lung volumes and capacities
- Fatigue or muscle weakness with impending respiratory failure
- Presence of acute, severe bronchospasm or exacerbated COPD that fails to respond to other therapy (consider MDI with spacer or holding chamber first)
- With demonstrated effectiveness, the patient's preference for a positive pressure device should be honored

ASSESSMENT OF OUTCOME

- A minimum delivered tidal volume of at least one-third of predicted IC ($\frac{1}{3} \times 50$ ml/kg) has been suggested
- FEV_1 or peak flow increase
- Cough more effective with treatment
- Secretion clearance enhanced as a consequence of deep breathing and coughing
- Chest radiograph improved
- Breath sounds improved
- Favorable patient subjective response

MONITORING

Items from the following list should be chosen as appropriate for the specific patient:

- Machine performance (trigger sensitivity, peak pressure, flow settings, FiO_2, inspiratory time, expiratory time, plateau pressure, PEEP)
- Respiratory rate and volume
- Peak flow or FEV_1/FVC
- Pulse rate and rhythm from electrocardiogram if available
- Patient subjective response to therapy (pain, discomfort, dyspnea)
- Sputum production (quantity, color, consistency, and odor)
- Mental function
- Skin color
- Breath sounds
- Blood pressure
- Arterial hemoglobin saturation by pulse oximetry (if hypoxemia is suspected)
- ICP in patients for whom ICP is of critical importance
- Chest radiograph

**For complete guidelines, see American Association for Respiratory Care: Intermittent positive pressure breathing—2003 revision and update. Respir Care 48:540, 2003.*

or exacerbations of lung disease.[12,15-17] CPAP or NIV may be the more appropriate treatments for patients with clinically diagnosed atelectasis unresponsive to other therapies, such as IS. IPPB should not be used as a single treatment modality for a patient with absorption atelectasis because of excessive airway secretions. Appropriate systemic hydration and airway clearance techniques should be used to assist in removal of excessive secretions.

In concept, IPPB treatment should provide the patient with augmented tidal volumes, achieved with minimal effort. There is no data to support the use of IPPB as a method of preventing or expanding atelectasis. However both the use of CPAP and NIV have shown promise in the management of postoperative respiratory complications.[7,18]

Contraindications

There are several clinical situations in which IPPB should not be used (Box 42-6). With the exception of untreated tension pneumothorax, most of these contraindications are relative. As with all procedures, a sound knowledge of the patient's condition tempered with good clinical insight should guide the RT in the decision-making process. A patient with any of the conditions listed in Box 42-6 should be carefully evaluated before a decision is made to begin IPPB therapy.

Hazards and Complications

As with any clinical intervention, certain hazards and complications are associated with IPPB. These potential problems should be addressed in the initial stages of planning for IPPB. In addition, hazards and complications must be considered throughout the course of therapy as part of the process of assessing the patient for unwanted side effects. The most common complication associated with IPPB is the inducement of respiratory alkalosis. Respiratory alkalosis is induced when the patient hyperventilates during the treatment. Deep, fast breathing leads to a sharp decrease in PCO_2 and an equally marked increase in arterial pH. The patient usually feels light-headed and numb around the mouth. Arrhythmias are also possible if the alkalosis is severe or if the patient has significant heart disease. This problem is easily avoided through proper coaching of the patient before and during treatment.

Another potential complication of IPPB is gastric distention; this occurs when gas from the IPPB device passes directly into the esophagus. Gastric distention is uncommon in an alert patient but is a significant risk for a neurologically obtunded patient. Normally, the esophagus does not open until a pressure of about 20 to 25 cm H_2O has been reached. Gastric distention represents the greatest risk in patients receiving IPPB at high pressures. The major hazards and complications of IPPB are listed in Box 42-7.

Administration

Effective IPPB requires careful preliminary planning, individualized patient assessment and implementation, and thoughtful follow-up. In all three phases of the process, the RT should work closely with the prescribing physician to determine patient need, select the appropriate therapeutic approach, and assess patient progress toward predefined clinical outcomes.

Preliminary Planning. During preliminary planning, the need for IPPB is determined, and desired therapeutic outcomes are established. The outcomes chosen for a patient are based on diagnostic information that supports the need for IPPB therapy. In addition, therapeutic outcomes should be as explicit and measurable as possible. Box 42-8 lists potential accepted and

Box 42-6 Clinical Situations Contraindicating Intermittent Positive Airway Pressure Breathing Therapy

- Tension pneumothorax
- ICP >15 mm Hg
- Hemodynamic instability
- Active hemoptysis
- Tracheoesophageal fistula
- Recent esophageal surgery
- Active, untreated tuberculosis
- Radiographic evidence of blebs
- Recent facial, oral, or skull surgery
- Singultus (hiccups)
- Air swallowing
- Nausea

Box 42-7 Hazards and Complications of Intermittent Positive Airway Pressure Breathing

- Increased airway resistance and work of breathing
- Barotrauma, pneumothorax
- Nosocomial infection
- Hypocarbia
- Hemoptysis
- Gastric distention
- Impaction of secretions (associated with inadequately humidified gas mixture)
- Psychologic dependence
- Impedance of venous return
- Exacerbation of hypoxemia
- Hypoventilation or hyperventilation
- Increased mismatch of ventilation and perfusion
- Air trapping, auto-PEEP, overdistention

Box 42-8 Potential Outcomes of Intermittent Positive Airway Pressure Breathing Therapy

- Improved VC
- Increased FEV_1 or peak flow
- Enhanced cough and secretion clearance
- Improved chest radiograph
- Improved breath sounds
- Improved oxygenation
- Favorable patient subjective response

desired outcomes of IPPB therapy. Not all the outcomes listed in Box 42-8 apply to every patient. For example, for a patient exhibiting clinical signs and symptoms of postoperative atelectasis, the following outcomes might be set: improved patient comfort, increased aeration on auscultation, decreased respiratory rate and work of breathing, and improvement in the chest radiograph.

Evaluating Alternatives. Before starting IPPB, the RT and prescribing physician must determine therapeutic objectives for the treatment and whether simpler and less costly methods might be as effective in achieving the desired outcomes.

Baseline Assessment. Before beginning therapy, a baseline patient assessment should be conducted. This information helps individualize the treatment and allows objective evaluation of the patient's subsequent response to therapy. Together with the patient's medical history, this baseline assessment also alerts the RT to possible problems or hazards associated with administering IPPB to the patient. The baseline assessment includes a general evaluation of the patient's clinical status and a specific assessment related to the chosen therapeutic goals. The general assessment, common to all patients for whom IPPB is ordered, includes (1) measurement of vital signs, (2) observational assessment of the patient's appearance and sensorium, and (3) breathing pattern and chest auscultation.

Discontinuation and Follow-up

Depending on the goals of therapy and condition of the patient, IPPB treatments typically last 10 to 15 minutes. Follow-up activities include posttreatment assessment of the patient, recordkeeping, and equipment maintenance.

Posttreatment Assessment. At the end of a treatment session, the patient assessment is repeated. As with the baseline assessment, this follow-up evaluation has two components. The general follow-up evaluation of the patient's clinical status should focus on determining any pertinent changes in vital signs, sensorium, and breath sounds, with emphasis on identifying possible untoward effects. The more specific follow-up assessment provides information relevant to evaluating progress toward achieving the chosen goals of therapy.

Treatment frequency should be determined by assessing patient response to therapy (Box 42-9). For acute care patients, orders should be reevaluated based on patient response to therapy at least every 72 hours or with any change of patient status.

Other Therapies

There are other therapies available to the respiratory therapist with the aim of secretion clearance and possible treatment of postoperative pulmonary complications: intrapulmonary percussive ventilation (IPV), and high-frequency chest wall compression (HFCWC). There is a lack of supporting evidence for the effectiveness of either of these therapies, although each is similar to techniques previously discussed within this chapter. IPV is similar to IPPB with a high respiratory rate, and HFCWC is similar to CPT using a pneumatic vest that the patient wears. These modalities are mentioned for completeness, although the evidence supporting them is low-level, or anectdotal.[3,19]

Box 42-9 Monitoring Intermittent Positive Airway Pressure Breathing Therapy

MACHINE PERFORMANCE
- Sensitivity
- Peak pressure
- Flow setting
- FiO_2
- I : E ratio

PATIENT RESPONSE*
- Breathing rate and expired volume
- Peak flow or FEV_1/FVC%
- Pulse rate and rhythm (from electrocardiogram if available)
- Sputum quantity, color, consistency, and odor
- Mental function
- Skin color
- Breath sounds
- Blood pressure
- SpO_2 (if hypoxemia is suspected)
- ICP (in patients for whom ICP is important)
- Chest radiograph (when appropriate)
- Subjective response to therapy

*Items should be chosen as appropriate for the specific patient.

Positive Airway Pressure Therapy

Similar to IPPB, positive airway pressure (PAP) adjuncts use positive pressure to increase the P_{TP} gradient and enhance lung expansion. In contrast to IPPB, PAP therapy requires no complex machinery. Some methods do not even need a source of pressurized gas.

Physiologic Basis

There are three current approaches to PAP therapy: PEP, flutter, and CPAP. All three techniques are effective in treating atelectasis in most postsurgical patients.[20,21] Because PEP and flutter are used most often as part of airway clearance, they are described in Chapter 43. This chapter describes the intermittent use of CPAP for the treatment of atelectasis.

PEP and flutter valves create expiratory positive pressure only, whereas CPAP maintains a positive airway pressure throughout both inspiration and expiration. Figure 42-6 compares the alveolar and P_{pl} changes occurring during a normal spontaneous breath (Figure 42-6, *A*) and CPAP (see Figure 42-6, *B*). As can be seen, CPAP elevates and maintains high alveolar and airway pressures throughout the full breathing cycle; this increases P_{TP} gradient throughout both inspiration and expiration. Typically, a patient on CPAP breathes through a pressurized circuit against a threshold resistor, with pressures maintained between 5 cm H_2O and 20 cm H_2O. To maintain system pressure throughout the breathing cycle, CPAP requires a source of pressurized gas.

The following factors involving PAP, flutter, and CPAP therapy contribute to the beneficial effects: (1) recruitment of

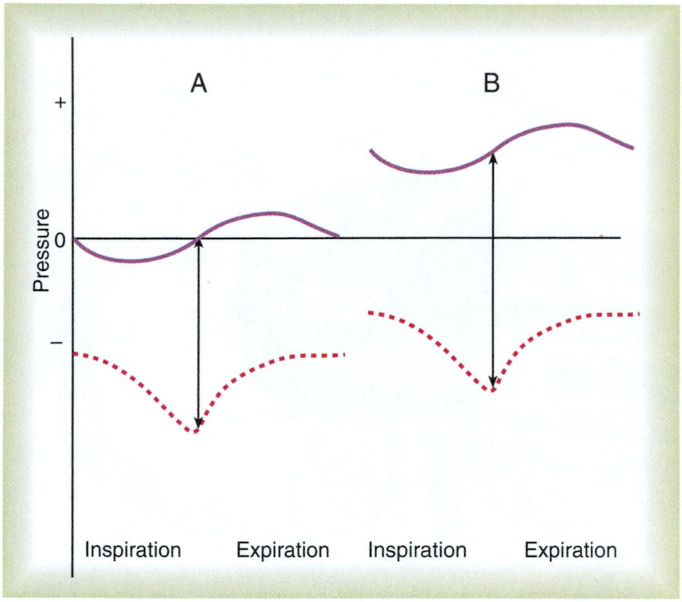

FIGURE 42-6 Alveolar *(solid lines)* and pleural *(dotted lines)* pressures during spontaneous breathing *(A)* and CPAP *(B)*. Note the difference in P_{TP} gradients *(double arrows)*.

collapsed alveoli via an increase in FRC, (2) decreased work of breathing secondary to increased compliance or elimination of intrinsic positive end expiratory pressure (PEEP), (3) improved distribution of ventilation through collateral channels (e.g., pores of Kohn), and (4) increase in the efficiency of secretion removal.

Indications

Although evidence exists to support the use of CPAP therapy in the treatment of postoperative atelectasis, as with all mechanical techniques, the duration of beneficial effects appears limited. The corresponding increase in FRC may be lost within 10 minutes after the end of the treatment. For this reason, it has been suggested that CPAP should be used on a continuous basis until the patient recovers.

CPAP by mask also has been used to treat cardiogenic pulmonary edema. In such patients, CPAP reduces venous return and cardiac filling pressures, which is helpful in reducing pulmonary vascular congestion. Lung compliance is improved, and the work of breathing is decreased.

Contraindications

Intermittent use of CPAP for the correction of atelectasis is contraindicated when certain clinical situations exist. A patient who is hemodynamically unstable is unlikely to tolerate CPAP for even a short period. A patient who is suspected to have hypoventilation is not a good candidate for CPAP because it does not ensure ventilation, but the patient may be an ideal candidate for consideration of NIV. Other problems that may indicate CPAP is not an appropriate therapy include nausea, facial trauma, untreated pneumothorax, and elevated intracranial pressure (ICP).

Hazards and Complications

Most hazards and complications associated with CPAP are caused by either the increased pressure or the apparatus. The increased work of breathing caused by the apparatus can lead to hypoventilation and hypercapnia. In addition, because CPAP does not augment spontaneous ventilation, patients with an accompanying ventilatory insufficiency may hypoventilate during application. Barotrauma is a potential hazard of CPAP and is more likely to occur in a patient with emphysema and blebs. Gastric distention may occur especially if CPAP values greater than 20 cm H_2O are needed. This condition may lead to vomiting and aspiration in a patient with an inadequate gag reflex.

Equipment

CPAP is most commonly delivered using either specialized CPAP machines (Figure 42-7), or ventilators. These devices allow for a more consistent level of positive pressure and provide the benefit of some level of patient monitoring. In the case where ICU-level ventilators are used, this includes monitoring of respiratory rate, airway pressures, and alarms. In the event of a disconnect, or if the patient becomes apneic, the ventilator can provide a measure of safety not realized with a high-flow system and resistor valve.

Administering Intermittent Continuous Positive Airway Pressure

As with all respiratory care, effective CPAP therapy requires careful planning, individualized patient assessment and implementation, and thoughtful follow-up.

Planning. During planning, the need for PAP therapy should be determined, and desired therapeutic outcomes should be set. Specifically, an improvement in breath sounds, improvement in vital signs (e.g., lower respiratory rate), resolution of abnormal radiograph findings, and restoration of normal oxygenation all would indicate that the therapy has achieved its goal.

Procedures. Whether used on an intermittent or continuous basis, CPAP is a complex and potentially hazardous approach to patient management. As with all therapies, the appropriate CPAP level for a patient must be determined on an individual basis. Initial application and monitoring require a broader range of knowledge and skill than required for simpler modes of lung expansion therapy.

Monitoring and Troubleshooting

CPAP poses a danger of hypoventilation. Experience with long-term CPAP shows that patients must be able to maintain adequate excretion of carbon dioxide on their own if the therapy is to be successful. For these reasons, patients receiving CPAP must be closely and continuously monitored for untoward effects. In addition, it is vital that the CPAP device be equipped with a means to monitor the pressure delivered to the airways and alarms to indicate the loss of pressure owing to system disconnect or mechanical failure. There should also be a device allowing for excessive pressure to be released (pop-off). These are essential components of any CPAP device.

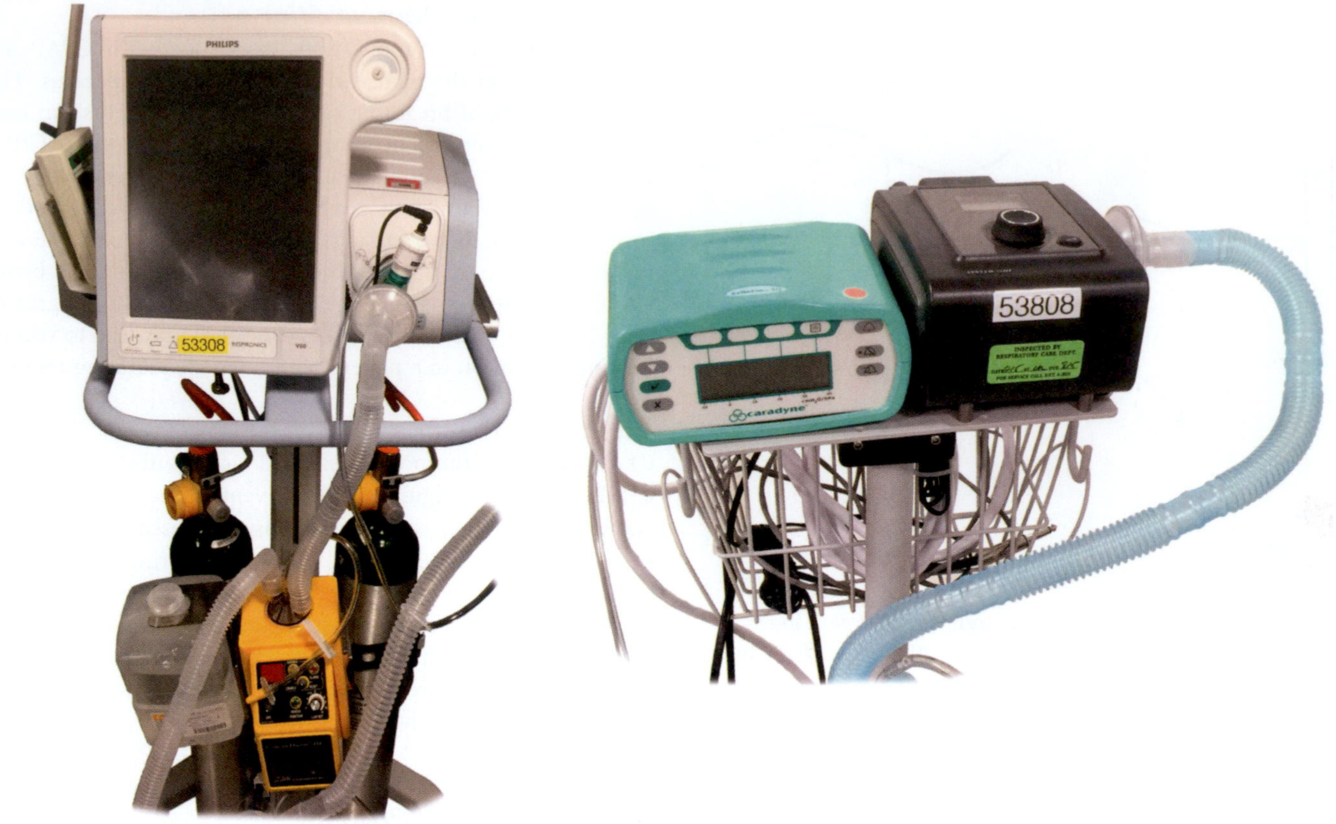

FIGURE 42-7 Various CPAP systems. See text for description.

The most common problem with PAP therapies is system leaks. When using a mask, a tight seal must be maintained to keep pressure levels above atmospheric levels. Any significant leaks in the system result in the loss of PAP. Because a tight seal requires a tight-fitting mask, pain and irritation may occur in some patients, especially if the therapy is prolonged.

The development of new CPAP units and improvement on the interface itself have addressed some of the comfort issues and correction of leakage associated with CPAP. The RT must also ensure that the flow is adequate to meet the patient's needs with the use of CPAP systems. Flow adjustments are made by carefully observing the airway pressure. Flow generally can be considered adequate when the system pressure decreases no more than 1 to 2 cm H_2O during inspiration.

SELECTING AN APPROACH

The best approach for achieving a given clinical goal is always the safest, simplest, and most effective method for an individual patient. Selecting an approach for lung expansion therapy requires in-depth knowledge of both the methods available and the specific condition and needs of the patient being considered for therapy.

Figure 42-8 presents a sample protocol for selecting an approach to lung expansion therapy. As indicated in the algorithm, the patient first must meet the criteria for therapy by having one or more of the indications previously specified. For patients meeting the inclusion criteria, the RT first determines the degree of alertness. Because an obtunded patient cannot be expected to cooperate with IS or PEP or EPAP therapy, IPPB or NIV is initiated with appropriate monitoring.

For a patient having no difficulty with secretions, if the VC exceeds 15 mℓ/kg of lean body weight or the IC is greater than 33% of predicted, IS is given. If either the VC or the IC is less than these threshold levels, IPPB is initiated, with the pressure gradually manipulated from the initial setting to deliver at least 15 ml/kg.

If excessive sputum production is a compounding factor, a trial of PEP therapy is substituted for IS. Based on patient response, bronchodilator therapy and bronchial hygiene measures may be added to this regimen. If monitoring fails to reveal improvement and atelectasis persists, a trial of CPAP should be considered. Because evidence of the effectiveness of CPAP is still contradictory, its use should be limited to treating atelectasis after alternative approaches have been tried without success.

Early Mobilization of the ICU Patient

Whether or not to keep critically ill patients on complete bed rest is being critically examined in the literature.[22-25] The complications of prolonged bed rest include cardiovascular, pulmonary, gastrointestinal, and skin integrity issues. Pulmonary issues include those that have been the focus of this chapter: development of atelectasis, pneumonia, and pulmonary emboli (PE).[23-25] Rates of early mobilization for ICU patients have been

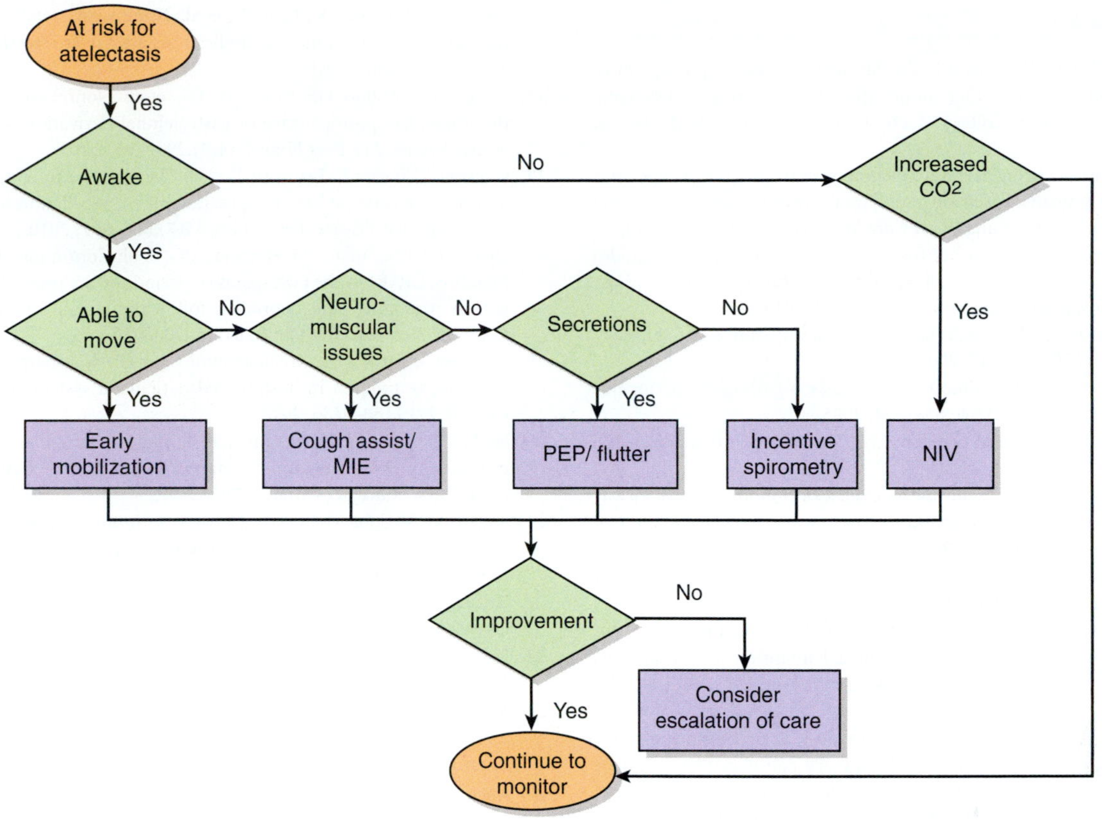

FIGURE 42-8 Protocol for selecting an approach for lung expansion therapy. See text for details.

increasing in both Europe and the United States along with the emphasis on decreasing morbidity in the ICU. Mobilization does not only include walking, but also sitting, standing, and getting out of bed into a chair. As the patient changes body position, his or her breathing changes as well as gas distribution within the lung. Improvements in ventilation result in less alveolar collapse.

Because of the beneficial pulmonary effects from early mobilization of the post–abdominal surgery patient, it has been suggested that mobilization should be considered as early as the day of surgery.[26] Recently, there has been a shift in the mindset that critically ill patients should be on complete bedrest. With the increasing knowledge of the benefits of early mobilization, the paradigm must change from thinking that a patient is too sick to get out of bed, to one in which we must think that a patient is too sick to stay in bed.[25]

In order to move the patient from the bed, it is important that they are not completely sedated. Along with early mobilization, there are other benefits of lighter sedation, and even "sedation vacations" when all sedation for the patient is temporarily discontinued in order to re-assess the need for sedation. Having a patient who is able to respond to the caregiver allows for better pain control with decreased risk of sedation-related complications.[27,28]

Although early mobilization does not classify as a procedure, it does have distinct benefits in decreasing morbidity and mortality. Early mobilization is the only true multidisciplinary approach requiring the various members of the health care team (respiratory therapist, nurse, physical therapist) to be present at the same time.

SUMMARY CHECKLIST

- Atelectasis is caused by persistent ventilation with small tidal volumes or by resorption of gas distal to obstructed airways.
- Patients who have undergone upper abdominal or thoracic surgery are at greatest risk for atelectasis.
- A history of lung disease or significant cigarette smoking increases the risk for atelectasis.
- Patients with atelectasis usually have rapid, shallow breathing; fine, late-inspiratory crackles; and abnormalities on chest radiograph.
- Lung expansion therapy corrects atelectasis by increasing the P_{TP} gradient; this can be accomplished by deep spontaneous breaths or by the application of positive pressure.
- The most common problem associated with lung expansion therapy is the onset of respiratory alkalosis, which occurs when the patient breathes too quickly.
- RTs are responsible for implementing, monitoring, and documenting results of lung expansion therapy.

References

1. Lawrence VA, Cornell JE, Smetana GW: Strategies to reduce postoperative pulmonary complications after noncardiothoracic surgery: systematic review for the American College of Physicians. *Ann Intern Med* 144:596, 2006.
2. Gulati G, Novero A, Loring SH, et al: Pleural pressure and optimal positive end-expiratory pressure based on esophageal pressure versus chest wall elastance: incompatible results*. *Crit Care Med* 41(8):1951–1957, 2013.
3. Strickland SL, Rubin BK, Drescher GS, et al: AARC clinical practice guideline: effectiveness of nonpharmacologic airway clearance therapies in hospitalized patients. *Respir Care* 58(12):2187–2193, 2013.
4. Duggan M, Kavanagh BP: Atelectasis in the perioperative patient. *Curr Opin Anaesthesiol* 20(1):37–42, 2007.
5. Duggan M, Kavanagh BP: Pulmonary atelectasis: a pathogenic perioperative entity. *Anesthesiology* 102(4):838–854, 2005.
6. Brower RG: Consequences of bed rest. *Crit Care Med* 37(10 Suppl):S422–S428, 2009.
7. Ferreyra GP, Baussano I, Squadrone V, et al: Continuous positive airway pressure for treatment of respiratory complications after abdominal surgery. *Ann Surg* 247(4):617–626, 2008.
8. Braga M, Vignali A, Zuliani W, et al: Laparoscopic versus open colorectal surgery. *Ann Surg* 242(6):890–896, 2005.
9. Polignano FM, Quyn AJ, de Figueiredo RS, et al: Laparoscopic versus open liver segmentectomy: prospective, case-matched, intention-to-treat analysis of clinical outcomes and cost effectiveness. *Surg Endosc* 22(12):2564–2570, 2008.
10. do Nascimento Junior P, Modolo SPN, Andrade S, et al: Incentive spirometry for prevention of postoperative pulmonary complications in upper abdominal surgery. *Cochrane Database Syst Rev* 2:2014, CD006058.
11. Hassanzadeh H, Jain A, Tan EW, et al: Postoperative incentive spirometry use. *Orthopedics* 35(6):e927–e931, 2012.
12. Restrepo RD, Wettstein R, Wittnebel L, et al: Incentive spirometry: 2011. *Respir Care* 56(10):1600–1604, 2011.
13. Freitas RFSE, Soares GOB, Cardoso JR, et al: Incentive spirometry for preventing pulmonary complications after coronary artery bypass graft. *Cochrane Database Syst Rev* 9:2012, CD004466.
14. Sorenson HM, Shelledy DC: AARC clinical practice guidelines: intermittent positive pressure breathing—2003 revision & update. *Respir Care* 48(5): 2003.
15. Narita M, Tanizawa K, Chin K, et al: Noninvasive ventilation improves the outcome of pulmonary complications after liver resection. *Intern Med* 49(15):1501–1507, 2010.
16. Pessoa KC, Araujo GF, Pinheiro AN, et al: Noninvasive ventilation in the immediate postoperative of gastrojejunal derivation with Roux-en-Y gastric bypass. *Rev Bras Fisioter* 14(4):290–295, 2010.
17. Guérin C, Vincent B, Petitjean T, et al: The short-term effects of intermittent positive prrssure breathing treatments on ventilation in patients with neuromuscular disease. *Respir Care* 55(7):866–872, 2010.
18. Ireland CJ, Chapman TM, Herbison PG, et al: Continuous positive airway pressure (CPAP) in the postoperative period for the prevention of postoperative morbidity and mortality following major abdominal surgery. *Cochrane Database Syst Rev* 2:2012, CD008930.
19. Andrews J, Sathe NA, Krishnaswami S, et al: Nonpharmacologic airway clearance techniques in hospitalized patients: a systematic review. *Respir Care* 58(12):2160–2186, 2013.
20. Sehlin M, Ohberg F, Johansson G, et al: Physiological responses to positive expiratory pressure breathing: a comparison of the PEP bottle and the PEP mask. *Respir Care* 52(8):1000–1005, 2007.
21. Squadrone V, Coha M, Cerutti E, et al: Continuous positive airway pressure for treatment of postoperative hypoxemia: a randomized controlled trial. *JAMA* 293(5):589–595, 2005.
22. Bell L: Achieving early mobility in mechanically ventilated patients. *Am J Crit Care* 18(3):222, 2009.
23. Kalisch BJ, Dabney BW, Lee S: Safety of mobilizing hospitalized adults. *J Nurs Care Qual* 28(2):162–168, 2013.
24. McWilliams D, Weblin J, Atkins G, et al: Enhancing rehabilitation of mechanically ventilated patients in the intensive care unit: a quality improvement project. *J Crit Care* 30(1):13–18, 2015.
25. Kress JP: Sedation and mobility. *Crit Care Clin* 29(1):67–75, 2013.
26. Havey R, Herriman E, O'Brien D: Guarding the gut. *Crit Care Nurs Q* 36(1):63–72, 2013.
27. Jackson JC, Girard TD, Gordon SM, et al: Long-term cognitive and psychological outcomes in the Awakening and Breathing Controlled trial. *Am J Respir Crit Care Med* 182(2):183–191, 2010.
28. Girard TD, Kress JP, Fuchs BD, et al: Efficacy and safety of a paired sedation and ventilator weaning protocol for mechanically ventilated patients in intensive care (Awakening and Breathing Controlled trial): a randomised controlled trial. *Lancet* 371(9607):126–134, 2008.

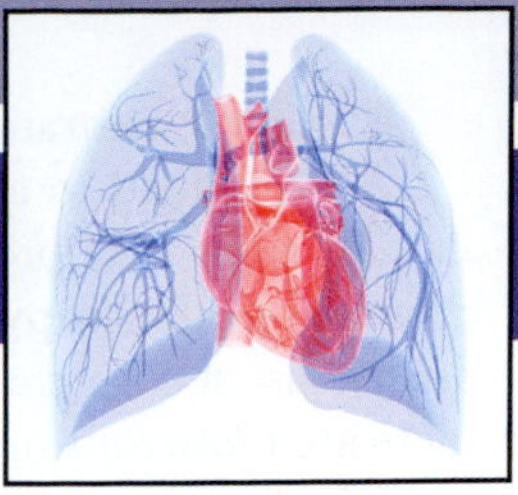

CHAPTER 43

Airway Clearance Therapy (ACT)

DAVID L. VINES AND DONNA D. GARDNER

CHAPTER OBJECTIVES

After reading this chapter you will be able to:

- Describe the normal airway clearance mechanisms and the factors that impair their function.
- Identify pulmonary diseases associated with abnormal secretion clearance.
- State the goals and clinical indications for airway clearance therapy.
- Describe the proper technique and potential benefit of each of the following:
  - Chest physical therapy
  - Directed coughing and related expulsion techniques
  - Vibratory positive expiratory pressure therapy
  - High-frequency positive airway pressure devices
  - High-frequency compression/oscillation devices
  - Mobilization and exercise
- Evaluate a patient's response to airway clearance therapy.
- Modify airway clearance therapies on the basis of patient response.

CHAPTER OUTLINE

Physiology of Airway Clearance Therapies (ACT)
- Normal Clearance
- Abnormal Clearance
- Diseases Associated With Abnormal Clearance

General Goals and Indications
- Airway Clearance Therapy for Acute Conditions
- Airway Clearance Therapy for Chronic Conditions
- Airway Clearance Therapy to Prevent Retention of Secretions

Determining the Need for Airway Clearance Therapy

Airway Clearance Methods
- Chest Physical Therapy
- Coughing and Related Expulsion Techniques
- Active Cycle of Breathing Technique
- Autogenic Drainage
- Mechanical Insufflation-Exsufflation
- Positive Airway Pressure Adjuncts
- High-Frequency Chest Wall Oscillation
- Exercise, Mobilization and Physical Activity

Selecting Airway Clearance Techniques
- Selection Factors
- Protocol-Based Airway Clearance

KEY TERMS

active cycle of breathing technique (ACBT)
autogenic drainage (AD)
bronchiectasis
chest physical therapy (CPT)
ciliary dyskinetic syndromes
forced expiratory technique (FET)
Hertz (Hz)
high-frequency chest wall compression (HFCWC)
high-frequency positive airway pressure devices (HFPAP)
huff coughing
inspissation
intrapulmonary percussive ventilation (IPV)
mechanical insufflation-exsufflation (MIE)
mucous plugging
oscillation
positive expiratory pressure (PEP)
splinting

Airway clearance therapy uses noninvasive techniques designed to assist in mobilizing and removing secretions to improve gas exchange.[1,2] Historically, the term **chest physical therapy** (**CPT**) described the primary techniques used to assist with clearing secretions from the airways. Today there are numerous options related to airway clearance including CPT, breathing retraining techniques, positive expiratory therapy (PEP), vibratory PEP, high-frequency positive pressure devices, high-frequency chest wall compression devices, and various exercise protocols.[1-4] This chapter focuses on airway clearance therapies or techniques used to mobilize secretions and noninvasively assist in their removal. The primary *invasive* method for removing airway secretions is suctioning, and is discussed in Chapter 36. Successful outcomes in airway clearance techniques require knowledge of normal and abnormal physiology, understanding of how clearance devices work, careful patient evaluation, rigorous application of evidence-based methods, and ongoing assessment targeted at achieving therapeutic goals.[1-6]

PHYSIOLOGY OF AIRWAY CLEARANCE THERAPIES (ACT)

To apply airway clearance therapies (ACT) properly, one first must understand how normal airway clearance mechanisms work and what can impair their function.

Normal Clearance

Normal airway clearance requires patent airways, a functional mucociliary escalator, adequate hydration, and effective coughs.[4,6] The mucociliary clearance happens from the larynx down to the respiratory bronchioles. Mucus is produced by secretory (Clara, goblet, and serous) cells and submucosal glands.[6] Ciliated epithelial cells move this mucus via a coordinated wave of ciliary motion toward the trachea and larynx, where secretions can be swallowed or expectorated. Healthy individuals produce 10 to 100 mL of secretions in the airway on a daily basis that are cleared by this mucociliary escalator.[1,4,6]

The cough is one of the most important protective reflexes.[1,2,4,6] Coughing clears the larger airways of excessive mucus and foreign matter, assists normal mucociliary clearance, and helps ensure airway patency. As shown in Figure 43-1, there are four distinct phases to a normal cough: *irritation, inspiration, compression,* and *expulsion*. In the initial irritation phase, an abnormal stimulus provokes sensory fibers in the airways to send impulses to the medullary cough center in the brain. This stimulus normally is inflammatory, mechanical, chemical, or thermal. Infection is a good example of an *inflammatory* process that can stimulate a cough. Foreign bodies can provoke a cough through *mechanical* stimulation. Inhaling irritating gases (e.g., cigarette smoke) can result in coughing through *chemical* stimulation. Finally, cold air may cause *thermal* stimulation of sensory nerves, producing a cough.

When these afferent impulses are received, the cough center generates a reflex stimulation of the respiratory muscles to initiate a deep inspiration (the second phase). In normal adults, this inspiration averages 1 to 2 L.

During the third or compression phase, reflex nerve impulses cause glottic closure and a forceful contraction of the expiratory muscles. This compression phase is normally about 0.2 second and results in a rapid increase in pleural and alveolar pressures, often greater than 100 mm Hg.

At this point, the glottis opens, initiating the expulsion phase. With the glottis open, a large pressure gradient between the lungs and the atmospheric pressure exists. Together with the continued contraction of the expiratory muscles, this pressure gradient causes a violent, expulsive high velocity of airflow from the lungs. This high-velocity gas flow, combined with dynamic airway compression, creates huge shear forces that displace mucus from the airway walls into the air stream. Mucus

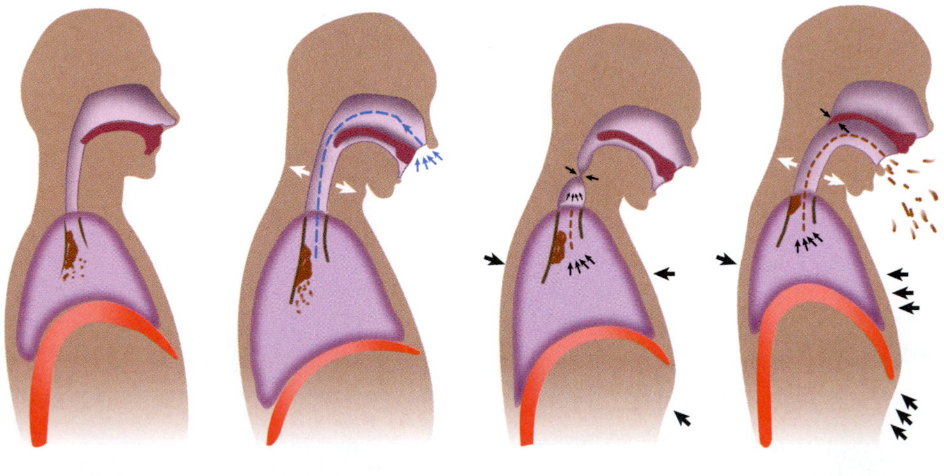

FIGURE 43-1 The cough reflex. (Modified from Cherniack RM, Cherniack L: Respiration in health and disease, ed 3, Philadelphia, 1983, WB Saunders.)

and foreign material are expelled from the lower airways to the upper airway, where they can be expectorated or swallowed.

Abnormal Clearance

Any abnormality that alters airway patency, mucociliary function, strength of the inspiratory or expiratory muscles, thickness of secretions, or effectiveness of the cough reflex can impair airway clearance leading to retention of secretions.[1,2,4-7] In addition, some therapeutic interventions, especially interventions used in critical care, such as an endotracheal tube, can result in abnormal clearance.

Retention of secretions can result in full or partial airway obstruction. Full obstruction, or **mucous plugging**, can result in atelectasis which causes hypoxemia due to shunting. A partial obstruction restricts airflow, increasing work of breathing and possibly leading to air trapping, lung overdistention, and ventilation/perfusion ($\dot{V}/\dot{Q}$) imbalances. In the presence of pathogenic organisms, retention of secretions can also lead to infections. Infectious processes provoke an inflammatory response and the release of chemical mediators. These chemical mediators, including leukotrienes, proteases, and elastases, can damage the airway epithelium and increase mucus production, resulting in a vicious cycle of worsening airway clearance.[6]

In patients with retained secretions, interference with one of the four phases of cough can result in ineffective airway clearance. This occurs in patients post thoracic or upper abdominal surgery, in the intensive care unit, or with neuromuscular diseases (NMD) such as amyotrophic lateral sclerosis (ALS), myasthenia gravis (MG), or spinal cord injuries.[4,7] Table 43-1 provides examples of factors that can impair the normal cough reflex.

As indicated in Box 43-1, additional factors can impair airway clearance in critically ill patients with artificial airways, the most important of which is the airway itself.[8] The presence of the tube in the trachea increases mucus secretion, and the cuff of the tube mechanically blocks the mucociliary escalator. In addition, movement of the tube tip and cuff can cause erosion of the tracheal mucosa leading to further impairment of the mucociliary escalator. The endotracheal tube also impairs the compression phase of the cough reflex by preventing closure of the glottis (see Table 43-1). Although suctioning is used to aid secretion clearance, it too can cause damage to the airway mucosa and impair mucociliary transport. Inadequate humidification can cause thickening or **inspissation** of secretions, mucous plugging, and airway obstruction.[9] High fractional inspired oxygen (FiO_2) concentrations can impair cilia function, resulting in retained secretions. Retained secretions can lead to acute tracheobronchitis. Several common drugs, including some general anesthetics and narcotic-analgesics, may also depress mucociliary transport.[10]

TABLE 43-1

Mechanisms Impairing Cough Reflex

Phase	Examples of Impairments
Irritation	Anesthesia CNS depression Narcotic-analgesics
Inspiration	Pain Neuromuscular dysfunction Pulmonary restriction Abdominal restriction
Compression	Laryngeal nerve damage Artificial airway Abdominal muscle weakness Abdominal surgery
Expulsion	Airway compression Airway obstruction Abdominal muscle weakness Inadequate lung recoil (e.g., emphysema)

CNS, Central nervous system.

Diseases Associated With Abnormal Clearance

Several diseases are associated with abnormal airway clearance, including diseases affecting airway patency, composition and production of mucus, ciliary structure and function, and normal cough reflex.[1,2,4,6,7] Internal obstruction or external compression of the airway lumen can impair airway clearance. Examples include foreign bodies, tumors, and congenital or acquired thoracic anomalies such as kyphoscoliosis. Internal obstruction also can occur with mucus hypersecretion, inflammatory changes, or bronchospasm that narrows the lumen. Examples include asthma, chronic bronchitis, and/or acute infections.

Diseases that alter normal mucociliary clearance also can cause retention of secretions. In cystic fibrosis (CF) the solute concentration of the mucus is altered because of abnormal sodium and chloride transport.[5,6] This alteration increases the viscosity of mucus and impairs its movement up the respiratory tract. Although less common, there are several conditions in which the respiratory tract cilia do not function properly.[6] These **ciliary dyskinetic syndromes** also can contribute to ineffective airway clearance. **Bronchiectasis** is permanently damaged and dilated airways that are prone to obstruction due to retained secretions.[6,11] Bronchiectasis is a common finding in CF and ciliary dyskinetc syndromes.[11,12]

Mucociliary function may be normal, but lack of an effective cough alters airway clearance leading to retained secretions,

Box 43-1 Causes of Impaired Mucociliary Clearance in Intubated Patients

- Endotracheal or tracheostomy tube
- Tracheobronchial suction
- Inadequate humidification
- High FiO_2 values
- Drugs
- General anesthetics
- Opiates
- Narcotics
- Underlying pulmonary disease

mucous plugs, obstructions, and atelectasis. The most common conditions affecting the cough reflex are musculoskeletal and NMDs,[6,7] including muscular dystrophy, ALS, spinal muscular atrophy, myasthenia gravis, poliomyelitis, and cerebral palsy (see Chapter 32).

GENERAL GOALS AND INDICATIONS

The primary goal of airway clearance therapy is to assist the patient to mobilize and remove retained secretions. Removal of these retained secretions may improve gas exchange, promote alveolar expansion, and reduce the work of breathing. Box 43-2 lists general indications for ACT.[1,2,4,7]

Airway Clearance Therapy for Acute Conditions

Patients with acute conditions in whom ACT may be indicated include (1) acutely or chronically ill patients with copious secretions; (2) patients with retained secretions or ineffective cough (coarse crackles, worsening oxygenation and/or ventilation, volume loss on chest radiograph); and possibly (3) patients with acute lobar atelectasis or (4) patients with $\dot{V}/\dot{Q}$ abnormalities.[13] In treating acute respiratory conditions, inhaled bronchodilator therapy before airway clearance therapy may improve the overall effectiveness of the treatment both by opening the airways and by increasing the mucociliary activity.[6] For acute pulmonary infections, inhaled antibiotics after airway clearance therapy can lead to improved deposition of the antibiotic.[14] Acute conditions for which airway clearance therapy is probably not indicated include (1) routine care of COPD, (2) pneumonia without clinically significant sputum production, (3) routine postoperative care, and (4) uncomplicated asthma.[1]

Airway Clearance Therapy for Chronic Conditions

Airway clearance therapy has proved effective in secretion clearance and improving pulmonary function in chronic conditions associated with copious sputum production, including CF, bronchiectasis, and ciliary dyskinetic syndromes, and COPD patients with retained secretions.[1,2,4,5,14] Generally, sputum production must exceed 20 to 30 ml/day for airway clearance therapy to improve secretion removal significantly.[2]

Box 43-2 Indications for Airway Clearance Therapy

ACUTE CONDITIONS
- Copious secretions
- Inability to mobilize secretions
- Ineffective cough

CHRONIC CONDITIONS
- CF
- Bronchiectasis
- Ciliary dyskinetic syndromes
- COPD patients with retained secretions

MINI CLINI

Assessing a Patient's Cough Clearance

PROBLEM: The RT is called by a nurse to determine a care plan to assist a patient who is having difficulty clearing secretions. The patient is an alert, obese, 45-year-old man who underwent general anesthesia and surgery for gallbladder removal 3 hours earlier. Physical signs indicate retention of secretions, but there is no history of lung disease. Auscultation reveals coarse expiratory crackles. The patient is breathing spontaneously, however, his breathing is shallow and he has a very weak cough. Visual clues indicate the patient has severe pain in the epigastric area. The patient was given an injection of morphine to assist with the pain 1 hour earlier.

Discussion: Even without lung disease, it is no surprise that this patient is having difficulty clearing secretions. Recent anesthesia and the narcotic-analgesic potentially are impairing his cough. In addition, obesity (abdominal restriction), weakness, and pain are impairing the inspiration, compression, and expulsion phases of his cough effort.

The patient should immediately be started on an ACT and hyperinflation or lung expansion therapies. Judicious use of pain medication, coinciding with therapies, should continue. Cough instruction including incisional splinting should be part of the plan. Early mobilization should be considered. Although the most common postoperative complication is atelectasis, pneumonia may also occur. The head of the patient's bed should be elevated at least to 30 to 45 degrees to minimize the risk of aspiration.

RULE OF THUMB

Patients with copious secretions (20 to 30 mL/day) or inability to mobilize and expectorate secretions may benefit from airway clearance therapy.

Airway Clearance Therapy to Prevent Retention of Secretions

Airway clearance therapy has been used as preventive therapy in various disorders. Current evidence is not supportive of this approach.[1,3] The best-documented preventive uses of airway clearance therapy include (1) body positioning and patient mobilization to prevent retained secretions in acutely ill patients and (2) ACT combined with physical activity to maintain lung function in patients with CF.[1,3,5] Other preventive applications of airway clearance therapy have not proved to be useful.[1,3,5]

DETERMINING THE NEED FOR AIRWAY CLEARANCE THERAPY

Effective airway clearance therapy requires proper initial and ongoing patient assessment (Chapter 16). Formulation of the respiratory care plan depends on review of the patient's medical

Box 43-3 Initial Assessment of Need for Airway Clearance Therapy

MEDICAL RECORD

History of pulmonary problems causing increased secretions
Admission for upper abdominal or thoracic surgery; consider:
- Age (elderly)
- History of COPD
- Obesity
- Nature of procedure
- Type of anesthesia
- Duration of procedure

Presence of artificial tracheal airway
Chest radiograph indicating atelectasis or infiltrates
Results of pulmonary function testing
Arterial blood gas values or O_2 saturation

PATIENT

Posture, muscle tone
Effectiveness of cough
Sputum production
Breathing pattern
General physical fitness
Breath sounds
Vital signs, heart rate and rhythm

history and interview for current symptoms, physical assessment, laboratory testing (including pulmonary function tests), and radiologic evaluation. Box 43-3 lists the key factors that must be considered when assessing a patient's need for airway clearance therapy.[1,2,5] Physical findings such as a loose, ineffective cough; labored breathing pattern; decreased or bronchial breath sounds; coarse inspiratory and expiratory crackles; tachypnea; tachycardia; or fever may indicate a potential problem with retained secretions.

AIRWAY CLEARANCE METHODS

Five general approaches to ACT, which can be used alone or in combination, include (1) CPT; (2) coughing and related expulsion techniques (including manual insufflation-exsufflation [MIE]); (3) positive airway pressure (PAP) adjuncts (**positive expiratory pressure [PEP]**, vibratory PEP, high-frequency positive airway pressure devices); (4) high-frequency compression/oscillation methods; and (5) mobilization and physical activity. Table 43-2 provides a brief description and limitations associated with these airway clearance therapies. Appropriate use of these techniques requires an understanding of their underlying principles, relative efficacy, and methods of application.

Chest Physical Therapy

CPT has long been considered a standard of care in patients with CF. Evidence suggests that these therapies benefit mucus transport and assist in the expectoration of secretions.[1,2,4,5] This therapy includes postural drainage (PD) and percussion or vibration.

CPT involves the use of positioning, gravity, and mechanical energy to help mobilize secretions. PD places the body in various positions that are intended to drain secretions from each of the patient's lung segments into the central airways, where they can be removed by cough or suctioning.[4,5] This drainage is accomplished by simply placing the segmental bronchus to be drained in a more vertical position, permitting gravity to assist in the process. Positions generally are held for 3 to 15 minutes (longer in special situations such as CF) and modified as the patient's condition and tolerance warrant.[13] Cough methods are used with CPT and are discussed separately.

The indications for CPT (and other ACT) in a patient are copious secretions, inability to mobilize and expectorate the secretions, and pulmonary disorders associated with retained secretions (CF, bronchiectasis, and ciliary dyskinetic syndromes).[1,2,4,5] This therapy does require a trained caregiver's assistance for it to be performed correctly. CPT may be most effective in conditions characterized by excessive sputum production that is not cleared by deep breathing and coughing. For maximum effect with PD, head-down positions should exceed 25 degrees below horizontal.[14,15] If the patient can not be placed in appropriate positions for the areas affected, other ACT should be considered. In spontaneously breathing patients, frequency should be determined by assessing patient response to therapy. Critically ill patients, especially patients being mechanically ventilated, should have their positions changed every 2 hours.[16]

Technique

On the basis of a preliminary assessment of the patient and review of the physician's order, the RT should identify the appropriate lobes and segments for drainage. The RT may need to choose a different method for ACT in patients with unstable cardiovascular status, hypertension, cerebrovascular disorders, or dyspnea. To avoid gastroesophageal reflux and the possibility of aspiration, treatment times should be scheduled before or at least 2 hours after meals or tube feedings.[10] If the patient assessment indicates that pain may hinder treatment implementation, the RT should consider coordinating the treatment regimen with prescribed pain medication. Contraindications for CPT are listed in Box 43-4.

Before positioning, the procedure (including adjunctive techniques) should be explained to the patient. The RT should inspect for incisions, monitoring leads, intravenous tubing, and oxygen (O_2) therapy equipment connected to the patient and, if necessary, make adjustments to ensure continued function during the procedure or choose a different ACT method. Before starting, during, and after the procedure, the RT should measure the patient's vital signs, auscultate the chest, and measure SpO_2 if hypoxemia is suspected. These simple assessments serve as baseline measurements for monitoring the patient's response during the procedure and can assist in determining outcomes. The following items should also be monitored before, during, and after CPT: subjective responses (pain, discomfort, dyspnea, response to therapy), arrhythmias, breathing pattern, sputum production (quantity, color, consistency, odor), skin color, and ICP if monitored.[13]

TABLE 43-2
Techniques and Devices Used for Airway Clearance Therapy

Techniques/Devices	Description	Potential Limitations
Chest Physiotherapy (CPT) includes Percussion and Postural Drainage	Manually striking the chest wall with cupped hands in a rhythmic fashion or vibrating it with a mechanical device to loosen secretions from the airways and propel them forward while placing the patient in various positions so gravity can assist in draining the secretions from lung segment to larger airways to be cleared.	There is no age limitation but it requires help of a caregiver. CPT's effectiveness may be dependent on appropriate positioning, and patients with shortness of breath may not tolerate Trendelenburg position. Patients are unable to perform concurrent aerosol therapy.
Active Cycle of Breathing	The patient alternates cycles of deep breathing, relaxed breathing, and forced expiration technique to mobilize secretions.	Begin to introduce the concept at 3 to 4 years of age and continue coaching until approximately 10 years of age. It is difficult to perform during exacerbations or when patients are unable to take a deep breath.
Autogenic Drainage	The patient uses series of breathing patterns from a low volume that loosens secretions to start, then a normal tidal volume breath to begin to move secretions, and finally a larger volume breath at higher peak flows to move secretions into the larger airways so they can be expelled with a cough.	Patients need to be approximately 10 to 12 years of age to perform correctly. It requires a coordinated breathing effort from the patients. It is difficult to perform during exacerbations or when patients are unable to take a deep breath.
Mechanical Insufflator-Exsufflator (MIE)	This device applied with a mask provides inspiratory positive airway pressure to augment the patient's tidal volume and then switches to a negative pressure to assist with expulsion of secretions.	Usually requires an additional caregiver. May worsen airway collapse in obstructive disorders. It is contraindicated when untreated pneumothorax, hemodynamic instability, increased intracranial pressure, recent maxillofacial surgery or trauma, active hemoptysis, or ruptured tympanic membrane exists or is suspected.
Positive Expiratory Pressure (PEP) or Vibratory PEP	The PEP devices use a fixed or variable orifice expiratory flow resistor to generate expiratory pressures of 10 to 20 cm H_2O as the patient actively exhales through the device. Vibratory or oscillatory PEP incorporates flow interruptions during the active expiration to create flow oscillations in addition to the PEP.	It is limited to children and adults who can take a deep breath and generate high enough flow rates to create PEP and vibrations. It is contraindicated when untreated pneumothorax, hemodynamic instability, increased intracranial pressure, recent maxillofacial surgery or trauma, active hemoptysis, or ruptured tympanic membrane exists or is suspected.
High-Frequency Positive Airway Pressure Devices or Intrapulmonary Percussive Ventilation (IPV)	IPV devices provide short, rapid positive airway pressure pulses as the patient breathes in and actively exhales against these pulsations to loosen secretions and move then forward. If patients don't actively exhale, exhalation occurs due to chest wall's elastic recoil.	It is limited to children and adults. It is contraindicated when untreated pneumothorax, hemodynamic instability, increased intracranial pressure, recent maxillofacial surgery or trauma, active hemoptysis, or ruptured tympanic membrane exists or is suspected.
High-Frequency Chest Wall Compression (HFCW)	High-frequency, small volumes are applied to the chest wall through a vest. These pulses of air create chest wall compressions that result in small expiratory flows in the airways that move secretions forward.	Used in children that are at least 2 to 3 years of age. Indwelling catheters and chest tubes should be avoided when this device is used.
Mobilization and Physical Activity	Physical activity that results in increased tidal ventilation, heart rate, and cardiac output, and improved physical conditioning.	Patients' medical condition must be such that they can safely participate in physical exercise, or medical supervision would be required to monitor for desaturations. Patients with reactive airways have a risk of developing bronchospasms.

Modified from Volsko T: Airway clearance therapy: finding the evidence. Respir Care 58(10):1669–1678, 2013.

Figure 43-2 depicts the primary positions used to drain the various lung lobes and segments. Generally, to obtain the proper head-down position, the RT must lower the head of the bed by at least 16 to 18 inches to achieve the desired 25-degree angle. In the ambulatory care setting, a tilt table can be used in lieu of a hospital bed. A tilt table allows precise positioning at head-down angles up to 45 degrees. When angles this large are used, shoulder supports must be provided to prevent the patient from sliding off the tilt table.

After the patient is positioned, the RT confirms the patient's comfort and ensures proper support of all joints and bony areas with pillows or towels. The indicated position is maintained for a minimum of 3 minutes if tolerated and longer if good sputum production results. Between positions, pauses for relaxation and

Box 43-4 Contraindications to the Use of CPT

The decision to use postural drainage requires assessment of potential benefits vs potential risks. Therapy should be provided for no longer than necessary to obtain the desired therapeutic results. Listed contraindications are relative unless marked as absolute *(A)*.

Positioning: All positions are contraindicated for:

- Head and neck injury until stabilized *(A)*
- Active hemorrhage with hemodynamic instability *(A)*
- Intracranial pressure (ICP) greater than 20 mm Hg
- Recent spinal surgery or acute spinal injury
- Active hemoptysis
- Empyema
- Bronchopleural fistula
- Pulmonary edema associated with congestive heart failure
- Aged, confused, or anxious patients who do not tolerate position changes
- Pulmonary embolism
- Rib fracture, with or without flail chest
- Surgical wound or healing tissue
- Large pleural effusions

Trendelenburg position contraindicated for:

- Recent gross hemoptysis related to recent lung carcinoma treated surgically or with radiation therapy
- ICP greater than 20 mm Hg
- Uncontrolled hypertension
- Distended abdomen
- Patients in whom increased ICP is to be avoided (e.g., neurosurgery, aneurysms, eye surgery)
- Uncontrolled airway at risk for aspiration (tube feeding or recent meal)
- Esophageal surgery

External manipulation of the thorax contradinciations (in addition to contraindications previously listed):

- Subcutaneous emphysema
- Recent epidural spinal infusion or spinal anesthesia
- Recently placed transvenous pacemaker or subcutaneous pacemaker
- Lung contusion
- Osteomyelitis of the ribs
- Coagulopathy
- Recent skin grafts, or flaps, on the thorax
- Burns, open wounds, and skin infections of the thorax
- Suspected pulmonary tuberculosis
- Bronchospasm
- Osteoporosis
- Complaint of chest wall pain

Excerpts from the American Association for Respiratory Care: Clinical practice guideline: postural drainage therapy. Respir Care 36:1418, 1991.

breathing control are useful and can help prevent hypoxemia. Because postural drainage therapy can increase O_2 consumption, critically ill patients should be given supplemental O_2 during the procedure if SpO_2 decreases.

During the procedure, the patient is continually observed for any side effects or complications. Moderate changes in vital signs are expected during treatment. Table 43-3 lists complications and recommended interventions. Significant problems may require immediate intervention.

MINI CLINI

Postural Drainage, Percussion, and Vibration

PROBLEM: A physician's progress note indicates a potential bacterial pneumonia localized to a patient's right middle lobe. The patient has coarse breath sounds on the right midlung and a nonproductive cough. The physician orders CPT four times daily "until radiograph clears." What positions should the RT select for postural drainage, and where should the RT provide percussion?

Discussion: The correct position for draining the right middle lobe would be head down (foot of bed raised about 12 inches), with the patient rotated about 45 degrees left from supine (modified left side-lying position). Percussion should be performed on the right anterior chest wall, between the fourth and sixth ribs (see Chapter 16 for external anatomic landmarks).

Also, the RT should ensure that the patient uses appropriate coughing technique during and after positioning. When using the head-down position, the patient should avoid strenuous coughing because this markedly increases intracranial pressure. Rather, the patient should use the forced expiration technique (described later in this chapter). Generally, total treatment time should not exceed 15 minutes for a routine treatment and 30 minutes for extended treatment. Both the patient and the RT should understand that postural drainage does not always result in the immediate production of secretions. More often, secretions are simply mobilized toward the trachea for easier removal by coughing. If the procedure causes vigorous coughing, have the patient sit up until the cough subsides.

After the procedure, the patient is repositioned to the pretreatment position, and the RT ensures the patient's stability and comfort. Immediate posttreatment assessment includes repeat vital signs, confirmation of satisfactory arterial saturation, chest auscultation, and questioning the patient regarding his or her subjective response to the procedure.

RULE OF THUMB

Generally, whenever you observe any patient adverse effects or complications during postural drainage, follow the "triple S rule": **stop** the therapy, return patient to original resting position, and **stay** with the patient until he or she is **stabilized**.

Outcome Assessment

Specific outcome criteria indicating a positive response to postural drainage are listed in Box 43-5. Generally, achievement of one or more of these outcomes indicates that the therapy is meeting its objectives and should be continued. Not all criteria are required to justify continuing postural drainage. Because

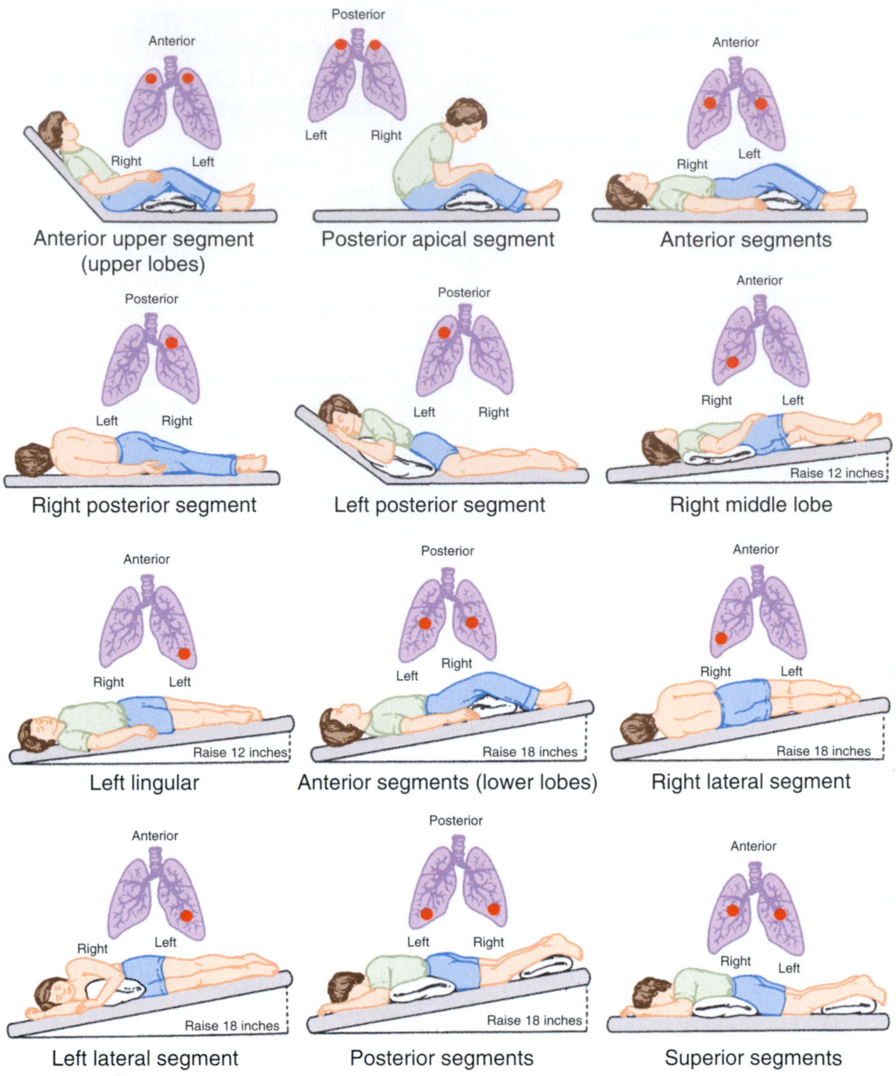

FIGURE 43-2 Patient positions for postural drainage. (Modified from Potter PA, Perry AG: Fundamentals of nursing: concepts, process and practice, ed 4, St Louis, 1997, Mosby.)

TABLE 43-3

Complications of Postural Drainage Therapy and Recommended Interventions

Complication	Action to Be Taken/Possible Intervention
Hypoxemia	Administer higher FiO_2 during procedure if potential for or observed hypoxemia exists. If patient becomes hypoxemic during treatment, administer 100% O_2, stop therapy immediately, return patient to original position, and consult physician
Increased intracranial pressure	Stop therapy, return patient to original resting position, and consult physician
Acute hypotension during procedure	Stop therapy, return patient to original resting position, and consult physician
Pulmonary hemorrhage	Stop therapy, return patient to original resting position, and call physician immediately. Administer O_2 and maintain an airway until physician responds
Pain or injury to muscles, ribs, or spine	Stop therapy that appears directly associated with pain or problem, exercise care in moving patient, and consult physician
Vomiting and aspiration	Stop therapy, clear airway and suction as needed, administer O_2, maintain airway, return patient to previous resting position, and contact physician immediately
Bronchospasm	Stop therapy, return patient to previous resting position, and administer or increase O_2 delivery while contacting physician. Administer physician-ordered bronchodilators
Arrhythmias	Stop therapy, return patient to previous resting position, and administer or increase O_2 delivery while contacting physician

Box 43-5 Assessment Outcomes after CPT

The following items represent individual criteria that indicate a positive response to therapy (and support continuation of therapy). Not all criteria are required to justify continuation of therapy (e.g., a ventilated patient may not have sputum production >30 ml/day but have improvement in breath sounds, chest radiograph, or increased compliance or decreased resistance).

- Change in sputum production
- Change in breath sounds of lung fields being drained
- Patient subjective response to therapy
- Change in vital signs
- Change in chest radiograph
- Change in arterial blood gas values or O_2 saturation
- Change in ventilator variables

Excerpts from the American Association for Respiratory Care: Clinical practice guideline: postural drainage therapy. Respir Care 36:1418, 1991.

secretion clearance is affected by patient hydration, the RT may need to wait for at least 24 hours after optimal systemic hydration has been achieved to see any evidence of increased sputum production. In the interim, tracheobronchial clearance may be enhanced in some patients by adding bland aerosol therapy.[17,18]

Breath sounds may seem to "worsen" after therapy by changing from diminished breath sounds before therapy to coarse crackles. This change is due to the loosening of secretions and their movement into the larger airways, an intended purpose of the therapy. These coarse crackles should clear after coughing or suctioning.

In terms of the patient's subjective response to therapy, the patient should be encouraged to report any pain, discomfort, shortness of breath, dizziness, or nausea during or after therapy. Any of these adverse effects may be grounds for either modifying or stopping treatment. Patient reports of easier clearance or increased volume of secretions after therapy support continuing therapy.

On the basis of assessment results, CPT orders should be reevaluated for need at least every 2 to 3 days for hospitalized patients. Patients receiving home care should be reevaluated at least every 3 months or whenever their status changes.

Documentation and Follow-Up

The chart entry should include the positions used, time of treatment, patient tolerance, pre and post vital signs and breath sounds, subjective and objective indicators of treatment effectiveness (including amount, color, and consistency of sputum produced), and any adverse effects observed.

Percussion and Vibration

Percussion and vibration involve application of mechanical energy to the chest wall by the use of either hands or various electrical or pneumatic devices. Both methods are designed to augment secretion clearance.[14] In theory, percussion should help loosen secretions from the tracheobronchial tree, making

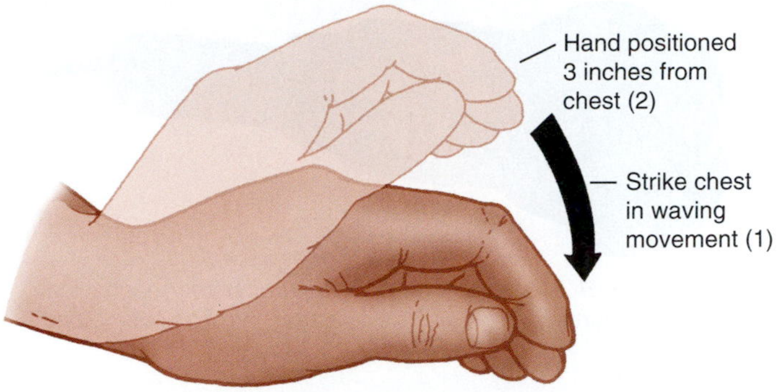

FIGURE 43-3 Movement of cupped hand at wrist, to percuss chest.

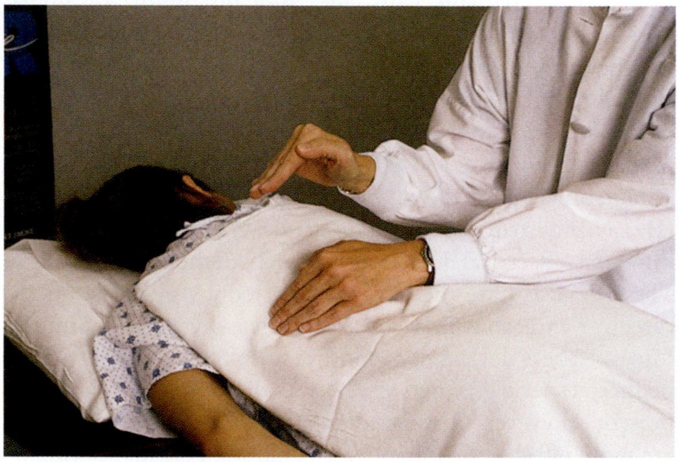

FIGURE 43-4 Hand placement for CPT. (From Harkreader H, Hogan M, Thobaben M: Fundamentals of nursing, caring and clinical judgment, ed 3, St Louis, 2007, Saunders.)

them easier to remove by coughing or suctioning. The effectiveness of percussion as an adjunct to postural drainage remains unclear.[2,3] This controversy is due to variability in practice and the difficulty related to performing these trials since percussion is only a part of the treatment regimen.

Manual Percussion. The therapist performs manual percussion with his or her hands in a cupped position, with fingers and thumb closed (Figure 43-3). This technique compresses air between the hand and chest wall. This technique should be applied against a thin layer of cloth, such as a hospital gown or bed sheet to help improve patient comfort. This technique involves the therapist's cupped hands rhythmically striking the chest wall in a waving motion, using both hands alternately in sequence with the elbows partially flexed and wrists loose (see Figure 43-3). Slower, more relaxing rates are better tolerated by the patient and the therapist. This technique requires practice to determine the appropriate force and maintain a rhythmic pattern during this therapy (Figure 43-4). Ideally, the RT should percuss back and forth in a circular pattern over the localized area for 3 to 5 minutes. Care should be taken to avoid tender areas or sites of trauma or surgery, and one should never percuss

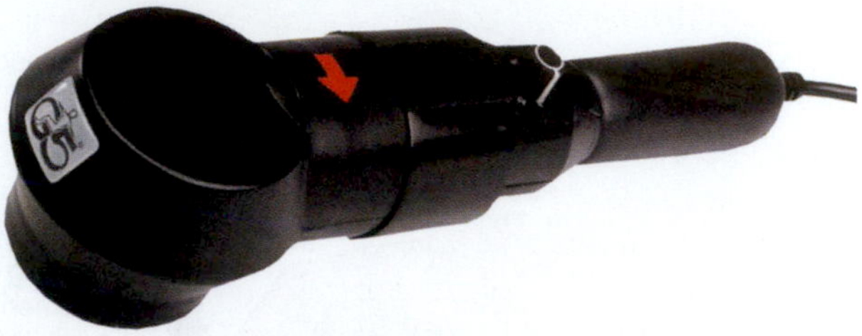

FIGURE 43-5 Example of an electrically powered mechanical percussor. (Courtesy General Physiotherapy, Inc. St Louis, MO.)

directly over bony prominences, such as the clavicles, vertebrae or sternum. Hands should be positioned parallel to the ribs.

Mechanical Percussion and Vibration. Mechanical vibration sometimes is used as an alternative to manual percussion in acutely ill patients with chest wall discomfort or injury. Various electrical and pneumatic devices have been developed to generate and apply the energy waves used during percussion and vibration. Typically, these devices have both a frequency and a percussion force control (Figure 43-5). Most units provide frequencies up to 20 to 50 cycles per second (20 to 50 Hz). Other sonic or acoustic devices may provide up to 120 **Hertz (Hz)**. Noise, excess force, and mechanical failure all are potential problems. Electrical devices also pose a potential shock hazard. These devices have the advantage of reducing fatigue on the caregiver and can deliver consistent rates, rhythms, and impact forces.[14] These devices may improve hospitalized patients' compliance, especially when chest wall discomfort or injury is present. However, there is no firm evidence that such devices are more effective than manual techniques. For this reason, the selection of manual or mechanical methods should be based on individual patient factors such as age, condition, and tolerance which are similar to other ACT modalities.[4]

Coughing and Related Expulsion Techniques

Most airway clearance therapies help only to move secretions into the central airways. Clearance of these secretions requires either coughing or suctioning. In this respect, an effective cough (or alternative expulsion measure) is an essential component of all ACT. These expulsion methods are also useful in obtaining sputum specimens for diagnostic analysis.

RULE OF THUMB

Clinicians should coach an effective cough with most airway clearance techniques to fully clear secretions.

Directed Cough

Directed cough is a deliberate maneuver that is taught, supervised, and monitored. It aims to assist in creating a productive cough in patients unable to clear secretions with an effective spontaneous cough.

In patients with copious secretions, directed coughing is an effective clearance method clearing secretions from the central, but not peripheral, airways.[1,2,19, 20] In addition to aiding in the removal of retained secretions from central airways, it should be a routine part of all ACT and may be helpful in obtaining sputum specimens for diagnostic analysis.[19]

Box 43-6 lists the relative contraindications and potential complications associated with directed cough. These patients should be monitored for pain, discomfort, dyspnea, pulse rate, cardiac rhythm (if electrocardiogram is available), breath sounds, pulse oximetry if desaturation is suspected, breathing pattern, skin color, sputum production, and ICP if elevated. To determine the effectiveness of directed cough techniques, therapists should evaluate the patient for any of the following outcome changes: increased sputum production, decreased pulse and respiratory rate, clearing of the breath sounds, improved oxygen saturation, and possibly clearing of infiltrates on the chest radiograph.[19]

Box 43-6 Directed Cough

CONTRAINDICATIONS

Directed cough is rarely contraindicated. The contraindications listed must be weighed against potential benefit in deciding to eliminate cough from the care of the patient. Listed contraindications are relative:

- Inability to control possible transmission of infection from patients suspected or known to have pathogens transmittable by droplet nuclei (e.g., *Mycobacterium tuberculosis*)
- Presence of elevated ICP or known intracranial aneurysm
- Presence of reduced coronary artery perfusion, such as in acute myocardial infarction
- Acute unstable head, neck, or spine injury
- Manually assisted directed cough with pressure to the epigastrium may be contraindicated in the presence of increased potential for regurgitation or aspiration, acute abdominal pathology, abdominal aortic aneurysm, hiatal hernia, pregnancy, bleeding diathesis, or untreated pneumothorax
- Manually assisted directed cough with pressure to the thoracic cage may be contraindicated in the presence of osteoporosis or flail chest

HAZARDS AND COMPLICATIONS

- Reduced coronary artery perfusion
- Reduced cerebral perfusion
- Incontinence
- Fatigue
- Rib or costochondral fracture
- Headache
- Visual disturbances, including retinal hemorrhage
- Bronchospasm
- Muscular damage or discomfort
- Incisional pain, evisceration
- Anorexia, vomiting
- Gastroesophageal reflux
- Spontaneous pneumothorax
- Pneumomediastinum
- Subcutaneous emphysema
- Cough paroxysms
- Chest pain
- Central line displacement

Excerpts from the American Association for Respiratory Care: Clinical practice guideline: directed cough. Respir Care 38:495, 1993.

Standard Technique. After the clinical need for directed coughing has been established, the RT should assess the patient for any factors that could limit the success of directed cough and relative contraindications. An effective directed cough is impossible with unresponsive, paralyzed, or uncooperative patients. In addition, some patients with severe COPD or severe restrictive disorders (including neurologic, muscular, or skeletal abnormalities) may be unable to generate an effective spontaneous cough. Pain, systemic dehydration, tenaciously thick secretions, artificial airways, or use of central nervous system depressants can also impact efforts to implement an effective directed cough. If any of these limitations exist, the RT should recommend an alternative to directed cough such as an assisted cough, which is discussed later in this chapter.

Patient education is a critical part of developing an effective directed cough. The three most important aspects in teaching a patient to have an effective cough are (1) instruction on proper positioning, (2) instruction on breathing control, and (3) exercises to strengthen the expiratory muscles.[21] These activities are modified according to the patient's underlying clinical problem.

First, patients are taught to assume a sitting position with one shoulder rotated inward and the head and spine slightly flexed to aid exhalation and allow easy thoracic compression. It is difficult to generate an effective cough in the supine position. The patient's feet should be supported to provide abdominal and thoracic support for the patient. If the patient is unable to sit up, the RT should raise the head of the bed and ensure that the patient's knees are slightly flexed with the feet braced on the mattress.

Breathing control measures help ensure that the inspiration, compression, and expulsion phases of the cough are maximally effective and coordinated. For effective inspiration, the patient should be taught to inspire slowly and deeply through the nose, using the diaphragm. In patients with copious amounts of sputum, such breaths alone may stimulate coughing by loosening secretions in the larger airways.

After confirming that the patient can take a good, deep inspiration, the RT has the patient bear down against the glottis, in much the same manner as would occur with straining when lifting weights or during a bowel movement. For patients with pain or patients subject to bronchial collapse, it is probably best that they be shown how to "stage" their expiratory effort into two or three short bursts. For these patients, this method is generally less fatiguing and more effective in producing sputum than a single violent expulsion. Effective breathing control and effective coughing are best taught by demonstration. The RT demonstrates the various phases of the cough sequence while emphasizing the correct technique. The RT explains how to avoid common errors, such as simple throat clearing.

Proper positioning and breathing control alone may not result in an effective cough and clear secretions. This limitation often is due to weak breathing muscles. Muscle weakness is common in patients with neuromuscular disease, patients with COPD, and patients needing long-term ventilatory support. These muscles may atrophy due to disease progression, lack of appropriate nutrition, or lack of use during mechanical ventilation. In these cases, either suctioning or using the **mechanical insufflation-exsufflation** (MIE) device may be effective in clearing these secretions.

Modifications to Directed Cough Technique. Modifying the normal directed cough to the needs of the individual patient may lead to a productive cough effort. Good clinical examples of the need to modify directed cough are seen in surgical patients, patients with COPD, and patients with neuromuscular disorders.

In surgical patients, preoperative training in deep breathing and directed cough can help prepare the patient for the postoperative regimen. This preparation can minimize the anxiety related to pain that commonly impairs an effective cough in these patients. In addition, coordinating the coughing sessions with prescribed pain medication and **splinting** the operative site can enhance these sessions. The RT can use his or her hands to support the area of incision during the expiratory phase of the cough. Eventually, the patient can learn to use a pillow or blanket roll to splint the incision site. The **forced expiratory technique** (**FET**) (discussed subsequently) may also be valuable in these patients.

In some patients with COPD, the high pleural pressures during a forced cough may compress the smaller airways and limit the cough's effectiveness. In this situation, the patient is placed in the sitting position previously described. The patient is instructed to take in a moderately deep breath slowly through the nose. To help enhance expulsion, the patient should exhale with moderate force through pursed lips, while bending forward. This forward flexion of the thorax enhances expiratory flow by upward displacement of the abdominal contents. After three or four repetitions of this maneuver, the patient is encouraged to bend forward and initiate short staccato-like bursts of air. This technique relieves the strain of a prolonged hard cough, and the staccato rhythm at a relatively low velocity minimizes airway collapse. These staccato-like bursts of air against an open glottis are referred to as *huffing*.[1,2,21] With this technique the patient is instructed to make the sound "huff, huff, huff" rapidly with the mouth and glottis open. **Huff coughing** is also referred to as FET.

Forced Expiratory Technique

As stated above, FET consists of one or two forced expirations of middle to low lung volume without closure of the glottis, followed by a period of diaphragmatic breathing and relaxation.[19] The goal of this method is to help clear secretions with less change in pleural pressure and less likelihood of bronchiolar collapse. To help keep the glottis open during FET, the patient is taught to phonate or "huff" during expiration. The period of diaphragmatic breathing and relaxation following the forced expiration is essential in restoring lung volume and minimizing fatigue. Comparative clinical studies on the effectiveness of FET have shown favorable results. The technique is particularly useful in patients prone to airway collapse during normal coughing, such as patients with COPD, CF, or bronchiectasis.[1,2,21]

Manual Assisted Cough

Patients with neuromuscular conditions present a special challenge in cough management. These patients typically are unable to generate the forceful expulsion needed to move secretions toward the trachea.[23] If this problem results in retained secretions, there are only three options: (1) placement of an artificial airway and removal of secretions by tracheobronchial suctioning (see Chapter 36), (2) manually assisted cough, and/or (3) MIE.

Manually assisted cough is external application of pressure to the thoracic cage or epigastric region, coordinated with forced exhalation.[19] In this technique, the patient takes as deep an inspiration as possible, assisted as needed by the application of positive pressure via a self-inflating bag or intermittent positive pressure breathing device. At the end of the patient's inspiration, the RT begins exerting pressure on the lateral costal margins or epigastrium. This pressure increases the force of compression throughout expiration; this mimics the normal cough mechanism by generating an increase in the velocity of the expired air and may be helpful in moving secretions toward the trachea, where they can be removed by suctioning. Assisted cough with pressure to the lateral costal margins is contraindicated in patients with osteoporosis or flail chest.[19] Assisted cough using epigastric pressure is contraindicated in unconscious patients with unprotected airways, in pregnant women, and in patients with acute abdominal pathology, abdominal aortic aneurysm, or hiatal hernia.[19]

MINI CLINI

Modifications to Directed Cough

PROBLEM: A patient who has been diagnosed with ALS who has been attending your multidisciplinary clinic for the last few years returns for a follow-up visit. The patient states she has noticed her cough is not as powerful as it has been and that she is "winded" when walking distances. The respiratory therapist assesses the patient and finds: pulse rate of 80, respiratory rate of 24, and breath sounds of scattered wet crackles in both lungs. The patient performs spirometry and maximum inspiratory and expiratory pressure maneuvers (MIP/MEP). Her FVC is 70% of predicted, MIP is negative 50 cm H_2O and MEP is 55 cm H_2O sitting, and MIP is negative 40 cm H_2O and MEP is 40 cm H_2O supine. The therapist reviews the values from the previous visit 3 months earlier and finds FVC was 75% of predicted and MIP was a negative 65 cm H_2O and the MEP was 70 cm H_2O both sitting and supine.

Discussion: Based on this assessment, the patient's lung volumes and muscle strength have declined. She also has retained secretions and would benefit from airway clearance therapy and possibly MIE to assist with secretion removal. The patient began high-frequency chest wall compressions to mobilize these secretions and MIE to assist in expectorating the secretions. This therapy should take place a minimum of twice a day.

Active Cycle of Breathing Technique

To emphasize that FET should include breathing exercises, the originators of this technique modified the procedure and renamed it the **active cycle of breathing technique (ACBT)**.[14,24] ACBT consists of repeated cycles of breathing control, thoracic expansion, and FET (Box 43-7). *Breathing control* involves gentle diaphragmatic breathing at normal tidal volumes for 5 to 10 seconds with relaxation of the upper chest and shoulders. This phase is intended to help prevent bronchospasm. The thoracic expansion exercises involve deep inhalation, approaching vital capacity, with relaxed exhalation, which may be accompanied by percussion, vibration, or compression. The *thoracic expansion* phase is designed to help loosen secretions, improve the distribution of ventilation, and provide the volume needed for FET. The subsequent FET moves secretions into the central airways. Postoperative patients may require splinting at the thoracic or abdominal incision site. Although ACBT can be performed in the sitting position, it is most beneficial when combined with postural drainage. When ACBT is compared with similar methods of secretion clearance, studies indicate that ACBT can provide comparable results in terms of both sputum production and distribution of ventilation.[24,25] ACBT is not useful with young children (<2 years old) or critically ill patients. Caution should be taken in patients with reactive airways during ACBT.

Autogenic Drainage

Autogenic drainage (AD) is another modification of directed coughing, designed as an airway clearance mechanism that can be performed independently by trained patients.[7,11,14,24] During AD, the patient uses diaphragmatic breathing to mobilize secretions by varying lung volumes and expiratory airflow in three distinct phases (Figure 43-6).[14,24] For maximum benefit, the patient should be in the sitting position. Patients are taught to control their expiratory flows to prevent airway collapse while trying to achieve a mucous "rattle" rather than a wheeze. Coughing should be suppressed until all three breathing phases are completed.

In patients with CF, AD provides sputum clearance comparable to PDPV but is less likely to produce O_2 desaturation. In addition, AD seems to be tolerated better by patients and has the advantage of being performed without assistance from a caregiver.[2,21,24-26]

Box 43-7 Active Cycle of Breathing Technique Sequence

1. Relaxation and breathing control
2. Three or four thoracic expansion exercises
3. Relaxation and breathing control
4. Repeat three to four thoracic expansion exercises
5. Repeat relaxation and breathing control
6. Perform one or two FETs (huffs)
7. Repeat relaxation and breathing control

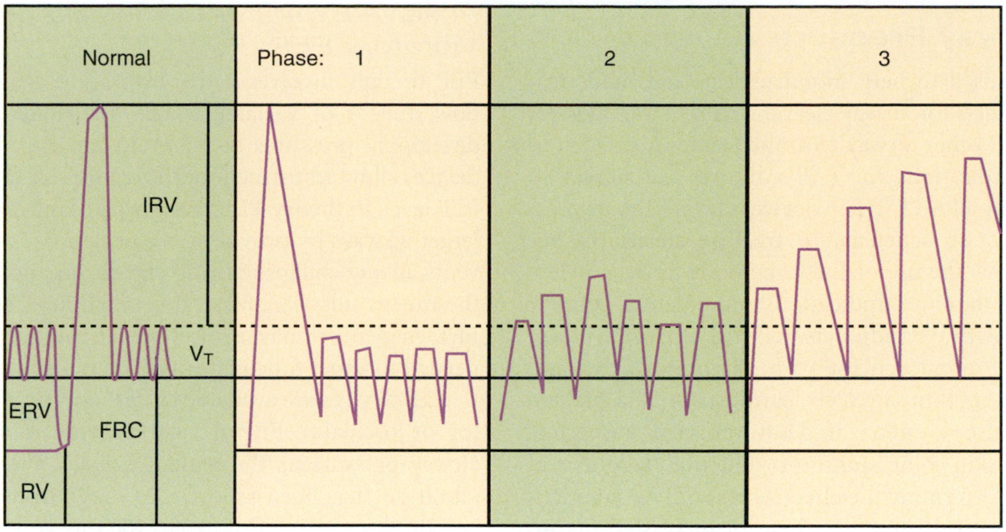

FIGURE 43-6 Spirogram of lung volumes during three phases of autogenic drainage. Phase 1 involves a full inspiratory capacity maneuver, followed by breathing at low lung volumes. This phase is designed to "unstick" peripheral mucus. Phase 2 involves breathing at low to middle lung volumes to collect mucus in the middle airways. Phase 3 is the evacuation phase, in which mucus is readied for expulsion from the large airways. (Modified from Hardy KA, Anderson BD: Respir Care Clin North Am 2:323, 1996.)

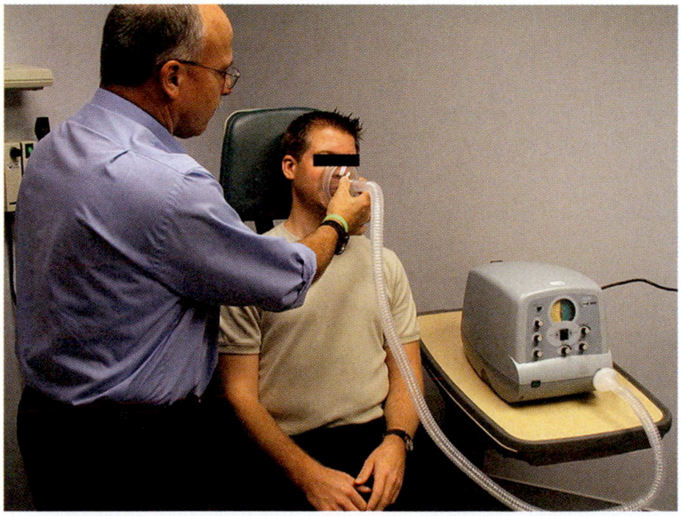

FIGURE 43-7 MIE device. (From Mason R, Broaddus V, Martin T, et al: Murray & Nadel's textbook of respiratory medicine, ed 10, Philadelphia, 2010, Saunders.)

Mechanical Insufflation-Exsufflation

The MIE device (also called *cough-assist device* or "coughlator") has gained popularity in its use to manage secretions in patients with certain neuromuscular disorders (Figure 43-7).[2,7,14] The reason is growing evidence that MIE helps prevent respiratory complications in patients with neuromuscular disorders by helping them generate sufficient expiratory flow rates needed for effective secretion clearance.[1,7,27]

NMD patients who are not able to demonstrate a peak cough flow greater than 180 L/min or not able to generate an effective cough may benefit from MIE.[7] The AARC clinical practice guideline for ACT recommends cough assist techniques when peak cough flows are less than 270 L/min in NMD patients.[1]

The MIE device delivers a positive pressure breath of 30 to 50 cm H_2O over a 1- to 3-second period via a face mask or artificial airway. The airway pressure is abruptly reversed to −30 to −50 cm H_2O and maintained for 2 to 3 seconds. Peak expiratory "cough" flows obtained with this device are in the normal range (mean 7.5 L/sec); far better than can be achieved with manually assisted coughing. Expiratory flows remain high in the immediate postexsufflation period, indicating that MIE does not promote airway collapse. Newer MIE devices have incorporated oscillation during inspiration or expiration to assist in mobilizing secretions.

A typical treatment session with the MIE consists of about five cycles (inspiration and expiration) followed by a period of normal spontaneous or assisted breathing (to avoid hyperventilation). This process is repeated five or more times until secretions are cleared from the airway and the patient is able to either suction or spit them out.

MIE via an oronasal mask is effective, provided that there is no fixed airway obstruction or glottic collapse during exsufflation. For patients with severe restrictive disease and NMD who are not able to take deep breaths, insufflation pressures should be increased gradually based on the patient and their assessment to avoid chest wall muscle strains. Abdominal distention is infrequent and reduced by decreasing airway pressures during insufflation, not exsufflation. The effectiveness of MIE in persons with airway obstructions such as COPD is less clear, and MIE may be detrimental because it may increase the amount of air trapping and auto-PEEP.[2]

Precautions should be observed using MIE with patients with known cardiac instability. It may be beneficial to monitor heart rate and O_2 saturation closely in these patients. MIE is contraindicated in patients with a history of bullous emphysema or previous barotraumas such as pneumothorax or pneumomediastinum.

Positive Airway Pressure Adjuncts

PAP adjuncts are used to help mobilize secretions and treat atelectasis. As adjuncts for airway clearance, these methods are usually paired with other airway clearance techniques such as directed cough. Indications for PAP adjuncts are similar to those listed early for all ACT. These devices elevate airway pressure and may also be beneficial in treating atelectasis. See Chapter 42 to review the use of these methods to treat atelectasis. Box 43-8 lists the contraindications and potential complications associated with PAP adjuncts. As with other ACT, these patients should be monitored for pain, discomfort, dyspnea, pulse rate, cardiac rhythm (if electrocardiogram is available), breath sounds, pulse oximetry if desaturation is suspected, breathing pattern, skin color, sputum production, fatigue, and ICP if elevated. To determine the effectiveness of PAP adjuncts, the therapist should evaluate the patient for increased sputum production, decreased pulse and respiratory rate, clearing of the breath sounds, improved oxygen saturation, and possibly clearing of infiltrates on the chest radiograph.[28] The following discussion will focus on the use of PAP devices for secretion clearance.

Box 43-8 Positive Airway Pressure (PAP) Adjuncts for Airway Clearance Therapy

CONTRAINDICATIONS

Although no absolute contraindications to the use of PAP adjuncts have been reported, the following should be carefully evaluated before initiating therapy:

- Patients unable to tolerate increased work of breathing (acute asthma, COPD)
- Intracranial pressure (ICP) greater than 20 mm Hg
- Hemodynamic instability
- Acute sinusitis
- Active hemoptysis
- Untreated pneumothorax
- Known or suspected tympanic membrane rupture or other middle ear pathology
- Recent facial, oral, or skull surgery or trauma
- Epistaxis
- Esophageal surgery
- Nausea

HAZARDS AND COMPLICATIONS INCLUDE

- Pulmonary barotraumas
- Increased ICP
- Cardiovascular compromise (myocardial ischemia, decreased venous return)
- Skin breakdown and discomfort from mask
- Air swallowing, vomiting, and aspiration
- Claustrophobia
- Increased work of breathing that may lead to hypoventilation and hypercapnia

Excerpts from the American Association for Respiratory Care: Clinical practice guideline: use of PAP adjuncts to bronchial hygiene therapy. Respir Care 38:516, 1993.

Positive Expiratory Pressure (PEP) and Vibratory PEP

PEP therapy involves active expiration against a fixed orifice flow resistor or variable orifice threshold resistor capable of developing pressures of 10 to 20 cm H_2O. Most fixed orifice devices allow adjustment of the orifice size to achieve a targeted PEP level. In theory, PEP therapy helps move secretions into the larger airways by providing a constant back-pressure that prevents airway collapse during expiration and the airway behind the mucus fills via collateral ventilation. A subsequent huff or FET maneuver may allow the patient to generate the flows needed to expel mucus from blocked airways.

PEP devices are available as PEP only or vibrator PEP. Vibrator or oscillator PEP devices provide rapid fluctuations in airway pressure as the patient exhales. The frequency of the vibrations has been reported to range from 10 to 30 Hz with amplitudes ranging from 20 to 100 torr at flows of 10 and 25 L/min.[29] Clinical studies of PEP and vibratory PEP therapy improved secretion clearance in hospitalized,[3] CF,[2,5,30,31] and COPD patients with secretion retention,[1] but is not beneficial in preventing postoperative atelectasis.[1] Generally, compared with other airway clearance methods (PDPV, AD, ACBT) in patients with CF, PEP therapy provides comparable mucociliary clearance, with the added advantages of being potentially self-administered and cost-effective.[2,32] Patients may prefer PEP over CPT.[5] PEP therapy cannot be used in young children (<3 years old). Patients must also be able to take a deep breath (>10-12 mL/kg) to generate adequate pressure, oscillations, and prolonged exhalations.

There are several available PEP and vibratory PEP devices on the market and manufacturer instructions on recommended application are included with each device (Figure 43-8). Most of these are single-use commercial devices. A general clinical procedure for application of PAP therapy is presented in Box 43-9.[16] Regardless of the equipment used, it is important that actual intended PEP levels are reached so initial monitoring of patient for correct use is essential.

Common strategies for PEP therapy vary, with frequency determined by assessment of patient response. Studies provide conflicting results related to the amount of time and intervals of therapy sessions during acute exacerbations associated with CF and COPD. Twice to four times daily are common frequencies used for PEP therapy.[28] Aerosol drug therapy may be added to a PEP session using either an in-line hand-held nebulizer or a metered dose inhaler attached to the one-way valve inlet of the system. The combination of aerosol drug therapy with PEP seems to improve the efficacy of bronchodilator administration because of better distribution to the peripheral airways.[17] Some PEP devices can be modified to incorporate a mask for patients with ALS, toddlers, or stroke patients who are unable to use a mouthpiece.

High-frequency vibrations or **oscillations** refer to the rapid vibratory movement of small volumes of air back and forth in the respiratory tract. At frequencies of 12 to 25 Hz these oscillations are thought to physically loosen secretions and move them toward the larger airways, which enhances airway

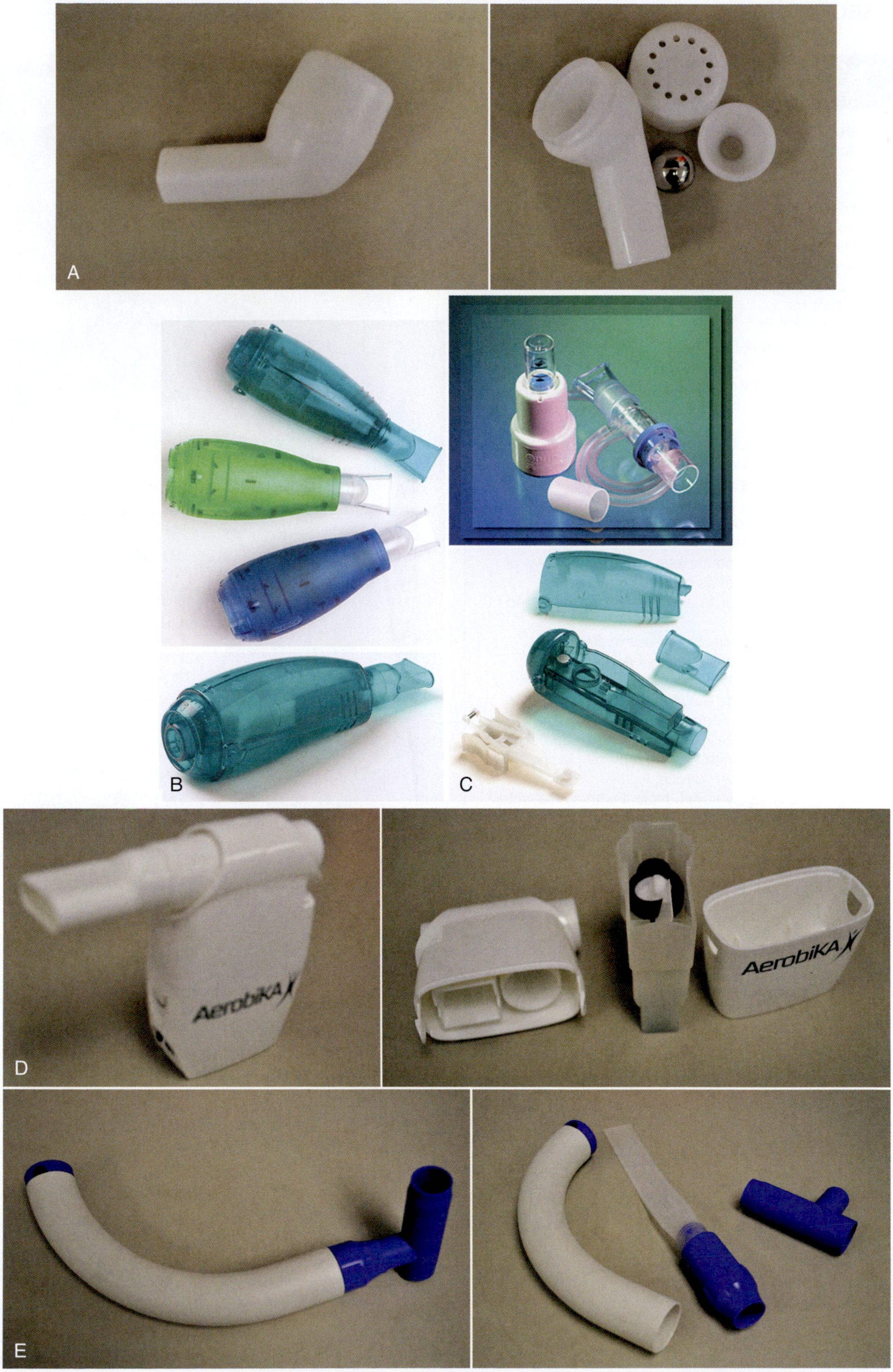

FIGURE 43-8 Positive expiratory devices: **A,** Flutter. **B,** TheraPEP. **C,** Acapella (Choice is used for a range of flows. Green is used for flows higher than 15 L/min. Blue is used for flows less than 15 L/min.). **D,** Aerobika. **E,** RC-Cornet.

Box 43-9 Clinical Procedure for Positive Airway Pressure Therapy

1. Assess need for PAP therapy and design a treatment program to accomplish treatment objectives.
   a. Bring equipment to bedside and provide initial therapy to patient, adjusting pressure settings to meet patient need.
   b. After initial patient treatment or training, communicate treatment plan to physician and nurse, and provide instruction to nursing staff if required.
2. Explain purpose of PAP therapy to patient; teach patient "huff" (directed cough procedure).
3. Instruct patient to:
   a. Sit comfortably.
   b. If using a mask, apply it tightly but comfortably over the nose and mouth. If mouthpiece is used, place lips firmly around it and breathe through mouth.
   c. Take in a breath that is larger than normal, but do not completely fill lungs.
   d. Exhale actively, but not forcefully, creating a PAP of 10 to 20 cm H_2O during exhalation (determined with manometer during initial therapy sessions). Length of inhalation should be approximately one-third of the total breathing cycle (inspiratory-to-expiratory ratio of 1 : 3 to 1 : 4).
   e. Perform 10 to 20 breaths.
   f. Remove the mask or mouthpiece, and perform two or three "huff" coughs; rest as needed.
   g. Repeat above cycle four to eight times, not to exceed 20 minutes.
4. Evaluate patient for the ability to self-administer.
5. When appropriate, teach patient to self-administer. Observations on several occasions of proper technique, uncoached, should precede allowing the patient to self-administer without supervision.
6. When patients are also receiving bronchodilator aerosol, administer in conjunction with PAP therapy by placing a nebulizer in line with the PAP device.
7. When PAP device is visibly soiled, rinse it with sterile water and shake or air dry; leave within reach at patient's bedside in a clear plastic bag.
8. Send the PAP device (if single-patient use) home with the patient, or discard it on discharge. If device is nondisposable, send in-house for high-level disinfection.
9. Document in the patient's medical record procedures performed (including device, settings used, pressure developed, number of breaths per treatment, and frequency), patient response to therapy, patient teaching provided, and patient ability to self-administer.

clearance. There are two general approaches: airway application of oscillation methods such as vibratory PEP discussed above or **high-frequency positive airway pressure devices (HFPAP)**, or external (chest wall) application referred to as **high-frequency chest wall compression (HFCWC)**. It is thought that the mucus moves as a result of the vibrations of the airways crated when the oscillation frequency resembles the resonance frequency of the pulmonary system.[22,29]

High-Frequency Positive Airway Pressure Devices

High-frequency positive airway pressure devices are also referred to as **intrapulmonary percussive ventilation (IPV)**.

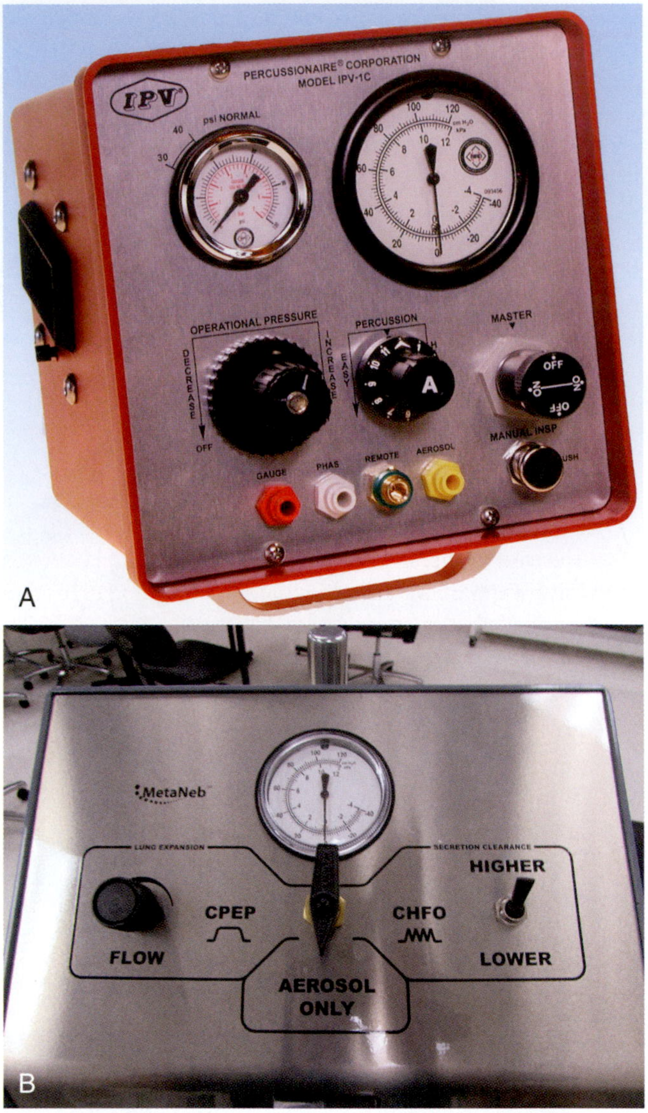

FIGURE 43-9 Intrapulmonary Percussive Ventilator, IPV. (Courtesy Percussionaire, SandPoint, Idaho, and MetaNeb.)

HFPAP or IPV devices (Figure 43-9) use a pneumatic device to deliver a rapid series of pressurized gas minibursts at rates of 100 to 225 cycles per minute (1.7 to 5 Hz) to the airway. During the percussive cycle, the patient can inhale and exhale through the device as this oscillating airway pressure is applied. These devices also deliver aerosolized medication, and rely on chest wall recoil or an active patient exhalation. Comparative studies show that IPV is equivalent to other airway clearance strategies in enhancing sputum expectoration in patients.[2,3,5] The therapy is well tolerated by stable patients and may provide a more effective alternative for airway clearance in patients unable to take a deep inspiration.

High-Frequency Chest Wall Oscillation

High-frequency chest wall oscillation (HFCWO) devices are passive oscillatory devices. These devices use a two-part system: (1) a variable air-pulse generator and (2) a nonstretch inflatable vest that wraps around the patient's entire torso (Vest Airway Clearance Systems, Hill-Rom Services, Inc., Batesville, IN). See Figure 43-10. Either one or two large-bore tubing(s) connect the vest to the air-pulse generator. Table 43-4 lists the devices, air-pulse waveforms, and hose configurations. The generator inflates and deflates the vest, creating pressure pulses against the thorax resulting in chest wall oscillations and moving secretions forward. These devices are used in hospital or home settings. The therapy is typically performed for a 30-minute session 2 to 6 times per day at oscillatory frequencies between 5 to 25 Hz. These therapy sessions depend on patient need and response.

Clinical trials with HFCWO have reported better or equivalent secretions clearance compared to other ACT in CF patients.[2,5] Studies in other populations have shown some improvement, as measured by patient perception, increased compliance, or outcome.[7,22]

The Biphasic Cuirass Ventilation (BCV) device is an alternative to the vest devices. This device may be used to provide noninvasive ventilation and/or cough assist. It uses a chest cuirass or shell that encompasses the anterior chest wall. The shell is connected to the generator that controls both phases of the respiratory cycle. The chest wall will expand when the negative pressure is applied. This device is capable of a frequency range between 1 and 999 oscillations per minute, I:E ratios of 1:6 and 6:1 and inspiratory and expiratory pressures of −70 to 70 cm H_2O. The recommended application is two sets of cycles that include a few minutes at a frequency between 600 and 700 at an I:E of 1:1, followed by a higher frequency at an inverse I:E ratio.[22] The therapy will ultimately depend on the patient's response.

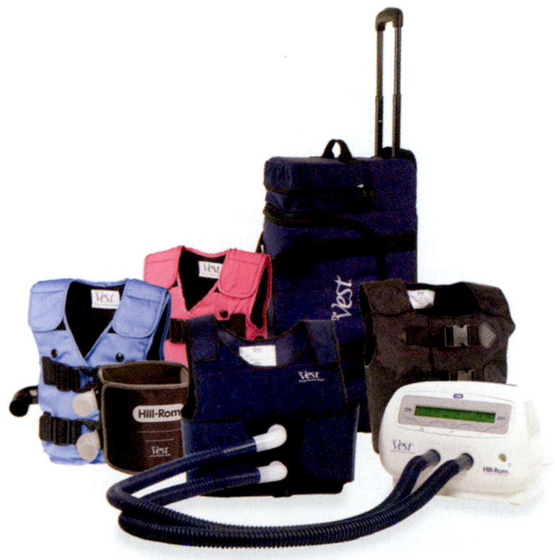

FIGURE 43-10 Patient using the Vest Airway Clearance System for high-frequency chest wall oscillation. (Copyright 2011 Hill-Rom Services, Inc., Batesville, IN. Reprinted with permission. All rights reserved.)

TABLE 43-4

High-Frequency Chest Wall Oscillator (HFCWO) Device Comparison

Company	Device	Air Pulse	Hose Configuration
Hill Rom	Vest™	Sine waveform	Single hose
Electromed	SmartVest™	Sine waveform	Double hose
RespirTech	InCourage™	Triangle waveform	Double hose

Exercise, Mobilization and Physical Activity

Immobility is a major factor contributing to complications in chronic disease and hospitalized patients. Early mobilization is recommended to reduce complications in hospitalized patients and is recommended as adjunctive therapy along with another ACT in CF to aid airway clearance and overall health benefits.[1,5,33,34] Physical activity may also improve lung function, exercise tolerance, quality of life, and adherence to therapy.[5] For more on the use of exercise in ambulatory patients with severe lung disease see Chapter 55.

SELECTING AIRWAY CLEARANCE TECHNIQUES

Selection Factors

Box 43-10 specifies many factors therapists should consider when selecting an airway clearance strategy. The correct application and patient motivation to perform the ACT are critical components regardless of the setting. No ACT is successful if it is abandoned by the patient. Likewise, no routine strategy is likely to be followed without results. In this regard, increased sputum production, less shortness of breath, and perhaps improved physical activity are a few outcomes that can be used to motivate patients and gain their ongoing cooperation.

Age, disease process, available resources, and patient preference often affect the choice of ACT. Patient and caregiver goals

Box 43-10 Key Factors in Selecting an Airway Clearance Strategy

- Patient's motivation
- Patient's goals
- Patient's ability to comprehend—literacy and cognition levels
- Patient's physical limitations
- Physician/caregiver goals
- Effectiveness of technique
- Ease of learning and teaching
- Skill of therapists
- Patient fatigue associated or work required to use device
- Need for assistance to use the equipment
- Limitations of technique based on disease type and severity
- Costs (direct and indirect)
- Desirability of combining methods

for treatment should be discussed jointly, with the intent of choosing the method that best fits the patient's goals and lifestyle. The RT's skill and patience in teaching the ACT is also a factor in determining the therapy's success. The patient's learning needs and barriers to learning should also be considered.

Because patients reject methods that are fatiguing, this should be considered in method selection. In addition, the patient's disease either may suggest the best approach or may impose certain limitations that preclude using a particular method. Cost is a critical factor in selecting all treatment strategies. There are multiple inexpensive options that are effective. Patient or caregiver education also plays an important role in the therapy's effectiveness (see Chapter 54).

MINI CLINI

Recommending Airway Clearance Strategies

PROBLEM: The RT is asked to evaluate and recommend an appropriate airway clearance therapy regimen for a 7-year-old active girl with CF who is being cared for in her home by elderly grandparents.

Discussion: Generally, appropriate secretion clearance strategies for this patient include exercise, vibratory PEP, CPT, ACBT, HFCWO, and IPV. CPT would be difficult to implement in this patient's home setting (elderly caregivers), so emphasis should be placed on either vibratory PEP with ACBT or HFCWO and FET. An exercise plan should also be incorporated into the overall strategy. Dietary and medication considerations are also important.

Protocol-Based Airway Clearance

Numerous RT-driven protocols have been published for airway clearance therapy. All of these protocols involve rigorous assessment of the patient both to establish preliminary need and to determine continuation of or modification in therapy. Figure 43-11 is an algorithm used in one such protocol. Changes in therapy occur throughout and are based on the patient's response and therapist's evaluation.

SUMMARY CHECKLIST

- Normal airway clearance requires a patent airway, a functional mucociliary escalator, and an effective cough.
- Patients with copious secretions (20 to 30 mL/day) or inability to mobilize and expectorate secretions may benefit from airway clearance therapy.
- The primary goal of airway clearance therapy is to help mobilize and remove retained secretions, improve gas exchange, and reduce the work of breathing.
- Retained secretions can increase the work of breathing, cause air trapping, worsen $\dot{V}/\dot{Q}$ imbalance, promote atelectasis and shunting, and increase the incidence of infection.
- Disorders associated with abnormal secretion clearance include foreign bodies, tumors, congenital or acquired thoracic anomalies, asthma, chronic bronchitis, CF, bronchiectasis, and acute infections.
- Musculoskeletal and neurologic disorders can impair coughing and lead to mucous plugging, airway obstruction, and atelectasis.
- Both mechanical and treatment factors impair mucociliary clearance in intubated patients.
- Clinical signs consistent with retained secretions include ineffective cough, absent or increased sputum production, a labored breathing pattern, abnormal or adventitious lung sounds (e.g., coarse crackles, decreased breath sounds), tachypnea, tachycardia, and fever.
- Turning promotes lung expansion, improves oxygenation, and prevents retention of secretions.
- Postural drainage involves placing the segmental bronchus to be drained in a vertical position relative to gravity and holding the position for 3 to 15 minutes.
- Cough methods must be modified in surgical patients, patients with COPD, and patients with neuromuscular disorders.
- FET, or huff cough, consists of one or two forced expirations of middle to low lung volume without closure of the glottis, followed by a period of diaphragmatic breathing and relaxation.
- ACBT consists of repeated cycles of breathing control, thoracic expansion, and FET.
- During AD, the patient uses diaphragmatic breathing to mobilize secretions by varying lung volumes and expiratory airflow in three distinct phases.
- MIE involves delivery of a positive pressure breath followed by the quick application of negative pressure; positive expiratory flows exceed flows developed by manually assisted coughing.
- PEP or vibratory therapy is a self-administered clearance technique involving active expiration against a variable-flow resistance, followed by FET; patients frequently prefer PEP over other methods.
- At high frequencies (12 to 25 Hz), airway oscillations enhance cough clearance of secretions.
- Airway oscillations can be created externally (HFCWC) or at the airway opening (flutter valve, IPV).
- Adding physical activity to mobilization and coughing enhances mucus clearance, improves overall aeration and $\dot{V}/\dot{Q}$ matching, and improves pulmonary function.
- If performed correctly, no airway clearance therapy has been proven better than another.
- Numerous factors must be considered in trying to select the best airway clearance strategy for a given patient.

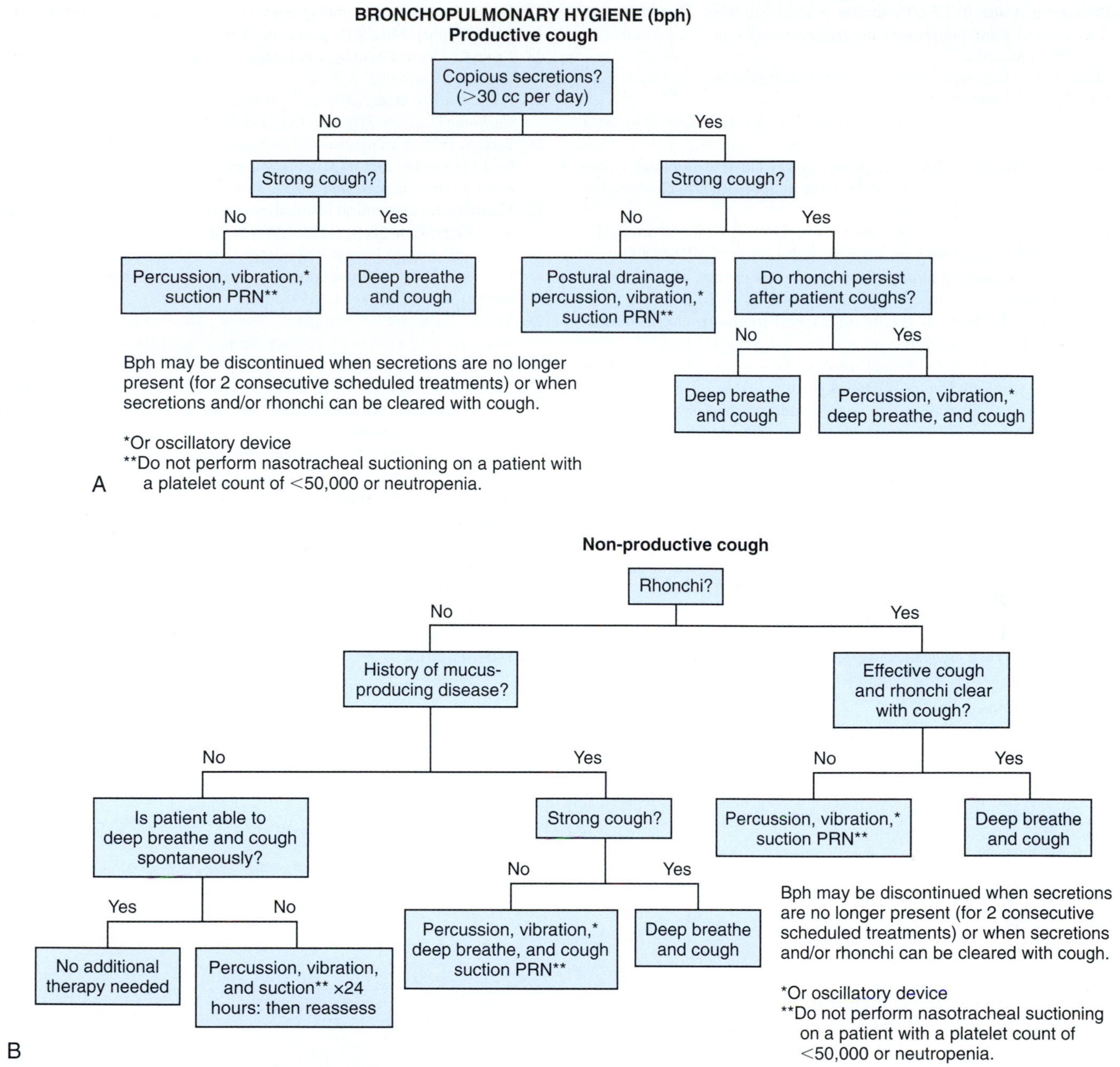

FIGURE 43-11 Example of algorithm underlying an airway clearance protocol. (Bronchial Hygiene Algorithm from the Cleveland Clinic Respiratory Therapy Consult Service Handbook. Courtesy of the Cleveland Clinic.)

References

1. Strickland S, Rubin B, Dresher G, et al: AARC clinical practice guideline: effectiveness of nonpharmacologic airway clearance therapies in hospitalized patients. *Respir Care* 58(12):2187–2193, 2013.
2. McCool F, Rosen M: Nonpharmacologic airway clearance therapies. ACCP evidence-based clinical practice guidelines. *CHEST Suppl* 129(1):250S–259S, 2006.
3. Andrews J, Sathe NA, Krishnaswami S, et al: Nonpharmacologic airway clearance techniques in hospitalized patients: a systemic review. *Respir Care* 58(12):2187–2193, 2013.
4. Volsko TA: Airway clearance therapy: finding the evidence. *Respir Care* 58:1669–1678, 2013.
5. Flume P, Mogayzel P, Robinson K, et al: Concise clinical review. Cystic fibrosis pulmonary guidelines. Airway clearance therapies. *Am J Respir Crit Care Med* 53(4):522–537, 2009.
6. Fahy JV, Dickey BF: Airway mucus function and dysfunction. *New Engl J Med* 363:2233–2247, 2010.
7. Miller RG, Jackson CE, Kasarskis EJ, et al: Practice parameter update: the care of the patient with amyotrophic lateral sclerosis: drug, nutritional and respiratory therapies (an evidence—based review) Report of the quality standards subcommittee of the American Academy of Neurology. *Neurol* 73(15):1218–1226, 2009.
8. Warwick WJ: Mechanisms of mucous transport. *Eur J Respir Dis Suppl* 64(Suppl 127):162–167, 1983.

9. Restrepo R, Walsh BK: AARC clinical practice guideline. Humidification during invasive and noninvasive mechanical ventilation: 2012. *Respir Care* 57(5):782–788, 2012.
10. Stiller K: Physiotherapy in intensive care: towards an evidence-base practice. *Chest* 118:1801, 2013.
11. Moulton BC, Barker AF: Pathogenesis of bronchiectasis. *Clin Chest Med* 33:211–217, 2012.
12. Barbato A, Frischer T, Kuehni C, et al: Primary ciliary dyskinesia: A consensus statement on diagnostic and treatment approaches in children. *Eur Respir J* 34(5):1264–1276, 2009.
13. American Association for Respiratory Care: AARC clinical practice guideline. Postural drainage therapy. *Respir Care* 36(12):1418–1426, 1991.
14. Hillegas E: *Essentials of cardiopulmonary physical therapy*, ed 3, St. Louis, 2011, Saunders.
15. Wong JW, et al: Effects of gravity on tracheal transport rates in normal subjects and in patients with cystic fibrosis. *Pediatrics* 60:146, 1977.
16. Winkelman C, Chiang L: Manual turns in patients receiving mechanical ventilation. *Crit Care Nurs* 30(4):36–44, 2010.
17. Conway JH, et al: Humidification as an adjunct to chest physiotherapy in aiding tracheobronchial clearance in patients with bronchiectasis. *Respir Med* 86:109, 1992.
18. American Association for Respiratory Care: Clinical practice guideline: bland aerosol administration. *Respir Care* 48:529, 2003.
19. American Association for Respiratory Care: AARC clinical practice guideline: directed cough. *Respir Care* 38(5):495–499, 1993.
20. Hasani A, et al: The effect of unproductive coughing/FET on regional mucus movement in the human lungs. *Respir Med* 85:23, 1991.
21. Fink JB: Forced expiratory technique, directed cough and autogenic drainage. *Respir Care* 52:1210, 2007.
22. Chatburn RL: High-frequency assisted airway clearance. *Respir Care* 52: 1224, 2007.
23. Guion L: *Respiratory management of ALS: amyotrophic lateral sclerosis*, ed 1, Sudbury, MA, 2010, Jones and Barlett.
24. Lapin C: Airway physiology, autogenic drainage, and active cycle of breathing. *Respir Care* 47:778, 2002.
25. Robinson KA, et al: Active cycle of breathing technique for cystic fibrosis. *Cochrane Database Syst Rev* (11):CD007862, 2012.
26. Savci S, et al: A comparison of autogenic drainage and the active cycle of breathing techniques in patients with chronic obstructive pulmonary diseases. *J Cardiopulm Rehabil* 20:37, 2000.
27. Homnick D: Mechanical insufflation-exsufflation for airway mucus clearance. *Respir Care* 52(10):1296–1305, 2007.
28. American Association for Respiratory Care: AARC clinical practice guideline. Use of positive airway pressure adjuncts to bronchial hygiene therapy. *Respir Care* 38(5):516–521, 1993.
29. Volsko T, DiFiore J, Chatburn RL: Performance comparison of two oscillating positive expiratory pressure devices: Acapella versus flutter. *Respir Care* 48(2):124–130, 2003.
30. Elkins MR, Jones A, van der Schans C: Positive expiratory pressure physiotherapy for airway clearance in people with cystic fibrosis. *Cochrane Database Syst Rev* (2):2006.
31. Morrison L, Agnew J: Oscillating devices for airway clearance in people with cystic fibrosis. *Cochrane Database Syst Rev* (7):CD006842, 2014.
32. Myers T: Positive expiratory pressure and oscillatory positive expiratory pressure therapies. *Respir Care* 52:1308, 2007.
33. Perme C, Chandrashekar R: Early mobility and walking program for patients in intensive care units: creating a standard of care. *Am J Crit Care* 18:212, 2009.
34. Cassidy MR, et al: I COUGH: Reducing postoperative pulmonary complications with a multidisciplinary patient care program. *JAMA Surg* 148(8): 740–745, 2013.

SECTION VI

ACUTE AND CRITICAL CARE

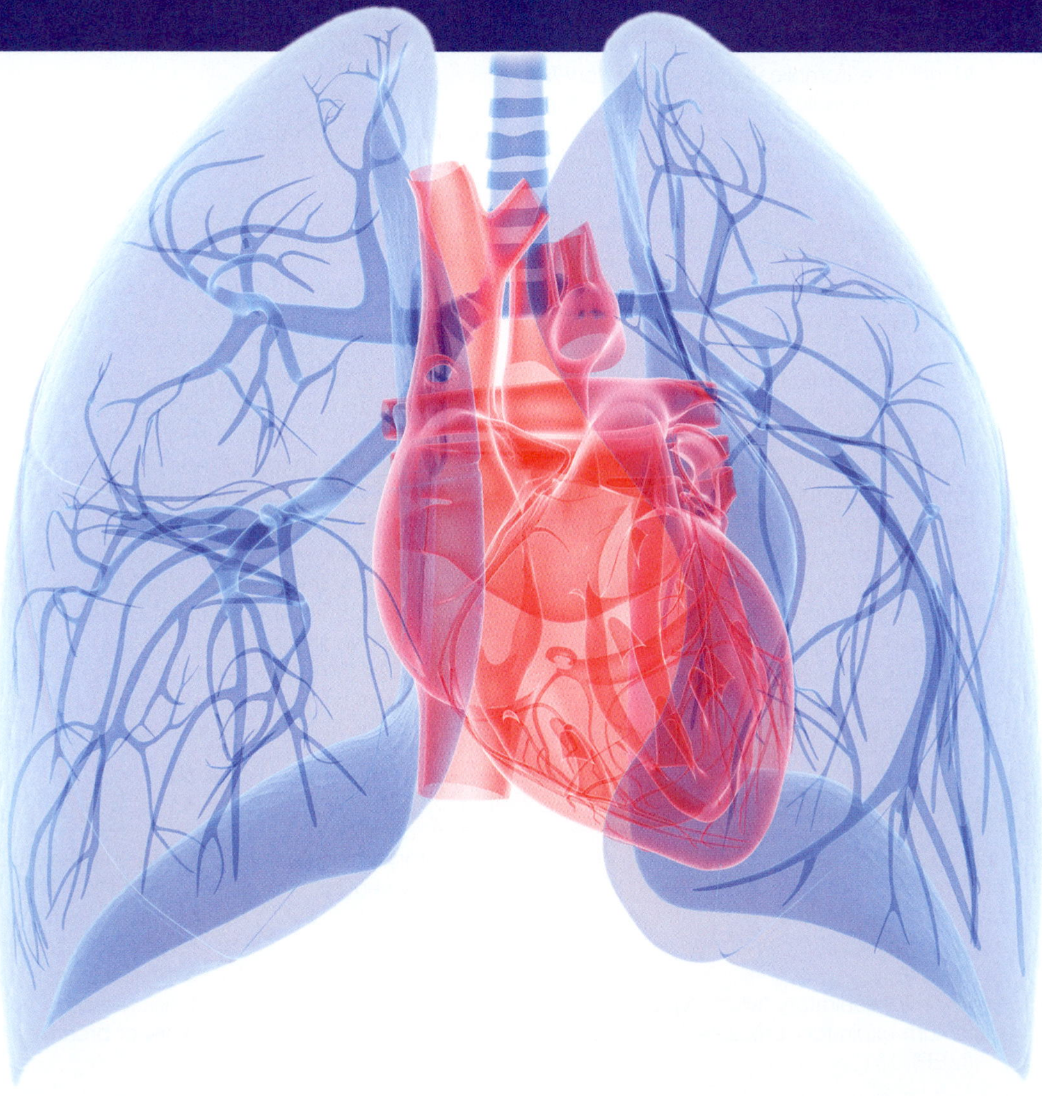

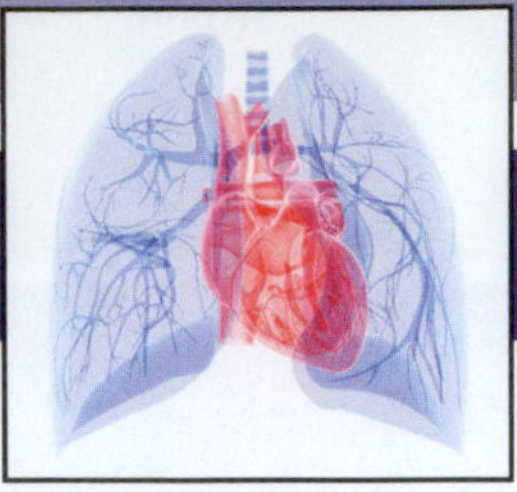

CHAPTER 44

Respiratory Failure and the Need for Ventilatory Support

LOUTFI S. ABOUSSOUAN

CHAPTER OBJECTIVES

After reading this chapter you will be able to:

- Define acute respiratory failure.
- Differentiate between hypoxemic respiratory failure (type I) and hypercapnic respiratory failure (type II).
- Discuss the causes of acute respiratory failure.
- Discuss the differences between chronic respiratory failure and acute-on-chronic respiratory failure.
- Identify the complications of respiratory failure.
- Discuss the indications for ventilatory support.
- Discuss general management principles of hypoxemic and hypercapnic respiratory failure.
- Discuss indications for noninvasive ventilation.

CHAPTER OUTLINE

Hypoxemic Respiratory Failure (Type I)
- Ventilation/Perfusion Mismatch
- Shunt
- Alveolar Hypoventilation
- Diffusion Impairment
- Perfusion/Diffusion Impairment
- Decreased Inspired Oxygen
- Venous Admixture
- Differentiating the Causes of Acute Hypoxemic Respiratory Failure

Hypercapnic Respiratory Failure (Type II)
- Insidious Exposure
- Increased Carbon Dioxide Production
- Impairment in Respiratory Control
- Impairment in Respiratory Effectors

Chronic Respiratory Failure (Type I and Type II)
- Acute-on-Chronic Respiratory Failure
- Complications of Acute Respiratory Failure
- Clinical Presentation
- Indications for Ventilatory Support

Assessment of Respiratory Fatigue, Weakness, and Failure and Work of Breathing
- Respiratory Muscle Weakness
- Respiratory Muscle Fatigue
- Respiratory Failure
- Work of Breathing

Choosing a Ventilatory Support Strategy for Different Causes of Respiratory Failure
- Noninvasive Ventilation
- Noninvasive Ventilation in Acute Conditions
- Noninvasive Ventilation in Chronic Conditions
- Invasive Ventilatory Support

KEY TERMS

auto-PEEP
barotrauma
dynamic hyperinflation
hypercapnic respiratory failure (type II)
hypoxemic respiratory failure (type I)
maximum expiratory pressure (MEP)
maximum inspiratory pressure (MIP)
maximum voluntary ventilation (MVV)
muscle fatigue
noninvasive ventilation (NIV)
orthodeoxia
platypnea
positive end-expiratory pressure (PEEP)
pressure control ventilation
respiratory alternans
sniff nasal inspiratory pressure
tension-time index
work of breathing

Respiratory failure is a clinical problem that all respiratory care practitioners must be skilled at identifying, assessing, and treating. The mortality of patients requiring intensive care unit (ICU) admission with respiratory failure was 44% in 1995, and only marginally improved to 34.5% in 2010.[1,2] The need for oxygen (O_2) delivery, mechanical ventilation, and other modalities in the management of such patients makes the respiratory therapist's (RT) role indispensable.

Respiratory failure is the "inability to maintain either the normal delivery of O_2 to the tissues or the normal removal of carbon dioxide (CO_2) from the tissues"[3] and often results from an imbalance between respiratory workload and ventilatory strength or endurance. Criteria for respiratory failure based on arterial blood gases (ABGs) were established by Campbell[4] and generally define *failure* as arterial partial pressure of oxygen (PaO_2) less than 60 mm Hg (also referred to as **hypoxemic** or **type I respiratory failure**), alveolar partial pressure of carbon dioxide ($PaCO_2$) greater than 50 mm Hg (**hypercapnic** or **type II respiratory failure**), or both, in otherwise healthy individuals breathing room air at sea level. Respiratory failure can be an acute or a chronic process. Hypercapnic respiratory failure is also known as *ventilatory failure* or "bellows" failure. Patients with baseline acid-base derangement (e.g., chronic obstructive pulmonary disease [COPD], neuromuscular disease, thoracic or parenchymal restrictive lung disease) may be chronically hypercapnic and in chronic ventilatory failure. Although ABG analysis is helpful in distinguishing hypoxemic (type I) and hypercapnic (type II) respiratory failure, many patients in acute respiratory failure develop both hypoxemia and hypercapnia.

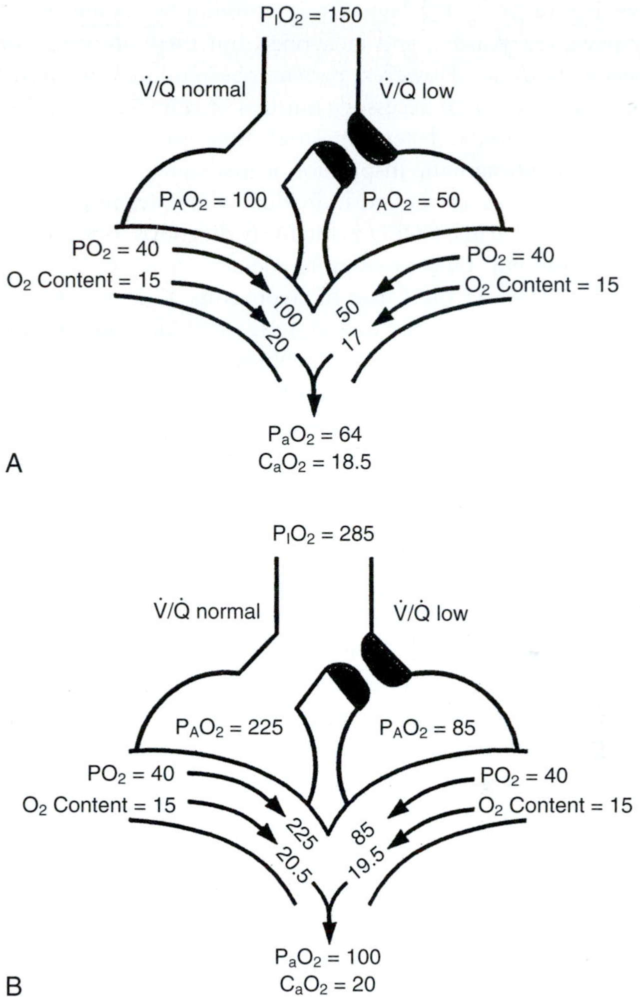

FIGURE 44-1 Hypoxemia caused by $\dot{V}/\dot{Q}$ mismatch showing the effect of supplemental O_2. $\dot{V}/\dot{Q}$ is normal on the left side of each idealized lung unit and low on the right. Only O_2 exchange is shown, and $P(A - a)O_2$ is assumed to be zero. **A,** With room air, not enough O_2 reaches the poorly ventilated alveolus to saturate its capillary blood fully. **B,** With 40% O_2, PaO_2 in this alveolus is increased enough to make capillary PO_2 nearly normal. PaO_2 in the mixed blood from the two capillaries is determined by the average of the O_2 contents of the two streams of blood, not by the PaO_2 values. (Modified from Pierson DJ, Kacmarek RM: Foundations of respiratory care, New York, 1992, Churchill Livingstone.)

HYPOXEMIC RESPIRATORY FAILURE (TYPE I)

The primary causes of hypoxemia are the following:

- Ventilation/perfusion ($\dot{V}/\dot{Q}$) mismatch
- Shunt
- Alveolar hypoventilation
- Diffusion impairment
- Perfusion/diffusion impairment
- Decreased inspired O_2
- Venous admixture

These entities are briefly discussed here and are discussed in more detail in Chapters 11 and 12.

Ventilation/Perfusion Mismatch

There are regions in healthy lungs where ventilation and perfusion are not evenly matched, so it seems logical that this is the most common cause of hypoxemia. RTs are familiar with this concept through the work of West,[5] which described a high $\dot{V}/\dot{Q}$ ratio at the apex of the lungs and a low ratio at the bases. This concept can be oversimplified and stated as there being more air than blood at the apexes and more blood than air at the bases.

Pathologic $\dot{V}/\dot{Q}$ mismatch occurs when disease disrupts this balance, and hypoxemia results (Figure 44-1, *A*). Most commonly, areas of low $\dot{V}/\dot{Q}$ ratio are seen in which ventilation is compromised despite adequate blood flow. Obstructive lung diseases are frequent causes. The bronchospasm, mucous plugging, inflammation, and premature airway closure that signal asthmatic or emphysematous exacerbations worsen ventilation and create $\dot{V}/\dot{Q}$ mismatch. Infection, heart failure, and inhalation injury may lead to partially collapsed or fluid-filled alveoli, also resulting in decreased ventilation and reduced blood O_2 levels.

Clinical Presentation

Because patients present with hypoxemia, the initial goal is always to treat the low PaO_2 or SpO_2 (arterial O_2 saturation by pulse oximeter). $\dot{V}/\dot{Q}$ mismatch responds to supplemental O_2

(see Figure 44-1, *B*). Hypoxemia commonly manifests with dyspnea, tachycardia, and tachypnea, but these are very nonspecific findings. However, patient observation is extremely valuable. The use of accessory muscles of respiration (scalene, pectoralis major, and sternomastoid) is an important sign that normal diaphragmatic inspiration is inadequate. In an elderly, cachectic, or barrel-chested individual who is leaning forward on his or her arms, COPD is the likely diagnosis. Nasal flaring may be present. Lower extremity edema is more indicative of cardiac failure as the cause of hypoxemia. Cyanosis may be peripheral and primarily due to decreased blood flow. Central cyanosis, seen most easily as a bluish tint around the lips, occurs when greater than 5 g/dl of unsaturated hemoglobin is present. This finding is more common in patients with polycythemia but may be subject to wide observer variability. More severe hypoxemia can lead to significant central nervous system (CNS) dysfunction, ranging from irritability to confusion to coma.

Auscultation and percussion are very useful when added to patient observation. Bilateral wheezing, especially in a young patient in respiratory distress, often identifies the bronchospasm of asthma. Upper airway disease or fluid-filled airways may also result in wheezing. Breath sounds that are diminished bilaterally with increased resonance on percussion are common in emphysema. Unilateral abnormalities are significant. Wheezing in one lung may identify an endobronchial lesion, whereas the absence of breath sounds and decreased resonance on one side of the chest may reflect collapse, infection, edema, or effusion as potential causes of $\dot{V}/\dot{Q}$ mismatch. Discordant exam findings with increased resonance on percussion and decreased breath sounds on the same side may signal a pneumothorax. Unilateral crackles and decreased resonance on percussion generally indicate an alveolar filling process (mass, infection, fluid).

Radiographically, $\dot{V}/\dot{Q}$ mismatch can manifest as a "black" radiograph, with large or hyperinflated lungs as in the case of obstructive disease. A "white" chest radiograph is evident when alveoli are partially occluded. The "blackness" or "whiteness" of the lung fields on the plain chest radiograph has important diagnostic value in assessing a patient with acute respiratory failure.

Shunt

Shunt is an extreme version of $\dot{V}/\dot{Q}$ mismatch in which there is no ventilation to match perfusion ($\dot{V}/\dot{Q} = 0$). About 2% to 3% of the blood supply is shunted via the bronchial and thebesian veins that feed the lungs and heart; this is normal anatomic shunt. Pathologic anatomic shunt occurs as a result of right-to-left blood flow through cardiac openings (e.g., atrial or ventricular septal defects) or in pulmonary arteriovenous malformations. Physiologic shunt leads to hypoxemia when alveoli collapse or are filled with fluid or exudate. Common etiologies of physiologic shunting include atelectasis, pulmonary edema, and pneumonia. In contrast to $\dot{V}/\dot{Q}$ mismatch, shunt does not respond to supplemental O_2 because the gas-exchange unit (the alveolus) is not open (Figure 44-2, *A*).

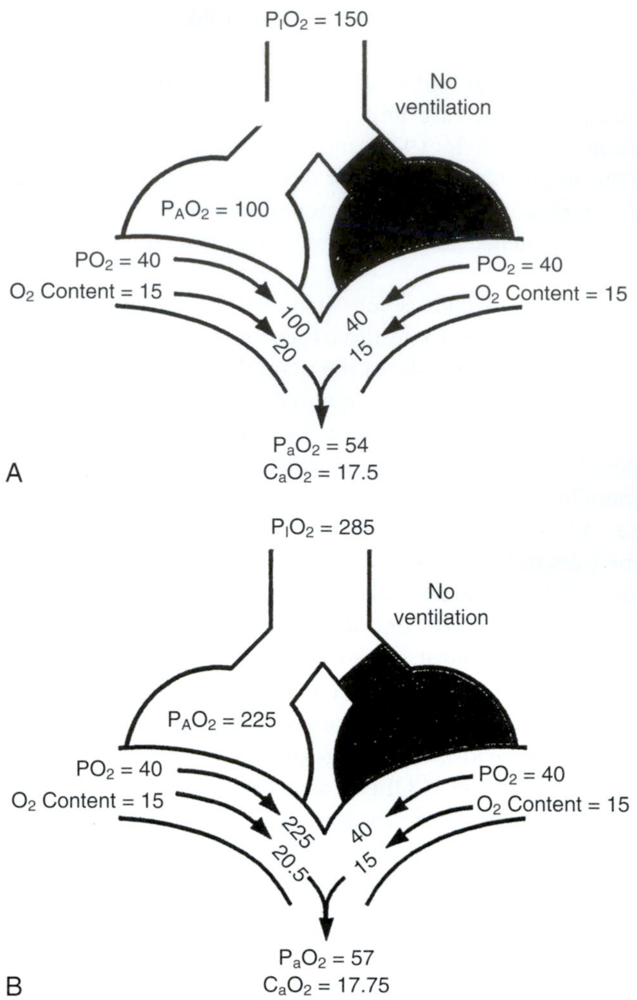

FIGURE 44-2 Alveolar-capillary diagram of intrapulmonary (capillary) shunting showing why supplemental O_2 fails to correct hypoxemia. Only O_2 exchange is shown, and $P(A - a)O_2$ is assumed to be zero. **A,** With room air, although blood leaving the normal alveolar-capillary unit is normally saturated, blood passing the capillary on the right "sees" no O_2 because its alveolus is unventilated, and it leaves the unit unsaturated. When the two streams of blood mix, the resulting PaO_2 is determined by the average of the O_2 contents, not by the PO_2 values. **B,** Addition of 40% O_2 fails to correct the hypoxemia because O_2 content is not significantly increased in the normal unit, and capillary blood in the unventilated unit still "sees" no O_2. Even 100% O_2 could not completely reverse the oxygenation defect in this example; this is very different from the effect with low $\dot{V}/\dot{Q}$ as illustrated in Figure 44-1. (Modified from Pierson DJ, Kacmarek RM: Foundations of respiratory care, New York, 1992, Churchill Livingstone.)

Clinical Presentation

The clinical presentation and patient observations in shunting are very similar in many ways to the presentation of $\dot{V}/\dot{Q}$ mismatch. Bilateral or unilateral crackles are common owing to the alveolar filling process. Unilateral absence of breath sounds may indicate significant collapse, mass, or effusion; these conditions require treatment before oxygenation can improve. The parenchyma on chest radiograph may be "white" with physiologic causes of shunting as may occur in the acute respiratory distress syndrome (ARDS). Anatomic shunts may be harder to diagnose as the chest radiograph may appear normal, but can be diagnosed by using 100% O_2 breathing techniques, contrast-enhanced echocardiography, macroaggregated albumin scanning, or pulmonary angiography.[6] Shunt is differentiated from $\dot{V}/\dot{Q}$ mismatch by the lack of increase in PO_2 as fractional inspired oxygen (FiO_2) is increased (see Figure 44-2, *B*).

Alveolar Hypoventilation

Alveolar hypoventilation is discussed subsequently in the section on hypercapnic respiratory failure (Type II).

Diffusion Impairment

Diffusion refers to movement of gas across the alveolar-capillary membrane along a pressure gradient. Although diffusion impairment is rarely a cause of significant hypoxemia at rest, its effects become more pronounced with exercise, which limits the time for gas exchange. Diffusion impairment in interstitial lung disease (e.g., pulmonary fibrosis, asbestosis, sarcoidosis), in which the thickening and scarring of the interstitium undermine normal gas exchange, may contribute 20% to 30% of the widening in the alveolar-arterial O_2 gradient during exercise.[7] Emphysema, with its inherent alveolar destruction, also has subnormal transfer of O_2 and CO_2 between the alveolus and the capillary. The reduced ventilation in both diseases implies that $\dot{V}/\dot{Q}$ mismatch also plays a role in the resulting hypoxemia.

Pulmonary vascular abnormalities can also lead to diffusion impairment. Anemia, pulmonary hypertension, and pulmonary embolus all may reduce capillary blood flow, resulting in diminished gas transfer.

Clinical Presentation

Signs and symptoms are related to the specific disease. Interstitial lung disease may be the diagnosis of a dyspneic patient with a dry cough and fine, basilar crackles on auscultation, and clubbing of the nail beds. Rheumatologic manifestations may be present if the underlying cause is a connective tissue disorder. Joint abnormalities, Raynaud disease, and *telangiectasia* (a vascular lesion formed by dilation of a group of small blood vessels) may be observed. The pallor of anemia can be a clue to poor gas exchange, although chronic hypoxemia may lead to polycythemia and possibly cyanosis. Pulmonary hypertension may manifest with signs of right-sided heart failure, such as edema, jugular venous distention, and a louder pulmonary component of the second heart sound.

Diffusion impairment can also manifest with multiple, varied radiographic forms. The hyperinflated, dark radiograph of emphysema was mentioned earlier. Interstitial disease may manifest with reduced lung volumes with interstitial markings. Enlarged right ventricle and pulmonary arteries may be evident in secondary pulmonary hypertension.

Perfusion/Diffusion Impairment

Perfusion/diffusion impairment is a cause of hypoxemia in individuals with liver disease complicated by the hepatopulmonary syndrome.[6] In this condition, right-to-left intracardiac shunt combines with dilated pulmonary capillaries resulting in impaired gas exchange because the normal alveolar partial pressures of O_2 may be insufficient to drive the O_2 molecules to the center of the dilated pulmonary vasculature. Cirrhosis is the most common liver disease, and portal hypertension is usually present. Although shunt is a component of the syndrome, significant supplemental O_2 can overcome the hypoxemia, so this is commonly called a *perfusion/diffusion defect.*

Clinical Presentation

Obvious signs of liver disease (e.g., ascites, jaundice, and spider nevi) may or may not be present. Digital clubbing can occur in hepatopulmonary syndrome. **Platypnea**, which is the sensation of dyspnea when moving to the upright position from the supine position, may be a patient complaint. **Orthodeoxia**, an actual decrease in the measured O_2 level, may parallel this subjective sensation.

Decreased Inspired Oxygen

Also clinically uncommon, hypoxemia may develop when the inspired O_2 is less than body requirements. The most common situation is at high altitude, where hypoxemia occurs not because of a decrease in the fraction of oxygen in the ambient air (which remains 21%) but from barometric pressure decreases, which results in a decrease in the partial pressure of inspired O_2. Even with pressurized airplanes, air travelers with chronic hypoxemia may still need supplemental O_2.[8] Similarly, mountain climbers sometimes require O_2 masks. Cases of patient-O_2 disconnects and delivery of an incorrect gas source are also included in this category.

Inspired O_2 less than 21% can be used diagnostically and therapeutically. The Hypoxia Altitude Simulation Test replicates inspired partial pressure of O_2 (PiO_2) during air travel by asking the potential traveler to inhale a hypoxic mixture. Inhaling at FiO_2 of 15% replicates the PiO_2 found at an altitude of 8000 feet (108 mm Hg). For a lower altitude of 5400 feet, an equivalent FiO_2 of 17% can be calculated.[8] Infants with certain cyanotic congenital heart defects (e.g., hypoplastic left ventricle) may benefit from FiO_2 below room air level. In the preoperative state, low FiO_2 helps to prevent pulmonary dilation and the excessive pulmonary blood flow, which could flood the lungs.

Clinical Presentation

The signs and symptoms of hypoxemia may be present, with the cause related to the patient environment such as the altitude.

Venous Admixture

A decrease in mixed venous O_2 increases the gradient by which O_2 needs to be stepped up as it passes through the lungs and can contribute to the development of hypoxemia. Congestive heart failure with low cardiac output is the most common cause of low mixed venous O_2, owing to increased peripheral extraction of O_2, and there are therefore other, more important coexisting determinants of hypoxemia, such as $\dot{V}/\dot{Q}$ mismatch and shunting.[3] Other causes include low hemoglobin concentration and increased O_2 consumption. A low mixed venous O_2 may have a significant effect on the ultimate arterial O_2 tension in the presence of lung disease.

Clinical Presentation

Signs and symptoms of congestive heart failure or underlying lung disease, or both, may be present and typically overshadow the clinical presentation.

Differentiating the Causes of Acute Hypoxemic Respiratory Failure

It is important to recognize the physiologic basis of each of the three main causes of hypoxemic respiratory failure (hypoventilation, $\dot{V}/\dot{Q}$ mismatch, and shunt). Hypoventilation differs from the other causes in manifesting with a normal alveolar-to-arterial PO_2 difference [$P(A - a)O_2$] indicating normal lung parenchyma (Table 44-1). A clinical determination of this difference is made by subtracting PaO_2 from PAO_2 (partial pressure of alveolar O_2) derived from the alveolar air equation:

$$PAO_2 = FiO_2(P_B - P_{H_2O}) - PaCO_2/R$$

where P_B is barometric pressure, P_{H2O} is water vapor tension, and R is the respiratory exchange ratio (0.8).

The $P(A - a)O_2$ ranges from 10 mm Hg in young patients to approximately 25 mm Hg in elderly patients while breathing room air (see the accompanying Rule of Thumb). In patients with hypoxemia caused by hypoventilation, treatment can be focused on improving ventilation because the hypoxemia is purely a result of alveolar displacement of O_2 by elevated CO_2.

RULE OF THUMB

The mean alveolar-to-arterial difference [$P(A - a)O_2$] in PO_2 increases slightly with age and can be estimated with the following equation:

$$\text{Mean age-specific } P(A - a)O_2 = (\text{age}/4) + 4$$

Example: A 76-year-old person living at sea level:

$$P(A - a)O_2 = (76/4) + 4 = 19 + 4 = 23 \text{ mm Hg}$$

A $\dot{V}/\dot{Q}$ mismatch and shunt both result in elevated $P(A - a)O_2$ levels, indicating that the resultant hypoxemia is due to an abnormality of lung tissue, requiring treatment to address that abnormality. When the RT encounters an increased $P(A - a)O_2$, a $\dot{V}/\dot{Q}$ mismatch and shunt can be differentiated by means of O_2 administration (see Figures 44-1 and 44-2). A significant response to applying even small amounts of O_2 identifies $\dot{V}/\dot{Q}$ mismatch as the cause of hypoxemia because altered $P(A - a)O_2$ has not been totally obliterated. True shunt shows little or no improvement in oxygenation even with 100% FiO_2 (see Table 44-1). As a result, treatment of intrapulmonary shunt must be directed toward opening collapsed alveoli or clearing fluid or exudative material before O_2 can be beneficial at below toxic levels. Testing to rule out anatomic shunt should be done in the right clinical setting (e.g., clear or black parenchyma on the chest radiograph).

TABLE 44-1
Differentiating the Cause of Hypoxemia

Cause	$P(A - a)O_2$	Response to Increased FiO_2
Hypoventilation	Normal	Marked
Shunt	Increased	Minimal
$\dot{V}/\dot{Q}$ mismatch	Increased	Marked

HYPERCAPNIC RESPIRATORY FAILURE (TYPE II)

Hypercapnic respiratory failure (type II), also known as *pump, bellows* or *ventilatory failure,* is characterized by an elevated $PaCO_2$, creating an uncompensated respiratory acidosis (whether acute or acute-on-chronic). $PaCO_2$ and alveolar ventilation ($\dot{V}_A$) are inversely related, meaning that alveolar and arterial PCO_2 levels are doubled when alveolar ventilation is halved. This is illustrated by the metabolic hyperbola relationship:

$$PaCO_2 = (0.863\ \dot{V}CO_2)/\dot{V}_A$$
$$\dot{V}_A = MV\ (1 - V_D/V_T)$$

where $\dot{V}_A$ is alveolar ventilation (L/min), MV is minute ventilation, V_D/V_T is dead space-to-tidal volume ratio, and $\dot{V}CO_2$ is CO_2 production (ml/min).

This equation demonstrates a rectangular hyperbola relation between the $PaCO_2$ and ventilation (Figure 44-3). Patients with chronic hypercapnia and low ventilation are on a steeper section of the metabolic hyperbola such that a minor drop in ventilation results in a significant increase in $PaCO_2$, making them more susceptible to developing a sudden, further increase in $PaCO_2$ in the context of even minor respiratory exacerbations. Additionally, with chronically elevated arterial $PaCO_2$, the ventilatory response to a further increase in $PaCO_2$ is more blunted.[9] This leads to an *acute ventilatory failure superimposed on chronic ventilatory failure.*

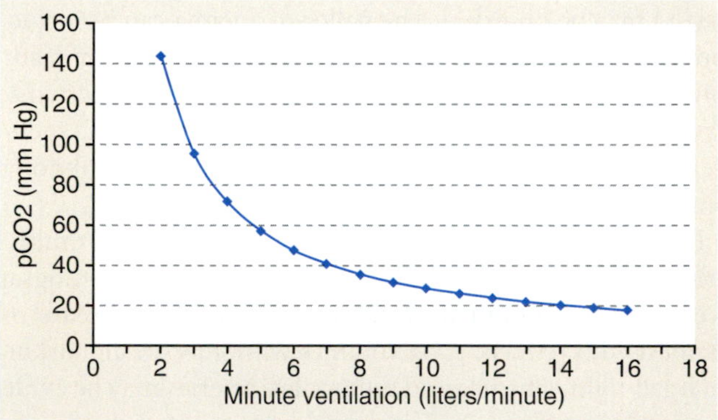

FIGURE 44-3 The metabolic hyperbola. Due to the hyperbolic relationship between the pCO_2 and ventilation, a minor drop of ventilation occurring at an already low minute ventilation results in a significantly greater increase in the pCO_2 relative to an equivalent drop occurring at a higher minute ventilation.

MINI CLINI

Differentiating Causes of Hypoxemia

PROBLEM: Two patients present with the following ABG values at sea level:

Patient A		Patient B	
pH	7.45	pH	7.21
$PaCO_2$	33 mm Hg	$PaCO_2$	72 mm Hg
PaO_2	40 mm Hg	PaO_2	53 mm Hg
HCO_3^-	22 mEq/L	HCO_3^-	28 mEq/L
SaO_2	70%	SaO_2	81%
FiO_2	0.21	FiO_2	0.21

1. Define the respiratory condition indicated by each ABG analysis.
2. What is the $P(A - a)O_2$ for each blood gas?
3. Identify the type of respiratory failure in each case.
4. In which case would administration of 100% FiO_2 help determine therapy?

Discussion:

1. Patient A exhibits uncompensated respiratory alkalosis with hypoxemia. Patient B exhibits partially compensated respiratory acidosis with hypoxemia.
2. Patient A:
   $PAO_2 = 0.21\ (760 - 47) - 33/0.8 = 108$ mm Hg
   $PaO_2 = 40$ mm Hg
   $P(A - a)O_2 = 108 - 40 = 68$ mm Hg on room air
   Patient B:
   $PAO_2 = 0.21\ (760 - 47) - 72/0.8 = 60$ mm Hg
   $PaO_2 = 53$ mm Hg
   $P(A - a)O_2 = 60 - 53 = 7$ mm Hg on room air
   The normal values for $P(A - a)O_2$ range from 10 mm Hg in young people to approximately 25 mm Hg in elderly people while breathing room air.
3. Patient A has hypoxemic respiratory failure (type I) as characterized by below-normal PaO_2 (40 mm Hg). $PaCO_2$ is also below normal (33 mm Hg), indicating hyperventilation is occurring in an effort to improve the oxygenation. Patient B has hypercapnic respiratory failure (type II) as characterized by above-normal $PaCO_2$ (72 mm Hg) indicating hypoventilation (ventilatory failure) is occurring. There is also an elevation of HCO_3^- (28 mEq/L), indicating that the acute ventilatory failure is superimposed on chronic ventilatory failure. This patient is also hypoxemic (53 mm Hg).
4. Patient A has hypoxemic respiratory failure with $P(A - a)O_2$ of 68 mm Hg, which is well above normal, indicating an oxygenation defect. The administration of 100% O_2 in this case would help to determine the cause of the defect. Significant response to 100% FiO_2 would point to $\dot{V}/\dot{Q}$ mismatch as the cause, whereas shunt would be implicated if PaO_2 did not respond to the increase in delivered O_2. In the latter condition, some form of PEEP would be necessary to improve gas exchange by improving functional residual capacity. Patient B has hypercapnic respiratory failure (ventilatory failure) with hypoxemia, but with $P(A - a)O_2$ of 7 mm Hg, which is within the normal range. A pure ventilatory defect is the cause of hypoxemia, and administration of 100% FiO_2 would not help to determine therapy. Depending on the full patient scenario, this patient may require non-invasive mechanical ventilation or intubation and invasive mechanical ventilation to restore normal acid-base status.

Similarly, this relationship shows that $PaCO_2$ may increase as dead space (V_D/V_T) rises or as CO_2 production ($\dot{V}CO_2$) increases. Additionally, a change in the $\dot{V}/\dot{Q}$ distribution of the lung toward lower ratios not only causes hypoxemia, as shown in Figures 44-1 and 44-2, but also to a lesser extent can cause an elevation of $PaCO_2$ by reducing the CO_2 discharge from the pulmonary circulation to the alveoli. However, increased dead space, increased $\dot{V}CO_2$, and shifts in the $\dot{V}/\dot{Q}$ distribution toward lower ratios all are usually matched by a corrective increase in ventilation because respiratory control mechanisms tend to maintain the $PaCO_2$ constant. The following sections describe mechanisms of hypercarbia caused by an imbalance between CO_2 exposure (external or internal) and CO_2 clearance (central and respiratory effector mechanisms). Hypoxemia may often accompany pump failure simply because of the displacement of alveolar PO_2 (PAO_2) by the increased $PaCO_2$ from alveolar hypoventilation. This situation is identified on a room air ABG assessment by a normal $P(A - a)O_2$ as discussed previously. The presence of an increased $P(A - a)O_2$ indicates that concomitant hypoxemia is present, most likely as a result of $\dot{V}/\dot{Q}$ mismatch or shunt. The disorders responsible for hypercapnic respiratory failure (ventilatory failure) are discussed next.

Insidious Exposure

Although most cases of increased $PaCO_2$ are due to hypoventilation, an insidious exposure can occur in certain situations.

Clinical Presentation

These insidious exposures follow unusual clinical scenarios including defective CO_2 scrubbers in the settings of anesthesia machines or life-support systems in scuba units, airtight chambers, spacecrafts, or submersible crafts. Occupational exposures also occur in spelunkers in caves (from groundwater seepage), individuals who work with dry ice (dry ice is a solid form of CO_2), miners, and firefighters.

Increased Carbon Dioxide Production

Fever, agitation, exertion, shivering, hypermetabolism, and excess caloric intake all can result in an increase in $\dot{V}CO_2$, with consequent hypercapnia in patients with additional impairment in respiratory control and effector mechanisms.

Clinical Presentation

The most common clinical scenario involving increases in CO_2 production probably involves mechanically ventilated patients with an already compromised lung function, in whom attempts to liberate from artificial ventilation are complicated by type II respiratory failure. Recognition and management of fever, agitation, hypermetabolic states, and excess caloric intake, particularly with carbohydrate-rich enteral solutions, may contribute to a favorable outcome.

Impairment in Respiratory Control

Both central (medullary) and peripheral (aortic and carotid bodies) chemoreceptors responding to CO_2 tension and O_2 tension stimulate the drive to breathe.[9] This ventilatory drive can be diminished by various factors, such as drugs (overdose or sedation), bilateral carotid endarterectomy with incidental resection of the carotid bodies, brainstem lesions, diseases of the CNS (multiple sclerosis, Parkinson disease, or elevated intracranial pressure), hypothyroidism, morbid obesity (e.g., obesity-hypoventilation), and sleep apnea. Other, less common potential causes include metabolic alkalosis, metabolic encephalopathy, malnutrition, and sleep deprivation.[10] Patients at risk of having a decreased ventilatory drive usually can be identified by their clinical situation (e.g., CNS insult, overdose of sedative medications), and the clinician should be attentive to reversible causes.

Clinical Presentation

The hallmark of the clinical scenario of decreased ventilatory drive is bradypnea and perhaps ultimately apnea. A respiratory rate is usually no less than 12 breaths/min in adults. Drug overdose or a brain disorder can manifest with an altered level of consciousness ranging from merely lethargic to obtunded and comatose, with decreased respirations. Evidence of drug use by history or toxicity screen confirms the diagnosis of drug overdose. Evidence of head trauma and brain computed tomography (CT) scan abnormalities are important in the diagnosis of a brain disorder. Although hypothyroidism classically manifests with fatigue, weight gain, hyporeflexia, and constipation, it can progress to significant hypoventilation and myxedema coma. Patients with obesity-hypoventilation may have a rapid, shallow breathing pattern, which results from decreased compliance and microatelectasis. Although these patients may also have nighttime sleep apnea, daytime $PaCO_2$ is also elevated because of a decrease in the drive to breathe or an increase in the **work of breathing**.[11] See Figure 44-3 for the relationship between PCO_2 and minute volume.

Impairment in Respiratory Effectors

Neurologic Diseases

The lungs inhale and exhale under the guidance of the CNS. In some patients, the CNS signal does not reach its goal, resulting in neuromuscular dysfunction. Examples include spinal trauma, motor neuron disease in which lesions of the anterior horn cells may gradually lead to progressive ventilatory failure (e.g., amyotrophic lateral sclerosis or poliomyelitis), motor nerve disorders (including Guillain-Barré syndrome and Charcot-Marie-Tooth disease), disorders of the neuromuscular junction (e.g., myasthenia gravis and botulism), and muscular diseases (including muscular dystrophy, myositis, critical care myopathy, and metabolic disorders).[12]

Clinical Presentation. Although hypercapnia may be a common end point, these diseases have varied clinical presentations. Patient observation is a key skill. Drooling, dysarthria, and weak cough are common bulbar signs in amyotrophic lateral sclerosis and myasthenia gravis. As muscle wasting and weakness become more severe, diaphragmatic insufficiency develops, and supine paradoxical breathing is common.[13] Guillain-Barré syndrome commonly manifests with lower extremity weakness progressing to the respiratory muscles in one-third of patients.[14] Weak cough and gag may be seen, which can threaten airway patency and lead to microatelectasis, hypoxemia, and uncompensated respiratory acidosis. Myasthenia gravis does not always result in respiratory failure.[15] These diseases are quite different in clinical course, but there is much overlap in their presentations, and they commonly result in respiratory **muscle fatigue** and failure and elevated $PaCO_2$.

Increased Work of Breathing

Despite normal respiratory drive, nerve transmission, and neuromuscular response, hypercapnic respiratory failure can still occur if the imposed workload cannot be overcome.[3,16] Most commonly, this situation occurs when increased dead space accompanies COPD, or elevated airway resistance accompanies asthma. Both of these obstructive airway diseases may increase respiratory work requirements excessively secondary to the presence of intrinsic **positive end-expiratory pressure (auto-PEEP)**. Increased workload can also result from thoracic abnormalities such as pneumothorax, rib fractures with a flail chest, pleural effusions, and other conditions creating a restrictive burden on the lungs. Finally, requirements for increased minute ventilation can arise when increased CO_2 production accompanies hypermetabolic states, such as in extensive burns.

Clinical Presentation. The RT must be alert to the possibility of respiratory failure when a heavy load is imposed on the respiratory system. Patients with asthma or COPD should present with hyperventilation in an exacerbation, but if breathing becomes more rapid but shallow, it may indicate impending failure. This increased V_D/V_T ratio leads to hypercapnia because the significant airway obstruction does not resolve with treatment. Diminished breath sounds in a young patient with asthma likewise can be an ominous sign. Irritability, confusion, and ultimately coma are possible signs in worsening hypercapnia, as they are in hypoxemic respiratory failure. More subtle findings include muscle tremor owing to catecholamine release and papilledema resulting from cerebral vasodilation in states of elevated arterial PCO_2.[17]

In summary, hypercapnic (type II) respiratory failure, also known as *ventilatory failure*, develops when ventilation is impaired secondary to intrinsically or extrinsically increased CO_2 exposure; impairment in respiratory control; or impairment in respiratory effector mechanisms, including neurologic

TABLE 44-2

Causes of Respiratory Failure

Type I (Hypoxemic)	Type II (Hypercapnic)			
	Increased Exposure	**Impaired Respiratory Control**	**Neurologic Disease**	**Increased Work of Breathing**
ARDS	Extrinsic	Drug overdose	Spinal cord trauma	Obstructive lung disease
Pulmonary embolism	Defective CO_2 scrubbers (anesthesia or life-support systems)	Bilateral endarterectomy with carotid body resection	Motor neuron	COPD
Pulmonary edema	Occupational exposure (miners, spelunkers, dry-ice workers, firemen)	Central sleep apnea	Poliomyelitis	Asthma
Septic shock	Intrinsic	Hypocapnia	Amyotrophic lateral sclerosis	Upper airway obstruction
Pulmonary infection	Fever	Cheyne-Stokes	Motor nerve	Obesity-hypoventilation
Viral	Shivering	Acromegaly	Phrenic nerve	Pneumothorax
Bacterial	Hypermetabolism	Hypothyroid	Guillain-Barré	Severe burns
Fungal	Agitation	Brainstem lesions	Charcot-Marie-Tooth	Chest wall disorders
Inhalation	Excess caloric intake	Cerebrovascular accident	Neuromuscular junction	Kyphoscoliosis
Smoke		Encephalitis	Myasthenia gravis	Ankylosing spondylitis
Chemical		Multiple sclerosis	Botulism	
Water		Parkinson disease	Muscular	
Pleural effusion		Metabolic alkalosis	Muscular dystrophy	
Interstitial lung disease		Primary alveolar hypoventilation	Myositis	
Obstructive lung disease		(Ondine's curse)	Myopathy	
Aspiration		Congenital central hypoventilation	Acid maltase	
Primary pulmonary hypertension		Carotid body resection	Metabolic	
		Obesity-hypoventilation		

disease or pulmonary and chest wall disorders associated with increased work of breathing (Table 44-2).

CHRONIC RESPIRATORY FAILURE (TYPE I AND TYPE II)

For some patients with pulmonary disease and respiratory failure, the condition has developed over weeks to months to years and has become a chronic state, allowing compensatory adaptive mechanisms to develop. Most commonly, chronic hypercapnic respiratory failure accompanying COPD or obesity-hypoventilation syndrome elicits a renal response, and the kidneys retain bicarbonate to elevate the blood pH. However, this compensatory metabolic alkalosis would not be expected to restore the pH to normal. Chronic hypercapnic respiratory failure is also known as *chronic ventilatory failure.*

RULE OF THUMB

Chronic and acute hypercapnic respiratory failure can be differentiated by the severity of change in pH.[16]

- Acute hypercapnic failure (acute ventilatory failure): pH decreases 0.08 for every 10-mm Hg increase in $PaCO_2$
- Chronic hypercapnic failure (chronic ventilatory failure): pH decreases 0.03 for every 10-mm Hg increase in $PaCO_2$

Similarly, polycythemia may result from prolonged hypoxemic respiratory failure (e.g., sleep apnea) when O_2 delivery to the tissues is compromised, and erythropoietin levels increase to elicit erythrocytosis. Hemoglobin also releases O_2 more easily as the O_2 dissociation curve shifts to the right in the face of acidosis. Finally, O_2 delivery to the brain is enhanced when hypercapnia results in increased cerebral blood flow.[17]

Acute-on-Chronic Respiratory Failure

Chronic respiratory failure can be complicated by acute setbacks that create acute-on-chronic respiratory failure. Patients with chronic hypercapnic respiratory failure are at significant risk for this condition, as indicated by the fact that COPD is now the third leading cause of death in the United States.[18] Acute-on-chronic respiratory failure can also be the presenting manifestation of neuromuscular disease in the setting of a concurrent pulmonary infection.[19] Most common precipitating factors include bacterial or viral infections, congestive heart failure, pulmonary embolus, pneumothorax, chest wall dysfunction, and medical noncompliance.[19-21] In these patients, the presence of respiratory failure cannot be judged by the normal ABG criteria but by a significant change from the baseline $PaCO_2$ to a level having the potential for morbidity and mortality.

Treatment goals include normalizing pH (avoiding mechanical ventilation if possible), elevating SaO_2 to 90% (if hypoxemia is also present), improving airflow, treating infection, monitoring and maintaining fluid status, and preventing or treating complications as necessary.[16,20,21] Deaths are less due to respiratory failure, and more associated with dysfunction of other organs, older age, significant baseline disease, a severe precipitating illness, severity of acidosis, and presence of complications.[22] Episodes of acute respiratory failure in these patients seem to have a significant long-term influence with mortality rates reaching 45% within the year after an exacerbation requiring mechanical ventilation and tracheostomy.[23]

Patients with chronic hypoxemic respiratory failure (type I) are at similar risk for acute deterioration of hypoxemia. Infection and heart failure can result in worsening of the tenuous oxygenation status of patients with interstitial pulmonary fibrosis or primary pulmonary hypertension.

Complications of Acute Respiratory Failure

Although respiratory failure is life-threatening by itself, complications frequently arise that can add significantly to morbidity and mortality. Especially in patients with ARDS, more deaths are due to complications (e.g., sepsis, multiorgan failure) than to the primary disease.[24] Modern ICUs with sophisticated mechanical ventilation can prolong but may not preserve life. Pulmonary complications such as emboli, **barotrauma**, and infection may be secondary to treatment strategies such as catheters, mechanical ventilation, and endotracheal tubes. A wide array of nonpulmonary complications may develop, including bacteremia, malnutrition, psychosis secondary to prolonged ICU stays, cardiac disorders (e.g., arrhythmias, hypotension), gastrointestinal ailments (e.g., hemorrhage, dysmotility), and renal disturbances (e.g., acute renal failure, positive fluid balance).

Clinical Presentation

Clinically, a patient with respiratory muscle fatigue shows an initially increased respiratory rate followed by *bradypnea* (slowed respiratory rate) and apnea as fatigue ensues. **Respiratory alternans**, which is a phasic alternation between rib cage and abdominal breathing, may also occur. Opinions vary on the sensitivity and specificity of abdominal motion paradox in patients with respiratory muscle weakness, but at least some investigators suggest that respiratory muscle paradox is an early sign (see Chapter 16). When ventilatory failure is full-blown, ABG results show hypercapnia with acidosis. As mentioned earlier, the presence of hypercapnia with acidosis can also indicate that the respiratory center is not responding properly.[25]

Tachypnea is the cardinal sign of increased work of breathing. Tachypnea occurs when the respiratory center increases breathing frequency in an attempt to lessen respiratory excursion and reduce the amount of work performed by the respiratory muscles.[26] Overall workload is reflected in the minute volume needed to maintain normocapnia.

Indications for Ventilatory Support

For each type of oxygenation and ventilatory failure, the goal of mechanical ventilation is either to support the patient until the underlying problem resolves or to maintain support of the patient with chronic ventilatory problems. These goals may be achieved by improving alveolar ventilation and arterial oxygenation, increasing lung volume, or reducing work of breathing.[27] This section discusses the indications for mechanical ventilation for hypoxemic (type I) and hypercapnic (type II) respiratory failure. Hypoxemic respiratory failure is divided into processes that require short-term and long-term ventilatory support. Hypercapnic respiratory failure is broken down into

MINI CLINI

Acute or Chronic Hypercapnic Respiratory Failure

PROBLEM: A 55-year-old man presents to the emergency department complaining of increased shortness of breath and yellow-green sputum production for 1 week. He is alert and oriented. He has a 60 pack-year smoking history. Vital signs are blood pressure 165/90 mm Hg, pulse 120 beats/min, respirations 25 breaths/min, and temperature 100.5° F oral.

ABG values on room air are as follows:

pH	7.28
$PaCO_2$	70 mm Hg
PaO_2	35 mm Hg
HCO_3^-	36 mm Hg
SaO_2	66%

1. Define the respiratory condition indicated by the ABG results.
2. What is the $P(A - a)O_2$?
3. What type of respiratory failure is present?
4. What kind of therapy is indicated?

Discussion

1. The ABG values indicate a partially compensated respiratory acidosis with hypoxemia.
2. $PAO_2 = 0.21\ (760 - 47) - 70/0.8 = 62$ mm Hg
   $PaO_2 = 35$ mm Hg
   $P(A - a)O_2 = 62 - 35 = 27$ mm Hg on room air
3. This is hypercapnic respiratory failure (type II), also known as *ventilatory failure*. However, in acute failure, the pH decreases 0.08 for every 10-mm Hg increase in $PaCO_2$. In this patient, $PaCO_2$ has increased 30 mm Hg (70 – 40), and the pH has decreased 0.12. The pH would be expected to decrease 0.24 (3 × 0.08) if this were acute ventilatory failure. This is a case of acute-on-chronic failure. HCO_3^- of 36 mEq/L (normal 22 to 26 mEq/L) also indicates renal compensation has occurred, which takes days to achieve. $P(A - a)O_2$ is 27 mm Hg, which is above normal, indicating that hypoxemia cannot be explained fully by hypoventilation.
4. Because the patient is alert, conservative therapy to improve lung function is indicated. O_2 administration to achieve SaO_2 of at least 90% is required. If PaO_2 does not respond to O_2 administration, shunt is present, and positive airway pressure may be necessary. Antibiotics are indicated for the probable infection (fever, discolored sputum), and bronchopulmonary hygiene (bronchodilators, steroids, cough assist) is indicated to improve ventilation.

unstable ventilatory drive, muscle fatigue, excessive work of breathing, and alveolar hypoventilation.

Parameters Indicating Need for Ventilatory Support

Although various measurements have been proposed to help decide if a patient needs mechanical ventilation, the clinical status of the patient is the most important criterion. Table 44-3 and the discussion that follows review common physiologic indicators for initiating support by the underlying cause of respiratory failure.

Hypoxemic Respiratory Failure. Severe, refractory hypoxemia is a common indication for intubation and ventilator support. Table 44-3 lists different measures of hypoxemia that have been used to assess the need for ventilatory support. Most commonly, PaO_2 is compared with FiO_2 as with the PaO_2/FiO_2 ratio or the alveolar-arterial O_2 difference $[P(A-a)O_2]$. Indicators of profoundly impaired oxygenation suggesting the need for intubation, high inspired O_2 administration, and PEEP include $P(A-a)O_2$ value of 350 mm Hg on FiO_2 of 1.0 or a PaO_2/FiO_2 value of less than 200. These values are useful for all causes of hypoxemic respiratory failure (type I) but cannot help distinguish if the process is a readily reversible one, such as pulmonary edema or atelectasis, or a process that resolves more slowly, such as acute lung injury. Frequently, patients have a combination of hypoxemic and hypercapnic respiratory failure.

Hypercapnic Respiratory Failure (Ventilatory Failure). As previously discussed, hypercapnic (type II) respiratory failure or ventilatory failure can be caused by increased ventilatory dead space, increased CO_2 production, or decreased alveolar ventilation. All of these processes cause an increase in $PaCO_2$.[25] Assessment of the pH allows a determination of whether the problem is acute or chronic. Chronic hypoventilation is compensated by the kidneys' retention of bicarbonate, although this response requires several days. The following example shows the importance of pH in interpreting the significance of elevated $PaCO_2$.

	Patient A	Patient B
$PaCO_2$	60 mm Hg	60 mm Hg
Serum HCO_3^-	25 mEq/L	36 mEq/L
pH	7.25	7.38

Although both patients in this example have the same level of hypercapnia, only patient A exhibits acute ventilatory failure with an elevated $PaCO_2$ but normal serum bicarbonate (25 mEq/L). Patient B has a compensated respiratory acidosis from chronic hypercapnic respiratory failure, as indicated by the normal pH and elevated serum bicarbonate (36 mEq/L). This condition is also known as *chronic ventilatory failure*. The distinction between acute and chronic ventilatory failure is very important in respiratory care and emphasizes the need to use both $PaCO_2$ and pH as indicators for ventilatory support. The trend in pH and $PaCO_2$ values is also useful in assessing the effects of therapies in correcting acute ventilatory failure.

Significance of Elevated Alveolar Partial Pressure of Carbon Dioxide. Because elevated $PaCO_2$ increases ventilatory drive in healthy subjects, the existence of hypoventilation suggests other problems with the respiratory apparatus. Specifically, the presence of acute respiratory acidosis indicates one of three major problems: (1) The respiratory center is not responding normally to elevated $PaCO_2$; (2) the respiratory center is responding normally, but the signal is not getting through to the respiratory muscles; or (3) despite normal neurologic response mechanisms, the lungs and chest bellows are incapable of providing adequate ventilation because of parenchymal lung disease or muscular weakness.[28]

TABLE 44-3

Physiologic Indicators for Ventilatory Support, Classified by Mechanism Underlying Respiratory Failure

Mechanism	Normal Values	Support Indicated
Inadequate Alveolar Ventilation		
$PaCO_2$ (mm Hg)	35-45	>55
pH	7.35-7.45	<7.20
Inadequate Lung Expansion		
Tidal volume (V_T) ml/kg	5-8	<5
Vital capacity (VC) ml/kg	65-75	<10
Respiratory rate	12-20	>35
Inadequate Muscle Strength		
Maximum inspiratory pressure (cm H_2O)	–80-100	≥–20
Vital capacity (VC, ml/kg)	65-75	<10
Maximum voluntary ventilation (MVV, L/min)	120-180	<2× VE
Increased Work of Breathing		
Minute ventilation (V_E)	5-6	>10
V_D/V_T (%)	0.25-0.40	>0.6
Hypoxemia		
$P(A-a)O_2$ on 100% O_2 (mm Hg)	25-65	>350
PaO_2/FiO_2	350-450	<200

VE, Minute ventilation.

ASSESSMENT OF RESPIRATORY FATIGUE, WEAKNESS, FAILURE, AND WORK OF BREATHING

Respiratory Muscle Weakness

Respiratory muscle weakness refers to the decreased capacity of a rested muscle to generate force and decreased endurance.[29] Respiratory muscle weakness occurs most commonly in patients with neuromuscular disease. Other conditions that lead to muscle weakness by increasing demand include COPD, kyphoscoliosis, and obesity.

The most commonly used tests to assess respiratory muscle strength at the bedside are **maximum inspiratory pressure (MIP)** and **maximum expiratory pressure (MEP)**,[30] forced vital capacity, and **maximum voluntary ventilation (MVV)** (see Table 44-3). MIP of –30 cm H_2O or less (more negative) usually indicates adequate respiratory muscle strength to continue spontaneous breathing, but the overall trend needs to be considered. This consideration is especially important in patients with myasthenic crisis or Guillain-Barré syndrome, where values of MIP that are becoming less negative may be the only clue to impending respiratory failure. The MVV maneuver can be performed at the bedside with a hand-held spirometer, but its use in the critical care setting is limited because substantial patient cooperation is required. The **sniff nasal inspiratory pressure** may also be used to assess inspiratory muscle strength. Advantages include ease of performance even in patients with advanced disease and its prognostic value.[31]

Respiratory Muscle Fatigue

Fatigue is usually defined as a condition in which there is loss of the capacity to develop force or velocity of a muscle resulting from muscle activity under load, which is reversible by rest.[32] Fatigue can be assessed by measuring the loss of force in response to repeated stimulations. It can be caused by both specific demands placed on the muscle and reduced supply of necessary nutrients. The demand on a muscle is increased by increased work of breathing, increased strength of muscle contraction, and decreased muscle efficiency. Hypoxemia, decreased inspiratory muscle blood flow, poor nutrition, and inability of a muscle to extract energy from supplied substrates can lead to fatigue as well.[29]

There are three types of respiratory **muscle fatigue**. (1) Central muscle fatigue is an exertion-induced, reversible decrease in central respiratory drive; (2) transmission muscle fatigue is an exertion-induced, reversible impairment in the transmission of neural impulses; and (3) contractile muscle fatigue is a reversible impairment in the contractile response to a neural impulse in an overloaded muscle.[28]

Respiratory Failure

Respiratory failure is an unfavorable imbalance between a respiratory workload, on the one hand, and ventilatory muscle strength and endurance, on the other hand. The **tension-time index** takes into account the fact that respiratory muscle endurance depends both on the magnitude of the respiratory load in relation to respiratory strength (P_{di}/P_{dimax}) and on the duration of the inspiratory effort in relation to total breath time (the duty cycle, or T_i/T_{tot}). This index $(P_{di}/P_{dimax}) \times (T_i/T_{tot})$ determines whether a respiratory load can be tolerated without development of failure: Values less than 0.15 are generally tolerated for a long period, whereas indices greater than 0.18 usually result in fatigue and respiratory failure within 45 minutes.[33] Comparing the spontaneous minute ventilation with MVV is also a helpful index because fatigue and failure are both likely to occur if the minute ventilation exceeds 60% of MVV.[34]

These closely related concepts of weakness, fatigue, and failure usually overlap and can result in acute or chronic respiratory failure. Respiratory muscle weakness can predispose to ventilatory muscle fatigue. Whether fatigue consistently leads to failure has historically been the subject of much debate.[35] In one study, weaning failure was not accompanied by fatigue of the diaphragm despite the presence of diaphragm weakness.[36] Alternatively, fatigue of the diaphragm lasting for 24 hours is reliably present after hyperventilation at 60% of MVV or greater until task failure.[34,37]

Work of Breathing

Work of breathing is the amount of pressure needed to move a given volume into the lung with a relaxed chest wall. Excessive work of breathing is the most common cause of respiratory muscle fatigue. Work of breathing is due to physiologic work and imposed work. Physiologic work involves overcoming the elastic forces during inspiration and overcoming the resistance of the airways and lung tissue. Normal work of breathing is 0.3 to 0.6 J/L. Airway and pulmonary parenchymal abnormalities can increase the physiologic work of breathing. In intubated patients, sources of imposed work of breathing include the endotracheal tube, ventilator circuit, and **auto-PEEP** secondary to **dynamic hyperinflation** with airflow obstruction, as is commonly seen in a patient with COPD.[26] Increased work of breathing can also be an impediment to weaning.[38] Measurement of work of breathing with an esophageal balloon catheter and a flow transducer has been used to determine work of breathing and break it down into physiologic and imposed components.[38] Kirton and colleagues[39] showed that 96% of patients with a physiologic work of breathing less than 0.8 J/L were successfully weaned and extubated from ventilatory support.

CHOOSING A VENTILATORY SUPPORT STRATEGY FOR DIFFERENT CAUSES OF RESPIRATORY FAILURE

The remainder of this chapter briefly discusses current ventilatory strategies for hypoxemic and hypercapnic respiratory failure. The clinical application of specific modes of mechanical ventilation is described in Chapters 45 and 48, and noninvasive ventilation (NIV) is reviewed in more detail in Chapter 49. When it has been determined that the patient needs ventilatory support, the initial decision is whether to intubate or to ventilate noninvasively. In the acute setting, this decision is sometimes based on the underlying process, the type of respiratory failure, and how rapidly the underlying process can be reversed.

Noninvasive Ventilation

A consensus report supports the use of noninvasive support of ventilation to reduce the morbidity and possibly the mortality of both hypoxemic and hypercarbic respiratory failure.[40] In this context, **noninvasive ventilation (NIV)** can be defined as any mode of ventilatory support that is provided without endotracheal intubation, encompassing continuous positive airway pressure (CPAP) alone or in combination with any mode of pressure-limited or volume-limited ventilation.[40] NIV can improve hypoxemia and hypercarbia via several mechanisms including but not limited to (1) compensating for the inspiratory threshold load imposed by intrinsic PEEP,[41] (2) supplementing a reduced tidal volume,[42] (3) partial or complete unloading of the respiratory muscles,[42] (4) reducing venous return and left ventricular afterload,[43,44] (5) alveolar recruitment,[45] (6) preventing intermittent narrowing and collapse in patients with concomitant obstructive sleep apnea hypopnea syndrome by acting as a pneumatic splint during sleep,[46] and (7) improving lung function (particularly functional residual capacity) and daytime gas exchange in obstructive sleep apnea hypopnea syndrome.[47] NIV currently has indications in both acute[48] and chronic[49] respiratory failure.

Noninvasive Ventilation in Acute Conditions

Exacerbations of Chronic Obstructive Pulmonary Disease

NIV is considered to be a standard of care in patients with exacerbations of COPD.[50] For instance, NIV combined with usual care in exacerbations of COPD reduces treatment failure (defined as mortality, need for intubation, or intolerance) such that the number needed to treat (NNT) to prevent 1 treatment failure was 5, intubations (NNT = 5), mortality (NNT = 8), complications (NNT = 3), and hospital length of stay by about 3 days.[50]

Recommendations are to initiate NIV when the $PaCO_2$ is greater than 45 mm Hg but before the development of severe acidosis in the course of a COPD exacerbation.[50] Otherwise, in patients with mild COPD exacerbations (pH >7.35), NIV was no more effective than standard medical therapy.[51] Nearly 50% of the patients did not tolerate NIV.[51]

Cardiogenic Pulmonary Edema

NIV is a recommended option in the management of acute respiratory failure in the setting of cardiogenic pulmonary edema. Studies showed that either CPAP or NIV in these patients significantly reduced dyspnea score, heart rate, acidosis, and hypercapnia within the first hour after the start of treatment.[52,53] In the largest study, mortality, rates of intubation, rate of admission to the critical care unit, or mean length of hospital stay were not improved,[52] but smaller trials showed decreased intubation and mortality rates with NIV.[53] Selection and methodologic criteria may explain the difference, see Chapter 49.

Acute Asthma

Studies have shown that NIV in asthma associated with acute respiratory failure progressively improved pH and $PaCO_2$ over 12 to 24 hours, reduced the respiratory rate, improved lung function, resolved the attack faster, and reduced the need for hospitalization.[54-55] Despite those promising results, the use of NIV in status asthmaticus remains controversial, and large, prospective, randomized controlled trials are needed to confirm the role of NIV in that setting.[56]

Acute Lung Injury and Acute Respiratory Distress Syndrome

NIV in the settings of acute lung injury and ARDS has been disappointing with a 50% to 84% failure rate.[57-59] A prospective study showed that NIV was successful in improving gas exchange and avoiding intubation in 54% of patients, with consequent reduction in ventilator-associated pneumonia and lower ICU mortality rate.[60] Factors that may be associated with NIV failure in these settings include the presence of shock, metabolic acidosis, severe hypoxemia, a Simplified Acute Physiology Score (SAPS) II greater than 34, and a PaO_2/FiO_2 less than 175 after 1 hour of NIV.[58-60]

Noninvasive Ventilation in Chronic Conditions

Obesity-Hypoventilation Syndrome

Obesity-hypoventilation syndrome refers to the presence of daytime hypercapnia ($PaCO_2 > 45$ mm Hg) in obese individuals when no other cause of hypoventilation is present. Factors associated with daytime hypercapnia include body mass index, the presence of nocturnal apnea hypopnea, mean overnight O_2 saturation, and severity of restrictive pulmonary function.[11] Average volume-assured pressure support, a form of NIV in which pressure support is automatically adjusted to reach a set tidal volume, lowers $PaCO_2$ compared with bilevel positive airway pressure alone but without improving oxygenation, sleep quality, or quality of life.[61]

Stable Chronic Obstructive Pulmonary Disease

NIV in patients with severe COPD and $PaCO_2$ greater than 46 mm Hg improves survival, but adherence to NIV is low, some quality of life indices appear to show worsening with NIV, and there was no reduction in hospitalization rates,[62] perhaps owing to selection of inspiratory pressures that were insufficient to reduce hypercapnia. For instance, compared with low-intensity NIV (mean inspiratory positive airway pressure 14 cm H_2O, backup rate 8/min), the use of settings that aimed to reduce $PaCO_2$ maximally (mean inspiratory positive airway pressure 29 cm H_2O with backup rate 17.5/min) increased the daily use of NIV by 3.6 hr/day and improved exercise-related dyspnea, daytime $PaCO_2$, forced expiratory volume in 1 second, vital capacity and health-related quality of life.[63]

Neuromuscular Diseases and Thoracic Cage Abnormalities

Several studies show that even in progressive neuromuscular disorders, NIV can prolong survival, improve quality of life, enhance cognitive function, and reduce pneumonia and hospitalization rates.[12] Other NIV techniques using rocking beds, pneumobelts, and negative pressure ventilation are much less frequently used and are becoming less easily available.

Invasive Ventilatory Support

Patients with profound hypoxemia from a process that is expected to resolve slowly, such as acute lung injury, usually require intubation and mechanical ventilation. Other indications for intubation include conditions where NIV may be poorly tolerated or even deleterious, such as the presence of upper airway obstruction, inability to clear secretions and protect airway, inability to achieve a proper mask fit, and intolerance of the intervention. Both hypoxemic and hypercarbic

MINI CLINI

Indications for Continuous Positive Airway Pressure versus Continuous Mechanical Ventilation With Positive End Expiratory Pressure

PROBLEM: A patient in the ICU is severely tachypneic and hypoxemic. The respiratory rate is 30 breaths/min. On approximately 50% O_2 by mask at sea level, PaO_2 is 50 mm Hg, $PaCO_2$ is 30 mm Hg, pH is 7.51, and HCO_3^- is 23 mEq/L. The patient is in distress but alert and able to cooperate and follow instructions.

1. What is this patient's $P(A - a)O_2$?
2. What type of respiratory failure is this?
3. What is the appropriate initial therapy?

Discussion: This patient does not have hypercapnic respiratory failure, as is confirmed by $PaCO_2$ of 30 mm Hg. The patient does have a serious oxygenation defect, as confirmed by $P(A - a)O_2$.

$$PAO_2 = 0.50\,(713) - 30/0.8 = 318 \text{ mm Hg}$$
$$P(A - a)O_2 = 318 - 50 = 268 \text{ mm Hg}$$

The elevated $P(A - a)O_2$ indicates the presence of severe intrapulmonary shunt. Shunts this severe can occur only when significant airway closure and atelectasis are present. The mode of therapy should be aimed at reinflating collapsed alveoli and keeping the alveoli open throughout the breathing cycle. In this patient, alveolar ventilation is not impaired ($PaCO_2$ = 30 mm Hg). CPAP alone may be effective in reducing shunt. (CPAP does not ventilate the patient; all breaths are patient-initiated and spontaneous.) CPAP may be applied noninvasively via face mask, as would be indicated in this alert, cooperative patient. If hypercapnia and acidemia develop, mechanical ventilation with PEEP would be indicated.

MINI CLINI

Acute Hypercapnic Respiratory Failure

PROBLEM: A patient with COPD presents to the emergency department in moderate respiratory distress. He is alert and cooperative. Respiratory rate is 26 breaths/min. Lung examination shows poor air entry with expiratory wheezing. Room air ABGs show pH 7.24, $PaCO_2$ 60 mm Hg, and PaO_2 60 mm Hg.

1. What type of respiratory failure is this?
2. How should the patient be managed?

Discussion: ABGs show an acute respiratory acidosis with normal $PAO_2 - PaO_2$ gradient.

$$PAO_2 = 0.21\,(713) - 60/0.8 = 74$$
$$P(A - a)O_2 = 74 - 60 = 14 \text{ mm Hg}$$

This patient has hypercapnic respiratory failure related to obstructive lung disease, also known as *ventilatory failure.* In addition to bronchodilators and corticosteroids, the RT should aim to improve ventilation to reverse the respiratory acidosis. In this patient, who is alert and cooperative, NIV via face mask may be tried. Initial mask ventilation can start in the pressure support ventilation mode with a level of support of 10 cm H_2O and 5 cm H_2O PEEP. Tidal volume should be maintained at approximately 6 to 8 ml/kg. If this patient deteriorates despite therapy, he will need to be intubated and mechanically ventilated.

types of respiratory failure can be managed effectively by invasive mechanical ventilation.

There are several ventilator variables, some independently set by the operators and others that are dependent on the set variables. Independent and dependent variables vary with the mode of ventilation. FiO_2 and **PEEP** are independently set variables regardless of mode of ventilation used to manage hypoxemia. In volume-controlled or flow-controlled ventilation, tidal volume, flow, and respiratory rate are independently set variables. In **pressure control ventilation**, driving pressure, inspiratory time, and respiratory rate are independently set variables. Other modes and strategies include inverse ratio ventilation, liquid ventilation, prone positioning, and airway pressure release ventilation. Considerations in selected cases of respiratory failure requiring invasive ventilatory support are briefly reviewed.

Acute Respiratory Distress Syndrome

Profound hypoxemic respiratory failure is often due to severe pneumonia and ARDS. Patients with these conditions have very noncompliant lungs. Volume-cycled ventilation in patients with ARDS frequently leads to high peak airway and plateau pressures. Ventilating these patients with small tidal volumes (about 6 ml/kg) reduces complications associated with mechanical ventilation and improves survival.[64]

Increased Intracranial Pressure

Hyperventilation applied acutely and for short periods may be used to reduce ICP. The goal is to lower $PaCO_2$ to between 25 mm Hg and 30 mm Hg, which causes alkalosis, which in combination with hypocapnia helps reduce cerebral blood flow until ICP can be controlled by other measures. Ongoing ventilatory support should maintain PCO_2 in the range of 30 to 40 mm Hg. By maintaining PCO_2 in this range, sudden increases in ICP can be quickly controlled by short-term hyperventilation. Although reducing blood flow can reduce brain swelling and ICP, cerebral ischemia can also result. Another concern in ventilating patients with elevated ICP is using PEEP to manage hypoxemia. There is a concern that increased intrathoracic pressure secondary to PEEP would cause decreased cerebral venous return leading to increased ICP and that PEEP can decrease cerebral perfusion by limiting cardiac output. The use of PEEP in patients with elevated ICP may require invasive monitoring of ICP because the combination of decreased cerebral perfusion and elevated ICP can narrow cerebral perfusion pressure.[65] Elevation of the head of the bed can offset the increased ICP associated with the application of PEEP.

Obstructive Lung Disease

Patients with obstructive lung disease have markedly increased airway resistance that leads to a decrease in the rate of expiratory flow with resulting hyperinflation. These patients frequently have problems with elevated airway pressure or dynamic hyperinflation (auto-PEEP), which can cause barotrauma and increased dyssynchrony, especially ineffective triggering of the ventilator.[66]

The management goal for patients with obstructive lung disease and respiratory failure is to oxygenate and ventilate the patient successfully, while avoiding dyssynchrony and dynamic hyperinflation. In these patients, lower tidal volumes (6 to 8 ml/kg), moderate respiratory rates, and high sustained (square wave) inspiratory flow rates (70 to 100 L/min) are recommended to avoid dynamic hyperinflation.[67] These maneuvers reduce inspiratory time and prolong expiratory time, which allows a patient with obstructive lung disease to have a longer time to exhale.

Another consideration in patients with obstructive lung disease is the inspiratory threshold load imposed by auto-PEEP resulting in increased patient inspiratory work.[41] In this case, applied (or extrinsic) PEEP can compensate for this threshold load and reduce the work of breathing for patient-triggered breaths in any assisted ventilatory mode.[41]

Ventilatory Support in Chronic Hypercapnic Respiratory Failure

The goal of therapy in hypercapnic respiratory failure (acute ventilatory failure) is to guarantee a set minute ventilation. In treating patients with chronic ventilatory failure, the goal is to normalize the pH but not the $PaCO_2$. Correction of $PaCO_2$ in a patient with chronic hypoventilation from diverse causes can lead to a posthypercapnic metabolic alkalosis, which can produce hypokalemia, seizures, and arrhythmias.

SUMMARY CHECKLIST

- Acute respiratory failure is identified by PaO_2 less than 60 mm Hg or $PaCO_2$ greater than 50 mm Hg, or both, in otherwise healthy individuals at sea level.
- Hypoxemic respiratory failure is most commonly due to $\dot{V}/\dot{Q}$ mismatch, shunt, or hypoventilation.
- Hypercapnic respiratory failure, also known as *ventilatory failure*, results from decreased ventilatory drive, neurologic disease, or increased work of breathing.
- Chronic respiratory failure may manifest with hypercapnia and evidence of a compensatory metabolic alkalosis (chronic ventilatory failure) or with polycythemia reflecting chronic hypoxemia.
- The clinical status of the patient is the most important factor determining the need for ventilatory support.
- Excessive work of breathing is the most common cause of respiratory muscle fatigue.
- The beneficial role of NIV in the acute setting has been best established in acute exacerbations of COPD and in cardiogenic edema.
- Increased FiO_2 and PEEP are the main therapies for severe hypoxemia.
- The goal of therapy in hypercapnic respiratory failure (acute ventilatory failure) is to normalize the pH.

References

1. Vasilyev S, Schaap RN, Mortensen JD: Hospital survival rates of patients with acute respiratory failure in modern respiratory intensive care units: an international, multicenter, prospective survey. *Chest* 107:1083–1088, 1995.
2. Wunsch H, Linde-Zwirble WT, Angus DC, et al: The epidemiology of mechanical ventilation use in the United States. *Crit Care Med* 38:1947–1953, 2010.
3. Greene KE, Peters JI: Pathophysiology of acute respiratory failure. *Clin Chest Med* 15:1–12, 1994.
4. Campbell EJ: Respiratory failure. *BMJ* 5448:1451–1460, 1965.
5. West JB: *Respiratory physiology: the essentials*, ed 7, Philadelphia, 2005, Lippincott Williams & Wilkins.
6. Aboussouan LS, Stoller JK: The hepatopulmonary syndrome. *Baillieres Best Pract Res Clin Gastroenterol* 14:1033–1048, 2000.
7. American Thoracic Society: Idiopathic pulmonary fibrosis: diagnosis and treatment. International consensus statement. American Thoracic Society (ATS), and the European Respiratory Society (ERS). *Am J Respir Crit Care Med* 161(2 Pt 1):646–664, 2000.
8. Aboussouan LS, Stoller JK: Traveling with supplemental oxygen for patients with chronic lung disease. In Maurer JR, editor: *Non-neoplastic advanced lung disease*, New York, 2003, Marcel Dekker, pp 711–730.
9. Caruana-Montaldo B, Gleeson K, Zwillich CW: The control of breathing in clinical practice. *Chest* 117:205–225, 2000.
10. Dick CR, Sassoon CS: Patient-ventilator interactions. *Clin Chest Med* 17:423–438, 1996.
11. Kaw R, Hernandez AV, Walker E, et al: Determinants of hypercapnia in obese patients with obstructive sleep apnea: a systematic review and meta-analysis of cohort studies. *Chest* 136:789–796, 2009.
12. Aboussouan LS: Respiratory disorders in neurologic diseases. *Cleve Clin J Med* 72:511–520, 2005.
13. Kaplan LM, Hollander D: Respiratory dysfunction in amyotrophic lateral sclerosis. *Clin Chest Med* 15:675–681, 1994.
14. Teitelbaum JS, Borel CO: Respiratory dysfunction in Guillain-Barre syndrome. *Clin Chest Med* 15:705–714, 1994.
15. Zulueta JJ, Fanburg BL: Respiratory dysfunction in myasthenia gravis. *Clin Chest Med* 15:68–691, 1994.
16. Curtis JR, Hudson LD: Emergent assessment and management of acute respiratory failure in COPD. *Clin Chest Med* 15:481–500, 1994.
17. Jozefowicz RF: Neurologic manifestations of pulmonary disease. *Neurol Clin* 7:605–616, 1989.
18. Hoyert DL, Xu J: Deaths: preliminary data for 2011. *Natl Vital Stat Rep* 61(6):1–51, 2012.
19. Chen R, Grand'Maison F, Strong MJ, et al: Motor neuron disease presenting as acute respiratory failure: a clinical and pathological study. *J Neurol Neurosurg Psychiatry* 60:455–458, 1996.
20. MacIntyre N, Huang NC: Acute exacerbations and respiratory failure in chronic obstructive pulmonary disease. *Proc Am Thorac Soc* 5:530–535, 2008.
21. Song JW, Hong S-B, Lim C-M, et al: Acute exacerbations of idiopathic pulmonary fibrosis: incidence, risk factors and outcome. *Eur Respir J* 37:356–363, 2011.
22. Flaatten H, Gjerd S, Guttormsen AB, et al: Outcome after acute respiratory failure is more dependent on dysfunction in other vital organs than on the severity of the respiratory failure. *Crit Care* 7:R72–R77, 2003.
23. Kojicic M, Li G, Ahmed A, et al: Long-term survival in patients with tracheostomy and prolonged mechanical ventilation in Olmsted County, Minnesota. *Respir Care* 56:1765–1770, 2011.

24. Stapleton RD, Wang BM, Hudson LD, et al: Causes and timing of death in patients with ARDS. *Chest* 128:525–532, 2005.
25. Roussos C: Respiratory muscle fatigue and ventilatory failure. *Chest* 97 (3 Suppl):89S–96S, 1990.
26. Banner MJ: Respiratory muscle loading and the work of breathing. *J Cardiothorac Vasc Anesth* 9:192–204, 1995.
27. Slutsky AS: Consensus conference on mechanical ventilation—January 28-30, 1993 at Northbrook, Illinois, USA. Part I. European Society of Intensive Care Medicine, the ACCP and the SCCM. *Intensive Care Med* 20:64–79, 1994.
28. Mador MJ: Respiratory muscle fatigue and breathing pattern. *Chest* 100:1430–1435, 1991.
29. Stoller JK: Physiologic rationale for resting the ventilatory muscles. *Respir Care* 36:290–296, 1991.
30. Gibson GJ: Measurement of respiratory muscle strength. *Respir Med* 89:529–535, 1995.
31. Morgan RK, McNally S, Alexander M, et al: Use of Sniff nasal-inspiratory force to predict survival in amyotrophic lateral sclerosis. *Am J Respir Crit Care Med* 171:269–274, 2005.
32. NHLBI Workshop summary: Respiratory muscle fatigue. Report of the Respiratory Muscle Fatigue Workshop Group. *Am Rev Respir Dis* 142:474–480, 1990.
33. Bellemare F, Grassino A: Effect of pressure and timing of contraction on human diaphragm fatigue. *J Appl Physiol* 53:1190–1195, 1982.
34. Mador JM, Rodis A, Diaz J: Diaphragmatic fatigue following voluntary hyperpnea. *Am J Respir Crit Care Med* 154:63–67, 1996.
35. Macklem PT, Roussos CS: Respiratory muscle fatigue: a cause of respiratory failure? *Clin Sci Mol Med* 53:419–422, 1977.
36. Laghi F, Cattapan SE, Jubran A, et al: Is weaning failure caused by low-frequency fatigue of the diaphragm? *Am J Respir Crit Care Med* 167:120–127, 2003.
37. Laghi F, D'Alfonso N, Tobin MJ: Pattern of recovery from diaphragmatic fatigue over 24 hours. *J Appl Physiol* 79:539–546, 1995.
38. Petros AJ, Lamond CT, Bennett D: The Bicore pulmonary monitor: a device to assess the work of breathing while weaning from mechanical ventilation. *Anaesthesia* 48:985–988, 1993.
39. Kirton OC, DeHaven CB, Morgan JP, et al: Elevated imposed work of breathing masquerading as ventilator weaning intolerance. *Chest* 108:1021–1025, 1995.
40. International Consensus Conferences in Intensive Care Medicine: Noninvasive positive pressure ventilation in acute respiratory failure. *Am J Respir Crit Care Med* 163:283–291, 2001.
41. MacIntyre NR, Cheng KC, McConnell R: Applied PEEP during pressure support reduces the inspiratory threshold load of intrinsic PEEP. *Chest* 111:188–193, 1997.
42. MacIntyre NR, Leatherman NE: Ventilatory muscle loads and the frequency-tidal volume pattern during inspiratory pressure-assisted (pressure-supported) ventilation. *Am Rev Respir Dis* 141:327–331, 1990.
43. Lenique F, Habis M, Lofaso F, et al: Ventilatory and hemodynamic effects of continuous positive airway pressure in left heart failure. *Am J Respir Crit Care Med* 155:500–505, 1997.
44. Naughton MT, Rahman MA, Hara K, et al: Effect of continuous positive airway pressure on intrathoracic and left ventricular transmural pressures in patients with congestive heart failure. *Circulation* 91:1725–1731, 1995.
45. De Michele M, Grasso S: Measurement of PEEP-induced alveolar recruitment: just a research tool? *Crit Care* 10:148, 2006.
46. Sullivan CE, Berthon-Jones M, Issa FG: Remission of severe obesity-hypoventilation syndrome after short-term treatment during sleep with nasal continuous positive airway pressure. *Am Rev Respir Dis* 128:177–181, 1983.
47. Verbraecken J, Willemen M, De Cock W, et al: Continuous positive airway pressure and lung inflation in sleep apnea patients. *Respiration* 68:357–364, 2001.
48. Aboussouan LS, Ricaurte B: Noninvasive positive pressure ventilation: increasing use in acute care. *Cleve Clin J Med* 77:307–316, 2010.
49. Theerakittikul T, Ricaurte B, Aboussouan LS: Noninvasive positive pressure ventilation for stable outpatients: CPAP and beyond. *Cleve Clin J Med* 77: 705–710, 2010.
50. Lightowler JV, Wedzicha JA, Elliott MW, et al: Non-invasive positive pressure ventilation to treat respiratory failure resulting from exacerbations of chronic obstructive pulmonary disease: Cochrane systematic review and meta-analysis. *BMJ* 326:185, 2003.
51. Keenan SP, Sinuff T, Cook DJ, et al: Which patients with acute exacerbation of chronic obstructive pulmonary disease benefit from noninvasive positive-pressure ventilation? A systematic review of the literature. *Ann Intern Med* 138:861–870, 2003.
52. Gray A, Goodacre S, Newby DE, et al: Noninvasive ventilation in acute cardiogenic pulmonary edema. *N Engl J Med* 359:142–151, 2008.
53. Ho KM, Wong K: A comparison of continuous and bi-level positive airway pressure non-invasive ventilation in patients with acute cardiogenic pulmonary oedema: a meta-analysis. *Crit Care* 10:R49, 2006.
54. Meduri GU, Cook TR, Turner RE, et al: Noninvasive positive pressure ventilation in status asthmaticus. *Chest* 110:767–774, 1996.
55. Soroksky A, Stav D, Shpirer I: A pilot prospective, randomized, placebo-controlled trial of bilevel positive airway pressure in acute asthmatic attack. *Chest* 123:1018–1025, 2003.
56. Lim WJ, Mohammed Akram R, Carson KV, et al: Non-invasive positive pressure ventilation for treatment of respiratory failure due to severe acute exacerbations of asthma. *Cochrane Database Syst Rev* CD004360, 2012.
57. Agarwal R, Aggarwal AN, Gupta D: Role of noninvasive ventilation in acute lung injury/acute respiratory distress syndrome: a proportion meta-analysis. *Respir Care* 55:1653–1660, 2010.
58. Thille AW, Contou D, Fragnoli C, et al: Non-invasive ventilation for acute hypoxemic respiratory failure: intubation rate and risk factors. *Crit Care* 17:R269, 2013.
59. Rana S, Jenad H, Gay PC, et al: Failure of non-invasive ventilation in patients with acute lung injury: observational cohort study. *Crit Care* 10:R79, 2006.
60. Antonelli M, Conti G, Esquinas A, et al: A multiple-center survey on the use in clinical practice of noninvasive ventilation as a first-line intervention for acute respiratory distress syndrome. *Crit Care Med* 35:18–25, 2007.
61. Storre JH, Seuthe B, Fiechter R, et al: Average volume-assured pressure support in obesity hypoventilation: a randomized crossover trial. *Chest* 130:815–821, 2006.
62. McEvoy RD, Pierce RJ, Hillman D, et al: Nocturnal non-invasive nasal ventilation in stable hypercapnic COPD: a randomised controlled trial. *Thorax* 64:561–566, 2009.
63. Dreher M, Storre JH, Schmoor C, et al: High-intensity versus low-intensity non-invasive ventilation in patients with stable hypercapnic COPD: a randomised crossover trial. *Thorax* 65:303–308, 2010.
64. Acute Respiratory Distress Syndrome Network: Ventilation with lower tidal volumes as compared with traditional tidal volumes for acute lung injury and the acute respiratory distress syndrome. *N Engl J Med* 342:1301–1308, 2000.
65. Borel C, Hanley D, Diringer MN, et al: Intensive management of severe head injury. *Chest* 98:180–189, 1990.
66. Mellott KG, Grap MJ, Munro CL, et al: Patient ventilator asynchrony in critically ill adults: frequency and types. *Heart Lung* 43:231–243, 2014.
67. Shapiro JM: Management of respiratory failure in status asthmaticus. *Am J Respir Med* 1:409–416, 2002.

CHAPTER 45

Mechanical Ventilators

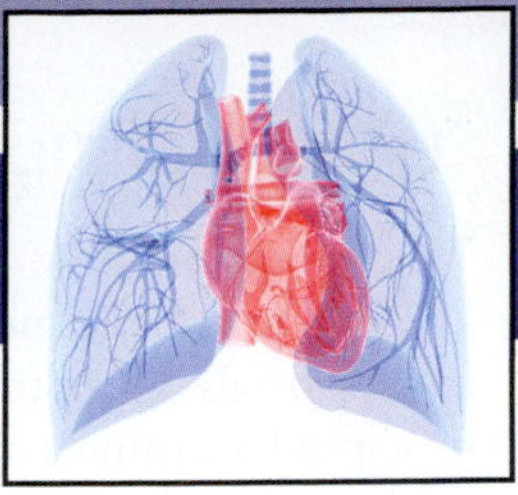

ROBERT L. CHATBURN AND TERESA A. VOLSKO

CHAPTER OBJECTIVES

After reading this chapter you will be able to:

- Define a mechanical ventilator.
- Differentiate between automatic resuscitators and mechanical ventilators.
- Describe the key design features of mechanical ventilators.
- Describe the 10 maxims used to develop a standardized ventilator taxonomy.
- Describe the operating characteristics of mechanical ventilators used along the continuum of care.
- List the basic ways to present monitored data.
- List the three main goals of mechanical ventilator support.

CHAPTER OUTLINE

KEY TERMS

assisted breath
continuous mandatory ventilation (CMV)
continuous spontaneous ventilation (CSV)
control system
cycle
elastance
intermittent mandatory ventilation (IMV)
loaded breathing
mandatory
mode
pressure-control ventilation
resistance
spontaneous breath
time constant
trigger
trigger variable
volume-control ventilation

To safely and effectively initiate and manage a mechanical ventilator, the respiratory therapist must thoroughly understand (1) ventilator design, classification, and operation; (2) appropriate clinical application of ventilatory modes (i.e., the proper matching of ventilator capability with physiologic need); and (3) the physiologic effects of mechanical ventilation, including gas exchange and pulmonary mechanics. This chapter focuses on the first of these. It explains classification terminology and outlines a framework for understanding current and future ventilatory support devices.[1-3]

HOW VENTILATORS WORK

To understand how ventilators work, one must have some knowledge of basic mechanics. A ventilator is a machine, which is a system designed to alter, transmit, and direct applied energy in a predetermined manner to perform useful work.[4] These complex machines deliver an array of medical gas mixtures such as nitric oxide, helium, and oxygen. Sophisticated software and advanced monitoring systems make it possible to deliver mechanical breaths from conventional or normal physiologic to high frequency rates.

Ventilators used along the continuum of care, from intensive care units to patient transport to long-term and home care, require energy in the form of either electricity or compressed gas to function. The energy is transmitted or transformed (by the ventilator's drive mechanism) in a predetermined manner (by the control circuit) to augment or replace the patient's muscles in performing the work of breathing (the desired output). Thus, to understand mechanical ventilators, their four basic functions must be understood:

- Input power
- Power transmission and conversion
- Control system
- Output (pressure, volume, and flow waveforms)

This simple outline format can be expanded to add as much detail about a given ventilator as desired.

Input Power

The power source for a ventilator comes from either electrical energy (energy = volts × amperes × time) or compressed gas (energy = pressure × volume).

Electrical Energy

An electrically powered ventilator uses voltage from an electrical line outlet. In the United States, this line voltage is normally 110 to 115 volts alternating current (AC) (60 Hz). In addition to powering the ventilator, this AC voltage may be reduced and converted to direct current (DC). This DC source can then be used to power delicate electronic control circuits.

Some ventilators, notably portable ventilators used for transport or to provide mechanical ventilation in the home, have rechargeable batteries to be used as a source of power if AC is not available. The length of time power is provided from an internal or external battery depends on the ventilator's drive mechanism, the ventilator settings, the load of the respiratory system, and the type of battery used to provide power. Lithium ion and nickel metal hydride batteries are more compact, weigh less, and have higher power with shorter recharging times compared with similar-sized lead/acid batteries. Battery power becomes essential when providing mechanical ventilation out of the acute care setting. Although portable ventilators have an internal battery that provides power on a limited basis, the availability of an external battery can be an essential lifesaving feature in the event of an extended power outage.

Pneumatic Energy

A pneumatically powered ventilator uses compressed gas as its power source. Most modern intensive care unit (ICU) ventilators are pneumatically powered. Ventilators powered by compressed gas usually have internal pressure-reducing valves so that the normal operating pressure is lower than the source pressure. This allows uninterrupted operation from hospital-piped gas sources, which are usually regulated to 50 psi (pounds per square inch) but are subject to periodic fluctuations.

Most pneumatically powered ICU ventilators still require electrical power to support their control functions (see the following section on control mechanisms). However, a few pneumatically powered ventilators can function without electrical power, using compressed gas to power lung inflation and the ventilator's control circuitry. Pneumatically powered ventilators are ideal in situations where electrical power may be unavailable (e.g., during patient transport), in a mass casualty situation where the influx of patient are triaged and stabilized in an area where electrical power is scarce (e.g., parking lot located adjacent to an emergency department), or as a back-up to electrically powered ventilators in case of extended power failures. They are also particularly useful where electrical power is undesirable, such as near magnetic resonance imaging (MRI) equipment. It is essential to understand how the ventilator consumes compressed gas, especially in settings where the compressed gas source may be limited, such as air or ground transport. Weight restrictions, especially on air transport, affect the number and size of the gas cylinders used. Therefore, it is essential for the respiratory therapist to anticipate the total amount of compressed gas needed (air, oxygen, and specialty gas). Since the compressed gas source is limited during interhospital transport, the respiratory therapist must ensure the compressed gas supply will not deplete and cause the ventilator to fail on the way to the transport team's final destination.

RULE OF THUMB

For patient transport, you must use either a pneumatically powered ventilator or one that can run solely on batteries. Always take along a manually powered bag-valve mask resuscitator, and for long transports be sure to have back-up power available (extra cylinders or batteries).

Power Transmission and Conversion

The power transmission and conversion system consists of the drive and output control mechanisms. The drive mechanism generates the actual force needed to deliver gas under pressure. The output control consists of one or more valves that regulate gas flow to the patient.

Drive Mechanism

The ventilator's drive mechanism converts the input power to useful work. The characteristic flow and pressure patterns the ventilator produces are determined, in part, by the type of drive mechanism it contains. Drive mechanisms can be either (1) a direct application of compressed gas through a pressure-reducing valve or (2) an indirect application by an electrical motor or compressor. Descriptions of these devices are given in textbooks devoted to respiratory care equipment.[5]

Output Control Valve

The output control valve regulates the flow of gas to the patient. Early ventilators had simple on/off exhalation valves. For most modern ventilators, the output control valve can shape the output waveform, as in the Maquet SERVO-i (Maquet, Bridgewater, NJ). Commonly used output control valves include the pneumatic diaphragm, electromagnetic poppet/plunger valve, and proportional valve.[6]

Control System

To manipulate pressure, volume, and flow, a ventilator must have a **control system**. A control system measures and directs the output of the ventilator and operates the exhalation manifold. A ventilator control circuit may include mechanical, pneumatic, electrical, electronic, or fluidic components. Most modern ventilators combine two or more of these subsystems to provide user control.

Mechanical control circuits use devices such as levers, pulleys, and cams. These types of circuits were used in the early manually operated ventilators illustrated in history books.[7] Pneumatic control is provided using gas-powered pressure regulators, needle valves, jet entrainment devices, and balloon-valves. Some transport ventilators use pneumatic control systems.

Electrical control circuits use only simple switches, rheostats (or potentiometers), and magnets to control ventilator operation. Electronic control circuits use devices such as resistors, capacitors, diodes, and transistors as well as combinations of these components in the form of integrated circuits. The most sophisticated electronic systems, incorporated into ventilators used in critical care, use microprocessors and complex software algorithms to manage monitoring and control ventilator function.

Fluidic logic-controlled ventilators, such as the Bio-Med MVP-10 (Bio-Med Devices, Stanford, CT) also use pressurized gas to regulate the parameters of ventilation. However, instead of simple pressurized valves and timers, these ventilators use fluidic logic circuits that function much like electrical circuit boards.[8] Fluidic control mechanisms have no moving parts and low gas consumption, which make them useful for patient transport. Additionally, fluidic circuits are immune to failure from surrounding electromagnetic interference, as can occur around MRI equipment. It is important to note that the MVP-10 does not have an alarm system to alert the clinician of a patient disconnect, or changes in the patient's lung mechanics that will affect minute ventilation. It is essential for the clinician to rely on information from noninvasive (e.g., pulse oximetry and end-tidal carbon dioxide monitoring) and cardiopulmonary monitoring (e.g., heart rate, respiratory rate, blood pressure) to evaluate and optimize the patient–ventilator interaction.

The Operator Interface

The ventilator's operator interface has undergone extensive evolution over the last 35 years. Originally, the displays on ventilators were analog. Operator inputs, or settings, were accomplished with hard-wired knobs, buttons, and dials. The ventilator outputs, such as alarm conditions and ventilating pressure, were displayed with bulbs, light emitting diodes (LEDs), and meters. Some simple transport ventilators still use analog displays (Figure 45-1). The development of inexpensive microprocessors has led manufacturers to use digital displays almost exclusively on all types of ventilators. Digital interfaces use LED or LCD screens for visual display of ventilator data along with some multipurpose hard-wired buttons. More advanced displays use dedicated special-purpose buttons and dials (Figure 45-2). The most advanced interfaces use the concept of the "virtual" instrument, meaning that knobs, buttons, dials, and meters are simulated on a computer screen (sometimes a touch screen) and often incorporate a single mechanical dial that is used to set multiple parameters (Figure 45-3). Computer screens allow graphic displays of alarm settings as, for example, bar graphs along with pressure, volume, and flow waveforms as scalars or loops.

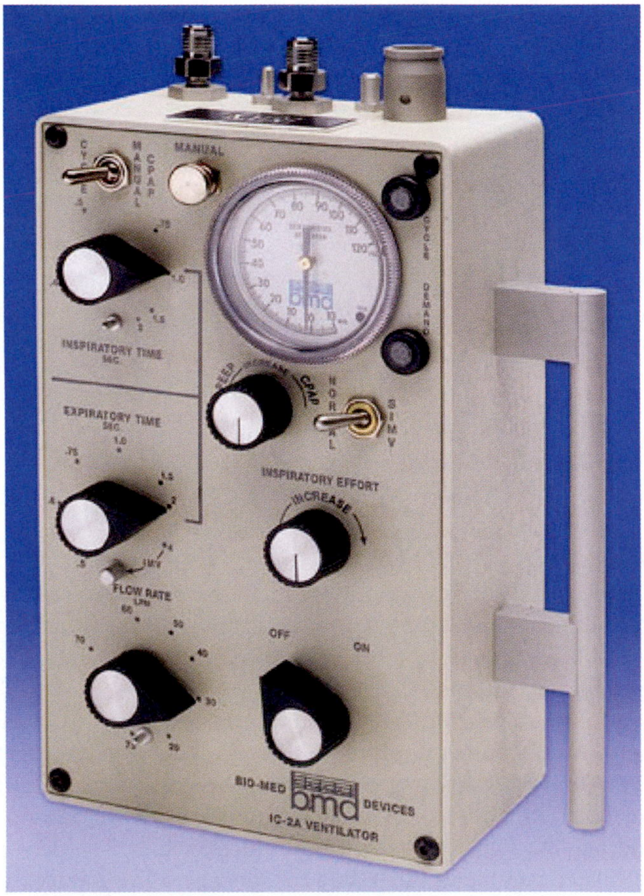

FIGURE 45-1 Transport ventilator with a simple operator interface. (Courtesy Airon Corp.)

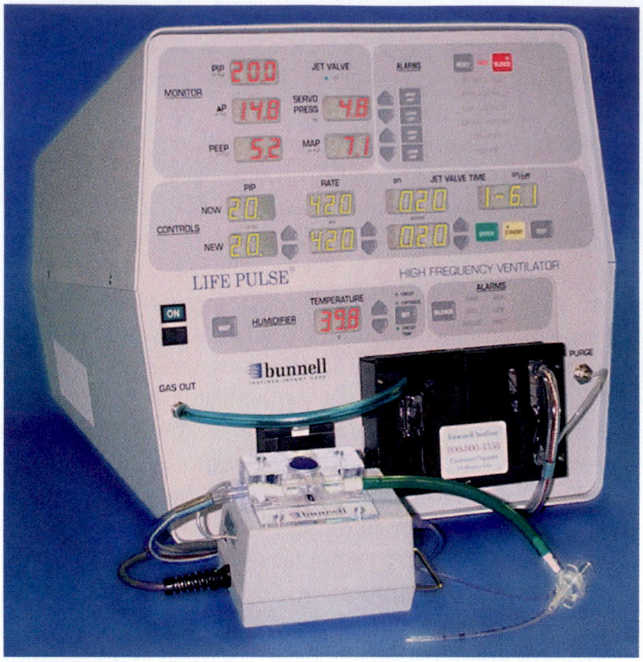

FIGURE 45-2 Covidien Newport e360 ventilator. (Courtesy Bunnel.)

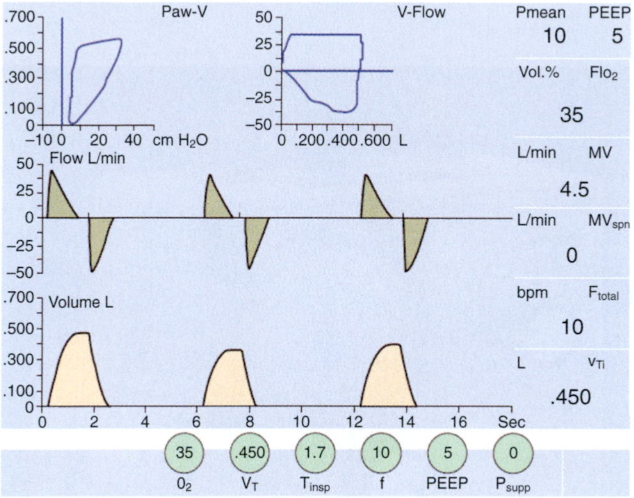

FIGURE 45-3 Operator interface of Dräger V500 ventilator. (© Drägerwerk AG & Co. KGaA, Lübeck.)

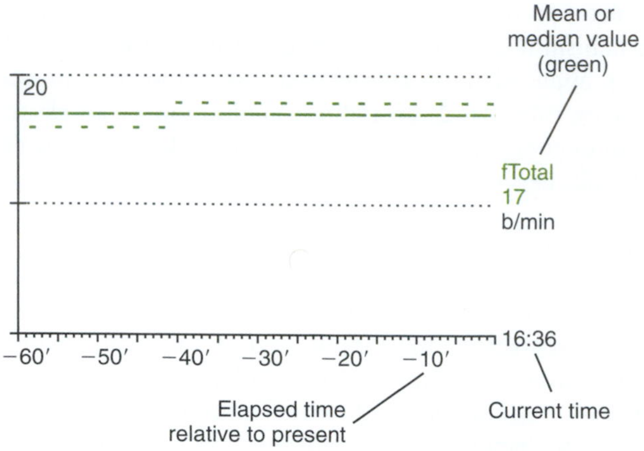

FIGURE 45-4 Trend screen display from the Hamilton G5 ventilator. (Courtesy Hamilton Medical.)

Ventilator Displays

The output displays of monitored data have also evolved significantly over the last 30 years. Ventilator and patient data are available as alphanumeric values, waveforms, trend lines, and even picture graphics.

Alphanumeric Values. Measured or calculated data in the form of alphanumeric values are presented in numbers or text. Typically F_IO_2, pressures (mean, baseline, peak, and plateau), volumes (inhaled/exhaled tidal volume, minute ventilation), and frequency are represented as numeric values. A variety of calculated parameters including I : E ratio, peak inspiratory and expiratory flow, percent leak, resistance, and compliance may also be displayed.

Trends. Trends provide clinicians with measured or calculated data related to ventilatory support over time (Figure 45-4). Gradual or sudden changes in the patient's ventilatory status can be identified by evaluating trends. Alarm logs can also be accessed and provide an additional layer of detail important for adjusting alarm limits to minimize nuisance alarms and enhance safety. Alarm logs can be invaluable in the event of a suspected ventilator failure and may be used as evidence in a legal investigation if significant patient harm has occurred.

Waveforms and Loops. Graphic displays of pressure, volume, and flow convey a wealth of information. Not only is it possible to determine the mode of ventilation by examining these graphics but one can also determine the causes of patient–ventilator asynchrony, including flow asynchrony, delayed or premature cycling, and missed triggers. Graphic representations of respiratory mechanics are helpful for identifying the ventilator parameters to be adjusted to improve the ventilator-patient interaction.[9,10] When pressure, volume, or flow is graphed on the vertical axis with time on the horizontal axis, a waveform or "scalar" display (Figure 45-5) is the result. Loop displays plot one variable against another as *x-y* graphs (Figure 45-6). Pressure-volume (PV) loops can be used to set optimal PEEP and tidal volume levels (Figure 45-7).[11] PV loops are created by using a "super syringe" to inject discrete volumes of gas and then measuring static pressures (static pressure–volume curve) or by using a ventilator at very low constant inspiratory flows (less than 10 L/min) or slow pressure ramps to minimize the pressure due to flow resistance and create what are called *quasi-static* loops. It is usually necessary to heavily sedate and/or paralyze the patient to avoid errors due to the patient's inspiratory efforts or minimize patient anxiety and discomfort during the maneuver. For volume control modes, pressure-volume loops are useful in displaying overdistention. Flow-volume loops are helpful in identifying the need for suctioning and/or response to bronchodilator therapy. An example of a composite display showing numeric values, waveforms, and loops is shown in Figure 45-8.

Picture Graphics. An interesting development in ventilator displays involves the use of picture graphics to represent useful

MINI CLINI

The Use of Trending Data to Optimize the Application of Mechanical Ventilation

PROBLEM: A patient with respiratory distress is ventilated with the following settings:

Mode: PC-CMV
Set frequency: 12/minute
Inspiratory pressure: 28 cm H_2O
PEEP: 8 cm H_2O
F_IO_2: 0.60
Inspiratory time: 1 second
The following trends are available:

Date	8/8	8/8	8/8	8/8	8/8	8/8
Time	0000	0200	0400	0600	0800	1000
V_T (mL)	420	415	390	385	373	362
Total frequency (Breaths/minute)	12	12	12	12	12	12
Minute ventilation (L/minute)	5.04	4.98	4.68	4.62	4.48	4.34

What value does the trend monitoring provide for the clinician? What additional data are needed for the clinician to optimize ventilation?

Answer: The data shows that the patient has had no respiratory effort over the recorded time period monitored. This can be seen by comparing the set frequency to the total frequency. The trends also show that the tidal volume has decreased over time. This can be attributed to an increase in airway resistance or a reduction in lung compliance (or both) because the mode was a form of pressure ventilation. Accessing the trends for airways resistance will enable the clinician to differentiate between airways resistance and lung compliance problems. If the airways resistance has remained relatively stable, the pulmonary compliance has decreased. Additional testing, such as chest radiography and arterial blood gas monitoring, may be required to determine pathologic changes such as atelectasis as well as aberrancies in acid-base balance.

information about the patient–ventilator system. Obstructed endotracheal tubes and auto-PEEP problems are detected more quickly and treated sooner with graphic rather than conventional displays.[12] Clinicians also perceive lower subjective workloads when using picture graphics.

Hamilton Medical was the first to make use of innovative picture graphics on their G5 ventilator. They created a graphic representation of the lungs, called a *dynamic lung panel,* that visually displays information about resistance and compliance by the shape and color of the lungs and airways (Figure 45-9). In addition, they have created a unique graphic representation called the *vent status panel* which displays key parameters (e.g., oxygenation, ventilation, and spontaneous breathing activity) and shows when each item is in or out of an acceptable zone and for how long. This makes weaning status, for example, easy to identify. Dräger Medical followed with a similar graphic display called the *Smart Pulmonary View,* which is a graphic display of respiratory system compliance and resistance as well as of the spontaneous and mandatory minute volume (Figure 45-10).

Alarm Settings

The purpose of ventilator alarms is to bring events to the attention of the clinician. *Events* are conditions or occurrences that require clinician awareness or intervention. Events can be classified according to four levels of priority.[13] Level 1 events are immediately life threatening. These include things such as insufficient or excessive gas delivery to the patient, exhalation valve failure, control circuit failure, or loss of power. Alarm indicators in this category should be mandatory (cannot be turned off by the operator), redundant, and noncanceling. Level 2 events range from mild irregularities in machine function to dangerous situations that could threaten patient safety if left unattended. These include failure of the air-oxygen blending system, inadequate or excessive PEEP, auto-triggering, circuit leak, circuit occlusion, inappropriate I:E ratio, and failure of the humidification system. Alarms in this category are not necessarily redundant and may be self-canceling (i.e., automatically turned off if the event ceases). Level 3 events reflect changes in the level of ventilatory support. Examples include changes in the patient's ventilatory drive or respiratory system mechanics and the presence of auto-PEEP. Level 3 events often trigger the same alarms as Levels 1 and 2. Level 4 events are focused entirely on the patient. These include changes in gas exchange, dead space, oxygenation, and cardiovascular functions. Many ventilators do not warn of these events, and external monitors are thus required for surveillance.

Ventilators do not display alarm settings in terms of levels of priority. Instead, they tend to lump them all together on the screen (Figures 45-11 and 45-12). The actual setting of alarm thresholds is a complicated topic that has been studied but for which little information is available regarding mechanical ventilation. The basic goal is to maximize true alarms and minimize false alarms. A high false alarm rate leads to clinicians ignoring warnings. False alarms can also lead to inappropriate responses. On average, ICU alarms occur 6 times per hour with only a small percentage indicating an actual urgent clinical situation (23%) and a high percentage being false positive alarms (44%).[14,15] Although studies have not addressed mechanical ventilator alarms specifically, it is not hard to imagine similar

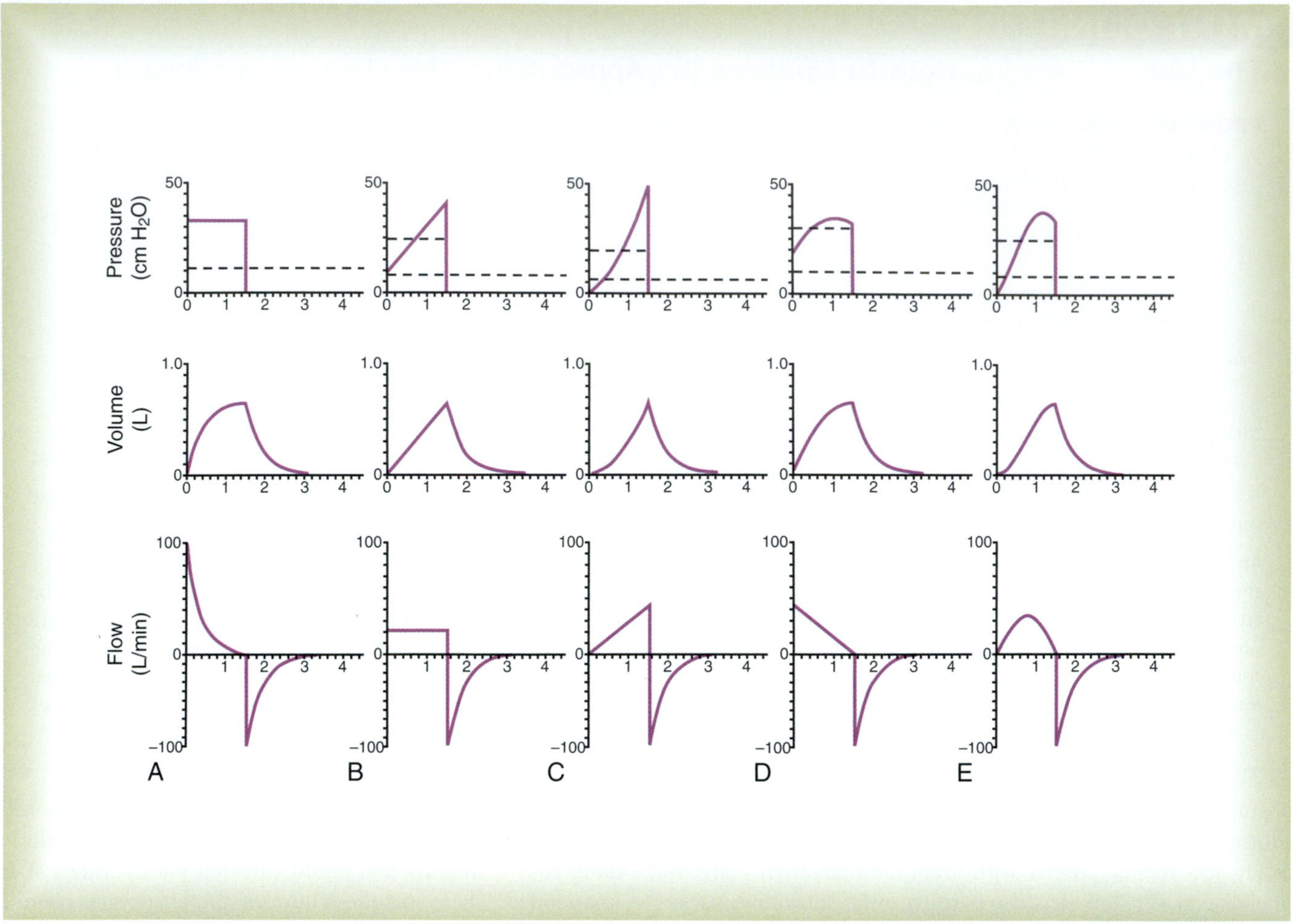

FIGURE 45-5 Model pressure, volume, and flow waveforms generated with a computer using the equation of motion. **A,** Pressure-controlled inspiration with a rectangular pressure waveform (identical to flow-controlled inspiration with an exponential decay flow waveform). **B,** Flow-controlled inspiration with a rectangular flow waveform (identical to volume-controlled inspiration with an ascending ramp volume waveform). **C,** Flow-controlled inspiration with an ascending ramp flow waveform. **D,** Flow-controlled inspiration with a descending ramp flow waveform. **E,** Flow-controlled inspiration with a sinusoidal flow waveform. The short dotted lines represent mean inspiratory pressure, while the long dotted lines represent mean airway pressure (assuming zero PEEP). Note that for the rectangular pressure waveform in **A,** the mean inspiratory pressure is the same as the PIP. For all waveforms, V_T = 644 ml, compliance = 20 ml/cm H_2O, and resistance = 20 cm H_2O/L/sec.

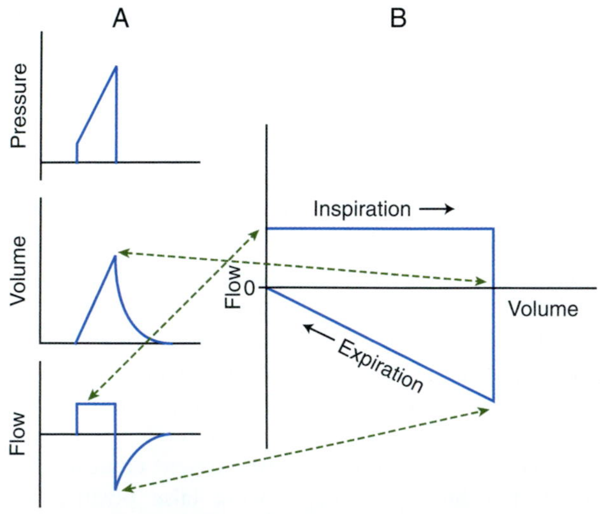

FIGURE 45-6 Idealized waveforms (**A**) for volume control ventilation with corresponding idealized dynamic (not static or quasi-static) pressure-volume loop (**B**). The dotted line arrows show the correspondence between the waveform display and the loop display for the initial pressure rise, peak pressure, and tidal volume. (Courtesy Mandu Press Ltd.)

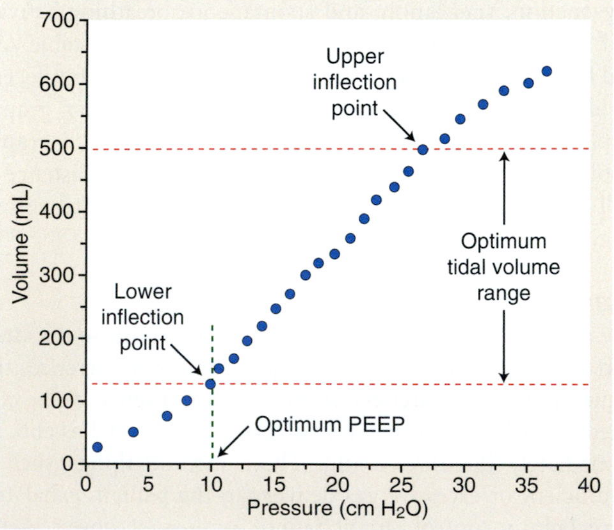

FIGURE 45-7 Static pressure-volume loop. (Courtesy Mandu Press Ltd.)

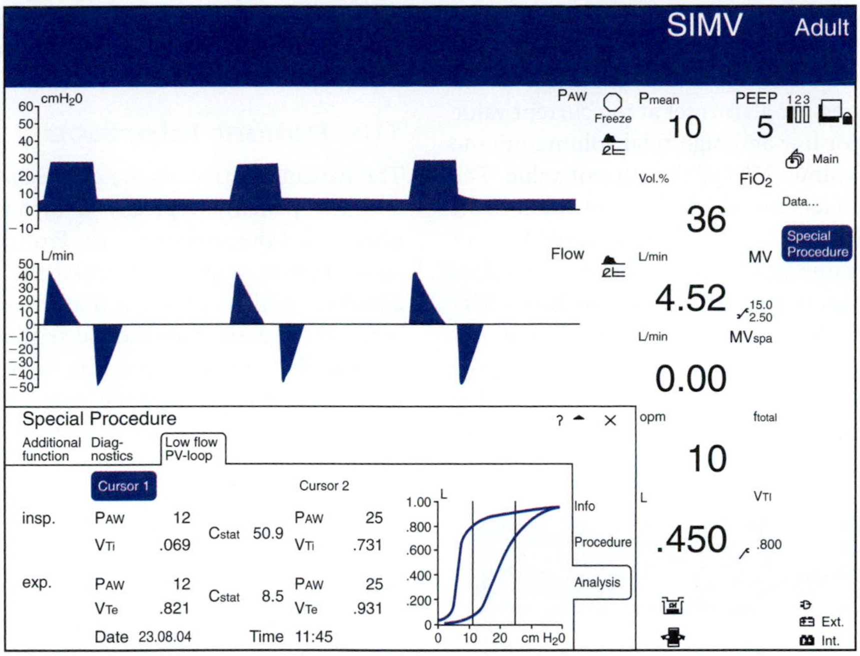

FIGURE 45-8 Portion of display screen on the Dräger Evita XL ventilator. (Courtesy Dräger Medical.)

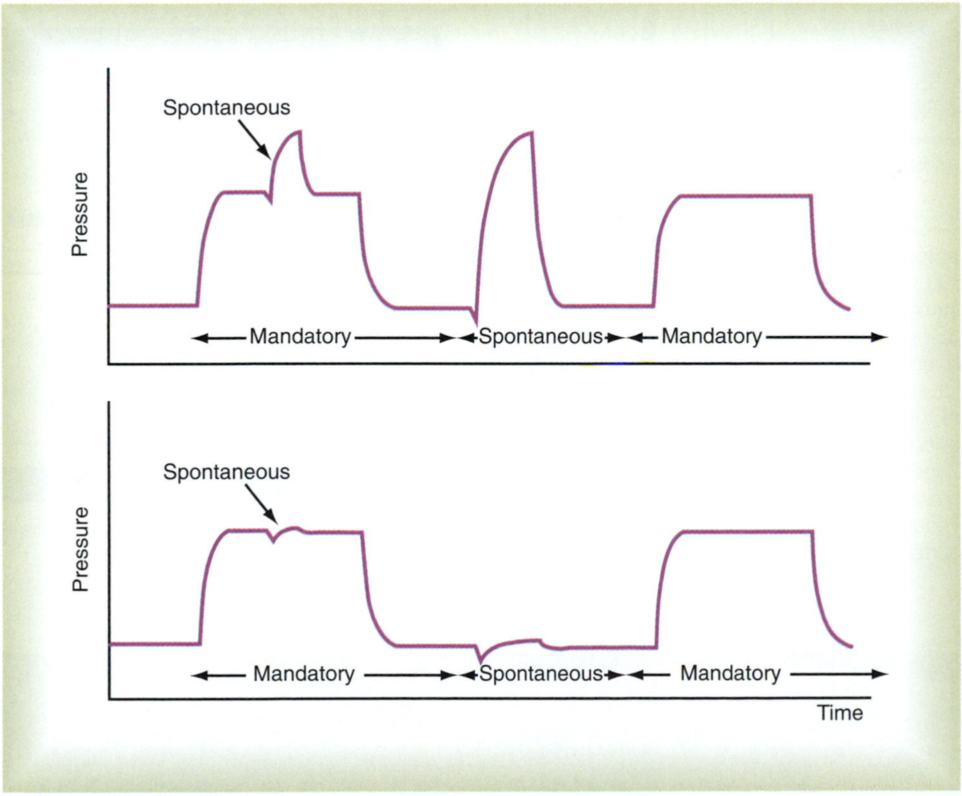

FIGURE 45-9 Picture graphic display from the Hamilton G5 ventilator showing the dynamic lung panel and the vent status panel. (Courtesy Hamilton Medical.)

results for such a study. Ventilator alarms are usually set by the operator (or as default values by the ventilator) as either a set value or a set percentage of the current value. Examples would be low and peak airway pressure alarms set at the current value plus or minus 5 cm H_2O or low and high tidal volume/minute ventilation set at plus or minus 25% of the current value. The problem is that the parameters for which clinicians want to set alarms, and these three in particular, are highly variable, with significant portions of readings at extreme values. Therefore limits set as absolute values or percentages may reduce safety for some extreme values while increasing nuisance events for other values. An alternative approach might be to reference the alarm limits to the current value of the parameter such that extreme values have tighter limits. Further research is needed to identify optimization algorithms (i.e., minimize both harmful and nuisance events) for intelligent targeting schemes to automatically set alarms during mechanical ventilation.

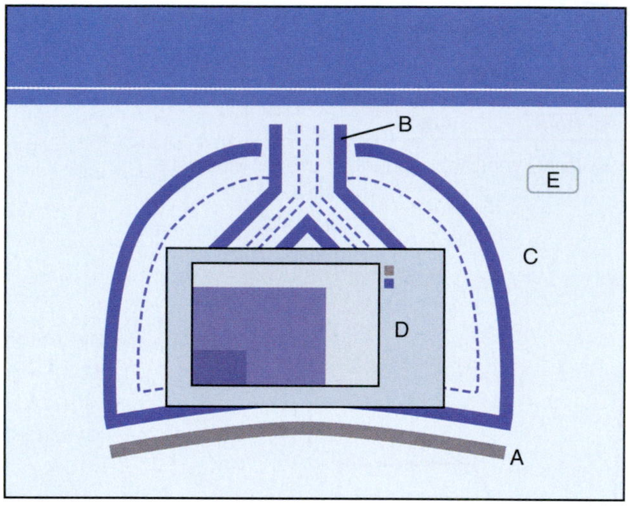

FIGURE 45-10 Example of picture graphic display from the Dräger Evita Infinity V500 ventilator showing the Smart Pulmonary View. **A,** The movement of the diaphragm indicates synchronized mandatory breaths or supported (triggered) breaths. **B,** The blue line around the trachea indicates the resistance (R). The higher the resistance, the thicker the line. The numeric value is also displayed. **C,** The blue line around the lungs indicates the compliance (Cdyn). The higher the compliance, the thinner the line. The numeric value is also displayed. **D,** Diagram displaying the relationship between spontaneous breathing and mandatory ventilation. The following parameters are displayed in different colors: $V_{T,spon}$ and RR_{spon}, $V_{T,mand}$ and RR_{mand}. (Courtesy Dräger Medical.)

The Patient Interface

The patient interface is the connection between the ventilator and the patient—typically a system of plastic hoses, and often called the *patient circuit*. From the perspective of understanding how ventilators work, the important thing to know about the patient circuit is that it contributes to discrepancies between the desired and actual ventilator output values. This is because the patient circuit has its own compliance and resistance. Thus, the pressure measured on the inspiratory side of a ventilator will always be higher than the pressure at the airway opening due to patient circuit resistance. In addition, the volume and flow coming out of the ventilator will exceed that delivered to the patient because of the compliance of the patient circuit.

Using an analogy to electrical circuits, compliance of the delivery circuit can be shown to be connected in series with the compliance of the respiratory system (that is, both elements sharing the same driving pressure). Consequently, the total compliance of the ventilator-patient system is simply the sum

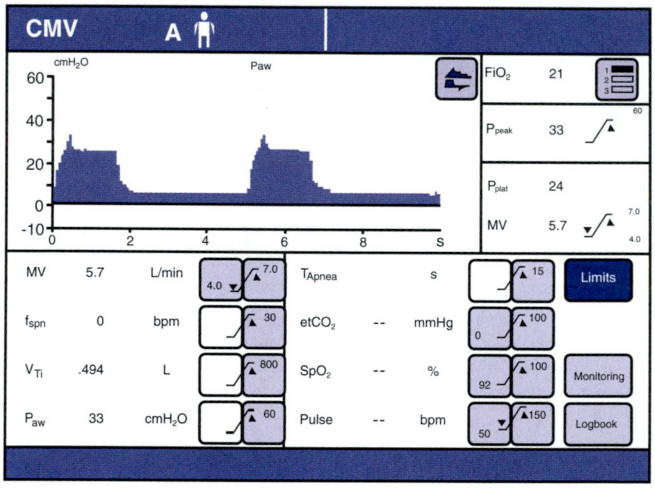

FIGURE 45-12 Alarm panel of Dräger Evita XL ventilator. (Courtesy Dräger Medical.)

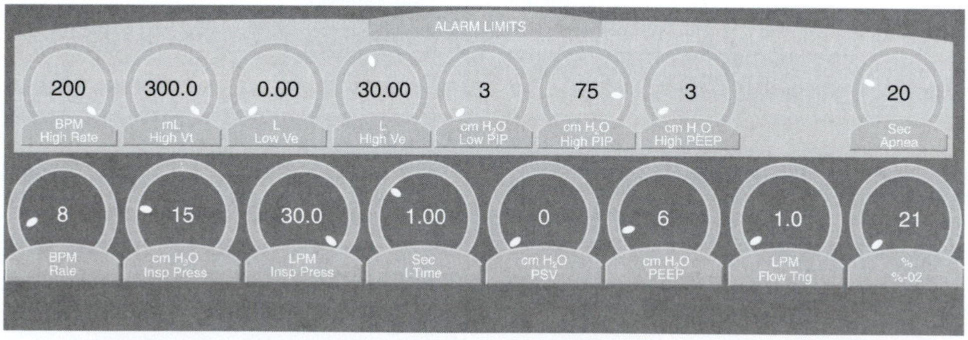

FIGURE 45-11 Alarm panel of CareFusionAvea ventilator. (Courtesy CareFusion.)

of the two compliances. Similarly, the resistance of the delivery circuit is connected in series with the respiratory system resistance (that is, both elements sharing the same flow) so that the total resistance is the sum of the two. Based on these assumptions, the relationship between the volume input to the patient (at the point of connection to the patient's airway opening) and the volume output from the ventilator (at the point of connection to the patient circuit) can be described by the following equation:

$$\text{Volume input to patient} = \frac{\text{Volume output from ventilator}}{1 + C_{pc}/C_{rs}}$$

Equation 45-1

where C_{pc} is the compliance of the patient circuit, and C_{rs} is the total compliance of the patient's respiratory system. The equation shows that the larger the patient circuit compliance compared with the patient's respiratory system, the larger the denominator on the right-hand side of the equation. Hence, the smaller the delivered tidal volume is compared with the volume coming from the ventilator's drive mechanism.

Assuming that the volume exiting the ventilator is the set tidal volume, the patient circuit compliance (C_{pc}) is calculated as follows:

$$C_{pc} = \frac{\text{Set tidal volume}}{P_{plat} - \text{PEEP}}$$

Equation 45-2

where P_{plat} is the pressure measured during an inspiratory hold maneuver with the Y-piece of the patient circuit occluded (patient not connected), and PEEP is end-expiratory pressure (that is, baseline pressure). Most authors recommend the use of PIP for P_{plat} in this equation, which is acceptable but may lead to a slight underestimation of patient circuit compliance. P_{plat} is slightly lower than PIP because of the flow-resistive pressure drop of the patient circuit if pressure is not measured at the Y-piece. This difference is greatest in small-bore, corrugated patient circuit tubing but is probably insignificant.

The effects of patient circuit compliance are most troublesome during volume-controlled ventilation. For example, in neonatal ventilation the patient circuit compliance can be as much as three times that of the respiratory system, even with small-bore tubing and a small-volume humidifier. Thus in an attempt to deliver a preset tidal volume, the volume delivered to the patient may be as little as 25% of that exiting the ventilator, whereas 75% is compressed in the patient circuit.

During pressure-control ventilation the compliance of the patient circuit has the effect of rounding the leading edge of a rectangular pressure waveform, which reduces the peak flow and could reduce the volume delivered to the patient. This effect is prevented if the pressure limit is maintained for at least 5 time constants of the respiratory system.

For both pressure- and volume-control ventilation the patient circuit compliance and resistance, along with the resistance of the exhalation valve (in series with the patient circuit and respiratory system resistance) increase the expiratory time constant. Thus a large circuit compliance coupled with a short expiratory time can lead to inadvertent or auto-PEEP.

In summary, the set values for pressure, volume, and flow may be different from the output (from ventilator) values due to calibration errors and the effects of the patient circuit. Thus two general sources of error cause discrepancies between the desired and actual patient values.

IDENTIFYING MODES OF MECHANICAL VENTILATION

Ventilator manufacturers coin unique names for modes available on their respective devices, primarily as marketing tools. As a result, there have been no industry standards for naming modes of ventilation. This makes it difficult for clinicians to understand how the various modes of ventilation function. In some cases, ventilator modes function in the same way but have very different names. For example, Pressure-Control Ventilation Plus Adaptive Pressure Ventilation on the Hamilton Galileo is the same as Pressure Regulated Volume Control on the Siemens Servo 300. Volume control continuous mandatory ventilation (VC-CMV) on the Maquet SERVO-i ventilator and the PB 840 have identical names, and function very differently.[16]

The 10 Maxims for Understanding Modes

A formal taxonomy for classifying modes of ventilation is now available.[17,18] This portion of the chapter will explain the derivation of this taxonomy in the form of 10 fundamental maxims (concise statements of scientific principles). These fundamental constructs of ventilator design and function are a culmination of data from an international survey[19] and more than 30 years of mechanical ventilation teaching experience.

1. A Breath is One Cycle of Positive Flow (Inspiration) and Negative Flow (Expiration) Defined in Terms of the Flow-Time Curve.

Breath delivery is one of the most basic functions a mechanical ventilator performs. A breath can simply be defined as one cycle of inspiratory flow followed by a matching expiratory flow (Figure 45-13). These flows are paired by size, meaning approximately equal inspiratory and expiratory volumes. However, there are some modes of ventilation in which inspiration is not followed immediately by the matching expiration. Airway pressure release ventilation provides an example of this. During this mode of ventilation the transition from low pressure to high pressure results in a large mandatory breath during inspiration, followed by a few small spontaneous inspirations and expirations during the low-pressure phase, which contribute to a smaller exhaled volume. The transition from high pressure to low pressure results in the matching mandatory exhalation. It is also possible to have many small mandatory breaths superimposed on larger spontaneous breaths, as seen during high-frequency oscillatory ventilation.

Inspiratory time and expiratory time are the two most basic definitions in reference to a breath. Inspiratory time is defined as the period from the start of inspiratory flow to the start of expiratory flow. Inspiratory time is equal to inspiratory flow

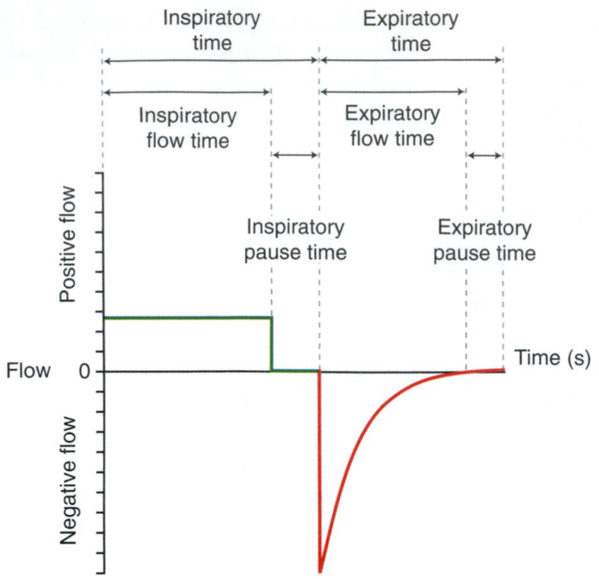

FIGURE 45-13 A breath is defined in terms of the flow-time waveform. (Courtesy Mandu Press Ltd.)

time plus inspiratory hold time. Inspiratory hold or pause time is the period from the cessation of inspiratory flow (into the airway opening) to the start of expiratory flow during mechanical ventilation. On some ventilators, the operator can directly set inspiratory hold time. On others, hold time is the difference between the preset inspiratory time and the inspiratory flow time due to the preset tidal volume at the preset inspiratory flow (i.e., inspiratory flow time = tidal volume/inspiratory flow). An inspiratory pause is often used to improve oxygenation by increasing mean airway pressure. It may also be used to create a static airway pressure also known as *plateau pressure*. During an inspiratory pause, the flow of gas to and from the patient ceases. Therefore, the pressure displayed during the inspiratory pause, or plateau pressure, can be used to calculate respiratory system resistance and compliance. The period from the start of expiratory flow to the start of inspiratory flow is known as *expiratory time*.

2. A Breath is Assisted If the Ventilator Provides Some or All of the Work of Breathing.

Ventilators are designed to assist with the patient's work of breathing. Work is defined in terms of the pressure necessary to deliver the tidal volume to the respiratory system. In the simplest case, work is the pressure change during inspiration times the volume change (i.e., tidal volume).[20] An **assisted breath**, therefore, is one for which the ventilator does some work on the respiratory system. Pressure is generated either by the patient's inspiratory muscles (P_{mus}) or the ventilator (P_{vent}), which causes an increase in the pressure difference across the respiratory system, called *inspiratory pressure* on some ventilators.[21]

On a ventilator graphic display, an assisted breath is identified as one in which airway pressure rises above baseline during inspiration (from Maxim 1, inspiration is identified by flow above zero). A drop in airway pressure below baseline during inspiration indicates that the patient is doing work against the ventilator. We say the breath is "loaded" rather than assisted. Some loading is unavoidable if the patient must signal to the ventilator when to start inspiratory flow by a drop in airway pressure, called *triggering* (see below).[22] Optimization of ventilator settings minimizes **loaded breathing** by maximizing the synchrony between the ventilator output and the patient's demand.

3. A Ventilator Assists Breathing Using Either Pressure Control or Volume Control Based on the Equation of Motion for the Respiratory System.

To understand how a ventilator assists breathing, we make use of a very important model of patient–ventilator interaction called the *equation of motion for the respiratory system*.[23] This equation is a mathematical model describing a physical model composed of a single flow conducting tube (representing the airways) and a single elastic compartment (representing the lungs and chest wall) as shown in Figure 45-14. There are many versions of this equation, but the simplest version, as it relates to ventilator mode classification, is as follows:

$$P_{vent}(t) + = EV(t) + R\dot{V}(t) \qquad \textbf{Equation 45-3}$$

Where $P_{vent}(t)$ is inspiratory pressure generated by the ventilator as a function of time, E is the **elastance** of the respiratory system ($\Delta P/\Delta V$), V(t) is volume as a function of time, R is respiratory-system **resistance** ($\Delta P/\Delta\dot{V}$), and $\dot{V}(t)$ is flow as a function of time. *Note that all these variables are measured relative to their end expiratory values.* Under normal circumstances these values are P_{vent} = set PEEP, V = end expiratory lung volume (functional residual capacity if PEEP = 0), and $\dot{V}$ = 0. Sometimes the equation is written with compliance (C = $\Delta V/\Delta P$) instead of elastance, in which case the term EV(t) becomes V(t)/C. If the patient is spontaneously triggering the ventilator, the left side of Equation 45-3 becomes $P_{muscles} + P_{vent}$, indicating that the work of breathing is shared in some way between the patient and the ventilator. However, if the patient is breathing independent of the ventilator, the left side of Equation 45-3 is simply $P_{muscles}$.

A plot of $P_{vent}(t)$, V(t), and $\dot{V}(t)$ versus time yields the waveforms seen on ventilator displays (Figure 45-15). If the shape of the pressure waveform is predetermined by the ventilator settings, independent of changes in respiratory system mechanics, the ventilator is providing *pressure control* (PC). One way to think about this is that the ventilator controls the left-hand side of Equation 45-1. That means for a given pressure waveform [i.e., graph of $P_{vent}(t)$], volume and flow are dependent on E and R. In more practical terms, if the operator sets inspiratory pressure, or inspiratory pressure is controlled by the ventilator to be proportional to some measure of the patient's inspiratory effort, then we say the mode of ventilation is a form of pressure control.

One very confusing issue with **pressure-control ventilation** is that sometimes the operator sets the magnitude of the

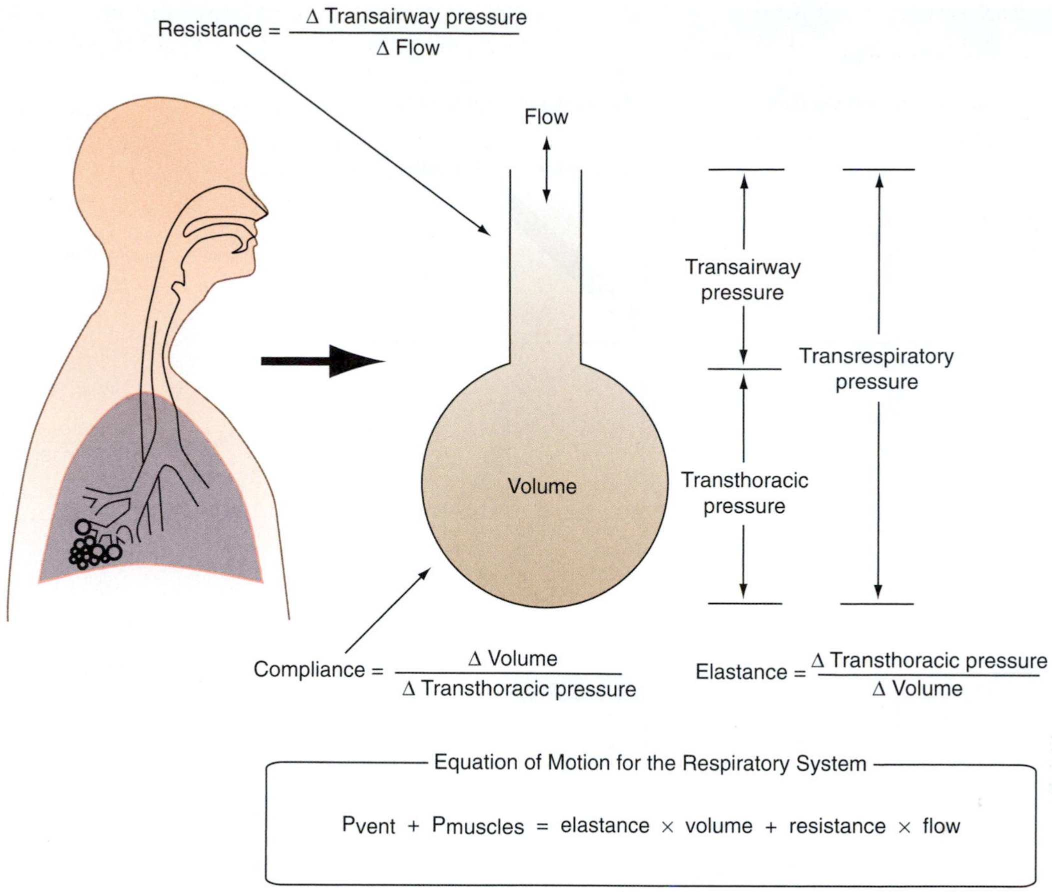

FIGURE 45-14 The respiratory system can be modeled as a single-flow conducting tube connected to a single elastic compartment. This physical model can be described by a mathematical model called the *equation of motion* for the respiratory system. In this model, pressure, volume, and flow are variables (i.e., functions of time), whereas resistance and elastance (or compliance) are constants.

pressure waveform relative to atmospheric pressure (called *peak inspiratory pressure*) and other times the magnitude is set relative to positive end expiratory pressure (PEEP), in this case simply termed inspiratory pressure.[24]

Refer again to Figure 45-15. If the shapes of the volume and flow waveforms are predetermined by the ventilator settings, and are unaffected by respiratory system mechanics, the ventilator is providing *volume control* (VC). In other words, the ventilator controls the right-hand side of Equation 45-1. That means for a given flow waveform [i.e., the graph of $\dot{V}(t)$], the volume waveform [i.e., the graph of $V(t)$] will be predetermined (because volume is simply a function of flow and time). Furthermore, the pressure waveform [i.e., the graph of $P_{vent}(t)$], will be dependent on E and R. In more practical terms, if the tidal volume *and* inspiratory flow are preset, then we say the mode of ventilation is a form of volume control. The term *volume control* is used rather than *flow control* merely for historical reasons. Note that during **volume-control ventilation,** *both* volume and flow are preset prior to inspiration. We emphasize this because there are some *pressure control modes* that allow the operator to set a target tidal volume but allow the ventilator to determine the flow. There are also pressure-control modes that allow the operator to set the maximum inspiratory flow, but not the tidal volume. In this case, tidal volume delivery depends on the operator-set inspiratory pressure target and the patient's respiratory system mechanics.

In some rare cases of nonconventional ventilation, inspiratory flow, inspiratory volume, and inspiratory pressure are all dependent on respiratory system mechanics. As no parameters of the pressure, volume, or flow waveforms are preset, the only control of the breath is the timing (i.e., inspiratory and expiratory times). When this happens the mode is called a form of *time control.* Examples of this are high-frequency oscillatory ventilation (3100ventilator, CareFusion, San Diego, Calif.) and volumetric diffusive respiration (Percussionaire, Sagle, Idaho).

One way to compare volume-control and pressure-control modes of ventilation is to first recognize that the aim is to control the patient's minute ventilation (because minute ventilation determines the $PaCO_2$ for a given rate of metabolic CO_2 production). Next, we can relate the operator-set variables that control minute ventilation for VC versus PC. A convenient way to do this is with influence diagrams, which are graphic illustrations that show how things are interrelated by using circles to represent (in this case) ventilator settings and lines to represent relationships. Figure 45-16 shows the influence diagram for volume-control ventilation and Figure 45-17 shows the influence diagram for pressure-control ventilation. The equations that relate the ventilator settings are given in Table 45-1.

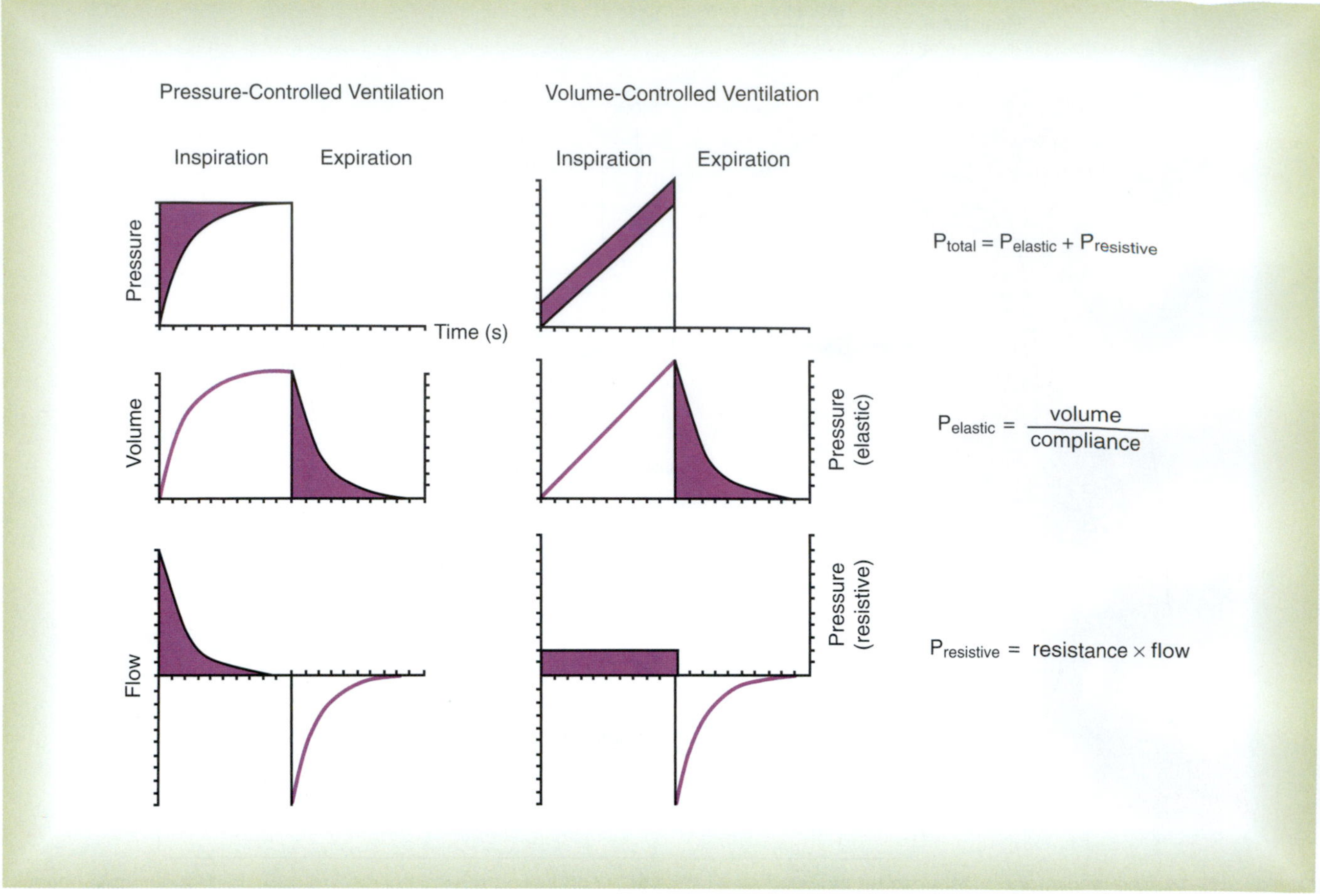

FIGURE 45-15 Idealized waveforms for volume-control ventilation and pressure-control ventilation. Note that the volume waveform has the same shape as the transthoracic or lung pressure waveform (i.e., pressure due to elastic recoil). The flow waveform has the same shape as the transairway pressure waveform (i.e., pressure due to airway resistance). The shaded areas represent pressures due to resistance; the open areas represent pressure due to elastic recoil. The dotted lines represent mean airway pressure. Note that the mean pressure at the airway is the same as that in the lung and that mean pressure for volume-control ventilation is less than that for pressure-control ventilation.

In summary:

Volume control means that *both* volume and flow are preset prior to inspiration.

Pressure control means that inspiratory pressure is preset to some constant value (e.g., Pressure Support mode) or is proportional to inspiratory effort (e.g., Proportional Assist Ventilation and Neurally Adjusted Ventilatory Assist modes).

Time control means that pressure, volume, and flow are all dependent on changing respiratory system mechanics and nothing is predetermined except inspiratory and expiratory times (e.g., high-frequency oscillatory ventilation).

4. Breaths Are Classified According to the Criteria That Trigger (Start) and Cycle (Stop) Inspiration.

The definition of a breath (Maxim 1) implies that the ventilator knows when to start (**trigger**) and when to stop (**cycle**) inspiratory flow. There are several signals that can be used to trigger inspiration, including time, and changes in airway pressure, volume, or flow. An electrical signal from the diaphragm can also be used to trigger inspiration. Common cycle signals are the same as those for triggering. *Sensitivity* is a term used to describe the amount that the trigger or cycle signal must change before inspiration starts or stops.

Trigger and cycle events are key definitions in the development of a classification system for **modes** of ventilation. They are used to define **mandatory** and spontaneous breaths (see Maxim 6). Mandatory and spontaneous breaths are used to describe ventilatory patterns (Maxim 7), and they form the basis for the mode taxonomy (see Maxim 10). Figure 45-18 shows an algorithm that can be used to identify trigger and cycle variables.

5. Trigger Variable and Cycle Events Can Be Either Patient or Machine Initiated.

There are instances when disease processes weaken the diaphragm or medications, such as sedation or paralytic agents, interfere with the patient's ability to generate trigger and cycle signals. Hence it is important to have a backup machine trigger system. However, when a patient's ability to generate trigger and cycle signals is intact, it is important to deliver inspiratory flow in synchrony with the patient's breathing efforts. Trigger and cycle capabilities are built into the mode of ventilation. The trigger variable can be either time, pressure, flow, or volume.

Inspiration may be triggered after a preset time interval (e.g., because of a preset breathing frequency). In this instance, inspiration has started regardless of any inspiratory efforts made by the patient. During such a breath, therefore, we say that inspiration is machine triggered. Minute ventilation threshold is another signal a ventilator can use to machine-trigger inspiration. Minute ventilation is calculated by dividing the tidal volume by the time for one breath cycle (equivalent to

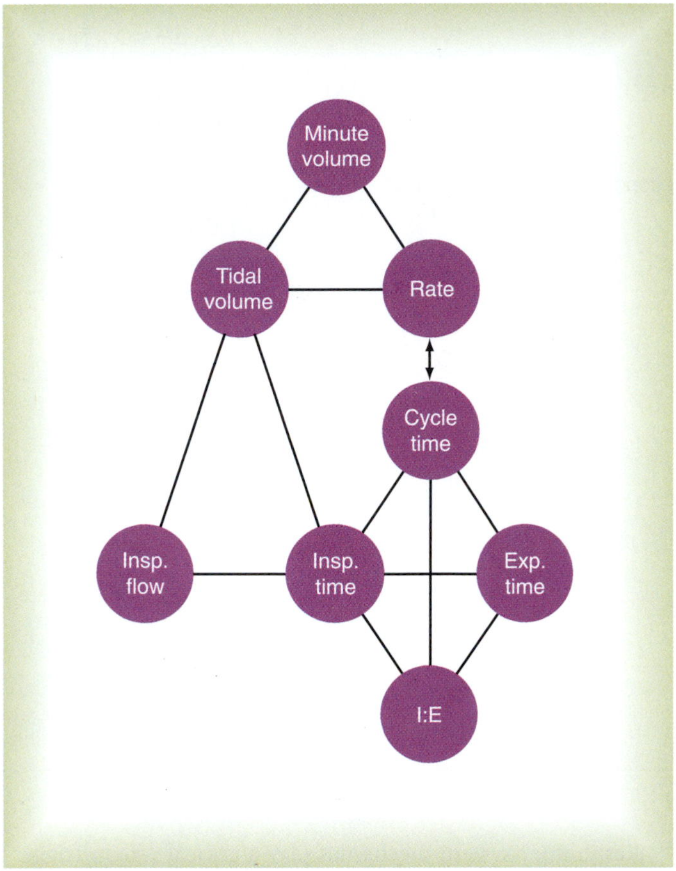

FIGURE 45-16 Influence diagram for volume-control ventilation. Variables are connected by straight lines such that if any two are known, the third can be calculated (see Table 45-1).

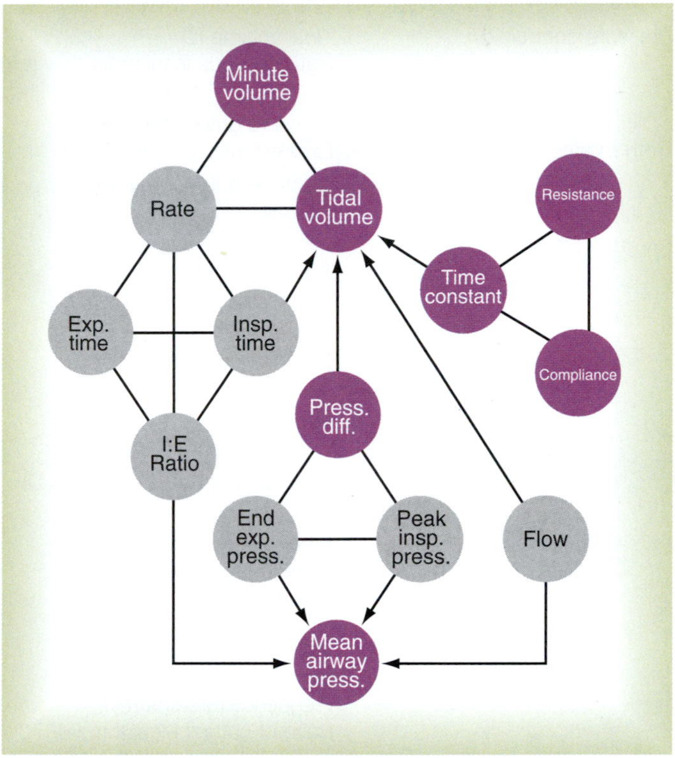

FIGURE 45-17 Influence diagram for pressure-control ventilation. Variables are connected by *straight lines* such that if any two are known, the third can be calculated (see Table 45-1). *Arrows* represent relations that are more complex. *Purple circles* represent variables that are directly controlled by ventilator settings. *Gray circles* show indirectly controlled variables.

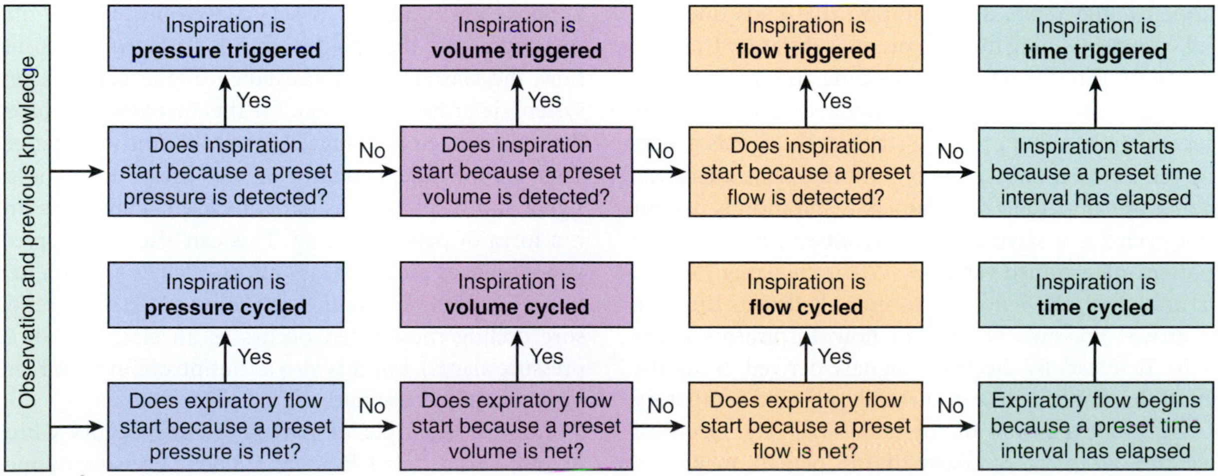

FIGURE 45-18 Algorithm for determining the trigger and cycle variables during a breath on a mechanical ventilator.

TABLE 45-1

Equations Relating the Important Parameters for Volume-Controlled and Pressure-Controlled Ventilation

Mode	Parameter	Symbol	Equation
Volume-controlled	Tidal volume (L)	V_T	$V_T = \dot{V}_E \div f$ $V_T = \dot{V}_I \times T_I$
	Mean inspiratory flow (L/min)	$\bar{\dot{V}}_I$	$\bar{\dot{V}}_I = 60 \times V_T \div T_I$ $\bar{\dot{V}}_1 = \frac{\dot{V}_E \times TCT}{T_1}$
Pressure-controlled	Tidal volume (L)	V_T	$V_T = \Delta P \times C \times (1 - e^{-t/\tau})$
	Instantaneous inspiratory flow (L/min)	$\dot{V}_1$	$\dot{V}_1 = \left(\frac{\Delta P}{R}\right) e^{-t/\tau}$
	Pressure gradient (cm H_2O)	ΔP	$\Delta P = PIP - PEEP$
Both modes	Exhaled minute ventilation (L/min)	$\dot{V}_E$	$\dot{V}_E = V_T \times f$
	Total cycle time or ventilatory period (seconds)	TCT	$TCT = T_I + T_E = 60 \div f$
	I:E ratio	I:E	$I:E = T_1 : T_E = \frac{T_1}{T_E}$
	Time constant (seconds)	τ	$\tau = R \times C$
	Resistance (cm H_2O/L/sec)	R	$R = \frac{\Delta P}{\Delta \dot{V}}$
	Compliance (L/cm H_2O)	C	$C = \frac{\Delta V}{\Delta P}$
	Elastance	E	$E = \frac{1}{C}$
	Mean airway pressure (cm H_2O)	$\bar{P}_{aw}$	$\bar{P}_{aw} = \left(\frac{1}{TCT}\right) \int_{t=0}^{t=TCT} P_{aw} dt$
Primary variables	Pressure (cm H_2O)	P	
	Volume (L)	V	
	Flow (cm H_2O/L/sec)	$\dot{V}$	
	Time (sec)	τ	
	Inspiratory time (sec)	T_I	
	Expiratory time (sec)	T_E	
	Frequency (breaths/min)	f	
	Base of natural logarithm (≈2.72)	e	

multiplying tidal volume by frequency). Depending on the brand of ventilator used, the clinician may be able to set a minimum threshold for minute ventilation. In this case, inspiration is triggered when minute ventilation drops below a preset threshold.

A variety of signals may be used to machine cycle inspiration. Volume cycling refers to inspiration that ends due to a preset tidal volume. Cycling due to a preset inspiratory time (or inspiratory pause time) is referred to as time cycling.

Patient triggering or cycling implies that inspiration starts or stops independent of any preset trigger or cycle signals generated by the ventilator. In the equation of motion, P_{mus}, elastance, and resistance are all patient determined. Inspiration is patient triggered or cycled if it starts or stops because of one or more of these patient-determined variables. When the patient makes an inspiratory effort, the ventilator commonly detects this by a change in airway pressure, volume, or flow. Inspiratory effort may also be detected by electrical signals derived from the movement of the diaphragm (e.g., neurally adjusted ventilatory assist [NAVA]) or expansion of the chest wall (e.g, electrical impedance tomography). Similarly, if the patient makes an expiratory effort, then inspiration may be cycled off.

Respiratory system mechanics play a critical role in triggering and cycling. These factors are easiest to understand in the passive patient ($P_{mus} = 0$). Let us first consider the cycling of inspiration. If the ventilator delivers a constant inspiratory flow, then peak airway pressure is determined by the preset flow and the elastance and resistance of the patient's respiratory system. Suppose the ventilator is set to cycle inspiration off when a preset pressure threshold is met; for a given preset inspiratory flow, the elastance and resistance of the patient's respiratory system determines the time for this threshold. If these patient-determined factors change, inspiratory time will change. Cycling thus occurs independently of any preset machine-generated signal and inspiration is patient cycled. Thus, pressure cycling is a form of patient cycling. This can also be observed when a patient makes an expiratory effort, such as a cough in response to airway irritation by the device interface or secretions. Pressure cycling most often occurs as an alarm condition (high pressure alarm), but it is also a routine cycling mechanism used in automatic resuscitators.[25]

Another example of patient cycling occurs with a mode of ventilation called *Pressure Support*. Pressure Support delivers pressure-controlled breaths to spontaneously breathing patients. During Pressure Support, inspiration is triggered by patient effort and cycled when the decaying flow signal meets a preset threshold (usually expressed as a percentage of the peak inspiratory flow), which in turn determines the inspiratory time. If P(t) in the equation of motion is set to be constant (i.e., preset constant inspiratory pressure), inspiratory flow can be calculated as a function of time. The solution is:

$$\dot{V}(t) = \frac{\Delta P}{R}(e^{-t/RC}) \qquad \textbf{Equation 45-4}$$

The term RC in above equation is known as the respiratory **time constant**, or the time at which an exponential function attains 63% of its steady state value in response to a step input (ΔP). In other words, in this case, it is the time necessary for inspiratory flow to drop to 63% of its peak value (Figure 45-19). The time constant, for a passive patient, determines how long it will take to reach the cycle threshold. The time constant thus determines the inspiratory time independent of any cycle signal generated by the ventilator, and we say the inspiration is patient cycled. Interestingly, a passive patient can trigger inspiration by the same mechanism, except in this case the trigger threshold is based on the decay of expiratory pressure (an exponential flow through a constant expiratory resistance gives an exponential pressure waveform). This is the mechanism used in some automatic resuscitators.[25]

As a further refinement, patient triggering can be defined as starting inspiration based on a patient signal (i.e., a measurement indicating the patient's breathing motion) occurring in a *trigger window*, independent of a machine trigger signal. A trigger window comprises the entire expiratory time minus a short refractory period required to reduce the risk of triggering a breath before exhalation is complete. If a signal from the patient (i.e., some measured variable indicating an inspiratory effort) occurs within this trigger window, inspiration starts and is defined as a patient-triggered event.

A *synchronization window* is a short period during which a patient signal may be used to synchronize the beginning or ending of inspiration to the patient's actions. The synchronization window occurs at the end of a preset expiratory time or at the end of a preset inspiratory time. If a patient signal occurs during an expiratory time synchronization window, inspiration starts and is defined as a machine-triggered event initiating a mandatory breath. The breath is defined in this manner because the mandatory breath would have been time triggered regardless of whether the patient signal had appeared or not. This distinction is necessary to avoid logical inconsistencies in defining mandatory and spontaneous breaths, which are the foundation of the mode taxonomy. A synchronization window may be used at the end of the inspiratory time of a pressure-controlled, time-cycled breath. An example of this would be when a patient signal occurs during the inspiratory time synchronization window and expiration starts, which is defined as a machine-cycled event, ending a mandatory breath.

Some ventilators offer the mode called *airway pressure release ventilation* (APRV). In this mode of ventilation both expiratory and inspiratory synchronization windows can be used. This mode provides us with an example of the importance of distinguishing between trigger/cycle windows (allowing

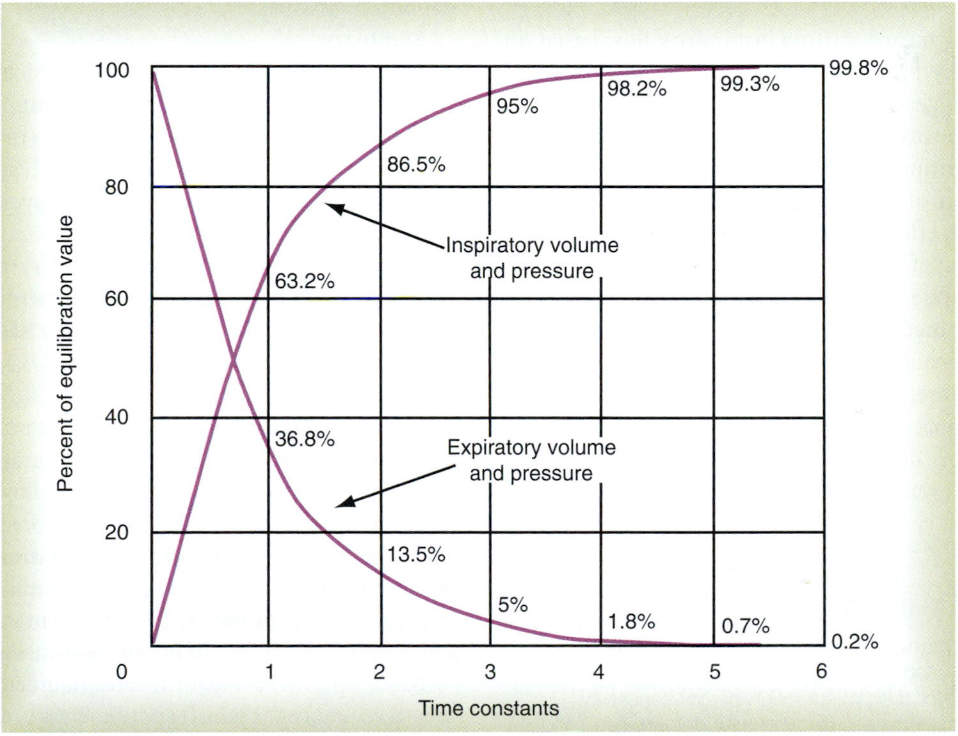

FIGURE 45-19 The time constant is a measure of how long the respiratory system takes to passively inflate or deflate in response to a sudden change in transrespiratory system pressure. The time constant is calculated as the product of resistance times compliance and is expressed in units of time, usually seconds.

for patient-triggered breaths) and synchronization windows (allowing for patient-synchronized, machine-triggered breaths). APRV is intended to provide a set number of releases or drops from a high-pressure level to a low-pressure level. Spontaneous breaths can occur at the high and low-pressure levels (although there may not be enough time to accomplish this if the duration of the low pressure is too short). Using the standardized vocabulary, these releases (paired with their respective rises) are actually mandatory breaths because, as originally described, they were time triggered and time cycled. There are ventilators that have synchronization windows added to both the expiratory time (to synchronize the transition to the high pressure with a patient inspiratory effort) and inspiratory time (to synchronize cycling with the expiratory phase of a spontaneous breath taken during the high-pressure level). If both triggering and cycling occurred with patient signals in the synchronization window, and if these events were called *patient-triggered* and *patient-cycled,* the result would be the ambiguous possibility of having spontaneous breaths (i.e., synchronized) occurring during spontaneous breaths (unsynchronized breaths during the high-pressure level).

On modes that are classified as forms of IMV (such as APRV), the operator must distinguish between the mandatory minute ventilation and the spontaneous minute ventilation (to gauge the level of mechanical support); this cannot be done if the definition of mandatory and spontaneous breaths are in any way ambiguous.

In summary:

Patient triggering means starting inspiration based on a signal from the patient independent of a machine trigger signal.

Machine triggering means starting inspiratory flow based on a signal (usually time) from the ventilator, independent of a patient trigger signal.

Patient cycling means ending inspiratory time based on signals representing the patient-determined components of the equation of motion (i.e., elastance or resistance) and including effects due to inspiratory effort. Flow cycling is a form of patient cycling because the rate of flow decay to the cycle threshold, and hence the inspiratory time, is determined by patient mechanics.

Machine cycling means ending inspiratory time independent of signals representing the patient-determined components of the equation of motion.

An algorithm for distinguishing between machine and patient trigger/cycle events is shown in Figure 45-20.

RULE OF THUMB

When initiating mechanical ventilatory support it is important to ensure that trigger sensitivity is set appropriately for the patient. High or low sensitivity thresholds may cause a delay in flow delivery or auto-triggering, respectively, which can ultimately increase a patient's work of breathing.

6. Breaths are Classified as Spontaneous or Mandatory Based on Both the Trigger and Cycle Events.

The terms *spontaneous* and *mandatory* as types of breaths are fundamental concepts for the classification of modes. The dictionary definition of *spontaneous* is "without premeditation or external stimulus." If we apply this definition to breathing, it implies that the patient retains substantial control over timing. Therefore, **spontaneous breaths** are those for which the patient determines the start and end of inspiration, independent of any machine settings for inspiratory time and expiratory time. In terms of the previous two maxims then, a spontaneous breath is one for which inspiration is both triggered and cycled by the patient. A spontaneous breath may occur during a mandatory breath (e.g., airway pressure release ventilation).

Some authors use the term spontaneous breath to refer only to unassisted breaths. But that is an unnecessary limitation that prevents the word from being used as a key term in the mode taxonomy. The definition given here applies for assisted and unassisted breathing. For unassisted breathing, the brain provides the trigger and cycle signals. For assisted breathing, the signals may come from the brain or the ventilator.

A mandatory breath is a breath for which the patient has lost control over timing (i.e., frequency or inspiratory time). During a mandatory breath, the start and/or end of inspiration is determined by the ventilator, independent of the patient. Again, in terms of the previous two maxims, a mandatory breath is one for which the machine triggers or cycles inspiration (or both). A mandatory breath can occur during a spontaneous breath (e.g., high-frequency jet ventilation). A mandatory breath is, by definition, assisted.

Summary:

A *spontaneous breath* is one for which inspiration is both triggered and cycled by the patient.

A *mandatory breath* is anything else (machine triggered and patient cycled; patient triggered and machine cycled; machine triggered and machine cycled).

7. There Are Three Basic Breath Sequences: Continuous Mandatory Ventilation, Intermittent Mandatory Ventilation, and Continuous Spontaneous Ventilation.

Spontaneous and mandatory breaths come out of a ventilator like dots and dashes come out of a telegraph machine. Because there are only two types of breaths, it follows that there are only three possible breath sequences: all breaths are mandatory, called **continuous mandatory ventilation** (**CMV**); there are both mandatory and spontaneous breaths, called **intermittent mandatory ventilation** (**IMV**); and all breaths are spontaneous, called **continuous spontaneous ventilation** (**CSV**).

More specifically, continuous mandatory ventilation is a breath sequence for which spontaneous breaths are not possible between mandatory breaths because every patient trigger signal in the trigger window produces a machine-cycled inspiration (i.e., a mandatory breath). Continuous mandatory ventilation

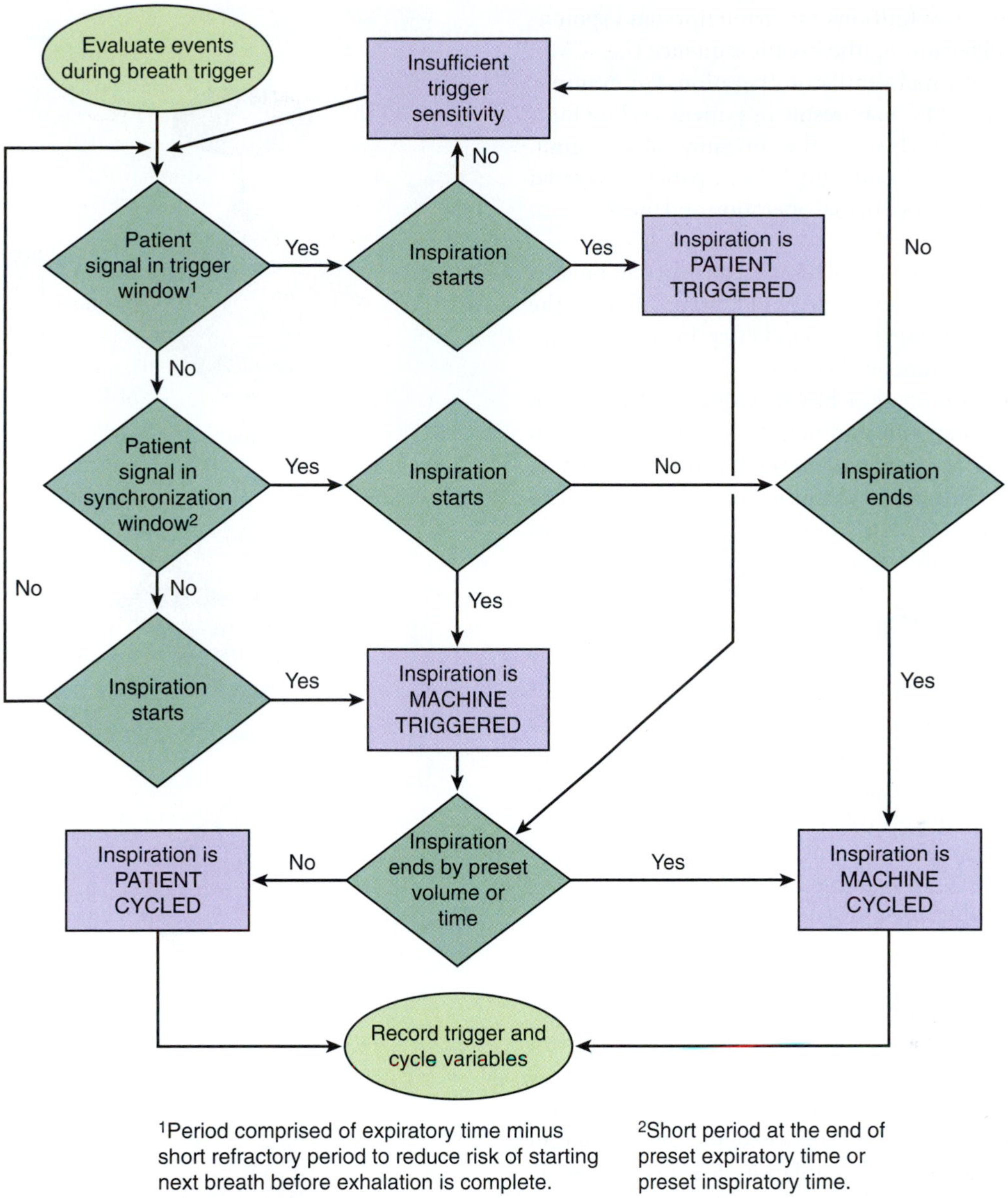

FIGURE 45-20 An algorithm for distinguishing between machine vs. patient events for triggering and cycling. (Courtesy Mandu Press Ltd.)

is commonly referred to as Assist/Control. Machine-triggered mandatory breaths may be delivered at a preset frequency with this breath sequence. The mandatory breath frequency for CMV is the set *minimum* value for the frequency. The total frequency may be higher than the set frequency but never below it. In some pressure controlled modes on ventilators with an active exhalation valve, spontaneous breaths may occur during mandatory breaths, but the defining characteristic of CMV is that spontaneous breaths are not permitted between mandatory breaths. Note that trigger windows are used to create CMV whereas synchronization windows are used for IMV.

Intermittent mandatory ventilation has three variations.

1. Mandatory breaths are always delivered at the set frequency (e.g., SIMV Volume Control mode on the Covidien PB 840 ventilator). When a synchronization window is used, the actual ventilatory period for a mandatory breath may be shorter than the set period. Some ventilators, such as the Dräger Evita XL, will add the difference to the next mandatory period to maintain the set mandatory breath frequency.
2. Mandatory breaths are delivered only when the spontaneous breath frequency falls below the set frequency. One example is the S/T mode on the Philips Respironic BiPAP noninvasive ventilator.
3. Mandatory breaths are delivered only when the measured minute ventilation (i.e., product of breath frequency and tidal volume) drops below a preset threshold. Examples of this variation include Dräger's Mandatory Minute Volume Ventilation mode and Hamilton's Adaptive Support Ventilation mode.

In contrast to CMV, in IMV the mandatory breath frequency can never be higher than the set rate, but it may be lower (i.e., the set frequency is a *maximum* value).

Note that use of the definitions for mandatory and spontaneous breaths for determining the breath sequence (i.e., CMV, IMV, CSV) assumes normal ventilator operation. For example, coughing during VC-CMV may result in patient cycling for a patient-triggered breath due to the pressure alarm limit. Although inspiration for that breath is both patient triggered and patient cycled, this is not normal operation and the sequence does not turn into IMV.

Continuous spontaneous ventilation means that all breaths are spontaneous. Alternatively, you could think of it as the opposite of CMV, meaning that mandatory breaths are not permitted between spontaneous breaths.

Note that the definition of a breath sequence depends on the definition of spontaneous and mandatory breaths (Maxim 6) and those definitions rely on the definitions of machine versus patient triggering and cycling (Maxims 4 and 5). The distinctions between CMV, IMC, and CSV are illustrated in Figure 45-21.

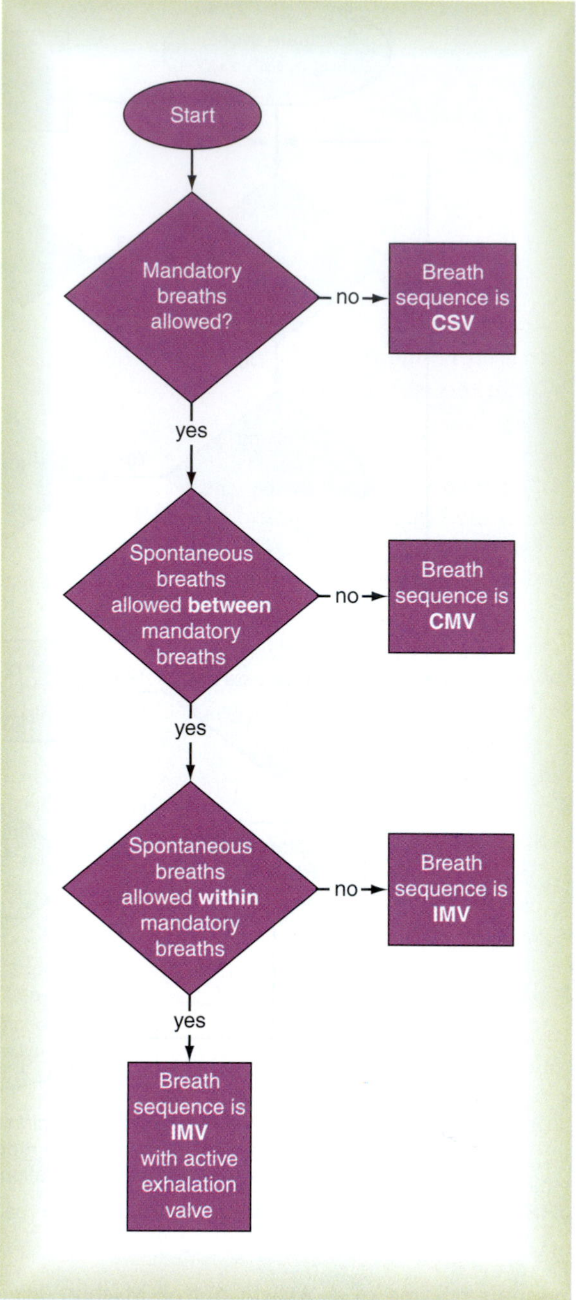

FIGURE 45-21 Algorithm distinguishing among CSV, CMV, and IMV.

8. There Are Five Basic Ventilatory Patterns: VC-CMV, VC-IMV, PC-CMV, PC-IMV, and PC-CSV.

A ventilatory pattern is a sequence of breaths (CMV, IMV, or CSV) with a designated control variable (volume or pressure) for the mandatory breaths (or the spontaneous breaths for CSV). Thus, with two control variables and three breath sequences, there are five possible ventilatory patterns: VC-CMV, VC-IMV, PC-CMV, PC-IMV, and PC-CSV. The VC-CSV combination is not possible because volume control implies that inspiration ends when the preset tidal volume is delivered, which implies ventilator cycling, and ventilator cycling makes every breath mandatory, not spontaneous (Maxim 6).

For completeness, we include the possibility of a time control (TC) ventilatory pattern such as TC-IMV. Although this is uncommon and nonconventional, it is possible, as demonstrated by modes such as high-frequency oscillatory ventilation and intrapulmonary percussive ventilation. Because any mode of ventilation can be associated with one and only one ventilatory pattern, the ventilatory pattern serves as a simple mode classification system.

Ventilatory patterns are a simple mode classification system that offers practical advantages in clinical situations. We can use it to describe different modes a patient may experience without using the names for modes that vary depending on the ventilator manufacturer. For example, during surgery there may be no need to worry about patient–ventilatory synchrony and thus we might say VC-CMV was used (instead of saying Volume Assist/Control or CMV, names that relate to specific ventilators). Postoperatively, we could say we switched to PC-CMV to allow unrestricted inspiratory flow when the patient begins to make some breathing effort (instead of saying Pressure Assist/Control or Pressure Control; again names of modes on specific ventilators). When the patient is evaluated for extubation, a "spontaneous breathing trial" may be attempted using PC-CSV (instead of saying Pressure Support or Volume Support). Referring to modes in terms of breathing patterns instead of specific names on particular ventilators simplifies both verbal communication, and perhaps more important, documentation in the patient's record.

9. Within Each Ventilatory Pattern There Are Several Types That Can Be Distinguished by Their Targeting Schemes (Set-Point, Dual, Bio-Variable, Servo, Adaptive, Optimal, and Intelligent).

Although the concept of ventilatory patterns may serve as a simple classification system in some cases, a better way to

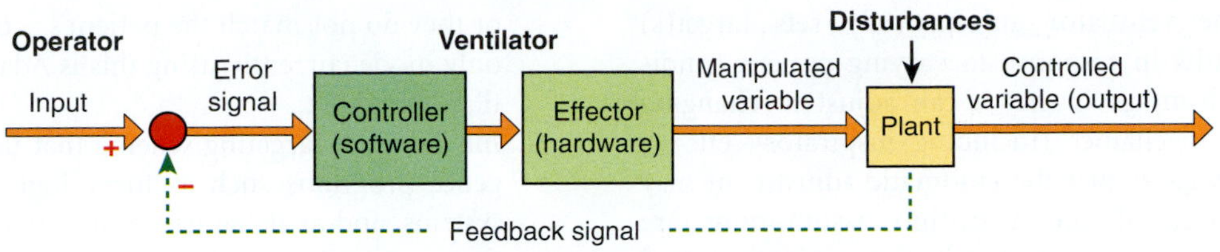

FIGURE 45-22 Schematic of a closed loop feedback control scheme for a ventilator. (Courtesy Mandu Press Ltd.)

identify the differences among modes is necessary. To do this, we need a deeper understanding of the feedback control schemes used by engineers who design modes. We refer to these as *targeting schemes*.

Targeting Schemes. Figure 45-22 illustrates a basic schematic of a closed-loop or feedback control scheme. The operator sets a desired *input*, for example, inspiratory pressure. The software sends control signals to the flow control and exhalation valves. The manipulated variable (typically flow) is delivered to the patient. The resulting inspiratory pressure (the *output*) is measured as a feedback signal and compared to the input setting. A variety of disturbances, such as patient circuit characteristics, leaks, patient ventilatory efforts, and respiratory system mechanics, to name a few, can affect the output. Any difference between the input and output generates an error signal that is passed on to the control valves to bring the output closer to the input. This system is referred to as a targeting scheme in this chapter as it relates to modes of ventilation.

The targeting scheme is a key component of a mode description. A target is basically a predetermined goal of ventilator output. Pressure, volume, and flow waveforms are called *within-breath* targets. Inspiratory pressure, rise time, inspiratory flow and tidal volume (set-point and dual targeting), and constant of proportionality between inspiratory pressure and patient effort (servo targeting) are examples of within-breath targets. Preset values within a breath that end inspiration, such as tidal volume, inspiratory time, or percent of peak flow, may also be considered cycle variables.

There may also be *between-breath targets.* These serve to modify the within-breath targets or the overall ventilatory pattern. Between-breath targets are used with more advanced targeting schemes, where targets act over multiple breaths. A simple example of a between-breath target is comparing actual exhaled volume to a preset between-breath tidal volume to automatically adjust the within-breath constant pressure or flow target for the next breath. Average tidal volume (for adaptive targeting), percent minute ventilation (for optimal targeting), and combined PCO_2, volume, and frequency values describing a zone of comfort (for intelligent targeting) are examples of between-breath targets and targeting schemes.

There are at least seven targeting schemes used on commercially available ventilators:[26]

1. *Set-point:* The operator sets all parameters of the pressure waveform (pressure control modes) or volume and flow waveforms (volume control modes) and the ventilator makes no automatic adjustments to targets. The advantage is simplicity. The disadvantage is that changing patient condition may make the settings inappropriate, so that frequent manual adjustments are necessary. An example mode name is Volume Assist/Control.
2. *Dual:* The ventilator can automatically switch between volume control and pressure control during a single inspiration. The advantage is the ability to adjust to changing patient condition and assure either a preset tidal volume or peak inspiratory pressure, whichever is deemed most important. The disadvantage is that some forms are complicated, difficult to set, and need constant readjustment. The original mode using dual targeting was called *Volume Assured Pressure Support.* In this mode, inspiration started off in pressure control but changed to volume control if flow decayed to the preset value before the tidal volume was delivered.[27] An example of the opposite approach, such as switching from volume control to pressure control, is Flow Adaptive Volume Control on the Maquet SERVO-i ventilator. If the patient makes little or no inspiratory efforts the mode looks like VC-CMV (e.g., Assist/Control). But if the patient makes strong enough efforts, the mode looks like PC-CSV (e.g., Pressure Support).[16]
3. *Bio-variable:* Studies have shown that varying tidal volume breath-by-breath to mimic normal breathing improves gas exchange.[28,29] Currently this biologically variable targeting scheme is available in only one mode, Variable Pressure Support on the Dräger V500 ventilator. The operator sets a target inspiratory pressure and a percent variability from 0% to 100%. A setting of 0% means the preset inspiratory pressure will be delivered for every breath. A 100% variability setting means that the actual inspiratory pressure varies randomly from PEEP/CPAP level to double the preset pressure support level.
4. *Servo:* The output of the ventilator (pressure/volume/flow) automatically follows a varying input. In current modes, this means that the inspiratory pressure is proportional to the patient's inspiratory effort; the more assistance the patient demands, the more the ventilator delivers. No other targeting scheme does this. The disadvantage is that it requires estimates of artificial airway and/or respiratory system mechanical properties or special equipment to monitor the respiratory effort signal. Example mode names include Automatic Tube Compensation (ATC), Proportional Assist Ventilation (PAV), and Neurally Adjusted Ventilatory Assist (NAVA).

5. *Adaptive:* The ventilator automatically sets target(s) between breaths in response to varying patient conditions. The advantage is that it can adjust to changing patient lung mechanics (including inspiratory effort). The disadvantage is that the automatic adjustment may be inappropriate if the algorithm assumptions are violated or they do not match the patient's actual physiology.[30] The first mode to use this was called *Pressure Regulated Volume Control.*
6. *Optimal:* The ventilator automatically adjusts the targets of the ventilatory pattern to either minimize or maximize some overall performance characteristic. The advantage is that it can adjust to changing patient condition. The disadvantage is that the automatic adjustment may be inappropriate if the algorithm assumptions are violated or they do not match the patient's actual physiology. The only mode currently using this is Adaptive Support Ventilation (ASV).
7. *Intelligent:* A targeting scheme that uses artificial intelligence programs such as fuzzy logic, rule-based expert systems, and artificial neural networks. The advantage is that it can adjust to changing patient condition. The disadvantage is that the automatic adjustment may be inappropriate if the algorithm assumptions are violated or they do not match the patient's actual physiology. The only modes currently using this scheme are SmartCare/PS and IntelliVent (not available in the United States).

These targeting schemes along with example modes that use them are summarized in Table 45-2.

TABLE 45-2
Specifications for Some Modes Found on the Draeger Evita XL Ventilator

Name (Abbreviation)	Description	Advantage	Disadvantage	Example Mode Name	Ventilator (Manufacturer)
Set-point (s)	The operator sets all parameters of the pressure waveform (pressure control modes) or volume and flow waveforms (volume control modes)	Simplicity	Changing patient conditions may make settings inappropriate	Volume control CMV	Evita Infinity V500 (Drager)
Dual (d)	The ventilator can automatically switch between volume control and pressure control during a single inspiration	It can adjust to changing patient conditions and ensure either a pre-set VT or peak inspiratory pressure, whichever is deemed most important	It may be complicated to set correctly and may need constant readjustment if not automatically controlled by the ventilator	Volume control	Servo-I (Maquet)
Servo (r)	The output of the ventilator (pressure/volume/flow) automatically follows a varying input	Support by the ventilator is proportional to inspiratory effort	It requires estimates of artificial airway and/or respiratory system mechanical properties	Proportional assist ventilation	PB840 (Covidien)
Adaptive (a)	The ventilator automatically sets target(s) between breaths in response to varying patient conditions	It can maintain stable VT delivery with pressure control for changing lung mechanics or patient inspiratory effort	Automatic adjustment may be inappropriate if algorithm assumptions are violated or if they do not match physiology	Pressure-regulated volume control	Servo-I
Bio-variable (b)	The ventilator automatically adjusts the inspiratory pressure or VT randomly	It simulates the inspiratory time or V_T observed during normal breathing and may improve oxygenation or mechanics	Manually set range of variability may be inappropriate to achieve goals	Variable pressure support	Evita Infinity V500
Optimal (o)	The ventilator automatically adjusts the targets of the ventilator pattern to either minimize or maximize some overall performance characteristic (e.g., work or rate of breathing)	It can adjust to changing lung mechanics or patient inspiratory effort	Automatic adjustment may be inappropriate if algorithm assumptions are violated or if they do not match physiology	ASV	GS (Hamilton Medical)
Intelligent (i)	This is a targeting scheme that uses artificial intelligence programs such as fuzzy logic, rule-based expert systems, and artificial neural networks	It can adjust to changing lung mechanics or patient inspiratory effort	Automatic adjustment may be inappropriate if algorithm assumptions are violated or if they do not match physiology	SmartCare/PS IrdelliVent-ASV	Evita Infinity V500 S1 (Hamilton Medical)

Limitations of Automatic Targeting Schemes. As targeting schemes have evolved, they have become more automated and, as a result, more complicated. Automation relies on various assumptions—for example, that compliance and resistance are linear or that a patient's carbon dioxide production is a particular number of mL per minute. If the underlying assumptions of a targeting scheme are violated, unexpected and possibly unwanted results may result. Set-point targeting provides an example. This targeting scheme assumes constant respiratory system mechanics. If respiratory system mechanics change rapidly, either peak airway pressure (during volume control ventilation) or tidal volume (during pressure control ventilation) may become unstable and drift out of acceptable ranges.

Dual targeting assumes that mechanics may change but may be useless without careful setting of the criteria for switching between volume- and pressure-control breaths. Servo control requires accurate data for respiratory system mechanical properties, such as resistance and elastance; if the data are unavailable, the mode cannot be used. Some forms of adaptive targeting assume that changes in respiratory system mechanics are related only to compliance. The ventilator is unable to distinguish between patient inspiratory effort and an increase in compliance. The targeting scheme is fooled into decreasing support when the patient needs it most.[30]

Optimal targeting is based on mathematical models (e.g., the relations among power of breathing, lung mechanics, frequency, and tidal volume). When the models do not match the actual physiology of the patient, they may instruct the ventilator to do inappropriate things (e.g., hyper/hypoventilate the patient or increase risk of ventilator-induced lung damage).

Intelligent targeting systems may rely on rules in the form of "if...then" statements; "if the patient does this, then the ventilator should do that." Ventilator algorithms or operational rules are derived from the consensus of clinical experts. These rules currently cover a very small set of actual clinical scenarios. Assumptions upon which the artificially intelligence system are based may be easily violated by actual patient conditions. For example, the targeting scheme might assume that the patient can be aggressively weaned when in fact the patient is not ready. Awareness of these drawbacks of ventilator technology should prompt the clinician to fully understand both the capabilities and limitations of the modes used.

10. A Mode of Ventilation is Classified According to Its Control Variable, Breath Sequence, and Targeting Scheme(s).

In general terms, a mode of ventilation is a predefined pattern of interaction between the ventilator and the patient. Historically, modes have been referred to by the names coined by ventilator manufacturers, who use them as marketing devices. As a consequence, there are now so many different names that understanding and comparing all modes has become nearly impossible. The solution is to use a *taxonomy* or formal classification system. The use of a taxonomy may make it easier (1) to compare research reports and facilitate the development of evidence-based clinical practice; (2) for clinicians to select the most appropriate modes, making optimal ventilator management more likely; and (3) for manufacturers to communicate with clients, thus improving the effectiveness of both sales and training.

The taxonomy of modes is based on the concepts of the control variable, the breath sequence, and the targeting scheme, as described in the previous nine maxims.

The Taxonomy for Mechanical Ventilation

A taxonomy is a hierarchy (outline) of concepts starting with the most general and progressing to more specific with each successive level of the outline. The ventilator mode taxonomy has four hierarchical levels (analogous to the order, class, genus, and species used in biology)[17,18]

1. Control variable (pressure or volume)
    A. Breath sequence (CMV, IMV, or CSV)
        i. Primary breath targeting scheme (for CMV or CSV)
            a. Secondary breath targeting scheme (for IMV)

The "primary breath" is either the only breath there is (mandatory for CMV and spontaneous for CSV) or it is the mandatory breath in IMV. The targeting schemes can be represented by single, lower case letters: set-point = s, dual = d, servo = r, bio-variable = b, adaptive = a, optimal = o, intelligent = i. For example, on the Covidien PB 840 ventilator there is a mode called *A/C Volume Control*. This mode is classified as volume control, continuous mandatory ventilation with set-point targeting, represented by VC-CMVs. A mode with the same functionality on the Dräger Evita XL ventilator is called *Continuous Mandatory Ventilation*. On that ventilator, you can alter the targeting scheme by activating a feature called *AutoFlow*. This changes the mode to pressure control continuous mandatory ventilation with adaptive targeting, PC-CMVa. Finally, some modes represent compound targeting schemes. For example, some ventilators offer Tube Compensation, a feature that increases inspiratory pressure in proportion to flow to support the resistive load of breathing through an artificial airway. This is a form of servo targeting. On the Dräger Evita XL, you can add Tube Compensation to CMV with AutoFlow to get a mode classified as PC-CMVar (*ar* represents the compound targeting scheme composed of servo added to set-point). A mode classified as pressure control intermittent mandatory ventilation with set-point control for both primary (mandatory) and secondary (spontaneous) breaths would have a tag that looks like this: PC-IMVs,s. If you added Tube Compensation to the spontaneous breaths (e.g., Covidien PB 840) the tag would change to PC-IMVs,sr. If you added it to both mandatory and spontaneous breaths (e.g., Dräger Evita XL), the tag would change to PC-IMVsr,sr.

The structure of this mode classification system is reminiscent of the taxonomy of biological organisms comprised of order (control variable), family (breath sequence), genus (primary targeting scheme), and species (secondary targeting scheme). Modes in the same "species" can be further differentiated by describing their "species variety" in term of their phase variables (i.e., trigger and cycle variables plus the within- and between-breath targets and control algorithms). An example of the use of a "species variety" description is to distinguish between Proportional Assist Ventilation and Neurally Adjusted Ventilatory Assist, both of which are forms of PC-CSVr. They can be distinguished simply by noting that PAV breaths are triggered and cycled with flow signals whereas NAVA is triggered and cycled with an electrical signal representing diaphragm activation. Of course there are a great many other distinguishing features (e.g., targeting algorithms) but these are better described in the operator's manuals than, for example, in a general classification table.

How to Classify Modes

Translating the name of a mode into a mode classification using the taxonomy we have described is a simple three-step procedure:

Step 1: Identify the control variable. Simply put, if you set inspiratory pressure, or if pressure is proportional to inspiratory effort, then the control variable is pressure. On the contrary, if you set tidal volume and inspiratory flow, then the control variable is volume. Figure 45-23 shows the decision algorithm with a few refinements to accommodate dual targeting.

Step 2: Identify the breath sequence. Figure 45-24 shows the decision rubric.

Step 3: Identify the targeting schemes for the primary and (if applicable) secondary breaths (see Table 45-2).

Examples

To demonstrate these steps, we will classify some of the most commonly used modes in intensive care units, starting with A/C Volume Control (Covidien PB 840). For this mode, both

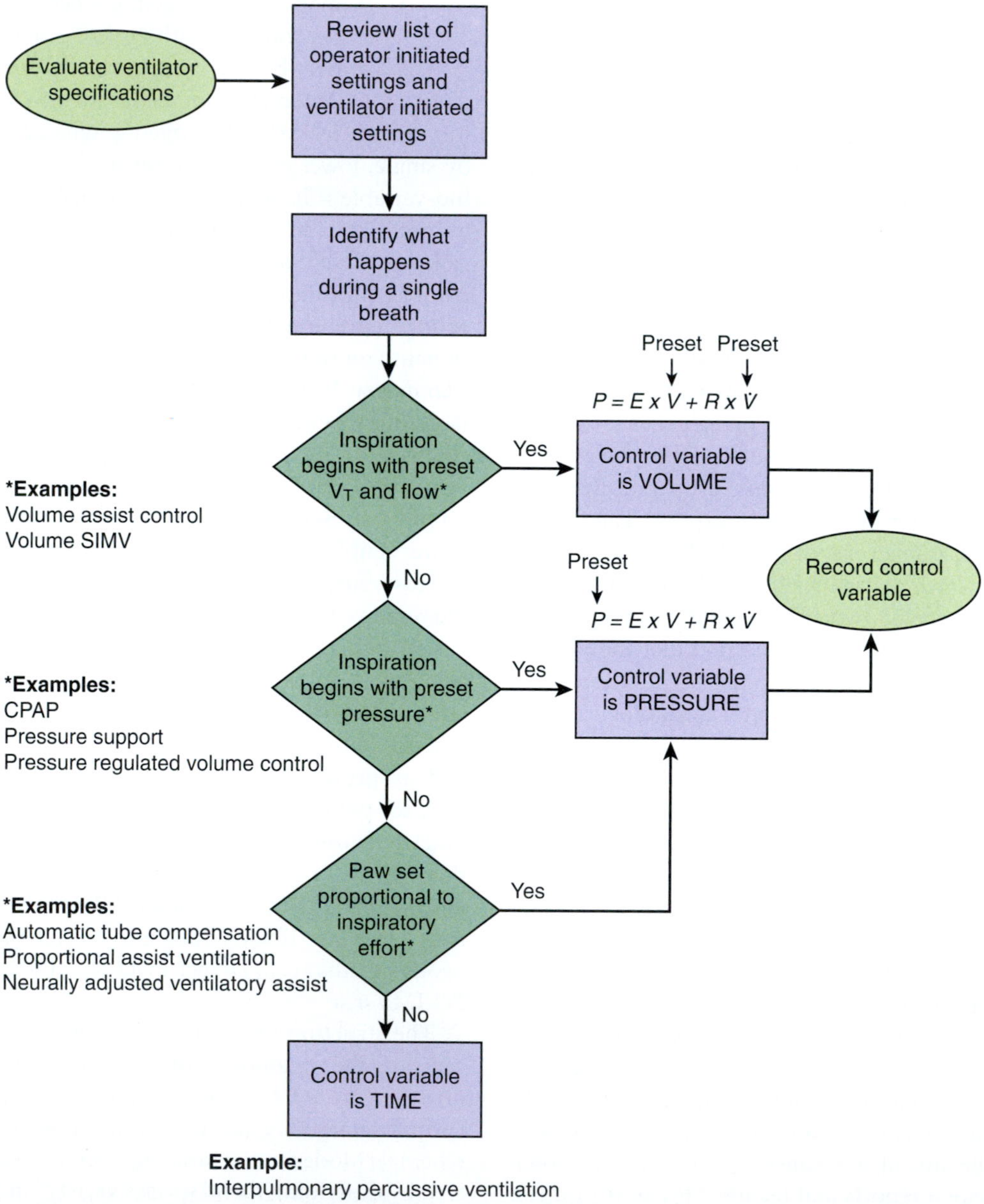

FIGURE 45-23 Algorithm for determining the control variable of a mode. (Courtesy Mandu Press Ltd.)

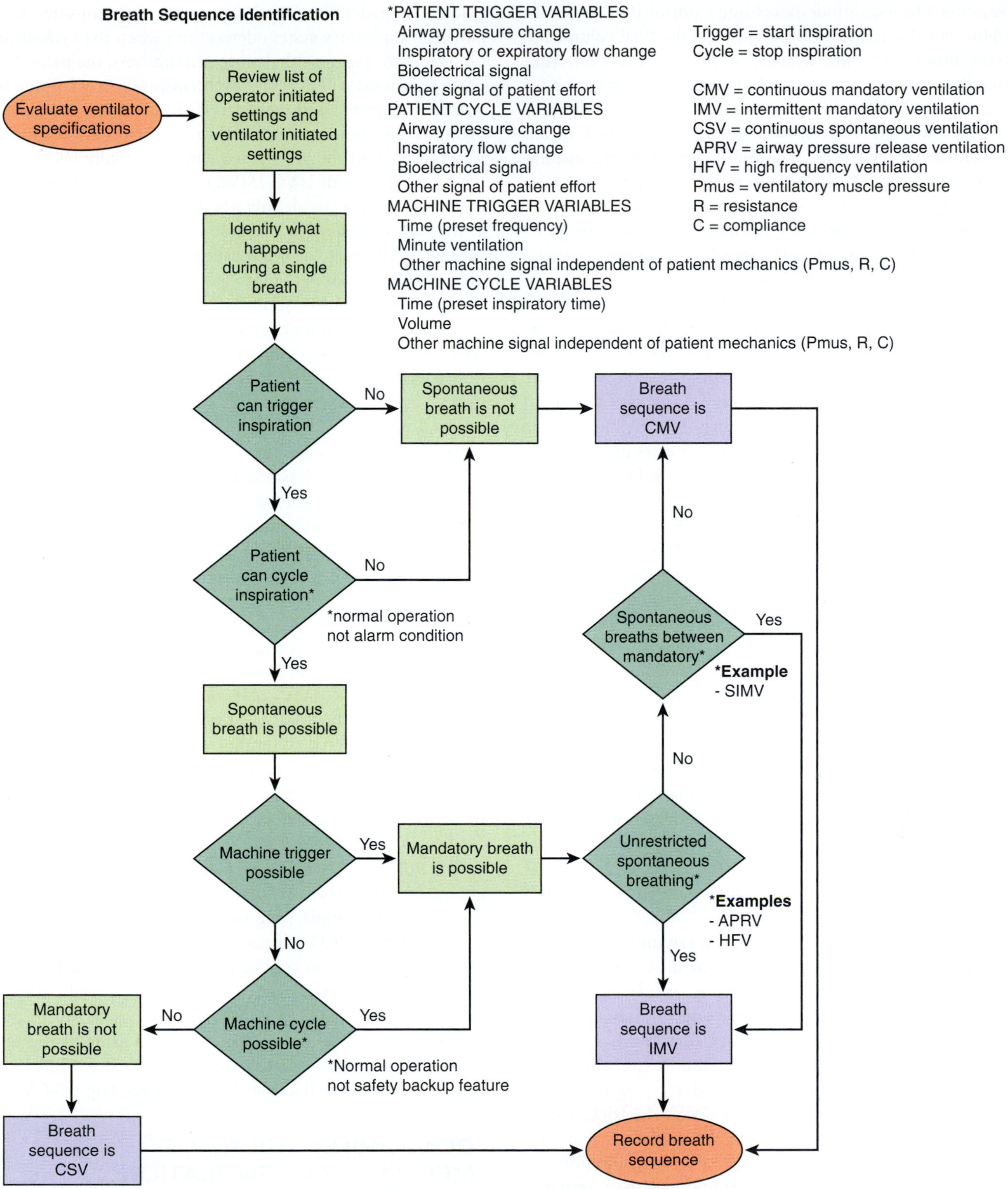

FIGURE 45-24 Algorithm for determining the breath sequence of a mode. (Courtesy Mandu Press Ltd.)

inspiratory volume and flow are preset, so the control variable is volume. Every breath is volume cycled, which is a form of machine cycling. Any breath for which inspiration is machine cycled is classified as a mandatory breath. Hence, the breath sequence is continuous mandatory ventilation. Finally, the operator sets all the parameters of the volume and flow waveforms, so the targeting scheme is set-point. Thus, the mode is classified as volume control continuous mandatory ventilation with set-point targeting (the tag or abbreviation is thus VC-CMVs).

Another common mode is Volume Control Plus (Covidien PB 840). For this mode, the operator sets the tidal volume but not the inspiratory flow. Because setting volume alone (like setting flow alone) is a necessary but not sufficient criterion for volume control, the control variable is pressure. Spontaneous breaths are allowed between mandatory breaths, which means the breath sequence is IMV. The ventilator adjusts the inspiratory pressure of mandatory breaths to achieve an average preset tidal volume, making the primary targeting scheme adaptive. Spontaneous breaths between mandatory breaths are either CPAP or Pressure Support, so the targeting scheme is set-point. The mode tag is thus PC-IMVa,s.

A very common mode for spontaneous breathing trials (or for assistance of spontaneous breaths in IMV modes) is Pressure Support. For this mode, the operator sets an inspiratory pressure, so the control variable is pressure. All breaths are patient triggered and patient cycled (note what was said about flow cycling above), so the breath sequence is CSV. Because the ventilator does not adjust any of the parameters of the breath, the targeting scheme is set-point and the tag is PC-CSVs.

If carefully applied, the taxonomy has the power to clarify and unmask hidden complexity in a mode that has a cryptic name. Take for example the mode called *CMV+AutoFlow* on the Dräger Evita XL ventilator. While "CMV" on this ventilator is the same as "Volume Assist/Control" described above, adding the "AutoFlow" feature changes it to a completely different mode. For CMV+AutoFlow, the operator sets a target tidal volume but not inspiratory flow. Indeed, inspiratory flow is highly variable because the ventilator actually sets the inspiratory pressure within a breath. Thus, the control variable, according to the equation of motion, is pressure. Every inspiration is time cycled and hence every breath is mandatory and the breath sequence is continuous mandatory ventilation (CMV). The ventilator adjusts the inspiratory pressure between breaths to achieve an average tidal volume equal to the preset value using an adaptive targeting scheme. Thus, the mode is classified as pressure control continuous mandatory ventilation with adaptive targeting (PC-CMVa).

On the other hand, the taxonomy also can unmask the complexity in an apparently simple mode. The mode called *Volume Control* (Maquet SERVO-i) allows setting of tidal volume and inspiratory time. Setting both volume and inspiratory time is equivalent to setting mean inspiratory flow (flow = volume/time), hence the control variable is volume. Every breath is normally time cycled and hence mandatory, so our initial thought is that the breath sequence is CMV. The tricky part is the targeting scheme. The operator's manual states that "if a pressure drop of 3 cm H_2O is detected during inspiration, the ventilator (switches) to Pressure Support with a resulting increase in inspiratory flow." This indicates dual targeting as described in maxim 9. Noting that the breath may switch to Pressure Support alerts us that the breath sequence is not what it first seemed to be. A breath may be patient triggered with a patient inspiratory effort, and if the effort is large enough and long enough, inspiration is flow cycled, not time cycled. Flow cycling (at a certain percentage of peak inspiratory pressure) is a form of patient cycling because the time constant of the patient's respiratory system determines when the cycle threshold is met for passive exhalation. Alternatively, the patient may make an expiratory effort that cycles inspiration off. Either way, a patient-triggered and patient-cycled breath is a spontaneous breath. Thus, spontaneous breaths may occur between mandatory breaths and the breaths sequence is actually IMV. Finally, the tag for this mode is VC-IMVd,d. Note that with dual targeting modes we need to identify which control variable is in effect at the start of inspiration (Figure 45-23) and in this case it is volume. In contrast, the mode called *Pressure A/C with Machine Volume* (CareFusionAvea) incorporates dual targeting, it starts out in pressure control and may switch to volume control.

Finally, some modes are comprised of compound targeting schemes. For example, some ventilators offer Tube Compensation, a feature that increases inspiratory pressure in proportion to flow to support the resistive load of breathing through an artificial airway. This is a form of servo targeting. On the Dräger Evita XL, Tube Compensation can be added to CMV with AutoFlow to get a mode classified as PC-CMVar (*ar* represents the compound targeting scheme composed of servo added to set-point, with no comma because there are only primary breaths). A mode classified as pressure control intermittent mandatory ventilation with set-point control for both primary (mandatory) and secondary (spontaneous) breaths would have a tag that looks like this: PC-IMVs,s (with a comma to denote primary and secondary breaths). If you added Tube Compensation to the spontaneous breaths (e.g., Covidien PB 840) the tag would change to PC-IMVs,sr. If you added it to both mandatory and spontaneous breaths (e.g., Dräger Evita XL) the tag would change to PC-IMVsr,sr. Another example is IntelliVent mode (Hamilton G5 ventilator), which uses optimal targeting to minimize the work rate and intelligent targeting to establish lung protective limits and adjust PEEP and FiO_2. The tag for this mode is PC-CMVoi,oi.

The utility of this taxonomy becomes evident when comparing modes on different ventilators (e.g., for making a purchase decision). For example, suppose your hospital has standardized on two common ICU ventilators, the Covidien PB 840 and the Maquet SERVO-i. You could construct a simple pocket card to show how the different names of modes are actually the same by classification (Table 45-3); the mode called *Assist/Control Volume Control Plus* on the PB 840 is the same as the mode called *Pressure Regulated Volume Control* on the SERVO-i, as indicated by the fact that they have the same tag: PC-CMVa.

COMPARING MODES OF MECHANICAL VENTILATION

The use of the ventilator mode taxonomy allows clinicians to appropriately match the technology to the patients' needs. Clinicians must not only know what tool to use but how to use it. Knowing how to use a mode involves understanding the technological capabilities of the mode and how they serve the goals of mechanical ventilation. These goals are safety, comfort, and liberation. *Safety* means maintaining adequate gas exchange

TABLE 45-3

Example of Pocket Card Comparing Mode Names from Two Common ICU Ventilators

Covidien PB 840	Mode Tag
A/C Volume Control	VC-CMVs
SIMV Volume Control with Pressure Support	VC-IMVs, s
SIMV Volume Control with Tube Compensation	VC-IMVs, r
A/C Pressure Control	PC-CMVs
A/C Volume Control Plus	PC-CMVa
SIMV-Pressure Control with Pressure Support	PC-IMVs, s
SIMV-Pressure Control with Tube Compensation	PC-IMVs, r
Bilevel with Pressure Support	PC-IMVs, s
Bilevel with Tube Compensation	PC-IMVs, r
SIMV Volume Control Plus with Pressure Support	PC-IMVa, s
SIMV Volume Control Plus with Tube Compensation	PC-IMVa, r
Spont Pressure Support	PC-CSVs
Spont Tube Compensation	PC-CSVr
Spont Proportional Assist	PC-CSVr
Spont Volume Support	PC-CSVa
Maquet Servo-1	**Mode Tag**
Volume Control	VC-IMVd, d
SIMV (Volume Control)	VC-IMVd, d
Automode (Volume Control to Volume Support)	VC-IMVd, a
Pressure Control	PC-CMVs
Pressure Regulated Volume Control	PC-CMVa
SIMV (Pressure Control)	PC-IMVs, s
Bi-Vent	PC-IMVs, s
Automode (Pressure Control to Pressure Support)	PC-IMVs, s
SIMV Pressure Regulated Volume Control	PC-IMVa, s
Automode (Pressure Regulated Volume Control to Volume Support)	PC-IMVa, a
Spontaneous/CPAP	PC-CSVs
Pressure Support	PC-CSVs
Neurally Adjusted Ventilatory Assist	PC-CSVr
Volume Support	PC-CSVa

S, Set-point; *d*, dual; *r*, servo; *a*, adaptive.

MINI CLINI

Calculate the Expiratory Time Setting from the Frequency and Inspiratory Time

PROBLEM: You are assigned to the neonatal intensive care unit (NICU) and have successfully intubated a newborn term infant diagnosed with respiratory distress syndrome. You are manually ventilating the infant with a flow-inflating bag at a frequency of 25 breaths per minute. An inline manometer indicates the PIP is approximately 24 cm H_2O and the PEEP is 4 cm H_2O. The infant's vital signs (heart rate, respiratory rate, and blood pressure) are within normal limits and Spo_2 is 95%. The pressure and frequency you are using manually will serve as the initial ventilator settings on an infant ventilator. With this particular ventilator, however, setting the inspiratory and expiratory times determines the frequency. The attending physician has requested an inspiratory time (T_I) of 0.3 seconds. Calculate the expiratory time (T_E) necessary to give the desired frequency.

Discussion: *Step 1:* Compute the total cycle time (TCT) using the frequency (f):

$$TCT = \frac{1}{f} = T_I + T_E$$

$$f = \frac{25\text{ breaths}}{\text{minute}} \times \frac{1\text{ minute}}{60\text{ seconds}} = \frac{25\text{ breaths}}{60\text{ seconds}}$$

$$TCT = \frac{1}{25\text{ breaths}/60\text{ seconds}} = \frac{60\text{ seconds}}{25\text{ breaths}} = \frac{2.4\text{ seconds}}{\text{breath}}$$

Step 2: Compute the expiratory time:

$$T_E = TCT - T_I = 2.4 - 0.3 = 2.1\text{ seconds}$$

Step 3: Check the digital display to verify the set frequency remains at 25/minute.

and hemodynamics while avoiding harm in the form of atelectrauma and volutrauma. *Comfort* means optimizing synchrony between the patient and the ventilator. *Liberation* means getting the patient off the ventilator in the shortest time with the fewest adverse events.

These goals can be further refined into specific objectives and clinical aims that may then be applied to individual patients. Goals, objectives, and aims are the product of a clinical assessment. After identifying the patient's need, the clinician simply matches those needs to the technological capabilities of the available modes of ventilation.[31]

TYPES OF VENTILATORS

Conventional Versus High-Frequency Ventilators

Ventilators may be divided into categories according to type and the setting in which the ventilator will be used. The two categories ventilators may be divided into are conventional and nonconventional. Conventional ventilators produce breathing patterns that are at or near physiologic normal values for the intended population (e.g., adult, pediatric, and infant). There are also manufacturing limits on the maximum breath rate a conventional ventilator may deliver. The Food and Drug Administration places a maximum breath rate limit of 150 breaths per minute for conventional ventilators. Tidal volumes that are either operator set or delivered to the patient as a result of a preset pressure through a conventional ventilator are sufficient or large enough to clear anatomic dead space. Conversely, high-frequency ventilators typically produce respiratory frequencies or breathing rates that are much higher than physiologically possible and tidal volumes that are less than anatomic dead space.

Conventional Ventilators

Conventional ventilators may be used with a variety of interfaces in the critical care setting. Options are available on this type of ventilator for use with an artificial airway (endotracheal or tracheostomy tube) or noninvasively with a variety of

MINI CLINI

Calculate Inspiratory Hold Time Given Set Inspiratory Time, Tidal Volume, and Flow

PROBLEM: You are performing a ventilator check on an ICU patient with a blunt chest trauma. The ventilator is set to deliver volume control SIMV. The physician wants the minimum mean airway pressure for the given level of ventilation to preserve the patient's already low cardiac output. She asks you to make sure the night shift therapist removed the inspiratory hold. Determine from the ventilator settings alone whether there is an inspiratory hold, and if so, make the appropriate changes to eliminate it.

Ventilator settings are:

Tidal volume: 500 ml = 0.5 L

Inspiratory flow: 60 L/min = 1 L/sec

Inspiratory time: 0.8 second

Frequency: 10 breaths per minute

Discussion: *Step 1:* Calculate the inspiratory flow time (TIF) using appropriate unit conversions:

$$T_{IF} = \frac{\text{tidal volume}}{\text{inspiratory flow}}$$

$$= \frac{500\text{ mL}}{60\text{ L/minute}} \times \frac{1\text{ L}}{1{,}000\text{ mL}} \times \frac{60\text{ seconds}}{1\text{ minute}} = 0.5\text{ seconds}$$

Step 2: Compare the set inspiratory time (0.8 second) with the flow time resulting from the tidal volume and flow settings (0.5 second). Inspiratory time lasts longer than inspiratory flow. Because inspiration is time cycled, this means that there is an inspiratory hold of duration equal to 0.8 − 0.5 = 0.3 second.

Step 3: You could eliminate the inspiratory hold either by decreasing the inspiratory flow or decreasing the inspiratory time. Your goal is to minimize the mean inspiratory pressure. You choose to decrease inspiratory time for two reasons: (1) it decreases the I:E ratio and may allow more time for spontaneous breaths to occur, thus lowering mean intrathoracic pressure; (2) decreasing inspiratory flow may make tidal volume delivery slower than the patient demands, thus decreasing patient–ventilator synchrony.

interfaces (e.g., nasal, oronasal, or full face masks). The availability of the noninvasive option eliminates the need for a standalone noninvasive ventilator. However, standalone noninvasive ventilators do have applications and are also used in the critical care setting. Detail will be given to this type of ventilator in the latter portion of this chapter. Ventilators used in the critical care environment have the capability to assess and monitor complex ventilator–patient interactions. Work of breathing and the intricacies of breath delivery may be examined by evaluating numerically or graphically displayed data. Many ventilators also apportion automatic adjustments to breath delivery in response to changes in lung mechanics and parameters preset by the operator. In addition to universal patient population applications, some critical care ventilators are manufactured with an internal battery. The SERVO-i, for example has a plug-in battery module. This ventilator can provide at least 3 hours of uninterrupted power supply when six rechargeable 12-volt batteries are used in the module. Uninterrupted ventilatory assistance may then be provided not only in the critical care setting, but during interhospital transport. Minimizing circuit disconnections can enhance safety by reducing the risks for derecruitment, hemodynamic instability, and factors contributing to nosocomial infections. The aforementioned features provide a platform through which clinicians may optimize the patient–ventilator interaction.

High-Frequency Ventilators

The availability of sophisticated devices such as jet ventilators and high-frequency oscillators facilitates ventilatory management of infants, children, and adults in the PC-IMV mode who fail to maintain adequate oxygenation and acid-base balance with conventional ventilatory support. High-frequency jet ventilators, such as the Bunnell Life Pulse (Bunnell Inc., Salt Lake City, UT), deliver short bursts, or jet pulses, of mixed gas through a special adaptor for endotracheal tubes or a specially designed endotracheal tube. High-frequency jet ventilators require a high pressure source (20 to 50 psig) to function. This type of ventilator consists of a system for regulating inlet pressure (psig), a cycling mechanism, and a device such as an air-oxygen blender for controlling F_IO_2. The small volumes of gas are delivered at rapid rates (4 to 250 times the normal respiratory rate). The benefits of rescue and elective use of high-frequency jet ventilation (HFJV) as a treatment for acute lung disease and adult respiratory distress syndrome are unclear. However, the literature supports its effectiveness in maintaining alveolar ventilation and reducing morbidity during surgical repair of tracheal and airway anomalies.

High-frequency oscillation (HFO) also allows very small tidal volumes to be delivered at rapid frequencies (180 to 1200 cycles per second). High-frequency oscillators utilize a piston or diaphragm to produce the airflow oscillations. Tidal volume is dependent on the force and distance the piston moves from baseline. A special endotracheal tube is not required to implement this form of PC-IMV. The SensorMedics 3100A and 3100 B high-frequency oscillators (CareFusion, San Diego, CA) are approved and commercially available for use in neonatal/pediatric (<35 kg) and pediatric/adult populations (>35 kg), respectively.

Classification of Ventilators by Use

Ventilators may also be categorized by the setting in which they are used, specifically critical care, subacute, home care and long-term care, and transport. Their designs match the needs of the population as well as the unique characteristics of the setting in which they are used. Ventilator manufacturers have paid particular attention to economic constraints health care facilities are facing. Innovations in ventilator design have broadened their use across settings. An example of this is the use of ventilators for different patient ages. Although ventilators will not be subcategorized as adult or pediatric in this chapter, is it crucial for the practitioner to be aware of the factors such as minimal tidal volume limits, trigger sensitivity, response time, and availability of leak compensation when selecting a ventilator for use with the pediatric population.

Critical Care Ventilators

Critical care ventilators provide clinicians with sophisticated methods for breath delivery. This class of ventilators also provides advanced monitoring capabilities and tools that enable clinicians to readily assess the patient–ventilator interaction. Calculations of lung mechanics parameters including auto-PEEP, static and dynamic compliance, inspiratory/expiratory resistance, rapid shallow breathing index, time constant, and work of breathing are integrated into ventilators used in this environment. Integrated physiologic noninvasive and invasive assessment tools, such as esophageal pressure monitoring and end-tidal CO_2 monitoring are also commercially available. The availability of these features equips bedside caregivers with the tools needed to assess patient–ventilator interaction and match ventilator capability with physiologic need.

Subacute Care Ventilators

Generally, mechanically ventilated patients in this setting have a stable cardiopulmonary status. Their condition is such that the care provided in this setting does not depend heavily on high-technology monitoring or complex diagnostic procedures. Rather, the focus is on coordinated services aimed at managing complex medical conditions, liberation from ventilatory support, and rehabilitation services. Ventilators used in this care venue have less sophisticated monitoring systems and mode options. Subacute care may be rendered in freestanding facilities or within a specialized unit within a hospital. As a result, the design of ventilators used in this environment bridge the gap between those designed specifically for critical care and those designed for home care and extended skilled care. As one example of this category of ventilators, The Savina (Dräger Medical, Telford, PA) offers some features of critical care ventilators, such as graphic display of pressure, volume, and flow waveforms, and the availability of a noninvasive ventilation mode of operation. The availability of a low-pressure oxygen option enables oxygen delivery independent of a central gas supply. An oxygen concentrator can be used to supply oxygen to the patient breathing circuit. This is analogous to oxygen delivery methods used by ventilators in the home care and long-term care environment.

Home Care Ventilators

Patients with chronic respiratory failure from primary pulmonary disease, trauma, or neuromuscular disease may require ventilatory assistance to augment or replace spontaneous breathing and maintain life. Ventilators designed for use in the home or at long-term care institutions facilitate the transition of patients from the acute and subacute care environment to one focusing on enhancing the individual's quality of life, and provision of services to sustain or improve physical and physiologic function in a cost-efficient manner. Ventilators must be able to support the ventilatory needs of the patient and provide supplemental oxygen in a venue where compressed gas resources are limited, power supply interruptions may occur, and patient mobility needs must be met. The interface on this type of ventilator is much simpler than those found on ventilators used in critical or subacute care. The availability of a low-pressure input port is an essential feature that allows supplemental oxygen to be delivered by stationary and portable devices commonly used in the home, such as oxygen concentrators, small high-pressure tanks, and portable liquid oxygen reservoirs. Machine dimensions are also an important consideration, and this type of ventilator is generally compact in nature. The option to lock operator-set parameters minimizes the occurrence of inadvertent setting changes and concomitant alterations in alveolar ventilation and acid-base balance.

Ventilators used in home care and extended care facilities require not only an internal battery for brief power interruptions, but connections for an external battery when the power supply is interrupted for extended periods of time due to natural disasters, man-made occurrences, and participation in academic, employment, or recreational activities. The Carina home ventilator (Dräger Medical) is an example of a home ventilator that can provide invasive or noninvasive ventilation. Although the ventilator's primary power source is 100-V or 240-V AC, the internal battery provides patients with approximately 2 hours of power. There is also an external battery pack that offers an additional 10-hour power supply when fully charged.

Transport Ventilators

Transport ventilators share attributes common to ventilators used in the home and critical care environments. It is necessary for this ventilator type to be lightweight, compact, durable, maintained on a reliable power supply, and have low compressed gas consumption. The ventilator interface should be easy to navigate, allowing the clinician to set or change parameters prior to or during movement to and from a prescribed destination. Operator-set and monitored data should be visible under optimal conditions or conditions of low ambient light. These characteristics enhance patient safety and minimize the potential for complications or adverse effects to occur during air or ground transport. Monitoring is also an important consideration. Clinical practice guidelines recommend the level of monitoring during patient transport be analogous with that provided to the patient during stationary care. Modern transport ventilators provide the ability to display scalar waveforms and numerical data. The BioMed Crossvent 4+ (BioMed Devices, Inc. Guilford, Conn.) is an example of a ventilator that can be used to transport critically ill patients of any age, from infant to adult. This particular ventilator may be configured with a blender, to allow for the delivery of a range of oxygen concentrations from 21% to 100% or with an air-entrainment unit that delivers either 50% or 100% oxygen without the need for an external air supply source. Pressure-controlled and volume-controlled ventilation may be provided in the CMV, IMV, or CSV mode. Tidal volumes may be adjusted from 5 to

2500 mL and flow delivered at rates up to 120 L/minute. The internal battery offers 6 hours of uninterrupted power when fully charged. This unit is small (28 cm × 25.4 cm × 14 cm) and weighs less than 5 kg. The unit's main display screen is color and backlit for enhanced visibility.

Noninvasive Ventilators

Noninvasive ventilation is used across the continuum of care—from critical care to home care—with individuals of any age. As previously mentioned, a noninvasive ventilation feature may be incorporated in critical care ventilators (e.g., SERVO-i and Puritan Bennett 840), subacute ventilators (Savina), and home care ventilators (Carina). However, standalone noninvasive ventilators exist and are extensively used in a variety of settings from the hospital to home. In the acute and critical care setting, noninvasive ventilators have been used to reduce complications associated with diagnostic procedures, such as bronchoscopy, as well as in the treatment of acute respiratory insufficiency, respiratory failure and prevention of postextubation failure. This technology has also been associated with positive outcomes in the outpatient setting. The literature reports the use of noninvasive ventilation to restore and maintain adequate alveolar ventilation with individuals compromised by neuromuscular disorders, congestive heart failure, chronic obstructive lung disease, and sleep-disordered breathing.

There are features common to home and hospital-grade units that enhance patient comfort and promote adherence to therapy. Ramp time allows the clinician to program a delay in the initiation of a delivered inspiratory pressure. Ramp time is usually adjustable (e.g., 0 to 45 minutes), during which the patient breathes at a preset or operator-set expiratory pressure (e.g., 4 cm H_2O). Likewise, rise time can be altered to reduce pressure overshoot and enhance breath delivery. The ability to detect and quantify interface leak, estimated tidal volume, and minute ventilation delivery are additional helpful tools. Hospital-grade units have the capability to display patient data in graphic and numeric form. Clinicians are able to view pressure, flow, and scalar waveforms, for example, on the BiPAP Vision (Respironics Inc., Murrysville, PA). As with critical care ventilators, careful analysis of waveforms may assist clinicians in the identification and correction of patient–ventilator synchrony.

SUMMARY CHECKLIST

- Ventilators can be described in terms of their input power requirements (e.g., electrical or pneumatic) and how the input power is transformed into desired outputs of pressure, volume, and flow.
- A key feature of a ventilator is the variety of modes of ventilation it offers.
- A mode of ventilation is a predetermined pattern of interaction with the patient. Modes are given many confusing names but they can be understood using a simple classification system.
- Mode classification is based on identifying 3 main components: the primary control variable, the breath sequence, and the targeting schemes used for mandatory and spontaneous breaths.
- Pressure control means that pressure delivery is predetermined by a targeting scheme such that inspiratory pressure is either proportional to patient effort or has a particular waveform regardless of respiratory system mechanics. Volume control means that inspiratory flow and volume delivery are predetermined by a targeting scheme to have particular waveforms independent of respiratory system mechanics.
- A spontaneous breath is one for which the timing and size of the breath is determined by the patient (i.e., inspiration is patient triggered and patient cycled). A mandatory breath is one for which the patient cannot determine the timing and/or size of the breath (i.e., inspiration is machine triggered and/or machine cycled).
- Spontaneous breaths may be assisted (meaning that the ventilator provides some portion of the work of breathing) or unassisted. Mandatory breaths are generally assisted.
- The breath sequence of a mode is the pattern of mandatory versus spontaneous breaths. Continuous spontaneous ventilation (CSV) means that all breaths delivered by the ventilator are spontaneous. Intermittent mandatory ventilation (IMV) means that spontaneous breaths can occur between mandatory breaths. Continuous mandatory ventilation means that spontaneous breaths cannot occur between mandatory breaths.
- The targeting scheme is a description of the relation between operator settings and ventilator outputs for a mode. Currently, all modes can be classified as having one of six targeting schemes (set-point, dual, servo, adaptive, optimal, and intelligent).
- Ventilators can also be categorized by the settings in which they are used. Examples include: critical care, subacute care, home care, transport, and noninvasive ventilators.

References

1. Chatburn RL, Primiano FP, Jr: A new system for understanding modes of mechanical ventilation. *Respir Care* 46:604, 2001.
2. Chatburn RL: Classification of ventilator modes: update and proposal for implementation. *Respir Care* 52(3):301–323, 2007.
3. Chatburn RL: Understanding mechanical ventilators. *Expert Rev Respir Med* 4(6):809–819, 2010.
4. Morris W: *The American heritage dictionary of the English language*, Boston, 1975, American Heritage and Houghton Mifflin.
5. Volsko TA, Chatburn RL, El-Khatib MF: *Equipment for respiratory care*, ed 1, Sudbury, MA, 2014, Jones and Bartlett.
6. Chatburn RL: Classification of mechanical ventilators. In Tobin MJ, editor: *Principles and practice of mechanical ventilation*, ed 3, New York, 2012, McGraw-Hill.
7. Morch ET: History of mechanical ventilation. In Kirby RR, Smith RA, Desautels DA, editors: *Mechanical ventilation*, New York, 1985, Churchill Livingstone.
8. Russell DF, Ross DG, Manson HJ: Fluidic cycling devices for inspiratory and expiratory timing in automatic ventilators. *J Biomech Eng* 5:227, 1983.
9. de Wit M: Monitoring of patient-ventilator interaction at the bedside. *Respir Care* 56:61–72, 2011.
10. Henderson WR, Sheel AW: Pulmonary mechanics during mechanical ventilation. *Respir Physiol Neurobiol* 180:162–172, 2012.

11. Grooms DA, Sibole SH, Tomlinson JR, et al: Customization of an open-lung ventilation strategy to treat a case of life-threatening acute respiratory distress syndrome. *Respir Care* 56:514–519, 2011.
12. Wachter SB, Johnson K, Albert R, et al: The evaluation of a pulmonary display to detect adverse respiratory events using high resolution human simulator. *J Am Med Inform Assoc* 13(6):635–642, 2006.
13. MacIntyre NR, Branson RD: *Mechanical ventilation*, ed 2, St. Louis, 2009, Saunders Elsevier.
14. Görges M, Markewitz BA, Westenskow DR: Improving alarm performance in the medical intensive care unit using delays and clinical context. *Anesth Analg* 108(5):1546–1552, 2009.
15. Siebig S, Kuhls S, Imhoff M, et al: Intensive care unit alarms—how many do we need? *Crit Care Med* 38(2):451–456, 2010.
16. Volsko TA, Hoffman J, Conger A, et al: The effect of targeting scheme on tidal volume delivery during volume control mechanical ventilation. *Respir Care* 57(8):1297–1304, 2012.
17. Chatburn RL, Carlo WA: A taxonomy for mechanical ventilation. In Berhardt LV, editor: *Advances in biology and medicine* (vol 78). Hauppange, NY, 2014, Nova Scientific Publishers, Inc. (eBook).
18. Chatburn RL, Khatib ME, Mireles-Cabodevila E: A taxonomy for mechanical ventilation: 10 fundamental maxims. *Respir Care* 2014. [Epub ahead of print]; pii: respcare.03057.
19. Chatburn RL, Volsko TA, Hazy J, et al: Determining the basis for a taxonomy of mechanical ventilation. *Respir Care* 57:514–524, 2012.
20. Marini JJ, Rodriguez RM, Lamb V: The inspiratory workload of patient-initiated mechanical ventilation. *Am Rev Respir Dis* 134(5):902–909, 1986.
21. Chatburn RL, Daoud EG: Ventilation. In Kacmarek RM, Stoller JK, Heuer AH, editors: *Egan's fundamentals of respiratory care*, ed 10, St. Louis, 2012, Mosby Elsevier.
22. Sassoon CSH: Triggering of the ventilator in patient-ventilator interactions. *Respir Care* 56:39–48, 2011.
23. Rodarte JR, Rehder K: Dynamics of respiration. In Fishman AP, Macklem PT, Mead J, et al, editors: *Handbook of Physiology. The Respiratory System. Volume III, Mechanics of Breathing, Part 1*, Bethesda, Md, 1986, American Physiological Society.
24. Chatburn RL, Volsko TA: Documentation issues for mechanical ventilation in pressure-control modes. *Respir Care* 55:1705–1716, 2011.
25. Babic MD, Chatburn RL, Stoller JK: Laboratory evaluation of the Vortran Automatic Resuscitator Model RTM. *Respir Care* 52:1718–1727, 2007.
26. Chatburn RL, Mireles-Cabodevila E: Closed-loop control of mechanical ventilation: description and classification of targeting schemes. *Respir Care* 56:85–102, 2011.
27. Amato MB, Barbas CS, Bonassa J, et al: Volume-assured pressure support ventilation (VAPSV). A new approach for reducing muscle workload during acute respiratory failure. *Chest* 102:1225–1234, 1992.
28. Mutch WA, Harms S, Ruth GM, et al: Biologically variable or naturally noisy mechanical ventilation recruits atelectatic lung. *Am J Respir Crit Care Med* 162:319–323, 2000.
29. Spieth PM, Güldner A, Beda A, et al: Comparative effects of proportional assist and variable pressure support ventilation on lung function and damage in experimental lung injury. *Crit Care Med* 40:2654–2661, 2012.
30. Mireles-Cabodevila E, Chatburn RL: Work of breathing in adaptive pressure control continuous mandatory ventilation. *Respir Care* 54:1467–1472, 2009.
31. Mireles-Cabodevila E, Hatipoglu U, Chatburn RL: A rational framework for selecting modes of ventilation. *Respir Care* 58(2):348–366, 2013.

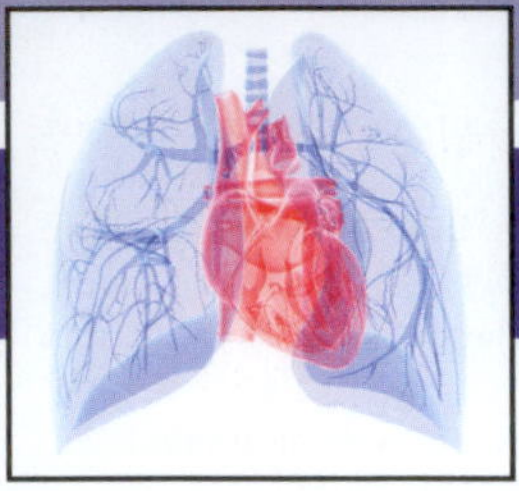

CHAPTER 46

Physiology of Ventilatory Support

ROBERT M. KACMAREK

CHAPTER OBJECTIVES

After reading this chapter you will be able to:

- Discuss the pressures and pressure gradients that affect gas delivery during spontaneous breathing, negative pressure ventilation (NPV), and positive pressure ventilation (PPV).
- Identify the effects of mechanical ventilation on oxygenation, ventilation, and lung mechanics.
- Describe the currently available modes of mechanical ventilation.
- Discuss the indications and physiologic effect of positive end expiratory pressure (PEEP).
- Describe the cardiovascular effects of PPV and NPV.
- Describe the effects of PPV on intracranial pressure, renal function, liver and splanchnic perfusion, gastrointestinal function, and central nervous system.
- Identify and list the complications and hazards of providing mechanical ventilatory support.
- Discuss how to minimize adverse effects of mechanical ventilation.

CHAPTER OUTLINE

Pressure and Pressure Gradients
- Airway, Alveolar, and Intrathoracic Pressure, Volume, and Flow During Spontaneous Ventilation
- Airway, Alveolar, and Intrathoracic Pressure, Volume, and Flow During Negative Pressure Mechanical Ventilation
- Airway, Alveolar, and Intrathoracic Pressure, Volume, and Flow During Positive Pressure Mechanical Ventilation

Effects of Mechanical Ventilation on Ventilation
- Minute Ventilation
- Increased Alveolar Ventilation
- Ventilation/Perfusion Ratio
- Alveolar and Arterial Carbon Dioxide
- Acid-Base Balance

Effects of Mechanical Ventilation on Oxygenation
- Inspired Oxygen
- Alveolar Oxygen and Alveolar Air Equation
- Arterial Oxygenation and Oxygen Content
- Decreased Shunt
- Increased Tissue Oxygen Delivery

Effects of Positive Pressure Mechanical Ventilation on Lung Mechanics
- Time Constants
- Increased Pressure
  - *Mean Airway Pressure*
  - *Effect of Peak Airway Pressure on Lung Recruitment*
- Increased Lung Volume: Tidal Volume
- Increased Functional Residual Capacity
- Pressure-Volume Curve and Lung Recruitment in Acute Respiratory Distress Syndrome
- Increased Dead Space
- Decreased Work of Breathing

Minimizing Adverse Pulmonary Effects of Positive Pressure Mechanical Ventilation
- Decreasing Pressure
- Positive End Expiratory Pressure or Continuous Positive Airway Pressure
- Effects of Ventilatory Pattern
- Trigger Site and Work of Breathing

Physiologic Effects of Ventilatory Modes
- Volume-Controlled Ventilation Versus Pressure-Controlled Ventilation
- Continuous Mandatory Ventilation
  - *Volume-Controlled Continuous Mandatory Ventilation*
  - *Pressure-Controlled Continuous Mandatory Ventilation*
  - *Pressure-Controlled Inverse Ratio Ventilation*
- Intermittent Mandatory Ventilation

KEY TERMS

aerophagia
autoregulation
atelectrauma
barotrauma
biotrauma
mean airway pressure
passive
patient-ventilator asynchrony
time constant
transairway pressure
transalveolar pressure
trans–chest wall pressure
transdiaphragmatic pressure
transpulmonary pressure
transrespiratory pressure
transthoracic pressure
volutrauma

Mechanical ventilation can be beneficial or detrimental depending on how it is applied and modified as the patient's condition changes. Respiratory therapists (RTs) must be able to anticipate the physiologic effects of mechanical ventilation and respond appropriately when complications arise. This chapter familiarizes the reader with (1) the physiologic effects of mechanical ventilation on lung and cardiovascular function and other body systems, (2) the basic approaches to providing mechanical ventilation, and (3) the complications and hazards of mechanical ventilation. A solid understanding of the normal physiology of breathing is essential for all RTs, especially when working with patients receiving mechanical ventilation. RTs must understand intrathoracic pressure changes associated with spontaneous, negative pressure, and positive pressure breathing. Intrathoracic pressure changes are necessary for ventilation to occur; however, large changes in these pressures may also induce physiologic changes in other systems.

PRESSURE AND PRESSURE GRADIENTS

For gas to flow through the airway, a pressure gradient must exist. The airways begin at the mouth and end at the alveoli, so mouth pressure (*pressure at the airway opening* [P_{awo}]) and *alveolar pressure* (P_{alv}) are important in describing gas flow, as are *intrapleural pressure* (P_{pl}) and *body surface pressure* or atmospheric pressure (P_{bs}). In addition, *intraabdominal pressure* (P_{ab}) affects the impact of P_{pl} change on diaphragm movement. P_{pl} is the pressure in the pleural space, the virtual space between the visceral and parietal pleurae, and is usually negative in relation to P_{alv}. Figure 46-1 shows a graphic model of the respiratory system with these pressures identified as points in space. The respiratory system is everything that exists between the airway opening and the body surface. The associated pressure difference is **transrespiratory pressure** (P_{TR}), defined as $P_{awo} - P_{bs}$. The components of transrespiratory pressure correspond to the

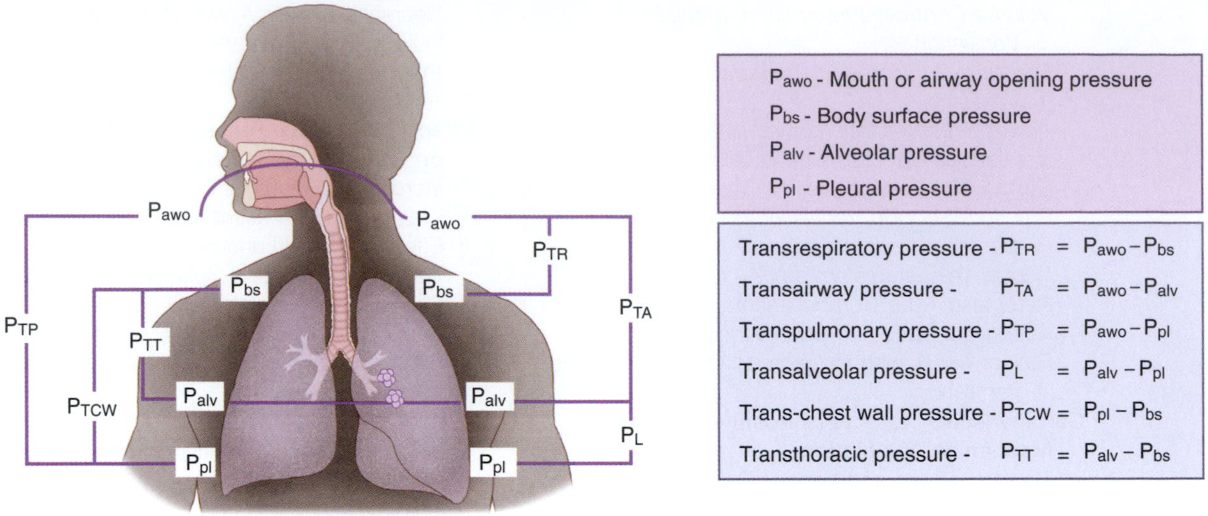

FIGURE 46-1 Pressures and pressure gradients in the lung. Airflow is a function of the transairway pressure (P_{ta}), which is the pressure gradient between the airway (P_{awo}) and the alveoli (P_{alv}). Transalveolar pressure (P_L) maintains alveolar inflation, and transpulmonary pressure (P_{tp}) is the pressure needed to expand the lungs and chest wall.

TABLE 46-1

Changes in Airway Pressure Gradients during Spontaneous, Negative, and Positive Pressure Ventilation

Pressure (cm H_2O) Ventilation Type	Transpulmonary Pressure	Transthoracic Pressure	Transairway Pressure	Transrespiratory Pressure
Spontaneous				
Inspiration	Small increase (+)	Increase (+)	Increase (+)	Constant (–)
Expiration	Small increase (–)	Increase (–)	Increase (–)	Constant (+)
Negative (NPV)				
Inspiration	Small increase (+)	Increase (+)	Increase (+)	Constant (–)
Expiration	Small increase (–)	Increase (–)	Increase (–)	Constant (+)
Positive (PPV)				
Inspiration	Small increase (+)	Increase (+)	Increase (+)	Increase (+)
Expiration	Decrease (–)	Decrease (–)	Decrease (–)	Decrease (–)

components of the graphic model. The airways are represented by **transairway pressure** (P_{TA}), defined as $P_{awo} - P_{alv}$. The lungs are represented by the **transalveolar pressure:** ($P_L = P_{alv} - P_{pl}$). However, clinically what can be measured is **transpulmonary pressure:** ($P_{TP} = P_{awo} - P_{pl}$). The chest wall is represented by **trans–chest wall pressure:** ($P_{TCW} = P_{pl} - P_{bs}$). If the lungs and chest wall are lumped together, they can be represented by **transthoracic pressure:** ($P_{TT} = P_{alv} - P_{bs}$).

Another pressure gradient not defined in Figure 46-1 that also affects gas movement is the **transdiaphragmatic pressure** (P_{di}). This pressure gradient is the difference between intraabdominal pressure and pleural pressure and affects diaphragmatic movement: ($P_{pl} - P_{ab}$).

Airway, Alveolar, and Intrathoracic Pressure, Volume, and Flow During Spontaneous Ventilation

Spontaneous breathing is normally an autonomic phenomenon. In other words, we do not think about breathing; it is controlled by the autonomic nervous system. Not until our breathing is stressed do we consider the effort to breathe or the energy expended. At end-exhalation, intrapleural pressure is slightly negative. Alveolar, mouth, and body surface pressures are zero. The diaphragm contracts in response to stimulation of the phrenic nerve via the respiratory center in the medulla of the brain. When the diaphragm contracts, it descends into the abdominal cavity, decreasing intrapleural pressure. When intrapleural pressure becomes more negative, alveolar pressure becomes negative as well. The effects of spontaneous breathing on the pressure gradients are shown in Table 46-1. Under normal circumstances, a decrease in intrapleural pressure results in decreased alveolar pressure, increased transairway pressure, and inspiration of the tidal volume (V_T) (Figure 46-2).

At end-inspiration, alveolar pressure returns to zero when the muscles of inspiration stop contracting. Lung recoil causes a sudden increase in alveolar pressure in relation to pressure at the mouth, reversing the transairway pressure gradient, and air

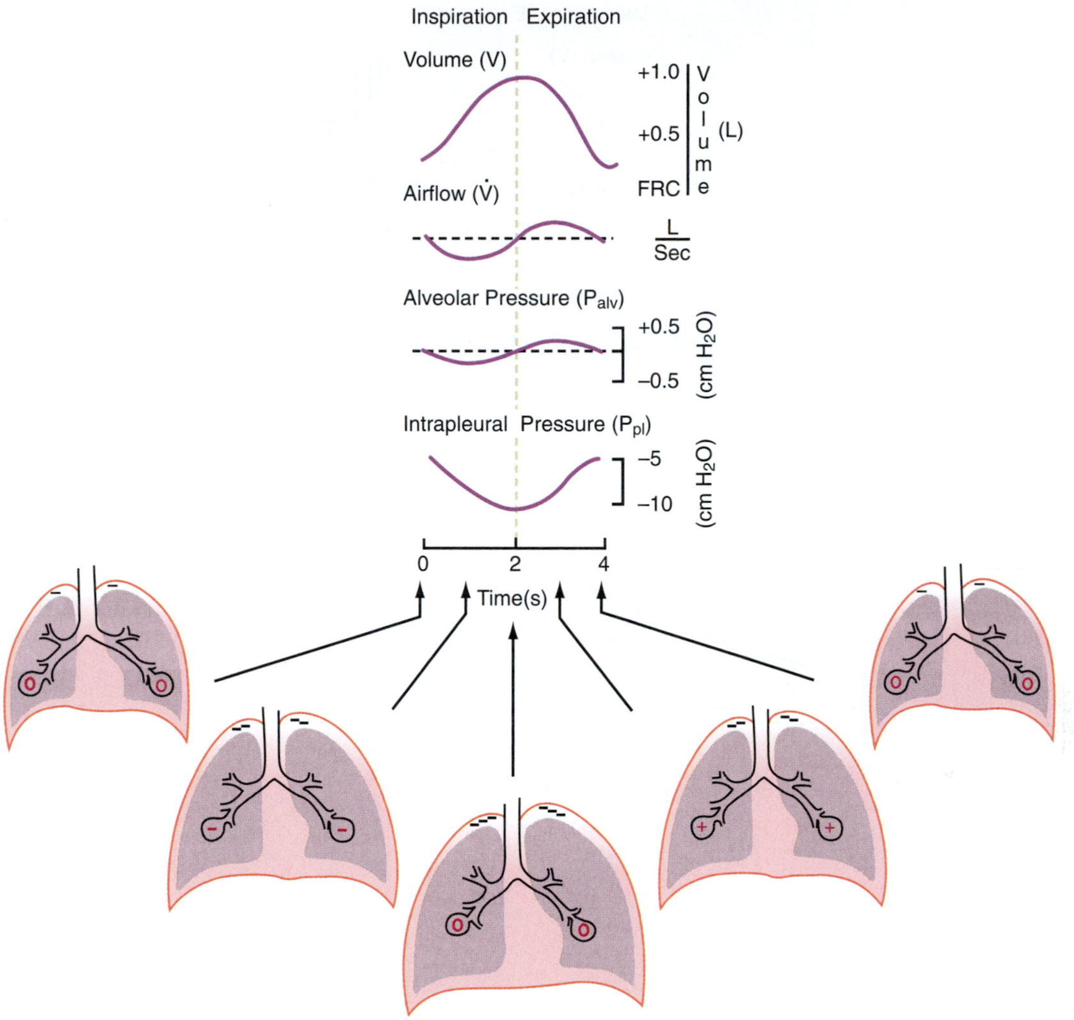

FIGURE 46-2 Changes in pressure, volume, and flow during a single spontaneous breath. (Modified from Martin L: Pulmonary physiology in clinical practice: the essentials for patient care and evaluation, St Louis, 1987, Mosby.)

flows out of the lungs. Normally, there is a short end expiratory pause before the next inspiration.

V_T and flow during spontaneous ventilation may be described by the equation of motion.[1,2] The equation of motion describes the relationship between muscle pressure (analogous to pleural pressure in spontaneous breathing), compliance, resistance, flow, and volume as follows:

$$P_{musc} = \text{Volume/Compliance} + (\text{Resistance} \times \text{Flow})$$

where P_{musc} is muscle pressure (P_{tp}), volume is tidal volume, compliance is lung-thorax compliance, resistance is airway resistance, and flow is gas flow through the airway. When the equation is rearranged, volume inhaled during spontaneous ventilation is proportional to muscle pressure and lung-thorax compliance and inversely related to the product of airway resistance and flow:

$$\text{Volume} = [P_{musc}/(\text{Resistance} \times \text{Flow})] + \text{Compliance}$$

Ventilation (owing to transpulmonary pressure) is the sum of the pressure needed to move gas through the airways (transairway pressure) and the pressure needed to inflate the alveoli (transalveolar pressure):

$$\text{Transpulmonary pressure} = P_{ta} + P_{alv}$$

Airway, Alveolar, and Intrathoracic Pressure, Volume, and Flow During Negative Pressure Mechanical Ventilation (NPV)

Mechanical NPV is similar to spontaneous breathing. NPV decreases pleural pressure (P_{pl}) during inspiration by exposing the chest to subatmospheric pressure. Negative pressure at the body surface (P_{bs}) is transmitted first to the pleural space and then to the alveoli (P_{alv}). Because the airway opening remains exposed to atmospheric pressure during NPV, a transairway pressure gradient is created. Gas flows from the relatively high pressure at the airway opening (zero) to the relatively low pressure in the alveoli (negative). As with spontaneous breathing, alveolar expansion during NPV is determined by the magnitude of the transpulmonary pressure gradient. During expiration in

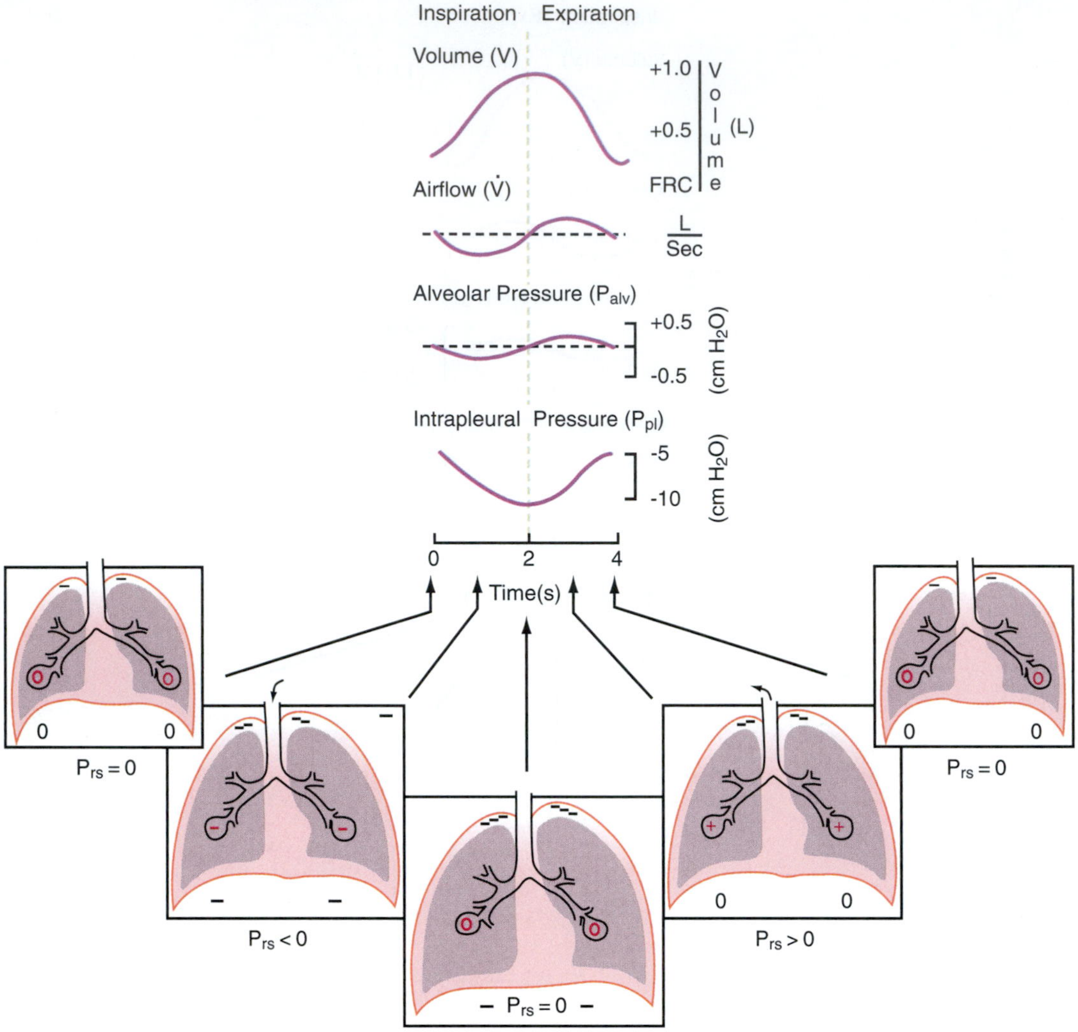

FIGURE 46-3 Changes in pressure, volume, and flow during a single mechanical negative pressure breath. The box surrounding the lungs represents the enclosure formed by the negative pressure ventilator. *Prs,* Pressure of the respiratory system. (Modified from Martin L: Pulmonary physiology in clinical practice: the essentials for patient care and evaluation, St Louis, 1987, Mosby.)

both spontaneous breathing and NPV, the lungs and chest wall passively recoil to their resting end expiratory levels. As this recoil occurs, pleural pressure becomes less negative, and alveolar pressure increases above atmospheric pressure (Figure 46-3). This increase in alveolar pressure reverses the transairway pressure gradient. As P_{alv} becomes greater than P_{awo}, gas flows from the alveoli to the airway opening. The effects of NPV on the pressure gradients are shown in Table 46-1.

Volume and flow during NPV also are described by the equation of motion except transairway pressure developed by the ventilator fully or partially replaces the patient's respiratory muscle pressure as follows:

$$P_{musc} + P_{vent} = \text{Volume/Compliance} + (\text{Resistance} \times \text{Flow})$$

In this equation, P_{vent} is the pressure the ventilator develops to overcome the patient's lung-thorax compliance and airway resistance to deliver the V_T. In this case, P_{vent} is negative but is the driving force behind decreasing the intrapleural pressure and increasing the transairway and transpulmonary pressures.

Physiologic complications associated with NPV are uncommon because NPV simulates normal spontaneous breathing. The most common problems with NPV are related to interference with caring for the patient caused by the device surrounding the chest (the iron lung or chest cuirass). Supplemental oxygen (O_2) cannot be provided to the patient through the negative pressure ventilator. Depending on patient need, low-flow or high-flow O_2 delivery devices must be used to provide O_2 therapy. Immediate access to patients requiring routine or emergent medical care may be difficult in systems that enclose the entire thorax and lower body, such as the iron lung and Porta-Lung (Respironics Inc, Murrysville, PA) (see Chapter 49). These systems may impede venous return by creating a negative pressure in the abdomen and lower half of the body, which may lead to hypotension, a phenomenon known as "tank shock." The risk of glottis closure and the development of obstructive sleep apnea have been reported in association with NPV of patients with chronic obstructive pulmonary disease (COPD) and neuromuscular dysfunction.

Airway, Alveolar, and Intrathoracic Pressure, Volume, and Flow During Positive Pressure Mechanical Ventilation (PPV)

PPV causes air to flow into the lungs because of an increase in airway pressure, not a decrease in pleural pressure as occurs during spontaneous breathing and NPV (Figure 46-4). However, similar to spontaneous breathing and NPV, PPV causes an increase in P_{tp}, which allows gas to flow into the lungs. Gas flows into the lungs because pressure at the airway opening (P_{awo}) is positive, and alveolar pressure (P_{alv}) is initially zero or less positive. Alveolar pressure rapidly increases during the inspiratory phase of PPV. The increased alveolar pressure expands the airways and alveoli. Because alveolar pressure is greater than pleural pressure (P_{pl}) during PPV, positive pressure is transmitted from the alveoli to the pleural space, causing pleural pressure to increase during inspiration. Depending on the compliance and resistance of the lungs, pleural pressure may markedly exceed atmospheric pressure during a portion of inspiration. These changes in pleural pressure during PPV can lead to significant physiologic changes (see later section). Pressure gradients during PPV are similar to pressure gradients during spontaneous breathing and NPV except that they are created by a positive pressure at the airway opening instead of a negative pressure in the pleural space (see Table 46-1). All pressure gradients change in the same direction as during NPV and spontaneous breathing except the transrespiratory pressure, which changes in the opposite direction.

Similar to spontaneous breathing, the recoil force of the lungs and chest wall, stored as potential energy during the positive pressure breath, causes passive exhalation. As gas flows from the alveoli to the airway opening, alveolar pressure decreases to atmospheric level, while pleural pressure is restored to its normal subatmospheric level (see Figure 46-4).

Volume and flow during PPV are also described by the equation of motion. The magnitude of P_{vent} not only depends on the patient's lung mechanics but also on the P_{musc} of the patient. If the patient makes no effort, P_{vent} is responsible for all volume and flow. During volume-controlled ventilation, as muscle

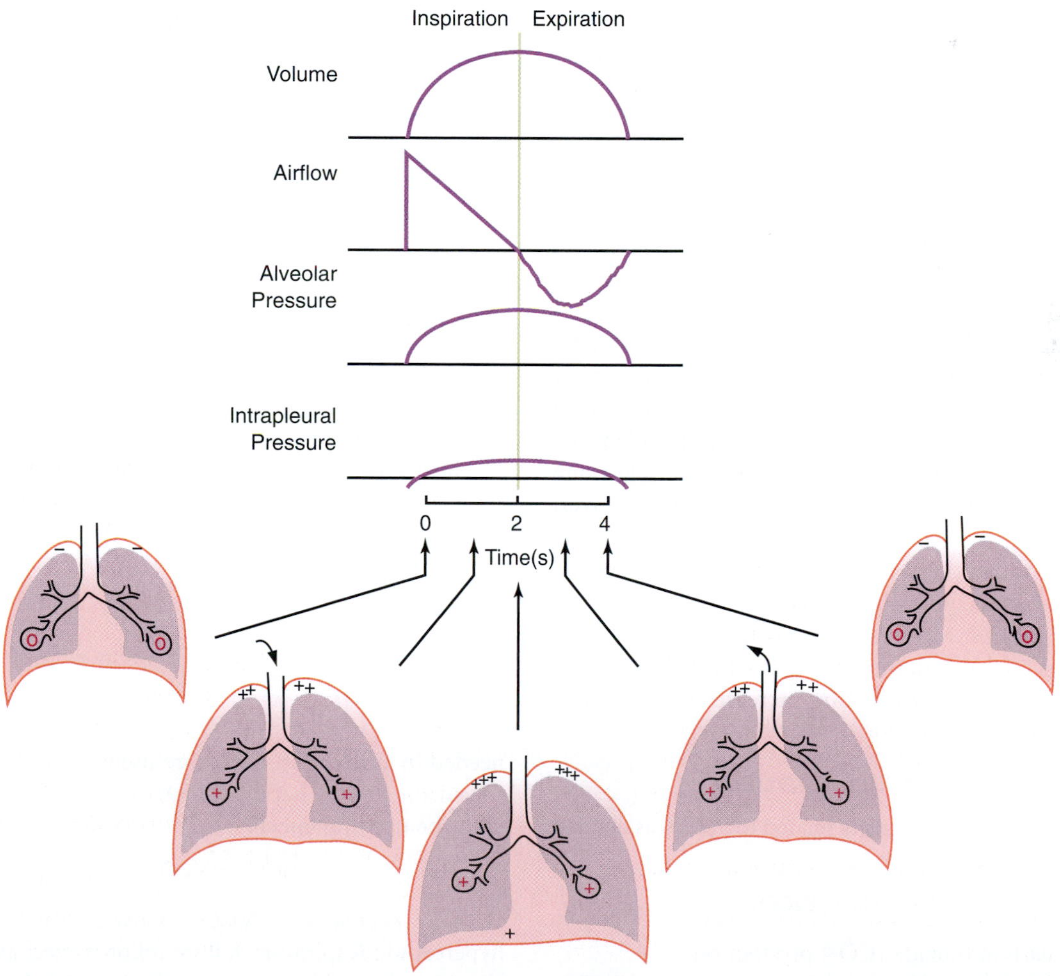

FIGURE 46-4 Changes in pressure, volume, and flow during a single decelerating flow, positive pressure breath. *Arrows* into and out of the trachea represent airflow. (Modified from Martin L: Pulmonary physiology in clinical practice: the essentials for patient care and evaluation, St Louis, 1987, Mosby.)

effort increases, P_{vent} decreases, and V_T remains constant. During pressure-controlled ventilation, as P_{musc} increases, V_T increases, and P_{vent} remains unchanged.

RULE OF THUMB

Ideally, the tranpulmonary pressure should be as low as possible during mechanical ventilation. A transpulmonary pressure less than about 28 cm H_2O minimizes the development of ventilator-induced lung injury. If the plateau pressure is kept less than 28 cm H_2O, the transalveolar pressure can never exceed this level during controlled ventilation.

EFFECTS OF MECHANICAL VENTILATION ON VENTILATION

Minute Ventilation

The primary indication for mechanical ventilation is *hypercapnic respiratory failure,* also known as *ventilatory failure.* For patients with acute ventilatory failure, the goal of mechanical ventilation is improving alveolar ventilation to compensate for the patient's inability to maintain normal $PaCO_2$. $PaCO_2$ is inversely related to alveolar ventilation, which is related to minute ventilation. Minute ventilation ($\dot{V}_E$) is the product of tidal volume (V_T) and ventilatory rate (f):

$$\dot{V} = V_T \times f$$

Use of a mechanical ventilator usually implies a change in V_T, ventilatory rate, or both from preintubation values. A normal spontaneous V_T is approximately 5 to 7 ml/kg. The currently accepted V_T for mechanical ventilation in acute respiratory failure is 4 to 8 ml/kg predicted body weight (PBW). These volumes are based on predicted body weight. The mechanical ventilator rate depends on the patient's status. For postoperative ventilation, a rate of 12 to 20 breaths/min may be adequate. Conditions that necessitate a higher initial rate include acute respiratory distress syndrome (ARDS), pulmonary fibrosis, acutely increased intracranial pressure (ICP) (with caution; see later), and metabolic acidosis. Conditions that may necessitate a lower rate include acute asthma exacerbation, to allow an increased expiratory time to minimize air trapping. When an appropriate V_T is established, the set rate is adjusted to achieve desired $PaCO_2$. Mechanical ventilation increases minute ventilation by increasing V_T, ventilator rate, or both.

Increased Alveolar Ventilation

Alveolar ventilation ($\dot{V}_A$) is inversely related to $PaCO_2$ as defined by the following relationship:

$$\dot{V}_A = (\dot{V}CO_2 \times 0.863)/PaCO_2$$

where $\dot{V}CO_2$ is carbon dioxide (CO_2) production.[2]

As alveolar ventilation decreases, $PaCO_2$ increases. As CO_2 production increases, alveolar ventilation must increase to maintain the same $PaCO_2$. Mechanical ventilation may be needed in either case. It is more useful to look at this equation solved for $PaCO_2$ because changes in $PaCO_2$ usually correlate with the need for mechanical ventilation:

$$PaCO_2 = (\dot{V}CO_2 \times 0.863)/\dot{V}_A$$

If $\dot{V}_A$ decreases or $\dot{V}CO_2$ increases, $PaCO_2$ increases, and hypercapnic respiratory failure follows; mechanical ventilation may be indicated in this setting. Because mechanical ventilation increases ventilation, $PaCO_2$ can be decreased to the desired level depending on the total ventilatory rate.

MINI CLINI

Alveolar, Transpulmonary, and Transalveolar Pressures

PROBLEM: Mr. Jones is 58 years old, 5 feet 8 inches tall, and weighs 410 lb and is being ventilated because of ARDS. His current ventilator settings are pressure control mode, peak pressure 35 cm H_2O, PEEP 20 cm H_2O, FiO_2 0.50, respiratory rate 30 breaths/min, and V_T 400 ml. At the end of expiration gas flow returns to zero about 100 msec before the end of the breath. What are the alveolar, transpulmonary, and transalveolar pressures for Mr. Jones?

Solution: Because there is a short end inspiratory pause, it is reasonable to assume that the peak airway pressure in pressure control is equal to the average peak alveolar pressure. The average is used because alveolar units have different time constants and as a result different peak pressure, but when there is end inspiratory equilibration of pressure, the resulting value is the average pressure across all lung units. To be more confident of this value, an additional end inspiratory pause can be added for a single breath to determine better the end inspiratory pause pressure or plateau pressure.

To determine the transpulmonary pressure ($P_{awo} - P_{pl}$) and transalveolar pressure ($P_{alv} - P_{pl}$), an estimate of pleural pressure must be made. The ideal method is to measure the esophageal pressure. Although not exactly equal to the pleural pressure, it accurately reflects changes in pleural pressure. Some authors have also recommended evaluation of bladder pressure, which changes in the same manner as esophageal pressure. The reading from the esophageal catheter at the time an end inspiratory pause was applied was 10 cm H_2O. The transpulmonary pressure and transalveolar pressure are the same: 35 − 10 cm H_2O or 25 cm H_2O. This is because Mr. Jones was ventilated in pressure control, and there was a short end inspiratory pause, so both peak and plateau pressures were equal. However, if he was ventilated in volume ventilation and the peak airway pressure was 45 cm H_2O, while the plateau pressure remained 35 cm H_2O when an end inspiratory pause was added, the transalveolar pressure and transpulmonary pressure would still be the same: 35 − 10 cm H_2O or 25 cm H_2O.

Mr. Jones is receiving lung protective ventilation because his transalveolar pressure is only 25 cm H_2O. The high airway pressures are needed because of his stiff chest wall, which minimizes the transmission of pressure across the lung, reducing lung stretch.

Ventilation/ Perfusion Ratio

Spontaneous ventilation results in gas distribution mainly to the dependent and peripheral zones of the lungs. Controlled PPV tends to reverse this normal pattern of gas distribution, and most of the delivered volume is directed to nondependent lung zones (Figure 46-5). This phenomenon is caused partly by the inactivity of the diaphragm and chest wall during controlled PPV. Although these structures actively facilitate gas movement during spontaneous breathing, inactivity of these structures during controlled PPV impedes ventilation to dependent lung zones. An increase in ventilation to the nondependent zones of the lung, where there is less perfusion, increases the ventilation/perfusion ($\dot{V}/\dot{Q}$) ratio, effectively increasing physiologic dead space. The increase in $P(A - a)O_2$ often observed with PPV is caused by areas of low $\dot{V}/\dot{Q}$ ratio.

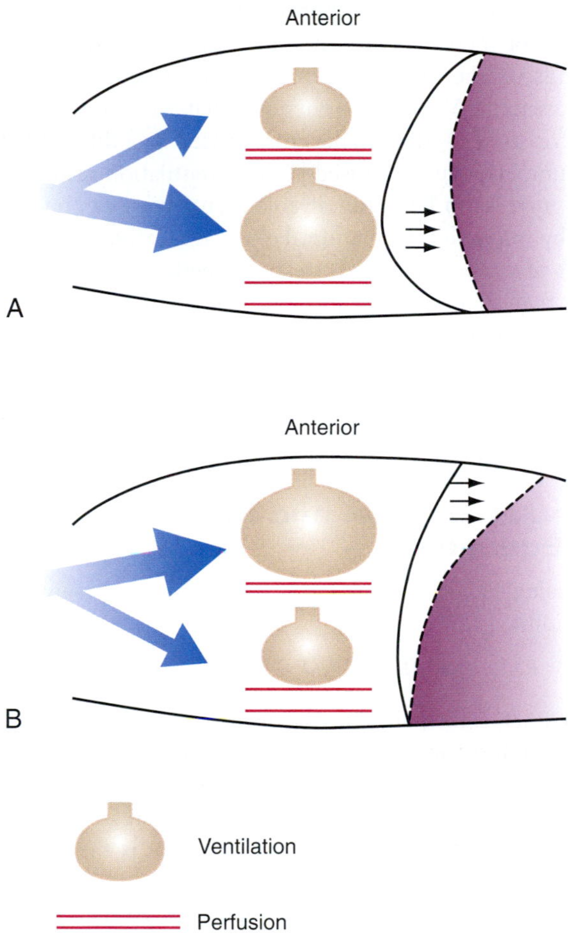

FIGURE 46-5 Effect of spontaneous ventilation and PPV on gas distribution in a supine subject. **A,** During spontaneous ventilation, diaphragmatic action distributes most ventilation to the dependent zones of the lungs, where perfusion is greatest. The result is a nearly normal $\dot{V}/\dot{Q}$ ratio. Partly because of diaphragmatic inactivity, PPV reverses this normal pattern of gas distribution, and most delivered volume is directed to the upper lung zones. **B,** An increase in ventilation to the upper lung zones, where there is less perfusion, increases the $\dot{V}/\dot{Q}$ ratio, effectively increasing physiologic dead space. At the same time, higher alveolar pressure in the better ventilated upper lung zones diverts blood flow away from these areas to the areas receiving the least ventilation. The result is areas of low $\dot{V}/\dot{Q}$ ratio and impaired oxygenation. (Modified from Kirby RR: Clinical application of ventilatory support, New York, 1990, Churchill Livingstone.)

PPV decreases the $\dot{V}/\dot{Q}$ ratio in the bases and dependent lung zones mainly as a result of ventilation being primarily distributed to nondependent lung zones. The $\dot{V}/\dot{Q}$ ratio may also increase in nondependent lung zones because of the effect of PPV on perfusion. PPV can compress the pulmonary capillaries. This compression increases pulmonary vascular resistance and decreases perfusion. Minimal blood flow perfuses the areas with the greatest V_T and contributes to a further increase in dead space. Conversely, blood intended for these areas is diverted to regions with lower vascular resistance—generally more dependent lung regions. Pulmonary blood flow during PPV tends to perfuse the least well-ventilated lung regions. This perfusion decreases the $\dot{V}/\dot{Q}$ ratio in those areas and increases the $P(A - a)O_2$.

Alveolar and Arterial Carbon Dioxide

Normal alveolar carbon dioxide tension ($PACO_2$) is 40 mm Hg, whereas mixed venous blood typically has a $P\bar{v}CO_2$ of 45 mm Hg. Under normal circumstances, CO_2 moves out of the blood at the pulmonary capillary interface; the result is a $PaCO_2$ of 40 mm Hg. In the event of a decrease in alveolar ventilation or an increase in CO_2 production, $PaCO_2$ increases. Mechanical ventilation can increase minute volume and alveolar ventilation and reduce $PACO_2$ and $PaCO_2$. With an increase in V_D/V_T, $PaCO_2$ increases if there is no change in minute volume; this may occur when alveolar blood flow is decreased by acute pulmonary embolism, an excessive level of positive end expiratory pressure (PEEP), or advanced dead space–producing disease such as emphysema or pulmonary embolism.

When excessive PEEP is used, blood flow is diverted from ventilated alveoli to hypoventilated alveoli; the result is an increased $\dot{V}/\dot{Q}$ ratio. In emphysema, formation of bullae is coincident with the destruction of pulmonary capillaries; the result is large areas of poorly perfused but ventilated alveoli. Pulmonary emboli may completely occlude pulmonary vessels; the result is lack of perfusion to alveoli distal to the blockage.

Acid-Base Balance

Respiratory acidemia, defined by a $PaCO_2$ greater than 45 mm Hg and a pH less than 7.35, occurs when minute ventilation and alveolar ventilation per minute ($\dot{V}_A$) are inadequate to meet the needs of the body. Respiratory acidemia can occur when the V_T is low, even though an accompanying mandatory rate is high.

Volume delivery also decreases if high airway pressures develop secondary to volume loss as a result of ventilator circuit tubing compliance (compressible volume loss). Ventilator circuits may have compliance of 1 to 3 ml/cm H_2O, which effectively reduces V_T:

$$\text{Volume lost} = \text{Tubing compliance} \times (\text{Peak pressure} - \text{PEEP})$$

Tubing compliance was a concern with older ventilators; however, most intensive care unit (ICU) ventilators in use at the present time allow the user to compensate for compressible volume loss as a result of tubing compliance. When activated, the volume set is the volume delivered to the patient. This issue is discussed in more detail later in the chapter.

An increase in V_D/V_T ratio can cause a reduction in alveolar ventilation, even though minute ventilation may be normal or increased. These problems emphasize the importance of proper selection of V_T and mandatory rate. When respiratory acidemia exists, the patient may become restless and anxious, resulting in **patient-ventilator asynchrony** (see Chapter 47). A communicative patient may complain of dyspnea. If these symptoms are observed, especially when $PaCO_2$ is increased, minute ventilation generally should be increased.

Respiratory alkalemia occurs if the minute ventilation is too high. It is recognized when $PaCO_2$ is less than 35 mm Hg and pH is greater than 7.45. A patient who is dyspneic, anxious, or in pain may develop this condition; the usual manifestations are an increased ventilatory rate or patient-ventilator asynchrony or both. The ventilator can cause respiratory alkalemia secondary to an inappropriately high V_T or rate. Regardless, the result is excessive minute and alveolar ventilation. This condition requires that the RT adjust the ventilator appropriately and address the patient's pain or anxiety to avoid the systemic effects of a prolonged alkalosis.

Metabolic acidemia in a patient receiving mechanical ventilation is recognized by a normal $PaCO_2$, with a decreased pH (<7.35), decreased bicarbonate level (<22 mEq/L), and increased base excess (<–2 mEq/L). With metabolic acidemia, the patient tries to compensate by increasing minute ventilation to blow off CO_2 in an effort to increase the pH. The resulting increase in work of breathing (WOB) may lead to ventilatory muscle fatigue and continued respiratory failure. The best therapy for metabolic acidosis is to manage the underlying cause while supporting the patient's ventilation as needed. Many patients cannot be liberated from mechanical ventilation until the underlying acidosis is controlled.

Bicarbonate has been used as therapy for metabolic acidosis. If it is administered, bicarbonate quickly combines with hydrogen ions and dissociates to form CO_2 and water, a reaction that may increase WOB. Generally, bicarbonate administration is not recommended until acidosis is severe (pH <7.2). When necessary, bicarbonate is administered according to the following formula:[2]

$$NaHCO_3^- \text{ required} = [\tfrac{1}{4}\text{ Body weight (kg)} \times \text{Base deficit}]/2$$

A temporary measure to compensate partially for metabolic acidosis is to increase minute ventilation during therapy to control the acidosis with the goal of a pH greater than 7.20.

Metabolic alkalemia is defined as a normal $PaCO_2$ with an elevated pH (>7.45) and an increased bicarbonate level (>26 mEq/L) and base excess (>+2 mEq/L). With metabolic alkalemia, in an effort to compensate for the increased pH, the patient tries to decrease minute ventilation. If weaning is attempted when the patient has a metabolic alkalemia, the patient may continue to hypoventilate, and weaning may fail. As with metabolic acidemia, the underlying cause should be determined and managed. Common causes of metabolic alkalosis include hypochloremia or hypokalemia secondary to gastrointestinal loss, diuretics, or steroid administration. See Chapter 14 for details on acid-base balance.

EFFECTS OF MECHANICAL VENTILATION ON OXYGENATION

Inspired Oxygen

Mechanical ventilators usually deliver an increased fractional inspired oxygen (FiO_2) ranging from room air (0.21) to 100% O_2 (1.0). As a result, the alveolar partial pressure of oxygen (PAO_2) and arterial partial pressure of oxygen (PaO_2) may be restored to normal with appropriate management. The effectiveness of increased FiO_2 in the management of hypoxemia depends on the cause of hypoxemia. Hypoxemia caused by a decrease in the $\dot{V}/\dot{Q}$ ratio or hypoventilation is more responsive to increased FiO_2 than hypoxemia caused by a diffusion defect or shunt. Hypoxemia caused by hypoventilation responds well to an increase in FiO_2, but alveolar ventilation can be restored only by improved ventilation. Hypoxemia caused by diffusion defect and shunt generally respond better to an increase in PEEP than to an increase in FiO_2. The fact that PaO_2 responds well to increased FiO_2 generally indicates that a low $\dot{V}/\dot{Q}$ ratio is the cause of hypoxemia. If the patient is receiving mechanical ventilation and has adequate alveolar ventilation, failure of the PaO_2 to respond to increased FiO_2 likely means that hypoxemia is due to a diffusion defect or shunt.

Alveolar Oxygen and Alveolar Air Equation

Increasing FiO_2 increases PAO_2, according to the alveolar air equation:[2]

$$P_AO_2 = [FiO_2(P_B - 47)] - P_aCO_2 \times [FiO_2 + (1 - FiO_2/R)]$$

where PAO_2 is the partial pressure of oxygen in the alveoli; FiO_2 is the fractional inspired oxygen; P_B is the barometric pressure in mm Hg; 47 is the partial pressure of water vapor in the alveoli in mm Hg at 37° C; $PaCO_2$ is the partial pressure of carbon dioxide in arterial blood in mm Hg; and R is the respiratory exchange ratio ($\dot{V}CO_2/\dot{V}O_2$), normally 0.8.

When FiO_2 is increased, PAO_2 increases as well, if there is no change in $PaCO_2$ or the respiratory exchange ratio. $PaCO_2$ may change with a change in alveolar ventilation or metabolic rate. O_2 consumption and CO_2 production increase with an increase in metabolic rate, such as with fever or overfeeding. If metabolic rate and alveolar ventilation are constant, an increase in FiO_2 results in a proportional increase in PAO_2.

Arterial Oxygenation and Oxygen Content

Mechanical ventilation at FiO_2 of 0.21 may restore arterial oxygenation if the only cause of hypoxemia was hypoventilation. Hypoventilation may be the sole cause with central nervous system depression, apnea, and neuromuscular disease. With other causes of hypoxemia, an increase in FiO_2 is needed to increase arterial O_2 content.

O_2 content is directly related to arterial oxygenation and hemoglobin concentration, defined by the equation for arterial oxygen content (CaO_2):[2]

$$CaO_2\ (vol\%) = (1.34 \times Hb \times SaO_2) + (PaO_2 \times 0.003\ ml\ O_2/mm\ Hg)$$

where 1.34 is a constant for the amount of O_2 carried by each fully saturated gram of hemoglobin (1.34 ml O_2/1 g hemoglobin), Hb is the hemoglobin concentration in g/dl, SaO_2 is the oxygen saturation of hemoglobin, and 0.003 is the amount of O_2 carried in the plasma in ml/mm Hg PaO_2. Under circumstances of normal diffusion, FiO_2, and hemoglobin concentration, the arterial content is normal at approximately 19.8 ml O_2/100 ml blood. As defined by this equation, CaO_2 decreases if hemoglobin concentration, arterial saturation, or PaO_2 decreases.

Decreased Shunt

Mechanical ventilation alone does not decrease shunt. Otherwise, it would be much easier to restore PaO_2 in patients with ARDS. Administration of PEEP with mechanical ventilation or to a spontaneously breathing patient in the form of continuous positive airway pressure (CPAP) helps to maintain open alveoli and stabilize small, collapsed, or fluid-filled alveoli. The results are an increase in alveolar surface area for diffusion and improvement in $\dot{V}/\dot{Q}$ matching and arterial oxygenation.

PEEP or CPAP should be used judiciously (see later in this chapter and Chapter 48). High pressure can overdistend alveoli and redistribute pulmonary blood flow to capillaries surrounding poorly ventilated alveoli, resulting in increased shunt.

Increased Tissue Oxygen Delivery

When a mechanical ventilator is used to improve arterial oxygenation by increasing FiO_2 or PEEP, CaO_2 increases. However, the increase in CaO_2 represents only part of tissue O_2 delivery because O_2 delivery is defined by CaO_2 and cardiac output, as follows:[2]

$$DO_2\ (\text{tissue oxygen delivery in ml/min}) = CaO_2\ (\text{ml } O_2/100\ \text{ml blood}) \times \text{Cardiac output (L/min)} \times 10$$

where 10 is a constant for converting deciliters to milliliters.

Normal tissue O_2 delivery is approximately 990 ml/min because the normal CaO_2 is approximately 20 vol%, and the normal cardiac output is approximately 5 L/min. When PaO_2, CaO_2, and cardiac output are adequate, so is tissue O_2 delivery. When PEEP is needed to improve PaO_2, it must be used cautiously because PEEP increases intrathoracic pressure. When intrathoracic pressure is increased, pleural pressure around the heart also increases, and the increase can affect the mechanical activity of the heart and impede venous return and decrease cardiac output. As discussed in Chapter 48, careful titration of PEEP must include monitoring the cardiovascular status of the patient. *Optimal PEEP* provides adequate arterial oxygenation and tissue O_2 delivery.

MINI CLINI

Oxygen Delivery

PROBLEM: Oxygen delivery (DO_2) depends on PaO_2, hemoglobin concentration, and cardiac output. The formula for DO_2 is:

$$DO_2 = CaO_2 \times \text{Cardiac output (L/min)} \times 10$$

where CaO_2 is the arterial oxygen content, and 10 is the conversion factor between deciliters and milliliters. Normal DO_2 is 990 ml/min. DO_2 is normal when the hemoglobin concentration is 15 g/dl, cardiac output is 5.0 L/min, and PaO_2 is 100 mm Hg:

$$DO_2 = [15\ g\ Hb \times 1.34\ ml\ O_2/g\ Hb \times 0.97\ (SaO_2) + 0.003 \times 100\ mm\ Hg] \times (5.0\ L/min) \times 10 = 19.8\ (CaO_2) \times 5\ (L/min) \times 10 = 990\ ml/min$$

When the practitioner calculates DO_2 and determines it to be low, the component of the formula that is low denotes the problem and the therapeutic target. If CaO_2 is low because of a low hemoglobin concentration, increasing the hemoglobin concentration with blood transfusion is indicated. If CaO_2 is low because of low PaO_2 or SaO_2, increasing PaO_2 and SaO_2 with O_2 or PEEP is indicated. If cardiac output is low, the cause (decreased preload, increased afterload, decreased contractility, or bradycardia) is determined, and appropriate therapy is initiated. Frequently, a decrease in CaO_2 results in an increase in the cardiac output to compensate for decreased DO_2.

Example: Given PaO_2 of 65 mm Hg, hemoglobin concentration of 10 g/dl, SaO_2 of 91%, and cardiac output of 4.8 L/min, what increase in cardiac output is necessary to maintain DO_2 of 900 ml/min?

$$DO_2\ \text{at given values is}\ [(1.34 \times 10 \times 0.97) + (0.003 \times 65)] \times 4.8 \times 10 = 633\ ml/min$$

An increase in cardiac output to 6.8 L/min results in DO_2 that is close to normal: $[(1.34 \times 10 \times 0.97) + (0.003 \times 65)] \times 6.8 \times 10 = 897$ ml/min. However, an increase in cardiac output to 6.8 L/min increases myocardial work. Because the cause of decreased DO_2 in this patient is hypoxemia and anemia, the goal of therapy should be to increase PaO_2. This strategy allows cardiac output and work to return to normal while adequate DO_2 is maintained. Increasing the hemoglobin concentration is normally not performed by transfusion unless the hemoglobin concentration is less than 8 to 10 g/dl because of the adverse effects associated with transfusions.

EFFECTS OF POSITIVE PRESSURE MECHANICAL VENTILATION ON LUNG MECHANICS

Time Constants

The time necessary for **passive** inflation and deflation of the lung or each alveolus is determined by the product of compliance and resistance. This product is the **time constant** of the lung or alveolar unit. The compliance of a "normal" lung is 0.1 L/cm H_2O, and resistance of a normal lung is 2.5 cm H_2O/L/sec. The time constant for a normal lung is 0.25 second (1.0 L/cm $H_2O \times 0.25$ cm H_2O/L/sec). For patients with normal lungs, 95% of the alveoli are inflated within three time constants (i.e., within 0.25 second). In four time constants (1.0 second), 98% of alveoli are inflated, and in five time constants (1.25 second), 99.3% of alveoli are inflated. The same numbers apply for exhalation.

The two major factors that affect alveolar time constants are changes in compliance and changes in resistance. If compliance or resistance decreases, the time constant for a given lung unit decreases, and the lung fills and empties faster. If compliance or resistance increases, the time constant increases, and it takes more time to fill and empty the lung.

There are clinical implications for patients with disorders consistent with abnormal time constants. A longer inspiratory time may be needed for patients with asthma because airway resistance is increased. Attempting to ventilate these patients with a normal inspiratory time may result in inadequate volume to affected lung units because the airways are obstructed, and volume is likely to travel to airways with the lowest resistance. Inspiratory time in severe asthma needs to be set between about 1.0 second to 1.5 seconds to ensure adequate gas delivery. The primary limiting factor is that the airways are also obstructed during exhalation. The expiratory time must also be longer to allow as complete an exhalation as possible.

Asthma is very different from COPD, in which the inspiratory time constant is normal, but the expiratory time constant is long. In general, asthma requires very slow respiratory rates with longer than normal inspiratory and expiratory times to account for the altered time constants during both inspiration and expiration. Patients with COPD generally tolerate a more rapid rate because only the expiratory time constant is lengthened. In both of these situations, air trapping is very common because of the long time constants. In patients with COPD, inspiratory times are generally short (about 0.7 to 0.9 second). In patients with ARDS or acute lung injury (ALI), time constants are very short, and as a result inspiratory times can also be very short. Most patients with ARDS require an inspiratory time of only 0.5 to 0.8 second. Expiratory time constants are also short—hence the ability to ventilate these patients rapidly with small V_T. Respiratory rates greater than 30 breaths/min are frequently well tolerated by patients with ARDS. The major concern with patients with ARDS and their short time constants is that any disruption of the airway rapidly results in loss of lung volume. Atelectasis occurs with disconnections from the ventilator of only 1 or 2 seconds. As a result, *all* patients with ARDS should be suctioned *only* with inline suction catheters, and any circuit disconnection should be avoided. Ventilator management in the care of patients with COPD, asthma, and ARDS is described in detail in Chapter 48.

Increased Pressure

Peak inspiratory pressure (PIP) is the highest pressure produced during the inspiratory phase. It is the sum of the pressures necessary to overcome airway resistance and lung and chest wall compliance. PIP is also known as *peak pressure* or *peak airway pressure*.

Plateau pressure (P_{plat}) is the pressure observed during a period of inflation hold or end inspiratory pause. To obtain a plateau pressure, the RT initiates an inspiratory pause time of 0.5 to 2.0 seconds. During inspiration, the peak pressure is reached and then immediately followed by the inspiratory pause. During the pause, pressure decreases to a pressure plateau. When a valid plateau pressure value is obtained, the inspiratory pause time is returned to zero. Plateau pressure represents the average peak alveolar pressure (P_{alv}). In volume-controlled ventilation, plateau pressure is always lower than peak pressure because the peak pressure is the sum of the alveolar pressure and the pressure needed to overcome airway resistance. When flow is delivered by a square waveform, the difference between plateau pressure and peak pressure is the pressure necessary to overcome airway resistance. If the V_T is divided by the difference between the plateau pressure and PEEP, the quotient is the quasistatic lung-thorax compliance:[3]

$$C_{static} = V_T/(P_{plat} - PEEP)$$

This value is referred to as the lung-thorax compliance because the compliance of the lungs and the compliance of the rib cage are being calculated as a unit. The lung compliance cannot be determined without the use of an esophageal balloon.[3] Ideally, the volume lost owing to tubing compliance should be subtracted from the V_T if the ventilator has not compensated for it, making the equation:[3]

$$C_{static} = \text{Adjusted } V_T/P_{plat} - \text{total PEEP})$$

In addition, the total PEEP should be subtracted from the P_{plat}. That is the total of applied PEEP plus any auto-PEEP present. The reason for this is that the baseline pressure prior to the start of inspiration is the total PEEP, not the applied PEEP.[3]

It may be more useful to follow trends in lung compliance, rather than making judgments on only one calculation. A downward trend in compliance means that the lungs or chest wall is stiffer, as in ARDS.

Airway resistance (R_{aw}) during volume ventilation is estimated by the difference between PIP and P_{plat} divided by the inspiratory flow ($\dot{V}_I$) in L/sec, provided that the flow is constant (square waveform):[3]

$$R_{aw} = (PIP - P_{plat})/\dot{V}_I$$

During mechanical ventilation, the plateau pressure should be less than 28 cm H_2O.[4,5] At levels greater than 28 cm H_2O, alveolar damage from overdistention is likely. This form of *ventilator-induced lung injury (VILI)* is referred to as **volutrauma** (see later). This trauma can result in air leakage from alveoli, the release of inflammatory mediators, and multisystem organ failure (MSOF). When the plateau pressure approaches 28 cm H_2O during either volume or pressure ventilation, the pressure limit or the V_T should be decreased. This approach to ventilation is referred to as *lung protective ventilation*.[3-5]

RULE OF THUMB

When measuring lung mechanics, airway resistance and compliance always use the same ventilator settings to make comparisons from one point in time to another much easier. In adults, settings are volume ventilation, V_T 500 ml, square wave flow, and peak flow set at 60 L/min.

Mean Airway Pressure

Mean airway pressure is the average pressure across the total cycle time (TCT). The mean airway pressure ($P_{\overline{AW}}$) can be calculated manually if the flow is constant, as follows:[3]

$$P_{\overline{AW}} = \tfrac{1}{2}(\text{PIP} - \text{PEEP}) \times (\text{Inspiratory time}/\text{TCT}) + \text{PEEP}$$

Mean airway pressure is computed by the ventilator as the integral of the pressure signal over the total cycle time (as a rolling average), so the RT can record the ventilator computed value, rather than manually calculating it. Because expiratory (baseline) pressure is lower than inspiratory pressure, the mean pressure is between peak and end expiratory pressure. The variables affecting mean pleural and mean airway pressure are summarized in Box 46-1. For a given minute volume, partial ventilatory support modes such as synchronized intermittent mandatory ventilation (SIMV) result in lower mean airway and pleural pressures than continuous mandatory ventilation (CMV) modes. For a specific mandatory breath, as peak pressure increases, so does mean pressure. Likewise, long inspiratory times increase mean pressure. Prolonging expiratory time has the opposite effect on mean airway pressure. Generally, the harmful cardiovascular effects of PPV are more likely to occur when $P_{\overline{AW}}$ or inspiratory-to-expiratory (I : E) ratio increases (e.g., >1 : 1).

The pressure waveform of a mandatory breath affects mean pressure. In Figure 46-6, for a given inspiratory time, the constant pressure pattern (curve *A*) results in the greatest area under the airway pressure curve and the highest mean airway pressure. A constant pressure pattern is normally produced by a pressure targeted breath that provides decreasing (descending ramp) flow. The effect of PEEP on mean airway pressure is simple: Every 1 cm H_2O of applied PEEP increases the mean airway pressure 1 cm H_2O.

Box 46-1 Factors That Increase Mean Airway Pressure

- Absence of spontaneous ventilation
- Increasing positive pressure
- Increasing duration of inspiration
- Decreasing duration of expiration
- Nature of inspiratory waveform
- Increasing level of PEEP
- Decreasing compliance, increasing airways resistance

Effect of Peak Airway Pressure on Lung Recruitment

As peak airway pressure increases, previously collapsed, small, or fluid-filled alveoli are recruited, that is, reopened.[6] This reopening of alveoli increases alveolar surface area and restores functional residual capacity (FRC). At the alveolar level, the surface area available for diffusion is increased. As a result, PaO_2 increases, consistent with Fick's law. The use of extrinsic PEEP maintains the airways and recruited open alveoli. Extrinsic PEEP is controlled directly by the PEEP control on the ventilator, and the RT always knows how much extrinsic PEEP is present. Several factors, including inverse ratio ventilation (IRV), may add intrinsic PEEP or auto-PEEP by starting the next breath before the previous exhalation has ended. The amount of intrinsic PEEP added by IRV can be measured by implementing an end expiratory pause, which stops the next breath from being delivered. During this end expiratory pause, alveolar and mouth pressures equilibrate, and the total PEEP is now presented by the ventilator. The amount of auto-PEEP present is the difference between the total PEEP and the extrinsic PEEP:

$$\text{Intrinsic PEEP (auto-PEEP)} = \text{Total PEEP} - \text{Extrinsic PEEP}$$

Increased Lung Volume: Tidal Volume

The volume delivered during pressure-controlled modes varies with changes in set pressure, patient effort, and lung mechanics. For all pressure-targeted modes, the volume delivered at a given pressure decreases as compliance decreases. An increase in resistance, active exhalation, or muscle tensing by the patient during inspiration also decreases delivered volume in pressure ventilation.

If pressure serves as the limit variable instead of the cycle variable, changes in airway resistance during pressure-limited ventilation may or may not affect delivered volume. In this case, the key factor is the time available for pressure equilibration. Volume can remain constant even if airway resistance increases, as long as there is sufficient time for alveolar and airway

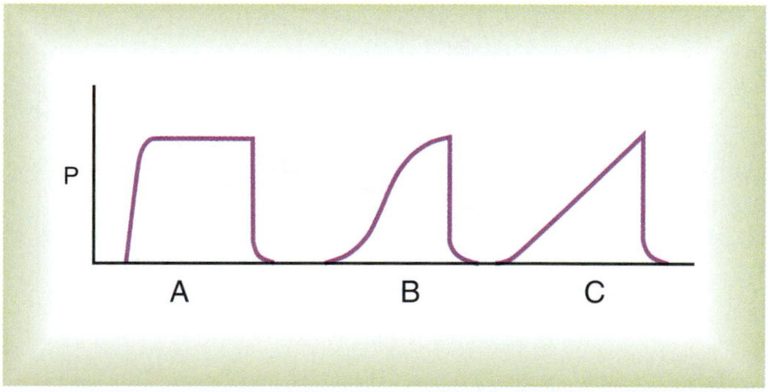

FIGURE 46-6 Pressure patterns resulting from a descending ramp flow waveform *(A)*, a sine wave flow waveform *(B)*, and a constant flow waveform *(C)*. Because waveform *A* has the highest pressure for the longest inspiratory time, it also has the greatest mean airway pressure.

pressures to equilibrate. However, if insufficient time is available for pressure equilibration, delivered volume decreases as airway resistance increases. The length of time needed for pressure equilibration is usually at least three times greater than the time constant for the respiratory system. In pressure modes, ventilator-delivered flow varies with patient effort and lung mechanics; this tends to avoid patient-ventilator asynchrony.[7]

Increased Functional Residual Capacity

FRC is not known to change significantly with the application of PPV alone because passive exhalation allows the end expiratory pressure to return to atmospheric pressure with each breath. If an increase in FRC is to be achieved, end expiratory pressure must be increased. This increase is commonly achieved with PEEP or CPAP. PEEP or CPAP does not recruit collapsed lung units but prevents lung units that have been opened from collapsing at end expiration. Peak airway pressure recruits lung volume. The magnitude of the increase in FRC sustained by PEEP or CPAP is proportional to the lung-thorax compliance. With acute restriction, as PEEP is increased, lung compliance improves. Initially, the FRC gain as PEEP is added is small. However, as FRC and compliance increase, additional increments of PEEP tend to result in larger increases in FRC up to the point at which overdistention occurs. At that point, as PEEP is increased, increases in FRC decline, as does compliance. There is no practical way of measuring FRC in all patients, so other methods of determining an increase in FRC are used, such as improving PaO_2 at a constant FiO_2, increasing PaO_2/FiO_2 ratio, decreasing shunt fraction, or decreasing FiO_2 while maintaining PaO_2. The management of PEEP is described in more detail in Chapter 48.

Pressure-Volume Curve and Lung Recruitment in Acute Respiratory Distress Syndrome

Figure 46-7 depicts the pressure-volume (P-V) relationship of the lung-thorax in an idealized patient with ARDS.[8] On the inflation P-V curve, there are two points of inflection: the lower inflection point referred to as P_{flex} or *lower corner pressure,* and an upper inflection point, also referred to as *upper corner pressure*. These two points represent defined changes in compliance. The lower inflection point represents an abrupt increase in lung-thorax compliance as collapsed or atelectatic lung begins to be recruited.[9] The upper deflection point represent the point where the rate of lung recruitment decreases and overinflation begins.[9] It is most important to realize from this graph that the lung is recruited by pressure and that the higher the peak airway pressure, the greater the potential for lung to be recruited. The maximum pressure needed to recruit a given patient's lung is unknown; however, pressures up to 50 cm H_2O most likely are safe with most patients when applied for short (1 to 3 minutes)

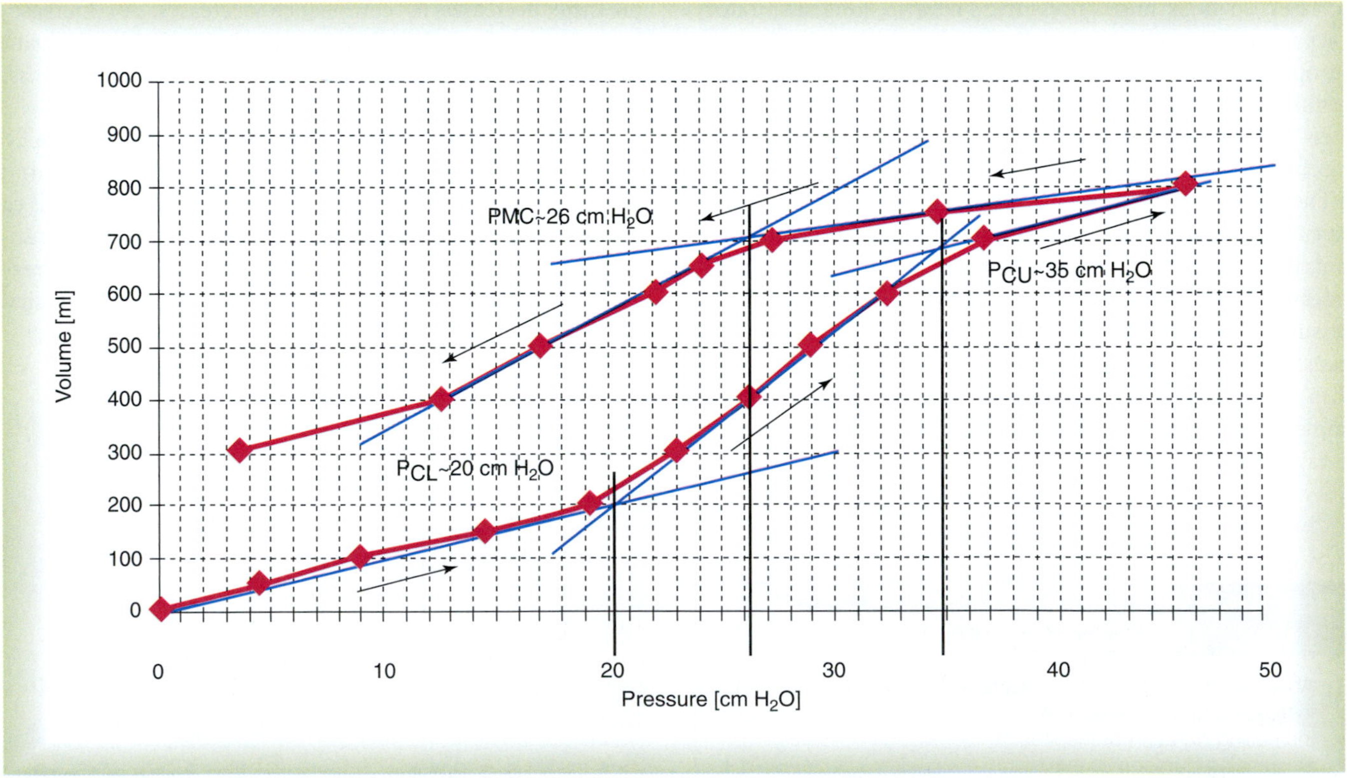

FIGURE 46-7 P-V curve of the lung-thorax indicating the inflation and deflation limbs. *Arrows* indicate direction of flow. P_{CL}, Lower corner pressure or P_{flex} or lower inflection point; P_{CU}, upper corner pressure or upper inflection point; P_{MC}, point of maximum compliance change. (Modified from Godon S, Fujino Y, Hromi JM, et al: Optimal mean airway pressure during high frequency oscillation. Anesthesiology 94:862-868, 2001.)

periods.[10-12] If these pressures were applied for longer periods, lung injury would most likely result.

The deflation limb of the P-V curve is similar in shape to the inflation limb but is separated from the inflation limb. This hysteresis (separation) is a result of surfactant and surface tension interactions. Basically, less pressure is required to keep the lung open on the deflation limb of the P-V curve than on the inflation limb; this is obvious on examination of the volume maintained in the lung at P_{flex}, or 20 cm H_2O. On the inflation limb, lung volume increases about 200 ml at 20 cm H_2O, but on the deflation limb, lung volume increases about 550 ml. The goal of an open lung approach to ventilation that has been proposed by many authors is to open the lung and then to ventilate the patient on the deflation limb of the P-V curve.[10-12]

Figure 46-7 is an idealized P-V curve; actual patient P-V curves in ARDS are not as well defined. In 10% to 20% of patients with ARDS, P_{flex} cannot be identified on the inflation P-V curve. As a result, despite two positive randomized controlled trials using P_{flex} to set PEEP,[13,14] the use of P-V curves clinically has not become common practice; a second reason for this is the difficulty of measuring the P-V curve. However, many newer ICU ventilators are including algorithms that allow P-V curves to be performed by the ventilator with the ventilator identifying P_{flex}. This option may increase the use of the P-V curve for the management of patients with ARDS.

The approach to setting PEEP that assures ventilation on the deflation limb of the P-V curve and the minimal PEEP to sustain the benefit of lung recruitment is a decremental PEEP trial immediately after a lung recruitment maneuver (RM).[12,13,15] Many different approaches to performing lung RMs have been published, but the approach that is considered the safest and most efficacious is the use of pressure-controlled continuous mandatory ventilation (PV-CMV).[12,13,15] To perform a lung RM with PC-CMV, high enough PEEP must be set to avoid derecruitment after each inspiration. Essentially, a minimum of 20 cm H_2O PEEP is required during the RM. Peak pressure is usually started at 35 to 40 cm H_2O, and if the patient tolerates the pressure hemodynamically, it may be increased to 50 cm H_2O, ensuring a driving pressure of no more than 15 cm H_2O (Box 46-2). Inspiratory time is increased to about 1.5 to 2.0 seconds, and respiratory rate is decreased to about 15 to 20 breaths/min. The maneuver is applied for 1 to 3 minutes. During the RM, the patient must be sedated to apnea to avoid fighting the ventilator.

Before any RM, the patient must be hemodynamically stable. RMs should not be performed in patients with existing **barotrauma** or with a high likelihood of developing barotrauma (blebs or bullae) or in patients who are hemodynamically unstable. In addition, RMs are most effective and result in the least adverse reaction if performed early in the course of ARDS. During and after the RM, the patient must be carefully monitored for hemodynamic and oxygenation instability and the development of barotrauma.

After an RM, the best way to identify the minimum effective PEEP level that maintains the lung open is to perform a decremental PEEP trial.[12,13,15] This trial is performed by changing the mode from PC-CMV to volume-controlled continuous mandatory ventilation (VC-CMV), V_T 4 to 6 ml/kg, inspiratory time 1.0 second or less, PEEP 20 to 25 cm H_2O, and rate set at the maximum that does not cause auto-PEEP.[8] After stabilization (3 to 5 minutes), dynamic compliance is measured.[8] PEEP is then decreased 2 cm H_2O, the patient is stabilized (3 to 5 minutes), and measurement of dynamic compliance is repeated; this is continued until the PEEP level at which the compliance decreases is identified. Generally, compliance at 20 to 25 cm H_2O PEEP is low, and it increases as PEEP is decreased; compliance then decreases as PEEP is decreased further. Open lung PEEP is the PEEP associated with the highest compliance. Set PEEP is open lung PEEP plus 2 cm H_2O.

After open lung PEEP is identified, the lung is again recruited because during the decremental PEEP trial derecruitment occurred. After recruitment, PEEP is set at the identified level, ventilation is adjusted using a lung protective V_T (4 to 8 ml/kg), and rate is adjusted to normalize PCO_2. After all is set, FiO_2 is decreased to the level that maintains PaO_2 in the range of 55 to 70 mm Hg. Repeat RMs may be needed if the patient did not respond to the initial RM or if the patient is disconnected from

Box 46-2 Performance of Recruitment Maneuver and Decremental Positive End Expiratory Pressure Trial

Pressure control ventilation settings are:
- PEEP 20-30 cm H_2O
- Peak inspiratory pressure 35-50 cm H_2O
- Driving pressure no greater than 15 cm H2O
- Inspiratory time 1-2 sec
- Rate about 15-20 breaths/min
- Time 1-3 min

After completing RM, set PEEP at 20 or 25 cm H_2O, ventilate with VC, V_T 4 to 6 ml/kg ideal body weight, increase rate, avoid auto-PEEP.

Measure dynamic compliance after 3 to 5 minutes of stabilization.

Decrease PEEP 2 cm H_2O.

Measure dynamic compliance after 3 to 5 minutes of stabilization.

Repeat until maximum compliance is determined.

Optimal PEEP = maximum compliance PEEP + 2 cm H_2O.

Repeat RM and set PEEP at the identified settings; adjust ventilation.

After PEEP and ventilation are set and stabilized, decrease FiO_2 until PO_2 is in target range.

If response is poor and the patient tolerates the procedure well, repeat RM with PEEP 25 cm H_2O and peak pressure 40 cm H_2O after a period of stabilization.

If response is still poor and the patient tolerates the procedure well, repeat RM with PEEP 30 cm H_2O and peak pressure 45 cm H_2O.

If response is still poor and the patient tolerates the procedure well, repeat RM with PEEP 35 cm H_2O and peak pressure 50 cm H_2O.

Do not exceed 50 cm H_2O peak airway pressure during RM.

the ventilator and derecruitment occurs. A successful RM is one that allows the FiO_2 to be reduced to less than 0.5.

The use of RM has been documented in many case series; however, no data have been published indicating that outcome is improved as a result of RMs and decremental PEEP settings. Research is ongoing.

RULE OF THUMB

A lung RM is most likely to be successful if it is performed early in the course of ARDS. Ideally, if indicated, a lung RM should be performed once the patient is fully stabilized after intubation and initiation of mechanical ventilation. The longer the patient is mechanically ventilated, the less likely it is that the RM would be successful.

Increased Dead Space

The dead space fraction is increased with the institution of mechanical ventilation owing to inspiratory mechanical bronchodilation and the preferential ventilation of more apical, nondependent alveoli, the reduction of blood flow away from ventilated alveoli, and the continued perfusion of basilar or dependent alveoli (see Figure 46-5). This increase is concurrent with a decrease in $\dot{V}/\dot{Q}$ ratio.

Decreased Work of Breathing

Although improper ventilator management can increase WOB (poor patient-ventilator interaction, see Chapter 47 for details), one of the primary objectives of mechanical ventilation is to decrease WOB. PPV can significantly reduce WOB in patients with actual or impending respiratory muscle fatigue. RTs frequently see patients relax as the ventilator assumes a major portion of their WOB. To lessen WOB, ventilation must be sufficient to meet the patient's needs. Otherwise, a spontaneously breathing patient tends to resist the ventilator, and an asynchronous breathing pattern develops. Inappropriately applied PPV can result in alveolar hypoventilation and consequently a considerable increase in the patient's WOB.

Mode, trigger setting, and inspiratory flow have an effect on WOB. WOB consists of two components: (1) ventilator work (WOB_{vent}) occurring as the ventilator forces gas into the lungs and (2) patient work (WOB_{pt}) as the inspiratory muscles draw gas into the lungs. The magnitude of WOB_{pt} depends on compliance, resistance, and ventilatory drive and on ventilator variables, such as trigger sensitivity, peak flow, cycling coordination, and V_T.[16,17]

Regardless whether flow or pressure triggering is selected, either should always be set as sensitive as possible without causing autotriggering. The less sensitive the setting, the greater the patient effort. In older generation ventilators, flow triggering was shown to require less effort than pressure triggering.[18] However, with the newest generation of ICU ventilators, both are equally effective.

As described in Chapter 45, a mode of ventilation is a ventilatory pattern that can be described by identifying the control variable, breath sequence, and targeting scheme. The breath sequence may be thought of as being on a continuum from assuming very little to assuming all WOB. As the breath sequence is changed from continuous spontaneous ventilation (CSV) to CMV, the ventilator assumes more WOB. An example of this transition would be from CPAP to pressure support to CMV. In CPAP, a continuous spontaneous mode of ventilation, the patient assumes all WOB. The ventilator merely provides positive pressure throughout the patient's breathing cycle. The ventilator assumes more WOB during CMV. Pressure support is also an example of CSV. During pressure support ventilation (PSV), the patient determines breath timing (length of inspiration and expiration) and frequency. Depending on the set inspiratory pressure, the clinician may program the ventilator to provide a minimal to a maximal amount of WOB. In instances where the patient has no spontaneous efforts, all breaths during CMV are time triggered, and all work performed is WOB_{vent}. Although it may be advantageous for the ventilator to assume all WOB for a while, extended periods of passive ventilation may cause diaphragmatic atrophy, which may unnecessarily prolong the need for mechanical ventilation and delay weaning. At initiation of patient-triggered pressure or volume modes, WOB_{pt} resumes.

During assisted ventilation, pressure-targeted modes are generally more capable of meeting patient ventilatory demands and minimizing WOB_{pt}.[19] As pressure level is increased, ventilatory muscles are unloaded, V_T increases for a given amount of patient effort, and WOB_{pt} decreases. Most clinicians increase pressure level until the breathing pattern approaches normal—that is, until the spontaneous ventilatory rate is 15 to 25 breaths/min and the spontaneous V_T is normal (5 to 8 ml/kg).

Measuring WOB is technically difficult. It is often accomplished by esophageal balloon monitoring, in which a balloon is placed in the distal third of the esophagus, and a pneumotachometer is attached to the airway (see Chapter 51). WOB is the integral of the esophageal pressure and V_T. Normal WOB is 0.6 to 0.9 J/L.[20]

MINIMIZING ADVERSE PULMONARY EFFECTS OF POSITIVE PRESSURE MECHANICAL VENTILATION

Decreasing Pressure

The main objective of mechanical ventilation is to provide a minute ventilation appropriate to achieve adequate alveolar ventilation and supplemental O_2 and PEEP to provide adequate arterial oxygenation.

Peak pressure is the result of the pressure required to overcome system resistance and compliance. Although there is no absolute maximum pressure, most practitioners try to avoid peak pressures greater than 40 cm H_2O. As the peak pressure approaches 40 cm H_2O, it is important to consider the causes. Factors that increase airway resistance include airway edema, bronchospasm, and secretions. The RT can manage or avoid these problems by ensuring adequate humidity, bronchial

MINI CLINI

Overcoming an Increase in the Work of Breathing

PROBLEM: A patient's WOB is minimal during mechanical ventilation with an appropriate V_T and rate. As the ventilator support is gradually discontinued and the patient is expected to take over more of WOB, airway resistance associated with breathing through an endotracheal tube may become clinically important. The RT must be able to recognize this problem readily and know how to correct it.

A patient has received mechanical ventilation in volume-controlled CMV mode for the past week. The patient's condition is now clinically stable, and ventilation is provided by PSV. As the PSV pressure level is reduced to 8 cm H_2O, the patient begins using accessory muscles to breathe, the spontaneous respiratory rate increases to 30 breaths/min, and the patient reports shortness of breath. Blood gas values are acceptable, and no abnormal lung sounds are present. What is the problem, and what should the RT do?

Solution: The patient may be experiencing excessive WOB because of airway resistance associated with the endotracheal tube; a small sized tube or partial obstruction of the tube with secretions may be the problem. Other possibilities that should be considered include deterioration in the patient's cardiopulmonary status, but the normal blood gas values and lung sounds suggest the problem is not the lungs. Passing a suction catheter through the tube may help to identify the problem. If the catheter does not pass easily, the tube may be partially obstructed. Two options exist: change the tube or extubate the patient. Because the tube would need to be removed regardless of the choice, a trial extubation should be considered. Because this patient is at risk immediately after extubation, noninvasive ventilation should be started. If the patient cannot tolerate extubation, an appropriate-sized endotracheal tube can be reinserted.

hygiene (suctioning, airway care), and administration of bronchodilators and antiinflammatory drugs. Factors that increase the pressure needed to inflate the lung and overcome compliance include alveolar and interstitial edema, atelectasis, fibrosis, and chest wall restriction.

Plateau pressure reflects mean maximum alveolar pressure. Plateau pressures of 28 cm H_2O or greater have an increased likelihood of causing lung injury.[3,4,5] If plateau pressure approaches 28 cm H_2O during volume ventilation, the V_T should be decreased so that the plateau pressure is less than 28 cm H_2O, or with pressure ventilation, target pressure should be set less than 28 cm H_2O.[4,21]

Mean airway pressure is decreased by decreasing inspiratory time, V_T, respiratory rate, PEEP, or PIP. Increased mean airway pressure reduces venous return and may reduce cardiac output.

Positive End Expiratory Pressure or Continuous Positive Airway Pressure

PEEP is the application of positive pressure at end-exhalation. PEEP is used primarily to improve oxygenation in patients with

TABLE 46-2
Physiologic Effects of Positive End Expiratory Pressure

Beneficial Effects of Appropriate PEEP	Detrimental Effects of Inappropriate PEEP
Restored FRC, avoids derecruitment	Increased pulmonary vascular resistance
Decreased shunt fraction	Potential decrease in venous return and cardiac output
Increased lung compliance	Decreased renal and portal blood flow
Decreased WOB	Increased ICP
Increased PaO_2 for a given FiO_2	Increased dead space

refractory hypoxemia. As a rule, refractory hypoxemia exists when PaO_2 cannot be maintained at greater than 50 to 60 mm Hg with FiO_2 0.50 or greater. PEEP improves oxygenation in these patients by maintaining alveoli open, restoring FRC, and decreasing physiologic shunting. The improved alveolar volume provided by PEEP allows a lower FiO_2. Other values such as lung compliance, shunt fraction, and PaO_2/FiO_2 ratio also may improve when PEEP is appropriately applied. PEEP may be indicated in the care of patients with COPD who have dynamic hyperinflation (auto-PEEP).[22,23] (See discussion later in this chapter.)

Beneficial and harmful effects are associated with the use of PEEP (Table 46-2). Detrimental effects of inappropriately high levels of PEEP include decreased cardiac output, increased pulmonary vascular resistance, and increased dead space. When one or more of these problems occur, PEEP is decreased to the previous level or to a value between the current level and the previous level. If cardiac output decreases and an increase in PEEP is necessary to maintain oxygenation, intravenous fluid, inotropic cardiac drugs, or both are administered to restore cardiac output.

PEEP is contraindicated in the presence of a tension pneumothorax. PEEP should be applied cautiously in patients with severe unilateral lung disease because PEEP would overinflate the lung with higher compliance. The result is lung overdistention and compression of adjacent pulmonary capillaries. Independent lung ventilation can be used to apply separate inspiratory and baseline pressures to the right and the left lung when severe unilateral lung disease is present.[24] PEEP is contraindicated in the care of patients with increased ICP only if the application of PEEP increases ICP further.

RULE OF THUMB

Refractory hypoxemia exists when PaO_2 cannot be maintained at greater than 50 to 60 mm Hg with FiO_2 0.50 or greater. This situation is an indication for PPV with PEEP or CPAP because an increased end expiratory pressure with either of these modalities improves oxygenation by decreasing physiologic shunting.

Effects of Ventilatory Pattern

The most commonly used inspiratory flow patterns are constant or square and descending ramp during volume-controlled ventilation and exponential decay during pressure-controlled ventilation. In mechanical and computer models, a descending ramp (volume-controlled ventilation) flow pattern improves gas distribution to lung units with long-time constants. The literature often refers to the descending ramp as a decelerating flow pattern. Similar findings in humans have been reported. Compared with a square flow waveform, a descending ramp has been shown to reduce peak pressure, inspiratory work, V_D/V_T, and $P(A-a)O_2$ without affecting hemodynamic values.[25] Compared with volume-controlled ventilation with a square flow waveform, pressure-controlled ventilation with an exponential decay flow waveform may result in a higher PaO_2, lower $PaCO_2$, and lower PIPs. However, mean airway pressure is higher with pressure-controlled ventilation compared with volume-controlled ventilation because pressure increases to the set inspiratory pressure and remains constant throughout inspiration. During pressure-controlled ventilation, flow is responsive to patient demand. The ventilator delivers flow to the patient in proportion to patient need. Flow is also greater at the onset of inspiration, resulting in V_T delivery at a time when the lungs are most compliant, the beginning of the breath. As a breath ends, flow is least, and the volume delivered is small. The result is a lower peak airway pressure for any given V_T.

In most spontaneously breathing persons, lower inspiratory flows improve gas distribution. However, during PPV, low inspiratory flow may lead to lengthy inspiratory times and air trapping if expiratory time is too short. High ventilator inspiratory flow allows more time for exhalation and reduces the incidence of air trapping. Avoidance of air trapping improves gas exchange and reduces WOB in patients with high ventilatory demands.[17,26]

An inflation hold also affects gas exchange. By momentarily maintaining lung volume under conditions of no flow, an inflation hold allows additional time for gas redistribution between lung units with different time constants. In both animal and human studies, increasing the length of an inflation hold decreases the V_D/V_T, $PaCO_2$, and inert gas washout time. Adding an inflation hold effectively increases total inspiratory time, shortening the time available for exhalation and predisposes patients with airway obstruction to auto-PEEP. In practice, an inflation hold should be used only to obtain P_{plat} values. Because the technique prevents the onset of exhalation, asynchrony occurs if the patient is actively breathing.

Trigger Site and Work of Breathing

Studies have examined the effects of sensing a patient's inspiratory effort at the tip of the endotracheal tube rather than in the ventilator circuit, as is done with all ventilators. Triggering and managing gas delivery by measurement of pressure at the tip of the endotracheal tube decreases patient effort and improves synchrony; however, no practical system has been designed.[27] In addition, the efficiency of ventilator flow and pressure triggering seems to improve with each new generation of mechanical ventilator.

PHYSIOLOGIC EFFECTS OF VENTILATORY MODES

Volume-Controlled Ventilation Versus Pressure-Controlled Ventilation

Figure 45-5 illustrates the important variables for volume ventilation modes. The figure shows that the primary variable to be controlled is the patient's minute ventilation. A particular ventilator may allow the operator to set minute ventilation directly. More frequently, minute ventilation is adjusted by means of a set V_T and frequency. V_T is a function of the set inspiratory flow and the set inspiratory time. Inspiratory time is affected by the set frequency and, if applicable, the set I : E ratio. The mathematical relationships among all these variables are shown in Table 46-3.

With pressure-controlled ventilation, the goal is also to maintain adequate minute ventilation. However (as the equation of motion shows), when pressure is controlled, V_T and minute ventilation are determined not only by the ventilator's pressure settings but also by the elastance and resistance of the patient's respiratory system. Minute ventilation and hence gas exchange are less stable in pressure-controlled modes than in volume-controlled modes. Figure 45-6 shows the important variables for pressure-controlled ventilation. V_T is not operator set on the ventilator. It is the result of the set inspiratory pressure, the patient's lung mechanics, and the inspiratory time. On most ventilators, the speed with which inspiratory pressure is achieved (i.e., the pressure rise time) is adjustable. That adjustment affects the shape of the pressure waveform and the mean airway pressure.

Continuous Mandatory Ventilation

CMV (also referred to as *assist/control*) is a mode of ventilation in which total ventilatory support is provided by the mechanical ventilator. All breaths are mandatory and delivered by the ventilator at a preset volume or pressure, breath rate, and inspiratory time. If the patient has spontaneous respiratory efforts, the ventilator delivers a patient-triggered breath. If patient efforts are absent, the ventilator delivers time-triggered breaths. The clinician needs to set an appropriate trigger level and flow rate for the patient in this mode of ventilation. There is a potential for the ventilator to autotrigger when the trigger level is set too sensitive. As a result, hyperventilation, air trapping, and patient anxiety often ensue. However, if the trigger level is not sensitive enough, the ventilator does not respond to the patient's inspiratory efforts, which results in increased WOB.

Occasionally, all attempts to optimize patient comfort, reduce WOB, and achieve the goals of this mode of ventilation are futile. In cases in which this mode is poorly tolerated and spontaneous triggering is counterproductive to the goals set for a particular patient, sedation or paralysis or both may be

TABLE 46-3

Equations Relating the Important Parameters for Volume-Controlled and Pressure-Controlled Ventilation

Mode	Parameter	Symbol	Equation
Volume-controlled	Tidal volume (L)	V_T	$V_T = \dot{V}_E \div f$ $V_T = \dot{V}_I \div T_I$
	Mean inspiratory flow (L/min)	$\bar{\dot{V}}_I$	$\dot{V}_I = 60 \times V_T \div T_I$ $\bar{\dot{V}}_I = \dfrac{\dot{V}_E \times TCT}{T_I}$
Pressure-controlled	Tidal volume (L)	V_T	$V_T = \Delta P \times C \times (1 - e^{-t/\tau})$
	Instantaneous inspiratory flow (L/min)	$\dot{V}_I$	$\dot{V}_I = \left(\dfrac{\Delta P}{R}\right) e^{-t/\tau}$
	Pressure gradient (cm H_2O)	ΔP	$\Delta P = PIP - PEEP$
Both modes	Exhaled minute ventilation (L/min)	$\dot{V}_E$	$\dot{V}_E = V_T \times f$
	Total cycle time or ventilatory period (sec)	TCT	$TCT = T_I + T_E = 60 \div f$
	I : E ratio	I : E	$I:E = T_I : T_E = \dfrac{T_I}{T_E}$
	Time constant (sec)	τ	$\tau = R \times C$
	Resistance (cm H_2O/L/sec)	R	$R = \dfrac{\Delta P}{\Delta \dot{V}}$
	Compliance (L/cm H_2O)	C	$C = \dfrac{\Delta V}{\Delta P}$
	Elastance	E	$E = \dfrac{1}{C}$
	Mean airway pressure (cm H_2O)	$\bar{P}_{aw}$	$\bar{P}_{aw} = \left(\dfrac{1}{TCT}\right) \int_{t=0}^{t=TCT} P_{aw} dt$
Primary variables	Pressure (cm H_2O)	P	
	Volume (L)	V	
	Flow (cm H_2O/L/sec)	$\dot{V}$	
	Time (sec)	τ	
	Inspiratory time (sec)	T_I	
	Expiratory time (sec)	T_E	
	Frequency (breaths/min)	f	
	Base of natural logarithm (≈2.72)	e	

required. These agents may be used to minimize patient effort and normalize WOB.

Volume-Controlled Continuous Mandatory Ventilation

Volume-controlled continuous mandatory ventilation (VC-CMV) is indicated when a precise minute ventilation or blood gas parameter, such as $PaCO_2$, is therapeutically essential to the care of patients.[26] Theoretically, volume control (with a constant inspiratory flow) (Figure 46-8) results in a more even distribution of ventilation (compared with pressure control) among lung units with different time constants where the units have equal resistances but unequal compliances (e.g., ARDS).[27]

During VC-CMV, volume is guaranteed, but airway pressure varies depending on changes in the patient's lung mechanics. A reduction in lung compliance or an increase in resistance causes higher peak airway pressures. Care should also be taken when setting the inspiratory flow. Avoid setting a flow that fails to match patient needs or exceeds patient demand. An insufficient flow rate would result in an imposed increase in the patient's WOB and a concomitant increase in O_2 consumption. The inspiratory phase may be prematurely shortened if the set inspiratory flow exceeds patient demands. Meticulous patient monitoring and use of VC-CMV allow the clinician to achieve precise and predictable physiologic results.

Example. Perhaps the most common application of VC-CMV is its use to ventilate patients in the immediate postoperative period. Patients are often sedated to minimize their response to noxious stimuli and ventilator asynchrony. VC-CMV can achieve fairly precise regulation of gas exchange.

Pressure-Controlled Continuous Mandatory Ventilation

Similar to VC-CMV, pressure-controlled continuous mandatory ventilation (CMV) can be used as a basic mode of ventilatory support. The primary difference between volume-controlled and pressure-controlled ventilation is the control variable with which the clinician is most concerned.[28,29] Theoretically, pressure control (with a constant inspiratory pressure) (Figure 46-9) results in a more even distribution of ventilation (compared with volume control) among lung units with different

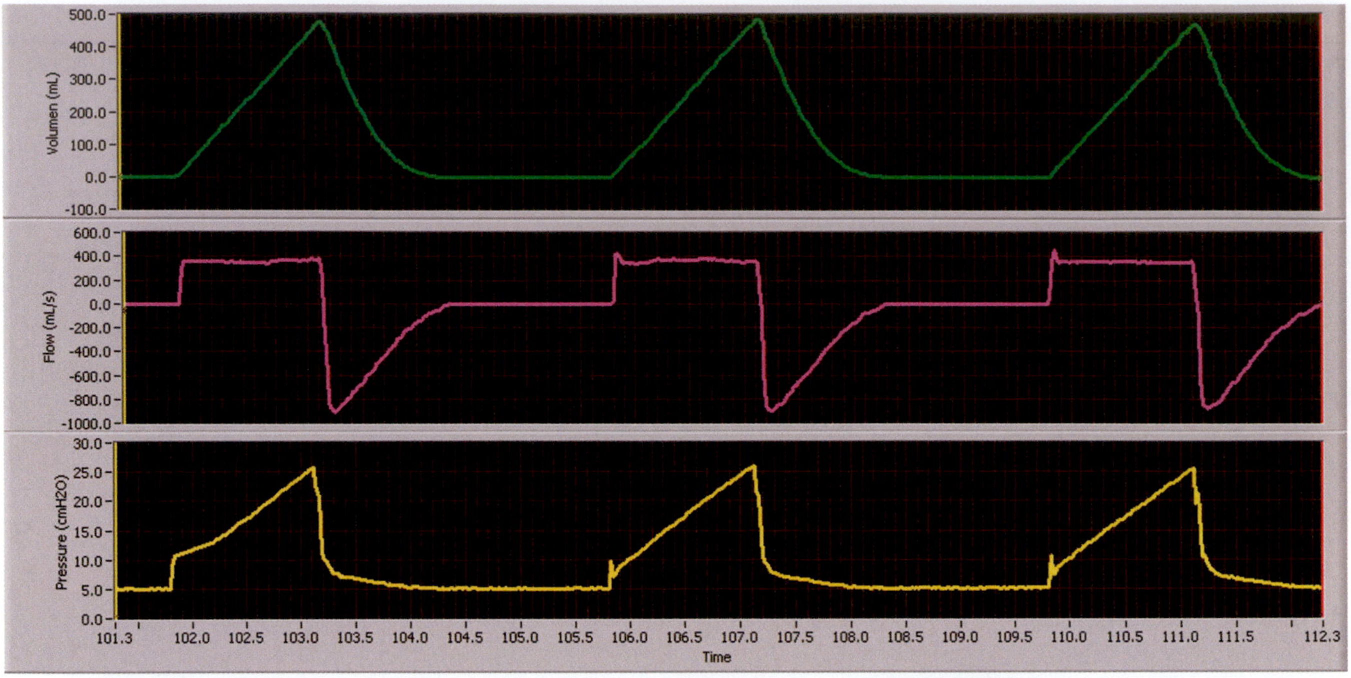

FIGURE 46-8 VC-CMV. *Top,* V_T; *middle,* flow; *bottom,* airway pressure waveform.

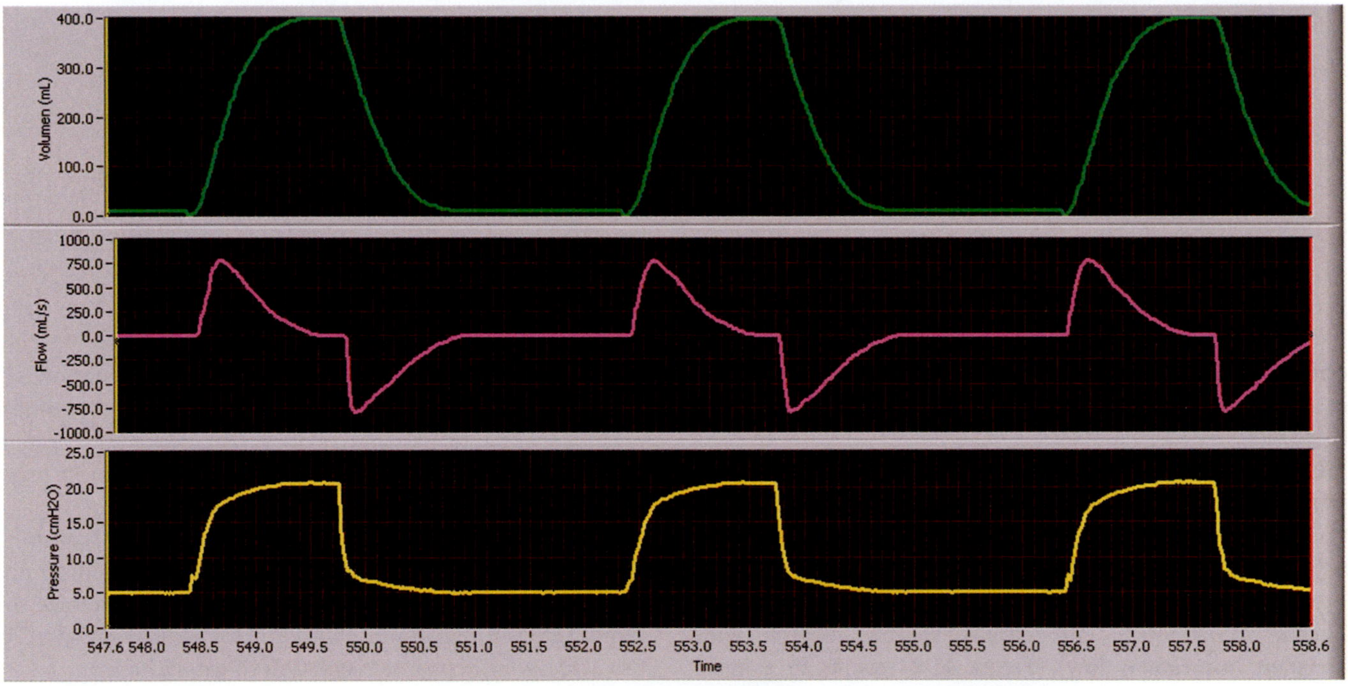

FIGURE 46-9 PC-CMV. *Top,* V_T; *middle,* flow; *bottom,* airway pressure waveform.

time constants when units have equal compliances but unequal resistances (e.g., status asthmaticus).[27] The instability of V_T caused by airway leaks can be minimized by using pressure-controlled rather than volume-controlled ventilation. Increased V_T stability may lead to better gas exchange and lower risk of pulmonary volutrauma.[30]

Use of a rectangular pressure waveform opens alveoli earlier in the inspiratory phase during PC-CMV and results in a higher mean airway pressure than VC-CMV with a rectangular flow waveform, allowing more time for oxygenation to occur.[31] In PC-CMV, however, inspiratory flow is not a parameter set by the clinician. It is variable and dependent on patient effort and lung mechanics, improving patient comfort and patient-ventilator synchrony. However, as lung mechanics or patient effort or both change, volume delivery (V_T and minute ventilation) changes.

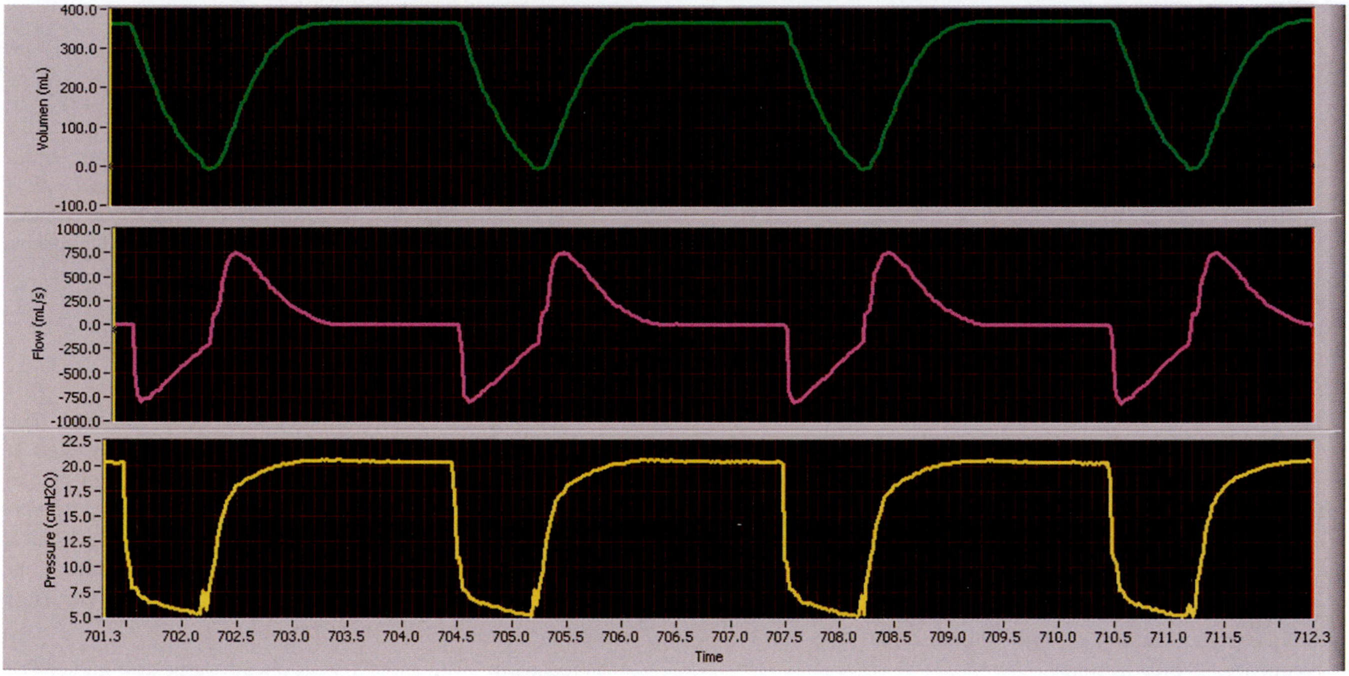

FIGURE 46-10 PC-IRV. The flow waveform for any breath does not return to baseline before the next breath, resulting in auto-PEEP and an increase in mean airway pressure. *Top,* V_T; *middle,* flow; *bottom,* airway pressure waveform.

Because V_T is not directly controlled, the pressure gradient (PIP – PEEP) is the primary parameter used to alter the breath size and CO_2 tensions. Typically, PIP is adjusted to provide the patient with a V_T within the desired range.[32] As with VC-CMV, the mandatory breath rate set by the clinician depends on the presence of ventilatory muscle activity and the severity of lung disease. When higher mandatory breath rates are needed (>30 breaths/min), it is essential for the clinician to provide a sufficient expiratory time and prevent air trapping.

As long as lung mechanics and patient effort remain constant, the volume and peak flow delivered to the patient remain unchanged.[33] When a decrease in patient effort, decrease in compliance, or increase in resistance occurs, less volume is delivered for the preset pressure for each breath. Conversely, improvements in patient effort and mechanics can dramatically increase the volume delivery to the patient in this mode. Close V_T monitoring is required to avoid ventilator-induced hyperventilation or hypoventilation.

The patient's cardiac index and O_2 consumption should be closely monitored as well. Higher mean airway pressures may impair cardiac output. In addition, PC-CMV with IRV can lead to the development of auto-PEEP, which can impair venous return, compromise O_2 delivery to the tissues, and result in marked air trapping.[34]

Pressure-Controlled Inverse Ratio Ventilation

PC-CMV may be used to accomplish pressure-controlled inverse ratio ventilation (PC-IRV), by increasing the inspiratory time directly or by increasing the I : E ratio to the desired value. PC-IRV is defined as pressure-controlled ventilation with an I : E ratio greater than 1 : 1 (Figure 46-10). Although some studies have shown improvement in oxygenation with PC-IRV versus CMV with PEEP, others have shown concurrent decreases in cardiac output.[28,35] Generally, if applied PEEP in normal ratio ventilation is equal to total PEEP (applied and intrinsic PEEP) in PC-IRV, the oxygenation benefits are equivalent without the marked depression in cardiac output.

Intermittent Mandatory Ventilation

As a partial support mode, IMV allows or requires the patient to sustain some WOB. The level of mechanical support needed depends on the specific physiologic process causing the need for mechanical ventilation, presence or degree of ventilatory muscle weakness, and presence and severity of lung disease. In this mode, mandatory breaths are delivered at a set rate. Between the mandatory breaths, the patient can breathe spontaneously at his or her own V_T and rate (Figure 46-11). Breaths can occur separately (e.g., IMV); breaths can be superimposed on each other (e.g., spontaneous breaths superimposed on mandatory breaths, as in bilevel positive airway pressure [bilevel PAP] or airway pressure release ventilation [APRV]); or mandatory breaths can be superimposed on spontaneous breaths, as in high-frequency ventilation administered during spontaneous breathing. Spontaneous breaths may be assisted (e.g., PSV) (Figure 46-12) or unassisted (e.g., PEEP or CPAP).

When the mandatory breath is patient-triggered, modern-day ventilators deliver the mandatory breath in synchrony with the patient's inspiratory effort. If no spontaneous efforts occur, the ventilator delivers a time-triggered breath. Because

MINI CLINI

Using Pressure-Controlled Ventilation

PROBLEM: The RT is caring for a 20-year-old patient with ARDS. The patient has no respiratory effort. Current ventilator settings are as follows:

Mode: VC-CMV
V_T: 400 ml
Frequency: 25 breaths/min
PEEP: 14 cm H_2O
FiO_2: 1
PIPs monitored on the ventilator: 40 to 50 cm H_2O
Mean airway pressure: 22 to 24 cm H_2O
Plateau pressure: 30 cm H_2O

An arterial blood gas is obtained, which reveals pH 7.28, PCO_2 41 mm Hg, and PO_2 50 mm Hg. The physician would like to employ pressure-controlled ventilation. What are the appropriate initial settings in PC-CMV mode to maintain the current minute ventilation?

Solution: Initial ventilator setting would be as follows:

Ventilator frequency, PEEP, and FiO_2: the same
Frequency: 25 breaths/min
PEEP: 14 cm H_2O
FiO_2: 1

To keep the minute ventilation constant, the RT needs to set the PIP high enough to deliver the same V_T as in volume control (400 ml).

1. Calculate the patient's respiratory system compliance:

$$\begin{aligned} \text{Compliance} &= V_T/\text{Plateau pressure} - \text{PEEP} \\ &= 400\ \text{ml}/30\ \text{cm H}_2\text{O} - 14\ \text{cm H}_2\text{O} \\ &= 25\ \text{ml/cm H}_2\text{O} \end{aligned}$$

2. Calculate the pressure limit in PC-CMV mode to achieve the target V_T. Because the pressure limit is measured relative to PEEP on this ventilator, the equation is:

$$\begin{aligned} \text{Ventilating pressure} &= V_T/\text{Compliance} \\ &= 400\ \text{ml}/25\ \text{ml/cm H}_2\text{O} \\ &= 16\ \text{cm H}_2\text{O} \end{aligned}$$

$$\text{PIP} = \text{Ventilating pressure (PC setting 16 cm H}_2\text{O)} + \text{PEEP (14 cm H}_2\text{O) or 30 cm H}_2\text{O}$$

A shortcut is to realize that the required pressure limit is the plateau pressure on VC-CMV. The PIP (relative to atmospheric pressure) is 30 cm H_2O.

MINI CLINI

Determining Appropriate Ventilator Rate

PROBLEM: A 36-year-old woman with traumatic brain injury was intubated in the emergency department with a 7-mm endotracheal tube and transferred to the RT in the neurointensive care unit. She is paralyzed and sedated. Her current ventilator settings are as follows:

Mode: VC-CMV
V_T: 405 ml
Frequency: 15 breaths/min
FiO_2: 0.5

The pulse oximeter displays 97%, and end-tidal CO_2 monitor is reading 49. The patient's weight is estimated at 45 kg. End-tidal CO_2 is stable and 4 mm Hg higher than $PaCO_2$. The clinical goal is to minimize ICP. Because intracranial blood flow is inversely proportional to $PaCO_2$, ventilation should be increased to maintain $PaCO_2$ at about 35 to 40 mm Hg. The RT needs to make appropriate ventilator changes to achieve the target $PaCO_2$.

Discussion: The current V_T is already large at 8 ml/kg. The increase in ventilation must be achieved by increasing frequency. Because the patient is paralyzed, the ventilation level is controlled by the set frequency, and $PaCO_2$ is predictable. The new frequency required is calculated using the following equation:

$$\text{Required frequency} = \text{Current frequency} \times \text{Current PaCO}_2/\text{Desired PaCO}_2$$

$$\begin{aligned} \text{Required frequency} &= 15\ \text{breaths/min} \times 49\ \text{mm Hg}/35\ \text{mm Hg} \\ &= 21\ \text{breaths/min} \end{aligned}$$

spontaneous breaths decrease pleural pressure, ventilatory support with IMV usually results in a lower mean intrathoracic pressure than CMV, which can result in a higher cardiac output.[36]

When used to wean a patient from mechanical ventilation, the intent of IMV is to provide respiratory muscle rest during the mandatory breaths and exercise during spontaneous breaths. However, studies have shown that IMV weaning prolongs the duration of mechanical ventilation compared with PSV and spontaneous breathing trials.[37,38]

Volume-Controlled Intermittent Mandatory Ventilation

Volume-controlled intermittent mandatory ventilation (VC-IMV) has been advocated for patients with relatively normal lung function recovering from sedation or rapidly reversing respiratory failure.[39] However, the use of IMV has greatly decreased over the years in favor of VC-CMV, PC-CMV, and PSV, and there are no specific situations in adults where IMV would be the optimal mode.

Example. VC-IMV has been usually selected for patients with neuromuscular disorders, such as Guillain-Barré syndrome. Typically, normal lung function and an intact ventilatory drive characterize these patients. As the disease progresses, ascending muscle weakness eventually affects the patient's ventilatory muscles. Mechanical ventilation is considered when it is difficult for the patient to sustain V_T and minute ventilation. The degree of support depends on the patient's inherent muscle strength. Large V_T (6 to 8 ml/kg) and high peak flow (>80 L/min) may be needed to alleviate dyspnea and maximize patient comfort.[40] As respiratory muscle function improves, mandatory breath support can be reduced.

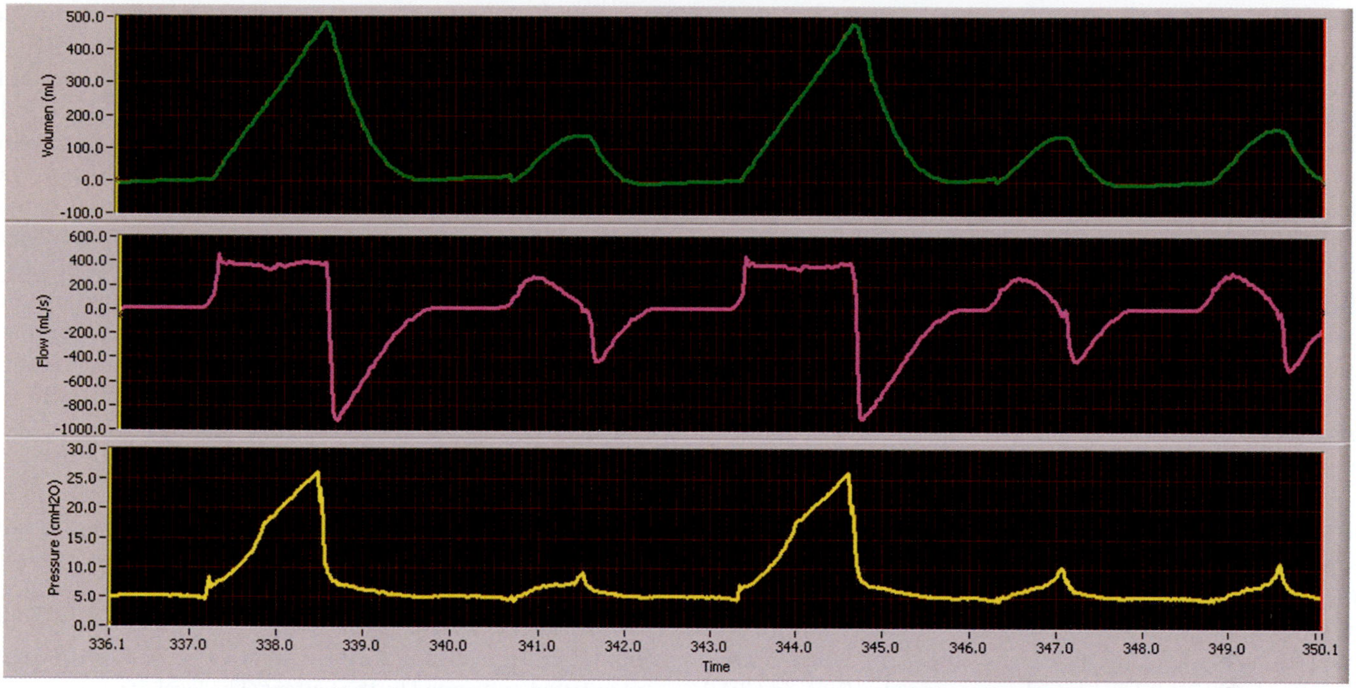

FIGURE 46-11 VC-SIMV + CPAP. *Top,* V_T; *middle,* flow; *bottom,* airway pressure waveform.

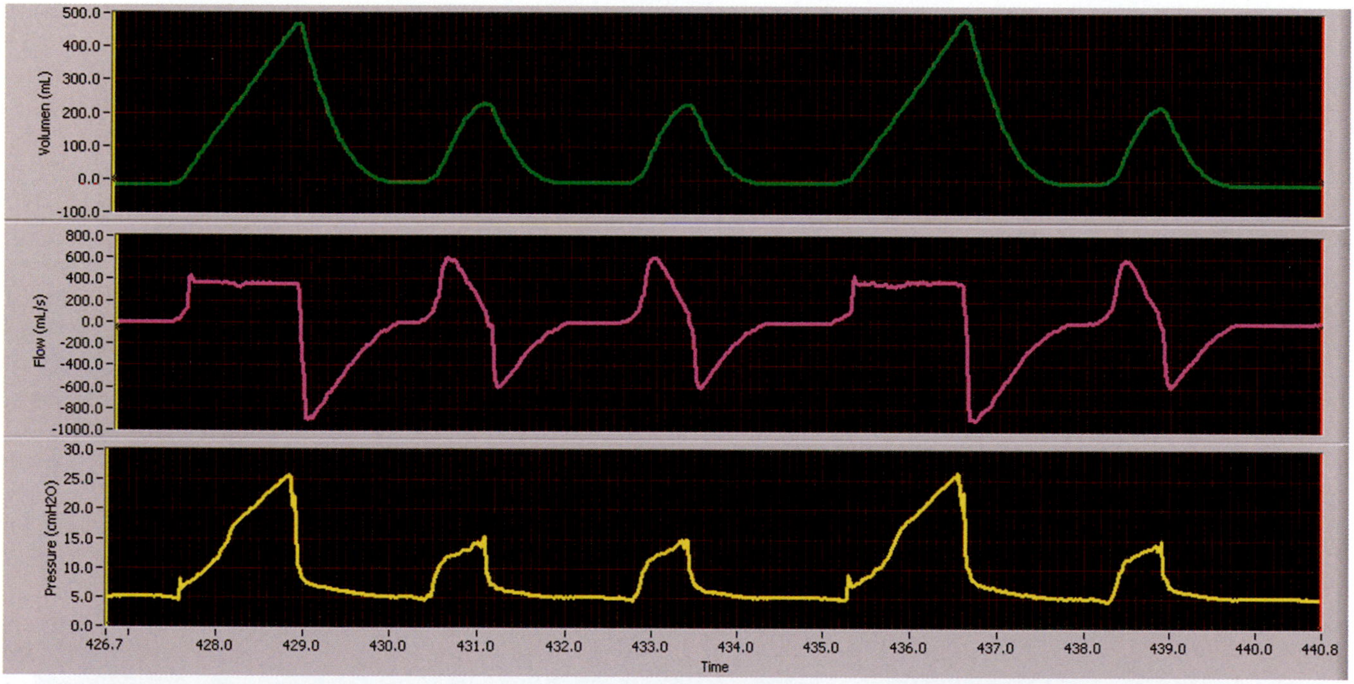

FIGURE 46-12 VC-SIMV + PSV. The addition of PSV to the spontaneous breaths increases spontaneous V_T. *Top,* V_T; *middle,* flow; *bottom,* airway pressure waveform.

Pressure-Controlled Intermittent Mandatory Ventilation

Pressure-controlled intermittent mandatory ventilation (PC-IMV) is indicated when preservation of the patient's spontaneous efforts is important and patient-ventilatory synchrony is a concern.[41] PC-IMV has been traditionally associated with mechanical ventilation of infants not only because of their oxygenation problems but also because traditionally it had been difficult to control V_T at such small values.[42]

Liberation from this mode involves the gradual reduction of the PIP and the mandatory breath rate. As lung compliance improves, adjustments in PIP are necessary to prevent overdistention of the lung. Adjustments in PIP and set mandatory breath rate are critical to prevent hyperventilation.

Example. Perhaps the most familiar scenario is the application of PC-IMV in premature infants with respiratory distress syndrome. Initially, because of a noncompliant lung, compliant chest wall, and poor respiratory effort, the infant may require a relatively high mandatory breath rate to achieve acceptable V_T and acid-base balance. Mandatory breath rates are set to provide adequate minute ventilation.

With PC-IMV, the infant can breathe spontaneously between or during the mandatory breaths, at his or her own rate and V_T. Liberation from this mode of partial support ventilation involves the gradual reduction of the PIP and mandatory breath rate. As the infant's lung compliance improves and spontaneous ventilatory efforts become more effective, lower PIPs and mandatory breath rates are needed to deliver adequate minute ventilation.

Airway Pressure Release Ventilation

A mode related to both PC-IRV and PC-IMV is APRV, in which the patient breathes spontaneously throughout periods of high and low applied CPAP (Figure 46-13).[43] APRV intermittently decreases or "releases" the airway pressure from an upper pressure (P_{high}) or CPAP level to a lower pressure (P_{low}) or CPAP level. The pressure release usually lasts about 0.2 to 1.5 seconds depending on whether or not air trapping is desired. In Figure 46-13, inspiratory time is longer than expiratory time, and spontaneous breaths are superimposed on this mandatory pattern of pressurization and release. Spontaneous breaths are supplemented by PSV. This is a feature of APRV available on some ventilators, where APRV is referred to as *bilevel ventilation.* In APRV, the I : E ratio is usually greater than 1 : 1, which is similar to PC-IRV, but APRV offers the advantage of allowing spontaneous breathing throughout the periods of inspiratory and expiratory positive pressure.[44]

APRV also provides ventilation and oxygenation without adversely affecting hemodynamic values because of the periodic reductions in intrathoracic pressure during the spontaneous breaths. In addition, peak airway pressure during APRV may be less than with VC-IRV for comparable oxygenation and ventilation.[45] APRV compared with conventional volume-controlled or pressure-controlled SIMV showed that with APRV there was a decrease in peak airway pressures, improved hemodynamics, and a decreased need for vasopressor and intropic support.[46] However, the cost of these potential benefits is patient effort; WOB is markedly increased and transpulmonary pressure is excessive, potentially inducing lung injury during APRV.[44] There are no data to indicate a better outcome with APRV than with other approaches to ventilatory support when a similar approach to managing oxygenation is used. Specific indications for APRV are unclear.

Continuous Spontaneous Ventilation

Spontaneous breath modes include modes in which all breaths are initiated and ended by the patient. The level of support these modes of ventilation provide determines the amount of WOB the patient ultimately assumes. CPAP, PSV,[47] automatic tube compensation (ATC), proportional assist ventilation (PAV), and neurally assisted ventilatory assist (NAVA) are continuous spontaneous breath modes.[48]

Continuous Positive Airway Pressure

CPAP is spontaneous breathing at an elevated baseline pressure (Figure 46-14). Breaths are patient-triggered and cycled.[49,50] V_T

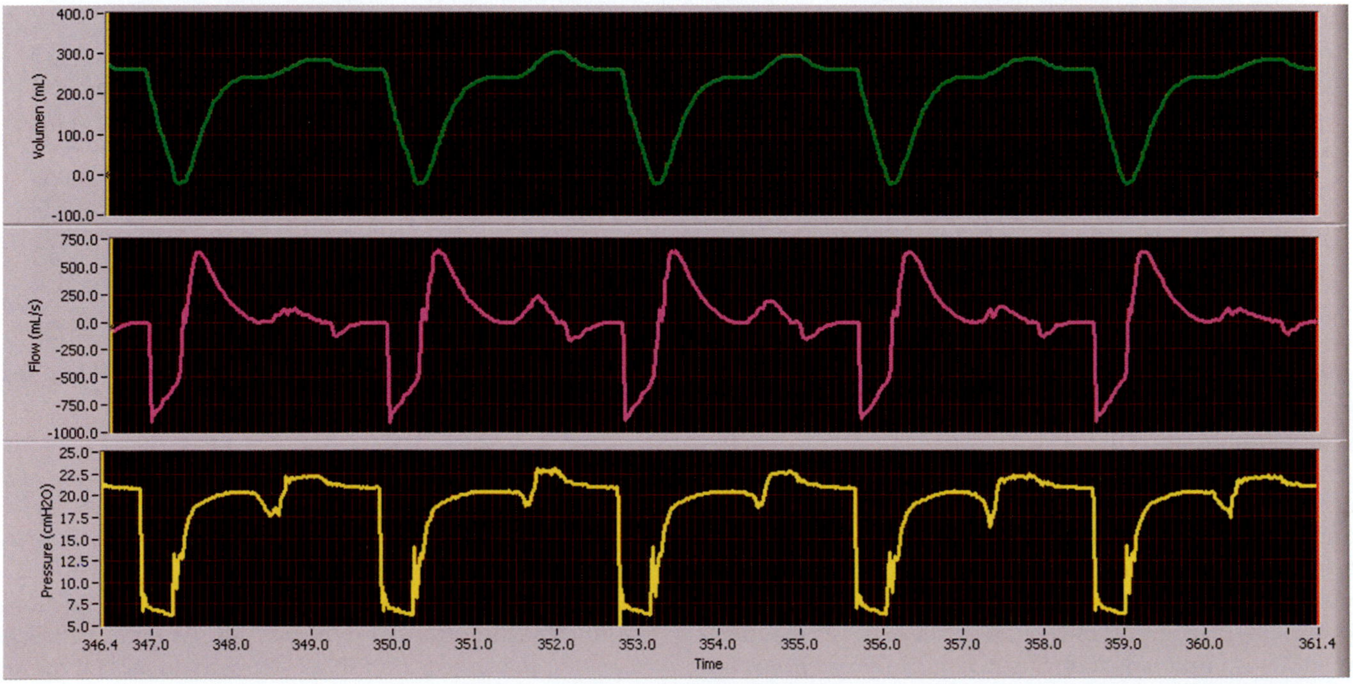

FIGURE 46-13 APRV. In APRV, the patient is able to breathe spontaneously throughout the total cycle time. *Top,* V_T; *middle,* flow; *bottom,* airway pressure waveform.

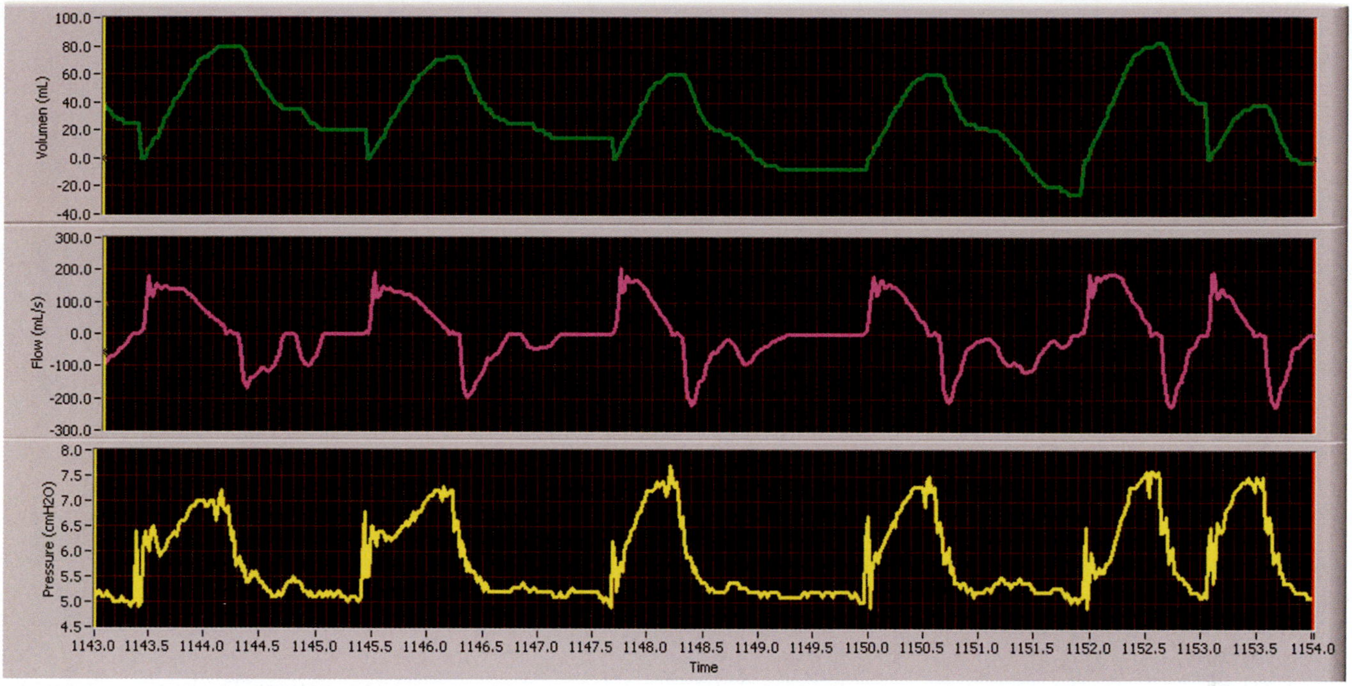

FIGURE 46-14 CPAP. *Top,* V_T scalar; *middle,* flow scalar; *bottom,* airway pressure scalar.

depends on patient effort and lung mechanics. CPAP increases alveolar pressure and maintains alveoli open. In contrast to NPV and PPV, airway pressure with CPAP is theoretically constant (baseline pressure ±2 cm H_2O) throughout the respiratory cycle. Because airway pressure does not change, CPAP does not provide ventilation. For gas to move into the lungs during CPAP, the patient must create a spontaneous transairway pressure gradient. Although NPV and PPV produce the pressure gradients needed for gas flow into the lungs, CPAP maintains alveoli at greater inflation volume, restoring FRC. An important physiologic feature of CPAP is that as alveoli are maintained open, FiO_2 needed to maintain adequate PaO_2 may decrease. Oxygenation becomes more efficient at any given FiO_2, as measured by PaO_2/FiO_2 ratio and shunt fraction. The potential side effects associated with PPV also exist for CPAP but usually to a lesser degree.

Pressure Support Ventilation

PSV is a form of PC-CSV that assists the patient's inspiratory efforts (Figure 46-15). At very low levels of support, this mode unloads WOB the ventilator circuitry imposes on the respiratory muscles.[51] If the level of support is maximized, the ventilator may assume all WOB.[52] The result of high levels of support is a reduction in the respiratory rate, reduction in respiratory muscle activity and fatigue, reduction in O_2 consumption, and improvement or stabilization of spontaneous V_T.[53,54] However, the positive attributes of this mode of ventilation can be negated if ventilator parameters are not properly set. The ventilator must be able to detect spontaneous patient effort. It is critical for the clinician to adjust the trigger sensitivity correctly. Of equal importance is the clinician-set rise time, the time required for the ventilator to reach the inspiratory pressure limit, and termination criteria, the minimal flow resulting in cycling to exhalation (see Chapter 47). Ventilator graphics are often helpful when adjusting these parameters and optimizing patient-ventilator synchrony.

Regardless of the level of support provided, the patient has primary control over the breath rate and inspiratory time and flow rate delivered during this mode of assisted ventilation. The V_T resulting from a PSV breath depends on the preset pressure level, patient effort, and mechanical forces opposing ventilation (lung–chest wall compliance and airway resistance). Of all of the classic modes of ventilation, PSV exerts the least control over the patient's ventilatory pattern and as a result should improve patient-ventilator synchrony. Since the first description of PSV in 1982, it has been used either to overcome the imposed resistance associated with the artificial airway or to provide ventilatory support with minimal control.[55] PSV is useful in any patient with an intact ventilatory drive and a stable ventilatory demand.

Bilevel PAP (BiPAP; Respironics, Inc, Murrysville, PA) is simply PSV with PEEP applied noninvasively.[56] With bilevel PAP, inspiratory positive airway pressure (or PSV) and expiratory positive airway pressure (PEEP) are set. The duration of inspiratory positive airway pressure and expiratory positive airway pressure can be independently adjusted to set the I : E ratio. Although it was originally developed to enhance the capabilities of home CPAP systems used for management of obstructive sleep apnea, bilevel PAP has been successfully used in the home and the hospital for noninvasive ventilatory support of patients with acute and chronic respiratory failure.[57]

Example. An example of the use of PC-CSV is noninvasive PSV and PEEP in the management of a patient with COPD in an acute exacerbation. As described in detail in Chapter 49, PSV

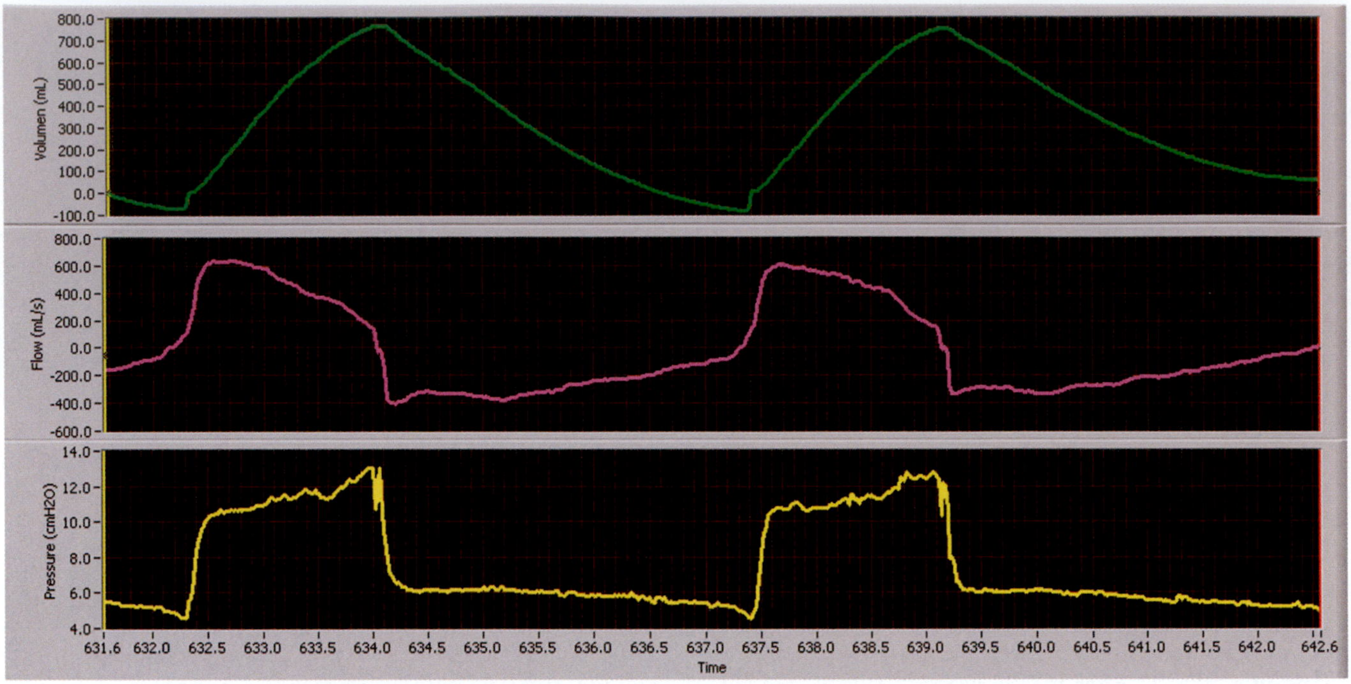

FIGURE 46-15 PSV. *Top,* V_T; *middle,* flow; *bottom,* airway pressure waveform.

has been shown in this setting to decrease the frequency of intubation, length of mechanical ventilation, development of ventilator-associated pneumonia, and patient mortality.

Proportional Assist Ventilation

PAV is based on both the mechanics of the total respiratory system and the resistive properties of the artificial airway; that is, the ventilator delivers a pressure assist in proportion to the patient's desired V_T (volume assist) and to the patient's instantaneous inspired flow (flow assist). The response of these two aspects of ventilatory assistance is automatically adjusted to meet changes in the patient's ongoing ventilatory demand. This algorithm is based on the law of motion as it applies to the respiratory system:

$$P_{musc} + P_{appl} = (\text{Volume} \times E) + (\text{Flow} \times R)$$

where P_{musc} is pressure generated by the respiratory muscles, P_{appl} is pressure applied by the ventilator, and E and R are elastic and resistance properties of the respiratory system. Assuming that E and R are linear during inspiration, the instantaneous flow and volume to be delivered are proportional to the resistive and elastic WOB. The ventilator continuously measures the instantaneous flow and volume and periodically measures the E and R. Using this information, the ventilator software adjusts gas delivery by estimating P_{musc} and assisting P_{musc} in a proportional manner, the percent set by the clinician. The patient is the determinant of the ventilatory pattern. Patients are given the freedom to select a ventilatory pattern that is rapid and shallow or slow and deep. If the patient desires a small V_T, a low level of pressure is applied, and if a large V_T is desired, a high pressure is applied. The ventilator does not force any control variable except the unloading of E and R in a proportional manner. See Chapter 45 for details on operation of PAV.

Numerous studies have evaluated the effect of PAV during noninvasive PPV.[58-62] Most of these comparisons were between PAV and PSV,[58,62] and in almost all of these comparisons the patients evaluated had chronic respiratory failure and were in an acute exacerbation. Patients managed with PAV had a lower refusal rate, had a more rapid reduction in respiratory rate, and developed fewer complications.[60,61] In these studies, gas exchange and respiratory pattern did not differ between PSV and PAV, but the patients ventilated with PAV were more comfortable. PAV has also been shown to be essentially equivalent to PSV in stable patients with chronic ventilatory failure[59] and in patients with acute cardiogenic pulmonary edema.[62]

PAV has been most widely studied during invasive mechanical ventilation.[63-65] As with the evaluation of PAV in other settings, most of the comparisons focused on the physiologic response observed when PSV is changed to PAV. Generally, during invasive ventilation, the change from PSV to PAV results in lower V_T, more rapid respiratory rate, lower peak airway pressure, and lower mean airway pressure without significant changes in gas exchange or hemodynamics.[66-68] In a randomized comparison of PAV versus PSV each for a 48-hour period in a series of critically ill patients,[65] the percentage of patients' failing the transition to PAV or PSV differed, 11% failing PAV versus 22% failing PSV. In addition, the proportion of patients developing asynchrony was greater with PSV versus PAV. The current data on PAV indicates it can sustain the same patients as PSV—patients who can breathe spontaneously and manage their ventilator drive normally.

Neurally Adjusted Ventilatory Assist

From a conceptual perspective, NAVA is essentially the same as PAV except that PAV responds to changes in airway pressure and flow, whereas NAVA responds to changes in diaphragmatic EMG activity. However, for NAVA to function properly, a specially designed nasogastric catheter with a 10-cm length of EMG electrodes must be in place. Both PAV and NAVA respond to patient effort providing ventilatory support in a proportional manner. The clinician does not set pressure, volume, flow, or time in either mode. The only parameter set is the proportion of effort unloaded by the ventilator; in NAVA, this is set as the number of cm H_2O applied per microvolt of diaphragmatic EMG activity.

NAVA responds similarly to PAV, when compared to pressure support—NAVA results in low airway pressures, smaller tidal volumes, more rapid rates, and increased patient-ventilator synchrony.[69,70] PEEP titration also affects baseline diaphragmatic EMG activity. As PEEP is increased EMG activity decreases. Minimal EMG activity seems to correspond to optimal PEEP level.[71]

NAVA application in neonates results in similar outcomes as observed in adults.[72,73] After the change to NAVA, V_T tends to decrease, respiratory rate to increase, and peak diaphragmatic EMG activity to decrease. In addition, despite the open ventilating system (uncuffed artificial airway), triggering and cycling were still primarily neurally activated.[72,73]

The most important advantage of PAV and NAVA over traditional modes of ventilation is improved synchrony. The specific indications for PAV and NAVA are not fully established; however, both can be reasonably used in any patient with an intact ventilatory drive. The primary indication would be a patient with a significant level of asynchrony.

Automatic Tube Compensation

ATC is similar to the flow assist aspect of PAV but considers only the resistance of the endotracheal tube.[74] ATC is an adjunct that automatically adjusts the airway pressure to compensate for endotracheal tube resistance to gas flow by maintaining tracheal pressure constant at the baseline level.[74] The goal is to eliminate WOB imposed by the endotracheal tube. In ATC, the RT inputs into the ventilator the type and size of artificial airway (endotracheal tube or tracheostomy tube) and the percent compensation desired (10% to 100%). The ventilator continuously measures flow and calculates the amount of pressure needed to overcome the resistance of the airway (pressure = resistance × flow). As a result, the greater the inspiratory demand, the greater the pressure applied. Pressure varies throughout the breath.

ATC may be applied during inspiration (positive airway pressure) or during both inspiration and expiration (negative airway pressure). However, expiratory ATC may result in early airway closure and increased air trapping. ATC has been referred to as *electronic extubation,* meaning that if the airway pressure is low during inspiration (5 to 7 cm H_2O), it is simply overcoming the resistance of the endotracheal tube with a normal inspiratory effort.[75] Consequently, many clinicians consider this an indication that spontaneous ventilation can be maintained without ventilatory support and the patient should be considered for extubation. Although in theory the use of ATC to wean patients appears ideal, no data to date have indicated that ATC weans patients faster than spontaneous breathing trials.

Adaptive Modes and Dual Control

The first adaptive control/dual control mode was described by Amato and colleagues.[76] Their major finding was that the ventilatory workload imposed on the inspiratory muscles during volume-assured PSV was significantly reduced by the use of dual control. In this mode, pressure support is combined with volume control. However, this benefit was due to the fact that inspiration started out in pressure support and stayed there unless the V_T target was not met. The improvement was mostly a result of the improved synchrony between the patient and the machine. These investigators did not show a specific benefit of the actual dual nature of the mode (i.e., switching from pressure support to volume control), and no evidence has been published in the literature since then supporting this mode. Anecdotal reports indicate that it is difficult to adjust pressure, volume, and flow settings to make the mode work properly, in particular, if the mechanical properties of the patient's respiratory system are changing rapidly.

Pressure-regulated volume control (PRVC), or PC-CMV, and *volume support (VS)*, or PC-CSV, are examples of adaptive control/dual control modes. PRVC is based on pressure-controlled ventilation, and VS is based on PSV. In both modes, the ventilator attempts to maintain a target V_T by adjusting the pressure level based on the previous breath. When a clinician places a patient in PRVC, a target V_T, breath rate, and maximum (i.e., alarm) pressure limit are clinician set, whereas for a patient placed in VS, a target V_T and maximum (i.e., alarm) pressure limit are clinician set. In both modes, once the patient is connected to the ventilator, the patient-ventilator interaction that occurs in the first few breaths is critical. Initially, the ventilator calculates total system compliance. On the succeeding three or four breaths, the ventilator monitors the peak airway pressures and expiratory V_T. The ventilator determines the pressure level necessary to deliver the clinician-set "target" V_T, for the given total system compliance. ("Target" is used because the ventilator aims to deliver it, over the course of several breaths, but may not hit the mark if the maximum pressure limit is set too low.)

The patient-ventilator interaction is monitored on a breath-by-breath basis. If the patient's lung compliance improves (or patient effort increases), the ventilator delivers subsequent mandatory breaths at a lower pressure level to maintain the target V_T. This adjustment by the ventilator reduces the risk of alveolar overdistention and volutrauma. Conversely, the ventilator responds to worsening pulmonary compliance (or decreasing patient effort) by increasing the pressure limit until the V_T is achieved. The ventilator makes pressure level changes in small increments, 1 to 3 cm H_2O per breath, and does not exceed the maximum pressure limit set by the clinician. These automatic ventilator responses to changes in a patient's lung mechanics minimize the risk of ventilator-induced hyperventilation or hypoventilation. The desired outcome is a stable or consistent minute ventilation and enhanced patient comfort. However, the major problem with these modes is that the ventilator cannot distinguish between the patient improving and heightened levels of ventilator demand. If patient demand results in a larger V_T, the ventilator ventilates less.[77]

In most ventilators, pressure can be decreased all the way to the PEEP level. This situation can lead to ventilatory failure.[77] Both RPVC and VS should be used very cautiously in all patients with a normal or increased ventilatory demand. Randomized comparison between these modes and other, more traditional, modes failed to show any outcome benefit.[78,79]

Example. PRVC or VS has been used in infants with respiratory distress syndrome.[80] Rapidly changing pulmonary mechanics from surfactant administration are associated with complications such as pulmonary air leaks, intraventricular hemorrhage, and bronchopulmonary dysplasia. These adaptive modes respond to changes in a patient's lung mechanics and may reduce the incidence of these common complications.

Adaptive support ventilation (ASV), or PC-IMV, is an example of optimal control in adaptive ventilation. Adaptive support ventilation is a pressure-targeted mode that optimizes the relationship between V_T and respiratory frequency based on lung mechanics as predicted by Otis.[81] ASV uses a pressure ventilation format establishing a ventilatory pattern that minimizes WOB and auto-PEEP, while limiting peak airway pressure. In this regard, ASV is similar to PC-CMV and PRVC in its gas delivery format. It differs from PC-CMV and PRVC by its additional algorithmic control of the ventilatory pattern.[82] ASV automatically determines the V_T and respiratory rate that best maintains the peak pressure below the target level.[83] The clinician inputs the patient's ideal body weight, high pressure limit, PEEP, FiO_2, inspiratory rise time, flow cycle percentage, and percentage of predicted minute volume desired. The ventilator periodically measures dynamic compliance and the respiratory time constant and determines the desired mandatory rate. Ideal body weight is used by the ventilator to calculate the minute volume, which is divided by the rate for determination of V_T.[84] The newest adaption to ASV is referred to as Intellivent. With this adaption the ventilator operates the same as with ASV but in addition has the ARDSnet PEEP/FIO_2 tables programmed into the ventilator algorithm. Thus, as the patient's SpO_2 changes PEEP and FIO_2 are adjusted as dictated by the ARDSnet protocols.

When ASV is compared to VC-IMV, ASV decreases inspiratory load and improves patient-ventilator synchrony.[85] Others have shown that ASV resulted in a shorter duration of intubation than VC-IMV in postoperative cardiac patients with no complications.[86] More recently, Belliato and colleagues[87] comparing PC-IMV (optimal) to ASV showed that the ventilator was able to differentiate between patient types and select appropriate settings.[88] Using a lung model, Sulemanji and coworkers[89] determined that ASV could provide better lung protection than a fixed V_T of 6 ml/kg ideal body weight. ASV control has been adapted to respond to end-tidal CO_2 levels.[89] This new adaptation allows specific algorithms to be selected based on patient diagnosis: ARDS, COPD, brain injury, or healthy lung. This mode is the most sophisticated of the closed loop control modes available on ICU ventilators at the present time. However, additional study is needed to determine fully the type of patient in whom ASV is most useful. Current data would indicate ASV works very well in patients under controlled approaches to ventilatory support, but additional data in spontaneously ventilated patients are needed before it can be recommended in these patients.

RULE OF THUMB

Most patients requiring ventilatory support can be effectively ventilated with volume assist/control, pressure assist/control, and PSV modes.

Patient Positioning to Optimize Oxygenation and Ventilation

Patients receiving mechanical ventilation are turned frequently, usually at least every 2 hours, unless turning is contraindicated. Kinetic beds continually rotate patients and are designed to help prevent atelectasis, hypoxemia, secretion retention, and pressure sores. When patients are kept immobile, pooling of secretions in dependent lung zones can promote nosocomial pneumonia, and shrinking of dependent alveoli leads to decreases in ventilation and hypoxemia. However, the use of rotating kinetic beds is controversial in the prevention of nosocomial pneumonia.[90] No data are available to indicate that these very expensive beds improve patient outcome.

Patients with unilateral lung disease benefit from being placed in positions that promote matching of ventilation and perfusion. In unilateral lung disease, only one lung is affected by atelectasis, consolidation, or pneumonia. If the affected lung is placed in the dependent position, blood flow follows. The resultant poor $\dot{V}/\dot{Q}$ ratio in the affected lung contributes to venous admixture and hypoxemia. However, if the patient is rotated so that the good lung is in the dependent position, these relationships are reversed. With the good lung down, blood flows to well-ventilated alveoli, and $\dot{V}/\dot{Q}$ matching and arterial blood gas values improve. An added benefit of this maneuver is that the affected lung is placed in a postural drainage position, which promotes gravity drainage of retained secretions so that they can be removed.

A similar phenomenon has been described in ARDS. In a supine patient with ARDS, alveoli in the bases and posterior segments become atelectatic. Shunt increases, and the patient requires a high FiO_2 and PEEP for adequate oxygenation. If the patient is rotated into the prone position, several mechanisms have been proposed to improve oxygenation.[91] Blood flow is redistributed to areas that are better ventilated. This redistribution improves $\dot{V}/\dot{Q}$ relationships. Prone positioning removes the weight of the heart from its position over the lungs while the patient is supine. Pleural pressure in the now nondependent collapsed lung becomes more negative, improving alveolar recruitment. In addition, the stomach no longer lies over the dependent basilar posterior segments of the lower lobes.

A number of studies have demonstrated some benefit of prone positioning.[92-95] However, several persons are needed to "flip" the patient while ensuring monitoring lines and catheters are not disrupted and the patient is not inadvertently extubated. Wound dehiscence, facial or upper chest wall necrosis despite extensive padding, cardiac arrest immediately after movement to the prone position, dependent edema of the face, and corneal abrasion have been reported.[93] A recent meta-analysis of existing randomized controlled trials indicated no outcome benefit from prone positioning in patients with ARDS.[94] However, this meta-analysis also found that patients with PaO_2/FiO_2 less than 100 mm Hg were the group most likely to benefit from prone positioning. A recent randomized controlled trail showed the same results.[95] Considering the complications associated with prone positioning, only patients with very severe hypoxemia (PaO_2/FiO_2 <100 mm Hg) should be placed prone.

RULE OF THUMB

Patients who have unilateral or dependent consolidation or atelectasis and severe hypoxemia may benefit from positioning with the affected lung or segments in the nondependent position to promote improvement in $\dot{V}/\dot{Q}$ relationships. Prone positioning is indicated only if the PaO_2/FiO_2 is less than 100 mm Hg. When positioning the patient, great care should be taken to avoid the hazards associated with prone positioning.

CARDIOVASCULAR EFFECTS OF POSITIVE PRESSURE MECHANICAL VENTILATION

Thoracic Pump and Venous Return During Spontaneous and Mechanical Ventilation

The lungs and heart have a close functional relationship, and impaired performance of one affects the other. For this reason, the RT must fully understand what happens to cardiovascular function when a patient receives ventilatory support.

Early studies of the effect of PPV on the cardiovascular system showed an early, small, and transient increase in cardiac output that was followed almost immediately by a marked reduction in left ventricular outflow. Generally, the reduced cardiac output in these cases was directly related to the amount of pressure applied. More specifically, the decrease in left ventricular output corresponded to the increase in pleural pressure that occurred with PPV. Figure 46-16 compares the effects of spontaneous inspiration with the effect observed during PPV. Negative pleural pressure during spontaneous inspiration normally enhances venous return, increases right atrial filling, and improves pulmonary blood flow (see Figure 46-16, *A*). In combination, these factors increase left atrial and left ventricular filling and left ventricular stroke volume.

However, during PPV, pleural pressure can become positive (see Figure 43-16, *B*). Positive pleural pressure compresses the intrathoracic veins and increases central venous and right atrial filling pressures. As these pressures increase, venous return to the heart is impeded, and right ventricular preload and stroke volume decrease, as does pulmonary blood flow. Blood already

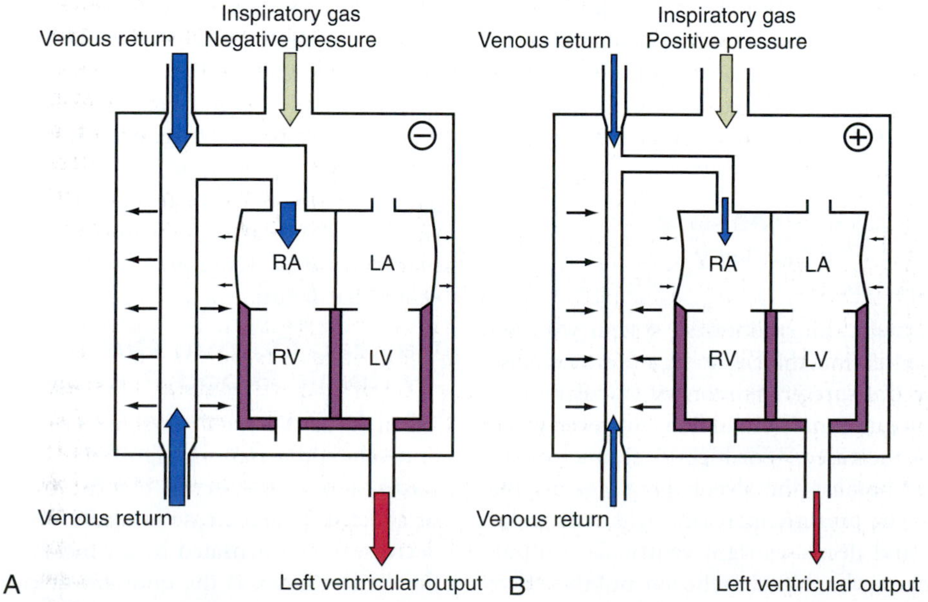

FIGURE 46-16 Relationship between pleural pressure and cardiac output in spontaneous **(A)** and positive pressure **(B)** breathing. *LA,* Left atrium; *LV,* left ventricle; *RA,* right atrium; *RV,* right ventricle.

in the pulmonary circulation is initially displaced into the left side of the heart and causes a transient increase in filling pressure and output. This initial effect lasts for only a few heartbeats. If positive pressure is continued, flow both to and from the left side of the heart decreases.

The high impedance encountered by blood returning to the right heart causes venous pooling, mainly in the capacitance vessels of abdominal viscera. This process effectively removes a large volume of blood from the circulation, which can further impair left ventricular output. These interactions are magnified when pleural pressure is increased further or circulating blood volume is low.[96] The venous impedance caused by PPV is not limited to blood flow coming from the abdomen. An increase in central venous pressure can restrict return flow from the brain. Impedance to venous return from the brain can increase ICP and reduce cerebral perfusion pressure (CPP). In combination with a decrease in left ventricular output, an increase in ICP during PPV can significantly impair cerebral perfusion and possibly result in cerebral ischemia and cerebral hypoxia.

In healthy individuals, the effects of PPV on cerebral blood flow (CBF) are minimized by autoregulatory mechanisms that maintain cranial perfusion pressures within a narrow range. However, patients with preexisting cerebrovascular problems and patients who already have an elevation in ICP may be at risk of decreased cerebral perfusion with PPV. Examples include neurosurgical patients and patients with head injuries, intracranial tumors, or cerebral edema from any cause. ICP monitoring may be necessary in the care of these patients.

Compensation in Healthy Persons

A decrease in cardiac output or blood pressure is rare among individuals with a normal cardiopulmonary system who are receiving mechanical ventilation. Compensatory mechanisms used to counter the decrease in stroke volume include increased heart rate, increase in systemic vascular and peripheral venous resistance, and shunting of blood away from the kidneys and lower extremities, which results in a consistent blood pressure. Because these compensatory mechanisms function by reflexes, the reflexes must be intact. Factors that block or blunt these vascular reflexes include sympathetic blockade, spinal anesthesia, spinal cord transection, and polyneuritis.

Pulmonary Vascular Pressure, Blood Flow, and Pulmonary Vascular Resistance

In patients with a normal cardiopulmonary system who are receiving mechanical ventilation, there is no significant increase in pulmonary vascular pressure or pulmonary vascular resistance and no decrease in pulmonary blood flow. However, when alveoli are distended by increased V_T or high PEEP, pulmonary blood flow is impeded because the alveoli press against the pulmonary capillaries. The pressure increases right ventricular afterload and volume and decreases right ventricular output. The ventricular septum may be shifted to the left, but this effect is more consistent with a high PEEP. This condition decreases left ventricular filling and output. The magnitude of these changes is proportional to lung compliance. As lung compliance decreases, the stiffer lungs can retain the increased pressure imposed by PEEP. In other words, the increased pressure in the lung is not transmitted to the vasculature to impede right ventricular output. An increase in intrapleural pressure secondary to an increase in lung pressure impedes venous return and decreases cardiac output further.

Right and Left Ventricular Function

Under conditions of a normal cardiovascular system with normal ventilation values, there are no significant changes in right or left ventricular function. Otherwise, mechanical ventilation would be difficult to manage, and the mortality and morbidity among patients receiving ventilation would be much higher. Right or left ventricular dysfunction appears to occur if the patient is hypovolemic, is receiving an excessive V_T, or is receiving more than optimum PEEP. The common factor is excessive alveolar pressure, enough to overcome or impede pulmonary blood flow or venous return.

Effect on Left Ventricular Dysfunction

PPV can improve cardiac output in some patients. In patients with left ventricular failure, application of PPV can increase both the left ventricular ejection fraction and the cardiac output. These improvements occur because PPV decreases left ventricular afterload in these patients. Afterload is an important factor in determining cardiac output, as is the resistance of the systemic vasculature. When afterload increases, cardiac output decreases (heart failure). When afterload is decreased by PPV or pharmacologic therapy, cardiac output may increase. This phenomenon explains why the cardiovascular status of some patients deteriorates when PPV is discontinued or treatment is changed from full to partial ventilatory support.

Endocardial Blood Flow

Blood flow in the coronary arteries depends on the gradient between the systemic diastolic pressure and the left ventricular end-diastolic pressure (represented by the pulmonary capillary wedge pressure). Any factor that decreases systemic diastolic pressure or increases wedge pressure decreases endocardial perfusion pressure. The factors of PPV that may decrease the systemic diastolic pressure are high mean airway pressure owing to a high PEEP, large V_T, or long inspiratory time. Factors that may increase the wedge pressure include excessive PEEP and left ventricular failure.

Cardiac Output, Cardiac Index, and Systemic Blood Pressure

When the cardiovascular system is normal with normal ventilation values, there are no significant changes in cardiac output, cardiac index, or systemic blood pressure. Cardiac output can be affected by a decrease in stroke volume with PPV, but this decrease is compensated by an increase in heart rate. Because the cardiac index is the quotient of cardiac output and body surface area (cardiac index = cardiac output in liters per minute/body surface area in square meters), a change in cardiac output would be reflected in the cardiac index. Systemic arterial pressure remains stable because of reflex compensation, which increases systemic vascular resistance. Cardiac output, cardiac index, and arterial pressure decrease only when mean airway pressure is high and intrapleural pressure increases precipitously. Hypotension owing to PPV alone is rare because clinicians do all that is necessary to prevent it, including adequate fluid administration, proper management of mean airway pressure and PEEP, and use of vasoconstricting drugs. Most cases of hypotension during mechanical ventilation are caused by sepsis and the accompanying vascular collapse.

RULE OF THUMB

Patients most likely to experience hemodynamic effects of mechanical ventilation are patients with a normal or increased lung compliance associated with decreased chest wall compliance. In this setting, there is little lung stretch but maximum transmission of ventilating pressure to the intrathoracic space.

MINIMIZING CARDIOVASCULAR EFFECTS OF POSITIVE PRESSURE MECHANICAL VENTILATION

The effect of PPV on the circulatory system depends primarily on two major factors: mean pleural pressure and cardiovascular status.

Mean Pleural Pressure

Pleural pressure is the pressure in the virtual pleural space. At the bedside, pleural pressure usually is measured indirectly as the esophageal pressure through an esophageal balloon connected to a pressure transducer. Because the esophagus is close to the pleurae, separated by only the flexible esophageal wall, change in esophageal pressure reflects change in pleural pressure but may not equal actual pleural pressure. An alternative to measuring pleural pressure is measuring mean airway pressure. Mean airway pressure is linearly related to mean pleural pressure and can be used clinically for monitoring of pressure changes.[97]

The effect of PEEP on pleural pressure is complex and depends on the patient's lungs and thoracic mechanics. Some of the pressure generated by a ventilator reaches the alveoli, where it is transmitted across the alveolar walls to the pleural space. How much of this alveolar pressure is transmitted to the pleural space depends on lung and thoracic mechanics.

Generally, for a given alveolar pressure, the more compliant the lung, the greater is the increase in pleural pressure. A patient with a disease causing a loss of elastic tissue, such as emphysema, is more subject to the cardiovascular effects of positive pressure than a person with normal lungs. In contrast, a lung with low compliance transmits less pressure to the pleural space; this explains, in part, why high levels of PEEP often are used with minimal cardiovascular effects on patients with low lung compliance (e.g., ARDS).

When the compliance of the chest wall is reduced, expansion of the thorax is limited, and more alveolar pressure is transmitted to the pleural space. Patients who have normal lungs but have thoracic restriction, as caused by kyphoscoliosis and spondylitis, are more subject to the cardiovascular effects of positive pressure than individuals with normal chest wall compliance. A similar effect can occur in patients with normal thoracic compliance who actively oppose a mandatory breath by contracting the expiratory muscles (as might occur in patient-ventilator asynchrony). Contraction of the expiratory muscles effectively decreases thoracic compliance and causes more alveolar pressure to be transmitted to the pleural space.

If resistance to airflow is high, less of the pressure generated at the airway reaches the alveoli. The high peak airway pressure common in patients with obstructive disorders is not reflected in high pleural pressure.

The effects of moderate increases in pleural pressure on cardiac output in healthy persons are minimal. In healthy persons, as left ventricular stroke volume decreases, compensatory responses increase both the cardiac rate and the tone of the venous capacitance vessels. These normal responses ensure adequate blood flow and perfusion pressure. However, if the patient already is hypovolemic or has lost peripheral venomotor tone, cardiovascular compensation may be impossible. In these cases, even a small increase in pleural pressure may result in a marked decrease in cardiac output.

Decreasing Mean Airway Pressure

Mean airway pressure is affected by respiratory rate, V_T, inspiratory time, inspiratory pause, expiratory time, I : E ratio, peak pressure, baseline pressure (PEEP or CPAP), and inspiratory flow waveform. If a decrease in mean airway pressure is necessary, altering any factor that contributes to mean airway pressure has an effect. If the PaO_2 is high, one of the most effective changes is a decrease in PEEP because it has a 1 : 1 relationship with mean airway pressure. If a decrease in PEEP is indicated, the RT must ensure that desaturation does not occur when the decrease has been accomplished. If the patient is being hyperventilated, a decrease in mandatory rate or V_T also decreases mean airway pressure.

The best way to determine the magnitude of the change is to use the mean airway pressure monitor on the ventilator. The peak pressure usually decreases with a decrease in VT. In pressure-controlled modes, the peak pressure may be decreased directly. The plateau pressure is a reflection of mean peak alveolar pressure. In volume-controlled ventilation, a decrease in V_T decreases plateau pressure. In pressure-controlled ventilation, the pressure setting may be reduced to limit plateau pressure. Efforts that increase lung compliance, such as PEEP or administration of diuretics to decrease interstitial edema, also may affect plateau pressure. Inspiratory time, expiratory time, and I : E ratio affect mean airway pressure. As inspiratory time lengthens or expiratory time decreases, mean airway pressure increases.

Fluid Management and Cardiac Output

The relationship between cardiac output and preload (end-diastolic volume) is described by the Frank-Starling phenomenon, which states, "in the normal heart, the diastolic volume (preload) is the principal force that governs the strength of ventricular contraction."[98] As preload (stretch) increases, so does force and presumably stroke volume. Stroke volume continues to increase with preload until the heart is distended by excess preload, after which stroke volume decreases. Another cause of a decrease in stroke volume is the decrease in ventricular contractility that occurs when afterload increases as the result of hypertension. With hypertension comes dilation and distention of the ventricles, which make the heart structurally abnormal. In an abnormal heart, it takes much less preload to put the heart into failure. Failure in this case is defined as decreased stroke volume despite increased preload (Figure 46-17).

When a patient receives PPV, there is risk of a decrease in venous return (preload) because of the increase in intrapleural pressure. Stroke volume may decrease, but the decrease is compensated for by a reflex increase in heart rate and vasomotor tone. Because of these compensatory mechanisms, most patients with a normal cardiopulmonary status who receive mechanical ventilation do not need additional fluid to maintain cardiac output. However, certain conditions can increase the risk of relative or actual hypovolemia, and the increase can decrease stroke volume, even if normal reflex compensation is present. These conditions include hypovolemic shock (owing to trauma and blood loss), sepsis (in which the normal reflex compensation is not present), and high PEEP and high mean airway pressure. In these conditions, fluid or blood administration may be necessary to maintain cardiac output and end-organ perfusion. In some patients who receive PPV with PEEP, an increase in PEEP can decrease cardiac output as discussed earlier. In this case, the outcome of PEEP in terms of improved tissue oxygenation ($DO_2 = CaO_2 \times$ cardiac output) should be determined. If tissue O_2 delivery decreases because of a decrease in cardiac output, but CaO_2 increases, fluid administration may be indicated to restore cardiac output by increasing preload.

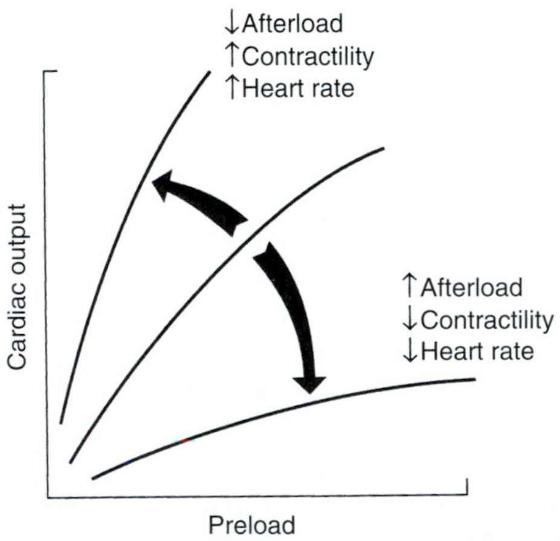

FIGURE 46-17 Effects of preload, afterload, contractility, and heart rate on cardiac output function curve. (Modified from Green JF: Fundamental cardiovascular and pulmonary physiology, ed 2, Philadelphia, 1987, Lea & Febiger.)

Pharmacologic Maintenance of Cardiac Output and Blood Pressure

First-line therapy for decreased cardiac output and blood pressure is fluid administration, unless the patient has congestive heart failure. In heart failure, inotropic therapy is indicated for decreased myocardial contractility, and vasodilators and diuretics are used to control hypertension, which decreases afterload. Diuretics are used to control fluid overload and to decrease preload to the distended heart. These factors in combination may return the heart to a more optimal portion of the Frank-Starling curve and improve stroke volume.

EFFECTS OF POSITIVE PRESSURE MECHANICAL VENTILATION ON OTHER BODY SYSTEMS

Increased Intracranial Pressure (ICP)

Perfusion of the brain is quantified by the cerebral perfusion pressure (CPP). The CPP is the difference between mean arterial pressure (MAP) and ICP. CPP may decrease in any case in which MAP decreases or ICP increases. If CPP decreases, cerebral blood flow (CBF) decreases. The result is cerebral ischemia and a decrease in cerebral O_2 metabolism. The cerebral circulation has the ability to maintain CBF even when CPP changes, a process called *cerebral autoregulation*. Cerebral **autoregulation** is a function of cerebral vascular resistance. If CPP decreases, cerebral vascular resistance decreases to maintain CPP. Cerebral autoregulation functions as long as CPP is in the range of 60 to 150 mm Hg and is limited by the ability of the cerebral arterioles to constrict and dilate. Under normal conditions, cerebral O_2 delivery and CPP exceed the metabolic needs of the brain for O_2 and glucose.

Normal MAP is 93 mm Hg if arterial pressure is 120/80 mm Hg. Normal ICP is less than 10 mm Hg, so normal CPP is about 80 to 85 mm Hg. CPP decreases when MAP decreases or ICP increases. Conditions leading to a decrease in MAP are shock, high PEEP, and high mean airway pressure. Increases in ICP are caused by traumatic brain injury (TBI), cerebral hemorrhage, cerebrovascular accident (stroke), and tumors. A CPP greater than 60 mm Hg maintains CBF and cerebral O_2 metabolism.

CO_2 is a potent cerebral vasodilator and an important regulator of the cerebral arteriolar diameter. As $PaCO_2$ decreases from 40 mm Hg, systemic pH increases. CO_2 concurrently diffuses across the blood-brain barrier. The result is an increased cerebrospinal fluid (CSF) pH. Although $PaCO_2$ is monitored in patients with TBI, the CSF pH modulates cerebral vascular resistance in an effort to decrease the ICP. When mechanical hyperventilation is used, cerebral vascular resistance increases, and the result is decreased ICP; this is why hyperventilation has been used in the management of TBI and acute increased ICP. However, in the presence of an already decreased CPP, CBF may decrease to the point at which cerebral ischemia is likely; this is the problem with immediate hyperventilation of a patient with TBI. In addition, prolonged hyperventilation allows renal excretion of bicarbonate, which allows the CSF pH to return to normal and negates any positive effect of hyperventilation on ICP. The effect of hyperventilation on the reduction of ICP lasts 1 hour. If hyperventilation is withdrawn and arterial pH and $PaCO_2$ return to normal values, the CSF pH decreases. Subsequent CSF acidosis leads to cerebral vasodilation and a rebound increase in CBF and ICP that exceeds the values before hyperventilation. For these reasons, hyperventilation must be used cautiously in the treatment of patients with TBI.[99]

Treatment of a Patient With a Closed Head Injury

Guidelines for the management of severe TBI were developed by neurosurgeons in the Joint Section on Neurotrauma and Critical Care.[100] The recommendation is as follows: "The use of prophylactic hyperventilation ($PaCO_2 < 35$ mm Hg) during the first 24 hours after TBI should be avoided because it can compromise cerebral perfusion during a time when CBF is reduced. Hyperventilation therapy may be necessary for brief periods when there is acute neurologic deterioration or for longer periods if there is intracranial hypertension refractory to sedation, paralysis, CSF drainage, and osmotic diuretics." The Joint Section further noted that "in the absence of increased ICP, chronic, prolonged hyperventilation therapy ($PaCO_2 <$ 35 mm Hg) should be avoided after TBI." These findings have resulted in several recommendations regarding the care of patients with TBI, as follows:

1. Patients with TBI may have transient, short periods of increased ICP, called *plateau waves*. Plateau waves may be caused by suctioning, repositioning, or other noxious stimuli. During a plateau wave, acute hyperventilation can control ICP until the pressure returns to baseline, at which time ventilation is resumed at the previous rate.
2. Hyperventilation should be avoided after TBI other methods can be employed to decrease elevated ICP. These methods include ventriculostomy for drainage of CSF, craniotomy for removal of mass lesions, osmotic diuretics, sedation, placing the patient in the semi-Fowler position, and paralysis. CPP should be maintained at greater than 70 mm Hg.
3. Intubation should be attempted only after the patient has been sedated, to prevent the associated increase in ICP. Exhaled partial pressure of end-tidal carbon dioxide ($PETCO_2$) should be monitored to maintain a constant $PaCO_2$ after arterial blood gas values are determined to find the correlation between $PaCO_2$ and $PETCO_2$.
4. ICP should be maintained at <20 mm Hg.[100]

Effect on Renal Function

Some patients receiving long-term PPV retain salt and water. In critically ill patients, water retention usually is evident when rapid weight gain occurs. In addition, such patients may have a reduced hematocrit, which is also consistent with hypervolemia secondary to water retention. These early observations are attributed to the direct and indirect effects of PPV on renal function.

In terms of direct effect, PPV can reduce urinary output 30% to 50%. This reduced urinary output during PPV is associated with a simultaneous reduction in renal blood flow, glomerular filtration rate, and sodium and potassium excretion.

Decreases in MAP to less than 75 mm Hg reduce renal blood flow, glomerular filtration rate, and urinary output. However, MAP this low seldom is caused by PPV alone, and kidney autoregulatory mechanisms generally can keep renal perfusion pressure within normal limits over a wide range of arterial pressures. Because restoring cardiac output to normal does not entirely restore urinary output compromised by PPV, other mechanisms must be involved. Impaired renal function during PPV is better associated with a decrease in intravascular volume.

The indirect effect of PPV on renal function may be most important. PPV has a marked effect on the water-retaining and sodium-retaining hormonal systems. Specifically, long-term PPV increases plasma renin activity, plasma aldosterone level, and level of vasopressin (urinary antidiuretic hormone). In addition, PPV decreases atrial natriuretic hormone levels (Figure 46-18).

Decreased right atrial transmural pressure is primarily responsible for the decrease in atrial natriuretic hormone, which leads to sodium retention. Similarly, vasopressin secretion may be enhanced by stimulation of the left atrial stretch receptors, which innervate the posterior pituitary gland. Increased secretion of vasopressin (antidiuretic hormone) and activation of the renin-angiotensin-aldosterone system lead to a decrease in urine output.

Decreased Liver and Splanchnic Perfusion

The effects of PPV on the liver and intestine are related to its effects on the cardiovascular system. Hepatic dysfunction with PPV can occur in patients with otherwise normal livers and manifests as an increase in serum bilirubin level. These effects appear to be directly related to the reduction in hepatic blood flow that occurs with PPV. Regardless of cause, these effects are aggravated by PEEP but can be reversed when cardiac output is returned to pre-PEEP levels with intravascular volume infusions.

Decreased Gastrointestinal Function

An increase in splanchnic resistance can contribute to gastric mucosal ischemia and helps explain the high incidence of gastrointestinal bleeding and stress ulceration in patients receiving long-term PPV. Stress ulcers (erosions of the gastric mucosa) are common among patients with life-threatening illness. Impaired blood flow inhibits the ability of the gastric mucosa to replace itself normally every 2 or 3 days. Stress ulcers are caused by impaired blood flow, not gastric acidity. Gastroduodenal motility also is severely impaired in mechanically ventilated patients.[101] These factors may result in translocation of

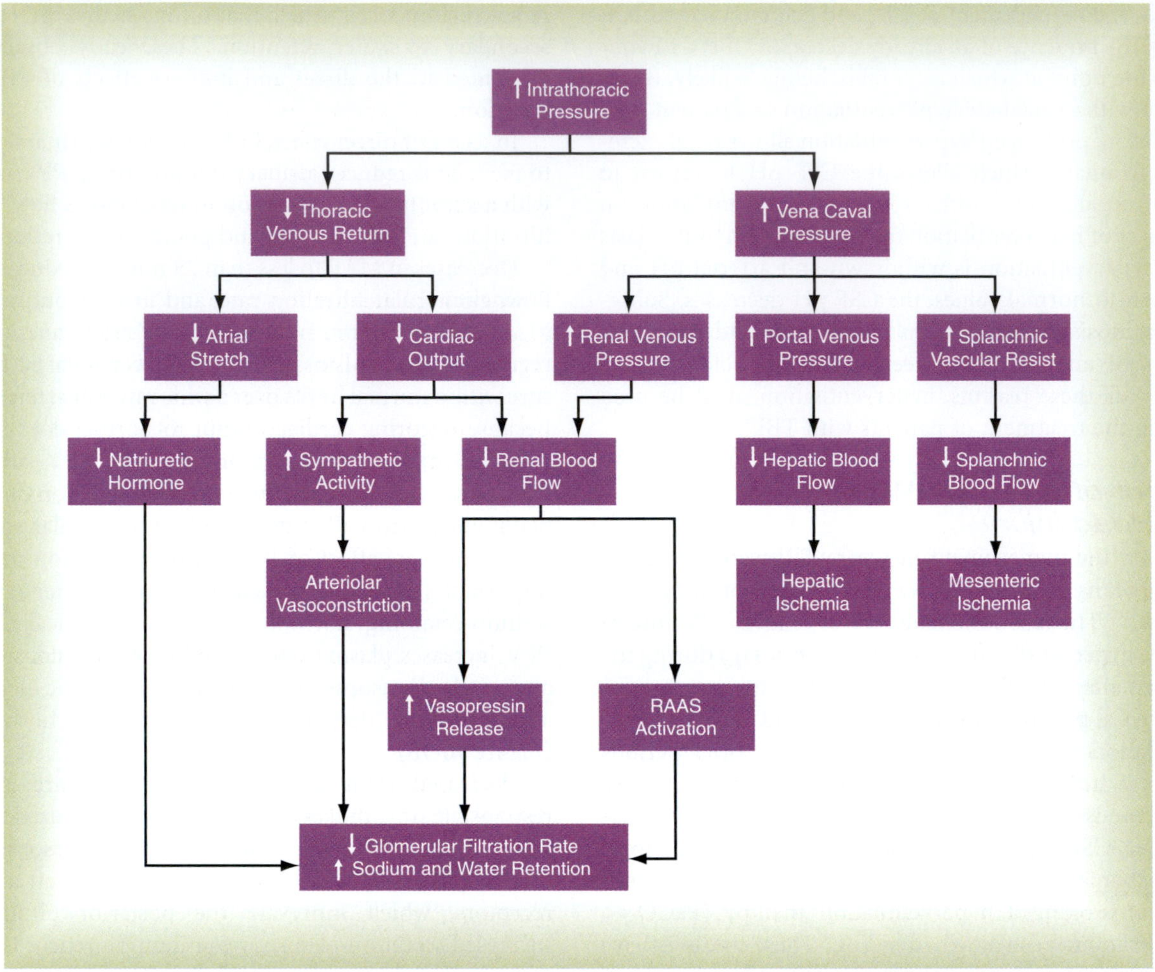

FIGURE 46-18 Cardiac, renal, hepatic, and splanchnic effects associated with increased intrathoracic pressure caused by PPV. *RAAS,* Renin-angiotensin-aldosterone system; ↑, increased; ↓, decreased. (Modified from Florete OG, Gammage GW: Complications of ventilatory support. In Kirby RR, Banner MI, Downs JB, editors: Clinical applications of ventilatory support, New York, 1990, Churchill Livingstone.)

bacteria from the intestine to the blood and nosocomial septicemia. Mechanical ventilation for more than 48 hours and most other conditions necessitating ICU admission are considered indications for stress ulcer prophylaxis. Optimal prophylaxis for stress ulcers is restoration of mesenteric blood flow. Pharmacologic approaches include administration of a cytoprotective agent (sucralfate) and an acid suppression agent (cimetidine or ranitidine).[98]

Gastric distention can be caused by **aerophagia** secondary to an artificial airway cuff leak or by the use of mask ventilation (pressure >20 to 25 cm H_2O). The RT can prevent this complication by taking great care to ensure that the cuff is properly inflated. If patients being ventilated noninvasively are swallowing air, an artificial airway may be considered. In the case of aerophagia and gastric distention, a nasogastric tube may be inserted to evacuate the air.

Bleeding from erosion through the surface vessels of the gastric mucosa is one consequence of stress ulceration. The incidence of bleeding from stress ulcers is almost 100%, but only approximately 5% of bleeding is clinically apparent hemorrhage, and less than 1% to 2% necessitates blood transfusion.

Because patients receiving mechanical ventilation often have an artificial airway or are obtunded, a nutritional deficit may exist. Even in a normal metabolic state, intravenous solutions of saline and dextrose provide only a fraction of the required calories and micronutrients. Patients in the ICU often are hypermetabolic and need two to three times the normal calories. See Chapter 23 for details on nutritional support.

Effect on Central Nervous System

Patients in the ICU are placed into an artificial environment over which they have little control. From the start, the patient loses autonomy. When mechanical ventilation is introduced, the patient is sedated and possibly paralyzed and may not return to a normal, awake level of consciousness until discharged from the ICU. Instead, the patient is kept somnolent (easily aroused and aware) or is stuporous (arousable with difficulty and impaired awareness) or comatose (arousable but unaware).[98] The presence of an artificial airway makes communication

Box 46-3 Modified Ramsay Sedation Scale

1. Agitated, anxious, restless
2. Calm, cooperative, oriented, tranquil
3. Responds to verbal commands
4. Brisk response to light touch
5. Unable to be assessed (paralyzed)

difficult. Caregivers should make a paper tablet and pen, communication board, or communication cards available to patients who are aware enough to write or use them.

Sedatives, Hypnotics, and Neuromuscular Blocking Agents

Sedation is necessary for the management of the nearly inevitable agitation, fear, and anxiety associated with the ICU environment, pain, invasive and noninvasive procedures, and loss of normal sleep pattern. The Society of Critical Care Medicine has published guidelines for sedation and analgesia in the care of critically ill patients.[102]

The level of sedation is monitored with the Modified Ramsay Sedation Scale (Box 46-3). Sedation is titrated to achieve a level of 2 to 3 on the Ramsay scale. This way the patient is responsive, yet not restless or agitated and not paralyzed or comatose.

According to the Society of Critical Care Medicine, facilitation of mechanical ventilation in severe ARDS is the most common reason for prolonged neuromuscular blockade. Neuromuscular blocking agents are used with mechanical ventilation to improve gas exchange, to avoid ICP spikes, to avoid hemodynamic instability, and to prevent bodily injury. Because they paralyze but do not sedate, neuromuscular blocking agents always are used in conjunction with appropriate sedative or analgesic agents (see earlier). In the absence of a sedative, a patient under the influence of a neuromuscular blocking agent is paralyzed and fully aware of the surroundings. During neuromuscular blockade, patients should be assessed for the degree of blockade that is being sustained.[102] The patient is observed for ventilatory effort, and train-of-four stimulation is performed. Neuromuscular blockade should be allowed to dissipate daily so that clinical evaluation, assessment of concomitant sedation and analgesia, and evaluation of the need for continued paralysis can be conducted.

COMPLICATIONS OF MECHANICAL VENTILATION

Negative Pressure Ventilation

Pulmonary

Hypoventilation during NPV can be caused by a decrease in the transairway pressure owing to inadequate negative pressure or leaks in the ventilator or patient-ventilator interface. Iron lung negative pressure ventilators rely on a tight seal at the patient's neck and at all access ports in the tank. Chest cuirass ventilators rely on a tight seal between the cuirass and thorax. Poncho-type ventilators must remain free of leaks or tears. When there is a leak at any of these points, transairway pressure decreases, and the result is a decrease in minute ventilation.

Hyperventilation can occur if the pressure is more negative than is necessary. The results are increased transairway pressure, increased V_T, and increased minute ventilation.

Cardiovascular

Abdominal blood pooling can occur in patients receiving NPV in an iron lung. The negative pressure exerted on the thorax also is exerted on the more compliant abdominal wall. When the pressure in the iron lung becomes negative, the abdominal wall is pulled outward and with it the viscera and associated blood supply. Venous return to the heart, cardiac output, and systemic blood pressure decrease; the result is a condition called "tank shock."

Positive Pressure Ventilation: Artificial Airway Complications

Chapter 36 describes complications related to artificial airways.

Complications Related to Pressure

Ventilator-associated lung injury is the term used to define lung injury in humans owing to mechanical ventilation. These are complications resulting from high pressure, infection, and patient-ventilator asynchrony. High ventilation pressure has long been associated with barotrauma. Barotrauma is categorized as pneumothorax, pneumomediastinum, pneumopericardium, and subcutaneous emphysema (Figure 46-19). All of these complications are descriptions of extraalveolar air. High ventilatory pressure can cause gas to escape through ruptured alveoli. The eventual location of the escaping gas defines the type of barotrauma. If gas escapes through ruptured alveoli into the pleural space, pneumothorax occurs. Gas escaping along perivascular sheaths to the mediastinum produces pneumomediastinum. Further dissection from the mediastinum to tissue planes in the neck and chest wall results in subcutaneous emphysema and potentially pneumomediastinum and pneumoperitoneum.

Pneumothorax is identified by observation of a decrease in chest movement, hyperresonance on percussion, possible deviation of the trachea away from the affected side, and decreased or absent breath sounds over the affected side. In nonintubated patients, there may also be a decrease in vocal fremitus over the affected side. A line separating lung tissue from air is observed on the chest radiograph, although the line sometimes is difficult to see in a small (<20%) pneumothorax. Respiratory distress increases with increasing pneumothorax, as does hypoxemia. Normally, in spontaneously breathing patients, intrapulmonary and pleural pressures are equal in pneumothorax. PPV can cause intrapleural pressures to increase (tension pneumothorax).

Tension pneumothorax is life-threatening, because it tends to develop very rapidly in patients who are mechanically ventilated and shifts the mediastinum, heart, and great

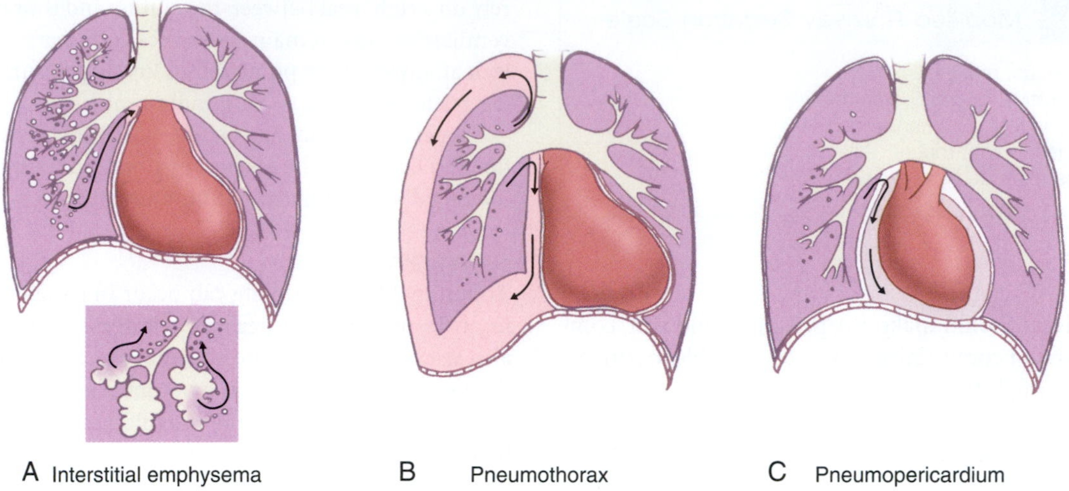

FIGURE 46-19 Pulmonary barotrauma. **A,** Ruptured alveoli are indicated in framed alveoli at bottom. Air dissects from alveoli along vascular sheaths to the hilum and then to the pleural space. **B,** Pneumothorax. Origin of air in lung tissue and its pathway to inflate the pleural space are indicated. The heart shifts to the left because of high pressure in the right side of the chest. **C,** Course of air from the lung to pericardial space. The distended pericardial space causes cardiac tamponade. (Modified from Korones SB: High-risk newborn infants, ed 4, St Louis, 1986, Mosby.)

vessels; the results are a decrease in cardiac output and hypotension. Tension pneumothorax is a medical emergency; it is relieved by insertion of a large-bore needle into the pleural space through the anterior second or third interspace above the rib. This maneuver is followed by chest tube insertion. While waiting for needle decompression, the patient may be ventilated with 100% O_2 at a low V_T and airway pressure. Pneumomediastinum and pneumoperitoneum are identified on a chest radiograph by the presence of air in these locations.

Complications Related to Volume

Ventilator-induced lung injury (VILI) has been defined as the application of pressure, positive or negative, to the lungs causing damage. The damage has been described as an increase in permeability of the alveolar-capillary membrane, pulmonary edema, cell wounding and necrosis, and diffuse alveolar damage as the result of using an inappropriate ventilation strategy. Several more recent reviews summarize understanding of the mechanisms, effects, and means to prevent VILI.[103-105]

It has been shown that overdistention, as opposed to volume or pressure per se, is an important determinant of lung damage. Animals ventilated with large V_T (>30 ml/kg) develop severe injury—hence the term **volutrauma**. The degree of alveolar distention is determined by the transpulmonary pressure (plateau pressure minus the pleural pressure), which must be approximated by the esophageal pressure. As plateau pressure increases, so does transpulmonary pressure, increasing the likelihood of lung damage. Lung damage may also occur when ventilating at low V_T, if alveoli are allowed to deflate and reinflate repeatedly with each breath. This injury is called **atelectrauma**. These two factors have led to the recommendation that lungs should be opened ("recruited") and kept open by an appropriate PEEP level and ventilated to a plateau pressure of no more than 28 cm H_2O by decreasing V_T. This technique is called the *open lung technique* and is described in detail in Chapter 48.

Factors that predispose a patient to VILI include underlying lung disease (injured lungs are more susceptible to VILI), systemic inflammation, surfactant dysfunction, aspiration, pulmonary edema, extremes of age, and heterogeneous lung ventilation. An important factor is the uneven distribution of ventilation, especially in ARDS. Because ARDS is a heterogeneous disorder, there are areas of both low and normal compliance. A given pressure in an area of low compliance may allow lung units to open and close with each breath, causing atelectrauma. The same pressure in an area of normal compliance may cause overdistention and stretch injury. Pulmonary edema is a prominent feature of VILI, owing to an increase in alveolar-capillary membrane permeability. Microvascular damage is characterized by separation of capillary endothelial cells, disruption of alveolar epithelium, and destruction of alveolar type I cells.

VILI occurs via two mechanisms, as shown in Figure 46-20.[106] One mechanism is the physical disruption of tissues and cells *(biophysical injury)*. Physical disruption of the tissues occurs as air ruptures across the alveolar epithelial surface and tracks along the bronchovascular sheath. Air tracks into the interstitium causing pulmonary interstitial emphysema, into the pleural space causing pneumothorax, and into the pericardium causing pneumopericardium. The pulmonary capillary epithelium also fails in response to high-volume ventilation, resulting in hemorrhage and edema. Another factor in biophysical injury is the interdependence of adjacent alveoli and terminal bronchi. When the lung is unevenly expanded, alveolar collapse increases the traction forces between alveoli. This recruitment-derecruitment develops pressures up to 140 cm H_2O across lung units, resulting in air-filled cavities and pseudocysts. Finally, injurious ventilation causes surfactant to become dysfunctional or deficient or both.

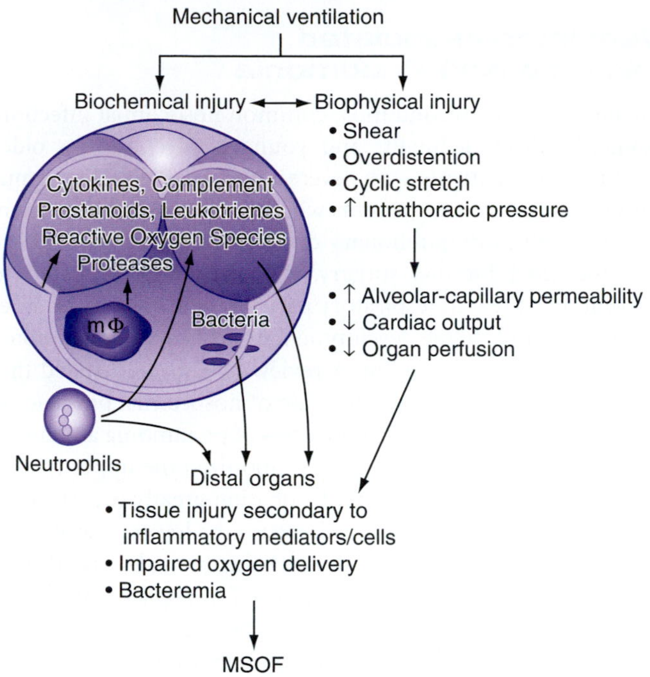

FIGURE 46-20 Mechanisms by which mechanical ventilation might contribute to MSOF. (From Mason RJ, Broaddus VC, Murray JF, et al: Murray and Nadel's textbook of respiratory medicine, ed 4, Philadelphia, 2005, Saunders.)

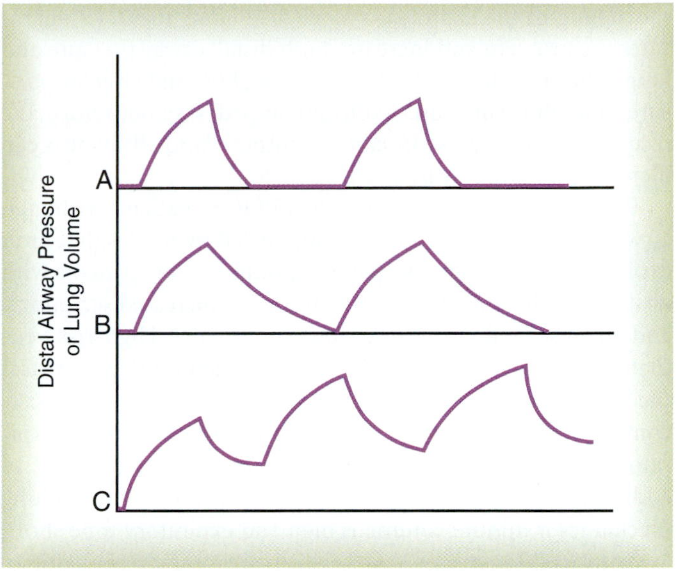

FIGURE 46-21 Causes of auto-PEEP. **A,** When airway resistance is normal and expiratory time is long enough, distal airway pressure and lung volume return to normal after a positive pressure breath. **B,** High expiratory resistance prolongs exhalation to the point at which air-trapping begins and causes auto-PEEP. **C,** Shortening the expiratory time aggravates the problem and worsens auto-PEEP. (Modified from Benson MS, Pierson DJ: Auto-PEEP during mechanical ventilation of adults. Respir Care 33:557, 1988.)

The second mechanism is the release of inflammatory mediators *(biochemical injury)*. When the lungs are abnormally stretched, this is detected by cells and converted into biochemical signals, a process called *mechanotransduction*. These biochemical signals cause the release of cytokines, complement, prostanoids, leukotrienes, reactive O_2 species, and proteases. The release of these substances has been called **biotrauma**. These mediators go on to the terminal organs and cause tissue inflammation, impairment of O_2 delivery, and bacteremia (see 29), leading to multisystem organ failure (MSOF). As mentioned earlier in the chapter, hyperinflation during mechanical ventilation causes bacteria to "spill over" from the gut into the bloodstream, a process called *translocation*. In this manner, translocation contributes to MSOF, as bacteria migrate into the blood and then to terminal organs. Other factors contributing to MSOF are an increase in circulating cell death (apoptotic) factors, suppression of the peripheral immune response, and individual genetic variability.

Alveolar distention occurs when the lungs are stiff and the chest wall is normal or when one or both lungs are ventilated with a high plateau pressure. Plateau pressure ideally should be maintained at less than 28 cm H_2O in all patients. However, in patients with a stiff chest wall (marked obesity, fluid overload, increased abdominal pressure), higher plateau pressure can be tolerated without injury because of the reduction in transpulmonary pressure caused by the stiff chest wall.

Human studies have compared high and low V_T ventilation, using ICU mortality, ventilator-free days, and overall mortality as outcome variables. The consensus is that a low V_T strategy, with PEEP adequate to keep lungs open to avoid atelectrauma, results in a significantly better outcome. In studies in which inflammatory mediators were also measured, high V_T groups had a higher level of inflammatory mediators.[107,108] VILI is related to both mechanical and chemical factors. On one hand, overstretch directly injures the alveolar epithelium and capillary endothelium. On the other hand, through mechanotransduction, cells release many inflammatory mediators into the blood, leading to MSOF.

Auto-Positive End Expiratory Pressure

Air trapping occurs with incomplete emptying of lung units. Lung units prone to air trapping are units with long-time constants (i.e., with high resistance or high compliance). Air trapping during PPV is often referred to as *dynamic hyperinflation, auto-PEEP, occult PEEP,* or *intrinsic PEEP*. This problem associated with air trapping cannot be determined by simple observation of airway pressure. Auto-PEEP often goes unrecognized.

Figure 46-21, *A*, shows the generation of auto-PEEP. As long as airway resistance is normal and expiratory time is sufficiently long, distal airway pressure and lung volume return to baseline during PPV breaths. Alone or in combination, three factors account for the development of auto-PEEP. First, by effectively increasing the time constant of the lung, high expiratory resistance prolongs exhalation to the point at which air trapping begins (see Figure 46-21, *B*). Second, any increase in the minute ventilation increases the likelihood of auto-PEEP. Third, any shortening of the expiratory time (see Figure 46-21, *C*) aggravates the problem and increases both distal airway pressure and lung volume (auto-PEEP). By increasing FRC and alveolar pressure, auto-PEEP increases WOB and impedes venous return, the result being a decrease in cardiac output. Auto-PEEP also can increase pulmonary vascular resistance.

Patients at greatest risk for auto-PEEP are patients with high airway resistance who are being supported by modes that limit expiratory time. High-risk patient groups include patients with obstructive disease, any disease producing increased secretions, and any disease that increases lung compliance. High-risk ventilatory support techniques include any method that increases the I : E ratio, especially CMV at a high rate or in the assist-control mode, and approaches that purposefully shorten expiratory time, such as IRV or the use of low inspiratory flow. In addition, auto-PEEP can develop in patients with normal lung mechanics if minute volume is high and expiratory time short.

Auto-PEEP increases WOB. This increase in WOB is due to two factors. First, hyperinflation caused by auto-PEEP stretches the lung, and the stretching impairs the contractile action of the diaphragm. Second, the high alveolar pressure caused by auto-PEEP must be overcome before any airway pressure change can occur. This situation effectively reduces machine sensitivity and increases response time. Increased effort is required by the patient before the ventilator recognizes the flow or pressure change and triggers to inspiration. The effect of auto-PEEP on WOB can be minimized by applied PEEP. However, applied PEEP is effective only if auto-PEEP is a result of dynamic airway obstruction. Essentially, PEEP should be applied in increments of 1 to 2 cm H_2O until every patient inspiratory effort is capable of triggering the ventilator.

Oxygen Toxicity

O_2 toxicity causes lung tissue damage and an increase in the permeability of the alveolar-capillary membrane. As suggested in Chapter 41, factors associated with the development of O_2 toxicity include elevated FiO_2, long duration of exposure, and patient susceptibility. FiO_2 of 0.6 or more for longer than 24 to 48 hours is associated with the development of O_2 toxicity. In the presence of a high concentration of O_2, O_2 free radicals are produced. These radicals are the hydroxyl (OH^-), perhydroxyl (HO_2), and superoxide (O_2^-) radicals. Free radicals normally are rapidly detoxified by the enzyme superoxide dismutase, which is produced by alveolar type II cells. With higher FiO_2, the presence of free radicals is greater, and type II cells are less likely to produce superoxide dismutase. The presence of free radicals increases the permeability of the alveolar-capillary membrane. The combination of direct injury by free radicals and decreased surfactant production leads to exudation of fluid into the alveoli and a subsequent decrease in compliance. Every effort should be made to decrease FiO_2 whenever it exceeds 0.6. The decrease usually is accomplished with application of PEEP or CPAP. However, the evidence supporting the development of O_2 toxicity in critically ill patients is poor, and oxygenation should never be sacrificed for the purpose of avoiding O_2 toxicity.

Ventilator-Associated (Nosocomial) Pneumonia

Pneumonia is the second most common nosocomial infection, primarily affecting infants and young children, adults older than 65 years, patients with severe underlying disease, immunosuppressed patients, patients who have depressed sensorium, patients with cardiopulmonary disease, and patients who have had thoracoabdominal surgery. RTs should be prepared to prevent this threat to respiratory patients, who are 6 to 21 times more susceptible to the development of nosocomial pneumonia than the general population. A review by Craven[109] stated that health care costs related to each case of nosocomial pneumonia are about $40,000. Most of these cases of pneumonia are caused by aspiration of bacteria that have colonized the upper gastrointestinal tract or oropharynx. Intubation greatly increases the risk of nosocomial pneumonia because the lower airway is left exposed, and normal protective mechanisms are bypassed. This type of pneumonia has been known for years as *ventilator-associated pneumonia*. This name has been challenged because it is not the ventilator, but rather the microaspiration of microorganisms in oral or gastrointestinal secretions, that causes the infection. Secretions that sit on the top of the endotracheal or tracheostomy tube cuff are aspirated via the small folds in the cuff. Most cases of pneumonia are polymicrobial, consisting of gram-negative organisms. However, methicillin-resistant *Staphylococcus aureus* has been common in the past 10 years. The endotracheal or tracheostomy tube is a site of bacterial growth, and these bacteria become encased in what is referred to as a *biofilm*. The use of a silver-coated endotracheal tube,[110] use of endotracheal tubes with alternative cuff designs,[111] use of subglottic suction airways,[112] proper cuff care,[113] the use of devices to remove biofilm from the inside of the ETT,[114] and avoidance of lavaging when suctioning all reduce the risk of aspiration. See Chapter 36 for details. Another source of infection is the endotracheal tube lumen.

Prevention of Ventilator-Associated Pneumonia

In addition to standard precautions, specific infection control procedures apply to the use of endotracheal tubes and ventilators. These ventilator bundles for prevention of ventilator-associated pneumonia include the following:[113]

- Perform appropriate hand hygiene. Hands should be disinfected with a sanitizer (e.g., Cal-Stat hand sanitizer) before entering any patient's room regardless of the reason and when leaving the patient's room regardless of the activities that occurred in the room.
- Perform gentle suctioning (presumably to help prevent coughing, aspiration, and sloughing of biofilm).
- Place the patient in a semirecumbent position (30- to 45-degree head elevation).
- Do not routinely change ventilator circuits.
- Drain and discard inspiratory tube condensate away from the patient, or prevent its formation by using heated wire circuits or heat and moisture exchangers.

- Use a metered dose inhaler rather than a nebulizer for medication administration. If a small volume nebulizer is used, it should be replaced after each treatment (i.e., one nebulizer = one treatment). However, the new vibrating disc nebulizers are as protective as meter dose inhalers.
- Interrupt sedatives daily to evaluate patient readiness to wean from the ventilator—this is effective in decreasing the length of intubation and mechanical ventilation.
- Assess daily the ability of the patient to perform a spontaneous breathing trial.
- Use noninvasive ventilation whenever possible to avoid intubation.
- Perform regular oral hygiene at least every 4 hours.

Early tracheostomy has been evaluated as a possible preventive measure, but several studies and meta-analyses showed no advantage of tracheostomy in preventing ventilator-associated pneumonia.[109] Other measures that may decrease the likelihood of nosocomial infection include the use of closed suction systems (although the benefit remains unproved); use of disposable resuscitation bags; and high-level disinfection of ventilators, O_2 analyzers, and other equipment between patients.

Ventilator Malfunction

Ventilator malfunction can be categorized as a failure in the patient circuit or a failure in the ventilator. Failures in the patient circuit include failures related to the endotracheal tube: cuff rupture, main stem intubation, laryngeal intubation, esophageal intubation, soft tissue erosion because the cuff pressure is too high, and disconnection from the circuit (Figure 46-22). Failures in the tubing circuit include leaks anywhere there is a tubing connection; a leak at the site of a nebulizer or metered dose inhaler; humidifier malfunctions that include failure to fill the reservoir, overheating, or mechanical failure; and exhalation valve failure. These failures are recognized by the ventilator as changes in respiratory rate, airway pressure, or V_T outside the limits set on the alarms.

Airway and ventilator malfunctions can be avoided with proper care of the endotracheal tube (taping the tube snugly), ensuring equal breath sounds, checking to ensure the tubing is patent and free of leaks, and ensuring that all connections are firmly made. If patient activity is the cause of ventilator disconnection, patient teaching to refrain from attempting to disconnect the ventilator or pulling on or biting the tube or sedation or restraint may be necessary. Failures related to the ventilator include electrical failure, microprocessor failure, exhalation valve failure, internal volume leakage, gas supply failure, and any failure that could result in an increase or decrease in minute ventilation or FiO_2. Ventilators have alarms that alert the RT to these dysfunctions.

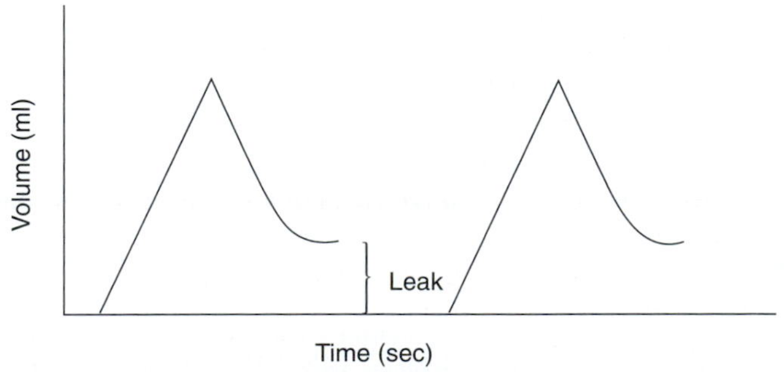

FIGURE 46-22 Volume-time waveform illustrating a leak in the ventilator circuit. Note the abrupt end of expiration before the tracing reaches the baseline.

Patient safety is always the primary concern when a malfunction is detected. For this reason, a manual resuscitator always should be placed near the bedside. If the reason for the patient's distress is clear, such as disconnection at the endotracheal tube, the connection is reestablished, and patient comfort and ventilation are ensured. If the reason is not obvious, the patient is ventilated with a manual ventilator while the cause of the malfunction is investigated. The steps for managing sudden distress in a patient receiving ventilatory support are listed in Table 46-4.

RULE OF THUMB

Always have a manual ventilator (bag-valve-mask device [Ambu bag]) at the bedside of a patient receiving mechanical ventilation. Ensure that the manual ventilator is connected to an O_2 source. If the patient is receiving PEEP, ensure that the manual ventilator is equipped with a PEEP valve that provides PEEP equivalent of that being administered to the patient with the ventilator. Keep the patient connection of the manual ventilator clean and covered and the valve free of secretions.

Operator Error

The provision of mechanical ventilation is highly complex, the equipment used is very sophisticated, and the potential options to be applied to a given patient increase each year. As a result, clinician error is an ongoing concern. To minimize the possibility of error, a clinician should never make an adjustment to a mechanical ventilator unless he or she has been properly trained to operate the ventilator and the clinician's skills at using the machine have been assessed by an independent evaluator. It is essential for the operator to document ventilator settings in a consistent manner and to understand the terminology used when documenting the ventilator-patient interaction in a paper chart or electronic medical record. Appropriate operation of the mechanical ventilator should be assessed on a regular basis based on the severity and criticality of the patient's clinical presentation. To minimize errors, any adjustment should be checked to ensure that the appropriate change was actually made and that the patient responded as expected. A clinician should never leave the bedside of a patient until the clinician is assured that the patient is being ventilated as ordered and that the ventilator is responding as expected. Patient safety should always be the primary concern of all RTs.

TABLE 46-4

Causes of Sudden Respiratory Distress and Remedies in a Patient Receiving Ventilatory Support

Cause	Remedy
Patient Related	
Artificial airway problems	Assessment of cuff, airway position (see Chapter 36)
Pneumothorax	Chest tube insertion
Bronchospasm	Bronchodilator therapy
Secretions	Suctioning, tracheobronchial hygiene
Pulmonary edema	Therapy directed at cause of pulmonary edema
Auto-PEEP	Decreased minute volume, tracheobronchial hygiene, decrease in I : E
Abnormal respiratory drive	Therapy directed at cause, possible sedation or paralysis
Alteration in body posture	Repositioning of patient
Abdominal distention	Therapy directed at cause, insertion of nasogastric tube
Anxiety	Reassurance, anxiolytics, assessment of minute ventilation
Patient-ventilator asynchrony	Assessment of flow and sensitivity, auto-PEEP, change of mode to accommodate patient's pattern of ventilation
Ventilator Related	
System leak	Assessment of connections in the ventilator circuit
Circuit malfunction	Assessment of circuit with test lung, replace if necessary
Inadequate FiO_2	Assessment of SpO_2, assessment of FiO_2 with analyzer, increase in FiO_2, or replacement of blender or ventilator if malfunction is found
Inadequate ventilatory support	Review of therapeutic strategy for the patient (see Chapter 48)
Improper flow-trigger setting	Adjust trigger and flow to patient demand

SUMMARY CHECKLIST

- Response to an increase in FiO_2 helps determine the cause of hypoxemia.
- Hypoxemia responsive to an increase in FiO_2 is likely caused by a low $\dot{V}/\dot{Q}$ ratio.
- Hypoxemia unresponsive to increased FiO_2 is likely caused by a diffusion defect or shunt.
- Alveolar ventilation and CO_2 production determine $PaCO_2$.
- Mechanical ventilation should increase alveolar ventilation and may decrease CO_2 production when WOB is relieved. These factors decrease $PaCO_2$.
- Mechanical ventilation with positive pressure increases dead space and increases $\dot{V}/\dot{Q}$ ratio.
- Inspiratory or expiratory time can be manipulated to improve oxygenation and alveolar emptying in disorders that affect alveolar time constants.
- Physiologic benefits of PPV include improved oxygenation and ventilation, alveolar expansion, decreased WOB and cardiac work, and improved O_2 delivery.
- No outcome differences have been identified among the various modes of ventilation except that SIMV prolongs the weaning process. However, modes of ventilation that allow the patient control over the process of gas delivery have been shown to improve patient-ventilator synchrony.
- No single flow pattern has been shown to be the most physiologically beneficial. However, research results indicate better oxygenation, ventilation, and patient-ventilator synchrony with the decelerating flow compared with the square wave flow pattern.
- A decelerating flow waveform tends to have a lower peak and a higher mean airway pressure, whereas a square wave tends to have a higher peak and a lower mean airway pressure.
- Flow triggering appears to decrease WOB compared with pressure triggering on older generation ventilators.
- PEEP is used to restore FRC in acute restrictive disease and to splint the airways in obstructive disease.
- WOB is decreased by the appropriate application of mode, trigger variable, and flow.
- PPV is detrimental to the $\dot{V}/\dot{Q}$ ratio primarily by shifting ventilation to areas that are less perfused. PPV can cause hyperventilation, tissue damage, and barotraumas if not carefully managed.
- PPV can decrease venous return and cardiac output, especially when it increases intrapleural and mean airway pressures.
- PPV can cause renal, hepatic, and gastrointestinal malfunction primarily owing to decreased perfusion of the capillary tissue beds.
- Elevation of the head, osmotic diuretics, and CSF drainage are effective means of decreasing ICP in TBI. Acute hyperventilation should be used only temporarily until other, more effective means can be employed.
- Ventilator bundles should always be adhered to during mechanical ventilation to minimize the development of ventilator-associated pneumonia.
- Patient safety and error-free patient care are the first priority when caring for any patient.

References

1. Chatburn RL: Classification of mechanical ventilators. In Tobin MJ, editor: *Principles and practice of mechanical ventilation*, ed 3, New York, 2012, McGraw-Hill.
2. Beachy W: *Respiratory care anatomy and physiology: foundations for clinical practice*, St Louis, 2007, Mosby.

3. Hess DR, Kacmarek RM: *Essentials of mechanical ventilation*, New York, 2014, McGraw-Hill.
4. The ARDSnet: Ventilation with low tidal volume compared with traditional tidal volumes for acute lung injury and the acute respiratory distress syndrome. *N Engl J Med* 342:1301–1308, 2000.
5. Chiumello D, Carlesso E, Cadringher P, et al: Lung stress and strain during mechanical ventilation for acute respiratory distress syndrome. *AJRCCM* 178:346–355, 2008.
6. Lachman B: Open up the lung and keep it open. *Intensive Care Med* 18:319–321, 1992.
7. MacIntyre NR: Patient-ventilator interactions. In MacIntyre NR, Branson RD, editors: *Mechanical ventilation*, Philadelphia, 2001, Saunders.
8. Goddon S, Fujino Y, Hromi JM, et al: Optimal mean airway pressure during high frequency oscillation. *Anesthesiol* 94:862–868, 2001.
9. Hickling KG: Best compliance during a decremental, but not incremental, positive end-expiratory pressure trial is related to open-lung positive end expiratory pressure: a mathematical model of acute respiratory distress syndrome lungs. *Am J Respir Crit Care Med* 163:69–78, 2001.
10. Borges JB, Okamoto VN, Matos GFJ, et al: Reversibility of lung collapse and hypoxemia in early acute respiratory distress syndrome. *Am J Respir Crit Care Med* 174:268–278, 2006.
11. Kacmarek RM, Villar J: Lung recruitment maneuvers during acute respiratory distress syndrome: is it useful? *Minerva Anesthesiol* 76:1–2, 2010.
12. Girgis K, Hamed H, Khater Y, et al: A decremental PEEP trial identifies the PEEP level that maintains oxygenation post lung recruitment. *Respir Care* 51:1132–1140, 2006.
13. Amato MBP, Barbas CSV, Medeiros DM, et al: Effect of a protective-ventilation strategy on mortality in the acute respiratory distress syndrome. *N Engl J Med* 338:347–354, 1998.
14. Villar J, Kacmarek RM, Perez-Mendez L, et al: ARIES Network: A high positive end-expiratory pressure, low tidal volume ventilatory strategy improves outcome in persistent acute respiratory distress syndrome: a randomized, controlled trial. *Crit Care Med* 34:1311–1318, 2006.
15. Suarez-Sipmann F, Bohm SH, Tusman G, et al: Use of dynamic compliance for open lung positive end-expiratory pressure titration in an experimental study. *Crit Care Med* 35:214–221, 2007.
16. Haas CF, et al: Patient-determined inspiratory flow during assisted mechanical ventilation. *Respir Care* 40:716, 1995.
17. Trille AW, Cabello B, Galia F, et al: Reduction of patient-ventilator asynchrony by reducing tidal volume during pressure support ventilation. *Intensive Care Med* 34:1477–1486, 2008.
18. Sassoon CS, et al: Influence of pressure and flow triggered synchronous intermittent mandatory ventilation on inspiratory muscle work. *Crit Care Med* 22:1933, 1994.
19. MacIntyre NR: Respiratory system mechanics. In MacIntyre NR, Branson RD, editors: *Mechanical ventilation*, Philadelphia, 2001, Saunders.
20. Banner MJ, et al: Partially and totally unloading respiratory muscles based on real-time measurements of work of breathing: a clinical approach. *Chest* 106:1835, 1994.
21. MacIntyre NR: Mechanical ventilation strategies for parenchymal lung injury. In MacIntyre NR, Branson RD, editors: *Mechanical ventilation*, Philadelphia, 2001, Saunders.
22. Ranieri VM, et al: Physiologic effects of positive end-expiratory pressure in patients with chronic obstructive pulmonary disease during acute ventilatory failure and controlled mechanical ventilation. *Am Rev Respir Dis* 147:5, 1993.
23. Chiumello D, Polli F, Tallarini F, et al: Effect of different cycling-off criteria and positive end-expiratory pressure during pressure support ventilation in patients with chronic obstructive pulmonary disease. *Crit Care Med* 35:2547–2552, 2007.
24. Ost D, Corbridge T: Independent lung ventilation. *Clin Chest Med* 17:591, 1996.
25. Al Saady N, Bennett ED: Decelerating inspiratory flow waveform improves lung mechanics and gas exchange in patients on intermittent positive-pressure ventilation. *Intensive Care Med* 11:68, 1985.
26. Rattenborg CC, Via-Reque E: *Clinical use of mechanical ventilation*, St Louis, 1981, Mosby.
27. Chatburn RL, El-Khatib MF, Smith PG: Respiratory system behavior during mechanical inflation with constant inspiratory pressure and flow. *Respir Care* 42:979, 1994.
28. Natalini G, et al: Pressure-controlled versus volume controlled ventilation with mask airway. *J Clin Anesth* 13:436, 2001.
29. Slutsky AS: Consensus conference on mechanical ventilation. *Intensive Care Med* 20:64, 1994.
30. Chatburn RL, Volsko TA, El-Khatib M: The effect of airway leak on tidal volume during pressure- or flow-controlled ventilation of the neonate: a model study. *Respir Care* 41:728, 1996.
31. Finney SJ, Evans TW: Mechanical ventilation in acute respiratory distress syndrome. *Curr Opin Anesthesiol* 14:165–171, 2001.
32. Gillette MA, Hess DR: Ventilator-induced lung injury and the evolution of lung protective strategies in acute respiratory distress syndrome. *Respir Care* 46:130, 2001.
33. Kacmarek RM, Dimas S, Mack C: *Essentials of respiratory care*, ed 4, St Louis, 2005, Elsevier.
34. McCarthy MC, et al: Pressure control inverse ratio ventilation in the treatment of adult respiratory distress syndrome in patients with blunt chest trauma. *Am Surg* 6:1027, 1999.
35. Demling R, Riessen R: Pulmonary dysfunction after cerebral injury. *Crit Care Med* 18:768, 1990.
36. Weisman JM, et al: Intermittent mandatory ventilation. *Am Rev Respir Dis* 127:641, 1983.
37. Brochard L, et al: Comparison of three methods of gradual withdrawal from ventilatory support during weaning from mechanical ventilation. *Am J Respir Crit Care Med* 150:896, 1994.
38. Esteban A, Frutos F, Tobin MJ, et al: A comparison of four methods of weaning patients from mechanical ventilation. *N Engl J Med* 332:345–350, 1995.
39. Calzia E, et al: Stress response during weaning after cardiac surgery. *Br J Anaesth* 87:490, 2001.
40. Hahn AF: The challenge of respiratory dysfunction in Guillain-Barré syndrome. *Arch Neurol* 58:893, 2001.
41. Roze JC, et al: Oxygen cost of breathing and weaning process in newborn infants. *Eur Respir J* 10:2583, 1997.
42. Sinha SK, Donn SM: Volume-controlled ventilation: variations on a theme. *Clin Perinatol* 28:547, 2001.
43. Putensen C, Zech S, Wrigge H, et al: Long-term effects of spontaneous breathing during ventilatory support in patients with acute lung injury. *Am J Respir Crit Care Med* 164:43, 2001.
44. Newman P, Golisch J, Strohmeyer A, et al: Influence of different release times on spontaneous breathing pattern during pressure release ventilation. *Intensive Care Med* 28:1742, 2002.
45. Davis K, et al: Airway pressure release ventilation. *Arch Surg* 128:1348, 1993.
46. Sydow M, et al: Long term effects of two different ventilatory modes on oxygenation in acute lung injury. *Am J Respir Crit Care Med* 149:1550, 1994.
47. Murias G, Villagra A, Blanch L: Patient-ventilator dyssynchrony during assisted invasive mechanical ventilation. *Minerva Anesthesiol* 79:434–444, 2013.
48. Kacmarek RM: Proportional assist ventilation and neurally adjusted ventilatory support. *Respir Care* 56:140–148, 2011.
49. Klerk AM, Klerk RK: Nasal continuous positive airway pressure and outcomes or preterm infants. *Neonatal Intensive Care* 14:58, 2001.
50. Dinger J, et al: Effect of positive end expiratory pressure on functional residual capacity and compliance in surfactant-treated preterm infants. *Neonat Intensive Care* 14:26, 2001.
51. Brochard L, Pluskwa F, Lemaire F: Improved efficacy of spontaneous breathing with inspiratory pressure support. *Am Rev Respir Dis* 136:411, 1987.
52. MacIntyre NR: Pressure support ventilation: effects on ventilatory reflexes and ventilatory muscle workload. *Respir Care* 32:447, 1987.
53. Brochard L, et al: Pressure support decreases work of breathing and oxygen consumption during weaning from mechanical ventilation (abstract). *Am Rev Respir Dis* 135:A51, 1987.

54. Grande CM, Kahn RC: The effect of pressure support ventilation on ventilatory variables and work of breathing (abstract). *Anesthesiol* 65:A84, 1986.
55. MacIntyre NR: Respiratory function during pressure support ventilation. *Chest* 89:677–683, 1986.
56. Sassoon CSH, Mahutte CK, Light RW: Ventilator modes: old and new. *Crit Care Clin* 6:605, 1990.
57. Hill NS, Brennan J, Garpestad E, et al: Noninvasive ventilation in acute respiratory failure. *Crit Care Med* 35:2402–2407, 2007.
58. Gay PC, Hess DR, Hill NS: Noninvasive proportional assist ventilation for acute respiratory insufficiency: comparison with pressure support ventilation. *Am J Respir Crit Care Med* 164:1606–1611, 2001.
59. Porta R, Appendini L, Vitacca M, et al: Mask proportional assist vs. pressure support ventilation in patients in clinically stable condition with chronic ventilatory failure. *Chest* 122:479–488, 2002.
60. Wysocki M, Richard JC, Meshaka P: Noninvasive proportional assist ventilation compared with noninvasive pressure support ventilation in hypercapnic acute respiratory failure. *Crit Care Med* 30:323–329, 2002.
61. Serra A, Polese G, Braggion C, et al: Non-invasive proportional assist and pressure support ventilation in patients with cystic fibrosis and chronic respiratory failure. *Thorax* 57:50–54, 2002.
62. Rusterholtz T, Bollaert PE, Feissel M, et al: Continuous positive airway pressure vs. proportional assist ventilation for noninvasive ventilation in acute cardiogenic pulmonary edema. *Intensive Care Med* 34:840–846, 2008.
63. Ranieri VM, Grasso S, Mascia L, et al: Effects of proportional assist ventilation on inspiratory muscle effort in patients with chronic obstructive pulmonary disease and acute respiratory failure. *Anesthesiol* 86:79–91, 1997.
64. Grasso S, Puntillo F, Mascia L, et al: Compensation for increase in respiratory workload during mechanical ventilation. *Am J Respir Crit Care Med* 16:819–826, 2000.
65. Xirouchaki N, Kondili E, Vaporidi K, et al: Proportional assist ventilation with load-adjustable gain factors in critically ill patients: comparison with pressure support. *Intensive Care Med* 34:2026–2034, 2008.
66. Wrigge H, Golisch W, Zinserling J, et al: Proportional assist versus pressure support ventilation: effects on breathing pattern and respiratory work of patients with chronic obstructive pulmonary disease. *Intensive Care Med* 25:790–798, 1999.
67. Passam F, Hoing S, Prinianakis G, et al: Effect of different levels of pressure support and proportional assist ventilation on breathing pattern work of breathing and gas exchange in mechanically ventilated hypercapnic COPD patients with acute respiratory failure. *Respiration* 70:355–361, 2003.
68. Delaere S, Roeseler J, D'hoore W, et al: Respiratory muscle workload in intubated, spontaneously breathing patients without COPD: pressure support vs. proportional assist ventilation. *Intensive Care Med* 29:949–954, 2003.
69. Colombo D, Cammarota G, Bergamaschi V, et al: Physiologic response to varying levels of pressure support and neurally adjusted ventilatory assist in patients with acute respiratory failure. *Intensive Care Med* 34:1010–2018, 2008.
70. Sgahija J, de Marchie M, Albert M, et al: Patient-ventilator interaction during pressure support ventilation and neurally adjusted ventilatory assist. *Crit Care Med* 38:518–526, 2010.
71. Passath C, Takala J, Tuchscherer D, et al: Physiological response to changing positive end-expiratory pressure during neurally adjusted ventilatory assist in sedated, critically ill adults. *Chest* 138:578–587, 2010.
72. Beck J, Reilly M, Grasselli G, et al: Patient-ventilator interaction during neurally adjusted ventilatory assist in low birth weight infants. *Pediatr Res* 65:663–668, 2009.
73. Bengtsson JA, Edberg KE: Neurally adjusted ventilatory assist in children: an observational study. *Pediatr Crit Care Med* 11:253–257, 2010.
74. Gutman J, Eberhard L, Fabry B: Continuous calculation of intratracheal pressure in tracheally intubated patients. *Anesthesiol* 79:503–511, 1993.
75. Fabry B, Haberthur C, Zappe D: Breathing pattern and additional work of breathing in spontaneously breathing patients with different ventilatory demands during inspiratory pressure support and automatic tube compensation. *Intensive Care Med* 23:545–552, 1997.
76. Amato MB, et al: Volume assure pressure support ventilation: a new approach for reducing muscle workload during acute respiratory failure. *Chest* 102:1225, 1992.
77. Jaber S, Delay JM, Matecki S, et al: Volume-guaranteed pressure support ventilation facing acute changes in ventilatory demand. *Intensive Care Med* 31:1181–1188, 2005.
78. Piotrowski A, Sobala W, Kawczynski P: Patient-initiated, pressure-regulated, volume-controlled ventilation compared with intermittent mandatory ventilation in neonates: a prospective, randomised study. *Intensive Care Med* 23:975–981, 1987.
79. Randolph AG, Wypig D, Venkataraman S, et al: Effect of mechanical ventilator weaning protocols on respiratory outcomes in infants and children: a randomized controlled trial. *JAMA* 288:2561–2568, 2002.
80. McCallion N, Davis PG, Morley CJ: Volume-targeted versus pressure-limited ventilation in the neonate. *Cochrane Database Syst Rev* (3):CD003666, 2005.
81. Otis AB: The work of breathing. *Physiol Rev* 34:449–458, 1954.
82. Branson RD, Chatburn RL: Controversies in the critical care setting: should adaptive pressure control modes be utilized for virtually all patients receiving mechanical ventilation? *Respir Care* 52:478–485, 2007.
83. Thompson BT, Hayden D, Matthay MA, et al: Clinicians' approaches to mechanical ventilation in acute lung injury and ARDS. *Chest* 120:1622–1627, 2001.
84. Hamilton Medical: Adaptive support ventilation. <www.hamilton-medical.com>, (Accessed August 2011).
85. Tassaux D, Dalmas E, Gratadour P, et al: Patient-ventilator interactions during partial ventilatory support: a preliminary study comparing the effects of adaptive support ventilation with synchronized intermittent mandatory ventilation plus inspiratory pressure support. *Crit Care Med* 30:801–807, 2002.
86. Sulzer CF, Chiolero R, Chassot PG, et al: Adaptive support ventilation for fast tracheal extubation after cardiac surgery: a randomized controlled study. *Anesthesiol* 95:1339–1345, 2001.
87. Belliato M, Palo A, Pasero D, et al: Evaluation of adaptive support ventilation in paralyzed patients and in a physical lung model. *Int J Artif Organs* 27:709–716, 2004.
88. Sulemanji D, Marchese A, Garbarini P, et al: Adaptive support ventilation: an appropriate mechanical ventilation strategy for acute respiratory distress syndrome? *Anesthesiol* 111:863–870, 2009.
89. Sulemanji DS, Marchese A, Wysocki M, et al: *Adaptive support ventilation with end-tidal CO_2 closed loop control vs. conventional ventilation (in normal settings, ARDS, COPD and brain injury)*, San Diego, January 2011, Society of Critical Care Medicine 40th Critical Care Congress.
90. Bouadma L, Wolff M, Lucet JC, et al: Ventilator associated pneumonia and its prevention. *Curr Opin Infect Dis* 25:395–404, 2012.
91. Taccone P, Pesenti A, Latini R, et al: Prone positioning in patients with moderate and severe acute respiratory distress syndrome: a randomized controlled trial. *JAMA* 302:1977–1984, 2009.
92. Guerin C: Prone position. *Curr Opin Crit Care* 20:92–97, 2014.
93. Mancebo J, Fernandez R, Blanch L, et al: A multicenter trial of prolonged prone ventilation in severe acute respiratory distress syndrome. *Am J Respir Crit Care Med* 173:1233–1239, 2006.
94. Sud S, Friedrich JO, Taccone P, et al: Prone ventilation reduces mortality in patients with acute respiratory failure and severe hypoxemia: systematic review and meta-analysis. *Intensive Care Med* 36:585–599, 2010.
95. Guerin C, Reignier J, Richard JC, et al: Prone positioning in severe acute respiratory distress syndrome. *New Engl J Med* 368:2159–2168, 2013.
96. Pinsky MR: The effects of mechanical ventilation on the cardiovascular system. *Crit Care Clin* 6:663, 1990.
97. Marini JJ, Ravenscraft SA: Mean airway pressure: physiologic determinants and clinical importance, I: physiologic determinants and measurements. *Crit Care Med* 20:1461, 1992.
98. Marino PL: *The ICU book*, ed 3, Philadelphia, 2005, Lippincott Williams & Wilkins.
99. Yundt KD, Diringer MN: The use of hyperventilation and its impact on cerebral ischemia in the treatment of traumatic brain injury. *Crit Care Clin* 13:163, 1997.

100. Bratton SL, Chestnut RM, Ghajar JP, et al: Guidelines for the management of severe tramatic brain injury. X. Hyperventilation. *J Neuortrauma* 249(Suppl 1):S87–S90, 2007.
101. Dive A, et al: Gastroduodenal motility in mechanically ventilated critically ill patients: a manometric study. *Crit Care Med* 22:441, 1994.
102. Barr J, Fraser GL, Puntillo K, et al: Clinical practice guidelines for the management of pain, agitation, and delirium in adult patients in the intensive care unit. *Crit Care Med* 41:263–306, 2013.
103. Whitehead T, Slutsky AS: The pulmonary physician in critical care. 7: ventilator-induced lung injury. *Thorax* 57:635–642, 2002.
104. Tremblay LN, Slutsky AS: Ventilator-induced lung injury: from the bench to the bedside. *Intensive Care Med* 32:24–33, 2006.
105. Plötz FB, Slutzsky AS, van Vught AJ, et al: Ventilator-induced lung injury and multiple system organ failure: a critical review of facts and hypotheses. *Intensive Care Med* 30:1865–1872, 2004.
106. Slutzky AS, Tremblay LN: Multiple system organ failure: is mechanical ventilation a contributing factor? *Am J Respir Crit Care Med* 157:1721–1725, 1998.
107. Ranieri VM, Suter PM, Tortella C, et al: Effect of mechanical ventilation on inflammatory mediators in patients with acute respiratory distress syndrome: a randomized controlled trial. *JAMA* 282:54–61, 1999.
108. Parsons P, Eisner MD, Thompson T, et al: Lower tidal volume ventilation and plasma cytokine markers of inflammation in patients with acute lung injury. *Crit Care Med* 33:1–6, 2005.
109. Craven DE: Preventing ventilator associated pneumonia in adults. *Chest* 130:251–260, 2006.
110. Kollef MH, Bekele A, Anzueto A: Silver-coated endotracheal tubes and incidence of ventilator-associated pneumonia: the NASCENT randomized trial. *JAMA* 300:805–813, 2008.
111. Dezfulian C, Shojania K, Collard HR, et al: Subglottic secretion drainage preventing ventilator associated pneumonia: a meta-analysis. *Am J Respir Crit Care Med* 118:11–18, 2005.
112. Pitts R, Fisher D, Sulemanji D, et al: Variables affecting leakage past endotracheal tube cuffs: a bench study. *Intensive Care Med* 36:2066–2073, 2010.
113. Torres A, Ewig S, Lode H, et al: European HAP working group: defining, treating and preventing hospital acquired pneumonia: European experience. *Intensive Care Med* 35:9–29, 2009.
114. Mietto C, Foley K, Salerno L, et al: Removal of endotracheal tube obstruction with a secretion clearance device. *Respir Care* 59(9):e122–e126, 2014.

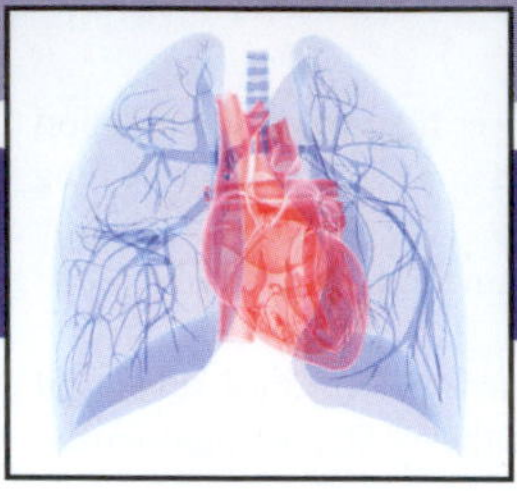

CHAPTER 47

Patient-Ventilator Interactions

ROBERT M. KACMAREK

CHAPTER OBJECTIVES

After reading this chapter you will be able to:

- Discuss the reasons why appropriate patient-ventilator interactions are critical to ensuring safe and effective mechanical ventilation.
- Discuss those clinical issues that can result in poor patient-ventilator interaction.
- Discuss and define the different types of asynchronies commonly observed during mechanical ventilation.
- Discuss the control variables that affect appropriate patient-ventilator interaction and identify the modes of ventilation that are most likely to result in asynchrony.
- Discuss the steps that should be taken to determine the cause of asynchrony before sedation is ordered.
- Discuss what should be done to modify or eliminate flow asynchrony.
- Discuss what should be done to modify double triggering.
- Discuss what should be done to modify missed triggering.
- Discuss what should be done to modify delayed triggering.
- Discuss what should done to modify autotriggering.
- Discuss the setting of rise time during pressure-targeted ventilation.
- Discuss the setting of expiratory cycling criteria during pressure support ventilation.
- Discuss the reasons why proportional assist ventilation (PAV) and neurally adjusted ventilatory assist (NAVA) modes are most likely to result in the least asynchrony.

CHAPTER OUTLINE

Effects of Poor Patient-Ventilator Interaction on Outcome
Causes of Poor Patient-Ventilator Interactions
- Change in Clinical Status
- Artificial Airways
- Pneumothorax
- Airway Emergencies
- The Mechanical Ventilator

Variables Controlled During Mechanical Ventilation
Types of Asynchrony
Causes of Asynchrony
Flow Asynchrony
- Volume Ventilation
- Pressure Ventilation

Trigger Asynchrony
- Auto-PEEP/Missed Triggering
- Trigger Delay
- Autotriggering
- Double triggering
- Reverse Triggering

Cycle Asynchrony
Mode Asynchrony

KEY TERMS

atrophy
autotriggering
cycle asynchrony
diaphragmatic dysfunction
double triggering
fatigue
endobronchial intubation
expiratory cycling criteria
innominate artery rupture
missed triggering
mode asynchrony
neurally adjusted ventilatory assist (NAVA)
patient-ventilator asynchrony
proportional assist ventilation (PAV)
reverse triggering
rise time
tension pneumothorax
tracheal malasia
tracheal stenosis
tracheoesophageal fistula
trigger asynchrony
trigger delay

In general, it is relatively easy to set and adjust controlled mechanical ventilation because the patient does not actively interact with the mechanical ventilator. Controlled mechanical ventilation is entirely a result of the adjustments made by the managing clinician. This is not true during assisted patient-triggered ventilation or partial ventilatory support. In this setting the patient and the ventilator must intimately interact, the ventilator must be set to meet the ventilatory demand of the patient, and the patient must be capable of adjusting to the settings of the ventilator. In most modes of mechanical ventilation the patient must follow the lead of the ventilator—that is, adjust to the way the ventilator is set and breathe with a ventilatory pattern that is consistent with the parameters defined by the mode of ventilation applied and the specific settings.[1] When this interaction is not good, **patient-ventilator asynchrony** occurs or the patient is characterized as "fighting the ventilator." However, it must be noted that there are many other clinical/technical issues that can result in poor patient-ventilator interaction. In this chapter all aspects of patient-ventilator interaction will be discussed with a focus on what should be done to improve the interaction. It is important to remember that sedation of the patient is **ALWAYS** the last intervention to be used to improve patient-ventilator interaction. Careful assessment of the patient, the airway, and the ventilator should be made and necessary adjustments carried out before the decision that sedation is necessary to improve the patient-ventilator interaction.[2]

RULE OF THUMB

Appropriate patient-ventilator interaction during patient-triggered assisted ventilation requires intimate coordination between the demands of the patient's respiratory center and the settings of the mechanical ventilator.

Patient-ventilator interaction refers to patient comfort, work of breathing (WOB), and synchrony during ventilator-assisted breaths. Generally, ventilatory support should be initially adjusted to minimize the WOB and to allow the ventilatory muscles to rest.[3,4] **Diaphragmatic dysfunction** often accompanies ventilatory failure, and a sustained increase in workload can lead to structural injury to the ventilatory muscles.[5] When the ventilatory muscles become fatigued, at least 24 hours is required for recovery.[6] Complete rest of the diaphragm, as in controlled ventilation, may lead to diaphragmatic deconditioning, weakness, and atrophy in 48 hours.[6] In the presence of spontaneous breathing, inappropriate ventilator settings may increase patient work and **fatigue** further.[2] However, careful selection of ventilator settings can reduce the workload to a normal range without resulting in deconditioning and **atrophy** of the respiratory muscles.[2]

EFFECTS OF POOR PATIENT-VENTILATOR INTERACTION ON OUTCOME

Regardless of the cause of the poor patient interaction, the result is negative for the patient. At minimum, hemodynamics, ventilatory pattern, and gas exchange are adversely affected. Patients may become hypotensive, hypertensive, tachycardic, or bradycardic. Their ventilatory pattern may markedly change to a rapid shallow pattern or they may attempt to inhale large tidal volumes at a slow rate when their ventilatory drive is affected by pharmacologic agents. Normally, poor patient-ventilator interaction results in hypoxemia as a result of poor matching of ventilation and perfusion or increased true shunt. Both hypercarbia and hypocarbia may result, based on the stimulus. Those who experience hypoxemia will frequently respond with hyperventilation. However, if hemodynamic compromise is present hypocarbia is normally the result.[2]

Most causes of poor patient-ventilator interaction are of rather short duration because the continuation of the cause frequently has significant negative short-term effects. For example, a tension pneumothorax during mechanical ventilation must be corrected quickly or the result is cardiac arrest. Obstruction of the airway, even if partial, normally results in marked changes in airway pressure or tidal volumes that rapidly alert clinicians of a problem. Bronchospasm or pulmonary edema are usually rapidly recognized by the changes in clinical presentation and alterations in patient response to the ventilator. Patient-ventilatory asynchrony is a more subtle problem that can be difficult to identify and can persist for the entire time that the patient is mechanically ventilated. Identification of asynchrony requires careful patient and ventilator waveform assessment and sometimes requires a lengthy observation of waveforms. Although asynchrony is more subtle than other causes of poor patient-ventilator interaction its effects in the long term can be very serious. Recent data indicate that asynchrony occurs in all patients receiving assisted patient-triggered ventilation, is most significant during the morning when clinician-patient interaction is greatest, is present even during periods of sedation, and varies from mild to very severe.[7] What is most important to remember is that asynchrony has been associated with increased length of mechanical ventilation, ICU and hospital length of stay, the need for trachestomy, and ICU and hospital mortality.[7,8,9] At this time it cannot be said that asynchrony causes an increase in mortality but that patients who have high levels of asynchrony have greater ICU and hospital mortality than patients who have a low level of asynchrony. As a result, careful review of ventilator settings should occur during every patient-ventilator assessment and adjustments should be made to minimize the level of asynchrony.

RULE OF THUMB

Asynchrony has been associated with increased length of mechanical ventilation, ICU and hospital length of stay, the need for trachestomy, and ICU and hospital mortality.

MINI CLINI

Management of Emergency Airway Issues

PROBLEM: Mr. Smith is a 36-year-old motor vehicle accident victim presenting with massive head and chest trauma. He is immediately intubated in the emergency department and mechanically ventilated in the volume control mode. He has received sedation and paralysis and is ventilated with the following settings. Tidal volume 500 ml (6 ml/kg PBW), rate 22/min, peak flow 40 liters/min, inspiratory time 0.66 sec. He has 10 cm H_2O PEEP and an F_IO_2 of 60%. At these settings his SpO_2 is 95%, pulse is 78/min, and arterial blood pressure is 110/70. His peak airway pressure is 24 cm H_2O and his plateau pressure is 18 cm H_2O. He has received a total of 4 liters of fluid.

As you are standing at the bedside you observe a breath-by-breath increase in his peak airway pressure and the high-pressure alarm sounds at 50 cm H_2O. His SpO_2 has decreased to 88% and appears to be decreasing breath by breath. His pulse is 140/min and blood pressure is 80/50. You observe that his trachea is deviated to the left, and on auscultation note an absence of breath sounds on the left. His percussion note is hyperresonant on the left side and on palpitation you note a rise only of the right chest. What should you do?

Solution: Clearly some dramatic change in your ability to ventilate the patient has rapidly occurred. This presentation is most likely the result of an airway obstruction, a mainstem intubation, or a tension pneumothorax. Immediately disconnect the patient from the ventilator and suction the endotracheal tube. This will eliminate obstruction of the airway and the ventilator as the problem. It is most likely not a mainstem intubation because most mainstem intubations are into the right mainstem bronchus and the fact that breath sounds are absent on the right eliminates this. In addition, his presentation is more consistent with a tension pneumothorax; rapid deterioration, hyperresonant on the affected side, deviated trachea way from the affected side, and an increase in peak airway pressure with each breath.

Immediate decompression of the chest with a 19-gauge needle is indicated, followed by insertion of a chest tube. Decompression is done by sliding the needle over the third rib at the mid-nipple line. Blood vessels and nerves run along the lower border of the ribs, not the upper border. During these procedures very gentle ventilation with a manual ventilator should occur with 100% oxygen and a rapid shallow pattern minimizing pressure to avoid extending the pneumothorax.

CAUSES OF POOR PATIENT-VENTILATOR INTERACTIONS

The primary causes of poor patient-ventilator interaction are listed in Table 47-1. It is important to note that most of these issues also result in sudden respiratory distress. Except for asynchrony, the causes listed in Table 47-1 can occur in patients under both controlled and assisted ventilated.

TABLE 47-1
Causes of Poor Patient-Ventilation Interaction

Patient-related Causes
Abnormal respiratory drive
Abdominal distension
Alteration in body posture
Artificial airway problems
Agitation
Bronchospasm
Drug-induced problems
Dynamic hyperinflation
Fever
Hemodynamic compromise
Hypoxemia
Pneumothorax
Pulmonary edema
Pulmonary embolism
Secretions
Ventilator-related Causes
Circuit malfunction
Inadequate F_IO_2
Inadequate ventilator support
System leak
Patient-ventilator asynchrony

Change in Clinical Status

One of the primary causes of poor patient interaction with the mechanical ventilator is a change in the patient's clinical status.[2] Excessive secretions, bronchospasm, and agitation are the most common and regularly seen causes of poor patient-ventilator interaction, and these issues should be assessed at every patient-ventilator assessment. In addition, fever, hypoxemia, and hemodynamic compromise are also regular causes of poor patient-ventilator interaction (Table 47-1). When these issues are present the cause should be identified and rapidly corrected. In addition, artificial airway problems, pneumothorax, pulmonary edema, pulmonary embolism, dynamic hyperinflation, alterations of body position, drug administration, and abdominal distension can all cause poor patient-ventilator interaction.[2]

Artificial Airways

Artificial airway problems are a common cause of sudden respiratory distress. As outlined in Chapter 36, a number of problems can suddenly occur with artificial airways. Of primary concern is the development of biofilm on the internal surface of the endotracheal tube, as illustrated in Figure 47-1. Biofilm develops on all endotracheal tubes but the extent of the development is based on the clinical presentation of the patient.[10] Patients who are aspirating oral secretions around the endotracheal tube or who have excessive lower airway secretion production can easily develop obstructions that occupy more than 50% of the lumen of the endotracheal tube, which can rapidly progress to complete occlusion if proper humidification is not provided.[11] If the lumen of the endotracheal tube is nearly totally obstructed, airway resistance markedly increases, resulting in an

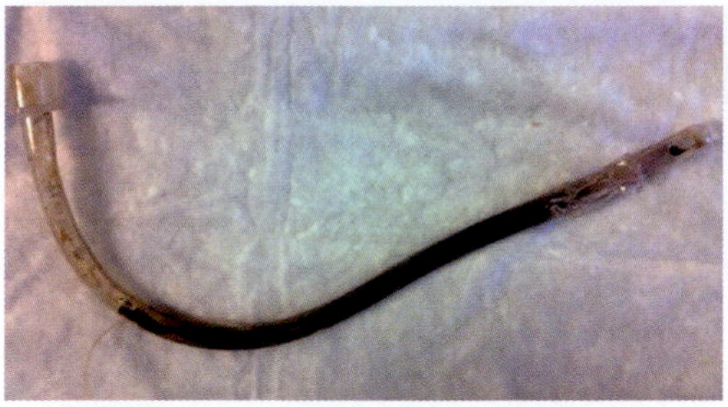

FIGURE 47-1 Picture of an endotracheal tube with biofilm/secretions partially occluding greater than ½ of the airway. (From: Mietto C, Foley K, Salerno L, et al: Removal of endotracheal tube obstruction with a secretion clearance device. Respir Care 59: e122–e126, 2014.)

increase in peak airway pressure during volume ventilation and a decrease in tidal volume in pressure ventilation. This is an airway emergency requiring immediate action. Either the endotracheal tube needs to be changed or the secretion must be removed. A number of devices are currently on the market designed to remove secretions form the lumen of the artificial airway (Figure 47-2). These mucus shaver devices can prevent the need to change the airway and dramatically improve ventilation.[12,13]

Another common problem with endotracheal tubes is movement of the airway into the oral pharynx or movement into the right mainstem bronchus. Both of these can be life threatening, although movement into the oral pharynx, essentially extubation, is the most life threatening. In some situations the airway can be moved back into the trachea, but in others reintubation is necessary. If movement of the airway occurs, adequate ventilation is generally impossible. Airway pressures and tidal volumes rapidly decrease and there is frequently gas leakage from the mouth and nose. Thus it is important to determine the location of the endotracheal tube at each patient-ventilator assessment. The tube should be positioned about 23 cm from the teeth (incisors) in men and 21 cm in women. In addition, following intubation the location of the tip of the tube in relation to the carina must be evaluated. In adults the tip of the tube should be 3 to 5 cm above the carina and its length at the teeth should be noted and regularly reassessed to ensure proper placement. A right mainstem intubation presents with sudden increases in airway pressure and absent breath sound on the right side of the chest. Depending on the patient's status, hypoxemia, hypercarbia, and hemodynamic compromise may be present. Careful movement of the tube to the proper position at the teeth corrects this problem but following adjustment a chest x-ray should always be performed to assure proper position. Flexion and extension of the head and neck always results in movement of the tip of the endotracheal tube. Extension of the head and neck moves the tip closer to the carina and flexion moves the tip closer to the pharynx. This movement on average is 1 to 3 cm in either direction.

Other potential problems with artificial airways include cuff herniation, the unequal expansion of the cuff causing part of

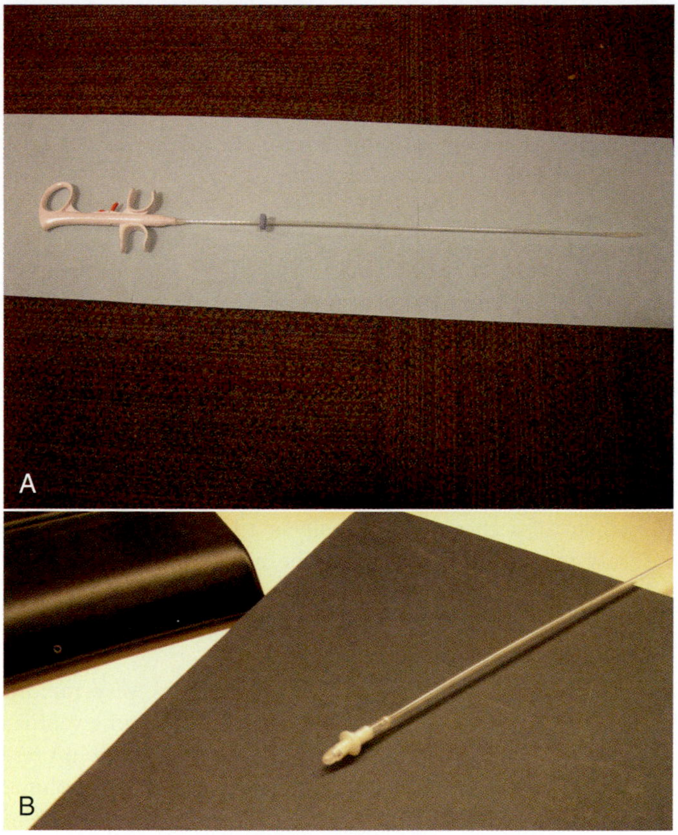

FIGURE 47-2 **A,** Picture of a mucus shaver device. This device is designed to remove biofilm/secretions from the inside of an artificial airway. **B,** Shows the dilated tip of the mucus shaver inflated to remove secretion.

the cuff to partially occlude the tip of the artificial airway. This can occur with both endotracheal and tracheostomy tubes. It is usually identified based on difficulty passing a suction catheter past the tip of the airway, which is resolved by deflating the cuff. If cuff herniation is present, the airway requires replacement. Cuffs can rupture, resulting in an inability to effectively ventilate with large oral/nasal leaks and the inability of the cuff to hold pressure. Again, the airway requires replacement.

Kinking of the endotracheal tube is also a potential problem. This usually occurs in a patient with a well-secured endotracheal tube that the patient is actively trying to move out of their airway by biting and "tonguing" the tube. This causes the tube to move toward the oral pharynx, but because it is well secured it kinks. The result is increased airway resistance. Inability to pass a suction catheter more than a short distance into the airway and visualization of the tube in the mouth and pharynx identifies this problem. Repositioning of the tube is indicated. Differentiation of tube kinking from tube obstruction can be difficult but biofilm and secretion obstruction usually occur in the lower third of the airway and kinking the middle to the first third of the airway.

Long-term artificial airway placement can also result in the development of **tracheal stenosis**, **tracheal malasia**, **tracheo-esophageal fistula**, and **innominate artery rupture**. Of these, innominate artery rupture is the most devastating. It requires surgical intervention and can be fatal. It is difficult to identify the problem until the rupture actually occurs. However, in some patients the tracheostomy tube will start to pulsate with eroding of the tracheal wall toward the innominate artery, allowing the pulse to be counted from the pulsation.

Pneumothorax

Another life-threatening situation during mechanical ventilation is the development of a pneumothorax, which in most circumstances is a tension pneumothorax. That is, with every positive pressure breath more gas moves into the pleural space but is unable to exit the space. As a result the pressure in the pleural space continues to increase, causing lung collapse and eventually causing complete cardiovascular collapse and cardiac arrest. Treatment is decompression of the pleural space and the placement of a chest tube. Initially, a 19-gauge needle can be inserted to relieve the pressure. The needle is inserted at the mid-nipple line, sliding over the top of the third rib or the highest point of the thoracic cage, allowing the gas to exit and relieving the tension.

A tension pneumothorax typically develops very rapidly. Airway pressure increases with each breath in volume ventilation, whereas tidal volume decreases with each breath in pressure ventilation. The change is more dramatic in volume ventilation than in pressure ventilation because the pressure in the pleural space can increase only to the peak pressure set by the clinician in pressure ventilation, whereas in volume ventilation pressure can increase to the pressure limit setting, which may be set very high. As pressure increases, the affected side's lung collapses and begins to compress the unaffected side. In severe cases the mediastium and trachea are shifted away from the side with the pneumothorax. Patients rapidly become hemodynamically unstable. Breath sounds are absent on the side of the pneumothorax, the percussion note is hyperresonnent on the affected side, and palpitation of the chest generally shows a rise and fall only of the side of the chest opposite the pneumothorax.

RULE OF THUMB

A tension pneumothorax causes increasing airway pressure with each breath in volume ventilation and decreasing tidal volume with each breath in pressure ventilation. As pressure in the pleural space increases, lung collapse occurs.

Airway Emergencies

A rapid deterioration in the patient's clinical status associated with increased airway pressure and decreased tidal volume associated with progressive hemodynamic compromise and deteriorating gas exchange should always alert clinicians to the possibility of three problems: tension pneumothorax, airway obstruction, and right mainstem intubation. Box 47-1 lists the steps that should be taken to identify the cause of the problem. Removing the patient from the ventilator and manually ventilating (ambuing) with rapid shallow breaths will eliminate the ventilator as the cause of the concern. Rapid suctioning of the airway will determine if airway obstruction is the problem. If obstruction is not the problem, then **endobronchial intubation** or a **tension pneumothorax** is the cause. If assessment of the patient is consistent with a tension pneumothorax and the tube is at the correct length at the teeth, the problem is almost always a tension pneumothorax. Severe hemodynamic compromise and continued increasing of airway pressure are not normally seen in a right mainstem intubation.

Box 47-1 Management of Sudden Respiratory Distress

1. Remove the patient from the ventilator.
2. Initiate manual ventilation using a self-inflating bag delivering 100% oxygen.
3. Perform a rapid physical examination and assess monitored indices.
4. Check patency of the airway (pass a suction catheter).
5. If death is imminent, consider and treat the most likely causes (e.g., pneumothorax, airway obstruction).
6. After the patient is stabilized, undertake more detailed assessment and management.

The Mechanical Ventilator

A potential but infrequent cause of poor patient-ventilator interaction is malfunction of the mechanical ventilator. Poor responsiveness and ventilator circuit issues can be a problem, but with the newest generation of mechanical ventilators these technical malfunctions are rarely the cause of poor patient-ventilator interaction. However, the ventilator settings should be checked to ensure that an appropriate tidal volume, respiratory rate, and F_IO_2 are being delivered.

RULE OF THUMB

The percentage of breaths on average that are asynchrous is about 3% but at some period of time in many patients over 50% of the breaths may be asynchronous!

VARIABLES CONTROLLED DURING MECHANICAL VENTILATION

During spontaneous ventilation the individual has complete control over the process of gas movement into and out of the lungs. In health, normal breathing is a process that generally goes unnoticed; we breathe without conscious thought of breathing and without any effort. As we know from the equation of motion (discussed in detail in Chapter 46), all of the

MINI CLINI

Assist/Control Volume Ventilation Square Wave

PROBLEM: Mrs. Jones, a 68-year-old with COPD, presented in the emergency department in an acute exacerbation. She was initially managed with noninvasive pressure support at 8 cm H_2O and 8 of PEEP. However, after 24 hrs she was intubated and mechanically ventilated in volume assist/control (A/C). She was started at a tidal volume of 300 ml (5 ml/kg PBW) with an inspiratory time of about 1.0 sec and a peak square wave flow of 20 L/min. Her PEEP level is set at 8 cm H_2O and F_IO_2 at 50%. Her SpO_2 is 90%, pulse 120/min, blood pressure 150/100, and respiratory rate 30/min. You study her airway pressure and flow waveforms and observe the following:

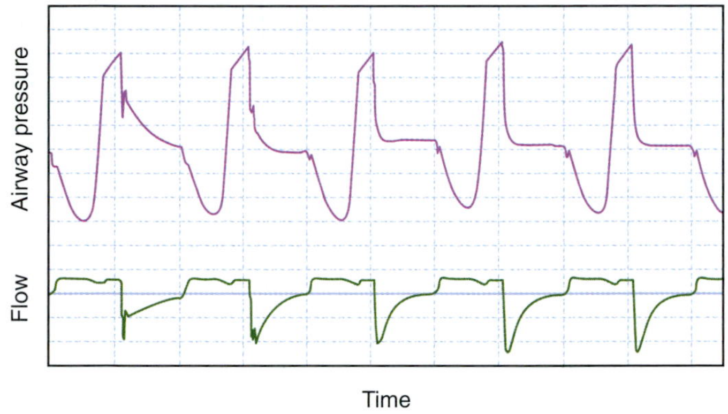

Solution: The shape of the airway pressure versus time curve would indicate that there is marked flow asynchrony. The airway pressure during triggering is below baseline for a considerable period of time and the rise in the airway pressure curve is concave and does not reach peak pressure until more than halfway through the inspiratory time. To try to correct this, peak flow should be increased to 50 l/min and the inspiratory time decreased to 0.6 sec. When this is done the following airway pressure and flow waveforms are obtained. These much more closely resemble the ideal waveforms during controlled ventilation.

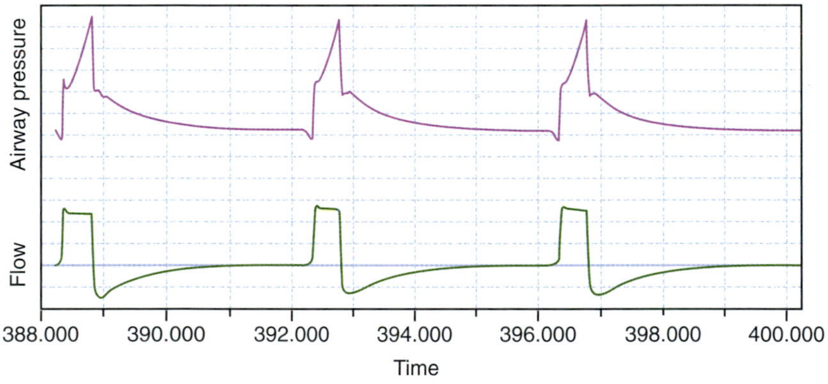

work of breathing is provided by the individual in spontaneous breathing. During controlled ventilation the patient has absolutely no control over the process of ventilation. The ventilator moves gas into and out of the lungs based on how the clinician decides to set the mechanical ventilator. Thus, from the patient's perspective no active work is performed and no concern exists for coordination between what the respiratory center desires versus how the clinician sets the ventilator. Of course to achieve controlled ventilation the patient must be pharmacologically medicated to apnea. Assisted mechanical ventilation is very different from either spontaneous breathing or controlled ventilation. In this case the patient and the ventilator must intimately interact. Ideally the ventilator is set to meet the neurologic output from the respiratory center and there is no competition between the respiratory center and the ventilator. However, this is rarely achieved in critically ill patients. The percentage of breaths on average that are asynchrous is about 3% but at some time in many patients over 50% of the breaths are asynchronous.[7]

Generally, the more control exerted by the ventilator the greater the likelihood that the patient will be asynchronous. Remember that with the classic modes of ventilation the

TABLE 47-2

Variables Controlled During Mechanical Ventilation
Possible Variables Controlled: Pressure, Flow, Volume, and Time

Volume A/C	Volume Flow Time
Pressure A/C	Pressure Time
Pressure Support	Pressure
PAV and NAVA	None

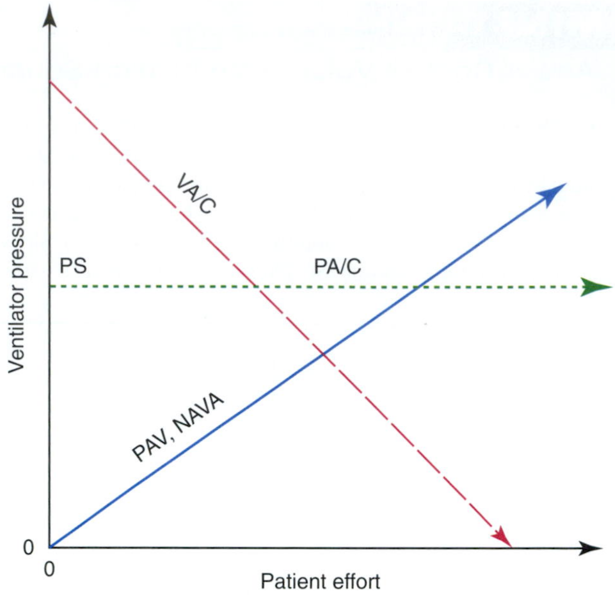

FIGURE 47-3 Relationship between ventilator pressure and patient effort during various forms of ventilatory support. During volume ventilation, there is always an indirect relationship between ventilator pressure and patient effort; the greater the patient effort, the less the ventilator pressure, and the greater the potential asynchrony. With pressure ventilation, airway pressure theoretically does not change as patient effort increases; there is equal ventilator work regardless of patient effort. During PAV and NAVA, ventilator pressure and patient effort are directly related. That is, as patient effort increases, ventilatory pressure increases. With PAV and NAVA, all the clinician sets is the distribution of effort between ventilator and patient. (Modified from Younes M: Proportional assist ventilation, a new approach to ventilatory support. Theory. Am Rev Respir Dis 145:114–117, 1992.)

ventilator leads and the patient must follow. Specifically, if the clinician sets the inspiratory time at 1.0 sec or the tidal volume at 400 ml this is what the patient must accommodate to. This accommodation is difficult and as a result asynchrony occurs. Depending on the mode of ventilation, the ventilator can control one or more of the following gas delivery variables: pressure, flow, volume or time (Table 47-2). The more variables controlled the greater the likelihood of asynchrony. Volume ventilation is the most controlling mode of ventilation because the ventilator in some way controls volume, flow, and time. The only variable the patient can control is pressure. As a result, the likelihood of asynchrony is greater with volume A/C than any other mode of ventilation. With pressure A/C the ventilator only controls pressure and time; less control means less likelihood of asynchrony. In pressure support only the pressure is controlled; thus, of all the classic modes of ventilation the mode that is least likely (if set properly) to cause asynchrony is pressure support. However, as is well documented in the literature,[14-17] **proportional assist ventilation (PAV)** and **neurally adjusted ventilatory assist (NAVA)** are the modes of ventilation that are least likely to cause asynchrony because they do not exert any control over the patient. These modes do not control pressure, flow, volume or time. What they do is provide a proportional assist based on patient demand (see Chapters 45 and 46). They do not require the patient to conform to the settings of the clinician, but instead they require the ventilator to follow the output of the respiratory center, and as a result the patient's respiratory center controls the ventilatory pattern—thus, less asynchrony.

Figure 47-3, modified from the original figure of Magdy Younes, depicts the response of different modes of ventilation to patient demand.[18] As noted, when patient demand (effort) increases in volume ventilation the ventilator provides less support, and an inverse relationship between patient effort and ventilator pressure is established. In pressure ventilation, when patient demand increases the ventilator support remains unchanged. However, in PAV and NAVA as patient effort increases ventilatory support increases, and as patient effort decreases ventilatory support decreases. Control is by the patient's respiratory center, creating greater synchrony than any other approaches to ventilatory support.

RULE OF THUMB

The ventilator can control one or more of the following gas delivery variables: pressure, flow, volume, or time. The more of these variables controlled by the ventilator, the greater the likelihood of asynchrony.

TYPES OF ASYNCHRONY

Table 47-3 lists the types of asynchrony and the subcategories of **trigger asynchrony. Flow asynchrony** occurs when the flow from the ventilator does not match the flow demand of the patient.[19-21] This can occur in any mode of ventilation but most commonly occurs in volume ventilation because the clinician sets the tidal volume, peak flow, flow waveform, and inspiratory time. Thus, the patient's respiratory center must demand exactly the same gas delivery each and every breath or there will be flow asynchrony.

There are several forms of trigger asynchrony and each can occur in any mode of ventilation. The most common form of trigger asynchrony is **trigger delay**, in which the length of time between the beginning of neuro-inspiration and activation of

TABLE 47-3
Types of Asynchrony

Flow asynchrony	Inadequate flow at onset and during inspiration to meet patient demand	
Trigger asynchrony	Poor coordination of patient's initiation of inspiration and ventilator response	Trigger delay Double trigger Missed trigger Auto trigger Reverse triggering
Cycling asynchrony	Poor coordination of patient's desire to exhale and ventilator response	Inappropriately short inspiratory time Inappropriately long inspiratory time
Mode Asynchrony	Inappropriate mode	

TABLE 47-4
Causes of Asynchrony

Inappropriately Set Sensitivity	
Inappropriately set PEEP	
Auto-PEEP	
Volume A/C	Inadequate peak flow Inappropriate inspiratory time Inadequate or excessive tidal volume
Pressure A/C or Pressure Support	Inappropriate rise time Inappropriate inspiratory time or inappropriate inspiratory termination criterion Inadequate or excessive driving pressure
Inappropriate Mode of Ventilation	

the ventilator is excessive.[22] Under normal circumstances, trigger delay should not exceed 100 milliseconds to avoid patient perception of the delay and an increase in ventilatory drive.[23-25] Another common form of trigger asynchrony is **missed triggering**, in which the patient is unable to trigger the ventilator with each inspiratory effort. Frequently a pattern of missed triggering and triggering is established.[26] That is, for every 2 or 3 inspiratory efforts the ventilator is only triggered once.[27] **Double triggering** is usually a result of the patient's ventilatory center desiring a larger breath or a longer inspiratory time than is set on the ventilator.[28] This causes the patient to continue inspiration when the ventilator transitions into the expiratory phase, resulting in the ventilator triggering a second time. The biggest problem with double triggering is that there is no exhalation after the first breath, so that the actual delivered tidal volume may be up to double what is set on the ventilator. Double triggering is most common with volume A/C because of the precise setting of the tidal volume. **Autotriggering** is a much less frequent form of trigger asynchrony. It is the seemingly automatic triggering of the ventilator without any patient inspiratory effort.[29]

The most recently described from of trigger asynchrony is **reverse triggering**. With reverse triggering a controlled mechanical breath results in stimulation of the respiratory center, which then triggers the subsequent breath.[30,31] This form of asynchrony occurs only during controlled ventilation. Most of the other forms of asynchrony occur only during assisted ventilation.

Cycle asynchrony occurs when the ventilator ends the breath at a time different from when the patient's respiratory center wants to end the breath.[32,33,34] It is more common in pressure-targeted than in volume-targeted ventilation, but it can occur in all modes of ventilation. Cycle asynchrony is described in two forms: asynchrony that results in an inappropriately long inspiratory time and asynchrony that results in an inappropriately short inspiratory time.

Mode asynchrony is the selection of a mode of ventilation that simply is highly unlikely to meet a patient's inspiratory demand. As should be obvious from Table 47-2, during assisted ventilation it is most likely that mode asynchrony occurs with volume A/C, followed by pressure A/C, and then pressure support. It is least likely to occur with PAV and NAVA.

CAUSES OF ASYNCHRONY

Table 47-4 summarizes the major causes of asynchrony. Across all modes of ventilation, inappropriately set sensitivity, inappropriate selection of PEEP, and the presence of auto-PEEP result in asynchrony. The one exception to this is NAVA; because NAVA is controlled by the diaphragmatic EMG signal the presence of auto-PEEP does not affect the function of this mode.[35] All other modes are triggered by airway pressure, flow or volume and are dramatically affected by auto-PEEP. In volume ventilation, poor matching of the ventilator settings to the patient's ventilatory drive results in asynchrony. Specifically, inadequate peak flow and inadequate or excessive inspiratory time result in asynchrony. In pressure A/C or pressure support ventilation asynchrony is caused by inappropriately set rise time, inappropriately set inspiratory time (pressure A/C) or termination criteria (pressure support), and inadequate or excessive tidal volume. Finally, selection of an inappropriate mode can cause asynchrony (see Chapters 46 and 48).

RULE OF THUMB

Asynchrony is a result of inappropriate matching of the ventilator's settings and the patient's ventilatory demand or the presence of auto-PEEP.

FLOW ASYNCHRONY

Volume Ventilation

Flow asynchrony can occur in any mode of ventilation but is more common in volume A/C because a precise flow pattern and peak flow is set, resulting in the selected tidal volume being delivered in a precise inspiratory time. This is not physiologic; with normal spontaneous breathing there is a large variability in the ventilatory pattern from breath to breath.

MINI CLINI

Assist/Control Pressure Targeted Ventilation

PROBLEM: Mr. Garcia is a 72-year-old patient with severe COPD who has been intubated and mechanically ventilated for the last 3 days. The ventilator is set with a PEEP of 5 cm H_2O, F_IO_2 of 0.4, and volume A/C tidal volume of 480 ml (6.5 ml/kg PBW). The ventilator respiratory rate is 18/min. The patient's pulse is 105/min, blood pressure 130/90, and SpO_2 92%. When you look at the ventilator you notice the following airway pressure and flow waveforms:

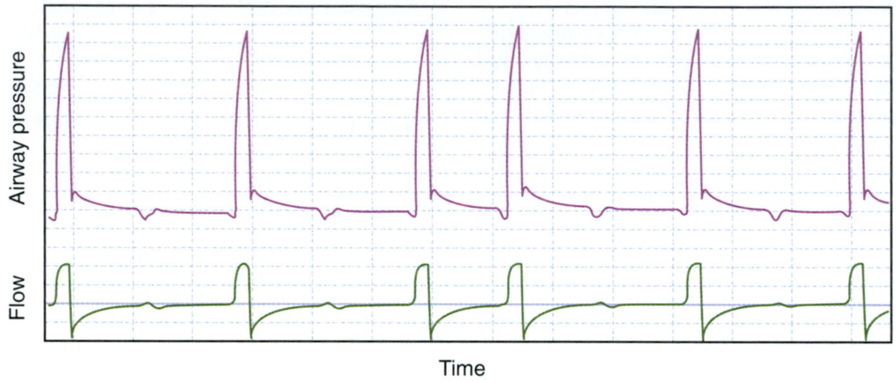

In addition, when you palpate the patient's diaphragm you note that the diaphragm is contracting at a rate of 36 times per minute with the ventilator only responding at a rate of 18 times per minute.

Solution: The expiratory flow does not return to baseline before the patient attempts to inspire. As a result, Mr. Garcia has auto-PEEP. The level must be fairly high since he is mistriggering at a ratio of two breaths to one ventilator-triggered breath. To correct this, either Mr. Garcia's tidal volume should be decreased or applied PEEP should be increased. Since his tidal volume is at 6.5 Ml/kg PBW it is unlikely that a further change will affect the level of auto-PEEP. Because he has dynamic airway obstruction from his severe COPD, adding PEEP to balance the auto-PEEP across the dynamic airway obstruction should decrease the pressure gradient to trigger the ventilator. PEEP should be increased in 1 to 2 cm H_2O steps until Mr. Garcia can trigger the ventilator with every inspiratory effort. At an applied PEEP level of 12 cm H_2O the mistriggering disappeared.

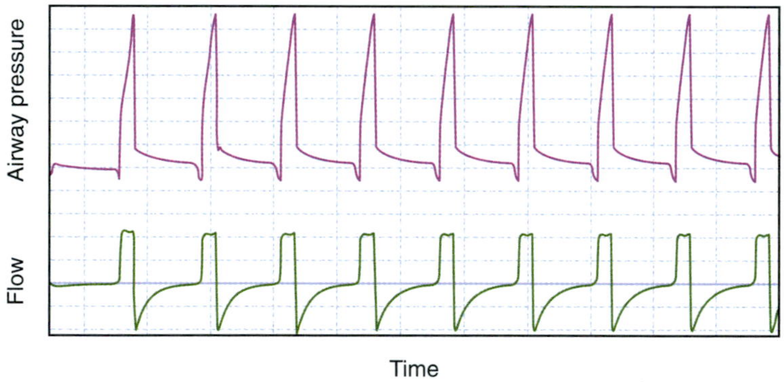

If a patient is spontaneously triggering the ventilator, peak flow delivery during volume ventilation should match the patient's inspiratory flow demand.[19-21] Most adult patients with moderate to strong ventilatory demands require a peak flow of 60 L/min or greater. As shown by Marini and colleagues,[19,20] if the peak flow does not meet the patient's inspiratory demand, the WOB performed by the patient increases (see Figure 47-4). In this setting, the efficiency of the work may be greater than during spontaneous breathing, but the overall patient work may be similar.[19,20] In volume ventilation, there is always an indirect relationship between the work provided by the ventilator and the patient's WOB (Figure 47-3). The more work the patient does, the less work the ventilator performs for the patient. If the patient is triggering the positive pressure breaths, the WOB is shared between the patient and the ventilator. For this reason, patients initially receiving assisted ventilation show altered gas delivery patterns after they are sedated to apnea. With the transition to controlled ventilation, the peak airway pressure usually increases during volume ventilation.[36] Because the patient no longer performs a portion of the WOB, the work performed by the ventilator must increase. The opposite is also true in volume ventilation when the patient's ventilatory demand is high—the

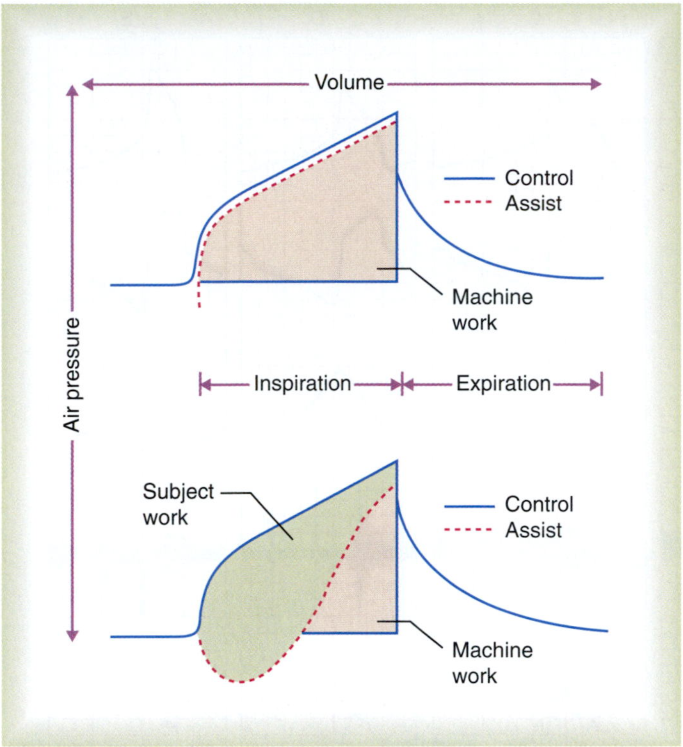

FIGURE 47-4 Plot of an ideal pressure-time waveform during volume-targeted ventilation *(top).* Plot of actual pressure-time curve *(dotted line)* is superimposed on the ideal curve *(bottom).* The scooped-out actual pressure waveform is evident. *Green area* reflects the work performed by the patient during assisted volume-targeted ventilation. This type of actual pressure waveform is indicative of inadequate peak inspiratory flow or too lengthy an inspiratory time. The peak flow should be increased, normally to between 60 L/min and 90 L/min to minimize patient effort during volume-limited ventilation. (Modified from Marini JJ, Rodriguez M, Lamb V: The inspiratory workload of patient-initiated mechanical ventilation. Am Rev Respir Dis 134:902, 1986.)

patient can be doing a disproportionate amount of work if the ventilator is not set to meet the patient's inspiratory demand.

Most ventilators during volume A/C can deliver gas flow in a decelerating or square wave flow pattern. If the patient is triggering inspiration, we recommend a decelerating flow pattern, especially when a small V_T is being delivered.[36,37] A decelerating flow pattern allows a high peak flow to be delivered but also ensures that the inspiratory time can be adequately set. In patients who are sedated and who are not triggering the ventilator, the choice of flow waveform is unimportant, and the setting of peak flow depends on the inspiratory time and V_T desired by the clinician.

If a patient is triggering every breath, the set inspiratory time should equal the patient's neuro-inspiratory time.[38] As illustrated in Figure 47-5, when the ventilator's inspiratory time is decreased to equal the patient's desired inspiratory time and peak flow is increased to match the patient's demand, the patient's WOB and effort correspondingly decrease (Box 47-2). This improvement in asynchrony can be performed without changing the tidal volume, as illustrated in Figure 47-5. A patient with a moderate to high ventilatory demand rarely desires an inspiratory time greater than 1 second.[36] Many adults with moderate or high ventilatory demands desire an inspiratory time between 0.6 second and 0.9 second.[37] Carefully matching the ventilator's inspiratory time with the patient's inspiratory time generally markedly improves patient-ventilator synchrony.

In general, the airway pressure waveform during volume A/C ventilation should be similar to the airway pressure waveform during controlled ventilation (Figure 47-4). The greater the actual waveform differs from the ideal, the greater the patient WOB and the greater the asynchrony.[19,20] If the ventilator cannot be set to meet patient demand and all other potential causes of asynchrony have been ruled out, the patient will require sedation or a change in the mode of ventilation. In general, the mode should be changed before the patient is markedly sedated.

Box 47-2 Flow Asynchrony: ***Volume Ventilation***

To correct flow asynchrony:
- Change to decelerating flow
- Increase peak flow (>60 L/min)
- Match ventilator's inspiratory time to patient's inspiratory time
- Ensure that the airway pressure waveform is as similiar as possible to the ideal airway pressure waveform during controlled volume ventilation

RULE OF THUMB

Flow asynchrony can occur in any mode of ventilation but is more common in volume A/C since a precise flow pattern and peak flow is set, resulting in the selected tidal volume being delivered in a precise inspiratory time.

Pressure Ventilation

Flow asynchrony occurs in pressure ventilation but it is less likely than in volume ventilation if the ventilator is set properly. All newer generation critical care ventilators include an inspiratory pressure **rise time** or pressure slope control. This control functions only with pressure-limited breaths (PSV, PCV, PRVC, volume support, airway pressure release ventilation, pressure SIMV). The purpose of this control is to adjust the rate at which flow increases from baseline to peak[38-40] (Figure 47-6). Generally, rise time should be set at a value that ensures adequate inspiratory gas flow (meeting or exceeding patient demand) without an excessive "overshoot" of the pressure at the beginning of inspiration. A slow or low rise time increases the patient's WOB[38-40] (Figure 47-7). If the rise time is inadequate to meet the patient's demand a concavity during the initial part of inspiration is noted, similar to what occurs in volume A/C with inadequate flow.[41] As in volume ventilation, the rise time should be set to ensure the actual airway pressure waveform matches the ideal airway pressure waveform (Box 47-3).

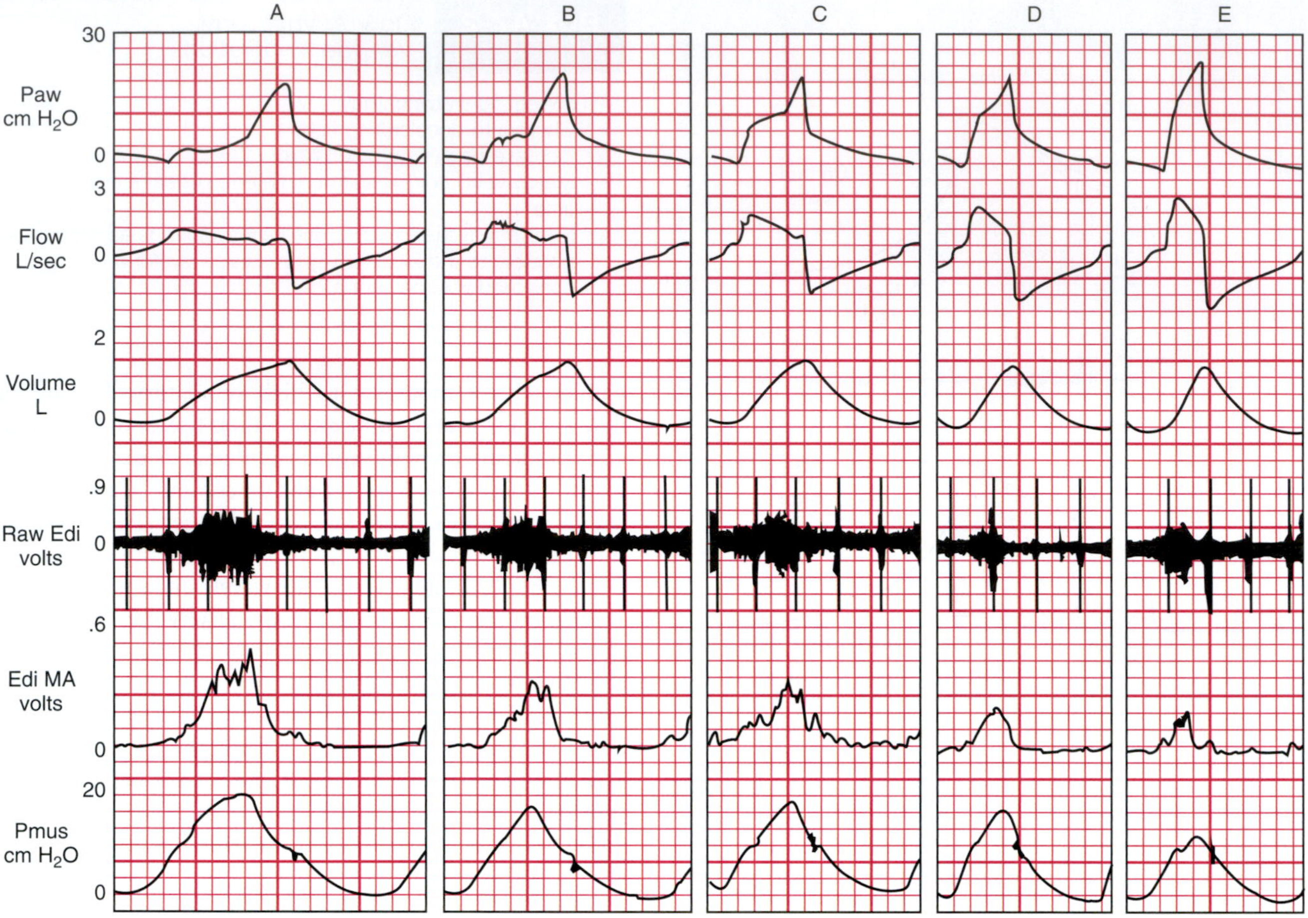

FIGURE 47-5 Airway pressure (P_{aw}), flow, volume, raw (R_{aw}) electromyographic activity of the diaphragm (E_{di}), integrated E_{di}, and muscular work of the diaphragm (P_{mus}) in volume ventilation during varying inspiratory flow and inspiratory time settings (columns *A, B, C, D, E*). As peak flow is increased and inspiratory time is decreased (left to right), indices of patient effort and work are decreased. Ideal settings of flow and inspiratory time generally can be identified by observing the airway pressure curve during volume ventilation. The closer the airway pressure curve is to the ideal curve (*D* and *E*), the less the patient's work. (From Fernandez R, Mendez M, Younes M: Effect of ventilator flow rate on respiratory timing in normal humans. Am J Respir Crit Care Med 159:710–719, 1999.)

Box 47-3 Flow Asynchrony: *Pressure Ventilation*

To correct flow asynchrony:
- Adjust rise time until the initial airway pressure rises rapidly without any concavity but does not exceed the set pressure at the beginning of inspiration
- If inadequate flow: initial concavity in airway pressure, increase rise time
- If excessive flow: initial airway pressure exceeds the set level, decrease rise time

RULE OF THUMB

Flow asynchrony can be greatly improved in volume ventilation by increasing peak flow and decreasing inspiratory time. In pressure ventilation flow asynchrony can be corrected by adjusting rise time.

TRIGGER ASYNCHRONY

As noted in Table 47-3, there are numerous types of trigger asynchrony and of these missed triggering is a common cause of asynchrony. However, the single most important variable affecting trigger asynchrony is the presence of auto-PEEP.

Auto-PEEP/Missed Triggering

As illustrated in Figure 47-8, auto-PEEP is a result of air trapped in the lung at the end of exhalation.[42] This is most commonly caused by dynamic airway obstruction[43] but it is also caused by the delivery of excessive minute ventilation/tidal volume.[44] In dynamic airway obstruction because of airways disease the structural integrity of the airways is compromised. A loss of smooth muscle causes the airway diameter to change from inspiration to expiration. During expiration the elastic recoil of the lung and thorax causes these damaged airways to at least partially collapse and in some cases totally collapse, trapping gas behind the obstruction or limiting flow to the point that at

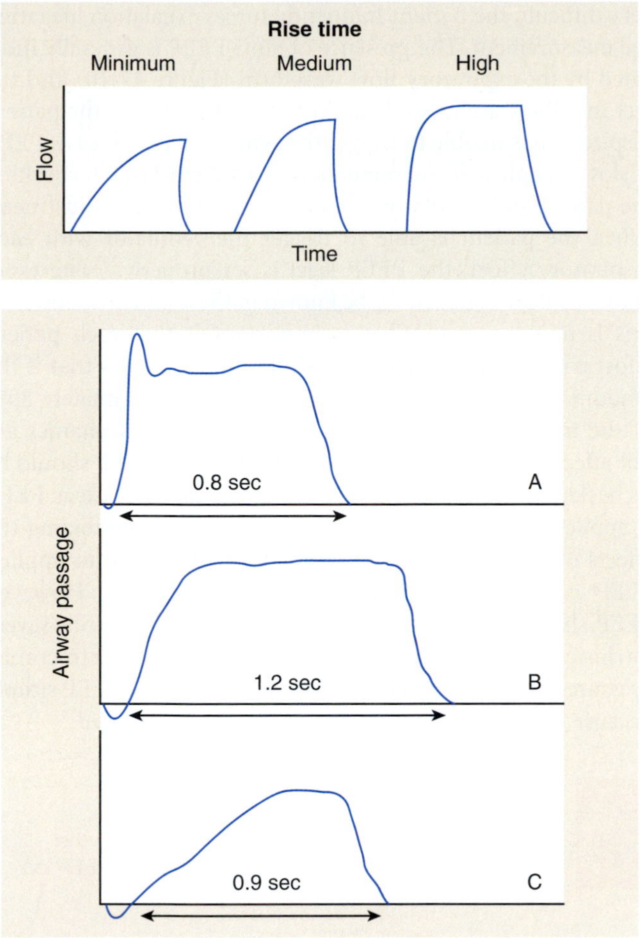

FIGURE 47-6 The effect of different rise time settings is illustrated. When rise time is adjusted the slope of the flow acceleration from zero to peak flow is altered. A slow rise time indicates that peak flow will not be achieved until sometime after the midpoint of the breath. A high rise time indicates that peak flow will be obtained early in the breath. A medium rise time is somewhere in between. The actual setting variation is manufacturer dependent.

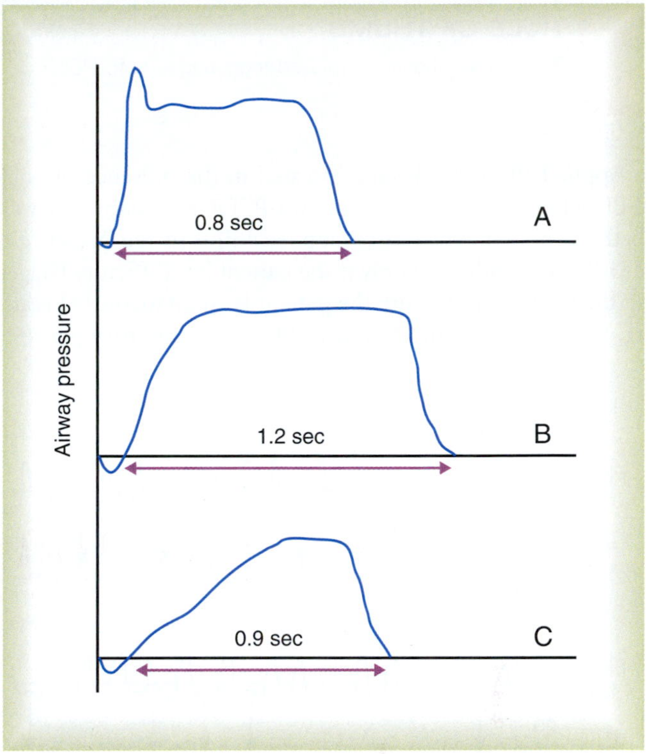

FIGURE 47-7 Effect of changing rise time during pressure-targeted breaths for a patient who prefers a moderate flow. *A,* Flow exceeds patient demand, and a pressure spike and short inspiratory time result. *B,* As flow is decreased, inspiratory time lengthens, and the pressure spike disappears. Machine output matches patient demand. *C,* When flow is reduced further, patient demand exceeds machine flow; the result is deformation of the pressure waveform and a decrease in inspiratory time. (Modified from Branson RD, Campbell RS, Davis K, et al: Altering flow rate during maximum pressure support ventilation [PSV_{max}]: effect on cardiorespiratory function. Respir Care 35:1056–1069, 1990.)

end-exhalation there is gas in the lung periphery under pressure or the presence of auto-PEEP.[42,43] The presence of auto-PEEP is not uniform. In some lung units no auto-PEEP is present, and in others there are varying levels of auto-PEEP. When auto-PEEP is measured it is the average level of auto-PEEP that is determined.

Auto-PEEP can develop in any patient who is mechanically ventilated if the minute ventilation/tidal volume is excessive and cannot be passively exhaled in the expiratory time defined by the respiratory center.[44] Auto-PEEP essentially has the same effect as applied PEEP but only in the lung units where auto-PEEP develops. In reference to asynchrony, auto-PEEP is the primary reason why missed triggering occurs. Essentially the patient cannot decompress the auto-PEEP with every inspiratory effort, and missed triggering occurs. In COPD patients auto-PEEP can be greater than 15 cm H_2O and frequently shows a pattern of 1 triggered breath to 1, 2, or 3 missed triggered breaths[27] (Figure 47-9).

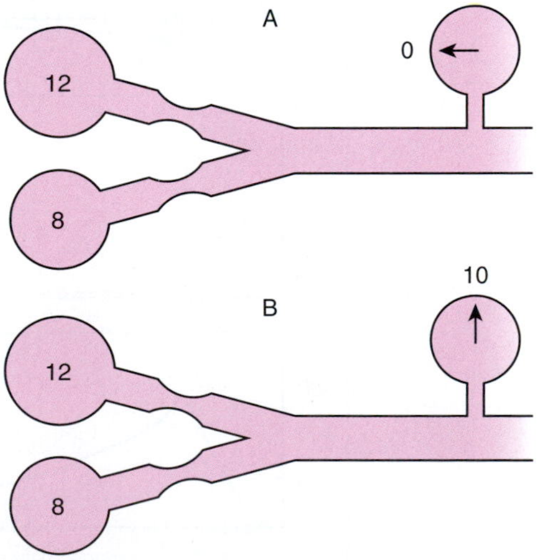

FIGURE 47-8 **A,** Shows two alveoli with different auto-PEEP levels and no end expiratory pause. **B,** Shows the same alveoli with an end expiratory pause. Note that in **A** the end expiratory pressure is zero since the system is open at end exhalation, while in **B** the average auto-PEEP level (10 cm H_2O) is indicated on the manometer because of the end expiratory pause.

RULE OF THUMB
The primary cause of missed triggering is auto-PEEP.

Applied PEEP has been advocated in the presence of auto-PEEP when the cause of the auto-PEEP is dynamic airways obstruction.[34] In this setting applied PEEP in the presence of auto-PEEP is indicated only if the patient has difficulty triggering the ventilator. Because the patient is spontaneously breathing, the measurement of auto-PEEP (end expiratory pause) is very difficult; the patient frequently forces exhalation, negating the measurement. The presence of auto-PEEP is generally indicated by the expiratory flow waveform (Figure 47-10) and the fact that there are missed triggered breaths. That is, the patient inspires but is unable to trigger the ventilator. In this case, PEEP is slowly applied in increments of 1 to 2 cm H_2O, rechecking the patient and ventilator response rate with each adjustment. When the patient is able to trigger the ventilator with each inspiratory effort, the PEEP level is set properly.[29] The exact auto-PEEP level may never be known in these patients; however, this is unimportant. What is important is that each patient effort triggers the ventilator. The literature indicates that if the amount of PEEP applied does not exceed approximately 80% of the measured auto-PEEP, the patient's lung mechanics are not affected by the application of PEEP.[45] Auto-PEEP should be rechecked to ensure intrinsic PEEP does not increase as PEEP is applied. Box 47-4 summarizes methods for minimizing the effects of auto-PEEP. An absolute contraindication to applied PEEP is an uncontrolled tension pneumothorax. However, PEEP should be cautiously applied in any patient with severe intrinsic lung disease, hypotension, and elevated intracranial pressure. During controlled ventilation, increasing PEEP simply because of the presence of auto-PEEP is not indicated.

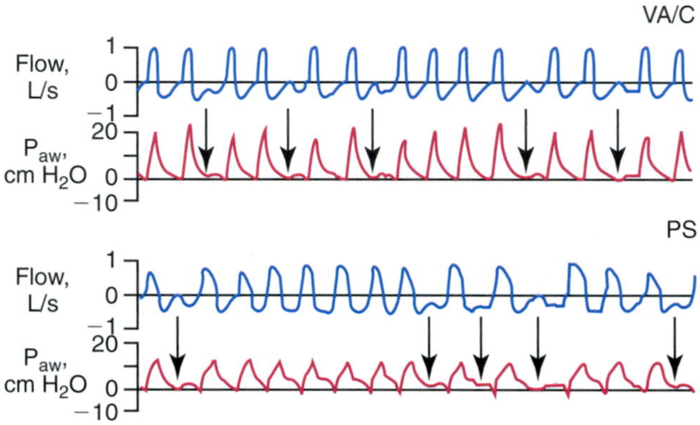

FIGURE 47-9 Airway pressure and flow waveforms during *VA/C* and pressure support *(PS)* ventilation in which frequent missed triggers are observed. (Modified from Leung P, Jubran A, Tobin MJ: Comparison of assisted ventilator modes on triggering, patient effort, and dyspnea. Am J Respir Crit Care Med 155:1387, 1997.)

RULE OF THUMB
In the presence of dynamic airways obstruction the application of PEEP offsets the effect of auto-PEEP on missed triggering.

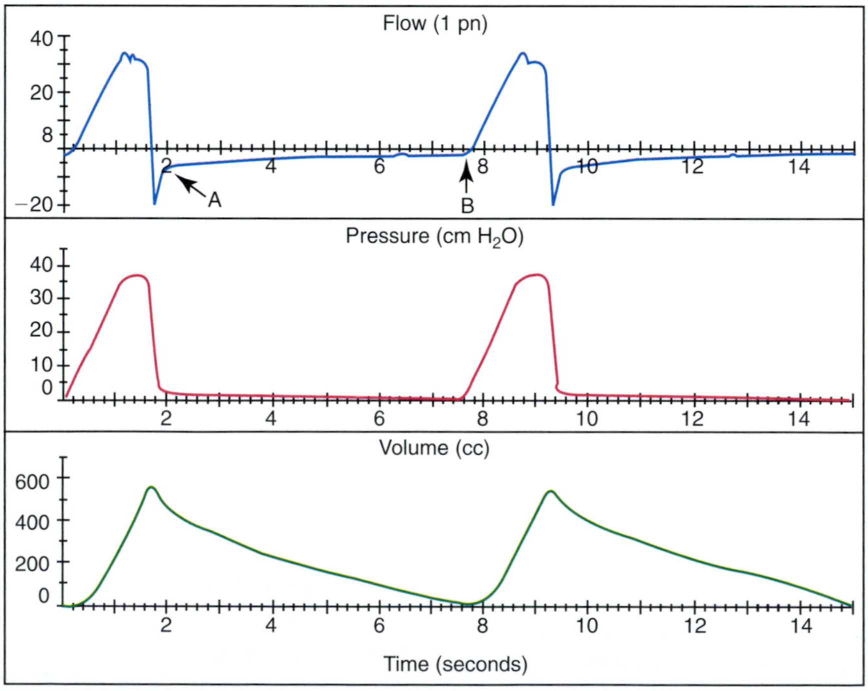

FIGURE 47-10 Airway flow, pressure, and volume in a patient with severe airflow obstruction and auto-PEEP. There is a rapid decrease in expiratory flow at the onset of exhalation because of the obstruction *(arrow A)*, and there is a lack of return of flow to baseline at the end of the breath *(arrow B)*. This type of expiratory flow pattern, regardless of the expiratory time, indicates auto-PEEP. The amount of auto-PEEP cannot be determined from this example, but anytime end expiratory flow is greater than zero, auto-PEEP is present.

In patients without intrinsic lung disease who develop auto-PEEP, dynamic airways obstruction is not present. Auto-PEEP is a result of excessive minute ventilation/tidal volume. Usually returning the tidal volume to the recommended 4 to 8 ml/kg PBW level eliminates the auto-PEEP and as a result the missed triggering.[44]

Box 47-4 Techniques for Minimizing Effects of Auto-PEEP

- Decrease airflow obstruction
- Secretion management
- Aggressive bronchodilation
- Larger sized endotracheal tubes
- Modify ventilatory pattern
- Decrease inspiratory time
- Increase inspiratory flow (on ventilators with inspiratory peak flow control)
- Decrease percentage inspiratory time (on ventilators with %T_i control)
- Decrease VT
- Increase expiratory time
- Decrease rate
- Use low-compressible volume circuit
- Apply PEEP or CPAP to balance auto-PEEP

Outside of auto-PEEP the only other factor that can result in missed triggering is inappropriately set sensitivity. In general, sensitivity should be set as sensitive as possible without causing autotriggering. Should flow or pressure sensitivity be used? With older generation ICU ventilators pressure sensitivity was less effective than flow sensitivity.[46,47] But in today's generation of ICU ventilators both function equivalently.[25] When both are set appropriately neither should be the cause of missed triggering.

RULE OF THUMB

Excessive minute ventilation/tidal volume in patients without dynamic airways obstruction results in auto-PEEP. Decreasing tidal volume to the 4 to 6 ml/kg PBW range generally eliminates the auto-PEEP.

Trigger Delay

Trigger delay is caused by an inappropriately set sensitivity and auto-PEEP insufficient to cause mistriggering.[25,39] Normally the trigger delay should be minimal, less than 100 milliseconds. When it exceeds 150 milliseconds the cause should be determined. Adjusting the sensitivity, setting the tidal volume

MINI CLINI

Volume Targeted A/C Ventilation

PROBLEM: Mr. King is 54-year-old with acute pancreatitis who has developed ARDS. He is currently being ventilated in volume A/C mode with a tidal volume of 6 ml/kg PBW (400 ml). His respiratory rate is 26/min, inspiratory time is 0.5 sec. Gas is being delivered in a square wave flow pattern with a peak flow of 48 liters/min. The patient is tachycardic, pulse rate 118/min, blood pressure 138/98, and SpO_2 92%. Visual assessment of the patient's ventilatory pattern indicates he is using his accessory muscles with every breath. You observe the following waveform on the ventilator:

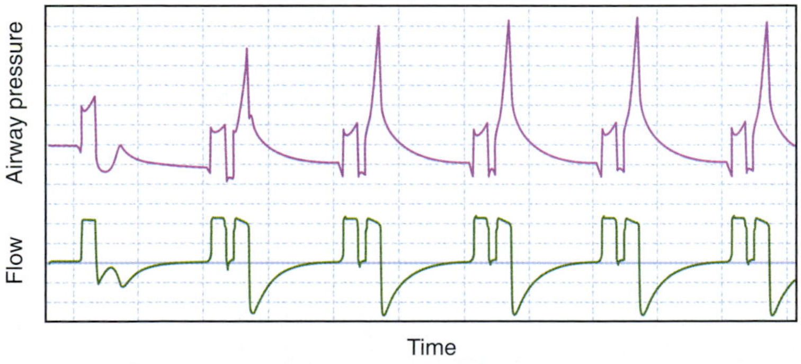

Solution: Assessment of the pressure and flow waveforms indicate that there is frequent double triggering. You have a number of choices on how to eliminate the double triggering: sedation, increasing the tidal volume to 8 ml/kg PBW, increasing the inspiratory time while changing the waveform to decelerating flow, changing to pressure support, or performing a number these changes. Changing to pressure support at a pressure level that maintains the tidal volume <8 ml/kg PBW may be the best option if the patient can maintain his ventilatory pattern. This would allow the patient to determine his tidal volume needs on a breath-by-breath basis. The tidal volume can simply be increased; this may work in some patients but in others the constant tidal volume may still be a problem. Inspiratory time can be increased with the waveform changed to decelerating flow and the tidal volume increased to 8 ml/kg PBW. This may also be a very viable option. Sedation is always the last choice and may not eliminate the double triggering until the patient is sedated to total apnea.

appropriately, and/or applying PEEP should correct delayed triggering unless there is a true malfunction of the ventilator (Box 47-5).

Autotriggering

Setting the sensitivity control to be overly sensitive will cause autotriggering. In addition, autotriggering can be caused by the movement of water accumulated in the ventilator circuit. The back and forth movement of fluid in the circuit can cause triggering of the ventilator. Leaks in the ventilator circuit are the most likely cause of autotriggering. The most easily missed cause of autotriggering is in the post–cardiac surgical patient who is in a hyperdynamic state.[29] The forceful contraction of the heart can trigger the ventilator. Careful assessment of diaphragmatic contraction and readjustment of the sensitivity setting are indicated (Box 47-6).

Box 47-5 Correcting Trigger Delay

Trigger delay is caused by:
- Auto-PEEP
- Poor sensitivity setting
- Ventilator malfunction

Correct by:
- Minimizing auto-PEEP
    - Apply PEEP
    - Decrease minute volume/tidal volume
    - Appropriately set sensitivity
    - Replace ventilator

Box 47-6 Autotriggering

Caused by:
- Circuit leaks
- Water in circuit
- Inappropriately set sensitivity
- Hyperdynamic cardiac contractions

Corrected by:
- New ventilator circuit
- Removal of water from the circuit
- Appropriate setting of sensitivity

Double Triggering

Double triggering most commonly occurs in volume A/C when the tidal volume delivered is less than the patient demands or the inspiratory time set on the ventilator is less than the neuro-inspiratory time.[28] Double triggering is a problem because, as demonstrated in Figure 47-11, in most cases of double triggering there is no exhalation between the two breaths. Thus, the tidal volume during the double triggered breath is twice the set tidal volume. A patient with a lung protective tidal volume of 6 ml/kg PBW would periodically be receiving a tidal volume of 12 ml/kg PBW, which is clearly not a lung protective tidal volume.[48,49] Double triggering can usually be corrected by increasing the tidal volume (but not greater than 8 ml/kg PBW), increasing the inspiratory time, or changing from volume A/C to pressure A/C or pressure support.[48,49] If none of these changes eliminate the double triggering, sedation is indicated (Box 47-7).

RULE OF THUMB

Double triggering is most commonly observed in volume ventilation when the set tidal volume and inspiratory time are less than the patient's demand. Increasing tidal volume or inspiratory time, or changing to pressure-targeted ventilation can correct double triggering.

Reverse Triggering

Reverse triggering is a form of double triggering that occurs during controlled ventilation. It has primarily been described

Box 47-7 Double Triggering

Caused by:
- Inadequate tidal volume
- Short inspiratory time
- Inappropriate mode of ventilation

Corrected by:
- Increased tidal volume (≤8 ml/kg PBW)
- Increased inspiratory time to match patient's inspiratory time
- Mode changed to pressure support

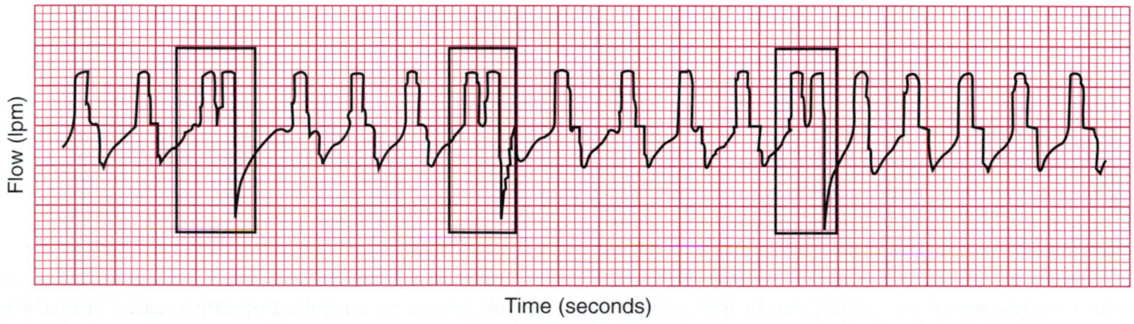

FIGURE 47-11 Double triggering in VA/C ventilation. (Modified from Pohlman MC, McCallister KE, Schweickert WD, et al: Excessive tidal volume from breath stacking during lung-protective ventilation for acute lung injury. Crit Care Med 36:3019–3023, 2008.)

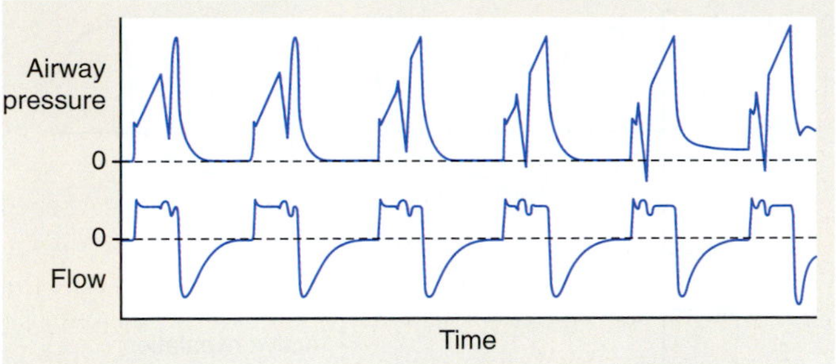

FIGURE 47-12 These waveforms illustrate reverse triggering. Note that the volume targeted breaths are all machine triggered, no patient effort. However, within each machine breath there is a patient inspiratory effort. Reverse triggering is the stimulation of a patient effort following a machine-controlled breath.

in patients with ARDS in which a controlled mechanical breath stimulates the respiratory center via stretch receptors to attempt a spontaneous breath.[30,31] The reverse trigger can occur in any mode of ventilation and can occur within the controlled breath or during the subsequent expiratory phase (Figure 47-12). Little is known about why reverse triggering develops or its effects on the patient, except that it can cause double triggering and the periodic delivery of excessive tidal volumes. If reverse triggering occurs, alteration of tidal volume or inspiratory time should be attempted. Since the patient is already sedated, sedation is not the solution. More research is needed to determine the potential harm of reverse triggering, its causes, and treatment.

CYCLE ASYNCHRONY

Cycle asynchrony is a result of a difference between the inspiratory time of the patient and the inspiratory time of the ventilator.[34] Thus, cycle asynchrony can result in excessively long inspiratory times (Figure 47-13) or excessively short inspiratory times (Figure 47-14). Theoretically, cycle asynchrony can occur in any mode of ventilation but is by far most commonly seen in pressure ventilation.[33] If the ventilator's inspiratory time is excessive compared to the patient's inspiratory time, a spike in pressure above the set level is commonly observed at the end of the pressure-targeted breath (Figure 47-13). If the ventilator inspiratory time is too short, a double trigger will occur every breath (Figure 47-14).

During pressure support cycle asynchrony can be corrected by adjusting the variable that terminates inspiration or the **expiratory cycling criteria.**[36,37] Normally, pressure support is terminated when the peak flow decreases to a predetermined level. Historically, this level was 25% of peak flow.[39] However, not all patients choose to terminate inspiration at this 25% setting (Figure 47-15). Patients with marked respiratory distress and patients with chronic pulmonary disease choose to end inspiration at high terminal flows.[33] In our experience, these patients require a termination criterion set at 50% or higher. Figure 47-16 depicts the problem encountered by patients if the termination criterion is set at a lower percentage than that at which the patient chooses to end inspiration; specifically, the patient's neuro-inspiratory time is shorter than the ventilator's inspiratory time.[33] When this happens, the patient activates accessory muscles of expiration to force the ventilator into exhalation. In Figure 47-16 abdominal muscles are activated midway through the ventilator inspiratory phase; that is, the patient starts to exhale in the middle of the ventilator's inspiratory phase. The clinician can identify that this is happening by an increase in the set pressure at the end of inspiration. This increase indicates that the breath is terminated by the pressure support secondary termination criterion, an increase in airway pressure above the

MINI CLINI

Pressure Support Ventilation

PROBLEM: Mrs. Gonzalez is a 68-year-old female with COPD presenting with an acute exacerbation. She has failed noninvasive ventilation and has been intubated and invasively ventilated in the pressure support mode. Her pressure support level is 12 cm H_2O with 8 cm H_2O PEEP delivering an average tidal volume of 6.5 ml/kg PBW (350 ml). F_IO_2 is 0.5 and respiratory rate is 28/min. She appears to be working hard to interact with the ventilator; she is using her accessory muscles to breath. Her SpO_2 is 90% and her blood gases are PO_2 59 mmHg, PCO_2 55 mmHg, with a pH of 7.34. You note the following pressure and flow waveforms on the ventilator.

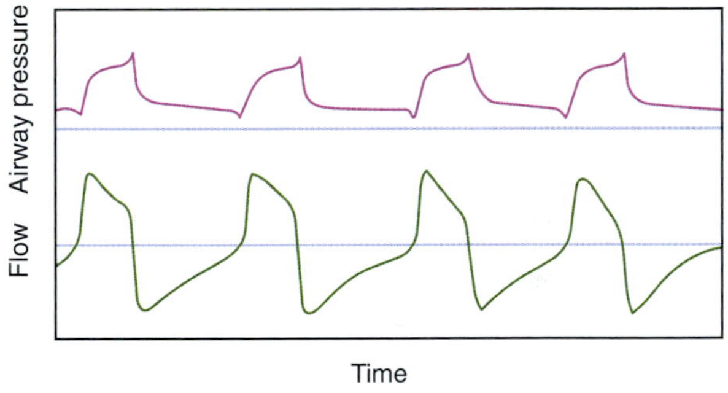

Solution: The patient and the ventilator are not ending inspiration at the same time. The patient is choosing to begin exhalation during the pressure support breath. This is shown on the airway pressure waveform as an increase in the airway pressure at the end of the pressure support breath. In addition, upon palpation of the diaphragm you note that Mrs. Gonzalez is contracting her abdominal muscles during the inspiratory phase of the ventilator, trying to force exhalation. To correct this, the expiratory cycling criterion must be properly set. It is currently set at 25% of peak flow but needs to be set at a much higher percentage. You should slowly increase the expiratory cycling criterion until the airway pressure waveform does not show a spike in airway pressure at the end of the breath. To do this, slowly increase the expiratory cycling criterion in 5% increments, observing the effect on the airway pressure curve. The lowest percentage that eliminates the pressure spike is the correct setting. When set properly, the patient's respiratory rate should decrease and contraction of her abdominal muscles during inspiration should end.

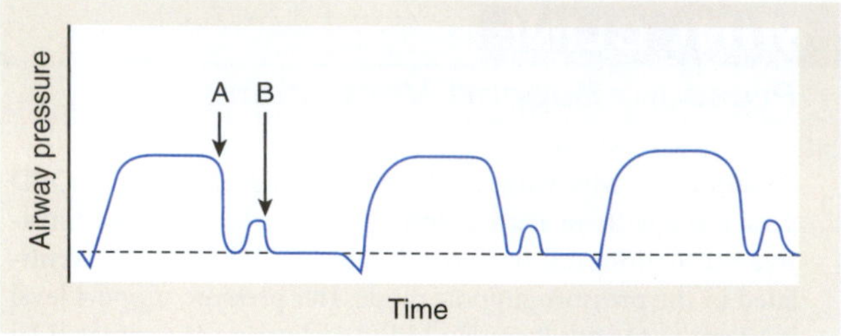

FIGURE 47-13 Cycling asynchrony in pressure ventilation is illustrated. In this figure the patient's inspiratory time is longer than the ventilator's inspiratory time. *A* indicates the end of the ventilator's inspiratory time, and *B* indicates the end of the patient's inspiratory time. To correct this the ventilator's inspiratory time must be increased to equal the patient's inspiratory time. In pressure support this is done by decreasing the percent cycle sensitivity and in pressure control breath by directly increasing the set inspiratory time.

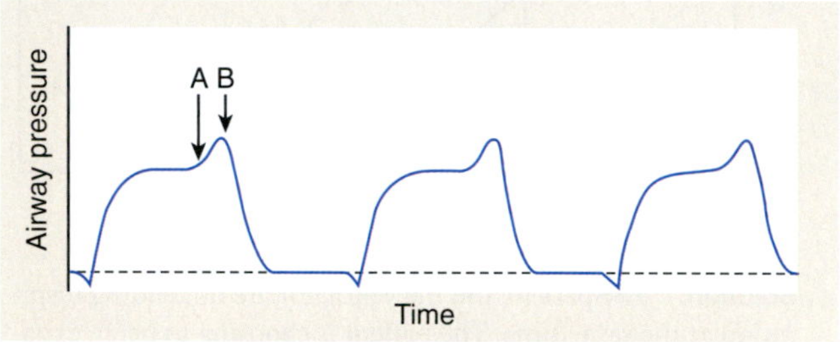

FIGURE 47-14 Cycling asynchrony in pressure ventilation is illustrated. In this figure the patient's inspiratory time is shorter than the ventilator's inspiratory time. *A* indicates the end of the patient's inspiratory time, and *B* indicates the end of the ventilator's inspiratory time. To correct this the ventilator's inspiratory time must be decreased to equal the patient's inspiratory time. In pressure support this is done by increasing the percent cycle sensitivity and in pressure control breath by directly decreasing the set inspiratory time.

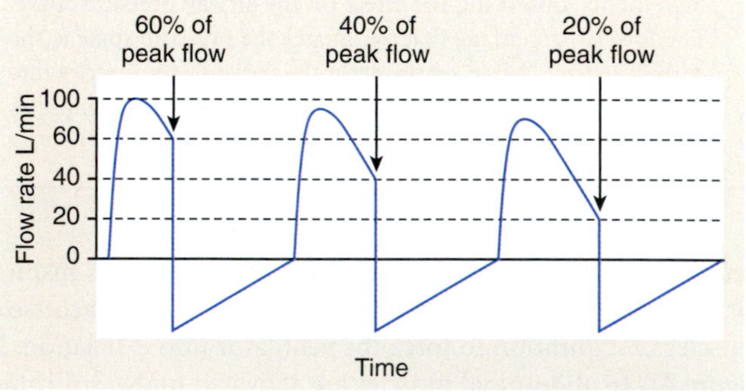

FIGURE 47-15 Function of cycling (termination) sensitivity (criterion). In all three breaths the peak flow is 100 liters/min. However, the first breath has the shortest inspiratory time, cycling criterion 60% (60% of peak flow). The middle breath has a longer inspiratory time, cycling criterion 40% (40% of peak flow). The last breath has the longest inspiratory time, cycling criterion 20% (20% of peak flow).

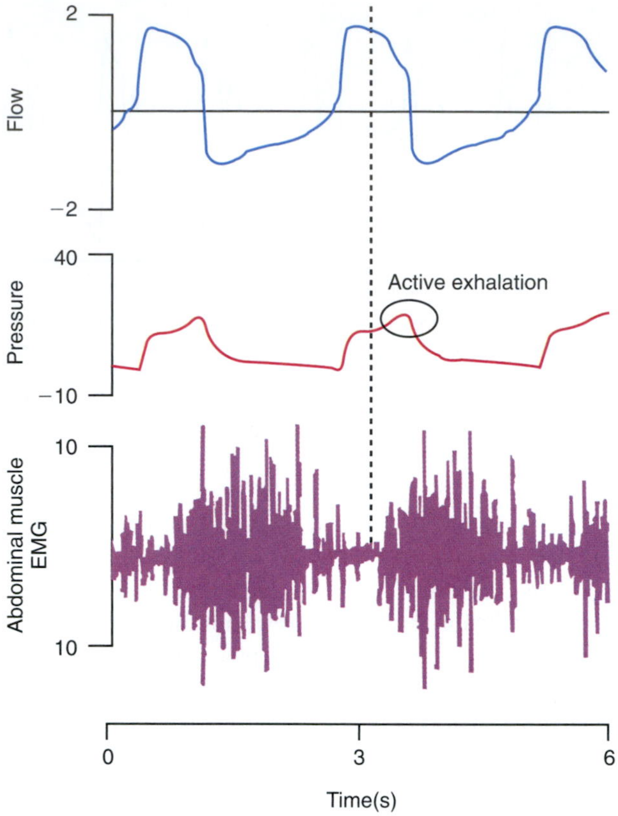

FIGURE 47-16 Airway flow, airway pressure, and abdominal muscle electromyographic (EMG) activity during pressure support ventilation with an inappropriately set termination criterion. *Dotted line* indicates the point where the patient initiates expiration. However, the ventilator does not cycle to exhalation until the spike in airway pressure *(circle)*. In this case, inspiration is cycled to exhalation by the ventilator's secondary cycling mechanism by an increase in airway pressure. Termination criterion should be increased until the spike in airway pressure is eliminated and the time at which the patient terminates the breath is equal to the time the ventilator terminates the breath. (From Parthasarathy S, Jubran A, Tobin MJ: Cycling of inspiratory and expiratory muscle groups with the ventilator in airflow limitation. Am J Respir Crit Care Med 158:1471–1478, 1998.)

set level. This level is ventilator-specific.[39] If the breath is ended by a spike in pressure, the termination criterion needs to be increased slowly until there is a smooth decrease in pressure. If the ventilator does not have the ability to adjust the termination criterion, the problem can be corrected by switching to PA/C. PA/C essentially operates during assisted breaths the same as PSV except that inspiration terminates at a set time.[33] If there is a spike in pressure at the end of a PA/C breath, the inspiratory time setting needs to be decreased until the spike disappears. In all other pressure modes inspiratory time or termination criteria can be adjusted to ensure patient and ventilator end the breath at the same time.

In patients with relatively healthy lungs if the termination criterion is set too high or inspiratory time too short, double triggering can occur every breath.[50,51] These are primarily post-operative patients or overdose patients (Figure 47-14). In these

Box 47-8 Cycle Asynchrony

Caused by:
- Pressure A/C or SIMV
  - Ventilator inspiratory time to short
  - Ventilator inspiratory time to long
- Pressure support
  - Expiratory cycling criteria percentage too high
  - Expiratory time criteria percentage too low

Corrected by:
- If ventilator inspiratory time too long
  - Decrease ventilator inspiratory time in pressure A/C or SIMV to eliminate the pressure spike at the end of the breath
  - Increase expiratory cycling criteria percentage so that the breath ends sooner, eliminating the pressure spike at the end of the breath
- If ventilator inspiratory time too short
  - Increase ventilator inspiratory time in pressure A/C or SIMV to eliminate the double tigger at the end of the breath
  - Decrease expiratory cycling criteria percentage so that the breath ends sooner, eliminating the double tigger at the end of the breath

patients the termination criterion is decreased until the double trigger is eliminated. As opposed to the patient with high ventilatory demand who requires a termination criteria of >50%, these patients frequently require the termination criteria be set at only 10% to 15%. In this setting, termination criterion is slowly decreased followed by careful assessment until the double triggering is gone. In pressure A/C and pressure SIMV where inspiratory time is set, inspiratory time is slowly increased until the double triggering is eliminated (Box 47-8).

RULE OF THUMB

Cycle asynchrony occurs most commonly in pressure ventilation when the patient's neuro-inspiratory time and the ventilator's inspiratory time are not equal.

MODE ASYNCHRONY

Mode asynchrony implies that an inappropriate mode of ventilation has been selected for a given patient. There are many biases regarding mode of ventilation and little data to support any relationship between mode and patient outcome. See Chapters 45, 46, and 48 for detailed discussion regarding modes of ventilation. However, it is increasingly clear that asynchrony is highest in volume ventilation because of its control over the variables associated with ventilation. Of all the classic modes of ventilation, pressure support is the least confining and should result in little asynchrony. PAV and NAVA, however, can be expected to result in the least asynchrony because those modes do not control any gas delivery variable and follow the patient's desires rather than dictating to the patient the required ventilatory pattern.[14-17] However, for clinicians to accept these modes of ventilation they must be willing to accept the resultant ventilatory pattern. Most patient's respiratory centers when experiencing respiratory distress/failure select a ventilatory pattern resulting in rapid shallow breathing, that is, tidal volumes in the 4 to 6 ml/kg PBW and respiratory rate >25/min. In spite of this pattern both PAV and NAVA have been shown to reduce asynchrony.[14-17]

The mode of ventilation that can be the most problematic is SIMV. This is because of the variation in ventilatory load between mechanical and spontaneous breaths (see Chapters 46 and 48 for details). As the percentage of the total spontaneous breaths increase, the work of breathing also increases, not only in the spontaneous breaths increase but also in the mechanical breaths.[52,53] Essentially, the respiratory center cannot distinguish between mechanical and spontaneous breaths once around 50% of the breaths are spontaneous, resulting in the same level of patient work exerted during both spontaneous and mechanical breaths.[52,53] This is a major reason why SIMV has been shown to be the mode least effective in weaning patients from ventilatory support.[54,55]

SUMMARY CHECKLIST

- Patient-ventilator interaction is not a problem during controlled ventilation because the patient is not interacting with the ventilator, but is always a major issue during patient-triggered ventilation.
- Poor patient-ventilator interaction has been associated with increased length of mechanical ventilation, length of ICU stay, need for a tracheotomy, and mortality.
- A change in patient status is commonly the reason for the development of poor patient-ventilator interaction.
- Artificial airway issues can cause marked changes in patient-ventilator interaction.
- The development of a pneumothorax or tension pneumothorax is a major cause of markedly deteriorating patient-ventilator interaction.
- Whenever there is an acute severe change in the ability to provide ventilatory support the three most probable causes are tension pneumothorax, airway obstruction, and right mainstem bronchus intubation.
- Malfunction of the mechanical ventilator can be a cause of poor patient-ventilator interaction but it is a high unlikely cause with today's mechanical ventilators.
- The four variables that can be controlled during classic modes of mechanical ventilation are pressure, flow, volume, and time.
- The less control exerted by the mechanical ventilator on the patient's ventilatory pattern, the less likely it is that the patient will develop patient-ventilator asynchrony.
- The general types of asynchrony are flow asynchrony, trigger asynchrony, cycle asynchrony, and mode asynchrony.
- Asynchrony can be caused by inappropriately set sensitivity, PEEP, flow, tidal volume, and inspiratory time.

- Flow asynchrony is a result of the flow provided by the ventilator being inadequate to match the patient's inspiratory demand.
- Trigger asynchrony can manifest as missed triggering, delayed triggering, autotriggering, double triggering, and reverse triggering.
- Missed triggering and delayed triggering are normally a result of auto-PEEP.
- Autotriggering is normally a result of circuit leaks or fluid moving back and forth in the ventilator circuit, but can also be caused by hyperdynamic contractions of the myocardium.
- Flow asynchrony is a result of the ventilator providing less flow then the patient's respiratory center requires.
- Mode asynchrony occurs when the selected mode of ventilation does not match the patient's ventilatory demands.
- Volume ventilation can be expected to cause the most asynchrony because it controls volume, flow, and time.
- Pressure support should result in the least asynchrony of the commonly used modes of ventilation.
- PAV and NAVA cause the least asynchrony because they do not force a ventilatory pattern but follow the ventilatory pattern selected by the patient.

References

1. Kacmarek RM: Proportional assist ventilation and neurally adjusted ventilatory assist. *Respir Care* 56:140–148, 2011.
2. Tobin MJ: *Principles and practice of mechanical ventilation*, ed 2, New York, 2006, McGraw-Hill.
3. MacIntyre N: Of Goldilocks and ventilatory muscle loading. *Crit Care Med* 28:588–594, 2000.
4. Kacmarek RM: The cost in some is an increase in the work of breathing: is it too high? (editorial). *Respir Care* 50:1624–1626, 2005.
5. Tobin MJ: Advances in mechanical ventilation. *N Engl J Med* 344:1986–1992, 2001.
6. Laghi F, D'Alfonso N, Tobin MJ: Pattern of recovery from diaphragmatic fatigue over 24 hours. *J Appl Physiol* 79:539–546, 1995.
7. Blanch L, Villagra A, Sales B, et al: Asynchronies during mechanical ventilation are associated with mortality. *Intensive Care Med* 41:633–641, 2015.
8. Thille AW, Rodriguez P, Cabello B, et al: Patient-ventilator asynchrony during assisted mechanical ventilation. *Intensive Care Med* 32:1515–1522, 2006.
9. de Wit M, Miller KB, Green DA, et al: Ineffective triggering predicts increased duration of mechanical ventilation. *Crit Care Med* 37:2740–2748, 2009.
10. Mietto C, Pinciroli R, Piriyapatsom A, et al: Tracheal tube obstruction in mechanically ventilated patients assessed by high-resolution computed tomography. *Anesthesiology* 121:1226–1235, 2014.
11. Gil-Perotin S, Ramirez P, Marti V, et al: Implications of endotracheal tube biofilm in ventilator-associated pneumonia response: a state of concept. *Crit Care* 16:R93, 2012.
12. Mietto C, Foley K, Salerno L, et al: Removal of endotracheal tube obstruction with a secretion clearance device. *Respir Care* 59:e122–e126, 2014.
13. Pinciroli R, Mietto C, Berra L: Respiratory therapy device modifications to prevent ventilator-associated pneumonia. *Curr Opin Infect Diss* 26:175–183, 2013.
14. Xirouchaki N, Kondili E, Vaporidi K, et al: Proportional assist ventilation with load-adjustable gain factors in critically ill patients: comparison with pressure support. *Intensive Care Med* 34:2026–2034, 2008.
15. Kondili E, Prinianakis G, Alexopoulou C, et al: Respiratory load compensation during mechanical ventilation–proportional assist ventilation with load-adjustable gain factors versus pressure support. *Intensive Care Med* 32:692–699, 2006.
16. Piquilloud L, Tassaux D, Bialais E, et al: Neurally adjusted ventilatory assist (NAVA) improves patient-ventilator interaction during non-invasive ventilation delivered by face mask. *Intensive Care Med* 38:1624–1631, 2012.
17. de la Oliva P, Schuffelmann C, Gomez-Zamora A, et al: Asynchrony, neural drive, ventilatory variability and COMFORT: NAVA versus pressure support in pediatric patients. A non-randomized crossover trial. *Intensive Care Med* 38:838–846, 2012.
18. Younes M: Proportional assist ventilation, a new approach to ventilatory support theory. *Am Review Respir Dis* 145:114–120, 1992.
19. Marini JJ, Rodriguez RM, Lamb V: The inspiratory workload of patient-initiated mechanical ventilation. *Am Rev Respir Dis* 134:902–910, 1986.
20. Marini JJ, Capps JS, Culver BH: The inspiratory work of breathing during assisted mechanical ventilation. *Chest* 87:612–618, 1985.
21. McIntyre NR, McConnell R, Cheng KC, et al: Patient-ventilator flow dyssynchrony: flow-limited versus pressure-limited breaths. *Crit Care Med* 25:1671–1677, 1997.
22. Sassoon CSH: Mechanical ventilator design and function: the trigger variable. *Respir Care* 37:1056–1062, 1992.
23. Branson RD: Flow-triggering systems. *Respir Care* 39:138–146, 1994.
24. Holbrook PJ, Guiles SP: Response time of four pressure support ventilators: effect of triggering method and bias flow. *Respir Care* 42:952–960, 1997.
25. Oto J, Chenelle CT, Marchese AD, et al: A comparison of leak compensation in acute care ventilators during noninvasive and invasive ventilation: a lung model study. *Respir Care* 58:2027–2037, 2013.
26. Hill LL, Pearl RG: Flow triggering, pressure triggering and auto triggering during mechanical ventilation. *Crit Care Med* 28:579, 2000.
27. Fabry B, Guttmann J, Eberhard L, et al: An analysis of desynchronization between the spontaneously breathing patient and ventilator during inspiratory pressure support. *Chest* 107:1387–1394, 1995.
28. Liao K-M, Ou C-Y, Chern C-W: Classifying different types of double triggering based on airway pressure and flow deflection in mechanically ventilated patients. *Respir Care* 56:460–466, 2011.
29. Noujeim C, BouAkl I, El-Khatib M, et al: Ventilator auto-cycling from cardiogenic oscillation: case report and review of literature. *Nursing Crit Care* 18:222–228, 2013.
30. Simon PM, Zurob AS, Wies WM, et al: Entrainment of respiration in humans by periodic lung inflations. *Am J Respir Crit Care Med* 160:950–960, 1999.
31. Akoumianaki E, Lyazidi A, Rey N, et al: Mechanical ventilation-induced reverse-triggered breaths. *Chest* 143:927–938, 2013.
32. Tassaux D, Gainnier M, Battisti A, et al: Impact of expiratory trigger setting on delayed cycling and inspiratory muscle workload. *Am J Respir Crit Care Med* 172:1283–1289, 2005.
33. Parthasarathy S, Jubran A, Tobin MJ: Cycling of inspiratory and expiratory muscle groups with the ventilator in airflow limitation. *Am J Respir Crit Care Med* 158:1471–1478, 1998.
34. Achour L, Letellier C, Cuvelier A, et al: Asynchrony and cyclic variability in pressure support noninvasive ventilation. *Computers Biol Med* 37:1308–1320, 2007.
35. Sinderby C, Navalesi P, Beck J, et al: Neural control of mechanical ventilation in respiratory failure. *Nature Med* 5:1433–1436, 1999.
36. Hess DR, Kacmarek RM: *Essentials of mechanical ventilation*, ed 3, New York, 2013, McGraw-Hill.
37. Kacmarek RM, Dimas S, Mack C: *Essentials of respiratory care*, ed 4, St Louis, 2005, Mosby.
38. Fernandez R, Mendez M, Younes M: Effect of ventilator flow rate on respiratory timing in normal humans. *Am J Respir Crit Care Med* 159:710–719, 1999.
39. Williams P, Muelver M, Kratohvil J, et al: Pressure support and pressure assist/control: are there differences? An evaluation of the newest ICU ventilators. *Respir Care* 45:1169–1181, 2000.

40. Bonmarchand G, Chevron V, Menard JF, et al: Effects of pressure ramp slope values on the work of breathing during pressure support ventilation in restrictive patients. *Crit Care Med* 27:715–722, 1999.
41. Branson RD, Campbell RS, Davis K, et al: Altering flow rate during maximum pressure support ventilation (PSVmax): effect on cardiorespiratory function. *Respir Care* 35:1056–1069, 1990.
42. Pepe PE, Marini JJ: Occult positive end-expiratory pressure in mechanically ventilated patients with airflow obstruction: the auto-PEEP effect. *Am Rev Respir Dis* 126:166–170, 1982.
43. Smith TC, Marini JJ: Impact of PEEP on lung mechanics and work of breathing in severe airflow obstruction. *J Appl Phys* 64:1488–1496, 1988.
44. Thille AW, Cabello B, Galia F, et al: Reduction of patient-ventilator asynchrony by reducing tidal volume during pressure-support ventilation. *Intensive Care Med* 34:1477–1486, 2008.
45. Seith J, Siegel MD: Mechanical ventilation in chronic obstructive lung disease. *Clin Chest Med* 21:799–812, 2000.
46. Ranieri VM, Mascia L, Petruzzelli V, et al: Inspiratory effort and measurement of dynamic intrinsic PEEP in COPD patients: effect of ventilator triggering systems. *Intensive Care Med* 21:896–903, 1995.
47. Goulet R, Hess D, Kacmarek RM: Pressure vs. flow triggering during pressure support ventilation. *Chest* 111:1649–1654, 1997.
48. Chanques G, Kress JP, Pohlman A, et al: Impact of ventilator adjustment and sedation—analgesia practices on severe asynchrony in patients ventilated in assist-control mode. *Crit Care Med* 41:2177–2187, 2013.
49. Pohlman MC, McCallister KE, Schweickert WD, et al: Excessive tidal volume from breath spacing during lung-protective ventilation for acute lung injury. *Crit Care Med* 36:3019–3023, 2008.
50. Nilsestuen JO, Hargett KD: Using ventilator graphics to identify patient-ventilator asynchrony. *Respir Care* 50:202–232, 2005.
51. Pierson DJ: Patient-ventilator interaction. *Respir Care* 56:214–228, 2011.
52. Marini JJ, Smith TC, Lamb VJ: External work output and force generation during synchronized intermittent mechanical ventilation. Effect of machine assistance on breathing effort. *Am Review of Respir Dis* 138:1169–1179, 1988.
53. Imsand C, Feihl F, Perret C, et al: Regulation of inspiratory neuromuscular output during synchronized intermittent mechanical ventilation. *Anes* 80:13–22, 1994.
54. Brochard L, Rauss A, Benito S, et al: Comparison of three methods of gradual withdrawal from ventilatory support during weaning from mechanical ventilation. *Am J Respir Crit Care Med* 150:896–903, 1994.
55. Estaban A, Frutos F, Tobin MJ, et al: A comparison of four methods of weaning patients from mechanical ventilation. *N Engl J Med* 332:345–350, 1995.

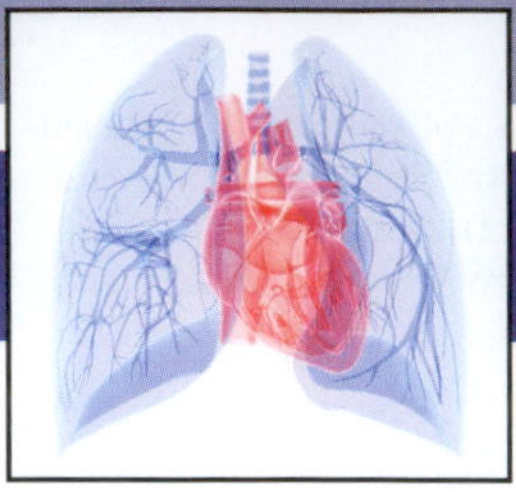

CHAPTER 48

Initiating and Adjusting Invasive Ventilatory Support

ROBERT M. KACMAREK

CHAPTER OBJECTIVES

After reading this chapter you will be able to:

- Discuss the goals of ventilatory support.
- Describe how to choose an appropriate ventilator to begin ventilatory support.
- Explain how to select an appropriate mode of ventilation given a patient's specific condition and ventilatory requirements.
- Choose appropriate initial ventilator settings, based on patient assessment.
- Describe how to assess a patient after initiation of ventilation.
- Discuss how to adjust ventilatory support based on oxygenation and ventilation status.
- Discuss how to ventilate using the concept of lung protective ventilation.
- Explain how to adjust the ventilator on the basis of the patient's response.

CHAPTER OUTLINE

KEY TERMS

assist/control volume ventilation
controlled ventilation
full ventilatory support
high-frequency oscillatory ventilation (HFOV)
lung protective ventilatory strategy
neurally adjusted ventilatory assist (NAVA)
partial ventilatory support
plateau pressure (P_{plat})
pressure-controlled ventilation (PCV)
pressure-regulated volume control (PRVC)
pressure support ventilation (PSV)
proportional assist ventilation (PAV)
synchronized intermittent mandatory ventilation (SIMV)
transpulmonary pressure
volume-controlled ventilation
volume support

Mechanical ventilation entails the use of sophisticated life-support technology aimed at maintaining tissue oxygenation and removal of carbon dioxide (CO_2). At its most basic level, mechanical ventilation supports or replaces the normal ventilatory pump, moving air into and out of the lungs. The primary function of a mechanical ventilator is simply to ventilate. The main indication for mechanical ventilation is inadequate or absent spontaneous breathing.

Mechanical ventilation is not without risk, and the complications and hazards can be life-threatening. The decision to initiate mechanical ventilatory support is a serious one that requires sound clinical judgment and a clear understanding of the various approaches to ventilatory support. This chapter reviews and describes the initial set-up of the ventilator. After ventilator initiation, adjustments in ventilatory support are made on the basis of the patient's response. Techniques for patient stabilization; methods for optimizing oxygenation, ventilation, and acid-base balance; and methods for minimizing harmful side effects are described.

GOALS OF MECHANICAL VENTILATION

The goals of mechanical ventilatory support are to maintain adequate alveolar ventilation and oxygen (O_2) delivery, restore acid-base balance, and reduce the work of breathing (WOB) with minimum harmful side effects and complications.[1] Mechanical ventilation also may reduce increased myocardial work secondary to hypoxemia and an increased WOB.[1] Other physiologic objectives of mechanical ventilatory support include increasing or maintaining lung volume with positive end expiratory pressure (PEEP) and continuous positive airway pressure (CPAP) for promotion, improvement, or maintenance of lung recruitment.[1]

A **lung protective ventilatory strategy** is an approach to mechanical ventilation that includes the use of small tidal volume (V_T) and appropriate levels of PEEP.[2] This approach was first described in patients with acute lung injury (ALI) or the acute respiratory distress syndrome (ARDS). However, the concept of lung protection should be applied to all patients requiring ventilatory support for acute respiratory failure. Lung injury is primarily caused by an elevated transpulmonary pressure during positive pressure ventilation.[3] **Transpulmonary pressure** is the difference between alveolar pressure and pleural pressure. A safe transpulmonary pressure during mechanical ventilation is not firmly established, but most clinicians would agree that the lower the transpulmonary pressure, the less likely the development of ventilator-induced lung injury.[4] On a theoretical basis, Chiumello et al. arguing from the perspective of stress and strain applied to the lungs during ventilatory support, identify 27 cm H_2O as the maximum transpulmonary pressure without increasing the risk of significant lung injury.[4] Thus, most recommend that plateau pressure should be maintained ≤28 cm H_2O. See Chapter 51 for a discussion of esophageal and transpulmonary pressure measurements. High transpulmonary pressures are associated with alveolar overdistention and lung injury.[3]

Plateau pressure (P_{plat}), the end inspiratory equilibration pressure, measures the mean peak alveolar pressure and is the best bedside clinical reflection of transpulmonary pressure.[2,4,5] Although P_{plat} is not an accurate measurement of transpulmonary pressure, the transpulmonary pressure during controlled ventilation never exceeds the P_{plat}.[4] P_{plat} provides an excellent bedside assessment of the level of potentially dangerous ventilating pressure. Limiting P_{plat} reduces the likelihood of ventilator-induced lung injury. Generally, the lower the P_{plat}, the better the patient outcome.[2,5] Ideally, P_{plat} should be less than 28 cm H_2O.[5] However, a P_{plat} greater than 28 cm H_2O may be applied in patients with a decreased thoracic compliance without resulting in overdistention[5] because a decrease in chest wall compliance (obesity, massive fluid resuscitation, abdominal distention, elevated bladder pressure) increases the pleural pressure, decreasing the transpulmonary pressure. Generally, the lowest possible P_{plat} is maintained by selecting a V_T of 4 to 8 ml/kg of ideal body weight (IBW). The higher the P_{plat}, the smaller the V_T should be. Generally, V_T greater than 10 ml/kg IBW is never indicated in critically ill patients.

Lung injury can also be caused by repetitive opening and closing of unstable lung units.[6] The application of an appropriate level of PEEP ensures that unstable lung units are maintained in the open position reducing the likelihood of additional lung injury.

Driving pressure, the difference between the peak airway pressure and PEEP has been recently linked to mortality. It has recently been demonstrated that driving pressures greater than 15 cm H_2O increase mortality.[8] Thus, the keys to lung protection are:

1. Transpulmonary pressure ≤27 cm H_2O; this usually corresponds to a plateau pressure of ≤28 cm H_2O unless there is a decrease in chest wall compliance.
2. A driving pressure of <15 cm H_2O.
3. A tidal volume of 4 to 8 ml/kg of IBW.
4. A PEEP set to avoid derecruitment during exhalation.

Specific clinical objectives of mechanical ventilation include reversal of hypoxemia, hypercapnia, and associated respiratory acidosis and prevention or reversal of ventilatory muscle dysfunction. The general trajectory of pH, PCO_2, and PO_2 during the progression of acute respiratory failure is depicted in Figure 48-1. Mechanical ventilation may be used to allow sedation or paralysis for certain procedures, to decrease myocardial and ventilatory muscle O_2 consumption to maximize O_2 delivery to the tissues, to decrease intracranial pressure acutely in the presence of closed head injury or cerebral edema (by reducing $PaCO_2$ to 25 to 30 mm Hg for a short period and promoting cerebral vasoconstriction), to prevent or reverse atelectasis, and to stabilize the chest wall in the case of a massive flail or chest wall resection. Table 48-1 lists the most common causes of acute respiratory failure leading to ventilatory support in the United States and Canada. Hazards of mechanical ventilation include decreased venous return and cardiac output, patient-ventilatory asynchrony, and ventilatory muscle dysfunction owing to inappropriate ventilator settings, ventilator-associated pneumonia, and ventilator-induced lung injury.[1] Box 48-1 lists the goals of ventilatory support, and Box 48-2 lists specific objectives of mechanical ventilation.

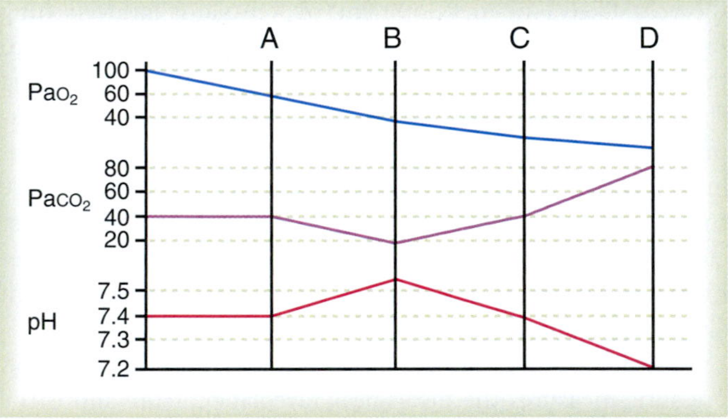

FIGURE 48-1 Typical progression of acute respiratory failure. Initially, there is a decline in arterial O_2 tension and saturation. When PaO_2 decreases to approximately 60 mm Hg *(A)*, the patient begins to breathe more, $PaCO_2$ decreases, and pH increases. Early in the progression, arterial blood gas results show acute alveolar hyperventilation (uncompensated respiratory alkalosis) secondary to hypoxemia. As the patient's condition worsens, increases in ventilatory workload typically lead to the adoption of a rapid, shallow breathing pattern; although minute ventilation may remain high, effective ventilation decreases, $PaCO_2$ begins to increase, and pH begins to decrease *(B)*. At point *C*, arterial blood gas results may show normal $PaCO_2$ and pH with moderate to severe hypoxemia. If mechanical ventilation is not initiated, the patient's condition may progress to acute ventilatory failure, severe hypoxemia, and corresponding severe respiratory acidosis *(D)*.

TABLE 48-1

Most Common Causes of Acute Respiratory Failure Requiring Mechanical Ventilation in the United States and Canada

Condition	Rank	Percentage
Postoperative respiratory failure	1	17
Sepsis	1	17
Other	2	16
Heart failure	3	13
Pneumonia	3	13
Trauma	3	13
ARDS	4	9
Aspiration	5	3

Modified from Esteban A, Anzueto A, Alia I, et al: How is mechanical ventilation employed in the intensive care unit? An international utilization review. Am J Respir Crit Care Med 161:1450, 2000.

Box 48-1 Physiologic Goals of Ventilatory Support

- Support or manipulate gas exchange
- Maintain alveolar ventilation ($PaCO_2$ and pH)
- Maintain arterial oxygenation (PaO_2, SaO_2, SpO_2, CaO_2, and DO_2)
- Increase end expiratory lung volume, functional residual capacity (FRC)
- Reduce or manipulate WOB
- Minimize cardiovascular impairment
- Ensure patient-ventilatory synchrony
- Avoid ventilator-induced lung injury

Box 48-2 Specific Clinical Objectives of Ventilatory Support

- To reverse hypoxemia
- To reverse acute respiratory acidosis
- To prevent or reverse atelectasis
- To reverse ventilatory muscle dysfunction
- To decrease systemic or myocardial O_2 consumption
- To maintain or improve cardiac output
- To reduce intracranial pressure
- To stabilize the chest

VENTILATOR INITIATION

When the decision to begin mechanical ventilatory support is made, one must choose the mode of ventilation, select an appropriate device, and establish the initial ventilator settings. In the selection of initial ventilator settings, the goal is to optimize the patient's oxygenation, ventilation, and acid-base balance, while avoiding harmful side effects. This goal is achieved by choosing an appropriate mode of ventilation, fractional inspired oxygen (FiO_2), V_T (volume ventilation) or pressure level (pressure ventilation), rate, peak flow and flow waveform, inspiratory time, and PEEP level. Appropriate trigger sensitivity, pressure limit, alarms, backup ventilation, and humidification must be selected. After initial ventilator setup, adjustments must be made on the basis of the patient's response and the patient-specific clinical objectives of ventilatory support. Most patients who need mechanical ventilatory support receive invasive positive pressure ventilation; however, an increasing number of patients are being ventilated noninvasively (see Chapter 49). Next, the clinician must choose the mode of ventilation (e.g., volume assist/control [VA/C], pressure assist/control [PA/C], pressure support ventilation [PSV], **pressure-regulated volume control** [PRVC], **volume support**, adaptive support ventilation, **proportional assist ventilation** [PAV], or **neurally adjusted ventilatory assist** [NAVA]) and initial ventilator settings (e.g., rate, V_T or pressure level, FiO_2, PEEP). Finally, the clinician must choose appropriate alarm and apnea settings. Box 48-3 summarizes key decisions that must be made as a part of initial ventilator setup.

Box 48-3 Initial Ventilator Setup

Initial ventilator setup includes the following key decisions:

- Noninvasive vs. invasive ventilation
- Type and method of establishment of an airway
- Partial vs. full ventilatory support
- Choice of ventilator
- Mode of ventilation
- Assist/control ventilation (volume vs. pressure) vs. SIMV (with or without pressure support)
- Pressure support
- Other newer modes and adjuncts to ventilation

Next, the clinician must consider key ventilatory values:

- Trigger method (pressure or flow trigger) and sensitivity
- V_T (volume ventilation) or pressure level (pressure support and PA/C)
- Rate
- Inspiratory flow, inspiratory time, expiratory time, or I:E ratio
- Inspiratory flow waveform
- FiO_2
- PEEP

Last, the clinician must choose appropriate alarm and backup values:

- Low-pressure, low PEEP alarms
- High-pressure limit and alarm
- Volume alarms (low V_T/high V_T, high and low minute ventilation)
- High rate and low rate alarms
- Apnea alarm and apnea ventilation values
- High/low O_2 alarm
- High/low temperature alarm
- I:E ratio limit and alarm

Noninvasive Ventilation

Although more than 75% to 80% of all patients receiving ventilatory assistance receive it invasively, the use of noninvasive ventilation should be considered in select patients requiring ventilatory assistance. Noninvasive ventilation is preferred in some patients because the outcomes are better. Chapter 49 provides details on all aspects on noninvasive ventilation.

Establishment of the Airway

Conventional mechanical ventilatory support requires the establishment of an artificial airway. Initially, nearly 100% of patients receiving positive pressure ventilation are intubated, and of these, 99% have oral endotracheal tubes, and only about 1% are intubated nasally.[7] Approximately 5% to 10% of patients receiving mechanical ventilation have a tracheotomy performed at some point.[7] Airway management is described in detail in Chapter 36.

Pressure-Controlled Versus Volume-Controlled Ventilation

The next decision to be made regarding initiation of mechanical ventilation is whether to use a primarily pressure-targeted or volume-targeted mode of ventilation. Volume-targeted ventilation essentially includes VA/C and synchronized intermittent mandatory ventilation (SIMV). Pressure ventilation includes PA/C, SIMV, PRVC, volume support, and airway pressure release ventilation. In addition, the clinician can select the patient-controlled modes PAV or NAVA. However, most patients are initially ventilated with pressure or volume forms of ventilation. The operational capabilities of these modes are described in detail in Chapter 45, and the indications, benefits, and concerns regarding these modes are discussed in Chapter 46.

Full Ventilatory Support Versus Partial Ventilatory Support

Full ventilatory support can be defined as the application of mechanical support such that all or most of the energy necessary for effective alveolar ventilation is provided by the ventilator.[9] When a ventilator is set to deliver full ventilatory support, the patient is either passive or simply triggers the breath to initiate inspiration allowing the ventilator to perform most of the work of breathing. However, it is very difficult to set the ventilator to assume all of the work of breathing without significantly sedating the patient. In most patient-triggered approaches to ventilatory support, patient-ventilatory synchrony is a major issue, and very careful titration of the ventilator settings is necessary to ensure synchrony and minimize patient WOB. See Chapter 47 for details on patient-ventilatory synchrony.

Partial ventilatory support implies that only a percentage of the WOB is provided by the ventilator.[9] Normally, when partial ventilatory support is indicated, SIMV, PSV, volume support, PAV, and NAVA are the modes of choice. However, as with full ventilatory support, care in setting the ventilator is critical to ensure that patient-ventilator synchrony is maximized. Partial ventilatory support strategies minimize the loss of ventilatory muscle function, require less sedation, assist in recruiting and stabilizing alveolar units, and generally move patients closer to ventilator discontinuance than full ventilatory support approaches.

Choice of a Ventilator

After the decision is made to initiate mechanical ventilator support, the clinician must select an appropriate ventilator. This decision should be guided by considering the features, modes available, pressure and flow capabilities, alarms and monitoring systems included, and reliability. However, the most important feature is the clinician's familiarity with the equipment. Only a ventilator with which the clinician is totally familiar with every feature should ever be used.

INITIAL VENTILATOR SETTINGS

Initial ventilator settings are chosen based on the patient's clinical presentation and the need to provide full or partial ventilator support.

Choice of Mode

Most modern critical care ventilators include VA/C, PA/C, SIMV, and PSV and many of the newer modes of ventilation. However, some modes of ventilation are found only on a specific type of ventilator, such as PAV PB 840 and PB 980 (Covidien-Nellcor, Boulder, Colorado), adaptive support ventilation and Intellivent Hamilton ventilators (Hamilton Medical, Bonaduz, Switzerland), NAVA Servo-i ventilator (Maquet, Inc, Wayne, New Jersey), and SmartCare Draeger ventilators (Draeger Medical, Inc, Telford, Pennsylvania).

Assist/Control Ventilation (Patient-Triggered or Time-Triggered Continuous Mandatory Ventilation)

Assist/control ventilation can be delivered in either pressure-targeted or volume-targeted ventilation. Suggested initial settings for **assist/control volume ventilation** in the care of adults are listed in Box 48-4. Advantages of assist/control volume ventilation include the assurance that a minimum safe level of ventilation is achieved, yet the patient can still set his or her own breathing rate. In the event of sedation or apnea, a minimum safe level of ventilation is guaranteed by the selection of an

MINI CLINI

Selecting Initial Ventilator Settings

PROBLEM: A 52-year-old man, 5 ft 10 in (178 cm) tall and weighing 200 lb (91 kg), is being returned from the operating room after coronary artery bypass surgery. He is being manually (bag-tube) ventilated with supplemental O_2 by the anesthesiologist en route to the ICU. He is apneic at this time. The patient has no history of lung disease and has never smoked cigarettes. Heart rate and blood pressure are stable, and SpO_2 during manual ventilation is 99%. What initial mode, V_T, rate, and FiO_2 should the RT select when starting ventilatory support for this patient?

Solution: The patient is apneic at this time but is likely to resume spontaneous breathing as the anesthetic wears off and sedation is reduced. Because the patient is expected to resume breathing spontaneously, volume ventilation or pressure ventilation in assist/control or SIMV is appropriate.

Initial V_T and rate should be selected to provide full ventilatory support. Generally, initial V_T of approximately 6 to 8 ml/kg IBW or pressure control setting to establish this V_T with a rate of 12 to 20 breaths/min provides an adequate starting minute ventilation for most adult patients. The formulas for estimating IBW are:

$$\text{IBW in kilograms (men)} = [106 + 6(H - 60)]/2.2$$
$$\text{IBW in kilograms (women)} = [105 + 5(H - 60)]/2.2$$

where H is height in inches.

For this patient:

$$\text{IBW} = [106 + 6(70 - 60)]/2.2 = 75.5 \text{ kg}$$

On the basis of IBW of 75.5 kg, initial V_T can be set at about 450 ml. Initial inspiratory flow should be set at 60 L/min with a decreasing ramp flow waveform to achieve an inspiratory time of approximately 0.8 second. Initially, rate can be set at 12/min. Because the patient has a normal respiratory system and it is usual to return from the operating room with a below-normal body temperature, a low initial control rate is indicated. Trigger sensitivity (assist/control or SIMV) should be set so that minimal patient effort triggers the ventilator without autocycling.

Initial FiO_2 should be set at 1.0, but because of the patient's history and the presence of normal lung function, it is expected that it will be reduced rapidly as the patient recovers. Initial PEEP is set at 5 cm H_2O. If the SIMV mode is chosen, PSV should be started at 10 cm H_2O and adjusted as needed when the patient resumes spontaneous breathing.

In summary, appropriate initial ventilator settings for this patient are:

Mode: Assist/control (volume or pressure) or SIMV (volume or pressure) with PSV

V_T: 6 ml/kg, 450 ml

f_{mach}: 12 breaths/min

PSV: 10 cm H_2O (SIMV mode only)

FiO_2: 1.0 followed by immediate assessment and SpO_2 observation with titration downward as indicated

Inspiratory flow and time: 60 L/min, decreasing ramp, inspiratory time approximately 0.8 second

Pressure limit: Adjust to 10 to 15 cm H_2O above PIP after patient connection

Humidification: Heated humidifier to achieve temperature >35° C at the airway or an appropriate HME

Box 48-4 Typical Values for Ventilator Initiation for Adults Receiving Volume or Pressure Assist/Control Ventilation

- Trigger sensitivity: –0.5 to –1.5 cm H_2O or 1 to 2 L/min set to minimize trigger work without autocycling
- V_T: Volume ventilation 6 to 8 ml/kg IBW; pressure ventilation, pressure level to achieve 6 to 8 ml/kg IBW
- Rate: Backup rate of ≥12 to 14 breaths/min if providing assisted ventilation
- Inspiratory flow: Volume ventilation 60 to 80 L/min to achieve inspiratory time of approximately <1 second and I : E ratio of ≤1 : 2; inspiratory flow ≥80 L/min may be required to meet or exceed the patient's spontaneous inspiratory flow demand
- Flow waveform volume ventilation: Decreasing ramp
- Inspiratory time pressure ventilation: <1.0 second
- PEEP: 5 cm H_2O
- Pressure limit: Start at 30 to 40 cm H_2O depending on approach (volume 40 cm H_2O, pressure 30 cm H_2O) and adjust after patient connection to 10 to 15 cm H_2O above PIP
- Humidification: Begin with heated humidifier to provide temperature 35° C at the airway connection or appropriate HME

Box 48-5 Advantages and Disadvantages of Pressure-Controlled Ventilation

ADVANTAGES

- Variable flow results in square pressure waveform and improves gas distribution
- Ensures that P_{plat} cannot exceed set pressure control level
- All alveoli are placed under the same sustained inspiratory pressure, which decreases hyperinflation of more compliant alveoli compared with volume ventilation square wave flow
- Sustained inspiratory pressure may result in more alveolar recruitment
- Improved gas distribution allows for lower V_T
- Lower PIP is achieved compared with that achieved with volume ventilation with a square flow waveform

DISADVANTAGES

- Higher mean airway pressure can decrease venous return and decrease cardiac output if preload is inadequate
- V_T varies depending on lung compliance, resistance, and patient effort
- If V_T or minute ventilation alarms are not set properly, alveolar hypoventilation and acidosis may not be detected

appropriate backup rate, usually approximately 4 to 6 breaths/min less than the patient's assist rate but not less than the rate necessary to provide a minimum safe level of ventilation (e.g., a backup rate of at least 12 to 14 breaths/min).[9]

Because assist/control ventilation usually provides full ventilatory support, it may result in less WOB than partial support modes. However, less WOB should not be assumed just because the patient is in assist/control ventilation. Trigger work may be significant if inappropriate sensitivity settings are selected. In addition, when a breath is triggered, inspiratory muscle activity persists.[10,11] If the inspiratory flow rate during volume ventilation does not meet or exceed the patient's inspiratory demand, or inspiratory time is too lengthy, the patient's WOB may be greater or equaling the work of a spontaneous unassisted breath.[10,11] In pressure ventilation, lengthy inspiratory times, inadequate rise time, and improperly set pressure levels can also cause asynchrony (see Chapter 47).

If properly applied and tolerated by the patient, assist/control ventilation may provide ventilatory muscle rest that allows the ventilatory muscles to recover from ventilatory muscle dysfunction. Disadvantages of assist/control mode include an increase in WOB if not applied properly.[9,12] Assist control also may be poorly tolerated by awake, nonsedated patients. The patient may fight the ventilator, or asynchronous patient-to-ventilator breathing patterns may develop. Because flow is based on patient demand in pressure-targeted ventilation, synchrony is generally better achieved during PA/C than with VA/C ventilation. Advantages and disadvantages of **pressure-controlled ventilation (PCV)** are described in Box 48-5.

Assist/control volume ventilation is the most common ventilator mode used throughout the world as the primary initial mode of ventilatory support.[7,13] Regardless of the indication for ventilatory support or underlying disease, this mode is able when properly adjusted and the patient is properly managed to provide adequate ventilatory support for all indications for ventilatory support.[6,13]

Controlled Ventilation (Time-Triggered Continuous Mandatory Ventilation)

Controlled ventilation, pressure or volume, is achieved using the assist/control mode when the patient is apneic because of a medical condition, anesthesia, or use of sedative drugs and paralytic agents. Ventilators in use today do not prevent a patient with sufficient effort from triggering the ventilator, a situation always to be avoided. Controlled ventilation can be achieved only with pharmacologic agents. Advantages of controlled ventilation include eliminating WOB and complete control over the patient's ventilatory pattern. In cases in which WOB is high, controlled ventilation may allow for ventilatory muscle rest, reduce O_2 consumption of the ventilatory muscles, and "free up" O_2 for delivery to the tissues.[9]

Controlled ventilation is a common initial approach in situations of severe acute respiratory failure, especially if the primary problem is hypoxemia. Figure 48-2 depicts the effects of inspiratory time on V_T during controlled ventilation. Disadvantages of controlled ventilation include the need for sedatives and perhaps paralytic drugs. All patients given paralytic drugs must be sedated adequately because paralysis does not alter the patients' perception of their surroundings. All patients' senses are active; none are affected by paralysis; only voluntary muscles are paralyzed. In addition, in the care of apneic patients, ventilator malfunction or disconnection can lead to death.

Synchronized Intermittent Mandatory Ventilation

Synchronized intermittent mandatory ventilation (SIMV) may be used as a means of providing partial or full ventilatory support.[9] With SIMV, the machine breath may be volume or pressure targeted; in adults, it is typically a volume-targeted

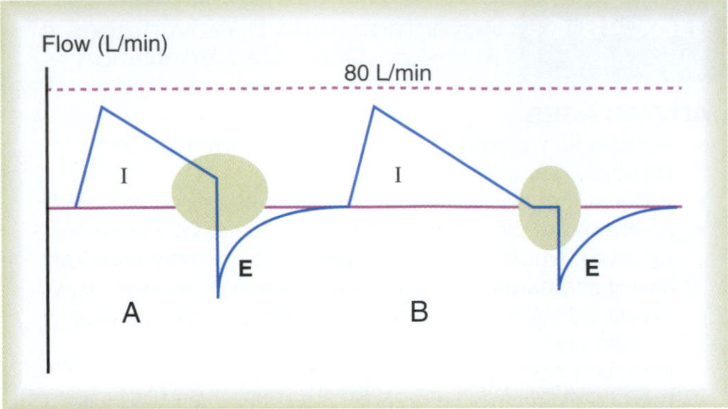

FIGURE 48-2 Flow versus time waveform during PCV. *Curve A* shows a flow pattern during controlled ventilation in which inspiratory time is inadequate to ensure maximum V_T has been delivered. During inspiration, flow does not decrease to zero before exhalation occurs, so the preset pressure has not equilibrated to that in the lung. *Curve B* shows an increase in inspiratory time from *curve A*. Inspiratory flow reaches zero maximizing V_T delivery and allows the preset pressure to equilibrate in the lungs. Exhaled V_T is greater for *curve B* than for *curve A* despite the pressure setting not changing.

TABLE 48-2
Advantages and Disadvantages of Synchronized Intermittent Mandatory Ventilation

Advantages	Disadvantages
Lower mean airway pressure may result than is achieved with assist/control ventilation	SIMV with PSV may increase mean airway pressure
Ventilatory muscle activity, strength, and coordination are maintained	Ventilatory muscle fatigue may occur
Level of support to maintain adequate levels of alveolar ventilation is easy to titrate	Acute hypoventilation may occur, especially with lower machine rates (<8-10 breaths/min)
Weaning protocols are easy to apply	Weaning is prolonged
Spontaneous breathing, which is physiologic, is incorporated	Addition of pressure support often is required to overcome WOB_I
Patients tend not to hyperventilate and may not fight the ventilator, as they may do with assist mode	Patients may have difficulty adjusting to the ventilator; breath stacking is possible with intermittent mandatory ventilation
Sedation or paralysis is not required, as it is in control mode	Patients may experience or continue a rapid, shallow breathing pattern or continue to make spontaneous breathing efforts during delivery of a "machine breath"
Full or partial ventilatory support and level of support can be titrated according to patient's need	Patient's workload increases considerably when SIMV rate decreases to approximately 50% of full ventilatory support value

breath. SIMV often is combined with pressure support to overcome the imposed work of breathing (WOB_I) during spontaneous breathing owing to the artificial airway. SIMV allows the clinician to vary the amount of support provided from minimal to full ventilatory support. Disadvantages of SIMV include possible development of respiratory muscle dysfunction, especially in patients with rapid, shallow spontaneous breathing patterns; acute hypoventilation with use of low rates if patients do not continue to do their share of breathing; and an increase in WOB secondary to lack of ventilatory support during spontaneous breaths unless pressure support is applied.[9] SIMV also delays weaning compared with spontaneous breathing trials or pressure support.[14,15] The advantages and disadvantages of assist/control and SIMV modes are summarized in Table 48-2. Outside of the United States, SIMV is an infrequently used mode of ventilation because of the above-mentioned problems.

Pressure Support Ventilation

Pressure support ventilation (PSV) assumes minimal control over the patient's ventilatory pattern. Specifically, only the level of pressure applied is controlled by the ventilator, and all other aspects of gas delivery are controlled by the patient. However, PSV is very similar to PA/C. The primary difference is that in PSV flow terminates the breath, whereas in PA/C time terminates the breath. Other than this, PA/C has a backup rate, and with pressure support an apnea mode of ventilation is set.[16] PSV can reduce work of breathing and may improve patient-ventilator synchrony by placing more control with the patient.[17] Many clinicians use PSV simply to overcome WOB imposed by the artificial airway.[17] The PSV level needed to overcome WOB_I may be estimated as follows:

$$PSV = \frac{(PIP - P_{plat}) \times \dot{V}_I \text{ spontaneous}}{\dot{V} \text{ ventilator}}$$

where PSV is the pressure support level needed to overcome WOB_I, PIP is the peak inspiratory pressure during a volume-control machine breath, P_{plat} is the plateau pressure after an inspiratory pause (usually >1 second), $\dot{V}_I$ is the patient's spontaneous peak inspiratory flow (L/sec), and $\dot{V}$ ventilator is the ventilator peak inspiratory flow rate (L/sec) with a square wave inspiratory flow waveform. An example of the calculations for PSV needed to overcome WOB_I is presented in Box 48-6.

PSV can and is increasingly being used as a primary mode of ventilation. PSV is essentially the only mode of ventilation used during noninvasive ventilation. It is also an acceptable mode of ventilation for any patients capable of triggering ventilatory support who have an intact ventilatory drive. Many clinicians use this mode in the initial phases of ventilatory support and following the most acute phase of ventilatory failure. The actual PSV level needed is based on the desired V_T. PSV is adjusted to ensure the desired V_T is delivered, and rise time and termination criteria are set to avoid asynchrony. Few clinicians at the present time attempt to calculate PSV level based on the previously listed formula.

High-Frequency Oscillatory Ventilation

High-frequency oscillatory ventilation (HFOV) is the primary approach to high-frequency ventilation used in adults. Respiratory rates range from about 3 Hz (180/min) to about 8 Hz

Box 48-6 Calculation of Pressure Support Ventilation Level Needed to Overcome Imposed Work of Breathing and during Synchronized Intermittent Mandatory Ventilation

- Machine delivered V_T during VA/C: 450 ml
- Machine inspiratory flow rate: 50 L/min (1 L/sec)
- Flow pattern: Square wave
- PIP: 25 cm H_2O
- P_{plat}: 23 cm H_2O
- Patient's spontaneous inspiratory flow rate: 30 L/min (0.5 L/sec)

$$PSV = \frac{(PIP - P_{plat}) \times \dot{V}_1 \text{ spontaneous}}{\text{Ventilator inspiratory flow}}$$
$$= \frac{(40 - 30 \text{ cm } H_2O) \times 0.5 \text{ L/s}}{1 \text{ L/s}}$$
$$= \frac{10 \text{ cm } H_2O \times 0.5 \text{ L/s}}{\text{L/s}} = 5 \text{ cm } H_2O$$

(480/min), and very small V_T, often approaching anatomic dead space, is delivered.[18] Gas transport during HFOV is due to conventional bulk flow, longitudinal (Taylor) dispersion, pendelluft, asymmetric velocity profiles, cardiogenic mixing, or enhanced molecular diffusion.[18] Although high-frequency ventilation has been shown to be safe and effective in maintaining oxygenation and ventilation in various patients,[18-20] HFOV has not been shown to be superior to conventional ventilation. In fact, two recent randomized controlled trials indicate that HFO in adults may negatively affect outcome.[21,22] In one of these trials those ventilated with HFO had a higher mortality than patients managed with conventional ventilation.[21] The primary setting where HFOV has been used is in the treatment of ARDS.

Initial Choice of Mode

Most patients who need mechanical ventilation in the acute care setting initially are managed with volume or pressure ventilation in the assist/control mode or with PSV.[7,13] SIMV may also be used, but it has no advantage over these modes, and it has considerable disadvantages. However, there is no evidence suggesting any of the modes are more beneficial in terms of patient outcomes except that weaning is delayed with SIMV.[14,15] Consequently, the choice of initial ventilator mode is primarily one of clinician preference and patient tolerance. Once the patient is stabilized on a ventilator mode, decisions can be made regarding the use of other, newer modes of ventilation, such as PRVC, volume support, adaptive support ventilation, PAV, or NAVA.

RULE OF THUMB

For most patients, begin mechanical ventilatory support with VA/C, PA/C, or PSV. When the patient is stabilized, other modes of ventilation can be considered.

Tidal Volume and Rate

V_T and machine rate should be chosen concurrently because these are the two major determinants of minute ventilation. Normal spontaneous V_T for unstressed adults is on average 6.3 ml/kg IBW (approximately 5 to 7 ml/kg IBW) with a respiratory rate of 12 to 18 breaths/min establishing a minute ventilation of approximately 100 ml/kg IBW per minute.[23] In the past, the Radford nomogram was used to estimate V_T and rate on the basis of estimated body weight (Figure 48-3). In modern practice, acceptable V_T for mechanical ventilation usually ranges from 4 to 8 ml/kg IBW,[1,5] V_T larger than 8 ml/kg IBW is harmful in patients with ALI/ARDS[2,24,25] and is mostly harmful to any patient in acute respiratory failure regardless of the cause of the failure.

Generally, regardless of mode, an initial V_T of 6 to 8 ml/kg IBW with a rate of 12 to 16 breaths/min is suggested for patients without acute restrictive disease.[5,26] After initiation of ventilation, the P_{plat} can be assessed, and V_T can be adjusted downward, as needed, for maintenance of a P_{plat} less than 28 cm H_2O and driving pressure less than 15 cm H_2O. A smaller initial V_T (4 to 6 ml/kg IBW) is appropriate for patients with ALI/ARDS[2,23,24] and a high P_{plat} and is usually necessary in patients with severe acute asthma. Table 48-3 lists V_T values for men and women according to calculated IBW.

RULE OF THUMB

When starting ventilatory support for most adult patients, use an initial V_T of 6 to 8 ml/kg (IBW) and a respiratory rate of 12 to 16 breaths/min.

V_T times rate (f) determines minute ventilation ($\dot{V}_E$). As a rule, for adult patients, the resultant minute ventilation should be approximately 100 ml/kg IBW per minute.[9] A 70-kg adult (IBW) would have a minute ventilation of approximately 7000 ml/min. Patients with elevated CO_2 production ($\dot{V}CO_2$) or increased physiologic dead space (V_{Dphys}) need a larger minute ventilation to maintain acceptable $PaCO_2$. Minute volume should be increased by increasing the rate, not the V_T.

In SIMV, the total minute ventilation is composed of spontaneous tidal volume (V_{Tsp}), spontaneous rate (f_{sp}), machine tidal volume (V_{Tmach}), and machine rate (f_{mach}). For SIMV, total minute ventilation ($\dot{V}_{E\,TOT}$) is described as follows:

$$\dot{V}_{E\,TOT} = \dot{V}_E \text{ machine} + \dot{V}_E \text{ spontaneous}$$

and

$$\dot{V}_E = (V_{Tmach} \times f_{mach}) + (V_{Tsp\text{-}average} \times f_{sp})$$

For PA/C or PSV, the delivered V_T depends on the pressure limit, the inspiratory time, and the patient's lung mechanics. Generally, the pressure limit is increased or decreased to achieve a target V_T while a P_{plat} of less than 28 cm H_2O and a driving pressure less than 15 cm H_2O is maintained. A good initial pressure setting is to start at 10 cm H_2O (above baseline pressure) and observe the resulting V_T. Pressure is increased or decreased

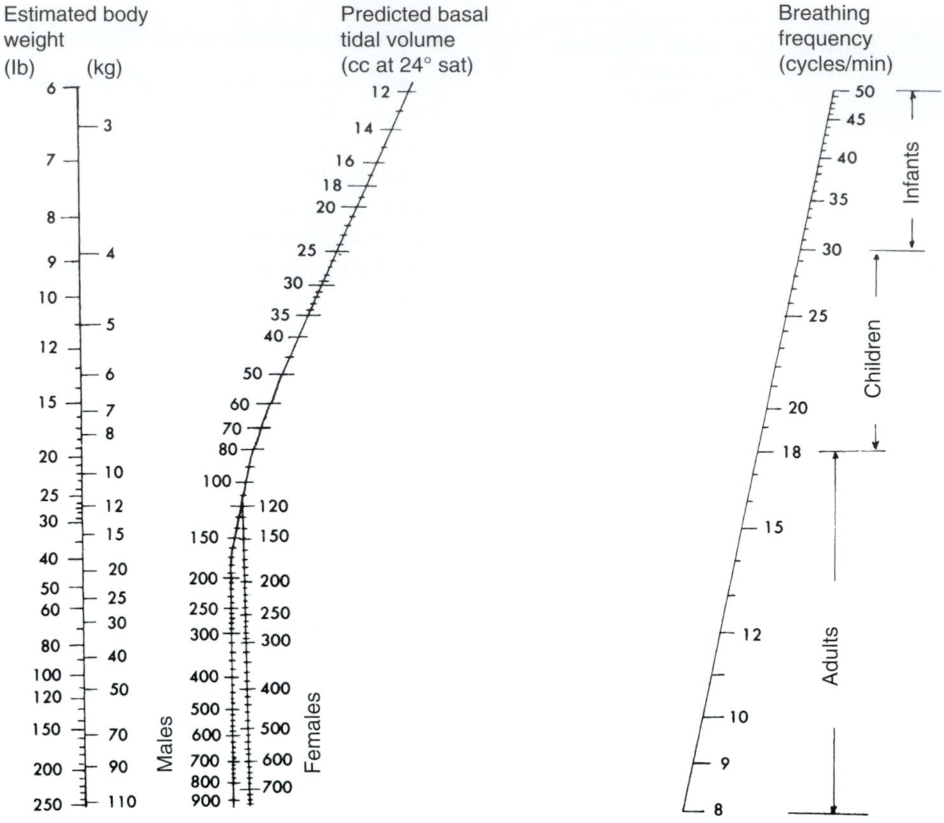

Corrections of predicted basal tidal volumes.
- For patients not in coma: add 10%
- Fever: add 5% for each °F above 99 (rectal)
  add 9% for each °C above 37 (rectal)
- Altitude: add 5% for each 2000 feet above sea level
  add 8% for each 1000 meters above sea level
- Intubation: subtract volume equal to one-half body weight in pounds
  subtract 1 cc/kg of body weight
- Dead space: add equipment dead space

FIGURE 48-3 Radford nomogram. Although first published in 1955, normal resting V_T can still be accurately predicted using this nomogram. (Modified from Radford EP Jr: Ventilation standards for use in artificial respiration. J Appl Physiol 7:451–460, 1955.)

to achieve the desired volume. As with VA/C, minute ventilation with PA/C is simply rate multiplied by V_T ($\dot{V}_E = f \times V_T$). Recommended initial V_T and frequency for various patient types are described in Table 48-4.

Patients with ALI/ARDS may need lower V_T to avoid further lung injury and a higher rate to maintain effective alveolar ventilation while P_{plat} is maintained less than 28 cm H_2O and driving pressure less than 15 cm H_2O. Results of multicenter studies suggest V_T of 4 to 8 ml/kg IBW for patients with ARDS.[2,23,24] Machine rates of 25 to 35 breaths/min may be needed in patients with ALI/ARDS to maintain adequate minute ventilation. Box 48-7 summarizes the ARDS Clinical Network guidelines for initial ventilator setup.[2]

Trigger Sensitivity

Trigger sensitivity should be set at the most sensitive level avoiding autotriggering to minimize trigger work and missed triggering. With flow triggering, the trigger should be set at 1 to 2 L/min, and with pressure triggering, the range is generally −0.5 to −1.5 cm H_2O. However, because of pin holes in disposable ventilator circuits, the sensitivity may need to be adjusted to 3 or 4 L/min or −2 cm H_2O to avoid autotriggering. The increased use of ventilator graphics packages has led to the recognition that patients' inspiratory efforts often are insufficient to trigger the ventilator.[9] Factors that can prolong ventilator response time include large V_T, low trigger sensitivity, auto-PEEP, high bias circuit flow, and abdominal paradox (Box 48-8) (see Chapter 47).

Many ventilators offer the option of a pressure or a flow trigger. With older generation intensive care unit (ICU) ventilators, flow triggering offered slightly lower trigger work than pressure triggering,[27-29] although the gain in terms of the patient's total WOB was slight. Newer ventilators with fast pressure-triggering capabilities are as sensitive as flow-triggered

TABLE 48-3
Tidal Volume Based on Ideal Body Weight*

Height (in)	Height (ft)	Weight (lb)	Weight (kg)	6 ml/kg	8 ml/kg	10 ml/kg	12 ml/kg
Men							
58	4′10″	94	43	260	340	430	520
59	4′11″	100	45	270	360	450	540
60	5′0″	106	48	290	380	480	580
61	5′1″	112	51	310	410	510	610
62	5′2″	118	54	320	430	540	650
63	5′3″	124	56	340	450	560	670
64	5′4″	130	59	350	470	590	710
65	5′5″	136	62	370	500	620	740
66	5′6″	142	65	390	520	650	780
67	5′7″	148	67	400	540	670	800
68	5′8″	154	70	420	560	700	840
69	5′9″	160	73	440	580	730	880
70	5′10″	166	75	450	600	750	900
71	5′11″	172	78	470	620	780	940
72	6′0″	178	81	490	650	810	970
73	6′1″	184	84	500	670	840	1010
74	6′2″	190	86	520	690	860	1030
75	6′3″	196	89	530	700	890	1070
76	6′4″	202	92	550	740	920	1100
77	6′5″	208	95	570	760	950	1140
Women							
55	4′7″	80	36	220	290	360	430
56	4′8″	85	39	230	310	390	470
57	4′9″	90	41	250	330	410	500
58	4′10″	95	43	260	340	430	520
59	4′11″	100	45	270	360	450	540
60	5′0″	105	48	290	380	480	580
61	5′1″	110	50	300	400	500	600
62	5′2″	115	52	310	416	520	620
63	5′3″	120	55	330	440	550	660
64	5′4″	125	57	340	460	570	680
65	5′5″	130	59	350	470	590	710
66	5′6″	135	61	370	490	610	730
67	5′7″	140	64	380	510	640	770
68	5′8″	145	66	400	530	660	790
69	5′9″	150	68	410	540	680	820
70	5′10″	155	70	420	560	700	840
71	5′11″	160	73	440	580	730	876
72	6′0″	165	75	450	600	750	900

*Ideal body weight (lb): Men, 106 + [6(H – 60)]; women, 105 + [5(H – 60)], where H is height in inches.

devices.[30,31] However, no triggering mechanism can reduce the WOB that is a result of auto-PEEP. Auto-PEEP must be addressed by other means (see Chapter 47). Flow-trigger settings vary by ventilator. Generally, for flow triggering, the trigger flow should be set 1 to 2 L/min below baseline or bias flow.

Inspiratory Flow, Time, and Inspiratory-to-Expiratory Ratio for Volume Ventilation

Most modern critical care ventilators allow the clinician to select peak flow, V_T, and rate *or* inspiratory time (or percentage inspiratory time, V_T, and rate). For most adults, an initial inspiratory time of approximately 0.8 second (range 0.6 to 1.0 second) with a resultant inspiratory-to-expiratory (I:E) ratio of 1:2 or lower is a good starting point. This value corresponds to an initial peak flow setting of approximately 60 L/min (range 40 to 80 L/min) and a down ramp or square flow waveform. Higher flow (≤100 L/min) may improve gas exchange in patients with chronic obstructive pulmonary disease (COPD).[10]

Inspiratory flow rate should be adjusted to ensure that the flow provided meets or exceeds the patient's spontaneous inspiratory flow[1] (see Chapter 47). A less sensitive trigger level and lower ventilator inspiratory flow tend to increase the patient's WOB. Common ventilator configurations and related controls that determine inspiratory flow, time, and I:E ratio are described in Figure 48-4.

For ventilators with V_T, peak flow, and rate controls, inspiratory time is determined by V_T, peak flow, and flow pattern. To

Box 48-7 Initial Ventilator Setup and Management of Oxygenation, Plateau Pressure, and pH

1. Calculate predicted (ideal) body weight as follows:
   - Men: Weight in kilograms = 50 + 2.3 (height in inches – 60)
   - Women: Weight in kilograms = 45.5 + 2.3 (height in inches – 60)
2. Select assist/control mode.
3. Set V_T to 8 ml/kg of predicted body weight.
4. Reduce V_T by 1 ml/kg at intervals of ≤2 hours until V_T is 6 ml/kg.
5. Set initial rate to achieve baseline minute ventilation ($\dot{V}_E$). Rate only limited by the development of auto-PEEP.
6. Adjust V_T and rate to achieve pH of 7.30 to 7.45 while maintaining P_{plat} of ≤28 cm H_2O.
7. Set inspiratory flow rate above patient demand (may be >80 L/min).
8. For oxygenation to achieve PaO_2 of 55 to 80 mm Hg or SpO_2 88% to 95%, use the following incremental FiO_2/PEEP combinations. Higher PEEP options (lower row) decrease FiO_2 and may be preferred in patients with high FiO_2 who can tolerate higher PEEP (stable blood pressure, no barotrauma). Survival is similar with both PEEP approaches.

FiO_2	0.3	0.4	0.4	0.5	0.5	0.6	0.7	0.7
Low PEEP	5	5	8	8	10	10	10	12
High PEEP	12-14	14	16	16	18-20	20	20	20
FiO_2	0.7	0.8	0.9	0.9	0.9	1.0	1.0	1.0
Low PEEP	14	14	14	16	18	20	22	24
High PEEP	20	20-22	22	22	22	22	22	24

9. Check P_{plat}, SpO_2, respiratory rate, V_T, and pH (if available) at least every 4 hours and after each change in PEEP or V_T:
   - If P_{plat} is >28 cm H_2O, decrease V_T by 1-ml/kg steps (minimum 4 ml/kg)
   - If P_{plat} is <25 cm H_2O and V_T is <6 ml/kg, increase V_T by 1-ml/kg steps until P_{plat} is >25 cm H_2O or V_T is 6 ml/kg
   - If P_{plat} is <20 and breath stacking occurs, V_T may be increased in 1-ml/kg increments (maximum 8 ml/kg)
10. The pH goal is 7.30 to 7.45.
    For acidosis management (pH < 7.30):
    - If pH is 7.15 to 7.30, increase the rate until pH is >7.30 or $PaCO_2$ is <25 mm Hg; if rate is 35 and $PaCO_2$ is <25 mm Hg, $NaHCO_3$ may be given
    - If pH is <7.15, increase rate to 35; if pH remains <7.15 and $NaHCO_3$ is considered, V_T may be increased in 1-ml/kg steps until pH is >7.15 (P_{plat} target may be exceeded)

    For alkalosis management (pH > 7.45), decrease ventilator rate, if possible.

Adapted from National Institutes of Health (NIH) National Heart Lung and Blood Institute (NHLBI) ARDS Clinical Network Mechanical Ventilation Protocol Summary (Mechanical Ventilation Protocol Summary, revised 25 January 2005).

Box 48-8 Factors That Can Prolong Ventilator Response Time

- Low trigger sensitivity
- Large V_T (causing air trapping)
- Abdomen–rib cage paradox
- Auto-PEEP (dynamic hyperinflation)
- High tubing compliance
- High circuit dead space
- High bias flow in the circuit
- Mechanical malfunction

TABLE 48-4
Suggested Initial Tidal Volume and Frequency for Mechanical Ventilation Based on Disease State or Condition

Patient Type	Tidal Volume (ml/kg)	Frequency (breaths/min)
Adults		
Normal lungs	6-8	12-16
Neuromuscular disease, postoperative period, or with normal pulmonary mechanics in which maintaining lung volume is a concern	6-8	12-16
Acute restrictive disease, ALI/ARDS	4-8*	20-35
Obstructive lung disease (COPD)	6-8	10-12†
Acute severe asthma exacerbation	4-6	10-12
Children		
Age 8-16 yr	6-8	20-30
Age 0-8 yr	6-8	25-35

*For ALI/ARDS, maintain P_{plat} at <28 cm H_2O. V_T begins at 8 ml/kg and is gradually reduced to 6 ml/kg. V_T of 4 ml/kg may be required in the care of these patients to avoid ventilator-induced lung injury.

†For patients with obstructive disease, ensure a short inspiratory time and long expiratory time to avoid air trapping and minimize auto-PEEP. Lower V_T and rate may be necessary in acute asthma to avoid further lung overinflation.

decrease inspiratory time, one may increase peak flow, decrease V_T, or change from a down ramp to a square wave flow pattern. Expiratory time and I:E ratio are determined by inspiratory time and rate. To increase expiratory time (and decrease I:E ratio), one may decrease the inspiratory time as described earlier or increase the expiratory time by decreasing the rate.[1]

For ventilators with V_T (or minute ventilation), percentage inspiratory time, and rate controls, the inspiratory time and V_T determine the inspiratory flow rate. On these ventilators, one can directly increase or decrease the percentage inspiratory time. At the same rate, as inspiratory time (or percentage inspiratory time) decreases, expiratory time and inspiratory flow rate increase, and I:E ratio decreases. An increase in V_T at the same percentage inspiratory time and rate also increases inspiratory flow rate with no change in I:E ratio. Box 48-9 shows

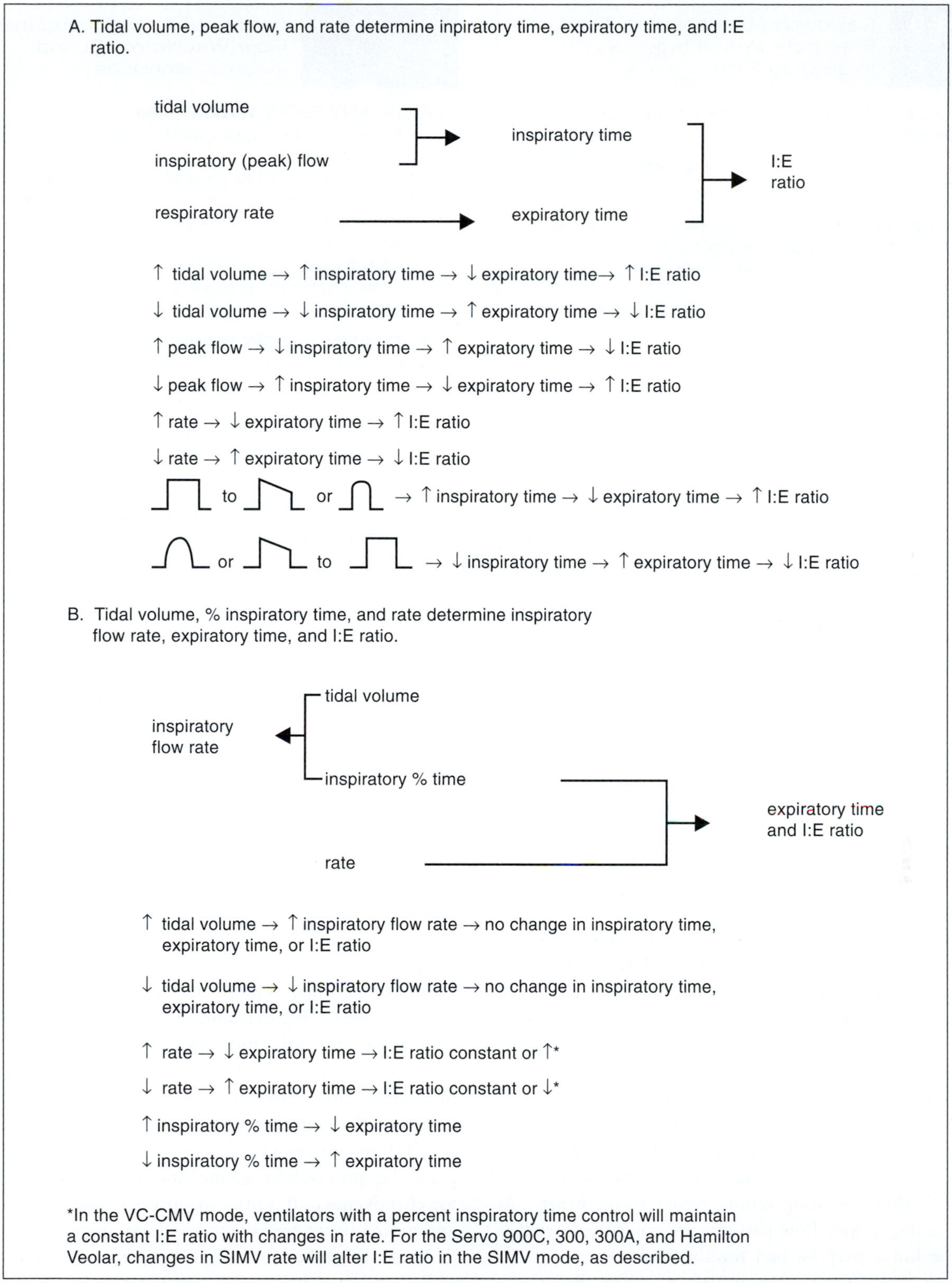

FIGURE 48-4 Relationship between V_T, inspiratory flow, inspiratory time, expiratory time, and I:E ratio in various ventilator systems. *A,* Effects of V_T, flow, and respiratory rate on inspiratory time, expiratory time, and I:E ratio. Some ventilators provide V_T, inspiratory flow, and rate control in volume control (VC) and SIMV modes. *B,* Effects of volume, inspiratory time, and rate on inspiratory flow, expiratory time, and I:E ratio. Other ventilators provide controls for inspiratory time (or percentage inspiratory time), V_T (or minute ventilation), and rate in the VC and SIMV modes. In the VC mode (controlled ventilation), ventilators with a percentage inspiratory time control maintain a constant I:E ratio with changes in respiratory rate. In the SIMV mode, changes in SIMV rate alter I:E ratio on these machines.

Box 48-9 Calculation of Inspiratory Flow Rate from Percentage Inspiratory Time

The effect of percentage inspiratory time on inspiratory flow rate can be estimated as follows:

$$\text{Inspiratory flow rate} = \frac{\text{Set minute ventilation}}{\text{Percentage inspiratory time} \times 0.01}$$

For example, a patient being treated with a Servo ventilator may have the following ventilator settings:

- Set minute ventilation = 12 L/min
- Set CMV rate = 20 breaths/min
- Resulting V_T = 12 L/20 breaths/min = 0.6 L or 600 ml
- Set time inspiratory percentage = 25%
- Set pause time percentage = 0%

$$\text{Inspiratory flow rate} = \frac{12\ \text{L/min}}{25\% \times 0.01} = \frac{12\ \text{L/min}}{0.25} = 48\ \text{L/min}$$

CMV, Continuous mechanical ventilation.

Box 48-10 Guidelines for Selecting Inspiratory Flow Waveforms During Volume Ventilation

CONSTANT FLOW WAVEFORM

- Alternative terms: Square wave, rectangular wave, constant flow generator
- Advantages: High flow provided with a reduced inspiratory time and improved I:E ratio; may decrease mean airway pressure, which may be helpful in terms of venous return and cardiac output in compromised patients
- Disadvantages: Increased PIP may lead to excessive pressure; lower mean airway pressure may affect oxygenation

DECREASING FLOW WAVEFORM

- Alternative terms: Down ramp, decelerating flow, descending ramp
- Advantages: Lower PIP and higher mean airway pressure; this flow waveform may improve gas distribution, oxygenation, and patient-ventilator synchrony
- Disadvantages: Increased mean airway pressure may impede venous return and cardiac output in compromised patients; in ventilators that have a peak flow control, the down ramp increases inspiratory time and I:E ratio and decreases expiratory time

the calculation of inspiratory flow rate based on percentage inspiratory time settings. To alter I:E ratio on these ventilators, one simply adjusts inspiratory percent time. Decreasing rate at the same inspiratory percent time setting does not affect I:E ratio, and both inspiratory time and expiratory time increase owing to a longer respiratory cycle. Changing the inspiratory flow waveform on these ventilators has no effect on inspiratory time, expiratory time, or I:E ratio; however, flow waveform changes affect peak and mean airway pressure.

Flow Waveform

Flow waveform options on mechanical ventilators vary from a preset square wave to seven adjustable waveforms on older ventilators. Common choices available on current generation ventilators for waveform are square or down ramp (decreasing or "decelerating" waveform). Pressure support and pressure-controlled modes also deliver decreasing flow waveforms, but the decrease is patient-specific and not programmed into the gas delivery. The literature on clinical application of specific waveforms is mixed.[32] However, as one moves from an increasing ("accelerating") flow waveform to a square wave to a decreasing flow waveform, while holding inspiratory time constant, there tends to be a predictable decrease in peak airway pressure and a corresponding increase in mean airway pressure.[32] Increases in mean airway pressure may improve oxygenation, while further impeding venous return to the heart.[32] At least as far as inspiratory flow patterns are concerned, what is good for the lungs may be bad for the heart. We suggest a decreasing, or down ramp, flow waveform when the goal is optimization of the distribution of inspired air and improvement in oxygenation. A square waveform may be useful in reducing mean airway pressure in patients with severe hypotension or cardiovascular instability. Figure 48-5 compares the effect of ventilator flow waveforms on peak and mean airway pressure. Box 48-10 describes guidelines for selecting flow waveform during volume ventilation.

During PCV or PSV, a decreasing flow waveform is delivered. The initial peak flow typically is reached rapidly. Flow decreases throughout inspiration until the breath is terminated. With PSV, inspiration ends when the flow decreases to a preset value, typically adjustable from 5% to 85% of the peak flow in some newer ventilators. With PCV, flow continues to decrease until the inspiratory time has elapsed. In the PCV mode, increasing inspiratory time tends to increase V_T until zero flow is reached at end inspiration. Further increases in inspiratory time do not increase V_T, although distribution of inspired air may improve, and mean airway pressure does increase.

Inspiratory Pause

In addition to inspiratory time or flow, most ventilators have an option for setting an inspiratory pause or hold in the volume-control mode. A brief inspiratory pause (up to 10%) has been recommended in the past for improving the distribution of the inspired air and PaO_2.[33] Use of an inspiratory pause has been suggested for administration of bronchodilators to improve medication delivery. However, in COPD patients, an inspiratory pause did not result in significant improvement in bronchodilator effectiveness.[9] If a brief inspiratory pause is used, I:E ratio and mean airway pressure increase. An inspiratory pause of 0.5 to 2 seconds applied for a single breath is used for measurement of P_{plat} and in estimation of airway resistance (Raw):

$$\text{Raw} = \text{PIP} - P_{plat}/\text{Inspiratory flow (L/sec)}$$

where PIP is peak inspiratory pressure. An inspiratory pause should never be set in a spontaneously breathing patient except for a single breath in attempts to measure P_{plat} because it increases the level of asynchrony causing the patient to fight the pause and to try to exhale during the pause.

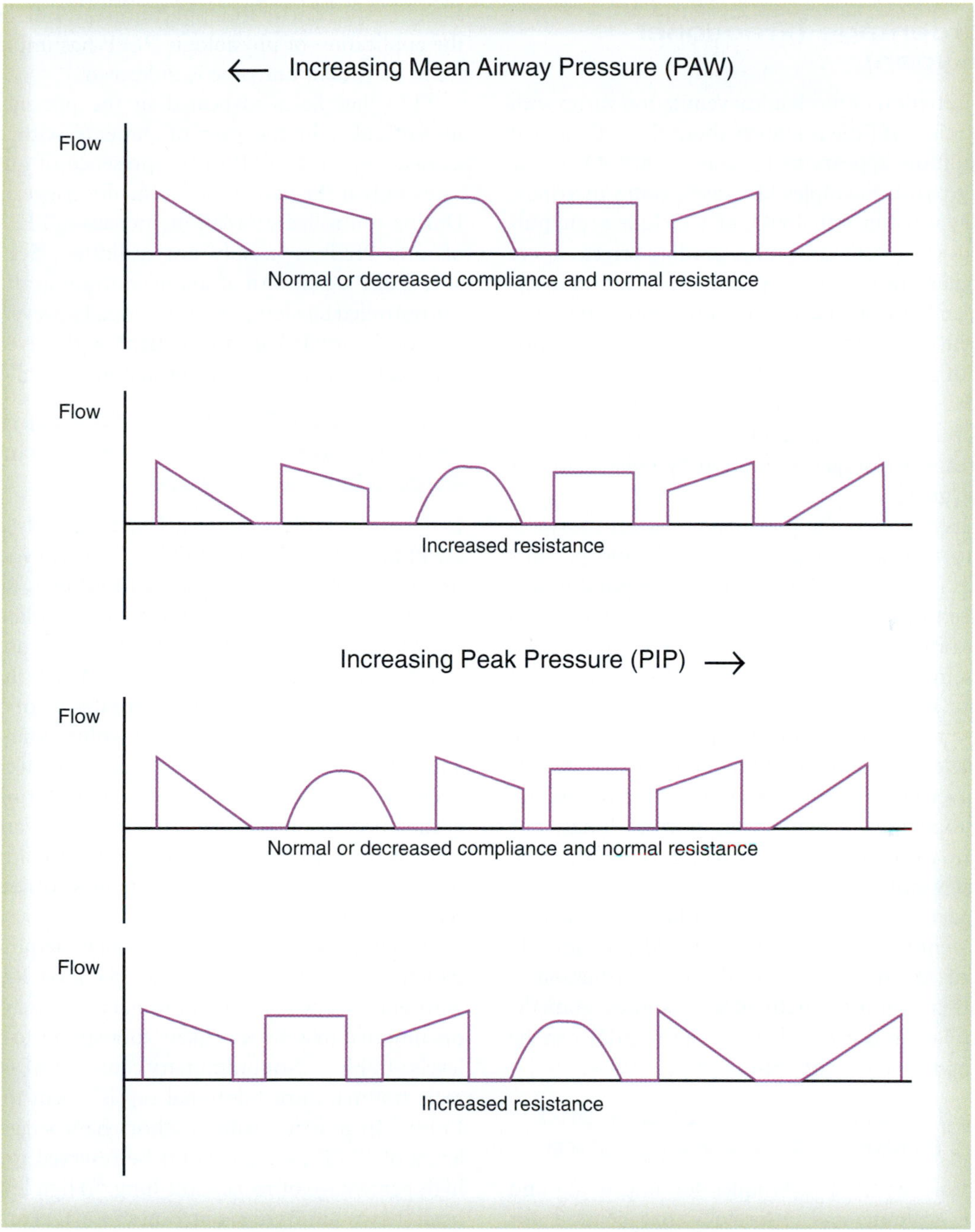

FIGURE 48-5 Effect of ventilator flow waveform on peak and mean airway pressure with changing lung mechanics. Generally, flow waveforms that tend to increase mean airway pressure also decrease peak pressure (PIP) and vice versa. Consequently, if increasing mean airway pressure is the goal, decelerating (down ramp) flow waveforms may be helpful. However, in the care of patients with cardiovascular compromise, in whom reducing mean airway pressure may be helpful, a square wave may be valuable. Accelerating flow waveforms are no longer available on newer critical care ventilators. (Modified from Rau JL, Shelledy DC: The effect of varying inspiratory flow waveforms on peak and mean airway pressures with a time-cycled volume ventilator: a bench study. Respir Care 36:347, 1991.)

An inspiratory pause can also be used to ensure a full inspiration before a chest radiograph is obtained, and this step may improve the quality of the resulting radiograph.[34] Use of an extended inspiratory pause should be limited because of the resultant increase in mean airway pressure and risk of impeding venous return and cardiac output, especially in patients who are hypovolemic or hypotensive or whose condition is hemodynamically unstable.

RULE OF THUMB

An end inspiratory pause should be used only to estimate the end inspiratory P_{plat}. It should never be applied continuously to a patient actively triggering the ventilator.

Oxygen Percentage (Fractional Inspired Oxygen)

FiO_2 selected on initiation of mechanical ventilation varies with the patient's condition. If little is known about the patient or if the patient's condition appears to be grave, 100% O_2 is the preferred starting point. Examples of disease states or conditions that typically warrant initial FiO_2 of 1 include acute pulmonary edema, ARDS, near drowning, cardiac arrest, severe trauma, suspected aspiration, severe pneumonia, carbon monoxide poisoning, and any disease state or condition resulting in a large right-to-left shunt. After initiation of mechanical ventilation with FiO_2 of 1, the FiO_2 should be reduced as soon as is practical to avoid O_2 toxicity and absorption atelectasis. In most patients, FiO_2 should always be adjusted to ensure PaO_2 of 60 mm Hg or greater or oxygen saturation by pulse oximeter (SpO_2) of 90% or greater.

Patients who have undergone previous blood gas measurement or oximetry who are doing well clinically and patients with disease states or conditions that normally respond to low to moderate concentrations of O_2 may begin ventilation with a lower O_2 concentration (50% to 70% O_2). These typically are patients with normal ventilation/perfusion ($\dot{V}/\dot{Q}$) or a $\dot{V}/\dot{Q}$ imbalance without shunt ($\dot{V}/\dot{Q}$ <1 but >0). Patients who often do well with low to moderate concentrations of O_2 include patients with acute exacerbation of COPD, emphysema, chronic bronchitis, drug overdose without aspiration, or neuromuscular disease and postoperative patients with normal lungs. For example, a patient with an acute exacerbation of COPD who needs mechanical ventilatory support may have had PaO_2 of 50 mm Hg with a nasal cannula at 4 L/min before intubation and mechanical ventilation. This patient would probably do well with FiO_2 of about 0.50 when adequate ventilation is restored. The patient can begin with 50% O_2 and be immediately assessed for assurance of adequate SpO_2. FiO_2 can be adjusted according to the patient's response.

Positive End Expiratory Pressure and Continuous Positive Airway Pressure

PEEP and CPAP are effective techniques for improving and maintaining lung volume and improving oxygenation for patients with acute restrictive disease such as pneumonia, pulmonary edema, and ARDS.[1,9] PEEP and CPAP should be cautiously applied in the treatment of patients with an already elevated FRC, such as patients with COPD or acute asthma, except at levels that are applied to offset auto-PEEP and air trapping.[9] Generally, the indication for PEEP or CPAP is inadequate arterial O_2 with moderate to high concentrations of O_2 caused by unstable lung units that are collapsed. PaO_2 less than 50 to 60 mm Hg with FiO_2 greater than 0.40 is a good general starting place for considering use of PEEP or CPAP.

In terms of ventilator initiation, initial PEEP or CPAP levels usually are 5 cm H_2O even in the absence of unstable lung units or auto-PEEP. Most experts advocate for the use of 5 cm H_2O "physiologic" PEEP for all patients who have an artificial airway in place. Intubation results in small reductions in FRC,[1,9] which can be balanced with the application of PEEP or CPAP. Whether the application of physiologic PEEP has important benefits in terms of patient outcome is unknown.

PEEP has been advocated in the presence of auto-PEEP, in particular, in the care of patients with obstructive lung disease.[35] Applied PEEP in the presence of auto-PEEP is indicated only if the patient has difficulty triggering the ventilator. During controlled ventilation, increasing PEEP in the presence of auto-PEEP is usually not indicated. See Chapter 47 for auto-PEEP details. An absolute contraindication to PEEP is an uncontrolled tension pneumothorax. However, PEEP should be cautiously applied in any patient with severe intrinsic lung disease, hypotension, and elevated intracranial pressure.

Open Lung Strategy, Recruitment Maneuvers, and Positive End Expiratory Pressure

In the care of patients with ARDS, it is usually necessary to initiate PEEP at 10 to 15 cm H_2O.[24,25,36,37] However, many clinicians use the ARDS Clinical Network PEEP/FiO_2 tables to set PEEP initially during the establishment of ventilatory support (see Box 48-7). When patients are stabilized, the use of an open lung ventilation strategy in early-stage ARDS has been recommended.[1,5] Such a strategy incorporates V_T of 4 to 8 ml/kg IBW with either pressure-targeted or volume-targeted ventilation and a PEEP level set after a lung recruitment maneuver using a decremental PEEP trial.[1,5,38] The lung recruitment maneuver is intended to open collapsed lung units, and the setting of PEEP using a decremental PEEP trial is intended to apply PEEP based on the patient's lung mechanics to keep the lung units recruited open.

Although all patients with ARDS require PEEP, not all patients with ARDS respond to low-level PEEP, and patients with pulmonary (vs. nonpulmonary) causes of ARDS, such as pneumonia, may be less likely to respond to low to moderate levels of PEEP.[12] Nonpulmonary causes of ARDS (e.g., extrathoracic trauma, intraabdominal sepsis) seem to respond well to PEEP.[12] In practice, some authors have suggested that higher levels of PEEP (>15 cm H_2O) be reserved for patients with a high percentage of recruitable lung.[39] High levels of PEEP have been shown to improve outcomes in ARDS in patients with the most severe forms of ARDS (PaO_2/FiO_2 < 150 mm Hg).[40,41] (See later section on the performance of recruitment maneuvers and the setting of PEEP by decremental trial.)

Pressure Rise Time or Slope

Most newer critical care ventilators include an inspiratory pressure rise time or pressure slope. This control functions only with pressure-limited breaths (PSV, PCV, PRVC, volume support, airway pressure release ventilation, pressure SIMV). The purpose of this control is to adjust the rate at which flow increases from baseline to peak.[42-44] See Chapter 47 for details.

Limits and Alarms

Ventilator alarms and limits warn of ventilator malfunction and changes in patient status. Ventilator malfunction alarms include power or gas supply loss and electronic or pneumatic malfunction. These alarms usually are preset by the manufacturer.

Patient status alarms usually are set by the respiratory therapist (RT). These include maximum inspiratory pressure, low-pressure and low-PEEP alarms, high-volume and low-volume and rate alarms, O_2 and humidification alarms, and apnea alarms. After initiation of ventilation, alarms and limits are readjusted as needed. Alarms usually are set so that they warn the clinician of important changes or problems. Without proper setting, these alarms can become a nuisance by falsely signaling problems that are not real.[9]

In volume ventilation, a pressure limit should be set. Generally, before the patient is connected to the ventilator, the limit should be set at 40 cm H_2O to avoid overpressuring the system when the patient is connected. After the patient is connected to the ventilator, the peak and plateau pressures should be assessed. If P_{plat} is greater than 30 cm H_2O, consideration should be given to decreasing the set V_T. If P_{plat} is less than 30 cm H_2O, the high pressure limit can be adjusted to 10 to 15 cm H_2O above PIP. One can decrease peak pressure by decreasing the peak flow rate, increasing the inspiratory time, changing the inspiratory flow waveform from a square to a down ramp, or decreasing the delivered V_T. For spontaneously breathing patients, inspiratory flow and time must meet or exceed the patient's inspiratory demand to ensure one does not increase the patient's WOB further (see Chapter 47 for details). Preset or adjustable alarms common to most ventilators include pressure (high-low), volume (high-low V_T, minute ventilation), apnea, O_2 percentage, and temperature. Suggested initial settings for these alarms and backup ventilator settings are presented in Table 48-5.

Humidification

Humidification is required during both invasive and noninvasive mechanical ventilation. A heated humidifier or a heat and moisture exchanger (HME) should provide a minimum of 30 mg/L of water with a temperature of 30° C or greater.[45] Use of HMEs should be avoided in the care of patients with secretion problems and patients with low body temperature (<32° C), high spontaneous minute ventilation (>10 L/min), or air leaks in which exhaled V_T is less than 70% of delivered V_T.[45] Heated humidifiers may be used to deliver 100% body humidity at 37° C. Current clinical practice guidelines suggest an inspired gas temperature of 35° C ± 2° C.[45] We prefer an optimal humidity approach and use of a heated humidifier to deliver gas in the range of 35° C to 37° C at the airway in most intubated patients and at a temperature consistent with patient comfort during noninvasive ventilation. However, in patients without primary pulmonary dysfunction and short-term ventilation, HMEs are very useful; generally, these are postoperative patients after elective surgery, patients in the emergency department, and patients recovering from an overdose.

TABLE 48-5

Alarm and Backup Ventilation Setting of Initial Ventilatory Setup (Adults)

Low pressure	5-10 cm H_2O below PIP
Low PEEP/CPAP	3-5 cm H_2O below PEEP
High pressure limit	50 cm H_2O, which is adjusted to 10-15 cm H_2O above PIP
Low exhaled V_T	100 ml or 50% below set V_T
Low exhaled minute ventilation	2-5 L/min or 50% below minimum SIMV or assist/control backup minute ventilation
High minute ventilation	50% above baseline minute ventilation
O_2 percentage (FiO_2)	5% above and below set O_2 percentage
Temperature	2° C above and below set temperature, high temperature not to exceed 37° C
Apnea delay	20 sec
Apnea values	V_T and rate set to achieve full ventilatory support (V_T 8-10 ml/kg; rate 10-12 breaths/min) with 100% O_2

Periodic Sighs

Constant, monotonous tidal ventilation at a small volume (<7 ml/kg) may result in progressive atelectasis.[9,46] Periodic deep breaths or sighs taken every 6 to 10 minutes reverse this trend.[9,46] During the 1960s and 1970s, it was common to ventilate patients with a smaller V_T (5 to 7 ml/kg) and no PEEP. As a result, an intermittent sigh function was incorporated into most volume ventilators. Sighs were programmed at 1½ to 2 times the set V_T at an interval of every 6 to 10 minutes. Sometimes multiple sighs were included at a preset interval of up to 10 times per hour. Because of the use of PEEP, sighs are no longer routinely included. PEEP prevents the formation of atelectasis in a patient on ventilation with constant small V_T. This is the primary reason why 5 cm H_2O of PEEP is routinely used on patients, including patients with healthy lungs. General guidelines for the initial ventilator settings for most adult patients are described in Box 48-11.

ADJUSTING VENTILATORY SUPPORT

After ventilator initiation, the patient should be carefully assessed and the ventilator adjusted so that patient-ventilator synchrony is ensured; WOB is minimized; and oxygenation, ventilation, and acid-base balance are optimized while harmful cardiovascular effects are minimized. Initial patient evaluation should include physical assessment, assessment of ventilator settings, cardiovascular assessment, oximetry, and measurement of arterial blood gases (Box 48-12).

Physical assessment should include general appearance, level of consciousness, signs of anxiety or dyspnea, color, extremities (temperature, edema, capillary refill), heart rate and blood pressure, respiratory rate and pattern, inspection of the neck for jugular venous distention, and chest examination. Cyanosis is associated with hypoxemia. Use of accessory muscles, tachypnea, retractions, or paradoxical abdomen movement may indicate increased WOB. Unilateral or unequal lung expansion is associated with bronchial intubation, pneumothorax, and other unilateral disorders.

Breath sounds should be assessed for good aeration, and absent, diminished, or abnormal breath sounds should be

Box 48-11 General Guidelines for Initial Ventilator Settings for Adult Patients

MODE
- Assist/control volume or pressure targeted
- Pressure support
- SIMV with or without pressure support volume or pressure targeted

TIDAL VOLUME
- 4 to 8 ml/kg IBW
- Avoid overdistention
- Maintain P_{plat} <28 cm H_2O
- For COPD, V_T 6 to 8 ml/kg IBW in assist/control or pressure support mode with adequate expiratory time for reducing air trapping is suggested
- For ARDS, begin at 6 to 8 ml/kg IBW; adjust as indicated to maintain P_{plat} <28 cm H_2O
- For acute asthma, V_T 4 to 6 ml/kg IBW is indicated to maintain P_{plat} <28 cm H_2O

RATE
- 18 (asthma) to 40 breaths/min
- Minimize auto-PEEP
- Set initial rate and V_T to maintain baseline minute ventilation (approximately 100 ml/kg IBW for most healthy adults)

PEEP
- 5 cm H_2O in most patients ventilated without acute lung injury
- 10 cm H_2O in patients with mild ARDS
- 15 to 20 cm H_2O in most patients with moderate to severe ARDS
- 5 cm H_2O in patients with COPD/asthma, adjust as indicated to offset effect of auto-PEEP on ventilator triggering
- Trigger sensitivity −0.5 to −1.5 cm H_2O or flow trigger 1 to 2 LPM; minimize trigger work without autocycle
- Inspiratory flow and time 60 to 100 L/min
- Inspiratory time 0.6 to 1.0 second; inspiratory flow must meet or exceed patient's spontaneous inspiratory flow demand
- Resultant I:E ratio should be ≤1:2

Box 48-12 Initial Assessment of Ventilatory Support

- Inspection, palpation, and auscultation
- Assessment of position of artificial airway and cuff inflation
- Assessment of pulse, blood pressure, oximetry, and electrocardiogram
- Inspection of patient-ventilator system breathing circuit, humidifier, ventilator settings, and findings
- Analysis of arterial blood gas values
- Inspection of chest radiograph

documented. Palpation should be performed as appropriate for tracheal position, chest wall motion, and presence of subcutaneous air. Percussion of the chest should be performed for assessment of resonance, dullness, or hyperresonance. Key findings at initial assessment of a patient undergoing ventilation are described in Table 48-6.

MINI CLINI

Humidification of the Airways During Mechanical Ventilation

PROBLEM: A mechanically ventilated patient is in the medical ICU recovering from acute respiratory failure secondary to aspiration pneumonia. The patient currently needs airway suctioning every 30 to 60 minutes according to the RT and staff nurse caring for the patient. Both caregivers note that the secretions are thick and copious. Current ventilator settings are as follows:

Mode: Assist/control volume ventilation
V_T: 500 ml (6.8 ml/kg IBW)
Preset rate: 16 breaths/min
Total rate: 26 breaths/min
FiO_2: 0.50
PIP: 31 cm H_2O
V_E: 13 L/min

The RT is asked to place an HME on the ventilator circuit at the "wye." Is this an appropriate action?

Solution: Humidification can be provided with either a heated humidifier or an HME. Although useful in some instances, placement of an HME would be contraindicated in this case for several reasons. Adequate humidification for a patient with an artificial airway is critical in preventing inspissation of airway secretions, injury to and destruction of the airway epithelium, and atelectasis.

The patient information in this clinical scenario points to several potential problems with use of an HME, the most obvious one being copious, thick airway secretions. The HME may not provide sufficient water vapor and heat output, and secretions could be retained. The airway secretions could be coughed into the HME, causing increased resistance to flow and possible obstruction. Because the patient has high ventilatory requirements, as evidenced by an elevated exhaled minute ventilation, it is important that the humidification system be able to maintain adequate heat and moisture output when demands dictate.

Other situations in which an HME should not be used are administration of aerosol treatments through the ventilator tubing circuit, high minute ventilation (>10 L/min), and body temperature less than 32° C.

Ventilator settings that should be assessed after initiation of mechanical ventilation include peak, plateau, and mean airway pressures; exhaled volumes (spontaneous and machine V_T, minute ventilation); respiratory rate (spontaneous and machine rate); baseline pressures (PEEP, CPAP, auto-PEEP); trigger effort; O_2 concentration; inspiratory time; flow; I:E ratio; humidification; airway temperature and airway cuff pressure. In addition, patient-ventilator interaction should be assessed to ensure that a spontaneously breathing patient is able to trigger a breath easily and that inspiratory flow and time are such that WOB is minimized. When using pressure ventilation, the patient should also be evaluated to ensure ease of cycling to expiration. Factors that may affect patient-ventilator interaction are discussed in detail in Chapter 47.

TABLE 48-6

Assessment of Ventilatory Support

Ancillary equipment in room	Crash cart (patient's condition unstable); cardiac monitor; chest tubes (pneumothorax, chest drainage, thoracic surgery); aortic balloon pump (heart failure); cooling blanket (fever); other
General appearance	Resting quietly, calm, relaxed (no distress); restless, anxious, distressed (pain, anxiety, inadequate oxygenation or ventilation)
Level of consciousness	Alert, awake, and oriented to person, place, and time (good mental status, neurologic function); confused (neurologic problems, hypoxia, low cardiac output, drugs); sleepy (tired, sedatives, narcotics); lethargic (exhaustion, impaired CNS status, sedation); somnolent (CNS impairment, sedation); coma (CNS malfunction, heavy sedation, severe hypoxia)
Extremities	Cyanosis (hypoxemia); pale, cold, and clammy (poor cardiac output, low blood pressure, shock); edema (fluid overload)
Respiratory rate and pattern	Normal (good cardiopulmonary status); tachypnea (pain, anxiety, hypoxemia, acidosis, CNS problems); bradypnea or apnea (severe hypoxia, CNS problems, heavy sedation, paralysis)
Head, eyes, ears, nose, and throat	Cyanotic lips and gums (hypoxemia); pupils dilated (drugs, severe hypoxia, low cardiac output, cardiac arrest); pupils dilated and fixed (brain death); pupils contracted (drugs, light); response to light (good if responsive)
Neck	Accessory muscle use (increased WOB, respiratory distress); jugular vein distention (right-sided heart failure, positive pressure impeding venous return)
Chest inspection	Right-left chest wall synchrony (normal); right-left chest wall asynchrony (right main stem intubation, pneumothorax, large unilateral pleural effusion, flail on one side); chest-diaphragm synchrony (normal); chest-diaphragm asynchrony—abdominal paradox (increased WOB, diaphragmatic fatigue)
Chest auscultation	Good bilateral breath sounds (normal); decreased breath sounds unilaterally (right main stem intubation, pneumothorax, unilateral lung disease); bilaterally decreased or absent breath sounds (inadequate or decreased ventilation, large leak, ventilator malfunction or disconnect, misplaced endotracheal tube); air leak around cuff (underinflation, cuff malfunction); wheezing (bronchospasm, tumor, narrowing of airway); bibasilar crackles in patients with congestive heart failure (pulmonary edema); rhonchi, coarse crackles (secretions in the larger airways); bronchial breath sounds (consolidation or microatelectasis)
Palpation	Subcutaneous air (pneumothorax, pneumomediastinum); tracheal shift (tension pneumothorax, large area of atelectasis); right-left chest motion symmetry (normal); right-left asymmetric breathing (unilateral disease, pneumothorax, bronchial intubation)
Percussion	Resonant over lung tissue (normal); dull (pleural effusion, lobar infiltrates, consolidation, atelectasis); hyperresonant (pneumothorax, overinflation—COPD, asthma exacerbation)
Vital signs	Normal heart rate and rhythm (normal); tachycardia (hypoxemia, pain, anxiety, distress); hypertension (anxiety, cardiovascular disease, head trauma); bradycardia (severe hypoxia, severe hypercapnia, cardiac disease); hypotension (blood loss, shock, gram-negative sepsis, heart failure)

CNS, Central nervous system.

The artificial airway should be assessed for proper placement, patency, and cuff inflation. Size, position, and depth of the endotracheal tube and cuff pressure, including volume used to inflate the cuff, should be recorded. An extra endotracheal tube or tracheostomy tube of the correct size should be placed at the patient's bedside, and the equipment needed to replace the airway must be available and easily accessible. A clean, functioning manual resuscitator with O_2 supply and suction equipment including an appropriate supply of suction catheters, sterile water or saline solution, and sterile gloves also must be placed near the bedside. Patients requiring high levels of PEEP (>5 cm H_2O) should have PEEP valves attached to the manual ventilator.

Cardiovascular assessment should include observation of heart rate, blood pressure, and electrocardiogram for the presence of arrhythmias. Tachycardia, ST segment elevation, and frequent premature ventricular contractions may indicate myocardial ischemia. If the patient has a central venous line or pulmonary arterial catheter, hemodynamic variables may be assessed, including central venous pressure, pulmonary arterial pressure, wedge pressure, and cardiac output.

Continuous monitoring with pulse oximetry is recommended for patients receiving mechanical ventilatory support in the ICU, and arterial blood gases should be measured 30 to 60 minutes after initiation of mechanical ventilation. A chest radiograph should be obtained to verify proper endotracheal tube placement and to evaluate the chest. After the initial assessment, the method and level of ventilatory support are adjusted to optimize oxygenation, ventilation, WOB, acid-base balance, and cardiovascular status. The ventilatory adjustments for each of these areas are discussed next.

Patient-Ventilator Interaction

Patient-ventilator interaction refers to patient comfort, WOB, and synchrony during ventilator-assisted breaths. Generally, ventilatory support should be initially adjusted to minimize the WOB and to allow the ventilatory muscles to rest.[47] See Chapter 47 for a detailed discussion.

OXYGENATION

Oxygen Concentration

Initiation of treatment for most patients in the acute care setting is with 100% O_2, unless detailed information identifying precise FiO_2 needed is available. FiO_2 is titrated to achieve PaO_2 of 60 to 80 mm Hg with SaO_2 or SpO_2 90% or greater. Estimate of O_2 needs can be derived as follows:

$$FiO_2 = \left(\frac{PaO_2 \text{ desired}}{PaO_2/PAO_2 \text{ ratio}} + PaCO_2 \times 1.25\right) \times \frac{1}{P_B - P_{H_2O}}$$

where FiO_2 required is the FiO_2 needed to achieve a desired PaO_2, PaO_2/PAO_2 is the initial PaO_2 divided by the initial alveolar partial pressure of oxygen (PAO_2), $PaCO_2$ is the initial $PaCO_2$, PB is barometric pressure, and P_{H_2O} is water vapor pressure. A simpler but less accurate calculation is the following:

$$\begin{array}{cc} \text{Initial} & \text{Desired} \\ PaO_{2(1)}/FiO_2(1) = & PaO_{2(2)}/FiO_2(2) \end{array}$$

Instead of a formula, a nomogram can be used to predict a patient's required FiO_2 (Figure 48-6). In either case, it is suggested that O_2 levels be titrated down from 100% to minimal FiO_2 required in decrements not to exceed 20%; titration is followed by oximetry or measurement of blood gases. When titrating FiO_2 downward, the clinician should wait at least 20 minutes between changes in FiO_2 to allow O_2 levels to stabilize. Patients with obstructive disease need a longer period for equilibration after a change in FiO_2.

When minimal FiO_2 is identified, further reduction in FiO_2 should be in steps of 5% to 10% followed by pulse oximetry measurements. Box 48-13 lists a conservative method of titrating O_2 concentration down from an initial FiO_2 of 1 on the basis of PaO_2.

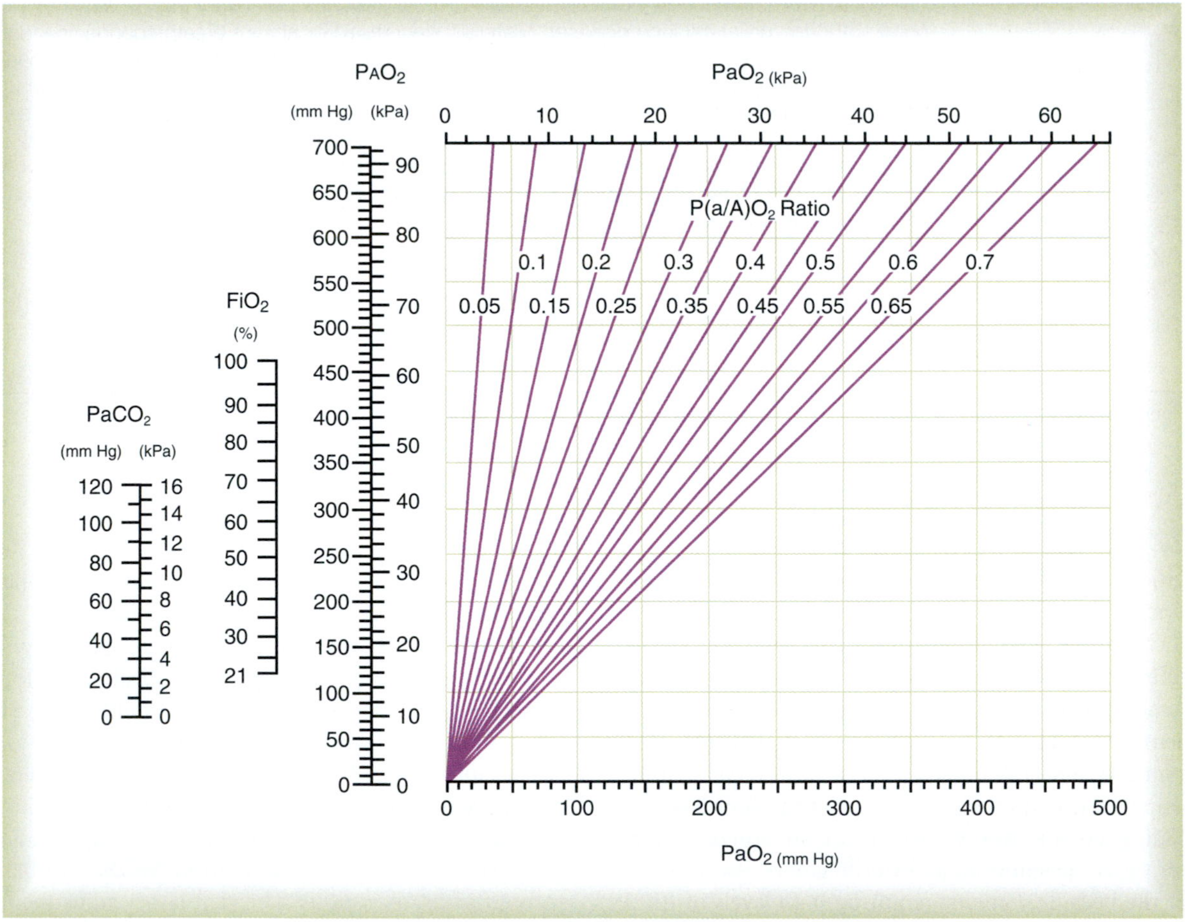

FIGURE 48-6 Nomogram for computing PaO_2/PAO_2 ratio and predicting FiO_2 required for desired PaO_2. To use the nomogram, first align the patient's current $PaCO_2$ and FiO_2 *(left two columns)* with a straight edge. This line intersects the vertical line corresponding to the patient's PAO_2 *(third column)*. Draw a horizontal line from this point to the vertical line corresponding to the patient's PaO_2. The diagonal line at this point (or one interpolated from the nearest diagonal lines bracketing it) is the PaO_2/PAO_2 ratio. $PaCO_2$ of 40 mm Hg and FiO_2 of 50% give PAO_2 of about 310 mm Hg. If PaO_2 is 50 mm Hg, PaO_2/PAO_2 is about 0.15. To predict FiO_2 required for PaO_2 of 70 mm Hg, follow the diagonal line representing 0.15 up to where it intersects the vertical line representing PaO_2 = 70 mm Hg. From this point, draw a horizontal line to the left intersecting the PAO_2 column at about 450 mm Hg. Connect this point to the present $PaCO_2$ (40 mm Hg) and note that the line passes through the required FiO_2 of about 70%. (From Chatburn RL, Lough MD: Handbook of respiratory care, Chicago, 1990, Year Book Medical Publishers.)

Box 48-13 Titrating Fractional Inspired Oxygen Down from an Initial Starting Point of 1.0 According to Initial PaO_2 and Pulse Oximetry Findings

Initial PaO_2 on FiO_2 1.0 (mm Hg)	FiO_2				
	Step 1	Step 2	Step 3	Step 4	Step 5
>300	0.80	0.60	0.50	0.40	0.35*
200-300	0.80	0.60	0.50	0.40*	—
150-199	0.80	0.60*	—	—	—
100-149	0.80*	—	—	—	—

Decrease FiO_2 to the target value in steps, and perform pulse oximetry or arterial blood gas measurements. Patients should continue to receive a given FiO_2 long enough to ensure equilibration and acceptable SpO_2 before further reductions are made in FiO_2. This procedure takes 20 minutes per FiO_2 change for most patients and up to 30 minutes for patients with obstructive disease. It usually is safe to continue to decrease FiO_2 as long as SpO_2 is greater than 95% (which should correspond to a PaO_2 > 90 mm Hg) for most patients. When SpO_2 is less than 95%, increase or decrease FiO_2 in steps of 0.05 per change.

*Target FiO_2 based on initial PaO_2.

Once the desired PaO_2 and saturation are reached, monitoring should be continued. Generally, O_2 levels are titrated up and down as needed with adjustments in FiO_2 of 0.05 to 0.10 to maintain PaO_2 of 60 to 80 mm Hg with SpO_2 of 90% to 95%. Titration is followed by pulse oximetry. SpO_2 of 88% to 90% may be acceptable for patients who need FiO_2 of 0.60 or more.

RULE OF THUMB

If a patient's oxygenation status is unknown, or if the patient's condition is unstable or critical, begin ventilatory support with FiO_2 of 1 until PaO_2, SaO_2, or SpO_2 can be assessed.

Positive End Expiratory Pressure and Continuous Positive Airway Pressure

Various approaches to adjusting PEEP or CPAP have been suggested over the years, including minimum PEEP, optimal or best PEEP, use of PEEP tables, PEEP titrated by compliance or pressure-volume curves, and decremental PEEP trials. With acute restrictive disease, as PEEP or CPAP levels are increased, PaO_2, SpO_2, and static compliance tend to improve until the point at which lung overinflation occurs.[47,48] As mean airway pressure increases, venous return decreases. The result may be a decrease in cardiac output. Figure 48-7 shows the physiologic factors that change during application of PEEP or CPAP. Several approaches to adjusting PEEP or CPAP are described later.

Minimum Positive End Expiratory Pressure

Minimum PEEP can be defined as the minimal PEEP needed to maintain recruited lung open and achieve adequate PaO_2 (and SpO_2) with FiO_2 less than 0.6. Generally, the PEEP level needed to achieve PaO_2 of at least 60 mm Hg (SpO_2 ≥90%) with FiO_2 of 0.40 to 0.50 or less is the minimum PEEP. With this approach, the least PEEP or CPAP level needed to achieve this therapeutic end point is applied.[1]

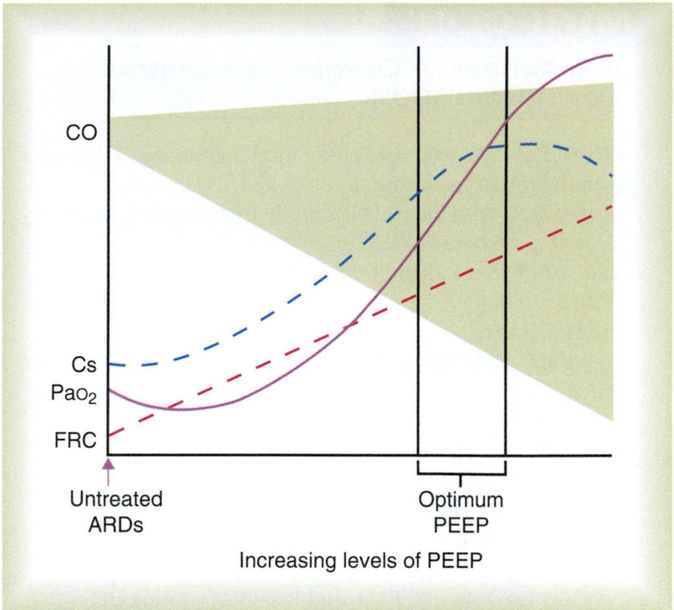

FIGURE 48-7 Curves represent the physiologic factors that change during the application of PEEP and CPAP. As PEEP level is increased, PaO_2, FRC, and static compliance (Cs) normally increase. Cardiac output (CO) *(shaded area)* can increase slightly, stay the same, or decrease. Optimum PEEP level can be expected to occur when PaO_2, FRC, and Cs are high. CO should be maintained near normal so that O_2 transport to the tissues remains high. (Modified from Pilbeam SP: Mechanical ventilation: physiological and clinical applications, ed 3, St Louis, 1998, Mosby.)

Optimal or Best Positive End Expiratory Pressure Based on Oxygen Delivery

Optimal or best PEEP may be defined as the PEEP that maximizes oxygen delivery (DO_2). Oxygen delivery is calculated as cardiac output ($\dot{Q}_T$) multiplied by oxygen content (CaO_2):

$$DO_2 = \dot{Q}_T \times CaO_2$$

For the optimal PEEP level, PEEP is increased in increments of 2 cm H_2O. Blood pressure, mixed venous O_2 levels (partial pressure of oxygen in mixed venous blood [$P\bar{v}O_2$], mixed venous oxygen saturation [$S\bar{v}O_2$], arteriovenous oxygen content difference [$C(a-\bar{v})O_2$]) cardiac output, and cardiac index are assessed. PEEP is increased incrementally until there is a decline in O_2 delivery, at which point the best or optimal PEEP has been exceeded. PEEP is adjusted down to the previous level that represents the "best" PEEP. Table 48-7 shows an example of a PEEP study for determining optimal PEEP based on O_2 delivery. In Table 48-7, as PEEP is increased from 8 cm H_2O to 10 cm H_2O to 12 cm H_2O, $P\bar{v}O_2$, $S\bar{v}O_2$, and O_2 delivery increase with

MINI CLINI

Adjustment of Oxygen Concentration Down from 100%

PROBLEM: At 9:00 AM, mechanical ventilation is initiated with the following settings for a 70-kg (IBW) patient:
Mode: VA/C with the patient actively triggering the ventilator
V_T: 420 ml/ 6.0 ml/kg /IBW
Rate: 20 to 26 breaths/min
FiO_2: 1
PEEP: 5 cm H_2O

An arterial blood gas is obtained 20 minutes after ventilator initiation:
FiO_2: 1
PaO_2: 225 mm Hg
pH: 7.42
$PaCO_2$: 40 mm Hg
HCO_3: 24 mEq/L
Base excess: +1 mEq/L

Calculated alveolar PAO_2 and PaO_2/PAO_2 ratios are:

$$PAO_2 = FiO_2\,(PB - P_{H_2O}) - PaCO_2 \times 1.25 = 663$$
$$PaO_2/PAO_2 = 225/663 = 0.34$$

What FiO_2 is needed to achieve a target PaO_2 of 80 mm Hg?

Solution: The following equation and normal barometric pressure ($P_B = 760$), lead to the calculation:

$$FiO_2\text{ required} = \left(\frac{PaO_2\text{ desired}}{PaO_2/PAO_2\text{ ratio}} + PaCO_2 \times 1.25\right) \times \frac{1}{P_B - P_{H_2O}}$$
$$= \left(\frac{80}{0.34} + 40 \times 1.25\right) \times \frac{1}{760 - 47} = 0.40$$

An alternative calculation would be:

$$\text{Initial} \qquad \text{Desired}$$
$$PaO_2/FiO_2 = PaO_2/FiO_2$$
$$225/1 = 80/FiO_2\text{ desired}$$
$$FiO_2\text{ desired} = 80 \times (1/225) = 80/225 = 0.36$$

What should the clinician do now?

The target O_2 concentration to achieve a PaO_2 in the range of 60 to 80 mm Hg (with 80 mm Hg as the specific target for the purpose of this calculation) would be approximately 40%. However, it is suggested that for adjusting down from 100% after initial ventilator setup, changes in FiO_2 be limited to 0.20 in the range of FiO_2 1 to 0.50 and 0.10 to 0.05 below FiO_2 of 0.50. Each change in FiO_2 should be followed by oximetry and patient assessment.

In this example, the FiO_2 can be decreased in a stepwise manner, as follows:

Time	FiO_2	SpO_2 (%)
9:30 AM	1	99
9:45 AM	0.80	99
10:00 AM	0.60	98
10:15 AM	0.50	97
10:30 AM	0.45	97
10:45 AM	0.40	95

Arterial blood gas on FiO_2 of 0.40 reveals a PaO_2 of 80 mm Hg.

MINI CLINI

Adjusting Fractional Inspired Oxygen

PROBLEM: A 65-kg (IBW) patient in the ICU is receiving mechanical ventilation in the VA/C mode. The patient's arterial blood gas values and related ventilator settings are:
Mode: VA/C the patient is not breathing spontaneously
FiO_2: 0.40
PaO_2: 50 mm Hg
V_T: 450 ml (7ml/Kg IBW)
pH: 7.4
Rate: 22 breaths/min
$PaCO_2$: 40 mm Hg
PEEP: 10 cm H_2O
HCO_3: 24 mEq/L
Base excess: +1 mEq/L

What FiO_2 would be required to increase this patient's PaO_2 to 60 mm Hg?

Solution: First, calculate the patient's current PAO_2 and PaO_2/PAO_2 ratio:

$$PAO_2 = FiO_2\,(PB - P_{H_2O}) - PaCO_2/0.8$$
$$= 0.40\,(760 - 47) - 40/0.8$$
$$= 285 - 50 = 235\text{ mm Hg}$$
$$PaO_2/PAO_2 = 50/235 = 0.21$$

Next, calculate the FiO_2 needed to achieve the desired PaO_2 of 60 mm Hg:

$$FiO_2\text{ required} = \left(\frac{PaO_2\text{ desired} + PaCO_2 \times 1.25 \times 1}{PaO_2/PAO_2\text{ ratio } P_B - P_{H_2O}}\right)$$
$$= \left(\frac{60 + (40 \times 1.25) \times 1}{0.21 760 - 47}\right)$$
$$= \frac{335.7 \times 1}{713} = 0.47$$

For this patient, if the FiO_2 is increased from 0.40 to 0.50, the PaO_2 should increase from 50 to 60 mm Hg. An alternative calculation, based on PaO_2/FiO_2 ratio, would be:

$$\text{Actual} \qquad \text{Desired}$$
$$PaO_2/FiO_2 = PaO_2/FiO_2$$

Solving for FiO_2, this becomes:

$$FiO_2\text{ required} = PaO_2\text{ desired} \times (FiO_2\text{ actual}/PaO_2\text{ actual})$$
$$= 60 \times (0.40/50) = 0.48$$

To increase this patient's PaO_2 to greater than 60 mm Hg would require increasing FiO_2 to approximately 0.50. Although FiO_2 of 0.50 or less is acceptable, as an alternative, the RT may consider increasing PEEP to 12 cm H_2O and then perform a clinical assessment, including evaluation of the effect of the increase on blood pressure, compliance, and arterial blood gases.

TABLE 48-7

Example of an Incremental Positive End Expiratory Pressure Study Including Ventilation, Oxygenation, and Hemodynamic Data*

Value	PEEP = 8	PEEP = 10	PEEP = 12	PEEP = 14	PEEP = 16
Time (min)	0	20	40	60	80
V_T (L)	0.6	0.6	0.6	0.6	0.6
f (breaths/min)	16	16	16	16	16
FiO_2 (%)	80	80	80	80	80
PEEP (cm H_2O)	0	5	10	15	20
I:E ratio	1:2.7	1:2.7	1:2.7	1:2.7	1:2.7
P_{peak} (cm H_2O)	30	32	35	42	50
P_{plat} (cm H_2O)	25	27	29	36	43
Cs (ml/cm H_2O)	24	27	32	29	26
$PaCO_2$ (mm Hg)	43	42	43	42	44
pH	7.38	7.37	7.39	7.35	7.32
PaO_2 (mm Hg)	52	66	87	90	97
SaO_2 (%)	86	92	96	97	98
$P\bar{v}O_2$ (mm Hg)	32	35	37	37	36
$S\bar{v}O_2$ (mm Hg)	61	66	71	69	64
Blood pressure (mm Hg)	131/78	133/82	130/79	125/74	110/69
Cardiac output (L/min)	5.9	5.7	5.9	5.4	4.8
DO_2 (ml/min)	989	1022	1105	1021	917

*When first reviewing a PEEP study, observe changes in the following: (1) airway pressure, (2) blood pressure, (3) arterial oxygen (PaO_2, SaO_2) and mixed venous oxygenation ($P\bar{v}O_2$, $S\bar{v}O_2$), and (4) oxygen transport (DO_2). With increases in PEEP, PaO_2 and saturation improve; airway pressure increases; compliance improves and then decreases at higher levels of PEEP; and oxygen transport (DO_2) improves and then declines. Optimum PEEP for this patient is 12 cm H_2O because it provides the best arterial oxygenation (PaO_2, SaO_2) without a decline in cardiac output.

no decline in cardiac output ($\dot{Q}_T$) or blood pressure. However, when PEEP is increased to 14 cm H_2O, $S\bar{v}O_2$, O_2 delivery, $\dot{Q}_T$, and blood pressure decline, indicating that optimal PEEP for this patient has been exceeded. The best PEEP for this patient would be 12 cm H_2O. Before determining PEEP using this approach, it is critical that the patient's hemodynamic status is stabilized. Patients with a compromised hemodynamic status generally do not tolerate PEEP titration without further compromise.

Compliance-Titrated Positive End Expiratory Pressure

With the compliance-titrated technique, PEEP is increased in increments of 2 cm H_2O, and the patient's estimated static compliance (Cs) is measured:

$$Cs = \frac{\text{Volume delivered (ml)}}{P_{plat} - P_{baseline}\ (\text{PEEP/CPAP})}$$

where total PEEP equals the sum of applied PEEP plus auto-PEEP.

Best PEEP has been exceeded at the point where an increase in PEEP is followed by a decrease in compliance. PEEP is reduced to the previous level, and this is optimal PEEP based on compliance.[48] For the example shown in Table 48-7, the best PEEP based on compliance would be 12 cm H_2O. Regional lung overdistention and declines in cardiac output can occur at levels less than compliance-titrated best PEEP, and consequently hemodynamic status should be optimized before any PEEP trial.

Positive End Expiratory Pressure Titrated With Pressure-Volume Curves as Part of a Lung Protective Strategy

A lung protective strategy that has been shown to improve outcome in ARDS includes use of a low V_T (4 to 8 ml/kg) and PEEP set 2 cm H_2O above the lower inflection point (P_{flex}) on a pressure-volume curve.[24,25] This strategy requires the use of static pressure-volume curves or slow-flow pressure-volume curves to determine best PEEP. To obtain a static pressure-volume curve, the RT passively inflates the patient's lungs with varying volumes in increasing increments of 50 to 100 ml. At each end point, static pressure is obtained by means of application of an end inspiratory pause, and the resultant pressure-volume curve is plotted (Figure 48-8). Upper and lower inflection points typically can be determined. The lower inflection point is thought to be the point at which alveolar recruitment begins. The upper inflection point indicates lung overdistention. PEEP is set at approximately 2 cm H_2O above the lower inflection point (P_{flex}). Determining PEEP level using the P_{flex} value may be done after a lung recruitment maneuver (see later). V_T is adjusted to ensure that the upper inflection point is not exceeded during inspiration.

Calculating the static pressure-volume curve is technically difficult and time-consuming.[12] An alternative is to use the slow-flow pressure-volume curve. A slow-flow curve (≤6 L/min) may also identify the lower inflection point for the purposes of setting PEEP (Figure 48-9). However, in either case, some patients do not have a lower inflection point. In about 25% of patients, the P_{flex} cannot be identified from the

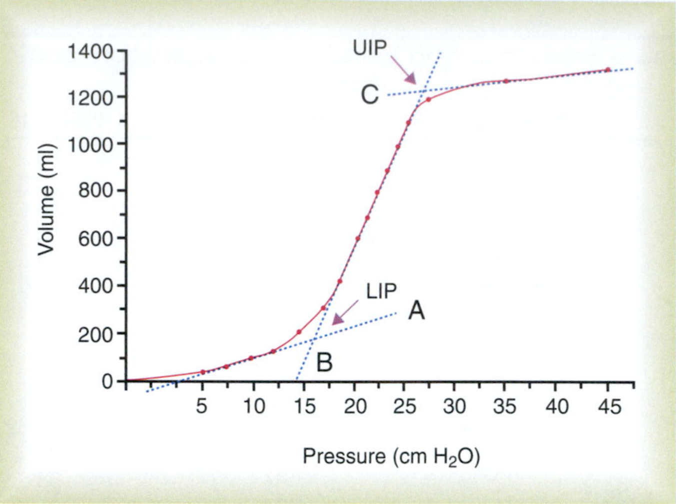

FIGURE 48-8 Static pressure-volume curve of a patient with ARDS. Volume is increased in increments of approximately 100 ml, inspiratory P_{plat} is measured, and a pressure-volume curve is plotted. Straight lines *(A, B,* and *C)* are drawn tangent to the curve, and the lower inflection point *(LIP)* and the upper inflection point *(UIP)* are identified. PEEP is adjusted to approximately 2 cm H_2O above the *LIP*.

Box 48-14 Performing a Lung Recruitment Maneuver and Decremental Positive End Expiratory Pressure Trial

- General approach: PCV
- PEEP: 20 to 25 cm H_2O
- Pressure control setting: 15 cm H_2O
- Inspiratory time: 1 to 2 seconds
- Rate: 15 to 20/min
- Duration 2 to 3 min

Immediately followed by a decremental PEEP trial

- Mode: Volume control
- PEEP: 20 to 25 cm H_2O
- V_T: 4 to 6 ml/kg IBW
- Rate: Highest rate avoiding auto-PEEP
- Ventilate until dynamic compliance stabilizes 1 to 2 minutes
- Record compliance
- Decrease PEEP by 2 cm H_2O
- Ventilate until dynamic compliance stabilizes 1 to 2 minutes
- Decrease PEEP by 2 cm H_2O
- Ventilate until dynamic compliance stabilizes 1 to 2 minutes
- Continue this until PEEP level that results in the best compliance is identified
- Repeat the recruitment maneuver
- Set PEEP at best compliance PEEP plus 2 to 3 cm H_2O

Before performing a recruitment maneuver, ensure that the patient is hemodynamically stable and sedated to apnea.

pressure-volume curve.[25] In addition, observer variability in identifying the lower inflection point can be significant.[50]

Positive End Expiratory Pressure and Lung Recruitment Maneuvers

Various lung recruitment maneuvers have been suggested for improving $\dot{V}/\dot{Q}$ and reducing shunting in patients with ARDS. These maneuvers include several variations that incorporate CPAP[25,51,52] or the use of PCV with high PEEP levels.[49,53] Regardless of approach, before any lung recruitment maneuver is performed, the patient must be hemodynamically stable and sedated to apnea. Neuromuscular paralysis is unnecessary, but the patient must be accepting of passive ventilation at high pressures. Hemodynamic stability is crucial because of the high intrathoracic pressures established during all recruitment maneuvers, although the few data that are available indicate that pressure control recruitment maneuvers are better tolerated than CPAP recruitment maneuvers.[54,55] The original recruitment techniques applied 40 to 45 cm H_2O CPAP for 30 to 40 seconds.[25,51,52] For recruitment maneuvers to be successful, they should be performed as early as possible after the patient is stabilized on the ventilator.[51-53] The longer the length of mechanical ventilation before the recruitment maneuver, the greater the likelihood that the maneuver will fail. See Box 48-14 for details on the performance of lung recruitment maneuvers and decremental PEEP trials.

The most widely accepted approach to recruiting the lung is the use of PCV. With this approach, PEEP is set higher than levels needed to maintain the recruited lung open, usually between 20 cm H_2O and 25 cm H_2O; a pressure control level 15 cm H_2O above this is then set. Ventilation is provided with an I:E of 1:1 to 1:2 at a rate of 15 to 20 per minute. All recruitment maneuvers are performed with 100% O_2. If this initial approach to lung recruitment does not open the lung, PEEP can be set higher in increments of 5 cm H_2O, and the recruitment repeated after the patient has totally stabilized from the previous maneuver (>30 minutes). The maximum safe peak pressure during a recruitment maneuver is 50 cm H_2O. Peak pressures greater than 50 cm H_2O increase the likelihood of barotraumas during the maneuver.[52,53]

The best method of establishing optimal PEEP after recruitment is a decremental PEEP trial.[49,51,53,56] It is best to perform the trial in volume ventilation because the easiest bedside method of identifying the optimal PEEP is to determine the best compliance PEEP. The best oxygenation PEEP can also be determined. It takes only about 1 to 2 minutes for the compliance to stabilize when PEEP is changed, but at least 20 minutes is required for PaO_2 to stabilize after a PEEP adjustment.

To perform the trial, PEEP should begin at 20 to 25 cm H_2O but always at PEEP higher than expected necessary to maintain the lung open. V_T during the decremental PEEP trial is usually set at 4 to 6 ml/kg IBW depending on P_{plat}. Inspiratory time is set at 0.6 to 0.8 second, and rate is at the highest level that does not result in auto-PEEP. First, the compliance is recorded at these settings after stabilization. Then the PEEP is decreased 2 cm H_2O, and the compliance again is allowed to stabilize. The process is continued until the best compliance PEEP can be identified. Generally, compliance is low at the starting PEEP (20 to 25 cm H_2O) because of overdistention. As PEEP is decreased, compliance improves until it peaks and then starts to decrease

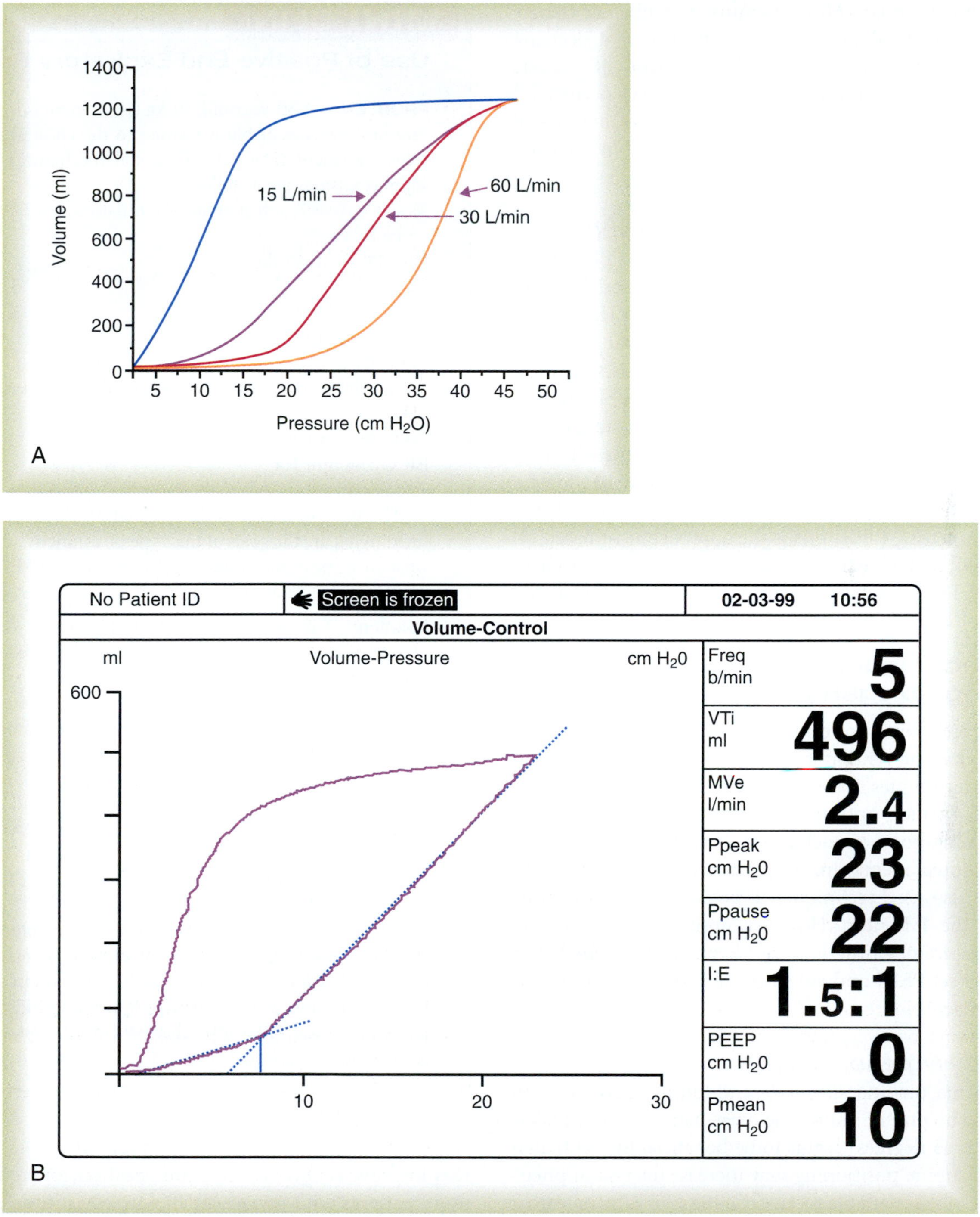

FIGURE 48-9 A, Pressure-volume curves generated by a ventilator graphics package with the flow set at 60 L/min, 30 L/min, and 15 L/min. As flow is decreased, the curve shifts to the left and more closely approximates a static pressure-volume curve. Flow of less than 6 L/min is recommended for identifying the lower inflection point *(LIP)* from a slow-flow pressure-volume curve. **B,** Slow-flow pressure-volume curve with use of a set rate of 5 breaths/min, I:E ratio of 1.5:1, and V_T of 500 ml. LIP is approximately 8 cm H_2O. The respiratory cycle time is 12 seconds (cycle time = 60/f = 60/5 = 12 seconds). An I:E ratio of 1.5:1 results in an inspiratory time of 4.8 seconds. Inspiratory flow is V_T/T_i = 0.5 L/4.8 sec = 0.104 L/sec, or approximately 6 L/min.

because of derecruitment and atelectasis.[49] The best compliance PEEP is increased by 2 to 3 cm H_2O because the best compliance PEEP underestimates the best oxygenation PEEP by 2 to 3 cm H_2O.[49] After identifying the optimal PEEP level, the lung must be recruited again because derecruitment occurred during the decremental PEEP trial. After this second recruitment, PEEP is set at the optimal level determined during the decremental trial.

A recruitment maneuver should be stopped if there is a decrease in SpO_2 to less than 85%, a significant change in heart rate (>140 beats/min or <60 beats/min), a significant change in mean arterial blood pressure (<60 mm Hg or a decrease >20 mm Hg from baseline), the development of cardiac arrhythmia, or any indication that barotraumas occurred.[51] More recent meta-analyses indicate that the use of high PEEP benefits patients with moderate to severe ARDS but does not benefit patients with mild ARDS.[40,41]

Positive End Expiratory Pressure Tables

The ARDS Clinical Network study used an FiO_2-PEEP table to adjust PEEP levels.[2] Using this approach, PEEP and FiO_2 are alternately adjusted to obtain PaO_2 of 60 to 80 mm Hg or SpO_2 90% or greater (see Box 48-7). The table offers higher and lower PEEP options. For the lower PEEP option, PEEP is set at 5 to 10 cm H_2O with FiO_2 of 0.30 to 0.70; the higher PEEP option sets PEEP at 12 to 20 cm H_2O in the same FiO_2 range. The higher PEEP option should be reserved for patients who may benefit from higher PEEP in terms of lung recruitment and who have a stable blood pressure and no barotrauma. Of all the approaches to setting PEEP, this is the approach least based on the physiology of the patient. It is a reasonable approach to establish initial PEEP, but it is generally a poor choice for further adjustment of PEEP.

Other Techniques for Improving Oxygenation

The primary techniques for optimizing oxygenation in patients receiving mechanical ventilatory support are adjusting FiO_2 and PEEP. Other techniques that may be helpful in improving arterial O_2 levels include optimizing the patient's hemodynamic status, providing good bronchial hygiene, prone positioning, and extracorporeal membrane oxygenation (ECMO). Some clinicians have also used techniques to prolong inspiratory time and reverse the I:E ratio. However, approaches focused on increasing inspiratory time have not been shown to be better than properly set PEEP and are associated with marked hemodynamic compromise.

Bronchial Hygiene

In many patients, turning, sitting up, and getting out of bed into a chair can be helpful in improving oxygenation. Upright positioning (30 to 45 degrees) seems to be beneficial for ventilated patients, and supine positioning may increase the risk of pneumonia, especially in patients receiving enteral feeding or with a decreased level of consciousness.[57] Elevation of the head of the bed greater than 30 degrees has been recommended in all ventilated patients to reduce the incidence of ventilator-associated pneumonia. Special rotational beds can be used to optimize PaO_2 in selected patients. Postural drainage, adequate humidification, and bronchodilator therapy all may improve oxygenation and should be considered in the care of ventilated patients when not specifically contraindicated.

Prone Positioning

Prone positioning may be an effective technique for improving oxygenation in some patients with ARDS.[58-61] Prone positioning may improve PaO_2, decrease shunt fraction, and reduce mortality in patients with severe ARDS when it is initiated early and applied for most of the day.[62] Although improvement in PaO_2 may be dramatic and sustained (up to 12 hours), not all patients benefit from prone positioning. The procedure is not without risk. Care must be taken to ensure that endotracheal tubes, intravenous lines, and catheters are not blocked or dislodged. The patient may also have skin breakdown at specific pressure points (face, sternum, hips, knees), and facial or eyelid edema may occur, although the latter is primarily a cosmetic concern that resolves quickly when the patient returns to a supine or sitting position.[63] The most serious complication is corneal abrasion necessitating corneal transplantation.[63,64] Prone positioning is labor-intensive, often requiring two nurses, an RT,

MINI CLINI

Use of Positive End Expiratory Pressure

PROBLEM: A 30-year-old, 80-kg (IBW) man is in the critical care unit because of blunt trauma to the chest after a motor vehicle accident. The patient's initial mechanical ventilatory support settings are as follows:

Mode: = Assist/control volume ventilation, V_T: 500 ml (6 ml/kg IBW)
Rate: 20 breaths/min
FiO_2: 0.70
PIP: 35 cm H_2O
P_{plat}: 30 cm H_2O
PEEP: 0

Arterial blood gas analysis yielded the following results:
pH: 7.38
PaO_2: 48 mm Hg
$PaCO_2$: 36 mm Hg
SaO_2: 81%

The RT considers a recommendation that PEEP be instituted. What are the goals of this type of adjunctive therapy, and what are some of the potential adverse effects of PEEP of which the RT should be aware?

Solution: The general goals of PEEP are to stabilize and maintain open alveolar units to achieve adequate oxygenation and to avoid potentially unsafe levels of FiO_2 and inflation pressure. Improvement is most commonly assessed with PaO_2 or SpO_2, compliance and measurement of blood pressure and cardiac output.

At least 5 cm H_2O PEEP should be used in all acutely ventilated patients unless the patient is too hemodynamically unstable to tolerate the use of PEEP. When PaO_2 does not respond to a high FiO_2, the condition is referred to as *refractory hypoxemia*. An appropriate initial PEEP for this patient would be 10 cm H_2O because of the patient PaO2/FiO2 ratio of 69, severe ARDS, and arterial blood gases, P_{plat}, and blood pressure, should be assessed. As the level of PEEP is increased, the RT must be alert for signs of decreased cardiac output. Measurement of effective compliance and P_{plat} is also indicated. In all cases, the lowest PEEP level that provides acceptable oxygenation should be selected.

and a physician to "flip" the patient. Numerous early randomized controlled trials have evaluated the impact of prone positioning on survival in ARDS[58-61]; however, none of the trials have shown improved outcome. A more recent meta-analysis indicated improved survival in patients with the most severe lung injury—patients with PaO_2/FiO_2 ratio less than 100 mm Hg.[62] A recent randomized control trial verified the meta-analysis finding.[65] As a result, prone positioning should be reserved for severe ARDS (PaO2/FiO2 < 100 mmHg) and after lung recruitment and appropriate PEEP titration has been preformed. Similar to all lung protective approaches to ventilatory support, prone positioning should be used early in the course of ARDS if it is to be beneficial.

The mechanism of action of prone positioning is unclear. In ARDS, dorsal lung injury tends to increase shunt and decrease $\dot{V}/\dot{Q}$, resulting in hypoxemia. Supine positioning tends to increase regional pressure in the dependent, or dorsal, portions of the lungs. Prone positioning may improve $\dot{V}/\dot{Q}$ and reduce shunting by removing the pressure of the heart on the dorsal regions, causing regional dorsal traction, which may promote lung opening. The recommended technique for prone positioning is outlined in Box 48-15.

VENTILATION

Alveolar ventilation is determined by respiratory rate, V_T, and dead space and is described by the following equation:

$$\dot{V}_A = (V_T - V_{Dphys})f$$

where $\dot{V}_A$ is alveolar ventilation, V_T is tidal volume, V_{Dphys} is physiologic dead space, and f is respiratory frequency or rate.

Box 48-15 Prone Positioning

Preparation for prone positioning includes the following:
- Adequate sedation of patient
- Clear assignment of responsibilities between team members
- Moving the patient to one side of the bed
- Checking all lines for length
- Checking the security of the endotracheal tube
- Endotracheal suctioning
- Preoxygenation with 100% O_2
- Checking all vital signs

The turn includes:
- Tipping the patient to the side
- Securing electrocardiogram leads
- Turning the patient prone
- Turning the patient's head toward the ventilator

Care after the turn includes:
- Checking artificial airway
- Checking all lines
- Checking ventilator pressure and volume
- Monitoring vital signs
- Repositioning and recalibrating pressure transducers
- The patient needs supports (pillows) for each side of chest and forehead so that the endotracheal tube and head are not compromised.

The relationship between arterial $PaCO_2$, alveolar ventilation ($\dot{V}_A$), and CO_2 production ($\dot{V}CO_2$) is described as follows:

$$PaCO_2 = (0.863)(\dot{V}CO_2)/\dot{V}_A$$

Arterial $PaCO_2$ is considered the best index of effective ventilation. Increases in $\dot{V}_A$ or decreases in $\dot{V}CO_2$ result in a decrease in $PaCO_2$, whereas increases in $\dot{V}CO_2$ or decreases in $\dot{V}_A$ result in an increase in $PaCO_2$. If there is no change in $\dot{V}CO_2$, the following relationships can be used to estimate the effect of changes in $\dot{V}_A$ on $PaCO_2$:

$$\begin{array}{cc} \text{Initial} & \text{Desired} \\ PaCO_{2(1)} \times \dot{V}_{A(1)} = & PaCO_{2(2)} \times \dot{V}_{A(2)} \end{array}$$

The foregoing predictive equation can be used during mechanical ventilation with the following modifications:

$$PaCO_{2(1)}(V_{T(1)} - V_{Dphys(1)})f_{(1)} = PaCO_{2(2)}(V_{T(2)} - V_{DSphys(2)})f_{(2)}$$

For changes in rate alone, if there is no change in $\dot{V}CO_2$ or V_{Dphys}, this becomes:

$$\begin{array}{cc} \text{Initial} & \text{Desired} \\ PaCO_{2(1)} \times f_{(1)} = & PaCO_{2(2)} \times f_{(2)} \end{array}$$

For changes in VT alone, this becomes:

$$\begin{array}{cc} \text{Initial} & \text{Desired} \\ PaCO_{2(1)} \times V_{T(1)} = & PaCO_{2(2)} \times V_{T(2)} \end{array}$$

A major goal of mechanical ventilatory support is optimization of the patient's ventilation and $PaCO_2$; however, this does not mean normalization of $PaCO_2$. Acceptable arterial pH and alveolar PCO_2 are assessed by P_{plat}. For many patients, the level of ventilatory support is adjusted to achieve a $PaCO_2$ of 35 to 45 mm Hg with a pH of 7.35 to 7.45. In the care of patients with acute exacerbation of COPD and accompanying chronic ventilatory failure, the clinician may target ventilatory support to achieve the patient's "normal" $PaCO_2$ and pH. For patients with COPD and chronic hypercapnia, the target $PaCO_2$ may be 50 to 60 mm Hg with a pH of 7.30 to 7.35. In patients with severe ARDS, a $PaCO_2$ of 70 mm Hg with an acidic pH may have to be accepted to protect the lung from ventilator-induced lung injury. The sicker the patient, the more likely the clinician is to accept oxygenation and acid-base values that greatly deviate from normal. Regardless of the patient's condition, optimizing pH is more important than targeting a specific $PaCO_2$ value.[1,9] Box 48-16 presents an example of the effect of change in $\dot{V}_A$ on $PaCO_2$.

Box 48-16 Example of the Effect of Change in $\dot{V}_A$ on $PaCO_2$

If a patient has an initial $PaCO_2$ of 50 mm Hg with a corresponding alveolar ventilation ($\dot{V}_A$) of 4 L/min, what level of alveolar ventilation is required to decrease the $PaCO_2$ to 40 mm Hg (if there is no change in $\dot{V}_ACO_2$)?

If the patient's $\dot{V}_A$ is increased from 4 L/min to 5 L/min, the $PaCO_2$ should decrease from 50 mm Hg to 40 mm Hg.

Adjusting Tidal Volume and Rate

V_T and rate may be adjusted for a desired level of ventilation as assessed by $PaCO_2$. V_T usually is based on specific patient considerations but ideally should never result in P_{plat} greater than 28 cm H_2O. Respiratory rate is adjusted to achieve the desired $PaCO_2$. Normal resting V_T of healthy individuals is 6.3 ml/kg IBW. In most critically ill patients, V_T should be in the range of 4 to 8 ml/kg IBW. In patients with improving respiratory function ready for extubation, V_T of 9 to 10 ml/kg IBW may be acceptable; however, V_T greater than 10 ml/kg IBW should never be selected for a critically ill patient.

Apnea (Controlled Ventilation)

In an apneic patient, precise control of $PaCO_2$ usually can be achieved with pressure or volume ventilation because the ventilator rate and V_T are determined directly or indirectly by the clinician.

Rate. In the care of apneic patients, the clinician has complete control over the patient's rate, and changes in ventilator rate can be used precisely to alter $PaCO_2$. For rate changes alone (V_T held constant):

Initial Desired

$$PaCO_{2(1)} \times f_{(1)} = PaCO_{2(2)} \times f_{(2)}$$

For example, if a patient's initial rate was 18 breaths/min and resultant $PaCO_2$ was 50 mm Hg, the rate change needed to decrease the patient's $PaCO_2$ to 40 mm Hg could be calculated as follows:

Initial Desired

$$PaCO_{2(1)} \times f_{(1)} = PaCO_{2(2)} \times f_{(2)}$$

$$50 \times 18 = 40 \times f_{(2)}$$

$$f_{(2)} = (50 \times 18)/40 = 23 \text{ breaths/min}$$

For this patient, an increase in machine rate from 18 to 23 breaths/min would decrease $PaCO_2$ from 50 mm Hg to 40 mm Hg. Two warnings must be kept in mind in the use of this predictive equation. First, it is assumed that $\dot{V}CO_2$ is constant. If there is an increase or decrease in $\dot{V}CO_2$, the resultant $PaCO_2$ would be different from the predicted value. Common causes of increased $\dot{V}CO_2$ in the ICU include pain, agitation, anxiety, fever, overfeeding, increased activity, and fighting the ventilator. Decreases in $\dot{V}CO_2$ may be caused by decreased activity, sedation, paralysis, anesthesia, or sleep. Second, the equation is based on the assumption that the patient is apneic. Patients who are triggering the ventilator in the assist/control mode determine their own $PaCO_2$ on the basis of the assist rate. Patients in the SIMV mode who are spontaneously breathing may simply increase or decrease their level of spontaneous breathing and make $PaCO_2$ prediction difficult. In addition, the primary factor that limits the selection of rate is the development of auto-PEEP. If auto-PEEP develops, plateau pressure increases in volume ventilation and tidal volume decreases in pressure ventilation.

Tidal Volume. Changes in V_T can be used to alter $PaCO_2$. For a patient 80 kg IBW receiving ventilation in the control mode with V_T of 600 ml (7.5 ml/kg) and resultant $PaCO_2$ of 30 mm Hg, the change in V_T to achieve a PaO_2 of 40 mm Hg would be calculated as follows:

Initial Desired

$$PaCO_{2(1)} \times V_{T(1)} = PaCO_{2(2)} \times V_{T(2)}$$

$$30 \times 600 = 40 \times V_{T(2)}$$

$$V_{T(2)} = (30 \times 600)/40 = 450 \text{ ml}$$

For this patient, a decrease in V_T from 600 ml to 450 ml results in an increase in $PaCO_2$ from 30 mm Hg to 40 mm Hg. This is directly altered in volume ventilation by changing the tidal volume or indirectly by decreasing the pressure control level in pressure ventilation. Several warnings should be kept in mind for changes in V_T. First, V_T should be within the preferred range for a given patient condition. In the example, new V_T (450 ml) represents 5.6 ml/kg IBW, which is an acceptable value. V_T should be small enough to avoid lung injury and maintain P_{plat} at less than 28 cm H_2O. Second, in this equation, $\dot{V}CO_2$ and V_{Dphys} are assumed to be constant because changes in $\dot{V}CO_2$ or V_{Dphys} affect $PaCO_2$. Activity, agitation, fever, and overfeeding may increase $\dot{V}CO_2$, whereas sedation, paralysis, or sleep may decrease $\dot{V}CO_2$. V_{Dphys} changes with changes in airway pressure, and increases in ventilator V_T may result in increased dead space. Development of pulmonary emboli or hemodynamic instability may abruptly increase V_{Dphys}.

Mechanical Dead Space. Mechanical dead space is defined as the volume of gas rebreathed as the result of a mechanical device. Large-bore tubing attached between the patient "wye" and the patient connection serves as mechanical dead space, and 6 inches (15 cm) of large-bore tubing represents a volume of approximately 50 to 70 ml.

For ventilation of tracheostomy patients, 6 inches (15 cm) of mechanical dead space often is used to keep the weight of the "wye" connection and tubing off of the tracheostomy tube and to give additional flexibility to the circuit for patient movement. Mechanical dead space usually is not used for endotracheally intubated patients, and the addition of mechanical dead space can serve as a cause for an increase in $PaCO_2$. Mechanical dead space is a primary concern in patients with severe ARDS in whom V_T is 4 to 6 ml/kg IBW, and as a result $PaCO_2$ is elevated. The simple removal of mechanical dead space in these patients in some cases can markedly improve CO_2 elimination. HME filters are another major cause of mechanical dead space. Depending on the brand, 80 ml of dead space can be added by these devices.

In healthy persons, V_{Dphys} and anatomic dead space are approximately the same and can be estimated at approximately 1 ml/lb or 2.2 ml/kg IBW. Although healthy persons have a dead space-to-tidal volume (V_D/V_T) ratio of approximately 0.20 to 0.40, a V_D/V_T ratio greater than 0.50 is common among ventilated patients.

Control of $PaCO_2$ in Synchronized Intermittent Mandatory Ventilation Mode

In the SIMV mode, machine breaths are interspersed with spontaneous breathing, and the spontaneous breaths may be

MINI CLINI

Adjusting $PaCO_2$ During Volume Ventilation

PROBLEM: A 22-year-old man, 5 ft 10 in (178 cm) tall, being treated for a drug overdose is being ventilated with the following settings:
Mode: VA/C
FiO_2: 0.40
V_T: 600 ml
Rate: 15 breaths/min
PIP: 20 cm H_2O
P_{plat}: 13 cm H_2O
PEEP: 5 cm H_2O

The patient's lungs are clear to auscultation, and there is no evidence of aspiration. Arterial blood gas values obtained 15 minutes ago were:
PaO_2: 80 mm Hg
$PaCO_2$: 30 mm Hg
SaO_2: 95%
HCO_3: 24 mEq/L
pH: 7.52
Base excess: +2 mEq/L

The physician asks the RT to normalize this patient's oxygenation and ventilatory status. What should the RT do?

Solution: At this time, the patient is making no spontaneous breathing efforts. The patients' oxygenation status is fine, and no adjustments are needed. In the absence of spontaneous breathing in the VA/C mode, $PaCO_2$ can be adjusted by changing machine rate (f) or V_T. Because the V_T is large (600 ml), the correct adjustment would be to decrease the V_T.

For prediction of the needed change in V_T to increase $PaCO_2$ to 40 mm Hg, the following calculation could be performed:

Actual Desired

$$V_{T(1)} \times PaCO_{2(1)} = V_{T(2)} \times PaCO_{2(2)}$$
$$V_{T(2)}\ \text{Desired} = (V_{T(1)} \times PaCO_{2(1)})/PaCO_{2(2)}$$
$$V_{T(2)}\ \text{Desired} = (600 \times 30)/40 = 458\ \text{ml}$$

If V_T is decreased to 450 ml, $PaCO_2$ and pH should normalize.

PSV. $PaCO_2$ can be decreased by increasing V_T, increasing PSV for spontaneous breaths, or increasing the machine rate. Levels of $PaCO_2$ may be increased by reducing the machine rate, decreasing V_T, or decreasing the level of PSV for spontaneous breaths. As with apneic (control) ventilation, an appropriate V_T should be selected on the basis of the patient's condition and with the goal of keeping P_{plat} less than 28 cm H_2O with V_T ideally 4 to 8 ml/kg IBW depending on the patient's pulmonary status. PSV level in the SIMV mode should be adjusted to overcome WOB_I; the usual range is 5 to 15 cm H_2O, although higher levels may be needed by patients with high resistance. PSV should be adjusted to ensure that during spontaneous breathing, WOB is not excessive. Accessory muscle use or suprasternal, intercostal, or substernal retractions during spontaneous breathing indicate the need to increase the PSV level. When appropriate V_T and PSV level are selected, the primary method for adjusting $PaCO_2$ is to increase or decrease SIMV rate.

After ventilator initiation, two different approaches may be taken. For full ventilatory support, an initial SIMV rate and V_T are selected to provide 100% of the patient's ventilatory requirements; for most adults, this means starting with V_T of 6 to 8 ml/kg IBW with SIMV rate of 15 to 20 breaths/min. Generally, a minute ventilation of approximately 100 ml/kg IBW is achieved with these initial settings. Arterial blood gas values are obtained 20 to 30 minutes after initiation of mechanical ventilation, and SIMV rate is titrated up or down in increments of 2 breaths/min until desired $PaCO_2$ is achieved. Monitoring is continued, and adjustments are made by increasing or decreasing SIMV rate to maintain full ventilatory support until the patient's condition improves and ventilator discontinuation is considered.

Partial ventilatory support in the SIMV mode requires a different initial approach. Ventilation begins with V_T and machine rate sufficient to provide full ventilatory support, and arterial blood gases are measured. If $PaCO_2$ is adequate, the patient is immediately challenged with a decrease in SIMV rate of 2 breaths/min. This procedure is followed by patient assessment and measurement of arterial blood gases, as indicated. If the resultant assessment values remain adequate, the patient continues to be challenged with decreases in SIMV rate until $PaCO_2$ increases. At that point, the patient's ventilatory capacity has been exceeded, and SIMV rate is returned to the previous value. Box 48-17 provides an example of titration of the SIMV rate for partial ventilatory support after ventilator initiation in a spontaneously breathing patient.

Assist/Control Mode Volume Ventilation and $PaCO_2$

Ventilator initiation in the VA/C mode begins with selection of initial V_T and backup control rate to ensure a safe minimum level of ventilation. In PA/C, a pressure control level sufficient to establish desired V_T is selected along with a backup as in VA/C. The patient is allowed to trigger the machine as often as desired above this backup rate, and the resultant assist rate is determined by the patient's ventilatory drive. If the respiratory drive is intact, patients tend to trigger the ventilator at an appropriate rate to achieve adequate $PaCO_2$ and pH. By allowing patients to set their own rates, the level of ventilation increases or decreases on the basis of the patient's physiologic needs. Should the patient become apneic owing to sedation or sleep, a minimum backup control rate is provided.

Because the patient determines the level of ventilation, $PaCO_2$ levels are regulated by the patient. However, problems arise when the patient triggers the ventilator at an inappropriately rapid rate. Pain, anxiety, hypoxemia, secretions in the airway, and metabolic acidosis may contribute to an excessive trigger rate. The result can be an inappropriate I : E ratio and an inadequate expiratory time. These abnormal values may increase mean airway pressure, reduce venous return, and result in auto-PEEP and overinflation and associated missed triggering of the ventilator, especially in patients with obstructive disease. Patients may fight the ventilator, resulting in high inspiratory

Box 48-17 Partial Ventilatory Support With Synchronized Intermittent Mandatory Ventilation

Mechanical ventilation is initiated in the SIMV mode for a 70-kg, spontaneously breathing 38-year-old man. Before initiation of ventilation, the patient's spontaneous rate was 30 breaths/min with a spontaneous V_T of 200 ml. Initial ventilator settings are:

V_T: 500 ml
SIMV rate: 14 breaths/min
FiO_2: 0.40
PSV: +8 cm H_2O
PIP: 24 cm H_2O
P_{plat}: 18 cm H_2O
PEEP: 8 cm H_2O

Arterial blood gases are obtained in 20 minutes, with the following results:

PaO_2: 88 mm Hg
SaO_2: 97%
pH: 7.38
$PaCO_2$: 40 mm Hg
HCO_3: 24 mEq/L
Base excess: +1 mEq/L

The decision is made to provide partial ventilatory support for this patient, and the SIMV rate is titrated as follows:

Time	V_T (ml)	SIMV Rate	Total Rate	$PaCO_2$ (mm Hg)
9:00 AM	600	14	20	40
9:30 AM	600	12	15	38
10:00 AM	600	10	18	38
10:30 AM	600	8	24	46
11:00 AM	600	10	18	42

The patient's condition should now be stabilized at a rate of 10 breaths/min with titration of SIMV to the patient's needs with observation and measurement of arterial blood gases. When the rate is decreased to 8 breaths/min, $PaCO_2$ begins to increase. The rate is increased to the previous setting of 10 breaths/min. Titrating the level of SIMV support to the patient's needs is not the same as weaning the patient. After improvement in the patient's condition, weaning may be tried (see Chapter 52) with a daily spontaneous breathing trial.

pressure. In the event that a patient receiving ventilation in the assist/control mode is triggering the ventilator at an inappropriately high rate, the first step the RT should take is to identify the cause of the increased rate. Patient anxiety may be diminished with simple reassurance and encouragement to relax and "let the machine breathe for you." Hypoxemia should be managed with appropriate O_2 therapy and PEEP, if indicated. Secretions should be removed by suctioning, and bronchial hygiene techniques should be applied. The cause of metabolic acidosis should be identified and managed, if possible.

In some patients, appropriate sedation improves the ventilatory rate. Patients who begin fighting the ventilator after a previous period of calm may have a new and potentially life-threatening complication. If a patient begins fighting the ventilator, a careful assessment should be made to identify the problem. Often, careful attention to the ventilator trigger sensitivity, flow rate, volume, and pressure is helpful, and administration of analgesic and sedative agents may be needed.[12] If sedation is required, the use of intermittent sedation with daily interruption using a sedation protocol may reduce the duration of mechanical ventilation.[66,67] A last resort is pharmacologic controlled ventilation.[12] In the presence of a metabolic acidosis, a sudden change from assisted ventilation at a rapid rate with the associated hyperventilation to controlled ventilation at a slower rate can result in severe acidosis, which can be life-threatening. Other problems with controlled ventilation include patient safety, ventilatory muscle atrophy, and prolonged muscle weakness if paralytic agents are used for a prolonged period.

Pressure Support Ventilation and $PaCO_2$

PSV is normally set at the level needed to establish a normal V_T of 4 to 8 ml/kg IBW. To increase or decrease V_T, the clinician simply increases or decreases the PSV level and observes the resultant V_T on the ventilator exhaled volume monitoring screen. Because PSV is an assist mode, the patient is allowed to trigger the ventilator as desired. The result should be an adequate $PaCO_2$ and pH. In patients with an unstable ventilatory drive or periods of apnea, PSV should be avoided.

Pressure-Controlled Ventilation and $PaCO_2$

Management of ventilation and $PaCO_2$ during PCV is similar to PSV; the only difference between these two modes in a spontaneously breathing patient is the method of breath termination. With PSV, the breath is terminated as a result of the patient's inspiratory flow decreasing to the termination cycling flow, whereas in PA/C, the breath is terminated when the inspiratory time is reached. No other real differences in these modes exist in a spontaneously breathing patient.

To increase or decrease $PaCO_2$ in the PCV mode, the RT can simply increase or decrease the pressure limit while observing the exhaled V_T on the ventilator display monitor until desired V_T is obtained. The most important problem with the use of V_T to adjust $PaCO_2$ in the PCV mode is that the peak pressure should not be increased greater than 28 cm H_2O to avoid ventilator-induced lung injury.

In a patient receiving PCV, a change in the rate affects $PaCO_2$ in the same manner as in **volume-controlled ventilation**. If V_T remains constant, an increase in rate decreases $PaCO_2$ and vice versa. However, in the PCV mode, percent inspiratory time ($\%T_i$) and I:E ratio may be fixed. If $\%T_i$ is constant, and respiratory rate is increased, actual inspiratory time decreases, and V_T also may decrease. Decreases in rate ($\%T_i$ and pressure limit constant) may result in an increase in delivered V_T. The following example shows this principle.

A patient receiving ventilation in the PCV mode has a pressure control setting of 15 cm H_2O, PEEP of 5 cm H_2O, $\%T_i$ of 50%, I:E ratio of 1:1, and rate of 20 breaths/min. In this example, respiratory cycle time can be calculated as follows:

$$\text{Respiratory cycle} = 60/f = 60/20 = 3 \text{ seconds}$$

Inspiratory time (T_i) would be:

$$T_i = \%T_i \times \text{Respiratory cycle} = 0.50 \times 3 = 1.5 \text{ seconds}$$

A pressure of 25 cm H_2O applied for 1.5 seconds might achieve V_T of 400 ml for this patient.

If the rate were increased to 30 breaths/min, what would happen to respiratory cycle time, inspiratory time, and delivered V_T? Respiratory cycle and inspiratory time are calculated for a rate of 30 breaths/min as follows:

$$\text{Respiratory cycle} = 60/f = 60/30 = 2 \text{ seconds}$$
$$T_i = \%T_i \times \text{Respiratory cycle} = 0.50 \times 2 = 1 \text{ second}$$

At a constant pressure control setting of 15 cm H_2O, a decrease in inspiratory time from 1.5 seconds to 1 second may reduce delivered V_T. An increase in respiratory rate may reduce delivered V_T and increase (rather than decrease) $PaCO_2$.

When using PCV, the RT should observe the effect of inspiratory time and pressure limit on the patient's flow and volume curves as displayed by a ventilator graphics monitoring package. Generally, as inspiratory time increases at a given pressure, volume also increases until an inspiratory plateau or hold is reached. This point can be identified by observing the inspiratory flow curve. If the inspiratory flow curve decreases to zero and holds that value for a time before exhalation begins, an inspiratory plateau is present (Figure 48-10). Further increases in inspiratory time do not result in additional V_T. Conversely, if an inspiratory plateau or hold is present, a decrease in inspiratory time does not decrease V_T (at the same pressure limit) until the inspiratory plateau is no longer present (see Figure 48-10). Table 48-8 summarizes methods of altering $PaCO_2$ during VCV and PCV.

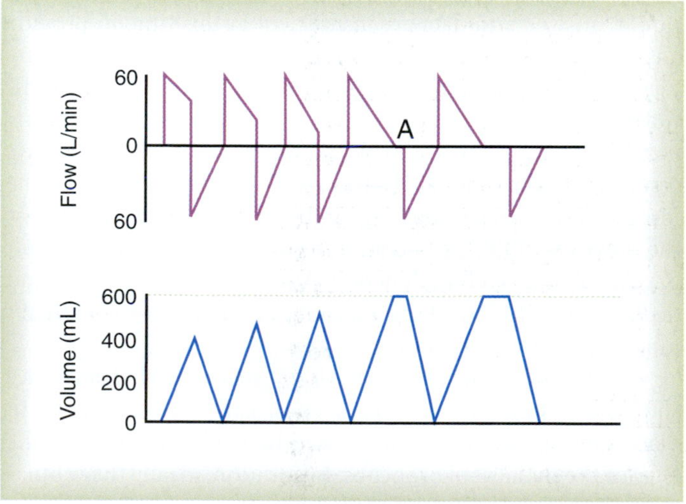

FIGURE 48-10 Effect of inspiratory time and inspiratory plateau on delivered V_T in the PCV mode. Initially, as inspiratory time is increased, V_T increases. When an inspiratory plateau *(A)* is achieved, a further increase in inspiratory time does not result in increased V_T. The same effect occurs as inspiratory time is decreased. Initially, with small decreases in inspiratory time, there would be no change in V_T as long as an end inspiratory plateau was maintained. When the inspiratory time is less than that needed for an inspiratory plateau, further decreases in inspiratory time result in a decrease in V_T at the same pressure.

$PaCO_2$ When Using Lung Protective Strategies for Acute Lung Injury and Acute Respiratory Distress Syndrome

Ventilation strategies for lung protection include low V_T, rapid respiratory rates, and permissive hypercapnia if necessary to avoid overdistention ($P_{plat} > 28$ cm H_2O).

Open Lung Approach

The use of a high PEEP, low V_T lung protective strategy using V_T of 4 to 8 ml/kg and PEEP set after a lung recruitment maneuver and decremental PEEP as discussed previously may improve mortality in patients with persistent ARDS.[24,25] Because V_T is reduced, respiratory rate should be increased incrementally up to 35 to 40 breaths/min. The limitation on rate is the development of auto-PEEP; if auto-PEEP does not develop, the rate can be increased. The primary concern in patients with severe ARDS is acidosis. However, most patients without severe sepsis, cardiovascular dysfunction, or renal failure can tolerate severe acidosis. The ARDS Clinical Network defined the limit for acidosis as pH less than 7.15.[2] $PaCO_2$, although important, should be allowed to increase before accepting V_T that results in P_{plat} greater than 28 mm Hg. The need to allow $PaCO_2$ to increase to avoid inducing lung injury is referred to as *permissive hypercapnia*. However, the goal is not to allow the $PaCO_2$ to increase but to avoid P_{plat} that may induce lung injury. With this approach in severe ARDS, V_T is frequently 4 to 5 ml/kg IBW, and $PaCO_2$ is greater than 60 mm Hg. Table 48-9 compares the effect of acute changes in $PaCO_2$ on pH.

TABLE 48-8

Changing Ventilation and $PaCO_2$

Mode Increase	Ventilation (↓ $PaCO_2$)	Decrease Ventilation (↑ $PaCO_2$)
Volume-Controlled Ventilation		
VC-CMV control	↑ V_T; ↑ f; remove V_{Dmach}	↓ V_T; ↓ f
VC-CMV assist control	↑ V_T; ↑ f (to greater than assist rate); remove V_{Dmach}	↓ VT; ↓ f (may require sedation, control mode)
SIMV	↑ VT; ↑ f; add/increase PSV; remove V_{Dmatch}	↓ VT; ↓ f; reduce PSV
Pressure-Controlled Ventilation		
PCV*	↑ ΔP; ↑ f (maintaining same T_i); remove V_{Dmatch}	↓ ΔP; ↓ f (maintaining same T_i)
PSV	↑ ΔP; remove V_{Dmatch}	↓ ΔP
Bilevel PAP	↑ IPAP (↑ ΔP); remove V_{Dmatch}	↓ IPAP (↓ ΔP)
APRV	↑ ΔP ↑ release frequency	↓ ΔP ↓ release frequency

Note: In assist (patient-triggered) mode, the patient may simply alter the trigger rate after a ventilator change, and it becomes difficult to predict the results of a ventilator change on $PaCO_2$ in the assist mode.

APRV, Airway pressure release ventilation; *IPAP,* inspiratory positive airway pressure.

*In PCV, if $\%T_i$ is preset, an increase in respiratory rate results in a decrease in inspiratory time and may reduce V_T. If $\%T_i$ is set at 50% in PCV mode, an increase in rate from 15 to 20 breaths/min causes inspiratory time to decrease from 2 seconds (50% of 4 seconds) to 1.5 seconds (50% of 3 seconds). If the pressure limit is not changed, V_T is likely to decrease.

MINI CLINI

Adjusting Ventilation in PA/C Mode

PROBLEM: A 70-kg (IBW) patient with ARDS is receiving PCV in the control mode with the following ventilator settings:
Pressure: 15 cm H_2O
Rate: 25 breaths/min
Inspiratory time: 0.8
FiO_2: 0.60
PEEP: 12 cm H_2O
V_T (exhaled): 425 ml

Arterial blood gas values with these ventilator settings are as follows:
PaO_2: 60 mm Hg
SaO_2: 90%
pH: 7.30
$PaCO_2$: 50 mm Hg
HCO_3: 23 mEq/L
Base excess: −2 mEq/L

The physician requests that the respiratory rate be increased to 18 breaths/min to decrease the patient's $PaCO_2$ to 40 mm Hg and normalize the pH. What should the RT do?

Solution: This patient has a PaO_2/FiO_2 ratio of 100 (60/0.60), which is consistent with the diagnosis of ARDS. Special considerations for the ventilatory management of ARDS include maintaining P_{plat} less than 28 cm H_2O. V_T is started at 8 ml/kg IBW and gradually reduced to 6 ml/kg IBW to achieve this goal and minimize ventilator-induced lung injury. Respiratory rate may be increased to maintain $PaCO_2$ and pH closer to normal, as long as volume and P_{plat} are acceptable. $PaCO_2$ may be allowed to increase if necessary to maintain P_{plat} less than 28 cm H_2O as long as pH is acceptable for the patient (usually >7.25). Oxygenation problems are managed initially with PEEP to achieve PaO_2 of 60 mm Hg or more with acceptable FiO_2. If PEEP fails to improve PaO_2, lung recruitment maneuvers and prone positioning may be used.

For this patient, the V_T is acceptable at approximately 6 ml/kg (70 kg × 6 ml/kg = 420 ml), and P_{plat} is 27 cm H_2O. $PaCO_2$ (50 mm Hg) and pH (7.30) are acceptable, and PEEP of 12 cm H_2O may be appropriate for a patient with ARDS. To decrease $PaCO_2$, the rate could be increased as follows:

$$\text{Initial} \qquad \text{Desired}$$
$$f_{(1)} \times PaCO_{2(1)} = f_{(2)} \times PaCO_2$$
$$25 \times 50 = f_{(2)} \times 40$$
$$f_{(2)}\ \text{Desired} = (25 \times 50/40) = 31.25$$

If V_T is maintained at 425 ml, a rate of 30 to 32 breaths/min should bring $PaCO_2$ and pH into normal range. However, if respiratory rate is increased, air trapping and auto-PEEP may develop. If auto-PEEP develops, V_T is likely to decrease. In pressure ventilation, an auto-PEEP increase is equal to an equivalent decrease in pressure control level, decreasing V_T. Rate should be increased cautiously, constantly evaluating the impact of the rate increase on V_T. More importantly, there is no reason to try to normalize $PaCO_2$ in this patient. $PaCO_2$ of 50 mm Hg with pH of 7.30 is acceptable.

TABLE 48-9
Effect of Acute Changes in $PaCO_2$ on pH

$PaCO_2$	pH
80	7.16
70	7.22
60	7.28
50	7.34
40	7.40
35	7.45
30	7.50
25	7.55
20	7.60

From Malley WJ: Clinical blood gases: assessment and intervention, ed 2, Philadelphia, 2005, Saunders.

When applying this approach, PEEP is set after it is determined by a lung recruitment maneuver and a decremental PEEP trial. V_T or pressure level is adjusted ensuring that P_{plat} or pressure control setting is less than 28 cm H_2O. Because V_T is small, inspiratory times can be short (frequently 0.6 to 0.8 second). The respiratory rate is set to achieve CO_2 elimination with its limit the development of auto-PEEP. Initially, FiO_2 is set to 1.0 but then titrated downward until PaO_2 is greater than 55 mm Hg. Generally, PEEP is sustained at the set level until FiO_2 is less than 0.5, and when PEEP is decreased, it should be decreased in increments of 2 cm H_2O no more frequently than about every 6 to 8 hours. If PaO_2 decreases when PEEP is decreased, the correct decision is to reestablish PEEP level, *not* increase FiO_2, because if this occurs, the lung is derecruited, and lung volume needs to be reestablished.

When to repeat a recruitment maneuver is a difficult question to answer, and data are insufficient at this time to provide an answer. However, if the PaO_2 does not decrease after the lung recruitment maneuver, there is no reason to perform an additional recruitment maneuver. Suctioning may cause derecruitment and hypoxemia, and ventilator discontinuation always results in derecruitment. If either of these situations occurs, the lung needs to be recruited again, but PEEP is reestablished at the previous PEEP level because the hypoxemia was *not* a result of deterioration in lung function. A recruitment maneuver and decremental PEEP trial should be repeated only if the patient's lung function deteriorates.

In all patients with severe ARDS, mechanical dead space should be eliminated, in-line suction catheters should be in place, and airway suctioning should be performed only to the level of the main stem bronchus. In addition, ideally the ventilator circuit should not be disconnected.

Other Lung Protective Strategies

Alternative techniques for facilitating CO_2 removal during lung protective ventilation in patients with ARDS include extracorporeal CO_2 removal (ECMO, see Chapter 50) reduction of CO_2 production by control of fever, avoidance of overfeeding, and neuromuscular paralysis. Patients with severe ARDS (PaO_2 < 150 mm Hg), should receive neuromuscular paralysis for the first 12 to 48 hours to allow for stabilization and titration of therapy. This has been shown to improve mortality in these patients.[68] Other authors have advocated the use of HFOV.[69-71] However, recent data in adults indicate that the use HFOV in ARDS patients results in poorer outcome then the continued use of conventional ventilation.[21,22] As a result, HFOV cannot be recommended in the management of ARDS.

SUMMARY CHECKLIST

- P_{plat} should ideally be maintained at less than 28 cm H_2O in all patients to prevent ventilator-induced lung injury.
- PEEP is used primarily to maintain lung volume resulting in improved oxygenation and lower FiO_2 in patients with severe oxygenation problems and refractory hypoxemia.
- Initially, all acutely ill patients should be ventilated with V_T of 4 to 8 ml/kg IBW with a respiratory rate to maintain adequate CO_2 removal.
- Patients with ARDS may begin mechanical ventilation with V_T of 8 ml/kg but may need volume adjusted to less than 6 ml/kg IBW to maintain P_{plat} less than 28 cm H_2O.
- Lung protective strategies in the management of ARDS include use of lower V_T (6 ml/kg), maintaining P_{plat} less than 28 cm H_2O, permissive hypercapnia, and PEEP set above the lower inflection point on the static pressure-volume curve.
- An open lung approach to mechanical ventilation includes the application of lung recruitment maneuvers, decremental PEEP trial, choosing V_T that maintains P_{plat} less than 28 cm H_2O, and accepting permissive hypercapnia.
- Inspiratory flow for most adult patients should be initially set at approximately 60 L/min or greater to achieve an inspiratory time of approximately 0.6 to 1 second.
- Patient ventilator synchrony is a major problem in patients during patient-triggered ventilation.
- In all modes of pressure ventilation, the pressure level should be set to ensure that V_T of 4 to 8 ml/kg IBW is delivered.
- When in doubt, initial FiO_2 should be set at 1.0.
- Auto-PEEP is a problem in patients with obstructive lung disease (COPD, asthma).
- In spontaneously breathing patients with COPD and auto-PEEP, applied PEEP should be added to ensure that all patient efforts result in triggering of the ventilator.
- An appropriate goal of PEEP would be to achieve PaO_2 60 to 80 mm Hg with FiO_2 less than 0.50.
- Alternative lung protective strategies in patients with ARDS include prone positioning and ECMO.
- Careful attention to acid-base homeostasis and the effect of $PaCO_2$ on pH is an essential part of ventilator management.

References

1. Hess DR, Kacmarek RM: *Essentials of mechanical ventilation*, ed 3, New York, 2013, McGraw-Hill.
2. The Acute Respiratory Distress Syndrome Network: Ventilation with lower tidal volumes as compared with traditional tidal volumes for acute lung injury and the acute respiratory distress syndrome. *N Engl J Med* 342:1301–1308, 2000.
3. Sutherasan Y, D'Antini D, Pelosi P: Advances in ventilator-associated lung injury: prevention is the target. *Expert Rev Respir Med* 8:233–248, 2014.
4. Chiumello D, Carlesso E, Cadringher P, et al: Lung stress and strain during mechanical ventilation for acute respiratory distress syndrome. *Am J Respir Crit Care Med* 178:346–355, 2008.
5. Kacmarek RM: The cost in some is an increase in the work of breathing: is it too high? (editorial). *Respir Care* 50:1624–1626, 2005.
6. Slutsky AS, Ranieri VM: Ventilator-induced lung injury. *N Engl J Med* 369:2126–2136, 2013.
7. Amoto MPB, Meade MO, Slutsky AS, et al: Driving pressure and survival in the acute respiratory distress syndrome. *N Engl J Med* 372:747–755, 2015.
8. Esteban A, Ferguson ND, Meade MO, et al: VENTILA Group: Evolution of mechanical ventilation in response to clinical research. *Am J Respir Crit Care Med* 177:170–177, 2008.
9. Tobin MJ: *Principles and practice of mechanical ventilation*, ed 2, New York, 2006, McGraw-Hill.
10. Marini JJ, Rodriguez RM, Lamb V: The inspiratory workload of patient-initiated mechanical ventilation. *Am Rev Respir Dis* 134:902, 1986.
11. Marini JJ, Capps JS, Culver BH: The inspiratory work of breathing during assisted mechanical ventilation. *Chest* 87:612, 1985.
12. Tobin MJ: Advances in mechanical ventilation. *N Engl J Med* 344:1986, 2001.
13. Esteban A, Anzueto A, Alia I, et al: How is mechanical ventilation employed in the intensive care unit? An international utilization review. *Am J Respir Crit Care Med* 161:1450, 2000.
14. Brochard L, Rauss A, Benito S, et al: Comparison of three methods of gradual withdrawal from ventilatory support during weaning from mechanical ventilation. *Am J Respir Crit Care Med* 150:896–903, 1994.
15. Estaban A, Frutos F, Tobin MJ, et al: A comparison of four methods of weaning patients from mechanical ventilation. *N Engl J Med* 332:345–350, 1995.
16. Williams P, Muelver M, Kratohvil J, et al: Pressure support and pressure assist/control: are there differences? An evaluation of the newest ICU ventilators. *Respir Care* 45:1169–1181, 2000.
17. Uchiyama A, Yoshida T, Yamanaka H, et al: Estimation of tracheal pressure and imposed expiratory work of breathing by the endotracheal tube, heat and moisture exchanger, and ventilator during mechanical ventilation. *Respir Care* 58:1157–1169, 2013.
18. Derdak S, Mehta S, Stewart TE, et al: High-frequency oscillatory ventilation for acute respiratory distress syndrome in adults: a randomized, controlled trial. *Am J Respir Crit Care Med* 166:801–808, 2002.
19. Bollen CW, Well G, Sherry T, et al: High frequency oscillatory ventilation compared with conventional mechanical ventilation in adult respiratory distress syndrome: a randomized controlled trial [ISRCTN2422669]. *Crit Care* 9:R430–R439, 2005.
20. Eastman A, Holland D, Higgins J, et al: High frequency percussive ventilation improves oxygenation in trauma patients with respiratory distress syndrome: a retrospective review. *Am J Surg* 192:191, 2006.
21. Ferguson ND, Cook DJ, Guyatt GH, et al: High-frequency oscillation in early acute respiratory distress syndrome. *N Engl J Med* 368:795–805, 2013.
22. Young D, Lamb SE, Shah S, et al: High-frequency oscillation for acute respiratory distress syndrome. *N Engl J Med* 368:806–813, 2013.
23. Jesus J, Kacmarek RM, Hedensternia G: From ventilator-induced lung injury to physician-induced lung injury: why the reluctance to use small tidal volumes? *Acta Anaesthesiol Scand* 48:267–271, 2004.
24. Amato MBP, Barbas CSV, Medeiros DM, et al: Effect of a protective-ventilation strategy on mortality in the acute respiratory distress syndrome. *N Engl J Med* 338:347–354, 1998.
25. Villar J, Kacmarek RM, Perez-Mendez L, et al: ARIES Network: A high positive end-expiratory pressure, low tidal volume ventilatory strategy improves outcome in persistent acute respiratory distress syndrome: a randomized, controlled trial. *Crit Care Med* 34:1311–1318, 2006.
26. Gajic O, Dara SI, Mendez JL, et al: Ventilator associated lung injury in patients without acute lung injury at the onset of mechanical ventilation. *Crit Care Med* 32:1817–1824, 2004.

27. Hill LL, Pearl RG: Flow triggering, pressure triggering and auto triggering during mechanical ventilation. *Crit Care Med* 28:579, 2000.
28. Sassoon CSH: Mechanical ventilator design and function: the trigger variable. *Respir Care* 37:1056, 1992.
29. Branson RD: Flow-triggering systems. *Respir Care* 39:138, 1994.
30. Oto J, Chenelle CT, Marchese AD, et al: A comparison of leak compensation in acute care ventilators during noninvasive and invasive ventilation: a lung model study. *Respir Care* 58:2027–2037, 2013.
31. Oto J, Chenelle CT, Marchese AD, et al: A comparison of leak compensation during pediatric noninvasive ventilation: a lung model study. *Respir Care* 59:241–251, 2014.
32. Rau JL, Shelledy DC: The effect of varying inspiratory flow waveforms on peak and mean airway pressures with a time-cycled volume ventilator: a bench study. *Respir Care* 36:347, 1991.
33. Lindahl S: Influence of an end inspiratory pause on pulmonary ventilation, gas distribution, and lung perfusion during artificial ventilation. *Crit Care Med* 7:540, 1979.
34. Langevin PB, Hellein V, Harms SM, et al: Synchronization of radiograph film exposure with the inspiratory pause: effect on the appearance of bedside chest radiographs in mechanically ventilated patients. *Am J Respir Crit Care Med* 160:2067, 1999.
35. Sethi J, Siegel MD: Mechanical ventilation in chronic obstructive lung disease. *Clin Chest Med* 21:799, 2000.
36. Mercat A, Richard JC, Vielle B, et al: Positive end-expiratory pressure setting in adults with acute lung injury and acute respiratory distress syndrome. *JAMA* 299:646–655, 2008.
37. Talmor D, Sarge T, Malhotra A, et al: Mechanical ventilation guided by esophageal pressure in acute lung injury. *N Engl J Med* 359:2095–2104, 2008.
38. Kacmarek RM, Villar J: Lung recruitment maneuvers during acute respiratory distress syndrome: is it useful? *Minerva Anestesiol* 77:85–89, 2011.
39. Gattinoni L, Caironi P, Cressoni M, et al: Lung recruitment in patients with acute respiratory distress syndrome. *N Engl J Med* 354:1175, 2006.
40. Phoenix SI, Paravastu S, Columb M, et al: Does a higher positive end expiratory pressure decrease mortality in acute respiratory distress syndrome? *Anesthesiology* 110:1098–1105, 2009.
41. Briel M, Meade M, Mercat A, et al: Higher vs lower positive end-expiratory pressure in patients with acute lung injury and acute respiratory distress syndrome: systematic review and meta-analysis. *JAMA* 303:865–873, 2010.
42. Bonmarchand G, Chevron V, Menard JF, et al: Effects of pressure ramp slope values on the work of breathing during pressure support ventilation in restrictive patients. *Crit Care Med* 27:715, 1999.
43. Branson RD, Campbell RS, Davis K, et al: Altering flow rate during maximum pressure support ventilation (PSV_{max}): effect on cardiorespiratory function. *Respir Care* 35:1056–1069, 1990.
44. Branson RD, Campbell RS: Pressure support ventilation, patient-ventilatory synchrony and ventilator algorithms. *Respir Care* 43:1045–1053, 1998.
45. American Association for Respiratory Care: AARC clinical practice guideline: humidification during mechanical ventilation. *Respir Care* 37:887, 1992.
46. Bendixen HH, Egbert LD, Hedley-Whyte J, et al: *Respiratory care*, St Louis, 1965, Mosby.
47. MacIntyre N: Of Goldilocks and ventilatory muscle loading. *Crit Care Med* 28:588, 2000.
48. Hickling KD: Best compliance during a decremental, but not incremental, positive end-expiratory pressure trial is related to open-lung positive end-expiratory pressure: a mathematical model of acute respiratory distress syndrome lung. *Am J Respir Crit Care Med* 163:69–78, 2001.
49. Suarez-Sipmann F, Bohm SH, Tusman G, et al: Use of dynamic compliance for open lung positive end-expiratory pressure titration in an experimental study. *Crit Care Med* 35:214–221, 2007.
50. O'Keefe GE, Gentilello LM, Erford S, et al: Imprecision in lower "inflection point" estimation from static pressure-volume curves in patients at risk for acute respiratory distress syndrome. *J Trauma* 44:1064, 1998.
51. Girgis K, Hamed H, Khater Y, et al: A decremental PEEP trial identifies the PEEP level that maintains oxygenation after lung recruitment. *Respir Care* 51:1132, 2006.
52. Medoff BD, Harris SR, Kesselman H, et al: Use of recruitment maneuvers and high positive end expiratory pressure in a patient with acute respiratory distress syndrome. *Crit Care Med* 28:1210, 2000.
53. Borges JB, Okamoto V, Gustavo M, et al: Reversibility of lung collapse and hypoxemia in early acute respiratory distress syndrome. *Am J Respir Crit Care Med* 174:268–278, 2006.
54. Lin SC, Alander A, Simonson DA, et al: Transient hemodynamic effects of recruitment maneuvers in three experimental models of acute lung injury. *Crit Care Med* 32:2371–2384, 2004.
55. Toth I, Leiner T, Mikor A, et al: Hemodynamic and respiratory changes during lung recruitment and descending optimal positive end-expiratory pressure titration in patients with acute respiratory distress syndrome. *Crit Care Med* 35:787–793, 2007.
56. Tugrul A, Akinci O, Ozcan PE, et al: Effects of sustained inflation and postinflation positive end-expiratory pressure in acute respiratory distress syndrome: focusing on pulmonary and extrapulmonary forms. *Crit Care Med* 31:738–744, 2003.
57. Drakulovic MB, Mm Hges A, Bauer TT, et al: Supine body position was a risk factor for nosocomial pneumonia in mechanically ventilated patients: a randomized trial. *Lancet* 354:1851, 1999.
58. Chatte G, Sab JM, Dubois JM, et al: Prone position in mechanically ventilated patients with severe acute respiratory failure. *Am J Respir Crit Care Med* 155:473–478, 1997.
59. Gattinoni L, Tognoni G, Pesnti A, et al: Effect of prone positioning on the survival of patients with acute respiratory failure. *N Engl J Med* 345:568–573, 2001.
60. Mancebo J, Fernandez R, Blanch L, et al: A multicenter trial of prolonged prone ventilation in severe acute respiratory distress syndrome. *Am J Respir Crit Care Med* 173:1233–1239, 2006.
61. Taccone P, Pesenti A, Latini R, et al: Prone positioning in patients with moderate and severe acute respiratory distress syndrome: a randomized controlled trial. *JAMA* 302:1977–1984, 2009.
62. Sud S, Friedrich JO, Taccone P, et al: Prone ventilation reduces mortality in patients with acute respiratory failure and severe hypoxemia: systematic review and meta-analysis. *Intensive Care Med* 36:585–599, 2010.
63. Curley MA: Prone positioning in patients with acute respiratory distress syndrome: a systematic review. *Am J Crit Care* 8:397, 1999.
64. Hirvela E: Advances in the management of acute respiratory distress syndrome: protective ventilation. *Arch Surg* 135:126, 2000.
65. Guérin C, Reignier J, Richard JC, et al: Prone positioning in severe acute respiratory distress syndrome. *N Engl J Med* 368:2159–2168, 2013.
66. Izurieta R, Rabatin J: Sedation during mechanical ventilation: a systematic review. *Crit Care Med* 30:2644–2648, 2002.
67. Girard TD, Kress JP, Fuchs BD, et al: Efficacy and safety of a paired sedation and ventilation weaning protocol for mechanically ventilated patients in intensive care (Awakening and Breathing Controlled trial): a randomized controlled trial. *Lancet* 371:126–134, 2008.
68. Papazian L, Forel JM, Gacouin A, et al: Neuromuscular blockers in early acute respiratory distress syndrome. *N Engl J Med* 363:1107–1116, 2010.
69. Derdak S, Mehta S, Stewart TE, et al: High-frequency oscillatory ventilation for acute respiratory distress syndrome in adults: a randomized, controlled trial. *Am J Respir Crit Care Med* 166:801–808, 2002.
70. Bollen CW, Well G, Sherry T, et al: High frequency oscillatory ventilation compared with conventional mechanical ventilation in adult respiratory distress syndrome: a randomized controlled trial [ISRCTN2422669]. *Crit Care* 9:R430–R439, 2005.
71. Mentzelopoulos SD, Malachias S, Tzoufi M, et al: High frequency oscillation and tracheal gas insufflation for severe acute respiratory distress syndrome. *Intensive Care Med* 33:S142, 2007.

CHAPTER 49

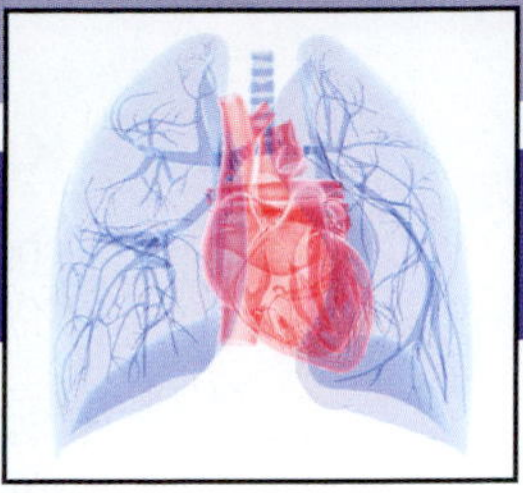

Noninvasive Ventilation

PURRIS F. WILLIAMS

CHAPTER OBJECTIVES

After reading this chapter you will be able to:

- List the goals and benefits of noninvasive ventilation (NIV).
- Discuss indications for NIV and the relative strength of the supporting evidence for each indication.
- List the selection and exclusion criteria for successful NIV.
- List the factors that predict successful NIV.
- Identify the types of patient interfaces available for NIV and how to choose an appropriate interface for a patient.
- Discuss the types of mechanical ventilators and ventilation modes used to provide NIV.
- Describe the role of the respiratory therapist during the initial application of NIV.
- Describe the ongoing ventilator management of NIV in the acute care setting.
- List potential complications associated with NIV, and suggest possible solutions.

CHAPTER OUTLINE

KEY TERMS

chest cuirass
continuous positive airway pressure (CPAP)
hypercapnic respiratory failure
hypoxemic respiratory failure
inspiratory positive airway pressure (IPAP)
iron lung
negative pressure ventilator
nocturnal hypoventilation
noninvasive positive pressure ventilation (NPPV)
noninvasive ventilation (NIV)
pneumobelt
rocking bed
Trendelenburg position

Noninvasive ventilation (NIV) is a means of delivering ventilatory support without using an invasive artificial airway, such as an endotracheal or tracheostomy tube. NIV can be provided by applying either negative or positive pressure to the airways. Almost any type of mechanical ventilator can be used to deliver NIV, and many noninvasive patient interfaces are available. However, at the present time, NIV is almost always delivered with a positive pressure ventilator designed specifically for noninvasive use or an ICU ventilator in conjunction with an oronasal or nasal mask. *NIV* is generally understood to include both **noninvasive positive pressure ventilation (NPPV)** and the noninvasive application of **continuous positive airway pressure (CPAP)**.

Interest in NIV has increased in recent years with the publication of findings from clinical trials using NIV in the management of respiratory failure. At the same time, technologically advanced noninvasive ventilators were introduced. Most intensive care unit (ICU) ventilators now include a specific noninvasive mode of ventilation. Improvements in the design of patient interfaces have made them more comfortable so that patients can tolerate NIV for longer periods. The net effect of these developments is that clinicians are using NIV more often than ever before in both acute and long-term care settings.[1] This chapter reviews the evidence supporting the use of NIV to manage various disease processes and makes recommendations on the types of patients and specific techniques for its successful application.

HISTORY AND DEVELOPMENT OF NONINVASIVE VENTILATION

Some early devices used for NIV relied on the intermittent application of abdominal pressure and the force of gravity to accomplish inspiration and expiration. These devices are most effective when used for patients with neuromuscular or neurologic disease in the absence of primary pulmonary disease. They are capable of generating tidal volume (V_T) in the range of 4 to 6 ml/kg predicted body weight (PBW) in appropriately selected patients.

First described in the 1930s, the **pneumobelt** consists of a rubber bladder that is strapped around the abdomen and connected to a positive pressure ventilator (Figure 49-1).[2] The pneumobelt is properly positioned above the pelvic arch and below the umbilicus. When inflated, the rubber bladder compresses the abdomen, pushes the diaphragm upward, and assists exhalation. On deflation of the rubber bladder, the abdominal contents and diaphragm move down, facilitating inspiration.[2] Because this device requires gravity to be effective, the patient must be sitting at an angle of at least 30 degrees.[3] Some abdominal mass is necessary for the pneumobelt to be effective. It does not work well in thin patients. Some patients with neuromuscular or neurologic disease and long-term dependence on a ventilator prefer the pneumobelt during daytime hours when they are out of bed and in a chair.[4]

The **rocking bed** (Figure 49-2) periodically rocks from the **Trendelenburg position** to reverse Trendelenburg position, using gravity to produce exhalation and inspiration. Rocking beds were used in the 1950s to wean patients from negative pressure ventilators and to provide long-term ventilatory support to patients following recovery from polio.[2] The main problem associated with the rocking bed is motion sickness. It can prevent patients from tolerating the device despite adequate ventilation.

Negative pressure ventilators were widely used from the late 1920s through the 1960s during the polio epidemic.[2] A **negative pressure ventilator** generates negative pressure within a chamber that surrounds the thorax. When pressure in the chamber decreases, the chest wall expands and intraalveolar pressure becomes negative, causing air to flow into the lung

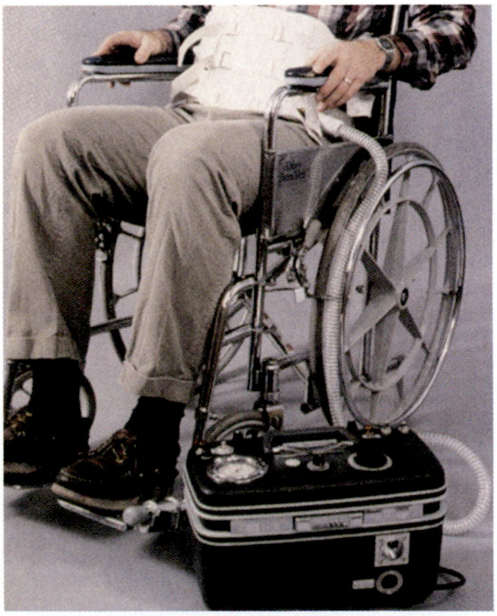

FIGURE 49-1 Pneumobelt, an intermittent abdominal pressure device. (From Albert RK, Spiro SG, Jett JR: Clinical respiratory medicine, ed 2, Philadelphia, 2004, Mosby.)

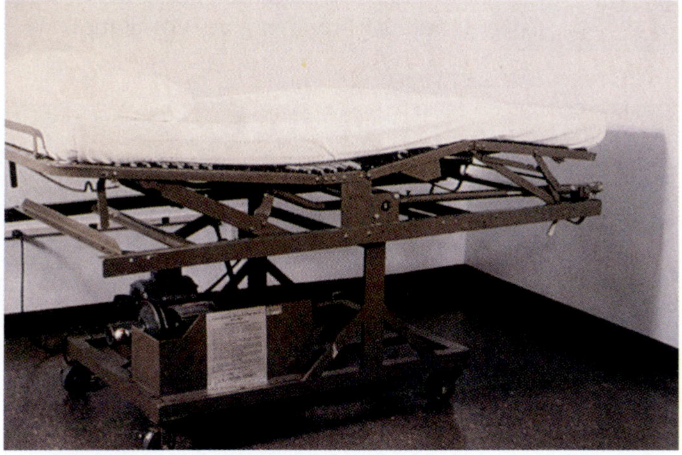

FIGURE 49-2 **A,** Rocking bed. **B,** Time-lapsed photography of the rocking bed in motion.

during inspiration. When the negative pressure is released, elastic recoil causes the lungs and chest wall to return to their normal size, resulting in passive exhalation. The first electrically powered negative pressure ventilator, known as the **iron lung** (Figure 49-3), surrounded the entire body from the neck down. Other designs were developed during that time, including the **chest cuirass**, which enclosed only the chest, the Porta-Lung, and the poncho wrap.[2] Effective negative pressure ventilation can be challenging to achieve if the device has air leaks or does not fit properly. Negative pressure ventilators that enclose the body limit caregiver access to the patient. In addition, collapse of the upper airway can occur during inspiration when excessive negative pressure is applied. With the development of positive pressure ventilators and the expanded use of NPPV, interest in negative pressure ventilation has greatly diminished.[2] Negative pressure ventilators are seldom seen in hospitals but some

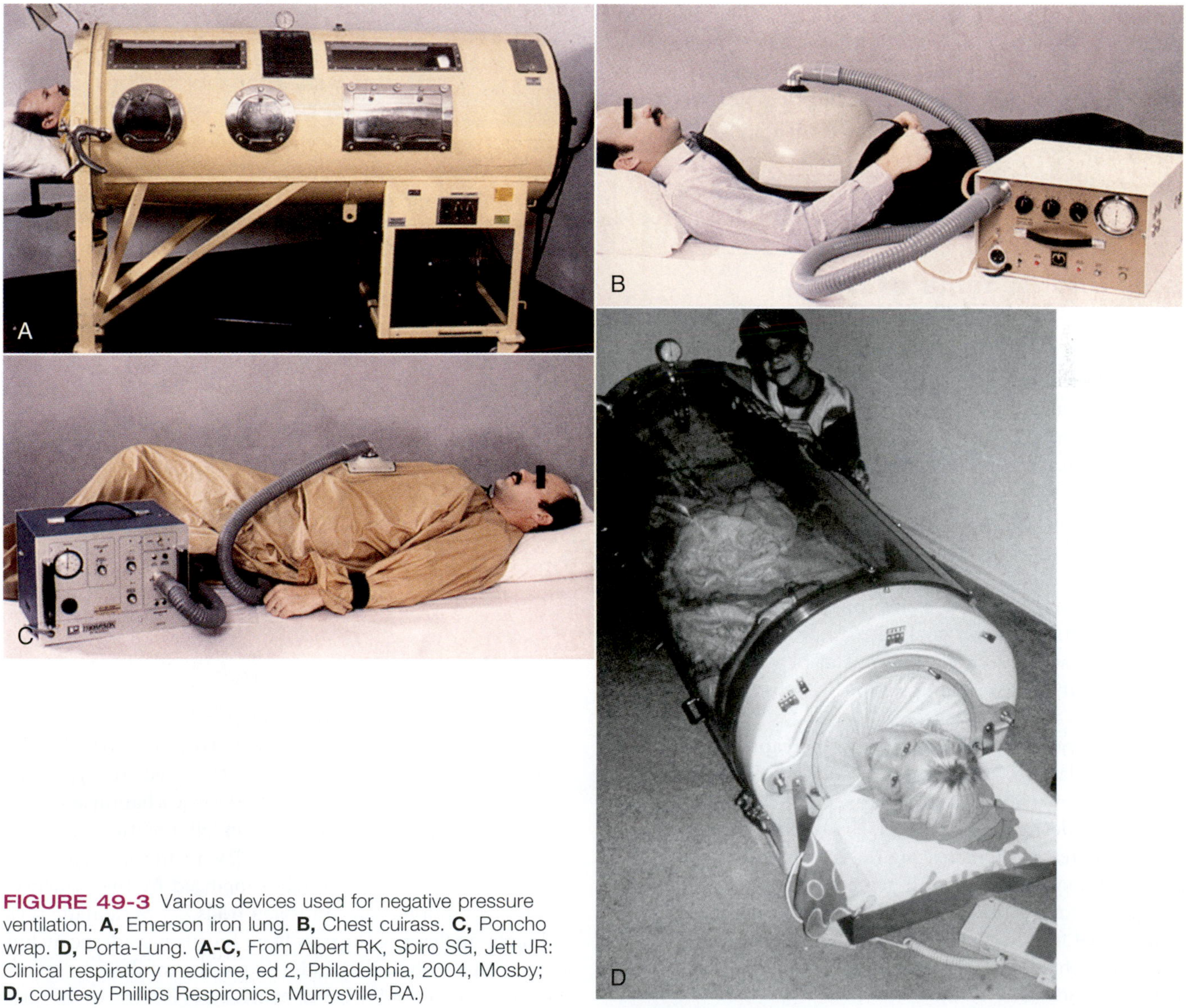

FIGURE 49-3 Various devices used for negative pressure ventilation. **A,** Emerson iron lung. **B,** Chest cuirass. **C,** Poncho wrap. **D,** Porta-Lung. (**A-C,** From Albert RK, Spiro SG, Jett JR: Clinical respiratory medicine, ed 2, Philadelphia, 2004, Mosby; **D,** courtesy Phillips Respironics, Murrysville, PA.)

continue to be used in the home by patients with chronic respiratory failure from neuromuscular diseases, such as polio.

The first reported use of NPPV was in 1780, when Chaussier used a bag and face mask during resuscitation.[1] However, widespread clinical use of NPPV did not begin until much later, with the introduction of intermittent positive pressure breathing in 1947.[1,2] Intermittent positive pressure breathing was primarily used to deliver aerosolized medications. The use of intermittent positive pressure breathing declined significantly in the mid-1980s[2] when the results of a randomized, controlled trial involving the treatment of patients with chronic obstructive pulmonary disease (COPD) showed no benefit compared to aerosol medication delivery with a small volume nebulizer.[5] Around this time, nasal mask CPAP was suggested as a therapy for obstructive sleep apnea.[6] Nasal masks also were used nocturnally in conjunction with positive pressure ventilators to provide rest for the respiratory muscles in patients with neuromuscular disorders.[7] In 1989, NPPV was used successfully to support 8 of 10 patients with acute respiratory failure (ARF).[8] Those positive findings renewed the interest in NIV that continues today. NIV has been used to treat a wide variety of clinical conditions in numerous trials during the past 20 years. The next section provides background and discussion focusing on the most relevant studies. Study findings are evaluated, and evidence-based recommendations for NIV are provided for each indication.

INDICATIONS FOR NONINVASIVE VENTILATION

Goals and Benefits of Using Noninvasive Ventilation

The hallmark of ARF is impaired gas exchange. The standard treatment to improve gas exchange in severe ARF is endotracheal intubation and mechanical ventilation. The primary goal of NIV is to improve gas exchange without endotracheal intubation. Significant complications associated with intubation can be prevented if NIV is applied successfully. The potential benefits of using NIV in the acute care setting include improving survival, decreasing the length of mechanical ventilation, decreasing the length of hospitalization, and decreasing the incidence of ventilator-associated pneumonia. In the long-term care setting, major goals are improving the patient's quality of life and relieving symptoms of hypoventilation. The goals of NIV in acute and long-term care settings are listed in Box 49-1.

The primary indication for NIV is **hypercapnic respiratory failure** secondary to COPD exacerbation. Hypercapnic ARF is characterized by inadequate alveolar ventilation, elevated arterial PCO_2 and decreased arterial pH. Hypoxemia may be present, but is easily treated by increasing the inspired oxygen concentration. Although patients with acute hypercapnic respiratory failure are the most likely to benefit from the use of NIV, it is also indicated for selected patients with hypoxemic respiratory failure or with respiratory failure resulting from numerous other conditions (Box 49-2).[2,9]

Box 49-1 Goals of Noninvasive Ventilation

ACUTE CARE SETTING
- Improve gas exchange
- Avoid intubation
- Decrease mortality
- Decrease length of time on ventilator
- Decrease length of hospitalization
- Decrease incidence of ventilator-associated pneumonia
- Relieve symptoms of respiratory distress
- Improve patient-ventilator synchrony
- Maximize patient comfort

LONG-TERM CARE SETTING
- Relieve or improve symptoms
- Enhance quality of life
- Avoid hospitalization
- Increase survival
- Improve mobility

Modified from Mehta S, Hill NS: Noninvasive ventilation. Am J Respir Crit Care Med 163:540, 2001.

Box 49-2 Acute and Chronic Disease Processes for Which Noninvasive Ventilation May Be Indicated

ACUTE CONDITIONS
- Hypercapnic respiratory failure
- COPD exacerbation
- Asthma
- Facilitation of extubation, especially in COPD
- Hypoxemic respiratory failure but cautiously
- Acute cardiogenic pulmonary edema
- Respiratory failure in immunocompromised patients
- End-of-life care and DNI orders
- Postoperative respiratory failure
- Prevention of reintubation in high-risk patients
- Postextubation respiratory failure

CHRONIC CONDITIONS
- Nocturnal hypoventilation
- Restrictive thoracic disease
- ALS
- COPD
- OHS

Acute Care Indications

Hypercapnic Respiratory Failure

Chronic Obstructive Pulmonary Disease. NIV should be considered the standard of care for treatment of hypercapnic respiratory failure secondary to COPD exacerbation and should be available as first-line therapy in all institutions treating patients with COPD. The use of NIV in the management of COPD exacerbation is strongly supported by the evidence in numerous randomized, controlled trials.[10-16] Systematic review and meta-analyses of the data from fourteen studies concluded that patients with COPD and ARF require intubation less often when they receive NIV. Other benefits of NIV use in this group of patients include lower risk of mortality, fewer complications and reduced length of hospital stay.[10-13]

Early intervention with NIV should be considered before severe respiratory acidosis develops. However, NIV can be used successfully and safely in much sicker patients. Successful application of NIV has occurred in patients with hypercapnic coma and in awake, noncomatose patients. Severe hypercapnea and decreased level of consciousness should not be considered absolute contraindications to a cautious trial of NIV in selected patients.

RULE OF THUMB

All patients with an acute COPD exacerbation should be evaluated for NIV as an alternative to intubation and invasive mechanical ventilation. NIV is the standard of care in these patients.

Asthma

The evidence for NIV use in the management of ARF caused by severe asthma is inconclusive. Meduri and colleagues[17] reported positive results in an uncontrolled study using NIV to treat 17 patients in status asthmaticus. Other studies have reported using NIV successfully to manage ARF in patients with asthma[18-21] but no randomized, controlled trials have been performed. The role of NIV in this patient population remains controversial because of weak supportive evidence. Routine management with NIV is not recommended in asthmatic patients with ARF. If patients with severe asthma receive a trial of NIV, they must be monitored closely. Significant improvement in the symptoms of respiratory failure should be evident within 1 to 2 hours, and if improvement is not evident, intubation should proceed without delay.

Facilitation of Weaning in Chronic Obstructive Pulmonary Disease

Several randomized controlled studies have reported success using NIV to facilitate weaning from mechanical ventilation in patients with COPD who failed at least one spontaneous breathing trial (SBT).[15,22,23,24] In addition, NIV was associated with more successful weaning and lower mortality after 60 days. There is reasonable evidence that difficult-to-wean patients with COPD who were intubated for ARF and subsequently failed SBTs should be considered for an elective trial extubation directly to NIV. Ideally, the patients selected should have used NIV previously and should meet none of the NIV exclusion criteria. The failure of NIV to prevent intubation does not preclude its successful use at a later time.

RULE OF THUMB

A trial extubation directly to NIV should be considered for patients with COPD and hypercapnic ARF who are likely to receive a tracheostomy for failure to wean.

Hypoxemic Respiratory Failure

Hypoxemic respiratory failure, defined by a PaO_2/fractional inspired oxygen (FiO_2) ratio less than 300, can result from several distinct causes. Clinical trials of NIV to manage acute hypoxemic respiratory failure have yielded conflicting results. The efficacy of NIV largely depends on the etiology of the hypoxemia. Further study is needed to determine clearly the types of patients who would benefit from NIV.

Acute Cardiogenic Pulmonary Edema

In 1991, mask CPAP was shown to improve hypoxemia and reduce the need for intubation in patients with severe cardiogenic pulmonary edema.[25] Similar findings in other randomized controlled trials provide strong evidence that both CPAP[25-27] and NPPV[28-30] improve outcomes in these patients compared with simple oxygen (O_2) therapy.[31-35] Mask CPAP of 8 to 12 cm H_2O and 100% O_2 is first-line therapy to treat hypoxemia associated with severe cardiogenic pulmonary edema. NPPV should be reserved for patients with both hypercapnia and hypoxemia. Extra caution is recommended for patients who present with cardiac ischemia, hemodynamic instability, arrhythmias, or depressed mental status. Patients with these risk factors should be intubated and invasively ventilated.[31]

RULE OF THUMB

CPAP of 8 to 12 cm H_2O with 100% O_2 should be considered first-line therapy in acute pulmonary edema. NPPV should be used only when hypercapnia is present.

Pneumonia

NIV has been used in the management of severe community-acquired pneumonia, but with mixed results. Similar to other applications of NIV for hypoxemic respiratory failure, care should always be exercised and clinicians should always error on the conservative side. That is, if the patient's status does not improve within a few hours of application, invasive ventilation should be initiated. Additional studies are needed. The current recommendation for the use of NIV in pneumonia is to limit its routine use to patients who also have COPD.[36]

Acute Lung Injury and Acute Respiratory Distress Syndrome

Several studies have reported failure rates greater than 50% when NIV is used to treat acute lung injury (ALI) and acute respiratory distress syndrome (ARDS).[37-40] Patients with risk factors such as hemodynamic instability, metabolic acidosis, or profound hypoxemia are more likely to fail NIV.[38] Survey data from centers in the United States and Europe with extensive experience using NIV indicate that more than 60% of patients with hypoxemic respiratory failure required intubation, with greater than 60% mortality.[40] More recently, positive findings were reported in a prospective multicenter survey that used NIV as the first-line intervention in selected patients with ALI/ARDS.[41] Results showed that 54% avoided intubation with improved outcome. Failure was predicted if PaO_2/FiO_2 ratio was less than 175 after the first hour of NIV. Three randomized controlled trials in patients with ALI/ARDS found that NIV decreased intubation rate and mortality, resulting in improved outcome.[40,42,43] However, a meta-analysis of these trials indicated that NIV did not decrease mortality despite a reduction in intubation rate,[42] and this analysis was consistent with other reports.[42]

Another randomized controlled trial[44] in patients with hypoxemic respiratory failure but no hypercapnia showed that mask CPAP significantly improved PaO_2/FiO_2 ratio within the first hour but failed to reduce the intubation rate, length of ICU stay, or hospital mortality. In this study, many patients who failed CPAP sustained cardiac arrest during intubation.[44] It is thought that clinicians delayed intubation because they did not readily accept the failure of NIV to correct hypoxemia in these patients. The evidence to date does not support routine NIV use in patients with ALI/ARDS, but randomized controlled trials focusing exclusively on ALI/ARDS are needed.[9] The data suggest that a closely monitored trial of NIV in carefully selected patients may be appropriate. If NIV does not markedly improve hypoxemia within 1 to 2 hours, patients should be intubated.

Respiratory Failure in Immunosuppressed Patients

The risk of developing nosocomial infections, including ventilator-associated pneumonia, is decreased when NIV is used compared with intubation and invasive mechanical ventilation. Randomized controlled trials involving immunosuppressed patients and patients awaiting solid organ transplantation[45-50] who developed hypoxemic respiratory failure found decreased intubation rates and mortality with NIV compared with standard therapy. NIV in patients with AIDS and *Pneumocystis carinii* pneumonia showed similar results.[49] Despite the small numbers of patients in these single-center trials, NIV is accepted as first-line therapy in immunosuppressed patients because it avoids the risk of infection[50-52] associated with intubation in a setting where an infection can have devastating consequences.

Palliative Care and Do-Not-Intubate Orders

The use of NIV in patients with do-not-intubate (DNI) orders and end-stage disease remains controversial. Patients with DNI orders may receive NIV either for supportive treatment of a nonterminal, reversible event or for palliative care. There is evidence that NIV in patients with end-stage disease provides an effective method of support with some relief from associated symptoms.[53] Two more recent case series[52,53] support the use of NIV in the management of ARF in patients with DNI orders. Schettino and colleagues[52] and Levy and coworkers[53] showed that more than 65% of patients with COPD or cardiogenic pulmonary edema and DNI status were successfully managed with NIV. Palliative care focuses on relieving the symptoms and stress from serious diseases. The goals of NIV in this setting are to minimize feelings of dyspnea and improve the patient's comfort. If the patient is not more comfortable with NIV, it should be discontinued.

The primary controversy over the use of NIV in patients with DNI orders involves patient consent. NIV can be beneficial in the care of patients with DNI orders if a patient understands that NIV is a form of life support and that its goal is either to reverse an acute disease process or to provide comfort at the end of life.[54] Clinicians should take the time to explain NIV and its goals as part of the discussion with the patient and family about wishes for life-sustaining treatment.

Postoperative Respiratory Failure

A number of investigators have used NIV in the postoperative period.[55-57] In these studies NIV was beneficial in the postoperative management of obese patients post gastroplasty, or following other major abdominal surgery and thoracic surgery.

MINI CLINIC

Noninvasive Ventilation to Treat Hypoxemic Acute Respiratory Failure

PROBLEM: A patient with acute hypoxemic respiratory failure is receiving NIV via nasal mask with a noninvasive ventilator. The ventilator is delivering PSV with peak inspiratory pressure set at 12 cm H_2O and end expiratory pressure set at 5 cm H_2O. O_2 at 6 L/min is flowing into the nasal mask. After 40 minutes on NIV, the patient continues to have signs of respiratory distress (dyspnea, tachypnea with respiratory rate 30, heart rate 120 beats/min, SpO_2 88%, and cyanosis). The patient is having difficulty keeping his mouth closed, and there is a large air leak as a result. An arterial blood gas was drawn, and PaO_2 is 50 mm Hg.

Solutions

1. Change the interface to a full-face mask to prevent the air leak and provide more effective ventilator support. A chin strap could be tried but is not likely to be successful. Dyspneic patients tend to breathe through their mouths preferentially.
2. Change to a ventilator that can provide precise, high FiO_2; displays graphics; calculates exhaled volumes; and has alarms. Bleeding in O_2 to the mask or circuit provides only low, inconsistent FiO_2. Additional information from waveforms and calculated values can help provide better assessments and interventions. For a patient this sick, alarms are an important consideration.
3. Increase PEEP to 8 to 10 to maintain alveoli open and improve severe hypoxemia; 5 cm H_2O is probably inadequate in this situation.
4. If these interventions do not result in significant improvement in oxygenation within 30 to 45 minutes, the patient should be electively intubated and ventilated. Delaying intubation is associated with greater risk of death during intubation. Such delays can result if clinicians do not recognize an unsuccessful NIV trial in the setting of hypoxemia.

Although the results of these studies are encouraging, additional randomized trials are needed to identify specific postoperative populations that would benefit from NPPV or CPAP. At the present time, there is insufficient evidence to support routine postoperative use of NIV.

Prevention of Reintubation in High-Risk Patients

Reintubation has been associated with increased mortality, longer hospital stay, and a greater need for long-term care than in patients who are initially successfully extubated. In recent studies, Nava and colleagues[58] and Ferrer and coworkers[59] randomly assigned patients at risk for reintubation to NIV or standard care; both studies showed lower reintubation rates with NIV. Patients with hypercapnia gained the most benefit from NIV. Risk factors associated with extubation failure included a diagnosis of COPD or congestive heart failure, age older than 65 years, ineffective cough and excessive secretions, upper airway obstruction, history of one or more weaning failures, one or more comorbid conditions, and Acute Physiology and Chronic Health Evaluation (APACHE) II score greater than 12 on the day of extubation.

Sufficient evidence exists to support selective application of NIV to avoid reintubation and its associated negative impact on outcome. NIV should be started after extubation of patients with multiple risk factors, especially patients with COPD, congestive heart failure, or hypercapnia. These patients should be monitored closely and reintubated promptly if NIV does not prevent respiratory distress.

Postextubation Respiratory Failure

The use of NIV to manage postextubation hypoxemic respiratory failure requires a cautious approach. Two randomized controlled trials[60,61] indicated no benefit or worse outcome when NIV was used to manage hypoxemic ARF. Keenan and associates[60] compared NIV and standard therapy in patients who developed hypoxemic respiratory failure during the first 2 days after extubation and observed a 70% reintubation rate in both groups. Esteban and colleagues[61] randomly assigned patients to standard therapy or NIV at the first sign of postextubation respiratory distress. Both groups had a 50% reintubation rate, but the group managed with NIV had higher mortality. This finding was attributed to the delay in reintubation that occurred in the NIV group. Relatively few patients with COPD were included in these two studies. The use of NIV to treat postextubation ARF generally should be reserved for patients with COPD and hypercapnic respiratory failure or patients with congestive heart failure. If hypoxemia does not significantly improve with NIV, these patients should be reintubated without delay.

RULE OF THUMB

Before using NIV in the management of ARF, be sure the process causing respiratory failure is reversible, selection criteria are met, and exclusion criteria are absent.

Long-Term Care Indications

Nocturnal Hypoventilation

Nocturnal hypoventilation is common with neuromuscular diseases, severe kyphoscoliosis, COPD, obesity, and central and obstructive sleep apnea.[62] Patients with these disorders are able to breathe spontaneously without assistance but typically have symptoms related to hypoventilation and sleep-disordered breathing. These symptoms may include excessive sleepiness during daytime hours; fatigue; morning headaches; and cognitive dysfunction, such as difficulty concentrating.[63]

Normally, the onset of sleep is characterized by a slight increase in $PaCO_2$ followed by a further increase in hypercapnia during rapid eye movement (REM) sleep. It is thought that the increased work of breathing associated with obesity and COPD or the muscle weakness caused by neuromuscular diseases results in greater levels of hypercapnia. Some of these patients are hyporesponsive to carbon dioxide (CO_2), which contributes to even more CO_2 retention. In response, the kidneys attempt to compensate by retaining bicarbonate, reducing respiratory drive further. This vicious cycle progressively worsens, leading to pulmonary hypertension, cor pulmonale, CO_2 narcosis, and eventually death.[64,65] There is strong evidence that the cycle can be stopped if breathing is assisted by NIV for 4 hours per night for 1 to 3 months.[66,67] One study suggested that NIV use during the daytime hours promotes similar improvement in gas exchange during periods of unassisted ventilation as seen when NIV is used at night.[68]

Three mechanisms have been proposed to explain the positive effects of NIV on nocturnal hypoventilation. First, it was thought that NIV rests fatigued respiratory muscles, improving their performance during the day.[69,70] Common sense supports this hypothesis, but few studies have been able to show significant or sustained improvement in muscle strength after using NIV.[71] Second, NIV reduces $PaCO_2$ and may reset the central ventilatory controller to a lower baseline $PaCO_2$. Current evidence suggests that NIV is effective because it prevents nocturnal hypoventilation and preserves ventilatory response to increases in CO_2 in patients with COPD or restrictive thoracic diseases.[65,68-71] Third, the improvements in lung compliance, lung volume, and dead space that result from NIV may be beneficial.[66]

Restrictive Thoracic Diseases

Restrictive thoracic diseases successfully managed with NIV include postpolio syndrome, neuromuscular diseases, chest wall deformities, spinal cord injuries, and severe kyphoscoliosis.[66] Patients with severe kyphoscoliosis showed improved nighttime and daytime gas exchange, fewer symptoms of hypoventilation, and increased spontaneous V_T and FVC after using NIV.[68-71] A study of eight patients with Pompe disease found that NIV corrected arterial blood gas abnormalities and resolved cor pulmonale 3 to 6 months after starting NIV.[72] Disease progression was not slowed by NIV. Diaphragmatic weakness is characteristic of this disease, in contrast to most other neuromuscular diseases.[72] In patients with Duchenne muscular dystrophy, a rapidly progressive neuromuscular disorder, nocturnal NIV failed to slow progression of the disease and was associated with a higher mortality.[73]

The current recommendation for patients with restrictive thoracic disorders is to initiate NIV when patients develop symptoms of nocturnal hypoventilation. There is little evidence to support prophylactic NIV in patients with most restrictive thoracic diseases.

Amyotrophic Lateral Sclerosis

Amyotrophic lateral sclerosis (ALS), also known as *Lou Gehrig's disease,* is a neurodegenerative disease that affects motor neurons, resulting in progressive skeletal muscle weakness and paralysis. Mean survival time is 3 to 5 years after diagnosis. All patients with ALS eventually need full ventilatory support to survive. NIV is probably effective in prolonging the lives of patients with ALS.[74]

In a randomized controlled trial, Bourke and associates[75] found that patients with ALS who used NIV gained a median survival benefit of 205 days but only in the absence of bulbar dysfunction. Evidence suggests that using NIV slows the rate of lung function decline as indicated by FVC measurement.[75,76] Lung function decline occurs more slowly and survival benefit increases when NIV is used for more than 4 hours per day.[76] Several factors influencing compliance with NIV of patients with ALS have been identified. Early intervention[77] and orthopnea[78] correlated with better tolerance of NIV, whereas bulbar involvement[75,79] and the presence of cognitive or executive dysfunction[80] negatively affected compliance with NIV.

In contrast to other restrictive thoracic diseases, there may be a survival benefit when NIV is initiated earlier in the course of ALS. In one study, patients experiencing more than 15 episodes of nocturnal O_2 desaturation per hour were started on NIV.[81] This "early" intervention resulted in survival lasting 11 months longer and suggested that NIV may also provide some benefit in patients with bulbar involvement.[81] More studies are needed to assess the effects of early NIV initiation.

Clinicians in the acute care setting have conflicting feelings about initiating NIV in patients with ALS, expressing concerns about the patients' quality of life and eventual dependence on NIV. Four studies found that NIV had a positive effect on patients' quality of life.[78,81,82,83] Positive changes associated with NIV included relief from dyspnea, increased energy and vitality, better concentration, less physical fatigue, and fewer symptoms of hypoventilation.[34] There was no difference in the perceived quality of life of patients using NIV compared with patients who received invasive mechanical ventilation through a tracheostomy.[83] However, invasive ventilation through a tracheostomy tube may have a negative effect on caregivers' quality of life. Most patients were comfortable with their decisions involving assisted ventilation with 94% of patients receiving NIV and 81% of patients with a tracheostomy indicating that they would choose ventilation again.[83]

There is good evidence that using NIV lengthens survival and slows the decline of lung function of patients with ALS. In its evidence-based Practice Parameters, the American Academy of Neurology recommended considering NIV for all patients with ALS and respiratory failure.[78] NIV is typically started when pulmonary function declines significantly (FVC < 50%). Although the evidence supporting early NIV initiation is weak, starting NIV at the first sign of nocturnal hypoventilation may be considered to improve compliance with NIV.

RULE OF THUMB

Patients with restrictive thoracic disorders should have symptoms of nocturnal hypoventilation before NIV is considered.

Chronic Obstructive Pulmonary Disease in Patients Needing Long-Term Care

There are two proposed hypotheses to explain how patients with severe COPD benefit from the use of NIV.[66] First, positive inspiratory pressure improves gas exchange and may unload the respiratory muscles, allowing them to recover, gain strength, and reduce fatigue resulting in improved quality of life. Second, NIV should decrease the symptoms of nocturnal hypoventilation and sleep-disordered breathing, improving sleep quality and daytime gas exchange.[66]

The use of NIV in the management of stable COPD is controversial. Struik and colleagues conducted a systematic review of 7 randomized controlled studies of NIV used by patients with stable COPD.[84] They found no significant improvement in $PaCO_2$ and PaO_2; pulmonary function measurements, exercise tolerance, or perceived quality of life after 3 or 12 months on NIV use. The authors did note that lower $PaCO_2$ was associated with high IPAP setting (18 cm H_2O), compliance with therapy (5 hours of NIV per night), and higher baseline $PaCO_2$ (55 mm Hg). At the present time, there is not enough evidence to support routine treatment with NIV in patients with stable COPD.[85,86]

RULE OF THUMB

NIV should be considered for management of respiratory failure in patients with ALS because it probably slows the rate of decline of lung function and lengthens survival.

Obesity-Hypoventilation Syndrome

Obesity-hypoventilation syndrome (OHS) is defined as chronic daytime hypoventilation ($PaCO_2$ >45 mm Hg) associated with obesity (body mass index >30 kg/m^2) when no other known cause for hypoventilation is present. Approximately 0.5% of women and 1% of men in the general population are estimated to have OHS.[87] Evidence suggests that OHS is a common yet underdiagnosed condition in extremely obese patients.[88] Obese patients consume many health care resources before a diagnosis of OHS is made,[89] which is a cause for concern as obesity becomes more prevalent in the United States. In a study of hospitalized obese patients, Nowbar and colleagues[90] found that hypercapnia with no other reason for hypoventilation was present in approximately one-third of patients with body mass index greater than 35 kg/m^2 and almost one-half of patients with body mass index greater than 50 kg/m^2.

Several studies showed improved daytime gas exchange and relief of symptoms associated with nocturnal hypoventilation within 1 to 4 months of initiation of NIV.[91-93] A randomized trial of CPAP versus NPPV in patients with OHS without severe nocturnal desaturations found that both modes were equally effective in decreasing daytime $PaCO_2$.[93] At the present time, nocturnal NPPV is recommended for OHS when nasal CPAP and other first-line therapies fail to alleviate the hypoventilation.[66,94]

MINI CLINI

Preventing a High-Risk Patient from Requiring Reintubation

PROBLEM: A 74-year-old man was intubated for hypercapnic respiratory failure 3 days ago. Past medical history is significant for hypertension, coronary artery disease, COPD, and former cigarette smoker ×35 years (quit 10 years ago). He is currently on low-level PSV (PSV 8, PEEP 5 cm H_2O, FiO_2 0.3). Vital signs are heart rate 80 beats/min, blood pressure 130/70 mm Hg, respiratory rate 16 breaths/min, and SpO_2 95%. Endotracheal suctioning has been performed every 2 to 3 hours for moderate to large amounts of yellow secretions. Ipratropium MDI, 2 puffs every 6 hours, is ordered. He was placed on a spontaneous breathing trial this morning and passed; however, his ability to clear secretions is a concern. After much discussion among the patient care team, the decision was made not to extubate as planned.

Solutions

1. Extubate and immediately start NIV. Evidence supports using NIV to prevent reintubation in high-risk patients. Patients with hypercapnia are most likely to benefit. Other factors associated with high risk of extubation failure are age older than 65, COPD, and excessive secretions.
2. Continue aerosolized bronchodilators by delivering the MDI to a collapsible holding chamber added to the NIV circuit. Place the chamber between the exhalation port and the mask. Coordinate MDI actuation as closely as possible to the patient's own inspiration. Shake the MDI canister between each actuation to mix the propellant and the drug. These three points are important to deliver maximum medication to the patient.

SELECTING APPROPRIATE PATIENTS FOR NONINVASIVE VENTILATION

Acute Care Setting

The success or failure of NIV depends to a large degree on the clinician's clinical judgment in choosing appropriate patients. The primary selection criterion is the need for ventilatory assistance resulting from ARF. Patients who are unable to ventilate adequately on their own typically show signs and symptoms of respiratory distress, including use of accessory muscles, paradoxical breathing, tachypnea, and dyspnea.[2,9] In addition, patients in ARF are unable to maintain normal gas exchange and usually develop respiratory acidosis or severe hypoxemia (Box 49-3).[2,9]

NIV exclusion criteria include apnea, hemodynamic or cardiac instability, lack of cooperation by the patient, conditions that preclude use of a noninvasive interface, copious amounts of secretions, and high risk of aspiration (Box 49-4).[2,9] Decreased level of consciousness should not be considered an exclusion criterion for NIV in patients with COPD.[95,96] If the selection criteria are met and there are no contraindications, NIV should be considered.

It is important to consider the cause of ARF because the efficacy of NIV varies depending on the underlying condition being treated. In the acute care setting, most evidence supports the use of NIV in patients with COPD exacerbations or acute cardiogenic pulmonary edema. There is less evidence supporting NIV for the other indications discussed earlier; however, it is being used more frequently for patients with DNI orders, to facilitate extubation of high-risk patients, and as a means of preventing extubation failure and reintubation. Several studies identified potential predictors of success during NIV (Box 49-5). Early initiation of NIV is encouraged in patients with

Box 49-3 Noninvasive Ventilation Selection Criteria for Patients With Acute Respiratory Failure

Two or more of the following should be present:

- Use of accessory muscles
- Paradoxical breathing
- Respiratory rate ≥25 breaths/min
- Moderate to severe dyspnea (increased dyspnea in COPD patients)
- $PaCO_2$ >45 mm Hg with pH <7.35
- PaO_2/FIO_2 ratio <200

Modified from Mehta S, Hill NS: Noninvasive ventilation. Am J Respir Crit Care Med 163:540, 2001.

Box 49-4 Exclusion Criteria for Noninvasive Ventilation in Patients With Acute Respiratory Failure

- Apnea
- Inability to protect airway/high aspiration risk
- Hemodynamic or cardiac instability
- Lack of patient cooperation
- Inability to use a noninvasive interface because of facial burns, trauma, or abnormal anatomy
- Excessive amounts of secretions

Modified from Mehta S, Hill NS: Noninvasive ventilation. Am J Respir Crit Care Med 163:540, 2001.

Box 49-5 Predictors of Noninvasive Ventilation Success in the Acute Care Setting

- Minimal air leak
- Low severity of illness
- Respiratory acidosis ($PaCO_2$ >45 mm Hg but <92 mm Hg)
- pH <7.35 but >7.22
- Improvement in gas exchange within 1 to 2 hours of initiation
- Improvement in respiratory rate and heart rate

Modified from Mehta S, Hill NS: Noninvasive ventilation. Am J Respir Crit Care Med 163:540, 2001.

ARF because severe hypercapnia and acidosis are predictors of NIV failure.[97] Significant improvements in $PaCO_2$ and pH after 30 to 120 minutes of NIV are predictive of success.[98-100] In some cases, clinical judgment precludes an NIV trial based on the severity of the respiratory failure or the presence of comorbid conditions that increase the likelihood of failure to respond to NIV. However, in many situations, a reasonable plan would be a trial of NIV for 1 to 2 hours, with periodic reassessment and plans to intubate if the patient's condition does not significantly improve. Successful application of NIV includes short-term goals of improving gas exchange and preventing endotracheal intubation and long-term goals of improved outcome, decreased length of stay, and decreased mortality.

Long-Term Care Setting

The current recommended selection guidelines for NIV in restrictive thoracic disease may be separated into two parts. First, patients should have symptoms of chronic hypoventilation and lack of sleep quality. Second, patients should meet one of the following measurable parameters: $PaCO_2$ 45 mm Hg or greater, nocturnal O_2 saturation less than 88% for 5 minutes, maximal inspiratory pressure less than 60 cm H_2O, or FVC less than 50% of predicted.[66] Although a decline in pulmonary function has been associated with CO_2 retention, more evidence is needed to support the use of a declining maximal inspiratory pressure or FVC as an indication for NIV.[2]

Recommendations for use of NIV in the management of nocturnal hypoventilation caused by disorders other than restrictive lung disease and COPD include documentation of a disorder that causes hypoventilation and failure of the disorder to respond to first-line therapy. First-line therapy includes weight loss, O_2 therapy, respiratory stimulants, and CPAP. NIV is recommended as the initial therapy for moderate to severe cases of nocturnal hypoventilation.[66]

Patients with COPD and signs and symptoms of chronic hypoventilation and poor quality of sleep should receive optimal medical treatment before NIV is recommended.[66] If symptoms remain despite optimal management, the presence of one of the following selection criteria indicates the need for NPPV: $PaCO_2$ 55 mm Hg or greater or $PaCO_2$ 50 to 54 mm Hg with recurrent hospitalizations or nocturnal desaturation.[66] Recurrent hospitalization is defined as two or more hospitalizations for hypercapnic respiratory failure in a 12-month period. Nocturnal desaturation is defined by a pulse oximeter reading of less than 89% for 5 minutes with administration of at least 2 L/min of O_2.[62]

In long-term care settings, a follow-up examination is suggested 1 month or so after starting NIV to help the patient acclimate to the device. A 2-month follow-up is recommended to determine compliance with NIV and to assess benefit.[66]

Exclusion Criteria for Noninvasive Ventilation in a Long-Term Care Setting

Relative contraindications for the use of NIV for restrictive thoracic disease, nocturnal hypoventilation, and chronic COPD include an unsupportive family, copious amounts of secretions, uncooperative behavior on the part of the patient, high risk of aspiration, and any anatomic abnormality that interferes with gas delivery.[2]

EQUIPMENT USED FOR NONINVASIVE VENTILATION

Many factors, including the choice of patient interface, ventilator, mode of ventilation, and initial ventilator settings, play a role in determining whether NIV will be successful in a given patient. This section discusses the equipment and modes of ventilation used in the application of NIV.

Patient Interfaces

Various devices are available to provide a noninvasive interface between the patient and the ventilator. When selecting an interface, clinicians should evaluate the fit and air leak associated with the interface. These factors have a major impact on the efficacy of NIV. Patient comfort is also an important consideration because it influences patient compliance with therapy, particularly in the long-term care setting. Other considerations include volume of dead space and position of the exhalation port in the interface and whether the interface functions properly with the type of ventilator to be used. The most common noninvasive patient interfaces used in the acute care setting are full-face or oronasal masks followed by nasal masks. An oronasal mask is usually the best choice when NIV is used to treat ARF.

Nasal and Oronasal Masks

Nasal and oronasal masks are typically manufactured in two parts. The body of these devices is made of clear, hard plastic. Surrounding the outer edge of the mask body is either a soft plastic or silicone lip or a cushion filled with hydrogel, silicone gel, or air. The best design has a soft inner lip that forms a seal with the patient's face. When a higher positive pressure is applied, the mask fits more closely to the face. The opposite effect occurs when resuscitation masks are used for positive pressure ventilation. Higher airway pressures tend to force this type of mask away from the face, increasing the air leak.

NIV masks incorporate straps and headgear to maintain and stabilize the mask's position on the face (Figure 49-4). It is

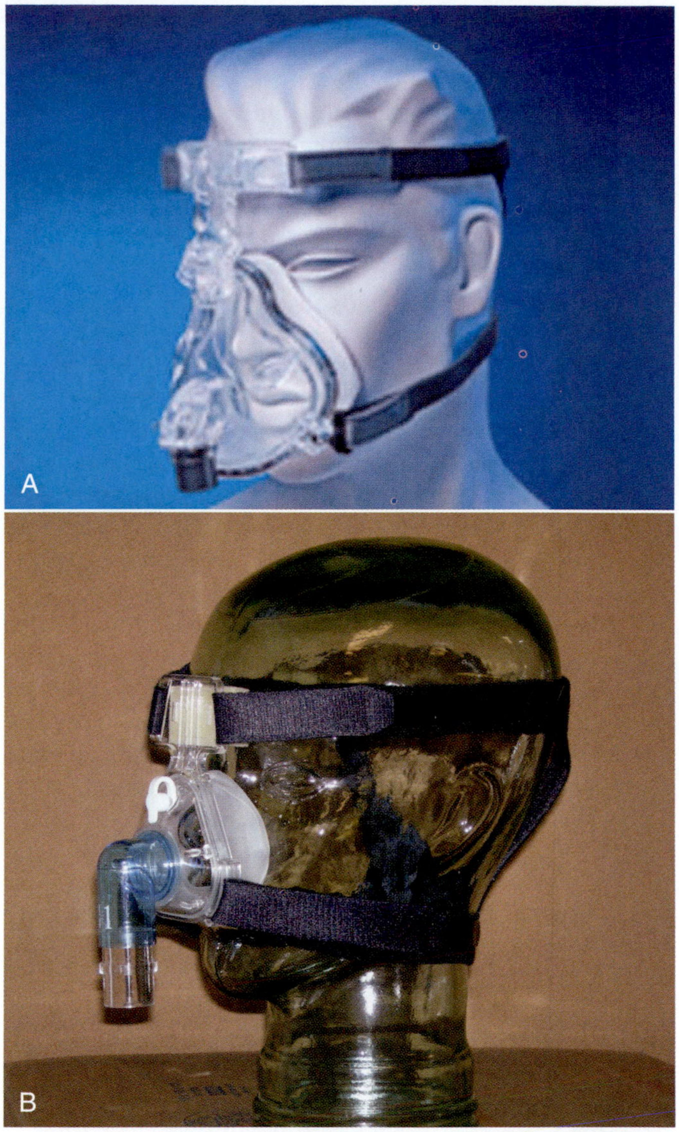

FIGURE 49-4 **A,** Nasal mask that incorporates adjustable forehead support to minimize pressure on the bridge of the nose. **B,** Nasal mask designed for small size and minimal facial contact. (**A,** Courtesy ResMed Corp, San Diego, CA. **B,** Courtesy of Phillips Respironics, Murrysville, PA.)

important to avoid tightening the straps more than necessary. A perfect seal between the mask and the face is not required because ventilators used for NIV are designed to function properly in the presence of small air leaks. Pulling the straps excessively tight is likely to result in pressure-related damage to the skin on the bridge of the nose or sometimes on the cheeks. Clinicians must be vigilant for early signs of skin damage and take steps to minimize damage and prevent development of pressure ulcers. An area of reddened skin that persists after removal of the mask is usually the first sign of pressure-related skin damage. A liquid skin barrier and a hydrocolloid patch may be applied to protect the reddened area.

To address the problem of skin breakdown, most masks incorporate some means of minimizing pressure on the skin.

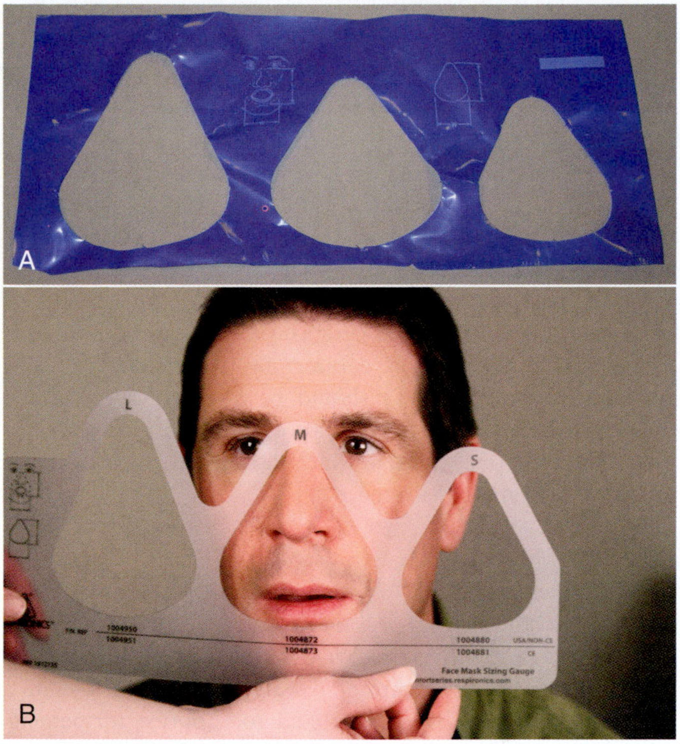

FIGURE 49-5 **A,** Templates help clinicians select an appropriately sized mask. **B,** Oronasal masks should rest on the bridge of the nose between the eyes and in the indentation between the chin and the lower lip. (Courtesy ResMed Corp. San Diego, CA.)

These include foam wedges used as spacers and adjustable mechanical controls that prevent the apex of the mask from being pulled too close to the face. Some masks have foam pads that rest on the forehead to help maintain proper mask positioning. An easy way to check for excessive tightness is to insert two fingers between the straps and the patient's face. If the straps are too tight it is not easy to do this, and they should be loosened slightly. A strategy for minimizing the risk of pressure ulcer formation is to alternate the use of two or more masks with different points of facial contact.

A key factor in patient tolerance and NIV efficacy is the choice of an appropriately sized mask. Most masks include sizing templates that can be used before removing the mask from its packaging (Figure 49-5). Nasal masks should be sized so that the cushion starts one-third of the way down from the top of the bridge of the nose and fits closely along the lateral aspects of the nose and rests above the upper lip, just under the nose. Oronasal masks fit similarly except the bottom of the mask rests in the depression above the chin and just below the lower lip. Mask sizes range from extra small to large, but for many individuals, a small or medium-small mask is a good fit. Ill-fitting masks can allow air leaks into the eyes, leading to poor tolerance. Small leaks around the mouth are generally less problematic because most ventilators used for NIV are designed to function with a baseline leak.

Nasal masks are more prone to air leaks than full-face masks, especially for patients who are mouth breathers. Chin straps are available that provide tension to help keep the mouth closed, but in practice, they seldom work well. Oronasal masks are less prone to mouth leaks because both the mouth and the nose are covered. Disadvantages associated with oronasal masks include increases in dead space, risk of aspiration, and feelings of claustrophobia. Nasal masks may be better tolerated by patients with claustrophobia. Oronasal masks interfere with patients' ability to communicate, eat, drink, and expectorate secretions without removing the mask.

In the past few years, new types of patient interfaces have been introduced in various designs, sizes, and shapes that are intended to promote more comfort and better tolerance. The respiratory therapist (RT) should be aware of all available designs to choose a relatively comfortable, well-tolerated, correctly fitted interface through which the needed level of ventilatory support can be delivered.

Nasal Pillows

Nasal pillows (Figure 49-6) are round, soft cushions that fit directly into the nares. Specially designed headgear holds the prongs in place. This interface is used most often during nasal CPAP by patients with chronic disease who do not tolerate a nasal mask. Nasal pillows are often a good option for patients with skin necrosis on the bridge of the nose or to deliver nocturnal CPAP to patients who prefer to sleep on their side. A newer design is the wedge-shaped mini-nasal mask that covers only the end of the nose. Another is the hybrid mask (Figure 49-7), which covers the mouth with a small mask and seals the nares with nasal pillows connected to the top. This interface allows ventilation with fewer leaks, similar to an oronasal mask that does not have contact with the skin on the bridge of the nose. Besides the advantage of decreased risk of tissue damage, this design allows patients to wear glasses during NIV.

Other Interfaces

The total face mask surrounds the entire face (Figure 49-8) without applying pressure to the bridge of the nose. For this reason, it is often a good choice for patients with severe skin breakdown. A soft, flexible layer around the edge of the mask forms a seal and prevents leaking when the mask is pressurized. The total face mask comes in one size, which allows quick application in the emergency department or critical care unit. Because it does not obstruct the patient's vision, this mask may help patients who feel claustrophobic when wearing other masks.

The helmet is an interface that is unavailable in the United States at the present time (Figure 49-9). This interface surrounds the entire head like a plastic bubble. The only point where the patient experiences stress is in the axillary area where the two straps holding the helmet in place cross. Numerous recent studies have evaluated the effectiveness of the helmet during CPAP and NPPV.[101-105] Results indicated that the helmet

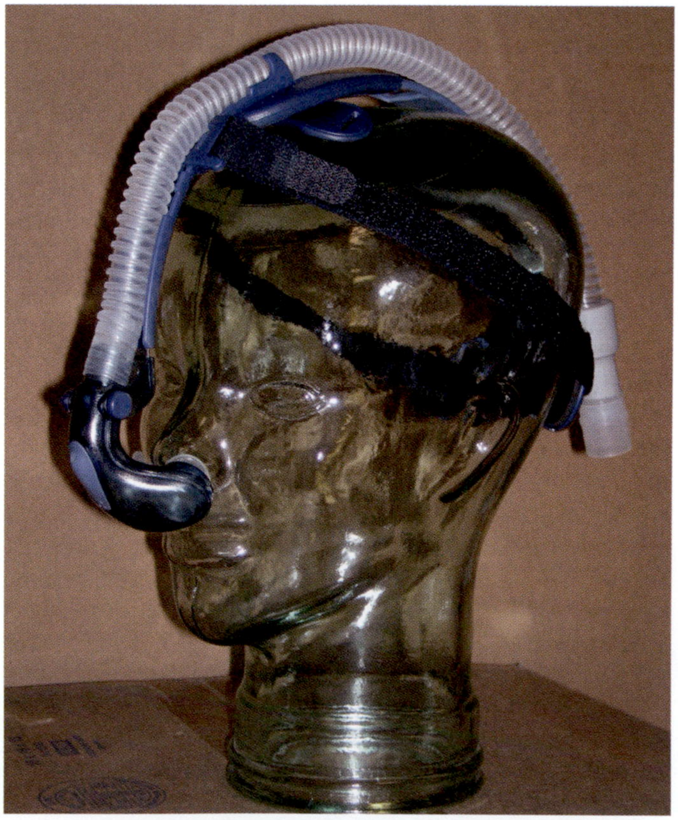

FIGURE 49-6 Nasal pillows are available in several designs and various sizes. (Courtesy ResMed Corp, San Diego, CA.)

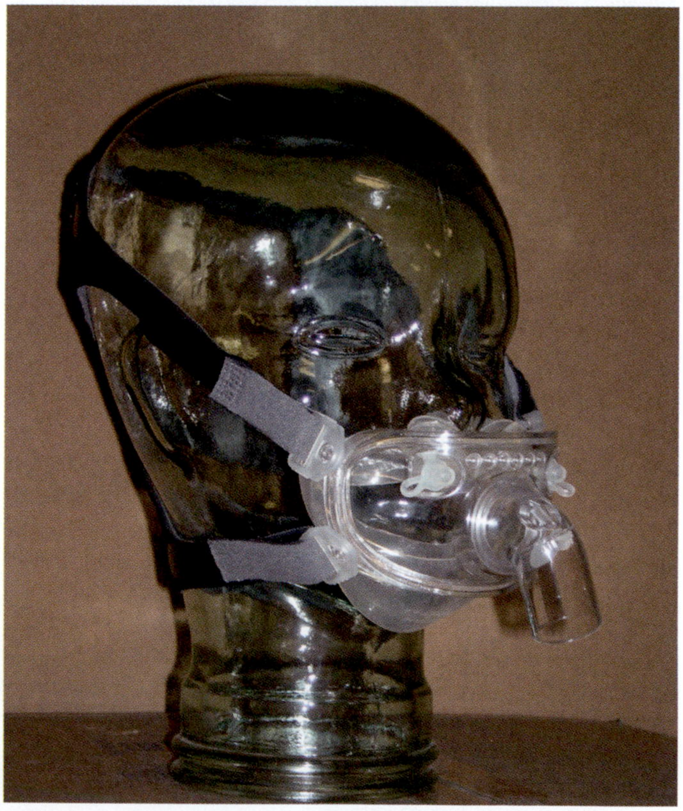

FIGURE 49-7 The hybrid mask covers the mouth and incorporates nasal pillows into the mask. (Courtesy InnoMed Technologies, Coconut Creek, FL.)

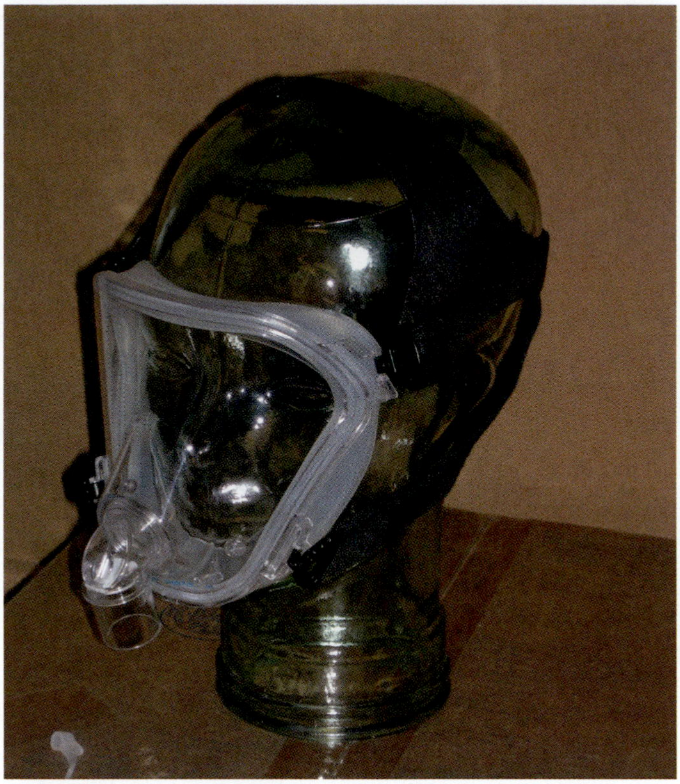

FIGURE 49-8 The Total Face Mask. (Courtesy Phillips Respironics, Murrysville, PA.)

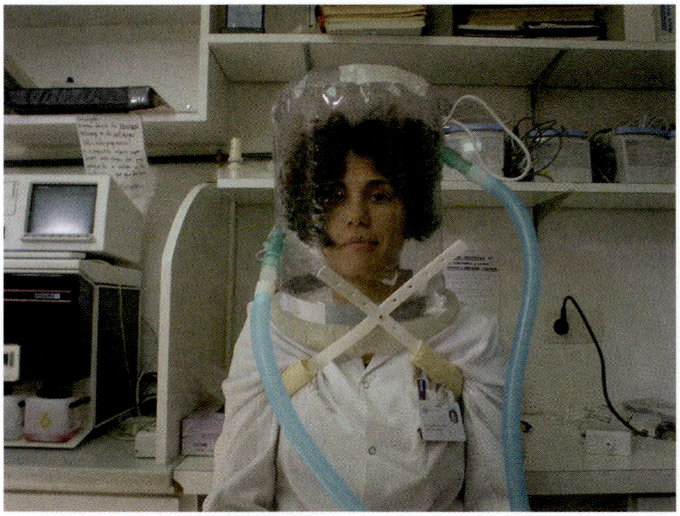

FIGURE 49-9 The helmet is used in Europe to provide continuous high-flow CPAP. (Courtesy Intersurgical Nederland, B.V.)

is more effective for CPAP than NPPV.[104] However, CPAP must be applied with a high continuous flow to prevent CO_2 from accumulating inside the helmet.[105] If CPAP is provided by a ventilator, the patient is likely to rebreathe CO_2 because of the large capacitance of the helmet.[105] During NIV with the helmet, CO_2 is not eliminated as effectively compared with full-face masks, and triggering and cycling the ventilator can be adversely affected.[104]

Face masks are specifically designed for use with either ICU or noninvasive ventilators (Figure 49-10). Face masks for noninvasive ventilators have entrainment valves that prevent asphyxia if the ventilator fails or the tubing becomes disconnected. Full-face masks designed for ICU ventilators do not have this feature. In addition, noninvasive ventilators using a single-limb circuit require a leak port either in the tubing or in the mask itself (Figure 49-11). Masks with leak ports should be used only with noninvasive ventilators because the leak interferes with the function of ICU ventilators.

Few data are available in the literature to help guide the choice of an interface for NIV. One study compared 30 minutes of full-face mask, nasal mask, and nasal pillows applied in random order to hypercapnic patients.[106] The investigators reported that the full-face mask and nasal pillows improved ventilation more than the nasal mask but that the nasal mask was better tolerated.[106] Use of a full-face mask also was associated with a significant increase in V_T compared with the nasal mask.[106] Similar findings were reported in a more recent study of 90 patients with hypercapnic ARF randomly assigned to full-face mask or nasal mask.[107] Both studies support the belief that full-face masks may be more effective for patients in the acute care setting.[106,107] There is no perfect NIV interface that meets the needs of every patient. Success is more likely if the interface can be tolerated for long periods and only a small air leak is present. A full-face mask is the interface of choice for patients requiring NIV for ARF. For patients who cannot tolerate a full-face mask, a nasal mask should be tried before accepting failure.

RULE OF THUMB

Use a full-face mask for patients in ARF. If the patient is unable to tolerate a full-face mask, try a nasal mask before accepting NIV failure.

Types of Mechanical Ventilators and Modes of Ventilation

Three types of ventilators are used for NIV: noninvasive ventilators, critical care ventilators, and portable home care ventilators. This section describes the characteristics and function of the three types of ventilators.

Noninvasive Ventilators

Most noninvasive ventilators are electrically powered, blower-driven, and microprocessor-controlled (Figure 49-12). These devices deliver a continuous but variable flow of gas to the patient through a single-limb circuit without an exhalation valve. To function properly, noninvasive ventilators must have a continuous air leak through one or more small ports either in the ventilator circuit or in the patient interface. The ports also provide the outlet through which the patient's exhaled gas is vented from the circuit. The main advantage of noninvasive ventilators over other types of ventilators is the ability to trigger

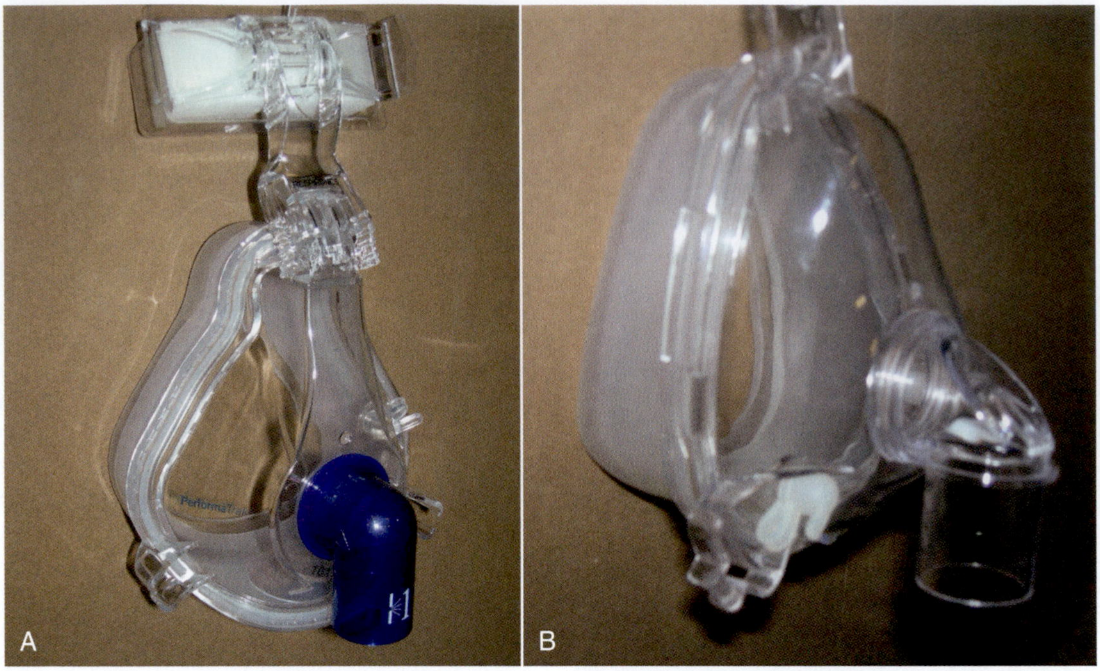

FIGURE 49-10 **A,** Oronasal mask designed for use with a critical care ventilator. **B,** Oronasal mask with anti-suffocation valve intended for use with a noninvasive ventilator. (**A,** Courtesy Phillips Respironics, Murrysville, PA, **B,** Pulmodyne, Indianapolis, IN.)

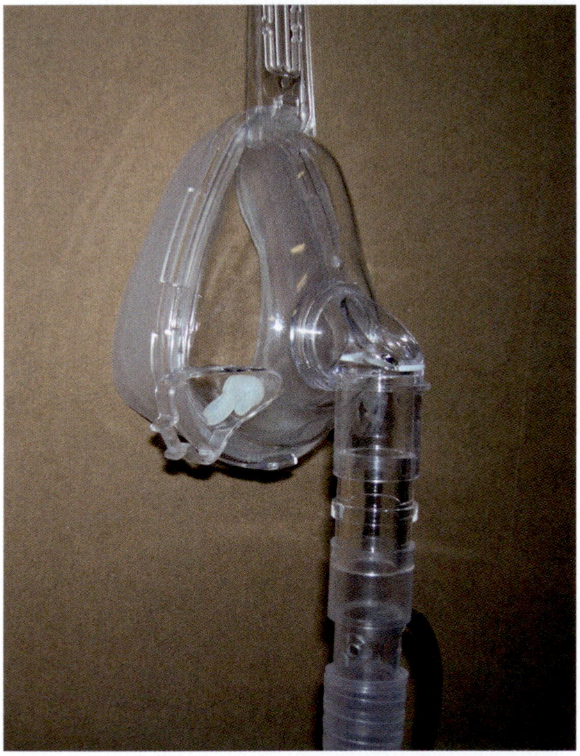

FIGURE 49-11 A leak port is required with noninvasive ventilators to ensure proper function, either as shown, in the ventilator circuit, or in the nasal or oronasal mask. Occlusion of the leak port will result in ventilator malfunction. (Courtesy Phillips Pulmodyne, Indianapolis, IN.)

MINI CLINI

Problems With Triggering During Noninvasive Ventilation

PROBLEM: A patient with COPD is receiving NIV with a noninvasive ventilator using a full-face mask. The ventilator settings are as follows: PSV mode, peak pressure 14 cm H_2O, PEEP 4 cm H_2O, backup rate 10 breaths/min. Arterial blood gas was obtained after 30 minutes on NIV. $PaCO_2$ was 75 mm Hg, essentially unchanged since NIV was initiated. The RT notices that the ventilator is not triggering with every patient effort, and his respiratory distress has not improved. What should the RT do?

Solutions

1. The problems of failure to trigger and ineffective ventilation could be caused by a large air leak. Determine if an air leak is present. If so, reposition, refit, or select a better fitting mask; adjust strap tension; and consider adding a forehead spacer to minimize the leak.
2. These two problems could be related to intrinsic PEEP. Carefully observe the patient and ventilator graphics, if available, for missed trigger attempts. The ventilator should trigger with every inspiratory effort by the patient. Try increasing PEEP slowly from 4 cm H_2O to 6 cm H_2O or 8 cm H_2O. If the applied PEEP from the ventilator is set to minimize the difference between end expiratory pressure and the patient's intrinsic PEEP, the ability to trigger should improve. In some ventilators, increasing or decreasing PEEP in pressure-targeted ventilation modes does not also affect the peak pressure. In this case, increasing PEEP could result in a decrease in the ventilating pressure and V_T. Check the peak pressure to determine if the ventilating pressure has changed, and increase the peak pressure by the same amount as PEEP is increased. Effective ventilation is usually achieved if the exhaled V_T is about 4 to 6 ml/kg.

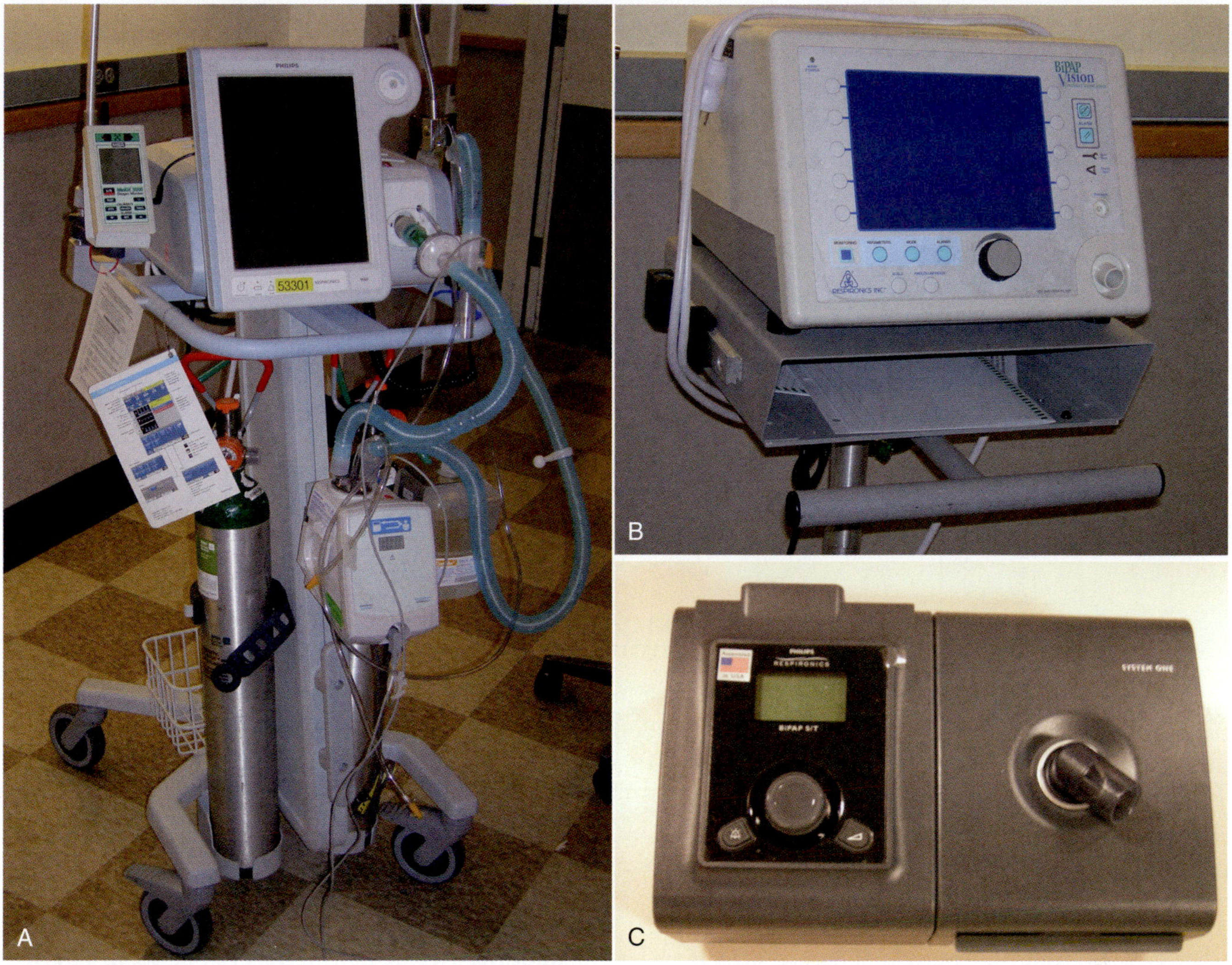

FIGURE 49-12 Examples of noninvasive ventilators with monitoring and alarm capabilities. (Courtesy Phillips Respironics, Murrysville, PA.)

and cycle appropriately when small to moderate air leaks are present.

The microprocessor controls gas delivery to the patient. Although flow and pressure are measured internally, the design of these ventilators maintains a low resistance between the patient and the ventilator at all times. Key factors are the absence of valves in the ventilator circuit, smooth internal lumen tubing for the circuit, and use of only low-resistance heated humidifiers. As a result, noninvasive ventilators are sensitive to changes in flow and pressure and can respond quickly to patient demands. Noninvasive ventilators used in the acute care setting for patients who would otherwise need intubation should meet a few safety requirements, including minimal CO_2 rebreathing and alarms for circuit disconnection, loss of power, and battery failure if a battery is present. An internal battery allows safe patient transport without interruption of NIV. Low baseline pressure settings have been associated with significant rebreathing of CO_2 in single-limb circuits.[108,109] A setting of at least 3 to 5 cm H_2O PEEP generates adequate flow to flush exhaled gas from the ventilator circuit and prevent rebreathing of CO_2.[108] For this reason, the expiratory pressure can be set no lower than 4 cm H_2O on many noninvasive ventilators. Masks used with noninvasive ventilators typically include an antiasphyxia valve that opens automatically in the event of power loss or circuit disconnection.

Ideally, noninvasive ventilators should have an internal blending device, capable of providing FiO_2 ranging from 0.21 to about 1. Simply adding an additional flow of O_2 into the ventilator circuit or mask results in maximum FiO_2 of about 0.5,[110] which is prone to wide fluctuations from variations in patient inspiratory flow rates, patient effort, and leaks. Other capabilities such as graphics monitoring; and display calculated volumes that estimate leak, V_T, and minute ventilation are useful when adjusting NIV settings to enhance patient-ventilator synchrony.

Modes available on noninvasive ventilators usually include CPAP, spontaneous (pressure support), and timed (pressure assist/control). Depending on the ventilator used, the ventilating pressure is referred to as **inspiratory positive airway pressure (IPAP)**, equal to peak airway pressure, or pressure support,

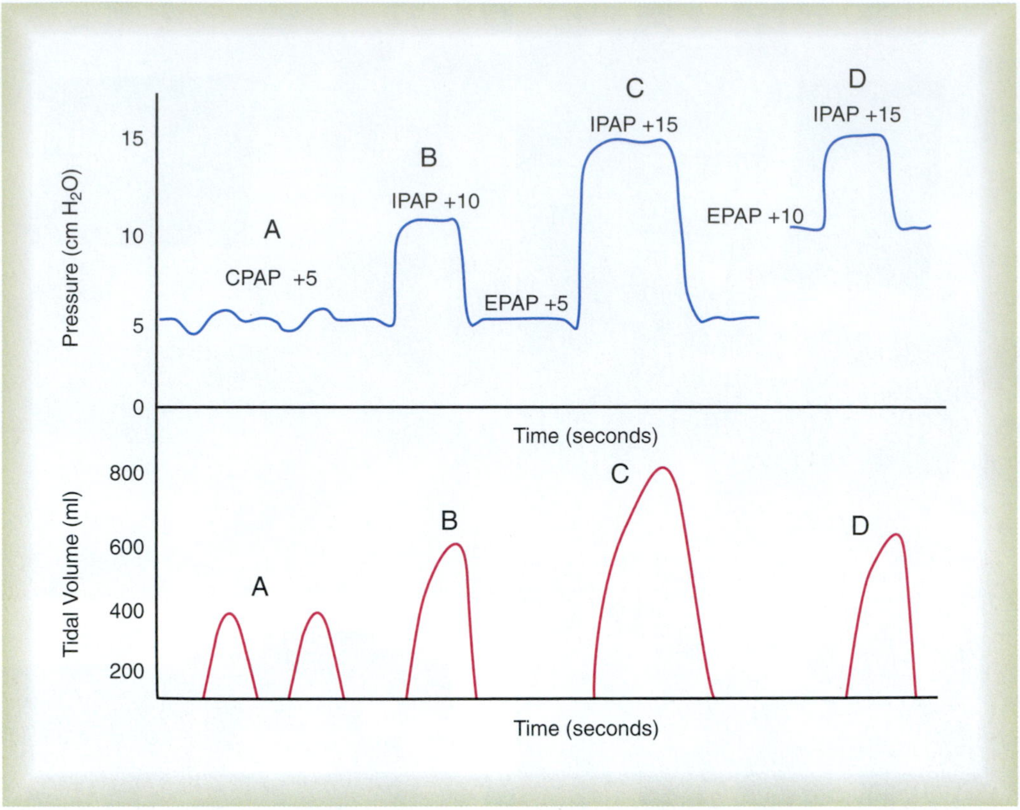

FIGURE 49-13 The effects of changing noninvasive ventilator settings (IPAP and EPAP). **A,** Spontaneous breathing on CPAP of 5 cm H_2O. **B,** Adding IPAP of 10 cm H_2O results in higher V_T. **C,** Increasing IPAP to 15 cm H_2O delivers even higher V_T. **D,** Increasing the baseline EPAP without a corresponding increase in IPAP results in lower V_T because the difference between IPAP and EPAP is less. (Copyright © 2015 Covidien. All rights reserved. Used with the permission of Covidien.)

which is the change in pressure above PEEP. In either case, this type of breath is usually pressure-limited and flow-cycled or time-cycled (Figure 49-13). With pressure support and spontaneous modes, inspiration is patient-triggered. With pressure assist/control or spontaneous-timed modes, inspiration is either patient-triggered or time-triggered.

Critical Care Ventilators

Critical care ventilators with noninvasive modes that compensate for leaks can be used to deliver NIV effectively but there is wide variability in their performance (Figure 49-14). These ventilators are equipped with internal air-oxygen blenders, graphics, and alarms, and are capable of delivering high inspiratory flow rates that meet patient demand. They generally use dual-limb circuits that prevent rebreathing of exhaled CO_2.

The main problem with using older critical care ventilators to provide NIV is their inability to compensate for leaks. Air leaks around the mask can cause problems including auto-triggering and failure to cycle. State-of-the-art critical care ventilators now have ventilation modes designed for noninvasive application. With a few models, the NIV mode activates only new alarms (low pressure) and deactivates low V_T and minute volume alarms. However, most models incorporate some level of leak compensation during triggering, cycling, or both. A common feature of NIV modes is the ability to set a maximum inspiratory time during PSV. This setting does not deactivate flow cycling but provides an additional limit for inspiration in the presence of a large leak.

To deliver NIV, ICU ventilators can be set in PSV mode, which is a patient-triggered, pressure-limited, flow-cycled mode. During inspiration, a high gas flow is delivered until the preset pressure limit is achieved. At that point, the flow begins to decrease until a predetermined level of flow is reached, cycling the breath to exhalation. Depending on the specific ventilator used, this flow level can be a fixed flow rate (e.g., 5 L/min) or a percentage of the peak flow (e.g., 25%). The flow-cycling mechanism of PSV can cause problems during NIV. In the presence of a large air leak, the flow may not decrease to the level necessary to cycle the breath to expiration. In this case, the patient may have to exhale actively, using abdominal muscles to increase airway pressure to cycle the ventilator to exhalation using secondary criteria.[111,112] This action increases work of breathing and can lead to failure of NIV.

Active exhalation can be recognized on the ventilator graphics by a spike in airway pressure at the end of the breath (Figure 49-15). There are two ways to correct this problem so that the patient can exhale passively again. First, inspiration can be time-cycled instead of flow-cycled by decreasing the maximum inspiratory time setting. Time-cycled (instead of flow-cycled), pressure-limited ventilation markedly improves patient-ventilator synchrony and patient comfort and compliance with therapy in the presence of air leaks.[113]

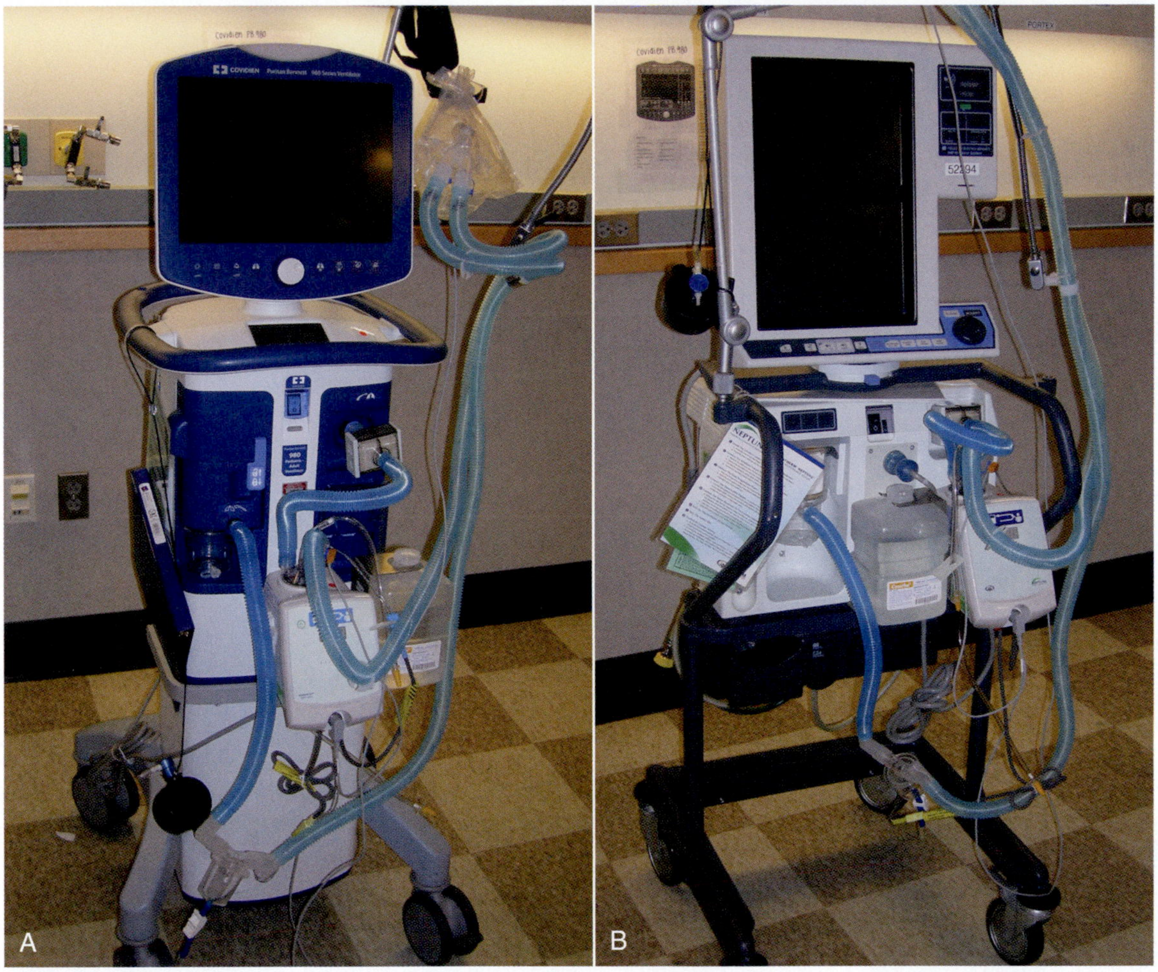

FIGURE 49-14 Examples of critical care ventilators that can be used to provide noninvasive ventilation. (Courtesy Medtronic, Boulder, CO.)

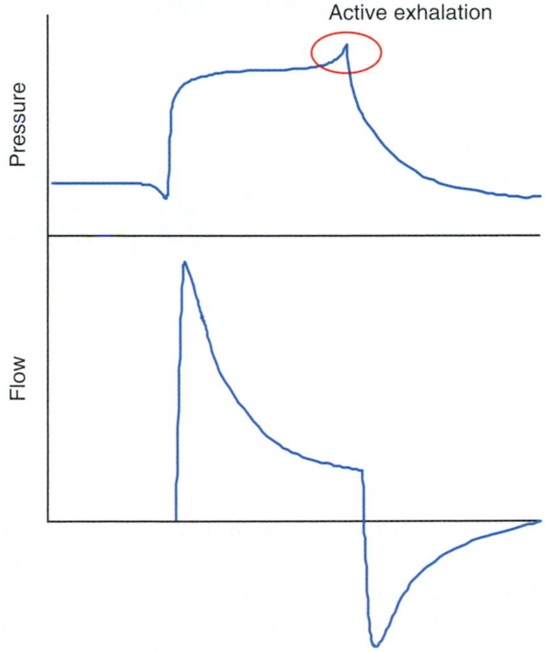

FIGURE 49-15 Active exhalation is recognized by the spike on the pressure waveform at the end of inspiration. The patient uses abdominal muscles to increase airway pressure and cycle the ventilator into exhalation.

The second option is to adjust the termination criterion[114] by changing the percentage of the peak inspiratory flow that terminates the breath. Most current generation ICU ventilators allow adjustment of the termination criterion setting over a wide range (Figure 49-16). To prevent active exhalation, the percentage is simply increased until the spike disappears from the pressure waveform. Proper adjustment of the termination criterion can markedly improve patient-ventilator synchrony during NIV.

PSV is the ventilation mode commonly used for NIV. Most RTs are familiar with using pressure-targeted ventilation for NIV on ventilators designed specifically for noninvasive application. The current recommendation by an international consensus conference on NIV in ARF is as follows: "Choice of mode should be based on local expertise and familiarity, tailored to the etiology and severity of the pathophysiological process responsible for ARF."[115] If a critical care ventilator is used for NIV, pressure ventilation makes sense because leak compensation is provided, triggering and cycling can be adjusted to suit patient needs, and minute ventilation and end expiratory pressures are preserved. Volume-controlled modes are not recommended for NIV. Inability to compensate for the decrease in minute ventilation and loss of pressure caused by large leaks are major problems when volume targeted modes are used for NIV.

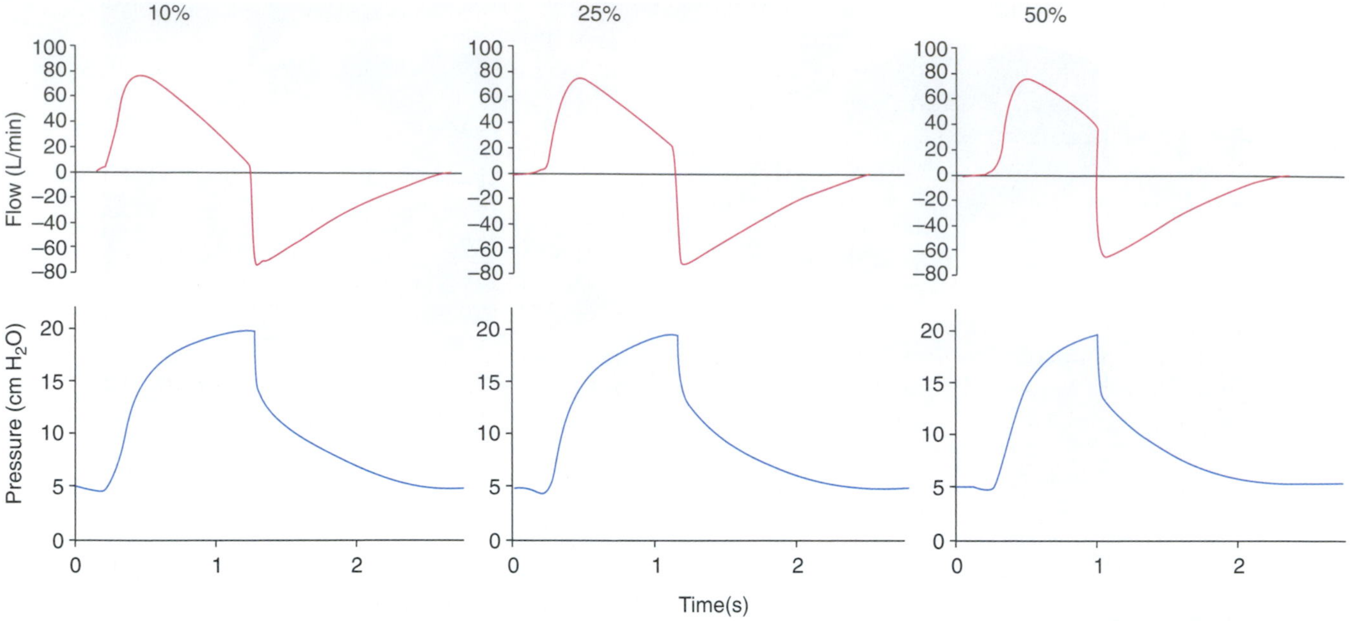

FIGURE 49-16 Effects of changing the termination criteria during PSV. Changing to a setting that ends inspiration at a higher percentage of peak flow results in shorter inspiratory time and lower tidal volume. This change is sometimes needed to improve patient-ventilator synchrony.

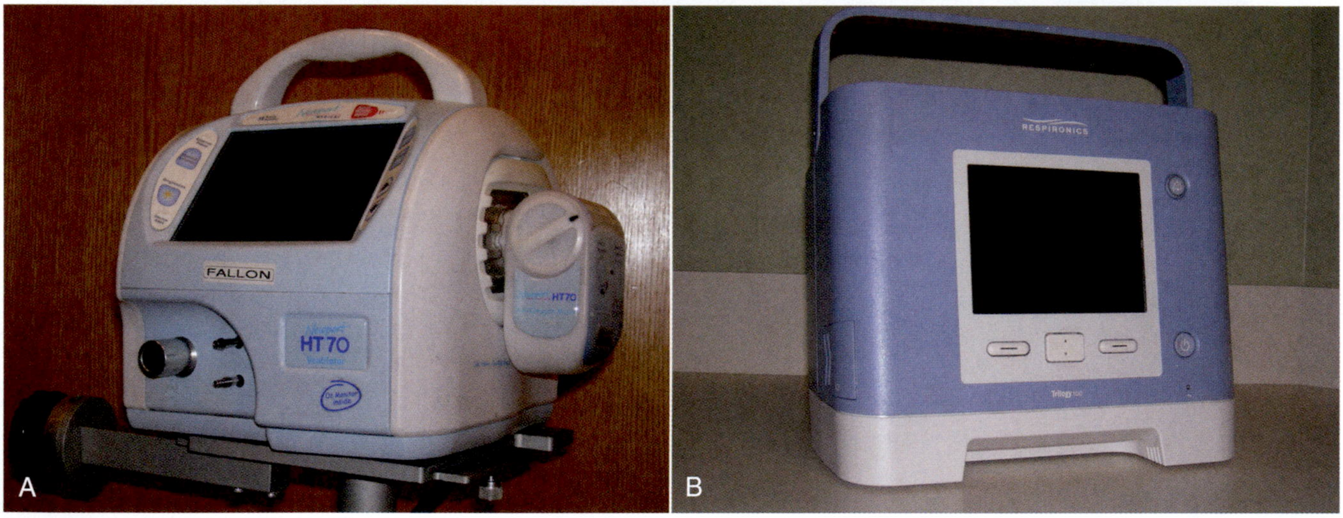

FIGURE 49-17 Two examples of new generation portable ventilators that can be used in acute care, home care, or transport settings. (**A,** Courtesy Covidien, courtesy Phillips Respironics, Murrysville, PA.)

In the long-term care setting, volume ventilation is sometimes used for patients with neuromuscular weakness.[3] Volume ventilation may allow a patient to stack breaths, increasing lung volume to near inspiratory capacity and resulting in improved cough peak flow. High cough peak flow should enhance secretion clearance. In patients with limited muscle strength, pressure-controlled ventilation does not allow breath stacking because inspiratory pressure is held constant, in contrast to volume ventilation, in which delivered V_T is constant. However, there is no proven advantage of one mode versus another in the long-term care setting.[2] Enhanced secretion clearance is easily provided using a mechanical cough-assist device.

Portable Home Care or Transport Ventilators

Most portable home care ventilators (Figure 49-17) are electrically powered and microprocessor-controlled. These devices can operate from alternating current (AC) or, if equipped with internal or external batteries, direct current (DC) power sources. The batteries usually can provide power for several hours. Batteries add a measure of safety in areas where AC power outages occur regularly. They also allow the patient to be more mobile, which may improve their quality of life. These ventilators use a single-limb or double-limb ventilator circuit with an exhalation valve that prevents rebreathing of CO_2. Updated technology has improved the performance characteristics of these ventilators to a level comparable to critical care ventilators with the added advantages of small size, light weight, and battery power that allow portability. Most newer models incorporate an NIV mode with the ability to compensate for leaks. Some models with adjustable bias flow settings improve the ability of the ventilator to sense patient triggering. Similar to critical care ventilators, additional features, such as variable termination criteria and maximum inspiratory time, are available on some of these devices to enhance breath termination in PSV.

Portable home care ventilators are currently recommended for patients who need continuous ventilatory support or high ventilating pressures, such as patients with severe chest wall deformities or obesity or for patients who want greater mobility.[2] For acute care, these ventilators could easily be used to initiate NIV in nontraditional locations and allow transport to an emergency department or ICU without the need to interrupt ventilation.

Heated Humidifiers

An increase in nasal resistance and congestion has been reported with CPAP in patients with mouth leaks.[116] The addition of heated humidity relieves nasal resistance and congestion. Cold passover humidification does not provide relief.[117,118] The use of heated humidity during nasal CPAP in patients with sleep apnea and nasal symptoms (sneezing, nasal draining, nasal and oral dryness, and nasal obstruction) has significantly improved patients' compliance with this therapy.[119] It seems likely that the same effect would occur in NPPV. To avoid the negative effect on patient compliance caused by this common complaint and the accumulation of dried retained secretions in the back of the oral pharynx, humidified gas, heated to a temperature that is comfortable to the patient (usually about 30° C), should be the standard when using NIV.

RULE OF THUMB

Heated humidity (about 30° C) should always be provided with NIV to avoid nasal symptoms, to avoid the accumulation of secretions in the back of the oral pharynx, and to enhance patient tolerance.

MANAGEMENT OF NONINVASIVE VENTILATION

Initial Application of Noninvasive Ventilation

Starting NIV requires the selection of a ventilator and an interface and a significant time commitment from the RT. The patient should be seated in a chair or bed at an angle of 30 degrees or greater (Box 49-6).[2] The RT should always explain the procedure and answer any questions about NIV before placing the mask on the patient. Clinicians should recognize that dyspnea can cause feelings of anxiety and fear. For this reason, the RT or the patient should hold the mask in place when applying the mask for the first time. Holding the mask allows it to be removed quickly if the patient begins to panic or wishes to communicate. A strategy of starting with low pressures can help patients adjust to NIV more readily. Ventilating pressures should be set as low as possible initially, especially if the patient is unfamiliar with the sensation of positive pressure ventilation. Then the ventilating pressures can be adjusted in small increments over 1 to 2 minutes until exhaled V_T is 4 to 6 mL/kg predicted body weight or respiratory distress improves. During this time, the RT should assess the patient frequently, adjusting the ventilator settings to synchronize breath delivery with the patient's breathing pattern and providing instructions and coaching as needed. The mask should not be strapped on until the patient is comfortable with the application of NIV and the RT has adjusted pressures to provide proper ventilation.

Box 49-6 Initiation of Noninvasive Ventilation

1. Choose a location with appropriate monitoring based on the severity of the patient's condition.
2. Position the patient with the head of the bed elevated ≥30 degrees.
3. Select a ventilator and an appropriately sized interface.
4. Turn on the ventilator and humidifier, and connect the interface.
5. Set initial settings at a low level of support: PEEP 0 to 4 cm H_2O, ventilatory pressure 2 to 4 cm H_2O.
6. Hold the mask on the patient's face or have the patient hold the mask until he or she is comfortable with the sensation of NIV.
7. Adjust FiO_2 or bleed in O_2 flow to keep SpO_2 >90%.
8. After the patient becomes comfortable with the initial settings, increase inspiratory pressure until V_T is about 4 to 6 ml/kg predicted body weight or signs of respiratory distress improve. Increase PEEP to reduce asynchrony from air trapping or to improve oxygenation.
9. Check for air leaks, especially around the eyes; adjust mask as needed.
10. Reassess frequently for tolerance and efficacy of NIV (at least every 30 minutes) for the first 1 to 2 hours.

The specific airway pressures needed to support the patient during NIV are best determined by bedside assessment of the patient's response and tolerance. They cannot be determined with accuracy before NIV is started. However, most patients require PEEP levels of 5 to 8 cm H_2O and ventilating pressure of 8 to 12 cm H_2O. Peak airway pressures greater than 20 cm H_2O are rarely needed. To avoid gastric distention, ventilating pressure should be less than the normal esophageal opening pressures of 20 to 25 cm H_2O.[120] If the patient has a nasogastric tube in place, the probability of gastric distention increases dramatically, as does the probability of NIV failure.

Final adjustment of the ventilator should deliver a V_T of about 4 to 6 ml/kg ideal body weight with a respiratory rate less than 30 breaths/min. The goal of NIV is not to deliver a large V_T but rather to maintain normal ventilatory patterns with acceptable gas exchange and decrease the work of breathing. FiO_2 should be titrated to PaO_2 of at least 60 mm Hg or SpO_2 88% to 95%.

RULE OF THUMB

Most patients with ARF can be stabilized with an expiratory pressure setting of 5 to 8 cm H_2O and ventilating pressure of 8 to 12 cm H_2O. Avoid using peak pressures greater than 20 cm H_2O.

Clinical Assessment Criteria to Identify Success or Failure of Noninvasive Ventilation

Careful monitoring and frequent reassessment are very important during the first 1 to 2 hours of NIV. Successful application of NIV is easy to recognize—gas exchange improves, $PaCO_2$ decreases, pH normalizes, and PaO_2 and SpO_2 increase. Along with improvement of these measured values, the patient's clinical presentation improves; respiratory rate decreases, V_T increases, accessory muscle use decreases or is eliminated, and pulse rate and blood pressure normalize. If clinical status and gas exchange have not improved after 1 to 2 hours of NIV, intubation should be considered. This is especially true if the indication for NIV was hypoxemic respiratory failure. Evidence suggests an increased risk of cardiac arrest in patients with hypoxemic respiratory failure who do not improve after a trial of NIV for 1 to 2 hours.[46]

Adjusting Noninvasive Ventilator Settings

Ventilator settings may need to be adjusted after the patient stabilizes and acclimates or when arterial blood gas analysis reveals gas exchange problems. Hypercapnia is addressed first by minimizing air leaks and if necessary, by increasing the ventilating pressure. The result is an increase in the delivered V_T and minute ventilation and a decrease in $PaCO_2$. NIV is typically delivered in a spontaneous mode, where all breaths are patient-triggered and none are mandatory, so adjusting the ventilator frequency is not an option. For patients with chronic hypercapnia, ventilation should be adjusted to maintain an acceptable pH. No attempt should be made to normalize the $PaCO_2$ in such patients.

Increasing PEEP increases the patient's functional residual capacity, mean airway pressure, and PaO_2. Higher PEEP should also improve trigger synchrony in the setting of air trapping. Decreasing PEEP theoretically should cause the opposite effects. In clinical practice, decreasing PEEP may not affect PaO_2 as the disease process resolves and alveolar stability improves.

If the assist/control mode is used for NIV, the rate should be set at a level below the patient's spontaneous rate, allowing the patient to trigger the ventilator as needed. Setting the rate in this manner provides a backup rate for safety if apnea occurs and avoids overventilating the patient. If the patient's disease process limits the ability to trigger or breathe spontaneously, as in some neuromuscular disorders, the set rate has a direct relationship to minute ventilation and an inverse relationship to $PaCO_2$. These relationships may not always be the case in clinical practice and in a spontaneously breathing patient. Table 49-1 summarizes ventilator adjustments during NIV.

TABLE 49-1
Expected Results of Changing Noninvasive Ventilator Settings

Setting	Adjustment	Anticipated Result
IPAP	↑	↑ V_T, ↑ minute ventilation, ↓ $PaCO_2$
	↓	↓ V_T, ↓ minute ventilation, ↑ $PaCO_2$
EPAP	↑	↑ FRC, ↑ PaO_2, ↓ V_T If intrinsic PEEP is present, fewer missed trigger attempts and improved patient-ventilator synchrony
	↓	↓ FRC, ↓ PaO_2, ↑ V_T, ↓ $PaCO_2$ Possible rebreathing of CO_2 if EPAP <4 cm H_2O
FiO_2	↑	↑ PaO_2; if bleeding O_2 into circuit, maximum expected FiO_2 is approximately 0.5; increasing O_2 flow >15 L/min may adversely affect triggering
	↓	↓ PaO_2
Rate control*	↑	↑ minute volume in timed modes, ↓ $PaCO_2$
	↓	↓ minute volume in timed modes, ↑ $PaCO_2$

FRC, Functional residual capacity.
*Rate control is generally set at 8 to 10 as a backup rate and not changed in spontaneous/timed mode.

Aerosolized Medication Delivery

For patients on intermittent NIV, aerosol medications are often administered while the patient is off the ventilator. Removal of assisted ventilation from patients in ARF makes little sense and is unnecessary. Aerosol therapy can be delivered in the usual manner through an ICU ventilator used for NIV. With a noninvasive ventilator, positioning the nebulizer between the exhalation port and mask maximizes drug delivery.[121] If the exhalation port is located in the mask or any other position distal to the nebulizer, much of the drug is lost via the exhalation port during both inspiration and expiration. A metered dose inhaler (MDI) can be administered by placing an adapter or collapsible holding chamber in the same position in the circuit. Drug delivery should improve because the MDI is actuated only during inspiration. However, dosing can safely be doubled and should be adjusted based on patient response to compensate for loss through leaks in the system and other inefficiencies.

Safe Delivery of Noninvasive Ventilation

Monitoring During Noninvasive Ventilation

In acute care or long-term care applications, clinicians must not lose sight of the goals of NIV.[2] The RT should confirm ventilator function and assess the patient on a regular basis for leaks, accessory muscle use, ventilator synchrony, comfort, and

MINI CLINI

Improving Patient-Ventilator Synchrony During Noninvasive Ventilation

PROBLEM: An oncology patient with DNI orders is receiving NIV from a critical care ventilator with a full-face mask. The ventilator is set in the PSV mode. Peak inspiratory pressure is 15 cm H_2O, PEEP is 5 cm H_2O, and flow trigger is 2 L/min. The patient has a nasogastric tube in place that is causing a large leak. The ventilator is self-triggering and fails to cycle into expiration when the patient exhales. The patient is dyspneic and appears uncomfortable.

Solutions Large leaks can cause patient-ventilator asynchrony with ventilators that do not have leak compensation. Triggering and cycling are affected because the ventilator is no longer sensitive to changes in flow or pressure changes generated by the patient.

1. Repositioning the mask and placing a flat piece of gauze or hydrocolloid dressing between the mask and the nasogastric tube and another between the nasogastric tube and the patient's face may help reduce the leak.
2. Change to a critical care ventilator with a noninvasive mode or a noninvasive ventilator designed for ICU use.
3. If switching ventilators is not feasible, and a large leak is still present, adjusting the termination criterion to a higher setting can shorten inspiratory time, allowing breath termination to occur at a higher percentage of the peak flow.
4. If termination criteria are not adjustable, change to pressure assist/control mode. Observe the ventilator graphics to determine the patient's desired inspiratory time, and set the inspiratory time on the ventilator accordingly. Typically, critically ill patients should have inspiratory times of about 0.7 to 1 second (in some cases, 0.5 second).

changes in vital signs and gas exchange. In the acute care setting, respiratory rate, heart rate, and gas exchange should improve within 1 to 2 hours after initiation of NIV. If there is no improvement after 1 to 2 hrs on optimal settings, intubation should be considered. At a minimum, SpO_2 must be continuously monitored. In the acute care setting, continuous monitoring of heart rate and blood pressure is the safest practice. A current consensus statement recommends a higher level of monitoring for patients with acute hypoxemia, worsening condition, involvement of nonrespiratory organ systems, or persistent acidosis.[122] If the patient cannot sustain ventilation independent of NIV for at least 1 hour, the same level of monitoring as any intubated patient should occur.

In the long-term care setting, improvement in gas exchange may require weeks to several months depending on daily use and compliance with the prescribed therapy.[2] Clinicians providing follow-up treatment in the long-term care setting should determine usage with the elapsed time indicator on the ventilator. The patient should be assessed for complications, symptoms of hypoventilation and poor sleep quality, patient-ventilator synchrony, and other factors that affect compliance.

Patient Location

NIV can be initiated in any acute care location, including the emergency department, ICU, or general care floor.[54] After NIV is initiated, patients should be transferred to an ICU or other inpatient location with continuous monitoring capabilities, skilled staff, and access to endotracheal intubation if needed.[2,54] Hypercapnic patients with COPD and a pH of 7.30 or greater and patients who can sustain ventilation without NIV for at least 1 hour can be managed safely on a general care floor.[54] It is important that staff members be adequately trained before caring for patients on NIV. Another consensus conference recommendation calls for one-to-one monitoring of NIV patients for the first few hours by a trained, experienced RT, nurse, or physician.[54]

Weaning from Noninvasive Ventilation

At the present time, there is no standard approach to weaning from NIV. One weaning strategy is to decrease high levels of inspiratory and baseline pressure gradually to minimal settings as the acute disease process resolves. The length of time off the ventilator can be increased gradually as tolerated. Another approach is to continue NIV until there is a need to remove the mask. Patients often request to remove the mask after several continuous hours of NIV. The patient's ability to ventilate adequately is reassessed after 5 to 30 minutes based on tolerance and NIV is either discontinued or restarted.

COMPLICATIONS OF NONINVASIVE VENTILATION

The reported failure rate of NIV ranges from 7% to 70%.[2] Serious complications such as aspiration or pneumothorax occur less than 5% of the time. The undesired side effects of NIV are less serious, although more common. These side effects can be grouped into categories related to the noninvasive interface and to gas flow and airway pressures. Table 49-2 lists the complications, frequency of occurrence, and suggested remedies.

Air leaks can cause several problems of various levels of concern, ranging from eye irritation and dry mouth to inability to trigger inspiration. Small air leaks should be expected during NIV. Large air leaks should be addressed immediately before they lead to patient-ventilator asynchrony or worsening gas exchange.[3] Air leaks often can be avoided by selecting an appropriately sized mask. If excessive airflow is leaking through the mouth, changing to a full-face mask should be helpful. If the problem persists, one can reposition the mask, add a forehead spacer, and readjust strap tension. Sometimes, ventilator settings must be adjusted if ventilation is adversely affected by the leak. Using a ventilator with leak compensation should resolve problems with leaks.

Mask-related side effects are the most common problems. Mask discomfort may be reported by up to 50%[2] of patients receiving NIV, and excessive discomfort decreases patient tolerance for NIV. Switching to a correctly sized mask or loosening the straps slightly is often all that it takes to resolve this issue. Skin damage is a problem that is only going to get worse if not

TABLE 49-2
Side Effects and Complications of Noninvasive Ventilation

	Incidence*	Possible Solutions
Interface-Related Side Effects		
Discomfort	Common	Loosen straps Refit, reposition, or change interface
Erythema	Common	Apply skin barrier or hydrocolloid dressing or both Loosen straps, adjust forehead support, or add spacer Alternate the use of 2 masks
Claustrophobia	Infrequent	Change interface Consider anxiolytic
Pressure ulcer	Infrequent	Apply hydrocolloid dressing Change interface
Skin rash	Infrequent	Apply topical steroid or antibiotic
Air Pressure–Related or Flow-Related Side Effects		
Nasal congestion	Common	Administer inhaled corticosteroid or decongestant
Nasal dryness	Common	Avoid by using heated humidification with NIV Administer saline nasal spray
Sinus or ear pain	Common	Decrease ventilating pressure
Eye irritation	Common	Refit, reposition, or change interface
Gastric distention	Infrequent	Administer simethicone Lower pressures
Serious Complications		
Aspiration	Rare	Avoid through careful patient selection Stop NIV, if status will allow
Pneumothorax	Rare	Decrease ventilating pressure Place chest tube, if tension pneumothorax
Hypotension	Rare	Decrease inflation pressure

From Mehta S, Hill NS: Noninvasive ventilation. Am J Respir Crit Care Med 163:540, 2001.
*Common—occurs in 30% to 50% of patients; infrequent—occurs in approximately 5% to 20% of patients; rare—occurs in <5% of patients.

addressed immediately for patients who need to continue using NIV. RTs should keep a watchful eye on reddened areas, usually on the bridge of the nose. A liquid skin barrier should be applied to protect the area. Applying "artificial skin" or a hydrocolloid dressing or patch is a good idea to provide further protection. These patches should also be used if a pressure ulcer forms. Taking steps to minimize pressure such as loosening the straps and adding a forehead spacer are important. Other strategies to reduce the risk of pressure ulcers include alternating use of two or more different masks and removing the mask every 4 to 6 hours for a few minutes if the patient can tolerate being off the ventilator without increased respiratory distress.

Complications related to air pressure and flow include nasal congestion, upper airway dryness, sinus and ear pain, eye irritation, and gastric insufflation.[2] Usually, nasal congestion and upper airway dryness can be prevented by using heated humidity whenever NIV is initiated. Decongestants and saline spray are sometimes needed to relieve symptoms of congestion. Sinus and ear pain may be related to high inspiratory pressure; use of the lowest effective inspiratory pressure may prevent or alleviate this problem.

Clinically significant gastric insufflation is a rare occurrence in patients using NIV.[2] Use of the lowest effective pressure may prevent gastric insufflation. Routine use of a nasogastric tube is not recommended. A nasogastric tube increases the risk of gastric insufflation, adversely affects mask fit, and usually causes a large air leak, increasing the likelihood of NIV failure.

Most major complications can be avoided with careful patient selection and use of the lowest inspiratory pressure that improves the patient's gas exchange and relieves symptoms. NIV should be avoided if the patient is a high aspiration risk or is hemodynamically unstable. The risk of aspiration increases if inspiratory pressures greater than 20 cm H_2O are used. In general, the head of the bed should be maintained at 30 degrees to reduce the risk of aspiration during NIV.

TIME AND COSTS ASSOCIATED WITH NONINVASIVE VENTILATION

The cost-effectiveness of NIV is linked to appropriate patient selection, familiarity of staff members with NIV, and the success or failure of NIV in preventing endotracheal intubation.[122,123] Staff time is one of the most valuable and expensive resources in hospitals. Time required by nurses and physicians during the first 48 hours of NIV is similar to the time required for invasive mechanical ventilation, but the time required by RTs for NIV is considerably greater than for invasive mechanical ventilation.[124] However, another study showed that the time required by RTs was significantly greater for the first 8 hours but significantly lower during the next 8 hours.[122] The increased time requirement associated with starting NIV is due to mask fitting, gradual upward adjustment of ventilator settings, and remaining at the bedside to provide coaching and encouragement to patients as they acclimate to NIV. After the patient begins to improve, the time required to maintain NIV should decrease to a level similar to invasive ventilation.

SUMMARY CHECKLIST

- NIV is the application of positive pressure ventilation or CPAP with a mask or other noninvasive interface to improve gas exchange or decrease the work of breathing.
- The use of NIV to manage ARF has improved patient outcomes.
- Evidence supports NIV as the standard of care for managing patients with COPD exacerbations and acute cardiogenic pulmonary edema. There is less evidence supporting other indications for NIV.
- NIV may be justified in the management of ARF if selection criteria (see Box 45-2) are present, exclusion criteria (see Box 45-3) are absent, and the disease process is reversible.
- Acute cardiogenic pulmonary edema should be managed initially with CPAP of 8 to 12 cm H_2O. NPPV should be considered only if hypercapnia is present.

- NIV is beneficial in the management of patients extubated but at risk of reintubation and patients with DNI orders.
- Patients with ALS should receive NIV because it probably prolongs their lives.
- Caution should be used in applying NIV to patients with acute hypoxemic respiratory failure.
- NIV is most successful in the acute care setting when air leaks are minimal, the patient's severity of illness is moderate, respiratory acidosis is present, and improvement in gas exchange and vital signs occurs within 1 to 2 hours after NIV initiation.
- When NIV is used for hypoxemic ARF, intubation and invasive ventilation should be initiated if gas exchange and patient presentation does not improve within 1 to 2 hrs of NIV.
- NIV is typically administered in the PSV mode with PEEP.
- Airway pressure during NIV should be kept as low as possible to achieve therapeutic goals (ideally <20 cm H_2O).
- Although any ventilator can be used for NIV, ventilators designed to compensate for leaks can be expected to perform best.
- Heated humidity (about 30° C) should always be provided with NIV.
- Aerosolized drugs can be administered without interrupting NIV.
- The initiation of NIV requires significant staff time, but after patients stabilize, the time required to maintain NIV is similar to invasive ventilation.

References

1. Pierson DJ: Noninvasive positive pressure ventilation: history and terminology. *Respir Care* 42:370, 1997.
2. Mehta S, Hill NS: Noninvasive ventilation. *Am J Respir Crit Care Med* 163:540, 2001.
3. Bach JR: The prevention of ventilatory failure due to inadequate pump function. *Respir Care* 42:403, 1997.
4. Bach JR, Alba AS: Intermittent abdominal pressure ventilation in a regimen of noninvasive ventilatory support. *Chest* 99:630, 1991.
5. Intermittent Positive Pressure Breathing Trial Group: Intermittent positive pressure breathing therapy of chronic obstructive pulmonary disease. *Ann Intern Med* 69:612, 1983.
6. Sullivan CE, Issa FG, Berthon-Jones M, et al: Reversal of obstructive sleep apnea by continuous positive airway pressure applied through the nares. *Lancet* 1:862–865, 1981.
7. Rideau Y, Gatin G, Bach J, et al: Prolongation of life in Duchenne's muscular dystrophy. *Acta Neurol Belg* 5:118–124, 1983.
8. Meduri GU, Conoscenti CC, Menashe P, et al: Noninvasive face mask ventilation in patients with acute respiratory failure. *Chest* 95:865–870, 1989.
9. Hill N, Brennan J, Garpestad E, et al: Noninvasive ventilation in acute respiratory failure. *Crit Care Med* 35:2402–2407, 2007.
10. Kramer N, Meyer TJ, Meharg J, et al: Randomized, prospective trial of noninvasive positive pressure ventilation in acute respiratory failure. *Am J Respir Crit Care Med* 151:1799–1806, 1995.
11. Brochard L, Mancebo J, Wysocki M, et al: Noninvasive ventilation for acute exacerbations of chronic obstructive pulmonary disease. *N Engl J Med* 333:817–822, 1995.
12. Celikel T, Sungur M, Ceyhan B, et al: Comparison of noninvasive positive pressure ventilation with standard medical therapy in hypercapnic acute respiratory failure. *Chest* 114:1636–1642, 1998.
13. Plant PK, Owen JL, Elliott MW: Noninvasive ventilation for acute exacerbations of chronic obstructive pulmonary disease on general respiratory wards: a multicentre randomized, controlled trial. *Lancet* 355:1931, 2000.
14. Bott J, Carroll MP, Conway JH, et al: Randomized, controlled trial of nasal ventilation in acute ventilatory failure due to chronic obstructive airways disease. *Lancet* 341:1555–1557, 1993.
15. Nava S, Ambrosino N, Clini E, et al: Noninvasive mechanical ventilation in the weaning of patients with respiratory failure due to chronic obstructive pulmonary disease: a randomized, controlled trial. *Ann Intern Med* 128: 721–728, 1998.
16. Keenan SP, Sinuff T, Cook DJ, et al: Which patients with acute exacerbation of chronic obstructive pulmonary disease benefit from noninvasive positive-pressure ventilation? A systematic review of the literature. *Ann Intern Med* 138:I27, 2003.
17. Meduri GU, Cook TR, Turner RE, et al: Noninvasive positive pressure ventilation in status asthmaticus. *Chest* 110:767–774, 1996.
18. Murase K, Tomdii K, Chin K, et al: The use of non-invasive ventilation for life-threatening asthma attacks: changes in the need for intubation. *Respirology* 15:714–720, 2010.
19. Carroll CL, Schramm CM: Noninvasive positive pressure ventilation for the treatment of status asthmaticus in children. *Ann Allergy Asthma Immunol* 96:454–459, 2006.
20. Ram FS, Wellington S, Row BH, et al: Noninvasive positive pressure ventilation for treatment of respiratory failure due to severe acute exacerbations of asthma. *Cochrane Database Syst Rev* (1):CD004360, 2005.
21. Rabatin JT, Gay PC: Noninvasive ventilation. *Mayo Clin Proc* 74:817–820, 1999.
22. Ferrer M, Esquinas A, Arancibia F, et al: Noninvasive ventilation during persistent weaning failure. *Am J Respir Crit Care Med* 168:70–76, 2003.
23. Girault C, Bubenheim M, Abroug F, et al: Noninvasive ventilation and weaning in patients with chronic hypercapnic respiratory failure: a randomized multicenter trial. *Am J Respir Crit Care Med* 184(6):672–679, 2011.
24. Vitacca M, Ambrosino N, Clini E, et al: Physiological response to pressure support ventilation delivered before and after extubation in patients not capable of totally spontaneous autonomous breathing. *Am J Respir Crit Care Med* 164:638–641, 2001.
25. Bersten AD, Holt AW, Vedig AE, et al: Treatment of severe cardiogenic pulmonary edema with continuous positive airway pressure delivered by face mask. *N Engl J Med* 325:1825–1830, 1991.
26. Lin M, Yang YF, Chiang HT, et al: Reappraisal of continuous positive airway pressure therapy in acute cardiogenic pulmonary edema. *Chest* 107:1379–1386, 1995.
27. Kelly CA, Newby DE, McDonagh TA, et al: Randomised controlled trial of continuous positive airway pressure and standard oxygen therapy in acute pulmonary oedema. *Eur Heart J* 23:1379–1386, 2002.
28. Masip J, Betbese AJ, Paez J, et al: Noninvasive pressure support ventilation versus conventional oxygen therapy in acute cardiogenic pulmonary oedema: a randomised trial. *Lancet* 356:2126–2132, 2000.
29. Levitt MA: A prospective, randomized trial of BiPAP in severe acute congestive heart failure. *J Emerg Med* 21:363–369, 2001.
30. Nava S, Carbone G, DiBattista N, et al: Noninvasive ventilation in cardiogenic pulmonary edema. *Am J Respir Crit Care Med* 168:1432–1437, 2003.
31. Bellone A, Monari A, Cortellaro F, et al: Myocardial infarction rate in acute pulmonary edema: noninvasive pressure support ventilation versus continuous positive airway pressure. *Crit Care Med* 32:1860–1865, 2004.
32. Bellone A, Vettorello M, Monari A, et al: Noninvasive pressure support ventilation versus continuous positive airway pressure in acute hypercapnic pulmonary edema. *Intensive Care Med* 31:807–811, 2005.
33. Park M, Lorenzi-Filho G, Feltrim MI, et al: Oxygen therapy, continuous positive airway pressure, or noninvasive bilevel positive pressure ventilation in the treatment of acute cardiogenic pulmonary edema. *Arq Bras Cardiol* 76:221–230, 2001.
34. Crane SD, Elliott MW, Gilligan P, et al: Randomised controlled comparison of continuous positive airways pressure, bilevel noninvasive ventilation, and standard treatment in emergency department patients with acute cardiogenic pulmonary oedema. *Emerg Med J* 21:155–161, 2004.

35. Park M, Sangean MC, Volpe Mde S, et al: Randomized, prospective trial of oxygen, continuous positive airway pressure, and bilevel positive airway pressure by face mask in acute cardiogenic pulmonary edema. *Crit Care Med* 32:2407–2415, 2004.
36. Jolliet P, Abajo B, Pasquina P: Non-invasive pressure support ventilation in severe community-acquired pneumonia. *Intensive Care Med* 27:797–799, 2001.
37. Rana S, Jenad H, Gay P, et al: Failure of non-invasive ventilation in patients with acute lung injury: observational cohort study. *Crit Care* 10:R79, 2006.
38. Antonelli M, Conti G, Moro ML, et al: Predictors of failure of noninvasive positive pressure ventilation in patients with acute hypoxemic respiratory failure: a multi-center study. *Intensive Care Med* 27:1718–1728, 2001.
39. Ferrer M, Esquinas A, Leon M, et al: Noninvasive ventilation in severe hypoxemic respiratory failure. *Am J Respir Crit Care Med* 168:1438–1444, 2003.
40. Antonelli M, Conti G, Esquinas A, et al: A multiple-center survey on the use in clinical practice of noninvasive ventilation as a first-line intervention for acute respiratory distress syndrome. *Crit Care Med* 35:18–25, 2007.
41. Martin TJ, Hovis JD, Costantino JP, et al: A randomized prospective evaluation of noninvasive ventilation for acute respiratory failure. *Am J Respir Crit Care Med* 161:807–813, 2000.
42. Keenan SP, Sinuff T, Cook DJ, et al: Does noninvasive positive pressure ventilation improve outcome in acute hypoxemic respiratory failure? A systematic review. *Crit Care Med* 32:2516–2523, 2004.
43. Schettino GPP, Hess D, Altobelli N, et al: Is noninvasive positive pressure ventilation (NPPV) effective outside of controlled trials? (abstract). *Am J Respir Crit Care Med* 165:A389, 2002.
44. Delclaux C, L'Her E, Alberti C, et al: Treatment of acute hypoxemic nonhypercapnic respiratory insufficiency with continuous positive airway pressure delivered by a face mask: a randomized, controlled trial. *JAMA* 284: 2352–2360, 2000.
45. Hilbert G, Gruson D, Vargas F, et al: Noninvasive ventilation in immunosuppressed patients with pulmonary infiltrates, fever, and acute respiratory failure. *N Engl J Med* 344:481–487, 2001.
46. Antonelli M, Conti G, Bufi M, et al: Noninvasive ventilation for treatment of acute respiratory failure in patients undergoing solid organ transplantation. *JAMA* 283:235–241, 2000.
47. Confalonieri M, Calderini E, Terraciano S, et al: Noninvasive ventilation for treating acute respiratory failure in AIDS patients with *Pneumocystis carinii* pneumonia. *Intensive Care Med* 28:1233–1238, 2002.
48. Nourdine N, Combes P, Carton MJ, et al: Does noninvasive ventilation reduce the ICU nosocomial infection risk? A prospective clinical survey. *Intensive Care Med* 25:567–573, 1999.
49. Girou E, Schortgen F, Delclaux C, et al: Association of noninvasive ventilation with nosocomial infections and survival in critically ill patients. *JAMA* 284:2361–2367, 2000.
50. Hill N: Noninvasive ventilation for immunocompromised patients. *N Engl J Med* 344:522, 2001.
51. Meduri GU, Fox RC, Abou-Shala N, et al: Noninvasive mechanical ventilation via face mask in patients with acute respiratory failure who refused endotracheal intubation. *Crit Care Med* 22:1584–1590, 1994.
52. Schettino G, Altobelli N, Kacmarek RM: Noninvasive positive pressure ventilation reverses acute respiratory failure in select "do-not-intubate" patients. *Crit Care Med* 33:1976–1982, 2005.
53. Levy M, Tanios MA, Nelson D, et al: Outcomes of patients with do-not-intubate orders treated with noninvasive ventilation. *Crit Care Med* 32: 2002–2007, 2004.
54. Curtis JR, Cook DJ, Sinuff T, et al: Noninvasive positive pressure ventilation in critical and palliative care settings: understanding the goals of therapy. *Crit Care Med* 35:932–939, 2007.
55. Joris JL, Sottiauz TM, Chiche JD, et al: Effect of bi-level positive airway pressure nasal ventilation on the postoperative pulmonary restrictive syndrome in obese patients undergoing gastroplasty. *Chest* 111:665–670, 1997.
56. Squadrone V, Coha M, Cerutti E, et al: Continuous positive airway pressure for treatment of postoperative hypoxemia. *JAMA* 293:589–595, 2005.
57. Kindgen-Milles D, Muller E, Buhl R, et al: Nasal-continuous positive airway pressure reduces pulmonary morbidity and length of hospital stay following thoracoabdominal aortic surgery. *Chest* 128:821–828, 2005.
58. Nava S, Gregoretti C, Fanfulla F, et al: Noninvasive ventilation for prevention of respiratory failure after extubation in high-risk patients. *Crit Care Med* 33:2465–2470, 2005.
59. Ferrer M, Valencia M, Nicolas JM, et al: Early noninvasive ventilation averts extubation failure in patients at risk. *Am J Respir Crit Care Med* 173:164–170, 2006.
60. Keenan SP, Powers C, McCormack DG, et al: Noninvasive positive-pressure ventilation for postextubation respiratory distress. *JAMA* 287:3238–3244, 2002.
61. Esteban A, Frutos-Vivar F, Ferguson ND, et al: Noninvasive positive-pressure ventilation for respiratory failure after extubation. *N Engl J Med* 350:2452–2460, 2004.
62. Ozsancak A, D'Ambrosio C, Hill N: Nocturnal noninvasive ventilation. *Chest* 133:1275–1285, 2008.
63. Clinical indications for noninvasive positive pressure ventilation in chronic respiratory failure due to restrictive lung disease, COPD, and nocturnal hypoventilation: a consensus conference report. *Chest* 116:521, 1999.
64. Schonhofer B, Polkey MI, Suchi S, et al: Effect of home mechanical ventilation on inspiratory muscle strength in COPD. *Chest* 130:1834–1838, 2006.
65. When should respiratory muscles be exercised? *Chest* 84:76–84, 1983.
66. Hill N: Noninvasive ventilation: does it work, for whom, and how? *Am Rev Respir Dis* 147:1050–1055, 1993.
67. Wijkstra PJ, Lacasse Y, Guyatt GH, et al: A meta-analysis of nocturnal noninvasive positive pressure ventilation in patients with stable COPD. *Chest* 124:337–343, 2003.
68. Hill NS, Eveloff SE, Carlisle CC, et al: Efficacy of nocturnal nasal ventilation in patients with restrictive thoracic disease. *Am Rev Respir Dis* 145:365–371, 1992.
69. Annane D, Quera-Salva MA, Lofasa F, et al: Mechanisms underlying the effects of nocturnal ventilation on daytime blood gases in neuromuscular diseases. *Eur Respir J* 13:157–162, 1999.
70. Nickol AN, Hart N, Hopkinson NS, et al: Mechanisms of improvement of respiratory failure in patients with restrictive thoracic disease treated with non-invasive ventilation. *Thorax* 60:754–760, 2005.
71. Ferris G, Servera-Pieras E, Vergara P, et al: Kyphoscoliosis ventilatory insufficiency: noninvasive management outcomes. *Am J Phys Med Rehabil* 79: 24–29, 2000.
72. Mellies U, Dohna-Schwake C, Ragette R, et al: Respiratory failure in Pompe disease: treatment with noninvasive ventilation. *Neurology* 64:1465–1467, 2005.
73. Raphael JC, Chevret S, Chastang C, et al: Randomized trial of preventive nasal ventilation in Duchenne muscular dystrophy. French Multicentre Cooperative Group on Home Mechanical Ventilation Assistance in Duchenne de Boulogne Muscular Dystrophy. *Lancet* 343:1600–1604, 1994.
74. Miller R, Jackson C, Kasarskis E, et al: Practice parameter update: the care of the patient with amyotrophic lateral sclerosis (an evidence-based review). Report of the Quality Standards Subcommittee of the American Academy of Neurology. *Neurology* 73:1218–1226, 2009.
75. Bourke S, Tomlinson M, Williams T, et al: Effects of non-invasive ventilation on survival and quality of life in patients with amyotrophic lateral sclerosis: a randomized controlled trial. *Lancet Neurol* 5:140–146, 2006.
76. Kleopa KA, Sherman M, Neal B, et al: Bipap improves survival and rate of pulmonary function decline in patients with ALS. *J Neurol Sci* 164:82–88, 1999.
77. Pinto A, de Carvalho M, Evangelista T, et al: Nocturnal pulse oximetry: a new approach to establish the appropriate time for non-invasive ventilation in ALS patients. *Amyotroph Lateral Scler Other Motor Neuron Disord* 4:31–35, 2003.
78. Bourke SC, Bullock RE, Williams TL, et al: Noninvasive ventilation in ALS: indications and effect on quality of life. *Neurology* 61:171–177, 2003.
79. Gruis KL, Brown DL, Schoennemann A, et al: Predictors of noninvasive ventilation tolerance in patients with amyotrophic lateral sclerosis. *Muscle Nerve* 32:808–811, 2005.
80. Olney RK, Murphy J, Forshew D, et al: The effects of executive and behavioral dysfunction on the course of ALS. *Neurology* 65:1774–1777, 2005.

81. Lyall RA, Donaldson N, Fleming T, et al: A prospective study of quality of life in ALS patients treated with noninvasive ventilation. *Neurology* 57:153–156, 2001.
82. Butz M, Wollinsky KH, Wiedemuth-Catrinescu U, et al: Longitudinal effects of noninvasive positive-pressure ventilation in patients with amyotrophic lateral sclerosis. *Am J Phys Med Rehabil* 82:597–604, 2003.
83. Kaub-Wittemer D, Steinbuchel N, Wasner M, et al: Quality of life and psychosocial issues in ventilated patients with amyotrophic lateral sclerosis and their caregivers. *J Pain Symptom Manage* 26:890–896, 2003.
84. Nocturnal noninvasive positive pressure ventilation in stable COPD: a systematic review and individual patient data meta-analysis. *Respir Med* 108(2):329–337, 2014.
85. Tuggery JM, Plant PK, Elliott MW: Domiciliary non-invasive ventilation for recurrent acidotic exacerbations of COPD: an economic analysis. *Thorax* 58:867–871, 2003.
86. Criner GJ, Brennan K, Travaline JM, et al: Efficacy and compliance with noninvasive positive pressure ventilation in patients with chronic respiratory failure. *Chest* 116:667–675, 1999.
87. Casey KR, Ortiz KO, Brown LK: Sleep-related hypoventilation/hypoxemic syndromes. *Chest* 131:1936–1948, 2007.
88. Olson AL, Zwillich C: The obesity hypoventilation syndrome. *Am J Med* 118:948–956, 2005.
89. Berg G, Delaive K, Manfreda J, et al: The use of health-care resources in obesity-hypoventilation syndrome. *Chest* 120:377–383, 2001.
90. Nowbar S, Burkart KM, Gonzales R, et al: Obesity-associated hypoventilation in hospitalized patients: prevalence, effects and outcome. *Am J Med* 116:1–7, 2004.
91. Masa JF, Celli BR, Riesco JA, et al: The obesity hypoventilation syndrome can be treated with noninvasive mechanical ventilation. *Chest* 119:1102–1107, 2001.
92. Perez de Llano LA, Golpe R, Ortiz Piquer M, et al: Short-term and long-term effects of nasal intermittent positive pressure ventilation in patients with obesity-hypoventilation syndrome. *Chest* 128:587–594, 2005.
93. Piper AJ, Wang D, Yee BJ, et al: Randomized trial of CPAP vs bilevel support in the treatment of obesity hypoventilation syndrome without severe nocturnal desaturation. *Thorax* 63:395–401, 2008.
94. Mokhlesi B, Tulaimat A: Recent advances in obesity hypoventilation syndrome. *Chest* 132:1322–1336, 2007.
95. Diaz GG, Alcaraz AC, Talavera JC, et al: Noninvasive positive-pressure ventilation to treat hypercapnic coma secondary to respiratory failure. *Chest* 127:952–960, 2005.
96. Scala R, Naldi M, Archinucci I, et al: Noninvasive positive pressure ventilation in patients with acute exacerbations of COPD and varying levels of consciousness. *Chest* 128:1657–1666, 2005.
97. Soo Hoo GW, Santiago S, Williams AJ: Nasal mechanical ventilation for hypercapnic respiratory failure in chronic obstructive pulmonary disease: determinants of success and failure. *Crit Care Med* 22:1253–1261, 1994.
98. Ambrosino N, Foglio K, Rubini F, et al: Noninvasive mechanical ventilation in acute respiratory failure due to chronic obstructive pulmonary disease: correlates for success. *Thorax* 50:755–757, 1995.
99. Poponick JM, Renston JP, Bennett RP, et al: Use of a ventilatory support system (BiPAP) for acute respiratory failure in the emergency department. *Chest* 116:166–171, 1999.
100. Meduri GU, Turner RE, Abou-Shala N, et al: Noninvasive positive pressure ventilation via face mask: first line intervention in patients with acute hypercapnic and hypoxemic respiratory failure. *Chest* 109:179–193, 1996.
101. Codazzi D, Nacoti M, Passoni M, et al: Continuous positive airway pressure with modified helmet for treatment of hypoxemic acute respiratory failure in infants and a preschool population: a feasibility study. *Pediatr Crit Care Med* 7:455–460, 2006.
102. Chiumello D, Pelosi P, Carlesso E, et al: Noninvasive positive pressure ventilation delivered by helmet versus standard face mask. *Intensive Care Med* 29:1671–1679, 2003.
103. Patroniti N, Foti G, Manfio A, et al: Head helmet versus face mask for noninvasive continuous positive airway pressure: a physiological study. *Intensive Care Med* 29:1680–1687, 2003.
104. Antonelli M, Pennisi MA, Pelosi P, et al: Noninvasive positive pressure ventilation using a helmet in patients with acute exacerbation of chronic obstructive pulmonary disease: a feasibility study. *Anesthesiology* 100:16–24, 2004.
105. Taccone P, Hess D, Caironi P, et al: Continuous positive airway pressure delivered with a "helmet": effects on carbon dioxide rebreathing. *Crit Care Med* 32:2090–2096, 2004.
106. Navalesi P, Fanfulla F, Frigerio P, et al: Physiologic evaluation of noninvasive mechanical ventilation delivered with three types of mask in patients with chronic hypercapnic respiratory failure. *Crit Care Med* 28:1785–1790, 2000.
107. Girault C, Briel A, Benichou J, et al: Interface strategy during noninvasive positive pressure ventilation for hypercapnic acute respiratory failure. *Crit Care Med* 37:124–131, 2009.
108. Ferguson GT, Gilmartin M: CO_2 rebreathing during BiPAP ventilatory assistance. *Am J Respir Crit Care Med* 151:1126–1135, 1995.
109. Lofaso F, Brochard L, Touchard D, et al: Evaluation of carbon dioxide rebreathing during pressure support ventilation with airway management system (BiPAP) devices. *Chest* 108:772–778, 1995.
110. Schwartz RA, Kacmarek RM, Hess DR: Factors affecting oxygen delivery with bi-level positive airway pressure. *Respir Care* 49:270–275, 2004.
111. Jurban A, Van de Graaff WB, Tobin MJ: Variability of patient-ventilator interaction with pressure support ventilation in patients in patients with chronic obstructive pulmonary disease. *Am J Respir Crit Care Med* 152:129, 1995.
112. Parthasarathy S, Jubran A, Tobin MJ: Cycling of inspiratory and expiratory muscle groups with the ventilator in airflow limitation. *Am J Respir Crit Care Med* 158:1471–1478, 1998.
113. Calderini E, Confalonieri M, Puccio PG, et al: Patient-ventilator asynchrony during noninvasive ventilation: the role of expiratory trigger. *Intensive Care Med* 25:662–667, 1999.
114. Branson RD, Campell RS: Pressure support ventilation, patient-ventilator synchrony, and ventilator algorithms. *Respir Care* 43:1045–1047, 1998.
115. Evans TW: International Consensus Conference in Intensive Care Medicine: noninvasive positive pressure ventilation. *Intensive Care Med* 27:166–178, 2001.
116. Richards GN, Cistulli PA, Ungar RG, et al: Mouth leak with nasal continuous positive airway pressure increases nasal airway resistance. *Am J Respir Crit Care Med* 154:182–186, 1996.
117. Hayes MJ, McGregor FB, Roberts DN, et al: Continuous nasal positive airway pressure with a mouth leak: effect on nasal mucosal blood flux and nasal geometry. *Thorax* 50:1179–1182, 1995.
118. Massie CA, Hart RW, Peralez K, et al: Effects of humidification on nasal symptoms and compliance in sleep apnea patients using continuous positive airway pressure. *Chest* 116:403–408, 1999.
119. Rakotonanahary D, Pelletier-Fleury N, Gagnadoux F, et al: Predictive factors for the need for additional humidification during nasal continuous positive airway pressure therapy. *Chest* 119:460–465, 2001.
120. Ho-Tai LM, Devitt JH, Noel AG, et al: Gas leak and gastric insufflation during controlled ventilation: face mask versus laryngeal mask airway. *Can J Anaesth* 45:206–211, 1998.
121. Chatmongkolchart S, Schettino GP, Dillman C, et al: In vitro evaluation of aerosol bronchodilator delivery during noninvasive positive pressure ventilation: effect of ventilator settings and nebulizer position. *Crit Care Med* 30:2515–2519, 2002.
122. Keenan SP, Gregor J, Sibbald WJ, et al: Noninvasive positive pressure ventilation in the setting of severe, acute exacerbations of chronic obstructive pulmonary disease: more effective and less expensive. *Crit Care Med* 28:2094–2102, 2000.
123. Jasmer RM, Matthay MA: Cost-effectiveness of noninvasive ventilation for acute chronic obstructive pulmonary disease: cashing in too quickly. *Crit Care Med* 28:2170–2171, 2000.
124. Nava S, Evangelisti I, Rampulla C, et al: Human and financial costs of noninvasive mechanical ventilation in patients affected by COPD and acute respiratory failure. *Chest* 111:1631–1638, 1997.

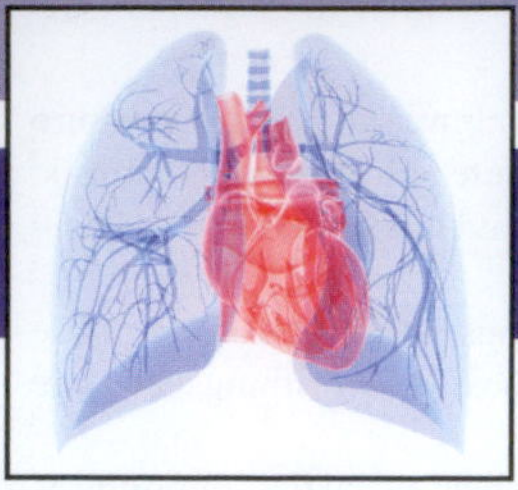

CHAPTER 50

Extracorporeal Life Support (ECLS)

CLORINDA SUAREZ AND PATRICIA ENGLISH

CHAPTER OBJECTIVES

After reading this chapter you will be able to:

- Describe two primary goals of extracorporeal membrane oxygenation (ECMO).
- List indications for initiating ECMO.
- Differentiate between venovenous (VV), venoarterial (VA), and arteriovenous (AV) ECMO.
- Discuss ECMO physiology.
- Identify components of a typical ECMO circuit and their functions.
- List risks and complications of ECMO.
- Discuss when and how to wean off of ECMO.
- Describe the respiratory therapist role as an ECMO specialist.
- Describe safety system incorporated in or added to ECMO systems.
- Identify typical sites for cannula placement for VA support.
- Identify typical sites for cannula placement in VV support.
- Describe the reasons ECMO patients need to be anticoagulated.
- Describe how anticoagulation is typically monitored during ECMO.
- Discuss the significance of ventilator support and management during ECMO.

CHAPTER OUTLINE

The Respiratory Therapist as ECMO Specialist
International Registry
Patients Receiving ECMO
  Newborns
  Pediatric and Adult Patients
Physiology
Equipment
Anticoagulation Management
Cannulas
Types of Support
  Venoarterial ECMO
  Venovenous ECMO
  Arteriovenous ECMO
Initiation of Support
Maintenance of an ECMO Run
Transporting a Patient on ECMO
Risks and Complications
Blood Products During ECMO
Weaning and Decannulation

KEY TERMS

activated clotting time
afterload
arteriovenous (AV)
extracorporeal life support (ECLS)
extracorporeal membrane oxygenation (ECMO)
cardiac output
cannulation
decannulation
membrane pressures
oxygen content
oxygen delivery
preload
pump flow
recirculation
sweep flow
tamponade
venoarterial (VA)
venous reservoir
venovenous (VV)

Extracorporeal life support (ECLS) encompasses several forms of mechanical support, all of which involve circulating blood from a patient to outside the body, through a mechanical gas exchanger, and returning it back to the patient. The most common form of ECLS is **extracorporeal membrane oxygenation (ECMO)**. There are three general types of ECMO support, **venoarterial (VA)**, **venovenous (VV)**, and the emerging **arteriovenous (AV)** support. Distinctions between the three types will be outlined later in this chapter.

ECMO is typically considered only in conditions when maximum conventional support has not been successful in delivering oxygen, removing CO_2 or providing adequate cardiac function. ECMO itself does not heal or fix the condition but rather is life-saving support for the most severe forms of acute heart and/or lung failure. Patients can be placed on ECMO for either cardiac or respiratory support, though at times both cardiac and respiratory support are indicated. ECMO will allow the heart and/or lungs to rest and help avoid the damage that can result from high levels of conventional treatments. The primary goals of ECMO are to provide adequate **oxygen delivery** and remove carbon dioxide while the lungs and/or heart recover, or in some cases until the lungs or heart can be transplanted.

RULE OF THUMB

ECMO is an option for the management of severe respiratory failure or cardiogenic shock refractory to conventional treatments for patients with reversible conditions or those eligible for transplantation.

THE RESPIRATORY THERAPIST AS ECMO SPECIALIST

ECMO is provided to patients with life-threatening conditions. These situations require intense monitoring by clinicians with good critical thinking skills, strong knowledge of cardiopulmonary physiology, and technical adeptness. Clinicians who perform this role are referred to as ECMO specialists. Respiratory therapists (RTs) are often viewed as ideal professionals for this role due to their primary training. RTs have a strong science background, a thorough understanding of cardiopulmonary physiology, and the ability to handle and manage highly technical equipment. In many ECMO centers RTs play a significant role in the ECMO program. They assist in the initiation of ECMO, provide hour-to-hour management of the ECMO support, and provide ECMO education for the many clinical services involved in the care of ECMO patients. Experienced RTs with good critical thinking skills receive additional training to take on the role of ECMO specialist. The specific role of a specialist varies among ECMO institutions but the essential education most often provided for this role follows the Extracorporeal Life Support Organization (ELSO) (see Box 50-1).

Box 50-1 ELSO Guidelines for Training of ECMO Specialists

- Introduction to ECMO
- Physiology of the diseases supported with ECMO
- Pre-ECMO procedures
- Criteria and contraindications for ECMO
- Physiology of coagulation
- ECMO equipment
- Physiology of VA and VV ECMO
- Daily patient and circuit management
- Emergencies and complications during ECMO
- Management of complex ECMO cases
- Weaning from ECMO
- Decannulation procedures
- Post-ECMO complications

TABLE 50-1
Number of Patients Reported to the ECLS Registry With Survival Rates in Each Category

	Total Patients	Survived ECLS		Survived to Dc or Transfer	
Neonatal					
Respiratory	27,728	23,358	84%	20,592	74%
Cardiac	5810	3600	62%	2389	41%
ECPR	1112	712	64%	449	40%
Pediatric					
Respiratory	6569	4327	66%	3760	57%
Cardiac	7314	4825	66%	3679	50%
ECPR	2370	1313	55%	976	41%
Adult					
Respiratory	7008	4587	65%	4026	57%
Cardiac	5603	3129	56%	2294	41%
ECPR	1657	639	39%	471	28%
Total	65,171	46,490	71%	38,636	59%

ECLS Registry Report, International Summary, January, 2015.

INTERNATIONAL REGISTRY

With the development of an international ECLS registry in the late 1980s, centers providing ECMO began submitting data on the patients supported in centers from around the world. Since that time patient information, including patient age, diagnosis, type of support, complications, and outcomes have been compiled by the registry. Table 50-1 shows a summary of patients entered into the registry and their outcomes.[1]

PATIENTS RECEIVING ECMO

Newborns

In the 1980s ECMO support was almost exclusively used for newborns with respiratory failure.[2] The primary conditions of patients placed on ECMO were meconium aspiration syndrome, respiratory distress syndrome, sepsis, congenital diaphragmatic hernia, and primary pulmonary hypertension.[2] Many of these patients also had pulmonary hypertension

Box 50-2 Indications for ECMO in Newborns

- Birth weight >2 kg
- Gestational age ≥34 weeks
- Maximum conventional ventilation
- Failure of optimal medical support including INO
- Lung disease considered reversible
- Absence of uncontrolled bleeding
- No uncorrectable cardiac anomalies
- No other lethal anomalies

Box 50-3 Indications for ECMO in Adult Patients

- Acute hypoxic or hypercarbic respiratory failure
    - Sat <88 on FiO_2 1.0 with PEEP 15 cm H_2O
    - With plateau pressure >30 and trail of INO or epoprostenol
    - Respiratory acidosis with pH ≤7.20
- Normal RV/LV function
- Murray Score >3

secondary to their primary condition. Improving oxygen delivery using ECMO support can greatly reduce pulmonary hypertension. ECMO often was the best option to improve oxygen delivery while the heart and lungs healed from the primary insult. According to the ECLS registry more than 27,000 newborns have received ECMO for respiratory failure with survival rates to hospital discharge from 51% to 94% depending on the specific diagnosis.[1] Criteria for ECMO in newborns with respiratory failure are well established and are outlined in Box 50-2.[3] Contraindications for offering ECMO in the newborn population fall into two categories: absolute and relative. Absolute contraindications include lethal congenital anomalies, severe irreversible brain damage, and Grade lll or higher intracranial hemorrhage (ICH).[4] Relative contraindications include birth weight <1.6 kg, gestational age <34 weeks, irreversible organ damage (unless a transplant candidate), mechanical ventilation with 100% oxygen for >13 days, and some coagulopathies.[4] The data collected over 25 years have been instrumental in establishing guidelines for newborn ECMO.

Development of less risky and less invasive therapies such as surfactants, nitric oxide, and improved ventilator strategies have decreased the number of newborns considered for ECMO.[5] ECMO support for newborn respiratory failure over the last few years has decreased significantly to only approximately 800 cases per year worldwide.[1]

Pediatric and Adult Patients

Although the number of newborns receiving ECMO continues to decline, ECMO cases in pediatric and adult patients are on the rise. This trend is likely due to improved strategies in ECMO management and advances in technology which has led to better equipment for long-term support. During the past five years the number of centers developing ECMO programs has increased greatly. Many new centers are providing ECMO primarily to pediatric and adult patients, with the largest increases in two categories: ECMO for cardiac support and ECMO as a bridge for lung transplant.[6] Unfortunately, guidelines for initiating ECMO support in pediatric and adult patients are less clear than the well-established guidelines for newborns. Criteria are generally associated with the type of support needed and are not always the same from center to center.[7] Box 50-3 provides an example of general indications for adult VA and VV ECMO. Contraindications for pediatric and adult patients generally fall into the absolute and relative categories. Absolute contraindications typically include acute ICH or stroke, mechanical ventilation >7 days, paralytics and steroids >48 hours, in hospital CPR >60 minutes, severe aortic insufficiency, end stage liver disease, BMI >40, contraindication to anticoagulation or refusal to receive blood products.[3] Relative contraindications are age >70 years old, active cancer, multiple suicide attempts, chronic kidney disease, and multiorgan system failure >3 organs.[3]

PHYSIOLOGY

To understand ECMO physiology it is essential to understand normal cardiopulmonary physiology. During normal circulation blood is pumped from the right side of the heart to the lungs where oxygen and carbon dioxide are exchanged. From the lungs, blood is returned to the left side of the heart. The left heart then pumps oxygenated blood to the major organs and tissues. The amount of oxygen contained in blood leaving the heart is the arterial oxygen content. The absolute amount of blood pumped from the heart is **cardiac output**. Oxygen content times cardiac output equals the amount of oxygen delivered to the tissues.

Oxygen content is rarely measured directly at the bedside but it is critical in managing severely ill patients. Oxygen is carried in the blood in two forms: dissolved in plasma and in red blood cells bound to hemoglobin (as a percentage of the maximum saturation). These two components make up the total **oxygen content** in the blood. The amount of oxygen dissolved in plasma is a very minor portion of the total oxygen content. The dissolved portion is represented by the PO_2 (mm Hg) × 0.003. The majority of oxygen is bound to hemoglobin and is represented by the equation Hb × % SaO_2 × 1.34. Total oxygen content is calculated using the following equation

$$O_2 \text{ Content}\left[(\text{P02}\times.003)+(\text{Hg}\times\text{SaO}_2\times1.34)\right]$$

Therefore with inadequate levels of hemoglobin, oxygen content is significantly diminished.

To understand the importance of hemoglobin, consider the following: A patient with a PO_2 of 40 mmHg, with a typical oxygen saturation of 70% and a normal hemoglobin level (15 gms) has more oxygen than a patient with a PO_2 of 100 (saturation 100%) and a low hemoglobin level (8 gms). See Chapter 12 for more complete details on oxygen content and oxygen delivery.

MINI CLINI

PROBLEM: Hemoglobin level in a patient who is bleeding has dropped from 15 to 10 g/dl. His PO_2 remains unchanged at 90 mm Hg. How much would his O_2 content change?

Calculate the change in O_2 content.

$$(PO_2 \times .003) \times (Hg \times SaO_2 \times 1.34)]$$

The O_2 content with a hemoglobin of 15 is 20.37.

The O_2 content with a hemoglobin of 10 is 13.67.

Discussion: This clearly demonstrates the importance of hemoglobin in providing adequate oxygen content. Delivery of oxygen is dependent on the oxygen content and the cardiac output. When oxygen content is low, the body will normally respond by increasing the cardiac output. Total delivered oxygen can be calculated using the following equation:

$$O_2\ \text{Delivery}\,[(PO_2 \times .003) + (Hg \times SaO_2 \times 1.34)] \times (HR \times SV) = DO_2$$

MINI CLINI

PROBLEM: The patient has a cardiac output of 5 L/min and is on 4 L/min of VA ECMO support. Eighty percent of the patient's cardiac output is therefore oxygenated by the artificial oxygenator and is 100% saturated. The patient has essentially no lung function. His SvO_2 is 65% with a PO_2 of 35 mm Hg. Twenty percent of the patient's cardiac output goes through the nonfunctional native lungs where no oxygen is added.

What is the patient's SaO_2 when blood from the ECMO-supported cardiac output and the native cardiac output mix?

Discussion: The combined saturation can be calculated by multiplying the % saturation of each portion of the cardiac output. This patient's combined saturation can be determined by multiplying the 80% (4 of 5 L/min) of the cardiac output that becomes 100% saturated by the ECMO oxygenator (0.8 x 1), and then multiplying the 20% (1 of 5 L/min) of the output that returns to the native lungs 65% saturated, (0.2 x 0.65) and adding the results of each

$$(0.8 \times 1) + (0.2 \times 0.65) = 0.93$$

The mixed saturation of this patient would be 93%. To achieve a higher saturation a larger portion of the cardiac output could be pumped through the oxygenator and saturated to 100%. The portion of cardiac output that would remain through the native lungs would decrease. With a smaller portion of blood saturated to only 65% the combined saturation would increase.

When cardiac function is impaired the ability to increase cardiac output is altered and will result in inadequate amounts of oxygen delivered to the tissues. When this happens, anaerobic metabolism occurs and lactic acid is produced. Alternatively, carbon dioxide is produced from systemic metabolism. With normal adequate lung function and normal blood flow through the lungs appropriate amounts of carbon dioxide are excreted and spontaneous ventilation keeps PCO_2 within acceptable ranges. When altered states of metabolism increase CO_2 production it is imperative that the lungs are able to remove more CO_2. In diseased lungs or conditions that alter blood flow to the lungs, higher levels of CO_2 remain in the blood. When maximum conventional support fails to provide adequate delivery of oxygen to the tissue or inadequate removal of carbon dioxide occurs, a patient who has no absolute contraindications can be considered for ECMO.

EQUIPMENT

ECMO systems are intended to temporarily support the cardiac and pulmonary function of the patient who cannot maintain adequate tissue oxygen delivery. Basically, ECMO has the task of pumping the blood, delivering oxygen to the blood, and removing CO_2. The circuit consists of polyvinylchloride (PVC) tubing segments that have different inner diameters depending on the patient's size: ¼-inch for a neonate to ⅜-inch for pediatric/adult sized patients. Some circuits contain a heparin-based coating to reduce the response of blood to nonendothelial surfaces and to decrease the risk of clot formation. The circuit is generally custom designed using the shortest amount of tubing necessary to allow less resistance to flow and to decrease circuit volume. This is of particular importance for the newborn population because larger circuit volumes result in hemodilution and require additional transfusion of blood products. Infusion ports can be added along the tubing for infusing medications in patients who have limited IV access. These ports can also be an option for access when continuous veno venous hemofiltration (CVVH) is required. Blood is drained from the patient into the circuit by either a centrifugal or roller pump. From the pump it goes through an artificial lung, referred to as an oxygenator, where oxygen is added and CO_2 removed (Figure 50-1).

In some systems a **venous reservoir**, referred to as a bladder, is placed before the pump to help with assessing available blood volume. The bladder is then connected to a pressure monitor which can be set to keep the pump from rotating too quickly and exerting an excessive negative pressure on the cannulated vessel (Figure 50-2). Newer systems that combine pressure monitors and servo regulation are more efficient and are eliminating the need for bladders. Bladders are most often used with roller pumps and are not typically needed with centrifugal pumps.

The ECMO system is powered by the blood pump. The pump function is to draw blood in, either from a venous reservoir (the bladder) or directly from the venous circulation, pump it through the oxygenator, and then back into the patient. The two types of pumps frequently used are the centrifugal (or vortex) pump and the roller (or occlusive) pump.

The centrifugal pump is made up of polycarbonate cones attached to a magnetic disk that is attached to a controller (Figure 50-3). The cones spin at an adjustable rate when

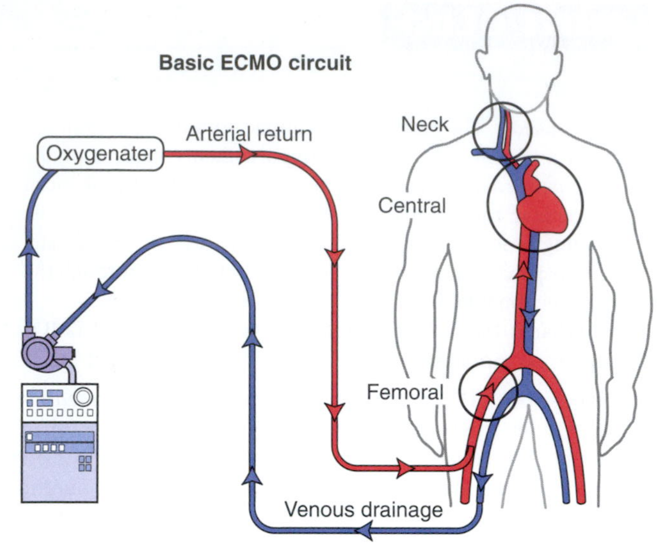

FIGURE 50-1 Illustration of the blood pathway of an ECMO circuit. Blood drains through the circuit to a blood pump which pushes it through an artificial lung oxygenating the blood and removing CO_2 before returning the blood to the body.

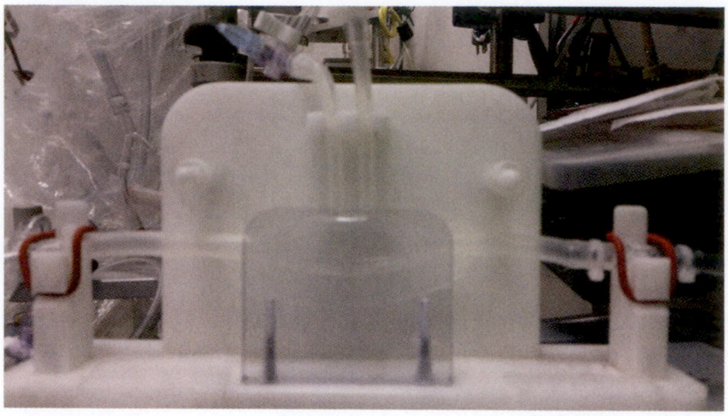

FIGURE 50-2 Venous bladder reservoir; some circuits incorporate a bladder which acts as a reservoir and helps to assess blood volume available for the pump.

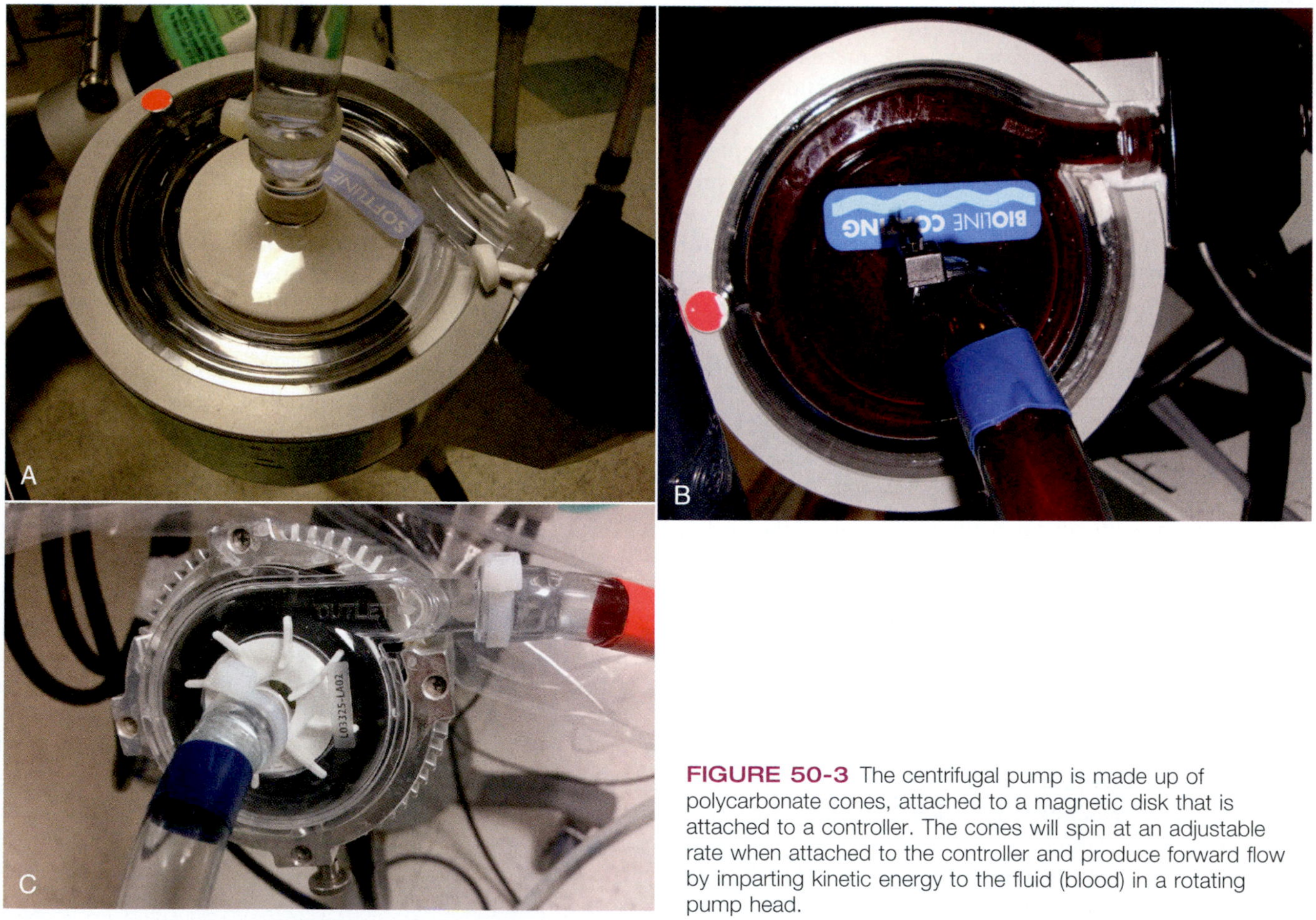

FIGURE 50-3 The centrifugal pump is made up of polycarbonate cones, attached to a magnetic disk that is attached to a controller. The cones will spin at an adjustable rate when attached to the controller and produce forward flow by imparting kinetic energy to the fluid (blood) in a rotating pump head.

attached to the controller and produce forward flow by imparting kinetic energy to the fluid (blood) in a rotating pump head. The **pump flow** provided is therefore dependent on both the patient's **preload** (the volume in the right side of the heart) and **afterload** (the resistance against the pump outlet from the left side of the heart). Because the centrifugal pump is not occlusive (like the roller pump), pump flow will vary despite a set rate per minute (RPM). A decrease in preload or increase in afterload can cause a decreased pump flow. Centrifugal pumps have the advantage of not being affected by gravity for drainage. However, pump flow can change drastically at a set RPM with changes in preload and afterload. Therefore a mechanism for monitoring pump flow changes is essential. Centrifugal pumps can operate at a wide range of RPMs—often as high as 5000—but higher RPMs can result in significant hemolysis.

The roller pump functions by occluding a segment of the circuit tubing called the *raceway*. Blood is drained by gravity from a venous cannula into the venous reservoir, and then pulled into the pump at a given RPM (Figure 50-4). The pump contains two rollers positioned opposite each other. Blood is displaced by the appropriate compression of the rollers on the tubing. This compression setting is called the *occlusion setting* and must be precisely set to produce an accurate flow. Blood is pumped forward under positive pressure. The pump flow is reliant on the diameter of the raceway tubing, the roller occlusion, and the set RPM. The pump will continue to spin despite a low blood volume state if not appropriately monitored. Servo regulation is commonly used as a safety mechanism to prevent excessive negative pressure on the right atrium in the presence of inadequate volume. This situation can result from hypovolemia, insufficient height of the patient (poor gravity-assisted flow), or a kink in the cannula or circuit tubing. The ECMO specialist must be vigilant that servo regulation is appropriately set to stop or slow the pump when there is inadequate blood volume. Without appropriate controls set the pump will continue to spin and cause cavitation, the formation of gas bubbles in the blood, causing significant risk of air embolization to the patient. Roller pumps work well for infants on relatively low flows because they are not affected by afterload and will provide a consistent pump flow.

Blood moves from the system pump to an oxygenator which functions as the lung of the ECMO system. The oxygenator contains hollow fibers for blood and gas to pass through. Gas flow referred to as the **sweep flow** is provided by a blender flowing in the opposite direction of blood flow (Figure 50-5). The blender is adjusted to ensure the hemoglobin of the blood leaving the oxygenator is 100% saturated with a PO_2 >250 mm Hg. As poorly saturated venous blood with very low partial pressure of oxygen is pumped into the oxygenator it traverses through fibers that are aligned with other fibers containing gas with a high partial pressure of oxygen. Oxygen diffuses from the fibers with a high concentration of oxygen to the blood with a lower concentration. There is no CO_2 in the sweep flow. Therefore the carbon dioxide in the blood diffuses into the

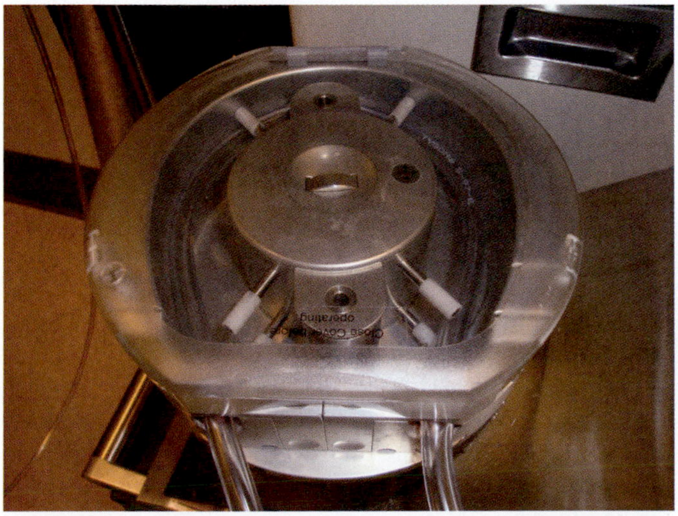

FIGURE 50-4 The roller pump contains two rollers positioned opposite each other. Blood is displaced by the appropriate compression of the rollers on the ECMO circuit, called the *occlusion*.

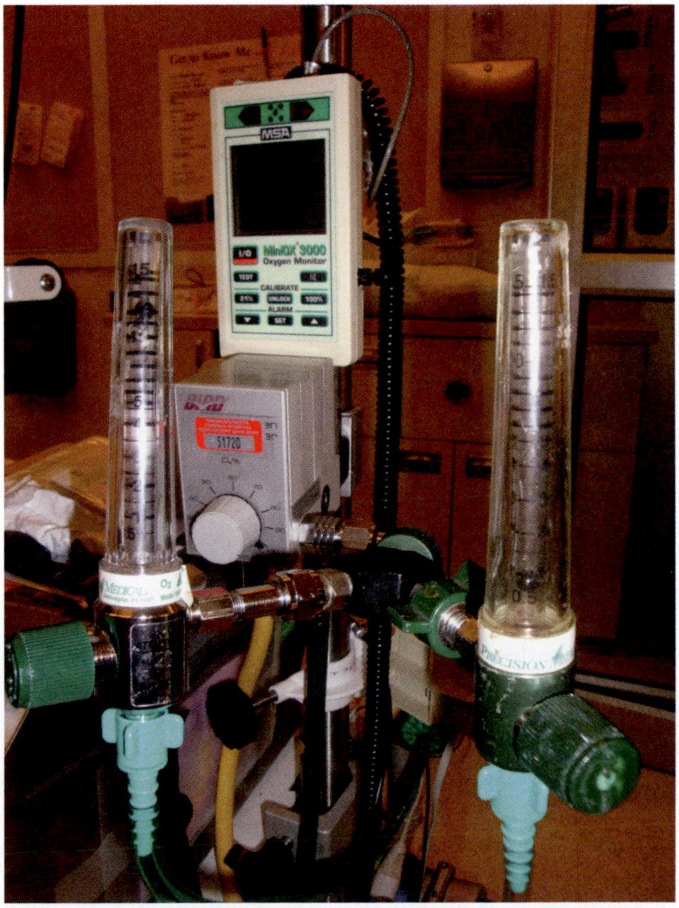

FIGURE 50-5 An oxygen flowmeter is connected to the circuit blender. Sweep flow is delivered into the artificial lung delivering up to 100% oxygen. A second flowmeter allows for analysis of the actual percent of oxygen delivered.

TABLE 50-2
Examples of Oxygenator Specifications

Oxygenator	Prime Volume	Maximum Sweep	Minimum Blood Flow	Maximum Blood Flow
Quadrox iD Adult	250 cc	15 lpm	500 cc/min	7 lpm
Quadrox iD Pediatric	81 cc	5.6 lmp	200 cc/m	2.8 lpm

sweep fibers and is flushed out of the oxygenator. The higher the sweep flow is set, the more CO_2 is eliminated. There is a range of effective sweep flows along with maximum blood flow for the different sizes of oxygenators (Table 50-2). From the oxygenator, fully saturated blood with the desired carbon dioxide level is pumped back to the patient either to a vein (VV support) or to an artery (VA support). The pump speed (RPM) is adjusted to allow the appropriate amount of the patient's blood volume to be oxygenated while the sweep flow rate is adjusted to maintain the desired CO_2 level.

RULE OF THUMB

The ratio of sweep flow to pump flow is often 1 : 1. When using 4 L/min pump flow, typically the sweep flow would be initiated at 4 L/min. The oxygenator functions to provide gas exchange much like native lungs perform gas exchange—oxygen diffuses into the blood from a gas source with a higher partial pressure and carbon dioxide diffuses out of the blood into a gas source with a lower partial pressure.

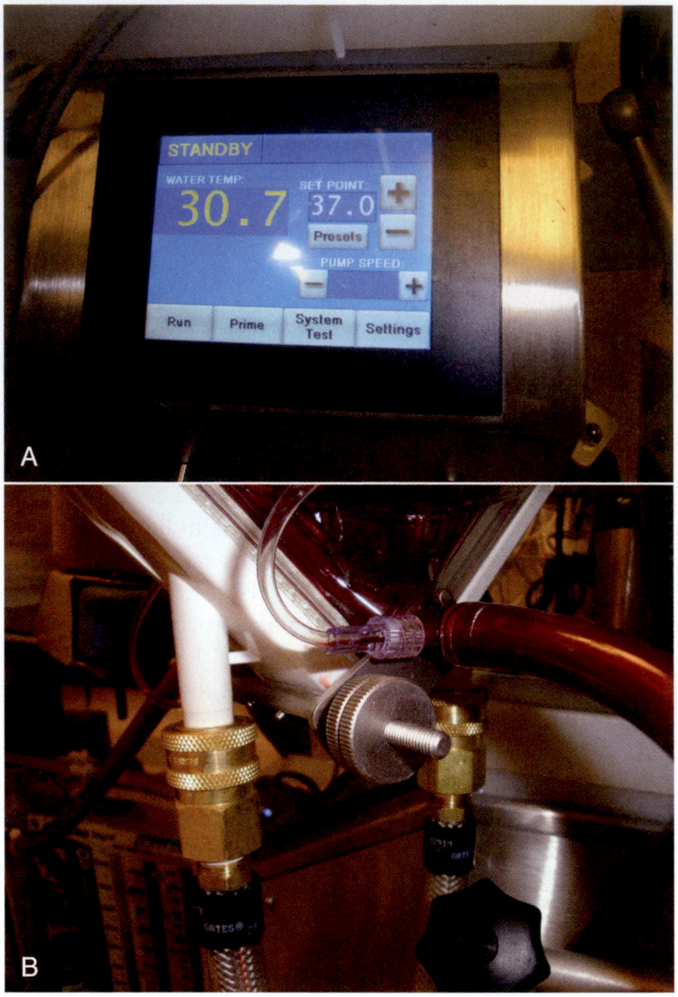

FIGURE 50-6 Blood warmer/cooler, a device that will warm or cool the blood, circulates sterile water **(A)** and sends the heated or cooled fluid through hoses attached to the artificial lung and surrounds the fibers containing the blood to warm or cool it **(B)** (right figure).

Additional equipment used with ECMO support includes a thermoregulation device referred to as the heater/cooler (Figure 50-6). As blood leaves the patient and circulates through the ECMO circuit, a considerable decrease in blood temperature can occur as the tubing that blood flows through is exposed to ambient temperature. Gas flow through the oxygenator is also cool, resulting in evaporative losses. Therefore, especially in neonates, active warming is required to maintain a normal body temperature. Temperature adjusted sterile water circulates around the fibers containing blood and allows appropriate temperature control of the blood returning to the patient. These devices have the potential to maintain hypothermic states when appropriate. Recent evidence has demonstrated that mild decreases in core temperature may have a salvaging effect on the brain[8] and can be easily achieved during ECMO support.

Pressure monitoring is a standard part of the circuit. Circuit pressures are measured before and after the oxygenator and indicate the absolute pressure in the circuit along with changes in resistance across the oxygenator (Figure 50-7). The change in resistance most often indicates development of clots within the oxygenator. Changes in pressures can alert the ECMO specialist to identify emerging situations such as kinks, clots, and in VA support, changes in hemodynamics.

RULE OF THUMB

Monitor pre and post oxygenator pressures frequently. Changes will alert clinicians to clots in the oxygenator. Increases in pre **membrane pressure** only = increased resistance within the oxygenator. Increases in pre AND post membrane pressures = increased resistance AFTER the oxygenator.

A pressure monitor can also be placed on the drainage line to detect excessive siphon on the system. Alarms and servo regulation can be used in association with these pressure monitors to create safer systems. Pressure monitoring is either integrated into the ECMO system or additional pressure transducers can be added.

As noted earlier, blood flow is regulated by dialing in a set RPM which results in flow. The flow is monitored using ultrasonic devices that are either incorporated into the system or

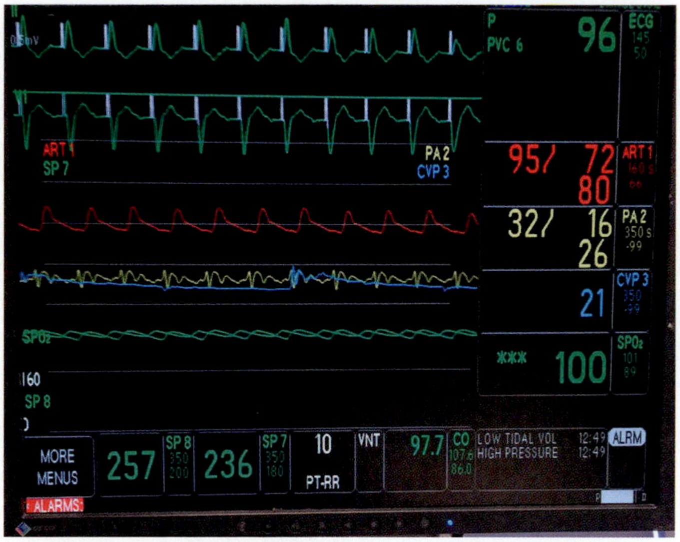

FIGURE 50-7 Oxygenator/pressure monitoring. Pressure transducers are attached to ports before and after the artificial lung with reading displayed on the bedside monitor. "SP5" indicates the pressure before the oxygenator and "SP6" indicates the pressure after the oxygenator. The difference between the two pressures is an indication of the resistance to blood flow through the oxygenator. Increases in pressure difference usually are a result of clot formation.

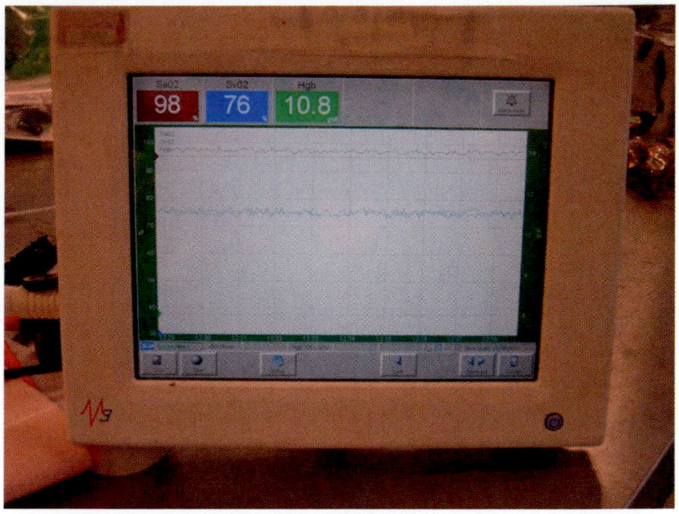

FIGURE 50-8 Example of inline oxygen saturation monitoring that can be used to trend the saturation of blood draining into the ECMO circuit.

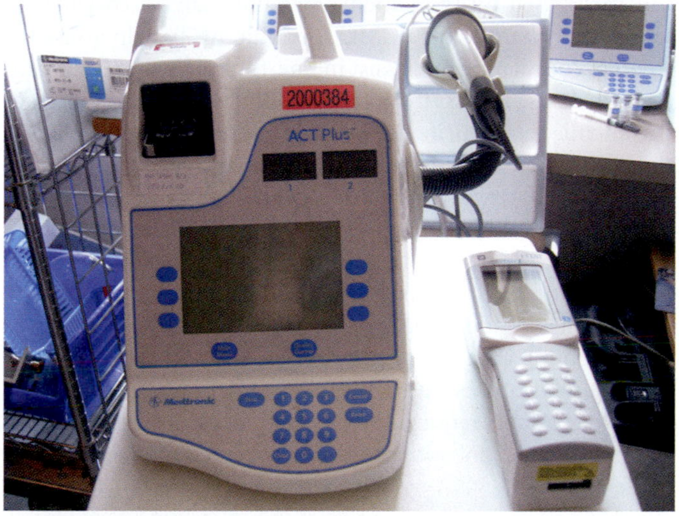

FIGURE 50-9 Two types of point of care activated clotting time (ACT) devices with their cartridges.

added to the circuit. Many systems will display a calculated flow but the accuracy of that flow is dependent on many factors. Flow is measured to assure appropriate occlusion when using roller pumps and to check variations in flow common with centrifugal pumps. Audible alarms are usually set to alert the ECMO specialist of changes in pump flow.

Air (bubble) detectors can be useful in identifying the presence of air in the ECMO circuit. They can be used on either the arterial or venous side of the circuit and detect inadvertent air passing through the system. These devices can function to stop support when air is detected or sound an alert. False alarms can be problematic because support to the patient is stopped and will often produce significant instability for the patient until support is resumed. The ECMO specialist must be able to immediately distinguish true presence of air bubbles from false alarms rapidly and take the appropriate action for either situation.

Additional blood parameter monitoring can be incorporated into an ECMO system by insertion of an indwelling optical cable. These devices help to trend continuous values such as venous saturations, arterial saturations, hemoglobin, hematocrit, and temperature (Figure 50-8). They are generally considered optional and the use of each varies from institution to institution.

Unlike some of the optional parameters monitored during ECMO support, monitoring of anticoagulation parameters on a routine basis is essential. The **activated clotting time** (ACT) is most often used as the primary test for anticoagulation at the bedside. The ACT is a low cost point of care test that gives a quick assessment of anticoagulation. There are several types of devices using a small volume of blood that can determine the number of seconds it takes for blood to clot (Figure 50-9). It is most often used in conjunction with other parameters to assess the patient's overall state of anticoagulation.

ANTICOAGULATION MANAGEMENT

Anticoagulation of the ECMO patient is a vital part of an ECMO run starting at **cannulation**. The blood's natural reaction is to activate coagulation when exposed to the nonbiologic surfaces of the cannulas and circuit. Therefore, anticoagulation is essential prior to cannula insertion and throughout the ECMO course. Heparin, the most commonly used anticoagulant, is easily reversed and widely available. It is prepared from bovine lung or porcine intestines and can be monitored at the bedside. Heparin inhibits the conversion of prothrombin

TABLE 50-3

Example of Anticoagulation Protocol

Laboratory Test	Frequency	Goals	Normal
ACT	Q1 until results in desired range ×2 hrs, then Q4 while on heparin	As ordered, typically 160-200 (as low as 140 in bleeding patients, 200-240 at pump flows <2 L/min	90-120 sec
ATIII	Pre-ECMO baseline Monday, Wednesday, and Friday at 8 AM	Level maintained >40%	40-100%
anti-Xa	Q 24 hrs at 8 AM	Target levels of 0.3-0.7 IU/mL	N/A
aPTT	Q 24 hrs	50-80 seconds	22-35 sec
PT	Q 24 hrs	Normal	11-14
Fibrinogen	Q 24 hrs	Keep in normal range (250-300 mg/dL)	250-300
Platelets	Q 6 hrs	>60,000/μL	150-400/μL

to thrombin and activates antithrombin III (ATIII). It does not break up clots, but rather decreases the risk of their occurrence. A bolus of heparin is administered just prior to cannulation. ACT levels are assessed shortly after to ensure the desired levels of anticoagulation have been achieved. The bolus dose can vary based on the patient's baseline state of coagulation. Once the patient is on ECMO, periodic ACTs help assess the trend in coagulation and assist in fine-tuning the heparin maintenance doses. The ACT can be affected by many factors including anemia, hypofibrinogenemia, hypothermia, hemodilution, thrombocytopenia, qualitative platelet abnormality, and other coagulation factor deficiencies. Reports in the literature[9] and the anticoagulation guidelines recently published from ELSO[10] suggest that using more than one parameter may be helpful in the assessment of anticoagulation during long-term support. Monitoring of additional parameters on a routine basis and implementing a guideline in response to the combined results may be useful in assessing the overall coagulation/anticoagulation status of patients requiring long-term extracorporeal support. An example of an anticoagulation protocol can be seen in Table 50-3.

MINI CLINI

PROBLEM: Patient is being maintained on a heparin infusion to achieve the prescribed ACT range of 180-200 seconds. Over the past 2 hours, chest tube output has increased significantly, resulting in a decrease in hemoglobin, necessitating multiple blood transfusions.

Discussion: The ECMO specialist recommends lowering the desired ACT range in order to decrease the amount of bleeding. This can be achieved by lowering the hourly heparin infusion rate and repeating the ACT to assess the change. Vigilance in assessing the circuit for evidence of increased clot formation in the circuit is essential.

Heparin levels (anti Xa) may more accurately assess heparin-induced anticoagulation and are less affected by abnormal physiologic states than are ACT values. ACT levels may better reflect the overall anticoagulation status of the patient, but are not specific for heparin effects versus clotting deficiencies. The two values may be used together to better assess appropriate heparin and blood product needs. A number of studies in ECLS patients have shown a superior correlation of the anti Xa assay to heparin dose.[11] The presence of antithrombin III (AT III) in blood is also essential to achieve the desired levels of anticoagulation. AT III levels may be increased by infusing fresh frozen plasma (FFP), a blood product that contains AT III, or using recombinant AT concentrate, a concentrated form of AT III that is more effective than FFP. However, AT concentrate is significantly more costly, therefore the cost-benefit ratio is often considered. Thermoelastogram (TEG) is an emerging method of assessing anticoagulation.[10] A small sample of blood is taken from a patient and rotated gently in a specific fashion to imitate sluggish venous flow and activate coagulation. TEG provides comprehensive whole blood hemostasis testing that can help assess bleeding and thrombotic risks, and also monitor antithrombotic therapies. Some more common coagulation values assessed during an ECMO run include prothrombin time (PT) and activated partial thromboplastin time (aPTT). The aPTT may not be as accurate at assessing anticoagulation during ECMO in newborns and small children when heparin is used as the anticoagulant.[12] However, it can be a better assessment of anticoagulation when direct thrombin inhibitors are used to anticoagulate ECMO patients who have a sensitivity to heparin.[13] Patients with sensitivity to heparin, identified by heparin-induced thrombocytopenia, may be managed on ECMO through the use of direct thrombin inhibitors, such as lipirudin and bivalrudin. When using these forms of direct thrombin inhibitors the accuracy of ACTs is less dependable. Despite diligence with maintaining appropriate levels of anticoagulation, clot formation within the circuit remains a major complication during ECMO.[1]

RULE OF THUMB

Patients receiving ECMO support require significant levels of anticoagulation making bleeding a risk and common complication incurring during ECMO.

CANNULAS

Cannulas are inserted to provide direct access to the patient. Cannula size is crucial to the amount of support an ECMO system can provide. The smaller the internal diameter of a cannula, the higher the resistance of the flow. When placing venous cannulas, the largest possible cannula should be placed to ensure adequate flows. Cannulas are sized by their outer diameter, in French units. All cannulas are tested for their pressure/flow relationship and an M number determined. The M number represents a resistive factor that can be used to approximate the expected flow at a specific pressure difference. Cannula characteristics vary in internal size, length, port placement, size, and number (Table 50-4). This information is important to know during the cannula selection process. Selection of the appropriate cannulas is dependent on the intended insertion sites, age/size of the patient, and the type and amount of support needed. They are designed to be placed through a surgical cut-down, via sternotomy or by percutaneous insertion.

TABLE 50-4
Flow Characteristics of Some Cannulas

Manufacturer	Size (Fr)	Length (cm)	M#	Flow @ 100 cm H20
Venous Cannulas (Single Lumen)				
Biomedicus	12	25	3.55	1.5
	14	25	3.35	2
	17	50	3.4	1.9
	19	50	3.15	2.6
	23	50	2.65	5
DLP	21	53	3.05	3
	28	65	2.5	5.5
RMI	20	52	3	3
	28	52	2.3	8
Venous Cannulas (Double Lumen)				
Origen	12	6	3.9V 4.7A	0.9
	15	8	3.5V 4.3A	1.6
	18	15	3.4V 3.8A	1.9
Jostra	15	3.6V 4.6A	1.4	
Coviden	14	10	3.5V 5.1A	1.6
Avalon		19	20	3.3V 3.8A
	23	29	3.1V 3.4A	2.6
	31	29	2.5V 2.8A	6
Arterial Cannulas				
Biomedicus	8	25	4.4	0.5
	10	25	4	0.9
	15	37	3.3	2.2
	17	37	3.05	3
	19	37	2.8	3.8
DLP	8	23	4.5	0.4
	14	23	3.3	2.2
	16	23	3	3
	17	17	2.95	3.2
RMI	18	15	3	3
	20	25	3	3
	20	15	2.8	3.8
	22	25	3.1	2.9

There are two types of venous cannulas: single and double lumen. Venous cannulas have several ports to allow for maximal drainage. Many are wire reinforced to decrease the potential for kinking. Some are coated to avoid an antiinflammatory response and decrease the risk of clot formation. Two types of double-lumen cannulas (DLC) are available for VV support (Figure 50-10). Newborn DLCs are inserted into a single vein and allow drainage of desaturated blood and return of oxygenated blood through the same vessel. They have multiple side ports to drain blood. The drainage lumen is typically larger than the return lumen, which allows for better drainage of venous blood. The return lumen has a single outlet and blood is pumped through the cannula by the positive pressure created from the pump's rotation.

The BiCaval DLC is another approach to VV support. It needs to be inserted under fluoroscopy or echocardiography guidance (Figure 50-11) because appropriate positioning is crucial and can be difficult without imaging. The drainage ports are positioned in both the superior and inferior vena cava with the return lumen positioned at the entry of the right atrium. These double-lumen cannulas are a single cannula with two lumens, the drainage lumen and the return lumen. Recirculation is expected when using a double-lumen cannula.

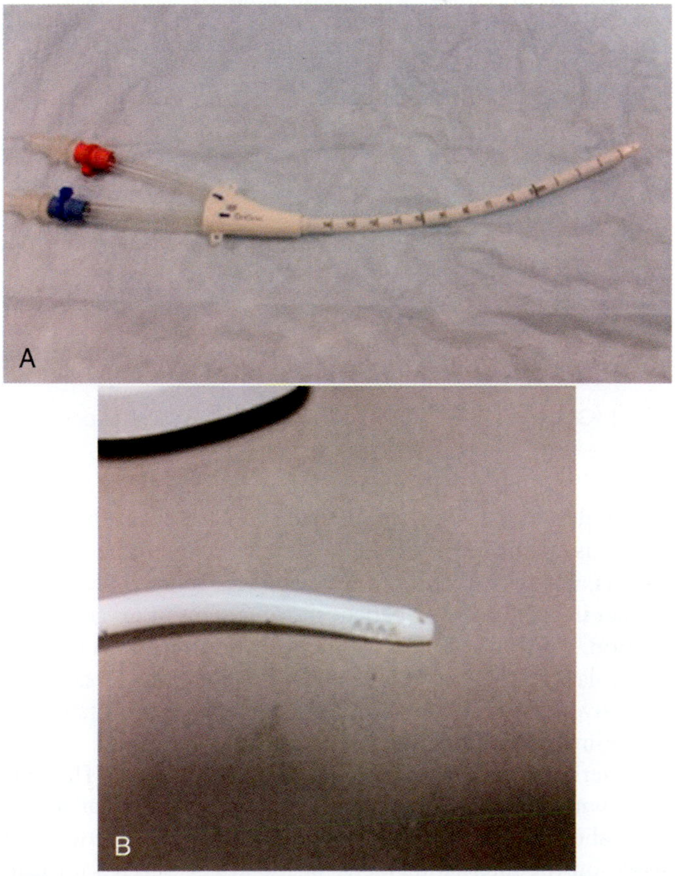

FIGURE 50-10 Double-lumen, single-vessel cannulas used for VV ECMO. **A,** Ports on one side of the cannula sit in the right atrium are used to drain blood into the circuit. **B,** The end return port is where blood is returned back into the RT Atrium and directed toward the tricuspid valve.

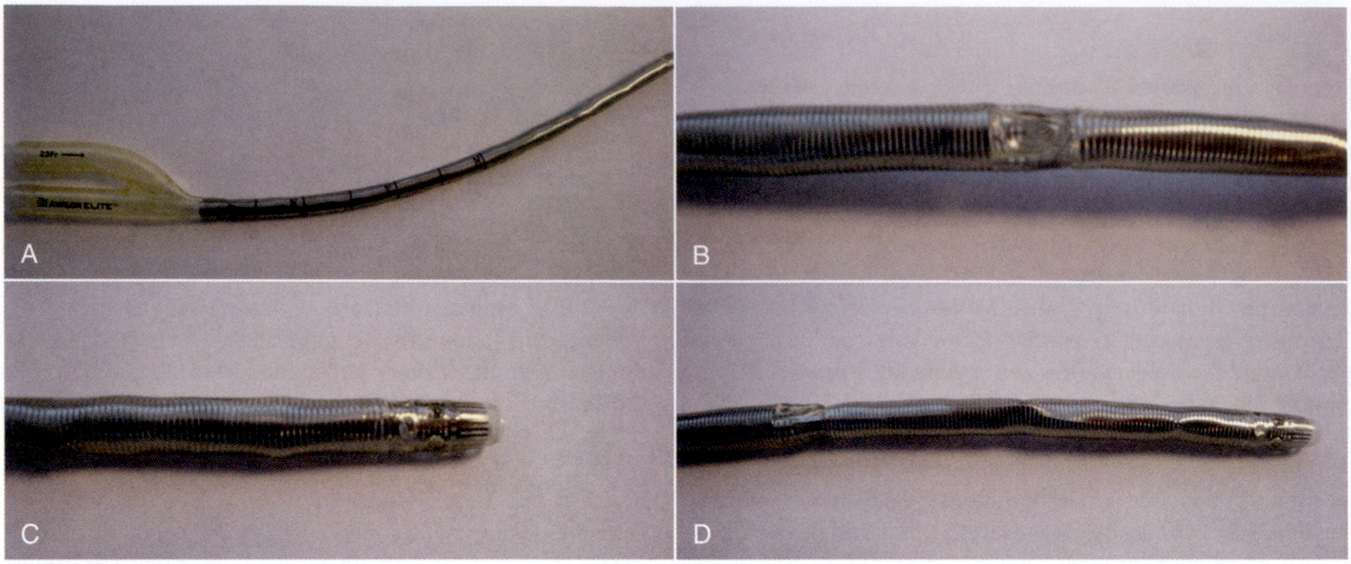

FIGURE 50-11 The BiCaval double-lumen cannula is inserted under fluoroscopy or echocardiography guidance. Drainage ports, seen on the right, are located in both the superior and inferior vena cava. The return lumen, seen on the left, is positioned in the right atrium across from the tricuspid valve.

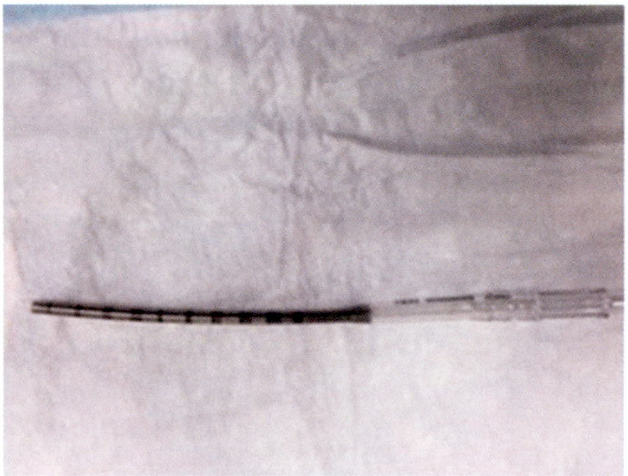

FIGURE 50-12 Arterial cannula with a single end port.

Recirculation occurs when oxygenated blood from the return lumen is siphoned back into the drainage side of the cannula. This is apparent when both drainage and return lines appear similar in color, with the patient showing signs of oxygen desaturation. Position is critical in a double-lumen cannula to avoid recirculation. Careful monitoring of the cannula is essential. Excessive recirculation will occur if the cannula is rotated out of optimal position, resulting in inadequate support.

Arterial cannulas typically have a single outlet. They are often wire reinforced and coated. Ideal arterial cannulas should be as short as possible and have thin walls. The size inserted is based on the internal diameter of the artery selected for cannulation. The narrow diameter of the arterial cannula creates the highest amount of resistance in the ECMO circuit. It is the conduit that allows for the return of oxygenated blood back to the patient's circulation (Figure 50-12).

TYPES OF SUPPORT

There are two primary types of ECMO support: VA and VV. VA support is partial cardiopulmonary bypass, providing both cardiac and pulmonary support. The degree of bypass depends on the underlying condition. VV does not bypass the cardiopulmonary circulation, thus only provides pulmonary support. A third, emerging type is AV ECMO, which is also referred to as pumpless ECMO. AV ECMO is primarily for CO_2 removal at low pump flows and requires the patient's own hemodynamics to pump blood through the oxygenator. This type of support is most effective at achieving adequate ventilation when native lung function is significantly impeded.[7]

Venoarterial ECMO

In VA ECMO a portion of the patient's blood volume is drained from the venous circulation to the ECMO circuit where gas exchange occurs (Figure 50-13). Fully saturated blood is returned through a cannula in the arterial circulation, which results in hemodynamic support. In VA ECMO a minimum of two cannulas are placed, with at least one in an artery and one in a vein. The cannulas can be placed via a surgical cut-down, through a sternotomy or percutaneously. The diameter, length, and position of the cannula will determine the potential flow that can be achieved. The typical artery accessed in the newborn would be the right common carotid artery. In larger patients placement can be in a left or right femoral artery, axillary artery or placed transthoracicly, directly into the aorta. When the femoral artery is cannulated, it is prudent to place a small reperfusion line to supplement blood flow to the lower leg and decrease the risk of limb ischemia (Figure 50-14). In some patients only a portion of their cardiac output is pumped through the ECMO circuit while some blood flow continues

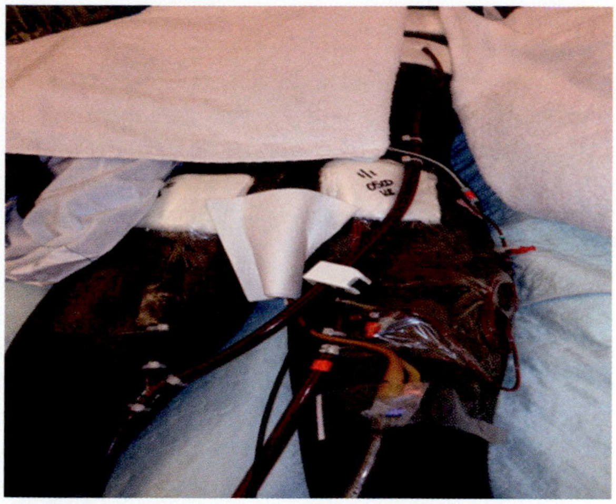

FIGURE 50-13 VA ECMO with drainage from the right femoral vein and right atrium with blood being returned to the left femoral artery.

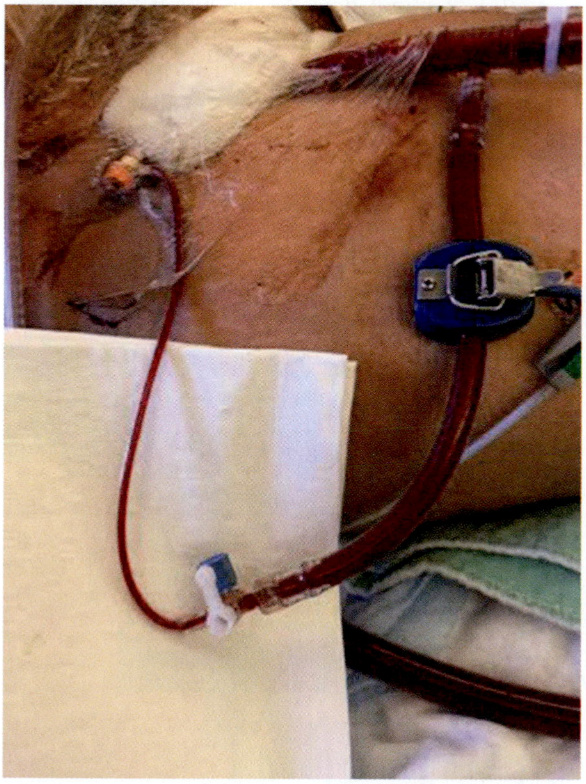

FIGURE 50-14 A secondary blood return line (reperfusion line) is placed in this femoral artery cannula to supplement blood flow to the lower limb and prevent limb ischemia.

through the native circulation. The blood from the ECMO circuit returns to the patient, bypassing the heart and lungs, and mixes with the native circulation. The total oxygen content depends on the proportions of blood through the two circulations. Similarly, the measured PCO_2 in the patient's arterial circulation will be a result of the combined relatively low PCO_2 returned from the ECMO circuit and the PCO_2 in the blood coming through the native circulation. The primary advantages

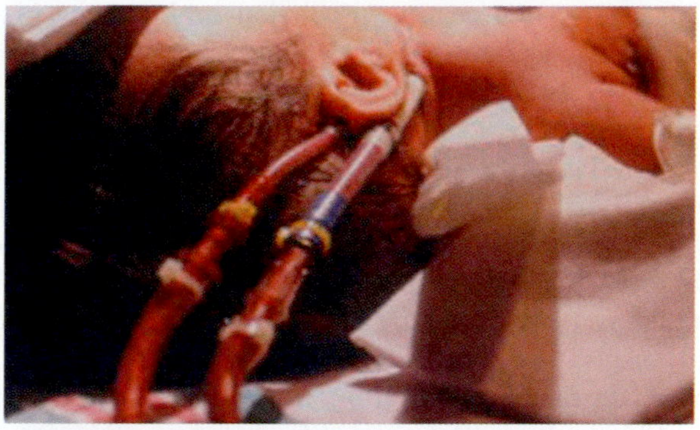

FIGURE 50-15 Common cannula used for VV ECMO support in newborns. Babies are often cannulated with a double-lumen cannula through the right internal jugular for VV ECMO.

Box 50-4 Characteristics of VA and VV Support

VENOARTERIAL ECMO
- Typically used for patients with cardiovascular failure
- Partial cardiopulmonary bypass
- Decreases preload
- Increases afterload
- Effects hemodynamics

VENOVENOUS ECMO
- Typically used for patients in respiratory failure
- Can be done with multiple cannnulas or a DLC
- Provides no hemodynamic support
- RV function may improve with increased S_VO_2

of VA ECMO are that it allows the heart to rest and reduces cardiac oxygen consumption while providing adequate systemic organ perfusion with oxygenated blood. There is no chance of recirculation and less ventilator support is needed. VA ECMO is best indicated for cardiogenic shock, as a bridge to a ventricular assist device or heart transplantation. A disadvantage of VA ECMO is the need to cannulate an artery which will require repair or ligation when support is no longer needed. See Box 50-4 for differences in VA and VV support.

Venovenous ECMO

As in VA ECMO, VV support involves a portion of the patient's blood volume being drained from the venous circulation to the ECMO circuit where gas exchange occurs. However, blood is returned back to the venous circulation either through the same cannula via the return lumen or via a separate cannula into another vein (Figure 50-15). The typical cannulation site for the newborn is in the right internal jugular vein. In larger patients, common sites are the right and left femoral veins, right internal jugular vein, pulmonary artery, or right atrium. Pulmonary artery and right atrium cannulations involve cannula placement via hemisternotomy or open chest surgery. Unlike VA ECMO, blood is returned to the venous circulation, therefore providing no direct cardiac support. Oxygenated blood that is lower in

CO_2 returns to the venous circulation and mixes with the remaining cardiac output. The total oxygen content and measured CO_2 is a result of this mix and can be affected by the patient's mechanical ventilation settings or spontaneous minute ventilation. Two distinct advantages of VV ECMO are lower risk of cerebral air embolism and no need to ligate or repair an artery. VV ECMO is often indicated for patients with acute respiratory failure due to viral or bacterial pneumonias.[14] VV is emerging as a bridge to lung transplant.[15] ECMO in the pre–lung transplant patient allows for improved gas exchange and decreases the risk of complications from high levels of mechanical ventilation. It can also prevent further deconditioning. The patient on VV ECMO can be extubated, awake, and ambulated while waiting for available lungs.[16]

Arteriovenous ECMO

AV ECMO is a more recent type of support. Unlike VA or VV support, AV support is low flow ECMO that provides gas exchange and relies on the patient's cardiac function to generate pump flow. It is a more compact system with shorter segments of circuit tubing that is attached to the oxygenator and blood is circulated via arterial blood pressure (Figure 50-16). The patients most likely to benefit from this type of support are COPD and pre–lung transplant patients.[7] In addition, ongoing clinical trials are determining if AV ECMO is useful in the management of patients with severe ARDS who require high airway pressure to adequately ventilate.[17] This form of ECMO requires that the patient has adequate cardiac function.

RULE OF THUMB

VA ECMO is primarily used to support patients with cardiac failure. VV ECMO is used primarily to support patients with respiratory failure.

INITIATION OF SUPPORT

ECMO is frequently initiated in the ICU. Specific circumstances may dictate ECMO being initiated in the operating room, cardiac catherization lab, emergency room or many other locations in the hospital. A formal activation guideline should be established so that access to the ECMO team and equipment can be rapidly deployed.

Cannulas are inserted in the appropriate vessels and then attached to an ECMO circuit. The circuit is assembled using sterile technique, de-aired, and crystalloid primed. Newborn circuits are often primed with blood to decrease the hemodilution effect that can be encountered with a crystalloid primed circuit. The circuit is attached to the cannulas and ECMO support commences. Pump flows are adjusted according to the type of support the patient is receiving and vary based on the underlying diagnosis. Patients needing cardiac support (VA) will often need a large portion of their cardiac output supported while patients on VV support may be maintained on a relatively lower amount of pump flow. As the pump flow increases, a larger portion of the patient's desaturated blood flows through the oxygenator and returns to the patient fully saturated. Box 50-5 shows sample target pump flows for different age groups. Once pump flow is at the desired level, alarms should be set appropriately to alert the ECMO specialist of any acute changes

Box 50-5 Target Pump Flows for Age Groups

- Infants: 120-150 cc/kg/min
- Children: 100-120 cc/kg/min
- Adults: 70-80 cc/kg/min
- Attempt to reach maximal flow early in run to determine buffer

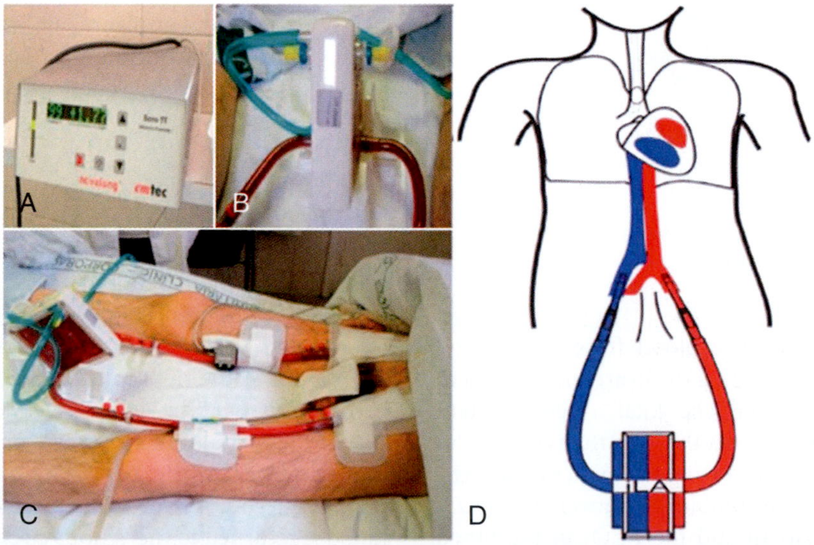

FIGURE 50-16 Arteriovenous ECMO without a pump; blood flow is maintained by the patient's "normally" functioning heart.

in pump support. Sweep flow is attached to the oxygenator and adjusted based on guidelines to achieve target CO_2.

RULE OF THUMB

The ratio of sweep flow to pump flow is often 1 : 1. When using 4 L/min pump flow, typically the sweep flow would be initiated at 4 L/min.

Consideration of adjustments in ventilator support is necessary to avoid hyper- and hypoventilation. Patients' ventilator settings can gradually be weaned to "rest settings" as the sweep flow is increased. Rest settings are intended to minimize lung trauma while avoiding atelectasis. Typically the FiO2 from the ventilator can be reduced to 0.4 to 0.6. The goal for some long-term patients (i.e., pre–lung transplant) is often extubation to allow for activities of daily living to be maintained in conjunction with physical therapy and ambulation while on ECMO support. Circuit temperature is adjusted to maintain patients at the intended body temperature. A chest x-ray is done to assess cannula placement. Serial blood gases and chemistries are obtained to ensure patient lab values are within acceptable ranges. Pump flow, sweep flow, and medications can be adjusted as needed. Blood products are transfused to maintain desired parameters. Baseline anticoagulation levels are obtained and a heparin infusion initiated at the dose necessary to achieve adequate anticoagulation. Sedation levels are adjusted to the appropriate level that will allow intermittent or continuous assessment of neurologic status. Levels of analgesia are provided as needed or as pain scores indicate. Emergency preparedness is an essential component of an ECMO start. Procedures to handle any complications during initiations should be developed for every ECMO center. Backup circuit components should be in a nearby location along with an alternative means to support the patient in the event of pump hardware failure.

MAINTENANCE OF AN ECMO RUN

ECMO runs can be expected to last from a few days to as long as several months. An established flow sheet to document key variables should record the trends in specific parameters. Monitoring the changes in these parameters allows the ECMO specialist to better assess a patient's progress, identify goals on a daily basis, and coordinate the best approach during the patient's course on ECMO (Box 50-6). Daily, the patient will receive a CXR to reaffirm cannula position and lung status. Periodic arterial blood gases are obtained as well as ACTs and other labs run at appropriate intervals to ensure values are maintained within desired range. Interdisciplinary team rounds occur at the bedside daily. Every discipline should be encouraged to contribute their perspective and together a well-defined strategy is formed. It is at these rounds that clear patient goals can be identified and a plan of care is established for the day. In addition to patient trends, documentation should also be maintained on various aspects of the active ECMO system (Box 50-7). Frequent circuit assessments, from the drainage cannula through the entire system and back to the return cannula, are essential. Specialists must be mindful of the many risks and potential complications associated with extracorporeal support. Diligence with frequent inspections and evaluation of components as well as ensuring the proper backup equipment should be part of the daily task of an ECMO specialist.

Certain categories of ECMO patients may require procedures unique to their condition. Open chest cardiac patients might need to travel to the OR for a chest washout or explorations to stop bleeding and, depending on the urgency, some surgical procedures may have to be done at the bedside. Bedside echocardiograms are done to assess any changes in cardiac function and sometimes to rule out **tamponade**. Cardiac catherization lab visits may also be necessary for procedures required during the ECMO run. Bronchoscopies and bronchial lavages are a little more common in patients being supported for respiratory failure. As with any ICU run there is a potential need to travel to CT scan or interventional radiology for diagnostic testing.

TRANSPORTING A PATIENT ON ECMO

Most ECMO systems are designed for intrahospital transport. However, detailed guidelines should be followed when preparing for transport. These should include a fully charged battery, adequate gas supply, transport ventilator, cardiac monitors, and defibrillator. A travel kit is advisable that includes connectors, clamps, additional medications, IV fluid, and other items that might be needed on route or at the destination. Provisions for temperature control may be necessary because the blood warmer/cooler may not be supported during the transport. Travelling on ECMO carries significant risks, and team work is essential to successful travel. Roles should be established prior to moving. It is wise to minimize the time of the transport by clearing hallways in advance and gaining easy access to elevators. During the transport, constant assessment of the patient along with battery charge level, gas supply, and close monitoring of the circuit should be practiced. When the destination is reached, close attention to detail should be made and reestablishment of piped gas and AC power obtained as soon as possible. Intrahospital transport includes elective patient ambulation in the ICU.

Preparing a patient to ambulate on ECMO takes collaboration among all services involved (Box 50-8). An agreement must be made on destination and maximum duration of time out of the patient's room. Roles of all providers should be clear. All necessary equipment should be identified and checked for function prior to beginning ambulation. There should be specific reasons to abort the exercise such as tachycardia, desaturation, patient fatigue or concerns for equipment or patient safety.

RISKS AND COMPLICATIONS

ECMO poses significant risks. The complications can be classified as mechanical as a result of equipment failure or patient from clinical issues. Box 50-9 outlines ECMO complications.[1]

Box 50-6 ECMO Flow Sheet for Monitoring Trends in Flows, Pressures, Hemodynamics, and Pertinent Lab Values

Date													
Time													
Heart rate (beats/minute)													
Arterial pressure Sys/dia (mm Hg)													
Mean arterial pressure (mm Hg)													
PA pressure Sys/dia (mm Hg)													
Mean PA pressure (mm Hg)													
Central venous pressure (mm Hg)													
Respiratory rate (breaths/min)													
FiO_2 / flow													
SPO_2 (%)													
SVO_2 (%)													
PO_2 / Hb													
PCO_2 / pH													
ECLS flow L/minin													
RPM													
Sweep flow L/minin													
Sweep blender %O_2													
Color change													
Oxygenator press Pre/post (mm Hg)													
Pre/post pressure differential (mm Hg)													
Venous drain pressure (mm Hg)													
Water bath temp (°C) set/measured													
Heparin infusion (units/hr)													
Activated clotting time (ACT) sec													
Initials													

ACT Range ____________	MAP ______	SPO_2 ______	☐Alarms appropriate, check Q shift +initial ______

Cannulation Date/Time	**Date Current Oxygenator Initiated**	**ECLS Type: _____ VA _____ VV**
		List cannula type, size, and site:
Signature:	Signature:	
Signature:	Signature:	

Box 50-7 Safety Shift Checklist to Verify Availability of Appropriate Alarms and Backup Equipment

ROTAFLOW SHIFT CHECK LIST (COMPLETE DURING THE FIRST HOUR OF EACH SHIFT)										
Date	Time	Mode	Cream tube on Rotaflow	External drive ready for use	Back up equipment available	Change out kit	ACT cartridges exp date?	Dash alarms appropriate H/L	Initials	Comments

ECMO specialists are clinicians specifically trained in all aspects of ECMO. It is essential that the ECMO specialist have a thorough understanding of ECMO physiology and ECMO patient management. These individuals must have critical thinking skills and be technically adept at assessing all components of the ECMO circuit. Monitoring and frequent inspection of the circuit and evaluating circuit functions are among the primary roles of the ECMO specialist. The risk of the many complications inherent in providing ECMO support diminishes with diligence on the part of the specialist.

Box 50-8 Guidelines for Ambulating With Patients on VV ECMO (Central-Peripheral)

I. Patient Assessment:
  a. Patient is able to participate in care
  b. Patient is able to be safely directed
  c. Demonstrates stability on ECMO
    1. Consider the following parameters
    2. Discuss with medical team if falls outside criteria
II. Prepare for Ambulation:

Hematologic	ECMO	General Considerations
No sign of bleeding over 12 hrs	Stability of flow, speed & sweep for 6hrs	Airway clearance
		Afebrile
Plts > 50	Cannulas: sites have been stable—no migration or bleeding	Tolerated HOB up, dangling, OOB to chair
Hgb ≥ 8-9		
ACT at goal		

  a. Obtain MD order for ambulation after assessment by RN, PT, RT
  b. Ensure ECMO cannulas, airway and all other lines are secured
  c. Equipment checklist:
    1. Full O_2 tank
    2. Clamps
    3. Portable SpO_2 monitor
    4. Wheelchair/recliner
    5. ECMO emergency equipment
    6. Assess battery life for all equipment
  d. Contingency plan:
    1. Identify red plug outlets
    2. Identify location of backup circuit
  e. Team discussion prior to take off to include destination & roles*
    - RN: IVs, tubing, chest tubes
    - RT: ECMO pump/cannula (circuit), monitor flow/speed, airway
    - PT: manages patient mobility
    - A minimum of 3 staff must be present during ambulation
    - *Each discipline to monitor hemodynamic parameters and alert team members if significant changes noted
  f. Ensure hallways are clear of obstruction
  g. Limit ambulation to within the ICU
III. Ambulate
IV. Documentation per each discipline's standards

Box 50-9 Common Complications

MECHANICAL COMPLICATIONS
- Pump failure
- Tubing rupture
- Cannula problems
- Oxygenator failure

PHYSIOLOGIC COMPLICATIONS
- Seizures
- Hemolysis
- Renal failure
- Bleeding; intracranial, surgical site
- Neurologic complications
- Arrhythmias
- Pneumothorax

The most common mechanical complication during ECMO is clot formation.[1] Clot can occur anywhere in the circuit but more frequently occurs in the oxygenator, at connectors, in the circuit bladder or any place with relatively low flow. Clots can result in increased resistance and may impede flow, limiting support of the patient. Clot formation within the fibers of the oxygenator will reduce gas exchange and if significant may require the oxygenator to be replaced (Figure 50-17). Inadvertent **decannulation** and pump failure are other significant complications that can cause circuit interruption and require immediate attention. These conditions might result in the need for an entire circuit to be replaced. Replacement of oxygenators or circuits requires the patient to be briefly removed from support. Practitioners trained in this procedure need to maintain competency to efficiently change out the oxygenator or circuit in the least amount of time to minimize patient decompensation from interruption of support. Proper coordination with the team caring for the patient is essential during this loss of support.

Air in the circuit is a major risk during ECMO. Despite the ECMO system being a closed system, air emboli can occur when air is entrained into the system. This can occur inadvertently through cavitation—air being pulled out of a solution due to increased negative pressure—if venous return is inadequate. It can occur from drainage ports of a cannula migrating out of a vessel or from access lines, such as through the CVVH port, infusion lines or other monitoring lines. The presence of air in the circuit, if not redirected or withdrawn, may enter the patient's circulation. In VA ECMO this is particularly life threatening because air will not be filtered through the pulmonary circulation as it is in VV ECMO. As with most mechanical complications, prevention is vital.

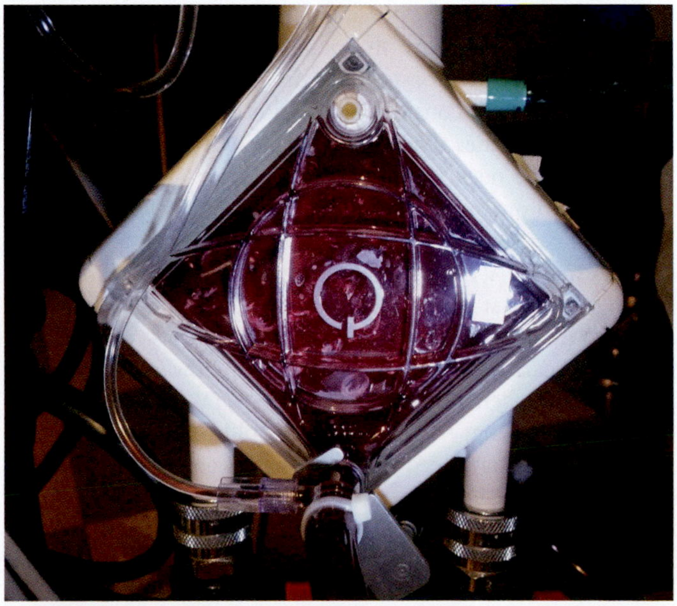

FIGURE 50-17 Oxygenator with significant clot accumluation.

Bleeding is a common risk of ECMO due to anticoagulation and the multiple surgical sites where bleeding can easily occur. Bleeding in the chest can lead to the complication of cardiac tamponade, an emergency needing immediate intervention, without which the patient will not likely survive. Cannula placement in the awake and active patient on ECMO can also contribute to the occurrence of tamponade. Loss of pump flow, hemodynamic changes with a narrowing of pulse pressure, arrhythmias, and decreases in hemoglobin and hematocrit levels are symptomatic of tamponade. Bleeding from any source resulting in low pump flow not only causes risks to the patient but to the circuit as well. Lower flows result in higher potential for clot formation in a circuit. The drop in hemoglobin is also a major concern because the oxygen carrying capacity is greatly reduced. Bleeding can occur from any surgical site, including cannula sites, chest tubes, or IVs. Bleeding becomes a risk with any venopuncture, NG or OG tube placement, rectal tube placement, suctioning, or anything that might cause mild trauma to the tissues. Internally, intracranial hemorrhage, GI and pulmonary bleeding are also bleeding risks associated with ECMO.

BLOOD PRODUCTS DURING ECMO

The most common blood product used during an ECMO run is packed red blood cells (PRBCs). PRBCs are transfused to maintain adequate levels of hemoglobin to ensure adequate oxygen carrying capacity. Typically hemoglobin is maintained at approximately 8 to 10 g/dl. Platelets, fresh frozen plasma, and cryoprecipitate are often used to target specific clotting factors. Protocols identify when transfusion of each individual product is indicated. Albumin may also be used intermittently throughout the run for volume expansion.

WEANING AND DECANNULATION

Daily assessments for the possibility of weaning should be made first by considering why the patient was initially placed on ECMO and whether or not the problem has been resolved. Other questions to consider are if additional issues have been identified that either indicate the necessity to continue support or identify the need to discontinue support. Throughout the run the team must consider if the risks of ECMO outweigh the benefits. The process of weaning off of ECMO is different in VA support than in VV support. During VA weaning, the function of the heart must be assessed as increased blood flow is redirected to the native circulation. This evaluation is often accomplished via cardiac ultrasound while pump flow is decreased. At the same time, hemodynamic stability, RV, LV function, and the degree of pulmonary hypertension should be evaluated. Ventilator support may need to be adjusted as pump flows are decreased, particularly ventilator FiO_2 to supplement the decrease in pump flow. At this time, the risk of clots developing in the circuit at the low flow states is present. Therefore, the duration of the wean should be limited to no more than an hour with close attention to anticoagulation.

For the patient who requires VA ECMO for both cardiac and pulmonary support, there is the option to convert to VV ECMO if the heart function recovers before adequate lung function is achieved. The patient can be supported on VV ECMO until there is further evidence of lung improvement. Patients on VV ECMO must demonstrate improvement in their pulmonary status before weaning can be considered. This includes an increase in lung compliance, improved aeration on CXR, and the ability for effective gas exchange on conventional ventilator settings that are not likely to produce lung injury. A test to evaluate the native lung's ability to oxygenate can be achieved while maintaining the same ECMO support and obtaining an arterial blood gas with the ventilator FiO_2 at 1.0. A daily assessment using this "100% gas" can demonstrate the improvement in oxygenation. Early stages of support will not reveal much change, but as the lungs improve significant increases in the PaO_2 will be obvious. The process of weaning off of VV ECMO involves maintaining pump flow and weaning sweep flow to assess the native lung's ability to remove CO_2. Adjustments in ventilator support to accommodate the decrease in sweep flow should be made at this time. Once there is an improvement in ventilation evidenced by reasonable levels of PCO_2 on moderate ventilator settings with an improvement in the 100% oxygen gas, the sweep flow can be removed. The pump flow continues while a period of assessment off of ECMO occurs to determine if the patient is ready for decannulation. The decannulation approach will be determined by the cannulation sites. Percutaneously inserted cannulas may be simply withdrawn at the bedside if vascular repair is not anticipated. If surgical repair or reconstruction of the vessel is needed or if the patient is centrally cannulated, decannulation typically will take place in the operating room. Post-decannulation anticoagulation is most often discontinued or adjusted to desired levels.

MINI CLINI

PROBLEM: A patient is cannulated for VV ECMO due to acute lung injury secondary to H1N1 flu. The patient initially required a pump flow of 4 L/min and sweep of 10 L/min to achieve the desired gas exchange. After 5 days on resting ventilator settings, an improvement in both CXR and lung compliance is noted. Additionally, PaO_2 with the ventilator FiO_2 at 1.0 is markedly improved: on day 1 it had been 50 mm Hg and after 5 days is now 220 mm Hg. What changes should be made to assess the patient's readiness to wean off of VV support?

Discussion: Gradual decreases in sweep flow will allow assessment of the patient's native lung ability to effectively ventilate. Simultaneously, ventilator adjustments should be made to support the transition when ECMO is discontinued. The patient is ready to be decannulated when gas exchange can be maintained without sweep flow and ventilator settings that will not induce any further lung injury (i.e., plateau pressures less than 30 and FiO_2 less than 0.6).

RULE OF THUMB

Weaning from VA support is accomplished by turning down the pump flow and assessing hemodynamics. Weaning from VV support is accomplished by turning down the sweep flow and assessing gas exchange.

SUMMARY CHECKLIST

- ECMO is an option for newborn, pediatric, and adult patients with severe cardiac or respiratory failure who meet the criteria outlined in Boxes 50-2 and 50-3 and who otherwise have no absolute contraindications.
- The primary goals of ECMO are to deliver adequate amounts of oxygen, remove carbon dioxide, and in cases of VA ECMO, provide hemodynamic support. ECMO physiology mimics native cardiopulmonary physiology in that it allows oxygen to diffuse into the blood and carbon dioxide to be removed. This is accomplished through a circuit that contains a pump and an artificial oxygenator.
- The patient is cannulated with either a double-lumen cannula or multiple single-lumen cannulas.
- During VV support cannulas are usually placed in the right internal jugular vein, right atrium, left or right femoral veins. In VA support, the venous cannulas are placed in the same locations as with VV support with the arterial cannula inserted into the aorta or either femoral artery.
- Blood is either drained or siphoned into the pump, which propels it forward into an oxygenator. The oxygenator provides gas exchange before returning the blood to the patient containing hemoglobin that is fully saturated and has the desired carbon dioxide level.
- A blood warmer/cooler keeps the blood at the desired temperature and additional monitors provide clinicians with valuable information regarding circuit pressures, flows, and additional lab values. Several of the monitors can be set to sound audible alarms when the values of certain parameters are outside of the acceptable range.
- The circuit and cannulas are made of materials foreign to blood. These surfaces will cause the normal activation of blood clotting reactions. Anticoagulation is necessary to decrease the risk of clots in the circuit, cannulas, and most importantly in the patient.
- Bedside coagulation testing is typically performed at regular intervals to keep a close watch on the level of anticoagulation, along with frequent inspection for clot development in any of the circuit components.
- A major advantage of ECMO is that ventilator support can be decreased once ECMO is initiated, thus reducing the potential of ventilator-induced lung injury. At times the ventilator can even be discontinued, reducing the potential of ventilator-associated pneumonia and allowing the patient to more actively participate in activities of daily living. This is of particular importance in the pretransplant patient.
- As technology advances and proper candidate selection is achieved, ECMO is certain to be more frequently utilized in ICU management of the critically ill patient.

References

1. *ECLS Registry Report International Summary: Extracorporeal Life Support Organization*; Ann Arbor, MI. Available at: <www.elso.org/Registry/Statistics.aspx>, Accessed January 2015.
2. *ELSO Guidelines for all Extracorporeal Life Support Cases: Neonatal Respiratory Failure v 1.3*, Ann Arbor, MI. Available at: <www.elsonet.org/Resource/guidelines.aspx>, December 2013.
3. *ELSO Guidelines for Neonatal Respiratory Failure v1.3*, Ann Arbor, MI. Available at: <www.elso.org/Resource/guidelines.aspx>.
4. ECMO: *Extracorporeal cardiopulmonary support in critical care*, ed 4, Ann Arbor, MI, 2012, Extracorporeal Life Support Organization.
5. Hintz SR, Suttner DM, Sheehan AM, et al: Decreased use of neonatal extracorporeal membrane oxygenation (ECMO): how new treatment modalities have affected ECMO utilization. *Pediatrics* 106:1339–1343, 2000.
6. Abrams D, Brody D: Emerging indications for ECMO in adults with respiratory failure. *Ann Am Thorac Soc* 10:371–377, 2013.
7. Martinez G, Vuylsteke A: Extracorporeal membrane oxygenation in adults. *Cont Edu Anaesth Crit Care Pain* 12:57–61, 2012.
8. Turner DA, Cheifetz IM: Extracorporeal membrane oxygenation for adult respiratory failure. *Respir Care* 58(June):1038–1052, 2013.
9. Esper SA, Levy J, Waters J, et al: ECMO in the adult: a review of anticoagulation monitoring and transfusion. *Anesth Analg* 118:731–743, 2014.
10. *ELSO Anticoagulation Guidelines 2014. Extracorporeal Life Support Organization*. Available at: <elso.net/resources/guidelines>, Oct. 1, 2014.
11. Liveris A, Bello RA, Friedmann P, et al: Antifactor Xa assay is a superior correlate of heparin dose than activated partial thromboplastin time or activated clotting time in pediatric extracorporeal membrane oxygen. *Pediatr Crit Care Med* 15:e72–e79, 2014.
12. Betit P: Are contraindications to extracorporeal membrane oxygenation slowly vanishing? *Respir Care* 56:1054–1055, 2011.
13. Randucci M, Ballotta A, Kandil H, et al: Bivalirudin-based versus conventional heparin anticoagulation for postcardiotomy extracorporeal membrane oxygenation. *Crit Care* 15:R275, 2011.
14. Olsson KM, Simon A, Strueber M, et al: Extracorporeal membrane oxygenation in nonintubated patients as bridge to lung transplantation. *Am J Transplant* 10:2173–2178, 2013.
15. Hayanga AJ, Aboagye J, Esper S, et al: Extracorporeal membrane oxygenation as a bridge to lung transplantation in the United States: an evolving strategy in the management of rapidly advancing pulmonary disease. *J Thorac Cardiovasc Surg* 149:291–296, 2015.
16. Garcia JP, Kon ZN, Evans C, et al: Ambulatory veno-venous extracorporeal membrane oxygenation: innovation and pitfalls. *J Thorac Cardiovasc Surg* 142:755–761, 2011.
17. Liu C, Lin Y, Du B, et al: Extracorporeal membrane oxygenation as a support for emergency bronchial reconstruction in a traumatic patient with severe hypoxaemia. *Interact Cardiovasc Thorac Surg* 19:699–701, 2014.

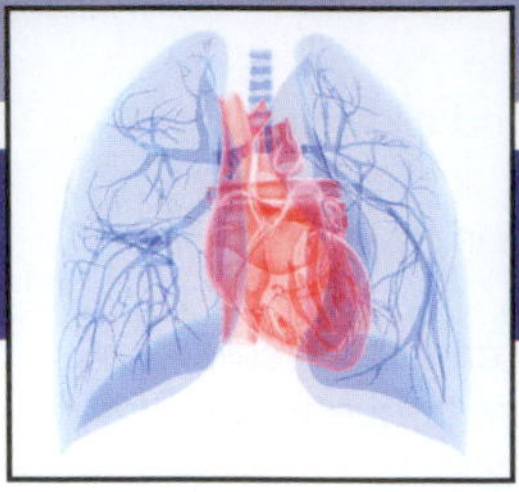

CHAPTER 51

Monitoring the Patient in the Intensive Care Unit

THOMAS PIRAINO

CHAPTER OBJECTIVES

After reading this chapter you will be able to:

- Discuss the principles of monitoring the respiratory system, cardiovascular system, neurologic status, renal function, liver function, and nutritional status of patients in intensive care.
- Identify the risks and benefits of intensive care unit (ICU) monitoring techniques.
- Explain why the caregiver is the most important monitor in the ICU.
- Describe how to evaluate measures of patient oxygenation in the ICU.
- Explain why $PaCO_2$ is the best index of ventilation for critically ill patients.
- Describe the approach used to evaluate changes in respiratory rate, tidal volume, minute ventilation, $PaCO_2$, and end-tidal PCO_2 values for monitoring purposes.
- Identify monitoring techniques used in the ICU to evaluate lung and chest wall mechanics and work of breathing.
- Describe the importance of measuring transpulmonary pressure in select patients.
- Discuss the importance of monitoring peak and plateau pressures in patients receiving mechanical ventilatory support.
- Identify monitoring techniques that have become available more recently, such as lung stress and strain, functional residual capacity, stress index, electrical impedance tomography, and acoustic respiratory monitoring.
- Describe the approach used to interpret the results of ventilator graphics monitoring.
- Describe the cardiovascular monitoring techniques used in the care of critically ill patients and how to interpret the results of hemodynamic monitoring.
- Discuss the importance of monitoring neurologic status in the ICU and the variables that should be monitored.
- Discuss evaluation of renal function, liver function, and nutritional status in the ICU.
- List and discuss the use of composite and global scores to measure patient status in the ICU, such as the APACHE severity of illness scoring system.
- Discuss monitoring and troubleshooting of the patient-ventilator system in the ICU.

CHAPTER OUTLINE

KEY TERMS

acoustic respiratory monitoring (ARM)
afterload
alveolar and arterial oxygen tension difference ($P(A - a)O_2$)
APACHE scoring system
artifacts
bladder pressure
capnography
capnometry
cardiac output
contractility
dead space/tidal volume (V_D/V_T) ratio
driving pressure
electrical impedance tomography (EIT)
esophageal balloon
factitious events
Fick equations
frequency/tidal volume (f/V_T) ratio
Glasgow Coma Scale (GCS)
Harris-Benedict equation
lung ultrasonography
lung stress and strain
maximal inspiratory pressure (MIP)
maximum voluntary ventilation (MVV)
mean airway pressure (MAP)
Murray lung injury score
oxygen consumption ($\dot{V}O_2$)
PaO_2/FiO_2 ratio
physiologic shunt ($\dot{Q}_S/\dot{Q}_T$)
preload
pressure-time product (PTP)
respiratory inductive plethysmography
stress index
Swan-Ganz catheter
systematic errors
tissue oxygen sensing
transpulmonary pressure
venous admixture
vital capacity (VC)

When patients are admitted to the intensive care unit (ICU) it is generally for the purpose of providing interventions that require continuous or periodic monitoring of physiologic parameters. Patients may require medications, fluid resuscitation to treat severe hypotension, or require noninvasive or invasive ventilatory support for respiratory failure. The monitoring of these patients is essential to assess the effectiveness of treatment in the ICU and to minimize, limit, or prevent adverse events.

Although diagnostic procedures such as radiographic imaging can be used to monitor the progression of disease over time, this chapter will focus on the periodic and/or continuous monitoring of the respiratory system, cardiovascular system, neurologic function, renal function, liver function, and nutritional status of patients in the ICU.

PRINCIPLES OF MONITORING

Monitoring options in the ICU always carry the risk of providing incorrect values, or having their values misinterpreted. Other risks of monitoring depend on the level of invasiveness. Noninvasive monitoring is monitoring that may or may not come in contact with the body, whereas invasive monitoring involves placement of the monitoring device/probe within the body. The best monitoring options provide detailed, easily interpreted data, obtained noninvasively. A monitoring tool that is highly invasive and carries a certain level of risk with use must provide a high level of valuable and required information to make the benefit of using it outweigh the risk.

New advancements in technology aim to make monitoring less invasive and at the same time provide the most clinically relevant data. The data provided should be accurate (reflect the true value) and precise (not vary widely when repeated). Many devices may require zeroing or calibration to minimize **systematic errors**.

Monitoring techniques utilized in the ICU also need to be validated and continually evaluated for their usefulness in guiding therapy and practice. When monitoring results of blood test values, interpretation may seem as simple as determining whether the values are within normal range. However, these acceptable ranges may change when new research becomes available, and generally require an understanding of the patient's "global status" to truly understand their relevance. When monitoring involves images, graphs, or waveforms, the data must be easily distinguishable from **artifacts**, **factitious events**, or normal variation, and still require an understanding of the overall status of the patient to understand their significance. Generally, the interpretation of monitored values requires skill and training to understand when something is considered abnormal and requires intervention. Interpretation also requires the use of multiple monitoring tools to help piece together more complicated conditions.

The best monitor in the ICU is the caregiver who understands how to use and interpret the various monitoring tools and techniques available to them. Caregivers may be the best monitors, but they cannot stand at the bedside continuously. Also, monitoring devices allow us to "see" the unseen. Values such as cardiac rhythms (ECG), respiratory system compliance, or alveolar ventilation would not be known using basic physical examination. Monitoring devices may require alarms to alert caregivers when values are outside of acceptable ranges for the patient. However, the skilled caregiver must understand the most appropriate setting for these alarms, and also be able to distinguish false alarms from those requiring immediate action. Devices also may prioritize alarms into low, medium, and high priority and alert clinicians with different sounds and visuals to assist with recognition in an environment filled with a variety of noise.

As monitoring devices become more advanced there is an increased risk of the clinicians ignoring the importance of physical assessment. Observing a monitor while ignoring the patient does not take into consideration the global status of the patient. We must combine the "seen" with the "unseen" to truly understand the patient (Box 51-1).

RULE OF THUMB

The caregiver must understand and interpret the information provided through monitoring. The key to proper interpretation of information is understanding how it applies to the global status of the individual patient.

PATHOPHYSIOLOGY AND MONITORING

The problem often faced at the bedside when presented with monitoring data is that clinicians may begin treating the numbers rather than the underlying pathophysiology. For example, when a patient is mechanically ventilated and the SpO_2 level drops you may improve the SpO_2 by increasing FiO_2, but adjusting the positive end expiratory pressure (PEEP) may be more appropriate if the SpO_2 drop was secondary to a change in lung mechanics. Treating the patient rather than the number requires the clinician to consider the underlying cause rather than implement a quick fix.

Box 51-1 Monitors and Monitoring Data

- Monitored values can exhibit physiologic and instrument variability.
- Monitoring devices can be noninvasive or invasive.
- Alarm systems should be set to alert caregivers properly yet avoid false alarms.
- Monitors can run continuously and measure what caregivers cannot see.
- The best monitors are caregivers who can assess and make decisions based on understanding the global status of the patient.

RESPIRATORY MONITORING

The function of the lungs is the uptake of oxygen and the removal of carbon dioxide. The arterial blood gas (ABG) gives valuable information regarding the effectiveness of the exchange (discussed in Chapter 19). Although ABGs can be drawn at the bedside, they usually require processing outside of the patient's room, either at a point-of-care machine or by the hospital laboratory. The most common bedside monitoring surrogates for O_2 uptake and CO_2 clearance are the SpO_2 (oxygen saturation) and respiratory rate (minute ventilation when the patient is mechanically ventilated). Both monitoring options have benefits, but with considerable limitations.

Monitoring Oxygenation

Tissue oxygenation depends on FiO_2, inspired partial pressure of oxygen (PiO_2), alveolar oxygen tension (PAO_2), arterial oxygenation (PaO_2, SaO_2, oxygen content of arterial blood [CaO_2]), oxygen delivery, tissue perfusion, and O_2 uptake.

Arterial Pulse Oximetry

Pulse oximetry uses a color spectrum measurement of pulsing arterial blood for continuous assessment of arterial oxygenation (SpO_2). ABG analysis has been the accepted method of detecting hypoxemia in critically ill patients, but obtaining arterial blood can be painful and cause complications, and ABG analysis does not provide immediate or continuous data. For these reasons, SpO_2 has become the standard for a continuous, noninvasive assessment of SaO_2. However, SpO_2 does not measure $PaCO_2$, and patients breathing an elevated FiO_2 can retain CO_2 (increased $PaCO_2$), although SpO_2 values are acceptable. Ventilatory failure may go unnoticed unless ABGs are measured.

SpO_2 measurements are based on spectrophotometric principles, which are based on the law of Beer-Lambert. Lightweight probes direct filtered light of specific wavelengths (usually two) through a digit, the bridge of the nose, or an earlobe or reflected from a forehead sensor. The relative absorption of these spectrophotometric beams after passing through the tissue (which differs for O_2 saturated and desaturated blood) is converted into the appropriate saturation value with processor-stored algorithms.

Tissue O_2 sensors designed to measure SaO_2 of muscle or the brain were developed more recently.[1] Brain oxygenation is crucial, and deep muscle tissue in compartment syndromes can become deoxygenated. This **tissue oxygen sensing** technique involves positioning of an emitter and detector (of usually four wavelengths) on the skin surface over the tissue or organ of interest. Light from the emitter reflects from tissue at a depth of one-third the distance between the emitter and detector. The light received by the detector is read, and algorithms determine tissue oxygenation, not SpO_2.

RULE OF THUMB

There are two very important problems with relying on SpO_2 to monitor adequate respiratory function: (1) SpO_2 values reflect oxygenation, not ventilation; and (2) SpO_2 measurement is susceptible to numerous factors that can produce false values.

Although SpO_2 has been universally adopted, it does have limitations (Box 51-2).[2,3] Motion artifact is an important problem, resulting in inaccurate readings and false alarms. Motion artifacts are common because of shivering, seizure activity, pressure on the sensor, or transport of the patient. The choice of probe site may also affect accuracy. Finger probes appear to be more accurate than forehead, nose, or earlobe probes during low perfusion states. Intense daylight and fluorescent, incandescent, xenon, and infrared light sources have caused errors in SpO_2 readings. Anemia and deeply pigmented skin can affect the accuracy of SpO_2; however, the effect of anemia is not clinically significant until the hemoglobin level is markedly reduced. Carboxyhemoglobin and methemoglobin can produce falsely high SpO_2 values, and some colors of nail polish, particularly blue, green, and black, interfere with light transmission and absorbency, as do some blood-borne dyes, such as indocyanine green and methylene blue, which tend to produce falsely low SpO_2 values. Although rare, exposure to numerous toxins and drugs, including topical benzocaine, can elevate methemoglobin and produce falsely elevated SpO_2 values.

Box 51-2 Values Affecting Pulse Oximetry

- Motion artifact
- Environmental light (e.g., sunlight, fluorescence)
- Anemia
- Deeply pigmented skin
- Carboxyhemoglobin, methemoglobin
- Nail polish
- Blood-borne dyes

MINI CLINI

Trusting the Pulse Oximeter

PROBLEM: A 32-week-gestation newborn is intubated and receiving CPAP therapy. The patient appears to be in mild to moderate respiratory distress, yet SpO_2 is 98%. Hurricane spray (20% benzocaine) had been used to reduce the irritation of the endotracheal tube. Analysis of ABG values reveals PaO_2 325 mm Hg, and the cooximeter shows a methemoglobin value of 38%.

Solution: The most common problems with the fidelity of pulse oximeter readings are motion artifacts, interference by external light sources, or malposition of the sensor. Each of these problems can be easily and quickly assessed. In this case, the clinical symptoms did not correlate with an acceptable SpO_2 value. Because adequate O_2 delivery is the ultimate goal, CO and O_2-carrying ability must be considered as causes of the respiratory distress. The high methemoglobin value necessitates immediate therapy with methylene blue dye. Although the pulse oximeter has provided an excellent, safe means of monitoring blood oxygenation, there must be a wary vigilance about trusting the values.

Oxygen Consumption

Oxygen consumption ($\dot{V}O_2$) is the volume of O_2 consumed by the body in milliliters per minute. Normal resting $\dot{V}O_2$ is approximately 250 ml/min, and $\dot{V}O_2$ increases with activity, stress, and temperature. The acquisition of O_2 from the lungs into the circulatory system is described by the **Fick equations**:

$$\dot{V}O_2 = \dot{Q}_T\,(CaO_2 - C\bar{v}O_2)\ \textit{or}\ \dot{Q}_T = \dot{V}O_2/(CaO_2 - C\bar{v}O_2)$$

in which $\dot{Q}_T$ is cardiac output (CO), and CaO_2 and $C\dot{V}O_2$ are arterial and mixed venous oxygen contents. If the values for $\dot{Q}_T$, CaO_2, and $C\dot{V}O_2$ are normal, this becomes:

$$\begin{aligned}\dot{V}O_2 \text{ in ml/min} &= \dot{Q}_T\,(CaO_2 - C\bar{v}O_2)\\ &= (5000\ \text{ml/min})\,(20\ \text{ml/100 ml} - 15\ \text{ml/100 ml})\\ &= (5000\ \text{ml/min})\,(5\ \text{ml/100 ml})\\ &= 250\ \text{ml/min}\end{aligned}$$

Simply stated, deoxygenated venous blood is converted to oxygenated arterial blood when O_2 in the alveoli diffuses into mixed venous blood flowing by at the pace of CO.

An alternative calculation for $\dot{V}O_2$ that does not require an arterial or mixed venous blood sample or measurement of **cardiac output** (CO) is:

$$\dot{V}O_2 = [(FiO_2)(\dot{V}_I)] - [(F_{\bar{E}}O_2)(\dot{V}_E)]$$

where FiO_2 and F_EO_2 are the mean inspired and expired fractional concentrations of oxygen, and $\dot{V}_I$ and $\dot{V}_E$ are the inspired and expired minute ventilations. If $\dot{V}_I$ equals $\dot{V}_E$ (normally $\dot{V}_I$ is slightly greater than $\dot{V}_E$, but the difference is small), this becomes:

$$\dot{V}O_2 = (FiO_2 - F_{\bar{E}}O_2)\,\dot{V}_E$$

If the values for minute ventilation and inspired and expired gas concentrations are normal, this becomes:

$$\dot{V}O_2 = (0.21 - 0.168)\,(6\ L/min) = 0.252\ L/min,$$
$$\text{or approximately } 250\ ml/min$$

A normal resting $\dot{V}O_2$ of 250 ml/min represents approximately 25% of normal O_2 delivery (1000 ml/min). The blood carries a large reservoir of O_2 that can diffuse into deoxygenated tissues under high O_2 demand conditions.

$\dot{V}O_2$ may be useful in determining nutritional requirements and adequacy of O_2 delivery and may occasionally help determine the cause of a high ventilation requirement. If there is a stable tissue demand for O_2, measurements of $\dot{V}O_2$ may be used to follow the hemodynamic response to therapeutic interventions.

Alveolar-Arterial Oxygen Tension Difference

The **alveolar and arterial oxygen tension difference (P(A – a) O2)** is a useful measurement of the efficiency of gas exchange. A healthy person breathing room air has $P(A - a)O_2$ of approximately 5 to 15 mm Hg. This value increases with age to approximately 10 to 20 mm Hg in elderly adults. $P(A - a)O_2$ also increases normally with an increase in FiO_2. A healthy person has $P(A - a)O_2$ of 5 to 15 mm Hg while breathing room air; however, $P(A - a)O_2$ increases to 100 to 150 mm Hg when the person is breathing 100% O_2.

Most importantly, an abnormal increase in $P(A - a)O_2$ is associated with gas-exchange problems. If PaO_2 is 80 mm Hg while the patient is breathing 100% O_2, a significant gas-exchange problem is present even though oxygenation seems acceptable.

If PaO_2 is 80 mm Hg, $PaCO_2$ is 40 mm, FiO_2 is 1, and barometric pressure (PB) is 760 mm Hg, then:

$$PAO_2 = PiO_2 - (PaCO_2)(1.25)$$
$$PiO_2 = [(PB - P_{H_2O})(FiO_2)] = 713$$
$$PAO_2 = [(760 - 47)(1)] - (40)(1.25) = 663\ mm\ Hg$$
$$P(A - a)O_2 = PAO_2 - PaO_2 = 663 - 80$$
$$P(A - a)O_2 = 583\ mm\ Hg$$

where P_{H2O} is water vapor pressure. $P(A - a)O_2$ is markedly elevated considering that normal $(A - a)O_2$ is 100 to 150 mm Hg while the patient is breathing 100% O_2. $(A - a)O_2$ also can be used to give a rough estimate of percentage shunt, where:

$$\text{Shunt} \cong \frac{[P(A - a)O_2 \text{ on } 100\%\ O_2]}{20}$$

In this example, percentage shunt would be approximately 29%: $P(A - a)O_2/20 = 583/20 = 29.2\%$.

$P(A - a)O_2$ takes into account $PaCO_2$ and eliminates hypoventilation and hypercapnia from consideration as the sole cause of hypoxemia. Although $P(A - a)O_2$ is infrequently calculated, astute experienced clinicians consciously or subconsciously can estimate $P(A - a)O_2$ from a blood gas value.

PaO_2/FiO_2 Ratio

The **PaO_2/FiO_2 ratio** has become important for the determination of the extent of acute respiratory distress syndrome (ARDS) in multicenter collaborative studies.[4,5] A normal PaO_2/FiO_2 ratio while breathing room air is about 400 to 500 mm Hg. The PaO_2/FiO_2 ratio provides an index for the effect of O_2 on PaO_2 when a range of FiO_2 settings may be prescribed. The index allows comparisons of severity between patients or if FiO_2 is changed in the same patient. The PaO_2/FiO_2 ratio is easy to calculate and a reliable index of gas exchange. The level of applied **mean airway pressure (MAP)**, which is strongly affected by PEEP, must also be considered as an independent factor that influences the PaO_2/FiO_2 ratio. This is done by calculating the oxygenation index (OI). Evidence suggests that the OI seems to have an independent effect on mortality when considering the use of rescue strategies in neonates.[6] In addition, a change in the FiO_2 can also affect the PaO_2/FiO_2 ratio. Some recommend that in ARDS the PaO_2/FiO_2 ratio should be determined at a specific FiO_2 and PEEP level.

RULE OF THUMB

The Berlin definition of ARDS includes:

- Bilateral infiltrates on chest radiograph
- Absence of left ventricular failure
- PaO_2/FiO_2 200 to 300 mm Hg for mild ARDS (previously considered acute lung injury or ALI)
- PaO_2/FiO_2 100 to 200 mm Hg for moderate ARDS
- PaO_2/FiO_2 less than 100 mm Hg for severe ARDS

Oxygenation Index

Calculation of oxygenation index (OI) by the following equation provides an index that accounts for FiO_2 and MAP:

$$OI = \frac{FiO_2 * MAP}{PaO_2}$$

Quantification of Shunt

The most accurate and reliable measure of oxygenation efficiency is direct computation of the **physiologic shunt** ($\dot{Q}_S/\dot{Q}_T$). The physiologic shunt is computed as follows:

$$\dot{Q}_S/\dot{Q}_T = (CcO_2 - CaO_2)/(CcO_2 - C\bar{v}O_2)$$

Where CcO_2 is the oxygen content of alveolar capillary blood, CaO_2 is the oxygen content of arterial blood, and $C\dot{V}O_2$ is the oxygen content of mixed venous blood, all expressed in milliliters of O_2 per 100 ml of blood. When the patient is breathing 100% O_2, $\dot{Q}_S/\dot{Q}_T$ can be estimated as follows:

$$\dot{Q}_S/\dot{Q}_T = [(P(A - a)O_2)][0.003]/[(P(A - a)O_2)][0.003]$$
$$+ [CaO_2 - C\bar{v}O_2]$$

For measurement of physiologic shunt, both an arterial and a mixed venous blood sample must be obtained. A true mixed venous blood sample can be obtained only from the distal sample port of an indwelling pulmonary arterial catheter. The total O_2 content of the arterial, mixed venous blood, and pulmonary capillary blood (CaO_2, $C\dot{V}O_2$, CcO_2) is calculated in the same manner as any O_2 content calculations:

$$O_2\ \text{content} = (1.34)(\text{Hb})(SO_2) + (0.003)(PO_2)$$

where Hb is the hemoglobin concentration, SO_2 is the oxygen saturation, and PO_2 is the partial pressure of oxygen. If the patient is breathing 100% O_2, the capillary saturation is 100%, the PCO_2 (capillary PO_2) being the calculated PAO_2 value. Samples should be obtained and analyzed quickly to avoid error from continued metabolism. Similar to $P(A-a)O_2$, $\dot{Q}_S/\dot{Q}_T$ is influenced by $\dot{V}/\dot{Q}$ mismatching and by fluctuations in mixed venous oxygen saturation ($S\bar{v}O_2$) and FiO_2. A "shunt" calculation when FiO_2 is less than 1.0 is defined as **venous admixture**. If venous admixture is elevated but all alveoli are patent, venous admixture decreases toward the normal value (<5%) as FiO_2 is increased. Conversely, if increased venous admixture is caused by a true shunt such as an intracardiac defect or atelectasis, there would be no change in venous admixture as FiO_2 is increased.

Murray Lung Injury Score

ARDS is a syndrome of severe lung injury that was originally described by Ashbaugh and Petty in 1970.[7] Evaluating and treating a patient with ARDS is a primary challenge for the ICU clinician. To monitor the severity of this disease, Murray and colleagues[8] developed a lung injury score that is often calculated in studies of ARDS. The **Murray lung injury score** quantifies the injury level using the following four factors: chest radiographic findings, PaO_2/FiO_2 ratio, positive end expiratory pressure (PEEP) setting, and compliance. The Murray lung injury score is an example of a composite score that allows quantification of lung status according to different aspects of the injury—gas exchange, radiographic findings, and mechanics. This score is used as an index of the effectiveness of therapy or for interstudy comparisons. The method for calculating the Murray lung injury score is shown in Box 51-3. Other measures of lung injury are listed in Box 51-4.

Monitoring Ventilation

Similar to oxygenation, the adequacy and efficiency of ventilation is routinely evaluated in the ICU (Box 51-5). Monitoring of patients receiving mechanical ventilatory support in the ICU includes measurement of the patient's tidal volume (V_T), respiratory rate (f), and minute ventilation ($\dot{V}_E$) where:

$$\dot{V}_E = (f) * (V_T)$$

However, effective ventilation depends on alveolar ventilation ($\dot{V}_A$), as follows:

$$\dot{V}_A = (V_T - V_{Dphys})(f)$$

where V_{Dphys} is physiologic dead space, and:

$$\dot{V}_A = (0.863 * \dot{V}CO_2)/PaCO_2$$

Box 51-3 Murray Lung Injury Score

Component	Value
1. Chest Radiograph	
No alveolar consolidation	0
Alveolar consolidation confined to 1 quadrant	1
Alveolar consolidation confined to 2 quadrants	2
Alveolar consolidation confined to 3 quadrants	3
Alveolar consolidation in all 4 quadrants	4
2. Hypoxemia Score	
$PaO_2/FiO_2 > 300$	0
PaO_2/FiO_2 225-299	1
PaO_2/FiO_2 175-224	2
PaO_2/FiO_2 100-174	3
$PaO_2/FiO_2 < 100$	4
3. PEEP Score (When Ventilated)	
PEEP ≤5 cm H_2O	0
PEEP 6-8 cm H_2O	1
PEEP 9-11 cm H_2O	2
PEEP 12-14 cm H_2O	3
PEEP > 15 cm H_2O	4
4. Respiratory System Compliance Score (When Available)	
Compliance ≥80 ml/cm H_2O	0
Compliance 60-79 ml/cm H_2O	1
Compliance 40-59 ml/cm H_2O	2
Compliance 20-39 ml/cm H_2O	3
Compliance ≤19 ml/cm H_2O	4

The final value is obtained by dividing the aggregate sum by the number of components used.

SCORE

No lung injury—0
Mild to moderate lung injury—0.1-2.5
Severe lung injury (ARDS) —>2.5

Box 51-4 Measures of Decreased Blood Oxygenation or Lung Injury

↓ SpO_2
↓ PaO_2
↑ $P(A-a)O_2$ – (PAO_2 – PaO_2)
↓ P/F ratio – (PaO_2/FiO_2)
↑ Shunt/venous admixture
↑ Murray lung injury score

Box 51-5 Monitoring the Adequacy of Ventilation

- Respiratory volume and rate (V_T, f, $\dot{V}_E$)
- $PaCO_2$
- V_D/V_T
- Capnometry (not for routine use but in special situations, such as ensuring tracheal intubation and cardiac blood flow in resuscitation efforts)

where $\dot{V}CO_2$ is CO_2 production in milliliters per minute, and 0.863 is a conversion factor. With a normal $PaCO_2$ and $\dot{V}CO_2$, this becomes:

$$\dot{V}_A = (0.863 * 200\ \text{ml/min})/40\ \text{mm Hg} = 4.3\ \text{L/min}$$

Ventilation is adequate if $PaCO_2$ is associated with a normal arterial pH. For healthy persons, $PaCO_2$ is between 35 mm Hg and 45 mm Hg, resulting in an arterial pH of 7.35 to 7.45. An elevated $PaCO_2$ with normal pH is common in patients with chronic obstructive pulmonary disease (COPD). It is generally accepted that pH becomes the goal during mechanical ventilation of the critically ill patient rather than $PaCO_2$. However, it is important to consider the acceptance of a lower pH level (7.25 to 7.35) when approaching the safe upper limits of mechanical ventilation that can occur in patients with ARDS.

Capnography

Capnometry is the measurement of CO_2 at the airway opening during the ventilatory cycle. **Capnography** refers to plotting CO_2 concentration against time or against exhaled volume. The normal CO_2 waveform is displayed in Figure 51-1. The height of the capnogram (the peak value) indicates the end-tidal CO_2 value. $P_{ET}CO_2$ normally is 1 to 5 mm Hg less than $PaCO_2$, ranging between 35 mm Hg and 43 mm Hg. Because $P_{ET}CO_2$ in healthy persons closely approximates $PaCO_2$, this measure is a potentially useful noninvasive index of the adequacy of ventilation.[9] Abnormal waveform contours can indicate changes in the distribution of ventilation and perfusion, or airway obstruction. These changes typically are an irregular increase in CO_2 level and a lower than normal end-tidal CO_2 level. Positive pressure ventilation (especially with PEEP), pulmonary embolism, cardiac arrest, and pulmonary hypoperfusion also may cause an increase in $PaCO_2$ to $P_{ET}CO_2$ difference $[P(a-ET)CO_2]$.[10] Exercise and a large V_T can reverse the $P(a-ET)CO_2$ difference, and $P_{ET}CO_2$ can exceed $PaCO_2$ temporarily.

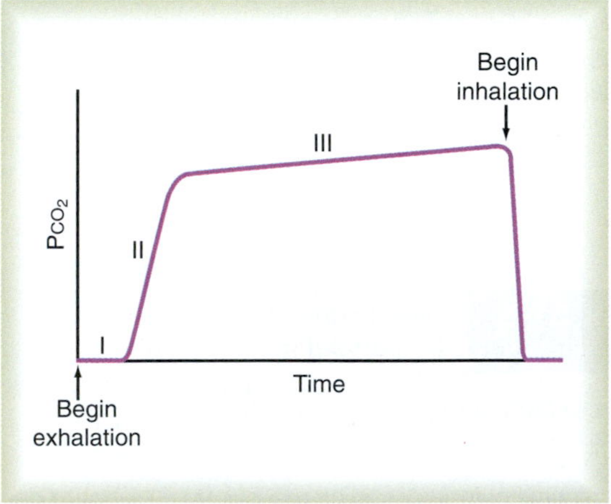

FIGURE 51-1 Time-based capnograph. *Phase I,* Anatomic dead space; *phase II,* transition from anatomic dead space to alveolar plateau; *phase III,* the alveolar plateau.

Patients for whom capnometry may be a useful monitoring tool include patients with normal lungs but an unstable ventilatory drive who are breathing spontaneously or receiving low-level ventilatory support. In these patients, capnometry readings should initially be validated by comparison with $PaCO_2$. Changes in $P_{ET}CO_2$ can be used to alert the clinician to potential changes in patient ventilation. Thereafter, periodic reevaluation should be performed as the patient's clinical state changes. Capnometry has been extremely useful in emergency situations, such as verification of endotracheal intubation and assessment of blood flow during or after cardiac arrest. Small in-line CO_2 monitors that employ colorimetry are now routinely used to verify endotracheal intubation.[11]

Although $P_{ET}CO_2$ and $PaCO_2$ values tend to correlate at a single point in time, correlation between changes in $P_{ET}CO_2$ and changes in $PaCO_2$ tend to be weaker.[12] Decreases in ventilation are reflected by increases in $P_{ET}CO_2$ and $PaCO_2$. However, with very small V_T, $PaCO_2$ increases, whereas $P_{ET}CO_2$ may decrease. Although the appropriate role of capnometry in critical care may be unclear, integration of capnometry into modern ventilators is reasonable because the primary role of the ventilator is CO_2 elimination. As a guide for clinicians, the American Association for Respiratory Care (AARC) has created clinical practice guidelines for the use of capnometry in ventilated patients.[13] Box 51-6 lists common causes of changes in monitored $P_{ET}CO_2$ values.

Volumetric CO_2 monitoring holds promise in the continuous monitoring of ventilation efficiency. VCO_2 can be continuously monitored in a patient being weaned from mechanical ventilation as an indicator of adequate or improving ventilatory efficiency.[14] The volumetric capnogram has been examined as a potential tool for detecting a pulmonary embolism,[15] tracking the efficiency of mechanical ventilation,[15] and calculating dead space.[17] The relationship between VCO_2 and dead space also makes it a valuable tool in PEEP optimization.

Box 51-6 Causes of Increased and Decreased End-Tidal Carbon Dioxide Values

INCREASED $P_{ET}CO_2$
- Decreased effective ventilation (↓ V_T, ↓ $\dot{V}_E$, ↓ $\dot{V}_A$, ↑ $PaCO_2$)
- Increased CO_2 production ($\dot{V}CO_2$) (agitation, stress, shivering, fighting the ventilator, pain, anxiety, recovery from sedation or paralysis)

DECREASED $P_{ET}CO_2$
- Increased effective ventilation (↑ V_T, ↑ $\dot{V}_E$, ↑ $\dot{V}_A$, ↓ $PaCO_2$)
- Marked decrease in effective ventilation (↓↓V_T approaching dead space volume; rapid shallow breathing)
- Decreased CO_2 production ($\dot{V}CO_2$) (sedation, sleep, cooling)
- Decrease in lung perfusion (pulmonary embolus, decreased CO)

ABSENT $P_{ET}CO_2$
- Apnea
- Cardiac arrest
- Ventilator disconnect or malfunction
- Airway obstruction

Dead Space

The **dead space/tidal volume (VD/VT) ratio** is a measure of the efficiency of gas exchange. This ratio is an estimate of the proportion of ventilation participating in diffusion of CO_2. V_D/V_T can be calculated from the Enghoff modification of the Bohr equation as follows:

$$V_D/V_T = (PaCO_2 - P_ECO_2)/PaCO_2$$

Where P_ECO_2 is the CO_2 concentration in mixed expired gas. A rapid response capnometry or exhaled flow analysis provides a volumetric CO_2 method for attaining P_ECO_2 values.[7] Research has shown that using the fraction of VCO_2 to exhaled minute ventilation (V_E) can be used to estimate P_ECO_2 using the following equation (assuming PB is 760 mm Hg)[17]:

$$P_ECO_2 = (760 - 47) \times VCO_2/V_E$$

When P_ECO_2 is determined, a specimen of arterial blood should be drawn for ABG analysis. When the gas and blood samples are analyzed, the preceding formula can be used to calculate V_D/V_T.

In healthy persons who are sitting, the V_D/V_T ratio is 0.20 to 0.40. This value varies little with age, position, exercise, V_T, or breath holding. In the setting of critical illness, however, the V_D/V_T ratio commonly exceeds 0.6. Frequently, the V_D/V_T ratio is increased in patients with congestive heart failure, pulmonary embolism, ARDS, or pulmonary hypertension and in patients undergoing mechanical ventilation. The V_D/V_T ratio has been used to evaluate patients being considered for weaning from mechanical ventilation. A V_D/V_T ratio greater than 0.60 generally requires continuation of ventilatory support. Increased V_D/V_T in the early phase of ARDS has been associated with an increased risk of death.[8,10]

Monitoring of Inspired and Exhaled Gas Volumes

Although the best index of effective ventilation is measurement of $PaCO_2$, measurement of inspired and expired gas volumes is an important aspect of monitoring patients receiving mechanical ventilatory support. For patients receiving controlled mechanical ventilation, minute ventilation ($\dot{V}_E$), respiratory rate (f), and V_T are assessed by:

$$\dot{V}_E = (V_T)(f) \textit{ and } V_T \text{ average} = \dot{V}_E/f$$

With an adequate V_T, increases in minute ventilation tend to increase alveolar ventilation and decrease $PaCO_2$, whereas decreases in minute ventilation tend to have the opposite effect. However, in the presence of rapid shallow breathing with normal or elevated minute ventilation, a decrease in effective ventilation can result in an increase in $PaCO_2$. This effect is caused by ineffective shallow tidal breaths that are at or below dead space volume. Spontaneous respiratory rate often is a sensitive indicator of the need for mechanical ventilation. Rates greater than 20 breaths/min may indicate distress, and a rate greater than 30 breaths/min with a spontaneous V_T of less than 300 ml often indicates the need for mechanical ventilatory support in adults because a large proportion of ventilatory effort is being expended to move dead space gases.

Inspired Versus Expired Tidal Volume

Normal inspired V_T and expired V_T should be nearly the same. However, in the presence of an air leak, inspired V_T may be larger than expired V_T, and measurement of delivered V_T versus exhaled V_T may be useful in detecting and quantifying the size of a leak—a situation that may require immediate attention.

Monitoring Lung and Chest Wall Mechanics

Ventilation of the lungs involves overcoming the flow-resistive, inertial, and elastic properties of the respiratory system. In a ventilated patient, change in airway pressure during ventilation is used to determine the compliance of the total respiratory system. Pressure changes measured by an esophageal balloon reflect compliance of the chest wall. The difference between the compliance of the respiratory system and chest wall is the lung compliance (lung compliance can also be measured in the passively ventilated patient using the change in transpulmonary pressure).

One method to assess the compliance of the respiratory system and its relation to lung volume is through the use of a P-V curve. There is normally a difference in the P-V relationship during inflation and deflation. However, a large difference between inflation and deflation, called *hysteresis*, typically implies lung units have been recruited after a threshold level of pressure was applied.

To measure a static P-V curve of a ventilated patient from resting (at functional residual capacity [FRC]) to total lung capacity, a calibrated syringe, referred to as a *supersyringe* ranging from 1.5 to 3 L, was used until more recently to inject 50- to 100-ml increments into the lungs while airway pressure was recorded. A P-V curve can be measured more easily by the continuous delivery of a low flow of gas into the lung (<5 L/min) with the simultaneous recording of system pressure change. Current ICU ventilators allow the determination of an inflation P-V curve using this approach. The P-V curve is plotted as part of the ventilator graphics package with cursors available to identify specific points on the curve. Patients should be sedated during the maneuver mostly because the flow delivered would be insufficient to satisfy patient demand. Also, the amount of pressure or volume applied during the maneuver would likely cause discomfort.

The inflation P-V curve often, but not always, reveals two points at which the slope of the curve changes. The lower point at which the slope changes is called the *lower inflection point*. As depicted in Figure 51-2 , a lower inflection point may occur over the lower range of volumes, indicating a pressure above which total respiratory system compliance is improved owing to the beginning of alveolar recruitment or the peripheralization of secretions.[16] A recommended strategy is to set PEEP slightly above the lower inflection point with the goal of maintaining recruitment and stabilization of dependent alveoli that may otherwise sustain injury from repetitive opening, closing, and

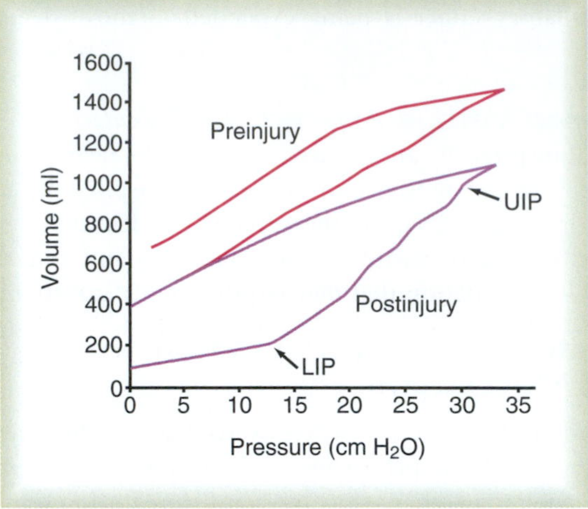

FIGURE 51-2 P-V curves generated by a normal lung (preinjury) and after oleic acid injury (postinjury). In the preinjury curve, the linear relationship between pressure and volume with minimal hysteresis is evident. The postinjury curve displays marked hysteresis and two changes in compliance on the inspiratory limb: a lower inflection point *(LIP)* and upper inflection point *(UIP)*.

reopening during tidal ventilation. The other pressure change in the slope, called an *upper deflection point,* may be seen at a higher volume, indicating where compliance decreases owing to alveolar overdistention or a slowing of lung recruitment. Although the risk of alveolar overdistention is generally reduced if the end inspiratory plateau pressure (P_{plat}) is less than 30 cm H_2O in patients with ARDS.[18] More recently, attention has been focused on the deflation area of the curve and what is called the *critical closing pressure,* the area of the deflation curve where there is significant loss in compliance.[19] The rationale for this is that when there is a significant amount of recruitment (showing as hysteresis), the amount of pressure required to maintain an open lung may be lower than during the inflation curve. The deflation area of the curve will be further discussed later in this chapter.

Respiratory System Compliance

Respiratory system compliance should be routinely monitored in all ventilated patients. To attain an accurate assessment of compliance (static compliance), two maneuvers must be performed: an end inspiratory hold, and an end expiratory hold. An end inspiratory hold maneuver in a passive, ventilated patient allows equilibration of pressure across the lung and an estimation of peak alveolar pressure or the end inspiratory P_{plat}. An end expiratory hold is required to assess the total PEEP ($PEEP_{-T}$) when auto-PEEP is present. Compliance (C) is calculated as follows:

$$C = \Delta V/\Delta P$$

Where V_T (corrected for tubing compliance) is ΔV and ΔP is $P_{plat} - PEEP_T$.

Normal compliance ranges from 60 to 100 ml/cm H_2O. Diseases of the lung parenchyma, such as pneumonia, pulmonary edema, and any chronic disease causing fibrosis, cause decreased effective compliance. Acute changes, such as atelectasis, pulmonary edema, ARDS, and lung compression caused by tension pneumothorax cause a rapid decrease in compliance. Compliance is often less than 25 to 30 ml/cm H_2O in patients with ARDS. Common causes of changes in respiratory system compliance are listed in Box 51-7. Several ventilators report breath-to-breath compliance and resistance values dynamically without the use of pause maneuvers. Monitoring these estimates can indicate impedance problems, and are useful for trending during ventilator setting titration (such as PEEP), but absolute values should be verified by static maneuver calculations.

Box 51-7 Common Causes of Changes in Compliance and Resistance in Mechanically Ventilated Patients

DECREASED COMPLIANCE

↓ Lung compliance (atelectasis, pneumonia, pulmonary edema, ARDS, pneumothorax, fibrosis, bronchial intubation)
↓ Thoracic compliance (obesity, ascites, chest wall deformity)

INCREASED COMPLIANCE

↑ Lung compliance (improvement in any of the above-listed conditions, pulmonary emphysema)
↑ Thoracic compliance (improvement in any of the above-listed conditions; flail chest; position change—sitting patient up)

INCREASED RESISTANCE

Small endotracheal tube, secretions plugging endotracheal tube, biting on endotracheal tube
↑ Bronchospasm, mucosal edema
↑ Secretions
↑ Airway obstruction
High gas flow rate (or ↑ gas flow)

DECREASED RESISTANCE

↓ Improvement in any of the above-listed conditions
↓ Bronchodilator administration
↓ Suctioning and airway care
↓ Use of lower inspiratory gas flow rate

Chest Wall Compliance

In a significant proportion of patients, chest wall compliance can influence the P-V relationship during ventilation. Poor respiratory system compliance may be largely due to external pathologies of the chest wall. Normal chest wall compliance accounts for approximately 20% of the respiratory compliance, but can commonly reach 50% or greater in critically ill patients. Chest wall abnormalities (including the abdomen) may cause an increase in pleural pressure both at rest and during positive pressure ventilation. Direct measurement of pleural pressure at the bedside is highly invasive, and this is why **esophageal balloon pressure** measurement are used as a surrogate (Box 51-8). Chest wall compliance (C_{CW}) by definition using esophageal pressure is as follows:

$$C_{CW} = \Delta V/P_{esipp} - P_{esexp}$$

where P_{esipp} is the esophageal pressure during an end inspiratory hold and P_{esexp} is the esophageal pressure during an end expiratory hold.

Box 51-8 Esophageal Pressure Monitoring

Esophageal pressure is used clinically as a surrogate for pleural pressure. The measurements are used to determine chest wall and lung compliance, measure work of breathing, determine the appropriateness of PEEP, and calculate lung stress. A thin esophageal catheter (approximately 2-mm diameter) is simple to insert, and poses little risk of esophageal perforation. Appropriate placement is achieved by first passing it into the stomach, then inflating the 10-cm long balloon with approximately 0.5 to 1.0 ml of air. The catheter is carefully withdrawn until the final position of the balloon is within the lower third of the esophagus, as verified by the presence of cardiac oscillations within the pressure tracing. In adults this is approximately 35 to 40 cm from the teeth when inserted orally. Proper placement can also be confirmed by occluding the airway (done with an expiratory hold on the ventilator) and measuring the simultaneous deflections in pressure at the airway opening and esophageal pressure either during spontaneous efforts or by a gentle push on the chest or abdomen. The change in pressure in the airway during occlusion should be the same as the pressure change that occurs in the esophageal pressure.

Box 51-9 Common Causes of Elevated Pleural Pressure in ICU Patients

- Obesity
- Intraabdominal hypertension
- Massive fluid resuscitation

Poor chest wall compliance (high chest wall elastance) may buffer the lung-damaging effect of elevated airway pressure by reducing end-inspiratory transpulmonary pressure (Ptp). Higher airway pressures may be required to ventilate these patients, but without the same risk of barotrauma as in patients with low pleural pressure or normal chest wall compliance. One of the most common causes of poor chest wall compliance is intraabdominal hypertension. Regular monitoring of **bladder pressure** can be useful at confirming issues of poor chest wall compliance in the absence of esophageal pressure monitoring. Some causes of elevated pleural pressure (resulting in poor chest wall compliance) are listed in Box 51-9.

Transpulmonary Pressure

Airway pressure as measured by the ventilator does not take into consideration the pleural pressure or chest wall compliance of the patient. True distending pressure of the lung (the pressure that stretches the lung) is the **transpulmonary pressure**. The appropriateness and safety of the airway pressures delivered by the ventilator, both at end-exhalation (PEEP) and end-inspiration (P_{plat}), depends on the resulting trasnspulmonary pressure.[20]

The estimation of transpulmonary pressure is commonly done through the use of esophageal pressure monitoring using the simple equation:

$$P_{airway} - P_{es} = Ptp$$

Where P_{airway} is the airway pressure and P_{es} is the esophageal pressure. Two variations are used in clinical practice, one for end-exhalation and one for end-inspiration. These variations are as follows:

$$P_{PEEP} - P_{esexp} = Ptp_{PEEP}$$
$$P_{plat} - P_{esinsp} = Ptp_{plat}$$

where the first equation is the transpulmonary pressure during an end expiratory hold and the second equation is the transpulmonary pressure during an end inspiratory hold. Lung compliance (C_L) can be derived from these measurements as follows:

$$C_L = \Delta V / Ptp_{plat} - Ptp_{PEEP}$$

End inspiratory Ptp can be monitored to evaluate global lung stress and the potential for overdistention—usually allowing some liberty in accepting higher P_{plat} to deliver adequate ventilation in patients with elevated pleural pressures (stiff chest walls). Current practice is to limit this end-inspiratory Ptp to less than 20 cm H_2O of pressure. For patients with a large degree of lung inhomogeneity any attempt to maintain an even lower end-inspiratory Ptp should be taken. The monitoring of end-expiratory Ptp has been used more recently as a rationale for setting PEEP.[21] A negative Ptp probably indicates lung closure (dependent lobe) during expiration that can result in lung opening and closing during the ventilatory cycle. Adequate or "optimal" PEEP when measuring Ptp is the PEEP level that avoids a negative Ptp_{PEEP}. (See Chapter 48 for details.)

Resistance

Depending on the **driving pressure** measured, various resistances can be calculated, including airway, pulmonary, chest wall, and total respiratory system resistance. An airway resistance (Raw) can be determined dynamically from simultaneous measurements of airflow and the pressure difference between the airway opening (P_{ao}) and the alveoli (P_{alv}) by Raw = (P_{ao} − P_{alv})/flow. Because resistance changes throughout inspiration and expiration, and expiratory resistance generally is greater than inspiratory resistance, instantaneous measures of resistance are not performed clinically. Inspiratory resistance can be calculated simply during constant flow, volume ventilation. This allows monitoring of airway status over time or after the effects of bronchodilator therapy and is determined by dividing the pressure change by the flow rate:

$$Raw = \Delta P / \Delta F = (P_{peak} - P_{plat}) / flow$$

where P_{peak} is peak airway pressure and P_{plat} is plateau pressure. Automated methods of measuring expiratory resistance have been integrated into some ventilators.

In ventilated patients, a significant component of the total flow resistance is from endotracheal tubes.[22] In healthy persons, flow is relatively laminar during tidal ventilation and becomes turbulent only with increasing ventilatory demands. The flow resistance offered by the endotracheal tube increases markedly with increasing flow and varies with the size of the tube. Normal airway resistance is approximately 1 to 2 cm H_2O/L per second;

however, intubated patients receiving mechanical ventilatory support typically have an airway resistance of 5 to 10 cm H_2O/L per second or more. Automated tube compensation modes have been added to mechanical ventilators to deliver flow that accounts for the added resistance of the endotracheal tube. Common causes of changes in airway resistance in mechanically ventilated patients are listed in Box 51-7.

Peak and Plateau Pressures

The maximum value of airway pressure at the airway opening during a ventilatory cycle is routinely monitored in the ICU. Peak airway pressure greater than 50 to 60 cm H_2O is generally discouraged because high values of peak pressure carry increased risk of barotrauma and hypotension.[23] During volume-targeted modes of ventilation, an increase in peak pressure results from increased resistive pressure or increased elastic pressure from decreased lung or chest wall compliance. During pressure-targeted modes of ventilation, increased resistive pressure or increased elastic pressure results in a decrease in delivered tidal volume rather than the increase in peak or plateau pressure. Measurement of end inspiratory P_{plat} helps to differentiate between the resistive and elastic components. The P_{plat} level should be monitored for all ventilated patients. P_{plat} ideally should not exceed 28 cm H_2O because elevated P_{plat} increases the likelihood of developing ventilator-induced lung injury. However, the limit for P_{plat} depends on the resulting lung stress and strain.

Lung Stress and Strain

During mechanical ventilation, the lungs are exposed to positive pressure that exerts more stress and strain on the lungs than experienced during spontaneous ventilation. This **lung stress and strain** may cause injury or extend existing lung injury along the injury/normal tissue border. When positive pressure becomes injurious, it is referred to as *ventilator-induced lung injury*. However, the concepts of stress and strain as applied to the lungs are not clearly defined. The physical definition of stress is a force per unit area. Strain is the deformation of a structure compared with its overall size. Hooke's law associates the two factors by the following relationship: stress = k * strain.

Working definitions for stress and strain applied to the lungs have been studied.[24] *Stress* (Ptp_{plat}) is defined as follows:[20]

$$Ptp_{plat} = Ptp_{PEEP} + E_L \times Vt$$

which can be simplified to:

$$Ptp_{plat} = Ptp_{PEEP} + \Delta Ptp$$

Driving pressure, as previously discussed, may be an alternative measure of stress. However, when chest wall compliance is poor it may be difficult to determine the potential for injury without measuring lung stress. *Strain* has been defined as V_T (the deformation) divided by FRC (the resting size of the lungs). These definitions have been associated as stress = 13.5 * strain, predicting that a stress of 27 cm H_2O (Ptp of 27 cm H_2O) and a strain of 2 (V_T of twice the FRC) approach the limits of safe ventilation.[24] The measurement of lung stress requires placement of an esophageal catheter. To measure strain, automated FRC determinations have become available on some modern ventilators.[25] Stress can also occur at lower pressures if lung units are opening and closing during the ventilator cycle.

Stress Index

Another index involving the dynamic measurement of stress has been reported.[26] The **stress index** is a value derived from the airway pressure-time curve during constant flow delivery of a tidal breath. During constant flow (when resistance is constant), the slope of the pressure-time tracing is analyzed to evaluate the elastic properties of the lungs. The index is calculated by performing a curve fit of the slope of the pressure-time tracing, where pressure = a * $time^b$ + c. Ideally, a slope (b) of 1 indicates normal filling during lung expansion, whereas a slope greater than 1 indicates overdistention, and a slope less than 1 indicates lung recruitment (Figure 51-3). This measure can be calculated for each delivered tidal breath, although an acceptance criterion should be used to exclude analysis of artifacts and factitious breaths. Although the index may not determine a threshold for excessive stress or strain, it may be a useful indicator of lung response to positive pressure. If the chest wall contributes variably to airway pressure, the calculated index can be altered and deceptive.[27]

Driving Pressure

Driving pressure is a measure of the pressure difference between P_{plat} and total PEEP (PEEP plus auto-PEEP). The swing in pressure from end-expiration to end-inspiration may be an independent stress factor on the lungs. Consider driving pressure as the amount of *energy* applied to the lung, the higher the energy applied to the lung, the greater the potential for lung injury. In general, the driving pressure should be kept less than or equal to 15 cm H_2O.

Auto-Positive End Expiratory Pressure (Intrinsic Positive End Expiratory Pressure)

PEEP is the pressure maintained in the airway by the ventilator at end-exhalation. An alveolar pressure that exists above the applied or extrinsic PEEP level at end-exhalation is termed *intrinsic PEEP* or *auto-PEEP*. At the bedside, *total PEEP* is the sum of extrinsic PEEP and intrinsic PEEP. Intrinsic or auto-PEEP is sometimes misunderstood when one considers "trapped" air versus breath-stacking that can occur when a patient is being passively ventilated with insufficient time to exhale. Intrinsic or auto-PEEP is often the result of small airway collapse and can also occur when excessive tidal volume is delivered to a patient with a high ventilatory demand, causing dynamic hyperinflation when the patient has difficulty exhaling all of the excess volume.

Numerous factors, both internal and external to the patient, contribute to the development of auto-PEEP. Expiratory muscle activity can increase auto-PEEP and may interfere with attempts at assessment of auto-PEEP based solely on dynamic hyperinflation. Patients receiving mechanical ventilation for obstructive airways disease have a large degree of inhomogeneity in the

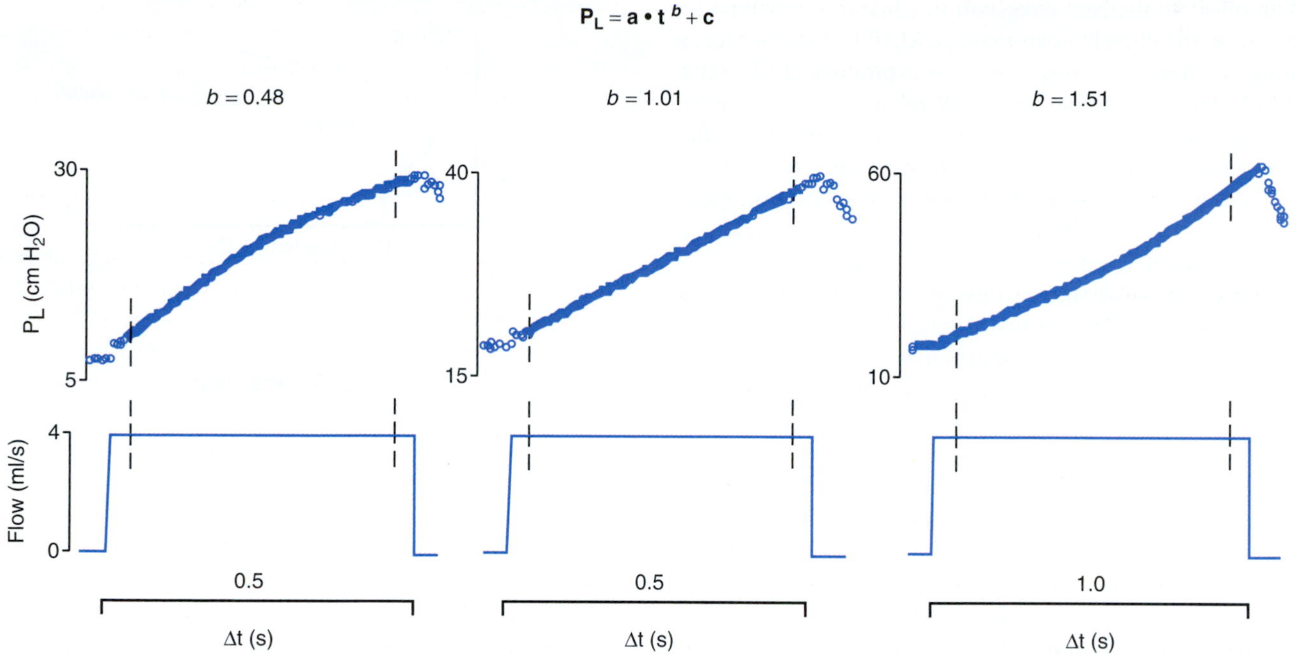

FIGURE 51-3 Conceptional illustration of the dynamic pressure-time (p-t) curve. *Left,* Convex curve indicating recruitment during the breath. *Center,* Linear relationship between pressure and time indicating no recruitment or overdistention. *Right,* Concave curve indicating overdistention. (From Formenti P, Graf J, Santos A, et al: Non-pulmonary factors strongly influence the stress index. Intensive Care Med 37:594–600, 2011.)

emptying of lung units, and auto-PEEP can develop even at relatively low minute ventilation. Auto-PEEP is common in mechanically ventilated patients receiving high minute ventilation and occurs in patients with ARDS.[28] An increase in mean alveolar pressure owing to auto-PEEP may exacerbate the hemodynamic effects of positive pressure ventilation and increase the likelihood of barotrauma in a manner similar to the application of PEEP. In addition, the presence of auto-PEEP makes it more difficult for the patient to trigger a ventilator-assisted breath.

Finally, if unrecognized, auto-PEEP leads to erroneous calculation of static lung compliance by underestimation of total PEEP. Decreasing minute volume can reduce or eliminate auto-PEEP; however, minimal auto-PEEP can be benign. In addition, increasing expiratory time allows more time for airways to empty normally, decreasing auto-PEEP. The use of extrinsic PEEP, when set appropriately, can partially overcome the trigger sensitivity problem seen with auto-PEEP and may provide a "stent" to allow more complete lung emptying and a decrease in patient effort.[29]

Methods for Determining Auto–Positive End Expiratory Pressure. Dynamically, auto-PEEP varies throughout the lungs; however, all measurements of auto-PEEP reflect an average auto-PEEP level throughout the lungs. Assessment of auto-PEEP involves first its detection and then a measurement. Auto-PEEP is suspected if flow continues at end-expiration as seen on ventilator graphics monitoring. In this case, auto-PEEP must be present unless there is active contraction of the expiratory muscles producing end expiratory flow. The following methods are used to estimate auto-PEEP level.

End Expiratory Hold by the Ventilator. Either automated or manual, end expiratory hold by the ventilator closes the expiratory valve at end-exhalation. The hold period must extend until the end expiratory pressure is stabilized or the value is an underestimate of auto-PEEP.

An **esophageal balloon** is used to measure the deflection in the pleural space required to trigger the ventilator. The change in esophageal pressure from baseline to the pressure initiating flow at the airway is equal to the total PEEP that must be overcome to trigger a breath.

Matching Auto–Positive End Expiratory Pressure With Positive End Expiratory Pressure. PEEP can be applied to a level (this is possible in some patients) that results in flow at end-exhalation being closer to zero. The concept involves stenting of the airways by PEEP to allow lung emptying and a better equilibration of end expiratory alveolar pressure with end expiratory ventilatory circuit pressure minimizing the pressure needed to decompress the alveoli and trigger the ventilator.[29] This maneuver is essentially performed by slowly increasing applied PEEP until every patient effort triggers a ventilator breath.

Mean Airway Pressure

MAP represents the average airway pressure over the total ventilatory cycle. Correct measurement of this value requires continuous sampling of airway pressure at the airway opening—this is an automated feature of modern ventilators. MAP is related to mean lung volume, which correlates with oxygenation if perfusion is adequate. When MAP is increased, arterial O_2 levels often improve, but venous return and subsequently arterial pressure can be adversely affected.

In an effort to increase oxygenation while monitoring arterial pressure, the clinician can manage MAP by several means, including V_T, frequency, inspiratory-to-expiratory (I : E) ratio, and PEEP. The management of MAP relates to a concern for improving oxygenation balanced against its detrimental influence on venous return to the chest. Normally, expiratory resistance is greater than (twice) inspiratory resistance, and mean alveolar pressure normally is greater than MAP. For patients with COPD and elevated expiratory resistance, high mean alveolar volume can be significant during mechanical ventilation. For patients with ARDS, airway resistance is more typically low, so MAP and mean alveolar pressures may be similar.

There is an understandable caution while increasing MAP, usually by increasing PEEP, yet two ventilator modes apply dramatic increases in MAP—high-frequency oscillation and airway pressure release ventilation. The marked improvements in oxygenation seen with these modes can be attributed to high MAP. In the case of high-frequency oscillation, the lungs are never allowed to derecruit between breaths. Airway pressure release ventilation is more complicated because the lung deflates to varying unknown alveolar volumes on exhalation. In the use of either mode, end expiratory alveolar lung volume status cannot be easily determined, but oxygenation is often improved.

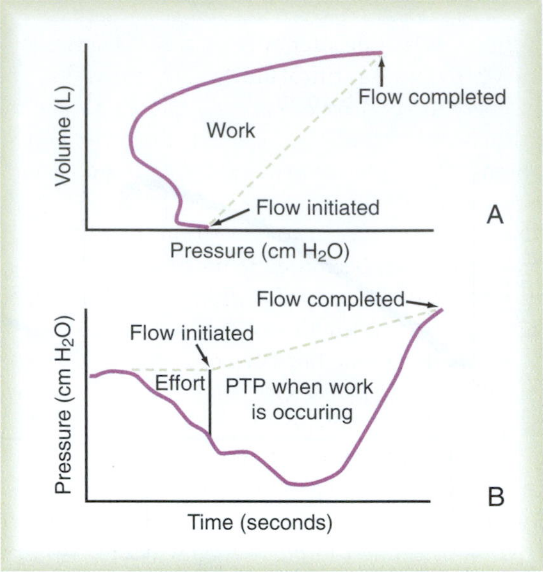

FIGURE 51-4 WOB **(A)** and PTP **(B)** from the same spontaneous breath of a patient receiving ventilatory support. *Dashed lines* represent a tracing of passive inflation by a ventilator-supported breath. Areas of work and PTP are not directly comparable because WOB units (P-V) and PTP units (pressure-time) differ. The area of effort in the total PTP area occurs before (and in addition to) the work measurement.

Monitoring Breathing Effort and Patterns

Work of Breathing

Work of breathing (WOB) is often increased in critically ill patients. Commercially available systems are available for measuring WOB in ventilated patients. For computation of WOB, changes in Ptp must be measured. The procedure requires an assessment of pleural pressure, which is normally estimated by esophageal pressure after placement of an esophageal balloon catheter. The measurement is estimated from the esophageal pressure-versus-volume curve (Figure 51-4).

For healthy persons, average total WOB ranges from 0.030 to 0.050 kg/m/L (0.3 to 0.6 J/L).[30] Patients with severe obstructive or restrictive lung disease "work" at levels two to three times this normal value at rest, with marked increases in work at higher minute ventilation. How much work a patient can tolerate before the ventilatory muscles fatigue is unclear. Maintaining adequate spontaneous ventilation is impossible in many patients when the workload exceeds 0.15 kg/m/L (1.5 J/L).

Monitoring WOB may be valuable in certain situations, such as weaning. Clinicians are expected to assess a patient's WOB continually and to take appropriate action if WOB becomes excessive. Because a direct measurement of WOB requires esophageal manometry, simpler indicators are sought. Monitoring the patient's spontaneous breathing rate, V_T, and **frequency/tidal volume (f/VT) ratio** provides useful surrogates for WOB during ventilator weaning trials. Assessment of the patient's overall clinical presentation also is useful in assessing the WOB. Increased WOB is associated with a rapid shallow breathing pattern, rapid pulse rate, hypertension, and use of accessory muscles of ventilation.

Pressure-Time Product. The **pressure-time product (PTP)** is the area encompassed by the esophageal pressure-time tracing during inspiration as shown in Figure 51-4. PTP is simpler to measure than WOB because it does not require simultaneous measurement of volume. PTP values parallel changes in effort and the O_2 cost of breathing because PTP includes a measure of the "isometric" component of muscle contraction.[31] This index includes work and effort components that may indicate endurance during a weaning trial.

Oxygen Cost of Breathing

The amount of O_2 consumed by the ventilatory muscles ($\dot{V}Q_2R$) is an estimate of respiratory effort at its most basic level. $\dot{V}Q_2R$ can be estimated by measurement of O_2 consumption during active breathing compared with the patient being fully supported in the control mode:

$$\dot{V}O_2R = \dot{V}O_2 \text{ active breathing} - \dot{V}O_2 \text{ apnea}$$

Normal $\dot{V}Q_2R$ is approximately 2% to 5% of total O_2 consumption; however, $\dot{V}Q_2R$ can be 30% of total O_2 consumption during hyperventilation owing to severe dyspnea. Theoretically, $\dot{V}Q_2R$ accounts for all factors that tax the respiratory muscles—that is, the external workload and the efficiency of the conversion between cellular energy and useful work. $\dot{V}Q_2R$ is difficult to measure if the patient's condition is unstable. Other measures of respiratory muscle function are sought to assess the cost of breathing.

Assessing Ventilatory Drive

Until more recently, little attention was paid to measurement of respiratory drive during critical illness. During machine-assisted breathing, ventilatory drive can play an important role in determining the energy expenditure of the patient. One study showed that patients not being weaned from mechanical ventilation often have an elevated drive to breathe and a limited ability to respond to increases in ventilatory load (e.g., increased $PaCO_2$).[32]

A measure that has been used to index drive is $P_{0.1}$. $P_{0.1}$ is the pressure recorded 100 msec after initiation of an inspiratory effort against an occluded airway. $P_{0.1}$ is influenced by muscle strength and lung volume but does not depend on respiratory mechanics. Elevated $P_{0.1}$ (>6 cm H_2O) indicates a continuing need for mechanical ventilation.

In a sophisticated, commercially available system, a direct measure of the neural drive to breathe from the phrenic nerve can be measured by a catheter positioned within the esophagus. This signal is integrated into a feedback circuit in a modern ventilator. As a mode within the ventilator, flow delivery is coordinated and augmented in response to the neural drive to breathe; this is known as *neurally adjusted ventilatory assist.* (See Chapters 45 and 46 for details.)

Rapid Shallow Breathing Index

When muscular strength is limited, patients tend to meet minute ventilation ($\dot{V}_E$) requirements by increasing frequency (f) while decreasing V_T. Although smaller breaths require less effort, rapid shallow breathing increases dead space ventilation causing a need for higher minute ventilation to eliminate CO_2. A very high and continuously increasing frequency (>30 breaths/min) is a sign of ventilatory muscle decompensation and, potentially, impending fatigue.

Considerable attention has been focused on the rapid shallow breathing index (f/V_T ratio), a simple bedside index that indicates whether mechanically ventilated patients can breathe without mechanical assistance.[29] The f/V_T ratio is easy to measure and is independent of the patient's effort and cooperation. Discontinuation of ventilator support is likely to prove successful if the f/V_T ratio is less than 105 breaths/min per L within the first minute of a brief trial of fully spontaneous breathing.[33]

Respiratory Inductive Plethysmography

Respiratory inductive plethysmography is a noninvasive means of monitoring frequency, V_T, fractional duration of inspiration (T_i/T_{tot}), and respiratory muscle coordination. With this technique, loose elastic bands encircle the chest and abdomen. Band expansion and contraction during ventilation (spontaneous or supported) provides a volume-time plot that can also reflect short-term shifts in actual lung volume.

Monitoring Strength and Muscle Endurance

Two values commonly used for bedside assessment of respiratory muscle strength are **vital capacity (VC)** and **maximal inspiratory pressure (MIP)**. A VC maneuver can be performed at the bedside with a simple respirometer connected to the patient's airway. Because VC is effort-dependent, accurate measurements can be obtained only when the patient is conscious and cooperative. Because of an expected variability in bedside VC, three measurements should be obtained, and the best result should be reported. Healthy persons are able to generate a VC of approximately 70 ml/kg. A VC less than 10 to 15 ml/kg indicates considerable muscle weakness, which indicates an inability to breathe spontaneously.

MIP is a more specific measure than VC. MIP provides information based solely on maximum output of the inspiratory muscles. A maximum stimulus is provided by total occlusion of the airway. In contrast to the VC maneuver, the MIP maneuver can be performed on unconscious or uncooperative patients. Measurement of MIP at the bedside requires an aneroid manometer with a maximum value indicator. In an effort to make the measurements more reliable, Marini and colleagues[34] described a modified technique in which a one-way valve is attached to the airway to ensure that inspiratory effort is made at a low lung volume. Maintaining an occlusion for 20 seconds, the values with the one-way valve in place were approximately one-third more negative than values without an occlusion (Figure 51-5).

Endurance: Maximum Voluntary Ventilation

Respiratory muscle fatigue (lack of endurance) may be a cause of respiratory failure. **Maximum voluntary ventilation (MVV)** is a measure used to assess respiratory muscle reserve, endurance, or fatigue. VC is measured to assess the patient's coordinated muscle function from a single breath; MVV is measured to determine the ability of a patient to sustain ventilation over time. Similar to the VC maneuver, the MVV procedure can be performed with a respirometer attached to the patient's airway as the patient is encouraged to breathe as deeply and as fast as possible over a predefined time interval (10 or 15 seconds). The value is extrapolated to a full minute.

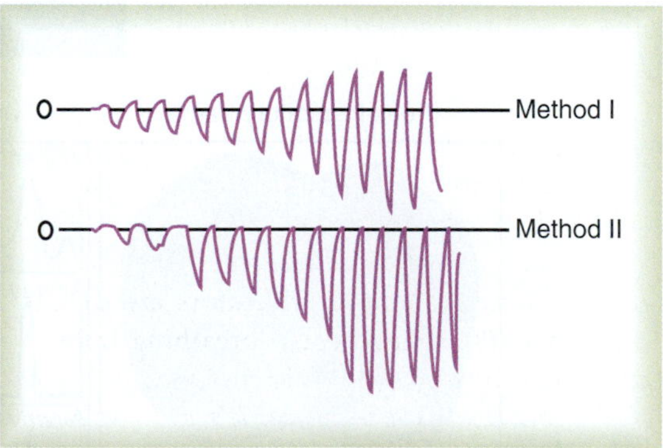

FIGURE 51-5 Measurement of MIP during 25 seconds of airway occlusion. *Method I* is occlusion by sealing the airway to allow no movement of air. *Method II* occludes inspiratory flow but allows expiratory flow through a unidirectional valve.

> **RULE OF THUMB**
>
> To wean from mechanical ventilation, the patient must have adequate gas exchange, respiratory muscle strength and endurance, and WOB that is not excessive. The original cause of respiratory failure must be partially, if not completely, resolved. Although numerous values have been studied to indicate the probability of successful weaning, a frequency-to-V_T ratio less than 105 has been the best index of ability to wean.

Normal MVV values for adults range from 120 to 180 L/min. Values less than twice the spontaneous minute ventilation are associated with difficulty in maintaining spontaneous ventilation without mechanical assistance.[35]

Lung Mapping

The extent of gas-exchange abnormalities is revealed by ABG values and SpO_2, but the location or source of the disorder remains unknown. The source, but not the extent or type of the pathologic process, can be assessed by auscultation. Localization of the disorder within the lungs is more precisely evaluated by static images obtained by radiographic techniques, such as chest x-ray or computed tomography (CT). These assessments are key to directing therapeutic approaches and for tracking changes in pathology (see Chapter 21). However, thorough imaging studies frequently require transportation of the patient to a radiology suite, and transport presents risks to the patient.[36] Also, the imaging is often static, not dynamically obtained throughout the ventilator cycle.

Mapping techniques that can actively locate regions of interest have been developed more recently. Two techniques are available that allow mapping of the lungs during ventilation: **electrical impedance tomography (EIT)** and **acoustic respiratory monitoring (ARM)**. Each technique produces a two-dimensional video or graphic representation of ventilation distribution throughout the lung and allows a regional assessment of the extent of injury. With EIT and ARM, there is an opportunity to perform at the bedside a real-time evaluation of the effects of PEEP, recruitment maneuvers, or other changes in ventilatory support (Figure 51-6).

Electrical Impedance Tomography (EIT)

EIT requires placement of electrodes around the chest (minimum of 16 electrodes). Recent designs utilize an expandable rubber belt (of various sizes) that has built-in electrodes. The belt is connected to a cable which is then connected to the EIT device. Impedance is measured between the electrodes rapidly and in a circular motion, capturing images that are reconstructed into a real-time graphic on the screen. Ventilation is displayed on the screen and various regions can be isolated

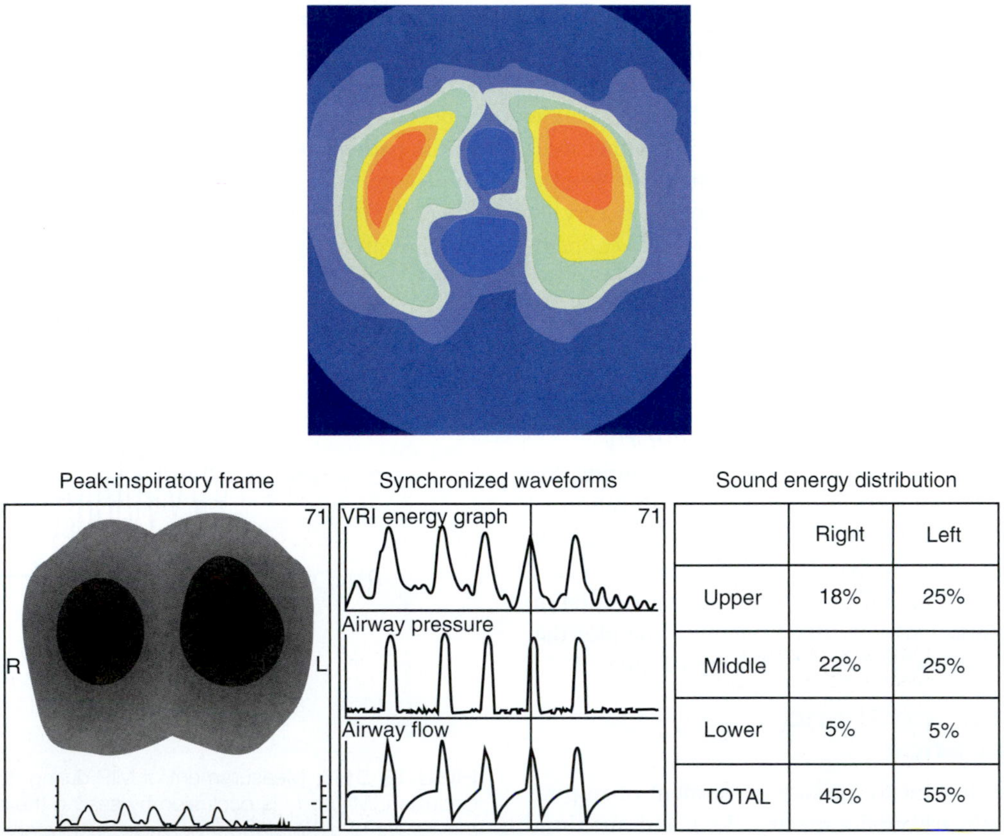

FIGURE 51-6 Mapping of ventilation by EIT. *Bottom,* Mapping of ventilation by acoustic respiratory monitoring.

for close monitoring of changes during normal ventilation cycles or during adjustment of ventilator parameters. The ability to regionally monitor areas within the lung is of most use with patients presenting with heterogeneous lung disease. Visualizing the effects of ventilator setting adjustment on the various regions of the lung can help balance ventilation and minimize overdistension.[37] Modern EIT devices have the ability to trend lung distribution over time, as well as trend changes in end expiratory lung impedance (EELI). Changes in EELI would represent changes in end expiratory lung volume (EELV), an important trend when titrating PEEP.

Acoustic Respiratory Monitoring (ARM)

ARM involves placement of a series of stethoscopes around the chest. The sounds during ventilation are localized, and, similarly, a map of sounds (ventilation) is reconstructed. Specific characteristics of crackles from interstitial pulmonary fibrosis compared with congestive heart failure have been differentiated by ARM.[38]

Lung Ultrasonography

Ultrasound technology is not as helpful for imaging the lungs because air-filled lung tissue is not penetrated by ultrasound. However, pathologic processes outside the lungs can be seen by ultrasound, such as pleural fluids, air, or lesions. Pneumothorax, empyema, and pleural effusions are most frequently located by **lung ultrasonography**; their extent can be defined and treated with the use of ultrasound. As a diagnostic tool, lung ultrasonography is relatively inexpensive, can be performed in 15 minutes, and does not emit ionizing radiation. There is potential for ultrasonography to evaluate the lung expansion effects on atelectatic lung tissue using recruitment maneuvers.

Monitoring Patient-Ventilator System

Monitoring of a patient during mechanical ventilatory support should include a physical examination (inspection, palpation, percussion, auscultation), assessment of oxygenation and ventilation, and assessment of ventilatory load and capacity. Table 51-1 lists key physiologic monitoring data and acceptable values

TABLE 51-1
Physiologic Monitoring Data (Respiratory Values)

Function Assessed	Description of Value	Symbol/Formula	Acceptable Value
Oxygenation			
Lung Exchange (External)			
Adequacy	Arterial oxygen pressure	PaO_2	60-100 mm Hg
	Arterial oxygen saturation	SaO_2	≥90%
	Oxygen saturation by pulse oximeter	SpO_2	≥90%
	Transcutaneous oxygen partial pressure	$PtcO_2$	60-100 mm Hg
Efficiency	Alveolar to arterial oxygen tension gradient	$P(A-a)O_2$	<350 mm Hg (100% O_2)
	Arterial to alveolar	PaO_2/PAO_2	>0.6
	Respiratory index	$P(A-a)O_2/PaO_2$	<5
	P/F ratio	PaO_2/FiO_2	>300
	Percentage shunt	$\dot{Q}_S/\dot{Q}_T$	<15%-20%
Time exchange (internal)	Mixed venous oxygen content	$C\bar{v}O_2$	>10.0 ml/dl
	Mixed venous oxygen partial pressure	$P\bar{v}O_2$	>30 mm Hg
	Mixed venous oxygen saturation	$S\bar{v}O_2$	>65%
	Arterial-venous oxygen content difference	$C(a-\bar{v}O_2)$	<7 ml/dl
Ventilation			
Adequacy	Minute ventilation	$\dot{V}_E$	5-10 L/min
	Arterial carbon dioxide	$PaCO_2$	35-45 mm Hg (normal pH)
	Transcutaneous carbon dioxide partial pressure	$PtcCO_2$	35-45 mm Hg (normal pH)
	End-tidal carbon dioxide partial pressure	$PETCO_2$	35-43 mm Hg (4.6%-5.6%)
Efficiency	Dead space/tidal volume ratio	V_D/V_T	<0.6
	Minute ventilation vs. carbon dioxide partial pressure	$\dot{V}_E$ vs. $PaCO_2$	$\dot{V}_E$ <10 L/min with normal $PaCO_2$
Ventilatory Load			
Total impedance	Dynamic compliance	$(V_T - V_C)/(PIP - PEEP)$	35-50 ml/cm H_2O
Compliance	Effective compliance	$C_{eff} = \dfrac{(V_T - V_C)}{P_{plat} - PEEP}$	60-100 ml/cm H_2O
WOB	Work = kg × m/L or J/L	Work = P × V	<0.15 kg × m/L <1.5 J/L
Ventilatory Capacity			
Drive	Occlusion pressure	P0.1	<6 cm H_2O
	Mean inspiratory flow	V_T/T_i	Not established
Strength	Vital capacity	VC	>10-15 mL/kg
	Maximal inspiratory pressure	MIP; PI_{max}	<–20 to –30 cm H_2O
Endurance	Maximum voluntary ventilation	MVV	>20 L/min or 2 × $\dot{V}_E$
	Ratio of minute ventilation to MVV	$\dot{V}_E$/MVV	<1 : 2
	Pressure-time index	$(Pdi/Pmax)*TI/T_{tot}$	<0.15

for patients receiving mechanical ventilation. Monitoring of all aspects of the patient-ventilator system is an important responsibility that must be clearly delineated within the ICU. Monitoring a ventilated patient is the primary responsibility of the RT. Important areas of this responsibility include the following:

- Assessing the integrity of the airway and circuitry, including secretion clearance
- Maintaining the prescribed settings and assessing their appropriateness
- Ensuring acceptable gas-exchange values
- Monitoring of respiratory system mechanics
- Evaluating the comfort and synchrony of breathing of the patient
- Setting of alarms
- Caring for any other safety issues, such as risk of extubation

A system of ensuring and documenting all aspects of safe and appropriate care must be in place. This system usually includes a manual or, more frequently, an electronic recording of all important settings, alarms, and ABG values at regular intervals. This monitoring process has been called *patient-ventilator assessments*. An example of a recording form used for this purpose is shown in Figure 51-7. Increasingly, electronic

Adult Mechanical Ventilation Flow Sheet

Patient ______	Cuff pressure (volume) ______
Physician ______	□ M.O.V. □ Minimal leak
Diagnosis ______	Ventilator ______ Vent. day ______
Age ______ Height ______	Circuit change (Date / Time) ______
Weight ______ Ideal body weight ______	Tape change (Date / Time) ______
ET tube / trach tube size ______	Other therapy ______
Tube Position (length) ______	______

Patient ID

	Date						
	Time						
	Mode (A/C; SIMV, PSV, PCV, etc.)						
	Set Tidal Volume / Delivered Tidal Volume						
	Spontaneous Tidal Volume						
	Machine Rate / Total Rate						
	Minute Volume						
	Peak Pressure / Static Pressure						
	Mean Airway Pressure						
	PEEP / CPAP [IPAP / EPAP]						
	Auto PEEP						
	Support / Pressure Control Level (cmH_2O)						
	Sensitivity or Flowtrigger (Flowby)						
	FIO2 Set / Analyzed						
	Inspiratory Flow / Time						
	Wave Form (⎍ ◺ ⎍)						
	I : E Ratio						
	Sigh Volume / Sigh Frequency						
	Airway Temperature						
	Static Compliance / Dynamic Compliance						
	Airway Resistance [(PIP - PLAT / Insp. Flow L/Sec)]						
	Apnea Parameters Check (Y / N)						
ALARMS	Pressure High / Low						
	Low VT						
	High / Low VE						
	High rate						
BLOOD GASES	pH						
	PaO2						
	PaC02						
	Sa02 / Oximetry (Sp02)						
	Hb						
	HC03-						
	B.E.						
	Ca02						
	Pv02						
	Sv02						
	Ca02 - Cv02						
	Qs / Qt						
	Vd / Vt						
	P (ET) C02						
HEMO DYNAMICS	Pulse						
	Blood Pressure (Systolic / Diastolic)						
	CVP						
	PAP (Systolic / Diastolic)						
	PCWP						
	Cardiac Output / Cardiac Index						
	SVR						
	PVR						
SPONTANEOUS	MIP / MEP						
	Vital Capacity (VC)						
	Spontaneous Volumes (VT / VE)						
	Spontaneous Rate (f)						
	RSBI (f/VT)						
	Other						
	Initials						

A

FIGURE 51-7 Ventilator flow sheet.

Adult Mechanical Ventilation Flow Sheet

Respiratory Care Progress Notes

S: (pt Awareness, response, sedations / paralytics) Responds ☐ Non-responsive ☐ Sedated ☐ Paralytics ☐ See comment ☐

O: (WOB, Color, Chest Expansion, BBS, Sputum Production, latest x-ray, pertinent pt assessment concerns, lab values, fluids)

General Skin Color
- ☐ Pink
- ☐ Ashy
- ☐ Cyanotic
- ☐ Jaundice

Skin Characteristics
- ☐ Warm
- ☐ Dry
- ☐ Diaphoretic
- ☐ Cool
- ☐ Moist

Mucous Membranes
- ☐ Pink
- ☐ Ashy
- ☐ Cyanotic

Work of Breathing
- ☐ Normal
- ☐ Mild
- ☐ Moderate
- ☐ High
- ☐ Absent

Chest Excursion
- ☐ Bilateral
- ☐ Unilateral
- ☐ Diminished
- ☐ Paradoxical/Flail

Chest Configuration
- ☐ Normal
- ☐ Other________

- ☐ Subcutaneous Emphysema
- ☐ Tactile Fremitus
- ☐ Tracheal Deviation
- ☐ Abdominal Distention

Nailbeds
- ☐ Pink
- ☐ Ashy
- ☐ Cyanotic

Capillary Refill
- ☐ Rapid
- ☐ Sluggish

Auscultation
1) Clear
2) Wheeze
3) Crackles
4) Rhonchi

Anterior

Posterior
A. Good Aeration
B. Diminished
C. Absent

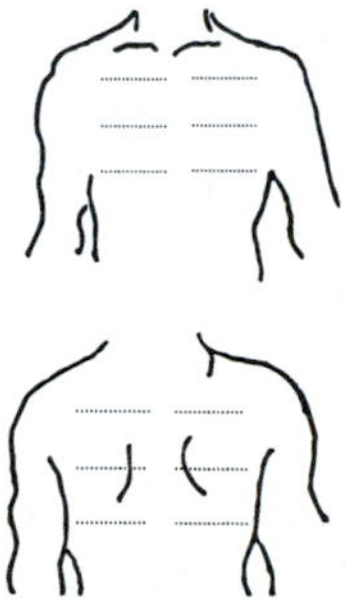

A: (Pt history, Admit dx. & date, events leading to intubation/trach/ventilation, significant problems, etc.)

P: (Care plan , standing orders, treatments)

WEANING MECHANICS		
TIME		
VC		
I/E FORCES		
VT		
RR		
VE		
f/VT		

Pt. EVENTS/CHANGES	Time	(Reasons for changes, significant pt. events, CT Scan, chest tube placement, BP problems, codes, etc.)

Signature ________ Initials ________

B

FIGURE 51-7, cont'd

transfer of ventilator settings and monitored data is being added to the electronic medical record. The responsibility of the RT is much greater than the task of recording values. This responsibility is care of a critically ill, vulnerable patient with respiratory failure who is being supported with a lifesaving machine. The procedure for performing a patient-ventilator system assessment is outlined in Table 51-2. Although the importance of monitoring the patient-ventilator system has increased, the necessity of entry and transcription of numbers into an assessment sheet is decreasing. The era of electronic transfer of monitored data directly to the patients' charts will soon become the standard. All modern ventilators have the capacity for data transfer, but until standardized transfer protocols, charting formats, and archiving methods are established, electronic monitoring of the patient-ventilator system will continue to be customized to the local setting.

Graphics Monitoring

Monitoring of graphic tracings generated during mechanical ventilation has become widely available and accepted in the ICU. A visual display of pressure, flow, and volume tracings is available on all modern ventilators. Graphic displays are possible through the development of improvements in sensing technology, integrated circuitry, and graphic-user interface. Ventilators measure inspiratory and expiratory flow and circuit pressure with pneumotachometers and transducers. The volume displays are generated through calculation of an integral of the flow tracings. All three values (flow, pressure, and volume)

TABLE 51-2
Performing a Patient-Ventilator System Assessment

Step	Key Points
Gather correct equipment and supplies	Respirometer, O_2 analyzer, stethoscope, and watch with second indicator are needed. *Note:* Most modern ventilators incorporate volume-measuring devices into the system Additional auxiliary equipment may include pulse oximeter, cuff pressure manometer, suction and airway equipment, and sterile distilled water
Review patient record	Note patient's admitting diagnosis or problem list, physician orders, medications, vital signs, history and physical examination findings, progress notes, results of laboratory studies, chest radiograph, blood gases, and respiratory care notes
Enter patient area; wash hands and put on gloves	Inattention to proper handwashing and poor aseptic technique are associated with nosocomial infection
Identify the patient	Wristbands sometimes may be attached to the patient's leg or to the foot of the bed If there is no attached name band, check with the patient's nurse
Explain what you are doing	Communication with the patient is important; even patients who appear unaware of their surroundings may be able to hear and understand Use broad terms, such as "I'm here to assess your breathing"
Observe overall situation and note general patient condition, including level of consciousness, condition of extremities, presence of pallor, skin color, capillary refill, airway patency, circuit connection and patency, and ECG findings	Note general appearance, sensorium, color, and level of activity Note equipment in use, including ventilator, circuit, airway type, humidification, manual resuscitation bag, and related equipment and supplies Ensure that the patient's condition appears stable and that ventilation is adequate
Drain tubing and service humidifier, if needed	This procedure should be done before the actual ventilator check, if possible
Attend to patient's airway, if necessary	Suctioning and other airway manipulation should be done before actual ventilator check, if possible; after suctioning, note volume and character of secretions Note endotracheal or tracheostomy tube stability and position; measure tube cuff pressure and volume to inflate If ventilator check is performed first and the patient circuit or airway is disrupted, errors may not be caught, and one of the purposes of ventilator monitoring, patient safety, is defeated
Inspect chest and note accessory muscle use, retractions, jugular vein engorgement, bilateral symmetric chest wall movement, symmetric diaphragm–chest wall movement, respiratory rate and rhythm, and chest wall stability (flail)	Be alert for signs of respiratory distress, increased WOB or patient-ventilatory asynchrony Observe patient effort to ensure adequate trigger sensitivity and inspiratory flow rate
Auscultate chest	Always move stethoscope from side to side to compare right and left sides of chest Note adventitious breath sounds (crackles, rhonchi, wheezing, bronchovesicular breath sounds) Note diminished or absent breath sounds; if breath sounds are absent, attempt to ascertain cause immediately Water in the tubing, use of chest tubes, or PEEP may result in adventitious sounds
Percuss chest for dullness, resonance, or hyperresonance	Dullness may be caused by pleural effusion, atelectasis, or consolidation Resonance is the percussion note found over normal lung tissue Hyperresonance is associated with excess air in the chest (pneumothorax, pulmonary hyperinflation)
Note location of trachea	Tracheal shift is associated with severe atelectasis and tension pneumothorax
Note peak pressure, static or plateau pressure (P_{plat}), baseline pressure (PEEP/CPAP), pressure support level, MAP, and presence of auto-PEEP	Sudden increase in peak airway pressure is associated with pneumothorax, secretions in the airway, bronchospasm, fighting the ventilator, biting the endotracheal tube, occlusion of the airway, and bronchial intubation Sudden decrease in peak airway pressure is associated with reversal of any of the above-mentioned conditions, a leak in the system, or patient disconnection MAP may be useful in predicting a decrease in CO or barotraumas; the lowest possible MAP needed to achieve adequate ventilation and oxygenation should be used P_{plat} >28 cm H_2O is associated with the development of ventilator-induced lung injury; if P_{plat} is ≥28 cm H_2O, consider reducing delivered V_T
Record exhaled volume (ml/kg predicted body weight) and respiratory frequency	Ensure ventilator compensates for compressible volume If volume is measured at the exhalation valve, volume loss caused by tubing compliance may be calculated and subtracted from the measured volume

TABLE 51-2
Performing a Patient-Ventilator System Assessment—cont'd

Step	Key Points
If intermittent mandatory ventilation (IMV)/SIMV system is in use, calculate delivered volume per machine breath, spontaneous volume between machine breaths, machine rate, total rate, patient spontaneous rate, and minute ventilation	For IMV/SIMV: $V_{ISP} = \frac{\dot{V}_{Etot} - \dot{V}_{Emech}}{f_{tot} - f_{mach}}$ For assist/control: $\text{Average } V_T = \frac{\dot{V}_{Etot}}{f_{tot}}$
If a ventilator graphics package is in use, observe pressure-time, flow-time, volume-time, and P-V curves	Mode of ventilation, patient trigger, adequacy of machine inspiratory flow, and patient-ventilator synchrony can be evaluated with a ventilator graphics package Slow flow P-V curve can be used to assess lower and upper inflection points Overdistention can be elevated with use of dynamic P-V curve Flow-volume curve may be helpful in assessing effect of bronchodilator
Note delivered FiO_2	FiO_2 should be analyzed
Record other ventilatory values	Ventilatory values include inspiratory flow, inspiratory time, I : E ratio, inspiratory and expiratory positive airway pressures (IPAP and EPAP), sigh volume and rate, airway temperature, compliance and resistance, and alarm settings Many departments chart endotracheal tube size, tube length, cuff pressure or volume, use of minimal occluding volume or minimal leak, ventilator day, circuit change, and other therapy
Record blood gas values and related data, as appropriate	These data may include pH, PaO_2, $PaCO_2$, SaO_2, hemoglobin level, HCO_3^- level, IPAP, base excess, and CaO_2 Blood gas data should be recorded in such a way that the corresponding FiO_2, PEEP, V_T, frequency, mode, and other ventilator settings on which the sample was obtained are noted
Record results of other physiologic monitoring of cardiopulmonary system, as appropriate	These values may include SpO_2, $PETCO_2$, $PtcCO_2$, $PtcO_2$, $\dot{Q}_S/\dot{Q}_T$, and V_D/V_T
Record hemodynamic data, as appropriate	These values may include heart rate, blood pressure, CVP, PAP, PCWP, $\dot{Q}_T$, cardiac index, $S\bar{v}O_2$, $P\bar{v}O_2$, $CaO_2 - C\bar{v}O_2$, pulmonary vascular resistance, and systemic vascular resistance
Record weaning values as appropriate	These values may include spontaneous frequency, V_T, f/V_T ratio, $\dot{V}_E$ VC, and inspiratory force (MIP)
Return all alarm systems to optimal condition. Complete charting using appropriate departmental forms or computer entry systems	Alarms include low pressure, high pressure, disconnection, and volume Apnea values should be reviewed. Apnea values usually are set to deliver an adequate V_T, f_{mach}, and FiO_2 (100%) in the event of apnea development

can be displayed and plotted against time or each other (Figure 51-8).

RULE OF THUMB

Modern mechanical ventilators routinely display tracings of flow, pressure, and volume versus time. Ventilator graphics monitoring is a convenient visual method for monitoring patient-ventilator interaction. The graphic patterns allow rapid determination of mode of ventilation, breathing pattern, auto-PEEP, excessive pressure, secretions in the airway, synchrony, and triggering efforts.

Ventilator manufacturers have developed the graphic displays that allow astute clinicians to base decisions on many more factors than gas-exchange values (Box 51-10). However, the study and verification of features observed in ventilator graphics have not developed at the pace of the technology. Ventilator graphics show many important patient-ventilator interactions, such as presence of auto-PEEP, elevated airway pressure, presence of secretions, and general pattern and dependability of supported ventilation (Figure 51-9). The potential for expanded use of ventilator graphics awaits further investigation of the clinical importance of the graphic displays. For more details, see Chapter 47.

Box 51-10 Purposes of Graphics Monitoring

- Confirm mode functions
- Detect inadequate flow in volume ventilation
- Detect too lengthy an inspiratory time
- Set appropriate rise time and termination criteria in pressure ventilation
- Detect auto-PEEP
- Determine patient-ventilator synchrony
- Assess and adjust trigger levels
- Measure WOB
- Adjust V_T and minimize overdistention
- Assess effect of administration of bronchodilators
- Detect equipment malfunction
- Determine appropriate PEEP level

Monitoring During Lung Protective Ventilation

A lung protective ventilation strategy that reduces the risk of pressure injury to the lungs has evolved from numerous animal studies and several key clinical studies.[39] Meticulous monitoring of the status of patients with ARDS or patients at risk of ARDS is necessary to avoid ventilator-induced lung injury. Three principles have been confirmed: (1) reduce the risk of high-pressure exposure by limiting P_{plat} to less than 28 cm H_2O, (2) reduce V_T ventilation to 4 to 8 ml/kg, and (3) maintain adequate end expiratory lung volume with PEEP to avoid opening/closing injury. The AARC created a clinical practice guideline on patient-ventilator system assessment; excerpts from this guideline appear in Clinical Practice Guideline 51-1.

Other considerations have received attention in monitoring patients with ARDS. Although P-V curves have been automated in ventilator algorithms, the clinical significance of curves determined from PEEP of 0 cm H_2O is questionable. However, current recommendations are to maintain ventilation on the

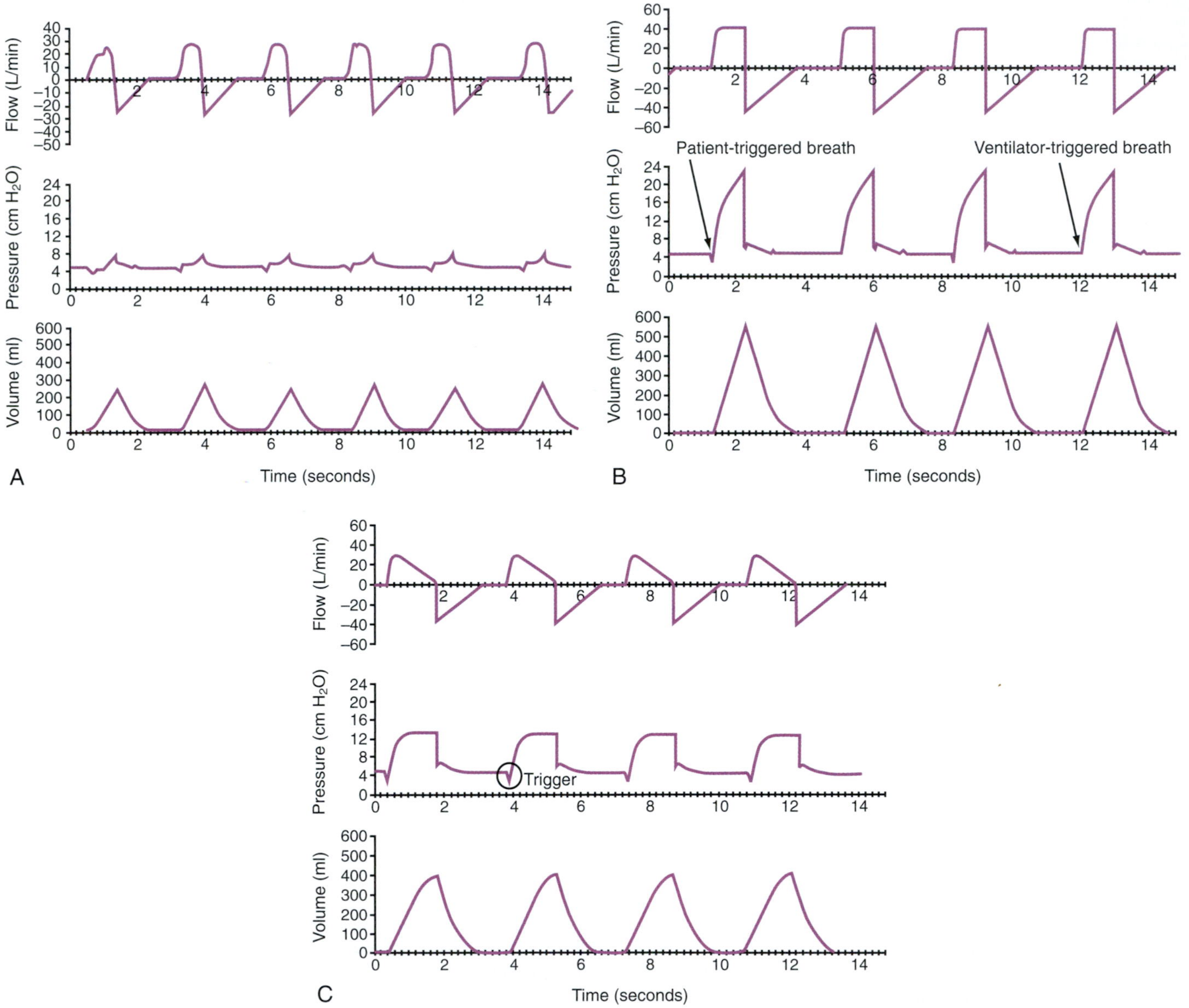

FIGURE 51-8 Ventilator graphics: flow, pressure, and volume tracings. **A,** Spontaneous breathing at an elevated baseline pressure (continuous positive airway pressure [CPAP]). Flow, pressure, and volume curves show spontaneous breathing with a CPAP level of approximately 5 cm H_2O. The flow curve is sinusoidal, the pressure curve fluctuates approximately 1 to 3 cm H_2O around the baseline pressure, and the volume delivered varies. These are typical observations during spontaneous breathing. **B,** Volume ventilation in the assist/control mode. Some breaths are time triggered, and others are patient triggered. There is a square wave flow pattern, and volume is constant, breath to breath. **C,** Pressure support breaths (pressure support ventilation). The patient trigger for each breath is evident. Flow is decelerating, and the pressure waveform approaches a square wave.

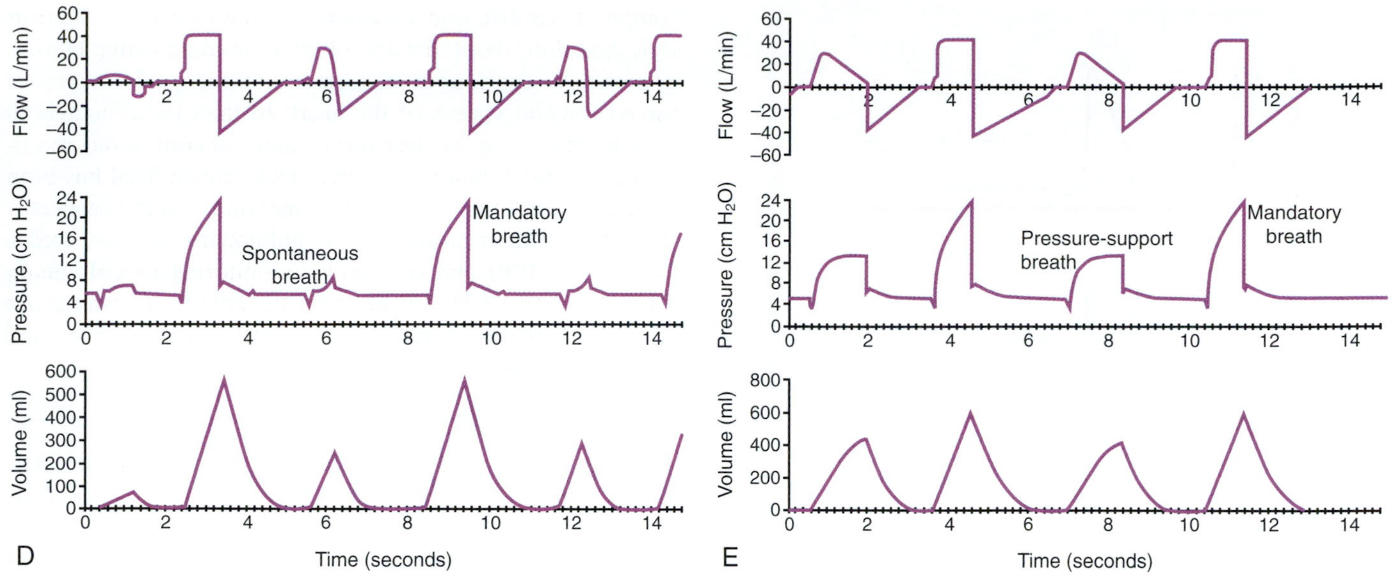

FIGURE 51-8, cont'd **D,** SIMV with an elevated baseline (PEEP). Spontaneous breathing and machine mandatory breaths are interspersed. Spontaneous volume varies, but the SIMV breaths are constant at 600 ml. The square wave flow pattern for mandatory breaths and the sinusoidal flow during spontaneous breathing are evident. The baseline pressure (PEEP) is elevated at approximately 5 cm H_2O. **E,** SIMV with pressure support. Mandatory breaths have a square flow waveform with a constant volume of 600 ml. The pressure support breaths have a decelerating flow waveform and a pressure pattern approaching a square wave. In this example, there is also an elevated baseline of approximately +5 cm H_2O (PEEP).

MINI CLINI

Ventilator Graphics

PROBLEM: The ventilator graphic display of a patient with COPD receiving mechanical ventilation is showing two distinct features: (1) a pressure-time tracing with spikes and dips that is generally irregular and (2) a flow-time tracing that does not reach zero flow at end expiration.

Solution: Graphic displays of pressure and flow allow rapid identification of the presence of secretions, auto-PEEP, and asynchrony. The irregular tracing implies the presence of airway secretions. Auscultation of the lungs should be performed to assess the need for endotracheal suctioning. Without an active expiratory effort, the existence of flow at end expiration confirms the presence of auto-PEEP. Auto-PEEP can be detected in many COPD patients receiving mechanical ventilation. However, intervention to reduce or eliminate auto-PEEP may be unnecessary. Auto-PEEP should be estimated regularly. More important, the effects of auto-PEEP on the ability to trigger the ventilator or on cardiovascular dynamics (caused by reduced venous return) should be monitored. For reduction or elimination of auto-PEEP, adjusting the ventilator settings or bronchodilator therapy may be required. If the patient is unable to trigger every breath because of the auto-PEEP, apply PEEP in steps of 1 to 2 cm H_2O until the patient is able to trigger the ventilator with every inspiratory effort.

upper portion of the deflation limb of the P-V curve to avoid alveolar derecruitment even though this position with the P-V hysteresis curve of a patient may be difficult to determine. A primary concern is to achieve adequate oxygenation in patients with lung injury, but this target can be deceptive if the price of adequate oxygenation is pressure injury to the lungs. An acceptable practice in ventilating these patients is permissive hypercapnia or pressure-protective ventilation that allows $PaCO_2$ to drift upward. This strategy is a higher frequency–lower V_T approach with the predictable effect of decreasing pH (by increasing $PaCO_2$) that requires careful monitoring.

As previously discussed, poor chest wall or abdominal compliance must also be considered during lung protective ventilation. This concern can be significant in obese patients. Essentially, the stiffer the chest wall or abdomen, the greater is the P_{plat} that can be established without inducing lung injury. Meta-analysis of higher versus lower PEEP suggests the use of higher levels of PEEP with patients suffering from moderate to severe ARDS, and high levels of PEEP should be used cautiously when treating mild ARDS.[40] Setting PEEP levels greater than 15 cm H_2O is often necessary in patients with moderate to severe ARDS to maintain oxygenation.[19] Elevated PEEP places greater importance on monitoring cardiovascular performance and development of barotrauma.

CARDIAC AND CARDIOVASCULAR MONITORING

The cardiovascular system is routinely monitored in the critical care setting because patient survival depends on reliable,

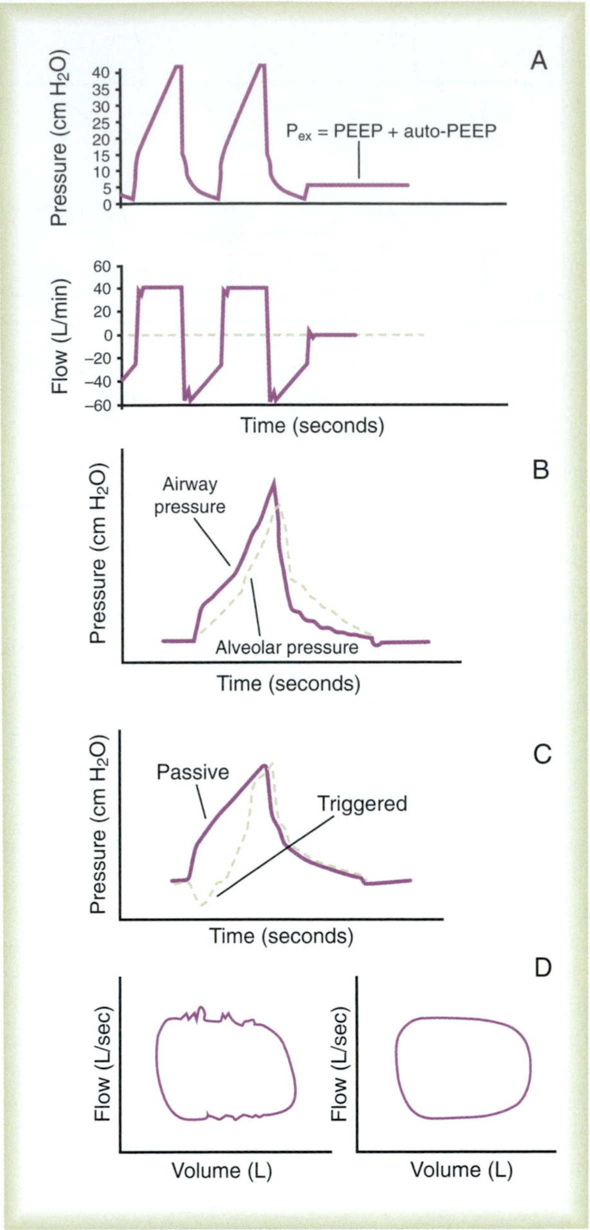

FIGURE 51-9 Patient-ventilator interactions easily identified from tracings of continuous monitoring of pressure, volume, and flow. **A,** Auto-PEEP. Flow and pressure tracings during ventilator-supported breaths and during end expiratory occlusion. The airway pressure during the end expiratory occlusion is an auto-PEEP estimate. **B,** Overdistention. The upper concavity of the airway pressure-time tracing is indicative of overdistention. This example also shows alveolar pressure and its corresponding overdistention. **C,** Patient effort. This is an example of mechanically ventilated passive inflation pressure and the airway pressure-time tracing deformation caused by effort by the patient. **D,** Presence of secretions. P-V tracing of a ventilator-supported breath displays the presence of secretions. The inspiratory and expiratory limbs are irregular (not smooth) when secretions are present. An irregular airflow-time tracing also can indicate the presence of secretions.

competent cardiac and cardiovascular performance. There is little question about the importance of monitoring ECG, a noninvasive, continuous assessment of the performance of the conduction system of the heart. In the care of acutely ill patients, there may be clear justification for continuous monitoring of arterial blood pressure. More controversial has been the assessment of left ventricular function by right heart catheterization with measurement of pulmonary capillary wedge pressure (PCWP) and continuous monitoring of pulmonary artery pressure (PAP) (Figure 51-10). Table 51-3 summarizes cardiovascular monitoring criteria with normal ranges and abnormal values.

Electrocardiography

The conduction system of the heart is monitored in the ICU with a purpose different from that of the standard 12-lead ECG examination (see Chapter 18). The standard 12-lead ECG can be used to analyze disturbances in the conductive pathway that allow location and extent of injury or the source of arrhythmia. The ECG in the ICU is used primarily to detect and manage arrhythmias such as tachycardia, bradycardia, atrioventricular dissociation, ventricular tachycardia, atrial flutter, premature ventricular contractions, and ventricular fibrillation. For this purpose, there is a need for only three electrodes: right arm (or shoulder or right upper chest), left arm (or shoulder or left upper chest), and left lower chest. The deflections usually represent lead II of a standard 12-lead ECG. The direction or amplitude of the waves is of lesser concern than the rhythms being displayed.

When any arrhythmia is detected, therapy or intervention should be considered. The source of the arrhythmia often necessitates management of the underlying cause, such as O_2 therapy for hypoxia or changes or addition to infusion therapy for fluid and electrolyte disturbances. In the ICU, certain interventions may be necessary and must be immediately available. A defibrillator must be available when ventricular fibrillation is detected.

Arterial Blood Pressure Monitoring

Arterial blood pressure is a crucial measurement for assessing the integrity of cardiovascular tone and the probability that O_2 delivery is dependable. Regulation of cardiovascular tone is under the influence of the autonomic nervous system, but there are other factors that affect blood pressure, such as fluid status or the effects of medications. Major concerns include the adequacy of O_2 delivery during hypotension and the risks of hypertension, such as increased hydrostatic pressure or stroke. Continuous monitoring of the actual blood pressure is performed by placement of a catheter usually in the femoral or radial artery. Because fluid is not compressible, the catheter and connecting tubing are filled with saline solution so that the arterial pressure is transmitted to a transducer that allows display of the arterial pressure tracing (Figure 51-11). The transducer must be properly zeroed and calibrated to reflect the true values of the deflections. The arterial line also provides access for obtaining arterial blood for ABG analysis.

51-1 Patient-Ventilator System Assessment

AARC Clinical Practice Guideline (Excerpts)*

INDICATIONS

A patient-ventilator system assessment must be performed on a scheduled basis, which is institution-specific, for any patient requiring mechanical ventilation for life support. An assessment also should be performed in the following circumstances:

- Before obtaining blood samples for analysis of blood gases and pH
- Before obtaining hemodynamic or bedside pulmonary function data
- After any change in ventilator settings
- As soon as possible after an acute deterioration of the patient's condition
- Any time ventilator performance is questionable

CONTRAINDICATIONS

There are no absolute contraindications to performance of a patient-ventilator system assessment.

ASSESSMENT OF NEED

Because of the complexity of mechanical ventilators and the numerous factors that can adversely affect patient-ventilator interaction, routine assessments of patient-ventilator system performance are mandatory.

ASSESSMENT OF OUTCOME

Routine patient-ventilator system assessments should prevent untoward incidents; warn of impending events; and ensure that proper ventilator settings, according to the physician's orders, are maintained.

FREQUENCY

A patient-ventilator system assessment should be performed at regularly scheduled intervals and in the following circumstances:

- After any change in ventilator settings
- Before obtaining any blood gas samples
- Before obtaining hemodynamic or pulmonary function data
- As soon as possible after an acute deterioration of the patient's condition, in particular, when this occurs after a violation of the ventilator alarm threshold

INFECTION CONTROL ISSUES

- Condensation from the patient circuit should be considered infectious waste and disposed of according to hospital policy.
- Universal precautions should be observed.

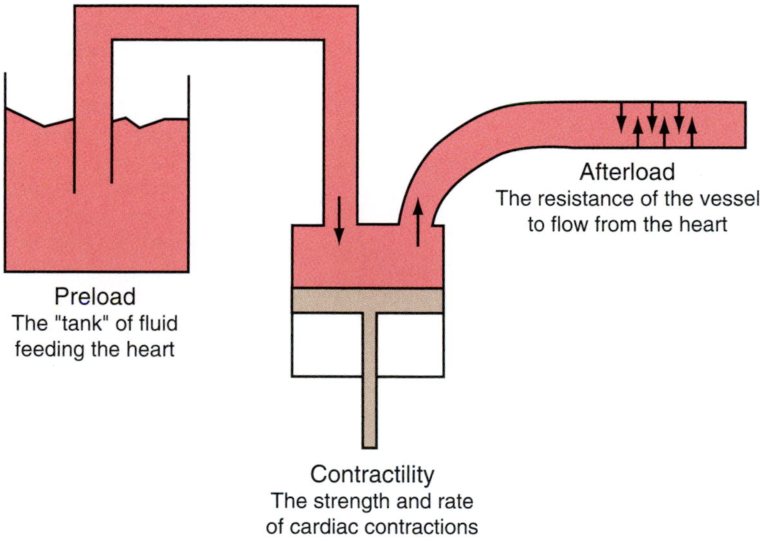

FIGURE 51-10 Preload contractility and afterload.

Central Venous Pressure–Right Atrial Pressure Monitoring

Right atrial pressure or CVP is monitored in the ICU by placement of a central venous catheter. Right atrial pressure normally is the lowest of all the heart chamber pressures, ranging from 2 to 6 mm Hg. Mean right atrial pressure is the same as CVP. CVP is a measure of right atrial preload. Atrial preload is determined by the balance between the capacity of the cardiovascular system, its circulating volume, and the amount of venous return to the heart (see Chapter 10). Right atrial pressure also is a reflection of right ventricular preload under normal circumstances. As a result, abnormally low right atrial pressure suggests inadequate filling of the right ventricle and is common in

TABLE 51-3
Cardiovascular Monitoring Criteria

Criterion	Normal Value (Range)	Abnormal Value
Heart rate (HR)	80 beats/min (60-100 beats/min)	>100 beats/min (tachycardia) <60 beats/min (bradycardia)
Arterial blood pressure (ABP)	120/80 mm Hg (90-140/60-90 mm Hg)	<140/90 mm Hg (hypertension) <90/60 mm Hg (hypotension)
Mean arterial blood pressure ($\overline{MAP}$)	90 mm Hg (80-100 mm Hg)	<80 mm Hg (hypotension) >100 mm Hg (hypertension)
ECG	Normal heart rate and rhythm	PR interval >0.2 sec (tachycardia, bradycardia, heart block [first, second, or third degree], premature ventricular contractions, premature atrial contractions, atrial fibrillation, atrial flutter, elevated ST segment, inverted T wave, ventricular tachycardia, ventricular fibrillation, asystole)
Central venous pressure (CVP)	2-6 mm Hg	>6 mm Hg (fluid overload, right ventricular failure, pulmonary hypertension, valvular stenosis, pulmonary embolus, cardiac tamponade, pneumothorax, positive pressure ventilation, PEEP, left ventricular failure) <2 mm Hg (hypovolemia, blood loss, shock, peripheral vasodilation, cardiovascular collapse)
Pulmonary artery pressure (PAP)	25/10 mm Hg (20-35/5-15 mm Hg)	>35/15 mm Hg (pulmonary hypertension, left ventricular failure, fluid overload) <20/5 mm Hg (pulmonary hypotension, hypovolemia, cardiovascular collapse)
Mean pulmonary artery pressure ($\overline{PAP}$)	15 mm Hg (10-20 mm Hg)	>20 mm Hg (same as ↑ PAP) <10 mm Hg (same as ↓ PAP)
Pulmonary capillary wedge pressure (PCWP)	5-10 mm Hg (<18 mm Hg)	>18 mm Hg (left ventricular failure, fluid overload) >20 mm Hg (interstitial edema) >25 mm Hg (alveolar filling) >30 mm Hg (frank pulmonary edema) <5 mm Hg (hypovolemia, shock, cardiovascular collapse)
Cardiac output ($\dot{Q}_T$ or CO)	5 L/min (4-8 L/min)	>8 L/min (elevated) (see Cardiac index) <4 L/min (decreased) (see Cardiac index)
Cardiac index (CI)	2.5-4 L/min per m^2	>4 L/min per m^2 (elevated owing to stress, septic shock, fever, hypervolemia, or drugs [dobutamine, dopamine, epinephrine, isoproterenol, and digitalis]) <2.5 L/min per m^2 (left ventricular failure, myocardial infarction, pulmonary embolus, high levels of positive pressure ventilation, PEEP, pneumothorax, blood loss, hypovolemia)
Systemic vascular resistance (SVR)	900-1400 dynes-sec/cm^5 (11.25-17.5 mm Hg/L per min)	>1400 dynes-sec/cm^5 (increased owing to vasoconstrictors [dopamine, norepinephrine, and epinephrine], hypovolemia, late septic shock) <900 dynes-sec/cm^5 (decreased owing to vasodilators [nitroglycerin, nitroprusside, and morphine] or early septic shock)
Pulmonary vascular resistance (PVR)	110-250 dynes-sec/cm^5 (1.38-3.13 mm Hg/L per min)	>250 dynes-sec/cm^5 (hypoxemia, ↓ pH, $PaCO_2$, vasopressors, emboli, emphysema, interstitial fibrosis, pneumothorax) <110 dynes-sec/cm^5 (pulmonary vasodilators, nitric oxide, O_2, calcium blockers)

CI = $\dot{Q}_T$ /Body surface area.
SVR = [($\overline{MAP}$ − CVP)/CO] × 80 = dynes-sec/cm^5.
PVR = [($\overline{PAP}$ − PCWP)/CO] − 80 = dynes-sec/cm^5.

hypovolemia. Causes of abnormal right atrial pressure or CVP are summarized in Box 51-11.

Pulmonary Artery Pressure Monitoring

Placement of a right heart/pulmonary artery catheter (**Swan-Ganz catheter**) is invasive and is associated with risk of pneumothorax, hemothorax, and arrhythmias. Placement of the balloon-tipped 7.5F catheter (Figure 51-12) must be performed aseptically by an experienced clinician. The catheter is guided into the pulmonary artery while the clinician visualizes waveforms with a fluid-filled system identical to the arterial pressure monitoring system (Figure 51-13).

Placement of a Swan-Ganz catheter allows determination of CVP, PAP, and PCWP. Data gathered with a Swan-Ganz catheter can be used to calculate thermodilution CO, pulmonary and arterial vascular resistance, and other associated indices (see Table 51-3). PAP monitoring may be helpful in the presence of shock (cardiogenic, hypovolemic, septic), left ventricular failure, myocardial infarction, pulmonary vascular disease, pulmonary edema, and ARDS. The reading and interpretation of Swan-Ganz catheter tracings can be inconsistent. There has been considerable controversy because of the risk-benefit ratio of the procedure.[41] The use of a pulmonary artery catheter in patients without primary cardiovascular disease has decreased markedly in more recent years.

Preload

Preload is defined as the pressure that stretches the ventricular walls at the onset of ventricular contraction. Preload can be approximated by measurement of PCWP. PCWP is an estimate of left atrial pressure, which reflects left ventricular end-diastolic pressure. During left-sided heart failure, preload increases; the increase is reflected in elevated PCWP. Symptoms of congestive heart failure usually can be controlled with diuretic therapy.

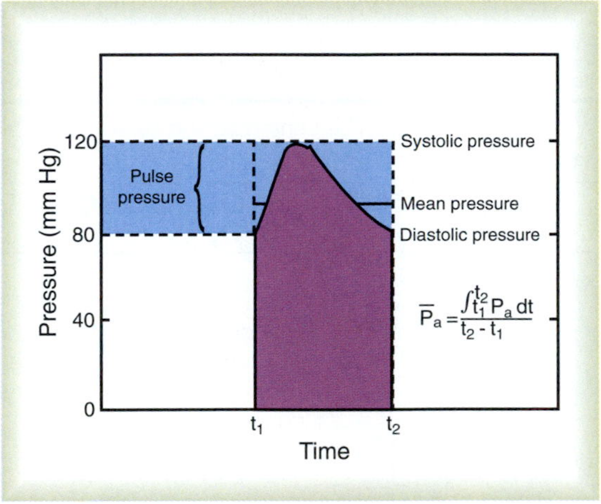

FIGURE 51-11 Arterial pressure wave form systolic pressure, diastolic pressure, MAP, and pulse pressure.

Box 51-11 Causes of Increased Right Atrial and Central Venous Pressure

- Right ventricular failure (myocardial infarction, cardiomyopathy)
- Pulmonary valvular stenosis
- Tricuspid stenosis and regurgitation
- Pulmonary hypertension
- Pulmonary embolism
- Volume overload
- Compression around the heart, constrictive pericarditis, cardiac tamponade
- Increased large vessel tone throughout the body, resulting in venoconstriction
- Arteriolar vasodilation, which increases blood supply to the venous system
- Increased intrathoracic pressure (positive pressure breath or pneumothorax)
- Placement of transducer below the patient's right atrial level
- Infusion of solution, especially with pressure infusion pumps, into CVP line
- Left-sided heart failure

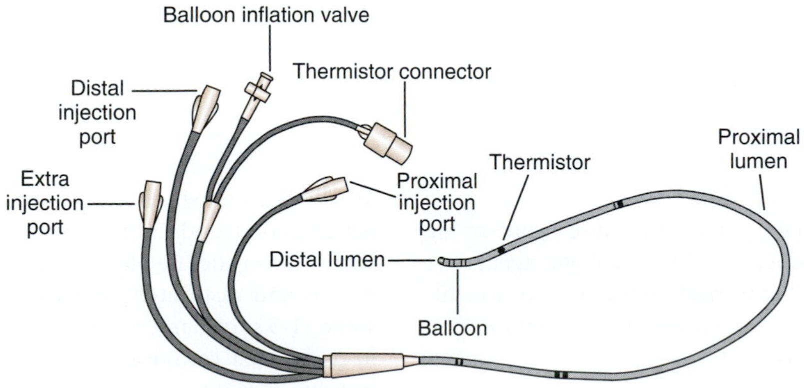

FIGURE 51-12 Quadruple-channel pulmonary artery catheter. The distalmost channel (distal injection port) is for measurement of PAP. Blood can be aspirated from this channel for mixed venous O_2 measurements. A second channel (balloon inflation valve) is used to inflate or deflate the distal balloon. A third channel (proximal injection port), which exits 30 cm from the catheter tip, is used for CVP (right atrial pressure) monitoring and fluid infusion. The fourth channel (extra injection port), which is not present on all catheters, can be used for continuous infusion of hyperalimentation fluid.

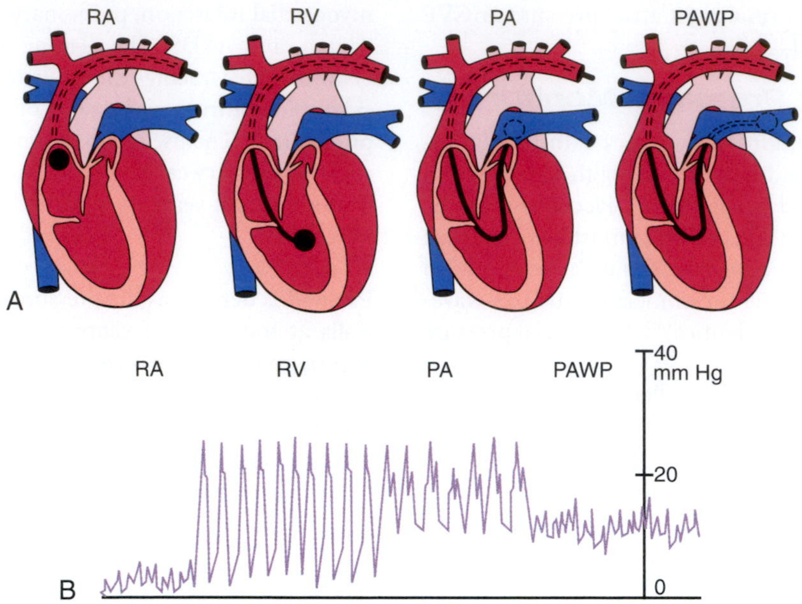

FIGURE 51-13 **A,** Position of pulmonary arterial catheter in the heart. **B,** As monitored by pressure tracings. *PA,* Pressure tracing from pulmonary artery; *PAWP,* pulmonary artery wedge pressure tracing; *RA,* pressure tracing from right atrium; *RV,* pressure tracing from right ventricle.

TABLE 51-4

Common Alterations in Hemodynamic Variables

	VARIABLE							
Condition	**Infiltrate on Chest Radiograph**	**BP**	**Cardiac Output**	**CVP**	**PAP**	**PCWP**	**$P\bar{v}O_2$ and $S\bar{v}O_2$**	**$C(a-\bar{v}O_2)$**
Shock								
Hypovolemic	—	↓	↓	↓	Variable	↓	↓	↑
Septic	None, one, or both sides	↓	↑	↓	N or ↓	N or ↓	N or ↑	N or ↑
Cardiogenic	One or both sides	↓	↓	↓↑	↑↑	↑↑	↓	↑
Left Ventricular Failure								
Mild	One or both sides	N or ↓	↓	N	↑	↑↑	↓	↑
Severe	One or both sides	↓	↓	N or ↑	↑↑	↑↑	↓	↑
Hypervolemic—fluid overload	One or both sides	N or ↑	N or ↑	N or ↑	↑	↑	N or ↑	N or ↓
Pulmonary embolus	None	N	Variable	↑	↑↑	N or ↓	Variable	Variable
ARDS	Both sides	Variable	Variable	Variable	Variable	N or ↓	Variable	Variable
Mechanical ventilation/PEEP	Variable	N or ↓	N or ↓	N or ↑	N or ↓	↑	N or ↓	N or ↑
Pulmonary hypertension	None	N or ↓	N or ↓	↑↑	↑↑	N	Variable	Variable

BP, Blood pressure; *N*, normal or little or no change.

Contractility

Contractility is the forcefulness of the heart muscle contracting under a constant load. Numerous pharmacologic agents are used to cause a modest increase in ejection fraction (contractility) and are associated with improvement in symptoms in patients with congestive heart failure.

Afterload

Afterload usually is defined as the load against which the ventricles must contract. An increase in systemic vascular resistance increases left ventricular afterload. Although increased afterload usually is equated with increased blood pressure, the cause is better understood as the muscle tension required by the left ventricle to generate blood flow. Table 51-4 lists common conditions and associated alterations in hemodynamic variables. Table 51-5 summarizes steps to take in troubleshooting changes in monitored cardiovascular values and vital signs, including possible causes and appropriate corrective action.

Cardiac Output

Cardiac performance is affected by preload, contractility, and afterload and is evaluated by the measurement of CO. The effect

TABLE 51-5

Troubleshooting Changes in Vital Signs

Clue	Possible Problem	Advice
Hypotension	Hypovolemia, pump failure	Evaluate fluid balance and possible need for intravenous fluids or inotropic agents
Hypertension	Anxiety; response to decreased PaO_2, decreased $PaCO_2$ or pain	Reassure, alleviate fear, check patient-ventilatory system; if not easily correctable, obtain and evaluate ABGs
Alteration of blood pressure with breathing	Decreased venous return (caused by changes in intrathoracic pressure)	If systolic/diastolic pressures are less than adequate perfusion levels, evaluate fluid balance; consider intravenous fluids
New arrhythmias, tachycardia, bradycardia	Anxiety	Reassure, alleviate fear
	Decreased PaO_2, decreased $PaCO_2$, increased $PaCO_2$	Check patient-ventilator system; if not quickly correctable, obtain and evaluate ABGs
Large swings in CVP or PCWP	Decreased venous return	Evaluate other hemodynamic values for adequacy of perfusion
Decreased urinary output	Decreased CO	Evaluate other hemodynamic values for adequacy of perfusion
	Hypovolemia	
Fever	Infection	Control infection; review preventive measures
	Atelectasis	Check patient-ventilator system for secretions, plugs, slippage of tube into right main stem bronchus
	Overheated humidifier	Check humidifier heater temperature
Weight gain	Fluid retention	Evaluate hemodynamic values for adequacy of perfusion; consider diuresis
Changes in respiratory rate	Altered settings	Check patient-ventilator settings
	Change in metabolic needs	Evaluate metabolic rate
	Anxiety	Reassure, alleviate fear
	Sleep	Normal; metabolic rate is decreased
Use of accessory muscles or paradoxical breathing	Increased WOB	Increase support level; check and change inspiratory flow
	Patient-ventilator asynchrony	Provide pressure support ventilation Increase sensitivity
	Auto-PEEP	Eliminate auto-PEEP

of cardiac pathology, medications, or mechanical ventilation on CO can be critical monitoring information. An accurate assessment of CO presents a challenge to the clinician. The physical examination (see Chapter 16) can reveal signs and symptoms of impaired cardiac performance, but a composite number provided by CO can provide more direct insight into problem and treatment options.

CO as determined by thermodilution via the use of a Swan-Ganz catheter was the primary method of CO assessment for three decades. The invasiveness of this method and inaccuracies in reading and interpretation led to a decrease in use of the Swan-Ganz catheter. Other methods of CO determination have become available based on algorithms that analyze the arterial pressure waveform and a Fick principle rebreathing method. The waveform analysis methods can be "calibrated" by lithium dilution or by thermodilution. Each technique has been studied and found to be accurate in relatively stable patients.[42-44]

NEUROLOGIC MONITORING

Monitoring of the nervous system is most frequently overlooked in the ICU for several reasons. The first and most important reason is lack of knowledge of proper assessment of the nervous system of a ventilated, restrained, and often sedated patient in the ICU. Neurologic dysfunction is difficult to recognize in a sedated patient. Proper clinical assessment of the nervous system emphasizes neurologic history and examination (Box 51-12).

History

Obtaining a history from a critically ill patient, in particular, a patient with altered state of consciousness, can be difficult. However, attempting to obtain a history by speaking with the patient or family members can provide extremely useful information in the ICU.

Medical conditions with neurologic symptoms can be revealed through history and appropriate clinical tests. A history of an evolving focal deficit occurring over days to weeks before loss of consciousness suggests abscess, tumor, or subdural hematoma, whereas a progression to coma over minutes to hours favors a metabolic cause. Problems such as hypothyroidism, renal failure, cirrhosis, or psychiatric illness suggest greater likelihood of a metabolic cause. Uncontrolled hypertension can induce metabolic (e.g., hypertensive encephalopathy) or structural (e.g., intracerebral hemorrhage) coma.

Box 51-12 Neurologic Monitoring

One of the most important, and frequently overlooked, areas of monitoring is the neurologic examination, which includes the following:

- History
- Assessment of mental status
- Pupillary response
- Eye movement assessment
- Corneal response
- Gag reflex
- Respiratory rate and pattern
- General motor and sensory evaluations

Neurologic Examination

The neurologic examination of a patient in the ICU should address several key issues. In addition to determination of level of consciousness, the primary goal is to determine the presence of focal neurologic signs so that the clinician can localize the lesion anatomically and generate a differential diagnosis and treatment plan.

Mental Status

The mental status examination should determine whether the patient has an altered state of consciousness. Terms such as *lethargy, confusion,* and *disorientation* lack precise definitions. A brief description of the applied stimulus and arousal pattern is preferred. The mental status examination in the ICU varies if the patient is intubated and cannot vocalize responses or speak. The earliest sign of abnormal mental status often is the patient's inability to follow a conversation or complex commands. Subtle changes in mental status often are the earliest signs of central nervous system dysfunction.

Pupillary Response

Pupil size, congruency, and response to light and accommodation should be described. Pupillary light reflexes provide information regarding the status of the brain and of the sympathetic and parasympathetic nervous systems. Pupillary function is controlled by the midbrain. If pupillary function is normal, the cause of coma is either metabolic or a structural lesion located above the midbrain. Small "pinpoint" pupils usually result from pontine hemorrhage or from ingestion of narcotics or organophosphates. Pupillary responses almost always remain intact in metabolic causes of coma. Dilated and fixed (unresponsive to light) pupils are seen in patients who have been given atropine. Midposition and fixed pupils often indicate severe cerebral damage.

Eye Movements

Abnormalities of extraocular movement have prognostic importance in the ICU. Normal movement of the eyes requires an intact pontomedullary-midbrain connection. The resting position of the gaze, the presence of nystagmus, and the response to head movements and cold tympanic membrane stimulation should be identified. Cervical spine stability must be ensured before oculocephalic maneuvers are performed. If rotation of the head (oculocephalic) and vestibular stimulation (calorics) produce no change in eye position, the pons is nonfunctional. If only the eye ipsilateral to the stimulus abducts, a lesion of the medial longitudinal fasciculus should be suspected.

Corneal Responses

The corneal reflex is used to test the afferent fifth and the efferent seventh cranial nerves. This test is performed by lightly touching the cornea with a cotton swab; the patient should blink both eyes in response. The presence of this response implies an intact ipsilateral fifth cranial nerve, intact central pons, and intact bilateral seventh cranial nerve. Testing must be performed bilaterally to evaluate both afferent components of the fifth cranial nerve.

Gag Reflex

The gag reflex is tested by using a tongue blade to stimulate one side of the posterior pharynx of an intubated patient. Each side should be tested separately. A normal response is bilateral movement of the posterior pharyngeal muscles and implies intact ninth and tenth cranial nerves. The ability to cough on suctioning can be tested in an intubated patient and implies an intact tenth cranial nerve. This test should not be attempted on nonintubated patients in the ICU because of the risk of aspiration.

Respiratory Rate and Pattern

The brainstem is the primary site of the central control of respiration. This control occurs at a subconscious level and results in rhythmic contraction and relaxation of the respiratory muscles. The most common abnormal respiratory pattern seen in patients with neurologic disorders is Cheyne-Stokes respiration, which consists of phases of hyperpnea that regularly alternate with episodes of apnea. Breathing waxes in a smooth crescendo and when a peak is reached wanes in an equally smooth decrescendo. Cheyne-Stokes respiration usually has an intracranial cause, although it can be caused by hypoxemia and cardiac failure. Ataxic breathing is a marker of severe brainstem dysfunction. Despite the nonspecificity of most breathing patterns, the respiratory pattern can provide valuable clues to the cause of coma.

Motor Evaluation

A thorough motor evaluation should be performed for all patients. The systematic approach described earlier is key to localization of the site of a pathologic process. The symmetry and pattern of the motor response to noxious stimuli and associated neurologic symptoms should be documented for all patients.

Sensory Evaluation

The assessment of light touch, pinprick, and temperature sensation can be achieved by applying a cotton swab, a clean pin, and a cold or warm object to various parts of the upper and lower extremities. Symmetry of responses between sides and between upper and lower extremities should be documented and is valuable in localizing the site of a pathologic process.

Intracranial Pressure Monitoring

There are three primary reasons to measure intracranial pressure (ICP): (1) to monitor patients at risk of life-threatening intracranial hypertension, (2) to monitor for evidence of infection, and (3) to assess the effects of therapy aimed at reducing ICP. Mean ICP of a supine patient is normally 10 to 15 mm Hg, and the ICP waveform normally undulates gently in time with the cardiac cycle. Fluctuations of the ICP waveform (>10 mm Hg) suggest a position near the critical inflection point of the cranial P-V curve. Elevations in ICP to 15 to 20 mm Hg compress the capillary bed and compromise microcirculation. At ICP levels of 30 to 35 mm Hg, venous drainage is impeded, and edema develops in uninjured tissue. Even when autoregulatory mechanisms are intact, cerebral perfusion cannot be maintained if ICP increases to within 40 to 50 mm Hg of the mean arterial pressure. When ICP approximates mean arterial pressure, perfusion stops, and the brain dies.

Two categories of ICP monitoring techniques are available at the present time. Fluid-filled systems have external transducers, such as an intraventricular catheter and subarachnoid bolts. Solid-state systems have miniature pressure transducers that can be inserted in the lateral ventricle, brain parenchyma, or subarachnoid or epidural space.

Glasgow Coma Scale Score

The most widely used scoring system for acute neurologic disorders is the **Glasgow Coma Scale (GCS)** (Table 51-6). The GCS score is used to test best motor response, best verbal response, and opening of the eyes. The scale goes from 3 to 15 and can be used for rapid triage. Patients with head injury and GCS scores of 13 to 15 often are admitted to a non-ICU observational unit unless neurologic examination or a CT scan reveals a lesion or abnormality that warrants ICU admission. Scores of 9 to 13 on the GCS signify a significant insult with depressed level of consciousness. Patients with head injury and GCS scores of 8 and less need monitoring of ICP.

TABLE 51-6
Glasgow Coma Scale

Eyes	Open	Spontaneous	4
		To verbal command	3
		To pain	2
		No response	1
Best motor response	To verbal command	Obeys	6
	To painful stimulus	Localized pain	5
		Flexion—withdrawal	4
		Flexion—decorticate	3
		Flexion—decerebrate	2
		No response	1
Best verbal response		Oriented, converses	5
		Disoriented, converses	4
		Inappropriate words	3
		Incomprehensible sounds	2
		No response	1
Total			*3-15*

MONITORING RENAL FUNCTION

The kidney is the main filter of waste products and the principal regulator of the volume and electrolyte composition of body fluid. Because the kidney is the primary excreter of nitrogenous waste, plasma concentrations of blood urea nitrogen (BUN) and creatinine are used to track renal function. As a general guideline, the BUN level increases 10 to 15 mg/dl per day, and the creatinine level increases 1 to 2.5 mg/dl per day after abrupt renal failure. The serum potassium level usually increases 0.5 mEq/L per day, and bicarbonate (HCO_3^-) level decreases approximately 1 mEq/L per day. Under the catabolic stress of burns, trauma, rhabdomyolysis (an acute and sometimes fatal disease in which products of skeletal muscle destruction produce acute renal failure), sepsis, or starvation, the rates of change in these values can double. In contrast to BUN, daily production of creatinine is relatively constant. An increasing creatinine level indicates that the rate of production exceeds clearance by means of glomerular filtration. A stable elevation in creatinine level implies a new steady state has been achieved at a decreased glomerular filtration rate. Until the creatinine level stabilizes, the severity of acute renal dysfunction cannot be assessed reliably. The most common method of estimating glomerular filtration rate (renal function) is measurement of plasma creatinine and creatinine clearance rate. Although calculation of creatinine clearance is more accurate, the procedure entails 24-hour urine collection. The most important factor is whether glomerular filtration rate is changing or stable, and plasma creatinine level is tracked for most patients.

Urine volume usually reflects kidney perfusion. *Polyuria* and *oliguria* refer to a daily urine output of more than 3 L and less than 0.4 L in average-sized adults. *Anuria* is present when urine output is less than 50 ml/day. Polyuria should not be confused with urinary frequency, in which multiple small voidings occur, but total output is less than 3 L/day.

MONITORING LIVER FUNCTION

Adequate liver function is essential for survival of critically ill patients. The liver must detoxify wastes from metabolism and digestion and process poisons. Elevated results of liver function tests reflect the occurrence of liver parenchymal damage. Hepatic dysfunction may precipitate or worsen ARDS.[45] Routine indications for liver function testing in the treatment of critically ill patients include abdominal pain, jaundice, unexplained fever, nausea, malaise, failure to thrive, weight loss, and leukocytosis. Additional indications are facilitation of acuity scoring and definition of the contribution of the liver to multisystem organ failure.

Batteries of biochemical studies are routine in the evaluation of critically ill patients, but they reflect liver function minimally. Acute liver disease can develop in critically ill patients receiving total parenteral nutrition.[46] Liver disease may manifest as increased liver size and tenderness. When abnormal results of liver function tests have been obtained, it is essential to determine the cause. Elevations in levels of canalicular enzymes and bilirubin necessitate a search for mechanical obstruction and appropriate radiographic investigations. Elevations of transaminase levels are unusual in cholestatic processes, unless there is a superimposed ischemic event—a confounding factor in many critically ill patients. Elevated levels of aspartate aminotransferase and alanine aminotransferase suggest hepatic inflammation. Ischemia, viral hepatitis, and autoimmune hepatitis should be considered in the differential diagnosis.

NUTRITIONAL MONITORING

Assessment and monitoring of nutrition are required in the care of some critically ill patients because nutritional disorders are frequent and important determinants of outcome. Nutritional support is commonly needed by patients who have been critically ill for an extended period and patients with increased metabolic demands and limited nutritional reserve.

Assessment of Nutritional Status

Early detection of malnutrition in critically ill patients, whether preexisting or a result of acute illness, enables prompt and aggressive intervention with supplemental nutrition. No single measurement or assessment tool can adequately characterize nutritional status, and the diagnosis of malnutrition is subjective. However, both functional and biochemical factors should be examined to identify whether a patient is at increased risk of malnutrition and its complications.

Functional Assessment

The functional nutritional assessment consists of the medical history, physical examination, and appraisal of muscle and organ function. Identification of preexisting malnutrition should be attempted by careful attention to the history of present illness, the relevant medical and surgical history, medications, social habits, and a dietary history. Obtaining this information from a critically ill patient frequently is impossible, but the patient's family may be able to provide data on recent dietary habits and weight loss. Historical data should be used to estimate the nutritional consequences of the current hospitalization. Prehospitalization weight should be documented, and any weight changes since hospitalization should be documented and evaluated in the context of diuresis or fluid supplementation. Critically ill patients frequently have volume overload, which makes changes in dry weight difficult to assess.

The physical examination findings may suggest the presence of nutritional and metabolic deficiencies. Temporal muscle wasting, sunken supraclavicular fossae, and decreased adipose stores are easily recognized signs of starvation. Careful inspection of the hair, skin, eyes, mouth, and extremities can reveal protein-calorie malnutrition or vitamin and mineral deficiencies. An assessment of muscle mass and function can provide information about a patient's protein reserves and overall nutritional status. An estimation of muscle mass and fat stores can be obtained from anthropometric measurements such as arm circumference.

The function of the cardiovascular, respiratory, and gastrointestinal systems should be evaluated both for evidence of malnutrition-related dysfunction and because functional deficits may affect the ability of the patient to tolerate nutritional supplementation. The large fluid volumes associated with parenteral nutrition may not be tolerated in the setting of impaired cardiovascular function, and a distended abdomen makes tolerance of enteral supplementation less likely.

Metabolic Assessment

Serum albumin concentration is the most frequently used laboratory measure of nutritional status; a value less than 2.2 g/dl generally reflects severe malnutrition. Although albumin level is popular as an indicator of nutritional status, the reliability of albumin as a marker of visceral protein status is compromised by its long half-life of 14 to 20 days, making it less responsive to acute changes in nutritional status. Serum albumin concentration increases rapidly in response to exogenously administered albumin and is altered regardless of nutritional status in conditions such as dehydration, sepsis, trauma, and liver disease.

Serum chemistry values are important in determining the specifics of nutritional support but do not directly reflect nutritional status. Sodium, potassium, chloride, total CO_2, BUN, glucose, prothrombin time, partial thromboplastin time, iron, magnesium, calcium, and phosphate should be measured at admission and rechecked periodically.

Estimating Nutritional Requirements

The first step in calculating the nutritional prescription is to estimate the energy or caloric needs of the patient. Determining energy needs requires calculating basal energy expenditure (BEE). The BEE is the amount of energy required to perform metabolic functions at rest and is influenced by body size and illness. The BEE classically is estimated with the **Harris-Benedict equation**, as follows:[47]

$$\text{Men: BEE} = 66 + (13.7)(\text{Weight}) + (5)(\text{Height}) - (6.8)(\text{Age})$$
$$\text{Women: BEE} = 65 + (9.6)(\text{Weight}) + (1.8)(\text{Height}) - (4.7)(\text{Age})$$

where weight is expressed in kilograms; height, in centimeters; and age, in years.

The weight in these equations should be the usual or actual weight of a patient without significant weight loss, current weight for a patient with marked weight loss, and ideal body weight for an obese patient. The use of this measurement in the care of a critically ill patient has traditionally involved multiplication by a stress factor of 0.5 to 2.5. The use of the stress factor may result in overfeeding and may predispose the patient to fatty degeneration of the liver (steatosis), hyperglycemia, electrolyte imbalances, respiratory embarrassment owing to increased CO_2 production, and macrophage dysfunction. Use of the baseline Harris-Benedict equation without the stress factor in determining the BEE of critically ill patients yields an average estimate of 25 kcal/kg body weight.

GLOBAL MONITORING INDICES

Organizing the flood of information made available by monitoring instruments is a skill and responsibility of critical care practitioners. In the ICU, the immediate concern is the welfare of the patient. Decisions frequently are based on prognosis with respect to the appropriate tests, treatments, and medications prescribed. Guiding these decisions is the weighing of risks and benefits to the patient and the responsible use of resources. Although the physician makes such decisions with all current information, specific data on the probability of survival can be estimated. In the past 30 years, prognostic indices have been derived from large clinical data sets that provide an indication of the seriousness of the patient's condition. These indices (Acute Physiology and Chronic Health Evaluation [APACHE I, II, III, and IV], Acute Physiology Score, Therapeutic Intervention Scoring System, and Burns Weaning Assessment Program) are determinations of scores from numerous monitored values obtained from isolated observations of the patient's condition, usually during the first 24 hours after hospital admission. A score may be assigned for that patient at that time, and risk of mortality can be calculated (Box 51-13).

The value of severity of illness scoring for individual patients is limited, and the accuracy and usefulness of physiology scoring often are questioned. Imposing a scoring system to judge intent to treat places too much emphasis on the validity of the system. Scoring systems have not been clearly associated with important outcomes such as length of stay or time on mechanical ventilation. At the present time, as a bedside tool in the care of an individual patient, scoring systems have limited value. A specific condition may "score" a 17% risk of death, but a patient has two possible outcomes: life (0%) and death (100%). The decision to withdraw or limit care would rarely be based on a "score" because many other factors are involved in such a decision. Inaccuracies in predicting mortality are frequently reported. Discrepancies are probably due to patient mix differences, hospital factors, admission policies, data collection methods, and differences in quality of care. At the present time, the global indices have limited use in care of individual patients.

Box 51-13 Global Monitoring Indices

Indices (scores) have been developed that take into account several monitored values.

These scoring systems provide an estimate of illness acuity level and an estimate of the risk of mortality.

For clinical studies, scoring systems are required to ensure that the control and experimental groups are similar.

Scoring systems can be useful as a longitudinal monitor of acuity or a means of evaluating the effect of changes in services.

At this time, scoring systems have little value in the care of individual patients. The most commonly used acuity of illness scoring system is APACHE II.

Global monitoring has a definite role in research. Global indices are valuable in the study of the effectiveness of new medications or therapy and the establishment of guidelines for care. When control and experimental (new treatment) groups are compared in a randomized, controlled trial, the severity scores of the groups must be similar, or differences in baseline condition may account for differences in results. As a tracking tool, scoring has significant value; the increasing severity of causes of ICU admissions can be followed over time with severity of illness scoring. The consequences of changes in services or policies or interhospital comparisons can be crudely tracked with the use of expected mortality calculations from APACHE scores. Some institutions calculate severity of illness scores for all patients.

Acute Physiology and Chronic Health Evaluation (APACHE)

The **APACHE scoring system** was developed in 1981 to monitor severity of illness in clinical studies.[48] Studies have referenced a risk of mortality estimate as calculated from APACHE scoring, and the studies can be compared with similar studies in which the APACHE scoring system is used. The APACHE II scoring system assigns points to physiologic variables on the basis of whether the values are high abnormal, low abnormal, or normal. Variables rated include temperature, mean arterial pressure, heart rate, respiratory rate, PaO_2 [or $P(A - a)O_2$], pH, sodium level, potassium level, creatinine level, hematocrit, white blood cell count, and GCS score. Assigned points are added to derive a total APACHE score. There is an imprecision to estimating a risk of mortality. To emphasize the importance of the neurologic examination, the scoring system is weighted toward the importance of the GCS score. Refinements of APACHE are ongoing, although the APACHE II system continues to be used more often than other systems.[49]

TROUBLESHOOTING

Identification and correction of patient-related and ventilator-related problems during mechanical ventilatory support are primary responsibilities of the RT. Under ideal circumstances, potential problems are identified before they occur, or before they can cause harm to the patient. Potential problems with the patient include anxiety, agitation, altered mental status, fighting the ventilator, hypoxemia, hypoventilation, and development of metabolic acidosis. The patient may experience acute changes in respiratory rate, heart rate, blood pressure, and CO.

Other common patient-related problems include excessive secretions, bronchospasm, and other causes of decreased compliance or increased resistance. Recognition of signs of pneumothorax, pneumomediastinum or subcutaneous emphysema, airway malfunction or leaks, and chest tube leaks should lead to prompt attention to the problem.

Problems associated with the ventilator include leaks or malfunctions in the system, inappropriate ventilator settings (including trigger sensitivity and inspiratory flow rate),

Box 51-14 Causes of Sudden Respiratory Distress in a Patient Receiving Ventilatory Support

PATIENT-RELATED CAUSES

- Artificial airway problems
- Movement of endotracheal tube
- Cuff herniation
- Cuff leak
- Kinking of endotracheal tube
- Foreign body
- Transesophageal fistula
- Innominate artery rupture
- Malpositioned nasogastric tube
- Secretions
- Bronchospasm
- Pneumothorax
- Pulmonary edema
- Pulmonary embolism
- Acute hypoxemia
- Blood in endotracheal tube
- Dynamic hyperinflation
- Abnormal respiratory drive
- Alteration in body posture
- Drug-induced problems
- Abdominal distention
- Agitation

VENTILATOR-RELATED CAUSES

- Ventilator malfunction
- Circuit malfunction
- Leaks or disconnects
- Condensate
- In-line nebulizers
- Inadequate ventilatory support
- Patient-ventilator asynchrony

From Tobin MJ, Alex CJ, Fahey PJ: Fighting the ventilator. In Tobin MJ, editor: Principles and practice of mechanical ventilation, New York, 2006, McGraw-Hill.

Box 51-15 Steps for Managing Sudden Distress in a Patient Receiving Ventilatory Support

1. Remove the patient from the ventilator.
2. Initiate manual ventilation with 100% O_2.
3. Patient improvement indicates that the ventilator is the cause of distress.
4. Lack of improvement indicates the problem is within the patient.
5. If death appears imminent, consider and manage the most likely causes, check for airway obstruction (by passing a suction catheter), a dislodged endotracheal tube, or a pneumothorax.
6. If death is not imminent, wait until the patient's condition is stable before attempting a more detailed assessment including a chest radiograph.

Modified from Tobin MJ, Alex CJ, Fahey PJ: Fighting the ventilator. In Tobin MJ, editor: Principles and practice of mechanical ventilation, New York, 2006, McGraw-Hill.

development of auto-PEEP, and improper humidification. Box 51-14 lists causes of sudden respiratory distress in patients receiving mechanical ventilatory support. Box 51-15 lists steps for managing sudden respiratory distress. Table 51-7 summarizes troubleshooting of the patient-ventilator system.

If medical and mechanical problems have been excluded and the patient continues to fight the ventilator or exhibit high levels of agitation or distress, sedation should be considered. Agents commonly used for sedation in the ICU include benzodiazepines (lorazepam, midazolam), opiates (fentanyl, morphine), haloperidol, and propofol.

Pharmacologic paralysis should be considered only when no other alternatives are effective. The one exception to this guideline is the patient presenting with severe ARDS (PaO_2/FiO_2 <100 mm Hg). In order to gain control of the patient's physiologic status it is now recommended to paralysis these patients for up to 48 hours. The use of neuromuscular blocking agents can mask other patient problems, and ventilator malfunction or disconnection in the care of a paralyzed patient can be catastrophic. In addition, some patients receiving neuromuscular blocking agents in the ICU may experience prolonged neuropathy. Pharmacologic agents used to produce sedation or paralysis in the ICU are listed in Box 51-16.

Box 51-16 Pharmacologic Agents Used to Produce Sedation or Paralysis

I. Benzodiazepine tranquilizing agents
   A. Diazepam (Valium)
   B. Lorazepam (Ativan)
   C. Midazolam (Versed)
II. Sedative hypnotics and miscellaneous agents
   A. Sodium thiopental (Pentothal)
   B. Etomidate (Amidate)
   C. Haloperidol (Haldol)
   D. Propofol (Diprivan)
   E. Dexmedetomidine (Precedex)
III. Narcotic analgesics
   A. Morphine
   B. Fentanyl (Sublimaze)
IV. Neuromuscular blocking agents
   A. Nondepolarizing (competitive)
      1. Steroidal agents
         Pancuronium (Pavulon)
         Pipecuronium (Arduan)
         Rocuronium (Zemuron)
         Vecuronium (Norcuron)
      2. Benzylisoquinolinium esters
         Atracurium (Tracrium)
         Cisatracurium (Nimbex)
         Doxacurium (Nuromax)
         Metocurine (Metubine)
         Mivacurium (Mivacron)
         Tubocurarine (Tubarine)
   B. Depolarizing
      1. Succinylcholine (Anectine, Quelicin)
      2. Decamethonium (Syncurine)

TABLE 51-7
Troubleshooting the Patient-Ventilator System

Clue to Problem	Possible Cause	Corrective Action
Decreased minute ventilation or V_T	Leak around endotracheal or chest tube	Check all connections for leaks
	Decreased patient-triggered respiratory rate	Evaluate patient Check sensitivity Measure auto-PEEP Increase set rate Change mode
	Decreased lung compliance	Evaluate patient
	Airway secretions	Clear airway of secretions
	Altered settings	Check patient-ventilator system
	Malfunctioning volume monitor	Check with external respirometer
Increased minute ventilation or V_T	Increased patient-triggered respiratory rate	Check respiratory rate Check sensitivity Change mode
	Altered settings	Check patient-ventilator system
	Hypoxia	Evaluate patient Consider ABG and SpO_2 values
	Increased lung compliance	Decrease pressure Decrease inspiratory time
	Malfunctioning volume monitor	Check with external respirometer
Change in respiratory rate	Altered setting	Check patient-ventilator system
	Increased metabolic demand	Evaluate patient
	Hypoxia	Evaluate patient Consider ABG and SpO_2 values
Sudden increase in peak airway pressure	Coughing	Alleviate uncontrolled coughing
	Airway secretions or plugs	Clear airway secretions
	Ventilator tubing kinked or filled with water	Check for kinks and water
	Changes in patient position	Consider repositioning patient
	Endotracheal tube in right main stem bronchus	Verify position
	Patient-ventilator asynchrony	Correct asynchrony Check for adequate peak flow Verify with waveforms
	Bronchospasm	Identify cause and treat
	Pneumothorax	Insert chest tubes
Gradual increase in peak airway pressure	Diffuse, reactive, or obstructive process	Evaluate for problems, such as atelectasis, increasing lung water, bronchospasm
Sudden decrease in peak airway pressure	Volume loss from leaks in the system	Check patient-ventilator systems for leaks Verify with waveforms Check for active inspirations Evaluate patient
FiO_2 drift	O_2 analyzer error	Calibrate analyzer Change O_2 sensor
	Blender piping failure	Correct failure
	O_2 source failure	Correct failure
	O_2 reservoir leak	Check ventilator reservoir
I : E ratio too high or too low	Altered inspiratory flow	Check flow setting and correct
	Alteration in other settings that control I : E ratio	Check settings and correct
	Alteration in sensitivity setting	Check setting and correct
	Airway secretions (pressure ventilator)	Clear airway of secretions
	Subtle leaks	Measure minute ventilation
Inspired gas temperature too high	Addition of cool water to humidifier	Wait
	Altered settings	Correct temperature control setting
	Adding cool gas by small-volume nebulizer treatment	Turn off heater during treatment
	Thermostat failure	Replace heater
Changes in PEEP	Change in V_T	Adjust PEEP level
	Change in compliance	Adjust PEEP level
	Altered settings	Check settings and correct
Changes in static pressure	Changes in lung compliance	Evaluate patient and correct if possible
Changes in ventilator setting	Changes in these settings resulting from deliberate or accidental adjustment of dials or knobs	Determine whether current settings are the intended ones

Modified from Martz K, Joiner JW, Shepherd RM: Management of the patient-ventilator system: a team approach, ed 2, St. Louis, 1994, Mosby.

SUMMARY CHECKLIST

- Caregivers must be experienced at filtering the noise from the changes in monitored variables that require attention. Caregivers need to recognize false alarms. They also need to discriminate real pathophysiologic changes from normal physiologic variations and from variations inherent in the data.
- Because only caregivers can make choices about altering care, caregivers continue to be the most important monitors.
- Monitoring of the respiratory system includes assessment of ventilation, gas exchange, and respiratory system mechanics and function.
- Ventilation is monitored by measurement of V_T, respiratory rate, and minute ventilation and by assessment of dead space and alveolar ventilation.
- Gas exchange is routinely monitored with ABG analysis and pulse oximetry. Derived values such as V_D/V_T, $P(A - a)O_2$ difference, PaO_2/FiO_2 ratio, shunt, and lung injury score can clarify the nature and severity of gas-exchange abnormality. Arterial $PaCO_2$ is the best index of alveolar ventilation.
- Respiratory system mechanics are routinely monitored by tracking peak pressure, P_{plat}, auto-PEEP, compliance, and resistance.
- When mechanically ventilating any patient, ideally, the tidal volume should be 4 to 8 ml/kg PBW and the plateau pressure should be less than 28 cm H_2O.
- Monitoring of transpulmonary pressure is becoming increasingly important in the management of patients with decreased chest wall compliance and patients with severe ARDS requiring high PEEP levels.
- Factors such as WOB, f/V_T, VC, MIP, and MVV can be extremely helpful in assessing the need to increase ventilatory support or in assessing the potential for weaning.
- Advanced monitoring techniques include EIT, ARM, lung stress and strain, stress index, and esophageal pressure monitoring.
- The most important responsibility of the RT in the ICU is monitoring of the patient-ventilator system.
- Monitoring of the patient-ventilator system includes overall assurance of the integrity and safety of the system. Monitoring requires complete knowledge of the ventilator settings; all aspects of ventilator function; the circuitry; airway status; gas exchange; ventilator graphics; lung mechanics; alarms; and the overall care, safety, and comfort of the patient.
- Acute changes in cardiac performance, cardiovascular status, or impulse conduction (ECG) can be life-threatening; some form of monitoring of the heart, vascular system, and ECG is necessary in the care of nearly all patients in the ICU.
- Hemodynamic monitoring requires the use of invasive pulmonary arterial, central venous, and arterial catheters. Values obtained with these monitoring lines must be carefully interpreted by experienced caregivers. All ICU patients should receive ECG monitoring.
- Monitoring of changes in neurologic status is extremely important and is more often overlooked than monitoring of other organ systems.
- The neurologic examination includes assessment of mental status, pupillary response, eye movements, corneal response, gag reflex, and respiratory rate and pattern and a general motor and sensory evaluation. ICP monitoring may be needed to detect or manage elevated ICP.
- Global index monitoring is calculation of an illness level score that is an estimate of the risk of mortality from numerous monitoring values. Illness scores are not used in the care plan for an individual patient, but scoring systems are widely used in clinical studies. The APACHE II system is among the most popular of these estimates.
- Troubleshooting the patient-ventilator system is aimed at identifying and correcting problems before they harm the patient.

References

1. Cohn SM, Nathens AB, Moore FA, et al: StO_2 in Trauma Patients Trial Investigators: tissue oxygen saturation predicts the development of organ dysfunction during traumatic shock resuscitation. *J Trauma* 62:44–54, 2007.
2. Mendelson Y: Pulse oximetry: theory and applications for noninvasive monitoring. *Clin Chem* 38:1601–1607, 1992.
3. Cairo JN, Pilbeam SP: *Mosby's respiratory care equipment*, ed 7, St Louis, 2004, Mosby.
4. Girard TD, Bernard GR: Mechanical ventilation in ARDS: a state-of-the-art review. *Chest* 131:921–929, 2007.
5. Villar J, Blanco J, Kacmarek RM: Acute respiratory distress syndrome definition: do we need a change? *Curr Opin Crit Care* 17:13–17, 2011.
6. Bollen C, Uiterwaal C, van Vught A: Systematic review of determinants of mortality in high frequency oscillatory ventilation in acute respiratory distress syndrome. *Critical Care* 10(1):R34, 2006.
7. Petty TL, Ashbaugh DG: The adult respiratory distress syndrome: clinical features, factors influencing prognosis and principles of management. *Chest* 60:233–239, 1971.
8. Murray JF, Matthay MA, Luce JM, et al: An expanded definition of the adult respiratory distress syndrome. *Am Rev Respir Dis* 138:720–723, 1988.
9. Kallet RH: Capnography and respiratory care in the 21st century. *Respir Care* 53:860–861, 2008.
10. Nuckton TJ, Alonso JA, Kallet RH, et al: Pulmonary dead-space fraction as a risk factor for death in the acute respiratory distress syndrome. *N Engl J Med* 346:1281–1286, 2002.
11. Rabitsch W, Nikolic A, Schellongowski P, et al: Evaluation of an end-tidal portable ETCO2 colorimetric breath indicator (COLIBRI). *Am J Emerg Med* 22:4–9, 2004.
12. Hinkelbein J, Floss F, Denz C, et al: Accuracy and precision of three different methods to determine Pco2 (Paco2 vs. Petco2 vs. Ptcco2) during interhospital ground transport of critically ill and ventilated adults. *J Trauma* 65:10–18, 2008.
13. AARC Clinical practice guidelines: Capnography/capnometry during mechanical ventilation: revised 2003. *Respir Care* 48:534–539, 2003.
14. Anderson CT, Breen PH: Carbon dioxide kinetics and capnography during critical care. *Crit Care* 4:207–215, 2000.
15. Yem JS, Turner MJ, Baker AB: Sources of error in partial rebreathing pulmonary blood flow measurements in lungs with emphysema and pulmonary embolism. *Br J Anaesth* 97:732–741, 2006.
16. Hubmayr RD: Perspective on lung injury and recruitment: a skeptical look at the opening and collapse story. *Am J Respir Crit Care Med* 165:1647–1653, 2002.
17. Siobal M, Ong H, Valdes J, et al: Calculation of physiologic dead space: comparison of ventilator volumetric capnography to measurements by metabolic analyzer and volumetric CO2 monitor. *Respir Care* 58:1143–1151, 2013.

18. Villar J, Pérez-Méndez L, Basaldúa S, et al: A risk textiles model for predicting mortality in patients with acute respiratory distress syndrome: Age, plateau pressure and PaO2/FIO2 at ARDS onset predict outcome. *Respir Care* 56:420–428, 2011.
19. Gattinoni L, Carlesso E, Brazzi L, et al: Positive end-expiratory pressure. *Curr Opin Crit Care* 16:39–44, 2010.
20. Loring S, O'Donnell C, Behazin N, et al: Esophageal pressures in acute lung injury: do they represent artifact or useful information about transpulmonary pressure, chest wall mechanics, and lung stress? *J Appl Physiol* 108:515–522, 2010.
21. Talmoar D, Fessler H: Are esophageal pressure measurements important in clinical decision-making in mechanically ventilated patients? *Respir Care* 55:162–172, 2010.
22. Schumann S, Haberthuer C, Guttmann J: Compensating for endotracheal tube resistance. *Anesth Analg* 110:639–640, 2010.
23. Stewart TE, Meade MO, Cook DJ, et al: Evaluation of a ventilation strategy to prevent barotrauma in patients at high risk for acute respiratory distress syndrome. Pressure- and Volume-Limited Ventilation Strategy Group. *N Engl J Med* 338:355–361, 1998.
24. Chiumello D, Carlesso E, Cadringher P, et al: Lung stress and strain during mechanical ventilation for acute respiratory distress syndrome. *Am J Respir Crit Care Med* 178:346–355, 2008.
25. Graf J, Santos A, Dries D, et al: Functional residual capacity by nitrogen washin/washout and CT techniques agree in pleural effusion model. *Respir Care* 11:1464–1468, 2010.
26. Grasso S, Terragni P, Mascia L, et al: Airway pressure-time profile (stress index) detects tidal recruitment/hyperinflation in experimental acute lung injury. *Crit Care Med* 32:1018–1027, 2004.
27. Formenti P, Graf J, Santos A, et al: Non-pulmonary factors strongly influence the stress index. *Intensive Care Med* 37:594–600, 2011.
28. Mughal MM, Culver DA, Minai OA, et al: Auto-positive end-expiratory pressure: mechanisms and treatment. *Cleve Clin J Med* 72:801–809, 2005.
29. Blanch L, Bernabé F, Lucangelo U: Measurement of air trapping, intrinsic positive end-expiratory pressure, and dynamic hyperinflation in mechanically ventilated patients. *Respir Care* 50:110–123, 2005.
30. Layon J, Banner MJ, Kirby RR, et al: Partially and totally unloading respiratory muscles based on real-time measurements. *Chest* 106:1835–1842A, 1994.
31. Kapasi M, Fujino Y, Kirmse M, et al: Effort and work of breathing in neonates during assisted patient-triggered ventilation. *Pediatr Crit Care Med* 2:9–16, 2001.
32. Purro A, Appendini L, De Gaetano A, et al: Physiologic determinants of ventilator dependence in long-term mechanically ventilated patients. *Am J Respir Crit Care Med* 161:1115–1123, 2000.
33. Yang K, Tobin M: A prospective study of indexes predicting outcome of trials of weaning from mechanical ventilation. *N Engl J Med* 324:1445–1450, 1991.
34. Marini JJ, Smith TC, Lamb V: Estimation of inspiratory muscle strength in mechanically ventilated patients: the measurement of maximal inspiratory pressure. *J Crit Care* 191:323–326, 1986.
35. Adams A: Pulmonary function in the mechanically ventilated patient. *Respir Care Clin North Am* 3:322–331, 1997.
36. Kue R, Brown P, Ness C, et al: Adverse clinical events during intrahospital transport by a specialized team: a preliminary report. *Am J Crit Care* 20:153–161, 2011.
37. Costa E, Borges J, Melo A, et al: Bedside estimation of recruitable alveolar collapse and hyperdistension by electrical impedance tomography. *Intensive Care Med* 35:1132–1137, 2009.
38. Vyshedskiy A, Ishikawa S, Murphy R: Crackle pitch and rate do not vary significantly during a single examining session in patients with pneumonia, congestive heart failure, and interstitial pulmonary fibrosis. *Respir Care* 56:806–817, 2011.
39. Yilmaz M, Gajic O: Optimal ventilator settings in acute lung injury and acute respiratory distress syndrome. *Eur J Anaesthesiol* 25:89–96, 2008.
40. Briel M, Meade M, Mercat A, et al: Higher vs lower positive end-expiratory pressure in patients with acute lung injury and acute respiratory distress syndrome: systematic review and meta-analysis. *JAMA* 303:865–873, 2010.
41. Wiener RS, Welch HG: Trends in the use of the pulmonary artery catheter in the United States, 1993-2004. *JAMA* 298:423–429, 2007.
42. Saraceni E, Rossi S, Persona P, et al: Comparison of two methods for cardiac output measurement in critically ill patients. *Br J Anaesth* 106:690–694, 2011.
43. Geerts B, de Wilde R, Aarts L, et al: Cardiothoracic pulse contour analysis to assess hemodynamic response to passive leg raising. *Vasc Anesth* 25:48–52, 2011.
44. Young BP, Low LL: Noninvasive monitoring cardiac output using partial CO(2) rebreathing. *Crit Care Clin* 26:383–392, 2010.
45. TenHoor T, Mannino DM, Moss M: Risk factors for ARDS in the United States: analysis of the 1993 National Mortality Followback Study. *Chest* 119:1179–1184, 2001.
46. Nussbaum MS, Fisher JE: Pathogenesis of hepatic steatosis during total parenteral nutrition. *Surg Ann* 223:1–11, 1991.
47. MacArthur C: Nutritional assessment and support. In *Respiratory care: principles and practice*, Boston, 2010, Jones & Bartlett, p 685.
48. Wong DT, Knaus WA: Predicting outcome in critical care: the current status of the APACHE prognostic scoring system. *Can J Anesth* 38:374–383, 1991.
49. Wheeler MM: APACHE: an evaluation. *Crit Care Nurs Q* 32:46–48, 2009.

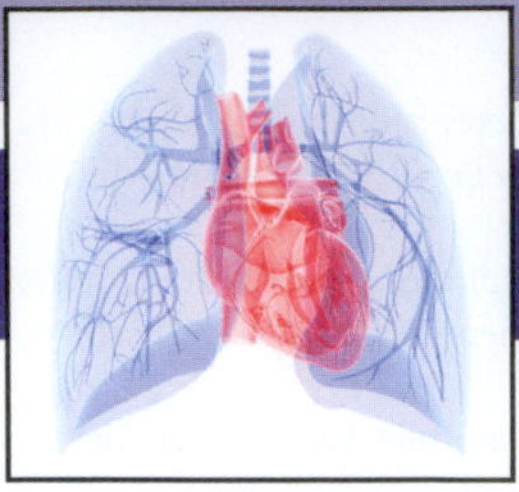

CHAPTER 52

Discontinuing Ventilatory Support

ROBERT M. KACMAREK

CHAPTER OBJECTIVES

After reading this chapter you will be able to:

- Discuss the relationship between ventilatory demand and ventilatory capacity as well as their relationship with ventilator discontinuance.
- List the factors associated with ventilator dependence.
- Explain how to evaluate a patient before attempting ventilator discontinuation or weaning.
- List acceptable values for specific weaning indices used to predict a patient's readiness for discontinuation of ventilatory support.
- Describe factors that should be optimized before an attempt is made at ventilator discontinuation or weaning.
- Describe techniques used in ventilator weaning, including daily spontaneous breathing trials, synchronized intermittent mandatory ventilation, pressure support ventilation, and other newer methods.
- Contrast the advantages and disadvantages associated with various weaning methods and techniques.
- Describe how to assess a patient for extubation.
- List the primary reasons why patients fail a ventilator discontinuance trial.
- Explain why some patients cannot be successfully weaned from ventilatory support.

CHAPTER OUTLINE

KEY TERMS

adaptive support ventilation (ASV)
airway occlusion pressure
automatic tube compensation (ATC)
continuous positive airway pressure (CPAP)
Intellivent
mandatory minute volume ventilation (MMV)
pressure support ventilation (PSV)
prolonged mechanical ventilation (PMV)
rapid, shallow breathing index (f/V_T)
spontaneous awaking trial (SAT)
spontaneous breathing trial (SBT)
synchronized intermittent mandatory ventilation (SIMV)

The purpose of mechanical ventilation is to support the patient until the disease state or condition that caused the need for support is alleviated or resolved. Ventilatory support can sustain life, but it cannot cure disease. Further, many complications and hazards are associated with mechanical ventilation. Consequently, ventilatory support should be withdrawn as soon as the patient is able to adequately resume spontaneous breathing.[1] All patients who are mechanically ventilated should be evaluated on a daily basis, beginning with the day of intubation, for their ability to wean from ventilatory support.[2,3] Frequently this evaluation is very quick, but it should be performed daily regardless of the patient's status.

After the problem or condition that caused the need for mechanical ventilation is resolved, most patients can be quickly and easily removed from ventilatory support. For example, for most patients who need mechanical ventilation as a result of drug overdose or severe asthma, for those who are recovering from postoperative anesthesia, and for those who have received ventilation for 72 hours or less, one may simply discontinue ventilation when the precipitating condition has resolved.[1,4] However, some patients require mechanical ventilation for longer periods. The term *ventilator dependent* is usually reserved for patients who need ventilatory support for lengthy periods (i.e., 2 weeks or more) or who have not responded to attempts at ventilator discontinuation. For these patients, a more prolonged ventilator discontinuation process is required.[1]

Ventilator discontinuation should be carefully timed. Premature removal from the ventilator may severely stress the cardiopulmonary system and delay the patient's recovery.[4] Premature discontinuation also exposes the patient to the hazards of reintubation. However, delays in discontinuing ventilation expose the patient to an increased risk of complications, including nosocomial pneumonia, myocardial infarction, and death.[4]

There are three basic methods for discontinuing ventilatory support[1]:

1. **Spontaneous breathing trials (SBTs)** alternating with mechanical ventilation
2. **Synchronized intermittent mandatory ventilation (SIMV)**
3. **Pressure support ventilation (PSV)**

Other techniques that may facilitate ventilator discontinuation include the use of volume-support ventilation (VSV); **adaptive support ventilation (ASV)/Intellivent**; automatic tube compensation (ATC); proportional assist ventilation (PAV), which is also known as *proportional pressure support* (PPS); neurally adjusted ventilatory assist (NAVA); and **continuous positive airway pressure (CPAP)**. However, little data exist that support the use of any of these techniques except for CPAP, which seems potentially beneficial during the ventilator discontinuation process.

Techniques for predicting when patients are ready for ventilator discontinuation and weaning have been studied extensively.[4] Many weaning indices designed to predict successful ventilatory discontinuation have been proposed. Despite this, there are no universally applicable indices for predicting success. Of all of the methods studied, SBTs and PSV have been shown to be the most effective methods for ventilator discontinuation and weaning. Evidence-based reviews recommend the use of at least daily SBTs.[1] Protocols for ventilator discontinuation administered by an interdisciplinary team of respiratory therapists, nurses, and physicians can be highly effective, and have been recommended.[1,4,5-9] Regardless of the method used, success is unlikely unless the precipitating problems that caused the ventilator dependency have been resolved.[1,4,9] After these problems are resolved, an organized plan or protocol should be followed, and variations should be based on each patient's response.[1,4,5]

Some patients cannot be successfully removed from mechanical ventilatory support. This group of ventilator-dependent patients poses clinical, economic, and ethical concerns.[10,11]

The term *weaning* has been used as a general term to refer to the process of discontinuing ventilatory support, regardless of the time frame or method involved. The term has also been used to refer to reductions in fractional inspired oxygen concentration (FiO_2), PEEP, and CPAP. Alternatively, the term *ventilator discontinuation* has been used to refer to the process of disconnecting a patient from mechanical ventilatory support. For the purposes of this chapter, the term *weaning* is defined as a gradual reduction in the level of ventilatory support, whereas *discontinuing ventilatory support* refers to the overall process of removing the patient from the ventilator, regardless of the method used. In general, patients who are being considered for removal from ventilatory support fall into one of five categories:

1. Those for whom removal is quick and routine, which is normally the vast majority of ventilated patients
2. Those who need a more systematic approach to discontinuing ventilatory support, which is normally about 15% to 20% of ventilated patients
3. Those who require days to weeks to wean from ventilatory support, which is usually less than 5% of ventilated patients
4. Those ventilator-dependent or "unweanable" patients, who compose less than 1% of patients who require ventilatory support
5. Those who have no chance for survival in whom the ventilator is discontinued while comfort measures are provided, normally referred to as terminal weaning.[12]

REASONS FOR VENTILATOR DEPENDENCE

Patients may require mechanical ventilation because of apnea, acute or impending ventilatory failure, or severe oxygenation problems that necessitate high levels of PEEP or CPAP. Regardless of the reason for initiating mechanical ventilation, patients remain dependent on the ventilator because of respiratory, cardiovascular, neurologic, or psychologic factors.[1]

Ventilatory Workload and Demand

Patients who need mechanical ventilation often have a ventilatory workload and demand that exceeds their ventilatory capacity. This is the most common cause of ventilator dependence.[1,4] The term *ventilatory workload* refers to the amount of work that the respiratory muscles are asked to perform to provide an appropriate level of ventilation. A patient's total ventilatory workload is primarily determined by the following: (1) the level of ventilation needed, (2) the compliance of the lungs and thorax, (3) the resistance to gas flow through the airways, and (4) any imposed work of breathing (WOB_I) due to ventilatory system mechanical factors.[1,4]

The level of ventilation required is determined by the following: (1) the metabolic rate; (2) the central nervous system (CNS) drive; and (3) the ventilatory dead space. Common causes of an increased demand for ventilation include increased carbon dioxide production (i.e., fever, shivering, agitation, trauma, or sepsis) and increased dead space (i.e., pulmonary emboli or chronic obstructive pulmonary disease [COPD]). Other common causes of increased ventilatory demand include metabolic acidosis, severe hypoxemia, pain, and anxiety.

Compliance is determined by the elastic nature of the lung–thorax system. Resistance is largely related to the nature of the conducting airways. Common causes of decreased lung compliance include atelectasis, pneumonia, pulmonary edema, acute lung injury, and acute respiratory distress syndrome. Thoracic compliance may be reduced because of obesity, ascites, or abdominal distention. Airway resistance increases with bronchospasm, excessive secretions, and mucosal edema.

Mechanical factors that can increase the work of breathing include artificial airways (i.e., endotracheal and tracheotomy tubes), partial obstruction of the airway, ventilator circuits, demand flow systems, auto-PEEP, and inappropriate ventilator flow and sensitivity settings. Factors that may increase ventilatory workload are summarized in Box 52-1.

Ventilatory Capacity

Ventilatory capacity is determined by CNS drive, ventilatory muscle strength, and ventilatory muscle endurance. Most patients who are being withdrawn from ventilatory support have a normal or an increased drive to breathe. Patients with neuromuscular disorders and those who are receiving sedatives, narcotics, or neuromuscular blocking agents may have a reduced drive to breathe or impaired neuromuscular transmission. Patients with metabolic alkalosis, hypothyroidism, and sleep deprivation also may have reduced ventilatory drive. Box 52-2 summarizes the factors that may reduce ventilatory drive.

Muscle strength is influenced by age, sex, muscle bulk, and overall health. Malnutrition, starvation, and electrolyte imbalances (especially involving calcium, magnesium, potassium, and phosphate) can lead to ventilatory muscle weakness. Critical illness myopathy, critical illness polyneuropathy, and the

Box 52-1 Factors That May Increase Ventilatory Workload

INCREASED VENTILATORY DEMAND: INCREASED LEVEL OF VENTILATION REQUIRED

- Increased CNS drive: hypoxia, acidosis, pain, fear, anxiety, and stimulation of J receptors (e.g., pulmonary edema)
- Increased metabolic rate: increased carbon dioxide production, fever, shivering, agitation, trauma, infection, and sepsis
- Increased dead space: COPD and pulmonary embolus

DECREASED COMPLIANCE

- Decreased lung compliance: atelectasis, pneumonia, fibrosis, pulmonary edema, and acute respiratory distress syndrome
- Decreased thoracic compliance: obesity, ascites, abdominal distention, and pregnancy

INCREASED RESISTANCE

- Increased airway resistance: bronchospasm, mucosal edema, and secretions
- Artificial airways: endotracheal tubes, tracheostomy tubes, and partial obstruction of the artificial airway or the patients airway
- Other mechanical factors: ventilator circuits, demand flow systems, and inappropriate ventilator flow or sensitivity settings

Box 52-2 Factors That May Reduce Ventilatory Drive

- Decreased $PaCO_2$ (respiratory alkalosis)
- Metabolic alkalosis
- Pain (visceral)
- Electrolyte imbalance
- Pharmacologic depressants (narcotics, sedatives)
- Fatigue
- Decreased metabolic rate
- Increased $PaCO_2$ associated with chronic carbon dioxide retention
- Neurologic or neuromuscular disease

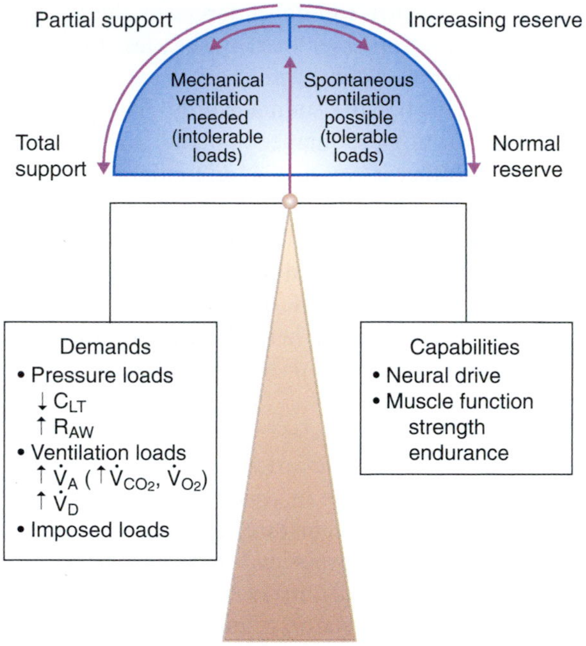

FIGURE 52-1 Ventilatory failure and the need for ventilatory support depend on the balance between ventilatory muscle demands (i.e., loads) and ventilatory muscle capabilities. C_{LT}, Lung–thorax compliance; *RAW,* airway resistance, $\dot{V}$, minute alveolar ventilation; $\dot{V}$, minute dead space ventilation. (Modified from MacIntyre NR: Respiratory factors in weaning from mechanical ventilatory support. Respir Care 40:244–259, 1995.)

prolonged use of neuromuscular blocking agents are major causes of the development of ventilatory muscle weakness in the intensive care unit (ICU).[13] Controlled ventilation for prolonged periods can result in ventilatory muscle discoordination and atrophy. Ventilatory muscle endurance is a function of energy supply versus demand. Energy supply is related to nutrition, perfusion, and cell use, whereas demand is related to the amount of work performed and is a function of minute ventilation, compliance, and resistance. Figure 52-1 summarizes the relationship between ventilatory demands and capabilities.

Global Criteria for Discontinuing Ventilatory Support

Success with the discontinuation of ventilatory support is related to the patient's condition in four main areas[1,2,3,4]:

1. Ventilatory workload versus ventilatory capacity
2. Oxygenation status
3. Cardiovascular function
4. Psychologic factors

Simply put, when ventilatory workload or demand exceeds ventilatory capacity, successful ventilator discontinuation is unlikely. Excessive ventilatory workload may lead to ventilatory muscle fatigue. When the ventilatory muscles fatigue, they must be rested for at least 24 hours to recover.[14] Ventilatory workload increases with decreased compliance, increased airway resistance, or an increased requirement for ventilation. Ventilatory capacity can be reduced by ventilatory muscle fatigue and by a loss of muscle strength and endurance.

Other factors that may contribute to ventilator dependence include inadequate arterial oxygenation, poor tissue oxygen delivery, myocardial ischemia, arrhythmias, low cardiac output, and cardiovascular instability. Neurologic problems that may contribute to ventilator dependence include decreased central drive to breathe and impaired peripheral nerve transmission. Psychologic issues that may contribute to ventilatory dependence include the fear of removal of the life-support system, anxiety, stress, depression, and sleep deprivation. Box 52-3 summarizes the major factors that contribute to ventilator dependence.

PATIENT EVALUATION

Careful patient assessment is required to determine which patients are ready to be removed from ventilatory support quickly, which patients may need a prolonged ventilator discontinuation phase, and which patients are not yet ready for the discontinuation of ventilatory support.

An important factor to consider as part of this assessment is the length of time that the patient has been receiving mechanical ventilation. In general, those who receive support for 72 hours or less often can be removed quickly from the ventilator.[15,16] Those who need a longer period of support may need a more prolonged approach. Current guidelines recommend that patients who need mechanical ventilation for more than 48 to 72 hours be carefully assessed to determine all of the possible causes of ventilator dependence.[1,4] These include the respiratory, cardiovascular, neurologic, and psychologic causes of ventilator dependence that are listed in Box 52-3. This recommendation is especially important for the care of patients who have had unsuccessful attempts at the discontinuation of ventilation.[1,4] Factors associated with readiness for the discontinuation of ventilatory support are summarized in Box 52-4.

The Most Important Criterion

The single most important criterion to consider when evaluating a patient for ventilator discontinuation or weaning is whether there has been significant alleviation or reversal of the disease state or condition that necessitated use of the ventilator in the first place.[1,4,9] The clinician should determine whether the patient's condition is improving, whether the initial reason for providing ventilatory support is improved or resolved, and

Box 52-3 Factors That Contribute to Ventilator Dependence

RESPIRATORY FACTORS

- Ventilatory workload exceeds ventilatory capacity
- Decreased compliance: lung or chest wall
- Increased resistance: artificial airways, bronchospasm, mucosal edema, secretions, and mechanical demand flow systems
- Increased dead space: pulmonary embolus and COPD
- Ventilatory muscle weakness or fatigue
- Oxygenation problems
  - ↓ $\dot{V}/\dot{Q}$
  - Increased shunt
  - ↓ DO_2
  - ↓ Oxygen extraction ratio

NONRESPIRATORY FACTORS

- Cardiovascular factors
- Myocardial ischemia
- Heart failure
- Hemodynamic instability, hypotension, and arrhythmias
- Neurologic factors
- Decreased or increased central drive to breathe
- Decreased peripheral nerve transmission
- Psychologic factors
- Fear and anxiety
- Stress
- Confusion or altered mental status
- Depression
- Poor nutrition
- Multiple-system organ failure
- Equipment shortcomings

Data from MacIntyre N: Respiratory factors in weaning from mechanical ventilatory support. Respir Care 40:244, 1995; Slutsky AS: Mechanical ventilation. American College of Chest Physicians' Consensus Conference. Chest 104:1833–1859, 1993; Pierson DJ: Nonrespiratory aspects of weaning from mechanical ventilation. Respir Care 40:263–270, 1995; MacIntyre NR, Cook DJ, Ely EW Jr, et al; American College of Chest Physicians; American Association for Respiratory Care; American College of Critical Care Medicine: Evidence-based guidelines for weaning and discontinuing ventilatory support: a collective task force facilitated by the American College of Chest Physicians; the American Association for Respiratory Care; and the American College of Critical Care Medicine. Chest 120(6 Suppl):375S–395S, 2001.

Box 52-4 Factors Associated With Readiness for the Discontinuation of Ventilatory Support

- Reversal or partial reversal of reason for instituting mechanical ventilation
- Good baseline functional status
- Ventilatory capacity that is capable of meeting ventilatory workload
- Good oxygenation status
- Good cardiovascular performance
- Good functional status of other organs and systems
- Short duration of the critical illness
- Short duration of mechanical ventilation
- No psychologic factors affecting current status

Modified from Pierson DJ: Nonrespiratory aspects of weaning from mechanical ventilation. Respir Care 40:263–270, 1995.

whether the patient's clinical condition is stable. The following specific questions for patient evaluation have been suggested[1]:

1. Is there evidence of improvement or reversal of the disease state or condition that caused the need for mechanical ventilation?
2. Is the patient's oxygenation status adequate? Specific criteria may include the following: PaO_2 of 60 mm Hg or more, FiO_2 of less than 0.40 to 0.50, PEEP of less than 5 to 8 cm H_2O; PaO_2/FiO_2 of 150 to 200 or more; and pH of 7.25 or more.
3. Is the patient medically and hemodynamically stable? Specific criteria may include the absence of acute myocardial ischemia or marked hypotension. Patients should have adequate blood pressure without vasopressor therapy or with only low-dose vasopressor therapy (i.e., less than 5 μg/kg/min of dopamine or dobutamine).
4. Can the patient breathe spontaneously? The patient must be able to breathe spontaneously and have a sufficient drive to breathe if ventilator discontinuation is being considered.

If the patient's condition is improving, if the alleviation or reversal of the precipitating disease state or condition has occurred, if the patient is capable of spontaneous breathing, and if the oxygenation status and hemodynamic values are stable, then ventilator discontinuation should be attempted.[1]

Weaning Indices

Mechanical ventilation is hazardous, and unnecessary delays in ventilator discontinuation increase the associated complication rate. Unfortunately, premature ventilator discontinuation may also cause serious problems, including difficulty with reestablishing the artificial airway and serious compromise of the patient's clinical status. Clinical judgment has been found to be a poor guide to determining whether a patient is ready for ventilator discontinuation, and more specific indicators have been sought. Specific indicators or weaning indices that clearly show whether a patient is ready to have the ventilator removed and help to avoid inappropriate ventilator discontinuation have been sought. Unfortunately, none of the current weaning indices are capable of predicting readiness for ventilator discontinuance with a high level of accuracy.[1,4]

Traditional discontinuation indices include the PaO_2/FiO_2 ratio, the alveolar-to-arterial partial pressure of oxygen difference $[P(A - a)O_2]$, the maximum inspiratory pressure (MIP), the vital capacity (VC), the spontaneous minute ventilation (V_{Esp}), and the maximum voluntary ventilation (MVV).[3,17] Newer indices include the **rapid, shallow breathing index (f/VT)**, **airway occlusion pressure** ($P_{0.1}$), and measures of WOB.[1,4] Although all of these values can be useful, there are enormous discrepancies in the literature regarding their accuracy with regard to the prediction of "weanability."[1,4] With respect to the more traditional discontinuation indices, vital capacity and MIP can be highly variable, whereas minute ventilation, respiratory rate (f), and f/V_T tend to be more reliable.[1,4] However, these measures may not correlate well with discontinuation success among all patients and especially among those receiving long-term ventilatory support, the elderly, and those with major pulmonary abnormalities.[1,4,18]

A comprehensive evidence-based review identified a possible role for 66 specific measurements as predictors of weaning success.[4] Of these, eight values were found to be the most useful for the prediction of successful ventilator discontinuation.[1,4] Useful predictive measures included spontaneous respiratory rate, spontaneous tidal volume, f/V_T, minute ventilation, MIP, $P_{0.1}$, $P_{0.1}$/MIP, and a combined index called the *CROP score* that included compliance, respiratory rate, oxygenation, and MIP.[1,4] Unfortunately, these measures all have limitations and relatively high false-positive predictions in specific settings.

It is doubtful that a single index will be found that can be used for consistent discrimination between discontinuation success and failure. Moreover, none of these traditional indicators alone has proved useful for the prediction of improvements in patient outcome or in the selection of a particular discontinuation method.[5] The likely explanation for this failure to identify any consistently powerful discontinuation predictor is that patients' conditions vary greatly and, for research purposes, clinicians already fully consider information from predictors when choosing patients for trials of the reduction or discontinuation of ventilatory support.[5,18]

Notwithstanding these limitations, the measurement of discontinuation indices in the difficult-to-wean patient may provide guidance with regard to the reasons that patients fail discontinuation trials. Many find it useful to trend these data on a daily basis for those patients who require lengthy weaning times.[10,15] Specific values for respiratory indices that are used to predict the successful discontinuation of ventilatory support are found in Table 52-1.

TABLE 52-1

Indices That Are Used to Predict the Success of Weaning and Ventilator Discontinuation

Measurement	Criterion
Oxygenation	
FiO_2	≤0.40 to 0.50
PEEP (cm H_2O)	≤5 to 8
PaO_2 (mm Hg)	≥60
SaO_2 (%)	≥90
SvO_2 (%)	≥60
PaO_2/PAO_2 ratio	≥0.35
PaO_2/FiO_2 ratio	>150 to 200
$P(A-a)O_2$ (mm Hg)	<350
$\dot{Q}_s\dot{Q}_T$ (% shunt)	<15% to 20%
No lactic acidosis, adequate $\dot{Q}_s\dot{Q}_T$, blood pressure	
Ventilation	
$PaCO_2$ (mm Hg)	<50
pH	≥7.35
Ventilatory Mechanics	
Respiratory rate (f) (breaths/min)	12 to 30
Tidal volume (V_T) (ml/kg)	>5
Vital capacity (VC) (ml/kg)	>10 to 15
Static compliance (ml/cm H_2O)	>25
f/V_T	<105
Respiratory Muscle Strength	
Maximum inspiratory force (MIF) (cm H_2O)	<–20 to –30
Ventilatory Drive (Demand)	
Minute ventilation ($\dot{V}_E$) for	
Normal PCO_2 (L/min)	<10
V_{DS}/V_T	<0.55 to 0.60
$P_{0.1}$ (cm H_2O)	<6
$P_{0.1}$/MIP	<0.30
Work of Breathing	
Spontaneous work of breathing	<1.6 kg·m/min (<0.14 kg·m/L)
Pressure-time index	<0.15 to 0.18
Ventilatory Reserve	
Maximum voluntary ventilation (MVV) (L/min)	>20; more than twice the $\dot{V}_E$

Data from MacIntyre NR, Cook DJ, Ely EW, et al: Evidence-based guidelines for weaning and discontinuing ventilator support: a collective task force facilitated by the American College of Chest Physicians, the American Association for Respiratory Care, and the American College of Critical Care Medicine. Chest 120:375S-395S, 2001; AHRQ publication no. 01-E010, Rockville, MD, 2000, Agency for Healthcare Research and Quality; American College of Chest Physicians: Chest 104:1833, 1993; Burns SM et al: Am J Crit Care 4:4, 1995; Sharar S: Resp Care 40:239, 1995; Bassili HR, Deitel M: JPEN J Parenter Enteral Nutr 5:161, 1981.

Ventilation

Increased thoracic cage movement during spontaneous breathing and asynchronous chest-wall-to-diaphragm movement are related to an increased workload that may lead to ventilatory muscle fatigue and failure. Tachypnea (i.e., more than 30 to 35 breaths/min in adults) is a sensitive marker of respiratory distress, but it can prolong intubation if it is used as an exclusive criterion. Irregular spontaneous breathing or periods of apnea indicate that the patient is at risk for weaning failure. Asynchronous and rapid, shallow breathing patterns—although not definitive—suggest respiratory decompensation.[18] However, decreased ventilatory variability over time (rate, V_T, minute ventilation) has been clearly shown to identify patients who will failure an SBT.[19,20]

The evaluation of patients for the presence of palpable scalene muscle use during inspiration, an irregular ventilatory pattern, palpable abdominal muscle tensing during expiration, and the inability to alter the ventilatory pattern on command can be helpful for the assessment of the potential for prolonged spontaneous ventilation. Patients with none of these signs have a very high probability of successful ventilator discontinuance. Patients with one or two of these signs usually need continued support. The presence of three or more of these signs can mean that the patient's condition is unstable and that the patient has a poor prognosis for ventilator removal.[21]

$P_{0.1}$ is the inspiratory pressure that is measured 100 milliseconds after airway occlusion.[1,4] The $P_{0.1}$ is effort independent, and it correlates well with central respiratory drive. Ventilator-dependent patients with COPD who have a $P_{0.1}$ of more than 6 cm H_2O tend to be difficult to wean.[1,4]

The f/V_T is the ratio of spontaneous breathing frequency (breaths/min) to tidal volume (liters), and it has been found to be a good predictor of discontinuation success for many patients who need mechanical ventilation.[1,4,18] The f/V_T has less predictive ability for patients who need ventilatory support for longer than 8 days, and it may be less useful for predicting discontinuation success among elderly patients.[1,4] Despite these limitations, an f/V_T of less than 105 can be an accurate and early predictor of weaning outcome, and an f/V_T of 80 is associated with an almost 95% probability of successful discontinuation.[18] The ratio must be calculated during 1 minute of unsupported spontaneous breathing, and the addition of pressure support during measurement significantly reduces the predictive value of the ratio.[18]

RULE OF THUMB

Adult patients with spontaneous respiratory rates in excess of 35 breaths/min and tidal volumes of less than 5 ml/kg PBW are difficult to wean.

The $P_{0.1}$/MIP ratio has been found to be a good early predictor of discontinuation success,[1,4] and it may be more useful than the MIP by itself. The f/V_T also has been found to be a better predictor of discontinuation success than the MIP alone.[1,4] However, even with f/V_T of less than 105, as many as 20% of patients have false-positive results (i.e., they cannot be discontinued from ventilation despite a favorable index) as a result of unpredictable factors such as congestive heart failure, aspiration, other comorbidities or the development of a new pulmonary lesion. In addition, some patients can be successfully discontinued from ventilatory support despite poor f/V_T values (>105).

MINI CLINI

Calculating and Interpreting the Rapid, Shallow Breathing Index

PROBLEM: You measure the following spontaneous breathing values for two patients who are being considered for weaning from mechanical ventilation:

Patient	Rate (f) (breaths/min)	V_T (L)
A	32	0.28
B	28	0.42

For which patient is successful weaning least likely?

Solution: First, compute the rapid, shallow breathing index for each patient as follows:

Patient	Rate (f) (breaths/min)	V_T (L)	f/V_T
A	32	0.28	114
B	28	0.42	67

Patient A clearly exceeds the threshold criterion of 105 breaths/min per liter, whereas patient B falls well below this criterion. All else being equal, patient A is least likely to be successfully weaned.

WOB would seem to be an excellent way to gauge spontaneous ventilatory workload. Successful weaning has been found to be less likely among patients with spontaneous WOB levels of more than 1.6 kg/m/min (16 J/min) or 0.14 kg/m/L (1.4 J/L).[1,4] However, WOB may not be predictive of weaning success for specific patients.[1,4] This may be because WOB does not take into account ventilatory muscle capacity or fatigue. Consequently, WOB may be less accurate than other conventional discontinuation indices, and it is very difficult to measure at the bedside.

Oxygen cost of breathing (OCB) is the difference between oxygen consumption during spontaneous breathing and oxygen consumption during apnea (i.e., during full ventilatory support), which is determined as follows:

$$OCB = VO_{2sp} - VO_2\ (\text{controlled ventilation})$$

After the OCB has been estimated, the relative proportion of oxygen consumed by the respiratory muscles as compared with the body as a whole can be calculated as follows:

$$\%VO_2\ (\text{Resp}) = (OCB/VO_{2sp}) \times 100$$

Both OCB and $\%VO_2$ have been correlated with the number of days required to wean patients. Patients with an OCB of 15% or less of the total VO_2 may be more likely to achieve discontinuation success.[1,4]

Pressure–time product (i.e., the area under the inspiratory pressure–time curve) and pressure–time index (PTI) may be the best measures of ventilatory workload of patients who are receiving mechanical support.[1] The PTI can be calculated as follows:

$$PTI = (\text{Mean inspiratory pressure}/MIP) \times T_i/T_{tot}$$

where MIP is maximum inspiratory pressure, T_i is the inspiratory time in seconds, and T_{tot} is the total respiratory cycle. The T_{tot} can be calculated by dividing 60 by the respiratory rate (f) (i.e., 60/f). A PTI of more than 0.15 to 0.18 has been associated with diaphragmatic fatigue, and a PTI of more than 0.15 cannot be sustained indefinitely.[1,4] There is currently no well accepted and reliable way to measure ventilatory muscle fatigue in patients who are receiving mechanical ventilation.

Oxygenation

Poor oxygenation status is associated with weaning failure. Arterial blood gas (ABG) analysis, pulse oximetry, and continuous mixed venous oximetry have been used to monitor and assess the oxygenation status of patients before and during a discontinuation trial. In general, a PaO_2 of more than 60 mm Hg (or of more than 55 mm Hg for patients with COPD with carbon dioxide retention) with an FiO_2 of less than 0.40 to 0.50 and a PEEP of 5 to 8 cm H_2O or less should be adequate for ventilator discontinuation. The PaO_2/FiO_2 ratio should be 150 to 200 mm Hg or more. With these values, a normal hemoglobin level, a normal oxygen saturation (SaO_2), and adequate cardiac output and tissue perfusion are assumed. Specific indices used to assess oxygenation status are found in Table 52-1.

Acid-Base Balance

Ideally the patient should have a normal acid-base balance (i.e., a pH of 7.35 to 7.45), and abnormalities in acid-base status have been corrected, if possible, before weaning. Patients with metabolic acidosis often have an increased ventilatory drive that can make weaning difficult. Patients who have metabolic alkalosis or those who have been mechanically hyperventilated for several days may have a reduced ventilatory drive. In these cases, a gradual method of discontinuing ventilatory support may be necessary.

Metabolic Factors

Metabolic factors primarily affect discontinuation in those patients who require long-term ventilatory support. Although nutritional factors are important for all patients, they are unlikely to affect discontinuation in those who only require short-term ventilatory support. Nutrition should be adequate to maintain respiratory muscle mass and contractile force. Feeding should be adjusted according to individual patient needs; most patients need 1.5 to 2.0 times their resting energy expenditure. In addition, protein intake should be between 1 and 1.5 g/kg per day. Excessive carbohydrate feeding can increase carbon dioxide production and may precipitate acute hypercapnic respiratory failure. Parenteral nutrition solutions that contain amino acid formulations (e.g., arginine/lysine) can cause metabolic acidosis and thus increase ventilatory demand. Metabolic rate can increase as a result of fever or sepsis. Increased WOB, shivering, seizures, and agitation can also increase oxygen demand and should be evaluated (see Chapter 23).

Renal Function and Electrolytes

Adequate renal function is required to maintain acid-base homeostasis, electrolyte concentrations, and fluid balance. The patient ideally should have an adequate urine output (i.e., more than 1000 ml/day), and there should be no inappropriate weight gain or edema.

Renal insufficiency can lead to metabolic acidosis, which increases respiratory drive. Electrolyte disorders can impair ventilatory muscle function. Key electrolytes should be normal (see Chapter 17 for details). Fluid overload can lead to congestive heart failure and pulmonary edema, which may impair pulmonary gas exchange.

Cardiovascular Function

Adequate cardiovascular function is needed to provide sufficient oxygen delivery to the tissues. Cardiac rate and rhythm and blood pressure should be evaluated. Tachycardia (i.e., a heart rate of more than 100 beats/min) and bradycardia (i.e., a heart rate of less than 60 beats/min) should be controlled. The presence of arrhythmias, hypotension (i.e., a blood pressure of less than 90/60 mm Hg), and severe hypertension (i.e., a blood pressure of more than 180/110 mm Hg) should be evaluated carefully before the discontinuation of ventilatory support is considered.

TABLE 52-2
Criteria for Confirming Cardiovascular Stability

Criterion	Normal Value	Values That May Be Inconsistent With Weaning
Heart rate (beats/min)	60 to 100	<60, >120
Blood pressure (mm Hg)	90/60 to 150/90	<90/60, >180/110
$\dot{Q}_t$ (L/min)	4 to 8	<4, >8
Cardiac index ($L/min^{-1} \cdot m^2$)	2.5 to 4	<2.1
Cardiac rhythm	No major arrhythmias present	Tachycardia, bradycardia, multiple premature ventricular contractions, heart block
Hemoglobin (g/dl)	12 to 15	Anemia, <8
Hematocrit	40% to 50%	<35%
No angina present		
No lactic acidosis		

Cardiac output and index measurements as well as central venous pressure measurements may be helpful for the evaluation of cardiovascular function. Left ventricular dysfunction, myocardial ischemia, and cardiovascular instability are associated with decreased discontinuation success.[1,4] Table 52-2 provides criteria for confirming cardiovascular stability.

Psychologic Factors and Central Nervous System Assessment

Adequate CNS function is needed to ensure stable ventilatory drive, adequate secretion clearance (i.e., coughing and deep breathing), and the protection of the airway (i.e., gag reflex and swallow). In addition, the level of consciousness, dyspnea, anxiety, depression, and motivation can affect discontinuation success.[1,4]

The patient ideally is awake and alert, free of seizures, and able to follow instructions. Patients should have an intact central drive to breathe and peripheral nerve function. Brainstem strokes, electrolyte disturbances, sedation, neuromuscular blocking agents, and narcotic drugs can impair the central neurologic control of ventilation. Mental status is a good predictor of discontinuation success, and patients who are not alert are at risk for upper airway obstruction, aspiration, and secretion retention. Obtunded patients should, at a minimum, have an adequate gag reflex and cough. Decreased levels of consciousness are associated with aspiration after extubation. The level of consciousness is affected by the use of narcotic, sedative, and analgesic drugs. Drugs with CNS depressant effects should be discontinued, if possible, before the withdrawal of ventilatory support and extubation. Protocols to reduce sedation and the daily cessation of sedative drugs may reduce weaning time[7,22,23] (see the section on Spontaneous Awaking Trials). Neuromuscular blocking agents to allow for controlled ventilation should only be administered when absolutely necessary to insure patient-ventilator interaction and for the shortest period possible.[24]

Psychologic factors may be among the most important nonrespiratory contributing factors that lead to ventilator dependence.[1,4] Fear, anxiety, pain, and stress should be minimized, and frequent communication among the staff, the patient, and the patient's family can be helpful. Box 52-5 summarizes nonrespiratory factors that affect discontinuation success.

Integrated Indices

Many factors are associated with discontinuation success. Integrated indices improve prediction by combining several measures of ability to breathe without ventilatory support. Current examples of integrated indices include the CROP score, the Adverse Factor/Ventilator Score, the weaning index, and the Burns Weaning Assessment Program.[1,4] The CROP score combines measures of ventilatory load, respiratory muscle strength, and gas exchange.

The Adverse Factor/Ventilator Score combines ratings of 15 adverse factors, including hemodynamic values, infection, nutrition, and neurologic/psychiatric state, with ratings of six ventilator factors, including FiO_2, compliance, minute ventilation, and rate.[1,4] The weaning index combines measures of ventilatory strength, endurance, and efficiency of gas exchange. A weaning index of less than 4 suggests successful discontinuation from mechanical ventilation. The Burns Weaning Assessment Program is a 26-item assessment that combines 12 general and 14 respiratory factors into a single score.[1,4] Although integrated indices appear promising, none of these indices has emerged as superior for use in diverse patient populations. Despite the success of these integrated indices in very specific settings, the best approach to determining if a patient can be successfully discontinued from ventilatory support is the patient's performance on a spontaneous breathing trial. All patients should be assessed daily, and their ability to breathe spontaneously should be the primary variable to determine if the ventilator can be discontinued.

Box 52-5 Nonrespiratory Factors That Affect Weaning

- Acid-base status
- Metabolic alkalosis: decreased ventilatory drive
- Metabolic acidosis: increased ventilatory demand
- Mineral and electrolyte balance
- Hypophosphatemia: ventilatory muscle weakness
- Hypomagnesemia: ventilatory muscle weakness
- Hypokalemia: ventilatory muscle weakness
- Hypothyroidism: decreased ventilatory drive and impaired muscle function
- Stability of other organs and systems
- Cardiac: excessive preload (e.g., overall volume overload, increased preload on discontinuation of positive pressure ventilation) and impaired contractility
- Renal: renal insufficiency and metabolic acidosis
- Hepatic: encephalopathy and protein synthesis
- Gastrointestinal: stress-related hemorrhage and ability to take enteral nutrition
- Neurologic: level of consciousness, ability to protect the airway, and clear secretions
- Effects of drugs: narcotics, benzodiazepines, other sedatives and hypnotics, muscle relaxants, and aminoglycosides
- Nutritional status
- Ventilatory muscle function
- Ventilatory drive
- Immune defense system
- Psychologic and motivational factors

Modified from Pierson DJ: Nonrespiratory aspects of weaning from mechanical ventilation. Respir Care 40:289, 1995.

MINI CLINI

Assessment of Readiness for a Spontaneous Breathing Trial

PROBLEM: A 64-year-old man who underwent a lung resection and who has a long history of COPD is now 24 hours postoperative, and he is being evaluated for readiness for an SBT. The data currently available for this patient include the following:

- Ventilator settings:
  - Mode pressure support 10 cm H_2O
  - Average V_T 450 ml (6.5 ml/kg ideal body weight)
- Respiratory rate of 28 breaths/min
- FiO_2 of 0.40
- PEEP of 5 cm H_2O

The patient is alert and cooperative.

The patient is not receiving any vasoactive drugs, and he is only receiving intermittent sedatives and narcotics.

Should this patient be placed on an SBT?

Solution: By 24 hours, the patient should have initially recovered from the effects of the surgical procedure. The patient's ventilator settings are offering minimal support. Because the patient is alert and able to breathe spontaneously and because he requires only intermittent sedatives or narcotics, it is very appropriate to perform an SBT on this patient at this time.

Evaluation of the Airway

The ability to maintain a patent natural airway and the likelihood of aspiration should be evaluated as a part of the process of discontinuing ventilatory support. It is important for the clinician to separate the decision to discontinue ventilatory support from the decision to extubate. The clinician must also be aware that most weaning indices do not evaluate airway patency or protection (see the section on Extubation). The inability to protect or maintain the natural airway is a clear contraindication to extubation. Some patients who can be successfully removed from a ventilator should not be extubated. Although controversial, evaluating if gas moves freely around the ETT with the cuff deflated may identify an increased likelihood of postextubation airway obstruction. If auscultation of the lateral neck does not identify gas flow around the EET, extubation should be delayed until airway edema is properly treated with steroids. Tracheotomy may be considered for patients who need artificial airways for an extended period.

Tracheotomy may improve patient comfort, allow for more effective suctioning, decrease airway resistance, enhance mobility, and allow the patient to eat and speak. Some patients also need high levels of sedation to tolerate the endotracheal tube. Consequently, tracheotomy should be considered for the care of patients who are likely to benefit and for those who need prolonged mechanical ventilatory support. See Chapter 36 for details about airway management and extubation.

Other patients with good airway patency and protection may be unable to maintain spontaneous breathing for prolonged periods without assistance.[29] These patients may be candidates for noninvasive ventilation (NIV) after extubation; see Chapter 49 for details.[25,26]

PREPARING THE PATIENT

Optimizing the Patient's Medical Condition

Before the removal of ventilatory support is attempted, the patient's oxygenation status, ventilation, cardiovascular status, and overall medical condition should be optimized. Disease-imposed ventilatory load is minimized with the management of infection, bronchospasm, and airway edema. Bronchodilator therapy should be maximized and the appropriate use of anti-inflammatory agents considered. Techniques to facilitate secretion clearance (e.g., suctioning, adequate humidification, bronchial hygiene techniques), good nutrition, and optimal positioning should be used. The patient should be rested and not fatigued or sleep deprived, which can be common in the ICU. The patient should be allowed to sleep at night while maintained on a level of ventilatory support that ensures ventilatory muscle rest.[27] Intrinsic PEEP during mechanical ventilation may increase trigger work, and small amounts of PEEP or CPAP can help to overcome this problem.[1,2] Box 52-6 lists factors that should be optimized before ventilatory support is discontinued.

Patients' Psychologic and Communication Needs

As many as 47% of patients who spend more than 5 days in an ICU may experience psychologic disturbances.[27] The cause may be the stress of critical illness, the interruption of nighttime sleep, or the use of sedatives, tranquilizers, hypnotics, narcotics, and other drugs that affect the CNS.[27] The patient's environment should be optimized, anxiety and depression should be evaluated, and communication should be maximized.

Environmental considerations that may improve the patient's sense of well-being and outlook include reducing extraneous noise and providing clocks, calendars, pictures, a radio, a television, and, if possible, a room with windows. Daily mobility should be considered, including getting the patient up in a chair or placing the patient in the hall in a chair. Patients whose condition has been stable can sometimes even be helped to walk

Box 52-6 Factors That Should Be Optimized Before the Discontinuation of Ventilatory Support Is Attempted

- Oxygenation
- PaO_2 and SaO_2
- Anemia, if present
- Atelectasis, pneumonia, and acute pulmonary disease
- Ventilation
- Humidification
- Secretion clearance (e.g., bronchial hygiene, suctioning)
- Bronchodilator therapy
- Respiratory alkalosis
- Imposed WOB
- Respiratory muscle fatigue or atrophy
- Acid-base balance and electrolytes
- Metabolic acidosis (e.g., lactic acidosis, ketoacidosis)
- Metabolic alkalosis (e.g., decreased serum potassium or chloride ions, nasogastric tube, vomiting)
- Low phosphate level
- Low magnesium level
- Cardiac and cardiovascular status
- Blood pressure and cardiac output
- Arrhythmias, if present
- Myocardial ischemia
- Left ventricular function
- Renal factors
- Kidney function
- Fluid balance
- Fever, infection, or sepsis
- Pain (i.e., minimize without oversedation)
- Sleep deprivation
- Drugs (narcotics, sedatives, tranquilizers, hypnotics, aminoglycosides, and neuromuscular blocking agents can depress or block the ventilatory drive)
- Psychologic status
- Level of consciousness (e.g., delirium, coma)
- Agitation
- Motivation
- Fear and anxiety
- Psychologic dependence on the ventilator
- Depression
- ICU psychosis
- Hypothyroidism
- Nutritional factors
- Overfeeding (i.e., increased carbon dioxide production)
- Malnutrition or protein loss
- Consider a high-fat, low-carbohydrate diet to minimize the production of carbon dioxide
- Gastrointestinal bleeding or obstruction
- Abdominal distention or ascites
- Time of day (avoid evenings, nights, and shift changes)
- Adequate staffing
- Interruptions and disruptions
- Technical factors

Modified from Hess DR, Kacmarek RM: Essentials of mechanical ventilation, ed 2, New York, 2003, McGraw Hill; Kacmarek RM, Mack CW, Dimus S: Essentials of respiratory care, ed 4, St. Louis, 2005, Mosby; and Tobin MJ: Principles and practice of mechanical ventilation, ed 2, McGraw Hill, 2006, New York.

with the use of an E cylinder for oxygen, a transport ventilator or ICU ventilator with appropriate battery support, and two or more health care workers for support.

A method for the patient to communicate with staff and visitors should be devised, if possible. Writing tablets, picture boards, and alphabet boards have been used effectively by patients to communicate with staff and visitors.

Anxiety and agitation should be minimized, and communication and encouragement may be helpful. The patient should be told what is planned and be given some control over the situation. Patients should be asked to participate and help in the weaning process. Depression or a lack of motivation may increase weaning time. If depression is present, assessment and treatment by an appropriate health care provider should be considered.

CAREGIVER PREPARATION

Just like careful patient preparation, caregiver preparation should occur before the onset on an SBT, the respiratory therapist needs to be properly prepared to perform the SBT. The orders should be checked and equipment should be gathered. Specifically, oxygen therapy, NIV, and reintubation equipment should be gathered and readied for use. The patient should be carefully assessed, the ventilator alarms properly set, and the patient emotionally prepared for the SBT. Patients should be aware that the SBT is a trial and that they may fail the trial. The patient should NOT consider a failed trial as a step backwards but as a part of a process to become independent of the ventilator and should know that a number of SBTs are commonly necessary before the ventilator is discontinued.

METHODS

There are three basic methods of discontinuing ventilatory support[1,4]:

1. Spontaneous breathing trials (via the mechanical ventilator or with a T-piece) alternating with mechanical ventilatory support
2. SIMV
3. PSV

Box 52-7 summarizes evidence-based criteria and related conclusions regarding methods for ventilator discontinuation.

Box 52-7 Agency for Healthcare Research and Quality Summary of Evidence for Criteria for Weaning from Mechanical Ventilation

- Differences in clinicians' intuitive thresholds for the reduction or discontinuation of ventilatory support have a far greater impact on the failure of SBTs and on reintubation than do modes of discontinuation. When clinicians set a high threshold, many patients who could tolerate weaning remain on mechanical support longer than is necessary.
- There may be an interaction between the threshold and the mode of discontinuation; in other words, one mode may be superior when the threshold is high, whereas another may be superior when the threshold is low.
- Research to date suggests that the best answer to the question of when to start discontinuation trials is to develop a protocol that can be implemented by nurses and respiratory therapists that begins testing for the opportunity to reduce support immediately after intubation and reduces support at every opportunity.
- For stepwise reductions in mechanical support, pressure support mode or multiple daily spontaneous breathing trials are superior to SIMV.
- For trials of unassisted breathing, low levels of pressure support may be beneficial in select patients.
- There may be substantial benefits to the use of noninvasive positive pressure ventilation immediately following discontinuation and extubation.
- After cardiac surgery, early extubation is achieved with a variety of interventions and ICU protocols.
- Although steroids can reduce postextubation stridor in children, the impact of steroids on reintubation in children and adults remains uncertain.
- Most theoretically plausible predictors of discontinuation and extubation success have no predictive power. Those with some predictive power include the rapid, shallow breathing index, which has been most intensively studied, the $P_{0.1}$/MIP ratio, and the CROP index. However, these are relatively weak predictors of discontinuation success.
- Tests are rarely useful for increasing the probability of discontinuation success; on occasion, the results can lead to moderate increases in the probability of success.
- In general, discontinuation predictors are probably found to perform poorly because physicians have already considered the results when they select patients for studies.

Modified from the Agency for Healthcare Research and Quality: Evidence report/technology assessment Number 23 (AHRQ Publication No. 01-E010), Rockville, Md, 2000, Agency for Healthcare Research and Quality.

Rapid Ventilator Discontinuation

When the precipitating disease state or condition that necessitates support has been significantly alleviated or reversed, most patients can be rapidly removed from mechanical ventilation.[1,4] These patients typically have acceptable blood gas levels with mechanical ventilation, adequate myocardial function, and no underlying cardiovascular, pulmonary, neurologic, or neuromuscular disorders. After a careful evaluation, patients in stable condition who have been treated with a ventilator for less than 72 hours and who have a good spontaneous respiratory rate and minute ventilation may undergo an SBT on the ventilator or with a T-piece for 30 to 120 minutes.[1,4,28] If the patient does well, the endotracheal tube can then be removed if there is no reason to maintain an artificial airway.

Today, most SBTs are performed with the patient attached to a ventilator that is set on zero PSV and zero CPAP. This allows for a stable FiO_2 and ongoing monitoring. Others have recommended treating the patient with a low level of PSV (i.e., 5 to 7 cm H_2O) to overcome the resistance caused by the ventilator circuit, the demand flow system, and the artificial airway.[1,4] Others may prefer simply using CPAP (i.e., 5 to 7 cm H_2O). These methods have the advantage of allowing the clinician to maintain ventilator alarm settings that can provide a margin of safety in the event of apnea or severe hypoventilation. Low levels of CPAP may be useful for maintaining lung volumes and overcoming intrinsic PEEP. Some experts recommend PSV in combination with PEEP or CPAP.[2] However, the most widely accepted guidelines recommend a simple spontaneous breathing trial for the first SBT using the ventilator at zero CPAP and zero PEEP or a T-piece.[1,4]

Patients Who Need Progressive Weaning of Ventilatory Support

Patients who have been receiving mechanical ventilation for more than 72 hours and those with marginal oxygenation, ventilatory, cardiovascular, or medical statuses may need a more prolonged period for ventilator discontinuation.[1,4] The most common method for accomplishing this is SBTs interspersed with continued ventilatory support.

Spontaneous Breathing Trials

The oldest discontinuation method is an SBT via either the ventilator or T-piece, which allows for spontaneous breathing several times per day interspersed with periods of mechanical ventilatory support. For gradual weaning, initial SBTs may last only 5 to 10 minutes. Full ventilatory support is resumed for a 1- to 4-hour rest period in the assist/control or pressure-support mode. The time off of the ventilator is gradually increased until the patient is able to stay off of the ventilator for an extended period. SBTs can progress rapidly to ventilator removal.

When weaning is very difficult, the process can last days or even weeks. When a T-piece is used instead of the ventilator, the patient must be more carefully monitored, because none of the ventilator alarms are active during the SBT. If distress occurs, mechanical ventilation is resumed. In no case should the patient be overstressed during the SBT, because exhaustion can delay weaning.[2,8] An example of an SBT is presented in Box 52-8.

Box 52-8 Steps for Spontaneous Breathing Trials

1. Prepare the patient psychologically.
2. Set the ventilator at zero PSV and zero CPAP.
3. Maintain the FiO_2 at the baseline FiO_2 that the patient is receiving.
4. Monitor the patient's appearance, pulse, oxygen saturation measured by pulse oximeter, and blood pressure; observe the cardiac monitor for arrhythmia. Use the ventilator to monitor respiratory rate, tidal volume, and minute ventilation.
5. If the patient tolerates the SBT for 30 to 120 minutes, consider extubation.
6. If the patient does not tolerate the SBT for at least 30 minutes, reestablish the ventilator settings, and allow the patient to rest for at least a few hours before reattempting another SBT.
7. If repeated SBTs over multiple days are needed, individualize the patient's schedule, depending on his or her condition. In general, the weaning schedule should be stopped during the night so that the patient can rest and sleep.

Advantages of SBTs include the early and frequent testing of the patient's ability to breathe spontaneously without support. The use of SBTs several times per day has become unpopular, because it requires a great deal of time on the part of ICU staff, and a single daily SBT seems to be just as effective for most patients.[1,4] PSV and CPAP are sometimes used during the SBT, and patients who tolerate spontaneous breathing with a low level of PSV (i.e., 7 cm H_2O or less) should be able to tolerate extubation.[29] Current recommendations suggest a single daily trial of spontaneous breathing may be preferable to other methods of weaning.[1,4] Results of randomized, controlled studies have shown SBTs to be faster than SIMV and at least as effective as PSV.[5,28,30] Furthermore, performing an SBT one time per day is as effective as performing SBTs several times per day, and 30-minute trials are as effective as 120-minute trials.[1,4]

A collective task force representing the American College of Chest Physicians, the American Association for Respiratory Care, and the American College of Critical Care Medicine published evidence-based guidelines for weaning and discontinuing ventilatory support.[1] These guidelines were based in part on a comprehensive review of the evidence collected under the direction of the U.S. Agency for Health Care Policy and Research.[4]

The task force made 12 specific recommendations (Box 52-9). These include the regular use of formal and carefully monitored SBTs to guide clinical decision making regarding the discontinuation of ventilatory support.[1] Specifically, the task force recommended that, for the care of patients who need mechanical ventilation for more than 24 hours, a search for all possible causes of ventilatory dependence should be conducted and an attempt should be made to reverse or optimize each condition. Spontaneously breathing patients with evidence of reversal of the underlying condition that necessitated the ventilatory support, adequate oxygenation, and hemodynamic stability should be assessed with an SBT. Table 52-3 lists criteria to be used when determining whether patients who are receiving high levels of ventilatory support can be considered for SBTs.

A daily screen that includes the assessment of oxygenation, PEEP, and the use of vasopressors and sedatives should be conducted. A PaO_2/FiO_2 ratio of more than 150 to 200, a PEEP value of less than 5 to 8 cm H_2O, and a lack of a continuous infusion of vasopressors or sedatives (i.e., less than 5 mg/kg/min of dopamine) were good predictors of successful extubation and survival.[31]

The formal SBT may be performed in combination with low levels of PSV (i.e., 5 to 7 cm H_2O), CPAP (i.e., 5 cm H_2O or less), or automatic tube compensation applied to just offset the imposed WOB caused by the endotracheal tube.[1] During the SBT, the patient is carefully observed for breathing comfort, anxiety, agitation, dyspnea, or diaphoresis. Respiratory rate, heart rate, blood pressure, and SpO_2 are monitored. The SBT is terminated if signs of distress are observed, including the following:

- Agitation, anxiety, diaphoresis, or a change in mental status
- A sustained respiratory rate of more than 35 breaths/min
- A sustained SpO_2 of less than 90%

Box 52-9 Evidence-Based Guidelines for Weaning and Discontinuing Ventilatory Support

Recommendation 1: For patients who need mechanical ventilation for more than 24 hours, a search for all of the causes that may be contributing to ventilatory dependence should be undertaken. This is particularly true for the patient who has failed attempts at withdrawing the mechanical ventilator. Reversing all possible ventilatory and nonventilatory issues should be an integral part of the ventilatory discontinuation process.

Recommendation 2: Patients who are receiving mechanical ventilation for respiratory failure should undergo a formal assessment of discontinuation potential if the following criteria are satisfied:

1. Evidence for some reversal of the underlying cause for respiratory failure;
2. Adequate oxygenation (e.g., PaO_2/FiO_2 ratio of more than 150 to 200; requiring PEEP of no more than 5 to 8 cm H_2O; FiO_2 of no more than 0.4 to 0.5) and pH of more than 7.25;
3. Hemodynamic stability as defined by the absence of active myocardial ischemia and the absence of clinically significant hypotension (i.e., a condition that necessitates no vasopressor therapy or therapy with only low-dose vasopressors such as dopamine or dobutamine [less than 5 μg/kg/min]); and
4. The capability to initiate an inspiratory effort. The decision to use these criteria must be individualized. Some patients who are not satisfying all of these criteria (e.g., patients with chronic hypoxemia values of less than the thresholds cited) may be ready for attempts at the discontinuation of mechanical ventilation.

Recommendation 3: Formal discontinuation assessments for patients who are receiving mechanical ventilation for respiratory failure should be performed during spontaneous breathing rather than while the patient is still receiving substantial ventilatory support. An initial brief period of spontaneous breathing can be used to assess the capability of continuing onto a formal SBT. The criteria with which to assess patient tolerance during SBTs are the respiratory pattern, the adequacy of gas exchange, hemodynamic stability, and subjective comfort. The tolerance of SBTs that last 30 to 120 minutes should prompt consideration for permanent ventilatory discontinuation.

Recommendation 4: The removal of the artificial airway from a patient who has successfully been discontinued from ventilatory support should be based on assessments of airway patency and the ability of the patient to protect the airway.

Recommendation 5: Patients who are receiving mechanical ventilation for respiratory failure who fail an SBT should have the cause of the failed SBT determined. After any reversible causes of failure are corrected and if the patient still meets the criteria listed in Table 52-3, subsequent SBTs should be performed every 24 hours.

Recommendation 6: Patients who are receiving mechanical ventilation for respiratory failure who fail an SBT should receive a stable, nonfatiguing, and comfortable form of ventilatory support.

Recommendation 7: Anesthesia and sedation strategies and ventilatory management that are aimed at early extubation should be used for postsurgical patients.

Recommendation 8: Weaning and discontinuation protocols that are designed for nonphysician health care professionals should be developed and implemented by ICUs. Protocols that are aimed at optimizing sedation should also be developed and implemented.

Recommendation 9: Tracheotomy should be considered after an initial period of stabilization on the ventilator when it becomes apparent that the patient needs prolonged ventilatory assistance. Tracheotomy should then be performed when the patient appears to be likely to gain one or more of the benefits ascribed to the procedure. Patients who may derive particular benefit from early tracheotomy include the following:

- Those who need high levels of sedation to tolerate translaryngeal tubes;
- Those with marginal respiratory mechanics (often manifested as tachypnea) in whom a tracheostomy tube with lower resistance may reduce the risk of muscle overload;
- Those who may derive psychological benefit from the ability to eat orally, communicate by articulated speech, and experience enhanced mobility; and
- Those in whom enhanced mobility may assist with physical therapy efforts.

Recommendation 10: Unless there is evidence for clearly irreversible disease (e.g., high spinal cord injury, advanced amyotrophic lateral sclerosis), a patient who requires prolonged mechanical ventilatory support for respiratory failure should not be considered permanently ventilator dependent until 3 months of weaning attempts have failed.

Recommendation 11: Critical care practitioners should familiarize themselves with facilities in their communities or units in hospitals that are staffed with individuals that specialize in managing patients who have prolonged dependence on mechanical ventilation. Such familiarization should include reviewing published peer-reviewed data from those units, if available. When they are medically stable for transfer, patients who have failed ventilatory discontinuation attempts in the ICU should be transferred to those facilities that have demonstrated success and safety with accomplishing ventilator discontinuation.

Recommendation 12: Weaning strategies in the patient who requires prolonged mechanical ventilation should be slow paced and should include gradually lengthening self-breathing trials.

Modified from MacIntyre NR, Cook DJ, Ely EW, Jr, et al; American College of Chest Physicians; American Association for Respiratory Care; American College of Critical Care Medicine: Evidence-based guidelines for weaning and discontinuing ventilatory support: a collective task force facilitated by the American College of Chest Physicians; the American Association for Respiratory Care; and the American College of Critical Care Medicine. Chest 120 (6 Suppl):375S–395S, 2001.

TABLE 52-3

Criteria Used to Determine Whether Patients Who Are Receiving Ventilatory Support Can Be Considered for Spontaneous Breathing Trials

Criteria	Description
Objective measurements	Adequate oxygenation (e.g., PO_2 of ≥60 mm Hg with an FiO_2 of ≤0.40 to 0.50; PEEP of ≤5 to 8 cm H_2O; PO_2/FiO_2 ratio of ≥150 to 200) Stable cardiovascular system (e.g., heart rate ≤100 beats/min; stable blood pressure; no [or minimal] pressors) Afebrile (i.e., temperature about 37° C) No significant respiratory acidosis Adequate hemoglobin (e.g., ≥8 to 10 g/dl) Adequate mentation (e.g., arousable, Glasgow coma score of ≥13, no continuous sedative infusions) Stable metabolic status (e.g., acceptable electrolyte levels)
Subjective clinical assessments	Resolution of acute phase of disease; physician believes discontinuation is possible; adequate cough

Modified from MacIntyre NR, Cook DJ, Ely EW, et al: Evidence-based guidelines for weaning and discontinuing ventilator support: a collective task force facilitated by the American College of Chest Physicians, the American Association for Respiratory Care, and the American College of Critical Care Medicine. Chest 120:375S–395S, 2001.

- A more than 20% increase or decrease in heart rate or a heart rate of more than 120 to 140 beats/min
- A systolic blood pressure of more than 180 mm Hg or of less than 90 mm Hg

Patients with unsuccessful results of an SBT are returned to full ventilatory support for 24 hours to allow the ventilatory muscles to recover. During this period, the causes of failure are identified and corrected, if possible, and the patient is then reevaluated. If the criteria listed in Table 52-3 continue to be met, SBTs are repeated every 24 hours.[3] Patients who tolerate the formal SBT for 30 to 120 minutes remain off of the ventilator, and extubation is considered. Box 52-10 is a sample protocol for an SBT for the discontinuation of ventilatory support.

Continuous Positive Airway Pressure

CPAP is used during an SBT in many facilities. CPAP has the advantages of maintaining the lung volume during the weaning phase and thus of improving the patient's oxygenation status. Minimal levels of CPAP may be useful for reducing WOB and compensating for auto-PEEP, particularly in patients with obstructive lung disease.[1,4] CPAP is usually provided through the use of the CPAP mode that is available on most mechanical ventilators. By using the ventilator in the CPAP mode, the clinician can take advantage of the alarm systems that are available. In fact, most institutions use the CPAP mode with zero CPAP level to take advantage of the ventilator alarms during weaning. This always provides an improved margin of safety as compared with the use of a T-piece and should be the standard approach to an SBT.

Box 52-10 Weaning Protocol for a Spontaneous Breathing Trial

1. Verify that the patient is a candidate for ventilator discontinuation.
   a. Is there evidence of the reversal or alleviation of the disease state or condition that required mechanical ventilatory support?
   b. Is the patient able to breathe spontaneously?
   c. Has the patient's medical condition been optimized (i.e., afebrile, adequate hemoglobin, and acceptable electrolyte levels)?
   d. Are oxygenation, ventilation, and blood gas values adequate?
      - PaO_2 of at least 60 mm Hg with FiO_2 of no more than 0.40 to 0.50 with PEEP/CPAP of no more than 5 to 8 cm H_2O
      - PaO_2/FiO_2 ratio of 150 to 200 mm Hg or more
      - pH of 7.25 or more
   e. Is the patient awake and alert, free of seizures, and able to follow instructions?
   f. Is there evidence of hemodynamic stability? Are vasopressors only administered intermittently?
2. Prepare the patient for the SBT.
   a. Be sure that adequate personnel are present.
   b. Ensure that there are no other ongoing procedures or other major activities.
   c. Eliminate or minimize respiratory depressants (e.g., sedatives, narcotics).
   d. Suction the airway, as needed.
   e. Sit the patient up in bed, if possible.
3. Set the ventilator at zero CPAP and zero pressure support.
4. Continuously monitor the patient.
5. If any of the following occurs and are sustained, return the patient to mechanical ventilatory support:
   a. Respiratory rate of at least 35 breaths/min
   b. Oxygen saturation measured by pulse oximeter of less than 90%
   c. 20% increase or decrease in heart rate or heart rate of more than120 beats/min
   d. Systolic blood pressure of more than 180 mm Hg or of less than 90 mm Hg
   e. Agitation, diaphoresis, or anxiety
6. Continue the trial for at least 30 minutes but not more than 2 hours. If no signs of intolerance develop (see step 5), consider extubation.

Modified from MacIntyre NR, Cook DJ, Ely EW, Jr, et al; American College of Chest Physicians; American Association for Respiratory Care; American College of Critical Care Medicine: Evidence-based guidelines for weaning and discontinuing ventilatory support: a collective task force facilitated by the American College of Chest Physicians; the American Association for Respiratory Care; and the American College of Critical Care Medicine. Chest 120(6 Suppl):375S–395S, 2001.

Synchronized Intermittent Mandatory Ventilation

SIMV can be used to provide full or partial ventilatory support. Weaning from SIMV involves the gradual reduction of the machine rate on the basis of the results of ABG analysis and patient assessment. Early claims that SIMV allowed for faster weaning times[8] have not been substantiated by subsequent studies.[28,29,30]

Patients who are receiving ventilation in the SIMV mode uncouple their breathing efforts from the support provided by the machine.[1,4] They continue to make spontaneous breathing efforts during the delivery of a "mandatory breath." Evidence also suggests that, once the machine cycling rate is reduced to approximately 50% of the full ventilatory support value, the patient breathes approximately as hard per cycle as when ventilatory support is completely withdrawn.[32,33] This additional work can be overcome with the use of pressure support (i.e., 5 to 10 cm H_2O). However, the addition of pressure support further complicates the weaning process. For initial ventilator setup, the SIMV rate and the tidal volume usually are set at values that are equivalent to those used during volume control-continuous mandatory ventilation (VC-CMV) or pressure control-continuous mandatory ventilation (PC-CMV). When the patient's condition has been stabilized, one of two approaches can be used. Some clinicians prefer to continue at these settings until the patient's precipitating disease state or condition has improved considerably. At that point, the rate is reduced in a stepwise manner until complete spontaneous breathing can be achieved. Other clinicians prefer to immediately reduce the level of mechanical ventilation to an SIMV rate of 4 to 8 per minute, thereby forcing the patient to perform additional WOB. From the beginning, attempts are made to reduce the SIMV rate, and the patient is challenged to provide a portion of the required ventilation. Unfortunately, research indicates that SIMV prolongs ventilatory support and that it is the least effective method of weaning from ventilatory support as compared with either SBT or PSV.[1,4,28,29,30]

Pressure Support Ventilation

PSV is a mode of ventilatory support that allows the patient to have significant control over the process of ventilatory support. The only gas-delivery variable directly controlled by the ventilator is peak airway pressure; see Chapters 45 and 48 for details.

For initial ventilator setup in the PSV mode, the beginning pressure level can be adjusted to deliver an appropriate tidal volume, which is usually approximately 4 to 8 ml/kg of the ideal body weight based on the patient's condition and the desired tidal volume. PSV is then gradually reduced to a minimal value that only compensates for the WOB imposed by the artificial airway.[28,29,30] Generally this is about 5 to 8 cm H_2O. After this reduction is accomplished, extubation can be performed directly from the low level pressure support, or an SBT may be conducted for 30 to 120 minutes.[1,4]

PSV allows the clinician to manipulate the level of patient work, but the benefit of this to weaning is questionable.[1,4] In general, patients who can spontaneously breathe comfortably at 5 to 8 cm H_2O of PSV can be extubated without problems. However, if upper airway edema is present, WOB after extubation may be about the same as that caused by the endotracheal tube. In these cases, low levels of pressure support may give a false impression about the patient's ability to tolerate extubation[1,4] (Box 52-11).

Box 52-11 Protocol for Pressure Support Weaning

1. Verify that the patient is a candidate for ventilator discontinuation:
   - Evidence of alleviation or reversal of the disease state or condition that necessitated ventilatory support
   - Stable, spontaneous breathing pattern without irregular breathing or periods of apnea
   - Optimization of the patient's medical condition
   - Adequate oxygenation, ventilation, and acid-base balance
2. Begin with a PSV level that achieves a tidal volume of 4 to 8 ml/kg of the ideal body weight. A PSV of more than 20 cm H_2O rarely is needed. The need for a high level of PSV indicates that the patient may not be ready for ventilator discontinuation.
3. Reduce the PSV 2 to 4 cm H_2O as tolerated, ideally at least twice daily, and reassess the patient for signs of intolerance:
   - Rate of at least 25 to 30 breaths/min
   - 20% or greater increase in heart rate or a heart rate of more than 120 beats/min
   - 20% or greater increase in systolic blood pressure or systolic blood pressure of more than 180 mm Hg or of less than 90 mm Hg
   - Agitation, anxiety, and diaphoresis
4. If the patient does not tolerate a reduction in PSV, return to the previous value, and reassess.
5. Continue to reduce PSV as tolerated at least twice per day and more frequently if the patient does not have signs of distress.
6. Consider extubation when the patient is able to tolerate a PSV of 5 to 8 cm H_2O for 2 hours with no apparent distress.

Modified from Esteban A, Frutos F, Tobin M, et al: A comparison of four methods of weaning patients from mechanical ventilation. Spanish Lung Failure Collaborative Group, N Engl J Med 332:345-350, 1995; and Brochard L, Rauss A, Benito S, et al: Comparison of three methods of gradual withdrawal from ventilatory support during weaning from mechanical ventilation. Am J Respir Crit Care Med 150:896–903, 1994.

Synchronized Intermittent Mandatory Ventilation With Pressure Support Ventilation

With SIMV, the addition of pressure support can overcome the WOB imposed during "spontaneous" breaths because of the presence of endotracheal and tracheostomy tubes, demand flow systems, and ventilator circuits. In this setting, pressure support is set to achieve the desired tidal volume during the spontaneous breaths (i.e., 4 to 8 ml/kg of the ideal body weight).

Although it is clear that the addition of PSV during SIMV can reduce or eliminate imposed work caused by mechanical factors, it has not been shown how this affects weaning. In one study, SIMV with PSV increased tidal volume and reduced respiratory rate but did not significantly reduce weaning time or success as compared with SIMV alone.[34] On the basis of all of the weaning trials, it can be concluded that this approach to weaning can only increase the length of ventilatory support. Current guidelines recommend the use of SBT to rapidly wean patients from ventilatory support.[1,4]

MINI CLINI

Setting Pressure Support Levels

PROBLEM: An intubated patient is receiving mechanical ventilation in the SIMV mode with the following settings:

- $V_T = 400$ ml
- Rate = 12 breaths/min
- Peak inspiratory pressure = 40 cm H_2O
- Plateau pressure (P_{plat}) = 20 cm H_2O
- Ventilator inspiratory flow ($\dot{V}$) = 60 L/min (1 L/s)

The patient is breathing spontaneously with a spontaneous rate of 12 breaths/min and a spontaneous peak inspiratory flow of 30 L/min (0.5 L/s). Find the level of PSV that is needed to overcome the imposed WOB.

Solution:

$$PSV = ([PIP - P_{plat}]/\dot{V}_{mach}) \times \dot{V}_{Imax}$$

$$PSV = ([40\ cm\ H_2O - 20\ cm\ H_2O]/1\ L/s) \times 0.5\ L/s$$

$$= 10\ cm\ H_2O$$

The calculated PSV level to overcome the imposed WOB for this patient is 10 cm.

Spontaneous Awaking Trials

Concern regarding the use of sedation in critically ill patients has increased markedly during the last few years. This concern has focused on the issue of delirium.[35] The indiscriminate use of sedatives in the ICU is considered inappropriate patient management. In general, sedatives should always be considered last when trying to handle an agitated patient (Chapter 47). Something has caused the patient's agitation, and it should be addressed and corrected, if possible, before sedation is administered. In addition, it is becoming clearer that the use of excessive sedation lengthens the time of mechanical ventilation. The use of **spontaneous awaking trials (SAT)** along with daily SBT results in the faster weaning of patients from ventilatory support as well as a decrease in mortality.[36] The decrease in mortality is attributed to patients being exposed for a shorter time to the complications of mechanical ventilation. Throughout the course of mechanical ventilation, sedation should be kept to the bare minimum necessary; patient sedation should be periodically carefully assessed before additional sedation is given.[36,37] In general, one of the currently available systems to rate the level of sedation should be in use on all mechanically ventilated patients (Riker/Sedation Agitation Scale (SAS), Ramsay Sedation Scale, or Richmond Agitation Scale (RASS).

NEWER TECHNIQUES FOR FACILITATING VENTILATOR DISCONTINUANCE

Mandatory Minute Volume Ventilation

Mandatory minute volume ventilation (MMV) was described and introduced in 1977.[38] With this mode of ventilation, the total minute volume is set, and the patient may elect to inspire all of the minute volume, part of the minute volume, or none of the minute volume spontaneously. The ventilator would automatically provide a clinician-set remainder of the minute volume. It was originally assumed that, as the patient's status improved, he or she would assume a greater and greater percentage of the set minute volume, eventually inspiring it all spontaneously. However, this did not occur; patients generally settled into a ventilator pattern where the overall WOB was shared between the patient and the ventilator, and the patient never assumed a greater percentage of the work.[39] There is no data to support the use of MMV over SBT or PSV to wean patients from ventilatory support.

Adaptive Support Ventilation/Intellivent

ASV is a newer mode of ventilation that maintains a minimum minute ventilation with an optimal breathing pattern (tidal volume and rate) that is based on the work of Otis;[40,41] see Chapters 45 and 48 for details. ASV automatically adjusts inspiratory pressure and ventilator breath rate to achieve the target minute volume set. As the patient's status improves, the target minute volume is reduced, and the level of pressure required each breath diminishes. When a minimal level is reached, the patient is considered weaned from ventilatory support and ready for extubation.

Preliminary studies of ASV for the care of patients who are recovering from cardiac surgery show a reduction in the duration of mechanical ventilation as compared with an SIMV weaning protocol.[41,42] Additional data about ASV indicates that it works very well for patients who are under controlled ventilation,[43] but data from large heterogeneous groups of patients will be necessary to determine if ASV truly improves the speed of ventilator discontinuation.

A recent upgrade of ASV is referred to as Intellivent.[44] With this modification the ventilator becomes a total closed loop controller of not only ventilation but also oxygenation. Incorporated into the management algorithm are the ARDSnet PEEP/F_IO_2 tables. Thus, all aspects of gas delivery are controlled. As with ASV, Intellivent works well on patients under control ventilation and those requiring simple postoperative ventilation, and has shown the ability to wean patients from ventilatory support.[45] However, no comparison to SBT is currently available. Intellivent use in the complex patient spontaneously triggering the ventilator is still controversial. However, one can expect this type of closed loop control of ventilation will begin to appear on other mechanical ventilators.

Computer-Based Weaning

Current versions of MMV and ASV/Intellivent are examples of computer-controlled mechanical ventilation. Several more complex systems have been developed, including Ventilation Manager, VQ-attending, ESTER, Continuous Respiratory Evaluator (CORE), KUSIVAR, and WEAN-PRO.[46] The desire to develop computer-based weaning protocols is based on two factors. First, weaning is a time-consuming and labor-intensive process. If computer control can expedite or simplify this process, considerable time and money can be saved. Second, because most weaning decisions are based on objective data, computer-based weaning protocols are relatively easy to develop.[46]

The most successful computerized application for weaning is the Smart Care approach.[47,48] The system adjusts pressure support on the basis of the patient's tidal volume, respiratory rate, and end-tidal carbon dioxide level. When the pressure support has been decreased to a predefined level, the ventilator automatically begins an SBT. If the patient fails the SBT, which is determined by changes in the patient's respiratory rate, tidal volume, and end-tidal carbon dioxide level, then the ventilator automatically reassumes ventilatory support. If the patient passes the SBT, the ventilator also returns to baseline ventilatory support but notifies the clinician that the patient is ready for ventilator discontinuation. Two randomized comparisons of SmartCare to clinician-controlled SBT have demonstrated that patients wean faster and both the total number of days that patients are maintained in the ICU and the need for postextubation NIV are reduced with SmartCare.[47,48] One criticism of this study was that the clinician-applied SBTs were not always performed consistently. However, this is clinical reality—in the ICU there is always good intention to do an SBT but emergencies, new admissions, and other distractions prevent clinicians from always performing the SBT in a timely manner. With SmartCare, if the patient meets criteria the SBT is performed regardless of the activity in the ICU. It should be noted that at least at the time of this revision the FDA only allows Smart Care in the United States to notify clinicians of the readiness for an SBT and the patient's status during the SBT. The clinician must adjust the ventilator into and out of the SBT. In the rest of the world this is performed automatically be the ventilator. It can be expected that automated weaning systems will increasingly have a place in the care of critically ill patients.

Automatic Tube Compensation

Automatic tube compensation (**ATC**) is an option on newer mechanical ventilators that compensates for the flow-dependent pressure decrease across the endotracheal tube during both inspiration and expiration; see Chapters 45 and 48 for details. ATC reduces WOB and may improve patient comfort.[49] Because it compensates for the imposed WOB caused by the artificial airway, ATC has been referred to as *electronic extubation*. Patients who are able to breathe adequately with the addition of ATC at low peak airway pressure (i.e., less than 8 cm H_2O) should tolerate extubation. ATC is similar to pressure support in that an inspiratory pressure is used to compensate for imposed WOB; however, ATC varies the pressure, depending on the size of the endotracheal tube and the patient's inspiratory flow rate. Alternatively, PSV delivers a preset inspiratory pressure that may overcompensate or undercompensate imposed WOB at any given point in time. However, no data are available to indicate that ATC weans patients faster than SBTs or PSV.

MINI CLINI

Response to a Spontaneous Breathing Trial

PROBLEM: A 70-year-old woman with a long history of congestive heart failure has been mechanically ventilated for 6 days. She has failed three previous SBTs, but today, at the end of a 45-minute SBT, her clinical presentation was as follows:

- Respiratory rate of 24 breaths/min
- Tidal volume of 300 ml (6 ml/kg ideal body weight)
- Pulse of 98 beats/min
- Blood pressure of 138/86 mm Hg

The patient did not appear to be short of breath, and she did not demonstrate excessive use of her accessory muscles of ventilation to breathe during the trial.

Should this patient's ventilatory support be discontinued?

Solution: On the basis of the given data, this patient passed her SBT and should be discontinued from ventilatory support and extubated if there is no reason for her to remain intubated. However, because of her age, history of congestive heart failure, and multiple failures of SBT, she should ideally be placed on NIV immediately after she is extubated and slowly transitioned to independent spontaneous breathing over the next 12 to 48 hours. See the following discussion below and Chapter 49.

Volume Support

VC is a newer mode of ventilation that combines pressure support and volume ventilation by allowing the level of pressure support to be automatically adjusted to maintain a target tidal volume. In the VC mode, inspiration is initiated by the patient. During the inspiratory phase, the pressure level is regulated to a value that is based on the previous breath's pressure-volume relationship as compared with a target tidal volume. The pressure-support level is automatically adjusted in a stepwise manner by up to ±3 cm H_2O from one breath to the next to maintain the target tidal volume.

A major problem with VC is the excessive reduction of airway pressure in the presence of high ventilatory demand, thereby increasing patient effort.[50] With most ventilators offering this mode, no lower limit to ventilating airway pressure is set, and inspiratory airway pressure can decrease all the way to the PEEP level. Volume support may offer a sort of automatic weaning from pressure support. As the patient's spontaneous tidal volume improves, the level of pressure support is automatically reduced. However, clinical trials indicate no benefit to the use of VC to wean patients.[51]

Proportional Assist Ventilation and Neurally Adjusted Ventilatory Assist

Proportional assist ventilation (PAV) and neurally adjusted ventilatory assist (NAVA) are two of the newest modes of ventilatory support.[52] These modes differ from all other modes of ventilation since they do NOT force a ventilatory pattern. Instead they follow the ventilatory pattern desired by the patient.

As a result, patient-ventilatory synchrony is greater with these modes than with any of the other ventilatory modes.[53,54,55] Unfortunately, there are no data regarding the use of these modes to facilitate ventilator discontinuation. At this time, regardless of how these modes improve patient-ventilator interaction, the decision to discontinue ventilatory support should be made based on performance of an SBT. Future research should be able to define if these modes have a greater role in discontinuation process.

Noninvasive Ventilation

A number of groups have studied the use of NIV as an adjunct to ventilator discontinuance. Essentially, NIV has been used in this setting in three different manners:

1. Transitioning patients with COPD who failed SBTs from invasive ventilation to spontaneous breathing[56-58]
2. Supporting patients who passed SBTs but who were considered to be at high risk for failing the extubation[25-26,59]
3. Supporting patients who developed hypoxemic respiratory failure after extubation[60,61]

The literature strongly supports the first two indications but does not support the third application. Refer to Chapter 49 for details regarding the application of NIV during weaning and the use of NIV in general.

Role of Mobility

If you do not move it, you lose it! This has become increasingly clear when it comes to patients in the process of weaning from ventilatory support. Mobilization of the mechanically ventilated patient should begin as soon as the patient is stabilized, requires minimal sedation, and is capable of interacting with the ventilator.[62,63] Mobilization may begin simply by sitting the mechanically ventilated patient at the side of the bed. However, in many cases it may mean that the patient is walked in the hallway while receiving ventilatory support. Of course this requires the cooperation of respiratory therapy, nursing, and physical therapy, and the use of equipment that facilitates mobilization: transport ventilator, portable suction, and walker/chair that maintains support of the patient but also allows the patient to sit and rest. Mobilization is increasingly important the longer the patient requires ventilatory support.

Respiratory-Therapist–Driven Protocols

A number of randomized, controlled clinical trials have demonstrated that patients are weaned faster with the use of protocols than with individual physician orders.[64-67] In all of these studies, the therapists, nurses, and physicians who normally manage patients in the unit developed the protocol. In addition, in the individual physician order group, the physicians who wrote the protocol also wrote the individual weaning orders. In all of these trials, patients who were randomized to the protocol group weaned faster and with fewer complications then the patients randomized to the individual physician group.[64-67]

What these results do not mean is that therapists wean patients better than physicians. However, what they do mean is that, when an evidence-based approach to patient management is developed and followed precisely, care is generally better than with individual physician orders. The reason for this is that protocols empower the clinician at the bedside to advance care when the patient meets specific criteria without waiting for the physician to come and write an order. In many community hospitals, the wait for the physician could be an hour or a whole shift or more. Thus, with protocols, care proceeds rapidly on the agreed-upon course. In addition, the individual bias of the caregiver does not affect the manner in which care is provided. Thus, the approach does not change from day to day depending on which physician is at the bedside. An example of a respiratory-therapist–directed ventilatory discontinuance protocol is presented in Box 52-12.

Box 52-12 Respiratory-Therapist–Directed Weaning Protocol

- The physician's written order identifies the patient as being eligible for the respiratory-therapist–directed weaning protocol.
- The timing of weaning initiation is defined as part of the protocol.
- All patients must undergo continuous oxyhemoglobin saturation monitoring by pulse oximetry.
- When the patient meets weaning criteria, the ventilator is set to zero CPAP and zero PEEP.
- The SBT continues for a minimum of 30 minutes to a maximum of 120 minutes if none of the following weaning failure conditions are present:
  - SaO_2 of less than 90% or diaphoresis
  - Spontaneous respiratory rate of at least 35 breaths/min that is sustained for at least 5 minutes
  - Agitation or a decreased level of consciousness
  - A heart rate increase of at least 20%
  - A blood pressure change of at least 20%
  - A cardiac output reduction of at least 30% or ventricular arrhythmia
- Results of the SBT are discussed with the unit physician
- If the SBT is well tolerated and there is no reason not to extubate the patient, the patient is extubated.

SELECTING AN APPROACH

Current evidence suggests that, for ventilator discontinuance and progressive weaning from mechanical support, it may be best to avoid SIMV.[1,4] It has also been suggested, regardless of approach used, that protocols administered by respiratory therapists and other health care workers be developed.[3,6,10] These protocols should be designed to begin testing for the opportunity to reduce support very soon after intubation and to reduce the level of ventilatory support at every opportunity.[1,66] The approach to weaning that seems to wean patients most rapidly is the SBT. This should be the approach that is used to identify readiness for ventilator discontinuance in the vast majority of patients.[1] In addition, NIV should be considered as part of the total ventilator discontinuance process.[65]

One area that requires additional research is the role of ventilatory muscle conditioning in patients who require long-term ventilatory support. Endurance conditioning of the ventilatory muscles can be achieved by the continuous repetition of low levels of ventilatory work. Strength conditioning can be achieved by maximal ventilatory effort for short periods. In theory, PSV would allow for improving ventilatory muscle endurance, whereas intermittent SBTs would favor the development of muscle strength. Inspiratory resistive training to improve ventilatory muscle strength has been tried as an adjunct to weaning for the care of patients undergoing long-term ventilation.[13] Unfortunately, the role of ventilatory muscle rest and load in the care of difficult-to-wean patients has not been established.[13]

In summary, a single daily SBT that lasts from 30 minutes to 2 hours has been recommended as the primary approach to weaning.[1,4] If the trial is successful, extubation is considered. If the trial is unsuccessful, a period of rest is provided before another trial is attempted.[1] There are advantages and disadvantages to each of the methods used to conduct ventilator weaning. Table 52-4 compares SBT, SIMV, and PSV as weaning techniques. The best approach currently supported by the literature is an SBT, but it may alternatively be the approach with which a given clinician is most familiar. It should be based on knowledge of the patient's condition, a sound rationale, and good clinical experience. The method chosen should include careful patient assessment, and the patient's condition should be optimized before weaning. For the vast majority of patients, a protocolized approach to ventilator discontinuance is most efficient.

MONITORING THE PATIENT DURING WEANING

Ventilatory Status

Respiratory rate and pattern are easy to monitor and may be the most reliable indicators of patient progress during weaning.[1,4] Weaning may proceed as quickly as the patient's respiratory rate and subjective tolerance allow. However, in no case should patients be pushed beyond their physiologic limits; to do so may result in diaphragmatic dysfunction and further delay the weaning process. If the patient is allowed to fatigue during a weaning trial, it will require at least 24 hours for the muscles to recover.[68,69] Dyspnea should be monitored during weaning and may be quantified with a visual analog scale or a modified Borg scale[70] (Table 52-5). The onset or worsening of discomfort, respiratory distress, fatigue, sweating, signs of increased WOB (e.g., accessory muscle use, abdominal paradox), deterioration in vital signs, or changes in mental status (e.g., agitation, anxiety, somnolence, coma) may be signs of intolerance of a weaning trial.[1]

The single best index of ventilation remains the measurement of $PaCO_2$. However, the assessment of a patient's tolerance of an SBT should be based on clinical presentation rather than $PaCO_2$. A patient with a $PaCO_2$ of 40 mm Hg but a clinical presentation defined by a rapid, shallow breathing pattern with abdominal paradox, tachycardia, and hypertension has not

TABLE 52-4
Comparison of Available Weaning Methods

Method	Advantages	Disadvantages
SBT	Tests patient's spontaneous breathing ability Allows periods of work and rest Weans faster than SIMV A single daily SBT may be as effective as multiple trials May be performed with 5 cm H_2O CPAP, 5 cm H_2O PSV, or both	More staff time Abrupt transition may be difficult for some patients May overstress the patient if not monitored carefully Requires careful supervision
SIMV	Less staff time Gradual transition Easy to use Minimum minute ventilation guaranteed Sophisticated alarm systems may be used May be used in combination with PSV or CPAP	Patient-ventilator asynchrony Prolongs weaning May worsen fatigue
PSV	Less staff time Gradual transition Prevents fatigue Maintains activity of diaphragm Increased patient comfort Weans faster than SIMV Overcomes resistive WOB caused by the following: Endotracheal and tracheostomy tubes Ventilator circuits Demand flow systems Patient can control cycle length, rate, and inspiratory flow Every breath is supported	Large changes in minute ventilation can occur Increased mean airway pressure as compared with SBT Tidal volume not guaranteed; low tidal volumes possible May prolong weaning

TABLE 52-5
Modified Borg Scale for Dyspnea

Grade	Degree of Dyspnea
0	None
0.5	Very, very slight (just noticeable)
1	Very slight
2	Slight
3	Moderate
4	Somewhat severe
5	Severe
6	Very severe
7	
8	
9	Very, very severe (almost maximal)
10	Maximal

Modified from Mahler DA: Dyspnea, Mt. Kisco, NY, 1990, Futura.

passed an SBT. The results of capnography should not be used to guide the weaning of patients. End-tidal PCO_2 values can be highly misleading as an estimate of effective ventilation in sick patients.[71] Gastric pH has been used as a predictor of patient status, and gastrointestinal acidosis may be an early sign of weaning failure.[72]

Oxygenation

During the SBT, FiO_2 should be the same as during ventilatory support or 10% higher. Continuous pulse oximetric (SpO_2) monitoring can provide a sensitive indicator of oxygenation status during weaning.[1] Arterial blood gas analysis for PaO_2 and SaO_2 and the calculation of the oxygen content of the arterial blood (CaO_2) may be performed after the patient has been considered a weaning failure to determine the extent of the failure. Success, however, can be based on the SpO_2 only. SpO_2 monitoring during the SBT is generally the standard of care.

Cardiovascular Status

Pulse, blood pressure, and cardiac rhythm should be monitored, and arrhythmias should be assessed to determine whether weaning should be continued. Tachycardia, bradycardia, and abnormalities in blood pressure should be promptly evaluated and the patient returned to ventilatory support or a higher level of support, if indicated. Silent myocardial ischemia may occur frequently in some postoperative patients during weaning.[73] Table 52-6 summarizes changes that may occur during the withdrawal of ventilatory support.

TABLE 52-6

Changes During the Withdrawal of Ventilatory Support

Expected Change	Deleterious Change
Respiratory	
Respiratory rate minimally increased	Respiratory rate of ≥35 breaths/min
Stable $\dot{V}$	Large increase or decrease in $\dot{V}_E$
SpO_2 ≥90%	Decrease in SpO_2 to ≤90%
5 to 10 mm Hg swing in PaO_2	PaO_2 of <60 mm Hg
5 to 10 mm Hg swing in $PaCO_2$	An increase of >10 mm Hg in $PaCO_2$
pH of >7.30 and <7.50	pH of <7.30
Minimal use of accessory muscles	Increased use of accessory muscles
No paradoxical breathing	Paradoxical breathing
	Diaphoresis
	Dyspnea
Cardiovascular	
Heart rate increased by 15 to 20 beats/min	Persistent tachycardia of ≥120 to 140 beats/min
Blood pressure increased 10 to 15 mm Hg	Hypotension (blood pressure of <90/60 mm Hg)
	Hypertension (systolic blood pressure of >180 mm Hg)
Increased cardiac index	Decreased cardiac index
Increased stroke volume	Decreased stroke volume
	Angina
	New arrhythmias
Other	
Mental status good (i.e., awake, alert, responsive)	Anxiety, agitation, somnolence, coma

EXTUBATION

Artificial Airways and Weaning

The effect on a patient of a properly sized artificial airway on WOB is controversial.[74] However, many endotracheal tubes are partially obstructed and as a result impose a significant increase in WOB. Removing the endotracheal tube may markedly improve the patient's clinical status. There is little difference in the airway resistance of healthy adults with low minute ventilation (i.e., <8 L/min) breathing through endotracheal tubes with an internal diameter (ID) of 7, 8, or 9 mm.[75] However, in critically ill patients decreases in ID and increases in minute ventilation increase WOB. Adults have a critical increase in workload when the tube has an ID of less than 7 mm.[75] It is thought that the added work due to the presence of an artificial airway may contribute to ventilator dependency among patients with borderline pulmonary function or ventilatory muscle weakness.[76]

Biofilm buildup on the inside of the endotracheal tube can cause dramatic increases in airway resistance, especially among infants and children.[77,78] Taking care to provide adequate humidification and careful suctioning can help to avoid this problem.

Tracheotomy may substantially reduce the WOB of patients who need mechanical ventilatory support. The short length of tracheotomy tubes results in an overall decrease in resistance as compared with the resistance of an endotracheal tube, even though the curvature of the tracheotomy tube is greater.[1] It appears that the performance of a tracheotomy improves airway resistance and reduces the load of the ventilatory muscles. It may be the ability to avoid secretions/biofilm buildup on the inside of the trachestomy tube that makes the difference.

Weaning and extubation should be separate decisions. Weaning indices are not predictive of the adequacy of airway patency or the need for the protection of the airway. The reintubation rate among patients with prolonged postoperative ventilation as a result of respiratory failure can range from 5% to 20%.[1,4]

Patients who have been successfully extubated generally have the following characteristics: (1) the resolution of the disease state or condition; (2) hemodynamic stability; (3) the absence of sepsis; (4) adequate oxygenation status with a decreased FiO_2 and decreased PEEP or CPAP; and (5) adequate ventilatory status and $PaCO_2$. The decision to extubate should be based on the assessment of upper airway patency and protection. No one indicator is 100% sensitive and specific with regard to the prediction of successful extubation. Practical guidelines for extubation are presented in Box 52-13. Regardless of the weaning technique used, an SBT is recommended before extubation to ensure that the patient can sustain spontaneous unsupported ventilation.[1]

Some patients may be successfully extubated even if extubation criteria are not met. If the patient is at risk, trained personnel who are able to perform reintubation must be immediately available before extubation is attempted. At a minimum, those who perform the extubation must be prepared to provide an airway and ventilatory support in the event that problems develop immediately after extubation. Extubation should be postponed when myocardial ischemia is present, when the patient has upper gastrointestinal hemorrhage, or when a procedure that necessitates reintubation is impending. If difficult reintubation is anticipated, trained personnel should be immediately available.

Many patients report hoarseness and sore throat after extubation, and patients should be advised that these symptoms may occur. Other common problems after extubation include airway obstruction, increased risk of aspiration, and difficulty with secretion clearance. Patients with neurologic or neuromuscular disorders and those with excessive secretions are at increased risk after extubation. The compression of the airway as a result of a traumatic or postoperative hematoma of the neck, infectious masses or abscesses, and malignant tumors or compression after major head or neck surgery can lead to upper airway obstruction after extubation. The cuff leak test may detect airway obstruction before extubation; however, results of studies addressing this are controversial.[79,80] An air leak of less than 11% to 12% or 110 to 130 ml has been shown to be predictive of stridor.[79,80] Box 52-13 provides a protocolized guide for extubation.

Box 52-13 Practical Guidelines for Extubation

- There is no immediate need for mechanical ventilation or intubation.
- The medical course does not suggest impending respiratory failure or other indications for mechanical ventilation.
- Procedures that require intubation and general anesthesia are not immediately planned.
- There is adequate oxygenation and ventilation with spontaneous ventilation.
- The patient's FiO_2 requirement can be achieved with a mask or a nasal cannula.
- The patient no longer needs mechanical ventilatory assistance.
- Weaning is successful.
- There is a minimal risk of upper airway obstruction.
- The patient has minimal edema or mass encroachment of the oropharynx and upper airway.
- There is adequate airway protection and a minimal risk of aspiration.
- The level of consciousness and neuromuscular function ensures a gag reflex and an adequate cough.
- Gastric contents are minimized by the discontinuation of tube feedings for 4 to 6 hours before extubation.
- A positive gag reflex is present.
- There is adequate clearance of pulmonary secretions.
- The level of consciousness and muscular strength allow for an effective cough.
- Secretion volume and thickness are not worsening.

After extubation, glottic edema can result in partial airway obstruction, which can cause mild to severe stridor. Postextubation stridor occurs in 2% to 16% of patients in the ICU and should be viewed with concern.[81] Severe edema after extubation can lead to complete airway obstruction. Children, patients with epiglottitis or angioedema (i.e., dermal, subcutaneous, or submucosal edema of the face or larynx), and patients who have sustained smoke inhalation are at greater risk. Postextubation edema occurs in as many as 47% of children with trauma injuries or burns.[1,4] See Chapter 36 for detailed information about airway management and postextubation care.

VENTILATOR DISCONTINUANCE FAILURE

As many as 25% of patients who have been removed from ventilatory support experience respiratory distress that is severe enough to necessitate the reinstitution of mechanical ventilation. In patients who are unlikely to be successfully weaned, rapid, shallow breathing begins almost immediately after the ventilator is disconnected. As spontaneous breathing continues, respiratory mechanics worsen in these patients for reasons that are not clearly understood. Approximately half of patients who have poor results after the discontinuation of ventilation experience marked hypercapnia as a result of rapid, shallow breathing. An unsuccessful SBT also causes considerable cardiovascular stress. Myocardial ischemia may occur frequently among ventilator-dependent patients, and it has been associated with weaning failure.[82] Critical illness polyneuropathy has been cited as a frequent cause of neuromuscular weaning failure among critically ill patients.[83] Unsuspected neuromuscular disease may be an important factor in ventilator dependency.

Inability to wean can sometimes be attributed to psychologic dependence, poor oxygenation status, or cardiovascular instability (i.e., congestive heart failure or ischemia).[1,4] However, the most common cause of the inability to wean is an imbalance between ventilatory capability and ventilatory demand. Inability to wean is usually caused by a concurrent pathologic process that necessitates treatment. Common causes of weaning failure are summarized in Box 52-14.

PROLONGED MECHANICAL VENTILATION

Prolonged mechanical ventilation (**PMV**) may be required for 3% to 7% of patients who are receiving mechanical ventilation.[1,4] Patients who require a lengthy course of ventilatory support after the acute phase of their disease has resolved may be suffering from some of the items listed in Table 52-7. Any patient who is repeatedly failing SBTs should undergo a complete review of all systems to determine if something has been overlooked that may add to the patient's workload, thereby preventing them from weaning. In many patients, their pulmonary mechanics have not been optimized and thus they are

Box 52-14 Common Causes of Weaning Failure

- Poor respiratory mechanics or wheezing
- Untreated cardiac disease
- Electrolyte imbalances
- Anxiety
- Secretions
- Aspiration
- Alkalosis
- Neuromuscular weakness
- Sepsis
- Excessive sedation
- Inadequate nutrition
- Opiates
- Obesity
- Thyroid disease

MINI CLINI

Patient Who Requires Long-Term Weaning

PROBLEM: A 68-year-old man with a history of COPD was hospitalized after a motor vehicle accident. Over the course of the next 2 weeks, the patient became septic and developed acute respiratory distress syndrome. For the last week, the patient has met the criteria for an SBT, but he has failed every attempt. How should this patient's ventilator care progress from this point forward?

Solution: This patient should be classified as a difficult-to-wean patient who would benefit from a program that has been designed specifically for patients who are failing to wean. This program should systematically evaluate all systems to determine the cause of weaning failure and include the assistance of other health care providers, specifically physical therapy, occupational therapy, and speech and language pathology; he may also benefit from the efforts of social services. Ideally, this should take place in a unit that has been specifically designed for the difficult-to-wean patient.

unable to assume the workload required of spontaneous breathing. In others, underlying cardiac disease may not have been properly treated. Always a concern is the patient's acid-base status. If a patient had baseline compensated respiratory acidosis, then he or she will not be able to wean if the compensation has been eliminated. Every time these patients are trialed on an SBT, their carbon dioxide levels will rise, and they will develop respiratory failure. If this is the problem, the baseline acid-base status must be slowly reestablished if these patients are to wean. In other patients, sedation, opiates, nutritional status, electrolytes, and other underlying issues many be the concern. The more carefully all systems are reviewed, the greater the likelihood that the problem will be identified and the patient weaned from ventilatory support.

Box 52-15 Goals for Weaning After Long-Term Mechanical Ventilation

- Reduce the amount of support.
- Decrease the invasiveness of any support.
- Increase independence from mechanical devices.
- Preserve function.
- Maintain medical stability.

From Pierson DJ: Nonrespiratory aspects of weaning from mechanical ventilation. Respir Care 40:289, 1995.

CHRONICALLY VENTILATOR-DEPENDENT PATIENTS

Chronically ventilator-dependent patients (i.e., less than 1% of those requiring ventilatory support) present ethical, economic, and practical problems.[84] From an economic point of view, the long-term care of ventilator-dependent patients in an ICU is prohibitively expensive. Often these patients are transferred to subacute or long-term care facilities, where they can be cared for in an environment that is less intrusive and more like home (see Chapter 56).[84] For cases in which the family has adequate resources, the patient may be cared for in the home. Regional weaning centers have been developed and have reported success with weaning most patients who are undergoing long-term mechanical ventilation.[1,84] Current guidelines suggest that, unless there is clear evidence of an irreversible cause of ventilator dependency (e.g., a high spinal cord injury, amyotrophic lateral sclerosis), patients should not be considered permanently ventilator dependent until 3 months of weaning attempts have failed. If the patient is unweanable, the goal should be to restore the patient to the highest level of independent function possible. For example, portable wheelchair-mounted ventilators have been effective for providing a surprising level of mobility and independence to persons who are quadriplegic. Table 52-7 describes the management of common problems among difficult-to-wean patients. Box 52-15 lists the goals for weaning of patients who are receiving long-term ventilation.

TERMINAL WEANING

The term *terminal weaning* has been used to refer to the discontinuation of mechanical ventilatory support in the face of a catastrophic and irreversible illness.[85] The decision to proceed with disconnecting the ventilator when such an act is likely to cause the death of a patient is fraught with ethical, emotional, and practical problems. The decision should be made by the family in consultation with the patient's physician and in accordance with established ethical and legal guidelines.[85] Determinants of the decision to withdraw ventilation include the patient's desire to not continue with life support, the predictions of a low chance of survival in the ICU (i.e., less than 10%), the likelihood that future cognitive function would be severely impaired, and the continuous need for inotropes or vasopressors to maintain blood pressure.[85] After the decision has been

TABLE 52-7

Management of Problems Among Difficult-to-Wean Patients

Problem	Management Strategy
Anemia	Transfuse when hemoglobin level is ≤10 g/dl and hematocrit level is ≤30% if these are thought to be factors in decreased tissue oxygenation.
Increased WOB	1. Tube related a. Apply pressure support or ATC. b. Change the size of the small endotracheal tube. c. Deflate the cuff if all breathing is spontaneous and the risk of aspiration is minimal. d. Consider tracheotomy. 2. Secretion related (see later) 3. Bronchospasm related a. Administer bronchodilators. • β_2-agonists • Anticholinergics • Steroids b. Apply CPAP to reduce auto-PEEP. c. Manage the cause. 4. Ventilator related a. Assure synchrony for machine breaths. b. Eliminate auto-PEEP. c. Use flow-by or flow-trigger ventilation with or without pressure support.
Secretions, atelectasis, or plugging	1. Systemically hydrate. 2. Provide adequate humidity (i.e., humidifier temperature 35° C to 37° C at airway connection). 3. Maximally bronchodilate when necessary. 4. Suction.
Dyspnea	1. Use positioning (i.e., out of bed, dangling, and leaning forward). 2. Reassure and communicate with the patient. 3. Increase endurance, alternate weaning with rest to promote endurance. 4. Provide distraction.
Malposition	1. Position the patient to maximize diaphragmatic excursion and to improve lung volume and gas exchange (i.e., sitting or dangling). 2. Use a rocking chair. 3. Follow $\dot{V}_E$, V_T, rate, values for optimum positioning.
Respiratory muscle fatigue	1. Direct management at the cause. 2. Ensure adequate oxygen transport and cardiac output. 3. Nourish the patient. 4. Replace depleted electrolytes. 5. Decrease the WOB. a. Administer supplemental oxygen. b. Clear secretions. c. Decrease airway resistance.
Hemodynamic and fluid problems	1. Administer volume replacement and drugs to increase contractility, increase or decrease preload, and decrease afterload. 2. Delay weaning until the patient's cardiovascular status is stable. 3. Use techniques and the mode of ventilation to decrease the mean airway pressure.
Infection	1. Identify potential sites of infection. 2. Remove lines early, or replace them periodically. 3. Control infection. 4. Nourish the patient.
Metabolic problems	1. Control the cause and postpone weaning if the patient has acidosis. 2. Keep the carbon dioxide level at baseline if the patient has COPD, or allow progressive renal compensation during long-term weaning. 3. Provide moderate carbohydrate loading with total parenteral nutrition.
Low magnesium level	4. Give supplements.
High magnesium level	5. Provide dialysis or calcium chloride.
Low calcium level	6. Control the cause before weaning.
Low phosphate level	7. Replace phosphate before weaning.
Nutrition	1. Assess weight, albumin, and total lymphocyte count at admission. 2. Label the degree of malnutrition, and calculate protein needs. 3. Nourish the patient.

TABLE 52-7

Management of Problems Among Difficult-to-Wean Patients—cont'd

Problem	Management Strategy
Exercise	1. Provide exercise therapy to increase muscle function, prevent contracture, and maintain joint integrity (i.e., passive-to-active range of motion and sitting to walking). 2. Increase strength during activities of daily living. 3. Secure a physiotherapy consultation. 4. Consider the use of an exercise bicycle. 5. Encourage wheelchair rides or walks with a portable ventilator. 6. Provide breathing retraining.
Psychologic problems	1. Secure early psychiatric consultation. 2. Allow for patient control. 3. Demonstrate staff accountability and honesty. 4. Provide a communication method. 5. Decrease environmental stress. 6. Teach relaxation methods. 7. Provide mental stimulation. 8. Provide recreation. 9. Provide rewards for reaching short-term goals. 10. Encourage self-care. 11. Allow other patients to visit. 12. Provide flexible visiting hours 13. Take the patient out of the ICU environment.
Sleep disturbances	1. Provide a quiet environment (i.e., dim lights), reposition the patient, give a back rub, and administer sedation. 2. Provide for uninterrupted sleep. 3. Avoid weaning at night. 4. Provide relaxation method (e.g., hypnosis, biofeedback, progressive muscle relaxation). 5. Prescribe short-acting sedative hypnotics.
Pain	1. Administer minimal analgesia.

Modified from Norton LC, Neureuter A: Weaning the long-term ventilator-dependent patient: common problems and management. Crit Care Nurse 9:42–52, 1989.

made, the process is generally one of ventilator disconnection rather than weaning. The method of terminal weaning should be as humane and as comfortable as possible and should not be done in a way that further burdens the family.[86]

SUMMARY CHECKLIST

- The most common cause of ventilator dependence is a ventilatory workload that exceeds the patient's ventilatory capabilities.
- Other common causes of ventilator dependence include oxygenation problems, cardiovascular instability, and psychologic factors.
- The most important criterion for determining whether a patient is ready for ventilator discontinuation or weaning is a significant improvement or reversal of the disease state or condition that caused the patient to need ventilatory support.
- Factors that should be optimized before weaning include oxygenation, ventilation, acid-base balance and electrolyte levels, cardiovascular status, kidney function and fluid balance, sleep deprivation, psychologic status, nutrition, and overall medical condition.
- Weaning techniques include spontaneous breathing trials, PSV, and SIMV.
- Spontaneous breathing trials and PSV result in faster discontinuation of ventilatory support as compared with SIMV.
- The ideal approach to weaning the vast majority of patients is a therapist-driven protocol that makes use of an SBT.
- The monitoring of the patient during weaning should include SpO_2, respiratory rate and pattern, dyspnea, cardiac rate and rhythm, and blood pressure assessments.
- The use of daily SATs or the maintenance of minimal sedation not only improves the speed of weaning but has also been shown to improve mortality.
- Before extubation, patients should be assessed for the ability to maintain and protect their airway and for the presence of upper airway edema.
- Common causes of weaning failure include an excessive ventilatory workload in the presence of ventilatory muscle weakness or fatigue, oxygenation problems, cardiovascular instability, the inability to clear secretions, poor mental status, and the presence of an underlying concurrent pathologic condition that necessitates treatment.
- The goals of the weaning of long-term ventilator-dependent patients include reducing the amount of support, reducing the invasiveness of support, and increasing the patient's level of independent function.
- Only <1.0% of patients that require mechanical ventilation end up long-term ventilator-dependent patients.
- The decision to terminally wean a patient should be made by the family in consultation with the patient's medical team and in accordance with established ethical and legal guidelines.

References

1. MacIntyre NR, Cook DJ, Ely EW, et al: Evidence-based guidelines for weaning and discontinuing ventilator support: a collective task force facilitated by the American College of Chest Physicians, the American Association for Respiratory Care, and the American College of Critical Care Medicine. *Chest* 120:375S–395S, 2001.
2. Tobin M: Medical progress: advances in mechanical ventilation. *N Engl J Med* 344:1986–1996, 2001.
3. Clement JM, Buck EA: Weaning from mechanical ventilatory support. *Dimens Crit Care Nurs* 15:114–129, 1996.
4. Agency for Healthcare Research and Quality: *Criteria for weaning from mechanical ventilation, evidence report/technology assessment No. 23 (AHRQ publication no. 01-E010)*, Rockville, MD, 2000, Agency for Healthcare Research and Quality.
5. Meade MO, Guyalt H, Cook DJ: Weaning from mechanical ventilation: the evidence from clinical research. *Respir Care* 46:1408–1415, 2001.
6. Grap MJ, Strickland D, Tormey L, et al: Collaborative practice: development, implementation, and evaluation of a weaning protocol for patients receiving mechanical ventilation. *Am J Crit Care* 12:454–460, 2003.
7. Tonnelier JM: Impact of a nurses' protocol-directed weaning procedure on outcomes in patients undergoing mechanical ventilation for longer than 48 hours: a prospective cohort study with a matched historical control group. *Crit Care* 9:R83–R89, 2005.
8. Smyrnios NA, Connolly A, Wilson MM, et al: Effects of a multifaceted, multidisciplinary, hospital-wide quality improvement program on weaning from mechanical ventilation. *Crit Care Med* 30:1224–1230, 2002.
9. Ramachandran V, Grap MJ, Sessier CN: Protocol-directed weaning: a process of continuous performance improvement. *Crit Care* 9:138–140, 2005.
10. Loni NI, Walsh TS: Prolonged mechanical ventilation in critically ill patients: epidemiology, outcome and modeling the potential cost consequences of establishing a regional weaning unit. *Criti Care* 15:102–109, 2011.
11. Hannan LM, Tan S, Hopkinson K, et al: Inpatient and long term outcomes of individuals admitted for weaning from mechanical ventilation at a specialized ventilator weaning unit. *Respirology* 18:154–160, 2013.
12. Bigatello LM, Stelfox HT, Berra L, et al: Outcome of patients undergoing prolonged mechanical ventilation after critical illness. *Crit Care Med* 35:2491–2497, 2007.
13. Deem S: Intensive-care-unit-acquired muscle weakness. *Respir Care* 51:1042–1052, 2006.
14. Laghi F, D'Alfonso N, Tobin MJ: Pattern of recovery from diaphragmatic fatigue over 24 hours. *J Appl Physiol* 79:539–546, 1995.
15. Thille AW, Cortes-Puch I, Estaban A: Weaning from the ventilator and extubation in the ICU. *Curr Opin Crit Care* 19:57–64, 2013.
16. Tobin MJ: Of principles and protocols and weaning. *Am J Respir and Crit Care Med* 169:66–72, 2004.
17. Hanneman SK, Ingersoll GL, Knebel AR, et al: Weaning from short term mechanical ventilation: a review. *Am J Crit Care* 3:421–441, 1994.
18. Yang KL: Reproducibility of weaning parameters: a need for specialization. *Chest* 102:1829–1832, 1992.
19. Bien MY, Shui Lin Y, Shih CH, et al: Comparisons of predictive performance of breathing pattern variability measured during T-piece, automatic tube compensation, and pressure support ventilation for weaning intensive care unit patients from mechanical ventilation. *Crit Care Med* 39:2253–2262, 2011.
20. Shikora PA, Benotti PN, Johannigman JA: The oxygen cost of breathing may predict weaning from mechanical ventilation better than respiratory rate to tidal volume ratio. *Arch Surg* 129:269–274, 1994.
21. Hess DR: Mechanical ventilation of the adult patient: initiation, management and weaning. In Burton GG, Hodgkin JE, Ward JJ, editors: *Respiratory care: a guide to clinical practice*, Philadelphia, 1997, Lippincott Williams & Wilkins.
22. Kress JP, Pohlman AS, O'Connor MF, et al: Daily interruption of sedative infusions in critically ill patients undergoing mechanical ventilation. *N Engl J Med* 342:1471–1477, 2000.
23. Sessler CN: Wake up and breathe. *Crit Care Med* 32:1413–1414, 2004.
24. Arroliga A, Frutos-Vivar F, Hall J, et al: Use of sedatives and neuromuscular blockers in a cohort of patients receiving mechanical ventilation. *Chest* 128:496–506, 2005.
25. Nava S, Gregoretti C, Fanfulla F, et al: Noninvasive ventilation for prevention of respiratory failure after extubation in high-risk patients. *Crit Care Med* 33:2465–2470, 2005.
26. Ferrer M, Valencia M, Nicolas JM, et al: Early noninvasive ventilation averts extubation failure in patients at risk. *Am J Respir Crit Care Med* 173:164–170, 2006.
27. MacIntyre NR: Psychological factors in weaning from mechanical ventilatory support. *Respir Care* 40:277–281, 1995.
28. Esteban A, Frutos F, Tobin MJ, et al: A comparison of four methods of weaning patients from mechanical ventilation. *N Engl J Med* 332:345–350, 1995.
29. Esteban A, Alia I, Gordo F, et al: Extubation outcome after spontaneous breathing trial with T-piece or pressure support ventilation. *Am J Respir Crit Care Med* 156:459–465, 1997.
30. Brochard L, Rauss A, Benito S, et al: Comparison of three methods of gradual withdrawal from ventilatory support during weaning from mechanical ventilation. *Am J Respir Crit Care Med* 150:896–903, 1994.
31. Ely EW, Baker AM, Evans GW, et al: The prognostic significance of passing a daily screen of weaning parameters. *Intensive Care Med* 25:581–587, 1999.
32. Marini JJ, Smith TC, Lamb VJ: External work output and force generation during synchronized intermittent mechanical ventilation. *Am Rev Respir Dis* 138:1169–1177, 1988.
33. Imsand C, Feihl F, Perret C, et al: Regulation of inspiratory neuromuscular output during synchronized intermittent mechanical ventilation. *Anesthesiology* 80:13–22, 1994.
34. Jounieaux V, Duran A, Levi-Valensi P: Synchronized intermittent mandatory ventilation with and without pressure support ventilation in weaning patients with COPD from mechanical ventilation. *Chest* 105:1204–1210, 1994.
35. Heymann A, Radtke F, Schiemann A, et al: Delayed treatment of delirium increases mortality rate in intensive care unit patients. *J Int Med Res* 38:1584–1595, 2010.
36. Girard TD, Kress JP, Fuchs BD, et al: Efficacy and safety of a paired sedation and ventilation weaning protocol for mechanically ventilated patients in intensive care (awaking and breathing control trial): a randomized controlled trial. *Lancet* 371:126–134, 2008.
37. Mehta S, Burry L, Cook D, et al: Daily sedation interruption in mechanically ventilated critically ill patients cared for with a sedation protocol: a randomized controlled trial. *JAMA* 308:1985–1992, 2012.
38. Hewlett AW, Plott AS, Terry VG: Mandatory minute ventilation. *Anesthesia* 32:163–169, 1977.
39. Davis S, Potgieter PD, Linton DM: Mandatory minute volume weaning in patients with pulmonary pathology. *Anaesth Intensive Care* 17:170–174, 1989.
40. Campbell RS, Branson RD, Johannigman JA: Adaptive support ventilation. *Respir Care Clin N Am* 7:425–440, 2001.
41. Sulzer CF, Chiolero R, Chassot P, et al: Adaptive support ventilation for fast tracheal extubation after cardiac surgery: a randomized controlled study. *Anesthesiology* 95:1339–1345, 2001.
42. Cassina T, Chioléro R, Mauri R, et al: Clinical experience with adaptive support ventilation for fast tract anesthesia. *J Cardiothorac Vasc Anesth* 17:571–575, 2003.
43. Armal JC, Wysocki M, Nafati C, et al: Automatic selection of breathing pattern using adaptive support ventilation. *Intensive Care Med* 34:75–81, 2008.
44. Arnal JM, Garnero A, Novonti D, et al: Feasibility study on full closed-loop control ventilation (IntelliVent-ASV™) in ICU patients with acute respiratory failure: a prospective observational comparative study. *Crit Care* 17:R196–R203, 2013.
45. Arnal JM, Wysocki M, Novotni D, et al: Safety and efficacy of a fully closed-loop control ventilation (IntelliVent-ASV®) in sedated ICU patients with acute respiratory failure: a prospective randomized crossover study. *Intensive Care Med* 38:781–787, 2012.

46. Iregui M, Ward S, Clinikscale D, et al: Use of a handheld computer by respiratory care practitioners to improve the efficiency of weaning patients from mechanical ventilation. *Crit Care Med* 30:2038–2043, 2002.
47. Lellouche F, Mancebo J, Jolliet P, et al: A multicenter randomized trial of computer-driven protocolized weaning from mechanical ventilation. *Am J Respir Crit Care Med* 174:849–851, 2006.
48. Burns KE, Lellouche F, Nisenbaum R, et al: Automated weaning and SBT systems versus non-automated weaning strategies for weaning time in invasively ventilated critically ill adults. *Cochrane Database Syst Rev* (9):CD008638, 2014.
49. Guttmann J, Haberthur C, Mols G: Automatic tube compensation. *Respir Care Clin N Am* 7:475–501, 2001.
50. Jabar S, Delay JM, Matecki S, et al: Volume guaranteed pressure support ventilation facing acute changes in ventilatory demand. *Intensive Care Med* 31:1181–1188, 2005.
51. Randolph AJ, Wypij D, Venkataraman S, et al: Effects of mechanical ventilation on respiratory outcome in infants and children. *JAMA* 288:2561–2568, 2002.
52. Kacmarek RM: Proportional assist ventilation and neurally adjusted ventilatory assist. *Respir Care* 56:140–152, 2011.
53. Xirouchaki N, Kondili E, Vaporidi K, et al: Proportional assist ventilation with load-adjustable gain factors in critically ill patients: comparison with pressure support. *Intensive Care Med* 34:2026–2034, 2008.
54. de la Oliva P, Schüffelmann C, Gómez-Zamora A, et al: Asynchrony, neural drive, ventilatory variability and COMFORT: NAVA versus pressure support in pediatric patients: A non-randomized cross-over trial. *Intensive Care Med* 38:838–846, 2012.
55. Piquilloud L, Tassaux D, Bialais E: Neurally adjusted ventilatory assist (NAVA) improves patient-ventilator interaction during non-invasive ventilation delivered by face mask. *Intensive Care Med* 38:1624–1632, 2012.
56. Nava S, Ambrosino N, Enrico C, et al: Noninvasive ventilation in the weaning of patients with respiratory failure due to chronic obstructive pulmonary disease: a randomized controlled trial. *Ann Intern Med* 128:721–728, 1998.
57. Girault C, Daudenthua I, Chevron V, et al: Noninvasive ventilation as a systematic extubation and weaning technique in acute-on-chronic respiratory failure: a prospective randomized controlled study. *Am J Respir Crit Care Med* 160:86–92, 1999.
58. Ferrer M, Esquinas A, Arancibia F, et al: Noninvasive ventilation during persistent weaning failure. *Am J Respir Crit Care Med* 168:70–76, 2003.
59. Ferrer M, Sellares J, Valencia M, et al: Noninvasive ventilation after extubation in hypercarbic patients with chronic respiratory disorders: a randomized controlled trial. *Lancet* 374:1082–1088, 2009.
60. Keenan SP, Powers C, McCormack DG, et al: Noninvasive positive pressure ventilation for post-extubation respiratory distress. *JAMA* 287:2338–2344, 2002.
61. Esteban A, Frutos-Vivar F, Ferguson ND, et al: Noninvasive positive pressure ventilation for respiratory failure alter extubation. *N Engl J Med* 350:2452–2460, 2004.
62. Patel BK, Pohlman AS, Hall JB, et al: Impact of early mobilization on glycemic control and ICU-acquired weakness in critically ill patients who are mechanically ventilated. *Chest* 146:583–589, 2014.
63. Abrams D, Javidfar J, Farrand E, et al: Early mobilization of patients receiving extracorporeal membrane oxygenation: a retrospective cohort study. *Crit Care* 18:R38, 2014.
64. Krishnan JA, Moore D, Robeson C: A prospective, controlled trial of a protocol-based strategy to discontinue mechanical ventilation. *Am J Respir Crit Care Med* 169:673–678, 2004.
65. Wood G, MacLeod B, Moffatt S: Weaning from mechanical ventilation: physician-directed vs a respiratory-therapist-directed protocol. *Respir Care* 40:219–224, 1995.
66. Ely W, Baker AM, Dunagan DP, et al: Effects on the duration of mechanical ventilation of identifying patients capable of breathing spontaneously. *N Engl J Med* 335:1864–1869, 1996.
67. Marlich G, Murin S, Battistella F, et al: Protocol weaning of mechanical ventilation in medical and surgical patients by respiratory care practitioners and nurses. *Chest* 118:459–467, 2000.
68. Sassoon C, Ehu Z, Caiozzo VJ: Assist-control mechanical ventilation attenuates ventilator-induced diaphragmatic dysfunction. *Am J Respir Crit Care Med* 170:626–632, 2004.
69. Jubran A: Critical illness and mechanical ventilation: effects on the diaphragm. *Respir Care* 51:1054–1061, 2006.
70. Marini JJ: Dyspnea during weaning. *Respir Care* 40:271–276, 1995.
71. Morley TF, Giaimo J, Maroszan E, et al: Use of capnography for assessment of the adequacy of alveolar ventilation during weaning. *Am Rev Respir Dis* 148:339–344, 1993.
72. Mohsenifar Z, Hay A, Hay J, et al: Gastric intramural pH as a predictor of success or failure in weaning patients from mechanical ventilation. *Ann Intern Med* 119:794–798, 1993.
73. Abalos A, Leibowitz AB, Distefano D, et al: Myocardial ischemia during the weaning period. *Am J Crit Care* 1:32–36, 1992.
74. Straus C, Louis B, Isabey D, et al: Contribution of the endotracheal tube and the upper airway to breathing workload. *Am J Respir Crit Care Med* 157:23–30, 1998.
75. Sharar S: The effects of artificial airways on airflow and ventilatory mechanics: basic concepts and clinical relevance. *Respir Care* 40:257–262, 1995.
76. Diehl JL, El Atrous S, Touchard D, et al: Changes in the work of breathing induced by tracheotomy in ventilatory-dependent patients. *Am J Respir Crit Care Med* 159:383–388, 1999.
77. Mietto C, Pinciroli R, Piriyapatsom A, et al: Tracheal tube obstruction in mechanically ventilated patients assessed by high-resolution computed tomography. *Anesthesiology* 12:1226–1235, 2014.
78. Mietto C, Foley K, Salerno L, et al: Removal of endotracheal tube obstruction with a secretion clearance device. *Respir Care* 59:1222–1226, 2014.
79. Miller RL, Cole RP: Association between reduced cuff leak volume and postextubation stridor. *Chest* 110:1035–1040, 1996.
80. Sandhu RS, Pasquale MD, Miller K, et al: Measurement of endotracheal tube cuff leak to predict postextubation stridor and need for reintubation. *J Am Coll Surg* 190:682–687, 2000.
81. Jaber S, Chanques G, Matecki S, et al: Post-extubation stridor in intensive care unit patients. Risk factors evaluation and importance of the cuff-leak test. *Intensive Care Med* 29:69–74, 2003.
82. Hurford WE, Favorito F: Association of myocardial ischemia with failure to wean from mechanical ventilation. *Crit Care Med* 23:1475–1480, 1995.
83. Hund EF, Fogel W, Krieger D, et al: Critical illness polyneuropathy: clinical findings and outcomes of a frequent cause of neuromuscular weaning failure. *Crit Care Med* 24:1328–1333, 1996.
84. Management of patients requiring prolonged mechanical ventilation: report of a NAMDRC Consensus Conference. *Chest* 128:3937–3954, 2005.
85. Shekleton ME, Burns SM, Clochesy JM, et al: Terminal weaning from mechanical ventilation: a review. *AACN Clin Issues Crit Care Nurs* 5:523–533, 1994.
86. Cook D, Rocker G, Marshall J, et al: Withdrawal of mechanical ventilation in anticipation of death in the intensive care unit. *N Engl J Med* 349:1123–1132, 2003.

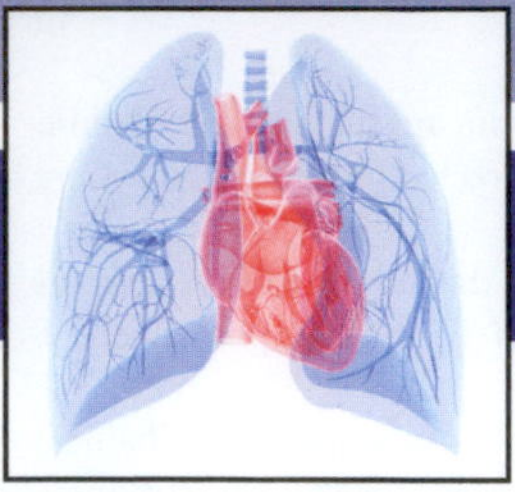

CHAPTER 53

Neonatal and Pediatric Respiratory Care

DANIEL W. CHIPMAN

CHAPTER OBJECTIVES

After reading this chapter you will be able to:

- Describe the correct approach to assessment of the fetus and newborn infant.
- Discuss the use of oxygen therapy, bronchial hygiene therapy, aerosol drug therapy, airway management, and resuscitation approaches in the care of infants and children.
- List the components of an Apgar Score.
- Identify the different S_pO_2 target ranges for preterm and full term infants and those with primary pulmonary hypertension.
- Describe the correct approach to assessment of the pediatric patient.
- Discuss the use of high flow nasal cannulas in infants and children.
- Discuss the use of continuous positive airway pressure and the basics of mechanical ventilation including high-frequency ventilation in the care of infants and children.
- Discuss the use of noninvasive ventilation in infants and children.
- List clinical situations where nitric oxide is used, and discuss its basic application.
- Explain the correct approach to ventilator management for a patient in status asthmaticus.
- Discuss the use of heliox for a patient with asthma.
- Discuss the steps to ventilator discontinuance for infants and children including a safety screen and assessment of ability to breathe spontaneously.

CHAPTER OUTLINE

KEY TERMS

- Apgar score
- appropriate for gestational age (AGA)
- continuous positive airway pressure (CPAP)
- extremely low birth weight (ELBW)
- grunting, flaring, and retracting
- high-frequency ventilation (HFV)
- inhaled nitric oxide (INO)
- large for gestational age (LGA)
- meconium
- patent ductus arteriosus (PDA)
- primary pulmonary hypertension of the newborn (PPHN)
- retinopathy of prematurity (ROP)
- small for gestational age (SGA)
- surfactant
- very low birth weight (VLBW)

Caring for infants and children is one of the most challenging and rewarding aspects of respiratory care. Competent clinical practice in this area requires knowledge of the many pathophysiologic differences among infants, children, and adults. Understanding the unique pathophysiology involved in neonatal and pediatric respiratory disorders (see Chapter 34) can assist the respiratory therapist (RT) in providing quality care to infants and children. A thorough understanding of how the respiratory system develops in the fetus is the first step toward acquiring the specialized knowledge needed to practice neonatal respiratory care (see Chapter 9). This chapter begins with an overview of neonatal and pediatric patient assessment and then describes respiratory care modalities used to treat these patients.

ASSESSMENT OF THE NEWBORN

Assessment of the newborn begins before birth with assessment of the maternal history, the maternal condition, and the status of the fetus.

Maternal Factors

Maternal risk factors include many medical, physical, and social conditions. Maternal health and individual physiology, pregnancy complications, and maternal behaviors affect the health of the fetus. Any condition that causes an interference with placental blood flow or the transfer of oxygen (O_2) to the fetus can result in an adverse outcome. The clinician must be prepared for the possibility of resuscitation at delivery. This possibility is best anticipated by identifying risk factors that relate to neonatal compromise. Table 53-1 lists maternal risks and related outcomes of which the team preparing to receive the infant should be aware when the infant is delivered.

Fetal Assessment

Fetal assessment is performed with ultrasonography, amniocentesis, fetal heart rate monitoring, and fetal blood gas analysis. Ultrasonography uses high-frequency sound waves to obtain an image of the infant in utero. This image allows the physician to view the position of the fetus and placenta, measure fetal growth, identify possible anatomic anomalies, and assess the amniotic fluid qualitatively.

Amniocentesis involves direct sampling and quantitative assessment of amniotic fluid. Amniotic fluid may be inspected for **meconium** (fetal bowel contents) or blood. In addition, sloughed fetal cells can be analyzed for genetic normality. Lung maturation can be assessed with amniocentesis. The lecithin-to-sphingomyelin ratio (L:S ratio) involves measurement of two phospholipids, lecithin and sphingomyelin, synthesized by the fetus in utero. As shown in Figure 53-1, the L:S ratio increases with increasing gestational age. At approximately 34 to 35 weeks' gestation, this ratio abruptly increases to greater

TABLE 53-1
Maternal Condition and Neonatal Outcomes

Maternal Condition	Fetal or Neonatal Outcome
Previous pregnancy complication	Same outcome as previous fetus
Diabetes mellitus	LGA, congenital malformations, RDS, hypoglycemia
Pregnancy-induced hypertension	Prematurity, SGA (preeclampsia)
Maternal age <17 years	Low birth weight, prematurity
Maternal age >35 years	Prematurity, chromosomal defects
Placenta previa	Prematurity, bleeding, SGA
Abruptio placentae	Fetal asphyxia, bleeding
Alcohol consumption	SGA, CNS dysfunction, mental retardation, facial dysmorphology
Smoking	SGA, prematurity, mental retardation, SIDS
Drug use	Placental abruption, IUGR, prematurity, CNS abnormalities, withdrawal disorders

IUGR, Intrauterine growth restriction; *RDS,* respiratory distress syndrome; *SIDS,* sudden infant death syndrome.

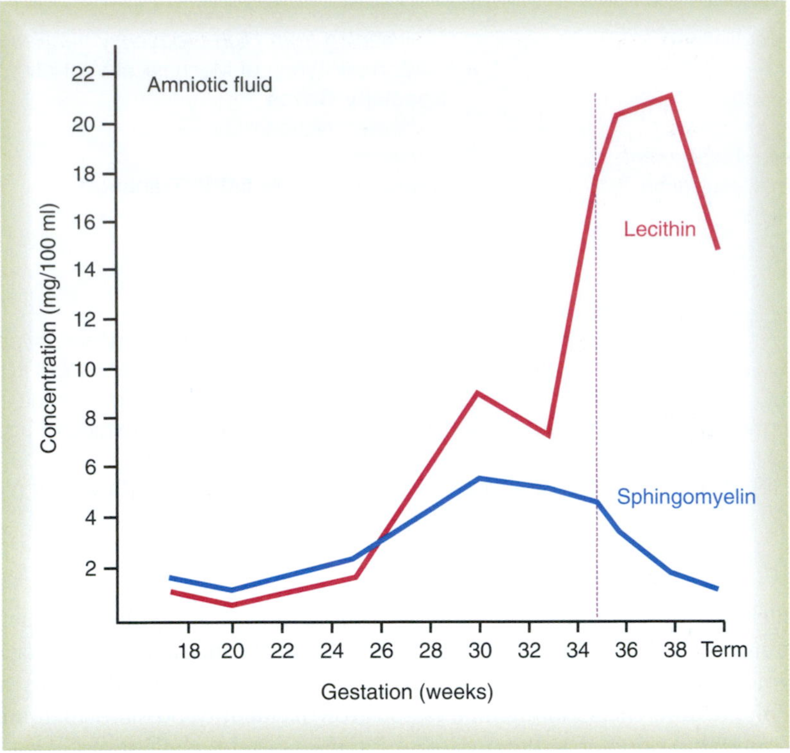

FIGURE 53-1 Lecithin *(red line)* and sphingomyelin *(blue line)* concentrations plotted against gestational age. L:S ratio rises to 1.2 at 28 weeks and to 2 or more at 35 weeks, indicating maturation of the fetal lung. (Modified from Gluck L, et al: Am J Obstet Gynecol 109:440, 1971.)

than 2:1. An L:S ratio greater than 2:1 indicates stable **surfactant** production and mature lungs.[1] Phosphatidylglycerol is another lipid found in the amniotic fluid that is used to assess fetal lung maturity. Phosphatidylglycerol first appears at approximately 35 to 36 weeks' gestation. If phosphatidylglycerol is more than 1% of the total phospholipids, the risk of respiratory distress syndrome is less than 1%.[2] Fetal heart rate monitoring includes the measurement of fetal heart rate and uterine contractions during labor. Examination of fetal heart rate changes related to uterine contractions identifies a fetus in distress. Fetal well-being is obtained by examining the variability and reactivity of the fetal heart rate. A normal fetal heart rate ranges from 120 to 160 beats/min. Fetal tachycardia can be a sign of fetal hypoxemia or could be related to other factors, such as prematurity or maternal fever. Temporary declines in fetal heart rate are called *decelerations* and can be mild (<15 beats/min), moderate (15 to 45 beats/min), or severe (>45 beats/min). Decelerations are classified by their occurrence in the uterine contraction cycle.

Figure 53-2 illustrates the three common patterns of early decelerations, late decelerations, and variable decelerations. Early decelerations occur when the fetal heart rate decreases in the beginning of a contraction. This type of deceleration is benign and in most cases is caused by a vagal response related to compression of the fetal head in the birth canal. A late deceleration occurs when the heart rate decreases 10 to 30 seconds after the onset of contractions. A late deceleration pattern indicates impaired maternal-placental blood flow, or uteroplacental insufficiency. With variable decelerations, there is no clear relationship between contractions and heart rate. This pattern is the most common of the three and probably related to umbilical cord compression. Short periods of cord compression are generally benign, but prolonged periods of compression result in impaired umbilical blood flow and can lead to fetal distress. Fetal heart rate variability is the beat-to-beat variation in rate that occurs because of normal sympathetic or parasympathetic influences. A completely monotonous heart rate tracing may be indicative of fetal asphyxia. Fetal heart rate reactivity is the ability of the fetal heart rate to increase in response to movement or external stimuli. A healthy fetus has two accelerations within a 20-minute period.

In utero, the fetus receives its blood supply from the placenta. Only a small portion of the blood that enters the fetal right heart flows through the lungs. This is a result of fetal pulmonary blood vessels being constricted with a high resistance to blood flow. There are two openings in the fetal heart through which most fetal blood flows. These normal anatomic shunts in the fetus are called *patent foramen ovale* and *patent ductus arteriosus (PDA)*. Blood flows through these openings and into the umbilical vessels before returning to the mother. Pressure in the umbilical vessels is low. During the transition from fetal life to newborn life, the umbilical cord is clamped, and the infant's systemic blood pressure is increased. The infant begins to breathe, and O_2 enters the infant's blood. Oxygenated blood

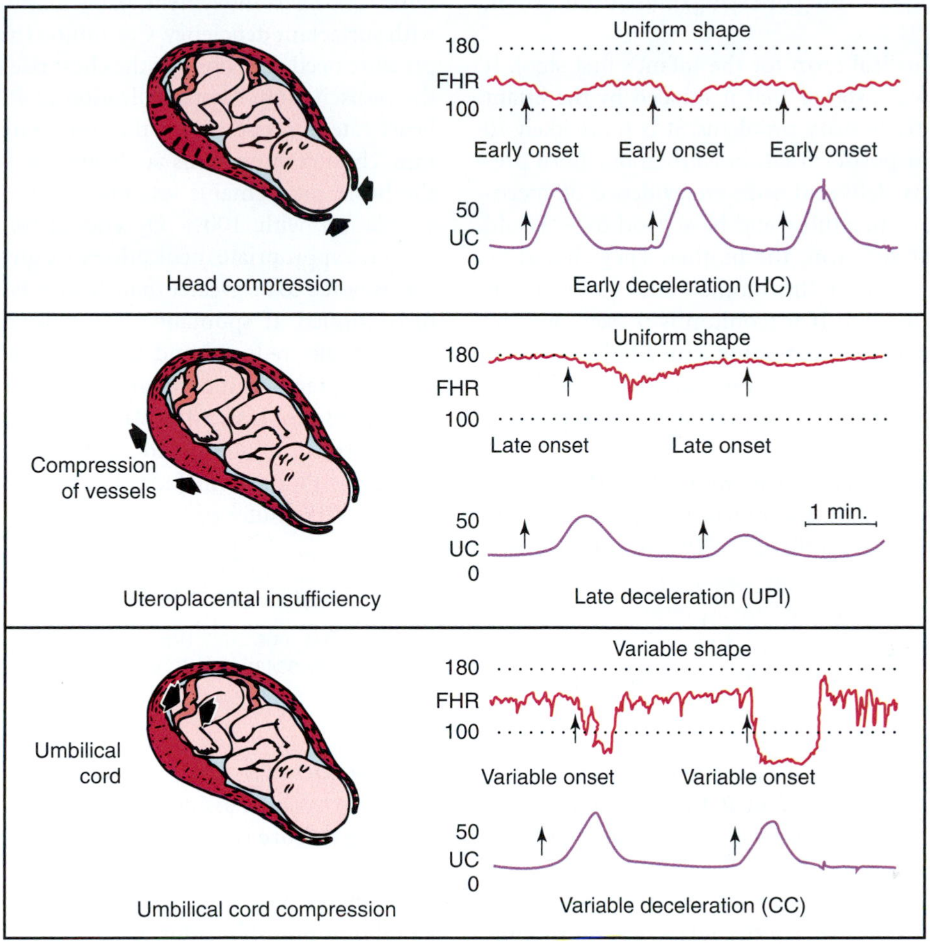

FIGURE 53-2 Fetal heart rate patterns. (Modified from Avery GB, editor: Neonatology: pathophysiology and management of the newborn, ed 2, Philadelphia, 1981, JB Lippincott.)

entering the pulmonary vessels causes the vessels to dilate and decreases pulmonary resistance. With higher systemic resistance and lower pulmonary resistance, less blood flows through the anatomic openings, and these openings begin to close. Evidence of normal transitional circulation is noted as the infant's skin turns from a bluish hue to pink over the first several minutes of life.

> **RULE OF THUMB**
>
> Infants presenting with a monotonous heart rate or a fetal scalp pH less than 7.2 may be experiencing asphyxia.

Fetal Blood Gas Analysis

When other factors indicate potential problems during labor and delivery, fetal blood pH can be used to determine severity. Normally, fetal blood is obtained from a capillary sample taken from the presenting body part, usually the scalp. Normal fetal capillary pH ranges from 7.35 to 7.25, with the lower values occurring late in labor. A pH less than 7.20 may indicate that the fetus is experiencing asphyxia. There is no direct correlation between fetal scalp and arterial blood pH; scalp pH should be used only to assist in interpreting clinical signs of fetal distress.

Evaluation of the Newborn

All newborns should be assessed immediately on delivery. Most newborns (>90%) do not need intervention when transitioning from intrauterine to extrauterine life. The two categories of newborns most likely to need intervention are infants born with evidence of meconium in their airway and premature infants. The need for intervention is determined by assessing for the presence of meconium, breathing or crying, muscle tone, color, and gestational age.

Meconium is the medical term for the infant's first stool. It is a sticky green-black substance that if inhaled by the infant can cause significant respiratory problems. It is more likely to be present in a term or postterm newborn than one born prematurely. Term infants delivered without evidence of meconium who are crying or breathing and have good tone should not routinely be separated from the mother. They should be dried, covered, and given to the mother and observed for breathing, activity, and color. If meconium is present and the infant is vigorous, pharyngeal suctioning with a bulb suction is appropriate. Simultaneously the infant should be dried and placed under a warmer and assessed for signs of respiratory distress.

If meconium is present in a nonvigorous infant, stimulation should be avoided. Immediate endotracheal intubation before beginning positive pressure ventilation (PPV) is indicated as a means to clear meconium from the airway. The endotracheal tube should be attached to a meconium aspirator, and a suction device should be regulated for −70 to −100 mm Hg. As soon as the endotracheal tube is inserted, suction should be applied to the tube, and then the endotracheal tube is withdrawn. Reintubation and repeat suctioning may be necessary if meconium is still visible in the airway. Frequent assessment of the heart rate is indicated during this process, and if the heart rate is less than 100 beats per minute, bag-mask ventilation should be performed.

Preterm infants frequently need intervention. The more preterm the infant, the more likely the infant will need some level of resuscitation. If an infant is preterm, is not breathing, is not vigorous, or does not have good tone, resuscitation efforts should be initiated. Efforts are directed at warming the infant because cold stress may increase O_2 consumption and impair all subsequent resuscitation efforts.

After the infant is dried and warmed, the infant is positioned supine, with the head in a neutral position or slightly extended. A bulb syringe or 8F to 10F suction catheter may be used for secretion removal; however, in the absence of blood or meconium, catheter suctioning should be limited because aggressive pharyngeal suctioning may cause laryngospasm or bradycardia. Suction pressure should not exceed −100 mm Hg. Once the infant is suctioned, dried, and warmed, if apnea or inadequate respirations are present, tactile stimulation may be used to encourage spontaneous breathing. Many infants respond to stimulation and need no further resuscitative efforts. If after 30 seconds the infant has a heart rate of less than 100 beats/min or is apneic, bag-mask ventilation at a rate of 40 to 60 beats/min should be initiated.

The *most* important and effective action in neonatal resuscitation is effective ventilation. Recommendations from the American Academy of Pediatrics are to attach a pulse oximeter to the infant, begin resuscitation efforts using room air, and assess carefully the amount of O_2 needed.[3] Effective PPV usually results in rapid improvement of heart rate. Initial ventilating pressures of 30 to 40 cm H_2O may be necessary to achieve noticeable chest movement, particularly in a preterm newborn with surfactant deficiency. Continuous assessment of the lowest pressure needed to observe the chest rise is essential throughout the resuscitation. After application of PPV for 30 seconds, the heart rate is reassessed. If the heart rate is less than 60 beats/min, chest compressions are begun, and PPV is maintained. If the heart rate remains less than 60 beats/min after adequate ventilation with 100% O_2 and chest compressions for 30 seconds, appropriate medications are given. As soon as the heart rate is noted to be greater than 100 beats/min, compressions are discontinued. If spontaneous breathing is present, PPV may be gradually reduced and then discontinued. If spontaneous breathing remains inadequate or if heart rate remains less than 100 beats/min, assisted ventilation is continued via bag-mask or endotracheal tube. Figure 53-3 outlines a newborn resuscitation algorithm and includes the targeted saturation levels for the first 10 minutes of life.

RULE OF THUMB

The most important and effective action in neonatal resuscitation is to ventilate.

Apgar Score

An Apgar score is assigned at 1 minute and 5 minutes of life. The **Apgar score** is an objective scoring system used to evaluate a newborn rapidly. As shown in Table 53-2, the score has five components: heart rate, respiratory effort, muscle tone, reflex irritability, and skin color. Each component is rated according to standard definitions, resulting in a composite assessment score. Generally, infants scoring 7 or higher at 1 minute are responding normally. An infant with a score of 7 may require supportive care, such as O_2 or stimulation to breathe. Infants

TABLE 53-2

Apgar Scoring System for Newborn Assessment

	SCORE		
Sign	**0**	**1**	**2**
Heart rate	Absent	<100/min	>100/min
Respirations	Absent	Slow, irregular	Good, crying
Muscle tone	Limp	Some flexion	Active motion
Reflex irritability (catheter in nares, tactile stimulation)	No response	Grimace	Cough, sneeze, cry
Color	Blue or pale	Pink body with completely blue extremities	Pink

From Koff PB, Eitzman DV, Neu J: Neonatal and pediatric respiratory care, ed 2, St Louis, 1993, Mosby.

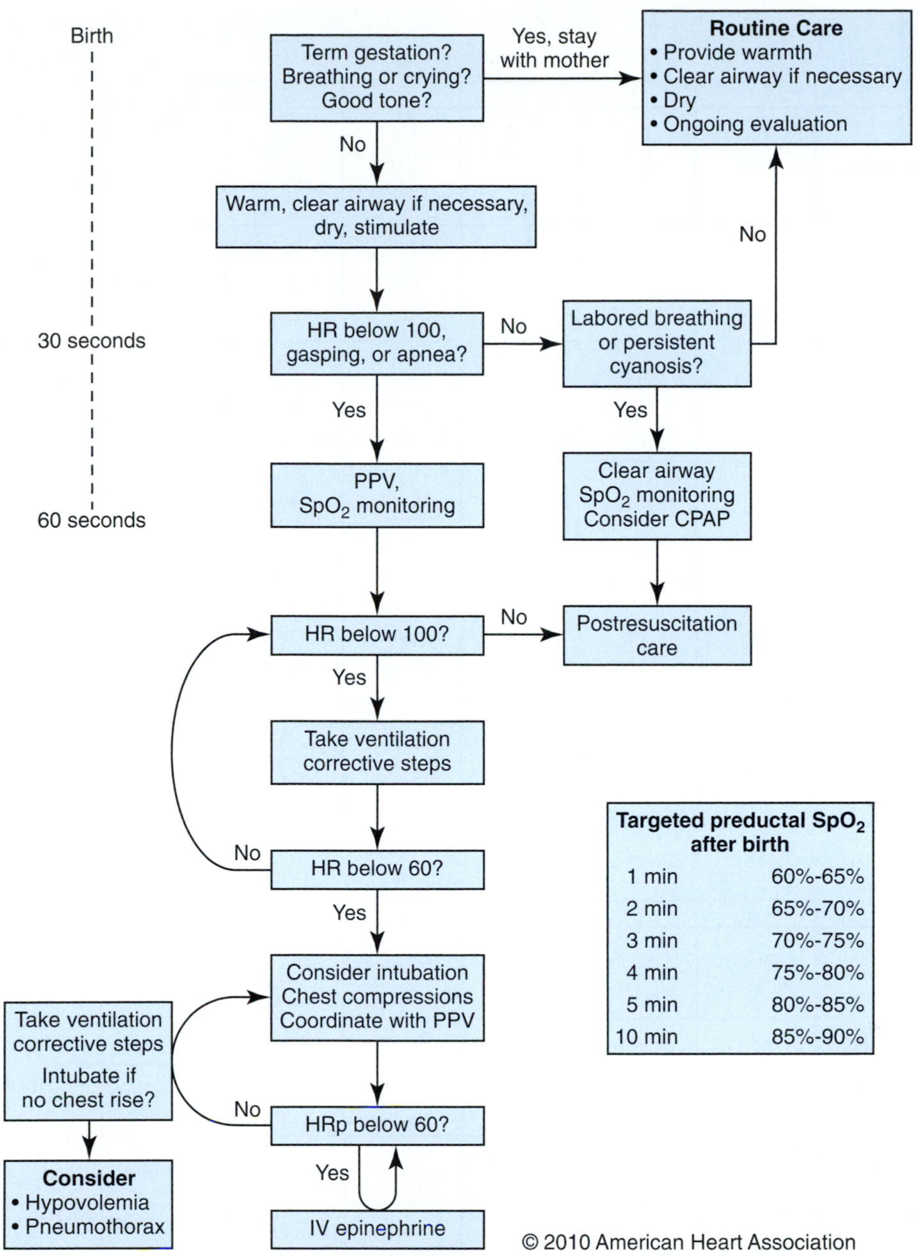

FIGURE 53-3 Neonatal resuscitation algorithm. Neonatal Resuscitation: 2010. American Heart Association Guidelines for Cardiopulmonary Resuscitation and Emergency Cardiovascular Care. © 2010 American Heart Association, Inc.

with a 1-minute Apgar score of 6 or lower may require more aggressive support.

Assessment of Gestational Age

Gestational age assessment and assessment of relationship of weight to gestational age are performed shortly after delivery. Determination of gestational age involves assessment of multiple physical characteristics and neurologic signs. Two common systems are used to determine gestational age: the Dubowitz scales and the Ballard scales. The Dubowitz scales involve assessment of 11 physical and 10 neurologic signs.[4] Physical criteria include assessment of skin texture, skin color, and genitalia. Neurologic criteria include posture and arm and leg recoil. The Ballard scales are a simplified version of the Dubowitz scales and include six physical and six neurologic signs as illustrated in Figure 53-4. Soon after delivery, the newborn is stabilized and weighed, followed by determination of gestational age. Infants born between 38 weeks and 42 weeks are considered term gestation. Infants born before 38 weeks are preterm. Infants born after 42 weeks are postterm.

All newborns weighing less than 2500 g are considered low birth weight. Newborns weighing less than 1500 g are considered **very low birth weight (VLBW)** Newborns weighing less than 1000 g are considered **extremely low birth weight (ELBW)** A newborn with a weight that is either too large or too small or who has been born preterm or postterm has a higher risk of

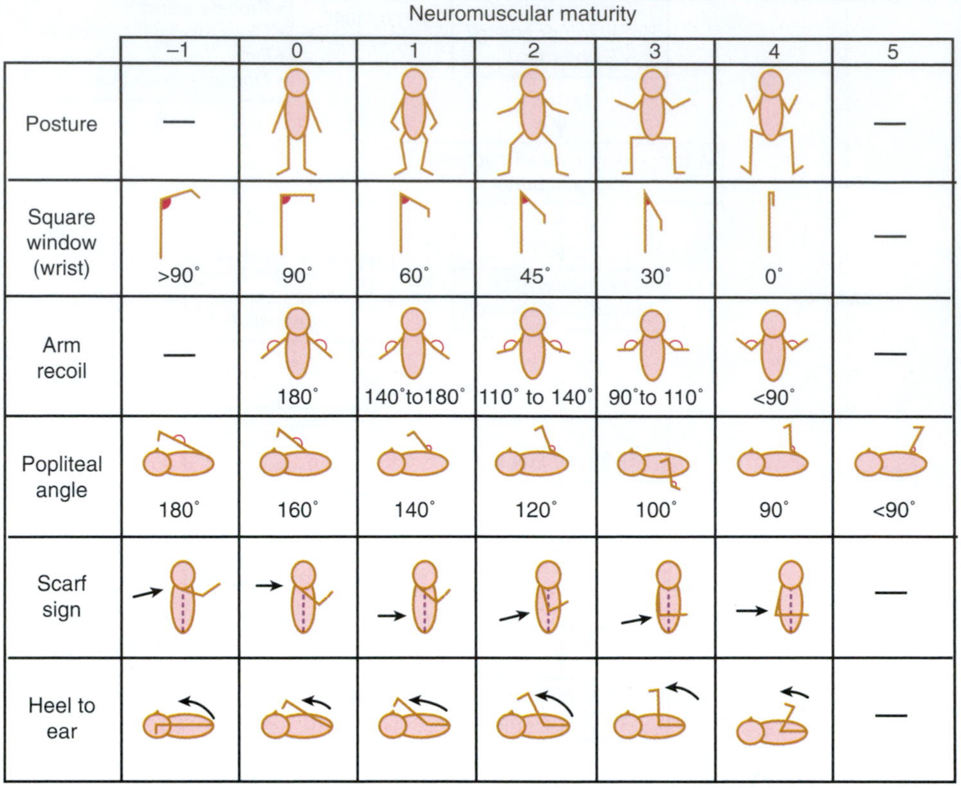

Physical maturity

	–1	0	1	2	3	4	5
Skin	Sticky, friable, transparent	Gelatinous, red, translucent	Superficial peeling or rash; few visible vessels	Superficial peeling or rash; few visible vessels	Cracking; pale areas; rare visible vessels	Parchment-like; deep cracking; no visible vessels	Leathery, cracked, wrinkled
Lanugo	None	Sparse	Abundant	Thinning	Bald areas	Mostly bald	—
Plantar surface	Heel-toe 40 to 50 mm: –1; <40mm: –2	>50 mm; no crease	Faint, red marks	Anterior transverse crease only	Creases over anterior two-thirds	Creases over entire sole	—
Breast	Imperceptible	Barely perceptible	Flat areola; no bud	Stippled areola; 1- to 2-mm bud	Raised areola; 3- to 4-mm bud	Full areola; 5- to 10-mm bud	—
Eye and ear	Lids fused, loosely: –1; tightly: –2	Lids open; pinna flat, stays folded	Slightly curved pinna; soft, slow recoil	Well curved pinna; soft but ready recoil	Formed and firm; instant recoil	Thick cartilage; ear stiff	—
Genitalia, male	Scrotum flat, smooth	Scrotum empty; faint rugae	Testes in upper canal; rare rugae	Testes descending; few rugae	Testes down; good rugae	Testes pendulous; deep rugae	—
Genitalia, female	Clitoris prominent; labia flat	Prominent clitoris; small labia minora	Prominent clitoris; enlarging minora	Major and minora equally prominent	Majora large; minora small	Majora cover clitoris and minora	—

Maturity rating

Score	–10	–5	0	5	10	15	20	25	30	35	40	45	50
Weeks	20	22	24	26	28	30	32	34	36	38	40	42	44

FIGURE 53-4 The Ballard gestational age assessment. (Modified from Ballard JL, et al: J Pediatr 95:769, 1979.)

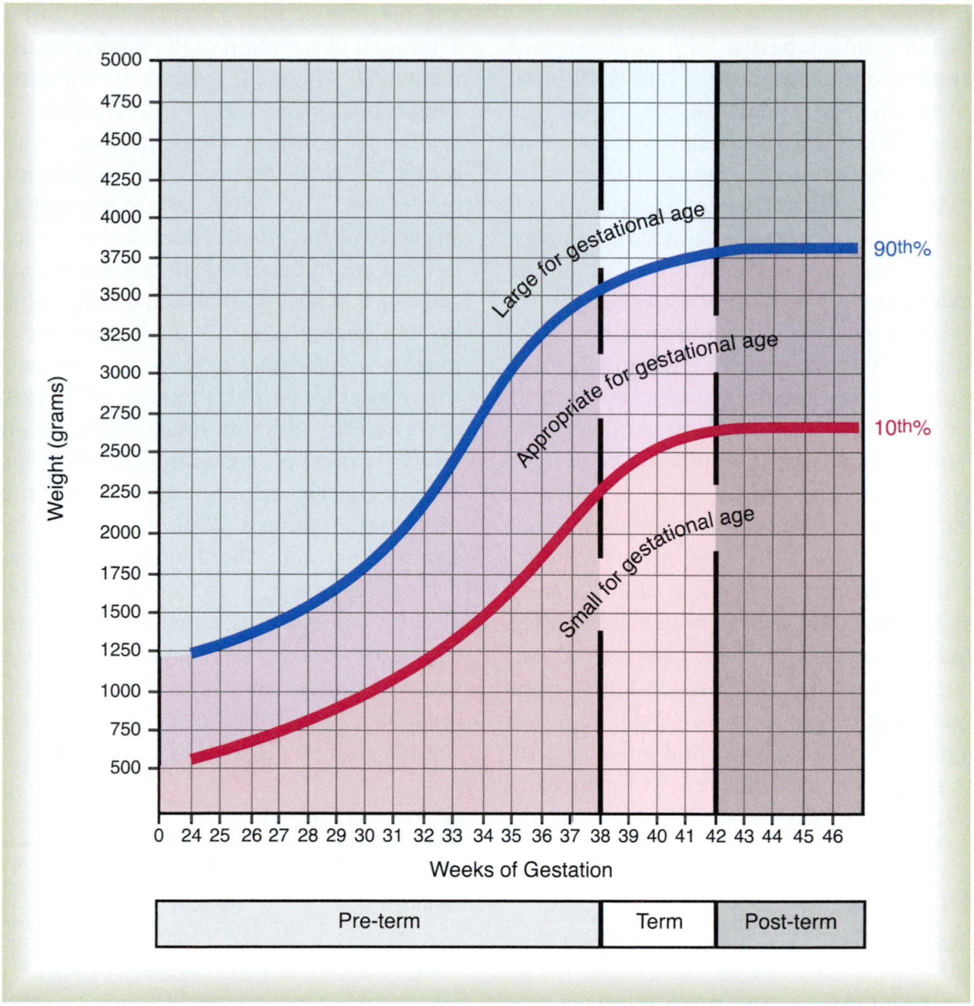

FIGURE 53-5 Colorado intrauterine growth chart. (Modified from Avery GB, editor: Neonatology: pathophysiology and management of the newborn, ed 4, Philadelphia, 1994, JB Lippincott.)

morbidity and mortality. As shown in Figure 53-5, by plotting the infant's gestational age against weight, the newborn's relative developmental status can be classified. Infants whose weight falls between the 10th and 90th percentiles are **appropriate for gestational age (AGA)** Infants whose weight is above the 90th percentile are **large for gestational age (LGA)** Infants whose weight is below the 10th percentile are **small for gestational age (SGA)**.

RULE OF THUMB

Infants weighing less than 2500 g are normally considered low birth weight neonates. Infants weighing less than 1500 g are considered VLBW neonates, and neonates weighing less than 1000 g are considered ELBW neonates.

By classifying infants into one of the combined categories, such as "preterm, AGA," the clinician can help identify infants at highest risk and predict the nature of the risks involved and the likely mortality rate. Small, preterm infants are at highest risk. Compared with term infants, the lungs of these infants are not yet fully prepared for gas exchange. In addition, their digestive tracts cannot normally absorb fat, and their immune systems are not yet capable of warding off infection. Small, preterm infants also have a very large surface area-to-body weight ratio; this increases heat loss and impairs thermoregulation. Finally, the vasculature of these small infants is underdeveloped, increasing the likelihood of hemorrhage (especially in the ventricles of the brain).

RULE OF THUMB

Infants born before 38 weeks' gestation are considered preterm.

Respiratory Assessment of the Infant

Not all respiratory problems occur at birth; many respiratory disorders develop after birth and may develop slowly or suddenly. RTs are commonly called on to help assess and treat infants who develop respiratory distress after birth.

Physical Assessment

Physical assessment of the infant begins with measurement of vital signs. A normal newborn respiratory rate is 40 to 60 breaths/min. The lower the gestational age, the higher the normal respiratory rate will be. A 28-week gestational age infant may normally breathe 60 times a minute, whereas the rate more typical of a term newborn is 40 breaths/min. Tachypnea (>60 breaths/min) can occur because of hypoxemia, acidosis, anxiety, or pain. Respiratory rates less than 40 breaths/min should be interpreted with previous trends of the newborn's respiratory rate. A baseline respiratory rate of 36 breaths/min in a term newborn is within normal limits; however, a respiratory rate of 36 breaths/min in a preterm newborn previously breathing at 70 breaths/min may indicate compromise. Causes of slow respiratory rates include medications, hypothermia, or neurologic impairment.

Normal infant heart rates rang from 100 to 160 beats/min. Heart rate can be assessed by auscultation of the apical pulse, normally located at the fifth intercostal space, midclavicular line. Alternatively, the brachial and femoral pulses may be used. Weak pulses indicate hypotension, shock, or vasoconstriction. Bounding peripheral pulses occur with major left-to-right shunting through a **patent ductus arteriosus (PDA)**.[5] A strong brachial pulse in the presence of a weak femoral pulse suggests either PDA or coarctation of the aorta. Table 53-3 lists normal ranges of blood pressure for neonates of different sizes.

RULE OF THUMB

The normal respiratory rate for a full-term infant is 40 to 60 breaths/min.

Chest examination in an infant is more difficult to perform and interpret than in an adult because of the small chest size and the ease of sound transmission through the infant chest. Thorough observation of the infant greatly enhances the assessment data obtained. Infants in respiratory distress typically exhibit one or more key physical signs: nasal flaring, cyanosis, expiratory grunting, tachypnea, retractions, and paradoxical breathing. Nasal flaring is seen as dilation of the ala nasi on inspiration. The extent of flaring varies according to facial structure of the infant. Nasal flaring coincides with an increase in the work of breathing. In concept, nasal flaring decreases the resistance to airflow. It also may help stabilize the upper airway by minimizing negative pharyngeal pressure during inspiration.[6] Cyanosis may be absent in infants with anemia, even when arterial partial pressure of oxygen (PaO_2) levels are decreased. In addition, infants with elevated fetal hemoglobin levels may not become cyanotic until PaO_2 decreases to less than 30 mm Hg. Hyperbilirubinemia, common among newborns, may mask cyanosis. Grunting occurs when infants exhale against a partially closed glottis. By increasing airway pressure during expiration, grunting helps prevent airway closure and alveolar collapse. Grunting is most common in infants with respiratory distress syndrome, but it is also seen in other respiratory disorders associated with alveolar collapse. Figure 53-6 illustrates the Silverman score, which is a system of grading severity of lung disease.

TABLE 53-3
Normal Neonatal Blood Pressures

Weight (g)	Systolic (mm Hg)	Diastolic (mm Hg)
750	35-45	14-34
1000	39-59	16-36
1500	40-61	19-39
3000	51-72	27-46

From Whitaker K: Comprehensive perinatal and pediatric respiratory care, ed 3, Albany, NY, 2001, Delmar.

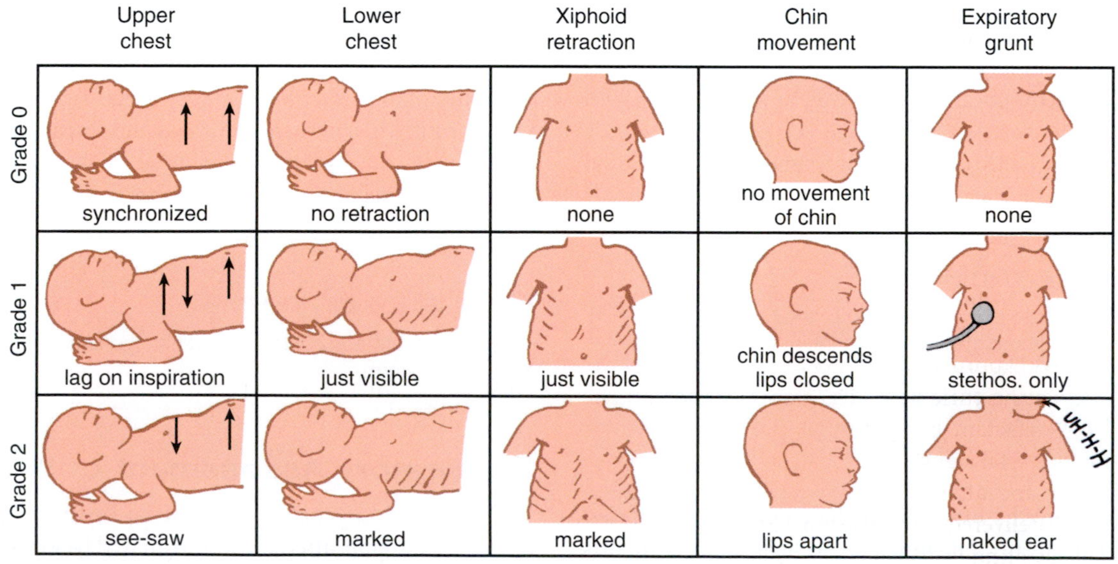

FIGURE 53-6 Silverman score—a system for grading severity of underlying lung disease. (Modified from Silverman WA, Anderson DH: Pediatrics 17:1, 1956.)

Retractions refer to the drawing in of chest wall skin between bony structures. Retractions can occur in the suprasternal, substernal, and intercostal regions. Retractions indicate an increase in the work of breathing, especially because of decreased pulmonary compliance. Paradoxical breathing in infants differs from paradoxical breathing normally seen in adults. Instead of drawing the abdomen in during inspiration, an infant with paradoxical breathing tends to draw in the chest wall. This inward movement of the chest wall may range in severity. As with retractions, paradoxical breathing indicates an increase in ventilatory work. Applying continuous positive airway pressure (CPAP) to a newborn exhibiting signs of respiratory distress including **grunting, flaring, and retracting** may help to increase lung volume by preventing alveolar collapse and improve gas exchange. The benefits of CPAP in children are discussed in more detail later.

Surfactant

Surfactant production begins around the 24th week of gestation and continues through gestation. Surfactant contributes to the stability of the alveolar sacs by reducing the surface tension of the fluids that coat the alveoli. Surfactant deficiency places an infant at increased risk for respiratory distress. By about 34 weeks' gestation, most infants have produced enough surfactant to keep the alveoli from collapsing. There are two specific approaches to preventing and treating surfactant deficiency. Surfactant deficiency is due to lung immaturity. When a premature delivery is anticipated, steroids are given to the mother to help promote lung maturation. In addition, infants born before 35 weeks' gestation, especially infants born very prematurely (<30 weeks), should be assessed clinically for the need to receive exogenous surfactant. The need for surfactant is determined by assessing the infant's lung volume on chest x-ray, evaluating the inspired O_2 concentration to maintain O_2 saturations greater than approximately 88%, and clinically assessing the infant's work of breathing.

Recent evidence supports early surfactant replacement, immediately following delivery, for infants less than 27 weeks' gestation. Infants 27 to 30 weeks' gestation should be placed on CPAP and evaluated clinically for the need to receive surfactant.[7-9]

Surfactant administration has also been shown to be useful in conditions in which surfactant structure and/or function has been altered. These conditions include meconium aspiration, neonatal pneumonia, pulmonary hemorrhage, and primary surfactant deficiency. Administration of surfactant requires intubation. It is essential to ensure the endotracheal tube is properly positioned, approximately 0.5 to 1 cm above the carina, before delivering surfactant. The dose depends on the specific brand of surfactant being administered. Close monitoring of the infant's vital signs, O_2 saturation, and compliance is necessary during and after surfactant administration. Soon after surfactant is delivered, the infant's compliance should begin to increase resulting in improved gas exchange. Ventilating pressures and fractional concentration of inspired oxygen (FiO_2) need to be decreased to avoid lung injury and excessive partial pressure of O_2. The ventilating pressure should be decreased to the level that maintains a tidal volume (V_T) of 5 to 7 ml/kg. FiO_2 should be decreased to maintain an oxygen saturation level (SpO_2) of approximately 89% to 94% in preterm infants and to the lowest FiO_2 possible to maintain SpO_2 >92% in term or postterm infants. Those with primary pulmonary hypertension should have SpO_2 >95% (see Clinical Practice Guideline 53-1).

Blood Gas and Pulse Oximetry Analysis

Blood gas analysis is helpful in assessing respiratory distress in an infant. Many noninvasive techniques, such as transcutaneous partial pressure of oxygen ($PtcO_2$), transcutaneous partial pressure of carbon dioxide ($PtcCO_2$), end-tidal carbon dioxide (CO_2), and pulse oximetry (SpO_2), are used to obtain comparable data, although blood gas analysis is more precise when results are critical. An infant blood gas sample can be obtained from an artery or capillary. Chapter 19 summarizes the advantages, disadvantages, and complications of these sampling methods. Care must be taken in assessing the results of capillary sampling. Capillary blood gases provide only information regarding ventilation and acid-base status, and accuracy is highly dependent on technique.[10] Normal values for infant blood gases are listed in Table 53-4.

Monitoring O_2 saturation using a pulse oximeter is a standard of care for sick newborns. Saturation probes must be carefully placed on the newborn; the most common sites are the wrist, the medial surface of the palm, or the foot. Sufficient cardiac output and skin blood flow are essential to provide an accurate saturation value. The pulse rate indicated on the oximeter should correlate with the infant's actual pulse before any conclusions regarding saturation can be drawn. Intracardiac shunting and intrapulmonary shunting are causes of decreased saturation in sick infants. When interpreting saturation levels in a newborn, it is important to consider where the saturation is being monitored. Saturation probes placed on the right hand assess preductal saturations. Probes placed on other extremities indicate postductal saturation levels. Infants at risk for pulmonary hypertension should have saturation probes placed to monitor preductal and postductal saturations. A large difference (>5%) between the two readings should prompt the clinician to consider pulmonary hypertension as a potential concern. Conditions that prevent the closing of the ductus arteriosus and foramen ovale result in decreased saturation. Many congenital heart defects result in significant intracardiac shunting. Interpreting adequate saturation for a newborn requires knowledge of any cardiac defect along with the infant's pulmonary condition.

Respiratory Assessment of the Pediatric Patient

Normal breathing in children is evidenced by quiet inspiration and passive expiration at an age-appropriate rate. Respiratory rates are rapid in neonates and decrease in toddlers and older children. Table 53-5 lists normal respiratory rates. The initial assessment of a pediatric patient starts with evaluating airway

53-1 Surfactant Replacement Therapy

AARC Clinical Practice Guideline (Excerpts)

INDICATIONS

- Prophylactic surfactant administration is indicated in (1) infants at high risk of developing respiratory distress syndrome (RDS) because of short gestation (<32 weeks) or low birth weight (<1300 g) and (2) infants with known surfactant deficiency
- Rescue therapy is indicated in preterm or full-term infants who (1) require intubation and mechanical ventilation secondary to increased work of breathing and O_2 requirements and (2) have clinical evidence of RDS

CONTRAINDICATIONS

Relative contraindications to surfactant administration are the following:

- Presence of congenital anomalies incompatible with life beyond the neonatal period
- Respiratory distress in infants with laboratory evidence of lung maturity

HAZARDS AND COMPLICATIONS

- Procedural complications resulting from the administration of surfactant
  - Plugging of endotracheal tube by surfactant
  - Administration of surfactant to only one lung
  - Hemoglobin desaturation or need for extra O_2
  - Drug dosing errors
  - Bradycardia secondary to hypoxia
  - Tachycardia secondary to agitation, with reflux of surfactant into endotracheal tube
  - Pharyngeal deposition of surfactant
- Physiologic complications of surfactant replacement therapy
  - Apnea
  - Increased necessity for treatment for PDA
  - Pulmonary hemorrhage
  - Marginal increase in ROP
  - Mucous plugs
  - Barotrauma with increased lung compliance

ASSESSMENT OF NEED

Determine that valid indications are present:

- Assess lung immaturity before prophylactic administration of surfactant (see Contraindications)
- Establish the diagnosis of RDS in the presence of short gestation or low birth weight

ASSESSMENT OF OUTCOME

- Reduction of FiO_2 requirement or work of breathing or both
- Improvement in lung volumes and lung fields as indicated by chest radiograph
- Improvement in pulmonary mechanics (e.g., compliance, airway resistance, V_T, VE, FRC, transpulmonary pressure)
- Reduction in ventilator requirements (PIP, PEEP, Paw)
- Improvement in ratio of arterial to alveolar PO_2 (a/A PO_2), oxygenation index

MONITORING

The following should be monitored as part of surfactant replacement therapy:

- Variables to be monitored during surfactant administration
  - Proper placement of delivery device
  - Position of patient (i.e., head direction)
  - FiO_2 and ventilator settings
  - Chest wall movement
  - Reflux of surfactant into endotracheal tube
  - O_2 saturation by pulse oximetry
  - Heart and respiratory rate, chest expansion, skin color, and vigor
- Variables to be monitored after surfactant administration
  - Arterial blood gases
  - Pulmonary mechanics and volumes
  - Chest radiography
  - Breath sounds
  - Ventilator PIP, PEEP, Paw, FiO_2
  - Blood pressure
  - Heart and respiratory rate, chest expansion, skin color, and vigor

For complete guideline, see American Association for Respiratory Care: Clinical practice guideline: surfactant replacement therapy. Respir Care 39:824, 1994.
VE, *Minute ventilation.*

TABLE 53-4
Age-Related Values Commonly Reported for Normal Blood Gases

	Normal Preterm Infants (at 1-5 Hours)	Normal Term Infants (at 5 Hours)	Normal Preterm Infants (at 5 Days)	Children, Adolescents, and Adults
pH (range)	7.33 (7.29-7.37)	7.34 (7.31-7.37)	7.38 (7.34-7.42)	7.40 (7.35-7.45)
PCO_2 (range)	47 (39-56)	35 (32-39)	36 (32-41)	40 (35-45)
PO_2 (range)	60 (52-68)	74 (62-86)	76 (62-92)	95 (85-100)
HCO_3^- range	25 (22-23)	19 (18-21)	21 (19-23)	24 (22-26)
BE range	−4 (−5 to −2.2)	−5 9 (−6 to −2)	−3 (−5.8 to −1.2)	0 (−2 to +2)

Modified from Orzalesi MM, Mendicini M, Bucci G, et al: Arterial oxygen studies in premature newborns with and without mild respiratory disorders. Arch Dis Child 42:174, 1967. From Koff PB, Eitzman DV, Neu J: Neonatal and pediatric respiratory care, ed 2, St Louis, 1993, Mosby.
BE, Base excess; *HCO_3^-*, bicarbonate.

MINI CLINI

Neonatal Ventilation

PROBLEM: A 1.8-kg, 28-week newborn is transported from the delivery room to the neonatal ICU. The patient was apneic and bradycardic at birth and failed to respond to initial stimulation and resuscitation. He was intubated with a 3.0 uncuffed endotracheal tube. His heart rate increased to 120 and he has been manually ventilated with a T-piece resuscitator at a PIP of 25 cm H_2O and PEEP of 5 cm H_2O during transport. When the neonate is admitted to the neonatal ICU, the RT is asked to recommend appropriate ventilator settings.

Solution:

- Mode—A/C pressure ventilation
- PIP—20 cm H_2O
- PEEP—5 cm H_2O
- Set respiratory rate—40 breaths/min
- Inspiratory time—0.3 sec
- FiO_2—0.4

Because the patient was manually ventilated during transport, it is unclear what V_T has been delivered. Initial PIP of 20 cm H_2O and PEEP of 5 cm H_2O are safe and common settings. Immediate observation of the chest would allow the RT to evaluate chest expansion and adjust PIP as required. Over the next several minutes if V_T monitoring is available, targeting V_T of 6 to 8 ml/kg would guide subsequent settings.

Set respiratory rate of 40 breaths/min is at the lower end of the normal range for this patient; however, use of the A/C mode with a time-cycled, pressure-limited breath and appropriately set trigger sensitivity would allow the patient to establish a more comfortable respiratory rate. Adjustment of the inspiratory time may also be necessary to increase patient comfort and improve patient-ventilator synchrony. Further adjustments may be guided by $PaCO_2$. Because this patient was born prematurely, rapid assessment of SpO_2 is essential, and FiO_2 should be adjusted to maintain SpO_2 between 88% and 92%.

This patient should receive surfactant replacement therapy. The clinician may consider volume-targeted, pressure-limited ventilation (e.g., pressure-regulated volume control, volume guarantee) during and immediately after surfactant delivery. This modality may help prevent lung overdistention until compliance has stabilized.[11,12]

TABLE 53-5

Normal Respiratory and Heart Rates by Age

Age	Breaths/Minute	Heart Rates
Infants (<1 yr)	30-60	90-120
Toddler (1-3 yr)	24-40	80-100
Preschooler (4-5 yr)	22-34	70-90
School age (6-12 yr)	18-30	70-90
Adolescent (13-18 yr)	16-22	60-80

patency. Normal heart rates are higher in younger children and decrease with age. In assessing a pediatric patient, establishing if the airway is patent or has any obstructive component is essential. Signs that suggest upper airway obstruction include increased inspiratory effort with retractions or inspiratory efforts with no airway or breath sounds.

The clinician observes for movement of the chest or abdomen. The clinician listens for breath sounds focusing on both inspiratory sounds and expiratory sounds. Chest or abdominal movement without breath sounds may indicate total airway obstruction, and basic life-support maneuvers are indicated. High-pitched sounds heard on inspiration (stridor) are often indicative of upper airway conditions, whereas expiratory noises are more often associated with lower airway obstruction.

Causes of stridor in children can be infections, such as croup; foreign body aspiration, particularly in a small child; congenital or acquired airway abnormalities; allergic reactions; or edema after a procedure. Inhaled epinephrine via nebulizer and intravenous steroids are commonly used to treat stridor. Common causes of lower airway obstruction are bronchiolitis and asthma. When wheezing is noted, inhaled bronchodilators are indicated. If the patient is able to use a metered dose inhaler (MDI), repeated inhalations can act quickly to improve aeration. When the patient is unable to use the MDI appropriately or when severe symptoms are present, delivering a bronchodilator with a nebulizer can bring relief. More than one nebulizer treatment often is necessary to relieve airway inflammation. A common approach is to deliver three consecutive treatments. If the patient continues to be symptomatic, continuous bronchodilator therapy may be delivered with a nebulizer attached to an infusion pump set to administer a bronchodilator continuously. Tachycardia secondary to the beta-1 effect of inhaled bronchodilators may occur. Frequent reassessment of any patient receiving continuous bronchodilator therapy is essential. Heliox, an inhaled mixture of helium and O_2 (described in the section on specialty gases), has been shown to be beneficial in cases of some airways conditions in children.

As noted in the section describing newborn assessment, use of accessory muscles, grunting, flaring, and retracting all can be signs of respiratory distress. Head bobbing, noted by chin up and neck extended during inspiration with chin falling during expiration, and seesaw respirations, indicated by the chest retracting and the abdomen expanding during inspiration, are signs of impending respiratory failure. Assessing the child's level of alertness is essential. Levels of alertness range from fully awake, agitated, minimally responsive, to unresponsive. A child's ability to protect his or her airway should be questioned in a minimally responsive or unresponsive child.

RESPIRATORY CARE

Respiratory care of infants and children incorporates approaches taken from adult practice. Important physiologic and age-related differences between adults and children require variations in the provision of respiratory care. This section focuses on neonatal and pediatric O_2 therapy, bronchial hygiene, humidity and aerosol therapy, airway management, and resuscitation.

Oxygen Therapy

Goals and Indications

O_2 should be administered as any other drug, using the lowest dose necessary to achieve the intended goal. The goal of O_2 therapy is to provide adequate tissue oxygenation. However, O_2 therapy is most frequently adjusted according to O_2 saturation levels. A clear understanding of the limitation of O_2 saturation is needed to interpret the saturation reading and make appropriate decisions. Infants and children receiving O_2 therapy have variable O_2 saturation target ranges depending on age and underlying condition.

Lower saturation levels are targeted in infants less than 32 weeks' gestation. There is evidence that exposure to supplemental O_2 in a premature infant is a risk factor for the development of **retinopathy of prematurity (ROP)** ROP is caused by an abnormal vascularization of the retina, which in the most severe cases leads to retinal detachment. Preterm neonates weighing less than 1500 g are most susceptible. Hyperoxia is not the only factor associated with ROP, but close monitoring and adjusting of O_2 therapy to avoid hyperoxia is crucial to decrease the risk of ROP. A specific saturation goal of 88% to 94% should be established for this age group, and O_2 should be adjusted to maintain the intended target. Avoiding very high or very low saturation levels is critical. Adjusting the delivered O_2 concentration by small increments avoids large swings in saturation levels.[13-17]

In a term infant with **primary pulmonary hypertension of the newborn (PPHN)** a higher targeted saturation level is desired to avoid further pulmonary constriction associated with hypoxemia. The position of the saturation probe needs to be considered when interpreting saturation. Intracardiac shunting can occur in the presence of PPHN. One saturation probe positioned on the upper right extremity represents preductal saturations and is indicative of the saturation of blood being delivered to the brain. O_2 saturation measured on other extremities is considered postductal and represents saturation to other parts of the body.

Newborns with certain cardiac anomalies are dependent on their intracardiac shunt through the ductus arteriosus to survive. An increased saturation in newborns promotes constriction of the ductus arteriosus. Although this constriction is normally a positive response, it may cause premature closure of the ductus arteriosus in infants with ductal-dependent congenital heart defects. An infant born with hypoplastic left heart syndrome, a defect in which the left-sided heart structures are poorly developed, relies on the patency of the ductus arteriosus for systemic blood supply. In addition, hyperoxia can increase aortic pressures and systemic vascular resistance, decreasing the cardiac index and O_2 transport in children with acyanotic congenital heart disease. The emphasis for O_2 therapy for all newborns should be to provide only as much O_2 as indicated by the infant's condition. O_2 therapy should be administered using a written care plan with specified clinical outcomes (e.g., titrate flow/FiO_2 to maintain SpO_2 88% to 92%, notify physician if FiO_2 is >0.40).

Methods of Administration

The effectiveness of O_2 devices depends on the performance characteristics of the device (delivered FiO_2, flow rate, relative humidity), the interface of the device, and the tolerance of the patient for using the device. Children are often frightened and combative, making it impractical to use some O_2 administration devices. Selection of an O_2 device must be based on the degree of hypoxemia and the emotional and physical needs of the child and family. O_2 can be administered to infants and children by mask, cannula, high-flow nasal cannula, or oxyhood. Table 53-6 compares the advantages and disadvantages of standard O_2 delivery methods.

TABLE 53-6
Oxygen Delivery Devices

Device	Age	FDO_2	Advantages	Disadvantages
Air entrainment mask	≥3 yr	High flow; 0.24-1	Precise FiO_2; good for transport; ease of application	Low relative humidity; pressure necrosis to face; difficult to fit and maintain on active child, not recommended for infants; risk of aspiration
Nasal cannula	Premature infants to adult	Low flow; 25 ml/min-6.0 L/min	Tolerated well by all ages	Inaccurate FiO_2; low relative humidity; excessive flows may cause inadvertent CPAP in infants; precise FiO_2 may be achieved with O_2 blender
Incubator	Newborns ≤28 days	<0.40 FiO_2, combine use with cannula or hood for precise FiO_2	Low FiO_2 for stable infants; neutral thermal environment for premature infants	Varying FiO_2; long stabilization time; limits access to child for patient care
Oxyhood	Premature infants to ≤6 mo	0.21-1 FiO_2 with O_2 blender maintained at 30° C to 34° C	Warmed and humidified gas at stable FiO_2 during routine patient care	Overheating may cause apnea and dehydration; underheating may cause O_2 consumption; inadequate flow causes CO_2 buildup; noise produced by humidification device may cause hearing loss

FDO_2, Delivered oxygen concentration.

Secretion Clearance Techniques

Secretion clearance techniques that can be applied to infants and children include chest physiotherapy, positive expiratory pressure therapy, autogenic drainage, flutter therapy, and mechanical insufflation-exsufflation.[18,19] Secretion clearance techniques are considered when accumulated secretions impair pulmonary function and an infiltrate is visible on a chest radiograph. Secretion retention is common in children who have pneumonia, bronchopulmonary dysplasia, cystic fibrosis, bronchiectasis, and some neuromuscular diseases. Figure 53-7 shows postural drainage and percussion positions for infants and children.

Methods

Infants and young children cannot cough on command. For this reason, secretions often must be removed by suctioning. For older children with excessive secretions, directed deep breathing and coughing may help improve pulmonary clearance. The use of mechanical insufflation-exsufflation in children with neuromuscular disease can be helpful in clearing secretions. Adjunctive therapy devices such as positive expiratory pressure, flutter, or intermittent percussive ventilation therapy have been effective in secretion clearance in patients with cystic fibrosis.[20]

Monitoring

Given the instability of most critically ill infants and children, a thorough initial assessment and ongoing patient evaluation during and after treatment are mandatory. Traditional assessment of vital signs, blood pressure, color, and breath sounds before, during, and after treatment should be supplemented with pulse oximetry monitoring if hypoxemia is suspected.

Humidity and Aerosol Therapy

Key differences in humidity and aerosol therapy in infants and children include assessment of patient response to therapy, age-related physiologic changes, and equipment application.

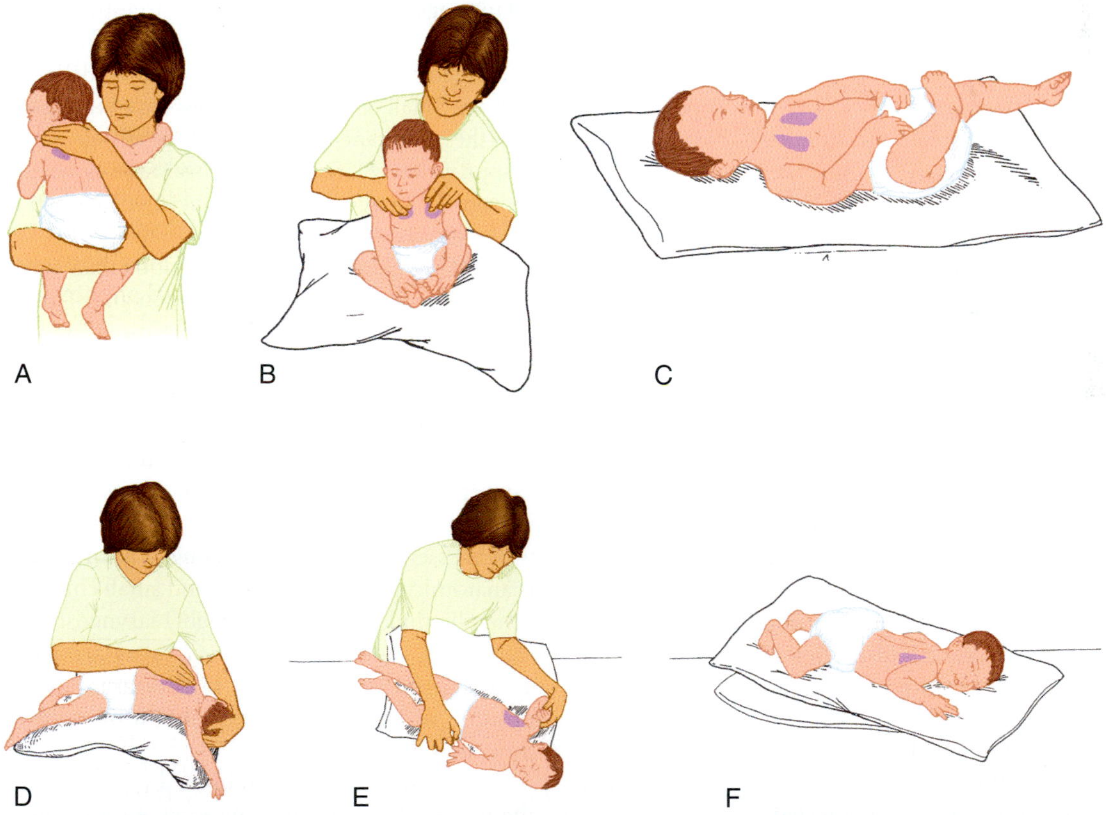

FIGURE 53-7 Postural drainage and percussion positions for infant and child. Angles of drainage for infant are not as obtuse as those for child. **A,** Posterior segments of right and left upper lobes are drained with patient in upright position at 30-degree angle forward. Percuss over upper posterior thorax. **B,** Apical segments of right and left upper lobes are drained with patient in upright position, leaning forward 30 degrees. Percuss over area between clavicle and tip of scapula on each side. **C,** Anterior segments of right and left upper lobes are drained with patient in flat, supine position. Percuss anterior side of chest directly under clavicles to around nipple area *(shaded).* Avoid direct pressure on sternum. **D,** Right and left lateral basal segments of lower lobes are drained at 30 degrees Trendelenburg. Patient lies on appropriate side, rotated 30 degrees forward. Percuss over uppermost portions of lower ribs. **E,** Right and left anterior basal segments of lower lobes are drained at 30 degrees Trendelenburg. Patient lies on appropriate side with a 20-degree turn backward. Percuss above anterior lower margin of ribs. **F,** Right and left superior segments of lower lobes are drained at 15 degrees Trendelenburg, with patient in prone position. Percuss below scapula in midback area.

Humidity Therapy

In children with an intact upper airway, O_2 therapy devices, such as low-flow nasal cannulas, do not routinely need to be humidified. However, any time the upper airway is bypassed by intubation, supplemental humidification must be provided using a heated humidifier. Humidification of inspired gases for infants and children receiving mechanical ventilation is commonly provided by a servo-controlled humidifier. Ideal features for these systems include the following: (1) low internal volume and constant water level to minimize compressed volume loss; (2) closed, continuous feed water supply to avoid contamination; (3) distal airway temperature sensor and high/low alarms. Common problems with humidifier systems include condensation in the tubing, inadequate humidification, and hazards associated with the heating coil.[21,22] Using heated wire circuits can also reduce condensation in the circuit. Frequent evaluation of the humidification system is necessary to increase the potential of adequate humidity delivered to the airway. Inadequate humidification occurs in nonheated circuits when the humidifier temperature probe is placed too far upstream from the airway connector. Variable humidification problems occur when ventilator circuits pass through an environment and then into a warmed enclosure, such as an incubator or radiant warmer.

Aerosol Drug Therapy

Drug action in infants and children differs significantly from drug action in adults because of differences in physiology, which may include immature enzyme systems, immature receptors, and variable gastrointestinal absorption. Dosing may be imprecise, and systemic effects may be hard to predict. Table 53-7 lists aerosolized medications commonly used in children.

Small volume nebulizers (SVNs), vibrating mesh nebulizers, MDIs, and dry powder inhalers (DPIs) can be used to deliver aerosolized drugs via mouthpiece or face mask to infants and children.[23] Continuous aerosol drug therapy is also used for patients unresponsive to intermittent SVN treatments. Aerosol drug administration to intubated infants and children is challenging because of the decreased deposition from baffling of small endotracheal tubes in these patients, which prevents approximately 90% of the drug from entering the lungs, regardless of delivery system. In addition, careful adjustments must be made to the ventilator so that nebulizer flows do not alter delivered V_T and inspiratory pressure and interfere with triggering efforts.[24] Newer vibrating mesh type nebulizers provide a more stable particle size and do not add additional flow to the breathing circuit. As a result, there is no change in the delivered tidal volume and patient triggering is not affected.

Airway Management

Airway management methods in infants and children are unique because of the anatomic differences between neonates and adults. Specifically, equipment and technique must be tailored to each child according to his or her size, weight, and postpartum age. Masks, resuscitation bags, oral airways, suction catheters, laryngoscope blades, and endotracheal tubes in a wide selection of infant and child sizes are needed to account for variations in patient age and weight. Table 53-8 provides recommendations regarding endotracheal tube and suction catheter sizes for infants and children.

Box 53-1 Complications and Hazards of Endotracheal Intubation in Infants and Children

- Palatal grooving (neonates)
- Incisal enamel hypoplasia (neonates)
- Accidental extubation
- Tube blockage
- Tracheal stenosis
- Esophageal perforation
- Tracheal perforation

Intubation

Endotracheal intubation is a generally safe method of airway management in infants and children, even when used for extended periods.[25,26] Complications and hazards associated with intubation in these age groups are listed in Box 53-1. The infant's age or weight can be used to estimate proper endotracheal tube size and depth of insertion. If the tube is too small in diameter, a leak may result, decreasing delivered minute ventilation. Small endotracheal tubes have high resistance, increasing the spontaneous work of breathing for the child. An inappropriately large endotracheal tube can cause mucosal and laryngeal damage that is evident after extubation, resulting in upper airway obstruction.[27]

Most neonatal and pediatric endotracheal tubes are uncuffed. The narrowest point of the airway in an infant and small child is the cricoid cartilage. When an appropriately sized uncuffed tube is positioned in the airway, the fit of the tube in the airway "seals" the airway enough so that adequate ventilation can usually be maintained. Cuffed endotracheal tubes are an option if a large leak persists around the tube and stable ventilation cannot be maintained. Similar to adults when a cuffed tube is used, careful attention to the pressure of the cuff on the tracheal wall is essential. Because the tongue is large and the epiglottis is anatomically high in infants and small children, practitioners generally find the Miller (straight) laryngoscope blade best for intubation. Infant endotracheal tubes are small and can be easily kinked or obstructed. In addition, slight changes in the position of the endotracheal tube in movement can result in bronchial intubation.[28]

Once a tube is inserted, immediate securing of the tube to the infant's face and ongoing evaluation of the security of the tube are essential. Proper head positioning and avoidance of cumbersome connecting apparatus help reduce the potential of accidental extubation. Estimates of the distance the tube should be inserted into the airway based on patient weight are provided in Table 53-9. Further confirmation of correct tube position should be evaluated with a chest x-ray. Noting the infant's head position when the chest x-ray is obtained is helpful in assessing appropriate tube position in the airway. Slight changes in head

TABLE 53-7

Commonly Used Aerosolized Medications

Medication Name	Dosage Form	Usual Child Dose	Comments
Bronchodilators			
Beta-2 Agonists			
Albuterol (Proventil, Ventolin)	MDI (90 mcg/puff)	1-2 puffs MDI q 15 min to q 6 hr ± PRN	May be used 15 min before exercise to prevent exercise-induced bronchospasm; should be used as a rescue medication
	Nebs (0.5%, 5 mg/ml)	0.01-0.05 ml/kg/dose (maximum 1 ml/dose) neb q 15 min to q 6 hr ± PRN	
	Rotohaler (200 mcg caps)	1-2 caps inhaled q 15 min to q 6 hr ± PRN	
Levalbuterol (Xopenex)	Nebs (0.63 mg/3 ml, 1.25 mg/3 ml)	0.32-1.25 mg neb q 6-8 hr ± PRN	May still cause extrapulmonary side effects including tachycardia and hypokalemia
Salmeterol (Serevent)	MDI (21 mcg/puff) DPI-Diskus (50 mcg/inhalation)	2 puffs inhalation q 12 hr 1 inhalation q 12 hr	Not to be used as a rescue medication; long-acting beta-2 agonist; QT_C prolongation has occurred in overdose
Anticholinergic			
Ipratropium (Atrovent)	MDI (18 mcg/puff) Nebs (0.02%)	2 puffs inhalation q 4-6 hr ± PRN 0.25-0.5 mg neb q 4-6 hr ± PRN	MDI is contraindicated in patients with peanut allergy; for neonates, use 25 mcg/kg/dose neb tid; may cause mydriasis if aerosolized drug gets into the eye
Antiinflammatory Agents			
Corticosteroids			
Beclomethasone (Beclovent, Vanceril)	MDI (42 mcg/puff)	1-2 puffs inhalation qid or 2-4 puffs inhalation bid	Start at lower end of dosing range if patient not previously on steroids; titrate to lowest dose that is effective; always rinse mouth after each treatment
	MDI double strength (84 mcg/puff)	2 puffs inhalation bid	
Budesonide (Pulmicort)	DPI-Turbuhaler (200 mcg/inhalation)	1-2 puffs inhalation bid	May take several weeks to see benefit; not to be used as a rescue medication
	Nebs-Respules (0.25 mg/2 ml, 0.5 mg/2 ml)	0.25-0.5 mg neb bid *or* 0.5-1 mg neb qd	
Flunisolide (Aerobid, Aerobid-M)	MDI (250 mcg/puff)	2-3 puffs inhalation bid	
Fluticasone (Flovent)	MDI (44 mcg/puff, 110 mcg/puff, 220 mcg/puff)	2 puffs inhalation bid (maximum 880 mcg/day)	
	Rotadisk (50 mcg/blister)	50-100 mcg inhalation bid	
Triamcinolone (Azmacort)	MDI (100 mcg/puff)	1-2 puffs inhal qid	
Mast Cell Stabilizers			
Cromolyn (Intal)	MDI (800 mcg/puff) Nebs (20 mg/2 ml)	2 puffs inhalation qid 20 mg neb qid	May take several weeks to see benefit; not to be used as a rescue medication
Nedocromil (Tilade)	MDI (1.75 mg/puff)	2 puffs inhalation qid	
Mucolytics			
N-acetylcysteine (Mucomyst)	Nebs (20%, 200 mg/ml)	3-5 ml neb qid	Consider pretreatment with albuterol 15 min before *N*-acetylcysteine secondary to bronchospasm
Dornase alfa (Pulmozyme)	Nebs (2.5 mg/2.5 ml)	2.5 mg neb qid-bid	May cause hemoptysis
Antiinfectives			
Pentamidine (Pentam)	Nebs (300 mg)	8 mg/kg/dose (maximum 300 mg/dose) neb q month	Used for PCP prophylaxis
Ribavirin (Virazole)	Powder (6 g vial)	2 g over 2 hr neb q 8 hr × 3-7 days *or* 6 g over 12-18 hr neb q 24 hr × 3-7 days	Used for RSV treatment; mutagenic, teratogenic
Tobramycin (TOBI)	Nebs (300 mg/5 ml)	300 mg neb q 12 hr	Used for pseudomonal infection of the lungs

Neb, Nebulizer; *PCP, Pneumocystis jiroveci* pneumonia; *RSV,* respiratory syncytial virus.

TABLE 53-8

Endotracheal Tube and Suction Catheter Sizes for Infants and Children

Age or Weight	Endotracheal Tube ID (mm)	Oral Tube Length (cm)	Nasal Tube Length (cm)	Suction Catheter (F)
Newborn				
<1000 g	2.5	9-11	11-12	6
1000-2000 g	3	9-11	11-12	6
2000-3000 g	3.5	10-12	12-14	6
>3000 g	4	11-12	13-14	8
Children				
6 mo	3-4	11-12	12-14	6-8
18 mo	3.5-4.5	11-13	13-15	8
2 yr	4-5	12-14	14-16	8-10
3-5 yr	4.5-5.5	12-15	14-17	8-10
6 yr	5.5-6	14-16	16-18	10
8 yr	6-6.5	15-17	17-19	10-12
12 yr	6-7	17-19	19-21	10-12
16 yr	6.5-7.5	19-21	21-23	10-12

Estimating formula for tube internal diameter (ID) in mm:
Tube ID = (Age + 16)/4
Tube ID = Height (cm)/20
Estimating formula for tube length in cm:
Oral: 12 + (Age/2)
Nasal: 15 + (Age/2)

TABLE 53-9

Approximate Distance from Infant's Lip to End of Inserted Oral Endotracheal Tube

Weight (kg)	Mark at Lip (cm)
<1	6.5
1	7
2	8
3	9
4	10

position can result in the tube position sitting too high or too low in the airway. In very small infants, slight flexion of the head can move the tube into the right main stem bronchus.

Breath sounds may be of limited value in infants and small children for evaluation of tube position. Portable end-tidal CO_2 monitoring devices may be used to help assess tracheal versus esophageal intubation, although they should be used only as additional assessment tools with recognition of their limitations. Factors associated with accidental extubation of infants include tension on the tube from the ventilator circuit, patient agitation, suctioning, head turning, chest physiotherapy, too short a tube distance between lip and adapter, moving the patient during procedures, and inadequately taped endotracheal tube.[23,29] Recently, infant-sized endotracheal tube holders have become available.

Laryngeal mask airways (LMAs) are available as an alternative to intubation. LMAs are typically used in children when a short-term airway is indicated, such as during some surgical procedures or when endotracheal intubation cannot be accomplished and an airway needs to be established. Table 53-10 outlines appropriate sizes and maximum cuff volumes of LMAs for varying weights.

TABLE 53-10

Appropriate Sizes and Maximum Cuff Volumes of Laryngeal Mask Airways for Varying Weights

LMA Size	Patient Weight (kg)	Maximum Cuff Volume
1	1-5	4
1.5	5-10	7
2	10-20	10
2.5	20-30	14
3	30-40	20

Box 53-2 Indications for Suctioning

ABSOLUTE INDICATIONS
- Secretions visible in endotracheal tube
- Aspiration of gastrointestinal or oropharyngeal contents
- Inadvertent water aspiration from ventilator circuit

RELATIVE INDICATIONS
- Rhonchi noted during auscultation raising suspicion of retained secretions
- Change in compliance (↓ V_T at same peak pressure or ↑ pressure for same V_T)
- ↑ Work of breathing
- ↓ SpO_2 with same or ↑ FiO_2

Suctioning Intubated Pediatric Patients

The goal of suctioning is to remove secretions from large airways and stimulate a cough. Although suctioning can be beneficial, significant risks are associated with the procedure, including lung derecruitment, hypoxia, hypertension, increased intracranial pressure, tracheal trauma, and infection. Absolute and relative indications for suctioning are listed in Box 53-2.

Additional considerations include the use of closed suction catheters for all mechanically ventilated patients. The closed suctioning technique helps to minimize derecruitment, which is more likely to occur during ventilator disconnections. An increase in O_2 concentration after suctioning may be necessary but should be evaluated for each patient. To reduce the risk of tracheal trauma, suction catheters should not be inserted further than 1 cm beyond the tip of the endotracheal tube or tracheostomy tube. Routine instillation of normal saline is not recommended. Increasing ventilator support to regain volume lost during the procedure may be necessary but should be assessed each time the patient is suctioned. Because of the risks associated with suctioning, the procedure should be performed only when a clinical indication exists, not on a fixed interval.

Suctioning. Nasopharyngeal and tracheal suctioning helps minimize aspiration, prevents endotracheal tube occlusion, and reduces airway resistance in infants and children.[2,30] Suctioning

Box 53-3 Complications and Hazards of Tracheal Suctioning in Infants and Small Children

- Infection
- Lung derecruitment
- Accidental extubation
- Atelectasis
- Blood pressure instability
- Increased intracranial pressure
- Cerebral vasodilation or increased blood volume
- Arterial hypoxemia
- Cerebral hypoxemia
- Hypercapnia
- Bradycardia
- Pneumothorax
- Mucosal damage

is a hazardous procedure, and complications can occur. Box 53-3 lists the common complications and hazards associated with tracheal suctioning of infants and children. Tracheal suctioning of preterm infants and neonates should be performed only when clinical signs indicate a need.[25,31,32]

Oral and pharyngeal suctioning of infants can be done with a bulb syringe. A DeLee trap or a mechanical vacuum source with catheter may be used for nasopharyngeal and nasotracheal suctioning of neonates. Equipment for suctioning larger infants and children is similar to the equipment used with adults with modifications in vacuum pressure and catheter size. Recommended suction pressures for neonates range from approximately −60 to −80 mm Hg. With large infants and children, pressures in the range of −80 to −100 mm Hg are generally safe and effective. Catheter sizes are chosen according to the age of the patient and the size of the tracheal airway (see Table 53-8). Other techniques for averting hypoxemia include use of endotracheal tube adapters that allow preoxygenation and suctioning without disconnection of the ventilator and use of closed tracheal suction systems.[27,33,34]

CONTINUOUS POSITIVE AIRWAY PRESSURE

Spontaneous breathing can be supported with **continuous positive airway pressure (CPAP)** a breathing mode that maintains a constant pressure above baseline throughout inspiration and expiration. Newborn infants have increased chest wall compliance along with decreased lung compliance, which makes them prone to developing atelectasis. CPAP maintains inspiratory and expiratory pressures above ambient, which improves functional residual capacity (FRC) and static lung compliance.[35] It is essential that the patient is able to maintain adequate minute volume while breathing spontaneously because ventilatory support is not provided.

CPAP is indicated when arterial oxygenation is inadequate despite elevated FiO_2. This condition is usually accompanied by certain signs of respiratory distress. CPAP is commonly used

Box 53-4 Indications for Continuous Positive Airway Pressure in Children

RESPIRATORY DISTRESS
- Tachypnea
- Retractions or accessory muscle use
- Grunting
- Nasal flaring
- Head bobbing

ABNORMAL BREATHING PATTERNS
- Apnea of prematurity
- Obstructive sleep apnea

LUNG DISEASE
- Decreased lung volumes on chest radiograph
- Pneumonia
- Tracheomalacia
- Pulmonary edema
- PaO_2 <50 mm Hg with FiO_2 ≥0.60

OTHER
- Postextubation failure

when PaO_2 is less than 50 mm Hg while the infant is breathing an FiO_2 of 0.60 or greater, provided that the $PaCO_2$ is less than or equal to 50 mm Hg and the pH is greater than 7.25. The indications for CPAP are described in Box 53-4.

Methods of Administration

The application of CPAP is most commonly accomplished noninvasively. In preterm and term neonates, short nasal prongs or oronasal masks are preferred over nasopharyngeal tubes which were traditionally used. Continued improvement of interface devices has led to more consistent CPAP delivery, better patient comfort, and reduced incidence of pressure ulcers (Figure 53-8). These interfaces include nasal masks, soft, pliable nasal CPAP cannulas, and the RAM cannula, all of which provide a comfortable interface without applying excessive pressure to maintain an effective seal. The American Association for Respiratory Care (AARC) has published Clinical Practice Guideline: Application of CPAP to Neonates via Nasal Prongs, Nasopharyngeal Tube, or Nasal Mask. Excerpts from this guideline appear in Clinical Practice Guideline 53-2.

For larger children, nasal masks, oronasal masks, nasal pillows, and other interfaces similar to interfaces used in adults may be used. In all patients, it is important to assess the patient-device interface at regular intervals to allow prevention or early detection and intervention in the event of pressure ulcers.

CPAP may be delivered using a mechanical ventilator in the CPAP mode, a CPAP driver, or continuous flow system with an underwater seal, also referred to as bubble CPAP. Mechanical ventilators provide better patient monitoring and may be connected to a central alarm system. CPAP drivers have the capability of adjusting flow to maintain set CPAP in the presence of a leak and/or increased patient inspiratory demand, and typically have some type of built in disconnect alarm. The continuous flow bubble CPAP systems are the simplest and least expensive

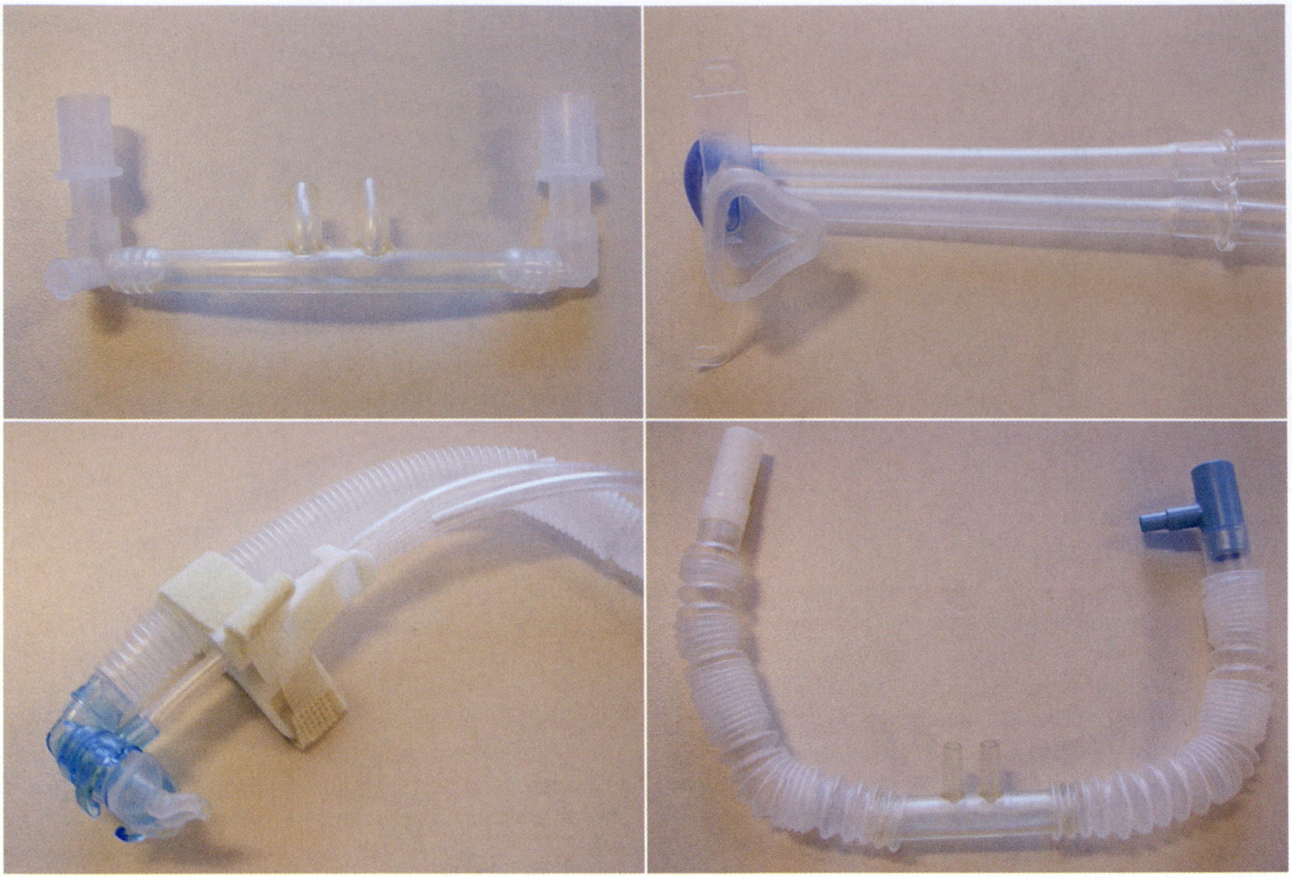

FIGURE 53-8 Patient interfaces for CPAP or NPPV.

of all the devices, but generally lack the ability to automatically adjust flow and do not have an integrated alarm system in the event of a patient disconnect. All are equally effective as long as the interface is appropriately sized and fitted to the patient. The choice of one device over another is often based on equipment availability or user or institutional bias.

CPAP levels are selected based on clinical observation. Initial CPAP levels are usually 5 to 7 cm H_2O and are adjusted in increments of 1 to 2 cm H_2O. The patient's SpO_2, respiratory rate, work of breathing, breath sounds, and blood pressure are monitored. The appropriate CPAP level is achieved when the respiratory rate decreases to near-normal ranges, signs of respiratory distress are lessened, and SpO_2 increases while O_2 requirements are reduced. Arterial and capillary blood gas analysis may provide additional information in determining the effectiveness of CPAP, and chest radiographs are obtained to determine the degree of lung inflation.

Weaning and eventually discontinuing CPAP is considered when oxygenation is adequate at FiO_2 less than 0.30 to 0.40, there is a sustained reduction in work of breathing, and chest radiograph and clinical assessment indicate resolution of the underlying disorder. The use of CPAP for prolonged periods in preterm infants helps reduce the work of breathing and prevent intubation. Long-term and intermittent use of CPAP is indicated in children with obstructive airway problems, chronic lung disease, and neuromuscular disorders.

High-Flow Nasal Cannula

Supplemental O_2 administration by nasal cannula is the most comfortable and simplest means of providing O_2 for infants and children. Evidence in preterm and term neonates indicates that using a nasal cannula at flow rates of 2 to 8 L/min may be as effective as and is easier to apply than a nasal CPAP system.[36-39]

Specially designed humidification systems have been developed and allow the use of nasal cannulas at flow rates of 2 to 30 L/min.[38] These devices maximize humidification and minimize condensation accumulating in the small-diameter supply tubing. The gas should always be conditioned (warmed and humidified) for approximately 5 to 10 minutes before it is connected to the patient. High-flow nasal cannula systems have been used successfully in neonates for the same indications that CPAP has been used. Instead of titrating levels of CPAP, the flow rate is incrementally adjusted. However, the amount of positive pressure that the high-flow nasal cannula potentially produces cannot be measured, and inadvertent high levels may occur, particularly if the nasal cannula fits snugly in the nares.[33,40-42] To prevent inadvertent high levels of CPAP from developing, the nasal prongs should not occupy more than 50% of the patient's nares.

High-flow nasal cannula systems have the potential for maximizing supplemental O_2 administration because the O_2

53-2 Application of Continuous Positive Airway Pressure to Neonates via Nasal Prongs, Nasopharyngeal Tube, or Nasal Mask

AARC Clinical Practice Guideline (Excerpts)*

INDICATIONS

- Abnormalities on physical examination—tachypnea, substernal and suprasternal retractions, grunting, and nasal flaring; the presence of pale or cyanotic skin color; agitation
- Inadequate oxygenation (PaO_2 <50 mm Hg with FiO_2 ≤0.60, provided that VE is adequate as indicated by $PaCO_2$ ≤50 mm Hg and pH ≥7.25)
- Presence of poorly expanded or infiltrated lung fields on chest radiograph
- Presence of a condition thought to be responsive to CPAP, including:
  - Respiratory distress syndrome
  - Recent extubation
  - Pulmonary edema
  - Transient tachypnea of the newborn
  - Atelectasis
  - Apnea of prematurity
  - Tracheomalacia or other similar abnormality of the lower airways

CONTRAINDICATIONS

- Although nasal CPAP has been used in bronchiolitis, this application may be contraindicated
- Need for intubation or mechanical ventilation or both as evidenced by the presence of:
  - Upper airway abnormalities that contraindicate nasal CPAP (e.g., choanal atresia, tracheoesophageal fistula)
  - Severe cardiovascular instability and impending arrest
  - Unstable respiratory drive with frequent apneic episodes resulting in desaturation or bradycardia or both
  - Ventilatory failure as indicated by the inability to maintain $PaCO_2$ <60 mm Hg and pH >7.25
  - Application of nasal CPAP to patients with untreated congenital diaphragmatic hernia may lead to gastric distention and further compromise of thoracic organs

HAZARDS AND COMPLICATIONS

Hazards and complications associated with equipment include the following:

- Obstruction of nasal prongs from mucous plugging or kinking may interfere with delivery of CPAP and result in a decrease in FiO_2 through entrainment of room air via opposite naris or mouth.
- Inactivation of airway pressure alarms
  - High resistance through nasal appliances can maintain pressure in the system even after decannulation; this can result in failure of low airway pressure or disconnect alarms to respond
  - Complete obstruction of nasal prongs and nasopharyngeal tubes results in continued pressurization of CPAP system without activation of low or high airway pressure alarms
- Activation of a manual breath (commonly available on infant ventilators) may cause gastric insufflation and patient discomfort, particularly if the peak pressure is set inappropriately high

Hazards and complications associated with the patient's clinical condition include the following:

- Lung overdistention causing barotrauma, $\dot{V}/\dot{Q}$ mismatch, hypercapnia, including work of breathing
- Impedance of pulmonary blood flow (increased pulmonary vascular resistance, decreased cardiac output)
- Gastric insufflation and abdominal distention potentially leading to aspiration
- Nasal irritation with septal distortion
- Skin irritation and pressure necrosis
- Nasal mucosal damage owing to inadequate humidification

ASSESSMENT OF OUTCOME

CPAP is initiated at levels of 4 to 5 cm H_2O and may be gradually increased up to 10 cm H_2O to provide the following:

- Stabilization of FiO_2 requirement ≤0.60 with PaO_2 levels >50 mm Hg or the presence of clinically acceptable noninvasive monitoring of O_2 ($PtcO_2$), while maintaining an adequate VE as indicated by $PaCO_2$ of ≤50 to 60 mm Hg and pH ≥7.25
- Reduced work of breathing as indicated by decreased respiratory rate, retractions, grunting, nasal flaring
- Improvement in lung volumes and appearance of lung as indicated by chest radiograph
- Improvement in patient comfort as assessed by bedside caregiver

MONITORING

Patient-ventilator system assessments should be performed at least every 2 to 4 hours and should include documentation of ventilator settings and patient assessments:

- O_2 and CO_2 monitoring, including periodic sampling of ABG values and continuous noninvasive monitoring (e.g., transcutaneous O_2 and CO_2 monitoring, pulse oximetry)
- Continuous monitoring of electrocardiogram and respiratory rate
- Continuous monitoring of proximal airway pressure, PEEP, and $\bar{P}aw$
- Continuous monitoring of FiO_2
- Periodic physical assessment of breath sounds and signs of increased work of breathing
- Periodic evaluation of chest radiographs

**For complete guideline, see American Association for Respiratory Care: Clinical practice guideline: application of continuous positive airway pressure to neonates via nasal prongs, nasopharyngeal tune, nasal mask: 2004 revision and update. Respir Care 49:1100, 2004.*
VE, *Minute ventilation.*

concentration delivered to the patient should approximate the set FiO_2. This approximation occurs because the anatomic reservoir of the upper airway is continuously flushed, greatly reducing the entrainment of room air. High-flow nasal cannula systems may be beneficial in stabilizing acute respiratory failure caused by hypoxemia, which may reduce the need for noninvasive or invasive assisted ventilation, such as in the case of a pulmonary exacerbation in a patient with bronchiolitis, cystic fibrosis or congestive heart failure.

RULE OF THUMB

When using a high-flow nasal cannula, the nasal prong should not occupy greater than 50% of the opening to patient's nares.

MECHANICAL VENTILATION

Early attempts to provide assisted ventilation to infants and children were largely derived from the experiences gained in adults, including the type of ventilators used and the associated techniques. Recognition of the physiologic differences of neonates and children led to further advances in ventilator design and modes and a wider range of capabilities. Although the classic "infant ventilator" is still used in some centers, modern microprocessor ventilators offer an ever-evolving array of options capable of supporting the full range of patient sizes and physiologic conditions.[43] Respiratory therapists caring for infants and children need to be familiar with their physiologic differences to select and modify the appropriate ventilatory strategy.[44-46]

Basic Principles

Conventional mechanical ventilation is the delivery of a bulk flow of humidified gas into and out of the lungs. The removal of CO_2, typically measured by PCO_2, is directly related to alveolar ventilation (frequency $\times$ V_T). Gas moves from the ventilator across an artificial airway in response to a change in pressure or pressure gradient. The magnitude of pressure required to move a particular amount of volume is derived from the compliance of the pulmonary system and the resistance of the airways.

Compliance is a measure of the distensibility of the lungs and is expressed as the volume change per unit of pressure change ($C = \Delta V/\Delta P$). *Resistance* is the tendency for airflow across the tracheobronchial tree to be impeded at a particular pressure per unit of gas flow ($R = \Delta P/\text{flow}$). The product of compliance and resistance is the respiratory time constant, or the measure of time necessary for the equilibration of a change in airway pressure ($TC = C \times R$). A patient with stiff or noncompliant lungs, such as a preterm infant with surfactant deficiency, has short time constants, meaning less time is required for equilibration, and filling and emptying of lungs occur faster, requiring shorter inspiratory and expiratory times. A patient with a disease characterized by impaired airflow or high resistance, such as a child with asthma, has longer time constants, in which more time is required for filling and emptying, thus longer inspiratory and expiratory times are needed.

Goals of Mechanical Ventilation

The basic goals of mechanical ventilation are to improve O_2 delivery to meet metabolic demand and eliminate CO_2, while reducing the work of breathing. The basic aim of assisted ventilation is to meet the goals while minimizing the associated deleterious effects. One approach to mechanical ventilation begins with the selection of an appropriate breath type, either pressure-controlled or volume-controlled, and a mode that best meets the physiologic needs of the patient's condition.[47] Box 53-5 lists the indications for mechanical ventilation in infants and children.

Modes of Ventilation and Breath Delivery Types

Historically, the most common mode of ventilation used in neonates and children was intermittent mandatory ventilation. Because early infant ventilators were unable to respond to the small triggering efforts of these patients, mandatory timed breaths were superimposed over a continuous flow of gas. These asynchronous, mandatory breaths provided most of the ventilation, while the patient was allowed to breathe spontaneously from the continuous gas source. Eventually, technologic improvements resulted in triggering devices that provided synchronization of the mandatory breaths with patient effort (synchronized intermittent mandatory ventilation [SIMV]) followed by the ability to provide assist/control (A/C) and pressure support ventilation (PSV). Despite evidence that SIMV is more likely to result in patient-ventilator asynchrony,[48,49] most

Box 53-5 Indications for Mechanical Ventilation

APNEA

Respiratory Failure
- PaO_2 <50 mm Hg
- $PaCO_2$ >65 mm Hg

Pulmonary Disease
- Respiratory distress syndrome
- PPHN
- Meconium aspiration syndrome
- Pneumonia
- ARDS

NEUROLOGIC AND NEUROMUSCULAR
- Asphyxia
- Head trauma
- Spinal muscle atrophy
- Muscular dystrophy

CONGENITAL ABNORMALITIES
- Congenital diaphragmatic hernia
- Congenital heart disease

POSTSURGERY
- Thoracic surgery

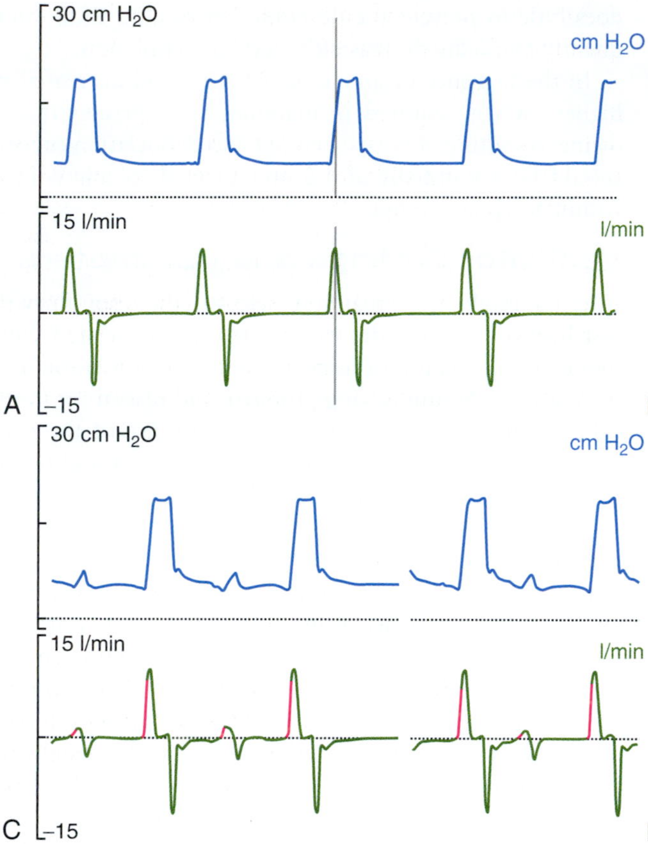

FIGURE 53-9 Airway graphics. **A,** Patient is apneic. Regardless of SIMV or A/C mode all breaths are mandatory at set rate. **B,** A/C mode. Total respiratory rate is determined by patient's spontaneous rate. **C,** SIMV mode. Mechanical breaths are delivered at a set rate. Patient is allowed to breathe spontaneously in between mandatory breaths. **D,** PSV mode. There are no set mandatory breaths. All breaths are pressure supported at patient's spontaneous rate.

neonatal and pediatric patients are managed by using one of these three modes or a combination (i.e., SIMV + PSV). The most common triggering device for infant ventilators is a pneumotachygraph placed in the ventilator circuit, often proximal to the airway, which in many cases also serves as a monitoring device. The pneumotachygraph allows for the integration of a flow signal, which can be displayed as inhaled and exhaled V_T and minute ventilation. Figure 53-9 displays graphic representations of A/C, SIMV, and PSV. Another mode of ventilation increasingly used in neonates and small children is called *neurologically adjusted ventilatory assist* (NAVA) in which the ventilator responds to electrical activity of the diaphragm (Eadi). This requires use of a special gastric tube with electrodes that sense Eadi. In this highly responsive mode ventilation is provided by adjusting the amount of airway pressure applied per 1 microvolt change in Eadi.

In almost all cases of neonatal ventilation, the mechanical breaths delivered during SIMV and A/C are time-cycled, pressure-limited breaths.[50] Inspiration is initiated by patient effort or as a result of the set respiratory rate (whichever comes first). Based on the available flow—continuous, demand, or both—the set inspiratory pressure is reached early in the inspiratory phase and maintained throughout the remainder of the inspiratory time, after which the ventilator cycles to expiration. In many cases, appropriate setting of the *inspiratory rise time* (the speed in which gas flow is delivered controlling how rapidly set airway pressure is achieved) improves patient-ventilator synchrony. Most current-generation ventilators are capable of providing volume-targeted, pressure-limited ventilation, often referred to as *pressure-regulated volume control* or *volume guarantee*. In this dual mode of ventilation, the inspiratory V_T is compared with a preset target V_T, and the inspiratory pressure on the next breath is adjusted up or down in an attempt to meet the target volume. True volume-controlled breaths are rarely used for ventilating neonatal patients. (See Chapter 45 for details.)

RULE OF THUMB

When ventilating neonates, choose time-cycled, pressure-limited mechanical breaths.

Pediatric patients may be ventilated with either volume-controlled or pressure-controlled breaths. The choice may be based on health care team or institutional preference, prior experience, and equipment availability or may be evidence-based for specific diseases (e.g., asthma).

MINI CLINI

Pediatric Ventilation

PROBLEM: A 12-year-old girl with asthma is admitted to the emergency department. She was intubated in the field by paramedics and is currently ventilated with a transport ventilator at the following settings:

- Mode—SIMV
- V_T—10 ml/kg
- PIP—90 cm H_2O
- PEEP—0 cm H_2O
- Set respiratory rate—16 breaths/min
- Total respiratory rate—20 breaths/min
- Inspiratory time—0.25 sec
- FiO_2—1.0

The paramedics inform the RT that since the patient has been placed on the mechanical ventilator, PIP has steadily increased, blood pressure has begun to decrease, and breaths sounds consisting of bilateral inspiratory and expiratory wheezes have become increasingly diminished. What should the RT recommend?

Solution: The ventilator circuit should be immediately disconnected from the endotracheal tube allowing the patient to exhale fully. This patient should be fully sedated and possibly paralyzed to allow the RT to set and control ventilation. The ventilator settings should be set as follows:

- Mode—A/C
- Breath delivery type—volume controlled
- V_T—4 to 6 ml/kg
- Plateau pressure—maintain at ≤30 cm H_2O
- Respiratory rate—set at whatever rate allows ventilation without an increase in auto-PEEP or increased plateau pressure or both
- Inspiratory time—1.0 sec
- PEEP—5 cm H_2O
- FiO_2—1.0

Patients with severe status asthmaticus are among the most challenging patients to ventilate. The pulmonary time constants are increased such that it is equally difficult to inflate the lungs as it is for the patient to exhale. The inspiratory flow rate must be controlled by the clinician by means of volume-controlled ventilation, and sufficient time must be provided to allow the lungs to inflate. Expiratory time must be sufficient to allow exhalation, preventing the accumulation of trapped gas or auto-PEEP. The result is a decrease in minute ventilation, which leads to permissive hypercapnia as a lung protective strategy. $PaCO_2$ should be allowed to increase as long as the pH is greater than or equal to 7.10.

The inspiratory time must be increased (up to 1 second for this patient and longer in older teenagers) to allow inspiratory gas flow to the patient. Although this increase in inspiratory time may seem counterintuitive in a patient with prolonged expiratory time constants, it is necessary to deliver gas on inspiration. Decreasing the inspiratory time to less than 1 second does little to prevent the development of auto-PEEP and frequently markedly decreases the level of ventilation.

In the presence of an elevated $PaCO_2$ and decreased pH, a higher FiO_2 is required to maintain SpO_2 greater than 90% owing to shifting of the oxyhemoglobin dissociation curve. FiO_2 should be set initially at 1.0 and titrated to maintain SpO_2 within acceptable range.

Ventilator Settings and Parameters

After the mode of ventilation is selected, the respiratory therapist begins to adjust the various settings associated with the mode, while keeping in mind the goals of ventilation and the patient's weight, underlying problem, and reason for mechanical ventilation. The RT often can get a sense of the patient's compliance by manually ventilating the patient and observing the pressure needed to make the chest rise.

Peak Inspiratory Pressure

For time-cycled, pressure-limited breaths, the peak inspiratory pressure (PIP) is set according to predetermined criteria (e.g., 20 to 25 cm H_2O) or by observing the pressure required to move the chest during manual ventilation with a flow inflating bag or T-piece resuscitator. The delivered V_T is monitored, and adjustments may be made. Increasing the PIP normally results in an increase in V_T, whereas a decrease in PIP results in decreased V_T. In the absence of V_T monitoring, PIP may be adjusted based on subjective assessment of chest movement and auscultation of breath sounds. Efforts should be made to maintain the lowest possible PIP that delivers the target V_T because PIP greater than 28 cm H_2O in time-cycled, pressuresimited (pressure controlled) breaths has been shown to increase the likelihood of ventilator-induced lung injury.

RULE OF THUMB

Always strive to maintain PIP less than or equal to 28 cm H_2O.

Positive End Expiratory Pressure

Positive end expiratory pressure (PEEP), referred to as the *baseline pressure,* is used to prevent alveolar collapse at end-expiration. PEEP results in improved oxygenation for a given O_2 concentration. If the PEEP is set too low, alveolar collapse may occur, resulting in decreased FRC, altered ventilation/perfusion ($\dot{V}/\dot{Q}$ matching), and hypoxemia. If the PEEP is set too high, overdistention may occur, increasing the likelihood of lung injury. Typically, PEEP is set between 5 cm H_2O and 6 cm H_2O, although higher levels may be used if necessary. PEEP is set in conjunction with PIP, and the difference between the two is often referred to as the delta P *or driving pressure.* As the delta P is increased, either by increasing PIP or decreasing PEEP, the V_T will most likely increase as well (unless overdistention occurs). Conversely, decreasing the delta P results in lower V_T. Ideally the delta pressure or driving pressure should not be greater than 15 cm H_2O.

Tidal Volume

When selecting V_T, the clinician must consider a volume that provides adequate lung inflation without overstretching the alveoli. Setting V_T that is too high most likely would result in lung injury. V_T of 6 to 8 ml/kg is generally considered safe in most patients. However, in some patients with extremely low lung compliance, such as patients with severe acute respiratory distress syndrome (ARDS), it may be necessary to reduce V_T to 4 to 5 ml/kg.

If the clinician chooses to deliver volume-controlled breaths, V_T is set as a control variable. Every mechanical breath delivers an identical V_T at either a preset inspiratory time or a preset flow rate. Set V_T, inspiratory time, and flow all are interrelated. If V_T is set at 300 ml, and flow rate is 30 L/min (0.5 L/sec), the inspiratory time is 0.6 second. See formulas in Box 53-6.

When ventilating patients with pressure-controlled breaths, V_T is not set, but it should be monitored. The clinician must compare the monitored V_T with a predetermined target and adjust the delta P to meet that target.

Regardless of whether the clinician chooses volume-controlled or pressure-controlled breaths, he or she must recognize that some of the V_T is compressed in the circuit and not delivered to the patient; this is referred to as *compressible volume loss*. Most current-generation ventilators automatically compensate for compressible volume loss and adjust the delivered and displayed (monitored) V_T accordingly. With older ventilators and current, less sophisticated ventilators, such as those used for transport, during volume-controlled breaths, the clinician must calculate the compressible volume loss and increase the set V_T to deliver the desired volume to the patient. During both volume-controlled and pressure-controlled breaths, the calculated compressible volume loss must be subtracted from the ventilator displayed exhaled V_T. See Box 53-7 for calculation of compressible volume loss.

Box 53-6 Interrelationship of Tidal Volume, Flow, and Time

$$V_T = \text{Flow in L/sec} \times \text{Inspiratory time}$$
$$\text{Inspiratory time} = V_T/\text{Flow rate}$$

Box 53-7 Determining Effective or Corrected Tidal Volume

$$\text{Effective } V_T = \text{Delivered } V_T - \text{Compressible volume}$$
$$\text{Compressible volume} = \text{Compressible factor} \times (\text{PIP} - \text{PEEP})$$

Example: A 12-year-old child weighing 28 kg requires assisted ventilation. V_T is set at 240 ml, PIP is 25 cm H_2O, and PEEP is 5 cm H_2O. The compressible factor for the ventilator is 2 ml/cm H_2O.

$$\text{Compressible volume} = (2\text{ ml/cm } H_2O) \times (25 - 5\text{ cm } H_2O) = 40\text{ ml}$$
$$\text{Effective } V_T = 240\text{ ml} - 40\text{ ml} = 200\text{ ml}$$
$$\text{Effective } V_T/\text{kg} = 200\text{ ml} \div 28\text{ kg} = 7.1\text{ ml/kg}$$

RULE OF THUMB

Large V_T (>8 ml/kg) is likely to overstretch the lung, resulting in acute lung injury, and should be avoided. Patients with severe ARDS may require even lower V_T (4 to 5 ml/kg). In addition, PIP and/or plateau pressure should be maintained <28 cm H_2O and delta P ≤15 cm H_2O.

MINI CLINI

Pediatric Ventilation

PROBLEM: A 10-year-old boy with a complex medical history including history of trisomy 21, intractable infantile spasms, seizure disorder, and developmental delay (nonverbal), is admitted with increased difficulty breathing. His temperature on admission is 101° F, and a chest x-ray shows a left lower lobe infiltrate consistent with pneumonia. His home regimen includes nocturnal NIV via nasal mask with an inspiratory pressure of 8 cm H_2O, 3 cm PEEP, and 2 L/min of O_2 added to the breathing circuit. On admission, the patient complains of shortness of breath. His respiratory rate is 40 breaths/min, and SpO_2 is 88% on a nonrebreathing mask. What should the RT suggest?

Solution:

- NIV—consider beginning NIV via oronasal mask
- PIP—10 to 12 cm H_2O
- PEEP—3 to 5 cm H_2O
- Set respiratory rate—12 breaths/min
- FiO_2—1.0

Although this patient receives NIV for nocturnal support when stable, he currently has an acute infection superimposed on chronic restrictive lung disease. Beginning NIV now may provide sufficient support to prevent intubation during this acute condition. Initial PIP of 10 to 12 cm H_2O titrated to patient comfort may provide additional support, increasing V_T and allowing respiratory rate to return to baseline. Choosing an oronasal mask may prove to be a more efficient interface than the patient's usual nasal mask at this time. The set respiratory rate of 12 breaths/min is intended to be a backup rate because this patient is spontaneously breathing and should be allowed to establish his own breathing pattern. FiO_2 should be adjusted to maintain an acceptable SpO_2.

Ventilator Rate

The ventilator rate is the set number of breaths delivered in 1 minute. During A/C ventilation, the set respiratory rate is the minimum number of breaths the patient will receive and is increased if the patient triggers the ventilator at a respiratory rate faster than that which is set. The actual or total respiratory rate multiplied by V_T determines the minute ventilation, which is directly related to alveolar ventilation and PCO_2. Because V_T is usually set according to the patient's ideal or calculated body weight, adjusting minute ventilation is most often accomplished by changing the respiratory rate. The clinician must be aware of the total respiratory rate when making changes to adjust minute ventilation. If the set respiratory rate is 16, but the total respiratory rate is 22 because of patient triggering, decreasing the set rate to 12 or increasing the set rate to 18 would have no effect on minute ventilation.

Inspiratory Time

The inspiratory time is often defined as the time required to deliver V_T; however, this may be misleading. As described earlier, with volume-controlled breaths, the inspiratory time is determined by V_T and inspiratory flow rate and is the time required to deliver the preset V_T at the preset flow rate. However, with pressure-controlled breaths, the inspiratory time is set by the clinician and may be shorter, longer, or equal to the time required to deliver the breath. In the case of increased airway resistance, such as a patient with asthma, if the inspiratory time is not set long enough, flow delivery to the patient may not decelerate to zero by the end of the set inspiratory time. Under these circumstances, increasing inspiratory time would result in an increase in delivered V_T. Conversely, under the same conditions, shortening the inspiratory time would result in a decrease in delivered V_T. In the case of decreased compliance, as in pneumonia, increasing inspiratory time beyond the time necessary to allow full flow deceleration would result in an inspiratory pause or breath-hold, which may not be tolerated by the patient.

RULE OF THUMB

Inspiratory time is usually set between 0.2 second and 0.4 second for neonates and up to 1.0 second in teenagers. With patients who are awake and have spontaneous breathing efforts, inspiratory time must be set at a level that matches patient demand to avoid patient-ventilator asynchrony.

Oxygen Concentration

The O_2 concentration or FiO_2 is kept as low as possible to avoid the risk of O_2 toxicity. Although the precise mechanisms are not understood, the best approach is to maintain the lowest FiO_2 possible. The immature lung is particularly susceptible to O_2 toxicity, which can result in the development of bronchopulmonary dysplasia. In a preterm infant, FiO_2 is titrated to a narrow SpO_2 range (e.g., 88% to 94%) so that retinal damage (ROP), which is caused by elevated PO_2, does not develop.[17]

RULE OF THUMB

O_2 is considered a drug and should be used appropriately. High O_2 concentrations are potentially injurious and may cause O_2 toxicity in the immature lung and retinal damage in preterm infants.

Mean Airway Pressure

Mean airway pressure ($\overline{P}aw$) is the average airway pressure during a 1-minute period. It is affected by changes in PIP, PEEP, inspiratory time, and respiratory rate. An increase in $\overline{P}aw$ is often associated with improved oxygenation but is not without hazards. Increasing PEEP would result in increased $\overline{P}aw$ and potentially increased oxygenation. However, if the PEEP is set too high, the alveoli may become overinflated resulting in worsening $\dot{V}/\dot{Q}$ matching, and lung injury may occur.

Noninvasive Ventilation

Noninvasive ventilation (NIV), also known as *noninvasive positive pressure ventilation,* has become more popular recently in neonatal patients. In the past, use of NIV was limited by the lack of available interfaces; however, these are becoming more readily available. Figure 53-8 shows various interfaces that may be used for NIV (or CPAP) in neonates. NIV for neonates has been used successfully for premature infants in the delivery room and as an accepted mode of ventilation in the NICU where it has been used to prevent initial intubation or secondarily to prevent reintubation in the setting of extubation failure. NIV has also been used as a primary mode of ventilation for patients with acute respiratory failure.[51-53] However, there is scant evidence to support the use of NIV over CPAP or as a method of reducing the incidence of bronchopulmonary dysplasia. Patient triggering may be problematic given the large leaks that may occur with most patient interfaces, even with some current ventilators' "Noninvasive Modes," which generally include various forms of sophisticated leak compensation. However, there is ample evidence to support the use of both synchronized and nonsynchronized NIV in the NICU.[54,55]

Outside the NICU, NIV has been used extensively in patients of all ages, including pediatric patients.[56-59] Indications may include short-term support of hypoxemic respiratory failure, such as that seen with pulmonary edema associated with left-sided heart failure; prevention of intubation; postextubation support; and long-term support of patients with neuromuscular disease. Some limitation of available interfaces persists, particularly in smaller patients; however, most patients can be fitted without too much difficulty. As with CPAP and other noninvasive interface devices, care must be taken to prevent or minimize patient injury owing to iatrogenic pressure ulcers from a tight or poorly fitted device.

NIV may be provided with simple, single-limb devices such as bilevel positive airway pressure generators, or sophisticated ICU ventilators. Care must be taken whenever a single-limb circuit is employed to provide sufficient PEEP in the system to prevent rebreathing of gases (see Chapter 51).

Monitoring Mechanical Ventilation

The RT should develop a systematic approach to monitoring the effects of mechanical ventilation. Components of a ventilator assessment should include an evaluation of the artificial airway, physical examination, assessment of patient-ventilator interaction,[60] analysis of laboratory and radiographic data, adjunct ventilator monitoring, and a systematic ventilator safety assessment including alarm function and assessment of humidification. Alarms should be connected to a central monitoring system to alert clinicians away from the bedside of a change the patient's condition.

A flow sheet is used to prompt the user and guide the clinician through the process of assessing the patient, while serving as documentation of the ventilator settings and outputs. In the past, these flow sheets were paper and were maintained as part of the patient's medical record. Currently, most flow sheets are integrated into an electronic medical record that is readily available to the entire patient care team. Although many elements of the patient-ventilator assessment may be automatically entered via an electronic interface and require validation only by the clinician, some data must still be entered by hand. As standardization improves and these systems become more sophisticated and interchangeable, all of the data, including ventilator information, laboratory values, and radiographic and other imaging data, should automatically download, eliminating transcription errors, providing a more comprehensive assessment, and allowing the clinician to focus on the patient and patient-ventilator interaction.

MINI CLINI

Pediatric Mechanical Ventilation

PROBLEM: A 14-month-old child, who weighs 13 kg and has a history of chronic lung disease (bronchopulmonary dysplasia), requires mechanical ventilation after surgery for correction of gastric reflux. The surgeon requests that the RT select ventilator parameters and develop a weaning plan for this child. The child has an uncuffed 4.5 oral endotracheal tube in place. SpO_2 is 100% with manual ventilation and 100% O_2. Sedation is prescribed to keep the child comfortable but allow spontaneous breathing.

This child needs a ventilatory strategy that takes into account his age, disease process, amount of sedation, and current ventilation needs. What would be the appropriate choices for his initial ventilator management in terms of mode, V_T, set rate, FiO_2, and PEEP level?

Solution:

- Mode—Pressure A/C
- Pressure level set to ensure V_T 6 to 8 ml/kg or 100 to 130 ml
- Respiratory rate—20 to 30 breaths/minute
- FiO_2—1.0 then titrated to an acceptable SpO_2
- PEEP—5 cm H_2O

If this child had previously been mechanically ventilated, reviewing the presurgery settings may be helpful in deciding a ventilator plan. If not, a rationale for the suggested parameters follows.

By using the Pressure A/C mode, patient-ventilator synchrony can be more easily achieved; this reduces the need for sedation later, after the pain of surgery has dissipated. The initial V_T is based on current recommendations. The ventilator rate is determined by the normal respiratory rate for the age of the child, the desired PCO_2 level, and the number of assisted or triggered breaths the child is having. Because this child has chronic lung disease, a higher PCO_2 may be optimal at this time. A younger child with a higher PCO_2 and with a decreased respiratory rate may have a higher set rate. Initial FiO_2 is usually reflective of the amount currently being delivered with hand ventilation but quickly titrated to maintain normal SpO_2. FiO_2 of 0.40 after surgery would not be unusual in the child. In addition, plateau pressure should not be greater than 28 cm H_2O and the delta P should not be higher than 15 cm H_2O.

Physical Examination

Examination of the patient can yield quick and useful information. The chest is examined for adequacy of chest rise, the presence of asymmetric movement and deformities, and signs of increased work of breathing such as retractions. Breath sounds are helpful in gauging the degree of air entry, verifying bilateral aeration, and identifying airflow problems and areas of diminished aeration. Skin appearance can also give the clinician a sense of the patient's perfusion—an indirect measure of cardiac output. A mottled appearance, poor capillary refill, and pale or gray color indicate poor perfusion.

Patient-Ventilator Interaction

The patient-ventilator interaction is the assessment used to determine the ease with which the patient can trigger and interact with the ventilator throughout the complete ventilatory cycle. This assessment is made by simultaneously observing the trigger indicator, waveforms, and the patient. Refinements in the trigger threshold may need to be made if there is a leak present or the work to trigger or initiate a breath is too great. Most ventilators may be flow triggered or pressure triggered. There is little difference between the two as long as they are set correctly. The trigger sensitivity should be set as sensitive as possible without auto-triggering. The manner in which the breath is terminated is also assessed. Pressure-supported breaths are flow cycled based on the patient's spontaneous inspiratory time and flow demand. Mechanical breaths are time cycled. Theoretically, flow-cycled, pressure-supported breaths should be more comfortable and promote improved patient-ventilator synchrony because the patient has more control over the breath than with mechanical breaths. Together, patient synchrony and comfort are determined. Patient-ventilator asynchrony occurs when the patient's efforts to breathe are unmatched with the preselected ventilator support. Airway graphics are also helpful in identifying nuances and refining ventilator settings.[61] Airway graphics routinely displayed are scalar waveforms of flow, airway pressure, and volume. Additionally, each of these parameters can be plotted against the others. Pressure-volume and flow-volume loops can be particularly helpful in assessing alterations in work of breathing, overdistention of the lung, and compliance. See Chapter 47 for more detail on patient-ventilator interaction.

Additional Monitoring

The use of noninvasive monitors, particularly measurements of end-tidal CO_2 and SpO_2, has become routine. Periodic blood gas analysis is a useful tool to quantify acid-base status and to refine ventilator settings further. Other laboratory data, such as electrolytes and hematologic information, are also assessed.

Periodic chest radiographs are obtained to identify suspected problems and to assess the progress of lung disease.

Patient-Ventilator Periodic Assessment

A systematic patient-ventilator assessment should be conducted periodically.[61] Prescribed ventilator settings are confirmed and documented along with verification of ventilator outputs. Measurements of mandatory and spontaneous V_T values are made and expressed per the patient's weight to determine if targets are being achieved. Alarms must be set and tested and should minimally detect loss of pressure, high pressure, and patient disconnection. Additional alarms should alert the clinician to changes in tidal volume, minute ventilation, respiratory rate, and PEEP.

The humidification system is evaluated including airway temperature and the presence of condensation in the ventilator circuit. Some visible condensation or "rain-out" is important because a completely dry circuit may be a sign of inadequate humidification, which results in thickened secretions and possible airway obstruction.

> **RULE OF THUMB**
>
> Routine monitoring of ventilated patients is essential and should include an assessment of the patient's physiologic status including vital signs and a systematic assessment of the patient-ventilator interaction.

Weaning from Mechanical Ventilation

Weaning or, more appropriately, liberation from mechanical ventilation is a topic that that has become more standardized over the past several years in pediatric patients.[62-64] Clear guidelines for "assessment of readiness to extubate" and "spontaneous breathing trials" have become standard practice.[65] However, some controversy remains and this assessment has not yet become standard practice in neonatal patients even though there is considerable literature available to guide clinicians in this area.[66-68] Considerable variation in practice exists among institutions and even among clinicians within institutions. Nevertheless, these patients should be assessed daily to determine their readiness for liberation from mechanical ventilation. Some general considerations for extubation are presented in Box 53-8. Once it is agreed that a patient may be ready for extubation, a systematic coordinated approach should be undertaken. This includes a safety screen followed by some agreed-upon evaluation of the patient's ability to breathe spontaneously without ventilatory assistance. Box 53-9. If a spontaneous breathing trial is attempted, it should be coordinated with a reduction in the level of sedation, often referred to as a *spontaneous awakening trial.* However, in some cases this may not be feasible as a reduction in sedation may result in the

Box 53-8 Considerations for Extubation

- Spontaneous respiratory rate appropriate for age and weight
- Presence of apnea or periodic breathing
- FiO_2 requirement ≤0.4
- Ability to protect airway
- Normal work of breathing
- Acceptable amount and consistency of respiratory secretions
- Normal vital signs
- Minimal sedation needs
- SpO_2 >90%
- Spontaneous V_T >4-5 ml/kg

Box 53-9 Pediatric/Neonatal Ventilator Discontinuance Protocol

STEP 1

Safety Screen (lack of the following)

- Brain death, ICP >15 mm Hg, suspected high ICP, or difficult to control ICP
- Neuromuscular blockade
- Significant hemoptysis (significant amounts of blood from endotracheal tube or tracheostomy)
- Hemodynamic instability
- Unstable airway
- FiO_2 >0.6
- PEEP ≥8 cm H_2O
- Lack of ICU team consensus
- Extracorporeal life support
- Chronic disease requiring ventilation

Issues to Address Before Extubation

- Fluid overload
- Secretions
- Neurologic impairment
- Medication requirement precludes safe extubation
- NPO time insufficient
- Unstable, unsafe, swollen airway
- Imminent procedure
- Psychosocial factors (e.g., unclear code status, assent)
- Imminent return to home hospital

STEP 2

If none of the above conditions exist, the pediatric ICU team discusses the feasibility of extubation.

Consider the Following

- Stage of ventilation
  I—initial or acute stage (escalation)
  II—ventilator management stage (plateau)
  III—discontinuance stage (deescalation)
- Immediate extubation (may include reversal of sedation)
- Spontaneous breathing trial (may include some level of pressure support)
- Reduction of ventilator settings

If Spontaneous Breathing Trial Is Performed, Stop Trial At Any Point for the Following

- Tachypnea, bradypnea, apnea (age appropriate)
- Excessive use of accessory muscles, nasal flaring present, subjective dyspnea (consider baseline)
- Significant, unresolved change in agitation or anxiety
- Significant tachycardia or bradycardia
- Hemodynamic changes
- Unacceptable decrease in SpO_2

STEP 3

Critical care team discusses extubation plan.

ICP, Intracranial pressure; *NPO,* nothing per mouth.

patient pulling the endotracheal tube (and intravenous lines, etc.) and unplanned extubation may occur. Whenever a patient is extubated, either planned or unplanned, there should be appropriate supplies, equipment, and personnel immediately available to reintubate if necessary. (See Chapter 52 for details on weaning.)

High-Frequency Ventilation

High-frequency ventilation (HFV) is a form of invasive mechanical ventilation that uses small V_T values (less than dead space) at rapid frequencies, up to 900 breaths/min (15 Hz). The primary goal of HFV is to provide adequate ventilation and oxygenation, while limiting the incidence of lung injury. HFV has been used as a primary mode of ventilation as well as a rescue therapy for patients determined to be failing conventional mechanical ventilation. Although early studies showed a beneficial effect on gas exchange compared with conventional ventilation, there has been no demonstrated improvement in outcome compared with current lung protective strategies.[69-75] In fact, recent studies have shown a trend toward increased mortality in patients treated with high-frequency ventilation.[76,77] Despite the lack of evidence supporting its use, HFV remains a controversial mode of ventilation for pediatric and neonatal patients but should be used only by clinicians expert in its clinical application and knowledgeable about its physiologic effects.

There are three basic types of HFV: high-frequency oscillatory ventilation, high-frequency jet ventilation, and high-frequency percussive ventilation. High-frequency oscillatory ventilation is the most common form of HFV. Oxygenation is achieved by inflating the patient's lungs to a high resting level, or FRC, by establishing a high mean airway pressure, similar to CPAP, at levels typically ranging from 16 to 30 cm H_2O. This "recruitment" improves the $\dot{V}/\dot{Q}$ ratio by opening previously collapsed alveoli. Ventilation is provided by the to-and-fro movement of a large piston in the ventilator circuit that results in high-frequency oscillations in the patient's airways. Gas exchange results from a combination of six mechanisms: bulk flow of gas, longitudinal dispersion, pendelluft, asymmetric velocity profiles, cardiogenic mixing, and molecular diffusion.

Gas exchange during high-frequency jet ventilation is believed to occur via two mechanisms—convection and diffusion. Fresh gas is injected into the endotracheal tube at a high velocity and travels down the mid-portion of the airways, reducing dead space. Bidirectional flow occurs as gas simultaneously travels up the outer lumen of the airways. Diffusion occurs in the lower airways as cross-sectional area increases and velocity decreases, similar to conventional ventilation.

During high-frequency percussive ventilation, a series of small, rapid breaths accompanied by air trapping are delivered that result in a steady increase in airway pressure, similar to a conventional breath. This is followed by a release phase to allow exhalation. The rapid "percussive" breaths are maintained through the entire breathing cycle, which facilitates gas exchange and simultaneously promotes movement of secretions to larger airways and eventually the trachea where they may be more easily removed.

Cardiovascular Effects

The cardiovascular effects of HFV vary with the strategy employed. Using the high lung volume strategy, lung volume is recruited, and $\overline{P}aw$ can be slowly reduced while maintaining alveolar ventilation. This strategy limits the adverse side effects of PPV on cardiovascular performance and may result in increased systemic blood flow. However, if $\overline{P}aw$ greater than that used during conventional ventilation is required during HFV, cardiovascular compromise may occur. Increases in intravascular volume and use of vasoactive drugs help support mean arterial blood pressure, cardiac output, and O_2 delivery. Increases in central venous pressure or decreases in mean arterial pressure indicate decreases in systemic blood flow as a result of overdistention of the lung and inappropriately high $\overline{P}aw$ after adequate intravascular volume has been established.

Weaning from High-Frequency Ventilation

When FiO_2 is equal to or less than 0.6, $\overline{P}aw$ is weaned slowly. When $\overline{P}aw$ is less than 15 to 18 cm H_2O, the patient may be trialed off or transitioned to conventional ventilation. Alternatively, the patient may be extubated directly from HFV once the mean airway pressure and F_IO_2 have been reduced to 8 to 9 cm H_2O and 0.3 respectively.

Complications of Mechanical Ventilation

Box 53-10 summarizes the most common complications associated with mechanical ventilation in newborns and other pediatric patients.

SPECIALTY GASES

Inhaled Nitric Oxide

Inhaled nitric oxide (INO) is a selective pulmonary vasodilator used to treat newborns who require mechanical ventilation for hypoxic respiratory failure.[78,79] INO improves oxygenation and reduces the need for extracorporeal membrane oxygenation (ECMO). See Chapter 50 for details. The approved indications for INO are listed in Box 53-11. INO also has been studied in preterm infants with the aim to reduce the incidence of chronic lung disease. These clinical investigations showed a modest improvement in pulmonary outcomes, but other problems associated with prematurity, such as intracranial hemorrhage, were unchanged. At the present time, INO is not routinely used in the management of respiratory failure associated with prematurity.

INO is administered in conjunction with mechanical ventilation via a specially designed delivery and monitoring system that provides precision drug dosing and safety features (Figure 53-10). The recommended INO dose is 20 parts per million (ppm) with an optimal response achieved when lung inflation is maximized.[80,81] When a response has been achieved and

Box 53-10 Complications of Mechanical Ventilation in Infants and Children

- Ventilator-induced injuries
- Air leak syndromes
- Pneumothorax
- Pneumomediastinum
- Pneumopericardium
- Pneumoperitoneum
- Pulmonary interstitial emphysema
- Subcutaneous emphysema
- Parenchymal lung damage
- Bronchopulmonary dysplasia
- Cardiovascular complications
- Decreased venous return
- Decreased cardiac output
- Increased pulmonary vascular resistance
- Increased intracranial pressure
- Increased incidence of intraventricular hemorrhage
- O_2-induced injuries
- O_2 toxicity
- ROP
- Airway complications
- Accidental extubation
- Atelectasis
- Inadequate humidification
- Endobronchial intubation
- Equipment contamination
- Postintubation stridor
- Endotracheal tube plugging or kinking
- Tracheal lesions
- Infection
- Ventilator-associated pneumonia

Box 53-11 Indications for Inhaled Nitric Oxide

Term and near-term neonates (>34 weeks' gestation) with PPHN
  Gradient between preductal and postductal SpO_2
  Echocardiographic evidence
Congenital diaphragmatic hernia
Oxygenation index (OI) >25
  $OI = (\bar{P}aw \times FiO_2/PaO_2)$

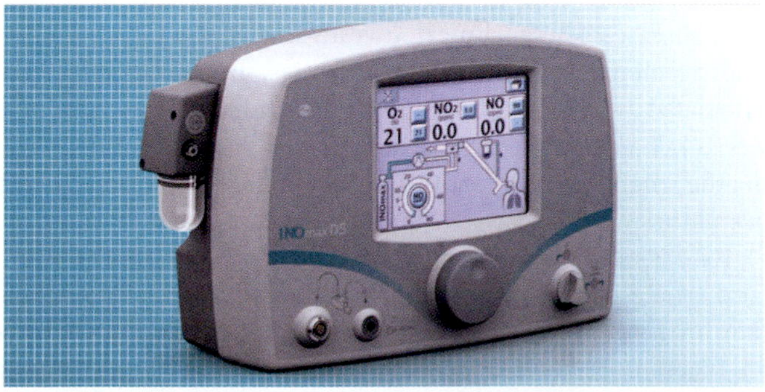

FIGURE 53-10 Nitric oxide delivery system (Ikaria INOmax DS_{ir} Operator's Manual, Ikaria, Inc. 2010).

sustained, the INO dose is gradually reduced, typically by 50% each step, to a final dose of 1 ppm, at which point the drug is discontinued. During withdrawal of INO, FiO_2 is increased to minimize any recurrence of pulmonary hypertension.[82]

During INO therapy, concentrations of nitric oxide and O_2 are continuously monitored. The combined exposure of nitric oxide and O_2 leads to the formation of nitrogen dioxide, which is potentially toxic and is continuously monitored. INO doses typically used are considered to be very low and have a good safety profile. A metabolite of INO is the formation of methemoglobin as the nitric oxide molecule is bound to hemoglobin. During INO administration, the patient's ability to metabolize methemoglobin is assessed by periodically monitoring methemoglobin levels.[83]

INO should be available in any hospital that has a level III intensive care nursery. INO should be an integral part of any high-risk transport team, and it is important that non-ECMO centers have a plan for treatment failure that takes into account the distance to an ECMO center.[84] INO therapy has also been used for diagnosing and treating certain congenital heart diseases; although used in the management of ARDS, it has no effect on outcome and the oxygenation benefit is normally lost within 48 hrs.[85] The AARC has published a clinical practice guideline on INO therapy. Excerpts from this guideline appear in Clinical Practice Guideline 53-3.[86]

Heliox

Heliox is a gas mixture of O_2 and helium. Typical concentration of a tank of heliox is 80%/20% or 70%/30% (helium/oxygen). Helium is less dense than air. Inhaling a less-dense gas can reduce the pressure needed to overcome airway resistance and results in decreased work of breathing. In patients with a high O_2 requirement, helium is less effective. Heliox has been used in conjunction with other therapies in the treatment of partial large airway obstruction and asthma where airway resistance is high. It may be used to deliver bronchodilators but due to its lower density is not as efficient as air or oxygen so a higher flow rate should be employed. Heliox may serve as a temporizing measure while steroids are administered to reduce airway swelling. When high O_2 concentrations are necessary, heliox is not likely to be effective as the amount of inspired helium is diminished. Signs of decreased work of breathing, decreased use of accessory muscles, improved aeration, and decreased respiratory rate after initiating heliox are indications of its effectiveness.

NEONATAL AND PEDIATRIC TRANSPORT

Treatment of a critically ill infant or child is usually provided at a tertiary care facility. Many of these facilities have established transport teams that go to the referring facility, initiate ICU-type support, and transport the patient back to the tertiary care center. The composition of transport teams varies from one institution to another; however, typical team members include some combination of registered nurse, RT, paramedic, nurse

53-3 Inhaled Nitric Oxide Therapy

AARC Clinical Practice Guideline (Excerpts)*

1. A trial of INO is recommended in newborns (>34 weeks' gestation, 14 days of age) with PaO_2 100 mm Hg on FiO_2 1.0 or an oxygenation index >25, or both. (Grade 1A)
2. It is recommended that INO therapy be instituted early in the disease course, which potentially reduces the length of mechanical ventilation, O_2 requirement, and stay within the ICU. (Grade 1A)
3. INO should not be used routinely in newborns with congenital diaphragmatic hernia. (Grade 1A)
4. INO therapy should not be used routinely in newborns with cardiac anomalies dependent on right-to-left shunts, congestive heart failure, and lethal congenital anomalies. (Grade 2C)
5. There are insufficient data to support the routine use of INO therapy in postoperative management of hypoxic term or near-term infants with congenital heart disease. (Grade 2C)
6. The recommended starting dose for INO is 20 ppm. (Grade 1A)
7. Response to a short trial (30-60 minutes) of INO should be judged by an improvement in PaO_2 or oxygenation index; if there is no response, INO should be discontinued. (Grade 1A)
8. For a newborn with parenchymal lung disease, optimal alveolar recruitment should be established before initiation of INO therapy. (Grade 1A)
9. For newborns with a response to INO therapy, the dose should be weaned to the lowest dose that maintains that response. (Grade 1A)
10. It is recommended that INO should not be discontinued until there is an appreciable clinical improvement, that the INO dose should be weaned to 1 ppm before an attempt is made to discontinue, and that FiO_2 should be increased before discontinuation of INO therapy. (Grade 1A)
11. INO delivery systems approved by the U.S. Food and Drug Administration should be used to ensure consistent and safe gas delivery during therapy. (Grade 1C)
12. During conventional mechanical ventilation, the INO gas injector module should be placed on the dry side of the humidifier. (Grade 2C)
13. During conventional ventilation, the sampling port should be placed in the inspiratory limb of the ventilator, downstream from the site of injection, no greater than 15 cm proximal to the patient connection/interface. (Grade 2C)
14. FiO_2 should be measured downstream from the injection of INO into the circuit. (Grade 2C)
15. The patient-ventilator system should be continuously monitored for changes in ventilation parameters, with adjustments to maintain desired settings during INO therapy. (Grade 2C)
16. The lowest effective doses of INO and O_2 should be used to avoid excessive exposure to nitric oxide, nitrogen dioxide (NO_2), and methemoglobinemia. (Grade 2C)
17. The INO delivery system should be properly purged before use to minimize inadvertent exposure to NO_2. (Grade 2C)
18. The high NO_2 alarm should be set at 2 ppm on the delivery system to prevent toxic gas exposure to the lungs. (Grade 2C)
19. Methemoglobin should be monitored approximately 8 hours and 24 hours after therapy initiation and daily thereafter. (Grade 2C)
20. The INO dose should be weaned or discontinued if methemoglobin increases to >5%. (Grade 2C)
21. It is suggested that continuous pulse oximetry and hemodynamic monitoring be used to assess patient response to INO therapy. (Grade 2C)
22. Scavenging of exhaled and unused gases during INO therapy is *not* necessary. (Grade 2C)

**For complete guideline, see DiBlasi RM, Myers TR, Hess DR: Evidence based clinical practice guideline: inhaled nitric oxide for neonates with acute hypoxic respiratory failure. Respir Care 55:1741, 2010.*

practitioner, and physician. Regardless of the composition of the team, there are some characteristics that all transport teams should have in common.[87] All members should have exquisite assessment and critical thinking skills. They should be technically adept and have good communication skills. Each team develops minimum criteria that a team member must possess. Many teams cross-train multiple disciplines to perform certain technical tasks. Establishing proficiency and maintaining proficiency with all skills is a must for team members.

The team essentially functions as an extension of the ICU. To do this, much of the same equipment used in the ICU is taken to the referring hospital. Establishing responsibility for assessing function and maintaining appropriate inventory is essential. Many centers use elaborate checklists to be certain not to be without necessary equipment, disposables, or medications. Teams generally prepare for the worst. Many times when the team arrives at the referring facility, the patient's condition is not the same as when the initial call for help was made. Being prepared for the worst helps in stabilizing the patient for transport. The American Academy of Pediatrics has guidelines for all ages and common conditions requiring transport to a tertiary facility. Box 53-12 lists the basic equipment and supplies needed to provide respiratory care during neonatal and pediatric transport.

Box 53-12 Equipment and Supplies Needed to Provide Respiratory Care During Neonatal and Pediatric Transport

EQUIPMENT
- Adequate supply of O_2 and compressed air
- Air-O_2 blender
- Mechanical ventilator with circuit
- Manual resuscitator capable of giving 100% O_2 with PEEP
- Noninvasive O_2 monitor (SpO_2 or $PtcO_2$)
- O_2 analyzer
- Airway pressure monitor (electronic or mechanical)
- Electrocardiograph monitor
- Portable suction apparatus
- Laryngoscope handle
- Laryngoscope blades (sizes newborn to adult)
- Extra laryngoscope bulbs and batteries
- Stethoscope

SUPPLIES
- Resuscitation masks (sizes 0, 1, 2, 3, 4)
- Feeding tubes (sizes 6F, 8F, and 10F)
- Disposable O_2 hood
- O_2 connecting tubing
- Disposable hand-held nebulizer with tubing (for bronchodilators)
- Cloth adhesive tape for taping endotracheal tubes
- Tincture of benzoin for taping endotracheal tubes
- Pulse oximeter probes (at least two, in case one fails)
- Endotracheal tubes (sizes 2.5-7)
- Stylet
- Forceps
- Suction apparatus

RULE OF THUMB

A high-risk transport team must be prepared to provide the same level of care and highly trained personnel as would be available in the ICUs they are transporting patients to and from.

SUMMARY CHECKLIST

- Neonatal and pediatric care is one of the most sophisticated specialty areas in the field of respiratory care. Competent practice in this area requires a firm understanding of the many anatomic and physiologic differences between infants, children, and adults.
- A critical component in the respiratory management of infants and children is thorough clinical assessment. Because of the significant anatomic and physiologic differences between adults and infants, many of the assessment techniques useful with adults do not apply to infants.
- General assessment of the infant begins before birth and involves the maternal history and the fetal and newborn status. As a child grows and develops, more of the assessment methods used with adults become applicable.
- Respiratory care plan development is based on accurate patient information, detailed knowledge of the disease process, and current treatment guidelines and recommendations.
- Respiratory care modalities provided to pediatric and neonatal patients enclude: O_2, aerosol and humidity, airway care, and mechanical ventilation.
- CPAP is commonly used to overcome atelectasis and oxygenation problems.
- Using high-flow nasal cannulas has become common practice; however, care must be taken to prevent the delivery of higher than expected levels of CPAP.
- Noninvasive ventilation has become an acceptable choice of ventilation.
- Improved design of nasal masks and nasal prongs should help prevent the development of pressure ulcers during CPAP and noninvasive ventilation.
- For mechanically ventilated patients, plateau pressure or PIP during pressure-targeted ventilation should not exceed 28 cm H_2O and delta P should not exceed 15 cm H_2O.
- V_T should be maintained between 4 ml/kg and 8 ml/kg.
- Compressible volume loss may account for a significant portion of the small V_T used for infants and small children.
- Infants and children can be effectively managed with conventional ventilation. The use of HFV has become increasingly controversial. Mechanically ventilated infants and children should be assessed daily for readiness for liberation from mechanical ventilation.
- Nitric oxide is now considered standard therapy for the management of term infants who present with PPHN and should be available in all level III neonatal ICUs.
- Surfactant replacement has become the standard of care for preterm (gestation <32 weeks) or low birth weight infants (<1300 g) and infants with known surfactant deficiency.
- Highly specialized transport teams are available to transport newborn and pediatric patients to tertiary care facilities.

References

1. Simon NV, et al: Prediction of fetal lung maturity by amniotic fluid fluorescence polarization, L:S ratio, and phosphatidyl glycerol. *Obstet Gynecol* 57:295–300, 1981.
2. Hallman M, Kulovich M, Kirkpatrick E, et al: Phosphatidyl-inositol and phosphatidylglycerol in amniotic fluid: Indices of lung maturity. *Am J Obstet Gynecol* 125:613, 1976.
3. American Association of Pediatrics: Guidelines for cardiopulmonary resuscitation and emergency cardiovascular care. *Pediatrics* 126:e1400, 2010.
4. Dubowitz LMS, Dubowitz D, Goldberg C: Clinical assessment of gestational age in the newborn infant. *J Pediatr* 77:110, 1970.
5. Shenoi A, Narang A, Bhakoo ON, et al: Clinical profile and management of symptomatic patent ductus arteriosus in premature newborns. *Indian Pediatr* 28:125, 1991.
6. Carlo WA, Martin RJ, Bruce EN, et al: Alae nasi activation (nasal flaring) decreases nasal resistance in preterm infants. *Pediatrics* 72:338, 1983.
7. Sundri F, Plavka R, Ancora G, et al: Prophylactic or early selective surfactant combined with nCPAP in very preterm infants. *Pediatrics* 125:e1402–e1409, 2010.
8. Dunn M, Kaempf J, de Klerk A, et al: Randomized trial comparing 3 approaches to the initial respiratory management of preterm neonates. *Pediatrics* 128:e1069–e1076, 2011.
9. Morley C, Davis P, Doyle L, et al: Nasal CPAP or intubation at birth for very preterm infants. *N Engl J Med* 358:700–708, 2008.

10. Courtney SE, Weber KR, Breakie LA, et al: Capillary blood gases in the neonate: a reassessment and review of the literature. *Am J Dis Child* 144:168, 1990.
11. Mrozek JD, Bendel-Stenzel EM, Meyers PA, et al: Randomized controlled trial of volume-targeted synchronized ventilation and conventional intermittent ventilation following initial exogenous surfactant therapy. *Pediatr Pulmonol* 29:11, 2000.
12. Cheema IU: Ahluwailia JS: Feasibility of tidal volume-guided ventilation in newborn infants: a randomized, crossover trial using the volume guaranteed modality. *Pediatrics* 107:1323, 2001.
13. American Association for Respiratory Care: Clinical practice guideline: infant/toddler pulmonary function tests. *Respir Care* 40:761, 1995.
14. American Association for Respiratory Care: Clinical practice guideline. Oxygen therapy in the acute care hospital. *Respir Care Clin North Am* 36:1410, 1991.
15. Walsh M: Oxygen therapy through nasal cannula to preterm infants: can practice be improved. *Pediatrics* 116:857, 2005.
16. Chow LC, Wright KW, Sola A: Can changes in clinical practice decrease the incidence of severe retinopathy of prematurity in very low birth weight infants? *Pediatrics* 111:339, 2003.
17. Minghua L, Chen H, Guo L: High or low oxygen saturation and severe retinopathy of prematurity: a meta-analysis. *Pediatrics* 125:e1483, 2010.
18. Perrotta C, Ortiz Z, Roque M: Chest physiotherapy for acute bronchiolitis in pediatric patients between 0 and 24 months old. *Cochrane Database Syst Rev* (1):CD004873, 2007.
19. Hess DR: The evidence for secretion clearance techniques. *Respir Care* 46:1276, 2001.
20. Mahlmeister MJ, Fink JB, Hoffman GL, et al: Positive expiratory pressure mask therapy: theoretical and practical considerations and a review of the literature. *Respir Care Clin N Am* 36:1218, 1991.
21. Emergency Care Research Institute: Heated wires can melt disposable breathing circuits. *Health Devices* 18:174, 1989.
22. Levy H, Simpson Q, Duval D: Hazards of humidifiers with heated wires. *Crit Care Med* 21:477, 1993.
23. Mellon M, Leflein B, Walton-Bowen C, et al: Comparable efficacy of administration with face mask or mouthpiece of nebulized budesonide inhalation suspension for infants and young children with persistent asthma. *Am J Respir Crit Care Med* 162:593, 2000.
24. Cole CH: Special problems in aerosol delivery: neonatal and pediatric considerations. *Respir Care* 45:646, 2000.
25. Veldman A, Trautschold T, Weib K, et al: Characteristics and outcome of unplanned extubation in ventilated preterm and term newborns on a neonatal intensive care unit. *Pediatr Anesth* 16:968, 2006.
26. McMillan DD, Rademaker AW, Buchan KA, et al: Benefits of orotracheal and nasotracheal intubation in neonates requiring ventilatory assistance. *Pediatrics* 77:39, 1986.
27. Black AE, Hatch DJ, Nauth-Misir N: Complications of tracheal intubation in neonates, infants and children: a review of 4 years' experience in a children's hospital. *Br J Anaesth* 65:461, 1990.
28. Roopchand R, Roopnarinesingh S, Ramsewak S: Instability of the tracheal tube in neonates: a postmortem study. *Anaesthesia* 44:107, 1989.
29. Brown MS: Prevention of accidental extubation in newborns. *Am J Dis Child* 142:1240, 1988.
30. Prendiville A, Thomson A, Silverman M: Effect of tracheobronchial suction on respiratory resistance in intubated preterm babies. *Arch Dis Child* 61: 1178, 1986.
31. Gardner D, Shirland L: Neonatal evidence-based guideline for suctioning the intubated neonate and infant. *Neonatal Netw* 28:281–302, 2009.
32. Shah AR, Kurth CD, Gwiazdowski B, et al: Fluctuations in cerebral oxygenation and blood volume during endotracheal suctioning in premature infants. *J Pediatr* 120:769, 1992.
33. Kalyn A, Blatz S, Feuerstake S, et al: Closed suctioning of intubated neonates maintains better physiologic stability: a randomized trial. *J Perinatol* 23:218–222, 2003.
34. El Masry A, Williams PF, Chipman DW, et al: The impact of closed endotracheal suctioning systems on mechanical ventilator performance. *Respir Care* 50:345–353, 2005.
35. American Association for Respiratory Care: Clinical practice guideline: application of continuous positive airway pressure to neonates via nasal prongs, nasopharyngeal tube, nasal mask: 2004 revision and update. *Respir Care* 49:1100, 2004.
36. Juretschke R, Spoula R: High flow nasal cannula in the neonatal population. *Neonatal Intensive Care* 17:20, 2004.
37. Sreenan C, Lemke RP, Hudson-Mason A, et al: High-flow nasal cannulae in the management of apnea of prematurity: a comparison with conventional nasal continuous positive airway pressure. *Pediatrics* 107:1081, 2001.
38. Locke RG, Wolfson MR, Shaffer TH, et al: Inadvertent administration of positive end-distending pressure during nasal cannula flow. *Pediatrics* 91:135, 1993.
39. Yoder B, Stoddard R, Li M, et al: Heated, humidified high-flow nasal cannula versus nasal cpap for respiratory support in neonates. *Pediatrics* 131:e1482–e1490, 2013.
40. Waugh JB, Granger WM: An evaluation of 2 new devices for high-flow gas therapy. *Respir Care* 49:902, 2004.
41. Sreenan C, Lemke RP, Hudson-Mason A, et al: High-flow nasal cannulae in the management of apnea of prematurity: a comparison with nasal continuous positive airway pressure. *Pediatrics* 107:1081–1083, 2001.
42. Holleman-Duray D, Kaupie D, Weiss M: Heated humidified high-flow nasal cannula: use and a neonatal early extubation protocol. *J Perinatol* 27:772–775, 2007.
43. Marchese AD, Chipman D, de le Oliva P, et al: Adult ICU ventilators to provide neonatal ventilation: a lung simulator study. *Intensive Care Med* 35:631, 2009.
44. Donn SM, Sinha SK: Invasive and noninvasive neonatal mechanical ventilation. *Respir Care* 48:426, 2003.
45. Cheifetz IM: Invasive and noninvasive pediatric mechanical ventilation. *Respir Care* 48:442, 2003.
46. Cannon ML, Cornell J, Tripp-Hamel DS, et al: Tidal volumes for ventilated infants should be determined with a pneumotachometer placed at the endotracheal tube. *Am J Respir Crit Care Med* 162:2109, 2000.
47. Mehta NM, Arnold JH: Mechanical ventilation in children with acute respiratory failure. *Curr Opin Crit Care* 10:7, 2004.
48. Greenough A, Milner AD, Dimitriou G: Synchronized mechanical ventilation for respiratory support in newborn infants. *Cochrane Database Syst Rev* (3):CD000456, 2005.
49. Kapasi M, Fujino Y, Kirmse M, et al: Effort and work of breathing in neonates during assisted patient-triggered ventilation. *Pediatr Crit Care Med* 2:9, 2001.
50. American Association for Respiratory Care: Clinical practice guideline: neonatal time-triggered, pressure-limited, time-cycled mechanical ventilation. *Respir Care* 39:808, 1994.
51. BiBlasi R: Neonatal noninvasive ventilation techniques: do we really need to intubate? *Respir Care* 56:1273–1294, 2011.
52. Bhandari V: Noninvasive respiratory support in the preterm infant. *Clin Perinatol* 39:497–511, 2012.
53. Menesis J, Bhabdari V, Alves J, et al: Noninvasive ventilation for respiratory distress syndrome : a randomized controlled trial. *Pediatrics* 127:300–307, 2011.
54. Bhandari V, Finer NN, Ehrenkranz RA, et al: Synchronized nasal intermittent positive-pressure ventilation and neonatal outcomes. *Pediatrics* 124: 517, 2009.
55. Chang H, Claure N, D'Ugard C, et al: Effects of synchronization during nasal ventilation in clinically stable preterm infants. *Pediatr Res* 69:84–89, 2011.
56. Hess DR: The evidence for non-invasive positive-pressure ventilation in the care of patients in acute respiratory failure: a systematic review of the literature. *Respir Care* 49:810, 2004.
57. Hess DR: Noninvasive ventilation in neuromuscular disease: equipment and application. *Respir Care* 51:896, 2006.
58. Panitch HB: Respiratory issues in the management of children with neuromuscular disease. *Respir Care* 51:885, 2006.
59. Padman R, Lawless ST, Kettrick RG: Noninvasive ventilation via bilevel positive airway support in pediatric practice. *Crit Care Med* 26:169, 1998.

60. Nilsestuen JO, Hargett KD: Using airway graphics to identify patient-ventilator asynchrony. *Respir Care* 50:202, 2005.
61. Wilson BG: Using airway graphics to optimize mechanical ventilation in neonates with respiratory distress syndrome. *Neonatal Netw* 16:71, 1997.
62. AARC Clinical Practice Guideline: Patient-ventilator system checks. *Respir Care* 37:882, 1992.
63. Randolph AG, Pediatric Acute Lung Injury and Sepsis Investigators Network: Effects of mechanical ventilator weaning protocols on respiratory outcomes in infants and children. *JAMA* 288:2561, 2002.
64. Newth C, Venkataraman S, Wilson D, et al: Weaning and extubation readiness in pediatric patients. *Pediatr Crit Care Med* 10:1–11, 2009.
65. Venkataraman S, Khan N, Brown A: Validation of predictors of extubation success and failure in mechanically ventilated infants and children. *Crit Care Med* 28:2991–2996, 2000.
66. Ferguson L, Walsh B, Munhall D, et al: A spontaneous breathing trial with pressure support overestimates readiness for extubation in children. *Pediatr Crit Care Med* 12:e330–e335, 2011.
67. Vento G, Tortorolo L, Zecca E, et al: Spontaneous minute ventilation is a predictor of extubation failure in extremely low birth weight infants. *J Matern Fetal Med* 15:147–154, 2004.
68. Kamlin C, Davis P, Argus B, et al: A trial of spontaneous breathing to determine the readiness to extubate in very low birth weight infants: a prospective evaluation. *Arch Dis Child Fetal Neonatal Ed* 93:F305–F306, 2008.
69. Szymankiewicz M, Vidyasagar D, Gadzinowski J: Predictors of successful extubation of preterm low birth weight infants with respiratory distress syndrome. *Pediatr Crit Care Med* 6:44–49, 2005.
70. Henderson-Smart DJ, Bhuta T, Cools F: Elective high frequency oscillatory ventilation versus conventional ventilation for acute pulmonary dysfunction in preterm infants. *Cochrane Database Syst Rev* (3):CD000104, 2005.
71. Bhuta T, Henderson-Smart DJ: Elective high frequency jet ventilation versus conventional ventilation for respiratory distress syndrome in preterm infants. *Cochrane Database Syst Rev* (3):CD000328, 2005.
72. Arnold JH, Anas NG, Luckett P: High-frequency oscillatory ventilation in pediatric respiratory failure: a multicenter experience. *Crit Care Med* 28:3913, 2000.
73. Thome UH, Carlo WA, Pohlandt F: Ventilation strategies and outcome in randomized trials of high frequency ventilation. *Arch Dis Fetal Neonatal Ed* 90:F466, 2005.
74. Courtney SE, Durand DJ, Asselin JM: High-frequency oscillatory ventilation versus conventional ventilation for very-low-birthweight infants. *N Engl J Med* 347:643, 2002.
75. Grenier B, Thompson J: High-frequency oscillatory ventilation in pediatric patients. *Respir Care Clin North Am* 2:545, 1996.
76. Bollen CW, Uiterwaal CS, van Vught AJ: Cumulative metaanalysis of high-frequency versus conventional ventilation in premature neonates. *Am J Respir Crit Care Med* 168:1150, 2003.
77. Ferguson N, Cook D, Guyatt G, et al: High frequency oscillation in early acute respiratory distress syndrome. *N Engl J Med* 368:795–805, 2013.
78. Gupta P, Green JW, Tang X, et al: Comparison of high-frequency oscillatory ventilation and conventional mechaical ventilation in pediatric respiratory failure. *JAMA pediatr* 168:243–249, 2014.
79. Ichinose F, Roberts JD, Zapol WM: Inhaled nitric oxide: a selective pulmonary vasodilator: current uses and therapeutic potential. *Circulation* 109: 3106, 2004.
80. Finer NN, Barrington KJ: Nitric oxide for respiratory failure in infants born at term or near term. *Cochrane Database Syst Rev* (3):2009.
81. Christou H, VanMarter LJ, Wessel DL, et al: Inhaled nitric oxide reduces the need for extracorporeal membrane oxygenation in infants with persistent pulmonary hypertension of the newborn. *Crit Care Med* 28:3722, 2000.
82. Guthrie SO, Walsh WF, Clarke RH, et al: Initial dosing of inhaled nitric oxide in infants with hypoxic respiratory failure. *J Perinatol* 24:387, 2004.
83. Sokol GM, Fineberg NS, Wright LL, et al: Changes in arterial oxygen tension when weaning neonates from inhaled nitric oxide. *Pediatr Pulmonol* 32:14, 2001.
84. American Academy of Pediatrics Committee on Fetus and Newborn: Use of inhaled nitric oxide. *Pediatrics* 2:344, 2000.
85. Sebald M, Friedlich P, Burns C, et al: Risk of the need for extracorporeal membrane oxygenation in neonates with congenital diaphragmatic hernia treated with inhaled nitric oxide. *J Perinatol* 24:143, 2004.
86. DiBlasi RM, Myers TR, Hess DR: Evidence based clinical practice guideline: inhaled nitric oxide for neonates with acute hypoxic respiratory failure. *Respir Care* 55:1741, 2010.
87. Waren J, From R, Orr RA, et al: American College of Critical Care Medicine: guidelines for the inter- and intrahospital transport of critically ill patients. *Crit Care Med* 32:256, 2004.

SECTION VII

PATIENT EDUCATION AND LONG-TERM CARE

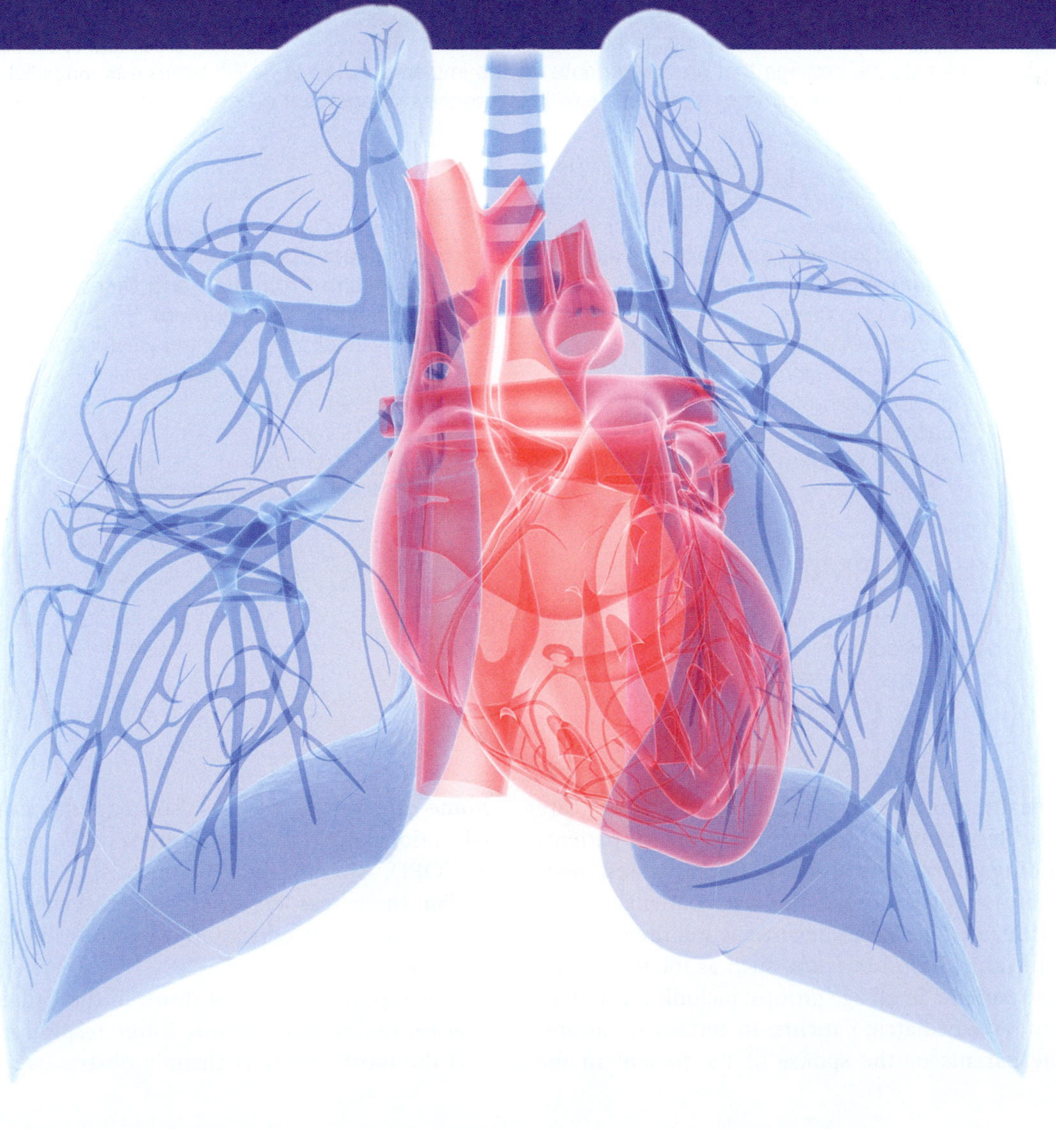

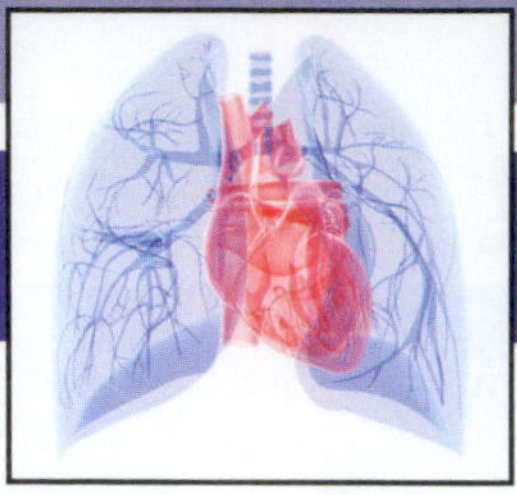

CHAPTER 54

Patient Education and Health Promotion

DONNA D. GARDNER

CHAPTER OBJECTIVES

After reading this chapter you will be able to:

- Write learning objectives in the cognitive, affective, and psychomotor domains.
- Compare and contrast how adults and children learn.
- Describe the methods that are used to evaluate patient education.
- Explain the importance of health education.
- Identify the settings that are appropriate for the implementation of health promotion activities.
- Describe the respiratory therapist's role in a disease management program.

CHAPTER OUTLINE

Patient Education
- Cultural Diversity and Health Literacy
- Performance Objectives
- Learning Domains
- *Cognitive Domain*
- *Psychomotor Domain*
- *Affective Domain*
- Teaching Tips
- Teaching Children As Compared With Teaching Adults
- Evaluation of Patient Education

Health Education

Health Promotion and Disease Prevention

Disease Management
- Implications for the Respiratory Therapist
- *Health Care Institutions*
- *Work Site*
- *Home*
- *Community*
- *Educational Institutions*

KEY TERMS

affective domain
cognitive domain
disease management
health education
health promotion
psychomotor domain
health literacy

Effective health education is invaluable to the health care of society. Respiratory therapists (RTs) educate patients by providing information about disease processes, medications, and treatment procedures. They teach patients how to perform diagnostic tests like basic spirometry, and they educate patients about health promotion issues such as tobacco cessation. RTs educate patients in all age groups, including geriatric, adult, adolescent, and pediatric patients. In certain situations, RTs educate the parents or the spouse of the patient in the home-care setting. RTs are also frequently called on to provide educational programs to patients with pulmonary diseases such as COPD, asthma and cystic fibrosis.

For these reasons, this chapter reviews important issues related to patient education, disease management, and health promotion.

The top three causes of death in the United States are heart disease, cancer, and chronic lower respiratory system disease, and the most deadly is chronic obstructive lung disease (i.e., bronchitis and emphysema).[1] Public education about risk factors is the key to the prevention of these diseases and probably has the greatest potential for making an impact on health care in this country. Therefore, the emphasis in health care should be on health promotion and disease prevention. RTs will need to play a greater role in health promotion and prevention in the future.

PATIENT EDUCATION

If we think of patient care as customer service—which it indeed is—then we cannot ignore education as a crucial component of that service. Whether we buy a car or a television set, we expect the salesperson to educate us about the essential aspects of our purchase. We also expect this information to be provided in writing. Likewise, education is an essential component of patient care. For patients to assume or resume control of their health, they must be educated. Because they rely on the health care practitioner to provide this education, every respiratory care education program should include instruction regarding patient education.

Cultural Diversity and Health Literacy

Culture refers to patterns of beliefs and behaviors shared by members of a population. Patients use their culture in the way they view health and the need for health care interventions. Successful respiratory therapy patient teaching must include patient cultural values that are appreciated and respected to better understand the patient's behaviors.

Some cultures do not recognize illness when symptoms are not present, such as with a chronic illness. Therefore, the ongoing need for care is a challenge when teaching patients whose symptoms have subsided. This occurs with asthma disease management. When asthma is under control the patient may not have symptoms and therefore the patient may stop taking his or her medication. There is risk associated with patients misunderstanding therapy or medications. This is not related to patients' ability to read; it is about patients' culture and their ability to comprehend information well enough to follow the instructions to take a medication, know when to reorder a medication, and how to complete a therapy necessary for lung disease.

Health literacy is the degree to which individuals have the capacity to obtain, process, and understand basic health information and services needed to make appropriate health decisions.[2] Health care information such as medication instruction is complex and often requires critical thinking skills. Health literacy encompasses educational, social, and cultural factors that influence an individual.

Respiratory therapists must understand where the patient is coming from in regards to the patient's beliefs, values, and cultural norms to influence the education provided. Low health literacy affects patient safety and the ability for the patient to participate in care, and results in poor health outcomes.

Respiratory patients will not be able to be self-directed and navigate the health care system if they do not have the ability to follow the educational programs and instructions provided. Reading and comprehension may not always go hand in hand. Patients often will not voluntarily admit that they do not understand to avoid embarrassment. Therefore, to determine whether or not a patient understands, it is important to look for the following clues that indicate reading or writing is a concern and to be sensitive to prevent any feelings of shame.

- Patient repeatedly is noncompliant
- Patient uses the excuse of being too busy, tired, or sick to maintain attention when given instruction
- Claims that the patient did not feel like reading the information, gave the information to a family member, or lost or forgot their glasses
- Insistence on taking the information home to read
- Demonstrates nervousness and stress, confused about the materials
- Talks about something else and not on topic
- Returns documents that are not complete or illegible

Respiratory therapy patient educators must assess readiness to learn from the patient's point of view to ensure patient compliance. Patients must believe the change in behavior is possible and beneficial before they will make a behavior change.

Performance Objectives

Initially it is helpful for the RT to develop learning objectives that are appropriate for the specific patient education topic to be addressed. These learning objectives will help to clarify the teaching strategies that are needed for patient education sessions. Objectives should be stated in measurable terms so that the RT and the patient can recognize when the objective has been accomplished. Clear objectives describe what is to be accomplished and how evaluation will occur.

The format for writing an objective is as follows:

1. Begin with the phrase, "At the end of the lesson, the patient will.…"
2. Write the action verb (e.g., "list," "describe," "demonstrate").
3. Write a condition, if needed (e.g., with or without the use of notes).
4. Write a standard, if needed (e.g., how fast, how accurate).

For example: At the end of the session, the patient will be given a metered-dose inhaler and spacer and be able to demonstrate the correct technique for using it without error.

Action verb: "demonstrate" (from the psychomotor domain; the relevant domains are discussed later in this chapter)

Condition: "given a metered-dose inhaler and spacer"

Standard: "without error "

Learning Domains

Learning occurs in three domains: **cognitive**, **psychomotor,** and **affective**. Some learning sessions will involve only one domain, whereas others may involve all three. The cognitive domain is very important, because it will address the knowledge that a patient needs regarding his or her illness and how to manage it. The psychomotor domain addresses the skills that the patient will need to acquire to perform specific treatment modalities (e.g., the use of metered-dose inhalers). The affective domain involves teaching patients about the necessary attitudes and motivations for successfully living with their diseases.

MINI CLINI

Developing Learning Objectives for the Use of an Albuterol Metered-Dose Inhaler

PROBLEM: Your 31-year-old patient is newly diagnosed with asthma, and she is being discharged tomorrow. She requires instruction regarding how to properly use her controller medication, Advair diskus, and the reliever medication albuterol metered-dose inhaler. Develop learning objectives for her, and address each learning domain.

Solution: Use a variety of learning objectives, including the following:

Cognitive domain: Describe the action of albuterol on the bronchial smooth muscle; recognize when it is necessary to seek medical attention.

Affective domain: Agree that it is important not to skip a dose; verbalize willingness to use the Advair diskus daily; feel satisfaction by controlling the disease.

Psychomotor domain: Demonstrate the ability to assemble the metered-dose inhaler and spacer; inhale slowly and deeply with an inspiratory hold.

Cognitive Domain

The cognitive domain is probably the easiest to translate into learning objectives because it involves the facts and concepts that the RT wants the patient to know and apply by the end of the education session. Objectives for the cognitive domain might include the following:

1. List the indications for oxygen therapy.
2. Discuss the importance of using the prescribed liter flow.
3. Explain the relationship between oxygen and combustion.

Any factual information that you expect the patient to understand and apply falls under the cognitive domain. Action verbs for the cognitive domain are included in Table 54-1.[3]

Psychomotor Domain

Repetition and active involvement are important when teaching a psychomotor skill. RTs who teach new skills to patients need to provide plenty of opportunity for the patient to practice the activity. Simple demonstration of the skill to the patient is not enough. To confirm performance in the psychomotor domain, have your patients provide a return demonstration. Be sure to provide help and encouragement as needed. Be patient; not everyone develops skills at the same rate.

Examples of action verbs for the psychomotor domain are included in Table 54-2.[3]

TABLE 54-1

Verbs for the Cognitive Domain

Purpose	Example Verbs
Knowledge	Cite, define, read, identify, list, label, name, outline, recognize, select, state
Comprehension	Convert, describe, defend, explain, illustrate, interpret, give examples of, predict, paraphrase, summarize, translate
Application	Apply, compute, construct, demonstrate, change, calculate, use, estimate, modify, present, prepare, solve, proceed, relate, utilize
Analysis	Analyze, associate, compare, contrast, determine, diagram, differentiate, discriminate, distinguish, outline, illustrate, separate
Synthesis	Categorize, combine, compile, compose, create, design, develop, devise, integrate, modify, organize, plan, propose, rearrange, reorganize, revise, rewrite, translate, write
Evaluation	Appraise, assess, compare, conclude, contrast, critique, discriminate, make a decision, support, evaluate, judge, weigh

Modified from French D, Olrech N, Hale C, et al: Blended learning: an ongoing process for Internet integration, Victoria, Canada, 2003, Trafford Publishing.

TABLE 54-2

Verbs for the Psychomotor Domain

Purpose	Example Verbs
Perception: prepares and recognizes sensory cues to want to respond	Detect, distinguish, differentiate, identify, isolate, relate, recognize, observe, perceive, see, watch
Ready to act and respond	Begin, explain, move, react, show, state, establish a body position, place, posture, assume a stance, sit, stand, position
Guided response: imitate and practice; rough sequencing of events	Copy, duplicate, imitate, manipulate, operate, try, practice, dismantle
Efficiency: smooth sequencing of events	Assemble, calibrate, construct, display, fasten, fix, grind, manipulate, measure, mix, sketch, demonstrate, execute, increase speed, improve, make, show dexterity, pace, produce
Perform alone: modifies, responds as needed	Act habitually, advance confidently, control, excel, guide, manage, master, organize, perform quickly and more accurately
Creates a new or original model	Adapt, alter, rearrange, reorganize, revise

Modified from French D, Olrech N, Hale C, et al: Blended learning: an ongoing process for Internet integration, Victoria, Canada, 2003, Trafford Publishing.

RULE OF THUMB

People learn by doing. Get the learner involved.

Affective Domain

The patient's attitudes and motivations influence his or her ability to learn. It is important to remember that, with patient education, timing is everything. Patients who have recently been given a poor prognosis or who are in pain are not in an optimal position to learn. Maslow suggested a hierarchy of needs, and he identified physiologic needs as the most basic of human needs, followed by safety, love, esteem, and self-actualization.[4] Lower-level needs must first be satisfied before moving on to higher-level needs. For example, if a patient is dyspneic or in pain, he or she will probably not be receptive to learning the steps that are involved in cleaning a small-volume nebulizer. It is important for RTs to assess a patient's readiness to learn by talking with the patient and his or her family and by listening to the patient's concerns. It is important to develop a relationship of trust and to be empathetic with the patient.

The RT should begin with easy-to-master facts and skills. After the patient conquers these, motivation should increase, and the patient will have a feeling of accomplishment. Motivation is also enhanced by presenting material clearly with the use of a variety of teaching methods and by relating the facts and skills to practical applications. Getting patients to see how these skills will benefit them is the key to motivation. Communicating to the patient that there is something that he or she can do to maintain or improve his or her health and sense of well-being is important.

Objectives in the affective domain—using the oxygen therapy example mentioned earlier—might include the following:

1. Express genuine concern for yourself by using your oxygen therapy correctly.
2. Commit to learn by being an active participant in the program.

Affective domain action verbs are included in Table 54-3.[3]

Teaching Tips

Following is a list of time-honored suggestions for improving patient education:

- Address the patient's immediate concerns first.
- Create an optimal learning environment. Teach in a quiet and relaxed setting.
- Have patients use as many of their senses as possible during their learning session. Whenever possible, include hearing, seeing, smelling, speaking, touching, and doing.
- Keep sessions short. If the material is complex, break it down into brief segments.
- Repeat, repeat, repeat!
- Provide many opportunities for the patient to practice psychomotor skills.
- Be prepared.
- Be organized. People learn more quickly when they are presented with information that is well organized.
- Demonstrate enthusiasm for what you are doing. The learner can always sense your level of motivation.
- Evaluate in a nonthreatening manner, and provide helpful feedback. Use evaluation as a learning tool.

TABLE 54-3
Verbs for the Affective Domain

Purpose	Example Verbs
Receive: becoming aware of	Accept, acknowledge, alert, choose, give, attend, notice, perceive, tolerate, select
Respond: interested in or doing something about something	Agree, assist with, aid, answer, assist, comply, conform, communicate, consent, label, obey, cooperate, follow, read, report, visit, volunteer, study
Value: concerned about, developing an attitude	Adopt, assume, behave, choose, demonstrate, commit, desire, initiate, join, exhibit, express, prefer, seek, share
Organize: arranging systematically, confirming	Adapt, adjust, arrange, classify, conceptualize, group, rank, validate, verify, strengthen, substantiate, corroborate, confirm
Characterize: internalizing a set of values, championing	Demonstrate a change in lifestyle, discriminate, defend, influence, invite, listen, preach, qualify, question, serve, act upon, advocate, devote, expose, justify, support

Modified from French D, Olrech N, Hale C, et al: Blended learning: an ongoing process for Internet integration, Victoria, Canada, 2003, Trafford Publishing.

Teaching Children as Compared With Teaching Adults

Teaching children is often very different than teaching adults. Children are more motivated by external factors (e.g., prizes) as compared with adults, who tend to have internal motivating factors. This suggests that adults will learn quicker if they can easily see the intrinsic value of knowing more about their illness. Alternatively, children may need a more obvious reward system in place before learning can take place. Adults, however, are more independent, and they do not like being dependent on others. This suggests that adults should be more involved in setting program goals and that they will readily learn skills that make them more independent. Other important issues related to differences between children and adult learners are listed in Box 54-1, and allocated time for teaching is given by age in Box 54-2.[5]

Evaluation of Patient Education

The critical question that remains when all of the patient education sessions are complete is, "Has the patient learned?" Evaluation is the process that answers that question. The method used to evaluate learning is determined by the measurable learning objectives (i.e., cognitive, affective, or psychomotor). Cognitive objectives are often evaluated with the use of a written examination. Objectives in the affective and psychomotor domains are evaluated with the use of performance checklists.

Informal evaluation should occur during the educational process. The RT can ask simple questions along the way to identify whether the patient has comprehended the information. If the patient provides an answer that is not correct, the RT should view this as an opportunity to repeat previous

Box 54-1 Learning Differences Between Children and Adults

CHILD
- Motivated by external factors like grades
- Directed by others
- Learning is a big part of his or her life
- Trusts teacher
- Has limited experience
- Learns for the future
- Learns quickly
- Tends to learn in accordance with his or her developmental stage
- Has no problem with a slow pace of learning
- Subject oriented

ADULT
- Motivated internally
- Is self-directed
- Learning is only one part of his or her life
- Questions the teacher
- Has rich life experiences
- Learns for the present
- May learn more slowly
- Varies with regard to learning ability
- Dislikes a slow pace of learning
- Problem oriented

Box 54-2 Attention Spans for Different Ages

- Toddlers: about 2 to 3 minutes
- School-aged children: about 10 to 15 minutes
- Adolescents and adults: about 20 to 30 minutes

discussions or to present the material with a new approach. The RT must never convey disappointment or frustration when patients are having trouble learning new material.

RULE OF THUMB

Evaluation results reflect the quality of instruction as much as the degree of learning.

HEALTH EDUCATION

Health education may have been the earliest form of organized health promotion in the United States. Health programs in schools is a result of Lemuel Shattuck's report in 1850 to the Sanitary Commission of Massachusetts, which described the value of schools helping to contain communicable diseases. However, it was not until 1875 that health education became widespread. During that year, the Women's Christian Temperance Union lobbied for alcohol education in the schools. As a result of these efforts, 38 states passed legislation to require this education, which later turned into tobacco, alcohol, and drug education. From that time, health education has been enhanced and expanded in schools. There are public health agencies at the local, state, national, and international levels that provide health education and care for those who would otherwise have none.

MINI CLINI

Metered-Dose Inhaler Instruction for a Pediatric Patient

PROBLEM: How would you change the approach to the metered-dose inhaler situation described in the previous Mini Clini if your patient was a 7-year-old boy with asthma?

Solution: Although the learning objectives may remain the same, the methods may be different. You may compare the slow, deep inspiration to getting ready to blow out the candles on a birthday cake. You may use swimming under water as an image to encourage breath holding. Use simple diagrams to show how the medication will act on the patient's lungs. If he likes sports, tell him about athletes who compete well despite having asthma (you may also use this illustration to stress the importance of controlling asthma). An abundance of resource materials are available for children with asthma; make use of them. Many local, state, and national lung associations (www.ala.org) offer such learning aids as age-appropriate books, coloring books, and puppets to make the learning process more fun for children.

Health education is a process of planned learning that is designed to enable individuals to make informed decisions and to take responsible actions regarding their health. The primary goal of health education is behavior change, and it is designed to promote, maintain, and improve both individual and community health. Health education covers the continuum between health and disease and between prevention and treatment.

Health promotion helps people change their lifestyles in a variety of settings, from the home or school to the workplace or the health care agency or institution. To be effective, health education must be combined with strategies for health promotion; the two are strongly linked. The American Association for Respiratory Care has created a statement for health promotion and disease prevention (Box 54-3).[7]

Although individuals must ultimately assume responsibility for their own health, promoting healthy behaviors through education is an important part of being an RT. In this capacity, the RT should serve as a role model for the public. Unless health care professionals model healthy behaviors, successful health outcomes cannot be expected from the public. To this end, the American Association for Respiratory Care has created a role-model statement to encourage RTs to set a positive example for the public (Box 54-4).[7]

Providing a good example is not enough to ensure successful health education programming. For the desired outcomes to be achieved, certain conditions must first be met. The components are remarkably similar to patient education requirements. The essential components of effective health education are as follows:

1. Program participants must be actively engaged in the learning process.

54-1 AARC Clinical Practice Guideline (Excerpts)*

Providing Patient and Caregiver Training

American Association for Respiratory Care Clinical Practice Guideline (Excerpts)* updated June of 2010. www.rcjournal.com/cpgs/pdf/06.10.0765.pdf.

INDICATIONS

Patients who need to increase knowledge and understanding of health status and therapy; improve skills needed for safe and effective health care; and develop a positive attitude, strong motivation, and increased compliance. Patients need to know the answers to "Ask Me 3": What is my main problem? What do I need to do? Why is it important for me to do this?

CONTRAINDICATIONS

None.

COMPLICATIONS

Omission of essential steps concerning care, presentation of inconsistent information, or failure to validate the learning process can lead to unfavorable results. Lack of cultural competence, and information appropriate in the language other than English will result in less than desirable outcomes. Lack of trust.

LIMITATIONS

- For the patient: Lack of motivation; impairment (physical, mental, or emotional); inability to understand instruction; illiteracy; language barriers; religious and/or cultural beliefs that are at odds with the material presented. Lack of health literacy, despite educational completed and conflicts of religious and/or cultural practices.
- For the RT: Lack of a positive attitude or flexibility; limited knowledge of skill being taught; inadequate assessment of patient's readiness to learn; cultural or religious practices that may affect learning; inability to personalize the material; insufficient time; inadequate communication skills, and inadequate knowledge of cultural or religious practice.
- For the system: Hospital stay too brief; lack of interdisciplinary communication and/or cooperation; inconsistent information presented; lack of an interpreter.
- Other factors: Lack of support system for the patient; reimbursement issues; interruptions, distractions, or noise; inadequate lighting, heat, or space; poorly chosen resources including inappropriate reading level and vocabulary.

ASSESSMENT OF NEED

Determine the knowledge gap between what the patient knows and what he or she needs to know. Apply this to cognitive, psychomotor, and affective domains.

ASSESSMENT OF OUTCOME

Evaluate knowledge gained, skills mastered, patient should return demonstration without assistance, reassess patient outlook, attitude and life style changes.

RESOURCES

Access trained interpreters, ensure the written materials are readable at a fifth or sixth grade level, materials should be available in a variety of formats (audio and visual), use demonstration models, reevaluate the skills.

MONITORING

The monitoring of the training processes should include awareness of the patient's verbal and nonverbal responses, including eye contact, listening skills, and participation in discussion.

**For the complete guideline, see the American Association for Respiratory Care: AARC Clinical Practice Guidelines. Providing patient and caregiver training 2010. Respir Care 55(6):765–769, 2010.*

2. Activities must incorporate the values and beliefs of the learner. Familial, cultural, societal, and economic factors must be considered.
3. The role of the health educator is to facilitate behavioral change. Thus, the learning process should be approached together by both the learner and the educator.
4. The process of predisposing an individual toward improved health as well as enabling and reinforcing health attitudes requires effort, which will only reap results over time.
5. The health care educator must be willing to listen nonjudgmentally to the concerns of the learners. Empathy and understanding are necessary to foster a trusting relationship.
6. The level of the learners' self-esteem and self-concept may either enhance or inhibit their ability to make decisions about their own health. The health care educator should be willing to provide emotional support as necessary.
7. The health care educator's personal characteristics have a direct impact on the outcome of the educational program. Generally, successful outcomes occur as a result of a confident and professional approach.

For RTs to assist patients, caregivers, or the public with regard to the development of healthier lifestyles, greater emphasis must be placed on health promotion and disease prevention strategies.

HEALTH PROMOTION AND DISEASE PREVENTION

In 2012, the United States spent $2.8 trillion, or $8,915 per person, on health care.[9] The top three causes of death in the United States are heart disease, cancer, and chronic obstructive pulmonary disease (COPD). All three lead to chronic

54-2 AARC Clinical Practice Guideline (Excerpts)*

Training of the Health Care Professional (HCP) for the Role of Patient and Caregiver Educator

American Association for Respiratory Care Clinical Practice Guideline (Excerpts)*

INDICATIONS

- HCPs who must educate patients and caregivers about knowledge, skills, and motivation necessary to effectively participate in health care.
- Evidence that HCPs lack the knowledge about educational principles and practices needed to:
  - Assess educational needs
  - Prepare educational objectives tailored to individuals or groups
  - Accomplish learning objectives
  - Prepare educational materials
  - Supervise practice of skills
  - Give feedback and assess outcomes
  - Modify educational efforts according to individual or group response

CONTRAINDICATIONS

None.

COMPLICATIONS

Inadequate training of the HCP may cause harm to the patient or inhibit the patient's ability to participate in the management of his or her own health.

LIMITATIONS

- Of the HCP: Lack of educational preparation; unreceptive or inept; lack of interdisciplinary cooperation; inability to modify learning objectives based on age, culture, or religion; inability to communicate effectively
- Of the system: Inadequate time, space, or financial resources; insufficient faculty for training program; inconsistent information provided to the HCP
- Of the patient or caregiver: Negative attitude; lack of basic education; presence of a language barrier or perception of cultural conflict

ASSESSMENT OF NEED

HCPs who provide education should be periodically assessed for adequate knowledge and skills by observation in a patient education setting and by a specialist.

ASSESSMENT OF OUTCOME

Evaluate verbally and in writing; observe HCP in teaching setting; evaluate whether goals set concerning knowledge, skills, compliance, and attitude have been met; evaluate long-term through institutional quality improvement indicators.

MONITORING

HCP training should include evidence of classes and in-service training; availability of written and audiovisual resources; and evaluation of training effectiveness.

For complete guideline, see Training the health care professional for the role of patient and caregiver educator. Respir Care 41(7):654–657, 1996; or www.rcjournal.com/cpgs/thcpcpg.html.

conditions and might be preventable by avoiding tobacco use, poor diet, and physical inactivity.

Current medical practice is designed to respond to the acute problems of patients; its focus is on diagnosing and treating the presenting symptoms rather than focusing on the prevention of disease by identifying risk factors and providing methods for behavioral changes. Only focusing on the acute or episodic health problems creates a discrepancy when using this model of care to care for chronic conditions that may be prevented or managed. Preventative health care is very different from chronic care.

With this in mind, a quote from Rufus Howe is appropriate: "What a rare privilege it is to be in a position to improve the lives of others."

A patient with asthma goes to the emergency department and is treated effectively and efficiently. The patient received good quality care, and, in many people's minds, the patient was "fixed." However, asthma is manageable to the point that the patient should not have to be in the emergency department. There are excellent national guidelines (www.NAEPP.org) that outline how to manage asthma, and there are medications that control asthma and keep the patient out of this situation. Usually the reason for the emergency visit is that the patient's asthma is not in control; this may occur because the patient is not using inhaled steroids, because he or she has a poor understanding of the disease and how to manage it, because the national guidelines are not being used, or because of a combination of all of these issues. Either way, this chronic disease can be self-managed by a patient with the proper multidisciplinary education and follow up.

However, the public health model attempts to reduce disease in the nation as a whole through mass education campaigns. Examples include education about the hazards of drinking and driving, tobacco use (both smokeless and smoking) education, and food labeling to indicate fat and cholesterol content. This is known as *health promotion and disease prevention.*[10] By participating in public education programs, RTs have the potential to affect the health of individuals and of the population as a whole.

Recent efforts such as Healthy People 2020 have attempted to place the focus on the health of the population rather than on that of the individual.[11] The four broad goals of the Healthy

Box 54-3 American Association for Respiratory Care Health Promotion and Disease Prevention Statement

HEALTH PROMOTION AND DISEASE PREVENTION

- The AARC acknowledges that respiratory therapists in both the civilian and uniformed/military services are integral members of the health care team, in hospitals, home health care settings, pulmonary laboratories, rehabilitation programs and all other environments (including ICUs and critical care transport) where respiratory care is practiced.
- The AARC recognizes that education and training of the respiratory therapist is the best method by which to instill the ability to improve the patient's quality and longevity of life, and that such information should be included in their formal education and training in CoARC accredited programs.
- The AARC recognizes the respiratory therapist's responsibility to participate in pulmonary disease teaching, smoking cessation programs, pulmonary function studies for the public, air pollution alerts, allergy warnings, and sulfite warnings in restaurants, as well as research in those and other areas where efforts could promote improved health and disease prevention. Furthermore, the respiratory therapist is in a unique position to provide leadership in determining health promotion and disease prevention activities for students, faculty, practitioners, patients, and the general public in both civilian and uniformed service environments.
- The AARC recognizes the need to 1) provide and promote consumer education related to the prevention and control of pulmonary disease; 2) establish a strong working relationship with other health agencies, educational institutions, Federal and state government, businesses, military and other community organizations; and 3) monitor such activities. Furthermore, the AARC supports efforts to develop personal and professional wellness models and action plans that will inspire and encourage all respiratory therapists to cooperate on health promotion and cardiorespiratory disease prevention.

Effective 1985.
Revised 2000.
Revised 2005.
From the American Association for Respiratory Care: Position statement (website): www.aarc.org/resources/position_statements/rms.html.

Box 54-4 American Association for Respiratory Care Role Model Statement

- As health care professionals engaged in the performance of cardiopulmonary care, RTs must strive to maintain the highest personal and professional standards.
- In addition to upholding the code of ethics, the RT shall serve as a leader and advocate of public health.
- The RT shall participate in activities leading to awareness of the causes and prevention of pulmonary disease and the problems associated with the cardiopulmonary system. The RT shall support the development and promotion of pulmonary disease awareness programs, to include smoking cessation programs, pulmonary function screenings, air pollution monitoring, allergy warnings, and other public education programs.
- The RT shall support research to improve health and prevent disease.
- The RT shall provide leadership in determining health promotion and disease prevention activities for students, faculty, practitioners, patients, and the general public.
- The RT shall serve as a physical example of cardiopulmonary health by abstaining from tobacco use and shall make a special personal effort to eliminate smoking and the use of other tobacco products from the home and work environment.
- The RT shall strive to be a model for all members of the health care team by demonstrating responsibility and cooperating with other health care professionals to meet the health needs of the public.

Effective 3/90.
Revised 3/00.
From the American Association for Respiratory Care: Position statement (website): www.aarc.org/resources/position_statements/rms.html.

People 2020 program are as follows: (1) to promote quality of life, healthy development, and healthy behaviors across all life stages; (2) to achieve health equity, eliminate disparities, and improve the health of all groups; (3) to attain high-quality, longer lives free of preventable disease, disability, injury, and premature death; and (4) to create social and physical environments that promote good heatlh for all.[11] These goals encompass the essential elements of health promotion and disease prevention, which are the prevention of premature death, disease, and disability as well as the improvement of the quality of life.

The recognition that allied health professionals such as RTs play vital roles in these activities prompted professional organizations to develop policy statements about health promotion and disease prevention. The American Association for Respiratory Care policy statement appears in Box 54-5.[6]

RTs can take an active role in the development of educational materials to assist both the public and other health professionals with regard to health promotion activities. Many medical manufacturers have also developed asthma education kits of various types that include peak flow meters, spacers, and educational materials. These kits are generally developed with input from the medical community and in particular from RTs. An example of an asthma program is given in Table 54-4.[12] Respiratory care educational programs need to be diligent when incorporating health promotion and disease prevention activities into all learning domains as part of their curricula.

Another specific area of health promotion that receives much attention in both hospital and public health settings is nicotine intervention. Hospitalized patients are more motivated to try to quit smoking for two reasons: the illness that resulted in the patient being in the hospital may have been made worse due to tobacco use, and hospitals have smoke-free environments. Therefore, RTs should use this opportunity to promote nicotine treatments.

Nicotine intervention is a progressive, comprehensive program that incorporates a series of steps from risk identification to maintenance support. Smoking is the leading cause of preventable disease and death in the US. January 11, 2014

Box 54-5 Health Promotion and Disease Prevention

- The AARC submits this paper to identify and illustrate the involvement of the RT in the promotion of health and prevention of disease and supports these activities. The AARC realizes that RTs are integral members of the health care team, in hospitals, home health care settings, pulmonary laboratories, rehabilitation programs, and all other environments where respiratory care is practiced.
- The AARC recognizes that education and training of the RT is the best method by which to instill the ability to improve the patient's quality and longevity of life, and that such information should be included in their formal education and training.
- The AARC recognizes the RT responsibility to participate in pulmonary disease teaching, smoking cessation programs, pulmonary function studies for the public, air pollution alerts, allergy warnings, and sulfite warnings in restaurants, as well as research in those and other areas where efforts could promote improved health and disease prevention. Furthermore, the RT is in a unique position to provide leadership in determining health promotion and disease prevention activities for students, faculty, practitioners, patients, and the general public.
- The AARC recognizes the need to provide and promote consumer education related to the prevention and control of pulmonary disease and to establish a strong working relationship with other health agencies, educational institutions, federal and state government, businesses and other community organizations and to monitor such. Furthermore, the AARC supports efforts to develop personal and professional wellness models and action plans that will inspire and encourage all RT to cooperate on health promotion and disease prevention.

Effective 7/85.
Revised 3/00.
From the American Association for Respiratory Care: Position statement (website): www.aarc.org/resources/position_statements/hpdp.html.

marked the fiftieth anniversary of the first Surgeon General Report on smoking and health that linked smoking with lung cancer and heart disease and the thirty-second Surgeon General Report,"The Health Consequences of Smoking— 50 years of progress: A report of the Surgeon General," which presents new data on the consequences of smoking.[13] The Affordable Care Act's (ACA) Public Health and Prevention Fund expanded access to smoking cessation services through most insurance companies to include Medicaid. The ACA supports community-based programs and public education campaigns promoting prevention and helping people to quit; 1.6 million smokers have made an attempt to quit.[13] Safe and effective tobacco treatment enhances the success for quitting. Nicotine replacement therapies (NRT) such as nicotine gum, lozenges, or patches are available over the counter. NRT combined with behavioral therapy is more effective for tobacco cessation. Varenicline tartrate (Chantix) and bupropirion (Zyban) do not contain nicotine. They are both available by prescription only.[14] Chantix interacts at the sites in the brain that are influenced by nicotine.

National, state, and local agencies such as the American Cancer Society, the American Lung Association, and the American Heart Association offer educational materials and behavioral counseling. The educational materials that these agencies offer are available via mail, telephone, and the Internet. In 2004, the U.S. Department of Health and Human Services established a nationwide toll-free number (800-QUIT-NOW [800-784-8669]) to serve as an access point for smokers who are seeking assistance with quitting. Components of the Office of Surgeon General's tobacco cessation program are included in Tables 54-5 and 54-6.[15]

DISEASE MANAGEMENT

The most recent data show that more than 145 million people—which is approximately half of all Americans—live with chronic disease.[16] Half of those with chronic illness have more than one chronic condition or comorbidity. The prevalence of chronic disease has increased due to tobacco use, physical inactivity, poor nutrition choices, obesity, and the aging of the population during the same time the cost of care has markedly risen. These chronic diseases are extremely expensive and lead to unnecessary admissions and readmissions (recidivism). Chronic care models have been used since the 1990s. A chronic care model is patient centered; it encourages multidisciplinary focus on self-management and continuous quality control. Wagner originally presented the chronic care model that is illustrated in Figure 54-1.[17]

Wagner explains the model as follows: "Patients and families who struggle with chronic illness require planned, regular interactions with their caregivers, with a focus on function and prevention of exacerbations. This interaction includes systematic assessments, attention to treatment guidelines, and behaviorally sophisticated support for the patient's role as a self manager. These interactions must be linked through time by clinically relevant information and continuing follow-up."[17]

As with **disease management**, which is a method of applying the best health care practices to a population with a chronic illness one person at a time,[10] the goals of this type of program include improving the health of the person, improving patient satisfaction, reducing mortality, improving quality of life, and eliminating unnecessary medical treatment to reduce the cost of health care.[10] There is no one definition of disease management. However, the Care Continuum Alliance defines disease management as a coordinated system of interventions for people who have conditions that require significant self-care.[18] Disease management is measured by its impact on costs, clinical outcomes, and quality of life. The programs have similar components, including a coordinated comprehensive interdisciplinary care team with a process for measuring improvement. Health insurance companies, pharmaceutical companies, and the federal government all pay for disease management programs.[10] Most programs have the following attributes:

- The provision of interdisciplinary comprehensive care (i.e., health promotion, prevention, and acute care involving

TABLE 54-4
Components of an Asthma Disease Management Program

Component 1: Assessment and monitoring	Assessment: • Detailed patient history • Thorough physical examination • Spirometry to document the reversibility of airflow obstruction Monitoring: Periodic assessment and ongoing monitoring of asthma to determine if goals are being met • Minimal or no chronic and troublesome symptoms, day or night • Normal or near-normal pulmonary function • No limitations on activities • Minimal or no recurrent exacerbations of asthma • Optimal medications with minimal or no adverse side effects • Satisfaction with asthma care
Component 2: Control of the factors that contribute to asthma	Identify the allergens and irritants • House dust mites, cockroach feces, molds, and animal dander • Tobacco smoke, emissions from wood-burning stoves, strong odors and sprays such as perfume and hairspray • Nitrogen dioxide and sulfur dioxide • Rhinitis and sinusitis • Gastroesophageal reflux disease • Viral respiratory infections • Aspirin • Sulfites Reduce exposure to the allergens and irritants, and provide medications or immunotherapy
Component 3: Pharmacologic therapy: managing asthma for the long term	Classify the asthma severity into one of the four levels on the basis of the severity of recurrent symptoms and lung function Prescribe medications for the level of asthma • All patients with asthma need a quick-relief medication (i.e., short-acting β2-agonists) • Those with persistent asthma need daily long-term control medications to achieve control (e.g., an inhaled corticosteroid) • Start treatment in a stepwise approach (i.e., begin at a higher level to achieve rapid control; when control is achieved and sustained, cautiously step down treatment)

Component 4: Patient education for a partnership in asthma care	Patient education begins at the time of diagnosis.
	• Provide basic facts about asthma
	• Identify the roles of the medications
	• Skills: correct use of the medication delivery devices, the peak flow meter, and the symptom diary
	• Discuss environmental control measures
	• Discuss when and how to take rescue actions
	Education techniques
	• Basic facts about asthma
	  • Describe the contrast between asthmatic and normal airways
	  • Describe what happens to the airways during an asthma attack
	• Describe the roles of the medications
	  • How the medications work
	  • Long-term control: medications that prevent symptoms, often by reducing inflammation
	  • Quick relief: short-acting bronchodilators relax muscles around the airways
	Stress the importance of long-term control medications, and emphasize that the patient should not expect quick relief
	• Skills
	  • Inhaler use (patient demonstration)
	  • Spacer and holding chamber use
	  • Symptom monitoring, peak flow monitoring, and recognizing early signs of deterioration
	• Environmental control measures
	  • Identifying and avoiding environmental precipitants or exposures
	  • When and how to take rescue actions
	• Responding to changes in asthma severity (i.e., daily self-management plan and action plan)

TABLE 54-5
The "5 As" Model for Treating Tobacco Use and Dependence as a Chronic Disease

Ask about tobacco use	Identify and document the tobacco use status of every patient at every visit • Expand the vital signs to include tobacco use
Advise to quit	Strongly urge all tobacco users to quit Advice should be clear, strong, and personalized
Assess every tobacco user's willingness to make a quit attempt	Ask every tobacco user if he or she is willing to make a quit attempt: "Are you willing to give quitting a try?" • If the patient is willing, provide assistance • If the patient is unwilling, provide a motivational intervention • If the patient is a member of a special population (e.g., pregnant, adolescent, minority), consider providing him or her with additional information
Assist by providing counseling and medication	• Set a quit date that is ideally within 2 weeks • Tell family and friends about quitting • Anticipate challenges, including nicotine withdrawal symptoms • Remove tobacco products from the environment Recommend the use of approved medications, except when they are contraindicated or if the patient is a member of a specific population (e.g., pregnant women, smokeless tobacco users, adolescents) • Explain how the medications work to increase success with quitting and to reduce withdrawal symptoms The medications approved for this purposed by the U.S. Food and Drug Administration include the following: • Bupropion SR • Nicotine gum • Nicotine inhaler • Nicotine lozenge • Nicotine nasal spray • Nicotine patch • Varenicline Provide practical counseling (i.e., problem solving, skills training): • Abstinence: striving for total abstinence is essential (i.e., "not one puff after the quit date") • Anticipate triggers and challenges: determine how the patient will successfully overcome these (i.e., avoid the triggers) • Alcohol should be avoided because it is associated with relapse (however, reducing alcohol intake could precipitate withdrawal in alcohol-dependent persons) • Other smokers in the home: quitting is more difficult when there is another smoker in the home; patients should encourage all to quit with them or to not smoke in their presence Provide intratreatment social support • Provide a supportive clinical environment while encouraging the patient in his or her quit attempt (i.e., "My office staff and I are here to assist you") Help the patient to obtain extra social support during treatment • Help the patient to develop social support in his or her environment outside of the treatment by asking the patient's spouse or partner, friends, and coworkers to support the quit attempt Provide supplementary materials, including information about quit lines • Sources: Federal agencies, nonprofit agencies, national quit line network (1-800-QUIT-NOW), and local/state/tribal health departments and quit lines • Type: culturally, racially, educationally, and age appropriate for the patient • Location: readily available Recommend counseling (there are three types): Practical counseling (i.e., problem solving, skills training) • Recognize danger situations • Develop coping skills • Provide basic information Supportive treatment counseling • Encourage the patient to quit • Communicate caring and concern • Encourage the patient to talk about quitting
Arrange for follow-up contacts, either in person or via the telephone	Timing: Follow-up contact should begin soon after the quit date, preferably during the first week; a second follow up is recommended within the first month, and follow up should be scheduled as indicated • Actions to take during the follow-up contacts: for all patients, identify problems that have been encountered, and anticipate challenges Assess the medication use and any associated problems: • Remind the patient of the support offered by quit lines • Address tobacco use at the next clinical visit • When patients have been abstinent, congratulate them on their success

TABLE 54-6

Components of a Tobacco Education Program for Those Who Are Unwilling to Quit Enhancing Motivation to Quit Tobacco: The "5 Rs"

Relevance	Encourage the patient to indicate why quitting is personally relevant and to be as specific as possible. Motivational information has the greatest impact if it is relevant to a patient's disease status or risk, to a family or social situation (e.g., having children in the home), or to health concerns, age, gender, and other important patient characteristics (e.g., prior quitting experience, personal barriers to cessation).
Risk	Ask the patient to identify potential negative consequences of tobacco use and suggest those that seem to be the most relevant to the patient. Emphasize that smoking low-tar or low-nicotine cigarettes or using other forms of tobacco (e.g., smokeless tobacco, cigars, pipes) will not eliminate these risks. Examples of risks include the following: • Acute risks: shortness of breath, exacerbation of asthma, harm to a pregnancy, impotence, infertility • Long-term risks: heart attack, stroke, lung and other cancers, chronic obstructive pulmonary disease, disability, need for extended care • Environmental risks: increased risk of lung cancer and heart disease in spouse, increased rates of smoking among children of tobacco users, sudden infant death syndrome, respiratory infections in the children of smokers
Rewards	Ask the patient to identify the potential benefits of stopping tobacco use: • Improved health • Food will taste better • Save money • Feel better • Home, car, clothing, and breath will smell better • Can stop worrying about quitting • Set an example for children • Have healthier babies and children • Reduce wrinkling and aging of skin
Roadblocks	Ask the patient to identify barriers to quitting: • Withdrawal symptoms • Fear of failure • Weight gain • Lack of support • Depression • Enjoyment of tobacco
Repetition	Repeat the motivational intervention information every time that an unmotivated patient is seen.

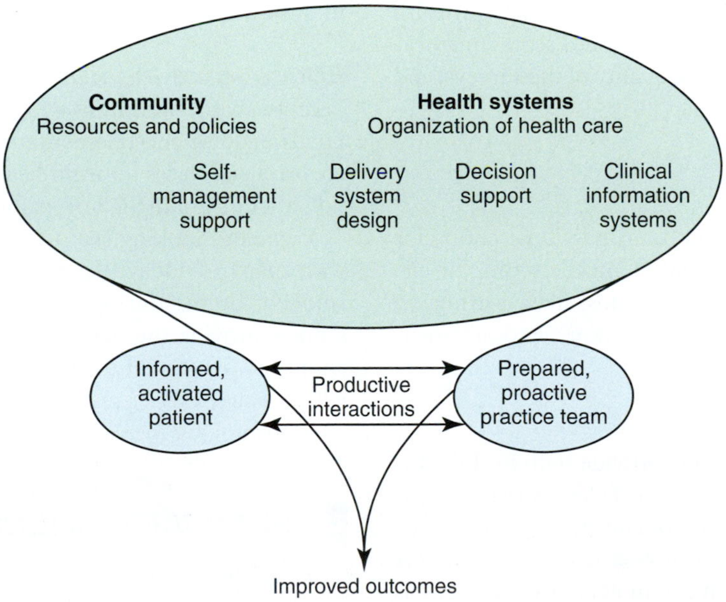

FIGURE 54-1 Illustration of a chronic care model that is focused on productive interactions and improved patient outcomes. (Modified from Wagner E: System changes and interventions: delivery system design. Improving chronic illness care, Orlando, Fl, 2001, Institute for Healthcare Improvement National Forum.)

interdisciplinary or multidisciplinary teams—physician, RT, nurse, PT, OT, pharmacist, and other health team members)

- A population-identification process (for a specific disease or condition)
- The use of evidence-based guidelines, protocols, and pathways
- Collaborative and coordinated components of care
- Active patient self-management and education (e.g., empowerment, behavior modification)
- Quality improvement methods to include outcomes measurement and evaluation
- The use of information technology to create a routine reporting and feedback loop

If you were interested in creating a disease management program, you would want to make sure to include these components. There are many disease management programs offered to patients with chronic diseases such as COPD, asthma, amyotrophic lateral sclerosis, and cystic fibrosis. RTs are ideal to create, coordinate, and participate as members of a disease management program. The patients whom RTs care for have chronic diseases, and these individuals need to be taught about the health risks associated with the disease, the prophylactic measures used to maintain quality health, and disease-specific respiratory therapy. For example, in a disease management program for a patient with COPD, RTs would provide one-on-one counseling for tobacco cessation education (if the patient continued to use these products); discuss pulmonary rehabilitation that included exercise as well as strength and endurance training; and recognize and manage an acute situation and appropriate medication management. The RT would work with the patient to establish personal goals, including changing the person's behaviors and reducing the risks associated with the chronic disease. Outcomes would be measured to include health care utilization or hospital admissions, dyspnea scores, medication use, missed work or school days, quality of life surveys, and number of ER visits.

Implications for the Respiratory Therapist

Because the RT can practice as both an individual counselor and a public health advocate, depending on the setting or circumstances, it is useful to examine the most likely settings in which the RT's health promotion and disease prevention knowledge can be put to good use.

Health Care Institutions

Health care institutions in which RTs provide both health education and promotion include inpatient facilities (e.g., hospitals, skilled nursing facilities) and ambulatory care centers (e.g., physicians' offices, clinics, health insurance organizations). RTs may practice in outpatient or long-term acute care settings as well as in corporate wellness programs for staff and patients that are aimed at improving cardiopulmonary health through disease management education that includes nutrition, medication management, and exercise (e.g., pulmonary rehabilitation, asthma management education programs).

Work Site

Healthier workers are absent from work less often; they are also more satisfied with their jobs and more productive. This all translates into a more cost-effective workplace. RTs may find themselves involved in work-site wellness by participating in the following: (1) performing pulmonary function or blood pressure screenings; (2) developing and implementing stress management or nicotine intervention programs; and (3) consulting on policies related to smoking and occupational or environmental exposure to foreign dusts (e.g., silica, asbestos) or noxious fumes (e.g., smog).

Home

Home health care continues to be a rapidly growing segment of the health care industry. It has been proved repeatedly to be more cost-effective than hospital care. RTs can perform a wide variety of services in the patient's home, including oxygen therapy and mechanical ventilation on either a temporary or long-term basis. Generally the focus is on prevention (i.e., preventing further decline). Patient education is of primary importance in the home so that the patient may become as self-reliant as possible (see Chapters 55 and 56).

Community

Most of the health promotion activities described earlier pertain to the individual. At the community level, the focus is on the group. Community health promotion activities provided by the RT may include the following: pulmonary function screening at health fairs, smoking cessation programs, family asthma management education programs, and COPD (i.e., better breathing) support groups. RTs, who are certified in basic cardiac life-support instruction, may also volunteer to perform certification in this practice for various groups.

Educational Institutions

Because many unhealthy behaviors begin during early childhood or adolescence, elementary, middle, and secondary schools are excellent places to begin health education activities. Education about smoking is one example.

Cigarette smoking is a primary risk factor that is associated with many of today's leading causes of death. Because most smoking begins during late childhood or early adolescence, schools provide the best setting in which to educate children about the dangers of tobacco. RTs are trained to provide these educational experiences. It is never too early to begin sending the antismoking message.

SUMMARY CHECKLIST

- Patient education and general approaches to health promotion are key issues in health care today.
- Incorporating health literacy and cultural beliefs into patient education programs affects patient compliance.
- Educators should use learning objectives to direct teaching strategies toward individuals or large groups of patients.

- Learning objectives call for the use of an action verb to define the performance that is expected of the patient at the end of instruction.
- Learning occurs in three domains: cognitive (knowledge), psychomotor (skills), and affective (attitudes).
- Patients tend to learn by doing. Passive participation usually does not cause a change in behavior.
- Evaluate the cognitive domain objectives with written tests. Evaluate psychomotor and affective domain objectives with a skills checklist.
- The clinician should evaluate his or her teaching in an effort to improve.
- The RT can have an impact on several areas of health education and health promotion, including tobacco cessation programs, asthma education programs, pulmonary rehabilitation and community health screenings.
- RTs can be key players in disease management programs because of their understanding of the manifestations of the chronic cardiopulmonary diseases and their abilities to teach patients self-management with the use of the patient education tools discussed in this chapter.

References

1. National Vital Statistics Report, Vol 61, No 6, October 10, 201. In Hoyert DL, Xu J, editors: *Deaths: preliminary data for 2011. National vital statistics reports; vol 61 no 8*, Hyattsville, MD, 2012, National Center for Health Statistics.
2. Institute of Medicine: *Health literacy: a prescription to end confusion*, Bethesda, 2004, National Academies Press.
3. French D, Olrech N, Hale C, et al: *Blended learning: an ongoing process for Internet integration*, Victoria, Canada, 2003, Trafford Publishing.
4. Maslow AH: A theory of human motivation. *Psychol Rev* 50:370–385, 1943.
5. The American Academy of Allergy, Asthma & Immunology: Pediatric asthma: promoting best practices; patient education. Retrieved March 14, 2007, From: <http://www.aaaai.org/members/resources/initiatives/pediatricasthmaguidelines/default.stm>.
6. American Association for Respiratory Care: Position statement: Health promotion and disease prevention. Retrieved on March 14, 2007, From: <http://www.aarc.org/resources/position_statements/hpdp.html>.
7. American Association for Respiratory Care: *Position statement: AARC role model statement*, Dallas, March 2000, American Association for Respiratory Care.
8. Martin AB, Hartman M, Whittle L, et al: National Health Spending in 2012: Rate of health Spending Growth Remained Low for the Fourth consecutive Year. *Health Aff* 33(1):67–77, 2014. doi: 10.1377/hlthaff.2013.1254.
9. Howe R: *The disease manager's handbook*, Boston, 2005, Jones and Bartlett.
10. U.S. Department of Health and Human Services: *Healthy People 2010: understanding and improving health*, ed 2, Washington, DC, November 2000, U.S. Government Printing Office. Retrieved from: <http://www.healthypeople.gov/document/pdf/uih/2010uih.pdf>.
11. Healthy People 2020. US Department of Health and Human Services. Last updated September 15, 2014. Retrieved from: <http://www.healthypeople.gov/2020/about/default.aspx>.
12. U.S. Department of Health and Human Services: *Making a difference in the management of asthma: a guide for respiratory therapists*, Bethesda, May 2003, National Institutes of Health, NIH publication No. 02-1964, May 2003.
13. US Department of Health and Human Services: *The health consequences of smoking: 50 years of progress: a report of the Surgeon General*, Atlanta, GA, 2014, US Department of Health and Human Services, Centers for Disease Control and Prevention, National Center for Chronic Disease Prevention and Health Promotion, Office on Smoking and Health. Printed with corrections, January 2014.
14. National Institute on Drug Abuse: *Research report: tobacco addiction*, Bethesda, 2006, National Institutes of Health, NIH publication No. 06-4342.
15. Fiore MC, Jaén CR, Baker TB, et al: *Treating tobacco use and dependence: 2008 update. Quick reference guide for clinicians*, Rockville, MD, 2009, U.S. Department of Health and Human Services. Public Health Service. Retrieved from: <http://www.ahrq.gov/clinic/tobacco/tobaqrg.htm#table4>.
16. Centers for Disease Control and Prevention: Public health and aging: trends in aging—United States and worldwide. *MMWR* 52(06):101–106, 2003.
17. Wagner E: *System changes and interventions: delivery system design*, Improving Chronic Illness Care, Orlando, FL, 2001, IHI National Forum.
18. Care Continuum Alliance (CCA) Definition of Disease Management. Available at: <http://www.carecontinuum.org/dm_definition.asp>.

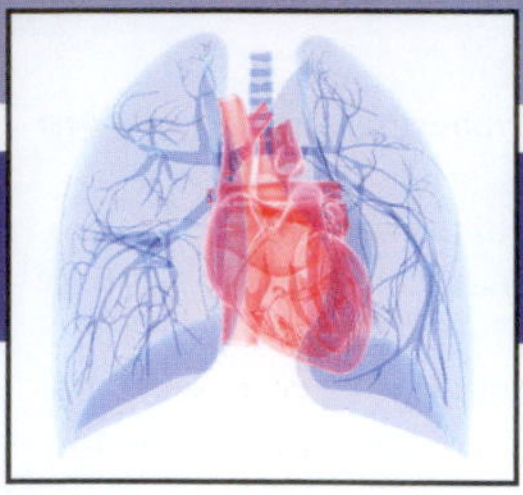

CHAPTER 55

Cardiopulmonary Rehabilitation

KENNETH A. WYKA

CHAPTER OBJECTIVES

After reading this chapter you will be able to:

- State the definition and general goals of pulmonary rehabilitation programs.
- Explain the rationale for exercise conditioning and psychosocial support of patients with chronic pulmonary disease.
- Describe how to evaluate and select patients for pulmonary rehabilitation.
- Describe pulmonary rehabilitation program design including format and content.
- List the educational content to be addressed in a pulmonary rehabilitation program.
- Describe the implementation of a pulmonary rehabilitation program, including staffing, facilities, scheduling, class size, equipment, costs, and reimbursement.
- Discuss the outcome measures that can be used to evaluate pulmonary rehabilitation programs.
- Identify the potential hazards associated with pulmonary rehabilitation.
- Compare the focus of pulmonary rehabilitation to that of cardiac rehabilitation.

CHAPTER OUTLINE

Definitions and Goals
Historical Perspective
Scientific Basis
Physical Reconditioning
Psychosocial Support
Structure of a Pulmonary Rehabilitation Program
Program Goals and Objectives
Patient Evaluation and Selection
Patient Evaluation
Patient Selection
Program Design
Format
Content
Physical Reconditioning
Educational Component
Psychosocial and Behavioral Components
Program Implementation
Staffing
Facilities
Scheduling
Class Size
Equipment
Cost, Fees, and Reimbursement
Program Results
Potential Hazards
Cardiac Rehabilitation
Conclusion

KEY TERMS

6- or 12-minute walk
aerobic exercises
cardiopulmonary exercise evaluation (CPX)
comprehensive outpatient rehabilitative facilities (CORFs)
Karvonen's formula
onset of blood lactate accumulation (OBLA)
Patient Protection and Affordable Care Act (PPACA)
progressive resistance
psychosocial support needs
pulmonary rehabilitation
reconditioning
target heart rate
ventilatory threshold

Steady improvements in acute care have resulted in improved patient survival and increasing numbers of individuals with chronic disorders. These chronic disorders are associated with a wide spectrum of physiologic, psychologic, and social disabilities. Foremost among these disorders is chronic obstructive pulmonary disease (COPD), which is now the third leading cause of death in the United States.[1]

Although differences in diagnoses can have an impact on treatment outcomes and survival, patients with chronic pulmonary disorders have much in common. All of these patients have difficulty coping with the physiologic limitations of their diseases and these physiologic limitations result in many psychosocial problems. The end result often is an unsatisfactory quality of life. The high incidence of repeated hospitalizations and the progressive disability of these patients require well-organized programs of rehabilitative care. With the passage in 2010 of the **Patient Protection and Affordable Care Act (PPACA)**, the reduction of early hospital readmissions for various chronic diseases, including COPD, is a major concern and focus of health care today. This chapter provides foundational knowledge regarding the goals, methods, and issues involved in providing planned programs of rehabilitation for individuals with chronic pulmonary disorders.

DEFINITIONS AND GOALS

The Council on Rehabilitation defines rehabilitation as "the restoration of the individual to the fullest medical, mental, emotional, social, and vocational potential of which he or she is capable."[2] The overall goal is to maximize functional ability and to minimize the impact the disability has on the individual, the family, and the community. **Pulmonary rehabilitation** is the "art of medical practice wherein an individually tailored, multidisciplinary program is formulated, which through accurate diagnosis, therapy, emotional support and education stabilizes or reverses both the physio- and psychopathology of pulmonary diseases and attempts to return the patient to the highest possible functional capacity allowed by his or her pulmonary handicap and overall life situation."[3]

The general goals of pulmonary rehabilitation are to control and alleviate symptoms, restore functional capabilities as much as possible, and improve quality of life.[4] Pulmonary rehabilitation does not reverse or stop progression of the disease, but it can improve a patient's overall quality of life.

HISTORICAL PERSPECTIVE

Pulmonary rehabilitation is not a new concept. In 1952, Barach and colleagues recommended reconditioning programs for patients with chronic lung disease to help improve their ability to walk without dyspnea.[5] Decades passed before clinicians paid any attention to this concept. Instead of having their patients participate in reconditioning programs, most physicians simply prescribed oxygen (O_2) therapy and bed rest. The result was a vicious cycle of skeletal muscle deterioration, progressive weakness and fatigue, and increasing levels of dyspnea including at rest. Patients became homebound, then room-bound and eventually bed-bound. Improved avenues of therapy and rehabilitation were needed.

In 1962, Pierce and associates published results confirming Barach's insight into the value of reconditioning. They observed that patients with COPD who participated in physical reconditioning exhibited lower pulse rates, respiratory rates, minute volumes, and carbon dioxide (CO_2) production during exercise. However, they also found that these benefits occurred without significant changes in pulmonary function.[6] Soon thereafter, Paez and associates showed that reconditioning could improve both the efficiency of motion and O_2 consumption in patients with COPD.[7] Subsequently, Christie showed that the benefits of reconditioning could be achieved on an outpatient basis with minimal supervision.[8] Since Christie's work in 1968, other investigators have continued to research the benefits of pulmonary rehabilitation.

The available evidence at the present time consistently indicates that pulmonary rehabilitation benefits patients with chronic obstructive and restrictive pulmonary diseases.[9-12] When combined with smoking cessation, optimization of blood gas results (arterial pO_2, pCO_2, and pH), and proper medication use, pulmonary rehabilitation offers the best treatment option for patients with symptomatic pulmonary disease. Programs for pulmonary rehabilitation must be founded on the sound application of current knowledge in the clinical and social sciences. In fall 2006, the American College of Chest Physicians (ACCP) and the American Association of Cardiovascular and Pulmonary Rehabilitation (AACVPR) released their evidence-based guidelines relating to pulmonary rehabilitation aimed at improving the way pulmonary rehabilitation programs are designed, implemented, and evaluated through patient outcomes.[13]

SCIENTIFIC BASIS

Rehabilitation must focus on the patient as a whole and not solely on the underlying disease. For this reason, effective pulmonary rehabilitation programs combine knowledge from both the clinical and the social sciences. Knowledge from the clinical sciences can help quantify the degree of physiologic impairment and establish outcome expectations for reconditioning. Application of the social sciences is helpful in determining the psychological, social, and vocational impact of the disability on the patient and family and in establishing ways to improve the patient's quality of life.

Physical Reconditioning

At rest, an individual maintains homeostasis by balancing external, internal, and cellular respiration. Physical activity, such as **aerobic exercises**, increases energy demands. To maintain homeostasis during exercise, the cardiorespiratory system must keep pace. Figure 55-1 shows how the body responds to exercise. Ventilation and circulation increase to supply tissues and cells with additional O_2 and to eliminate the higher levels of CO_2 produced by metabolism.

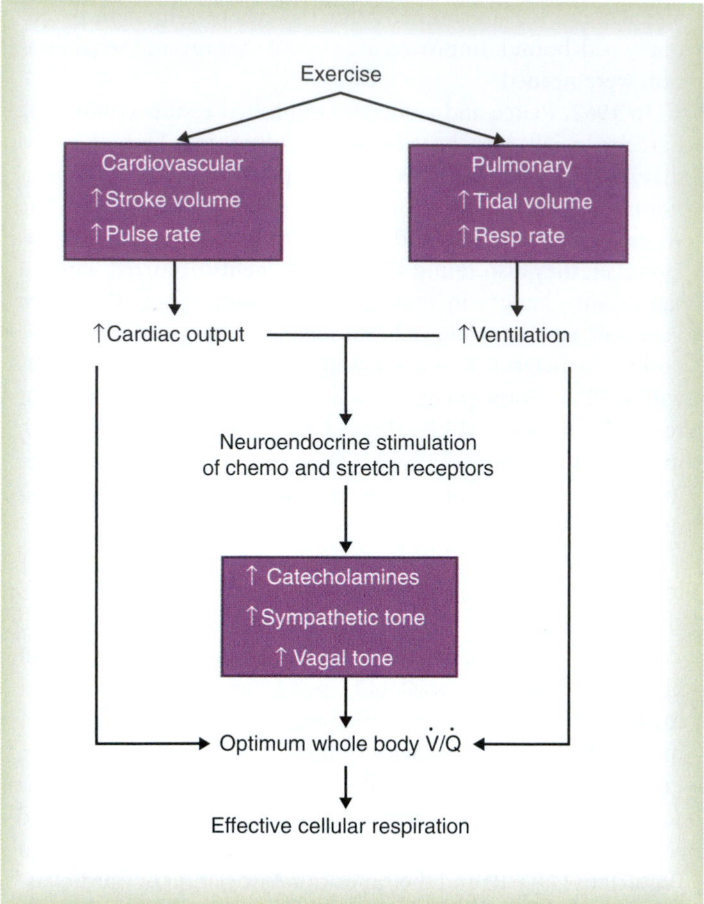

FIGURE 55-1 The body's response to increased levels of activity such as exercise.

As depicted in Figure 55-2, O_2 consumption and CO_2 production also increase in linear fashion as exercise intensity increases. If the body cannot deliver sufficient O_2 to meet the demands of energy metabolism, blood lactate levels increase above normal. In exercise physiology, this point is called the **onset of blood lactate accumulation (OBLA)**. As this excess lactic acid is buffered, CO_2 levels increase and the stimulus to breathe increases. The result is an abrupt upswing in both CO_2 and $\dot{V}_E$ (referred to as the **ventilatory threshold**). Beyond this point, metabolism becomes anaerobic, the efficiency of energy production decreases, lactic acid accumulates and fatigue sets in.

RULE OF THUMB

A good estimate of a patient's maximum voluntary ventilation (MVV) is derived by multiplying the FEV_1 (forced expiratory volume in 1 second) by a factor of 35. To estimate the MVV of a patient with FEV_1 of 1.5 L, multiply 1.5 L by 35:

$$MVV = FEV_1 \times 35$$
$$MVV = 1.5\,L \times 35 = 52.5\,L/min$$

Box 55-1 Benefits from Exercise Reconditioning

ACCEPTED BENEFITS

- Increased physical endurance
- Increased maximum O_2 consumption
- Increased activity levels with:
  - Decreased ventilation
  - Decreased $\dot{V}O_2$
  - Decreased heart rate
  - Increased ventilatory threshold
  - Improved blood lipids

POTENTIAL BENEFITS

- Increased sense of well-being
- Improved secretion clearance
- Increased hypoxic drive
- Improved cardiac function

UNPROVEN BENEFITS

- Prolonged survival
- Improved pulmonary function test results
- Decreased pulmonary artery pressure
- Improved blood gases
- Change in muscle O_2 extraction
- Change in step desaturation

Data from references 15 and 16.

Patients with COPD who lack adequate pulmonary function have severe limitations to their exercise capabilities. Their high rate of CO_2 production during exercise results in respiratory acidosis and a shortness of breath out of proportion to the level of activity. In addition, as ventilation increases, the rate of O_2 consumption in a patient with COPD increases significantly as depicted in Figure 55-3. Together, these factors limit patient tolerance for any significant increase in physical activity.

Pulmonary rehabilitation must include efforts to recondition patients physically and increase their exercise tolerance. **Reconditioning** involves strengthening essential muscle groups, improving overall O_2 utilization and enhancing the body's cardiovascular response to physical activity as noted in Box 55-1.

Psychosocial Support

If the overall goal of pulmonary rehabilitation is to improve the quality of patients' lives, physical reconditioning alone is insufficient. Psychosocial indicators generally are good predictors of morbidity in patients with COPD. Studies show that the relative success of reconditioning plays less of a role in determining whether patients complete a program than meeting their **psychosocial support needs.**[14]

There is a well-established relationship between physical, mental, and social well-being in humans. However, emotional states such as anxiety and stress can aggravate an existing physical problem. Likewise, physical manifestations of disease, such as recurrent dyspnea, can increase an individual's stress level.

The progressive nature of COPD can negatively affect the patient's overall outlook on his or her disease and reduce motivation to adapt to its consequences. The best medical care

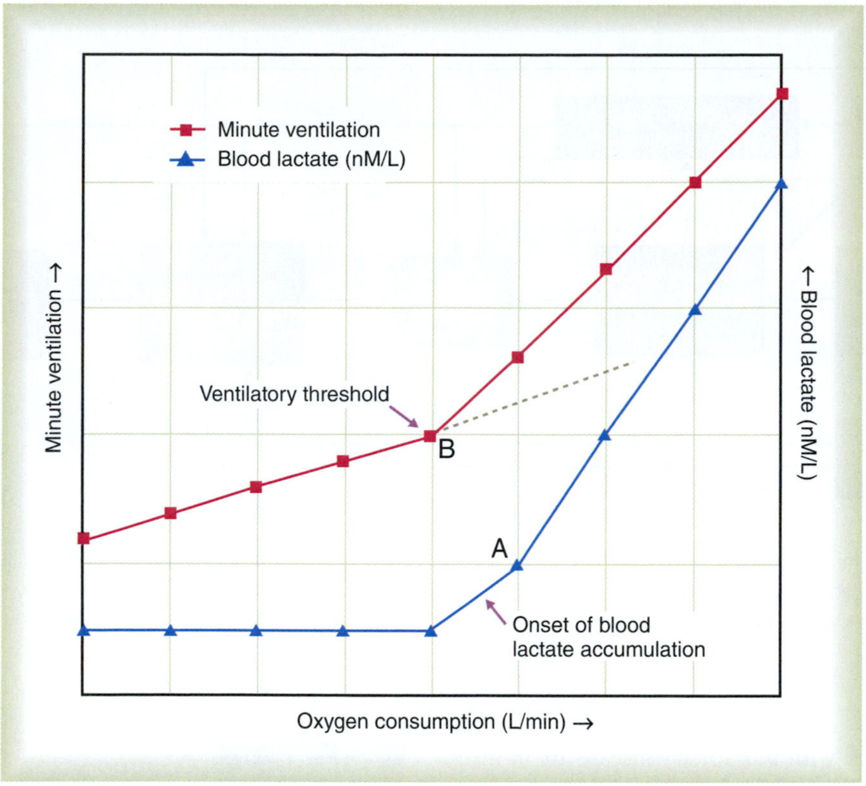

FIGURE 55-2 Minute ventilation, blood lactate, CO_2 production, and O_2 consumption during graded exercise to maximum. The dashed line represents the linear extrapolation between $\dot{V}E$ and $\dot{V}O_2$ during submaximal exercise. Point A represents OBLA. At the same time, $\dot{V}E$ and $\dot{V}CO_2$ "break" from their extrapolated rate of increase and abruptly rise (point B). This is referred to as the ventilatory threshold. (Modified from McArdle WD, Katch FI, Katch VL: Exercise physiology: energy, nutrition and human performance, ed 6, Baltimore, 2007, Williams & Wilkins.)

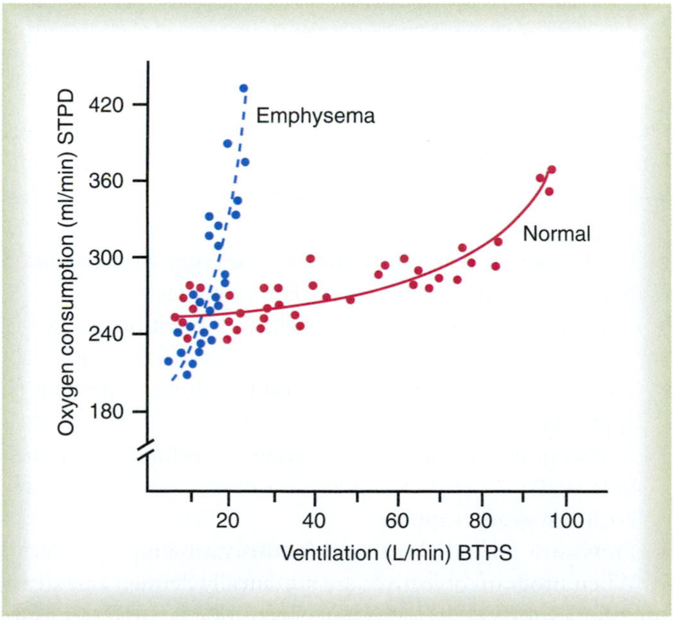

FIGURE 55-3 Changes in O_2 consumption with increasing ventilation in a normal subject and in a patient with emphysema. BTPS, Body temperature, body pressure saturated; STPD, volume of dry gas at 0° C and 760 mm Hg atmospheric pressure. (Modified from Cherniack RM, Cherniack L, Naimark A: Respiration in health and disease, ed 3, Philadelphia, 1984, Saunders.)

available can be negated and a patient can experience a progressively downhill course because of an unfavorable mental state. Patients with COPD often have a tendency to develop severe anxiety, hostility, and stress as a direct consequence of their disability.[15] Because patients are fearful of economic loss and death, they can develop hostility toward the disease and often toward the people around them. In terms of social function, the physiologic impairment of chronic lung disease combined with other variables can severely restrict a patient's ability to perform routine tasks requiring physical exertion. Moreover, patients' potential loss of confidence in their ability to care for themselves reduces feelings of dignity and self-worth.

Figure 55-4 presents elements of how chronic lung disease and other variables can have an impact on a patient's quality of life. It is here that the link between the physical reconditioning and psychosocial support components of rehabilitation becomes most evident. By reducing exercise intolerance and enhancing the body's cardiovascular response to physical activity, patients can develop a more independent and active lifestyle. For some patients, simply being able to walk to the market or play with their grandchildren can contribute to a greater feeling of social importance. For others, physical conditioning may allow a return to near-normal levels of activity, including vocational pursuits.

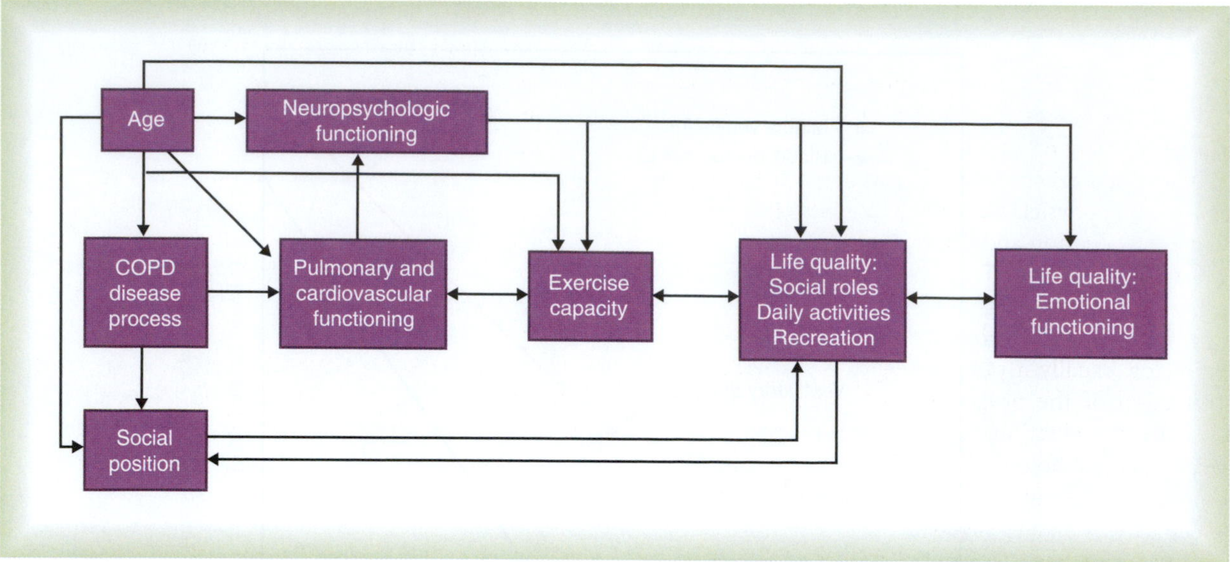

FIGURE 55-4 Model describing the relationship between physical and psychological dysfunction in patients with chronic lung disease. (Modified from McSweeney AJ, Grant I, Heaton RK, et al: Life quality of patients with chronic obstructive pulmonary disease. Arch Intern Med 142:473, 1982.)

Many patients disabled with pulmonary disease are in their economically productive years and are anxious to return to economic self-sufficiency. For these patients, occupational retraining and job placement are key ingredients in a good rehabilitation program. An occupational therapist can play a vital role here and should be included, if possible, as a member of the interdisciplinary rehabilitation team and in the pulmonary rehabilitation program. The pulmonary rehabilitation program should be based on the individual needs and expectations of each patient. Evaluation and placement of the rehabilitation patient may require the skills of vocational counselors and occupational therapists along with the cooperation of business and industry.

Box 55-2 Common Goals for Pulmonary Rehabilitation Programs

- Control of respiratory infections
- Basic airway management
- Improvement in ventilation and cardiac status
- Improvement in ambulation and other types of physical activity
- Reduction in overall medical costs
- Reduction in hospitalizations
- Psychosocial support
- Occupational retraining and placement (when and where possible)
- Family education, counseling, and support
- Patient education, counseling, and support
- Control of respiratory infections

STRUCTURE OF A PULMONARY REHABILITATION PROGRAM

Program Goals and Objectives

Pulmonary rehabilitation programs vary in their design and implementation but generally share common goals. Examples of these common goals are listed in Box 55-2. These general goals assist planners in formulating more specific program objectives. When determining objectives, both patients and members of the rehabilitation team should have input. These objectives should always be stated in measurable terms because this helps facilitate the determination of both patient outcomes and the therapeutic success and value of pulmonary rehabilitation. Depending on the specific needs of the participants, program objectives can include the following:

- Development of diaphragmatic breathing skills
- Development of stress management and relaxation techniques
- Involvement in a daily physical exercise regimen to condition both skeletal and respiratory-related muscles
- Adherence to proper hygiene, diet, and nutrition
- Smoking cessation (if applicable)
- Proper use of medications, O_2, and breathing equipment (if applicable)
- Application of airway clearance techniques (when indicated)
- Focus on group support
- Provisions for individual and family counseling

When program objectives are specifically defined and structured in a measurable way, strategies can be tailored to ensure the maximum results and benefit. Demonstration of program effectiveness also becomes easier and more acceptable by the medical community. However, benefits realized by participating patients are not always easy to identify and may be controversial.

Patient Evaluation and Selection

Before beginning a pulmonary rehabilitation program, clinicians need to define and establish criteria for entry or selection. They need to be aware of any comorbidity a patient may have along with the effects exercise may have on blood chemistry and a patient's overall physical status. Patient selection requires comprehensive evaluation and testing.[16]

Patient Evaluation

Pulmonary rehabilitation programs must have a qualified medical director, usually a pulmonologist, to provide overall medical direction of the program and to screen prospective patients.[17] Patient evaluation begins with a complete patient history—medical, psychological, vocational, and social. A well-designed patient questionnaire and interview form assist with this step. The patient history should be followed by a complete physical examination (see Chapter 16). A recent chest film, resting electrocardiogram (ECG), complete blood count, serum electrolytes, and urinalysis provide additional information on the patient's current medical status (see Chapter 17).

To determine the patient's cardiopulmonary status and exercise capacity, both pulmonary function testing and a cardiopulmonary exercise evaluation may be performed. Pulmonary function testing includes assessment of pulmonary ventilation, lung volume determinations, diffusing capacity (DLCO), and spirometry before and after bronchodilator use (see Chapter 20).

The **cardiopulmonary exercise evaluation (CPX)** serves two key purposes in pulmonary rehabilitation. First, it quantifies the patient's initial exercise capacity. This quantification provides the basis for the exercise prescription (including setting a **target heart rate**) and yields the baseline data for assessing a patient's progress over time. In addition, the evaluation helps determine the degree of hypoxemia or desaturation that can occur with exercise; this provides the objective basis for titrating O_2 therapy during the exercise program. To guide practitioners in implementing exercise evaluation, the American Association for Respiratory Care (AARC) has published clinical practice guidelines on exercise testing for evaluation of hypoxemia or desaturation or both[18] and pulmonary rehabilitation. Excerpts from these guidelines appear in Clinical Practice Guidelines 55-1 and 55-2.[19]

The exercise evaluation procedure involves serial or continuous measurements of several physiologic parameters during various graded levels of exercise on either an ergometer or a treadmill as described in Box 55-3. To allow for steady-state equilibration, these graded levels are usually spaced at 3-minute intervals. Work levels are increased progressively until either (1) the patient cannot tolerate a higher level or (2) an abnormal or hazardous response occurs.

Blood gas and arterial saturation measures are obtained at rest and at peak exercise. Samples from single arterial punctures are as good as samples drawn from indwelling catheters. If the peak exercise puncture is unsuccessful, a sample drawn within 10 to 15 seconds of test termination usually suffices. Owing to inherent problems, pulse oximetry has a limited but nonetheless important role in exercise evaluation. The best use of pulse oximetry is as a monitor to warn clinicians of gross desaturation events during testing. In addition, the pulse oximeter can be used to assess the patient's response to supplemental O_2 during exercise.

Relative contraindications to exercise testing include the following:

- Inability or unwillingness of patient to perform the test
- Severe pulmonary hypertension or cor pulmonale
- Known electrolyte disturbances (hypokalemia, hypomagnesemia)
- Resting diastolic blood pressure greater than 110 mm Hg or resting systolic blood pressure greater than 200 mm Hg
- Neuromuscular, musculoskeletal, or rheumatoid disorders exacerbated by exercise
- Uncontrolled metabolic disease (e.g., diabetes)
- SaO_2 or SpO_2 less than 85% with the subject breathing room air
- Untreated or unstable asthma
- Angina with exercise

Exercise evaluation also can help differentiate among patients with primary respiratory or cardiac limitations to increased

Modified Borg Dyspnea Scale (With Dyspnea Descriptors)

10	Maximal (worst possible you can imagine)
9	Very, very severe
8	Very, very severe
7	Very severe
6	Very severe
5	Severe
4	Somewhat severe
3	Moderate
2	Slight
1	Very slight
0.5	Very, very slight (just noticeable)
0	None at all

Box 55-3 Common Physiologic Parameters Measured During Exercise Evaluation

- Blood pressure
- Heart rate
- ECG
- Respiratory rate
- Arterial blood gases/O_2 saturation
- Maximum ventilation ($\dot{V}E_{max}$)
- O_2 consumption (either absolute $\dot{V}O_2$ or METS)
- CO_2 production ($\dot{V}E/\dot{V}CO_2$)
- Respiratory quotient (RQ)
- O_2 pulse ($\dot{V}O_2$:heart rate)

METS, Metabolic equivalents of O_2 consumption.

55-1 Exercise Testing for Evaluation of Hypoxemia, Desaturation, or Both

AARC Clinical Practice Guidelines (Excerpts)*

INDICATIONS

- The need to assess and quantify arterial oxyhemoglobin (HbO_2) levels during exercise in patients with suspected desaturation
- The need to quantify the response to therapeutic intervention
- The need to titrate the optimum level of O_2 therapy during activity
- The need for preoperative assessment for lung resection or transplant
- The need to assess the degree of impairment for disability evaluation

CONTRAINDICATIONS

Absolute contraindications include the following:

- Acute ECG changes indicating myocardial ischemia or serious cardiac dysrhythmias
- Unstable angina
- Acute pericarditis
- Aneurysm of the heart or aorta
- Uncontrolled systemic hypertension
- Recent (within prior 4 weeks) myocardial infarction or myocarditis
- Second-degree or third-degree heart block
- Recent systemic or pulmonary embolus
- Acute thrombophlebitis or deep venous thrombosis

Relative contraindications to exercise testing include the following:

- Inability or unwillingness of patient to perform the test
- Severe pulmonary hypertension or cor pulmonale
- Known electrolyte disturbances (hypokalemia, hypomagnesemia)
- Resting diastolic blood pressure >110 mm Hg or resting systolic blood pressure >200 mm Hg
- Neuromuscular, musculoskeletal, or rheumatoid disorders exacerbated by exercise
- Uncontrolled metabolic disease (e.g., diabetes)
- SaO_2 or SpO_2 <85% with the subject breathing room air
- Untreated or unstable asthma

PRECAUTIONS AND POSSIBLE COMPLICATIONS

Indications for ending testing include the following:

- ECG abnormalities (e.g., dangerous dysrhythmias, ventricular tachycardia, ST-T wave changes)
- Severe desaturation (SaO_2 <80% or SpO_2 <83% or 10% fall from baseline values)
- Angina
- Hypotensive responses
- Decrease of >20 mm Hg in systolic pressure, occurring after the normal exercise increase
- Decrease in systolic blood pressure below preexercise level
- Lightheadedness
- Request from patient to terminate test

Abnormal responses that may require discontinuation of exercise include (1) increase in systolic blood pressure to >250 mm Hg or diastolic pressure to >120 mm Hg, (2) increase in systolic pressure of >20 mm Hg from resting level, (3) mental confusion or headache, (4) cyanosis, (5) nausea or vomiting, (6) muscle cramping.

ASSESSMENT OF NEED

Indications for exercise testing to evaluate hypoxemia or desaturation or both include the following:

- History and physical examination indicators suggesting hypoxemia or desaturation or both
- The presence of abnormal diagnostic test results (e.g., DLCO, FEV_1, arterial blood gases)
- The need to titrate or adjust a therapy

MONITORING

The following should be monitored during testing:

- Physical assessment (chest pain, leg cramps, color, perceived exertion, dyspnea)
- Respiratory rate
- SpO_2
- Cooperation and effort level
- Borg or Modified Borg Dyspnea Scale
- Blood gas sampling site and technique
- Heart rate, rhythm, and ST-T wave changes
- Blood pressure

**For the complete guidelines, see American Association for Respiratory Care: AARC clinical practice guideline: exercise testing for evaluation of hypoxemia and/or desaturation. Respir Care 46:514, 2001.*
Refer to the Modified Borg Dyspnea Scale (immediately following).

work capacity. Table 55-1 summarizes these key similarities and differences. Besides helping to differentiate between the underlying cause of exercise intolerance, test results can assist in placing patients in the appropriate type of rehabilitation program.

To minimize patient risk during exercise evaluation, certain safety measures are implemented. First, the patient should undergo a physical examination just before the test, including a resting ECG. Second, a qualified physician should be present throughout the entire test. Third, emergency resuscitation equipment (cardiac crash cart with monitor, defibrillator, O_2, cardiac drugs, suction equipment, and airway equipment) must be readily available. Fourth, staff conducting and assisting with the procedure should be certified in basic and advanced life-support techniques. Last, the test should be terminated promptly whenever indicated.

55-2 Pulmonary Rehabilitation

AARC Clinical Practice Guideline (Excerpts)*

SETTINGS

Pulmonary rehabilitation (PR) may take place in any of the following sites:

- Inpatient setting, including medical center, skilled nursing facility, or rehabilitation hospital
- Outpatient setting, including outpatient hospital-based clinic, CORF, physician's office, alternative or extended care facility, or patient's home

INDICATIONS

Indications for PR include any of the following:

- Dyspnea during rest or exertion
- Hypoxemia or hypercapnia
- Reduced exercise tolerance
- Unexpected deterioration or worsening of symptoms against a background of chronic dyspnea and reduced but stable exercise tolerance
- Need for surgical intervention
- Chronic respiratory failure
- Ventilator dependence
- Increasing need for acute care intervention (i.e., emergency department visits, hospitalizations, or unscheduled physician office visits)

CONTRAINDICATIONS

Contraindications for PR include any of the following:

- Ischemic cardiac disease
- Acute cor pulmonale
- Severe pulmonary hypertension
- Significant hepatic dysfunction
- Metastatic cancer
- Renal failure
- Severe cognitive deficit
- Psychiatric disease affecting memory and compliance
- Substance abuse without the desire to cease use of substance
- Physical limitations, such as poor eyesight, impaired hearing, speech impediment, or orthopedic impairment, that may require modification of the PR setting but should not interfere with participation in the program

HAZARDS AND COMPLICATIONS

Hazards and complications are primarily related to the exercise portion of the program. During exercise, the cardiovascular and ventilatory systems must be able to respond to increased demands. Also, exercise can lead to muscle or ligament injuries.

ASSESSMENT OF NEED

Patients should be under the care of a physician for the pulmonary condition requiring PR. Appropriate members of the PR team participate in patient assessment. The initial evaluation should include medical history; diagnostic tests; assessment of current symptoms; physical assessment; determination of psychological, social, and vocational needs; assessment of nutritional status; assessment of exercise tolerance; determination of educational needs; and assessment of the patient's ability to carry out activities of daily living.

MONITORING

Patients should be monitored at baseline and at appropriate intervals to ensure validity of results and appropriateness of intervention. Monitoring should include the following:

- Patient's response to progressive and general reconditioning exercises in conjunction with breathing techniques
- Patient's O_2 requirements at rest and with exercise
- Knowledge and skills acquisition
- Patient's subjective comments
- Progress in achieving goals
- Patient appearance
- Vital signs
- Cardiac telemetry (if needed)
- Perceived exertion and dyspnea (use of Borg or Modified Borg Dyspnea Scale)

**For the complete guidelines, see American Association for Respiratory Care: AARC clinical practice guideline: pulmonary rehabilitation. Respir Care 47:617, 2002.*

With regard to test preparation, patients should fast 8 hours before the procedure. If the purpose of the test is to formulate an exercise prescription, the patient can take his or her regular medications. The patient should wear comfortable, loose-fitting clothing and footwear with adequate traction for treadmill or ergometer activity. The mouthpiece or face mask used during the test should be sized properly and fit comfortably with no leaks. Test conditions should be as standardized as possible to allow for comparison of results before and after rehabilitation periodically from year to year as the patient is treated and followed.

Patient Selection

Patients most likely to benefit from participation in pulmonary rehabilitation are patients with persistent symptoms caused by COPD who have low maximum O_2 uptakes at baseline. Pulmonary rehabilitation should be a part of the discharge planning process when a patient is released from the hospital after an exacerbation of the existing chronic respiratory condition. The feasibility of rehabilitation should be reviewed with the patient, physician, and respiratory therapist (RT). Other indications for pulmonary rehabilitation are listed in Box 55-4. Regardless of underlying conditions, patients also should be ex-smokers. Any

TABLE 55-1
Exercise Parameters Distinguishing Cardiac and Ventilatory (Chronic Obstructive Pulmonary Disease) Limitations

Parameter*	Cardiac†	COPD†
Maximum $\dot{V}O_2$	↓	↓
Maximum HR	N or ↓	↓
O2 pulse	↓	N
Maximum $\dot{Q}$	↓	↓
$\dot{Q}/\dot{V}O_2$	↓	N
PaO_2	N	↓
$PaCO_2$	↓	↑
$\dot{V}E/\dot{V}CO_2$	↑	↑
VT	↓	N

Modified from Lane EE, Walker JF: Clinical arterial blood gas analysis, St Louis, 1987, Mosby.
*HR, Heart rate; $\dot{Q}$, cardiac output; $\dot{V}E/\dot{V}CO_2$, ratio of minute ventilation to CO_2 production; $\dot{V}O_2$, oxygen consumption; VT, ventilatory threshold.
†N, Normal; ↑, increased; ↓, decreased.

Box 55-4 Indications and Contraindications for Pulmonary Rehabilitation

INDICATIONS
Symptomatic patients with COPD—usually GOLD stage III (severe) and stage IV (very severe), but stage II (moderate) may also be considered
Patients with bronchial asthma and associated bronchitis (asthmatic bronchitis)
Patients with combined obstructive and restrictive ventilatory defects
Patients with chronic mucociliary clearance problems
Patients with exercise limitations because of severe dyspnea

CONTRAINDICATIONS
Cardiovascular instability requiring cardiac monitoring (consider cardiac rehabilitation)
Malignant neoplasms involving the respiratory system
Severe arthritis or neuromuscular abnormalities (a relative contraindication—refer to physical therapy for case-by-case review)

patients who smoke should enroll in a smoking cessation program before starting pulmonary rehabilitation. Patients are excluded from pulmonary rehabilitation activities if (1) concurrent problems limit or preclude participation in exercise or (2) their condition is complicated by malignant neoplasms, such as lung cancer (see Box 55-4).

Objectively, candidates considered for inclusion in a pulmonary rehabilitation program generally fall into one of the following groups[20]:

- Patients in whom there is a respiratory limitation to exercise resulting in termination at a level less than 75% of the predicted maximum O_2 consumption ($\dot{V}O_{2max}$)
- Patients in whom there is significant irreversible airway obstruction with a forced expiratory volume in 1 second (FEV_1) of less than 2 L or an $FEV_{1\%}$ (ratio of FEV_1 to forced vital capacity [FVC]) of less than 60% (refer to the Global Initiative on Obstructive Lung Disease [GOLD] standards for COPD severity)
- Patients in whom there is significant restrictive lung disease with a total lung capacity (TLC) of less than 80% of predicted and single breath carbon monoxide diffusing capacity (DL_{CO}) of less than 80% of predicted
- Patients with pulmonary vascular disease in whom single breath DL_{CO} is less than 80% of predicted or in whom exercise is limited to less than 75% of maximum predicted O_2 consumption (predicted $\dot{V}O_{2max}$)

Groups or classes for pulmonary rehabilitation should be kept homogeneous. Placing individuals in a program who are at different stages of cardiopulmonary disability can be very defeating. Individuals with mild to moderate impairment may become discouraged on how severe lung disease can become, and individuals with severe impairment may feel they cannot keep up with or maintain the level of activity exhibited by others with less severe impairment.

Program Design

A good design helps achieve specific programming objectives with the selected group of participating patients. Key design considerations involve both format and content, with emphasis on patient reconditioning and education.

Format

Programs can use either an open-ended or a closed design, with or without planned follow-up sessions. With an open-ended format, patients enter the program and progress through it until they achieve certain predetermined objectives. There is no set time frame. Depending on his or her condition, needs, motivation, and performance, an individual patient can complete an open-ended program over weeks or months. This format is good for self-directed patients or patients with scheduling difficulties. It also may be the best format for patients requiring individual attention. The major drawback of the open-ended format is the lack of group support and involvement. In addition, insurance reimbursement may be a factor when the program is open-ended.

The more traditional closed design uses a set time period to cover program content. These programs usually run 6 to 16 weeks, with classes meeting one to three times a week. However, insurance coverage may dictate how many sessions make up the program. Medicare covers 36 initial sessions with possible coverage of another 36 sessions if the patient qualifies and would benefit from the additional rehabilitation sessions. Class sessions usually last up to 2 hours. Presentations are more formal and group support involvement is encouraged. A major drawback to this format is that the schedule determines program completion, rather than the objectives. However, most programs allow patients to reenroll if the anticipated improvements are not achieved.

Regardless of the format used, long-term improvements cannot be expected without planned follow-up.[21] Follow-up must be ongoing and available to all patients who complete the

TABLE 55-2

Sample Pulmonary Rehabilitation Session

Component	Focus	Time Frame
Educational	Welcome (group interaction)	5 min
	Review of program diaries (activities of past week)	20 min
	Presentation of educational topic	20 min
	Questions, answers, and group discussion	15 min
Physical reconditioning	Physical activity and reconditioning	45 min
	Individual goal setting and session summary	15 min
Total session		120 min (2 hr)

program. Frequently, this essential element of the process is difficult, especially when it is not covered by most insurance plans, but program coordinators must ensure that it is routinely scheduled. Follow-up or reinforcement could be open-ended (available during regular rehabilitation sessions and offering open attendance) or could be scheduled weekly, monthly, bimonthly, or quarterly. The important thing is to have some type of follow-up available.[22,23]

Content

The content of the rehabilitation program usually combines physical reconditioning with education activities. Table 55-2 outlines a sample session incorporating these two complementary components. Programs providing reconditioning or education alone are unlikely to be effective.

As shown in Table 55-2, the ideal rehabilitation session should last about 2 hours. Group size, available equipment, and group interaction dictate session length. Patients should arrive 10 to 15 minutes before a scheduled session to allow for informal group interaction and support. Classes should begin on time and conclude promptly as scheduled. Educational presentations should be brief and to the point. The use of audiovisuals or demonstrations should enhance understanding. To facilitate patient comprehension, the language should be simple and unnecessary technical terms or concepts should be avoided. Handouts that enhance certain points made during a presentation are both useful and desirable. A folder or notebook in which program activities may be recorded and handout materials kept should be maintained by each patient.

Physical Reconditioning

The physical reconditioning component of the pulmonary rehabilitation program consists primarily of an exercise prescription with target heart rate based on the results of the patient's initial exercise evaluation. For most patients, an initial target heart rate is set using **Karvonen's formula**, or estimated as 20 beats/min greater than resting rate. Because of the severity of ventilatory impairment, some patients begin exercise reconditioning without a prescribed target heart rate.

MINI CLINI

Patient Selection for Pulmonary Rehabilitation

PROBLEM: A patient is being evaluated for possible inclusion in a pulmonary rehabilitation program. The patient undergoes a complete history and physical examination and pulmonary function testing, arterial blood gas analysis, and exercise evaluation. During the exercise test, the patient develops severe hypertension and premature ventricular contractions. The physician recommends that the patient be admitted to pulmonary rehabilitation and prescribes a modified exercise routine. The RT performing the test disagrees. How should the RT proceed?

Solution: The RT should contact the department medical director for intervention. Although this patient could possibly be admitted to pulmonary rehabilitation, there is a high risk that some type of adverse response might occur during the exercise component of the program. The best direction would be to treat the cardiac manifestations first. After identifying the causes of the exercise-induced hypertension and arrhythmia, these problems can be properly treated. When the patient's cardiac manifestations are under control, the patient may be admitted to pulmonary rehabilitation and safely participate in and complete the program. Any underlying condition should be treated and managed first before pulmonary rehabilitation begins.

RULE OF THUMB

To set a target heart rate for patient exercise, use Karvonen's formula:

$$\text{Target heart rate} = [(\text{MHR} - \text{RHR}) \times (50\% - 70\%)] + \text{RHR}$$

where MHR is maximum heart rate at limit of exercise tolerance and RHR is resting heart rate.

A good target exercise heart rate for a patient with COPD with MHR of 150 beats/min and RHR of 90 beats/min would be $[(150 - 90) \times 0.60] + 90 = 126$ beats/min.

Typically, the exercise prescription includes the following four related components:[24,25]

1. Lower extremity (leg) aerobic exercises
2. Timed walking (**6- or 12-minute walk**)
3. Upper extremity (arm) aerobic exercises
4. Ventilatory muscle training

To ensure success with physical reconditioning, patients must actively participate both at the rehabilitation facility and at home. While exercising at the facility, patients should be monitored by pulse oximetry. Blood pressure measurements may also be made, but these are usually done at the start and end of each session unless a patient's condition dictates otherwise. In addition, exercise sessions should be upbeat. Lively

Patient Log Week # _______

Day	Flow Resistive Device	6-min or 12-min Walk	Exercycle	Other Activity	Remarks
	Setting ____________ Duration ____________	Distance __________ No. of stops ________	Distance ______ Duration ______	Type ________ Duration _____	
	Setting ____________ Duration ____________	Distance __________ No. of stops ________	Distance ______ Duration ______	Type ________ Duration _____	
	Setting ____________ Duration ____________	Distance __________ No. of stops ________	Distance ______ Duration ______	Type ________ Duration _____	
	Setting ____________ Duration ____________	Distance __________ No. of stops ________	Distance ______ Duration ______	Type ________ Duration _____	
	Setting ____________ Duration ____________	Distance __________ No. of stops ________	Distance ______ Duration ______	Type ________ Duration _____	
	Setting ____________ Duration ____________	Distance __________ No. of stops ________	Distance ______ Duration ______	Type ________ Duration _____	
	Setting ____________ Duration ____________	Distance __________ No. of stops ________	Distance ______ Duration ______	Type ________ Duration _____	

FIGURE 55-5 Sample log or diary form on which a patient in a pulmonary rehabilitation program records daily physical reconditioning activities and exercises.

music helps to maintain a positive atmosphere. Clinicians must remember that these patients are ill and require a nurturing attitude from team members, family, and the group itself.

To ensure compliance with the program, a daily log or diary sheet is completed. Figure 55-5 depicts a sample log sheet that makes up a section of the patient manual. These log or diary forms are reviewed each time the patient attends a session. Based on this information, further individualized reconditioning goals are set.

Lower extremity exercises may include either walking or bicycling. Patients can walk on a stationary treadmill (with set goals for distance or time and grade) or on a flat, smooth surface. Patients can bicycle on an exercise cycle. With the treadmill or stationary bicycle, patients are required to cover a certain distance or duration every day that they are in the program. Commonly, the duration is set to 30 minutes daily, with patients encouraged to increase both their distance and equipment tension or resistance as tolerated. Patients with significant orthopedic disabilities can participate in aerobic aquatic exercises.

Walking also improves overall conditioning; this usually takes the form of a 6- or 12-minute walk performed once a day, depending on the patient's condition and tolerance. These walk exercises are a convenient way for patients to carry out a well-defined amount of activity with increasing vigor and results over a number of weeks. During the 6 or 12 minutes, patients should walk on flat ground for as far as possible. If dyspnea occurs, they should stop and rest, with the rest time included as part of the time interval. After resting briefly, they should try to continue walking at a comfortable pace. The objective is to walk as far as possible during the allotted time. Landmarks such as telephone poles, city blocks, or actual distance measures can be used to quantify progress. Under adverse weather conditions, walking can be done indoors in shopping malls, stores, or long hallways. Patients should record their progress in their manuals or diaries.

Aerobic upper extremity exercises improve rehabilitation outcomes for patients whose regular activities involve lifting or raising the arms.[24,26] Arm ergometers or rowing machines are available for this purpose; however, simple calisthenics using either a broomstick or free weights (by prescription and with training) are a satisfactory alternative. Upper body endurance generally is more limited, with many patients capable of only 2 to 3 minutes of daily activity to start. This limitation usually is related to the fact that patients may revert to using accessory muscles for breathing while doing the upper body exercise. Patients need to breathe diaphragmatically and perform the exercises at the same time. Arm exercises should get progressively longer, up to 20 minutes if possible. Upper body conditioning helps patients perform numerous useful activities at home and can increase overall physical endurance. As with other activity, patients should record daily results in their logs or manuals.

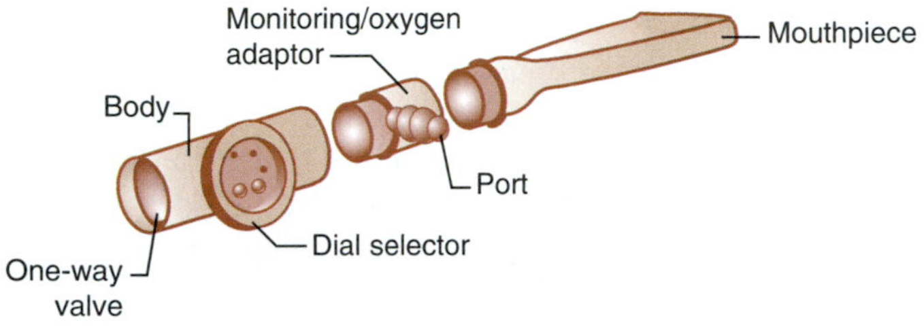

FIGURE 55-6 Flow-resistive breathing device.

Although controversy exists, ventilatory muscle training probably can enhance the benefits of these more traditional exercises.[27] Ventilatory muscle training is based on the concept of **progressive resistance**. By imposing progressively greater loads on the inspiratory muscles (mainly the diaphragm) over time, the patient's strength and endurance should increase. These improvements should increase the patient's exercise tolerance.

Figure 55-6 shows a typical inspiratory resistance breathing device. The device is an adjustable flow resistor with a one-way breathing valve. The inspiratory load is created by forcing the patient to inhale through a restricted orifice. Varying the size of this orifice varies the inspiratory load, as do changes in the

TABLE 55-3

Normal Maximum Inspiratory Pressure by Age and Sex

Age Group (yr)	PI_{MAX} FROM RESIDUAL VOLUME ($CM\ H_2O$), MEAN ± SD	
	Male	Female
9-18	96 ± 35	90 ± 25
19-50	127 ± 28	91 ± 25
51-70	112 ± 20	77 ± 18
>70	76 ± 27	66 ± 18

From Rochester DF, Hyatt RE: Respiratory muscle failure, Med Clin North Am 67:573, 1983.

patient's inspiratory flow. During expiration, gas flows unimpeded out the one-way exhalation valve. Other types of devices are also available. One model replaces the variable size orifice with an adjustable spring-loaded valve. This valve ensures a constant load regardless of how quickly or slowly the patient breathes.

Because variations in breathing strategy during ventilatory muscle training can affect outcomes, proper patient evaluation, training and follow-up are required. The RT initially measures the patient's maximum inspiratory pressure (PI_{max}) using a calibrated pressure manometer. The RT next compares the patient's maximum with established norms as noted in Table 55-3. This preliminary measure of inspiratory pressure helps to establish initial loads and provides the basis for the subsequent monitoring of patient progress.

Before beginning ventilatory muscle training, the patient should assume a position that relaxes the abdominal muscles, such as the position used for cough training. If using a flow resistive device, the RT begins at the maximum orifice setting, while measuring the inspiratory pressure generated through monitoring using the O_2 adapter (a second adapter may be needed if the patient is receiving supplemental O_2). The RT encourages the patient to breathe slowly through the device, at a rate no greater than 10 to 12 breaths/min. If the patient's inspiratory pressure is less than 30% of the measured PI_{max}, the next smaller orifice is selected, with this procedure repeated until the 30% effort is consistently achieved.

At this point, the RT instructs the patient to exercise with the device in one or two regular daily sessions lasting 10 to 15 minutes. As the level of resistance becomes more tolerable over time, the patient should progressively increase session duration up to 30 minutes. A self-maintained log of treatment times can help motivate the patient and assist the RT in subsequent progress monitoring.

Educational Component

The educational portion of the program covers topics that are both useful and necessary to the patient. Table 55-4 lists examples of topics covered during a 12-week rehabilitation program. Recommendations regarding the best facilitators for each session are included. Naturally, other topics can be included depending on the program schedule, but in terms of relative importance, the ones listed in Table 55-4 generally have the highest priority.

TABLE 55-4

Typical Educational Topic Schedule for a 12-Week Pulmonary Rehabilitation Program

Session (Week)	Topic(s)	Recommended Facilitator(s)
1	Introduction and welcome; program orientation	Program administrator or rehabilitation team
2	Respiratory structure, function, and pathology	Physician or RT
3	Breathing control methods	PT or RT
4	Relaxation and stress management	Clinical psychologist
5	Proper exercise techniques and personal routines	PT or RT
6	Methods to aid secretion clearance (bronchial hygiene)	PT or RT
7	Home oxygen and aerosol therapy	RT
8	Medications—their use and abuse	Pharmacist, physician, or nurse practitioner
9	Medications—use of MDIs and spacers	RT
10	Dietary guidelines and good nutrition	Dietitian or nutritionist
11	Recreation and vocational counseling Activities of daily living	Occupational therapist
12	Follow-up planning and program evaluation Graduation	Rehabilitation team

MDIs, Metered dose inhalers; *PT*, physical therapist; *RT*, respiratory therapist.

These topics should be presented in an orderly, coherent fashion using supplementary audiovisual tools and demonstrations, where appropriate. Team members should allocate sufficient time both for the class sessions themselves and for setup and breakdown of equipment.

The program facilitator or leader must ensure that sessions begin on time and encourage maximum participation by each patient. If available, health care professionals such as dietitians, occupational therapists, physical therapists, and psychologists should be invited to present their respective topics and discuss the subject matter with the group. However, this may add to the overall operating costs of the pulmonary rehabilitation program. In addition to technical knowledge, session leaders must possess group facilitation skills and be able to motivate patients to participate both in class and at home and to adhere to program guidelines. This task is not an easy one, but it can be accomplished with patience and persistence. The desired end result is to help patients lead more productive lives with decreased hospitalizations.

Respiratory Structure, Function, and Pathology, Including a Discussion of Dyspnea. This presentation lays the groundwork for the program and gives each patient some basic information about the cardiorespiratory system and related disorders. The causes of shortness of breath are presented.

Breathing Control Methods. This presentation serves as the cornerstone for the physical reconditioning effort. Patients must learn how to control their breathing efforts to ensure maximum result (ventilation) at a minimum of effort (energy expenditure). Diaphragmatic breathing with pursed lips helps to accomplish this, but this technique requires daily practice on the part of the patient and continued reinforcement throughout the entire program by the group facilitator.

Methods of Relaxation and Stress Management. Patients must learn to avoid aggravation and upsetting circumstances and to adopt a more relaxed attitude about their particular life circumstances. This attitude can help to reduce unnecessary O_2 use, conserve energy, and avoid undesirable cardiovascular and nervous responses to stress.

Exercise Techniques and Personal Routines. The rationale for and value of exercise should be discussed with suggestions for the adoption of personal exercise routines after the rehabilitation program is over.

Secretion Clearance and Bronchial Hygiene Techniques. This topic is especially helpful to patients who have secretion clearance problems associated with chronic bronchitis and bronchiectasis. Family members and friends may be invited to attend this session to acquire basic skills with these procedures.

Home Oxygen and Aerosol Therapy. An RT with home care experience should provide this session. The focus should be on the care and use of home care equipment and self-administration of therapy. Patients who have not yet been prescribed this type of therapeutic regimen may have questions or fears and be unreceptive to the concept. Presenting the modalities available and having patients discuss their positive experiences with respiratory home care personnel can help alleviate the fears and anxieties of others.

Medications. This is another topic about which patients have numerous questions and concerns. Content should emphasize proper use of medications, along with possible abuses and adverse effects. Participants' current prescriptions should dictate which specific drugs to cover. Common categories include beta-adrenergic agents, anticholinergic agents, steroids, diuretics, and methylxanthines. The session leader should demonstrate proper use of metered dose inhalers including spacers or holding chambers, dry powder inhalers and hand-held nebulizers. Sufficient time should be provided for questions and answers. Two sessions should be allotted for this topic.

Dietary Guidelines. This subject focuses on weight management and good nutrition as it relates to cardiopulmonary health. Emphasis should be on the importance of a sound high-protein, low-carbohydrate diet. The facilitator also should cover proper eating habits, methods of gaining and losing weight, foods to avoid, ways to increase appetite, adequate hydration, and daily menu planning. This session can stimulate patients to eat better and supply their bodies with the necessary fuel for increased energy production.

Recreational and Vocational Counseling. This session should motivate participants to participate in recreational activities and, according to ability, return to work. This topic is often presented at the end of the program when patients have increased their physical endurance and are preparing for a more active and productive lifestyle. The class may brainstorm ideas for recreational or physical activities, from which members can generate action plans.

Psychosocial and Behavioral Components

Psychological and emotional stress is a common problem for patients with moderate to severe chronic lung disease. Pulmonary rehabilitation programs can bring in experts to implement psychosocial and behavioral therapies that provide patients with the opportunity to learn coping strategies. This component is most useful for patients with anxiety or depression or both.

Program Implementation

In 1987, the AARC and the AACVPR jointly conducted the first national survey of pulmonary rehabilitation programs. This National Pulmonary Rehabilitation Survey was published in 1988 and showed the variation existing in rehabilitation program structure, content, staffing, and cost throughout the United States.[28] In 2006, the ACCP, in conjunction with the AACVPR, released new evidence-based guidelines pertaining to the design and implementation of pulmonary rehabilitation programs.[13]

Staffing

Pulmonary rehabilitation is a multidisciplinary endeavor. Team care is enhanced by involving various health care professionals in the planning, implementation, and evaluation components of the program as illustrated in Figure 55-7. It is recommended that any staff conducting pulmonary rehabilitation program sessions be certified in basic life support or advanced cardiac life support through the American Heart Association. In addition to professional involvement, family members are needed to provide feedback and ensure that instructions and the exercise prescription are carried out at home.

Facilities

Location and quality of facilities can directly affect patient attendance. Patients are less likely to attend programs that are inaccessible to public transportation, have poor parking arrangements, or are physically difficult to reach. The facility must be wheelchair accessible. For elderly patients who do not drive, arrangements can be made with community organizations to provide transportation to and from the program. Ideally, the facility should provide two separate rooms for the program—one room for educational activities and one room for physical reconditioning. Rooms should be spacious and comfortable with adequate lighting, ventilation, and temperature control. Chairs should be comfortable with good back support. Restroom facilities need to be readily accessible. A room for individual counseling is helpful, but any private office would suffice. It is also preferable to have pulmonary function testing and blood gas analysis capabilities on site. If this space

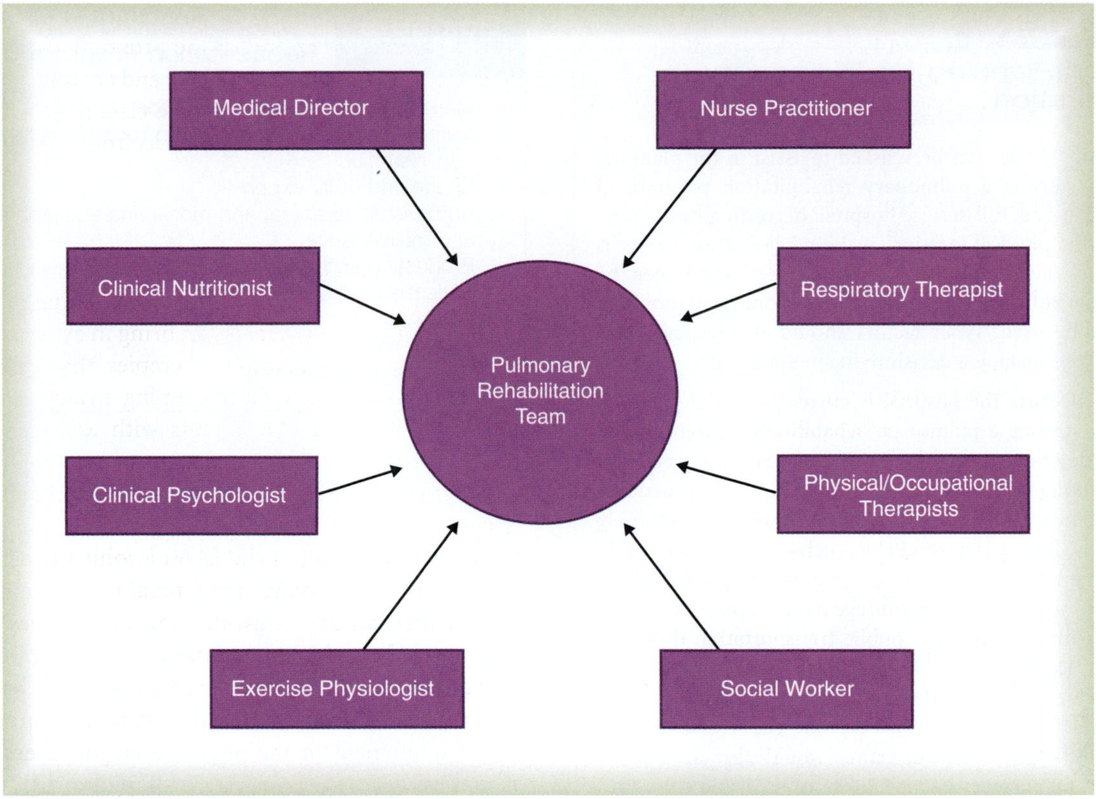

FIGURE 55-7 Multidisciplinary nature of pulmonary rehabilitation.

is used by other departments for other functions, proper scheduling of rehabilitation sessions needs to be considered.

Scheduling

Another aspect of program implementation involves timely scheduling of the rehabilitation sessions. Most sessions are scheduled one to three times per week for 1 to 2 hours, with programs running 8 to 16 weeks. The length of the program often depends on insurance coverage and expected reimbursement for sessions attended. Class times need to be scheduled when the largest number of patients can attend. Traffic patterns, bus schedules, and availability of rides are concerns that need to be addressed. Sessions can be conducted in the morning, afternoon, or evening and on weekends if necessary. Proper scheduling helps to encourage participation and removes potential stumbling blocks, which could undermine the rehabilitation process.

Class Size

Class size is another issue that must be addressed. Theoretically, class size for a rehabilitation program could range from 1 to 15 participants, depending on available space, equipment, staff, and patient condition/needs. However, to foster group identity, interaction, and support, small group discussions are encouraged. The ideal class size should range from 3 to 10 participants. Keeping the class size manageable facilitates vital group interaction processes and allows for more individualized attention. These factors help sustain motivation, reducing the likelihood of participant attrition.

Naturally, economic concerns surface when class size is considered. Although program quality must be the first priority, program viability realistically depends on the number of participants. Programs generally should be conducted with a class size that is comfortable with regard to space and staffing and that is economically feasible. Such an approach helps ensure that programs produce meaningful patient outcomes.

Equipment

Both the instruction and the reconditioning component of the program require equipment. To meet the educational needs of the program, a whiteboard or flipchart, computer with a PowerPoint projector screen, overhead projector, and/or CD player are needed. A DVD player with monitor may also be helpful, especially if individualized instruction or commercially available programs are used. Also, videos and formal learning packages dealing with the educational topics covered during the rehabilitation program should be available for group and individualized presentation. These can be purchased from outside sources or designed and developed in-house.

For physical reconditioning, stationary bicycles, treadmills, rowing machines, upper extremity ergometers, weights, pulse oximeters, and inspiratory resistance breathing devices constitute the minimum equipment requirements. The quantity of equipment needed depends on class size, scheduling, and

MINI CLINI

Facilities Planning for Pulmonary Rehabilitation

PROBLEM: The RT has been asked to assist in the planning process for starting a pulmonary rehabilitation program to support a 350-bed, full-service hospital. According to the strategic plan, the physical location of the rehabilitation center is about 3 blocks away from the hospital. The RT has not seen the proposed site but was asked to approve a recommendation that the facility be used. What factors should the RT take into account before making a decision on site selection?

Solution: Because the hospital is currently in the planning process for starting a pulmonary rehabilitation program and has not made a final facility selection, the RT is in a key position to assess, among other areas, issues related to the proposed site. Patient attendance and participation would be adversely affected if the facility is unreachable, such as at the top of a hill. If the location is in a high crime or unsafe area with little or no security, this too would discourage patients from attending. As is true with any program, public transportation that does not permit accessibility to the proposed facility would be a limiting factor, as would little or no available parking. Numerous other facility considerations outside the actual physical location of the rehabilitation center would also need to be addressed. The current square footage of available space and room for future expansion would need to be evaluated relative to anticipated needs, as would whether the facility itself is wheelchair accessible with no barriers present.

available space. Sufficient equipment should be on hand to keep all patients exercising and to monitor their activity. Emergency O_2 and bronchodilator medications should also be maintained in the rehabilitation area. Equipment guidelines for a class of 6 to 10 participants include the following: five stationary bicycles, two treadmills, two rowing machines, two upper extremity ergometers, five pulse oximeters for monitoring heart rate and O_2 saturation, one emergency O_2 cylinder (E), and bronchodilator medications. In addition, each patient should be supplied with an inspiratory resistance breathing device.

Because equipment can be expensive, care must be taken in its selection and purchase. Devices and appliances should be durable, easy and safe to use, simple to maintain, and not overly expensive. Initially, basic items are purchased. As a program develops and expands, equipment resources can be enhanced. Other program needs include the following:

- Maintaining individual patient manuals, including daily log forms or activity diaries
- Providing light refreshments for program participants
- Developing a communication network to announce schedule changes because of emergencies or cancellation of class sessions because of illness or weather
- Identifying available durable medical equipment providers for participants in need of specialized home care equipment

Box 55-5 Factors Affecting Pulmonary Rehabilitation Program Costs

- Marketing and program promotion
- Number of personnel involved in program facilitation and administration
- Space and utility expenses
- Audiovisual, exercise, and monitoring equipment (purchase and maintenance)
- Production and duplication of course materials
- Patient supplies
- Office supplies
- Refreshments
- Miscellaneous expenses

- Developing a system of charges and mechanism for patient payment

By considering all of the factors needed for effective implementation of pulmonary rehabilitation, programs have lower patient attrition and a greater chance for overall success. As programs are conducted, regular evaluations must be made by both patients and staff. Needed changes should be implemented on an ongoing basis. Only in this manner can one expect continued refinement of the process and improvement in patient outcomes.

Cost, Fees, and Reimbursement

Rehabilitation programs usually project their fees based on the average cost per participant. According to regional labor and material prices, costs vary throughout the United States. Several factors must be considered when projecting program costs as noted in Box 55-5. The larger the class size and the more participants involved in the overall program, the lower the cost would be per patient. The aim should be to offer and conduct the highest quality program possible at a reasonable cost that meets any existing budgetary constraints.

When determining patient charges, consideration must also be given to the type and amount of funding that has been received to offset program expenses and available insurance reimbursement. Preprogram and postprogram testing and evaluations naturally generate revenues but should not be included in the formulation of program charges. However, payments for pulmonary function testing, exercise testing, arterial blood gas analysis, and other evaluations may help to keep a pulmonary rehabilitation program financially viable.

Charges for an entire program or for each session must be structured in a way that does not deter patient attendance. Many patients with a chronic pulmonary disease are on a fixed income and have other living and medical expenses. A happy medium between a patient's ability to pay and program expenses must be identified. Funding from local charitable organizations, foundations, or agencies such as the American Lung Association and the COPD Foundation can help ease the financial burden. The most comprehensive and effective program available can have no impact if patients are unwilling or unable to attend and participate because of financial limitations.

Along with health care costs in general, the cost of providing pulmonary rehabilitation has increased over the years. Nationwide charges for pulmonary rehabilitation vary, depending on program length and, most importantly, insurance coverage. With most insurance plans reimbursing programs at 80% after a deductible, each patient would be responsible for the remaining 20% or copayment. Additional or supplemental medical coverage may cover this balance.

Charges for participation in these programs and inpatient rehabilitation reimbursement policies vary throughout the United States. In 1982, the Centers for Medicare and Medicaid Services (CMS), formerly the Health Care Financing Administration or HCFA, published the final rules for Medicare reimbursement guidelines for **comprehensive outpatient rehabilitative facilities (CORFs)**. Under Part B of Medicare, the scope of services of a CORF includes reimbursement for outpatient activities and one home visit. Reimbursement requires that the CORF meet the conditions of participation established in section 933 of Public Law 96-499; this also includes provisions for certification of the program. To establish reimbursement mechanisms, each CORF must present its program description and anticipated results to local third-party payers.[29] The AACVPR has also developed guidelines for program design, implementation, and recognition.

By following recognized guidelines, Medicare has established an allowable charge for pulmonary rehabilitation and reimburses 80% of this rate after the patient meets the annual prescribed deductible. In the past, inpatient and outpatient pulmonary rehabilitation programs obtained reimbursement from third-party payers by charging for rehabilitation sessions as physical therapy exercises for COPD, reconditioning exercise sessions, office visits with therapeutic exercises, serial pulse oximetry determinations, or physician office visits. The goal was to obtain as much insurance reimbursement as possible, decreasing the financial burden on the patient. Box 55-6 lists all possible sources of reimbursement.[30,31]

Box 55-6 Sources of Reimbursement for Pulmonary Rehabilitation Programs

- Nongovernment health insurance programs—private, single, or group health insurance plans
  - Health maintenance organizations (HMOs)
  - Preferred provider organizations (PPOs)
  - Medicare supplement
- Federal and state health insurance programs
  - Medicare
  - Medicaid
  - Uncompensated services (Hill-Burton)
  - CORF
  - Veterans Administration benefits
  - Civilian Health and Medical Programs of the Uniformed Services (CHAMPUS)
  - Federal workers insurance
- Ancillary liability and casualty insurance programs
  - Automobile insurance—related to automobile accidents
  - Workers' compensation—related to accidents on the job
  - Business insurance coverage—related to injuries sustained on business premises
  - Homeowner's insurance—related to injuries sustained on the owner's premises
  - Malpractice insurance on providers of health care
  - Product and service liability insurance—related to injuries caused by a product or service
- Other options of reimbursement
  - Senior care
  - Rehabilitation hospitals
  - Grants

RULE OF THUMB

To help ensure adequate reimbursement for pulmonary rehabilitation, identify patient goals and objectives; formulate and implement an effective exercise prescription for each patient; use diagnostic codes from the International Classification of Diseases, Ninth Revision, Clinical Modification (ICD-9-CM); use current and proper CPT (Current Procedural Terminology) coding; and document, document, document. Please note that ICD-9-CM will be replaced by ICD-10-CM beginning with FY 2015, which changes disease-related coding.

There is now a national coverage policy for pulmonary rehabilitation under Medicare, which took effect on January 1, 2010, as a result of the passage of HR 6331. Programs have to obtain reimbursement from their Medicare beneficiaries following accepted protocol, policies, and provisions specified by Medicare. Coverage is for patients with stage II, III, and IV COPD (moderate to very severe according to the GOLD standards). Pulmonary rehabilitation programs must include five components which must be documented in the patient's medical record. The five components include the following:

1. Physician-prescribed exercise, including aerobic exercise performed during each session
2. Education and training that relate to an individual patient's needs
3. Psychosocial assessment
4. Outcomes assessment
5. Treatment plan that details how these components are used for each individual patient[31]

According to CMS, claims for Medicare patients should be submitted to Medicare Part A for any component of pulmonary rehabilitation performed during a hospital stay and claims for rehabilitation components provided on an outpatient basis must be submitted to Medicare Part B. As with other forms of therapy covered by CMS, other insurance providers have already or will follow Medicare policy for reimbursement of pulmonary rehabilitation. This payment mechanism has already undergone changes and it is anticipated that Medicare will continue to change its reimbursement policy for pulmonary rehabilitation in the future. It is incumbent on clinicians who provide pulmonary rehabilitation to stay abreast of any changes in reimbursement policy and procedure and to make necessary adjustments to receive payment.

At the present time, there is provision to reimburse pulmonary rehabilitation programs for two 1-hour rehabilitation sessions per patient per day up to 36 sessions. An additional 36 sessions over an extended period can be approved by the individual Medicare contractor based on patient need for continued rehabilitation and physician referral. Documentation of programs is essential for payment of services rendered. Current coding for pulmonary rehabilitation under Medicare Part B uses the HCPCS G0424 code. Provision has been made for face-to-face patient sessions and for group (two or more patients) sessions. Individual sessions must be at least 31 minutes in length. If two sessions are performed on the same day, services may be reported only if the duration of the combined treatments is at least 91 minutes. It is essential that the practitioner who conducts pulmonary rehabilitation is familiar with all current practices so that therapy provided and billed for complies with current Medicare policy, is properly documented for each patient, and is submitted in a timely manner.[31-33]

MINI CLINI

Obtaining Insurance Payment for Pulmonary Rehabilitation

PROBLEM: The RT is asked to design and implement a pulmonary rehabilitation program on an outpatient basis at her hospital. After completing the first class that ran for 12 weeks, the hospital scheduled another one. However, although the institution had been submitting bills on a timely basis to numerous insurance providers, including Medicare, no payment has been received. What is the problem and how can it be corrected?

Solution: The insurance companies apparently either have denied claims or have not responded to the claims being submitted. This problem is often associated with improper or inaccurate claim filing. The RT should work closely with the billing department at the hospital to ensure that all information is complete for each patient (i.e., correct patient identification numbers), that the hospital has the correct addresses to submit claims, and that diagnoses and procedures have been properly coded. Some insurance companies have their own coding schemes and these must be followed accordingly. Managed care companies also require preauthorization, which must be obtained before entering any patient with a managed care plan into pulmonary rehabilitation. Finally, follow-up telephone calls are always helpful and should be conducted if payment is not received in a timely fashion.

Box 55-7 Evaluation of Rehabilitation Program Outcomes

- Changes in exercise tolerance
- Before and after 6- or 12-minute walking distance
- Before and after pulmonary exercise stress test
- Review of patient home exercise logs
- Strength measurement
- Flexibility and posture
- Performance on specific exercises (e.g., ventilatory muscle, upper extremity)
- Changes in symptoms
- Dyspnea measurement comparison
- Frequency of cough, sputum production, or wheezing
- Weight loss or gain
- Psychological test instruments
- Other changes
- Activities of daily living changes
- Postprogram follow-up questionnaires
- Preprogram and postprogram knowledge tests
- Compliance improvement with pulmonary rehabilitation medical regimen
- Frequency and duration of respiratory exacerbations
- Frequency and duration of hospitalizations
- Frequency of emergency department visits
- Return to productive employment

Program Results

Patient and program outcomes must be evaluated at the conclusion of the program and periodically thereafter as described in Box 55-7. This evaluation must compare patient status before the program with current patient status and may include physiologic, psychological, and sociologic data. Common outcome measures include exercise tolerance, levels of dyspnea at rest and with exertion, and quality-of-life surveys.

Results of pulmonary rehabilitation must be communicated to the patient, family, referring physician, and home care company, if appropriate. Further goals and objectives for continued improvement may be established to provide the basis for follow-up and reinforcement activities. Quality of life for patients with chronic lung diseases is an outcome measure that many pulmonary rehabilitation programs are documenting.[34] A major predictor for improvement in health-related quality of life of a patient with COPD is frequent attendance in a maintenance program.[3,35]

If no improvements in physical or psychosocial measures occur within a class or group, program deficiencies are the most likely cause. Specifically, insufficient professional training in rehabilitation methods, a lack of uniformity in approach, inadequate program length, and lack of follow-up are the major reasons for unsatisfactory outcomes.

Finally, pulmonary rehabilitation has become recognized as a prerequisite for certain patients with emphysema who are able to undergo lung volume reduction (LVR) surgery. Physical reconditioning and patient education before the procedure help to increase the chances for a successful outcome. Pulmonary rehabilitation appears to have favorable results with this specific patient population because of added patient and practitioner commitment and focus. Patients who do not complete the presurgical rehabilitation protocol are at higher risk for postsurgical complications.[36-39]

Potential Hazards

Although most patients with COPD can expect to realize benefits through physical reconditioning and pulmonary rehabilitation, certain potential hazards do exist, as follows:

I. Cardiovascular abnormalities
   A. Cardiac arrhythmias (can be reduced with supplemental O_2 during exercise)
   B. Systemic hypotension and hypertension
II. Blood gas abnormalities
   A. Arterial desaturation
   B. Hypercapnia
   C. Acidosis
III. Muscular abnormalities
   A. Functional or structural injuries
   B. Diaphragmatic fatigue and failure
   C. Exercise-induced muscle contracture
IV. Miscellaneous
   A. Exercise-induced asthma (more common in young patients with asthma than in patients with COPD)
   B. Hypoglycemia
   C. Dehydration

Proper patient selection, education, supervision, and monitoring are key factors in reducing possible hazards.

MINI CLINI

What to Expect from Pulmonary Rehabilitation

PROBLEM: The RT is asked to consult on a 63-year-old man hospitalized with severe COPD for possible participation in an outpatient pulmonary rehabilitation program. During the patient interview, the patient tells the RT that if the program will not cure him, he sees no reason to participate. How should the RT respond to the patient, keeping in mind his expectations of what pulmonary rehabilitation should accomplish?

Solution: It is crucial for all RTs and other caregivers involved in pulmonary rehabilitation to recognize that the focus of any program should attempt to treat the patient as a whole and not solely the underlying disease. A well-constructed pulmonary rehabilitation program should be able both to quantify the extent of physiologic impairment and to assist in establishing outcome expectations for physical reconditioning. Regardless of setting or design, such programs must address the psychological, social, and vocational impact of the disability on the patient and family and seek ways to improve the patient's quality of life. In this case, the RT should describe the benefits of pulmonary rehabilitation outside the traditional measures of pulmonary function. Although pulmonary rehabilitation cannot affect the progressive deterioration in lung function that occurs with COPD, both education and exercise may improve the patient's ability to perform activities of daily living and exercise tolerance. In addition, effective breathing techniques may lessen the frequency and severity of "panic breathing" episodes.

CARDIAC REHABILITATION

Patients with primary cardiac disease are often referred to cardiac rehabilitation programs where the focus is on improving cardiovascular fitness. Cardiac rehabilitation is defined as a comprehensive exercise and educational program designed for patients with cardiovascular diseases. Similar to pulmonary rehabilitation, good cardiac rehabilitation programs are multidisciplinary in approach and focus. Goals include patient education promoting heart-healthy living, physical reconditioning to improve work capacity, weight loss, and a return to work.

Enrollment in a cardiac rehabilitation program is based on a thorough cardiovascular evaluation and related parameters. The goal of a structured cardiac rehabilitation program is to assist patients in developing a regular pattern of safe exercise to achieve greater cardiovascular performance during activity. Most cardiac rehabilitation programs are conducted within a hospital facility. Programs are generally divided into monitored and maintenance segments, with home options available. Exercise prescriptions are individualized for participating patients to maximize outcomes and reduce the likelihood of adverse effects.

Pulmonary and cardiac rehabilitation share many similarities and differences. Similarities include the need for patient evaluation before program enrollment, patient education, the focus on exercises to increase fitness and stamina, and the need to monitor patients during exercise and for compliance. Differences include disease focus, patient age (most cardiac patients range in age from late 30s to 60s and 70s, whereas pulmonary patients for the most part are ≥50 years), and exercises used within the program. Many cardiac patients can walk for up to 1 hour, whereas this may be virtually impossible for most pulmonary patients. Breathing exercises to improve ventilation are essential to the pulmonary patient but are not that important to cardiac patients.

Reimbursement varies between the two types of programs with cardiac rehabilitation being more recognized by insurance payers, including Medicare. Because cardiac rehabilitation has existed longer than pulmonary rehabilitation and because outcomes tend to have greater validity and acceptance, insurance reimbursement has been more readily available. There are four phases to cardiac rehabilitation from program introduction to the ongoing fitness aspect. Patient reimbursement depends on the phase of cardiac rehabilitation the patient is in. This division into phases does not currently exist for patients in pulmonary rehabilitation.

Finally, respiratory involvement in cardiac rehabilitation is significantly less. For the most part, the RT is involved with instruction on O_2 use and may assist with patient exercise sessions during cardiac rehabilitation. Most often, the cardiologist and cardiac nurse specialist are involved with program facilitation and administration. Other health care providers who may be involved include a dietitian, physical therapist or occupational therapist or both, and a psychologist.

MINI CLINI

Reacting to Adverse Outcomes

PROBLEM: A 73-year-old man with stage III COPD was accepted into a pulmonary rehabilitation program. Because of the severity of his disease, his preprogram cardiopulmonary exercise evaluation was stopped after 5 minutes because of excessive dyspnea and oxygen desaturation. He was placed on O_2 but was unable to complete the study. However, because of the desire of the patient's physician to get him into a program of pulmonary rehabilitation and the patient's desire to participate, the patient was put on home O_2 and admitted to the program. While exercising on a treadmill with supplemental O_2, the patient complained of headache and nausea. The RT stopped the exercise session and documented a significant increase in the patient's blood pressure (220/130 mm Hg). How should the RT proceed in this case?

Solution: The RT should document the elevated blood pressure and notify the physician overseeing the pulmonary rehabilitation program and the patient's prescribing physician (if different) immediately. It is likely that the preprogram cardiopulmonary exercise test was stopped before the excessive increase in blood pressure was noted. While in pulmonary rehabilitation, the patient (on supplemental O_2) was able to exercise to a level greater than that during the exercise test. This elevated blood pressure will result in the patient going on some type of antihypertensive therapy and being reevaluated during another exercise test to determine the extent of his hypertensive condition. Depending on the instability of the patient's hypertension, it is also possible that this patient will be admitted to cardiac rehabilitation first before returning to the pulmonary rehabilitation program. This case shows the importance of a thorough and complete assessment of a patient's status before any admission to pulmonary rehabilitation.

CONCLUSION

A properly planned and implemented pulmonary rehabilitation program can produce positive and measurable patient outcomes. Goals and objectives of pulmonary rehabilitation should be written in these measurable terms and explained to the patient in a clear, concise fashion to achieve optimum therapeutic outcomes. The success of pulmonary rehabilitation depends on this along with careful application of current clinical knowledge and the use of a multidisciplinary approach throughout all phases of program organization, implementation, and evaluation. Within this context, pulmonary rehabilitation will continue to gain greater acceptance and the role of the RT in pulmonary rehabilitation will be increasingly more important.

SUMMARY CHECKLIST

- Pulmonary rehabilitation has two major aims: (1) to control and alleviate disease symptoms and (2) to help patients achieve optimal levels of activity.
- Patients best able to benefit from pulmonary rehabilitation are patients with symptomatic COPD; patients with unstable cardiovascular disorders should be referred for cardiac rehabilitation.
- Effective rehabilitation programming requires a multidisciplinary approach and combines physical reconditioning with education and psychosocial support.
- Rehabilitation does not alter the progressive deterioration in pulmonary function that occurs with chronic lung disease.
- Increased exercise tolerance, decreased intensity of symptoms, and improved activity levels are the best-documented benefits of pulmonary rehabilitation.
- The exercise evaluation provides the basis for the exercise prescription, yields the baseline data needed to assess a patient's progress, and helps determine the degree of hypoxemia or need for supplemental O_2 during exercise.
- Reconditioning should combine lower extremity and upper extremity aerobic exercises with ventilatory muscle training.
- The educational portion of a rehabilitation program should provide patients with knowledge they can use to help cope with their disease and manage symptoms better.
- Decisions regarding facilities, scheduling, class size, and equipment all can affect rehabilitation program outcomes.
- Patient charges should be based on projected costs, as offset by external funding or available insurance reimbursement.
- Cardiac rehabilitation should be considered first if a patient with pulmonary disease also has an underlying cardiac condition that needs to be addressed and appropriately managed.

References

1. COPD International: COPD statistics. <COPD International.com>, Accessed March 16, 2004.
2. Council on Rehabilitation: *Definition of rehabilitation*, Chicago, 1942, Council on Rehabilitation.
3. Petty TL: Pulmonary rehabilitation. *Basics RD* 4:1, 1975.
4. Harris PL: A guide to prescribing pulmonary rehabilitation. *Prim Care* 12:253, 1985.
5. Barach AL, Bickerman HA, Beck G: Advances in the treatment of nontuberculous pulmonary disease. *Bull N Y Acad Med* 28:353, 1952.
6. Pierce AK, et al: Responses to exercise training in patients with emphysema. *Arch Intern Med* 113:28, 1964.
7. Paez PN, et al: The physiological basis of training patients with emphysema. *Am Rev Respir Dis* 95:944, 1967.
8. Christie D: Physical training in chronic obstructive lung disease. *BMJ* 2:150, 1968.
9. Jastrzebski D, Gumola A, Gawlik R, et al: Dyspnea and quality of life in patients with pulmonary fibrosis after six weeks of respiratory rehabilitation. *J Physiol Pharmacol* 4:139–148, 2006.
10. Guell R, Resqueti V, Sangenis M: Impact of pulmonary rehabilitation on psychosocial morbidity in patients with severe COPD. *Chest* 129:899–904, 2006.
11. Naji NA, Conner MC, Donnelly SC, et al: Effectiveness of pulmonary rehabilitation in restrictive lung disease. *J Cardiopulm Rehabil* 26:237–243, 2006.

12. Lacasse Y, Goldstein R, Lasserson TJ: Pulmonary rehabilitation for chronic pulmonary disease. *Cochrane Database Syst Rev* (4):CD003793, 2006.
13. Ries AL, Bauldoff GS, Carlin BW, et al: Pulmonary rehabilitation. Joint ACCP/AACVPR evidence-based clinical practice guidelines. *Chest* 131:1S–42S, 2007.
14. California Pulmonary Rehabilitation Collaborative Group: Effects of pulmonary rehabilitation on dyspnea, quality of life, and health care costs in California. *J Cardiopulm Rehabil* 24:52–62, 2004.
15. Hughes RL, Davison R: Limitations of exercise in COPD. *Chest* 83:241, 1983.
16. Stoedefalke K: Effects of exercise training on blood lipids and lipoproteins in children and adolescents. *J Sports Sci Med* 6:313–318, 2007.
17. Hill NS: Pulmonary rehabilitation. *Proc Am Thorac Soc* 3:66–74, 2006.
18. American Association for Respiratory Care: AARC clinical practice guideline: exercise testing for evaluation of hypoxemia and/or desaturation. *Respir Care* 46:514, 2001.
19. American Association for Respiratory Care: AARC clinical practice guideline: pulmonary rehabilitation. *Respir Care* 47:617, 2002.
20. Porszasz J, Emtner M, Whipp BJ, et al: Endurance training decreases exercise-induced dynamic hyperinflation in patients with COPD. *Eur Respir J* 22:205s, 2003.
21. Wijkstra PJ, Ten Vergert EM, van Altena R, et al: Long-term benefits of rehabilitation at home on quality of life and exercise tolerance in patients with chronic obstructive pulmonary disease. *Thorax* 50:824, 1995.
22. Heppner PS, Morgan C, Kaplan RM, et al: Regular walking and long-term maintenance of outcomes after pulmonary rehabilitation. *J Cardiopulm Rehabil* 26:44–53, 2006.
23. Cockram J, Cecins N, Jenkins S: Maintaining exercise capacity and quality of life following pulmonary rehabilitation. *Respirology* 11:98–104, 2006.
24. Nici L, Donner C, Wouters E, et al: American Thoracic Society/European Respiratory Society statement on pulmonary rehabilitation. *Am J Respir Crit Care Med* 173:1390–1413, 2006.
25. Global strategy for diagnosis, management, and prevention of chronic obstructive pulmonary disease. 2008. Retrieved from <www.globalcopd.com/guidelineitem.asp?1=2&12=1&intld=2003>, Accessed November 23, 2009.
26. Lake FR, Henderson K, Briffa T, et al: Upper-limb and lower-limb exercise training in patients with chronic airflow obstruction. *Chest* 97:1077, 1990.
27. Weiner P, Azgad Y, Ganam R: Inspiratory muscle training combined with general exercise reconditioning in patients with COPD. *Chest* 102:1351, 1992.
28. Bickford LS, Hodgkin JE: National pulmonary rehabilitation survey. *Respir Care Clin N Am* 33:1030, 1988.
29. Medicare Learning Network: Comprehensive outpatient rehabilitation facility—fact sheet. ICN 904085. Department of Health and Human Services. Centers for Medicare and Medicaid Services (CMS), Bethesda, August 2011.
30. Hilling LR: Reimbursement for pulmonary rehabilitation remains elusive. RT for Decision Makers in Respir Care, editorial. 2005. <www.rtmagazine.com/issues/articles/2005-12_06.asp>, Accessed on March 15, 2010.
31. Mackaman D: New Medicare Part B services for 2010: pulmonary rehabilitation, HCPro, Medicare Find. 2010. <blogs.hcpro.com/medicarefind/2010/01/new-medicare-part-b-services>, Accessed on March 15, 2010.
32. American Thoracic Society: Pulmonary rehabilitation: final rule sets Medicare coverage and reimbursement policy. <www.thoracic.org/sections/about-ats/advocacy/washington-letter/letters/September-7-2009.html>.
33. CMS: Correction notice to the OPSS final rule (for pulmonary rehabilitation). Federal Register, December 31, 2009.
34. Kaplan RM, Ries AL: Quality of life as an outcome measure in pulmonary diseases. *J Cardiopulm Rehabil* 25:321–331, 2005.
35. Nishiyama O, Taniguchi H, Kondoh Y, et al: Factors in maintaining long-term improvements in health-related quality of life after pulmonary rehabilitation for COPD. *Qual Life Res* 14:2315–2321, 2005.
36. Varnell M: Therapists may benefit from NETT's rehab project. *Ad J Respir Care Pract* 12:7, 1999.
37. Foss CM: Lung volume reduction surgery: what's up with "NETT"? *AARC Times* 25:42, 2001.
38. National Emphysema Treatment Trial Research Group: A randomized trial comparing lung volume reduction surgery with medical therapy for severe emphysema. *N Engl J Med* 348:2059–2073, 2003.
39. National Emphysema Treatment Trial Research Group: Cost-effectiveness of lung volume reduction surgery for patients with severe emphysema. *N Engl J Med* 348:2092–2102, 2003.

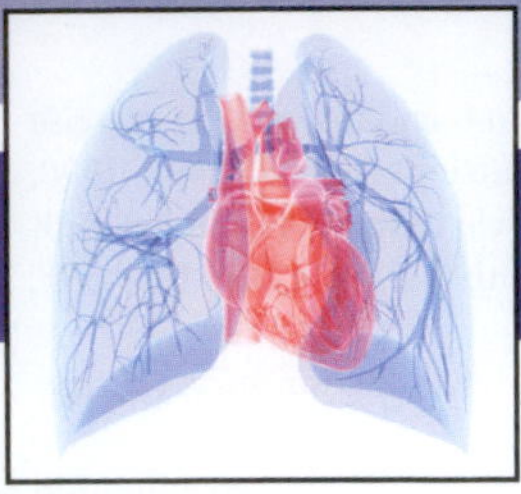

CHAPTER 56

Respiratory Care in Alternative Settings

ALBERT J. HEUER

CHAPTER OBJECTIVES

After reading this chapter you will be able to:

- Describe alternative care settings in which respiratory care is often performed.
- Discuss more recent developments and trends in respiratory care at alternative sites.
- Identify who regulates alternative care settings.
- List the standards that apply to the delivery of respiratory care in alternative settings.
- Describe how to help formulate an effective discharge plan.
- List factors to evaluate when assessing alternative care sites and support services.
- Discuss how to justify, provide, evaluate, and modify oxygen (O_2) therapy in alternative care settings.
- Explain how to select, assemble, monitor, and maintain O_2 therapy equipment in alternative settings.
- Identify the special challenges that exist in providing ventilatory support outside an acute care hospital.
- Describe how to instruct patients or caregivers and confirm their ability to provide care in alternative settings.
- Identify which patients benefit the most from ventilatory support outside acute care hospitals.
- Explain how to select, assemble, monitor, and maintain portable ventilatory support and continuous positive airway pressure equipment, including applicable interfaces or appliances.
- Describe proper documentation regarding patient evaluation and progress in alternative settings.
- State how to ensure safety and infection control in alternative patient care settings.

CHAPTER OUTLINE

KEY TERMS

alternative (nonacute) care
Centers for Medicare and Medicaid Services (CMS)
conditions of participation
durable medical equipment (DME) supplier
inexsufflator
long-term acute care hospitals (LTACHs)
molecular sieve
noninvasive ventilation (NIV)
O_2-conserving device
skilled nursing facility (SNF)
transtracheal oxygen therapy (TTOT)

Although home care remains the most common alternative site for providing health care, numerous other **alternative (nonacute) care** settings, including subacute facilities, **long-term acute care hospitals (LTACHs)**, rehabilitation facilities, and **skilled nursing facilities (SNFs)**, provide respiratory care to patients.[1] Alternative health care settings offer advantages over acute care facilities which include lower costs and enhanced patient comfort. In general, caring for respiratory patients in alternative sites can reduce patient care cost by as much as four- to five-fold.[1] However, improper or premature discharging of patients to alternative care settings and poor care plan implementation can erase these benefits and result in short-term readmission.

This chapter summarizes recent policy developments, discusses aspects of optimal discharge and patient care planning, and reviews various therapeutic respiratory modalities in alternative care sites. A major alternative site is the sleep laboratory where respiratory therapists (RTs) may conduct polysomnography, or sleep studies. However, the pathophysiology, diagnosis, and treatment of disorders of sleep is covered in Chapter 33.

MORE RECENT DEVELOPMENTS AND TRENDS

There have been several developments in the area of respiratory care in alternative sites. Such changes range from governmental initiatives affecting reimbursement, to enhancements involving respiratory equipment used in such settings.

Over the past two decades, an assortment of legislation and regulations was enacted that has reduced reimbursement for respiratory care in alternative settings. Furthermore, with the exceptions described below, reimbursement for RT time spent setting up the equipment and assessing and administering prescribed treatment to patients is not generally recognized. This has presented challenges to organizations and agencies attempting to provide quality care in alternative settings.[2-5]

The Patient Protection and Affordable Care Act (ACA) of 2010 has expanded health care coverage to many uninsured Americans, prohibits the exclusion of preexisting conditions, and increases the scope of coverage for certain types of preventive care. This law also encourages the formation of Accountable Care Organizations (ACOs), which are groups of doctors, hospitals, and health care providers who voluntarily come together to deliver coordinated patient care. However, many provisions of this law are still being modified and others are just beginning to be implemented. Consequently, the exact impact of this bill on respiratory care in general, and in alternative settings, is still somewhat unclear.[6]

Even more recently, some states have and continue to review and pilot programs to reimburse for certain therapies and education done by RTs in alternative settings. Specifically, some states' Medicaid programs are planning to begin reimbursement for certain types of education done by RTs for purposes such as asthma management. Furthermore, the American Association for Respiratory Care (AARC), through its Government Affairs initiatives, continues to promote legislation and sponsor efforts to expand the recognition of RTs.[7]

A further development stemming mainly from the aging U.S. population is a significant increase in the popularity of another form of alternative care site known as *assisted living facilities*. These facilities permit residents, who are generally elderly or disabled, to live in their own units either alone or with a companion. These arrangements permit residents to live relatively independently with the convenience and safety of routine health services nearby. A growing number of home care and other alternative sites have RTs providing care to their patients at such locations.

Other changes affecting RTs in alternative sites have resulted from research study outcomes. Starting in the late 1990s, there has been a small but growing body of research indicating that patients in alternative settings have better outcomes when treated by RTs.[8,9] It is hoped that this trend continues and encourages public agencies and private health care payers to recognize the value of RTs in alternative care settings and shape policies accordingly.

RELEVANT TERMS AND GOALS

As the elderly population increases and managed care becomes the dominant delivery model, more health care services are being provided outside the acute care hospital in such settings as SNFs, LTACHs, and at home. Rather than representing distinct entities, these alternative settings are part of an evolving continuum of care, are often elements of ACOs, and share the common goal of providing appropriate medical services cost-effectively and at settings suitable to a patient's condition.

Similar to the acute care setting, alternative care settings accomplish this goal through a coordinated team effort among many disciplines. The patient care team in alternative settings uses various specialized respiratory care services and equipment, including continuous O_2 therapy, long-term mechanical ventilation, aerosol drug administration, airway care, sleep apnea monitoring and treatment, and pulmonary rehabilitation. Each of the major alternative settings, the respiratory equipment used within them, and other relevant considerations including patient and family education are discussed in subsequent sections of this chapter.

Long-Term Subacute Care Hospitals

Advances in technology, research, and clinical specialization have permitted more acutely ill patients to be treated outside of large-scale, acute care hospitals. Over the past decade, LTACHs have become more prevalent. These facilities provide highly focused care to patients with complex medical conditions, including patients who have been ventilator-dependent and difficult to wean. Generally, LTACHs employ a highly experienced clinical staff, including RTs, to provide integrated interdisciplinary care using the latest equipment and protocols. During the 20- to 30-day typical length of stay at an LTACH, patients commonly experience significant improvement, including successful ventilator weaning and increased functionality.[10]

Subacute Care

According to the National Association of Subacute/Post Acute Care, *subacute care* is a comprehensive level of inpatient care for stable patients who (1) have experienced an acute event resulting from injury, illness, or exacerbation of a disease process; (2) have a determined course of treatment; and (3) require diagnostic or invasive procedures but not those requiring acute care.[10] Typically, the severity of the patient's condition requires active physician direction with frequent on-site visits, professional nursing care, significant ancillary services, and an outcomes-focused interdisciplinary approach employing a professional team.

The goal of acute care is to apply intensive resources to stabilize patients after severe episodic illness, whereas subacute care aims to restore the whole patient back to the highest practical level of function—ideally self-care. This holistic approach requires goal-oriented interdisciplinary team care, with frequent assessment of progress and a time-limited plan of care.[11]

Although most patients receiving subacute care are elderly, all age groups can be found at these sites. Pediatric, adolescent, and adult patients requiring ventilatory support or extensive care, depending on their diagnosis, are also cared for at these sites.

Home Care

Currently, most respiratory care in the alternative setting is provided in the home. The primary goal of home care is to provide quality health care services to patients in their home setting, minimizing their dependence on institutional care. In regard to respiratory home care, several specific objectives are evident.[12] Respiratory home care can contribute to the following:

- Supporting and maintaining life
- Improving patients' physical, emotional, and social well-being
- Promoting patient and family self-sufficiency
- Ensuring cost-effective delivery of care
- Maximizing patient comfort near the end of life

Most patients for whom respiratory home care is considered have chronic respiratory diseases. Applicable categories of disorders include the following:

- COPD
- Cystic fibrosis
- Chronic neuromuscular disorders
- Chronic restrictive conditions
- Carcinomas of the lung

Although not all aspects of respiratory home care have proven effective, various studies have shown that carefully selected treatment regimens can be of significant benefit to patients. These benefits include increased longevity, improved quality of life, increased functional performance, and a reduction in the individual and societal costs associated with hospitalization.[13,14]

STANDARDS

Standards for the delivery of respiratory care in the subacute and home settings are derived from several different sources. First, the Clinical Practice Guidelines created and published by the AARC offer RTs an evidence-based clinical framework for performing numerous respiratory procedures, including many procedures used in alternative care settings. Several of these guidelines are described throughout this chapter. Other standards are established by federal and state laws and private-sector accreditation.

Regulations

Most reimbursement for care in alternative settings is through either the federal Medicare program or federal or state Medicaid programs. As the largest purchaser of health services, the federal government (in connection with state and local governments) plays a major role in setting standards and regulating this industry. The federal agency responsible for the overall administration of Medicare and Medicaid is the **Centers for Medicare and Medicaid Services (CMS)**. Created in 1997, CMS oversees the framework for providing health coverage to elderly adults, disabled adults, and many disadvantaged young children in the United States.[5,6]

As part of this structure, CMS created the Medicare Provider Certification Program. This program ensures that institutional providers that serve Medicare beneficiaries, including hospitals, SNFs, LTACHs, home health agencies, and assisted living facilities, meet minimum health and safety requirements. These requirements are called **conditions of participation**. Current conditions of participation emphasize quality indicators, outcome measures, and cost efficiency designed to improve the quality and effectiveness of care provided to beneficiaries.[5,6] Institutions undergo certification surveys by either state survey agencies or private accrediting organizations, such as The Joint Commission (TJC), which is discussed in more detail in the following section.[15,16]

State survey agencies are partners with the federal government and principal agents in performing institutional certification. Typically, a state survey agency is either the state department of health or state licensing authority for health care facilities. The main function of the state survey agency is to ensure that facilities providing Medicare or Medicaid services comply with state and federal health, safety, and quality standards, as determined by periodic on-site inspections.

In addition to federal Medicare and Medicaid conditions of participation, most states set additional regulations that govern licensing of providers of care in alternative settings. Because these regulations are different in each state, readers should contact their state health department for details.

Private Sector Accreditation

The primary organization responsible for standard setting and voluntary accreditation of care providers in alternative settings is TJC. To assist hospitals and health care organizations with the accreditation process and overall performance improvement, TJC develops and publishes standards and National Patient Safety Goals for long-term and subacute care, home care, and assisted living facilities. The standards and goals relate to the delivery of quality patient care and the process and structure needed to do so. These categories include patient rights, ethics, and assessment and organizational leadership and management of information. The patient safety goals target for improvement common problem areas for health care organizations, such as proper patient identification, medication safety, and infection control.[15,16]

Approximately 90% of all hospitals and other health care organizations voluntarily subscribe to TJC accreditation and as a result are surveyed at least every 3 years. Insufficient or unsatisfactory compliance is flagged and requires formal follow-up to ensure correction. In certain circumstances, such unfavorable results may translate into a facility or an organization failing to maintain TJC accreditation.[15,16]

TRADITIONAL ACUTE CARE VERSUS ALTERNATIVE SETTING CARE

For the RT, working in the alternative care setting is distinctly different from working in an acute care hospital. Key differences involve resource availability, supervision and work schedules, documentation and assessment, and provider-patient interaction (Table 56-1).[17] Although some practitioners do not like the alternative work settings, many find the greater independence,

TABLE 56-1

Major Differences between Traditional Acute Care Setting and Alternative Settings for Delivery of Respiratory Care Services

Area	Traditional Setting (Acute Care Hospital)	Alternative Settings (Long-Term Acute Care, Subacute Care, Home Care)
Diagnostic resources	In-house laboratory, x-ray, ABG analysis, PFT	Must rely on outside vendors to provide diagnostic tests
Equipment support	Extensive; supported by piped-in O_2 and suctioning	Limited availability; must use portable O_2 and suctioning systems
Travel requirements	None; remain in one facility	Must travel between facilities or residences
Level of supervision	Direct supervision	Respiratory care provider works independently with minimal supervision
Patient assessment	Moderate—primarily provided by attending physician or residents	Heavy—core responsibility related to care planning
Documentation requirements	Moderate—limited to medical record keeping	Heavy—includes initial justification, ongoing follow-up, and often detailed financial record keeping
Work schedule	Specific hours	Varied work schedule, often including "on-call" off hours coverage
Time constraints	More than one shift to deliver therapy	Must complete all therapy during shift or visit
Patient-family interaction	Limited treatment time available; little family interaction	One-on-one therapy; intensive family interaction
Provider interaction	Primarily attending physicians and patient's nurses	Continuous interaction with all members of professional team

ABG, Arterial blood gas; *PFT*, pulmonary function testing.

professional team orientation, creativity, and higher level of patient and family interaction quite rewarding.

DISCHARGE PLANNING

Effective discharge planning provides the foundation for quality care in the alternative care setting. A properly designed and implemented discharge plan guides the multidisciplinary team in successfully transferring a respiratory care patient from the health care facility to an alternative site of care.[18] Effective implementation of the discharge plan also ensures the safety and efficacy of the patient's continuing care. In addition, Medicare's Readmission Reduction Program, which is part of the ACA, penalizes hospitals that have high short-term readmission rates for selected conditions, including COPD and CHF. Hence, it has become essential for hospitals and other health care providers to adopt and evaluate the effectiveness of evidence-based discharge protocols. In general, the key elements of such protocols include the following:

- Proper patient screening and evaluation
- Early identification of patients at high risk for short-term readmission
- Intensive patient and family education
- Multidisciplinary discharge planning that addresses all major potential barriers
- Patient follow-up.[4]

To guide practitioners in providing quality care, the AARC has published Clinical Practice Guideline: Discharge Planning for the Respiratory Care Patient.[4,19] Excerpts from this guideline appear in Clinical Practice Guideline 56-1.

Multidisciplinary Team

Although a physician normally initiates an order to discharge a patient to an alternative site, many other health care professionals are involved in the discharge process. Table 56-2 identifies these key professionals and their major responsibilities.[18] As with pulmonary rehabilitation (see Chapter 55), a team approach produces the best patient results. Communication and mutual respect for the talents and abilities of each team member are two key elements in making patient care in the alternative care setting work. Any breakdown in the system may delay or adversely affect patient discharge and the patient's physical health and mental well-being.

TABLE 56-2
Members of Patient Care Team in Alternative Settings

Discipline	Responsibilities
Utilization review	Advises or recommends consideration of patient discharge. Documents patient's in-hospital care
Discharge planning (social service or community or public health)	Brings all the needed elements together and ensures that a patient can be discharged to alternative care sites. Makes contacts with outside agencies that may assist with patient care
Physician	Writes order for patient discharge. Evaluates patient's condition and prescribes needed care. Establishes therapeutic objectives
Respiratory care	Evaluates patient and recommends appropriate respiratory care. Provides care and follow-up
Nursing	Writes and implements nursing care plan for patient. Assesses patient's status and provides necessary follow-up
Dietary and nutrition	Assesses patient's nutritional needs and writes dietary plan for patient. Makes arrangements for meals as necessary
Physical and occupational therapy	Provides necessary physical therapy and recommends any additional modalities or procedures
Psychiatry or psychology	Assesses patient's emotional status and provides any needed counseling or support
DME supplier or home care company	Provides needed equipment and supplies and handles any emergency situations involving delivery or equipment operation

Site and Support Service Evaluation

The primary factors determining the appropriate site for discharge are the goals and needs of the patient. These goals and needs should be met in an optimal and cost-effective manner using the resources available at the proposed site. In terms of institutional personnel, the staff of the selected facility must have all the competencies required to meet the patient's respiratory needs, be able to provide other needed health care services (e.g., physical therapy), and provide adequate 24-hour coverage.[17,19]

For a successful discharge to the home, it is essential that the ability of caregivers to learn and perform the required care be evaluated before transfer. Caregivers must clearly demonstrate and have documented the competencies required to care for the specific patient and, in combination, provide 24-hour coverage.[17,19]

RULE OF THUMB

To help ensure a successful discharge and confirm that a nonprofessional caregiver can perform a particular skill, the RT must go beyond demonstration and verbal confirmation of the caregiver's understanding. The RT must observe a return demonstration, whereby the caregiver properly performs the same procedural steps the RT demonstrated. In addition, providing the caregiver with written information relating to the procedural sets and equipment setup, maintenance, and basic troubleshooting can help reinforce key areas and ensure caregiver mastery of the competency.

Beyond the performance of a particular skill, it is imperative for the discharge team to ensure that an adequate number of professional and nonprofessional caregivers are part of the care plan to provide appropriate patient care coverage; this is particularly true when more complicated modes, such as

56-1 Discharge Planning for the Respiratory Care Patient

AARC Clinical Practice Guideline (Excerpts)*

INDICATIONS

Discharge planning is indicated for all respiratory care patients being considered for discharge or transfer to alternative sites. The plan should be developed and implemented as early as possible before transfer.

CONTRAINDICATIONS

There are no contraindications to the development of a discharge plan.

PRECAUTIONS AND POSSIBLE COMPLICATIONS

Undesirable or unexpected outcomes may occur if the patient is discharged before the full implementation of the plan. Undesirable or unexpected patient outcomes may also occur because of (1) the natural course of the disease or (2) other factors beyond the control of the discharge planning process.

METHOD

Discharge planning and implementation should begin as early as possible. The complexity of the plan is determined by the patient's medical condition, needs, and goals. The steps in the planning process are:

- Patient evaluation
  - Patient's medical condition
  - Psychosocial condition of patient and family
  - Respiratory and ventilatory support required
  - Desires for medical and ventilator care of patient and family
  - Patient's physical and functional ability and activities of daily living
  - Goals of care (patient and family, physician, health care professionals, bedside caregivers)
- Site evaluation for continuing care
  - Personnel
  - Physical environment (safety and suitability)
  - Equipment and supplies
  - Financial resources
- Development of multidisciplinary plan of care based on the patient's needs and goals
  - Plan for integration into the community
  - Medication administration
  - Plan for patient self-care as appropriate
  - Method for ongoing assessment of outcomes
  - Roles and responsibilities of team members for daily care management
  - Method to assess growth and development of pediatric patients
  - Documented mechanism for securing and training additional caregivers
  - Mechanism for communication among all members of health care team
  - Alternative emergency and contingency plan
  - Follow-up (e.g., medical, respiratory care) plans
  - Plan for use, maintenance, and troubleshooting of equipment
  - Plan for monitoring and appropriately responding to changes in patient's medical condition
  - Time frame for implementation
- Education and training with clear demonstration and documentation of competencies must occur before discharge and address key elements of the plan of care

ASSESSMENT OF NEED

All patients with a respiratory diagnosis should be assessed for a discharge plan.

ASSESSMENT OF OUTCOME

The desired outcome of the discharge plan is determined by the following:

- No readmission occurs because of discharge plan failure
- The equipment meets the patient's needs
- All treatments and modalities are performed satisfactorily by caregivers as instructed
- Caregivers are able to assess the patient, troubleshoot, and solve problems as they arise
- The treatment meets the patient's needs and goals
- The patient and family are satisfied
- The site provides the necessary services

MONITORING

The discharge plan coordinator and the physician should monitor the progress of the discharge plan. Each team member should participate in regularly scheduled team conferences to assess the progress of the discharge plan. Modifications may be made according to the goals and needs of the individual patient.

**For the complete guideline, see American Association for Respiratory Care: Clinical practice guideline: discharge planning for the respiratory care patient. Respir Care Clin N Am 40:1308, 1995.*

mechanical ventilation, or multiple therapies are required by the patient. Generally, substantial caregiver strain is associated with the care of such patients in alternative settings. Proper assessment of the capabilities and number of potential caregivers in light of the therapy needed at home and appropriate training of such individuals can help address this concern.

Equipment support and selected clinical services for patients receiving respiratory home care are often provided by a **durable medical equipment (DME) supplier**. DME suppliers range in size from multimillion-dollar national corporations offering a broad range of services to small local companies. Both large and small companies usually provide the following services:

- Service 24 hours, 7 days a week
- Third-party insurance processing
- Home instruction and follow-up by an RT
- Most forms of respiratory care

MINI CLINI

Minimizing Short-term Readmissions

PROBLEM: A COPD patient who was admitted to the hospital for an exacerbation, is now improving and targeted for discharge in two days. Due to patient quality-of-life considerations and newer financial penalties for excessive short-term readmissions, the patient care team wishes to help minimize the likelihood of a short-term (30-day) readmission for this individual and similar patients. What are some of the major considerations that should be addressed in the discharge plan for this patient to help avoid a short-term readmission?

Solution: COPD patients, especially those with moderate to severe disease, may often be deemed more clinically "fragile" and therefore especially prone to short-term readmissions. Hence, it is imperative for the multidisciplinary patient care team to quickly recognize the predisposition and to carefully plan to address the major risks. Education and patient follow-up are at the core of most short-term readmission reduction protocols. In this case, the education should focus on the pathophysiology of COPD and, more important, the purpose and importance of each element of the care plan. Reinforcing proper medication use such as bronchodilators and steroids as well as safe use of home oxygen are priorities. Phone, computer-aided or in-person patient follow-up should focus on continued compliance with the treatment plan, adherence to scheduled physician visits, and participation in any prescribed pulmonary rehabilitation programs. Barriers such as those related to transportation issues and assistance with activities of daily living should also be promptly identified and addressed. In some instances, transportation to physician visits and pulmonary rehabilitation sessions, or certified home-health aids, can be arranged in advance by the discharge planning team or patient follow-up clinicians.

When selecting a DME supplier from the available choices, the patient and family members and other members of the discharge planning team should consider the company's accreditation status, cost and scope of services, dependability, location, personnel, past track record, and availability. Charges should be reasonable and competitive, and clinical respiratory services should generally be provided by credentialed RTs.[17]

Finally, the selected site must meet basic safety standards and be suitable for managing the patient's specific condition. It should be free of fire, health, and safety hazards; provide adequate heating, cooling, and ventilation; provide adequate electrical service; and provide for patient access and mobility with adequate patient space (room to house medical and adaptive equipment) and storage facilities. The selected site must be capable of operating, maintaining, and supporting all equipment needed by the patient; including both respiratory and ancillary equipment and supplies as needed, such as the ventilator, suction, O_2, intravenous therapy, nutritional therapy, and adaptive equipment.[17,19] Box 56-1 lists key factors one should assess in planning the discharge of a respiratory care patient to the home environment.

Box 56-1 Assessing the Home Environment

ACCESSIBILITY
- In and out of house or apartment
- Accessibility between rooms
- Doorway width and threshold heights
- Stairways
- Wheelchair mobility
- Bathroom
- Kitchen
- Carpeting

EQUIPMENT
- Available space
- Electrical power supply
- Amperage
- Grounded outlets
- Presence of hazardous appliances

ENVIRONMENT
- Heating and ventilation
- Humidity
- Lighting
- Living space

A variety of equipment is available when a patient with a pulmonary disorder is discharged to an alternative setting. The most common types of respiratory therapy equipment used in alternative settings are discussed in the following sections.

MINI CLINI

Assessing the Home Environment

PROBLEM: A wheelchair-bound patient with a tracheostomy who requires mechanical ventilation is being discharged to the home care setting. Inspection of the two-story home reveals front and rear elevated porch entrances with all bedrooms upstairs. All room floors (except the kitchen and bathrooms) are covered with high pile carpeting. The largest bedroom is 12 ft by 14 ft. The electrical service is rated at 75 amps, and the only grounded outlets are in the kitchen and garage. Heating is provided by a forced hot-air system; there is a single window air conditioner in the patient's bedroom.

What problems do you see, and what changes would you recommend to provide the proper home environment for this patient?

Solution: Although wheelchair-bound, this patient is still mobile. Both the elevated porch entrances and the high pile carpeting restrict mobility. A ramp entrance needs to be constructed, and the carpeting needs to be removed or covered with a flat, hard surface material. Given the size of the patient's upstairs room and the obstacle of the stairwell, it would be best to identify a large first-story room for conversion to a bedroom. Because the patient is likely to need at least an electrical bed, ventilator, and suction machine, the electrical service capacity is inadequate and needs upgrading to ensure at least 15 to 20 amps in the patient area, with 200 amps overall. Appliance, counter, sink, and toilet heights need to be assessed for easy patient access.

OXYGEN THERAPY IN ALTERNATIVE SETTINGS

O_2 therapy is the most common mode of respiratory care in alternative care settings. This high use is based on the fact that O_2 therapy improves both survival and quality of life in selected patient groups, especially patients with advanced COPD.[20, 21] In particular, studies have shown improved nocturnal O_2 saturation, reduced pulmonary artery pressure, and lower pulmonary vascular resistance with appropriate outpatient O_2 therapy.[22,23]

To guide practitioners in providing quality care, the AARC has published a Practice Guideline on Oxygen Therapy in the Home or Extended Care Facility.[24] Excerpts from the AARC guideline, including the indications, contraindications, precautions and possible complications, method, assessment of need, assessment of outcome, and monitoring, appear in Clinical Practice Guideline 56-2.

Oxygen Therapy Prescription

As indicated in Clinical Practice Guideline 56-2, O_2 prescriptions must be based on documented hypoxemia, as determined by either arterial blood gas analysis or oximetry. Prescriptions for O_2 therapy no longer can be based simply on patient diagnosis or signs and symptoms. In addition, as-needed O_2 therapy is no longer acceptable in the alternative care setting.

When the need for O_2 therapy is established, the physician writes a prescription. A prescription for O_2 therapy in the alternative care setting must include the following elements:[25]

- Flow rate in L/min or concentration or both
- Frequency of use in hours per day and minutes per hour (if applicable)
- Duration of need
- Diagnosis (severe primary lung disease, secondary conditions related to lung disease and hypoxia, related conditions or symptoms that may improve with O_2)
- Laboratory evidence (arterial blood gas analysis or oximetry under the appropriate testing conditions); home care companies cannot provide this testing
- Additional medical documentation (no acceptable alternatives to home O_2 therapy)

For home use, the ordering physician must authorize O_2 therapy using the CMS Certification of Medical Necessity form for O_2. After the need for long-term therapy is documented, repeat arterial blood gas analysis or SpO_2 measurements are not needed. However, blood O_2 levels may still be measured when the need arises to assess changes in the patient's condition.[26]

Supply Methods

Most alternative care sites do not have bulk O_2 storage or delivery systems. In these settings, O_2 normally is supplied from one of the following three sources:[27] (1) compressed O_2 cylinders, (2) liquid O_2 systems, or (3) O_2 concentrators. Table 56-3 summarizes the major advantages and disadvantages of each system.

Compressed Oxygen Cylinders

For practical reasons, the primary use of compressed O_2 cylinders in alternative settings is either for ambulation (small cylinders) or as a backup to liquid or concentrator supply systems (H/K cylinders). Safety measures for cylinder O_2 are the same as those discussed in Chapters 40 and 41. For home use, the RT should thoroughly review these safety measures with both the patient and family members. After instruction, the RT should always confirm and document abilities of caregivers to use the delivery system safely.

TABLE 56-3
Advantages and Disadvantages of Major Alternative Oxygen Supply Systems

System	Advantages	Disadvantages
Compressed O_2	Good for small volume user	Large cylinders are heavy and bulky
	No waste or loss	High-pressure safety hazard
	Stores O_2 indefinitely	Provides limited volume
	Widespread availability	Requires frequent deliveries
	Portability (small cylinders)	Tight valves can be a problem
Liquid O_2 system	Provides large volumes	Must be delivered as needed
	Low-pressure system (20-25 psi)	Loss of O_2 because of venting of system when not in use
	Portable units can be refilled from reservoir (up to 8-hr supply at 2 L/min)	Low temperature safety hazard
		Cannot operate ventilators or other high-pressure devices
	Valuable for rehabilitation	Some difficulty in filling portable unit
O_2 concentrator	No waste or loss	Disruption in electrical service renders system inoperable
	Low-pressure system (15 psi)	Backup O_2 is needed
	Cost-effective when continual supply of O_2 is needed	Cannot operate ventilators or other high-pressure devices
		FiO_2 decreases with increasing flow
	Eliminates need for deliveries	High electrical costs possible

56-2 Oxygen Therapy in the Home or Alternative Site Health Care Facility

AARC Clinical Practice Guideline (Excerpts)*

INDICATIONS

- Documented hypoxemia
- Adults, children, and infants >28 days old: PaO_2 ≤55 mm Hg or SaO_2 ≤88% (room air)
- PaO_2 56 to 59 mm Hg or SaO_2 ≤89% in association with specific clinical conditions (e.g., cor pulmonale, congestive heart failure, or erythrocythemia with hematocrit >56%)
- Patients who do not qualify for O_2 therapy at rest may qualify during ambulation, sleep, or exercise if SaO_2 decreases to <89% during these specific activities

CONTRAINDICATIONS

No absolute contraindications to O_2 therapy exist when indications are present.

PRECAUTIONS AND POSSIBLE COMPLICATIONS

- In spontaneously breathing hypoxemic patients with COPD, O_2 therapy may increase $PaCO_2$
- Problems may occur if the patient fails to comply with the physician's orders or receives inadequate instruction
- Complications may result from use of nasal cannulas or transtracheal catheters
- Fire hazard is increased in the presence of increased O_2 concentrations
- Bacterial contamination associated with certain nebulizers and humidifiers may occur
- Physical hazards include unsecured cylinders, ungrounded equipment, and liquid O_2 burns
- Power or equipment failure can lead to an inadequate O_2 supply

ASSESSMENT OF NEED

- Initial need is determined by documented hypoxemia at rest or during activity (see Indications)
- Additional measurements of blood gas tension or saturation by invasive or noninvasive methods may be indicated whenever there is a major change in clinical status that may be cardiopulmonary related
- Blood gases should be repeated after 1 to 3 months to determine the need for long-term O_2 therapy
- Once the need for long-term O_2 therapy has been documented, repeated measures are unnecessary other than to follow the course of the disease, to assess changes in clinical status, or to facilitate changes in the O_2 prescription

ASSESSMENT OF OUTCOME

Outcome is determined by clinical and physiologic assessment to establish adequacy of patient response to therapy.

MONITORING

- Patient
    - Initial and ongoing clinical assessment of patient's need for O_2 therapy should be performed by licensed or credentialed RTs (RRT or CRT) or other professional persons with equivalent training and documented ability to perform the tasks as part of a patient-specific plan of care/plan of service
    - Care plans should be developed at the initiation of O_2 therapy based on the needs of the individual patient and updated as necessary
    - Measurement of baseline O_2 tension or saturation is essential before O_2 therapy is begun. Measurements should be repeated when clinically indicated or to follow the course of the disease, as determined by the attending physician
    - Measurements of O_2 saturation also should be made to determine appropriate O_2 flow for ambulation, exercise, or sleep
- Equipment
    - All O_2 delivery equipment should be checked at least once daily by the patient or caregiver. Facets to be assessed include proper function of the equipment, prescribed flow rates, remaining liquid or compressed gas content, and backup supply
    - O_2 equipment should be serviced and maintained in accordance with the manufacturer's specification and consistent with all federal, state, and local laws and regulations
    - In the event there are no manufacturer specifications or guidance, O_2 equipment should be checked for proper function and performance by an appropriately trained or credentialed person no less than once per year

**For the complete guideline, see American Association for Respiratory Care: Clinical practice guideline: oxygen therapy in the home or alternate site health care facility. Respir Care 52:1063, 2007.*

In addition to the cylinder gas, a pressure-reducing valve with flowmeter is needed to deliver O_2 at the prescribed flow. Standard clinical flowmeters deliver flows up to 15 L/min; however, flows used in alternative settings are typically in the 0.25 to 5 L/min range. For this reason, the RT should select a calibrated low-flow flowmeter whenever possible (see Chapter 40).

As in the hospital, there is usually no need to humidify nasal O_2 at flows of 4 L/min or less.[24] If humidification is needed, a simple unheated bubble humidifier can be used. Because the mineral content of tap water may be high (hard water), water used in these humidifiers should be distilled. Otherwise, the porous diffusing element may become occluded. Although complete blockage is unlikely, occlusion of the diffusing element can impair humidification and alter flow.

Liquid Oxygen Systems

Though the higher cost of liquid O_2 delivery systems versus other systems has greatly reduced its use, such systems offer some advantages over others and are therefore still used under certain conditions in alternative settings. One of the main advantages of liquid O_2 systems relates to the fact that 1 cubic ft of liquid O_2 equals 860 cubic ft of gas and therefore it is possible to store large quantities in small spaces. As shown in Figure 56-1, a typical personal liquid O_2 system is a miniature version of a hospital liquid oxygen system. Similar to its larger counterpart, this system consists of a reservoir unit similar in design to a thermos bottle. The inner container of liquid O_2 is suspended in an outer container, with a vacuum in between. The liquid O_2 is kept at approximately −300° F. Because of constant vaporization, gaseous O_2 always exists above the liquid. When the cylinder is not in use, this vaporization maintains pressures between 20 psi and 25 psi. When pressures increase above this level, gas vents out the pressure relief valve.

When flow is turned on, gaseous O_2 passes through a vaporizing coil, where it is warmed by exposure to room temperature. It leaves the system through an outlet, where it is metered by a flow control valve. These metering devices are usually calibrated in 0.5-L/min units and limited to a maximum flow of 5 to 8 L/min.

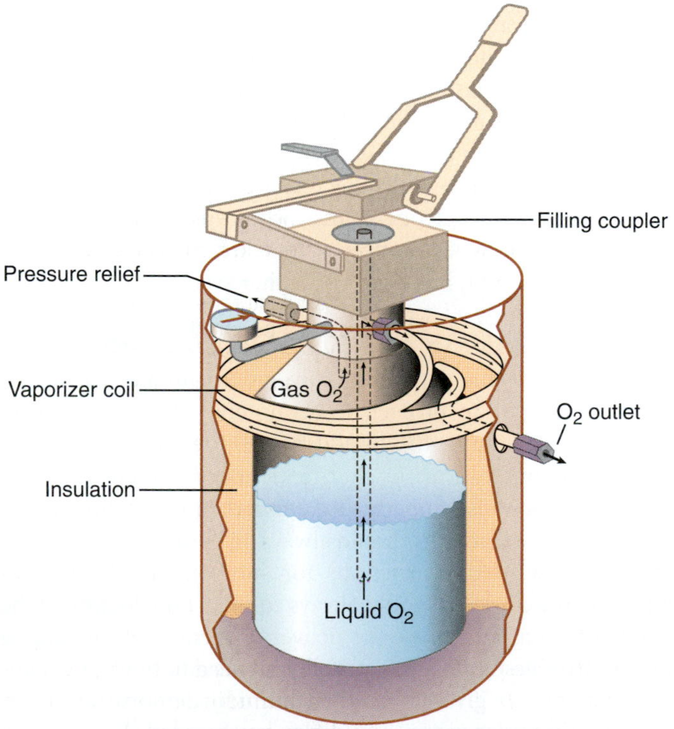

FIGURE 56-1 Diagram of a personal liquid oxygen supply system. (Modified from Lampton LM: Home and outpatient oxygen therapy. In Brashear RE, Rhodes ML, editors: Chronic obstructive lung disease, St Louis, 1978, Mosby.)

Depending on manufacturer and model, small liquid O_2 cylinders hold 45 to 100 lb of liquid O_2. To calculate duration of flow of a liquid O_2 system, one first converts the weight of liquid O_2 in pounds to the equivalent volume of gaseous O_2 in liters. At normal liquid cylinder operating pressures, 1 lb of liquid O_2 equals approximately 344 L of gaseous O_2. The accompanying Mini Clini provides an example of how the clinician can compute the duration of flow in a liquid O_2 system.

MINI CLINI

Computing Duration of Flow of a Liquid Oxygen System

PROBLEM: A home care patient receives nasal O_2 at 2 L/min from a 100-lb liquid O_2 system. The system gauge indicates that the cylinder is half full. Approximately how long will this system last until empty?

Solution:

Step 1: Compute the available liquid O_2 (in lb)

$$100 \times 0.5 = 50\ \text{lb}$$

Step 2: Compute the available gaseous O_2

$$\text{Weight (lb) remaining} \times \text{factor}$$
$$50\ \text{lb} \times 344\ \text{L/lb} = 17{,}200\ \text{L}$$

Step 3: Divide the available volume of gaseous O_2 by the prescribed liter flow

$$\text{Duration of flow (min)} = \frac{\text{Volume of gaseous } O_2 \text{ (L)}}{\text{Liter flow (L/min)}}$$

$$\text{Duration of flow (min)} = \frac{17{,}200\ \text{L}}{2\ \text{L/min}} = 8600\ \text{min} = 143.3\ \text{hr}$$
$$= 6\ \text{days}$$

To help avoid these computations, many manufacturers provide simple conversion charts. Table 56-4 is an example of a conversion chart for a typical 100-lb personal liquid O_2 system.

Many personal liquid O_2 systems also come with smaller portable units (Figure 56-2). This system is suitable for an

TABLE 56-4

Conversion Chart for Computing Duration of Flow for 100-lb (40-L) Liquid Oxygen Reservoir

Gauge reading	1	2	3	4	4
Weight (lb)	12.5	25	50	75	100
Liquid liters	5	10	20	30	40
Gaseous liters	4303	8606	17,212	25,818	34,424
Duration of Flow (Hours)					
Flow (L/min)					
1	72	143	287	430	574
2	36	72	143	215	287
3	24	48	96	143	191
4	18	36	72	108	143
5	14	29	57	86	115

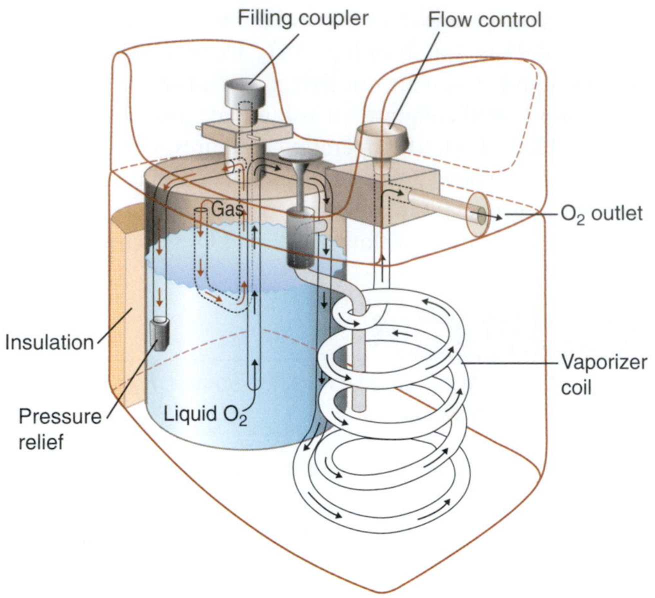

FIGURE 56-2 Diagram of a portable liquid oxygen unit. (Modified from Lampton LM: Home and outpatient oxygen therapy. In Brashear RE, Rhodes ML, editors: Chronic obstructive lung disease, St Louis, 1978, Mosby.)

Box 56-2 Steps for Filling a Portable Liquid Oxygen Unit from the Reservoir

1. Check the gauge on the reservoir unit to ensure there is enough liquid O_2 in the reservoir to fill the portable unit.
2. Check the connectors on both units to ensure that they are clean and dry. Moisture on these connectors could cause the connectors to freeze together.
3. Connect the portable unit to the reservoir according to the manufacturer's instructions, generally by engaging the fittings on the portable unit and reservoir, then carefully twisting the portable unit until it "seats." The flow-rate controller should be turned off.
4. Open the portable unit vent. Allow the portable unit to fill. The portable unit is filled when excess O_2 begins venting and the sound emitted from the unit changes. Close the vent valve.
5. Disengage the portable unit according to the manufacturer's instructions, generally by carefully twisting the portable tank until it is released from the liquid reservoir.

ambulatory patient who is capable of physical activity. Typical portable units weigh 5 to 14 lb and can be refilled directly from the stationary reservoir. Most portable units come with a carrying case or small cart and can provide 5 to 8 hours of O_2 at a flow of 2 L/min. Either an adjustable flow restrictor or a Bourdon-type gauge is used to meter flow, with a weight gauge used to indicate O_2 contents. The functional use time of portable liquid O_2 units can be extended with O_2-conserving devices, including the demand-flow systems discussed later in this chapter.

Because of the extremely low temperature of liquid O_2, patients and caregivers must be extremely careful when refilling these portable systems. Box 56-2 lists the steps needed to fill a portable liquid O_2 unit from a reservoir.[27]

Oxygen Concentrators

An O_2 concentrator is an electrically powered device that physically separates the O_2 in room air from nitrogen. These systems are much more common than either gaseous tanks or liquid systems. The most common type of concentrator uses a **molecular sieve** to extract O_2.[27]

The molecular sieve concentrator uses a pump to compress and deliver filtered room air to one of two sets of sieves (Figure 56-3). These sieves contain sodium-aluminum silicate pellets that absorb nitrogen, carbon dioxide (CO_2), and water vapor. To remove these unwanted gases from the pellets, an automatic pressure swing cycle switches back and forth between the sieve sets. One set is pressurized to produce O_2, and the other is depressurized to purge nitrogen, CO_2, and water vapor.

Gas leaving the sieves is stored in a small accumulator. At flows of 1 to 2 L/min, the typical molecular sieve concentrator provides between 92% and 95% O_2. At 5 L/min or greater, O_2 concentrations are between 85% and 93%.[27] The output of many concentrator models has been limited to 5 L/min. However, more recently, models capable of delivering 10 L/min, have been introduced. In addition, technologic advances have accounted for other enhancements to O_2 production and delivery devices in alternative care settings. One example is portable battery-powered concentrators with demand-flow conserving capabilities. These units afford patients receiving low-flow O_2 increased mobility and have been approved for use in most commercial aircraft.

O_2 concentrators are the most cost-efficient supply method for patients in alternative care settings who need continuous low-flow O_2. For home use, a concentrator running 24 hours/day increases the average monthly electrical bill by only 5% to 10%. Depending on the season, heat given off by the concentrator's compressor can also affect energy usage by increasing room temperature. Nonetheless, when used with patients receiving low-flow O_2, concentrators are just as effective in increasing blood O_2 levels as most other systems.

Problem Solving and Troubleshooting

Technical problems with O_2 supply systems in alternative settings are similar to problems encountered in the acute care hospital (see Chapter 40). In addition to these technical problems, situations can arise when patients or caregivers fail to follow instructions properly. To avoid communication problems, verbal instructions should always be reinforced by providing simple written instructions for subsequent reference. In addition, the clinician should always confirm and document the ability of caregivers to use the delivery system safely, including how to troubleshoot simple problems. The ability of caregivers and patients to give an adequate return demonstration on proper equipment usage should also be recorded.[24]

To avoid problems before they occur, the patient or caregiver should be instructed to check all O_2 delivery equipment at least once a day.[18] The proper function of all equipment, including

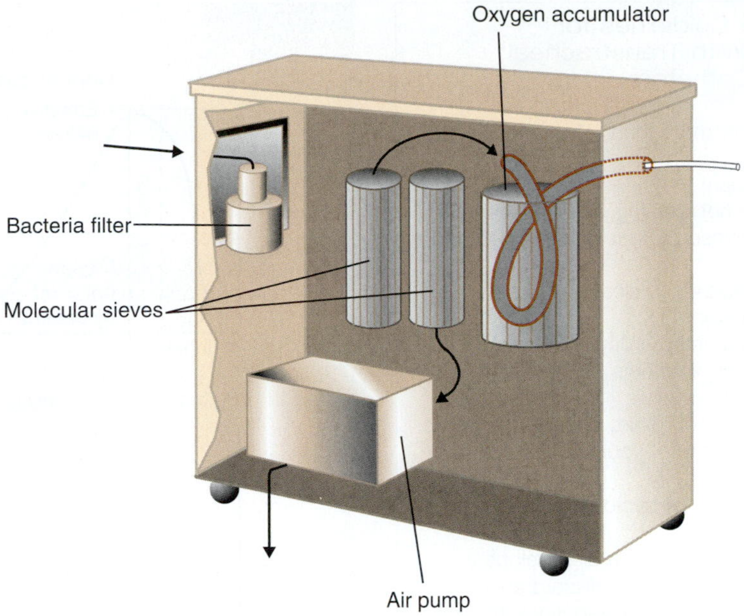

FIGURE 56-3 A molecular sieve oxygen concentrator.

liter flow, connections, and fractional inspired oxygen (FiO_2) levels, should also be confirmed. If the FiO_2 is less than the manufacturer's specification at the given flow, the pellet canisters are probably exhausted and should be replaced.[28, 29] Last, concentrator air inlet filters must be cleaned weekly. In the home setting, providing the patient or caregiver with a simple checklist form can help ensure that these important tasks are performed regularly.

In contrast to the hospital setting, O_2 supply problems in the alternative care setting cannot always be addressed immediately. For this reason, the clinician must ensure that all such systems have an emergency backup supply. This backup supply is normally provided by a large H/K gaseous cylinder, or at a minimum, an E cylinder. If the primary O_2 supply of a home care patient is by concentrator, the home care RT should notify the electric power company in writing that life-support equipment is in use; in the event of a power outage, many utility companies will try to give priority to that location. For patients in more remote geographic areas, an emergency gasoline electrical generator is often recommended.

Possible physical hazards to patients and caregivers include unsecured cylinders, ungrounded equipment, mishandling of liquid (resulting in burns), and fire.[24] Careful preliminary instruction, followed by ongoing assessment of the environment, can help minimize these problems. Bacterial contamination of nebulizer or humidification systems is another potential problem.[24] Infection control procedures designed to minimize bacterial contamination are discussed later in this chapter.

RULE OF THUMB

If an O_2 concentrator cannot supply at least 85% O_2 at 5 L/min, the pellet canisters are probably exhausted and should be replaced.

Delivery Methods

The most common O_2 delivery system for long-term care is the nasal cannula. Simple O_2 masks and air entrainment masks may also be used but are much less common. To decrease O_2 use and costs, numerous O_2-conserving devices have been developed, including transtracheal O_2 catheter, reservoir cannula, and demand or pulsed-dose O_2 delivery systems.

RULE OF THUMB

O_2-conserving devices exhibit performance comparable to a nasal cannula at approximately one-third to one-half the flow. Based on this knowledge, when switching a patient from a nasal cannula at 2 L/min to an O_2-conserving device, the RT would start out at half the original flow, in this case, 1 L/min. The RT would then assess the response using a pulse oximeter and adjust the flow accordingly.

The performance characteristics, advantages, and disadvantages of transtracheal O_2 catheters and reservoir cannulas are described in detail in Chapter 41. We focus here on the application of the transtracheal O_2 catheter and the technical aspects of demand-flow systems.

Transtracheal Oxygen Therapy

Transtracheal oxygen therapy (TTOT) is O_2 delivered via a catheter with a small orifice that is inserted through the skin and neck tissue into the trachea. Although uncommon, as described in Chapter 41, this delivery method offers advantages of improved cosmetic appearance and lower flows to achieve the same therapeutic effect. However, not all long-term O_2 patients are good candidates for TTOT, and only those who

Box 56-3 Self-Care Guidelines for Patients With Transtracheal Oxygen Catheters

- Never remove the catheter for more than a few minutes to avoid tract closure.
- Always keep the catheter clean.
- If you believe the catheter is not working properly even after cleaning it or if you cannot reinsert it, put on a nasal cannula and call your physician.
- If your humidifier pop-off is sounding, clear any hose blockage and clean the catheter.
- Never remove or insert the catheter while O_2 is flowing.
- Do not use antibiotics or other ointments at the site of catheter insertion.
- Try to keep the O_2 hose under your shirt, blouse, T-shirt, or pajama top and clipped to the top of your pants, skirt, or pajama bottom.
- Treat the O_2 hose as your lifeline by avoiding abuse or damage.
- If the equipment becomes split or broken or develops a permanent kink or foul odor, immediately discard and replace it. Catheters and hoses should be routinely replaced every 3 months.
- Always take catheter cleaning supplies, a nasal cannula, and a spare catheter when traveling.

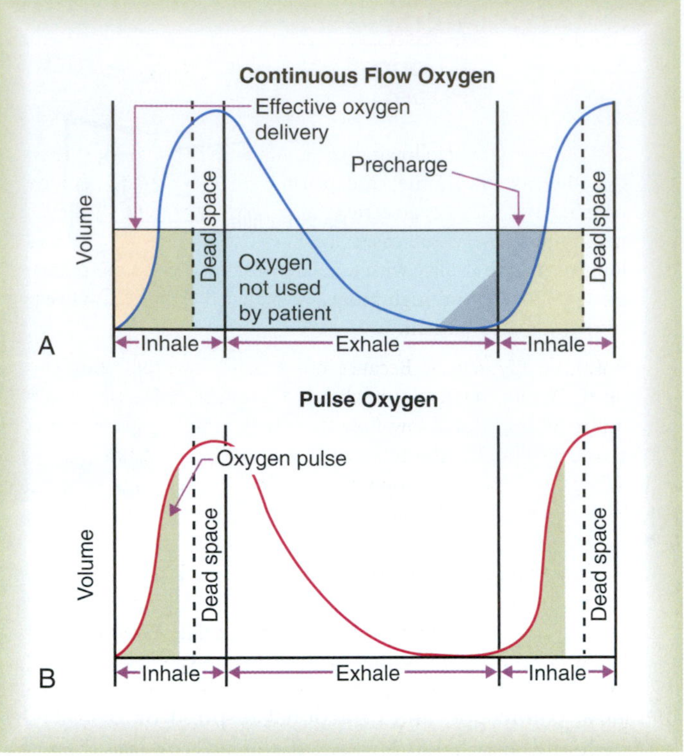

FIGURE 56-4 Demand-flow oxygen delivery. With continuous flow **(A),** most oxygen is delivered during the first half of inhalation, with the remainder wasted. With a coordinated pulse **(B),** most oxygen is delivered during the first 25% of inspiration, and no waste occurs. (Modified from O'Donohue WJ: The future of home oxygen therapy. Respir Care 33:1125, 1988.)

meet one or more of the following criteria should be considered: (1) cannot be adequately oxygenated with standard approaches, (2) do not comply well when using other devices, (3) exhibit complications from nasal cannula use, (4) prefer TTOT for cosmetic reasons, and (5) have need for increased mobility.[30]

As with most modalities in alternative care settings, the success of TTOT depends mainly on effective patient education and ongoing self-care with professional follow-up. Key patient responsibilities include routine catheter cleaning and recognizing and troubleshooting common problems. Box 56-3 describes key self-care guidelines for patients with transtracheal O_2 catheters.

Demand-Flow Oxygen Systems

A demand-flow O_2 delivery device, also known as a pulsed-dose **O2-conserving device**, uses a flow sensor and valve to synchronize gas delivery with the beginning of inspiration.[31] As indicated in Figure 56-4, *A,* with continuous O_2 flow, most of the effective O_2 delivery occurs during the first half of inspiration. All the O_2 delivered during the latter half of inspiration and throughout most of expiration is wasted. Figure 56-4, *B,* shows the effect of a synchronized pulse of O_2 delivered at the beginning of inspiration. Ideally, this O_2 pulse should occur during the first quarter of inspiration. Under these conditions, a pulsed O_2 system can produce SaO_2 levels equal to levels seen with continuous flow, while using 60% less O_2.[32]

In theory, demand-flow O_2 systems provide the greatest savings in O_2 use for a given level of arterial saturation. Recent improvements to demand-flow systems have made them more reliable and user-friendly, addressing the major disadvantages of earlier versions. As a result of these improvements and the ability of these devices to increase the duration of flow by two or three times, they have now gained wide acceptance.[31,33]

Selecting a Long-Term Oxygen Delivery System

As when selecting hospital-based O_2 therapy systems, the "three P's" should always be considered when selecting a long-term O_2 system: purpose, patient, and performance. The goal is always to match the *performance* of the equipment to both the objectives of therapy *(purpose)* and the *patient's* special needs. Patients requiring low-flow home O_2 and enhanced mobility should be considered for a portable concentrator alone, or one with a conserving feature or a liquid O_2 setup with a pulsed-dose O_2-conserving device.

Problem Solving and Troubleshooting

Most problems with long-term O_2 delivery systems are related to people. Patients and caregivers often fail to follow instructions or comply with the prescribed therapeutic or maintenance regimen.[24] Generally, caregivers should be allowed to operate and maintain O_2 delivery devices only after they have been instructed by credentialed RTs and have demonstrated the appropriate level of skill. In no case should the patient or caregiver be allowed or instructed to alter flow settings. Instead,

MINI CLINI

Selecting a Long-Term Oxygen Delivery System

PROBLEM: The following three patients require long-term O_2: (1) a stable home care patient with restricted activity needing low FiO_2; (2) an active home care patient with low FiO_2 needs who desires increased mobility; and (3) a patient in a long-term care facility with a tracheostomy who needs moderate levels of O_2 and high humidity. Select the best O_2 delivery system for each patient.

Solution: *Patient 1:* Because most home care patients who need O_2 are relatively stable, and because FiO_2 needs are minimal, traditional low-flow therapy by nasal cannula (using a concentrator) is the most common and accepted approach. When combined with a portable gas cylinder (for backup and limited walking), this combination is ideal for patients with restricted activity.

Patient 2: For an active patient with low FiO_2 needs who desires increased mobility, a conserving device used in conjunction with a portable concentrator (coupled with a home-based concentrator) is the ideal choice. Given that selected models of reservoir cannulas are poorly accepted by some patients, the choice of conserving device usually narrows to a transtracheal catheter or a demand-flow/pulse-dosed system. Patients who meet the criteria for TTOT and can provide meticulous self-care should be considered for TTOT. Alternatively, demand-flow/pulsed-dose systems are also a viable choice.

Patient 3: Patients with artificial airways in alternative sites who need O_2 present a special problem. Because of high O_2 use and infection concerns, an O_2-powered air entrainment nebulizer is unsatisfactory. Instead, a compressor-driven humidifier with supplemental O_2, bled in at low flows from a concentrator or liquid system, should be used. In this case, the RT must confirm the FiO_2 by calibrated analyzer.

when in doubt, they should be taught to switch to the backup supply at the same liter flow.

Technical problems are most common with TTOT and demand-flow systems. Most problems with TTOT are related to initial catheter insertion or ongoing maintenance. Most problems with demand-flow systems are based on the current limits of this technology.

The most common complications of TTOT are listed in Box 56-4. Although these problems occur infrequently, the clinician must be on constant guard for their occurrence. In particular, the RT should immediately report any evidence of tract tenderness, fever, excessive cough, increased dyspnea, or subcutaneous emphysema to the patient's physician.

To avoid complications or product failure, catheters and their tubing should be replaced every 3 months, at which time a checkup by the physician is also recommended. The patient or caregiver should clean the catheter every day, per the self-care guidelines listed within this chapter. Patients should be instructed always to put on a nasal cannula and to call the physician if any major problem occurs.

Similarly, there can be problems with the use of demand-flow or pulsed-dose O_2-conserving systems. Although improvements to these devices have significantly increased their use, these units tend to add to the weight of portable setups, and they can easily be damaged. These and other potential problems with demand-flow O_2 delivery systems are listed in Box 56-5.[33]

Box 56-4 Complications of Transtracheal Oxygen Therapy

- Bleeding*
- Pneumothorax*
- Bronchospasm*
- Subcutaneous emphysema
- Catheter dislodgment or lost tract
- Increased sputum production
- Blockage by inspissated mucus
- Infection or abscess
- Extensive self-care and cleaning to avoid infection or blockage
- Tract tenderness

*Complications associated mainly with insertion.

Box 56-5 Potential Problems With Demand-Flow Oxygen Delivery Systems

- The devices can be cumbersome and cosmetically unattractive.
- The initial and maintenance costs of equipment can be high and not fully reimbursed.
- Earlier devices may possess poor response times and delays in valve opening or closing.
- The devices tend to be fragile and can be damaged easily if they fall.
- Most units require a battery, which needs to be charged or replaced.
- The catheters and sensors may malfunction because of sensor dislodgment or plugging or changes in breathing problems.

VENTILATORY SUPPORT IN ALTERNATIVE SETTINGS

Providing successful ventilatory support outside the acute care hospital requires careful patient selection and good discharge planning.[34] Key factors include an interdisciplinary team approach, effective caregiver and family education, thorough assessment and preparation of the environment, and careful selection of needed equipment and supplies. Properly planned ventilatory support delivered in alternative settings can provide major benefits for both the patient and family, with substantial savings in health care costs.[35]

Patient Selection

Most patients needing ventilatory support outside the acute care hospital fall into one of the following three broad categories:[36]

1. Patients unable to maintain adequate ventilation over prolonged periods (in particular, noninvasive nocturnal or intermittent use)
2. Patients requiring continuous mechanical ventilation for long-term survival
3. Patients who are terminally ill with short life expectancies

Table 56-5 provides more detailed profiles of these patient groups. In addition to adults, a growing number of ventilator-assisted children are being managed in alternative settings. The same basic principles of discharge planning and patient care for adult patients should be followed for ventilator-assisted children.[37]

Regardless of diagnosis, patients being considered for ventilatory support in alternative settings must be medically and psychologically stable. In regard to assessing patient stability, Box 56-6 outlines the criteria developed by the American College of Chest Physicians (ACCP).[38]

Settings and Approaches

The most common setting for ventilatory support outside the acute care hospital is the home. Additional sites include long-term care facilities, including specialized long-term units such as LTACHs, designed specifically for ventilator patients.[38,39]

Based on individual evaluation of patient need, one of the following two major support approaches may be considered: (1) invasive or (2) noninvasive support. In alternative settings, invasive ventilatory support always involves application of positive pressure ventilation by tracheotomy. Noninvasive approaches include positive pressure and negative pressure ventilation via an intact upper airway or abdominal displacement methods.[40,41]

Standards and Guidelines

Standards and guidelines for ventilatory support outside the acute care hospital continue to evolve.[38,42] The AARC developed a clinical practice guideline on long-term invasive mechanical ventilation in the home.[43] Excerpts from these guidelines appear in Clinical Practice Guideline 56-3.

Special Challenges in Providing Home Ventilatory Support

Institutions that provide ventilatory support in alternative settings differ from acute care facilities mainly in their level of technology support. The home setting not only lacks this support but also must depend extensively on nontechnical, nonprofessional caregivers. For these reasons, providing ventilatory support in the home presents many special challenges.

Prerequisites

For home ventilatory support to be successful, several prerequisites must be met, including the following:[44]

- Willingness of family to accept responsibility
- Adequacy of family and professional support
- Overall viability of the home care plan
- Stability of patient
- Adequacy of home setting

In regard to the home setting, the same factors listed in Box 56-1 should be evaluated for patients being considered for home ventilatory support.

TABLE 56-5
Profiles of Patient Groups Requiring Ventilatory Support in Alternative Settings

Group Description	Diseases Involved
Profile 1	
Mainly composed of neuromuscular and thoracic wall disorders; particular stage of disease process allows patient certain periods of spontaneous breathing time during day; generally requires only nocturnal mechanical support	Amyotrophic lateral sclerosis Multiple sclerosis Kyphoscoliosis and related chest wall deformities Diaphragmatic paralysis Myasthenia gravis
Profile 2	
Requires continuous mechanical ventilatory support associated with long-term survival rates	High spinal cord injuries Apneic encephalopathies Severe COPD Late-stage muscular dystrophy
Profile 3	
Usually returns home at request of patient and family; patient's condition is terminal, life expectancy is short, and patient and family wish to spend remaining time at home; patients usually pose management problems in the home because of their rapidly deteriorating conditions	Lung cancer End-stage COPD Cystic fibrosis

Box 56-6 Criteria to Determine Patient Stability for Ventilatory Support in Alternative Care Settings

- Ability to tolerate mechanical ventilation
- Acceptable arterial blood gas results and other blood chemistry (e.g., complete blood count)
- Relatively low FiO_2 needs (generally ≤40%)
- Psychological stability
- Absence of life-limiting comorbidities, including cardiac dysfunction and arrhythmias
- PEEP should not exceed 10 cm H_2O
- Ability to clear airway secretions by cough, suction, or cough-assist device
- Tracheostomy tube, as opposed to endotracheal tube, for invasive ventilation
- No readmissions expected for >1 month

56-3 Long-Term Invasive Mechanical Ventilation in the Home

AARC Clinical Practice Guideline (Excerpts)*

INDICATIONS

Patients requiring invasive long-term ventilatory support have shown:

- Inability to be completely weaned from invasive ventilatory support *or*
- Progression of disease etiology that requires increasing ventilatory support

Conditions that meet these criteria may include but are not limited to:

- Ventilatory muscle disorders
- Alveolar hypoventilatory syndrome
- Primary respiratory disorders
- Obstructive diseases
- Restrictive diseases
- Cardiac disorders including congenital anomalies

CONTRAINDICATIONS

Contraindications to long-term home mechanical ventilation include:

- Unstable condition that requires a level of care or resources unavailable in the home
    - FiO2 requirement >0.40
    - PEEP >10 cm H_2O
    - Need for continuous invasive monitoring (adults)
    - Lack of mature tracheostomy
- Patient's choice not to receive home mechanical ventilation
- Lack of an appropriate discharge plan
- Unsafe physical environment as determined by the patient's discharge planning team
    - Presence of fire, health, or safety hazards, including unsanitary conditions
    - Inadequate basic utilities (e.g., heat, air conditioning, electricity)
- Inadequate resources for care in the home
    - Financial
    - Personnel (e.g., inadequate medical follow-up, inability of patient to care for self, inadequate respite care for caregivers, inadequate numbers of competent caregivers)

PRECAUTIONS AND POSSIBLE COMPLICATIONS

Deterioration or acute change in clinical status of patient. The following may cause death or require rehospitalization for acute treatment:

- *Medical:* Hypocapnia, respiratory alkalosis, hypercapnia, respiratory acidosis, hypoxemia, barotrauma, seizures, hemodynamic instability, airway complications, respiratory infection, bronchospasm, exacerbation of underlying disease, or natural course of the disease
- *Equipment-related:* Failure of the ventilator, malfunction of equipment, inadequate warming and humidification of the inspired gases, inadvertent changes in ventilator settings, accidental disconnection from ventilator, accidental decannulation
- *Psychosocial:* Depression, anxiety, loss of resources (caregiver or financial), detrimental change in family structure or coping capacity

ASSESSMENT OF NEED

- Determination that indications are present and contraindications are absent
- Determination that one or more of the following goals can be met
    - To sustain and extend life and enhance quality of life
    - To reduce mortality
    - To improve or sustain physical and psychological function and enhance growth and development of pediatric patients
    - To provide cost-effective care
- Determination that no continued need exists for higher level of services
    - Determination that frequent changes to the plan of care will not be needed

ASSESSMENT OF OUTCOME

At least the following aspects of patient management and condition should be evaluated periodically as long as the patient receives mechanical ventilation in the home:

- Implementation and adherence to plan of care
- Quality of life
- Patient satisfaction
- Resource satisfaction
- Growth and development in the pediatric patient
- Change in prognosis
- Unanticipated morbidity, including need for higher level site of care
- Unanticipated mortality

MONITORING

Frequency of monitoring should be determined by the ongoing individualized care plan and be based on the patient's current medical condition. The ventilator settings, proper function of equipment, and the patient's physical condition should be monitored and verified (1) with each initiation of invasive ventilation to the patient, including altering the source of ventilation, as from one ventilator or resuscitation bag to another ventilator; (2) with each ventilator setting change; (3) after moving the patient; (4) on a regular basis as specified by individualized plan of care.

All appropriately trained caregivers, both professional and appropriately trained lay caregivers, should follow the care plan and implement the monitoring that has been prescribed. After being trained and evaluated on their level of knowledge and ability to respond to each intervention, lay caregivers, with documented competency, may operate equipment, perform routine maintenance tasks, monitor equipment, and perform personal care required.

After completing training and demonstrating competency and if directed in the plan of care, lay caregivers should monitor the following:

- Patient's physical condition
    - Respiratory rate
    - Heart rate
    - Color changes
    - Chest excursion
    - Diaphoresis
    - Lethargy
    - Blood pressure
    - Body temperature

Continued

56-3 Long-Term Invasive Mechanical Ventilation in the Home—cont'd

AARC Clinical Practice Guideline (Excerpts)*

- Ventilator settings (frequency should be specified in the plan of care)
  - Peak pressures
  - PEEP level (if applicable)
  - Preset tidal volume
  - Appropriate humidification of inspired gases
  - Frequency of ventilator breaths
  - Temperature of inspired gases (if applicable)
  - Verification of FiO_2
  - Heat and moisture exchanger function
- Equipment function (frequency should be specified in the plan of care)
  - Appropriate configuration of circuit
  - Internal and external battery power levels
  - Alarm function
  - Overall condition of all equipment
  - Cleanliness of filters—according to manufacturer's recommendation
  - Self-inflating bag-valve-mask—cleanliness and function

Health care professionals should perform a thorough, comprehensive assessment of the patient and the patient-ventilator system on a regular basis as prescribed by the plan of care. In addition, the health care professional should implement, monitor, and assess results of other interventions as indicated by the clinical situation and anticipated in the care plan.

- Pulse oximetry—should be used to assess patients requiring a change in prescribed FiO_2 or in patients with a suspected change in condition; a physician's order for pulse oximetry must be obtained before testing is performed
- End-tidal CO_2—may be useful for establishing trends in CO_2 levels; a physician's order for end-tidal CO_2 monitoring must be obtained before it is performed
- Ventilator settings
- Exhaled tidal volume
- Analysis of fraction of inspired O_2

Health care professionals are also responsible for maintaining interdisciplinary communication concerning the plan of care. Health care professionals should integrate the respiratory plan of care into the patient's total care plan. The plan of care should include:

- All aspects of patient's respiratory care
- Ongoing assessment and education of the caregivers involved

**For the complete guideline, see American Association for Respiratory Care: Clinical practice guideline: long-term invasive mechanical ventilation in the home—2007 revision and update. Respir Care 52:1056, 2007.*

Planning

Successful home ventilatory support requires extensive planning, education, and follow-up by all members of the home care team. Basic steps in the discharge process for a ventilator-dependent patient include the following:

1. Family is consulted regarding feasibility.
2. Physician writes appropriate orders.
3. Discharge planner coordinates efforts of team members and discharge plan is formulated.
4. Physician and other team members discuss plan with family and caregivers.
5. Education and training are initiated and completed.
6. Patient and family are prepared for discharge.
7. Home layout is assessed with necessary changes made.
8. Equipment and supplies are readied.
9. Discharge planner meets with team and makes final preparations.
10. Patient is discharged (with trial period, if necessary).
11. Local power company is notified regarding the presence of life-support equipment; appropriate backup power (battery or compressed gas source) is made available.
12. Ongoing and follow-up care is provided by visiting nurse, RT, and other health care professionals (as necessary).

Caregiver Education

To prepare patients, family members, and other caregivers properly for home discharge, a comprehensive educational program must be undertaken and completed. Essential skills that must be taught include the following:[34]

- Simple patient assessment
- Airway management, including tracheostomy and stoma care, cuff care, suctioning, cough-assist, changing artificial airways or ties
- Chest physical therapy techniques, including percussion, vibration, and coughing
- Medication administration, including oral and aerosol
- Patient movement and ambulation
- Equipment operation and maintenance
- Equipment troubleshooting
- Cleaning and disinfection
- Emergency procedures

Emergency situations that caregivers must be trained to recognize and deal with properly include the following:

- Ventilator or power failure
- Ventilator circuit problems
- Airway emergencies
- Cardiac arrest

All caregivers should successfully complete this educational process. Training generally requires a minimum of 1 to 2 weeks, over which time several education sessions can take place and cover instruction, demonstration, caregiver practice, and evaluation. Caregivers should be strongly encouraged to complete a course in basic life support, such as is offered by the American Heart Association, before the patient is discharged. Ideally, the patient should have a trial period on the actual home ventilator before discharge. In the early stages after discharge, patient follow-up by an RT likely should occur every day. As patient and caregivers become more familiar with the equipment and procedures, follow-up visits generally decrease to about once per month.[45,46]

Invasive Versus Noninvasive Ventilatory Support

Until recently, invasive positive pressure ventilation by tracheostomy was the default standard for long-term mechanical ventilation, especially for patients requiring 24-hour support. However, long-term tracheostomy is associated with some potential problems, including secretion retention, infection, aspiration, and ventilator-associated pneumonia, as well as communication difficulties between caregivers and patients. Because many long-term care facilities treat a tracheostomy as an open wound, patient placement at certain sites is prohibited.[47] Last, invasive ventilation by tracheostomy poses significant limits on the patient's quality of life. For these reasons, noninvasive support is becoming increasingly popular. Noninvasive ventilatory support involves any method designed to augment alveolar ventilation without an endotracheal airway. **Noninvasive ventilation (NIV)** is usually the first choice. Any individual requiring mechanical ventilation can be supported with NIV if the following conditions are met:[47]

- The patient is mentally competent, cooperative, and not using heavy sedation or narcotics.
- Supplemental O_2 therapy is generally minimal (FiO_2 ≤40%).
- SaO_2 can be maintained at greater than 90% by aggressive airway clearance techniques.
- Bulbar muscle function is adequate for swallowing and airway protection.
- No history exists of substance abuse or uncontrollable seizures.
- Unassisted or manually assisted peak expiratory flows during coughing exceed about 3 L/sec.
- No conditions are present that interfere with NIV interfaces (e.g., facial trauma, inadequate bite for mouthpiece, presence of orogastric or nasogastric tube, or facial hair that can hamper an airtight seal).

Patients who can benefit from NIV generally fall into one of two categories.[48] Patients in the first category have conditions in which cessation of ventilation could lead to imminent death. This category includes both acutely ill patients (patients with asthma, acute exacerbation of COPD, or pulmonary edema) and patients requiring long-term, 24-hour support (some patients with quadriplegia or patients with certain neuromuscular disorders). Patients in the second category have conditions in which NIV may offer clinical benefit, but cessation is not life-threatening. These patients generally require only intermittent or nocturnal support. Patients in this category include patients with chronic neuromuscular and chest wall diseases, such as muscular dystrophy and kyphoscoliosis. The application of long-term NIV for patients with obstructive disorders such as end-stage COPD or cystic fibrosis is much less common.[48] Relative contraindications to NIV include severe upper airway dysfunction, copious secretions that cannot be cleared by spontaneous or assisted cough, and O_2 concentration requirements exceeding 40%.[48]

Equipment

Box 56-7 lists the essential equipment and supplies needed for ventilator-dependent patients in alternative settings.[34,37]

Selecting Appropriate Ventilator

The choice of ventilator for a patient in an alternative care setting should be based on the patient's clinical need and the

Box 56-7 Essential Equipment and Supplies for Ventilator-Dependent Patients in Alternative Care Settings

EQUIPMENT
- Ventilator(s)
- Manual resuscitator (bag-valve-mask unit)
- Heated ventilator humidifier with thermostat and heat and moisture exchanger
- Monitoring or alarm devices (including remote where necessary)
- 12-V battery and battery charger
- Air compressor
- O_2 source
- Power strip or surge protector
- Suction machine with backup (manual or battery)
- Stethoscope and sphygmomanometer
- O_2 analyzer
- Pulse oximeter
- Hospital bed with table
- Patient lift
- Bedside commode, urinal, or bedpan
- Wheelchair

SUPPLIES
- O_2
- O_2 delivery devices, including manual resuscitator
- Airway interface (masks, mouthpieces, tracheostomy tubes)
- Tracheostomy tube inner cannulas
- Extra tracheostomy tubes including a tube one size smaller
- Tracheostomy care kits
- Ventilator circuits
- Bacterial filters
- Connecting tubing (aerosol, O_2, suction)
- Suction catheters
- Disposable gloves
- Distilled or sterile water
- Small volume nebulizer or metered dose inhaler with ventilator adapters, if appropriate
- Cleaning and disinfection supplies (10-ml syringe, 15- to 22-mm tubing adapters)

Box 56-8 Absolute Contraindications Against Using Noninvasive Ventilation

- Need for immediate intubation
- Hemodynamic instability
- Uncooperative patient
- Facial burns or trauma
- Inadequate airway protection
- Patent tracheoesophageal fistula

available support resources. In some cases, patient needs may dictate that more than one ventilator be provided.[43] A second backup ventilator should be provided for patients who cannot maintain spontaneous ventilation for more than 4 consecutive hours, for patients living in an area where a replacement ventilator cannot be secured within about 2 hours, and for patients whose care plan requires mechanical ventilation during mobility.[48]

Generally, ventilators chosen for care in alternative settings must be dependable and easy for caregivers to operate. If mobility is an essential element of the patient's care plan, the ventilator system selected should be portable. If the patient is receiving continuous ventilatory support in any alternative setting, external battery backup is required, and emergency AC power by way of a generator is recommended.

If invasive ventilation by tracheostomy is the selected approach, the best choice is a positive pressure ventilator. The invasive route also requires a humidification system, preferably a servo-controlled heated humidifier with alarms. Patients with a tracheostomy without retained secretions may use a heat and moisture exchanger during transport or to enhance their mobility.[43] For patients with an intact upper airway, a device capable of NIV is the first choice, unless contraindicated (Box 56-8 lists the absolute contraindications against using NIV).[49] In patients with an intact upper airway for whom NIV is contraindicated or unsuccessful, a negative pressure ventilator may be considered.

Positive Pressure Ventilators

Table 56-6 lists the essential, recommended, and optional features of positive pressure ventilators used in alternative care settings. An *essential* feature is basic to safe and effective operation in most patient care settings. A *recommended* feature helps provide optimal patient management. An *optional* feature is possibly useful in limited situations but not needed for most patients.[42,50]

As in the acute care setting, the use of volume-cycled versus pressure-limited ventilators is debated in alternative settings. Although volume-cycled ventilation has been the predominant mode of support in these settings, pressure-limited ventilation is gaining popularity for use in selected patients.

As shown in Figure 56-5, there are many new positive pressure ventilators designed for use in alternative settings. These ventilators can be used on adults or pediatric patients weighing at least 5 kg. Some are approximately the size and weight of a laptop computer and have many of the capabilities of much larger mechanical ventilators used in alternative sites and in acute care. These new ventilators offer ventilator-dependent patients the advantages of greater mobility and space conservation. Many of these models also offer pressure support and can provide positive end expiratory pressure (PEEP) without having to add an adapter to the ventilator circuit.[51-53]

TABLE 56-6 Essential, Recommended, and Optional Features of a Positive Pressure Ventilator for Use in an Alternative Care Setting

Feature	Necessity
Positive pressure tidal breaths	Essential
Mandatory rate	Essential
Flow or inspiratory-to-expiratory or inspiratory time	Recommended*
Expiratory pressure (PEEP)	Recommended*
FiO_2 to 1	Optional
Patient spontaneous breath (e.g., CPAP, intermittent mandatory ventilation)	Optional
Breath-triggering mechanism (flow or pressure sensors to initiate ventilator breath)	Recommended*
Flow-timing interaction (e.g., pressure support)	Optional
Feedback control (e.g., mandatory minute ventilation)	Optional

*Essential if the patient has intact ventilatory drive and respiratory muscles or if the possibility of partial or complete ventilator independence is anticipated.

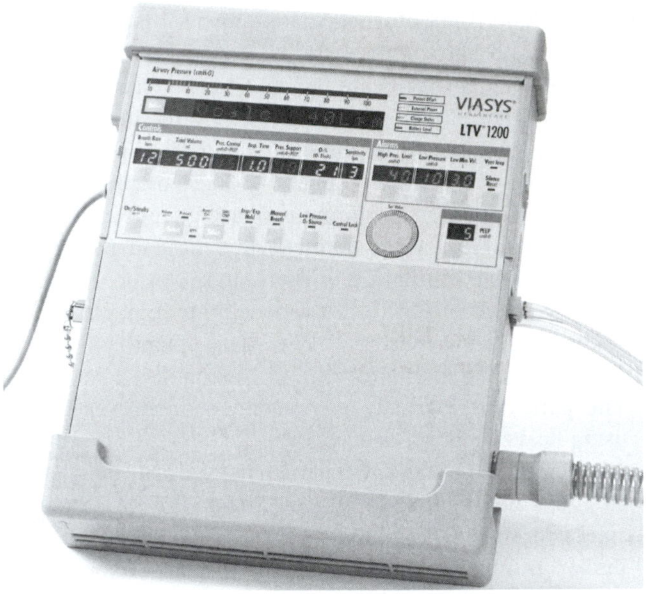

FIGURE 56-5 CareFusion LTV 1200 ventilator. (Courtesy CareFusion, Inc., Yorba Linda, CA.)

Many new positive pressure ventilators designed for alternative care settings (see Figures 56-5 and 56-6) have an internal battery, which can provide several hours of use in the event of a power failure. For longer periods of use away from AC line power, many of these devices can run for 10 to 12 hours using an external battery.

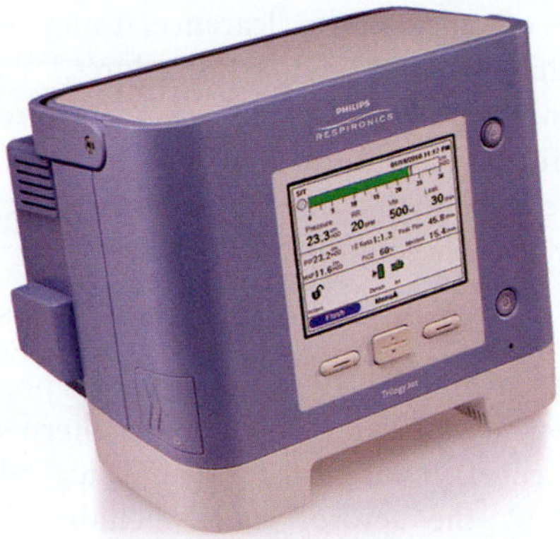

FIGURE 56-6 Philips-Respironics Trilogy 202 ventilator. (Used with permission of Philips Respironics, Murrysville, PA.)

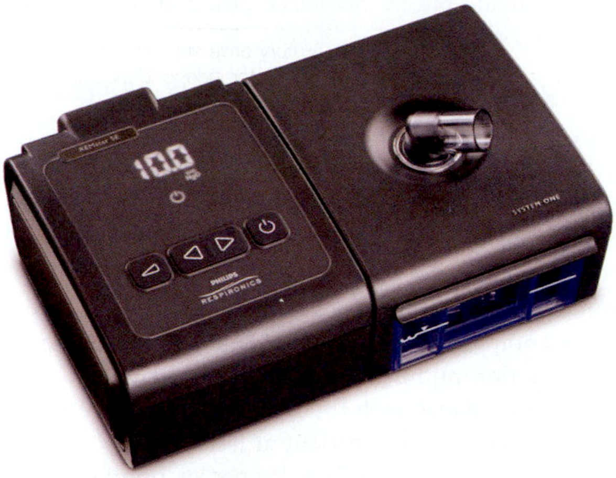

FIGURE 56-7 Respironics REMstar SE. (Used with permission of Philips Respironics, Murrysville, PA.)

Additionally, time-triggered or patient-triggered, pressure-limited, flow-cycled devices (pressure support with timed backup) have been successfully applied in alternative settings.[41,54,55] Many units are currently available (Figure 56-7) that are specifically designed to provide this type of support, usually noninvasively by nasal or oronasal (full-face) masks.[41,56,57]

Most positive pressure ventilators can be used to provide NIV.[48,58] NIV is normally provided by pressure-targeted ventilation regardless of the cause of ventilatory failure. The newest generation of these ventilators include alarm capabilities and internal battery backup.[56]

The biggest challenge with NIV is not selecting the right ventilator but getting a good, comfortable, minimal leak interface. Interfaces commonly found in alternative care settings include oronasal (full-face) masks; nasal masks; nasal "pillows"; and simple, flanged, or custom mouthpieces. For long-term use, some patients prefer alternating between devices. A patient may prefer a simple mouthpiece for easy accessibility during the day, with a nasal mask providing support at night.[48] Table 56-7 summarizes common problems associated with NIV interfaces and how to correct them.[41,59]

TABLE 56-7

Adverse Effects of Noninvasive Ventilation Interfaces and Possible Corrective Actions

Interface	Adverse Effect	Remedy
Nasal and oronasal masks	Discomfort	Proper fit, adjust strap tension, change mask type
	Nasal bridge redness, pressure sores, conjunctivitis	Reduce strap tension, use forehead spacer, try nasal pillow, use artificial skin
	Acneiform rash	Cortisone cream, alternative (gel) mask
Oronasal masks	Impede speech and eating	Permit periodic removal if tolerated by the patient
	Claustrophobia	Choose clear masks with minimal bulk
	Aspiration	Exclude patients unable to protect airway; nasogastric tubes for patient with nausea and abdominal distention
Mouthpieces/ lip seals	Interference with swallowing, salivary retention	Coaching, adaptation
	Pressure on lips, cheeks	Proper fit, strap adjustment
	Dental deformity	Orthodontic consultation
	Aerophagia	Simethicone, coaching
	Allergic reactions	Change prosthetic materials
	Nasal air leaking	Nose clips
	Accidental disconnection	Appropriate alarms in ventilator-dependent patients

All positive pressure ventilators used in alternative settings must have an alarm to indicate loss of power (pneumatic or electrical). Portable volume-cycled ventilators should also incorporate a high-pressure alarm or cycle override. For patients with conditions in which cessation of ventilation would cause death, a patient-disconnect alarm (low-pressure or low-exhaled volume) must be provided.[43,48] In some settings, a remote alarm or secondary disconnect alarm, or both, may be needed. A secondary alarm may be based on chest wall impedance and cardiac activity, exhaled volume, end-tidal CO_2, or pulse oximetry with alarm capabilities.[43] For patients in alternative settings who require only intermittent NIV, a loss-of-power alarm is generally sufficient.[48]

Negative Pressure Ventilators

Compared with NIV, negative pressure ventilation is harder to apply, more cumbersome, and less well tolerated (because of poor breath synchronization). Negative pressure ventilation tends to limit patient mobility and can worsen upper airway obstruction in susceptible patients. Nonetheless, negative pressure ventilation may be appropriate in patients who are unable to use NIV or who have failed NIV trials.[41] Negative pressure ventilation may also be considered for patients who require frequent airway access for suctioning.[47,60]

The original negative pressure ventilator was the *iron lung*, used for patients needing ventilator assistance after poliomyelitis. For practical reasons, the cumbersome iron lung was essentially replaced by the chest cuirass and wrap or "pneumosuit."

The chest cuirass (a rigid shell) and wrap-type systems (nylon fabric surrounding a semicylindrical tentlike support) are simply enclosures that allow application of negative pressure to the thorax. These devices require a separate electrically powered negative pressure generator. An example of a negative pressure generator used to power cuirass or wrap-type systems is the Philips-Respironics NEV-100 (Phillips-Respironics, Murrysville, PA).[60]

Evaluation and Follow-Up

Patient parameters to be monitored during positive pressure ventilation are essentially the same parameters that are assessed in the acute care setting, with an emphasis on simplicity.[61] The caregiver should assess the patient's vital signs, lung sounds, and sputum production on a daily basis; arterial blood gas analysis (by the RT) may be conducted monthly or only when changes in the care plan appear to be needed. Likewise, compliance and resistance measures are performed only when other evidence indicates the need.

Routine follow-up visits by the RT help ensure the success of patient management within the home and proper equipment maintenance and functioning. The patient's status should be carefully assessed, and appropriate care plan modifications should be recommended to the prescribing physician. Follow-up visits should occur about monthly, and a report documenting the status of the patient and equipment and progress toward care plan goals should be completed after each visit and maintained as part of the patient record.

OTHER MODES OF RESPIRATORY CARE IN ALTERNATIVE SITES

In addition to O_2 therapy and ventilatory support, other modes of respiratory care are now common in the alternative care setting. These may represent the primary therapy or may be used to supplement other modes of care. Included for discussion here are bland aerosol therapy, aerosol drug administration, airway care and clearance methods, nasal CPAP, and apnea monitoring.

Bland Aerosol Therapy

The delivery of bland aerosols has been common in alternative sites for many years. According to the AARC's Clinical Practice Guideline, bland aerosol therapy includes the delivery of sterile water or various concentrations of saline solution in aerosol form.[62] The aerosol can be produced by either an ultrasonic or jet (large volume) nebulizer. If using a jet nebulizer, a 50-psi air compressor is also required. Supplemental O_2 is provided by either a concentrator or liquid supply system.

Depending on the patient's condition and therapeutic objectives, bland aerosol therapy may be either continuous or intermittent. Though bland aerosol alone may have little effect on the properties of mucus or its clearance, it may be useful as an adjunct to other airway clearance procedures.[62,63]

The potential problem is infection from contaminated equipment. To reduce the incidence of infection, equipment and patient delivery systems must be cleaned and changed regularly, as noted elsewhere in this chapter.

Aerosol Drug Administration

As in the acute care setting, the aerosol route is popular for drug administration to respiratory patients in alternative care settings. As described in Chapter 39, drug categories commonly administered by the aerosol route include beta-adrenergic bronchodilators, anticholinergic agents, and antiinflammatory drugs.

Most pulmonary drugs are available in either metered dose inhaler or dry powder inhaler form. Alternatively, the caregiver can use a small volume nebulizer powered by a low output diaphragm compressor.[64]

Airway Care and Clearance Methods

Patients in alternative care settings with tracheostomies require both daily stoma care and tracheobronchial secretion clearance. Tracheostomy care can be provided by any trained caregiver, but tube changes should generally be performed only by an RT or a physician.

In most alternative care settings, tracheobronchial clearance is often accomplished by suctioning using a portable electrically powered suction pump with collection bottle and connection tubing. In accordance with the AARC Clinical Practice Guideline for suctioning of the patient at home, some patients may be taught to suction themselves. Proper suctioning procedures should also be taught to caregivers. Education and training on proper suctioning methods may begin before patient discharge from the acute care setting, with reinforcement and follow-up as needed.[65] Because many of these systems measure pressure in inches of mercury (in Hg), care must be taken to teach proper adjustment according to patient age. Daily maintenance and cleaning are required. In an alternative care setting, a single suction catheter commonly may be used for up to 24 hours but to prevent bacterial growth, catheters are often placed in a disinfecting solution between suctioning attempts.

RULE OF THUMB

For portable suction units calibrated in inches of mercury (in Hg), the following vacuum ranges are recommended (adjustment may be needed based on volume and viscosity of secretions):

Patient Category	Vacuum Setting (in Hg)
Infants	5-7
Children	7-12
Adults	12-15

Numerous methods are available for patients in an alternative care setting with an intact upper airway who need help with secretion clearance. These methods include both patient-independent and caregiver-dependent techniques.[66] Patients can be taught to apply independently coughing, forced exhalation, active cycle of breathing, and autogenic drainage methods. Caregiver assistance is required with traditional postural drainage, percussion and vibration, and directed or assisted cough. Additional assistance can be provided by mechanical devices such as positive expiratory pressure mask, flutter valve, intrapulmonary percussive ventilator, and high-frequency chest compression vest.

Another airway clearance method involves the use of cough-assist devices such as the Emerson mechanical **inexsufflator**, or "coughlator." The inexsufflator uses alternating positive and negative pressure to simulate a cough as a form of lung expansion and airway clearance therapy. These devices can be especially effective with patients receiving NIV. The application of secretion clearance devices or techniques by nonprofessional caregivers should involve good preliminary instruction and ongoing follow-up by the RT working in any alternative site.[66] See Chapter 36 for more in-depth discussion of the inexsufflator and other secretion clearance devices.

Nasal Continuous Positive Airway Pressure Therapy

Nasal CPAP therapy has become an accepted form of home care used to treat sleep apnea-hypopnea syndrome. For Medicare reimbursement of home nasal CPAP equipment, the diagnosis of sleep apnea must be confirmed by polysomnography, also known as a *sleep study*. With proper application and patient compliance, CPAP therapy can dramatically lessen or resolve the many problems associated with sleep apnea-hypopnea syndrome (morning headaches, daytime hypersomnolence, cognitive impairment). The patient's quality of life can be enhanced, and more severe complications, such as systemic and pulmonary hypertension and cor pulmonale, may be reduced.[67]

Equipment

A typical nasal CPAP apparatus consists of a flow generator capable of establishing varying levels of PEEP or CPAP, a circuit, and a patient interface (e.g., nasal mask, nasal pillows). One of the most common interfaces in alternative settings is the nasal mask (Figure 56-8). However, many patients requiring nocturnal CPAP do prefer to use a full-face mask instead of a nasal mask. Most systems provide manually adjustable pressures in the range of 2.5 to 30 cm H_2O. Most units have a ramp feature that gradually increases the pressure to the prescribed level over a time interval to increase comfort and therapy compliance.

Some patients with sleep apnea require NIV. The difference in PEEP and peak airway pressure aids the patient's inspiratory effort, improving ventilation. NIV in these patients may also reduce the adverse effects associated with nasal CPAP therapy and improve patient tolerance.[68]

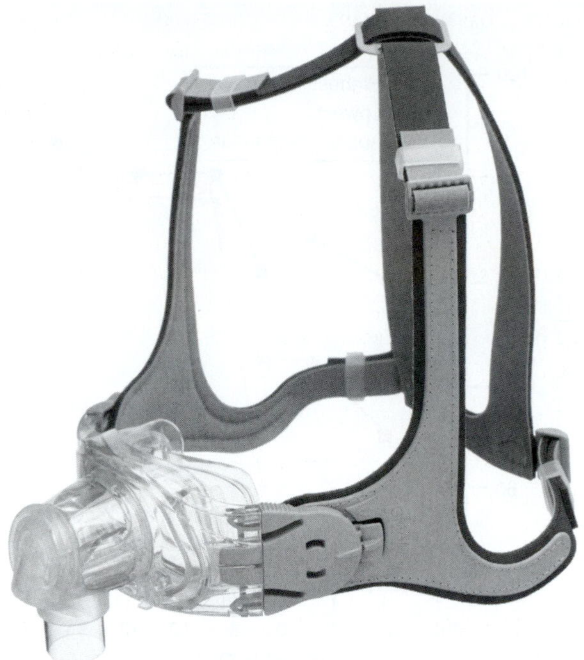

FIGURE 56-8 An example of a nasal mask. (Mirage Kidsta Mask, Courtesy ResMed Inc, San Diego, CA.)

Determining Proper Continuous Positive Airway Pressure Level

The proper CPAP level for a patient is determined by one of several methods. The most common method is to conduct the sleep study, titrating different levels of CPAP. Observed changes in the apnea-hypopnea index are correlated with the various CPAP levels. The prescribed level of CPAP is the lowest pressure at which apneic episodes are reduced to an acceptable frequency and duration.

More recently, CPAP units that automatically adjust the pressures to maintain airway patency are commonly used. These self-titrating or auto-CPAP devices generally result in use of the lowest effective pressures and better patient compliance, while reducing the need for a subsequent sleep study and titration.[69]

Alternatively, CPAP may be titrated against pulse oximetry data (Figure 56-9). In this case, the goal is to use the lowest CPAP that maintains adequate arterial saturation (SpO_2 <90%).

Use and Maintenance

Once proper CPAP level is determined, the patient is fitted for a mask and trained in the proper use, cleaning, and maintenance of the equipment. Typical patient instructions for self-administration of nasal or full-face mask CPAP therapy are provided in Box 56-9.

Problem Solving and Troubleshooting

Patient problems associated with nasal or full-face mask CPAP therapy include skin irritation, conjunctivitis, epistaxis, and nasal discomfort (dryness, burning, and congestion). Skin irritation is usually because of tight mask straps or a dirty patient interface. Persistent redness on the face or around the nose is the primary sign. Adjusting the straps (while maintaining a good mask seal) can help prevent irritation. In addition, the patient interface should be cleaned daily to remove dirt and

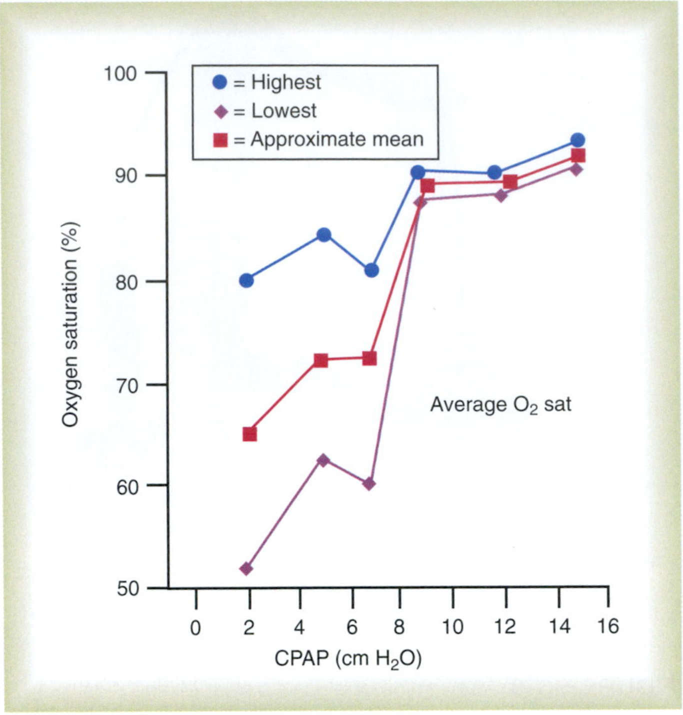

FIGURE 56-9 Illustration of CPAP levels and corresponding oxygen saturations while patient was asleep and using nasal CPAP. (Modified from Sleeper GP, Strohl KP, Armeni MA: Nasal CPAP for at-home treatment of obstructive sleep apnea: a case report. Respir Care Clin N Am 30:90, 1985.)

facial oils. Even with proper care, masks and nasal pillows should be replaced approximately every 3 to 6 months or sooner if leakage or discomfort occurs.

Conjunctivitis probably is the result of mask leakage around the bridge of the nose, which is easily corrected by ensuring a good seal in this area. Epistaxis and nasal discomfort are associated with drying of the nasal mucosa—a particular problem in cold, dry winter climates. Methods used to overcome excessive drying include in-line humidifiers, chin straps (to decrease loss of upper airway moisture), and saline nasal sprays.[70] Because none of these methods have proved satisfactory for all patients, selection should be based on individual patient acceptance and observed improvement in comfort. However, almost all patients receiving nocturnal CPAP therapy benefit from the addition of an in-line humidifier.

The most common problem with the CPAP apparatus is an inability to reach or maintain the set pressure. This problem is usually due to either inadequate flow or, more commonly, system leaks. Common causes of leaks include inappropriate patient interface (mask vs. nasal pillows) or pressure loss through an open mouth. As part of their initial training, patients and caregivers should be taught how to recognize and correct these common problems. Box 56-10 outlines the procedures patients or caregivers can use to troubleshoot inadequate flows and system leaks.[71]

Follow-up with patients soon after they begin CPAP therapy is important to resolve complications promptly. If left

Box 56-9 Typical Patient Instructions for Self-Administration of Nasal or Full-Face Mask Continuous Positive Airway Pressure Therapy

EQUIPMENT PREPARATION

1. Place blower unit on a level surface (table or nightstand) close to where you sleep.
2. Ensure that the air exhaust and inlet vents are not obstructed.
3. Plug machine into a standard grounded (three-prong) electrical outlet.
4. Check air inlet filter to ensure it is in place and free of dust.
5. Connect one end of the tubing to the interface (e.g., mask, nasal pillows).
6. Attach interface to the nose or face.
7. Adjust headgear strap tightness to seat interface firmly onto the nose or face.
8. Turn on the blower and verify a flow of air.
9. Ensure proper fit and adjustment of mask and headgear. Air should not be leaking out around the bridge of the nose into the eyes or from the mask to upper lip.
10. CPAP therapy is now fully functional, but minor adjustments may be needed as use continues.

IN THE MORNING

1. Remove mask by slipping strap off back of head (you may leave the head strap connected between cleaning).
2. Turn off blower.
3. Wash interface every morning with a mild detergent, then rinse it with water.
4. Once dry, store interface in a plastic bag to keep it clean.

WEEKLY

1. Wipe off the blower unit with a clean, damp cloth.
2. Wash the head strap and circuit tubing.
3. Service the filters according to the instructions in your patient manual.

Box 56-10 Patient and Caregiver Instructions for Troubleshooting Continuous Positive Airway Pressure Equipment

INADEQUATE FLOW

1. Ensure that unit is plugged into a working electrical outlet.
2. Confirm that unit is turned on.
3. Ensure all connections are tight.
4. Confirm that airflow is coming from blower.
5. Ensure that the intake/exhaust vents are not obstructed.
6. Check the blower inlet filter to confirm that air can easily enter unit. If the filter appears obstructed, wash or replace it.
7. If there is still no flow, contact your home care provider.

AIR LEAKS

1. Check interface fit, and readjust mask or headgear if necessary.
2. Request a chin strap to help keep mouth closed.
3. If problem is not resolved, contact the home care provider for adjustments or a different interface such as nasal pillows.

unresolved, these issues often discourage the patient and result in decreased compliance and a return of original symptoms.[71]

MINI CLINI

Troubleshooting Nasal Dryness With Continuous Positive Airway Pressure

PROBLEM: A 43-year-old obese man with documented obstructive sleep apnea has been advised by his attending physician that home CPAP therapy at night is needed. The home care RT makes an appointment with the patient to assess his tolerance to the CPAP unit. During the visit, the patient notes that he has been experiencing nasal discomfort. How can the RT assist in problem solving with this specific complaint, and what are some of the other potential patient problems associated with CPAP therapy that the clinician should be alerted to?

Solution: CPAP devices use some type of patient interface such as a nasal mask or pillows, or full-face mask with supporting headgear. Complaints of nasal discomfort are common and are most likely due to the effects of dry airflow through the CPAP unit blower. However, other factors may aggravate the sensation of nasal irritation. Poor systemic hydration could worsen nasal mucosal drying. In addition, environmental humidity may be a factor. Cold, dry, winter climates can aggravate symptoms, as can dry, forced-air heating systems. In these cases, the RT might recommend increasing oral intake of fluids (if no restrictions on fluid intake), the installation of a room or heating system humidifier or the as-needed use of a saline nasal spray. Also, almost all patients receiving nocturnal CPAP therapy benefit from the addition of an in-line humidifier.

In addition to the above-mentioned factors, large leaks in the system can significantly increase flows and worsen the drying effect of these devices. Often such leaks originate from a poorly fitting patient interface. Consequently, these problems can be remedied by ensuring a proper fit via repositioning the interface or switching to one of the many alternative masks or nasal pillows available today.

Apnea Monitoring

Apnea monitors alert clinicians and caregivers of certain life-threatening events, most notably recurrent apnea, bradycardia, and hypoxemia. At-risk infants are frequently set up on apnea monitors while they are in the hospital. After extensive family instruction in both equipment use and resuscitation, some of these infants may be discharged to the home with this equipment.[72]

Most apnea monitors detect both respirations and heart rate and activate audio and visual alarms when preset high or low limits are reached. Follow-up visits by the RT are usually frequent at first but occur less often as the family becomes skilled with the equipment and monitoring routine. Some models record each alarm event and can be useful in monitoring the patient's progress. The "memory" of such monitors can be monitored continuously via an Internet connection or via periodic downloading. Apnea monitors are usually discontinued after an infant has a negative pneumocardiogram (sleep study) or when recorded memory reveals no events during a prescribed time frame—often 2 to 4 months from the initial setup.[72]

PATIENT ASSESSMENT AND DOCUMENTATION

Alternative care sites demand extensive patient assessment and documentation. These requirements are based on both stringent reimbursement criteria and the rehabilitation orientation characterizing these settings.

Institutional Long-Term Care

In institutions providing long-term care, the assessment and documentation process involves four key components: screening, treatment planning, ongoing assessment, and discharge (Figure 56-10).

Screening

On admission to a long-term care facility, all patients with a respiratory-related admitting diagnosis should be screened by an RT.[17] This screening is often accomplished mainly by a medical record review. During screening, the RT reviews the pertinent respiratory diagnosis, onset and severity of symptoms, current radiograph results, pulmonary function tests, arterial blood gas values, and other nonrespiratory treatment orders (e.g., physical therapy).

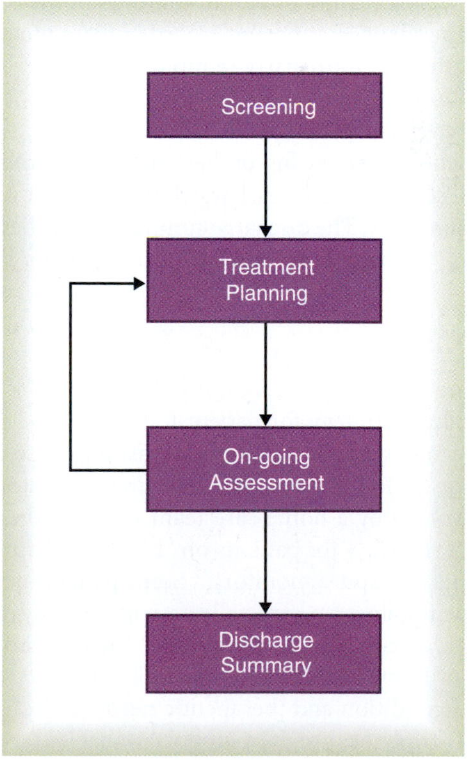

FIGURE 56-10 The assessment and documentation process in institutional subacute or long-term care.

If the review indicates the need for a more in-depth assessment, the RT can recommend a more complete evaluation. On receipt of the appropriate orders, the RT interviews the patient and conducts a physical assessment, including inspection, palpation, auscultation, and percussion. Key clinical findings include description of breath sounds; rate, depth, and pattern of respirations; heart rate; signs of dyspnea; cough; sputum production; level of consciousness; and ability of the resident to understand and follow commands. Also noteworthy are the resident's prior respiratory status, use of supplemental O_2, pulse oximetry, skin turgor, and medications.[17,18]

Treatment Planning and Ongoing Assessment

Based on the information obtained during the initial screening process, the RT designs a specific treatment plan. A typical treatment plan includes patient demographics, assessment information, short-term and long-term goals reflective of overall rehabilitation potential, and measures to be used to achieve such goals. A treatment plan for a resident of a long-term care facility with moderate to severe COPD would likely reflect the treatment goal of correcting hypoxemia through the use of low-flow O_2 and patient monitoring.[17,18]

After therapy has been initiated, the RT uses several other tools to monitor a patient's progress. In addition to regular treatment documentation, the RT should document a regular summary on each patient. This summary provides a synopsis of progress toward goal attainment, including changes in respiratory status, results of any additional tests, explanation of any patient education, and recommendations for additional therapy. Additionally, treatment plans and progress summaries become part of the resident's permanent record and are often required documentation for third-party reimbursement.[17,18]

Discharge Summary

When a patient reaches his or her maximum potential, has attained all set goals, or is discharged, the RT must complete a discharge summary. The discharge summary describes the complete course of respiratory therapy, including its success or failure.[17-19]

Home Care

A home care plan must specify not only the types of care provided but also a strategy for patient follow-up. The individual making the follow-up visits is often the visiting nurse, a physical therapist, or an RT. For patients receiving respiratory care at home, follow-up by a home care team member should occur regularly, particularly for patients on "hi-tech" equipment such as ventilators and apnea monitors.[12] Some patients may require more frequent follow-up, especially patients recently discharged or patients requiring ventilatory support. Factors relevant to the frequency of home visits include the following:

- Patient's condition and therapeutic needs (objectives)
- Level of family or caregiver support available
- Type and complexity of home care equipment
- Overall home environment
- Ability of the patient to provide self-care
- Third-party reimbursement for such visits

When a visit is made by the RT, numerous functions must be performed, including the following:

- Patient assessment (objective/subjective data and pretreatment/posttreatment data)
- Patient's compliance with prescribed respiratory home care
- Equipment assessment (operation, cleanliness, and need for related supplies)
- Identification of any problem areas or patient concerns
- Statement related to patient goals and therapeutic plan

A standard written report, consistent with the care plan, should be completed by the visiting RT. Copies are often sent to the patient's physician, the home care referral source, and any other member of the patient care team requiring this information. The report should become part of the patient's medical record and should be referred to when following the patient's course and overall progress.[12,16]

EQUIPMENT DISINFECTION AND MAINTENANCE

With many patients receiving respiratory care outside the hospital, the danger of infection caused by direct contact with caregivers and visitors or indirect contact with contaminated articles has grown. To help minimize home-related infection, guidelines for disinfecting home respiratory care equipment have been established. Accepted infection control techniques are based on clinical evidence, such as the evidence outlined in several of the AARC Clinical Practice Guidelines that pertain to respiratory care provided in alternative settings.[24,43,62,65,73]

Collectively, these guidelines focus on sources of infection, basic principles of infection control, patients at high risk, disinfection methods, equipment processing, and care of solutions and medications. Procedures focus significantly on surveillance, prevention, and control of infection.[15,16]

In regard to infection control, all guidelines and procedures mandate proper hand hygiene techniques by all caregivers—proper handwashing and use of antiseptic hand lotions. In addition, visits to the patient by friends or relatives with respiratory infections are discouraged. Relating to medical equipment suppliers, the guidelines suggest that all permanent equipment (e.g., ventilator circuits, O_2 delivery equipment, and aerosol systems) be sterilized or receive high-level disinfection before being supplied to another patient. Disposable or single-patient use equipment must be used by one patient only. It is recommended that all equipment be completely disassembled and washed first in water, followed by a soak in warm soapy water for several minutes, with equipment scrubbed as needed to remove any remaining organic material. Following this step, the equipment must be thoroughly rinsed to remove any residual soap and drained of excess water. Air drying on a clean surface or rack is recommended to minimize recontamination.

Additionally, the broad bactericidal activity exhibited by many premanufactured disinfectant solutions makes them the first choice. Other disinfection solutions to be considered include a 1 : 50 dilution of 5.25% to 6.15% sodium hypochlorite (household bleach) with water for a minimum of 3 minutes.

In regard to using water for humidification or nebulization, it is recommended that distilled water be used as a first choice. However, boiled water, cooled in a refrigerator and discarded after 24 hours, is also generally acceptable. It is recommended that manufacturers' guidelines for the proper handling of specific medications be strictly followed. Detailed instructions for patients and caregivers on how to clean and disinfect selected respiratory care equipment are generally available from most manufacturers.[73-74]

PALLIATIVE CARE

This chapter would not be complete without some discussion of palliative respiratory care in alternative settings. Although the primary goal of home care involves minimizing a patient's dependence on institutional care, an additional goal is to maximize the comfort and well-being of a terminally ill patient near the end of life.

The definition of *palliative care* by the World Health Organization involves the control of pain and other symptoms such as dyspnea of terminally ill patients and maximizing the psychological, social, and spiritual well-being of family members and patients nearing the end of life.[75] Many terminally ill patients have respiratory dysfunction directly or indirectly resulting from their terminal illness. Some of these patients choose to experience the remainder of their life at home. Hospice is a philosophy of care that helps support the efforts of such patients by providing clinician coverage and equipment to these patients at home.[75]

Respiratory modalities, such as O_2 therapy and mechanical ventilation or aerosol drug administration, can be combined with other therapies, such as pain management, to increase patients' comfort and permit them to die at home with their family and friends nearby. The RT can help such patients and families by providing training on the proper use and maintenance of such equipment. The presence of the RT can also be a supportive influence for patients and their families. Although such cases can place a psychological strain on the RT, maximizing the comfort of terminally ill patients can be rewarding, and not easily forgotten.

SUMMARY CHECKLIST

- An increasing number of health services are being provided in alternative care settings.
- Subacute care aims achieve the highest level of patient functioning—ideally self-care.
- Standards for subacute and home health care derive from federal and state laws and private-sector accreditation, mainly TJC.
- Acute and alternative care settings differ in regard to resource availability, supervision and work schedules, documentation and assessment, and professional-patient interaction.
- Effective discharge planning (1) guides the multidisciplinary team in transferring patients to alternative sites of care and (2) ensures the safety and efficacy of the patient's continuing care.
- Alternative site caregivers must have all the competencies required to meet the patient's ventilatory and respiratory needs and provide adequate 24-hour coverage. The selected site also must be safe and suitable for the patient's specific condition.
- O_2 prescriptions for patients in alternative settings must be based on documented hypoxemia, as determined by either blood gas analysis or oximetry.
- In most alternative care sites, O_2 normally is most often supplied by concentrators with gaseous cylinders as backup and for portability.
- Most patients in alternative care settings needing O_2 use a nasal cannula; conserving devices such as transtracheal catheter, reservoir cannula, and demand-flow O_2 system can decrease O_2 use and costs and provide greater patient mobility.
- Because most problems with long-term O_2 therapy are "people" problems, caregivers should be allowed to operate and maintain O_2 delivery devices only after they have been properly instructed by credentialed RTs.
- Key factors needed for successful ventilatory support in alternative sites include (1) careful patient selection, (2) effective discharge planning, (3) interdisciplinary team approach, (4) effective caregiver and family education, (5) thorough assessment and preparation of the environment, and (6) careful selection of needed equipment and supplies.
- Patients being considered for ventilatory support in alternative settings must be medically and psychologically stable.
- Most patients requiring mechanical ventilation in alternative settings can be supported with NIV if they are alert and cooperative, can maintain acceptable oxygenation without high FiO_2, and have intact airway reflexes and adequate clearance mechanisms.
- Positive pressure ventilators used in alternative settings should be electrically powered, easy to operate, and portable (run on both AC and DC power). Loss-of-power alarms are essential, high-pressure alarms are needed on volume-cycled ventilators, and patient-disconnect (low-pressure) alarms should be provided.
- Negative pressure ventilators, such as the chest cuirass and "pneumosuit," are a second-line choice for ventilatory support in alternative care settings.
- Patients with tracheostomies in alternative care settings require both daily stoma care and secretion clearance; tube changes should be performed only by a qualified health professional.
- A typical nocturnal CPAP system consists of a flow generator or blower, PEEP or CPAP valve, and nasal or full-face mask; some units can increase pressure to the prescribed level over time (ramping); others can autoadjust the CPAP level in response to apnea, hypopnea, airflow limitation, or snoring.
- The proper CPAP level can be determined by polysomnography, continuous monitoring of hemoglobin saturation, or by an auto-CPAP system.

- A common problem with nocturnal CPAP systems is an inability to reach or maintain the set pressure, usually because of either inadequate flow or system leaks.
- Proper caregiver hand hygiene, limiting visits by persons with respiratory infections, providing sterile or disposable clean equipment, and proper equipment processing are the keys to infection control in such settings.
- Providing palliative care to keep terminally ill patients as comfortable as possible is an important aspect of respiratory care in alternative sites.

References

1. Lipsitz LA: The 3-night hospital stay and Medicare coverage for skilled nursing care. *JAMA* 14:1441, 2013.
2. Ottenbacher KJ, Karmarkar A, Graham JE, et al: Thirty-day hospital readmission following discharge from postacute rehabilitation in fee-for-service Medicare patients. *JAMA* 311:604, 2014.
3. Fan VS, Gaziano JM, Lew R, et al: A comprehensive care management program to prevent chronic obstructive pulmonary disease hospitalizations: a randomized, controlled trial. *Arch Intern Med* 156:673, 2012.
4. Sharma G, et al: Outpatient follow-up visit and 30-day emergency department visit and readmission in patients hospitalized for chronic obstructive pulmonary disease. *Arch Intern Med* 170:1664, 2010.
5. U.S. Department of Health and Human Services: Centers for Medicare & Medicaid Services: Skilled nursing facility prospective payment system—Fact Sheet. Bethesda, 2013.
6. Shaffer ER: The affordable care act: the value of systemic disruption. *Am J Public Health* 103:969, 2013.
7. Center for Medicare & Medicaid Services: Home health prospective payment system. *Medicare Learning Network*, Bethesda, 2012.
8. Bunch D: 1999 Muse study shows respiratory therapists' positive impact on SNF patient outcomes and Medicare cost savings. *AARC Times* 23:20–27, 1999.
9. Courtois DR, Lamouroux AD, Delpierre S, et al: Home-based respiratory rehabilitation in adult patients with moderate or severe persistent asthma. *J Asthma* 51:552, 2014.
10. National Association of Subacute/Post Acute Care: *NASPAC frequently asked questions*, Washington, DC, 2010, National Association of Subacute/Post Acute Care.
11. Dajczman E, Robitaille C, Ernst P, et al: Integrated interdisciplinary care for patients with chronic obstructive pulmonary disease reduces emergency department visits, admissions and costs: a quality assurance study. *Can Respir J* 20:351, 2013.
12. American Association for Respiratory Care: *Home respiratory care services. An official position statement by the AARC, American Association for Respiratory Care—Revised*, Irving TX, 2010, AARC.
13. Utens CM, Goossens LM, Smeenk FW, et al: Early assisted discharge with generic community nursing for chronic obstructive pulmonary disease exacerbations: results of a randomized controlled trial. *BMJ Open* 2:1684, 2012.
14. Utens CM, et al: Effectiveness and cost-effectiveness of early assisted discharge for chronic obstructive pulmonary disease exacerbations: the design of a randomized controlled trial. *BMC Public Health* 10:618, 2010.
15. Joint Commission: *2014 Comprehensive accreditation manual for long term care*, Oakbrook Terrace, IL, 2013.
16. The Joint Commission: *Facts about home care accreditation: 2014 standards for home medical equipment and clinical respiratory*, Oakbrook Terrace, IL, 2013.
17. Huang TT, Peng JM: Role adaptation of family caregivers for ventilator-dependent patients transition from respiratory care ward to home. *J Clin Nurs* 19:1686, 2010.
18. Abad-Corpa E, et al: Evaluation of the effectiveness of hospital discharge planning and follow-up in the primary care of patients with chronic obstructive pulmonary disease. *J Clin Nurs* 22:669, 2013.
19. American Association for Respiratory Care: Clinical practice guideline: discharge planning for the respiratory care patient. *Respir Care Clin N Am* 40:1308, 1995.
20. Dunne PJ: The clinical impact of new long-term oxygen therapy technology. *Respir Care* 54:1100, 2009.
21. Godoy I, Tanni SE, Hernandez C: The importance of knowing the home conditions of patients receiving long-term oxygen therapy. *Int J Chron Obstruct Pulmon Dis* 7:421, 2012.
22. Qaseem A, Wilt TJ, Welnberger SE, et al: Diagnosis and management of stable obstructive pulmonary disease: a clinical practice guideline update. *Annals Internal Med* 155:191, 2011.
23. Ruiz OF, Lobato DS, Iturri JB, et al: Continuous home oxygen therapy. *Arch Bronconeumol* 50:185, 2014.
24. American Association for Respiratory Care: Clinical practice guideline: oxygen therapy in the home or alternate site health care facility. *Respir Care* 52:1063, 2007.
25. Kent CL, Porte P: Topics in practice management: long-term oxygen therapy. *Chest* 139:430, 2011.
26. U.S. Department of Health and Human Services, Centers for Medicare & Medicaid Services: Certificate of medical necessity CMS 484 oxygen. *Fed Reg* 71:44082, 2007.
27. Goldbart J, Yohannes AM, Woolrych R, et al: "It is not going to change his life but it has picked him up": a qualitative study of perspectives on long term oxygen therapy for people with chronic obstructive pulmonary disease. *Health Qual Life Outcomes* 11:124, 2013.
28. McCoy RW: Options for home oxygen therapy equipment: storage and metering of oxygen in the home. *Respir Care* 58:65, 2013.
29. COPD Working Group: Long term oxygen therapy for patients with chronic obstructive pulmonary disease (COPD). *Ont Health Technol Assess Ser* 12:1, 2012.
30. Christopher KL, Schwartz MD: Transtracheal oxygen therapy. *Chest* 139:435, 2011.
31. Palwai A, et al: Critical comparisons of the clinical performance of oxygen-conserving devices. *Am J Respir Crit Care Med* 181:1061, 2010.
32. Marti S, Pajares V, Morante F: Are oxygen-conserving devices effective for correcting exercise hypoxemia? *Respir Care* 58:1606, 2013.
33. Chatburn RL, Lewarski JS, McCoy RW: Nocturnal oxygenation using pulsed-dose oxygen-conserving device compared to continuous flow. *Respir Care* 51:252, 2006.
34. Marti S, Pajares V, Morante F: Are oxygen-conserving devices effective for correcting exercise hypoxemia? *Respir Care* 58:1606, 2013.
35. King AC: Long-term home mechanical ventilation in the United States. *Respir Care* 57:921, 2012.
36. Murphy P, Hart N: Who benefits from home mechanical ventilation? *Clin Med* 9:160, 2009.
37. Kun SS, et al: How much do primary care givers know about tracheostomy and home mechanical ventilation emergency care? *Pediatr Pulmonol* 45:270, 2010.
38. American Association for Respiratory Care: *Delivery of respiratory therapy services in skilled nursing facilities providing ventilator and/or high acuity respiratory care. An official position statement by the AARC, American Association for Respiratory Care—Revised*, Irving TX, 2013, AARC.
39. Szubski CR, Tellez A, Klika AK, et al: Predicting discharge to a long term acute care hospital after admission to an intensive care unit. *Am J Crit Care* 23:46, 2014.
40. Oppersma E, Doorduin J, Heijden EH, et al: Noninvasive ventilation and the upper airway: should we pay more attention? *Crit Care* 17:245, 2013.
41. Hess DR: Noninvasive ventilation in neuromuscular disease: equipment and application. *Respir Care* 51:896, 2006.
42. White AC: Long-term mechanical ventilation: management strategies. *Respir Care* 57:889, 2012.
43. American Association for Respiratory Care: Clinical practice guideline: long-term invasive mechanical ventilation in the home—2007 revision and update. *Respir Care* 52:1056, 2007.

44. Guentner K, et al: Preferences for mechanical ventilation among survivors of prolonged mechanical ventilation and tracheostomy. *Am J Crit Care* 15:65, 2006.
45. Sinderby C, Lui S, Colombo D: An automated and standardized neural index to quantify patient-ventilator interaction. *Crit Care* 17:239, 2013.
46. Tsay SF, Mu PF, Lin S: The experience of adult ventilator-dependent patients: a meta-synthesis review. *Nurs Health Sci* 15:525, 2013.
47. Hess DR: The growing role of noninvasive ventilation in patients requiring prolonged mechanical ventilation. *Respir Care* 57:900, 2012.
48. Ugurlu AO, Sidhom SS, Khodabandeh A: Use and outcomes of noninvasive positive pressure ventilation in acute care hospitals in Massachusetts. *Chest* 145:964, 2014.
49. Riario CG, Scarpazza P, Incorvaia C: Role of noninvasive ventilation in elderly patients with hypercapnic respiratory failure. *Clin Ter* 163:47, 2012.
50. Senent C, et al: Home mechanical ventilators: the point of view of the patients. *J Eval Clin Pract* 16:832, 2010.
51. Cairo JM: *Mosby's respiratory equipment*, ed 9, St Louis, 2013, Mosby.
52. Dybwik K, Nielsen EW, Brinchmann BS: Home mechanical ventilation and specialized health care in the community: between a rock and a hard place. *BMC Health Serv Res* 11:115, 2011.
53. *LTV 1200/1150 ventilator user manual*, Minneapolis, MN, 2009, Pulmonetic Systems, Inc.
54. Murphy PB, Davidson C, Hind MD: Volume target versus pressure support non-invasive ventilation in patients with super obesity and chronic respiratory failure: a randomized controlled trial. *Thorax* 67:727, 2012.
55. Theerakittikul T, Ricaurte B, Aboussouan LS: Noninvasive positive pressure ventilation for stable outpatients: CPAP and beyond. *Cleve Clin J Med* 77:705, 2010.
56. Blakeman TC, Branson RD: Evaluation of 4 new generation portable ventilators. *Respir Care* 58:264, 2013.
57. Blakeman TC, Rodriguez D, Hanseman D: Bench evaluation of 7 home care ventilators. *Respir Care* 56:1791, 2011.
58. Bhatt SP, Peterson MW, Wilson JS, et al: Noninvasive positive pressure ventilation in subjects with stable COPD: a randomized trial. *Int J Chron Obstruct Pulmon Dis* 8:581, 2013.
59. Ryan S, et al: Nasal pillows as an alternative interface in patients with obstructive sleep apnea syndrome initiating continuous positive airway pressure therapy. *J Sleep Res* 28:114, 2010.
60. Engelberts D, Malhotra A, Butler JP: Relative effects of negative versus positive pressure ventilation depend on applied conditions. *Intensive Care Med* 38:879, 2012.
61. Simmons FM, Ferro J, Thomas-Nelson S: Discharging the ventilator-dependent patient to home—part 1. *Prof Case Manag* 15:296, 2010.
62. American Association for Respiratory Care: Clinical practice guideline: bland aerosol administration. *Respir Care* 48:529, 2003.
63. Milne RJ, Hockey H, Rea H: Long-term air humidification therapy is cost effective for patients with moderate or severe chronic obstructive pulmonary disease or bronchiectasis. *Value Health* 17:320, 2014.
64. Dolovich MB, et al: Device selection and outcomes of aerosol therapy: evidence-based guidelines. *Chest* 127:335, 2005.
65. American Association for Respiratory Care: Clinical practice guideline: suctioning of the patient at home. *Respir Care* 44:99, 1999.
66. American Association of Respiratory Care: Clinical practice guideline: effectiveness of nonpharmacologic airway clearance therapies in hospitalized patients. *Respir Care* 58:2186, 2013.
67. Park J, William J, Johnson J, et al: Does therapeutic continuous positive airway pressure predict success with an oral appliance in the treatment of obstructive sleep apnea. *Chest* 144:978, 2013.
68. Antonescu-Turcu A, Parthasarthy S: CPAP and bi-level PAP therapy: new and established roles. *Respir Care* 55:1216, 2010.
69. Xu T, Li T, Wei D, et al: Effect of automatic versus fixed continuous positive airway pressure for the treatment of obstructive sleep apnea: an up-to-date meta-analysis. *Sleep Breath* 16:1017, 2012.
70. Esquinas RM, Scala R, Soroksky A, et al: Clinical review: humidifiers during non-invasive ventilation—key topics and practical implications. *Crit Care* 16:203, 2012.
71. Ruthle KH, Franke KJ, Domanski U, et al: Quality of life, compliance, sleep and nasopharyngeal side effects during CPAP therapy with and without controlled heated humidification. *Sleep Breath* 15:479, 2011.
72. Strehle EM, Gray WK, Gopisetti S, et al: Can home monitoring reduce mortality in infants at increased risk of sudden infant death syndrome? A systemic review. *Acta Pediatr* 101:8, 2012.
73. Busa T, et al: Hygiene of nasal masks used at home for non-invasive ventilation in children. *J Hosp Infect* 76:187, 2010.
74. Attia F, Whitener CJ, Hnatuck P, et al: Monitoring of cleaning practices for portable multiuse medical equipment. *Infect Control Hosp Epidemiol* 34:1331, 2013.
75. Brown-Saltzman K, et al: An intervention to improve respiratory therapists' comfort with end-of-life care. *Respir Care* 55:858, 2010.

Glossary

A

AARC abbreviation for the *American Association for Respiratory Care*, the primary voluntary professional association for respiratory therapists. (Chapter 1)

abdominal compartment syndrome the abdomen has become a fixed compartment with increased pressure resulting in ischemia and organ dysfunction. (Chapter 16)

abdominal paradox abnormal breathing pattern seen as a sinking inward motion of the abdomen with each inspiratory effort; a sign of diaphragm fatigue. (Chapter 16)

abdominal thrust external pressure forcefully exerted on the abdomen, under the diaphragm, to expel obstructing objects from the upper airway. (Chapter 37)

absolute humidity actual mass or content of water in a measured volume of air, usually expressed in grams per cubic meter or pounds. (Chapter 6)

absorption atelectasis atelectasis resulting from the absorption of O_2 from obstructed or partially obstructed alveoli with high O_2 concentrations. (Chapter 11)

A/C alternative abbreviation for *assist/control ventilation;* see *assist/control.* (Chapter 42)

accessory muscles of breathing muscles of the neck, back, and abdomen that may assist the diaphragm and the internal and external intercostal muscles in respiration, especially in some breathing disorders or during exercise. (Chapter 9)

accountable care organizations (ACOs) are groups of doctors, hospitals, and health care providers who voluntarily come together to deliver coordinated patient care. (Chapter 56)

acid compound that yields hydrogen ions (H^+) when dissolved in an aqueous solution. (Chapter 13)

acidemia state in which arterial blood is more acidic than normal (pH < 7.35). (Chapter 14)

acid-fast of or pertaining to a bacterial stain that does not decolorize easily when washed with an acid solution; also refers to certain bacteria (especially mycobacteria) that retain red dyes after an acid wash. (Chapter 17)

acid-fast bacterium type of bacteria that resists decolorizing by acid after accepting a stain. (Chapter 17)

acinus any small, saclike structure, particularly one found in a gland. (Chapter 9)

acoustic respiratory monitoring (ARM) provides imaging of ventilation that allows localization of the injury and an assessment of the extent of injury. The technique produces a two-dimensional video or graphic representation of ventilation; quiet regions without ventilation are not "seen." With this technique there is an opportunity at the bedside to perform a real-time evaluation of the effects of positive end expiratory pressure, recruitment maneuvers, or other changes in ventilatory support. (Chapter 51)

activated clotting time the amount of time it takes blood to form a clot. (Chapter 28)

active cycle of breathing (ACB) airway clearance strategy consisting of repeated cycles of breathing control and thoracic expansion, followed by the forced expiratory technique. (Chapter 40)

active transport movement of molecules across membranes in a direction opposite that expected because of diffusion or osmotic pressure. (Chapter 13)

acute chest syndrome a syndrome developed in patients with sickle cell disease. The chief complaints are acute chest pain, cough, and shortness of breath caused by the sickling of red blood cells. (Chapter 12)

acute exacerbation of COPD state of worsening of chronic obstructive pulmonary disease (COPD), often defined by the need to increase medication or to escalate care. (Chapter 25)

acute hypoxemic respiratory failure (AHRF) respiratory compromise characterized by severely decreased oxygenation that develops over a relatively short period of time. (Chapter 29)

acute lung injury (ALI) condition characterized by alveolar flooding caused by an acute insult (e.g., sepsis). Normally a rapidly developing bilateral pulmonary process of noncardiac origin with a PaO_2 to FiO_2 ratio greater than 200 mm Hg but less than 300 mm Hg. (Chapter 29)

acute respiratory distress syndrome (ARDS) respiratory disorder characterized by respiratory insufficiency and hypoxemia; triggers include gram-negative sepsis, O_2 toxicity, trauma, pneumonia, and systemic inflammatory responses. (Chapter 29)

adaptive support ventilation (ASV) mode of ventilation guided by evaluation of the patient's lung mechanics; the ventilator tries to impose a ventilatory pattern that results in the least amount of patient work. (Chapter 52)

adenocarcinoma type of cancer characterized by glandular structures. (Chapter 31)

adhesion band of scar tissue that binds anatomic surfaces that normally are separate from each other. Adhesions most commonly form in the abdomen, after abdominal surgery, inflammation, or injury. (Chapter 6)

adrenergic of or pertaining to the sympathetic nerve fibers of the autonomic nervous system that use epinephrine or epinephrine-like substances as neurotransmitters; any chemical or drug that mimics the effect of these neurotransmitters. Also called a *sympathomimetic drug; catecholamine.* (Chapter 35)

Advanced Cardiac Life Support (ACLS) emergency medical procedures beyond basic life support; includes intravenous fluid line establishment, defibrillation, drug administration, control of cardiac arrhythmias, and use of ventilation equipment. ACLS usually requires direct or indirect supervision by a physician. (Chapter 37)

advanced directive document in which an individual specifies what medical care he or she desires to receive in the future, should he or she no longer be able to make decisions about medical treatment; may be in the form of a living will or durable power of attorney. (Chapters 5, 16)

adventitious lung sounds abnormal lung sounds. (Chapter 16)

aerobic exercise any physical activity that requires increased cardiac output and ventilation to meet the increased O_2 demands of the skeletal muscles. (Chapter 55)

aerophagia swallowing of air. (Chapter 46)

aerosol suspension of solid or liquid particles in a gas. (Chapter 39)

aerosol medications any medication that is delivered by aerosol via the respiratory tract. (Chapter 1)

aerosol output weight or mass of aerosol particles produced by a nebulizer per unit time or volume. (Chapter 39)

affective domain a learning domain addressing the area of emotion, mood, or feeling. (Chapter 54)

afterload load against which an activated muscle must try to shorten; greater afterloads result in lower velocities. (Chapters 10, 51)

ageing growing older. (Chapter 39)

agonist of or pertaining to a chemical substance or drug that has affinity for a receptor and exerts a desired or expected effect (as opposed to an antagonist). (Chapter 35)

air bronchograms lucent tubular shadows running through areas of consolidation. (Chapter 21)

airway hyperresponsiveness state of airways that causes them to constrict abnormally in response to stress or insults (e.g., exercise, inhaled materials such as dust or allergens). (Chapter 25)

airway inflammation localized protective response to pathogens occurring within the routes for passage of air into and out of the lungs and involving the release of mediators including mast cells, eosinophils, macrophages, epithelial cells, and T lymphocytes. (Chapter 25)

airway management the process of ensuring that the upper airway is free of foreign substances and patent to gas flow. (Chapter 1)

airway obstruction state of abnormally slowed expiration, characterized most commonly by a decrease in FEV_1. (Chapter 25)

airway occlusion pressure inspiratory pressure generated 100 msec after airway occlusion; P0.1 is effort-independent and is thought to be a good measure of central respiratory drive. (Chapter 52)

airway pressure release ventilation (APRV) form of pressure ventilation that uses two levels of continuous positive airway pressure in an intermittent mandatory ventilation breathing pattern. (Chapter 29)

airway resistance measure of the impedance to ventilation caused by the movement of gas through the airways; abbreviated as Raw, airway resistance is computed as the change in pressure along a tube divided by the flow. (Chapter 11)

airway stents devices designed for internal splinting of the airway lumen to help reduce airway obstruction from malignant or benign processes that compress the airway from the outside. (Chapter 22)

alae the lateral surface of the external nose; the alae may flare out during respiratory distress. (Chapter 9)

algorithm predetermined group of directions to solve a problem in a finite number of steps. (Chapter 2)

alkalemia a decreased hydrogen ion concentration in the blood; as applied to arterial blood, denotes pH greater than 7.45. (Chapter 14)

alveolar-arterial oxygen tension difference ($P(A - a)O_2$) difference between the alveolar and arterial PO_2, usually about 5 to 10 mm Hg when breathing room air. (Chapter 51)

alveolar-capillary membrane tissue that separates air from blood in the lung; consists of alveolar epithelium, basement membrane, and capillary endothelium, along with their associated structures. (Chapter 9)

alveolar dead space alveoli that are ventilated but are not perfused. The condition may exist when pulmonary circulation is obstructed, as by a thromboembolus. (Chapters 11, 12)

alveolar shunt alveolar units that are closed to ventilation but are still perfused. (Chapter 12)

alveoli small outpouching of walls of alveolar space through which gas exchange between alveolar air and pulmonary capillary blood occurs. (Chapter 9)

alveolopleural fistula an abnormal communication between the alveoli and the pleura, often associated with pneumothorax. (Chapter 27)

ambulation process of helping a bedridden patient begin to sit up, stand, and walk around independently. (Chapter 3)

American Association for Respiratory Care (AARC) profenssional association of respiratory therapists. (Chapter 1)

American Respiratory Care Foundation (ARCF) a nonprofit organization formed for the purpose of supporting research, education, and charitable activities in respiratory care. (Chapter 1)

American Society for Testing and Materials (ASTM) nongovernment agency that establishes performance standards for various equipment and materials. (Chapters 33, 38)

American standard safety system (ASSS) specifications adopted in the United States and Canada for threaded high-pressure connections between compressed gas cylinders and their attachments. (Chapter 40)

amniocentesis process of direct sampling and quantitative assessment of the amniotic fluid. (Chapter 53)

ampere basic unit of electrical energy current; equivalent to the amount of electrons flowing when 1 V of electromotive force is applied to a circuit with 1 ohm of resistance. (Chapter 3)

amyotrophic lateral sclerosis (ALS) degenerative disease of the motor neurons often characterized by atrophy of the muscles of the hands, forearms, and legs and eventually involving most of the body, including the muscles of respiration. (Chapter 32)

analyte a chemical substance that is being measured as in a broad test. (Chapter 19)

analyzer a person or device that evaluates some submitted material (e.g., a machine that measures blood chemistry components). (Chapter 19)

anemia abnormal condition characterized by a reduction in the number of circulating red blood cells or the amount of normal hemoglobin available to carry O_2. (Chapter 17)

anergy lack of activity; an immunodeficient condition characterized by a lack of or diminished reaction to an antigen or group of antigens. This state may be seen in advanced tuberculosis and other serious infections, AIDS, and some malignancies. (Chapter 23)

angina spasmodic, cramplike choking feeling. (Chapter 16)

angle of Louis slightly oblique angle where the manubrium articulates with the body of the sternum. (Chapter 9)

anion a negative ion that migrates to the anode (positive electrode) in an electrolyte solution; a negative ion. (Chapter 13)

ankylosing spondylitis chronic inflammatory disease of unknown origin, first affecting the spine and adjacent structures and commonly leading to eventual fusion (ankylosis) of the involved joints. (Chapter 32)

antagonist in pharmacology, a drug that has affinity but produces no effect; an antagonist can be competitive (forms reversible bond with receptor) or noncompetitive (forms irreversible bond). (Chapter 35)

anterior nares opening to the nose. (Chapter 9)

anthropometrics science of measuring the human body—height, weight, and size of component parts, including skin folds—to study and compare the relative proportions under normal and abnormal conditions. Also called *anthropometric measurement.* (Chapter 23)

antiadrenergic pertaining to blocking of the effects of impulses transmitted by the adrenergic postganglionic fibers of the sympathetic nervous system. (Chapter 35)

antibiotic therapy treatment of infections with antimicrobial agents, such as the penicillins. (Chapter 24)

anticholinergic of or pertaining to blockade of acetylcholine receptors that results in the inhibition of transmission of parasympathetic nerve impulses. (Chapter 35)

antiseptic tending to inhibit growth and reproduction of microorganisms. (Chapter 4)

APACHE scoring system *Acute Physiology and Chronic Health Evaluation* scoring system; severity of illness scoring system used with critically ill patients. (Chapter 51)

Apgar score evaluation of an infant's physical condition, usually performed 1 minute and 5 minutes after birth, based on a rating of five factors that reflect the infant's ability to adjust to extrauterine life. (Chapter 53)

apices uppermost portions of the lungs. (Chapter 9)

apnea absence of spontaneous breathing. (Chapter 15)

apnea of prematurity disorder of preterm infants, probably of central nervous system origin, characterized by frequent apneic pauses lasting longer than 20 seconds and often associated with cyanosis, pallor, hypotonia, or bradycardia. (Chapter 34)

apneustic breathing pattern of respirations characterized by a prolonged inspiratory phase followed by expiratory apnea. (Chapters 15, 32)

apneustic center localized collection of neurons in the pons located at the level of the vestibular area that moderates the rhythmic activity of the medullary respiratory centers. (Chapter 15)

appropriate for gestational age (AGA) refers to a newborn whose size, growth, and maturation are normal for gestational age, whether delivered prematurely, at term, or later than term. (Chapter 53)

ARCF abbreviation for *American Respiratory Care Foundation,* a philanthropic agency that promotes the field of respiratory care through grants and awards. (Chapter 1)

argon plasma coagulation a medical endoscopic procedure used to stop bleeding or to remove tumor tissue. (Chapter 22)

arterialized blood blood that resembles the blood in arteries (e.g., from the finger or earlobe capillaries). (Chapter 19)

arteriovenous anastomosis communication between an artery and a vein, either as a congenital anomaly or as a surgically produced link between vessels. (Chapter 10)

artifacts an aberration as a result of interference or technical failure. These changes do not represent a normal or so-called physiologic change. (Chapter 51)

asbestosis restrictive lung disease caused by prolonged exposure to asbestos fibers; associated with a high incidence of malignant lung tumors and pleural abnormalities. (Chapter 26)

assault any conduct that creates a reasonable apprehension of being touched in an injurious manner; no actual touching is required to prove assault. (Chapter 5)

assist/control (A/C or ACV) volume ventilation continuous mandatory ventilation (CMV) in which the minimum breathing rate is predetermined, but the patient can initiate mechanical ventilation at an increased rate. (Chapter 48)

assisted breath a breath whose delivery is aided by a mechanical device. (Chapter 45)

asthma respiratory disorder characterized by recurring episodes of paroxysmal dyspnea, wheezing on expiration or inspiration caused by constriction of the bronchi, coughing, and viscous mucoid bronchial secretions. The episodes may be precipitated by inhalation of allergens or pollutants, infection, cold air, vigorous exercise, or emotional stress. Also called *bronchial asthma*. (Chapter 25)

ataxic breathing type of breathing associated with a lesion in the medullary respiratory center and characterized by a series of increasing and decreasing inspirations and expirations. (Chapter 32)

atelectasis collapse of distal lung parenchyma. (Chapters 21, 42)

atelectrauma lung injury as a result of alveolar collapse secondary to inappropriate PEEP settings. (Chapter 46)

atmospheric pressure absolute (ATA) measure of pressure used in hyperbaric medicine; 1 ATA equals 760 mm Hg or 101.32 kPa. (Chapter 41)

atomizer device that produces an aerosol suspension of liquid particles without using baffles to control particle size. (Chapter 39)

atrial kick the propulsion of blood that results from contraction of the atrium heart chamber. (Chapter 18)

atrophy the loss of muscle mass as a result of disuse. (Chapter 47)

ATPS abbreviation for *ambient temperature, ambient pressure, saturated* (with water vapor). (Chapter 6)

attending title applied to the responsible most senior physician caring for the patient in an academic medical center. (Chapter 3)

atypical pathogens select organisms in *Legionella* species, *Chlamydophila pneumoniae,* and *Mycoplasma pneumoniae* that cause pneumonia. (Chapter 24)

auditory pertaining to the sense of hearing. (Chapter 3)

autogenic drainage (AD) modification of directed coughing, beginning with low lung volume breathing, inspiratory breath holds, and controlled exhalation and progressing to increased inspired volumes and expiratory flows. (Chapter 40)

automatic external defibrillator (AED) portable automatic device to perform defibrillation on patients outside a hospital. (Chapter 37)

automatic tube compensation (ATC) mode of ventilation that attempts to maintain tracheal pressure equal to end expiratory pressure during both inspiration and expiration. (Chapter 52)

automaticity refers to the heart's ability to generate its own intrinsic electrical rhythm. (Chapters 10, 18)

autonomy quality of having the ability or tendency to function independently. (Chapter 5)

auto-PEEP pressure above atmospheric remaining in the alveoli at end-exhalation due to air trapping. Also called *intrinsic PEEP*. (Chapter 44)

autoregulation automatic control of a mechanical or physiologic system; necessitates both a sensing mechanism (to measure what is regulated) and a feedback loop (to respond to changes). (Chapter 46)

auto-triggering triggering of a ventilator by any phenomenon that is not a result of the patient making an inspiratory effort. Most commonly a result of a small circuit leak. (Chapter 47)

Avogadro's law law in physics stating that equal volumes of all gases at a given temperature and pressure contain the identical number of molecules. (Chapter 5)

axiology the study of values (e.g., the way patients give priority to a choice). (Chapter 5)

azotemia buildup of excess nitrogenous waste products in the blood, usually secondary to renal failure. (Chapter 23)

B

bactericidal substances with the ability to kill microorganisms. (Chapter 4)

bacteriostatic ability to restrain the growth of microorganisms. (Chapter 4)

baffle surface in a nebulizer designed specifically to cause impaction of large aerosol particles, causing either further fragmentation or removal from the suspension via condensation back into the reservoir. (Chapter 39)

baffling process of removing large water particles from suspension in a jet nebulizer so that the particles entering the patient's airways are of a uniform therapeutic size. (Chapter 38)

bands bundle of fibers, as seen in striated muscle that encircles a structure or binds one part of the body to another. (Chapter 17)

baroreceptor one of the pressure-sensitive nerve endings in the walls of the atria of the heart, the vena cava, the aortic arch, and the carotid sinus. (Chapter 10)

barotrauma physical injury sustained as a result of exposure to ambient pressures above normal, most commonly secondary to positive pressure ventilation (e.g., pneumothorax, pneumomediastinum). (Chapters 29, 44, 46)

barrel chest abnormal increase in the anteroposterior diameter of the chest caused by hyperinflation of the lungs. (Chapter 16)

basal metabolic rate (BMR) amount of energy used in a unit of time by a fasting, resting subject. BMR, determined by the amount of O_2 used, is expressed in calories consumed per hour per square meter of body surface area or per kilogram of body weight. Also called *basal energy expenditure (BEE)*. (Chapter 23)

base compound that yields hydroxyl ions [OH^-] when dissolved in an aqueous solution. (Chapter 13)

base excess (BE) difference between the normal buffer base (NBB) and the actual buffer base (BB) in a whole-blood sample, expressed in mEq/L; a normal BE is +2 mEq/L. (Chapter 14)

basic chemistry panel (BCP) or basic metabolic panel includes the predominant electrolytes sodium (Na^+), potassium (K^+), chloride (Cl^-), and total CO_2/bicarbonate (CO_2) and glucose. (Chapter 17)

basic life support (BLS) cardiopulmonary resuscitation designed to reinstitute either circulatory or respiratory function without equipment or drugs. (Chapter 37)

battery (legal) an unconsented touching of an individual that causes injury. (Chapter 5)

Becker muscular dystrophy chronic degenerative disease of the muscles, characterized by progressive weakness; occurs in children 8 to 20 years old. (Chapter 32)

benchmarking establishing the relationship between an organization's ability to perform at a given level to that of other comparable organizations. (Chapter 7)

beneficence principle that requires that health providers go beyond doing no harm and actively contribute to the health and well-being of their patients. (Chapter 5)

benevolent deception actions in which the truth is withheld from the patient for his or her own good. (Chapter 5)

bias the state of having your opinion markedly affected by past experience or knowledge; an oblique or a diagonal line. (Chapter 8)

bibliographic database a collection of reference sources often used in research. (Chapter 8)

bilevel positive airway pressure (bilevel PAP) spontaneous breath mode of ventilatory support that allows separate regulation of the inspiratory and expiratory pressures. (Chapter 33)

Biot respiration breathing characterized by irregular periods of apnea alternating with periods in which four or five breaths of identical depth are taken. (Chapter 15)

biotrauma inflammation of the lungs in response to inappropriate mechanical ventilation that promotes alveolar overdistention in inspiration and derecruitment on exhalation. (Chapter 46)

bladder pressure pressure that is established in the bladder. (Chapter 51)

blood-brain barrier anatomic-physiologic feature of the brain thought to consist of walls of capillaries in the central nervous system and surrounding astrocytic glial membranes. The barrier separates the parenchyma of the central nervous system from blood. The blood-brain barrier prevents or slows the passage of some drugs and other chemical compounds, radioactive ions, and disease-causing organisms such as viruses from the blood into the central nervous system. (Chapter 15)

blunt trauma nonpenetrating trauma that may result in pulmonary contusion. (Chapter 30)

Board of Medical Advisors (BOMA) the medical advisory group for the American Association for Respiratory Care. (Chapter 1)

body humidity absolute humidity in a volume of gas saturated at a body temperature of 37° C; equivalent to 43.8 mg/L of water in the air. (Chapter 38)

body mass index (BMI) formula for determining obesity, calculated by dividing a person's weight in kilograms by the square of the person's height in meters. (Chapter 23)

Bohr effect effect of variations in blood pH on the affinity of hemoglobin for O_2. (Chapter 12)
Borg dyspnea scale validated scale used by patients to quantify the severity of dyspnea. (Chapter 20)
Bourdon gauge fixed orifice, variable pressure flowmeter. (Chapter 40)
BPF abbreviation for *bronchopleural fistula*. (Chapter 27)
brachytherapy a method to deliver short distance radiation therapy to a tumor via a bronchoscope. (Chapter 22)
bradycardia abnormally decreased heart rate. (Chapter 16)
bradypnea abnormal decrease in breathing rate. (Chapter 16)
breach of contract failure, without legal excuse, to carry out the terms of a legal agreement. (Chapter 5)
breath-actuated nebulizer aerosol device that is responsive to the patient's inspiratory effort and reduces or eliminates aerosol generation during exhalation. (Chapter 39)
breath-enhanced nebulizer nebulizers that entrain room air in direct relationship to the inspiratory flow of the patient. (Chapter 39)
breathing pattern the ventilation pattern assumed by a patient during normal or mechanical ventilation. (Chapter 42)
breathlessness distressful sensation of uncomfortable breathing that may be caused by certain heart conditions, strenuous exercise, or anxiety. (Chapter 16)
bronchial washings and brushings material sampled during bronchoscopy, specifically from instilling and withdrawing saline into the lung (washings) or inserting a brush into the lung. (Chapter 22)
bronchiectasis abnormal condition of the bronchial tree characterized by irreversible dilation and destruction of the bronchial walls. (Chapters 25, 40)
bronchiolitis acute infection of the lower respiratory tract causing expiratory wheezing, respiratory distress, inflammation, and obstruction of the bronchioles; bronchiolitis is usually caused by respiratory syncytial virus (RSV) and is most common in infants younger than 2 years old. (Chapter 33)
bronchoalveolar lavage (BAL) technique used to obtain specimens from the alveolar level of the lung. BAL is performed by instilling a small volume (up to 50 mL) of normal saline solution deep into the airways and then suctioning it back. (Chapter 22)
bronchodilator substance, especially a drug, that relaxes contractions of the smooth muscle of the bronchioles to improve ventilation to the lungs. Pharmacologic bronchodilators are prescribed to improve aeration in asthma, bronchiectasis, bronchitis, and emphysema. (Chapter 25)
bronchophony abnormal voice sounds heard over lung consolidation. (Chapter 16)
bronchopleural fistula any air communication from the lung to the pleural space. (Chapter 27)
bronchopneumonia acute inflammation of the lungs and bronchioles, characterized by chills, fever, high pulse and respirator rates, bronchial breathing, cough with purulent bloody sputum, and chest pain. (Chapter 41)
bronchopulmonary dysplasia (BPD) chronic respiratory disorder characterized by scarring of lung tissue, thickened pulmonary arterial walls, and mismatch between lung ventilation and perfusion. It often occurs in infants who have been dependent on long-term mechanical ventilation. (Chapters 33, 41)
bronchoscopy process of passing a bronchoscope into the airways for diagnostic testing or therapeutic purposes. (Chapter 36)
bronchospasm abnormal contraction of the smooth muscle of the bronchi, resulting in acute narrowing and obstruction. (Chapter 25)
BTPS abbreviation for *body temperature, ambient pressure, saturated* (with water vapor). (Chapter 6)
buffer base total blood buffer capable of binding hydrogen ions; normal buffer base (NBB) ranges from 48 to 52 mEq/L. (Chapter 14)
buffering the process of removing H^+ or OH^- in solution to minimize change in pH. (Chapter 13)
business intelligence (BI) a set of tools that permit capture, storage, and transformation of data into useful and actionable information. (Chapter 7)

C

cachexia general ill health and malnutrition characterized by weakness and emaciation. (Chapter 16)
cachexic the state of being of general ill health and suffering from malnutrition. (Chapter 23)
calibration media types of equipment used to test and ensure that the output of an analyzer (blood gas) is both accurate and linear across the range of measured values. (Chapter 19)
cannulation the process of placing a catheter in an artery or vein. (Chapters 19 and 20)
capnography process of obtaining a tracing of the proportion of CO_2 in expired air using a capnograph. (Chapters 19, 51)
capnometry measurement of CO_2 in a volume of gas, usually by methods of infrared absorption or mass spectrometry. (Chapters 19, 51)
capped-rental items eligible for reimbursement under the Medicare prospective payment system for only a predetermined number of months, after which the equipment is deemed owned by the patient and rental payments cease. (Chapter 51)
carbon monoxide poisoning exposure to carbon monoxide that allows the attachment of carbon monoxide to hemoglobin, preventing the attachment of O_2 to hemoglobin. (Chapter 30)
carboxyhemoglobin compound produced by the chemical combination of hemoglobin with carbon monoxide. (Chapter 12)
cardiac output volume of blood pumped per minute by the heart. (Chapters 10, 51)
cardiac tamponade compression of the heart caused by the collection of blood, fluid, or gas under pressure in the pericardium. (Chapter 10)
cardiopulmonary exercise evaluation (CPX) exercise-based assessment of a patient before pulmonary rehabilitation designed to determine the patient's exercise capacity and risk for desaturation. (Chapter 55)
cardiopulmonary resuscitation (CPR) basic emergency procedure for life support, consisting of artificial respiration and manual external cardiac massage. (Chapter 37)
cardiopulmonary system the combination of the respiratory and cardiac systems. (Chapter 1)
cardioversion using electrical energy to correct an abnormal heart rhythm to normal. (Chapter 37)
carina bifurcation of the trachea into the right and left main stem bronchi. (Chapter 9)
catecholamine any one of a group of sympathomimetic compounds composed of a catechol molecule and the aliphatic portion of an amine. (Chapter 35)
cation positively charged ion. (Chapter 13)
Centers for Medicare and Medicaid Services (CMS) federal agency within the U.S. Department of Health and Human Services that administers the Medicare program and works in partnership with state governments to administer Medicaid. (Chapter 56)
central cyanosis abnormal discoloration of the skin distributed in central structures like the nose and lips. (Chapter 16)
central neurogenic hyperinflation hyperinflation caused by a neurologic progress generally resulting in a markedly increased minute ventilation. (Chapter 32)
central sleep apnea absence of breathing as the result of medullary depression that inhibits respiratory movement, which becomes more pronounced during sleep. (Chapter 33)
cephalization refers to increased visualization of pulmonary blood vessels on a chest radiograph in the nondependent regions of the lung; often a sign of left heart failure. (Chapter 21)
channel passageway or groove that conveys fluid, such as the central channels that connect the arterioles with the venules. (Chapter 3)
chemoreceptor sensory nerve cell activated by changes in the chemical environment surrounding it; the chemoreceptors in the carotid artery are sensitive to PCO_2 in the blood, signaling the respiratory center in the brain to increase or decrease ventilation. (Chapters 10, 15)
chemotherapy treatment of infections and other diseases with chemical agents. (Chapter 32)
chest cuirass device to deliver negative pressure ventilation that fits over the thorax. (Chapter 45)
chest physical therapy (CPT) collection of therapeutic techniques designed to aid clearance of secretions, improve ventilation, and enhance the conditioning of the respiratory muscles; includes positioning techniques, chest percussion and vibration, directed coughing, and various breathing and conditioning exercises. (Chapter 40)
chest radiograph x-ray image of the chest; a posteroanterior view and a lateral, or side, view are routinely obtained. (Chapter 21)
Cheyne-Stokes respiration abnormal breathing pattern with periods of progressively deeper

breaths alternating with periods of shallow breathing and apnea. (Chapters 15, 32)

CHF abbreviation for *congestive heart failure;* an abnormal condition that reflects impaired cardiac output, caused by myocardial infarction, ischemic heart disease, or cardiomyopathy. (Chapters 10, 29)

chlorofluorocarbons (CFCs) gaseous chemical compounds that were originally used to power metered dose inhalers but currently phased out of use. (Chapter 39)

cholinergic of or pertaining to nerve fibers that elaborate acetylcholine at the myoneural junctions. (Chapter 35)

chronic bronchitis common debilitating pulmonary disease, characterized by greatly increased production of mucus by the glands of the trachea and bronchi that results in a cough with expectoration for at least 3 months of the year for more than 2 consecutive years. (Chapter 25)

chronic cough cough that persists, sometimes defined as greater than 8 weeks (to distinguish from acute cough [<3 weeks] and subacute cough [3-8 weeks]). (Chapter 16)

chyle cloudy liquid products of digestion taken up by the small intestine. Consisting mainly of emulsified fats, chyle passes through finger-like projections in the small intestine, called *lacteals,* and into the lymphatic system for transport to the venous circulation at the thoracic duct in the neck. (Chapter 27)

chylothorax pleural fluid collection that is high in triglycerides, usually from disruption of the thoracic duct. (Chapter 27)

cilia tiny hairlike projections that line mucus-producing structures. Generally they operate in a wavelike motion moving mucous along the structure. (Chapter 9)

ciliary dyskinetic syndromes conditions in which respiratory tract cilia do not function properly. (Chapter 40)

circulatory failure the failure of the circulatory system to maintain normal cardiac output. (Chapter 37)

clinical decision support (CDS) health information technology functionality that builds on the foundation of an electronic health record to provide specific information, which is intelligently filtered and organized, at appropriate times, to enhance health and health care. (Chapter 7)

clinical queries search filter in PubMed effective in retrieving valid research studies. (Chapter 7)

clinical simulation the simulation of an actual clinical scenario using actors, manikins, and paper and pencil. (Chapter 7)

closed buffer system buffer system in which all components of acid-base reactions remain in the system. Products accumulate and reach equilibrium with reactants, and chemical activity ceases (no further buffering activity can take place). Closed buffer systems in the body include nonbicarbonate buffers, such as plasma proteins, hemoglobin, and phosphates. (Chapter 14)

closed-loop control control circuit that receives feedback from a measured variable that automatically adjusts a gas delivery variable based on the feedback. (Chapter 42)

clubbing bulbous swelling of the terminal phalanges of the fingers and toes, often associated with certain chronic lung diseases. (Chapter 16)

Coanda effect phenomenon in hydrodynamics whereby a fluid in motion may be attracted or held to a wall. (Chapter 6)

cognitive domain area of the mental processes of comprehension, judgment, memory, and reasoning. (Chapter 54)

cohesion attractive force between like molecules. (Chapter 6)

cohorting grouping individuals who share a common characteristic, such as the same age or the same sex or a common infection. (Chapter 4)

cold shock cardiorespiratory reflexes reflexes activated by water temperature less than 25° C. A breathing pattern characterized by gasping followed by hyperventilation and shallow breathing at total lung capacity. (Chapter 30)

collateral circulation redundant circulation in an area of tissue or an organ that supplies blood to the tissue through more than one path. (Chapter 19)

colloids substances that contains large molecules that attract and hold water; also a dispersion or a gel. (Chapter 13)

Committee on Accreditation for Respiratory Care (CoARC) committee that establishes standards and overseas approval of educational programs in respiratory care. (Chapters 1, 2)

competencies measurable or observable skills, knowledge, behaviors, or abilities to perform a job or task. (Chapters 2, 3)

community-acquired pneumonia acute inflammation of the lungs contracted from the environment (as distinguished from nosocomial, or hospital-acquired, pneumonia). (Chapter 24)

compensatory justice calls for the recovery of damages that were a result of the action of others. (Chapter 5)

complete blood count a determination of the number of red and white blood cells per cubic millimeter of blood. A complete blood count is one of the most routinely performed tests in a clinical laboratory and one of the most valuable screening and diagnostic techniques. (Chapter 17)

compliance volume change per unit in applied pressure. (Chapters 11, 20)

Comprehensive outpatient rehabilitation facilities (CORF) Medicare-approved facilities that provides a broad scope of ambulatory rehabilitation services as defined in section 933 of Public Law 96-499. (Chapter 55)

compressed volume volume of gas compressed in the ventilator circuit and not delivered to the patient during a positive pressure breath. (Chapter 45)

compression atelectasis collapse of a part of the lung as a result of an external force compressing the lung. (Chapter 41)

computed tomography (CT) radiographic technique that produces a film that represents a detailed cross section of tissue structure. (Chapters 21, 30)

computerized physician order entry (CPOE) a system by which medical orders can be electronically transmitted to the electronic health record saving time and reducing transcription errors resulting from illegible handwriting. (Chapter 7)

condensation change of state from gas to liquid, as with water vapor condensation. (Chapter 6)

conditions of participation a certificate awarded institutions that meet specific standards of quality and safety as determined by the Centers for Medicare and Medicaid Services. (Chapter 51)

conduction transfer of heat by the direct interaction of atoms or molecules in a hot area that contact atoms or molecules in a cooler area. (Chapter 6)

confidentiality nondisclosure of certain information except to another authorized person. (Chapter 5)

congestive heart failure (CHF) abnormal condition that reflects impaired cardiac pumping; caused by myocardial infarction, ischemic heart disease, or cardiomyopathy that results in either pulmonary or systemic edema. (Chapters 10, 29)

conjugate base the base associated with the weak acid in a buffer system. (Chapter 14)

conjunctivitis inflammation of the conjunctiva, caused by bacterial or viral infection, allergy, or environmental factors. (Chapter 45)

connective tissue disease group of acquired disorders that have in common diffuse immunologic and inflammatory changes in small blood vessels and connective tissue. The cause of most of these diseases is unknown. Also called *collagen vascular disease.* (Chapter 26)

consequentialism idea of judging an act to be right; an ethical viewpoint in which decisions are based on the assessment of consequences. (Chapter 5)

conservative fluid management a strategy of administering fluids that attempt to minimize fluid excess over output. (Chapter 29)

contact precautions safeguards designed to reduce the risk for transmission of epidemiologically important microorganisms by direct or indirect contact. (Chapter 4)

continuing respiratory care education education sought by respiratory therapists after graduation. (Chapter 7)

continuous mandatory ventilation (CMV) system of mechanical ventilation in which the patient is allowed to initiate breathing, but the ventilator delivers a set volume or pressure with each breath. The ventilator also can be programmed to initiate breathing if the patient's breathing slows beyond a certain point or stops altogether. (Chapter 45)

continuous positive airway pressure (CPAP) method of ventilatory support whereby the patient breathes spontaneously without mechanical assistance against threshold resistance, with pressure above atmospheric maintained at the airway throughout breathing. (Chapters 33, 42, 45, 51, 53)

continuous quality improvement (CQI) aa process-based data driven approach that attempts to enhance the quality of care and patient safety. (Chapter 7)

continuous spontaneous ventilation (CSV) method of delivering ventilatory support in which the patient determines when a breath is initiated and when it is terminated. (Chapter 45)

contractility property of muscle tissue to shorten in response to a stimulus, usually electrical. (Chapters 10, 51)

control system the system used to determine how a mechanical ventilator delivers gas (e.g., targeting schemes). (Chapter 45)

control variable primary variable that the ventilator controls to provide inspiration: pressure, volume, time, or flow. (Chapter 42)

controlled ventilation use of an intermittent positive pressure breathing unit or other respirator that has an automatic cycling device that replaces spontaneous respiration. (Chapter 48)

convection heat transfer through the mixing of fluid molecules at different temperature states via thermal currents. (Chapter 6)

corticosteroid any one of the natural or synthetic hormones associated with the adrenal cortex, which influences or controls key processes of the body, such as carbohydrate and protein metabolism, electrolyte and water balance, and function of the cardiovascular system and kidneys. (Chapter 26)

costal cartilage fibrous tissues that connect the ribs to the sternum and to each other anteriorly. (Chapter 9)

costophrenic angle acute angle where the costal pleura meets the diaphragm. (Chapter 9)

cough forceful expiratory effort designed to expel mucus and other foreign material from the upper airway. (Chapter 16)

crackles discontinuous type of adventitious lung sound. (Chapter 16)

cricoid cartilage ring of cartilage that forms the lower border of the larynx. (Chapter 9)

critical illness myopathy a heterogeneous constellation of symptoms commonly occurring in the intensive care unit in which patients develop flaccid weakness of proximal muscles. Risk factors include corticosteroids, use of paralytic agents, hyperglycemia, hyperthyroidism, and possibly a systemic inflammatory response without sepsis. (Chapter 32)

critical illness polyneuropathy the development of muscle weakness and atrophy, loss of deep tendon reflexes, and loss of peripheral sensation to pinprick and touch in patients with severe sepsis. (Chapter 32)

critical pressure pressure exerted by a vapor in an evacuated container at its critical temperature. (Chapter 6)

critical temperature highest temperature at which a substance can exist as a liquid, regardless of pressure. (Chapter 6)

critical test value a test result that requires immediate communication of the result with a physician. (Chapter 17)

cross-training process of providing health care professionals with multiple skills in areas that span disciplines; for example, training a respiratory care practitioner to take chest radiographs. (Chapter 3)

croup infectious disorder of the upper airway occurring chiefly in infants and children that normally results in subglottic swelling and obstruction. (Chapters 33, 41)

CRT abbreviation for *certified respiratory therapist;* a respiratory therapist who has successfully completed the technician (entry-level) certification examination of the NBRC. (Chapter 1)

cryogenic related to very low temperature. (Chapter 40)

cryotherapy treatment using the application of cold temperatures, as for airway lesions during bronchoscopy. (Chapter 22)

current a flowing or streaming movement; a flow of electrons along a conductor in a closed circuit; an electric current. (Chapter 3)

cuvette small transparent tube or container with specific optical properties. The chemical composition of the container determines the vessel's use, such as Pyrex glass for examining materials in the visible spectrum or silica for examining materials in the ultraviolet range. (Chapter 19)

cyanide toxicity a result of the inhalation of gas produced by the burning of nitrogenous material. Cyanide combines with cytochrome oxide, the last receptor of the electron transport chain, which prevents the utilization of O_2. (Chapter 30)

cyanocobalamin chemical that reduces the half-life of the toxic compound that results from the reaction of cyanide with cytochrome oxide. (Chapter 30)

cyanosis abnormal bluish discoloration of the skin or mucous membranes. (Chapter 16)

cycle a complete breath of inspiration and expiration. (Chapter 45)

cytochrome oxidase the final electron acceptor on the electron transport chain in the mitochondrion. (Chapter 30)

cycle asynchrony a lack of coordination of the ending of a patient's inspiration with the ending of the ventilator inspiration. (Chapter 47)

cycle variable variable that terminates inspiration during mechanical ventilation. (Chapter 42)

cyclic guanosine 3,5-monophosphate (cGMP) substance that mediates the action of certain hormones in a manner similar to cyclic adenosine monophosphate. (Chapter 41)

cystic fibrosis autosomal recessive disease characterized by pancreatic insufficiency, abnormally thick secretions from the exocrine glands, and increased concentration of sodium and chloride in the sweat glands; known in Europe as *mucoviscidosis.* (Chapters 25, 34)

D

Dalton's law in physics, law stating that the total pressure exerted by a mixture of gases is equal to the sum of the pressures exerted by the individual gases if they were present alone in the container. (Chapter 6)

DataArc secure, password-protected, web-based database management system for documenting and reporting clinical educational activities for nursing and allied health professions, including respiratory care. (Chapter 7)

dead space respired gas volume that does not participate in gas exchange; may be anatomic, alveolar, or mechanical. (Chapter 12)

dead space/tidal volume ratio (V_D/V_T) percentage of tidal volume that does not participate in gas exchange, usually approximately 30% to 35%. (Chapter 51)

decannulation removal of a cannula or tube that may have been inserted during a therapeutic or surgical procedure. (Chapter 36)

decremental PEEP trial progressively decreasing the amount of PEEP to assess oxygenation and hemodynamic status immediately following a recruitment maneuver. (Chapter 30)

deep breathing/directed cough movements used to improve pulmonary gas exchange or to maintain respiratory function, especially after prolonged inactivity or general anesthesia. (Chapter 42)

deep venous thrombosis (DVT) blood clot forming in the deep veins, usually of the legs. (Chapter 28)

defendant person denying the party against whom relief or recovery is sought in an action or suit; also, the accused in a criminal case. (Chapter 5)

defibrillation termination of ventricular fibrillation by delivering a direct electrical countershock to the patient's precordium. (Chapter 37)

depolarization reduction of a membrane potential to a less negative value; in cardiac fibers, this results in the release of calcium ions into the myofibrils and activates the contractile process. (Chapter 18)

deposition testimony of a witness taken on interrogatories, either oral or in writing. (Chapter 39)

dermatomyositis condition characterized by inflammation of the muscles and/or skin. (Chapter 32)

dew point temperature at which water vapor condenses back to its liquid form. (Chapter 6)

diagnosis identifying the underlying cause for signs and symptoms, as in naming a disease the patient has. (Chapter 16)

diameter-indexed safety system (DISS) specifications established to prevent accidental interchange of low-pressure (<200 psig) medical gas connectors. DISS is used in respiratory care to connect equipment to a low-pressure gas source. (Chapter 40)

diaphoresis secretion of sweat, especially profuse secretion associated with an elevated body temperature, physical exertion, exposure to heat, and mental or emotional stress. (Chapter 16)

diaphragm large dome-shaped muscle that separates the thorax from the abdomen; the primary muscle of ventilation. (Chapter 9)

diaphragmatic dysfunction an inability of the diaphragm to contract normally. (Chapter 47)

diastolic pressure baseline blood pressure in the arteries during ventricular relaxation. (Chapter 16)

diffusing capacity of the lung (DL) number of milliliters of gas that transfer from the lungs to the pulmonary blood per minute for each 1 mm Hg partial pressure difference between the alveoli and pulmonary capillary blood. (Chapter 20)

diffusing capacity of the lung to alveolar volume ratio ($DLCO/V_A$) index of the diffusing capacity for each 1 L of lung volume and an index of the functional alveolar surface area available for diffusion. (Chapter 20)

diffusing capacity of the lung-to–effective total lung capacity ratio index of the diffusing capacity normalized to the total lung capacity, useful to distinguish between interstitial lung disease and extrathoracic causes of restriction. (Chapter 20)

diluent substance, generally a fluid, that makes a solution or mixture less concentrated, less viscous, or more liquid. (Chapter 13)

dilute solution a solution that contains a small amount of solute in relation to solvent. (Chapter 13)

dilution equation an equation used to determine the final concentration of a solution in which the original volume multiplied by the original concentration are equal to the final volume multiplied by the final concentration. (Chapter 13)

disease management an integrated process for the care of patients with a particular chronic disease. Generally, a multidisciplinary group of practitioners providing care, most of which are non-physicians. (Chapters 3, 54)

disinfection process of destroying at least the vegetative phase of pathogenic microorganisms by physical or chemical means. (Chapter 4)

distributive justice refers to proper allotment of the benefits and burdens in a society, such as taxes and subsidies. (Chapter 5)

dorsal respiratory groups (DRGs) groupings of cells in the medulla oblongata that are active in controlling inspiration. (Chapter 15)

double effect the understanding that many good actions have both a good and bad effect. (Chapter 5)

double triggering the activation of a second ventilator-delivered breath without exhalation after the first breath. Normally occurs when tidal volume is too small and inspiratory time is too short. (Chapter 47)

downstream relative reference to a point more distal from the source in a stream of flowing fluid. (Chapter 40)

driving pressure the pressure that is driving a fluid from one point to another. During mechanical ventilation, this is the difference between plateau pressure and PEEP. (Chapter 51)

droplet nuclei residue of evaporated water droplets; owing to their small size (0.5 to 12 mm), droplet nuclei can remain suspended in the air for long periods. (Chapter 4)

droplet precautions safeguards designed to reduce the risk for droplet transmission of infectious agents. (Chapter 4)

drug signaling mechanism by which a drug exerts its effect on receptors. (Chapter 35)

dry drowning drowning without water entry into the lungs, occurs as a result of reflex laryngeal spasm. (Chapter 30)

dual-control mode of ventilation in which the control variable (pressure, volume, flow) switches during a breath. (Chapter 45)

Duchenne muscular dystrophy (DMD) abnormal congenital condition characterized by progressive symmetric wasting of the leg and pelvic muscles; predominantly affects males and accounts for 50% of all muscular dystrophy diseases. (Chapter 32)

ductus arteriosus vascular channel in the fetus that joins the pulmonary artery directly to the descending aorta; it normally closes after birth. (Chapters 9, 34)

ductus venosus vascular channel in the fetus passing through the liver and joining the umbilical vein with the inferior vena cava; before birth, it carries highly oxygenated blood from the placenta to the fetal circulation. (Chapter 9)

durable medical equipment (DME) supplier a company that provides medical equipment to patients in the home. (Chapter 51)

dynamic compression collapse of airways caused by a pressure gradient that occurs with breathing or forced breathing and normally occurs in diseased airways. (Chapter 11)

dynamic hyperinflation increase in functional residual capacity (FRC) above the elastic equilibrium volume of the respiratory system; causes include increased flow resistance, short inspiratory time, and increased postinspiratory muscle activity; see also *auto-PEEP*. (Chapters 11, 44)

dysoxia abnormal metabolic state in which the tissues are unable to use properly the O_2 made available to them. (Chapter 12)

dyspnea difficult or labored breathing as perceived by the patient. (Chapter 16)

E

ECLS extracorporeal lung support, the same process as ECMO. (Chapter 29)

ECMO extracorporeal membrane oxygenation is the process whereby blood is removed from the body, pumped through a membrane to exchange CO_2 for O_2, and then returned to the body. (Chapter 29)

ectopic beat impulse that originates in the heart at a site other than the sinus node. (Chapter 18)

ectopic focus origination of a heartbeat from some place in the heart other than the sinoatrial node. (Chapter 18)

edema excess fluid in the interstitial spaces between cells; in the lungs, edema fluid may also be present in the airways and alveolar spaces. (Chapter 29)

effective total lung capacity (V_A) single-breath technique distributes a gas mixture through unobstructed airways to an alveolar volume. (Chapter 20)

egophony physical examination finding of increased resonance of voice sounds when auscultating the chest (e.g., due to lung consolidation). (Chapter 16)

elastance tendency of matter to resist a stretching force and recoil or return to its original size or form after deformation or expansion; the reciprocal of compliance. Also called *elasticity*. (Chapters 11, 45)

elasticity ability of tissue to regain its original shape and size after being stretched, squeezed, or otherwise deformed. Muscle tissue is generally regarded as elastic because it is able to change size and shape and return to its original condition. (Chapter 11)

electrical impedance tomography (EIT) the process by which mapping of the lung is obtained by a series of electrodes placed around the chest that sequentially emit low level current. The variability among the impedance to the current between electrodes is used to map lung volume. (Chapter 51)

electrocardiogram (ECG) an important diagnostic tool used to measure the electrical activity of the heart. (Chapter 18)

electrochemical refers to processes where electrical changes drive chemical processes. (Chapter 19)

electromagnetic navigational bronchoscopy a bronchioscopic technique that facilitates accurate navigation to sample peripheral pulmonary target lesions. (Chapter 22)

electronic health record (EHR) the sum of all medical records produced for a patient during the different encounters with various health care entities throughout their lifetime, and which are available across the continuum of care in all geographic locations. These data are stored in an electronic system. (Chapter 7)

electronic medical record (EMR) a system for which the medical record is stored in a computer (rather than on paper records). (Chapter 7)

E-medicine is the term that relates to the use of computerized or digital technology to enhance efficiency and effectiveness of health care in general and more specifically patient care. (Chapter 7, 22)

emitted dose describes the mass of drug leaving the mouthpiece of a nebulizer or inhaler as aerosol. (Chapter 39)

emphysema destructive process of the lung parenchyma leading to permanent enlargement of the distal air spaces; classified as either centrilobular (CLE), which mainly involves the respiratory bronchioles, or panlobular (PLE), which can involve the entire terminal respiratory unit. (Chapter 25)

empyema pus within the pleural space. A pleural fluid Gram stain that shows bacteria. (Chapters 21, 27)

end-diastolic volume (EDV) volume of blood remaining in the ventricles just prior to contraction. (Chapter 10)

end-systolic volume (ESV) volume of blood in the ventricles at the end of contraction, or systole. (Chapter 10)

endobronchial biopsy a sampling of an abnormality seen within the bronchus on bronchoscopy. (Chapter 22)

endobronchial intubation the purposeful or accidental placement of an endotracheal tube into a main stem bronchus, usually the right main stem bronchus. (Chapter 47)

endotracheal tubes artificial airways that pass through the oropharynx or nasopharynx into the trachea. (Chapter 36)

enterprise software packages computer software that is used by a whole health system. (Chapter 7)

epiglottis flat cartilage that extends from the base of the tongue backward and upward. (Chapter 9)

epiglottitis acute, often life-threatening infection of the upper airway, which causes severe obstruction secondary to supraglottic swelling; caused primarily by *Haemophilus influenzae* type B and affecting mainly children younger than 5 years old. (Chapter 34)

epistaxis to bleed from the nose. (Chapter 9)

equal pressure point (EPP) during forced exhalation, the point along an airway where the pressure inside its wall equals the intrapleural pressure; upstream beyond this point, the pleural pressure exceeds the pressure inside the airway, tending to promote bronchiolar collapse. (Chapter 11)

equilibrium constant a constant determined by the amount of a buffer that dissociates in solution. Identifies the pH at which the buffer is most effective. (Chapter 14)

equivalent weight weight of an element in any given unit (e.g., grams) that displaces a unit weight of hydrogen from a compound or combines with or replaces a unit weight of hydrogen. (Chapter 13)

erythrocyte red blood cell. (Chapter 17)

esophageal balloon a catheter with an elongated balloon placed in the esophagus used to measure pressure change that is reflective of pleural pressure change. (Chapter 51)

eustachian tubes bilateral tubes that connect the nasopharynx to the middle ear and mastoid sinus. (Chapter 9)

evaporation change in state of a substance from liquid to gaseous form occurring below its boiling point. (Chapter 6)

evidence-based medicine (EBM) is an approach to medical practice intended to optimize decision-making by emphasizing the use of evidence from well designed research projects. (Chapter 2)

expiratory cycling criteria the criteria employed by the ventilator to transition from inspiration to exhalation. In pressure support ventilation, this is usually flow. (Chapter 47)

expiratory positive airway pressure (EPAP) application of positive pressure to the airway during exhalation. Compare with *inspiratory positive airway pressure.* (Chapter 45)

expiratory reserve volume (ERV) total amount of gas that can be exhaled from the lung after a quiet exhalation. (Chapter 20)

external nares the external opening of the nasal passages. (Chapter 9)

external oblique abdominal muscle group that functions as an accessory muscle of ventilation. (Chapter 9)

external respiration part of the respiratory process that involves the exchange of gases in the alveoli of the lungs. (Chapter 9)

extracorporeal carbon dioxide removal ($ECCO_2R$) procedure whereby blood is passed from the patient through an external membrane, which filters CO_2 to support ventilation. (Chapter 29)

extracorporeal membrane oxygenation (ECMO) procedure whereby venous blood is pumped outside the body to a heart-lung machine for oxygenation and returned to the body. (Chapter 29)

extremely low birth weight (ELBW) a neonate weighting less than 1 kilogram at birth. (Chapter 53)

extubation process of withdrawing a tube from an orifice or cavity of the body. (Chapter 36)

exudate the fluid that oozes from cells and tissues. (Chapters 30, 41)

exudative relating to the oozing of fluid and other materials from cells and tissues, usually as a result of inflammation or injury. (Chapter 41)

exudative pleural effusion any pleural effusion high in protein or lactate dehydrogenase, which implies inflammation or vascular injury on the pleural surface. (Chapter 27)

ex vivo pertaining to outside of the body. (Chapter 18)

F

factitious events values that are real but "out-of-range" and often are temporary, such as the elevation in airway pressure during a cough. (Chapter 51)

false ribs of the 12 pairs of ribs forming a large part of the thoracic skeleton, the first 7 are called *true ribs,* and the next 5 are called *false ribs;* the first 3 attach to the ribs above, and the last 2 are free. (Chapter 9)

fatigue the inability of a muscle to carry its normal load. (Chapter 46)

fasciotomy a surgical procedure that cuts away the fascia to relieve tension or pressure. Used to treat burn patients with severe scar formation. (Chapter 30)

febrile to have a fever. (Chapter 16)

feedback in communication theory, information produced by a receiver and perceived by a sender that informs the sender of the receiver's reaction to the message. Feedback is a cyclic part of the process of communication that regulates and modifies the content of messages. (Chapter 3)

Fellow of the American Association for Respiratory Care (FAARC) a person who has been recognized for the AARC for sustained and substantial contributions to the field of respiratory care. (Chapter 1)

fenestrated an opening into a structure; from the Latin *fenestra,* meaning "window." (Chapter 36)

fetal hemoglobin (HbF) hemoglobin variant that has a greater affinity for O_2 than adult hemoglobin; HbF is gradually replaced over the first year of life by HbA. (Chapter 12)

fetid foul-smelling. (Chapter 16)

fever abnormal elevation of body temperature owing to disease. (Chapter 16)

fever of unknown origin (FUO) a fever for which the cause is not known nor attributable to common causes such as infection. (Chapter 16)

fiberoptic bundles individual coated fibers (or fibers formed into ribbons or bundles) that have a tough resin buffer layer which are used to transmit light from a light source to view the airways through a bronchoscope. (Chapter 22)

Fick equation equation for computing cardiac output based on knowledge of O_2 consumption and the arterial-venous O_2 content difference. (Chapters 12, 51)

Fick's first law of diffusion law for determining the rate of gaseous diffusion across biologic membranes. (Chapter 12)

filling density ratio between the weight of liquid gas put into a cylinder and the weight of water the cylinder could contain if full. (Chapter 40)

fine-particle fraction particles that are small enough to reach the lower respiratory tract. (Chapter 39)

fissures narrow clefts or slits; the lines that divide or separate the lobes of the lung glottis. (Chapter 9)

fixed acid titratable, nonvolatile acid representing the by-product of protein catabolism; examples include phosphoric acid and sulfuric acid. (Chapter 14)

flail chest traumatic chest injury in which a portion of the rib cage becomes unstable because of multiple rib fractures or costochondral separation; typically, the flail region exhibits paradoxical movement during inspiration, contributing to a maldistribution of ventilation. (Chapter 32)

flammable the ability of a substance to burn or ignite, causing fire or combustion. (Chapter 40)

flange rim used to strengthen an object, to help guide it, and to facilitate its attachment to another object. (Chapter 33)

flexible bronchoscopy a bronchoscopy that is flexible in structure, allowing it to be placed deep into the respiratory tract. (Chapter 32)

floating ribs last two rib pairs that are free at their ventral extremities. (Chapter 9)

flow asynchrony asynchrony as a result of the ventilator not providing sufficient flow to meet the patient's inspiratory demand. Most commonly occurs in volume ventilation. (Chapter 47)

flowmeter device operated by a needle valve that controls and measures gas flow according to the principles of viscosity and density. (Chapter 40)

flow resistance difference in pressure between the two points along a tube, divided by the actual flow. (Chapter 6)

fluid entrainment use of the Bernoulli effect to draw a second fluid into a stream of flow. (Chapter 6)

fluvial or brackish water sea water used in reference to drowning. (Chapter 30)

fomite nonliving material, such as bed linens or equipment, which may transmit pathogenic organisms to a person who comes into contact with the object. (Chapters 4, 24)

foramen ovale opening in the septum between the right and the left atria in the fetal heart. This opening provides a bypass for blood that would otherwise flow to the fetal lungs. After birth, the foramen ovale functionally closes. (Chapter 9)

forced expiration technique (FET) modification of the normal cough sequence designed to facilitate clearance of bronchial secretions, while minimizing the likelihood of bronchiolar collapse. (Chapter 43)

forced expiratory flow between 200 ml and 1200 ml ($FEF_{200-1200}$) measure of average expiratory flow during the early phase of exhalation; specifically, it is a measure of the flow rate for the 1000 ml of expired gas immediately following the first 200 ml of expired gas. Formerly called *maximum expiratory flow rate (MEFR)*. (Chapter 20)

forced expiratory flow between 25% and 75% of forced vital capacity ($FEF_{25\%-75\%}$) measure of average expiratory flow during the middle half of forced vital capacity. (Chapter 20)

forced expiratory flow between 75% and 85% of forced vital capacity ($FEF_{75\%-85\%}$) measure of average expiratory flow during the end of forced vital capacity. (Chapter 20)

forced expiratory volume in half of a second ($FEV_{0.5}$) maximum volume of gas that the patient can exhale during the first half second of a forced vital capacity maneuver. (Chapter 20)

forced expiratory volume in 1 second (FEV_1) maximum volume of gas that the patient can exhale during the first second of the forced vital capacity maneuver. (Chapter 20)

forced expiratory volume in 1 second–to–vital capacity ratio (%FEV_1/FVC) percent of the measured forced vital capacity that can be exhaled in 1 second. (Chapter 20)

forced vital capacity (FVC) maximum volume of gas that the subject can exhale as forcefully and as quickly as possible. (Chapter 20)

formalism ethical viewpoint that relies on rules and principles. (Chapter 5)

fractional distillation process of separating the components of a liquid mixture according to their boiling points via the application of heat; the primary commercial process used to produce O_2. (Chapter 40)

Frank-Starling principle the more a muscle fiber is stretched, the greater is the tension the muscle fiber generates when contracted. (Chapter 10)

frequency/tidal volume ratio (f/V_T) ratio of the tidal volume in ml divided by the respiratory rate. (Chapter 51)

full ventilatory support ventilatory support modes in which the ventilator provides all the minute ventilation requirements of the patient. (Chapter 48)

functional residual capacity (FRC) total amount of gas left in the lungs after a resting expiration. (Chapter 20)

G

gallop rhythm abnormal heart sound that resembles the gallop of a horse, most often indicates heart failure. (Chapter 16)

gantry examination table used for computed tomography (CT) scans. (Chapter 21)

gas absorption atelectasis collapsing of airways due to hyperoxygenation and nitrogen washout. (Chapter 42)

gasping the process of breathing periodically with a labored forced inspiration. (Chapter 32)

gastric inflation introduction of air into the stomach and intestines. (Chapter 37)

gastroesophageal reflux disease (GERD) condition characterized by abnormal movement of stomach contents into the esophagus or mouth; acid from the stomach may be aspirated into the lung and cause asthma-like symptoms. (Chapter 34)

geometric standard deviation (GSD) describes the variability of particle size in an aerosol distribution set at 1 standard deviation above and below the median. (Chapter 39)

gladiolus the body of the sternum. (Chapter 9)

Glasgow Coma Scale (GCS) scale used to provide a score to classify the level of conscious awareness in patients suspected to have an acute brain injury. (Chapters 30, 51)

glomerular filtration rate the volume of water filtered out of the plasma through glomerular capillary walls into Bowman's capsule in the kidney per unit of time. (Chapter 30)

glottis variable opening between the vocal cords. (Chapter 9)

Graham law law stating that the rate of diffusion of a gas through a liquid (or the alveolar-capillary membrane) is directly proportional to its solubility coefficient and inversely proportional to the square root of its density. (Chapter 6)

ground connection between the electrical circuit and the ground, which becomes a part of the circuit. (Chapter 3)

grunting, flaring, and retracting (GFR) the respiratory pattern observed in infants in marked respiratory distress. The neonate makes a grunting sound during breathing with flaring of the nostrils. (Chapter 53)

Guillain-Barré syndrome idiopathic, peripheral polyneuritis characterized by lower extremity weakness that progresses to the upper extremities and face; may lead to flaccid paraplegia and marked respiratory muscle weakness. (Chapter 32)

H

Haldane effect influence of hemoglobin saturation with O_2 on CO_2 dissociation. (Chapter 12)

Hamburger phenomenon the shifting of Cl ions out of the red blood cell as HCO ion is formed in the cell by hydrolysis (combination of CO_2 with H_2O). (Chapter 12)

Harris-Benedict equation equation used to estimate the caloric expenditure in normal individuals under conditions of minimal activity. (Chapter 51)

health care–associated infection (HAI) is an infection which develops from a hospital or other health care environment. (Chapter 4)

health care–associated pneumonia (HCAP) pneumonia occurring in any patient hospitalized for 2 or more days in the past 90 days in an acute care setting or who, in the past 30 days, has resided in a long-term care or nursing facility; attended a hospital or hemodialysis clinic; or received intravenous antibiotics, chemotherapy, or wound care. (Chapter 24)

Health Care Infection Control Practices Advisory Committee (HICPAC) federal advisory committee composed of 14 external infection control experts who provide advice and guidance to the U.S. Centers for Disease Control and Prevention (CDC) and the Secretary of the Department of Health and Human Services regarding the practice of health care infection control and strategies for surveillance and prevention and control of health care–associated infections in U.S. health care facilities. (Chapter 4)

health education process of planned learning opportunities designed to enable individuals to make informed decisions about and act to promote their own health. (Chapter 54)

health informatics the systematic application of information and computer science and technology to clinical or public health practice. (Chapter 7)

***Health Information Technology for Economic and Clinical Health Act* (HITECH Act)** part of a national strategy for building a national health information infrastructure that, among other things, began providing incentives to hospitals, physicians, and other health service providers who demonstrate that they are meaningfully using their electronic health records by meeting predefined standards. (Chapter 7)

health literacy is the degree to which individuals can obtain, process and understand basic health information to make appropriate health decisions and recommendations. (Chapter 54)

health promotion combination of educational, organizational, economic, and environmental support necessary for behavior conducive to health; includes both disease prevention and wellness activities. (Chapter 54)

heart rate (HR) number of heart beats per unit of time, usually expressed as beats per minute (beats/min). (Chapter 10)

heat and moisture exchanger (HME) a device which recirculates moisture from exhaled gas to humidify the next inhaled breath. (Chapter 38)

heave a precordial impulse that may be felt (palpated) in patients with cardiac or respiratory disease. (Chapter 16)

heliox low-density therapeutic mixture of helium with at least 20% O_2; used in some centers to treat large airway obstruction. (Chapter 40)

heliox therapy used to reduce the work of breathing, especially in patients with severe acute asthma or upper airway obstructions, until the primary problem can be resolved. (Chapter 41)

hematemesis vomiting blood. (Chapter 16)

hematocrit packed red blood cell volume in relation to total blood volume, expressed as a percentage. (Chapter 17)

hematology branch of medicine involved in the study of blood morphology, physiology, and pathology. (Chapter 17)

hemolysis rupture of red blood cells. (Chapter 16)

hemoptysis the coughing up of blood from the lungs. (Chapter 16)

hemothorax accumulation of blood in the pleural cavity. (Chapter 27)

Henderson-Hasselbalch (H-H) equation the determination of pH as a measure of acidity (using pK_a, the negative log of the acid dissociation constant) in biological and chemical systems. (Chapter 14)

Henry law in physics, law stating that the solubility of a gas in a liquid is proportional to the pressure of the gas if the temperature is constant and if the gas does not chemically react with the liquid. (Chapter 6)

HEPA (high-efficiency particulate air/aerosol) filter filtration device, usually capable of 99.99% efficacy on particulate matter down to 0.3 mm in size. (Chapter 4)

hepatomegaly abnormal enlargement of the liver; usually a sign of disease. (Chapter 16)

Hering-Breuer inflation reflex parasympathetic inflation reflex mediated via the lung's stretch receptors that appears to influence the duration of the expiratory pause occurring between breaths. (Chapter 15)

heterodisperse referring to an aerosol consisting of particles of varying diameters and sizes. (Chapter 39)

high-flow nasal cannula (HFNC) a variation of the standard nasal cannula that can deliver both FiO_2 and relative humidity greater than 90% by using heated, humidified O_2 with flows up to 50 L/min. These systems have been shown to successfully treat moderate hypoxemia through a combination of a high FiO_2, distending positive airway pressure and meeting or exceeding the patient's minute ventilation. (Chapter 41)

high-flow system O_2 therapy equipment that supplies inspired gases at a consistent preset O_2 concentration. (Chapter 41)

high-frequency chest wall compression (HFCC) mechanical technique for augmenting secretion clearance; small gas volumes are alternately injected into and withdrawn from a vest by an air-pulse generator at a fast rate, creating an oscillatory motion against the patient's thorax. (Chapter 43)

high-frequency oscillatory ventilation (HFOV) is a type of mechanical ventilation which utilizes a respiratory rate greater than 4 times the normal value and very small tidal volumes. (Chapters 29, 48)

high-frequency ventilation (HFV) ventilatory support provided at rates significantly higher than normal breathing frequencies. (Chapters 44, 53)

hilum vertical opening on either side of the mediastinum through which all the airways and pulmonary vessels pass. (Chapter 9)

homeostasis relative constancy in the internal environment of the body, naturally maintained by adaptive responses that promote healthy survival. (Chapter 17)

Hoover sign inward movement of the lower lateral margins of the chest wall with each inspiratory effort owing to a low, flat diaphragm as seen in emphysema. (Chapter 16)

hospital-acquired or nosocomial infection infection acquired at least 72 hours after hospitalization, often caused by *Candida albicans, Escherichia coli,* hepatitis viruses, herpes zoster virus, *Pseudomonas,* or *Staphylococcus.* (Chapter 4)

hospital-acquired pneumonia (HAP) lower respiratory tract infection that develops in hospitalized patients more than 48 hours after admission and excludes community-acquired infections that are incubating at the time of admission. (Chapter 24)

huff cough type of forced expiration with an open glottis to replace coughing when pain limits normal coughing. (Chapter 43)

humidifier device that adds molecular water to gas. (Chapter 38)

hydrofluoroalkane (HFA) the current gaseous chemical compound used to power metered dose inhalers. (Chapter 39)

hydrophilic drugs drugs with strongly polar groups that readily interact with water. (Chapter 30)

hydrophobic pertaining to the property of repelling water molecules, a quality possessed by nonpolar radicals or molecules that are more soluble in organic solvents than in water. (Chapter 38)

hydropneumothorax a pneumothorax that is partially fluid filled. (Chapter 21)

hydrostatic relating to the pressure of fluids or to their properties when in equilibrium. (Chapter 27)

hydrostatic pressure pressure caused by the weight of fluid; related to the volume of fluid in a container and the effects of gravity. (Chapter 13)

hydrostatic pulmonary edema pulmonary edema that is caused by an increase in hydrostatic (water) pressure. (Chapter 29)

hydrothorax noninflammatory accumulation of serous fluid in one or both pleural cavities. (Chapter 20)

hygrometer instrument that directly measures relative humidity of the atmosphere or the proportion of water in a specific gas or gas mixture, without extracting the moisture. (Chapter 38)

hygroscopic attracting or absorbing moisture from the air. (Chapters 38, 39)

hyperbaric oxygen therapy therapeutic application of O_2 at pressures greater than 1 atm (or 760 mm Hg). Also called *hyperbaric oxygenation.* (Chapter 41)

hypercalcemia greater than normal amounts of calcium in the blood, most often resulting from excessive bone resorption and release of calcium, as occurs in hyperparathyroidism, metastatic tumors of bone, Paget disease, and osteoporosis. (Chapter 15)

hypercapnia abnormal presence of excess amounts of CO_2 in the blood (in arterial blood, $PCO_2 > 45$ mm Hg). (Chapter 14)

hypercapnic respiratory failure type II inability to maintain normal removal of CO_2 from the tissues; may be indicated by $PaCO_2$ greater than 50 mm Hg in an otherwise healthy individual. See *ventilatory failure.* (Chapter 44)

hyperglycemia is an abnormally elevated blood glucose level most often resulting from either diabetes or severe sepsis. (Chapter 17)

hyperkalemia greater than normal amounts of potassium in the blood. (Chapters 13, 17)

hypernatremia greater than normal concentration of sodium in the blood, caused by excessive loss of water and electrolytes secondary to polyuria, diarrhea, excessive sweating, or inadequate water intake. (Chapter 17)

hypersensitivity pneumonitis inflammatory form of interstitial pneumonia that results from an immunologic reaction in a hypersensitive person. The reaction may be provoked by various inhaled organic dusts, often containing fungal spores. The disease can be prevented by avoiding contact with the causative agents. Also called *extrinsic allergic alveolitis.* (Chapter 26)

hypertension persistently high blood pressure. (Chapter 16)

hypertonic saline hypertonic saline refers to a greater concentration of salt than what is found in normal saline solution and is often used to mobilize secretions. (Chapter 13)

hyperventilation ventilation greater than necessary to meet metabolic needs; signified by PCO_2 less than 35 mm Hg in the arterial blood. (Chapter 11)

hypocapnia presence of lower than normal amounts of CO_2 in the blood (in arterial blood, $PCO_2 < 35$ mm Hg). (Chapter 14)

hypoglycemia less than normal amount of glucose in the blood, usually caused by administration of too much insulin, excessive secretion of insulin by the islet cells of the pancreas, or dietary deficiency (normal blood glucose levels range from 70 to 105 mg/dl). (Chapter 17)

hypokalemia condition in which an inadequate amount of potassium, the major intracellular cation, is found in the circulating bloodstream. (Chapter 17)

hyponatremia less than normal concentration of sodium in the blood, caused by inadequate excretion of water or by excessive water in the circulating bloodstream. (Chapter 17)

hypopharynx lower portion of the upper airway between the oropharynx and the larynx. (Chapter 9)

hypotension abnormal condition in which the blood pressure is inadequate for normal perfusion and oxygenation of the tissues. (Chapter 16)

hypothermia abnormal and dangerous condition in which the temperature of the body is less than 32° C, usually caused by prolonged exposure to cold. (Chapters 16, 38)

hypothesis is a proposed explanation for a phenomenon to be proven or disproven through well founded research. (Chapter 8)

hypotonic having a tonicity less than normal saline (0.9% NaCl). (Chapter 13)

hypoventilation ventilation less than necessary to meet metabolic needs; signified by PCO_2 greater than 45 mm Hg in the arterial blood. (Chapter 11)

hypovolemia abnormally low circulating blood volume. (Chapter 16)

hypoxemia abnormal deficiency of O_2 in the arterial blood. (Chapter 12)

hypoxemic respiratory failure inability to maintain normal oxygenation in the arterial blood. (Chapters 44, 45)

hypoxia abnormal condition in which the O_2 available to the body cells is inadequate to meet metabolic needs. (Chapter 12)

hysteresis failure of two associated phenomena to coincide, as in the observed difference between the inflation and deflation volume-pressure curves of the lung. (Chapter 11)

I

idiopathic pulmonary fibrosis formation of scar tissue in the connective tissue of the lungs without known cause resulting in severe chronic restrictive lung disease. (Chapter 26)

immunocompromised hosts individuals who have a weakened immune system and are more predisposed to infection. (Chapter 4)

imprecision implying a level of inaccuracy in a particular measurement. (Chapter 18)

impulse-conducting system Purkinje fibers within the heart muscle that conduct impulses controlling the contractions of the atria and ventricles. (Chapter 18)

incentive spirometry process of encouraging a bedridden patient to take deep breaths to avoid atelectasis; most often done with the use of an incentive spirometer that provides feedback to the patient when a predetermined lung volume is reached during inspiration. (Chapter 42)

inclusion body myositis inflammatory myopathy of unknown cause. (Chapter 32)

indirect calorimetry measurement of the amount of energy a body consumes (in kcal) by determining the consumption of O_2 and production of CO_2. (Chapter 23)

inertial impaction deposition of particles by collision with a surface; primary mechanism for pulmonary deposition of particles greater than 5 mm in diameter. (Chapter 39)

infiltrate fluid that passes through body tissues into a space or virtual space as seen in the lung. (Chapter 21)

inhaled mass the mass of the particles inhaled from an aerosol. (Chapter 39)

inhaled nitric oxide (INO) gas that is administered to decrease pulmonary hypertension. (Chapter 53)

innominate artery rupture a rupture of the innominate artery usually a result of a tracheostomy tube eroding the tissue leading to the artery and eventually causing the artery to rupture. (Chapter 47)

inspiratory capacity (IC) maximum amount of air that can be inhaled from the resting end expiratory level or FRC; sum of the tidal volume and inspiratory reserve volume. (Chapter 20)

inspiratory-to-expiratory ratio (I/E) the relationship between the time devolved to inhalation versus that related to the exhalation portion of the breathing cycle, expressed as a proportion. (Chapter 29)

inspiratory positive airway pressure (IPAP) application of positive pressure to the airway during inspiration. (Chapter 45)

inspiratory reserve volume (IRV) maximum volume of air that can be inhaled after a normal quiet inspiration. (Chapter 20)

inspissated (of a fluid) thickened or hardened through the absorption or evaporation of the liquid portion, as can occur with respiratory secretions when the upper airway is bypassed. (Chapters 38, 40)

insufflator-exsufflator mechanical device that provides an artificial cough by alternately applying positive pressure and negative pressure to the airway. (Chapter 51)

Intellivent the ability of a mechanical ventilator to utilize programmed algorithms to either make or recommend setting changes, including those related to weaning and discontinuance. (Chapter 52)

intercostal of or pertaining to the space between two ribs.

intercostal muscles referring to the muscle groups between the ribs. (Chapter 9)

intercostal nerves the nerves serving the intercostal muscles. (Chapter 9)

intermittent mandatory ventilation (IMV) mode of mechanical ventilatory support in which the patient receives a preset number of machine breaths per minute set by time. The patient is allowed to breathe spontaneously as often as desired in between machine breaths. Depending on the base rate, IMV can provide partial or full ventilatory support. (Chapter 45)

intermittent positive pressure breathing (IPPB) application of positive pressure breaths to a patient for a relatively short period (10 to 20 minutes). (Chapter 42)

internal oblique abdominal muscle group that functions as an accessory muscle of ventilation. (Chapter 9)

internal respiration the exchange of O_2 and CO_2 at the tissue level. (Chapter 9)

International Council for Respiratory Care (ICRC) a diverse group of worldwide health professionals addressing issues affecting educational, medical, and professional trends in the global respiratory care community. (Chapter 1)

International Standards Organization (ISO) nongovernment agency that sets standards for various technical equipment and procedures. (Chapter 38)

interstitial fluid fluid between cells but outside of the vascular spaces. (Chapter 13)

interstitial lung disease (ILD) respiratory disorder characterized by a dry, unproductive cough and dyspnea on exertion. X-ray films usually show fibrotic infiltrates in the lung tissue, usually in the lower lobes. (Chapters 21, 26)

intrapulmonary percussive ventilation (IPV) airway clearance technique that uses a pneumatic device to deliver a series of pressurized small volume breaths at high rates (1.6 to 3.75 Hz) to the respiratory tract, usually via a mouthpiece; usually combined with aerosolized bronchodilator therapy. (Chapter 40)

intubation passage of a tube into a body aperture; commonly refers to the insertion of an endotracheal tube within the trachea. (Chapter 36)

intuitionism an ethical viewpoint that holds that there are certain self-evident truths, usually based on moral maxims such as "treat others fairly." (Chapter 5)

invasive characterized by a tendency to spread or infiltrate; also refers to the use of diagnostic or therapeutic methods requiring access to the inside of the body. (Chapter 19)

in vivo (of a biologic reaction) occurring in a living organism. (Chapter 18)

ionic electrovalent; relating to or containing matter in the form of charged atoms or groups of atoms. (Chapter 13)

iron lung full-body negative pressure ventilator. (Chapter 45)

isohydric buffering a buffering process where the H ion produced by one buffer system is immediately buffered by another, such as the buffering of H ion by hemoglobin when H ion is formed by the combination of CO_2 and H_2O in the red blood cell. (Chapter 14)

isothermic saturation boundary (ISB) point at which inspired gas becomes fully saturated to 100% relative humidity at body temperature. (Chapter 38)

isotonic (of a solution) having the same concentration of solute as another solution and exerting the same amount of osmotic pressure as that solution, such as an isotonic saline solution that contains an amount of salt equal to that found in the extracellular fluid. (Chapter 13)

J

J-receptors vagal sensory sites that are located in the alveolar units; so named because they are found primarily in juxtaposition to the pulmonary capillaries. (Chapter 15)

Joint Commission private nongovernment agency that establishes guidelines for the operation of hospitals and other health care facilities, conducts accreditation programs and surveys, and encourages the attainment of high standards of institutional medical care in the United States; formerly Joint Commission on Accreditation of Healthcare Organizations (JCAHO). (Chapter 2)

jugular venous distention abnormal distention of the jugular veins, most often caused by heart failure. (Chapter 16)

justice principle of fair and equal treatment for all, with due reward and honor. (Chapter 5)

K

Karvonen formula simple formula used to set a target heart rate for patients during exercise. (Chapter 55)

Kerley B lines thin lines seen near the pleural edge on a chest film as a result of increased pulmonary capillary pressures. (Chapter 21)

key performance indicators specific measures which are used to determine the level of quality outcomes within a health care setting. (Chapter 7)

kinetic energy energy a body possesses by virtue of its motion. (Chapter 6)

Kussmaul respiration hyperpnea associated with diabetic ketoacidosis. (Chapter 16)

Kussmaul sign paradoxical increase in venous pressure with distention of the jugular veins during inspiration, as seen in constrictive pericarditis or mediastinal tumor. (Chapter 16)

kwashiorkor protein-energy malnutrition resulting from the stress of disease and the resulting increase in catabolic rate. (Chapter 23)

kyphoscoliosis abnormal condition characterized by anteroposterior and lateral curvature of the spine. (Chapter 32)

L

lactate anion of lactic acid. (Chapter 17)

Lambert-Eaton syndrome disorder of neuromuscular conduction commonly associated with an underlying malignancy that leads to muscle weakness frequently with sensory deficits that can often be improved by repetitive muscle contraction against pressure. (Chapter 32)

laminar flow pattern of flow consisting of concentric layers of fluid flowing parallel to the tube wall at linear velocities that increase toward the center. (Chapter 6)

Laplace law principle of physics that the tension on the wall of a sphere is the product of the pressure times the radius of the chamber, and the tension is inversely related to the thickness of the wall. (Chapter 6)

large cell carcinoma type of lung cancer characterized by large cells. (Chapter 32)

large for gestational age (LGA) refers to an infant whose fetal growth was accelerated and whose size and weight at birth are above the 90th percentile of appropriate-for-gestational-age infants, whether delivered prematurely, at term, or later than term. (Chapter 53)

laryngectomy the surgical removal of the larynx. (Chapter 36)

laryngopharynx one of the three regions of the throat, extending from the hyoid bone to the esophagus. (Chapter 9)

larynx organ of the voice that is part of the upper air passage connecting the pharynx with the trachea. It accounts for a large bump in the neck called the *Adam's apple* and is larger in men than in women, although it remains the same size in boys and girls until puberty. (Chapter 9)

laser photocoagulation a means of using a laser with a bronchoscope to stop the bleeding in the airway. (Chapter 22)

latent heat of fusion the amount of heat at a substance's melting point required to change 1 gram of the substance from a solid to a liquid. (Chapter 6)

latent heat of vaporization the amount of heat at a substances boiling point required to change 1 gram of the substance from a liquid to a gas. (Chapter 6)

law of continuity velocity of a fluid moving through a tube varies inversely with the available cross-sectional area. (Chapter 6)

law of mass action states that acids and bases in solution freely dissociate and reassociate in a solution at a constant rate relative to the structure of the acid and the temperature of the solution. (Chapter 13)

laws of thermodynamics laws that describe the relation between temperature and the kinetics of matter changing its state. (Chapter 6)

learning management systems computerized, web-based platforms which are used to offer courses and other learning resources. (Chapter 7)

leukocyte white blood cell. (Chapter 17)

leukocytopenia abnormal decrease in white blood cells.

leukocytosis abnormal increase in the number of circulating white blood cells. (Chapter 17)

leukopenia a low white blood cell count. (Chapter 17)

leukotriene class of biologically active compounds that occur naturally in leukocytes and produce allergic and inflammatory reactions similar to histamine. They are thought to play a role in the development of allergic and autoallergic diseases such as asthma, rheumatoid arthritis, inflammatory bowel disease, and psoriasis. (Chapter 35)

libel false accusation written, printed, or typewritten or presented in a picture or a sign that is made with malicious intent to defame the reputation of a person who is living or the memory of a person who is dead, resulting in public embarrassment, contempt, ridicule, or hatred. (Chapter 5)

lipophilic drugs drugs that can readily dissolve in lipid substances. (Chapter 30)

living will advance declaration by a patient that indicates agreement between a patient and physician to withhold heroic measures if the patient's condition is found to be irreversible. (Chapter 5)

lobar atelectasis a collapsing of the airways and or alveoli which is limited to a lung segment. (Chapter 42)

lobes major divisions of the lungs; the right lung has three lobes, and the left lung has two lobes. (Chapter 9)

long-term subacute care hospitals (LTACHs) facilities that provide highly focused care to patients with complex medical conditions outside of traditional acute care hospitals, including patients who have been ventilator-dependent and difficult to wean. (Chapter 56)

loud P-2 abnormally loud closure of the pulmonic valve as part of S_2; usually caused by pulmonary hypertension. (Chapter 16)

Lou Gehrig disease popular name for amyotrophic lateral sclerosis (ALS), a disease characterized by progressive muscle weakness secondary to nerve deterioration. (Chapter 32)

lower respiratory tract infection any infectious disease of the left and right bronchi and the alveoli. (Chapter 24)

low-flow system variable performance O_2 therapy device that delivers O_2 at a flow that provides only a portion of the patient's inspired gas needs. Also called *variable performance system*. (Chapter 41)

L/T ratio refers to aerosol, it is the lung availability of an aerosol divided by the total system availability of the aerosol. (Chapter 35)

lung protective ventilation (LPV) the use of low tidal volumes to help prevent ventilator induced lung injury. (Chapter 29)

lung protective ventilatory strategy approach to mechanical ventilation that attempts to avoid overdistention of the lung and recruitment and derecruitment of unstable lung units with each breath. (Chapter 48)

lung strain is the deformation of a structure compared to its overall size. As applied to the respiratory system it is equal to the tidal volume. (Chapter 51)

lung stress the force applied per unit area. As applied to the respiratory system it is equal to transpulmonary pressure. (Chapter 51)

lung ultrasonography the use of ultrasound technology to view lung structures. (Chapter 51)

lymphadenopathy of or pertaining to a disease of the lymph nodes; refers also to the visualization of enlarged lymph nodes on radiographs. (Chapter 16)

lymphangioleiomyomatosis (LAM) lung abnormality most commonly observed in women and characterized by abnormal proliferation of smooth muscle cells in the interstitium, dyspnea, abnormal radiographic findings, and commonly pneumothorax. (Chapter 26)

lymphatic drainage system the main conduit for the removal of filtered fluid and protein from the lung. (Chapter 27)

M

macroshock shock from an electrical current of 1 mA or greater that is applied externally to the skin. (Chapter 3)

magnetic resonance imaging (MRI) imaging technique using magnetic disturbance of tissue to obtain images. (Chapter 30)

Mallampati classification is one of the most commonly used methods to identify the ability to visualize the vocal cords and glottis and therefore assess the degree of difficulty clinicians may encounter during intubation. (Chapter 22)

malpractice in law, professional negligence that is the proximate cause of injury or harm to a patient, resulting from a lack of professional knowledge, experience, or skill that can be expected in others in the profession or from a failure to exercise reasonable care or judgment in the application of professional knowledge, experience, or skill. (Chapter 5)

mandatory breath ventilatory support breath either initiated or ended by the machine. (Chapter 45)

mandatory minute volume ventilation (MMV) variation of the intermittent mandatory ventilation mode of ventilatory support in which the ventilator keeps the total minute volume constant. (Chapter 52)

manifold pipe with many connections; in medical gas storage, a collection of gas cylinders linked together for purposes of bulk storage and usually including at least one reserve bank and other safety systems, such as low-pressure alarms. (Chapter 40)

manubrium upper triangular portion of the sternum. (Chapter 8)

marasmus protein-energy malnutrition caused by starvation. (Chapter 23)

mass physical property of matter that gives it weight and inertia; aggregate of cells clumped together, such as a tumor. (Chapter 32)

mass median aerodynamic diameter (MMAD) measure of central tendency that describes the particle diameter in micrometers in medical aerosols and pertains to cascade impaction. (Chapter 39)

maximum expiratory pressure (MEP) measure of the output of the expiratory muscles against a maximum stimulus, measured in cm H_2O positive pressure. (Chapter 44)

maximum inspiratory pressure (MIP) measure of the output of the inspiratory muscles against a maximum stimulus, measured in cm H_2O negative pressure. Also known as *negative inspiratory force (NIF)* or *maximum inspiratory force (MIF)*. (Chapters 44, 51)

maximum voluntary ventilation (MVV) maximum volume of air in L/min that a patient can breathe during a 12- to 15-second period. It is a very patient-dependent test. Formerly called the *maximum breathing capacity (MBC)*. (Chapters 20, 44, 51)

mean airway pressure average pressure applied to the airway. (Chapters 46, 51)

mechanical insufflation-exsufflation mechanical device that provides an artificial cough by alternately applying positive pressure and negative pressure to the airway, also referred to as an *in-exsufflator*. (Chapter 40)

mechanical ventilator an artificial device to assist a patient to breathe. (Chapter 1)

meconium material that collects in the intestines of a fetus and forms the first stools of a newborn. (Chapter 53)

meconium aspiration syndrome inhalation of meconium by a fetus or newborn; can block the air passages and cause failure of the lungs to expand. (Chapter 34)

mediastinum portion of the thoracic cavity lying in the middle of the thorax (between the two pleural cavities); extends from the vertebral column to the sternum and contains the trachea, esophagus, heart, and great vessels of the circulatory system. (Chapter 9)

melting point characteristic temperature at which the solid and liquid forms of a substance are in equilibrium. (Chapter 6)

membrane pressures the pressure across an oxygenator used in an ECMO circuit. (Chapter 50)

metabolic acidosis nonrespiratory processes resulting in acidemia. (Chapter 14)

metabolic alkalosis nonrespiratory processes resulting in alkalemia. (Chapter 14)

methemoglobin abnormal form of hemoglobin in which the iron component has been oxidized from the ferrous to the ferric state. (Chapter 12)

methemoglobinemia abnormal condition characterized by high levels of methemoglobin in the blood and reduction in O_2-carrying capacity; may be caused by nitrite poisoning or ingestion of a certain oxidizing agent or a genetic defect in the enzyme NADH methemoglobin reductase (an autosomal dominant trait). (Chapters 12, 22)

micrognathia underdevelopment of the jaw, especially the mandible. (Chapter 31)

microshock shock from a usually imperceptible electrical current (<1 mA) that is allowed to bypass the skin and follow a direct, low-resistance pathway into the body. (Chapter 3)

minute ventilation total lung ventilation per minute, the product of tidal volume and respiration rate. It is measured by expired gas collection for a period of 1 to 3 minutes; normal rate is 5 to 10 L/min. (Chapters 20, 52)

misallocation process of prescribing diagnostic or treatment services when not indicated, consisting both of overordering and underordering services. (Chapter 2)

missed triggering the inability of a patient to trigger the ventilator during a particular inspiratory effort. Usually a result of auto-PEEP or too large a tidal volume with a rapid respiratory rate. (Chapter 47)

mode (ventilatory) any one of many categories of mechanical ventilation that are determined by a number of characteristics, including how the breath is initiated and how the inhalation ceases and exhalation starts. (Chapter 45)

mode asynchrony the selection of a mode of ventilation that does not synchronously interact with the patient's inspiratory efforts. (Chapter 47)

moderate (conscious) sedation a form of sedation used for certain procedures such a bronchoscopy, whereby patients can respond to verbal stimuli and maintain protective airway reflexes. (Chapter 22)

modified Allen test most common technique to determine the adequacy of ulnar circulation. (Chapter 19)

molecular sieve crystalline chemical separation device with molecular size pores that adsorbs small but not large molecules. (Chapter 51)

monitor to observe and evaluate a function of the body closely and constantly; mechanical device that provides a visual or audible signal or a graphic record of a particular function, such as a cardiac monitor or a fetal monitor. (Chapter 19)

monodisperse referring to an aerosol in which particles are of uniform size. (Chapter 39)

morbid obesity a state of having a body mass index (BMI) of greater than 45 kg/m^2. (Chapter 30)

mucociliary escalator a term used to define the process in which the cilia of the airways continually move mucus from the lower respiratory tract to the oral cavity. (Chapter 9)

mucoid resembling mucus. (Chapter 16)

mucous plugging the partial or complete occlusion of the airway by thick mucus. (Chapter 40)

multiple organ dysfunction syndrome (MODS) condition in which dysfunction of many different organs occurs, usually accompanying acute lung injury. (Chapter 29)

murmur abnormal heart sound created by turbulent blood flow through a narrowed or incompetent heart valve. (Chapter 16)

Murray lung injury score a score used to define the severity of injury in patients with ARDS. (Chapter 51)

muscarinic stimulating the postganglionic parasympathetic receptor; pertaining to the poisonous activity of muscarine. (Chapter 35)

muscle fatigue condition involving loss of the capacity to develop force or velocity of a muscle resulting from muscle activity overload, which is reversible by rest. (Chapter 44)

myasthenia gravis disorder of neuromuscular conduction that leads to muscle weakness of the skeletal muscles, particularly the muscles of the face, throat, and respiratory system. Weakness and respiratory failure can occur rapidly as muscle strength decreases with repetitive contraction against a load. (Chapter 32)

mydriasis dilation of the pupil of the eye. (Chapter 32)

myopathy abnormal condition of skeletal muscle leading to muscle weakness, wasting, and histologic changes in the muscle tissue, as seen in muscular dystrophies. (Chapter 32)

myositis inflammation of the muscle. (Chapter 32)

myotonic dystrophy type of muscular dystrophy. (Chapter 32)

N

nanomole a quantity equal to 10^{-9} of a mole. (Chapter 13)

narrow band imaging an imaging technique for used in conjunction with bronchoscopy, where light of specific blue and green wavelengths is used to enhance the detail of certain aspects of the surface of the mucosa. (Chapter 22)

nasal flaring dilation of the alar nasi on inspiration; an early sign of an increase in ventilatory demands and the work of breathing, especially in infants. (Chapter 34)

nasopharynx upper portion of the airway behind the nasal and oral cavities. (Chapter 9)

National Board for Respiratory Care (NBRC) national credentialing agency for respiratory care practitioners and pulmonary function technologists. (Chapters 1, 2)

nebulizer device that produces an aerosol suspension of liquid particles in a gaseous medium using baffling to control particle size. (Chapters 38, 39)

needle capping device safety device used to prevent or minimize needlestick injuries when capping a syringe needle (as required after blood gas sampling). (Chapter 19)

negative feedback loop when the output of a system acts to oppose changes to the input of the system, with the result that the changes are attenuated and output is balanced. (Chapter 10)

negative inotropism decrease in contractility of the heart. (Chapter 10)

negative-pressure ventilation approach to ventilation in which negative pressure is intermittently applied to the chest surface in an effort to cause inflation of the lungs. (Chapter 45)

negligence omission to do something that a reasonable person, guided by ordinary considerations, would do. (Chapter 5)

neovascularization formation of new capillary beds. (Chapter 41)

neurally adjusted ventilatory assistance (NAVA) an approach to ventilation based on the electromyelographic (EMG) activity of the diaphragm. Airway pressure is increased proportional to the change in EMG activity. No control variable is set. (Chapters 47, 48)

neuropathy refers to abnormal conditions characterized by inflammation or degeneration of the nerves. (Chapter 32)

neutral thermal environment (NTE) ambient environment that prevents or minimizes the loss of body heat. (Chapter 41)

neutropenia abnormal decrease in the number of neutrophils in the blood. (Chapters 17, 35)

nitric oxide (NO) an inhaled gas used to reduce pulmonary artery pressure and improve arterial oxygenation. (Chapter 41)

nocturnal hypoventilation elevated $PaCO_2$ and accompanying decline in O_2 saturation that occurs in response to a progressive decrease in minute ventilation occurring during sleep, most often in the REM stage. (Chapter 45)

nodule small node; small nodelike structure. (Chapter 32)

nonflammable unable to support combustion. (Chapter 40)

nonhydrostatic pulmonary edema pulmonary edema that is caused by something other than an increase in blood pressure. (Chapter 29)

noninvasive pertaining to a diagnostic or therapeutic technique that does not require the skin to be broken or a cavity or organ of the body to be entered, such as obtaining a blood pressure reading by auscultation with a stethoscope and sphygmomanometer. (Chapter 19)

noninvasive positive pressure ventilation (NPPV) (also referred to as **noninvasive ventilation** or **NIV**) positive pressure ventilation without endotracheal intubation or tracheotomy, usually via a form-fitting mask. (Chapters 41, 45)

noninvasive ventilation mechanical ventilation performed without intubation or tracheostomy, usually with mask ventilation. (Chapters 25, 42, 44, 51)

nonmaleficence principle that obligates health care providers to avoid harming patients and actively to prevent harm where possible. (Chapter 5)

non–small cell carcinoma major category of histologic types of lung carcinomas, including adenocarcinoma of the lung, large cell carcinoma, and squamous cell carcinoma. Treatment depends on the stage of development of the cancer at the time of initial presentation. The treatment of choice for otherwise physically fit patients with early stages of disease is resection. (Chapter 32)

normal solution solution that contains the gram-equivalent weight of a reagent per liter; denoted by the symbols *N/l* or *N*. (Chapter 13)

normometabolic the normal level of metabolic function in a healthy individual. (Chapter 23)

nosocomial pneumonia infectious inflammatory process of the lung parenchyma that is contracted in the hospital. (Chapter 24)

O

O_2-conserving device an O_2 delivery system that minimizes the amount of O_2 actually delivered to a patient while also maintaining the FiO_2. (Chapter 51)

obesity hypoventilation general syndrome involving chronic hypercapnia and hypoxemia, sleep apnea, and decreased respiratory center responsiveness to CO_2. Complications, primarily owing to chronic hypoxemia, include polycythemia, pulmonary hypertension, and cor pulmonale. (Chapter 33)

obstructive pulmonary disease any respiratory disease characterized by decreased airway size and increased airway secretions. (Chapter 20)

obstructive sleep apnea (OSA) condition in which five or more apneic periods (lasting at least 10 seconds each) occur per hour of sleep and characterized by occlusion of the oropharyngeal airway with continued efforts to breathe. (Chapter 33)

obturator device used to block a passage or a canal or to fill in a space, such as the obturator used to insert a tracheostomy tube. (Chapter 36)

Occupational Safety and Health Administration (OSHA) a federal agency of the United States that regulates workplace safety and health. (Chapter 4)

occupational interstitial lung disease (ILD) interstitial lung disease resulting from an occupational exposure; asbestosis is a common example. (Chapter 26)

ohm unit of measurement to report the resistance to the flow of electricity. (Chapter 3)

Ondine curse apnea caused by loss of automatic control of respiration (derived from the name of a fabled water nymph). (Chapter 32)

onset of blood lactate accumulation (OBLA) point at which blood lactate levels increase above normal when the body cannot deliver sufficient O_2 to meet the demands of energy metabolism; term used in exercise physiology. (Chapter 55)

open buffer system the bicarbonate buffer system is an open buffer system because H_2CO_3 can be removed as CO_2, is broken down into H_2O and CO_2 as long as ventilation removes CO_2. (Chapter 14)

open loop control system in which there is no control over the delivered variable. (Chapter 42)

optical fluorescence the use of fluorescent dyes that are illuminated with light of a specific wavelength for the measurement of respiratory gases. (Chapter 19)

optode fluorescent chemosensor useful in measuring pH or gas tensions in arterial or mixed venous blood. (Chapter 19)

organizing pneumonia (OP) is the new term for bronchiolitis obliterans organizing pneumonia, that generally occurs in the setting of connective tissue disease. (Chapter 26)

oropharynx the portion of the pharynx which is located most closely to the mouth. (Chapter 9)

orthodeoxia decrease in PaO_2 owing to changes in position. (Chapter 16)

orthopnea labored breathing in the reclining position. (Chapter 16)

oscillation back-and-forth motion; vibration or the effects of mechanical or electrical vibration. (Chapter 40)

OSHA abbreviation for the Occupational Safety and Health Administration, a branch of the U.S. Department of Labor responsible for regulations pertaining to on-the-job safety. (Chapter 4)

osmolality is a measure of the concentration of a solute in a solution. (Chapter 13)

osmolarity osmotic pressure of a solution expressed in osmoles or mOsm/kg of the solution.

osmotic pressure force produced by solvent particles across semipermeable membranes. (Chapter 13)

oxidizing to combine or cause to combine with O_2, to remove hydrogen, or to increase the valence of an element through the loss of electrons. (Chapter 40)

oximetry a non-invasive method for monitoring how saturated a persons hemoglobin is with oxygen and other gases. (Chapter 19)

oxygen consumption ($\dot{V}O_2$) the amount of O_2 consumed per minute; normal value 200 ml/min. (Chapter 51)

oxygen therapy any procedure in which O_2 is administered to a patient to relieve hypoxemia. (Chapter 1)

oxyhemoglobin chemical combination resulting from the covalent bonding of O_2 to the ferrous iron pigment in hemoglobin. (Chapter 12)

P

P_{50} quantifies variations in the affinity of Hb for O_2. It is the partial pressure of O_2 at which the Hb is 50% saturated, standardized to a pH level of 7.40. (Chapter 12)

pack-years a method of determining the quantity of cigarettes a patient smoked over time. The number of packs of cigarettes a person smoked divided by the number of years they smoked. (Chapter 16)

palate bony plate that separates the nasal cavity from the oral cavity. (Chapter 9)

Pancoast syndrome combination of signs associated with a tumor in the apex of the lung; signs include neuritic pain in the arm, atrophy of the muscles of the arm and the hand, and Horner syndrome and are caused by the damaging effects of the tumor on the brachial plexus and sympathetic ganglia. (Chapter 32)

PaO_2/FiO_2 ratio the PaO_2 divided by the FiO_2, indicative of the severity of lung injury. (Chapter 51)

paradoxical motion movement of the thoracic cavity where the cavity bows out with expiration and collapses inward during a spontaneous breath. The movement is associated with a decreased pressure gradient to drive inspiration and expiration and can result in respiratory failure. (Chapter 32)

paraneoplastic syndrome effect of tumors remote from the tumor site and often mediated by reactions to tumor products or immune response to the tumor. (Chapter 32)

paresthesia any subjective sensation, experienced as numbness, tingling, or a "pins and needles" feeling. (Chapter 14)

parietal pleura thin membrane covering the surface of the chest wall, mediastinum, and diaphragm that is continuous with the visceral pleura around the lung hilum. (Chapters 9, 27)

partial ventilatory support modes of ventilatory support in which the patient must contribute to the total minute volume with spontaneous breathing. (Chapter 48)

Pascal principle law stating that a confined liquid transmits pressure equally in all directions. (Chapter 6)

passive (exhalation) the release of previously stored energy from the elastic recoil of the chest wall and lungs to facilitate exhalation. (Chapter 46)

patent ductus arteriosus (PDA) common cardiovascular anomaly of infants in which the ductus arteriosus either fails to close or reopens after birth. (Chapter 53)

***Patient Protection and Affordable Care Act* (ACA) of 2010** legislation that changed many aspects of the American health care system by expanding health care coverage to many uninsured people, prohibiting the exclusion of preexisting conditions, creating an exchange for purchasing health insurance coverage, increasing the scope of coverage for certain types of preventive care and many other provisions. (Chapter 56)

patient-ventilator asynchrony lack of coordinated gas delivery between the patient and the ventilator. (Chapters 46, 47)

peak expiratory flow rate (PEFR) maximum expiratory flow rate in L/sec. (Chapter 20)

pedal edema swelling of the ankles usually secondary to heart failure. (Chapter 16)

penetrating trauma chest trauma that is the result of bullet, knife, etc. that makes a singular entry into the chest. Normally pulmonary contusion does not occur with penetrating trauma. (Chapter 30)

percent total body surface area (%TBSA) that percent of the body surface that is affected. Normally used to identify the extent of body surface burns. (Chapter 30)

performance improvement measuring the results of a process and then changing it to enhance future results. (Chapters 2, 3)

pericardium fibrous, serous sac that surrounds the heart and roots of the great vessels. (Chapter 10)

peripheral cyanosis a bluish tinge of the extremities often caused by low arterial blood oxygen content or poor circulation. (Chapter 16)

periodic breathing abnormal pattern of respiration, characterized by alternating periods of apnea and deep, rapid breathing. (Chapter 32)

persistent pulmonary hypertension of the newborn (PPHN) clinical syndrome seen in infants soon after birth and characterized by abnormally increased pulmonary vascular resistance. (Chapter 33)

pharmacodynamic phase mechanisms of drug action that cause effects on the body. (Chapter 35)

pharmacokinetic phase time, course, and disposition of a drug in the body. (Chapter 35)

pharyngeal airways devices that maintain the patency of the pharyngeal structure. (Chapter 36)

pharynx the throat—tubular structure approximately 13 cm long that extends from the base of the skull to the esophagus and is situated immediately in front of the cervical vertebrae. The pharynx serves as a passageway for the respiratory and digestive tracts and changes shape to allow the formation of various vowel sounds. (Chapter 9)

phase variable signal that is measured and used by the ventilator to begin some part (phase) of the breathing cycle. (Chapter 42)

phlegm mucus from the tracheobronchial tree. (Chapter 16)

photoplethysmography light-emitting technology used to detect changes in blood flow. (Chapter 19)

phrenic nerves paired nerves that originate as branches of spinal nerves C3-5, pass down along the mediastinum, and innervate the diaphragm. (Chapter 9)

psychomotor domain the skills associated with the ability to physically manipulate an object. (Chapter 54)

physician assistant (PA) individual academically and clinically prepared to practice medicine under the supervision of a licensed doctor of medicine or osteopathy. Within the physician-PA relationship, PAs exercise autonomy in medical decisions and provide a wide range of diagnostic and therapeutic services. Training programs average 25 to 27 months. National certification is available to graduates of approved training programs. (Chapter 1)

physiologic dead space area in the respiratory system that includes the anatomic dead space together with the space in the alveoli occupied by air that does not contribute to the O_2-CO_2 exchange. (Chapter 11)

physiologic shunt (Q_s/Q_T) percentage of the cardiac output that does not participate in gas exchange in the lung. (Chapter 51)

picture archiving and communication systems a medical imaging technology which permits storage and convenient access to images. (Chapter 7)

piezoelectric crystal transducer capable of converting electrical energy into the physical energy of high-frequency vibrations. (Chapter 38)

pin-indexed safety system (PISS) part of the American standard safety system, these specifications apply only to the valve outlets of small cylinders, up to and including size E, that use a yoke-type connection. (Chapter 40)

plaintiff person who brings an action; a person who seeks remedial relief for an injury to his or her rights. (Chapter 5)

plasma watery, colorless fluid portion of the blood and lymph in which cellular elements are suspended. (Chapter 12)

plasma colloid osmotic pressure (oncotic pressure) osmotic pressure exerted by the colloid suspended in the blood. (Chapter 13)

plateau pressure (P_{plat}) pressure in the patient's airway during mechanical ventilation resulting from the application of an end inspiratory hold. This is equal to the average peak alveolar pressure. (Chapter 48)

plate (or platelike) atelectasis lung collapse that appears in distinct platelike structures. (Chapter 20)

platypnea opposite of orthopnea; an abnormal condition characterized by difficult breathing in the standing position that is relieved in the lying or recumbent position. (Chapter 16)

plethysmograph device for measuring pressure; in pulmonary physiology, a chamber in which the subject sits to measure lung pressures and volumes. (Chapter 11)

pleural effusion abnormal collection of fluid in the pleural space. (Chapters 21, 27)

pleurisy pain that comes from the pleural surface; usually a direct result of viral infections but has been generalized to any condition (e.g., pulmonary embolism) causing pleural pain. Synonymous with *pleurodynia*. (Chapter 27)

pleurodesis procedure of fusing the parietal and visceral pleura to prevent formation of pleural fluid or recurrence of pneumothorax. (Chapter 27)

pneumobelt ventilatory assist device that applies positive pressure to the abdominal contents during expiration. (Chapter 45)

pneumomediastinum presence of air or gas in the mediastinal tissues, which may lead to pneumothorax or pneumopericardium. (Chapter 21)

pneumonia inflammatory process of the lung parenchyma, usually infectious in origin. (Chapter 24)

pneumotachometer any device for measuring gas flow. (Chapter 11)

pneumotaxic center center in the upper part of the pons that rhythmically inhibits inspiration independently of the vagi. (Chapter 15)

pneumothorax presence of air or gas in the pleural space of the thorax; if this air or gas is trapped under pressure, tension pneumothorax exists. (Chapters 16, 21, 27)

point-of-care testing analysis of body fluids at the bedside, as opposed to conventional laboratory testing. (Chapters 7, 19)

Poiseuille's law the physical law which describes the difference in pressure required to produce a given flow under conditions of laminar flow, through a smooth tube of a fixed size. (Chapter 6)

polycythemia abnormal increase in the number of erythrocytes in the blood; termed *secondary* if attributable to defined causes other than direct stimulation of the bone marrow, such as occurs in chronic hypoxemia. (Chapter 17)

polymyositis condition characterized by inflammation of many muscles. (Chapter 32)

pores of Kohn small openings between adjacent alveoli. (Chapter 9)

portals a means by which authorized users can gain access to computerized medical records and health resources. (Chapter 8)

positive end expiratory pressure (PEEP) application and maintenance of pressure above atmospheric at the airway throughout the expiratory phase of positive pressure mechanical ventilation. (Chapters 29, 44)

positive expiratory pressure (PEP) airway clearance technique in which the patient exhales against a fixed-orifice flow resistor to help move secretions into the larger airways for expectoration via coughing or swallowing. (Chapters 42, 40)

positive inotropism increase in the contractility of muscle tissue. (Chapter 10)

positron emission tomography (PET) computerized radiographic technique that uses radioactive substances to examine the metabolic activity of various body structures. The patient either inhales or is injected with a metabolically important substance such as glucose, carrying a radioactive element that emits positively charged particles, or positrons. When the positrons combine with electrons normally found in the cells of the body, gamma rays are emitted. The electronic circuitry and computers of the PET device detect the gamma rays and construct color-coded images that indicate the intensity of metabolic activity throughout the organ involved. (Chapter 31)

postural hypotension sudden decrease in arterial blood pressure caused by a change in position; most often occurs when a hypovolemic patient moves from the reclining position to the upright position. (Chapter 16)

potential energy energy contained in a body as a result of its position in space, internal structure, and stresses imposed on it. (Chapter 6)

preanalytic error error that occurs outside of that actual testing procedure. (Chapter 19)

precision the accuracy of an instrument during the measurement of a particular substance. (Chapter 19)

preload pressure stretching the ventricular walls at the onset of ventricular contraction. (Chapters 10, 51)

premature ventricular contractions are abnormal and bizarre ECG rhythms that are much wider than normal. (Chapter 18)

preoperative of or pertaining to the period of time preceding a surgical procedure. (Chapter 39)

pressure controlled ventilation (PCV) mode of ventilatory support in which mandatory support breaths are delivered to the patient at a set inspiratory pressure. (Chapters 44, 45, 48)

pressure gradient the pressure difference between two points in a system. (Chapter 11)

pressure-regulated volume control (PRVC) pressure limited ventilation in which inspiratory time and a backup rate are set and a tidal volume is targeted. (Chapter 48)

pressure support ventilation (PSV) mode of ventilatory support designed to augment spontaneous breathing; patient-triggered, pressure-limited, flow-cycled ventilation. (Chapters 48, 52)

pressure-time product product of pressure over a time interval, usually pleural pressure times inspiratory time during breathing. (Chapter 51)

primary lobule the terminal bronchiole and the cluster of respiratory bronchioles that it supplies. (Chapter 9)

primary pulmonary hypertension of the newborn form of pulmonary hypertension that occurs in the absence of other heart or lung diseases and is characterized by diffuse narrowing of the pulmonary arterioles without obvious reason. (Chapter 53)

primary spontaneous pneumothorax pneumothorax that occurs without underlying lung disease. (Chapter 27)

problem-oriented medical record (POMR) method of recording data about the health status of a patient in a problem system. (Chapter 3)

process control a method of quality control which uses detailed information about a process to optimize outcomes. (Chapter 3)

prodrug inactive or partially active drug that is metabolically changed in the body to an active drug. (Chapter 35)

proficiency testing (PT) process of comparing measurements of a known value from different sources to establish a level of accuracy. (Chapter 19)

progressive resistance method of increasing the strength of a weak or injured muscle by gradually increasing the resistance against which the muscle works, such as by using graduated weights over a period. Also called *graduated resistance*. (Chapter 55)

prolonged mechanical ventilation a lengthy process of mechanical ventilatory support. No precise length has been determined but most would consider longer than 3 weeks prolonged ventilatory support. (Chapter 52)

prone positioning when a patient is placed in a face down position, often during mechanical ventilation to help improve ventilation and oxygenation. (Chapter 29)

propellant something that propels or provides thrust, as the propellant in a metered dose inhaler. (Chapter 39)

proportional assist ventilation (PAV) mode of ventilation without any control variable that delivers gas in proportion to the patient's actual inspiratory effort. (Chapters 47, 48)

protein-energy malnutrition (PEM) wasting condition resulting from a diet deficient in either protein or energy (calories) or both. (Chapter 23)

pseudostratified epithelia of or pertaining to an epithelial cell type that appears to be organized in layers but in which each cell actually contacts the basement membrane. (Chapter 9)

psig abbreviation for pounds per square inch-gauge—the pressure above atmospheric registered on a meter or gauge. (Chapter 40)

psychomotor domain area of observable performance of skills that require some degree of neuromuscular coordination. (Chapter 54)

psychosocial support needs of or pertaining to the mental, emotional, and social aspects of human existence or development. (Chapter 55)

PubMed a free, computerized search engine which facilitates access to peer-reviewed articles, abstracts and references related to life sciences. (Chapter 8)

pulmonary arterial hypertension an increase above normal levels in blood pressure in the pulmonary vasculature. (Chapter 28)

pulmonary contusion the internal pulmonary bleeding and edema that result from blunt trauma. Generally it is localized to the area adjacent to the trauma. (Chapter 30)

pulmonary edema condition in which excessive amounts of plasma enter the pulmonary interstitium and alveoli; usually accompanied by severe respiratory distress, tachypnea, and hypoxemia. (Chapter 29)

pulmonary embolism (PE) blockage of a pulmonary artery by foreign matter. The obstruction may be fat, air, tumor tissue, or a thrombus that usually arises from a peripheral vein (most frequently arising from the deep veins of the legs). Pulmonary embolism is detected by chest x-ray, pulmonary angiography, and radioscanning of the lung fields. (Chapter 28)

pulmonary function testing (PFT) procedure for determining the capacity of the lungs to exchange O_2 and CO_2 efficiently. There are two general kinds of pulmonary function tests: one measures ventilation, or the ability of the bellows action of the chest and lungs to move gas in and out of alveoli; the other kind measures the diffusion of gas across the alveolar capillary membrane and the perfusion of the lungs by blood. (Chapters 1)

pulmonary hypertension (PH) condition characterized by abnormally high pulmonary artery pressures (i.e., mean pulmonary artery pressures > 22 mm Hg). (Chapter 28)

pulmonary Langerhans cell histiocytosis (PLCH) condition characterized by abnormal proliferation of Langerhans cells, accompanied by interstitial markings on the chest film and dyspnea. (Chapter 26)

pulmonary rehabilitation an organized multidisciplinary approach to improve the functional status of patients with chronic obstructive pulmonary disease, usually including education, exercise, aerosolized medication, and O_2 therapy. (Chapter 55)

pulmonary surfactant a surface active lipoprotein formed by Type II cells which reduces surface tension and facilitates alveolar expansion during inhalation. (Chapter 9)

pulseless electrical activity (PEA) a serious condition characterized by a disassociation between the electrical and mechanical activity of the heart. In essence, the electrical ECG pattern on the monitor neither generates mechanical activity of the heart nor a pulse. (Chapter 18)

pulse co-oximetry a pulse oximetry that is capable of measuring carboxyhemoglobin and methemoglobin. (Chapter 19)

pulse deficit discrepancy between the ventricular rate auscultated at the apex of the heart and the arterial rate of the radial pulse. (Chapter 16)
pulse pressure difference between systolic blood pressure and diastolic blood pressure. (Chapter 16)
pulsus alternans alternating between strong and weak heartbeats. (Chapter 16)
pulsus paradoxus abnormal decrease in pulse pressure with each inspiratory effort. (Chapter 16)
pump flow the flow of blood pumped through on ECMO system in liters per minute. (Chapter 50)
purulent consisting of or containing pus. (Chapter 16)

Q

quality the extent to which a process, structure, product and/or organization adheres to current best-practices, is free of errors and achieves intended outcomes. (Chapter 2)
quality assurance any evaluation of services provided and the results achieved compared with accepted standards. (Chapters 2, 3)
quality control planned, systematic approach to designing, measuring, assessing, and improving performance. (Chapter 19)
quality improvement the enhancement of a process, structure, product and/or organization to more closely adhere to best-practices, reduce errors and achieve intended outcomes. (Chapter 3)

R

radiation treatment of neoplastic disease by using x-rays or gamma rays, usually from a cobalt source, to deter the proliferation of malignant cells by decreasing the rate of mitosis or impairing deoxyribonucleic acid synthesis. (Chapter 6)
radiograph x-ray image. (Chapter 21)
radiolucent of or pertaining to a substance or tissue that readily permits the passage of x-rays or other radiant energy. Compare with *radiopaque*. (Chapter 21)
radiopaque of or pertaining to a substance or tissue that does not readily permit the passage of x- rays or other radiant energy. Compare with *radiolucent*. (Chapters 21, 36)
radiotherapy treatment with radiation. (Chapter 31)
rales an abnormal breath sound also known as "crackles" and which is discontinuous and can be further characterized as "fine rales" associated with congestive heart failure or "coarse rales" most often associated with air moving through secretions in the airways. (Chapter 16)
random error variability of a measurement outside of accepted limits that occurs in a nonreproducible fashion. (Chapter 19)
rapid shallow breathing index (f/V_T) patient's spontaneous respiratory rate (f) in breaths per minute divided by the spontaneous tidal volume in liters. Values greater than 100 are associated with poor weaning outcomes. (Chapter 52)
recirculation the movement of blood from one cannula to another in an ECMO circuit. Specifically blood being infused in to a patient by a venous return catheter that is immediately removed from the patient by the venous drainage catheter during venovenous ECMO. (Chapter 50)
reconditioning physical activity to strengthen essential muscle groups, improve overall O_2 use, and enhance the cardiovascular response of the body to physical activity. (Chapter 55)
recruitment maneuvers a intermittent intervention used on mechanically ventilated patients involving the very brief, but repeated use of high ventilation pressures to expand previously collapsed alveoli. (Chapter 30)
rectus abdominis abdominal muscle group that functions as an accessory muscle of ventilation. (Chapter 9)
reducing valve valve that reduces gas pressure. (Chapter 40)
reexpansion pulmonary edema pulmonary edema that forms after rapid reexpansion of a lung that has been compressed with pleural fluid or pneumothorax. (Chapter 27)
reference range the acceptable range for a laboratory value measured during calibration or validation of operation. (Chapter 17)
regulator device that controls both pressure and flow. (Chapter 40)
regurgitation backward flow of blood through an incompetent valve of the heart. (Chapter 10)
relative humidity (RH) amount of moisture in the air compared with the maximum the air could contain at the same temperature. (Chapter 6)
repolarization process by which the cell is restored to its resting potential. (Chapter 18)
research protocol a documented procedure which described each step in conducting a research study. (Chapter 8)
reservoir system O_2 delivery system that provides a reservoir O_2 volume that the patient taps into when the patient's inspiratory flow exceeds the device flow. (Chapter 41)
residual drug volume medication that remains in a small-volume nebulizer after the device is no longer producing mist. (Chapter 39)
residual volume (RV) volume of gas remaining in the lungs after a complete exhalation. (Chapter 20)
res ipsa loquitur "the thing speaks for itself"; rule of evidence whereby negligence of an alleged wrongdoer may be inferred from the fact that the accident happened. (Chapter 5)
resistance impedance to flow in a tube or conduit; quantified as ratio of the difference in pressure between the two points. (Chapter 3)
respirable mass proportion of aerosolized drug of the proper particle size to reach the lower respiratory tract. (Chapters 39, 42)
respiratory acidosis hypoventilation resulting in acidemia. (Chapter 14)
respiratory alternans alternating between use of the diaphragm for short periods and use of the accessory muscles to breathe; indicative of end-stage respiratory muscle fatigue. (Chapters 16, 44)
x **respiratory care** health care discipline that specializes in the promotion of optimal cardiopulmonary function and health. Also called *respiratory therapy*. (Chapter 1)
respiratory care management information systems an information system specifically designed for managing data regarding the respiratory care provided to patients. (Chapter 7)
respiratory care practitioner health professional with special training and experience in the treatment and rehabilitation of patients with respiratory disorders. The respiratory care practitioner typically does not diagnose but must be competent with patient assessment in various clinical settings. (Chapter 1)
respiratory care protocol specification of actions that allows respiratory care practitioners to initiate and adjust therapy independently, within guidelines previously established by medical staff. Also called *therapist-driven protocol*. (Chapter 2)
respiratory distress syndrome (RDS) condition of respiratory distress in newborns, usually caused by inadequate surfactant production (owing to immaturity). (Chapter 33)
respiratory hygiene a state in which the respiratory tract is kept as free as possible from containments such as bacteria and other microbes. (Chapter 4)
respiratory inductive plethysmography device that, by measuring the change in the diameter of the chest and abdomen, can estimate inhaled and exhaled tidal volume. (Chapter 51)
respiratory therapist (RT) graduate of a CAAHEP/CoARC accredited school designed to qualify the graduate for the registry examination of the National Board for Respiratory Care (NBRC). (Chapter 1)
respiratory therapy any treatment that maintains or improves the ventilatory function of the respiratory tract. (Chapter 1)
respiratory therapy consult service program in which respiratory care services are determined by respiratory care practitioners based on prescribed guidelines or algorithms. Also called *evaluate-and-treat program*. (Chapter 2)
respondeat superior "let the master answer"; the master is liable in certain cases for the wrongful acts of his servant, meaning that a physician may be liable for the wrongful acts of someone working under the physician's supervision. The doctrine is inapplicable where injury occurs while the servant is acting outside the legitimate scope of authority. (Chapter 5)
resting energy expenditure (REE) caloric needs of the body estimated from O_2 consumption and CO_2 production, usually expressed in kcal/24 hr. (Chapter 23)
restrictive lung disease broad category of disorders with widely variable causes but all resulting in a reduction in lung volumes, particularly the inspiratory and vital capacities; categorized according to origin—skeletal/thoracic, neuromuscular, pleural, interstitial, and alveolar. (Chapter 20)
retinopathy of prematurity (ROP) abnormal ocular condition that occurs in some premature or low-birth-weight infants who receive O_2.

Previously called *retrolental fibroplasias*. (Chapters 41, 53)

retractions sinking inward of the skin around the chest cage with each inspiratory effort. (Chapter 16)

reverse triggering the stimulation of the respiratory center to inspire after the delivery of a controlled positive pressure breath in a sedated patient. (Chapter 47)

Reynold's number a dimensionless number used to determine if flow is laminar or turbulent. If the Reynold's number is above 2000 flow is turbulent. It is determined by multiplying the diameter of the system by the velocity of gas flow times the density of the gas divided by the viscosity of the gas. (Chapter 6)

rhonchi a discontinuous, abnormal breath sound, also known as coarse crackles or rales, caused by air moving through airways which have excessive mucous. (Chapter 16)

right-to-left shunt anatomic bypass in which blood flows from the venous to the arterial side of the circulation, bypassing the lungs; this lowers both the O_2 content and PO_2 of the arterial blood. (Chapter 12)

rise time the time it takes for the ventilator flow to reach its maximum flow. Rise time is a control variable available in all pressure-targeted modes. Functionally it changes the slope of the flow increase from baseline to maximum. (Chapter 47)

rocking bed bed that rocks back and forth moving the abdominal contents up and down facilitating inspiration and expiration. (Chapter 45)

roentgenogram an x-ray image. (Chapter 21)

root-cause analysis is a process by which the underlying primary, secondary, and other notable causes of a medical error or other safety issue are identified, and then an action plan is created and implemented. (Chapters 7, 20)

rule utilitarianism moral reasoning approach based not on which act has the greatest utility but on which rule would promote the greatest good if it were generally followed. (Chapter 5)

S

sarcoidosis chronic disorder of unknown origin characterized by the formation of tubercles of nonnecrotizing epithelioid tissue. (Chapter 26)

saturated solution solution in which the solvent contains the maximum amount of solute it can take up. (Chapter 13)

scalenes referring to the three muscles arising from the cervical vertebrae, inserting into the first and second ribs; accessory muscles of ventilation. (Chapter 9)

scintigraphy photograph showing the distribution and intensity of radioactivity in various tissues and organs after administration of a radiopharmaceutical. (Chapter 36)

screening preliminary procedure, such as a test or examination, to detect the most characteristic sign or signs of a disorder that may require further investigation. (Chapter 31)

secondary spontaneous pneumothorax pneumothorax that occurs because of underlying lung disease. (Chapter 27)

sedimentation primary mechanism for deposition of particles 1 to 5 mm in diameter in the central airways, when particles slow and settle out of suspension. (Chapter 39)

segments minor divisions of the lung; each segment is associated with a major branch of the airway. (Chapter 9)

segs refers to segmented neutrophils the mature form of circulating neutrophils. (Chapter 17)

sensorium general term referring to the relative state of a patient's consciousness or alertness. (Chapter 16)

servo-controlled heating system in a humidifier, heating unit that monitors the temperature of gas delivered to the patient, adjusting the power to the heater based on the difference between the temperature setting and the temperature monitored by a thermistor probe placed downstream from the humidifier, at or near the patient airway connection. (Chapter 38)

severe obesity the state of having a body mass index of greater than 40 kg/m^2. (Chapter 30)

shock condition in which perfusion to vital organs is inadequate to meet metabolic needs; includes hypovolemic, cardiogenic, septic, anaphylactic, and neurogenic forms. (Chapter 16)

sickle cell hemoglobin the presence of hemoglobin S causing the hemoglobin cell to form a sickle shape. (Chapter 12)

signs the objective manifestation of illness such as increased respiratory rate. (Chapter 16)

silicosis lung disorder caused by continued, long-term exposure to the dust of an inorganic compound, silicon dioxide, which is found in sands, quartzes, and many other stones; chronic silicosis is marked by widespread fibrotic nodular lesions in both lungs. (Chapter 26)

six or twelve-minute walk (6- or 12-minute) a test which involves walking and an established protocol to assess a patient's level of physical conditioning. (Chapter 55)

skilled nursing facility (SNF) institution or part of an institution that meets criteria for accreditation established by the sections of the *Social Security Act* that determine the basis for Medicaid and Medicare reimbursement for skilled nursing care. Skilled nursing care includes rehabilitation and various medical and nursing procedures. (Chapter 51)

slander any words spoken with malice that are untrue and prejudicial to the reputation, professional practice, commercial trade, office, or business of another person. (Chapter 5)

sleep-disordered breathing periods of an absence of attempts to breathe during sleep. (Chapter 33)

small cell cancer malignant, usually bronchogenic epithelial neoplasm consisting of small; tightly packed; round, oval, or spindle-shaped epithelial cells that stain darkly and contain neurosecretory granules and little or no cytoplasm. Many malignant tumors of the lung are of this type. Also called *oat cell carcinoma* or *small cell carcinoma*. (Chapter 31)

SOAP in a problem-oriented medical record, abbreviation for *subjective, objective, assessment,* and *plan,* the four parts of a written account of the health problem. (Chapter 3)

soft palate structure composed of mucous membrane, muscular fibers, and mucous glands, suspended from the posterior border of the hard palate forming the roof of the mouth. (Chapter 9)

solitary pulmonary nodule (SPN) a pulmonary parenchymal opacity smaller than 3 cm in diameter that is totally surrounded by aerated lung. (Chapter 21)

solubility coefficient (gas) volume of gas that can be dissolved in 1 ml of a given liquid at standard pressure and specified temperature. (Chapter 6)

solute substance dissolved in a solution. (Chapter 13)

solution mixture of one or more substances dissolved in another substance. The molecules of each of the substances disperse homogeneously and do not change chemically. A solution may be a gas, a liquid, or a solid. (Chapter 13)

solvent any liquid in which another substance can be dissolved. (Chapter 13)

specific gravity ratio of the density of a substance to the density of another substance accepted as a standard. The usual standard for liquids and solids is water. A liquid or solid with a specific gravity of 4 times as dense as water at the same temperature. Hydrogen is the usual standard for gases. (Chapter 6)

spectrophotometry measurement of color in a solution by determining the amount of light absorbed in the ultraviolet, infrared, or visible spectrum, widely used in clinical chemistry to calculate the concentration of substances in solution. (Chapter 19)

splinting process of immobilizing, restraining, or supporting a body part. (Chapter 40)

spontaneous awaking trial a trial of sedation removal or reduction preformed prior to a spontaneous breathing trial. (Chapter 47)

spontaneous breath ventilatory support breaths initiated and ended by the patient. (Chapter 45)

spontaneous breathing trial (SBT) trial of spontaneous breathing independent of the ventilator. (Chapter 47)

sporicidal destructive to the spore form of bacteria. (Chapter 4)

sputum mucus from the respiratory tract that has passed through the mouth. (Chapter 16)

squamous cell carcinoma type of lung cancer characterized by cells that appear platelike. (Chapter 31)

staging system See *TNM staging.* (Chapter 31)

standard bicarbonate plasma concentration of HCO_3^- in mEq/L that would exist if PCO_2 were normal (40 mm Hg). (Chapter 14)

standard precautions guidelines recommended by the U.S. Centers for Disease Control and Prevention to reduce the risk of transmission of blood-borne and other pathogens in hospitals. Standard precautions apply to (1) blood; (2) all body fluids, secretions, and excretions, excluding sweat, regardless of whether they contain blood; (3) nonintact skin; and (4) mucous membranes. (Chapter 4)

Starling equilibrium the filtration of fluid across a membrane is a result of equilibration of osmotic and hydrostatic forces across the membrane. (Chapter 13)

stenosis narrowing of a valve or vessel. (Chapters 10, 36)

sterilization complete destruction of all microorganisms, usually by heat or chemical means. (Chapter 4)

sternal angle the fused connection between the manubrium and the body of the sternum is known as the sternal angle or angle of Louis. (Chapter 9)

sternocleidomastoid muscles muscle of the neck that is attached to the mastoid process of the temporal bone and superior nuchal line and by separate heads to the sternum and clavicle; sternocleidomastoid muscles function together to flex the head. (Chapter 9)

sternum elongated flattened bone forming the middle portion of the anterior thorax. (Chapter 9)

stomata small holes within the parietal pleura that are the main route for pleural fluid to exit. (Chapter 27)

STPD conditions of a volume of gas at 0° C and 760 mm Hg and containing no water vapor (dry). It should contain a calculable number of moles of a particular gas. (Chapter 6)

strain-gauge pressure transducers a pressure measuring device that records pressures by the expansion and contraction of a flexible metal diaphragm connected to electrical wires. (Chapter 6)

stress index an index used to determine if during mechanical controlled inhalation there is over distention or recruitment of collapse lung; determined by the slope change in the airway pressure curve during volume controlled square wave ventilation. (Chapter 51)

strict liability theory in tort law that can be used to impose liability without fault, even in situations where injury occurs under conditions of reasonable care; the most common cases of strict liability involve the use of dangerous products or techniques. (Chapter 5)

stridor high-pitched, continuous type of adventitious lung sound heard from the upper airway. (Chapter 16)

stroke condition characterized by the sudden onset of a neurologic deficit. (Chapter 32)

stroke volume volume of blood ejected by the left ventricle during each contraction. (Chapter 10)

sub-atmospheric below atmospheric; used to describe pressures below ambient. (Chapter 11)

subcutaneous emphysema accumulation of air in the subcutaneous tissues owing to leakage from the lung. (Chapter 16)

suctioning process of mechanically aspirating airway secretions. (Chapter 36)

sudden infant death syndrome (SIDS) leading cause of death in infants less than 1 year old in the United States. Commonly called *crib death.* (Chapter 33)

super obesity the state of having a body mass index of greater than 50 kg/m^2. (Chapter 30)

supplemental oxygen O_2 delivered at concentrations exceeding 21% to increase the amount of O_2 circulating in the blood. (Chapter 25)

suprasternal above the sternum. (Chapter 9)

surface tension tendency of a liquid to minimize the area of its surface by contracting. This property causes liquids to rise in a capillary tube, effects the exchange of gases in the pulmonary alveoli, and alters the ability of various liquids to wet another surface. (Chapters 6, 11)

surfactant surface-acting agent that forms a monomolecular layer over pulmonary alveolar surfaces. These agents prevent alveolar collapse at lower lung volumes by reducing alveolar surface tension. (Chapter 53)

surgical resection the partial removal of an organ or tissues by surgical means. (Chapter 31)

surveillance (bacteriologic) ongoing process designed to ensure that infection control procedures are working; generally involves equipment, microbiologic identification, and epidemiologic investigation. (Chapter 4)

suspensions dispersion of large particles suspended in a fluid medium; without physical agitation, the particles eventually settle out. (Chapter 13)

Swan-Ganz catheter catheter that is positioned in the pulmonary artery to measure pressures in the heart and pulmonary circulation and can be used to determine the patient's circulatory status. (Chapter 51)

sweep flow the flow of gas in a direction opposite the flow of blood through an ECMO oxygenator to remove CO_2 and add O_2. Normally the gas is O_2 but on occasion small amounts of CO_2 are added. (Chapter 50)

symptoms the sensation or subjective experience of some aspect of an illness, such as breathlessness. (Chapter 16)

synchronized cardioversion countershock synchronized with the heart's electrical activity. (Chapter 37)

synchronous intermittent mandatory ventilation (SIMV) mode of ventilatory support using periodic assisted ventilation with spontaneous breathing in between. Assisted breaths are responsive to patient demand. (Chapters 48, 52)

syncope temporary unconsciousness; fainting. (Chapter 16)

synthesized database a set of computerized records or data which have been reviewed, interpreted and categorized in relation to an area of research. (Chapter 8)

systematic error nonrandom statistical error that affects the mean of a population of data and defines the bias between the means of two populations. (Chapters 19, 51)

systolic pressure peak blood pressure occurring in the arteries during ventricular contraction. (Chapter 16)

T

tachycardia abnormally elevated heart rate. (Chapter 16)

tachyphylaxis phenomenon in which the repeated administration of some drugs results in a marked decrease in effectiveness. (Chapter 35)

tachypnea abnormal elevation of breathing rate. (Chapter 16)

tamponade (cardiac) the accumulation of blood in the pericardial sac, increasing pericardial pressure and reducing cardiac output. (Chapter 30)

target heart rate heart rate achieved at 65% of a patient's maximum O_2 consumption during an exercise evaluation, used for aerobic conditioning. (Chapter 55)

target variable a variable that can be reached and maintained at a preset level before inspiration ends but does not terminate inspiration. (Chapter 42)

targeting scheme the approach used by a particular mode to achieve the various targets active during ventilation. (Chapter 42)

telemedicine refers to the use of electronic and telecommunication technologies to support health care at a geographically different location from the patient, thus increasing access to specialty patient care. (Chapter 7)

telemonitoring monitoring a patient's clinical condition through a computerized connection to a health care facility. (Chapter 7)

tension pneumothorax air in the pleural space that exceeds atmospheric pressure causing outward expansion of the ribs, downward depression of the diaphragm, mediastinal shift, and hypotension. (Chapters 27, 30, 47)

tension-time index product of contractile force (ratio of diaphragmatic pressure to maximum diaphragmatic pressure) and contractile duration (ratio of inspiratory time to total breathing cycle time) used to indicate a level of contraction associated with fatigue. (Chapter 44)

tetralogy of Fallot congenital cardiac anomaly that consists of four defects: pulmonic stenosis, ventricular septal defect, malposition of the aorta so that it arises from the septal defect or the right ventricle, and right ventricular hypertrophy. (Chapter 33)

therapeutic index difference between the minimum therapeutic and minimum toxic concentrations of a drug. (Chapter 39)

therapist-driven protocol specification of actions that allow respiratory care practitioners to initiate and adjust therapy independently, within guidelines previously established by medical staff. Also called *respiratory care protocol.* (Chapter 2)

thermal conductivity measure of gas concentrations in a sample calculated by detecting the rate at which different gases conduct heat. (Chapter 6)

thermodynamics science of the interconversion of heat and work. (Chapter 6)

thiosulfate a compound ($S_2O_3^{2-}$) that is an oxyanion of sulfur used in treating carbon monoxide poisoning. (Chapter 30)

thoracentesis surgical perforation of the chest wall and pleural space with a needle for diagnostic or therapeutic purposes or for the removal of a specimen for biopsy. (Chapter 27)

thoracic flap or flail chest two or more ribs broken in two or more places creating an unstable segment of the chest wall. (Chapter 30)

thoracic gas volume (TGV) technique that measures lung volume. (Chapter 20)

Thorpe tube variable orifice, constant pressure flowmeter. (Chapter 40)

thrill fine palpable vibration felt accompanying a cardiac or vascular murmur. (Chapter 16)

thrombocytes smallest cells in the blood; they are formed in the red bone marrow, and some are stored in the spleen. Platelets are disc-shaped, contain no hemoglobin, and are essential for the coagulation of blood and in maintenance of hemostasis. (Chapter 16)

thrombocytopenia abnormal condition in which the number of blood platelets is reduced, usually associated with neoplastic diseases or an immune response to a drug. (Chapter 17)

tidal volume (V_T) volume of air that is inhaled or exhaled from the lungs during effortless breath. (Chapters 11, 20)

time constant mathematical expression describing the relative efficacy of lung unit filling and emptying and computed as the product of compliance times resistance (measured in seconds). (Chapters 11, 45, 46)

tissue oxygen sensing the monitoring of the O_2 saturation or PO_2 at the tissue level. (Chapter 51)

tort legal wrong committed on a person or property independent of contract. (Chapter 5)

total lung capacity (TLC) total amount of gas in the lungs after a maximum inspiration. (Chapter 19)

trachea large main intrathoracic airway. (Chapter 9)

tracheal tugging effect of an aortic aneurysm in which the trachea is pulled downward with each heart contraction. (Chapter 16)

tracheoesophageal fistula a congenital malformation or an abnormality associated with disease in which there is an abnormal tubelike passage between the trachea and the esophagus. (Chapters 36, 47)

tracheoinnominate fistula a fistula (connection between the trachea and the innominate artery). (Chapter 36)

tracheal malacia softening of the tracheal cartilages. (Chapters 36, 47)

tracheal stenosis a narrowing of the tracheal diameter. (Chapter 47)

tracheostomy opening through the neck into the trachea, through which an indwelling tube may be inserted. (Chapter 36)

tracheostomy tubes artificial airways that are surgically placed directly into the trachea. (Chapter 36)

tracheotomy procedure by which an incision is made into the trachea through the neck below the larynx to gain access to the lower airways. (Chapter 36)

transairway pressure difference between airway pressure and alveolar pressure. (Chapters 11, 46)

transalveolar pressure difference between alveolar pressure and pleural pressure. (Chapters 11, 46)

transbronchial biopsy a lung tissue specimen which is obtained through a needle insertion, bronchoscopy or surgery. (Chapter 22, 31)

transbronchial needle aspiration technique of sampling lung tissue through a bronchoscope that involves passing a thin needle through a bronchus. (Chapters 22, 31)

trans–chest wall pressure difference between the pleural space and the body surface. Also called *transthoracic pressure*. (Chapters 11, 46)

transdiaphragmatic pressure (P_{di}) the pressure change across the diaphragm associated with breathing. (Chapter 46)

transtracheal oxygen therapy (TTOT) low-flow O_2 delivered via a catheter with a small orifice that is inserted through the skin and neck tissue into the trachea through the anterior tracheal wall. (Chapter 56)

transient tachypnea of the newborn (TTN) the periodic increase in respiratory rate that is commonly observed in low-birth-weight infants. (Chapter 34)

transposition of the great arteries congenital cardiac condition characterized by an anatomic abnormality in which the aorta arises from the right ventricle and the pulmonary artery arises from the left ventricle. (Chapter 34)

transpulmonary of or pertaining to the difference in a parameter (e.g., pressure) between the alveoli and pleural space. (Chapter 10)

transpulmonary pressure the difference between the alveolar pressure and intrapleural pressure of the lungs. (Chapters 46, 48, 51)

transpulmonary pressure difference difference between intraalveolar and intrapleural pressure, or the pressure acting across the ling from the pleural space to the alveoli. (Chapters 11)

transrespiratory across the respiratory system; of or pertaining to the difference in a parameter (e.g., pressure) between the alveoli and the body surface.

transrespiratory pressure the difference between the alveolar pressure and pressure on the body surface. (Chapter 46)

transrespiratory pressure gradient pressure differential between the mouth and the alveoli that causes gas to flow in and out of the lungs. (Chapters 43)

transthoracic across the thorax; of or pertaining to the difference in a parameter (e.g., pressure) between the pleural space and body surface.

transthoracic needle biopsy technique of obtaining a biopsy specimen of lung tissue by which a needle is passed into the chest, often guided by imaging. (Chapter 31)

transthoracic pressure of or pertaining to the difference in a parameter (such as pressure) between the pleural space and body surface. (Chapter 46)

transthoracic pressure difference (P_{TT}) difference between the pleural space and the body surface. Also called *trans–chest wall pressure*. (Chapter 11)

transtracheal oxygen therapy (T_{TOT}) administration of O_2 via a low-flow catheter inserted directly into the trachea. (Chapter 51)

transudate the fluid that moves out of a cell or tissue as a result of a concentration/pressure gradient. (Chapter 30)

transudative pleural effusion pleural effusion low in protein and lactate dehydrogenase, usually caused by congestive heart failure, nephrosis, or cirrhosis. (Chapter 27)

traumatic brain injury general term referring to any class of either focal or diffuse lesions that can result from head trauma; these lesions include injury to the nerve body (axon), hypoxic brain damage, swelling, hemorrhage, contusions, laceration, and infection. (Chapter 32)

Trendelenburg position position in which the head is low and the body and legs are on an inclined plane. (Chapter 45)

trepopnea shortness of breath which is experienced by a patient while lying on one side or the other. (Chapter 16)

trigger the inspiratory force a patient must generate to initiate a breath on a mechanical ventilator. (Chapter 45)

trigger asynchrony a lack of coordination between the patient's inspiratory effort and the response of the mechanical ventilator. (Chapter 47)

trigger delay a delay in ventilator response to a patient's inspiratory effort. (Chapter 47)

trigger variable variable that initiates inspiration during mechanical ventilation. (Chapter 45)

tripodding breathing technique most often used by patients with chronic obstructive pulmonary disease in which they lean forward and place their elbows on a table or arms of a chair to support breathing with the accessory muscles. (Chapter 16)

troponin protein in the striated cell ultrastructure that modulates the interaction between actin and myosin molecules. It is believed to be part of the calcium-binding complex of the thin myofilaments. The level of blood troponin is used to identify the presence of a myocardial infarction. (Chapter 17)

troponin I protein similar to CPK-2; troponin I levels peak 12 to 16 hours after myocardial infarction. It is associated with cardiac muscle damage. (Chapter 17)

true ribs the first seven ribs on each side of the thorax are called *true ribs*. (Chapter 9)

tuberculosis chronic granulomatous infection caused by an acid-fast bacillus, *Mycobacterium tuberculosis*. It is generally transmitted by the inhalation or ingestion of infected droplets and usually affects the lungs, although infection of multiple organ systems occurs. (Chapter 24)

tumor, node, metastasis (TNM) staging staging system based on a size of the tumor *(T)*, the presence and position of abnormal lymph nodes *(N)*, and the presence or absence of metastasis (or spread beyond the primary tumor site) *(M)*. (Chapter 28)

turbinates bony structures that extend from the lateral walls of the interior nasal passages. (Chapter 9)

turbulent flow flow of a fluid that does not occur in a straight line; flow in which molecules tumble over each other. (Chapter 6)

12-minute walk usually a part of a pulmonary rehabilitation program, performed once per day for the duration of the program. The objective is for the patient to walk on a flat, smooth surface as far as possible during the 12 minutes, stopping as necessary and quantifying the total distance covered. (Chapter 55)

type I pneumocyte cuboidal, secretory epithelia that line the blind tubules of the acinus cells. (Chapter 9)

type II pneumocyte pneumocyte granular cells that are highly active and form part of the lining of the alveoli. These cells secrete surfactant and other substances. (Chapter 9)

U

ultrasonic nebulizer (USN) aerosol generator in which an electrical signal is used to produce high-frequency vibrations in a container of fluid. The vibrations break up the fluid into aerosol particles. (Chapter 38)

ultrathin bronchoscopy a bronchoscope which has a smaller than usual diameter and circumference to permit insertion into small airways. (Chapter 22)

upper airway stimulation a newer way of treating obstructive sleep apnea which involves implantation of a nerve stimulator to maintain upper airway patency. (Chapter 33)

upstream relative reference to a point closer to the source in a stream of flowing fluid. (Chapter 40)

uvula small cone-shaped process suspended in the mouth from the middle of the posterior border of the soft palate. (Chapter 9)

uvulopalatopharyngoplasty (UVPPP) surgical procedure used in treating severe obstructive sleep apnea, which involves shortening of the soft palate and removal of the uvula and tonsils. (Chapter 33)

V

VA ECMO venous arterial extracorporeal membrane oxygenation, the removal of blood from a vein that then moves to an O_2 and CO_2 exchanger before returning to the patient via an artery. VA ECMO is used to provide support for both the respiratory and cardiovascular system. (Chapter 50)

vagovagal reflexes reflexes caused by stimulation of parasympathetic receptors in the airways that can result in laryngospasm, bronchoconstriction, hyperpnea, and bradycardia; often associated with mechanical stimulation, as during procedures such as tracheobronchial aspiration, intubation, or bronchoscopy. (Chapter 15)

vallecula the anatomic depression immediately beyond the base of the tongue. (Chapter 9)

value-based purchasing (VBP) system is a system of reimbursement by the government CMS to hospitals and health care providers that is partially based on their ability to meet a predefined set of standards. (Chapter 7)

vaporization process whereby matter in its liquid form is changed into its vapor or gaseous form. (Chapter 6)

vasoconstriction narrowing of the blood vessels. (Chapter 10)

vasodilation widening or distention of blood vessels, particularly arterioles, usually caused by nerve impulses or certain drugs that relax smooth muscle in the walls of the blood vessels. (Chapter 10)

vasopressor a medication which causes constriction of the blood vessels, generally used to increase blood pressure. (Chapter 35)

VCV acronym for *volume-controlled ventilation,* a mode of ventilatory support in which volume (or flow × time) serves as the cycle variable. (Chapters 3, 27, 45, 48)

venous admixture mixing of venous blood with arterial blood, resulting in a decrease in the O_2 content of the latter; occurs in anatomic and physiologic shunting. (Chapters 12, 51)

venous reservoir the capacity of the venous system to pool large volumes of blood. (Chapter 10)

venous thromboembolism (VTE) clot that spreads from one venous bed to another, such as from the leg veins to the lung. (Chapter 28)

ventilation molecular exchange of O_2 and CO_2 within the body's tissues. (Chapter 11)

ventilation/perfusion ($\dot{V}/\dot{Q}$) ratio ratio of pulmonary alveolar ventilation to pulmonary capillary perfusion, both measured quantities being expressed in the same units. (Chapter 12)

ventilator-associated pneumonia lower respiratory tract infection that develops more than 48 to 72 hours after endotracheal intubation. (Chapter 24)

ventilator-induced lung injury (VILI) lung injury which occurs as a result of excessive pressure and/or volume during mechanical ventilation. (Chapter 29)

ventilatory threshold during exercise, the point at which increased levels of lactic acid result in increased CO_2 production and minute ventilation; the respiratory quotient equals or exceeds 1.0, indicating that CO_2 production equals or exceeds O_2 consumption; at this point, metabolism becomes anaerobic, decreasing energy production and increasing muscle fatigue. (Chapter 55)

ventral respiratory groups (VRGs) groupings of cells in the medulla oblongata that are active in controlling both inspiration and expiration. (Chapter 15)

ventricular fibrillation (VF) the most life-threatening electrocardiographic arrhythmia characterized by erratic quivering of the ventricular muscle mass. (Chapter 18)

ventricular tachycardia (VT) a run of three or more premature ventricular contractions that is usually easy to recognize as a series of wide, bizarre QRS complexes that have no preceding P wave. (Chapter 18)

veracity principle that binds the health provider and the patient to tell the truth, creating an environment of trust and mutual sharing of information. (Chapter 5)

very low birth weight (VLBW) a newborn who weights less than the 95% percentile of weight for newborns. (Chapter 53)

virtue ethics viewpoint that asks what a virtuous person would do in a similar circumstance; it is based on personal attributes of character or virtue, rather than on rules or consequences. (Chapter 5)

virucidal agent that destroys or inactivates viruses. (Chapter 4)

visceral pleura thin membrane covered by mesothelial cells that covers the entire surface of the lung, dipping into the lobar fissures. (Chapter 9, 27)

viscosity internal force that opposes flow of a fluid, either liquids or gases. (Chapter 6)

vital capacity (VC) total amount of air that can be exhaled after a maximum inspiration; the sum of the inspiratory reserve volume, tidal volume, and expiratory reserve volume. (Chapters 20, 51)

volatile acid acid that can be excreted in its gaseous form; physiologically, carbonic acid is a volatile acid; approximately 24,000 mmol/L CO_2 is eliminated from the body daily via normal ventilation. (Chapter 14)

voltage expression of electromotive force in terms of volts. (Chapter 3)

volume-controlled ventilation (CMV) a mode of ventilatory support in which a specific tidal volume is set and delivered for each breath under control ventilation conditions. (Chapters 3, 27, 45, 48)

volume-limited ventilation same as CMV, the primary control variable is tidal volume. (Chapter 27)

volume-median diameter (VMD) the median diameter of an aerosol particle measured in units of volume. (Chapter 39)

volume support pressure-limited ventilation in which tidal volume is targeted. (Chapter 48)

volumetric capnography a way of measuring the volume of exhaled carbon dioxide to assess the a patient's ventilatory status. (Chapter 19)

volutrauma alveolar overdistention and damage caused by ventilation with high peak inflation pressures. (Chapters 29, 46)

VV ECMO venovenous extracorporeal membrane oxygenation, the removal of blood from a vein which then moves to an O_2 and CO_2 exchanger before returning to the patient via a vein. VV ECMO is used to provide support for the respiratory system but not the circulatory system. (Chapter 50)

W

water vapor pressure the pressure exerted by water in its gaseous state. (Chapter 6)

wet drowning drowning that is a result of a large amount of water entering the lungs. (Chapter 30)

wheezes high-pitched, continuous type of adventitious lung sound. (Chapter 16)

work of breathing (WOB) amount of force needed to move a given volume into the lung with a relaxed chest wall; mathematically, work is the integral of pressure times volume. (Chapter 44)

X

xiphoid process pointed lower portion of the sternum. (Chapter 9)

Z

zone valve on/off piping valve that controls medical gas distribution to a prespecified zone of a building. (Chapter 40)

Index

Note: Page numbers followed by "f" refer to illustrations; page numbers followed by "t" refer to tables; page numbers followed by "b" refer to boxes.

B

C

F

G

H

O

W

N-SiPAP	nasal positive airway pressure with periodic (sigh) bilevel positive airway pressure breaths or bilevel nasal continuous positive airway pressure
NTE	neutral thermal environment
O_2	oxygen
O_2Hb	oxygenated hemoglobin
OH^-	hydroxide ions
OHDC	oxyhemoglobin dissociation curve
OSA	obstructive sleep apnea
P	pressure
ΔP	change in pressure
P_{50}	PO_2 at which 50% saturation of hemoglobin occurs
P_{100}	pressure on inspiration measured at 100 msec
Pa	arterial pressure
PA	pulmonary artery
$P(A-a)O_2$	alveolar-to-arterial partial pressure of oxygen
P(A-awo)	pressure gradient from alveolus to airway opening
$PACO_2$	partial pressure of carbon dioxide in the alveoli
$PaCO_2$	partial pressure of carbon dioxide in the arteries
P_{al}	alveolar pressure
PAO_2	partial pressure of oxygen in the alveoli
PaO_2	partial pressure of oxygen in the arteries
PaO_2/FiO_2	ratio of arterial PO_2 to FiO_2
PaO_2/PAO_2	ratio of arterial PO_2 to alveolar PO_2
PAOP	pulmonary artery occlusion pressure (Also known as pulmonary capillary wedge pressure [PCWP])
PAP	pulmonary artery pressure
$\overline{PAP}$	mean pulmonary artery pressure
$P(a-et)CO_2$	arterial-to-end-tidal partial pressure of carbon dioxide
PAGE	perfluorocarbon associated gas exchange
P_{aug}	pressure augmentation
PAV	proportional assist ventilation
P_{aw}	airway pressure
$\overline{P_{aw}}$	mean airway pressure
P_{awo}	airway opening pressure
PAWP	pulmonary artery wedge pressure
PB	barometric pressure
PBW	predicted body weight
P_{bs}	pressure at the body's surface
PC-CMV	pressure-controlled continuous mandatory ventilation
PCEF	peak cough expiratory flow
PCIRV	pressure control inverse ratio ventilation
PCO_2	partial pressure of carbon dioxide
PC-IMV	pressure-controlled intermittent mandatory ventilation
PC-SIMV	pressure-controlled synchronized intermittent mandatory ventilation
POCT	point of care testing
PCV	pressure-controlled ventilation
PCWP	pulmonary capillary wedge pressure
$PCWP_{tm}$	transmural pulmonary capillary wedge pressure
PDA	patent ductus arteriosus
PE	pulmonary embolism
PE_{max}	maximal expiratory pressure
PEA	pulseless electrical activity
$P_{\bar{E}}CO_2$	partial pressure of mixed expired carbon dioxide
PEEP	positive end expiratory pressure
$PEEP_E$	extrinsic PEEP (set-PEEP)
$PEEP_I$	intrinsic PEEP (auto-PEEP)
$PEEP_{total}$	total PEEP (sum of intrinsic and extrinsic PEEP)
PEFR	peak expiratory flow rate
P_{es}	esophageal pressure
$PetCO_2$	partial pressure of end-tidal carbon dioxide
P_{flex}	pressure at the inflection point of a pressure/volume curve
PFT	pulmonary function test(ing)
P_{ga}	gastric pressure
pH	relative acidity or alkalinity of a solution
P_{high}	high pressure during APRV
PHY	permissive hypercapnia
PIE	pulmonary interstitial edema
PIF	pulmonary interstitial fibrosis
PI_{max}	maximum inspiratory pressure (also MIP, MIF, NIF)
P_{inside}	inside pressure
$P_{intrapleural}$	intrapleural pressure (also Ppl)
PiO_2	partial pressure of inspired oxygen
PIP	peak inspiratory pressure (also P_{peak})
PISS	pin-indexed safety system
P_L	transpulmonary pressure
P_{low}	low pressure during APRV
PLV	partial liquid ventilation
P_M	mouth pressure
pMDI	pressurized metered dose inhaler
P_{mus}	muscle pressure
PO_2	partial pressure of oxygen
$P_{outside}$	pressure outside
P_{peak}	peak inspiratory pressure (also PIP)
PPHN	primary pulmonary hypertension of the neonate
P_{pl}	intrapleural pressure
$P_{plateau}$	plateau pressure
ppm	parts per million
PPST	premature pressure support termination
PPV	positive pressure ventilation
PRA	plasma renin activity
PRVC	pressure regulated volume control
PS	pressure support
PSB	protected specimen brush
P_{set}	set pressure
psi	pounds per square inch
psig	pounds per square inch gauge
PS_{max}	maximum pressure support
P_{st}	static transpulmonary pressure at a specified lung volume
PSV	pressure support ventilation
P_{TA}	transairway pressure
$PtcCO_2$	transcutaneous PCO_2
$PtcO_2$	transcutaneous PO_2
P_{tm}	transmural pressure
P_{TR}	transrespiratory pressure
PTSD	posttraumatic stress disorder
P_{TT}	transthoracic pressure (also Pw)
P-V	pressure-volume
PV	pressure ventilation
PVC(s)	premature ventricular contraction(s)
$P\bar{v}O_2$	partial pressure of oxygen in mixed venous blood
PVR	pulmonary vascular resistance
PVS	partial ventilatory support
P_w	transthoracic pressure (also P_{TT})
Q	blood volume
$\dot{Q}$	blood flow
$\dot{Q}_{c'}$	pulmonary capillary blood flow
q2h	every 2 hours
$\dot{Q}_T$	cardiac output
$\frac{\dot{Q}_s}{\dot{Q}_t}$	shunt
$\dot{Q}sp$	physiologic shunt flow (total venous admixture)
R	resistance (i.e., pressure per unit flow)
$\bar{R}$	mean total resistance
RAM	random access memory
RAP	right atrial pressure
R_{aw}	airway resistance